CANADIAN MATERNITY and PEDIATRIC Nursing

Jessica Webster, RN, MN, PNC(C)
Senior Teaching Associate
Faculty of Nursing
University of New Brunswick
Fredericton, New Brunswick

Caroline Sanders, MBE, PhD, RCN, RN, PGD, PGC
Associate Professor
University of Northern British Columbia
Prince George, British Columbia

Susan Scott Ricci, ARNP, MSN, MEd, CNE
College of Nursing Faculty
University of Central Florida
Orlando, Florida
Former Nursing Program Director and Faculty
Lake Sumter State College
Leesburg, Florida

Terri Kyle, DNP, CPNP-PC, CNE
Adjunct Faculty
University of West Florida
Pensacola, Florida

Susan Carman, MSN, MBA
Professor of Nursing
Most recently, Edison Community College
Fort Myers, Florida

Edition 2

Wolters Kluwer

Philadelphia • Baltimore • New York • London
Buenos Aires • Hong Kong • Sydney • Tokyo

Vice President and Publisher: Julie K. Stegman
Director, Nursing Education: Renee Gagliardi
Director of Product Development: Jennifer K. Forestieri
Senior Development Editor: Michael Kerns
Editorial Coordinator: David Murphy
Senior Marketing Manager: Sarah Schuessler
Editorial Assistant: Leo Gray
Design Coordinator: Elaine Kasmer
Art Director, Illustration: Jennifer Clements
Production Project Manager: Kim Cox
Manufacturing Coordinator: Karin Duffield
Prepress Vendor: Aptara, Inc.

2nd Edition

9 8 7 6 5 4 3 2 1

Printed in China

Library of Congress Cataloging-in-Publication Data

Names: Webster, Jessica, author. | Sanders, Caroline, author. | Ricci, Susan
    Scott, author. | Kyle, Terri, author. | Carman, Susan, author.
Title: Canadian maternity and pediatric nursing / Jessica Webster, Caroline
    Sanders, Susan Scott Ricci, Terri Kyle, Susan Carman.
Description: Second edition. | Philadelphia : Wolters Kluwer, [2020] |
    Preceded by Canadian maternity and pediatric nursing / Jean Chow…
    [et al.]. c2013. | Includes bibliographical references and index.
Identifiers: LCCN 2019018144 | ISBN 9781496386090 (hardback)
Subjects: | MESH: Maternal-Child Nursing | Women's Health | Pediatric Nursing
    | Obstetric Nursing | Canada
Classification: LCC RG951 | NLM WY 157.3 | DDC 618.92/00231–dc23
LC record available at https://lccn.loc.gov/2019018144

CCS0719

Jessica Webster

Jessica Webster earned a baccalaureate degree in Nursing as well as a Diploma in University Teaching from the University of New Brunswick, and a Masters in Nursing also from the University of New Brunswick. She has earned and maintained certification in perinatal nursing through the Canadian Nurses Association since 2004. Her expertise and areas of interest within perinatal nursing are women's reproductive and sexual health as well as breastfeeding. Jessica has been involved in the Baby-Friendly Initiative work in New Brunswick for over a decade, and currently chairs the NB BFI Steering Committee. Jessica has 20 years' clinical expertise both in inpatient perinatal care as well as community-based sexual health care.

In recent years, Jessica has devoted significant study to her interests in health assessment, cultural sensitivity, and international nursing. For the past five years, Jessica has supervised nursing students in an annual independent study in Malawi, Africa, focusing on perinatal and reproductive health.

Jessica has been recognized as a leader in nursing education, receiving the first Excellence in Teaching Award within the Nursing faculty, as well as the Dr. Allan P. Stuart award which honours outstanding teaching achievement at the University of New Brunswick. She is currently a Senior Teaching Associate in the Faculty of Nursing, at the University of New Brunswick.

Caroline Sanders

Caroline Sanders earned a Bachelor of Science in Nursing from the University of Manchester, United Kingdom, and a PhD in Nursing from University of Central Lancashire. She is a registered nurse practicing in pediatric nursing for over 30 years, having had opportunities to serve children and their families in a variety of diverse settings. Caroline was awarded an MBE in 2014 for services to pediatric nursing.

She has experience in tertiary inpatient pediatrics, community care, and more recently engaged in working in community hospitals in Rural Canada. Caroline has worked as a pediatric nurse consultant in the United Kingdom in pediatric specialty clinics. She has been involved in specialist teaching and more recently RN teaching for over 20 years with experience in both graduate and undergraduate education. Caroline is a member of the Canadian Association of Paediatric Nursing.

With the changing education portfolio across Canada, Caroline recognized the need for a maternity and pediatric nursing textbook that was accessible for those students who may have limited opportunities to learn about this aspect of nursing at the undergraduate level. Caroline, similar to the U.S. authors of this text, believes in a concept-based approach for learning nursing that helps students develop clinical decision-making skills.

Susan Scott Ricci

Susan Scott Ricci earned a diploma in nursing from the Washington Hospital Center School of Nursing, and went on to receive a BSN and MSN in Maternal—Infant Nursing, from the Catholic University of America in Washington, DC. She also obtained an MEd in Counseling from the University of Southern Mississippi, along with a recent national certification as a nurse educator. She has worked in a variety of women's health care settings, including labour and birth, postpartum, prenatal, and family planning ambulatory care clinics. Susan is a certified women's health care nurse practitioner who has spent 30+ years in nursing education teaching in LPN, ADN, and BSN programs. She is involved in several professional nursing organizations and holds application of knowledge within nursing practice.

Terri Kyle

Terri Kyle earned a Bachelor of Science in Nursing from the University of North Carolina at Chapel Hill, a Master of Science in Nursing from Emory University in Atlanta, Georgia, and a Doctorate of Nursing Practice with a focus in educational leadership from American Sentinel University. She is a certified pediatric nurse practitioner, and practicing pediatric nursing for over 30 years, she has had the opportunity to serve children and their families in a variety of diverse settings. Terri also holds the credential of certified nurse educator.

She has experience in inpatient pediatrics, in pediatric and neonatal intensive care units, newborn nursery, specialized pediatric units, and community hospitals. She has worked as a pediatric nurse practitioner in pediatric specialty clinics and primary care. She has been involved in teaching nursing for over 25 years with experience in both graduate and undergraduate education. Terri is a fellow in the National Association of Pediatric Nurse Practitioners and a member of the Sigma Theta Tau International Honor Society of Nursing, the National League for Nursing, and the Society of Pediatric Nurses.

With the limited time allotted to the topic of maternity and pediatric nursing in nursing programs, Terri recognized the need for a textbook that "got to the point." She strongly believes in a concept-based approach for learning nursing—that is, to teach the basics to students in a broad, contextual format so that they can apply that knowledge in a variety of situations. The concept-based approach to nursing education is time efficient for nursing educators and fosters the development of critical thinking skills in student nurses.

Susan Carman

Susan Carman earned a Bachelor of Science in Nursing from the University of Wisconsin-Madison and a Master of Science in Nursing and Master in Business Administration from the University of Colorado-Denver. As a pediatric nurse for over 20 years, Susan has had the opportunity to care for children in a variety of diverse settings and in many of the major children's hospitals throughout the United States. She also has provided volunteer nursing care in a variety of settings including the Dominican Republic and India. She has been involved in teaching nursing for the past 15 years and enjoys watching students transform into competent nurses with strong critical thinking skills. She is a member of Sigma Theta Tau and Beta Gamma Sigma.

Contributors to the Second Canadian Edition

Linda Adams, RN, BScN, MN, CNCCP(C)
Clinical Nurse Specialist
Pediatric Palliative Care
Canuck Place Children's Hospice
Vancouver, British Columbia

Linlea Armstrong, MD, FRCPC, CCMG
Clinical Associate Professor
Department of Medical Genetics
The University of British Columbia
Vancouver, British Columbia

Leigh Baetz-Craft, RN, MN, IBCLC, PNC(C)
Advanced Practice Nurse Clinician
Maternal/Newborn and Child Health Services
Michael Garron Hospital
Toronto, Ontario

Kathryn Banks, PhD, MSN, RN
Assistant Professor
School of Nursing
Thomson Rivers University
Kamloops, British Columbia

Davina Banner, PhD, RN
Associate Professor
School of Nursing
University of Northern British Columbia
Prince George, British Columbia

Keri-Ann Berga, RN, BScN, MScN, IBCLC, PNC
Assistant Professor
Department of Nursing Science, Faculty of Nursing
MacEwan University
Edmonton, Alberta

Rebecca Brooke, RN, BSN
Endocrine Clinic Nurse
Pediatric Endocrine and Diabetes
BC Children's Hospital
Vancouver, British Columbia

Chantell Canessa, MN-NP
Adjunct Faculty
School of Nursing
University of British Columbia
Vancouver, British Columbia

Aimee Castro, MA
Master of Science (Applied) in Nursing—Direct Entry
    Candidate
Ingram School of Nursing
McGill University
Montreal, Quebec

Khadidja Chougui, BA
Shriners Hospitals for Children
Canada

Genevieve Currie, RN, MN
Associate Professor
Mount Royal University
Calgary, Alberta

Heidi Dodenberg, BScN, MScN (p), RN
Instructor
School of Nursing
University of Northern British Columbia
Prince George, British Columbia

Jennifer Dunlop, MSN, NP (P)
Pediatric Nurse Practitioner
Orthopaedics
BC Children's Hospital
Vancouver, British Columbia

Julie Easley, BA, MA, PhD
Research Associate
Family Medicine Teaching Unit
Dalhousie University
Fredericton, New Brunswick

Kathi Evans, RN, BSN, CGN (C)
Nurse Clinician
Division of Gastroenterology
BC Children's Hospital
Vancouver, British Columbia

Heather Ezurike, RN, MN, PNC(C)
Perinatal Nurse Consultant
Reproductive Care Program of Nova Scotia
IWK Health Centre
Halifax, Nova Scotia

Christine C. Finnbogason, RN, BSc, BN, MN, PNC(C)
Clinical Nurse Specialist
Women's Health
Women's Hospital, Health Science Centre
Winnipeg, Manitoba

Darlene Fjellgaard, BScN
Clinical Nurse Educator
Pediatric Services
University Hospital of Northern British Columbia
Prince George, British Columbia

Sarah Fox-Smith, RN, BScN, MN, CPHON
Faculty
School of Nursing
University of Regina
Regina, SK Canada

Lucy Gilmore, RN MScN
Clinical Nurse Specialist
Women's and Children's Program
Headwaters Health Care Centre
Orangeville, Ontario

Jeanne Hagreen, RN, BSN, IBCLC, RLC
Lactation Consultant
Maternal Child, Lactation Support Department
University Hospital of Northern British Columbia
Prince George, British Columbia

Beverly Haight, RN, BScN
Sessional Instructor
Pediatrics
University of Northern British Columbia
Prince George, British Columbia

Cindy Hardy, MD, PhD
Hardy Psychological Services
Prince George, British Columbia

Ngoc Huynh, RN, BA, PGDip, MN
Senior Lab Instructor III/Teaching Associate
School of Nursing
University of Northern British Columbia
Prince George, British Columbia

Megan Ireland, NP-F, MScN-FNP
Nurse Practitioner
Primary Care Department
Three Bridges Community Health Centre
Vancouver, British Columbia

Lauren Irving, MN-NP(F)
Adjunct Professor
UNBC School of Nursing
University of Northern British Columbia
Family Nurse Practitioner
Northern Health
Prince George, British Columbia

Andrea Kennedy, RN, PhD
Associate Professor
School of Nursing and Midwifery
Faculty of Health, Community and Education
Mount Royal University
Calgary, Alberta

Amy Klepetar, RN, MScPH
Assistant Professor & Coordinator
School of Nursing
University of Northern British Columbia-Terrace
Terrace, British Columbia

Tanya Levit, RN, MScN
Clinical Resource Leader Paediatrics/Special Care
    Nursery
Michael Garron Hospital
Toronto, Canada

Nicole Lewis-Power, RN, BN, MN
Lecturer
Faculty of Nursing
Memorial University of Newfoundland & Labrador
St. John's, Newfoundland

Jenny Lindstrom, BSN
Registered Nurse
MHSU Community Crisis Response Team
Interior Health
William Lake
Mental Health Clinical Nurse Educator
BC Children's Hospital
Vancouver, British Columbia

Jennifer Marandola, RN, MN, IBCLC, PNC(C)
Advanced-Practice Nurse Consultant
Maternal Child Program
CIUSSS West-Island of Montreal
Montreal, Quebec

Kathy Martin, RN, BScN, MEd
Faculty
British Columbia Institute of Technology
Burnaby, British Columbia

Gisele Martins, RN, PhD
Associate Professor
Department of Nursing
Faculty of Health Sciences
University of Brasilia (UnB)
Brazil

Tracey McCaig-Beattie, RN, MN
Faculty
School of Nursing
Saskatchewan Polytechnic
Saskatoon, SK Canada

Susan McRae, MN, ACNP, NP (P)
Adjunct Professor
School of Nursing
University of British Columbia
Pediatric Nurse Practitioner
Nurse Practitioner
Child and Youth Primary Care Clinic
British Columbia Children's Hospital
Vancouver, Canada

Lucia New, RN, MBA
Faculty
School of Nursing
Saskatchewan Polytechnic
Saskatoon, SK Canada

Robert Pammett, BSP, MSc
Research and Development Pharmacist—Primary Care
Pharmacy
University Hospital of Northern British Columbia
Prince George, British Columbia

Mary C. Paone, MSN
Adjunct Professor (Ret)
Department of Nursing
UBC School of Nursing
Nursing Lead for Transition (Ret)
Youth Health
BC Children's Hospital
Vancouver, British Columbia

Lisa Papau, MN, Pediatric NP, CPNP
Pediatric Nurse Practitioner
Specialty Medicine
BC Children's Hospital
Vancouver, British Columbia

Kaethe Patterson, BSc, RD
Registered Dietitian
Pediatrics NICU Maternity
University Hospital of Northern
Prince George, British Columbia

Renee Petersen, RN, BScN
Nursing Instructor
College of New Caledonia
University of Northern British Columbia

Dr. Natasha Prodan-Bhalla, BScN, MN/NP (A), DNP
British Columbia Women's Hospital
Health Centre
Vancouver, British Columbia, Canada

Leslie Raffin, RN, BSN, CCRP
Pediatric Nurse Clinician
Department of Cardiology
Children's Heart Centre
British Columbia Children's Hospital
Vancouver, British Columbia

Danielle Raiser, MScN-FNP, BScN
Pender Community Health Centre
Vancouver Coastal Health
Vancouver

Tami Rowe, BScN
Sessional Instructor
School of Nursing
University of Northern British Columbia
Prince George, British Columbia

Kristine H. Rowswell, MSCN – FPN
Family Nurse Practitioner
Primary Care Services
Northern Health
Instructor
University of Northern British Columbia
Prince George, British Columbia

Catharine Schiller, RN, BScN, MSc, JD, PhD (C)
Assistant Professor
School of Nursing
University of Northern British Columbia
Prince George, British Columbia

Ruth Schofield, RN, MSc(T)
Assistant Professor
Faculty of Health Sciences
McMaster University
Hamilton, Ontario

Maia Siedlikowski, MSc
Research Assistant
Clinical Research
Shriners Hospitals for Children—Canada
Montreal, Quebec

Mable Tan, RN, MSN
Nurse Clinician
Endocrine & Diabetes Unit
BC Children's Hospital
Vancouver, British Columbia

Dr. Jonathan Thursfield, D. Clin. Psych
Clinical Psychologist
Prince George, British Columbia

Argerie Tsimicalis, RN, PhD
Assistant Professor
Ingram School of Nursing
McGill University
Montreal, Quebec

Kimberly Wartak, BA, CCLS
Child Life Specialist
Child & Youth Services
Surrey Memorial Hospital
Surrey, British Columbia

Amy Wright, MScN, PhD
Neonatal Intensive Care Unit
McMaster Children's Hospital
Hamilton, Ontario

Reviewers to the Canadian Edition

Christina Barnes, RN, BSN
Sessional Instructor
University of Northern British Columbia
Prince George, British Columbia

Marianne Cochrane, MHSc(N)
Professor
Faculty of Health Sciences
University of Ontario Institute of Technology
Oshawa, Ontario

Kim Derksen, RN, BN, BA, MEd candidate
Department of Nursing
University of Lethbridge
Lethbridge, Alberta

Shelley Doerksen, MSc, SLP(C), RSLP
Speech Language Pathologist
Student Support Services
John McInnis Service Centre
Prince George, British Columbia

Alison Everett
Child Life Specialist
Child & Youth Services
Surrey Memorial Hospital
Surrey, British Columbia

Kim Foster, BSc, PT
Physiothcrapist-Paediatrics & NICU
University Hospital of Northern British Columbia
Prince George, British Columbia

Lisa Goldberg, PhD
Associate Professor and Caritas Coach
Department of Nursing
Dalhousie University
Halifax, Nova Scotia

Mona Haimour, BScN, MScN
Assistant Professor
Department of Nursing
MacEwan University
Edmonton, Alberta

Amandah Hoogbruin, PhD
BSN Faculty
Faculty of Health
Kwantlen Polytechnic University
Surrey, British Columbia

Kelly Kidd, MN
Professor
Department of Health and Community Studies
Algonquin College
Pembroke, Ontario

Sandra Klinck, DEC
Professor, Nursing Program
Champlain College Lennoxville
Sherbrooke, Quebec

Cynthia Mannion, PhD, MSc(A)
Associate Professor
Department of Nursing
University of Calgary
Calgary, Alberta

Natalie Matthews, MSN, RN
Senior Instructor
University of British Columbia
Kelowna, British Columbia

Candi Muise, MN, BScN, RN
Nursing Instructor
Department of Nursing and Allied Health
Keyano College
Fort McMurray, Alberta

Pamela Pastirik, MSN, BN, PNC(C)
Senior Teaching Associate
Department of Nursing and Health Sciences
University of New Brunswick Saint John
Saint John, New Brunswick

Suzette Roy, MN
Assistant Professor
Department of Nursing
MacEwan University
Edmonton, Alberta

Gwen Schmidt, BA
Nursing Instructor
Bow Valley College
Calgary, Alberta

Dorothy Wurst-Thurn, MEd
LPN Instructor
Practical Nursing Program
Northern Lakes College
Grande Prairie, Alberta

Reviewers to the Canadian Edition

Christina Barnes, RN, BN

Maralobe Cochrane, MHScN

Kim Derksen, RN, RN, BA, MA Candidate
Department of Nursing
University of Lethbridge
Lethbridge, Alberta

Shelley MacEwen, RN, SPNC, BST

Alison Farrell

Kim Fraser, RN, PT

Lisa Goldberg, PhD
Associate Professor and Graduate Coordinator
Department of Nursing
Dalhousie University
Halifax, Nova Scotia

Mona Hatzeras, RN, MScN
Assistant Professor
Department of Nursing
University of Lethbridge
Edmonton, Alberta

Amandah Hoogbruin, PhD

Kelly Kidd, RN
Professor
Department of Social and Community Studies
Algonquin College
Pembroke, Ontario

Sandra Killick, RN
Professor, Pre-care Program
Champlain College, Lennoxville
Sherbrooke, Quebec

Cynthia Mannion, PhD, MScN
Associate Professor
Department of Nursing
University of Calgary
Calgary, Alberta

Natalie Mathews, RN, MN
Senior Instructor
University of British Columbia
Kelowna, British Columbia

Carol Maire, MN, BScN, RN
Nursing Instructor
Department of Nursing and Allied Health
Keyano College
Fort McMurray, Alberta

Pamela Parrish, MN, RN, RNCHE
Senior Teaching Associate
Department of Nursing and Health Sciences
University of New Brunswick Saint John
Saint John, New Brunswick

Suzette Roy, RN
Assistant Professor
Department of Nursing
McEwan University
Edmonton, Alberta

Gwen Schmidt, RN
Nursing Instructor
Bow Valley College
Calgary, Alberta

Dorothy Worth-Thurn, MN
University Lecturer
Practical Nurse Program
Northern Lakes College
Grande Prairie, Alberta

Reviewers to the Third U.S. Edition

Dolores Holland, MSN, RN, CNOR
McLennan Community College
Waco, Texas

Terri Kahle, MSN, RNC, CNE
Instructor
Southeast Missouri Hospital College of Nursing
   and Health Sciences
Cape Girardeau, Missouri

Deborah Raines, PhD, EdS, RN, ANEF
Associate Professor
State University of New York at Buffalo
Buffalo, New York

Leslie S. Reifel, MSN, RN, CPNP, CNE
Associate Professor
Sentara College of Health Sciences
Chesapeake, Virginia

Valerie Taylor-Haslip, PhD, RN, FNP
Associate Professor
Chairperson
Department of Nursing
York College
City University of New York
Jamaica, New York

Diane Tinker, RN, MNSc, CNM
Lead Faculty
Obstetrical Nursing
Brookline College
Phoenix, Arizona

Elaine Webber, MS, RNCS, IBCLC
Assistant Professor
University of Detroit Mercy
Huntington Woods, Michigan

Barbara Morrison Wilford, DNP, MBA/HCA, CKC, RN
Associate Professor
Allied Health and Nursing
Lorain County Community College
Elyria, Ohio

Reviewers to the Third U.S. Edition

Preface

Many nursing curricula combine and teach maternity and pediatrics in tandem. This can be viewed as a *natural fit* of two content areas that belong together. Nursing education in general is founded upon the principle of mastering simpler concepts first and incorporating those concepts into the student's knowledge base. The student is then able to progress to problem solving in more complex situations. In today's education climate with reduced class time devoted to specialty courses, it is particularly important for nursing educators to focus on key concepts, rather than attempting to cover everything within a specific topic.

The intent of *Canadian Maternity and Pediatric Nursing* is to provide the nurse the basis needed for sound nursing care of women and children, with a focus on Canadian population. The content in the book will enable the reader to guide women and children toward higher levels of wellness throughout the life cycle. In addition, the focus of the textbook will allow the reader to anticipate, identify, and address common problems and provide timely, evidence-based interventions to reduce long-term sequelae.

This textbook is designed as a practical approach to understanding the health of women and children. The main objective is to help the student build a strong knowledge base and assist with the development of critical thinking skills. Women in our society are becoming empowered to make informed and responsible choices regarding their health and that of their children, but to do so they need the encouragement and support of nurses who care for them. This textbook focuses on women and children throughout their life span, covering a broad scope of topics with emphasis placed upon common issues. Maternity nursing content coverage is comprehensive, yet presented in a concise and straightforward manner. The pediatric nursing content presents the important differences when caring for children compared with caring for adults. A nursing process approach provides relevant information in a concise and nonredundant manner.[1]

Organization

Each chapter of *Canadian Maternity and Pediatric Nursing* focuses on a different aspect of maternity and/or

[1]Nursing Process Overview contains NANDA-I approved nursing diagnoses. Material related to nursing diagnoses is from T. Heather Herdman/Shigemi Kamitsuru (Eds.), NANDA International, Inc. *Nursing Diagnoses: Definitions and Classification 2018-2020*, Eleventh Edition © 2017 NANDA International, ISBN 978-1-62623-929-6. Used by arrangement with the Thieme Group, Stuttgart/New York. In order to make safe and effective judgments using NANDA-I nursing diagnoses it is essential that nurses refer to the definitions and defining characteristics of the diagnoses listed in Appendix G of this text.

pediatric nursing care. The book is divided into 11 units, beginning with general concepts related to maternity and pediatric nursing care, progressing from women's health, pregnancy and birth, through child health promotion and nursing management of alterations in children's health.

Unit 1: Introduction to Maternity and Pediatric Nursing

Unit 1 helps build a foundation for the student beginning the study of the care of women, infants, and children. This unit explores contemporary issues and trends in maternity and pediatric nursing. Perspectives on women's health and pediatric nursing, core concepts of maternal and pediatric nursing, including, family-centred and atraumatic care, and communication, and community-based nursing are addressed.

Unit 2: Women's Health Throughout the Life Span

Unit 2 introduces the student to selected women's health topics, including structure and function of the reproductive system, common reproductive concerns, sexually transmitted infections, problems of the breast, and benign disorders and cancers of the female reproductive tract. This unit encourages the student to assist women in maintaining their quality of life, reducing their risk of disease, and becoming active partners with their health care professional.

Unit 3: Pregnancy

Unit 3 addresses topics related to normal pregnancy, including fetal development, genetics, and maternal adaptation to pregnancy. Nursing management during normal pregnancy is addressed, encouraging application of basic knowledge to nursing practice. Nursing management includes maternal and fetal assessment throughout pregnancy, interventions to promote self-care and minimize common discomforts, and patient education.

Unit 4: Labour and Birth

Unit 4 begins with an explanation of the normal labour and birth process, including maternal and fetal adaptations. This is followed by content focusing on the nurse's role during normal labour and birth, which includes maternal and fetal assessment, pharmacologic and non-pharmacologic comfort measures and pain management, and specific nursing interventions during each stage of labour and birth.

Unit 5: Postpartum Period

Unit 5 focuses on maternal adaptation during the normal postpartum period. Both physiologic and psychological aspects are explored. Paternal adaptation is also considered. This unit also presents related nursing management, including assessment of physical and emotional status, promoting comfort, assisting with elimination, counselling about sexuality and contraception, promoting nutrition, promoting family adaptation, and preparing for discharge.

Unit 6: The Newborn

Unit 6 covers physiologic and behavioural adaptations of the normal newborn. It also delves into nursing management of the normal newborn, including immediate assessment and specific interventions as well as ongoing assessment, physical examination, and specific interventions during the early newborn period.

Unit 7: Childbearing at Risk

Unit 7 shifts the focus to at-risk pregnancy, childbirth, and postpartum care. Pre-existing conditions of the woman, pregnancy-related complications, at-risk labour, emergencies associated with labour and birth, and medical conditions and complications affecting the postpartum woman are all covered. Treatment and nursing management are presented for each medical condition. This organization allows the student to build on a solid foundation of normal material when studying the at-risk content.

Unit 8: The Newborn at Risk

Unit 8 continues to centre on at-risk content. Issues of the newborn with birth weight variations, gestational age variations, congenital conditions, and acquired disorders are explored. Treatment and nursing management are presented for each medical condition. This organization helps cement the student's understanding of the material.

Unit 9: Health Promotion of the Growing Child and Family

Unit 9 provides information related to growth and development expectations of the well child from newborn through adolescence. Although not exhaustive in nature, this unit provides a broad knowledge base related to normal growth and development that the nurse can draw on in any situation. Common concerns related to growth and development and client/family education are included in each age-specific chapter.

Unit 10: Foundations of Pediatric Nursing

Unit 10 covers broad concepts that provide the foundation for providing nursing care for children. Rather than reiterating all aspects of nursing care, the unit focuses on specific details needed to provide nursing care for children in general. The content remains focused upon differences in caring for children compared with adults. Topics covered in this unit include atraumatic care, anticipatory guidance, and routine well child care (including immunization and safety), health assessment, nursing care of the child in diverse settings, including the hospital and at home, concerns common to special needs children, pediatric variations in medication and intravenous fluid delivery and nutritional support, and pain management in children.

Unit 11: Nursing Care of the Child With a Health Disorder

Unit 11 focuses on children's responses to health disorders. This unit provides comprehensive coverage of illnesses affecting children and is presented according to broad topics of disorders organized with a body systems approach. It also includes infectious, genetic, and mental health disorders as well as pediatric emergencies. Each chapter follows a similar format in order to facilitate presentation of the information as well as reduce repetition. The chapters begin with a nursing process overview for the particular broad topic, presenting differences in children and how the nursing process applies. The approach provides a general framework for addressing disorders within the chapter. Individual disorders are then addressed with attention to specifics related to pathophysiology, nursing assessment, nursing management, and special considerations. Common pediatric disorders are covered in greater depth than less common disorders. The format of the chapters allows for the building of a strong knowledge base and encourages critical thinking. In addition, the format is nursing process driven and consistent from chapter to chapter, providing a practical and sensible presentation of the information.

Recurring Features

In order to provide the instructor and student with an exciting and user-friendly text, a number of recurring features have been developed.

Key Terms

A list of terms that are considered essential to the chapter's understanding is presented at the beginning of each chapter. Each key term appears in boldface, with the definition included in the text.

Learning Objectives

Learning Objectives included at the beginning of each chapter guide the student in understanding what is important and why, leading the student to prioritize information for learning. These valuable learning tools also provide opportunities for self-testing or instructor evaluation of student knowledge and ability.

Threaded Case Studies

Real-life scenarios present relevant woman, child, and family information that are intended to hone the student's caregiving skills. Questions about the scenario provide an opportunity for the student to critically evaluate the appropriate course of action.

Evidence-Based Practice

The consistent promotion of evidence-based practice is a key feature of the text. Throughout the chapters, pivotal questions addressed by current research have been incorporated into Evidence-Based Practice displays, which cite studies relevant to chapter content.

Atraumatic Care

These highlights, located throughout the pediatric sections of the book, provide tips for providing atraumatic care to children in particular situations in relation to the topic being discussed.

Thinking About Development

The content featured in these boxes in chapters related to the care of children will encourage student to think critically about special developmental concerns relating to the topic being discussed.

Teaching Guidelines

An important tool for achieving health promotion and disease prevention is health education. Throughout the textbook, Teaching Guidelines raise awareness, provide timely and accurate information, and are designed to ensure the student's preparation for educating women, children, and their families about various issues.

Consider This

In every chapter the student is asked to *Consider This*. These first-person narratives engage the student in real-life scenarios experienced by their clients. The personal accounts evoke empathy and help the student to perfect caregiving skills. Each box ends with an opportunity for further contemplation, encouraging the student to think critically about the scenario.

Take Note!

The *Take Note!* feature draws the student's attention to points of critical emphasis throughout the chapter. This feature is often used to stress life-threatening or otherwise vitally important information.

Safety Checks

In several chapters the student is asked to review goals linked to the safe use of medications. These brief safety checks emphasize harm reduction when using high-risk medications.

Drug Guides

Drug guide tables summarize information about commonly used medications. The actions, indications, and significant nursing implications presented assist the student in providing optimum care to women, children, and their families.

Common Laboratory and Diagnostic Tests

The Common Laboratory and Diagnostic Tests tables in many of the chapters provide the student with a general understanding of how a broad range of disorders is diagnosed. Rather than reading the information repeatedly throughout the narrative, the student is then able to refer to the table as needed.

Common Medical Treatments

The Common Medical Treatments tables in many of the nursing management chapters provide the student with a broad awareness of how a common group of disorders is treated either medically or surgically. The tables serve as a reference point for common medical treatments.

Nursing Care Plans

Nursing Care Plans provide concrete examples of each step of the nursing process and are included in numerous chapters. The Nursing Care Plans summarize issue- or system-related content, thereby minimizing repetition.

Comparison Charts

These charts compare two or more disorders or other easily confused concepts. They serve to provide an explanation that clarifies the concepts for the student.

Nursing Procedures

Step-by-step Nursing Procedures are presented in a clear, concise format to facilitate competent performance of relevant procedures as well as to clarify pediatric variations when appropriate.

Icons

 WATCH AND LEARN

A special icon throughout the book directs students to free video clips locate on thePoint that highlight growth and development, communicating with children, and providing nursing care to the child in the hospital.

 CONCEPTS IN ACTION ANIMATIONS

These unique animations, also located on thePoint bring physiologic and pathophysiologic concepts to life and enhance student comprehension.

Tables, Boxes, Illustrations, and Photographs

Abundant tables and boxes summarize key content throughout the book. In addition, beautiful illustrations and photographs help the student to visualize the content. These features allow the student to quickly and easily access information.

Key Concepts

At the end of each chapter, Key Concepts provide a quick review of essential chapter elements. These bulleted lists help the student focus on the important aspects of the chapter.

References and Helpful Websites

References used in the development of the text are provided at the end of each chapter. These listings enable the student to further explore topics of interest. Many online resources are provided on thePoint as a means for the student to electronically explore relevant content material. These resources can be shared with women, children, and their families to enhance patient education and support.

Chapter Worksheets

Chapter worksheets at the end of each chapter assist the student in reviewing essential concepts. Chapter worksheets include:

- **Multiple Choice Questions**—These review questions are written to test the student's ability to apply chapter material. Questions cover maternal-newborn, women's health, and pediatric content that

the student might encounter on the national licensing exam (NCLEX®).
- **Critical Thinking Exercises**—These exercises challenge the student to incorporate new knowledge with previously learned concepts and reach a satisfactory conclusion. They encourage the student to think critically, problem solve, and consider his or her own perspective on given topics.
- **Study Activities**—These interactive activities promote student participation in the learning process. This section encourages increased interaction/learning via clinical, online, and community activities.

Teaching–Learning Package
Instructor's Resources

Tools to assist you with teaching your course are available upon adoption of this text on thePoint.

- An **E-Book** on thePoint gives you access to the book's full text and images online.
- A **Test Generator** that features hundreds of questions within a powerful tool to help the instructor create quizzes and tests.
- **PowerPoint presentations** with **Guided Lecture Notes** provide an easy way for you to integrate the textbook with our students' class-room experience, either via slide shows or handouts. Multiple choice and true/false questions are integrated into the presentations to promote class participation and allow you to use i-clicker technology.
- An **Image Bank** lets you use the photographs and illustrations from this textbook in your PowerPoint slides or as you see fit in your course.
- **Case Studies** with related questions (and suggested answers) give students an opportunity to apply their knowledge to a client case similar to one they might encounter in practice.
- **Pre-Lecture Quizzes** (and answers) are quick, knowledge-based assessments that allow you to check students' reading.
- **Discussion Topics** (and suggested answers) can be used as conversation starters or in online discussion boards.
- **Assignments** (and suggested answers) include group, written, clinical, and web assignments.
- Sample **Syllabi** provide guidance for structuring your pediatric nursing courses and are provided for four different course lengths: 6, 8, 10, and 15 weeks.
- **Journal Articles,** updated for the new edition, offer access to current research available in Lippincott Williams & Wilkins journals.

Contact your sales representative or check out LWW.com/Nursing for more details and ordering information.

Student Resources

An exciting set of free resources is available to help students review material and become even more familiar with vital concepts. Students can access all these resources on thePoint using the codes printed in the front of their textbooks.

- **NCLEX-Style Review Questions** for each chapter help students review important concepts and practice for NCLEX. **Over 700 questions** are included, more than twice as many as last edition!

- **Multimedia Resources** appeal to a variety of learning styles. Icons in the text direct readers to relevant videos and animations:
  - **Watch and Learn Videos** highlight growth and development, communicating with children, and providing nursing care to the child in the hospital.
  - **Concepts in Action Animations** bring physiologic and pathophysiologic concepts to life and enhance student comprehension.
- **Journal Articles** offer access to current research available in Lippincott Williams & Wilkins journals.

Contents in Brief

Contents

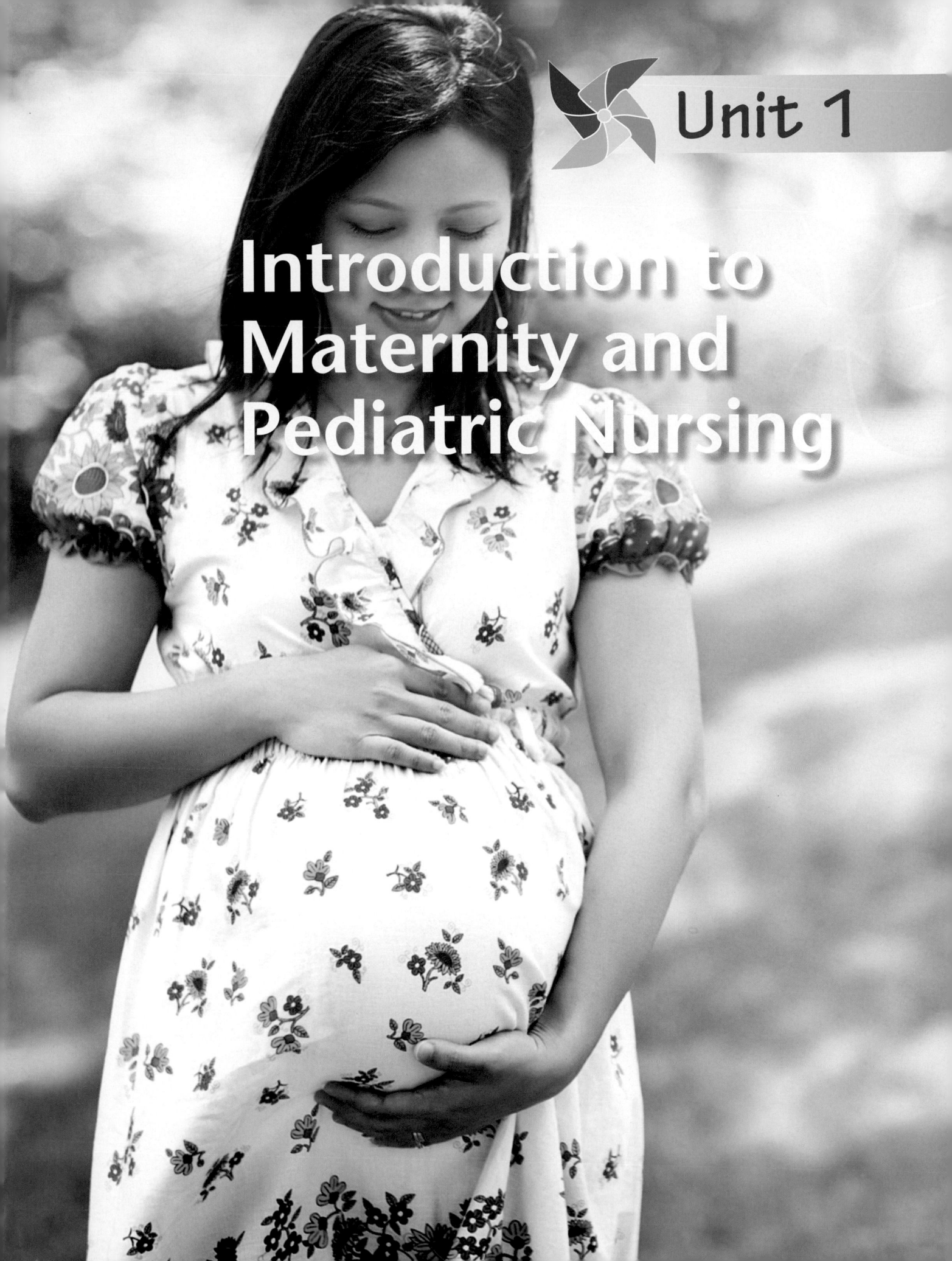

Unit 1

Introduction to Maternity and Pediatric Nursing

Perspectives on Maternal and Child Health Care

Learning Objectives

Upon completion of the chapter, you will be able to:

1. Analyze the key milestones in the history of maternal, newborn, and child health and health care.

2. Outline the evolution of maternal, newborn, and pediatric nursing.

3. Compare the past definitions of health and illness to the current definitions, as well as the measurements used to assess health and illness in children.

4. Assess the factors that affect maternal and child health.

5. Differentiate the structures, roles, and functions of the family and how they affect the health of women and children.

6. Evaluate how society and culture can influence the health of women, children, and families.

7. Appraise the health care barriers affecting women, children, and families.

8. Research the ethical and legal issues that may arise when caring for women, children, and families.

Sophia Greenly, a 38-year-old woman pregnant with her third child, comes to the prenatal clinic for a routine follow-up visit. Her mother, Betty, accompanies her because Sophia's husband is out of town. Sophia lives with her husband and two children, ages 4 and 9. She works part-time as a lunch aide in the local elementary school. What factors may play a role in influencing the health of Sophia and her family?

INTRODUCTION

A person's ability to lead a fulfilling life and to participate fully in society depends largely on their health status. This is especially true for women, who commonly are responsible for not only their own health, but also that of others: their children and families. Thus, it is important to concentrate on the health of women, children, and families (Government of Canada, 2019; Human Early Learning Partnership [HELP], 2019). Although the overall health of children has improved and the rates of death and illness in some areas have decreased (Raising Canada, 2018), the need to focus on the health of women and children remains a priority at government and provincial levels (i.e., Provincial Council for Maternal and Child Health [PCMCH], 2019). Habits and practices established during pregnancy and early childhood can have profound effects on a person's health and illness throughout life (Gonzalez et al., 2018). As a society, creating a population that cares about women, children, and families while promoting accessible health care and lifestyle choices is crucial.

Maternity care is an integrated care process, which consists of different services (prenatal, intranatal, and postnatal), involves different professionals, and covers extended time frames. Maternal and newborn nursing encompasses a wide scope of practice typically associated with childbearing. It includes care of the individual before pregnancy, care of the person and fetus during pregnancy, care of the client after pregnancy, and care of the newborn, usually during the first 6 weeks after birth. The overall goal of maternal and newborn nursing is to promote and maintain optimal health of the individual and the family. Providing quality maternity care includes client satisfaction and achieving best evidence-based outcomes with the fewest interventions.

Child health nursing, commonly referred to as pediatric nursing, involves the care of the child from infancy through adolescence. In Canada, there are approximately 7.9 million children under the age of 18 years, accounting for 22.4% of the population; 51.3% male to 48.7% female (Statistics Canada, 2016). The overall goal of pediatric nursing practice is to promote and assist the child in maintaining optimal levels of health, while recognizing the influence of the family on the child's well-being. This goal involves health promotion and disease, illness, and injury prevention as well as assisting with care during illness across a continuum of settings (Children's Healthcare Canada, 2018). The common thread in both of these is the care of the family (Children's Healthcare Canada, 2018).

This chapter presents a general overview of the health care of women, children, and families and describes the major factors affecting maternal and child health. Nurses need to be knowledgeable about these concepts and factors to ensure that they provide professional care.

HISTORICAL DEVELOPMENT

The health care of women and children has changed over the years due in part to changes in childbirth methods, devastating epidemics, social trends in our country, changes in the health care system, and federal and provincial regulations. By reviewing historical events, nurses can gain a better understanding of the current and future status of maternal and child health and how maternal and pediatric nursing care has evolved.

The History of Maternal and Newborn Health and Health Care

Childbirth in colonial North America was a difficult and dangerous experience. During the 17th and 18th centuries, women giving birth often died as a result of exhaustion, dehydration, infection, hemorrhage, or seizures. Approximately 50% of all children died before age 5 (Norman, 2015), compared with the 0.45% infant mortality rate in Canada today (World Health Organization [WHO], 2018).

There was a time when nearly every infant that came into this world was attended by a midwife (Relyea, 1992). Centuries ago, "granny midwives" handled the normal birthing process for most families. These lay midwives learned their skills through an apprenticeship with a more experienced midwife. Physicians usually were called only in extremely difficult cases, and all births took place at home. The medicalization of birth in the 19th century drove midwifery to the periphery, but within the last century, midwifery has reemerged as an organized profession, appearing everywhere from home births to hospital labour units (Plummer, 2000). Those who laboured and gave birth at home were traditionally attended to by relatives and midwives. Having continuous support during childbirth yields better outcomes (Evidence-Based Practice 1.1).

During the early 1900s, physicians attended about half the births in the North America. Midwives often cared for those who could not afford a doctor (Rooks, 2014). Many people were attracted to hospitals for birthing because this showed affluence and provided pain management, which was not available with home births. In the 1950s, "natural childbirth" practices advocating birth without medication and focusing on relaxation techniques were introduced. These techniques opened the door to childbirth education classes and helped bring the father back into the picture. Both partners could participate by taking an active role in pregnancy, childbirth, and parenting (Fig. 1.1).

Box 1.1 shows a time line of childbirth in North America. In many ways, childbirth practices in Canada have come full circle, as we see the return of **licensed midwives** and **doulas**. Regulated midwifery care is available in nearly all provinces and territories, with the exception of Newfoundland, Prince Edward Island, and the Yukon territory (Canadian Association of Midwives

EVIDENCE-BASED PRACTICE 1.1   CONTINUOUS SUPPORT DURING CHILDBIRTH

STUDY

Throughout history, women have been helping other women in labour by providing emotional support, comfort measures, information, and advocacy. However, in recent years this practice has waned, and facilities frequently adhere to strict specific routines that may leave the pregnant individual feeling "dehumanized." A study was done to assess the effects on mothers and their newborns of continuous, one-to-one intrapartum care in comparison to usual care. The study also evaluated routine practices and policies in the birth environment that might affect a woman's autonomy, freedom of movement, and ability to cope with labour; who the caregiver was, whether or not a staff member of the facility; and when the support began, early or late in labour.

All published and unpublished randomized clinical trials (23) comparing continuous support during labour with usual care were examined involving 15,000 women. One author and one research assistant used standard methods for data collection and analysis and extracted the data independently. Clinical trial authors provided additional information. The researchers used relative risk for categorical data and weighted mean difference for continuous data.

Findings

Women receiving continuous intrapartum support had a greater chance of a spontaneous vaginal delivery (including without forceps or vacuum extraction). They also had a slight decrease in the length of labour and required less analgesia during this time. These women also reported increased satisfaction with their labour and childbirth experience. Overall, the support, when provided by someone other than a facility staff member and initiated early in labour, proved to be more effective.

Nursing Implications

Based on this research, it is clear that individuals in labour benefit from one-to-one support during that experience. Nurses can use the information gained from this study to educate clients about the importance of support persons during labour and delivery. Nurses can also act as client advocates in facilities where they work to foster an environment that encourages the use of support persons during the intrapartum period. The focus of nursing needs to be individualized, supportive, and collaborative with the family during their childbearing experience. In short, nurses should place the needs of the client and family first in providing a continuum of care.

Although the study found that support is more effective when provided by someone other than a staff member, support from an individual is essential. Assigning the same nurse to provide care to the couple throughout the birthing experience also fosters a one-to-one relationship that helps meet the couple's needs and promotes feelings of security. By meeting the couple's needs, the nurse is enhancing their birthing experience.

Bohren, M. A., Hofmeyr, G. J., Sakala, C., Fukuzawa, R. K., & Cuthbert, A. (2017). Continuous support for women during childbirth. *Cochrane Database of Systematic Reviews*, *7*, CD003766. doi: 10.1002/14651858.CD003766.pub6

[CAM], 2019a). Today, childbirth choices are often based on what works best for the parents and family. Political discourses continue, linked to "evacuation" birthing, or the need for women on rural and remote reserves to leave home communities (Lawford, Giles & Bourgeault, 2018; Olson & Couchie, 2013).

The History of Child Health and Child Health Care

Canada's history of public health dates back to well before the arrival of European settlers. Indigenous people inhabiting this land practiced traditional methods of

FIGURE 1.1 Today fathers and partners are encouraged to take an active role in the pregnancy and childbirth experience. **A.** A couple can participate together in childbirth education classes. (Photo by Gus Freedman.) **B.** Fathers and partners can assist the pregnant partner throughout the labour and birth. (Photo by Joe Mitchell.)

BOX 1.1

CHILDBIRTH IN NORTH AMERICA: A TIME LINE

1700s   Men did not attend births because it was considered indecent.
Women faced birth not with joy and ecstasy but with fear of death.
Female midwives attended the majority of all births at home.

1800s   There is a shift from using midwives to doctors among middle-class women.
The word *obstetrician* was formed from the Latin, meaning "to stand before."
Puerperal (childbed) fever was occurring in epidemic proportions.
Louis Pasteur demonstrated that streptococci were the major cause of puerperal fever that was killing mothers after delivery.
The first cesarean section was performed in Boston in 1894.
The x-ray was developed in 1895 and was used to assess pelvic size for birthing purposes.

1900s   Twilight sleep (a heavy dose of narcotics and amnesiacs) was used on women during childbirth in the United States.
50% to 75% of all births took place in hospitals by 1940.
Nurseries were started because mothers could not care for their baby for several days after receiving chloroform gas.
Dr. Grantly Dick-Read (1933) wrote *Childbirth Without Fear,* which reduced the "fear–tension–pain" cycle women experienced during labour and birth.
Dr. Fernand Lamaze (1984) wrote *Painless Childbirth: The Lamaze Method,* which advocated distraction and relaxation techniques to minimize the perception of pain.
Amniocentesis was first performed to assess fetal growth in 1966.
In the 1970s the cesarean section rate was about 5%. In 2011, it rose to 32%, where it stands currently.
The 1970s and 1980s see a growing trend to return birthing back to the basics—nonmedicated, nonintervening childbirth.
In the late 1900s, freestanding birthing centres—LDRPs—were designed, and the number of home births began to increase.

2000s   One in three women undergoes a surgical birth (caesarean).
Registered midwives once again assist couples at home, in hospitals, or in freestanding facilities with natural childbirths. Research shows that midwives are the safest birth attendants for most women, with lower infant mortality and maternal rates, and fewer invasive interventions such as episiotomies and caesareans.
Childbirth classes of every flavour abound in most communities.
According to the latest available data, Canada ranks 161st in the world in maternal deaths. The maternal mortality ratio is approximately 7 in 100,000 live births.
According to the latest available data, Canada ranks 180th in the world (compared to 224 other countries) in infant mortality rates. The infant mortality rate is approximately 4.5 in 1,000 live births.

Adapted from CIA World Factbook. (2019a). *Country comparison: Infant mortality rate.* Retrieved from https://www.cia.gov/library/publications/the-world-factbook/rankorder/2091rank.html; CIA World Factbook. (2019b). *Country comparison: Maternal mortality rate.* Retrieved from https://www.cia.gov/library/publications/resources/the-world-factbook/fields/353rank.html; and Cox, K. J., & King, T. L. (2015). Preventing primary cesarean births: Midwifery care. *Clinical Obstetrics and Gynecology, 58*(2), 282–293.

---

balancing health through sensitive and intentional respect of the earth and each other. Europeans brought diseases to this land, for which Indigenous people had little protection (Public Health Agency of Canada [PHAC], 2008).

In the 18th and 19th centuries, the health of people living in Canada was poor: mortality rates were high and life expectancy was short. Infectious diseases were rampant, and unsanitary food sources contributed to illness in children. Devastating epidemics of smallpox, diphtheria, scarlet fever, and measles hit children and Indigenous communities the hardest. During this period, the dominant colonial view was that children were a commodity; their role was to increase the population and share in the work to be done. This view changed over the years. Public schools were established, and the court

system began viewing children as minors. The health of children began to receive more and more attention.

A grievous practice in Canadian history during this time was the implementation of the residential school program for Indigenous children. Over 150,000 First Nations, Inuit, and Métis children were removed from their homes and families over the course of a century. These children were forced to live in English-speaking federally funded colonial schools, many of which were jointly operated through Anglican, Presbyterian, Catholic, or United Churches, in efforts to assimilate the children into the dominant settler culture. Inside these residential schools, many children endured years of physical, emotional, and sexual abuse. The loss of Indigenous people's language, culture, and familial relationships continues to have a direct impact on the health and wellness of Indigenous families and children in Canada today (Hanson, 2009).

Take Note!

In 2008, the Prime Minister of Canada, Stephen Harper, issued a formal apology to Indigenous families and community members, stating that: "Today, we recognize that this policy of assimilation was wrong, has caused great harm, and has no place in our country" (Government of Canada, 2013, para 2).

In the late 19th and early 20th centuries, public health improvements such as sanitation services, treated municipal water, and improvements in hygiene led to great improvements in the health of Canadian populations. Water-borne diseases such as cholera and typhoid began to take less of a toll on children (PHAC, 2008). The turn of the 20th century brought new knowledge about nutrition, sanitation, bacteriology, pharmacology, medication, and psychology. Penicillin, corticosteroids, and increased numbers of vaccines, which were developed during this time, assisted with the fight against communicable diseases. Thus, by the end of the 20th century, unintentional injuries surpassed disease as the leading cause of death for children greater than 1 year old (Epstein, 2011).

A steady decline in infant mortality over the last six decades has resulted in a rate of 4.5 deaths per 1,000 live births (Raising Canada, 2018). Continued focus on lowering mortality and morbidity focuses on public health approaches aimed at injury prevention (Yanchar, Warda, & Fuselli, 2012) as well as wider health promotion and population health strategies.

Technologic advances have significantly affected all aspects of health care and led to increased survival rates in children. However, many children who survive illnesses that were previously considered fatal can be left with chronic disabilities. For example, before the 1960s, extremely premature infants did not survive because of the immaturity of their lungs. Mechanical ventilation and the use of medications to foster lung development have increased survival rates in premature infants, but survivors are often faced with a myriad of chronic illnesses such as chronic lung disease (bronchopulmonary dysplasia), retinopathy of prematurity, cerebral palsy, or developmental delay. This increased survival has resulted in a significant increase in chronic illness relative to acute illness as a cause of hospitalization and mortality (Kelly, 2010).

In recent years advances in biomedicine have created a trend toward earlier diagnosis and treatment of disorders and diseases. Additionally, in utero gene therapy, fetoscopy, and maternal pharmacologic treatments have been targeted toward pathophysiologic processes with an aim to reduce maternal and child morbidity (Ulivi & Breeze, 2018). In addition, early genetic defect identification allows for appropriate counselling.

In addition to improvement in technology and biomedicine, a number of national and international organizations have been formed in recent years to protect children's rights both in Canada (i.e., Children First Canada, 2018; Children's Healthcare Canada, 2018) and worldwide (UNICEF Canada, 2019). These organizations focus on such issues as basic rights, violence and abuse, child labour and soldiering, juvenile justice, child immigrants and orphaned children, and abandonment and homelessness—all of which have a negative impact on children's health. A child whose rights are restored and upheld has an improved opportunity for growth, development, education, and health.

The gains in child health have been huge but, unfortunately, these gains are not shared equally among all children. Certain health concerns such as asthma, obesity, poor nutrition, environmental toxin exposure, and learning or behavioural disorders affect children from families with socioeconomic challenges at higher rates than those from affluent and middle-class families (HELP, 2019; Seith & Isakson, 2011). Children from Indigenous families face a higher rate of acute and chronic illnesses (Anderson, Lyons, Luke, & Reich, 2017) and greater differences between birth outcomes than non-Indigenous people (Philpott, 2018; Shapiro et al., 2018; Sheppard et al., 2017).

Evolution of Maternal and Newborn Nursing

The history of maternity nursing is characterized by innovations that became common practice in later years. These innovations include fetal monitoring, mother/baby care, and early postpartum discharge. The driving forces behind changes in care within the social context of the times were scientific/medical developments and families' desires for the best possible childbearing experience.

Prior to World War II, Canadian women moved from home to the hospital for childbirth in part because they were convinced that setting would improve birth outcomes. Hospitals were the major employers of maternity nurses. Early ambulation and rooming-in induced changes in the focus of care for the growing numbers of mothers and infants. Maternity nurses' focus shifted away from carrying out tasks and performing procedures to teaching mothers about self and infant care. Improved staffing patterns within hospitals meant longer hospital stays for the mothers, which allowed maternity nurses to spend more time with mothers for teaching purposes. Maternity nursing has changed dramatically since the Baby Boom era. The natural childbirth movement became a catalyst to bring about a change in nursing practice on the postpartum nursing units.

Other innovations that came later included breastfeeding and rooming-in to facilitate maternal–newborn bonding. Maternity nurses were then able to help the new mothers learn better how to care for their infants, to promote breastfeeding and bonding. The mid-1960s and early 1970s ushered in a consumer revolt which brought back home births, prepared childbirth, birth centres, the father/partner's involvement in the birthing process, and midwives—which had all but disappeared from the health care system (Stapleton, 2017). Maternal–infant bonding became recognized as an essential part of postnatal care, and maternity nurses took a lead role to facilitate it.

With innovations becoming commonplace, maternity nursing practice has become more complex. How maternity nurses approach present-day challenges of increasing technology of birth, looming threats of litigation, and providing care under time and economic restraints is continuing to evolve.

A regulated midwife has a baccalaureate education in the care of normal pregnancy and delivery and is registered with their provincial regulating body, overseen by CAM. Midwives are primary care providers for women with a special emphasis on pregnancy, childbirth, and reproductive health. They are committed to providing ethical, individualized, evidence-based care for all women throughout their prenatal, birth, and postnatal care (CAM, 2019b).

A doula is a nonmedical birth companion who provides continuous emotional, physical, and educational support to the pregnant client and family during childbirth and the postpartum period. Doulas do not perform clinical or medical tasks; they are there to comfort and support the mother and partner with a view to enhance communication between the mother and medical professionals (DONA International, 2019). Many nurses working in labour and birth areas today are credentialed in their specialty so that they can provide optimal care to the woman and her newborn. The Canadian Nurses Association (CNA) offers a self-study and examination program for certification in perinatal nursing. This certification shows a commitment to lifelong learning and the ability to stay up to date in the rapidly changing health care environment (CNA, 2019).

Evolution of Pediatric Nursing

Much of nursing's approach to pediatric care in Canada has been informed by the United States. In 1870, the first pediatric professorship for a physician was awarded in the United States to Abraham Jacobi, known as the father of pediatrics. For the first time, the medical community realized the need to provide specialized training and education about children to health care providers. In the early 1900s, Lillian Wald established the Henry Street Settlement House in New York City; this was the start of public health nursing. This facility provided medical and other services to poor families. These services included home nurse visits to teach mothers about health care.

During this time, health care personnel were trained to take care of children in hospitals, but parents of hospitalized children were discouraged from visiting to prevent the spread of infection. Restricting parents from being involved in their child's care was also thought to minimize emotional stress. However, this shifted in the mid-1960s with the emergence of child- and family-centred care within pediatric nursing (Coyne, Hallström, & Söderbäck, 2016; Shields, 2015). The CNA (2005) has long identified the goal of nursing as family centred which includes acute, community, and school settings for the care of children and their families. While some countries have specific nurse training for pediatric nursing, North America is at the stage of exploring the feasibility of further specific pediatric examinations with the CNA currently taking the lead supported by Children's Healthcare Canada and the Canadian Association of Paediatric Nurses.

HEALTH STATUS OF WOMEN AND CHILDREN

At one time, health was defined simply as the absence of disease. Health was measured by monitoring the mortality and morbidity of a group. Over the past century, however, the focus on health has shifted to disease prevention, health promotion, and wellness. The WHO (2019a) defines health as "a state of complete physical, mental, and social well-being, and not merely the absence of disease or infirmity." The definition of health is complex. It is not merely the absence of disease or an analysis of mortality and morbidity statistics but also linked to the conditions in which people live (Canadian Foundation for Healthcare Improvement, 2019).

There are specific health topic areas, including women and children's health topics, which serve as a method for evaluation of progress made in public health (Box 1.2). These topic areas also serve as focal points to coordinate the national health improvement efforts as linked to a range of outcomes—health promoting approaches, social determinants of health, and maternal and infant mental health and wellbeing (PHAC, 2019).

Measuring health status is not always a simple process. For example, some women and children with chronic illnesses do not see themselves as "ill" if their disease is under control. A traditional method of measuring health is to examine mortality and morbidity data. This information is collected and analyzed to provide an objective description of the nation's health.

Mortality

Mortality is the incidence or number of people who have died over a specific period. This statistic is presented as rates per 1,000 live births and is calculated from a sample of death certificates (Raising Canada, 2018; Statistics Canada, 2018c).

BOX 1.2

FOUR FOUNDATIONAL HEALTH MEASURES

1. General Health Status
   • Measures include:
     • Life expectancy
     • Healthy life expectancy
     • Years of potential life lost
     • Physically and mentally unhealthy days
     • Self-assessed health status
     • Limitation of activity
     • Chronic disease prevalence
2. Health-Related Quality of Life and Well-Being
   • Measures include:
     • Physical, mental, and social health-related quality of life
     • Well-being/satisfaction
     • Participation in common activities
3. Key Determinants of Health (a range of personal, social, economic, and environmental factors that influence health status)
   • Include:
     • Income and social status
     • Social support networks
     • Education and literacy
     • Employment/working conditions
     • Social environments
     • Physical environments
     • Personal health practices and coping skills
     • Healthy child development
     • Biology and genetic endowment
     • Health services
     • Gender
     • Culture
4. Disparities
   • Measures include differences in health status based on demographics, health behaviours, and environmental contexts including:
     • Race/ethnicity
     • Gender
     • Physical and mental ability
     • Geography

Adapted from Health Canada. (2016). *Government of Canada health portfolio*. Retrieved from https://www.150.statcan.gc.ca/n1/pub/82-229-x/2009001/demo/int1-eng.htm

Maternal Mortality

The maternal mortality ratio is the annual number of deaths from any cause related to or aggravated by pregnancy or its management (excluding accidental or incidental causes) during pregnancy and childbirth or within 42 days of termination of pregnancy, irrespective of the duration and site of the pregnancy, per 100,000 live births, for a specified year. In Canada, there are approximately 6.1% maternal deaths per 100,000 deliveries. The rate of maternal mortality in Canada has decreased in the last decade but continues to be studied as a significant proportion of these deaths are preventable (Maron, 2015). The most common diagnosis linked to maternal death includes postpartum

hemorrhage, hypertension, disease of the digestive system, and mental health difficulties (PHAC, 2017).

In Canada, the maternal mortality ratio is mixed depending on ethnic background. Indigenous women suffer maternal mortality ratios far higher than any other ethnic group.

During the past several decades, mortality and morbidity have dramatically decreased as a result of an increased emphasis on hygiene, good nutrition, exercise, and prenatal care for all women. However, women are still experiencing complications at significant rates (PHAC, 2017). **Maternal mortality** is defined as the number of maternal deaths in pregnancy, during birth, up to 42 days postnatal or termination of pregnancy (PHAC, 2017). Increasing childbearing age, diversity of demographics (i.e., refugee and immigration trends), rurality, and wider social economic factors impact morbidity and mortality risk for women (Khanlou, Haque, Skinner, Mantini, & Kurtz Landy, 2017).

The perinatal and newborn mortality rates for Indigenous populations in Canada are nearly two times higher than that of the rest of the population (Verstraeten, Mijovic-Kondejewski, Takeda, Tanaka, & Olson, 2015). Suspected causes of the higher maternal mortality rates for minority women include low socioeconomic status, bias among health care providers (which may foster distrust), and quality of care available in the community. Language and legal barriers may also explain why some newcomers to Canada do not receive good prenatal care (Khanlou et al., 2017). Lack of care during pregnancy is a major factor contributing to a poor outcome. Prenatal care is well known to prevent complications of pregnancy and to support the birth of healthy infants, but not all pregnant individuals receive the same quality and quantity or experience of maternity of health care services (PHAC, 2009b). Eliminating racial and ethnic disparities in maternal–child health care requires enhanced efforts at preventing disease, promoting health, and delivering appropriate and timely care.

Fetal Mortality

The fetal mortality rate or fetal death rate refers to the spontaneous intrauterine death of a fetus at any time during pregnancy per 1,000 live births. Fetal deaths later in pregnancy (>20 weeks of gestation) are also referred to as stillbirths. Fetal mortality may be attributable to maternal factors (e.g., malnutrition, disease, or preterm cervical dilation) or fetal factors (e.g., chromosomal abnormalities or poor placental attachment) (Centers for Disease Control and Prevention [CDC], 2018a).

Fetal mortality is a major, but often overlooked, public health problem. **Fetal mortality** refers to spontaneous intrauterine death at any time during pregnancy. Much of the public concern regarding reproductive loss has concentrated on infant mortality, as less is known about fetal mortality. However, the impact of fetal mortality on Canadian families is considerable, as it provides an overall picture of the quality of maternal health and prenatal care.

Neonatal and Infant Mortality

The **neonatal mortality** rate is the number of infant deaths occurring in the first 28 days of life per 1,000 live births. A mortality rate of 5.7 per 1,000 births for perinatal deaths appears to range between 5.7 and 6.0 per 1,000 over a 5-year period (2012–2016) (Statistics Canada, 2019a). Furthermore, the burden is inequitably carried by the poor. Evidence-based strategies are urgently needed to reduce the burden of intrapartum-related deaths and effective interventions to address these problems must be incorporated into policy decisions (Oza, Lawn, Hogan, Mathers, & Cousens, 2015). The reliability of the neonatal mortality estimates depends on accuracy and completeness of reporting and recording of births and deaths. Underreporting and misclassification are common, especially for deaths occurring early on in life.

Perinatal mortality encompasses late and early neonatal mortality and is defined as the number of stillbirths and deaths in the first week of life per 1,000 live births; it is also a useful indicator for population health. The perinatal mortality is the sum of the fetal mortality and the neonatal mortality. Work is ongoing to improve estimates of stillbirth rates, a major component of perinatal mortality (WHO, 2019b). Data on fetal mortality rates in Canada is not routinely collected, however the stillbirth rate is reported as 3,159 in 2017 (Statistics Canada, 2019b).

The **infant mortality rate** is the number of deaths occurring in the first 12 months of life (Fig. 1.2) or as the number of deaths of infants younger than 1 year of age per 1,000 live births. Neonatal mortality and postneonatal mortality (covering the remaining 11 months of the first year of life) are reflected in the infant mortality rate. The infant mortality rate is used as an index of the general health of a country. The rate of infant mortality remains relatively stable in Canada (Statistics Canada, 2019a).

However, the infant mortality rate varies greatly by province and territory and between certain populations within Canada. The Canadian Perinatal Surveillance System (CPSS) aims to strengthen health surveillance as part of PHAC. The CPSS is a multidisciplinary and multisectoral approach to data reporting to drive policy change. The main causes of early infant death in Canada include problems occurring at birth or shortly thereafter such as prematurity, low birth weight, congenital and chromosomal anomalies, sudden infant death syndrome (SIDS), respiratory distress syndrome, unintentional injuries, bacterial sepsis, and necrotizing enterocolitis (Osterman, Kochanek, MacDorman, Strobino, & Guyer, 2015).

Take Note!

Indigenous infants have consistently had higher infant mortality rates than other Canadian ethnic groups as a result of various factors including pre-existing maternal medical conditions, childbearing age, and access to health care (Sheppard et al., 2017).

Congenital anomalies and chromosomal abnormalities remain the leading cause of infant mortality in Canada (Statistics Canada, 2019a). In addition, low birth weight and prematurity are major indicators of infant health and significant predictors of infant mortality (Griffin, Lee, Profit, & Tancedi, 2015). The lower the birth weight, the higher the risk of infant mortality. The percentage of infants born preterm in Canada is about 8% therefore increasing the risk of higher rates of mortality and morbidity for this group (Shah et al., 2018).

After birth, other health promotion strategies can significantly improve an infant's health and chances of survival. Breastfeeding has been shown to reduce rates of infection in infants and to improve their long-term health. Human milk also reduces the risk for allergic and autoimmune diseases, and the risk of obesity and its complications (Wilson, Nizet, Maldonado, Remington, & Klein, 2016). Emphasizing the importance of placing an infant on his or her back to sleep reduces the incidence of SIDS. In addition, parents/partners are encouraged to practice safe sleeping behaviours to minimize risk (Adams, Ward, & Garcia, 2015). Encouraging mothers or caregivers to join support groups to prevent postpartum depression and learn sound child-rearing practices can improve the health of both mothers and their infants.

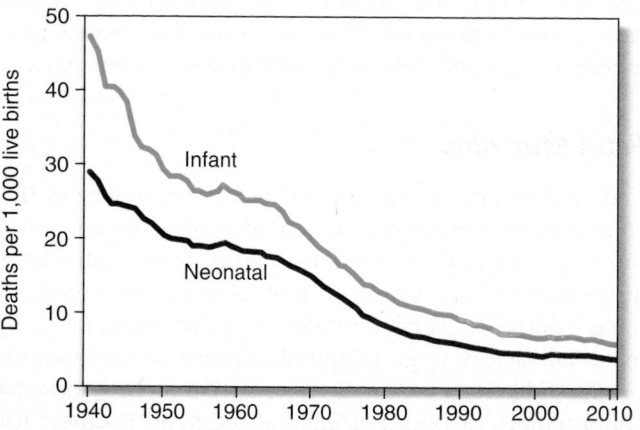

NOTE: Rates are infant (under 1 year) and neonatal (under 28 days) deaths per 1,000 live births in specified group.
SOURCE: CDC/NCHS, National Vital Statistics System, Mortality

FIGURE 1.2 Infant and neonatal mortality from 1940 to 2011. (Adapted from Kochanek, K. D., Sherry, L., Murphy, S. L., & Xu, J. Q. [2015]. Deaths: Final data for 2011. *National Vital Statistics Reports, 63*(3), 1–120. Hyattsville, MD: National Center for Health Statistics. Retrieved from http://www.cdc.gov/nchs/data/nvsr/nvsr63/nvsr63_03.pdf.)

Childhood Mortality

The **childhood mortality rate** is the number of deaths per 100,000 population in children 1 to 19 years of age (Statistics Canada, 2019c). Other causes of childhood mortality include suicide, homicide, accidents (unintentional injury), malignant neoplasms, influenza, and pneumonia.

Even as research continues into the preventable nature of childhood injuries, unintentional injury (e.g., motor vehicle accidents, fires, drowning, bicycle or pedestrian accidents, poisoning, falls) remains a leading cause of mortality and morbidity in children. Specific populations have a higher rate of unintentional injury—accidents linked to SDH, rurality, and population (Fridman, Fraser-Thomas, Pike, & Macpherson, 2018). These injuries have far-reaching consequences for children, families, and society in general. Risk factors associated with childhood injuries include young age, male gender, low socioeconomic status, parents who are unmarried or single, low maternal education level, poor housing, parental drug or alcohol abuse, and low support within the family. These deaths can often be prevented through education about the value of using car seats and seat belts, the dangers of driving under the influence of alcohol and other substances, and the importance of pedestrian and bicycle safety, fire safety, water safety, and home safety.

Take Note!

In Canada, children from Indigenous families, as well as those living in rural settings, are most vulnerable to unintended injury (Canadian Paediatric Society [CPS], 2012). Nurses' supportive education for all families is essential in keeping Canadian children safe and healthy.

Morbidity

Morbidity is the measure of the prevalence of a specific illness in a population at a particular time. It is presented in rates per 1,000 population. Morbidity is often difficult to define and record because the definitions used vary widely. For example, morbidity may be defined as visits to the physician or diagnosis for hospital admission. Also, data may be difficult to obtain. Morbidity statistics are revised less frequently because of the difficulty in defining or obtaining the information.

Women's Health Indicators

Cisgender women face not only diseases of genetic origin but also diseases that arise from poor health choices. Even though women represent 51% of the population, only recently have researchers and the medical community focused on their special health needs.

Cardiovascular disease (CVD) is the number-one cause of death in Canadian cisgender women over the age of 55 (PHAC, 2009a). More women than men die each year from CVD. More than 31,000 women die annually of CVD in Canada (Heart and Stroke Foundation of Canada, 2018). More than 8.6 million women die from CVD globally each year (World Heart Federation [WHF], 2017). Women who have a heart attack are more likely than men to die. Heart attacks in women are often more difficult to diagnose than in men because of their vague and varied symptoms. Heart disease is still thought of as a "man's disease," and thus a heart attack may not be considered in the differential diagnosis when a woman presents to the emergency room.

Nurses need to look beyond the obvious "crushing chest pain" textbook symptom that heralds a heart attack in cisgender men. Risk factors of heart disease differ between men and women in several other ways—for example, menopause (associated with a significant rise in coronary events); diabetes, high cholesterol levels, and left ventricular hypertrophy; and repeated episodes of weight loss and gain (increased coronary morbidity and mortality) (WHF, 2017). Clinical manifestations of a heart attack observed in women include nausea, dizziness, irregular heartbeat, unusual fatigue, sleep disturbances, indigestion, anxiety, shortness of breath, pain or discomfort in one or both arms, and weakness (Brown, 2015). The prevalence, mortality, lack of warning signs in some women, and decreased awareness within this population make it imperative for nurses to assume an active role in assessing these clients, evaluating risk factors, and advocating for prevention of CVD in all women.

Cancer is a major public health problem in Canada and globally. It is the second leading cause of death among women and is expected to surpass heart disease as the leading cause of death in the next few years (Siegel, Miller, & Jemal, 2015). Although much attention is focused on cancer of the reproductive system, lung cancer is common (Canadian Cancer Society [CCS], 2018). Lung cancer is largely the result of smoking and secondhand smoke. Lung cancer has no early symptoms, making early detection difficult. For women in Canada lung and bronchus cancer is reported as having a 20% 5-year net survival rate, with a lifetime probability rate of developing cancer reported as 1 in 14 (CCS, 2018).

Breast cancer is the most common cancer in cisgender women in Canada, with 1 in 8 at risk throughout their life time (CCS, 2018). It is estimated that about 26,300 new cases of invasive breast cancer will be diagnosed among women in Canada. An estimated 5,000 women are expected to die from the disease in 2017 (CCS, 2018). Although a positive family history of breast cancer, aging, and irregularities in the menstrual cycle at an early age are major risk factors, other risk factors include excess weight or obesity, not having children, oral contraceptive use, excessive alcohol consumption, a high-fat diet, sedentary lifestyle, and long-term use of hormone therapy after menopause. While breast cancer 5-year net survival rates are reported as 87% in 2018 (CCS, 2018), early detection and treatment continue to offer the best chance for a cure, and reducing the risk of cancer by decreasing avoidable risks continues to be the best preventive plan.

Pregnant individuals are by no means immune to any of the health issues presented thus far. Many individuals begin a pregnancy with existing health conditions, including hypertension, obesity, CVD, diabetes, inflammatory processes, autoimmune diseases, anemia, asthma, sexually transmitted infections, depression, or cancer. Although the majority of pregnant people are young and fairly healthy, the incidence of certain chronic health issues in them is increasing secondary to the obesity epidemic in the North America (Cancello, 2015).

Health is a complex issue, and no single policy is going to change the overall state of health among populations. Although progress in science and technology has helped reduce the incidence of, and improve the survival rates for, several diseases, many health issues continue to have an impact on our society. By eliminating or decreasing some of the risk factors and causes for prevalent diseases and illnesses, society and science could minimize certain chronic health problems. Focusing on the causes and effects of particular illnesses could help resolve many women's health issues of today.

Childhood Morbidity

The health of Canadian children is linked to key indicators as well as being influenced by events in childhood that impact morbidity (Raphael, 2010). The *Health Status of Canadians 2016* (Health Canada, 2017) includes information linked to children and youth, while the *Canadian Health Survey on Children and Youth* (Statistics Canada, 2019d) is designed to offer insight into the well-being as linked to physical and mental health. While nationally healthy behaviours linked to childhood and adolescence are reported via Public Health Agency Canada, much work happens at the provincial level. The diversity of populations, levels of poverty, and exposure to environmental risks vary depending on geography as well as access to health care and provincial political factors.

A key indicator of morbidity is the degree of disability it produces. While in children this is the number of days missed from school or confined to bed, it is difficult to determine national figures. Various reasons exist for missed school days, for example, bullying, mental health difficulties, and gender-related issues. Furthermore, home schooling rates vary across provinces. Nurses would be well placed to examine local data which can often be sourced via government health systems such as health, education, and social care.

While improvements have occurred in child health as a result of infant immunizations, morbidity and disability from some conditions, such as asthma, diabetes, attention-deficit/hyperactivity disorder, and obesity, have increased in recent decades. As such, common health problems in children include respiratory disorders such as asthma; gastrointestinal disturbances, which lead to malnutrition and dehydration; and injuries. Asthma is the leading chronic disease in children with a prevalence of between 11% and 16% (Senthilselvan et al., 2015; Subbarao et al., 2015). Diseases of the respiratory system, such as asthma and pneumonia, can result in hospital admission for children and youth. Preschoolers have the highest rate of emergency department visits linked to asthma symptoms and management (Canadian Paediatric Society [CPS], 2015).

An increasing trend globally is the challenges children and youth are reporting linked to their mental health as well as complexities linked to emotional, social, or behavioural problems. The Mental Health Commission of Canada reports that 1 in 12 youth received treatment for mental health needs (Raising Canada, 2018). These problems result in increased emergency room visits, hospitalization, and pharmacologic treatments which together may limit the child's educational success. They also increase the child's risk for significant mental health problems later in life or emotional problems and possible use of firearms, reckless driving, risky sexual activity, and substance abuse during adolescence. Overall, these behavioural, social, and educational problems can interfere with children's social and academic development.

FACTORS AFFECTING MATERNAL AND CHILD HEALTH

From conception, children are shaped by a myriad of factors, such as genetics, social epigenetics, and the environment. As members of a family, they are also members of a specific population, community, culture, and society. As they learn and grow, they are affected by multiple, complex, and ever-changing influences around them. For example, dramatic demographic changes in Canada have led to shifts in majority and minority population groups. Globalization has led to an international focus on health. Access to health care and the types of health care have changed due to modifications in health care delivery and financing. The factors affecting health discussed in this section include family, genetics, society, culture, health status and lifestyle, access to health care, improvements in diagnosis and treatments, and empowerment of health care consumers.

These factors may affect the person positively, by promoting healthy growth and development, or negatively, by increasing the person's health risks. Nurses, especially those working with women and children, need to understand how these influences affect the quality of nursing care and health outcomes. They must examine the impact of these variables to gain the knowledge and skills needed to plan effective care, thereby achieving the best possible outcomes for women, children, and families.

Family

The family is considered as the basic social unit and linked to the dwelling in which care is provided (Statistics Canada, 2015). Earlier definitions of family emphasize the legal ties or genetic relationships of people living in the same household with specific roles. Given the diversity of families in today's society, however, some believe that family should be defined as whatever the client says it is (Fig. 1.3) (Holtzman, 2011; Patterson, 1995).

The family greatly influences the development and health of its members. For example, children learn health care activities, health beliefs, and health values from their family. The family's structure, the roles assumed by family members, and social changes that affect the family's life can influence the woman's and child's health status. Families are unique; each one has different views and requires distinct methods for support CPS (2019).

Various theories and models have been generated to explain the concept of family. They have influenced the definition of family, the understanding of the structure and function of the family, and the way family coping and adaptation are assessed. Table 1.1 summarizes some of the major theories related to family.

Take Note!

The lifestyle of the parents basically is the lifestyle of the children. For instance, parents who are inactive and eat poorly will have children who do the same, and the problems associated with these unhealthy habits, such as diabetes, obesity, and early heart disease, are showing up earlier in children and adolescents. It is important for parents, where possible, to serve as role models for proper nutrition and physical activity (through sports, hobbies, or other activities).

Family Structure

Family structure is the composition of people who interact with one another on a regular, recurring basis in socially sanctioned ways. It involves how the family unit is organized, which often influences the relationship of the members of the family. Family members can be gained or lost through events such as divorce, marriage, birth, death, abandonment, displacement, and incarceration. All of these events can alter the family structure, leading to roles being redefined or redistributed. Table 1.2 provides examples of the types of family structures found in today's society.

The traditional nuclear family is no longer considered the dominant family structure. From 1980 to 2012, the percentage of children who were living with their

(text continues on page 18)

FIGURE 1.3 Nurses must take into account family dynamics when providing health care. There are many different family structures, and they influence the client's needs. **A.** The traditional nuclear family is composed of two parents and their biologic or adopted children. **B.** The extended family includes the nuclear family plus other family members, such as grandparents, aunts, uncles, and cousins. **C.** Gay and lesbian families comprise two people of the same sex sharing a committed relationship with or without children.

TABLE 1.1   SUMMARY OF MAJOR THEORIES RELATED TO FAMILY

Theory	Description	Key Components
Friedman's structural functional theory	Emphasizes the social system of family, such as the organization or structure of the family and how the structure relates to the function	Identified five functions of families: • Affective function: meeting the love and belonging needs of each member • Socialization and social placement function: teaching children how to function and assume adult roles in society • Reproductive role: continuing the family and society in general • Economic function: ensuring the family has necessary resources with appropriate allocation • Health care function: involving the provision of physical care to keep family healthy
Duvall's developmental theory	Emphasizes the developmental stages that all families go through, beginning with marriage; the longitudinal career of the family is also known as the family life cycle	Described eight chronologic stages with specific predictable tasks that each family completes: • Marriage: beginning of family • Childbearing stage • Family with preschool children • Family with school-age children • Family with adolescents • Family with young adults • Middle-age parents • Family in later years
Von Bertalanffy: general system theory applied to families	Emphasizes the family as a system with interdependent, interacting parts that endure over time to ensure the survival, continuity, and growth of its components; the family is not the sum of its parts but is characterized by wholeness and unity	Used to define how families interact with and are influenced by the members of their family and society and how to analyze the interrelationships of the members and the impact that change affecting one member will have on other members
Family stress theory	Addresses the way families respond to stress and how the family copes with the stress as a group and how each individual member copes	Described elements of stress as occurring internally within the family (e.g., values, beliefs, structure) that the family can control or change or externally from outside the family (e.g., culture of the surrounding community, genetics, the family's current time or place) over which the family has no control Mobilization of family resources resulting in either a positive response of constructive coping or negative response of a crisis Identified the main determinant of adequate coping based on the meaning of the stressful event to the family and its individual members
Resiliency model of family stress and family adjustment, and adaptation response model	Addresses the way families adapt to stress and can rebound from adversity	Identified the elements of risks and protective factors that aid a family in achieving positive outcomes
Calgary Family Assessment Model	Provides a framework for nurses working, and performing assessments, with families to build on families' strengths in supporting positive changes	Rooted in systems, cybernetics, change, and communication theories to observe, describe, and support the structural, development, and functional components of a family

Adapted from Friedman, M. M. (1998). *Family nursing: Theory and practice* (4th ed.). Stanford, CT: Appleton & Lange; Duvall, E. (1997). *Marriage and family development* (5th ed.). Philadelphia, PA: J. B. Lippincott; Von Bertalanffy, L. (1968). *General systems theory*. London: Penguin Press; Boss, P. (2001). *Family stress management*. Newbury Park, CA: Sage; Patterson, J. (2002). Integrating family resilience and family stress theory. *Journal of Marriage and Family, 64*(2), 349–360; and Wright, L. M., & Leahy, M. (2013). *Nurses and families: A guide to family assessment and intervention* (6th ed.). Philadelphia, PA: F.A. Davis.

TABLE 1.2	TYPES OF FAMILY STRUCTURES	
Structure	**Description**	**Specific Issues**
Nuclear family	Husband, wife, and children living in same household	May include natural or adopted children Once considered the traditional family structure; now decreased due to trends in divorce rates or other social situations such as nonmarital childbearing
Binuclear family	Child who is member of two families due to joint custody; parenting is considered a joint venture	Always works better when the interests of the child are put above the parents' needs and desires
Single-parent family	One parent responsible for care of children	May result from death, divorce, desertion, birth outside marriage, or adoption Likely to encounter several challenges because of economic, social, and personal restraints; one person as homemaker, caregiver, and financial provider
Commuter family	Adults in the family living and working apart for professional or financial reasons, often leaving the daily care of children to one parent	Similar to single-parent family, but without as much economic challenge
Step or blended family	Adults with children from previous marriages or from the new marriage	May lead to family conflict due to different expectations for the child and adults; may have different views and practices related to child care and health
Extended family	Nuclear family and grandparents, cousins, aunts, and uncles	Need to determine decision maker as well as primary caretaker of the children May be encouraged and supported by some cultures, such as Hispanic and Asian cultures
LGBTQ+ family (includes same-sex couples, or those with one or both transgender partners)	Adults of the same sex or who identify as transgender or gender nonconforming, living together with or without children	May face prejudice against those with different lifestyles
Communal family	Group of people living together to raise children and manage household; unrelated by blood or marriage	May face prejudice against those with different lifestyles Need to determine the decision maker and caretaker of children
Foster family	A temporary family for children who are placed away from their parents to ensure their emotional and physical well-being	May include foster family's children and other foster children in the home Foster children are more likely to have unmet health needs and chronic health problems because they may have been living in a variety of settings
Grandparents-as-parents families	Grandparents raising their grandchildren if parents are unable to do so	May increase the risk for physical, financial, and emotional stress on older adults May lead to confusion and emotional stress for child if biologic parents are in and out of the child's life
Adolescent families	Young parents still mastering the developmental tasks of their own childhood	Teenagers have greater risk for health problems during pregnancy and delivery of premature infants, leading to risk of subsequent health and developmental problems Probably still need support from their family related to financial, emotional, and school issues

own married parents decreased steadily from 77% to 64% (Federal Interagency Forum on Child and Family Statistics, 2013). By understanding clients' family structure and any changes that may occur, nurses can provide them with support to alleviate or prevent dysfunctional alterations in family coping and adaptation.

Families today face complex challenges as they try to nurture, develop, and socialize their members. Family structure changes such as divorce, blending families, adoption, or foster care can have wide-ranging and lifelong effects. These special situations require astute assessment and proactive intervention to minimize the risk to the family.

DIVORCED FAMILY

Divorce is a common reason why the family structure changes. Today, over 40% of marriages end in divorce and many of these marriages include children (Serwint, 2011). Divorce can have a great impact on the child, with chronic and devastating results. Typically, divorce is not a single event. Changes have most likely been occurring in the family for years, and children may have been exposed to turmoil, violence, or changes in structure before the actual divorce. Children feel scared and confused by the threat divorce poses on their security. The initial response of children to divorce depends on their age; problems are most apparent the year after the divorce and diminish over the next couple of years (Kim, 2011). However, regardless of family type, children whose parents had a hostile interparental relationship tended to have poorer emotional well-being than children whose parents had a nonhostile relationship (Baxter, Weston, & Lixia, 2011; CPS, 2018a).

Parents need to understand the impact that divorce can have on their children so that they can place the children's interests in the forefront. The loss of a parent through divorce can leave children vulnerable to physical and mental illnesses (CPS, 2018b). Changes in households can result in dysfunction, a shift in the financial stability, physical violence, or even neglect (Government of Canada, 2017). A combination of these factors can place the child at risk for adverse childhood events (ACEs), which are known to have later adult health impact (CPS, 2015). However, by appropriately utilizing family strengths and providing care and attention, children can be helped to deal constructively with divorce. Parents can use the rules in Box 1.3 to help reduce tension and conflict, thereby minimizing the impact of separation and divorce on their children. Health care providers can offer support, guidance, and resources to help make the strain of divorce easier on the entire family.

SINGLE-PARENT FAMILIES

Single-parent families can result from divorce or separation, death of a spouse, an unmarried woman or man raising his/her own child, or adoption by an unmarried

---

BOX 1.3

RULES FOR DIVORCING PARENTS

1. Tell your children about the divorce and the reasons for the divorce in terms that they can understand. Be sure that you and your spouse are present together when telling the children; tell all the children at the same time.
2. Reassure your children that the divorce is not their fault. Repeat this as often as possible and as necessary.
3. Inform the children well in advance of anyone moving out of the house (except when abuse is present or there are concerns for immediate safety).
4. Clearly inform the children about the family structure after the divorce, such as who will live with whom and where; also discuss visitation clearly and honestly.
5. Do not make your children be or act like adults. Seek support from other adults in your life.
6. Do not discuss money or finances with your children.
7. Minimize unpredictable schedules and maintain routines, rules, and discipline, and be consistent in this area.
8. Never force or allow your children to take sides.
9. Avoid belittling your former spouse when the children can hear. However, do not lie to cover up for irresponsible behaviour by the other parent.
10. Never put your children in the middle between you and your ex-spouse.
11. Keep each parent involved in the child's life. Write letters, emails, phone calls, and text messages to continue communication. This shows the child they remain important to you even when they are with the other parent.
12. Communicate directly with the other parent. Avoid making the child your messenger.

Adapted from New, M. (2011). Helping your child through a divorce. KidsHealth for Parents. Retrieved from http://kidshealth.org/parent/positive/talk/help_child_divorce.html#; Kemp, G., Smith, M., & Segal, J. (2018). *Children and divorce.* Retrieved from http://www.helpguide.org/articles/family-divorce/children-and-divorce.htm; and Government of Canada Department of Justice. (2017). *Voice and support: Programs for children experiencing parental separation and divorce.* Retrieved from http://www.justice.gc.ca/eng/rp-pf/fl-lf/divorce/2004_2/p.3.html

---

man or woman. In 2016 one in five children under 1 year (20.7%) were living with a single parent or in a stepfamily without their parent (Statistics Canada, 2017a). For children of ages 0 to 14 there continues to be an increase in lone parenting; from 17.8% in 2001 to 19.2% in 2016 (Statistics Canada, 2017a).

Single-parent families have several concerns that can affect the health of the children. Life in a single-parent household can be stressful for both the adult and the children. The single parent may feel overwhelmed with no one to share the day-to-day responsibilities of juggling the care of the children, maintaining a job, and keeping up with the home and finances. These issues may be compounded by other pressures, such as custody problems, decreased time available to spend with children, continuing conflicts between parents who are separated or divorced, or changes in relationships with extended family members.

Communication and support are essential to the optimal functioning of the single-parent family. The parent and children need to be able to express their feelings and work through the problems together. Single parents must provide greater support for their children. Even though a single parent may feel alone they need to ensure they treat their children as children and not a substitute for a partner. Support and comfort need to come from outside resources. Community resources can be helpful.

BLENDED FAMILIES

Before the age of 14, 1 in 10 children in Canada was part of a stepfamily (Statistics Canada, 2017a). Creating a blended family (parents and their stepchildren), even though considered a form of "normal" these days, it can be stressful for the parents and children alike. Although it creates a structure and stability and reduces some of the financial stresses of single parenthood, making the transition to a blended family takes time. Children may feel jealous of the stepparent or feel disloyal toward the previous biologic parent. There may be competition or rivalry among the stepchildren. The child may fear that the stepparent is interfering with the child's relationship with the parent or taking away his or her source of love, affection, and attention.

Mutual respect and open, honest communication among all individuals involved are key, and this should include the previous biologic parent when possible. Responsibilities for parenting must be shared, including decisions about expectations, limits, and discipline. The continued role of the previous biologic parent and the role of the stepparent in the child's life are important to address.

ADOPTED FAMILIES

Adoption can occur domestically (through an agency or intermediary such as an attorney in the family's own area or country), or the family may choose to adopt a child from another country. The child may be of a different culture, race, or ethnicity (Fig. 1.4). The number of children eligible for adoption in Canada varies but detailed information can be sourced at the Adoption Council of Canada (see the**Point**).

The amount of contact between the child and the birth mother can vary. In a closed adoption there is no contact between the adoptive parents, the adopted child, and the birth mother. In an open adoption there is as much contact among the individuals as desired. Regardless of the method used to adopt a child, adoptive families may be faced with unique issues. Some adopted children

FIGURE 1.4 **An adoptive family with children from a different culture.**

have complex medical, developmental, behavioural, educational, and psychological issues (Faver & Alanis, 2012). They may have been exposed to poverty, neglect, infectious diseases, food insecurity, clothing, shelter, and nurturing, placing them at risk for medical problems, physical growth and development delays or abnormalities, and behavioural, cognitive, and emotional problems. The adoptive parents may know about these problems, but in other situations little if any history may be available.

Differences in culture, ethnicity, or race can further influence the adopted child's sense of identity (Faver & Alanis, 2012). Children may be subjected to social injustices. Extended family members may not accept the child as part of the family. Parents need to emphasize that the adopted child is their child and is as much a part of the family as any other member. Parents need to openly recognize racial differences that exist between them and their child. Parents should encourage and assist the child to learn about their heritage, culture, and ethnic group (Jones, Schulte, & Committee on Early Childhood, Council on Foster Care, Adoption, and Kinship Care, 2012). Adopted adolescents and adults may feel a need to identify their biologic parents. Children adopted from other countries may travel to the country of their birth, and children adopted domestically may search for biologic relatives. Although this search is an indicator of healthy emotional growth, it can upset the adoptive parents, who may feel rejected.

As the adopted child grows older, he or she may feel the loss of a birth family or may question what he or she did that led to the birth parents' decision to proceed with adoption. Attachment to the adoptive family is important. In order to attach in future relationships children must appropriately grieve past losses. This can be particularly complex and difficult for older children and children previously living in foster care or orphanages.

Take Note!

Adolescents face vast challenges adjusting to adoption at this age because of the added complexity of identity issues facing this age group (Jones et al., 2012).

Clear, open, honest communication and discussion are essential to promote a healthy, strong relationship. Support, guidance, and open communication are key for all parties involved. Open acknowledgement of the adoptive relationship helps to nurture trust, security, and a child's self-esteem as he or she learns to understand what it means to be part of a family through adoption (Jones et al., 2012).

The pediatric nurse needs to be sensitive, understanding, and supportive when interacting with adopted children and their families. "Positive" adoption language should be used. This includes saying "birth parent" when referring to biologic parents instead of "natural" or "real parent" and just "parents" when talking about adoptive parents (Jones et al., 2012). Also, do not refer to the child as their "adopted child" or other children as "natural child" (Jones et al., 2012). When discussing adoption using terms such as "make an adoption plan," instead of "give away" or "give up for adoption," is preferred (Jones et al., 2012). The nurse also needs to provide reassurance and understanding regarding missing health information and provide appropriate resources and referrals to resources that are knowledgeable about adoption and sensitive to the issues that may arise.

FOSTER CARE FAMILY

Foster care is a situation in which a child is cared for in an alternative living situation apart from his or her parents or legal guardians. The child may be placed in this living situation due to difficulties in the family situation, such as abuse, neglect, abandonment, or the parents' inability to meet the child's needs, due to illness, substance abuse, or death. The child may be sent to live with relatives (kinship care) or foster parents, who are strangers providing protection and shelter in a province-approved foster home.

From the last reported census data there were approximately 28,030 children (0.5%) living in foster care with a further 22,610 (0.4%) living with other relatives and 32,505 (0.6%) with grandparents (Statistics Canada, 2017a). The goal of foster care is to provide temporary services until the child can return home to his or her family or be adopted. Unfortunately, children may remain in foster care for several years or longer and may be moved from one foster family to another.

Many children who are placed in foster care have been the victims of abuse or neglect. Children in foster care are more likely to exhibit a wide range of medical, emotional, behavioural, dental, educational, or developmental problems (Bernedo, Salas, García-Martín, & Fuentes,

2012). However, children are very resilient and most children in foster care are determined to live their lives, but they may struggle with certain issues, including the following:

- Unmet health care needs
- Significant mental health problems, such as depression, social problems, anxiety, and posttraumatic stress disorder due to trauma, loss, and unpredictability
- Behavioural problems such as substance use, problems with the law, and self-destructive behaviours
- Interruptions in developmental stages and developmental delay
- Educational obstacles due to frequent moves and educational difficulties
- Self-blame and feelings of guilt
- Feelings of being unwanted
- Feelings of helplessness and powerlessness
- Insecurity about the future
- Ambivalent feelings related to foster parents; feelings of being disloyal to birth parents (Zlotnick, Tam, & Soman, 2012)

Individual attention to the child in foster care is essential. A multidisciplinary approach to care that includes the birth parents, foster parents, child, health care professionals, and support services is important to meet the child's needs for growth and development. Nurses play a key role in advocating for the child.

Family Roles and Functions

Regardless of the structure of the family, the role of the family in caring for the child includes not only providing physical and emotional care but also imparting the rules and expected behaviours of society through teaching and discipline techniques. These expected behaviours depend on the culture, values, and beliefs of the family and the child's developmental stage and physical and cognitive abilities. Roles and functions are further defined by each family's own traditions and values and the family's set of standards for interaction within and outside the family. For instance, some families may value privacy more than others. These family members may tend to be more self-protective and secretive.

CAREGIVER–CHILD INTERACTION

The caregiver–child interaction is critical to the survival and healthy development of a young child (WHO, 2016; Xu, 2011). Typically, the primary caregivers are the parents. Ideally, parents nurture their children and provide them with an environment in which they can become competent, productive, self-directed members of society. For young children in particular, growth, health, and their very personhood itself depend on the ability of the adults in their life to understand and respond to them (Groark & McCall, 2011; WHO, 2016).

PARENTAL ROLES

Parenting is an enormous responsibility and takes a lot of time as well as physical and mental energy. Parental roles are vast and numerous. Typical parental roles include nurturer/caregiver, financial provider, decision maker, schedule manager, financial manager, problem solver, counsellor, teacher, behaviour support and manager, and health manager. Parenting is a responsibility which changes over the life span for both the parent and the child (Ponzetti, 2015). Parenting roles are also frequently gendered, impacted by occupation, income, time, and many other factors (Horvath, Lee, & Bax, 2015).

CHANGES IN PARENTAL ROLES OVER TIME

Parental roles evolve due to societal and economic changes as well as individual family changes. Traditionally, the role of provider was assigned to the father. However, with increased numbers of women in the workplace and more households with two parents working, today both parents are often the providers as well as the nurturers to their children. Technologic innovations have provided parents with opportunities to work at home, allowing some parents to maintain the provider role while simultaneously fulfilling the nurturer and health manager roles. Fathers are taking on greater responsibilities related to household management and child care. Within some communities the number of children being raised by their grandparents is common and therefore this population may require access to additional community supports (CPS, 2018a). Moreover, as baby boomers age, parents may find themselves caring for both their children and their aging parents.

> **Recall Sophia, the pregnant woman described at the beginning of the chapter. Identify the parental roles Sophia would assume. How might these roles be different from those of her mother when she was Sophia's age?**

PARENTING STYLES

Beginning in the 1960s with a psychologist named Baumrind, and later in the 1980s with Maccoby and Martin, parenting styles have been well-studied over the years. Four major parenting styles have been suggested: authoritarian, authoritative, permissive, and uninvolved or rejecting-neglecting (as cited in Cherry, 2018). The styles are defined by the amount of support and control exerted over the child during parenting. Many parents may use more than one parenting style and may fall somewhere in between styles instead of adhering strictly to one style. Also, some parents may change parenting styles as the child ages and matures. Whatever the style, sensitive and responsive caregiving is needed to promote appropriate physical, neurophysiologic, and psychological development (Beers, 2011). Nurses need to recognize different parenting styles and provide support to parents by discussing the effects of different parenting models and teaching parenting skills.

Authoritarian. The *authoritarian* parent expects obedience from the child and discourages the child from questioning the family's rules. The parent provides low support and high control over the child (Cherry, 2018). The rules and standards set forth by the parents are strictly enforced and firm. The parents expect the child to accept the family's beliefs and values and demand respect for these beliefs. The parents are the ultimate authority and allow little, if any, participation by the child in making decisions. Behaviour that does not adhere to the family's rules and standards is punished. This parenting style is associated with negative effects on self-esteem, happiness and social skills, increased aggression, and defiance (Cherry, 2018; Hamon & Schrodt, 2012).

Authoritative. The *authoritative* or democratic parent shows some respect for the child's opinions. Although parents still have the ultimate authority and expect the child to adhere to the rules, authoritative parents allow children to be different and believe that each child is an individual. They exhibit warmth and consistently, fairly, and firmly enforce the family's rules and standards without emphasizing punishment. This type of parenting is associated with increased independence, happiness, self-confidence, and socially responsible individuals (Cherry, 2018; Piko & Balázs, 2012).

Permissive. Permissive or laissez-faire parents have little control over the behaviour of their children. Rules or standards may be inconsistent, unclear, or nonexistent. Permissive parents allow their children to determine their own standards and rules for behaviour. Discipline can be lax, inconsistent, or absent. Parents can be warm, cool, or uninvolved. There are more negative than positive effects associated with this style of parenting. Negative effects include children being impulsive, low happiness, poor school performance, problems with authority, lacking responsibility and independence (Cherry, 2018; Hamon & Schrodt, 2012).

Uninvolved or Rejecting-Neglecting. Uninvolved parents are indifferent. They do not provide rules or standards. The child's basic needs are often met but the parent is disconnected from the child's life. In some cases the parents may neglect or reject the child. They can be cold and uninterested in meeting the child's needs. They minimize their interactions and time with the children. This type of parenting is associated with negative effects such as the child lacking interest in school, lacking interest in the future, and lacking emotional and self-control

(Cherry, 2018). This type of parenting may also lead to lack of trust, low self-esteem, and anger toward others (Cherry, 2018; Kawabata, Alink, Tseng, van Ijzendoorn, & Crick, 2011).

DISCIPLINE

Much of parenting involves increasing desirable behaviour and decreasing or eliminating undesirable behaviour, a process generally known as **discipline**. There are various opinions across our society about the best or most effective method of discipline while achieving the "hoped for" child outcomes (Grusec, Danyliuk, Kil, & O'Neill, 2017). Each child and family is unique. Discipline that works with one child or within one family may not work for another family. Discipline should focus on the development of the child while ensuring to preserve their self-esteem and dignity. It should be based on age-appropriate expectations with clear, consistent guidelines while offering meaningful choices when possible. Discipline involves teaching and it is ongoing, not something that is done just when the child misbehaves.

The American Academy of Pediatrics (AAP, 2018) suggests various strategies for effective discipline (see also Teaching Guidelines 1.1), including:

- Maintaining a positive, supportive, nurturing caregiver–child relationship
- Using positive reinforcement to increase desirable behaviours
- Removing positive reinforcements or using punishment to reduce or eliminate undesirable behaviours

Teaching Guidelines 1.1
PROMOTING EFFECTIVE DISCIPLINE

- Set clear, consistent, and developmentally appropriate expected behaviours; offer choices whenever possible.
- Maintain consistency in responding to behaviours; provide encouragement and affection.
- Role-model appropriate behaviours.
- Provide an age-appropriate explanation of the consequence if the child demonstrates unacceptable behaviour.
- Always administer the consequence soon after the unacceptable behaviour.
- Keep the consequence appropriate to the age of the child and the situation.
- Stay calm but firm without showing anger when administering the consequence.
- Always praise the child for displaying appropriate behaviour (positive reinforcement).
- Set the environment to assist the child in accomplishing the appropriate behaviour; remove temptations that may lead to inappropriate behaviour.
- Reinforce that the child's behaviour was "bad" but the child was not "bad."

- Use extinction to reduce or eliminate reinforcement for an inappropriate behaviour (e.g., ignore a temper tantrum).
- When using time-out, use 1 minute per year of the child's age. Do not exceed 5 minutes.
- Maintaining a positive, supportive, nurturing caregiver–child relationship.
  - Using positive reinforcement to increase desirable behaviours
  - Using extinction or punishment to reduce or eliminate undesirable behaviours

POSITIVE REINFORCEMENT

Attention from parents is a very powerful form of positive reinforcement and can help increase desirable behaviours. The key is to focus on the child's appropriate behaviours rather than emphasize the inappropriate ones. Immediate, consistent, and frequent feedback is crucial. This feedback can be in the form of smiles, praise, special attention, or rewards such as extra privileges or a special token or activity. Providing the feedback immediately is important so that the child learns to associate the feedback with the appropriate behaviour, thereby reinforcing the behaviour.

EXTINCTION

Another form of discipline is extinction, which focuses on reducing or eliminating the positive reinforcement for inappropriate behaviour. Examples are ignoring the temper tantrums of a toddler, withholding or removing privileges, and requiring "time-out." Withholding or removing privileges such as TV, music device, computer, or cell phone use is most effective for older children and adolescents. The adolescent may be grounded for a short time or not allowed to drive the car. To be effective, the privilege being withheld or removed must be something that the child values.

Time-out is an extinction discipline method that is most effective with toddlers, preschoolers, and early school-age children. It involves removing the child from the problem area and placing him or her in a neutral, nonthreatening, safe area where no interaction occurs between the child and parents or others for a specifically determined period (Fig. 1.5).

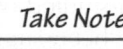
Take Note!
The amount of time that a child spends in time-out is typically 1 minute per year of age. For example, a 3 year old would spend 3 minutes in time-out (Sege et al., 2018).

PUNISHMENT

Discipline is often confused with punishment, but **punishment** involves a negative or unpleasant experience or consequence for doing or not doing something.

FIGURE 1.5 Although he might not like it, quiet solitude helps the child develop inner control.

Although punishment is sometimes a necessary element of discipline, to be an effective tool it must be coupled with rewards for good behaviour (Flaskerud, 2011).

Punishment may be verbal or corporal. Verbal punishment commonly takes the form of reprimands or scolding (the use of disapproving statements). The statements are intended to change or eliminate the inappropriate behaviour. Verbal reprimands can be effective in the short term if they are used sparingly and are focused on the child's specific behaviour. If verbal reprimands are used frequently and indiscriminately, they lose their effectiveness, can provoke anxiety in the child, and encourage the child to ignore the parent. Frequent use also may reinforce the behaviour by providing the child with attention (Sege et al., 2018).

Corporal punishment involves the use of physical pain as a means to decrease inappropriate behaviour. The most common form of corporal punishment is spanking (the use of an open hand to the buttocks or an extremity with the intention of modifying behaviour without causing injury) (Sege et al., 2018). Research shows that many parents have spanked their children at some point, with 90% of parents having spanked their child at least once (Perron et al., 2014). Over the past two decades a growing body of research has suggested that corporal punishment can cause an increase in behaviour problems and have lasting effects into adulthood (Lansford, Wager, Bates, Pettit, & Dodge, 2012). "What's wrong with spanking?" is a campaign initiative

by PHAC (2016b). The use of reasonable force within Canada to keep children safe, manage behaviour, and protect people from danger is situated with Criminal Law, section 43 of the *Criminal Code* (2016). Note that "using reasonable force with children aged 2–12 years as a restraint may be considered as acceptable in some circumstances" (Government of Canada Department of Justice, 2016).

> **Take Note!**
>
> Other forms of discipline, if used incorrectly, can also cause problems for the child and interfere with the caregiver–child relationship. For example, disapproval using tone of voice, facial expression, or gestures can be effective in stopping inappropriate behaviour, but if the disapproval comes in the form of verbal statements that attack the child rather than the behaviour, negative consequences may occur (Sege et al., 2018).

Genetics

Genetics, the study of heredity and its variations, is a field that has applications to all stages of life and all types of diseases. The child's biologic traits, including gender, race, some behavioural traits, and the presence of certain diseases or illnesses, are directly linked to genetic inheritance. Heredity is the process of transmitting genetic characteristics from parent to offspring.

Gender

The terms *sex* and *gender* are often used interchangeably, however they are distinct concepts linked to physical (genetic and biologic process, for sex) and wider social discourses (sense of self, behaviours, and belonging, for gender). A person's gender can be expressed in many ways and influence many aspects, such as physical characteristics and personal attributes, attitudes, and behaviours. A person's gender identity is typically established by age 4 (Rafferty, 2018). Transgender identity in adults as well as children and youth are growing areas of study, with nurses and other providers becoming increasingly sensitive to the need of avoiding cisnormativity (the assumption that people identify as the gender assigned at birth) in our approaches to clients and families (Newhook et al., 2018). Some diseases or illnesses are more common in one sex; for example, scoliosis is more common in cisgender females and colour blindness in cisgender males (Lewis, 2011).

In addition to the specific biologic and physical traits related to gender are the social effects. Children develop specific gender attitudes and behaviours that are appropriate in their own culture. Interactions with family members and peers as well as activities and societal values affect how children perceive themselves as a specific gender (Fig. 1.6).

FIGURE 1.6 Interactions with family members and peers as well as activities and societal values affect how children perceive themselves as a certain gender.

Race

Race refers to the physical features that distinguish members of a particular group, such as skin colour, bone structure, or blood type. Some of the physical variations may be normal in a particular race but may be considered an identifying characteristic of a disorder in other races. For example, epicanthal folds (the vertical folds of skin that partially or completely cover the inner canthi of the eye) are normal in Asian children but may occur in children with Down syndrome or renal agenesis in other races. In addition, certain malformations and diseases are found more commonly in specific races. For example, sickle cell anemia occurs more often in people of African descent (Long, Thomas, Grubs, Gettig, & Krishnamurti, 2011).

Public awareness is important in educating couples at genetic risk about the benefits of screening programs and proactively seeking preconceptual genetic counselling to consider options that could include preimplantation genetic diagnosis (the use of in vitro fertilization [IVF] technology to screen for unaffected embryos) (Rafi & Kai, 2011). The lack of engagement by ethnic minorities might simply reflect a lack of genetic awareness. Nurses can take the lead in assisting couples to gain that needed awareness to be empowered to make intelligent reproductive decisions.

Temperament

Temperament is the manner in which a child interacts with the environment. The way a child experiences a particular event will be influenced by his or her temperament, and the child's temperament will influence the responses of others, including the parents, to the child. Early on, infants demonstrate differences in their behaviour in response to stimuli. These responses are an integral part of the infant's developing personality and individuality. Although a child's temperament is intrinsic and relatively resistant to change, it does stabilize as the child matures (Crawford, Schrock, & Woodruff-Borden, 2011). Knowing a child's temperament can help parents understand and accept the characteristics of the child without feeling responsible for having caused them.

The classic temperament theory proposes nine parameters of temperament: activity level, rhythmicity, approach and withdrawal, adaptability, threshold of responsiveness, intensity of reaction, quality of mood, distractibility, and attention span and persistence (Feigelman, 2011). This theory seeks to identify behavioural characteristics that lead the child to respond to the world in specific ways. Using the nine parameters, children's temperaments may be categorized into three major groups: easy, difficult, and slow to warm up; various temperaments are a combination of these groups (Feigelman, 2011; Kiff, Lengua, & Zalewski, 2011). Easy children are even tempered and have regular biologic functions, predictable behaviour, and a positive attitude toward new experiences. Difficult children are irritable, highly active, and intense; they react to new experiences by withdrawing and are frustrated easily. Children in the slow-to-warm-up category are moody and less active and have more irregular reactions; they react to new experiences with mild but passive resistance and need extra time to adjust to new situations.

A child's temperament may cause problems in the family if it conflicts with that of the parents (e.g., a difficult 2 year old with slow-to-warm-up parents). If parents want and expect their child to be predictable, but predictability is not in the child's style, parents may perceive the child to have problems; this conflict may then affect the child's health. The key is not to label the child but to recognize the strengths and limitations of each group. Understanding a child's temperament can help parents understand a child's characteristics and behaviours and allow parents to adjust their parenting style.

Genetically Linked Diseases

New technologies in molecular biology and biochemistry have led to better understanding of the mechanisms involved in hereditary transmission, including those associated with genetic disorders. These advances are now leading to better diagnostic tests and management options.

Reproductive genetic testing, counselling, and other genetic services can be valuable components in the reproductive health care of women and their families. These services have the potential to increase knowledge about possible pregnancy outcomes that may occur if a woman decides to reproduce; to provide reassurance during pregnancy; and to enhance the developing relationship between the woman, her expected child, and others (Edwards et al., 2015). This awareness can provide each woman with an opportunity to have access to desired genetic services in a way that will improve her control over the circumstances of her reproductive life, her pregnancies, childbearing, and parenting, within a framework that is sensitive to her needs and values. Nurses can be a vital facilitator in this process and to these services.

Two major areas of study in genetics that are important to pediatrics are cytogenetics and the Human Genome Project. Cytogenetics is the study of genetics at the chromosome level. Since the genetic code was deciphered, much has been learned about the chromosomal structure shared by all human organisms. Chromosomal anomalies occur in 0.4% of all live births and are the most prevalent cause of cognitive impairment and congenital anomalies or birth defects (Ferguson-Smith, 2015). Anomalies are even more common among spontaneous abortions and stillbirths. The Human Genome Project was an international research effort involving the localization, isolation, and characterization of human genes and investigation of the function of the gene products and their interaction with one another. It was considered one of the most ambitious and successful international research collaborations in the history of biology. Completion of this project provided scientists with greatly enhanced information about how DNA shapes species development and genetic diseases to aid in developing new ways to identify, treat, cure, or even prevent them. Chapters 10 and 49 offer more detailed discussions of genetics.

Society

Society has a major impact on the health of women, children, and families. Major components of a society that influence children and their health include social roles, socioeconomic status, the media, their experiences of "charity" and social injustices, and the expanding global nature of society. Each of these areas may influence a person's self-concept, the communities where they live, their choice of lifestyle, and their health. Nurses need to assess these areas and their influence on the child and family so that individualized strategies can be designed and implemented to enhance the positive effects and minimize the negative effects on the child's and family's health. More recently there has been an emergence of advocacy services for children and youth to promote their civil and legal rights, their human rights to health (Tobin, 2019), as well as ensuring their voices are heard when decisions are being made "about them" (Boylan & Dalrymple, 2011). Promoting the rights and well-being of Indigenous children and youth in Canada focuses on narrowing the gap between health disparities with a view to promoting equity (Greenwood & de Leeuw, 2012).

Social Roles

Society often prescribes specific patterns of behaviours: certain behaviours are permitted and others are prohibited. These social roles are often an important factor in the development of self-concept. Social roles influence a person's ideas about self. Social roles are generally carried out in groups with which the individual has intimate daily contact, such as the family, school, workplace, or peer groups.

Socioeconomic Status

Another dominant influence is a person's socioeconomic status, meaning their relative position in society. This includes the family's economic, occupational, and educational levels. Children are raised differently by parents of different educational levels, occupations, and incomes. Low socioeconomic status typically has an adverse influence on an individual's health. Supplemental health care costs are continuing to rise, as are the costs of healthy foods and many physical activities. The family may not be able to afford food, health care, and housing; meals may be unbalanced, erratic, or insufficient. Housing may be overcrowded or have poor sanitation. These families may not understand the importance of preventive care or may simply not be able to afford it. As a result, they may be exposed to health risks such as lead poisoning or may not be immunized against communicable diseases. Studies have documented that children who come from low socioeconomic environments are more likely to suffer from acute and chronic conditions experiencing more limitations from these, as well as injuries and mental health conditions (Allin & Stabile, 2012; HELP, 2019).

Take Note!

Research studies have shown that lower socioeconomic status was associated with increased cortisol levels over time (Chen, Cohen, & Miller, 2010). Cortisol plays a role in psychiatric and physical illnesses; therefore, findings of elevated cortisol levels in children from a low socioeconomic status may help explain why low socioeconomic status is negatively related to health (Chen et al., 2010).

POVERTY

Poverty is a measurement based on the specific monetary income of a family. Nearly five million Canadians (roughly one in seven) live in poverty, one quarter of whom are children (Canada Without Poverty, 2019). Children with disabilities are almost twice as likely to be living in homes that rely on social benefits assistance (Canada Without Poverty, 2019). Initiatives aimed at addressing poverty are configured at national and provincial levels with local directives implemented to try to bring about change.

Despite the many global economic gains that have been made during the past century, poverty continues to grow and the gap between rich and poor is widening. Major gaps continue between the economic opportunities and status afforded to women and those offered to men. A disproportionate share of the burden of poverty rests on women's shoulders, and this undermines their health. However, poverty, particularly for women, is more than monetary deficiency. Women continue to lag behind men in control of cash, equal pay, credit, and collateral. Other forms of impoverishment may include deficiencies in literacy, health care access, education, skills, employment opportunities, mobility, and political representation, as well as pressures on time and energy linked to their responsibilities. These poverty factors may affect a person's health (Robinson, Stoffel, & Haider, 2015).

The effects of poverty on children's health can be wide ranging. The family may be able to afford only substandard housing or a house or apartment in a dangerous neighbourhood (e.g., unsanitary conditions, toxins, violence). Poverty may also lead to homelessness.

Basic financial stability enhances the general health and well-being of children, and thus an important negative influence on children's health is poverty. Children living in poverty are more likely to have poor health, be retained in a grade or drop out of school, become teen parents, experience violent crimes, and become adults who live in poverty (Da Fonseca, 2012). They have greater rates of death and illness from almost all causes, except suicide and motor vehicle accidents (Da Fonseca, 2012).

HOMELESSNESS

It is impossible to measure homelessness with 100% accuracy. Therefore, looking at trends is important to demonstrate if progress is being made or not. Homelessness occurs in large urban areas and midsize cities as well as suburban and rural areas. The principal causes of homelessness in families are poverty and lack of affordable housing. Other causes include cutbacks in public welfare programs, mental health issues, and traumatic events such as unemployment, illness, or accidents and personal crises such as divorce, domestic violence, or substance abuse. Children may be forced out of their house or choose to run away and become homeless because they have been abused or neglected, lived in foster homes, or were placed in residential treatment or juvenile detention centres. Over the course of a year figures suggest that as many as 40,000 Canadian youth experience episodes of homelessness (Gaetz, O'Grady, Kidd, & Schwan, 2016). Marginalized groups such as LGBTQ+, minority populations such as Black youth, and those experiencing extreme poverty are overrepresented with between 25% and 40% experiencing homelessness (Abramovich, 2013).

Homelessness can have a negative impact on health and well-being in numerous ways, including the following:

• Increased mental health issues such as anxiety, depression, or aggressive behaviour

• Higher incidence of chronic health problems and trauma-related injuries
• Problems related to nutritional deficiencies, affecting fetal or child growth and development
• Participation in behaviours such as illegal substance use or unprotected sex with multiple partners
• Limited access to health care services such as preventive care, prenatal care, or dental care
• Inability to attend school consistently, because the environment is not conducive to learning; may result in learning problems, socialization issues, or behavioural issues

Media

Today's children are inundated with various forms of media, such as television, video and computer games, iPods, iPads, the Internet, social media, such as Facebook, movies, magazines, books, and newspapers (Fig. 1.7). Media has both positive and negative effects on the development of children and much depends on the content to which they are exposed (CPS, 2017). Some of the images and information are not always in the best interests of children. Children may identify with, and mimic, characters who engage in risk-taking behaviours or lifestyles. Health risk behaviours, such as excessive caloric intake, physical inactivity, smoking, underage drinking, and violent behaviour have been linked to media exposure (CPS, 2017; Strasburger, 2011). Research has established a strong link between media violence and violent, aggressive behaviour (Martins & Wilson, 2012). If an image or type of behaviour is portrayed as the norm, children may view this as acceptable behaviour without examining the potential health risks or other long-term consequences. For example, thinness is portrayed as the body type that is identified with beauty, leading some children to develop unhealthy dieting or other behaviours to develop that body type. For the child who has a

FIGURE 1.7 Computer games can be fun and educational, but the child should be monitored while using the computer and other forms of media to minimize negative effects.

body type that does not fit the ideal, depression or self-esteem issues may develop.

Overall, the images children view every day will affect their behaviour and possibly their health, and pediatric nurses should take this into account when working with children and their families.

The media's influence relates not only to the content but also to the total viewing time. For example, excessive TV viewing has been linked to obesity, poor cognitive skills, and irregular sleep patterns. Overuse of computer or video games may lead to poor school performance. Media has become a major factor in children's lives with TV remaining the dominant medium (CPS, 2017). Young children spend more time on media then they do in school. It is the leading activity other than sleeping. Media can be a positive influence, such as when it offers educational programming or public service messages on the negative effects of substance abuse, smoking, or gang involvement. Also, public broadcasting networks offer valuable programming.

Obtaining a media history provides helpful and important information. The nurse is encouraged to ask questions regarding the amount of recreational screen time and if the child has a television or Internet-connected device in their bedroom. It is important for parents to set limits and know what their children are viewing, whether it is on the TV, computer, tablet, or phone.

Take Note!

The CPS (2016) offers guidance to providers and parents. The campaign 4Ms: Minimize, Mitigate, be Mindful, Model focuses on health promotion behaviours and digital technologies. For further information see the**Point**.

Widespread access to the Internet has fostered a connection to other areas of the world that would not have been possible in previous years. Children are no longer limited to their immediate surroundings, and they have access to a wealth of information. The Internet can be a valuable resource for parents and children to access information, learn new things, and communicate with friends and family. However, online threats exist that can affect the child's health and safety such as sexual predators, pornography, violence, and racism. Parents need to be alert to these hazards and set up safety guidelines (Teaching Guidelines 1.2).

Teaching Guidelines 1.2
PROMOTING SAFE INTERNET USE

- Determine a specific time limit that your child can spend online each day or week. Be consistent in enforcing this time limit.
- Ensure that Internet use does not replace or interfere with homework, friends, or household or school activities.
- Tell your child NEVER to share personal information with anyone online unless you are sure of the person and the child has your permission to do so.
- Urge your child NEVER to share his or her password with anyone, even friends.
- Review Internet sites with your child, and explain what information and websites are appropriate. Use safety and parental controls offered by your Internet service provider.
- Avoid placing the computer in the child's room. Instead, place the computer in a public area of your home, such as the den or kitchen, so that you can monitor your child's use.
- Discuss with your child the need for maintaining safety while using the Internet. Explain potential hazards in terms the child can understand.
- Advise your child to immediately close any sites or stop any communication that makes him or her confused or uncomfortable. Tell your child NEVER to arrange any face-to-face meeting with persons he or she meets online. Urge your child to seek you out if he or she encounters such a situation.
- Teach the child NEVER to open email from any unknown senders.
- Be aware of computer use policies in your child's school.

Global Society

The world is connected in many ways today: People travel from one nation to another easily, new products and immigrants arrive each day, and the Internet makes worldwide communication simple. The United Nations International Children's Emergency Fund (UNICEF) and the WHO lead the world in dealing with the issues of children. Every year about 6.3 million children die around the world, 5.4 million of whom were under the age of 5 (WHO, 2018). Hundreds of thousands of children born in developing countries and their families are moving to more developed nations including Canada as refugees, immigrants, or international adoptees. These families become part of this nation.

Nurses need to be aware of the impact of worldwide events, such as natural and human-made disasters, on families. Families can be displaced by events such as hurricanes or wars, placing them at increased risk for problems such as infectious diseases, malnutrition, and psychological trauma.

Young children bear the brunt of the global burden of disease but progress has been made in reducing mortality in children less than 5 years old (WHO, 2018). The UNICEF and the WHO have identified major problems affecting child growth and development and survival:
- Acute respiratory infections, such as pneumonia
- Malnutrition, including micronutrient deficiency
- HIV/AIDS

- Diarrhea related to lack of clean water and sanitation
- Vaccine-preventable diseases such as measles
- Malaria
- Preterm birth complications
- Poor health care of pregnant and nursing mothers (UNICEF, 2019; WHO, 2018)

These organizations work to propose ways to eradicate these conditions by improving the case management skills of providers with adapted guidelines; improving the health systems with good district health planning and management as well as appropriate supplies, medications, information systems, and referral systems; and improving the family and community practices (WHO, 2016).

Today, families, children, and society as a whole have concerns over world threats and safety. The increase in stressors such as war, terrorism, school violence, and natural disasters puts women, children, and their families at risk for experiencing mental health difficulties. Children who have experienced these events are at risk for issues such as posttraumatic stress disorder, behavioural problems, depression, anxiety, sleep disturbances, restlessness, irritability, aggression, bullying, physiologic responses such as gastrointestinal symptoms, changes in academic performance, social isolation, and safety and security concerns (American Psychological Association [APA], 2015). Children's coping abilities may be reduced and alterations in growth and development may be seen. Children's reactions depend on age and developmental level and are highly influenced by the emotional state of their caregivers. Nurses must be aware of the effects of world threats on women and children so that they can assess for alterations and intervene to promote security and stability.

Violence

Violence can occur in any setting and can involve any person. Gender-based and intimate partner violence (IPV) is a major health concern—affecting thousands of lives and costs the health care system millions of dollars. Violence affects families, women, and children of all ages, ethnic backgrounds, races, educational levels, and socioeconomic levels. Pregnancy is often a time when physical abuse starts or escalates, resulting in poorer outcomes for the pregnant individual and the baby. The effects of IPV on health include insufficient or inconsistent prenatal care, poor nutrition, substance abuse, inadequate weight gain, and depression. Adverse neonatal outcomes include low birth weight, preterm birth, and small-for-gestational-age infants (Alhusen, Ray, Sharps, & Bullock, 2015). Many of these can lead to maternal or neonatal morbidity or mortality.

There are many opportunities within the current health care system for screening and early intervention during routine prenatal care or during episodic care in a hospital setting. The nurse is responsible for assessing for and following up on any abuse. Due to the potential

---

BOX 1.4
RADAR
R—Routinely screen every client for abuse.
A—Ask direct, supportive, and nonjudgmental questions.
D—Document all findings.
A—Assess your client's safety.
R—Review options and provide referrals.

---

impact of gender-based violence and IPV on individuals, children, and families, it is essential to identify any violent situation via a thorough assessment. All nurses need to include "RADAR" in every client visit (Box 1.4). Nurses serve their clients well—by not rescuing them, but by helping them build on their strengths and providing support. For example, in promoting strength-based interventions, recognizing reliance, and strengthening protective factors. Essentially, nurses empower their clients to help themselves. Providing referrals to community and wider resources, that is, shelters and child advocacy centres and intervening to assist women and children in dealing with this issue are paramount.

INTIMATE PARTNER VIOLENCE

IPV is a major public health concern globally and in Canada. It is linked to intergenerational violence and histories of trauma and colonization (Burczycka, 2018). This violence is known as intimate partner abuse, family violence, wife beating, battering, marital abuse, or partner abuse, but regardless of the term used, its effects are widespread and most commonly perpetrated by males (Burczycka, 2018).

Children who are exposed to stressors such as domestic violence or who are victims of **child abuse or neglect** are at high risk for short- and long-term problems in both childhood and adult life. Such events are referred to as adverse child events (ACEs) (Hughes et al., 2017). These problems will manifest differently based on the child's age and developmental ability; the younger the child, and the longer the exposure, the more serious the problems seen. Short-term problems include sleep disturbances, headaches, stomach aches, depression, asthma, enuresis, aggressive behaviours such as increased peer aggression and bullying, decreased social competencies, withdrawal, avoidant attachment, developmental regression, fears, anxiety, and learning problems. Long-term problems may include poor school performance, truancy, absenteeism, and difficulty with adult relationships and tasks. There is a strong correlation between the number of exposures to adverse events and negative behaviours such as early initiation of smoking, sexual activity, and illicit drug use, adolescent pregnancies, and suicide attempts (CDC, 2016; Cotter & Young, 2018).

Take Note!
Witnessing and being exposed to violence in childhood result in a higher tolerance, and greater use, of violence as an adult (Child Trends, 2019).

Not all children exposed to violence suffer negative consequences. Children have resilience, and preliminary studies have identified protective factors that can help buffer children from the effects of violence and reduce the risk that the child will develop violent behaviours (Futures Without Violence, 2016). Examples of protective factors include the following:

- Feelings of connectedness or a secure attachment to a nonviolent parent or caregiver
- Strong commitment to school and academic performance
- Involvement in social activities
- Social and community support
- Positive sibling and peer relationships
- Ability to discuss problems with parents or a supportive adult
- Consistent presence of a parent at least once during the day, such as in the morning on awakening, when getting home from school, at dinnertime, or when going to bed
- Positive view of self
- Strong cultural and/or spiritual identity

Thus, interventions need to focus on reducing children's exposure to violence and fostering protective factors.

YOUTH VIOLENCE

Youth violence affects the community as well as the child and family. Studies have shown that youth violence is associated with a disruption in social services, an increase in health care costs, and a decline in property values (CDC, 2016). Research continues to show that children exposed to violence suffer serious consequences, such as problems with development, behaviour, and physical and mental health issues that last a lifetime (Finkelhor, Turner, Shattuck, & Hamby, 2013).

VIOLENT CRIMES

Violent crimes include murder, rape, robbery, and aggravated assault. A snapshot of youth at risk and youth offending in Canada can be found on thePoint. Statistics from Public Safety Canada (2018) report that 37% of youth have engaged in delinquent behaviours in their lifetime.

SUICIDE

Suicide is a serious public health problem affecting young people today. While in the United States suicide is the third-leading cause of death in people of ages 10 to 14 years, with 56.9% due to firearms and 34.8% due to poisoning (CDC, 2018b). Of these reported suicides, boys (77.9%) were much more likely than girls to die from suicide (CDC, 2018b). Within Canada females are three to four times more likely to attempt suicide, resulting in increased hospital admission rates. Most males commit suicide by hanging (46%) with an increasing number of youth committing suicide; a quarter of all youth deaths are attributed to suicide. These numbers have increased from 9% to 23% between 1974 and 2009 (Statistics Canada, 2017b).

SCHOOL VIOLENCE

In recent years, due to several high-profile cases of school shootings, much attention has been directed at school violence and concern for student and staff safety. While statistics in Canada are limited, US research indicates that between 1% and 2% of school-age homicides occur on the way to or from school, at school events, or during school hours (CDC, 2018c). Students are much less likely to be victims of crime at school than away, but some schools continue to have serious crime and violence problems (CDC, 2018c).

School violence often involves situations of bullying, which is repeated negative actions that are clearly malicious and unwarranted by one or more persons directed at a victim. Verbal, written, or social media violence must be taken seriously (Royal Canadian Mounted Police [RCMP], 2016). Public health or school nurses need to be aware of the impact of violence in and outside schools and offer support, guidance, and intervention when necessary to the students and staff. Working collaboratively with community teams, imbedding healthy school policies and attending to local risks are important ways in which nurses can be involved in promoting a culture of safety (RCMP, 2016).

Safe schools are essential for student learning, growth and development, development of healthy relationships, and overall health of our children. Violence in schools has a negative effect not only on students but also on the school and the entire community. The continued coordination among schools, law enforcement, social services, and mental health systems and the development of effective programs will help to reduce these risk behaviours (RCMP, 2016).

Community

Community encompasses a broad range of concepts, from the nation where a person lives, to a particular neighbourhood or group. The surrounding community affects many aspects of a person's health and general welfare. The quality of life within the community has a great influence on a person's ability to develop and become a functional member of society. Community influences include the school, which is a community in itself, and peer groups. The support and assistance offered to individuals, children, and families from other areas of the community, such as school programs and community centres, can improve the person's overall health and well-being.

SCHOOLS AND OTHER COMMUNITY CENTRES

Children spend more time in child care settings and are involved in various community centres and activities. By age 3 or 4, many children are in an "early years," kindergarten, or preschool program for several hours a day (Government of Canada, 2017). Some children spend more awake time in school and child care settings than in their family home. Thus, schools and child care settings have become major influences on children.

School also provides a means of socialization. School rules about attendance and authority relationships and the system of sanctions and rewards based on achievement help to teach children behavioural expectations that they will need for future employment and relationships in the adult world. Although the primary role of schools has always been academic education, today schools are performing more health-related functions. Schools play an important role in promoting healthy behaviours and educating children about proper exercise, nutrition, safety, sex, drugs, and mental health.

Academic success is linked to healthy behaviours. Academic success is a good indicator of child well-being and is a predictor of adult health outcomes (HELP, 2019). Because in many families both parents need to work, many children are enrolled in child care and after-school programs. Thus, the socialization process begins earlier and involves a larger percentage of the child's waking hours (Fig. 1.8).

After-school hours are a critical time where children may participate in risky health behaviours if they are not provided with supervised, structured activity where they can learn and grow. Community centres and after-school programs can provide an opportunity for children to learn new skills, have new experiences, and develop relationships with caring adults in a safe and supportive environment.

FIGURE 1.8 Daycare centres provide socialization and support for young children.

PEER GROUPS

A child's friends can have a major influence, positive or negative, on his or her growth and development. Peer group relationships often begin early and are a large part of the child's world, particularly with school-age children and adolescents. This influence starts in playgroups in preschool or elementary school. The child is confronted with a variety of values and belief systems from interactions with friends. To be accepted, the child must conform to the specific values and beliefs of the group. When these values and beliefs differ from those of the adults in the child's world, conflicts can occur, possibly separating children from the adults and strengthening their sense of belonging to the peer group.

When the child's friends are successful in school or other activities, the growth and development of the child continues in a healthy and positive way. When these groups demonstrate healthy behaviours, the influence is very positive, but peer groups can also exert negative influences on the child. Thus, it is vital to identify the important peer groups in a child's life and the positive or negative behaviours connected with these groups.

Culture

Culture (the view of the world and implementation of a set of traditions that are used by a specific social group in order to pass these traditions along to the next generation) plays a critical role in shaping a woman, child, or family including their health and health practices (Stanhope & Lancaster, 2011). Culture is a complex phenomenon involving the integration of many components such as beliefs, values, language, time, personal space, and view of the world, all of which shape a person's actions and behaviours. Individuals learn these patterns of cultural behaviours from their family and community through a process called **enculturation**, which involves acquiring knowledge and internalizing values (Adams-Leander & Rector, 2014; Yoon, Hacker, Hewitt, Abrams, & Cleary, 2012).

Culture is learned first in the family, then in school, and then in the community and other social organizations. Culture influences every aspect of development and is reflected in childbearing and child-rearing beliefs and practices designed to promote healthy adaptation (Andrews & Boyle, 2015).

With today's changing demographic patterns, nurses must be able to incorporate cultural knowledge into their interventions so that they can care effectively for culturally diverse individuals, children, and families. They must be aware of the wide range of cultural traditions, values, and ethics that exist in Canada today. All nurses must consider how to work toward meaningful **cultural competence** and cultural safety when working with children and families (CNA, 2018).

The nurse should know about various cultural groups, ethnicity, culture-based health practices, and how they may affect children, as well as the demographics of the local population. The goal is for the nurse to view culture as a point of congruence rather than a potential source of conflict.

Cultural Groups

A cultural group is a self-defined group of people who share a commonality such as religion, language, nationality, ethnicity, race, or a physical trait. In a society there are typically dominant and minority groups. The dominant group, often the largest group, has the greatest authority to control the values and sanctions of the society (Adams-Leander & Rector, 2014; Kersey-Matusiak, 2012). As a result, the dominant culture may have the largest impact on the individual's health, whereas minority cultural groups may still maintain some of their own traditions and values.

The relationship of culture to health care can become obscured by the use of broad group titles. In reality, there are many distinct cultural groups, and within a group there may be many subcultures. Geographic differences also can occur as well as diversity with urban neighbourhoods (HELP, 2019).

Nurses should also be aware of the traditional health care values and practices that are passed along from one generation to the next. For example, some cultures believe in consulting healers, and this belief may have a major influence on children's health (Table 1.3). The nurse must remember that diversity exists within cultures and this is as important as the diversity between cultures. Every person is a unique individual with his or her own beliefs, values, and history. Nurses must avoid stereotyping, which can lead to misconceptions.

Ethnicity

Ethnicity, a term sometimes used synonymously with culture, involves group membership by virtue of common ancestry–shared culture and identity. The basic groups are differentiated by their customs, characteristics, language, or similar distinguishing factors. Ethnic groups have their own family structures, languages, food preferences, moral codes, and health care practices. Children learn the accepted mode of behaviour by observing and imitating those around them. The influences of culture and ethnicity on individuals, children, and families are highly variable and dynamic. Probably the most important characteristic of ethnicity is the sense of shared identity felt by members (Nagle & Clancy, 2012).

Children who come from a minority group may experience conflict and difficulties with interactions, including health care providers, because their native customs are different from those of the dominant culture.

Stereotyping or labelling can result from **ethnocentrism**, a belief that one's own ethnic group is superior to other ethnic groups. This attitude can lead to a slanted view of the world, and it may hinder the nurse's ability to provide culturally competent care.

Cultural Health Practices

Health practices are often the result of health beliefs derived from a person's culture. For example, does the child and family view health and illness as the result of natural forces, supernatural forces, or the imbalance of forces? Most cultures have remedies that people may use or consider before they seek professional health care. Asian Canadians may consult a practitioner who specializes in traditional Asian therapies such as acupuncture, acupressure, and moxibustion. These healers are often very powerful in their community, speak the language, and are very familiar with the culture's spiritual or religious aspects.

Pediatric integrative medicine (PIM) explores evidence-informed approaches to using alternative therapies with medical treatments (Loo, 2009; Vohra et al., 2017). More recently clinical trials are being developed to explore safety and provider training is being examined in various areas, such as chiropractic and naturopathic in acute and community settings.

Take Note!

Nurses can help to shape a person's lifelong perceptions of health and health services. An understanding of how the individual's, child's, and family's culture affects their health practices gives the nurse an opportunity to incorporate appropriate and beneficial health practices into the family's cultural milieu, providing sources of strength rather than areas of conflict.

Changing Cultural Demographics

The ethnocultural diversity in Canada is continuing to increase with one in five people identifying as a member of a visible minority. This becomes more evident in larger cities, as 96% of Canadians who belong to a visible minority group live in more urban areas, such as Toronto, Vancouver, and Montréal (Statistics Canada, 2018b). The largest visible minority group is South Asian, which by 2031 may account for up to 28% of the Canadian population. As expected with a wide scope of ethnocultural diversity, Canada is a multilingual society even beyond the official English and French languages.

Approximately 4.3% of people in Canada identify as having an Aboriginal identity: 60.8% as First Nation, 32.3% as Métis, and 4.2% as Inuit (note that some people identify with more than one group; see Statistics Canada, 2018a). Children represent over a quarter of the Indigenous population (28%). Historical determinants have

TABLE 1.3	TRADITIONAL BELIEFS AND PRACTICES OF SELECTED CULTURAL GROUPS
Cultural Group	**Beliefs and Practices Affecting Children's Health**
African Canadians	Strong extended family relationships; mother as head of household; elder family members valued and respected Food as a symbol of health and wealth View of health as harmony with nature, illness as disruption in harmony Use of folk healing and home remedies common to treat body, mind, and spirit Strong church/religious affiliation Belief in illnesses as natural (due to natural forces that the person hasn't protected self against) and unnatural (due to person or spirit) Individuals vulnerable to external forces
Asian Canadians	Strong loyalty to the family; father head of household Family as the centre, with members expected to care for one another Preserving family pride and dignity is important Use of complementary modalities with Western health care practices View of life as a cycle, with everything connected to health Health viewed as a balance between the forces of *yang (hot)* and *yin (cold)* resulting in *qi* (pronounced chee), which is a balanced state of harmony Respect for authority emphasized
Arab Canadians	Women subordinate to men; young individuals subordinate to older persons Family loyalty is primary Modesty is a core value Disease and illness attributed to the will of Allah Good health associated with eating properly, consuming nutritious foods, and fasting to cure disease Illness due to inadequate diet, shifts in hot and cold, exposure of stomach while sleeping, emotional or spiritual distress, and "evil eye" Cleanliness important for prayer
Indigenous, First Nations, Métis	High value on family and tribe; respect for elders Family as an extended network providing care for newborns and children Women as the verbal decision makers and story holders Celebrations to mark the stages of growth and development Use of food to celebrate life events and in healing and religious ceremonies Health as harmony with nature; illness due to disharmony, evil spirits; purification rituals (immersion in water, sweat lodges) to cleanse the body and spirit and maintain harmony with nature Prefer restoration of physical, mental, and spiritual balance through herbal medicines and healing ceremonies
Hispanic Canadians	Family important; father as the source of strength, wisdom, and self-confidence Mother as the caretaker and decision maker for health View of children as persons to continue the family and culture Use of food for celebrations and socialization Health as God's will maintainable with a balance of hot and cold food intake Cope with illness through prayer and faith in God Freedom from pain indicative of good health; pain tolerated stoically due to belief that it is God's will Folk medicine practices and prayers, herbal teas, and poultices for illness treatment

Adapted from Adams-Leander, S., & Rector, C. (2014). Chapter 5: Transcultural nursing in the community. In J. A. Allender, C. Rector, & K. D. Warner (Eds.). *Community & public health nursing. Promoting the public's health* (8th ed., pp. 115–149). Philadelphia, PA: Wolters Kluwer Health/Lippincott Williams & Wilkins.

shaped Aboriginal women's status and subsequently access to health services, resulting in fragmented care and inequality (Halseth, 2013). Nurses must be mindful of lessons learned from the past when working with culturally diverse populations. The six National Collaborating Centres for Public Health (NCCPH) across Canada link public health work, research, and knowledge translation by providing an array of evidence-informed resources, access to training, and multimedia tools (NCCPH, 2018).

Immigration

Canada has one of the highest levels of immigration in the world. While employment and economic opportunities, expanded human rights, educational opportunities, and other types of freedoms and opportunities encourage many foreigners to move to Canada, other migrants are displaced peoples, such as refugees. Of the growing number of immigrants, approximately 20% of new permanent residents are children (CPS, 2018c). The majority of immigrants to the country live in Ontario, British Columbia, Alberta, and Quebec. Newcomers to Canada face a range of challenges and barriers linked to health access as a result of finance, pre-existing health conditions, language and literacy difficulties, and factors linked to gender and culture (CPS, 2018c).

By helping newcomers understand the Interim Federal Health Program administered by Medavie Blue Cross, as well as explaining other requirements and local policies, nurses can position themselves to break down barriers to quality care. Nurses as providers must become familiar with using culturally competent care when working with immigrant populations as well as being able to identify health risks, such as uncommon Canadian infectious diseases and mental health trauma (CPS, 2018c). In addition, the health status of immigrant children may be compromised due to the lack of at-birth and early childhood screenings, which may manifest with problems such as inborn errors of metabolism, lack of preventive care, no immunizations, and no dental care.

Inability to speak English can hinder an immigrant person's educational attainment, economic opportunities, and ability to participate in the mainstream of society. Often children serve as translators for their parents who may speak or understand little English. This is an additional and often hidden burden for children. Furthermore, immigrant parents who do not speak English may have trouble accessing health care and supplemental health insurance, through accessing work or better-paying jobs.

Spirituality and Religion

Spirituality is a basic human quality involving the belief in something greater than oneself and a faith that affirms life positively. It is a major influence in many people's lives, providing a meaning or purpose to life and a foundation for and source of love, relationships, and service. Spirituality is considered a universal human phenomenon with an assumption of the wholeness of people and their connectedness to a higher being. During life-changing events and crises, such as a serious illness or the birth of a child with a congenital defect, families often turn to spirituality for hope, comfort, and relief.

The word *religion* is often used interchangeably with spirituality in our society. However, spirituality is a more private and individual belief, whereas religion is an organized way of sharing beliefs and practicing worship. Therefore, spirituality and religion are an important focus when working with women, children, and their families. A person's reaction to health and illness may be affected by these beliefs. In some religions, illness is seen as a punishment for sin or wrongdoing. Other religions view illness as a test of strength (Adams-Leander & Rector, 2014).

People appreciate the recognition of, and respect for, their beliefs. Therefore, identifying the individual's and family's religious beliefs and customs is important. People may adhere to special dietary restrictions, rituals such as baptism or holy communion, use of amulets or icons, or practices related to dying that can be incorporated into the plan of care. Using open-ended questions and observing for the use of religious articles during assessment can provide clues to the family's beliefs and practices. Visits from spiritual leaders, Elders, may also be noted. Table 1.4 identifies some of the ways in which tenets of major religious beliefs may affect children's health.

Take Note!

Never make assumptions about a family's religious or spiritual affiliation. Although they may belong to a particular religion, family members may not adhere to all of its beliefs or participate in all aspects of the religion. Be alert for clues that would provide insight into their specific beliefs.

Health Status and Lifestyle

Obviously, the general health status of a person and specific lifestyle can influence that person's health. Health status may be a factor soon after birth. Societal shifts, triggered by a greater focus on education and careers, have resulted in a trend toward delayed childbearing in Canadian women (Statistics Canada, 2018d). This timing has increased the incidence of multiple births due to the increased use of IVF and other assisted reproductive technologies along with women delaying childbearing until they are older (Crawford & Steiner, 2015). Potential complications of multiple births include prematurity and intrauterine growth retardation, which may lead to chronic health problems in the child. Children with chronic health conditions may also have developmental delays, especially in acquiring skills related to cognition, communication, adaptation, social functioning, and motor functioning. Thus, the beginning health status of a child may affect his or her long-term health and development.

Developmental Level and Disease Distribution

Developmental level has a major impact on a person's health status. In general, the distribution of diseases or illnesses varies with age. For example, adolescents who become pregnant are at a higher risk for certain complications, such as anemia, hypertension, preterm labour, cephalopelvic disproportion, and postpartum hemorrhage. Pregnant adolescents also experience higher rates of IPV and substance abuse. Moreover, substance abuse can contribute to low birth weight, intrauterine growth restriction, preterm births, newborn addiction, and sepsis (Wong, Ordean, & Kahan, 2011). Women who become

TABLE 1.4	SELECTED RELIGIOUS BELIEFS AFFECTING CHILDREN'S HEALTH		
Religion	**Beliefs About Health and Illness**	**Dietary Practices**	**Beliefs About Birth and Death**
Buddhism	Illness from karmic causes (ignorant craving) Illness as an opportunity to develop the soul Ultimate goal of achieving nirvana (state of supreme tranquility, purity, and stability) No restrictions for medications, vaccines, nutritional therapies, or other therapeutic interventions	Moderation in diet encouraged Some sects vegetarian; some branches have strict dietary regulation; therefore, it is important to inquire about client's preferences	No baptism Last rite chanting at bedside soon after death; if there is hope for recovery and continuing the pursuit of enlightenment all means of intervention are encouraged Organ donation acceptable Cremation common
Christian Science	Disease viewed as error of human mind that can be dispelled by spiritual truth Health viewed within a spiritual framework; healing through prayer and spiritual regeneration Possible contact of own healing ministry (Christian Science practitioners) if child is hospitalized General opposition to human interventions with drugs or other therapies except for legally required immunizations Usually do not use blood or blood components, seek transplants or act as donors, seek biopsies or physical examination	No special requirements or restrictions	No baptism or last rites Unlikely to seek medical means to prolong life, use of prayer for recovery. Disposal of body in death left to family to decide
Hindu	Illness due to sins committed in previous life Acceptance of most medical practice/care Nonviolent approach to life	Meat consumption forbidden (especially beef) Some are strict vegetarians	No baptism View of death as a step in an ongoing cycle to reach nirvana Certain prescribed rites after death, such as washing the body by family and restrictions on who touches the body Cremation common
Islam	Belief that God cures but will accept treatment Compulsory prayers at dawn, noon, afternoon, after sunset, and after nightfall	Ingestion of pork and pork products and alcohol forbidden Fasting (by boys from age 7, girls from age 9, and adults) required during Ramadan (ninth month of Islamic year) (exceptions for pregnant/nursing mothers, elderly, or very ill)	No baptism Special party (*Aqeeqa*) to celebrate birth Specific burial rituals (rinsing and washing, wrapping, special prayers, and burial)

TABLE 1.4	SELECTED RELIGIOUS BELIEFS AFFECTING CHILDREN'S HEALTH (continued)		
Religion	**Beliefs About Health and Illness**	**Dietary Practices**	**Beliefs About Birth and Death**
Judaism (orthodox and conservative)	Illness as possible reason for violating some dietary restrictions No treatments or procedures on Sabbath (which begins 18 minutes before sunset on Friday and ends 42 minutes after sunset on Saturday) or holy days	Ingestion of blood (such as raw meat) prohibited Kosher dietary laws; highly individualized observance Abstinence from ingestion of pork and predatory fowl and no mixing of milk dishes with meat dishes; ingestion of only fish with fins and scales; no shellfish (strict followers) Fasting during Yom Kippur, and matzo replaces leavened bread during Passover week	No baptism Ritual circumcision of male infants on eighth day of life Ritual of washing body after death; family and close friends remain with the deceased for a period of time No cremation
Mormon (Church of Jesus Christ of Latter-Day Saints)	Belief in divine health via laying on of hands. Medical therapy not prohibited Common use of herbal folk remedies	Ingestion of caffeinated tea, coffee, and alcohol and use of tobacco prohibited Fasting (no food or drink including water) once a month for 24 hours on a designated day, exceptions made (pregnant women, very young or old, and ill)	Baptism at older age (approximately 8 years old); infant blessed by church official after the birth Death believed to be another step in eternal progression Cremation discouraged, but not forbidden
Roman Catholic	Care of sick encouraged Misuse of any substance considered harmful to the body and a sin Eucharist as the food of healing and health	Moderation in diet encouraged Fasting and abstinence from meat and meat products on Ash Wednesday and Good Friday Abstinence on Fridays during Lent, but exceptions made if ill	Infant baptism; sacrament of the sick if prognosis is poor while child is alive; anointing of the sick Burial and treatment of the body with respect and honour Cremation is acceptable in certain circumstances

Adapted from Andrews, M. M., & Boyle, J. (2015). *Transcultural concepts in nursing care* (7th ed.). Philadelphia, PA: Lippincott Williams & Wilkins; Hanson, P. A., & Andrews, M. M. (2012). Chapter 13: Religion, culture and nursing. In M. M. Andrews, & J. S. Boyle (Eds.). *Transcultural concepts in nursing care* (6th ed., pp. 351–402). Philadelphia, PA: Wolters Kluwer Health/Lippincott Williams & Wilkins.

pregnant after age 35 are at risk for hypertension, dystocia, and postpartum hemorrhage. Older pregnant women are also more likely to have a pre-existing condition that could complicate the pregnancy. Moreover, fetuses of older pregnant women are at risk for chromosomal abnormalities. While data indicate that Canadians overall are delaying childbirth, women in Indigenous populations are continuing to have children at younger ages (Statistics Canada, 2018d).

Certain communicable diseases are more commonly associated with certain age groups. Roseola, which is a viral illness resulting in high fevers and rash, is most often seen in infants 6 to 15 months; scarlet fever, a group A streptococci infection, is a disease that primarily affects children between 4 and 8 years of age. The physiologic immaturity of an infant's body systems increases the risk for infection. Ingestion of toxic substances and poisoning are major health concerns for toddlers as they become more mobile and inquisitive. Because preschool and school-age children are generally quite active, they are more prone to injury and accidents. Adolescents are establishing their identity, which may lead them to distance themselves from their family values and traditions for a period of time and conform more with their peers. This journey may lead to risky behaviours, resulting in injuries or other situations that may impair their health.

Nutrition

Nutrition provides the body with the calories and nutrients to sustain life and promote growth, as well as the essentials required to maintain health and prevent illness.

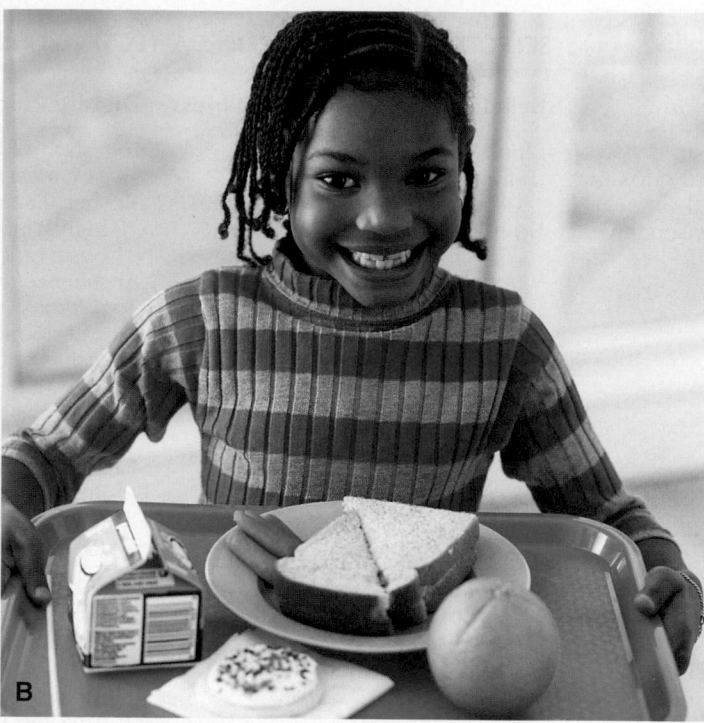

FIGURE 1.9 **A.** This pregnant client is eating a healthy meal to ensure adequate nutrition. **B.** The dietary habits established early in life can have a long-lasting impact on the child's health and quality of life.

Nutritional deficiencies, such as iron-deficiency anemia, or excesses, such as the increasing incidence of childhood obesity, are still common problems in Canada. Effective obesity prevention and treatment interventions targeting children and their families are needed to help curb the obesity epidemic (Seburg, Olson-Bullis, Bredeson, Hayes, & Sherwood, 2015). Some factors contributing to poor nutrition include inadequate food intake, nutritionally unsound social and cultural food practices, the easy accessibility of processed and nutritionally inadequate foods, lack of nutrition education in homes and schools, and the presence of illness that interferes with ingestion, digestion, and absorption of food.

During pregnancy, additional calories are needed to support fetal growth and development as well as to support the pregnant individual's own needs, and an adequate intake of folic acid is important to prevent neural tube defects (Fig. 1.9). For the child, inadequate nutrition is associated with lowered cognitive ability, poor or altered emotional and mental health, increased susceptibility to childhood illnesses, and stunted physical growth (Miller & Scott, 2015). The so-called fast food or junk food that is prevalent in today's society is a key factor in the epidemic of childhood obesity and increases in the prevalence of childhood type 2 diabetes. Nutrition and its effects on health status are integrated throughout this text.

Lifestyle Choices

Lifestyle choices that affect a person's health include patterns of eating; amount and type of exercise; use of tobacco, drugs, or alcohol; and methods of coping with stress. Most health problems that arise today are due to a person's lifestyle. For children, the lifestyle of the parents can become the modelled behaviour for the child. Inactive parents who eat poorly commonly have children with similar habits, which can result in diabetes, obesity, and early heart disease. These typically adult problems are being diagnosed more frequently in children and adolescents today. Parents should first self-evaluate their own dietary and activity habits, make changes where necessary, and then strive to encourage healthy eating habits and an appropriate level of physical activity in the child's life through sports, hobbies such as dancing, or family activities.

Environmental Exposure

Some environmental exposures can jeopardize health. In utero, the child can be affected by poor nutrition, infections, or use of alcohol, tobacco, and drugs. Nurses caring for pregnant clients should be aware of the risks to the fetus posed by certain drugs, chemicals, and dietary agents, as well as illnesses. These agents, known as teratogens, may be linked to birth defects in children.

Not all drugs or agents are associated with fetal effects, however, and research is necessary to identify the correlations between teratogens and other variables.

The environment continues to affect a child's health after birth. Exposure to air pollution, tobacco, and water or food contaminants can impair a child's health status. Safety hazards in the home or community can contribute to falls, burns, drowning, or other accidents. Exposure to second-hand smoke and other pollutants, such as from radiation or chemicals, is a health hazard for children. Because children are smaller and still developing, environmental exposures can cause them additional health problems. For example, lead exposure is a common preventable poisoning in children, especially children less than 6 years of age. Due to their rapidly developing nervous system, young children are more sensitive to the effects of lead. Sources include lead-contaminated dust and lead contained in soil and water. Lead exposure can result in developmental and behavioural problems ranging from inattentiveness and hyperactivity to permanent brain damage and death, depending on the level of exposure.

Take Note!

A recent study found that residual tobacco smoke and carcinogens remain after a cigarette is extinguished (referred to as third-hand smoke). These toxins cling to the smoker's hair and clothes and can be present on any surface in the house, such as carpet and cushions. Children are particularly susceptible to third-hand smoke since they breathe near, crawl, touch, and mouth contaminated surfaces (Karim et al., 2015).

Stress and Coping

Stressors such as war, terrorism, school violence, and natural disasters may decrease a person's coping ability (Yahav, 2011) and lead to alterations in growth and development (Masten & Narayan, 2012). Exposure to traumatic events and violence may have long-term effects on an individual's psychosocial development and status. Some children can adapt and respond to the stress, while others do not. The term **resilience** refers to the qualities that enable a person to cope with significant adverse events or stresses and still function competently (Masten & Narayan, 2012).

Exposure to stress is not limited to disasters or traumatic events. Stress (or adverse events) can also include financial hardship in the family or community, family crises such as divorce, inadequate support systems, illness, or violence. Stress can also be associated with the normal problems associated with growth and development, such as entering a new classroom, learning a new skill, or being teased by a classmate. Similar to disasters and traumatic events, the effects of these stressors can dramatically affect the health status of a woman, child, or family.

Recall Sophia, the 38-year-old pregnant woman who has come to the prenatal clinic for a visit. While talking with the nurse, Sophia mentions that her children are very involved in activities. She says, "My husband is busy at work, so I do most of the running around. Sometimes I feel like the people at the drive-thru know me by name! My husband helps out on the weekends, but during the week, it's all me." What factors may be influencing Sophia's health? How might these factors be influencing the health of the children and the family?

Access to Health Care

Dynamic reform in health care will continue across Canada. Universal hospital care was introduced following World War II with publicly funded acute care and diagnostic services (Government of Canada, 2018a). Universal physician and service insurance plans came into effect by 1972 as a result of the *Medical Care Act* (1966). Ongoing reforms such as the *Canada Health Act* (1985) and the *10-Year Plan to Strengthen Health Care* (Health Canada, 2004) continue to shape services. Within Canada the roles and responsibilities for delivering health care are divided between federal, provincial, and territorial governments. Taxes and levies support public funding while insurance schemes are often linked to employers. Public health (infectious disease, sanitation, etc.) is shared between federal, provincial/territories while often coordinated and delivered locally. The federal government provides health service funding for specific groups including First Nations living on reserve, Inuit, those in the armed forces, and incarcerated people. The majority of health care is delivered at the provincial and territory level. Insurance plans, assistance, and benefits are available for certain groups (e.g., low-income, seniors) yet medication prescribed outside of a hospital setting, hearing, vision, and dental care costs are not covered under the *Canada Health Act* (Government of Canada, 2018a).

Preventive Care Focus

The emphasis on cost reduction also led to an emphasis on preventive care and services. Anticipatory guidance is vital during each health contact with women, children, and families. Education of the family includes everything from keeping the home safe to preventing illness.

The Continuum of Care Emphasis

A "continuum of care" strategy is cost effective and provides more efficient and effective services. This continuum extends from acute care settings such as hospitals to outpatient settings such as ambulatory care clinics, primary care settings, rehabilitative units, community care settings, long-term facilities, homes, and even schools. For example, the hospital stay is now integrated into a continuum that allows the client to complete therapy at home, school, or other community settings, while reentering the hospital for short periods for specific treatments or illnesses.

Improvements in Diagnosis and Treatments

Because of the tremendous improvements that have been made in technology and biomedicine, disorders and diseases are being diagnosed and treated earlier. The 1990s witnessed a remarkable and productive connection between genetics and various pathophysiologic processes. Many genetic defects are being identified so counselling and treatment may occur early. With these improved diagnoses and treatments, nurses will be caring for people who have survived experiences that were at one time fatal. In addition, people treated for illness in childhood are living with chronic conditions and making decision about having a family of their own. For example, at one time individuals with congenital heart disease did not live long enough to become pregnant. However, with new surgical techniques to correct such defects in childhood, many of these people survive and become pregnant, progressing through their pregnancy without significant problems.

While positive and exciting, these advances and trends also pose new challenges for the health care community. For example, as health care for premature newborns improves and survival rates increase, the incidence of long-term chronic conditions such as respiratory airway dysfunction or developmental delays has also increased. As a result, nurses are faced with caring for clients at all stages along the health–illness continuum, such as well children, those who are occasionally ill, and women, children, and families with chronic and sometimes life-limiting conditions.

Empowerment of Health Care Consumers

Due to the influence of managed care, the focus on prevention, a more educated population, and technologic advances, individuals and families have taken an increased responsibility for their own health. The consumers of health care are now better informed, and they want to play a greater role in managing health and illness. Families want access to evidence-informed information about health and disease management in order to be informed and participate in making decisions about treatment options. As client advocates valuing family-centred care, nurses are instrumental in promoting this empowerment. To do this, the nurse should respect the family's views and concerns, address all issues and concerns, consider the family members as important participants, and always include the woman, child, and family in the decision-making process.

BARRIERS TO HEALTH CARE

Women are major consumers of health care services, in many cases arranging not only their own care but also that of family members. Compared with men, research indicates that women have more health problems, longer life spans, and more significant reproductive health needs (Davis, 2014). Access to care can be jeopardized by lower incomes and greater responsibilities (juggling work and family). Barriers to health care include health literacy, lack of finances; sociocultural barriers, including lack of transportation, no babysitters, and language; and health care delivery system barriers, including inconvenient clinic hours and poor attitudes by health care workers. These barriers often discourage clients from seeking health care (Patel & Rushefsky, 2015).

Finances

Financial barriers are one of the most important factors that limit care. Fertility treatments and childbirth have associated health care costs. IVF is largely coordinated by private clinics with the cost burden falling to the hopeful parent(s). The Medicare system for Canadian citizens or residents supports the cost of having a baby, while private or midwifery services can be purchased. Tourists and visitors to Canada will have to pay or use their travel insurance to cover the cost which can range between $5,000 and $8,000 for a vaginal birth to $10,000 to $12,000 for a C-section. Birth tourism is a topic which is debated within the scope of the *Citizenship Act* and is linked to the citizenship status of the child when born in Canada to parents who are not citizens.

Sociocultural Barriers

Lack of transportation and the need for both parents to work poses barriers to seeking health care. It can be difficult to attend all recommended prenatal health care visits or well-child visits, especially if the woman has other small children who must be taken along on the visit. These challenges can reduce the adherence to scheduled appointments and follow-up. Knowledge barriers (e.g., lack of understanding of the importance of prenatal care or preventive health care), language barriers (e.g., speaking a different language than the health care providers), or spiritual barriers (e.g., religious beliefs discouraging some forms of treatment) also exist. For women living in rural communities, access to services can be limited by their rurality as well as weather conditions and transport difficulties should they need to travel.

Health Care Delivery System Barriers

The health care delivery system itself can create barriers. A reduction in traditional approaches to birthing for Indigenous peoples has resulted in births happening away from family and community. Furthermore, studies examining the perinatal experiences for women with disabilities have identified attitudinal barriers from staff, financial constraints, and limited access to appropriate health information (Vanier Institute of the Family, 2017). Furthermore, limited number of Indigenous nurses as well as Indigenous-speaking health care workers influences access, communication, and health outcome for people.

Organizational factors must be considered when providing care, for example, clinic hours must meet the needs of the clients, not the health care providers who work there. Evening or weekend hours might be needed to meet the schedules of working clients. Clinic personnel should evaluate the availability and accessibility of the services they offer.

Unfortunately, some health care workers exhibit negative attitudes toward underprivileged or culturally diverse families, and this could deter these clients from seeking health care. Long delays, hurried examinations, and rude comments by staff discourage clients from returning.

Consider This

I was a 17-year-old pregnant newcomer to Canada needing prenatal care. Although my English wasn't good, I was able to show the receptionist my "big belly" and ask for services. All the receptionist seemed interested in was a health card—which I did not have. She proceeded to ask me personal questions concerning who the father was and commented on how young I looked. The receptionist then "ordered" me in a loud voice to sit down and wait for an answer by someone in the back, but never contacted anyone that I could see. It seemed to me like all eyes were on me while I found an empty seat in the waiting room. After sitting there quietly for over an hour without any attention or answer, I left.

Thoughts: Why did she leave before receiving any health care service? What must she have been feeling during her wait? Would you come back to this clinic again?

LEGAL AND ETHICAL ISSUES IN PERINATAL AND CHILD HEALTH CARE

Law and ethics are interrelated and affect all aspects of nursing. Professional nurses must understand their scope of practice, standards of care, institutional or agency policies, and provincial laws. Every nurse is responsible for knowing current information regarding ethics and laws related to their practice. Numerous federal programs have had a major impact on women's and children's health. These include abortion, substance abuse, fetal therapy, maternal–fetal conflict, stem cell research, umbilical cord blood banking, informed consent, client rights, and confidentiality.

Abortion

Abortion remains a controversial legal, social, and political issue. It has been legal in Canada since 1988 when the Supreme Court of Canada removed restrictive abortion laws, citing violations to Section 7 of the *Canadian Charter of Rights and Freedoms*. The regulation of abortion health care services is governed by the Canada Health Act (1985). Canada, like many other countries, has seen a shift in the legalization of abortion over the last century. Abortions can be safely performed in hospital settings as well as private outpatient clinics.

Abortion is consistently a hotly debated political issue that separates people into two camps: pro-choice and pro-life. The pro-choice group supports the right of any person to make decisions about their own reproductive functions based on their moral and ethical beliefs. The pro-life group believes that abortion is murder and deprives the fetus of the right to life. Both sides will continue to debate this very emotional issue for years to come.

The termination of a pregnancy may be induced either medically or surgically. Over 95% of the 100,000 abortions performed in Canada each year are done surgically, and two thirds of these procedures are completed within the first 13 weeks of pregnancy, meaning within the first trimester (Costescu, Guilbert, & SOGC Surgical Abortion Working Group, 2018). The Society of Obstetricians and Gynaecologists of Canada (SOGC) state that clients may seek an abortion for a variety of personal reasons, each of which is valid. All clients undergoing abortion need emotional support, a stable environment in which to recover, and nonjudgmental care throughout the experience (Costescu et al., 2018).

Abortion is a complex issue, and the controversy is not only in the public arena; many nurses struggle with the conflict between their personal convictions and their professional duty. Nurses are taught to be supportive client advocates and to interact with a nonjudgmental attitude under all circumstances even when personal and political views differ from those of their clients.

With advances in abortion care, this points toward greater nursing involvement. Although this bodes well for person-centred care, the burden on nurses is likely to increase incrementally. Nurses need to clarify their personal values and beliefs on this issue and must be able to provide nonbiased care before assuming responsibility for clients who might be in a position to consider abortion. Their decision to care for or refuse to care for such clients affects staff unity, influences staffing decisions, and challenges the ethical concept of duty (McLemore, Kools, & Levi, 2015).

The CNA's *Code of Ethics for Registered Nurses* describes the nurse's responsibility to provide safe, accountable nursing care: "If nursing care is requested that is in conflict with the nurse's moral beliefs and values but in keeping with professional practice, the nurse provides safe, compassionate, competent and ethical care until alternative care arrangements are in place to meet the person's needs or desires" (CNA, 2017, p. 17). Open communication and acceptance of the personal beliefs of others can promote a comfortable working environment.

Substance Abuse

Substance use disorder (SUD) for any person is a problem, but when it involves a pregnant individual, substance use can cause fetal injury and thus health and ethical implications. Substance use during pregnancy may cause fetal anomalies, preterm birth, placental abruption, and central nervous system developmental alterations (Viteri et al., 2015). In the United States, many states have laws requiring reporting any evidence of prenatal drug exposure, which may lead to charges of negligence and child endangerment against the pregnant person. However, incarceration, or threat of it, has no effect in reducing cases of alcohol or drug abuse (Malinowska-Sempruch & Rychkova, 2015). The punitive approach to fetal injury in the United States raises ethical and legal questions about the degree of governmental control that is appropriate in the interests of child safety.

Nurses should employ a flexible approach to the care of clients who are struggling with substance use, and nurses should encourage clients to seek support from all available community resources. Nurses should counsel clients about the risks of preconception, antepartum, and postpartum substance abuse in a calm, supportive, and nonjudgmental manner (Galante, French, & Grace, 2015).

Intrauterine Therapy

Progress in prenatal diagnosis can lead to the diagnosis of severe fetal abnormalities which previously would have led to a fatal outcome or the development of severe disability. Intrauterine therapy can now be offered in these selected cases and also in the treatment of fetal obstructive uropathy (anomalies of the fetal urinary tract), intrauterine transfusions for fetal anemia, spina bifida repair, and stem cell transplantation. Intrauterine therapy is a procedure that involves opening the uterus

during pregnancy, performing a surgery, and replacing the fetus in the uterus. Although the risks to the fetus and the pregnant person are both great, fetal therapy may be used to correct anatomic lesions (Yuan, 2015). Some argue that medical technology should not interfere with nature, and thus this intervention should not take place. Others would argue that the surgical intervention improves the child's quality of life. For many people, these are the subjects of debates and intellectual discussions, but for nurses, these procedures may be part of their daily routine.

Nurses play an important supportive role in caring and advocating for clients and their families. As the use of technology grows, situations will surface more frequently that test a nurse's belief system. Encouraging open discussions to address emotional issues and differences of opinion among staff members is healthy and increases tolerance for differing points of view.

Maternal–Fetal Conflict

In perinatal nursing, the ethical principles of beneficence and autonomy provide the fundamental framework that guides the management of all pregnant individuals. As there is the need for consideration of the fetus, autonomy can become a complex issue, which gives rise to what is sometimes called the **maternal–fetal conflict**.

Fetal care becomes problematic when what is required to benefit one member of the dyad will cause an unacceptable harm to the other. When a fetal condition poses no health threat to the pregnant person, caring for the fetus will always carry some degree of risk to the pregnant person, without direct therapeutic benefit for them. The ethical principles of beneficence ("be of benefit") and nonmaleficence ("do no harm") can come into conflict.

Because these two are biologically linked, both, or neither, must be treated alike. It would be unethical to recommend fetal therapy as if it were medically indicated for both clients. Still, given a recommendation for fetal therapy, most often pregnant clients will consent to treatment, which promotes fetal health. When pregnant individuals decline therapeutic interventions, health care providers must remember that the ethical injunction against harming one client in order to benefit another is virtually absolute.

Stem Cell Research

Stem cells constitute one of the most promising tools for regenerative medicine. They can grow into any cell type in the body and have been touted as a potential cure for everything from type 1 diabetes to stroke. The goal of stem cell research is a relief of human suffering, which ethically is good. Benefits of stem cell research include therapies for Parkinson disease, regeneration of diseased body tissues, repair of spinal cord injuries, and the growing of needed organs for transplant.

It would seem morally compelling to explore all the sources that might provide us with them, but the ethical concerns surrounding stem cell research vary depending on the origin of the stem cells. Adult stem cells are found in adults, who can replace old cells by reproducing new ones (e.g., blood and liver cells). Bone marrow transplants are examples of the use of adult stem cells in medical therapy. Embryonic stem cells are derived from the inner cell mass of an early embryo. They aren't without controversy; the process of obtaining these cells results in the destruction of the embryo. However, they hold huge promise too (de Miguel-Beriain, 2015).

Some people feel that the destruction of the human embryo constitutes the killing of a human being and reject this practice on religious grounds. Views about when life begins and whether the early embryo is considered a person with moral status are the heart of the ethical deliberations related to embryonic stem cells. Everyone has to decide based on their own personal values and ethical background. In Canada, the use of stem cells, including embryonic cells, for the purpose of research requires careful ethical review. The Federal Panel on Research Ethics developed the *Tri-Council Policy Statement: Ethical Conduct for Research Involving Humans* (Government of Canada, 2014b) which sets the standards for federally funded research through the three major federal funding agencies: Canadian Institutes of Health Research (CIHR), Natural Sciences and Engineering Research Council of Canada (NSERC), and Social Sciences and Humanities Research Council of Canada (SSHRC).

Umbilical Cord Blood Banking

Umbilical cord blood, the remaining blood in the umbilical cord at birth, can be collected and be a source of stem cells for an individual in need of a bone marrow transplant later in life. It can also be used for admission laboratory studies in neonates and also for a transfusion if needed (Carroll & Christensen, 2015). The extraordinary scientific and technologic advance of contemporary medicine constantly leads toward the introduction of new treatments. Umbilical cord blood is a potential vast source of primitive hematopoietic stem and progenitor cells available for clinical application. Cord blood can be used as an alternative source for bone marrow transplantation and its use is developing into a new field of treatment for pediatric and adult clients presenting with hematologic disorders, immunologic defects, and specific genetic diseases (Roura, Pujal, Gálvez-Montón, & Bayes-Genis, 2015).

Blood from a newborn's umbilical cord, once considered a waste product that was routinely discarded along with the placenta, is now recognized to contain potentially life-saving stem cells. Private banks were initially developed to store cord blood stem cells from newborns, for a fee, for potential future use by the same child or a family member if the child developed disease later in life. Today, there are public banks that store, for free, stem cells that can be used by anyone needing them, similar to how public blood banks work.

Pregnant individuals should be aware that stem cells from cord blood cannot currently be used to treat inborn errors of metabolism or other genetic diseases in the same individual from which they were collected because the cord blood would have the same genetic mutation. Cord blood collected from a newborn that later develops childhood leukemia cannot be used to treat that leukemia for much the same reason (Lubin, 2018). Umbilical cord banks are a central component, as umbilical cord tissue providers, in both medical treatment and scientific research with stem cells. But, whereas the creation of umbilical cord banks is seen as successful practice, others perceive it as ethically risky.

The fact that private cord banks offer their services as "biologic insurance" in order to obtain informed consent by promising the parents that the tissue that will be stored to insure the health of their child in the future raises the issue of whether the consent is freely given or given under coercion. Another consideration that must be made in relation to privately owned cord banks involves the ownership of the stored umbilical cord. Conflicts between moral principles and economic interests (e.g., many private blood banks are owned by physicians) cause dilemmas in the clinical practice of umbilical cord blood storage and use, especially in privately owned banks (Ballen, Verter, & Kurtzberg, 2015).

In Canada, the SOGC (Armson, Allan, & Casper, 2015) advocates for health professionals to support parents' informed decision making which includes a clear discussion of potential benefits, as well as limitations of both private and public banks. The Clinical Practice Guideline also indicates that health care providers must disclose any financial interests or conflict of interest involving private cord blood banking. In Canada, there are three types of cord blood banks: public, private, and biobanks. Public banks allow parents to donate their child's cord blood for use by anyone who needs it (allogenic use) across the country. There are no fees associated with public cord blood banking, however collection is currently limited to four locations in Canada: Ottawa and Brampton, Ontario; Edmonton, Alberta; and Vancouver, British Columbia (Canadian Blood Services, 2019). Private banks allow parents to keep their cord blood for their own personal use, if their child was to need it later in life (autologous use). Biobanks store and use stem cells for research and pharmacotherapy development (Government of Canada, 2018b). Nurses need to provide unbiased education about this topic with all pregnant clients and their families to allow informed choices to be made.

Informed Consent

Most care given in a health care setting is covered by the initial consent for treatment signed when the person becomes a client at that office or clinic, or by the consent to treatment signed upon admission to the hospital or other inpatient facility. Certain procedures, however, require a specific process of informed consent. Procedures that require informed consent vary but often include major and minor surgery; invasive procedures such as amniocentesis, internal fetal monitoring, lumbar puncture, or bone marrow aspiration; treatments placing the person at higher risk, such as chemotherapy or radiation therapy; procedures or treatments involving research; application of restraints; and photography involving the person.

Informed consent (knowing about what is involved), proxy consent (given by a parent on behalf of a child), assent (child's agreement to participate, usually in research) are examples of the consent language used in health care (Alderson, 2007). The physician has a role in determining a child's mental capacity or competence to provide informed consent. Maturity and competency are complex issues tied to concepts of freedom in decision making and taking (Alderson & Goodey, 1998). Therefore, consent is linked to ethics and involves others (usually medical staff and or parents) assessing the child's ability, understanding, and intelligence in relation to making and taking decisions (Alderson & Goodey, 1998). When conflict (dissent) exists between a child and parent legal advice or counsel may be necessary.

Take Note!

Never assume that the adult accompanying the child is the parent or legal guardian. Always clarify the relationship of the accompanying adult.

The informed consent process, which must be done before the procedure or specific care, addresses the legal and ethical requirement of informing the person about the procedure. Note that while consent is often described as an ongoing process, ensuring how this happens in practice can be difficult (Moore, McArthur & Noble-Carr, 2018). It originates from the right of the child and family to direct their care and the ethical responsibility of health care providers to involve the child and family in health care decisions. Nurses should involve children and adolescents in the decision-making process by facilitating dialogue and providing opportunity to explore understanding (Alderson, 2007). Where the parent has responsibility for giving or sharing consent in normalizing surgical approaches, that is, cleft lip surgeries, differences of sex development (or intersex) surgeries (Davis & Evans, 2018) further care must be taken in the decision-making process. The physician or advanced practitioner providing or performing the treatment and/or procedure is responsible for informing the child and family about the procedure and obtaining

---

> ### BOX 1.5
>
> #### KEY ELEMENTS OF INFORMED CONSENT (COLLECTED BY A PHYSICIAN OR NURSE PRACTITIONER)
>
> - The decision maker must be of legal age in that province (or be considered to have autonomy, understanding, and intelligence) with full civil rights, and must be competent (have the ability to make the decision).
> - Present information that is simple, concise, and appropriate to the level of education and language of the individual responsible for making the decision.
> - The decision must be voluntary, and without coercion, force, or influence of duress.
> - Have a witness to the process of informed consent.
> - Have the witness sign the consent form.

informed consent by providing a detailed description of the procedure or treatment, the potential risks and benefits, and alternative methods available.

The nurse's responsibility related to informed consent includes the following:

- Ensuring that the consent form is completed with signatures from the client (or parents or legal guardians if the client is a child and unable to provide consent)
- Serving as a witness to the signature process
- Determining whether the client or parents or legal guardians understand what they are signing by asking them pertinent questions

Box 1.5 describes the key elements of informed consent, although laws vary across the provinces.

Nurses must become familiar with the provincial and wider country mandates and laws as well as the policies and procedures of the health care agency. Treating children without obtaining proper informed consent violates their rights, and the physician and/or facility may be held liable for any damages (Murray, 2012).

Special Situations to Informed Consent

There are special situations related to informed consent. If the parent is not available, then the person in charge (relative, babysitter, or teacher) may give consent for emergency treatment if that person has a signed form from the parent or legal guardian allowing him or her to do so. During an emergency situation, a verbal consent via the telephone may be obtained. Two witnesses must be listening simultaneously and will sign the consent form, indicating that consent was received via telephone. Health care providers can provide emergency treatment to a child without consent if they have made reasonable attempts to contact the child's parent or legal guardian. Most health providers will have systems in place to guide such decisions; comprehensive documentation is imperative in such situations. For those children receiving care by court order a social worker is involved in the process of consent.

Exceptions to Parental Consent Requirement

In some provinces, a **mature minor** may give consent to certain medical treatment. The health care provider must determine that the adolescent (usually over 14 years of age) is sufficiently mature and intelligent to make the decision for treatment. The provider also considers the complexity of the treatment, its risks and benefits, and whether the treatment is necessary or elective before obtaining consent from a mature minor (Wright, 2011).

Provincial laws vary in relation to the definition of an **emancipated minor** and the types of treatment that may be obtained by an emancipated minor (without parental consent). The nurse must be familiar with the particular province's legislation. Emancipation may be considered in any of the following situations, depending on the provincial laws:
- Membership in a branch of the armed services
- Marriage
- Court-determined emancipation
- Financial independence and living apart from parents
- Pregnancy
- Mother less than 18 years of age
- Homeless youth (Gaetz, O'Grady, Buccieri, Karabanow, & Marsolais, 2013)

The emancipated minor is considered to have the legal capacity of an adult and may make his or her own health care decisions (AAP Committee on Bioethics [CB], 2016; Wright, 2011).

Many provinces do not require consent or notification of parents or legal guardians when providing specific care to minors. Depending on the provincial regulations, health care may be provided to minors for certain conditions, in a confidential manner, without including the parents. These types of care may include pregnancy counselling, prenatal care, contraception, testing for and treatment of sexually transmitted infections and communicable diseases (including HIV), substance abuse, and mental illness counselling and treatment (Brooke, 2011). These exceptions allow children to seek help in a confidential manner in situations where they might otherwise avoid care if they were required to inform their parents or legal guardian. Again, laws vary by province, so the nurse must be knowledgeable about the laws, resources, and local policies.

Assent

Assent means agreeing to something. In pediatric health care, the term **assent** refers to the child's participation in the decision-making process about health care

(Coughlin, 2018). The age of assent depends on the child's developmental level, maturity, and psychological state. The CPS recommends that children and adolescents are actively involved in discussions about their health care and kept informed in an age-appropriate manner (Coughlin, 2018). As a child gets older, assent or dissent should be given more serious consideration. The pediatric client needs to be empowered by health care providers to the extent of their capabilities, and as children mature and develop over time they should become the primary decision maker regarding their own health care (Sirbaugh & Diekema, 2011). The CPS recommends that health care decisions for the pediatric population follow the same three guiding principles as informed consent in the adult population: (1) the person/child has the capacity to make the decision, (2) the person/child is adequately informed, and (3) that the final decision is voluntary and free of coercion (Coughlin, 2018).

When determining capacity and obtaining assent, first help the child to understand his or her health condition, considering the child's developmental capacity and their experience of illness or disease (Alderson, 2007). Next, inform the child of the treatment planned and discuss what he or she should expect. Then determine what the child understands about the situation and make sure he or she is not being unduly influenced to decide one way or another. Finally, ascertain the child's willingness to participate in the treatment or research (Coughlin, 2018). Assent is an ongoing process and should continue throughout the course of treatment or research protocol.

The converse of assent is **dissent** (disagreeing with the treatment plan), and it may be ethically binding (Coughlin, 2018). If the health care provider is not going to honour the pediatric client's dissent, then the argument can be made that the provider should not ask for the client's assent. In some cases, such as in those of significant morbidity or mortality, dissent may need to be overridden. These cases need to be looked at on an individual basis, and legal counsel can be sought. If the decision is made to move forward with treatment despite the child's dissent, then this decision must be explained to the child in developmentally appropriate terms.

There has been an increased emphasis on including children in research studies. Children are not little adults but 70% of medicines given to children have only been tested on adults (Children and Clinical Studies, 2019). In research studies investigators and investigation review boards (IRBs)/research ethics boards (REBs) are responsible for ensuring measures are taken to protect the children in the studies (Government of Canada, 2014a). The nurse caring for these children also has the responsibility to ensure protection at all stages of the research process. Nurses can become members of ethics boards; they should also become familiar with studies that have been approved in their work setting to help ensure their pediatric clients are protected.

Take Note!

Whenever possible, obtain assent for participation from the child.

Refusal of Medical Treatment

All clients have the right to decline medical treatment (Evans, 2016). Ideally, medical care without informed consent should be used only when the client's life is in danger. Clients may refuse treatment if it conflicts with their religious or cultural beliefs (Brudney & Lantos, 2011). An example would be a Jehovah's Witness. Individuals of this faith have strong beliefs based upon passages from the Bible that are interpreted as prohibiting the "consumption" of blood. Their beliefs prevent them from accepting transfusion of whole blood or its primary components. With recent advances and use of biologic hemostats that aid coagulation and reduce blood loss, major surgery can be performed safely in the Jehovah's Witness who refuses blood transfusion by utilizing these devices (Darwish, 2011). In these cases, it is important to educate the client and family about the importance of the recommended treatment without coercing or forcing the client to agree. Sometimes common ground may be reached between the family's religious or cultural beliefs and the health care team's recommendations. Communication and education are key in these situations.

In the case of a child, parental autonomy (the right to decide for or against medical treatment) is a fundamental, constitutionally protected right, but not an absolute one. The general assumption is that parents act in the best interests of their children. Ideally, medical care without informed consent should be given only when the child's life is in danger. In some cases, parents may refuse medical treatment for their child. This refusal may arise when treatment conflicts with their religious or cultural beliefs or the parents' (or child's) traditional or alternative medicine choices. The nurse should be aware of some of these common beliefs as well as how such decisions are reported in the media and debated within legal circles. Some religions, such as Christian Science, Pentecostal, Church of the First Born, and Followers of Christ, prefer prayer or faith healing over allopathic medicine (Bingham, 2012; Hall, 2013). The Muslim culture advocates vegan diets and refuses pork-based medicines or treatments. People from an Islamic background may refuse the use of any potentially addictive substances such as narcotics or medicines containing alcohol. People of Hindu faith may refuse beef-based foods and medicines (Leever, 2011). Sometimes common ground may be reached between the family's religious or cultural beliefs and the health care team's recommendations.

Take Note!

Do not assume what a family's beliefs are based on religious affiliation. Assess each family and child views on an individual basis.

In other cases, parents may refuse treatment if they perceive that their child's quality of life may be significantly impaired by the medical care that is offered. The health care team must appropriately educate the family and communicate with them on a level that they can understand. The child and family should be informed of what to expect with certain tests or treatments. The health care team should make a clinical assessment of the child's and family's understanding of the situation and their reasons for refusing treatment. Active, compassionate listening may allow the health care provider to address the concerns, fears, or reservations the family may have regarding their child's care.

Refusal of medical care may be considered a form of child neglect. If providing medical treatment may prevent substantial harm and suffering, or save a child's life, health care providers and the judicial system strive to advocate for the child. The province has an overriding interest in the health and welfare of the child and can order that medical treatment to proceed without signed informed consent; this is referred to as *parens patriae* (the province as well as the federal government has a right and a duty to protect children). If the parents refuse treatment and the health care team feels the treatment is reasonable and warranted, the case should be referred to the institution's ethics committee. If the issue remains unresolved, or in complex cases, the judicial system may become involved (AAP, 2012).

Advance Directives

For children and youth requiring complex care as a result of chronic life-limiting conditions advanced care planning may be warranted. Such planning involves a multidisciplinary approach and involves the drafting of formal advance directives (Tsai, 2018).

Advanced care planning happens largely in intensive care contexts and for those children with complex and life-limiting condition (Tsai, 2018). Life-sustaining care may include antibiotics, chemotherapy, dialysis, ventilation, cardiopulmonary resuscitation, and artificial nutrition and hydration. Some families may choose to withdraw these treatments if they are already in place or to not begin them should the need arise. **Do not attempt resuscitation (DNAR) orders** are in place for some children, particularly when planning end-of-life care within the context of palliative services. Some institutions have started using the term AND (Allow Natural Death). No matter what term is used, these orders should include specific instructions regarding the child's and family's wishes (e.g., some families may desire oxygen but not chest compressions or code medications).

When the child is hospitalized, the DNAR order must be documented in the physician orders and updated according to the facility's policy. DNAR orders may also be in place in the home, but only a few states allow emergency medical services to honour a child's DNAR order in the home. Children with DNAR orders may also still be attending school. In that case, the health care professionals involved should meet with the school officials (the board of education and its legal counsel) to discuss how the DNAR request can be upheld in the school setting (McGowan, 2011). The health care provider should help educate the school about the child's condition, potential complications, and health care goals. They should work with the school and family on developing an individualized health care plan that will include what to do instead of CPR such as comfort measures (AAP & CSHCB, 2013).

Health care providers must continue to work with parents of extremely sick or premature infants to ensure they are accurately informed about the condition of their child and the risks and benefits of treatment. Health care providers must also be aware of federal, provincial, and hospital policy regarding care of very ill, premature, and/or disabled newborns. Medical assistance in dying (MAID) has been passed in Canada, but this does not extend to infants/children (Davies, 2018). The complexity of MAID and its place within pediatric care is presently under consultation and review. For children and youth with life-limiting conditions access to quality, evidence-informed pediatric palliative care is essential (Davies, 2018).

The nurse must be knowledgeable about the laws related to health care of children in the province where he or she practices as well as the policies of the health care institution. The nurse must be sensitive to the various ethical situations that he or she may become involved in and should apply knowledge of laws as well as concepts of ethics to provide appropriate care.

Confidentiality

Privacy and confidentiality laws within Canada are the responsibility of various government organizations including the Office of the Privacy Commissioner of Canada (2018). Two federal laws the *Privacy Act* (1985) and the *Personal Information Protection and Electronic Document Act* (*PIPEDA,* 2000) govern how personal information is gathered, stored, and used. While provincial laws share similar elements linked to health information and privacy, confidentially and health records, the nurse needs to be aware of provincial health privacy laws (Office of the Privacy Commissioner of Canada, 2018).

With the increased use of electronic medical records (EMRs) and electronic billing came the increased possibility that personal health information might be inappropriately distributed. Client confidentiality and privacy must be maintained in the same manner as it is with paper documentation. Nurses can ensure that privacy is maintained when using computerized documentation and EMRs by doing the following:

- Always maintain the security of personal log-in information; nurses should never share it with other health care providers or other persons.
- Always log off when leaving the computer.
- Do not leave client information visible on a monitor screen when the computer/monitor is unattended.
- Use safeguards, such as encryption, when using alternative means of communication such as email.

Exceptions to confidentiality exist. For example, suspicion of physical or sexual abuse and injuries caused by a weapon or criminal act must be reported to the proper authorities. Abuse cases are reported to the appropriate welfare authorities, whereas criminal acts are reported to the police. In addition, if the minor is a threat to self, then information may need to be disclosed to protect the child. The health care provider must also follow public health laws that require reporting certain infectious diseases to the local health department (e.g., tuberculosis, hepatitis, HIV, and other sexually transmitted infections). Finally, there is a duty to warn third parties when a specific threat is made to an identifiable person.

Health care providers must strike a balance between confidentiality and required disclosure. Even if disclosure is required it is recommended that the health care provider attempt to gain consent for the disclosure and when possible inform the minor of the limits to confidentiality and consent prior to the initiation of care (Murray, Calhoun, & Philipsen, 2011).

IMPLICATIONS FOR NURSES

The health care system is intricately woven into the political and social structure of our society, and nurses should understand social, legal, and ethical health care issues so that they can play an active role in meeting the health care needs of women, children, and families. Nurses need to take a proactive role in advocating for and empowering their clients. For example, nurses can help individuals to increase control over the factors that affect health, thereby improving their health status. A woman may become empowered by developing skills not only to cope with her environment, but also to change it. Nurses also can assume this mentoring role with children and families, thus helping them to improve their overall health status and health outcomes.

Nurses must have a solid knowledge base about the factors affecting maternal and child health and barriers to health care. They can use this information to provide anticipatory guidance, health counselling, and teaching for women, children, and families. It also is useful in identifying high-risk groups in order for enhanced services to be accessed (HELP, 2019).

When caring for women, children, and families, the nurse operates within the framework of the nursing process, which is applicable to all health care settings. Maternal and child health nursing is everchanging as globalization and the exchange of information expands. Nurses must remain up to date about new technologies and treatments and integrate high-quality, evidence-informed interventions into the care they provide.

KEY CONCEPTS

- One method to establish the aggregate health status of women, infants, and children is with statistical data, such as mortality and morbidity rates.

- The family is considered the basic social unit. The family greatly influences the development and health of its members. Members learn health care activities, health beliefs, and health values from their family.

- Social roles are often an important factor in the development of one's self-concept, which can have a very positive influence on health or present various limitations and problems, possibly resulting in a negative influence on health.

- Culture influences every aspect of development and is reflected in childbearing and child-rearing beliefs and practices designed to promote healthy adaptation.

- Spirituality, a major influence for many individuals, provides a meaning and purpose to life and is a foundation for and a source of love, relationships, and service. Spiritual and religious beliefs and views can provide strength and support to individuals, children, and their families during times of stress and illness.

- Other factors impacting the health of both children and adults include health status and lifestyles, improved diagnosis and treatment, and health care consumer empowerment. Finances, transportation, language, culture, and the health care delivery system can provide barriers to health care.

- Advances in science and technology have led to increased ethical dilemmas in health care.

- The nurse must be knowledgeable about the laws related to health care of women and children in the specific province of nursing practice as well as the specific policies of the health care institution.

REFERENCES AND RECOMMENDED READINGS

Abramovich, A. I. (2013). *No fixed address: Young, queer, and restless.* Toronto: Canadian Observatory on Homelessness. Retrieved from http://homelesshub.ca/resource/23-no-fixed-address-young-queer-and-restless.

Adams, S. M., Ward, C. E., & Garcia, K. L. (2015). Sudden infant death syndrome. *American Family Physician, 91*(11), 778–783.

Adams-Leander, S., & Rector, C. (2014). Chapter 5: Transcultural nursing in the community. In J. A. Allender, C. Rector, & K. D. Warner (Eds.). *Community & public health nursing. Promoting the public's health* (8th ed., pp. 115–149). Philadelphia, PA: Wolters Kluwer Health/Lippincott Williams & Wilkins.

Alderson, P. (2007). Competent children? Minors' consent to health care treatment and research. *Social Science & Medicine, 65*(11), 2272–2283.

Alderson, P., & Goodey, L. (1998). Theories of consent. *BMJ Clinical Research, 317*(7168), 1313–1315.

Alhusen, J. L., Ray, E., Sharps, P., & Bullock, L. (2015). Intimate partner violence during pregnancy: Maternal and neonatal outcomes. *Journal of Women's Health, 24*(1), 100–106.

Allin, S., & Stabile, M. (2012). Socioeconomic status and child health: What is the role of health care, health conditions, injuries and maternal health? *Health Economics, Policy, and Law, 7*(2), 227–242.

American Academy of Pediatrics (AAP). (2013). Policy statement: Children, adolescents, and the media. *Pediatrics, 132*(5), 958–961.

American Academy of Pediatrics (AAP). (2018). *What's the best way to discipline my child?* Retrieved from http://www.healthychildren.org/english/family-life/family-dynamics/communication-discipline/pages/disciplining-your-child.aspx.

American Academy of Pediatrics (AAP) Committee on Bioethics (CB). (2016). Informed consent in decision-making in pediatric practice. *Pediatrics, 138*(2). Retrieved from http://pediatrics.aappublications.org/content/pediatrics/138/2/e20161484.full.pdf.

American Psychological Association (APA). (2015). *The impact of terrorism and disasters on children.* Retrieved from https://www.apa.org/topics/disasters/index.

Anderson, I., Lyons, J. G., Luke, J. N., & Reich, H. S. (2017). Health determinants and educational outcomes for Indigenous children. In M. Walter, K. L. Martin, & G. Bodkin-Andrews (Eds.). *Indigenous children growing up strong.* London: Palgrave Macmillan. https://doi.org/10.1057/978-1-137-53435-4_12

Andrews, M. M., & Boyle, J. (2015). *Transcultural concepts in nursing care* (7th ed.). Philadelphia, PA: Lippincott Williams & Wilkins.

Armson, B. A., Allan, D. S., & Casper, R. F. (2015). SOGC Clinical practice guideline No. 328, Umbilical cord blood: Counselling, collection, and banking. *Journal of Obstetrics & Gynaecology Canada, 37*(9), 832–855. Retrieved from https://sogc.org/wp-content/uploads/2015/09/gui328CPG1509E1.pdf

Ballen, K. K., Verter, F., & Kurtzberg, J. (2015). Umbilical cord blood donation: Public or private? *Bone Marrow Transplantation, 50*(10), 1271–1278.

Baxter, J., Weston, R., & Lixia, Q. (2011). Family structure, co-parental relationship quality, post-separation paternal involvement and children's emotional well-being. *Journal of Family Studies, 17*(2), 86–109.

Beers, M. (2011). Strategies for intervention: Guiding parents of young children in sensitive caregiving. *Brown University Child & Adolescent Behavior Letter, 27*(12), 1–7.

Bernedo, I. M., Salas, M. D., García-Martín, M. A., & Fuentes, M. J. (2012). Teacher assessment of behavior problems in foster care children. *Children & Youth Services Review, 34*(4), 615–621.

Bingham, S. (2012). Refusal of treatment and decision-making capacity. *Nursing Ethics, 19*(1), 167–172.

Bohren, M. A., Hofmeyr, G. J., Sakala, C., Fukuzawa, R. K., & Cuthbert, A. (2017). Continuous support for women during childbirth. *Cochrane Database of Systematic Reviews, 7,* CD003766.

Boylan, J., & Dalrymple, J. (2011). Advocacy, social justice and children's rights. *Practice, 23*(1), 19–30.

Brooke, P. (2011). Legal questions. Informed consent: Take time to ask. *Nursing, 41*(8), 12.

Brown, N. (2015). How the American Heart Association helped change women's heart health. *Circulation: Cardiovascular Quality and Outcomes, 8*(2 suppl 1), S60–S62.

Brudney, D., & Lantos, J. (2011). Agency and authenticity: Which value grounds patient choice? *Theoretical Medicine and Bioethics, 32*(4), 217–227.

Burczycka, M. (2018). *Section 2, Police-reported family violence in Canada: An overview.* Retrieved from https://www150.statcan.gc.ca/n1/pub/85-002-x/2018001/article/54893/02-eng.htm.

Canada Without Poverty. (2019). *Just the facts.* Retrieved from http://www.cwp-csp.ca/poverty/just-the-facts/.

Canadian Association of Midwives (CAM). (2019a). *Midwifery across Canada.* Retrieved from https://canadianmidwives.org/midwifery-across-canada/#1467634074483-f50b550d-db87.

Canadian Association of Midwives (CAM). (2019b). *Mission and vision.* Retrieved from https://canadianmidwives.org/mission-vision/.

Canadian Blood Services. (2019). *Cord blood donation process.* Retrieved from https://blood.ca/en/stem-cells/donating-cord-blood/donation-process.

Canadian Cancer Society (CCS). (2018). *Canadian cancer statistics: A 2018 special report on cancer incidence by stage.* Retrieved from http://www.cancer.ca/~/media/cancer.ca/CW/cancer%20information/cancer%20101/Canadian%20cancer%20statistics/Canadian-Cancer-Statistics-2018-EN.pdf?la=en.

Canadian Foundation for Healthcare Improvement. (2019). *Better together.* Retrieved from https://www.cfhi-fcass.ca/WhatWeDo/better-together.

Canada Health Act. (1985). *Canada Health Act.* Retrieved from https://laws-lois.justice.gc.ca/eng/acts/C-6/.

Canadian Nurses Association (CNA). (2005). *Children's health and nursing: A summary of the issues.* Retrieved from https://www.cna-aiic.ca/~/media/cna/page-content/pdf-en/bg2_childrens_health_and_nursing_e.pdf.

Canadian Nurses Association (CNA). (2017). *Code of ethics for registered nurses.* Retrieved from https://www.cna-aiic.ca/-/media/cna/page-content/pdf-en/code-of-ethics-2017-edition-secure-interactive.pdf.

Canadian Nurses Association (CNA). (2018). *Position statement: Promoting cultural competence in nursing.* Retrieved from https://www.cna-aiic.ca/-/media/cna/page-content/pdf-en/position_statement_promoting_cultural_competence_in_nursing.pdf?la=en&hash=4B394DAE5C2138E7F6134D59E505DCB059754BA9.

Canadian Nurses Association (CNA). (2019). *CNA certification program.* Retrieved from https://www.cna-aiic.ca/en/certification

Canadian Paediatric Society (CPS). (2012). *Position statement, Child and youth injury prevention: A public health approach.* Retrieved from https://www.cps.ca/en/documents/position/child-and-youth-injury-prevention.

Canadian Paediatric Society (CPS). (2015). *Position statement, Diagnosis and management of asthma in preschoolers: A Canadian Thoracic Society and Canadian Paediatric Society position paper.* Retrieved from https://www.cps.ca/en/documents/position/asthma-in-preschoolers.

Canadian Paediatric Society (CPS). (2016). *Childhood lasts forever: The need to invest in the early years.* Retrieved from https://www.cps.ca/en/blog-blogue/childhood-lasts-forever-the-need-to-invest-in-the-early-years.

Canadian Paediatric Society. (2017). *Screen time and young children: Promoting health and development in a a digital world.* Retrieved from https://www.cps.ca/en/documents/position/screen-time-and-young-children.

Canadian Paediatric Society (CPS). (2018a). *Community resources.* Retrieved from https://www.cps.ca/en/first-debut/community-resources.

Canadian Paediatric Society (CPS). (2018b). *Supporting the mental health of children and youth of separating parents.* Retrieved from https://www.cps.ca/en/documents/position/mental-health-children-and-youth-of-separating-parents.

Canadian Paediatric Society (CPS). (2018c). *Caring for kids new to Canada.* Retrieved from https://www.kidsnewtocanada.ca/care/overview.

Canadian Paediatric Society (CPS). (2019). *Relationships matter: How clinicians can support positive parenting in the early years.* Retrieved from https://www.cps.ca/cn/documents/position/positive-parenting

Cancello, R. (2015). Obesity and inflammation in pregnancy. In E. Ferrazzi & B. Sears (Eds.). *Metabolic syndrome and complications of pregnancy* (pp. 65–75). New York: Springer International Publishing.

Carroll, P. D., & Christensen, R. D. (2015). New and underutilized uses of umbilical cord blood in neonatal care. *Maternal Health, Neonatology and Perinatology, 1*(1), 16–23.

Centers for Disease Control and Prevention (CDC). (2016). *Adverse childhood experiences (ACEs).* Retrieved from https://www.cdc.gov/violenceprevention/acestudy/index.html.

Centers for Disease Control and Prevention (CDC). (2018a). *Fetal deaths.* Retrieved from https://www.cdc.gov/nchs/nvss/fetal_death.htm.

Centers for Disease Control and Prevention (CDC). (2018b). *Suicide prevention.* Retrieved from https://www.cdc.gov/violenceprevention/suicide/index.html.

Centers for Disease Control and Prevention (CDC). (2018c). *About school violence.* Retrieved from http://www.cdc.gov/violenceprevention/youthviolence/schoolviolence/data_stats.html.

Centers for Disease Control and Prevention (CDC), National Center for Health Statistics. (2017). *Child health.* Retrieved from http://www.cdc.gov/nchs/fastats/child-health.htm.

Chen, E., Cohen, S., & Miller, G. E. (2010). How low socioeconomic status affects 2-year hormonal trajectories in children. *Psychological Science, 21*(1), 31–37.

Cherry, K. (2018). *Why parenting styles matter when raising children*. Retrieved from https://www.verywellmind.com/parenting-styles-2795072.

Child Trends. (2019). *Children's exposure to violence*. Retrieved from http://www.childtrends.org/?indicators=childrens-exposure-to-violence.

Child Trends. (2018). *Infant, child, and teen mortality*. Retrieved from https://www.childtrends.org/indicators/infant-child-and-teen-mortality.

Children and Clinical Studies. (2019). *The importance of children in clinical studies*. Retrieved from http://www.childrenandclinicalstudies.org/.

Children First Canada. (2018). *Canadian children's charter*. Retrieved from https://www.childrenfirstcanada.com/canadian-childrens-charter/.

Children's Healthcare Canada. (2018). *Patient and family centred care*. Retrieved from https://www.childrenshealthcare-canada.ca/patient-and-family-centred-care/?rq=patient.

CIA World Factbook. (2019a). *Country comparison: Infant mortality rate*. Retrieved from https://www.cia.gov/library/publications/the-world-factbook/rankorder/2091rank.html.

CIA World Factbook. (2019b). *Country comparison: Maternal mortality rate*. Retrieved from https://www.cia.gov/library/publications/resources/the-world-factbook/fields/353rank.html.

Costescu, D., Guilbert, E., & SOGC Surgical Abortion Working Group. (2018). SOGC Clinical practice guideline No. 360-Induced abortion: Surgical abortion and second trimester medical methods. *Journal of Obstetrics and Gynaecology Canada, 40*(6), 750–783. Retrieved from https://www.jogc.com/article/S1701-2163(17)31309-9/pdf.

Cotter, J., & Yung, A. R. (2018). Exploring the impact of adverse childhood experiences on symptomatic and functional outcomes in adulthood: Advances, limitations and considerations. *Irish Journal of Psychological Medicine, 35*(1), 5–7.

Couglin, K. W. (2018). Position statement, Medical decision-making in paediatrics: Infancy to adolescence. *Paediatrics & Child Health, 23*(2), 138–146. Retrieved from https://www.cps.ca/en/documents/position/medical-decision-making-in-paediatrics-infancy-to-adolescence.

Cox, K. J., & King, T. L. (2015). Preventing primary cesarean births: Midwifery care. *Clinical Obstetrics and Gynecology, 58*(2), 282–293.

Coyne, I., Hallström, I., & Söderbäck, M. (2016). Reframing the focus from a family-centred to a child-centred care approach for children's healthcare. *Journal of Child Health Care, 20*(4), 494–502. https://doi.org/10.1177%2F1367493516642744.

Crawford, N. A., Schrock, M., & Woodruff-Borden, J. (2011). Child internalizing symptoms: Contributions of child temperament, maternal negative affect, and family functioning. *Child Psychiatry & Human Development, 42*(1), 53–64.

Crawford, N. M., & Steiner, A. Z. (2015). Age-related infertility. *Obstetrics and Gynecology Clinics of North America, 42*(1), 15–25.

Da Fonseca, M. A. (2012). The effects of poverty on children's development and oral health. *Pediatric Dentistry, 34*(1), 32–38.

Darwish, A. (2011). Liver transplant in Jehovah's Witnesses patients. *Current Opinion in Organ Transplantation, 16*(3), 326–330.

Davies, D. (2018). Medical assistance in dying: A paediatric perspective. *Paediatrics & Child Health, 23*(2), 125–130. Retrieved from https://www.cps.ca/en/documents/position/medical-assistance-in-dying.

Davis, K. E. (2014). *Statistical brief #461: Access to health care of adult men and women, ages 18–64*. Retrieved from http://meps.ahrq.gov/mepsweb/data_files/publications/st461/stat461.shtml.

Davis, G., & Evans, M. J. (2018). Surgically shaping sex: A gender structure analysis of the violation of intersex people's human rights. In B. J. Risman, C. M. Froyum, & W. J. Scarborough (Eds.). *Handbook of the sociology of gender* (pp. 273–284). Cham: Springer.

de Miguel-Beriain, I. (2015). The ethics of stem cells revisited. *Advanced Drug Delivery Reviews, 82*, 176–180.

DONA International. (2019). *What is a doula?* Retrieved from https://www.dona.org/what-is-a-doula/.

Duvall, E. (1997). *Marriage and family development* (5th ed.). Philadelphia, PA: J. B. Lippincott.

Edwards, J. G., Feldman, G., Goldberg, J., Gregg, A. R., Norton, M. E., Rose, N. C., . . . Watson, M. S. (2015). Expanded carrier screening in reproductive medicine—Points to consider: A joint statement of the American College of Medical Genetics and Genomics, American College of Obstetricians and Gynecologists, National Society of Genetic Counselors, Perinatal Quality Foundation, and Society for Maternal-Fetal Medicine. *Obstetrics & Gynecology, 125*(3), 653–662.

Edwards, J. D., Kun, S. S., Graham, R. J., & Keens, T. G. (2012). End-of-life discussions and advanced care planning for children on long-term assisted ventilation with life-limiting conditions. *Journal of Palliative Care, 28*(1), 21–27.

Egbe, A., Lee, S., Ho, D., Uppu, S., & Srivastava, S. (2015). Racial/ethnic differences in the birth prevalence of congenital anomalies in the United States. *Journal of Perinatal Medicine, 43*(1), 111–117.

Epstein, R. H. (2011). *Get me out: A history of childbirth from the Garden of Eden to the sperm bank*. New York: W.W. Norton & Company.

Evans, K. G. (2016). *Consent: A guide for Canadian physicians*. The Canadian Medical Protective Association. Retrieved from https://www.cmpa-acpm.ca/en/advice-publications/handbooks/consent-a-guide-for-canadian-physicians.

Faver, C. A., & Alanis, E. (2012). Fostering empathy through stories: A pilot program for special needs adoptive families. *Children & Youth Services Review, 34*(4), 660–665.

Federal Interagency Forum on Child and Family Statistics. (2013). *America's children: Key national indicators of well-being, 2013*. Washington, DC: U.S. Government Printing Office.

Feigelman, S. (2011). Chapter 6: Overview and assessment of variability. In R. M. Kleigman, B. F. Stanton, J. W. St. Geme III, N. F. Schor, & R. E. Behrman (Eds.). *Nelson textbook of pediatrics* (19th ed., p. 26). Philadelphia, PA: Saunders.

Ferguson-Smith, M. A. (2015). History and evolution of cytogenetics. *Molecular Cytogenetics, 8*(1), 19–27.

Finkelhor, D., Turner, H. A., Shattuck, A., & Hamby, S. L. (2013). Violence, crime, and abuse exposure in a national sample of children and youth: An update. *JAMA Pediatrics*, *167*(7), 614–621.

Flaskerud, J. H. (2011). Discipline and effective parenting. *Issues in Mental Health Nursing*, *32*(1), 82–84.

Fridman, L., Fraser-Thomas, J., Pike, I., & Macpherson, A. K. (2018). An interprovincial comparison of unintentional childhood injury rates in Canada for the period 2006–2012. *Canadian Journal of Public Health*, *109*(4), 573–580.

Friedman, M. M. (1998). *Family nursing: Theory and practice* (4th ed.). Stanford, CT: Appleton & Lange.

Futures Without Violence. (2016). *Protective factors & resiliency.* Retrieved from http://promising.futureswithoutviolence.org/what-do-kids-need/supporting-parenting/protective-factors-resiliency/.

Gaetz, S., O'Grady, B., Buccieri, K., Karabanow, J., & Marsolais, A. (2013). *Youth homelessness in Canada: Implications for policy and practice.* Toronto: Canadian Homelessness Research Network Press. Retrieved from https://www.homelesshub.ca/sites/default/files/attachments/YouthHomelessnessweb.pdf.

Gaetz, S., O'Grady, B., Kidd, S., & Schwan, K. (2016). *Without a home: The National Youth Homelessness Survey.* Toronto: Canadian Observatory on Homelessness Press.

Galante, L., French, C., & Grace, K. B. (2015). Nursing perspectives in managing patients with substance abuse. In *Substance abuse* (pp. 229–248). New York: Springer Publishers.

Gonzalez, A., Catherine, N., Boyle, M., Jack, S. M., Atkinson, L., Kobor, M., . . . MacMillan, H. L. (2018). Healthy Foundations Study: A randomised controlled trial to evaluate biological embedding of early-life experiences. *BMJ Open*, *8*(1), e018915.

Government of Canada. (1985). *Privacy act.* Retrieved from https://laws-lois.justice.gc.ca/PDF/P-21.pdf.

Government of Canada. (2013). *Statement of apology to former students of Indian residential schools.* Retrieved from http://publications.gc.ca/collections/collection_2017/aanc-inac/R5-142-2013-eng.pdf.

Government of Canada. (2014a). *Requirements for informed consent documents.* Retrieved from https://www.canada.ca/en/health-canada/services/science-research/science-advice-decision-making/research-ethics-board/requirements-informed-consent-documents.html.

Government of Canada. (2014b). *Tri-council policy statement: Ethical conduct for research involving humans.* Retrieved from http://www.pre.ethics.gc.ca/pdf/eng/tcps2-2014/TCPS_2_FINAL_Web.pdf.

Government of Canada. (2017). *Elementary and secondary education.* Retrieved from https://www.canada.ca/en/immigration-refugees-citizenship/services/new-immigrants/new-life-canada/enrol-school/elementary-secondary.html.

Government of Canada. (2018a). *Canada's health care system.* Retrieved from https://www.canada.ca/en/health-canada/services/health-care-system/reports-publications/health-care-system/canada.html.

Government of Canada. (2018b). *Thinking about banking your child's cord blood?* Retrieved from https://www.canada.ca/en/health-canada/services/healthy-living/healthy-pregnancy/banking-cord-blood.html.

Government of Canada. (2019). *Healthy living.* Retrieved from https://www.canada.ca/en/health-canada/services/healthy-living.html.

Government of Canada Department of Justice. (2016). *The criminal law and managing children's behaviour.* Retrieved from https://www.justice.gc.ca/eng/rp-pr/cj-jp/fv-vf/mcb-cce/index.html.

Government of Canada Department of Justice. (2017). *Voice and support: Programs for children experiencing parental separation and divorce.* Retrieved from https://www.justice.gc.ca/eng/rp-pr/fl-lf/divorce/2004_2/index.html.

Greenwood, M. L., & de Leeuw, S. N. (2012). Social determinants of health and the future well-being of Aboriginal children in Canada. *Paediatrics & Child Health*, *17*(7), 381–384.

Griffin, I. J., Lee, H. C., Profit, J., & Tancedi, D. J. (2015). The smallest of the small: Short-term outcomes of profoundly growth restricted and profoundly low birth weight preterm infants. *Journal of Perinatology*, *35*(7), 503–510.

Groark, C. J., & McCall, R. B. (2011). Implementing changes in institutions to improve young children's development. *Infant Mental Health Journal*, *32*(5), 509–525.

Grusec, J. E., Danyliuk, T., Kil, H., & O'Neill, D. (2017). Perspectives on parent discipline and child outcomes. *International Journal of Behavioral Development*, *41*(4), 465–471.

Hall, H. (2013). Faith healing: Religious freedom vs. child protection. *Science Based Medicine.* Retrieved from http://www.sciencebasedmedicine.org/faith-healing-religious-freedom-vs-child-protection/.

Halseth, R. (2013). *Aboriginal women in Canada: Gender, socio-economic determinants of health, and initiatives to close the wellness gap.* Prince George, BC: National Collaborating Centre for Aboriginal Health. Retrieved from https://www.ccnsa-nccah.ca/docs/determinants/RPT-Aboriginal-WomenCanada-Halseth-EN.pdf.

Hamon, J. D., & Schrodt, P. (2012). Do parenting styles moderate the association between family conformity orientation and young adults' mental well-being? *Journal of Family Communication*, *12*(2), 151–166.

Hanson, E. (2009). *The residential school system.* Retrieved from http://indigenousfoundations.arts.ubc.ca/the_residential_school_system/.

Hanson, P. A., & Andrews, M. M. (2012). Chapter 13: Religion, culture and nursing. In M. M. Andrews, & J. S. Boyle (Eds.). *Transcultural concepts in nursing care* (6th ed., pp. 351–402). Philadelphia, PA: Wolters Kluwer Health/Lippincott Williams & Wilkins.

Health Canada. (2004). *First minister's meeting on the future of health care 2004: A 10-year plan to strengthen health care.* Ottawa: Author. Retrieved from https://www.cna-aiic.ca/-/media/cna/page-content/pdf-en/brief_10_year_plan_e.pdf?la=en&hash=D6B333AD9AA01C7ADD3F054A0C5E10449FCDC3D3

Health Canada. (2017). *Government of Canada health portfolio.* Retrieved from https://www.canada.ca/en/health-canada/corporate/health-portfolio.html.

Heart and Stroke Foundation of Canada. (2018). *Heart: Women's unique risk factors.* Retrieved from http://www.heartandstroke.ca/heart/risk-and-prevention/womens-unique-risk-factors.

Holtzman, M. (2011). Nonmarital unions, family definitions, and custody decision making. *Family Relations*, *60*(5), 617–632.

Horvath, C. A., Lee, C. M., & Bax, K. (2015). How similar are mothers and fathers of young children in their parenting responses and goals? *Journal of Child and Family Studies, 24*(12), 3542–3551.

Hughes, K., Bellis, M. A., Hardcastle, K. A., Sethi, D., Butchart, A., Mikton, C., . . . Dunne, M. P. (2017). The effect of multiple adverse childhood experiences on health: A systematic review and meta-analysis. *The Lancet Public Health, 2*(8), e356–e366.

Human Early Learning Partnership (HELP). (2019). *Early development instrument*. Retrieved from http://earlylearning. ubc.ca/edi/.

Jones, V. F., Schulte, E. E., & Committee on Early Childhood, Council on Foster Care, Adoption, and Kinship Care. (2012). The pediatrician's role in supporting adoptive families. *Pediatrics, 130*(4), e1040–e1049.

Karim, Z. A., Alshbool, F. Z., Vemana, H. P., Adhami, N., Dhall, S., Espinosa, E. V., . . . Khasawneh, F. T. (2015). Third hand smoke: Impact on hemostasis and thrombogenesis. *Journal of Cardiovascular Pharmacology, 66*(2), 177–182.

Kawabata, Y., Alink, L. A., Tseng, W., van Ijzendoorn, M. H., & Crick, N. R. (2011). Maternal and paternal parenting styles associated with relational aggression in children and adolescents: A conceptual analysis and meta-analytic review. *Developmental Review, 31*(4), 240–278.

Kelly, M. M. (2010). Prematurity. In P. J. Allen, J. A. Vessey, & N. A. Schapiro (Eds.). *Primary care of the child with a chronic condition* (5th ed.). St. Louis, MO: Mosby.

Kemp, G., Smith, M., & Segal, J. (2018). *Children and divorce*. Retrieved from http://www.helpguide.org/articles/family-divorce/children-and-divorce.htm.

Kersey-Matusiak, G. (2012). Culturally competent care: Are we there yet? *Nursing, 42*(2), 49–52.

Khanlou, N., Haque, N., Skinner, A., Mantini, A., & Kurtz Landy, C. (2017). Scoping review on maternal health among immigrant and refugee women in Canada: Prenatal, intrapartum, and postnatal care. *Journal of Pregnancy*. Retrieved from https://www.hindawi.com/journals/jp/2017/8783294/abs/.

Kiff, C. J., Lengua, L. J., & Zalewski, M. (2011). Nature and nurturing: Parenting in the context of child temperament. *Clinical Child and Family Psychology Review, 14*(3), 251–301.

Kim, H. (2011). Consequences of parental divorce for child development. *American Sociological Review, 76*(3), 487–511.

Kim, M., Han, S., & Shin, M. (2015). Influencing factors on the cord-blood donation of post-partum women. *Nursing & Health Sciences, 17*(2), 269–275.

Kochanek, K. D., Murphy, S. L., & Xu, J. Q. (2015). Deaths: Final data for 2011. *National Vital Statistics Reports, 63*(3), 1–120. Hyattsville, MD: National Center for Health Statistics. Retrieved from http://www.cdc.gov/nchs/data/nvsr/nvsr63/nvsr63_03.pdf.

Lansford, J. E., Wager, L. B., Bates, J. E., Pettit, G. S., & Dodge, K. A. (2012). Forms of spanking and children's externalizing behaviors. *Family Relations, 61*(2), 224–236.

Lawford, K. M., Giles, A. R., & Bourgeault, I. L. (2018). Canada's evacuation policy for pregnant First Nations women: Resignation, resilience, and resistance. *Women and Birth, 31*(6), 479–488. https://doi.org/10.1016/j.wombi.2018.01.009.

Leever, M. G. (2011). Culture competence: Reflection on patient autonomy and patient good. *Nursing Ethics, 18*(4), 560–570.

Lewis, R. (2011). *Human genetics: Concepts and applications* (10th ed.). New York: McGraw-Hill Publishers.

Long, K., Thomas, S., Grubs, R., Gettig, E., & Krishnamurti, L. (2011). Attitudes and beliefs of African-Americans toward genetics, genetic testing, and sickle cell disease education and awareness. *Journal of Genetic Counseling, 20*(6), 572–592.

Loo, M. (2009). *Integrative medicine for children*. St. Louis, MO: Elsevier Health Sciences.

Lubin, B. H. (2018). Collection and storage of umbilical cord blood for hematopoietic cell transplantation. *UpToDate*. Retrieved from https://www.uptodate.com/contents/collection-and-storage-of-umbilical-cord-blood-for-hematopoietic-cell-transplantation.

Malinowska-Sempruch, K., & Rychkova, O. (2015). *The impact of drug policy on women*. Retrieved from https://www.opensocietyfoundations.org/reports/impact-drug-policy-women.

Maron, D. F. (2015). *Has maternal mortality really doubled in the US?* Scientific American. Retrieved from http://www.scientificamerican.com/article/has-maternal-mortality-really-doubled-in-the-u-s/.

Martins, N., & Wilson, B. J. (2012). Social aggression on television and its relationship to children's aggression in the classroom. *Human Communication Research, 38*(1), 48–71.

Masten, A. S., & Narayan, A. J. (2012). Child development in the context of disaster, war, and terrorism: Pathways of risk and resilience. *Annual Review of Psychology, 63*(1), 227–257.

McGowan, C. (2011). Legal aspects of end-of-life care. *Critical Care Nurse, 31*(5), 64–69.

McLemore, M. R., Kools, S., & Levi, A. J. (2015). Calculus formation: Nurses' decision-making in abortion-related care. *Research in Nursing & Health, 38*(3), 222–231.

Mental Health Commission of Canada. (2018). *Children and youth*. Retrieved from https://www.mentalhealthcommission.ca/English/what-we-do/children-and-youth.

Medical Care Act (1966). *Canada's health care system*. Retrieved from https://www.canada.ca/en/health-canada/services/health-care-system/reports-publications/health-care-system/canada.html.

Miller, J., & Scott, J. (2015). Newborn and infant (0–12 months). In S. Croxford, C. Itsiopoulos, R. Belski, A. Thodis, S. Shepherd, A. Forsyth, & A. Tierney (Eds.). *Food and nutrition throughout life: A comprehensive overview of food and nutrition in all stages of life* (p. 117). London, UK: Allen & Unwin Publishers.

Moore, T. P., McArthur, M., & Noble-Carr, D. (2018). More a marathon than a hurdle: Towards children's informed consent in a study on safety. *Qualitative Research, 18*(1), 88–107.

Murray, B. (2012). Informed consent: What must a physician disclose to a patient? *American Medical Association Journal of Ethics, 14*(7), 563–566.

Murray, T. L., Calhoun, M., & Philipsen, N. C. (2011). Privacy, confidentiality, HIPAA, and hightech: Implications for the health care practitioner. *Journal for Nurse Practitioners, 7*(9), 747–752.

Nagle, J., & Clancy, M. A. C. (2010). *Shared society or benign apartheid?: understanding peace-building in divided societies*. Palgrave Macmillan.

National Collaborating Centres for Public Health (NCCPH). (2018). *About us*. Retrieved from http://nccph.ca/about-us.

Newhook, J. T., Winters, K., Pyne, J., Jamieson, A., Holmes, C., Feder, S., . . . Sinnott, M. L. (2018). Teach your parents and providers well: Call for refocus on the health of trans and gender-diverse children. *Canadian Family Physician, 64*(5), 332–335.

Norman, A. (2015). *The complicated birth of midwifery.* Retrieved from http://all-that-is-interesting.com/midwife-history.

Office of the Privacy Commissioner of Canada. (2018). Office of the privacy commissioner. Retrieved from https://www.priv.gc.ca/en/.

Olson, R., & Couchie, C. (2013). Returning birth: The politics of midwifery implementation on First Nations reserves in Canada. *Midwifery, 29*(8), 981–987. https://doi.org/10.1016/j.midw.2012.12.005.

Osterman, M. J., Kochanek, K. D., MacDorman, M. F., Strobino, D. M., & Guyer, B. (2015). Annual summary of vital statistics: 2012–2013. *Pediatrics, 135*(6), 1115–1125.

Oza, S., Lawn, J. E., Hogan, D. R., Mathers, C., & Cousens, S. N. (2015). Neonatal cause-of-death estimates for the early and late neonatal periods for 194 countries: 2000–2013. *Bulletin of the World Health Organization, 93*(1), 19–28.

Patel, K., & Rushefsky, M. E. (2015). *Health care in America: Separate and unequal.* New York: Routledge.

Patterson, J. (1995). Promoting resilience in families experiencing stress. *Pediatric Clinics of North America, 42*(1), 47–63.

Patterson, J. (2002). Integrating family resilience and family stress theory. *Journal of Marriage and Family, 64*(2), 349–360.

Perron, J. L., Lee, C. M., LaRoche, K. J., Ateah, C., Clément, M. È., & Chan, K. (2014). Child and parent characteristics associated with Canadian parents' reports of spanking. *Canadian Journal of Community Mental Health, 33*(2), 31–45.

Personal Information Protection and Electronic Document Act (PIPEDA). (2000). *Office of the Privacy Commissioner.* Retrieved from https://www.priv.gc.ca/en/privacy-topics/privacy-laws-in-canada/02_05_d_15/#heading-0-0-3-1.

Philpott, J. (2018). Canada's efforts to ensure the health and wellbeing of Indigenous peoples. *The Lancet, 391*(10131), 1650–1651. https://doi.org/10.1016/S0140-6736(18)30179-X

Piko, B. B., & Balázs, M. M. (2012). Control or involvement? Relationship between authoritative parenting style and adolescent depressive symptomatology. *European Child & Adolescent Psychiatry, 21*(3), 149–155.

Plummer, K. (2000). From nursing outposts to contemporary midwifery in 20th century Canada. *Journal of Midwifery & Women's Health, 45*(2), 169–175.

Ponzetti Jr, J. J. (2015). Overview and history of parenting education. In *Evidence-based parenting education* (pp. 29–37). Routledge.

Provincial Council for Maternal and Child Health (PCMCH). (2019). *PCMCH strategies and initiatives.* Retrieved from http://www.pcmch.on.ca/health-care-providers/maternity-care/pcmch-strategies-and-initiatives/.

Public Health Agency of Canada (PHAC). (2008). *The Chief Public Health Officer's report on the state of public health in Canada 2008: Canada's public health history.* Retrieved from https://www.canada.ca/en/public-health/corporate/publications/chief-public-health-officer-reports-state-public-health-canada/report-on-state-public-health-canada-2008/chapter-2b.html.

Public Health Agency of Canada (PHAC). (2009a). *Are women at risk for heart disease?* Retrieved from https://www.canada.ca/en/public-health/services/chronic-diseases/cardiovascular-disease/women-risk-heart-disease.html.

Public Health Agency of Canada (PHAC). (2009b). *What mothers say: The Canadian maternity experiences survey.* Retrieved from http://www.phac-aspc.gc.ca/rhs-ssg/pdf/survey-eng.pdf.

Public Health Agency of Canada (PHAC). (2015). *Canadian best practices portal: Maternal infant health (0-2 years).* Retrieved from http://cbpp-pcpe.phac-aspc.gc.ca/public-health-topics/maternal-infant-health/.

Public Health Agency of Canada (PHAC). (2016a). *Health status of Canadians 2016.* Retrieved from http://healthy-canadians.gc.ca/publications/department-ministere/state-public-health-status-2016-etat-sante-publique-statut/alt/pdf-eng.pdf.

Public Health Agency of Canada (PHAC). (2016b). *What's wrong with spanking?* Retrieved from https://www.canada.ca/en/public-health/services/publications/healthy-living/pamphlet-what-s-wrong-with-spanking.html.

Public Health Agency of Canada (PHAC). (2017). *Perinatal health indicators for Canada 2017: A report from the Canadian perinatal surveillance system.* Retrieved from http://publications.gc.ca/collections/collection_2018/aspc-phac/HP7-1-2017-eng.pdf.

Public Health Agency of Canada (PHAC). (2019). *Canadian best practices portal.* Retrieved from http://www.cbpp-pcpe.phac-aspc.gc.ca.

Public Safety Canada. (2018). *A statistical snapshot of youth at risk and youth offending in Canada.* Retrieved from https://www.publicsafety.gc.ca/cnt/rsrcs/pblctns/ststclsnpsht-yth/index-en.aspx.

Rafferty, J. (2018). Gender identity development in children. *American Academy of Pediatrics.* Retrieved from http://www.healthychildren.org/English/ages-stages/gradeschool/pages/Gender-Identity-and-Gender-Confusion-In-Children.aspx.

Rafi, I., & Kai, J. (2011). Genetics and ethnicity. *Pulse, 71*(6), 22–23.

Raising Canada. (2018). *A report on children in Canada, their health and wellbeing.* Retrieved from https://obrieniph.ucalgary.ca/files/iph/raising-canada-report.pdf.

Raphael, D. (2010). The health of Canada's children. Part I: Canadian children's health in comparative perspective. *Paediatrics & Child Health, 15*(1), 23–29.

Relyea, M. J. (1992). The rebirth of midwifery in Canada: An historical perspective. *Midwifery, 8*(4), 159–169.

Robinson, N., Stoffel, C., & Haider, S. (2015). Global women's health is more than maternal health: A review of gynecology care needs in low-resource settings. *Obstetrical & Gynecological Survey, 70*(3), 211–222.

Rooks, J. P. (2014). The history of midwifery. *Our Bodies Ourselves.* Retrieved from https://www.ourbodiesourselves.org/book-excerpts/health-article/history-of-midwifery/.

Roura, S., Pujal, J. M., Gálvez-Montón, C., & Bayes-Genis, A. (2015). The role and potential of umbilical cord blood in an era of new therapies: A review. *Stem Cell Research & Therapy, 6*(1), 1–11.

Royal Canadian Mounted Police (RCMP). (2016). *School violence.* Retrieved from http://www.rcmp-grc.gc.ca/cycp-cpcj/violence/sv-ve/index-eng.htm.

Seburg, E. M., Olson-Bullis, B. A., Bredeson, D. M., Hayes, M. G., & Sherwood, N. E. (2015). A review of primary care-based childhood obesity prevention and treatment interventions. *Current Obesity Reports, 4*(2), 157–173.

Sege, R. D., Siegel, B. S.; AAP Council on Child Abuse and Neglect; AAP Committee on Psychosocial Aspects of Child and Family Health. (2018). Effective discipline to raise healthy children. *Pediatrics, 142*(6), e20183112. Retrieved from https://pediatrics.aappublications.org/content/pediatrics/142/6/e20183112.full.pdf.

Seith, D., & Isakson, E. (2011). *Who are America's poor children? Examining health disparities among children in the United States.* New York: National Center for Children in Poverty.

Senthilselvan, A., Niruban, S. J., King, M., Majaesic, C., Veugelers, P., Laing, L., & Rowe, B. H. (2015). Prevalence and risk factors of asthma in First Nations children living on reserves in Canada. *Canadian Journal of Public Health, 106*(8), e483–e488.

Serwint, J. R. (2011). Chapter 16: Separation, loss & bereavement. In R. M. Kleigman, B. F. Stanton, J. W. St. Geme III, N. F. Schor, & R. E. Behrman (Eds.). *Nelson textbook of pediatrics* (19th ed., p. 45). Philadelphia, PA: Saunders.

Shah, A. (2011). Today, over 21,000 children died around the world. *Global Issues.* Retrieved from http://www.globalissues.org/article/715/today-over-26500-children-died-around-the-world.

Shah, P. S., McDonald, S. D., Barrett, J., Synnes, A., Robson, K., Foster, J., . . . Pechlivanoglou, P. (2018). The Canadian preterm birth network: A study protocol for improving outcomes for preterm infants and their families. *CMAJ Open, 6*(1), E44. Retrieved from https://www.ncbi.nlm.nih.gov/pmc/articles/PMC5878956/.

Shapiro, G. D., Sheppard, A. J., Bushnik, T., Kramer, M. S., Mashford-Pringle, A., Kaufman, J. S., & Yang, S. (2018). Adverse birth outcomes and infant mortality according to registered First Nations status and First Nations community residence across Canada. *Canadian Journal of Public Health, 109*(5-6), 692–699. https://doi.org/10.17269/s41997-018-0134-6.

Sheppard, A. J., Shapiro, G. D., Bushnik, T., Wilkins, R., Perry, S., Kaufman, J. S., . . . Yang, S. (2017). Birth outcomes among First Nations, Inuit and Métis populations. *Health Reports, 28*(11), 11–16.

Shields, L. (2015). What is "family-centred care"? *European Journal for Person Centered Healthcare, 3*(2), 139–144. http://ubplj.org/index.php/ejpch/article/view/993.

Siegel, R. L., Miller, K. D., & Jemal, A. (2015). Cancer statistics, 2015. *CA: A Cancer Journal for Clinicians, 65*(1), 5–29.

Sirbaugh, P. E., & Diekema, D. S. (2011). Policy statement-consent for emergency medical services for children and adolescents. *Pediatrics, 128*(2), 427–433.

Stanhope, M., & Lancaster, J. (2011). *Public health nursing: Population-centered health care in the community* (8th ed.). St. Louis, MO: Mosby Elsevier.

Stapleton, S. (2017). Birth centers. *UpToDate.* Retrieved from http://www.uptodate.com/contents/birth-centers.

Statistics Canada. (2015). *Census family.* Retrieved from http://www23.statcan.gc.ca/imdb/p3Var.pl?Function=Unit&Id=32746.

Statistics Canada. (2017). Population size and growth in Canada: Key results from the 2016 Census. Retrieved from https://www150.statcan.gc.ca/n1/daily-quotidien/170208/dq170208a-eng.htm.

Statistics Canada. (2017a). *Portrait of children's family life in Canada in 2016.* Retrieved from https://www12.statcan.gc.ca/census-recensement/2016/as-sa/98-200-x/2016006/98-200-x2016006-eng.pdf.

Statistics Canada. (2017b). *Suicide rates: An overview.* Retrieved from https://www150.statcan.gc.ca/n1/pub/82-624-x/2012001/article/11696-eng.htm.

Statistics Canada. (2018a). *Aboriginal peoples in Canada: First Nations people, Métis and Inuit.* Retrieved from https://www12.statcan.gc.ca/nhs-enm/2011/as-sa/99-011-x/99-011-x2011001-eng.cfm.

Statistics Canada. (2018b). *Ethnic diversity and immigration.* Retrieved from https://www150.statcan.gc.ca/n1/pub/11-402-x/2011000/chap/imm/imm-eng.htm.

Statistics Canada. (2018c). *Mortality: Overview 2014 to 2016.* Retrieved from https://www150.statcan.gc.ca/n1/pub/91-209-x/2018001/article/54957-eng.htm.

Statistics Canada. (2018d). Fertility: Overview, 2012 to 2016. Retrieved from https://www150.statcan.gc.ca/n1/pub/91-209-x/2018001/article/54956-eng.htm.

Statistics Canada. (2019a). *Table: 13-10-0714-01 Perinatal mortality (late fetal deaths and early neonatal deaths).* Retrieved from https://www150.statcan.gc.ca/t1/tbl1/en/tv.action?pid=1310071401.

Statistics Canada. (2019b). *Table: 13-10-0428-01 Live births and fetal deaths (stillbirths), by type of birth (single or multiple).* Retrieved from https://www150.statcan.gc.ca/t1/tbl1/en/tv.action?pid=1310042801.

Statistics Canada. (2019c). *Table 13-10-0394-01 Leading causes of death, total population, by age group.* Retrieved from https://www150.statcan.gc.ca/t1/tbl1/en/tv.action?pid=1310039401&pickMembers%5B0%5D=2.21&pickMembers%5B1%5D=3.1.

Statistics Canada (2019d). Canadian Health Survey on Children and Youth. Retrieved from http://www23.statcan.gc.ca/imdb/p2SV.pl?Function=getSurvey&SDDS=5233.

Strasburger, V. (2011). Children, adolescents, obesity, and the media. *Pediatrics, 128*(1), 201–208.

Subbarao, P., Anand, S. S., Becker, A. B., Befus, A. D., Brauer, M., Brook, J. R., . . . Kozyrskyj, A. L. (2015). The Canadian Healthy Infant Longitudinal Development (CHILD) Study: Examining developmental origins of allergy and asthma. *Thorax, 70*(10), 998–1000.

Tobin, J. (2019). Children's right to health. *International Human Rights of Children,* 277–298. doi: 10.1007/978-981-10-4184-6_12.

Tsai, E. (2018). Advanced care planning for paediatric patients (reaffirmed). *Paediatric Child Health, 13*(9), 791–796.

Tucker, B., Fager, C., Srinivas, S., & Lorch, S. (2011). Racial and ethnic differences in use of intubation for periviable neonates. *Pediatrics, 127*(5), e1120–e1127.

Ulivi, G., & Breeze, A. C. (2018). Advances in fetal therapy. *Obstetrics, Gynaecology & Reproductive Medicine.* Retrieved from https://doi.org/10.1016/j.ogrm.2018.04.002.

UNICEF Canada. (2019). *Child advocacy.* Retrieved from https://www.unicef.ca/en/discover/advocacy.

The United Nations International Children's Emergency Fund (UNICEF). (2019). *What we do.* Retrieved from http://www.unicef.org/what-we-do.

Vanier Institute of the Family. (2017). *In context: Understanding maternity care in Canada*. Retrieved from https://vanierinstitute.ca/context-understanding-maternity-care-canada/.

Verstraeten, B. S., Mijovic-Kondejewski, J., Takeda, J., Tanaka, S., & Olson, D. M. (2015). Canada's pregnancy-related mortality rates: Doing well but room for improvement. *Clinical and Investigative Medicine, 38*(1), E15–E36. Retrieved from https://cimonline.ca/index.php/cim/article/download/22410/18194/.

Viteri, O. A., Soto, E. E., Bahado-Singh, R. O., Christensen, C. W., Chauhan, S. P., & Sibai, B. M. (2015). Fetal anomalies and long-term effects associated with substance abuse in pregnancy: A literature review. *American Journal of Perinatology, 32*(5), 405–416.

Vohra, S., Schlegelmilch, M., Jou, H., Hartfield, D., Mayan, M., Ohinmaa, A., . . . Grundy, P. (2017). Comparative effectiveness of pediatric integrative medicine as an adjunct to usual care for pediatric inpatients of a North American tertiary care centre: A study protocol for a pragmatic cluster controlled trial. *Contemporary Clinical Trials Communications, 5*, 12–18.

Von Bertalanffy, L. (1968). *General systems theory*. London: Penguin Press.

Wilson, C. B., Nizet, V., Maldonado, Y., Remington, J. S., & Klein, J. O. (2016). *Remington and Klein's infectious diseases of the fetus and newborn infant*. Philadelphia, PA: Elsevier Health Sciences.

Wong, S., Ordean, A., & Kahan, M. (2011). Substance use in pregnancy. *Journal of Obstetrics and Gynecology Canada, 4*, 367–384.

World Health Organization (WHO). (2016). *Child maltreatment*. Retrieved from https://www.who.int/en/news-room/fact-sheets/detail/child-maltreatment.

World Health Organization (WHO). (2018). *Children: Reducing mortality*. Retrieved from https://www.who.int/en/news-room/fact-sheets/detail/children-reducing-mortality.

World Health Organization (WHO). (2019a). *Frequently asked questions*. Retrieved from https://www.who.int/suggestions/faq/en/.

World Health Organization (WHO). (2019b). *Maternal and perinatal health*. Retrieved from http://www.who.int/maternal_child_adolescent/topics/maternal/maternal_perinatal/en/.

World Heart Federation (WHF). (2017). *Women and CVD: Facts and tips*. Retrieved from https://www.world-heart-federation.org/resources/women-cvd-facts-tips/.

Wright, T. (2011). Consent and children: A practical summary. *Clinical Risk, 17*(5), 192–194.

Wright, L. M., & Leahy, M. (2013). *Nurses and families: A guide to family assessment and intervention* (6th ed.). Philadelphia, PA: F.A. Davis.

Xu, Y. (2011). The effects of teaching primary caregivers to conduct formative assessment on caregiver-child social interaction and children's developmental outcomes. *Early Child Development and Care, 181*(4), 549–571.

Yahav, R. (2011). Exposure of children to war and terrorism: A review. *Journal of Child & Adolescent Trauma, 4*(2), 90–108.

Yanchar, N. L., Warda, L. J., & Fuselli, P. (2012). Canadian Paediatric Society Position Statement, Injury Prevention Committee. Child and youth injury prevention: A public health approach. *Paediatrics & Child Health, 17*(9), 511. Retrieved from https://www.cps.ca/en/documents/position/child-and-youth-injury-prevention.

Yoon, E., Hacker, J., Hewitt, A., Abrams, M., & Cleary, S. (2012). Social connectedness, discrimination, and social status as mediators of acculturation/enculturation and well-being. *Journal of Counseling Psychology, 59*(1), 86–96.

Yuan, S. M. (2015). Fetal cardiac interventions. *Pediatrics & Neonatology, 56*(2), 81–87.

Zlotnick, C., Tam, T. W., & Soman, L. A. (2012). Life course outcomes on mental and physical health: The impact of foster care on adulthood. *American Journal of Public Health, 102*(3), 534–540.

CHAPTER **WORKSHEET**

MULTIPLE CHOICE QUESTIONS

1. When preparing a presentation for a local woman's group on health concerns, what would the nurse include as the number-one cause of mortality for women in Canada?
   a. Breast cancer
   b. Childbirth complications
   c. Injury resulting from violence
   d. Heart disease

2. Which factor would most likely be responsible for a pregnant individual's failure to receive adequate prenatal care in Canada?
   a. Belief that it is not necessary in a normal pregnancy
   b. Use of denial to cope with pregnancy
   c. Lack of access
   d. Inability to trust traditional medical practices

3. When caring for an adolescent, in which instance must the nurse share information with the parents?
   a. Pregnancy counselling
   b. Depression
   c. Contraception
   d. Tuberculosis

4. The nurse is preparing a class for a group of students about homelessness. Which factors contribute to homelessness? Select all that apply.
   a. Decrease in the number of people living in poverty
   b. Rises in unemployment
   c. Exposure to abuse or neglect
   d. Cutbacks in public welfare programs
   e. Development of community crisis centres

CRITICAL THINKING EXERCISES

1. As a nurse working in a low-income clinic offering women's health services, you are becoming increasingly frustrated with the number of "no-shows," or appointments missed in your prenatal clinic. Some clients come for their initial prenatal intake appointment and never come back. You realize that some just forget their appointments, but most don't even call to notify you. Many of the clients are high risk and thus are jeopardizing their health and the health of their future child.
   a. What changes might be helpful to address this situation?
   b. Outline what you might say at your next staff meeting to address the issue of clients making one clinic visit and then never returning.

   c. What strategies might you use to improve attendance and notification?
   d. Describe what cultural sensitivity might be needed.

2. A couple has adopted an 11-month-old infant girl from China and brought her to the health care facility for a developmental checkup. The couple had no contact with the infant's birth parents. The infant spent 7 months in an orphanage before being adopted. Describe the family structure and the issues that may affect this family.

3. You have been asked by the local school district to speak to a group of middle-school children and their parents about Internet safety. Describe the topics that you should address.

4. A 12-year-old is to undergo research treatment for a serious illness. Explain the concept of assent as it relates to this situation.

STUDY ACTIVITIES

1. Research a current policy, bill, or issue being debated on the community, provincial, or national level that pertains to the health and welfare of women, parents, or children. Summarize the major facts and supporting and opposing arguments, and prepare an oral report on your findings.

2. Within your clinical group, debate the following statement: Should access to health care be a right or a privilege?

3. Visit a local community health centre that offers services to families from various cultures. Interview the staff about any barriers to health care that they have identified. Investigate what the staff has done to minimize these barriers.

BRINGING IT ALL TOGETHER: A CASE STUDY

Maali, a 19-year-old Arab immigrant, presents at the local prenatal clinic accompanied by her husband Labib. The couple and their 18-month-old daughter, Labiba, have lived with relatives since arriving in Canada 5 months ago. During the prenatal interview, Maali reports that she is 4 months pregnant and is the primary caregiver for their daughter as well as caring for Labib's sister's toddler son while her sister-in-law is at work during the day.

Go to thePoint **to find questions to consider about this case.**

2

Family-Centred Community-Based Care

Learning Objectives

Upon completion of the chapter, you will be able to:

1. Identify the core concepts associated with the nursing management of women, children, and families.

2. Examine the major components and key elements of family-centred care.

3. Explain the different levels of prevention in nursing, providing examples of each.

4. Give examples of cultural issues that may be faced when providing nursing care.

5. Provide culturally sensitive and competent care to women, children, and families.

6. Outline the various roles and functions assumed by the nurse working with women, children, and families.

7. Demonstrate the ability to use excellent therapeutic communication skills when interacting with women, children, and families.

8. Explain the process of health teaching as it relates to parents, children, and families.

9. Examine the importance of discharge planning and case management in providing nursing care.

10. Explain the reasons for the increased emphasis on community-based care.

11. Differentiate community-based nursing from nursing in acute care settings.

12. Identify the variety of settings where community-based care can be provided to parents, children, and families.

Gabrielle was home a few days after giving birth to her first child. She had just changed her newborn son and placed him on his stomach for a nap when the community health nurse arrived for a postpartum visit. Because the nurse didn't speak Arabic and Gabrielle spoke very little English, a great deal of gesturing followed. After examining Gabrielle, the nurse then picked up her son and placed him on his back in the crib. How might the nurse have prepared for this home visit? What message did the nurse convey in changing the newborn's position?

INTRODUCTION

Now more than ever, nurses contribute to nearly every health care experience. Historically, people were born at home, cared for when ill at home, and then died at home surrounded by loved ones. Today, these events from birth to death, and every health care emergency in between, will likely involve the presence of a nurse. Involvement of a knowledgeable, supportive, comforting nurse often leads to a positive health care experience. Skilled nursing practice depends on a solid base of knowledge and clinical expertise delivered in a caring, holistic manner. Nurses, using their knowledge and passion, help meet the health care needs of their clients throughout the life span, whether the client is a pregnant individual, a fetus, a partner, a child, or the parents or family members of a child. Nurses fill a variety of roles in helping clients to live healthier lives by providing direct care, emotional support, comfort, information, advice, advocacy, support, and counselling. Nurses are often "in the trenches" advocating on various issues, drawing attention to the importance of health care for women, parents, and children, encouraging a focus on education and prevention, and assisting families who lack resources or access to health care.

Families receive a majority of their health care, both well and ill care, in the community setting. During the past several years, the health care delivery system has changed dramatically. With a focus on cost containment, people are spending less time in the hospital. Clients are being discharged "sicker and quicker" from their hospital beds (Hansen, 2015). The health care system has moved from reactive treatment strategies in hospitals to a proactive approach in the community, known as **primary health care** (PHC). This has resulted in an increasing need for health promotion and illness prevention within the community.

The Canadian Nurses Association (CNA) contends that nurses play an important role in the health and wellness of a community by continuing advocate for continued investments in these PHC measures (CNA, 2015). This is an exciting time for nurses delivering out-of-hospital care. The rising trend of delivering care in or near people's homes and away from acute care facilities will necessitate flexible ways of working and greater integration of community nursing roles (Massey, 2015). They not only meet the health care needs of the individual but also go beyond that to implement interventions that affect the community as a whole. Nurses practice in a variety of settings within a **community**, such as clinics and physician and nurse practitioner offices, schools, shelters, churches, health departments, community health centres, and homes. They promote the health of individuals, families, groups, communities, and populations and promote an environment that supports health.

This chapter describes the core concepts of maternal and child health nursing and community and community-based nursing. Nurses need to be knowledgeable about these concepts to ensure that they provide professional care.

CORE CONCEPTS OF MATERNAL AND CHILD HEALTH NURSING

Maternal and child health nursing focuses on providing evidence-based care to the client within the context of the family. This care involves the implementation of an interdisciplinary plan in a collaborative manner to ensure continuity of care that is cost effective, quality oriented, and outcome focused. Nurses provide this care by focusing on the family, using evidence-based practice (EBP), working collaboratively, providing atraumatic therapeutic care, communicating effectively, providing education, providing discharge planning and case management, providing advocacy and resource management, providing preventative care, providing culturally competent nursing care, and being knowledgeable about complementary and alternative medicine (CAM).

Family-Centred Care

Family-centred care refers to the collaborative partnership among the individual, family, and caregivers to determine goals, share information, offer support, and formulate plans for health care. It is generally understood to be an approach in which clients and their families are considered integral components of the health care decision-making and delivery processes. It recognizes the client and the family as the source of control and a full partner in their care (Roberts, 2015). It is based on mutual trust and collaboration between parents, children, families, and the health care professional. It is a partnership approach of families and their caregivers that recognizes the strength and integrity of the family.

The philosophy of family-centred care recognizes the family as the constant. The health and functioning of the family affect the health of the client and other members of the family. Family members support one another well beyond the health care provider's brief time with them, such as during the childbearing process or during a child's illness.

Family-centred care requires sensitivity to the client's and family's beliefs and those supporting their culture. This involves listening to the family's needs and a shift of the nurse's authoritarian role to the family to empower them to make their own decisions within the context of a supportive environment.

With family-centred care, support and respect for the uniqueness and diversity of families are essential, along with encouragement and enhancement of the family's strengths and competencies. It is important to create opportunities for families to demonstrate their abilities and skills. Families can also acquire new abilities and skills to maintain a sense of control and empowerment in meeting the needs of the client. Family-centred care promotes greater family self-determination, decision-making abilities, control, and self-efficacy, thereby enhancing the client's and family's sense of empowerment. When implementing family-centred care, nurses seek caregiver input. These suggestions and advice are incorporated into the client's plan of care as the nurse counsels and teaches the family appropriate health care interventions. Today, as nurses partner with various experts to provide high-quality and cost-effective care, one expert partnership that nurses must make is with the client's family.

The impact of family-centred care can be seen in the models of care delivery for families and children. From the 1980s to the present, there has been increased access to care for new parents and infants, with hospital redesigns (labour, birthing, and recovery rooms; labour, birthing, recovery, and postpartum spaces) aimed at keeping families together during the childbirth experience and to minimize interruptions in breastfeeding dyads (Ayers, Grassley, & Koprowski, 2015). This impact can also be seen in the care of children. For example, rooming-in and liberal visiting policies allow parents and other family members to participate in the child's care (Fig. 2.1).

Family-centred care works well in all arenas of health care, from preventive care to long-term care. Using a family-centred approach is associated with positive outcomes such as decreased anxiety, improved pain management, shorter recovery times, and enhanced confidence and problem-solving skills. Communication between the health care team and the family is also improved, leading to greater satisfaction for both health care providers and health care consumers (families). It is important for nurses to remain neutral to all they hear and see in order to enhance trust and maintain open communication lines with all family members. Nurses need to remember that clients are an expert of their own health, thus nurses should work within the clients' framework when planning health promotion interventions.

Evidence-Informed Care

Evidence-informed nursing practice involves the use of research or evidence in establishing a plan of care and then implementing that care. It is a clinical decision-making approach that involves the integration of the best scientific evidence, client values and preferences, clinical circumstances, and clinical expertise to promote best outcomes (Williamson, Almaskari, Lester, & Maguire, 2015). It is important that nurses develop the skills and knowledge necessary to ask pertinent clinical questions, search for current best evidence, analyze the evidence, integrate the evidence into practice when appropriate, and evaluate outcomes. EBP may lead to a decrease in variations in care while at the same time increasing quality and improving health care.

Scientific research findings help nurses not only stay current in their clinical specialties, but also in their choice of the most effective interventions. Many of the professional organizations such as the Canadian Association of Perinatal and Women's Health Nurses (CAPWHN), CNA, and Registered Nurses' Association of Ontario (RNAO) have developed evidence-based clinical practice guidelines for the safest and effective delivery of family-centred nursing care. Nurses should be diligent in seeking out these evidence-based guidelines to ensure excellence in their daily practice. When EBP is delivered in a context of caring and in a supportive organizational culture, the highest quality of care and best client outcomes can be achieved (Bridges, 2015; Makic, Rauen, Jones, & Fisk, 2015).

Collaborative Care

Nurses must embrace interprofessional collaborative care because health care reform has transformed health care delivery models that require team work. Nurses must transition from working in a silo to working with interprofessional teams. This transition is needed to provide high-quality, safe, and accountable care to achieve positive client outcomes (CNA, 2011; Lomax & White, 2015). Modern health care focuses on an interdisciplinary plan of care designed to meet a client's physical, developmental, educational, spiritual, and psychosocial needs. This interdisciplinary collaborative type of care is termed **case**

FIGURE 2.1 Providing an opportunity for the parent to interact with the child is an important component of family-centred nursing care.

management, a collaborative process involving assessment, planning, implementation, coordination, monitoring, and evaluation.

When the nurse effectively functions in the role as a case manager, client and family satisfaction is increased, fragmentation of care is decreased, and outcome measurement for a homogeneous group of clients is possible.

Atraumatic Pediatric Care

Children undergo a wide range of interventions, many of which can be traumatic, stressful, and painful. The various settings where the child receives care can be scary and overwhelming to the child and family. The child and family interact with various health care personnel, which leads to an increased potential for anxiety. A major component of the child health nursing philosophy is the importance of providing atraumatic care. **Atraumatic care** refers to the delivery of care that minimizes or eliminates the psychological and physical distress experienced by children and their families in the health care system (Wong-Baker FACES Foundation, 2016). The key principles of atraumatic care include the following:

- Preventing or minimizing physical stressors
- Preventing or minimizing separation of the child from the family
- Promoting a sense of control

Nurses must be alert for any situation that has the potential for causing distress and should be able to identify potential stressors. Pediatric nurses should minimize separation of the child from the family, should decrease the child's exposure to stressful situations, and should strive to prevent or minimize pain and injury. The importance of providing atraumatic care to children is integrated throughout this text and discussed in detail in Chapter 30.

Communication

Communication is a way of conveying messages to various people using a common system of symbols, signs, or behaviours. Infants start their first communication soon after birth when they cry to convey the message of discomfort or hunger. Effective therapeutic communication with parents, children, and families is essential to the provision of quality nursing care. Client- and family-centred communication increases satisfaction with nursing care and aids in improving knowledge and health care skills (Arnold & Boggs, 2016). The significance of communication revolves around its effectiveness and the climate in which communication occurs. Trust, respect, and empathy are three factors needed to create and foster effective therapeutic communication between people.

(See Chapter 30 for specifics on effective communication when working with children.)

Verbal Communication

Communicating through the use of words, either written or spoken, is termed **verbal communication**. Nurses use verbal communication throughout the day when interacting with clients. Good verbal communication skills are necessary when performing nursing assessments and providing child/family teaching. General guidelines for appropriate verbal communication include the following:

- Use open-ended questions that do not restrict the child's or parents' answers.
- Redirect the conversation to maintain focus.
- Use reflection to clarify the parents' feelings.
- Paraphrase the child's or parents' feelings to demonstrate empathy.
- Acknowledge emotions.
- Demonstrate active listening by using the child's or family's own words.

Remember that most parents are laypersons, so avoid using medical jargon. The abbreviations and shortened terms that health care providers use almost without thinking may sound scary or foreign to children and parents. When medical terminology is necessary, provide a definition using developmentally appropriate language.

Providing culturally sensitive care requires nurses to remember that communication is significantly influenced by a person's culture: comfort discussing aspects of the body or health, pacing and even volume of speech may be a reflection of the client's cultural background. Awareness of cultural differences helps nurses avoid making inaccurate assumptions related to the client's intended message.

Nonverbal Communication

Nonverbal communication, or body language, includes attending to others and active listening. The nurse should listen to the other person's verbal communication from the beginning of the interaction. When parents and children feel they are being heard, trust and rapport are established. Guidelines for appropriate nonverbal communication include the following:

- Relax; maintain an open posture, with the arms uncrossed.
- Sit opposite the family and lean forward slightly.
- Maintain eye contact.
- Nod your head to demonstrate interest.
- Note the child's or parent's posture, eye contact, and facial expressions.

Cultural influences on nonverbal communication can include variations in comfort with eye contact, facial expression, and touch.

Take Note!

People of all ages desire to be listened to without interruption (Gupta, Mehta, & Sagar, 2015).

Active listening is critical to the communication process. Listening may uncover fears or concerns that the nurse may not have discovered through questioning.

Paying attention while children and parents talk is a powerful communication tool. By not listening, the nurse may miss critical information and the family may be reluctant to share further. When interacting with the child and family, determine whether the messages sent by the child's or parents' verbal and nonverbal communication are congruent.

Recall Gabrielle, who recently was discharged from the hospital with her newborn son. How did the nurse communicate with Gabrielle? Did the nurse's actions during the visit promote the development of trust between Gabrielle and the nurse? What might have been done differently to foster trust?

Communicating Across Cultures

Understanding and respecting the client's and family's culture helps foster good communication and improves child and family education about health care. Culture, religion, and spirituality are intertwined concepts that affect the client's and family's communication styles, health status, and health beliefs. It is important to be aware of the family's background, lifestyle, and health care practices to meet their information needs.

Learning about the practices of various cultures is just the beginning; the nurse must assess each family's individual beliefs and practices, not generalize. The best way to assess the family's cultural practices is to ask and then listen. Determine the language spoken at home and observe the use of eye contact and other physical contact. Demonstrate a caring, nonjudgmental attitude and sensitivity to the client's and family's cultural diversity.

Working With an Interpreter

Attempting to communicate with a family who does not speak English can be one of the most frustrating situations in which health care providers find themselves. In this situation, trained interpreters are an invaluable aid and an essential component of client and family education. Whether working with an interpreter in person or over the phone, it is important to coordinate efforts so that both the family and the interpreter understand the information to be communicated. Working as a team, the nurse questions or informs and the interpreter conveys the information completely and accurately (College

of Nurses of Ontario, 2009). Well-trained translators can also help prevent cultural missteps and can help guide the health care provider to provide information in a more culturally accepted manner (Levetown; American Academy of Pediatrics Committee on Bioethics, 2011). Box 2.1 presents tips for working with an interpreter to maximize teaching efforts.

On the second visit to Gabrielle's home, the nurse brought an Arabic-speaking interpreter who explained the reason for the "back to sleep" position and demonstrated to Gabrielle several other useful positions for feeding and holding. Gabrielle was smiling when the nurse left and asking when she would be back. What made the difference in their relationship in the second visit? What interventions demonstrate culturally competent care?

Communicating With Deaf or Hearing-Impaired Clients and Families

Nearly one in four adult Canadians has some form of hearing loss, while approximately 10% of Canadians self-identify as deaf, oral deaf, deafened, or hard of hearing. Approximately 4 in 1,000 babies born in Canada have some degree of hearing loss or will develop early progressive childhood hearing loss (Canadian Hearing Society, 2013). Health care providers are under a duty to provide auxiliary aids and services to establish effective communication with their clients. Providing assistance to the hearing impaired in health care settings is critically important because, without assistance through auxiliary aids and services, health service providers run the risk of not understanding the client's symptoms, misdiagnosing the client's health problem, and prescribing inadequate or even harmful treatment (Smith, 2015b).

Hearing-impaired pregnant clients are often neglected mostly due to a lack of understanding of how best to care for people with different communication needs. Nurses have a key role in exchanging information and taking the time to understand their needs in order to act as an advocate and help them to overcome the barriers that can be created by deafness. In order to fulfill this role, nurses need to have an understanding of the problems faced by pregnant clients with altered hearing and their partners when accessing perinatal services (Jackson, 2011).

For the hearing impaired, determine the method of communication used: lip reading, American Sign Language (ASL), another method, or some combination. If the nurse is not proficient in ASL and the client or family uses it, then an ASL interpreter must be available if another adult family member is not present for

---

BOX 2.1

TIPS FOR WORKING WITH AN INTERPRETER

- **Seek the client's consent** to use an interpreter or any other arrangement for communication.
- **Help the interpreter prepare and understand what needs to be done ahead of time.** A few minutes of preparation may save a lot of time and help communication flow more smoothly in the long run.
- The interpreter may have valuable cultural or familial insight. **Ask the interpreter to share these insights**, and to identify them clearly as his or her insights and not as facts or the client's actual beliefs.
- **Introduce yourself to both parties.** It is the key to easy communication across the language barrier.
- **Physically place yourselves so that you are facing your client, and your client is facing you.** Place the interpreter physically close to both of you, but not in a position that breaks the line of sight between you and your client.
- **Speak to the client, not to the interpreter.** Maintain eye contact, as appropriate. This reinforces the message that the communication is between the provider and the client, assisted by the interpreter. This also allows you to assess the nonverbal reactions and responses.
- **Begin with a minute or two of light conversation to establish a rhythm before getting into the business at hand.** This establishes the quantity of speech in the conversation.
- **Explain** to the client and the interpreter **that confidentiality will be maintained**. The interpreter must not disclose client information to anyone.
- **Remember, the interpreter is the "communication bridge" and not the "content expert."** The nurse's presence at teaching sessions is vital.
- **Be patient. The interpreter's timing may not match that of others involved.** It often takes longer to say in some languages what has already been said in English; therefore, plan for more time than you normally would.

- **Speak slowly and clearly.** Avoid jargon. Use short sentences and be concise; short sentences can reduce the risk of error or omission. Avoid interrupting the interpreter.
- **Pause every few sentences so the interpreter can translate your information.** After 30 seconds of speaking, stop and let the interpreter express the information. Talk directly to the family, not the interpreter.
- **Give the family and the interpreter a break.** Sessions that last longer than 20 or 30 minutes are too much for anyone's attention span and concentration.
- **Express the information in two or three different ways if needed.** There may be cultural barriers as well as language and dialect differences that interfere with understanding. Interpreters may often know the correct communication protocols for the family.
- **Write down key points**, directions, appointment times, and any other material that has numbers or can easily be confused or forgotten. Giving the client a written record prevents the interpreter from having to rely entirely on memory.
- **Avoid side conversations during sessions.** These can be uncomfortable for the family and jeopardize client–provider relationships and trust.
- **Ask** the interpreter **if there was anything about the interaction that made it difficult to interpret**. This will allow you to assess the overall quality of the interaction.
- **Remember, just because someone speaks another language doesn't mean that he or she will make a good interpreter.** An interpreter who has no medical background may not understand or interpret correctly, no matter how good his or her language skills are.
- **Do not use children as interpreters.** Doing so can affect family relationships, proper understanding, and compliance with health care issues.

Adapted from College of Nurses of Ontario. (2018). *Culturally sensitive care*. Retrieved from http://www.cno.org/en/learn-about-standards-guidelines/educational-tools/ask-practice/culturally-sensitive-care/; Refugee Health Technical Assistance Center. (2011). *Best practices for communicating through an interpreter*. Retrieved from http://refugeehealthta.org/access-to-care/language-access/best-practices-communicating-through-an-interpreter/

---

translation. The Canadian Charter of Rights and Freedoms outlines the basic human rights of all Canadians, including the right to communication and information, as well as the right to language of their choice, including ASL or the presence of an interpreter who knows ASL (Canadian Charter of Rights and Freedoms, 1982, s. 14).

Education

Due to shortened hospital stays and decreased admissions, providing client and family education is a key role for nurses. Generally, teaching begins in the primary care setting and then continues in the community setting, especially the home. In the community-based setting, client teaching is often focused on assisting the client and family to achieve independence.

Regardless of the type of setting, nurses are in a unique position to help clients and families manage their own health care needs. Clients and families need to be knowledgeable about areas such as their condition, the health care management plan, and when and how to contact health care providers. With the limited time available in all health care arenas, nurses must focus on teaching goals and begin teaching at the earliest opportunity. Education and planning care are essential components of quality client care (Peter, Robinson, Jordan, Lawrence, Casey, & Salas-Lopez, 2015).

Client education occurs when nurses share information, knowledge, and skills with clients and families, thus empowering them to take responsibility for their health care. Through client education, clients and families can overcome feelings of powerlessness and helplessness and gain the confidence and capability to be active members in their plan of care.

Overall, client and family education allows clients and families to make informed decisions, ensures the presence of basic health care skills, promotes recognition of problem situations, promotes appropriate responses to problems, and allows for questions to be answered. When thorough and structured education begins in the hospital setting, it can carry over into the home setting, which can decrease hospital readmissions. Verification sheets can play an important role in aiding bedside nurses to provide early formal education for clients and families being discharged home with a new device so that safe care can be achieved in the home setting (Hamilton, 2011).

Take Note!

To cope effectively with illness, understand and participate in decisions about treatment plans, and maintain and improve health after treatment; clients and their families must have access to the specific knowledge and skills relevant to their conditions (CDC, 2016).

Steps of Client and Family Education

The steps of client and family education are similar to the steps of the nursing process. The nurse must assess the client, develop a plan, implement services needed, perform follow-up evaluation, and finally document education. Once the nurse achieves a level of comfort and experience with each of these steps, they all blend together into one harmonious whole that becomes an everyday part of nursing practice. Client education begins with the first client encounter and proceeds through discharge and beyond. Reassessment after each step or change in the process is critical to ensuring success.

ASSESSING TEACHING AND LEARNING NEEDS

Excellent nursing care begins with a thorough assessment of the client. In the same way, client and family education begins with a learning needs assessment that includes the client's and family's learning needs, learning styles and preferences, and potential barriers to learning. Based on the results of the assessment, an individualized plan can be developed to reduce the time and effort required for teaching while maximizing learning for the client and family. Although actual nursing care in pediatrics is given to the child, the educational process is targeted at both the child, when developmentally appropriate, and the adult members of the family. Therefore, it is advisable to conduct a learning needs assessment on both the adult caregivers and the child, when appropriate. Box 2.2 describes the components of a learning needs assessment. This is also a good time to establish rapport with the family, demonstrating your interest in them and your confidence in their ability to learn.

BOX 2.2

COMPONENTS OF LEARNING NEEDS ASSESSMENT

Assess

- Learner characteristics: Find out more about the child and family's life and how the child's illness has affected it. Learn more about the child and family's social, cultural, and spiritual values.
- Learner needs and readiness: Including what they want and need to know and what they know already; readiness and willingness to learn; motivation to learn and emotional concerns; capacity to learn such as physical or cognitive abilities including ability to read and developmental level.
- Learning style: How does the child and family learn best; preferred learning methods.
- Learning barriers: Cultural or language barriers; cognitive or physical disabilities; presence of pain; lack of support network.

Adapted from The Sentinel Watch: Nursing. (2014). *Improve your patient education skills to enhance care.* Retrieved from http://www.americansentinel.edu/blog/2014/12/17/improve-your-patient-education-skills-to-enhance-care/; and The Joint Commission (TJC). (2012). *Patient education.* Retrieved from http://www.mghpcs.org/eed_portal/Documents/PatientEd/JC_Standards_PatientEd.pdf

---

Share the assessment with all members of the interdisciplinary team so that the entire team can support the client's and family's learning. Initial assessments generally take place during the first or second meeting with the client and family and should continue with each encounter to check for any changes that may occur.

Malcolm Knowles outlined core learning principles to consider when teaching adults (Knowles, Holton, & Swanson, 2011). He found that instruction for adults needs to focus more on the process than on the content. Box 2.3 lists adult learner-centred principles.

CULTURAL IMPACT ON ASSESSMENT OF LEARNING NEEDS

In addition to determining the language spoken in the home and use of eye and physical contact, investigate the following during the assessment:

- Who is the person caring for the child at home?
- Who is the authority figure in the family?
- What is the social support structure?
- Are there any special dietary needs and concerns?
- Are any traditional health practices used (e.g., healers, shamans, talismans, folk remedies, and herbs)?
- Are any special clothes or other items used to help maintain health?
- What religious beliefs, ceremonies, and spiritual practices are important?

Learning needs can then be negotiated with the family and met based on the assessment. Issues encountered

---

BOX 2.3

SPECIFIC LEARNING PRINCIPLES RELATED TO PARENTS

- **Adults are self-directed.** Adults value independence and want to learn on their own terms. Teaching strategies that include such concepts as role playing, demonstration, and self-evaluation are most helpful. Using this model, nurses can partner with families to ensure that education is interactive and adopt the role of facilitator rather than lecturer.
- **Adults are problem focused and task oriented.** Adults learn best when they perceive there is a gap in their knowledge base and want information and skills to fill the gap. Providing a reason to learn can often motivate families that appear slow to comply with their child's care and education.
- **Adults are goal oriented.** Adults learn best at a time when learning meets an immediate need. Presenting information in an organized, sequential, and timely fashion can often help families understand the importance of learning a particular piece of information or task.
- **Adults value past experiences and beliefs.** Adults bring an accumulated wealth of experiences to each health care encounter; this provides a rich base for new learning. Education should take into account a wide range of backgrounds. Appreciating and using individual differences during teaching encounters can help improve compliance and reduce resistance to educational goals.

Knowles, M. S., Holton, III, E. F., & Swanson, R. A. (2011). *The adult learner* (7th ed.). Burlington, MA: Elsevier.

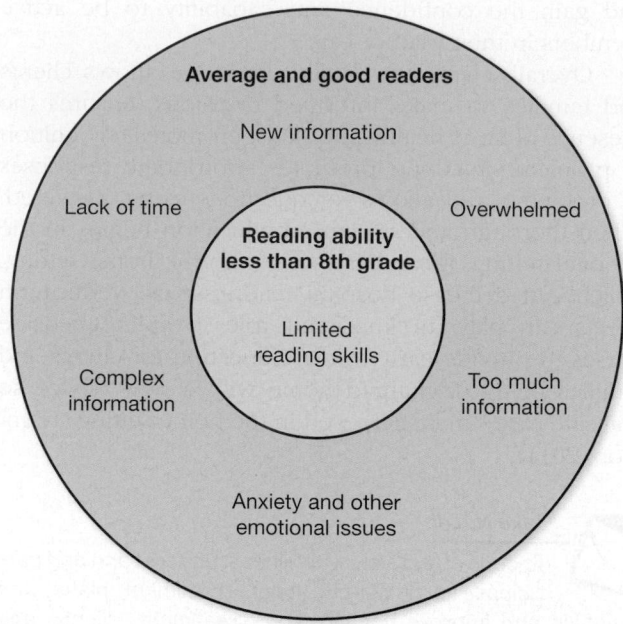

FIGURE 2.2 Factors contributing to poor health literacy.

when teaching immigrant or refugee families might include confusion regarding the use of the imperial versus the metric scale; preparing formulas and medicines using a "handful" or "pinch" of ingredients rather than specific measurements such as a measuring cup or syringe; access to refrigeration for liquid antibiotics; and breastfeeding practices.

LITERACY ISSUES

Adequate literacy skills are essential for client and family education, yet many people in this country have marginal reading capabilities. Approximately 17% of Canadians have low literacy abilities (Statistics Canada, 2013).

Even people with adequate literacy skills may have difficulty reading, understanding, and applying information to health care situations (Fig. 2.2). **Health literacy** is the ability to read, understand, and use health care information to make appropriate health care decisions and successfully navigate the health care system (Hersh, Salzman, & Snyderman, 2015). It is not simply having the ability to read the health care information, but also includes listening; displaying oral, analytic, and decision-making skills; using electronic technology; and applying these skills to health care situations. The inability to read and comprehend health care information is an enormous problem for

many Canadians today. Low health literacy affects people of all ages, races, and educational and income levels.

Take Note!

The Canadian Public Health Association (CPHA, 2008) reported that 55% of Canadians between the ages of 16 and 65 scored low in health literacy on the International Adult Literacy and Skills Survey, and that only approximately 12% of adults over age 65 have a functional level of health literacy. Other health literacy studies have suggested that people with inadequate health literacy have higher rates of hospitalization and longer hospital stays, higher usage of expensive emergency services, increased medication errors, and generally a higher level of illness (Centers for Disease Control and Prevention [CDC], 2016).

Medical information is becoming increasingly complex, while the amount of time nurses have to spend with clients is decreasing. Also, when unfamiliar information is introduced or when emotional distress is present, reading ability and understanding are further reduced. As a result, many studies have shown that persons with limited literacy skills cannot understand basic medical words and health concepts, verbal or written. For example, in one study it was noted that:

- One in four did not understand when their next appointment was scheduled.
- Almost half did not understand the instructions, "Take medication on an empty stomach."
- Three quarters misunderstood warnings on medication labels or the rights and responsibilities section of a Medicaid application (Duell, Wright, Renzaho, & Bhattacharya, 2015).

RECOGNIZING POOR HEALTH LITERACY SKILLS

Poor health literacy skills are difficult to recognize: appearance, verbal ability, employment status, and educational level cannot reliably detect persons who do not read well. Also, many people who do not read well go to great lengths to hide their disability: 68% of people with limited literacy skills have never told their spouse and 75% have never told their health care provider (Brega et al., 2015). Poor health literacy affects all segments of the population but certain groups such as the elderly, those with low income, members of minority groups, recent immigrants with limited English, and those who are born in this country but for whom English is an additional language are at higher risk (Zambrana, Meghea, Talley, Hammad, Lockett, & Williams, 2015).

Red flags that might indicate poor literacy skills include the following:

- Difficulty filling out registration forms, questionnaires, and consent forms; forms are incomplete, incorrect, or inaccurate
- Frequently missed appointments
- Noncompliance and lack of follow-up with treatment regimens
- History of medication errors
- Responses such as, "I forgot my glasses" or "I'll read this when I get home"
- Inability to answer common questions about their treatment or medicines
- Avoiding asking questions for fear of looking "stupid" (Brega et al., 2015)

Nurses need to provide understandable and accessible information to all clients, regardless of their literacy or education levels. This would include avoiding medical jargon, breaking down information or instructions into small concrete steps, limiting the focus of a visit to three key points or tasks, and assessing for comprehension. In addition, printed information should be written at or below a fifth to sixth grade reading level with plenty of visual aids or pictures (Hersh et al., 2015).

PLANNING EDUCATION

Once the assessment is completed, plan mutually agreed-upon, achievable learning goals and objectives. It is important that both the teacher and learner believe the goals can be accomplished. Finding common ground and building a bridge between the client's and family's concerns and what the health care team believes they need to know is a critical part of an education plan. This also is an excellent time to consider which client education materials and resources can be used to maximize learning and retention. No single teaching method will suit every client and family. Individualize educational methods to meet the learning needs and abilities of the audience that is being taught. Ensuring instructional methods are chosen based on educational outcomes is a key to success (Su, Herron, & Osisek, 2011).

A review of recent research on patient education found effective teaching strategies that include computer technology, audiotapes, videos, written materials prepared at an appropriate reading level for the general population, and demonstration (Friedman, Cosby, Boyko, Hatto-Bauer, & Turnbull, 2011). Verbal instruction was found to be least effective and should be used along with another teaching method (Friedman et al., 2011). Using multiple teaching strategies, such as using videos, dolls, play therapy, or computer-based instruction along with written material for future reference, is beneficial. Almost 67% of patients had better outcomes when multiple teaching methods were used (Friedman et al., 2011). Visual aids such as pictures and illustrations are very helpful and can assist those with low literacy. Education that is culturally appropriate, presented in a structured manner and specific to the individual has been found to be more effective (Friedman et al., 2011).

Planning client and family education should involve input from the entire interdisciplinary team when appropriate. Through good communication and collaboration, team members can work together to empower the child and family to become knowledgeable and skilful caregivers. Leaving behind the traditional path of teacher-centred education and providing family-centred education instead requires thought and skill.

PRACTICAL INTERVENTIONS TO ENHANCE LEARNING

The assessed needs and planned learning objectives lead to good teaching interventions. Evaluate these interventions frequently to ensure that the child and family are learning and meeting agreed-upon goals. Table 2.1 presents six techniques that can help improve learning.

HELPING CHILDREN AND FAMILIES WITH LOW HEALTH LITERACY SKILLS

Nurses are in an excellent position to create a "blame-free" environment and offer help. It is entirely appropriate to say to the child or family member, "Many people have a problem reading and remembering the information on this teaching sheet (booklet, manual). Is this ever a problem for you?" For children or family members with low health literacy, the nurse must adjust oral communication techniques and written materials to assist with learning, and should communicate this need to the entire interdisciplinary health care team.

TABLE 2.1	SIX TECHNIQUES TO IMPROVE LEARNING
Technique	**Explanation**
Slow down and repeat information often.	Since most of the education in a health care setting is done verbally, repeat important information at least four or five times.
Speak in conversational style using plain, nonmedical language.	When writing directions, write only several words, bullet points, or phrases. Use common, "living-room-type" language containing one or two syllables whenever possible.
Group information and teach it in small amounts using logical steps.	This is especially important when there are large amounts of complex information for the family to learn. Teach for 10 to 15 minutes, give the learner a break, and return later to teach again.
Prioritize information and teach "survival skills" first.	Due to time constraints and multiple demands on the part of staff, coupled with the rapid turnaround times of health care encounters for clients, there never seems to be enough time to teach. Nurses must provide the client and family with the necessary information to meet their immediate needs. This may include information about the following: • The child's medical condition • Treatment information • Why the information is important • Possible problems, adverse effects, or concerns • What to do if problems arise • Who to contact for further help, information, or supplies
Use visuals, such as pictures, videos, and models.	Use visual resources to enhance and reinforce learning when available. Drawing simple pictures and charts or using alternative methods such as colour-coding often allows learning to occur for families who are having difficulty grasping information or concepts.
Teach using an interactive, "hands-on" approach.	When the learner uses hands-on practice, or participates in care, learning occurs more quickly and easily. Learning first on a doll or model can ease anxiety and bolster self-confidence before actually performing care or procedures on the child.

If literacy problems are known or suspected, the nurse can take the following steps to enhance learning:
• Draw pictures or use medical illustrations.
• Use videos.
• Colour-code medications or the steps of a procedure.
• Record an audiotape.
• Repeat verbal information often and organize it into small groups.
• Teach a "back-up" family member.

EVALUATING LEARNING

Teaching, even when done well, does not necessarily mean that learning has occurred. Evaluation of learning is critical to ensure that the client and family have actually learned what was taught. In a health care setting, perform an evaluation with each educational encounter and adjust goals and interventions accordingly. The nurse, along with the rest of the interdisciplinary team, is responsible for client and family learning. Help ensure understanding by asking for feedback and offering an opportunity for questions. Also, assessing for signs of confusion, such as increased anxiety, can help evaluate learning. If they have not learned, the health care team ensures that teaching strategies are adjusted so that the client or family does learn.

Take Note!

The ultimate goal of education is a change in behaviour on the part of the child and family; this change can occur in their level of knowledge or skill, and often both.

Evaluation can occur in several different ways, depending on the topic and the method of teaching. The child or family may:
• Demonstrate a skill, often referred to as return demonstration. Learning can quickly and easily be identified using this method.
• Repeat back or teach back the information using their own words.
• Answer open-ended questions. Open-ended questions provide an opportunity to assess for missing or incorrect information. Open-ended questions are those that cannot be answered with a simple "yes" or "no."

Another option to evaluate learning is to provide a "pretend" scenario for the family, mentally placing them in their own home. Have them verbalize all the steps needed to care for their child, from routine care to handling an emergency situation. They will need to convey information accurately and completely as they walk through the steps necessary to provide care for their child independently at home.

DOCUMENTING EDUCATION FOR THE CHILD AND FAMILY

Documenting child care and education on the medical record is part of every nurse's professional practice. First and foremost, the child's medical record serves as a communication tool that the entire interdisciplinary team can use to keep track of what the child and family has learned already and what learning still needs to occur. It also serves to testify to the education the family has received, if and when legal matters arise.

Documentation of child and family education is imperative. It is the only way to ensure that the family's educational plan and objectives have been completed and that the family is ready for discharge. Documentation of child and family education should include topics such as the following:
- The learning needs assessment
- Information on the client's medical condition and plan of care
- Goals of client education; the date goal is met
- Teaching method used and how it was received by client and family
- Medications, including drug–drug and drug–food interactions
- Modified diets and nutritional needs
- Safe use of medical equipment
- Follow-up care and community resources discussed

Client and family education plays an essential role in promoting safe self-management practice. To ensure that clients and their families attain the required abilities, client and family education needs to be competency based. When developing and applying a competency-based education lesson/program, each nurse must identify essential competencies to be taught, optimal teaching methods, best method to evaluate achievement, and documentation of evidence of learning taken place (King, 2015).

Discharge Planner and Case Manager

Discharge planning involves the development and implementation of a comprehensive plan for the safe discharge of a client from a health care facility and for continuing safe and effective care in the community and at home. Case management focuses on coordinating health care services while balancing quality and cost outcomes. Due to the short length of stays in acute settings and the shift to community settings for clients with complex

health needs, discharge planning and case management have become an especially important nursing role in the community (Stanhope & Lancaster, 2015). Often clients requiring community-based care, especially home care, have complex medical needs that require an interdisciplinary team to meet their physical, psychosocial, medical, nursing, developmental, and education needs. The nurse plays an important role in initiating and maintaining the link between team members and the client to ensure that the client and family are receiving comprehensive, coordinated care. (See Chapter 33 for more information on discharge planning and case management for the pediatric population.)

Client Advocate and Resource Manager

Client advocate is another important role of the maternity and pediatric nurse to ensure that the client's and family's needs are being met. Advocacy also helps ensure that the client and family have available resources and appropriate health care services. For example, the pregnant client on bed rest at home may need help in caring for any older children, maintaining the household, or getting to health care appointments. Children with complex medical needs may require financial assistance through Medicaid or Medicaid waivers (state-run programs that use federal and state money to pay for the health care of individuals with certain medical conditions). They may also need assistance in obtaining needed equipment, additional services, and transportation. Nurses require a basic understanding of community, provincial, and federal resources to collaborate with the appropriate interprofessional colleagues in ensuring that clients and their families have access to those necessary for them. (See Chapter 33 for more information on advocacy and resource management in the pediatric population.)

Preventative Care

The concept of prevention is a key part of maternal and pediatric nursing. The emphasis on health care delivery has moved beyond primary preventive health care (e.g., well-child checkups, routine physical examinations, prenatal care, and treatment of common acute illnesses) and now encompasses secondary and tertiary care.

Primary Prevention

It is the responsibility of all nurses to incorporate health promotion and disease prevention activities into their professional roles. The concept of primary prevention involves preventing the disease or condition before it occurs through health promotion activities, environmental protection, and specific protection against disease or injury. Its focus is on health promotion to reduce the person's vulnerability to any illness by strengthening the person's capacity to withstand physical, emotional, and environmental stressors (Clark, 2014). It encompasses a vast array of areas, including nutrition, good hygiene, sanitation, immunizations, protection from ultraviolet rays, genetic counselling, bicycle helmets, handrails on bathtubs, drug education for school children, adequate shelter, smoking cessation, family planning, and the use of seat belts (Stanhope & Lancaster, 2015). See Figure 2.3 for examples.

In Canada, for every 10,000 births, approximately 5 infants are born with a neural tube defect (NTD), a group of anomalies related to the central nervous system (Public Health Agency of Canada [PHAC], 2017). Prevention of NTDs, such as anencephaly and spina bifida, is an example of primary prevention. The use of folic acid supplementation daily for 3 months before and 3 months after conception reduces the risk of first occurrence of an NTD. In the late 1990s, the rates of NTDs dropped after the introduction of folic acid–fortified flour in North America (PHAC, 2013). Pregnant individuals who get enough folic acid have a 50% to 70% reduced risk of having a baby with such a defect (CDC, 2018). Anyone who is planning to become pregnant should be advised to take 0.4-mg folic acid daily, and ti continue taking it throughout the pregnancy to prevent this devastating condition. Giving anticipatory guidance to parents about poison prevention and safety during play is another example of primary prevention.

Secondary Prevention

Secondary prevention is the early detection and treatment of adverse health conditions. This level of prevention is aimed at halting the disease, thus shortening its duration and severity to get the person back to a normal state of functioning. Health screenings are the mainstay of secondary prevention. Pregnancy testing, blood pressure evaluations, cholesterol monitoring, fecal occult blood testing, breast examinations, mammography screening, hearing and vision examinations, and Papanicolaou (Pap) smears are examples of this level of prevention. Such interventions do not prevent the health problem but are intended for early detection and prompt treatment to prevent complications (Smith, 2015a). If the health condition cannot be cured and further complications and disability moves in, then the tertiary level of prevention is needed.

Tertiary Prevention

Tertiary prevention is designed to reduce or limit the progression of a permanent, irreversible disease or disability. The purpose of tertiary prevention is to restore individuals to their maximum potential (Klemp, 2015). Tertiary

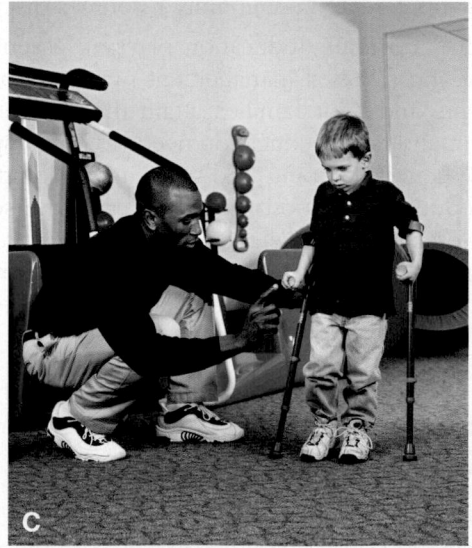

FIGURE 2.3 Levels of prevention. **A.** At the primary prevention level, the nurse provides anticipatory guidance and family teaching. **B.** At the secondary level of prevention, a woman undergoes a mammography screening for early detection of breast problems. **C.** At the tertiary level of prevention, a child with a developmental disability participates in a rehabilitation program.

intervention takes place only if the condition results in a permanent disability. Tertiary prevention measures are supportive and restorative. For example, tertiary prevention efforts would focus on minimizing and managing the effects of a chronic illness such as cerebrovascular disease or the chronic effects of sexually transmitted infections (e.g., herpes, human immunodeficiency virus [HIV], and untreated syphilis). Another example would involve working with women who have suffered long-term consequences of violence. Client education is the cornerstone of all disease management programs. The focus of the nurse would be to maximize the client's strengths through education, to help recover from the trauma and loss, and to build support systems.

The Nurse's Role in Preventive Care

All health professionals have a special role in health promotion, health protection, and disease prevention. Much of nursing involves prevention, early identification, and prompt treatment of health problems and monitoring for emerging threats that might lead to health problems. Nurses provide health care for parents and children at all three levels of prevention. This care often involves advocacy for services to meet their needs.

Culturally Competent Nursing Care

Canada is comprised of an ever-growing mix of cultural groups. This **population** is made up of numerous diverse cultural backgrounds arriving from every corner of the world into our country daily. In 2016, Canada welcomed over 296,000 new permanent residents, and maintains an ongoing target of 300,000 newcomers annually. A significant portion of these new Canadians were refugees, largely from Syria. That year saw the highest number of immigrant families reunited as well, following through with the Government of Canada's commitment to reunite more families, faster (Government of Canada, 2017).

This growing diversity has significant implications for the health care system. For years, nurses have endeavoured to provide optimal health care that meets the needs of women, children, and their families from varied cultures and ethnic groups. In addition to displaying competence in technical skills, nurses must also become competent in caring for clients from varied ethnic and racial backgrounds. Adapting to different cultural beliefs and practices requires flexibility and acceptance of others' viewpoints. Nurses must listen to clients and learn about their beliefs about health and wellness. To provide culturally appropriate care to diverse populations, nurses need to know, understand, and respect culturally influenced health behaviours. Chapter 1 provides a more detailed discussion of culture and its impact on the health of individuals and families.

Nurses must research and understand the cultural characteristics, values, and beliefs of the various people to whom they deliver care so that false assumptions and stereotyping do not lead to insensitive care. Time orientation, personal space, family orientation (patriarchal, matriarchal, or egalitarian), and language are important cultural concepts. Although the location might be different in community-based care, these principles apply to both inpatient and outpatient settings.

Nurses should possess an understanding of the perspectives, traditions, values, practices, and family systems of culturally diverse individuals, families, communities, and populations for whom they provide care, as well as knowledge of the complex variables that affect the achievement of health and well-being (USDHHS Office of Minority Health, n.d.). **Cultural competence** is a dynamic process during which nurses obtain and then apply cultural information. Nurses must look at clients through their own eyes and the eyes of clients and family members. Nurses must develop nonjudgmental acceptance of cultural differences in clients, using diversity as a strength that empowers them to achieve mutually acceptable health care goals. Nurses must integrate their client's cultural beliefs and practices into health prescriptions to eliminate or mitigate health disparities and provide client satisfaction. While the term "competence" might suggest an ultimate level of achievement of ability in cultural sensitivity, cultural competence is a dynamic, lifelong learning process. Understanding the process for assessing cultural patterns and factors that influence individual and group differences is critical in preventing overgeneralization and stereotyping (Harkess & Kaddoura, 2016). This cultural awareness allows nurses to see the entire picture and improves the quality of care and health outcomes (Box 2.4). Cultural competence does not appear suddenly; it must be developed through a series of steps, and cultivated throughout a nurse's career.

Barriers to Cultural Competence

Illness is culturally shaped in the sense that how we perceive, experience, and cope with disease is based upon our explanations of sickness. Awareness of how this might be of influence—instead of mere knowledge about the cultural practices or beliefs of specific ethnic groups—and an appreciation of this factor helps nurses deal effectively with cultural issues (RNAO, 2016). When a health care provider lacks knowledge of a client's cultural practices and beliefs or when the provider's beliefs differ from those of the client, the provider may be unprepared to respond when the client makes unexpected health care decisions. System-related barriers can occur if agencies that have not been designed for cultural diversity want all clients to conform to the established rules and regulations and attempt to fit everyone into the same mould.

BOX 2.4

STEPS TO DEVELOPING CULTURAL COMPETENCE

1. Cultural self-awareness
   - Become aware of, appreciate, and become sensitive to the values, beliefs, customs, and behaviours that have shaped one's own culture.
   - Engage in self-exploration beyond one's own culture and "see" clients from different cultures.
   - Health care has a multicultural environment.
   - Cultural diversity is awareness of the presence of differences among clients.
   - Examine personal biases and prejudices toward other cultures.
   - Become aware of differences in personal and clients' backgrounds.
2. Cultural knowledge
   - Obtain knowledge about various worldviews of different cultures, such as through reading about different cultures, attending continuing education courses on different cultures, accessing websites, and attending cultural diversity conferences.
   - Become familiar with culturally/ethnically diverse groups, worldviews, beliefs, practices, lifestyles, and problem-solving strategies.
3. Cultural skills
   - Learn how to perform a competent cultural assessment.
   - Assess each client's unique cultural values, beliefs, and practices without depending solely on written facts about specific cultural groups.
   - Embracing ethics empowers mutual respect, equality, and trust.
4. Cultural encounter
5. Engage in cross-cultural interactions with people from culturally diverse backgrounds, such as attending religious services or ceremonies and participating in important family events.
6. Participate in as many cultural encounters as possible to avoid cultural stereotyping.

Adapted from Harkess, L., & Kaddoura, M. (2015). Culture and cultural competence in nursing education and practice: The state of the art. *Nursing Forum, 51*(3), 211–222. doi: 10.1111/nuf.12140; and Darnell, L. K., & Hickson, S. V. (2015). Cultural competent patient-centered nursing care. *The Nursing Clinics of North America, 50*(1), 99–108.

Consider This

*O*ur medical mission took a team of nurse practitioners into the rural mountains of Guatemala to offer medical services to people who had never had any. One day, a distraught mother brought her 10-year-old daughter to the mission clinic, asking me if there was anything I could do about her daughter's right wrist. She had sustained a fracture a year ago and it had not healed properly. As I looked at the girl's malformed wrist, I asked if it had been splinted to help with alignment, knowing what the answer was going to be. The interpreter enlightened me by saying that this young girl would never marry and have children because of this injury. I appeared puzzled at the interpreter's prediction of this girl's future. It was later explained to me that if the girl couldn't make tortes from corn meal for her husband because of her wrist disability, she would not be worthy of becoming someone's wife and thus would probably live with her parents the rest of her life.

I reminded myself during the week of the medical mission not to impose my cultural values on the women for whom I was caring and to accept their cultural mores without judgment. These silent self-reminders served me well throughout the week, for I was open to learning about their lifestyles and customs.

Thoughts: *What must the young girl be feeling at the age of 10, being rejected for a disability that wasn't her fault? What might have happened if I had imposed my value system on this client? How effective would I have been in helping her if she didn't feel accepted? This incident ripped my heart out, for this young girl will be deprived of a fulfilling family life based on a wrist disability. This is just another example of female suppression that happens all over the world—such a tragedy—and yet a part of their culture, on which nurses should not pass judgment.*

Cultural competence does not mean replacing one's own cultural identity with another, ignoring the variability within cultural groups, or even appreciating the cultures being served. Instead, nurses skilled at cultural competence show a respect for difference, an eagerness to learn, and a willingness to accept multiple views of the world. Much of the process of developing cultural competence involves a reexamination of our values and the influence of these values on our beliefs, which affect our attitudes and actions. At the core of both client centredness and cultural competence is the importance of seeing the client as a unique person (Dauvrin & Lorant,

2015). It is important for all nurses to incorporate the client's traditional healing and health practices with conventional medicine by asking questions such as: Do you have treatment preferences you would like me to include in your care plan? Some clients may prefer certain foods or drinks when they are ill. In addition, during fasting and religious seasons, diets may be different and need to be considered during the process of determining the appropriate course of treatment. Some may have a different idea of what caused the illness. Spirituality, culture, and experience may have a significant role in the client's understanding and treatment of the illness.

Complementary and Alternative Medicine

Health Canada established the Natural and Non-prescription Health Products Directorate (NNHPD) which oversees all natural health products in Canada, including quality control testing and overseeing that manufacturing of these products meets the federal Natural Health Product Regulations (Health Canada, 2015). The PHAC reports that over 70% of Canadian regularly use CAM to help maintain their health and wellness (PHAC, 2008). *Complementary* medicine is used together with conventional medicine, such as using aromatherapy to reduce discomfort after surgery or to reduce pain during a procedure or during early labour. *Alternative* medicine is used in place of conventional medicine, such as eating a special natural diet to control nausea and vomiting or to treat cancer instead of undergoing surgery, chemotherapy, or radiation that has been recommended by a conventional doctor. *Integrative* medicine combines mainstream medical therapies and CAM therapies for which there is some scientific evidence of safety and effectiveness (National Center for Complementary and Integrative Health [NCCIH], 2018). These include acupuncture, reflexology, therapeutic touch, meditation, yoga, herbal therapies, nutritional supplements, homeopathy, naturopathic medicine, and many more used for the promotion of health and well-being (Holden, Gardiner, Birdee, Davis, & Yeh, 2015).

The philosophy of integrative medicine focuses on treating the whole person, not just the disease. The goal is to treat the mind, body, and spirit all at the same time. History has taught us that in science, application of the results is never determined by a single study, but by the weight of the evidence. It is right that medicine rests upon a foundation that begins with good clinical observations, case reports, and careful interpretations. Replication across scientists, which is the true hallmark of valid science, establishes whether those clinical observations are important and perhaps applicable. While some of the therapies used are nonconventional, a guiding principle within integrative medicine is to use therapies that have some high-quality evidence to support them (George, 2015). Integrative medicine combines conventional Western medicine with complementary treatments—all in the effort to treat the whole person. The nurse should avoid judgment and encourage the family to research all approaches that are evidence based that support healthy outcomes. Table 2.2 describes selected CAM therapies and treatments.

The theoretic underpinnings of complementary and alternative health practices propose that health and illness are complex interactions of the mind, body, and spirit. It is then surmised that many aspects of clients' health experiences are not subject to traditional scientific methods. This field does not lend itself readily to scientific study or to investigation and therefore is not easily

TABLE 2.2	SELECTED COMPLEMENTARY AND ALTERNATIVE THERAPIES
Therapy	**Description**
Aromatherapy	Use of essential oils to stimulate the sense of smell for balancing mind, body, and spirit
Homeopathy	Based on the theory of "like treats like"; helps restore the body's natural balance
Acupressure	Restoration of balance by pressing an appropriate point so self-healing capacities can take over
Feng shui (pronounced *fung shway*)	The Chinese art of placement. Objects are positioned in the environment to induce harmony with chi
Guided imagery	Use of consciously chosen positive and healing images along with deep relaxation to reduce stress and to help people cope
Reflexology	Use of deep massage on identified points of the foot or hand to scan and rebalance body parts that correspond with each point
Therapeutic touch	Balancing of energy by centring, invoking an intention to heal, and moving the hands from the head to the feet several inches from the skin
Herbal medicine	The therapeutic use of plants for healing and treating diseases and conditions
Spiritual healing	Praying, chanting, presence, laying on of hands, rituals, and meditation to assist in healing
Chiropractic therapy	Aimed at removing irritants to the nervous system to restore proper function—spinal manipulation done for musculoskeletal complaints
Massage therapy	Therapeutic stroking or kneading of the body to decrease pain, produce relaxation, and/or to improve circulation to that body part

Adapted from Hall, H. G., Griffiths, D., & McKenna, L. G. (2015). Complementary and alternative medicine: Interaction and communication between midwives and women. *Women and Birth, 28*(2), 137–142; National Center for Complementary and Integrative Health (NCCIH). (2018). *Complementary, alternative, or integrative health: What's in a name?* Retrieved from https://nccih.nih.gov/health/integrative-health.

embraced by many hard-core scientists (Ernst, 2015). Much of what is considered to be alternative medicine comes from the Eastern world, Indigenous traditions, folk medicine, and religious and spiritual practices. There is no unifying basic theory for the numerous treatments or modalities, except (as noted previously) that health and illness are considered to be complex interactions among the body, mind, and spirit.

Because of heightened interest in complementary treatments and their widening use, anecdotal efficacy, and growing supporting research evidence, nurses need to be sensitive to and knowledgeable enough to answer many of the questions clients ask and to guide them in a safe, objective way (Ernst, 2015). Nurses have a unique opportunity to provide services that facilitate wholeness. They need to understand all aspects of CAM, including costs, client knowledge, and drug interactions, if they are to promote holistic strategies for clients and families. With all of the enthusiasm in favour of CAM therapies, nurses must not forget their obligation to embrace the principles of EBP and critical evaluation before being misled into therapies that have no scientific basis to justify their use.

The growing use of complementary and alternative therapies during pregnancy and childbirth could be interpreted as a response to a need for autonomy and active participation in clients' health care during this time. Studies show that massage, acupuncture, vitamins, and herbs are the most frequently applied methods during pregnancy. In a recent study, only half of the pregnant women revealed their use of CAM to their health care provider during their prenatal visits (Holden et al., 2015).

Many clients who use complementary or alternative therapies do not reveal this fact to their health care provider. Therefore, one of the nurse's most important roles during the assessment phase of the nursing process is to encourage clients to communicate their use of these therapies to eliminate the possibility of harmful interactions and contraindications with current medical therapies. When assessing clients, ask specific questions about any nonprescription medications they may be taking, including vitamins, minerals, or herbs. Clients should also be asked about any therapies they are taking that have not been ordered by their primary care provider.

When caring for clients and their families who practice CAM, nurses need to:
- Be culturally sensitive to nontraditional treatments
- Acknowledge and respect different beliefs, attitudes, and lifestyles
- Keep an open mind, remembering that standard medical treatments do not work for all clients
- Accept CAM and integrate it if it brings comfort without harm
- Provide accurate information, not unsubstantiated opinions

- Advise clients how they can best monitor their condition using CAM
- Discourage practices only if they are harmful to the client's health
- Instruct the client to weigh the risks and benefits of CAM use
- Avoid confrontation when asking clients about CAM
- Be reflective, nonjudgmental, and open minded about CAM

The use of complementary therapies is widespread, especially by those desiring to alleviate the nausea and vomiting of early pregnancy. Ginger powder or tea, Sea-Bands (acupressure), hypnosis, and vitamin B_6 are typically used to treat morning sickness (Tyler & Nagtalon-Ramos, 2015). Although these may not cause any ill effects during the pregnancy, most substances ingested cross the placenta and have the potential to reach the fetus; so nurses should stress to all pregnant clients that it is better to be cautious when using CAM.

Individuals at risk for osteoporosis are seeking alternatives to menopausal hormone therapy since the Women's Health Initiative (WHI) study raised doubts about the benefit of estrogen. Some of the alternative therapies for osteoporosis include soy isoflavones, progesterone cream, magnet therapy, tai chi, and hip protectors (NCCIH, 2017). In addition, menopausal clients may seek CAM therapies for hot flashes. Once again, despite many claims, most of these therapies have not undergone scientific testing and thus could place the person at risk.

If clients are considering the use of or using CAM therapies, suggest they check with their health care provider before taking any "natural" substance. Offer clients the following instructions:
- Do not take for granted that because a substance is a natural herb or plant product, it is beneficial or harmless.
- Seek medical care when ill.
- Always inform the provider if you are taking herbs or other therapies.
- Be sure that any product package contains a list of all ingredients and amounts of each.
- Be aware that frequent or continual use of large doses of a CAM preparation is not advisable, and harm may result if therapies are mixed (e.g., vitamin E, garlic, and aspirin all have anticoagulant properties).
- Research CAM through resources such as books, websites, and articles (Chang & Chang, 2015).

All nurses, especially nurses working in the community, must educate themselves about the pros and cons of CAM and be prepared to discuss and help their clients make sense of it all. Expanding our consciousness by understanding and respecting diverse cultures and CAM will enable nurses to provide the best treatment for clients and their families receiving community-based care.

COMMUNITY-BASED CARE

Community may be defined as a specific group of people, often living in a defined geographical area, who share common interests, who interact with each other, and who function collectively within a defined social structure to address common concerns (Stanhope & Lancaster, 2015). The common features of a community may be common rights and privileges as members of a certain city or common ties of identity, values, norms, culture, language, or social support. Women are often caregivers to children, parents, spouses, and neighbours and provide important social support in these roles. The child's community consists of the family, school, neighbourhood, youth organizations, and other peer groups.

A person can be a part of many communities throughout their daily life. Examples might include area of residence (home, apartment, shelter), gender, place of employment (organization or home), language spoken (Spanish, Chinese, English), educational background or student status, culture (Indigenous, African Canadian, Syrian), career (nurse, businessperson, homemaker), place of worship (church or synagogue), and community memberships (garden club, YMCA, support group, school PTA, youth organizations, athletic teams).

A population is a group of people who share personal or environmental characteristics. Typically the most common characteristic is geographic location. Populations are made up of human beings within complex social and physical environments. The betterment of human populations remains the goal of community-based nursing care.

In community-based care, the community is the unit of service. The providers of care are concerned not only with the clients who present for service but also with the larger population of potential or at-risk clients.

Community Health Nursing

Community health nursing focuses on preventing illness and improving the health of populations and communities. Population is defined as a group of people who may or may not interact with each other within a defined geographic location (McMurray & Clendon, 2015). Community health nurses work in geographically and culturally diverse settings. They address current and potential health needs of the population or community. They promote and preserve the health of a population and are not limited to particular age groups or diagnoses. Public health nursing is a specialized area of community health nursing.

Epidemiology, the study of the causes, distribution, and control of disease in populations, can help determine the health and health needs of a population and assist in planning health services. Community health nurses perform epidemiologic investigations to help analyze and develop health policy and community health

initiatives. Community health initiatives can be focused on the community as a whole or a specific target population with specific needs. Health Canada's First Nations and Inuit Health strategies provide examples of national health initiatives aimed at improving specific aspects of health among Indigenous people, families, and communities in Canada. One of these programs is the Children's Oral Health Initiative, aimed to reduce the disparity of oral health among Indigenous children in this country. The strategy involves health promotion education targeted at three specific groups: pregnant individuals, preschool age children (ages 0 to 4 years), and school-age children (ages 5 to 7 years) (Health Canada, 2016).

The focus of health care initiatives today is on people and their needs, strengthening their abilities to shape their own lives. The emphasis has shifted away from dependence on health professionals toward personal involvement and personal responsibility, and this gives nurses the opportunity to interact with individuals in a variety of self-help roles. Nurses in the community can be the primary force in identifying the challenges and implementing changes in women's and children's health for the future.

Community-Based Nursing

In the past, the only community-based roles for nurses were community health nurses or public health nurses. This is now a subset of what is considered community-based nursing. The health needs of the society and consumer demand brought about community-based and community-focused services. The movement from an illness-oriented "cure" perspective in hospitals to a focus on health promotion and PHC in community-based settings has dramatically changed employment opportunities for today's nurses.

This shift in emphasis to PHC and outpatient treatment and management will likely continue. As a result, employment growth in a variety of community-based settings can be expected for properly educated nurses.

With the worldwide strategic shift of health care delivery from secondary to primary care settings, more newly qualified nurses are working in primary care, making exposure to the variety of roles available to nurses essential for future workforce development. The idea of nurses being change agents and thriving amid change may seem overwhelming, but all nurses need to be open to change. The time is now for nurses to be lifelong learners prepared for change in any health care setting (Orr & Davenport, 2015).

The Canadian Nurses Association (2019) reports the following statistics related to employment of registered nurses (RNs) in Canada:
- 63% of RNs work in the hospital setting.
- 16% work outside the hospital in a community health agency.
- 9% work in long-term care facilities or nursing homes.

Shift in Responsibilities From Hospital- to Community-Based Nursing

Many nurses find the shift from acute care nursing to a community setting challenging. Community care, especially home care, is a rapidly growing service in Canada. Nurses play an important role in the treatment and care of clients in the community and need to collaborate with acute care nurses to integrate appropriate community interventions along the continuum of care (Lemetti, Stolt, Rickard, & Suhonen, 2015). Community-based care has been shown to be a cost-effective method for providing care. An increase in disposable income and the increased longevity of people with chronic and debilitating health conditions have also contributed to the continued shift of health care to the community and home setting. Technology has advanced, allowing for improved monitoring of clients in community settings and at home as well as allowing complicated procedures to be done at home, such as intravenous administration of antibiotics, telehealth surveillance, and renal dialysis (Farrar, 2015).

Caring for children at home not only improves their physical health but also allows for adequate growth and development within their family. They are in a familiar environment with the comfort and support of family, which leads to improved care and quality of life.

Community-based nursing settings include ambulatory care, home health care, occupational health, school health, and hospice settings (Table 2.3). Clinical practice within the community may also include case management, research, quality improvement, and discharge planning. Nurses with advanced practice and experience may be employed in areas of staff development, program development, and community education.

Community-Based Nursing Interventions

Nursing interventions involve any treatment that the nurse performs to enhance the client's outcome. Nursing practice in the community uses the nursing process and is similar to that in the acute care setting, because assessing, performing procedures, administering medications, coordinating services and equipment, counselling clients and their families, and teaching about care are all part of the care administered by nurses in the community (Evidence-Based Practice 2.1). Box 2.5 highlights the most common nursing interventions used in community-based nursing practice.

Community-Based Nursing Challenges

Despite the benefits achieved by caring for families in their own homes and communities, challenges also exist.

TABLE 2.3	COMMUNITY-BASED PRACTICE SETTINGS	
Setting	**Description**
Ambulatory care	Doctors' and nurse practitioners' office settings Day surgery centres Family planning clinics Mobile mammography centres
Home health care services	High-risk pregnancy/neonate care Maternal/child newborn care Skilled nursing care Hospice care
Health Department services	Maternal/child health clinics Family planning clinics Sexually transmitted infection programs Immunization clinics Substance abuse programs Jails and prisons
Long-term care	Skilled nursing facilities Nursing homes Hospices Assisted living
Other community-based settings	Parish nursing programs Summer camps Childbirth education programs School health programs Occupational health programs

---

EVIDENCE-BASED PRACTICE 2.1

COMMUNITY-BASED INTERVENTION PACKAGES FOR REDUCING MATERNAL–NEONATAL MORBIDITY AND MORTALITY AND IMPROVING NEONATAL OUTCOMES

Maternal, infant, and under-five child mortality rates have declined significantly in the past decades, but newborn mortality rates have reduced more slowly. About half of all newborn deaths are preventable by using evidence-based interventions such as tetanus toxoid immunizations to mothers, clean and skilled care at birth, newborn resuscitation, exclusive breastfeeding, clean umbilical cord care, and management of newborn infections. A large portion of these maternal and newborn deaths and diseases can be addressed through community-based packaged interventions.

STUDY

The purpose of this study was to assess the effectiveness of community-based intervention packages in reducing maternal and neonatal morbidity and mortality to improve neonatal outcomes. The authors found 26 randomized and quasi-randomized controlled studies evaluating the impact of community-based intervention packages for the prevention of maternal illnesses and death and in improving newborn health outcomes.

Findings

A statistically significant reduction was observed in maternal morbidity, neonatal mortality, and perinatal mortality as a consequence of implemented community-based interventional care packages. It is found that the value of integrating maternal and newborn care in community settings through a range of interventions impacts the health of this vulnerable population positively.

Nursing Implications

This review highlights the importance of integrating maternal and newborn care in community settings through a range of interventions which can be delivered by community health nurses and health promotion groups. There is sufficient evidence to scale up community-based care. As this study pointed out—maternal–child care can't stop upon discharge from the hospital, it must continue in community health care settings and homes to impact maternal–neonatal outcomes positively. Community health nurses can take a lead role in facilitating this care to improve maternal–child outcomes.

Adapted from Lassi, Z. S., & Bhutta, Z. A. (2015). Community-based intervention packages for reducing maternal and neonatal morbidity and mortality and improving neonatal outcomes. *Cochrane Database of Systematic Reviews*, (3), CD007754. doi: 10.1002/14651858.CD007754.pub3.

BOX 2.5

COMMUNITY-BASED NURSING INTERVENTIONS

- Health screening—detecting unrecognized or preclinical illness among individuals so they can be referred for definitive diagnosis and treatment (e.g., mammogram or Pap smear, well-child vision and hearing checks)
- Health education programs—assisting clients in making health-related decisions about self-care, use of health resources, and social health issues such as smoking bans and motorcycle helmet laws (e.g., childbirth education or breast self-examination, child safety programs, poisoning prevention, youth drug awareness programs)
- Medication administration—preparing, giving, and evaluating the effectiveness of prescription and over-the-counter drugs (e.g., hormone replacement therapy in menopausal clients, childhood immunizations)
- Telephone consultation—identifying the problem to be addressed; listening and providing support, information, or instruction; documenting advice/instructions given to concerns raised by caller (e.g., consultation for a mother with a newborn with colic, interaction with a parent whose child has a fever or is vomiting)

- Health system referral—passing along information about the location, services offered, and ways to contact agencies (e.g., referring a woman for a breast prosthesis after a mastectomy, arranging for home tutoring for a child with a long-term illness)
- Instructional—teaching an individual or a group about a medication, disease process, lifestyle changes, community resources, or research findings concerning their environment (e.g., childbirth education class, basic life support classes for parents, child safety education classes)
- Nutritional counselling—demonstrating the direct relationship between nutrition and illness while focusing on the need for diet modification to promote wellness (e.g., counsellor interviewing a pregnant client with anemia; eating disorders program)
- Risk identification—recognizing personal or group characteristics that predispose people to develop a specific health problem, and modifying or eliminating them (e.g., genetic counselling of an older pregnant clients at risk for an infant with Down syndrome; genetic screening of family members for cystic fibrosis or Huntington disease)

Adapted from Wright, L. M., & Leahey, M. (2013). *Nurses and families: A guide to family assessment and intervention* (6th ed.). Philadelphia, PA: F.A. Davis Company.

Clients are being discharged from acute care facilities very early in their recovery course and present with more health care needs than in the past. As a result, nursing care and procedures in the home and community are becoming more complex and time consuming. Consider the example of a woman who developed a systemic infection, a pelvic abscess, and deep vein thrombosis in her leg after a cesarean birth who is being discharged from the hospital. The nurse's primary focus of care in this situation would be to administer heparin and antibiotics intravenously rather than educating her about child care and follow-up appointments. In the past, this woman would have remained hospitalized for treatment, but home infusion therapy is now less costly and allows the client to be discharged sooner.

This demand on the nurse's time may limit the amount of time spent on prevention measures, education, and the family's psychosocial issues. More time may be needed to help families deal with these issues and concerns. With large client caseloads, nurses may find it difficult to spend the time needed while meeting the time restrictions dictated by their health care agencies. Nurses need to plan the tasks to be accomplished (Box 2.6).

Nurses working in the community have fewer resources available to them compared with the acute care setting. Decisions often have to be made in isolation. The nurse must possess excellent assessment skills and the ability to communicate effectively with the family to be successful in carrying out the appropriate plan of care.

Nurses interested in working in community-based settings must be able to apply the nursing process in an environment that is less structured or controlled

---

BOX 2.6

HOME CARE VISITATION PLANNING

- Review previous interventions to eliminate unsuccessful ones.
  - Check previous home visit narrative to validate interventions.
  - Communicate with previous nurse to ask questions and clarify.
  - Formulate plan of interventions based on data received (e.g., client preference of IV placement or order of fluids).
- Prioritize client needs based on their potential to threaten the client's health status.
  - Use Maslow hierarchy of needs to set forth a plan of care.
  - Address life-threatening physiologic issues first (e.g., an infectious process would take precedence over anorexia).
- Develop goals that reflect primary, secondary, and tertiary prevention levels.
  - *Primary prevention*—Have the client consume adequate fluid to prevent dehydration.
  - *Secondary prevention*—Administer drug therapy as prescribed to contain and treat an existing infectious process.
  - *Tertiary prevention*—Instruct the client who has experienced a stroke how to exercise to minimize disability.
- Bear in mind the client's readiness to accept intervention and education.
  - Ascertain the client's focus and how she sees her needs.
  - Address client issues that might interfere with intervention (e.g., if the client is in pain, attempting to teach her about her care will be lost; her pain must be addressed first before she is ready to learn).
- Consider the timing of the visit to prevent interfering with other client activities.
  - Schedule all visits at convenient times per client if possible (e.g., if the client has a favourite television show to watch, attempt to schedule around that event, if possible).
  - Reschedule a home visit if a client event comes up suddenly.
- Outline nursing activities to be completed during the scheduled visit.
  - Know the health care agency's policy and procedures for home visits.
  - Consider the time line and other visits scheduled that day.
  - Research evidence-based best practices to use in the home to validate your intervention decisions.
- Obtain necessary materials/supplies before making the visit.
  - Assemble all equipment needed for any procedure in advance.
  - Secure any equipment that might be needed if a problem occurs (e.g., bring additional IV tubing and a catheter to make sure the procedure can be carried out without delay).
- Determine criteria to be used to evaluate the effectiveness of the home visit.
  - Revisit outcome goals to determine the effectiveness of the intervention.
  - Assess the client's health status to validate improvement.
  - Monitor changes in the client's behaviour toward health promotion activities and disease prevention (e.g., verify/observe that the client demonstrates correct hand-washing technique after instruction and reinforcement during the home care visit).

Adapted from Stanhope, M., & Lancaster, J. (2015). *Public health nursing: Population-centered health care in the community* (9th ed.). St. Louis, MO: Mosby Elsevier; de la Rosa, I. A., Perry, J., & Johnson, V. (2015). Pathways to resilience: Enhancing family well-being with a home visitation model. *Journal of Youth Development, 10*(1), 35–58; and Aston, M., Price, S., Etowa, J., Vukic, A., Young, L., Hart, C., … Randel, P. (2015). The power of relationships: Exploring how public health nurses support mothers and families during postpartum home visits. *Journal of Family Nursing, 21*(1), 11–34.

than those associated with acute care facilities. Nurses must be able to assimilate information well beyond the immediate physical and psychosocial needs of the client in a controlled acute care setting and deal with environmental threats, lifestyle choices, family issues, different cultural patterns, financial burdens, transportation challenges, employment hazards, communication barriers, limited resources, and client acceptance and compliance.

Although opportunities for employment in community-based settings are plentiful, many positions require a baccalaureate degree. Previous medical-surgical experience in an acute care setting is typically required by home health agencies because these nurses must function fairly independently within the home environment.

The nurse must also be familiar with and respectful of many different cultures and socioeconomic levels, remaining objective in dealing with such diversity and demonstrating an understanding of and appreciation for cultural differences. Nurses are increasingly working with clients from diverse cultural backgrounds with different cultural values pertaining to their health. Interventions must be individualized to address the cultural, social, and economic diversity among clients in their own environment (Darawsheh & Chard, 2015).

Community-Based Nursing Care Settings for Women, Parents, and Children

Community-based nursing takes place in a variety of settings, including physicians' and nurse practitioners' offices, clinics, health departments, urgent care centres, hospital outpatient centres, schools, camps, churches, shelters, and clients' homes. Nurses provide well care, episodic ill care, and chronic care. They work to promote, preserve, and improve the health of the women, parents, children, and families in these settings.

Due to technologic advances, cost containment, and shortened hospital stays, the home is a common care setting for families today. Home care is geared toward the needs of the client and family. Private duty nursing care is used when more extensive care is needed; it may be delivered hourly (several hours per day) or on a full-time, live-in basis. Periodic nursing visits may be used for intermittent interventions, such as IV antibiotic administration, follow-up with client teaching, and monitoring. The goals of nursing care in the home setting include promoting, restoring, and maintaining the health of the client.

Home care focuses on minimizing the effects of the illness or disability along with providing the client with the means to care for the illness or disability at home. Nurses in the home care setting are direct care providers, educators, advocates, and case managers.

Prenatal Care

Early, adequate prenatal care has long been associated with improved pregnancy outcomes (March of Dimes, 2015). Adequate prenatal care is a comprehensive process in which any problems associated with pregnancy are identified and treated. Basic components of prenatal care are early and continuing risk assessment, health promotion, medical and psychosocial interventions, and follow-up. Within the community setting, several services are available to provide health care for pregnant individuals (Box 2.7).

Not all clients are aware of the community resources available to them. Most public health services are available for consultation, local hospitals have "hotlines" for questions, and public libraries have pregnancy-related resources as well as Internet access. Nurses can be a very helpful link to resources for all clients regardless of their economic status.

Technologically advanced care has been shown to improve maternal and child outcomes. The advanced technology found in perinatal regional centres and community-based prenatal surveillance programs have resulted in better risk-adjusted mortality rates. Regionalized systems of perinatal care are recommended to ensure that each mother and newborn achieve optimal outcomes.

BOX 2.7

MATERNAL–CHILD COMMUNITY HEALTH CARE SERVICES

- Many hospitals provide outpatient maternal–child health services, in the form of Breastfeeding Clinics or Mother-Baby Clinics. Many of these offer prenatal education classes.
- Some family physicians provide prenatal care throughout the duration of pregnancy; those who do not will refer to an OB/GYN or midwife.
- Freestanding birth centres offer prenatal care for low-risk mothers as well as childbirth classes to educate couples regarding the birthing process.
- Midwifery services are available across Canada, with the exception of Newfoundland, PEI, and the Yukon. Midwives provide care during pregnancy, birth, and for 6 weeks postpartum.
- Childbirth classes offer pregnant individuals and their partners a series of educational classes on childbirth preparation. Generally these take place in the last trimester of pregnancy. Some classes are free and some have a fee.
- Local La Leche League groups provide mother-to-mother support for breastfeeding, nutrition, and infant care problem-solving strategies. All parents who have an interest in breastfeeding are welcome to participate in the meetings, which are typically held in the home of a La Leche member.

Adapted from Canadian Association of Midwives. (2017). *What is a midwife?* Retrieved from https://canadianmidwives.org/what-midwife/; La Leche League Canada. (2019). *Who we are.* Retrieved from https://www.lllc.ca/

Labour and Birth Care

Pregnancy involves numerous choices: cloth or disposable diapers, breastfeeding or bottle feeding, doctor or midwife, and where to give birth—at a birthing centre, at home, or at a hospital. Deciding where to give birth depends on the client's pregnancy risk status. For the pregnant client who is at high risk as a result of medical or social factors, the hospital is considered the safest place for birth. Potential complications can be addressed because medical technology, skilled professionals, and neonatal services are available. For low-risk clients, a freestanding birthing centre or a home birth is an option.

The choice between a birthing centre, home birth, or hospital depends on the client's preferences, risk status, and distance from a hospital. Some clients choose an all-natural birth with no medications and no medical intervention, whereas others would feel more comfortable in a setting in which medications and trained staff are available if needed. Presenting the facts to clients and allowing them to choose in collaboration with their health care provider is the nurse's role. Client safety is paramount, but at the same time nurses must protect the individual's right to select birth options and should promote family-centred care in all maternity settings.

BIRTHING CENTRE

A birthing centre is a cross between a home birth and a hospital. Birthing centres offer a home-like setting but with close proximity to a hospital in case of complications. Midwives often are the sole care providers typically in freestanding birthing centres, with obstetricians as backups in case of emergencies. Birthing centres usually have fewer restrictions and guidelines for families to follow and allow for more freedom in making decisions about labour. The rates of cesarean birth and the costs are much lower than those of a hospital (Childbirth Connection, 2019). Midwife-led comprehensive care in a birthing centre using the same medical guidelines as in standard care in hospitals reduced medical interventions without jeopardizing maternal and infant health. Birthing centres are recognized as a natural alternative to a hospital, as well as a place of female empowerment and control. The normal discharge time after birth is usually measured in hours (4 to 24 hours), not days.

Birthing centres aim to provide a relaxing home environment and promote a culture of normalcy. Currently, we are seeing a rise in the number of birth centres being established, which is essential in the promotion of normality. It is in these birth centres that midwives will learn about normalcy, building the skills needed to support clients through labour, rather than managing labour. Birth is a normal physiologic process, and most centres use a noninterventional view of labour and birth. The range of services for the expectant family often includes prenatal care, childbirth education, intrapartum care, and postpartum care, including home follow-up and family planning (Fig. 2.4). One of the hallmarks of the freestanding birthing centre is that it can provide truly family-centred care by approaching pregnancy and birth as a normal family event and encouraging all family members to participate. Education is often provided by such centres, encouraging families to become informed and self-reliant in the care of themselves and their families (Steinberg & Sackmary, 2015).

Birthing centres provide an alternative for those who are uncomfortable with a home birth but who do not want to give birth in a hospital. Advantages of birthing centres include a noninterventional approach to obstetric care, freedom to eat and move around during labour, ability to give birth in any position, and the right to have any number of family and friends attend the birth. Disadvantages are that some centres have rigid screening criteria, which may eliminate healthy mothers from using birth centres; many have rigid rules concerning transporting the mother to the hospital (e.g., prolonged labour, ruptured membranes); and many have no pediatrician on staff if the newborn has special needs after birth (Childbirth Connection, 2019).

HOME BIRTH

For centuries parents have been giving birth to babies in their home. Many feel more comfortable and relaxed when giving birth in their own environment. Individuals who want no medical interventions and a very family-centred birth often choose to have a home birth. Home births are recommended for those who are considered to be at low risk for complications during labour and birth (Zielinski, Ackerson, & Low, 2015). Home birth is advantageous because it:

- Is the least expensive
- Allows the client to experience labour and birth in the privacy, comfort, and familiarity of home while surrounded by loved ones
- Permits the pregnant individual to maintain control over every aspect affecting her labour (e.g., positions, attire, support people)
- Minimizes interference and unnecessary interventions, allowing labour to progress normally
- Provides continuous one-on-one care by the midwife throughout the childbirth process
- Promotes the development of a trusting relationship with the midwife (American Pregnancy Association, 2015)

A home birth has certain disadvantages, however, including the limited availability of pain medication and danger to the mother and baby if an emergency arises (e.g., placenta abruptio, uterine rupture, cord prolapse, or a distressed fetus). Delay in getting to the hospital could jeopardize the life of the child or the mother. A backup plan for a health care provider and nearby hospital on

FIGURE 2.4 Birthing centres aim to provide a relaxing home environment and promote a culture of normality while offering a full range of health care services to the expectant family. (Photos by Gus Freedman.)

standby must be established should an emergency occur. The available evidence suggests that planned home birth is safe for healthy, low risk pregnant clients, when cared for by appropriately qualified and licensed midwives with access to timely transfer to a hospital if required (Hutton et al., 2016; Zielinski et al., 2015).

Postpartum and Newborn Care

Recent reforms in health care financing have reduced hospital stays significantly for new mothers. As a result, community-based nurses play a major role in extending care beyond the hospital setting. When new mothers are discharged from the hospital, most are still experiencing perineal discomfort and uterine cramping. They may still have pain from an episiotomy. They are fatigued and may be constipated. They may feel uncertain about feeding and caring for their newborn. These new mothers need to be made aware of community resources such as telephone consultation by nurses, outpatient clinics, home visits, neighbourhood mothers' support groups, and online new parent forums.

TELEPHONE CONSULTATION

Many hospitals offer telephone consultation services by their maternity nurses. The discharged mother is given the phone number of the nursing unit on the day of discharge and is instructed to call if she has any questions or concerns. Because the nurses on the unit are familiar with her birth history and the newborn, they are in a good position to assist her in adjusting to her new role. Although this service is usually free, not all families recognize a problem early or use this valuable informational resource.

OUTPATIENT CLINICS

Outpatient clinics offer another community-based site where the childbearing family can obtain services. In some cases, the mother has received prenatal care before giving birth and thus has established some rapport with the nursing staff there. The clinic staff is usually willing to answer any questions she may have about her health or that of her newborn. Appointments usually include an examination of the mother and newborn and instructions about umbilical cord care, postpartum and infant care, and nutrition for both mother and infant.

POSTPARTUM HOME VISITS

Home visits offer services similar to those offered at a scheduled clinic visit, but they also give the nurse an opportunity to assess the family's adaptation and dynamics and the home environment. During the past decade, hospital stays have averaged 24 to 48 hours or less for vaginal births and 72 to 96 hours for cesarean births; in 2016 the average length of stay in hospital after birth (vaginally and by cesarean) was 2.3 days (CIHI, 2017). These shortened stays have reduced the time available for educating new parents about caring for themselves and their newborns. Home visiting programs in general seek to promote child health/development, prevent child abuse/neglect, improve maternal well-being, and improve the parental capacity of mothers. Provincially funded postpartum home visiting programs vary across the country. Many provinces have screening tools to determine eligibility for these free services (Government of New Brunswick [GNB], 2018).

Postpartum care in the home environment usually includes the following:

- Monitoring the physical and emotional well-being of the family members (Fig. 2.5)

FIGURE 2.5 The nurse makes a postpartum home visit to assess the woman and her newborn. During the visit, the nurse assists the mother with breastfeeding.

- Identifying potential or developing complications for the mother and newborn
- Breast care during breastfeeding and engorgement
- Instruction on pelvic floor exercises, nutrition, and self-hygiene care
- Linking the family, as needed, to community social services, housing, and governmental programs
- Bridging the gap between discharge and ambulatory follow-up for mothers and their newborns (King, Brucker, Kriebs, Fahey, Gegor, & Varney, 2015)

SUPPORT GROUPS FOR NEW MOTHERS

Typically, these groups are locally led by a facilitator with previous experience in motherhood, breastfeeding, and infant care. Usually they are composed of 6 to 12 mothers who share information on breastfeeding techniques, infant sleeping patterns, child care issues, body image issues, and how to integrate the new baby into the family unit. The support group usually meets weekly and provides an avenue of support for new mothers on the same journey.

ONLINE MOTHERHOOD FORUMS/BLOGS

Support groups in online communities provide an anonymous place to exchange information and advice. Previous research has suggested that these groups offer a safe, nonjudgmental forum for new mothers to share experiences and interact anonymously. They serve as a safe, supportive space in which new mothers can better understand their new role of parenting. They offer a viable form of education for new parents, but caution must be used on advice provided on some websites to new mothers (Makinen & Tuominen, 2015).

HIGH-RISK NEWBORN HOME CARE

With the reduced lengths of stay, high-risk newborns are also being cared for in community settings. High-technology care once was provided only in the hospital. Now, however, the increasing cost of complex care and the influences of managed care have led to the provision of such care at home. Families have become "health care systems" by providing physical, emotional, social, and developmental home care for their technology-dependent infants. Suitable candidates for home care may include preterm infants who continue to need oxygen, low–birth-weight infants needing nutritional or hypercaloric formulas or adjunct feeding methods (e.g., tube feedings), or infants with hydrocephalus or cerebral palsy. Home care with prepared caregivers might contribute to earlier detection of significant residual/recurrent problems amenable to therapy (Smith & Stewart, 2019). A wide range of equipment may be used, including mechanical ventilation, electronic apnea monitors, home oxygen equipment, intravenous infusions, respiratory nebulizers, phototherapy, and suction equipment.

All family members must work together to provide 24-hour care. The parents must negotiate with insurers for reimbursement for durable medical equipment not covered by provincial health care, must be able to troubleshoot equipment problems, and must be able to manage inventories of supplies and equipment. In addition, they must be able to assess the infant for problems; determine the problem; decide when to call the nurse, pharmacist, or physical therapist; and interpret and implement prescriptions. Technology in the home requires nurses to focus on the family "home care system" to provide total care to the infant.

Nurses can play a key role in assisting families by preparing them for and increasing their confidence in caring for their infants at home. This adaptation begins before discharge from the hospital. Family members are active participants in the transition-to-home plan. Recognition of parental needs and addressing each area in the discharge plan will ease the transition home.

Assessment of the family's preparedness is essential. The following areas should be explored:

• *Parenting education*—assess the family's knowledge of positioning and handling of their infant, nutrition, hygiene, elimination, growth and development, immunizations needed, and recognition of illnesses. Asking questions in a sensitive manner will assist the nurse in identifying knowledge deficiencies, so they can be reinforced in the nurse's teaching plan.

• *Postpartum care*—determine the mother's concerns in areas of body image, weight loss, sleep/rest needs, discomfort, fatigue, and adjustment to her new role. Asking open-ended questions concerning these areas will help the nurse extract more information to include in the teaching plan. Targeting the mother's areas of concern will help the nurse focus on needed education to facilitate the mother's transition into her new role as a parent.

• *Support systems*—assess physical and emotional support for the new mother by asking questions about the availability of her immediate family, other relatives, and significant others to help out. If lacking, referrals may need to be made to community parenting programs, cooperative daycare, or other community resources needed to assist this family. Exploring these vital areas through sensitive questioning hopefully will convey the nurse's concern for the infant and family while obtaining a thorough assessment of the family's learning needs.

Once preparedness has been assessed, the nurse can intervene as necessary. For example, if the caretakers do not think they are prepared to maintain machinery, technology, medication, or developmental therapy, then the nurse can demonstrate the care to the family. The nurse provides instructions and hands-on experience within a supportive environment until the family's confidence increases. The nurse can also assist the family to anticipate the common problems that might occur (e.g., advising them to avoid running out of supplies, to have enough medication or special formula mixture to last throughout the weekend, and to keep backup batteries for powering machines or portable oxygen). The outcome of

the preparedness assessment and intervention is that the safety of the infant is established and maintained.

Nursing for families who are using complex home care equipment requires caring for the infant and family members' physical and emotional well-being as well as providing effective solutions to problems they may encounter. Home health nurses need to identify, mobilize, and adapt a myriad of community resources to support the family in giving the best possible care in the home setting. Preparing families for high-tech care before hospital discharge, with home health nurses continuing and reinforcing that focus, will help ease the burden of managing high-tech equipment in the home.

Women's Health Care

A cis-gender woman's reproductive years span half her lifetime, on average. This is not a static period, but rather one that encompasses several significant stages. As reproductive goals change, so do a woman's health care needs. Because of these changing needs, comprehensive community-centred care is critical.

Community-based women's health services have received increased emphasis during the past few decades simply because of economics. Women use more health care services than men, they make as many as 90% of health care decisions, and they represent the majority of the population (CDC, 2017). In 2016, the most commonly performed surgery in Canada was cesarean section (CIHI, 2017). Examples of community-based women's health care services that can be freestanding or hospital based include the following:

• Screening centres that offer mammograms, Pap smears, bone density assessments, genetic counselling, ultrasound, breast examinations, complete health risk appraisals, laboratory studies (complete blood count, cholesterol testing, thyroid testing, glucose testing for diabetes, follicle-stimulating hormone [FSH] levels), and electrocardiograms

• Educational centres that provide women's health lectures, instruction on breast self-examinations and Pap smears, and computers for research

• Counselling centres that offer various support groups: genetics, psychotherapy, substance abuse, sexual assault, and domestic violence

• Wellness centres that offer stress reduction techniques, massage therapy, guided imagery, hypnosis, smoking cessation, weight reduction, tai chi, yoga, and fitness/exercise classes

• Alternative/wholeness healing centres that provide acupuncture, aromatherapy, biofeedback, therapeutic touch, facials, reflexology, and herbal remedies

• Retail centres that offer specialty equipment for rental and purchase, such as breast prostheses

Clients have multiple choices regarding services, settings, and health care providers. In the past most women received health care services from physicians such as obstetricians, gynecologists, and family physicians, but today midwives and nurse practitioners are becoming more prevalent in providing well-women care.

Nurses who work in community-based settings need to be familiar with the many health issues commonly encountered by the members of those communities. All nurses who work in community-based settings, including the workplace, schools, practitioner offices, and clinics, should possess a thorough understanding of the scope of primary health care and should be prepared to intervene appropriately to prevent problems and to promote health.

Child Health Care

The majority of care for a child occurs in the community setting. The numerous settings may be broad or highly specialized. For example, one setting may provide well-child care as well as illness-related care. Another setting may be limited to providing well-child care; a third setting may be limited to diagnostic evaluation, emergency care, or surgical intervention. Other settings may focus on caring for children with specific conditions or diagnosis, such as diabetes or cancer. See Chapter 33 for specific community-based child health care settings.

KEY CONCEPTS

- Core concepts of maternal and pediatric nursing include family-centred care, EBP, collaborative care, atraumatic therapeutic care, communication, education, discharge planning and case management, advocacy and resource management, preventative care, culturally competent care, and being knowledgeable about CAM.

- Family-centred care recognizes the concept of the family as the constant. The health and functioning ability of the family influences and impacts the health of the client and other members of the family. Family-centred care recognizes and respects family strengths and individuality, encourages referrals for family support, and facilitates collaboration. It ensures flexible, accessible, and responsive health care delivery while incorporating developmental needs and implementing policies to provide emotional and financial support to women, parents, children, and families.

- Open, honest lines of communication are essential for nurses. The use of an interpreter may be necessary to ensure effective communication with women, children, and their families in the community setting. Maintaining confidentiality and privacy are key.

- A family's knowledge related to the client's health or illness is vitally important. Nurses play a major role in educating women, parents, children, and their families. For children, teaching is provided based on the child's developmental level.

- Discharge planning provides a comprehensive plan for the safe discharge of a client from a health care facility and for continuing safe and effective care in the community. Case management focuses on coordinating health care services while balancing quality and cost outcomes. Both contribute to improved transition from the hospital to the community for women, children, their families, and the health care team.

- Advocacy and resource management help ensure that the client and family have the necessary resources and appropriate health care services available to them.

- Health care delivery has moved from acute care settings out into the community, with an emphasis on health promotion and illness prevention (Clark, 2011). Community health nursing focuses on prevention and improvement of the health of populations and communities, addressing current and potential health needs of the population or community, promoting and preserving the health of a population regardless of a particular age group or diagnosis. Community health nurses perform epidemiologic investigations to help analyze and develop health policy and community health initiatives.

- Community-based nurses focus on providing personal care to individuals and families in the community. They focus on promoting and preserving health as well as preventing disease or injury. They help women, children, and their families cope with illness and disease. Community-based nurses are direct care providers as well as advocates and educators. They focus on minimizing and removing barriers to allow the client to develop to his or her full potential.

- Settings for community-based nursing include physicians' and nurse practitioners' offices, clinics, health departments, urgent care centres, clients' homes, schools, camps, churches, and shelters such as abuse, homeless, and disaster shelters. Nurses provide both well, episodic ill care, and chronic care to women, parents, children, and their families.

○ There has been a rise in home health care due to shorter hospital stays and cost containment along with an increase in income and longevity of people with chronic and debilitating health conditions. Technology also has improved, which allows clients to be monitored and to undergo complicated procedures at home.

REFERENCES AND RECOMMENDED READINGS

American Pregnancy Association. (2015). *Home birth.* Retrieved from http://americanpregnancy.org/labor-and-birth/home-birth/

American Speech-Language-Hearing Association. (2019). *Collaborating with interpreters.* Retrieved from https://www.asha.org/PRPSpecificTopic.aspx?folderid=8589935334&section=Key_Issues

Arnold, E. C., & Boggs, K. U. (2016). *Interpersonal relationships: Professional communication skills for nurses.* St. Louis, MO: Elsevier Health Sciences.

Aston, M., Price, S., Etowa, J., Vukic, A., Young, L., Hart, C., … Randel, P. (2015). The power of relationships: Exploring how public health nurses support mothers and families during postpartum home visits. *Journal of Family Nursing, 21*(1), 11–34.

Ayers, B., Grassley, J., & Koprowski, K. (2015). Pilot study of breastfeeding support on the night shift. *Clinical Lactation, 6*(2), 53–59.

Brega, A. G., Barnard, J., Mabachi, N. M., Weiss, B. D., DeWalt, D. A., Brach, C., … West, D. R. (2015). *AHRQ health literacy universal precautions toolkit* (2nd ed.). AHRQ publication no. 15–0023-EF. Rockville, MD: Agency for Healthcare Research and Quality.

Bridges, E. J. (2015). Research at the bedside: It makes a difference. *American Journal of Critical Care, 24*(4), 283–289.

Canadian Charter of Rights and Freedoms, Part I of the Constitution Act, 1982, being Schedule B to the Canada Act 1982 (U.K.) 1982, c.11. Retrieved from http://laws-lois.justice.gc.ca/eng/Const/page-15.html

Canadian Hearing Society. (2013). *Facts and figures.* Retrieved from https://www.chs.ca/facts-and-figures

Canadian Institute for Health Information (CIHI). (2017). *Inpatient hospitalizations, surgeries, newborns and childbirth indicators, 2015–2016.* Retrieved from https://secure.cihi.ca/free_products/cad_hospitalization_and_childbirth_snapshot_2015-2016_en.pdf

Canadian Nurses Association (CNA). (2011). *Position statement: Interprofessional collaboration.* Retrieved from https://www.cna-aiic.ca/~/media/cna/page-content/pdf-en/interproffessional-collaboration_position-statement.pdf?la=en

Canadian Nurses Association (CNA). (2015). *Position statement: Primary health care.* Retrieved from https://www.cna-aiic.ca/~/media/cna/page-content/pdf-en/primary-health-care-position-statement.pdf?la=en

Canadian Nurses Association. (2019). *Registered nurses profile (including Nurse Practitioners), Canada, 2017.* Retrieved from https://www.cna-aiic.ca/en/nursing-practice/the-practice-of-nursing/health-human-resources/nursing-statistics/canada

Canadian Public Health Association (CPHA). (2008). *A vision for a health literate Canada: Report of the expert panel on health literacy.* Retrieved from https://www.cpha.ca/sites/default/files/uploads/resources/healthlit/report_e.pdf

Centers for Disease Control and Prevention (CDC). (2016). *What is health literacy?* Retrieved from http://www.cdc.gov/healthliteracy/learn/index.html

Centers for Disease Control and Prevention (CDC). (2018). *Folic acid.* Retrieved from http://www.cdc.gov/ncbddd/folicacid/features/foic-acid-use-ntd.html

Centers for Disease Control and Prevention (CDC). (2017). *Access to health care.* Retrieved from http://www.cdc.gov/nchs/fastats/access-to-health-care.htm

Chang, H. Y., & Chang, H. L. (2015). A review of nurses' knowledge, attitudes, and ability to communicate the risks and benefits of complementary and alternative medicine. *Journal of Clinical Nursing, 24*, 1466–1478.

Childbirth Connection. (2019). *Choosing a place of birth.* Retrieved from http://www.childbirthconnection.org/healthy-pregnancy/choosing-a-place-of-birth/healthy-pregnancy/choosing-a-place-of-birth/

Clark, C. C. (2011). *Evidence based health promotion for nurses.* Sudbury, MA: Jones & Bartlett Learning.

Clark, M. J. (2014). *Community health nursing: Advocating for healthy populations* (6th ed.). Upper Saddle River, NJ: Prentice Hall.

Clark, C. C., & Paraska, K. K. (2012). *Health promotion for nurses.* Burlington, MA: Jones & Bartlett Learning.

College of Nurses of Ontario. (2018). *Culturally sensitive care.* Retrieved from http://www.cno.org/en/learn-about-standards-guidelines/educational-tools/ask-practice/culturally-sensitive-care/

Coyne, I., O'Neill, C., Murphy, M., Costello, T., & O'Shea, R. (2011). What does family-centered care mean to nurses and how do they think it could be enhanced in practice. *Journal of Advanced Nursing, 67*(12), 2561–2573.

Darawsheh, W., & Chard, G. (2015). Towards culturally competent professional practice: Exploring the concepts of independence and interdependence. *Social Services Research Group Journal: Research, Policy and Planning, 31*(1), 3–17.

Darnell, L. K., & Hickson, S. V. (2015). Cultural competent patient-centered nursing care. *The Nursing Clinics of North America, 50*(1), 99–108.

Dauvrin, M., & Lorant, V. (2015). Leadership and cultural competence of health care professionals: A social network analysis. *Nursing Research, 64*(3), 200–210.

de la Rosa, I. A., Perry, J., & Johnson, V. (2015). Pathways to resilience: Enhancing family well-being with a home visitation model. *Journal of Youth Development, 10*(1), 35–58.

Duell, P., Wright, D., Renzaho, A. M., & Bhattacharya, D. (2015). Optimal health literacy measurement for the clinical setting: A systematic review. *Patient Education and Counseling, 98*(11), 1295–1307.

Dykes, D. C., & White, III, A. A. (2011). Culturally competent care pedagogy: What works?. *Clinical Orthopedics & Related Research, 469*(7), 1813–1816.

Eisler, K. (2011). Executive director's report. Patient and family centered care: What does it mean for RNs?. *SRNA Newsbulletin, 13*(1), 4.

Ernst, E. (2015). How nurses can be misled about complementary and alternative medicine. *Journal of Advanced Nursing, 71*(2), 235–236.

Farrar, F. C. (2015). Transforming home health nursing with telehealth technology. *Nursing Clinics of North America, 50*(2), 269–281.

Friedman, A. J., Cosby, R., Boyko, S., Hatto-Bauer, J., & Turnbull, G. (2011). Effective teaching strategies and methods of delivery for patient education: A systematic review and practice guideline recommendations. *Journal of Cancer Education, 26*(1), 12–21.

George, M. (2015). Integrative medicine is integral to providing patient-centered care. *Annals of Allergy, Asthma & Immunology, 114*(4), 261–265.

Government of Canada. (2017). *2017 annual report to parliament on immigration*. Retrieved from https://www.canada.ca/en/immigration-refugees-citizenship/corporate/publications-manuals/annual-report-parliament-immigration-2017.html

Government of New Brunswick (GNB). (2018). *Healthy families, healthy babies program*. Retrieved from https://www2.gnb.ca/content/gnb/en/services/services_renderer.10795.Healthy_Families,_Healthy_Babies_Program.html

Gupta, D., Mehta, M., & Sagar, R. (2015). Interpersonal skills. In M. Mehta, & R. Sagar (Eds.). *A practical approach to cognitive behaviour therapy for adolescents* (pp. 91–107). India: Springer Publishers.

Hall, H. G., Griffiths, D., & McKenna, L. G. (2015). Complementary and alternative medicine: Interaction and communication between midwives and women. *Women and Birth, 28*(2), 137–142.

Hamilton, K. (2011). Family education: Development of a formal education process to ensure quality education prior to discharge. *Journal of Pediatric Nursing, 26*(2), e3.

Hansen, L. O. (2015). Passing beyond a wing and a prayer after hospital discharge. *Journal of General Internal Medicine, 30*(4), 390–391.

Harkess, L., & Kaddoura, M. (2016). Culture and cultural competence in nursing education and practice: The state of the art. *Nursing Forum, 51*(3), 211–222. doi: 10.1111/nuf.12140

Health Canada. (2015). *Natural and non-prescription health products*. Retrieved from https://www.canada.ca/en/health-canada/services/drugs-health-products/natural-non-prescription.html

Health Canada. (2016). *First Nations and Inuit health strategies and initiatives*. Retrieved from https://www.canada.ca/en/health-canada/corporate/about-health-canada/activities-responsibilities/strategies-initiatives/first-nations-inuit-health-strategies-initiatives.html

Hersh, L., Salzman, B., & Snyderman, D. (2015). Health literacy in primary care practice. *American Family Physician, 92*(2), 118–124.

Holden, S. C., Gardiner, P., Birdee, G., Davis, R. B., & Yeh, G. Y. (2015). Complementary and alternative medicine use among women during pregnancy and childbearing years. *Birth, 42*(3), 261–269.

Hutton, E. K., Cappelletti, A., Reitsma, A. H., Simioni, J., Horne, J., McGregor, C., & Ahmed, R. J. (2016). Outcomes associated with planned place of birth among women with low-risk pregnancies. *CMAJ: Canadian Medical Association Journal, 188*(5), E80–E90.

Jackson, M. (2011). Deafness and antenatal care: Understanding issues with access. *British Journal of Midwifery, 19*(5), 280–284.

The Joint Commission (TJC). (2012). *Patient education*. Retrieved from http://www.mghpcs.org/eed_portal/Documents/PatientEd/JC_Standards_PatientEd.pdf

Kelly, M. M., & Penney, E. D. (2011). Collaboration of hospital case managers and home care liaisons when transitioning patients. *Professional Case Management, 16*(3), 128–138.

King, S. B. (2015). Competency-based education. *JACC: Cardiovascular Interventions, 8*(2), 374–375.

King, T. L., Brucker, M. C., Kriebs, J. M., Fahey, J. O., Gegor, C. L., & Varney, H. (2015). *Varney's midwifery* (5th ed.). Burlington, MA: Jones & Bartlett Learning.

Klemp, J. R. (2015). Breast cancer prevention across the cancer care continuum. *Seminars in Oncology Nursing, 31*(2), 89–99.

Knowles, M. S., Holton, III, E. F., & Swanson, R. A. (2011). *The adult learner* (7th ed.). Burlington, MA: Elsevier.

La Leche League Canada. (2019). *Who we are*. Retrieved from https://www.lllc.ca/

Lassi, Z. S., & Bhutta, Z. A. (2015). Community-based intervention packages for reducing maternal and neonatal morbidity and mortality and improving neonatal outcomes. *Cochrane Database of Systematic Reviews*, (3), CD007754.

Lemetti, T., Stolt, M., Rickard, N., & Suhonen, R. (2015). Collaboration between hospital and primary care nurses: A literature review. *International Nursing Review, 62*, 248–266.

Levetown, M.; American Academy of Pediatrics Committee on Bioethics. (2011). Communicating with children and families: From everyday interactions to skill in conveying distressing information. *Pediatrics, 121*(5), e1441–e1460. doi: 10.1542/peds.2008-0565

Lomax, S. W., & White, D. (2015). Interprofessional collaborative care skills for the frontline nurse. *Nursing Clinics of North America, 50*(1), 59–73.

Makic, M. B., Rauen, C., Jones, K., & Fisk, A. C. (2015). Continuing to challenge practice to be evidence based. *Critical Care Nurse, 35*(2), 39–50.

Makinen, R., & Tuominen, P. (2015). Discussion frames in motherhood blogs: A case study on suburban mom. In M. H. Bilgin, H. Danis, E. Demir, & C. K. M. Lau (Eds.). *Innovation, finance, and the economy* (pp. 47–67). New York: Springer International Publishing.

March of Dimes. (2015). *Prenatal care*. Retrieved from http://www.marchofdimes.com/pregnancy/prenatalcare.html

Massey, M. T. (2015). New focus on community nurses. *Primary Health Care, 25*(4), 5–6.

McMurray, A., & Clendon, J. (2015). *Community health and wellness: Primary care in practice* (5th ed.). Chatswood, NSW: Elsevier Australia.

National Center for Complementary and Integrative Health (NCCIH). (2018). *Complementary, alternative, or integrative health: What's in a name?*. Retrieved from https://nccih.nih.gov/health/integrative-health

National Center for Complementary and Integrative Health (NCCIH). (2017). *Osteoporosis*. Retrieved from https://nccih.nih.gov/health/osteoporosis.

National Institutes of Health (NIH). (2015). *Health literacy*. Retrieved from http://www.nih.gov/clearcommunication/healthliteracy.htm.

National Network of Libraries of Medicine (NNLM). (2015). *Health literacy*. Retrieved from http://nnlm.gov/outreach/consumer/hlthlit.html

Orr, P., & Davenport, D. (2015). Embracing change. *Nursing Clinics of North America, 50*(1), 1–18.

Peter, D., Robinson, P., Jordan, M., Lawrence, S., Casey, K., & Salas-Lopez, D. (2015). Reducing readmissions using teach-back: Enhancing patient and family education. *Journal of Nursing Administration, 45*(1), 35–42.

Pierce, D., Pompe-Waltman, J., Stanton, N., & Bland, L. (2011). Congratulations on your new baby: A nursing model for successful family transitions. *JOGNN: Journal of Obstetric, Gynecologic & Neonatal Nursing, 40*, 83.

Public Health Agency of Canada (PHAC). (2008). *Complementary and alternative health*. Retrieved from http://www.phac-aspc.gc.ca/chn-rcs/cah-acps-eng.php

Public Health Agency of Canada (PHAC). (2013). *Congenital anomalies in Canada: A perinatal health surveillance report*. Retrieved from http://publications.gc.ca/collections/collection_2014/aspc-phac/HP35-40-2013-eng.pdf

Public Health Agency of Canada (PHAC). (2017). *Perinatal health indicators for Canada 2017: A report from the Canadian Perinatal Surveillance System*. Ottawa: Author.

Refugee Health Technical Assistance Center. (2011). *Best practices for communicating through an interpreter*. Retrieved from http://refugeehealthta.org/access-to-care/language-access/best-practices-communicating-through-an-interpreter/

Registered Nurses' Association of Ontario (RNAO). (2016). *Embracing cultural diversity in health care: Developing cultural competence [Best practice guideline]*. Retrieved from http://rnao.ca/bpg/guidelines/embracing-cultural-diversity-health-care-developing-culturalcompetence

Roberts, B. (2015). Person and family centered care. *Creative Nursing, 21*(1), 63–66.

The Sentinel Watch: Nursing. (2014). *Improve your patient education skills to enhance care*. Retrieved from http://www.americansentinel.edu/blog/2014/12/17/improve-your-patient-education-skills-to-enhance-care/

Shepperd, S., Doll, H., Angus, R. M., Clarke, M. J., Iliffe, S., Kalra, L., Wilson, A. D., & Gonçalves-Bradley, D. C. (2016). Admission avoidance hospital at home. *Cochrane Database of Systematic Reviews, 9*, CD007491. doi: 10.1002/14651858.CD007491.pub2.

Shorofi, S. (2011). Complementary and alternative medicine (CAM) among hospitalized patients: Reported use of CAM and reasons for use, CAM preferred during hospitalization, and the socio-demographic determinants of CAM users. *Complementary Therapies in Clinical Practice, 17*(4), 199–205.

Smith, G. N. (2015a). The maternal health clinic: Improving women's cardiovascular health. *Seminars in Perinatology, 39*(4), 316–319.

Smith, L. S. (2015b). Tune into safety for hearing-impaired patients. *Nursing, 45*(6), 64–66.

Smith, V. C., & Stewart, J. (2019). Discharge planning for high-risk newborns. *UpToDate*. Retrieved from http://www.uptodate.com/contents/discharge-planning-for-high-risk-newborns

Stanhope, M., & Lancaster, J. (2015). *Public health nursing: Population-centered health care in the community* (9th ed.). St. Louis, MO: Mosby Elsevier.

Statistics Canada. (2013). *Skills in Canada: First results from the Programme for the International Assessment of Adult Competencies, 2012 (final)*. Retrieved from http://www.statcan.gc.ca/daily-quotidien/131008/dq131008b-eng.htm

Steinberg, M., & Sackmary, B. (2015). Marketing in health services: A review of recent trends in obstetrics. In E. G. Thomas, & S. R. Rao (Eds.). *Proceedings of the 1988 International Conference of Services Marketing* (pp. 306–316). New York: Springer International Publishing.

Su, W. M., Herron, B., & Osisek, P. J. (2011). Using a competency-based approach to patient education: Achieving congruence among learning, teaching and evaluation. *Nursing Clinics of North America, 46*(3), 291–298.

Thomas, S. D., Hudgins, J. L., Sutherland, D. E., Ange, B. L., & Mobley, S. C. (2015). Perinatal program evaluations: Methods, impacts, and future goals. *Maternal and Child Health Journal, 19*, 1440–1446.

Tyler, S., & Nagtalon-Ramos, J. (2015). Managing nausea and vomiting of pregnancy. *Women's Healthcare, 3*(2), 7–14.

USDHHS Office of Minority Health. (n.d.). *Culturally competent nursing care: A cornerstone of caring*. Retrieved from https://ccnm.thinkculturalhealth.hhs.gov/Content/Introduction/Introduction1.asp.

Williamson, K. M., Almaskari, M., Lester, Z., & Maguire, D. (2015). Utilization of evidence-based practice knowledge, attitude, and skill of clinical nurses in the planning of professional development programming. *Journal for Nurses in Professional Development, 31*(2), 73–80.

Wong-Baker FACES Foundation. (2016). *Atraumatic care*. Retrieved from https://wongbakerfaces.org/atraumatic-care/

Wright, L. M., & Leahey, M. (2013). *Nurses and families: A guide to family assessment and intervention* (6th ed.). Philadelphia, PA: F.A. Davis Company.

Zambrana, R. E., Meghea, C., Talley, C., Hammad, A., Lockett, M., & Williams, K. P. (2015). Association between family communication and health literacy among underserved racial/ethnic women. *Journal of Health Care for the Poor and Underserved, 26*(2), 391–405.

Zielinski, R., Ackerson, K., & Low, L. K. (2015). Planned home birth: benefits, risks, and opportunities. *International Journal of Women's Health, 7*, 361–377.

CHAPTER **WORKSHEET**

MULTIPLE CHOICE QUESTIONS

1. When caring for children, how should the nurse best incorporate the concept of family-centred care?
   a. Encourage the family to allow the physician to make health care decisions for the child.
   b. Use the concepts of respect, family strengths, diversity, and collaboration with family.
   c. Advise the family to choose a primary health care provider.
   d. Recognize that families undergoing stress related to the child's illness cannot make good decisions.

2. A community-based nurse is involved in secondary prevention activities. Which activities might be included? Select all that apply.
   a. Fecal occult blood testing
   b. Hearing screening
   c. Smoking cessation program
   d. Cholesterol testing
   e. Hygiene program
   f. Pregnancy testing

3. A woman is to undergo a colonoscopy at a freestanding outpatient surgery centre. Which would the nurse identify as a major disadvantage associated with this community-based setting?
   a. Increased risk for infection
   b. Increased health care costs
   c. Need to be transferred if overnight stay is required
   d. Increased disruption of family functioning

4. When developing a teaching plan for a child and his or her parents, which action would the nurse do first?
   a. Decide which procedures and medications the child will be discharged on.
   b. Determine the child's and family's learning needs and styles.
   c. Ask the family if they have ever performed this type of procedure.
   d. Tell the child and family what the goals of the teaching session are.

5. The clinic nurse is concerned about the client's ability to understand the instructions given and the health literacy level of her client. Which of the following can the nurse employ to increase the client's understanding of the instructions?
   a. Draw pictures of the procedure and write down the steps to it.
   b. Instruct the client to call the nurse if they have questions.
   c. Discuss the instructions with an elderly family member in addition to the client.
   d. Question the client about their reading level and educational level.

CRITICAL THINKING EXERCISES

1. A 3-year-old girl from Saudi Arabia has become seriously ill while on a visit to Canada. It is projected that she will require a lengthy hospitalization. Describe the steps the nurse should take to communicate with and provide extensive health care teaching to this child's family.

2. A pregnant woman is discharged home from the hospital after admission due to preterm labour. The woman is to be on complete bed rest and will receive home health care through a local agency to assist her and her family and to monitor her health status. As the home health nurse assigned to this woman, what should your nursing assessment include?

STUDY ACTIVITIES

1. Shadow a nurse working in a community setting, such as a women's health clinic, birthing centre, camp, home care, or health department. Identify the role the nurse plays in the health of women, parents, children, and families in the setting and in the community.

2. Arrange for a visit to a community health centre that offers services to various cultural groups. Interview the staff about the strategies used to overcome communication barriers and different health care practices for the women and children in these groups.

3. Select one of the websites listed on thePoint and explore the information provided. How could a community-based nurse use this information?

BRINGING IT ALL TOGETHER: A CASE STUDY

Bianca, a 23-year-old Hispanic client, is about to give birth to her first child, a daughter that will be named Amelia. Her partner, Alejandro, has been supportive of Bianca during her labour and plans to be present during the birth but seems uneasy about the prospect of caring for his daughter claiming, "I'm not use to being around little babies." The birthing centre focuses on family-centred care and the nurse will plan the care of Bianca and Amelia as well as the support of Alejandro based on that model.

Go to thePoint **to find questions to consider about this case.**

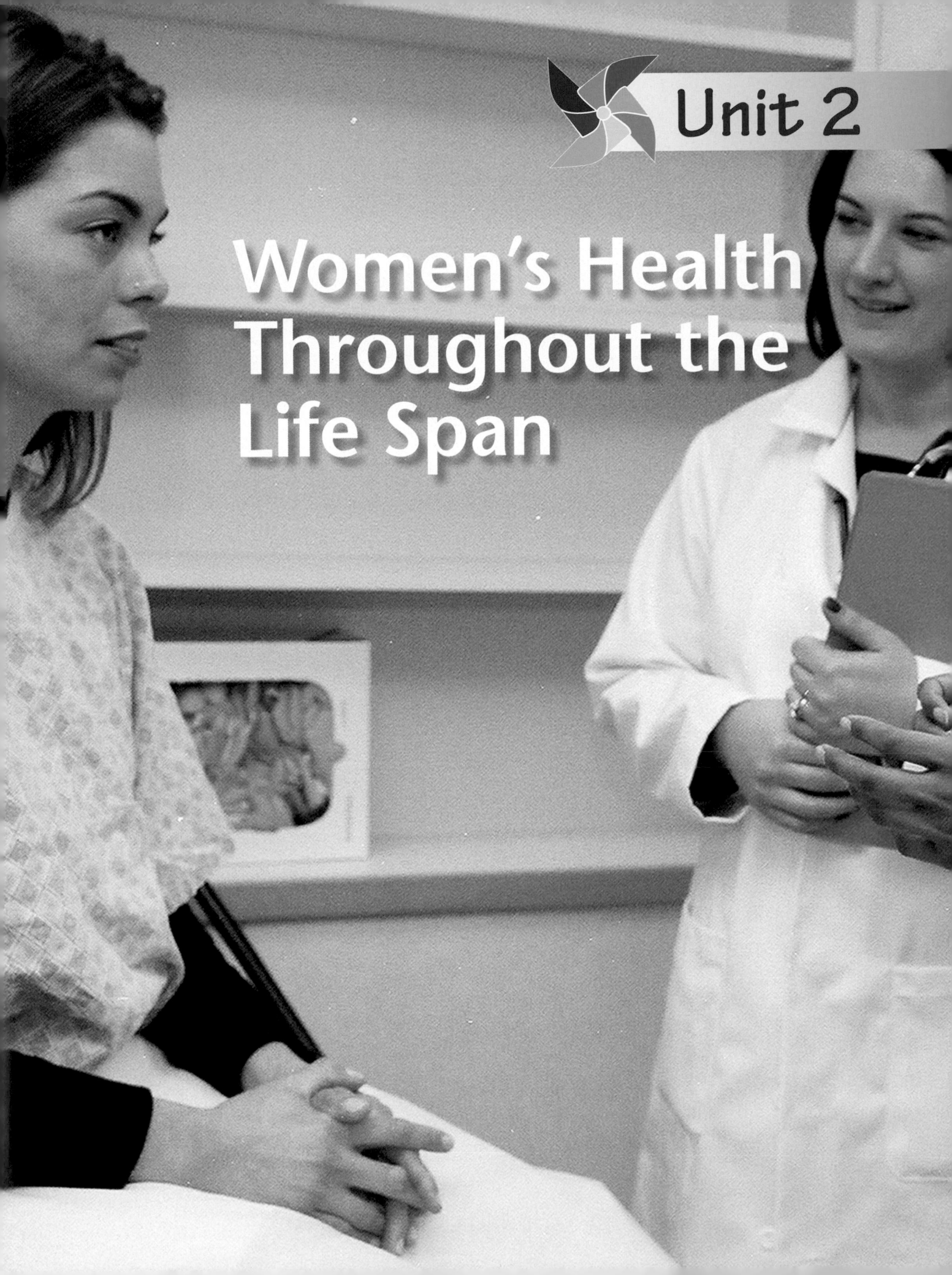

Women's Health Throughout the Life Span

3

Anatomy and Physiology of the Reproductive System

Learning Objectives

Upon completion of the chapter, you will be able to:

1. Contrast the structure and function of the major external and internal female genital organs.

2. Outline the phases of the menstrual cycle, the dominant hormones involved, and the changes taking place in each phase.

3. Classify external and internal male reproductive structures and the function of each in hormonal regulation.

Linda, 49, started menstruating when she was 12 years old. Her menstrual periods have always been regular, but now she is experiencing irregular, heavier, and longer ones. She wonders if there is something wrong or if this is normal.

INTRODUCTION

The reproductive system is a collection of organs that function in the production of offspring. Scientists argue that the reproductive system is among the most important systems in the entire body. Without the ability to reproduce, a species dies. The female reproductive system produces the female reproductive cells (the eggs, or ova) and contains an organ (**uterus**) in which development of the fetus takes place; the male reproductive system produces the male reproductive cells (the sperm) and contains an organ (**penis**) that deposits the sperm within a vagina. Nurses need to have a thorough understanding of the anatomy and physiology of the male and female reproductive systems to be able to assess the health of these systems, to promote reproductive system health, to care for conditions that might affect the reproductive organs, and to provide client teaching concerning the reproductive system. This chapter reviews the female and male reproductive systems and the menstrual cycle as it relates to reproduction.

When discussing "female" and "male" reproductive systems, health care professionals must be sensitive to the needs of transgender patients, as the anatomy of trans women and trans men will differ from their **cisgender** counterparts (those whose gender identities match the sex assigned at birth). The use of the terms "woman/female" and "man/male" in this chapter refer to cis-gender women, and cis-gender men.

FEMALE REPRODUCTIVE ANATOMY AND PHYSIOLOGY

The female reproductive system is composed of both external and internal reproductive organs. It consists of the paired ovaries and oviducts, the uterus, the vagina, the external genitalia, and the mammary glands. All of these structures have evolved for the important functions of **ovulation**, fertilization of an ovum by a sperm, support of the developing embryo and fetus, and the birth and care of a newborn.

External Female Reproductive Organs

The external female reproductive organs collectively are called the **vulva** (which means "covering" in Latin). The vulva serves to protect the urethral and vaginal openings and is highly sensitive to touch to increase the female's pleasure during sexual arousal (Patton & Thibodeau, 2016). The structures that make up the vulva include the mons pubis, the labia majora and minora, the clitoris and prepuce, the structures within the vestibule, and the perineum (Fig. 3.1).

FIGURE 3.1 **A.** The external female reproductive organs. **B.** Normal appearance of external structures. (Photo by B. Proud.)

Mons Pubis

The mons pubis is the elevated, rounded, fleshy prominence made up of fatty tissue that overlays the symphysis pubis. The skin of this fatty tissue is covered with coarse, curly pubic hair after puberty. The mons pubis protects the symphysis pubis during sexual intercourse.

Labia

The labia majora (large lips), which are relatively large and fleshy, are comparable to the scrotum in males. The labia majora contain sweat and sebaceous (oil-secreting) glands; after puberty, they are covered with hair. Their function is to protect the vaginal opening and provide cushioning during sexual activity. The labia minora (small lips) are the delicate hairless inner folds of skin; they can be very small or up to 2 in wide. They lie just inside the labia majora and surround the openings to the vagina and urethra. The labia minora grow down from the anterior inner part of the labia majora on each side.

These lips surround the vaginal opening and extend upward to form protection around both the clitoris and urethra. They are highly vascular and abundant in nerve supply. They lubricate the vulva, swell in response to stimulation, and are highly sensitive.

Clitoris and Prepuce

The clitoris is a small, cylindrical mass of erectile tissue and nerves. It is highly sensitive and is analogous to the head of the male's penis (the glans penis). Unlike the penis, however, the function of the clitoris is purely erogenous. Most of the components of the clitoris are buried under the skin and connective tissue of the vulva. It is located at the anterior junction of the labia minora. There are folds above and below the clitoris. The joining of the folds above the clitoris forms the prepuce, a hood-like covering over the clitoris; the junction below the clitoris forms the frenulum.

Take Note!

The hood-like covering over the clitoris is the site for female genital mutilation or cutting, which is a cultural ritual still practiced today in countries around the world. It is internationally recognized as a human rights violation against women, and the practice is illegal in Canada.

A rich supply of blood vessels gives the clitoris a pink colour. Like the penis, the clitoris is very sensitive to touch, stimulation, and temperature and can also become erect. For its small size, 9 to 11 cm, it has a generous blood and nerve supply. There are more free nerve endings of sensory reception located on the clitoris than on any other part of the body, and it is, unsurprisingly, the most erotically sensitive part of the genitalia for most females. Its function is sexual stimulation (Pauls, 2015).

Take Note!

The word clitoris is from the Greek word for "key"; in ancient times the clitoris was thought to be the key to a woman's sexuality.

Vestibule

The vestibule is an oval area enclosed by the labia minora laterally. It is inside the labia minora and outside of the hymen and is perforated by six openings. Opening into the vestibule are the urethra from the urinary bladder, the vagina, and two sets of glands. The opening to the vagina is called the introitus, and the half-moon–shaped area behind the opening is called the fourchette. Through tiny ducts beside the introitus, Bartholin's glands, when stimulated, secrete mucus that supplies lubrication for intercourse. Skene's glands are located on either side of the opening to the urethra. They secrete a small amount of mucus to keep the opening moist and lubricated for the passage of urine (Velkey, Hall, & Robboy, 2015).

The vaginal opening is surrounded by the hymen (maidenhead). The hymen is a tough, elastic, perforated, mucosa-covered tissue across the vaginal introitus. In a virgin, the hymen may completely cover the opening, but it usually encircles the opening like a tight ring. Because the degree of tightness varies among women, the hymen may tear at the first attempt at intercourse, or it may be so soft and pliable that no tearing occurs. In a woman who is not a virgin, the hymen usually appears as small tags of tissue surrounding the vaginal opening, but the presence or absence of the hymen can neither confirm nor rule out sexual experience (Acién & Acién, 2015).

Take Note!

Heavy physical exertion, use of tampons, or injury to the area can alter the appearance of the hymen in girls and women who have not been sexually active.

Perineum

The perineum is the most posterior part of the external female reproductive organs. This external region is located between the vulva and the anus. It is made up of skin, muscle, and fascia. The perineum can become lacerated or incised during childbirth and may need to be repaired with sutures. Incising the perineal area to provide more space for the presenting part is called an episiotomy. Although still a relatively common obstetric procedure, the use of episiotomy has decreased during the past 25 years. The procedure should be applied selectively rather than routinely. An episiotomy can add to postpartum discomfort and perineal trauma and can lead to fecal incontinence (King et al., 2015).

Internal Female Reproductive Organs

The internal female reproductive organs consist of the vagina, uterus, fallopian tubes, and ovaries (Fig. 3.2). These structures develop and function according to specific hormonal influences that affect fertility and childbearing.

Vagina

The **vagina** is a highly distensible canal situated anterior to the rectum and posterior to the bladder. It is a tubular, fibromuscular organ lined with mucous membrane that lies in a series of transverse folds called rugae. The rugae allow for extreme dilation of the canal during labour and birth. The vagina is a canal that connects the external genitals (vulva) to the cervix. It receives the penis and the sperm ejaculated during sexual intercourse, and it serves as an exit passageway for menstrual blood and for the

Ureter

Ovary

Fallopian tube

Urinary bladder

Symphysis pubis

Urethra

Clitoris

Prepuce of clitoris

Urethral orifice

Labia minora

Labia majora

Vaginal orifice

Rectum

Uterus

Posterior fornix of vagina

Rectouterine pouch

Cervix

Vagina

Anus

A

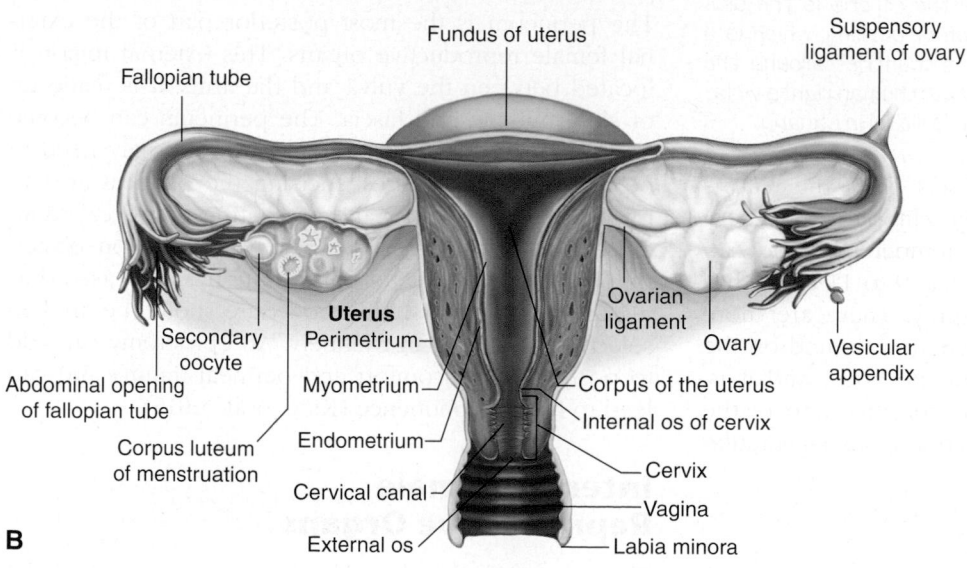

Fundus of uterus

Suspensory ligament of ovary

Fallopian tube

Uterus
Perimetrium

Secondary oocyte

Abdominal opening of fallopian tube

Corpus luteum of menstruation

Myometrium

Endometrium

Cervical canal

External os

Ovarian ligament

Ovary

Vesicular appendix

Corpus of the uterus

Internal os of cervix

Cervix

Vagina

Labia minora

B

FIGURE 3.2 The internal female reproductive organs. **A.** Lateral view. **B.** Anterior view. (Adapted from Anatomical Chart Company. [2001]. *Atlas of human anatomy.* Springhouse, PA: Springhouse.)

fetus during childbirth. The front and back walls normally touch each other so that there is no space in the vagina except when it is opened (e.g., during a pelvic examination or intercourse). In the adult, the vaginal cavity is 8 to 10 cm (3 to 4 in) long. Muscles that control its diameter surround the lower third of the vagina. The upper two thirds of the vagina lie above these muscles and can be stretched easily. During a woman's reproductive years, the mucosal lining of the vagina has a corrugated appearance and is resistant to bacterial colonization. Before puberty and after menopause (if the woman is not taking estrogen), the mucosa is smooth due to lower levels of estrogen (Farage, Miller, & Maibach, 2015).

The vagina has an acidic environment, which protects it against ascending infections. Antibiotic therapy, douching, perineal hygiene sprays, and deodorants upset the acid balance within the vaginal environment and can predispose women to infections.

Uterus

The uterus is an inverted, pear-shaped muscular organ at the top of the vagina. It lies behind the bladder and in front of the rectum and is anchored in position by eight ligaments, although it is not firmly attached or adherent to any part of the skeleton. A full bladder tilts the uterus backward; a distended rectum tilts it forward. The uterus alters its position by gravity or with change of posture, and is the size and shape of an inverted pear. It is the site of menstruation, receiving a fertilized ovum, development of the fetus during pregnancy, and contracting to help in the expulsion of the fetus and placenta. Before the first pregnancy, it measures approximately 8 cm long, 5 cm wide, and 2 to 3 cm thick. After a pregnancy, the uterus remains larger than before the pregnancy. After menopause, it becomes smaller and atrophies.

The uterine wall is relatively thick and composed of three layers: the **endometrium** (innermost layer), the myometrium (muscular middle layer), and the perimetrium (outer serosal layer that covers the body of the uterus). The endometrium is the mucosal layer that lines the uterine cavity in nonpregnant women. It varies in thickness from 0.5 to 5 mm and has an abundant supply of glands and blood vessels (Tambouret & Wilbur, 2015). The myometrium makes up the major portion of the uterus and is composed of smooth muscle linked by connective tissue with numerous elastic fibres. During pregnancy, the upper myometrium undergoes marked hypertrophy, but there is limited change in the cervical muscle content.

Anatomic subdivisions of the uterus include the convex portion above the uterine tubes (the fundus), the central portion (the corpus or body) between the fundus and the cervix, and the cervix, or neck, which opens into the vagina.

CERVIX

The **cervix**, the lower part of the uterus, is sometimes called the neck of the uterus. It opens into the vagina and has a channel that allows sperm to enter the uterus and menstrual discharge to exit. It is composed of fibrous connective tissue. During a pelvic examination, the part of the cervix that protrudes into the upper end of the vagina can be visualized. Like the vagina, this part of the cervix is covered by mucosa, which is smooth, firm, and doughnut shaped, with a visible central opening called the external os (Fig. 3.3). Before childbirth, the external cervical os is a small, oval opening. After childbirth, the opening is converted into a transverse slit that resembles lips (Fig. 3.4). Except during menstruation or ovulation, the cervix is usually a good barrier against bacteria. The cervix has an alkaline environment, which protects the sperm from the acidic environment in the vagina.

The canal or channel of the cervix is lined with mucus-secreting glands. This mucus is thick and impenetrable to sperm until just before the ovaries release an egg (ovulation). At ovulation, the consistency of the mucus changes so that sperm can swim through it, allowing fertilization. At the same time, the mucus-secreting glands of the cervix actually become able to store live sperm for 2 or 3 days. These sperm can later move up through the corpus and into the fallopian tubes to fertilize the egg; thus, intercourse 1 or 2 days before ovulation can lead to pregnancy. Because some women do not ovulate consistently, pregnancy can occur at varying times after the last menstrual period. During pregnancy, the cervix

FIGURE 3.3 **Appearance of normal cervix.** *Note:* This is the cervix of a multipara female. (Photo by B. Proud.)

is the vital mechanical barrier which resists compressive and tensile loads generated from a growing fetus. The channel in the cervix is too narrow for the fetus to pass through during pregnancy, but during labour it stretches to let the newborn through.

CORPUS

The corpus, or the main body of the uterus, is a highly muscular organ that enlarges to hold the fetus during pregnancy. The inner lining of the corpus (endometrium) undergoes cyclic changes as a result of the changing levels of hormones secreted by the ovaries: it is thickest during the part of the menstrual cycle in which a fertilized egg would be expected to enter the uterus and is thinnest just after menstruation. If fertilization does not take place during this cycle, most of the endometrium is shed and bleeding occurs, resulting in the monthly period. If fertilization does take place, the embryo attaches to the wall of the uterus, where it becomes embedded in the endometrium (about 1 week

A   B

FIGURE 3.4 **A:** Nulliparous cervical os. **B:** Parous cervical os.

after fertilization); this process is called implantation (Patton & Thibodeau, 2015). Menstruation then ceases throughout the 40 weeks (280 days) of pregnancy. During labour, the muscular walls of the corpus contract to push the baby through the cervix and into the vagina.

Fallopian Tubes

The **fallopian tubes**, also known as oviducts, are hollow, cylindrical structures that extend 5 to 7 cm from the upper edges of the uterus toward the ovaries. Each tube is about 7 to 10 cm long and approximately 0.7 cm in diameter. The end of each tube flares into a funnel shape, providing a large opening for the egg to fall into when it is released from the ovary. Cilia (beating, hairlike extensions on cells) line the fallopian tube and the muscles in the tube's wall. The fallopian tubes convey the ovum from the ovary to the uterus and sperm from the uterus toward the ovary. This movement is accomplished via ciliary action and peristaltic contraction. If sperm are present in the fallopian tube as a result of sexual intercourse or artificial insemination, fertilization of the ovum can occur in the distal portion of the tube. If the egg is fertilized, it will divide over a period of 4 days while it moves slowly down the fallopian tube and into the uterus, where it implants into the uterine lining.

Ovaries

The **ovaries** are a set of paired glands resembling unshelled almonds that are the organs of gamete production in the female. They are set in the pelvic cavity below and to either side of the umbilicus. They are usually pearl coloured, oblong, and have a lumpy surface. They are homologous to the testes. Each mature ovary weighs from 2 to 5 g and is about 4 cm long, 2 cm wide, and 1 cm thick (Jones & Lopez, 2014). The ovaries are not attached to the fallopian tubes but are suspended nearby from several ligaments, which help

hold them in position. The development and the release of the ovum and the secretion of the hormones **estrogen** and **progesterone** are the two primary functions of the ovary. The ovaries link the reproductive system to the body's system of endocrine glands, as they produce the ova (eggs) and secrete, in cyclic fashion, the female sex hormones estrogen and progesterone. After an ovum matures, it passes into the fallopian tubes.

Breasts

The two mammary glands, or **breasts**, are accessory organs of the female reproductive system that are specialized to secrete milk following pregnancy. They overlie the pectoralis major muscles and extend from the second to the sixth ribs and from the sternum to the axilla. Each breast has a nipple located near the tip, which is surrounded by a circular area of pigmented skin called the areola. Each breast is composed of approximately nine lobes (although the number can range between 4 and 18), which contain alveolar glands and a lactiferous duct that leads to the nipple and opens to the outside (Fig. 3.5). The lobes are separated by dense connective and adipose tissues, which also help support the weight of the breasts (Kandeel, 2014).

During pregnancy, placental estrogen and progesterone stimulate the development of the mammary glands. The breasts begin producing colostrum as early as 16 weeks in a pregnancy (Lawrence & Lawrence, 2011). Because of this hormonal activity, the breasts may double in size during pregnancy. At the same time, glandular tissue replaces the adipose tissue of the breasts.

Following childbirth and the expulsion of the placenta, levels of placental hormones (progesterone and lactogen) fall rapidly, and the action of prolactin (a milk-producing hormone) is no longer inhibited. Prolactin stimulates the production of milk within a few days after childbirth, but in the interim, colostrum is present. This early milk, colostrum, is a dark yellow colour, and

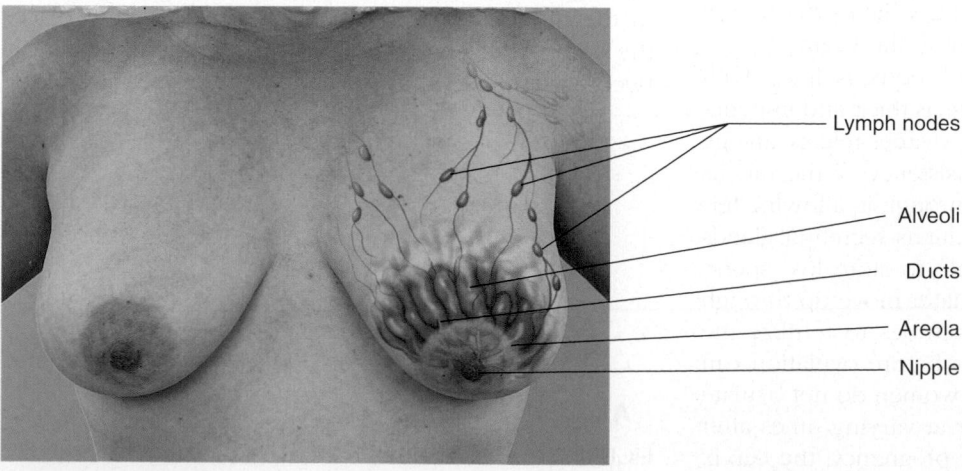

Lymph nodes

Alveoli

Ducts

Areola

Nipple

FIGURE 3.5 Anatomy of the breasts. (Photo by B. Proud.)

contains more minerals and protein, but less sugar and fat, than mature breastmilk. Colostrum secretion may continue for approximately a week after childbirth, with gradual conversion to mature milk. Colostrum is rich in maternal antibodies, especially immunoglobulin A (IgA), which offers protection for the newborn against enteric pathogens.

Female Sexual Response

The sexual response in both females and males is governed primarily by the nervous system rather than by hormones. The sexual response starts in a state of sexual neutrality, and the person's sexual desire is more of a reciprocal response than a spontaneous one (Housman & Odum, 2016). The sexual cycle is usually thought of as having five phases: desire, excitement, plateau, orgasm, and resolution:

1. *Desire:* starts with a desire for sexual intimacy, also known as *libido.*
2. *Excitement:* both partners have a heightened sexual awareness. When a female is sexually aroused, her brain coordinates a patterned sexual response cycle consisting of increased heart rate, respiratory rate, blood pressure, and general level of excitement (Sherwood, 2016). With sexual stimulation, tissues in the clitoris and breasts and around the vaginal orifice fill with blood and the erectile tissues swell. At the same time, the vagina begins to expand and elongate to accommodate the penis. As part of the whole vasocongestive reaction, the labia majora and minor swell and darken. As sexual stimulation intensifies, the vestibular glands secrete mucus to moisten and lubricate the tissues to facilitate insertion of the penis. Hormones play an integral role in the female sexual response as well. Adequate estrogen and testosterone must be available for the brain to sense incoming arousal stimuli. Research indicates that estrogen preserves the vascular function of female sex organs and affects genital sensation, and it also is believed to promote blood flow to these areas during stimulation. Testosterone is needed to stimulate sexual desire in women. Research findings also suggest that testosterone therapy improves sexual desire, arousal, orgasm frequency, and satisfaction in women (Davis, 2013).
3. *Plateau:* the heart rate, blood pressure, level of muscle tension, and respiration rate all increase. During this phase, the penile erection intensifies and the vagina constricts around the penis. Continued stimulation of the clitoris and penis with movement leads to the next phase of the sexual response—*orgasmic phase.*
4. *Orgasm:* women experience rhythmic contractions of the pelvic muscles and vaginal walls. In men, ejaculation occurs during the *orgasmic phase* and both sexes experience a peak of sexual pleasure at orgasm.

Typically, there is a warm and relaxed feeling after an orgasm. Within a short time after orgasm, the two physiologic mechanisms that created the sexual response, vasocongestion and muscle contraction, rapidly dissipate. The orgasmic experience varies from person to person and from time to time in the same person. Orgasm is an intense sensation of pleasure achieved by stimulation of erogenous zones. Women do not have a refractory period after each orgasm and can, therefore, experience multiple orgasms. Clitoral sexual response and the female orgasm are not affected by aging (Minkin, 2016). Some orgasms are intense, some are quiet, and some are gentle (Wheatley & Puts, 2015). At the completion of the sexual episode, the brain and body return to an unaroused state, which is termed *sexual resolution.* During this phase, the heart rate, blood pressure, and respirations slow; the muscles relax. Frequently, fatigue sets in for both partners.

THE FEMALE REPRODUCTIVE CYCLE

The female reproductive cycle is a complex process that encompasses an intricate series of chemical secretions and reactions to produce the ultimate potential for fertility and birth. The female reproductive cycle is a general term that includes the ovarian cycle, the endometrial (uterine) cycle, the hormonal changes that regulate them, and the cyclical changes in the breasts. The endometrium, ovaries, pituitary gland, and hypothalamus are all involved in the cyclic changes that help to prepare the body for fertilization. Absence of fertilization results in menstruation, the monthly shedding of the uterine lining. **Menstruation** (shedding of the endometrium) marks the beginning and end of the monthly cycle. Menopause is the naturally occurring cessation of menstrual cycles.

The menstrual cycle results from a functional hypothalamic–pituitary–ovarian axis and a precise sequencing of hormones that lead to ovulation. The ovarian cycle, during which ovulation occurs, and the endometrial cycle, during which menstruation occurs, are divided at midcycle by ovulation. Ovulation occurs when the ovum is released from its follicle; after leaving the ovary, the ovum enters the fallopian tube and journeys toward the uterus. If sperm fertilize the ovum during its journey, pregnancy occurs (Fig. 3.6).

Ovarian Cycle

The ovarian cycle is the series of events associated with a developing oocyte (ovum or egg) within the ovaries. Whereas men manufacture sperm daily, often into advanced age, women are born with a single lifetime supply of ova that are released from the ovaries

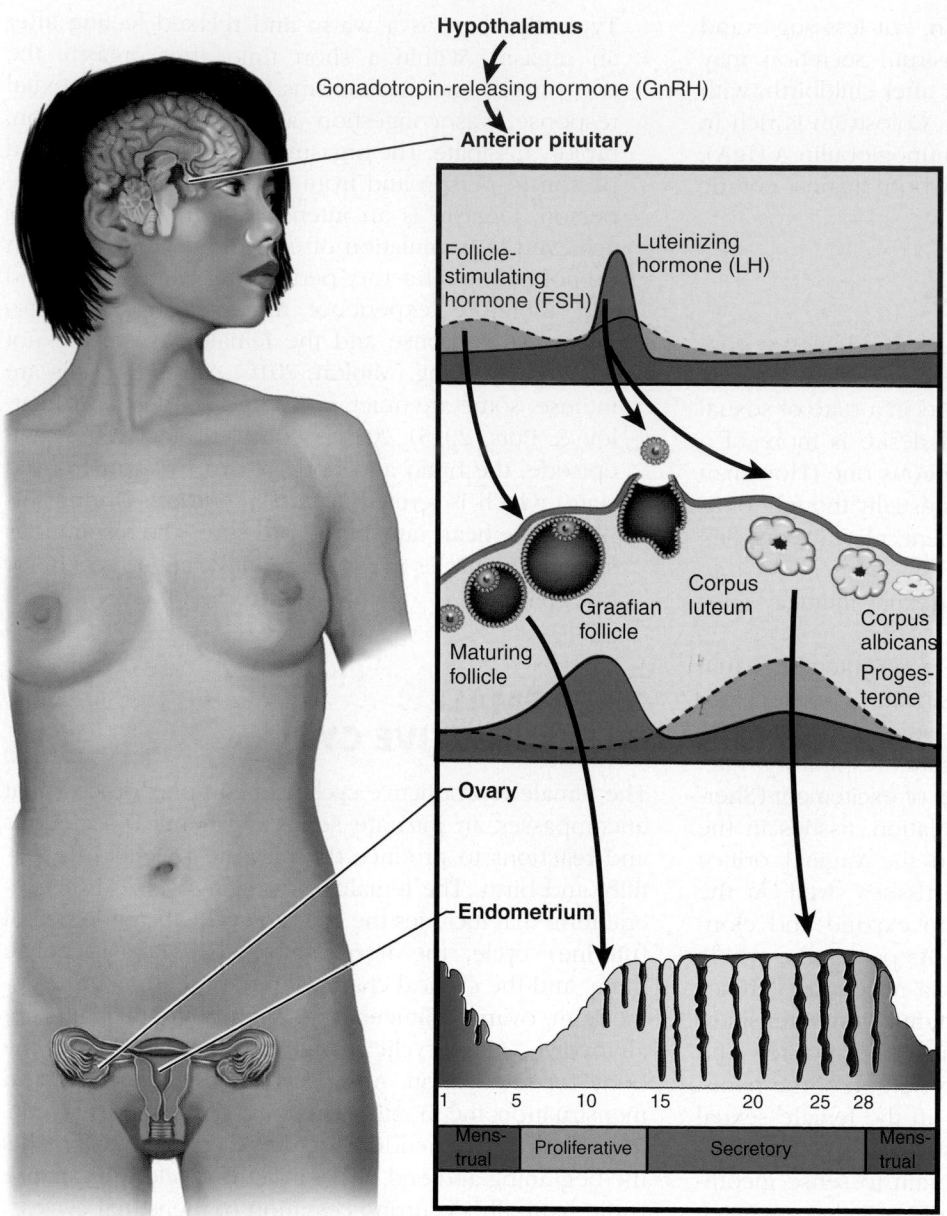

Hypothalamus

Gonadotropin-releasing hormone (GnRH)

Anterior pituitary

Follicle-stimulating hormone (FSH)

Luteinizing hormone (LH)

Maturing follicle

Graafian follicle

Corpus luteum

Corpus albicans

Proges-terone

Ovary

Endometrium

| 1 | 5 | 10 | 15 | 20 | 25 | 28 |

| Mens-trual | Proliferative | Secretory | Mens-trual |

FIGURE 3.6 Menstrual cycle summary based on a 28-day (average) menstrual cycle.

gradually throughout the childbearing years. In the female ovary, 1 million oocytes are present at birth, and about 200,000 to 400,000 follicles are still present at puberty. Typically, a woman ovulates one oocyte per month over an approximately 40-year reproductive life span. This accounts for the loss of 400 to 500 follicles. By age 35 she will have fewer than 100,000 follicles, and, by menopause, her follicular supply will be nearly depleted (Jones & Lopez, 2014). The ovarian cycle begins when the follicular cells (ovum and surrounding cells) swell and the maturation process starts. The maturing follicle at this stage is called a graafian follicle. The ovary raises many follicles monthly, but usually only one follicle matures to reach ovulation. The ovarian cycle consists of three phases: the follicular phase, ovulation, and the luteal phase.

Follicular Phase

This phase is so named because it is when the follicles in the ovary grow and form a mature egg. The goal of this phase is to produce an ovum for fertilization. This phase starts on day 1 of the menstrual cycle and continues until ovulation, approximately 10 to 14 days later. The follicular phase is not consistent in duration because of the time variations in follicular development. These variations account for the differences in menstrual cycle lengths (Sherwood, 2016). The hypothalamus is the initiator of this phase. Increasing levels of estrogen secreted from the maturing follicular cells and the continued growth of the dominant follicle cell induce proliferation of the endometrium and myometrium. This thickening of the uterine lining supports an implanted ovum if pregnancy occurs.

Prompted by the hypothalamus, the pituitary gland releases **follicle-stimulating hormone (FSH)**, which stimulates the ovary to produce 5 to 20 immature follicles. Each follicle houses an immature oocyte or egg. The follicle that is targeted to mature fully will soon rupture and expel a mature oocyte in the process of ovulation. A surge in **luteinizing hormone (LH)** from the anterior pituitary gland is actually responsible for affecting the final development and subsequent rupture of the mature follicle.

Ovulation

At ovulation, a mature follicle ruptures in response to a surge of LH, releasing a mature oocyte (ovum). No one single event causes ovulation. This usually occurs on day 14 in a 28-day cycle. When ovulation occurs, there is a drop in estrogen. Typically, ovulation takes place approximately 10 to 12 hours after the LH peak and 24 to 36 hours after estrogen levels peak (King et al., 2015). The distal ends of the fallopian tubes become active near the time of ovulation and create currents that help carry the ovum into the uterus. The life span of the ovum is only about 24 hours; unless it meets a sperm on its journey within that time, it will die.

During ovulation, the cervix produces thin, clear, stretchy, slippery mucus called spinnbarkeit which is designed to capture the man's sperm, nourish it, and help the sperm travel up through the cervix to meet the ovum for fertilization. Ovulation symptoms also include vaginal spotting, an increase in vaginal discharge giving the woman a "feeling of wetness," an increased libido leading to more desire to be intimate, a slight rise in basal body temperature, and lower abdominal cramping.

The one constant, whether a menstrual cycle is 28 days or 120 days, is that ovulation takes place 14 days before menstruation (Housman & Odum, 2016).

Take Note!

About one in five people who ovulate can feel a pain on one side of the abdomen around the time the egg is released. This midcycle pain is called mittelschmerz.

Luteal Phase

The luteal phase begins at ovulation and lasts until the menstrual phase of the next cycle. It typically occurs on days 15 through 28 of a 28-day cycle. After the follicle ruptures as it releases the egg, it closes and forms a corpus luteum. The corpus luteum secretes increasing amounts of the hormone progesterone, which interacts with the endometrium to prepare it for implantation. At the beginning of the luteal phase, progesterone induces the endometrial glands to secrete glycogen, mucus, and other substances. These glands become tortuous and have large lumens due to increased secretory activity.

The progesterone secreted by the corpus luteum causes the temperature of the body to rise slightly until the start of the next period. A significant increase in temperature, usually 0.3° to 0.6°C, is generally seen within a day or two after ovulation has occurred; the temperature remains elevated until 3 days before the onset on the next menstruation (Housman & Odum, 2016). This rise in temperature can be plotted on a graph and gives an indication of when ovulation has occurred. In the absence of fertilization, the corpus luteum begins to degenerate and consequently ovarian hormone levels decrease. As estrogen and progesterone levels decrease, the endometrium undergoes involution. In a 28-day cycle, menstruation then begins approximately 14 days after ovulation in the absence of pregnancy. FSH and LH are generally at their lowest levels during the luteal phase and highest during the follicular phase.

Endometrial (Uterine) Cycle

The endometrial (uterine) cycle occurs in response to cyclic hormonal changes. The four phases of the endometrial cycle are the proliferative phase, secretory phase, ischemic phase, and menstrual phase.

Proliferative Phase

The proliferative phase of the endometrial cycle corresponds to the follicular phase of the ovarian cycle. It starts with enlargement of the endometrial glands in response to increasing amounts of estrogen. The blood vessels become dilated and the endometrium increases in thickness dramatically from 0.5 to 5 mm in height and increases eightfold in thickness in preparation for implantation of the fertilized ovum (Oyelowo & Johnson, 2016). Cervical mucus becomes thin, clear, stretchy, and more alkaline, making it more favourable to sperm to enhance the opportunity for fertilization. The proliferative phase starts on about day 5 of the menstrual cycle and lasts to the time of ovulation. This phase depends on estrogen stimulation resulting from ovarian follicles, and this phase coincides with the follicular phase of the ovarian cycle.

Secretory Phase

The secretory phase begins at ovulation to about 3 days before the next menstrual period. Under the influence of progesterone released by the corpus luteum after ovulation, the endometrium becomes thickened and more vascular (growth of the spiral arteries) and glandular (secretion of more glycogen and lipids). These dramatic changes are all in preparation for implantation, if it were to occur. This phase typically lasts from day 15 (after ovulation) to day 28 and coincides with the luteal phase of the ovarian cycle. In the absence of fertilization by day 23 of the menstrual cycle, the corpus luteum begins to degenerate and consequently ovarian hormone levels decrease. As estrogen and progesterone levels decrease, the endometrium undergoes involution.

Ischemic Phase

If fertilization does not occur, the ischemic phase begins. Estrogen and progesterone levels drop sharply during this phase as the corpus luteum starts to degenerate. Changes in the endometrium occur with spasm of the arterioles, resulting in ischemia of the basal layer. The ischemia leads to shedding of the endometrium down to the basal layer, and menstrual flow begins.

Menstrual Phase

The menstrual phase begins as the spiral arteries rupture secondary to ischemia, releasing blood into the uterus, and the sloughing of the endometrial lining begins. If fertilization does not take place, the corpus luteum degenerates. As a result, both estrogen and progesterone levels fall and the thickened endometrial lining sloughs away from the uterine wall and passes out via the vagina. The beginning of the menstrual flow marks the end of one menstrual cycle and the start of a new one. Most women report menstrual bleeding for an average of 3 to 7 days. The amount of menstrual flow varies but averages 30 mL or a range of approximately 20 to 80 mL (2/3 to 2 2/3 oz) in volume per cycle (Thornhill & Gangestad, 2015).

Menstruation

Menstruation is a term derived from the Latin word *mensis,* meaning "month." It is the normal, predictable physiologic process whereby the inner lining of the uterus (endometrium) is expelled by the body. Typically, this occurs monthly. Menstruation has many effects on girls and women, including emotional and self-image issues. In Canada, the average age at **menarche** (the start of menstruation) is 12.7 years, with a range between 8 and 18. Genetics is the most important factor in determining the age at which menarche starts, but geographic location, nutrition, weight, general health, nutrition, cultural and social practices, the girl's educational level, attitude, family environment, and beliefs are also important (Krieger et al., 2015).

Pubertal events preceding the first menses have an orderly progression: thelarche, the development of breast buds; adrenarche, the appearance of pubic and then axillary hair, followed by a growth spurt; and menarche (occurring about 2 years after the start of breast development). In healthy pubertal girls, the menstrual period varies in flow heaviness and may remain irregular in occurrence for up to 2 years following menarche. After that time, the regular menstrual cycle should be established. Most women will experience 300 to 400

menstrual cycles within their lifetime (King et al., 2015). Normal, regular menstrual cycles vary in frequency and blood loss (Kandeel, 2014). Irregular menses can be associated with irregular ovulation, polycystic ovary syndrome, type 2 diabetes, weather conditions, stress, disease, and hormonal imbalances (Senie, 2014).

Think back to Linda, who was introduced at the beginning of the chapter. What questions might need to be asked to assess her condition? What laboratory work might be anticipated to validate her heavier flow?

Although menstruation is a normal process, various cultural groups have taken a wide variety of attitudes toward it, seeing it as everything from a sacred time to an unclean time. Folk culture surrounding menstrual-related matters has considerable implications for symptom expression and treatment-seeking behaviour. Research findings indicate the need for education to help adolescent girls manage menstrual symptoms and increase awareness of the benefit of treating them. Given that menstrual-related information comes from mothers, family, and social culture, negative attitudes toward their monthly cycles can be formed in young impressionable girls. Nurses, through formal instruction, can help young girls in shaping good menstrual attitudes and a more positive image of this natural physiologic process (Clark & Paraska, 2014).

Consider This

We had been married 2 years when my husband and I decided to start a family. I began thinking back to my high school biology class and tried to remember about ovulation and what to look for. I also used the Internet to find the answers I was seeking. As I was reading, it all started to come into place. During ovulation, a woman's cervical mucus increases and she experiences a wet sensation for several days midcycle. The mucus also becomes stretchable during this time. In addition, body temperature rises slightly and then falls if no conception takes place. Armed with this knowledge, I began to check my temperature daily before arising and began to monitor the consistency of my cervical mucus. I figured that monitoring these two signs of ovulation could help me discover the best time to conceive. After 6 months of trying without results, I wondered what I was doing wrong. Did I really understand my body's reproductive activity?

Thoughts: *What additional suggestions might the nurse offer this woman in her journey to conception? What community resources might be available to assist this couple? How does knowledge of the reproductive system help nurses take care of couples who are trying to become pregnant?*

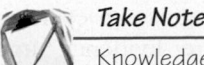

Menstrual Cycle Hormones

The menstrual cycle involves a complex interaction of hormones. The predominant hormones include gonadotropin-releasing hormone (GnRH), FSH, LH, estrogen, progesterone, and prostaglandins. Box 3.1 summarizes menstrual cycle hormones.

Gonadotropin-Releasing Hormone

GnRH is secreted from the hypothalamus in a pulsatile manner throughout the reproductive cycle. It pulsates slowly during the follicular phase and increases during the luteal phase. GnRH induces the release of FSH and LH to assist with ovulation.

Follicle-Stimulating Hormone

FSH is secreted by the anterior pituitary gland and is primarily responsible for the maturation of the ovarian follicle. FSH secretion is highest and most important during the first week of the follicular phase of the reproductive cycle.

Luteinizing Hormone

LH is secreted by the anterior pituitary gland and is required for both the final maturation of preovulatory follicles and luteinization of the ruptured follicle. As a result, estrogen production declines and progesterone secretion continues. Thus, estrogen levels fall a day before ovulation, and progesterone levels begin to rise.

Estrogen

Estrogen is secreted by the ovaries and is crucial for the development and maturation of the follicle. Estrogen is predominant at the end of the proliferative phase, directly preceding ovulation. After ovulation, estrogen levels drop sharply as progesterone dominates. In the endometrial cycle, estrogen induces proliferation of the endometrial glands. Estrogen also causes the uterus to increase in size and weight because of increased glycogen, amino acids, electrolytes, and water. Blood supply is expanded as well.

Progesterone

Progesterone is secreted by the corpus luteum. Progesterone levels increase just before ovulation and peak 5 to 7 days after ovulation. During the luteal phase, progesterone induces swelling and increased secretion of the endometrium. This hormone is often called the hormone of pregnancy because of its calming effect (reduces uterine contractions) on the uterus, allowing pregnancy to be maintained.

Prostaglandins

Prostaglandins are primary mediators of the body's inflammatory processes and are essential for the normal physiologic function of the female reproductive system. They are a closely related group of oxygenated fatty acids that are produced by the endometrium, with a variety of effects throughout the body. Although they have regulatory effects and are sometimes called hormones, prostaglandins are not technically hormones because they are produced by all tissues rather than by special glands (Jones & Lopez, 2014). Prostaglandins increase during follicular maturation and play a key role in ovulation by freeing the ovum inside the graafian follicle. Large amounts of prostaglandins are found in menstrual blood. Current research suggests that the pathogenesis of menstrual cramps/pain is due to prostaglandin F2a (PGF2a), a potent myometrial stimulant and vasoconstrictor, in the secretory endometrium. Elevated prostaglandin levels are found in the endometrial fluid of women with dysmenorrhea (painful menses) and correlates well with their degree of pain. Nonsteroidal anti-inflammatory drugs have been introduced as the primary choice of treatment for menstrual cramps (Nguyen, Humphrey, Kitchen, Rehman, & Norquist, 2015).

Perimenopause

Perimenopause or menopausal transition and menopause are biologic markers of the transition from young adulthood

---

BOX 3.1

SUMMARY OF MENSTRUAL CYCLE HORMONES

- Luteinizing hormone (LH) rises and stimulates the follicle to produce estrogen.
- As estrogen is produced by the follicle, estrogen levels rise, inhibiting the output of LH.
- Ovulation occurs after an LH surge damages the estrogen-producing cells, resulting in a decline in estrogen.
- The LH surge results in establishment of the corpus luteum, which produces estrogen and progesterone.
- Estrogen and progesterone levels rise, suppressing LH output.
- Lack of LH promotes degeneration of the corpus luteum.
- Cessation of the corpus luteum means a decline in estrogen and progesterone output.
- The decline of the ovarian hormones ends their negative effect on the secretion of LH.
- LH is secreted, and the menstrual cycle begins again.

to middle age. Neither of these is a symptom or disease, but rather a natural maturing of the reproductive system.

During the perimenopausal years (2 to 8 years prior to menopause), women may experience physical changes associated with decreasing estrogen levels, which may include vasomotor symptoms of hot flashes, irregular menstrual cycles, sleep disruptions, forgetfulness, irritability, mood disturbances, weight gain and bloating, irregular menses, headaches, decreased vaginal lubrication, night sweats, fatigue, vaginal atrophy, and depression (McNamara, Batur, & DeSapri, 2015). Vasomotor symptoms (hot flashes and night sweats) are the most common complaints for which women seek treatment. Several therapies can be considered to help manage these complaints. Choosing an appropriate treatment approach for the management of these symptoms requires careful assessment of the risk/benefit ratio of each alternative, as well as individual client preference (Schuiling & Likis, 2016).

Menopause

Menopause is a universal and irreversible part of the overall aging process involving a woman's reproductive system, after which she no longer menstruates. This naturally occurring phase of every woman's life marks the end of her childbearing capacity. The average age of natural menopause—defined as 1 year without a menstrual period—is 50 to 51 years old (Alexander, LaRosa, Bader, & Garfield, 2014). This period is frequently termed the *climacteric* or *perimenopause,* but mostly recently the *menopausal transition* has been used (Hoyt & Falconi, 2015). As the average life expectancy for women increases, the number of women reaching and living in menopause has escalated. Most women can expect to spend more than one third of their lives beyond menopause. It is usually marked by atrophy of the breasts, uterus, fallopian tubes, and ovaries (Crawford, 2015).

Many women pass through menopause without untoward symptoms. These women remain active and in good health with little interruption of their daily routines. Other women experience vasomotor symptoms, which give rise to sensations of heat, cold, sweating, headache, insomnia, and irritability. A recent study found that women experiencing menopausal symptoms reported significantly lower health-related quality of life and significantly high work impairment when compared to women without menopausal symptoms (Coney, 2018).

Until recently, hormone therapy was the mainstay of menopause pharmacotherapy, but with the recent results of the Women's Health Initiative trial and the Heart and Estrogen Replacement Study (HERS), the use of hormone therapy has become controversial. Many women have turned to nontraditional remedies to manage their menopausal symptoms. Common complementary and alternative medicine (CAM) remedies used for the treatment of menopausal symptoms include black cohosh, dong quai, St. John's wort, hops, wild yam, ginseng, evening primrose oil, exercise, and acupuncture. Evidence supporting the efficacy and safety of most CAM for relief of menopausal symptoms is limited and most of the reports of efficacy don't support use of them (Wicks & Mahady, 2015). Nurses can play a major role in assisting menopausal women by educating and counselling them about the multitude of options available for disease prevention and treatments for menopausal symptoms during this time of change in their lives. Menopause should be an opportunity for women to strive for a healthy, long life, and nurses can help to make this opportunity a reality. (See Chapter 4 for more information about menopause.)

> **Recall Linda, who was experiencing changes in her menstrual patterns. Which hormones might be changing, and which systems might they affect? What approach should the nurse take to enlighten Linda about what is happening to her?**

MALE REPRODUCTIVE ANATOMY AND PHYSIOLOGY

The male reproductive system, like that of the female, consists of those organs that facilitate reproduction. The male organs are specialized to produce and maintain the male sex cells, or sperm; to transport them, along with supporting fluids, to the female reproductive system; and to secrete the male hormone testosterone. The organs of the male reproductive system include the penis, scrotum, two **testes** (where sperm cells and testosterone are made), and accessory organs (epididymis, vas deferens, seminal vesicles, ejaculatory duct, urethra, bulbourethral glands, and prostate gland).

External Male Reproductive Organs

The penis and the scrotum form the external genitalia in the male (Fig. 3.7).

Penis

The penis is the organ for copulation and serves as the outlet for both sperm and urine. The penis becomes engorged with blood during sexual arousal and is inserted into the female vagina during intercourse for reproduction. The skin of the penis is thin, with no hairs. The prepuce (foreskin) is a circular fold of skin that extends over the glans unless it is removed by circumcision. The urinary meatus, located at the tip of the penis, serves as the external opening to the urethra (Fig. 3.8). The penis is composed mostly of erectile tissue. Most of the body of the penis consists of three cylindrical spaces (sinuses) of erectile tissue. The two larger ones, the corpora cavernosa, are side by side. The third sinus, the corpus spongiosum, surrounds the urethra. Erection results when nerve impulses from the autonomic nervous system dilate the arteries of the penis, allowing arterial blood to flow into the erectile tissues of the organ.

Scrotum

The scrotum is the thin-skinned sac that surrounds and protects the testes. The scrotum also acts as a climate-control system for the testes, because they need to be slightly cooler than body temperature to allow normal sperm development. The scrotum is covered with hair starting in puberty. The cremaster muscles in the scrotal wall relax or contract to allow the testes to hang farther from the body to cool or to be pulled closer to the body for warmth or protection (Patton & Thibodeau, 2015). A medial septum divides the scrotum into two chambers, each of which encloses a testis.

Internal Male Reproductive Organs

The internal structures include the testes, the ductal system, and accessory glands (Fig. 3.9).

Testes

The testes are oval bodies in the size of large olives that lie in the scrotum; usually the left testis hangs a

FIGURE 3.7 **The external male reproductive organs. (Photo by B. Proud.)**

Scrotum — Penis shaft — Glans penis

FIGURE 3.8 **The urinary meatus. (Photo by B. Proud.)**

FIGURE 3.9 Lateral view of the internal male reproductive organs. (Adapted from Anatomical Chart Company. [2001]. *Atlas of human anatomy*. Springhouse, PA: Springhouse.)

Prostate gland
Vas deferens
Corpus cavernosum
Corpus spongiosum
External urethral opening
Epididymis
Testis

Urinary bladder
Openings of ureter
Ampulla of vas deferens
Rectum
Seminal vesicle
Ejaculatory duct
Bulbourethral gland and duct
Urethra

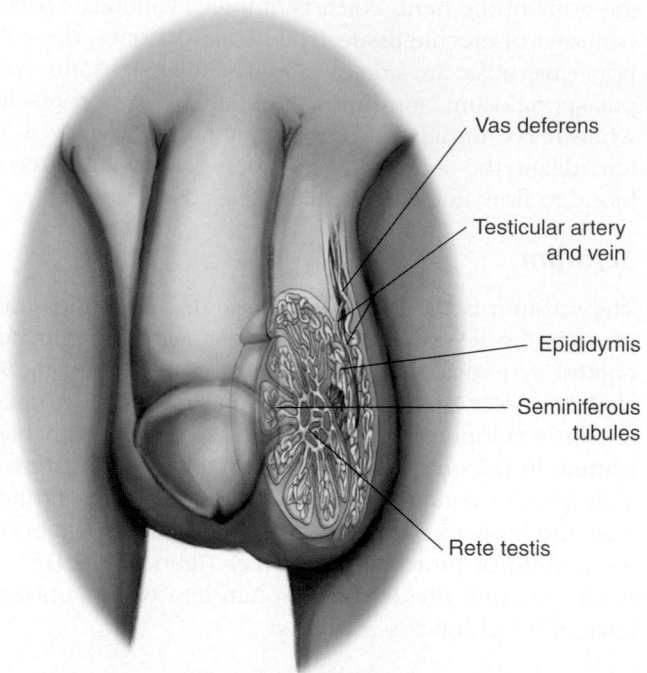

FIGURE 3.10 Internal structures of a testis.

little lower than the right one. These two nut-like structures are analogous to ovaries in the female. The testes have two functions: producing sperm, and synthesizing testosterone (the primary male sex hormone). Sperm is produced in the seminiferous tubules of the testes. Similar to the female reproductive system, the anterior pituitary releases the gonadotropins, FSH and LH. These hormones stimulate the testes to produce testosterone, which assists in maintaining spermatogenesis, increases sperm production by the seminiferous tubules, and stimulates production of seminal fluid (Jones & Lopez, 2014). The epididymis, which lies against the testes, is a coiled tube almost 20 ft long. It collects sperm from the testes and provides the space and environment for sperm to mature (Fig. 3.10).

The Ductal System

The vas deferens is a cord-like duct that transports sperm from the epididymis. One such duct travels from each testis up to the back of the prostate and enters the urethra to form the ejaculatory ducts. Other structures, such as blood vessels and nerves, also travel along with each vas deferens and together form the spermatic cord. The urethra is the terminal duct of the reproductive and urinary systems, serving as a passageway for semen (fluid containing sperm) and urine. It passes through the prostate gland and the penis and opens to the outside at the urethral meatus.

Accessory Glands

The seminal vesicles, which produce nutrient seminal fluid, and the prostate gland, which produces alkaline prostatic fluid, are both connected to the ejaculatory duct leading into the urethra. The paired seminal vesicles are convoluted pouch-like structures lying posterior to, and at the base of, the urinary bladder in front of the rectum. They secrete an alkaline fluid that contains fructose and prostaglandins. The fructose supplies energy to the sperm on its journey to meet the ovum, and the prostaglandins assist in sperm mobility.

The prostate gland lies just under the bladder in the pelvis and surrounds the middle portion of the urethra. Usually the size of a walnut, this gland enlarges with age. The prostate and the seminal vesicles above it produce fluid that nourishes the sperm. This fluid provides most of the volume of semen, the secretion in which sperm are expelled during ejaculation. Other fluid that makes up the semen comes from the vas deferens and from mucous glands in the head of the penis.

The bulbourethral glands (Cowper's glands) are two small structures about the size of peas, located inferior to the prostate gland. They are composed of several tubes whose epithelial linings secrete a mucus-like fluid. It is released in response to sexual stimulation and lubricates the head of the penis in preparation for sexual intercourse, in addition, neutralizes the acidity of the urethra to protect sperm during their journey out of the body during ejaculation. Their existence is said to be constant, but they gradually diminish in size with advancing age.

Male Sexual Response

Regardless of the type of sexual stimulation, the physiologic response in both men and women is similar and usually follows a five-phase pattern, as described earlier:
1. *Desire:* starts with a desire for sexual intimacy. This can also be termed libido.
2. *Excitement:* The man experiences sexual arousal with either thoughts or physical sexual stimuli which cause specific changes such as the heart beating faster, blood pressure rising, the testicles enlarging and more blood flowing into the penis, creating an erection.
3. *Plateau:* is the phase between excitement and orgasm in which the head of the penis enlarges and becomes more purplish in colour; the glands secrete semen into the urethra; and it is challenging to stop from having an orgasm.
4. *Orgasm:* is a total body response. The tension that built up during the previous two phases is released. It triggers a series of muscle spasms in the legs, stomach, arms, back, and penis. The feelings are intense and pleasurable. Ejaculation of semen occurs at this time.

5. *Resolution:* The body returns to the physiologic non-stimulated state. The blood flows out of the penis and erection ceases; an overall feeling of relaxation ensues, and the testes and scrotum return to their normal size (Housman & Odum, 2016).

Sexual behaviour involves the participation of autonomic and somatic nerves and the integration of numerous spinal sites in the central nervous system (CNS). The penile portion of the process that leads to erections represents only a single component. Penile erections are an integration of complex physiologic processes involving the CNS, peripheral nervous system, and hormonal and vascular systems (Sherwood, 2016). With sexual stimulation, the arteries leading to the penis dilate and increase blood flow into erectile tissues. At the same time, the erectile tissue compresses the veins of the penis, reducing blood flow away from the penis. Blood accumulates, causing the penis to swell and elongate and producing an erection. As in women, the culmination of sexual stimulation is an orgasm, a pleasurable feeling of physiologic and psychological release.

Orgasm is accompanied by emission (movement of sperm from the testes and fluids from the accessory glands) into the urethra, where the sperm and fluids are mixed to form semen. As the urethra fills with semen, the base of the erect penis contracts, this increases pressure. This pressure forces the semen through the urethra to the outside (ejaculation). During ejaculation, the ducts of the testes, epididymis, and vas deferens contract and cause expulsion of sperm into the urethra, where the sperm mixes with the seminal and prostatic fluids. These substances, together with mucus secreted by accessory glands, form the semen, which is discharged from the urethra.

KEY CONCEPTS

- The female reproductive system produces the female reproductive cells (the eggs, or ova) and contains an organ (uterus) where the fetus develops. The male reproductive system produces the male reproductive cells (the sperm) and contains an organ (penis) that deposits the sperm within the female.

- The internal female reproductive organs consist of the vagina, the uterus, the fallopian tubes, and the ovaries. The external female reproductive organs make up the vulva. These include the mons pubis, the labia majora and minora, the clitoris and prepuce, structures within the vestibule, and the perineum.

- The breasts are accessory organs of the female reproductive system that are specialized to produce and secrete milk following pregnancy.

- The main function of the reproductive cycle is to stimulate growth of a follicle to release an egg and prepare a site for implantation if fertilization occurs.

- Menstruation, the monthly shedding of the uterine lining, marks the beginning and end of the cycle if fertilization does not occur.

- The ovarian cycle is the series of events associated with a developing oocyte (ovum or egg) within the ovaries.

- At ovulation, a mature follicle ruptures in response to a surge of luteinizing hormone (LH), releasing a mature oocyte (ovum).

- The endometrial cycle is divided into four phases: the follicular or proliferative phase, the luteal or secretory phase, the ischemic phase, and the menstrual phase.

- The menstrual cycle involves a complex interaction of hormones. The predominant hormones are gonadotropin-releasing hormone (GnRH), follicle-stimulating hormone (FSH), LH, estrogen, progesterone, and prostaglandins.

- The organs of the male reproductive system include the penis, scrotum, two testes (where sperm cells and testosterone are made), and accessory organs (epididymis, vas deferens, seminal vesicles, ejaculatory ducts, urethra, bulbourethral glands, and prostate gland).

REFERENCES AND RECOMMENDED READINGS

Acién, M., & Acién, P. (2015). Normal embryological development of the female genital tract. In *Female genital tract congenital malformations* (pp. 3–14). London, UK: Springer.

Alexander, L. L., LaRosa, J. H., Bader, H., & Garfield, S. (2014). *New dimensions in women's health* (6th ed.). Sudbury, MA: Jones and Bartlett.

Clark, C. C., & Paraska, K. K. (2014). *Health promotion for nurses: A practical guide*. Burlington, MA: Jones & Bartlett Learning.

Coney, P. (2018). *Menopause. eMedicine*. Retrieved from http://emedicine.medscape.com/article/264088-overview

Crawford, S. L. (2015). What should women expect after stopping hormone therapy? *Menopause, 22*(4), 367–368.

Davis, S. R. (2013). Androgen therapy in women, beyond libido. *Climacteric, 16*, 18–24.

Farage, M. A., Miller, K. W., & Maibach, H. I. (2015). Post-menopausal vulva and vagina. In *Skin, mucosa and menopause* (pp. 385–395). Heidelberg, Berlin: Springer.

Housman, J., & Odum, M. (2016). *Alters & Schiff's essential concepts for healthy living* (7th ed.). Burlington, MA: Jones & Bartlett Learning.

Hoyt, L. T., & Falconi, A. (2015). Puberty and perimenopause: Reproductive transitions and their implications for women's health. *Social Science & Medicine, 132*, 103–112.

Jones, R. E., & Lopez, K. H. (2014). *Human reproductive biology* (4th ed.). Waltham, MA: Elsevier.

Kandeel, F. (2014). *Female reproductive and sexual medicine.* New York: Springer.

King, T. L., Brucker, M. C., Kriebs, J. M., Fahey, J. O., Gegor, C. L., & Varney, H. (2015). *Varney's midwifery* (5th ed.). Burlington, MA: Jones & Bartlett Learning.

Krieger, N., Kiang, M. V., Kosheleva, A., Waterman, P. D., Chen, J. T., & Beckfield, J. (2015). Age at menarche: 50-year socioeconomic trends among US-born black and white women. *American Journal of Public Health, 105*(2), 388–397.

Lawrence, R. A., Lawrence, R. M. (2011). *Breastfeeding, a guide for the medical profession* (7th ed.). Maryland Heights, Missouri: Elsevier Mosby.

McNamara, M., Batur, P., & DeSapri, K. T. (2015). In the clinic. Perimenopause. *Annals of Internal Medicine, 162*(3), ITC1–ITC15.

Minkin, M. J. (2016). Sexual health and relationships after age 60. *Matutitas, 83*, 27–32.

Nguyen, A. M., Humphrey, L., Kitchen, H., Rehman, T., & Norquist, J. M. (2015). A qualitative study to develop a patient-reported outcome for dysmenorrhea. *Quality of Life Research, 24*(1), 181–191.

Oyelowo, T., & Johnson, J. L. (2016). *A guide to women's health* (2nd ed.). Burlington, MA: Jones & Bartlett Learning.

Patton, K. T., & Thibodeau, G. A. (2015). *Anatomy & physiology* (9th ed.). St. Louis, MO: Mosby Elsevier.

Patton, K. T., & Thibodeau, G. A. (2016). *The Human Body in Health and Disease* (6th ed.). St. Louis, MO: Mosby Elsevier.

Pauls, R. N. (2015). Anatomy of the clitoris and the female sexual response. *Clinical Anatomy, 28*(3), 376–384.

Schuiling, K. D., & Likis, F. E. (2016). *Women's gynecologic health* (3rd ed.). Burlington, MA: Jones & Bartlett Learning.

Senie, R. T. (2014). *Epidemiology of women's health.* Burlington, MA: Jones & Bartlett Learning.

Sherwood, L. (2016). *Human physiology: From cells to systems* (9th ed.). Boston, MA: Cengage Learning.

Tambouret, R. H., & Wilbur, D. C. (2015). Normal histology and cytology of the endocervix and endometrium. In *Glandular lesions of the uterine cervix* (pp. 25–40). New York: Springer.

Thornhill, R., & Gangestad, S. W. (2015). The functional design and phylogeny of women's sexuality. In T. K. Shackelford & R. D. Hansen (Eds.), *Evolutionary psychology. The evolution of sexuality* (pp. 149–184). Cham, Switzerland: Springer International Publishing.

Velkey, J. M., Hall, A. H., & Robboy, S. J. (2015). Normal vulva: Embryology, anatomy, and histology. In *Vulvar pathology* (pp. 3–17). New York: Springer.

Wheatley, J. R., & Puts, D. A. (2015). Evolutionary science of female orgasm. In *The evolution of sexuality* (pp. 123–148). Springer International Publishing.

Wicks, S. M., & Mahady, G. B. (2015). Herbal and complementary medicines used for women's health. In *Medicines for women* (pp. 373–399). Springer International Publishing.

CHAPTER **WORKSHEET**

MULTIPLE CHOICE QUESTIONS

1. The predominant anterior pituitary hormones that orchestrate the menstrual cycle include:
   a. Thyroid-stimulating hormone (TSH)
   b. Follicle-stimulating hormone (FSH)
   c. Corticotropin-releasing hormone (CRH)
   d. Gonadotropin-releasing hormone (GnRH)

2. Which glands are located on either side of the female urethra and secrete mucus to keep the opening moist and lubricated for urination?
   a. Cowper's
   b. Bartholin's
   c. Skene's
   d. Seminal

3. What event occurs during the proliferative phase of the menstrual cycle?
   a. Menstrual flow starts
   b. Endometrium thickens
   c. Ovulation occurs
   d. Progesterone secretion peaks

4. Which hormone is produced in high levels to prepare the endometrium for implantation just after ovulation by the corpus luteum?
   a. Estrogen
   b. Prostaglandins
   c. Prolactin
   d. Progesterone

5. Sperm maturation and storage in the male reproductive system occur in the:
   a. Testes
   b. Vas deferens
   c. Epididymis
   d. Seminal vesicles

6. The nurse is preparing to teach a class to a group of middle-aged women regarding the most common vasomotor symptoms experienced during menopause and possible modalities of treatment available. Common vasomotor symptoms would include which of the following?
   a. Chronic fatigue and confusion
   b. Forgetfulness and irritability
   c. Night sweats and hot flashes
   d. Decrease in sexual response and appetite

CRITICAL THINKING EXERCISE

1. The school nurse was asked to speak to a 10th-grade biology class about menstruation. The teacher felt that the students did not understand this monthly event and wanted to dispel some myths about it. After the nurse explains the factors influencing the menses, one girl asks, "Could someone get pregnant if she had sex during her period?"
   a. How should the nurse respond to this question?
   b. What factor regarding the menstrual cycle was not clarified?
   c. What additional topics might this question lead to that might be discussed?

STUDY ACTIVITIES

1. Should sex education be taught in public schools, and if so, what topics should be addressed? Debate the pros and cons of teaching this and then outline which topics should be covered.

2. Respond to the following as a topic sentence: "When I was growing up, talking about sexual matters with my parents was _____ because _____ Now the situation is _____?

3. List the predominant hormones and their function in the menstrual cycle.

4. The ovarian cycle describes the series of events associated with the development of the _____ within the ovaries.

5. Sperm cells and the male hormone testosterone are made in which of the following structures? Select all that apply.
   a. Vas deferens
   b. Penis
   c. Scrotum
   d. Ejaculatory ducts
   e. Prostate gland
   f. Testes
   g. Seminiferous tubules
   h. Bulbourethral glands

BRINGING IT ALL TOGETHER: A CASE STUDY

A 53-year-old woman came to see her nurse practitioner for her annual examination. She had a hysterectomy 20 years ago for a prolapsed uterus and has been healthy up until now. She had a long list of symptoms that had been bothering her, but until recently just chalked them up to the aging process. She told the nurse practitioner that she was experiencing insomnia, weight gain around her middle despite not consuming additional calories, painful intercourse and hot flashes that were increasing in frequency throughout the day and night. She had been taking black cohosh for these distressing symptoms for the past several months, but was not getting any relief. She was concerned that something awful was wrong with her since this natural herb was not reducing her symptoms and they seemed to be getting worse.

1. What explanation should be offered to this woman regarding what is causing her distress?
2. What is the current thinking regarding natural herbs in the treatment of menopausal symptoms?
3. What treatment might be suggested for this woman?
4. What is the current principle concerning hormone therapy in the treatment of menopause?

4

Common Reproductive Issues

Learning Objectives

Upon completion of the chapter, you will be able to:

1. Examine common reproductive concerns in terms of symptoms, diagnostic tests, and appropriate interventions.

2. Identify risk factors and outline appropriate client education needed in common reproductive disorders.

3. Compare and contrast the various contraceptive methods available and their overall effectiveness.

4. Analyze the physiologic and psychological aspects of menopausal transition.

5. Delineate the nursing management needed for clients experiencing common reproductive disorders.

Izzy, **a 27-year-old, presents to her health care provider complaining of progressive severe pelvic pain associated with her monthly periods. She has to take off work and "dope up" with pills to endure the pain. In addition, she has been trying to conceive for over a year without any luck.**

INTRODUCTION

Good health throughout the life cycle begins with the individual. Women today can expect to live well into their 80s and need to be proactive in maintaining their own quality of life. Women need to take steps to reduce their risk of disease and need to become active partners with their health care professional to identify problems early, when treatment may be most successful (Teaching Guidelines 4.1). Nurses can assist clients in maintaining their quality of life by helping them to become more attuned to their body and its clues and can use the assessment period as an opportunity for teaching and counselling. Nurses are in a prime position to offer information that provides clients with the tools needed to maintain a healthy lifestyle and assist in altering behaviours that may cause harm or illness.

 Teaching Guidelines 4.1

TIPS FOR BEING AN ACTIVE PARTNER IN MANAGING YOUR HEALTH

- Become an informed consumer. Read, ask, and search.
- Know your family history and know factors that put you at high risk.
- Maintain a healthy lifestyle and let moderation be your guide.
- Schedule regular medical checkups and screenings for early detection.
- Ask your health care provider for a full explanation of any treatment.
- Seek a second medical opinion if you feel you need more information.
- Know when to seek medical care by being aware of disease symptoms.

Common reproductive issues addressed in this chapter that nurses might encounter in caring for clients include menstrual disorders, infertility, contraception, abortion, and the menopausal transition.

EQUITABLE HEALTH CARE FOR ALL

A group that has long been marginalized within many aspects of society including reproductive health care is the **transgender** community and those who identify as gender nonconforming (GNC). Nurses and health care professionals must always remain mindful that not all clients who identify as women will have health care needs involving reproductive organs of **cis-gender** females (those who are assigned the gender of female at birth, and who independently identify as female). And not all clients who have a vagina, cervix, uterus, fallopian tubes, and ovaries will identify as female; they may be GNC or a transgender man (assigned female gender at birth but identify as male). The assumption that all women have vaginas and all men have penises is a form of prejudice called *cis-normativity*, and should be avoided in professional practice. A growing body of evidence indicates that transgender clients access health care significantly less often than cis-gender clients, and face higher risks in many aspects of health (Giblon & Bauer, 2017). For example, transgender women have HIV infection rates 49 times higher than cis-gender women globally (Jones, 2016). Trans clients report a number of barriers to seeking health care, including institutional and social prejudices, substandard care, and even verbal abuse (Bauer & Sheim, 2015; Kosenko, Rintamaki, Raney, & Maness, 2013). The Society of Obstetricians and Gynecologists of Canada (SOGC, 2017), the Canadian Association of Midwives (2015), and the Canadian Association of Schools of Nursing (2017) have each declared the need for health care professionals to provide inclusive reproductive/sexual health care for all clients to avoid marginalizing gender minorities. Nurses and care providers must reflect on any personal biases and approach all clients in a caring manner, creating a safe space for all clients to feel welcome and supported in meeting their health care needs.

MENSTRUAL DISORDERS

Many clients sail through their monthly menstrual cycles with little or no concern. With few symptoms to worry about, their menses are like clockwork, starting and stopping at nearly the same times every month. For others, the menstrual cycle causes physical and emotional symptoms that initiate visits to their health care provider for consultation. The following menstruation-related conditions will be discussed in this section: amenorrhea, dysmenorrhea, abnormal uterine bleeding (AUB), premenstrual syndrome (PMS), premenstrual dysphoric disorder (PMDD), and endometriosis. To gain an understanding of menstrual disorders, nurses should know the terms used to describe them (Box 4.1).

Amenorrhea

Amenorrhea simply means absence of menses. Amenorrhea is normal in prepubertal, pregnant, postpartum, and postmenopausal females. The uterus, endometrial lining,

---

BOX 4.1

MENSTRUAL DISORDER VOCABULARY

- *meno* = menstrual related
- *metro* = time
- *oligo* = few
- *a* = without, none, or lack of
- *rhagia* = excess or abnormal
- *dys* = not or pain
- *rhea* = flow

ovaries, pituitary, and hypothalamus must function properly and in harmony for a menstrual cycle to occur. The two categories of amenorrhea are primary and secondary amenorrhea. Primary amenorrhea is defined as either the:

1. Absence of menses by age 14, with absence of growth and development of secondary sexual characteristics, or
2. Absence of menses by age 16, with normal development of secondary sexual characteristics (Schuiling & Likis, 2016).

In Canada, the average age at menarche is 12.7 years. Over 80% of young girls will begin menstruating by age 14 (Al-Sahab, Ardern, Hamadeh, & Tamim, 2010). Findings of recent studies indicate that age at menarche has overall declined since the 20th century (King et al., 2015). Once menarche has occurred, cycles may take up to 2 years to become regular, ovulatory cycles. Secondary amenorrhea is the absence of regular menses for three cycles or irregular menses for 6 months in those who have previously menstruated regularly.

Nurses need to consider the causes of amenorrhea as occurring in one of four anatomical areas: outflow area of the uterus and vagina; the ovaries; the pituitary gland; or the central nervous system. Outflow area problems are obstructive in nature and can be found on physical examination, whereas ovarian, pituitary, and central nervous system problems involve disruptions in the hypothalamic–pituitary–ovarian axis that controls the neuroendocrine processes required for a normal menstrual cycle and are generally found through laboratory analysis (King et al., 2015).

Etiology

Primary amenorrhea has multiple causes:
- Extreme weight gain or loss
- Congenital abnormalities of the reproductive system
- Stress from a major life event
- Excessive exercise
- Eating disorders (anorexia nervosa or bulimia)
- Cushing disease
- Polycystic ovary syndrome
- Hypothyroidism
- Turner syndrome—defective development of the gonads (ovary or testes)
- Imperforate hymen
- Chronic illness—diabetes, thyroid disease, depression
- Pregnancy
- Cystic fibrosis
- Congenital heart disease (cyanotic)
- Ovarian or adrenal tumours

Causes of secondary amenorrhea can include:
- Pregnancy
- Breastfeeding
- Emotional stress
- Pituitary, ovarian, or adrenal tumours
- Depression
- Hyperthyroid or hypothyroid conditions
- Malnutrition
- Hyperprolactinemia
- Rapid weight gain or loss
- Chemotherapy or radiation therapy to the pelvic area
- Vigorous exercise, such as long-distance running
- Kidney failure
- Colitis
- Chemotherapy, irradiation
- Use of tranquilizers or antidepressants
- Postpartum pituitary necrosis (Sheehan syndrome)
- Early menopause (Kovanci & Schutt, 2015)

Therapeutic Management

Therapeutic intervention depends on the cause of the amenorrhea. The treatment of primary amenorrhea involves the correction of any underlying disorders and estrogen replacement therapy to stimulate the development of secondary sexual characteristics (Moses, 2018a). If a pituitary tumour is the cause, it might be treated with drug therapy, surgical resection, or radiation therapy. Surgery might be needed to correct any structural abnormalities of the genital tract. Dopamine agonists are effective in treating hyperprolactinemia. In most cases, this treatment restores normal ovarian endocrine function and ovulation (Goswami, 2015). Therapeutic interventions for secondary amenorrhea can include:
- Cyclic progesterone, when the cause is anovulation, or oral contraceptives (OCs)
- Bromocriptine to treat hyperprolactinemia
- Nutritional counselling to address anorexia, bulimia, or obesity
- Gonadotropin-releasing hormone (GnRH), when the cause is hypothalamic failure
- Thyroid hormone replacement, when the cause is hypothyroidism (Creatsas & Creatsa, 2015)

Nursing Assessment

Nursing assessment for a client experiencing amenorrhea includes a thorough health history, physical examination, and several laboratory and diagnostic tests of selected hormone levels to help identify an underlying cause.

HEALTH HISTORY AND PHYSICAL EXAMINATION

A thorough history and physical examination are needed to determine the etiology. The history should include questions about the client's menstrual history; past illnesses; hospitalizations and surgeries; obstetric history; use of prescription and over-the-counter drugs; recent or past lifestyle changes; and history of present illness, with an assessment of anybody changes.

The physical examination should begin with an overall assessment of the client's nutritional status and general health. A sensitive and gentle approach to the pelvic examination is critical in young clients. Height, weight, and body mass index (BMI) should be taken, along with vital signs. Hypothermia, bradycardia, hypotension, and reduced subcutaneous fat may be observed in those with anorexia nervosa. Facial hair and acne might be evidence of androgen excess secondary to a tumour. The presence or absence of axillary and pubic hair may indicate adrenal and ovarian hyposecretion or delayed puberty. A general physical examination may uncover unexpected findings that are indirectly related to amenorrhea. For example, hepatosplenomegaly, which may suggest a chronic systemic disease or an enlarged thyroid gland, might point to a thyroid disorder as well as a reason for amenorrhea (Tharpe, Farley, & Jordan, 2016). Examination of the breasts also deserves careful attention because breast development is a reliable indicator of estrogen production. The Tanner stages of breast development should also be noted. The Tanner stages include:

- Stage I—Papilla elevation only
- Stage II—Breast buds palpable and areolae enlarge ~11 years old
- Stage III—Elevation of breast contour; areolae enlarge ~12 years old
- Stage IV—Areolae forms secondary mound on the breast ~13 years old
- Stage V—Adult breast contour; areola recesses to breast contour (Moses, 2018b)

Information gained from the history and physical examination clearly can exclude certain diagnostic possibilities, but first impressions also can be deceiving and lead to errors in judgment. A methodical, systematic approach to identify the etiology of amenorrhea is best.

LABORATORY AND DIAGNOSTIC TESTS

Common laboratory tests that might be ordered to determine the cause of amenorrhea include:

- Karyotype (might be positive for Turner syndrome)
- Ultrasound to detect ovarian cysts
- Quantitative human chorionic gonadotropin (hCG) test to rule out pregnancy
- Thyroid function studies to determine thyroid disorder
- Prolactin level (an elevated level might indicate a pituitary tumour)
- Follicle-stimulating hormone (FSH) level (an elevated level might indicate ovarian failure)
- Luteinizing hormone (LH) level (an elevated level might indicate gonadal dysfunction)
- 17-Ketosteroids (an elevated level might indicate an adrenal tumour) (Pagana, Pagana, & Pagana, 2015)

Nursing Management

Counselling and education are primary interventions and appropriate nursing roles. Address the diverse causes

of amenorrhea, the relationship to sexual identity, possible infertility, and the possibility of a tumour or a life-threatening disease. Evidence is mounting that loss of menstrual regularity is a risk factor for later development of osteoporosis and hip fractures, so treatment to restore regular menstrual cycles is essential (Carlson, 2015). In addition, inform the client about the purpose of each diagnostic test, how it is performed, and when the results will be available to discuss with her. Listening sensitively, interviewing, and presenting treatment options are paramount to gain the client's cooperation and understanding.

Nutritional counselling is also vital in managing this disorder, especially if the client has findings suggestive of an eating disorder. The relation between eating disorders and menstrual dysfunction has been identified in research studies. Careful evaluation of menstrual status is warranted for all clients with eating disorders. Timely intervention is important because shorter duration of illness is associated with improved outcomes (Golden et al., 2015). Although not all causes can be addressed by making lifestyle changes, emphasize maintaining a healthy lifestyle (Teaching Guidelines 4.2).

Teaching Guidelines 4.2
TIPS FOR MAINTAINING A HEALTHY LIFESTYLE

- Balance energy expenditure with energy intake to maintain ideal weight range.
- Modify your diet to maintain ideal weight to avoid becoming over weight.
- Avoid excessive use of alcohol and mood-altering or sedative drugs.
- Avoid cigarette smoking to prevent cardiovascular disease and lung cancer.
- Identify areas of emotional stress and seek assistance to resolve them.
- Balance work, recreation, and rest to reduce anxiety and stress in life.
- Maintain a positive outlook regarding the diagnosis and prognosis.
- Participate in ongoing care to monitor any medical conditions.
- Maintain bone density through:
  - Calcium intake (1,200 to 1,600 mg daily)
  - Vitamin D (600 to 1,000 International Units/daily)
  - Weightbearing exercise (30 minutes or more daily)
  - Hormone therapy for low risk, postmenopausal clients

Adapted from Centers for Disease Control and Prevention (CDC). (2016b). *Healthy eating for a healthy weight.* Retrieved from http://www.cdc.gov/healthyweight/healthy_eating/; Housman, J., & Odum, M. (2016). *Alters & Schiff's essential concepts for healthy living* (7th ed.). Burlington, MA: Jones & Bartlett Learning.

Dysmenorrhea

Dysmenorrhea refers to painful menstruation and is a common problem in adolescence. This condition has also been termed *cyclic perimenstrual pain.* Usually, pain starts along with the start of bleeding and lasts for 48 to 72 hours (Creatsas & Creatsa, 2015). The term *dysmenorrhea* is derived from the Greek words *dys*, meaning "difficult, painful, or abnormal," and *rrhea*, meaning "flow." Based on results of large epidemiologic studies, it is estimated that it may affect more than half of menstruating individuals. It is the leading cause of absenteeism of work and school and has adverse effects on the quality of life of young women (Joshi, Kural, Agrawal, Noor, & Patil, 2015). Another recent research study linked early smoking (<13 years old) to an increased risk for developing chronic dysmenorrhea (Weinberger et al., 2015). Uterine contractions occur during all periods, but in some clients these cramps can be frequent and very intense. It has a major impact on clients' quality of life, work productivity, and health care utilization. Dysmenorrhea is classified as primary (spasmodic) or secondary (congestive) (Calis, Popat, Dang, & Kalantaridou, 2017).

Etiology

Primary dysmenorrhea refers to painful menstrual bleedings in the absence of any detectable underlying pathology. It is caused by increased prostaglandin production by the endometrium in an ovulatory cycle. This hormone causes contraction of the uterus, and levels tend to be higher in clients with severe menstrual pain than those who experience mild or no menstrual pain. Dysmenorrhea is caused by an excess of prostaglandin production. These levels are highest during the first 2 days of menses, when symptoms peak (Maurice & Rosenzweig, 2015). This results in increased rhythmic uterine contractions from vasoconstriction of the small vessels of the uterine wall. This condition usually begins within a few years of the onset of ovulatory cycles at menarche.

Secondary dysmenorrhea is painful menstruation due to pelvic or uterine pathology. It may be caused by endometriosis, adenomyosis, fibroids, pelvic infection, an intrauterine system (IUS), cervical stenosis, or congenital uterine or vaginal abnormalities. Adenomyosis involves the ingrowth of the endometrium into the uterine musculature. Endometriosis involves ectopic implantation of endometrial tissue in other parts of the pelvis. It occurs most commonly in the third or fourth decades of life and affects 5% to 10% of Canadian (cis-gender) women of reproductive age. The pain is generally chronic, progressive, with relapsing episodes (Singh, Best, Dunn, Leyland, & Wolfman, 2013). Endometriosis is the most common cause of secondary dysmenorrhea and is associated with pain beyond menstruation, dyspareunia, low back pain, heavy or irregular bleeding, bloating, nausea, and vomiting, and infertility (Singh et al., 2013). Treatment is directed toward removing the underlying pathology.

> **Think back to Izzy from the chapter opener. Is her pelvic pain a common experience with menstruation?**

Therapeutic Management

The goal of treatment is to provide adequate pain relief to allow the client to perform normal activities. Current treatment is mainly based on surgery and ovarian suppressive agents (OCs, progestins, GnRH antagonist, levonorgestrel-releasing intrauterine system [LNG-IUS], and androgenic agents). Hormonal treatments are often associated with unwanted side effects and recurrence of symptoms when stopped. Severe dysmenorrhea can be distressing, adversely affecting social and occupational activities. Treatments vary from over-the-counter remedies to hormonal control. However, for some clients, satisfactory pain relief is difficult to achieve and, increasingly, they seek alternative options. Complementary therapies such as acupuncture (needles are used to stimulate certain points of the body to balance the flow of energy within the body) and acupressure (the use of fingers and hands to stimulate acupoints and maintain the balance of energy) are gaining popularity and the evidence base for their use is growing (Wicks & Mahady, 2015).

Therapeutic intervention is directed toward pain relief and building coping strategies that will promote a productive lifestyle. General measures for management include client education and reassurance. Treatment is supportive and should be guided by individual needs. Treatment measures usually include treating infections if present; suppressing the endometrium if endometriosis is suspected by administering low-dose OCs; administering prostaglandin inhibitors to reduce the pain; administering Depo-Provera to suppress ovulation, which thins the endometrial lining of the uterus with subsequent reduction of fluid contents of the uterus during menses; and initiating lifestyle changes (Schuiling & Likis, 2016). Table 4.1 lists selected treatment options for dysmenorrhea.

Nursing Assessment

As with any gynecologic concern, a thorough focused history and physical examination are needed to make the diagnosis of primary or secondary dysmenorrhea. In primary dysmenorrhea, the history usually reveals the typical cramping pain with menstruation, and the physical examination is completely normal. In secondary dysmenorrhea, the history discloses cramping pain starting after 25 years old with a pelvic abnormality, a history of infertility, heavy menstrual flow, irregular cycles, and

TABLE 4.1 TREATMENT OPTIONS FOR DYSMENORRHEA

Therapy Options	Dosage	Comments
Nonsteroidal anti-inflammatory drugs (NSAIDs)		NSAIDs prevent prostaglandin synthesis by inhibiting COX-1 and COX-2 conversion, reducing cramping
Ibuprofen (Advil, Motrin, Midol)	400–800 mg TID	Take with meals Do not take with aspirin
Naproxen (Anaprox, Naprosyn, Aleve)	250–500 mg TID	Avoid alcohol Watch for signs of GI bleeding Same as above
Hormonal contraceptives		Decrease prostaglandin synthesis; second-line treatment
Low-dose oral contraceptives	Taken daily—extended cycle formulas (84 days on, 7 days off)	Take active pills for an extended time to reduce number of monthly cycles
Depo-medroxyprogesterone (DMPA), Depo-Provera	150 mg IM every 12 weeks	Within 9–12 months of DMPA therapy, 75% of women will experience amenorrhea
Levonorgestrel-releasing IUS (Mirena, Jaydess, Kyleena)	Inserted into uterine cavity and may remain for 3–5 years	Inhibits ovulation and decreases thickness of endometrium Inhibits uterine contractions and reduces pain from menstrual cramps
Selective estrogen receptor modulators (SERMs)	Used for clients not responding to NSAIDs and oral contraceptives; dosage is individualized	Adverse effects include hot flashes, nausea and vomiting, and risk of thromboembolism
Raloxifene hydrochloride (Evista); tamoxifen citrate (Nolvadex)		Research is needed to validate effectiveness, doses, side effects, and contradictions
Complementary therapies		
Thiamine (vitamin B)		
Vitamin E (tocopherols)		
Magnesium		Gives sense of control over life
Omega-3 fatty acids (fish oil)		
Lifestyle changes		
Daily exercise		
Limited salty foods		
Weight loss		
Smoking cessation		
Relaxation techniques		

Adapted from Calis, K. A., Popat, V., Dang, D. K., & Kalantaridou, S. N. (2017). Dysmenorrhea. *eMedicine*. Retrieved from http://emedicine.medscape.com/article/253812-overview; King, T. L., Brucker, M. C., Kriebs, J. M., Fahey, J. O., Gegor, C. L., & Varney, H. (2015). *Varney's midwifery* (5th ed.). Burlington, MA: Jones & Bartlett Learning; Schuiling, K. D., & Likis, F. E. (2016). *Women's gynecologic health* (3rd ed.). Burlington, MA: Jones & Bartlett Learning.

little response to nonsteroidal anti-inflammatory drugs (NSAIDs), OCs, or both (Elnashar, 2015).

HEALTH HISTORY AND CLINICAL MANIFESTATIONS

Note past medical history, including any chronic illnesses and family history of gynecologic concerns. Determine medication and substance use, such as prescription medications, contraceptives, anabolic steroids, tobacco, marijuana, and cocaine, or other illegal drugs. A detailed sexual history is essential to assess for inflammation and scarring (adhesions) secondary to pelvic inflammatory disease (PID). Clients with a previous history of PID, sexually transmitted infections (STIs), low consumption of fruits and vegetables, depression, high stress level, multiple sexual partners, or unprotected sex are at increased risk (Tharpe et al., 2016).

During the initial interview, the nurse might ask some of the following questions to assess the client's history of dysmenorrhea:

- At what age did your menstrual cycles start?
- Have your cycles always been painful, or did the pain start recently?
- When in your cycle do you experience the pain?
- How would you describe the pain you feel?
- Are you sexually active?
- What impact does your cycle have on your physical and social activities?
- When was the first day of your last menstrual cycle?
- Was the flow of your last menstrual cycle a normal amount for you?
- Do your cycles tend to be heavy or last longer than 5 days?
- Are your cycles generally regular and predictable?
- What have you done to relieve your discomfort? Is it effective?
- Has there been a progression of symptom severity?
- Do you have any other symptoms?

Assess for clinical manifestations of dysmenorrhea. Affected clients experience sharp, intermittent spasms of pain, usually in the suprapubic area. Pain may radiate to the back of the legs or the lower back. Pain usually develops within hours of the start of menstruation and peaks as the flow becomes heaviest during the first day or second day of the cycle (King et al., 2015). Systemic symptoms of nausea, vomiting, diarrhea, fatigue, fever, headache, or dizziness are fairly common. Explore the history for physical symptoms of bloating, water retention, weight gain, headache, muscle aches, abdominal pain, food cravings, or breast tenderness.

PHYSICAL EXAMINATION

The physical examination performed by the health care provider centres on the bimanual pelvic examination. This examination is done during the nonmenstrual phase of the cycle. Explain to the client how it is to be performed, especially if it is her first pelvic examination. Prepare the client in the examining room by offering her a cover gown to put on and covering her lap with a privacy sheet on the examination table. Remain in the examining room throughout the examination to assist the health care provider with any procedures or specimens and to offer the client reassurance.

LABORATORY AND DIAGNOSTIC TESTS

Common diagnostic tests that may be ordered to determine the cause of dysmenorrhea can include:

- Complete blood count to rule out anemia
- Urinalysis to rule out a bladder infection
- Pregnancy test (hCG level) to rule out pregnancy
- Cervical culture to exclude STI
- Erythrocyte sedimentation rate to detect an inflammatory process

- Stool guaiac test to exclude gastrointestinal bleeding or disorders
- Pelvic and/or vaginal ultrasound to detect pelvic masses or cysts
- Diagnostic laparoscopy and/or laparotomy to visualize pathology that may account for the symptoms (Tharpe et al., 2016)

What diagnostic tests might be ordered to diagnose Izzy's pelvic pain?

Nursing Management

Educating the client about the normal events of the menstrual cycle and the etiology of the pain is paramount in achieving a successful outcome. Explaining the normal menstrual cycle will teach the client the correct terms to use so she can communicate her symptoms more accurately and will help dispel myths. Provide the client with monthly graphs or charts to record menses, the onset of pain, the timing of medication, relief afforded, and coping strategies used. This involves the client in the plan of care and provides objective information so that therapy can be modified if necessary.

The nurse should explain in detail the dosing regimen and the side effects of the medication therapy selected. Commonly prescribed drugs include NSAIDs such as ibuprofen (Motrin, Advil) or naproxen (Naprosyn). These drugs alleviate dysmenorrhea symptoms by decreasing intrauterine pressure and inhibiting prostaglandin synthesis, thus reducing pain (Skidmore-Roth, 2015). The primary goal of NSAID therapy of dysmenorrhea is to preempt the production of prostaglandins; thus starting the medication prophylactically and using sufficient doses to maximally suppress prostaglandin production are essential. If pain relief is not achieved in two to four cycles, a low-dose combination OC may be initiated. Client teaching and counselling should include information about how to take pills, side effects, and danger signs to watch for.

Encourage the client to apply a heating pad or warm compress to alleviate menstrual cramps. Additional lifestyle changes that the client can make to restore some sense of control and active participation in care are listed in Teaching Guidelines 4.3.

Teaching Guidelines 4.3
TIPS FOR MANAGING DYSMENORRHEA

- Exercise to increase endorphins and suppress prostaglandin release.
- Limit salty foods to prevent fluid retention.
- Increase water consumption to serve as a natural diuretic.

- Increase fibre intake with fruits and vegetables to prevent constipation.
- Use heating pads or warm baths to increase comfort.
- Take warm showers to promote relaxation.
- Sip on warm beverages, such as decaffeinated green tea.
- Keep legs elevated while lying down or lie on side with knees bent.
- Use stress management techniques to reduce emotional stress.
- Practice relaxation techniques to enhance ability to cope with pain.
- Stop smoking and decrease alcohol use which causes vasoconstriction.

Adapted from Burnett, M., & Lemyre, M. (2017). Clinical practice guideline No. 345: Primary dysmenorrhea consensus guideline. *Journal of Obstetrics and Gynecology Canada, 39*(7), 585–595; Calis, K. A., Popat, V., Dang, D. K., & Kalantaridou, S. N. (2017). Dysmenorrhea. *eMedicine.* Retrieved from http://emedicine.medscape.com/article/253812-overview; Smith, R. P., & Kaunitz, A. M. (2018). *Painful menstrual periods: Beyond the basics.* UpToDate. Retrieved from http://www.uptodate.com/contents/painful-menstrual-periods-dys-menorrhea-beyond-the-basics; ACOG. (2015b). *Dysmenorrhea: Painful periods.* FAQ046. Retrieved from www.acog.org/~/media/For Patients/faq046.ashx

Abnormal Uterine Bleeding

Disturbances of menstrual bleeding manifest in a wide range of presentations. **Abnormal uterine bleeding (AUB)** is the umbrella term used to describe any deviation from normal menstruation or from a normal menstrual cycle pattern. It can occur in clients with a uterus at any age. The key characteristics are regularity, frequency, volume or heaviness of flow, and duration of flow, but each of these may exhibit considerable variability.

AUB is a disorder that occurs most frequently the beginning and end of the reproductive years, affecting up to 30% of individuals with a uterus (Singh et al., 2013). AUB is defined as painless endometrial bleeding that is prolonged, excessive, and irregular and not attributed to any underlying structural or systemic disease (Creatsas & Creatsa, 2015). It is frequently associated with anovulatory cycles, which are common for the first year after menarche and is associated with immaturity of the hypothalamic–pituitary–ovarian axis. It also occurs later in life as clients approach menopause and experience irregular menstrual cycles.

The pathophysiology of AUB is related to a hormone disturbance. With anovulation, estrogen levels rise as usual in the early phase of the menstrual cycle. In the absence of ovulation, a corpus luteum never forms and progesterone is not produced. The endometrium moves into a hyperproliferative state, ultimately outgrowing its estrogen supply. This leads to irregular sloughing of the endometrium and excessive bleeding (King et al., 2015). If the bleeding is heavy enough and frequent enough,

anemia can result. AUB is similar to several other types of uterine bleeding disorders and sometimes overlaps these conditions. They include:

- Menorrhagia (abnormally long, heavy periods, prolonged bleeding)
- Oligomenorrhea (bleeding occurs at intervals of more than 35 days)
- Metrorrhagia (bleeding between periods, irregular bleeding)
- Menometrorrhagia (excessive uterine bleeding at and between menstrual periods)
- Polymenorrhea (too frequent periods)

Etiology

The possible causes of AUB may include:

- Adenomyosis
- Pregnancy
- Hormonal imbalance
- Fibroid tumours (see Chapter 7)
- Endometrial polyps or cancer
- Endometriosis
- IUSs
- Polycystic ovary syndrome
- Morbid obesity
- Steroid therapy
- Hypothyroidism
- Blood dyscrasias/clotting disorder
- Malignancy and hyperplasia
- Uterine polyps

Therapeutic Management

Treatment of AUB depends on the cause of the bleeding, the age of the client, and whether or not future fertility is desired. When known, the underlying cause of the disorder is treated. Otherwise, the goal of treatment is to normalize the bleeding, correct the anemia, prevent or diagnose early cancer, and restore quality of life (Schuiling & Likis, 2016).

Treatment options for AUB include combined OCs, progestogens, NSAIDs, tranexamic acid (antifibrinolytic), GnRH analogues, Danazol, and LNG-IUS (Bitzer, Heikinheimo, Nelson, Calaf-Alsina, & Fraser, 2015).

Management of AUB might include medical care with pharmacotherapy or insertion of a hormone-secreting IUS. OCs are used for cycle regulation as well as for contraception. They help prevent the risks associated with prolonged, unopposed estrogen stimulation of the endometrium. NSAIDs and progestin therapy (progesterone-releasing IUS [Mirena] or Depo-Provera) significantly decrease menstrual blood loss (Skidmore-Roth, 2015). The drug categories used in the treatment of AUB are:

- *Estrogens:* cause vasospasm of the uterine arteries to decrease bleeding

- *Progestins:* used to stabilize an estrogen-primed endometrium
- *OCs:* regulate the cycle and suppress the endometrium
- *NSAIDs:* inhibit prostaglandins in ovulatory menstrual cycles
- *Progesterone-releasing IUSs:* suppress endometrial growth
- *Androgens:* create a high-androgen/low-estrogen environment that inhibits endometrial growth
- *Antifibrinolytic drugs:* (tranexamic acid) prevent fibrin degradation to reduce bleeding
- *Iron replacement therapy:* replenish iron stores lost during heavy bleeding

If the client does not respond to medical therapy, surgical intervention might include dilation and curettage (D&C), hysteroscopic polypectomy, endometrial ablation, myomectomy, or hysterectomy. Surgery should be considered in clients for whom medical treatment has failed, cannot be tolerated, or is contraindicated (Kho & Mathur, 2015). Endometrial ablation is an alternative to hysterectomy, but both would be for the client no longer desiring fertility as both procedures can cause infertility. Techniques used for ablation include laser, electrosurgery excision procedure, freezing, heated fluid infusion, or thermal balloon ablation. Most clients will have reduced menstrual flow following endometrial ablation, and up to half will stop having periods. Younger clients are less likely than older clients to respond to endometrial ablation. Recent scientific evidence supports that up to one-quarter of clients treated with endometrial ablation require repeat ablation or subsequent hysterectomy to stop AUB. Hysterectomy should be considered a last resort for AUB (Singh et al., 2013).

Nursing Assessment

A thorough history should be taken to differentiate between AUB and other conditions that might cause vaginal bleeding, such as pregnancy and pregnancy-related conditions (abruptio placentae, ectopic pregnancy, abortion, or placenta previa); systemic conditions such as Cushing disease, blood dyscrasias, liver disease, renal disease, or thyroid disease; and genital tract pathology such as infections, tumours, or trauma (Schuiling & Likis, 2016).

Assess for clinical manifestations of AUB, which commonly include vaginal bleeding between periods, irregular menstrual cycles (usually less than 28 days between cycles), infertility, mood swings, hot flashes, vaginal tenderness, variable menstrual flow ranging from scanty to profuse, obesity, acne, stress, anorexia, thyroid disease, and diabetes. Signs of polycystic ovary syndrome might be present, because it is associated with unopposed estrogen stimulation, elevated androgen levels, and insulin resistance, and is a common cause of anovulation (Tharpe et al., 2016).

Measure orthostatic blood pressure and orthostatic pulse; a drop in pressure or pulse rate may occur with anemia. The health care provider, with the nurse assisting, performs a pelvic examination to identify any structural abnormalities.

Common diagnostic/lab tests that may be ordered to determine the cause of AUB include:
- Complete blood count to detect anemia
- Prothrombin time to detect blood dyscrasias
- Pregnancy test to rule out a spontaneous abortion or ectopic pregnancy
- Thyroid-stimulating hormone level to screen for hypothyroidism
- Transvaginal ultrasound to measure endometrium
- Pelvic ultrasound to view any structural abnormalities
- Endometrial biopsy to check for intrauterine pathology
- D&C for diagnostic evaluation

Nursing Management

Educate the client about normal menstrual cycles and the possible reasons for the abnormal pattern. Inform the client about treatment options. Do not suggest the client should simply "live with it." Instruct the client about any prescribed medications and potential side effects. For example, if high-dose estrogens are prescribed, the client may experience nausea. Teach her to take antiemetics as prescribed and encourage her to eat small, frequent meals to alleviate nausea. Adequate follow-up and evaluation are essential for clients who do not respond to medical management. See Nursing Care Plan 4.1: Overview of a Client With Abnormal Uterine Bleeding (at the end of chapter).

Take Note!

Complications such as infertility can result from lack of ovulation, severe anemia can result secondary to prolonged or heavy menses, depression and embarrassment may be secondary to the irregular and heavy bleeding, and endometrial cancer can occur associated with prolonged buildup of the endometrial lining without menstrual bleeding (Hoyt & Falconi, 2015).

Premenstrual Syndrome

Premenstrual syndrome (PMS) describes a constellation of recurrent symptoms that occur during the luteal phase or last half of the menstrual cycle and resolve with the onset of menstruation. A majority of cis-gender women in their reproductive years experience a variety of premenstrual symptoms that can alter their behaviour and well-being. Women have between 400 and 500 menstrual cycles over their reproductive years, and since premenstrual distress symptoms peak during 4 to 7 days prior to menses, consistently symptomatic women may spend up to 10 years of their lives in a state of compromised physical functioning and/or psychological well-being; thus it would constitute a major health problem for women (Tacani, Ribeiro, Barros Guimarães, Machado, & Tacani, 2015). A client experiencing PMS may have a wide variety of seemingly unrelated symptoms; for that reason, it is difficult to define and more challenging to diagnose. PMS affects millions of people during their reproductive years. Approximately 80% of (cis-gender) women will experience cyclic fluctuations in mood, sleep, and sense of well-being, related to their menstrual cycles (King et al., 2015). The exact cause of PMS is not known. It is thought to be related to the interaction between hormonal events and neurotransmitter function, specifically serotonin. Not all clients respond to serotonin reuptake inhibitors (SSRIs; Prozac, Paxil, Zoloft), however, which implies that other mechanisms may be involved (Skidmore-Roth, 2015).

As defined by the American Psychiatric Association, PMDD is a more severe variant of PMS affecting 5% to 8% of premenopausal women. Experts compare the difference between PMS and PMDD to the difference between a mild tension headache and a migraine. Risk factors identified that predispose to PMS/PMDD are age between 25 and 35 years, a psychiatric history, a family history of PMDD, unhealthy living habits, and stressful life events (Santamaria & Lago, 2015). PMDD markedly interferes with work, school, social activities, and relationships with others.

Therapeutic Management

Treatment of PMS is often frustrating for both clients and health care providers. Clinical outcomes can be expected to improve as a result of recent consensus on the diagnostic criteria for PMS and PMDD, data from clinical trials, and the availability of evidence-based clinical guidelines.

The management of PMS or PMDD requires a multidimensional approach because these conditions are not likely to have a single cause, and they appear to affect multiple systems within a person's body; therefore, they are not likely to be amenable to treatment with a single therapy (Naeimi, 2015). To reduce the negative impact of premenstrual disorders on a client's life, education, along with reassurance and anticipatory guidance, is needed for clients to feel they have some control over their condition.

Take Note!

Because there are no diagnostic tests that can reliably determine the existence of PMS or PMDD, the client must decide if help is needed during this time of the month. The client must embrace multiple therapies and become an active participant in the treatment plan to find the best level of symptom relief.

BOX 4.2

TREATMENT OPTIONS FOR PMS AND PMDD

- Lifestyle changes
  - Reduce stress
  - Exercise three to five times each week
  - Eat a balanced diet and increase water intake
  - Decrease caffeine intake
  - Stop smoking and limit the intake of alcohol
  - Attend a PMS support group
- Vitamin and mineral supplements
  - Multivitamin daily
  - Vitamin E, 400 units daily
  - Calcium, 1,200 to 1,600 mg daily
  - Magnesium, 200 to 400 mg daily
- Medications
  - NSAIDs taken a week prior to menses
  - Oral contraceptives (low dose)
  - Antidepressants (SSRIs)
  - Anxiolytics (taken during luteal phase)
  - Diuretics to remove excess fluid
  - Progestins
  - Gonadotropin-releasing hormone (GnRH) agonists
  - Danazol (an androgen hormone that inhibits estrogen production)

Adapted from Walsh, S., Ismaili, E., Naheed, B., & O'Brien, S. (2015). Diagnosis, pathophysiology and management of premenstrual syndrome. *The Obstetrician & Gynaecologist, 17*, 99–104; King, T. L., Brucker, M. C., Kriebs, J. M., Fahey, J. O., Gegor, C. L., & Varney, H. (2015). *Varney's midwifery* (5th ed.). Burlington, MA: Jones & Bartlett Learning; Htay, T. T., & Aung, K. (2016). Premenstrual dysphoric disorder. *eMedicine*. Retrieved from http://emedicine.medscape.com/article/293257-overview

---

Therapeutic interventions for PMS and PMDD address the symptoms because the exact cause of this condition is still unknown. Treatments may include vitamin supplements, diet changes, exercise, lifestyle changes, and medications (Box 4.2). Medications used in treating PMDD may include antidepressant and antianxiety drugs, diuretics, anti-inflammatory medications, analgesics, synthetic androgen agents, OCs, or GnRH agonists to regulate menses. Unlike the approach to the treatment of depression, antidepressants need not be given daily but can be effective when used cyclically, only in the luteal phase, or even limited to the duration of the monthly symptoms.

COMPLEMENTARY AND ALTERNATIVE THERAPIES

No single treatment is universally recognized as effective, and many clients often turn to therapeutic approaches outside of conventional medicine. Many clients use dietary supplements and herbal remedies for their menstrual health and treating their bleeding disorders, although there has been little research to demonstrate their efficacy. Alternative treatments for treating PMDD include calcium supplementation, vitex agnus castus (chaste tree berry), hypericum perforatum (St. John's wort), and cognitive/behavioural/relaxation therapies (Wicks & Mahady,

2015). Some other alternative therapies include the use of yoga, magnesium, vitamin B₆, evening primrose oil, vitex agnus castus, *Ginkgo biloba*, viburnum, dandelion, stinging nettle, burdock, raspberry leaf, and skullcap (Tremellen & Pearce, 2015). Although research has not validated the efficacy of these alternative therapies, it is important for the nurse to be aware of the alternative products that many clients choose to use.

Nursing Assessment

Although little consensus exists in the medical literature and among researchers about what constitutes PMS and PMDD, the physical and psychological symptoms are very real. The extent to which the symptoms debilitate or incapacitate a client is highly variable.

More than 150 symptoms are assigned to PMS, but irritability, food cravings, mood swings, tearfulness, depression, sleep disturbances, headache, back pain, fatigue, bloating, edema of the face, abdominal area, and extremities, tension, and dysphoria (a profound state of unease and anxiety) are the most prominent and consistently described (Tacani et al., 2015). To establish the diagnosis of PMS, elicit a description of cyclic symptoms occurring before the client's menstrual period. The client should chart symptoms daily for two cycles. These data will help demonstrate symptoms clustering around the luteal phase of ovulation, with resolution after bleeding starts. Ask the client to bring the list of symptoms to the next appointment. Symptoms can be categorized using the following:

• **A**—*anxiety:* difficulty sleeping, tenseness, mood swings, and clumsiness
• **C**—*craving:* cravings for sweets, salty foods, chocolate
• **D**—*depression:* feelings of low self-esteem, anger, easily upset
• **H**—*hydration:* weight gain, abdominal bloating, breast tenderness
• **O**—*other:* hot flashes or cold sweats, nausea, change in bowel habits, aches or pains, dysmenorrhea, acne breakout (Naeimi, 2015)

The American College of Obstetricians and Gynecologists (ACOG) diagnostic criteria for PMS consist of having at least one of the following affective and somatic symptoms during the 5 days before menses in each of the three previous cycles:

• Affective symptoms: depression, angry outbursts, irritability, anxiety
• Somatic symptoms: breast tenderness, abdominal bloating, edema, headache
• Symptoms relieved from days 4 to 13 of the menstrual cycle (American College of Obstetricians & Gynecologists [ACOG], 2015a)

In PMDD, the main symptoms are mood disorders such as depression, anxiety, tension, and persistent anger or irritability. Physical symptoms such as headache, joint and muscle pain, lack of energy, bloating, and breast tenderness are also present (Htay, 2016). It is estimated that up to 75% of reproductive-age cis-gender women experience premenstrual symptoms that meet the ACOG criteria for PMS and up to 5% meet the diagnostic criteria for PMDD (Pearlstein, 2015).

According to the American Psychiatric Association, a woman must have at least five of the typical symptoms to be diagnosed with PMDD (Pearlstein, 2015). These must occur during the week before and a few days after the onset of menstruation and must include one or more of the first four symptoms:

• Affective lability: sadness, tearfulness, irritability
• Anxiety and tension
• Persistent or marked anger or irritability
• Depressed mood, feelings of hopelessness
• Difficulty concentrating
• Sleep difficulties
• Increased or decreased appetite
• Increased or decreased sexual desire
• Chronic fatigue
• Headache
• Constipation or diarrhea
• Breast swelling and tenderness (Htay, 2016)

Nursing Management

Educate clients about the management of PMS or PMDD. Advise them that lifestyle changes often result in significant symptom improvement without pharmacotherapy. Encourage clients to eat a balanced diet that includes nutrient-rich foods to avoid hypoglycemia and associated mood swings. Encourage all clients to participate in aerobic exercise three times a week to promote a sense of well-being, decrease fatigue, and reduce stress. Administer calcium (1,200 to 1,600 mg/day), magnesium (400 to 800 mg/day), and vitamin B₆ (50 to 100 mg/day) as prescribed. In some studies, these nutrients have been shown to decrease the intensity of PMS symptoms. NSAIDs may be useful for painful physical symptoms, and spironolactone (Aldactone) may help with bloating and water retention. Herbs such as vitex agnus castus (chaste tree berry), evening primrose, and SAM-e (a dietary supplement used to enhance mood) may be recommended; although not harmful, not all herbs have enough clinical or research evidence to document their safety or efficacy. Nutritional treatments include a diet low in salt, alcohol, caffeine, and sugar (Schuiling & Likis, 2016).

A recent research study proposes calcium (1,600 mg/day) and vitamin D (400 International Units/day) supplementation in menstruating adolescents and adults in an effort to prevent PMS, but further research using a larger population needs to be conducted to validate this (Santamaria & Lago, 2015).

Explain to your client the relationship between cyclic estrogen fluctuation and changes in levels of serotonin

EVIDENCE-BASED PRACTICE 4.1   **THE EFFECT OF WHEAT GERM EXTRACT ON PREMENSTRUAL SYNDROME SYMPTOMS**

STUDY

Premenstrual syndrome is one of the most common disorders in women and impairs work and social relationships. Several treatment modalities have been proposed including herbal medicines. Herbal medicines are among the most common treatments because they are economical, safe, noninvasive, and have fewer side effects than do traditional medicines. Wheat germ contains magnesium, zinc, calcium, selenium, potassium, phosphorus, chromium, and vitamins A, E, C, B_{12}, B_6, niacin, and folic acid. Considering the properties of wheat germ, this study aimed to determine the effects of wheat germ extract on the symptoms of premenstrual syndrome.

Findings

This triple blind clinical trial was conducted on 84 women that completed daily records regarding their symptoms for two consecutive months while taking 400-mg capsules of wheat germ extract or placebo three times a day from day 16 until day 5 of the next menstrual cycle. The study found that wheat germ significantly reduced the severity of physical symptoms (64%), psychological symptoms (66%), and general symptoms (65%) when compared with the placebo group within the first month of treatment. No complications were observed in either group.

Nursing Implications

Based on the study results, it seems that using wheat germ extract reduces the severity of general, psychological, and physical symptoms of premenstrual syndrome in women that take it during their midcycle. Given the positive effects of taking B_6 and E, calcium, and magnesium in previous studies to reduce the symptoms of PMS, it makes sense that wheat germ which contains all of the compounds listed would help relieve PMS symptoms. Nurses can suggest using nontraditional modalities to women that request them and cite this study's results to validate them.

Adapted from Ataollahi, M., Akbari, S. A., Mojab, F., & Alavi Majd, H. (2015). The effect of wheat germ extract on premenstrual syndrome symptoms. *Iranian Journal of Pharmaceutical Research: IJPR, 14*(1), 159–166.

levels, and how the different management strategies help maintain serotonin levels, thus improving symptoms. It is important to rule out other conditions that might cause erratic or dysphoric behaviour. If the initial treatment regimen does not work, explain that the client should return for further testing. Behavioural counselling and stress management might help clients regain control during these stressful periods. Reassuring the client that support and help are available through many community resources/support groups can be instrumental in her acceptance of this monthly disorder. Nurses can be a very calming force for many clients experiencing PMS or PMDD. A holistic approach, including lifestyle modifications, pharmacotherapy, herbal therapies, and cognitive behavioural therapy, is most beneficial for symptom reduction, improvement in daily functioning, and quality of life. See Evidence-Based Practice 4.1.

Take Note!

Clients of any age who experience more extensive emotional symptoms with PMS should be evaluated for PMDD, because they may require antidepressant therapy.

Endometriosis

Endometriosis is one of the most common gynecologic diseases, affecting approximately 10% of the menstruating population (Davila et al., 2018). In this condition, for unknown reasons, bits of functioning endometrial tissue are located outside of their normal site, the uterine cavity.

This endometrial tissue is commonly found attached to the ovaries, fallopian tubes, the outer surface of the uterus, the bowels, the area between the vagina and the rectum (rectovaginal septum), and the pelvic side wall (Fig. 4.1). The places where the tissue attaches are called **implants**, or lesions. Endometrial tissue found outside the uterus responds to hormones released during the menstrual cycle in the same way as endometrial lining within the uterus.

At the beginning of the menstrual cycle, when the lining of the uterus is shed and menstrual bleeding begins, these abnormally located implants swell and bleed also. In short, the client with endometriosis experiences several "mini-periods" throughout the abdomen, wherever this endometrial tissue exists. In addition to cyclic bleeding outside the uterus, scarring and adhesion formation throughout the pelvis occur. Symptoms begin as early as adolescence and typically settle after menopause.

Think back to Izzy, with her progressive pelvic pain and infertility concerns. After a pelvic examination, her health care provider suspects she has endometriosis.

Etiology and Risk Factors

It is not currently known why endometrial tissue becomes transplanted and grows in other parts of the body. Several theories exist, but to date none has been scientifically

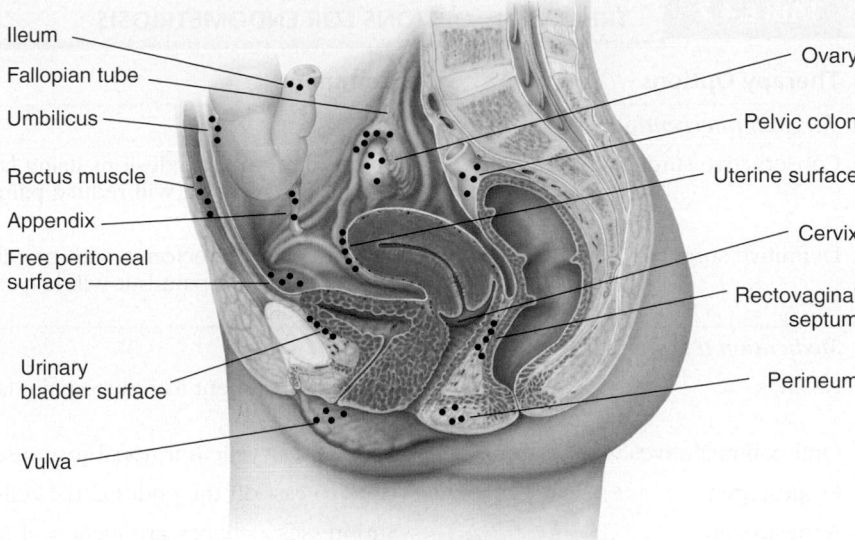

FIGURE 4.1 **Common sites of endometriosis formation.** (Asset provided by Anatomical Chart Co.)

proven. However, several factors that increase a client's risk of developing endometriosis have been identified:

- The aging process
- Family history of endometriosis in a first-degree relative
- Short menstrual cycle (less than 28 days)
- Long menstrual flow (more than 1 week)
- High dietary fat consumption
- Young age of menarche (younger than 12)
- Few (one or two) or no pregnancies (Johnston, Reid, & Hunter, 2015)

Therapeutic Management

Therapeutic management of the client with endometriosis needs to take into consideration the following factors: severity of symptoms, desire for fertility, degree of disease, and the client's therapy goals. The aim of therapy is to suppress levels of estrogen and progesterone, which cause the endometrium to grow. Current treatment of endometriosis is mainly based on surgery and ovarian suppressive agents (OCs, progestins, GnRH agonists, and androgenic agents). Approximately only half of clients with endometriosis experience pain relief from existing medial or surgical treatments (National Institute of Child Health and Human Development [NICHD], 2015). Treatment can include surgical removal of ectopic endometrial tissue or medications such as NSAIDs, OCs, Depo-Provera, synthetic testosterone, and GnRH agonists. Also, alternative therapies may be used, including acupuncture and supplements of vitamins, minerals, and fish oil (Elnashar, 2015). These interventions may control symptoms initially, but many have significant adverse effects and limits on duration of therapy (Table 4.2).

Nursing Assessment

Nurses encounter clients with endometriosis in a variety of settings: community health settings, schools, clinics, day surgical centres, and hospitals. Health care professionals must not trivialize or dismiss the concerns of these clients, because early recognition is essential to preserve fertility. The diversity of presenting symptoms and a low index of suspicion contribute to clients with endometriosis falling through the cracks and not being diagnosed promptly.

HEALTH HISTORY

Obtain a health history and elicit a description of signs and symptoms to determine risk factors. Endometriosis is often asymptomatic, but it can be a severe and debilitating condition. It typically is chronic and progressive. Ask specifically about menarche, history of menstrual problems, details of pregnancies, and difficulties with conception. Assess the client for clinical manifestations, which include:

- Infertility
- Back pain
- Pain before and during menstrual periods
- Pain during or after sexual intercourse
- Painful urination
- Depression
- Fatigue
- Painful bowel movements
- Chronic pelvic pain
- Hypermenorrhea (heavy menses)
- Pelvic adhesions
- Irregular and more frequent menses
- Premenstrual vaginal spotting (Schuiling & Likis, 2016)

TABLE 4.2	TREATMENT OPTIONS FOR ENDOMETRIOSIS
Therapy Options	**Comment**
Surgical intervention	
Conservative surgery	Removal of implants/lesions using laser, cautery, or small surgical instruments. This intervention will reduce pain and allows pregnancy to occur in the future
Definitive surgery	Abdominal hysterectomy, with or without bilateral salpingo-oophorectomy. Will eliminate pain but will leave a client unable to become pregnant in the future
Medication therapy	
NSAIDs	First-line treatment to reduce pain; taken early when premenstrual symptoms are first felt
Oral contraceptives	Suppresses cyclic hormonal response of the endometrial tissue
Progestogens	Used to cast off the endometrial cells and thus destroy them
Antiestrogens	Suppresses a client's production of estrogen, thus stopping the menstrual cycle and preventing further growth of endometrium
Gonadotropin-releasing hormone analogues (GnRH-a)	Suppresses endometriosis by creating a temporary pseudomenopause

Adapted from Davila, G. W., Kapoor, D. W., Alderman, E., Hiraoka, M. K., Ghoniem, G. M., & Peskin, B. D. (2018). Endometriosis. *eMedicine.* Retrieved from http://emedicine.medscape.com/article/271899-overview; Elnashar, A. (2015). Emerging treatment of endometriosis. *Middle East Fertility Society Journal, 20,* 61–69. Retrieved from http://www.sciencedirect.com/science/article/pii/S1110569014200562; King, T. L., Brucker, M. C., Kriebs, J. M., Fahey, J. O., Gegor, C. L., & Varney, H. (2015). *Varney's midwifery* (5th ed.). Burlington, MA: Jones & Bartlett Learning.

The two most common symptoms are infertility and pelvic pain. Endometriosis occurs in 38% of infertile cisgender women and in 71% to 87% of those with chronic pelvic pain (Davila et al., 2018). About 30% to 40% of women with this condition are infertile, making it one of the top three causes of female infertility (Brown & Farquhar, 2015).

What are the two most common symptoms experienced by women with endometriosis? Is Izzy's profile typical? As a nurse, what would be your role in Izzy's continued workup?

PHYSICAL EXAMINATION AND LABORATORY AND DIAGNOSTIC TESTS

The pelvic examination typically correlates with the extent of the endometriosis. The usual finding is nonspecific pelvic tenderness. The hallmark finding is the presence of tender nodular masses on the uterosacral ligaments, the posterior uterus, or the posterior cul-de-sac. The only definitive diagnosis is one made during surgery (Signorile & Baldi, 2015).

After a thorough history and a pelvic examination, the health care provider may suspect endometriosis, but the only certain method of diagnosing it is by seeing it.

Pelvic or transvaginal ultrasound is used to assess pelvic organ structures. However, a laparoscopy is needed to diagnose endometriosis. Laparoscopy is the direct visualization of the internal organs with a lighted instrument inserted through an abdominal incision. A tissue biopsy of the suspected implant taken at the same time and examined microscopically confirms the diagnosis (Society of Obstetricians and Gynecologists of Canada [SOGC], 2010).

Nurses can play a role by offering a thorough explanation of the condition and explaining why tests are needed to diagnose endometriosis. The nurse can set up appointments for imaging studies and laparoscopy.

Nursing Management

In addition to the interventions outlined above, the nurse should encourage the client to adopt healthy lifestyle habits with respect to diet, exercise, sleep, and stress management. Referrals to support groups and Internet resources can help the client to understand this condition and to cope with chronic pain. A number of organizations provide information about the diagnosis and treatment of endometriosis and offer support to clients and their families. Nurses are uniquely situated to improve client outcomes by assisting clients to make informed

BOX 4.3

ORGANIZATIONS AND WEB RESOURCES TO ASSIST THE CLIENT WITH ENDOMETRIOSIS

- Center for Endometriosis Care
  http://www.centerforendo.com
- Endometriosis Association
  http://www.endometriosisassn.org
  http://www.KillerCramps.org
- Endometriosis Association support groups
  e-mail: support@endometriosisassn.org
- Endometriosis Clinic at McMaster University
  http://www.endometriosisclinic.ca
- National Institute of Child Health and Human Development Information Resource Center
  http://www.nichd.nih.gov
  e-mail: NICHDClearinghouse@mail.nih.gov
- Society of Obstetricians and Gynecologists of Canada (SOGC)
  https://sogc.org/
- The Endometriosis Network of Canada
  http://endometriosisnetwork.com/
- Your Period, Endometriosis: SOGC
  https://www.yourperiod.ca/endometriosis

treatment decisions. A prompt diagnosis ensures appropriate care (Box 4.3).

INFERTILITY

Infertility is defined as the inability to conceive a child after 1 year of regular sexual intercourse unprotected by contraception for women under the age of 35, or 6 months of trying for women over the age of 35 (SOGC, 2018). Secondary infertility is the inability to conceive after a previous pregnancy. Many people take the ability to conceive and produce a child for granted, but infertility affects 1 in 6 heterosexual Canadian couples. Infertility is a widespread problem that has an emotional, social, and economic impact on couples. Although male infertility accounts for approximately 30% of infertility issues, infertility remains a woman's social burden. It affects relationships, leads to tension and anger between partners, and can result in severe sexual dysfunction and breakdown of the relationship. Nurses must recognize infertility and understand its causes and treatment options so that they can help couples understand the possibilities as well as the limitations of current therapies. Nurses have a central role in supporting couples through these stressful treatments. Couples will frequently confide in their nurse and can gain great benefit from a sympathetic and sensible discussion. Recent studies have found that women wish to be treated with respect and dignity and given appropriate information and support. Women want their distress recognized and they want to feel cared for and to have confidence in health care providers in situations where outcomes are uncertain. The caring aspect of professional nursing is an essential component of meeting the special needs of these couples (Whitman, 2015). Prevention of infertility through education should also be incorporated into any client–nurse interaction.

After completing several diagnostic tests, Izzy is diagnosed with endometriosis. She asks you about her chances of becoming pregnant and becoming pain-free. What treatment options would you explain to Izzy? What information can you give about her future childbearing ability?

Cultural Considerations

Infertility is not only a physiologic problem, but is one that can initiate a life crisis that is experienced with psychological, familial, social, and cultural consequences. Cross-culturally, the expectation for couples to reproduce is an accepted norm and the inability to conceive may be considered a violation of this cultural norm. In this context, infertility represents a crisis for the couple. The manner in which different cultures, ethnic groups, and religious groups perceive and manage infertility may be very different. For example, many African Canadians may believe that assisted reproductive techniques are unnatural and that they remove the spiritual or divine nature of creation from conception. For this reason, they may seek spiritual rather than medical assistance when trying to conceive. The Hispanic culture believes that children validate the marriage, so families are typically large. Like the African-Canadian culture, Hispanics are traditionally very spiritual and may consider infertility a test of faith and seek spiritual counselling. Disappointing one's spouse may be of greater concern to women of African descent, whereas avoiding the stigmatization of infertility may be of greatest concern to women of Asian descent (Inhorn & Patrizio, 2015).

Religion often influences cultural factors and for this reason may also be considered when pursuing treatment for infertility. In the Orthodox Jewish religion, procreation is considered to be a "mitzvah," a commandment to have children. However, even Orthodox Jews accept the use of contraceptives to prevent conception when it is not desired. Conservative and Reform Jews put no restrictions on contraception (McFarland & Wehbe-Alamah, 2015). Roman Catholics have a very restrictive view on the use of assisted reproductive technologies, since in their view procreation cannot be separated from the relationship between parents. Thus, God wants human life to begin through the "conjugal act" and not artificially. Most religious teachings speak to the significance of procreation; thus infertility can impact the self and relational identities of the couple wishing to become parents. Therefore, the risk is present for both a crisis of identity and of faith

(Dombo & Flood, 2015). Nurses must be cognizant of the client's cultural and religious background and how it may dictate which, if any, reproductive treatment options are chosen. Nurses need to include this awareness in their counselling of infertile couples.

Etiology and Risk Factors

Reproduction requires the interaction of the two complementary reproductive tracts, which involves (1) the release of a normal preovulatory oocyte, (2) the production of adequate spermatozoa, (3) the normal transport of the gametes to the ampullary portion of the fallopian tube (where fertilization takes place), and (4) the subsequent transport of the cleaving embryo into the endometrial cavity for implantation and development (Puscheck & Woodward, 2016).

Multiple known and unknown factors affect fertility. Female-factor infertility is detected in about 40% of cases, male-factor infertility in about 30% of cases. In 20% of infertility cases, the challenges are combined (both male and female factors), and approximately 10% of the time, infertility remains unexplained (Health Canada, 2013).

Consider This

We had been married for 3 years and wanted to start a family, but much to our dismay nothing happened after a year of trying. I had some irregular periods and was finally diagnosed with endometriosis and put on Clomid for three cycles. After that time without achieving a pregnancy, I went to a fertility expert. The doctor lasered the misplaced endometriosis tissue, sent carbon dioxide through my tubes to make sure they were patent, and put me back on Clomid, but still with no luck. Finally, 2 years later, we were put on an in vitro fertilization (IVF) waiting list and prayed we would have the money for the procedure. By then I felt a failure as a woman. We then decided that it was more important for us to be parents than it was for me to be pregnant, so we considered adoption. We tried for another year without any results.

We went to the adoption agency to fill out the paperwork for the process to begin. Our blood was taken and we waited for an hour, wondering the whole time why it was taking so long for the results. The nurse finally appeared and handed a piece of paper to me with the word "positive" written on it. I started to cry tears of joy, for a pregnancy had started and our long journey of infertility was finally ending.

Thoughts: *For many couples, the dream of having a child is not easily realized. Infertility can affect self-esteem, disrupt relationships, and result in depression. This couple experienced many years of frustration in trying to have a family. What help can be offered to couples during this time? What can be said to comfort a woman who feels she is a failure?*

In women, ovarian dysfunction (40%) and tubal/pelvic pathology (40%) are the primary contributing factors to infertility (ASRM, 2018).

Risk factors for infertility in women include:
- Overweight or underweight (can disrupt hormone function)
- Hormonal imbalances leading to irregular ovulation
- Uterine fibroids
- Tubal blockages
- Cervical stenosis
- Reduced oocyte quality
- Chromosomal abnormalities
- Congenital anomalies of the uterus
- Immune system disorders
- Chronic illnesses such as diabetes, thyroid disease, asthma
- STIs
- Ectopic pregnancy
- Age older than 27
- Endometriosis
- Turner syndrome
- Eating disorders
- History of PID
- Smoking and alcohol consumption
- Multiple miscarriages
- Menstrual abnormalities
- Exposure to chemotherapeutic agents
- Psychological stress (Senie, 2014)

Risk factors for infertility in men include:
- Exposure to toxic substances (lead, mercury, x-rays, chemotherapy)
- Cigarette or marijuana smoke
- Heavy alcohol consumption
- Use of prescription drugs for ulcers or psoriasis
- Exposure of the genitals to high temperatures (hot tubs or saunas)
- Hernia repair
- Obesity is associated with decreased sperm quality
- Cushing syndrome
- Frequent long-distance cycling or running
- STIs
- Undescended testicles (cryptorchidism)
- Mumps after puberty (Puscheck & Woodward, 2016)

Therapeutic Management

As noted earlier, the main causes of infertility are female factor (anovulation, tubal damage, endometriosis, and ovarian failure), male factor (low or absent numbers of motile sperm in the ejaculate, and erectile dysfunction), or unexplained infertility (Jin, 2015). The test results are presented to the couple and different treatment options are suggested. The majority of infertility cases are treated with drugs or surgery. Treatment options include lifestyle changes, such as weight loss

FIGURE 4.2 Artificial insemination. Sperm are deposited next to the cervix (**A**) or injected directly into the uterine cavity (**B**).

A **B**

and smoking cessation; taking clomiphene to promote ovulation; hormone injections to promote ovulation; intrauterine insemination; and IVF. Various ovulation-enhancement drugs and timed intercourse might be used for the clients with ovulation problems. The client should understand a drug's benefits and side effects before consenting to take it. Depending on the type of drug used and the dosage, some clients may experience multiple births. If the client's reproductive organs are damaged, surgery may be done to repair them. Still other couples might opt for the hi-tech approaches of artificial insemination (Fig. 4.2), IVF (Fig. 4.3), and egg donation or they may contract for a gestational carrier or surrogate (Jin, 2015). Table 4.3 lists selected treatment options for infertility.

Nursing Assessment

Infertile couples are under tremendous pressure and often keep the problem a secret, considering it to be very personal. Couples are often beset by feelings of inadequacy and guilt, and many are subject to pressures from both family and friends. As the problem becomes more chronic, they may begin to blame one another, with consequent discord in the relationship. Seeking help is often a very difficult step for them, and it may take a lot of courage to discuss something about which they feel deeply embarrassed or upset. The nurse working in this specialty setting must be aware of the conflict and problems couples present with and must be very sensitive to their needs.

A full medical history should be taken from both partners, along with a physical examination. The data needed for the infertility evaluation are very sensitive and of a personal nature, so the nurse must use professional and therapeutic interviewing skills.

Infertility has numerous causes and contributing factors, so it is important to use the process of elimination, determining what problems do not exist to better comprehend the problems that do exist. At the first visit, a plan of investigation is outlined and a complete health history is taken. This first visit forces many couples to

A **B** **C** **D**

FIGURE 4.3 Steps involved in in vitro fertilization. **A.** Ovulation. **B.** Capture of the ova (done here intra-abdominally). **C.** Fertilization of ova and growth in culture medium. **D.** Insertion of fertilized ova into uterus.

TABLE 4.3   SELECTED TREATMENT OPTIONS FOR INFERTILITY

Procedure	Comments	Nursing Considerations
Fertility drugs		
Clomiphene citrate (Clomid)	A nonsteroidal synthetic antiestrogen used to induce ovulation Clomid is typically discontinued after three cycles of use	Nurse can advise the couple to have intercourse every other day for 1 week starting after day 5 of medication
Human menopausal gonadotropin (HMG); Pergonal	Induces ovulation by direct stimulation of ovarian follicle	Same as above
Artificial insemination	The insertion of a prepared semen sample into the cervical os or intrauterine cavity Enables sperm to be deposited closer to improve chances of conception. Partner or donor sperm can be used	Advise couple that the procedure might need to be repeated if not successful the first time
Assisted reproductive technologies[a]		
In vitro fertilization (IVF)	Oocytes are fertilized in the lab and transferred to the uterus Usually indicated for tubal obstruction, endometriosis, pelvic adhesions, and low sperm counts	Educate clients regarding the need to take medication to stimulate ovulation so the mature ovum can be retrieved by needle aspiration
Gamete intrafallopian transfer (GIFT)	Oocytes and sperm are combined and immediately placed in the fallopian tube so fertilization can occur naturally Requires laparoscopy and general anesthesia, which increases risk	Inform couple of risks and have consent signed
Intracytoplasmic sperm injection (ICSI)	One sperm is injected into the cytoplasm of the oocyte to fertilize it. Indicated for male factor infertility	Inform the male that sperm will be aspirated by a needle through the skin into the epididymis
Donor oocytes or sperm	Eggs or sperm are retrieved from a donor and the eggs are inseminated; resulting embryos are transferred via IVF Recommended for clients older than 40 years and those with poor-quality eggs	Support couple in their ethical/religious discussions prior to deciding
Preimplantation genetic diagnosis (PGD)	Used to identify genetic defects in embryos created through IVF before pregnancy. This is done specifically when one or both genetic parents have a known genetic abnormality and testing is performed on an embryo to see if it also carries a genetic abnormality	Inform couple about this option and support them until test results return
Gestational carrier (surrogacy)	Laboratory fertilization takes place and embryos are transferred to the uterus of another person, who will carry the pregnancy. Or intrauterine insemination can be done with the male sperm Medical–legal issues have resulted over the "true ownership" of the resulting infant	Encourage an open discussion regarding implications of this method with the couple

[a]When other options have been exhausted, these are considered.

Adapted from American Society for Reproductive Medicine (ASRM). (2018). *Frequently asked questions about infertility*. Retrieved from http://www.asrm.org/detail.aspx?id=2322; Jin, J. (2015). Treatments for infertility. *Journal of the American Medical Association, 313*(3), 320; Puscheck, E. E., & Woodward, T. L. (2016). Infertility. *eMedicine*. Retrieved from http://emedicine.medscape.com/article/274143-overview

confront the reality that their desired pregnancy may not occur naturally. Alleviate some of the anxiety associated with diagnostic testing by explaining the timing and reasons for each test.

Assessing Sperm-Related Factors

The initial screening evaluation for the male partner should include a reproductive history and a semen analysis. From the male perspective, three things must happen for conception to take place: the number of sperm must be adequate; those sperm must be healthy and mature; and the sperm must be able to penetrate and fertilize the egg. Healthy males have more than 20 million sperm per millilitre with greater than 50% motility (World Health Organization [WHO], 2015). Semen analysis is the most important indicator of male fertility. The man should abstain from sexual activity for 24 to 48 hours before giving the sample. For a semen examination, the man is asked to produce a specimen by ejaculating into a specimen container and delivering it to the laboratory for analysis within 1 to 2 hours. When the specimen is brought to the laboratory, it is analyzed for volume, viscosity, number of sperm, sperm viability, motility, and sperm shape. If semen parameters are normal, no further male evaluation is necessary (Puscheck & Woodward, 2016).

A recent study shows that social strain and stress are highest among couples without a clear etiology for their infertility. These findings highlight the clinically significant negative sexual, personal, and social strains of a perceived infertility diagnosis for men (Cavallini, 2015). Nurses need to be very cognizant of this impact on males and address it.

The physical examination routinely includes:
- Assessment for appropriate male sexual characteristics, such as body hair distribution, development of the Adam's apple, and muscle development
- Examination of the penis, scrotum, testicles, epididymis, and vas deferens for abnormalities (e.g., nodules, irregularities, varicocele)
- Assessment for normal development of external genitalia (small testicles)
- Performance of a digital internal examination of the prostate to check for tenderness or swelling (Dohle, 2015)

Assessing Uterine-Related Factors

The initial assessment of the client should include a thorough history of factors associated with ovulation and the pelvic organs. Diagnostic tests to determine female infertility may include:
- Assessment of ovarian function
- Ovulation predictor kits used midcycle
- Urinary LH level
- Clomiphene citrate challenge test
- Assessment of pelvic organs
- Papanicolaou (Pap) smear to rule out cervical cancer or inflammation
- Cervical culture to rule out any STIs
- Ultrasound to assess pelvic structures
- Hysterosalpingography to visualize structural defects
- Laparoscopy to visualize pelvic structures and diagnose endometriosis (Dadhich, Ramasamy, & Lipshultz, 2015)

Laboratory and Diagnostic Testing

The diagnostic procedures that should be done during an infertility workup should be guided by the couple's history. They generally proceed from less to more invasive tests.

HOME OVULATION PREDICTOR KITS

Home ovulation predictor kits contain monoclonal antibodies specific for LH and use the ELISA test to determine the amount of LH present in the urine. A significant colour change from baseline indicates the LH surge and presumably the most fertile day of the month for the woman.

CLOMIPHENE CITRATE CHALLENGE TEST

The clomiphene citrate challenge test is used to assess a client's ovarian reserve (ability of the eggs to become fertilized). FSH levels are drawn on cycle day 3 and on cycle day 10 after the client has taken 100-mg clomiphene citrate on cycle days 5 through 9. If the FSH level is greater than 15, the result is considered abnormal and the likelihood of conception with her own eggs is very low (Schuiling & Likis, 2016).

HYSTEROSALPINGOGRAPHY

Hysterosalpingography is the gold standard in assessing patency (being open and unobstructed) of the fallopian tubes. Fallopian tube obstruction is among the most common causes of female factor infertility. Ultrasonography and magnetic resonance imaging (MRI) are used in this assessment. In hysterosalpingography, 3 to 10 mL of an opaque contrast medium is slowly injected through a catheter into the endocervical canal so that the uterus and tubes can be visualized during fluoroscopy and radiography. If the fallopian tubes are patent, the dye will ascend upward to distend the uterus and the tubes and will spill out into the peritoneal cavity (Hemingway & Trew, 2015; Fig. 4.4).

LAPAROSCOPY

A laparoscopy is usually performed early in the menstrual cycle. It is not part of the routine infertility evaluation. It is used when abnormalities are found on the ultrasound or the hysterosalpingogram. Because of the

FIGURE 4.4 Insertion of a dye for a hysterosalpingogram. The contrast dye outlines the uterus and fallopian tubes on an x-ray to demonstrate patency.

added risks of surgery, the need for anesthesia, and operative costs, it is only used when clearly indicated. During the procedure, an endoscope is inserted through a small incision in the anterior abdominal wall. Visualization of the peritoneal cavity in an infertile client may reveal endometriosis, pelvic adhesions, tubal occlusion, fibroids, or polycystic ovaries (Kodaman, 2015).

Nursing Management

Nurses play an important role in the care of infertile couples. They are pivotal educators about preventive health care. A number of potentially modifiable risk factors are associated with the development of impaired fertility, and clients need to be aware of these risks to institute change. The nurse is most effective when he or she offers care and treatment in a professional manner and regards the couple as valued and respected individuals. The nurse must be respectful and mindful that many clients may seek spiritual help for their infertility issues in addition to traditional medical modalities (King et al., 2015). The nurse's focus must encompass the whole person, not just the results of the various infertility studies. Throughout the entire process, the nurse's role is to provide information, anticipatory guidance, stress management, and counselling. The couple's emotional distress is usually very high, and the nurse must be able to recognize that anxiety and provide emotional support. The nurse may need to refer couples to a reproductive endocrinologist or surgeon, depending on the problem identified.

There is no absolute way to prevent infertility per se because so many factors are involved in conception. Nurses can be instrumental in educating couples about the factors that contribute to infertility. The nurse can also outline the risks and benefits of treatments so that the couple can make an informed decision. As couples struggle with infertility, they frequently turn to nurses for empathy, counselling, and support. By understanding the struggles and lived experiences of clients and couples experiencing infertility, the nurse can tailor his/her approach to better meet their needs so that the pregnancy and birth experience of these clients is healing, transformative, and positive.

With advances in genetics and reproductive medicine also come a myriad of ethical, social, and cultural issues that will affect the couple's decisions. With this in mind, provide an opportunity for the couple to make informed decisions in a nondirective, nonjudgmental environment. It is important to encourage couples to remain optimistic throughout investigation and treatment. Through the use of advocacy and anticipatory guidance, assist and support couples through the diagnosis and treatment of infertility (Ying & Loke, 2015).

Many infertile couples are not prepared for the emotional roller coaster of grief and loss that accompanies infertility treatments. Financial concerns and coping as a couple are two major areas of stress when treatment is undertaken. While the cost of fertility investigations is covered by provincial health care, only a few provinces (Quebec and Ontario) cover the cost of fertility treatments, such as IVF (Infertility Network, 2018). During the course of what may be months or even years of infertility care, it is essential to develop a holistic approach to nursing care. Stress management and anxiety reduction need to be addressed, and referral to a peer support group might be in order (Box 4.4).

BOX 4.4

ORGANIZATIONS AND WEB RESOURCES TO ASSIST THE CLIENT WITH INFERTILITY

- **Canadian Fertility and Andrology Society:** A multidisciplinary non-profit organization made up of reproductive specialists, scientists, and allied health professionals working in the field of Assisted Reproduction in Canada (https://cfas.ca/about-cfas/)
- **Fertility Matters Canada:** A national organization for support, building awareness, providing information and education, as well as promoting equitable access to fertility treatments in Canada (http://fertilitymatters.ca/)
- **Fertility, Health Canada** (https://www.canada.ca/en/public-health/services/fertility/fertility.html)
- **Infertility Network:** An international organization which strives to increase public understanding and awareness of infertility, reproductive technology, and related issues (https://www.infertilitynetwork.org)
- **American Society of Reproductive Medicine (ASRM):** Provides fact sheets and other resources on infertility, treatments, insurance, and other issues (http://www.asrm.org)
- **International Council on Infertility Information Dissemination (INCIID):** Provides information about infertility, support forums, and a directory of infertility specialists (http://www.inciid.org)

CONTRACEPTION

Contraception is any method that prevents conception or childbirth, including OCs, and male condoms, which are the most popular methods used in Canada (SOGC, 2015). Additional types of contraceptives are discussed later in this chapter.

The United Nations Population Fund (UNFPA, 2018) *State of the World Population 2018 Report* reported that over 7 billion people inhabit the earth now and over 80 million people are added to the world each year, more than half of whom are unintended.

In addition to unwanted pregnancies, which can result in abortion, some contraceptives also help prevent transmission of STIs and human immunodeficiency virus (HIV). The Public Health Agency of Canada (Public Health Agency of Canada [PHAC], 2015) reported that, in 2014, approximately 75,500 Canadians were living with HIV, with an estimated 2,570 new infections annually. Much of this suffering could be prevented by access to and consistent use of safe, efficient, appropriate, modern contraception for everyone who wants it, as well as proper education regarding benefits and instructions for use. In addition, climate change (extreme temperature changes and rising ocean levels) will interact with population growth in ways that put additional stress on already weak health systems and will exacerbate vulnerability to the adverse health effects of climate change. The damage done to the environment by modern society is perhaps one of the most inequitable health risks of our time (UNFPA, 2018).

Today, the voluntary control of fertility is of vital importance to modern society. From a global perspective, countries currently face a crisis of rapid population growth that has begun to threaten human survival. At the present rate, the population of the world will double in 40 years; in several of the more socioeconomically disadvantaged countries, populations will double in less than 20 years (UNFPA, 2018).

Types of Contraceptive Methods

Contraceptive methods can be divided into four types: behavioural methods, barrier methods, hormonal methods, and permanent methods. Clients must decide which method is appropriate for them to meet their changing contraceptive needs throughout their life cycles. Nurses provide education and assistance during this selection process. This part of the chapter will outline the most common birth control methods available.

In an era when many people wish to delay pregnancy and avoid STIs, choices are difficult. Numerous methods of contraception are available today, and many more will be offered in the near future. The ideal contraceptive method for many clients would have the following characteristics: ease of use, safety, effectiveness,

---

BOX 4.5

OUTLINE OF CONTRACEPTIVE METHODS

Reversible Methods
- **Behavioural**
  - Abstinence
  - Fertility awareness–based methods
  - Withdrawal (coitus interruptus)
  - Lactational amenorrhea method (LAM)
- **Barrier**
  - Condom (male and female)
  - Diaphragm
  - Cervical cap
  - Sponge
- **Hormonal**
  - Oral contraceptive
  - Injectable contraceptive
  - Transdermal patch
  - Vaginal ring
  - Implantable contraceptive (not currently available in Canada)
  - Intrauterine contraceptive
  - Emergency contraceptive

Permanent Methods
- Tubal ligation
- Vasectomy

---

minimal side effects, "naturalness," nonhormonal method, and immediate reversibility (Casey, 2018). Currently, no one contraceptive method offers everything. Box 4.5 outlines the contraceptive methods available today. Table 4.4 provides a detailed summary of each type, including information on failure rates, advantages, disadvantages, STI protection, and danger signs.

Sexual Abstinence

Sexual abstinence (not having vaginal or anal intercourse) is one of the least expensive forms of contraception and has been used for thousands of years. Basically, pregnancy cannot occur if sperm is kept out of the vagina. It also reduces the risk of contracting HIV/AIDS and other STIs, unless body fluids are exchanged through oral sex; however, some infections, such as herpes and human papilloma virus (HPV), can be passed by skin-to-skin contact. Dental dams can be used to prevent transmission, however. There are many pleasurable options for sex play without intercourse ("outercourse"), such as kissing, masturbation, erotic massage, sexual fantasy, sex toys such as vibrators, and oral sex.

Many people have strong feelings about abstinence based on religious and moral beliefs. There are many good and personal reasons to choose abstinence. For

(text continues on page 132)

| TABLE 4.4 | SUMMARY OF CONTRACEPTIVE METHODS |

Type	Description	Failure Rate	Pros	Cons	STI Protection	Danger Signs	Comments
Abstinence	Refrain from sexual activity	None	Costs nothing	Difficult to maintain	100%	None	Must be joint couple decision
Fertility awareness-based methods	Refrain from sex during fertile period	25%	No side effects; acceptable to most religious groups	High failure rate with incorrect use	None	None	Requires high level of couple commitment
Withdrawal (coitus interruptus)	Withdrawing the penis from the vagina before ejaculation	27%	Involves no devices and is always available	Requires considerable self-control by the man	None	None	Places partner in trusting and dependent role
Lactational amenorrhea method (LAM)	Uses lactational infertility for protection from pregnancy	1–2% chance of pregnancy in first 6 mo	No cost; not coitus linked	Temporary method; effective for only 6 months after giving birth	None	None	Involves breastfeeding on demand without supplementation for 6 mo
Male condom	Thin sheath placed over an erect penis, blocking sperm	15%	Widely available; low cost; physiologically safe	Decreased penile sensation; interferes with sexual spontaneity; breakage risk	Provides protection against STIs	Latex allergy	Couple must be instructed on proper use of condom
Female condom	Polyurethane sheath inserted vaginally to block sperm	21%	Use controlled by woman; eliminates postcoital drainage of semen	Expensive for frequent use; cumbersome; noisy during sex act; for single use only	Provides protection against STIs	Allergy to polyurethane	Couple must be instructed on proper use of condom
Diaphragm with spermicide	Shallow latex cup with spring mechanism in its rim to hold it in place in the vagina	16%	Does not use hormone; considered medically safe; provides some protection against cervical cancer	Requires accurate fitting by health care professional; increase in UTIs	None	Allergy to latex, rubber, polyurethane, or spermicide Report symptoms of toxic shock syndrome May become dislodged when in superior position	Client must be taught to insert and remove diaphragm correctly

Method	Description	Effectiveness	Advantages	Disadvantages		Side Effects/Risks	Nursing Considerations
Cervical cap with spermicide	Soft cup-shaped latex device that fits over base of cervix	24%	No use of hormones; provides continuous protection while in place	Requires accurate fitting by health care professional; odour may occur if left in too long	None	Irritation, allergic reaction; abnormal Pap test; risk of toxic shock syndrome	Instructions on insertion and removal must be understood by client
Sponge with spermicide	Disk-shaped polyurethane device containing a spermicide that is activated by wetting it with water	25%	Offers immediate and continuous protection for 24 hours; OTC	Can fall out of vagina with voiding; is not form-fitting in the vagina	None	Irritation, allergic reactions; toxic shock syndrome can occur if sponge left in too long	Caution client not to leave sponge in beyond 24 hours
Oral contraceptives (combination)	A pill that suppresses ovulation by combined action of estrogen and progestin	8%	Easy to use; high rate of effectiveness; protection against ovarian and endometrial cancer	User must remember to take pill daily; possible undesirable side effects; cost; prescription needed	None	Dizziness, nausea, mood changes, high blood pressure, blood clots, heart attacks, strokes	Each client must be assessed thoroughly for risk factors including smoking and history of thromboembolic disease
Oral contraceptives (progestin-only minipills)	A pill containing only progestin that thickens cervical mucus to prevent sperm from penetrating	8%	No estrogen-related side effects; may be used by lactating clients; may be used by those with history of thrombophlebitis	Must be taken with meticulous accuracy; may cause irregular bleeding; less effective than combination pills	None	Irregular bleeding, weight gain, increased incidence of ectopic pregnancy	Clients should be screened for history of functional ovarian cysts, previous ectopic pregnancy, and hyperlipidemia prior to giving prescription
Patch (Ortho Evra)	Transdermal patch that releases estrogen and progestin into circulation	8%	Easy system to remember; very effective	May cause skin irritation where it is placed; may fall off and not be noticed and thus provide no protection	None	Less effective in clients more than 200 lb	Instruct client to apply patch every week for 3 weeks and then not to wear one during week 4

(continued)

TABLE 4.4 | **SUMMARY OF CONTRACEPTIVE METHODS** (continued)

Type	Description	Failure Rate	Pros	Cons	STI Protection	Danger Signs	Comments
Ring (NuvaRing)	Vaginal contraceptive ring about 2 in in diameter that is inserted into the vagina; releases estrogen and progestin	8%	Easy system to remember; very effective	May cause a vaginal discharge; can be expelled without noticing and not offer protection	None	Similar to oral contraceptives	Instruct client to use a backup method if ring is expelled and remains out for more than 3 hours
Depo-Provera injection	An injectable progestin that inhibits ovulation	3%	Long duration of action (3 months); highly effective; estrogen-free; may be used by smokers; can be used by lactating individuals	Menstrual irregularities; return visit needed every 12 weeks; weight gain, headaches, depression; return to fertility delayed up to 12 months	None	If depression is a problem, this method may increase the depression	Inform client that fertility is delayed after stopping the injections
Implant (Nexplanon)	A time-release implant (one rod) of levonorgestrel for 3 years	0.05%	Long duration of action; low dose of hormones; reversible; estrogen-free	Irregular bleeding; weight gain; breast tenderness; headaches; difficulty in removal	None	If bleeding is heavy, anemia may occur	Before insertion, inform client that this method will produce about 3 years of infertility
Intrauterine contraceptives (IUCs)	A T-shaped device inserted into the uterus that releases copper or progesterone or levonorgestrel	1%	It is immediately and highly effective; allows for sexual spontaneity; can be used during lactation; return to fertility not impaired; requires no motivation by the user after insertion	Insertion requires a skilled professional; menstrual irregularities; prolonged amenorrhea; can be unknowingly expelled; may increase the risk of pelvic infection; user must regularly check string for placement; no protection against STIs; delay of fertility after discontinuing for possibly 6–12 months	None	Cramps, bleeding, pelvic inflammatory disease; infertility; perforation of the uterus	Instruct client how to locate string to check monthly for placement

Method	Description	Effectiveness	Advantages	Disadvantages		Side effects	Counseling considerations
Postcoital emergency contraceptives (ECs)	Combination of levonorgestrel-only pills; combined estrogen and progestin pills; or the copper IUS inserted within 72 hours after unprotected intercourse	80%	Provides a last chance to prevent a pregnancy	Risk of ectopic pregnancy if EC fails	None	Nausea, vomiting, abdominal pain, fatigue, headache	Inform client that ECs do not interrupt an established pregnancy, and the sooner they are taken, the more effective they are
Permanent sterilization							
Vasectomy	Sealing, tying, or cutting the vas deferens	<1%	One-time decision provides permanent sterility; short recovery time; low long-term risks	Procedures are difficult to reverse; initial cost may be high; chance of regret; some pain/discomfort after procedures	None for both		Counsel both as to permanence of procedure and urge them to think it through prior to signing consent
Tubal Ligation	Fallopian tubes are blocked to prevent conception	<1%					

Adapted from Raymond, E. G., & Cleland, K. (2015). Emergency contraception. New England Journal of Medicine, 372(14), 1342–1348; King, T. L., Brucker, M. C., Kriebs, J. M., Fahey, J. O., Gegor, C. L., & Varney, H. (2015). Varney's midwifery (5th ed.). Burlington, MA: Jones & Bartlett Learning; Ilic, K. (2015). Emergency contraception. In Medicines for women (pp. 203–225). Cham, Switzerland: Springer International Publishing; Casey, F. E. (2018). Contraception. eMedicine. Retrieved from http://emedicine.medscape.com/article/258507-overview; Schuiling, K. D., & Likis, F. E. (2016). Women's gynecologic health (3rd ed.). Burlington, MA: Jones & Bartlett Learning.

some people it is a way of life, whereas for others it is a temporary choice. Some people choose sexual abstinence because they want to:
- Wait until they are older
- Wait for a long-term relationship
- Avoid pregnancy or STIs
- Relieve feelings of depression or anxiety
- Follow religious or cultural expectations

Fertility Awareness–Based Methods

Fertility awareness refers to any natural contraceptive method that does not require hormones, pharmaceutical compounds, physical barriers, or surgery to prevent pregnancy. Fertility awareness–based (FAB) methods, or fertility awareness methods (FAM), use physical signs and symptoms that change with hormone fluctuations throughout a client's menstrual cycle to predict fertility. Ovulation occurs on 1 day during each menstrual cycle, and the several days preceding ovulation are when intercourse is most likely to result in pregnancy. Collectively, the potentially fertile days up to and including the day of ovulation are called the "fertile window." Awareness of fertility is a better fertility-producing method than contraceptives. The unifying theme of FAMs is that people can reduce their chance of pregnancy by abstaining from coitus or using barrier methods during times of fertility. These methods require couples to take an active role in preventing pregnancy through their sexual behaviours, and menstrual cycles must be regular for it to be effective. Couples agree to practice certain techniques, use calculations, and be observant of the "fertile" and the "safe" periods in a monthly menstrual cycle. Using these methods for birth control requires a strong commitment from both partners. The normal physiologic changes caused by hormonal fluctuations during the menstrual cycle can be observed and charted. This information can then be used to avoid or promote pregnancy. Fertility awareness methods rely on the following assumptions:

- A single ovum is released from the ovary 14 days before the next menstrual period. It lives approximately 24 hours.
- People using this method must have regular menstrual cycles for it to be effective.
- Sperm can live up to 5 days after intercourse. The "unsafe period" during the menstrual cycle is thus approximately 6 days: 3 days before and 3 days after ovulation. Because body changes start to occur before ovulation, the client can become aware of them and not have intercourse on these days or use another method to prevent pregnancy.
- The exact time of ovulation cannot be determined, so 2 to 3 days are added to the beginning and end to avoid pregnancy (SOGC, 2015).

Techniques used to determine fertility include the cervical mucus ovulation method, the basal body temperature (BBT) method, the symptothermal method, standard days method (SDM), and two-day method (Everett, 2014). Fertility awareness methods are moderately effective but are very unforgiving if not carried out as prescribed. Fertility awareness can be used in combination with coital abstinence or barrier methods during fertile days if pregnancy is not desired.

CERVICAL MUCUS OVULATION METHOD

Cervical mucus is a jelly-like vaginal discharge that comes from the cervix. The **cervical mucus ovulation method** is used to assess the character of the cervical mucus. Cervical mucus changes consistently during the menstrual cycle and plays a vital role in fertilization of the egg. Studies conducted by the WHO indicate that 93% of women, regardless of their education level, are capable of identifying and distinguishing fertile and infertile cervical secretions (Planned Parenthood, 2018a). In the days preceding ovulation, fertile cervical mucus helps draw sperm up and into the fallopian tubes, where fertilization usually takes place. It also helps maintain the survival of sperm. As ovulation approaches, the mucus becomes more abundant, clear, slippery, and smooth; it can be stretched between two fingers without breaking. Under the influence of estrogen, this mucus looks like egg whites. It is called *spinnbarkeit* mucus (Fig. 4.5). After ovulation, the cervical mucus becomes thick and dry under the influence of progesterone.

The cervical position can also be assessed to confirm changes in the cervical mucus at ovulation. Near ovulation, the cervix feels soft and is high/deep in the vagina, the os is slightly open, and the cervical mucus is copious and slippery (Bieber, Sanfilippo, Horowitz, & Shafi, 2015). This method works because clients become aware of their body changes accompanying ovulation. When these changes occur, the couple abstains from

FIGURE 4.5 Spinnbarkeit mucus is cervical mucus that can stretch a distance before breaking.

sexual intercourse or uses another method to prevent pregnancy. Each person is an individual, so everyone's unsafe time of the month is unique and thus must be individually assessed and determined.

BASAL BODY TEMPERATURE METHOD

The **basal body temperature (BBT)** refers to the lowest temperature reached on awakening. The client takes an oral temperature before rising and records it on a chart. Preovulation temperatures are suppressed by estrogen, whereas postovulation temperatures are increased under the influence of heat-inducing progesterone. Temperatures typically rise within a day or two after ovulation and remain elevated for approximately 2 weeks (at which point bleeding usually begins). If using this method by itself, the couples should avoid unprotected intercourse until the BBT has been elevated for 3 days. Nurses should instruct clients using the BBT method that it is important to keep in mind that illness and any drugs, including alcohol, can raise their body temperature and give a false reading. Other fertility awareness methods should be used along with BBT for better results (Fig. 4.6).

SYMPTOTHERMAL METHOD

The **symptothermal method** relies on a combination of techniques to recognize ovulation, including BBT, cervical mucus changes, alterations in the position and firmness of the cervix, and other symptoms of ovulation, such as increased libido, *mittelschmerz* (midcycle, lower abdominal pain at ovulation), pelvic fullness or tenderness, and breast tenderness (Planned Parenthood, 2018a). Combining all these predictors increases awareness of when ovulation occurs and increases the effectiveness of this method. A home predictor test for ovulation is also available in most pharmacies. It measures LH levels to pinpoint the day before or the day of ovulation. These tests are widely used for fertility and infertility regimens.

THE STANDARD DAYS METHOD AND THE TWO-DAY METHOD

The SDM and the two-day method are both natural methods of contraception developed by Georgetown University Medical Center's Institute for Reproductive Health. Both methods provide simple, clear instructions for identifying fertile days. Clients with menstrual cycles between 26 and 32 days long can use the SDM to prevent pregnancy by avoiding unprotected intercourse on days 8 through 19 of their cycles. Most SDM users utilize a visual aid—CycleBeads—to assist their correct use of SDM. An international clinical trial of the SDM showed that the method is more than 95% effective when used correctly (Wright, Iqteit, & Hardee, 2015). SDM identifies the 12-day "fertile window" of a client's menstrual cycle. These 12 days take into account the life span of the egg (about 24 hours) and the viability of the sperm (about 5 days) as well as the variation in the actual timing of ovulation

Basal body temperature

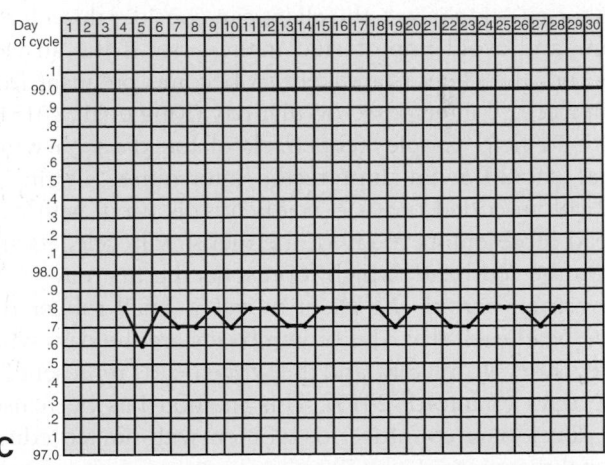

FIGURE 4.6 Basal body temperature graph. **A.** The person's temperature dips slightly at midpoint in the menstrual cycle, then rises sharply, an indication of ovulation. Toward the end of the cycle (the 24th day), the temperature begins to decline, indicating that progesterone levels are falling and that conception did not take place. **B.** The person's temperature rises at the midpoint in the cycle and remains at that elevated level past the time of normal menstrual flow, suggesting that pregnancy has occurred. **C.** There is no preovulatory dip and no rise of temperature anywhere during the cycle. This is the typical pattern of an individual who does not ovulate.

If your period does not start by the day after you move the ring to the last BROWN bead, your cycle is longer than 32 days.

The RED bead marks the first day of your menstrual period. On the day your period starts, move the ring to the red bead. Continue to move the ring one bead each day.

The DARK BROWN bead helps you know if your cycle is less than 26 days long. If your period starts before you move the ring to the dark brown bead, your cycle is shorter than 26 days.

All BROWN beads mark the days when you are not likely to get pregnant if you have unprotected sex.

All WHITE beads mark the days when you are likely to get pregnant. Do not have unprotected sex on the white bead days if you do not want to get pregnant.

FIGURE 4.7 CycleBeads help individuals use the Standard Days Method.

from one cycle to another. For the 2-day method, clients observe the presence or absence of cervical secretions by examining toilet paper or underwear or by monitoring their physical sensations. Every day, the client asks two simple questions: "Did I note any secretions yesterday?" and "Did I note any secretions today?" If the answer to either question is yes, the client can consider this a fertile time and avoid unprotected intercourse. If the answers are no, the client is unlikely to become pregnant from unprotected intercourse on that day (King et al., 2015).

To help people keep track of the days on which they should avoid unprotected intercourse, a string of 32 colour-coded beads (CycleBeads) is used, with each bead representing a day of the menstrual cycle. Starting with the red bead, which represents the first day of the menstrual period, the client moves a small rubber ring one bead each day. The brown beads are the days when pregnancy is unlikely, and the white beads represent fertile days (Stanford, 2015). This method has been used in developing countries for women with limited educational resources (Fig. 4.7).

Withdrawal (Coitus Interruptus)

In **coitus interruptus**, also known as withdrawal, ejaculation is controlled during sexual intercourse and takes place outside the vagina. It is better known colloquially as "pulling out in time" or "being careful." The Canadian Contraception Survey found that 12% of Canadians report using withdrawal as the primary method of contraception (SOGC, 2015). It is one of the oldest and most

widely used means of preventing pregnancy in the world and also one of the least effective methods in preventing pregnancy (Creatsas, 2015). The problem with this method is that the first few drops of the true ejaculate contain the greatest concentration of sperm, and if some pre-ejaculatory fluid escapes from the urethra before orgasm, conception may result. This method requires that the clients rely solely on the cooperation and judgment of the partner not ejaculating inside the vagina. Nurses might wish to discuss emergency contraceptives be available with this couple or use a more effective method of contraception.

Lactational Amenorrhea Method

The **lactational amenorrhea method** (LAM) is an effective temporary method of contraception when breastfeeding. It relies on physiologic changes associated with breastfeeding for contraception. Continuous breastfeeding usually can postpone ovulation and thus prevent pregnancy. Breastfeeding stimulates the hormone prolactin, which is necessary for milk production, and also inhibits the release of another hormone, gonadotropin, which is necessary for ovulation.

Breastfeeding as a contraceptive method can be fairly effective for up to 6 months after giving birth only if:
- Menstrual periods have not resumed since giving birth
- Infant is younger than 6 months of age
- The baby breastfeeds at least six times daily on both breasts
- Breastfeeding "on demand," at least every 4 hours
- Nighttime feedings are provided at least every 6 hours

The baby does not receive any other foods in addition to breastmilk (Planned Parenthood, 2018a).

Nurses can help couples to make a decision about family planning options available in the postpartum period by discussing the advantages and disadvantages of each, taking into consideration the demands of the postpartum period. The options they may consider include lactational amenorrhea, combined oral contraception, implants, IUSs, injectable methods, barrier methods, emergency contraception (EC), and sterilization (Hughes, 2015).

Barrier Methods

Barrier contraceptives are forms of birth control that prevent pregnancy by preventing the sperm from reaching the ovum. Mechanical barriers include condoms, diaphragms, cervical caps, and sponges. These devices are placed over the penis or cervix to physically obstruct the passage of sperm through the cervix. Chemical barriers called spermicides may be used along with mechanical barrier devices. They come in creams, jellies, foam, suppositories, and vaginal films. They chemically destroy the sperm in the vagina. These contraceptives are called barrier methods because they not only provide a physical barrier for sperm, but also protect against STIs. Since the HIV/AIDS epidemic started in the early 1980s, these methods have become extremely popular. Progress has been made in society's reaction to condom use as a disease prevention device now and not just as a contraceptive (Haddad, Philpott-Jones, & Schonfeld, 2015).

Many of these barrier methods contain latex. Allergy to latex was first recognized in the late 1970s, and since then it has become a major health concern, with increasing numbers of people affected. Health care workers in both the medical and dental environments face a higher incidence of latex allergies (approximately 10%), as well as specific groups of individuals including those with spina bifida, myelodysplasia, and food allergies (banana, kiwi, avocado, and others) are at increased risk of sensitization (over 7%) compared with the general population (approximately 4%) (Kim, 2015; Wu, McIntosh, & Liu, 2016). Teaching Guidelines 4.4 provides tips for individuals with latex allergy.

Teaching Guidelines 4.4
TIPS FOR INDIVIDUALS ALLERGIC TO LATEX

Symptoms of latex allergy include:
- Skin rash, itching, hives
- Itching or burning eyes
- Swollen mucous membranes in the genitals
- Shortness of breath, difficulty breathing, wheezing
- Anaphylactic shock
- Use of or contact with latex condoms, cervical caps, and diaphragms is contraindicated for men and women with a latex allergy
- If their partner is allergic to latex, instruct a male to apply a natural condom over the latex one
- If a male partner experiences penile irritation after condom use, try different brands or place the latex condom over a natural condom
- Use polyurethane condoms rather than latex ones
- Use female condoms; they are made of polyurethane
- Switch to another birth control method that is not made with latex, such as oral contraceptives, intrauterine systems, Depo-Provera, fertility awareness, and other nonbarrier methods. However, these methods do not protect against sexually transmitted infections.

Adapted from American Academy of Allergy, Asthma and Immunology (AAAAI). (2018). *Latex allergy: Tips to remember.* Retrieved from http://www.aaaai.org/conditions-and-treatments/library/allergy-library/latex-allergy.aspx; Kim, J. S. (2015). Latex allergy. In H. A. Sampson (Ed.). *Allergy and clinical immunology* (pp. 288–293). Chichester, UK: John Wiley & Sons; Occupational Health and Safety Administration (OSHA). (2018). *Latex allergy.* Retrieved from http://www.osha.gov/SLTC/latex-allergy

CONDOMS

Condoms are barrier methods of contraceptives made in forms to cover and protect both the penis and the vagina. The penile condom is made from latex or polyurethane or natural membrane and may be coated with spermicide. Penile condoms are available in many colours, textures, sizes, shapes, and thicknesses. When used correctly, the condom is put on over an erect penis before it enters the vagina and is worn throughout sexual intercourse (Fig. 4.8). It serves as a barrier to pregnancy by trapping seminal fluid and sperm and offers protection against STIs. Condoms are not perfect barriers, however, because breakage and slippage can occur. Emergency postcoital contraception may need to be sought to prevent a pregnancy. In addition, the nonlatex condoms have a higher risk of pregnancy and STIs than latex condoms (Everett, 2014).

The vaginal condom is a polyurethane pouch inserted into the vagina. It consists of an outer and inner ring that is inserted vaginally and held in place by the pubic bone. Some people complain that the vaginal condom is cumbersome to use and makes noise during intercourse. Vaginal condoms are readily available, are inexpensive, and can be carried inconspicuously. The female condom was the first woman-controlled method that offered protection against pregnancy and some STIs. Nurses can play a key role in educating clients on how to initiate and maintain use of the vaginal condom, an underused method for HIV/STI and pregnancy prevention. Providing a brief education session along with free samples would go a long way to promote increased use of this device to prevent STIs transmission as well as pregnancy (Boyd, Perkins, Lawrence, Sutherland, & Blake, 2015).

DIAPHRAGM

The **diaphragm** is a soft latex dome surrounded by a metal spring. Used in conjunction with a spermicidal jelly or cream, it is inserted into the vagina to cover the cervix (Fig. 4.9). The diaphragm may be inserted up to 4 hours before intercourse but must be left in place for at least 6 hours afterward. Diaphragms are available in a range of sizes and styles. The diaphragm is available only by prescription and must be professionally fitted by a health care provider. Clients may need to be refitted with a different-sized diaphragm after pregnancy, abdominal or pelvic surgery, or weight loss or gain of 10 lb or more. As a general rule, diaphragms should be replaced every 1 to 2 years. Recently, a single-sized diaphragm used with contraceptive jelly was introduced and studied for its effectiveness. The single-sized diaphragm was deemed safe and as effective as a standard individually fitted one based on a population sample of >400 women who participated in the research study (Schwartz et al., 2015). The diaphragm provides both a physical and chemical barrier to sperm (Tharpe et al., 2016).

FIGURE 4.8 **A.** Male condom. **B.** Applying a male condom. Leaving space at the tip helps to ensure the condom will not break with ejaculation. **C.** The female condom. **D.** Insertion technique.

Diaphragms are user-controlled, nonhormonal methods that are needed only at the time of intercourse, but they are not effective unless used correctly. Clients require thorough instruction about diaphragm use and should practice putting one in and taking it out before they leave the health care office (Fig. 4.10).

Results of a 2-year multisite study indicate that the effectiveness rates of the SILCS single-sized, contoured diaphragm are similar to those of traditional diaphragms, but they also provide a long-term controlled release of the lead candidate anti-HIV microbicide dapivirine. This would make it a new multipurpose prevention device (Schwartz et al., 2015). The biggest difference with this new device is that since it is single size, a pelvic examination to assess the size is not required, and it also releases an anti-HIV microbicide

that potentially is capable of preventing HIV transmission. Most women in the study were able to correctly insert, remove, and check correct position of the device by simply using the instructions (Schwartz et al., 2015).

CERVICAL CAP

The **cervical cap** is smaller than the diaphragm and covers only the cervix; it is held in place by suction. Caps are made from silicone or latex and are used with spermicide (Fig. 4.11). The cap may be inserted up to 36 hours before intercourse and provides protection for 48 hours. The cap must be kept in the vagina for 6 hours after the final act of intercourse and should be replaced every year of use. A refitting may also be necessary when a client experiences pregnancy, abortion, or weight changes.

FIGURE 4.9 Sample diaphragm used for measuring.

FIGURE 4.11 A cervical cap is placed over the cervix and used with a spermicidal jelly, the same as a diaphragm.

Inserting the diaphragm

A

Positioning the diaphragm

B

Removing the diaphragm

C

FIGURE 4.10 Application of a diaphragm. **A.** To insert, fold the diaphragm in half, separate the labia with one hand, then insert upward and back into the vagina. **B.** To position, make certain the diaphragm securely covers the cervix. **C.** To remove, hook a finger over the top of the rim and bring the diaphragm down and out.

The dome of the cap is filled about one third full with spermicide. Spermicide should not be applied to the rim because it might interfere with the seal that must form around the cervix. The cap is available only by prescription and must be fitted by a health care provider. Contraindications to the use of a cervical cap include cervical cancer, recent urinary tract infection, latex allergy, pelvic-organ prolapse, and history of toxic shock syndrome. Using the cervical cap during menstruation may increase the risk of toxic shock syndrome and, therefore, should be avoided (Schuiling & Likis, 2016).

CONTRACEPTIVE SPONGE

The **contraceptive sponge** is a nonhormonal, nonprescription device that includes both a barrier and a spermicide. The contraceptive sponge is a soft concave device that prevents pregnancy by covering the cervix and releasing spermicide. The sponge, made of polyurethane saturated with nonoxynol-9 (1,000 mg), releases 125 mg of the spermicide over 24 hours of use. Unlike the diaphragm, the sponge can be used for more than one coital act within 24 hours without the insertion of additional spermicide, and the sponge does not require fitting or a prescription from a health care provider (Zieman, 2015). While it was less effective than several other methods and does not offer protection against STIs, the sponge achieved a wide following among people who appreciated the spontaneity with which it could be used and its easy availability. When compared with the diaphragm in a recent study, the sponge was found to be less effective than the diaphragm in preventing pregnancy. Discontinuation rates were higher at 12 months as well (Sharma & Walmsley, 2015).

To use the sponge, the client first wets it with water, and then inserts it into the vagina with a finger, using a cord loop attachment. It can be inserted up to 24 hours before intercourse and should be left in place for at least 6 hours following intercourse. The sponge provides protection for up to 12 hours, but should not be left in for more than 30 hours after insertion to avoid the risk of toxic shock syndrome (Moses, 2018c).

Hormonal Methods

Several options are available to clients who want long-term but not permanent protection against pregnancy. These methods of contraception work by altering the hormones within the body. They rely on estrogen and progestin or progestin alone to prevent ovulation. When used consistently, these methods are a reliable way to prevent pregnancy. Hormonal methods include OCs, injectables, implants, vaginal rings, and transdermal patches.

ORAL CONTRACEPTIVES

As early as 1937, scientists recognized that the injection of progesterone inhibited ovulation in rabbits and provided contraception. The first hormonal pill, called *Enovid*, was approved by the U.S. FDA in May 1960. It contained high levels of estrogen to prevent ovulation. In Canada at that time, simply discussing birth control was illegal, so the oral contraceptive was marketed only for "cycle control." By 1969, contraception became decriminalized in Canada (Liao & Dollin, 2012). Since that time, the birth control pill has evolved through gradual lowering of estrogen and is now combined with many different progestins. Breakthrough bleeding was reported in early clinical trials in women, and the role of estrogen in cycle control was launched. This established the rationale for modern-combination OCs that contain both estrogen and progesterone (Stewart & Black, 2015).

Development of hormonal contraception marked a revolutionary step in social change that has improved the lives of people and families worldwide. Since the first OC was introduced, hormonal contraception has undergone various stages of advancement. Today, OC regimens are safer and more tolerable, with equal or improved efficacy, than the early formulations. Incremental decreases in the estrogen dosage helped to alleviate some of the unwanted side effects of the pill (Craik & Melvin, 2015). The most notable change in over 50 years of OC improvement has been the lowering of the estrogen dose to as low as 10 mcg and the introduction of new progestins.

Oral contraception is one of the most frequently used medications, being taken by ¾ of Canadian women at some point in their lives (Rotterman, Dunn, & Black, 2015; Fig. 4.12). Unlike the original OCs from decades ago, the new low-dose forms carry fewer health risks.

OC, although most commonly prescribed for contraception, has long been used in the management of a wide range of conditions and has many health benefits, such as:

• Reduced incidence of ovarian and endometrial cancer
• Prevention and treatment of endometriosis
• Decreased incidence of acne and hirsutism

FIGURE 4.12 **Oral contraceptive.**

- Decreased incidence of ectopic pregnancy
- Decreased incidence of acute PID and possible protection against PID
- Reduced incidence of fibrocystic breast disease
- Decreased perimenopausal symptoms
- Reduced risk of developing uterine fibroids
- Maintenance of bone mineral density (BMD)
- Improvement in asthmatic symptoms
- Delayed onset of multiple sclerosis and arthritis
- Increased menstrual cycle regularity
- Lower incidence of colorectal cancer
- Decreased number of pregnancy-related deaths by preventing pregnancy
- Reduced iron-deficiency anemia by treating menorrhagia
- Reduced incidence of dysmenorrhea (Evans & Sutton, 2015)

OCs work primarily by suppressing ovulation by adding estrogen and progesterone to the body, thus mimicking pregnancy. This hormonal level stifles GnRH, which in turn suppresses FSH and LH and thus inhibits ovulation. Cervical mucus also thickens, which hinders sperm transport into the uterus. Implantation is inhibited by suppression of the maturation of the endometrium and alterations of uterine secretions (Everett, 2014).

The combination pills are prescribed as monophasic pills, which deliver fixed dosages of estrogen and progestin, or as multiphasic ones. Multiphasic pills (e.g., biphasic and triphasic OCs) alter the amount of progestin and estrogen within each cycle. To maintain adequate hormonal levels for contraception and enhance adherence to the regimen, OCs should be taken at the same time daily.

OCs that contain progestin only are sometimes called mini-pills. Progestin-only pills (POPs) have both advantages and disadvantages when compared with combined pills. The pill-taking regimen is simple and fixed; no pill colour changes or days without pill-taking occur. These pills are appropriate for clients who cannot take estrogen in combined OCs, for example, older than 35 years and smoking cigarettes. They are prescribed for clients who cannot take estrogen at all. These OCs work primarily by thickening the cervical mucus to prevent penetration of the sperm and make the endometrium unfavourable for implantation. POPs must be taken at a certain time every 24 hours. Breakthrough bleeding and a higher risk of pregnancy have made these OCs less popular than combination OCs (Craik & Melvin, 2015).

Extended OC regimens have been used for the management of menstrual disorders and endometriosis for years but now are attracting wider attention. Surveys asking women about their willingness to reduce their menstrual cycles from 12 to 4 annually were returned with a resounding "yes!" (Zorbas, Economopoulos, & Vlahos, 2015). Research has confirmed that the extended use of active OC pills carries the same safety profile as the conventional 28-day regimens. OCs taken continuously or in long cycles offer benefits with regard to menstrual symptoms and the recurrence of symptoms related to endometriosis (Zieman, 2015). The extended regimen consists of 84 consecutive days of active combination pills, followed by 7 days of placebos. The client has four withdrawal-bleeding episodes a year. Seasonale and Seasonique, a combination OC, is on the market for clients who choose to reduce the number of periods that they have. In 2009, the makers of Seasonique came out with LoSeasonique. LoSeasonique consists of 84 orange tablets containing 0.1-mg levonorgestrel and 0.02-mg ethinyl estradiol and 7 yellow tablets containing 0.01-mg ethinyl estradiol. The risk profile is similar to those of its sister products, Seasonale and Seasonique; however, the risk of unplanned breakthrough bleeding is increased (Casey, 2018).

In the United States, Lybrel was the first FDA-approved OC with 365-day combination dosing in 2007; it was later approved in Canada in 2012. Since that time, generic versions of the drug have become available, causing the manufacturer to cease distribution under the Lybrel trade name. This oral contraception option contains a low combined daily dose of the hormones levonorgestrel and ethinyl estradiol (90 and 20 mcg, respectively). It provides clients with more hormonal exposure on a yearly basis (13 additional weeks of hormone intake per year) than conventional cyclic OCs that contain the same strength of synthetic estrogens and similar strength of progestins (Casey & Isaacs, 2015). There is no physiologic requirement for cyclic hormonal withdrawal bleeds while taking OCs (Skidmore-Roth, 2015).

A growing body of evidence indicates that an over-the-counter access to OC pills is safe and effective and that clients are interested in obtaining pills this way. With half of all pregnancies being unintended—a figure that has remained unchanged for decades—innovation is needed to address this statistic. Although an over-the-counter contraceptive pill may sound revolutionary, over-the-counter access is already a reality in more than 100 countries and has been for decades.

The balance between the benefits and the risks of OCs must be determined for each client when being assessed for this type of contraceptive. It is a highly effective contraceptive when taken properly but can aggravate many medical conditions, especially in women who smoke. Comparison Chart 4.1 lists advantages and disadvantages of OCs. A thorough history and pelvic examination, including a Pap smear, are not required before the medication is prescribed, but a regular medical follow-up is advised. Clients should also be counselled that the effectiveness of OCs is decreased when taking antibiotics; thus, an alternative or secondary method is necessary during this time to prevent pregnancy.

COMPARISON CHART 4.1 ADVANTAGES AND DISADVANTAGES OF ORAL CONTRACEPTIVES

Advantages	Disadvantages
Regulate and shorten menstrual cycle	Offer no protection against STIs
Decrease severe cramping and bleeding	Pose slightly increased risk of breast cancer
Reduce anemia	
Reduce ovarian and colorectal cancer risk	Modest risk for venous thrombosis and pulmonary emboli
Decrease benign breast disease	Increased risk for migraine headaches
Reduce risk of endometrial cancer, colorectal cancer, and ovarian cancer	
Improve acne and reduces incidence of menstrual headaches	Increased risk for myocardial infarction, stroke, and hypertension for women who smoke
Minimize perimenopausal symptoms	May increase risk of depression
Decrease incidence of rheumatoid arthritis	User must remember to take pill daily
Improve PMS symptoms	High cost for some women
Protect against loss of bone density and reduces risk of osteoporosis	

Adapted from Jick, S. (2015). Oral contraceptives and the risk of venous thromboembolism. In M. Harrison-Woolrych (Ed.). *Medicines for women* (pp. 181–201). Switzerland: Springer International Publishing; Zieman, M. (2015). *Managing contraception on the go* (13th ed.). New York: Ardnet Media; Everett, S. (2014). *Handbook of contraception and sexual health* (3rd ed.). New York: Routledge.

Nurses need to provide OC users with a great deal of education before they leave the health care facility. They need to be able to identify early signs and symptoms that might indicate a problem.

Take Note!

The mnemonic "ACHES" can help clients taking OCs to remember the early warning signs that necessitate a return to the health care provider (Box 4.6).

INJECTABLE CONTRACEPTIVE

Injectable contraception includes progestin-only and combination estrogen and progestin agents that provide

---

BOX 4.6

EARLY SIGNS OF COMPLICATIONS FOR USERS OF ORAL CONTRACEPTIVES

A = Abdominal pain may indicate liver or gallbladder problems.
C = Chest pain or shortness of breath may indicate a pulmonary embolus.
H = Headaches may indicate hypertension or impending stroke.
E = Eye problems may indicate hypertension or an attack.
S = Severe leg pain may indicate a thromboembolic event.

Adapted from Everett, S. (2014). *Handbook of contraception and sexual health* (3rd ed.). New York: Routledge.

---

safe and highly effective birth control for up to 3 months. Injectable agents are widely available and play an important role in family planning worldwide. They offer a discreet, convenient, reversible, and non–coital-dependent method of birth control.

Depo-Provera is the trade name for an intramuscular injectable of a progesterone-only contraceptive given every 12 weeks which contains 150 mg/mL. Depo-subQ Pronera is a lower-dose injection given subcutaneously delivering 104 mg/0.65 mL every 12 weeks. They are the only injectable agents available in Canada. Depo-Provera works by suppressing ovulation and the production of FSH and LH by the pituitary gland, and by increasing the viscosity of cervical mucus and causing endometrial atrophy. A single intramuscular injection of 150 mg acts like other progestin-only products to prevent pregnancy for 3 months at a time (Fig. 4.13). The primary side effect of Depo-Provera is menstrual cycle disturbance.

Recent clinical studies have raised concerns about whether Depo-Provera reduces BMD. This evidence has prompted the manufacturer to issue a warning about the long-term use (>2 years) of Depo-Provera and bone loss (Wolfe & Cansino, 2015). It is not entirely clear if this loss in BMD is reversible because there have not been any long-term prospective studies in current and past users. The SOGC recommends that health care professionals discuss the risks and benefits of injectable contraceptives, particularly in relation to BMD; however, there is

FIGURE 4.13 Injectable contraceptive.

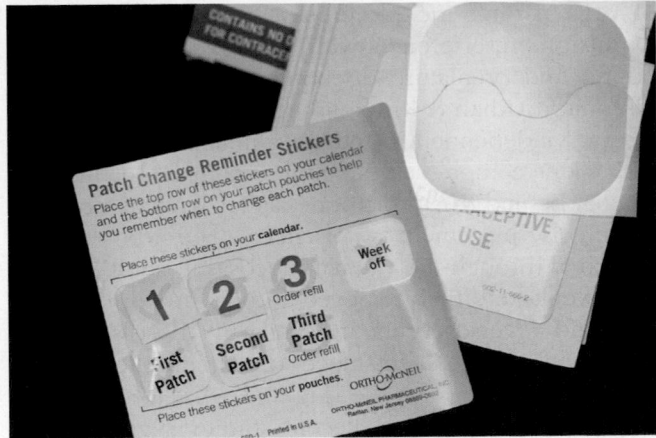

FIGURE 4.14 Transdermal patch.

no recommendation for increased BMD monitoring for these clients (SOGC, 2006).

TRANSDERMAL PATCHES

Transdermal delivery of contraceptive hormones avoids hepatic first-pass metabolism, allowing a lower total hormone doses when compared with that of oral products that are metabolized in the liver. A **transdermal patch**, Ortho Evra, is available in Canada. It is a matchbox-sized patch containing hormones that are absorbed through the skin when placed on the lower abdomen, upper outer arm, buttocks, or upper torso (avoiding the breasts). The patch is applied weekly for 3 weeks, followed by a patch-free week during which withdrawal bleeding occurs. The patch delivers continuous levels of progesterone and estrogen. Transdermal absorption allows the drug to enter the bloodstream directly, avoiding rapid inactivation in the liver known as first-pass metabolism. Because estrogen and progesterone are metabolized by liver enzymes, avoiding first-pass metabolism was thought to reduce adverse effects. However, recent evidence suggests that the risk of venous thrombosis and embolism is increased with the patch and the risk of skin burns occurring if undergoing an MRI, but still less than the risk of venous thromboembolism during pregnancy (Nelson, 2015). Additional studies are under way to understand the clinical significance of these latest findings, but in the interim, nurses need to focus on ongoing risk assessment and should be prepared to discuss current research findings with clients.

Adherence to the regimen of combination contraceptive patch use has been shown to be significantly greater than adherence with OCs. In addition, research suggests that overweight and obese women with weights exceeding 198 lb should be advised of the potentially decreased effectiveness of the patch and increase incidence of venous thromboembolism and weight gain (Pocius & Dutton, 2015). The patch provides combination hormone therapy (HT) with a side-effect profile similar to that of OCs (Fig. 4.14).

VAGINAL RINGS

The **vaginal ring** is a 54-mm, flexible, soft, transparent ring that contains both estrogen and progesterone hormones and is inserted by the user for a 3-week period of continuous use followed by a ring-free week to allow withdrawal bleeding (Fig. 4.15). Ethinyl estradiol and etonogestrel are rapidly absorbed through the vaginal epithelium and result in a steady serum concentration. Because the hormones are released directly into the vagina, a lower daily dose of hormones is required in comparison with OC doses. Studies have demonstrated that the efficacy and safety of the ring are equivalent to those of OCs. Clients report being highly satisfied with the vaginal ring and report fewer systemic side effects than do OC users. The ring provides effective cycle control as well as symptom relief for clients with menorrhagia, dysmenorrhea, and polycystic ovarian syndrome. Reported problems associated with the use

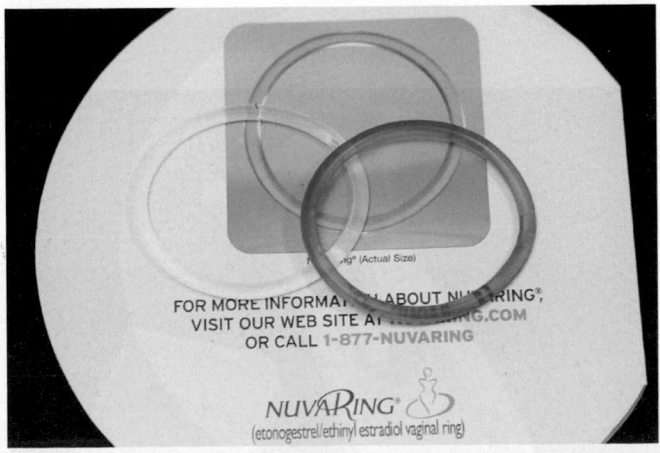

FIGURE 4.15 Vaginal ring. (NUVARING materials/images reproduced with permission of Merck Sharp & Dohme Corp., a subsidiary of Merck & Co., Inc., Kenilworth, New Jersey, U.S.A. All rights reserved.)

of vaginal rings include erosion of vaginal wall, ring expulsion, interference with coitus, unpleasant ring odour, and premature discontinuation due to vaginal discomfort (Khan & Krupanidhi, 2015). The ring can be inserted independently and does not have to be fitted. The client compresses the ring and inserts it into the vagina, behind the pubic bone, as far back as possible, but precise placement is not critical. The hormones are absorbed through the vaginal mucosa. It is left in place for 3 weeks and then removed and discarded. Effectiveness and adverse events are similar to those seen with combination OCs. Clients need to be counselled regarding timely insertion of the ring and what to do in case of accidental expulsion. Recent studies suggest that a vaginal ring containing etonogestrel and ethinyl estradiol used in an extended regimen is a safe contraceptive method that offers good cycle control and can be an option for clients who have gastric intolerance or other side effects when using oral hormonal contraceptives (King et al., 2015).

IMPLANTABLE CONTRACEPTIVES

The implant is a subdermal time-release method that delivers synthetic progestin that inhibits ovulation. Once in place, it delivers 3 years of continuous, highly effective contraception. Like POPs, implants act by inhibiting ovulation and thickening cervical mucus so sperm cannot penetrate. A single-rod progestin implant (Nexplanon) is currently available in the United States and European countries, but is not available in Canada. Nexplanon is 4 cm long and 2 mm in diameter, and contains 68 mg of the hormone progestin. The implant is radio-opaque and is over 99% effective (King et al., 2015). The side effects are also similar to those of POPs: irregular bleeding, headaches, weight gain, breast tenderness, and depression. Fertility is restored quickly after it is removed. Implants require a minor surgical procedure for both insertion and removal. The implants do not offer any protection against STIs.

Hormonal side effects are not exclusive to implants but tend to be a problem with all hormonal contraceptives. Preinsertion counselling by the nurse is essential to prepare the client for any such side effects. Expert counselling should cover the one-side effect most likely to cause discontinuation: initial irregular bleeding and the possibility of amenorrhea with longer use (Craik & Rowlands, 2015).

INTRAUTERINE CONTRACEPTIVES

Intrauterine contraceptives (IUCs) are classified as either hormonal or nonhormonal. Both types prevent pregnancy via inhibition of sperm mobility and sperm viability and change the speed of transport of the ovum in the fallopian tube. An IUC is a small plastic T-shaped object that is placed inside the uterus to provide contraception (Fig. 4.16). It prevents pregnancy by making the endometrium of the uterus hostile to implantation of a fertilized ovum by causing a nonspecific inflammatory reaction and inhibiting sperm and ovum from meeting (Wildemeersch, Goldstuck, Hasskamp, Jandi, & Pett, 2015). The hormonal IUC will make monthly periods lighter, shorter, and less painful, making this a useful method for clients with heavy, painful periods. The implants contain either copper or progesterone to enhance their effectiveness. One or two attached strings protrude into the vagina so that the user can check for placement.

Currently, there are four types of IUCs available in Canada: the copper intrauterine device (IUD) (nonhormonal), and three types of levonogestrel-releasing intrauterine systems (LNG-IUS), which release progestin in varying amounts (marketed as Mirena, Jaydess, and Kyleena). The copper IUD can remain in place for 10 years. Its mechanism of action is based on the release of copper ions, which alone are spermicidal. Additionally, the device causes an inflammatory action leading to a hostile uterine environment. The copper IUD is also approved for use as EC. The LG-IUSs release a small amount of levonorgestrel, a synthetic form of

Drug reservoir (progesterone)

Rate controlling membrane

Monofilament thread (string)

FIGURE 4.16 **A.** Intrauterine contraceptive. **B.** An IUC in place in the uterus.

progesterone, which thickens cervical mucus, thins the lining of the uterus, and inhibits movement of sperm. Mirena and Kyleena provide intrauterine contraception for 5 years. Jaydess, which contains the lowest concentration of levonorgestrel, has been approved for 3 years of pregnancy prevention (Island Sexual Health, 2017). The IUDS can also result in a major reduction in menstrual flow and dysmenorrhea, suggesting that they are viable alternative to hysterectomy and endometrial ablation in clients with menorrhagia (Atkin, Beal, Long-Middleton, & Roncari, 2015). An advantage of these hormonally impregnated IUSs is that they are relatively maintenance-free: users must consciously discontinue using them to become pregnant rather than making a daily decision to avoid conception (Alan Guttmacher Institute, 2018a).

The IUCs provide a safe, highly effective, long-lasting, yet reversible method of contraception. Expanding access to intrauterine contraception is an important measure to reduce the rate of unintended pregnancy in Canada. Nurses should consider including them in their discussion to appropriate candidates, including those who are nulliparous, adolescent, immediately postpartum, or postabortion and those who desire EC, and as an alternative to permanent sterilization. Barriers to obtaining intrauterine contraception such as requiring cervical cancer screening before insertion, routine testing for gonorrhea and chlamydial infection in low-risk clients, or scheduling insertion only during menses are unnecessary. IUC insertion can take place on any day of the menstrual cycle, if absence of pregnancy is confirmed (Cheng & Van Leuven, 2015). Box 4.7 highlights the warning signs of the potential complications of IUCs.

EMERGENCY CONTRACEPTION

Unplanned pregnancy is a major health, economic, and social issue. Approximately, one third of all unplanned pregnancies end in abortion (CDC, 2016a), and an estimated one third of Canadian women will undergo a therapeutic abortion at some point in their reproductive lives (SOGC, 2015). Using an emergency contraceptive

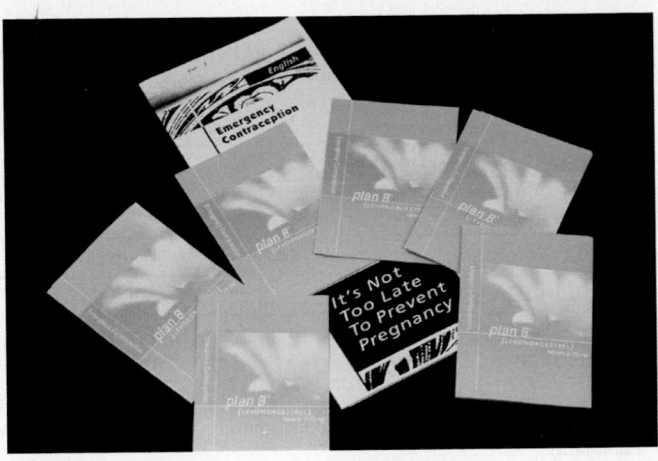

FIGURE 4.17 Emergency contraceptive kit.

provides a second chance to prevent an unintended pregnancy. EC reduces the risk of pregnancy after unprotected intercourse or contraceptive failure such as condom breakage (Raymond & Cleland, 2015). It is used within 72 hours of unprotected intercourse to prevent pregnancy. The sooner ECs are taken, the more effective they are. They reduce the risk of pregnancy for a single act of unprotected sex by almost 80% (Casey & Isaacs, 2015). The methods available in Canada are POPs, Plan B (Fig. 4.17), Norlevo, Option 2, and Next Choice; combined estrogen and progestin pills, or insertion of a copper-releasing IUS up to 7 days after unprotected intercourse. Ulipristal acetate (marketed as Ella) is a selective progesterone receptor modulator that, when taken as a single 30-mg dose, is a new, safe, and effective emergency contraceptive that can be used from the first day and up to 5 days following unprotected intercourse. The older progesterone-only emergency contraceptive, levonorgestrel, is taken as two 0.75-mg pills 12 hours apart (Next Choice; Watson Pharmaceuticals Inc.) or as a single 1.5-mg pill (Plan B One-Step; Watson Pharmaceuticals Inc.), and is approved for only 72 hours after unprotected intercourse (Mulligan, 2016).

EC is now available over-the-counter across Canada, and therefore available for purchase without a prescription, although some provinces (Saskatchewan and Quebec) keep these behind the counter for reimbursement purposes (SOGC, 2015).

Although access to EC has increased with nonprescription status and approval of Plan B One-Step without age restrictions, many barriers remain in public awareness and unintended pregnancies continue to rise. Because of the lack of awareness of EC and the politics surrounding it, EC is not used as widely as would be warranted by the incidence of unprotected coitus. Nurses need to educate their clients to bring about increased awareness of this second chance method. Table 4.5 lists recommended oral medication and intrauterine regimens.

BOX 4.7

WARNINGS FOR INTRAUTERINE SYSTEM USERS OF POTENTIAL COMPLICATIONS

P = Period late, pregnancy, abnormal spotting or bleeding
A = Abdominal pain, pain with intercourse
I = Infection exposure, abnormal vaginal discharge
N = Not feeling well, fever, chills
S = String length shorter or longer or missing

Adapted from King, T. L., Brucker, M. C., Kriebs, J. M., Fahey, J. O., Gegor, C. L., & Varney, H. (2015). *Varney's midwifery* (5th ed.). Burlington, MA: Jones & Bartlett Learning.

TABLE 4.5	EMERGENCY POSTCOITAL CONTRACEPTION OPTIONS	
Product	**Dosage (Within 72 hours)**	**Comments**
Combined estrogen and progestin pills (Yuzpe regimen)	OCs are taken in various formulations to prevent conception	Interfere with the cascade of events that result in ovulation and fertilization
Plan B One-Step	1.5-mg pill taken	Can cause nausea and vomiting
Intrauterine		
Copper-bearing IUS (ParaGard-TCu-380A)	Inserted within 5 days after unprotected sexual episode	Can be left in for long-term contraception (10 years)

Adapted from King, T. L., Brucker, M. C., Kriebs, J. M., Fahey, J. O., Gegor, C. L., & Varney, H. (2015). *Varney's midwifery* (5th ed.). Burlington, MA: Jones & Bartlett Learning; Ilic, K. (2015). Emergency contraception. In *Medicines for women* (pp. 203–225). Cham, Switzerland: Springer International Publishing.

Prime points to stress concerning ECs are:
- ECs do not offer any protection against STIs or future pregnancies.
- ECs should not be used in place of a regular birth control method, because they are less effective.
- ECs may delay the next menses, so evaluation for pregnancy is needed if menses does not occur within 3 weeks after EC use.
- Report any severe abdominal pain to health care provider immediately.
- ECs are regular birth control pills given at a higher dose.
- ECs are contraindicated during pregnancy (Ilic, 2015).

Take Note!

Contrary to popular belief, ECs do not induce abortion and are not related to mifepristone or mifegymiso, a prescription medication indicated for medically terminating a pregnancy up to 9 weeks gestation, which was approved by Health Canada in 2017.

Mifegymiso chemically induces abortion by blocking the body's progesterone receptors, which are necessary for pregnancy maintenance, and causes evacuation of the uterus. ECs simply prevent embryo creation and uterine implantation from occurring in the first place. There is no evidence that ECs have any effect on an already implanted ovum. The side effects are nausea and vomiting.

Sterilization

Sterilization is a permanent, safe, and highly effective method of contraception for those who are certain they do not want any or any more children. Vasectomy is the only highly reliable form of male contraception. Approximately 20,000 tubal occlusions and 55,000 vasectomies are performed in Canada annually, and over 220 million worldwide (Shoupe & Mishell, 2016). It is the most widely used method of family planning in the world in both developed and developing countries. Sterilization refers to surgical procedures intended to render the person infertile. Laparoscopic, abdominal, and hysteroscopic methods of female sterilization are available in Canada, with most of these procedures performed outside the hospital. Sterilization is a safe and effective form of permanent birth control. In Canada, it is the second most commonly used form of contraception for clients over 40 years of age (SOGC, 2015). More Canadian men undergo surgical sterilization than women (SOGC, 2015). Sterilization should be considered a permanent end to fertility because reversal surgery is difficult, expensive, and not always successful. Because these methods are intended to be irreversible, all couples should be appropriately counselled about the permanency of sterilization and the availability of highly effective, long-acting, reversible methods of contraception before their decision is made.

TUBAL LIGATION

Tubal ligation, a sterilization procedure, can be performed postpartum, after an abortion, or as an interval procedure unrelated to pregnancy. Mini-laparotomies and laparoscopies are the two most common techniques. In the laparoscopy procedure, the abdomen is filled with carbon dioxide gas so that the abdominal wall balloons away from the tubes and provide a view of the fallopian tubes. They are grasped and sealed with a cauterizing instrument or with rings, bands, or clips or cut and tied (Fig. 4.18).

ESSURE

Essure is a nonsurgical, nonhormonal, permanent birth control method that was available in Canada from 2001 to 2017, and is currently still available in the United States. This method is for clients who desire no more children as it is a permanent method of birth control. It offers advantages over a conventional tubal ligation: general anesthesia and incisions are not needed, thereby increasing safety, lowering costs, and improving access to sterilization. A tiny coil

FIGURE 4.18 Laparoscopy for tubal sterilization.

(Essure) is introduced and released into the fallopian tubes through the cervix. The coil promotes tissue growth in the fallopian tubes, and over a period of 3 months, this growth blocks the tubes. The buildup of tissue creates a barrier that keeps sperm from reaching the ovum, thus preventing conception (Thurkow, 2015). Sterilization does not occur immediately after this procedure, so clients must be educated to use additional contraception for 3 months until permanent tubal occlusion is verified. In 2017, the manufacturer withdrew the product from the Canadian market, citing dwindling sales following a class action lawsuit of 297 Canadian women reporting complications of the device, including emergency hysterectomies (McKnight, 2017).

VASECTOMY

Male sterilization is accomplished with a surgical procedure known as a **vasectomy**. Approximately 22% of Canadian couples rely on male vasectomy as their primary method of birth control (UN Department of Economic and Social Affairs, Population Division, 2014). It is usually performed under local anesthesia in a urologist's office, and most men can return to work and normal activities in a day or two. The procedure involves making a small incision into the scrotum and cutting the vas deferens, which carries sperm from the testes to the penis (Fig. 4.19). Complications from vasectomy are rare and minor in nature. Immediate risks include infection, hematoma, and pain. After vasectomy, semen no longer contains sperm. This is not immediate, though, and the man must submit semen specimens for analysis 8 to 16 weeks after a vasectomy until two specimens show that no sperm is present. When the specimen shows azoospermia, the man's sterility is confirmed (Whitaker, 2015).

Nursing Management of the Client Choosing a Contraceptive Method

The choice of a contraceptive method is a very personal one involving many factors. When approaching the topic of contraception with a client, nurses must first avoid prejudice through **heteronormativity**, or the assumption that

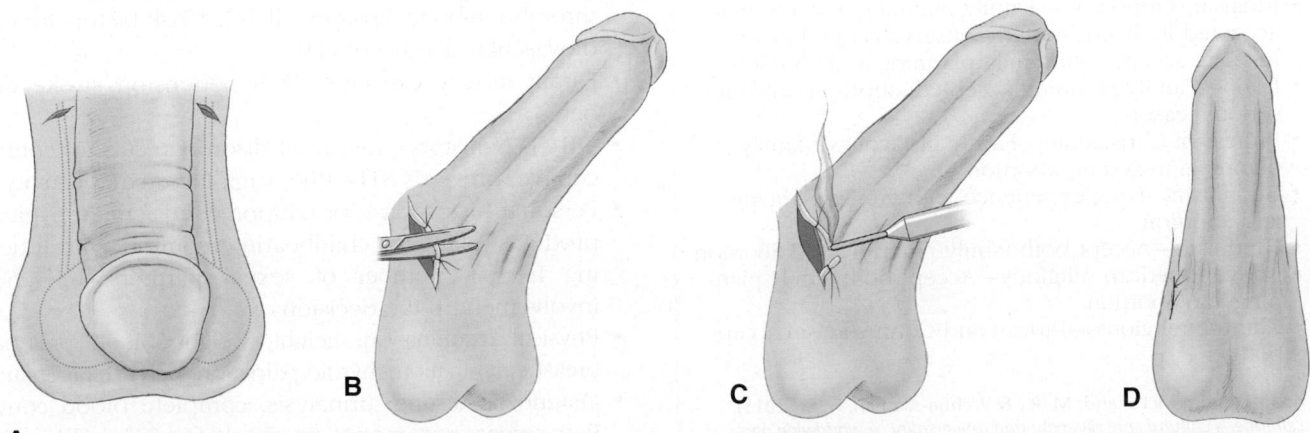

FIGURE 4.19 Vasectomy. **A.** Site of vasectomy incisions. **B.** The vas deferens is cut with surgical scissors. **C.** Cut ends of the vas deferens are cauterized to ensure blockage of the passage of sperm. **D.** Final skin suture.

all people are in heterosexual relationships. When a client discloses that they are sexually active, the nurse must sensitively inquire if the client has female or male partners, or both. This allows the nurse to understand the client's true contraceptive needs, if any. When making contraceptive choices, clients must balance their sexual lives, their reproductive goals, and each partner's health and safety. The search for a choice that satisfies all three objectives is challenging. A method that works for a sexually active teenage girl may not meet their needs later in life. Several considerations influence a person's choice of contraceptives:

- Motivation
- Cost
- Cultural and religious beliefs (Box 4.8)
- Convenience
- Effectiveness
- Side effects
- Desire for children in the future
- Safety of the method
- Comfort level with sexuality
- Protection from STIs
- Interference with spontaneity

If a contraceptive is to be effective, the client must understand how it works, must be able to use it correctly and consistently, and must be comfortable and confident with it. If a client cannot adhere to taking a pill daily, consider a method used once a week (transdermal patches), once every 3 weeks (transvaginal ring), or once every 3 months (Depo-Provera injection). Another option may be a progesterone IUC that lasts 3 to 5 years and reduces menstrual flow significantly.

BOX 4.8

SELECTED RELIGIOUS CHOICES FOR FAMILY PLANNING AND ABORTION

- Roman Catholic—Abstinence and natural family planning; no abortion
- Judaism (Orthodox)—Family planning and abortion accepted in first trimester. Conservative and Reform Judaism accept both family planning and abortion
- Islam—Family planning accepted; abortion only for serious reasons
- Protestant Christianity—Firmly in favour of family planning; mixed on abortion
- Buddhism—Long experience with family planning and abortion
- Hinduism—Accept both family planning and abortion
- Native American religions—Accept both family planning and abortion
- Chinese religions—Taoism and Confucianism accept both

Adapted from McFarland, M. R., & Wehbe-Alamah, H. B. (2015). *Leininger's cultural care diversity and universality: A worldwide nursing theory* (3rd ed.). Burlington, MA: Jones & Bartlett Learning; McFarlane, D. R. (2015). *Global population and reproductive health.* Burlington, MA: Jones & Bartlett Learning.

Regardless of which method is chosen, the client's needs should be paramount in the discussion. The nurse can educate clients about which methods are available and their advantages and disadvantages, efficacy, cost, and safety. Knowledge of contraceptive effectiveness is crucial to making an informed choice. The couple has to comprehend the pros and cons of the contraceptive methods being considered. Choice may be influenced by understanding the likelihood of pregnancy with each method and factors that influence effectiveness. Counselling can help the client and couple choose a contraceptive method that is efficacious and fits their preferences and lifestyle.

Nursing Assessment

When assessing which contraceptive method might meet the client's needs, the nurse might ask:

- Are your religious beliefs with a consideration for any methods?
- Will this method interfere with your sexual pleasure?
- Are you aware of the various methods currently available?
- Is cost a major consideration, or does your insurance cover it?
- Does your partner influence which method you choose?
- Are you in a stable, monogamous relationship?
- Have you heard anything troubling about any of the methods?
- How comfortable are you touching your own body?
- What are your future plans for having children?

Although deciding on a contraceptive is a very personal decision, nurses can assist in this process by performing a complete health history and physical examination, and by educating the client and partner about necessary laboratory and diagnostic testing. Areas of focus during the nursing assessment are as follows:

- Medical history: smoking status, cancer of reproductive tract, diabetes mellitus, migraines, hypertension, thromboembolic disorder, allergies, risk factors for cardiovascular disease (CVD)
- Family history: cancer, CVD, hypertension, stroke, diabetes
- OB/GYN history: menstrual disorders, current contraceptive, previous STIs, PID, vaginitis, sexual activity
- Personal history: use of tampons and female hygiene products, plans for childbearing, comfort with touching herself, number of sexual partners and their involvement in the decision
- Physical examination: height, weight, blood pressure, breast examination, thyroid palpation, pelvic examination
- Diagnostic testing: urinalysis, complete blood count, Pap smear, wet mount to check for STIs, HIV/AIDS tests, lipid profile, glucose level

Figure 4.20 shows an example of a family planning flow record that can be used during the assessment.

FAMILY PLANNING FLOW (VISIT) RECORD

Name: _____
ID #: _____
Date of Birth: _____

	Date:			Date:	
Current Method					
Reason for Visit					
LMP					
SUBJECTIVE DATA	**Pt.**	**Comments**		**Pt.**	**Comments**
Severe headaches					
Depression					
Visual abnormalities					
Dyspnea/chest pain					
Breast changes					
SBE					
Abdominal pain					
Nausea and vomiting					
Dysuria/frequency					
Menstrual irregularities					
Vaginal discharge/infections					
Leg pain					
Surgery, injury, infections, or serious illness since last visit					
Allergic reaction					
Pregnancy plans					
Other					
OBJECTIVE DATA	**Weight**	**B.P.**		**Weight**	**B.P.**
Other					
Lab					
ASSESSMENT					
Check here if assessment continues on progress notes	O			O	
PLAN					
Type of contraceptive given					
COUNSELLING/EDUCATION					
Next appointment					
SIGNATURE/TITLE					
SIGNATURE/TITLE					

O = normal   ✓ = abnormal

FIGURE 4.20 Family planning flow (visit) record.

After collecting the assessment data above, consider the medical factors to help decide if the client is a candidate for all methods or whether some should be eliminated. For example, if the client reports having multiple sex partners and a history of pelvic infections, an IUC would not be a safe option. Barrier methods (male or female condoms) of contraception might be recommended to this client to offer protection against STIs.

Nursing Diagnoses

A few nursing diagnoses that might be appropriate based on the nurse's assessment during the decision-making process include:
- Deficient knowledge related to:
  - Methods available
  - Side effects/safety
  - Correct use of method chosen
  - Previous myths believed
- Risk for infection related to:
  - Unprotected sexual intercourse
  - Past history of STIs
  - Methods offering protection

Nursing diagnoses applicable to the contraceptive would be:
- Health-seeking behaviours related to:
  - Perceived need for limiting number of children
  - Overall health relative to contraceptives
- Risk for ineffective health maintenance related to:
  - Not being familiar with the various contraceptive methods
  - Being unaware of high-risk sexual behaviour leading to STIs
- Fear related to:
  - Not understanding the correct procedure to use
  - Unintended pregnancy occurring if not used correctly
  - General health concerning the long-term side effects

Nursing Interventions

Contraception is an important issue for all couples, and the method used should be decided by the client and partner jointly. Facilitate this process by establishing a trusting relationship with the client and by providing unbiased, accurate information about all methods available. As a nurse, reflect honestly on your feelings about contraceptives while allowing the client's feelings to be paramount. Be aware of the practical issues involved in contraceptive use, and avoid making assumptions, making decisions on the client's behalf, and making judgments about the situation. To do so, it is important to keep up to date on the latest methods available and convey this information to clients. Encourage female clients to take control of their lives by sharing information that allows them to plan their futures.

FIGURE 4.21 The nurse demonstrates insertion of a vaginal ring during client teaching.

The following guidelines are helpful in counselling and educating the client or couple about contraceptives:
- Encourage the client/couple to participate in choosing a method.
- Provide client education. The client/couple must become informed users before the method is chosen. Education should be targeted to the client's level so it is understood. Provide step-by-step teaching and an opportunity for practice for certain methods (cervical caps, diaphragms, vaginal rings, and condoms). See Teaching Guidelines 4.5 and Figure 4.21.
- Obtain written informed consents, which are needed for IUCs, implants, abortion, or sterilization. Informed consent implies that the client is making a knowledgeable, voluntary choice; has received complete information about the method, including the risks; and is free to change her mind before using the method or having the procedure (Schuiling & Likis, 2016).
- Discuss contraindications for all selected contraceptives.
- Consider the client's cultural and religious beliefs when providing care.
- Address myths and misperceptions about the methods under consideration in your initial discussion of contraceptives.

 Teaching Guidelines 4.5
TIPS FOR THE USE OF CERVICAL CAPS, DIAPHRAGMS, VAGINAL RINGS, AND CONDOMS
Cervical Cap Insertion/Removal Technique
- It is important to be involved in the fitting process.
- To insert the cap, pinch the sides together, compress the cap dome, insert into the vagina, and place over the cervix.

- Use one finger to feel around the entire circumference to make sure there are no gaps between the cap rim and the cervix.
- After a minute or two, pinch the dome and tug gently to check for evidence of suction. The cap should resist the tug and not slide off easily.
- To remove the cap, press the index finger against the rim and tip the cap slightly to break the suction. Gently pull out the cap.
- The client should practice inserting and removing the cervical cap three times to validate comfort and proficiency with this device.

Client Teaching and Counselling Regarding the Cervical Cap
- Fill the dome of the cap up about one third full with spermicide cream or jelly. Do not apply spermicide to the rim, since it may interfere with the seal.
- Wait approximately 30 minutes after insertion before engaging in sexual intercourse to be sure that a seal has formed between the rim and the cervix.
- Leave the cervical cap in place for a minimum of 6 hours after sexual intercourse. It can be left in place for up to 48 hours without additional spermicide being added.
- Do not use during menses due to the potential for toxic shock syndrome. Use an alternative method such as condoms during this time.
- Replace the cervical cap after each year of use.
- Inspect the cervical cap prior to insertion for cracks, holes, or tears.
- After using the cervical cap, wash it with soap and water, dry thoroughly, and store in its container.

Diaphragm Insertion/Removal Technique
- Always empty the bladder prior to inserting the diaphragm.
- Inspect diaphragm for holes or tears by holding it up to a light source, or fill it with water and check for a leak.
- Place approximately a tablespoon of spermicidal jelly or cream in the dome and around the rim of the diaphragm.
- The diaphragm can be inserted up to 6 hours prior to intercourse.
- Select the position that is most comfortable for insertion:
  - Squatting
  - Leg up, raising the nondominant leg up on a low stool
  - Reclining position, lying on back in bed
  - Sitting forward on the edge of a chair
- Hold the diaphragm between the thumb and fingers and compress it to form a "figure-eight" shape.
- Insert the diaphragm into the vagina, directing it downward as far as it will go.

- Tuck the front rim of the diaphragm behind the pubic bone so that the rubber hugs the front wall of the vagina.
- Feel for the cervix through the diaphragm to make sure it is properly placed.
- To remove the diaphragm, insert the finger up and over the top side and move slightly to the side, breaking the suction.
- Pull the diaphragm down and out of the vagina.

Client Teaching and Counselling Regarding the Diaphragm
- Avoid the use of oil-based products, such as baby oil, because they may weaken the rubber.
- Wash the diaphragm with soap and water after use and dry thoroughly.
- Place the diaphragm back into the storage case.
- The diaphragm may need to be refitted after weight loss or gain or childbirth.
- Diaphragms should not be used by women with latex allergies.

Vaginal Ring Insertion/Removal Technique and Counselling
- Each ring is used for one menstrual cycle, which consists of 3 weeks of continuous use followed by a ring-free week to allow for menses.
- No fitting is necessary—one size fits all.
- The ring is compressed and inserted into the vagina, behind the pubic bone, as far back as possible.
- Precision placement is not essential.
- Backup contraception is needed for 7 days if the ring is expelled for more than 3 hours during the 3-week period of continuous use.
- The vaginal ring is left in place for 3 weeks, then removed and discarded.
- The vaginal ring is not recommended for people with uterine prolapse or lack of vaginal muscle tone (Schuiling & Likis, 2016).

Male Condom Insertion/Removal Technique and Counselling
- Always keep the condom in its original package until ready to use.
- Store in a cool, dry place.
- Spermicidal condoms should be used if available.
- Check expiration date before using.
- Use a new condom for each sexual act.
- Condom is placed over the erect penis prior to insertion.
- Place condom on the head of the penis and unroll it down the shaft.
- Leave a half-inch of empty space at the end to collect ejaculate.
- Avoid use of oil-based products, because they may cause breakage.
- After intercourse, remove the condom while the penis is still erect.
- Discard condom after use.

Female Condom Insertion/Removal Technique and Counselling

- Practice wearing and inserting prior to first use with sexual intercourse.
- Condom can be inserted up to 8 hours before intercourse.
- Condom is intended for one-time use.
- It can be purchased over-the-counter—one size fits all.
- Avoid wearing rings to prevent tears; long fingernails can also cause tears.
- Spermicidal lubricant can be used if desired.
- Insert the inner ring high in the vagina, against the cervix.
- Place the outer ring on the outside of the vagina.
- Make sure the erect penis is placed inside the female condom.
- Remove the condom after intercourse. Avoid spilling the ejaculate.

Education and Counselling of Clients Using Injectable Contraceptives

- Consume a diet high in calcium and vitamin D to prevent bone mineral loss
- Know the conditions that need to be reported to the health care provider
  - Significant headaches
  - Menorrhagia
  - Depression
  - Severe abdominal pain
- Awareness of any infection present at injection site

It is also important to clear up common misconceptions about contraception and pregnancy. Clearing up misconceptions will permit new learning to take hold and a better client response to whichever methods are explored and ultimately selected. Some common misconceptions include:

- Breastfeeding prevents pregnancy.
- Pregnancy can be avoided if the male partner "pulls out" before he ejaculates.
- Pregnancy cannot occur during menses.
- Douching after sex will prevent pregnancy.
- Pregnancy will not happen during the first sexual experience.
- Taking birth control pills protects against STIs.
- The client is too old to get pregnant.
- If both partners do not reach orgasm, conception is not likely.
- Irregular menstruation prevents pregnancy.

When discussing in detail each method of birth control, focus on specific information for each method outlined. Include information such as how this particular method works to prevent pregnancy under normal circumstances of use; the noncontraceptive benefits to overall health; advantages and disadvantages of all methods; the cost involved for each particular method; danger signs that need to be reported to the health care provider; and the required frequency of office visits needed for the particular method.

In addition, outline factors that place the client at risk for method failure. Contraceptives can fail for any of many reasons. Use Table 4.6 to provide client education concerning a few of the reasons for contraceptive failure. Help clients who have chosen abstinence or fertility awareness methods to define the sexual activities in which they do or do not want to participate. This helps them set sexual limits or boundaries. Help them to develop communication and negotiation skills that will allow them to be successful. Supporting, encouraging, and respecting a couple's choice of abstinence is vital for nurses.

After clients have chosen a method of contraception, it is important to address the following:

- Emphasize that a second method to use as a backup is always needed.
- Provide both oral and written instructions on the method chosen.
- Discuss the need for STI protection if not using a barrier method.
- Inform the client about the availability of ECs.

Steady progress in contraception research has been achieved over the past several years. Hormonal and nonhormonal contraceptives have improved people's lives by reducing different health conditions that contribute to morbidity. However, the contraceptives available today are not suitable to all users, and the need to expand contraceptive choices still exists. It is hoped that the introduction of newer methods in the near future with additional health benefits will continue to help clients and couples meet their family planning needs.

ABORTION

Abortion is defined as the expulsion of an embryo or fetus before it is viable (Alexander, LaRosa, Bader, & Garfield, 2014). Abortion can be a medical or surgical procedure. The purpose of abortion is to terminate a pregnancy. More than 40% of people who become pregnant will end a pregnancy by abortion at some time in their reproductive lives. In 2015, over 100,000 abortions were performed in Canada (Canadian Institute for Health Information [CIHI], 2015). Both in Canada and globally, more than one fifth of all known pregnancies end in abortion (McFarlane, 2015). Eighty-nine percent of abortions occur in the first 12 weeks of pregnancy (Alan Guttmacher Institute, 2018b). Both medical and surgical abortions are safe and legal in Canada; an abortion is considered a human right based on the 1982 Charter of Rights and Freedoms, according to the Supreme Court of Canada.

TABLE 4.6	CONTRACEPTIVE PROBLEMS AND EDUCATIONAL NEEDS
Contraceptive Failure Problem	**Client Education Needed**
Not following instructions for use of contraceptive correctly	Take pill the same time every day Use condoms properly and check condition before using Make sure diaphragm or cervical cap covers cervix completely Check IUD for placement monthly
Inconsistent use of contraceptive	Contraceptives must be used regularly to achieve maximum effectiveness All it takes is one unprotected act of sexual intercourse to become pregnant Two percent to 5% of condoms will break or tear during use
Condom broke during sex	Check expiration date Store condoms properly Use only a water-based lubricant Watch for tears caused by long fingernails Use spermicides to decrease possibility of pregnancy Seek emergency postcoital conception
Use of antibiotics or other herbs taken with OCs	Use alternative methods during the antibiotic therapy, plus 7 additional days. Implement on day 1 of taking antibiotics
Belief that you can't get pregnant during menses or that it is safe "just this one-time"	It may be possible to become pregnant on almost any day of the menstrual cycle

Since the landmark Supreme Court decision *R v. Morgentaler* decriminalized abortion in 1988, debate has continued over how and when abortions are provided, and access is varied across the country. New Brunswick, for example, only covers the cost of abortions provided in hospitals, not in outpatient clinics. In Ontario, some free-standing abortion clinics receive only partial funding. These regulations leave clients having to pay for some or all of the cost of abortion services out of pocket; a situation many argue is in violation of the Canada Health Act (Abortion Rights Coalition of Canada, 2017). Opponents of abortion continue to lobby for political influence through the introduction of various bills to bestow human rights on a fetus with the intent of superseding the person's right to bodily autonomy and therefore the right to terminate the pregnancy.

Surgical Abortion

Two types of surgical abortion are available: vacuum aspiration or dilation, and evacuation (D&C). Method selection is based on gestational age. It is an ambulatory procedure done under local anesthesia. The cervix is dilated prior to surgery and then the products of conception are removed by suction evacuation. The uterus may gently be scraped by curettage to make sure that it is empty. The entire procedure lasts about 10 minutes. The overall risk of complications is less than 1% for surgical termination (Upadhyay et al., 2015). The major risks and complications in the first trimester are infection, retained tissue, or hemorrhage, uterine perforation, retained products of conception, or

cervical tear (Udoh et al., 2015). For clients whose blood is Rh negative, *RhoGAM* is indicated prior to start of either medical or surgical termination to prevent potential Rh isoimmunization.

Medical Abortion

Global studies have indicated that in countries where medical abortions are available and accessible, the rates of complications from unsafe abortions are reduced, and there is no increase in frequency of abortions (Costescu et al., 2016). Medical abortions are achieved through administration of medication either vaginally or orally. The administration of medication occurs in the clinic or doctor's office, and may require two to four office visits (Planned Parenthood, 2018b). Three drugs are currently used to terminate a pregnancy during the first trimester. The first drug is methotrexate (an antineoplastic agent; Rheumatrex) followed by misoprostol (a prostaglandin agent; Cytotec) given as a vaginal suppository or in oral form 3 to 7 days later. Methotrexate induces abortion because of its toxicity to trophoblastic tissue, the growing embryo. Misoprostol works by causing uterine contractions, which helps to expel the products of conception. This method is 90% to 98% successful in completing an abortion (Patil & Edelman, 2015).

The second drug used to induce first-trimester abortions involves using a combination of mifepristone (a progesterone antagonist; RU-486) followed 48 hours later by misoprostol (a prostaglandin agent), which causes contractions of the uterus and expulsion of the uterine contents. This method was initially approved by Health Canada for safe termination of pregnancy up to 7 weeks gestation (49 days from the first day of the last menstrual period [LMP]); in 2017, the administration guideline was revised for use up to 9 weeks gestation, or 63 days after LMP (Health Canada, 2017). Another frequent method used includes the combination of methotrexate with misoprostol (Schuiling & Likis, 2016). Mifepristone, the generic name for RU-486, is sold under the brand names Mifeprex and Early Option. Mifepristone is an antiprogestin and blocks the action of progesterone, which is necessary for the maintenance of the pregnancy. This method is 95% effective when used within 49 days after the last menstrual cycle (Patil & Edelman, 2015).

Another drug frequently used is misoprostol (Cytotec), which is a prostaglandin analogue that softens the cervix and causes uterine contractions, which results in the expulsion of uterine contents. There is no standard protocol for use of misoprostol (Cytotec) alone for termination of early pregnancy, and it is not FDA-approved for this purpose (King et al., 2015). Complications of medical abortions include incomplete expulsion of uterine contents; uterine infection; and heavy bleeding (Ganatra, Guest, & Berer, 2015).

The assessment of the client with an unintended pregnancy should be performed with cautious sensitivity. It is essential to explore the client's feelings about pregnancy before offering congratulations or consolations. The encounter should be guided by the feelings of the client, not by the assumptions and values of the nurse.

Abortion is a very emotional, deeply personal issue. Give support and accurate information. If for personal, religious, or ethical reasons you feel unable to actively participate in the care of a client undergoing an abortion, you still have the professional responsibility to ensure that the client receives the nursing care and help required. This may necessitate a transfer to another area or a staffing reassignment. Nurses must keep in mind that all clients have the right to have access to unbiased, factual information about available reproductive health choices, whether they seek to end or start a pregnancy, from which they can then make informed decisions about their own reproductive health.

MENOPAUSAL TRANSITION

Menopause is a natural process that occurs as part of normal aging. *Meno* is derived from the Greek word for "month," and *pause* is derived from the Greek word for "pause" or "halt." Menopause is the technical term for a point in time at which menses and fertility cease (King et al., 2015). The change of life. The end of fertility. The beginning of freedom. Whatever people call it, menopause is a unique and personal experience for everyone.

The term **menopausal transition** refers to the transition from the reproductive phase of life to the final menstrual period. This period is also referred to as *perimenopause*. It is the end of menstruation and childbearing capacity. The average age of natural menopause—defined as 1 year without a menstrual period—is 51.4 years old. The average age of natural menopause has remained constant for the last several hundred years despite improvements in nutrition and health care (Alexander et al., 2014). With current female life expectancy at 84 years, this event comes in the middle of a woman's adult life. Many clients go through the menopausal transition with few or no symptoms, while some have significant or even disabling symptoms (Kessenich, 2017).

 Take Note!

Humans are virtually the only species to outlive their reproductive capacities.

Menopause signals the end of an era. It concludes the ability to reproduce, and some clients find advancing age, altered roles, and these physiologic changes to be overwhelming events that may precipitate depression and anxiety (Woods & Mitchell, 2015). Menopause does not happen in isolation. Midlife is often experienced as a time of change and reflection. Change happens in many arenas: children are leaving or returning home, employment pressures intensify as career moves or decisions are required, older adult parents require more care or the death of a parent may have a major impact, and partners are retrenching or undergoing their own midlife crises. Nurses offer support and guidance as clients negotiate all these changes in addition to menopause. Managing these stressful changes can be very challenging for many clients as they make the transition into midlife.

A cis-gender female is born with approximately 2 million ova, but only about 400 ever mature fully to be released during the menstrual cycle. The absolute number of ova in the ovary is a major determinant of fertility. Over the course of her premenopausal life, there is a steady decline in the number of immature ova (Wood, 2015). No one understands this depletion, but it does not occur in isolation. Maturing ova are surrounded by follicles that produce two major hormones: estrogen, in the form of estradiol, and progesterone. The cyclic maturation of the ovum is directed by the hypothalamus. The hypothalamus triggers a cascade of neurohormones, which act through the pituitary and the ovaries as a pulse generator for reproduction. This hypothalamic–pituitary–ovarian axis begins to break down long before there is any sign that menopause is imminent. Some scientists believe that the pulse generator in the hypothalamus simply degenerates; others speculate that the ovary becomes more resistant to the pituitary hormone FSH and simply shuts down (Schuiling & Likis, 2016). The final act in this well-orchestrated process is amenorrhea.

As menopause approaches, more and more of the menstrual cycles become anovulatory. This period of time, usually 2 to 8 years before cessation of menstruation, is termed *perimenopause* (McNamara, Batur, & DeSapri, 2015). In perimenopause, the ovaries begin to fail, producing irregular and missed periods and an occasional hot flash. When menopause finally appears, viable ova are gone. Estrogen levels plummet by 90%, and estrone, produced in fat cells, replaces estradiol as the body's main form of estrogen. The major hormone produced by the ovaries during the reproductive years is estradiol; the estrogen found in postmenopausal clients is estrone. Estradiol is much more biologically active than estrone (Hoyt & Falconi, 2015). In addition, testosterone levels decrease with menopause.

Menopausal transition, with its dramatic decline in estrogen, affects not only the reproductive organs, but also other body systems:

- Brain: hot flashes, disturbed sleep, mood and memory problems
- Cardiovascular: lower levels of HDL and increased risk of CVD
- Skeletal: rapid loss of bone density that increases the risk of osteoporosis
- Breasts: replacement of duct and glandular tissues by fat
- Genitourinary: vaginal dryness, stress incontinence, cystitis
- Gastrointestinal: less absorption of calcium from food, increasing the risk for fractures
- Integumentary: dry, thin skin and decreased collagen levels
- Body shape: more abdominal fat; waist size that swells relative to hips

Therapeutic Management

Menopausal transition should be managed individually. In the past, despite the wide diversity of symptoms and risks, the traditional reaction was to reach for the one-size-fits-all therapy: HT. Today the medical community is changing its thinking in light of the Women's Health Initiative (WHI) study and the Heart and Estrogen/Progestin Replacement Study Follow-Up (HERS II), which reported that long-term HT increased the risks of heart attacks, strokes, and breast cancer; in short, the overall health risks of HT exceeded the benefits (Kyvernitakis, Kostev, Hars, Albert, & Hadji, 2015). In addition, HT did not protect against the development of coronary artery disease (CAD), nor did it prevent the progression of CAD, as it was previously touted to do.

A recent research finding examined the timing of HT in relation to CAD in women and it found that the earlier initiation of HT was associated with less CAD in women with natural but not surgical menopause. A Cochrane Review study found that HT in postmenopausal women overall had little benefit in CAD prevention, but caused an increase in the risk of stroke and venous thromboembolic events (Boardman et al., 2015). As expected, the fallout from this study and others forced practitioners to reevaluate their usual therapies and tailor treatment to each client's history, needs, and risk factors. A current study, however, shows that the incidence of fractures among menopausal transition and postmenopausal women increased significantly in the 3 years after publication of the WHI and HERS II results. This trend followed a decline in the use of HT, concurrent with an increase in the use of other bone-modifying agents (Bakour & Williamson, 2015). There is considerable evidence that estrogen or HT reduces the risk of postmenopausal osteoporotic fracture of both the spine and hip (Mirkin, Archer, Pickar, & Komm, 2015).

A number of treatment options are available, but factors in the client's history should be the driving force when determining therapy. Clients need education about the latest research findings and collaborate with their health care provider on the right menopause therapy. The following factors should be considered in management:

- The risk/benefit ratio is highest in younger clients who begin HT not long after menopause.
- HT is approved for two indications: relief of vasomotor symptoms and prevention of osteoporosis.
- Research suggests that HT may be beneficial for preventing diabetes, improving mood, or avoiding urinary tract problems.
- Using HT long beyond menopause carries increased risks, which may be outweighed by the benefits (Bakour & Williamson, 2015).

Many menopausal clients consider nonhormonal therapies such as bisphosphonates and selective estrogen receptor modulators (SERMs). Consider weightbearing exercises, calcium and vitamin D intake, smoking cessation, and avoidance of alcohol to treat or prevent osteoporosis. Annual breast examinations and mammograms are essential. Local estrogen creams can be used for vaginal atrophy. Consider herbal therapies for symptoms, although none have been validated by rigorous research studies (Ismail et al., 2015).

The SOGC (2014) revised guidelines on treating menopausal symptoms. Their recommendations include systemic HT, with estrogen or estrogen plus progestin, which is the most effective approach for treating vasomotor symptoms; the lowest effective dose for the shortest duration is the best regimen; thromboembolic disease and breast cancer are risks for combined systemic HT; and local estrogen therapy is advised for isolated atrophic vaginal symptoms.

Although numerous symptoms have been attributed to menopause (Box 4.9), some of them are more closely related to the aging process than to estrogen deficiency. A few of the more common menopausal conditions and their management are discussed next.

BOX 4.9

COMMON SYMPTOMS OF MENOPAUSE

- Hot flashes or flushes of the head and neck
- Dryness in the eyes and vagina
- Personality changes
- Anxiety and/or depression
- Loss of libido
- Decreased lubrication
- Weight gain and water retention
- Night sweats
- Atrophic changes—loss of elasticity of vaginal tissues
- Fatigue
- Irritability
- Poor self-esteem
- Insomnia
- Stress incontinence
- Heart palpitations

Adapted from Coney, P. (2018). Menopause. *eMedicine*. Retrieved from http://emedicine.medscape.com/article/264088-overview; Kessenich, C. R. (2017). Inevitable menopause. *Nursing Spectrum*. Retrieved from http://ce.nurse.com/ce232–60/Inevitable-Menopause; Schuiling, K. D., & Likis, F. E. (2016). *Women's gynecologic health* (3rd ed.). Burlington, MA: Jones & Bartlett Learning.

Managing Hot Flashes and Night Sweats

The emergence of hot flashes and night sweats (also known as vasomotor symptoms) coincides with a period in life that is also marked by dynamic changes in hormone and reproductive function that interconnect with the aging process, changes in metabolism, lifestyle behaviours, and overall health (Wood, 2015). Hot flashes and night sweats are classic signs of estrogen deficiency and the predominant complaint of perimenopausal clients. A hot flash is a transient and sudden sensation of warmth that spreads over the body, particularly the neck, face, and chest. Hot flashes are caused by vasomotor instability. This instability causes inappropriate peripheral vasodilation of superficial blood vessels, which gives the sensation of heat. Nearly 85% of menopausal clients experience them (Alexander et al., 2014). Hot flashes are an early and acute sign of estrogen deficiency. These flashes can be mild or extreme and can last from 2 to 30 minutes and may occur as frequently as every hour to several times per week. On average, clients experience hot flashes for a period of 6 months to 2 years, but the symptoms may last up to 10 years or more. Severe vasomotor symptoms can have a significant and detrimental effect on quality of life. Factors that trigger vasomotor symptoms include caffeine and alcohol consumption, intake of hot drinks and spicy foods, hot environment, depression, stress, and anxiety (Avis et al., 2015).

Many options are available for treating hot flashes. Treatment must be based on symptom severity, the client's medical history, and the client's values and concerns. Although the gold standard in the treatment of hot flashes is estrogen, this is not recommended for all clients who have high-risk factors in their history.

TRADITIONAL THERAPIES FOR THE MANAGEMENT OF HOT FLASHES

The following are traditional therapies for the management of hot flashes:

- Pharmacologic options
- HT unless contraindicated
- Androgen therapy (potentiates estrogen)
- Estrogen and androgen combinations
- Progestin therapy (Depo-Provera injection every 3 months)
- Clonidine (central alpha-adrenergic agonist) weekly patch
- Neurontin (antiseizure) decreased hot flashes
- Propranolol (beta-adrenergic blocker)
- Brisdelle: FDA-approved nonhormonal medication
- Short-term sleep aids: Ambien, Dalmane
- Gabapentin (Neurontin): antiseizure drug
- SSRIs: venlafaxine (Effexor) and paroxetine (Paxil) have shown promise (King & Brucker, 2016)

COMPLEMENTARY AND ALTERNATIVE THERAPIES FOR MANAGEMENT OF HOT FLASHES

Many clients are choosing alternative treatments for managing menopausal symptoms. Bioidentical hormones have the ability to bind to receptors in the human body and function in the same way as natural hormones. They simulate three estrogens (estradiol, estriol, and estrone), as well as progesterone, testosterone, dehydroepiandrosterone (DHEA), thyroxine, and cortisol. Bioidentical hormones are not, however, natural hormones. The estrogens are derived via a chemical process from soybeans (*Glycine max*) and progesterone from Mexican yam (*Dioscorea villosa*). As with conventional hormones, however, bioidentical hormones are available only with a physician's prescription and through a pharmacy. Because of their natural origin, people may perceive that alternative treatments are safer. The interest in phytoestrogens came about because of the low prevalence of hot flashes in Asian women, which was attributed to their diet being rich in phytoestrogens. Recent studies have found that black cohosh, multibotanical herbs, and increased soy intake do not reduce the frequency or severity of menopausal hot flashes or night sweats.

Other remedies for easing menopausal symptoms might include red clover, motherwort, ginseng, sarsaparilla root, valerian root, L-tryptophan, calcium–magnesium, and kelp tablets (Ismail et al., 2015). Again, research thus far has been skeptical about their efficacy, but many clients report they ease their symptoms and their use has skyrocketed. Although some benefits may accrue from their use, evidence of the efficacy of alternative products in menopause is largely anecdotal. Small, preliminary clinical trials might demonstrate the safety of some of the nonpharmacologic products. Nurses should be aware of the purported action of these agents as well as any adverse effects or drug interactions.

The following are lifestyle changes and complementary alternative medicine (CAM) therapies for the treatment of hot flashes:

- Lifestyle changes
- Lower room temperature; use fans
- Wear clothing in layers for easy removal
- Limit caffeine and alcohol intake
- Drink 8 to 10 glasses of water daily
- Stop smoking or cut back
- Avoid hot drinks and spicy food
- Take calcium (1,200 to 1,600 mg) and vitamin D (400 to 600 International Units)
- Exercise daily, but not just before bedtime
- Maintain a healthy weight
- Identify stressors and learn to manage them
- Keep a diary to identify triggers of hot flashes
- Phytoestrogens: isoflavones, ligands, coumestrol
- Black cohosh
- Chamomile: mild sedative to alleviate insomnia
- Unopposed transdermal progesterone
- Compounded bioidentical hormones
- Try relaxation techniques, deep breathing, and meditation
- Acupuncture may reduce the frequency of hot flashes
- Vitamin E: 100 mg daily
- DHEA
- Chaste tree berry (vitex): balances progesterone and estrogen
- Dong quai: acts as a form of phytoestrogen
- Ginseng: purported to improve memory
- St. John's wort: reduces depression and fatigue
- Wild yam: treats menopausal symptoms
- Valerian root: induces sleep and relaxation (Wood, 2015)

Managing Urogenital Changes

Menopausal transition can be a physically and emotionally challenging time for many clients. In addition to the psychological burden of leaving behind the reproductive phase of life and the stigma of an aging body, sexual difficulties resulting from urogenital changes are troublesome but are frequently not addressed. Sexual desire is affected by endocrine and psychosocial factors. Menopausal hormonal changes are relevant to the causes of sexual dysfunction during reproductive aging. The frequency of sexual intercourse declines as people enter midlife. While partner availability and function probably play a role, menopausal symptoms, such as vaginal dryness, are also present (Comhaire & Depypere, 2015).

Vaginal atrophy occurs during menopause because of declining estrogen levels. These changes include thinning of the vaginal walls, an increase in pH, irritation, increased susceptibility to infection, **dyspareunia** (difficult or painful sexual intercourse), loss of lubrication

with intercourse, vaginal dryness, and a decrease in sexual desire related to these changes. Decreased estrogen levels can also influence a client's sexual function as well. Delayed clitoral reaction, decreased vaginal lubrication, diminished circulatory response during sexual stimulation, and reduced contractions during orgasm have all been linked to low estrogen levels (Coney, 2018).

Management of these changes might include the use of estrogen vaginal tablets (Vagifem) or Premarin cream; Estring, an estrogen-releasing vaginal ring that lasts for months; testosterone patches; and over-the-counter moisturizers and lubricants (such as Astroglide) (King et al., 2015). A positive outlook on sexuality and a supportive partner are also needed to make the sexual experience enjoyable and fulfilling. Nurses can improve the sexual health and quality of life in menopausal clients by educating them about their symptoms and offering them choices about managing them.

Take Note!

Sexual health is an important aspect of the human experience. By keeping an open mind, listening, and providing evidence-based treatment options, the nurse can help improve quality of life for menopausal clients.

Preventing and Managing Osteoporosis

Osteoporosis has been recognized as a significant worldwide public health problem. As the world's population ages, both in Canada and internationally, the prevalence of osteoporosis is expected to increase significantly. Osteoporosis is the state of diminished bone density. This disorder is a systemic skeletal disease characterized by low bone mass and microarchitectural deterioration of bone tissue with a consequent increase in bone fragility and susceptibility to fracture (National Osteoporosis Foundation [NOF], 2018).

Osteoporosis is a major medical problem that affects nearly 20% of women over the age of 50 and approximately 3% of men over 50; beyond age 70, the numbers are even higher: over 31% of women and approximately 6% of men will be diagnosed with osteoporosis; this represents 1.5 million Canadians (Garriguet, 2011; PHAC, 2010). Approximately one in five people living with osteoporosis report having experienced a facture, most commonly in the wrist, upper arm, spine, pelvis, or hip (PHAC, 2010). In fact, factures in seniors are more common than heart attack, stroke, and breast cancer combined (Osteoporosis Canada, 2018). In 2010, the cost of health care for osteoporosis was calculated to be $2.3 billion, which amounts to over 1.3% of the entire health care spending (Tarride et al., 2012). With the rapidly aging population, the problem of osteoporosis is now reaching epidemic proportions. Baby boomers make up nearly 30% of the

FIGURE 4.22 Skeletal changes associated with osteoporosis. (John Radcliffe Hospital/Science Source.)

Canadian population and are entering the stage in their lives when they are most at risk for osteoporosis (Statistics Canada, 2015). One half of all women and one third of all men will sustain a fragility fracture during their lifetimes. Osteoporosis continues to be underdiagnosed and undertreated because it is often not recognized until the first fracture occurs.

Women are greatly affected by osteoporosis after menopause. Osteoporosis is a condition in which bone mass declines to such an extent that fractures occur with minimal trauma. Bone loss begins in the third or fourth decade of a woman's life and accelerates rapidly after menopause (Alexander et al., 2014). This condition puts many women into long-term care, with a resulting loss of independence. Figure 4.22 shows the skeletal changes associated with osteoporosis.

Most individuals with osteoporosis do not know they have the disease until they sustain a fracture, usually of the wrist or hip. Risk factors include:
- Increasing age
- Postmenopausal status without hormone replacement
- Small, thin-boned frame
- Low BMD
- White or Asian with small bone frame
- Impaired eyesight that would increase risk of falling
- Rheumatoid arthritis
- Family history of osteoporosis
- Sedentary lifestyle
- History of treatment with:
  - Antacids with aluminum
  - Heparin

- Long-term use of steroids >3 months
- Thyroid replacement drugs
- Smoking and consuming alcohol
- Low calcium and vitamin D intake
- Excessive amounts of caffeine
- Personal history of nontraumatic fracture
- Anorexia nervosa or bulimia (NOF, 2018)

Currently, no method exists for directly measuring bone mass. Instead, a BMD measurement is used. BMD is a two-dimensional measurement of the average content of mineral in a section of bone. BMD evaluations are made at the hip, femoral neck, and spine. There is a significant relationship between BMD and fracture: as BMD is reduced, the risk of fracture increases (Sullivan et al., 2015). Screening tests to measure bone density are not good predictors for young clients who might be at risk for developing this condition. Dual-energy x-ray absorptiometry (DXA or DEXA) is a screening test that calculates the mineral content of the bone at the spine and hip. It is highly accurate, fast, and relatively inexpensive. The DEXA scan is the gold standard radiologic method for identifying osteoporosis through measuring BMD (NOF, 2019a).

Hip fracture is the most devastating of the fragility fractures secondary to osteoporosis. A number of medical, social, and economic consequences follow a hip fracture. Of women older than 50 years, on average, 24% die within the first year after hip fracture (Wang et al., 2015). The concern surrounding osteoporosis is not the rate of fracture alone but also the potential for lifelong disability secondary to fracture. The incidence of hip fracture is estimated to double by the year 2025 and nearly double again by 2050. For women, this is a projected 240% increase (NOF, 2018).

The best management for this painful, crippling, and potentially fatal disease is prevention.

Clients can modify many risk factors by doing the following:
- Engage in daily weightbearing exercise, such as walking, to increase osteoblast activity.
- Increase calcium and vitamin D intake.
- Avoid smoking and excessive alcohol (more than two drinks per day).
- Discuss bone health with a health care provider.
- When appropriate, have a bone density test and take medication if needed (NOF, 2019b).

Medications that can help in preventing and managing osteoporosis include:
- HT (Premarin)
- SERMs (raloxifene [Evista])
- Calcium and vitamin D supplements (Tums)
- Estrogen agonist/antagonist (SERM) (Evista)
- Bisphosphonates (Actonel, Fosamax, Boniva, or Reclast)
- Parathyroid hormone (Forteo)
- Calcitonin (Miacalcin) (King & Brucker, 2016).

Preventing and Managing Cardiovascular Disease

Despite the dramatic decrease in annual CVD mortality and total cardiovascular mortality, CVD remains the number one cause of premature death for Canadian women, accounting for over 31,000 women annually. Five times as many women die of heart disease each year than of breast cancer. The prevalence of heart disease is likely due to increased rates of obesity, sedentary lifestyle, diabetes, and high cholesterol levels (Chomistek et al., 2015). One woman dies every 20 minutes in this country of CVD, with strokes accounting for about 20% of the deaths (Heart & Stroke Foundation of Canada, 2018). While men's mortality from CVD has decreased since the 1980s, women's mortality from CVD has climbed. This has resulted in a sex-related CVD mortality gap, with women having higher mortality than men since 1984. There is also a gender imbalance in current clinical research in this area: two thirds of clinical research in heart disease is focused on men (Heart & Stroke Foundation of Canada, 2017). Contributing to this mortality gap is a lack of awareness among women and their physicians of the risk for CVD. Awareness campaigns, such as the Heart Truth and the Red Dress symbol, appear to have improved recognition of CVD risk in women. Further, female-specific guidelines have been developed to prevent and reduce CVD. Though the current understanding of the role of menopause in CVD is controversial, studies suggest that menopause does not exacerbate CVD independent of aging, and HT is not effective for secondary prevention of CVD (Hale & Shufelt, 2015).

For the first half of a woman's life, estrogen seems to be a protective substance for the cardiovascular system by smoothing, relaxing, and dilating blood vessels. It even helps boost HDL and lower LDL levels, helping to keep the arteries clean from plaque accumulation. But when estrogen levels plummet as women age and experience menopause, the incidence of CVD increases dramatically. Women are more likely to have atypical cardiovascular symptoms compared with men. This may lead to a delayed diagnosis or misdiagnosis of CAD and suboptimal treatment. These symptoms may include:

- A—Angina (chest pain)
- B—Breathlessness
- C—Chronic fatigue
- D—Dizziness
- E—Edema of hands and feet
- F—Fluttering of the heart
- G—Gastric upset
- H—Heavy pain in back and shoulders

Menopause is not the only factor that increases a woman's risk for CVD. Lifestyle and medical history factors such as the following play a major role:

- Smoking
- Obesity
- High-fat diet
- Sedentary lifestyle
- High cholesterol levels
- Family history of CVD
- Hypertension
- Apple-shaped body
- Diabetes

Two of the major risk factors for coronary heart disease are hypertension and dyslipidemia. Both are modifiable and can be prevented by lifestyle changes and, if needed, controlled by medication. This is why prevention is essential. In addition, clients who experience early menopause lose the protection afforded by endogenous estrogen to the cardiac system and are at greater risk for more extensive atherosclerosis. Major preventive strategies include a healthy diet, increased activity, exercise, smoking cessation, decreased alcohol intake, and weight reduction.

Nurses, particularly those caring for clients during their reproductive years, are uniquely positioned to provide education and support for long-term cardiovascular health. Raising awareness of heart disease in women is an essential role for nurses. The good news is that CVD is largely preventable. Because CVD is a chronic disease that develops over time, primary prevention lifestyle modification interventions are most effective if initiated before the development of overt disease. Stressing the importance of lifestyle modifications must begin early in life and should be reinforced from the beginning of a young woman's reproductive years through menopause (CDC, 2016b). Nurses are in an ideal position to teach the importance of good nutrition, healthy weight, and daily exercise before CVD becomes clinically evident.

Nursing Assessment

Menopausal transition is a universal and irreversible part of the overall aging process involving the reproductive system. Although not a disease state, menopausal transition does place a client at greater risk for the development of many conditions of aging. Nurses can help the client become aware of her risk for postmenopausal diseases, as well as strategies to prevent them. The nurse can be instrumental in assessing risk factors and planning interventions in collaboration with the client. These might include:

- Screening for osteoporosis, CVD, and cancer risk
  - Assessment of blood pressure to identify hypertension
  - Blood cholesterol test to identify hyperlipidemia risk
  - Mammogram to find a cancerous lesion
  - Pap smear to identify cervical cancer
  - Pelvic examination to identify endometrial cancer or masses
  - Digital rectal examination to assess for colon cancer
  - Bone density testing as a baseline at menopause to identify osteopenia (low bone mass), which might lead to osteoporosis

- Assessing lifestyle to plan strategies to prevent chronic conditions:
  - Dietary intake of fat, cholesterol, and sodium
  - Weight management
  - Calcium intake
  - Use of tobacco, alcohol, and caffeine
  - Amount and type of daily exercise routines

Nursing Management

There is no "magic bullet" in managing menopause. Nurses can counsel clients about their risks and help them to prevent disease and debilitating conditions with specific health maintenance education. Clients must make their own educated decisions, but the nurse is responsible for making sure they are armed with the facts to do so intelligently. Nurses can offer a thorough explanation of the menopausal process, including the latest research findings, to help clients understand and make decisions about this inevitable event.

If the client decides to use HT to control menopausal symptoms, after being thoroughly educated, frequent reassessments will be needed. There are no hard-and-fast rules that apply to meeting a client's individual needs. The nurse can provide realistic expectations of the therapy to reduce the client's anxiety and concern.

It is also useful to emphasize the value of friends to gain support and share information and resources. Often just talking about emotional difficulties such as the death of a parent or problematic relationships helps solve problems. It also shows the client that any emotional responses are valid.

Healthy lifestyles and stress management techniques are vital to health and longevity, and it is important to keep these on the client's agenda when discussing menopause (North American Menopause Society, 2018). Evidence-based interventions include lifestyle modifications, risk management therapies, and preventive drug interventions, such as the following:

- Participate actively in maintaining health.
- Exercise regularly to prevent CVD and osteoporosis.
- Take supplemental calcium and eat appropriately to prevent osteoporosis.
- Stop smoking to prevent lung and heart disease.
- Reduce caffeine and alcohol intake to prevent osteoporosis.
- Monitor blood pressure, lipids, and diabetes (drug therapy management).
- Use low-dose aspirin to prevent blood clots.
- Reduce dietary intake of fat, cholesterol, and sodium to prevent CVD.
- Maintain a healthy weight for body frame.
- Perform breast self-examinations for breast awareness.
- Control stress to prevent depression (Houseman & Odum, 2016; Worel & Hayman, 2015).

These life approaches may seem low-tech, but they can stave off menopause-related complications such as CVD, osteoporosis, and depression. These tips for healthy living work well, but the client needs to be motivated to stick with them.

NURSING CARE PLAN 4.1

Overview of a Client With Abnormal Uterine Bleeding

Stacy, a 52-year-old obese woman, comes to her gynecologist with the complaint of heavy erratic bleeding. Her periods were fairly regular until about 4 months ago, and since that time they have been unpredictable, excessive, and prolonged. Stacy reports she is tired all the time, can't sleep, and feels "out of sorts" and anxious. She is fearful she has cancer.

NURSING DIAGNOSIS: Fear related to current signs and symptoms possibly indicating a life-threatening condition

Outcome Identification and Evaluation

The client will acknowledge her fears as evidenced by statements made that fear and anxiety have been lessened after explanation of diagnosis.

Interventions: *Reducing Fear and Anxiety*

- Distinguish between anxiety and fear to determine appropriate interventions.
- Check complete blood count and assess for possible anemia secondary to excessive bleeding to determine if fatigue is contributing to anxiety and fear. Fatigue occurs because the oxygen-carrying capacity of the blood is reduced.

NURSING CARE PLAN 4.1

Overview of a Client With Abnormal Uterine Bleeding (continued)

- Reassure client that symptoms can be managed to help address her current concerns.
- Provide client with factual information and explain what to expect to assist client with identifying fears and help her to cope with her condition.
- Provide symptom management to reduce concerns associated with the cause of bleeding.
- Teach client about early manifestations of fear and anxiety to aid in prompt recognition and to minimize escalation of anxiety.
- Assess client's use of coping strategies in the past and reinforce use of effective ones to help control anxiety and fear.
- Instruct client in relaxation methods, such as deep-breathing exercises and imagery, to provide her with additional methods for controlling anxiety and fear.

NURSING DIAGNOSIS: Deficient knowledge related to menopausal transition and its management

Outcome Identification and Evaluation

The client will demonstrate understanding of her symptoms as evidenced by making health-promoting lifestyle choices, verbalizing appropriate health care practices, and adhering to measures and complying with therapy.

Interventions: *Providing Client Education*

- Assess client's understanding of menopausal transition and its treatment to provide a baseline for teaching and developing a plan of care.
- Review instructions about prescribed procedures and recommendations for self-care, frequently obtaining feedback from the client to validate adequate understanding of information.
- Outline link between anovulatory cycles and excessive buildup of uterine lining in menopausal transition clients to assist client in understanding the etiology of her bleeding.
- Provide written material with pictures to promote learning and help client visualize what is occurring to her body during menopausal transition.
- Inform client about the availability of community resources and make appropriate referrals as needed to provide additional education and support.
- Document details of teaching and learning to allow for continuity of care and further education, if needed.

KEY CONCEPTS

- Establishing good health habits and avoiding risky behaviours early in life will prevent chronic conditions later in life.
- PMS has more than 150 symptoms, and at least two different syndromes have been recognized: PMS and PMDD.
- Endometriosis is a condition in which bits of functioning endometrial tissue are located outside their normal site, the uterine cavity.
- Infertility is a widespread problem that has an emotional, social, and economic impact on couples.
- More than half of all unintended pregnancies occur in clients who report using some method of birth control during the month of conception.
- Hormonal methods include OCs, injectables, implants, vaginal rings, and transdermal patches.
- Recent studies have shown that the extension of active extended cycle OC pills carries the same

safety profile as the conventional 28-day regimens (Shoupe & Mishell, 2016).

- Currently, four IUCs are available in Canada: the copper ParaGard-TCu-380A, and three LNG-IUSs marketed as Mirena, Jaydess, and Kyleena (Island Sexual Health, 2017).

- OCs, sterilization, and male condoms are the most popular methods of contraception in the Canada and worldwide (Alan Guttmacher Institute, 2018a).

- Menopause, with a dramatic decline in estrogen levels, affects not only the reproductive organs but also other body systems.

- Most women with osteoporosis do not know they have the disease until they sustain a fracture, usually of the wrist or hip (NOF, 2018).

- Over 31,000 women die annually in Canada of CVD, with strokes accounting for about 20% of the deaths (Alexander et al., 2014).

- Nurses should aim to have a holistic approach to the sexual health of clients from menarche through menopause.

REFERENCES AND RECOMMENDED READINGS

Abortion Rights Coalition of Canada. (2017). *Position Paper #1: Abortion is a "medically necessary" service and cannot be delisted.* Retrieved from http://www.arcc-cdac.ca/postionpapers/01-Abortion-Medically-Required.pdf

Alan Guttmacher Institute. (2018a). *Contraceptive use in the United States.* Retrieved from http://www.guttmacher.org/pubs/fb_contr_use.html

Alan Guttmacher Institute. (2018b). *Induced abortion in the United States.* Retrieved from https://www.guttmacher.org/fact-sheet/induced-abortion-united-states

Alexander, L. L., LaRosa, J. H., Bader, H., & Garfield, S. (2014). *New dimensions in women's health* (6th ed.). Sudbury, MA: Jones & Bartlett.

Al-Sahab, B., Ardern, C. I., Hamadeh, M. J., Tamim, H. (2010). Age at menarche in Canada: Results from the National Longitudinal Survey of Children & Youth. *BMC Public Health, 10,* 736.

American Academy of Allergy, Asthma and Immunology (AAAAI). (2018). *Latex allergy: Tips to remember.* Retrieved from http://www.aaaai.org/conditions-and-treatments/library/allergy-library/latex-allergy.aspx

American College of Obstetricians & Gynecologists (ACOG). (2015a). *Premenstrual syndrome.* Retrieved from https://www.acog.org/Patients/FAQs/Premenstrual-Syndrome-PMS

American College of Obstetricians & Gynecologists (ACOG). (2015b). *Dysmenorrhea: Painful periods.* FAQ046. Retrieved from https://www.acog.org/Patients/FAQs/Dysmenorrhea-Painful-Periods?IsMobileSet=false

American Society for Reproductive Medicine (ASRM). (2018). *Frequently asked questions about infertility.* Retrieved from https://www.reproductivefacts.org/faqs/frequently-asked-questions-about-infertility/

Ataollahi, M., Akbari, S. A., Mojab, F., & Alavi Majd, H. (2015). The effect of wheat germ extract on premenstrual syndrome symptoms. *Iranian Journal of Pharmaceutical Research, 14*(1), 159–166.

Atkin, K., Beal, M. W., Long-Middleton, E., & Roncari, D. (2015). Long-acting reversible contraceptives for teenagers: Primary care recommendations. *The Nurse Practitioner, 40*(3), 38–46.

Avis, N. E., Crawford, S. L., Greendale, G., Bromberger, J. T., Everson-Rose, S. A., Gold, E. B., … Thurston, R. C. (2015). Duration of menopausal vasomotor symptoms over the menopause transition. *JAMA Internal Medicine, 175*(4), 531–539.

Bakour, S. H., & Williamson, J. (2015). Latest evidence on using hormone replacement therapy in the menopause. *Obstetrician & Gynecologist, 17*(1), 20–28.

Bauer, G. R., & Scheim, A. I. (2015). *Transgender people in Ontario, Canada: Statistics to inform human rights policy.* Retrieved from https://www.rainbowhealthontario.ca/wp-content/uploads/woocommerce_uploads/2015/09/Trans-PULSE-Statistics-Relevant-for-Human-Rights-Policy-June-2015.pdf

Bieber, E. J., Sanfilippo, J. S., Horowitz, I. R., & Shafi, M. I. (2015). *Clinical gynecology* (2nd ed.). Cambridge, UK: Cambridge University Press.

Bitzer, J., Heikinheimo, O., Nelson, A. L., Calaf-Alsina, J., & Fraser, I. S. (2015). Medical management of heavy menstrual bleeding: A comprehensive review of the literature. *Obstetrical & Gynecological Survey, 70*(2), 115–130.

Black, D. M., & Rosen, C. J. (2016). Postmenopausal osteoporosis. *New England Journal of Medicine, 374,* 254–262.

Boardman, H. M., Hartley, L., Eisinga, A., Main, C., Roqué i Figuls, M., Bonfill Cosp, X., … Knight, B. (2015). Hormone therapy for preventing cardiovascular disease in postmenopausal women. *Cochrane Database of Systematic Reviews,* (3), CD002229.

Boyd, K., Perkins, P., Lawrence, K., Sutherland, J., & Blake, K. (2015). The female condom: Knowledge, image, and power. *Journal of Black Sexuality and Relationships, 1*(3), 97–112.

Brown, J., & Farquhar, C. (2015). An overview of treatments for endometriosis. *Journal of the American Medical Association, 313*(3), 296–297.

Calis, K. A., Popat, V., Dang, D. K., & Kalantaridou, S. N. (2017). Dysmenorrhea. *eMedicine.* Retrieved from http://emedicine.medscape.com/article/253812-overview

Canadian Association of Midwives. (2015). *A statement on gender inclusivity & human rights.* Retrieved from https://canadianmidwives.org/wp-content/uploads/2016/06/CAM-GenderInclusivity-HumanRights-Sept2015.pdf

Canadian Association of Schools of Nursing. (2017). *Entry-to-practice competencies for nursing care of the childbearing family for baccalaureate programs in nursing.* Retrieved from https://www.casn.ca/wp-content/uploads/2016/09/FINAL-CHILDBEARING-FAMILY-COMPETENCIES-revised.pdf

Canadian Institute for Health Information. (2015). Induced abortions reported in Canada in 2015. Retrieved from https://www.cihi.ca/sites/default/files/document/induced-abortion-can-2015-en-web.xlsx

Carlson, J. L. (2015). The menstrual cycle. In C. M. Gordon & M. S. LeBoff (Eds.). *The female athlete triad: A clinical guide* (pp. 29–38). Philadelphia, PA: Springer Publishers.

Casey, F. E. (2018). Contraception. *eMedicine.* Retrieved from http://emedicine.medscape.com/article/258507-overview

Casey, F., & Isaacs, C. (2015). Are we getting the word out about emergency contraception? *Contemporary OB/GYN, 60*(2), 18–19.

Cavallini, G. (2015). General therapeutic approach to male infertility. In G. Cavallini & G. Beretta (Eds.). *Clinical management of male infertility* (pp. 33–39). Switzerland: Springer International Publishing.

Centers for Disease Control and Prevention (CDC). (2016a). *Contraceptive use.* National Center for Health Statistics. Retrieved from https://www.cdc.gov/nchs/fastats/contraceptive.htm

Centers for Disease Control and Prevention (CDC). (2016b). *Healthy eating for a healthy weight.* Retrieved from http://www.cdc.gov/healthyweight/healthy_eating/

Centers for Disease Control and Prevention (CDC). (2017). U.S. selected practice recommendations for contraceptive use, 2016. Retrieved from https://www.cdc.gov/mmwr/volumes/65/rr/rr6504a1.htm

Cheng, S. C., & Van Leuven, K. A. (2015). Intrauterine contraception and the facts for college health. *The Journal for Nurse Practitioners, 11*(4), 417–423.

Chomistek, A. K., Chiuve, S. E., Eliassen, A. H., Mukamal, K. J., Willett, W. C., & Rimm, E. B. (2015). Healthy lifestyle in the primordial prevention of cardiovascular disease among young women. *Journal of the American College of Cardiology, 65*(1), 43–51.

Comhaire, F. H., & Depypere, H. T. (2015). Hormones, herbal preparations and nutraceuticals for a better life after the menopause: Part II. *Climacteric: The Journal of the International Menopause Society, 18*, 364–371.

Coney, P. (2018). Menopause. *eMedicine.* Retrieved from http://emedicine.medscape.com/article/264088-overview

Costescu, D., Guilbert, E., Bernardin, J., Black, A., Dunn, S., Fitzsimmons, B., … Reeves, M. (2016). Medical abortion. *Journal of Obstetrics and Gynecology Canada, 38*(4), 366–389.

Craik, J., & Melvin, L. (2015). Oral contraceptives: Benefits and risks. In M. Harrison-Woolrych (Ed.). *Medicines for women* (pp. 141–180). Switzerland: Springer International Publishing.

Craik, J., & Rowlands, S. (2015). Contraceptive devices for women: Implants, intrauterine devices and other products. In M. Harrison-Woolrych (Ed.). *Medicines for women* (pp. 227–270). Switzerland: Springer International Publishing.

Creatsas, G. K. (2015). Prevention of adolescent pregnancies. In A. R. Genazzani & M. Brincat (Eds.). *Frontiers in gynecological endocrinology* (pp. 41–45). Switzerland: Springer International Publishing.

Creatsas, G. K., & Creatsa, M. (2015). Disorders of the menstrual cycle during adolescence. In A. R. Genazzani & M. Brincat (Eds.). *Frontiers in gynecological endocrinology* (pp. 3–9). Switzerland: Springer International Publishing.

Dadhich, P., Ramasamy, R., & Lipshultz, L. I. (2015). The male infertility office visit. *The Italian Journal of Urology and Nephrology.* Retrieved from http://europepmc.org/abstract/med/25604696

Davila, G. W., Kapoor, D. W., Alderman, E., Hiraoka, M. K., Ghoniem, G. M., & Peskin, B. D. (2018). Endometriosis. *eMedicine.* Retrieved from http://emedicine.medscape.com/article/271899-overview

Dohle, G. R. (2015). Male factors in couple's infertility. In V. Mirone (Ed.). *Clinical uro-andrology* (pp. 197–201). Berlin: Springer Publishers.

Dombo, E. A., & Flood, M. (2015). *Spirituality infertility counseling. Fertility counseling* (Vol. 11, pp. 74–85). Cambridge, UK: Cambridge University Press.

Elnashar, A. (2015). Emerging treatment of endometriosis. *Middle East Fertility Society Journal.* Retrieved from http://www.sciencedirect.com/science/article/pii/S1110569014200562

Evans, G., & Sutton, E. L. (2015). Oral contraception. *Medical Clinics of North America, 99*(3), 479–503.

Everett, S. (2014). *Handbook of contraception and sexual health* (3rd ed.). New York: Routledge

Foster, D. G., Biggs, M. A., Phillips, K. A., Grindlay, K., & Grossman, D. (2015). Potential public sector cost-savings from over-the-counter access to oral contraceptives. *Contraception, 91*, 373–379.

Ganatra, B., Guest, P., & Berer, M. (2015). Expanding access to medical abortion: Challenges and opportunities. *Reproductive Health Matters, 22*(44), 1–3.

Garriguet, D. (2011). Bone health: Osteoporosis, calcium and vitamin D. Statistics Canada Catalogue no. 82-003-X. Retrieved from http://www.statcan.gc.ca/pub/82-003-x/2011003/article/11515-eng.pdf

Giblon, R., & Bauer, G. R. (2017). Health care availability, quality, and unmet need: A comparison of transgender and cisgender residents of Ontario, Canada. *BMC Health Services Research, 17*, 283.

Golden, N. H., Katzman, D. K., Sawyer, S. M., Ornstein, R. M., Rome, E. S., Garber, A. K., … Kreipe, R. E. (2015). Update on the medical management of eating disorders in adolescents. *Journal of Adolescent Health, 56*(4), 370–375.

Goswami, D. (2015). Primary ovarian insufficiency: The paradox of menopause in young women. *MAMC Journal of Medical Sciences, 1*(1), 3.

Haddad, L. B., Philpott-Jones, S., & Schonfeld, T. (2015). Contraception and prevention of HIV transmission: A potential conflict of public health principles. *Journal of Family Planning and Reproductive Health Care, 41*(1), 20–23.

Hale, G. E., & Shufelt, C. L. (2015). Hormone therapy in menopause: An update on cardiovascular disease considerations. *Trends in Cardiovascular Medicine, 25*(6), 540–549.

Health Canada. (2013). *Fertility.* Retrieved from https://www.canada.ca/en/public-health/services/fertility/fertility.html

Health Canada. (2017). *Mifegymiso (mifepristone and misoprostol tablets): Updates to product monograph and risk management plan.* Retrieved from http://healthycanadians.gc.ca/recall-alert-rappel-avis/hc-sc/2017/65030a-eng.php

Heart & Stroke Foundation of Canada. (2017). *MsUnderstood: 2018 Heart report.* Retrieved from http://www.heartand-stroke.ca/-/media/pdf-files/canada/2018-heart-month/hs_2018-heart-report_en.ashx

Heart & Stroke Foundation of Canada. (2018). *Women's unique risk factors.* Retrieved from http://www.heartand-stroke.ca/heart/risk-and-prevention/womens-unique-risk-factors

Hemingway, A. P., & Trew, G. H. (2015). Hysterosalpingography. In G. F. Grimbizis, R. Campo, B. C. Tarlatzis, & S. Gordts (Eds.). *Female genital tract congenital malformations* (pp. 49–61). London: Springer Publishers.

Housman, J., & Odum, M. (2016). *Alters & Schiff's essential concepts for healthy living* (7th ed.). Burlington, MA: Jones & Bartlett Learning.

Hoyt, L. T., & Falconi, A. M. (2015). Puberty and perimeno-pause: Reproductive transitions and their implications for women's health. *Social Science & Medicine, 132*, 103–112.

Htay, T. T. (2016). Premenstrual dysphoric disorder. *eMedicine*. Retrieved from http://emedicine.medscape.com/article/293257-overview

Hughes, H. (2015). Postpartum contraception. *Journal of Family Health Care, 19*(1), 9–10.

Ilic, K. (2015). Emergency contraception. In M. Harrison-Woolrych (Ed.). *Medicines for women* (pp. 203–225). Switzerland: Springer International Publishing.

Infertility Network. (2018). *Insurance/IVF funding*. Retrieved from https://www.infertilitynetwork.org/Insurance-Canada

Inhorn, M. C., & Patrizio, P. (2015). Infertility around the globe: New thinking on gender, reproductive technologies and global movements in the 21st century. *Human Reproduction Update, 21*, 411–426.

Island Sexual Health. (2017). Comparing IUDs: Copper, Mirena, Kyleena, and Jaydess at a glance. Retrieved from https://www.islandsexualhealth.org/wp-content/uploads/2017/07/IUD-handout-and-comparison-chart.pdf

Ismail, R., Taylor-Swanson, L., Thomas, A., Schnall, J. G., Cray, L., Mitchell, E. S., & Woods, N. F. (2015). Effects of herbal preparations on symptom clusters during the menopausal transition. *Climacteric, 18*(1), 11–28.

Jick, S. (2015). Oral contraceptives and the risk of venous thromboembolism. In M. Harrison-Woolrych (Ed.). *Medicines for women* (pp. 181–201). Switzerland: Springer International Publishing.

Jin, J. (2015). *JAMA* patient page. Treatments for infertility. *Journal of the American Medical Association, 313*(3), 320–321.

Johnston, J. L., Reid, H., & Hunter, D. (2015). Diagnosing endometriosis in primary care: Clinical update. *British Journal of General Practice, 65*(631), 101–102.

Jones, A. M. (2016). A picture of trans Canadians' health and access to healthcare. *University of British Columbia Medical Journal, 7*(2), 40–41. Retrieved from http://med-fom-ubcmj.sites.olt.ubc.ca/files/2016/03/v7i2-news-and-letters-5.pdf

Joshi, T., Kural, M. R., Agrawal, D. P., Noor, N. N., & Patil, A. (2015). Primary dysmenorrhea and its effect on quality of life in young girls. *International Journal of Medical Science and Public Health, 4*(3), 381–385.

Kessenich, C. R. (2017). Inevitable menopause. *Nursing Spectrum*. Retrieved from https://www.nurse.com/ce/inevitable-menopause

Khan, A. B., & Krupanidhi, C. S. (2015). A review on vaginal drug delivery system. *RGUHS Journal of Pharmaceutical Sciences, 4*(4), 142–147.

Kho, C. L., & Mathur, M. (2015). Uterine artery embolization for acute dysfunctional uterine bleeding with failed medical therapy: A novel approach to management. *BMJ Case Reports*. doi:10.1136/bcr-2014-204446

Kim, J. S. (2015). Latex allergy. In H. A. Sampson (Ed.). *Allergy and clinical immunology* (pp. 288–293). Chichester, UK: John Wiley & Sons.

King, T. L., & Brucker, M. C. (2016). *Pharmacology for women's health* (2nd ed.). Sudbury, MA: Jones & Bartlett Learning.

King, T. L., Brucker, M. C., Kriebs, J. M., Fahey, J. O., Gegor, C. L., & Varney, H. (2015). *Varney's midwifery* (5th ed.). Burlington, MA: Jones & Bartlett Learning.

Kodaman, P. H. (2015). Current strategies for endometriosis management. *Obstetrics and Gynecology Clinics of North America, 42*(1), 87–101.

Kosenko, K., Rintamaki, L., Raney, S., & Maness, K. (2013). Transgender patient perceptions of stigma in health care contexts. *Medical Care, 51*(9), 819–822.

Kovanci, E., & Schutt, A. K. (2015). Premature ovarian failure: Clinical presentation and treatment. *Obstetrics and Gynecology Clinics of North America, 42*(1), 153–161.

Kreitzer, R. J. (2015). Politics and morality in state abortion policy. *State Politics & Policy Quarterly, 15*(1), 41–66.

Krieger, N., Kiang, M. V., Kosheleva, A., Waterman, P. D., Chen, J. T., & Beckfield, J. (2015). Age at menarche: 50-year socioeconomic trends among US-born Black and White women. *American Journal of Public Health, 105*(2), 388–397.

Kyvernitakis, I., Kostev, K., Hars, O., Albert, U., & Hadji, P. (2015). Discontinuation rates of menopausal hormone therapy among postmenopausal women in the post-WHI Study ERA. *Climacteric: The Journal of the International Menopause Society, 18*, 737–742. doi:10.3109/13697137.2015.1037267.

Liao, P. V., & Dollin, J. (2012). Half a century of the oral contraceptive pill. *Canadian Family Physician, 58*(12), e757–e760.

Maurice, J. M., & Rosenzweig, B. A. (2015). Acute gynecologic pelvic pain. In T. J. Saclarides, J. A. Myers, & K. W. Millikan (Eds.). *Common surgical diseases* (pp. 319–322). New York: Springer Publishers.

McFarland, M. R., & Wehbe-Alamah, H. B. (2015). *Leininger's cultural care diversity and universality: A worldwide nursing theory* (3rd ed.). Burlington, MA: Jones & Bartlett Learning.

McFarlane, D. R. (2015). *Global population and reproductive health*. Burlington, MA: Jones & Bartlett Learning.

McKnight, Z. (2017). Controversial Essure birth control device will no longer be sold in Canada. *The Star*. Retrieved from https://www.thestar.com/life/health_wellness/2017/06/17/controversial-essure-birth-control-device-will-no-longer-be-sold-in-canada.html

Mclaren, A., & Marshall, T. R. (2013). Henry Morgentaler. *The Canadian Encyclopedia*. Retrieved from http://www.thecanadianencyclopedia.ca/en/article/henry-morgentaler/

McNamara, M., Batur, P., & DeSapri, K. T. (2015). In the clinic. Perimenopause. *Annals of Internal Medicine, 162*(3), ITC1–ITC15.

Mirkin, S., Archer, D. F., Pickar, J. H., & Komm, B. S. (2015). Recent advances help understand and improve the safety of menopausal therapies. *Menopause, 22*(3), 351–360.

Moses, S. (2018a). Primary amenorrhea. *Family Practice Notebook*. Retrieved from http://www.fpnotebook.com/gyn/Menses/PrmryAmnrh.htm

Moses, S. (2018b). Female Tanner stage. *Family Practice Notebook*. Retrieved from http://www.fpnotebook.com/endo/exam/fmltnrstg.htm

Moses, S. (2018c). Contraceptive sponge. *Family Practice Notebook*. Retrieved from http://www.fpnotebook.com/gyn/contraception/CntrcptvSpng.htm

Mulligan, K. (2016). Access to emergency contraception and its impact on fertility and sexual behavior. *Health Economics, 25*, 455–469.

Naeimi, N. (2015). The prevalence and symptoms of premenstrual syndrome under examination. *Journal of Biosciences and Medicines, 3*, 1–8.

National Institute of Child Health and Human Development (NICHD). (2015). *Endometriosis.* Retrieved from https://www.nichd.nih.gov/sites/default/files/publications/pubs/Documents/endometriosis-2002.pdf#search=NIH-Pub.-No.-02-2413

National Osteoporosis Foundation (NOF). (2018). *Bone health basics: Get the facts.* Retrieved from https://www.nof.org/preventing-fractures/general-facts/

National Osteoporosis Foundation (NOF). (2019a). *Bone density exam/Testing.* Retrieved from https://www.nof.org/patients/diagnosis-information/bone-density-examtesting/

National Osteoporosis Foundation (NOF). (2019b). *Prevention and healthy living.* Retrieved from https://www.nof.org/preventing-fractures/prevention/prevention-and-healthy-living/

Nelson, A. L. (2015). Transdermal contraception methods: Today's patches and new options on the horizon. *Expert Opinion on Pharmacotherapy, 16*(6), 863–873.

North American Menopause Society. (2018). Menopause FAQs: Your health after menopause. Retrieved from http://www.menopause.org/for-women/menopause-faqs-your-health-after-menopause

Occupational Health and Safety Administration. (2018). *Latex allergy.* Retrieved from http://www.osha.gov/SLTC/latexallergy

Osteoporosis Canada. (2018). *About the disease.* Retrieved from https://osteoporosis.ca/about-the-disease

Pagana, K. D., Pagana, T. J., & Pagana, T. N. (2015). *Mosby's diagnostic and laboratory test reference* (12th ed.). St. Louis, MO: Elsevier Mosby.

Patil, E., & Edelman, A. (2015). Medical abortion: Use of mifepristone and misoprostol in first and second trimesters of pregnancy. *Current Obstetrics and Gynecology Reports, 4*(1), 69–78.

Pearlstein, T. (2015). Depressive disorders: Premenstrual dysphoric disorder. In A. Tasman, J. Kay, J. A. Lieberman, & M.B. First (Eds.). *Psychiatry* (4th ed., pp. 966–980). Chichester, UK: John Wiley & Sons.

Planned Parenthood. (2018a). *Fertility awareness-based methods.* Retrieved from http://www.plannedparenthood.org/health-topics/birth-control/fertility-awareness-4217.htm

Planned Parenthood. (2018b). *The abortion pill.* Retrieved from http://m.plannedparenthood.org/mt/www.plannedparenthood.org/health-topics/abortion/abortion-pill-medication-abortion-4354.asp

Planned Parenthood. (2018c). *Cervical cap.* Retrieved from https://www.plannedparenthood.org/learn/birth-control/cervical-cap

Pocius, K. D., & Dutton, C. R. (2015). Update on hormonal contraception and obesity. *Current Obstetrics and Gynecology Reports, 4,* 61–68.

Public Health Agency of Canada. (2010). *What is the impact of osteoporosis in Canada and what are Canadians doing to maintain healthy bones?* Retrieved from http://www.phac-aspc.gc.ca/cd-mc/osteoporosis-osteoporose/pdf/osteoporosis.pdf

Public Health Agency of Canada. (2015). *Summary: Estimates of HIV incidence, prevalence and proportion undiagnosed in Canada, 2014.* Retrieved from http://www.catie.ca/sites/default/files/2014-HIV-Estimates-in-Canada-EN.pdf

Puscheck, E. E., & Woodward, T. L. (2016). Infertility. *eMedicine.* Retrieved from http://emedicine.medscape.com/article/274143-overview

Raymond, E. G., & Cleland, K. (2015). Emergency contraception. *New England Journal of Medicine, 372*(14), 1342–1348.

RESOLVE (National Infertility Association). (2015). *What is infertility?* Retrieved from http://www.resolve.org/infertility-overview/what-is-infertility

Rotterman, M., Dunn, S., & Black, A. (2015). *Oral contraceptive use among women aged 15 to 49: Results from the Canadian Health Measures Survey.* Retrieved from http://www.statcan.gc.ca/pub/82-003-x/2015010/article/14222-eng.htm

Santamaría, M., & Lago, I. (2015). Premenstrual experience premenstrual syndrome and dysphoric disorder. In M. Saenz-Herrero (Ed.). *Psychopathology in women* (pp. 423–449). Switzerland: Springer International Publishing.

Schuiling, K. D., & Likis, F. E. (2016). *Women's gynecologic health* (4th ed.). Burlington, MA: Jones & Bartlett Learning.

Schwartz, J. L., Weiner, D. H., Lai, J. J., Frezieres, R. G., Creinin, M. D., Archer, D. F., … Mauck, C. K. (2015). Contraceptive efficacy, safety, fit, and acceptability of a single-size diaphragm developed with end-user input. *Obstetrics and Gynecology, 125*(4), 895–903.

Senie, R. T. (2014). *Epidemiology of women's health.* Burlington, MA: Jones & Bartlett Learning.

Sharma, M., & Walmsley, S. L. (2015). Contraceptive options for HIV-positive women: Making evidence-based, patient-centered decisions. *HIV Medicine, 16,* 329–336.

Shoupe, D., & Mishell, D. R. (2016). *The handbook of contraception: A guide for practical management* (2nd ed.). Switzerland: Springer International Publishing.

Signorile, P. G., & Baldi, A. (2015). New evidence in endometriosis. *The International Journal of Biochemistry & Cell Biology, 60,* 19–22.

Singh, S., Best, C., Dunn, S., Leyland, N., & Wolfman, W. L. (2013). Abnormal uterine bleeding in pre-menopausal women: Clinical practice guideline. *Journal of Obstetrics and Gynecology Canada, 35*(5 eSuppl), S1–S28. Retrieved from https://sogc.org/wp-content/uploads/2013/07/gui292CPG1305E.pdf

Skidmore-Roth, L. (2015). *Mosby's 2015 nursing drug reference* (28th ed.). St. Louis, MO: Elsevier Mosby.

Smith, R. P., & Kaunitz, A. M. (2018). Treatment of primary dysmenorrhea in adult women. *UpToDate.* Retrieved from http://www.uptodate.com/contents/treatment-of-primary-dysmenorrhea-in-adult-women

Society of Obstetricians and Gynecologists of Canada. (2006). Canadian contraception consensus: Update on depot medroxyprogesterone acetate (DMPA). *Journal of Obstetrics and Gynecology Canada.* Retrieved from https://sogc.org/wp-content/uploads/2013/01/174E-CONS-April20061.pdf

Society of Obstetricians and Gynecologists of Canada. (2010). Endometriosis: Diagnosis and management, practice guideline. *Journal of Obstetrics and Gynecology Canada, 32*(7), S1–S32. Retrieved from https://sogc.org/wp-content/uploads/2013/01/gui244CPG1007E.pdf

Society of Obstetricians and Gynecologists of Canada. (2014). Clinical practice guideline: Managing menopause. *Journal of Obstetrics and Gynecology Canada, 36*(9), S1–S74. Retrieved from https://sogc.org/wp-content/uploads/2014/09/gui311CPG1505Erev.pdf

Society of Obstetricians and Gynecologists of Canada. (2015). Clinical practice guideline: Canadian contraception consensus. *Journal of Obstetrics and Gynecology Canada, 37*(10), 936–942. Retrieved from https://sogc.org/wp-content/uploads/2015/11/gui329Pt1CPG1510E.pdf

Society of Obstetricians and Gynecologists of Canada. (2017). *Gender-inclusive language policy: SOGC to promote LGBTQ+ inclusivity.* Retrieved from https://sogc.org/files/Gender%20 Inclusive%20Language%20Policy_web.pdf

Society of Obstetricians and Gynecologists of Canada. (2018). *Pregnancy info: Fertility.* Retrieved from https://www.pregnancyinfo.ca/before-you-conceive/fertility/

Stanford, J. B. (2015). Revisiting the fertile window. *Fertility and Sterility, 103,* 1152–1153.

Statistics Canada. (2015). *Generations in Canada.* Retrieved from http://www12.statcan.gc.ca/census-recensement/2011/as-sa/98-311-x/98-311-x2011003_2-eng.cfm

Stewart, M., & Black, K. (2015). Choosing a combined oral contraceptive pill. *Australian Prescriber, 38*(1), 6–11.

Sullivan, S. D., Lehman, A., Thomas, F., Johnson, K. C., Jackson, R., Wactawski-Wende, J., … Howard, B. V. (2015). Effects of self-reported age at nonsurgical menopause on time to first fracture and bone mineral density in the Women's Health Initiative Observational Study. *Menopause (New York, N.Y.), 22*(10), 1035–1044.

Tacani, P. M., Ribeiro, D. O., Barros Guimarães, B. E., Machado, A. P., & Tacani, R. E. (2015). Characterization of symptoms and edema distribution in premenstrual syndrome. *International Journal of Women's Health, 7,* 297–303.

Tarride, J. E., Hopkins, R. B., Leslie, W. D., Morin, S., Adachi, J. D., Papaioannou, A., … Goeree, R. (2012). The burden of illness of osteoporosis in Canada. *Osteoporosis International, 23,* 2591–2600.

Tharpe, N. L., Farley, C. L., & Jordan, R. G. (2016). *Clinical practice guidelines for midwifery & women's health* (5th ed.). Burlington, MA: Jones & Bartlett Learning.

Thurkow, A. L. (2015). Hysteroscopic sterilization. In *Minimally invasive gynecological surgery* (pp. 49–59). Berlin: Springer.

Tremellen, K., & Pearce, K. (2015). *Nutrition, fertility, and human reproductive function.* Boca Raton, FL: CRC Press Taylor & Francis Group.

Turchi, P. (2015). Prevalence, definition, and classification of infertility. In G. Cavallini & G. Beretta. *Clinical management of male infertility* (pp. 5–11). Switzerland: Springer International Publishing.

Udoh, A., Effa, E. E., Oduwole, O., Okusanya, B. O., Okafo, O., & Iya, J. (2015). Antibiotics for treating septic abortion. *Cochrane Database of Systematic Reviews, 2,* CD011528.

UN Department of Economic and Social Affairs, Population Division. (2014). *World contraceptive patterns wall chart 2013.* Retrieved from http://www.un.org/en/development/desa/population/publications/pdf/family/worldContraceptivePatternsWallChart2013.pdf

UNFPA. (2018). *The state of the world population 2018 report.* Retrieved from https://www.unfpa.org/sites/default/files/pub-pdf/UNFPA_PUB_2018_EN_SWP.pdf

Upadhyay, U. D., Desai, S., Zlidar, V., Weitz, T. A., Grossman, D., Anderson, P., & Taylor, D. (2015). Incidence of emergency department visits and complications after abortion. *Obstetrics and Gynecology, 125*(1), 175–183.

Walsh, S., Ismaili, E., Naheed, B., & O'Brien, S. (2015). Diagnosis, pathophysiology and management of premenstrual syndrome. *The Obstetrician & Gynaecologist, 17,* 99–104.

Wang, Q., Chen, D., Cheng, S. M., Nicholson, P., Alen, M., & Cheng, S. (2015). Growth and aging of proximal femoral bone: A study with women spanning three generations. *Journal of Bone and Mineral Research, 30*(3), 528–534.

Weinberger, A. H., Smith, P. H., Allen, S. S., Cosgrove, K. P., Saladin, M. E., Gray, K. M., … McKee, S. A. (2015). Systematic and meta-analytic review of research examining the impact of menstrual cycle phase and ovarian hormones on smoking and cessation. *Nicotine & Tobacco Research, 17*(4), 407–421.

Whitaker, T. (2015). Vasectomy. In A. L. Halverson & D. C. Borgstrom (Eds.). *Advanced surgical techniques for rural surgeons* (pp. 251–254). New York: Springer.

Whitman, M. (2015). Patient education: What worries the patient most? *Nursing, 45*(1), 52–54.

Wicks, S. M., & Mahady, G. B. (2015). Herbal and complementary medicines used for women's health. In M. Harrison-Woolrych (Ed.). *Medicines for women* (pp. 373–399). Switzerland: Springer International Publishing.

Wildemeersch, D., Goldstuck N., Hasskamp T., Jandi, S., & Pett, A. (2015). Intrauterine device quo vadis? Why intrauterine device use should be revisited particularly in nulliparous women? *Open Access Journal of Contraception, 6,* 1–12.

Wolfe, K., & Cansino, C. (2015). Injectable contraception: Current practices and future trends. *Current Obstetrics and Gynecology Reports, 4*(1), 26–36.

Wood, D. (2015). Inevitable menopause. *Nurse.Com Nursing Spectrum (Philadelphia Tri-State), 24*(3), 26–31.

Woods, N. F., & Mitchell, E. S. (2015). The menopausal transition and women's health. In M. A. Farage, K. W. Miller, N. F. Woods, & H. I. Maibach (Eds.). *Skin, mucosa and menopause: Management of clinical issues* (pp. 433–452). Berlin: Springer.

Worel, J. N., & Hayman, L. L. (2015). Cardiovascular disease prevention in women: Reducing the major threat to women's health. *Journal of Cardiovascular Nursing, 30*(1), 5–7.

World Health Organization (WHO). (2015). *Fertility and infertility: Assisting couples and individuals.* Retrieved from http://www.who.int/reproductivehealth/topics/infertility/en/

Wright, K., Iqteit, H., & Hardee, K. (2015). Standard Days Method of contraception: Evidence on use, implementation, and scale-up. In *Working paper.* Washington, DC: Population Council, The Evidence Project.

Wu, M., McIntosh, J., & Liu, J. (2016). Current prevalence rate of latex allergy: Why it remains a problem? *Journal of Occupational Health, 58*(2), 138–144.

Ying, L. Y., & Loke, A. Y. (2015). An analysis of the concept of partnership in the couples undergoing infertility treatment. *Journal of Sex & Marital Therapy, 42,* 243–256.

Zieman, M. (2015). *Managing contraception on the go* (13th ed.). New York: Ardnet Media.

Zorbas, K. A., Economopoulos, K. P., & Vlahos, N. F. (2015). Continuous versus cyclic oral contraceptives for the treatment of endometriosis: A systematic review. *Archives of Gynecology and Obstetrics, 292,* 37–43.

MULTIPLE CHOICE QUESTIONS

1. Under the age of 35, a couple is considered infertile after how many months of trying to conceive?
   a. 6 months
   b. 12 months
   c. 18 months
   d. 24 months

2. A couple reports that their condom broke while they were having sexual intercourse last night. What would you advise to prevent pregnancy?
   a. Inject a spermicidal agent into the vagina immediately.
   b. Obtain emergency contraceptives and take them immediately.
   c. Douche with a solution of vinegar and hot water tonight.
   d. Take a strong laxative now and again at bedtime.

3. Which of the following combination contraceptives has been approved for extended continuous use?
   a. Seasonale
   b. Triphasil
   c. Ortho Evra
   d. Mirena

4. Which of the following measures helps prevent osteoporosis?
   a. Supplementing with iron
   b. Sleeping 8 hours nightly
   c. Eating lean meats only
   d. Walking daily

5. Which of the following activities will increase a person's risk of cardiovascular disease if taking oral contraceptives?
   a. Eating a high-fibre diet
   b. Smoking cigarettes
   c. Taking daily multivitamins
   d. Drinking alcohol

6. The nurse is preparing to teach a class to a group of middle-aged women regarding the most common vasomotor symptoms experienced during menopause and possible modalities of treatment available. Which of the following would be a vasomotor symptom experienced during menopause?
   a. Weight gain
   b. Bone density
   c. Hot flashes
   d. Heart disease

7. Throughout life, a person's most proactive activity to promote health would be to engage in:
   a. Consistent exercise
   b. Socialization with friends
   c. Quality quiet alone time
   d. Consuming water

8. What comment by a client would indicate that a diaphragm is not the best contraceptive option?
   a. "My husband says it is my job to keep from getting pregnant."
   b. "I have a hard time remembering to take my vitamins daily."
   c. "Hormones cause cancer and I don't want to take them."
   d. "I am not comfortable touching myself down there."

9. The most common cause of menstrual abnormality in a reproductive-age client is:
   a. Ectopic pregnancy
   b. Coagulopathy
   c. Carcinoma
   d. Anovulation

CRITICAL THINKING EXERCISE

1. Maria London, age 25, comes to your family planning clinic requesting to have an intrauterine contraceptive (IUC) inserted because "birth control pills give you cancer." In reviewing her history, you note she has been into the STI clinic three times in the past year with vaginal infections and was hospitalized for PID last month. When you question her about her sexual history, she reports having sex with multiple partners and not always using protection.
   a. Is an IUC the most appropriate method for her? Why or why not?
   b. What myths/misperceptions will you address in your counselling session?
   c. Outline the safer sex discussion you plan to have with her.

STUDY ACTIVITIES

1. Develop a teaching plan for an adolescent with premenstrual syndrome and dysmenorrhea.

2. Arrange to shadow a nurse working in family planning for the morning. What questions does the nurse ask to ascertain the kind of family planning method that is right for each client? What teaching goes along with each method? What follow-up care is needed? Share your findings with your classmates during a clinical conference.

3. Surf the Internet and locate three resources for couples experiencing infertility to consult that provide support and resources.

4. Sterilization is one of the most prevalent methods of contraception used by married couples in Canada. Contact a local urologist and gynecologist to learn about the procedure involved and the cost of a male and female sterilization. Which procedure poses less risk?

5. Take a field trip to a local drugstore to check out the variety and costs of male and female condoms. How many different brands did you find? What was the range of costs?

6. Noncontraceptive benefits of combined oral contraceptives include which of the following? Select all that apply.
   a. Protection against ovarian cancer
   b. Protection against endometrial cancer
   c. Protection against breast cancer
   d. Reduction in incidence of ectopic pregnancy
   e. Prevention of functional ovarian cysts
   f. Reduction in deep venous thrombosis
   g. Reduction in the risk of colorectal cancer

BRINGING IT ALL TOGETHER: A CASE STUDY

L.H. is a 66-year-old White female who presents to the Women's Health Primary Care Clinic for her annual gynecologic examination. She states that she is fairly healthy with no active medical conditions other than hypertension controlled with medication. She is postmenopausal and feels she is doing well, but has a few questions and concerns. Her primary concern is that she is bothered by vaginal dryness and pain with sexual intercourse. Over-the-counter lubricants and moisturizers have not been useful. She never took HT since her hot flashes were not severe, but asks if she should start taking it now to reduce her vaginal dryness.

ASSESSMENT

L.H.'s family history includes an aunt who had breast cancer at the age of 60 and her mother who died of a heart attack at the age of 71. L.H. is a nonsmoker and drinks a glass of wine at dinner daily. Her last DXA bone scan indicated osteopenia and her pelvic examination demonstrated extensive atrophic changes in her vulvovaginal tissue. Her vital signs were within normal range; her weight was 125 lb; her height was 5 ft 2 in. She states she seemed to be taller previously as her slacks seem to be too long and she needs to hem them now.

1. What is this woman's chief complaint today? What is the etiology of it?

2. Any concerns about this woman's history or her family history?

3. Based on her height and weight, is there a health concern here?

L.H. has significant vulvovaginal atrophy that is not responding to OTC lubricants and is not likely to improve with anything other than estrogen therapy. She has an unfavourable family history of cancer and cardiovascular disease. Her bone density results indicate osteoporosis.

PLAN

1. What health issues should the nurse address with this woman after her examination?

2. What health promotion measures are needed to reduce her risk of osteoporosis?

3. What medications might be prescribed for this woman?

4. When would you have this woman return for follow-up care?

The nurse should discuss vaginal estrogen products such as vaginal cream, tablets, and the vaginal ring to address L.H.'s vaginal atrophy. It should be up to the client to decide which form of estrogen she is comfortable with. These therapies provide local, vaginal effects, not systemic effects, which may place her at risk based on her family history.

To build or maintain bone health, the nurse should encourage her to take 1,200 to 1,600 mg of calcium and 600 to 1,000 IU of vitamin D, through diet and/or supplements. She should also be instructed to walk daily with a gradual increase in distance.

L.H. is also a candidate for osteoporosis pharmacotherapy. The risks and benefits should be discussed. The initial drug prescribed might be a bisphosphonate. An annual return appointment is needed with a repeat DXA in 2 years to monitor her response to therapy.

5

Sexually Transmitted Infections

KEY TERMS

bacterial vaginosis

cervicitis

chlamydia

genital/vulvovaginal
   candidiasis

gonorrhea

pelvic inflammatory
   disease (PID)

sexually transmitted
   infection (STI)

syphilis

trichomoniasis

vaginitis

Learning Objectives

Upon completion of the chapter, you will be able to:

1. Evaluate the spread and control of sexually transmitted infections.

2. Identify risk factors and outline appropriate client education needed in common sexually transmitted infections.

3. Describe how contraceptives can play a role in the prevention of sexually transmitted infections.

4. Analyze the physiologic and psychological aspects of sexually transmitted infections.

5. Outline the nursing management needed for clients with sexually transmitted infections.

Sandy, a 19-year-old, couldn't imagine what these "things" were that appeared "down there" in her genital area last week. She was too embarrassed to tell anyone, so she stopped by the college health service today to find out what they were.

INTRODUCTION

Sexually transmitted infections (STIs) are a significant global health challenge. STIs are bacterial, viral, and parasitic infections of the reproductive tract caused by microorganisms transmitted through vaginal, anal, or oral sexual intercourse. STIs pose a serious threat not only to client's sexual health, but also to the general health and well-being of millions of people worldwide. STIs are responsible for genital tract infections that may lead to later complications such as pelvic inflammatory disease (PID) or infertility. They may also cause chronic liver diseases and cancer due to hepatitis B virus (HBV) and hepatitis C virus (HCV) infections: genital cancer associated with human papillomavirus (HPV), and AIDS caused by human immunodeficiency virus (HIV). STIs constitute an epidemic of tremendous magnitude globally with approximately 500 million new cases of curable STIs each year. The Public Health Agency of Canada (PHAC) reports that the rates of STIs in Canada have continued to rise since the year 2000 (PHAC, 2017a).

STIs are biologically sexist, presenting greater risk and causing more complications among cisgender women than among cisgender men. After only a single exposure, women are twice as likely as men to acquire infections from pathogens causing gonorrhea, chlamydia infection, hepatitis B, HPV, and syphilis (Oyelowo & Johnson, 2016). STIs may contribute to cervical cancer, infertility, ectopic pregnancy, chronic pelvic pain,

and death. Certain infections can be transmitted in utero to the fetus or during childbirth to the newborn (Table 5.1). STIs know no class, racial, ethnic, or social barriers—all individuals are vulnerable if exposed to the infectious organism. Safer-sex practices that include limiting the number of sexual partners and using latex condoms during sexual activity must be recommended to all sexually active individuals. The problem of STIs has still not been tackled adequately on a global scale, and until this is done, numbers worldwide will continue to increase.

A special section on STIs and adolescents is presented next, followed by discussion of specific STIs categorized according to the Centers for Disease Control and Prevention (CDC) framework. The CDC groups STIs according to the major symptom manifested (Box 5.1). The CDC classifies STIs according to their clinical symptoms (see Box 5.1 for the categories). A section on preventing STIs is included at the end of the chapter.

SEXUALLY TRANSMITTED INFECTIONS AND ADOLESCENTS

Individuals aged 15 to 24 years represent almost half of all cases of new STIs acquired. Today, 4 in 10 sexually active teen girls have an STI that can cause infertility and even death. Adolescent males make up more than three fourths of HIV diagnosis among 13 to 19 year olds (U.S. Department of Health and Human Services Office

TABLE 5.1	EFFECTS OF SEXUALLY TRANSMITTED INFECTIONS ON THE FETUS OR NEWBORN
STI	**Effects on Fetus or Newborn**
Chlamydia	Newborn can be infected during delivery Eye infections (neonatal conjunctivitis), pneumonia, low birth weight, increased risk of premature rupture of the membranes (PROM), preterm birth, and stillbirth
Gonorrhea	Newborn can be infected during delivery. Increased risk of miscarriage, PROM, and preterm birth Rhinitis, vaginitis, urethritis, inflammation of sites of fetal monitoring Gonococcal ophthalmia neonatorum can lead to blindness and sepsis (including arthritis and meningitis)
Herpes type II (genital herpes)	Contamination can occur during birth. Newborn may develop skin or mouth sores Mental retardation, premature birth, low birth weight, blindness, death
Syphilis	Can be passed in utero Can result in fetal or infant death Congenital syphilis symptoms include skin ulcers, rashes, fever, weakened or hoarse cry, swollen liver and spleen, jaundice and anemia, various deformations
Trichomoniasis	Low birth weight, increased risk of PROM, and preterm birth
Venereal warts	May develop warts in throat (laryngeal papillomatosis); uncommon but life threatening

Adapted from Public Health Agency of Canada (PHAC). (2017f). Section 6-4: Canadian guidelines on sexually transmitted infections, specific populations—Pregnancy. Retrieved from https://www.canada.ca/en/public-health/services/infectious-diseases/sexual-health-sexually-transmitted-infections/canadian-guidelines/sexually-transmitted-infections/canadian-guidelines-sexually-transmitted-infections-41.html

BOX 5.1

CDC CLASSIFICATION OF STIs

- Infections characterized by vaginal discharge
  - Vulvovaginal candidiasis
  - Trichomoniasis
  - Bacterial vaginosis
- Infections characterized by cervicitis
  - Chlamydia
  - Gonorrhea
- Infections characterized by genital ulcers
  - Genital herpes simplex
  - Syphilis
- Pelvic inflammatory disease (PID)
- Human immunodeficiency virus (HIV)
- Human papillomavirus (HPV) infection
- Vaccine-preventable STIs
  - Hepatitis A
  - Hepatitis B
- Ectoparasitic infections
- Pediculosis pubis
- Scabies

of Adolescent Health, 2016). In Canada, teens who are sexually active experience high rates of STIs, and some groups are at higher risk, including Indigenous and youths living in poverty, and those with limited educational attainment.

Take Note!

It is estimated that before graduating from high school, 25% of adolescents will contract an STI.

Biologic, social, and behavioural factors place teenagers at high risk. Heterosexual female adolescents are more susceptible to STIs due to their anatomy. During adolescence and young adulthood, the columnar epithelial cells are especially sensitive to invasion by sexually transmitted organisms, such as chlamydia and gonococci, because they extend out over the vaginal surface of the cervix, where they are unprotected by cervical mucus; these cells recede to a more protected location as women age. Social factors such as poverty, lack of education, social inequality, and limited access to health care services impact the prevalence of STIs in this high-risk population. Adolescent females may perceive that they have limited power over when and where intercourse occurs with their partners. They typically lack negotiating skills and self-confidence needed to successfully negotiate for safer-sex practices and thus are exposed to STIs (Petrova & Garcia-Retamero, 2015).

Behaviourally, adolescents and young adults tend to think they are invincible and deny the risks of their behaviour. This risky behaviour exposes them to STIs and HIV/AIDS. Adolescents frequently have unprotected

intercourse, they engage in partnerships of limited duration, and they face many obstacles that prevent them from using the health care system (CDC, 2018f).

Nursing Assessment

Many health care providers fail to assess adolescent sexual behaviour and STI risks, to screen for asymptomatic infection during clinic visits, or to counsel adolescents on STI risk reduction. Nurses need to remember that they play a key role in the detection, prevention, and treatment of STIs in adolescents. Table 5.2 discusses clinical manifestations of common STIs in adolescents.

Nursing Management

Nurses working with adolescents need to convey their willingness to discuss sexual habits. Provide effective guidance that promotes sexual health so that primary and/or repeat infections can be avoided. Adolescents bear disproportionate burdens when it comes to STIs, so nurses need to educate them to protect their client's reproductive futures.

Encourage the client to complete the antibiotic prescription (specific management for each type of STI is discussed further in the chapter).

Prevention of STIs among adolescents is critical. Health care providers have a unique opportunity to provide counselling and education to their clients. Adapt the style, content, and message to the adolescent's developmental level. Identify risk factors and risk behaviours and guide the adolescent to develop specific individualized actions of prevention. The nurse's interaction and conversation with the adolescent need to be direct, nonjudgmental, and inclusive. Nurses should avoid making assumptions about an adolescent's gender or sexuality, and instead ask respectful questions in a caring and sensitive manner.

Encourage adolescents to postpone initiation of sexual activity for as long as possible, but if they choose to be sexually active, explain the necessity of using barrier methods, such as male and female condoms (Teaching Guidelines 5.1). For teens who have already had sexual intercourse, the clinician can encourage abstinence at this point. If adolescents are sexually active, they should be directed to teen clinics where contraceptive options can be explained. In areas where specialized teen clinics are not available, nurses should feel comfortable discussing sexuality, safety, and contraception with teens. Encourage adolescents to minimize their lifetime number of sexual partners, to use barrier methods consistently and correctly, and to be aware of the connection between drug and alcohol use and the incorrect use of barrier methods. Table 5.3 discusses barriers to condom use and means to overcome them.

(text continues on page 174)

TABLE 5.2	SEXUALLY TRANSMITTED INFECTIONS COMMON IN ADOLESCENTS

Disease	Causative Organism	Transmission Mode	Diagnostic Testing and Recommended Screening for Sexually Active Adolescent
Chlamydia Curable STI Seen frequently among sexually active adolescents and young adults	*Chlamydia trachomatis* (bacteria)	Vaginal, anal, and oral sex and by childbirth	Culture fluid from urethral swabs in males or endocervical swabs for females Noninvasive, non–culture-based testing is available using nucleic acid amplification and testing (NAAT) from urine—single test can test for chlamydia and gonorrhea Conjunctival secretions in neonates Females: screen annually Males: screen high-risk adolescents
Gonorrhea Curable STI Adolescent often coinfected with *C. trachomatis*	*Neisseria gonorrhoeae* (bacteria)	Vaginal, anal, and oral sex and by childbirth	Gram stain or culture directly for the bacterium or same noninvasive, non–culture-based test, NAAT, as chlamydia Females: screen annually Males: screen high-risk adolescents
Herpes type 2 (genital herpes) Lifelong recurrent viral disease Most people have not been diagnosed There is no cure	Herpes simplex virus 1 and 2 (HSV-1 and HSV-2)	HSV-1 is spread through oral secretions; can be spread to genitals through poor handwashing of infected person or oral-genital contact HSV-2 is spread by having sexual contact (vaginal, oral, or anal) with someone who is shedding the herpes virus either during an outbreak or during a period with no symptoms; can be spread to an infant through childbirth	Visual inspection and symptoms or culture from swabs taken from lesions (success depends on stage of lesion—optimum is during vesicular stage) Polymerase chain reaction is more sensitive than culture Serologic tests, such as antibody-based testing (herpes Western blot assay is the most sensitive) Type-specific laboratory testing important Routine screening not recommended

Female Symptoms	Male Symptoms	Recommended Treatment
May be asymptomatic Dysuria, urinary frequency, dyspareunia Cervical discharge (mucus or pus) Endocervicitis May lead to pelvic inflammatory disease, ectopic pregnancy, infertility Can cause inflammation of the rectum and conjunctiva Can infect the throat from oral sexual contact with an infected partner	May be asymptomatic Dysuria, urethral itching Penile discharge (mucus or pus) Urethral tingling May lead to epididymitis and sterility Can cause inflammation of the rectum and conjunctiva Can infect the throat from oral sexual contact with an infected partner	Azithromycin (Zithromax) Doxycycline (Vibramycin) Erythromycin (EES) Levofloxacin Ofloxacin (Floxin) Sexual partners need evaluation, testing, and treatment also Abstinence from sexual activity until therapy complete and symptoms no longer present Retesting in 3 months to rule out recurrence
May be asymptomatic or no recognizable symptoms until serious complications such as pelvic inflammatory disease Dysuria Urinary frequency Vaginal discharge (yellow and foul) Dyspareunia Endocervicitis Arthritis May lead to pelvic inflammatory disease, ectopic pregnancy, infertility Symptoms of rectal infection include discharge, anal itching, and occasional painful bowel movements with fresh blood	Most produce symptoms, but can be asymptomatic Dysuria Penile discharge (pus) Arthritis May lead to epididymitis and sterility Symptoms of rectal infection include discharge, anal itching, and occasional painful bowel movements with fresh blood	At this time, due to concerns about *N. gonorrhoeae* resistance to certain antimicrobials, the CDC currently recommends only one regimen, dual therapy with ceftriaxone and azithromycin Sexual partners need evaluation, testing, and treatment also Abstinence from sexual activity until therapy complete and symptoms no longer present Retesting in 3 months to rule out recurrence
Initial symptoms include itching, tingling, and pain in genital area followed by small pustules and blister-like genital lesions that then crust over and gradually heal. Recurrence episodes are usually milder than the initial episode Dysuria, dyspareunia, and urine retention Fever, headache, malaise, muscle aches	Same as female	Antivirals used to treat first episode, recurrence, and suppression Acyclovir, valacyclovir, and famciclovir mainstay in treatment Does not cure; just controls symptoms Counselling important to help adolescent cope and to prevent transmission Sexual partners benefit from evaluation and counselling. If symptomatic, need treatment If asymptomatic, offer testing and education

(continued)

TABLE 5.2	SEXUALLY TRANSMITTED INFECTIONS COMMON IN ADOLESCENTS (continued)

Disease	Causative Organism	Transmission Mode	Diagnostic Testing and Recommended Screening for Sexually Active Adolescent
Syphilis	*Treponema pallidum* (spirochete bacteria)	Sexual contact with an infected person	Serologic testing mainstay for diagnosis Venereal Disease Research Laboratory (VDRL), rapid plasma reagin (RPR), and treponemal tests (e.g., fluorescent treponemal antibody absorbed [FTA-ABS]) can lead to a presumptive diagnosis and are useful for screening. Use of two tests required Dark-field examination and direct fluorescent antibody tests of lesion exudate or tissue provide definitive diagnosis of early syphilis New tests are in development such as enzyme immunoassay Screen based on epidemiology and personal risk factors
Trichomoniasis	*Trichomonas vaginalis* (protozoa)	Vaginal intercourse with an infected partner May be picked up from direct genital contact with damp or moist objects, such as towels or wet clothing	Highly sensitive and specific testing available and recommended, such as NAAT Microscopic evaluation of vaginal secretions or culture still common but less sensitive
Venereal warts (condylomata acuminata) One of the most common STIs in the United States Could lead to cancers of the cervix, vulva, vagina, anus, or penis No cure; warts can be removed but virus remains	Human papillomavirus (HPV)	Vaginal, anal, or oral sex with an infected partner	Visual inspection Abnormal pap smear may indicate cervical infection of HPV

Adapted from Centers for Disease Control and Prevention (CDC). (2015a). Sexually transmitted diseases treatment guidelines, 2015. *Morbidity and Mortality Weekly Report (MMWR), 64*(3), 1–137. Retrieved from http://www.cdc.gov/std/tg2015/tg-2015-print.pdf; Grossman, L. C. (2014). Chapter 55: Sexually transmitted infections. In S. Grossman, & C. M. Porth (Eds.). *Porth's Pathophysiology: Concepts of altered health states* (9th ed., pp. 1416–1429). Philadelphia, PA: Wolters Kluwer Health/Lippincott Williams & Wilkins.

Female Symptoms	Male Symptoms	Recommended Treatment
Course of disease divided into stages **Primary infection:** • Chancre on place of entrance of bacteria (usually vulva or vagina but can develop in other parts of the body) **Secondary infection:** • Maculopapular rash (hands and feet) • Sore throat • Lymphadenopathy • Flu-like symptoms **Latent infection:** • No symptoms • Can be infective during first 1–2 years of latency • Many people if not treated will suffer no further signs and symptoms Some people will go on to develop tertiary or late syphilis **Tertiary infections:** • Tumours of skin, bones, and liver • Central nervous system symptoms • Cardiovascular symptoms • Usually not reversible at this stage	Course of disease divided into stages **Primary infection:** • Chancre on place of entrance of bacteria (usually on penis but can develop in other parts of the body) **Secondary, latent, and tertiary infections:** All similar to female symptoms	Benzathine penicillin G injection (if penicillin allergy, doxycycline, tetracycline, or erythromycin) Sexual partners need evaluation and testing
Many women have symptoms but some may be asymptomatic Dysuria Frequency Vaginal discharge (yellow, green, or grey and foul odour) Dyspareunia Irritation or itching of genital area	Most men infected are asymptomatic Dysuria Penile discharge (watery white)	Metronidazole (Flagyl) or tinidazole Sexual partners need evaluation, testing, and treatment also Sexual abstinence is recommended until medical treatment is complete
Wart-like lesions that are soft, moist, or flesh coloured and appear on the vulva and cervix, and inside and surrounding the vagina and anus Sometimes appear in clusters that resemble cauliflower-like bumps, and are either raised or flat, small or large	Wart-like lesions that are soft, moist, or flesh coloured and appear on the scrotum or penis. They sometimes appear in clusters that resemble cauliflower-like bumps, and are either raised or flat, small or large	May disappear without treatment Treatment is aimed at removing the lesions rather than HPV itself No optimal treatment has been identified, but there are several ways to treat depending on size and location Most methods rely on chemical or physical destruction of the lesion: Imiquimod cream 20% Podophyllin antimitotic solution 0.5% Podofilox solution 5% 5-Fluorouracil cream Trichloroacetic acid (TCA) Small warts can be removed by: • Freezing (cryosurgery) • Burning (electrocautery) • Laser treatment • Surgical excision Large warts that have not responded to treatment may be removed surgically Vaccination recommended starting around age 12 and may lead to decrease in cancer associated with HPV Abstinence from sexual activity during treatment to promote healing

Teaching Guidelines 5.1
PROPER CONDOM USE

- Use latex condoms.
- Use a new condom with each act of vaginal, anal, or oral sex. Never reuse a condom.
- Handle condoms with care to prevent damage from sharp objects such as fingernails and teeth.
- Ensure condom has been stored in a cool, dry place away from direct sunlight. Do not store condoms in wallet or automobile or anywhere where they would be exposed to extreme temperatures.
- Do not use a condom if it appears brittle, sticky, or discoloured. These are signs of aging.
- Put condom on before any genital contact.
- Put condom on when the penis is erect with rolled side out. Ensure it is placed so it will readily unroll.
- Hold the tip of the condom while unrolling. Ensure there is a space at the tip for semen to collect (about ½ in), but make sure no air is trapped in the tip (air bubbles can cause breakage).
- Ensure adequate lubrication during intercourse. If external lubricants are used, use only water-based lubricants such as KY jelly with latex condoms. Oil- or petroleum-based lubricants, such as body lotion, massage oil, or cooking oil, can weaken latex condoms.

- If you feel the condom break, stop immediately, withdraw, remove broken condom, and replace.
- Withdraw while penis is still erect, and hold condom firmly against the base of the penis. Remove carefully to ensure no semen spills out. Dispose of properly.

Adapted from Centers for Disease Control and Prevention (CDC). (2013). *Condom fact sheet in brief.* Retrieved from http://www.cdc.gov/condomeffectiveness/docs/condomfactsheetinbrief.pdf

Think back to Sandy, who was introduced at the beginning of the chapter. How should the nurse handle Sandy's anxious state? What specific questions should the nurse ask Sandy to determine the source of the possible infection in her genital area?

INFECTIONS CHARACTERIZED BY VAGINAL DISCHARGE

Vaginitis is a generic term that means inflammation and infection of the vagina. There can be hundreds of causes for vaginitis, but more often than not the cause is infection by one of three organisms:
- Candida, a fungus
- Trichomonas, a protozoa
- Gardnerella, a bacterium

TABLE 5.3	BARRIERS TO CONDOM USE AND MEANS TO OVERCOME THEM
Perceived Barrier	**Intervention Strategy**
Decreases sexual pleasure (sensation) *Note:* Often perceived by those who have never used a condom	• Encourage client to try • Put a drop of water-based lubricant or saliva inside the tip of the condom or on the glans of the penis before putting on the condom • Try a thinner latex condom or a different brand or more lubrication
Decreases spontaneity of sexual activity	• Incorporate condom use into foreplay • Remind client that peace of mind may enhance pleasure for self and partner
Embarrassing, juvenile, "unmanly"	• Remind client that it is "manly" to protect himself and others.
Poor fit (too small or too big, slips off, uncomfortable)	• Smaller and larger condoms are available.
Requires prompt withdrawal after ejaculation	• Reinforce the protective nature of prompt withdrawal and suggest substituting other postcoital sexual activities.
Fear of breakage may lead to less vigorous sexual activity	• With prolonged intercourse, lubricant wears off and the condom begins to rub. Have a water-soluble lubricant available to reapply.
Nonpenetrative sexual activity	• Condoms have been advocated for use during fellatio; unlubricated condoms may prove best for this purpose due to the taste of the lubricant • Other barriers, such as dental dams or an unlubricated condom, can be cut down the middle to form a barrier; these have been advocated for use during certain forms of nonpenetrative sexual activity (e.g., cunnilingus and anolingual sex)
Allergy to latex	• Polyurethane male and female condoms are available • A natural skin condom can be used together with a latex condom to protect the man or woman from contact with latex

Adapted from Public Health Agency of Canada (PHAC). (2016). *Canadian guidelines on sexually transmitted infections.* Retrieved from http://www.phac-aspc.gc.ca/std-mts/sti-its/

The complex balance of microbiologic organisms in the vagina is a key element in the maintenance of health. Subtle shifts in the vaginal environment may allow organisms with pathologic potential to proliferate, causing infectious symptoms.

The nurse's role in managing vaginitis is one of primary prevention and education to limit recurrences of these infections. Primary prevention begins with changing the sexual behaviours that increase risk for infection. In addition to assessing for the common signs and symptoms and risk factors, the nurse can help clients to avoid vaginitis or to prevent a recurrence by teaching them to take the precautions highlighted in Teaching Guidelines 5.2.

 Teaching Guidelines 5.2
PREVENTING VAGINITIS

- Avoid douching to prevent altering the vaginal environment.
- Use condoms to avoid spreading the organism.
- Avoid tights, nylon underpants, and tight clothes.
- Wipe from front to back after using the toilet.
- Avoid powders, bubble baths, and perfumed vaginal sprays.
- Wear clean cotton underpants.
- Change out of wet bathing suits as soon as possible.
- Become familiar with the signs and symptoms of vaginitis.
- Choose to lead a healthy lifestyle.

Genital/Vulvovaginal Candidiasis

Genital/vulvovaginal candidiasis (VVC) is one of the most common causes of vaginal discharge. It is also referred to as yeast, monilia, and a fungal infection. It is not considered an STI because Candida is a normal constituent in the vagina and becomes pathologic only when the vaginal environment becomes altered. An estimated 75% of women will have at least one episode of VVC, and 40% to 50% will have two or more episodes in their lifetime (CDC, 2017a).

Therapeutic Management

Treatment of candidiasis includes one of the following medications:
- Miconazole cream or suppository
- Clotrimazole tablet or cream
- Fluconazole oral tablet (CDC, 2015a)

Most of these medications are used intravaginally in the form of a cream, tablet, or suppositories for 3 to 7 days. If fluconazole is prescribed, a 150-mg oral tablet is taken as a single dose.

Topical azole preparations are effective in the treatment of VVC, relieving symptoms and producing negative cultures in 80% to 90% of women who complete therapy (CDC, 2015a). If VVC is not treated effectively during pregnancy, the newborn can develop an oral infection known as thrush during the birth process; that infection must be treated with a local azole preparation after birth.

Nursing Assessment

Assess the client's health history for predisposing factors for VVC, which include:
- Pregnancy
- Use of oral contraceptives with a high estrogen content
- Use of broad-spectrum antibiotics
- Diabetes mellitus
- Obesity
- Use of steroid and immunosuppressive drugs
- HIV infection
- Wearing tight, restrictive clothes and nylon underpants
- Trauma to vaginal mucosa from chemical irritants or douching

Assess the client for clinical manifestations of VVC. Typical symptoms, which can worsen just before menses, include:
- Pruritus
- Vaginal discharge (thick, white, curd like)
- Vaginal soreness
- Vulvar burning
- Erythema in the vulvovaginal area
- Dyspareunia
- External dysuria

Figure 5.1 shows the typical appearance of VVC.

Speculum examination will reveal white plaques on the vaginal walls. The vaginal pH remains within normal range. Definitive diagnosis is made by a wet smear, which reveals the filamentous hyphae and spores characteristic of a fungus when viewed under a microscope.

Nursing Management

Teach preventive measures to clients with frequent VVC infections, including:
- Reduce dietary intake of simple sugars and soda.
- Wear white, 100% cotton underpants.
- Avoid wearing tight pants or exercise clothes with spandex.
- Shower rather than taking tub baths.
- Wash with a mild, unscented soap and dry the genitals gently.
- Avoid the use of bubble baths or scented bath products.
- Wash underwear in unscented laundry detergent and hot water.
- Dry underwear in a hot dryer to kill the yeast that clings to the fabric.
- Remove wet bathing suits promptly.
- Practice good body hygiene.
- Avoid vaginal sprays/deodorants.

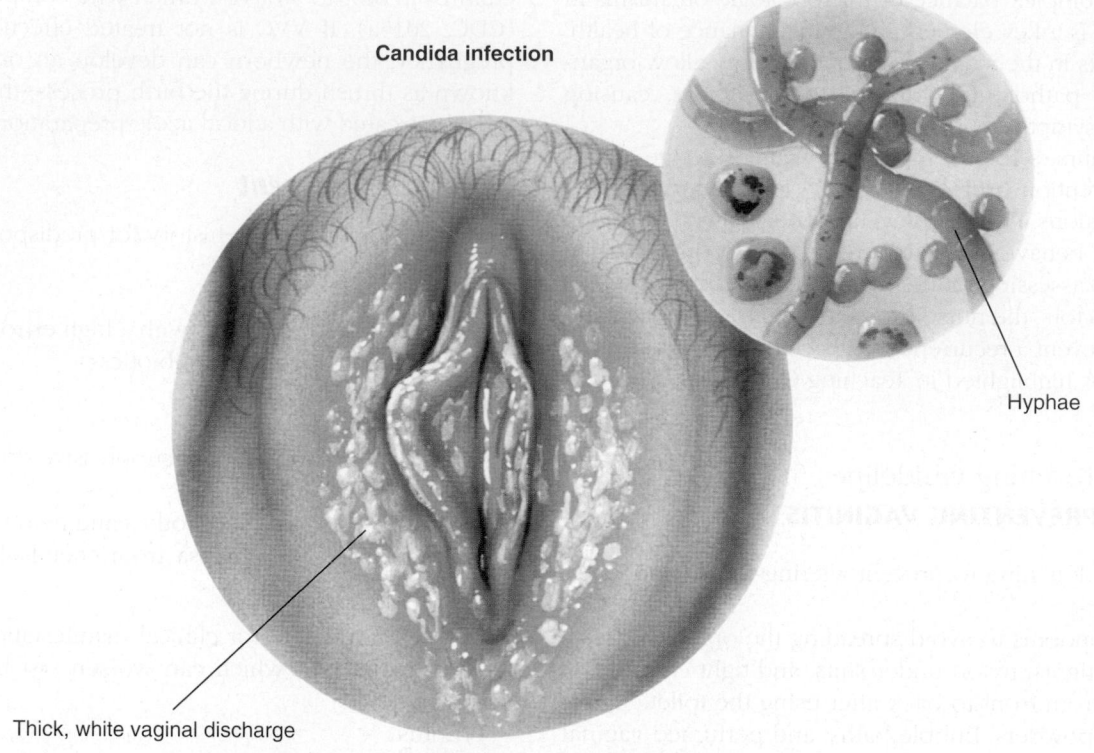

Candida infection

Hyphae

Thick, white vaginal discharge

FIGURE 5.1 Vulvovaginal candidiasis. (Asset provided by Anatomical Chart Co.)

- Avoid wearing pantyhose (or cut out the crotch to allow air circulation).
- Use white, unscented toilet paper and wipe from front to back.
- Avoid douching (which washes away protective vaginal mucus).
- Avoid the use of super-absorbent tampons (use pads instead).

Trichomoniasis

Trichomoniasis is another common vaginal infection that causes a discharge, but is not always sexually transmitted. The organism can live on damp/wet surfaces and poorly cleaned/maintained hot tubs and drains. The client may be markedly symptomatic or asymptomatic. When symptoms are present, they include vulvar itching and a malodourous foamy vaginal discharge. Cisgender men can be asymptomatic carriers. Although this infection is localized, there is increasing evidence of preterm birth and postpartum endometritis in perinatal clients with this vaginitis (CDC, 2015a). The high prevalence of this infection globally and frequency of coinfection with other STIs make trichomoniasis a public health concern. Notably, research finds that an infection with trichomoniasis increases the risk of HIV transmission in both men and women (Smith & Ramos, 2018). *Trichomonas vaginalis* is an ovoid, single-cell protozoan parasite that can be observed under the microscope making a jerky swaying motion.

Therapeutic Management

A single 2-g dose of oral metronidazole or tinidazole for both partners is a common treatment for this infection. Sexual partners of those with trichomoniasis should be treated to avoid recurrence of infection.

Nursing Assessment

Assess the client for clinical manifestations of trichomoniasis, which include:
- A heavy yellow/green or grey frothy or bubbly discharge
- Vaginal pruritus and vulvar soreness
- Dyspareunia
- Cervix may bleed on contact
- Dysuria
  - Vaginal odour, described as foul
  - Vaginal or vulvar erythema
- Petechiae on the cervix

Note, however, that 10% to 50% of clients with trichomoniasis will be asymptomatic (PHAC, 2013a).

Figure 5.2 shows the typical appearance of trichomoniasis.

The diagnosis is confirmed when a motile flagellated trichomonad is visualized under the microscope. In addition, a vaginal pH of greater than 4.5 is a typical finding. Tests for trichomoniasis include OSOM Trichomonas Rapid Test (Genzyme Diagnostics, Cambridge, Massachusetts), an immunochromatographic capillary flow dipstick technology, and the Affirm VP III (Becton

Microscopic view
of the organism

Greenish-gray cervical
discharge

FIGURE 5.2 Trichomoniasis. (Asset provided by
Anatomical Chart Co.)

Dickenson, San Jose, California), a nucleic acid probe test that evaluates for *Trichomonas vaginalis, Gardnerella vaginalis,* and *Candida albicans.* Each of these tests, which are performed on vaginal secretions, has a sensitivity of 83% and a specificity of 97%. Both tests are considered point-of-care diagnostics (CDC, 2015a).

Nursing Management

Instruct clients to avoid sexual activity until they and their sexual partners are cured (i.e., when therapy has been completed and both partners are symptom free) and also to avoid consuming alcohol during treatment because mixing the medications and alcohol causes severe nausea and vomiting (CDC, 2015a). In addition, it is important to provide information regarding infection cause and transmission, effects on reproductive organs and future fertility, and the need for partner notification and treatment. Follow-up testing is not indicated if symptoms resolve with treatment. See Evidence-Based Practice 5.1 for interventions for trichomoniasis in pregnancy.

EVIDENCE-BASED PRACTICE 5.1   **ANTENATAL LOWER GENITAL TRACT INFECTION SCREENING AND TREATMENT PROGRAMS FOR PREVENTING PRETERM DELIVERY**

A genital tract infection during pregnancy can cross into the amniotic fluid and result in prelabour rupture on the membranes and is associated with preterm births. Preterm births are associated with poor infant health, admissions to NICUs in the first weeks of life, prolonged hospital stays, and long-term neurologic disabilities.

STUDY

In this review, 4,155 women were randomly assigned to either an intervention group whereby they were treated for bacterial vaginosis, trichomoniasis, and candidiasis, or into a control group where they received screening but results were not revealed and treatment not instituted.

Findings

There was evidence that infection screening and treatment for pregnant women before 20 weeks' gestation reduced preterm births and low-weight infants. Infection screening and treatment programs are associated with cost savings when used for prevention of preterm births. The numbers of low-weight infants were significantly lower in the intervention group when compared with the control group.

Nursing Implications

A simple infection screening and treatment program done during routine prenatal care may reduce preterm births and preterm low-weight infants. Nurses can apply this study's findings when educating women preconceptually how important prenatal care is and screening for vaginal infections that may be asymptomatic. It is important to establish a link between preterm birth prevention measures to improve maternal–infant outcomes in all pregnant women.

Sangkomkamhang, U. S., Lumbiganon, P., Prasertcharoensuk, W., & Laopaiboon, M. (2015). Antenatal lower genital tract infection screening and treatment programs for preventing preterm delivery. *Cochrane Database of Systematic Reviews, 2,* CD006178. doi: 10.1002/14651858.CD006178.pub3.

Bacterial Vaginosis

A third common infection of the vagina is **bacterial vaginosis** caused by the gram-negative bacillus *G. vaginalis*. It is the most prevalent cause of vaginal discharge or malodour, but up to 50% of clients are asymptomatic. Bacterial vaginosis is a sexually associated infection characterized by alterations in vaginal flora in which lactobacilli in the vagina are replaced with high concentrations of anaerobic bacteria. The cause of the microbial alteration is not fully understood, but is associated with having multiple sex partners, douching, and lack of vaginal lactobacilli. Bacterial vaginosis can increase a person's susceptibility to other STIs such as HIV, herpes, chlamydia, and gonorrhea (CDC, 2015a). Research suggests that bacterial vaginosis is associated with preterm labour, premature rupture of membranes (PROM), chorioamnionitis, postpartum endometritis, and PID (CDC, 2015a).

Therapeutic Management

Treatment for bacterial vaginosis includes metronidazole (oral or gel) or clindamycin cream. Treatment of the male partner has not been beneficial in preventing recurrence because sexual transmission of bacterial vaginosis has not been proven (CDC, 2015a).

Nursing Assessment

Assess the client for clinical manifestations of bacterial vaginosis. Primary symptoms are a thin, white homogeneous vaginal discharge and a characteristic "stale fish" odour. Figure 5.3 shows the typical appearance of bacterial vaginosis.

To diagnose bacterial vaginosis, three of the four criteria must be met:
- Thin, white homogeneous vaginal discharge
- Vaginal pH 4.5
- Positive "whiff test" (secretion is mixed with a drop of 10% potassium hydroxide on a slide, producing a characteristic stale fishy odour)
- The presence of clue cells on wet mount examination (CDC, 2015a)

Nursing Management

The nurse's role is one of primary prevention and education to limit recurrences of these infections. Primary prevention begins with changing the sexual behaviours that place clients at risk for infection. In addition to assessing for common signs, symptoms, and risk factors, the nurse can help clients to avoid vaginitis or to prevent a recurrence by teaching them to take the precautions highlighted in Teaching Guidelines 5.2.

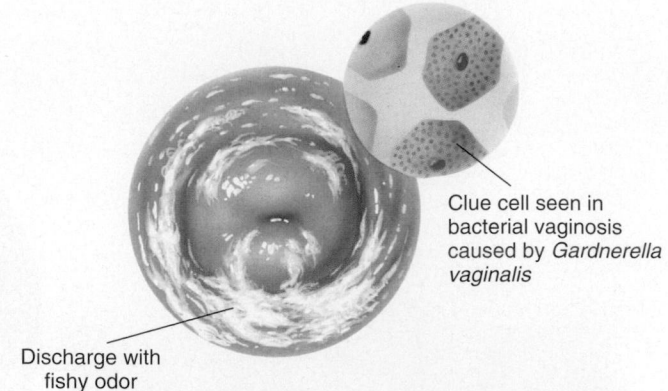

Clue cell seen in bacterial vaginosis caused by *Gardnerella vaginalis*

Discharge with fishy odor

FIGURE 5.3 Bacterial vaginosis. (Illustration provided by Anatomical Chart Co. Photograph from Sweet, R. L., Gibbs, R. S. [2005]. *Atlas of infectious diseases of the female genital tract.* Philadelphia, PA: Lippincott Williams & Wilkins.)

INFECTIONS CHARACTERIZED BY CERVICITIS

Cervicitis is a catchall term that implies the presence of inflammation or infection of the cervix. It is used to describe everything from symptomless erosions to an inflamed cervix that bleeds on contact and produces quantities of purulent discharge containing organisms not ordinarily found in the vagina. Cervicitis is usually caused by gonorrhea or chlamydia, as well as almost any pathogenic bacterial agent and a number of viruses. The treatment of cervicitis involves the appropriate therapy for the specific organism that has caused it.

Chlamydia

Chlamydia is the most commonly reported bacterial STI in Canada, with rates steadily increasing since the late 1990s (Choudhri, Miller, Sandhu, Leon, & Aho, 2018). In recent years, the PHAC reports over a hundred thousand new cases annually, which amounts to an average of 325 cases per 100,000 people (Choudhri et al., 2018). While rates have increased among nearly all age groups, the highest rates of infection are among those aged 15 to 19 years, mainly because their sexual relations are often unplanned and are sometimes the result of pressure or force, and typically happen before they have the experience and skills to protect themselves. The rates are highest among this group regardless of demographics or location (CDC, 2017b). The young have the most to lose from acquiring STIs, since they will suffer the consequences the longest and might not reach their full reproductive potential. The most common risk factors associated with chlamydia are age less than 25 years, recent change in sexual partner or multiple sexual partners, poor socioeconomic conditions, exchange of sex for money, being a person of colour, single status, and lack of use of barrier contraception. In Canada, the health care costs associated with chlamydial infections have been estimated at over $51 million annually (Tuite et al., 2012). Worldwide, it is likely the most common infectious cause of infertility in women. An estimated 106 million cases of chlamydia occur globally among both men and women each year, so the global burden is substantial (Brunham, 2015).

Asymptomatic infection is common among both men and women. Cisgender men primarily develop urethritis. In cisgender women, chlamydia is linked with cervicitis, acute urethral syndrome, salpingitis, ectopic pregnancy, PID, and infertility (Qureshi, 2018). The CDC (2017b) recommends yearly chlamydia testing of all sexually active women aged 25 years or younger, older women with risk factors for chlamydial infections (those who have a new sex partner or multiple sex partners), and all pregnant clients.

Chlamydia trachomatis is the bacterium that causes chlamydia. It is an intracellular parasite that cannot produce its own energy and depends on the host for survival. It is often difficult to detect, and this can pose problems for women due to the long-term consequences of untreated infection. Moreover, lack of treatment provides more opportunity for the infection to be transmitted to sexual partners. Newborns of infected mothers may develop conjunctivitis which occurs in 25% to 50% of all newborns. Ophthalmia neonatorum is an acute mucopurulent conjunctivitis occurring in the first month of birth, acquired from exposure during the birth process (Thomas, Bates, & Mathew, 2015).

Therapeutic Management

Antibiotics are usually used in treating this STI. The PHAC (2017b) treatment options for chlamydia include doxycycline 100 mg orally (PO) twice a day for 7 days or azithromycin 1 g PO in a single dose. Because of the common coinfection of chlamydia and gonorrhea, a combination regimen of ceftriaxone with doxycycline or azithromycin is prescribed frequently (CDC, 2015a). Additional CDC guidelines for client management include annual screening of all sexually active clients aged 20 to 25 years old; screening of all high-risk people; and treatment with antibiotics effective against both gonorrhea and chlamydia for anyone diagnosed with a gonococcal infection (CDC, 2017b). Except in pregnant women, test-of-cure (repeat testing 3 to 4 weeks after completing therapy) is not recommended, unless therapeutic compliance is in question, symptoms persist, or reinfection is suspected (CDC, 2015a).

Nursing Assessment

Assess the health history for significant risk factors for chlamydia, which may include:
- Being an adolescent
- Having multiple sex partners
- Having a new sex partner
- Engaging in sex without using a barrier contraceptive (such as a condom)
- Using oral contraceptives
- Being pregnant
- Having a history of another STI (King et al., 2015)

Assess the client for clinical manifestations of chlamydia. The majority of those infected (70% to 80%) are asymptomatic (CDC, 2017b). If the client is symptomatic, clinical manifestations include:
- Mucopurulent vaginal discharge
- Urethritis
- Bartholinitis
- Endometritis
- Salpingitis
- Dysfunctional uterine bleeding

The diagnosis can be made by urine testing or swab specimens collected from the endocervix or vagina. Culture, direct immunofluorescence, enzyme immunoassay (EIA), or nucleic acid amplification methods such as Gen-Probe or PACE 2 are highly sensitive and specific when used on urethral and cervicovaginal swabs. They can also be used with good sensitivity and specificity on first-void urine specimens (Qureshi, 2018). The chain reaction tests are the most sensitive and cost effective. The CDC (2015b) strongly recommends screening of asymptomatic clients at high risk in whom infection would otherwise go undetected.

Chlamydia is an important preventable cause of infertility and other adverse reproductive health outcomes. Effective prevention interventions are available to reduce the burden of chlamydia and its sequelae, but they are underutilized. Although many prevention programs are available, improvements can be made in raising awareness about chlamydia, increasing screening coverage, and enhancing partner services. In addition, nurses can focus their efforts on reaching disproportionately affected racial/ethnic groups. To break the cycle of chlamydia transmission in Canada, health care providers should encourage annual chlamydia screening for all sexually active females aged >25 years and maximize use of effective partner treatment services (CDC, 2015b; PHAC, 2017b).

Gonorrhea

Gonorrhea is a serious, and potentially very severe, bacterial infection. It is the second most commonly reported infection in Canada and is an urgent problem globally because it is now capable of developing resistance to multiple antibiotic classes. Gonorrhea is highly contagious and is a reportable infection to the health department authorities. Gonorrhea increases the risk for PID, infertility, ectopic pregnancy, and HIV acquisition and transmission (PHAC, 2017c). It is rapidly becoming more and more resistant to cure. In Canada, an estimated 16,000 new gonorrhea infections occur annually (PHAC, 2017c). In common with all other STIs, it is an equal-opportunity infection—no one is immune to it, regardless of race, creed, sex, age, or sexual orientation.

The cause of gonorrhea is an aerobic gram-negative intracellular diplococcus, *Neisseria gonorrhoeae*. The site of infection is the columnar epithelium of the endocervix. Gonorrhea is almost exclusively transmitted by sexual activity. In pregnant clients, gonorrhea is associated with chorioamnionitis, premature labour, PROM, and postpartum endometritis (Ross, Tao, Patton, & Hoover, 2015). It can also be transmitted to the newborn in the form of ophthalmia neonatorum during birth by direct contact with gonococcal organisms in the cervix. Ophthalmia neonatorum is highly contagious and if untreated leads to blindness in the newborn.

Therapeutic Management

Gonorrhea can be cured with the right treatment. The PHAC now recommends dual therapy (i.e., using two drugs as the treatment for gonorrhea). Dual therapy is recommended to prevent drug resistance and is also effective against chlamydia. The treatment of choice for uncomplicated gonococcal infections is a cephalosporin and a macrolide, in the form of 250-mg ceftriaxone injected intramuscularly (IM) and azithromycin 1 g PO as a first-line treatment for uncomplicated anogenital and pharyngeal infections in adults (PHAC, 2017d).

Pregnant clients with gonorrhea should not be treated with quinolones or tetracyclines. Pregnant clients with a positive test for gonorrhea should be treated with the same recommended dual therapy of ceftriaxone with either azithromycin or amoxicillin (CDC, 2015a). To prevent gonococcal ophthalmia neonatorum, a prophylactic agent should be instilled into the eyes of all newborns; this procedure is still mandated in some provinces; however, most now require parents' consent. Erythromycin or tetracycline ophthalmic ointment in a single application is recommended (King et al., 2015). With use of recommended treatment, follow-up testing to document

eradication of gonorrhea is no longer recommended. Instead, rescreening in 2 to 3 months to identify reinfection is suggested (CDC, 2015a).

Nursing Assessment

Assess the client's health history for risk factors, which may include low socioeconomic status, living in an urban area, single status, inconsistent use of barrier contraceptives, age under 20 years, and multiple sex partners. Assess the client for clinical manifestations of gonorrhea, keeping in mind that between 50% and 90% of cisgender women infected with gonorrhea are totally symptom free (Wong, 2018). Because this group is so frequently asymptomatic, they are regarded as a major factor in the spread of gonorrhea. If symptoms are present, they might include:

• Abnormal vaginal discharge
• Dysuria
• Cervicitis
• Enlarged lymph glands locally
• Abnormal vaginal bleeding
• Bartholin abscess
• PID
• Neonatal conjunctivitis in newborns
• Mild sore throat (for pharyngeal gonorrhea)
• Rectal infection (itching, soreness, bleeding, discharge)
• Perihepatitis (King et al., 2015)

Sometimes, a local gonorrhea infection is self-limiting (there is no further spread), but usually the organism ascends upward through the endocervical canal to the endometrium of the uterus, further on to the fallopian tubes, and out into the peritoneal cavity. When the peritoneum and the ovaries become involved, the condition is known as PID. The scarring to the fallopian tubes is permanent. This damage is a major cause of infertility and is a possible contributing factor in ectopic pregnancy (Heller, 2015).

If gonorrhea remains untreated, it can enter the bloodstream and produce a disseminated gonococcal infection. This severe form of infection can invade the joints (arthritis), the heart (endocarditis), the brain (meningitis), and the liver (toxic hepatitis). Figure 5.4 shows the typical appearance of gonorrhea.

The CDC recommends screening for all women at risk for gonorrhea. Pregnant women should be screened at the first prenatal visit and again at 36 weeks of gestation. Nucleic acid hybridization tests (Gen-Probe) are used for diagnosis. Any client suspected of having gonorrhea should be tested for chlamydia also because coinfection (45%) is extremely common (CDC, 2015e).

Nursing Management of Chlamydia and Gonorrhea

The prevalence of chlamydia and gonorrhea is increasing dramatically, and these infections can have long-term

FIGURE 5.4 Gonorrhea. (From Jensen, S. [2015]. *Nursing health assessment: A best practice approach* [2nd ed.]. Philadelphia, PA: Wolters Kluwer.)

effects on people's lives. Sexual health is an important part of a person's physical and mental health, and nurses have a professional obligation to address it. Be particularly sensitive when addressing STIs because clients are often embarrassed or feel guilty. There is still a social stigma attached to STIs, so clients need to be reassured about confidentiality.

The nurse's knowledge about chlamydia and gonorrhea should include treatment strategies, referral sources, and preventive measures. It is important to be skilled at client education and counselling and to be comfortable talking with, and advising, clients diagnosed with these infections. Provide education about risk factors for these infections. High-risk groups include single women, younger than 25 years, those with a history of STIs, having new or multiple sex partners, inconsistent use of barrier contraception, and living in communities with high infection rates (Wong, 2018). Assessment involves taking a health history that includes a comprehensive sexual history. Ask about the number of sex partners and the use of safer-sex techniques. Review previous and current symptoms. Emphasize the importance of seeking treatment and informing sex partners. The four-level P-LI-SS-IT model (Box 5.2) can be used to determine interventions for various clients because it can be adapted to the nurse's level of knowledge, skill, and experience. Of utmost importance is the willingness to listen and show interest and respect in a nonjudgmental manner.

In addition to meeting the health needs of clients with chlamydia and gonorrhea, the nurse is responsible for educating the public about the increasing incidence of these infections. This information should include high-risk behaviours associated with these infections, signs and symptoms, and the treatment modalities available. Stress that both of these STIs can lead to infertility and long-term sequelae. Teach safer-sex practices to people in nonmonogamous relationships. Know the physical and psychosocial responses to these STIs to prevent transmission and the disabling consequences. Nurses must also inform their pregnant clients that they should avoid quinolones or tetracyclines to prevent hepatotoxicity and pancreatitis as well as risks associated with malformation of teeth, bones, and joints in the fetus (King et al., 2015).

Take Note!

If the epidemic of chlamydia and gonorrhea is to be halted, nurses must take a major front-line role now.

INFECTIONS CHARACTERIZED BY GENITAL ULCERS

The majority of young, sexually active clients who have genital ulcers have genital herpes, syphilis, or chancroid. The frequency of each condition differs by geographic area and client population; however, genital herpes is the most prevalent of these diseases. More than one of these diseases can be present in a client who has genital ulcers. All three of these diseases have been associated with an increased risk for HIV infection. Not all genital ulcers are caused by STIs.

Genital Herpes Simplex

Genital herpes is a recurrent, lifelong viral infection that has the potential for transmission throughout the lifespan.

The CDC estimates that one out of six people 14 to 49 years old have genital herpes simplex virus (HSV) infection, with 500 million worldwide new cases annually (CDC, 2015d). Two serotypes of HSV have been identified: HSV-1 and HSV-2. Today, a smaller portion of genital herpes infections is thought to be caused by HSV-1 and the bulk of them by HSV-2. HSV-1 mostly causes the familiar fever blisters or cold sores on the lips, eyes, and face. HSV-2 typically invades the mucous membranes of the genital tract and is known as herpes genitalis. Most people infected with HSV-2 have not been diagnosed.

HSV is transmitted by contact of mucous membranes or breaks in the skin with visible or nonvisible lesions. Most genital herpes infections are transmitted by individuals unaware that they have an infection. Many have mild or unrecognized infections but still shed the herpes virus intermittently. HSV is transmitted primarily by direct contact with an infected individual who is shedding the virus. Kissing, sexual contact (including oral sex), and vaginal birth are means of transmission. The virus replicates at the site of infection, then travels to the dorsal root ganglia and remains latent until stimuli such as fever, stress, ultraviolet radiation, or immunosuppression occur and reactivates it (Selim, Parra, Sangueza, Requena, & Sangueza, 2015).

Having sex with an infected partner places the individual at risk for contracting HSV. Clients must be educated about the real potential of transmission even when no active lesions are present. Research has indicated that as much as 70% of HSV infections have resulted from sexual contact during times of asymptomatic viral shedding (Albrecht, 2018). After the primary outbreak, the virus remains dormant in the nerve cells for life, resulting in periodic recurrent outbreaks. Recurrent genital herpes outbreaks are triggered by precipitating factors such as emotional stress, menses, and sexual intercourse, but more than half of recurrences occur without a precipitating cause. Immunocompromised clients have more frequent and more severe recurrent outbreaks than healthy hosts (Silasi et al., 2015).

Living with genital herpes can be difficult due to the erratic, recurrent nature of the infection, the location of the lesions, the unknown causes of the recurrences, and the lack of a cure. Further, the stigma associated with this infection may affect the individual's self-esteem and interaction with partners. Potential psychosocial consequences may include emotional distress, isolation, fear of rejection by a partner, fear of transmission of the disease, loss of confidence, and altered interpersonal relationships (Alexander, LaRosa, Bader, & Garfield, 2014).

Along with the increase in the incidence of genital herpes has been an increase in neonatal HSV infections, which are associated with a high incidence of mortality and morbidity. The risk of neonatal infection with a primary maternal outbreak is between 30% and 50%; it is less than 1% with a recurrent maternal infection (CDC, 2015d).

Therapeutic Management

No cure exists, but antiviral drug therapy helps to reduce or suppress symptoms, shedding, and recurrent episodes. Advances in treatment with acyclovir 400 mg PO three times daily for 7 to 10 days, famciclovir 250 mg PO three times daily for 7 to 10 days, and valacyclovir 1 g PO twice daily for 7 to 10 days have resulted in an improved quality of life for those infected with HSV. However, these drugs neither eradicate latent virus nor affect the risk, frequency, or severity of recurrences after the drug is discontinued (CDC, 2015a). Suppressive therapy is recommended for individuals with six or more recurrences per year. The natural course of the disease is for recurrences to be less frequent over time.

The management of genital herpes includes antiviral therapy. The safety of antiviral therapy has not been established during pregnancy. Disclosure of this lifelong viral infection is often a challenge for individuals living with genital herpes. Therapeutic management also includes counselling regarding the natural history of the disease, the risk of sexual and perinatal transmission, and the use of methods to prevent further spread. The following are a few guidelines to delivering information in a time-limited environment: (a) after determining the client's literacy level, use all available client reading and resource materials; (b) have another knowledgeable staff member in the office who can spend extra time with women who need it; (c) refer clients to good and accurate websites such as the Society of Obstetricians and Gynaecologists of Canada (SOGC) *Sex and U* website (www.sexandu.ca/); (d) know the phone numbers of herpes support groups in your area; (e) educate the client to abstain from all sexual activity until HSV lesions resolve; (f) use good handwashing technique to prevent spread; (g) educate that there is no cure, and that practicing safe sex (using barrier methods) with every sex act is essential to prevent transmission; and (h) encourage all clients to inform their current sex partners that they have genital herpes and to inform future partners before initiating a sexual relationship. Finally, use a sympathetic, nonjudgmental approach in all discussions. The nurse can state in clear terms that having herpes does not change the core of the person or make them less worthwhile (Myers, Buhi, Marhefka, Daley, & Dedrick, 2015).

Nursing Assessment

Assess the client for clinical manifestations of HSV. Clinical manifestations can be divided into the primary episode and recurrent infections. The first or primary episode is usually the most severe, with a prolonged period of viral shedding. Primary HSV is a systemic disease characterized by multiple painful vesicular lesions, mucopurulent discharge, superinfection with candida, fever, chills, malaise, dysuria, headache, genital irritation,

Herpetic lesions on labia majora

FIGURE 5.5 Genital herpes simplex. (Illustration provided by Anatomical Chart Co. Photograph courtesy of Stephen Ludwig, MD.)

inguinal tenderness, and lymphadenopathy. Without treatment, symptoms may last 2 to 4 weeks (Albrecht, 2018). The lesions in the primary herpes episode are frequently located on the vulva, vagina, and perineal areas. The vesicles will open and weep and finally crust over, dry, and disappear without scar formation (Fig. 5.5). This viral shedding process usually takes up to 2 weeks to complete.

Recurrent infection episodes are usually much milder and shorter in duration than the primary one. Tingling, itching, pain, unilateral genital lesions, and a more rapid resolution of lesions are characteristics of recurrent infections. Recurrent herpes is a localized disease characterized by typical HSV lesions at the site of initial viral entry. Recurrent herpes lesions are generally fewer in number, less painful, and resolve more rapidly (Albrecht, 2018).

Diagnosis of HSV is often based on clinical signs and symptoms and is confirmed by viral culture of fluid from the vesicle. Papanicolaou (Pap) smears are an insensitive and nonspecific diagnostic test for HSV and should not be relied on for diagnosis. The client should be tested for all common STIs, especially if risk factors are present, such as a new sexual partner or partners.

Syphilis

Syphilis is a chronic, multistage, curable bacterial infection caused by the spirochete *Treponema pallidum* that is typically transmitted sexually with an infected partner or congenitally from an infected mother to her fetus. It is a serious systemic disease that can lead to disability and death if untreated. Rates of syphilis in Canada have been increasing rapidly since 2001, and it is currently the third most common reported STI behind chlamydia and gonorrhea (Choudhri et al., 2018). Of primary and secondary syphilis cases, 75% occur in men who have sex with men (CDC, 2018e; Choudhri et al., 2018). It continues to be one of the most important STIs both because of its biologic effect on HIV acquisition and transmission and because of its impact on infant health. Because there is no vaccine to prevent syphilis, control is mainly dependent on the identification and treatment of infected individuals and their contacts with penicillin G, the first-line drug for all stages of syphilis (Stamm, 2015).

The spirochete rapidly penetrates intact mucous membranes or microscopic lesions in the skin and within hours enters the lymphatic system and bloodstream to produce a systemic infection long before the appearance of a primary lesion. The site of entry may be vaginal, rectal, or oral (Chandrasekar, 2017). The syphilis spirochete can cross the placenta at any time during pregnancy. Maternal infection consequences include spontaneous abortion, low birth weight, fetal growth restriction, prematurity, stillbirth, and multisystem failure of the heart, lungs, spleen, liver, and pancreas, as well as structural bone damage and nervous system involvement and mental retardation (Chen et al., 2015). Most newborns born with congenital syphilis are exposed in utero after the 4th month of pregnancy, although syphilis acquired late in the third trimester can also be transmitted to an infant through exposure to an active genital lesion at the time of birth. If untreated, syphilis is a lifelong infection progressing in orderly staging. The five stages of syphilis infection are (1) primary, (2) secondary, (3) early latent, (4) late latent, and (5) tertiary. The primary, secondary, and early latent stages are considered the most infectious: The estimated risk of per person transmission is 60% (PHAC, 2018).

Therapeutic Management

Fortunately, there is effective treatment for syphilis. Benzathine penicillin G, administered by either the IM or intravenous (IV) route, is the preferred drug for all stages of syphilis. For pregnant or nonpregnant women with syphilis of less than 1 year's duration, the CDC recommends 2.4 million units of benzathine penicillin G IM in a single dose. If the syphilis is of longer duration (more than 1 year) or of unknown duration, 2.4 million units of benzathine penicillin G is given IM once a week for 3 weeks. The preparations used, the dosage, and the length of treatment depend on the stage and clinical manifestations of disease (CDC, 2015a). Other medications, such as doxycycline, are available if the client is allergic to penicillin.

Clients should be reevaluated at 3, 6, and 12 months after treatment for primary, secondary, or early latent syphilis with additional serologic testing. Clients with late latent syphilis should be followed clinically and serologically at 12 and 24 months and also tested for HIV (PHAC, 2018).

Nursing Assessment

Assess the client for clinical manifestations and staging of syphilis. Primary syphilis is characterized by a chancre (painless ulcer) at the site of bacterial entry that will disappear within 1 to 6 weeks without intervention (Fig. 5.6). Motile spirochetes are present on dark-field examination of ulcer exudate. In addition, painless bilateral adenopathy is present during this highly infectious period. If left untreated, the infection progresses to the secondary stage. Secondary syphilis appears 2 to 6 months after the initial exposure and is manifested by flu-like symptoms and a maculopapular rash of the trunk, palms, and soles. Alopecia and adenopathy are both common during this stage. In addition to rashes, secondary syphilis may present with symptoms of fever, pharyngitis, weight loss, and fatigue (Chandrasekar, 2017). The secondary stage of syphilis lasts about 2 years. Once the secondary stage subsides, the latency period begins. This stage is characterized by the absence of any clinical manifestations of disease,

FIGURE 5.6 Chancre of primary syphilis. (From Sweet, R. L., Gibbs, R. S. [2005]. *Atlas of infectious diseases of the female genital tract*. Philadelphia, PA: Lippincott Williams & Wilkins.)

although the serology is positive. This stage can last as long as 20 years. If not treated, tertiary or late syphilis occurs, with life-threatening heart disease and neurologic disease that slowly destroys the heart, eyes, brain, central nervous system, and skin.

Clients with a diagnosis of HIV or another STI should be screened for syphilis, and all pregnant clients should be screened at their first prenatal visit. Dark-field microscopic examinations and direct fluorescent antibody tests of lesion exudate or tissue are the definitive methods for diagnosing early syphilis. A presumptive diagnosis can be made by using two serologic tests:

- Nontreponemal tests (Venereal Disease Research Laboratory [VDRL] and rapid plasma reagin [RPR]).
- Treponemal tests (fluorescent treponemal antibody absorbed [FTA-ABS] and *Treponema pallidum* particle agglutination [TP-PA]). Dark-field microscopic examinations and direct fluorescent antibody tests of lesion exudate or tissue are the definitive methods for diagnosing early syphilis (CDC, 2015f).

Nursing Management of Herpes and Syphilis

Genital ulcers from either herpes or syphilis can be devastating to clients, and the nurse can be instrumental in helping them through this difficult time. Referral to a support group for additional social support may be helpful. Address the psychosocial aspects of these STIs with clients by discussing appropriate coping skills, acceptance of the lifelong nature of the condition (herpes), and options for treatment and rehabilitation. Teaching Guidelines 5.3 highlights appropriate teaching points for the client with genital ulcers.

Teaching Guidelines 5.3
CARING FOR GENITAL ULCERS

* Abstain from intercourse during the prodromal period and when lesions are present.
* Wash hands with soap and water after touching lesions to avoid autoinoculation.
* Use comfort measures such as wearing nonconstricting clothes, wearing cotton underwear, urinating in water if urination is painful, taking lukewarm sitz baths, and air-drying lesions with a hair dryer on low heat.
* Avoid extremes of temperature such as ice packs or hot pads to the genital area as well as application of steroid creams, sprays, or gels.
* Use condoms with all new or noninfected partners.
* Inform health care professionals of your condition.

PELVIC INFLAMMATORY DISEASE

PID is an infection-induced inflammation of the female upper reproductive tract. PID rates remain unacceptably high. While exact numbers are unknown because reporting of PID is not mandatory in Canada, approximately 100,000 new cases are identified in this country annually (PHAC, 2013b). PID may involve the uterine lining (endometritis), the connective tissue adjacent to the uterus (parametritis), the fallopian tubes (salpingitis), or the serous membrane that lines part of the abdominal cavity and viscera (peritonitis), or it may manifest as tubo-ovarian abscess (Brunham, Gottlieb, & Paavonen, 2015). PID results from an ascending polymicrobial infection of the upper reproductive tract, frequently caused by untreated chlamydia or gonorrhea (Fig. 5.7). Complications include

Spread of gonorrhea or chlamydia

FIGURE 5.7 Pelvic inflammatory disease. Chlamydia or gonorrhea spreads up the vagina into the uterus and then to the fallopian tubes and ovaries.

ectopic pregnancy, pelvic abscess, subfertility, recurrent or chronic episodes of the disease, chronic abdominal pain, pelvic adhesions, and depression (Gilbert, 2015). Because most PID cases are secondary to STIs, especially chlamydia, the most effective approach to control it is prevention. Nurses can be instrumental in advocating for health promotion and educational initiatives to inform communities and screen for STIs, to reduce PID within populations.

Therapeutic Management

Broad-spectrum antibiotic therapy is generally required to cover chlamydia, gonorrhea, and/or any anaerobic infection. The current recommended treatment from PHAC (2014a) is cefoxitin 2 g IV every 6 hours plus doxycycline 100 mg IV or PO every 12 hours, changing to oral administration after 24 hours when the client shows clinical improvement, and continuing for a total of 14 days of treatment. PID in pregnancy is uncommon, particularly in areas where STI testing is standard with prenatal care, but when diagnosed, a combination of cefotaxime, azithromycin, and metronidazole for 14 days may be used. The client is treated on an ambulatory basis with a single-dose injectable antibiotic or is hospitalized and given antibiotics IV. The decision to hospitalize a client is based on clinical judgment and the severity of her symptoms (e.g., severely ill with high fever, a tubo-ovarian abscess is suspected, immunocompromised or presents with protracted vomiting). Treatment then includes IV antibiotics, increased oral fluids to improve hydration, bed rest, and pain management. Follow-up is needed to validate that the infectious process is gone to prevent the development of chronic pelvic pain.

Nursing Assessment

Nursing assessment of the client with PID involves a complete health history and assessment of clinical manifestations, physical examination, and laboratory and diagnostic testing.

Health History and Clinical Manifestations

Explore the client's current and past medical health history for risk factors for PID, which may include:

* Adolescence or young adulthood
* Women of colour
* Having multiple sex partners
* Early onset of sexual activity
* History of PID or STI
* Sexual intercourse at an early age
* Alcohol or drug use
* Having intercourse with a partner who has untreated urethritis
* Recent insertion of an intrauterine contraceptive (IUC)

- Nulliparity
- Cigarette smoking
- Recent termination of pregnancy
- Lack of consistent condom use
- Lack of contraceptive use
- Douching
- Sex work (Hay et al., 2016)

Assess the client for clinical manifestations of PID, keeping in mind that because of the wide variety of clinical manifestations of PID, clinical diagnosis can be challenging. To reduce the risk of missed diagnosis, the CDC has established criteria to establish the diagnosis of PID. Minimal criteria (all must be present) are lower abdominal tenderness, adnexal tenderness, and cervical motion tenderness. Additional supportive criteria that support a diagnosis of PID are:

- Abnormal cervical or vaginal mucopurulent discharge
- Oral temperature above 38°C (101°F)
- Cervical motion tenderness
- Elevated erythrocyte sedimentation rate (inflammatory process)
- Elevated C-reactive protein level (inflammatory process)
- *N. gonorrhoeae* or *C. trachomatis* infection documented (causative bacterial organism)
- White blood cells on saline vaginal smear
- Prolonged or increased menstrual bleeding
- Dysmenorrhea
- Dysuria
- Painful sexual intercourse
- Nausea
- Vomiting (CDC, 2017e)

Physical Examination and Laboratory and Diagnostic Tests

Inspect the client for presence of fever (usually over 38°C) or vaginal discharge. Palpate the abdomen, noting tenderness over the uterus or ovaries. However, the only way to diagnose PID definitively is through an endometrial biopsy, transvaginal ultrasound, or laparoscopic examination.

Nursing Management

If the client with PID is hospitalized, maintain hydration via IV fluids if necessary, and administer analgesics as needed for pain. Semi-Fowler positioning facilitates pelvic drainage. A key element to treatment of PID is education to prevent recurrence. Depending on the clinical setting (hospital or community clinic) where the nurse encounters the client diagnosed with PID, a risk assessment should be done to ascertain what interventions are appropriate to prevent a recurrence. To gain the client's cooperation, explain the various diagnostic tests needed. Discuss the implications of PID and the risk factors

for the infection; sexual partner(s) should be included if possible. Sexual counselling should include practicing safer sex, using barrier contraceptives consistently, avoiding vaginal douching, considering another contraceptive method if currently using an intrauterine system (IUS) and has multiple sexual partners, and completing the course of antibiotics prescribed (Shepherd, 2017). Review the serious sequelae that may occur if the condition is not treated or if the client does not comply with the treatment plan. Ask the client to have any partners go for evaluation and treatment to prevent a repeat infection. The management of clients with PID is considered inadequate unless their sexual partners are also clinically evaluated (PHAC, 2014a). Provide nonjudgmental support while stressing the importance of barrier contraceptive methods and follow-up care. Teaching Guidelines 5.4 gives further information related to PID prevention.

Teaching Guidelines 5.4
PREVENTING PELVIC INFLAMMATORY DISEASE
- Advise sexually active girls and women to insist their partners use condoms.
- Discourage routine vaginal douching, as this may lead to bacterial overgrowth.
- Encourage regular STI screening.
- Emphasize the importance of having each sexual partner receive antibiotic treatment.

VACCINE-PREVENTABLE STIs

Some STIs can be effectively prevented through preexposure vaccination. Vaccines are under development or are undergoing clinical trials for certain STIs, including HIV and HSV. However, the only vaccines currently available are for prevention of hepatitis A virus (HAV), HBV, and HPV infection. Vaccination efforts focus largely on integrating the use of these available vaccines into STI prevention and treatment activities (CDC, 2017c).

Human Papillomavirus

HPV is the most common viral infection in Canada and worldwide (PHAC, 2017e). Estimates indicate that at least 70% of sexually active Canadians will experience an HPV infection at some point in their lives. Many of these infections occur asymptomatically, and will resolve without treatment (PHAC, 2017e). Genital warts or condylomata (Greek for "warts") are caused by HPV. Clinical studies have confirmed that HPV is the cause of essentially all cases of cervical cancer, which is the fourth most common cancer in women in the United States, following lung, breast, and colorectal cancer (American Cancer Society [ACS], 2018). HPV-mediated oncogenesis is responsible for up to 95% of cervical squamous cell carcinomas and nearly all preinvasive cervical neoplasms (Gearhart, Higgins, Randall, & Buckley, 2018). More than 30 types of HPV can infect the genital tract. HPV is most prevalent in young women between the ages of 20 and 24 years, followed closely by the 15- to 19-year-old age group (Callahan, 2016).

Take Note!

Most sexually active Canadians will get HPV at some point in their lives. This means everyone is at risk (PHAC, 2017e).

Nursing Assessment

Nursing assessment of the woman with HPV involves a complete health history and assessment of clinical manifestations, physical examination, and laboratory and diagnostic testing.

HEALTH HISTORY AND CLINICAL MANIFESTATIONS

Assess the client's health history for risk factors for HPV, which include having multiple sex partners, age 15 to 25 years old, sex with a male who has had multiple sexual partners, and first intercourse at 16 years or younger (Dillner, 2015). Risk factors contributing to the development of cervical cancer include smoking, few or no screenings for cervical cancer, multiple sex partners, immunosuppressed state, nulliparity, long-term contraceptive use

(more than 2 years), coinfection with another STI, pregnancy, nutritional deficiencies, and early onset of sexual activity (Coffey, Beral, Green, Reeves, & Barnes, 2015).

Assess the client for clinical manifestations of HPV. Most HPV infections are asymptomatic, unrecognized, or subclinical. Visible genital warts are usually caused by HPV types 6 or 11. In addition to the external genitalia, genital warts can occur on the cervix and in the vagina, urethra, anus, and mouth. Depending on the size and location, genital warts can be painful, friable, and pruritic, although most are typically asymptomatic (Fig. 5.8). The strains of HPV associated with genital warts are considered low risk for development of cervical cancer, but other HPV types (16, 18, 31, 33, 45, 52, and 58) have been strongly associated with cervical cancer (CDC, 2017d).

PHYSICAL EXAMINATION AND LABORATORY AND DIAGNOSTIC TESTS

Clinically, visible warts are diagnosed by inspection. The warts are fleshy papules with a warty, granular surface. Lesions can grow very large during pregnancy, affecting urination, defecation, mobility, and descent of the fetus (CDC, 2017d). Large lesions, which may resemble cauliflowers, exist in coalesced clusters and bleed easily.

Serial Pap smears are performed for low-risk cisgender women and transgender men. These regular Pap smears will detect the cellular changes associated with HPV. The HPV-specific test may be a helpful addition to the Pap test for general screening of clients aged 30 years and above. While HPV is very common in clients under age 30, most of these infections will not

Genital warts on perineum

FIGURE 5.8 Genital warts. (Illustration provided by Anatomical Chart Co. Photograph from Gorbach, S. L., Bartlett, J. G., Blacklow, N. R. [2004]. *Infectious diseases*. Philadelphia, PA: Lippincott Williams & Wilkins.)

develop into cervical cancer, as clients in this age group are most likely to clear the infections (Canadian Cancer Society, 2018). The HPV test is a diagnostic test that can determine the specific HPV strain, which is useful in discriminating between low- and high-risk HPV types. A specimen for testing can be obtained with a fluid-phase collection system such as ThinPrep. The HPV test can identify 13 of the high-risk types of HPV associated with the development of cervical cancer and can detect high-risk types of HPV even before there are any conclusive visible changes to the cervical cells. If the test is positive for the high-risk types of HPV, the client should be referred for colposcopy.

> Upon physical examination, it is determined that Sandy has genital warts. The nurse finds out that Sandy engaged in high-risk behaviour with a stranger she "hooked up" with recently at university. She couldn't imagine that he would give her an STI because "he looked so clean-cut." She wonders how she could possibly have genital warts. What information should be given to Sandy about STIs in general? What specific information about HPV should be stressed?

Therapeutic Management

There is currently no medical treatment or cure for HPV. Instead, therapeutic management focuses heavily on prevention through the use of the HPV vaccine and education and on the treatment of lesions and warts caused by HPV. Health Canada has approved three HPV vaccines to prevent cervical cancer: Cervarix, Gardasil, and Gardasil 9. All three are prophylactic HPV vaccines designed primarily for cervical cancer prevention. Cervarix is effective against HPV-16, 18, 31, 33, and 45, the five most common cancer-causing types, including most causes of adenocarcinoma for which we cannot screen adequately. Gardasil is effective against HPV-16, 18, and 31, three common squamous cell cancer–causing types. In addition, Gardasil is effective against HPV-6 and 11, causes of genital warts and respiratory papillomatosis. The most important determinant of vaccine impact to reduce cervical cancer is its duration of efficacy. Cervarix is used only in females, whereas Gardasil 9 is used for both boys and girls. Gardasil 9 is effective against HPV types 6, 11, 16, 18, 31, 33, 45, 52, and 58. The newest vaccine (Gardasil 9) can potentially prevent about 90% of cervical, vulvar, vaginal, and anal cancers (Gearhart et al., 2018). The National Advisory Committee on Immunization (NACI) recommends HPV immunization for clients aged 9 to 26 years for the prevention of cervical cancer and pre-cancerous lesions, and may be administered to those 27 years of age and older at ongoing risk of exposure to HPV. They also recommend vaccinating males

aged 9 to 26 years with either Gardasil or Gardasil 9 for the prevention of anal cancers, pre-cancerous lesions, and anogenital warts, and may be administered to men 27 years of age and older at ongoing risk of exposure to HPV (NACI, 2017). Prophylactic HPV vaccines are safe, well tolerated, and highly efficacious in preventing persistent infections and cervical diseases associated with vaccine-HPV types among young females.

The vaccine is administered IM in three separate 0.5-mL doses. The first dose may be given to any individual 9 to 26 years old prior to initiation of sexual activity. The second dose is administered 2 months after the first, and the third dose is given 6 months after the initial dose. The deltoid region of the upper arm or anterolateral area of the thigh may be used. The most common vaccine side effects include pain, fainting, redness, and swelling at the injection site; fatigue; headache; muscle and joint aches; and gastrointestinal distress. The vaccine is given in a series of three injections over a 6-month period (CDC, 2017d).

If the cisgender woman or transgender man doesn't receive primary prevention with the vaccine, then secondary prevention would focus on education about the importance of receiving regular Pap smears and, for those over age 30 years, including an HPV test to determine whether there is a latent high-risk virus that could lead to precancerous cervical changes. Finally, treatment options for precancerous cervical lesions or genital warts caused by HPV are numerous and may include:

- Topical trichloroacetic acid 80% to 90%
- Liquid nitrogen cryotherapy
- Topical imiquimod 5% cream
- Topical podophyllin 10% to 25%
- Sinecatechins 15% ointment
- Laser carbon dioxide vaporization
- Client-applied podofilox 0.5% solution or gel
- Simple surgical excision
- Loop electrosurgical excisional procedure (LEEP)
- Intralesional interferon therapy (CDC, 2015a)

The goal of treating genital warts is to remove the warts and induce wart-free periods for the client. Treatment of genital warts should be guided by the preference of the client and available resources. No single treatment has been found to be ideal for all clients, and most treatment modalities appear to have comparable efficacy. Because genital warts can proliferate and become friable during pregnancy, they should be removed using a local agent. A cesarean birth is not indicated solely to prevent transmission of HPV infection to the newborn, unless the pelvic outlet is obstructed by warts (Gearhart et al., 2018).

Nursing Management

An HPV infection has many implications for the client's health, but many people are unaware of HPV and its role in cervical cancer. The average age of sexual debut is in early adolescence; therefore, it is important to target this population for use of the HPV/cervical cancer vaccine.

Key nursing roles are teaching about prevention of HPV infection and client education and promotion of vaccines and screening tests in order to reduce the morbidity and mortality associated with cervical cancer caused by HPV infection. Teach all clients that the only way to prevent HPV is to refrain from any genital contact with another person. Although the effect of condoms in preventing HPV infection is unknown, latex condom use has been associated with a lower rate of cervical cancer. Teach clients about the link between HPV and cervical cancer. Explain that, in most cases, there are no signs or symptoms of infection with HPV. Strongly encourage all young people aged between 9 and 26 years to consider getting Gardasil 9, the vaccine against HPV. For all cisgender women and transgender men, promote the importance of obtaining regular Pap smears and, for those over 30 years, suggest an HPV test to rule out the presence of a latent high-risk strain of HPV.

Education and counselling are important aspects of managing clients with genital warts. Teach the client that:
- Even after genital warts are removed, HPV still remains and viral shedding will continue.
- The likelihood of transmission to future partners and the duration of infectivity after treatment for genital warts are unknown.
- The recurrence of genital warts within the first few months after treatment is common and usually indicates recurrence rather than reinfection (CDC, 2015a).

Hepatitis A and B

Hepatitis is an acute, systemic, viral infection that can be transmitted sexually. The viruses associated with hepatitis or inflammation of the liver are hepatitis A, B, C, D, E, and G. HAV is spread via the gastrointestinal tract. It can be acquired by drinking polluted water, by eating uncooked shellfish from sewage-contaminated waters or food handled by a hepatitis carrier with poor hygiene, and from oral/anal sexual contact. A person with hepatitis A can easily pass the disease to others within the same household. People infected with HAV can have a wide range of effects, varying from no symptoms to fever, loss of appetite, stomach cramps, fatigue, dark urine, and jaundice. Approximately 10% to 15% of people who do not show symptoms can still carry the disease for up to 6 months (Health Canada, 2015).

HBV is transmitted through saliva, blood serum, semen, menstrual blood, and vaginal secretions. The incubation period from the time of exposure to onset of symptoms is 6 weeks to 6 months (CDC, 2018b). In the early 2000s, transmission among heterosexual partners accounted for 40% of infections, and transmission among men who have sex with men accounted for 20% of infections. The World Health Organization (WHO) estimates that the prevalence of hepatitis B worldwide is 2 billion people, with about 240 million chronically infected with it. Worldwide, hepatitis B has the highest death rate of any STI except HIV (WHO, 2018b). Risk factors for infection include having multiple sex partners, engaging in unprotected receptive anal intercourse, and having a history of other STIs (CDC, 2018b). The most effective means to prevent the transmission of hepatitis A or B is pre-exposure immunization. Vaccines are available for the prevention of HAV and HBV, both of which can be transmitted sexually. Every person seeking treatment for an STI should be considered a candidate for hepatitis B vaccination, and some individuals (e.g., men who have sex with men, and injection drug users) should be considered for hepatitis A vaccination (CDC, 2018b).

Therapeutic Management

Unlike other STIs, HBV and HAV are preventable through immunization. HAV is usually self-limiting and does not result in chronic infection. HBV can result in serious, permanent liver damage. Treatment is generally supportive. No specific treatment for acute HBV infection exists.

Nursing Assessment

Assess the client for clinical manifestations of hepatitis A and B. Symptoms of hepatitis B are similar to those of hepatitis A, but with less fever and skin involvement. The diagnosis of hepatitis A cannot be made based on clinical manifestations alone and requires serologic testing. The presence of IgM antibody to HAV is diagnostic of acute HAV infection. Hepatitis B is detected by a blood test that looks for antibodies and proteins produced by the virus and is positively diagnosed by the presence of hepatitis B surface antibody (HBsAb) (Pyrsopoulos & Reddy, 2018).

Nursing Management

Nurses should encourage all clients having their regular Pap smear screening to be screened for hepatitis at the same time, or sooner if high-risk behaviour is identified. Nurses should also encourage clients to undergo HBV screening at their first prenatal visit and repeat screening in the last trimester for those at higher risk (Lee & Lok, 2018). Nurses can also explain that hepatitis B vaccine is recommended for all infants after birth in most hospitals. The vaccination consists of a series of three injections given within 6 months. The vaccine has been shown to be safe and well tolerated by most recipients (CDC, 2015a). Hepatitis A vaccine is strongly encouraged for children between 12 and 23 months; persons 1 year of age and older traveling to countries with a high prevalence of hepatitis A, such as Central or South America, Mexico, Asia, Africa, and eastern Europe; men who have sex with men; persons who use street drugs; and persons with chronic liver disease (CDC, 2018a). For others, hepatitis A vaccine series (two doses 6 months apart) may be started whenever a person is at risk of infection.

Hepatitis C

Although HCV is not transmitted sexually, it deserves a brief mention here because of its inclusion in the category of sexually transmitted and blood borne infections (STBBI). Clients at high risk include those with a history of injection drug use, sexual partners who use injection drugs, and those with a history of blood transfusion before 1992 (CDC, 2018c). The majority of infected clients are not aware they have HCV because they are not clinically ill. Perinatal transmission of HCV is relatively rare, except in those who are immunocompromised (HIV/AIDS) (Mattson & Smith, 2015).

ECTOPARASITIC INFECTIONS

Ectoparasites are a common cause of skin rash and pruritus throughout the world, affecting people of all ages, races, and socioeconomic groups. Overcrowding, delayed diagnosis and treatment, and poor public education contribute to the prevalence of ectoparasites in both industrial and nonindustrial nations. Approximately 300 million ectoparasitic cases are reported worldwide each year (CDC, 2015c). These infections include infestations of scabies and pubic lice. Since these parasites are easily passed from one person to another during sexual intimacy, clients should be assessed for them when receiving care for other STIs. Scabies is an intensely pruritic dermatitis caused by a mite. The female mite burrows under the skin and deposits eggs, which hatch. The lesions start as a small papule that reddens, erodes, and sometimes crusts. Diagnosis is based on history and appearance of burrows in the webs of the fingers and the genitalia (Guenther & Maguiness, 2018). Aggressive infestation can occur in immunodeficient, debilitated, or malnourished people, but healthy people do not usually suffer sequelae.

Clients with pediculosis pubis (pubic lice) usually seek treatment because of the pruritus, because of a rash brought on by skin irritation from scratching, or because they notice lice or nits in their pubic hair, axillary hair, abdominal and thigh hair, and sometimes in the eyebrows, eyelashes, and beards. Infestation is usually asymptomatic until after a week or so, when bites cause pruritus and secondary infections from scratching (Fig. 5.9). Diagnosis is based on history and the presence of nits (small, shiny, yellow, oval, dewdrop-like eggs) affixed to hair shafts or lice (a yellowish, oval, wingless insect) (Monsel & Chosidow, 2015).

Treatment is directed at the infested area, using permethrin 1% cream rinse and pyrethrin with piperonyl

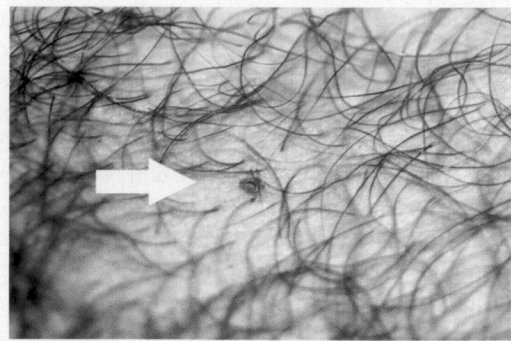

FIGURE 5.9 Pubic lice. A small brown living crab louse is seen at the base of hairs (*arrow*). (From Goodheart, H. [2009]. *Goodheart's photoguide of common skin disorders.* Philadelphia, PA: Lippincott Williams & Wilkins.)

butoxide, which are FDA approved for treating head lice. Both are available as over-the-counter (OTC) preparations. Repeat treatment in 1 week is advised to eradicate eggs that may have hatched after treatment started (King et al., 2015). Bedding and clothing should be washed in hot water to decontaminate it. Sexual partners should be treated also, as well as family members who live in close contact with the infected person.

Nursing care of a client infested with lice or scabies involves a three-tiered approach: eradicating the infestation with medication, removing nits, and preventing spread or recurrence by managing the environment. OTC products are safe for use and kill the active lice or mites. Nurses should provide education about these products (Teaching Guidelines 5.5). The nurse can follow these same guidelines to prevent the health care facility from becoming infested.

 Teaching Guidelines 5.5

TREATING AND MINIMIZING THE SPREAD OF SCABIES AND PUBIC LICE

- Use the medication according to the manufacturer's instructions.
- Remove nits with a fine-toothed nit comb.
- Do not share any personal items with others or accept items from others.
- Treat objects, clothing, and bedding and wash them in hot water.
- Meticulously vacuum carpets to prevent a recurrence of infestation.

HUMAN IMMUNODEFICIENCY VIRUS

There are 34 million people around the world currently living with HIV, including over 63,000 Canadians. According to the Canadian AIDS Treatment Information

Exchange (CATIE), the prevalence of people living with HIV in Canada is 173 per 100,000 (CATIE, 2018a). In terms of epidemiology, fatality rate, and its social, legal, ethical, and political aspects, HIV infection became a global public health crisis over 20 years ago and has generated more concern than any other infectious disease in modern medical history (Oyelowo & Johnson, 2016). To date, there is no cure for this fatal viral infection.

The HIV virus is transmitted by intimate sexual contact, by sharing needles for IV drug use, from an infected person to their fetus during pregnancy, or by transfusion of infected blood or blood products. Men who have sex with men represent the largest proportion of new infections in Canada (approximately 52%), followed by men and women infected through heterosexual sex (approximately 32%) (CATIE, 2018a). Twenty-three percent of people living with HIV infection in Canada are women (CATIE, 2018a). HIV infection disproportionately affects Indigenous people in Canada. Indigenous people make up approximately 5% of the total Canadian population, but data from 2016 showed that 11.3% of new infections were among Indigenous peoples, making the incidence 2.7 times higher than among Canadians of other ethnicities (CATIE, 2018a).

AIDS is a breakdown in the immune function caused by HIV, a retrovirus. The infected person develops opportunistic infections or malignancies that become fatal. Progression from HIV infection to AIDS varies within individuals. HIV affects CD4 cells in two ways: by depleting them and by impairing the remaining ones. This invasion of CD4 cells results in a gradual loss of immune function. If nothing is done to stop this invasion of CD4 cells, HIV can destroy as many as 1 billion CD4 cells daily (King et al., 2015).

Over 35 years have passed since HIV/AIDS began to affect our society. Since then, 1 million people have been infected by the virus, with AIDS being the fourth leading cause of death globally (CDC, 2018e). The morbidity and mortality of HIV continue to hold the attention of the medical community. While there has been a dramatic improvement in both morbidity and mortality with the use of antiretroviral therapy (ART), the incidence of HIV infection continues to be a public health challenge.

Take Note!

Once the HIV infection has progressed to AIDS, the survival period is usually less than 2 years in untreated clients (Bennett & Gilroy, 2018).

The fetal and neonatal effects of acquiring HIV through perinatal transmission can be devastating. If the HIV-infected infant goes untreated, progression to AIDS and eventual fatality will occur. A pregnant person who is HIV-positive can transmit the infection to the newborn before or during birth and through breast milk. Current incidence of perinatal transmission is less than 1% if the HIV-positive pregnant client is taking antiretroviral (ARV) medication during pregnancy (CDC, 2018e).

Human Immunodeficiency Virus and Adolescents

As a typical function of development, adolescents may view themselves as invincible, and thus delay seeking health care. They may be embarrassed or lacking access to health care or may delay or refuse treatment if a diagnosis of HIV infection is made. Though the rates of HIV infection among adolescents have remained stable since 2006, the effects of HIV infection in this population continue to be of concern (CDC, 2018d). On average, the development of AIDS occurs about 11 years after infection; so most young adults with AIDS were infected during adolescence (Fairlie, Sipambo, Fick, & Moultrie, 2015).

Most HIV-infected adolescents are exposed to the virus through heterosexual or homosexual contact. The majority of HIV-infected adolescent males are infected through sex with other males, while female teenagers are mostly exposed through heterosexual contact. Injected drug use accounts for a small percentage of HIV infection among adolescents. More than 2 million adolescents between the ages of 10 and 19 are living with HIV around the world today, and many do not receive the care and support they need to stay in good health.

Clinical Manifestations

HIV infection undergoes three distinct phases—acute seroconversion, asymptomatic infection, and then progresses to AIDS. When a person is initially infected with HIV, they go through an acute primary infection period for about 3 weeks. The HIV viral load drops rapidly because the host's immune system works well to fight this initial infection. The onset of the acute primary infection occurs 2 to 6 weeks after exposure. Symptoms include fever, pharyngitis, rash, and myalgia. Most people do not associate this flu-like condition with HIV infection. After initial exposure, there is a period of 3 to 12 months before seroconversion. The person is considered infectious during this time.

After the acute phase, the infected person becomes asymptomatic, but the HIV virus begins to replicate. Even though there are no symptoms, the immune system runs down. A healthy person has a CD4 T-cell count of 450 to 1,200 cells per μL. When the CD4 T-cell count reaches 200 or less, the person has reached the stage of AIDS. The immune system begins a constant battle to fight this viral invasion, but over time it falls behind. A viral reservoir occurs in T cells that can store various stages of the virus. The onset and severity of the disease correlate directly with the viral load: The more HIV virus that is present, the worse the person will feel.

As profound immunosuppression begins to occur, an opportunistic infection will occur, qualifying the person for the diagnosis of AIDS. The diagnosis is finally confirmed when the CD4 count is below 200. As of now, AIDS will eventually develop in everyone who is HIV-positive.

WHO (2018a) now recommends earlier initiation of ART for adults and adolescents, the delivery of more client-friendly ARV drugs, and prolonged use of ARVs to reduce the risk of mother-to-child transmission of HIV. ART should be started when the CD4 count reaches the 350 to 500 range. Also, WHO (2018c) recommends that HIV-positive mothers or their infants take ARVs while breastfeeding to prevent HIV transmission for up to 12 months after birth.

Diagnosis

HIV testing is regarded as the gateway to prevention and treatment. Several types of tests are approved to detect antigens, antibodies, or RNA. Screening for HIV infection is paramount, since infected individuals may remain asymptomatic for years while the infection progresses. Currently, there are two categories of screening methods: rapid HIV tests and confirmatory tests. The rapid tests allow for screening at the point of care and offer quick results. Quick tests for HIV produce results in 10 to 20 minutes and also lower the health care worker's risk of occupational exposure by eliminating the need to draw blood. A positive result is followed up with a confirmatory test called the Geenius HIV-1/2 Confirmatory Assay, available in all provinces across Canada. Some provinces also have access to nucleic acid amplification tests (NAATs) and/or p24 antigen testing (CATIE, 2018b).

Fewer than half of adults between the ages of 18 and 64 have ever had an HIV test, according to the CDC. The PHAC estimates that 25% of people who are infected with HIV in Canada do not know they are infected (PHAC, 2014b). This means they are not receiving treatment that can prolong their lives, and they may be unknowingly infecting others. In addition, even when people do get tested, one in three failed to return to the testing site to learn their results when there was a 2-week wait. The CDC hopes that the new "one-stop" approach to HIV testing changes that pattern.

People who are infected with HIV but not aware of it are not able to take advantage of the therapies that can keep them healthy and extend their lives, nor do they have the knowledge to protect their sexual or drug-use partners from becoming infected. Knowing whether one is positive or negative for HIV confers great benefits in healthy decision making.

Rapid point of service HIV tests are becoming powerful screening tools in various health care settings because they offer the opportunity to not only screen for HIV, but also to educate the person regarding risk factors, and discuss their test results—all in one clinical visit. Most use a finger stick drop of blood or a swab of saliva taken from the mouth. Results are typically ready within 10 to 20 minutes. Home HIV testing kits are available for purchase online or OTC in some countries, including the United States. However, no self-tests have been approved for use in Canada (CATIE, 2018b).

If the confirmation test (Geenius, NAAT, or p24 antigen test) is positive, the person is infected with HIV and is capable of transmitting the virus to others. The HIV rapid testing methods have a high sensitivity (99.9%), meaning that the test can correctly indicate that an HIV-positive person has the virus. The specificity, or the ability to correctly identify a negative result, is slightly lower (99.5%), indicating a slightly higher potential of a false-positive result. Therefore, all positive results on rapid tests are sent for a confirmatory Geenius assay (CATIE, 2018b).

Therapeutic Management

The goals of HIV drug therapy are to:
• Decrease the HIV viral load below the level of detection
• Restore the body's ability to fight off pathogens
• Improve the client's quality of life
• Reduce HIV morbidity and mortality (King et al., 2015)

Highly active antiretroviral therapy (HAART), which combines at least three ARV drugs, has dramatically improved the prognosis of HIV/AIDS. Treatment with HAART should begin for any person with an AIDS-defining illness or with a history of a CD4 count less than 350 cells/mm (WHO, 2018d). The current HAART standard is a triple combination therapy, but some clients may be given a fourth or fifth agent.

Current therapy to prevent the transmission of HIV to the newborn includes a three-part regimen of having the mother take an oral ARV agent at 14 to 34 weeks of gestation; it is continued throughout pregnancy. During labour, an ARV agent is administered IV until delivery. An ARV syrup is administered to the infant within 12 hours after birth.

Dramatic new treatment advances with ARV medications have turned a disease that used to be a death sentence into a chronic, manageable one for individuals who live in countries where ART is available. Despite these advances in treatment, however, only a minority of HIV-positive people in the United States who take ARV medications are receiving the full benefits because they are not adhering to the prescribed regimen. Successful ART requires nearly perfect adherence to a complex medication regimen; less-than-perfect adherence leads to drug resistance (King et al., 2015).

Adherence is difficult because of the complexity of the regimen and the lifelong duration of treatment. A typical ARV regimen may consist of three or more medications taken twice daily. Adherence is made even more difficult because of the unpleasant side effects, such as nausea and diarrhea. Women in early pregnancy already experience these, and the ARV medication only exacerbates them.

Nursing Management

Nurses can play a major role in caring for the HIV-positive clients by helping them accept the possibility of a shortened lifespan, cope with others' reactions to a stigmatizing illness, and develop strategies to maintain their physical and emotional health. Educate the client about behavioural changes to prevent spreading HIV to others, and refer to appropriate community resources such as HIV medical care services, substance abuse, mental health services, and social services. See Nursing Care Plan 5.1: Overview of the Woman Who Is HIV-Positive (at the end of the chapter).

Providing Education About Drug Therapy

The goal of ART is to suppress viral replication so that the viral load becomes undetectable by diagnostic tests. This is done to preserve immune function and delay disease progression but is a challenge because of the side effects of nausea and vomiting, diarrhea, altered taste, anorexia, flatulence, constipation, headaches, anemia, and fatigue. Although not everyone experiences all of the side effects, the majority do have some of them. Current research has not documented the long-term safety of exposure of the fetus to ARV agents during pregnancy, but collection of data is ongoing.

Help to reduce the development of drug resistance and thus treatment failure by identifying the barriers to adherence; identifying these barriers can help the client to overcome them. Some of the common barriers include:

- A lack of understanding of the link between drug resistance and nonadherence
- Fears of revealing the HIV status by being seen taking medication
- Not having adjusted emotionally to the HIV diagnosis
- Not understanding the dosing regimen or schedule
- Experiencing unpleasant side effects frequently
- Feeling anxious or depressed (Abdurakhmanov & Zandman-Goddard, 2015)

Educate the client about the prescribed drug therapy and stress, and that it is very important to take the regimen as prescribed. Offer suggestions about how to cope with anorexia, nausea, and vomiting by:

- Separating the intake of food and fluids
- Eating dry crackers upon arising
- Eating six small meals daily
- Using high-protein supplements (such as Boost or Ensure) to provide quick and easy protein and calories
- Eating "comfort foods," which may appeal when other foods do not

Promoting Compliance

Remaining compliant with drug therapy is a huge challenge for many HIV-infected people. Compliance becomes difficult when the same pills that are supposed to thwart the disease are making the person sick. Nausea and diarrhea are just two of the possible side effects. It is often difficult to increase the client's quality of life when so much oral medication is required. The combination medication therapy is challenging for many people, and staying compliant over a period of years is extremely difficult. Stress the importance of taking the prescribed ARV drug therapies by explaining that they help prevent replication of the retroviruses and subsequent progression of the disease, as well as decreasing the risk of perinatal transmission of HIV. In addition, provide written materials describing diet, exercise, medications, and signs and symptoms of complications and opportunistic infections. Reinforce this information at each visit.

Preventing Human Immunodeficiency Virus Infection

The lack of information about HIV infection and AIDS causes great anxiety and fear of the unknown. It is vital to take a leadership role in educating the public about risky behaviours in the fight to control this disease. The core of HIV prevention is to abstain from unsafe sex, and to use condoms. This is all good advice for many clients, but some simply do not have the economic and social power or choices or control over their lives to put that advice into practice. Recognize that fact, and address the factors that will give clients more control over their lives by providing anticipatory guidance, giving ample opportunities to practice negotiation techniques and refusal skills in a safe environment, and encouraging the use of female condoms to protect against this deadly virus. Prevention is the key to reversing the current infection trends.

Providing Care During Pregnancy and Childbirth

Voluntary counselling and HIV testing should be offered to all pregnant clients as early in the pregnancy as possible to identify HIV infection so that treatment can be initiated early. Once a pregnant client is identified as being HIV-positive, the risk for perinatal infection must be discussed. The risk of perinatal transmission of HIV from an infected person to the newborn is about 25%. This risk falls to less than 1% if the client receives ART during pregnancy (Adam, 2015). HIV can be spread to the infant through breastfeeding so that when acceptable alternative infant formulas are readily available, HIV-infected parents should be counselled to avoid breastfeeding and use formula instead. WHO (2018e) recommendations indicate that transmission of HIV via breast milk is decreased when the mother is undergoing ART.

In addition, the client needs instructions on ways to enhance the immune system by following these guidelines during pregnancy:

- Getting adequate sleep each night (7 to 9 hours)
- Avoiding infections (e.g., staying away from crowds, handwashing)
- Decreasing life stressors
- Consuming adequate protein and vitamins
- Increasing fluid intake to 2 L daily to stay hydrated
- Planning rest periods throughout the day to prevent fatigue

Despite the dramatic reduction in perinatal transmission, hundreds of infants will be born infected with HIV. The birth of each infected infant is a missed prevention opportunity. To minimize perinatal HIV transmission, identify HIV infections, preferably before pregnancy; provide information about disease prevention; and encourage HIV-infected clients to follow the prescribed drug therapy.

Providing Appropriate Referrals

The HIV-infected client may have difficulty coping with the normal activities of daily living due to having less energy and a decreased physical endurance. The client may be overwhelmed by the financial burdens of medical and drug therapies and the emotional responses to a life-threatening condition, as well as concern about the infant's future, if pregnant. A case management approach is needed to deal with the complexity of needs during this time. Be an empathetic listener and make appropriate referrals for nutritional services, counselling, homemaker services, spiritual care, and local support groups. Many community-based organizations have developed programs to address the numerous issues regarding HIV/AIDS. Go to thePoint for link to the Canadian AIDS Society's list of provincial HIV information hotlines. Table 5.4 provides a summary of perinatal effects of STIs during pregnancy.

TABLE 5.4	MATERNAL AND FETAL EFFECTS FROM STIs	
STI	**Maternal Effects**	**Fetal Effects**
Candidiasis	Resistant to treatment during pregnancy; Uncomfortable localized genital itching and discharge	Can acquire thrush in the mouth during birthing process if mother infected
Trichomoniasis	Has been implicated to cause PROM and preterm births	Risk of prematurity
Bacterial vaginosis	Increases risk for spontaneous abortion, PROM, chorioamnionitis, postpartum endometritis, and preterm labour	Risk of neonatal sepsis
Chlamydia	Postpartum endometritis, PROM, and preterm birth	Conjunctivitis, which can lead to blindness; Low birth weight; and pneumonitis
Gonorrhea	Chorioamnionitis, preterm birth, PROM, fetal growth restriction, postpartum sepsis	Eye infection *gonococcal ophthalmia* which can cause blindness
Genital herpes	Spontaneous abortion, intrauterine infection, preterm labour, PROM, fetal growth restriction	Birth anomalies; transplacental infection
Syphilis	Spontaneous abortion, preterm birth, stillbirth	Congenital syphilis: multisystem organ failure, structural damage; mental retardation
Human papillomavirus (HPV)	May cause dystocia if large lesions	None known
Hepatitis B	May cause preterm birth; can be transmitted to fetus if active in last trimester	Can become chronic carrier of hepatitis B which may lead to liver cancer or cirrhosis
HIV	Fatigue, nausea, weight loss	Transmission can occur transplacentally, during childbirth or through breast milk

Callahan, T. L. (2016). *Tarascon OB/GYN pocketbook*. Burlington, MA: Jones & Bartlett Learning; King, T. L., Brucker, M. C., Kriebs, J. M., Fahey, J. O., Gegor, C. L., & Varney, H. (2015). *Varney's midwifery* (5th ed.). Burlington, MA: Jones & Bartlett Learning; Queenan, J. T., Spong, C. Y., & Lockwood, C. J. (2015). *Protocols for high-risk pregnancies: An evidence-based approach* (6th ed.). Somerset, NJ: John Wiley & Sons; and Silasi, M., Cardenas, I., Kwon, J. Y., Racicot, K., Aldo, P., & Mor, G. (2015). Viral infections during pregnancy. *American Journal of Reproductive Immunology, 73*(3), 199–213.

PREVENTING SEXUALLY TRANSMITTED INFECTIONS

Education about safer-sex practices—and the resulting increase in the use of condoms—can play a vital role in reducing STI rates all over the world. Clearly, knowledge and prevention are the best defences against STIs. The prevention and control of STIs is based on the following concepts (CDC, 2017c).

1. Education and counselling of people at risk about safer sexual behaviour
2. Identification of asymptomatic infected people and of symptomatic people unlikely to seek diagnosis and treatment
3. Effective diagnosis and treatment of infected people
4. Evaluation, treatment, and counselling of sex partners of people who are infected with an STI
5. Pre-exposure vaccination of people at risk for vaccine-preventable STIs

Nurses play an integral role in identifying and preventing STIs. They have a unique opportunity to educate the public about this serious public health issue by communicating the methods of transmission and symptoms associated with each condition, tracking the updated Health Canada treatment guidelines, and offering clients strategic preventive measures to reduce the spread of STIs.

It is not easy to discuss STI prevention when globally we are failing at it. Knowledge exists on how to prevent every single route of transmission, but the incidence continues to climb. Challenges to prevention of STIs include lack of resources and difficulty in changing the behaviours that contribute to their spread. Regardless of the challenging factors involved, nurses must continue to educate and meet the needs of all clients to promote their sexual health. Successful treatment and prevention of STIs are impossible without education. Successful teaching approaches include giving clear, accurate messages that are age appropriate and culturally sensitive.

Primary prevention strategies include education of all clients, especially adolescents, regarding the risk of early sexual activity, the number of sexual partners, and STIs. Sexual abstinence is ideal but often not practiced; therefore, the use of barrier contraception (condoms) should be encouraged (see Teaching Guidelines 5.1).

Secondary prevention involves the need for regular pelvic examinations with Pap smears for all sexually active clients, regardless of age. Many people with STIs are asymptomatic, so regular screening examinations are paramount for early detection. Understanding the relationship between poor socioeconomic conditions and poor patterns of sexual and reproductive self-care is significant in disease prevention and health promotion strategies.

Every successful form of prevention requires a change in behaviour. The nursing role in teaching and rendering quality health care is invaluable evidence that

---

BOX 5.3

SELECTED NURSING STRATEGIES TO PREVENT THE SPREAD OF STIs

- Provide basic information about STI transmission.
- Outline safer sexual behaviours for people at risk for STIs.
- Refer clients to appropriate community resources to reduce risk.
- Screen asymptomatic persons with STIs.
- Identify barriers to STI testing and remove them.
- Offer pre-exposure immunizations for vaccine-preventable STIs.
- Respond honestly about testing results and options available.
- Counsel and treat sexual partners of persons with STIs.
- Educate school administrators, parents, and teens about STIs.
- Support youth development activities to reduce sexual risk taking.
- Promote the use of barrier methods (condoms, diaphragms) to prevent the spread of STIs.
- Assist clients to gain skills in negotiating safer sex.
- Discuss reducing the number of sexual partners to reduce risk.

the key to reducing the spread of STIs is through behavioural change. Nurses working in these specialty areas have a responsibility to educate themselves, their clients, their families, and the community about STIs, and to provide compassionate and supportive care to clients. Some strategies nurses can use to prevent the spread of STIs are detailed in Box 5.3.

Consider This

I was thinking of my carefree college days, when the most important thing was having an active social life and meeting guys. I had been raised by very strict parents and was never allowed to date under their watch. Since I attended a university in another province, I figured that my parents' outdated advice and rules no longer applied. Abruptly, my thoughts of the past were interrupted by the HIV counsellor asking about my feelings concerning my positive diagnosis. What was there to say at this point? I had a lot of fun but never dreamed it would haunt me for the rest of my life, which was going to be shortened considerably now. I only wish I could turn back the hands of time and listen to my parents' advice, which somehow doesn't seem so outdated now.

Thoughts: All of us have thought back on our lives to better times and wondered how our lives would have changed if we had made better choices or gone down another path. It is a pity that we have only one chance to make good, sound decisions at times. What would you have changed in your life if given a second chance? Can you still make a change for the better now?

Behaviour Modification

Research validates that changing behaviours do result in a decrease in new STIs, but it must encompass all levels—governments, community organizations, schools, churches, parents, and individuals. Nurses can advocate for the development and implementation of educational initiatives to increase awareness of STIs (Alexander, Jemmott, Teitelman, & D'Antonio, 2015). Education must address ways to prevent becoming infected, ways to prevent transmitting infection, symptoms of STIs, and treatment. At this point in the STI epidemic, nurses do not have time to debate the relative merits of prevention versus treatment: both are underused and underfunded, and one leads to the other. But being serious about prevention and focusing on the strategies outlined above will bring about a positive change on everyone's part.

Contraception

The spread of STIs could be prevented by access to safe, efficient, appropriate, modern contraception for everyone who wants it. Nurses can play an important role in helping clients to identify their risk of STIs and to adopt preventive measures through the dual protection that contraceptives offer.

Nurses can expand their scopes in either setting by discussing dual protection by use of a male or female condom alone or by use of a condom along with a nonbarrier contraceptive. Because barrier methods are not the most effective means of fertility control, they have not been typically recommended as a method alone for dual protection. Unfortunately, the most effective pregnancy prevention methods—sterilization, hormonal methods, and intrauterine devices—do not protect against STIs. Dual-method use protects against both STIs and pregnancy.

NURSING CARE PLAN 5.1

Overview of the Woman Who Is HIV-Positive

Annie, a 28-year-old woman, is HIV-positive. She acquired HIV through unprotected sexual contact. She has been inconsistent in taking her antiretroviral medications and presents today stating she is tired and doesn't feel well.

NURSING DIAGNOSIS: Ineffective protection, related to risk of infection secondary to inadequate immune system as manifested by client stating she has been inconsistent in taking her antiretroviral therapy medications.

Outcome Identification and Evaluation

Client will remain free of opportunistic infections as evidenced by temperature within acceptable parameters and absence of signs and symptoms of opportunistic infections.

Interventions: *Minimizing the Risk of Opportunistic Infections*

- Assess CD4 count and viral loads *to determine disease progression* (CD4 counts 500/L and viral loads >10,000 copies/L = increased risk for opportunistic infections).
- Assess complete blood count *to identify presence of infection* (>10,000 cells/mm³ may indicate infection).
- Assess oral cavity and mucous membranes for painful white patches in mouth *to evaluate for possible fungal infection*.
- Teach client to monitor for general signs and symptoms of infections, such as fever, weakness, and fatigue, *to ensure early identification*.
- Provide information explaining the importance of avoiding people with infections when possible *to minimize risk of exposure to infections*.
- Teach importance of keeping appointments so her CD4 count and viral load can be monitored *to alert*

the health care provider about her immune system status.
- Instruct her to reduce her exposure to infections via:
  - Meticulous handwashing
  - Thorough cooking of meats, eggs, and vegetables
  - Wearing shoes at all times, especially when outdoors
- Encourage a balance of rest with activity throughout the day *to prevent overexertion*.
- Stress importance of maintaining prescribed antiretroviral drug therapies *to prevent disease progression and resistance*.
- If necessary, refer Annie to a nutritionist to help her understand what constitutes a well-balanced diet with supplements *to promote health and ward off infection*.

NURSING CARE PLAN 5.1

Overview of the Woman Who Is HIV-Positive (continued)

NURSING DIAGNOSIS: Deficient knowledge related to HIV infection and possible complications.

Outcome Identification and Evaluation

Client will demonstrate increased understanding of HIV infection as evidenced by verbalizing appropriate health care practices and adhering to measures to comply with therapy and reduce her risk of further exposure and reduce risk of disease progression.

Interventions: *Providing Client Education*

- Assess her understanding of HIV and its treatment *to provide a baseline for teaching.*
- Establish trust and be honest with Annie; encourage her to talk about her fears and the impact of the disease *to provide an outlet for her concerns.* Encourage her to discuss reasons for her noncompliance.
- Provide a nonjudgmental, accessible, confidential, and culturally sensitive approach *to promote Annie's self-esteem and allow her to feel that she is a priority.*
- Explain measures, including safer-sex practices and birth control options, to prevent disease transmission; determine her willingness to practice safer sex to protect others *to determine further teaching needs.*
- Discuss the signs and symptoms of disease progression and potential opportunistic infections *to promote early detection for prompt intervention.*
- Outline with the client the availability of community resources and make appropriate referrals as needed *to provide additional education and support.*
- Encourage Annie to keep scheduled appointments *to ensure follow-up and allow early detection of potential problems.*

KEY CONCEPTS

- Avoiding risky sexual behaviours may preserve fertility and prevent chronic conditions later in life.

- An estimated 65 million people live with an incurable STI, and another 20 million are infected each year.

- The most reliable way to avoid transmission of STIs is to abstain from sexual intercourse (i.e., oral, vaginal, or anal sex) or to be in a long-term, mutually monogamous relationship with an uninfected partner.

- Barrier methods of contraception are recommended because they increase protection from contact with urethral discharge, mucosal secretions, and lesions of the cervix or penis.

- The high rate of asymptomatic transmission of STIs calls for teaching high-risk clients the nature of transmission and how to recognize infections.

- Nurses should practice good handwashing techniques and follow standard precautions to protect themselves and their clients from STIs.

- Nurses are in an important position to promote sexual health. Nurses should make their clients and the community aware of the perinatal implications and lifelong sequelae of STIs.

REFERENCES AND RECOMMENDED READINGS

Abdurakhmanov, A., & Zandman-Goddard, G. (2015). HIV spectrum and autoimmune diseases. In Y. Shoenfeld, N. Agmon-Levin, & N. Rose (Eds.). *Infection and autoimmunity* (2nd ed., pp. 371–392). St. Louis, MO: Elsevier.

Adam, S. (2015). HIV and pregnancy: review. *Obstetrics and Gynecology Forum, 25*(2), 19–22. Sabinet Online.

Albrecht, M. A. (2018). Epidemiology, clinical manifestations, and diagnosis of genital herpes simplex virus infection. *UpToDate.* Retrieved from https://www.uptodate.com/contents/epidemiology-clinical-manifestations-and-diagnosis-of-genital-herpes-simplex-virus-infection

Alexander, K. A., Jemmott, L. S., Teitelman, A. M., & D'Antonio, P. (2015). Addressing sexual health behavior during emerging adulthood: A critical review of the literature. *Journal of Clinical Nursing, 24*(1–2), 4–18.

Alexander, L. L., LaRosa, J. H., Bader, H., & Garfield, S. (2014). *New dimensions in women's health* (6th ed.). Sudbury, MA: Jones and Bartlett Publishers.

American Cancer Society (ACS). (2018). *HPV (human papilloma virus)*. Retrieved from http://www.cancer.org/cancer/cancer-causes/othercarcinogens/infectiousagents/hpv/hpv-landing

Bennett, N. J., & Gilroy, S. A. (2018). *HIV infection and AIDS*. Retrieved from http://emedicine.medscape.com/article/211316-overview

Brunham, R. C. (2015). A Chlamydia vaccine on the horizon. *Science, 348*(6241), 1322–1323.

Brunham, R. C., Gottlieb, S. L., & Paavonen, J. (2015). Pelvic inflammatory disease. *New England Journal of Medicine, 372*(21), 2039–2048.

Callahan, T. L. (2016). *Tarascon OB/GYN pocketbook*. Burlington, MA: Jones & Bartlett Learning.

Canadian Cancer Society. (2018). *Human papillomavirus (HPV) test*. Retrieved from http://www.cancer.ca/en/cancer-information/diagnosis-and-treatment/tests-and-procedures/hpv-test/?region=on

CATIE. (2018a). *The epidemiology of HIV in Canada*. Retrieved from http://www.catie.ca/fact-sheets/epidemiology/epidemiology-hiv-canada

CATIE. (2018b). *HIV testing technologies*. Retrieved from http://www.catie.ca/en/fact-sheets/testing/hiv-testing-technologies

Centers for Disease Control and Prevention (CDC). (2013). *Condom fact sheet in brief*. Retrieved from http://www.cdc.gov/condomeffectiveness/docs/condomfactsheetinbrief.pdf

Centers for Disease Control and Prevention (CDC). (2015a). *2015 Sexually transmitted diseases treatment guidelines*. Retrieved from http://www.cdc.gov/std/tg2015/

Centers for Disease Control and Prevention (CDC). (2015b). *Chlamydial infections*. Retrieved from http://www.cdc.gov/std/tg2015/chlamydia.htm

Centers for Disease Control and Prevention (CDC). (2015c). *Ectoparasitic infections*. Retrieved from http://www.cdc.gov/std/tg2015/ectoparasitic.htm

Centers for Disease Control and Prevention (CDC). (2015d). *Genital herpes*. Retrieved from http://www.cdc.gov/std/herpes

Centers for Disease Control and Prevention. (2015e). *Gonorrhea*. Retrieved from http://www.cdc.gov/std/gonorrhea/default.htm

Centers for Disease Control and Prevention (CDC). (2015f). *Syphilis*. Retrieved from http://www.cdc.gov/std/tg2015/syphilis.htm

Centers for Disease Control and Prevention (CDC). (2017a). *Fungal diseases: Candidiasis*. Retrieved from http://www.cdc.gov/fungal/diseases/candidiasis/

Centers for Disease Control and Prevention (CDC). (2017b). *Chlamydia—CDC fact sheet*. Retrieved from http://www.cdc.gov/std/chlamydia/stdfact-chlamydia.htm

Centers for Disease Control and Prevention (CDC). (2017c). *What are STDs?* Retrieved from http://www.cdc.gov/std/general/default.htm

Centers for Disease Control and Prevention (CDC). (2017d). *Human papillomavirus (HPV)*. Retrieved from http://www.cdc.gov/std/hpv/default.htm

Centers for Disease Control and Prevention (CDC). (2017e). *Pelvic inflammatory disease (PID)—CDC fact sheet*. Retrieved from http://www.cdc.gov/std/pid/stdfact-pid-detailed.htm

Centers for Disease Control and Prevention (CDC). (2018a). *Hepatitis A questions and answers for health professionals*. Retrieved from http://www.cdc.gov/hepatitis/hav/havfaq.htm#general

Centers for Disease Control and prevention (CDC). (2018b). *Hepatitis B questions and answers for health professionals*. Retrieved from http://www.cdc.gov/hepatitis/hbv/hbvfaq.htm#overview

Centers for Disease Control and Prevention (CDC). (2018c). *Hepatitis C questions and answers for health professionals*. Retrieved from http://www.cdc.gov/hepatitis/hcv/hcvfaq.htm#section1

Centers for Disease Control and Prevention (CDC). (2018d). *HIV among youth*. Retrieved from http://www.cdc.gov/hiv/group/age/youth/index.html

Centers for Disease Control and Prevention (CDC). (2018e). *HIV/AIDS*. Retrieved from http://www.cdc.gov/hiv/basics/index.html

Centers for Disease Control and Prevention (CDC). (2018f). *Sexual risk behaviors: HIV, STD, & teen pregnancy prevention*. Retrieved from http://www.cdc.gov/healthyyouth/sexualbehaviors/

Chandrasekar, P. H. (2017). *Syphilis*. Retrieved from https://emedicine.medscape.com/article/229461-overview

Chen, M. Y., Klausner, J. D., Fairley, C. K., Guy, R., Wilson, D., & Donovan, B. (2015). Syphilis: A fresh look at an old foe. *Sexual Health, 12*(2), 93–95.

Choudhri, Y., Miller, J., Sandhu, J., Leon, A., & Aho, J. (2018). Surveillance: Chlamydia in Canada, 2010–2015. *CCDR, 44*(2). Retrieved from https://www.canada.ca/content/dam/phac-aspc/documents/services/reports-publications/canada-communicable-disease-report-ccdr/monthly-issue/2018-44/issue-2-february-1-2018/ccdrv44i02a03-eng.pdf

Coffey, K., Beral, V., Green, J., Reeves, G., & Barnes, I. (2015). Lifestyle and reproductive risk factors associated with anal cancer in women aged over 50 years. *British Journal of Cancer, 112*(9), 1568–1574. doi: 10.1038/bjc.2015.89

Dillner, J. (2015). Prevention of human papillomavirus–associated cancers. *Seminars in Oncology, 42*(2), 272–283.

Dore, M. (2015). Observations on home HIV testing. *AIDS, 29*(11), 1421–1422.

Fairlie, L., Sipambo, N., Fick, C., & Moultrie, H. (2015). Focus on adolescents with HIV and AIDS. *South African Medical Journal, 104*(12), 897–904.

Gearhart, P. A., Randall, T. C., Buckley, R. M., & Higgins, R. V. (2018). *Human papillomavirus (HPV)*. Retrieved from http://emedicine.medscape.com/article/219110-overview

Gilbert, L. (2015). Update on pelvic inflammatory disease. *Pathology, 47(Suppl 1)*, S49. doi: 10.1097/01.PAT.0000461451.11655.2 c

Guenther, L. C. C., & Maguiness, S. (2018). *Pediculosis and phthiriasis (lice infestation)*. Retrieved from http://emedicine.medscape.com/article/225013-overview

Hay, P. E., Kerry, S. R., Normansell, R., Horner, P. J., Reid, F., Kerry, S. M., … Oakeshott, P. (2016). Which sexually active young female students are most at risk of pelvic inflammatory disease? A prospective study. *Sexually Transmitted Infections, 92*(1), 63–66. doi: 10.1136/sextrans-2015–052063

Health Canada. (2015). *Hepatitis A.* Retrieved from https://www.canada.ca/en/public-health/services/food-poisoning/hepatitis-a.html

Heller, D. S. (2015). *Diseases of the fallopian tube. OB-GYN pathology for the clinician* (pp. 135–145). New York: Springer International Publishing.

King, T. L., Brucker, M. C., Kriebs, J. M., Fahey, J. O., Gegor, C. L., & Varney, H. (2015). *Varney's midwifery* (5th ed.). Burlington, MA: Jones & Bartlett Learning.

Lawrence, D., Cresswell, F., Whetham, J., & Fisher, M. (2015). Syphilis treatment in the presence of HIV: The debate goes on. *Current Opinion in Infectious Diseases, 28*(1), 44–52.

Lee, H., & Lok, A. S. F. (2018). Hepatitis B and pregnancy. *UpToDate.* Retrieved from http://www.uptodate.com/contents/hepatitis-b-and-pregnancy

Mattson, S., & Smith, J. E. (2015). *Core curriculum for maternal-newborn nursing* (5th ed.). St. Louis, MO: Saunders Elsevier.

Monsel, G., & Chosidow, O. (2015). 24. Scabies, lice, and myiasis. In S. David (Ed.). *Clinical infectious disease* (2nd ed., pp. 162–166). Cambridge: Cambridge University Press.

Myers, J. L., Buhi, E. R., Marhefka, S., Daley, E., & Dedrick, R. (2015). Associations between individual and relationship characteristics and genital herpes disclosure. *Journal of Health Psychology, 21*(10), 2283–2293. doi: 10.1177/1359105315575039.

National Advisory Committee on Immunization (NACI). (2017). *Updated recommendations on human papillomavirus (HPV) vaccines: 9-valent HPV vaccine 2-dose immunization schedule and the use of HPV vaccines in immunocompromised populations.* Retrieved from https://www.canada.ca/en/public-health/services/publications/healthy-living/updated-recommendations-human-papillomavirus-immunization-schedule-immunocompromised-populations.html

Oyelowo, T., & Johnson, J. L. (2016). *A guide to women's health* (2nd ed.). Burlington, MA: Jones & Bartlett Learning.

Petrova, D., & Garcia-Retamero, R. (2015). Effective evidence-based programs for preventing sexually-transmitted infections: A meta-analysis. *Current HIV Research, 13*(5), 432–438.

Public Health Agency of Canada (PHAC). (2013a). *Section 4–8: Canadian guidelines on sexually transmitted infections – management and treatment of specific syndromes – Vaginal discharge. In Canadian guidelines on sexually transmitted infections.* Retrieved from https://www.canada.ca/en/public-health/services/infectious-diseases/sexual-health-sexually-transmitted-infections/canadian-guidelines/sexually-transmitted-infections/canadian-guidelines-sexually-transmitted-infections-26.html

Public Health Agency of Canada (PHAC). (2013b). *Section 4-4: Pelvic inflammatory disease (PID). In Canadian guidelines on sexually transmitted infections.* Retrieved from https://www.canada.ca/en/public-health/services/infectious-diseases/sexual-health-sexually-transmitted-infections/canadian-guidelines/sexually-transmitted-infections/canadian-guidelines-sexually-transmitted-infections-22.html

Public Health Agency of Canada (PHAC). (2014a). *Supplementary statement for recommendations related to the diagnosis, management, and follow-up of pelvic inflammatory disease. In Canadian guidelines on sexually transmitted infections.* Retrieved from https://www.canada.ca/en/public-health/services/infectious-diseases/sexual-health-sexually-transmitted-infections/canadian-guidelines/sexually-transmitted-infections/canadian-guidelines-sexually-transmitted-infections-11.html

Public Health Agency of Canada (PHAC). (2014b). *Human immunodeficiency virus: HIV screening and testing guide.* Retrieved from https://www.canada.ca/en/public-health/services/hiv-aids/hiv-screening-testing-guide.html

Public Health Agency of Canada (PHAC). (2016). *Canadian guidelines on sexually transmitted infections.* Retrieved from http://www.phac-aspc.gc.ca/std-mts/sti-its/

Public Health Agency of Canada (PHAC). (2017a). *Report on sexually transmitted infections in Canada: 2013–2014.* Retrieved from https://www.canada.ca/en/public-health/services/publications/diseases-conditions/report-sexually-transmitted-infections-canada-2013-14.html

Public Health Agency of Canada (PHAC). (2017b). *Canadian guidelines on sexually transmitted infections, Section 5.2: Management and treatment of specific infections, chlamydial infections.* Retrieved from https://www.canada.ca/en/public-health/services/infectious-diseases/sexual-health-sexually-transmitted-infections/canadian-guidelines/sexually-transmitted-infections/canadian-guidelines-sexually-transmitted-infections-30.html

Public Health Agency of Canada (PHAC). (2017c). *Report on the enhanced surveillance of antimicrobial-resistant gonorrhea.* Retrieved from https://www.canada.ca/content/dam/phac-aspc/documents/services/publications/diseases-conditions/gonorrhea-alternate-treatment/gonorrhea-2014-pilot-surveillance-antimicrobial-resistant-eng.pdf

Public Health Agency of Canada (PHAC). (2017d). *Canadian guidelines on sexually transmitted infections: 2016 Updates summary.* Retrieved from https://www.canada.ca/content/dam/phac-aspc/migration/phac-aspc/std-mts/sti-its/assets/pdf/updates-summary-eng.pdf

Public Health Agency of Canada (PHAC). (2017e). *Human papillomavirus (HPV).* Retrieved from https://www.canada.ca/en/public-health/services/infectious-diseases/sexual-health-sexually-transmitted-infections/human-papillomavirus-hpv.html

Public Health Agency of Canada (PHAC). (2018). *Canadian guidelines on sexually transmitted infections: Section 5–10, syphilis.* Retrieved from https://www.canada.ca/en/public-health/services/infectious-diseases/sexual-health-sexually-transmitted-infections/canadian-guidelines/sexually-transmitted-infections/canadian-guidelines-sexually-transmitted-infections-27.html

Pyrsopoulos, N. T., & Reddy, K. R. (2018). *Hepatitis B.* Retrieved from http://emedicine.medscape.com/article/177632-overview

Queenan, J. T., Spong, C. Y., & Lockwood, C. J. (2015). *Protocols for high-risk pregnancies: An evidence-based approach* (6th ed.). Somerset, NJ: John Wiley & Sons.

Qureshi, S. (2018). *Chlamydia (chlamydial genitourinary infections).* Retrieved from http://emedicine.medscape.com/article/214823-overview

Ross, C. E., Tao, G., Patton, M., & Hoover, K. W. (2015). Screening for human immunodeficiency virus and other sexually transmitted diseases among US women with prenatal care. *Obstetrics & Gynecology, 125*(5), 1211–1216.

Sangkomkamhang, U. S., Lumbiganon, P., Prasertcharoensuk, W., & Laopaiboon, M. (2015). Antenatal lower genital tract infection screening and treatment programs for preventing preterm delivery. *Cochrane Database of Systematic Reviews, 2*, CD006178. doi: 10.1002/14651858.CD006178.pub3.

Selim, M. A., Parra, V., Sangueza, O. P., Requena, L., & Sangueza, M. A. (2015). Infectious diseases and infestations of the vulva. In P. H. Mai, & M. A. Selim (Eds.). *Vulvar pathology* (pp. 139–193). New York: Springer.

Shepherd, S. M. (2017). *Pelvic inflammatory disease.* Retrieved from http://emedicine.medscape.com/article/256448-overview

Silasi, M., Cardenas, I., Kwon, J. Y., Racicot, K., Aldo, P., & Mor, G. (2015). Viral infections during pregnancy. *American Journal of Reproductive Immunology, 73*(3), 199–213.

Smith, D. S., & Ramos, N. (2018). *Trichomoniasis.* Retrieved from http://emedicine.medscape.com/article/230617-overview

Society of Obstetricians and Gynaecologists of Canada (SOGC). (2013). *The prevention of early-onset neonatal group B streptococcal disease.* Clinical practice guideline number 298. Retrieved from https://sogc.org/wp-content/uploads/2013/09/October2013-CPG298-ENG-Online_Final.pdf

Stamm, L. V. (2015). Syphilis: Antibiotic treatment and resistance. *Epidemiology and Infection, 143*(08), 1567–1574.

Thomas, J., Bates, C. M., & Mathew, T. (2015). P251 treatment dilemma of chlamydia in pregnancy. *Sexually Transmitted Infections, 91*(Suppl 1), A98–A98.

Tuite, A. R, Jayaraman, G. C., Allen, V. G., Fisman, D. N. (2012). Estimation of the burden of disease and costs of genital Chlamydia trachomatis infection in Canada. *Sexually Transmitted Diseases, 39*(4), 260--267. doi: 10.1097/OLQ.0b013e31824717ae

U.S. Department of Health and Human Services Office of Adolescent Health. (2016). *Adolescent development and STDs.* Retrieved from http://www.hhs.gov/ash/oah/adolescent-health-topics/reproductive-health/stds.html

Wong, B. (2018). *Gonorrhea.* Retrieved from http://emedicine.medscape.com/article/218059-overview

World Health Organization (WHO). (2018a). *HIV/AIDS: Treatment and care.* Retrieved from http://www.who.int/hiv/topics/treatment/en/

World Health Organization (WHO). (2018b). *Hepatitis B.* Retrieved from http://www.who.int/mediacentre/factsheets/fs204/en/

World Health Organization (WHO). (2018c). *Updated recommendations on first-line and second-line antiretroviral regimens and post-exposure prophylaxis and recommendations on early infant diagnosis of HIV.* Retrieved from http://apps.who.int/iris/bitstream/handle/10665/273632/WHO-CDS-HIV-18.18-eng.pdf?ua=1

World Health Organization (WHO). (2018d). *Viral suppression for HIV treatment success and prevention of sexual transmission of HIV.* Retrieved from http://www.who.int/hiv/mediacentre/news/viral-supression-hiv-transmission/en/

World Health Organization (WHO). (2018e). *Infant and young child feeding.* Retrieved from http://www.who.int/news-room/fact-sheets/detail/infant-and-young-child-feeding

Zapata, L. B., Tregear, S. J., Curtis, K. M., Tiller, M., Pazol, K., Mautone-Smith, N., & Gavin, L. E. (2015). Impact of contraceptive counseling in clinical settings: A systematic review. *American Journal of Preventive Medicine, 49*(2), S31–S45.

CHAPTER **WORKSHEET**

MULTIPLE CHOICE QUESTIONS

1. Which of the following contraceptive methods offers protection against sexually transmitted infections (STIs)?
   a. Oral contraceptives
   b. Withdrawal
   c. Latex condom
   d. Intrauterine system

2. When teaching about HIV transmission, which of the following actions does the nurse explain cannot transmit the virus?
   a. Shaking hands
   b. Sharing drug needles
   c. Sexual intercourse
   d. Breastfeeding

3. A woman with HPV is likely to present with which nursing assessment finding?
   a. Profuse, pus-filled vaginal discharge
   b. Clusters of genital warts
   c. Single painless ulcer
   d. Multiple vesicles on genitalia

4. The nurse's discharge teaching plan for the woman with PID should reinforce which of the following potentially life-threatening complications?
   a. Involuntary infertility
   b. Chronic pelvic pain
   c. Depression
   d. Ectopic pregnancy

5. To confirm a finding of primary syphilis, the nurse would observe which of the following on the external genitalia?
   a. A highly variable skin rash
   b. A yellow-green vaginal discharge
   c. A nontender, indurated ulcer
   d. A localized gumma formation

6. A sexually active 19-year-old presents to the clinic with postcoital bleeding, dysuria, and a yellow discharge. Her cervix upon examination is red and friable. What might the nurse suspect?
   a. Cervical cancer
   b. A tampon injury
   c. Primary syphilis
   d. Chlamydia

CRITICAL THINKING EXERCISE

1. Sally, age 17, comes to the teen clinic saying that she is in pain and has some "crud" between her legs. The nurse takes her into the examining room and questions her about her symptoms. Sally states she had numerous genital bumps that had been filled with fluid, then ruptured and turned into ulcers with crusts. In addition, she has pain on urination and overall body pain. Sally says she had unprotected sex with several men when she was drunk at a party a few weeks back, but she thought they were "clean."
   a. Which STI would the nurse suspect?
   b. The nurse should give immediate consideration to which of Sally's reported symptoms?
   c. What should be the goal of the nurse in teaching Sally about STIs?

STUDY ACTIVITIES

1. Select a website at the end of the chapter to explore. Educate yourself about one specific STI thoroughly and share your expertise with your clinical group.

2. Contact your local Public Health Office and request current statistics regarding three STIs. Ask them to compare the current number of cases reported to last year's. Are they less or more? What may be some of the reasons for the change in the number of cases reported?

3. Request permission to attend a local STI clinic to shadow a nurse for a few hours. Describe the nurse's counselling role with clients and what specific information is emphasized to clients.

4. Two common STIs that appear together and commonly are treated together regardless of identification of the secondary one are _____ and _____.

5. Genital warts can be treated with which of the following? Select all that apply.
   a. Penicillin
   b. Podophyllin
   c. Imiquimod
   d. Cryotherapy
   e. Antiretroviral therapy
   f. Acyclovir

CHAPTER **WORKSHEET**

BRINGING IT ALL TOGETHER: A CASE STUDY

Charlotte, a 22-year-old, has presented at the local clinic with concerns of having contracted a sexually transmitted infection (STI). During the nursing interview Charlotte identifies that she has been sexually active since the age of 15 and has had "at least 5 different sex partners."

The health assessment confirms that Charlotte has been infected with pediculosis pubis (pubic lice) and treatment has been prescribed.

Go to thePoint **to find questions to consider about this case.**

6

Disorders of the Breasts

Learning Objectives

Upon completion of the chapter, you will be able to:

1. Identify the incidence, risk factors, screening methods, and treatment modalities for benign breast conditions.

2. Appraise reasons behind breast augmentation including the potential benefits and risks.

3. Outline preventive strategies for breast cancer through lifestyle changes and health screening.

4. Analyze the incidence, risk factors, treatment modalities, and nursing considerations related to breast cancer.

5. Develop an educational plan to teach BSE to a group of high-risk women.

Nancy hasn't been able to sleep well since she felt the lump in her left breast over a month ago, just after her 60th birthday. She knows she is at high risk because her mother died of breast cancer, but she can't bring herself to have it checked out.

INTRODUCTION

The breasts are modified sweat glands, lying over the pectoralis major muscles of the chest wall. Physiologically, the breast is an organ specialized for milk formation to nourish their offspring. Each breast extends approximately from the second to the sixth rib. The female breasts are closely linked to womanhood in North American culture. The development of breasts acts as a physical marker for transitions from one stage of life to another, and although the primary function of the breasts is lactation, they are perceived as a symbol of beauty and sexuality.

This chapter discusses assessments, screening procedures, and management of specific benign and malignant breast disorders. Nurses play a key role in helping individuals maintain breast health by providing education and screening. A good working knowledge of early detection techniques, diagnosis, and treatment options is essential.

BENIGN BREAST DISORDERS

A **benign breast disorder** is any noncancerous breast abnormality. Though not life-threatening, benign disorders can cause pain and discomfort, and they account for a large number of visits to primary care providers. Fully understanding benign breast disorders should enable the nurse to appropriately evaluate symptoms, determine which breast lesions require treatment, and identify clients who are at increased risk for breast cancer.

Depending on the type of benign breast disorder, treatment might or might not be necessary. Although these disorders are benign, the emotional trauma individuals experience is phenomenal. Fear, anxiety, disbelief, helplessness, and depression are just a few of the reactions that a person may have when a breast lump is discovered. Many people believe that all lumps are cancerous, but actually more than 80% of the lumps discovered are benign and need no treatment (Alexander et al., 2014). Patience, support, and education are essential components of nursing care.

The most commonly encountered benign breast disorders include fibrocystic changes of the breasts, fibroadenomas, and mastitis. Although these breast disorders are considered benign, fibrocystic changes of the breasts carry a cancer risk, with prolific masses and hyperplastic changes occurring within the breasts. Generally speaking, fibroadenomas and mastitis carry little cancer risk (Seetharam & Rodrigues, 2015). Table 6.1 summarizes benign breast conditions.

Fibrocystic Breast Changes

Fibrocystic breast changes, also known as *benign breast disease* (BBD), represent a variety of changes in the glandular and structural tissues of the breast. Because this condition affects 50% to 60% of all women at some point, it is more accurately defined as a "change" rather than a "disease." Fibrocystic changes are caused by an overgrowth of fibrous tissues in the connective tissues supporting the breasts. This is frequently accompanied by the presence of fluid-filled cysts, which contribute to the lumpy feeling experienced by individuals. In contrast to malignant breast lesions, the cysts that develop move freely when palpated and symptoms decline after menopause when levels of estrogen and progesterone drop (Sabel, 2018). Fibrocystic changes do not increase the risk

TABLE 6.1		SUMMARY OF BENIGN BREAST DISORDERS			
Breast Condition	**Nipple Discharge**	**Site**	**Characteristics/Age of Client**	**Tenderness**	**Diagnosis and Treatment**

Fibrocystic breast changes	+ or −	Bilateral; upper outer quadrant	Round, smooth
			Several lesions
			Cyclic, palpable
			30–50 years old
				+	Aspiration and biopsy
					Limit caffeine;
					  ibuprofen;
					  supportive bra

Fibroadenomas		Unilateral; nipple area or upper outer quadrant	Round, firm, movable Palpable, rubbery Well delineated Single lesion 15–30 years old	−	Mammogram "Watchful waiting" Aspiration and biopsy Surgical excision
Mastitis	−	Unilateral; outer quadrant	Wedge shaped Warmth, redness Swelling Nipple cracked Breast engorged	+	Antibiotics Warm shower Supportive bra Breastfeeding Increase fluids

Adapted from Alexander, L. L., LaRosa, J. H., Bader, H., & Garfield, S. (2014). *New dimensions in women's health* (6th ed.). Sudbury, MA: Jones & Bartlett; American Cancer Society (ACS). (2019). *Fibrosis and simple cysts in the breast.* Retrieved from https://www.cancer.org/cancer/breast-cancer/non-cancerous-breast-conditions/fibrosis-and-simple-cysts-in-the-breast.html; and Bope, E. T., & Kellerman, R. D. (2015). *Conn's current therapy 2015.* Philadelphia, PA: Saunders Elsevier.

of breast cancer for most people except when the breast biopsy shows "atypia" or abnormal breast cells. The cause for concern for many individuals with fibrocystic changes is that breast examinations and mammography become more difficult to interpret with multiple cysts present, and early cancerous lesions may occasionally be overlooked (American Cancer Society [ACS], 2018a).

Fibrocystic breast changes are most common in individuals between the ages of 20 and 50. The condition is rare in postmenopausal persons not taking hormone replacement therapy (HRT). According to the ACS (2018a), fibrocystic breast changes affect at least half of all women at some point in their lives and are the most common breast disorder today.

Therapeutic Management

Management of the symptoms of fibrocystic breast changes begins with self-care. For some individuals, diet and lifestyle changes help to reduce discomfort. Other options include wearing a supportive bra, taking over-the-counter pain relievers, and limiting salt consumption which can cause fluid retention (Files, Allen, & Pruthi, 2015). In severe cases drugs, including bromocriptine, tamoxifen, or danazol, can be used to reduce the influence of estrogen on breast tissue. However, several undesirable side effects, including masculinization, have been documented. Aspiration or surgical removal of breast lumps will reduce pain and swelling by removing the space-occupying mass.

Nursing Assessment

Nursing assessment consists of a health history, physical examination, and laboratory and diagnostic tests.

HEALTH HISTORY

Ask the client about common clinical manifestations, which include lumpy, tender breasts, particularly during the week before menses. Changes in breast tissue produce pain by nerve irritation from edema in connective tissue and by fibrosis from nerve pinching. The pain is cyclic and frequently dissipates after the onset of menses. The pain is described as a dull, aching feeling of fullness. Masses or nodularities usually appear in both breasts and are often found in the upper outer quadrants. Some individuals also experience spontaneous clear to yellow nipple discharge when the breast is squeezed or manipulated.

PHYSICAL EXAMINATION

It is best to examine a client's breast a week after menses, when swelling has subsided. The breast examination is performed using the Triple Touch Method in which the health care provider uses the pads of the middle three fingers and makes dime-sized overlapping circles to feel the breast tissue with three levels of pressure: light, medium, and firm (Jarvis, 2015). Observe the breasts for

fibrosis, or thickening of the normal breast tissues, which occurs in the early stages. Cysts form in the later stages and feel like multiple, smooth, well-delineated tiny pebbles or bumpy oatmeal under the skin (Fig. 6.1). On physical examination of the breasts, a few characteristics might be helpful in differentiating a cyst from a cancerous lesion. Cancerous lesions typically are fixed and painless and may cause skin retraction (pulling). Cysts tend to be mobile and tender and do not cause skin retraction in the surrounding tissue.

LABORATORY AND DIAGNOSTIC TESTS

Mammography can be helpful in distinguishing fibrocystic changes from breast cancer. Ultrasound is a useful adjunct to mammography for breast evaluation because it helps to differentiate a cystic mass from a solid one (Dixon & Macaskill, 2015). Ultrasound produces images of the breasts by sending sound waves through a gel applied to the breasts. Fine-needle aspiration biopsy can also be done to differentiate a solid tumour, cyst, or malignancy. A fine-needle aspiration biopsy uses a thin needle guided by ultrasound to the mass. In a method called stereotactic needle biopsy, a computer maps the exact location of the mass using mammograms taken from two angles, and the map is used to guide the needle.

Nursing Management

A nurse caring for clients with fibrocystic breast changes can teach them about the condition, provide tips for self-care (Teaching Guidelines 6.1), suggest lifestyle changes, and demonstrate how to perform monthly breast self-examination (BSE) after their menses to monitor the changes. Nursing Care Plan 6.1 (at the end of the chapter) presents a plan of care for a client with fibrocystic breast changes.

 Teaching Guidelines 6.1
RELIEVING SYMPTOMS OF FIBROCYSTIC BREAST CHANGES

- Wear an extra-supportive bra to prevent undue strain on the ligaments of the breasts to reduce discomfort.
- Take oral contraceptives, as recommended by a health care practitioner, to stabilize the monthly hormonal levels.
- Eat a low-fat diet rich in fruits, vegetables, and grains to maintain a healthy nutritional lifestyle and ideal weight.
- Apply heat to the breasts to help reduce pain via vasodilation of vessels.
- Take diuretics, as recommended by a health care practitioner, to counteract fluid retention and swelling of the breasts.
- Reduce salt intake to reduce fluid retention and swelling in the breasts.

FIGURE 6.1 **A.** Fibrocystic breast changes. **B.** Breast cysts. **C.** This gross study shows that most of the abnormal tissue is fibrous. Cysts are relatively inconspicuous in this example. **D.** The microscopic study shows dense fibrous tissue containing dilated ducts lined by hyperplastic epithelium. (Images A & B are from The Anatomical Chart Company. [2006]. *Atlas of pathophysiology*. Springhouse, PA: Springhouse Corporation. Images C & D courtesy of McConnell, T. H. [2014]. *The nature of disease pathology for the health professions* [2nd ed.]. Philadelphia, PA: Lippincott Williams & Wilkins.)

• Take over-the-counter medications, such as acetyl-salicylic acid (Aspirin) or ibuprofen (Motrin, Advil, Nuprin), to reduce inflammation and discomfort.
• Use thiamine and vitamin E therapy. This has been found helpful for some individuals, but research has failed to demonstrate a direct benefit from either therapy.

• Take medications as prescribed (e.g., bromocriptine, tamoxifen, or danazol).
• Discuss the possibility of aspiration or surgical removal of breast lumps with a health care practitioner.
• Avoid caffeinated drinks (coffee, tea, soda) which tend to trigger breast discomfort.

Fibroadenomas

Fibroadenomas are common benign solid breast tumours that occur in about 25% of all women and account for up to half of all breast biopsies. They are the most common mass in women aged 15 to 25 years (Seetharam & Rodrigues, 2015). They are considered hyperplastic lesions associated with an aberration of normal development and involution rather than a neoplasm. Fibroadenomas can be stimulated by external estrogen, progesterone, lactation, and pregnancy (Schuiling & Likis, 2016). They are composed of both fibrous and glandular tissue that feels round or oval, firm, rubbery and smooth, and is mobile and may be tender. They are usually unilateral, but may present in both breasts (Alexander et al., 2014). Giant fibroadenomas account for approximately 4% of cases. These masses are frequently larger than 5 cm and occur most often in pregnant or lactating individuals. These large lesions may regress in size once hormonal stimulation subsides (Janardhan, Venkateshwar, & Rao, 2015). Fibroadenomas are rarely associated with cancer.

Therapeutic Management

Treatment may include a period of "watchful waiting" because many fibroadenomas stop growing or shrink on their own without any treatment. Other growths may need to be surgically removed if they do not regress or if they remain unchanged. Cryoablation, an alternative to surgery, can also be used to remove a tumour. In this procedure, extremely cold gas is piped into the tumour using ultrasound guidance. The tumour freezes and dies. The current trend is toward a more conservative approach to treatment after careful evaluation and continued monitoring.

Nursing Assessment

Ask the client about clinical manifestations of fibroadenomas. These lumps are felt as firm, rubbery, well-circumscribed, freely mobile nodules that might or might not be tender when palpated.

Breast fibroadenomas are usually detected incidentally during clinical or self-examinations and are usually located in the upper outer quadrant of the breast; more than one may be present (Fig. 6.2). Several other breast lesions have similar characteristics, so every client with a breast mass should be evaluated to exclude cancer. A clinical breast examination (CBE) by a health care provider is critical. In addition, diagnostic studies include imaging studies (mammography, ultrasound, or both) and some form of biopsy, most often a fine-needle aspiration, core needle biopsy, or stereotactic needle biopsy. The core needle biopsy removes a small cylinder of tissue from the breast mass, more than the fine-needle aspiration biopsy. If additional tissue needs to be evaluated, the advanced breast biopsy instrument (ABBI) is

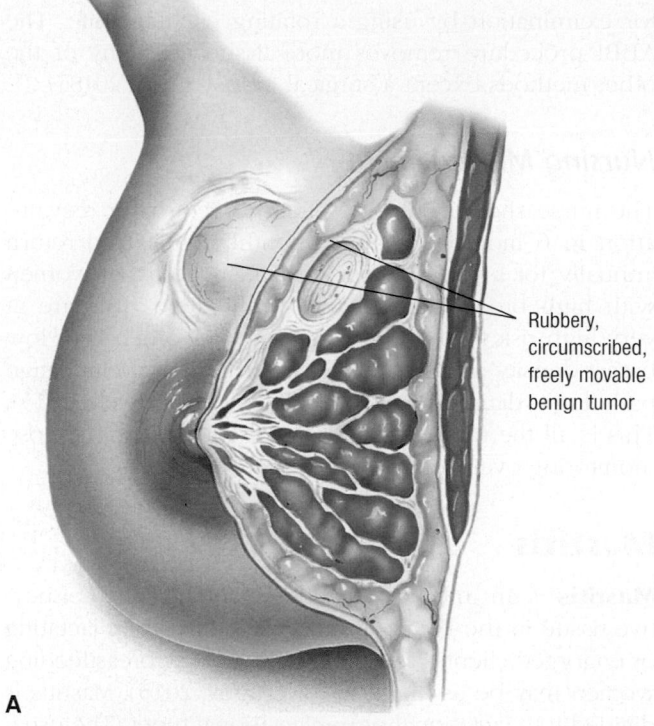

Rubbery, circumscribed, freely movable benign tumor

A

B

FIGURE 6.2 **A.** Fibroadenoma. (Asset provided by Anatomical Chart Co.) **B.** Spot compression view of a smoothly marinated mass proven to represent a fibroadenoma. Ultrasonography demonstrated a solid mass.

used. This instrument removes a larger cylinder of tissue for examination by using a rotating circular knife. The ABBI procedure removes more tissue than any of the other methods except a surgical biopsy (ACS, 2018a).

Nursing Management

The nurse should urge the client to return for reevaluation in 6 months, perform monthly BSEs, and return annually for a CBE. Recent studies suggest that women with high breast density and proliferative BBD are at very high risk for future breast cancer. Women with low breast density are at low risk, regardless of their benign pathologic diagnosis (Slanetz, Freer, & Birdwell, 2015). This is all the more reason for individuals to have close monitoring over time.

Mastitis

Mastitis is an infection or inflammation of the connective tissue in the breast that occurs primarily in lactating or engorged clients. The prevalence of it in breastfeeding women may be as high as 33% (Faguy, 2015). Mastitis is divided into lactational or nonlactational types. The usual causative organisms for lactational mastitis are *Staphylococcus aureus, Haemophilus influenzae,* and haemophilus and streptococcus species, the source of which is the baby's flora. Lactating mastitis typically occurs in the first 2 to 3 weeks of lactation, but can occur at any stage of lactation. One or more of the ducts drain poorly or become blocked, resulting in bacterial growth in the retained milk (Pluchinotta, 2015). The only evidence-based predisposing factor that may lead to mastitis is the development of milk stasis. However, other associated factors include damaged or cracked nipples, especially those colonized with *S. aureus;* irregular or missed feedings; failing to allow the infant to empty one breast completely before moving on to the next breast; poor latch and transfer of milk; illness of mother or infant; oversupply; a tight bra; blocked nipple pore or duct; being primiparous; and maternal stress and fatigue (Miller, Escamilla, & King, 2018).

Nonlactational mastitis can be caused by **duct ectasia,** which occurs when the milk ducts become congested with secretions and debris, resulting in periductal inflammation. It may be divided into central (periareolar) and peripheral breast lesions. Periareolar infections consist of active inflammation around nondilated subareolar breast ducts—a condition termed periductal mastitis. Peripheral nonlactating breast abscesses are less common than periareolar abscesses and are often associated with an underlying condition, such as diabetes, rheumatoid arthritis, steroid treatment, granulomatous lobular mastitis, and trauma (Faguy, 2015). Clients with these types of abscesses present with greenish nipple discharge, nipple retraction, and noncyclical pain.

Therapeutic Management

Effective milk removal, pain medication, and antibiotic therapy have been the mainstays of treatment. Management of both types of mastitis involves the use of oral antibiotics (usually a penicillinase-resistant penicillin or cephalosporin), warm compresses to the inflamed area of the breast, continued breastfeeding, and acetaminophen (Tylenol) for pain and fever (King et al., 2015).

Nursing Assessment

Assess the client's health history for risk factors for mastitis, which include poor hand hygiene ductal abnormalities, nipple cracks and fissures, lowered maternal defenses due to fatigue, tight clothing, poor support of pendulous breasts, failure to empty the breasts properly while breastfeeding, or missing breastfeedings.

The diagnosis of mastitis is made clinically on the basis of a localized, unilateral area of erythema with associated fever. Assess the client for clinical manifestations of mastitis, which include flu-like symptoms of malaise, nausea, headache, leukocytosis, fever, fatigue, and chills. Physical examination of the breasts reveals increased warmth, swollen area of one breast, redness, tenderness, and swelling. The nipple is usually cracked or abraded and the breast is distended with milk (Fig. 6.3). In a lactating person, severe engorgement can be differentiated from mastitis because engorgement is bilateral with general involvement of the whole breast. Ultrasound scans can be undertaken to differentiate between the types of mastitis or abscesses, but typically the diagnosis is made based on history and examination.

Nursing Management

Teach clients about the etiology of mastitis and encourage them to continue to breastfeed, emphasizing that it is safe for their infants to do so. Stress to all breastfeeding clients

FIGURE 6.3 Mastitis. (From Sweet, R. L., & Gibbs, R. S. [2009]. *Infectious diseases of the female genital tract.* Philadelphia, PA: Lippincott Williams & Wilkins.)

to check for medication safety before taking it. Drugs administered to breastfeeding clients can accumulate in the bodies of their infants and can alter infant's bowel flora, causing diarrhea. Clients should be warned about this to reduce their anxiety. Once it has been declared safe to do so, the nurse should urge them to take the medication as prescribed until completed. Continued emptying of the breast or pumping improves the outcome, decreases the duration of symptoms, and decreases the incidence of breast abscess. Thus, continued breastfeeding is recommended in the presence of mastitis (King et al., 2015).

Although 80% of breast biopsy results prove to be benign, increased surveillance is necessary because of the risk of cancer development. The recommended follow-up schedule is imaging (mammography or ultrasound) and a CBE by a surgeon at 6, 12, and 24 months after a benign breast biopsy finding (Tharpe, Farley, & Jordan, 2016). Instructions for the client with mastitis are detailed in Teaching Guidelines 6.2.

Teaching Guidelines 6.2
CARING FOR MASTITIS

- Take medications as prescribed to reduce inflammation and infection.
- Continue breastfeeding, as tolerated to keep the milk flowing.
- Begin feeding on most affected breast to allow it to be emptied first.
- Massage the breasts before and during breastfeeding to encourage milk extraction.
- Wear a supportive bra 24 hours a day to support the breasts for comfort.
- Increase fluid intake to stay hydrated.
- Gently massage toward nipple several times daily.
- Vary the infants breastfeeding position—cradle, side-lying, football, and belly to belly.
- Make sure infant is positioned correctly on the nipple to prevent discomfort.
- Practice good hand hygiene techniques to reduce risk of bacterial transfer.
- Apply warm compresses to the affected breast or take a warm shower before breastfeeding.
- Frequently change positions while nursing to improve milk flow.
- Get adequate rest and nutrition to support or improve the immune system.
- Instruct to contact their health care provider if fever returns, chills, or worsening symptoms.

Adapted from King, T. L., Brucker, M. C., Kriebs, J. M., Fahey, J. O., Gegor, C. L., & Varney, H. (2015). *Varney's midwifery* (5th ed.). Burlington, MA: Jones & Bartlett Learning; and Tharpe, N. L., Farley, C. L., & Jordan, R. G. (2016). *Clinical practice guidelines for midwifery & women's health* (4th ed.). Burlington, MA: Jones & Bartlett Learning.

MALIGNANT BREAST DISORDER

Breast cancer is a neoplastic disease in which normal body cells are transformed into malignant ones (National Cancer Institute [NCI], 2018a). It is the most common cancer in women and the second leading cause of cancer deaths (lung cancer is first) among Canadian women. It is estimated that one out of every eight Canadian women will develop the disease at some time during her life, and the mortality rate of those with breast cancer is 1 in 31 (Canadian Cancer Society's Advisory Committee on Cancer Statistics [CCACCS], 2017).

Breast cancer can also affect men, but less than 1% of all individuals diagnosed with breast cancer annually are men. In Canada, an estimated 26,300 cases of breast cancer were diagnosed in women in 2017, and 230 cases diagnosed in men (CCACCS, 2017). Because men are not routinely screened for breast cancer, the diagnosis is often delayed. The most common clinical manifestation of male breast cancer is a painless, firm, subareolar breast mass. Any suspicious breast mass in a male should undergo diagnostic biopsy. If a malignancy is diagnosed, typical treatment is mastectomy with assessment of the axillary nodes.

The cause of breast cancer, while not well understood, is thought to be a complex interaction between environmental, genetic, and hormonal factors. Breast cancer is a progressive rather than a systemic disease, meaning that most cancers grow from small size with low metastatic potential to larger size and greater metastatic potential. Tumour stage, size, and lymph node involvement are major predictors of metastatic potential (Arora et al., 2015).

Consider This

It was pouring down rain and I was driving alone along dark wet streets to my 8 AM appointment for a breast ultrasound. I recently had my annual mammogram and the radiologist thought he saw something suspicious on my right breast. I was on my way to confirm or refute his suspicions, and I couldn't keep focused on the road ahead. For the past few days I had been a basket case, fearing the worst. I was playing in my mind, what I would do if...? What changes would I make in my life and how would I react when told? I have been through such personal turmoil since that doctor announced he wanted "more tests."

Thoughts: *This woman is worrying and is emotionally devastated before she even has a conclusive diagnosis. Is this a typical reaction to a breast disorder? Why do people fear the worst? Many individuals use denial to mask their feelings and hope against hope the doctor made a mistake or misread their mammogram. How would you react if you or your sister, friend, or mother were confronted with a breast disorder?*

Pathophysiology

Cancer is not just one disease, but rather a group of diseases that result from unregulated cell growth. Without regulation, cells divide and grow uncontrollably until they eventually form a tumour. Extensive research has determined that all cancer is the result of changes in DNA or chromosome structure that cause the mutation of specific genes. Most genetic mutations that cause cancer are acquired sporadically, which means they occur by chance and are not necessarily due to inherited mutations (Shannon & Chittenden, 2015). Cancer development is thought to be clonal in nature, which means that each cell is derived from another cell. If one cell develops a mutation, any daughter cell derived from that cell will have that same mutation, and this process continues until a malignant tumour forms.

Breast cancer starts in the epithelial cells that line the mammary ducts within the breast. The growth rate depends on hormonal influences, mainly estrogen and progesterone. The two major categories of breast cancer are noninvasive and invasive. Noninvasive, or in situ, breast cancers are those that have not extended beyond their duct, lobule, or point of origin into the surrounding breast tissue. Conversely, invasive (infiltrating) breast cancers have extended into the surrounding breast tissue, with the potential to metastasize. Many researchers believe that most invasive cancers probably originate as noninvasive cancers (Cuzick & Thorat, 2015).

Breast cancer is considered to be a highly variable disease. While the process of metastasis is a complex and poorly understood phenomenon, there is evidence to suggest that new vascularization of the tumour plays an important role in the biologic aggressiveness of breast cancer (Toi et al., 2015). Breast cancer metastasizes widely and to almost all organs of the body, but primarily to the bone, lungs, lymph nodes, liver, and brain. The first sites of metastases are usually local or regional, involving the chest wall or axillary supraclavicular lymph nodes or bone (ACS, 2018a).

Invasive Ductal Carcinoma

By far the most common breast cancer is invasive ductal carcinoma, which represents 85% of all cases (ACS, 2018c). **Carcinoma** is a malignant tumour that occurs in epithelial tissue; it tends to infiltrate and give rise to metastases. The incidence of this cancer peaks in the sixth decade of life (>60 years old). It spreads rapidly to axillary and other lymph nodes, even while small. Infiltrating ductal carcinoma may take various histologic forms—well differentiated and slow growing, poorly differentiated and infiltrating, or highly malignant and undifferentiated with numerous metastases. This common type of breast cancer starts in the ducts, breaks through the duct wall, and invades the fatty breast tissue. This type of cancer accounts for 75% of all breast cancers (Stopeck, Chalasani, & Thompson, 2015).

Invasive Lobular Carcinoma

Invasive lobular carcinomas, which originate in the terminal lobular units of breast ducts, account for 10% of all cases of breast cancer. The peak incidence is in women aged 40 to 50 years old. It presents as an area of ill-defined thickening rather than a palpable mass. The tumour is frequently located in the upper outer quadrant of the breast, and by the time it is discovered the prognosis is usually poor (Selvi, 2015).

Other Invasive Carcinomas

Other invasive types of cancer include tubular carcinoma (29%), which is fairly uncommon and typically occurs in women aged 55 and older. Colloid carcinoma (2% to 4%) occurs in women 60 to 70 years of age and is characterized by the presence of large pools of mucus interspersed with small islands of tumour cells. Medullary carcinoma accounts for 5% to 7% of malignant breast tumours; it occurs frequently in younger women (<50 years of age) and grows into large tumour masses. Inflammatory breast cancer (<4%) often presents with skin edema, redness, and warmth and is associated with a poor prognosis. Paget disease (2% to 4%) originates in the nipple and typically occurs with invasive ductal carcinoma (Bope & Kellerman, 2015).

Staging of Breast Cancer

Breast cancers are classified into three stages based on:
1. Tumour size
2. Extent of lymph node involvement
3. Evidence of metastasis

The purposes of tumour staging are to determine the probability that the tumour has metastasized, to decide on an appropriate course of therapy, and to assess the client's prognosis. Table 6.2 gives details and characteristics of each stage (also Fig. 6.4). The overall 10-year survival rate for a woman with stage I breast cancer is 80% to 90%; for a woman with stage II, it is about 50%. The outlook is not as good for women with stage III or IV disease (Alexander et al., 2014).

There is no completely accurate way to know whether the cancer has micrometastasized to distant organs, but certain tests can help determine if the cancer has spread. A bone scan can be performed to assess the bones. Magnetic resonance imaging (MRI) can be used to detect metastases to the liver, abdominal cavity, lungs, or brain.

Risk Factors

An estimated 80% of women in whom breast cancer develops have no documented risk factors (Bope & Kellerman, 2015). Breast cancer is thought to develop in

TABLE 6.2	STAGING OF BREAST CANCER
Stage	**Characteristics**
0	Carcinoma in situ One of the following applies: • There are cancer cells only in the lining of a breast duct. This is called ductal carcinoma in situ (DCIS). • There is a buildup of abnormal cells in the breast lobules. This is called lobular carcinoma in situ (LCIS). • There is Paget disease of the breast without any invasive carcinoma, DCIS or LCIS.
1A	• The tumour is 2 cm or smaller
1B	• The tumour is 2 cm or smaller, or no tumour can be seen in the breast. A small number of cancer cells are found in the lymph nodes (micrometastases). Each lymph node with cancer cells in it is no larger than 2 mm.
2A	• The tumour is 2 cm or smaller, or no tumour can be seen in the breast. Cancer cells are found in 1–3 lymph nodes under the arm (axillary lymph nodes), in lymph nodes inside the chest around the breastbone (internal mammary lymph nodes) or in both areas. • Or the tumour is larger than 2 cm but not more than 5 cm.
2B	• The tumour is larger than 2 cm but not more than 5 cm. The cancer has also spread to 1–3 axillary lymph nodes, internal mammary lymph nodes or both areas. • Or the tumour is larger than 5 cm.
3A	• The tumour is 5 cm or smaller, or no tumour can be seen in the breast. Cancer cells are found in 4–9 axillary lymph nodes, or in internal mammary lymph nodes but not in axillary lymph nodes. • Or the tumour is larger than 5 cm. The cancer has also spread to 1–9 axillary lymph nodes or to internal mammary lymph nodes. Or it may have spread to 1-3 axillary lymph nodes and internal mammary lymph nodes.
3B	• The tumour has grown into the muscles of the chest wall or the skin or both. The cancer may have also spread to 1–9 axillary lymph nodes or to internal mammary lymph nodes. Or it may have spread to 1–3 axillary lymph nodes and internal mammary lymph nodes. • Or it is inflammatory breast cancer. Inflammatory breast cancer develops when cancer cells block the lymph vessels in the skin of the breast. It is called inflammatory because the breast becomes red and swollen.
3C	It is stage 3C when any of the following applies: • The cancer has spread to 10 or more axillary lymph nodes or to lymph nodes below the collarbone (infraclavicular lymph nodes). • The cancer has spread to more than 3 axillary lymph nodes and internal mammary lymph nodes. • The cancer has spread to lymph nodes above the collarbone (supraclavicular lymph nodes).
4	• The cancer has spread to other parts of the body (called distant metastasis), such as to the bone, liver, lungs or brain. This is also called metastatic breast cancer.

Adapted from Canadian Cancer Society. *Stages of Breast Cancer.* Retrieved from http://www.cancer.ca/en/cancer-information/cancer-type/breast/staging/?region=on#ixzz5DgYxyAu8

FIGURE 6.4 Stages I to IV of breast cancer.

response to a number of related factors: aging; gender (99% of cases occur in women, delayed childbearing or never bearing children, genetic influences); BRCA1 and BRCA2 genetic mutations; history of receiving ionizing radiation; high breast density; postmenopausal obesity; family history of cancer; hormonal factors such as early menarche <12 years, late menopause >50 years, first term pregnancy >30 to 35 years of age; HRT with estrogen plus progestin; and ingestion of two drinks or more alcohol each day (ACS, 2018b). Other factors might contribute to breast cancer but have not been scientifically proven.

In 1970, the lifetime risk for developing breast cancer was 1 in 10; since then, the risk has gradually risen (NCI, 2018b). This slight increase in incidence might be explained in a variety of ways: better detection and screening tools are available, which have identified more cases; people are living to an older age, when their risk increases; and lifestyle changes (having the first pregnancy at an older age, having fewer children, and using hormonal therapy to treat the symptoms of menopause) might have produced the higher numbers. Age is a significant risk factor. Because rates of breast cancer increase with age, estimates of risk at specific ages are more meaningful than estimates of lifetime risk. The probability of developing breast cancer in the subsequent 10 years at various ages is detailed in Table 6.3.

Risk factors for breast cancer can be divided into those that cannot be changed (nonmodifiable risk factors) and those that can be changed (modifiable risk factors). Nonmodifiable risk factors (ACS, 2018b) are:
- Gender (female)
- Aging (>50 years old)
- Genetic mutations (BRCA1 and BRCA2 genes)
- Personal history of ovarian or colon cancer
- Increased breast density increases the risk three- to fivefold
- Family history of breast cancer
- Personal history of breast cancer (three- to fourfold increase in risk for recurrence)

TABLE 6.3	PROBABILITY (%) OF DEVELOPING BREAST CANCER IN THE NEXT 10 YEARS AT SELECTED AGES
Age 30	0.4%
Age 40	1.3%
Age 50	2.3%
Age 60	3.3%
Age 70	3.6%
Age 80	2.9%

Adapted from: Canadian Cancer Society's Advisory Committee on Cancer Statistics (2017). *Canadian Cancer Statistics 2017*. Toronto, ON: Canadian Cancer Society. Retrieved from cancer.ca/Canadian-CancerStatistics-2017-EN.pdf Accessed April 2018.

- Race/ethnicity (studies in the United States and United Kingdom show that rates are higher in Caucasian women, but African-American women are more likely to die of it)
- Previous abnormal breast biopsy (atypical hyperplasia)
- Exposure to chest radiation (radiation damages DNA)
- Previous breast radiation (12 times normal risk)
- Early menarche (<12 years old) or late onset of menopause (>55 years old), which represents increased estrogen exposure over the lifetime

Modifiable risk factors related to lifestyle choices (ACS, 2018b) include:
- Not having children at all or not having children until after age 30—this increases the risk of breast cancer by not reducing the number of menstrual cycles
- Postmenopausal use of estrogens and progestins—the Women's Health Initiative study (2002) reported increased risks with long-term (>5 years) use of HRT
- Failing to breastfeed for up to a year after pregnancy—increases the risk of breast cancer because it does not reduce the total number of lifetime menstrual cycles
- Alcohol consumption—boosts the level of estrogen in the bloodstream
- Smoking—exposure to carcinogenic agents found in cigarettes
- Obesity and consumption of high-fat diet—fat cells produce and store estrogen, so more fat cells create higher estrogen levels
- Sedentary lifestyle and lack of physical exercise—increases body fat, which houses estrogen

The presence of risk factors, especially several of them, calls for careful ongoing monitoring and evaluation to promote early detection. Even though risk factors are important considerations, many individuals with newly diagnosed breast cancer have no known risk factors. Although routine mammography and self-examination are prudent for high-risk clients, these precautions may become lifesavers for early detection of cancerous lesions.

Consuming a low-fat diet with plenty of fruits, vegetables, legumes, and whole grains can provide all the vitamins and nutrients our bodies need and has been shown to significantly reduce the risk of developing many types of cancer. A plant-based diet can also reduce cancer recurrence: high-fibre, low-fat diets rich in fruits and vegetables, avoiding sugared beverages and calorie dense foods, and processed meats reduce breast cancer recurrence, according to Catsburg et al. (2015). They studied the effectiveness of a high-vegetable, low-fat diet, aimed at markedly raising circulating carotenoid concentrations from food sources, in reducing additional breast cancer events and early death in women with early-stage invasive breast cancer. It is a prescription for cancer prevention that has only positive side effects—lower cholesterol, weight loss, and a lower risk of heart disease. Adherence to a plant-based diet that limits red meat intake may be associated with reduced risk of breast cancer, particularly in postmenopausal women (Catsburg et al., 2015).

Screening for breast cancer begins with a routine history and physical examination. Nurses should take every opportunity to educate and emphasize the goal of breast cancer screening: early detection reduces mortality. Screening also includes a BSE, CBE, and mammography.

Diagnosis

Many studies can be performed to make an accurate diagnosis of a malignant breast lump. Diagnostic tests include:

- Diagnostic mammography or digital mammography
- Magnetic resonance mammography (MRM)
- Fine-needle aspiration
- Stereotactic needle-guided biopsy
- Sentinel lymph node biopsy
- Hormone receptor status
- Infrared thermal imaging
- DNA ploidy status
- Cell proliferative indices
- HER-2/neu genetic marker (Han et al., 2015)

Mammography

Mammography has become an accepted screening procedure that is sanctioned by most cancer organizations. Mammography serves a twofold purpose: to screen and to diagnose. Mammography involves taking x-ray pictures of a bare breast while it is compressed between two plastic plates. This procedure is a screening tool used to identify and characterize a breast mass and to detect an early malignancy. It remains the gold standard screening method for individuals at average risk for breast cancer. It is relatively inexpensive, requires only a low dose of radiation, and reliably identifies malignant tumours, especially those that are too small to feel. It can also be used to investigate breast lumps and other symptoms. A screening mammogram typically consists of four views, two per breast (Fig. 6.5). It can detect lesions as small as 0.5 cm (the average size of a tumour detected by a person practicing occasional BSE is approximately 2.5 cm) (Rifkin & Lazris, 2015).

A diagnostic mammogram is performed when a client has suspicious clinical findings on a breast examination or an abnormality has been found on a screening mammogram. A diagnostic mammogram uses additional views of the affected breast as well as magnification views. Diagnostic mammography provides the radiologist with additional detail to render a more specific diagnosis. Currently, digital mammography is being used to diagnose breast lesions.

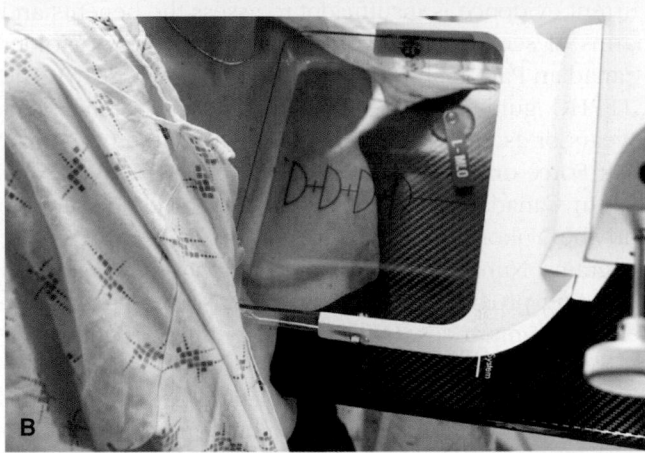

FIGURE 6.5 Mammography. **A.** A top-to-bottom view of the breast. **B.** A side view of the breast.

Most individuals find the 10-minute mammography procedure uncomfortable but not painful. Teaching Guidelines 6.3 offers tips for clients to follow before they undergo this procedure.

Teaching Guidelines 6.3
PREPARING FOR A SCREENING MAMMOGRAM

- Schedule the procedure just after menses, when breasts are less tender.
- Do not use deodorant or powder on the day of the procedure, because they can appear on the x-ray film as calcium spots.
- Acetaminophen (Tylenol) or acetylsalicylic acid (aspirin) can relieve any discomfort after the procedure.
- Remove all jewelry from around your neck, because the metal can cause distortions on the film image.

In 1994, the Canadian Task Force on Preventative Health (CTFPH) released guidelines recommending that women aged 50 to 69 years undergo screening for breast cancer with mammography and CBE every 1 to 2 years, and recommending against screening women aged 40 to 49. An update to these recommendations was released in 2001, stating that there is insufficient evidence to recommend for or against screening average-risk women aged 40 to 49 years. In 2011, the Task Force released a full update to its 1994 screening guidelines based on evidence that was reviewed by the U.S. Preventive Services Task Force (USPSTF). It is now recommended in Canada that average-risk individuals aged 50 to 74 years be screened with mammography every 2 to 3 years. It is also recommended that the decision to start screening mammography in women prior to age 50 years should be determined on an individual basis and concluded that current evidence is insufficient to assess the benefits and harms of screening in women 75 years of age or older (Canadian Partnership Against Cancer [CPAC], 2016). The CTFPHC guidelines are updated approximately every 5 years or as new evidence become available (Canadian Task Force on Preventive Health Care, 2011).

In Canada, all provinces, the Northwest Territories, and the Yukon have implemented organized screening programs. Nunavut does not currently have an organized screening program but does provide some screening in select circumstances. Organized screening programs use a centralized and systemic approach for the identification and invitation of the target population, provision of the screening examination using mammography, follow-up of abnormalities detected at screening, and recall after a normal or benign screening episode, all free of charge to the client (CPAC, 2016). Clients can also access breast cancer screening mammography through physician referral and by self-referral in some provinces.

Magnetic Resonance Mammography

MRM is a relatively new procedure that might allow for earlier detection because it can detect smaller lesions and provide finer detail. MRM is a highly accurate (>90% sensitivity for invasive carcinoma) but costly tool. Contrast infusion is used to evaluate the rate at which the dye initially enters the breast tissue. The basis of the high sensitivity of MRM is the tumour angiogenesis (vessel growth) that accompanies a majority of breast cancers, even early ones. Malignant lesions tend to exhibit increased enhancement within the first 2 minutes (Bhatti et al., 2015). Currently MRM is used as a complement to mammography and CBE because it is expensive, but recent research findings report that it is more accurate than mammography for size assessment of breast lesions (Poulos, 2015).

Fine-Needle Aspiration Biopsy or Core Biopsy

Fine-needle aspiration biopsy is done to identify a solid tumour, cyst, or malignancy. It is a simple office procedure that can be performed with or without anesthesia. A small (23- to 27-gauge) needle connected to a 10-mL or larger syringe is inserted into the breast mass and suction is applied to withdraw the contents. The aspirate is then sent to the cytology laboratory to be evaluated for abnormal cells.

A core needle biopsy is much like a fine-needle biopsy except that a larger needle is used to withdraw small cylinders or cores of tissue from the abnormal area of the breast. It takes longer than the fine-needle biopsy, but more tissue is sampled to be tested.

Stereotactic Needle-Guided Biopsy

This diagnostic tool is used to target and identify mammographically detected nonpalpable lesions in the breast. This procedure is less expensive than an excisional biopsy. The procedure takes place in a specially equipped room and generally takes about an hour. Individuals are required to lie prone and must be able to remain still for approximately 20 minutes while the biopsy is taken. When proper placement of the breast mass is confirmed by digital mammograms, the breast is locally anesthetized and a spring-loaded biopsy gun is used to obtain two or three core biopsy tissue samples. After the procedure is finished, the biopsy area is cleaned and a sterile dressing is applied.

Sentinel Lymph Node Biopsy

The status of the axillary lymph nodes is an important prognostic indicator in early-stage breast cancer. The presence or absence of malignant cells in lymph nodes is highly significant: the more lymph nodes involved and the more aggressive the cancer, the more powerful chemotherapy will have to be, both in terms of the toxicity of drugs and the duration of treatment (Tsujimoto, 2015). With a sentinel lymph node biopsy, the clinician can determine whether breast cancer has spread to the axillary lymph nodes without having to do a traditional axillary lymph node dissection. Experience has shown that the lymph ducts of the breast typically drain to one lymph node first before draining through the rest of the lymph nodes under the arm. The first lymph node is called the sentinel lymph node.

This procedure can be performed under local anesthesia. A radioactive blue dye is injected 2 hours before the biopsy to identify the afferent sentinel lymph node. The surgeon usually removes one to three nodes and sends them to the pathologist to determine whether cancer cells are present. The sentinel lymph node biopsy is usually performed before a lumpectomy to make sure the cancer has not spread. Removing only the sentinel lymph node can allow clients with breast cancer to avoid many of the side effects (lymphedema) associated with a traditional axillary lymph node dissection. This procedure is associated with less morbidity compared to the axillary lymph node dissection, which results in more accurate staging, better axillary tumour control and improved survival. It is considered a standard of care for initial evaluation of metastatic spread to the axillary lymph node chain (Chatterjee, Serniak, & Czerniecki, 2015).

Hormone Receptor Status

Normal breast epithelium has hormone receptors and responds specifically to the stimulatory effects of estrogen and progesterone. Most breast cancers retain estrogen receptors, and for those tumours estrogen will retain proliferative control over the malignant cells. It is therefore useful to know the hormone receptor status of the cancer to predict which women will respond to hormone manipulation. Hormone receptor status reveals whether the tumour is stimulated to grow by estrogen and progesterone. Postmenopausal individuals tend to be ER+; premenopausal individuals tend to be ER− (Kalinsky et al., 2015). To determine hormone receptor status, a sample of breast cancer tissue obtained during a biopsy or a tumour removed surgically during a lumpectomy or mastectomy is examined by a cytologist.

Therapeutic Management

Individuals diagnosed with breast cancer have many treatments available to them. Generally, treatments fall into two categories: local and systemic. Local treatments are surgery and radiation therapy. Effective systemic treatments include chemotherapy, hormonal therapy, and immunotherapy (Evidence-Based Practice 6.1).

Treatment plans are based on multiple factors, with the primary factors being whether the cancer is invasive or noninvasive, the tumour's size and grade, the number of cancerous axillary lymph nodes, the hormone receptor status, and the ability to obtain clear surgical margins (ACS, 2018e). A combination of surgical options and adjunctive therapy is often recommended.

Another consideration in making decisions about a treatment plan is genetic testing for BRCA1 and BRCA2 genetic mutations. This genetic testing became available in 1995 and can pinpoint individuals who have a significantly increased risk for breast and ovarian cancer, and contralateral breast cancer: individuals with BRCA1 and BRCA2 mutations have a 75% lifetime risk of breast cancer and a 30% lifetime risk of ovarian cancer. Most cases of breast and ovarian cancer are sporadic in nature, but approximately 10% of breast and ovarian cancers are thought to result from genetic inheritance (Li et al., 2015). DNA (from a blood or saliva sample) is needed

EVIDENCE-BASED PRACTICE 6.1 — COMBINATION (SEVERAL DRUGS AT A TIME) VERSUS SEQUENTIAL CHEMOTHERAPY (SAME DRUG GIVEN ONE AFTER THE OTHER) FOR METASTATIC BREAST CANCER

STUDY

Combination chemotherapy can cause greater tumour cell kill if the drug dose is not compromised, while sequential single-agent chemotherapy may allow for greater dose intensity and treatment time, potentially meaning greater benefit from each single agent. In addition, sequentially using single agents might cause less toxicity and impairment of quality of life, but it is not known whether this might compromise survival time. The purpose of this study was to assess the effect of combination chemotherapy compared to the same drugs given sequentially in women with metastatic breast cancer.

Findings

Randomized controlled trials of combination chemotherapy compared to the same drugs used sequentially in women with metastatic breast cancer in the first-, second-, or third-line setting were selected. Twelve trials reporting on 9 treatment comparisons (2,317 patients randomized) were identified. The findings concluded that sequential single-agent chemotherapy has a positive effect on progression-free survival, whereas combination chemotherapy has a

higher response rate and a higher risk of febrile neutropenia in metastatic breast cancer. There was no difference in overall survival time between these treatment strategies, but when drugs were given one at a time, there was more time before the tumours grew back again. However, combination chemotherapy caused tumours to shrink more. Generally, this study supports the recommendations by international guidelines to use sequential monotherapy unless there is rapid disease progression.

Nursing Implications

Although not entirely conclusive in its findings, nurses need to be aware of this study's findings to be able to counsel individuals when both therapies are being considered. This study suggests that accurate information about both therapies is needed for all individuals with metastatic breast cancer, for them to make an informed decision. Nurses need to remember that metastatic breast cancer is not currently curable, but can be effectively treated with chemotherapy. Average survival is about 2 years, but many individuals live much longer. The type of therapy chosen should take into consideration optimizing survival, minimizing side effects, and quality of life.

Adapted from Dear, R. F., McGeechan, K., Jenkins, M. C., Barratt, A., Tattersall, M. H. N., & Wilcken, N. (2015). Combination versus sequential single agent chemotherapy for metastatic breast cancer. *Cochrane Database of Systematic Reviews 2013*, 3:CD008792. doi: 10.1002/14651858.CD008792.pub2.

for mutation testing. The sample is sent to a laboratory for analysis. It usually takes about a month to get the results back. Testing positive for a BRCA1 or BRCA2 mutation can significantly alter health care decisions. In some cases, before genetic testing was available, lumpectomy with radiation or mastectomy was the treatment most often recommended. However, if the client is found to have a BRCA1 mutation, most likely the option of bilateral prophylactic mastectomy and possible bilateral oophorectomy will be offered. A recent study found that current evidence does not support worse breast cancer survival of BRCA1/2 mutation carriers in the adjuvant setting; differences if any are likely to be small when compared to non-BRCA1/2 mutation carriers (van den Broek et al., 2015).

Discovery of mutations in the breast and ovarian cancer susceptibility genes BRCA1 and BRCA2 can have emotional consequences for both the tested individual and his or her relatives.

Severe psychological distress can occur as a result of genetic testing. Their distress relates to family cancer history, relationships, coping strategies, communication patterns, and mutation status (Wevers et al., 2015). Nurses might find it useful to explore these issues in order to prepare clients before BRCA1/BRCA2 testing and to support them through shifts in family dynamics after disclosure of results. Also, many individuals perceive their breasts as intrinsic to their femininity, self-esteem, and sexuality, and the risk of losing a breast can provoke extreme anxiety (Alexander et al., 2014). Nurses need to address the physical, emotional, and spiritual needs of the individuals they care for, as well as their families, since this mutation is inherited in an autosomal dominant fashion. Nurses should identify the client's personal coping style which has an impact on the likelihood of experiencing distress after the diagnosis. Individuals who are emotionally expressive and/or have a "fighting spirit" usually experience lower levels of emotional distress. Based on Mendelian genetics, individuals with BRCA1 and BRCA2 mutations have a 5- to 20-fold increased risk of developing breast and ovarian cancer (Caple & Schub, 2015).

Surgical Options

Generally, the first treatment option for a person diagnosed with breast cancer is surgery. A few individuals with tumours larger than 5 cm or inflammatory breast cancer may undergo neoadjuvant chemotherapy or radiotherapy to shrink the tumour before surgical removal is attempted (Debled et al., 2015). The surgical options depend on the type and extent of cancer. The choices are typically either breast-conserving surgery (lumpectomy with radiation) or mastectomy with or without reconstruction. The overall survival rate with lumpectomy and radiation is about the same as that with modified radical mastectomy (ACS, 2018f). Research has shown that the survival rates in individuals who have had mastectomies versus those

who have undergone breast-conserving surgery followed by radiation are the same. However, lumpectomy may not be an option for some people, including those:

- Who have two or more cancer sites that cannot be removed through one incision
- Whose surgery will not result in a clean margin of tissue
- Who have active connective tissue conditions (lupus or scleroderma) that make body tissues especially sensitive to the side effects of radiation
- Who have had previous radiation to the affected breast
- Whose tumours are larger than 5 cm (2 in) (National Comprehensive Cancer Network [NCCN], 2018)

These decisions are made jointly between the individual and the surgeon. If mastectomy is chosen, because of either tumour characteristics or client preference, then discussion needs to include breast reconstruction and regional lymph node biopsy versus sentinel lymph node biopsy. The mastectomy techniques are a simple mastectomy with sentinel node biopsy or a radical mastectomy with regional node biopsy. Removal of numerous lymph nodes places the client at high risk for lymphedema.

BREAST-CONSERVING SURGERY

Breast-conserving surgery, the least invasive procedure, is the wide local excision (or lumpectomy) of the tumour along with a 1-cm margin of normal tissue. A lumpectomy is often used for early-stage localized tumours. The goal of breast-conserving surgery is to remove the suspicious mass along with tissue free of malignant cells to prevent recurrence. The results are less drastic and emotionally less scarring than having a mastectomy to the person. Individuals undergoing breast-conserving therapy receive radiation after lumpectomy with the goal of eradicating residual microscopic cancer cells to limit locoregional recurrence. In clients who do not require adjuvant chemotherapy, radiation therapy typically begins 2 to 4 weeks after surgery to allow healing of the lumpectomy incision site. Radiation is administered to the entire breast at daily doses over a period of several weeks (Corradini et al., 2015).

A sentinel lymph node biopsy may also be performed since the lymph nodes draining the breast are located primarily in the axilla. Theoretically, if breast cancer is to metastasize to other parts of the body, it will probably do so via the lymphatic system. If malignant cells are found in the nodes, more aggressive systemic treatment may be needed.

MASTECTOMY

A **simple mastectomy** is the removal of all breast tissue, the nipple, and the areola. The axillary nodes and pectoral muscles are spared. This procedure would be used for a large tumour or multiple tumours that have not metastasized to adjacent structures or the lymph system.

A **modified radical mastectomy** is another surgical option, conducive to breast reconstruction and results in greater mobility and less lymphedema (Alexander et al., 2014). This procedure involves removal of breast tissue, and a few positive axillary nodes. Breast-conserving surgeries do not increase the future risk of death from recurrent disease when compared with mastectomy (Schuiling & Likis, 2016).

In conjunction with the mastectomy, lymph node surgery (removal of underarm nodes) may need to be done to reduce the risk of distant metastasis and improve an individual's chance of long-term survival. For individuals with a positive sentinel node biopsy, 10 to 20 underarm lymph nodes may need to be removed. Complications associated with axillary lymph node surgery include nerve damage during surgery, causing temporary numbness down the upper aspect of the arm; seroma formation (fluid build-up) followed by wound infection; restrictions in arm mobility (some women need physiotherapy); and lymphedema (swelling related to the lymph glands). In many clients, lymphedema can be avoided by:

- Avoiding using the affected arm for drawing blood, inserting intravenous lines, or measuring blood pressure (can cause trauma and possible infection)
- Seeking medical care immediately if the affected arm swells
- Wearing gloves when engaging in activities such as gardening that might cause injury
- Wearing a well-fitted compression sleeve to promote drainage return

Individuals having mastectomies must decide whether to have further surgery to reconstruct the breast. If the person decides to have reconstructive surgery, it ideally is performed immediately after the mastectomy. The individual must also determine whether she wants the surgeon to use saline implants or natural tissue from her abdomen (TRAM flap method) or back (LAT flap method).

If reconstructive surgery is desired, the ultimate decision regarding the method will be determined by the individual's anatomy (e.g., is there sufficient fat and muscle to permit natural reconstruction?) and overall health status. Both procedures require a prolonged recovery period.

Some individuals opt for no reconstruction, and many of them choose to wear breast prostheses. Some prostheses are worn in the bra cup and others fit against the skin or into special pockets created into clothing.

Whether to have reconstructive surgery is an individual and very complex decision. Each person must be presented with all of the options and then allowed to decide. The nurse can play an important role here by presenting the facts to clients so that they can make an intelligent decision to meet their unique situations. Breast reconstruction surgery can help restore the look and feel of the breast after a mastectomy. Performed by a plastic surgeon, breast reconstruction can be done immediately after the mastectomy or at a later date. Breast reconstruction can be done with **breast implants** (filled with saline or silicone); natural tissue flaps (using skin fat and muscle from your own body); or a combination of both. Side effects or complications include risk of rupture, hardening of the tissues around the implant, infection, and pain. Nurses need to educate the client about these potential problems and make sure they understand before consenting to breast reconstruction. See Figure 6.6 for examples of a postmastectomy (A) and reconstruction breast Augmentation (B).

FIGURE 6.6 **After mastectomy (A)**, after postmastectomy **(B)** reconstruction.

BREAST AUGMENTATION

Breast augmentation is a common surgical procedure with individuals undergoing it with implants for a variety of reasons ranging from aesthetic to reconstructive surgery following a mastectomy. Saline- or silicone-filled implants are used in cosmetic enhancement and reconstructive surgeries. The exact anatomical placement of breast implants can vary, but the location typically is subglandular (over the pectoral muscle) or subpectoral (under the muscle). Breast implants are not lifetime devices, but most are guaranteed for approximately 10 years in case of rupture. Breast augmentation with implants is not without risks. Potential complications include capsular contracture, rippling, implant rupture, infection, or hematoma. Capsular contraction occurs when scar tissue forms, contracts, and hardens around the implant. Rippling most often occurs when wrinkles form in the implant or as a complication of contracture (Mugea, 2015).

Breast examination in clients with reconstructive surgery is done exactly the same way as for natural breasts. Breasts with implants in place usually feel firmer than normal breast tissue on palpation due to the formation of a fibrotic band or capsule around the implant. If implants are used, press firmly inward at the edges of the implant to feel the ribs beneath.

Adjunctive Therapy

Adjunctive therapy is supportive or additional therapy that is recommended after surgery. Adjunctive therapies include local therapy such as radiation therapy and systemic therapies using chemotherapy, hormonal therapy, and immunotherapy.

RADIATION THERAPY

Radiation therapy (also called radiotherapy) uses high-energy rays to destroy cancer cells that might have been left behind in the breast, chest wall, or underarm area after a tumour has been removed surgically. Usually serial radiation doses are given 5 days a week to the tumour site for 6 to 8 weeks postoperatively. Each treatment takes only a few minutes, but the dose is cumulative. Individuals undergoing breast-conserving therapy receive radiation to the entire breast after lumpectomy with the goal of eradicating residual microscopic cancer cells to reduce the chance of recurrence (Chu et al., 2015).

Side Effects. Side effects of traditional radiation therapy include inflammation, local edema, anorexia, swelling, and heaviness in the breast; sunburn-like skin changes in the treated area; and fatigue. Changes to the breast tissue and skin usually resolve in about a year in most people

(Lara et al., 2015). This type of therapy can be given several ways: external beam radiation, which delivers a carefully focused dose of radiation from a machine outside the body, or internal radiation, in which tiny pellets that contain radioactive material are placed into the tumour.

Several advances have taken place in the field of radiation oncology for the treatment of individuals with early-stage breast cancer that assist in reducing the side effects. The treatment position for external radiation has changed from supine to prone, with the arm on the affected side raised above the head, so that the treated breast hangs dependently through the opening of the treatment board. Treatment in the prone position improves dose distribution within the breast and allows for a decrease in the dose delivered to the heart, lung, chest wall, and other breast (NCCN, 2018).

High-dose brachytherapy is another advance that is an alternative to traditional radiation treatment. A balloon catheter is used to insert radioactive seeds into the breast after the tumour has been removed surgically. The seeds deliver a concentrated dose directly to the operative site; this is important because most cancer recurrences in the breast occur at or near the lumpectomy site (Chang et al., 2015). This allows a high dose of radiation to be delivered to a small target volume with a minimal dose to the surrounding normal tissue. This procedure takes 4 to 5 days as opposed to the 4 to 6 weeks that traditional radiation therapy takes; it also eliminates the need to delay radiation therapy to allow for wound healing. Brachytherapy is now used as a primary radiation treatment after breast-conserving surgery in selected individuals as an alternative to whole breast irradiation (Guinot et al., 2015). Side effects of brachytherapy include redness or discharge around catheters, fever, and infection. Daily cleansing of the catheter insertion site with a mild soap and application of an antibiotic ointment will minimize the risk of infection.

Intensity-modulated radiation therapy (IMRT) offers still another new approach to the delivery of treatment to reduce the dose within the target area while sparing surrounding normal structures. A computed tomography scan is used to create a three-dimensional model of the breast. Based on this model, a series of intensity-modulated beams is produced to the desired dose distribution to reduce radiation exposure to underlying structures. Acute toxicity is thus minimized (Muralidhar, Soubhagya, & Ahmed, 2015). Research is ongoing to evaluate the impact of all of these advances in radiation therapy.

CHEMOTHERAPY

Chemotherapy refers to the use of drugs that are toxic to all cells and interfere with a cell's ability to reproduce. They are particularly effective against malignant cells but affect all rapidly dividing cells, especially those of the skin, the hair follicles, the mouth, the gastrointestinal tract, and the bone marrow. Breast cancer is a systemic disease in which micrometastases are already present in other organs by the time the breast cancer is diagnosed. Chemotherapeutic agents perform a systemic "sweep" of the body to reduce the chances that distant tumours will start growing.

Chemotherapy may be indicated for clients with tumours larger than 1 cm, positive lymph nodes, or cancer of an aggressive type. Chemotherapy is prescribed in cycles, with each period of treatment followed by a rest period. Treatment typically lasts 3 to 6 months, depending on the dose used and the client's health status.

Different classes of drugs affect different aspects of cell division and are used in combinations or "cocktails." The most active and commonly used chemotherapeutic agents for breast cancer include alkylating agents, anthracyclines, antimetabolites, and vinca alkaloids. Fifty or more chemotherapeutic agents can be used to treat breast cancer; however, a combination drug approach appears to be more effective than a single drug treatment (ACS, 2018g). Refer to Evidence-Based Practice 6.1.

Side Effects. Side effects of chemotherapy depend on the agents used, the intensity of dosage, the dosage schedule, the type and extent of cancer, and the client's physical and emotional status. Nurses need to remain current in order to accommodate new treatments and the side-effect profiles. This knowledge is vital to providing evidence-based care for clients with breast cancer receiving these treatments (Bourdeanu & Lui, 2015). However, typical side effects include nausea and vomiting, diarrhea or constipation, hair loss, weight loss, stomatitis, fatigue, and immunosuppression. The most serious is bone marrow suppression (myelosuppression). This causes an increased risk of infection, bleeding, and a reduced red blood cell count, which can lead to anemia. Treatment of the side effects can generally be addressed through appropriate support medications such as antinausea drugs. In addition, growth-stimulating factors, such as filgrastim (Neupogen), help keep blood counts from dropping too low. Counts that are too low would stop or delay the use of chemotherapy.

An aggressive systemic option, when other treatments have failed or when there is a strong possibility of relapse or metastatic disease, is high-dose chemotherapy with bone marrow and/or stem cell transplant. This therapy involves the withdrawal of bone marrow before the administration of toxic levels of chemotherapeutic agents. The marrow is frozen and then returned to the client after the high-dose chemotherapy is finished. Clinical trials are still researching this experimental therapy (King et al., 2015).

HORMONAL THERAPY

One of estrogen's normal functions is to stimulate the growth and division of healthy cells in the breasts. However, in some individuals with breast cancer, this normal function contributes to the growth and division of cancer cells.

The objective of **endocrine therapy** is to block or counter the effect of estrogen. Estrogen plays a central role in the pathogenesis of cancer, and treatment with estrogen deprivation has proven to be effective. Approximately two thirds of individuals diagnosed with early-stage breast cancer have hormone-sensitive disease (estrogen receptor positive and/or progesterone receptor positive), and adjuvant hormone therapy plays an essential role in reducing the risk of recurrence and improving survival (Gradishar, 2015). Several different drug classes are used to interfere or block estrogen receptors. They include selective estrogen receptor modulators (SERMs), estrogen receptor downregulators, aromatase inhibitors, luteinizing hormone–releasing hormone, progestin, and biologic response modifiers (King et al., 2015). The current recommendations for most clients with ER+ breast cancer is to take a hormone-like medication—known as a SERM antiestrogenic agent—daily for up to 5 years after initial treatment. Certain areas in the female body (breasts, uterus, ovaries, skin, vagina, and brain) contain specialized cells called hormone receptors that allow estrogen to enter the cell and stimulate it to divide. SERMs enter these same receptors and act like keys, turning off the signal for growth inside the cell (King et al., 2015). The best-known SERM is tamoxifen (Nolvadex, 20 mg daily for 5 years). Although it works well in preventing further spread of cancer, it is also associated with an increased incidence of endometrial cancer, pulmonary embolus, deep vein thrombosis, hot flashes, vaginal discharge and bleeding, stroke, and cataract formation (Jager et al., 2015).

Another SERM is the antiosteoporosis drug raloxifene (Evista), which has shown promising results. It has antiestrogen effects on the breast and uterus. In recent studies involving postmenopausal individuals at high risk for breast cancer, raloxifene worked as well as tamoxifen in preventing breast cancer, but with fewer serious adverse effects. Both drugs cut the cancer risk in half (Bevers, 2015). It was originally marketed solely for the prevention and treatment of osteoporosis but is now used as adjunctive breast cancer therapy.

Another class of endocrine agents, aromatase inhibitors, works by inhibiting the conversion of androgens to estrogens. Aromatase inhibitors include letrozole (Femara, 2.5 mg daily), exemestane (Aromasin, 25 mg daily), and anastrozole (Arimidex, 1 mg daily for 5 years), all of which are taken orally. These are usually given to individuals with advanced breast cancer. In recent clinical studies in postmenopausal women with breast cancer, third-generation aromatase inhibitors were shown to be superior to tamoxifen for the treatment of metastatic disease (Bevers, 2015).

Side Effects. The side effects associated with these endocrine therapies include hot flashes, bone pain, bone thinning, insomnia, weight gain, depression, fatigue, nausea, cough, dyspnea, and headache (Breast Cancer Organization, 2018). Individuals with hormone-sensitive cancers can live for long periods without any intervention other than hormonal manipulation, but quality-of-life issues need to be addressed in the balance between treatment and side effects.

IMMUNOTHERAPY

Immunotherapy, used as an adjunct to surgery, represents an attempt to stimulate the body's natural defenses to recognize and attack cancer cells. Trastuzumab (Herceptin, 2 to 4 mg/kg intravenous infusion) is the first monoclonal antibody approved for breast cancer (NCCN, 2018). Some tumours produce excessive amounts of HER-2/neu protein, which regulates cancer cell growth. Breast cancers that overexpress the HER-2/neu protein are associated with a more aggressive form of disease and a poorer prognosis. Trastuzumab blocks the effect of this protein to inhibit the growth of cancer cells. It can be used alone or in combination with other chemotherapy to treat clients with metastatic breast disease. Although immunotherapy has shown some promise against the fight against cancer, recent data suggest that greater success will be achieved by combining it with other therapies, such as radiation (Leavy, 2015).

Take Note!

Tamoxifen is a selective estrogen receptor modulator used to prevent further spread of breast cancer in individuals with ER-positive breast cancer. Trastuzumab is a monoclonal antibody used in the treatment of breast cancer and is considered immunotherapy.

Side Effects. Adverse effects of trastuzumab include cardiac toxicity, vascular thrombosis, hepatic failure, fever, chills, nausea, vomiting, and pain with first infusion (Skidmore-Roth, 2015).

NURSING PROCESS FOR THE CLIENT WITH BREAST CANCER

When people are diagnosed with breast cancer, they face treatments that may alter their body shape, may make them feel unwell, and may not carry a certainty of cure. Nurses can support these individuals from the time of diagnosis, through the treatments, and through follow-up after the surgical and adjunctive treatments have been completed. Allowing clients time to ask questions and to discuss any necessary preparations for treatment is critical. As our understanding of breast disorders keeps improving, treatments continue to change.

Although the goal of treatment remains improved survival, increasing emphasis is being focused on prevention. Breast cancer prevention measures focus on evaluating and reducing risk factors. Approaches for reducing breast cancer risk include lifestyle modifications (diet and physical exercise), chemoprevention (SERMs and AIs), and prophylactic surgery (bilateral salpingo-oophorectomy and bilateral prophylactic mastectomy) (Euhus & Diaz, 2015). Nurses can have an impact on early detection of breast disorders, treatment, and symptom management. Individuals with a cancer diagnosis often experience negative emotions and nurses' empathic response can help alleviate their distress (Alexander et al., 2014). A nurse who is involved in the client's treatment plan from the beginning can effectively offer support throughout the whole experience.

Teamwork is important in breast screening and caring for individuals with breast disorders. Treatment is often fragmented between the hospital and community treatment centres, which can be emotionally traumatic for individuals and their families. The advances being made in the diagnosis and treatment of breast disorders mean that guidelines are constantly changing, requiring all health care providers to keep up to date. Informed nurses can provide support and information and, most importantly, continuity of care for the client undergoing treatment for a breast problem.

The nurse plays a particularly important role in providing psychological support and self-care teaching to clients with breast cancer. Nurses can influence both physical and emotional recovery, which are both important aspects of care that help in improving the individual's quality of life and the ability to survive. The nurse's role should extend beyond helping clients; spreading the word in the community about screening and prevention is a big part in the ongoing fight against cancer. The community should see nurses as both educators and valued sources of credible information. This role will help improve clinical outcomes while achieving high levels of client satisfaction.

Despite the new guidelines issued by various governmental agencies regarding BSEs, a CBE done by a professional health care provider is essential for good breast health for all individuals. See Box 6.1 for additional information.

Remember Nancy from the chapter opener? Is her response typical of many women upon discovering a lump in their breast? Nancy confides her discovery of the lump and her worries to you. What advice would you give her?

BOX 6.1

CLINICAL BREAST EXAMINATION BY HEALTH CARE PROVIDER

If the individual is deemed high risk, the nurse would then teach the individual to perform a BSE to enhance breast awareness.

Purpose: To Assess Breasts for Abnormal Findings

1. Inspect the breast for size, symmetry, and skin texture and colour. It is common for the left breast to be slightly larger than the right. Inspect the nipples and areola. Ask the client to sit at the edge of the examination table, with arms resting at the client's sides.

2. Inspect the breast for masses, retraction, dimpling, or ecchymosis.
   • The client places hands on the hips.

   • The client then raises arms over the head so the axillae can also be inspected.

• The client then stands, with hands on hips, and leans forward.

3. Palpate the breasts using the pads of your first three fingers and make a rotary motion on the breast. Assist the client into a supine position with the client's arms above the head. Place a pillow or towel under the client's head to help spread the breasts. Three patterns might be used to palpate the breasts:

• Spiral

- Pie-shaped wedges

- Vertical strip

4. Compress the nipple gently between the thumb and index finger to evaluate for masses and squeeze to check for any discharge.

5. Palpate the axillary area for any tenderness or lymph node enlargement. Have the client sit up and move to the edge of the examination table. While supporting the client's arm, palpate downward from the armpit, palpating toward the ribs just below the breast.

Adapted from Ball, J. W., Dains, J. E., Flynn, J. A., Soloman, B. S., & Stewart, R. W. (2015). *Seidel's guide to physical examination* (8th ed.). St. Louis, MO: Elsevier Saunders.

Assessment

Early breast cancer has no symptoms. The earliest sign of breast cancer is often an abnormality seen on a screening mammogram before the individual or the health care provider feels it. A healthy, asymptomatic presentation is typical. However, symptoms may include a lump in the breast that is usually nontender, fixed, and hard with irregular borders. In the person presenting with a breast disorder, take a thorough history of the problem and explore the person's risk factors for breast cancer. Assess the client for clinical manifestations of breast cancer, such as changes in breast appearance and contour, which become apparent with advancing breast cancer (ACS, 2018d). These changes include:

- Continued and persistent changes in the breast
- A lump or thickening in one breast
- Persistent nipple irritation
- Unusual breast swelling or asymmetry
- A lump or swelling in the axilla
- Changes in skin colour or texture
- Nipple retraction, tenderness, or discharge

Complete a breast examination to validate the clinical manifestations and findings of the health history and risk factor assessment. The CBE involves both inspection and palpation (Box 6.1). Helpful characteristics in evaluating palpable breast masses are described in Table 6.4. If a lump can be palpated, the cancer has been there for quite some time.

TABLE 6.4	CHARACTERISTICS OF BENIGN VERSUS MALIGNANT BREAST MASSES	
Benign Breast Masses Are Described As	**Malignant Breast Masses Are Described As**	
• Frequently painful • Firm, rubbery mass • Bilateral masses • Induced nipple discharge • Regular margins (clearly delineated) • No skin dimpling • No nipple retraction • Mobile, not affixed to the chest wall • No bloody discharge	• Hard to palpation • Painless • Irregularly shaped (poorly delineated) • Immobile, fixed to the chest wall • Skin dimpling • Nipple retraction • Unilateral mass • Bloody, serosanguineous, or serous nipple discharge • Spontaneous nipple discharge	

Be cognizant of the impact that breast cancer has on an individual's emotional state, coping ability, and quality of life. Individuals may experience sadness, vulnerability, loss of control, alteration of body image and integrity, anger, the illness's impact on relationships, fear of mortality, the need to reassess life priorities, and guilt as a result of having breast cancer. However, despite potential negative outcomes, many people have a positive outlook for their future and adapt to treatment modalities with a good quality of life (Kleban & Glaser, 2015). Closely monitor clients for their psychosocial adjustment to diagnosis and treatment and be able to identify those who need further psychological intervention. By giving practical advice, the nurse can help clients adjust to their altered body image and to accept the changes in their lives.

Because family members play a significant role in supporting individuals through breast cancer diagnosis and treatment, assess the emotional distress of both partners during the course of treatment and, if needed, make a referral for psychological counselling. By identifying interpersonal strains, negative psychosocial side effects of cancer treatment can be minimized.

Nursing Diagnosis

Appropriate nursing diagnoses for a person with a diagnosis of breast cancer might include:
• Disturbed body image related to:
  • Loss of body part (breast)
  • Loss of femininity
  • Loss of hair due to chemotherapy
• Fear related to:
  • Diagnosis of cancer
  • Prognosis of disease
• Deficient knowledge related to:
  • Cancer treatment options
  • Reconstructive surgery decisions
  • Breast self-examination

Nursing Interventions

Offer information, support, and perioperative care to individuals diagnosed with breast cancer who are undergoing treatment. Implement health promotion and disease prevention strategies to minimize the risk for developing breast cancer and to promote optimal outcomes.

> **Remember Nancy, who discovered a breast lump? You offer to go with her to the doctor. After a full examination and several diagnostic tests, the results come back positive for breast cancer. What treatment options does Nancy have, and what factors need to be considered in selecting those options?**

Providing Client Education

Help clients and their partners to prioritize the voluminous amount of information given to them so that they can make informed decisions. Explain all treatment options in detail so clients and their families understand them. By preparing an individualized packet of information and reviewing it with clients and their partners (if applicable), the nurse can help clients understand their specific type of cancer, the diagnostic studies and treatment options they may choose, and the goals of treatment. For example, nurses play an important role in educating people about the use of endocrine therapies, observing clients' experiences with treatment, and communicating those observations to their primary health care providers to make dosage adjustments, in addition to contributing to the knowledge base of endocrine therapy in the treatment of breast cancer.

Providing information is a central role of the nurse in caring for the client with a diagnosis of breast cancer. This information can be given via telephone counselling, one-to-one contact, and pamphlets. Telephone counselling with clients and their partners may be an effective method to improve symptom management and quality of life. Educate clients on living with risk, maintaining quality of life, and participating in support groups (Strayer & Schub, 2014).

PROVIDING EMOTIONAL SUPPORT

The diagnosis of cancer affects all aspects of life for individuals and their families. The threatening nature of the disease and feelings of uncertainty about the future can lead to anxiety and stress. Address the client's need for:

- Information about diagnosis and treatment
- Physical care while undergoing treatments
- Contact with supportive people
- Education about disease, options, and prevention measures
- Discussion and support by a caring, competent nurse

Reassure clients and their families that the diagnosis of breast cancer does not necessarily mean imminent death, a decrease in attractiveness, or diminished sexuality. Encourage clients to express their fears and worries. Be available to listen and address clients' concerns in an open manner to help them toward recovery. All aspects of care must include sensitivity to the client's personal efforts to cope and heal. Some individuals will become involved in organizations or charities that support cancer research; they may participate in breast cancer walks to raise awareness or become a *Peer Support Service* or *Cancer Connection* volunteer through the Canadian Cancer Society to help others. People cope in their own personal manner, and all of these efforts can be positive motivators for their own healing.

Providing Postoperative Care

For the client who has had surgery to remove a malignant breast lump or an entire breast, excellent postoperative nursing care is crucial. Tell the client what to expect in terms of symptoms and when they usually occur during treatment and after surgery. This allows clients to anticipate these symptoms and proactively employ management strategies to improve their cancer experience. Postoperative care includes immediate postoperative care, pain management, care of the affected arm, wound care, mobility care, respiratory care, emotional care, referrals, and educational needs.

IMMEDIATE POSTOPERATIVE CARE

Assess the client's respiratory status by auscultating the lungs and observing the breathing pattern. Assess circulation; note vital signs, skin colour, and skin temperature. Observe the client's neurologic status by evaluating the level of alertness and orientation. Monitor the wound for amount and colour of drainage.

Monitor the intravenous lines for patency, correct fluid, and rate. Assess the drainage tube for amount, colour, and consistency of drainage.

PAIN MANAGEMENT

Provide analgesics as needed. Reassure the client that the pain will be controlled. Teach the client how to communicate the pain intensity on a scale of 0 to 10, with 10 being the worst pain imaginable. Assess the client's pain level frequently and anticipate pain before assisting the client to ambulate.

AFFECTED ARM CARE

Elevate the affected arm on a pillow to promote lymph drainage. Make sure that no treatments are performed on the affected arm, including laboratory draws, intravenous lines, blood pressures, and so on. Place a sign above the bed to warn others not to touch the affected arm.

WOUND CARE

Observe the wound often and empty drainage reservoirs as needed. Tell the client to report any evidence of infection early, such as fever, chills, or any area of redness or inflammation along the incision line. Also tell the client to report any increase in drainage, foul odour, or separation at the incision site.

MOBILITY CARE

Perform active range-of-motion and arm exercises as ordered. Encourage self-care activities for successful rehabilitation. Perform dressing and drainage care; explain the care during the procedure.

RESPIRATORY CARE

Assist with turning, coughing, and deep breathing every 2 hours. Explain that this helps to expand collapsed alveoli in the lungs, promotes faster clearance of inhalation agents from the body, and prevents postoperative pneumonia and atelectasis.

EMOTIONAL CARE AND REFERRALS

Encourage clients to participate in their care. Assess their coping strategies preoperatively. Explain possible body image concerns after discharge. Promote the Canadian Cancer Society website, which provides the latest cancer therapy news. Encourage the client to attend local or online support groups for breast cancer survivors.

EDUCATIONAL NEEDS

Provide follow-up information about adjunctive therapy. Explain that radiation therapy may start within weeks postoperatively. Discuss chemotherapy, its side effects and cycles, home care during treatment, and future monitoring strategies. Explain hormonal therapy, including anti-estrogens or aromatase inhibitors. Teach progressive arm exercises to minimize lymphedema. Explain that ongoing surveillance is needed to detect recurrence of cancer or a new primary site and that the client will typically see the health care provider every 6 months.

> *Nancy* **underwent a mastectomy with radiation and chemotherapy. What follow-up care is needed? How can the nurse assist Nancy to cope with her uncertain future? What community resources might help her?**

Implementing Health Promotion and Disease Prevention Strategies

In the past, most people assumed that there was little they could do to reduce their risk of developing breast cancer, but since the 1970s significant advances have been made in the diagnosis and treatment of breast cancer. Mortality rates have decreased since 1990, particularly in women <50 years old. The declining incidence of breast cancer and lower mortality rates have been attributed to early detection, improved treatment, and research (Sestak & Cuzick, 2015). However, research has found that the choices individuals make concerning breast cancer screening, diet, exercise, and other health practices have a profound impact on cancer risk. In the fight against cancer, nurses often assume a variety of roles, such as educator, counselor, advocate, and role model. Nurses can offer education about the following:

- Prevention
- Early detection
- Screening
- Dispelling myths and fears
- Self-examination techniques if needed
- Individual risk status and strategies for risk reduction

It is important to be knowledgeable about the most current evidence-based practices and cognizant of how the media present this information. Offer prevention strategies within the context of an individual's life. Factors such as lifestyle choices, economic status, and multiple roles need to be taken into consideration when counselling clients. Advocate for healthy lifestyles and making sound choices to prevent cancer. Nurses, like all health care providers, should offer guidance from a comprehensive perspective that acknowledges the unique needs of each individual. Nurses need to not only be proficient in the postoperative physical care of clients who undergo mastectomy but also demonstrate advanced skills related to the educational needs of clients and their families and to ensure care is delivered in a manner that is client-centred and individualized. Nurses require advanced skills to meet the social and psychological care needs of clients and their families during this major life event (Fallowfield & Jenkins, 2015).

Like a black cloud hanging over their heads, with little regard for any victim, breast cancer stalks individuals everywhere they go. Many people are left with new health risks and lingering effects associated with treatment (e.g., limited mobility, memory problems, low social activity, and support). Many have a close friend or relative who is battling the disease; many have watched their mothers, sisters and friends die of this dreaded disease. Those with risk factors live with even greater anxiety and fear. No person wants to hear those chilling words: "The biopsy is positive. You have breast cancer." Provide clients with information about detection and risk factors, inform them about screening guidelines, instruct them on BSE, and outline dietary changes that might reduce their risk of breast cancer.

Awareness is the first step toward a change in habits. Raising the level of awareness about breast cancer is of paramount importance, and nurses can play an important role in health promotion, disease prevention, and education.

BREAST CANCER SCREENING

The three components of early detection are BSE, CBE, and mammography. People are exposed to multiple sources of cancer prevention information, and much of it may not be sound. Discuss the benefits, risks, and potential limitations of BSE, CBE, and mammography with each client and tailor the information to specific risk factors relevant to them (ACS, 2018b). Based on the guidelines, make clinical judgments as to the appropriateness of recommending BSE, and reevaluate the need to teach the procedure to all clients. The focus might instead be on encouraging regular mammograms (depending, of course, on the client's individual risk factors).

Breast Self-Examination

Breast self-examination (BSE) is a technique that enables individuals to detect any changes in their breasts. BSEs, once thought essential for early breast cancer detection, are now considered optional. Instead, breast awareness is stressed. Breast awareness refers to a person being familiar with the normal consistency of both breasts and the underlying tissue. This emphasis is now on awareness of breast changes, not just discovery of cancer. Research has shown that BSE plays a small role in detecting breast cancer compared with self-awareness. However, doing BSE is one way for individuals to know how their breasts normally feel so that they can notice any changes that do occur (ACS, 2018d).

If appropriate, there are two steps to conducting a BSE: visual inspection and tactile palpation. The visual part should be done in three separate positions: with the arms up behind the head, with the arms down at the sides, and bending forward. Instruct the client to look for:

- Changes in shape, size, contour, or symmetry
- Skin discolouration or dimpling, bumps/lumps
- Sores or scaly skin
- Discharge or puckering of the nipple

In the second part, the tactile examination, the health care provider feels the client's breasts in one of three specific patterns: spiral, pie-shaped wedges, or a vertical strip (up and down). When using any of the three patterns, the client should use a circular rubbing motion (in dime-sized circles) without lifting the fingers. The examiner checks not only the breasts but also between the breast and the axilla, the axilla itself, and the area above the breast up to the clavicle and across the shoulder. The pads of the three middle fingers on the right hand are used to assess the left breast; the pads of the three middle fingers on the left hand are used to assess the right breast. Instruct the client to use three different degrees of pressure:

- Light (move the skin without moving the tissue underneath)
- Medium (midway into the tissue)
- Hard (down to the ribs)

NUTRITION

Nutrition plays a critical role in health promotion and disease prevention. Cancer is considered to be a chronic disease that may be influenced at many stages by nutrition. These factors may affect prevention, progression, and treatment of the disease (Shrivastava, Shrivastava, & Ramasamy, 2015). Being overweight or obese is a risk factor for breast cancer in postmenopausal individuals. Excess body weight has been linked to an increased risk of postmenopausal breast cancer, and growing evidence also suggests that obesity is associated with poor prognosis in individuals diagnosed with early-stage breast cancer. Dozens of studies demonstrate that people who are overweight or obese at the time of breast cancer diagnosis are at increased risk of cancer recurrence and death compared with those who are leaner, and some evidence suggests that individuals who gain weight after breast cancer diagnosis may also be at increased risk of poor outcomes (Wright et al., 2015). Almost 65% of women over the age of 20 years are overweight; of these, 33.4% are obese (Carlson, 2015). A Mediterranean diet high in fruits, vegetables, and high-fibre carbohydrates and low in animal fats seems to offer protection against breast cancer as well as weight control. Women who followed these dietary guidelines decreased their risk of breast cancer. In addition, substantial evidence has shown that obesity, as measured by body mass index (BMI) is linked to breast cancer outcomes and greater mortality risks (Chan & Norat, 2015).

The Women's Health Initiative Dietary Modification Trial (Brasky et al., 2015) was designed to study a low-fat diet, a nutritional approach to prevention of chronic diseases. It found a marginally statistically significant reduction in breast cancer incidence among women in the low-fat dietary pattern group, and also disproved that "heart healthy eating" prevented future cardiac events in women.

The American Institute for Cancer Research, which conducts extensive research, made the following recommendations to reduce an individual's risk for developing breast cancer:

- Engaging in daily moderate exercise and weekly vigorous physical activity
- Consuming at least five servings of fruits and vegetables daily
- Not smoking or using any tobacco products
- Keeping a maximum BMI of 25 and limiting weight gain to no more than 11 lb since age 18
- Consuming seven or more daily portions of complex carbohydrates, such as whole grains and cereals
- Limiting intake of processed foods and refined sugar
- Limiting consumption of energy-dense foods and sugary drinks
- Avoiding use of dietary supplements which are unlikely to improve prognosis
- Restricting red meat intake to approximately 3 oz daily
- Limiting intake of fatty foods, particularly those of animal origin
- Restricting intake of salted foods and use of salt in cooking (Swisher et al., 2015)

The medical community is also starting to study the role of phytochemicals in health. The unique geographic variability of breast cancer around the world and the low rate of breast cancer in Asian countries compared with Western countries prompted this interest. This area of research appears hopeful for individuals seeking to prevent breast cancer as well as those recovering from it. Although the mechanism is not clear, certain foods demonstrate anticancer properties and boost the immune system. Phytochemical-rich foods include:

- Green tea and herbal teas
- Garlic
- Whole grains and legumes
- Onions and leeks
- Soybeans and soy products
- Tomato products (cooked tomatoes)
- Fruits (citrus, apricots, pumpkin, berries)
- Green leafy vegetables (spinach, collards, romaine)
- Colourful vegetables (carrots, squash, tomatoes)
- Cruciferous vegetables (broccoli, cabbage, cauliflower)
- Flax seeds (Bahadoran, Karimi, & Abedini, 2015)

Adopt a holistic approach when addressing the nutritional needs of individuals with breast cancer. Incorporate nutritional assessment into the general overall assessment of all women. Culturally sensitive nutritional assessment tools need to be developed and used to enhance this process. Providing examples of appropriate foods associated with the individual's current dietary habits, relating current health status to nutritional intake, and placing proposed modifications within a realistic personal framework may increase an individual's willingness to incorporate needed changes in nutritional behaviour. Be able to interpret research results and stay up to date on nutritional influences so that you can transmit this key information to the public.

NURSING CARE PLAN 6.1

Overview of the Woman With Fibrocystic Breast Changes

Sheree Rollins is a 37-year-old woman who comes to the clinic for her routine checkup. During the examination, she says, "Sometimes my breasts feel so heavy and they ache a lot. I noticed a couple of lumpy areas in my breast last week just before I got my period. Is this normal? Now they feel like they're almost gone. Should I be worried?" Clinical breast examination reveals two small (pea-sized), mobile, slightly tender nodules in each breast bilaterally. No skin retraction noted. Previous mammogram revealed fibrocystic breast changes.

NURSING DIAGNOSIS: Pain related to changes in breast tissue

Outcome Identification and Evaluation

The client will demonstrate a decrease in breast pain as evidenced by a pain rating of 1 or 2 on a pain rating scale of 0 to 10 with statements made that her pain is lessened.

Interventions: *Relieving Pain*

- Ask client to rate her pain using a numeric pain rating scale to establish a baseline.
- Discuss with client any measures used to relieve pain to determine effectiveness of the measures.
- Encourage use of a supportive bra to aid in reducing discomfort.
- Instruct client in use of over-the-counter analgesics to promote pain relief.

- Advise the client to apply warm compresses or allow warm water from the shower to flow over her breasts to promote vasodilation and subsequent pain relief.
- Tell client to reduce her intake of salt to reduce risk of fluid retention and swelling leading to increased pain.

NURSING DIAGNOSIS: Deficient knowledge related to fibrocystic breast changes and appropriate care measures

Outcome Identification and Evaluation

The client will verbalize understanding of condition as evidenced by statements about the cause of breast changes and appropriate choices for lifestyle changes, and demonstration of self-care measures.

Interventions: *Providing Client Education*

- Assess client's knowledge of fibrocystic breast changes to establish a baseline for teaching.
- Explain the role of monthly hormonal level changes and describe the signs and symptoms to promote understanding of this condition.
- Teach the client how to perform breast self-examination after a menstrual period to monitor for changes.
- Encourage client to report any changes promptly to ensure early detection of problems.
- Suggest client speak with her primary care provider about the use of oral contraceptives to help stabilize monthly hormonal levels.
- Review lifestyle choices, such as eating a low-fat diet rich in fruits, vegetables, and grains, and adhering to screening recommendations to promote health.
- Discuss measures for pain relief to minimize discomfort associated with breast changes.

KEY CONCEPTS

- Many people believe that all lumps are cancerous, but actually more than 80% of the lumps discovered are benign and need no treatment (Alexander et al., 2014).

- The most commonly encountered benign breast disorders in women include fibrocystic breasts, fibroadenomas, and mastitis (Bope & Kellerman, 2015).

- Current research suggests that women with fibrocystic breast disease or other benign breast conditions are more likely to develop breast cancer later only if a breast biopsy shows "atypia" or abnormal breast cells (ACS, 2018a).

- Fibroadenomas are common benign solid breast tumours that can be stimulated by external estrogen, progesterone, lactation, and pregnancy.

- Mastitis is an infection of the connective tissue in the breast that occurs primarily in lactating or engorged individuals; it is divided into lactational or nonlactational types.

- Management of both types of mastitis involves the use of oral antibiotics (usually a penicillinase-resistant penicillin or cephalosporin) and acetaminophen (Tylenol) for pain and fever (Miller, Escamilla, & King, 2018).

- Breast cancer is the most common cancer in women and the second leading cause of cancer deaths (lung cancer is first) among Canadian women (CCACCS, 2017).

- Breast cancer metastasizes widely and to almost all organs of the body, but primarily to the bone, lungs, lymph nodes, liver, and brain.

- The etiology of breast cancer is unknown, but the disease is thought to develop in response to a number of related factors: aging, delayed childbearing or never bearing children, high breast density, family history of cancer, late menopause, obesity, and hormonal factors.

- Breast cancer treatments fall into two categories: local and systemic. Local treatments are surgery and radiation therapy. Effective systemic treatments include chemotherapy, hormonal therapy, and immunotherapy.

- Women commonly perceive their breasts as intrinsic to their femininity, self-esteem, and sexuality, and the risk of losing a breast can provoke extreme anxiety.

- Nurses can influence both physical and emotional recovery, which are both important aspects of care that help in improving the individual's quality of life and the ability to survive.

- Providing up-to-date information and emotional support are central roles of the nurse in caring for the individuals with a diagnosis of breast cancer.

REFERENCES AND RECOMMENDED READINGS

Alexander, L. L., LaRosa, J. H., Bader, H., & Garfield, S. (2014). *New dimensions in women's health* (6th ed.). Sudbury, MA: Jones & Bartlett.

American Cancer Society (ACS). (2018a). *Breast cancer.* Retrieved from http://www.cancer.org/Cancer/BreastCancer/index

American Cancer Society (ACS). (2018b). *Risk factors for breast cancer.* Retrieved from http://www.cancer.org/cancer/breastcancer/detailedguide/breast-cancer-risk-factors

American Cancer Society (ACS). (2018c). *Understanding a breast cancer diagnosis.* Retrieved from http://www.cancer.org/cancer/breastcancer/detailedguide/breast-cancer-breast-cancer-types

American Cancer Society (ACS). (2018d). *Guidelines for the early detection of cancer.* Retrieved from http://www.cancer.org/healthy/findcancerearly/cancerscreeningguidelines/american-cancer-society-guidelines-for-the-early-detection-of-cancer

American Cancer Society (ACS). (2018e). *Cancer facts & figures.* Retrieved from http://www.cancer.org/acs/groups/content/@epidemiologysurveilance/documents/document/acspc-036845.pdf

American Cancer Society (ACS). (2018f). *Surgery for breast cancer.* Retrieved from http://www.cancer.org/cancer/breastcancer/detailedguide/breast-cancer-treating-surgery

American Cancer Society (ACS). (2018g). *Chemotherapy for breast cancer.* Retrieved from http://www.cancer.org/cancer/breastcancer/detailedguide/breast-cancer-treating-chemotherapy

American Cancer Society (ACS). (2019). *Fibrosis and simple cysts in the breast.* Retrieved from https://www.cancer.org/cancer/breast-cancer/non-cancerous-breast-conditions/fibrosis-and-simple-cysts-in-the-breast.html

Arora, R., Schmitt, D., Karanam, B., Tan, M., Yates, C., & Dean-Colomb, W. (2015). Inhibition of the Warburg effect with a natural compound reveals a novel measurement for determining the metastatic potential of breast cancers. *Oncotarget, 6*(2), 662–678.

Bahadoran, Z., Karimi, Z., & Abedini, S. (2015). Healthy dietary patterns and the risk of breast cancer: A review of current data. *American Journal of Life Sciences, 3*(2–1), 1–5.

Ball, J. W., Dains, J. E., Flynn, J. A., Soloman, B. S., & Stewart, R. W. (2015). *Seidel's guide to physical examination* (8th ed.). St. Louis, MO: Elsevier Saunders.

Bevers, T. B. (2015). Breast cancer risk reduction therapy: The low-hanging fruit. *Journal of the National Comprehensive Cancer Network, 13*(4), 376–378.

Bhatti, L., Hoang, J. K., Dale, B. M., & Bashir, M. R. (2015). Advanced magnetic resonance techniques: 3 T. *Radiologic Clinics of North America, 53*(3), 441–455.

Bope, E. T., & Kellerman, R. D. (2015). *Conn's current therapy 2015*. Philadelphia, PA: Saunders Elsevier.

Bourdeanu, L., & Liu, E. A. (2015). Systemic treatment for breast cancer: Chemotherapy and biotherapy agents. *Seminars in Oncology Nursing, 31*(2), 156–162.

Brasky, T. M., Rodabough, R. J., Liu, J., Kurta, M. L., Wise, L. A., Orchard, T. S., … Neuhouser, M. L. (2015). Long-chain ω-3 fatty acid intake and endometrial cancer risk in the Women's Health Initiative. *The American Journal of Clinical Nutrition, 101*(4), 824–834.

Breast Cancer Organization. (2018). *Hormonal therapy side effects*. Retrieved from http://www.breastcancer.org/treatment/hormonal/comp_chart

Canadian Cancer Society's Advisory Committee on Cancer Statistics. (2017). *Canadian Cancer Statistics 2017*. Toronto, ON: Canadian Cancer Society. Retrieved from cancer.ca/Canadian-CancerStatistics-2017-EN.pdf Accessed April 2018.

Canadian Partnership Against Cancer. (2016). *Breast Cancer Screening in Canada: Monitoring and Evaluation of Quality Indicators—Results Report, January 2011–December 2012*. Toronto, ON: Canadian Partnership Against Cancer.

Canadian Task Force on Preventive Health Care. (2011). Recommendations on screening for breast cancer in average-risk women aged 40–74 years. *Canadian Medical Association Journal, 183*(17), 1991–2001.

Caple, C., & Schub, T. (2015). Breast cancer: Psychological adjustment. *CINAHL Information Systems*. (Online 4/17/15) Evidence-based Care Sheet.

Carlson, R. H. (2015). Obesity and breast cancer: Research update. *Oncology Times, 37*(9), 33.

Catsburg, C., Kim, R. S., Kirsh, V. A., Soskolne, C. L., Kreiger, N., & Rohan, T. E. (2015). Dietary patterns and breast cancer risk: A study in 2 cohorts. *The American Journal of Clinical Nutrition, 101*(4), 817–823.

Chan, D. S., & Norat, T. (2015). Obesity and breast cancer: Not only a risk factor of the disease. *Current Treatment Options in Oncology, 16*(5), 1–17.

Chang, Z., Craciunescu, O., Xu, X., Steffey, B., Meltsner, S., Cai, J., … Chino, J. (2015). Evaluating radiation-induced changes with diffusion weighted imaging in patients with gynecologic cancers treated with combined external beam radiation radiotherapy and high-dose-rate brachytherapy: Initial results. *Brachytherapy, 14*, S75–S76.

Chatterjee, A., Serniak, N., & Czerniecki, B. J. (2015). Sentinel lymph node biopsy in breast cancer: A work in progress. *The Cancer Journal, 21*(1), 7–10.

Chu, Q. D., Caldito, G., Miller, J. K., & Townsend, B. (2015). Postmastectomy radiation for N2/N3 breast cancer: Factors associated with low compliance rate. *Journal of the American College of Surgeons, 220*(4), 659–669.

Corradini, S., Niyazi, M., Niemoeller, O. M., Li, M., Roeder, F., Eckel, R., … Belka, C. (2015). Adjuvant radiotherapy after breast conserving surgery—A comparative effectiveness research study. *Radiotherapy & Oncology, 114*(1), 28–34.

Cuzick, J., & Thorat, M. (2015). PG 6.02 Preventing invasive breast cancer in women at high risk based on benign/in situ pathology. *The Breast, 24*, S11.

Dear, R. F., McGeechan, K., Jenkins, M. C., Barratt, A., Tattersall, M. H., & Wilcken, N. (2015). Combination versus sequential single agent chemotherapy for metastatic breast cancer. *Cochrane Database of Systematic Reviews, 3*:CD008792.

Debled, M., MacGrogan, G., Breton-Callu, C., Ferron, S., Hurtevent, G., Fournier, M., … Tunon de Lara, C. (2015). Surgery following neoadjuvant chemotherapy for HER2-positive locally advanced breast cancer. Time to reconsider the standard attitude. *European Journal of Cancer, 51*(6), 697–704.

Dixon, J. M., & Macaskill, E. J. (2015). Management of benign breast disease. In A. Riker (Ed.), *Breast disease* (pp. 51–77). New York: Springer Publishers.

Euhus, D. M., & Diaz, J. (2015). Breast cancer prevention. *The Breast Journal, 21*(1), 76–81.

Faguy, K. (2015). Breast disorders in pregnant and lactating women. *Radiologic Technology, 86*(4), 419M–438M.

Fallowfield, L., & Jenkins, V. (2015). Psychosocial/Survivorship issues in breast cancer: Are we doing better? *Journal of the National Cancer Institute, 107*(1), 335.

Files, J. A., Allen, S. V., & Pruthi, S. (2015). Management of breast pain. In A. Riker (Ed.), *Breast disease* (pp. 79–91). New York: Springer Publishers.

Gradishar, W. J. (2015). Adjuvant therapy for breast cancer: Hormonal therapy. In A. Riker (Ed.), *Breast disease* (pp. 353–362). New York: Springer Publishers.

Guinot, J. L., Baixauli-Perez, C., Soler, P., Tortajada, M. I., Moreno, A., Santos, M. A., … Arribas, L. (2015). High-dose-rate brachytherapy boost effect on local tumor control in young women with breast cancer. *International Journal of Radiation Oncology, Biology, Physics, 91*(1), 165–171.

Han, F., Shi, G., Liang, C., Wang, L., & Li, K. (2015). A simple and efficient method for breast cancer diagnosis based on infrared thermal imaging. *Cell Biochemistry and Biophysics, 71*(1), 491–498.

Jager, N. G. L., Linn, S. C., Schellens, J. H., & Beijnen, J. H. (2015). Tailored tamoxifen treatment for breast cancer patients: A perspective. *Clinical Breast Cancer, 15*(4), 241–244.

Janardhan, J., Venkateshwar, P., & Rao, K. S. (2015). Giant fibroadenoma of the breast: Conservative surgery. *International Archives of Integrated Medicine, 2*(4), 156–160.

Jarvis, C. (2015). *Physical examination & health assessment* (7th ed.). St. Louis, MO: Elsevier Health Sciences.

Kalinsky, K., Mayer, J. A., Xu, X., Pham, T., Wong, K. L., Villarin, E., … Bischoff, F. Z. (2015). Correlation of hormone receptor status between circulating tumor cells, primary tumor, and metastasis in breast cancer patients. *Clinical and Translational Oncology, 17*(7), 539–546.

Khan, M. H., Allerton, R., & Pettit, L. (2015). Hormone therapy for male breast cancer. *Clinical Breast Cancer, 15*(4), 245–250.

King, T. L., Brucker, M. C., Kriebs, J. M., Fahey, J. O., Gegor, C. L., & Varney, H. (2015) *Varney's midwifery* (5th ed.). Burlington, MA: Jones & Bartlett Learning.

Kleban, R., & Glaser, S. (2015). The many dimensions of breast cancer: Determining the scope of needed services. In G. Christ, C. Messner, & L. Behar (Eds.), *Handbook of oncology social work: Psychosocial care for people with cancer* (pp. 93–99). New York: Oxford University Press.

Lara, P. C., López-Peñalver, J. J., Farias, V. A., Ruiz-Ruiz, M. C., Oliver, F. J., & Ruiz de Almodóvar, J. M. (2015). Direct and bystander radiation effects: A biophysical model and clinical perspectives. *Cancer Letters, 356*(1), 5–16.

Leavy, O. (2015). Immunotherapy: A triple blow for cancer. *Nature Reviews Cancer, 15*, 258–259.

Li, J., Holm, J., Bergh, J., Eriksson, M., Darabi, H., Lindström, L. S., … Czene, K. (2015). Breast cancer genetic risk profile is differentially associated with interval and screen-detected breast cancers. *Annals of Oncology, 26*(3), 517–522.

Miller, A. C., Escamilla, C., & King, A. R. (2018). Breast abscess and masses. *eMedicine*. Retrieved from http://emedicine.medscape.com/article/781116-overview#a0104

Mills, S. (2013). Performing a clinical breast exam. *Nursing, 43*(9), 68.

Mugea, T. T. (2015). Complications of breast augmentation. In T. T. Mugea & M. A. Shiffman (Eds.), *Aesthetic surgery of the breast* (pp. 425–512). Berlin, Heidelberg: Springer.

Muralidhar, K. R., Soubhagya, B., & Ahmed, S. (2015). Intensity modulated radiotherapy versus volumetric modulated arc therapy in breast cancer: A comparative dosimetric analysis. *International Journal of Cancer Therapy and Oncology, 3*(2), 1–6.

National Cancer Institute (NCI). (2018a). Breast cancer. Retrieved from http://www.cancer.gov/cancertopics/types/breast

National Cancer Institute (NCI). (2018b). Probability of breast cancer in American women. Retrieved from http://www.cancer.gov/cancertopics/factsheet/detection/probability-breast-cancer

National Comprehensive Cancer Network (NCCN). (2018). *Breast cancer treatment guidelines: NCCN patient guidelines*. Retrieved from http://www.nccn.org/patients/patient_gls/_english/_breast/5_treatment.asp

Pluchinotta, A. M. (2015). Inflammatory diseases of the breast. In A. M. Pluchinotta (Ed.), *The outpatient breast clinic* (pp. 169–195). Springer International Publishing.

Poulos, A. (2015). Diagnostic breast imaging: Mammography, sonography, magnetic resonance imaging, and interventional procedures. *Journal of Medical Radiation Sciences, 62*(1), 86–87.

Rifkin, E., & Lazris, A. (2015). Breast cancer screening: Mammograms. In E. Rifkin & A. Lazris (Eds.), *Interpreting health benefits and risks* (pp. 33–41). Springer International Publishing.

Sabel, M. S. (2018). Overview of benign breast disease. *UpToDate*. Retrieved from http://www.uptodate.com/contents/overview-of-benign-breast-disease

Schuiling, K. D., & Likis, F. E. (2016). *Women's gynecological health* (3rd ed.). Burlington, MA: Jones & Bartlett Learning.

Seetharam, P., & Rodrigues, G. (2015). Benign breast disorders: An insight with a detailed literature review. *Webmed Central Breast, 6*(1) doi: 10.9754/journal.wmc.2015.004806

Selvi, R. (2015). Invasive lobular carcinoma. In R. Selvi (Ed.), *Breast diseases: Imaging and clinical management* (pp. 281–286). India: Springer Publishers.

Sestak, I., & Cuzick, J. (2015). Update on breast cancer risk prediction and prevention. *Current Opinion in Obstetrics and Gynecology, 27*(1), 92–97.

Shannon, K. M., & Chittenden, A. (2015). Breast cancer genetics and risk assessment. In M. Shetty (Ed.), *Breast cancer screening and diagnosis* (pp. 1–21). New York: Springer Publishers.

Shrivastava, S. R., Shrivastava, P. S., & Ramasamy, J. (2015). Assessing the contribution of dietary factors in breast cancer. *Clinical Cancer Investigation Journal, 4*(1), 1–5.

Skidmore-Roth, L. (2015). *Mosby's 2015 nursing drug reference* (28th ed.). St. Louis, MO: Elsevier Health Science.

Slanetz, P. J., Freer, P. E., & Birdwell, R. L. (2015). Breast-density legislation—Practical considerations. *New England Journal of Medicine, 372*(7), 593–595.

Stopeck, A. T., Chalasani, P., & Thompson, P. A. (2015). Breast cancer. *eMedicine*. Retrieved from http://emedicine.medscape.com/article/1947145-overview

Strayer, D. A., & Schub, T. (2014). Breast cancer. Published by CINAHL Information Systems. Full Text, EBSCOhost

Swisher, A. K., Abraham, J., Bonner, D., Gilleland, D., Hobbs, G., Kurian, S., … Vona-Davis, L. (2015). Exercise and dietary advice intervention for survivors of triple-negative breast cancer: effects on body fat, physical function, quality of life, and adipokine profile. *Supportive Care in Cancer, 23*(10), 2995–3003.

Tharpe, N. L., Farley, C. L., & Jordan, R. G. (2016). *Clinical practice guidelines for midwifery & women's health* (5th ed.). Burlington, MA: Jones & Bartlett Learning.

Toi, M., Winer, E. P., Benson, J. R., & Klimberg, S. (2015). *Personalized treatment of breast cancer*. Japan: Springer Publishers.

Tsujimoto, M. (2015). Recent advances in sentinel node biopsy in breast surgery. *Breast Cancer, 22*(3), 211.

U.S. Preventive Services Task Force (USPSTF). (2016). *Screening for breast cancer*. Retrieved from https://www.uspreventiveservicestaskforce.org/Announcements/News/Item/final-recommendation-statement-screening-for-breast-cancer

van den Broek, A. J., Schmidt, M. K., van't Veer, L. J., Tollenaar, R. M., & van Leeuwen, F. E. (2015). Worse breast cancer prognosis of BRCA1/BRCA2 mutation carriers: What's the evidence? A systematic review with meta-analysis. *Plos ONE, 10*(3), 1–29.

Wevers, M. R., Ausems, M. M., Verhoef, S., Bleiker, E. A., Hahn, D. E., Brouwer, T., … Aaronson, N. K. (2015). Does rapid genetic counseling and testing in newly diagnosed breast cancer patients cause additional psychosocial distress? Results from a randomized clinical trial. *Genetics in Medicine: Official Journal of the American College of Medical Genetics, 18*(2), 137–144.

Wright, C. E., Harvie, M., Howell, A., Evans, D. G., Hulbert-Williams, N., & Donnelly, L. S. (2015). Beliefs about weight and breast cancer: An interview study with high risk women following a 12 month weight loss intervention. *Hereditary Cancer in Clinical Practice, 13*(1), 1.

Writing Group for the Women's Health Initiative Investigators. (2002). Women's Health Initiative Study. *JAMA, 288*(3), 321–333.

CHAPTER **WORKSHEET**

MULTIPLE CHOICE QUESTIONS

1. Breast self-examinations involve both touching of breast tissue and:
   a. Palpation of cervical lymph nodes
   b. Firm squeezing of both breast nipples
   c. Visualizing both breasts for any change
   d. A mammogram to evaluate breast tissue

2. Which of the following is the strongest risk factor for breast cancer?
   a. Advancing age and being female
   b. High number of children
   c. Genetic mutations in BRCA1 and BRCA2 genes
   d. Family history of colon cancer

3. A biopsy procedure that traces radioisotopes and blue dye from the tumour site through the lymphatic system into the axillary nodes is:
   a. Stereotactic biopsy
   b. Sentinel node biopsy
   c. Axillary dissection biopsy
   d. Advanced breast biopsy

4. The most serious potential adverse reaction from chemotherapy is:
   a. Thrombocytopenia
   b. Deep vein thrombosis
   c. Alopecia
   d. Myelosuppression

5. What suggestion would be helpful for the client experiencing painful fibrocystic breast changes?
   a. Increase caffeine intake.
   b. Take a mild analgesic when needed.
   c. Reduce intake of leafy vegetables.
   d. Wear a bra bigger than needed.

6. A postoperative mastectomy client should be referred to which of the following organizations for assistance upon discharge from the hospital?
   a. National Organization for Women (NOW)
   b. Food and Drug Administration (FDA)
   c. March of Dimes Foundation (MDF)
   d. Canadian Cancer Society (CCS)

7. Breast cancer that is localized is referred to as:
   a. Primary
   b. In situ
   c. Metastasized
   d. Localized

8. A 25-year-old woman presents with an asymptomatic breast mass. Which of the following is true concerning her diagnosis and treatment?
   a. All breast masses should be considered premalignant
   b. The breast mass should be surgically removed immediately
   c. Ultrasound is typically used to determine the diagnosis
   d. Since it is asymptomatic, just reassurance is needed now

CRITICAL THINKING EXERCISES

1. Mrs. Gordon, 48, presents to the community clinic where you work as a nurse. She is very upset and crying. She tells you that she found lumps in her breast: "I know that it's cancer and I will die." When you ask her about her problem, she says she does not check her breasts monthly and hasn't had a mammogram for years. She also describes the intermittent pain she experiences.
   a. What specific questions would you ask this client to get a clearer picture?
   b. What education is needed for this client regarding breast health?
   c. What community referrals are needed to meet this client's future needs?

2. Ruth Davis, 51, stops in at the urgent care facility with an anxious look on her face. She tells the nurse practitioner that she has green discharge coming from her right breast and discomfort intermittently. She can't understand how this would happen since she hasn't previously had any nipple discharge or pain.
   a. What benign breast condition might the nurse practitioner suspect based on her description?
   b. What specific information should the nurse practitioner give Mrs. Davis about duct ectasia?
   c. The typical treatment of this benign breast condition would include what?

STUDY ACTIVITIES

1. Discuss with a group of women what their breasts symbolize to them and to society. Do they symbolize something different to each one?

2. When an individual experiences a breast disorder, what feelings might that individual be experiencing and how can a nurse help sort these feelings out?

3. Interview a woman who has fibrocystic breast changes and find out how she manages this condition.

4. An infection of the breast connective tissue that frequently occurs in the lactating individual is _____.

CHAPTER **WORKSHEET**

BRINGING IT ALL TOGETHER: A CASE STUDY

A 67-year-old obese woman presented to her internist after a several year absence complaining of back pain that has persisted despite taking a nonsteroidal anti-inflammatory drug (NSAID) for several weeks. She also has recently noticed a 10-lb weight loss over the past 6 months and occasional right upper quadrant discomfort. She also states that she has been feeling tired over the last several months, but rationalized it as "old age" catching up with her.

ASSESSMENT

She has a family history of breast and colon cancer in her immediate family and both of her parents died from these (mother from breast cancer and father from colon cancer). Her aunt also had breast cancer, but is in remission now after treatment. She can't remember when the last time she had a Pap smear or mammogram. She admits that she doesn't keep up with her health checkups, since she babysits for her grandchildren and has difficulty scheduling them. She confesses that her diet hasn't been what it should be, since her grandchildren prefer fast food and sodas for meals, rather than home-cooked ones. Thus, she gives into them and eats what they want.

1. Based on her chief complaint, what might be a reason for her current back pain?

2. What is concerning about her family health history that might have a bearing on her present symptoms?

3. How does her poor dietary intake and weight status impact her overall health status?

   Breast cancer does metastasize to the bone and this could be the reason for her back pain that doesn't respond to anti-inflammatory medications. Since she has first-degree relatives that had cancer, she is at high risk for it herself. Research in nutrition and obesity and its link to cancer suggests that high consumption of processed foods (fast foods) and low consumption of fruits and vegetables in addition to being obese places people at risk for cancer.

PLAN

1. What diagnostic tests might be ordered to determine her diagnosis?

2. What treatment modalities are available to her if metastatic cancer is found?

3. What health promotion instructions are needed for this client?

4. How can the nurse provide an open forum for this woman to discuss her feelings?

   An MRI and a bone scan might be ordered to identify any "hot spots" or cancerous lesions on her bones as well as her liver, which are common areas cancer might have spread to. Depending on the extent of the metastasis, chemotherapy and radiation might be treatment modalities. Nutrition counselling and lifestyle changes to lose weight to promote better health are both health promotion areas that need to be addressed with this client. A thorough explanation of the treatments, their side effects and prognosis need to also be discussed to make sure she understands. Fear and anxiety are common feelings felt by anyone with a cancer diagnosis, so the nurse needs to be open and supportive to her and allow time for her to express her fears.

7

Benign Disorders of the Reproductive Tract

KEY TERMS

cystocele

enterocele

genital fistula

ovarian cyst

pelvic floor muscle
    exercises (Kegel
    exercises)

pelvic organ
    prolapse (POP)

pessary

polycystic ovary
    syndrome (PCOS)

polyps

rectocele

urinary
    incontinence (UI)

uterine fibroids

uterine prolapse

Learning Objectives

Upon completion of the chapter, you will be able to:

1. Characterize the major pelvic relaxation disorders in terms of etiology, management, and nursing interventions.

2. Outline the nursing management needed for common benign reproductive disorders.

3. Evaluate urinary incontinence in terms of pathology, clinical manifestations, treatment options, and effect on quality of life.

4. Compare the various benign growths in terms of their symptoms and management.

5. Analyze the emotional impact of polycystic ovarian syndrome and the nurse's role as a counsellor, educator, and advocate.

Liz, **a 26-year-old woman, presented to the clinic with hirsutism and facial acne and told the nurse she was concerned about her weight gain and irregular menstrual periods. She also said that recently the hair on top of her head seemed to be falling out. What diagnostic tests might the nurse anticipate with this client? How can the nurse prepare Liz for them?**

INTRODUCTION

The incidence of several benign pelvic disorders increases as cis-gender women and transgender men age. For instance, pelvic floor disorders related to pelvic relaxation or urinary incontinence (UI) increase with aging. These disorders generally develop after years of wear and tear on the muscles and tissues that support the pelvic floor—such as that which occurs with childbearing, chronic coughing, straining, surgery, or simply aging. In addition to pelvic floor disorders, individuals may also experience various benign neoplasms of the reproductive tract, such as cervical polyps, uterine leiomyomas (fibroids), ovarian cysts, genital fistulas, and Bartholin cysts. This chapter provides an overview of various pelvic floor disorders and benign neoplasms, discussing the assessment, treatment, and prevention strategies for each. The chapter also addresses female genital cutting in the context of it being a harmful practice that affects affected individuals' health. While the pelvic organs and conditions outlined in this chapter have historically been labelled as "female," these also pertain to transgender men who have not undergone surgical transition.

PELVIC FLOOR DISORDERS

Pelvic floor disorders such as pelvic organ prolapse (POP) or genital prolapse and urinary and fecal incontinence are common in aging cis-gender women. Age is closely linked to prevalence and the level of severity of all pelvic floor disorders (Hallock & Handa, 2016). Miedel, Tegerstedt, Moehle-Schmidt, Nyren, and Hammarstrom (2009) conducted a study which investigated over 5,400 women between the ages of 30 and 79 years with an intact uterus and a negative history of pelvic surgeries. They found that age had a profound impact on symptomatic POP (Miedel et al., 2009). Women in their 70s and 80s had a significant increase in bothersome symptoms as compared to those in their 50s (Kinman et al., 2017).

Pelvic floor disorders cause significant physical and psychological morbidity and can diminish a person's social interactions, emotional well-being, and overall quality of life. Because these disorders increase with age, the problem will grow worse as our population ages. The term "pelvic floor" refers to the group of muscles that form a sling or hammock across the pelvis. Together with their surrounding tissues, these muscles hold the pelvic organs (uterus, bladder, and bowel) in place so that they can function correctly. These disorders occur as a result of weakness of the connective tissue and muscular support of pelvic organs due to a number of factors: pregnancy, vaginal childbirth, obesity, lifting, chronic cough from smoking, straining at defecation secondary to constipation, radiation to the pelvis for cancer, and estrogen deficiency (American College of Obstetricians and Gynecologists [ACOG], 2017). The female anatomy is susceptible to the development of pelvic floor disorders because of its vertical structures placement. The bony pelvis has an exaggerated lumbar spinal curve and downward tilt to it. The bladder rests on the symphysis and the posterior organs rest on the sacrum and coccyx. The pelvis holds the organs, but a person's erect posture causes a funneling effect and constant downward pressure.

Pelvic Organ Prolapse

Pelvic organ prolapse (POP) (from the Latin *prolapsus,* "a slipping forth") refers to the abnormal descent or herniation of the pelvic organs from their original attachment sites or their normal position in the pelvis. POP occurs when structures of the pelvis shift and protrude into or outside of the vaginal canal. This disorder affects an individual's micturition, defecation, and sexual activity. The Egyptians were the first to describe prolapse of the genital organs. Hippocrates in 400 BC made reference to placing a pomegranate half into the vagina to treat organ prolapse. POP rarely results in severe morbidity or mortality but can affect a person's daily activities and quality of life (Brown, 2015). It is difficult to determine the incidence of POP, because the disorder is often asymptomatic and many affected individuals do not seek treatment. Each year, over 250,000 clients undergo surgery to repair the prolapse at a cost of over $1 billion for hospitalization and physician or nurse practitioner fees alone (Maher & Haya, 2015). As the older adult population is expected to double in number by 2030, POP and its associated symptoms will become more prevalent (Mukwege, El-Nashar, Rhodes, Dowdy, & Trabuco, 2015).

Obesity is associated with a high prevalence of pelvic floor disorders (Lee, Kerkhof, van Leijsen, & Heesakkers, 2017). Obesity can also aggravate symptoms of POP, fecal incontinence, sexual dysfunction, stress UI, and increase the risk of endometrial polyps and symptomatic fibroids. Weight reduction enhances reproductive outcomes, diminishes symptoms of UI, improves sexual dysfunction, and reduces morbidity following gynecologic surgery. Sustained and substantial weight loss, however, is difficult to achieve for many clients with their current lifestyle and dietary choices (Ramalingam & Monga, 2015).

The treatment and diagnosis of POP is challenging and problematic.

Types of Pelvic Organ Prolapse

The four most common types of pelvic or genital prolapse are cystocele, rectocele, enterocele, and uterine prolapse (Fig. 7.1):

- **Cystocele** occurs when the posterior bladder wall protrudes downward through the anterior vaginal wall.
- **Rectocele** occurs when the rectum sags and pushes against or into the posterior vaginal wall.

FIGURE 7.1 Types of pelvic prolapses. **A.** Normal. **B.** Rectocele
and cystocele. **C.** Enterocele.
D. Uterine prolapse.

- **Enterocele** occurs when the small intestine bulges through the posterior vaginal wall (especially common when straining).
- **Uterine prolapse** occurs when the uterus descends through the pelvic floor and into the vaginal canal. Multiparous individuals are at particular risk for uterine prolapse. The extent of uterine prolapse is classified in terms of stages:
  - *Stage 0:* No descent of pelvic structure during straining.
  - *Stage I:* The prolapsed descending organ is >1 cm above the hymenal ring.
  - *Stage II:* The prolapsed organ extends ~1 cm below the hymenal ring.
  - *Stage III:* The prolapsed organ extends 2 to 3 cm below the hymenal ring.
  - *Stage IV:* The vagina is completely everted or the prolapsed organ is >3 cm below the hymenal ring (Riss & Koch, 2015).

Etiology

Anatomic support of the pelvic organs is mainly provided by the levator ani muscle complex and the connective tissue attachments of the pelvic organ fascia. Dysfunction of one or both of these components can lead to loss of support and eventually POP. Weakened pelvic floor muscles also prevent complete closure of the urethra, resulting in urine leakage during physical stress. This problem is not limited to older clients: UI has been documented in cis-gender women of varying ages, including those under the age of 25 years (Walters, 2015).

Many risk factors for POP have been suggested, but the true cause is likely to be multifactorial. Causes might include:

- Constant downward gravity because of erect human posture
- Atrophy of supporting tissues with aging and decline of estrogen levels
- Weakening of pelvic support related to childbirth trauma
- Reproductive surgery, including hysterectomy
- Instrumental childbirth
- Multiparity
- Uncontrolled rapid birth
- Family history of POP
- Young age at first birth
- Connective tissue disorders

- Infant birth weight of more than 4,500 g
- Pelvic radiation
- Increased abdominal pressure secondary to:
  - Lifting of children or heavy objects
  - Straining due to chronic constipation
  - Respiratory problems or chronic coughing
  - Obesity (Rodriguez-Mias, Martínez-Franco, Aguado, Sánchez, & Amat-Tardiu, 2015)

Therapeutic Management

Treatment options for POP depend on the symptoms and their effect on the person's quality of life. Important considerations when deciding on nonsurgical or surgical options include the severity of symptoms, client's personal preferences, health status, age, suitability for surgery, and the presence of other pelvic conditions (urinary or fecal incontinence).

Conservative measures such as pelvic floor muscle exercises (PFMEs), or Kegel exercises, supplemented by lifestyle interventions such as weight loss, avoidance of straining (reducing lifting heavy weights, treatment of chronic cough and constipation) are recommended as first-line management. PFME is aimed to increase the strength and endurance of the pelvic floor supports, prevent or delay worsening of prolapse, and improve prolapse symptoms. PFME can help clients delay or avert the need for surgery and pre- and postoperatively have been found to improve outcomes after surgery.

When surgery is being considered, the nature of the procedure and the likely outcome must be fully explained and discussed with the client. Treatment options for POP include PFMEs, estrogen replacement therapy, dietary and lifestyle modifications, use of a **pessary** (a removable device placed into the vagina to support pelvic organs), and surgery (Evidence-Based Practice 7.1).

PELVIC FLOOR MUSCLE EXERCISES

Pelvic floor muscle exercises (PFME), also known as **Kegel exercises**, strengthen the pelvic floor muscles to support the inner organs and prevent further prolapse. PFMEs are generally accepted as first-line treatment for stress and urge UI and they are also widely used for anal incontinence. Over the past 30 years a wealth of research has proven the benefits of PFMEs in treating both UI and POP (McClurg, Gerrard, & Hove, 2015). The purpose of pelvic floor exercises is to increase the muscle volume, which will result in a stronger muscular contraction. PFMEs might limit the progression of mild prolapse and alleviate mild prolapse symptoms, including low back

---

EVIDENCE-BASED PRACTICE 7.1

PELVIC FLOOR MUSCLE TRAINING VERSES NO TREATMENT, OR INACTIVE CONTROL TREATMENTS, FOR URINARY INCONTINENCE

STUDY

Involuntary leakage of urine (urinary incontinence) affects cis-gender women of all ages, particularly older women who live in residential care such as nursing homes. Some individuals leak urine during exercise or when they cough or sneeze (stress urinary incontinence) and this may occur as a result of weakness of the pelvic floor muscles such as damage during childbirth. Others leak urine before going to the toilet when there is a sudden and compelling need to pass urine (urgency urinary incontinence). This may be caused by involuntary contraction of the bladder muscle. Mixed urinary incontinence is the combination of both stress and urgency urinary incontinence. Pelvic floor muscle training is a supervised physical therapy treatment and it involves muscle-clenching exercises to strengthen the pelvic floor muscles. It is a common treatment used by women to stop urine leakage. Other treatments are also available which can either be used alone or in combination with pelvic floor muscle training (PFMT).

PFMT is a conservative treatment for urinary incontinence. This systematic review evaluated the effects of PFMT when compared to no treatment, placebo, or other inactive control treatments for urinary incontinence in women.

This study was done to compare the effects of PFMT to no treatment, placebo, or other inactive control treatments in the management of women with urinary incontinence.

Findings

Randomized or quasi-randomized trials were used. Twenty-one trials (1,281 women) met the eligibility criteria for inclusion, comprising women with stress urinary incontinence (SUI), urgency urinary incontinence (UUI), or mixed urinary incontinence (MUI), and they compared PFMT added to no treatment, placebo, or other inactive control treatments.

This systematic review found support for the widespread recommendation that PFMT be included in first-line conservative management programs for women with stress and any type of urinary incontinence. In women with stress incontinence, there was high-quality evidence that PFMT is associated with improvement or cure.

Nursing Implications

Overall, according to this study, there is sufficient evidence to support the widespread recommendation that PFMT should be included in a first-line conservative management program for cis-gender women with stress, urge, or mixed urinary incontinence. Previous studies have validated that pelvic floor exercises do help in bringing tone to the muscles that control micturition. Nurses can continue to instruct clients with urinary incontinence to perform PFMT daily to improve their urinary control and their quality of life.

Adapted from Dumoulin, C., Hay-Smith, J., Habee-Seguin, G. M., & Mercier, J. (2015). Pelvic floor muscle training verses no treatment, or inactive control treatments, for urinary incontinence in women: A short version Cochrane systematic review with meta-analysis. *Neurourology and Urodynamics, 34*(4), 300–308.

pain and pelvic pressure. They will not, however, help severe uterine prolapse.

HORMONE REPLACEMENT THERAPY

Hormone replacement therapy, or HRT (orally, transdermally, low-dose vaginal ring, or vaginal cream) may improve the tone, natural thickness, and vascularity of the supporting tissue in perimenopausal and menopausal clients by increasing blood perfusion and the elasticity of the vaginal wall. HRT has many benefits, as well as risks. It is essential that the benefits are weighed out against the risks before this therapy is initiated.

Take Note!

Before hormone therapy is considered, a thorough medical history must be taken to assess a client's risk for complications (e.g., endometrial cancer, myocardial infarction, stroke, breast cancer, pulmonary emboli, and deep vein thrombosis). Because of these risks, estrogens, with or without progestins, should be given at the lowest effective dose and for the shortest duration consistent with the treatment goals and risks for the individual (ACOG, 2017).

DIETARY AND LIFESTYLE MODIFICATIONS

Dietary and lifestyle modifications may help prevent pelvic relaxation and chronic problems later in life. Specific lifestyle changes would include avoiding constipation, bladder irritants, heavy lifting, or high impact exercise, and focusing attention on healthy weight loss and smoking cessation. Dietary habits can exacerbate the prolapse by causing constipation and consequently chronic straining. Constipated stools are hard and dry, and typically cause straining while bearing down to defecate. This straining to pass a hard stool increases intra-abdominal pressure, which over time causes the pelvic organs to prolapse. Dietary modifications can help to establish regular bowel movements without discomfort and eliminate flatus and bloating. A weight loss regimen will also be recommended if the client is overweight.

PESSARIES

Vaginal pessaries are synthetic devices inserted in the vagina to provide support to the bladder and other pelvic organs as a corrective measure for UI and/or POP (Fig. 7.2). Today almost all pessaries are made of medical-grade silicone, which provides many advantages. Silicone pessaries are pliable and have a long shelf life; lack odour and secretion absorption; are biologically inert, nonallergenic, and noncarcinogenic; and they can be boiled or autoclaved for sterilization. Because most pessaries are made of silicone, pessary style and size are the main considerations when selecting a pessary (Colyar, 2015). Although many types and shapes are available, the most commonly used pessary is a firm ring that presses against the wall of the vagina and urethra to

FIGURE 7.2 **Examples of pessaries. A.** Various shapes and sizes of pessaries available. **B.** Insertion of one type of pessary.

help decrease leakage and support a prolapsed vagina or uterus. Pessaries are a low-risk treatment option with the advantage of being cost effective, minimally invasive while providing immediate relief of symptoms.

Indications for pessary use include uterine prolapse or cystocele, especially among elderly clients for whom surgery is contraindicated; younger clients with prolapse who plan to have additional children; and those with marked prolapse who prefer to use a pessary rather than undergo surgery (Ralph & Tamussino, 2015). Many clients use pessaries for only a short period of time and become free of symptoms. Long-term use can lead to pressure necrosis and the development of fistulas in some individuals; in this situation, other methods of support should be explored. Pessaries are fitted by trial and error; the client often needs to try several sizes or styles. The largest pessary that the person can wear comfortably is generally the most effective. The client should be instructed to report any discomfort or difficulty with urination or defecation while wearing the pessary and also to attend follow-up care appointments to check positioning.

Nurses need to be aware of the personal isolation and embarrassment and social and cultural implications that UI may cause as well as the subjective experiences of using a pessary. With appropriate support, vaginal pessaries can provide affected individuals with the freedom to lead active, engaged social lives.

SURGICAL INTERVENTIONS

Surgical interventions for pelvic or genital organ prolapse are designed to correct specific defects, with the goals being to restore normal anatomy and to preserve function. Surgery may not be an option for all clients. Those who are at high risk of suffering recurrent prolapse after a surgical repair or who have morbid obesity, chronic obstructive pulmonary disease, or medical conditions in which general anesthesia would be risky are not good candidates for surgical repair (Alexander, Shakespeare, Barradell, & Orme, 2015), and noninvasive treatment strategies should be discussed with them.

Surgical interventions might include anterior or posterior colporrhaphy (to repair a cystocele or rectocele) and vaginal hysterectomy (for uterine prolapse). This can be done laparoscopically whereby the uterus is removed through the vagina. An anterior and posterior colporrhaphy may be effective for a first-degree prolapse. This surgical procedure tightens the anterior and posterior vaginal wall, thus repairing a cystocele or rectocele. The pubocervical fascia (supportive tissue between the vagina and bladder) is folded and sutured to bring the bladder and urethra in proper position (Nilsson, 2015).

A vaginal hysterectomy is the treatment of choice for uterine prolapse because it removes the prolapsed organ that is bringing down the bladder and rectum with it. It can be combined with an anterior and posterior repair if a cystocele or rectocele is present.

Nursing Assessment

Nursing assessment for clients with POP includes a thorough health history, a physical examination, and several laboratory and diagnostic tests.

HEALTH HISTORY AND CLINICAL MANIFESTATIONS

A history and general assessment of the client is important to exclude pathology and evaluate various factors that may influence choice and success of management. Evaluation of systems such as bowel, urinary and sexual function, coexistent morbidities, medical and surgical history, any physical or mental impairment, and lifestyle are noticeably very important, particularly in older women. The client's social circumstances and support systems, desire for treatment, and expectations will have implications on the management options.

The cause of prolapse is multifactorial, with vaginal childbirth, advancing age, heavy work, poor nutrition, vaginal surgery, and increasing body mass index being the most consistent risk factors (Rodriguez-Mias et al., 2015). Assessment of risk factors (chronic straining, hysterectomy, normal aging, and abnormalities of connective tissue) in the person's history will assist the health care provider in the diagnosis and treatment of POP. The history should include questions about:

- The obstetrical history (number of pregnancies, weight of newborns, pregnancy spacing)
- Chronic respiratory condition (chronic coughing)
- Menopausal status
- Weight history (loss or gain)
- Constipation (frequency and chronicity)
- Age
- Work history (e.g., physical labour or light office work)
- Nutritional assessment
- Family history (family member with POP)
- UI
- Previous pelvic surgeries

Assess for clinical manifestations of POP. POP is often asymptomatic, but when symptoms do occur, they are often related to the site and type of prolapse. Symptoms common to all types of prolapses are a feeling of dragging, a lump in the vagina, or something "coming down." Clients with POP can present either with one symptom, such as vaginal bulging or pelvic pressure, or with several complaints, including many bladder, bowel, and pelvic symptoms. Symptoms associated with POP are summarized in Box 7.1.

Clients can present with varying degrees of uterine descent. Uterine prolapse is the most troubling type of pelvic relaxation because it is often associated with concomitant defects of the vagina in the anterior, posterior, and lateral compartments (Lazarou & Grigorescu, 2016).

PHYSICAL EXAMINATION

The pelvic examination performed by the health care provider includes an external genital inspection to visualize any obvious protrusion of the uterus, bladder, urethra, or vaginal wall occurring at the vaginal opening. Usually the client is asked to perform the Valsalva manoeuvre (bearing down) while the examiner notes which organ prolapses first and the degree to which it occurs. Any urine leakage during the examination is important to note. The client is asked to contract the pubococcygeal (PC) muscles; the health care provider inserts two fingers into the vagina to assess the strength and symmetry of the contraction. Because pelvic or genital organ prolapse can cause urinary symptoms such as incontinence, bladder function should be assessed by determining postvoid residual with a catheter. If the client has more than 100 mL of retained urine, a referral for further urodynamic evaluation and testing should be considered.

BOX 7.1

SYMPTOMS ASSOCIATED WITH PELVIC ORGAN PROLAPSE

- Urinary symptoms
  - Stress incontinence
  - Frequency (diurnal and nocturnal)
  - Urgency and urge incontinence
  - Hesitancy
  - Poor or prolonged stream
  - Feeling of incomplete emptying
- Bowel symptoms
  - Difficulty with defecation
  - Incontinence of flatus or liquid or solid stool
  - Urgency of defecation
  - Feeling of incomplete evacuation
  - Rectal protrusion or prolapse after defecation
- Sexual symptoms
  - Inability to have frequent intercourse
  - Dyspareunia
  - Lack of satisfaction or orgasm
  - Incontinence during sexual activity
- Other local symptoms
  - Pressure or heaviness in the vagina
  - Pain in the vagina or perineum
  - Low back pain after long periods of standing
  - Palpable bulge in the vaginal vault
  - Difficulty walking due to a protrusion from the vagina
  - Difficulty inserting or keeping a tampon in place
  - Vaginal-cervical mucosa hypertrophy, excoriation, ulceration, and bleeding
  - Abdominal pressure or pain

Adapted from American College of Obstetricians and Gynecologists (ACOG). (2017). *Pelvic support problems.* Retrieved from https://www.acog.org/Patients/FAQs/Pelvic-Support-Problems; Lazarou, G., & Grigorescu, B. A. (2016). Pelvic organ prolapse. *eMedicine.* Retrieved from http://emedicine.medscape.com/article/276259-overview.

LABORATORY AND DIAGNOSTIC TESTS

Common laboratory tests that may be ordered to determine the cause of POP include a urinalysis to rule out a bacterial infection, urine culture to identify the specific organism if present, visualization of urine loss during the pelvic examination, and measurement of postvoid urine volume.

Nursing Management

Help the client understand the nature of the condition, the treatment options, and the likely outcomes. Nursing considerations might include the following:

- Describe normal anatomy and causes of pelvic prolapse.
- Assess how this condition has affected the person's life.
- Outline the options, with the advantages and disadvantages of each.
- Allow clients to make the decision that is right for them.

- Provide education.
- Schedule preoperative activities needed for surgery.
- Reassure clients that there are solutions for the symptoms.
- Provide community education about genital prolapse.

Nursing Care Plan 7.1 (at the end of the chapter) provides an overview of care for a client with POP.

PROMOTE PREVENTION STRATEGIES

Limited data are available on ways to prevent POP, but a nurse needs first to understand its incidence, risk factors, prevalence, clinical implications, and treatment options to be an effective support. The nurse's understanding will not only improve his or her ability to treat this growing client population, but will also help in developing preventive strategies to address a client's suffering from this condition.

Approaches include lifestyle changes that reduce modifiable risk factors, such as losing weight, avoiding heavy lifting, and relieving constipation. Explore what factors in the client's lifestyle might be modified to reduce the risk of developing POP (primary prevention) or to improve quality of life after receiving treatment (secondary prevention).

ENCOURAGE PELVIC FLOOR MUSCLE TRAINING

Encourage the client to perform PFME daily (Teaching Guidelines 7.1). PFMEs allow clients to have the ability to make changes through exercises. Hormone therapy may not be appropriate for everyone. Discuss current research findings and educate about estrogen therapy, allowing the client to make the decision on whether to use hormones.

Teaching Guidelines 7.1
PERFORMING PELVIC FLOOR EXERCISES

- Squeeze the muscles in your rectum as if you are trying to prevent passing flatus.
- Stop and start urinary flow to help identify the pubococcygeus muscle.
- Tighten the pubococcygeus muscle for a count of three, and then relax it.
- Contract and relax the pubococcygeus muscle rapidly 10 times.
- Try to bring up the entire pelvic floor and bear down 10 times.
- Repeat pelvic floor muscle exercises at least five times daily.

ENCOURAGE DIETARY AND LIFESTYLE MODIFICATIONS

Instruct clients to increase dietary fibre and fluids to prevent constipation. A high-fibre diet with an increase in fluid intake alleviates constipation by increasing stool bulk and stimulating peristalsis. It is accomplished by replacing refined, low-fibre foods with high-fibre foods. The recommended daily intake of fibre is at least 25 g (Buyken et al., 2018; Health Canada, 2017; Meyer, 2015). In addition to increasing the amount of fibre in the diet, also encourage the client to drink eight 250-mL (8-oz) glasses of fluid daily and to engage in regular low-impact aerobic exercise, which promotes muscle tone and stimulates peristalsis.

Educate the client about other lifestyle changes that will assist with prolapse, such as:

- Achieve ideal weight to reduce intra-abdominal pressure and strain on pelvic organs, including pressure on the bladder.
- Wear a girdle or abdominal support to support the muscles surrounding the pelvic organs.
- Avoid lifting heavy objects to reduce the risk of increasing intra-abdominal pressure, which can push the pelvic organs downward.
- Avoid high-impact aerobics, jogging, or jumping repeatedly to minimize the risk of increasing intra-abdominal pressure, which places downward pressure on the organs.
- Give up smoking to minimize the risk for a chronic "smoker's cough," which increases intra-abdominal pressure and forces the pelvic organs downward.

PROVIDE TEACHING FOR PESSARY USE

Educate the client about pessary use. Discuss complications as part of the instruction. Although the pessary is a safe device, it is still a foreign body in the vagina. Because of this, the most common side effects of the pessary are increased vaginal discharge, urinary tract infections, vaginitis, and odour. Odours can be reduced by douching with dilute vinegar or hydrogen peroxide. Postmenopausal clients with thin vaginal mucosa are susceptible to vaginal ulceration with the use of a pessary. Advise the client to use estrogen cream to make the vaginal mucosa more resistant to erosion and to strengthen the vaginal walls.

The client must be capable of managing use of the pessary, either alone or with the help of a caretaker. The most common recommendations for pessary care include removing the pessary twice weekly and cleaning it with soap and water; using a lubricant for insertion; and having regular follow-up examinations every 6 to 12 months after an initial period of adjustment.

Besides cleaning, clients must properly reinsert the device into their vaginal cavity, and must also be willing to participate in all aspects of care of the pessary for this treatment option to be successful. All clients choosing this option must be instructed in the care of the pessary to feel comfortable with all aspects of it before leaving the health care facility. Health care visits should allow adequate time for clients to share their concerns, anxieties, and fears surrounding the transition to life with a pessary.

PROVIDE PERIOPERATIVE CARE

Prepare the client for surgery by reinforcing the risks and benefits of surgery and describing the postoperative course. Explain that a Foley catheter will be in place for up to 1 week, and that urinating may be difficult due to the swelling after the catheter has been removed. Provide home care instructions for the Foley catheter, including cleansing the perineal area daily with mild soap and water, especially around where the catheter enters the urinary meatus. If the client is provided with a leg bag to be worn during waking hours, provide instruction on emptying it frequently and keeping it below the level of the bladder to prevent backflow. The same principles are applied to the primary Foley bag when emptying it.

During the recovery period, instruct the client to avoid for several weeks activities that cause an increase in abdominal pressure, such as straining, sneezing, and coughing. In addition, advise against lifting anything heavy or straining to push anything. Explain that stool softeners and gentle laxatives might be prescribed to prevent constipation and straining with bowel movements. Avoiding vaginal intercourse will be recommended until the operative area is healed in 6 weeks.

Urinary Incontinence

Urinary incontinence (UI) is defined by the Canadian Continence Foundation (2018) as the involuntary loss of bladder control and general bladder weakness, which can have a dramatic impact on an individual's life. This disorder affects over 3.3 million people in Canada (Canadian Continence Foundation, 2018), but is underreported. It has been estimated that 50% of all cis-gender women experience UI at some time in their life, varying in severity from mild to severe (Files, Mayer, & Chutka, 2015). Total costs related to UI in Canada are estimated at approximately $2.6 billion annually (The Canadian Continence Foundation, 2014; Cassidy et al., 2017). The psychosocial costs and morbidities are even more difficult to quantify. Embarrassment and depression are common. The affected individual may experience a decrease in social interactions, excursions out of the home, and sexual activity (Su, Sun, & Jiann, 2015). It is more common than diabetes and Alzheimer disease, both of which receive a great deal of media attention. Despite the considerable impact of incontinence on quality of life, many individuals are unlikely to bring up the subject of their lack of bladder control and very few seek help or treatment for incontinence concerns. The following are several possible explanations for why clients do not talk about their bladder control issues. The client may:

- Feel that UI is inevitable and not amenable to treatment.
- Feel that UI is a "normal" part of aging.

COMPARISON CHART 7.1	URGE INCONTINENCE VERSUS STRESS INCONTINENCE	
	Urge Incontinence	**Stress Incontinence**
Description	Precipitous loss of urine, preceded by a strong urge to void, with increased bladder pressure and detrusor contraction	Accidental leakage of urine that occurs with increased pressure on the bladder from coughing, sneezing, laughing, or physical exertion
Etiology	Causes might be neurologic, idiopathic, or infectious	Develops commonly in individuals in their 40s and 50s, usually as the result of weakened muscles and ligaments in the pelvis following childbirth
Signs and Symptoms	Urgency, frequency, nocturia, and a large amount of urine loss	Involuntary loss of a small amount of urine in response to physical activity that raises intra-abdominal pressure

- Believe that UI is part of being "female." Cis-gender women tend to accept urinary symptoms such as UI more so than men.
- Feel embarrassment and try to deny that it is a real problem.
- Think that the only treatment option is surgical.
- The client may consider a UI a hygiene problem and not a medical condition.

Take Note!

Incontinence is preventable, treatable, and often curable. However, many people believe that loss of bladder function is a normal and expected part of aging.

Incontinence can have far-reaching effects. Some people experience anxiety, depression, social isolation, embarrassment, insomnia, fear, feelings of uncleanliness, worry, vulnerability, shame, limited ability to travel far from home or have social engagements, and disruptions in their self-esteem and dignity (Cameron Institute, 2014). UI can cause the individual to stop working, travelling, socializing, and enjoying sexual relationships. In addition, incontinence can create a tremendous burden for caretakers and is a common reason for admission to a long-term care facility. Depression and high levels of stress are typical in these clients (Kwak, Kwon, & Kim, 2016).

Individuals often try to cope with UI through lifestyle modifications such as wearing protective pads, avoiding certain activities, emptying the bladder frequently, and modifying diet/fluid intake. Those who experience UI are generally most distressed by the social implications and many go to great efforts to hide their symptoms. In some cultures, UI is abhorred to the point where those affected are shunned by their communities. A sense of control, normality, and self-esteem are central issues in living with UI. Generally, with time and worsening of symptoms, people will pursue medical evaluation and treatment (Waetjen, Xing, Johnson, Melnikow, & Gold, 2015).

The types of UI are defined based on their presenting symptoms and signs. The three most common types of incontinence are urgency UI (overactive bladder caused by detrusor muscle contractions), stress incontinence (inadequate urinary sphincter function), and mixed incontinence (involves both stress and urge incontinence) (King et al., 2015). Comparison Chart 7.1 details these types of UI.

Pathophysiology and Etiology

Urinary continence requires several factors, including effective functioning of the bladder, adequate pelvic floor muscles, neural control from the brain, and integrity of the neural connections that facilitate voluntary control. The bladder neck and proximal urethra function as a sphincter. During urination the sphincter relaxes and the bladder empties. The ability to control urination requires the integrated function of numerous components of the lower urinary tract, which must be structurally sound and functioning normally.

Incontinence can develop if the bladder muscles become overactive due to weakened sphincter muscles, if the bladder muscles become too weak to contract properly, or if signals from the nervous system to the urinary structures are interrupted. A major factor that contributes to urinary continence is the estrogen level, because this hormone helps maintain bladder sphincter tone. In perimenopausal or menopausal clients, incontinence can be a problem as estrogen levels begin to decline and genitourinary changes occur. In simple terms, the bladder is the reservoir, the urethra is the seal, and the levator ani muscle is the gate that holds pressure against the outflow of urine by supporting the urethra and bladder from below. When any of these three structures is not functioning normally, incontinence occurs.

Contributing factors in UI include:
- Fluid intake, especially alcohol, carbonated drinks, and caffeinated beverages

- Constipation: alters the position of the pelvic organs and puts pressure on the bladder
- Habitual "preventive" emptying: may result in training the bladder to hold only small amounts of urine
- Menopause and depletion of estrogen
- Chronic disease such as stroke, multiple sclerosis, or diabetes
- Smoking: nicotine increases detrusor muscle contractions
- Advancing age: age-related anatomic changes provide less pelvic support
- Pregnancy and childbirth: damage to pelvic structures during childbirth
- Obesity: increases abdominal pressure (Schuiling & Likis, 2016).

Therapeutic Management

Treatment options depend on the type of UI. In general, the least invasive procedure with the fewest risks is the first choice for treatment. Surgery is used only if other methods have failed. There is a widespread belief that UI is an inevitable problem of getting older and that little or nothing can be done to relieve symptoms or reverse it. Nothing is further from the truth, and attitudes must change so that women will feel comfortable seeking help for this embarrassing condition.

For many clients with urge incontinence, simple reassurance and lifestyle interventions might help. The promotion of a healthy weight can help to reduce incontinence related to obesity. However, if more than simple lifestyle measures are needed, effective treatments might include:

- Bladder training to establish normal voiding intervals (every 3 to 5 hours)
- PFMEs to strengthen the pelvic floor musculature
- Pessary ring to support pelvic structures that have weakened
- Pharmacotherapy to reduce the urge to void. Anticholinergic agents such as oxybutynin (Ditropan) or tolterodine (Detrol) or oxybutynin (Oxytrol) might be prescribed. The most common side effects of anticholinergic agents are dry mouth, blurred vision, constipation, nausea, dizziness, and headaches (King et al., 2015).

For clients with stress incontinence, treatment is not always a cure, but it can minimize the impact of this condition on quality of life. Some treatment options for stress incontinence might include:

- Weight loss if needed
- Avoidance of constipation
- Smoking cessation
- PFMEs to strengthen the pelvic floor
- Pessaries
- Weighted vaginal cones to improve the tone of pelvic floor muscles

- Periurethral injection (injecting a bulking agent [collagen] to form a bulge that brings the urethral walls closer together to achieve a better closure)
- Medications such as duloxetine (Cymbalta, Yentreve) to increase urethral sphincter contractions during the storage phase of the urination cycle
- Estrogen replacement therapy to improve bladder sphincter tone
- Surgery to correct genital prolapse and improve urethral and bladder tone

Consider This

Life can be complicated and embarrassing at times when we least expect it. I met a man in church who seemed interested in me, and he asked me out for coffee after Sunday services. I have been alone for 10 years and this prospect seemed exciting to me. We talked for hours over coffee and seemed to have a great deal in common, especially since both of us had lost our spouses to cancer. He asked me to go square dancing with him, since that was an activity we both had enjoyed in the past with our spouses. I hadn't been out or physically active for ages and didn't realize how my body had changed with age.

It was during the first dance that I noticed a wet sensation between my legs, which I was unable to control. I managed to continue on and pretend that all was fine, but then realized what many of my friends were talking about—stress incontinence. Not being able to control one's urine is very embarrassing and it complicates your life, but I made up my mind that it wasn't going to control me!

Thoughts: *Gravity and childbirth take a toll on person's reproductive organs by pushing them downward. This woman is not going to let stress incontinence curtail her outside activity, which demonstrates a good attitude. What can be done about her embarrassing accidents? Were there any preventive strategies she could have used at an earlier age?*

Nursing Assessment

The assessment of the client experiencing UI includes a history, physical examination, laboratory tests, and possibly urodynamic testing. The onset, frequency, severity, and pattern of incontinence should be determined, as well as any associated symptoms such as frequency, dysuria, urgency, and nocturia. Incontinence may be quantified by asking if the client wears a pad and how often the pad is changed. A review of current medications, including over-the-counter medications, should be included in the history.

A complete physical examination should be carried out by the health care provider; it should include a neurologic assessment and pelvic and rectal examinations. The presence of associated POP should be noted because it can contribute to voiding problems and may have an impact on diagnosis and treatment. A rectal examination is done to evaluate sphincter tone and perineal sensation. A "cough stress test" can be performed by asking the client to cough with a full bladder and subsequently observing for leakage of urine from the urethra can also help in assessing the client's ability to control voiding.

A urinalysis is performed to look for hematuria, pyuria, glucosuria, or proteinuria. A urine culture is done if there is pyuria or bacteriuria. Postvoid residual should be measured either with pelvic ultrasound or directly with a catheter. If the residual exceeds the limit set, urodynamic testing is then used to diagnose the incontinence.

Nursing Management

Incontinence can be devastating and can cause psychosocial concerns and isolation. Nurses can encourage clients with troublesome symptoms to seek help. Discuss the treatment options, including benefits and potential outcomes, and encourage the client to select the continence treatment best for their lifestyle. Provide education about good bladder habits and strategies to reduce the incidence or severity of incontinence (Teaching Guidelines 7.2). Provide support and encouragement to ensure adherence to the guidelines. Remember that aging can increase the risk of incontinence, but incontinence is not an inevitable part of aging. Review the anatomy and physiology of the urinary system and offer simple explanations to help the client cope with urinary alterations. Therapeutic listening is important. Be aware of the courage it takes for a person to disclose an embarrassing condition.

Take Note!

Simple diet and lifestyle alterations, combined with a proper pelvic floor muscle strengthening program, can often produce significant improvements for clients of all ages.

Teaching Guidelines 7.2
MANAGING URINARY INCONTINENCE

- Avoid drinking too much fluid (i.e., 1.5 L total daily limit), but do not decrease your intake of fluids.
- Reduce intake of fluids and foods that are bladder irritants and precipitate urgency, such as chocolate, caffeine, sodas, alcohol, artificial sweetener, hot spicy foods, orange juice, tomatoes, and watermelon.
- Increase fibre and fluids in your diet to reduce constipation.
- Control blood glucose levels to prevent polyuria.
- Treat chronic cough.
- Remove any barriers that delay you from reaching the toilet.

- Practice good perineal hygiene by using mild soap and water. Wipe from front to back to prevent urinary tract infections.
- Become aware of adverse drug effects.
- Take your medications as prescribed.
- Continue to do pelvic floor muscle exercises.

Adapted from Files, J. A., Mayer, A. P., & Chutka, D. S. (2015). Urinary incontinence: Not just a mid-laugh crisis. *Journal of Women's Health, 24*(1), 107–108; McClurg, D., Gerrard, J., & Hove, R. T. (2015). Reducing the incidence of incontinence. *British Journal of Midwifery, 23*(1), 17–20; and Vasavada, S. P., Carmel, M. E., & Rackley, R. (2017). Urinary incontinence. *eMedicine.* Retrieved from http://emedicine.medscape.com/article/452289-overview.

BENIGN GROWTHS

The most common benign growths of the reproductive tract include cervical, endocervical, and endometrial polyps; uterine fibroids (leiomyomas); genital fistulas; Bartholin cysts; and ovarian cysts.

Polyps

Polyps are small, usually benign growths. The incidence of malignancy in cervical polyps is 1 in 1,000. Malignancy is more common in perimenopausal or postmenopausal clients (Nelson, Papa, & Ritchie, 2015). The cause of polyp growth is not well understood, but they are frequently the result of infection. Polyps might be associated with chronic inflammation, an abnormal local response to increased levels of estrogen, or local congestion of the cervical vasculature (Stewart, 2018). Single or multiple polyps might occur. They are most common in multiparous individuals. Polyps can appear anywhere but are most common on the cervix and in the uterus (Fig. 7.3).

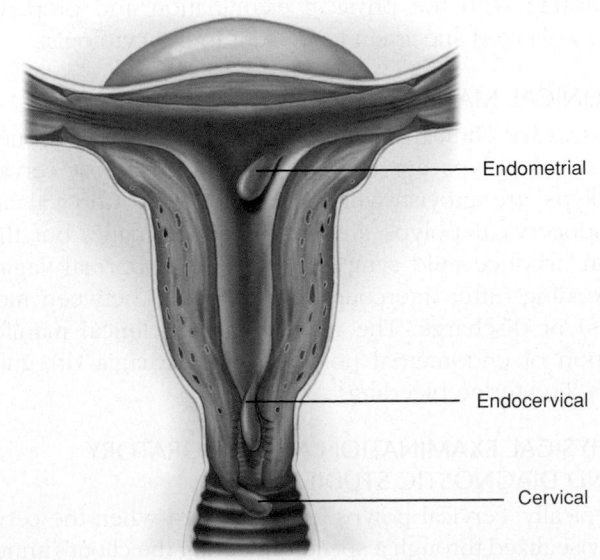

FIGURE 7.3 Cervical, endocervical, and endometrial polyps.

Cervical polyps often appear after menarche. They occur in 2% to 5% of cis-gender women, and approximately 2% of these polyps have cancerous changes (Schuiling & Likis, 2016). Endocervical polyps are commonly found in multiparous individuals aged 40 to 60 years. Endocervical polyps are more common than cervical polyps, with a stalk of varied width and length. Endometrial polyps are benign tumours or localized overgrowths of the endometrium. Most endometrial polyps are solitary, and they rarely occur in those younger than 20 years of age. The incidence of these polyps rises steadily with increasing age, peaks in the fifth decade of life, and gradually declines after menopause. They are present in up to 25% of clients being seen for abnormal vaginal/uterine bleeding (Lieng, 2015).

Therapeutic Management

Treatment of polyps usually consists of simple removal with small forceps done on an outpatient basis, removal during hysteroscopy, or dilation and curettage (D&C). The polyp base can be removed by laser vaporization. Because many polyps are infected, an antibiotic may be ordered after removal as a preventive measure or to treat early signs of infection.

Although polyps are rarely cancerous, a specimen should be sent after surgery to a pathology laboratory to exclude malignancy. A cervical biopsy typically reveals mildly atypical cells and signs of infection. Polyps rarely return after they are removed. Regularly scheduled Pap smears are suggested for clients with cervical polyps to detect any future abnormal growths that may be malignant.

Nursing Assessment

Nursing assessment for a client with polyps includes assisting with the physical examination and preparing the collected specimen to be sent to the cytologist.

CLINICAL MANIFESTATIONS

Assess for clinical manifestations of polyps. Most endocervical polyps are cherry red, whereas most cervical polyps are greyish-white (Heller, 2015). Cervical and endocervical polyps are often asymptomatic, but they can produce mild symptoms such as abnormal vaginal bleeding (after intercourse or douching, between menses) or discharge. The most common clinical manifestation of endometrial polyps is metrorrhagia (irregular, acyclic uterine bleeding).

PHYSICAL EXAMINATION AND LABORATORY AND DIAGNOSTIC STUDIES

Typically, cervical polyps are diagnosed when the cervix is visualized through a speculum during the client's annual gynecologic examination (Nelson et al., 2015). Endometrial polyps are not detected on physical examination, but

rather with ultrasound or hysteroscopy (introduction of a small camera through the cervix to visualize the uterine cavity).

Nursing Management

Nursing management of polyps involves explaining the condition and the rationale for removal and giving follow-up care instructions. The nurse also assists the health care provider with the removal procedure.

Uterine Fibroids

Uterine fibroids, also known as myomas or leiomyomas, are benign tumours composed of smooth muscle and fibrous connective tissue in the uterus. Unlike cancerous tumours, fibroids usually grow slower responding to present estrogen levels and their cells do not break away and invade other parts of the body. Fibroids are classified according to their position in the uterus and on the uterine layer most involved (Fig. 7.4):

- *Subserosal fibroids:* lie underneath the outermost peritoneal layer of the uterus and grow outside the uterus. They are attached to the uterus by a stalk or peduncle.
- *Intramural fibroids:* grow within the wall of the uterus and are the most common type.
- *Submucosal fibroids:* grow from immediately below the inner uterine surface (endometrium) into the uterine cavity (King et al., 2015).

FIGURE 7.4 Submucosal, intramural, and subserosal fibroids.

Fibroids are estrogen-dependent and thus grow rapidly during the childbearing years, when estrogen is plentiful, but they shrink during menopause, when estrogen levels decline. It is believed that these benign tumours develop in up to 70% of all cis-gender women over 30 years of age, but up to 50% are asymptomatic (Stewart, 2018). It is difficult to be precise because fibroids may cause no symptoms, and thus many affected individuals do not know they have them.

Fibroids are the most common gynaecologic tumour. Evidence has indicated that approximately 30% of cis-gender women of reproductive age are affected (Lefebvre, Allaire, Jeffrey, & Vilos, 2018).

Etiology

Although the cause of fibroids is unknown, several predisposing factors have been identified, including:
* Age (late reproductive years)
* Genetic predisposition
* African-American ethnicity
* Hypertension
* Nulliparity
* Obesity (Alexander, LaRosa, Bader, & Garfield, 2014; Lee et al., 2017).

Therapeutic Management

Treatment depends on the size of the fibroids and the client's symptoms, which can include heavy or painful menses, feeling "full" in the lower pelvis, urinating frequently, pain during sexual relations, lower back pain, and infertility (National Institutes of Health [NIH], 2018). Several treatment options exist, ranging from watchful waiting to surgery.

MEDICAL MANAGEMENT

The goals of medical therapy are to reduce symptoms and/or to reduce the tumour size. This can be accomplished with pain medications to treat mild or occasional pain from fibroids; birth control pills to control heavy menses; or gonadotropin-releasing hormone (GnRH) agonists such as leuprolide (Lupron), nafarelin (Synarel), or goserelin (Zoladex), which stop ovulation and the production of estrogen, or low-dose mifepristone, a progestin antagonist. Both have produced regression and reduced the size of the tumours without surgery, but long-term therapy is expensive and not tolerated by most women. The side effects of GnRH medications include hot flashes, headaches, mood changes, vaginal dryness, musculoskeletal malaise, bone loss, and depression (King et al., 2015; Vallerand & Sanoski, 2017). Long-term mifepristone therapy can result in endometrial hyperplasia, which increases the risk of endometrial malignancy. Once either therapy is stopped, the fibroids typically recur.

Uterine artery embolization (UAE) is an option in which polyvinyl alcohol pellets are injected into selected blood vessels via a catheter to block circulation to the fibroid, causing it to shrink and producing symptom resolution. The procedure is carried out by an interventional radiologist who makes a tiny incision in the groin, introduces a fine catheter into the main artery leading to the uterus, and injects tiny particles of plastic or gelatin sponge into the artery that supplies blood to the fibroid. These particles stop the flow of blood, causing the fibroid to shrink or disappear completely over time. UAE has short-term advantages over surgery. Over the mid and long term, the benefits were similar, except for a higher reintervention rate after UAE (Hehenkamp, Huirne, & Brölmann, 2015). There remains a need for a treatment that is noninvasive and that preserves fertility.

SURGICAL MANAGEMENT

For clients with large uterine fibroids or severe menorrhagia, surgery is preferred over medical treatment. Surgical management might involve myomectomy, laser surgery, or hysterectomy.

Myomectomy. Myomectomy involves removing the fibroid alone. A myomectomy is performed via laparoscopy, through an abdominal incision or through a vaginal approach. The advantage is that only the fibroid is removed; fertility is not jeopardized because this procedure leaves the uterine muscle walls intact. Myomectomy relieves symptoms but does not affect the underlying process; thus, fibroids grow back and further treatment will be needed in the future.

Laser Surgery. Laser surgery (or electrocauterization) involves destroying small fibroids with lasers. Laser therapy can be done using a vaginal approach or laparoscopically. The laser treatment preserves the uterus, but the process may cause scarring and adhesions, thus impairing fertility (Shigetomi, Oka, Seki, & Kobayashi, 2015). Fibroids can return after this procedure. Controversy remains as to whether laser treatment weakens the uterine wall and thus may contribute to uterine rupture in the future.

Hysterectomy. A hysterectomy is the surgical removal of the uterus. It is the most effective treatment for symptomatic fibroids with no recurrence. After cesarean section, it is the second most frequently performed surgical procedure for cis-gender women in Canada (Canadian Institute for Health Information, 2010). The top three conditions associated with hysterectomies are fibroids, endometriosis, and uterine prolapse (Centers for Disease Control and Prevention [CDC], 2017). A hysterectomy to remove fibroids eliminates both the symptoms and the risk of recurrence (Lefebvre et al., 2018), but it also terminates the client's ability to bear children. Three types

TABLE 7.1	SUMMARY OF TREATMENT OPTIONS FOR UTERINE FIBROIDS	
Method	**Advantages**	**Disadvantages**
Hormones	Noninvasive Reduces size of fibroids Symptom improvement	Serious side effects with long-term use Fibroids regrow when meds stopped
Uterine artery embolization	Minimally invasive Dramatic decrease in symptoms Future fertility possible	Procedure frequently painful Requires radiation and contrast dye Permanently implanted material Possible negative fertility impact
Myomectomy	Performed as minor surgery Uterus is preserved	Requires general anesthesia New growth of fibroids occurs
Hysterectomy	Complete removal of fibroids Immediate symptom relief	Requires general anesthesia Major surgery with associated risks Fertility not preserved
Laser surgery	Can be done as an outpatient procedure to destroy small fibroids	Vaporization process can cause scarring and adhesions, affecting future fertility

of hysterectomy surgeries are available: vaginal hysterectomy, laparoscopically assisted vaginal hysterectomy, and abdominal hysterectomy.

In a vaginal hysterectomy, the uterus is removed through an incision in the posterior vagina. Advantages include a shorter hospital stay and recovery time and no abdominal scars. The Society of Obstetricians and Gynaecologists of Canada (SOGC) recommends that vaginal hysterectomies should be considered as a first choice for all benign indications (Lefebvre et al., 2018). Disadvantages of this route include a limited operating space and poor visualization of other pelvic organs.

In a laparoscopically assisted vaginal hysterectomy, the uterus is removed through a laparoscope, through which structures within the abdomen and pelvis are visualized. Small incisions are made in the abdominal wall to permit the laparoscope to enter the surgical site. Advantages include a better surgical field, less pain, lower cost, and a shorter recovery time when compared to open laparotomy. Disadvantages include potential injury to the bladder and the inability to remove enlarged uteruses and scar tissue (Lefebvre et al., 2018).

In an abdominal hysterectomy, the uterus and other pelvic organs are removed through an incision in the abdomen. This procedure allows the surgeon to visualize all pelvic organs and is typically used when a malignancy is suspected or a very large uterus is present. Disadvantages include the need for general anesthesia, a longer hospital stay and recovery period, more pain, higher cost, and a visible scar on the abdomen.

Complications of hysterectomy vary based on route of surgery and technique. The most common complications include infection, venous thromboembolic, genitourinary and gastrointestinal injuries, and hemorrhage (Goldman, Lynch, Jones, Rutledge, & Burke, 2015;

Lefebvre et al., 2018). With astute nursing observations and assessments, these complications can be reduced or minimized. A summary of treatment options for uterine fibroids is presented in Table 7.1.

Nursing Assessment

Nursing assessment for the client with uterine fibroids includes a thorough health history, physical examination, and laboratory and diagnostic studies.

HEALTH HISTORY AND CLINICAL MANIFESTATIONS

The history should include questions about the client's menstrual cycle, including alterations in the menstrual pattern (e.g., pain or pressure, aggravating and alleviating factors), history of infertility, and any history of spontaneous abortion, which might indicate a space-occupying uterine lesion. Ask if any relatives have had uterine fibroids, because there is a familial predisposition. Assess for clinical manifestations of uterine fibroids. Symptoms of fibroids depend on their size and location and may include:

• Chronic pelvic pain
• Low back pain
• Iron-deficiency anemia secondary to bleeding
• Bloating
• Constipation
• Infertility (with large tumours)
• Dysmenorrhea
• Miscarriage
• Sciatica
• Dyspareunia
• Urinary frequency, urgency, incontinence
• Irregular vaginal bleeding (menorrhagia)
• Feeling of heaviness in the pelvic region

PHYSICAL EXAMINATION AND LABORATORY AND DIAGNOSTIC STUDIES

The bimanual examination performed by the health care provider typically shows an enlarged, irregular uterus. The uterus may be palpable abdominally if the fibroid is very large. Ultrasound may be used to confirm the diagnosis.

Nursing Management

The level of support that nurses can provide clients with fibroids depends on the type of treatment offered and her choice of them. Nurses should be able to explain any current treatment options and the implications of a diagnosis of fibroids. Many people have not heard of fibroids previously and need reassurance that they are both common and benign. If medication is prescribed, it is essential to explain the possible side effects and why medication can only be taken for a limited duration. If surgery is selected, verbal and written information about it and the aftercare should be addressed (Box 7.2).

A client undergoing a hysterectomy for the treatment of fibroids often needs special care and can benefit from presurgical and postsurgical support provided by nurses. Personalized nursing, tailored to the individual's needs, enhances the client's coping strategies and alleviates different adverse psychological sequelae following gynecologic surgery. Clients must cope with a variety of psychological adjustment difficulties, related to the changes in self-image, self-esteem, loss of femininity or identity, and sexual dysfunction. The incidence of postsurgical problems can be reduced greatly with proper client-centred perioperative nursing care.

Genital Fistulas

Genital fistulas are an underestimated problem worldwide and have devastating consequences. **Genital fistulas** are abnormal openings between a genital tract organ and another organ, such as the urinary tract or the gastrointestinal tract. A fistula can result from a congenital anomaly, surgical complications, Bartholin gland abscesses,

---

BOX 7.2

NURSING INTERVENTIONS FOR A CLIENT UNDERGOING A HYSTERECTOMY

Preoperative Care
- Instruct the client and family about the procedure and aftercare.
- Provide interventions to reduce anxiety (due to perceived threats to the client's self-concept and role functioning) and fear of alteration in body image, complications, and pain. Prepare the client for what to expect throughout her perioperative experience. Explain postoperative pain management procedures that will be used. Identify those at high risk to help reduce stress.
- Teach turning, deep breathing, and coughing before surgery to prevent postoperative atelectasis and respiratory complications such as pneumonia.
- Encourage the client to discuss their feelings. Some cis-gender women equate their femaleness with their reproductive capability, and loss of the uterus could evoke grieving.
- Complete all preoperative orders in a timely manner to allow for rest.

Postoperative Care
- Provide comfort measures.
- Administer analgesics promptly or use a patient-controlled anesthesia (PCA) pump.
- Administer antiemetics to control nausea and vomiting per order.
- Change the client's linens and gown frequently to promote hygiene.
- Change the client's position frequently and use pillows for support to promote comfort and pain management.

- Assess the incision, the dressing, and vaginal bleeding and report if bleeding is excessive (soaking perineal pad within an hour).
- Monitor elimination and provide increased fluids and fibre to prevent constipation and straining.
- Encourage ambulation and active range-of-motion exercises when in bed to prevent thrombophlebitis and venous stasis.
- Monitor vital signs to detect early complications.
- Be comfortable discussing sexual concerns with the client.

Discharge Planning
- Advise the client to reduce activity to avoid fatigue, which might inhibit healing.
- Advise the client to rest when feeling tired and to increase activity level slowly.
- Educate the client on the need for pelvic rest (nothing in the vagina) for 6 weeks.
- Instruct the client to avoid heavy lifting or straining for about 6 weeks to prevent an increase in intra-abdominal pressure, which could weaken her sutures.
- Teach the client the signs and symptoms of infection.
- Advise the client to take showers instead of tub baths to reduce the risk for infection.
- Encourage the client to eat a healthy diet with increased intake of fluids to prevent dehydration and fluid and electrolyte imbalance.
- Instruct the client to change perineal pads frequently to prevent infection.
- Explain and schedule follow-up care appointments as needed.
- Provide information about community resources for support/help.

radiation, or malignancy, but the majority of fistulas that occur worldwide are related to obstetrical trauma and female genital cutting (Spurlock, 2016). During normal labour, the bladder is displaced upward into the abdomen, and the anterior vaginal wall, the base of the bladder, and the urethra are compressed between the fetal head and the posterior pubis. When labour is obstructed or prolonged, this unrelieved compression causes ischemia, which causes pressure necrosis and subsequent fistula formation.

Common types of fistulas include:

- *Vesicovaginal:* communication between the bladder and genital tract
- *Urethrovaginal:* communication between the urethra and the vagina
- *Rectovaginal:* communication between the rectum or sigmoid colon and the vagina

The direct consequences of this damage include UI and fecal incontinence if the rectum is involved. This tragic condition has plagued women since the beginning of history (Taylor & Rakinic, 2017). Another major cause of genital trauma leading to the development of genital fistulas is female genital cutting. This cultural practice, primarily carried out in Africa and Asia, is receiving worldwide attention as part of the international public health agenda to move toward reducing its incidence. Reasons for continuing this practice include rite of passage, preserving chastity, ensuring marriageability, religion, hygiene, improving fertility, and enhancing sexual pleasure for men (Nour, 2015). Because of migration, health care professionals are increasingly confronted with the range of negative urogynecologic effects that result from this practice. Nurses need to have a deeper understanding of the history, cultural beliefs, medical complications, and methods of surgical reconstruction to provide culturally competent care to this unique group of clients. This cultural practice will be addressed in detail in Chapter 9.

Therapeutic Management

Many small fistulas will heal without treatment, but large fistulas often require surgical repair; surgery may be postponed until the edema or inflammation in the surrounding tissues has dissipated. Surgical repair of fistulas is associated with a high success rate if it is done in a timely manner, but larger fistulas and those of long duration have a poorer prognosis (Jellison & Raz, 2015).

Nursing Assessment

The history should include questions about any changes in the client's urinary and bowel patterns. Assess for common signs and symptoms of fistulas, which are related to the type of fistula. If the opening involves the rectum,

feces and flatus will leak through the vagina. If it involves the bladder, urine will leak from the vagina. Depending on the location and size of the fistula, the client may or may not experience discomfort. The health care provider can detect these abnormal openings through inspection and palpation during the pelvic examination. Diagnostic or laboratory tests are generally not ordered once this condition is found.

Nursing Management

Provide guidance and support. Offer information to help the client learn about the condition and, with appropriate intervention, to improve quality of life. Begin by making sure the client understands the anatomy and the reason behind such symptoms. Provide a thorough explanation of the treatment options so that the client can make an informed decision. Be sensitive to the client's feeling of shame and fear about incontinence; these feelings may be the reason for a delay in seeking treatment. Address all of the client's needs, both physical and emotional.

Bartholin Cysts

The Bartholin glands are two mucus-secreting glandular structures with duct openings bilaterally at the base of the labia minora near the opening of the vagina that provide lubrication during sexual arousal. A Bartholin cyst is a swollen, fluid-filled, sac-like structure that results when one of the ducts of the Bartholin gland becomes blocked. The cyst may become infected and an abscess may develop in the gland. Normally these glands cannot be felt or seen unless they are infected. Bartholin cysts are the most common cystic growths in the vulva, affecting approximately 2% of cis-gender women at some time in their life (Reif et al., 2015).

Therapeutic Management

Treatment can be conservative or surgical depending on the symptoms, the size of the cyst, and whether it is infected or not. Small asymptomatic cysts do not require treatment. Sitz baths along with analgesics are used to reduce discomfort. Antibiotics are prescribed if the gland is infected. The aim of treatment for a cyst or abscess is to create a fistulous tract from the dilated duct to the outside vulva by incision and drainage. However, cysts or abscesses tend to return if this option is used.

Other treatment options beyond incision and drainage include placement of a Word catheter or a small loop of plastic tubing secured in place to prevent closure and to allow drainage. The use of a carbon dioxide laser to remove the cyst is also possible. After the Word catheter is inserted, the balloon tip is inflated and it is left in place for 4 to 6 weeks. The follow-up of the plastic tubing for removal is in approximately 3 weeks. Both procedures are safe and effective alternatives to surgery (Prabhu & Gardella, 2015). Treatment for a pregnant client with a Bartholin cyst depends on the severity of the symptoms and whether an infection is present. Surgery may be delayed until after the client gives birth if there are no symptoms.

Nursing Assessment

Nursing assessment for the client with a Bartholin cyst includes a thorough health history, physical examination, and laboratory and diagnostic tests.

HEALTH HISTORY

The history should include questions about the client's sexual practices and protective measures used. Assess for common signs and symptoms of Bartholin cysts. The client may be asymptomatic if the cyst is small (less than 5 cm) and not infected. If infection is present, symptoms include varying degrees of pain, especially when walking or sitting; unilateral edema; redness around the gland; and dyspareunia. Extensive inflammation may cause systemic symptoms. Abscess formation occurs when the cystic fluid becomes infected. An abscess usually develops rapidly over a 2- to 3-day period and may spontaneously rupture. A history of sudden relief of pain following profuse discharge is highly suggestive of spontaneous rupture (Schuiling & Likis, 2016).

PHYSICAL EXAMINATION AND LABORATORY AND DIAGNOSTIC STUDIES

The diagnosis of Bartholin cysts or abscesses is primarily made during a physical examination when a protruding tender labial mass is located. In cis-gender women over the age of 40, there is an increased risk of malignancy, typically sarcomas which account for 2% of all invasive vulvar malignancies. They are characterized by rapid growth, high metastatic potential, frequent recurrences, aggressive behaviour, and high mortality rate (Chokoeva et al., 2015). Cultures of the purulent abscess fluid and of the cervix should be obtained for *Neisseria gonorrhoeae* and *Chlamydia trachomatis* to rule out a sexually transmitted infection.

Nursing Management

Nurses must be aware of and knowledgeable about vulvar cysts and treatment options. The client may be aware of a vulvar cyst secondary to the pain or may be unaware of it if it is asymptomatic. A Bartholin cyst may be an incidental finding during a routine pelvic examination. Explain the cause of the cyst and assist with cultures if needed. Provide reassurance and support.

Ovarian Cysts

An **ovarian cyst** is a fluid-filled sac that forms on the ovary (Fig. 7.5). These very common growths are benign 90% of the time and are asymptomatic in many affected individuals. The cysts are discovered incidentally during

Fallopian tube

Fimbriae

Opening of fallopian tube

Semitransparent, distended, fluid-filled cyst

FIGURE 7.5 Ovarian cyst. (Asset provided by Anatomical Chart Co.)

an ultrasound or routine pelvic examination. Ovarian cysts occur in 30% of cis-gender women with regular menses, 50% of those with irregular menses, and 7% of postmenopausal individuals (Templeman, 2015). When the cysts grow large and exert pressure on surrounding structures, clients often seek medical help.

Types of Ovarian Cysts

The most common benign ovarian cysts are follicular cysts, corpus luteum (lutein) cysts, theca lutein cysts, and polycystic ovarian syndrome (PCOS).

FOLLICULAR CYSTS

Small follicular cysts are commonly found in the ovaries of prepubertal girls and women of reproductive age, and in most cases, they are of no clinical significance. They are usually self-limiting and resolve spontaneously. Follicular cysts are caused by the failure of the ovarian follicle to rupture at the time of ovulation. Follicular cysts seldom grow larger than 5 cm in diameter; most regress and require no treatment. They can occur at any age and are rare after menopause. They are detected by vaginal ultrasound.

CORPUS LUTEUM (LUTEIN) CYSTS

A corpus luteum cyst forms when the corpus luteum becomes cystic or hemorrhagic and fails to degenerate after 14 days. These cysts might cause pain and delay the next menstrual period. A pelvic ultrasound helps to make this diagnosis. Typically these cysts appear after ovulation and resolve without intervention.

THECA LUTEIN CYSTS

Prolonged abnormally high levels of human chorionic gonadotropin (hCG) stimulate the development of theca lutein cysts. Although rare, these cysts are associated with hydatidiform mole, choriocarcinoma, polycystic ovary syndrome (PCOS), and Clomid therapy.

POLYCYSTIC OVARY SYNDROME

PCOS is the most common endocrine condition in cisgender women of reproductive age. It is a heterogeneous condition that involves the presence of multiple inactive follicle cysts within the ovary that interfere with ovarian function. It is a multifaceted disorder, and central to its pathogenesis are hyperandrogenemia and hyperinsulinemia, which are targets for treatment (King et al., 2015). It is associated with obesity, hyperinsulinemia, elevated luteinizing hormone levels (linked to ovulation), elevated androgen levels (virilization), hirsutism (dark coarse hair growth on the face, chest, and back), obstructive sleep apnea, follicular atresia (ovarian growth failure), ovarian growth and cyst formation, anovulation (failure to ovulate), infertility, type 2 diabetes, sleep apnea, amenorrhea (absence of menstruation or irregular periods), metabolic syndrome which is characterized by abdominal obesity

(waist circumference >35 in), dyslipidemia (triglyceride level >150 mg/dL, high-density lipoprotein cholesterol level <50 mg/dL), elevated blood pressure, a proinflammatory state characterized by an elevated C-reactive protein level, and a prothrombotic state characterized by elevated PAI-1 and fibrinogen levels. Recent studies also indicate that PCOS is associated with an increase in the risk of uterine fibroids, depression, adverse pregnancy outcomes, and neonatal complications. A recent meta-analysis found that individuals with PCOS demonstrated a significantly higher risk of developing gestational diabetes, gestational hypertension, preeclampsia, preterm birth, and had a higher cesarean section rate when compared to controls (Kyrou, Weickert, & Randeva, 2015). With an estimated prevalence of 5% to 10% of all cisgender females, PCOS is the most common cause of medically treatable infertility and is responsible for 70% of cases of anovulatory subfertility and up to 20% of couples' infertility cases (NIH, 2017).

Take Note!

Careful attention should be given to this condition because affected individuals are at increased risk for long-term health problems such as cardiovascular disease, hypertension, dyslipidemia, type 2 diabetes (found in half those affected), infertility, and cancer (endometrial, breast, and ovarian) (Moran, Norman, & Teede, 2015).

Initially PCOS was called Stein–Leventhal syndrome after its researchers, but it is now recognized to be an anabolic syndrome. Unfortunately, less than two thirds of affected individuals are aware of their diagnosis or the concomitant high risk for developing type 2 diabetes mellitus and cardiovascular disease related to metabolic syndrome. Its etiology is not clearly understood, but studies suggest a genetic (autosomal-dominant) component. People with PCOS have abnormalities in the metabolism of androgens and estrogen and in the control of androgen production. In addition, they have peripheral insulin resistance and hyperinsulinemia and obesity (Trikudanathan, 2015). All of these clinical manifestations must be addressed throughout the lifespan with an emphasis on prevention of cardiometabolic risks in the treatment plan.

Therapeutic Management

Treatment is centred on the clinical manifestations and should be initiated early to prevent or limit long-term complications such as metabolic syndrome, diabetes, endometrial carcinoma, and infertility (Ganie, Chakraborty, & Rehman, 2015). Oral contraceptives, antidiabetic agents, and statins are some of the common therapies used to address the symptoms of this complex hormonal condition. Weight loss and surgery may also be beneficial as nondrug options.

Treatment of ovarian cysts focuses on differentiating a benign cyst from a solid ovarian malignancy. Transvaginal ultrasound is useful in distinguishing fluid-filled cysts from solid masses. Laparoscopy may be needed to remove the cyst if it is large and pressing on surrounding structures. For smaller cysts, monitoring with repeat ultrasounds every 3 to 6 months might be in order (Lucidi, 2018). Oral contraceptives are often prescribed to suppress gonadotropin levels, which may help resolve the cysts. Pain medication is also prescribed if needed.

Medical management of PCOS is aimed at the treatment of metabolic derangements, anovulation, hirsutism, and menstrual irregularity. This includes both drug and nondrug therapy, along with lifestyle modifications. Goals of therapy focus on reducing the production and circulating levels of androgens, protecting the endometrium against the effects of unopposed estrogens, supporting lifestyle changes to achieve ideal body weight, lowering the risk of cardiovascular disease, avoiding the effects of hyperinsulinemia on the risk of cardiovascular disease and diabetes, and inducing ovulation to achieve pregnancy if desired (Evidence-Based Practice 7.2). Treatment modalities for PCOS are highlighted in Box 7.3.

BOX 7.3

TREATMENT MODALITIES FOR PCOS

- Oral contraceptives to treat menstrual irregularities and acne
- Mechanical hair removal (shaving, waxing, plucking, or electrolysis) to treat hirsutism
- Glucophage (metformin), which improves insulin uptake by fat and muscle cells, to treat hyperinsulinemia; thiazolidinediones (Actos, Avandia) to decrease insulin resistance
- Ovulation induction agents (Clomid) to treat infertility
- Lifestyle changes (including weight loss, exercise, balanced low-fat diet)
- Referral to support groups to help improve emotional state and build self-esteem

Adapted from King, T. L., Brucker, M. C., Kriebs, J. M., Fahey, J. O., Gegor, C. L., & Varney, H. (2015). *Varney's midwifery.* (5th ed.). Burlington, MA: Jones & Bartlett Learning; Kyrou, I., Weickert, M. O., & Randeva, H. S. (2015). Diagnosis and management of polycystic ovary syndrome (PCOS). In R. Ajjan & S. M. Orme (Eds.). *Endocrinology and diabetes* (pp. 99–113). London, England: Springer Publishers; and Lucidi, R. S. (2015). Polycystic ovarian syndrome. *eMedicine.* Available at: http://emedicine.medscape.com/article/256806-overview

EVIDENCE-BASED PRACTICE 7.2

IT'S NOT JUST PHYSICAL: THE ADVERSE PSYCHOSOCIAL EFFECTS OF POLYCYSTIC OVARY SYNDROME IN ADOLESCENTS

STUDY

The prevalence of depression and other psychological disorders in individuals with PCOS is high and varies in numerous studies. In particular, women with PCOS have been found to be at an increased risk of social phobia and suicide attempts. The reasons for a higher prevalence of psychological disorders in women with PCOS are likely complex. Some investigators suggest that physical symptoms experienced by those with PCOS are the likely cause of psychological distress. However, evidence is inconsistent. While acne, hirsutism, and obesity have been linked to increased psychological distress in some studies, no link is demonstrated in others. It is likely that multiple factors contribute to the high prevalence of psychosocial disorders in clients with PCOS.

This study sheds light on the fact that this gynecologic disorder of endocrine origin can be associated with a great number of psychological symptoms (e.g., depression, anxiety, body image dissatisfaction, eating and sexual disorders, and poor quality of life). The goal of the study was to address the prevalence of psychological disorders and determinants of well-being.

Findings

An overwhelming majority of scientific literature on PCOS has focused on the medical approach to analyze the disorder and only a few studies have investigated its predisposing psychological factors. The literature review revealed several psychological disorders that accompany this syndrome with limited attention given to them to help women cope. The symptoms typically associated with PCOS, including amenorrhea, oligomenorrhea, hirsutism, obesity, infertility, anovulation, and acne, can lead to symptoms of depression, withdrawal from society, emotional distress, embarrassment, lower self-esteem, anxiety, body image disturbances, eating disorders, marital and social maladjustment, and impaired sexual functioning.

Nursing Implications

PCOS is closely associated with psychological disorders with important implications that necessitate identification and treatment of the disorders. The high prevalence rate of these psychological disorders in this population suggests that initial evaluation of all clients with PCOS should also include an assessment of their mental health. Psychological support by nurses should take on an important role in the management of clients affected with PCOS. This should not suggest that medical treatment of PCOS is not required, but a thorough cooperation between medical treatment and psychological support would improve the situation of PCOS-affected individuals. The physical and psychosocial aspects of management of PCOS go hand in hand. Meeting physical management goals (e.g., weight loss, reduction in hyperandrogenism manifestations) can lessen some of the distressing psychosocial effects, and enhance self-esteem.

Adapted from Lee, J. S. (2015). It's not just physical: The adverse psychosocial effects of polycystic ovary syndrome in adolescents. *Women's Healthcare, 3*(1), 20–28.

Nursing Assessment

Nursing assessment for the client with PCOS includes a thorough health history, physical examination, and laboratory and diagnostic tests.

HEALTH HISTORY

The history should include questions about the client's symptoms, including onset, location, frequency, quality, intensity, and aggravating and alleviating factors of any discomfort. Note the last menstrual period and whether or not menstrual cycles are regular. Ask about overall general health and any changes recently noticed, such as a change in abdominal girth without a concomitant weight gain. Assess for common signs and symptoms of ovarian cysts. Findings might include:

- Hirsutism (face and chin, upper lip, areola, lower abdomen, and perineum)
- Alopecia (frontal region and crown of head)
- Virilization (clitoral hypertrophy, deepening of voice, increased muscle mass, breast atrophy, male-pattern baldness)
- Menstrual irregularity and infertility (menorrhagia, anovulation)
- Polycystic ovaries (12 or more follicles on ovaries)
- Obesity (occurs in more than 50% of those with PCOS; occurs in abdominal region, with an increase in the waist–hip ratio)
- Insulin resistance (chronic hyperinsulinemia leads to type 2 diabetes)
- Metabolic syndrome (elevated cholesterol, triglycerides, low-density lipoprotein; risk of cardiovascular disease)
- Increased risk for endometrial cancer, ovarian cancer, breast cancer
- Psychological impact (depression, frustration, anxiety, eating disorders)
- Acne (face and shoulders) (Lucidi, 2018)

PHYSICAL EXAMINATION AND LABORATORY AND DIAGNOSTIC STUDIES

The physical examination includes inspection, auscultation, and palpation of the abdomen because large ovarian masses may cause visible changes in the abdomen. A complete pelvic examination is performed to assess the location, size, shape, texture, mobility, and tenderness of any palpable mass.

Diagnostic tests include a pregnancy test to rule out ectopic pregnancy. Gonorrhea and chlamydia testing is warranted if an ovarian abscess is suspected. An ultrasound may be ordered to differentiate between functional or simple ovarian cysts and a solid tumour. Additional tests may be performed depending on the findings.

> **Remember Liz, the client with irregular menses, facial hair, and acne? Her glucose level is elevated, multiple cysts were felt on her ovaries during the pelvic examination, and laboratory tests found elevated lipid and lipoprotein levels. What education should the nurse provide Liz regarding her PCOS diagnosis? What medications might be prescribed to address her abnormal laboratory values?**

Nursing Management

Nursing care should include education about the condition, treatment options, diagnostic test arrangements, and referral for surgery if needed. Provide support and reassurance during the diagnostic period to allay anxiety in the client and family. Provide reassurance that the majority of ovarian cysts are benign, but stress the importance of follow-up care. Listen to the client's concerns about physical appearance including facial hair growth, and infertility. Explore options to help the client boost self-esteem and maximize health.

Nurses can have a positive impact on clients with PCOS through counselling and education. Provide support for those dealing with negative self-image secondary to the physical manifestations of PCOS. Through education, help the client understand the syndrome and its associated risk factors to prevent long-term health problems. Encourage the client to make positive lifestyle changes. Make community referrals to local support groups to help build coping skills.

> **Liz returns to the clinic a month later for re-evaluation of her PCOS. She has been taking metformin to reduce her insulin resistance and has followed her exercise regimen and reduced her caloric intake to lose weight, but she still complains about her facial hair and acne. What interventions might be helpful to address this problem? What medication might also be prescribed to regularize her menses and relieve the hirsutism?**

NURSING CARE PLAN 7.1

Overview of a Woman Client With Pelvic Organ Prolapse

Katherine, a 62-year-old multiparous woman, came to her gynecologist with reports of a chronic dragging or heavy painful feeling in her pelvis, lower backache, constipation, and urine leakage. Her symptoms increase when she stands for long periods. She has not had menstrual cycles for at least a decade. She tells you, "I'm not taking any of those menopausal hormones." She also states she is very self-conscious and embarrassed about her urine leakage and restricts her outside activities.

NURSING DIAGNOSIS: Disturbed body image related to relaxation of pelvic support and elimination difficulties

Outcome Identification and Evaluation

The client will report an improved body image after management of pelvic organ prolapse and improved urinary control.

Interventions: *Providing Pain Management*

- Obtain a thorough history, including ongoing embarrassing experiences, methods of urine control used, what worked, what didn't, any changes in sexual practices related to this, and the effect of this condition on her activities of daily living *to provide a baseline and enable a systematic approach to address it.*
- Assess the frequency, severity, precipitating factors, and aggravating/alleviating factors *to identify characteristics of the client's abnormal urinary patterns to plan appropriate interventions.*
- Educate client about any medications prescribed (correct dosage, route, side effects, and precautions)

to increase the client's understanding of the therapy and promote compliance.
- Assess problematic elimination patterns *to identify underlying factors from which to plan appropriate prevention strategies.*
- Encourage client to increase fluids and fibre in diet and increase physical activity daily *to promote peristalsis.*
- Assist client with establishing regular toileting patterns by setting aside time daily for bowel elimination *to promote regular bowel function and evacuation.*
- Urge client to avoid the routine use of laxatives *to reduce risk of compounding constipation.*

NURSING DIAGNOSIS: Deficient knowledge related to causes of structural disorders and treatment options

Outcome Identification and Evaluation

The client will demonstrate an understanding of current condition and treatments as evidenced by identifying treatment options, making health-promoting lifestyle choices, verbalizing appropriate health care practices, and adhering to treatment plan.

Interventions: *Providing Client Education*

- Assess client's understanding of pelvic organ prolapse and its treatment options *to provide a baseline for teaching.*
- Review information provided about surgical procedures and recommendations for healthy lifestyle, obtaining feedback frequently, *to validate client's understanding of instructions.*
- Discuss association between uterine, bladder, and rectal prolapse and symptoms *to help client understand the etiology of her symptoms and pain.*
- Have client verbalize and discuss information related to diagnosis, surgical procedure, preoperative routine, and postoperative regimen *to ensure adequate understanding and provide time for correcting or clarifying any misinformation or misconceptions.*

(continued)

NURSING CARE PLAN 7.1

Overview of a Woman Client With Pelvic Organ Prolapse (continued)

- Provide written material with pictures *to promote learning and help client visualize what has occurred to her body secondary to aging, weight gain, childbirth, and gravity.*
- Discuss pros and cons of hormone replacement therapy, osteoporosis prevention, and cardiovascular events common in postmenopausal women *to promote informed decision making by the client about available menopausal therapies.*
- Inform client about the availability of community resources and make appropriate referrals as needed *to provide additional education and support.*
- Document details of teaching and learning *to allow for continuity of care and further education, if needed.*

KEY CONCEPTS

- Pelvic floor disorders such as pelvic organ prolapse and urinary and fecal incontinence are prevalent conditions in aging cis-gender women. They cause significant physical and psychological morbidity, with obvious detriment to individual's social interactions, emotional well-being, and overall quality of life.

- The four most common types of genital prolapse are cystocele, rectocele, enterocele, and uterine prolapse.

- The purpose of pelvic floor muscle exercises is to increase the muscle volume, which will result in a stronger muscular contraction. These exercises might limit the progression of mild prolapse and alleviate mild prolapse symptoms, including low back pain and pelvic pressure.

- UI is the involuntary loss of urine sufficient enough to be a social or hygiene problem. It affects approximately 3.5 million women in Canada.

- The three most common types of incontinence are urge incontinence (overactive bladder caused by detrusor muscle contractions), stress incontinence (inadequate urinary sphincter function), and mixed incontinence (involves both stress and urge incontinence).

- The most common benign growths of the reproductive tract include cervical, endocervical, and endometrial polyps; uterine fibroids (leiomyomas); genital fistulas; Bartholin cysts; and ovarian cysts.

- Polycystic ovary syndrome (PCOS) involves the presence of multiple inactive follicle cysts within the ovary that interfere with ovarian function.

Hyperandrogenism, insulin resistance, and chronic anovulation characterize PCOS. Careful attention should be given to this condition because affected individuals are at increased risk for long-term health problems such as cardiovascular disease, hypertension, dyslipidemia, infertility, type 2 diabetes, and cancer (endometrial, breast, and ovarian).

REFERENCES AND RECOMMENDED READINGS

Alexander, L. L., LaRosa, J. H., Bader, H., & Garfield, S. (2014). *New dimensions in women's health* (6th ed.). Sudbury, MA: Jones & Bartlett.

Alexander, L., Shakespeare, K., Barradell, V., & Orme, S. (2015). Management of urinary incontinence in frail elderly women. *Obstetrics, Gynaecology and Reproductive Medicine, 25*(3), 75–82.

American College of Obstetricians and Gynecologists (ACOG). (2017). Pelvic support problems. *ACOG Educational Pamphlet.* Retrieved from https://www.acog.org/Patients/FAQs/Pelvic-Support-Problems

Brown, D. N. (2015). Pelvic organ prolapse: A consequence of nature or nurture?. *Menopause, 22*(5), 477–479.

Buyken, A. E., Mela, D. J., Dussort, P., Johnson, I. T., Macdonald, I. A., Stowell, J. D., & Brouns, F. J. P. H. (2018). Dietary carbohydrates: A review of international recommendations and the methods used to derive them. *European Journal of Clinical Nutrition, 72,* 1625–1643. Retrieved from https://www.nature.com/articles/s41430-017-0035-4#Tab3

Cameron Institute. (2014). *The impact of incontinence in Canada: A briefing for policy-makers.* Retrieved from http://www.canadiancontinence.ca/pdfs/en-impact-of-incontinence-in-canada-2014.pdf

Canadian Continence Foundation. (2014). *The impact of incontinence in Canada: A briefing document for policy-makers.* Retrieved from http://www.canadiancontinence.ca/pdfs/en-impact-of-incontinence-in-canada-2014.pdf

Canadian Continence Foundation. (2018). What is urinary incontinence?. Retrieved from http://www.canadiancontinence.ca/EN/what-is-urinary-incontinence.php

Canadian Institute for Health Information. (2010). Health care in Canada 2010. Retrieved from https://secure.cihi.ca/estore/productFamily.htm?pf=PFC1568&lang=en&media=0

Cassidy, T., Fortin, A., Kaczmer, S., Shumaker, J. T. L., Szeto, J., & Madill, S. J. (2017). Relationship between back pain and urinary incontinence in the Canadian population. *Physical Therapy, 94*(4), 449–454.

Centers for Disease Control and Prevention (CDC). (2017). *Women's reproductive health: Hysterectomy.* Retrieved from https://www.cdc.gov/reproductivehealth/womensrh/index.htm

Chokoeva, A. A., Tchernev, G., Cardoso, J. C., Patterson, J. W., Dechev, I., Valkanov, S., . . . Wollina, U. (2015). Vulvar sarcomas: Short guideline for histopathological recognition and clinical management. Part 1. *International Journal of Immunopathology and Pharmacology, 28*(2), 168–177.

Colyar, M. R. (2015). *Advanced practice nursing procedures.* Philadelphia, PA: F.A. Davis Company.

Dumoulin, C., Hay-Smith, J., Habee-Seguin, G. M., & Mercier, J. (2015). Pelvic floor muscle training verses no treatment, or inactive control treatments, for urinary incontinence in women: A short version Cochrane systematic review with meta-analysis. *Neurourology and Urodynamics, 34*(4), 300–308.

Files, J. A., Mayer, A. P., & Chutka, D. S. (2015). Urinary incontinence: Not just a mid-laugh crisis. *Journal of Women's Health, 24*(1), 107–108.

Ganie, M. A., Chakraborty, S., & Rehman, H. (2015). Treatment of polycystic ovary syndrome: Recent trial results. *Clinical Investigation, 5*(3), 337–350.

Goldman, N. A., Lynch, K., Jones, H., Rutledge, J., & Burke, W. M. (2015). Comparison of complications in patients undergoing robotic-assisted hysterectomy for large leiomyomas [107]. *Obstetrics and Gynecology, 125*, 40S.

Hallock, J. L., & Handa, V. L. (2016). The epidemiology of pelvic floor disorders and childbirth: An update. *Obstetrics and Gynecology Clinics, 43*(1), 1–3.

Health Canada. (2017). *Fibre.* Retrieved from https://www.canada.ca/en/health-canada/services/nutrients/fibre.html.

Hehenkamp, W. J., Huirne, J. A., & Brölmann, H. A. (2015). Uterine artery embolization and new ablation techniques. In A. Tinelli & A. Malvasi (Eds.). *Uterine myoma, myomectomy and minimally invasive treatments* (pp. 153–168). Springer International Publishing.

Heller, D. S. (2015). Diseases of the cervix. In D. S. Heller (Ed.). *OB-GYN pathology for the clinician* (pp. 91–106). Springer International Publishing.

Jellison, F. C., & Raz, S. (2015). Vaginal fistula repairs. In F. Firoozi (Ed.), *Female pelvic surgery* (pp. 145–163). New York: Springer Publishers.

King, T. L., Brucker, M. C., Kriebs, J. M., Fahey, J. O., Gegor, C. L., & Varney, H. (2015). *Varney's midwifery* (5th ed.). Burlington, MA: Jones & Bartlett Learning.

Kinman, C. L., Lemieux, C. A., Agrawal, A., Gaskins, J. T., Meriwether, K. V., & Francis, S. L. (2017). The relationship between age and pelvic organ prolapse bother. *International Urogynecology Journal, 28*(5), 751–755.

Kirby, A. C., Tan-Kim, J., & Nager, C. W. (2015). Dynamic maximum urethral closure pressures measured by high-resolution manometry increase markedly after sling surgery. *International Urogynecology Journal, 26*, 905–909.

Kwak, Y., Kwon, H., & Kim, Y. (2016). Health-related quality of life and mental health in older women with urinary incontinence. *Aging and Mental Health, 20*, 719–726.

Kyrou, I., Weickert, M. O., & Randeva, H. S. (2015). Diagnosis and management of polycystic ovary syndrome (PCOS). In R. Ajjan & S. M. Orme (Eds.). *Endocrinology and diabetes* (pp. 99–113). London, England: Springer Publishers.

Lazarou, G., & Grigorescu, B. A. (2016). Pelvic organ prolapse. *eMedicine.* Retrieved from http://emedicine.medscape.com/article/276259-overview.

Lee, J. S. (2015). It's not just physical: The adverse psychosocial effects of polycystic ovary syndrome in adolescents. *Women's Healthcare, 3*(1), 20–28.

Lee, U. J., Kerkhof, M. H., van Leijsen, S. A., & Heesakkers, J. P. (2017). Obesity and pelvic organ prolapse. *Current Opinion in Urology, 24*(5), 428–434.

Lefebvre, G., Allaire, C., Jeffrey, J., & Vilos, G. (2018). SOGC clinical practice guideline No. 109: Hysterectomy. *Journal of Obstetrics and Gynaecology Canada, 40*(7), e567–e579.

Lieng, M. (2015). Endometrial polyps. In O. Istre (Ed.). *Minimally invasive gynecological surgery* (pp. 61–73). Berlin, Heidelberg: Springer Publishers.

Lucidi, R. S. (2018). Polycystic ovarian syndrome. *eMedicine.* Retrieved from http://emedicine.medscape.com/article/256806-overview.

Maher, C., & Haya, N. (2015). Changing trends in pelvic organ prolapse surgery. *Obstetrics, Gynaecology and Reproductive Medicine, 25*(6), 147–151.

McClurg, D., Gerrard, J., & Hove, R. T. (2015). Reducing the incidence of incontinence. *British Journal of Midwifery, 23*(1), 17–20.

Meyer, D. (2015). Health benefits of prebiotic fibers. *Advances in Food and Nutrition Research, 74*, 47–91.

Miedel, A., Tegerstedt, G., Moehle-Schmidt, M., Nyren, O., & Hammarstrom, M. (2009). Nonobstetric risk factors for symptomatic pelvic organ prolapse. *Obstetrics and Gynecology, 113*, 1089–1097.

Moran, L. J., Norman, R. J., & Teede, H. J. (2015). Metabolic risk in PCOS: Phenotype and adiposity impact. *Trends in Endocrinology and Metabolism, 26*(3), 136–143.

Mukwege, A. A., El-Nashar, S. A., Rhodes, D., Dowdy, S. C., & Trabuco, E. C. (2015). Are demographic and clinical characteristics of women presenting with advanced pelvic organ prolapse different compared with women presenting in earlier stages? [374]. *Obstetrics and Gynecology, 125*, 116S–117S.

National Institutes of Health (NIH). (2017). *Polycystic ovarian syndrome.* Retrieved from http://www.nichd.nih.gov/health/topics/PCOS/Pages/default.aspx.

National Institutes of Health (NIH). (2018). *About uterine fibroids.* Retrieved from http://www.nichd.nih.gov/health/topics/uterine/conditioninfo/Pages/default.aspx.

Nelson, A. L., Papa, R. R., & Ritchie, J. J. (2015). Asymptomatic cervical polyps: Can we just let them be?. *Women's Health, 11*(2), 121–126.

Nilsson, C. G. (2015). Creating a gold standard surgical procedure: The development and implementation of TVT. *International Urogynecology Journal, 26*, 467–469.

Nour, N. M. (2015). Female genital cutting: Impact on women's health. *Seminars in Reproductive Medicine, 33*(1), 41–46.

Prabhu, A., & Gardella, C. (2015). Common vaginal and vulvar disorders. *Medical Clinics of North America, 99*(3), 553–574.

Ralph, G., & Tamussino, K. (2015). Conservative management of pelvic organ prolapse. In A. Tamilselvi & A. Rane (Eds.). *Principles and practice of urogynaecology* (pp. 115–122). India: Springer Publishers.

Ramalingam, K., & Monga, A. (2015). Obesity and pelvic floor dysfunction. *Best Practice and Research Clinical Obstetrics and Gynaecology, 29*(4), 541–547.

Reif, P., Ulrich, D., Bjelic-Radisic, V., Häusler, M., Schnedl-Lamprecht, E., & Tamussino, K. (2015). Management of Bartholin's cyst and abscess using the Word catheter: Implementation, recurrence rates and costs. *European Journal of Obstetrics and Gynecology and Reproductive Biology, 190*, 81–84.

Riss, P., & Koch, M. (2015). Evaluation of pelvic organ prolapse. In A. Tamilselvi & A. Rane (Eds.). *Principles and practice of urogynaecology* (pp. 107–114). India: Springer Publishers.

Rodríguez-Mias, N. L., Martínez-Franco, E., Aguado, J., Sánchez, E., & Amat-Tardiu, L. (2015). Pelvic organ prolapse and stress urinary incontinence, do they share the same risk factors?. *European Journal of Obstetrics and Gynecology and Reproductive Biology, 190*, 52–57.

Schuiling, K. D., & Likis, F. E. (2016). *Women's gynecologic health* (3rd ed.). Sudbury, MA: Jones & Bartlett.

Shigetomi, H., Oka, K., Seki, T., & Kobayashi, H. (2015). Design and preclinical validation of the composite-type optical fiberscope for minimally invasive procedure of intra-uterine disease. *Journal of Minimally Invasive Gynecology, 22*(6), 985–991.

Spurlock, J. (2016). Vesicovaginal fistula. *eMedicine*. Retrieved from http://emedicine.medscape.com/article/267943-overview#a0102.

Stewart, E. A. (2018). Endometrial polyps. *UpToDate*. Retrieved from http://www.uptodate.com/contents/endometrial-polyps.

Su, C. C., Sun, B. Y., & Jiann, B. P. (2015). Association of urinary incontinence and sexual function in women. *International Journal of Urology, 22*(1), 109–113.

Taylor, D., & Rakinic, J. (2017). Rectovaginal fistula. *eMedicine*. Retrieved from http://emedicine.medscape.com/article/193277-overview.

Templeman, C. (2015). Ovarian cysts. *Journal of Pediatric and Adolescent Gynecology, 17*, 297–298.

Trikudanathan, S. (2015). Polycystic ovarian syndrome. *Medical Clinics of North America, 99*(1), 221–235.

Vallerand, A. H., & Sanoski, C. A. (2017). *Davis's Canadian drug guide for nurses* (15th ed.). Philadelphia: PA: F. A. Davis Company.

Vasavada, S. P., Carmel, M. E., & Rackley, R. (2017). Urinary incontinence. *eMedicine*. Retrieved from http://emedicine.medscape.com/article/452289-overview.

Waetjen, L. E., Xing, G., Johnson, W. O., Melnikow, J., Gold, E. B., & Study of Women's Health Across the Nation (SWAN). (2015). Factors associated with seeking treatment for urinary incontinence during the menopausal transition. *Obstetrics and Gynecology, 125*(5), 1071–1079.

Walters, M. (2015). Urinary incontinence in women comes and goes, and reasons remain elusive. *BJOG: An International Journal of Obstetrics and Gynaecology, 122*, 824.

CHAPTER **WORKSHEET**

MULTIPLE CHOICE QUESTIONS

1. When you are interviewing a client with uterine fibroids, what subjective data would you expect to find in their history?
   a. Cyclic migraine headaches
   b. Urinary tract infections
   c. Chronic pelvic pain
   d. Chronic constipation

2. Conservative treatment options available for clients with pelvic organ prolapse are:
   a. Pessaries and PFM exercises
   b. External pelvic fixation devices
   c. Weight gain and yoga
   d. Firm panty-and-girdle garments

3. Which of the following dietary and lifestyle modifications might the nurse recommend to help prevent pelvic relaxation as clients age?
   a. Eat a high-fibre diet to avoid constipation and straining.
   b. Avoid sitting for long periods; get up and walk around frequently.
   c. Limit the amount of exercise to prevent overdeveloping muscles.
   d. Space children a year apart to reduce wear and tear on the uterus.

4. Individuals with polycystic ovarian syndrome (PCOS) are at increased risk for developing which of the following long-term health problems?
   a. Osteoporosis
   b. Lupus
   c. Type 2 diabetes
   d. Migraine headaches

5. Side effects experienced by clients taking gonadotropin-releasing hormone (GnRH) agonists for the treatment of fibroids closely resemble those of:
   a. Anorexia nervosa
   b. Osteoarthritis
   c. Depression
   d. Menopause

6. In securing a health history of a 65-year-old woman, which clinical manifestation described by the client would the nurse suspect is related to pelvic organ prolapse?
   a. Chronic abdominal pain
   b. Heavy feeling or dragging in vagina
   c. Uterine cramping and backache
   d. Weight gain and edema of ankles

CRITICAL THINKING EXERCISE

1. Faith, a 42-year-old multiparous woman, presents to the health clinic reporting a history of pelvic pain, menorrhagia, and vaginal discharge. She says she has been having these problems for several months. On examination, her uterus is enlarged and irregular in shape. Her blood studies reveal anemia.
   a. What condition might Faith have, based on her symptoms?
   b. What treatment options are available to address this condition?
   c. What educational interventions should the nurse discuss with Faith?

STUDY ACTIVITIES

1. Prepare an educational session to teach clients how to do pelvic floor muscle exercises to prevent stress incontinence and pelvic floor relaxation.

2. In a small group, discuss the personal, social, and sexual issues that might affect a client with pelvic organ prolapse. How might these issues affect socialization? How might a support group help?

3. List the symptoms that a client with uterine fibroids might have. Discuss how these symptoms might mimic a more frightening condition and why someone might delay seeking treatment.

4. A bladder that herniates into the vagina is a
   _____.

5. A rectum that herniates into the vagina is a
   _____.

BRINGING IT ALL TOGETHER: A CASE STUDY

Elizabeth, a 52-year-old woman, presented to the gynecologic clinic to discuss a "horrible personal problem" that was ruining her life. She appeared very distressed and only wanted to talk to the nurse in private about it. A few months ago when she was out walking her dog, she experienced a sudden rectal urgency that she thought was gas, but she expelled feces instead. Over the past few months, her fecal incontinence has increased in severity and frequency causing her extreme stress. To avoid embarrassment, she has had to cover and excuse herself from work situations and turn down social invitations. She now has to wear a protective pad and disposable pants.

ASSESSMENT

Elizabeth is otherwise healthy and takes no prescription medications presently. She has had five vaginal births with three episiotomies. She has a body mass index of 27, mild stress urinary incontinence, and a low-grade rectocele with slightly decreased anal sphincter tone. Her pelvic examination demonstrated pelvic organ prolapse. The digital rectal examination ruled out fecal impaction and any rectal mass. A detailed history of her incontinence episodes was also taken.

1. What risk factors are associated with fecal incontinence? Which does Elizabeth have?
2. Is her condition common in women of her age? If so, why?
3. What treatment options might help Elizabeth with her condition?

Risk factors for fecal incontinence include increasing age, anorectal procedures, obesity, urinary incontinence, vaginal births, pelvic organ prolapse, and cis-gender female. Fecal incontinence is not a disease state, but rather is a symptom of an underlying pelvic disorder such as POP. It is a nonfatal condition, but can greatly reduce the individual's quality of life. Treatment options include nonoperative interventions such as bulking agents to improve stool consistency, pelvic floor muscle exercises, antidiarrheal agents, and surgery.

PLAN

1. What specific health promotion strategy can the nurse discuss to reduce her symptoms?
2. How can the nurse improve Elizabeth's coping strategies?
3. What dietary changes might be helpful for Elizabeth?
4. How can the nurse offer client-centred care to Elizabeth?

Since Elizabeth has a high BMI; a weight loss intervention would be helpful in reducing the intra-abdominal pressure on her pelvic organs. Obesity is a risk factor for this condition. The nurse can discuss ways to reduce her weight through diet and exercise. Coping strategies should include a discussion of continence products available, providing emotional and psychological support to her, the use of anal plugs, skin-care, odour control, bowel training, laundry advice, and advice on preservation of dignity. Dietary changes might include starting a food and fluid diary to determine if there are food items increasing her stool frequency, advise her to modify one food at a time, and consuming foods that add bulk to her diet to increase formed stools. Management should be tailored to the needs of the individual. Information should be provided in a caring format in which Elizabeth can understand, so that she can participate in decisions about their treatment.

8

Cancers of the Female Reproductive Tract

Learning Objectives

Upon completion of the chapter, you will be able to:

1. Evaluate the major modifiable risk factors for reproductive tract cancers.

2. Analyze the screening methods and treatment modalities for cancers of the female reproductive tract.

3. Outline the nursing management needed for the most common malignant reproductive tract cancers.

4. Examine lifestyle changes and health screenings that can reduce the risk of or prevent reproductive tract cancers.

5. Assess at least three website resources available for a person diagnosed with cancer of the reproductive tract.

6. Appraise the psychological distress felt by clients diagnosed with cancer, and outline information that can help them to cope.

Carmella is an obese, 55-year-old woman who presents to her health care provider with vaginal bleeding. She has been through menopause and wonders why she is having a period again. Her history includes infertility and hypertension. Three years ago, she had a mastectomy for breast cancer, and she has been taking tamoxifen (Nolvadex) to prevent recurrent breast cancer since her surgery. What risk factors in Carmella's history might predispose her to a reproductive tract cancer? What additional information is needed to make a diagnosis?

INTRODUCTION

Cancer is the leading cause of death in Canada, responsible for 30% of all deaths, followed by cardiovascular diseases (heart disease and cerebrovascular diseases), lower respiratory diseases, and accidents (Statistics Canada, 2018). According to the Canadian Cancer Society, approximately half of all Canadians will develop cancer in their lifetime, and about one quarter of Canadians will die of the disease (Canadian Cancer Society's Advisory Committee on Cancer Statistics [CCACCS], 2017). However, the World Health Organization estimates that between 30% and 50% of cancers are preventable with a healthy diet, tobacco, and alcohol use reduction and a physically active lifestyle (World Health Organization, 2015). Certain cancers are related to infectious agents, such as hepatitis B virus (HBV), human papillomavirus (HPV), human immunodeficiency virus (HIV), and *Helicobacter pylori*, and can be prevented through behavioural changes, vaccines, or antibiotics (Herrington, Coates, & Duprex, 2015). In addition, many of the more than 2 million skin cancers that are diagnosed annually could be prevented by protecting the skin from the sun's rays and avoiding indoor tanning. Sunburns, especially if they occur repetitively in childhood, may lead to melanoma. Most melanomas are treated successfully if discovered early, but metastatic melanoma has no good treatment (Balk, 2015).

Nurses need to focus their energies on screening, education, and early detection to help reduce the numbers of premature deaths due to potentially preventable cancers. Because cancer risk is strongly associated with lifestyle and behaviour, screening programs are of particular importance for early detection. There is evidence that prevention and early detection have reduced cancer mortality rates and prevented reproductive cancers (CDC, 2015b).

This chapter begins with a nursing process overview of the care of clients with reproductive cancers. It then describes selected cancers of the reproductive system: ovarian, endometrial, cervical, vaginal, and vulvar cancer. The chapter discusses the nurse's role through diagnosis, intervention, and follow-up care. Cancer management requires a multidisciplinary approach, including specialists in surgical, medical, and radiation oncology. The nurse can provide guidance and support to clients as they find their way through the health care maze.

NURSING PROCESS OVERVIEW FOR THE PERSON WITH CANCER OF THE REPRODUCTIVE TRACT

The word *cancer* is laden with fear and dread. These feelings may worsen when the cancer involves a person's reproductive tract. The diagnosis of a reproductive tract cancer can have a profound impact on a person's sexuality because it can affect the individual's core concept of sexual identity. The loss of the reproductive body part as well as the possible loss of childbearing ability can have a significant effect on clients and their partners. Nurses need to remember this when counselling clients and their partners about cancer treatment and side effects and changes in gender roles and sexuality.

When a person is first diagnosed with a reproductive tract cancer, two primary needs arise: information and emotional support. When the diagnosis is made, the person typically has many questions, such as "What is going to happen to me?" "How will this change my life?" and "Will I survive?" Nurses can play a major role in helping clients find the answers to their questions and directing them to the resources they need. A reliable source of general cancer information is the Canadian Cancer Society, who can be reached via the Internet or by phone.

The nurse also plays a key role in offering emotional support, determining appropriate sources of support, and helping the client use effective coping strategies. A recent research study found that social support from family, friends, and coworkers is a strong predictor of coping (Garner et al., 2015). Implications for nurses working with clients following a cancer diagnosis include assessing the person's definition and availability of support; respecting varied needs for informational support; providing a supportive clinical environment; educating clinicians, family, and friends regarding unsupportive responses within the cultural context; and validating the client's control and balancing of support needs. Nurses are well positioned to provide clients with anticipatory guidance from diagnosis to the end of treatment (Shirvani & Alhani, 2015). Individuals without a social support network may need a social work referral or may need to be guided toward support groups to receive the emotional support they need.

In addition, clients diagnosed with cancer have a strong need for hope. Strategies for inspiring hope may include active listening, touch, presence, and helping clients overcome communication barriers. Often it is not what nurses say or do but just their presence that counts.

Assessment

Assessment of a person with cancer of the reproductive tract involves a thorough history and physical examination. In addition, various laboratory and diagnostic tests may be done to evaluate for malignancy.

Health History and Physical Examination

Interview clients carefully to determine any current or past factors that might increase their risk of cancer, such as early menarche, late menopause, sexually transmitted infections (STIs), use of hormonal agents,

COMMON LABORATORY AND DIAGNOSTIC TESTS 8.1

Test	Explanation	Indications	Nursing Implications
Clinical breast examination	Assessment of the breast for abnormal findings; client may discover lump; high-risk history for breast cancer	Identifies palpable mass, skin change, inverted nipple, or unresolved rash	• Educate client to perform breast self-examination and report any abnormalities if high risk • Reinforce need for frequent clinical breast examinations if risk factors are present
Mammography	Screening modality for breast cancer or any distortion in breast tissue architecture	Detects calcifications, densities, and nonpalpable cancer lesions	Stress importance of annual mammograms for all women after the age of 40 or 50, depending on their risk history
Pap smear	Cervical cytology screening to diagnose cervical cancers	Aids in detecting abnormal cells of the cervix (from squamocolumnar junction of the cervix; most cervical cancers arise here)	Encourage all sexually active individuals to receive a pelvic examination, including a Pap smear if they have a high-risk profile, to promote early detection of cervical cancer
Transvaginal ultrasound	Screening for pelvic pathology to assist in diagnosing endometrial cancers	Allows measurement of endometrial thickness to determine if endometrial biopsy is needed for postmenopausal bleeding	• Review the risk factors for the development of endometrial cancer and reason for this screening test • Assist in preparing the client for this examination
CA-125	Nonspecific blood test used as a tumour marker	Elevation of marker suggests malignancy but is not specific to ovarian cancer	• Review risk factors for ovarian cancer and explain that a series of diagnostic tests may be performed (transvaginal ultrasound, CT scan, CA-125) to assist in the diagnosis and treatment plan • Elevated marker levels are not specific to ovarian cancer; they can be elevated in other types of cancer

Adapted from American Cancer Society (ACS). (2015b). *American Cancer Society guidelines for the early detection of cancer.* Retrieved from http://www.cancer.org/Healthy/FindCancerEarly/CancerScreeningGuidelines/american-cancer-society-guidelines-for-the-early-detection-of-cancer; Centers for Disease Control and Prevention (CDC). (2015b). *Cancer prevention and control.* Retrieved from http://www.cdc.gov/cancer/dcpc/prevention/other.htm; and National Cancer Institute (NCI). (2015c). *General cancer prevention.* Retrieved from http://www.cancer.gov/cancertopics/prevention#General+Cancer+Prevention+Information

or infertility. Find out if the client has a family history of cancer. Be thorough in obtaining the client's past medical history, especially reproductive, obstetric, and gynecologic history. Ask about lifestyle and behaviours, including risky behaviours such as engaging in unprotected sexual intercourse or sexual intercourse with multiple partners. Find out if the client has had routine or recommended screening procedures.

Ask if the client has had any symptoms, such as abnormal vaginal bleeding or discharge or vaginal discomfort. Often the symptoms of cancer are vague and nonspecific and the person may attribute them to another problem, such as aging, stress, or improper diet.

Perform a complete physical examination, including a review of body systems and a pelvic examination. Observe for lesions or masses in the perineal area. Note any masses when palpating the abdomen or when performing the pelvic examination.

Laboratory and Diagnostic Testing

Some of the laboratory and diagnostic tests used to help diagnose cancer of the reproductive tract are discussed in Common Laboratory and Diagnostic Tests 8.1.

Nursing Diagnoses and Related Interventions

Upon completion of a thorough assessment, the nurse might identify several nursing diagnoses, including:
• Deficient knowledge
• Disturbed body image
• Anxiety
• Fear
• Pain

Nursing goals, interventions, and evaluation for the person with reproductive cancer are based on the nursing diagnoses. Nursing Care Plan 8.1 (at the end of the chapter) may be used as a guide in planning nursing care for the client with reproductive cancer. It should be individualized based on the client's symptoms and needs.

Nurses have traditionally served as advocates in the health care arena and should continue to be on the forefront of health education and diagnosis, acting as leaders in the fight against cancer. The public needs to know that not only are many cancer deaths preventable, but many of the cancers themselves are preventable. Nurses need to work to improve the availability and quality of cancer-screening services, making them accessible to underserved and socioeconomically disadvantaged clients. Through a unified effort by health care providers, health policy experts, government agencies, health insurance companies, the media, educational institutions, and clients themselves, along with consistency and continuity, nurses can offer quality care to all persons with cancer.

Educating to Prevent Cancer

Globally, there are nearly 13 million new cases of cancer and 8 million deaths from cancer each year. The most important cause of cancer is tobacco, which causes 30% of cancer deaths. Dietary factors, including obesity, are estimated to cause around 25% of cancer deaths, and alcohol about 6% of cancer deaths. All of these factors associated with cancer are preventable (Key, 2015). Nurses need to provide clients with information to help prevent disease and enhance quality of life. Educate clients about the importance of consistent and timely screenings to identify cancer early. Emphasize the importance of having routine cancer screening and follow-up screenings as recommended. Provide clients with information if further diagnostic testing is required. Nurses also play a key role in promoting cancer awareness, prevention, and control. Advocate improving the availability of cancer-screening services and work to provide public education about risk factors for cancer.

Nurses can be instrumental in helping individuals to identify and change behaviours that put them at risk for various reproductive tract cancers (Teaching Guidelines 8.1). Do not limit your interventions to providing preventive education only: inform clients about the consequences of doing nothing about their conditions and what the long-range outcomes might be without treatment. For example, stress the importance of visiting a health care provider if certain signs and symptoms appear:

- Blood in a bowel movement, which is considered abnormal
- Unusual vaginal discharge or chronic vulvar itching
- Persistent abdominal bloating or constipation
- Irregular vaginal bleeding

- Persistent low backache not related to standing
- Elevated or discoloured vulvar lesions
- Bleeding after menopause
- Pain or bleeding after sexual intercourse

Teaching Guidelines 8.1
REDUCING YOUR RISK FOR CANCER

- Do not smoke; smoking is linked to lung cancer development.
- Drink alcohol only in moderation (no more than one drink daily).
- Be physically active daily.
- Eat a healthy diet.
- Stay current with immunizations.
- Use a condom with every sexual encounter.
- Reach and maintain a healthy weight.
- Take preventive medicines if needed.
- Get recommended screening tests:
  - Body mass index (BMI) to identify obesity
  - Mammogram every 1 to 2 years starting at age 40
  - Pap smear every 3 years if sexually active, between the ages of 25 and 69
  - Cholesterol checked annually starting at age 45
  - Blood pressure checked at least every 2 years
  - Diabetes test if hypertensive or hypercholesterolemia
  - Check for STIs if sexually active

Adapted from Agency for Healthcare Research and Quality. (2014). *Cancer screening and treatment in women: Recent findings.* Retrieved from http://www.ahrq.gov/research/findings/factsheets/women/cancerwom/; American Cancer Society (ACS). (2015b). *American Cancer Society guidelines for the early detection of cancer.* Retrieved from http://www.cancer.org/Healthy/FindCancerEarly/CancerScreeningGuidelines/american-cancer-society-guidelines-for-the-early-detection-of-cancer; Mayo Clinic. (2015). *Cancer prevention: 7 steps to reduce your risk.* Retrieved from http://www.mayoclinic.org/cancer-prevention/art-20044816; National Cancer Institute (NCI). (2015c). *General cancer prevention.* Retrieved from http://www.cancer.gov/cancertopics/prevention#General±Cancer±Prevention±Information; World Health Organization. (2015). Cancer prevention and control. Retrieved from http://www.who.int/nmh/a5816/en/.

Teaching Clients About Their Diagnoses

Provide information about tests that may be required to confirm or rule out the diagnosis. Review with clients what has been told to them about their diagnoses and their understanding of the conditions. It is not unusual for clients to hear the diagnosis and then become overwhelmed by the thought of cancer, blocking out whatever is said after that. Answer any questions clients may have. Go slowly and repeat the information as necessary. Use written materials to explain and reinforce the teaching. Provide information about their conditions and recommended therapies. For example, if a client is undergoing surgery, discuss postoperative

issues such as incision care, pain, and activity level. Instruct clients on health maintenance activities after treatment and inform clients and their families about available support resources.

Providing Emotional Support

Once the diagnosis is made, provide clients and their families with emotional support. Validate feelings and provide realistic hope, using a nonjudgmental approach and therapeutic communication skills during all interactions. Nurses can be invaluable when assisting individuals who are coping with the uncertainty of their future by providing positive communication and support. Nurses need to focus on the physical, psychosocial, and economic concerns, from diagnosis through treatment and, if applicable, until the end of life, for all of the clients for whom they care. Individualize the care based on the client's cultural traditions and beliefs, as explained in the following section.

ENSURING CULTURALLY COMPETENT CANCER CARE

Cultural diversity in Canada is increasing, and as diverse cultures interact, conflicts inevitably ensue. These conflicts can affect health care outcomes. Providing culturally competent cancer care can improve outcomes and decrease disparities in care. If nurses are to meet the needs of ethnically diverse populations, they must be culturally sensitive, appreciative of differing health beliefs and practices, and very flexible in the way they approach health care. It is we who must adapt, expand, and learn.

Nurses have the opportunity to learn about diverse cultures, religions, and faith traditions that support clients and families during their cancer journey and while facing a serious life-limiting illness. Nurses' care practices embrace all clients with whom they come in contact and, by having a better understanding of diverse groups, nurses can build trust in clients seeking oncology care needs that range from detection to diagnosis and treatment possibly through palliative care and end of life.

Be aware of the client's cultural background, religion, migration history, degree of acculturation, living conditions, educational level, and legal status, because each of these factors can affect the client's understanding of her diagnosis and the eventual outcome. A person's reaction to a cancer diagnosis and decisions about treatment are influenced by an individual's cultural values and how the community views cancer. A diagnosis of cancer carries deep physical, psychosocial, and cultural implications. Sensitive cross-cultural communication and cultural competence are vital for all nurses to deliver equal care to all cancer clients. Nurses need to understand the disparities and the influence of those disparities on health outcomes. Persons with cancer reflect the demographic changes occurring in Canada and represent increasing differences in culture, religion, socioeconomic status, race, and lifestyle. Through embracing and learning from these differences, nurses become stronger care providers (Surbone, 2015).

In some cultures, sharing news of a serious illness like cancer is considered disrespectful and impolite. For example, some Europeans view such sharing as inhumane; the Asian culture views a cancer diagnosis as unnecessarily cruel. The Chinese, out of respect for aging family members, withhold discussions of serious illness to avoid causing unnecessary anxieties (Lofters, 2015). Integrate this knowledge in your care to ensure a culturally competent approach.

The Indigenous people of Canada are referred to as Aboriginal peoples and include three distinct groups: First Nations, Inuit, and Métis peoples of Canada (Cameron, Plazas, Salas, Bearskin, & Hungler, 2014). They represent the fastest growing population in Canada and possess rich and diverse traditions, distinct practices and beliefs, and unique understandings of health and wellness (Kewayosh et al., 2015). Health disparities exist between Indigenous and non-Indigenous populations in Canada. Cancer incidence rates are on the rise in this population and studies show that Indigenous people often have lower survival rates for cancer than non-Indigenous people (Withrow, Pole, Nishri, Tjepkema, & Marrett, 2017). Although more research is needed to determine the exact causes of this disparity, factors such as poor access to care, geographical isolation, language barriers, poor housing, existing comorbidities, high rates of tobacco and alcohol use, and low socio-economic status may all play a role (Kewayosh et al., 2015). Prevention and early detection are key areas where nurses can have an impact on the health outcomes for Indigenous peoples. Nurses can play a role in helping to educate Indigenous clients about risk factors and lifestyle modifications such as tobacco and alcohol use reduction, eating a healthy diet, and increasing physical activity. It is also important to encourage clients to participate in routine cancer screening and HPV vaccination programs.

> ***Take Note!***
>
> When a diagnosis of cancer is made, assessing an individual's strengths and weaknesses from a cultural perspective will help the nurse to provide culturally competent care.

As life becomes increasingly multilingual, multicultural, and multireligious, learning about clients' values and cultural beliefs becomes challenging. Be willing to learn about client preferences; doing so promotes caring and nurturing.

SUPPORTING THE PREGNANT CLIENT WITH CANCER

Pregnancy complicated by cancer is relatively rare, occurring in 1 out of every 1,000 pregnancies

(Cancer.Net, 2015a). The incidence is increasing because people in Western societies are tending to delay childbearing to the third and fourth decades of life; this phenomenon is going to be encountered more often in the future by nurses. The most frequent malignancies diagnosed during pregnancy are breast cancer, cervical cancer, hematologic malignancies (lymphomas and acute leukemia), and melanoma. Breast cancer is the most common cancer diagnosed in pregnant persons which affects approximately 1 in 3,000 pregnancies. Less common tumours during pregnancy include gastrointestinal, ovarian, urologic, and lung cancers (Amant et al., 2015).

Theoretically, changes in the immune system during pregnancy can increase the risk of malignancy because cell-mediated immunity, which is suppressed in pregnancy, normally protects against cancerous tumours (Kim & Chu, 2015). Some research has hinted at an increased rate of progression and decreased survival times in women who develop breast and cervical cancer and then become pregnant, but this generally has not been validated by research studies. With the cooperation of multidisciplinary teams, treatment of cancer during pregnancy with normal fetal outcome is feasible (Andersson, Johansson, Fredriksson, & Lambe, 2015).

Ovarian cancer during pregnancy is rare because the disease typically occurs in older populations. Because most pregnant persons receive frequent medical care, including pelvic examinations, most ovarian cancers in pregnant clients are found at early stages; this carries a good prognosis for both the mother and the newborn. The presence of ascites indicates advanced disease (de Haan, Verheecke, & Amant, 2015).

Endometrial cancer is the most common neoplasia of the female reproductive system, with the highest incidence among uterine malignancies. It is rarely associated with pregnancy. Adenocarcinoma associated with pregnancy is typically endometrioid, focal, well differentiated, and minimally invasive. Active treatment of endometrial cancer is incompatible with continuation of the pregnancy. Since routine screening for endometrial cancer is currently not recommended in the general population, few cases would be detected in the relatively young pregnant population (Cancer in Pregnancy, 2015a). Cervical cancer is more common in the pregnant population than other reproductive malignancies, and it can affect the person's health status and the pregnancy. Approximately 30% of individuals diagnosed with cervical cancer are in their reproductive years, whereas 3% of cervical cancers are diagnosed during pregnancy (Cancer in Pregnancy, 2015b). Management of cervical cancer during pregnancy depends on the following factors:

- Stage of the disease (and the tumour size)
- Nodal status
- Histologic subtype of the tumour
- Term of the pregnancy
- Whether the client wishes to continue her pregnancy
- Person's desire for future fertility

In clients with early-stage disease and absence of nodal involvement who are diagnosed during the first two trimesters of pregnancy, there is an increasing tendency to preserve the pregnancy while awaiting fetal maturity. The birth (when the fetal maturity is attained) should be performed using a cesarean section (ACS, 2015c). Treatment decisions are influenced by the stage of the cancer, the histologic type, the stage of the pregnancy, and the client's wishes. Both maternal and fetal safety and well-being have to be taken into account. Termination of pregnancy is not indicated in all cases. Pregnancy preservation in tumours diagnosed during early gestation is feasible in carefully selected cases. Discussions with clients and their families are essential and treatment has to be individualized (ACS, 2015c).

Nurses caring for young clients with cervical cancer must be aware of the surgical fertility preservation options, which clients are candidates for these surgeries, and the options for future assisted reproductive technology. Nurses need to be able to coordinate care for these clients with gynecologic oncologists and reproductive endocrinologists in order to facilitate optimal outcomes.

Individuals diagnosed with any malignancy during pregnancy must confront the reality of the disease and its impact on their future fertility and live with the risk of recurrence. The prognosis for a pregnant person with cancer is often the same as other individuals of the same age with the same type of cancer (Cancer. Net, 2015a). The wishes of the pregnant person and the family are of paramount importance when making decisions about continuing the pregnancy and undergoing cancer treatment. Some clients will decide to terminate the pregnancy for the sake of their own health; others will undergo treatment during the pregnancy to preserve the life of the unborn child. Regardless of the client's decision, provide support, hope, and education during treatment, birth, and beyond.

OVARIAN CANCER

Ovarian cancer is malignant neoplastic growth of the ovary (Fig. 8.1). It is the eighth most common cancer among women and the fifth most common cause of cancer deaths for women in Canada (CCSACCS, 2017). It accounts for more deaths than any other cancer of the reproductive system (Navaneelan, 2015). The risk of getting invasive ovarian cancer in the course of a lifetime is about 1 in 75. The lifetime chance of dying from invasive ovarian cancer is about 1 in 100 (ACS, 2015d). This

Uterus

Carcinoma of the left ovary

Fallopian tube

Ovary

Microscopic view of ovarian cancer cells

FIGURE 8.1 Ovarian cancer. (Asset provided by Anatomical Chart Co.)

cancer mainly develops in older individuals. About half of the people who are diagnosed with ovarian cancer are 63 years or older.

The most important variable influencing the prognosis is the extent of the disease. Survival depends on the stage of the tumour, grade of differentiation, gross findings at surgery, amount of residual tumour after surgery, and effectiveness of any adjunct treatment postoperatively. Many individuals with ovarian cancer will experience recurrence despite best efforts to eradicate the cancer through surgery, radiation, or chemotherapy to eliminate residual tumour cells. The likelihood of long-term survival in the event of recurrence is dismal (Matsumoto, Onada, & Yaegashi, 2015). The 5-year survival rates (the percentage of individuals who live at least 5 years after their diagnosis) are shown in Table 8.1 according to stage.

Pathophysiology

Ovarian cancer, the cause of which is unknown, can originate from different cell types. Most ovarian cancers are thought to originate in the ovarian epithelium. New insights now propose a pivotal role for the fallopian tube

during ovarian cancer pathogenesis. Increasing evidence suggests that serous ovarian cancer originates from the fimbriated distal end of the fallopian tube, whereas the ovary gets only involved at a later stage. These represent 50% to 60% of all epithelial ovarian cancers. Based on

TABLE 8.1	FIVE-YEAR SURVIVAL RATES FOR OVARIAN CANCER		
	Five-Year Relative Survival Rates		
Stage	*Epithelial (%)*	*Stromal Tumour (%)*	*Germ Cell (%)*
I	90	95	98
II	70	78	94
III	39	65	87
IV	17	35	69

Adapted from Canadian Cancer Society (CCS). (2018). *Survival statistics for ovarian cancer*. Retrieved from http://www.cancer.ca/en/cancer-information/cancer-type/ovarian/prognosis-and-survival/survival-statistics/?region=on this finding, a post-reproductive salpingectomy deserves consideration as a prophylactic intervention that may confer protection against an often deadly disease (Poole, Rice, Crum, & Tworoger, 2015).

Tumours usually present as solid masses that have spread beyond the ovary and seeded into the peritoneum prior to diagnosis. Thorough understanding of the true pathogenesis of this cancer's origin could lead to the development of new and more effective therapies as well as novel biomarkers in early detection.

Screening and Diagnosis

Individuals with ovarian cancer are typically diagnosed at a late stage, when the cancer has spread into the peritoneal cavity and complete surgical removal is challenging. Seventy-five percent of ovarian cancers are not diagnosed until the cancer has advanced to stage III or IV, primarily because there is still no adequate screening test. The 5-year survival time for individuals diagnosed at this stage is 30%, in contrast with a 5-year survival of 90% for those diagnosed at an early stage (Wright et al., 2015). The United States Preventive Services Task Force (USPSTF, 2015), along with the American College of Obstetricians and Gynecologists (ACOG), and the American Medical Association (AMA) recently reviewed the evidence for ovarian cancer screening and did not recommend screening for individuals at average risk. However, individuals with increased risk related to BRCA ½ mutations or a family history of ovarian cancer should be considered for genetic counselling to further evaluate their risk (Cliby et al., 2015).

Two genes, BRCA1 and BRCA2, are linked with hereditary breast and ovarian cancers. Blood tests can be performed to assess DNA in white blood cells to detect mutations in the BRCA genes. These genetic markers do not predict whether the person will develop cancer. Rather, they provide information regarding the risk of developing cancer: a person who is BRCA positive may have up to an 80% chance of developing breast cancer and a 40% chance of developing ovarian cancer (Liede, Sun, & Narod, 2015).

To assist in screening, researchers have developed an ovarian cancer symptom index that includes pelvic and abdominal pain, urinary frequency and urgency, increased abdominal size (bloating), and difficulty eating (feeling full). But this symptom index is not much helpful in detecting the disease early, as these symptoms tend to go unrecognized, leading to delays in diagnosis. When the presentation of such symptoms triggers a medical evaluation for ovarian cancer, the disease is diagnosed in only 1 in 100 women. The NCI reports that the present symptom index has a "low positive predictive value," especially for early-stage disease discovery (NCI, 2015d).

Specific clinical guidelines for ovarian cancer screening have not been developed, so the disease is often not diagnosed until it has metastasized. The USPSTF recommends against routine screening for ovarian cancer with serum CA-125 or transvaginal ultrasound because earlier detection would have a small effect, at best, on mortality. CA-125 is a biologic tumour marker associated with ovarian cancer. Although levels are elevated in many individuals with ovarian cancer, CA-125 is not specific for this cancer and levels may be elevated with other malignancies (pancreatic, liver, colon, breast, and lung cancers). Despite the discovery that CA-125 and other serum markers increase before the clinical onset of ovarian cancer, it has proven surprisingly difficult to devise a successful screening program for asymptomatic individuals with ovarian cancer. Currently, it is not sensitive enough to serve as a screening tool alone (Ebell, Culp, Lastinger, & Dasigi, 2015). The USPSTF (2015) reports that there is no supporting evidence that any screening test, including a CA-125, ultrasound, or pelvic examination, reduces mortality from ovarian cancer. Thus, they recommend against routine screening for ovarian cancer.

Therapeutic Management

Treatment options for ovarian cancer vary depending on the stage and severity of the disease. Usually, a laparoscopy (abdominal exploration with an endoscope) is performed for diagnosis and staging, as well as evaluation for therapy. In stage I, the cancer is limited to the ovaries. In stage II, the growth involves one or both ovaries, with pelvic extension. Stage III cancer has spread to the lymph nodes and other organs or structures inside the abdominal cavity. In stage IV, the cancer has metastasized to distant sites (Alexander et al., 2014). Figure 8.2 shows the likely metastatic sites for ovarian cancer.

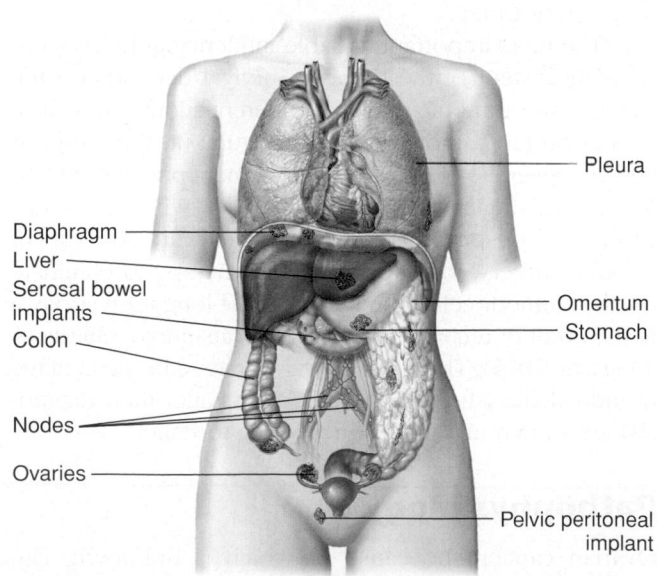

FIGURE 8.2 Common metastatic sites for ovarian cancer. (Asset provided by Anatomical Chart Co.)

Surgical intervention remains the mainstay of management of ovarian cancer. Surgery generally includes a total abdominal hysterectomy, bilateral salpingo-oophorectomy, peritoneal biopsies, omentectomy (excision of all or part of the omentum, which is a sheet of fat covered by the peritoneum that protects the abdominal structures), and pelvic para-aortic lymph node sampling to evaluate cancer extension (Nick, Coleman, Ramirez, & Sood, 2015). Because most individuals are diagnosed with advanced-stage ovarian cancer, aggressive management involving debulking or cytoreductive surgery is commonly performed. This surgery involves resecting all visible tumours from the peritoneum, taking peritoneal biopsies, sampling lymph nodes, and removing all reproductive organs and the omentum. This aggressive surgery has been shown to improve long-term survival rates.

Additional therapy with radiation may be warranted. Chemotherapy is recommended for all stages of ovarian cancer. Intraperitoneal chemotherapy, combined with surgery, has produced encouraging results for overall survivals at acceptable morbidity and mortality rates. Despite all of these therapies, virtually the only agreement about treatment for advanced disease is that surgery and chemotherapy play a role, and that current treatment is ineffective in far too many people (Helm, 2015a).

Nursing Assessment

Ovarian cancers are considered the worst of all the gynecologic malignancies, primarily because they develop slowly and remain silent without symptoms until the cancer is far advanced. It has been described as the "overlooked disease" or "silent killer" because individuals and health care providers often ignore or rationalize early symptoms. For example, a person may attribute gastrointestinal problems to stress and midlife changes. However, these vague complaints may precede more obvious symptoms by months. The most common early symptoms include abdominal bloating, early satiety, fatigue, vague abdominal pain, urinary frequency, diarrhea or constipation, malaise, and unexplained weight loss or gain. The later symptoms include anorexia, dyspepsia, ascites, a palpable abdominal mass, pelvic pain, and back pain (Goldstein, Susman, Lockwood, Medlin, & Behbakht, 2015).

Obtain a thorough history of the client's symptoms, including their onset, duration, and frequency. Review the client's history for risk factors such as:
- Nulliparity
- Early menarche (before 12 years old)
- Late menopause (after 55 years old)
- Increasing age (after menopause)
- High-fat diet
- Obesity
- Persistent ovulation over time
- First-degree relative with ovarian cancer
- Genetics (women of Ashkenazi Jewish decent)

- Use of perineal talcum powder or hygiene sprays
- Older than 30 years at first pregnancy
- Positive BRCA1 and BRCA2 mutations
- Personal history of breast, bladder, or colon cancer
- Hormone replacement therapy (HRT) for more than 10 years
- Infertility (CDC, 2015c)

Perform a complete physical examination. Inspect the abdomen, noting any distention or bloating. Palpate the abdomen. Be alert for a mass or pain on palpation. Anticipate further testing to confirm the diagnosis.

Nursing Management

The complexities of ovarian cancer make a multidisciplinary approach necessary for optimal management. With the subtle nature and high risk of recurrence and mortality of this condition, most people find it an emotionally exhausting and devastating experience. The presence of hope is essential for individuals at the time of the diagnosis; they want to believe in being cured and able to continue their life as usual with loved ones, friends, and relatives. Still, the newly received cancer diagnosis makes people oscillate between hope and hopelessness, and between positive expectations of getting cured and frightening feelings of the disease taking command. Nurses are invaluable resources in inspiring clients to find hope in life when diagnosed with cancer. Nursing management needs to focus on measures to promote early detection, educate the person about the disease and its treatments, and provide emotional support. Nurses should show a positive attitude that communicates understanding and reassurance.

Promoting Early Detection

Nurses need to ensure that clients are aware of the risk factors for ovarian cancer. Urge them not to dismiss seemingly innocuous symptoms as "just a part of aging." Encourage clients to describe such nonspecific complaints at health visits.

Assess the person's family and personal history for risk factors and encourage genetic testing for individuals with affected family members. Outline screening guidelines for clients with hereditary cancer syndrome and inform those at high risk about the appropriate screening strategies.

Urge clients to have yearly bimanual pelvic examinations and a transvaginal ultrasound to allow identification of ovarian masses in their early stages. After menopause, a mass on an ovary is not a cyst: physiologic cysts can arise only from a follicle that has not ruptured or from the cystic degeneration of the corpus luteum. Ovarian cancer is not always silent and may manifest with several vague gastrointestinal symptoms. Although screening the general population is not recommended, nurses need to know what factors place a person at high risk and really listen to the person's complaints to detect this type of cancer before it becomes advanced.

Take Note!

A small ovarian "cyst" found on ultrasound in an asymptomatic postmenopausal person should arouse suspicion. Any mass or ovary palpated in a postmenopausal client should be considered cancerous until proven otherwise (Helm, 2015b).

Educating the Client

Education is a major focus of nursing care. This teaching involves risk reduction and health promotion. Teach the client about risk reduction strategies; for instance, pregnancy, use of oral contraceptives, and breast-feeding reduce the risk of ovarian cancer. Instruct clients to avoid using talc and hygiene sprays on their genitals. Review the lifetime risks related to *BRCA1* and *BRCA2* genes and options available should the person test positive for these genes. Help to promote community awareness of ovarian cancer by educating the public about risk-reducing behaviours. See research on reproductive cancer risk factor (Evidence-Based Practice 8.1).

Instruct the client about the importance of healthy lifestyles. Stress the importance of maintaining a healthy weight to reduce risk. Encourage clients to eat a low-fat diet. Factors associated with a reduced risk of ovarian cancer include the use of oral contraceptives for 3 years or longer, pregnancy and breast-feeding before the age

of 30, bilateral tubal ligation, and removal of the ovaries (Memorial Sloan Kettering Cancer Center, 2015).

For the person who is diagnosed with ovarian cancer, describe in simple terms the tests, treatment modalities, and follow-up needed. For example, if the client will be having surgery, provide thorough teaching about what to expect before, during, and after surgery. Outline treatment options and the implications of choices. Assist clients and their families to decipher the myriad of information related to staging, tests, and treatments. Teach the client about additional treatment measures, such as radiation therapy or chemotherapy, including how to handle the common adverse effects of treatment.

Supporting the Client and Family

The diagnosis of ovarian cancer, like any cancer, can be overwhelming. In addition, the treatments and their effects can be highly stressful, both physically and emotionally. Provide one-to-one support for clients facing treatment for ovarian cancer. Ovarian cancer involves the reproductive system, which has a direct impact on the person's self-view. Encourage open discussion of sexuality and the impact of cancer. Listen and support the client and family as they try to cope with this disease. By being aware of clients' individual needs and different coping strategies, nurses can improve appropriate support in this vulnerable situation. Encourage the use of appropriate coping strategies to allow for the best quality of life. Try

---

EVIDENCE-BASED PRACTICE 8.1   **DOES OVARIAN STIMULATION FOR IVF INCREASE GYNECOLOGIC CANCER RISK? A SYSTEMATIC REVIEW AND META-ANALYSIS**

STUDY

Drugs to stimulate ovulation have been widely used for various types of subfertility since the early 1960s, and their use has increased in recent years. The use of assisted reproductive techniques is increasing, but the possible link between fertility drugs and reproductive cancer remains controversial. Subfertile individuals are commonly exposed to these agents, which may be administered at high doses for long periods of time during treatment for subfertility. There is uncertainty about the safety of these drugs and the potential risk of causing cancers associated with their use. The objective of this study was to evaluate the risk of reproductive cancer in individuals previously treated with ovulation-stimulating drugs for infertility.

Findings

A systematic review and meta-analysis was conducted. Clinical trials that examined the association between ovarian stimulation for IVF and gynecologic cancers were included. Twelve cohort studies with 178,396 women exposed to IVF were included. The meta-analysis found no

significant association between ovarian stimulation for IVF and increased ovarian, endometrial, cervical, and breast cancer risk. Ovarian stimulation for IVF, therefore, does not increase the gynecologic risk, whether hormone-dependent endometrial and breast cancer risk or non–hormone-dependent ovarian and cervical cancer. This study found no convincing evidence of an increased risk of reproductive cancer with fertility drug treatment.

Nursing Implications

Nurses can use the information from this study to reassure clients that having experienced infertility and undergone in vitro fertilization treatments in the past are not increasing their risk of having reproductive cancer later in life. When individuals are trying to decide to undergo fertility treatment using drug therapy, it can be very anxiety producing for them as well as their partners. Knowing that in vitro fertilization treatment will not increase their risk of reproductive cancer as they age, based on earlier exposure to ovulation-stimulating drug therapy, can reduce their anxiety regarding their decision.

Adapted from Li, Y., Zhao, J., Zhang, Q., & Wang, Y. (2015). Does ovarian stimulation for IVF increase gynecological cancer risk? A systematic review and meta-analysis. *Reproductive BioMedicine Online, 31*(1), 20–29.

to restore hope to clients with ovarian cancer, and stress treatment compliance. Nurses should not forget about the family caregivers who need help with managing emotions about prognosis, balancing their own and the client's needs, work, and decision-making when there is uncertainty. If appropriate, encourage participation in clinical trials to offer hope for all persons. Continue to offer support to clients and their family members as they experience sadness and grief.

Consider This

I felt I was a lucky woman because I had been in remission from breast cancer for 12 years, and I had been given the gift of life to share with my beloved family. Recently I became ill with stomach problems: pain, indigestion, bloating, and nausea. My doctor treated me for gastric reflux disease, but the symptoms persisted. I then was referred to a gastroenterologist, a urologist, and then a gynecologist, who did an ultrasound, which was negative. I received reassurance from all three that there was nothing wrong with me. As time went by, I experienced more pain, more symptoms, and increased frustration. Six months after seeing all three specialists, a repeat ultrasound revealed I had ovarian cancer, and I needed surgery as soon as possible. I underwent a complete hysterectomy and my surgeon found I was in stage III. Since then, I have undergone chemotherapy and participated in a clinical cancer study that wasn't successful for me, and now I am facing the fact that I am going to die soon.

Thoughts: *This woman has tried everything to save her life, but, alas, time has run out for her with advanced ovarian cancer. Women diagnosed with breast cancer are at a significant risk for developing ovarian cancer later in life. Of the string of doctors she saw, one has to ponder why none ordered more extensive testing, given her history of breast cancer. We are haunted with the question: If they had, would she be in stage III now? We will never know.*

ENDOMETRIAL CANCER

Endometrial cancer (also known as uterine cancer) is malignant neoplastic growth of the uterine lining. It is the most commonly diagnosed reproductive system cancer and accounts for 6.3% of all cancers in women in Canada (Navaneelan, 2015). Endometrial cancer is responsible for over 75,000 deaths annually among women worldwide (Siegel, Miller, & Jemal, 2015). It is uncommon before the age of 55, but as people age, their risk of endometrial cancer increases. Approximately 80% of these malignancies are carcinomas of the endometrium. Because endometrial cancer is usually diagnosed in the early stages, it has a better prognosis than cervical or ovarian cancer (ACS, 2015e).

The increasing incidence and prevalence of endometrial cancer can be explained by the increase in life expectancy, increased caloric intake, increased obesity rates, infertility, null parity (never bearing children), older age of first pregnancy, and long-term use of unopposed estrogens for HRT. Protection against endometrial cancer includes increased parity, daily physical activity, use of combined oral contraceptives, and increased age at last childbirth (Schmid et al., 2015).

Pathophysiology

Two mechanisms are believed to be involved in the development of endometrial cancer. A history of exposure to unopposed estrogen is the cause in approximately 80% of individuals. Those that are spontaneous and are unrelated to estrogen or endometrial hyperplasia represent the other 20% of endometrial cancers. There has been an increase in incidence over the past several decades associated with an increased use of estrogen replacement therapy (without progestin) and obesity (adipose fat converts androstenedione to estrone, thereby increasing circulating estrogen levels) (Temple, 2015).

Endometrial cancer may originate in a polyp or in a diffuse multifocal pattern. The pattern of spread partially depends on the degree of cellular differentiation. Well-differentiated tumours tend to limit their spread to the surface of the endometrium. Metastatic spread occurs in a characteristic pattern and most commonly involves the lungs, inguinal and supraclavicular nodes, liver, bones, brain, and vagina (NCI, 2015f). Early tumour growth is characterized by friable and spontaneous bleeding. Later tumour growth is characterized by myometrial invasion and growth toward the cervix (Fig. 8.3).

Adenocarcinoma of the endometrium is typically preceded by hyperplasia. Carcinoma in situ is found only on the endometrial surface. Type I carcinomas, the most common, begin as endometrial hyperplasia and progress to carcinomas. Giving estrogen preparations without progestin for HRT leads to an increased risk for endometrial cancer. Type I is generally found at an earlier stage and treatment results are more favourable.

Unlike type I endometrial carcinoma, type II carcinomas appear spontaneously, are associated with a poorly differentiated cell type, and have a poor prognosis. They account for less than 10% of all endometrial cancers but contribute to the majority of all endometrial deaths. This type is unrelated to estrogen or endometrial hyperplasia (ACS, 2015f).

> **Remember Carmella, the woman with postmenopausal bleeding? In postmenopausal persons, any bleeding is abnormal and warrants further assessment. What testing would the nurse anticipate as being ordered to confirm the diagnosis? What would be the nurse's role during this testing?**

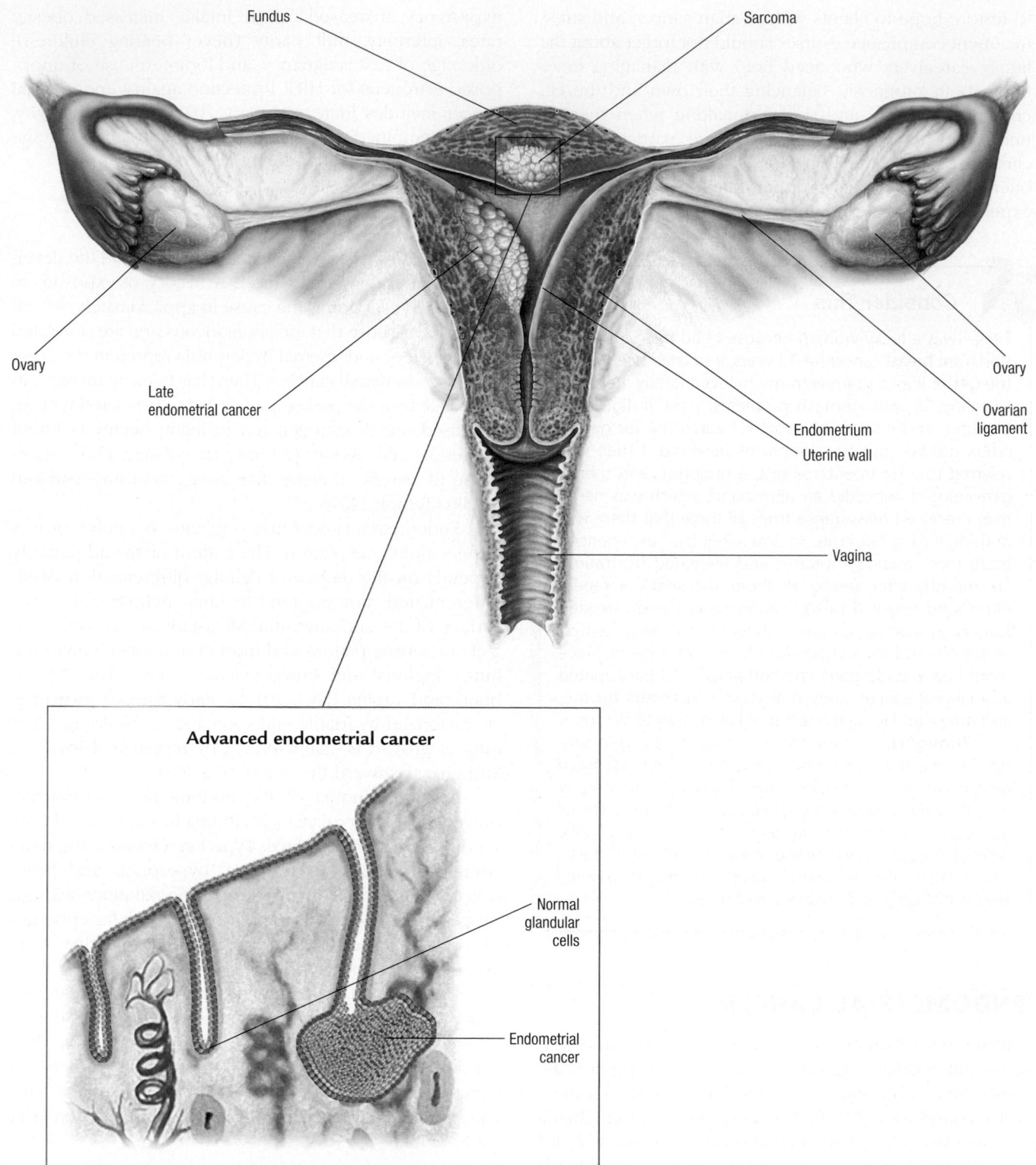

FIGURE 8.3 Progression of endometrial cancer. (Image 1 provided by Anatomical Chart Co.)

Screening and Diagnosis

There is no specific screening test currently available to detect endometrial cancer. Screening for endometrial cancer is not routinely done because it is not practical or cost-effective. The ACS (2015f) recommends that individ- uals be informed about the risks and symptoms of endo- metrial cancer at the onset of menopause and strongly encouraged to report any unexpected bleeding or spot- ting to their health care provider. A pelvic examination is frequently normal in the early stages of the disease.

Changes in the size, shape, or consistency of the uterus or its surrounding support structures may exist when the disease is more advanced.

During the past two decades, the role of ultrasound in the evaluation of postmenopausal bleeding has changed markedly, from little or no role to a major role today. In the intervening years, numerous studies have shown that ultrasound is at least as sensitive as endometrial biopsy for endometrial cancer and that ultrasound can reliably exclude cancer without the need for biopsy in some persons with postmenopausal bleeding. The depth of myometrium is an important diagnostic factor. In particular, numerous studies have shown that individuals with an endometrial thickness of 4 mm or less have an extremely low likelihood of endometrial cancer and thus do not need to undergo endometrial biopsy. Ultrasound can also help in the selection of an appropriate biopsy technique. In a person with postmenopausal bleeding and a thick endometrium, a sonohysterogram can determine whether the endometrium is diffusely thick or has focal areas of thickening. With diffuse thickening, an endometrial biopsy is appropriate. When one or more focal areas of thickening are present, hysteroscopic biopsy is likely to be the better choice. Typically, the noninvasive ultrasound is done first before an invasive endometrial biopsy is attempted (Dueholm, Marinovskij, Hansen, Møller, & Ørtoft, 2015).

Transvaginal ultrasound can be used to evaluate the endometrial cavity and measure the thickness of the endometrial lining. It can be used to detect endometrial hyperplasia. If the endometrium measures less than 4 mm, then the client is at low risk for malignancy. Large prospective studies have shown that an endometrial thickness of ≤4 mm on transvaginal ultrasound in postmenopausal individuals with bleeding has a low risk of malignancy. Thus, in postmenopausal clients with bleeding, biopsy is not indicted when endometrial thickness is ≤4 mm, thereby avoiding invasive diagnostics (Wong et al., 2015).

Endometrial biopsy is an office procedure that is also one of the first steps in the diagnosis of endometrial cancer in a person with postmenopausal bleeding. The biopsy is obtained through the use of an endometrial suction catheter that is inserted through the cervix into the uterine cavity and a tissue sample is taken. The sensitivity and specificity of the biopsy procedure tend to be in the range of 95% for detection of endometrial cancer or other pathologies (King et al., 2015).

As indicated earlier, staging is the process of looking at all of the information the doctors have learned about the tumour to determine how much the cancer may have spread. The stage of an endometrial cancer is the most important factor in choosing a treatment plan. It can spread *locally* to other parts of the uterus or *regionally* to nearby lymph nodes. The regional lymph nodes are found in the pelvis and farther away along the aorta. Finally, the cancer can spread (*metastasize*) to distant lymph nodes or organs such as lung, liver, bone, brain, and others.

In stage I, the tumour is confined to the corpus uteri. In stage II, it has spread to the cervix, but not outside the uterus. In stage III, it has spread locally and regionally. In stage IV, it has invaded the bladder mucosa, bowel with distant metastases to the lungs, liver, and bone (International Federation of Gynecology & Obstetrics, 2015).

Therapeutic Management

Typically, the stage of the disease directs treatment. It usually involves surgery with adjunct therapy based on pathologic findings. Surgery most often involves removal of the uterus (hysterectomy) and the fallopian tubes and ovaries (salpingo-oophorectomy). Removal of the fallopian tubes and ovaries is recommended because tumour cells spread early to the ovaries, and any dormant cancer cells could be stimulated to grow by ovarian estrogen. In more advanced cancers, radiation and chemotherapy are used as adjuncts to surgery. Routine surveillance intervals for follow-up care are typically every 3 to 4 months for the first 2 years, since 85% of recurrences occur in the first 3 years after diagnosis (Brennan et al., 2015).

Nursing Assessment

Obtain a thorough history from the client, ascertaining the primary complaint. Most commonly, the major initial symptom of endometrial cancer is abnormal and painless vaginal bleeding. Obtain a menstrual history and inquire if the client is taking any hormones. Also ascertain if there is a personal or family history of breast, ovarian, or colon cancer. These key pieces of information will assist in identifying the person at high risk for endometrial cancer.

 Take Note!

Any episode of bright-red bleeding that occurs after menopause should be investigated. Abnormal uterine bleeding is rarely the result of uterine malignancy in a young person, but in the postmenopausal person it should be regarded with suspicion.

Also, review the client's history for any risk factors, including:

- Nulliparity
- Obesity (more than 50 lb overweight)
- Liver disease
- Infertility
- Diabetes mellitus
- Hypertension
- History of pelvic radiation
- Polycystic ovary syndrome
- Early menarche (before 12 years old)
- High-fat diet

- Use of prolonged exogenous unopposed estrogen with an intact uterus
- Endometrial hyperplasia
- Family history of endometrial cancer
- Personal history of hereditary nonpolyposis colon cancer
- Personal history of breast, colon, or ovarian cancer
- History of uterine fibroids
- Late onset of menopause (after age 52 years)
- Tamoxifen use
- Chronic anovulation (Moses, 2015)

Assess the client for additional manifestations, such as dyspareunia, low back pain, purulent genital discharge, dysuria, pelvic pain, weight loss, and a change in bladder and bowel habits. These may suggest advanced disease.

Perform a physical examination or assist with, as appropriate, a pelvic examination. Observe for vaginal discharge. Note any changes in the size, shape, or consistency of the uterus or surrounding structures or client reports of pain during examination. Anticipate the need for transvaginal ultrasound to identify endometrial hyperplasia (usually greater than 4 mm) and endometrial biopsy to identify malignant cells.

Nursing Management

Ensure that the client understands all of the treatment options. Address any concerns the client expresses, including questions about sexuality. Ensure that follow-up appointments are scheduled appropriately. Refer the client to a support group. Offer the client and family explanations and emotional support throughout.

Educate clients about preventive measures or follow-up care if they have been treated for cancer. Education may be the most important tool currently available for the early detection of endometrial cancer. Many risk factors for endometrial cancer are modifiable or treatable, including obesity, hypertension, and diabetes. Educating clients about risk factors and ways to decrease the risks is essential so that they can learn about their own risk and can become partners in the fight against the number-one gynecologic cancer (Teaching Guidelines 8.2).

Teaching Guidelines 8.2
PREVENTIVE AND FOLLOW-UP MEASURES FOR ENDOMETRIAL CANCER
- Schedule regular pelvic examinations after the age of 25.
- Visit health care practitioner for early evaluation of any abnormal bleeding after menopause.
- Maintain a low-fat diet throughout life.
- Exercise daily.
- Manage weight to discourage hyperestrogenic states, which predispose to endometrial hyperplasia.

- Pregnancy serves as a protective factor by reducing estrogen.
- Ask your doctor about the use of combination estrogen and progestin pills.
- When combination oral contraceptives are taken to facilitate the regular shedding of the uterine lining, take risk reduction measures.
- Be aware of risk factors for endometrial cancer and make modifications as needed.
- Report any of the following symptoms immediately:
  - Bleeding or spotting after sexual intercourse
  - Bleeding that lasts longer than a week
  - Reappearance of bleeding after 6 months or more of no menses
- After cancer therapy, schedule follow-up appointments for the next few years.
- After cancer therapy, frequently communicate with your health care provider concerning your status.
- After surgery, maintain a healthy weight.

Carmella's endometrial biopsy indicates endometrial adenocarcinoma. Her health care provider recommends surgery and adjuvant radiation therapy. How long will Carmella need to follow up after surgery? What lifestyle changes will the nurse need to stress with Carmella?

CERVICAL CANCER

Cervical cancer is cancer of the uterine cervix. It is the third most common genital malignancy in women in Canada, after cancers of the endometrium and the ovary (Navaneelan, 2015). In 2017, an estimated 1,550 new cases of cervical cancer were diagnosed in Canada, making it the 13th most commonly diagnosed cancer in Canadian women (CCSACCS, 2017). Some researchers estimate that noninvasive cervical cancer (carcinoma in situ) is about four times more common than invasive cervical cancer. The 5-year survival rate for all stages of cervical cancer is 73% (CCSACCS, 2016). Cervical cancer is five to eight times more common in women affected with HIV or AIDS than those who do not have this virus.

Hispanic people are most likely to get cervical cancer, followed by African Americans, Asians and Pacific Islanders, and Whites. Cervical cancer remains a disease of socioeconomic disparity. The high mortality rates of minorities are indicative of barriers to health care among those living in poverty. Hispanic people also have the highest rates of poverty, poor access to health care, and language and cultural barriers. Barriers to screening and prevention of cervical cancer include procrastination, fear of finding out that they have cancer, and embarrassment about having a Papanicolaou (Pap) test. In addition, most have little to no knowledge about **HPV** (also known as genital warts) and its link with cancer (Strohl et al., 2015).

The incidence and mortality rates of cervical cancer have decreased noticeably in the past several decades, with most of the reduction attributed to the Pap test, which detects cervical cancer and some precancerous lesions. The Pap test (also known as a Pap smear) is a procedure used to obtain cells from the cervix for cytology screening. Cervical cancer is one of the most treatable cancers when detected at an early stage (ACS, 2015g; CCSACCS, 2016). Cervical cancer tends to occur in midlife. Most cases are found in individuals younger than age 50, with the highest incidence in women aged 40 to 49 (CCSACCS, 2016). It rarely develops in persons younger than age 20. Many older persons do not realize that the risk of developing cervical cancer is still present as they age.

Pathophysiology

Cervical cancer starts with abnormal changes in the cellular lining or surface of the cervix. Typically, these changes occur in the squamous–columnar junction of the cervix. Here, cylindrical secretory epithelial cells (columnar) meet the protective flat epithelial cells (squamous) from the outer cervix and vagina in what is termed the transformation zone. The continuous replacement of columnar epithelial cells by squamous epithelial cells in this area makes these cells vulnerable to taking up foreign or abnormal genetic material (ACS, 2015h). Figure 8.4 shows the pathophysiology of cervical cancer.

HPV infection must be present for cervical cancer to occur. HPV infections occur in a high percentage of sexually active individuals, but a successful immune response results in viral control or clearance of HPV. Most people who have HPV are asymptomatic and, therefore, do not realize they have the virus. More than 90% of squamous cervical cancers contain HPV DNA, and the virus is now accepted as a major causative factor in the development of cervical cancer and its precursor, **cervical dysplasia** (disordered growth of abnormal cells). Since only a small proportion of HPV infections progress to cancer, other factors must be involved in the process of carcinogenesis.

Screening and Diagnosis

Screening for cervical cancer is very effective because the presence of a precursor lesion, cervical intraepithelial neoplasia, helps determine whether further tests are needed. Lesions start as *dysplasia* and progress in a predictable fashion over a long period, allowing ample opportunity for intervention at a precancerous stage. Progression from low-grade to high-grade dysplasia takes an average of 9 years, and progression from high-grade dysplasia to invasive cancer takes up to 2 years. Three main factors have been postulated to influence the progression of low-grade dysplasia to high grade. These include the type and duration of viral infection, with high-risk HPV type and persistent infection predicting a higher risk for progression; host conditions that compromise immunity, such as multiparity or poor nutritional status; and environmental factors such as smoking, oral contraceptive use, or vitamin deficiencies. In addition, various gynecologic factors, including age of menarche, age of first intercourse, and number of sexual partners, significantly increase the risk for cervical cancer (Broadman & Matthews, 2015).

Widespread use of the **Pap test** is credited with saving tens of thousands of lives and decreasing deaths from cervical cancer. Routine Pap smear testing for all sexually active clients has been one of the primary screening methods for early detection of cervical irregularities

FIGURE 8.4 Cervical cancer. (Illustration is from The Anatomical Chart Company. [2009]. *Atlas of pathophysiology* [3rd ed.]. Philadelphia, PA: Lippincott Williams & Wilkins.)

related to HPV and is crucial for the prevention of cervical cancer.

Despite its outstanding record of success as a screening tool for cervical cancer (it detects approximately 90% of early cancer changes), the conventional Pap smear has a 20% false-negative rate. High-grade abnormalities missed by human screening are frequently detected by computerized instruments (NCI, 2015g). Thus, many technologies have been developed to improve the sensitivity and specificity of Pap testing, including:

• *Thin-Prep:* In this liquid-based technique, the cervical specimen is placed into a vial of preservative solution rather than on a glass slide.
• *Computer-assisted automated Pap test rescreening (Autopap):* An algorithm-based decision-making technology identifies slides that should be rescreened by cytopathologists by selecting samples that exceed a certain threshold for the likelihood of abnormal cells.
• *HPV-DNA typing (Hybrid Capture):* This system uses the association between certain types of HPV (16, 18, 31, 33, 35, 45, 51, 52, and 56) and the development of cervical cancer. This system can identify high-risk HPV types and improves detection and management.
• *Computer-assisted technology (Cytyc CDS-1000, Auto-Cyte, AcCell):* These computerized instruments can detect abnormal cells that are sometimes missed by technologists (CDC, 2015d; SOGC, 2007).

The high rate of false-negative results may also be due to other factors, including errors in sampling the cervix, in preparing the slide, and in client preparation. Although cytology-based nationwide cervical screening has been helpful in identifying abnormal cervical cells, the sensitivity of cytology for the detection of high-grade precursor lesions is limited. Additionally, adenocarcinoma and its precursors are often missed by cytology. The current insight that infection with HPV is the causative agent of cervical cancer and its precursors has led to the development of molecular tests for the detection of HPV. Strong evidence now supports the use of HPV testing in the prevention of cervical cancer. It is evident that HPV can be detected in urine-based testing which might eventually become a helpful tool in cervical cancer screening and HPV surveillance efforts. Nurses need to keep up to date on the latest research developments as well as the strengths and weaknesses of various screening methods (Fontenot, 2015).

The Canadian Task Force on Preventive Health Care (2013) recommended screening every 3 years for asymptomatic, sexually active individuals between the ages of 25 and 69 years. Subsequently, the Society of Obstetricians and Gynecologists of Canada (SOGC), the Society of Gynecologic Oncology of Canada (GOC), and the Society of Canadian Colposcopists (SCC) issued a position statement encouraging the initiation of screening at age 21 (SOGC, GOC, & SCC, 2013). Screening may cease

TABLE 8.2	CERVICAL CANCER SCREENING GUIDELINES
Ages 25–29	Recommend routine screening for cervical cancer every 3 years
Ages 30–69	Recommend routine screening for cervical cancer every 3 years
Age >70 years	For individuals aged 70 or over who have been adequately screened (i.e., three successive negative Pap tests in the last 10 years), it is recommended that routine screening may cease. For individuals aged 70 or over who have not been adequately screened, it is recommended to continue screening until three negative test results have been obtained

Canadian Task Force on Preventive Health Care. (2013). Recommendations on screening for cervical cancer. *Canadian Medical Association Journal, 185*(1), 35–45.

for individuals aged 70 years of age and older who have had three successive negative Pap tests in the previous 10 years. Clients who have had a hysterectomy should stop screening. Individuals who have received the HPV vaccine should be screened according to the same guidelines as those who have not been vaccinated. In addition, individuals must have a clear understanding of the results of Pap smear testing and follow-up guidelines. High-risk persons should continue to have annual Pap smears throughout their life (Table 8.2).

Pap smear results are classified using the Bethesda System (Box 8.1), which provides a uniform diagnostic terminology that allows clear communication between the laboratory and the health care provider. The information provided by the laboratory is divided into three categories: specimen adequacy, general categorization of cytologic findings, and interpretation/result (ACS, 2015h).

Therapeutic Management

Treatment for abnormal Pap smears depends on the severity of the results and the health history of the person. Therapeutic choices all involve destroying as many affected cells as possible. With the introduction of multimodality therapy for cervical cancer, many clients will be long-term survivors in need of comprehensive surveillance care. Obesity and smoking are significant comorbidities that may complicate care in cervical cancer survivors. Nurses can focus their interventions at modifying these risk factors to increase the quality of life for cervical cancer survivors. Box 8.2 describes treatment options.

BOX 8.1

THE BETHESDA SYSTEM FOR CLASSIFYING PAP SMEARS

Specimen Type: Conventional Pap smear vs. liquid-based

Specimen Adequacy: Satisfactory or unsatisfactory for evaluation

General Categorization: (optional)
- Negative for intraepithelial lesion or malignancy
- Epithelial cell abnormality; see interpretation/result

Automated Review: If case was examined by automated device or not

Ancillary Testing: Provides a brief description of the test methods and report results so health care provider understands

Interpretation/Result:
- Negative for intraepithelial lesion or malignancy
- Organisms: *Trichomonas vaginalis*; fungus; bacterial vaginosis; herpes simplex
- Other non-neoplastic findings: Reactive cellular changes associated with inflammation, radiation, intrauterine devices, atrophy
- Other: Endometrial cells in a woman >40 years of age
- Epithelial cell abnormalities:
- *Squamous cell*
  - Atypical squamous cells
    - Of undetermined significance (ASC-US)
    - Cannot exclude HSIL (ASC-H)
  - Low-grade squamous intraepithelial lesion (LSIL)
    - Encompassing HPV/mild dysplasia/CIN-1
  - High-grade squamous intraepithelial lesion (HSIL)
  - Encompassing moderate and severe dysplasia CIS/CIN-2 and CIN-3
  - With features suspicious for invasion
  - Squamous cell carcinoma
- Glandular cell: Atypical
  - Endocervical, endometrial, or glandular cells
    - Endocervical cells—favor neoplastic
    - Glandular cells—favor neoplastic
    - Endocervical adenocarcinoma in situ
  - Adenocarcinoma
    - Endocervical, endometrial, extrauterine
  - Other malignant neoplasms (specify)

Educational Notes and Suggestions: (optional)

Adapted from American Society of Cytopathology. (2015). *The Bethesda System for reporting cervical cytology: Definitions, criteria and explanatory notes.* Retrieved from http://www.cytopathology.org/the-bethesda-system-for-reporting-cervical-cytology-definitions-criteria-and-explanatory-notes-3rd-edition/; National Cancer Institute (NCI). (2015k). *Cervical cancer prevention.* Retrieved from http://www.cancer.gov/cancertopics/pdq/prevention/cervical/Patient/page3; Schuiling, K. D., & Likis, F. E. (2016). *Women's gynecologic health* (3rd ed.). Sudbury, MA: Jones & Bartlett.

BOX 8.2

TREATMENT OPTIONS FOR CERVICAL CANCER

- **Cryotherapy**—destroys abnormal cervical tissue by freezing with liquid nitrogen, Freon, or nitrous oxide. Studies show a 90% cure rate (NCI, 2015g). Healing takes up to 6 weeks, and the client may experience a profuse, watery vaginal discharge for 3 to 4 weeks.
- **Cone biopsy** or **conization**—removes a cone-shaped section of cervical tissue. The base of the cone is formed by the ectocervix (outer part of the cervix) and the point or apex of the cone is from the endocervical canal. The transformation zone is contained within the cone sample. The cone biopsy is also a treatment and can be used to completely remove any precancers and very early cancers. Two methods are commonly used for cone biopsies:
  - **LEEP (loop electrosurgical excision procedure)** or **LLETZ (large loop excision of the transformation zone)**—the abnormal cervical tissue is removed with a wire that is heated by an electrical current. For this procedure, a local anesthetic is used. It is performed in the health care provider's office in approximately 10 minutes. Mild cramping and bleeding may persist for several weeks after the procedure.
  - **Cold knife cone biopsy**—a surgical scalpel or a laser is used instead of a heated wire to remove tissue. This procedure requires general anesthesia and is done in a hospital setting. After the procedure, cramping and bleeding may persist for a few weeks.
- **Laser therapy**—destroys diseased cervical tissue by using a focused beam of high-energy light to vaporize it (burn it off). After the procedure, the woman may experience a watery brown discharge for a few weeks. Very effective in destroying precancers and preventing them from developing into cancers.
- **Hysterectomy**—removes the uterus and cervix surgically.
- **Radiation therapy**—delivered by internal radium applications to the cervix or external radiation therapy that includes lymphatics of the pelvis.
- **Chemoradiation**—weekly cisplatin therapy concurrent with radiation. Investigation of this therapy is ongoing (ACS, 2015h).

- *Atypical glandular cells (AGC) and adenocarcinoma in situ (AIS):* Immediate colposcopy; follow-up is based on the findings.

Colposcopy is a microscopic examination of the lower genital tract using a magnifying instrument called a colposcope. Specific patterns of cells that correlate well with certain histologic findings can be visualized.

Nursing Assessment

Obtain a thorough history and physical examination of all clients. Investigate their history for risk factors such as:
- Early age at first intercourse (within 1 year of menarche)
- Lower socioeconomic status
- Promiscuous partners

Using the Bethesda System, the following management guidelines for abnormal Pap results were developed by the NCI to provide direction to health care providers and clients:
- *ASC-US:* Repeat the Pap smear in 4 to 6 months or refer for colposcopy.
- *ASC-H:* Refer for colposcopy with HPV testing.

- Unprotected sexual intercourse
- Family history of cervical cancer (mother or sisters)
- Sexual intercourse with uncircumcised men
- Offspring of mothers who took diethylstilbestrol (DES)
- Infections with genital herpes or chronic chlamydia
- Multiple sex partners
- Cigarette smoking
- Immunocompromised state
- HIV infection
- Oral contraceptive use
- Moderate dysplasia on Pap smear within past 5 years
- HPV infection (CDC, 2015e)

Question the client about any signs and symptoms. Clinically, the first sign is abnormal vaginal bleeding, usually after sexual intercourse. Also be alert for reports of vaginal discomfort, malodorous discharge, and dysuria. In some cases, the woman is asymptomatic, with detection occurring at an annual gynecologic examination and Pap test.

Perform a physical examination. Inspect the perineal area for vaginal discharge or genital warts. Perform or assist with a pelvic examination, including the collection of a Pap smear as indicated (Nursing Procedure 8.1).

NURSING PROCEDURE 8.1

Assisting With Collection of a Pap Smear

Purpose: To Obtain Cells From the Cervix for Cervical Cytology Screening

1. Explain procedure to the client (Fig. A).
2. Instruct client to empty bladder.
3. Wash hands thoroughly.
4. Assemble equipment, maintaining sterility of equipment (Fig. B).

1. Position client on stirrups or foot pedals so that her knees fall outward.
2. Drape client with a sheet for privacy, covering the abdomen but leaving the perineal area exposed.
3. Open packages as needed.
4. Encourage client to relax.

5. Provide support to client as the practitioner obtains a sample by spreading the labia; inserting the speculum; inserting the cytobrush and swabbing the endocervix; and inserting the plastic spatula and swabbing the cervix (Figs. C–H).

NURSING PROCEDURE 8.1

Assisting With Collection of a Pap Smear (continued)

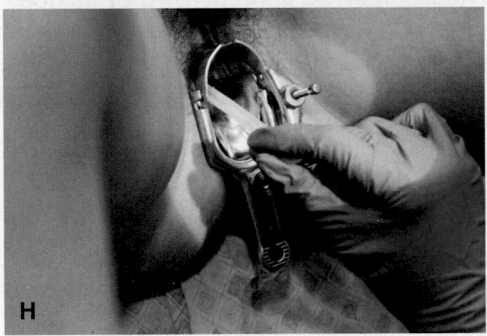

1. Transfer specimen to container (Fig. I) or slide. If a slide is used, spray the fixative on the slide holding the spray container about 12 in away from the slide.

2. Place sterile lubricant on the practitioner's fingertip when indicated for the bimanual examination.

3. Wash hands thoroughly.

4. Label specimen according to facility policy.

5. Rinse reusable instruments to prepare them for effective sanitizing/sterilizing, and dispose of waste appropriately (Fig. J).

6. Wash hands thoroughly.

7. Assist the client up after the examination is completed.

Adapted from King, T. L., Brucker, M. C., Kriebs, J. M., Fahey, J. O., Gegor, C. L., & Varney, H. (2015). *Varney's midwifery* (5th ed.). Burlington, MA: Jones & Bartlett Learning; Schuiling, K. D., & Likis, F. E. (2016). *Women's gynecologic health* (3rd ed.). Burlington, MA: Jones & Bartlett Learning.

Take Note!

Suspect advanced cervical cancer in individuals with pelvic, back, or leg pain, weight loss, anorexia, weakness and fatigue, and fractures.

Prepare the client for further diagnostic testing if indicated, such as a **colposcopy**. In a colposcopy, the person is placed in the lithotomy position and the cervix is cleansed with acetic acid solution. Acetic acid makes abnormal cells appear white, which is referred to as *acetowhite*. These white areas are then biopsied and sent to the pathologist for assessment. Although this test is not painful, has minor side effects (minor bleeding, cramping, and a risk of an infection developing after the biopsy), and can be performed safely in the clinic or office setting, individuals may be apprehensive or anxious about it because it is done to identify and confirm potential abnormal cell growth. Some health care providers request that the person premedicate with a mild analgesic such as ibuprofen prior to undergoing the procedure.

Nursing Management

The nurse's role involves primary prevention by providing education about risk factors and ways to prevent cervical dysplasia. Cervical cancer rates have decreased in Canada because of the widespread use of Pap testing, which can detect precancerous lesions of the cervix before they develop into cancer.

Take Note!

The key points to remember in cervical cancer prevention are smoking cessation, limiting alcohol consumption, and encouraging teens to refrain from early sexual activity.

Gardasil and Cervarix are vaccines approved by Health Canada to protect individuals from HPV and thus prevent cervical cancer. The vaccines prevent infection from four HPV types: HPV 6, 11, 16, and 18. These types are responsible for 70% of cervical cancers and 90% of genital warts (NCI, 2015h). Clinical trials indicate that the vaccine has high efficacy in preventing persistent HPV infection, cervical cancer precursor lesions, vaginal and vulvar cancer precursor lesions, and genital warts (NCI, 2015h). The vaccine is administered by intramuscular injection, and the recommended schedule is a three-dose series with the second and third doses administered 2 and 6 months after the first dose. The recommended age for vaccination is 9 to 26 years (Castle & Schmeler, 2015). The vaccines protect against infection with these types of HPV for 6 to 8 years. It is not known if the protection lasts longer. The vaccines do not protect individuals who are already infected with HPV (NCI, 2015h). However, the vaccine is not a substitute for routine cervical cancer screening, and individuals who have been vaccinated should have Pap smears as recommended.

Focus primary prevention education on the following:
- Identify high-risk behaviours in clients and teach them how to reduce such behaviours:
  - Take steps to prevent STIs.
  - Avoid early sexual activity.
  - Faithfully use barrier methods of contraception.
  - Avoid smoking and drinking.
  - Receive the HPV vaccine.
- Instruct individuals on the importance of screening for cervical cancer by having annual Pap smears. Outline the proper preparation before having a Pap smear (Teaching Guidelines 8.3). Reinforce specific guidelines for screening.

Teaching Guidelines 8.3
STRATEGIES TO OPTIMIZE PAP SMEAR RESULTS
- Schedule your Pap smear appointment about 2 weeks (10 to 18 days) after the first day of your last menses to increase the chance of getting the best sample of cervical cells without menses.
- Refrain from intercourse for 48 hours before the test because additional matter such as sperm can obscure the specimen.
- Do not douche within 48 hours before the test to prevent washing away cervical cells that might be abnormal.
- Do not use tampons, birth control foams, jellies, vaginal creams, or vaginal medications for 72 hours before the test, because they could cover up or obscure the cervical cell sample.
- Cancel your Pap appointment if vaginal bleeding occurs, because the presence of blood cells interferes with visual evaluation of the sample (Schuiling & Likis, 2016).

The identification and treatment of early precancerous lesions is critical to prevention of cervical cancer. Prevention measures should include educating clients that the risk of infection can be reduced by delaying the onset of sexual activity, decreasing the number of sexual partners, using condoms consistently, and never start smoking.

Secondary prevention focuses on reducing or limiting the area of cervical dysplasia. Tertiary prevention focuses on minimizing disability or the spread of cervical cancer. Explain in detail all procedures that might be needed. Encourage the client who has undergone any cervical treatment to allow the pelvic area to rest for approximately 1 month. Discuss this rest period with clients and their partners to gain their cooperation. Outline alternatives to vaginal intercourse, such as cuddling, holding hands, and kissing. Remind clients about any follow-up procedures that are needed and assist them with scheduling if necessary.

Tertiary prevention of cervical cancer involves the diagnosis and treatment of confirmed cases of cancer. Treatment is typically through surgery, radiotherapy, and frequently chemotherapy. Palliative care is provided to clients when the disease has already reached an incurable stage. Knowing that the client and the family have been told about the prognosis, the nurse is in a position to support them when the impact of the diagnosis is realized.

Throughout the process, provide emotional support to the client and family. During the decision-making process, the client may be overwhelmed by the diagnosis and all the information being presented. Refer the client and family to appropriate community resources and support groups as indicated. It is crucial for all persons to be given correct information regarding safe sexual practices, informed about the preventive role of the HPV vaccination, and become educated about the role of the Pap test as a secondary screening measure for cervical cancer. The emotional needs of the person diagnosed with cancer can best be met by a warm, friendly personality, an attitude of empathy rather than sympathy, and skilled communication. Nurses across all settings are in a powerful position to be advocates for safe health care practices through education at personal, community, and national levels.

VAGINAL CANCER

Vaginal cancer is a rare malignant tissue growth arising in the vagina. Only about 1 of every 1,000 individuals will develop vaginal cancer in their lifetime (Duarte-Franco & Franco, 2004). The peak incidence of vaginal cancer occurs at 60 to 65 years of age. The prognosis of vaginal cancer depends largely on the stage of disease and the type of tumour. The overall 5-year survival rate for squamous cell carcinoma is about 42%; that for adenocarcinoma is about 78% (NCI, 2015i). Vaginal cancer can be effectively treated, and when found early it is often curable.

Pathophysiology

The etiology of vaginal cancer has not been identified. Malignant diseases of the vagina are either primary vaginal cancers or metastatic forms from adjacent or distant organs. About 80% of vaginal cancers are metastatic, primarily from the cervix and endometrium. These cancers invade the vagina directly. Cancers from distant sites that metastasize to the vagina through the blood or lymphatic system are typically from the colon, kidneys, skin (melanoma), or breast. Tumours in the vagina commonly occur on the posterior wall and spread to the cervix or vulva (NCI, 2015i).

Squamous cell carcinomas that begin in the epithelial lining of the vagina account for about 85% of vaginal cancers. This type of cancer usually occurs in individuals over the age of 50. The squamous cell carcinomas develop slowly over a period of years, commonly in the upper third of the vagina. They tend to spread early by directly invading the bladder and rectal walls. They also metastasize through blood and lymphatics. The remaining 15% are adenocarcinomas, which differ from squamous cell carcinomas by an increase in pulmonary metastases and supraclavicular and pelvic node involvement (ACS, 2015j).

Therapeutic Management

Treatment of vaginal cancer depends on the type of cells involved and the stage of the disease. If the cancer is localized, radiation, laser surgery, or both may be used. If the cancer has spread, radical surgery might be needed, such as a hysterectomy, or removal of the upper vagina with dissection of the pelvic nodes in addition to radiation therapy.

Nursing Assessment

Begin the history and physical examination by reviewing for risk factors. Although direct risk factors for the initial development of vaginal cancer have not been identified, associated risk factors include advancing age (over 60 years old), previous pelvic radiation, exposure to DES in utero, vaginal trauma, history of genital warts (HPV infection), HIV infection, cervical cancer, chronic vaginal discharge, smoking, and low socioeconomic level (ACS, 2015k).

Question the client about any symptoms. Most individuals with vaginal cancer are asymptomatic. Those with symptoms have painless vaginal bleeding (often after sexual intercourse), abnormal vaginal discharge, dyspareunia, dysuria, constipation, and pelvic pain (NCI, 2015i). During the physical examination, observe for any obvious vaginal discharge or genital warts or changes in the appearance of the vaginal mucosa. Anticipate colposcopy with biopsy of suspicious lesions to confirm the diagnosis.

Nursing Management

Nursing management for this cancer is similar to that for other reproductive cancers, with emphasis on sexuality counselling and referral to local support groups. Clients undergoing radical surgery need intensive counselling about the nature of the surgery, risks, potential complications, changes in physical appearance and physiologic function, and sexuality alterations. Nurses should focus their care on education, pain and symptom management, communication with clients and their families, and coordination of care across of all settings.

VULVAR CANCER

Vulvar cancer is an abnormal neoplastic growth on the external female genitalia including the clitoris, vaginal lips, and opening to the vagina (Fig. 8.5). Vulvar cancer accounts for approximately 5% of all female genital malignancies, and is the fourth most common gynecologic cancer, after endometrial, ovarian, and cervical cancers

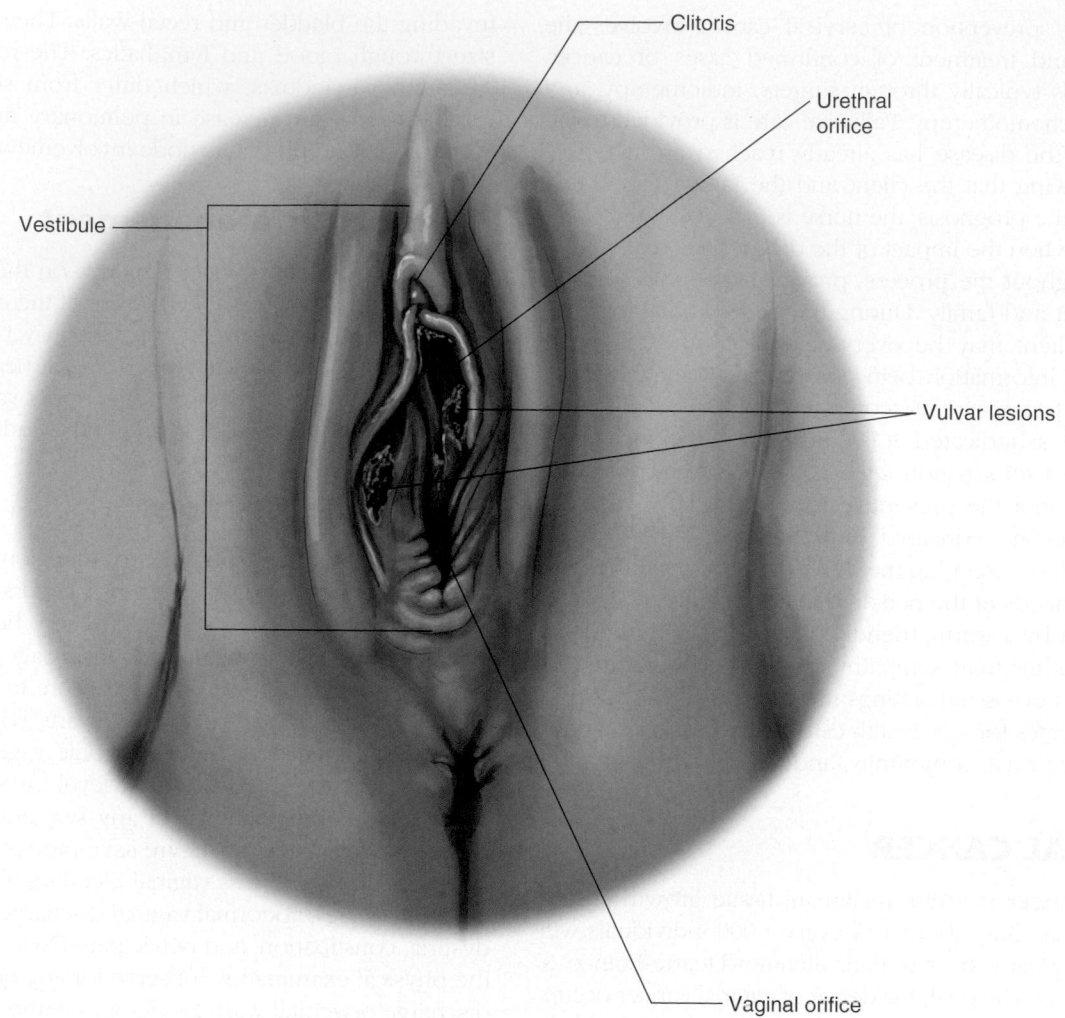

FIGURE 8.5 Vulvar cancer. (The Anatomical Chart Company. [2009]. *Atlas of pathophysiology* [3rd ed.]. Philadelphia, PA: Lippincott Williams & Wilkins.)

(NCI, 2015j). When detected early, it is highly curable. Typically, it can be advanced at diagnosis, though it is a visible cancer. Awareness is essential for early detection of this rare cancer.

Vulvar cancer is found most commonly in older persons in their mid-60s to mid-70s, but the incidence in individuals younger than 35 years old has increased during the past few decades. The overall 5-year survival rate when lymph nodes are not involved is 90%, but it drops to 50% to 70% when the lymph nodes have been invaded (ACS, 2015m).

Pathophysiology

Vulvar cancer can be classified into two groups according to predisposing factors: the first type correlates with a HPV infection and occurs mostly in younger persons. The second group is not HPV-associated and occurs in elderly individuals without cancerous disorders. Approximately 80% of vulvar tumours are squamous

cell carcinomas. This type of cancer forms slowly over several years and is usually preceded by precancerous changes. These precancerous changes are termed vulvar intraepithelial neoplasia (VIN). The two major types of VIN are classic (undifferentiated) and simplex (differentiated). Classic VIN, the more common one, is associated with HPV infection (genital warts due to types 16, 18, 31, 33, 35, 45, and 54) and smoking (Alkatout et al., 2015). It typically occurs in individuals between 30 and 40 years. In contrast to classic VIN, simplex VIN usually occurs in postmenopausal individuals and is not associated with HPV but chronic irritation over time (Cancer. Net, 2015b).

Screening and Diagnosis

Annual vulvar examination is the most effective way to prevent vulvar cancer. Careful inspection of the vulva during routine annual gynecologic examinations remains the most productive diagnostic technique. Liberal use of biopsies of any suspicious vulvar lesion is usually necessary to make the diagnosis and to guide treatment. However, many individuals do not seek health care evaluation for months or years after noticing an abnormal lump or lesion. Leading presenting complaints of clients with vulvar cancer include dyspareunia, long history of pruritus, ulcers on the "outside" genitalia, vulvar swelling, vulvar bleeding, and urinary problems (Alkatout et al., 2015). The diagnosis of vulvar cancer is made by a biopsy of the suspicious lesion, which is usually found on the labia majora.

Take Note!

Vulvar pruritus or a lump is present in the majority of women with vulvar cancer. Lumps should be biopsied even if the person is asymptomatic.

Therapeutic Management

Treatment varies depending on the extent of the disease. Laser surgery, cryosurgery, or electrosurgical incision may be used. Larger lesions may need more extensive surgery and skin grafting. The traditional treatment for vulvar cancer has been radical vulvectomy, but more conservative techniques are being used to improve psychosexual outcomes and less morbidity, without compromising survival (Forner, Dakhil, & Lampe, 2015).

Nursing Assessment

Typically, no single specific clinical symptom heralds this disease, so diagnosis is often delayed significantly. Therefore, it is important to review the client's history for risk factors such as:

- Exposure to HPV type 16
- Age over 50 years
- HIV infection
- VIN
- Lichen sclerosus (a patchy skin disorder)
- Melanoma or atypical moles
- Exposure to HSV type 2
- Multiple sex partners
- Smoking
- Herpes simplex
- History of breast cancer
- Immune suppression
- Hypertension
- Diabetes mellitus
- Obesity (ACS, 2015n)

In most cases, the client reports persistent vulvar itching, burning, and edema that do not improve with the use of creams or ointments. A history of condyloma, gonorrhea, and herpes simplex are some of the factors for greater risk for VIN. Diagnosis of vulvar carcinoma is often delayed. Individuals neglect to seek treatment for an average of 6 months from the onset of symptoms. In addition, a delay in diagnosis often occurs after the client presents to the physician or nurse practitioner. In many cases, a biopsy of the lesion is not performed until the problem fails to respond to numerous topical therapies. During the physical examination, observe for any masses or thickening of the vulvar area. A vulvar lump or mass most often is noted. The vulvar lesion is usually raised and may be fleshy, ulcerated, leukoplakic (looking like white patches), or warty. The cancer can appear anywhere on the vulva, although about three-fourths arise primarily on the labia (Vargo & Beriwal, 2015). Less commonly, the person may present with vulvar bleeding, discharge, dysuria, and pain.

Nursing Management

Persons with vulvar cancer must clearly understand their disease, treatment options, and prognosis. To accomplish this, provide information and establish effective communication with clients and their families. Act as an educator and advocate.

Teach clients about healthy lifestyle behaviours, such as smoking cessation and measures to reduce risk factors. For example, instruct clients how to examine their genital areas, urging them to do so monthly between menstrual periods. Tell them to look for any changes in appearance (e.g., whitened or reddened patches of skin); changes in feel (e.g., areas of the vulva becoming itchy or painful); or the development of lumps, moles (e.g., changes in size, shape, or colour), freckles, cuts, or sores on the vulva. Urge clients to report these changes to their health care provider (ACS, 2015m).

Teach clients about preventive measures such as not wearing tight undergarments and not using perfumes and dyes in the vulvar region. Also educate them about the use of barrier methods of birth control (e.g., condoms) to reduce the risk of contracting HIV, HSV, and HPV. Other prevention measures include delaying first sexual intercourse, avoiding sexual intercourse with multiple partners, not starting smoking or quitting if a smoker already, and getting the HPV vaccine available for individuals between 9 and 26 years.

For clients diagnosed with vulvar cancer, provide information and support. Discuss potential changes in sexuality if radical surgery is performed. Encourage them to communicate openly with their partners. Refer them to appropriate community resources and support groups. All nurses come in contact with persons in their clinical practices who have the potential to become cancer clients, already have suspicious signs or symptoms of cancer, are already undergoing cancer treatment, or are terminal cancer clients. The nurse will be involved with all aspects of cancer, from diagnosis through palliative care. Each nurse has an obligation to keep informed of current developments in the cancer field to function effectively and be able to educate clients and their families.

NURSING CARE PLAN 8.1

Overview of a Person With a Reproductive Tract Cancer

Molly, a thin 28-year-old woman, comes to the free health clinic complaining of a thin, watery vaginal discharge and spotting after sex. Molly says she has had multiple sex partners since the age of 15 years. She had an abnormal Pap smear "a while back" but did not return to the clinic for follow-up. Cervical cancer is suspected.

NURSING DIAGNOSIS: Anxiety related to uncertainty of diagnosis, possible diagnosis of cancer, and eventual outcome as evidenced by client's report of signs and symptoms and statements of being worried and not knowing what she would do

Outcome Identification and Evaluation

The client will demonstrate measures to cope with anxiety *as evidenced by statements acknowledging anxiety, use of positive coping strategies, and verbalization that anxiety has decreased.*

Interventions: *Reducing Anxiety*

- Encourage client to express feelings and concerns *to reduce anxiety and to determine appropriate interventions.*
- Assess the meaning of the diagnosis to the client, clarify misconceptions, and provide reliable, realistic information *to enhance understanding of the condition, subsequently reducing anxiety.*
- Assess client's psychological status *to determine degree of emotional distress related to diagnosis and treatment options.*
- Identify and address verbalized concerns, providing information about what to expect *to decrease uncertainty about the unknown.*

- Assess the client's use of coping mechanisms in the past and their effectiveness *to foster use of positive strategies.*
- Teach client about early signs of anxiety and help the client to recognize them (e.g., fast heartbeat, sweating, or feeling flushed) *to minimize escalation of anxiety.*
- Provide positive reinforcement that the client's condition can be managed *to relieve anxiety.*

NURSING DIAGNOSIS: Deficient knowledge related to diagnosis, prevention strategies, disease course, and treatment as evidenced by client's statements about hoping nothing bad is wrong, lack of follow-up for previous abnormal Pap test, and high-risk behaviours

Outcome Identification and Evaluation

The client will demonstrate an understanding of diagnosis, *as evidenced by making health-promoting lifestyle choices, verbalizing appropriate health care practices, describing condition once diagnosed, and adhering to measures to comply with therapy.*

Interventions: *Providing Client Teaching*

- Assess client's current knowledge about the diagnosis and proposed therapeutic regimen *to establish a baseline from which to develop a teaching plan.*
- Review contributing factors associated with development of reproductive tract cancer, including lifestyle behaviours, *to foster an understanding of the etiology of cervical cancer.*
- Review information about treatments and procedures and recommendations for healthy lifestyle, obtaining feedback frequently *to validate adequate understanding of instructions.*

NURSING CARE PLAN 8.1

Overview of a Person With a Reproductive Tract Cancer (continued)

- Discuss strategies, including using condoms and limiting the number of sexual partners, *to reduce the risk of transmission of STIs,* including HPV, which is associated with cervical cancer.
- Encourage client to obtain prompt treatment of any vaginal or cervical infections *to minimize the risk for cervical cancer.*
- Urge the client to have an annual Pap smear and/or HPV test *to allow screening and early detection.*
- Describe the treatment measures used *to provide client with knowledge of what may be necessary.*
- Provide written material with pictures *to allow for client review and to help her visualize what is occurring in her body.*
- Inform client about available community resources and make appropriate referrals as needed *to provide additional education and support.*
- Document details of teaching and learning *to allow for continuity of care and further education, if needed.*

NURSING DIAGNOSIS: Disturbed body image related to suspected reproductive tract cancer and impact on client's sexuality and sense of self as evidenced by statement of being worried about not being the same

Outcome Identification and Evaluation

The client will verbalize or demonstrate a positive self-esteem in relation to body image as evidenced by positive statements about self, sexuality, and participation in activities with others.

Interventions: *Promoting Healthy Body Image*

- Assess client's use of self-criticism *to determine client's current state of coping and adjustment.*
- Determine if the client's change in body image has contributed to social isolation *to provide a direction for care.*
- Provide opportunities for client to explore her feelings related to issues of sexuality, including past behaviours that may have placed the client at risk, *to minimize feelings of guilt about the condition.*
- Acknowledge the client's feelings about possible changes in the body and sexuality and the illness *to foster trust and allow client to ventilate feelings and concerns.*
- Facilitate contact with other clients with the same type of cancer *to promote sharing of feelings and decrease feelings of isolation.*
- Initiate referrals for counselling and community support groups as necessary *to assist client in gaining a positive self-image.*

KEY CONCEPTS

- In Canada, individuals have a one-in-two lifetime risk of developing cancer, and one out of every four deaths is from cancer; thus, nurses must focus on screening and educating all individuals regardless of risk factors.

- The nurse plays a key role in offering emotional support, determining appropriate sources of support, and helping the person use effective coping strategies when facing a diagnosis of cancer of the reproductive tract. Although reproductive tract cancer is rare during pregnancy, the person's vigilance and routine screenings should continue throughout.

- A person's sexuality and culture are inextricably interwoven, and it is essential that nurses working with clients of various cultures recognize this and remain sensitive to the vast changes that will take place when the diagnosis of cancer is made.

- Ovarian cancer is the eighth most common cancer among women and the fifth most common cause of cancer deaths for women in Canada, accounting for more deaths than any other cancer of the reproductive system.

- Ovarian cancer has been described as the "overlooked disease" or "silent killer" because individuals and health care practitioners often ignore or rationalize early symptoms. It is typically diagnosed in advanced stages.

- Unopposed endogenous and exogenous estrogens, obesity, nulliparity, menopause after the age of 52 years, and diabetes are the major etiologic risk factors associated with the development of endometrial cancer.

- Clients should be informed about risks and symptoms of endometrial cancer at the onset of menopause and strongly encouraged to report any unexpected bleeding or spotting to their health care providers.

- Malignant diseases of the vagina are either primary vaginal cancers or metastatic forms from adjacent or distant organs. Vaginal cancer tumours can be effectively treated and, when found early, are often curable.

- Cervical cancer incidence and mortality rates have decreased noticeably in the past several decades, with most of the reduction attributed to the Pap test, which detects cervical cancer and precancerous lesions.

- The nurse's role involves primary prevention of cervical cancer through client education regarding risk factors and preventive vaccines to avoid cervical dysplasia.

- Diagnosis of about 80% of vaginal cancers is metastatic, primarily from the cervix and endometrium. These cancers invade the vagina directly. Vulvar cancer is often delayed significantly because there is no single specific clinical symptom that heralds it. The most common presentation is persistent vulvar itching that does not improve with the application of creams or ointments.

REFERENCES AND RECOMMENDED READINGS

Agency for Healthcare Research and Quality. (2014). *Cancer screening and treatment in women: Recent findings.*

Retrieved from http://www.ahrq.gov/research/findings/fact-sheets/women/cancerwom/

Alexander, L. L., LaRosa, J. H., Bader, H., & Garfield, S. (2014). *New dimensions in women's health* (6th ed.). Sudbury, MA: Jones & Bartlett.

Alkatout, I., Schubert, M., Garbrecht, N., Weigel, M. T., Jonat, W., Mundhenke, C., & Günther, V. (2015). Vulvar cancer: Epidemiology, clinical presentation, and management options. *International Journal of Women's Health*, 7, 305–313.

Amant, F., Han, S. N., Gziri, M. M., Vandenbroucke, T., Verheecke, M., & Van Calsteren, K. (2015). Management of cancer in pregnancy. *Best Practice & Research Clinical Obstetrics & Gynecology*, 29(5), 741–753.

American Cancer Society (ACS). (2015a). *Key statistics about lung cancer.* Retrieved from http://www.cancer.org/cancer/lungcancer-non-smallcell/detailedguide/non-small-cell-lung-cancer-key-statistics

American Cancer Society (ACS). (2015b). *ACS guidelines for the early detection of cancer.* Retrieved from http://www.cancer.org/healthy/findcancerearly/cancerscreeningguidelines/american-cancer-society-guidelines-for-the-early-detection-of-cancer

American Cancer Society (ACS). (2015c). *Cervical cancer and pregnancy.* Retrieved from http://www.cancer.org/cancer/cervicalcancer/overviewguide/cervical-cancer-overview-treating-pregnancy

American Cancer Society (ACS). (2015d). *What are the key statistics about ovarian cancer?* Retrieved from http://www.cancer.org/cancer/ovariancancer/detailedguide/ovarian-cancer-key-statistics

American Cancer Society (ACS). (2015e). *What are the key statistics about endometrial cancer?* Retrieved from http://www.cancer.org/cancer/endometrialcancer/detailedguide/endometrial-uterine-cancer-key-statistics

American Cancer Society (ACS). (2015f). *Endometrial (uterine) cancer.* Retrieved from http://www.cancer.org/acs/groups/cid/documents/webcontent/003097-pdf.pdf

American Cancer Society (ACS). (2015g). *What are the key statistics about cervical cancer?* Retrieved from http://www.cancer.org/cancer/cervicalcancer/detailedguide/cervical-cancer-key-statistics

American Cancer Society (ACS). (2015h). *Cervical cancer.* Retrieved from http://www.cancer.org/acs/groups/cid/documents/webcontent/003094-pdf.pdf

American Cancer Society (ACS). (2015i). *What are the key statistics about vaginal cancer?* Retrieved from http://www.cancer.org/cancer/vaginalcancer/detailedguide/vaginal-cancer-key-statistics

American Cancer Society (ACS). (2015j). *Vaginal cancer.* Retrieved from http://www.cancer.org/cancer/vaginal-cancer/detailedguide/

American Cancer Society (ACS). (2015k). *What are risk factors for vaginal cancer?* Retrieved from http://www.cancer.org/cancer/vaginalcancer/detailedguide/vaginal-cancer-risk-factors

American Cancer Society (ACS). (2015l). *What are the key statistics about vulvar cancer?* Retrieved from http://www.cancer.org/cancer/vulvarcancer/detailedguide/vulvar-cancer-key-statistics

American Cancer Society (ACS). (2015m). *What is vulvar cancer?* Retrieved from http://www.cancer.org/cancer/vulvar-cancer/detailedguide/vulvar-cancer-what-is-vulvar-cancer

American Cancer Society (ACS). (2015n). *What are the risk factors for vulvar cancer?* Retrieved from http://www.cancer.org/cancer/vulvarcancer/detailedguide/vulvar-cancer-risk-factors

American Cancer Society (ACS). (2015o). *Survival rates for ovarian cancer by stage.* Retrieved from http://www.cancer.org/cancer/ovariancancer/detailedguide/ovarian-cancer-survival-rates

American Cancer Society (ACS). (2016). *Cancer facts & figures 2016.* Retrieved from http://www.cancer.org/research/cancerfactsstatistics/cancerfactsfigures2016/index

American College of Obstetricians and Gynecologists (ACOG). (2015). *The ACOG cervical cancer screening guidelines: Key changes.* Retrieved from https://www.hpv16and18.com/hcp/cervical-cancer-screening-guidelines/acog-guidelines.html

American Society of Cytopathology. (2015). *The Bethesda System for reporting cervical cytology: Definitions, criteria and explanatory notes.* Retrieved from http://www.cytopathology.org/the-bethesda-system-for-reporting-cervical-cytology-definitions-criteria-and-explanatory-notes-3rd-edition/

Andersson, T. M., Johansson, A. L., Fredriksson, I., & Lambe, M. (2015). Cancer during pregnancy and the postpartum period: A population-based study. *Cancer, 121*(12), 2072–2077.

Balk, S. J. (2015). Pediatricians can play role in reducing skin cancer epidemic. *AAP News, 36*(1), 8–9.

Brennan, D. J., Hackethal, A., Mann, K. P., Mutz-Dehbalaie, I., Fiegl, H., Marth, C., & Obermair, A. (2015). Serum HE4 detects recurrent endometrial cancer in patients undergoing routine clinical surveillance. *BMC Cancer, 15*(1), 33–36.

Broadman, C. H., & Matthews, K. J. (2015). Cervical cancer. *eMedicine.* Retrieved from http://emedicine.medscape.com/article/253513-overview

Cameron, B. L., Carmargo Plazas Mdel, P., Salas, A. S., Bourque Bearskin, R. L., & Hungler, K. (2014). Understanding inequalities in access to health care services for Aboriginal people: a call for nursing action. *Advances in Nursing Science, 37*(3), E1–E16.

Canadian Cancer Society's Advisory Committee on Cancer Statistics. (2016). *Canadian Cancer Statistics 2016.* Toronto, ON: Canadian Cancer Society; 2016.

Canadian Cancer Society's Advisory Committee on Cancer Statistics. (2017). *Canadian Cancer Statistics 2017.* Toronto, ON: Canadian Cancer Society. Retrieved from cancer.ca/Canadian-CancerStatistics-2017-EN.pdf. Accessed March 2018.

Canadian Task Force on Preventive Health Care. (2013). Recommendations on screening for cervical cancer. *Canadian Medical Association Journal, 185*(1), 35–45.

CancerCare Manitoba. (2017). *Pap test learning module for health care providers.* Retrieved from http://getcheckedmanitoba.ca/files/x-ptlm.pdf

Cancer in Pregnancy. (2015a). *Endometrial cancer.* Retrieved from http://www.cancerinpregnancy.org/node/103

Cancer in Pregnancy. (2015b). *Cervical cancer.* Retrieved from http://www.cancerinpregnancy.org/node/52

Cancer.Net. (2015a). *Cancer during pregnancy.* Retrieved from http://www.cancer.net/coping/emotional-and-physical-matters/sexual-and-reproductive-health/cancer-during-pregnancy

Cancer.Net. (2015b). *Vulvar cancer.* Retrieved from http://www.cancer.net/cancer-types/vulvar-cancer/risk-factors-and-prevention

Castle, P. E., & Schmeler, K. M. (2015). HPV vaccination: For women of all ages? *The Lancet, 384*(9961), 2178–2180.

Centers for Disease Control and Prevention (CDC). (2015a). *Cancer among women.* Retrieved from http://www.cdc.gov/cancer/dcpc/data/women.htm

Centers for Disease Control and Prevention (CDC). (2015b). *Cancer prevention and control.* Retrieved from http://www.cdc.gov/cancer/dcpc/prevention/other.htm

Centers for Disease Control and Prevention (CDC). (2015c). *Ovarian cancer risk factors.* Retrieved from http://www.cdc.gov/cancer/ovarian/basic_info/risk_factors.htm

Centers for Disease Control and Prevention (CDC). (2015d). *Cervical cancer screening.* Retrieved from http://www.cdc.gov/cancer/cervical/basic_info/screening.htm

Centers for Disease Control and Prevention (CDC). (2015e). *Cervical cancer risk factors.* Retrieved from http://www.cdc.gov/cancer/cervical/basic_info/risk_factors.htm

Cliby, W. A., Powell, M. A., Al-Hammadi, N., Chen, L., Miller, J. P., Roland, P. Y., … Bristow, R. E. (2015). Ovarian cancer in the United States: Contemporary patterns of care associated with improved survival. *Gynecologic Oncology, 136*(1), 11–17.

de Haan, J., Verheecke, M., & Amant, F. (2015). Management of ovarian cysts and cancer in pregnancy. *Facts, Views & Vision in ObGyn, 7*(1), 25–31.

Duarte-Franco, E., & Franco, E. L. (2004). Other gynecologic cancers: Endometrial, ovarian, vulvar and vaginal cancers. *BMC Women's Health, 4*(1), S14.

Dueholm, M., Marinovskij, E., Hansen, E. S., Møller, C., & Ørtoft, G. (2015). Diagnostic methods for fast-track identification of endometrial cancer in women with postmenopausal bleeding and endometrial thickness greater than 5 mm. *Menopause, 22*(6), 1.

Ebell, M. H., Culp, M., Lastinger, K., & Dasigi, T. (2015). A systematic review of the bimanual examination as a test for ovarian cancer. *American Journal of Preventive Medicine, 48*(3), 350–356.

Fontenot, H. B. (2015). Urine-based HPV testing as a method to screen for cervical cancer. *Nursing for Women's Health, 19*, 59–65.

Forner, D. M., Dakhil, R., & Lampe, B. (2015). Quality of life and sexual function after surgery in early stage vulvar cancer. *European Journal of Surgical Oncology (EJSO), 41*(1), 40–45.

Garner, M. J., McGregor, B. A., Murphy, K. M., Koenig, A. L., Dolan, E. D., & Albano, D. (2015). Optimism and depression: A new look at social support as a mediator among women at risk for breast cancer. *Psychooncology, 24*(12), 1708–1713.

Goldstein, C. L., Susman, E., Lockwood, S., Medlin, E. E., & Behbakht, K. (2015). Awareness of symptoms and risk factors of ovarian cancer in a population of women and healthcare providers. *Clinical Journal of Oncology Nursing, 19*(2), 206–212.

Helm, C. W. (2015a). Hyperthermic intraperitoneal chemotherapy for ovarian cancer: Is there a role? *Journal of Gynecologic Oncology, 26*(1), 1–2.

Helm, C. W. (2015b). Ovarian cysts. *eMedicine.* Retrieved from http://emedicine.medscape.com/article/255865-overview

Herrington, C., Coates, P., & Duprex, W. (2015). Viruses and disease: Emerging concepts for prevention, diagnosis and treatment. *Journal of Pathology, 235*(2), 149–152.

International Federation of Gynecology & Obstetrics. (2015). *Endometrial carcinoma staging.* Retrieved from http://www.figo.org/search/node/endometrial+cancer+staging

Kewayosh, A., Marrett, L., Aslam, U., Steiner, R., Lum-Kwong, M. M., Imre, J., & Amartey, A. (2015). Improving health equity for First Nations, Inuit and Métis people: Ontario's Aboriginal Cancer Strategy II. *Law & Governance, 17*(2).

Key, T. (2015). Cancer prevention and treatment. In D. M. Bier, J. Mann, D. H. Alpers, H. E. Vorster, & M. J. Gibney (Eds.). *Nutrition for the primary care provider* (pp. 111, 123–129). Oxford, UK: Karger Publishers.

Kim, R. H., & Chu, Q. D. (2015). Breast cancer during pregnancy. In Q. D. Chu, J. F. Gibbs, & G. B. Zibari (Eds.). *Surgical oncology: A practical and comprehensive approach* (pp. 163–168). New York: Springer Publishers.

King, T. L, Brucker, M. C., Kriebs, J. M., Fahey, J. O., Gegor, C. L., & Varney, H. (2015). *Varney's midwifery* (5th ed.). Burlington, MA: Jones & Bartlett Learning.

Li, Y., Zhao, J., Zhang, Q., & Wang, Y. (2015). Does ovarian stimulation for IVF increase gynecological cancer risk? A systematic review and meta-analysis. *Reproductive BioMedicine Online, 31*(1), 20–29.

Liede, A., Sun, P., & Narod, S. (2015). Effect of breast cancer after ovarian cancer on mortality for BRCA mutation carriers. *JAMA Surgery, 150*(5), 490–491.

Lofters, A. K. (2015). Ethnicity and breast cancer stage at diagnosis: An issue of health equity. *Current Oncology, 22*(2), 80–81.

Matsumoto, K., Onda, T., & Yaegashi, N. (2015). Pharmacotherapy for recurrent ovarian cancer: Current status and future perspectives. *Japanese Journal of Clinical Oncology, 45*(5), 408–410.

Mayo Clinic. (2015). *Cancer prevention: 7 steps to reduce your risk.* Retrieved from http://www.mayoclinic.org/cancer-prevention/art-20044816

Memorial Sloan Kettering Cancer Center. (2015). *Ovarian cancer risk factors.* Retrieved from http://www.mskcc.org/cancer-care/adult/ovarian/risk-factors

Moses, S. (2015). *Endometrial cancer risk factors. Family practice notebook.* Retrieved from http://www.fpnotebook.com/Gyn/HemeOnc/EndmtrlCncrRskFctr.htm

National Cancer Institute (NCI). (2015a). *SEER cancer statistics review.* Retrieved from http://seer.cancer.gov/csr/1975_2010/

National Cancer Institute (NCI). (2015b). *The burden of cancer.* Retrieved from http://www.cancer.gov/cancertopics/pdq/prevention/overview/HealthProfessional

National Cancer Institute (NCI). (2015c). *General cancer prevention.* Retrieved from http://www.cancer.gov/cancertopics/prevention#General+Cancer+Prevention+Information

National Cancer Institute (NCI). (2015d). *General information about ovarian epithelial cancer.* Retrieved from: http://www.cancer.gov/cancertopics/pdq/treatment/ovarianepithelial/healthprofessional

National Cancer Institute (NCI). (2015e). *Stat fact sheets: Endometrial cancer.* Retrieved from http://seer.cancer.gov/statfacts/html/corp.html

National Cancer Institute (NCI). (2015f). *Endometrial cancer.* Retrieved from http://www.cancer.gov/cancertopics/types/endometrial

National Cancer Institute (NCI). (2015g). *Screening and testing to detect cervical cancer.* Retrieved from http://www.cancer.gov/cancertopics/screening/cervical

National Cancer Institute (NCI). (2015h). *Human papillomavirus (HPV) vaccines.* Retrieved from http://www.cancer.gov/cancertopics/factsheet/prevention/HPV-vaccine

National Cancer Institute (NCI). (2015i). *General information about vaginal cancer.* Retrieved from http://www.cancer.gov/cancertopics/pdq/treatment/vaginal/Patient/page1

National Cancer Institute (NCI). (2015j). *General information about vulvar cancer.* Retrieved from http://www.cancer.gov/cancertopics/pdq/treatment/vulvar/HealthProfessional/page1

National Cancer Institute (NCI). (2015k). *Cervical cancer prevention.* Retrieved from http://www.cancer.gov/cancertopics/pdq/prevention/cervical/Patient/page3

National Institutes of Health (NIH). (2015). *Cervical cancer.* Retrieved from http://report.nih.gov/nihfactsheets/viewfactsheet.aspx?csid=76

Navaneelan, T. (2015). Trends in the incidence and mortality of female reproductive system cancers. Health at a Glance, Statistics Canada catalogue no. 82-624-X.

Nick, A. M., Coleman, R. L., Ramirez, P. T., & Sood, A. K. (2015). A framework for a personalized surgical approach to ovarian cancer. *Nature Reviews Clinical Oncology, 12*(4), 239–245.

Poole, E. M., Rice, M. S., Crum, C. P., & Tworoger, S. S. (2015). Salpingectomy as a potential ovarian cancer risk-reducing procedure. *Journal of the National Cancer Institute, 107*(2), dju490.

Sawaya, G. F., Kulasingam, S., Denberg, T., & Qaseem, A. (2015). Cervical cancer screening in average-risk women: Best practice advice from the clinical guidelines committee of the American College of Physicians. *Annals of Internal Medicine, 162*(12), 851–859.

Schmid, D., Behrens, G., Keimling, M., Jochem, C., Ricci, C., & Leitzmann, M. (2015). A systematic review and meta-analysis of physical activity and endometrial cancer risk. *European Journal of Epidemiology, 30*(5), 137–412.

Schuiling, K. D., & Likis, F. E. (2016). *Women's gynecologic health* (3rd ed.). Sudbury, MA: Jones & Bartlett.

Shirvani, H., & Alhani, F. (2015). Challenges nursing role on improving quality of life in women with breast cancer undergoing chemotherapy. *Journal of Clinical Nursing and Midwifery, 3*(4), 1–12.

Siegel, R. L., Miller, K. D., & Jemal, A. (2015). Cancer statistics, 2015. *CA: A Cancer Journal for Clinicians, 65*, 5–29.

Society of Obstetricians and Gynecologists of Canada. (2007). Canadian consensus guidelines on human papillomavirus. *Journal of Obstetrics and Gynaecology Canada, 29*(8). Retrieved from https://sogc.org/wp-content/uploads/2013/01/gui196CPG0708revised_000.pdf

Society of Obstetricians and Gynecologists of Canada, Society of Gynecologic Oncology of Canada, & Society of Canadian Colposcopists. (2013). Position statement: Recommendations on screening for cervical cancer. Retrieved from https://sogc.org/wp-content/uploads/2013/04/medCervicalCancer-ScreeningENG130220.pdf

Statistics Canada. (2018). Table 102–0561—Leading causes of death, total population, by age group and sex, Canada, annual, CANSIM (database). Last updated: February 23, 2018. Retrieved from http://www.statcan.gc.ca/tables-tableaux/sum-som/l01/cst01/hlth36c-eng.htm. Accessed March 21, 2018.

Strohl, A. E., Mendoza, G., Ghant, M. S., Cameron, K. A., Simon, M. A., Schink, J. C., & Marsh, E. E. (2015). Barriers to prevention: Knowledge of HPV, cervical cancer, and HPV vaccinations among African American women. *American Journal of Obstetrics and Gynecology, 212*(1), 65.e1–e5.

Surbone, A. (2015). A review of cultural attitudes about cancer. In K. D. Miller, & M. Simon (Eds.). *Global perspectives on cancer: Incidence, care, and experience [2 volumes]* (pp. 19–37). Santa Barbara, CA: ABC-CLIO Publisher.

Temple, S. V. (2015). Cancers of the reproductive system. In J. K. Itano, J. Brant, F. Conde, & M. Saria (Eds.). *Core curriculum for oncology nursing* (5th ed., pp. 103–116). St. Louis, MO: Elsevier.

U.S. Department of Health and Human Services. (2015). *Healthy People 2020*. Retrieved from http://www.healthypeople.gov/2020/topicsobjectives2020.

U.S. Preventive Services Task Force (USPSTF). (2015). *Screening for ovarian cancer. U.S. Preventive Services Task Force summary of recommendations.* Retrieved from http://www.ahrq.gov/clinic/pocketgd1011/gcp10s2.htm

Vargo, J. A., & Beriwal, S. (2015). Vulvar cancer. In N. Y. Lee, N. Riaz, & J. J. Lu (Eds.). *Target volume delineation for conformal and intensity-modulated radiation therapy* (pp. 349–358). New York: Springer Publishers.

Withrow, D. R., Pole, J. D., Nishri, E. D., Tjepkema, M., & Marrett, L. D. (2017). Cancer survival disparities between First Nation and non-aboriginal adults in Canada: follow-up of the 1991 census mortality cohort. *Cancer Epidemiology and Prevention Biomarkers, 26*(1), 145–151.

Wong, A. S., Lao, T. T., Cheung, C. W., Yeung, S. W., Fan, H. L., Ng, P. S., … Sahota, D. S. (2015). Reappraisal of endometrial thickness for the detection of endometrial cancer in postmenopausal bleeding: A retrospective cohort study. *BJOG: An International Journal of Obstetrics & Gynaecology, 123*(3), 439–446.

World Health Organization. (2015). *Cancer prevention and control.* Retrieved from http://www.who.int/nmh/a5816/en/

Wright, J. D., Chen, L., Tergas, A. I., Patankar, S., Burke, W. M., Hou, J. Y., … Hershman, D. L. (2015). Trends in relative survival for ovarian cancer from 1975 to 2011. *Obstetrics & Gynecology, 125*(6), 1345–1352.

CHAPTER **WORKSHEET**

MULTIPLE CHOICE QUESTIONS

1. When describing ovarian cancer to a local group of people, the nurse states that ovarian cancer often is not diagnosed early because:
   a. The disease progresses very slowly.
   b. The early stages produce very vague symptoms.
   c. The disease usually is diagnosed only at autopsy.
   d. Clients do not follow up on acute pelvic pain.

2. A postmenopausal person reports spotting which has started again. Which of the following would the nurse do?
   a. Instruct the client to keep a menstrual diary for the next few months.
   b. Tell her not to worry, since this a common but not serious event.
   c. Have her start warm-water douches to promote healing.
   d. Anticipate that the doctor will assess her endometrium thickness.

3. Which of the following would the nurse identify as the priority psychosocial need for a person diagnosed with reproductive cancer?
   a. Research findings
   b. Hand-holding
   c. Cheerfulness
   d. Offering of hope

4. When teaching a group of individuals about screening and early detection of cervical cancer, the nurse would include which of the following as most effective?
   a. Fecal occult blood test
   b. CA-125 blood test
   c. Pap smear and HPV test
   d. Sigmoidoscopy

5. After teaching a group of students about reproductive tract cancers, the nursing instructor determines that the teaching was successful when the students identify which of the following as the deadliest type of female reproductive cancer?
   a. Vulvar
   b. Ovarian
   c. Endometrial
   d. Cervical

6. The nurse is attempting to reassure her obese client about the discovery of an ovarian cyst after a pelvic examination. Which of the following statements is true concerning ovarian cysts? They are:
   a. Frequently seen in polycystic kidney disease
   b. Always painful and need to be removed surgically

c. A precursor to ovarian carcinoma
d. Part of a syndrome that includes hypertension and diabetes

7. Which of the following is considered a risk factor for vulvar cancer?
   a. Vitamin B_{12} deficiency
   b. Epstein–Barr virus
   c. Human papillomavirus
   d. Adenovirus

CRITICAL THINKING EXERCISES

1. A 27-year-old sexually active White woman visits the Health Department family planning clinic and requests information about the various available methods of contraception. In taking her history, the nurse learns that she started having sex at age 15 and has had multiple sex partners since then. She smokes two packs of cigarettes daily. Because she has been unemployed for a few months, her health insurance policy has lapsed. She has never previously obtained any gynecologic care.
   a. Based on her history, which risk factors for cervical cancer are present?
   b. What recommendations would you make for her and why?
   c. What are this client's educational needs concerning health maintenance?

2. A 60-year-old nulliparous woman presents to the gynecologic oncology clinic after her health care provider palpated an adnexal mass on her right ovary. In taking her history, the nurse learns that she has experienced mild abdominal bloating and weight loss for the past several months but felt fine otherwise. She was diagnosed with breast cancer 15 years ago and was treated with a lumpectomy and radiation. She has occasionally used talcum powder in her perineal area over the past 20 years. A transvaginal ultrasound reveals a complex mass in the right adnexa. She undergoes a total abdominal hysterectomy and bilateral salpingo-oophorectomy and lymph node biopsy. Pathology confirms a diagnosis of stage III ovarian cancer with abdominal metastasis and positive lymph nodes.
   a. Is this client's profile typical for a person with this diagnosis?
   b. What in her history might have increased her risk for ovarian cancer?
   c. What can the nurse do to increase awareness of this cancer for all individuals?

CHAPTER **WORKSHEET**

STUDY ACTIVITIES

1. During your surgical clinical rotation, interview a client undergoing surgery for a reproductive cancer. Ask the client to recall the symptoms that brought the client to the health care provider. Ask the client what thoughts, feelings, and emotions went through the mind before and after the diagnosis. Finally, ask the client how this experience will change life in the future.

2. Visit an oncology and radiology treatment centre to find out about the various treatment modalities available for reproductive cancers. Contrast the various treatment methods and report your findings to your class.

3. Visit one of the websites listed in the extensive list of websites provided to explore a topic of interest concerning reproductive cancers. How correct and current is the content? What is its level? Share your assessment with your classmates.

4. Taking oral contraceptives provides protection against _____ cancer.

5. Two genes, *BRCA1* and *BRCA2*, are linked with hereditary _____ and _____ cancers.

BRINGING IT ALL TOGETHER: A CASE STUDY

Jill, a 38-year-old obese female with a history of infertility and irregular bleeding, returned to her OB/GYN doctor for a follow-up appointment. She had a D&C the week before to stop a profuse bleeding episode. She is informed by the doctor that her pathology report came back from the D&C showing endometrial adenocarcinoma. She is in shock over the diagnosis at her young age.

ASSESSMENT

The nurse took Jill's history, which included irregular menstrual cycles since her menarche. She has a BMI of 32. She takes medication to manage her diabetes and hypertension. She had been previously diagnosed with polycystic ovary syndrome (PCOS) when she was a teenager. Her pelvic examination demonstrated an enlarged uterus. She had been to see her doctor several times because of her irregular bleeding, but she had been treated with medications until a D&C was done after months of unsuccessful drug therapy.

1. What risk factors for endometrial cancer does Jill have?

2. Is it unusual for a woman of Jill's age to have this diagnosis? Why or why not?

3. What treatment options might Jill need to consider after her diagnosis?

PLAN

Jill's histopathology at the time of surgery was reported as grade III adenocarcinoma with pelvic lymph node involvement. Jill underwent a total hysterectomy with bilateral salpingo-oophorectomy and went through three courses of chemotherapy also.

1. What health promotion instructions can the nurse impart to Jill when she returns for her postoperative office visit?

2. In what ways can the nurse assist Jill during this challenging time?

3. What is the "take-home" message learned from this case study?

9

Violence and Abuse

Learning Objectives

Upon completion of the chapter, you will be able to:

1. Examine the incidence of gender-based violence.

2. Characterize the cycle of violence and appropriate interventions.

3. Evaluate the various myths and facts about violence.

4. Explain how trauma-informed care techniques can improve the health care response to gender-based violence.

5. Analyze the dynamics of rape/sexual assault and sexual abuse.

6. Select the resources available for clients experiencing abuse.

7. Outline the role of the nurse who cares for survivors of abuse.

Dorothy came to the prenatal clinic with a complaint of recurring headaches. She had been in twice this week already, but insisted she be seen today and started to cry. When the nurse called her into the examination room, Dorothy's cell phone rang. She hurried to answer it and told the person on the other end that she was at the store. When the nurse asked if she was afraid at home, Dorothy answered "at times." What cues did the nurse pick up on to ask that question? How frequent is this problem in women?

INTRODUCTION

Imagine if you were subjected to assault, rape, sexual slavery, torture, verbal abuse, mutilation, even murder—all because of your gender. It is rarely acknowledged that violence against women and girls exists on the scale it does. Many of these females are brutalized from cradle to grave simply because of their gender. This abuse is the most pervasive human rights violation in the world today, and yet remains silent to many ears around the globe.

Gender-based violence is a term that encompasses abuse and violence directed toward women, men, or children, because of their gender. Gender-based violence is a major global public health and human rights problem and one that often goes unrecognized and unreported. It is a common source of physical, psychological, and emotional morbidity. It occurs in all countries, irrespective of social, economic, religious, or cultural group. It affects women across race, ethnicity, age, socioeconomic status, religion, sexual orientation, and geographic boundaries. No segments of society are immune from the vestiges of this problem. Due to the unequal power relations between men and women, women are violated either in the family, in the community, or in the country in which they live. The causes are multidimensional and are social, economic, cultural, political, and religious. Pregnancy is a time of unique vulnerability to intimate partner violence (IPV) victimization because of changes in women's physical, social, emotional, and economic needs during pregnancy. Although the true prevalence of violence during pregnancy is unclear, research suggests it is substantial and often continues into the postpartum period. Pregnancy has been recognized as a time when violence in the relationship can escalate and have lethal results. Programs such as *Gender-Based Violence: We All Can Help* or *Violence Evidence Guidance Action* (VEGA) are Canadian programs that promote **trauma-informed care**. Gender-based violence is one of the most rigorous challenges of women's health and well-being; it is a harrowing worldwide public health concern with serious consequences for individuals, families, and societies (Berthold, 2015).

Female-perpetrated violence against male partners receives little attention. Although women are victims of violence more frequently than men, the prevalence of violence among men nonetheless represents a significant public health concern. One out of every four men has experienced rape, physical violence, and/or stalking by an intimate partner, either male or female, in their lifetime (National Coalition Against Domestic Violence, 2015).

Although women can be violent in relationships with men, and also in same-sex partnerships, the overwhelming burden of partner violence is borne by women at the hands of men. The World Health Organization (WHO, 2017) reported that over one third of women, approximately 35%, have experienced rape, physical violence, and/or stalking in their lifetime, and as many as 38% of murders of women are committed by a male intimate partner. In North America, 40% to 60% of murders of women are committed by intimate partners (Federal Bureau of Investigation [FBI], 2015). Of all the strides women have made in societies around the world over the past 100 years, obliterating violence against themselves is not one of them. Violence against women is a growing problem and in many countries is still accepted as part of normal behaviour. Indigenous women face a greater risk of gender-based violence and barriers to accessing health care (Daoud et al., 2012; Public Health Agency of Canada [PHAC], 2016). Brownridge et al. (2017) identified that Indigenous people face a greater risk of experiencing both child maltreatment and IPV. Ongoing work around Truth and Reconciliation for Indigenous people in Canada has highlighted the high incidence of IPV and the associated trauma for women, children, and families (Truth and Reconciliation Commission [TRC], 2015). Initiatives such as the First Nations Health Authority in British Columbia (2017) *Position Statement on Cultural Humility*, and the Canadian Association of Perinatal and Women's Health Nurses (CAPWHN) *Position Statement on Cultural Safety/Humility* (2017) draw attention to ways to work with individuals and communities to change past practices. Nurses have a responsibility to provide culturally sensitive care to this vulnerable population, who have been historically marginalized in Canadian society. See Box 9.1 for effective nursing care for Indigenous survivors.

BOX 9.1

CULTURAL SENSITIVITY FOR INDIGENOUS SURVIVORS

A culturally humble approach to perinatal and women's/two spirit health nursing care includes:
- Providing health care in a way that respects Indigenous people as equal partners in their own care
- Understanding personal biases and developing and maintaining mutually respectful partnerships based on mutual trust through life-long process of self-reflection and self-critique
- Respecting the individual and family in the provision of care and respect for self as a life-long learner in coming to understand another person and community
- Challenging assumptions regarding other people's cultural experiences including the acknowledgement that an individual's culture is integral to identity or relevant to their health care
- Acknowledging that health care professionals can never be "expert" or "competent" in another person's culture or history, but can instead, demonstrate an openness to learning

Adapted from CAPWHN. (2017). *Position Statement on Cultural Safety/Humility*. Ottawa: Author. Retrieved from http://www.capwhn.ca/uploads/documents//CAPWHN_Position_Statement_on_Cultural_Safety_Humility_Final.pdf

Federal funding for the problem is trickling down to local programs, but it is not reaching victims fast enough. In Canada, funding for shelters and transition houses is provided by a combination of government and nonprofit societies. The various types of shelters sought by women experiencing IPV include transition houses, second-stage housing, women's emergency centres, emergency shelters, and safe home networks (Beattie & Hutchins, 2015). In the United States, there are three times more shelters for animals than for battered women (Bouchet & Braswell, 2015). In many cases, a victim escapes her abuser only to be turned away from a local shelter because it is full. The number of abused women is staggering: one woman is being battered every 12 seconds in the United States (Centers for Disease Control & Prevention [CDC], 2017a).

Nurses play a major role in assessing women who have suffered some type of violence. Nurses have a central ethic of caring and an agenda of early intervention and health promotion for their clients to improve their health status and well-being. Often, after a woman is victimized, she will complain about physical ailments that will give her the opportunity to visit a health care setting. A visit to a health care agency is an ideal time for women to be assessed for violence. Because nurses are viewed as trustworthy and sensitive about very personal subjects, women often feel comfortable confiding in them and discussing these issues with them. As a professional nurse, the act of screening women seen in every health care setting is often the first step for a victim to start thinking about a better future. Remember, your words carry weight with your client who looks to you for help, support, and encouragement.

The recent discussion about truth and reconciliation for Indigenous peoples in Canada is an ongoing discussion to address the abuse that many Indigenous people have suffered under colonial rule, which in turn have led to generations of family violence within many Indigenous families and communities (TRC, 2015).

Take Note!

Nurses will come in contact with violence and sexual abuse no matter what health care setting they work in. Nurses must be ready to ask the right questions and to act on the answers, because such action could be lifesaving.

This chapter addresses several types of gender-based violence: IPV, female genital cutting (FGC), human trafficking, and sexual abuse. All of these types of violence against women have devastating and costly consequences for all of society.

INTIMATE PARTNER VIOLENCE

IPV is actual or threatened physical or sexual violence or psychological/emotional abuse. Research suggests

FIGURE 9.1 Intimate partner violence has significant physical, psychological, social, and economic consequences. An important role of the health care provider is to identify abusive or potentially abusive situations as soon as possible and provide support for the victim.

that physical violence in intimate relationships is often accompanied by psychological abuse and in one third to over one half of cases by sexual abuse (CDC, 2017b). Intimate partners include individuals who are currently in dating, cohabitating, or marital relationships, or those who have been in such relationships in the past. Some of the common terms used to describe IPV are domestic abuse, spousal abuse, domestic violence, gender-based violence, and battering. IPV affects a distressingly high percentage of the population and has physical, psychological, social, and economic consequences (Fig. 9.1).

Because a nurse may be the first health care provider to assess and identify the signs of IPV, a nurse can have a profound impact on a woman's decision to seek help. Thus, it is important for nurses to be able to identify abuse and aid the victim. IPV can leave significant psychological scars, and a well-trained nurse can have a positive impact on the victim's mental and emotional health.

Incidence

Overall, lifetime, and 1-year estimates for sexual violence, stalking, and IPV are alarmingly high for adult Americans, with IPV alone affecting more than 12 million people each year. On average, 20 persons per minute are victims of rape, physical violence, or stalking by an intimate partner in the United States. Women are disproportionately affected. The estimated cost of violence in the United States exceeds $70 billion each year. Each year, IPV results in an estimated 2,500 deaths and 3 million injuries among women (CDC, 2014).

Women are at risk for violence at nearly every stage of their lives. Old, young, married, single—no woman is completely safe from the risk of IPV. IPV against women causes more serious injuries and deaths than automobile accidents, rapes, and muggings combined. IPV is expensive. The medical cost of IPV approaches $4.4 trillion each year globally to pay for medical and surgical care, counselling, child care, burden on the justice system, incarceration, attorney fees, and loss of work productivity (Lomborg, 2015).

IPV is pervasive and crosses all boundaries of sexual orientation, race, and class. The intimidation of another person through abusive acts and words is not a gender issue. Violence within these relationships may go unreported for fear of harassment or ridicule. The medical community's efforts to address IPV have often neglected members of the lesbian, gay, bisexual, and transgender (LGBT+) population. Heterosexual women are primarily targeted for IPV screening and intervention despite the similar prevalence of IPV in LGBT+ individuals and its detrimental health effects (Cannon & Buttell, 2015). Perhaps because of the multiple barriers that confront LGBT+ victims of abuse, and the invisibility of the problem in the context of IPV services, the role of the nurse as their advocate is all the more critical.

Little is known about the national prevalence of IPV, sexual violence, and stalking among the LGBT+ community. Research documents that rates of IPV among LGBT+ individuals are equal to or greater than rates observed among heterosexual individuals. Risk factors are also similar to those documented among heterosexual individuals, in addition to help-seeking leaving, and recovery process (Edwards, Sylaska, & Neal, 2015). Current findings also indicate some disparities in perceptions of what constitutes abuse among same and opposite sex couples (Russell & Chapleau, 2015). As individuals and society come to realize same-sex partner violence as an existing problem, there is hope.

Background

Until the mid-1970s, our society tended to legitimize a man's power and control over a woman. The legal and judicial systems considered intervention into family disputes wrong and a violation of the family's right to privacy. IPV was often tolerated and even socially acceptable. Fortunately, attitudes and laws have changed to protect women and punish abusers.

Characteristics of Intimate Partner Violence

Although more research is needed in this area, studies have found certain risk factors for IPV in men. These risk factors can be divided into four different categories: individual factors, relationship factors, community factors, and societal factors. Specific risk factors within each category are listed in Table 9.1.

Generation-to-Generation Continuum of Violence

Violence is a learned behaviour that, without intervention, is self-perpetuating. It is a cyclical health problem.

The long-term effects of violence on victims and children can be profound. Children who witness one parent abuse another are more likely to become delinquents or batterers themselves because they see abuse as an integral part of a close relationship. Thus, an abusive relationship between father and mother can perpetuate future abusive relationships. Violence in childhood and adolescence is linked to the child's perception of the family as a hostile environment and of violence against women as a corrective measure, and insults, swearing, and humiliation by their partner as acceptable (Song, Wenzel, Kim, & Nam, 2017). If one considers violence against children and spouses, the psychological consequences are huge, stemming from the paradox of the victim being abused by a member of the family with whom he or she expects to have a supportive, loving, and respectful relationship. Research has found that children who witness IPV are at risk for developing psychiatric disorders, posttraumatic stress disorder (PTSD), developmental problems, school failure, violence against others, and low self-esteem (Cater, Miller, Howell, & Graham-Bermann, 2015).

Childhood maltreatment is a major health problem that is associated with a wide range of physical conditions and leads to high rates of psychiatric morbidity and social problems in adulthood. Consequences of violence extend far beyond the physical and mental suffering of victims and their families and have an impact on schools, neighbourhoods, businesses, and the legal and health care systems. Women who were physically or sexually abused as children have an increased risk of victimization and fear of crime, poor general health, and in addition experience adverse mental health conditions such as depression, anxiety, and low self-esteem as adults (Barrios et al., 2015).

In many cases when a parent is abused, the children are abused as well. The lifetime economic cost to society due to childhood maltreatment is estimated to be $124 billion dollars (Jackson & Deye, 2015). Young children who live with family violence represent a disempowered group. Developmentally, young children have relatively limited verbal skills and emotional literacy. In addition, the environment becomes one of secrecy and intimidation, as well as reduced emotional availability from the child's main caretaker. Taken together, these factors severely restrict these young children's capacity and opportunity to make their voices and needs heard (Jackson & Deye, 2015). Exposure to violence has a negative impact on children's physical, emotional, and cognitive well-being. The cycle continues into another generation through learned responses and violent acting out. Although there are always exceptions, most children deprived of their basic physical, psychological, and spiritual needs do not develop healthy personalities. They grow up with feelings of fear, behavioural problems, substance abuse, relationship difficulties, inadequacy, anxiety, anger, hostility, guilt, and rage. They often lack

TABLE 9.1   COMMON MYTHS AND FACTS ABOUT VIOLENCE

Myths	Facts
Battering of women occurs only in lower socioeconomic classes.	Violence occurs in all socioeconomic classes.
Substance abuse causes the violence.	Violence is a learned behaviour and can be changed. The presence of drugs and alcohol can make a bad problem worse.
Men have the right to discipline their partners. Battering is not a crime.	In the past, our patriarchal legal system afforded men the right to physically chastise their wives and children; we no longer live under that system. Women and children are no longer considered the property of men, and violence against them is a crime in every state.
Violence occurs to only a small percentage of women.	One in four women will be victims of violence.
Intimate partner violence (IPV) is typically a one-time, isolated occurrence.	IPV is a pattern of coercion and control that one person exerts over another. It is repeated using a number of tactics, including intimidation, threats, physical injury, economic deprivation, isolation, and sexual abuse. The various forms of abuse utilized by batterers help to maintain power and control over their victims.
Women can easily choose to leave an abusive relationship.	Women stay in the abusive relationship because they feel they have no options.
Only men with mental health problems commit violence against women.	Abusers often seem "normal" and do not appear to suffer from personality disorders or other forms of mental illness.
Pregnant women are protected from abuse by their partners.	One in five women is physically abused during pregnancy. The effects of violence on infant outcomes can include preterm delivery, fetal distress, low birth weight, and child abuse.
Women provoke their partners to abuse them.	Women may be willing to blame themselves for someone else's bad behaviour, but nobody deserves to be beaten.
Violent tendencies have gone on for generations and are accepted.	The police, justice system, and society are beginning to make IPV socially unacceptable.
IPV is only a heterosexual issue.	There is as much IPV in the lesbian/gay/bisexual/transgender (LGBT+) population as in heterosexual relationships with the added psychological abuse of "outing" (when one partner threatens to disclose the others sexual preference in an effort to maintain power and control).

Adapted from Domestic Violence Organization. (2015a). *Common myths and why they are wrong*. Retrieved from http://www.domesticviolence.org/common-myths/; Tahoe Safe Alliance. (2017). *Myths about intimate partner violence in the LGBTQUA community*. Retrieved from http://tahoesafealliance.org/for-lgbtqtia/lgbtqiamyths/; and Medicine Net. (2016). *Domestic violence*. Retrieved from http://www.medicinenet.com/domestic_violence/page4.htm#what_are_the_causes_or_risk_factors_for_intimate_partner_violence

coping skills, blame others, demonstrate poor impulse control, have early delinquent behaviour, and generally struggle with authority (Huang, Vikse, Lu, & Yi, 2015). Unless this cycle is broken, more than half become abusers themselves (CDC, 2017d).

The Cycle of Violence

In an abusive relationship, the **cycle of violence** comprises three distinct phases: the tension-building phase, the acute battering phase, and the honeymoon phase (Lawrence, 2015). The cyclical behaviour begins with a time of tension-building arguments, progresses to violence, and settles into a making-up or calm period. This cycle of violence increases in frequency and severity as

it is repeated over and over again. The cycle can cover a long or short period of time. The honeymoon phase gradually shortens and eventually disappears altogether. Abuse in relationships typically becomes accelerated and thus more dangerous over time. The abuser no longer feels the need to apologize and indulge in a honeymoon phase as the woman becomes increasingly disempowered in the relationship.

PHASE 1: TENSION BUILDING

During the first—and usually the longest—phase of the cycle, tension escalates between the couple. Excessive drinking, jealousy, or other factors might lead to name-calling, hostility, and friction. The woman might sense that her partner is reacting to her more negatively, that he is on edge and reacts heatedly to any trivial frustration. A woman often will accept her partner's building anger as legitimately directed toward her. She internalizes what she perceives as her responsibility to keep the situation from exploding. In her mind, if she does her job well, her partner remains calm. But if she fails, the resulting violence is her fault.

PHASE 2: ACUTE BATTERING

The second phase of the cycle is the explosion of violence. The batterer loses control both physically and emotionally. This is when the woman may be assaulted or murdered. After a battering episode, most victims consider themselves lucky that the abuse was not worse, no matter how severe their injuries. They often deny the seriousness of their injuries and refuse to seek medical treatment.

PHASE 3: HONEYMOON

The third phase of the cycle is a period of calm, loving, contrite behaviour on the part of the batterer. He may be genuinely sorry for the pain he caused his partner. He attempts to make up for his brutal behaviour and believes he can control himself and never hurt the woman he loves. The victim wants to believe that her partner really can change. She feels responsible, at least in part, for causing the incident, and she feels responsible for her partner's well-being (Box 9.2).

BOX 9.2

CYCLE OF VIOLENCE (FEMALE SURVIVOR AND MALE ABUSER)

- *Phase 1—Tension building:* Verbal or minor battery occurs. Almost any subject, such as housekeeping or money, may trigger the buildup of tension. There is a breakdown of communication. The victim attempts to calm the abuser. Victim feels like "walking on egg shells" around the abuser.
- *Phase 2—Acute battering:* Characterized by uncontrollable discharge of tension. Violence is rarely triggered by the victim's behaviour: she is battered no matter what her response. The start of the battering episode is unpredictable and beyond the victim's control.
- *Phase 3—Reconciliation (honeymoon)/calm phase:* First, the abuser is ashamed of his behaviour. The batterer tries to minimize the abuse and blame it on the partner. The batterer becomes loving, kind, and apologetic and expresses guilt. Then the abuser works on making the victim feel responsible. This loving behaviour strengthens the bond between partners and will probably convince the victim, once again, that leaving the relationship is not necessary.

Adapted from Domestic Violence Organization. (2015b). Cycle of violence. Retrieved from http://www.domesticviolence.org/cycle-of-violence/; Focht, J & National Center for Health Research. (2018). *The cycle of domestic violence.* Retrieved from http://www.center4research.org/cycle-domestic-violence/

Types of Abuse

Abusers may use whatever it takes to control a situation—from emotional abuse and humiliation to physical assault. Victims often tolerate emotional, physical, financial, and sexual abuse. Many remain in abusive relationships because they believe they deserve the abuse.

Emotional Abuse

Emotional abuse includes:
- Promising, swearing, or threatening to hit the woman
- Forcing the victim to perform degrading or humiliating acts
- Threatening to harm children, pets, or close friends
- Humiliating the woman by name-calling and insults
- Threatening to leave her and the children
- Isolation from family and friends
- Destroying valued possessions
- Controlling the woman's every move

Physical Abuse

Physical abuse includes:
- Hitting or grabbing the woman so hard that it leaves marks
- Throwing things at the woman
- Slapping, spitting at, biting, burning, pushing, choking, or shoving the woman
- Kicking or punching the woman, or slamming her against things
- Attacking the woman with a knife, gun, rope, or electrical cord
- Controlling access to health care for injury

Financial Abuse

Financial abuse includes:
- Preventing the woman from getting a job
- Sabotaging a current job
- Controlling how all money is spent
- Failing to contribute financially

Sexual Abuse

Sexual abuse includes:
- Forcing the woman to have vaginal, oral, or anal intercourse against her will
- Biting the victim's breasts or genitals
- Forcefully inserting objects into the victim's vagina or anus
- Forcing the woman to do something sexual that she finds degrading or humiliating
- Forcing the victim to perform sexual acts on other people or animals

Myths and Facts About Intimate Partner Violence

Table 9.2 lists many of the myths about IPV. Health care providers should take steps to dispel these myths.

Abuse Profiles

Victims

Ironically, victims rarely describe themselves as abused. In battered woman syndrome, the woman has experienced deliberate and repeated physical or sexual assault by an intimate partner. She is terrified and feels trapped, helpless, and alone. She reacts to any expression of anger or threat by avoidance and withdrawal behaviour. Some women believe that the abuse is caused by a personality flaw or inadequacy in themselves (e.g., inability to keep the man happy). These feelings of failure are reinforced and exploited by their partners. After being told repeatedly that they are "bad," some women begin to believe it. Many victims were abused as children and may have poor self-esteem, poor health, PTSD, depression, insomnia, low education achievement, or a history of suicide attempts, injury, or drug and alcohol abuse (Barrios et. al., 2015).

Abusers

Abusers come from all walks of life and often feel insecure, powerless, and helpless, feelings that are not in line with the macho image they would like to project. The abuser expresses his feelings of inadequacy through violence or aggression toward others (Lawson, 2015).

TABLE 9.2 COMMON MYTHS AND FACTS ABOUT SEXUAL ASSAULT

Myths	Facts
Women who are sexually assaulted get over it quickly.	It can take several years to recover emotionally and physically from a sexual assault.
Most victims tell someone about it.	The majority of women never tell anyone about it. In fact, almost two thirds of survivors never report it to the police.
Once the sexual assault is over, a survivor can again feel safe in her life.	The survivor often feels vulnerable, betrayed, and insecure afterward.
If a woman does not want to be sexually assaulted, it cannot happen.	A woman can be forced and overpowered by most men.
Women who feel guilty after having sex then say they were raped.	Few women falsely cry "rape." It is very traumatizing to be a victim.
Victims should report the violence to the police and judicial system.	Only 1% of perpetrators are arrested and convicted. Factoring unreported sexual assaults together with the odds of being arrested and getting a felony conviction, only 6% of assailants will ever spend a day in jail. In other words: 15 of 16 rapists walk free.
Women blame themselves for the sexual assault, believing they did something to provoke it.	Women should never blame themselves for being the victim of someone else's violence.
When it comes to sex, men can be provoked to "a point of no return."	Men are physically able to stop at any point during sexual activity. Rape is not an act of impulsive, uncontrolled passion; it is a premeditated act of violence.
Women who wear tight, short clothes are "asking for it."	No victim invites sexual assault, and what she wears is irrelevant.
Women have rape fantasies and want to be raped.	Reality and fantasy are different. Dreams have nothing to do with the brutal violation of rape.
Only attractive women are sexually assaulted.	Anyone can be sexually assaulted. Children, the elderly, and people with physical and mental disabilities are easy targets for perpetrators because of their vulnerability.
Medication can help women forget about the sexual assault.	Initially medication may help, but counselling is needed.

Adapted from Centers for Disease Control and Prevention [CDC]. (2017e). *Preventing sexual violence.* Retrieved from https://www.cdc.gov/violenceprevention/pdf/SV-Factsheet.pdf; Rape Crisis. (2018). *Myths vs realities.* Retrieved from https://rapecrisis.org.uk/mythsvsrealities.php; Women Against Violence Against Women [WAVAW]. (2015). *Common myths about sexual assault.* Retrieved from http://www.wavaw.ca/wp-content/uploads/2014/05/FactSheet_Myths.pdf; WELLWVU The Student's Center of Health. (2018). *Rape myths.* Retrieved from https://well.wvu.edu/resources/sexual-assault/rape-myths

Violence typically occurs at home and is usually directed toward the man's intimate partner or the children who live there. Abusers refuse to share power and choose violence to control their victims. They often exhibit childlike aggression or antisocial behaviours. They may fail to accept responsibility or blame others for their own problems. They might also have a history of substance abuse problems, trouble with the justice system, few close relationships, being sensitive to criticism, having a tendency to hold grudges, involved in power struggles, emotionally dysregulated, lacking in insight, prone to feeling misunderstood, mistreated, or victimized, mental illness, arrests, troubled relationships, obsessive jealousy, controlling behaviours, generally violent behaviour, erratic employment history, and financial problems (Lawson, 2015).

Intimate Partner Violence During Pregnancy

Many think of pregnancy as a time of celebration and planning for the unborn child's future, but in a troubled relationship it can be a time of escalating violence. The strongest predictor of abuse during pregnancy is prior abuse. Violence against pregnant women seems to be more prevalent than diseases routinely investigated during prenatal care, such as preeclampsia and diabetes (Lévesque & Chamberland, 2016). For women who have been abused before, beatings and violence during pregnancy are likely to continue.

Women are at a higher risk for violence during pregnancy. Recent research findings indicate that having children does not protect women from IPV. On the contrary, the IPV appears to last longer if women have children, and this also seems to be the case even after the partnership has come to an end (Mauri, Nespoli, Persico, & Zobbi, 2015). Pregnant women are vulnerable during this time, and abusers can take advantage of it. An estimated 325,000 pregnant women are abused by their partners each year (CDC, 2017a). Abuse during pregnancy poses special risks and dynamics. Various factors may lead to battering during pregnancy, including:

- Inability of the couple to cope with the stressors of pregnancy
- Young age at time of pregnancy
- Having less than a high school education for both partners
- Unemployment for either or both in partnership
- Violence in the family of origin
- Cohabitation and single marital status
- Sexual proprietariness on the part of the male partner
- Heavy drinking by partner
- Resentment toward the interference of the growing fetus and change in the woman's shape
- Doubts about paternity or the expectant woman's fidelity during pregnancy

- Perception that the baby will be a competitor
- Outside attention the pregnancy brings to the woman
- Unwanted pregnancy
- The woman's new interest in herself and her unborn baby
- Insecurity and jealousy about the pregnancy and the responsibilities it brings
- Financial burden related to expense of pregnancy and loss of income
- Stress of role transition from adult man to becoming the father of a child
- Physical and emotional changes of pregnancy that make the woman vulnerable
- Previous isolation from family and friends that limit the couple's support system

Abuse during pregnancy threatens the well-being of the mother and fetus. Physical violence may involve injuries to the head, face, neck, thorax, breasts, and abdomen. The mental health consequences are also significant. Several studies have confirmed the relationship between abuse and poor mental health, especially depression and PTSD; poor quality of life; increased distress, fearfulness, anxiousness, and stressfulness; and increased use of tobacco, alcohol, and/or illicit drugs (Lawson, 2015). For the pregnant woman, many of these conditions most often manifest during the postpartum period.

 Take Note!

Frequently the fear of harm to her unborn child will motivate a woman to escape an abusive relationship.

Women assaulted during pregnancy are at risk for:
- Injuries to themselves and the fetus
- Depression
- Panic disorder
- Fetal and maternal deaths
- Chronic anxiety
- Miscarriage
- Stillbirth
- Poor nutrition
- Insomnia
- Placental abruption
- Uterine rupture
- Excessive weight gain or loss
- Smoking and substance abuse
- Delayed or no prenatal care
- Preterm labour
- Higher rate of surgical births
- Chorioamnionitis
- Vaginitis
- Sexually transmitted infections (STIs)
- Urinary tract infections
- Premature and low–birth-weight infants (Association of Women's Health, Obstetric and Neonatal Nurses [AWHONN], 2015)

EVIDENCE-BASED PRACTICE 9.1

EFFECTIVENESS OF HOME VISITING IN REDUCING PARTNER VIOLENCE FOR FAMILIES EXPERIENCING ABUSE: A SYSTEMATIC REVIEW

STUDY

Intimate partner violence against women is a major, global societal problem with tremendous health consequences both for mother and child. Home-visiting interventions by nurses for families at risk of abuse seem promising in decreasing IVP. In this systematic review the effectiveness of home visiting was assessed as an intervention to reduce IPV experienced by mothers.

Findings

A systematic review was conducted of 1,258 articles; 19 of them met the inclusion criteria and were examined in detail. Sixteen reported lower rates of physical assault with home visits by nurses and three studies showed no significant reduction of IPV. This systematic review found that home-visiting interventions that support abused women

during their pregnancy and beyond to stop IPV seem to be effective in reducing the incidence of IPV. However, it is not known whether these results are effective long term.

Nursing Implications

By nurses making home visits, a trusting relationship can be established between the client and nurse. By addressing factors that may increase the risk of IPV in general, such as stress as well as other contributing factors, IPV can be reduced and the cycle of violence can be broken. A major benefit of home-visiting interventions is that they succeed in reaching high-risk young pregnant women, who are notoriously hard to reach for regular prenatal services during a vulnerable stage in their lives. Nurses can see the home environment and can detect risk factors and plan interventions to address them.

Adapted from Prosman, G. J., Lo Fo Wong, S. H., van der Wouden, J. C., & Lagro-Janssen, A. L. (2015). Effectiveness of home visiting in reducing partner violence for families experiencing abuse: A systematic review. *Family Practice, 32*, 247–256.

Signs of abuse can emerge during pregnancy and may include poor attendance at prenatal visits, unrealistic fears, weight fluctuations, difficulty with pelvic examinations, and nonadherence to treatment. See Evidence-Based Practice 9.1 for an intervention utilized for pregnant women experiencing IPV.

Uncovering abuse in pregnant women requires a consistent and direct approach to every client by the nurse. Multiple assessments may enhance reporting by enabling the nurse to establish trust and rapport with the woman and identify changes in her behaviour. Once abuse is discovered in a pregnant woman, interventions should include safety assessment, emotional support, counselling, referral to community services, and ongoing prenatal care to avoid adverse health outcomes (Hewitt, 2015).

Violence Against Older Women

IPV affects women of all ages, but often the literature focuses on women in the childbearing years, ignoring the problems of aging women who experience abuse. Elder mistreatment (i.e., abuse and neglect) is defined as intentional actions that cause harm or create a serious risk of harm to a vulnerable elder by a caregiver or other person who stands in a trust relationship to the elder. It is estimated that 1 in 10 older adults experience abuse, but only 1 in 5 to as little as 1 in 24 are reported. Research suggests that female elders are abused at a higher rate than males and that the older one is, the more likely one is to be abused. Elder abuse is expected to increase as the population ages (Wang, Brisbin, Loo, & Straus, 2015).

Types of abuse experienced by the older woman may include physical abuse, neglect, emotional abuse, sexual abuse, and financial/exploitation abuse (National Center on Elder Abuse, 2017).

Although an injury may bring the older woman into the health care system, the physical and emotional sequelae of IPV may be subtler and may include depression, insomnia, chronic pain, difficulty trusting others, low self-esteem, thoughts of suicide, substance abuse, anger issues, atypical chest pain, or other kinds of somatic symptoms. Research suggests that older women usually have endured long-term abuse, have developed unhealthy strategies to cope (substance abuse, keeping the family together at all cost, and physical/mental health consequences), and shoulder blame from their adult children, yet have developed empowerment from within to be able to cope with the abuse (Policastro & Finn, 2017).

Accurate detection and assessment of abuse in older women are essential duties of all nurses. Nurses have frequent contact with older victims of abuse, providing them the opportunity to play a significant role in detecting, reporting, and intervening in such cases. As part of a thorough screening, nurses should determine what the client has done to attempt to resolve the abuse and the effectiveness of those strategies. Actions taken by the client, prior to revealing her abuse issue to the nurse, might have included passive acceptance, calling law enforcement, counselling, or other measures. In addition, taking time to establish rapport with older women builds a sense of trust, safety, and openness. Nurses must listen carefully and nonjudgmentally. Judging or criticizing the victim for her decisions might lead to the impression that she deserves the abuse or that she is to blame. Finally, nurses should attempt to stay current in their knowledge of referral resources to assist the older woman experiencing abuse. Some of these resources may be housing, transportation, medical services, employment, social services, and local support groups. A coordinated and comprehensive response to IPV is essential to reduce its sequelae.

Nursing Management of Intimate Partner Violence Survivors

Nurses encounter thousands of abuse survivors each year in their practice settings, but many survivors slip through the cracks. As universal violence assessment has increased in recent years, nurses need to be aware of not only how to screen for violence, but how to respond in a way that is helpful, sincere, nonjudgmental, and legally adequate. This will require nurses to move beyond a description of violence toward a response that is action oriented and evidence based, which includes safety planning and referrals. There are many things that nurses can do to help survivors. Early recognition and intervention can significantly reduce the morbidity and mortality associated with IPV. To stop the cycle of violence, nurses need to know how to assess for and identify IPV and implement appropriate actions.

Assessment

Routine screening for IPV is the first way to detect abuse. The nurse should build rapport by listening, showing an interest in the concerns of the woman, and creating an atmosphere of openness. Communicating support through a nonjudgmental attitude and telling the woman that no one deserves to be abused are first steps toward establishing trust and rapport. Rather than overlooking abused women as "chronic complainers," astute nurses need to be vigilant for subtle clues of abuse. Learning how to assess for abuse is critical. Some basic assessment guidelines follow.

SCREEN FOR ABUSE DURING EVERY HEALTH CARE VISIT

Screening for violence takes only a few minutes and can have an enormously positive effect on the outcome for the abused woman. Any woman could be a victim; no single sign marks a woman as an abuse victim, but the following clues may be helpful:

- Injuries: bruises on their chest and abdomen, scars from blunt trauma, minor lacerations or weapon wounds on the face, head, and neck
- Injury sequelae: headaches, hearing loss from ruptured ear drums, joint pain, sinus infections, teeth marks, clumps of hair missing, dental trauma, pelvic pain, breast or genital injuries

- Reported history of injury that is not consistent with the actual presenting problem
- Mental health problems: depression, anxiety, substance abuse, eating disorders, suicidal ideation or suicide attempts, anger toward health care provider, PTSD
- Frequent tranquilizer or sedative use
- Delay in seeking medical attention and patterns of repeated injury
- Bruises to the upper arm, neck and face, abdomen, or breasts
- Comments about emotional or physical abuse of "a friend"
- STIs or pelvic inflammatory disease
- Appears nervous, ashamed, or evasive when asked questions
- Frequent health care visits for chronic, stress-related disorders such as chest pain, headaches, back or pelvic pain, insomnia, injuries, anxiety, and gastrointestinal disturbances
- Partner's behaviour at the health care visit: appears overly solicitous or overprotective, is unwilling to leave her alone with the health care provider, answers questions for her, and attempts to control the situation (Ghandour, Campbell, & Lloyd, 2015)

Dorothy, who you met at the beginning of the chapter, has been frequenting the clinic with vague somatic complaints in recent weeks and admits she is sometimes afraid at home. She tells the nurse her partner doesn't want her to work, although he is only sporadically employed at low-paying jobs. What cues in her assessment might indicate abuse? What physical signs might the nurse observe?

ISOLATE CLIENT IMMEDIATELY FROM FAMILY

If abuse is detected, immediately isolate the woman to provide privacy and to prevent potential retaliation from the abuser. Asking about abuse in front of the perpetrator may trigger an abusive episode during the interview or at home. Ways to ensure the woman's safety would be to take the victim to an area away from the abuser to ask questions. The assessment can take place anywhere that is private and away from the abuser, for example, x-ray area, ultrasound room, elevator, private bathroom, or laboratory.

If abuse is detected, the nurse can do the following to enhance the nurse–client relationship:
- Educate the woman about the connection between the violence and her symptoms.
- Help the woman acknowledge what has happened to her and begin to deal with the situation.
- Offer her referrals so she can get the help that will allow her to begin to heal.

Dorothy returns to the prenatal clinic a month later with anemia, inadequate weight gain, bruises on her face and neck, and second-trimester bleeding. This time she is accompanied by her partner, who stays close to Dorothy. What questions should the nurse ask to assess the situation? Where is the appropriate location to ask these questions? What legal responsibilities does the nurse have concerning her observations?

ASK DIRECT OR INDIRECT QUESTIONS ABOUT ABUSE

Violence against women is often unseen, unknown, and hidden in families. Questions to screen for abuse should be routine and handled just like any other question. Many nurses feel uncomfortable asking questions of this nature, but broaching the subject is important even if the answer comes later. Opening up the possibility for women to express themselves about their experience of abuse to a nurse sends out a clear message that violence should never be tolerated and not kept hidden; it also conveys the message that nurses care about women's experiences and want to offer a best practice initial response. Just knowing that someone else knows about the abuse offers a victim some relief and may help her disclose it.

Ask difficult questions in an empathetic and non-threatening manner and remain nonjudgmental in all responses and interactions. Choose the type of question that makes you most comfortable. Direct and indirect questions produce the same results. "Does your partner hit you?" or "Have you ever been or are you now in an abusive relationship?" are direct questions. If that approach feels uncomfortable, try indirect questions: "We see many women with injuries or complaints like yours and often they are being abused. Is that what is happening to you?" or "Many women in our community experience abuse from their partners. Is anything like that happening in your life?" With either approach, nurses need to maintain a nonjudgmental acceptance of whatever answers the woman offers. The SAVE Model is a screening protocol that nurses can use when assessing women for violence (Box 9.3).

ASSESS IMMEDIATE SAFETY

It is essential to assist the woman by assessing her safety and the safety of her children. To do this, speak to the woman alone and ask her:

- Does she feel safe going home after her meeting with you?
- Does she need an immediate place of safety for herself or her children?
- Does she have a plan of escape if she becomes at risk for her safety?

BOX 9.3

SAVE MODEL

Screen all of your clients for violence by asking:

- Within the last year, have you been physically hurt by someone?
- Do you feel you are in control of your life?
- Within the last year, has anyone forced you to engage in sexual activities?
- Can you talk about your abuse with me now?
- In general, how would you describe your present relationship?

Ask direct questions in a nonjudgmental way:

- Begin by normalizing the topic to the woman.
- Make continuous eye contact with the woman.
- Stay calm; avoid emotional reactions to what she tells you.
- Never blame the woman, even if she blames herself.
- Do not dismiss or minimize what she tells you, even if she does.
- Wait for each answer patiently. Do not rush to the next question.
- Do not use formal, technical, or medical language.
- Avoid using leading questions; be direct and to the point.
- Use a nonthreatening, accepting approach.

Validate the client by telling her:

- You believe her story.
- You do not blame her for what happened.
- It is brave of her to tell you this.
- Help is available for her.
- Talking with you is a hopeful sign and a first big step.

Evaluate, educate, and refer this client by asking her:

- What type of violence was it?
- Is she now in any danger?
- How is she feeling now?
- Does she know that there are consequences to violence?
- Is she aware of community resources available to help her?

Adapted from U.S. Department of Health and Human Services (USDHHS). (2015c). Screening for domestic violence in health care settings. *Office of the Assistant Secretary for Planning and Evaluation.* Retrieved from http://aspe.hhs.gov/hsp/13/dv/pb_screeningdomestic.cfm; Association of Women's Health, Obstetric and Neonatal Nurses (AWHONN). (2015). Intimate partner violence. *Journal of Obstetric, Gynecologic, and Neonatal Nursing, 44*(3), 405–408; and Canadian Domestic Homicide Prevention Initiative. (2015). Domestic violence risk assessment: Informing safety planning & risk management brief. Retrieved from http://cdhpi.ca/domestic-violence-risk-assessment-informing-safety-planning-risk-management-brief

---

- Does she need to consider an alternative exit from this building?
- Who are the people she could contact for help or support?

BOX 9.4

DANGER ASSESSMENT TOOL

Several risk factors have been associated with increased risk of homicides (murders) of women and men in violent relationships. No one can predict what will happen in your case, but we would like you to be aware of the danger of homicide in situations of abuse and for you to see how many of the risk factors apply to your situation. ("He" refers to your husband, partner, ex-husband, ex-partner, or whoever is currently physically hurting you.)

_____1. Has the physical violence increased in severity or frequency over the past year?

_____2. Does he own a gun?

_____3. Have you left him after living together during the past year?

_____4. Is he unemployed?

_____5. Has he ever used a weapon against you or threatened you with a lethal weapon?

_____6. Does he threaten to kill you?

_____7. Has he avoided being arrested for domestic violence?

_____8. Do you have a child that is not his?

_____9. Has he ever forced you to have sex when you did not wish to do so?

_____10. Does he ever try to choke you?

_____11. Does he use illegal drugs? By drugs, I mean "uppers" or amphetamines, "meth," speed, angel dust, cocaine, "crack," street drugs, or mixtures.

_____12. Is he an alcoholic or problem drinker?

_____13. Does he control most or all of your daily activities? For instance: does he tell you who you can be friends with, when you can see your family, how much money you can use, or when you can take the car?

_____14. Is he violently and constantly jealous of you? (For instance, does he say "If I can't have you, no one can.")

_____15. Have you ever been beaten by him while you were pregnant?

_____16. Has he ever threatened or tried to commit suicide?

_____17. Does he threaten to harm your children?

_____18. Do you believe he is capable of killing you?

_____19. Does he follow or spy on you, leave threatening notes or messages on answering machine, destroy your property, or call you when you don't want him to?

_____20. Have you ever threatened or tried to commit suicide?

_____ Total "Yes" Answers

Thank you. Please talk to your nurse, advocate, or counsellor about what the Danger Assessment means in terms of your situation.

Source: March of Dimes Danger Assessment questionnaire. (From Campbell, J. C. [1986]. Nursing assessment for risk of homicide with battered women. _Advances in Nursing Science, 8_[4], 36–51.) Reprinted with permission from Jacquelyn C. Campbell, Ph.D., R.N. Copyright © 2003; update 2018; www.dangerassessment.com.

The Danger Assessment Tool (Box 9.4) helps women and health care providers assess the potential for homicidal behaviour in an ongoing abusive relationship. It is based on research that showed several risk factors for abuse-related murders:

- Increased frequency or severity of abuse
- Presence of firearms
- Sexual abuse
- Substance abuse
- Precipitated by arguments and conflicts
- Generally violent behaviour outside of the home
- Control issues (e.g., daily chores, friends, job, money)
- Physical abuse during pregnancy
- Suicide threats or attempts (victim or abuser)
- Child abuse (Sugg, 2015)

DOCUMENT AND REPORT YOUR FINDINGS

If the interview reveals a history of abuse, accurate documentation is critical because this evidence may support the woman's case in court. Documentation must include details about the frequency and severity of abuse; the location, extent, and outcome of injuries; and any treatments or interventions. When documenting, use direct quotes and be very specific: "He choked me." Describe any visible injuries and use a body map (outline of a woman's body) to show where the injuries are. Obtain photos (with informed consent) or document if the woman declines photos. Pictures or diagrams can be worth a thousand words. Figure 9.2 shows a sample documentation form for IPV.

Domestic Violence Screening/Documentation Form

DV Screen
☐ DV + (Positive)
☐ DV? (Suspected)

Date _____ Patient ID# _____

Patient Name _____

Provider Name _____

Patient Pregnant? ☐ Yes   ☐ No

Assess Patient Safety

☐ Yes   ☐ No   Is abuser here now?

☐ Yes   ☐ No   Is patient afraid of their partner?

☐ Yes   ☐ No   Is patient afraid to go home?

☐ Yes   ☐ No   Has physical violence increased in severity?

☐ Yes   ☐ No   Has partner physically abused children?

☐ Yes   ☐ No   Have children witnessed violence in the home?

☐ Yes   ☐ No   Threats of homicide?

By whom?_____

☐ Yes   ☐ No   Threats of suicide?

By whom?_____

☐ Yes   ☐ No   Is there a gun in the home?

☐ Yes   ☐ No   Alcohol or substance abuse?

☐ Yes   ☐ No   Was safety plan discussed?

Referrals

☐ Hotline number given

☐ Legal referral made

☐ Shelter number given

☐ In-house referral made

Describe:_____

☐ Other referral made

Describe:_____

Reporting

☐ Law enforcement report made

☐ Child Protective Services report made

☐ Adult Protective Services report made

Photographs

☐ Yes   ☐ No   Consent to be photographed?

☐ Yes   ☐ No   Photographs taken?

Attach photographs and consent form

FIGURE 9.2 Intimate partner violence documentation form. (Reprinted from Cassidy K. How to assess and intervene in domestic violence situations. *Home Healthcare Nurse, 17,* 644–672, Copyright 1999, with permission from Lippincott Williams & Wilkins.)

Laws require health care providers to alert the police to any injuries that involve knives, firearms, or other deadly weapons or that present life-threatening emergencies. If assessment reveals suspicion or actual indication of abuse, nurses can explain to the woman that they are required by law to report it.

Nursing Diagnosis

When violence is suspected or validated, the nurse needs to formulate nursing diagnoses based on the completed assessment. Possible nursing diagnoses related to violence against women might include the following:

- Deficient knowledge related to understanding the cycle of violence and availability of resources
- Anxiety related to threat to self-concept, situational crisis of abuse
- Situational low self-esteem related to negative family interactions
- Powerlessness related to lifestyle of helplessness
- Compromised family coping related to abusive patterns

Interventions

The response of nurses to battered women can have a profound effect on their willingness to open up or seek help. Some responses to assist successful communication in these circumstances could include:

- Listening—"I hear and understand what you are saying." Being listened to can be an empowering experience for a woman who has been abused.
- Communicating belief—"That must have been very frightening for you."
- Validating the decision to disclose—"It must have been difficult for you to talk about this today."
- Emphasizing the unacceptability of this violence—"You don't deserve to be treated this way."

If abuse is identified, nurses can undertake interventions that can increase the woman's safety and improve her health. The goal of intervention is to enable the victim to gain control of her life. Provide sensitive, predictable care in an acceptable setting. Offer step-by-step explanations of procedures. Provide educational materials about violence. Allow the victim to actively participate in her care and have control over all health care decisions. Pace your nursing interventions and allow the woman to take the lead. Communicate support through a nonjudgmental attitude. Carefully document all of your assessment findings and nursing interventions.

Take Note!

Although it is certainly important that the woman in an abusive situation is safe, it is most important for a woman to regain a sense of control in her life. A lack of control is what prevents a woman from escaping an abusive situation.

A public health approach to violence prevention requires input from and coordination across sectors, including health, education, social services, justice, and policy. The goal of public health is to improve the health of the entire community or society. Depending on when in the cycle of violence the nurse encounters the abused woman, goals may fall into three groups:

- *Primary prevention:* aimed at breaking the abuse cycle through community educational initiatives by nurses, physicians and nurse practitioners, law enforcement, teachers, and clergy
- *Secondary prevention:* focuses on screening high-risk individuals and dealing with victims and abusers in early stages, with the goal of preventing progression of abuse
- *Tertiary prevention:* activities are geared toward helping severely abused women and children recover and become productive members of society and rehabilitating abusers to stop the cycle of violence. These activities are typically long term and expensive.

A modified tool developed by Holtz and Furniss (1993)—the ABCDES—provides a framework for providing sensitive nursing interventions to abused women (Box 9.5). Specific nursing interventions for the abused woman include educating her about community services, providing emotional support, and offering a safety plan.

EDUCATE THE WOMAN ABOUT COMMUNITY SERVICES

A wide range of support services are available to meet the needs of victims of violence. Nurses should be prepared to help the woman take advantage of these opportunities. Services will vary by community but might include psychological counselling, legal advice, social services, crisis services, support groups, hotlines, housing, vocational training, and other community-based referrals.

Give the woman information about shelters or services even if she initially rejects it. The PHAC maintains a list of family violence supports and services in each province and territory (PHAC, 2015). ShelterSafe.ca is another national resource listing shelters available to women across the country.

PROVIDE EMOTIONAL SUPPORT

Providing reassurance and support to a victim of abuse is essential if the violence is to end. The physical, psychological, and emotional effects of IPV on women and their children can be severe and long lasting. Nurses in all clinical settings can help victims to feel a sense of personal power and provide them with a safe and supportive environment. Appropriate action can help victims to express their thoughts and feelings in constructive ways, manage stress, and move on with their lives. Appropriate interventions are:

BOX 9.5

THE ABCDES OF CARING FOR ABUSED WOMEN

- **A** is reassuring the woman that she is not alone. The isolation by her abuser keeps her from knowing that others are in the same situation and that health care providers can help her.
- **B** is expressing the belief that violence against women is not acceptable in any situation and that it is not her fault. Demonstrate by your actions and words that you believe her disclosure.
- **C** is confidentiality, since the woman might believe that if the abuse is reported, the abuser will retaliate. Interview her in private, without her partner or family members being present. Assure her that you will not release her information without her permission.
- **D** is documentation, which includes the following:
  - A clear quoted statement about the abuse in the woman's own words.
  - Accurate descriptions of injuries and the history of them.
  - Information on the first, the worst, and the most recent abusive incident.
  - Photos of the injuries (with the woman's consent).
- **E** is education about the cycle of violence and that it will escalate:
  - Educate about abuse and its health effects.
  - Help her to understand that she is not alone.
  - Offer appropriate community support and referrals.
  - Display posters and brochures to foster awareness of this public health problem.
- **S** is safety, the most important aspect of the intervention, to ensure that the woman has resources and a plan of action to carry out when she decides to leave.

Adapted from Centers for Disease Control & Prevention (CDC). (2017a). Preventing intimate partner violence. Retrieved from https://www.cdc.gov/violenceprevention/pdf/ipv-factsheet.pdf; Ghandour, R. M., Campbell, J. C., & Lloyd, J. (2015). Screening and counseling for intimate partner violence: A vision for the future. *Journal of Women's Health, 24*(1), 57–61.

- Strengthen the woman's sense of control over her life by:
  - Teach coping strategies to manage her stress
  - Assist with activities of daily living to improve her lifestyle
  - Allow her to make as many decisions as she can
  - Educate her about the symptoms of PTSD and their basis
- Encourage the woman to establish realistic goals for herself by:
  - Teaching problem-solving skills
  - Encouraging social activities to connect with other people
- Providing support and allow the woman to grieve for her losses by:
  - Listening to and clarifying her reactions to the traumatic event
  - Discussing shock, disbelief, anger, depression, and acceptance

- Explain to the woman that:
  - Abuse is never OK. She didn't ask for it and she doesn't deserve it
  - She is not alone and help is available
  - Abuse is a crime and she is a victim
  - Alcohol, drugs, money problems, depression, or jealousy does not cause violence, but these things can give the abuser an excuse for losing control and abusing her
  - The actions of the abuser are not her fault
  - Her history of abuse is believed
  - Making a decision to leave an abusive relationship can be very hard and takes time

OFFER A SAFETY PLAN

The choice to leave must rest with the woman. Nurses cannot choose a life for the woman; they can only offer choices. Leaving is a process, not an event. Women may try to leave their abusers as many as seven or eight times before succeeding. Frequently, the final attempt to leave may result in the death of the victim. Women planning to leave an abusive relationship should have a safety plan, if possible (Teaching Guidelines 9.1).

Teaching Guidelines 9.1

SAFETY PLAN FOR LEAVING AN ABUSIVE RELATIONSHIP

- When leaving an abusive relationship, take the following items:
  - Driver's license or photo ID
  - Social insurance number
  - Birth certificates for you and your children
  - Phone numbers for social services or women's shelter
  - The deed or lease to your home or apartment
  - Any court papers or orders
  - A change of clothing for you and your children
  - Pay stubs, chequebook, credit cards, and cash
  - Provincial health care cards
  - If you need to leave a domestic violence situation immediately, turn to authorities for assistance in gathering this material
- Develop a "game plan" for leaving and rehearse it

Adapted from Burnett, L. B. (2018). Domestic violence. *eMedicine.* Retrieved from http://emedicine.medscape.com/article/805546-overview; Murray, C. E., Horton, G. E., Johnson, C. H., Notestine, L., Garr, B., Pow, A. M., . . . Doom, E. (2015). Domestic violence service providers' perceptions of safety planning: A focus group study. *Journal of Family Violence, 30*(3), 381–392; and Chang, J. C. (2015). Domestic violence: Epidemiology and risk factors. In E. J. Bieber, J. S. Sanfilippo, I. R. Horowitz, & M. I. Shafi (Eds.). *Clinical Gynecology* (2nd ed., pp. 94–101), Cambridge, UK: Cambridge University Press.

Nurses need to remember that their role is that of a guide, not a saviour. A woman will make the best decision she sees fit at that moment in time. A nurse may be her most effective resource in her stress-filled environment. Just allowing the woman to talk may be the most valuable intervention. The impact of the nurse's presence and support will stay with the woman, no matter what decision she makes.

SEXUAL VIOLENCE

Sexual violence is both a public health problem and a human rights violation. Sexual violence includes IPV, human trafficking, incest, FGC, forced prostitution, bondage, exploitation, neglect, infanticide, and sexual assault. It occurs worldwide and affects up to one third of women over a lifetime (Bagwell-Gray, Messing, & Baldwin-White, 2015). Once every 2 minutes, or 30 times an hour, or 1,871 times a day, girls and women in North America are raped. One in 5 women and 1 in 71 men will be sexually assaulted during their lifetime (Rape, Abuse, and Incest National Network [RAINN], 2018a). Rape has been reported against females from age 6 months to 93 years, but it remains one of the most underreported violent crimes in the North America. Once every 2 minutes, a woman is sexually assaulted in the United States (RAINN, 2018a). The National Center for Prevention and Control of Sexual Assault estimates that two thirds of sexual assaults will not be reported (CDC, 2017e). The General Social Survey on Canadians' Safety (Victimization) found that the rates of self-reported sexual assault were 22 incidents for every 1,000 Canadians aged 15 and older in 2014. This represents approximately 636,000 reported incidents of sexual assault (Conroy & Cotter, 2017). Over the course of their lives, women may experience more than one type of violence.

Sexual violence can have a variety of devastating short- and long-term effects. Women can experience psychological, physical, and cognitive symptoms that affect them daily. They can include chronic pelvic pain, headaches, backache, STIs, pregnancy, anxiety, denial, fear, withdrawal, sleep disturbances, guilt, nervousness, phobias, substance abuse, depression, sexual dysfunction, and PTSD. Many contemplate suicide (CDC, 2017e). A traumatic experience not only damages a woman's sense of safety in the world, but it can also reduce her self-esteem and her ability to continue her education, to earn money and be productive, to have children and, if she has children, to nurture and protect them. Overall, sexually assaulted women exhibit lower functioning as adults afterward (MacGregor et al., 2015).

Take Note!

Sexual violence has been called a "tragedy of youth." Females aged 16 to 19 are four times more likely to be raped or sexually assaulted (RAINN, 2018b).

Characteristics of Assailants

Assailants, like their victims, come from all walks of life and all ethnic backgrounds; there is no typical profile. More than half are under the age of 25, and the majority are married and leading otherwise "normal" sex lives. Why do men rape? No theory provides a satisfactory explanation. So few assailants are caught and convicted that a clear profile remains elusive. What is known is that many assailants have trouble dealing with the stresses of daily life. Such men become angry and experience feelings of powerlessness. They become jealous easily; do not view women as equals; frequently are hot tempered; have a need to be reassured of their manhood; and do not handle stress in their lives well. They commit a sexual assault as an expression of power and control (Kilmartin, 2015).

Sexual Abuse

Sexual abuse occurs when a woman is forced to have sexual contact of any kind (vaginal, oral, or anal) without her consent. Current estimates indicate that one of five girls is sexually abused, and the peak ages of such abuse are from 8 to 12 years of age. At every age in the life span, females are more likely to be sexually abused by father, brother, family member, neighbour, boyfriend, husband, partner, or ex-partner than by a stranger or anonymous assailant. Sexual abuse knows no economic or cultural barriers (de Jong, Alink, Bijleveld, Finkenauer, & Hendriks, 2015). Marriage does not constitute a tacit agreement for a spouse to inflict one's demands on the other without permission.

Childhood sexual abuse is any type of sexual exploitation that involves a child younger than 18 years old. It might include disrobing, nudity, masturbation, fondling, digital penetration, forced performance of sexual acts on the perpetrator, and intercourse (Dutton, 2015). Childhood sexual abuse has a lifelong impact on its survivors. There is strong evidence that sexual assault in childhood or adolescence is a serious risk factor for mental illness (Brooker & Durmaz, 2015). Women who were sexually abused during childhood are at a heightened risk for repeat abuse. This is because the early abuse lowers their self-esteem and their ability to protect themselves and set firm boundaries. Childhood sexual abuse is a trauma that influences the way victims form relationships, deal with adversity, cope with daily problems, relate to their children and peers, protect their health, and live. See Evidence-Based Practice 9.2 for study regarding childhood sexual abuse. Studies have shown that the more victimization a woman experiences, the more likely it is she will be revictimized (Brenner & Ben-Amitay, 2015).

Interventions for sexually abused children or women should include referral for mental health counselling.

EVIDENCE-BASED PRACTICE 9.2 **SIBLING SEXUAL ABUSE: AN EXPLORATORY STUDY OF LONG-TERM CONSEQUENCES FOR SELF-ESTEEM AND COUNSELLING CONSIDERATIONS**

Today, health care providers recognize childhood sexual abuse within the family as a significant and widespread problem with consequences lasting long into adulthood. Despite this progression, the research related to interfamilial incest conducted by researchers has focused primarily on father to daughter incest, largely ignoring the experience of sibling sexual assault, although it is more common than parental incest. Clearly, sibling incest is a pandemic problem that requires more attention from health care providers.

STUDY

This study addresses experiencing sibling sexual abuse as a child and how it inversely affects the level of self-esteem in adulthood. One hundred college students were used as the sample size; 67% were female and 33% were male with a diverse cultural representation. The age of the students ranged from 20 to 59 years old. A survey with two sections was used. The first section addressed recollection of the prevalence and severity of sibling abuse; the second section of the survey addressed self-esteem using the Rosenberg Self-Esteem Scale. Reliability and validity of this tool reflected a Cronbach alpha coefficient of 0.82.

Findings

This study supported the likelihood that sibling sexual abuse could be the most common form of child sexual abuse in the United States. In spite of the apparent prevalence of this, it is disturbing how little has been done to address the complexity surrounding this form of abuse. Both survivors and offenders of sibling sexual abuse experience the lasting impact of the abuse as they become adults in their social interactions, school, work, and family life. In addition to a low self-esteem, other mental health issues experienced include symptoms of PTSD, anxiety disorders, depression, eating disorders, angry outbursts, self-injury, somatic complaints, and suicidal ideation. Many engage in at-risk behaviours such as unprotected sex, self-medication with drugs and alcohol, and dating violence. Clearly, ignoring the problem of sibling sexual abuse has a negative effect on a sense of well-being as these children become adults.

Nursing Implications

One of the most important aspects is to establish trust with these clients and create a safe environment. An important role for nurses is in primary prevention of sibling sexual abuse through educating parents. When parents understand how to promote positive parent–child relationships and sibling interactions, the risk of abuse in the entire family tends to be reduced. Nurses can take a lead role through promotion of structured parent education programs within their communities and referrals to national networks such as Family Support America.

Adopted from Morrill, M. (2014). Sibling sexual abuse: An exploratory study of long term consequences for self-esteem and counseling considerations. *Journal of Family Violence, 29*(2), 205–213.

Follow-up for any medical problems (e.g., genitourinary complaints) should be arranged with the child's or woman's primary care physician or nurse practitioner. If the community has an abuse referral centre, refer the victim there for follow-up care according to local protocol.

The medical consequences of sexual abuse require the prophylaxis and treatment of STIs, emergency contraception, and treatment of any injuries that resulted from the abuse. Victims with postassault bleeding require an emergent evaluation and may need emergency treatment by a gynecologist for repair of genital injury. The psychosocial aspects of sexual abuse must also be addressed because appropriate therapeutic follow-up is essential to the victim's future emotional well-being.

Incest

Incest is defined as sexual activity between persons so closely related that marriage between them is legally or culturally prohibited (Dorland, 2015). The exact incidence of child sexual victimization is unknown. Such sexual abuse is not only a crime but also a symptom of acute and irreversible family dysfunction. Childhood incest abuse involves any kind of sexual exploitation between a child and another person that violates the social taboos of family roles; children cannot yet understand these activities and cannot give informed consent. Adult women with a history of incest exhibit a clinical syndrome that includes low self-esteem, difficulty with intimate relationships, sexual dysfunction, flashbacks and nightmares, repeated victimization, as well as suicidality, depressive symptomatology, eating disorders, and substance abuse (Harkins, 2015). Survivors of incest are often tricked, coerced, or manipulated. All adults appear to be powerful to children. Perpetrators might threaten victims so that they are afraid to disclose the abuse or might tell them the abuse is their fault. Often these threats serve to silence victims.

Incestuous relationships in the home endanger not only the child's intellectual and moral development, but also the health of the child. Many children do not ask for help because they do not want to expose their "secret." For this reason, just the tip of the iceberg is statistically visible: serious injuries, internal damage, STIs, or pregnancy. Incest can have serious long-term effects on its victims, which may include eating disorders, sexual problems in adult life, difficulty in interpersonal relationships, anxiety, PTSD, intense guilt and shame, low self-esteem, depression, and self-destructive behaviour (National Center for Victims of Crime [NCVC], 2015a).

Whether an incest victim endured an isolated incident of abuse or ongoing assaults over an extended period, recovery can be painful and difficult. The recovery process begins with admission of abuse and the recognition that help and services are needed. Resources for incest victims include books, self-help groups, workshops, therapy programs, and possibly legal remedies. In addition to listening to and believing incest victims, nurses need to search for ways to prevent future generations from enduring such abuse and from continuing the cycle of abuse in their own family and relationships. Nurses have the ability and the responsibility to function within an interdisciplinary system responsible for the assessment and ongoing treatment of incestuous families. Nurses can fulfill their roles as advocates for children, while at the same time adding necessary referrals to social services and legal authorities. Forming this partnership with the social service and judicial communities will help protect the child from future abuse and ensure the child a safe environment in which to grow and develop.

Take Note!

Childhood sexual abuse is a trauma that can affect every aspect of the victim's life.

Sexual Assault

Sexual assault is an expression of violence, not a sexual act. Sexual assault distorts one of the most intimate forms of human interaction. It is not an act of lust or an overzealous release of passion: it is a violent, aggressive assault on the victim's body and integrity. Those who rape do so for a number of reasons, but they basically involve the motives of anger, power, eroticized cruelty, and opportunistic mating (Keygnaert, Vettenburg, & Temmerman, 2015). **Sexual assault** and **rape** are legal rather than medical terms. It denotes penile penetration of the vagina, mouth, or rectum of the female or male without consent. It may or may not include the use of a weapon. **Statutory rape** is sexual activity between an adult and a person under the age of 18 and is considered to have occurred even if the underage person was willing (RAINN, 2018b). Nine out of every 10 people who are sexually assaulted are female (Alexander, LaRosa, Bader, & Garfield, 2014). Enforcement of laws, education, and community empowerment are all needed to prevent sexual assault.

Consider This

At 53 years old, I stood and looked at myself in the mirror. The image staring back at me was one of a frightened, middle-aged, cowardly woman hiding her past. I had been sexually abused by my father for many years as a child and never told anyone. My mother knew of the abuse but felt helpless to make it stop. I married right out of high school to escape and felt I lived a "happy normal life" with my husband and three children. My children have left home and live away, and my husband recently died of a sudden heart attack. I am now experiencing dreams and thoughts about my past abuse and feeling afraid again.

Thoughts: This woman suppressed her abusive past for most of her life and now her painful experience has surfaced. What can be done to reach out to her at this point? Did her health care providers miss the "red flags" that are common to women with a history of childhood sexual abuse all those years?

Many people believe that sexual assault usually occurs on a dark night when a stranger assaults a provocatively dressed, promiscuous woman. They believe that rapists are sex-starved people seeking sexual gratification. Rape myths are destructive beliefs about sexual aggression (i.e., its scope, causes, context, and consequences) that serve to deny, downplay, or justify sexually aggressive behaviour that men commit against women. A sexual assault survivor's recovery is frequently complicated by the public's failure to believe the survivor and restore justice (Klaus, Buczkowski, & Wiktorska, 2015). Sexual assault/rape myths serve to blame survivors and exonerate perpetrators. Such myths and the facts are presented in Table 9.3.

Acquaintance Sexual Assault/Rape

In acquaintance sexual assault/rape, someone is forced to have sex by a person he or she knows. Sexual assault by a coworker, a teacher, a husband's friend, or a boss is considered acquaintance sexual assault. **Date rape,** an assault that occurs within a dating relationship or marriage without consent of one of the participants, is a form of acquaintance sexual assault/rape. Acquaintance and date assaults commonly occur on college campuses. One in four college women has been sexually assaulted—that is, has been forced, physically or verbally, actively or implicitly, to engage in sexual activity (Wilson & Miller, 2016).

These forms of sexual assault are physically and emotionally devastating for the survivors. Research has indicated that the survivors of acquaintance rape report similar levels of depression, anxiety, complications in subsequent relationships, and difficulty attaining pre-rape levels of sexual satisfaction to those reported by

TABLE 9.3	FOUR PHASES OF RAPE RECOVERY
Phase	**Survivor's Response**
Acute phase (disorganization)	Shock, fear, disbelief, anger, shame, guilt, feelings of uncleanliness; insomnia, nightmares, and sobbing
Outward adjustment phase (denial)	Appears outwardly composed and returns to work or school; refuses to discuss the assault and denies need for counselling
Reorganization	Denial and suppression do not work, and the survivor attempts to make life adjustments by moving or changing jobs and uses emotional distancing to cope
Integration and recovery	Survivor begins to feel safe and starts to trust others. She may become an advocate for other rape victims

Adapted from National Center for Victims of Crime [NCVC]. (2015b). *The trauma of victimization.* Retrieved from http://victimsofcrime.org/help-for-crime-victims/get-help-bulletins-for-crime-victims/trauma-of-victimization#ptsd; Rape, Abuse, and Incest National Network [RAINN]. (2018d). *Recovery from sexual violence.* Retrieved from https://www.rainn.org/recovering-sexual-violence

survivors of stranger rape. **Acquaintance rape** remains a controversial topic because there is lack of agreement on the definition of consent. Despite the violation and reality of physical and emotional trauma, survivors of acquaintance assault often do not identify their experience as sexual assault. Instead of focusing on the violation of the sexual assault, victims of acquaintance rape often blame themselves for the assault (RAINN, 2018c).

Although acquaintance rape and date rape do not always involve drugs, a rapist might use alcohol or other drugs to sedate his victim. In 1996, the federal government passed a law making it a felony to give an unsuspecting person a "date rape drug" with the intent of raping him or her. Even with penalties of large fines and up to 20 years in prison, the use of date rape drugs is growing (U.S. Department of Health and Human Services [USDHHS], 2015a). Date rape drugs are also known as "club drugs" because they are often used at dance clubs, fraternity parties, and all-night raves. The most common is Rohypnol (also known as "roofies," "forget pills," "mind erasers," and the "drop drug"). It comes in the form of a liquid or pill that quickly dissolves in liquid with no odour, taste, or colour. This drug is 10 times as strong as diazepam (Valium). The effects can be felt within 30 minutes and produces memory loss for up to 8 hours. Gamma hydroxybutyrate (GHB; called "liquid ecstasy" or "easy lay") produces euphoria, an out-of-body high,

sleepiness, increased sex drive, and memory loss. GHB takes effect in about 15 minutes and can last 3 to 4 hours. It comes in a white powder or liquid and may cause unconsciousness, depression, and coma. The third date rape drug, ketamine (known as "Special K," "vitamin K," or "super acid"), acts on the central nervous system very quickly to separate perception and sensation. Combining ketamine with other drugs can be fatal. Date rape drugs can be very dangerous, and women can protect themselves against them in a variety of ways (Teaching Guidelines 9.2).

Teaching Guidelines 9.2
PROTECTING YOURSELF AGAINST DATE RAPE DRUGS
• Never leave a drink of any kind unattended.
• Don't accept a drink from someone else.
• Accept drinks from a bartender or in a closed container only.
• If a drink is left unattended, pour it out, don't drink it.
• Don't drink anything that tastes or smells strange.
• Don't drink from a punch bowl or a keg.
• If you think someone drugged you, call 911.

Recovery from Rape/Sexual Assault

Survivors take a long time to heal from their traumatic experience. Some women never heal and never get professional counselling, but most can cope. Rape/sexual assault is viewed as a situational crisis that the survivor is unprepared to handle because it is an unforeseen event. Survivors typically go through four phases of recovery following rape/sexual assault (Table 9.4).

A significant proportion of women who are assaulted also experience symptoms of PTSD. PTSD develops when an event outside the range of normal human experience occurs that produces marked distress in the person. Symptoms of PTSD are divided into three groups:

• **Intrusion** (re-experiencing the trauma, including nightmares, flashbacks, recurrent thoughts)
• **Avoidance** (avoiding trauma-related stimuli, social withdrawal, emotional numbing)
• **Hyperarousal** (increased emotional arousal, exaggerated startle response, irritability)

Not every traumatized female develops full-blown or even minor PTSD. Symptoms usually begin within 3 months of the incident, but occasionally may only emerge years later. They must last more than a month to be considered PTSD. The condition varies from person to person. Some women recover within months, while others have symptoms for much longer. In some people, the condition becomes chronic (Darnell et al., 2015; Friedman, 2015).

TABLE 9.4	RISK FACTORS FOR INTIMATE PARTNER VIOLENCE IN MEN			
Individual Factors	**Relationship Factors**	**Community Factors**	**Societal Factors**	
Young age	Martial conflict	Weak sanctions against IPV	Traditional gender norms	
Heavy drinking	Economic stress	Poverty	Social norms supportive of violence	
Personality disorders	Dysfunctional family	Low social capital		
Depression	Marital instability			
Low academic achievement	Male dominance in family			
Witnessing violence as a child	Cohabitation			
Low income and/or unemployment	Having outside sexual partners			
Experiencing violence as a child				
Desire for power and control in all relationships				
Anger and hostility	Taking aggression out on others while growing up			

Adapted from Centers for Disease Control and Prevention [CDC]. (2017c) *Intimate partner violence: Risk and protective factors.* Retrieved from http://www.cdc.gov/violenceprevention/intimatepartnerviolence/riskprotectivefactors.html; Ghandour, R. M., Campbell, J. C., & Lloyd, J. (2015). *Screening and counseling for intimate partner violence: A vision for the future. Journal of Women's Health, 24*(1), 57–61.

Nursing Management of Survivors of Sexual Assault

Health care providers, along with sexual assault nurse examiners (SANE), can make a difference in the lives of survivors by understanding the facts, the effects this violence can have on mental and physical health, where to find information for themselves and their clients, and how to properly care for a survivor. Language is important and referring to the woman as a survivor rather than a victim of sexual assault starts to empower the woman and support her in her decision making. A SANE is a registered nurse specially trained to conduct sexual assault evidentiary exams for survivors of sexual assault. In addition to the collection of forensic evidence, they also provide access to crisis intervention, STI testing, and emergency contraception (International Association of Forensic Nurses, 2017).

Research has found that survivors undergo a profound and complex trauma. Exposure therapy has been used to help survivors confront their trauma-related memories, feelings, and stimuli that evoke fear and anxiety (Nacasch, Rachamim, & Foa, 2015). The survivor should be provided with a safe and comfortable environment for a forensic examination. Nursing care of the survivor should focus on providing supportive care, collecting and documenting evidence, assessing for STIs, preventing pregnancy, and assessing for PTSD. Once

initial treatment and evidence collection have been completed, follow-up care should include counselling, medical treatment, and crisis intervention. There is mounting evidence that early intervention and immediate counselling speed a survivor's recovery. By early intervention, it means interventions implemented in the initials hours, days, or weeks after the traumatic event (Bryant, 2015). Nursing Care Plan 9.1 (at the end of the chapter) highlights a sample plan of care for a survivor of sexual assault.

Take Note!
Many survivors seek treatment in the hospital emergency department if no sexual assault/rape crisis centre is available. Unfortunately, many emergency department doctors and nurses have little training in how to treat survivors or in collecting evidence. To make matters worse, if they have to wait for hours in public waiting rooms, survivors may leave the hospital, never to receive treatment or supply the evidence needed to arrest and convict their assailants.

PROVIDING SUPPORTIVE CARE
Establishing a therapeutic and trusting relationship will help the survivor describe her experience. Take the woman to a secure, isolated area away from family, friends, and other clients and staff so she can be open

and honest when asked about the assault. Provide a change of clothes, access to a shower and toiletries, and a private waiting area for family and friends.

COLLECTING AND DOCUMENTING EVIDENCE

The victim should be instructed to bring all clothing, especially undergarments, worn at the time of the assault to the medical facility. The survivor should not shower or bathe before presenting for care. Typically, a specially trained nurse will collect the evidence from the survivor.

ASSESSING FOR SEXUALLY TRANSMITTED INFECTIONS

As part of the assessment, a pelvic examination will be done to collect vaginal secretions to rule out any STIs. This examination is very emotionally stressful for most women and should be carried out very gently and sensitively.

PREVENTING PREGNANCY

An essential element in the care of survivors involves offering them pregnancy prevention. After unprotected intercourse, including sexual assault, pregnancy can be prevented by using an emergency contraceptive pill, sometimes called postcoital contraception. Emergency contraceptive pills involve high doses of the same oral contraceptives that millions of women take every day. The emergency regimen consists of one dose taken within 72 to 120 hours of the unprotected intercourse. Emergency contraception works by preventing ovulation, fertilization, or implantation. It does not disrupt an established pregnancy and should not be confused with mifepristone (RU-486), a drug approved by the Food and Drug Administration for abortion in the first 49 days of gestation. Emergency contraception is most effective if it is taken within 12 hours of the assault; it becomes less effective with every 12 hours of delay thereafter.

ASSESSING FOR POSTTRAUMATIC STRESS DISORDER

Nurses can begin to assess the extent to which a survivor is suffering from **PTSD** by asking the following questions:
- To assess the presence of intrusive thoughts:
  - Do upsetting thoughts and nightmares of the trauma bother you?
  - Do you feel as though you are actually reliving the trauma?
  - Does it upset you to be exposed to anything that reminds you of that event?
- To assess the presence of avoidance reactions:
  - Do you find yourself trying to avoid thinking about the trauma?
  - Do you stay away from situations that remind you of the event?
  - Do you have trouble recalling exactly what happened?
  - Do you feel numb emotionally?

- To assess the presence of physical symptoms:
  - Are you having trouble sleeping?
  - Have you felt irritable or experienced outbursts of anger?
  - Do you have heart palpitations and sweating?
  - Do you have muscle aches and pains all over? (NCVC, 2015b)

With a growing body of knowledge about rape-related PTSD, help is available through most sexual assault/rape crisis and trauma centres. Support groups have been established where survivors can meet regularly to share experiences to help relieve the symptoms of PTSD. For some survivors, medication prescribed along with therapy is the best combination to relieve the pain. Just as in the treatment of any other illness, at the first opportunity, the woman should be encouraged to talk about the traumatic experience. This ventilating provides a chance to receive needed support and comfort, as well as an opportunity to begin making sense of the experience. To diminish symptoms of PTSD, survivors must work on two fronts: coming to terms with the past and alleviating stress in the present (Bryant, 2015).

In order to have a better understanding of the aftermath of criminal victimization such as sexual assault, nurses must begin to accept the reality that crime is random, senseless, and can happen to anyone regardless of the precautions that are taken to prevent it. Nurses must also understand that a survivor's life is turned upside down when he or she becomes a victim of crime. In order to help survivors to trust society again and regain a sense of balance and self-worth, nurses must educate all those who come in contact with survivors to be sensitive to their needs.

Female Genital Cutting

FGC, also referred to as female genital mutilation (FGM) or female circumcision, is defined as a procedure involving any injury of the external female genitalia for cultural or nontherapeutic reasons. It confers severe health consequences for girls and women. The international community views this practice as a human rights violation (Gayle & Rymer, 2015). It is the surgical removal of a portion or portions of the genitalia of female infants, girls, and women, including the clitoris (type I), clitoris and labia minora (type II), and clitoris, labia minora, labia majora, and then suturing of the remaining tissue, known as fibulation, to leave only a small opening for urination, menstruation, intercourse, and childbirth (type III). There is a type IV, which encompasses all other mutilations of the female genital area such as pricking, piercing, cutting, cauterizing, and scraping of the vaginal tissue, incisions to the clitoris and vagina, and burning, scarring, or cauterizing of tissue with the aim of tightening or narrowing the vagina (Nour, 2015).

FGC is a worldwide practice that affects millions of women and girls. According to the WHO (2018) and UNICEF, 140 million women are victims of FGC with about 130 million girls between infancy and age 15 undergoing FGC every year. Countries where this is practiced include 30 African countries and parts of the Middle East and Asia. Prevalence in countries such as Sudan and Egypt has been estimated as high as 99% (Johnsdotter, 2015). The exact origins of FGC are not known. Although FGC may be interwoven into the culture, it is not mandated by any religion. This practice predates both Islam and Christianity (Gruenbaum & Wirtz, 2015). In some cultures, it is associated with feminine beauty and often signifies a rite of passage from childhood to adulthood. Female cutting is performed to decrease a woman's sexual desires and to ensure her chastity until marriage and receipt of a dowry from the prospective groom (Farage et al., 2015). Ultimately, the reality of being ostracized by the community and the possibility of being ineligible to marry create enormous social pressure to have FGC carried out, pressure that outweighs the known physical and emotional damage of this practice (Nour, 2015).

Complications vary, depending on the type of cutting and the way it was performed. It is frequently performed without anesthesia under nonsterile conditions. Cutting tools can be anything from razors blades to knives to pieces of glass or tin can lids. Complications can include infertility, dysmenorrhea, dyspareunia, sexual dysfunction, infection, hemorrhage after the procedure, vaginal stenosis, chronic vaginitis, pelvic inflammatory disease, chronic urinary tract infections, incontinence, genital fistulas, recurrent abscesses, transmission of HIV and hepatitis during the procedure, severe pain and shock after the procedure, difficulty walking or using stairs due to severe scarring, urinary retention, inability to experience orgasm, and difficulty in giving birth. Long-term complications related to FGC include chronic pain, dyspareunia, and difficult childbirth. The most common long-term complication is the formation of inclusion clitoral dermoid cysts and labial fusion. These become large as a grapefruit and can lead to difficulty in walking, sitting, and can cause psychological distress from the deformity. The psychological effects range from eating disorders, insomnia, depression, PTSD, and negative effects on the women's self-esteem and identity (Creighton, 2015).

As immigration to Canada increases, nurses are increasingly likely to encounter women affected by FGC and its complications. The psychological pressure and trauma of being torn between two cultures and feeling different may lie heavily on the women in a new setting where FGC is foreign and banned. Nurses need updated education regarding women with FGC so that appropriate care for this population can be provided for this very sensitive health care problem. Well-informed nurses are the best tool for providing culturally sensitive care to this population. Nurses are in a unique position to contact and educate women who have been cut or are at risk for mutilation. To advocate for these women, a thorough understanding of the practice of FGC, its cultural overtones, religious implications, and psychosocial effects is needed.

The Society of Obstetricians and Gynecologists of Canada published clinical practice guidelines regarding FGC in 2013. While health care professionals are advised not to stigmatize women who have had FGC and to be prepared to care for women who may need to manage complication, they are advised it is illegal to perform FGC in Canada.

Take Note!

From a Western perspective, FGC is hard to comprehend. Because it is not talked about openly in communities that practice it, women who have undergone it accept it without question and assume it is done to all girls (Gruenbaum & Wirtz, 2015).

Background

Reasons for performing the ritual reflect the ideology and cultural values of each community that practices it. Some consider it a rite of passage into womanhood; others use it as a means of preserving virginity until marriage. In cultures where it is practiced, it is an important part of culturally defined gender identity. In any case, all the reasons are cultural and traditional and are not rooted in any religious texts (Research Action and Information Network for the Bodily Integrity of Women [RAINBO], 2018). Since FGC has no health benefits and often leaves women with lifelong physical and emotional trauma, there is a human rights justification to end the practice. International pressure to end FGC has been mounting since 1997, when the WHO, UNICEF, and UNFPA issued a joint statement to call on governments to ban the practice (Borsand, Friedman, Mirzayan, & Borsand, 2015). Box 9.6 lists types of FGC procedures.

Nursing Management of the Client who Experienced Female Genital Cutting

Because of increasing migration, nurses throughout the world are increasingly exposed to women who have experienced these procedures and thus need to know about its impact on women's reproductive health. Helping women who have had an FGC procedure requires good communication skills and often an interpreter, since many may not speak English. As nurses, we are educated to provide comprehensive, culturally sensitive care regardless of our client's circumstances. Nurses must keep in mind that FGC is considered normal in many cultures and to not have it done would be unthinkable. Nurses have the opportunity to educate clients by providing accurate information and positive health care

FOUR MAJOR TYPES OF FEMALE GENITAL MUTILATION PROCEDURES

Type I: Excision of the prepuce with excision of part or the entire clitoris

Type II: Excision of the clitoris and part or all of the labia minora

Type III (Infibulation): Excision of all or part of the external genitalia and stitching/narrowing of the vaginal opening

Type IV: Pricking, piercing, or incision of the clitoris or labia

- Stretching of the clitoris and/or labia
- Cauterizing by burning the clitoris and surrounding tissues
- Scraping or cutting the vaginal orifice
- Introduction of a corrosive substance into the vagina
- Placing herbs into the vagina to narrow it

Adapted from World Health Organization (WHO). (2018). Female genital mutilation. Retrieved from http://www.who.int/news-room/fact-sheets/detail/female-genital-mutilation; Nour, N. M. (2015). Female genital cutting: Impact on women's health. *Seminars in Reproductive Medicine, 33*(1), 41–46; and Research Action and Information Network for the Bodily Integrity of Women (RAINBO). (2018). Caring for women with circumcision: Fact sheet for physicians. Retrieved from http://www.rainbo.org/factsheet.html

experiences. Make sure that you are comfortable with your own feelings about this practice before dealing with clients. Some guidelines are as follows:

- Let the client know you are concerned and interested and want to help.
- Speak clearly and slowly, using simple, accurate terms.
- Use the term or name for this practice that the recipient uses, not "FGC."
- Use pictures and diagrams to help the woman understand what you are saying.
- Be patient in allowing the client to answer questions.
- Include men in any education, as they are influential in this practice.
- Repeat back your understanding of the client's statements.
- Always look and talk directly to the client, not the interpreter.
- Place no judgment on the cultural practice.
- Maintain respect for older women who have experienced FGC.
- Encourage the client to express herself freely.
- Maintain strict confidentiality.
- Provide culturally attuned care to all clients.

In short, FGC is a form of violence against women, and it is only through education and empowerment of women that real changes in this practice can be made. Because this practice often defines a woman and becomes a part of her identity, nurses must understand this to be able to assist women who have had this done

to them. Only through intense education will the next generation of girls be saved from this practice.

Human Trafficking

The United Nations defines **human trafficking** as the recruitment, transportation, transfer, harbouring or receipt of persons, by means of the threat or use of force, of abduction, of fraud, or deception to achieve the consent of a person having control over another person, for the purpose of exploitation (United Nations Office on Drugs and Crime [UNODC], 2018).

A girl who was just 14 years old was held captive in a tiny trailer room, where she was forced to have sex with as many as 30 men a day. On her nightstand was a teddy bear that reminded her of her childhood in Mexico from where she was abducted and forced into sexual slavery.

This scenario describes human trafficking, the enslavement of immigrants for profit. Within our borders, thousands of foreign nationals and citizens, many of them children, are forced or coerced into sex work or various forms of labour every year (Weitzer, 2015). Human trafficking is both a global problem and a domestic problem. Canadian laws prohibit human trafficking for any exploitative purpose, regardless of whether the trafficking occurs within Canada or whether it involves individuals being brought into Canada (Public Safety Canada, 2018). Human trafficking is a modern form of slavery that affects nearly 1 million people worldwide. In 2017, the Royal Canadian Mounted Police (RCMP) Human Trafficking National Coordination Centre (HTNCC) reported 455 cases since 2005 where human trafficking-specific charges were laid; 433 of these were domestic, and 22 were international human trafficking cases (Public Safety Canada, 2018). In the United States, estimates indicate approximately 20,000 persons annually (U.S. Department of State, 2018). Women and children are the primary victims of human trafficking, many in the sex trade as described above and others through forced-labour domestic servitude. Poverty and lack of economic opportunity make women and children potential victims of traffickers associated with international criminal organizations. They are vulnerable to false promises of job opportunities in other countries. Many of those who accept these offers, from what initially appears to be legitimate sources, find themselves in situations where their legal documents are destroyed, they or their families are threatened with harm, or they are bound to their trafficker by a debt that they have no chance of repaying.

Trafficking persons is hugely profitable: one estimate places global profits at approximately $35 billion annually. Among illegal enterprises, trafficking is second only to drug dealing and is tied with the illegal arms industry in its ability to generate dollars (Aronowitz & Koning, 2015).

Canada and the United States are profitable destination countries for traffickers, and these profits contribute to the development of organized criminal enterprises worldwide. According to findings of the Victims of Trafficking and Violence Protection Act of 2000:

- Victims are primarily women and children who lack education, employment, and economic opportunities in their own countries.
- Traffickers promise victims employment as nannies, maids, dancers, factory workers, sales clerks, or models.
- Traffickers transport the victims from their counties to unfamiliar destinations away from their support systems.
- Once they are here, traffickers coerce them, using rape, torture, starvation, imprisonment, threats, or physical force, into prostitution, pornography, the sex trade, forced labour, or involuntary servitude.

These victims are exposed to serious and numerous health risks such as rape; physical injury such as cigarette burns, fractures, bruises; torture; HIV/AIDS; STIs; cervical cancer; violence; hazardous work environments; poor nutrition; and drug and alcohol addiction (Greenbaum et al., 2015). Health care is one of the most pressing needs of these victims, but no comprehensive care is available to undocumented immigrants. Nurses and other health care providers who encounter victims of trafficking often do not realize it, and opportunities to intervene are lost. Although no one sign can demonstrate with certainty when someone is being trafficked, clinicians should be aware of several indicators. It is important to be alert for trafficking victims in any setting and to recognize cues (Box 9.7).

Nursing interventions in the case of trafficking victims would include the following:
- Building trust is the number-one priority
- Take the time to listen and develop rapport
- Screen in a private place to ensure confidentiality and safety
- Reassure the potential victim
- One-on-one interactions are ideal
- Specifically ask about the client's safety
- Offer reworded stories
- Stay calm and on an even keel
- Understand the risk these victims are taking by disclosing their plight
- ALWAYS document your suspicion in your notes, at the very least

Human trafficking is a violation of human rights. Few crimes are more repugnant than the sex trafficking of helpless and innocent victims. Nurses are one of the few groups of professionals likely to interact with trafficked victims while they are still in captivity. They have the opportunity to screen, identify, intervene, and rescue these victims. If you suspect a trafficking situation, notify local law enforcement and a regional social

service organization that has experience in dealing with trafficking victims. It is imperative to reach out to these victims and stop the cycle of abuse by following through on your suspicions. Nurses can also reach out within their communities to bring about awareness through community education to human trafficking to uncover the hard truth about it to our nation's blind eyes.

SUMMARY

The causes of violence against women are complex. Previously, violence against women was largely invisible, natural, and trivial. Many laughed at the notion that intimate or community violence against women should be seen as a human rights violation. Raising awareness

---

BOX 9.7

IDENTIFYING VICTIMS OF HUMAN TRAFFICKING

Look beneath the surface and ask yourself: Is this person
- A female or a child in poor health?
- Foreign-born and doesn't speak English?
- Lacking immigration documents?
- Giving an inconsistent explanation of injury?
- Reluctant to give any information about self, injury, home, or work?
- Fearful of authority Figure or "sponsor" if present? ("Sponsor" might not leave victim alone with health care provider.)
- Living with the employer?

Sample questions to ask the potential victim of human trafficking:
- Can you leave your job or situation if you wish?
- Can you come and go as you please?
- Have you been threatened if you try to leave?
- Has anyone threatened your family with harm if you leave?
- What are your working and living conditions?
- Do you have to ask permission to go to the bathroom, eat, or sleep?
- Is there a lock on your door so you cannot get out?
- What brought you to the United States? Are your plans the same now?
- Are you free to leave your current work or home situation?
- Who has your immigration papers? Why don't you have them?
- Are you paid for the work you do?
- Are there times you feel afraid?
- How can your situation be changed?

Adapted from United Nations Office on Drugs and Crime (UNODC). (2018). Human trafficking. Retrieved from http://www.unodc.org/unodc/en/human-trafficking/what-is-human-trafficking.html; Sanchez, R., & Stark, S. (2014). The hard truth about human trafficking. *Nursing Management, 45*(1), 18–23; and Weitzer, R. (2015). Human trafficking and contemporary slavery. *Annual Review of Sociology, 41*(1), 223–242. Retrieved from https://www.annualreviews.org/doi/abs/10.1146/annurev-soc-073014-112506

and developing evidence-based programs, practices and policies to prevent IPV and sexual assault are essential in stopping violent behaviour before it starts. Many women will experience some type of violence in their lives, and it can have a debilitating effect on their health and future relationships. Nurses have the skills, professional experience, and perspective to be an important part of comprehensive violence prevention efforts in communities. Violence is a preventable public health problem if multiple sectors understand patterns of violence and implement prevention strategies to reduce it (Copelon, 2015).

Violence frequently leaves a "legacy of pain" to future generations. Nurses can empower women and encourage them to move forward and take control of their lives. When women live in peace and security, free from violence, they have an enormous potential to contribute to their own communities and to the national and global society. Nurses can play an important role in working toward the creation of a violence-free community, but they must first become informed. Nurses must insist that health care agencies that employ them accept this responsibility and work together to reach out to those being abused. The time is ripe for nurses to act and ensure serious inroads are made in improving the health and well-being of all women across the globe.

Violence against women is not normal, legal, or acceptable and it should never be tolerated or justified. It can and must be stopped by the entire world community. Early education and prevention provide the best hope for creating healthy futures and fostering a global society without violence.

NURSING CARE PLAN 9.1

Overview of the Woman Who is a Survivor of Sexual Assault

Lucia, a 20-year-old college junior, was admitted to the emergency room after police found her when a passerby called 911 to report an assault. She stated, "I was raped a few hours ago while I was walking home through the park." Assessment reveals the following: numerous cuts and bruises of varying sizes on her face, arms, and legs; lip swollen and cut; right eye swollen and bruised; jacket and shirt ripped and bloodied; hair matted with grass and debris; vital signs within acceptable parameters; client tearful, clutching her clothing, and trembling; perineal bruising and tearing.

NURSING DIAGNOSIS: Rape-trauma syndrome related to report of recent sexual assault

Outcome Identification and Evaluation

Client will demonstrate adequate coping skills related to effects of rape as evidenced by her ability to discuss the event, verbalize her feelings and fears, and exhibit appropriate actions to return to her precrisis level of functioning.

Interventions: *Promoting Adequate Coping Skills*

- Stay with the client to promote feelings of safety.
- Explain the procedures to be completed based on facility's policy to help alleviate client's fear of the unknown.
- Assist with physical examination for specimen collection to obtain evidence for legal proceedings.
- Administer prophylactic medication as ordered to prevent pregnancy and STIs.
- Provide care to wounds as ordered to prevent infection.
- Assist client with hygiene measures as necessary to promote self-esteem.

- Allow client to describe the events as much as possible to encourage ventilation of feelings about the incident; engage in active listening and offer nonjudgmental support to facilitate coping and demonstrate understanding of the client's situation and feelings.
- Help the client identify positive coping skills and personal strengths used in the past to aid in effective decision making.
- Assist client in developing additional coping strategies and teach client relaxation techniques to help deal with the current crisis and anxiety.
- Contact the counsellor in the facility to help the client deal with the crisis.

NURSING CARE PLAN 9.1

Overview of the Woman Who is a Survivor of Sexual Assault (continued)

- Arrange for follow-up visit with counsellor to provide continued care and to promote continuity of care.
- Encourage the client to contact a close friend, partner, or family member to accompany her home to provide support.

- Provide the client with the telephone number of a counselling service or community support groups to help her cope and obtain ongoing support.
- Provide written instructions related to follow-up appointments, care, and testing to ensure adequate understanding.

KEY CONCEPTS

- ◎ Gender-based violence is a major public health and social problem because it violates a person's very being and causes numerous mental and physical health sequelae.

- ◎ Abuse may be mental, physical, or sexual in nature or a combination of all of these.

- ◎ The cycle of violence includes three phases: tension building, acute battering, and honeymoon.

- ◎ Many individuals experience PTSD after being sexually assaulted. PTSD can inhibit a survivor from adapting or coping in a healthy manner.

- ◎ Intimate partner violence can increase before, during, or after pregnancy.

- ◎ FGC is practiced worldwide and nurses in Canada need to become knowledgeable about it and place no judgment on this cultural practice.

- ◎ Human trafficking is a violation against human rights, and nurses who suspect it should report it to stop the cycle of abuse against young children and women.

- ◎ The nurse's role in dealing with survivors of violence is to establish rapport; open up lines of communication; apply the nursing process to assess and screen all clients in all settings; and implement and intervene as appropriate.

REFERENCES AND RECOMMENDED READINGS

Alexander, L. L., LaRosa, J. H., Bader, H., & Garfield, S. (2014). *New dimensions in women's health* (6th ed.). Sudbury, MA: Jones & Bartlett.

Aronowitz, A. A., & Koning, A. (2015). Understanding human trafficking as a market system: Addressing the demand side of trafficking for sexual exploitation. *Revue Internationale de droit Pénal, 85*(3), 669–696.

Association of Women's Health, Obstetric and Neonatal Nurses (AWHONN). (2015). Intimate partner violence. *Journal of Obstetric, Gynecologic, and Neonatal Nursing, 44*(3), 405–408.

Bagwell-Gray, M. E., Messing, J. T., & Baldwin-White, A. (2015). Intimate partner sexual violence: A review of terms, definitions, and prevalence. *Trauma, Violence, and Abuse, 16*(3), 316–335.

Barrios, Y. V., Gelaye, B., Zhong, Q., Nicolaidis, C., Rondon, M. B., Garcia, P. J., . . . Williams, M. A. (2015). Association of childhood physical and sexual abuse with intimate partner violence, poor general health and depressive symptoms among pregnant women. *PLoS One, 10*(1), e0116609.

Beattie, S., & Hutchins, H. (2015). *Shelters for abused women in Canada, 2014. Catalogue no. 85-002-X.* Ottawa: Statistics Canada. Retrieved from https://www150.statcan.gc.ca/n1/pub/85-002-x/2015001/article/14207-eng.pdf

Berthold, S. M. (2015). Intimate partner violence and a rights-based approach to healing. In *Human rights-based approaches to clinical social work* (pp. 85–113). Springer International Publishing.

Borsand, M., Friedman, B., Mirzayan, N., & Borsand, A. (2015). Female genital cutting: An ancient practice embedded in an ever-evolving world. *American Journal of Cosmetic Surgery, 32*(1), 31–36.

Bouchet, S., & Braswell, K. (2015). *Beyond silence and violence.* Dunwoody, GA: Fathers Incorporated. www.fathersincorporated.com

Brenner, I., & Ben-Amitay, G. (2015). Sexual revictimization: The impact of attachment anxiety, accumulated trauma, and response to childhood sexual abuse disclosure. *Violence and Victims, 30*(1), 49–65.

Brooker, C., & Durmaz, E. (2015). Mental health, sexual violence and the work of Sexual Assault Referral centres (SARCs) in England. *Journal of Forensic and Legal Medicine, 31*, 47–51.

Brownridge, D. A., Taillieu, T., Afifi, T., Chan, K. L., Emery, C., Lavoie, J., & Elgar, F. (2017). Child maltreatment and intimate partner violence among indigenous and non-indigenous Canadians. *Journal of Family Violence, 32*, 607–619.

Bryant, R. A. (2015). Early intervention after trauma. In U. Schnyder, M. Cloitre (Eds.). *Evidence based treatments for* trauma-related psychological disorders (pp. 125–142). Cham, Switzerland: Springer International Publishing.

Burnett, L. B. (2018). Domestic violence. *eMedicine*. Retrieved from http://emedicine.medscape.com/article/805546-overview.

Canadian Association of Perinatal and Women's Health Nurses (CAPWHN). (2017). *Position Statement on Cultural Safety/Humility*. Ottawa: Author. Retrieved from http://www.capwhn.ca/uploads/documents//CAPWHN_Position_Statement_on_Cultural_Safety_Humility_Final.pdf

Canadian Domestic Homicide Prevention Initiative. (2015). *Risk assessment, risk management and safety planning*. Retrieved from http://www.learningtoendabuse.ca/cdhpi/risk-assessment-risk-management-and-safety-planning.

Cannon, C., & Buttell, F. (2015). Illusion of inclusion: The failure of the gender paradigm to account for intimate partner violence in LGBT relationships. *Partner Abuse, 6*(1), 65–70.

Cater, Å. K., Miller, L. E., Howell, K. H., & Graham-Bermann, S. A. (2015). Childhood exposure to intimate partner violence and adult mental health problems: Relationships with gender and age of exposure. *Journal of Family Violence, 30*(7), 875–886.

Centers for Disease Control & Prevention (CDC). (2014). *CDC grand rounds: A public health approach to prevention of intimate partner violence*. Retrieved from https://www.cdc.gov/mmwr/preview/mmwrhtml/mm6302a4.htm?s_cid=mm6302a4_w.

Centers for Disease Control & Prevention (CDC). (2017a). *Understanding intimate partner violence: Fact sheet*. Retrieved from https://www.cdc.gov/violenceprevention/pdf/ipv-factsheet.pdf.

Centers for Disease Control and Prevention (CDC). (2017b). *Preventing partner violence*. Retrieved from https://www.cdc.gov/violenceprevention/pdf/ipv-factsheet.pdf.

Centers for Disease Control & Prevention (CDC). (2017c). *Intimate partner violence: Risk and protective factors*. Retrieved from http://www.cdc.gov/violenceprevention/intimatepartnerviolence/riskprotectivefactors.html.

Centers for Disease Control and Prevention (CDC). (2017d). *Preventing intimate partner violence across the lifespan: A technical package of programs, policies, and practices*. Retrieved from https://www.cdc.gov/violenceprevention/pdf/ipv-technicalpackages.pdf.

Centers for Disease Control and Prevention (CDC). (2017e). *Preventing sexual violence*. Retrieved from https://www.cdc.gov/violenceprevention/pdf/SV-Factsheet.pdf.

Chang, J. C. (2015). Domestic violence: Epidemiology and risk factors. In E. J. Bieber, J. S. Sanfilippo, I. R. Horowitz, & M. I. Shafi (Eds.). *Clinical gynecology* (2nd ed., pp. 94–101), Cambridge, UK: Cambridge University Press.

Conroy, S., & Cotter, A. (2017). *Self-reported sexual assault in Canada, 2014. Catalogue no. 85-002-X*. Ottawa: Statistics Canada. Retrieved from https://www150.statcan.gc.ca/n1/en/pub/85-002-x/2017001/article/14842-eng.pdf?st=bK3tSvi5

Copelon, R. (2015). Violence against women: The potential and challenge of a human rights perspective. *Women's Health Journal*, (2–3), 62–67.

Creighton, S. M. (2015). Female genital mutilation (FGM) and the lower urinary tract. *International Journal of Urological Nursing, 9*(2), 69–73.

Daoud, N., Urquia, M. L., O'Campo, P., Heaman, M., Janssen, P., Smylie, J., & Thiessen, K. (2012). Prevalence of abuse and violence before, during, and after pregnancy in a national sample of Canadian women. *American Journal of Public Health, 102*(10), 1893–1901.

Darnell, D., Peterson, R., Berliner, L., Stewart, T., Russo, J., Whiteside, L., & Zatzick, D. (2015). Factors associated with follow-up attendance among rape victims seen in acute medical care. *Psychiatry, 78*(1), 89–101.

de Jong, R., Alink, L., Bijleveld, C., Finkenauer, C., & Hendriks, J. (2015). Transition to adulthood of child sexual abuse victims. *Aggression and Violent Behavior, 24*, 175–187.

Domestic Violence Organization. (2015a). *Common myths and why they are wrong*. Retrieved from http://www.domesticviolence.org/common-myths/

Domestic Violence Organization. (2015b). *Cycle of violence*. Retrieved from http://www.domesticviolence.org/cycle-of-violence/

Dorland, W. A. N. (2015). *Dorland's dictionary of medical acronyms & abbreviations* (7th ed.). Philadelphia, PA: Elsevier Health Sciences.

Dutton, M. A. (2015). Mindfulness-based stress reduction for underserved trauma populations. In *Mindfulness-oriented interventions for trauma: Integrating contemplative practices (Chapter 15)*. New York: The Guilford Press.

Edwards, K. M., Sylaska, K. M., & Neal, A. M. (2015). Intimate partner violence among sexual minority populations: A critical review of the literature and agenda for future research. *Psychology of Violence, 5*(2), 112–121.

Farage, M. A., Miller, K. W., Tzeghai, G. E., Azuka, C. E., Sobel, J. D., & Ledger, W. J. (2015). Female genital cutting: Confronting cultural challenges and health complications across the lifespan. *Women's Health, 11*(1), 79–94.

Federal Bureau of Investigation (FBI). (2015). *Intimate partner violence*. Retrieved from http://www.justice.gov/usao-cdca/victimwitness/domestic-violence-laws.

First Nations Health Authority. (2017). *All regulated health professions commit to a safer health system for First Nations and Aboriginal People*. Retrieved from http://www.fnha.ca/about/news-and-events/news/health-regulators-commit-to-cultural-safety

Focht & National Center for Health Research. (2018). *The cycle of domestic violence*. Retrieved from http://www.center4research.org/cycle-domestic-violence/.

Friedman, M. J. (2015). Overview of posttraumatic stress disorder (PTSD). In *Posttraumatic and acute stress disorders* (pp. 1–8). Springer International Publishing.

Gayle, C. M., & Rymer, J. M. (2015). Female genital mutilation. In E. J. Bieber, J. S. Sanfilippo, I. R. Horowitz, & M. I. Shafi (Eds.). *Clinical gynecology* (2nd ed., pp. 102–111). Cambridge, UK: Cambridge University Press.

Ghandour, R. M., Campbell, J. C., & Lloyd, J. (2015). Screening and counseling for intimate partner violence: A vision for the future. *Journal of Women's Health, 24*(1), 57–61.

Greenbaum, J., Crawford-Jakubiak, J. E., Christian, C. W., Flaherty, E. G., Leventhal, J. M., Lukefahr, J. L., . . . Hurley, T. P. (2015). Child sex trafficking and commercial sexual exploitation: Health care needs of victims. *Pediatrics, 135*(3), 566–574.

Gruenbaum, E., & Wirtz, E. (2015). Female genital cutting debates. *The International Encyclopedia of Human Sexuality*. (Online 4/20/15).

Harkins, G. (2015). Incest. *The International Encyclopedia of Human Sexuality.* 583–625.

Hewitt, L. N. (2015). Intimate partner violence: The role of nurses in protection of patients. *Critical Care Nursing Clinics of North America, 27*(2), 271–275.

Holtz, H., & Furniss, K. K. (1993). The health care provider's role in domestic violence. *Trends in Health Care Law and Ethics, 15*, 519–522.

Huang, C. C., Vikse, J. H., Lu, S., & Yi, S. (2015). Children's exposure to intimate partner violence and early delinquency. *Journal of Family Violence, 30*(8), 953–965.

International Association of Forensic Nurses. (2017). *Sexual assault nurse examiners.* Retrieved from http://www.forensicnurses.org/?page=aboutsane

Jackson, A. M., & Deye, K. (2015). Aspects of abuse: Consequences of childhood victimization. *Current Problems in Pediatric and Adolescent Health Care, 45*(3), 86–93.

Johnsdotter, S. (2015). Genital cutting, female. *The International Encyclopedia of Human Sexuality.* doi: 10.1002/9781118896877.wbiehs180

Joint Commission. (2015). *The Joint Commission accreditation manual for hospitals.* Chicago, IL: Author.

Keygnaert, I., Vettenburg, N., & Temmerman, M. (2015). Hidden violence is silent rape. *Culture, Health and Sexuality: An Introduction*, 189–206.

Kilmartin, C. (2015). Men's violence against women: An overview. In *Religion and Men's Violence against Women* (pp. 15–25). New York: Springer Publishers.

Klaus, W., Buczkowski, K., & Wiktorska, P. (2015). Empowering the victims of crime: A real goal of the criminal justice system or no more than a pipe dream?. In *Trust and Legitimacy in Criminal Justice* (pp. 65–91). Springer International Publishing.

Lawrence, D. (2015). Breaking the cycle of violence. *Nursing Standard, 29*, 18–21.

Lawson, D. M. (2015). *Family violence: Explanations and evidence-based clinical practice.* Hoboken, NJ: John Wiley & Sons.

Lévesque, S., & Chamberland, C. (2016). Intimate partner violence among pregnant young women: A qualitative inquiry. *Journal of Interpersonal Violence, 31*, 3282–3301.

Lomborg, B. (2015) *Why domestic violence costs more than war. World Economic Forum.* Retrieved from https://agenda.weforum.org/2015/09/domestic-violence-cost-war-development-goals/

MacGregor, K. E., Villalta, L., Clarke, V., Viner, R. M., Kramer, T., & Khadr, S. N. (2015). G146 A systematic review of mental health outcomes in young people following sexual assault. *Archives of Disease in Childhood, 100*(Suppl 3), A63.

Mauri, E. M., Nespoli, A., Persico, G., & Zobbi, V. F. (2015). Domestic violence during pregnancy: Midwives' experiences. *Midwifery, 31*(5), 498–504.

Medicine Net. (2016). *Domestic violence.* Retrieved from http://www.medicinenet.com/domestic_violence/page4.htm#what_are_the_causes_or_risk_factors_for_intimate_partner_violence

Morrill, M. (2014). Sibling sexual abuse: An exploratory study of long term consequences for self-esteem and counseling considerations. *Journal of Family Violence, 29*(2), 205–213.

Murray, C. E., Horton, G. E., Johnson, C. H., Notestine, L., Garr, B., Pow, A. M., . . . Doom, E. (2015). Domestic violence service providers' perceptions of safety planning: A focus group study. *Journal of Family Violence, 30*(3), 381–392.

Nacasch, N., Rachamim, L., & Foa, E. B. (2015). Prolonged exposure treatment. In M. P. Safir, H. S. Wallach, & A. Skip Rizzo (Eds.). *Future directions in post-traumatic stress disorder* (pp. 245–251). Philadelphia, PA: Springer Publishers.

National Center for Victims of Crime (NCVC). (2015a). *Incest.* Retrieved from http://www.victimsofcrime.org/

National Center for Victims of Crime (NCVC). (2015b). *The trauma of victimization.* Retrieved from http://victimsofcrime.org/help-for-crime-victims/get-help-bulletins-for-crime-victims/trauma-of-victimization#ptsd

National Center on Elder Abuse. (2017). *Research: Statistics/data.* Retrieved from https://ncea.acl.gov/whatwedo/research/statistics.html

National Coalition Against Domestic Violence. (2015). Fact sheet: National Statistics. Retrieved from http://www.ncadv.org/learn/statistics

Nour, N. M. (2015). Female genital cutting: Impact on women's health. *Seminars in Reproductive Medicine, 33*(1), 41–46.

Policastro, C., & Finn, M. A. (2017). Coercive control and physical violence in older adults: Analysis using data from the National Elder Mistreatment Study. *Journal of Interpersonal Violence, 32*, 311–330.

Prosman, G. J., Lo Fo Wong, S. H., van der Wouden, J. C., & Lagro-Janssen, A. L. (2015). Effectiveness of home visiting in reducing partner violence for families experiencing abuse: A systematic review. *Family Practice, 32*, 247–256.

Public Health Agency of Canada (PHAC). (2015). *Find services in your area: Family violence prevention services.* Retrieved from https://www.canada.ca/en/public-health/services/health-promotion/stop-family-violence/services.html

Public Health Agency of Canada (PHAC). (2016). *The chief public health officer's report on the state of public Health in Canada: A focus on family violence in Canada.* (Publication: 160152). Retrieved from https://www.canada.ca/en/public-health/services/publications/chief-public-health-officer-reports-state-public-health-canada/2016-focus-family-violence-canada.html

Public Safety Canada. (2018). *National consultations discussion paper: The way forward to end human trafficking.* Retrieved from https://www.publicsafety.gc.ca/cnt/rsrcs/pblctns/wy-frwrd-nd-hmn-trffckng-ppr/index-en.aspx

Rape, Abuse, and Incest National Network (RAINN). (2018a). *Statistics.* Retrieved from https://www.rainn.org/statistics

Rape, Abuse, and Incest National Network (RAINN). (2018b). *Children and teens: Statistics.* Retrieved from https://www.rainn.org/statistics/children-and-teens

Rape, Abuse, and Incest National Network (RAINN). (2018c). *Sexual assault.* Retrieved from https://www.rainn.org/articles/sexual-assault

Rape, Abuse, and Incest National Network (RAINN). (2018d). *Recovery from sexual violence.* Retrieved from https://www.rainn.org/recovering-sexual-violence

Research Action and Information Network for the Bodily Integrity of Women (RAINBO). (2018). *Caring for women with circumcision: Fact sheet for physicians.* Retrieved from http://www.rainbo.org/factsheet.html

Russell, B., & Chapleau, K. (2015). When is it abuse? How assailant gender, sexual orientation, and protection orders influence perceptions of intimate partner abuse. *Partner Abuse, 6*(1), 47–64.

Sanchez, R., & Stark, S. (2014). The hard truth about human trafficking. *Nursing Management, 45*(1), 18–23.

Snapshot of Family Violence in Canada - Infographic. (2015). *Government of Canada*. Retrieved from https://www.canada.ca/en/public-health/services/health-promotion/stop-family-violence/snapshot-family-violence-canada-infographic.html

Society of Obstetricians and Gynecologist of Canada (SOGC). (2013). *Clinical practice guidelines: Female genital cutting*. Publication 299. Retrieved from https://sogc.org/wp-content/uploads/2013/10/gui299CPG1311E.pdf

Song, A., Wenzel, S. L., Kim, J. Y., & Nam, B. (2017). Experience of domestic violence during childhood, intimate partner violence, and the deterrent effect of awareness of legal consequences. *Journal of Interpersonal Violence, 32*, 357–372.

Sugg, N. (2015). Intimate partner violence: Prevalence, health consequences, and intervention. *Medical Clinics of North America, 99*(3), 629–649.

TahoeSafe Alliance. (2017). Myths about intimate partner violence in the LGBTQUA community. Retrieved from http://tahoesafealliance.org/for-lgbqtia/lgbtqiamyths/

Truth and Reconciliation Commission (TRC). (2015). *Truth and Reconciliation Commission of Canada: Calls to Action Report*. Retrieved from http://www.trc.ca/websites/trcinstitution/File/2015/Findings/Calls_to_Action_English2.pdf

United Nations Office on Drugs and Crime (UNODC). (2018). *Human trafficking*. Retrieved from http://www.unodc.org/unodc/en/human-trafficking/what-is-human-trafficking.html

U.S. Department of Health and Human Services (USDHHS). (2015a). *Date rape drugs fact sheet. National Women's Health Information Center*. Retrieved from http://www.womenshealth.gov/publications/our-publications/fact-sheet/date-rape-drugs.html

U.S. Department of Health and Human Services (USDHHS). (2015b). *Healthy People 2020*. Retrieved from http://www.healthypeople.gov/document/HTML/Volume2/15Injury.htm#_Toc490549392

U.S. Department of Health and Human Services (USDHHS). (2015c). Screening for domestic violence in health care settings. *Office of the Assistant Secretary for Planning and Evaluation*. Retrieved from http://aspe.hhs.gov/hsp/13/dv/pb_screeningdomestic.cfm

U.S. Department of State. (2018). *What is modern slavery?*. Retrieved from http://www.state.gov/j/tip/what/index.htm

Victims of Trafficking and Violence Protection Act of 2000. (2000). *Pub. Law No. 106–386 [H.R. 3244] (2000)*. Retrieved from http://ojp.gov/vawo/laws/vawo2000/stitle_a.htm

Wang, X. M., Brisbin, S., Loo, T., & Straus, S. (2015). Elder abuse: An approach to identification, assessment and intervention. *Canadian Medical Association Journal, 187*(8), 575–581.

Weitzer, R. (2015). Human trafficking and contemporary slavery. *Annual Review of Sociology, 41*(1), 223–242. Retrieved from https://www.annualreviews.org/doi/abs/10.1146/annurev-soc-073014-112506

WELLWVU The Student's Center of Health. (2018). *Rape myths*. Retrieved from https://well.wvu.edu/resources/sexual-assault/rape-myths

Wilson, L. C., & Miller, K. E. (2016). Meta-analysis of the prevalence of unacknowledged rape. *Trauma, Violence, & Abuse, 17*, 149–159. (Online 3/17/15).

Women Against Violence Against Women (WAVAW). (2015). *Rape myths*. Retrieved from http://www.wavaw.ca/mythbusting/rape-myths/

World Health Organization (WHO). (2017). *Violence against women*. Retrieved from http://www.who.int/en/news-room/fact-sheets/detail/violence-against-women

World Health Organization (WHO). (2018). *Female genital mutilation*. Retrieved from http://www.who.int/news-room/fact-sheets/detail/female-genital-mutilation

CHAPTER **WORKSHEET**

MULTIPLE CHOICE QUESTIONS

1. The primary goal of intervention in working with abused women is to:
   a. Set up an appointment with a mental health counsellor for the victim
   b. Convince them to set up a safety plan to use when they leave
   c. Help them to develop courage and financial support to leave the abuser
   d. Empower them and improve their self-esteem to regain control of their lives

2. The first phase of the abuse cycle is characterized by:
   a. The woman provoking the abuser to bring about battering
   b. Tension building and verbal or minor battery
   c. A honeymoon period that lulls the victim into forgetting
   d. An acute episode of physical battering

3. Women recovering from abusive relationships need to learn ways to improve their:
   a. Educational level by getting a college degree
   b. Earning power so they can move to a better neighbourhood
   c. Self-esteem and communication skills to increase assertiveness
   d. Relationship skills so they will be better prepared to deal with their partners

4. Which of the following statements might empower abuse victims to take action?
   a. "You deserve better than this."
   b. "Your children deserve to grow up in a two-parent family."
   c. "Try to figure out what you do to trigger his abuse and stop it."
   d. "Give your partner more time to come to his senses about this."

5. If a woman thinks she is being stalked when driving, a good safety measure is to:
   a. Drive to a local police or fire department
   b. Take short cuts through back streets to lose them
   c. Wave a handgun to intimidate them
   d. Roll down her window and confront them

6. Nurses play an important role in screening and assessment of any client for abuse/violence. Which of the following statements is correct?
   a. Most clients are extremely reluctant to come forth with private matters.
   b. Any intimate partner violence questions should be asked in the presence of both partners.
   c. To invite disclosure, assure the woman that you won't document her statements.
   d. The best statement to make to the abused victim is: "You don't deserve this."

7. What should the nurse do if a victim of intimate partner violence chooses not to disclose information about her abusive relationship during your interview?
   a. Confront the victim with the physical evidence and telltale signs of abuse
   b. Contact family members to tell you about their abusive relationship
   c. Call the local police department to inquire about domestic disturbance calls
   d. Respect the client's right of self-determination and provide her with resources

CRITICAL THINKING EXERCISE

1. Mrs. Boggs has three children under the age of 5 and is 6 months pregnant with her fourth child. She has made repeated unscheduled visits to your clinic with vague somatic complaints regarding the children as well as herself but has missed several scheduled prenatal appointments. On occasion she has worn sunglasses to cover bruises around her eyes. As a nurse you sense there is something else bothering her, but she doesn't seem to want to discuss it with you. She appears sad and the children cling to her.
   a. Outline your conversation when you broach the subject of abuse with Mrs. Boggs.
   b. What is your role as a nurse in caring for a family in which you suspect abuse is occurring?
   c. What ethical/legal considerations are important in planning care for this family?

STUDY ACTIVITIES

1. Research the statistics about violence against women in your province. Are law enforcement and community interventions reducing the incidence of sexual assault and intimate partner violence?

2. Attend a dorm orientation at a local university to hear about measures in place to protect women's safety on campus. Find out the number of sexual assaults reported and what strategies the college uses to reduce this number.

3. Interview a local police officer, RCMP officer, or 911 dispatch operator about the frequency and trends of domestic violence calls.

4. Identify three community resources that could be useful to a victim of violence. Identify their sources of funding and the services they provide.

BRINGING IT ALL TOGETHER: A CASE STUDY

A 23-year-old pregnant female presents to the public health maternity clinic for the third time in a month with a myriad of vague complaints including insomnia, diffuse body aches and pains, poor appetite, fatigue, and constipation. This is her first pregnancy, and it was unplanned. Her recent obstetrical examination and laboratory survey are within normal limits. Her past medical history notes anxiety and depression. According to the client, she does not drink or smoke. She does not work outside of the home.

ASSESSMENT

On physical examination the nurse notes a well-dressed, pleasant, but anxious young female. Her husband of a year usually accompanies her to the office visits, but is absent today. She tends to avoid eye contact with the nurse when asked questions about her symptoms. Her vital signs and fetal heart rate are all within the normal range. On further examination, the nurse notices several bruises on her upper arms and thighs. When questioned about these marks, the client looks away.

QUESTIONS

1. Based on her frequent visits and diversity of symptoms with no abnormal findings, what might the nurse suspect?

2. What makes this woman vulnerable to IPV?

3. If she is experiencing abuse, what are the health consequences of it?

PLAN

1. What is the next step for the nurse in managing this client?

2. What information does the nurse need to know prior to questioning this client?

3. What important resource for abused clients is vital to inform her about for help?

4. What message does the nurse need to convey to any abused client?

Pregnancy

10

Fetal Development and Genetics

Learning Objectives

Upon completion of the chapter, you will be able to:

1. Characterize the process of fertilization, implantation, and cell differentiation.
2. Examine the functions of the placenta, umbilical cord, and amniotic fluid.
3. Outline normal fetal development from conception through birth.
4. Compare the various inheritance patterns, including nontraditional patterns of inheritance.
5. Analyze examples of ethical and legal issues surrounding genetic testing.
6. Research the role of the nurse in genetic counselling and genetic-related activities.

Robert and Kate Shafer have just received the good news that Kate's pregnancy test is positive. It had been a long and anxious 3 years of trying to start a family. Although both are elated about the prospect of becoming parents, they are concerned about the possibility of a genetic problem because Kate is 38 years old. What might be their first step in looking into their genetic concern? As a nurse, what might raise concerns for you?

INTRODUCTION

Human reproduction is one of the most intimate spheres of an individual's life. For conception to occur, a healthy ovum is released from the ovary, passes into an open fallopian tube, and starts its journey downward. Sperm is deposited into the vagina and swims approximately 7 in to meet the ovum at the outermost portion of the fallopian tube, the area where fertilization takes place. This process occurs in about an hour (Solomon, 2015). When one spermatozoon penetrates the ovum's thick outer membrane, pregnancy begins. All this activity may take place within a 5-hour time span.

Nurses caring for the childbearing family need to have a basic understanding of conception and prenatal development so they can identify problems or variations and can initiate appropriate interventions should any problems occur. This chapter presents an overview of fetal development, beginning with conception. It also discusses hereditary influences on fetal development and the nurse's role in genetic counselling.

FETAL DEVELOPMENT

Fetal development during pregnancy is measured in number of weeks after fertilization. The duration of pregnancy is about 40 weeks from the time of fertilization. This equates to 9 calendar months or approximately 266 to 280 calendar days. The three stages of fetal development during pregnancy are:

1. **Preembryonic stage:** fertilization through the second week
2. **Embryonic stage:** end of the second week through the eighth week
3. **Fetal stage:** end of the eighth week until birth

Fetal circulation is a significant aspect of fetal development that spans all three stages.

Preembryonic Stage

The preembryonic stage begins with fertilization, also called *conception*. **Fertilization** is the union of ovum and sperm, which is the starting point of pregnancy. Fertilization typically occurs around 2 weeks after the last normal menstrual period in a 28-day cycle (Mader & Windelspecht, 2015). Fertilization requires a timely interaction between the release of the mature ovum at ovulation and the ejaculation of enough healthy, mobile sperm to survive the hostile vaginal environment through which they must travel to meet the ovum. All things considered, the act of conception is difficult at best. To say merely that it occurs when the sperm unites with the ovum is overly simple because this union requires an intricate interplay of hormonal preparation and overcoming an overwhelming number of natural

barriers. A human being is truly an amazing outcome of this elaborate process.

Prior to fertilization, the ovum and the spermatozoon undergo the process of meiosis. The primary oocyte completes its first meiotic division before ovulation. The secondary oocyte begins its second meiotic division just before ovulation. Primary and secondary spermatocytes undergo meiotic division while still in the testes (Fig. 10.1).

Although more than 200 million sperm/mL are contained in the ejaculated semen, only one is able to enter the ovum to fertilize it. All others are blocked by the clear protein layer called the **zona pellucida.** The zona pellucida disappears in about 5 days. Once the sperm reaches the plasma membrane, the ovum resumes meiosis and forms a nucleus with half the number of chromosomes (23). When the nucleus from the ovum and the nucleus of the sperm make contact, they lose their respective nuclear membranes and combine their collective chromosomes. Because each nucleus contains a haploid number of chromosomes (23), this union restores the diploid number (46). The resulting zygote begins the process of a new life. The genetic information from both ovum and sperm establishes the unique physical characteristics of the individual. Sex determination is also determined at fertilization and depends on whether the ovum is fertilized by a Y-bearing sperm or an X-bearing sperm. Approximately half of the sperm carry the XX chromosome and the other half carries XY. An XX zygote will become genetically female and an XY zygote will become genetically male (Fig. 10.2). That is why it is scientifically correct to say that the sex of the infant is determined by the sperm and not by the ovum.

Fertilization takes place in the outer third of the ampulla of the fallopian tube. When the ovum is fertilized by the sperm (now called a **zygote**), a great deal of activity immediately takes place. Mitosis, or *cleavage,* occurs as the zygote is slowly transported into the uterine cavity by tubal muscular movements (Fig. 10.3). After a series of 4 cleavages, the 16 cells appear as a solid ball of cells, or **morula,** meaning "little mulberry." The morula reaches the uterine cavity about 72 hours after fertilization. As fluid from the uterine cavity, which provides nutrients, enters the morula, the blastocyst is formed (Mader & Windelspecht, 2015).

With additional cell division, the morula divides into specialized cells that will later form fetal structures. Within the morula, an off-centre, fluid-filled space appears, transforming it into a hollow ball of cells called a **blastocyst** (Fig. 10.4). The inner surface of the blastocyst will form the embryo and amnion. The outer layer of cells surrounding the blastocyst cavity is called a **trophoblast.** Eventually, the trophoblast develops into one of the embryonic membranes, the chorion, and helps to form the placenta.

At this time, the developing blastocyst needs more food and oxygen to keep growing. The trophoblast

FIGURE 10.1 The formation of gametes by the process of meiosis is known as gametogenesis. **A.** Spermatogenesis. One spermatogonium gives rise to four spermatozoa. **B.** Oogenesis. From each oogonium, one mature ovum and three abortive cells are produced. The chromosomes are reduced to one half the number characteristic for the general body cells of the species. In humans, the number in the body cells is 46, and that in the mature spermatozoon and secondary oocyte is 23.

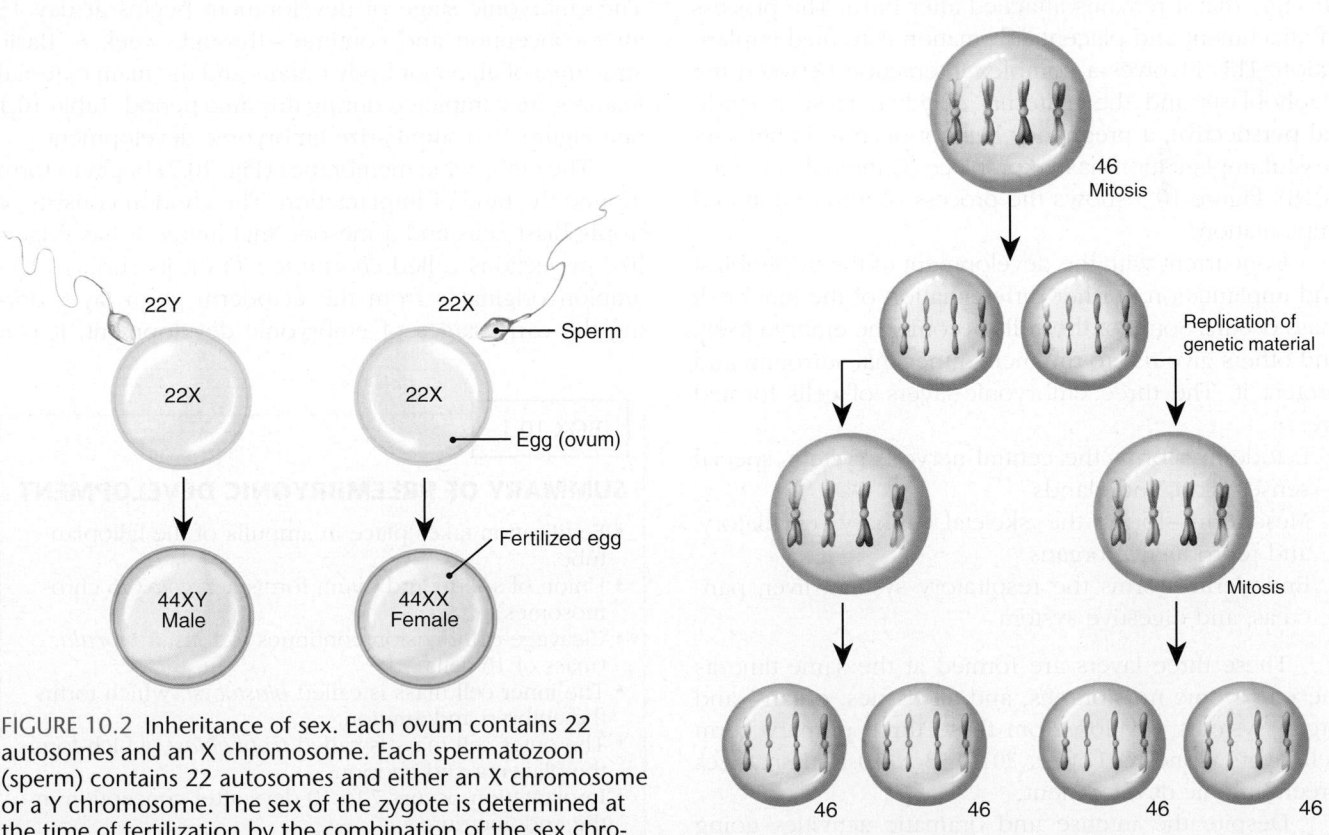

FIGURE 10.2 Inheritance of sex. Each ovum contains 22 autosomes and an X chromosome. Each spermatozoon (sperm) contains 22 autosomes and either an X chromosome or a Y chromosome. The sex of the zygote is determined at the time of fertilization by the combination of the sex chromosomes of the sperm (either X or Y) and the ovum (X).

FIGURE 10.3 Mitosis of the stoma cells.

FIGURE 10.4 **A.** Fertilized human egg (zygote) having reached the blastocyst stage. Zygote contains 20 to 30 eggs and a fluid-filled blastocele is beginning to form. **B.** Implantation. Stylized image showing a frontal view of a uterus with a blastocyst about to implant into endometrium of the uterus. (Images from LifeART image copyright (c) 2011 Lippincott Williams & Wilkins. All rights reserved.)

attaches itself to the surface of the endometrium for further nourishment. Normally, implantation occurs in the upper uterus (fundus), where a rich blood supply is available. This area also contains strong muscular fibers, which clamp down on blood vessels after the placenta separates from the inner wall of the uterus. Additionally, the lining is thickest here so the placenta cannot attach so strongly that it remains attached after birth. The process of attachment and placental formation is termed implantation. This involves a complex interaction between the trophoblasts and the maternal decidua. From a medical perspective, a pregnancy has not occurred until successful implantation has taken place (Cunningham et al., 2018). Figure 10.5 shows the process of fertilization and implantation.

Concurrent with the development of the trophoblast and implantation, further differentiation of the inner cell mass occurs. Some of the cells become the embryo itself, and others give rise to the membranes that surround and protect it. The three embryonic layers of cells formed are:

1. Ectoderm—forms the central nervous system, special senses, skin, and glands
2. Mesoderm—forms the skeletal, urinary, circulatory, and reproductive organs
3. Endoderm—forms the respiratory system, liver, pancreas, and digestive system

These three layers are formed at the same time as the embryonic membranes, and all tissues, organs, and organ systems develop from these three primary germ cell layers (Jones & Lopez, 2014). Box 10.1 summarizes preembryonic development.

Despite the intense and dramatic activities going on internally to create a human life, many childbearing individuals are unaware that pregnancy has begun. Several weeks will pass before even one of the presumptive signs of pregnancy—missing the first menstrual period—will take place.

Embryonic Stage

The embryonic stage of development begins at day 15 after conception and continues through week 8. Basic structures of all major body organs and the main external features are completed during this time period. Table 10.1 and Figure 10.6 summarize embryonic development.

The embryonic membranes (Fig. 10.7) begin to form around the time of implantation. The chorion consists of trophoblast cells and a mesodermal lining. It has finger-like projections called *chorionic villi* on its surface. The amnion originates from the ectoderm germ layer during the early stages of embryonic development. It is a

---

BOX 10.1

SUMMARY OF PREEMBRYONIC DEVELOPMENT

- Fertilization takes place in ampulla of the fallopian tube.
- Union of sperm and ovum forms a *zygote* (46 chromosomes).
- Cleavage cell division continues to form a *morula* (mass of 16 cells).
- The inner cell mass is called *blastocyst,* which forms the embryo and amnion.
- The outer cell mass is called *trophoblast,* which forms the placenta and chorion.
- Implantation occurs 7 to 10 days after conception in the endometrium.

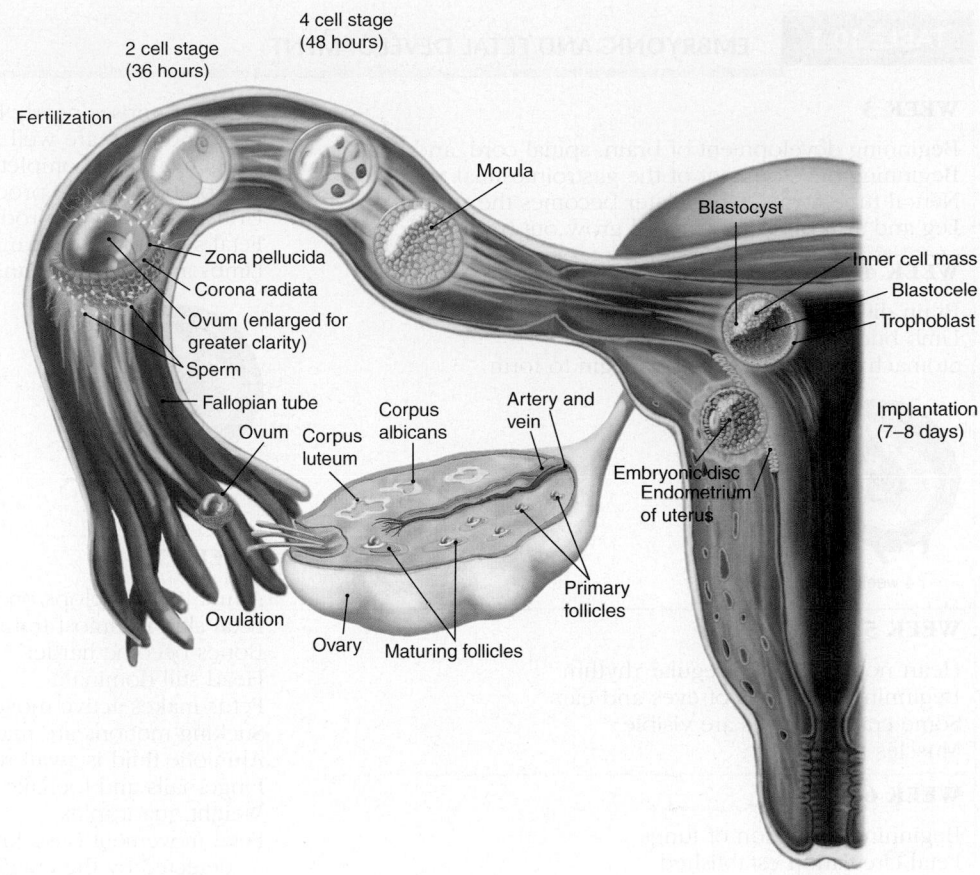

2 cell stage
(36 hours)

4 cell stage
(48 hours)

Fertilization

Morula

Blastocyst

Inner cell mass

Blastocele

Trophoblast

Zona pellucida

Corona radiata

Ovum (enlarged for greater clarity)

Sperm

Fallopian tube

Ovum

Corpus luteum

Corpus albicans

Artery and vein

Implantation (7–8 days)

Embryonic disc

Endometrium of uterus

Primary follicles

Ovulation

Ovary   Maturing follicles

FIGURE 10.5 Fertilization and tubal transport of the zygote. From fertilization to implantation, the zygote travels through the fallopian tube, experiencing rapid mitotic division (cleavage). During the journey toward the uterus the zygote evolves through several stages, including morula and blastocyst.

thin protective membrane that contains amniotic fluid. As the embryo grows, the amnion (inner layer) expands until it touches the chorion (outer layer). These two fetal membranes form the fluid-filled amniotic sac, or bag of waters, that protects the floating embryo (Cunningham et al., 2018).

Amniotic fluid surrounds the embryo and increases in volume as the pregnancy progresses, reaching approximately 1 L at term. Amniotic fluid is derived from two sources: fluid transported from the maternal blood across the amnion and fetal urine. Its volume changes constantly as the fetus swallows and voids. Sufficient amounts of amniotic fluid help maintain a constant body temperature for the fetus, permit symmetric growth and development, cushion the fetus from trauma, allow the umbilical cord to be relatively free from compression,

A

B

C

FIGURE 10.6 Embryonic development. **A.** 4-week embryo. **B.** 5-week embryo. **C.** 6-week embryo.

TABLE 10.1   EMBRYONIC AND FETAL DEVELOPMENT

WEEK 3

Beginning development of brain, spinal cord, and heart
Beginning development of the gastrointestinal tract
Neural tube forms, which later becomes the spinal cord
Leg and arm buds appear and grow out from body

WEEK 4

Brain differentiates
Limb buds grow and develop more
Stomach, pancreas, and liver begin to form

4 weeks

WEEK 5

Heart now beats at a regular rhythm
Beginning structures of eyes and ears
Some cranial nerves are visible
Muscles innervated

WEEK 6

Beginning formation of lungs
Fetal circulation established
Liver produces RBCs
Further development of the brain
Primitive skeleton forms
Central nervous system forms
Brain waves detectable

WEEK 7

Straightening of trunk
Nipples and hair follicles form
Elbows and toes visible
Arms and legs move
Diaphragm formed
Fetal heartbeat can be heard
Mouth with lips and early tooth buds

WEEK 8

Rotation of intestines
Facial features continue to develop
Heart development complete
Resembles a human being (Mattson & Smith, 2015).

8 weeks

WEEKS 9–12

Sexual differentiation continues
Buds for all 20 temporary teeth laid down
Digestive system shows activity

Head comprises nearly half the fetus size
Face and neck are well formed
Urogenital tract completes development
Red blood cells are produced in the liver
Urine begins to be produced and excreted
Fetal sex can be determined by week 12
Limbs are long and thin; digits are well formed

12 weeks

WEEKS 13–16

A fine hair develops on the head called lanugo
Fetal skin is almost transparent
Bones become harder
Head still dominant
Fetus makes active movement
Sucking motions are made with the mouth
Amniotic fluid is swallowed
Fingernails and toenails present
Weight quadruples
Fetal movement (also known as quickening) may be
    detected by the childbearing person

16 weeks

WEEKS 17–20

Rapid brain growth occurs
Fetal heart tones can be heard with stethoscope
Kidneys continue to secret urine into amniotic fluid
Vernix caseosa, a white greasy film, covers the fetus
Eyebrows and head hair appear
Sebaceous glands appear
Brown fat deposited to help maintain temperature
Nails are present on both fingers and toes
Muscles are well developed

20 weeks

TABLE 10.1   EMBRYONIC AND FETAL DEVELOPMENT (continued)

WEEKS 21–24

Eyebrows and eyelashes are well formed
Fetus has a hand grasp and startle reflex
Alveoli forming in lungs
Body is lean but fairly well proportioned
Skin is translucent and red
Lungs begin to produce surfactant

25 weeks

WEEKS 25–28

Fetus reaches a length of 15 in
Rapid brain development
Eyelids open and close
Nervous system controls some functions
Fingerprints are set
Blood formation shifts from spleen to bone marrow
Fetus usually assumes head-down position

28 weeks

WEEKS 29–32

Rapid increase in amount of body fat
Increased central nervous system control over body
  functions
Rhythmic practice breathing movements occur
Lungs are not fully mature
Fetus stores iron, calcium, and phosphorus

32 weeks

WEEKS 33–38

Testes are in scrotum of male fetus
Lanugo begins to disappear
Increase in body fat
Fingernails reach the ends of fingertips
Small breast buds are present on both sexes
Fetus receives antibodies against disease from the
  childbearing person
Fetus is considered full term at 38 weeks
Fetus fills uterus (El-Mazny, 2014)

37 weeks

and promote fetal movement to enhance musculoskeletal development. Amniotic fluid is composed of 98% water and 2% organic matter. It is slightly alkaline and contains albumin, urea, bile pigments, renin, glucose, hormones, uric acid, creatinine, bilirubin, lecithin, sphingomyelin, epithelial cells, vernix, and fine hair called lanugo. The composition of amniotic fluid changes with gestation. Adequate amniotic fluid volume is necessary for proper fetal growth and development (Magann & Ross, 2018).

The volume of amniotic fluid is important in determining fetal well-being. It gradually fluctuates throughout the pregnancy. Alterations in amniotic fluid volume can be associated with problems in the fetus. Too little amniotic fluid (<500 mL at term), termed *oligohydramnios,* is associated with uteroplacental insufficiency, fetal renal abnormalities, and a higher risk of surgical births and low birth weight infants. Too much amniotic fluid (>2,000 mL at term), termed *polyhydramnios,* is associated with maternal diabetes, neural tube defects, chromosomal deviations, and malformations of the central nervous system and/or gastrointestinal tract that prevent normal swallowing of amniotic fluid by the fetus. Polyhydramnios may threaten premature rupture of membranes due to uterine over distention (Moore, 2015).

FIGURE 10.7 **A.** The embryo is floating in amniotic fluid, surrounded by the protective fetal membranes (amnion and chorion). **B.** Longitudinal sonogram of a pregnant uterus at 11 weeks showing the intrauterine gestational sac (*black arrowheads*) and the amniotic cavity (AC) filled with amniotic fluid; the fetus is seen in longitudinal section with the head (H) and coccyx (C) well displayed. The myometrium (MY) of the uterus can be identified. (*Figure B is courtesy of L Scoutt.*)

While the placenta is developing (beginning at the end of the second week), the **umbilical cord** is also formed from the amnion. It is the lifeline to the growing embryo. It contains one large vein and two small arteries. Wharton's jelly (a specialized connective tissue) surrounds these three blood vessels in the umbilical cord to prevent compression, which would cut off fetal blood and nutrient supply. The cord reaches its maximum length by 30 weeks of gestation. Its length is determined by genetics and intrauterine space and fetal activity, which places tension on the cord. At term, the average umbilical cord is 56 cm (22 in) long and 2 to 3 cm (1 in) wide (King et al., 2015).

The precursor cells of the placenta—the trophoblasts—first appear 4 days after fertilization as the outer layer of cells of the blastocyst. These early blastocyst trophoblasts differentiate into all the cells that form the placenta. When fully developed, the **placenta** serves as the interface between the childbearing person and the developing fetus. As early as 3 days after conception, the trophoblasts make human chorionic gonadotropin (hCG), a hormone that ensures that the endometrium will be receptive to the implanting embryo. During the next few weeks the placenta begins to make hormones that control the basic physiology of the childbearing person in such a way that the fetus is supplied with the

nutrients and oxygen needed for growth. The placenta also protects the fetus from immune attack by the childbearing person, removes waste products from the fetus, induces the childbearing person to bring more food to the placenta and, near the time of childbirth, produces hormones that ready fetal organs for life outside the uterus. Placenta function depends on the maternal blood pressure supplying circulation. If there is an interference with blood flow to the placenta, it cannot carry out its functions to the embryo or fetus (Mattson & Smith, 2015).

Theoretically, at no time during pregnancy does the childbearing person's blood mix with fetal blood, because there is no direct contact between their bloods; layers of fetal tissue always separate the childbearing person's blood and the fetal blood. These fetal tissues are called the *placental barrier.* Materials can be interchanged only through diffusion. The uterine arteries deliver the nutrients to the placenta, which in turn provides nutrients to the developing fetus; the uterine veins carry fetal waste products away. The structure of the placenta is usually completed by week 12.

The placenta is not only a transfer organ but a hormone factory as well. Placental hormones have profound effects on the childbearing person's metabolism, initially building up energy reserves and then releasing these to support fetal growth in later pregnancy and lactation postnatally. Several hormones are produced that are necessary for normal pregnancy:

- hCG—preserves the corpus luteum and its progesterone production so that the endometrial lining of the uterus is maintained; this is the basis for pregnancy tests
- Human placental lactogen (hPL)—modulates the metabolism of the childbearing person and the fetus, participates in the development of breasts for lactation, and decreases the childbearing person's insulin sensitivity to increase its availability for fetal nutrition
- Estrogen (estriol)—causes enlargement of a childbearing person's breasts, uterus, and external genitalia; stimulates myometrial contractility
- Progesterone (progestin)—maintains the endometrium, decreases the contractility of the uterus, stimulates metabolism and breast development, provides nourishment for the early products of conception, or **conceptus**
- Relaxin—acts synergistically with progesterone to maintain pregnancy, causes relaxation of the pelvic ligaments, softens the cervix in preparation for birth (Freemark, 2015)

The placenta acts as a pass-through between the childbearing person and fetus, not a barrier. Almost everything the childbearing person ingests (food, alcohol, drugs) passes through to the developing conceptus. This is why it is so important to advise a pregnant person not to use unprescribed drugs, alcohol, and tobacco, because they can be harmful to the conceptus.

During the embryonic stage, the conceptus grows rapidly as all organs and structures are forming. During this critical period of differentiation, the growing embryo is most susceptible to damage from external sources, including **teratogens** (substances that cause birth defects, such as alcohol and drugs), infections (such as rubella or cytomegalovirus), radiation, and nutritional deficiencies.

Fetal Stage

The average pregnancy lasts 280 days from the first day of the last menstrual period. The fetal stage is the time from the end of the eighth week until birth. It is the longest period of prenatal development. During this stage, the conceptus is mature enough to be called a fetus. Although all major systems are present in their basic form, dramatic growth and refinement of all organ systems take place during the fetal period (see Table 10.1). Figure 10.8 depicts a 12- to 15-week-old fetus.

Fetal Circulation

Fetal circulation differs from adult circulation due to the presence of certain vessels and shunts. These shunts will close after birth and most of the vessels will be seen as remnants in the adult circulation. The function of these

FIGURE 10.8 Fetal development: 12- to 15-week fetus.

shunts is to direct oxygen-rich venous blood to the systemic circulation and to ensure that oxygen-depleted venous blood bypasses the underdeveloped pulmonary circulation. The lungs finish their development after birth. Prior to birth, the lungs' function is taken over by the placenta during fetal life (Finnemore & Groves, 2015). The circulation through the fetus during uterine life differs from that of a child or an adult. In the extrauterine world, oxygenation occurs in the lungs and oxygenated blood returns via the pulmonary veins to the left side of the heart to be ejected by the left ventricle into the systemic circulation. In contrast, fetal circulation oxygenation occurs in the placenta, and the fetal lungs are nonfunctional as far as the transfer of oxygen and carbon dioxide is concerned. For oxygenated blood derived from the placenta to reach the fetus's systemic circulation, it must travel through a series of shunts to accomplish this.

Thus, fetal circulation involves the circulation of blood from the placenta to and through the fetus, and back to the placenta. A properly functioning fetal circulation system is essential to sustain the fetus. Before it develops, nutrients and oxygen diffuse through the extraembryonic coelom and the yolk sac from the placenta. As the embryo grows, its nutrient needs increase and the amount of tissue easily reached by diffusion increases. Thus, the circulation must develop quickly and accurately (Jones & Lopez, 2014).

The circulatory system of the fetus functions much differently from that of a newborn. The most significant difference is that oxygen is received from the placenta during fetal life and via the lungs after birth. In addition, the fetal liver does not perform the metabolic functions that it will after birth because the pregnant body performs these functions. Three shunts also are present during fetal life:

1. Ductus venosus—connects the umbilical vein to the inferior vena cava
2. Ductus arteriosus—connects the main pulmonary artery to the aorta
3. Foramen ovale—anatomic opening between the right and left atrium

Take Note!

Fetal circulation functions to carry highly oxygen-ated blood to vital areas (e.g., heart, brain) while first shunting it away from less important ones (e.g., lungs, liver). The placenta essentially takes over the functions of the lungs and liver during fetal life. As a result, large volumes of oxygenated blood are not needed.

The oxygenated blood is carried from the placenta to the fetus via the umbilical vein. About half of this blood passes through the hepatic capillaries and the rest flows through the ductus venosus into the inferior vena cava. Blood from the vena cava is mostly deflected through the foramen ovale into the left atrium, then to the left ventricle, into the ascending aorta, and on to the head and upper body. This allows the fetal coronary circulation and the brain to receive the blood with the highest level of oxygenation.

Deoxygenated blood from the superior vena cava flows into the right atrium, the right ventricle, and then the pulmonary artery. Because of high pulmonary vascular resistance, only a small percentage (5% to 10%) of the blood in the pulmonary artery flows to the lungs; the majority is shunted through the patent ductus arteriosus and then to the descending aorta (American Heart Association, 2018). The fetal lungs are essentially nonfunctional because they are filled with fluid, making them resistant to incoming blood flow. They receive only enough blood for proper nourishment. Finally, two umbilical arteries carry the unoxygenated blood from the descending aorta back to the placenta.

At birth, a dramatic change in the fetal circulatory pattern occurs. The foramen ovale, ductus arteriosus, ductus venosus, and umbilical vessels are no longer needed. With the newborn's first breath, the lungs inflate, which leads to an increase in blood flow to the lungs from the right ventricle. This increase raises the pressure in the left atrium, causing a one-way flap on the left side of the foramen ovale, called the septum primum, to press against the opening, creating a functional separation between the two atria. Blood flow to the lungs increases because blood entering the right atrium can no longer bypass the right ventricle. As a result, the right ventricle pumps blood into the pulmonary artery and on to the lungs. Typically, the foramen ovale is functionally closed within 1 to 2 hours after birth. It is physiologically closed by 1 month with deposits of fibrin to seal the shunt. Permanent closure occurs by the sixth month of life.

The ductus venosus, which links the inferior vena cava with the umbilical vein, usually closes with the clamping of the umbilical cord and inhibition of blood flow through the umbilical vein. This fetal structure closes by the end of the first week. The ductus arteriosus constricts partly in response to the higher arterial oxygen levels that occur after the first few breaths. This closure prevents blood from the aorta from entering the pulmonary artery.

Functional closure of the ductus arteriosus in a term infant usually occurs within the first 72 hours after birth. Permanent closure occurs at 3 to 4 weeks of age. Frequently a functional or innocent murmur is auscultated by the nursery nurse when there are delayed fetal shunt closures, but they usually are not associated with a heart lesion (Lawford & Tulloh, 2015). All of these changes at birth leave the newborn with the typical adult pattern of circulation with right ventricle output equaling that of the left. Figure 10.9 shows fetal circulation. Go to thePoint for a web link to a video depicting fetal circulation.

GENETICS

Genetics is the study of heredity and its variation (Nussbaum, McInnes, & Willard, 2016). **Genomics,** a relatively new science, is the study of all genes and includes interactions among genes as well as interactions between genes and the environment. Genomics plays a role in complex conditions such as heart disease and diabetes. Another emerging area of research is that of pharmacogenomics, the study of genetic and genomic influences on pharmacodynamics and pharmacotherapeutics. It aims to use an individual's genetic information in order to treat diseases more efficiently and minimize adverse events (Meyer zu Schwabedissen, 2015). An individual's genetics influences wellness and health issues throughout that person's lifespan. The challenge for health care providers is to find the link between the client's genetic makeup and diseases (Brazeau, 2015).

According to the Public Health Agency of Canada (2013), congenital anomalies occur in about 4% of all infants born in Canada, or 1 in every 25 infants. Traditionally, genetics has been associated with making decisions about childbearing and caring for children with genetic disorders. Recently, genetic and technologic advances are expanding our understanding of how genetic changes affect human diseases such as diabetes, cancer, Alzheimer's disease, and other multifactorial diseases that are prevalent in adults. Today's genetic technologies are not yet a crystal ball for seeing a child's future, but scientists are closer to routinely glimpsing at the genetic blueprints of a fetus just months after sperm meets egg (Kumar, Kingsley, & DiStefano, 2015). Newborn screening is perhaps the most widely used application of genetics in perinatal and neonatal care. Our ability to diagnose genetic conditions is more advanced than our ability to cure or treat the disorders. However, accurate diagnosis has led to improved treatment and outcomes for those affected with these disorders.

Take Note!

Genetic science has the potential to revolutionize health care with regard to national screening programs, predisposition testing, detection of genetic disorders, and pharmacogenetics.

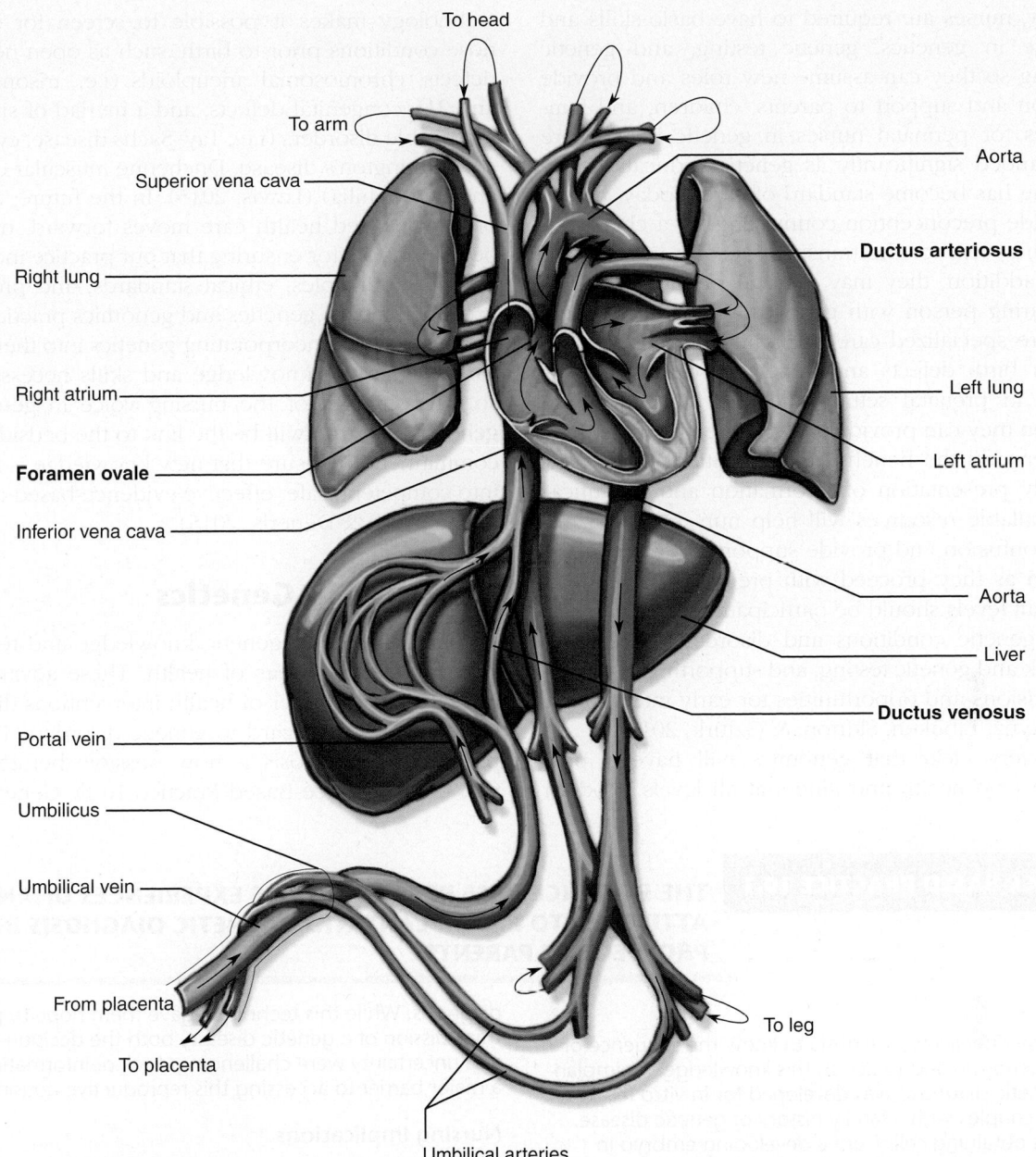

To head

To arm

Superior vena cava

Right lung

Right atrium

Foramen ovale

Inferior vena cava

Portal vein

Umbilicus

Umbilical vein

From placenta

To placenta

Umbilical arteries

Aorta

Ductus arteriosus

Left lung

Left atrium

Aorta

Liver

Ductus venosus

To leg

FIGURE 10.9 Fetal circulation. *Arrows* indicate the path of blood. The umbilical vein carries oxygen-rich blood from the placenta to the liver and through the ductus venosus. From there it is carried to the inferior vena cava to the right atrium of the heart. Some of the blood is shunted through the foramen ovale to the left side of the heart, where it is routed to the brain and upper extremities. The rest of the blood travels down to the right ventricle and through the pulmonary artery. A small portion of the blood travels to the nonfunctioning lungs, while the remaining blood is shunted through the ductus arteriosus into the aorta to supply the rest of the body.

Genetics has been a part of perinatal care for decades. Rapid development and implementation of advanced genetics technology in prenatal settings includes the ability to screen for and diagnose a broader range of diseases and conditions of the fetus in early gestational ages. Ultrasounds and maternal serum screening have become routine elements of prenatal care. Preconception carrier screening for conditions such as Tay–Sachs

disease has been in place among high-risk populations such as Ashkenazi Jews. Amniocentesis and chorionic villus sampling are diagnostic tests that may confirm a genetic anomaly in a developing fetus, but they are all invasive procedures. A fetal nuchal translucency (FNT) test, as seen on ultrasound, may be suggestive of the presence of trisomy 21 or Down syndrome if increased nuchal thickness is found (Lichtenbelt et al., 2015).

Today, nurses are required to have basic skills and knowledge in genetics, genetic testing, and genetic counselling so they can assume new roles and provide information and support to parents, children, and families. Roles for perinatal nurses in genetic health care have expanded significantly as genetics education and counselling has become standard of care. Today, nurses may provide preconception counselling for a childbearing person at risk for the transmission of a genetic disorder. In addition, they may provide prenatal care for a childbearing person with genetically linked disorders that require specialized care or participate in screening infants for birth defects and genetic disorders. Nurses employed in prenatal settings need to have accurate information they can provide to a childbearing person so they understand the benefits and limitations of screening. Timely presentation of information and identification of available resources will help nurses minimize a couple's confusion and provide support for a childbearing person as they proceed with pregnancy screening. Nurses at all levels should be participating in risk assessment for genetic conditions and disorders, explaining genetic risk and genetic testing, and supporting informed health decisions and opportunities for early intervention (Seven, Akyüz, Elbüken, Skirton, & Öztürk, 2015).

It is very clear that genomics will have a profound effect on health and illness at all levels. Modern technology makes it possible to screen for and diagnose conditions prior to birth, such as open neural tube defects, chromosomal aneuploids (i.e., trisomy 13, 18, and 21), congenital defects, and a myriad of single gene inheritable disorders (i.e., Tay–Sachs disease, cystic fibrosis, Huntington's disease, Duchenne muscular dystrophy, and hemophilia) (Lewis, 2015). In the future, as the era of personalized health care moves forward, nurses will be responsible for ensuring that our practice includes the scientific principles, ethical standards, and professional accountability of genetics and genomics practice. Nurses are increasingly incorporating genetics into their practice as they gain the knowledge and skills necessary to do so. The strength of the nursing voice in genetics and genomic research will be the link to the bedside and the commitment to ensure that new knowledge is translated into competent, safe, effective evidence-based client care (Latendresse & Deneris, 2015).

Advances in Genetics

Recent advances in genetic knowledge and technology have affected all areas of health. These advances have increased the number of health interventions that can be undertaken with regard to genetic disorders. For example, genetic diagnosis is now possible before conception (see Evidence-Based Practice 10.1). Genetic testing

EVIDENCE-BASED PRACTICE 10.1   **THE EVIDENCE BASE REGARDING THE EXPERIENCES OF AND ATTITUDES TO PREIMPLANTATION GENETIC DIAGNOSIS IN PROSPECTIVE PARENTS**

STUDY

Technology now allows scientists to know the sequence of people's genomes and to act on this knowledge. Preimplantation genetic diagnosis was developed for in vitro fertilization (IVF) couples with a family history of genetic disease. It involves obtaining cells from a developing embryo in culture, which is then subjected to genetic diagnostic analysis. The resulting information is used to guide which embryos are transferred into the uterus. Previous research has suggested that couples wishing to avoid having a child with an inherited genetic condition favor preimplantation genetic testing to prevent the need for pregnancy termination following a prenatal diagnosis of an affected fetus. The purpose of this study was to understand the experiences of couples who have used or considered this technique.

Findings

A systematic review was conducted using nine studies that met the inclusion criteria. Results of the studies were analyzed and synthesized with three main themes emerging: (1) motivating factors; (2) emotional labour; (3) choices and uncertainty. The review identified an emotional and difficult journey for couples pursing preimplantation genetic diagnosis. While this technique gave them hope to prevent transmission of a genetic disease, both the decision-making and uncertainty were challenging. Lack of information was a major barrier to accessing this reproductive option.

Nursing Implications

Based on the findings, more education is needed for nurses regarding various reproductive screening tests that are available for couples with a family history of a genetic disease or at risk for them. Being aware of the spectrum of genetic disorders and linking them with the appropriate genetic tests when counselling couples would assist them greatly. The nurse needs to know which genetic problems this option would help. They might include autosomal recessive diseases in which both parents are known carriers, such as cystic fibrosis, Tay–Sachs disease, or sickle cell disease; autosomal dominant diseases, such as Huntington's disease; genetic mutations with important consequences, such as BRCA gene (breast cancer); and X-linked diseases, such as hemophilia. With greater understanding and current knowledge of the various options available for couples, nurses can improve communication and provide psychological support to couples.

Source: Cunningham, J., Goldsmith, L., & Skirton, H. (2015). The evidence base regarding the experiences of and attitudes to preimplantation genetic diagnosis in prospective parents. *Midwifery, 31*(2), 288–296.

can identify presymptomatic conditions in children and adults, and provide carrier screening, prenatal diagnostic testing, newborn screening, confirmation of a diagnosis, forensic and identity testing, preimplantation genetic diagnosis and pharmacogenetic testing, which provides information on how an individual will respond to certain medications based on genetic variability (National Human Genome Research Institute [NHGRI], 2015a); National Institutes of Health [NIH], 2018a). Over 2,000 genetic tests are available for diseases such as Duchenne muscular dystrophy/Becker muscular dystrophy, cystic fibrosis, and sickle cell disease (NIH, 2018b). Gene therapy can be used to replace or repair defective or missing genes with normal ones. It is a promising treatment option for many inherited and incurable diseases; however, it currently remains an experimental treatment option (NGHRI, 2015b). Hundreds of clinical trials are underway to test gene therapy but currently it is only available in the research setting (NGHRI, 2017).

The Human Genome Project (HGP) and continued research by the National Human Genome Research Institute have helped foster much of this progress. The **genome** of an organism is its entire hereditary information encoded in the DNA. The HGP, in an international effort to produce a comprehensive sequence of the human genome, was coordinated by the U.S. Department of Energy and the National Institutes of Health in collaboration with over a dozen other countries including Canada, who joined in 1992. This work began in October 1990 and was completed in May 2003. Its goals included:

- Identify all of the approximately 20,500 genes in human DNA.
- Determine the sequences of the 3 billion chemical base pairs that make up human DNA.
- Store this information in databases to make it accessible for further study.
- Improve tools for data analysis.
- Transfer-related technologies to the private sector.
- Address the ethical, legal, and social implications of this discovery (U.S. Department of Energy Genome Programs, 2017).

The HGP has led to the discovery of the genetic basis for hundreds of disorders and has advanced our understanding of basic genetic processes at the molecular level. A link to additional information about the HGP is available at thePoint.

One goal of the HGP was to translate the findings into new and more effective strategies for the prevention, diagnosis, and treatment of genetic diseases and disorders.

Current and potential applications of the HGP to health care include rapid and more specific diagnosis of disease, with hundreds of genetic tests available in research or clinical practice; earlier detection of genetic predisposition to disease; less emphasis on treating the symptoms of a disease and more emphasis on looking at the fundamental causes of the disease; new classes of drugs; avoiding environmental conditions that may trigger disease; and repair or replacement of defective genes through gene therapy (Genome Canada, 2018; U.S. Department of Energy Genome Programs, 2018). This new genetic knowledge and technology, along with the commercialization of this knowledge, will change both professional and parental understanding of genetic disorders.

The potential benefits of these discoveries are vast, but so is the potential for misuse. These advances challenge all health care professionals to consider the many ethical, legal, and social ramifications of genetics in human lives. In the near future, risk profiling based on an individual's unique genetic makeup will be used to tailor prevention, treatment, and ongoing management of health conditions. This profiling will raise issues associated with privacy and confidentiality related to workplace discrimination and access to health insurance. Issues of autonomy are equally problematic as society considers how to address the injustices that will inevitably surface when disease risk can be determined years in advance of its occurrence. Nurses will play an important role in developing policies and providing direction and support in this arena, and to do so they will need a basic understanding of genetics, including inheritance and inheritance patterns. Visit thePoint for links to websites sharing additional information on the ethical, social, and legal issues surrounding human genetic research and advances.

Inheritance

The nucleus within the cell is the controlling factor in all cellular activities because it contains chromosomes, long continuous strands of deoxyribonucleic acid (DNA) that carry genetic information. Each chromosome is made up of genes. **Genes** are individual units of heredity of all traits and are organized into long segments of DNA that occupy a specific location on a chromosome and determine a particular characteristic in an organism.

DNA stores genetic information and encodes the instructions for synthesizing specific proteins needed to maintain life. DNA is double stranded and takes the form of a double helix. The side pieces of the double helix are made up of a sugar, deoxyribose, and a phosphate, occurring in alternating groups. The cross connections or rungs of the ladder are attached to the sides and are made up of four nitrogenous bases: adenine, cytosine, thymine, and guanine. The sequence of the base pairs as they form each rung of the ladder is referred to as the genetic code (Fig. 10.10) (Travers & Muskhelishvili, 2015).

Each gene has a segment of DNA with a specific set of instructions for making proteins needed by body cells for proper functioning. Genes control the types of proteins made and the rate at which they are produced (Snustad & Simmons, 2015). Any change in gene structure or location leads to a mutation, which may alter

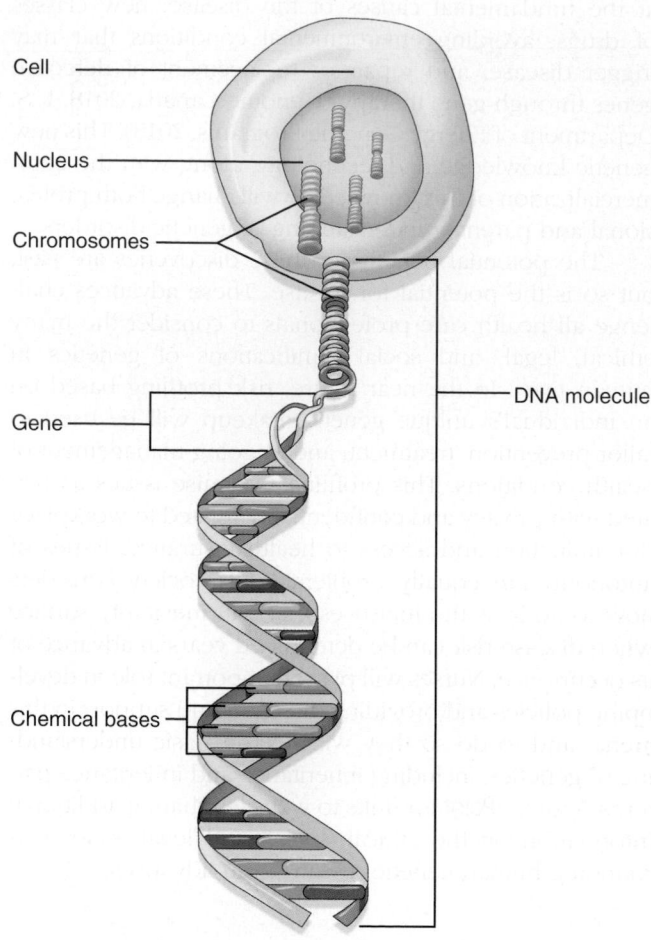

Cell

Nucleus

Chromosomes

Gene

DNA molecule

Chemical bases

FIGURE 10.10 DNA is made up of four chemical bases. Tightly coiled strands of DNA are packaged in units called chromosomes, housed in the cell's nucleus. Working subunits of DNA are known as genes. (From the National Institutes of Health and National Cancer Institute. [1995]. *Understanding gene testing [NIH Pub. No. 96–3905].* Washington, DC: U.S. Department of Human Services.)

the type and amount of protein produced (Fig. 10.11). Genes never act in isolation; they always interact with other genes and the environment. They are arranged in a specific linear formation along a chromosome.

The **genotype,** the specific genetic makeup of an individual, usually in the form of DNA, is the internally coded inheritable information. It refers to the particular **allele,** which is one of two or more alternative versions of gene at a given position or locus on a chromosome that imparts the same characteristic of that gene. For instance, each human has a gene that controls height, but there are variations of these genes, which are alleles, in accordance with the specific height for which the gene codes. A gene that controls eye colour may have an allele that can produce blue eyes or an allele that produces brown eyes. The genotype, together with environmental variation that influences the individual, determines the **phenotype,** or the observed, outward characteristics of an individual. A human inherits two genes, one from each parent. Therefore, one allele comes from the ovum and one from the sperm. These alleles may be the same for the characteristic (**homozygous**) or different (**heterozygous**). For example, WW stands for homozygous dominant; ww stands for homozygous recessive. Heterozygous would be indicated as Ww. If the two alleles differ, such as Ww, the dominant one will usually be expressed in the phenotype of the individual.

Human beings typically have 46 chromosomes. This includes 22 pairs of non-sex chromosomes or autosomes and 1 pair of sex chromosomes (2 X chromosomes in females, and an X chromosome and a Y chromosome in males). Offspring receive 1 chromosome of each of the 23 pairs from each of the ovum and sperm.

The pictorial analysis of the number, form, and size of an individual's chromosomes is termed the **karyotype.** This analysis commonly uses white blood cells and fetal cells in amniotic fluid. The chromosomes are numbered

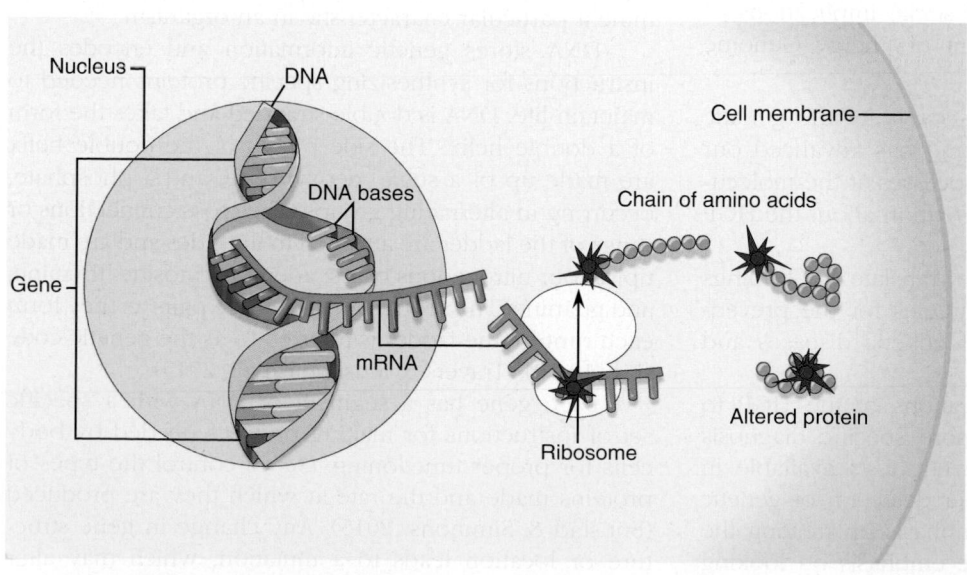

Nucleus

DNA

Cell membrane

Gene

DNA bases

Chain of amino acids

mRNA

Altered protein

Ribosome

FIGURE 10.11 When a gene contains a mutation, the protein encoded by that gene will be abnormal. Some protein changes are insignificant, while others are disabling. (From the National Institutes of Health and National Cancer Institute. [1995]. *Understanding gene testing [NIH Pub. No. 96–3905].* Washington, DC: U.S. Department of Human Services.)

FIGURE 10.12 Karyotype pattern. **A.** Normal female karyotype. **B.** Normal male karyotype.

from the largest to the smallest, 1 to 22, and the sex chromosomes are designated by the letter X or Y. A genetically female karyotype is designated as 46, XX and a genetically male karyotype is designated as 46, XY. Figure 10.12 illustrates an example of a karyotyping pattern.

Regulation and expression of the thousands of human genes is very complex and is the result of many intricate interactions within each cell. Alterations in gene structure, function, transcription, translation, and protein synthesis can influence an individual's health (Jones & Lopez, 2014). Gene **mutations** are a permanent change in the sequence of DNA. Some mutations have no significant effect, whereas others can have a tremendous impact on the health of the individual. Several genetic disorders can result from these mutations, such as cystic fibrosis, sickle cell disease, phenylketonuria, or hemophilia.

Patterns of Inheritance for Genetic Disorders

Patterns of inheritance demonstrate how genetic abnormalities can be passed on to offspring. Although diagnosis of a genetic disorder is usually based on clinical signs and symptoms or on laboratory confirmation of an altered gene associated with the disorder, accurate diagnosis can be aided by the recognition of the pattern of inheritance within a family. In addition, nurses must understand the patterns of inheritance so they can teach and counsel

families about the risks of genetic disorders occurring in future pregnancies. Some genetic disorders occur in multiple family members, while others may occur in only a single family member. A genetic disorder is caused by completely or partially altered genetic material, whereas a familial disorder is more common in relatives of the affected individual but may be caused by environmental influences and not genetic alterations. For a more detailed discussion of specific types of genetic disorders, see Chapter 49.

Mendelian or Monogenic Laws of Inheritance

Principles of inheritance of single-gene disorders are the same principles that govern the inheritance of other traits, such as eye and hair colour. These are known as Mendel's laws of inheritance, named for Gregory Mendel, an Austrian naturalist who conducted genetic research. These patterns occur because a single gene is defective and the disorders that result are referred to as monogenic or, sometimes, Mendelian disorders. If the defect occurs on the autosome, the genetic disorder is termed autosomal; if the defect is on the X chromosome, the genetic disorder is termed X linked. The defect also can be classified as dominant or recessive. Monogenic disorders include autosomal dominant, autosomal recessive, X-linked dominant, and X-linked recessive patterns.

AUTOSOMAL DOMINANT INHERITANCE DISORDERS

Autosomal dominant inherited disorders occur when a single gene in the heterozygous state is capable of producing the phenotype. In other words, the abnormal or mutant gene overshadows the normal gene and the person will demonstrate signs and symptoms of the disorder. The affected person generally will have inherited this genetic material from either the egg or the sperm. However, there are varying degrees of presentation among individuals in a family. For example, an individual with a mild form of the disorder could have a child with a more severe form (termed *variable expression*). In some autosomal dominant disorders there may be no history of an affected family member. This can be due to the child representing a new mutation or the result of incomplete or reduced penetrance, which means that a person with the genetic mutation does not develop phenotypic features of the disorder. Incomplete or reduced penetrance may result from a combination of genetic, environmental, and lifestyle factors, age, and gender.

Offspring of an affected individual will have a 50% chance of inheriting two normal genes (disorder free) and a 50% chance of inheriting one normal and one abnormal gene (and, thus, the disorder) (Fig. 10.13) (NIH, 2018b). Female karyotypes and male karyotypes are equally affected by autosomal dominant disorders and an affected male karyotype can pass the disorder on to their children with XY chromosomes (NIH, 2018b). This transmission is important in distinguishing autosomal dominant inheritance from X-linked inheritance. Common types of genetic disorders that follow the autosomal

dominant pattern of inheritance include neurofibromatosis (genetic disorders affecting the development and growth of neural cells and tissues), Huntington's disease (a genetic disorder affecting the nervous system characterized by abnormal involuntary movements and progressive dementia), achondroplasia (a genetic disorder resulting in disordered growth and abnormal body proportion), and polycystic kidney disease (a genetic disorder involving the growth of multiple, bilateral, grapelike clusters of fluid-filled cysts in the kidneys that eventually compress and replace functioning renal tissue).

AUTOSOMAL RECESSIVE INHERITANCE DISORDERS

Autosomal recessive inherited disorders occur when two copies of the mutant or abnormal gene in the homozygous state are necessary to produce the phenotype. In other words, two abnormal genes are needed for the individual to demonstrate signs and symptoms of the disorder. Both the egg and the sperm must be heterozygous carriers of the gene (clinically normal but carriers of the gene). Offspring of two carriers of the abnormal gene have a 25% chance of inheriting two normal genes; a 50% chance of inheriting one normal gene and one abnormal gene (carrier); and a 25% chance of inheriting two abnormal genes (and, thus, the disorder) (Fig. 10.14) (NIH, 2018b). Affected people are usually present in only one generation of the family. Female and male karyotypes are equally affected and an individual with a genetically male karyotype can pass the disorder on to offspring with XY chromosomes. The chance that any two genetic donors will both be carriers of the mutant

FIGURE 10.13 Autosomal dominant inheritance.

FIGURE 10.14 Autosomal recessive inheritance.

gene is increased if the couple has consanguinity (relationship by blood or common ancestry) (NIH, 2018b). Common types of genetic disorders that follow the autosomal recessive inheritance pattern include cystic fibrosis (a genetic disorder involving generalized dysfunction of the exocrine glands), phenylketonuria (a disorder involving a deficiency in a liver enzyme that leads to the inability to process the essential amino acid phenylalanine), Tay–Sachs disease (a disorder due to insufficient activity of the enzyme hexosaminidase, which is necessary for the breakdown of certain fatty substances in the brain and nerve cells), and sickle cell disease (a genetic disorder in which the red blood cells carry an ineffective type of hemoglobin instead of the normal adult hemoglobin).

X-LINKED INHERITANCE DISORDERS

X-linked inherited disorders are those associated with altered genes present on the X chromosome. They differ from autosomal disorders. If an individual with a male karyotype inherits an X-linked altered gene, they will express the condition. This is because they only have one X chromosome, therefore all the genes on the X chromosome will be expressed (the Y chromosome carries no normal allele to compensate for the altered gene). Individuals who inherit two X chromosomes can be either heterozygous or homozygous for any allele. Therefore, X-linked disorders in these individuals are expressed similarly to autosomal disorders.

X-LINKED RECESSIVE INHERITANCE

Most X-linked disorders demonstrate a recessive pattern of inheritance (Snustad & Simmons, 2015). There are more affected individuals with genetically male karyotypes than those with genetically female karyotypes because when a person has one X and one Y chromosomes all the genes on an X chromosome will be expressed (Snustad & Simmons, 2015). On the other hand, a person with two X chromosomes will need both to be abnormal to exhibit the disease, and one normal and one abnormal X chromosome to be a carrier of the disease. There is no XY-to-XY transmission (since no X chromosome from the male is transmitted to male offspring), but any individual with an XY chromosome who is affected with an X-linked recessive disorder will have carrier XX offspring. If an individual with XX chromosomes is a carrier, there is a 25% chance they will have an affected XY offspring, a 25% chance that their XX offspring will be a carrier, a 25% chance that they will have an unaffected XY offspring, and a 25% chance the XX offspring will be a noncarrier (Fig. 10.15) (Conley, 2014). Common types of genetic disorders that follow X-linked recessive inheritance patterns include hemophilia, colour blindness, and Duchenne muscular dystrophy (NIH, 2018b).

X-LINKED DOMINANT INHERITANCE

X-linked dominant inheritance occurs when an individual with XY karyotype has an abnormal X chromosome or

Healthy XY chromosome   Carrier XX chromosome

X Y   X X

Normal Male   Normal Female   Carrier Female   Affected male

FIGURE 10.15 X-linked recessive inheritance.

an individual with XX karyotype has one abnormal X chromosome. All of the offspring with XX chromosomes and none of the offspring with XY chromosomes of an affected XY donor will inherit the condition, while all of the offspring of an affected XX donor have a 50% chance of inheriting the condition (Fig. 10.16) (NIH, 2018b). Individuals with XY chromosomes are more severely affected

Healthy XY chromosome   Affected XX chromosome

X Y   X X

Normal Male   Affected Female   Affected Male   Normal Female

FIGURE 10.16 X-linked dominant inheritance.

than individuals with XX chromosomes. Many X-linked dominant disorders have lethal results in individuals with XY chromosomes (Slavotinek & Ali, 2015). In individuals with XX chromosomes, even though the gene is dominant, having a second normal X gene offsets the effects of the dominant gene to some extent resulting in decreasing severity of the disorder. X-linked dominant disorders are rare; examples include hypophosphatemic (vitamin D–resistant) rickets and fragile X syndrome. Fragile X syndrome causes a range of developmental problems including learning disabilities and cognitive impairment (Van Esch, 2018). A characteristic of X-linked dominant inheritance is that donors with an XY karyotype cannot pass X-linked traits to their offspring with XY chromosomes (no XY-to-XY transmission) (NGHRI, 2015b).

Multifactorial Inheritance Disorders

Many of the common congenital malformations, such as cleft lip, cleft palate, spina bifida, pyloric stenosis, clubfoot, congenital hip dysplasia, and cardiac defects, are attributed to multifactorial inheritance (Snustad & Simmons, 2015). These conditions are thought to be caused by multiple gene and environmental factors. That is, a combination of genes from both the ovum and the sperm, along with unknown environmental factors, produces the trait or condition. An individual may inherit a predisposition to a particular anomaly or disease. The anomalies or diseases vary in severity, and often a sex bias is present. For example, pyloric stenosis is seen more often in individuals with XY chromosomes, while congenital hip dysplasia is much more likely to occur in those with XX chromosomes. Multifactorial conditions tend to run in families, but the pattern of inheritance is not as predictable as with single-gene disorders. The chance of recurrence is also less than in single-gene disorders, but the degree of risk is related to the number of genes in common with the affected individual. The closer the degree of relationship, the more genes an individual has in common with the affected family member, resulting in a higher chance the individual's offspring will have a similar defect. In multifactorial inheritance the likelihood that both identical twins will be affected is not 100%, indicating that there are nongenetic factors involved.

Nontraditional Inheritance Patterns

Molecular studies have revealed that some genetic disorders are inherited in ways that do not follow the typical patterns of dominant, recessive, X-linked, or multifactorial inheritance. Examples of nontraditional inheritance patterns include mitochondrial inheritance and genomic imprinting. As the science of molecular genetics advances and more is learned about inheritance patterns, other nontraditional patterns of inheritance may be discovered or found to be relatively common.

MITOCHONDRIAL INHERITANCE

Certain diseases result from mutations in the mitochondrial DNA. Mitochondria (the part of the cell responsible for energy production) are inherited almost exclusively from the childbearing person. Therefore, mitochondrial inheritance is usually passed from the childbearing person to the offspring, regardless of the offspring's sex (differentiating mitochondrial inheritance from X-linked recessive inheritance). These mutations are often deletions and abnormalities and are often seen in one or more organs, such as the brain, eye, and skeletal muscle. They are often associated with energy deficits in cells with high energy requirements, such as nerve and muscle cells. These disorders tend to be progressive and the age of onset can vary from infancy to adulthood. There is an extreme amount of variability in symptoms within a family. Examples of disorders that follow mitochondrial inheritance include Kearns–Sayre syndrome (a neuromuscular disorder) and Leber's hereditary optic neuropathy (which causes progressive visual impairment).

GENOMIC IMPRINTING

Another nontraditional inheritance pattern results from a process called genomic imprinting. Genomic imprinting plays a critical role in fetal growth and development and placental functioning. It is a phenomenon by which the expression of a gene is determined by its parental origin. In genomic imprinting both donor alleles are present, but only one is expressed; the other is inactive. Genomic imprinting does not alter the genetic sequence itself, but affects the phenotype observed. In these cases, the altered genes in a certain region of the genome have very different expressions depending on which donor they were inherited from. Several human syndromes are known to be associated with defects in gene imprinting. Disorders that result from a disruption of imprinting usually involve a growth phenotype and include varying degrees of developmental problems. Common examples include Prader–Willi syndrome (a condition resulting in severe hypotonia and hyperphagia, leading to obesity and intellectual disability), Angelman syndrome (a neurodevelopmental disorder associated with intellectual disability, jerky movements, and seizures), and Beckwith–Wiedemann syndrome (characterized by somatic overgrowth, congenital malformations, and a predisposition to embryonic neoplasia).

Chromosomal Abnormalities

In some cases of genetic disorders, the abnormality occurs due to problems with the chromosomes. Chromosomal abnormalities do not follow straightforward patterns of inheritance. Although some chromosomal disorders can be inherited, most others occur due to random events during the formation of reproductive cells or in early fetal development. Most chromosomal abnormalities occur due to an error in the ovum or sperm. Therefore, the abnormality is present in every cell of the body. Some abnormalities can happen after fertilization, during mitotic cell division, and result in mosaicism. **Mosaicism** or the mosaic form is when the chromosomal abnormalities do not show up in every cell; only some cells or tissues carry the abnormality. In mosaic forms of the disorder the symptoms are usually less severe than if all the cells were abnormal.

Globally, chromosomal abnormalities occur in about 1 in 153 births (Verma & Puri, 2015). Congenital anomalies and intellectual disability are often associated with chromosomal abnormalities (Bacino & Lee, 2016). These abnormalities occur on autosomal or non-sex chromosomes as well as sex chromosomes and can result from abnormalities of either chromosome number or chromosome structure.

As mentioned, a karyotype is a pictorial analysis of chromosomes. It depicts a systematic arrangement of chromosomes of a single cell by pairs (see Fig. 10.12). Karyotyping is often used in prenatal testing to diagnose or predict genetic diseases.

Abnormalities of Chromosome Number

Chromosomal abnormalities of number often result due to nondisjunction (failure of separation of the chromosome pair during cell division, meiosis, or mitosis). Few chromosomal numerical abnormalities are compatible with full-term development and most result in spontaneous abortion (Snustad & Simmons, 2015).

There are some numerical abnormalities that do support development to term because the chromosome on which the abnormality is present carries relatively few genes (such as chromosome 13, 18, 21, or X). Two common abnormalities of chromosome number are monosomy and trisomy. In **monosomy**, there is only one copy of a particular chromosome instead of the usual pair (an entire single chromosome is missing). In these cases, all fetuses spontaneously abort in early pregnancy. Survival is seen only in mosaic forms of these disorders. In **trisomy,** there are three of a particular chromosome instead of the usual two (an entire single chromosome is added). The most common trisomies include trisomy 21 (Down syndrome), trisomy 18, and trisomy 13. Figure 10.17 shows the karyotype of a child with Down syndrome. (See Chapter 49 for a detailed discussion of these disorders.) Trisomies may be present in every cell or may present in the mosaic form.

Abnormalities of Chromosome Structure

Abnormalities of chromosome structure usually occur when there is a breakage and loss of a portion of one or more chromosomes, and during the repair process the broken ends are rejoined incorrectly. Structural abnormalities usually lead to having too much or too little

FIGURE 10.17 **Karyotype of a child with Down syndrome.**

genetic material. Altered chromosome structure can take on several forms. Deletions occur when a portion of the chromosome is missing or deleted, resulting in a loss of that portion of the chromosome. Duplications are seen when a portion of the chromosome is duplicated and an extra chromosomal segment is present. Clinical findings vary depending on how much chromosomal material is involved. Inversions occur when a portion of the chromosome breaks off at two points and is turned upside down and reattached; therefore, the genetic material is inverted. With inversion, there is no loss or gain of chromosomal material and carriers are phenotypically normal, but they do have an increased risk for miscarriage and having chromosomally abnormal offspring (NGHRI, 2017). Ring chromosomes are seen when a portion of a chromosome has broken off in two places and formed a circle or ring. The most clinically significant structural abnormality is a translocation. This occurs when a portion of one chromosome is transferred to another chromosome and an abnormal rearrangement is present.

Structural abnormalities can be balanced or unbalanced. Balanced abnormalities involve the rearrangement of genetic material with neither an overall gain nor loss. Individuals who inherit a balanced structural abnormality are usually phenotypically normal but are at a higher risk for miscarriages and having chromosomally abnormal offspring. Examples of structural rearrangements that can be balanced include inversions, translocation, and ring chromosomes. Unbalanced structural abnormalities are similar to numerical abnormalities because genetic material is either gained or lost. Unbalanced structural abnormalities can encompass several genes and result in severe clinical consequences.

Sex Chromosome Abnormalities

Chromosomal abnormalities can also involve sex chromosomes. These cases are usually less severe in their clinical effects than autosomal chromosomal abnormalities. Sex chromosome abnormalities are gender specific and involve a missing or extra sex chromosome. They affect sexual development and may cause infertility, growth abnormalities, and possibly behavioural and learning problems (Defendi, 2018). However, many affected people lead essentially normal lives. Examples are Turner syndrome in individuals with XY chromosomes and Klinefelter syndrome in individuals with XY chromosomes. (See Chapter 49 for a more detailed discussion of these disorders.)

GENETIC EVALUATION AND COUNSELLING

Genetic counselling is a communication and educational process where the genetic influence of health is explained along with information regarding a specific genetic disorder, its transmission, inheritance, and options available in management and family planning (Nussbaum et al., 2016). There are a variety of reasons a person should be referred for genetic counselling (Box 10.2). In many cases, geneticists and genetic counsellors provide information to families regarding genetic diseases. However, an experienced

family physician, pediatrician, or nurse who has received special training in genetics may also provide the information. A genetic consultation involves evaluation of an individual or a family. Its purpose is to confirm, diagnose, or rule out genetic conditions; identify medical management issues; calculate and communicate genetic risks to a family; discuss ethical and legal issues; and assist in providing and arranging psychosocial support. Genetic counsellors serve as educators and resource persons for other health care providers and the general public. Nurses have long been on the forefront of genetic counselling for their clients. The knowledge gained from the HGP is transforming the health care model, with implications for nurses in genetic counselling, practice, and research (International Society of Nurses in Genetics [ISONG], 2018).

The ideal time for genetic counselling is before conception. Preconception counselling allows individuals to identify and reduce potential pregnancy risks, plan for known risks, and establish early prenatal care. Unfortunately, many childbearing people delay seeking prenatal care until their second or third trimester, after the crucial time of organogenesis. Therefore, it is important that preconception counselling is offered to all individuals as they seek health care throughout their childbearing years, especially if they are contemplating pregnancy. This requires health care providers to take an active role. Consideration of genetics is rapidly becoming a part of routine health care, and all nurses need to be up to date and confident in their understanding of this topic.

BOX 10.2

THOSE WHO MAY BENEFIT FROM GENETIC COUNSELLING

- Maternal age 35 years or older when the baby is born
- Paternal age 50 years or older
- Previous child, parents, or close relatives with an inherited disease, congenital anomalies, metabolic disorders, developmental disorders, or chromosomal abnormalities
- Consanguinity or incest
- Pregnancy screening abnormality, including alpha-fetoprotein, triple/quadruple screen, amniocentesis, or ultrasound
- Stillborn with congenital anomalies
- Two or more pregnancy losses
- Exposure to drugs, medications, radiation, chemicals, or infection
- Teratogen exposure or risk
- Concerns about genetic defects that occur frequently in their ethnic or racial group (e.g., those of African descent are most at risk for having a child with sickle cell anemia)
- Abnormal newborn screening
- Couples with a family history of X-linked disorders
- Carriers of autosomal recessive or dominant diseases
- Child born with one or more major malformations in a major organ system
- Child with abnormalities of growth
- Child with developmental delay, intellectual disability, blindness, or deafness

Adapted from March of Dimes. (2018). Genetic counseling. Retrieved from http://www.marchofdimes.org/pregnancy/genetic-counseling.aspx; National Human Genome Research Institute. (2015b). Frequently asked questions about genetic counseling. Retrieved from http://www.genome.gov/19016905; Lewis, R. (2015). *Human genetics: Concepts and applications* (11th ed.). New York: McGraw-Hill Companies, Incorporated.

Consider This

As I waited for the genetic counsellor to come into the room, my mind was filled with numerous fears and questions. What does an inconclusive amniocentesis really mean? What if this pregnancy produced an abnormal baby? How would I cope with a special-needs child in my life? If only I had gone to the midwife sooner when I thought I was pregnant, but was still in denial. Why did I wait so long to admit this pregnancy and get prenatal care? If only I had started to take my folic acid pills when prescribed. Why didn't I research my family's history to know of any hidden genetic conditions? What about my sister's child with Down syndrome? What must I have been thinking? I guess I could play the "what-if" game forever and never come up with answers. It was too late to do anything about this pregnancy because I was in my last trimester. I started to pray silently when the counsellor opened the door....

Thoughts: *This person is reviewing the last several months, looking for answers to deep-seated fears. Inconclusive screenings can introduce emotional torment for many clients as they wait for validating results. Are these common thoughts and fears for many childbearing individuals facing potential genetic disorders? What supportive interventions might the nurse offer?*

Preconception counselling plays a key role in preparing for a pregnancy. In couples with a history of recurrent early pregnancy loss, counselling is of particular importance because these clients are invariably more distressed and require reassurance to avoid future pregnancy losses. Several interventions ranging from genetic testing to lifestyle changes and medications may have a positive effect on the chances of a successful pregnancy. Early pregnancy monitoring and support increases the chance of a live birth and helps to predict potential future pregnancy complications. Recent research suggests that events that occur in the uterine decidua, even before a person knows they are pregnant, may have a significant impact on fetal growth and the outcome of pregnancy. With this in mind, shifting future research and clinical practice to focus on the periconceptual period and the very early stages of pregnancy should offer significant benefits to the health of both the childbearing person and their infant. The overall aim should be to effectively use every pregnancy as the health care opportunity of two lifetimes (Lopes, de Omena Bomfim, & Floria-Santos, 2015).

Preconception screening and counselling can raise serious ethical and moral issues for a couple. The results of prenatal genetic testing can lead to the decision to terminate a pregnancy, even if the results are not conclusive but indicate a strong possibility that the child will have an abnormality. The severity of the abnormality may not be known, and some may find the decision to terminate unethical. Another difficult situation that provides an example of the ethical and moral issues surrounding genetic screening and counselling involves disorders that affect only one gender of offspring. A childbearing person may find they are a carrier of a gene for a disorder for which there is no prenatal screening test available. In these cases, the client or couple may decide to terminate any pregnancy where the fetus is the affected sex, even though there is a 50% chance that the child will not inherit the disorder. In these situations, the choice is up to the individual, and information and support must be provided in a nondirective, nonjudgmental manner.

Genetic counselling is particularly important if a congenital anomaly or genetic disease has been diagnosed prenatally or when a child is born with a life-threatening congenital anomaly or genetic disease. In these cases, families need information urgently so they can make immediate decisions. If a diagnosis with genetic implications is made later in life, if a couple with a family history of a genetic disorder or a previous child with a genetic disorder is planning a family, or if there is suspected teratogen exposure, urgency of information is not such an issue. In these situations, the family needs to take in all the information and explore their options. This may occur during several meetings over a longer period of time.

FIGURE 10.18 A pedigree is a diagram made using symbols that demonstrates the links between family members and focuses on medical and health information for each relative.

Genetic counselling involves extensive information gathering about birth history, past medical history, and current health status as well as a family history of congenital anomalies, mental retardation, genetic diseases, reproductive history, general health, and causes of death. A detailed family history is imperative and, in most cases, will include the development of a pedigree, which is like a family tree (Fig. 10.18). Information is ideally gathered on three generations, but if the family history is complicated, information from more distant relatives may be needed. Families receiving genetic counselling should be told that this information will be necessary so that they can discuss these sensitive issues with family members in advance. When necessary, medical records may be requested for family members, especially those who have a genetic disorder, to help ensure accuracy of the information. Sometimes the process of preparing a pedigree may reveal information that is not known by all family members, such as an adoption, a child conceived through in vitro fertilization, or a husband not being the father of a baby. Therefore, it is extremely important to take steps to maintain confidentiality. After careful analysis of the data obtained, referral to a genetic counsellor when indicated is appropriate.

Medical genetic knowledge has increased dramatically over the past few decades. This has greatly expanded the role of the genetic counsellor. It is possible not only to detect specific diseases with genetic mutations, but also to test for a genetic predisposition to various diseases or conditions and certain physical characteristics. This leads to complex ethical, moral, and social issues. Health care providers need to maintain privacy and confidentiality and administer care in a nondiscriminatory manner while maintaining sensitivity to cultural differences. It is essential to respect the individual's autonomy and present information in a nondirective manner.

Nursing Roles and Responsibilities

The nurse is likely to interact with the client in a variety of ways related to genetics—taking a family history, scheduling genetic testing, explaining the purposes of all screening and diagnostic tests, answering questions, and addressing concerns raised by family members. Nurses are often the first health care providers to encounter a childbearing individual or couple with preconception and prenatal issues. Nurses play an important role in beginning the preconception counselling process and referring clients and their partners for further genetic testing when indicated.

An accurate and thorough family history is an essential part of preconception counselling. Nurses in any practice setting can obtain a client's history during the initial encounter. The purpose is to gather client and family information that may provide clues as to whether the client has a genetic trait, inherited condition, or inherited predisposition (ISONG, 2018). At a basic level, all nurses should be able to take a family medical history to help identify those at risk for genetic conditions, and then initiate a referral when appropriate. Box 10.3 presents

examples of focused assessment questions that can be used. Box 10.4 and Figure 10.19 assist health care providers with completing a complete family history. Based on the information gathered during the history, the nurse must decide whether a referral to a genetic specialist is necessary or whether further evaluation is needed. Families identified with genetic issues need unique clinical care including management of acute illnesses, screening for long-term complications, discussion of the etiology of the condition, connections to social supports, and clarification of the recurrence risks, and prenatal testing and treatment options (ISONG, 2018). Prenatal testing to assess for genetic risks and defects might be used to identify genetic disorders. These tests are described in Common Laboratory and Diagnostic Tests 10.1.

Remember Robert and Kate Shafer? Based on the information gathered from their genetic history, they were referred to a genetic specialist. What prenatal tests might be ordered to assess their risk for genetic disorders? What would be the nurse's role related to genetic counselling?

Nurses working with families involved with genetic counselling typically have certain responsibilities. These include:

- Using interviewing and active listening skills to identify genetic concerns
- Knowing basic genetic terminology and inheritance patterns
- Explaining basic concepts of probability and disorder susceptibility
- Safeguarding the privacy and confidentiality of clients' genetic information
- Providing complete informed consent to facilitate decisions about genetic testing
- Discussing costs of genetic services and extent of provincial health care coverage for genetic services
- Recognizing and defining ethical, legal, and social issues
- Providing accurate information about the risks and benefits of genetic testing
- Providing culturally appropriate methods to convey genetic information
- Monitoring clients' emotional reactions after receiving genetic analysis
- Providing information on appropriate local support groups
- Knowing their own limitations and making appropriate referrals (Sermon & Viville, 2014)

Talking with families who have recently been diagnosed with a genetic disorder or who have had a child born with congenital anomalies is very difficult. Many times, the nurse may be the one who has first contact

---

BOX 10.3

FOCUSED HEALTH ASSESSMENT: GENETIC HISTORY

What was the cause and age of death for deceased family members?

Does any consanguinity exist between relatives?

Do any serious illnesses or chronic conditions exist? If so, what was the age of onset?

Do any female family members have a history of miscarriages, stillbirths, or diabetes?

Do any female members have a history of alcohol or drug use during pregnancy?

What were the ages of female members during childbearing, especially if older than 35?

Do any family members have mental retardation or developmental delays?

Do any family members have a known or suspected metabolic disorder such as PKU?

Do any family members have an affective disorder such as bipolar disorder?

Have any close relatives been diagnosed with any type of cancer?

What is your ethnic background (explore as related to certain disorders)?

Do any family members have a known or suspected chromosomal disorder?

Do any family members have a progressive neurologic disorder?

Source: Edelman, C. L., Kudzma, E. C., & Mandle, C. L. (2014). *Health promotion throughout the lifespan* (8th ed.). St. Louis, MO: Mosby Elsevier; Nussbaum, R. L., McInnes, R. R., & Willard, H. F. (2016). *Thompson & Thompson genetics in medicine* (8th ed.), Philadelphia, PA: Elsevier; Genetic Alliance. (n.d.). Family health history. Retrieved from http://www.geneticalliance.org/programs/genesinlife/fhh

---

BOX 10.4

TAKING A PRECONCEPTION HISTORY FOR ASSESSMENT AND COUNSELLING

REPRODUCTIVE, GENETIC, AND INFECTIOUS HISTORY

A thorough preconception history identifies couples who are genetically at risk. When clients and their partners are informed of the risks of having a baby with birth defects or a genetic disorder prior to pregnancy, they are then able to determine their options regarding a pregnancy (including contraception, artificial insemination, adoption, prenatal invasive testing, or no specific intervention.)

Reproductive History

Discuss past obstetric history, including early miscarriages; number of pregnancies; type of birth; length of labour; and specific complications, such as premature labour or delivery, gestational diabetes, pregnancy-induced hypertension, and postpartum depression.

Family History

Construct a three-generation pedigree.

Include assessment of genetic disorders, including muscular dystrophy, hemophilia, cystic fibrosis, fragile X syndrome, congenital heart disease, phenylketonuria, dwarfism, sickle cell anemia, and Tay–Sachs disease.

Include assessment of multifactorial congenital malformations, such as spina bifida, anencephaly, cleft palate and cleft lip, hypospadias, and congenital heart disease.

Include assessment of familial diseases with a major genetic component, such as developmental disability, premature atherosclerosis, diabetes mellitus, psychosis, epileptic disorders, hypertension, rheumatoid arthritis, deafness, and severe refractive disorders of the eye.

Age

Establish risks associated with age (e.g., pregnancy under age 15 or over age 35 may carry increased biologic risk).

Ethnic History

Establish risk for specific conditions related to ethnic origin, such as sickle cell anemia, Tay–Sachs disease, neural tube defects, beta-thalassemia, and alpha-thalassemia.

Infectious Conditions

Identify clients who are rubella or varicella susceptible. If they are not actively attempting pregnancy, offer a vaccination.

Identify and counsel clients at risk for hepatitis B. Routine preconception testing of all women with hepatitis B is not currently recommended.

Identify and counsel clients about the parasite risk and to avoid exposure to cat feces and raw and undercooked meats. Routine serologic testing for toxoplasmosis in the preconception period is not recommended.

Evaluate the client and partner's exposure to sexually transmitted disease (chlamydia, HIV, gonorrhea, syphilis).

HEALTH HISTORY

Gynaecologic History

Collect information about menstrual, contraceptive, and sexual histories; infertility; abnormal Pap smears; or in utero exposure to diethylstilbestrol.

Discuss menstrual difficulties, specifically excessive cycle bleeding, amenorrhea, and oligomenorrhea.

Discuss gynaecologic disease, such as endometriosis or pelvic inflammatory disease.

Chronic Conditions

Assess the presence of chronic conditions that can affect a client's ability to conceive, as well as the use of medications in treatment of chronic disease and their potential effect on pregnancy.

The following specific conditions should be considered: diabetes mellitus, anemias, thyroid disorders, gynaecologic disorders, hyperphenylalaninemia, asthma, sexually transmitted diseases, heart disease, hypertension, deep venous thrombosis, kidney disease, systemic lupus erythematosus, epilepsy, hemoglobinopathies, cancer, seizure disorders, tuberculosis, rheumatoid arthritis, neurodegenerative disorders, and mental health/psychiatric disorders.

Lifestyle Assessment

Assess lifestyle issues, including such factors as nutrition, physical activity, prescription and over-the-counter drug use; other substance use; and environmental exposures, current and past.

Source: Adapted from Wilson, R. D. (2017). Women's pre-conception evaluation: Genetic and fetal risk considerations for counselling and informed choice. *Journal of Obstetrics and Gynaecology Canada, 40*(7), 935–949.

---

with these parents and will be the one to provide follow-up care.

Genetic disorders are significant, life-changing, and possibly life-threatening situations. The information is highly technical and the field is undergoing significant technologic advances. Nurses need an understanding of who will benefit from genetic counselling and must be able to discuss the role of the genetic counsellor with families. The nurse wants to ensure that families at risk are aware that genetic counselling is available before they attempt to have another baby.

> **Based on the results of their genetic tests, Robert and Kate are placed at moderate risk for having an infant with an autosomal recessive genetic disorder. The couple asks the nurse what all of this means. What information should the nurse provide about concepts of probability and disorder susceptibility for this couple? How can the nurse help this couple to make knowledgeable decisions concerning their reproductive future?**

Primary factor   **History**   **Evaluate / Screen**

☐   Reproductive history   G   T   P   TA   SA   LB   SB   NND   Living

Genetic

☐   Family   - *3 generation pedigree*

☐   Maternal age >35
☐   Paternal age >40
☐   Specific disease - *personal or previous offspring*   **Maternal**   **Paternal**
                 Recessive   CF Caucasian / Thalessemia Asian-Mediterranean / SC African
                 Dominant   NF / HD / MS
                 X-linked   f-X / MD / Hemophilia

☐   Multi-factorial   congenital anomalies- *personal or previous offspring*
                                                    Maternal   *Paternal*

       Congenital anomalies Cardiac
                                 CNS
                                 Renal
                                 GI
                                 Respiratory
                                 MSK

       Familial association Diabetes
                                 Other endocrine
                                 Hypertension
                                 Autoimmune

☐   Ethnic / Consanguinous Recessive Genetic Risk African / Asian / Jewish / Amish / Mennonite
☐   Infectious conditions   *pregnancy routine*   **Immune or Vaccine status**: rubella / varicella

                                                    urine / swab : GC / syphilis / Chlamydia
       ***Other* vaccine or exposures**   immune status
            Hepatitis B / C   HIV   CMV   Parvo B19   Zika virus
            YES

Personal health   **Maternal**   **Paternal**   age
                                                                            other pregnancies

☐   Gynaecology / Medical / Surgical history

☐   Chronic conditions   Obesity
                          Endocrine / diabetes / thyroid
                          Cardiac / hypertension
                          Respiratory / asthma
                          Gastro-intestinal / Autoimmune
                          Epilepsy / seizures
                          Renal
                          Migraine

☐   Psycho-social conditions   Family history of mental health

☐   Lifestyle assessment   Smoking
                            Alcohol
                            Non prescription drug use
                            BMI / nutrition

☐   Other   maternal: Rh negative (with red cell antibodies)
            negative platelet typing (NAIT risk)

This checklist is meant to prompt and to summarize the important areas for reproductive consideration in planning but individual assessment and complete follow-up with counselling and recommendations is required.

FIGURE 10.19 SOG Preconception Checklist: for the assessment, evaluation, and management. (From Wilson, R. D. [2017]. Women's pre-conception evaluation: Genetic and fetal risk considerations for counselling and informed choice. *Journal of Obstetrics and Gynaecology Canada, 40*[7], 935–949.)

COMMON LABORATORY AND DIAGNOSTIC TESTS 10.1

PRENATAL TESTS TO ASSESS RISK FOR GENETIC DISORDERS

Test	Description	Indication	Timing
Alpha-fetoprotein	A sample of the pregnant client's blood is drawn to evaluate plasma protein that is produced by the fetal liver, yolk sac, and GI tract, and crosses from the amniotic fluid into the maternal blood	Increased levels might indicate a neural tube defect, Turner syndrome, tetralogy of Fallot, multiple gestation, omphalocele gastroschisis, or hydrocephaly. Decreased levels might indicate Down syndrome or trisomy 18	Typically performed between 15 and 18 weeks' gestation
Amniocentesis	Amniotic fluid aspirated from the amniotic sac; safety concerns include infection, pregnancy loss, and fetal needle injuries	To perform chromosome analysis, alpha-fetoprotein, DNA markers, viral studies, karyotyping, and identify inborn errors of metabolism	Usually performed between 15 and 20 weeks' gestation to allow for adequate amniotic fluid volume to accumulate; results take 2–4 weeks
Chorionic villus sampling	Removal of small tissue specimen from the fetal portion of the placenta, which reflects the fetal genetic makeup; main complications include severe transverse limb defects and spontaneous pregnancy loss	To detect fetal karyotype, sickle cell anemia, phenylketonuria, Down syndrome, Duchenne muscular dystrophy, and numerous other genetic disorders	Typically performed between 10 and 12 weeks' gestation, with results available in less than 1 week
Percutaneous umbilical blood sampling	Insertion of a needle directly into a fetal umbilical vessel under ultrasound guidance; two potential complications: fetal hemorrhage and risk of infection	Used for prenatal diagnosis of inherited blood disorders such as hemophilia A, karyotyping, detection of fetal infection, determination of acid–base status, and assessment and treatment of isoimmunization	Generally performed after 16 weeks' gestation
Fetal nuchal translucency (FNT)	An intravaginal ultrasound that measures fluid collection in the subcutaneous space between the skin and the cervical spine of the fetus	To identify fetal anomalies; abnormal fluid collection can be associated with genetic disorders (trisomies 13, 18, and 21), Turner syndrome, cardiac deformities, and/or physical anomalies. When the FNT is greater than 2.5 mm, the measurement is considered abnormal	Performed between 10 and 14 weeks' gestation
Level II ultrasound/fetal scan	Use of high-frequency sound waves to visualize the fetus	Enables evaluation of structural changes to be identified early	Typically performed after 18 weeks' gestation
Triple and quad screening tests	Triple screening includes alpha-fetoprotein, estriol, and beta-hCG; quad screening includes alpha-fetoprotein, estriol, beta-hCG, and inhibin A	To identify risk for Down syndrome, neural tube defects, and other chromosomal disorders. Elevated hCG combined with lower-than-normal estriol and MSAFP levels indicate increased risk for Down syndrome or other trisomy condition	Performed between 15 and 18 weeks' gestation
Preimplantation genetic diagnosis	Genetic testing of embryos produced through in vitro fertilization (IVF)	Identifies embryos carrying specific genetic alterations that can cause disease, and transfer those without genetic alterations into the woman's uterus to start a pregnancy; prevents inheritable genetic disease before implantation	Usually on day 3 after egg retrieval and 2 days after fertilization, a single blastomere is removed from the developing embryo to be evaluated
Cell-free fetal DNA (CffDNA)	A noninvasive prenatal test using maternal plasma which hold a mixture of maternal and fetal DNA after 4 weeks' gestation	Determines fetal sex in pregnancies at risk of sex-linked conditions; RhD genotyping in pregnancies at risk of hemolytic disease of the newborn and fetal chromosomal abnormalities such as Down syndrome	A maternal blood sample is taken and next generation sequencing is used to analyze the cffDNA at approximately 10 weeks' gestation

Source: Latendresse, G., & Deneris, A. (2015). An update on current prenatal testing options: First trimester and noninvasive prenatal testing. *Journal of Midwifery & Women's Health, 60*(1), 24–36; Dayal, M. B., & Athanasiadia, I. (2018). Preimplantation genetic diagnosis. Retrieved from http://emedicine.medscape.com/article/273415-overview; Khalil, A., & Coates, A. (2015). Prenatal diagnosis of chromosomal abnormalities. In F. Arias, A. Bhide, S. Arulkumaran, K. R. Damania, & S. N. Daftary (Eds.). *Arias' practical guide to high-risk pregnancy and delivery: A South Asian perspective* (4th ed., pp. 1–13). New Delhi, India: Elsevier; Van Leeuwen, A. M., & Bladh, M. L. (2015). *Davis's comprehensive handbook of laboratory & diagnostic tests with nursing implications* (6th ed.). Philadelphia, PA: F. A. Davis Company.

Nurses play an essential role in providing emotional support to the family through this challenging time. Genetics permeate all aspects of health care. Today, everyone is embracing quality and evidence-based care. Nurses who have an understanding of genetics and genomics will possess the foundation to provide quality, evidence-based care especially with follow-up counselling after the couple or family has been to the genetic specialist (Verklan & Walden, 2015).

Take Note!

Nurses need to be actively engaged with clients and their families and help them consider the facts, values, and context in which they are making decisions. Nurses need to be open and honest with families as they discuss these sensitive and emotionally laden choices.

The nurse is in an ideal position to help families review what has been discussed during the genetic counselling sessions and to answer any additional questions they might have. Referral to appropriate agencies, support groups, and resources, such as a social worker, a chaplain, or an ethicist, is another key role when caring for families with suspected or diagnosed genetic disorders. Couples need unique clinical care which includes screening for genetic disorders, discussion of the etiology of a potential condition, connections to social supports, and clarification of the recurrence risks, and prenatal testing and treatment options. Nurses need to be involved in all aspects of this care.

KEY CONCEPTS

- Fertilization, which takes place in the outer third of the ampulla of the fallopian tube, leads to the formation of a zygote. The zygote undergoes cleavage, eventually implanting in the endometrium about 7 to 10 days after conception.

- Three embryonic layers of cells are formed and include the ectoderm, which forms the central nervous system, special senses, skin, and glands; the mesoderm, which forms the skeletal, urinary, circulatory, and reproductive systems; and the endoderm, which forms the respiratory system, liver, pancreas, and digestive system.

- Amniotic fluid surrounds the embryo and increases in volume as the pregnancy progresses, reaching approximately 1 L in volume by term.

- At no time during pregnancy is there any direct connection between the blood of the fetus and the maternal blood supply, so there is no mixing of blood. A specialized connective tissue known as Wharton's jelly surrounds the three blood vessels in the umbilical cord to prevent compression, which would choke off the blood supply and nutrients to the growing life inside.

- The placenta protects the fetus from immune attack by maternal antibodies, removes waste products from the fetus, induces the childbearing person to bring more food to the placenta and, near the time of birth, produces hormones that mature fetal organs in preparation for life outside the uterus.

- The purpose of fetal circulation is to carry highly oxygenated blood to vital areas (heart and brain) while first shunting it away from less vital ones (lungs and liver).

- Humans have 46 paired chromosomes that are found in all cells of the body, except the ovum and sperm cells, which have just 23 chromosomes. Each person has a unique genetic constitution, or genotype.

- Research from the Human Genome Project has provided a better understanding of the genetic contribution to disease.

- Genetic disorders can result from abnormalities in patterns of inheritance or chromosomal abnormalities involving chromosomal number or structure.

- Autosomal dominant inheritance occurs when a single gene in the heterozygous state is capable of producing the phenotype. Autosomal recessive inheritance occurs when two copies of the mutant or abnormal gene in the homozygous state are necessary to produce the phenotype. X-linked inheritance disorders are those associated with altered genes present on the X chromosome. They can be dominant or recessive. Multifactorial inheritance is thought to be caused by multiple genetic and environmental factors.

- In some cases of genetic disorders, a chromosomal abnormality occurs. Chromosomal abnormalities do not follow straightforward patterns of inheritance. These abnormalities occur on autosomal as well as sex chromosomes and can result from changes in the number or structure of the chromosomes.

- Genetic counselling involves evaluation of an individual or a family. Its purpose is to confirm, diagnose, or rule out genetic conditions; identify medical management issues; calculate and communicate genetic risks to a family; discuss ethical and legal issues; and assist in providing and arranging psychosocial support.

○ Legal, ethical, and social issues can arise related to genetic testing and may include the privacy and confidentiality of genetic information, who should have access to personal genetic information, psychological impact, and stigmatization due to individual genetic differences, use of genetic information in reproductive decision-making and reproductive rights, and whether testing should be performed if no cure is available.

○ Preconception screening and counselling can raise serious ethical and moral issues for a couple. The results of prenatal genetic testing can lead to the decision to terminate a pregnancy.

○ Nurses play an important role in beginning the preconception counselling process and referring clients and their partners for further genetic information when indicated. Many times, the nurse is the one who has first contact with these clients and will be the one to provide follow-up care.

○ Nurses need to have a solid understanding of who will benefit from genetic counselling and be able to discuss the role of the genetic counsellor with families, ensuring that families at risk are aware that genetic counselling is available before they attempt to have another baby.

○ Nurses play an essential role in providing emotional support and referrals to appropriate agencies, support groups, and resources when caring for families with suspected or diagnosed genetic disorders. Nurses can further assist clients with their decision-making by referring them to a social worker, chaplain, or ethicist.

REFERENCES AND RECOMMENDED READINGS

American Heart Association. (2018). *Fetal circulation.* Retrieved from http://www.heart.org/en/health-topics/congenital-heart-defects/symptoms–diagnosis-of-congenital-heart-defects/fetal-circulation

Bacino, C. A., & Lee, B. (2016). Chapter 81: Cytogenetics. In R. M. Kleigman, B. F. Stanton, J. W. St. Geme III, & N. F. Schor (Eds.). *Nelson textbook of pediatrics* (20th ed., pp. 604–626). Philadelphia, PA: Elsevier.

Brazeau, G. (2015). Chapter 10: Pharmacogenomics/pharmacogenetics and interprofessional education and practice. In D. H. Lea, D. J. Cheek, D. Brazeau, & G. Brazeau (Eds.). *Mastering pharmacogenomics: A nurse's handbook for success* (pp. 191–204). Indianapolis, IN: Sigma Theta Tau International.

Burke, W., Tarini, B., Press, N. A., & Evans, J. P. (2011). Genetic screening. *Epidemiologic Reviews, 33*, 148–164.

Carcio, H. A., & Secor, M. C. (2010). *Advanced health assessment of women* (2nd ed.). New York: Springer Publishing Company, Inc.

Conley, Y. P. (2014). Chapter 4: Genetics and health applications. In S. M. Nettina (Ed.). *Lippincott manual of nursing practice* (10th ed., pp. 33–44). Philadelphia, PA: Wolters Kluwer Health/Lippincott Williams & Wilkins.

Cunningham, J., Goldsmith, L., & Skirton, H. (2015). The evidence base regarding the experiences of and attitudes to preimplantation genetic diagnosis in prospective parents. *Midwifery, 31*(2), 288–296.

Cunningham, F. G., Leveno, K. J., Bloom, S. L., Spong, C. Y., Dashe, J. S., Hoffman, B. L., … Spong, C. Y. (2018). *William's obstetrics* (25th ed.). New York: McGraw Education.

Dayal, M. B., & Athanasiadia, I. (2018). *Preimplantation genetic diagnosis.* Retrieved from http://emedicine.medscape.com/article/273415-overview

Defendi, G. L. (2018). *Klinefelter syndrome.* Retrieved from http://emedicine.medscape.com/article/945649-overview

Edelman, C. L., Kudzma, E. C., & Mandle, C. L. (2014). *Health promotion throughout the lifespan* (8th ed.). St. Louis, MO: Mosby Elsevier.

El-Mazny, A. (2014). *Human reproduction: Basic anatomy and physiology.* Charleston, SC: Amazon CreateSpace Publishers.

Finnemore, A., & Groves, A. (2015). Physiology of the fetal and transitional circulation. *Seminars in Fetal & Neonatal Medicine, 20*(4), 210–216.

Freemark, M. (2015). Placental hormones and the control of fetal growth. *International Journal of Pediatric Endocrinology, 2015*(Suppl 1), O13.

Genetic Alliance. (n.d.). *Family health history.* Retrieved from http://www.geneticalliance.org/programs/genesinlife/fhh

Genome Canada. (2018). *Genomics by sector: Health.* Retrieved from https://www.genomecanada.ca/en/why-genomics/genomics-sector/health

International Society of Nurses in Genetics. (2018). *What is a genetics nurse?* Retrieved from https://www.isong.org/page-1325153

Jones, R. E., & Lopez, K. H. (2014). *Human reproductive biology* (4th ed.). Waltham, MA: Elsevier Health Sciences.

Khalil, A., & Coates, A. (2015). Prenatal diagnosis of chromosomal abnormalities. In F. Arias, A. Bhide, S. Arulkumaran, K. R. Damania, & S. N. Daftary (Eds.). *Arias' practical guide to high-risk pregnancy and delivery: A South Asian perspective* (4th ed., pp. 1–13). New Delhi, India: Elsevier.

King, T. L., Brucker, M. C., Kriebs, J. M., Fahey, J. O., Gegor, C. L., & Varney, H. (2015). *Varney's midwifery* (5th ed.). Burlington, MA: Jones & Bartlett Learning.

Kumar, S., Kingsley, C., & DiStefano, J. K. (2015). The Human Genome Project: Where are we now and where are we going? In R. Dugurala, L. Almasy, S. Williams-Blangero, S. F. D. Paul, & C. Kole (Eds.). *Genome mapping and genomics in human and non-human primates* (pp. 7–31). New York: Springer-Verlag Berlin Heidelberg.

Latendresse, G., & Deneris, A. (2015). An update on current prenatal testing options: First trimester and noninvasive prenatal testing. *Journal of Midwifery & Women's Health, 60*(1), 24–36.

Lawford, A., & Tulloh, R. M. (2015). Cardiovascular adaptation to extra uterine life. *Pediatrics and Child Health, 25*(1), 1–6.

Lea, D., Skirton, H., Read, C. Y., & Williams, J. K. (2011). Implications for educating the next generation of nurses on genetics and genomics in the 21st century. *Journal of Nursing Scholarship, 43*(1), 3–12.

Lee, B. (2011). Chapter 72: Integration of genetics into pediatric practice. In R. M. Kliegman, B. F. Stanton, J. W. St. Geme, N. F. Schor, & R. E. Behrman, (Eds.). *Nelson's textbook of pediatrics* (19th ed., pp. 376–380). Philadelphia, PA: Saunders.

Lewis, R. (2015). *Human genetics: Concepts and applications* (11th ed.). New York: McGraw-Hill Companies, Incorporated.

Lichtenbelt, K. D., Diemel, B. D., Koster, M. P., Manten, G. T., Siljee, J., Schuring-Blom, G. H., & Page-Christiaens, G. C. (2015). Detection of fetal chromosomal anomalies: Does nuchal translucency measurement have added value in the era of non-invasive prenatal testing? *Prenatal Diagnosis, 35,* 663–668.

Lopes, L. C., de Omena Bomfim, E., & Flória-Santos, M. (2015). Genomics-based health care: Implications for nursing. *International Journal of Nursing Didactics, 5*(02), 11–15.

Mader, S., & Windelspecht, M. (2015). *Human biology* (14th ed.). New York: McGraw-Hill Higher Education.

Magann, E., & Ross, M. G. (2018). *Assessment of amniotic fluid volume.* Retrieved from http://www.uptodate.com/contents/assessment-of-amniotic-fluid-volume

March of Dimes. (2018). *Genetic counseling.* Retrieved from http://www.marchofdimes.org/pregnancy/genetic-counseling.aspx

Mattson, S., & Smith, J. E. (2015). *Core curriculum for maternal-newborn nursing* (5th ed.). St. Louis, MO: Saunders Elsevier.

Meyer zu Schwabedissen, H. E. (2015). The role of pharmacogenomics in individualized medicine. In T. Fischer, M. Langanke, P. Marschall, & S. Michl (Eds.). *Individualized medicine: Ethical, economical, and historical perspectives* (pp. 93–112). New York: Springer International Publishing.

Moore, T. R. (2015). Abnormal amniotic fluid. In J. T. Queenan, C. Y. Spong, & C. J. Lockwood (Eds.). *Protocols for high-risk pregnancies: An evidence-based approach* (6th ed., pp. 315–328). West Sussex, UK: Wiley Blackwell Publishers.

National Human Genome Research Institute. (2015a). *All about the Human Genome Project (HGP).* Retrieved from http://www.genome.gov/10001772

National Human Genome Research Institute. (2015b). *Frequently asked questions about genetic counseling.* Retrieved from http://www.genome.gov/19016905

National Human Genome Research Institute. (2017). *Frequently asked questions about genetic testing.* Retrieved from http://www.genome.gov/19516567

National Institutes of Health. (2018a). *Genetics home reference: Guide to understanding genetic conditions.* Retrieved from https://ghr.nlm.nih.gov/

National Institutes of Health. (2018b). *Genetic testing: How it is used for healthcare.* Retrieved from http://www.report.nih.gov/NIHfactsheets/ViewFactSheet.aspx?csid=43&key=G

Nussbaum, R. L., McInnes, R. R., & Willard, H. F. (2016). *Thompson & Thompson genetics in medicine* (8th ed.). Philadelphia, PA: Elsevier.

Public Health Agency of Canada. (2013). *Congenital anomalies in Canada 2013: A perinatal health surveillance report.* Ottawa. Retrieved from http://publications.gc.ca/collections/collection_2014/aspc-phac/HP35-40-2013-eng.pdf

Scott, D. A., & Lee, B. (2011). Chapter 80: Patterns of genetic transmission. In R. M. Kliegman, B. F. Stanton, J. W. St. Geme, & N. F. Schor (Eds.). *Nelson's textbook of pediatrics* (20th ed., pp. 593–603). Philadelphia, PA: Elsevier.

Sermon, K., & Viville, S. (2014). *Textbook of human reproductive genetics.* New York: Cambridge University Press.

Seven, M., Akyüz, A., Elbüken, B., Skirton, H., & Öztürk, H. (2015). Nurses' knowledge and educational needs regarding genetics. *Nurse Education Today, 35*(3), 444–449.

Slavotinek, A., & Ali, M. (2015). Recognizable syndromes in the newborn period. *Clinics in Perinatology, 42*(2), 263–280.

Snustad, D. P., & Simmons, M. J. (2015). *Principles of genetics* (7th ed.). New York: Wiley Publishers.

Solomon, E. P. (2015). *Introduction to human anatomy and physiology* (4th ed.). Philadelphia, PA: Elsevier Health Sciences.

Travers, A., & Muskhelishvili, G. (2015). DNA structure and function. *FEBS Journal, 282,* 2279–2295.

U.S. Department of Energy Genome Programs. (2017). *Human Genome Project information archive.* Retrieved from http://www.ornl.gov/sci/techresources/Human_Genome/home.shtml

U.S. Department of Energy Genome Programs. (2018). *Human Genome Project information: Gene testing.* Retrieved from http://doegenomestolife.org/program/index.shtml

Van Esch, H. (2018). *Fragile X syndrome: Clinical features and diagnosis in children and adolescents.* Retrieved from http://www.uptodate.com/contents/fragile-x-syndrome-clinical-features-and-diagnosis-in-children-and-adolescents

Van Leeuwen, A. M., & Bladh, M. L. (2015). *Davis's comprehensive handbook of laboratory & diagnostic tests with nursing implications* (6th ed.). Philadelphia, PA: F. A. Davis Company.

Verklan, M. T., & Walden, M. (2015). *Core curriculum for neonatal intensive care nursing* (4th ed.). St. Louis, MO: Saunders Elsevier.

Verma, I. C., & Puri, R. D. (2015). Global burden of genetic disease and the role of genetic screening. *Seminars in Fetal & Neonatal Medicine, 20,* 354–363.

Wilson, R. D. (2017). Women's pre-conception evaluation: Genetic and fetal risk considerations for counselling and informed choice. *Journal of Obstetrics and Gynaecology Canada, 40*(7), 935–949.

CHAPTER **WORKSHEET**

MULTIPLE CHOICE QUESTIONS

1. After teaching a group of students about fertilization, the instructor determines that the teaching was successful when the group identifies which as the usual site of fertilization?
   a. Fundus of the uterus
   b. Endometrium of the uterus
   c. Distal portion of fallopian tube
   d. Follicular tissue of the ovary

2. A client comes to the clinic for pregnancy testing. The nurse explains that the test detects the presence of which hormone?
   a. Human placental lactogen (hPL)
   b. Human chorionic gonadotropin (hCG)
   c. Follicle-stimulating hormone (FSH)
   d. Thyroid-stimulating hormone (TSH)

3. The nurse is counselling a couple, one of whom is affected by an autosomal dominant disorder. They express concerns about the risk of transmitting the disorder. What is the best response by the nurse regarding the risk that their baby may have for the disease?
   a. "You have a one in four (25%) chance."
   b. "The risk is 12.5%, or a one in eight chance."
   c. "The chance is 100%."
   d. "Your risk is 50%, or a one in two chance."

4. What is the first step in determining a couple's risk for a genetic disorder?
   a. Observing the client and family over time
   b. Conducting extensive psychological testing
   c. Obtaining a thorough family health history
   d. Completing an extensive exclusionary list

5. A nurse is working in a reproductive health clinic. Which client would genetic counselling be most appropriate for?
   a. Had their first miscarriage at 10 weeks
   b. Is 30 years old and planning to conceive
   c. Has a history with a close relative with Down syndrome
   d. Is 18 weeks pregnant with a normal triple screen result

6. Which of the following is an example of an autosomal dominant disorder?
   a. Phenylketonuria
   b. Tay–Sachs disease
   c. Polycystic kidney disease
   d. Cystic fibrosis

7. Which of the following is the major goal of genetic counselling?
   a. Diagnose and determine the role of heredity
   b. Reinforce previously presented test data
   c. Emphasize good communication skills
   d. Offer referral to community support groups

CRITICAL THINKING EXERCISE

1. Mr. and Mrs. Martin wish to start a family, but they can't agree on something important. Mr. Martin wants his wife to be tested for cystic fibrosis (CF) to see if she is a carrier. Mr. Martin had a brother with CF and watched his parents struggle with the hardship and the expense of caring for him for years, and he doesn't want to experience it in his own life. Mr. Martin has found out he is a CF carrier. Mrs. Martin doesn't want to have the test because she figures that once a baby is in their arms, they will be glad, no matter what.
   a. What information/education should this couple consider before deciding whether to have the test?
   b. How can you assist this couple in their decision-making process?
   c. What is your role in this situation if you don't agree with their decision?

STUDY ACTIVITIES

1. Select one of the websites listed in thePoint to explore the topic of genetics. Critique the information presented. Was it understandable to a layperson? What specifically did you learn? Share your findings with your classmates during a discussion group.

2. Draw your own family pedigree, identifying inheritance patterns. Share it with your family to validate its accuracy. What did you discover about your family's past health?

3. Select one of the various prenatal screening tests (alpha-fetoprotein, amniocentesis, chorionic villus sampling, or fetal nuchal translucency) and research it in depth. Role play with another nursing student how you would explain its purpose, the procedure, and potential findings to an expectant couple at risk for a fetal abnormality.

BRINGING IT ALL TOGETHER: A CASE STUDY

Rebecca and Jon are a couple seeking genetic counselling. Rebecca, 43 years old, is 10 weeks pregnant with their first baby. The couple is concerned about the possibility of their child demonstrating trisomy 21 (Down syndrome).

Go to thePoint **to find questions to consider about this case.**

11

Adaptations During Pregnancy

Learning Objectives

Upon completion of the chapter, you will be able to:

1. Differentiate between subjective (presumptive), objective (probable), and diagnostic (positive) signs of pregnancy.

2. Describe maternal physiologic changes that occur during pregnancy.

3. Summarize the nutritional needs of the pregnant client and the fetus.

4. Characterize the emotional and psychological changes that occur during pregnancy.

Marva, age 17, appeared at the health clinic complaining that she had a stomach virus and needed to be seen right away. When the nurse asked her additional questions about her illness, Marva reported that she had been sick to her stomach and "beat tired" for days. She had stopped eating to avoid any more nausea and vomiting.

INTRODUCTION

Pregnancy is a normal life event that involves considerable physical and psychological adjustments for the mother. A pregnancy is divided into three **trimesters** of 13 weeks each (Edelman, Kudzma, & Mandle, 2014). Within each trimester, numerous adaptations take place that facilitate the growth of the fetus. The most obvious are physical changes to accommodate the growing fetus, but pregnant people also undergo psychological changes as they prepare for parenthood. A thorough understanding of these numerous changes and adaptations is essential for all nurses caring for clients during pregnancy.

SIGNS AND SYMPTOMS OF PREGNANCY

Traditionally, signs and symptoms of pregnancy have been grouped into the following categories: presumptive, probable, and positive (Box 11.1). The only signs that can determine a pregnancy with 100% accuracy are positive signs.

What additional information is necessary to complete the assessment of Marva, the 17-year-old with nausea and vomiting? What diagnostic tests might be done to confirm the nurse's suspicion that she is pregnant?

Subjective (Presumptive) Signs

Presumptive signs are those signs that the mother can perceive. The most obvious presumptive sign of pregnancy is the absence of menstruation. Skipping a period is not a reliable sign of pregnancy by itself, but if it is

accompanied by consistent nausea, fatigue, breast tenderness, and urinary frequency, pregnancy would seem very likely.

Presumptive changes are the least reliable indicators of pregnancy because any one of them can be caused by conditions other than pregnancy (Shields, 2017). For example, amenorrhea can be caused by early menopause, endocrine dysfunction, malnutrition, anemia, diabetes mellitus, long-distance running, cancer, or stress.

Consider This

Jay and I decided to start our family, so I stopped taking the pill 3 months ago. One morning when I got out of bed to take the dog out, I felt queasy and light-headed. I sure hoped I wasn't coming down with the flu. By the end of the week, I was feeling really tired and started taking naps in the afternoon. In addition, I seemed to be going to the bathroom frequently, despite not drinking much fluid. When my breasts started to tingle and ache, I decided to make an appointment with my doctor to see what "illness" I had contracted.

After listening to my list of physical complaints, the office nurse asked me if I might be pregnant. My eyes opened wide: I had somehow missed the link between my symptoms and pregnancy. I started to think about when my last period was, and it had been 2 months ago. The office ran a pregnancy test and much to my surprise it was positive!

Thoughts: Many people stop contraceptives in an attempt to achieve pregnancy but miss the early signs of pregnancy. This person was experiencing several signs of early pregnancy—urinary frequency, fatigue, morning nausea, and breast tenderness. What advice can the nurse give this client to ease these symptoms? What additional education related to pregnancy would be appropriate at this time?

BOX 11.1		

SIGNS AND SYMPTOMS OF PREGNANCY

Presumptive (Time of Occurrence, weeks)	Probable (Time of Occurrence, weeks)	Positive (Time of Occurrence, weeks)
Fatigue (12)	Braxton Hicks contractions (16–28)	Ultrasound verification of embryo or fetus (4–6)
Breast tenderness (3–4)	Positive pregnancy test (4–12)	Fetal movement felt by experienced clinician (20)
Nausea and vomiting (4–14)	Abdominal enlargement (14)	Auscultation of fetal heart tones via Doppler (10–12)
Amenorrhea (4)	Ballottement (16–28)	
Urinary frequency (6–12)	Goodell's sign (5)	
Hyperpigmentation of the skin (16)	Chadwick's sign (6–8)	
Fetal movements (quickening; 16–20)	Hegar's sign (6–12)	
Uterine enlargement (7–12)		
Breast enlargement (6)		

Adapted from Bope, E. T., & Kellerman, R. D. (2015). *Conn's current therapy 2015.* Philadelphia, PA: Saunders Elsevier; Shields, A. D. (2017). Pregnancy diagnosis. *eMedicine.* Retrieved from http://emedicine.medscape.com/article/262591-overview; Jordan, R. G., Engstrom, J., Matrfell, J., & Farley, C. L. (2014). *Prenatal and postnatal care: A woman-centered approach.* Ames, IA: Wiley-Blackwell.

Nausea and vomiting can be caused by gastrointestinal disorders, food poisoning, acute infections, or eating disorders. Fatigue could be caused by anemia, stress, or viral infections. Breast tenderness may result from chronic cystic mastitis, premenstrual changes, or the use of oral contraceptives. Urinary frequency could have a variety of causes other than pregnancy, such as infection, cystocele, structural disorders, pelvic tumors, or emotional tension (Tharpe, Farley, & Jordan, 2016).

Objective (Probable) Signs

Physical Signs

Probable signs of pregnancy are those that can be detected on physical examination by a health care provider. Common probable signs of pregnancy include softening of the lower uterine segment or isthmus **(Hegar's sign),** softening of the cervix **(Goodell's sign),** and a bluish-purple colouration of the vaginal mucosa and cervix **(Chadwick's sign)**. Other probable signs include changes in the shape and size of the uterus, abdominal enlargement, Braxton Hicks contractions, and **ballottement** (the examiner pushes against the client's cervix during a pelvic examination and feels a rebound from the floating fetus).

Pregnancy Tests

Along with these physical signs, pregnancy tests are also considered a probable sign of pregnancy. In-home pregnancy testing became available in Canada, the United States, and some areas in Europe in the late 1970s. In-home testing appealed to the general public because of convenience, cost, and confidentiality. Several pregnancy tests are available (Table 11.1). The tests vary in sensitivity, specificity, and accuracy and are influenced by the length of gestation, specimen concentration, presence of blood, and the presence of some drugs. Human chorionic gonadotropin (hCG) is detectable in the serum of approximately 5% of clients 8 days after conception and in more than 98% of clients by day 11 (Shields, 2017). There are various different home pregnancy tests currently marketed in Canada. Most of these tests claim "99% accuracy" according to a U.S. Food and Drug Administration (FDA) guideline or make other similar statements on the packaging or product insert. The 99% accuracy statement in reference to the FDA guideline is misleading in that it has no bearing on the ability of the home pregnancy test to detect early pregnancy (Shields, 2017). The limitations of these tests must be understood so that pregnancy detection is not delayed significantly. Early pregnancy detection allows for the commencement of prenatal care, potential medication changes, and lifestyle changes to promote a healthy pregnancy.

hCG is a glycoprotein and the earliest biochemical marker for pregnancy. Many pregnancy tests are based on the recognition of hCG or a beta subunit of hCG. hCG levels in normal pregnancy usually double every 48 to 72 hours until they peak approximately 60 to 70 days after fertilization. At this point, they decrease to a plateau at 100 to 130 days of pregnancy. The hCG doubling time has been used as a marker by clinicians to differentiate normal from abnormal gestations. Low levels are associated with an ectopic pregnancy and higher-than-normal levels may indicate a molar pregnancy or multiple-gestational pregnancies (Zinaman, Johnson, & Marriott, 2015).

 Take Note!

This elevation of hCG corresponds to the morning sickness period of approximately 6 to 12 weeks during early pregnancy.

TABLE 11.1	SELECTED PREGNANCY TESTS		
Type	**Specimen**	**Example**	**Remarks**
Agglutination inhibition tests	Urine	Pregnosticon, Gravindex	If hCG is present in urine, agglutination does not occur, which is positive for pregnancy; reliable 14–21 days after conception; 95% accurate in diagnosing pregnancy
Immunoradiometric assay	Blood serum	Neocept, Pregnosis	Measures ability of blood sample to inhibit the binding of radiolabeled hCG to receptors; reliable 6–8 days after conception; 99% accurate in diagnosing pregnancy
Enzyme-linked immunosorbent assay (ELISA)	Blood serum or urine	Over-the-counter home/office pregnancy tests; precise	Uses an enzyme to bond with hCG in the urine if present; reliable 4 days after implantation; 99% accurate if hCG specific

Adapted from Jordan, R. G., Engstrom, J., Matrfell, J., & Farley, C. L. (2014). *Prenatal and postnatal care: A woman-centered approach.* Ames, IA: Wiley-Blackwell; King, T. L., Brucker, M. C., Kriebs, J. M., Fahey, J. O., Gegor, C. L., & Varney, H. (2015). *Varney's midwifery* (5th ed.). Burlington, MA: Jones & Bartlett Learning; Shields, A. D. (2017). Pregnancy diagnosis. *eMedicine.* Retrieved from http://emedicine.medscape.com/article/262591-overview

Although probable signs suggest pregnancy and are more reliable than presumptive signs, they still are not 100% reliable in confirming a pregnancy. For example, uterine tumors, polyps, infection, and pelvic congestion can cause changes to uterine shape, size, and consistency. And although pregnancy tests are used to establish the diagnosis of pregnancy when the physical signs are still inconclusive, they are not completely reliable, because conditions other than pregnancy (e.g., ovarian cancer, choriocarcinoma, hydatidiform mole) can also elevate hCG levels.

Positive Signs

Usually within 2 weeks after a missed period, enough subjective symptoms are present so that a person can be reasonably sure about being pregnant. However, an experienced health care provider can confirm the suspicion by identifying positive signs of pregnancy that can be directly attributed to the fetus. The positive signs of pregnancy confirm that a fetus is growing in the uterus. Visualizing the fetus by ultrasound, palpating for fetal movements, and hearing a fetal heartbeat are all signs that make the pregnancy a certainty.

If the pregnancy test is positive, the clinical visit should include an estimation of gestational age so that appropriate counseling can be provided. In addition, clients should receive information about the normal signs and symptoms of early pregnancy, and should be instructed to report any concerns to the health care provider for further evaluation. Once pregnancy has been confirmed, the health care provider will set up a schedule of prenatal visits to assess the client and the fetus throughout the entire pregnancy. Assessment and education begins at the first visits and continues throughout the pregnancy (see Chapter 12).

> Remember Marva, who thought she had a stomach virus? Her pregnancy test was positive. On questioning by the nurse, she acknowledged missing two menstrual periods and being sexually active with her boyfriend without using protection. What is the nurse's role at this point with Marva? What instructions might be given to her while she waits for her first prenatal visit?

PHYSIOLOGIC ADAPTATIONS DURING PREGNANCY

Every system of a person's body changes during pregnancy to accommodate the needs of the growing fetus, and these changes occur with startling rapidity. The physical changes of pregnancy can be uncomfortable, although every person reacts uniquely.

Reproductive System Adaptations

Significant changes occur throughout the client's body during pregnancy to accommodate the growing human being within her. Many have a protective role to maintain homeostasis and are essential to meet the demands of both the pregnant person and the fetus. Many adaptations are reversible after the client gives birth, but some persist for life.

Uterus

The uterus grows at a steady, predictable rate during pregnancy. During the first few months of pregnancy, estrogen stimulates uterine growth, and the uterus undergoes a tremendous increase in size, weight, length, width, depth, volume, and overall capacity throughout pregnancy. The weight of the uterus increases from 70 g to about 1,100 to 1,200 g at term; its capacity increases from 10 to 5,000 mL or more at term (King et al., 2015). The uterine walls thin to 1.5 cm or less; the shape changes from pear shape to a solid globe in the first trimester, and then expands to become a hollow vessel.

Uterine growth occurs as a result of both hyperplasia and hypertrophy of the myometrial cells, which do not increase much in number but do increase in size. In early pregnancy, uterine growth is due to hyperplasia of uterine smooth muscle cells within the myometrium; however, the major component of myometrial growth occurs after mid-gestation due to smooth muscle cell hypertrophy caused by mechanical stretch of uterine tissue by the growing fetus (Osol & Moore, 2014). Blood vessels elongate, enlarge, dilate, and sprout new branches to support and nourish the growing muscle tissue, and the increase in uterine weight is accompanied by a large increase in uterine blood flow, which is necessary to perfuse the uterine muscle and accommodate the growing fetus. As pregnancy progresses, 80% to 90% of uterine blood flow goes to the placenta, with the remainder distributed between the endometrium and myometrium. During pregnancy, the diameter of the main uterine artery approximately doubles in size. This enlargement from a narrow to a larger-caliber vessel enhances the capacity of the uteroplacental vessels to accommodate the increased blood volume needed to supply the placenta (Osol & Moore, 2014).

Uterine contractility is enhanced as well. Spontaneous, irregular, and painless contractions, called **Braxton Hicks contractions**, begin during the first trimester. These contractions continue throughout pregnancy, becoming especially noticeable during the last month, when they function to thin out or efface the cervix before birth (see Chapter 12 for more information).

The lower portion of the uterus (the isthmus) does not undergo hypertrophy and becomes increasingly thinner as pregnancy progresses, thereby forming the lower

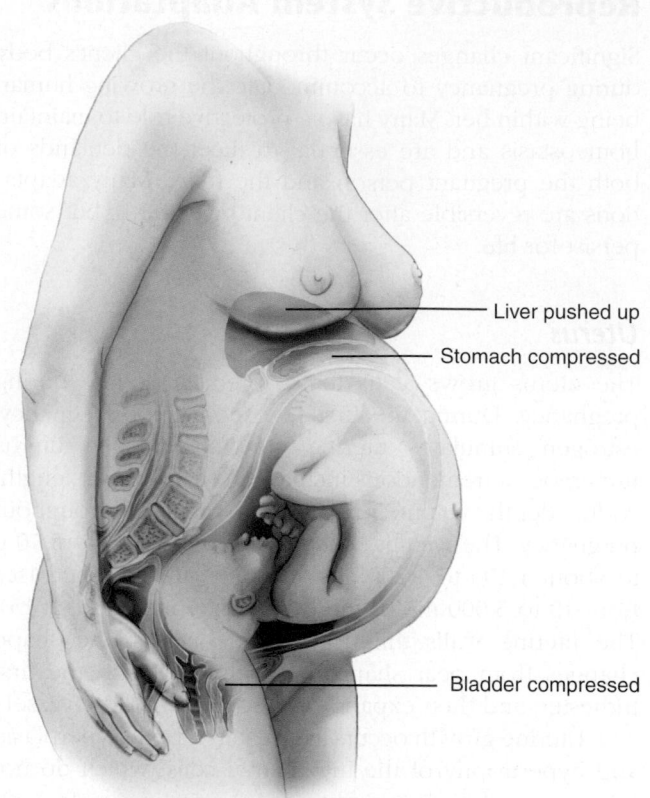

FIGURE 11.1 **The growing uterus in the abdomen.**

— Liver pushed up

— Stomach compressed

— Bladder compressed

Vena Cava
Aorta

Supine position

Side-lying position

FIGURE 11.2 **Supine hypotensive syndrome.**

uterine segment. Changes in the lower uterus occurring during the first 6 to 8 weeks of gestation produce some of the typical findings, including a positive Hegar's sign. This softening and compressibility of the lower uterine segment results in exaggerated uterine anteflexion during the early months of pregnancy, which adds to urinary frequency (Heffner & Schust, 2014).

The uterus remains in the pelvic cavity for the first 3 months of pregnancy, after which it progressively ascends into the abdomen (Fig. 11.1). As the uterus grows, it presses on the urinary bladder and causes the increased frequency of urination experienced during early pregnancy. In addition, the heavy gravid uterus in the last trimester can fall back against the inferior vena cava in the supine position, resulting in vena cava compression, which reduces venous return and decreases cardiac output and blood pressure, with increasing orthostatic stress. This occurs when the pregnant person changes position from recumbent to sitting to standing. This acute hemodynamic change, termed supine hypotensive syndrome, causes the client to experience symptoms of weakness, light-headedness, nausea, dizziness, or syncope (Fig. 11.2). These changes are reversed when the pregnant person is in the side-lying position, which displaces the uterus to the left and off the vena cava.

The uterus, which starts as a pear-shaped organ, becomes ovoid as length increases over width. By 20 weeks of gestation, the fundus, or top of the uterus, is at the level of the umbilicus and measures 20 cm. A monthly measurement of the height of the top of the uterus in centimeters, which corresponds to the number of gestational weeks, is commonly used to date the pregnancy.

Take Note!

Fundal height usually can be correlated with gestational weeks most accurately between 18 and 32 weeks. Obesity, hydramnios, and uterine fibroids interfere with the accuracy of this correlation.

The fundus reaches its highest level, at the xiphoid process, at approximately 36 weeks. Between 38 and 40 weeks, fundal height drops as the fetus begins to descend and engage into the pelvis. Because it pushes against the diaphragm, many people experience shortness of breath. By 40 weeks, the fetal head begins to descend and engage in the pelvis, which is termed *lightening*. For the client who is pregnant for the first time, lightening usually occurs approximately 2 weeks before the onset of labour; for the client who is experiencing a second or subsequent pregnancy, it usually occurs at the onset of labour. Although breathing becomes easier because of this descent, the pressure on the urinary bladder now increases and the client now experiences urinary frequency again, as in the first trimester of pregnancy.

Cervix

Between weeks 6 and 8 of pregnancy, the cervix begins to soften (Goodell's sign) due to vasocongestion and the influence of estrogen. Along with the softening, the endocervical glands increase in size and number and produce more cervical mucus. Under the influence of progesterone, a thick mucus plug is formed that blocks the cervical os and protects the opening from bacterial invasion. At about the same time, increased vascularization of the cervix causes Chadwick's sign, a cyanosis or bluish-purple discolouration. Cervical ripening (softening, effacement, and increased distensibility) begins about 4 weeks before birth. The connective tissues of the cervix undergo biochemical modifications in preparation for labour that result in changes to its elasticity and strength. These changes are mediated through several factors, including inflammation, cervical stretch, pressure of the fetal presenting part, and release of hormones, including oxytocin, relaxin, nitric oxide, and prostaglandins (Myers et al., 2015).

Vagina

During pregnancy, vascularity increases because of the influences of estrogen, resulting in pelvic congestion and hypertrophy of the vagina in preparation for the distention needed for birth. The vaginal mucosa thickens, the connective tissue begins to loosen, the smooth muscle begins to hypertrophy, and the vaginal vault begins to lengthen (Bope & Kellerman, 2015). Vaginal secretions become more acidic, white, and thick. Most pregnant people experience an increase in a whitish vaginal discharge, called leukorrhea, during pregnancy. This is normal except when it is accompanied by itching and irritation, possibly suggesting *Candida albicans,* a monilial vaginitis, which is a very common occurrence in this glycogen-rich environment (King et al., 2015). Symptomatic vulvovaginal candidiasis affects 15% of pregnant clients (Krapf, 2018). It is a benign fungal condition that is uncomfortable for the pregnant person and can be transmitted from an infected person to the newborn at birth. Neonates develop an oral infection known as thrush, which presents as white patches on the mucous membranes of their mouths. It is self-limiting and is treated with local antifungal agents.

Ovaries

The increased blood supply to the ovaries causes them to enlarge until approximately the 12th to 14th week of gestation. The ovaries are not palpable after that time because the uterus fills the pelvic cavity. Ovulation ceases during pregnancy because of the elevated levels of estrogen and progesterone, which block secretion of follicle-stimulating hormone (FSH) and luteinizing hormone (LH) from the anterior pituitary. The ovaries are very active in hormone production to support the pregnancy until about weeks 6 to 7, when the corpus luteum regresses and the placenta takes over the major production of progesterone.

Breasts

The breasts increase in fullness, become tender, and grow larger throughout pregnancy under the influence of estrogen and progesterone. The breasts become highly vascular, and veins become visible under the skin. The nipples become larger and more erect. Both the nipples and the areola become deeply pigmented, and tubercles of Montgomery (sebaceous glands) become prominent. These sebaceous glands keep the nipples lubricated for breastfeeding.

Changes that occur in the connective tissue of the breasts, along with the tremendous growth, lead to striae (stretch marks) in approximately half of all pregnant women (Jordan, Engstrom, Matrfell, & Farley, 2014). Initially they appear as pink to purple lines on the skin, but they eventually fade to a silver colour. Although they become less conspicuous in time, they never completely disappear.

Creamy, yellowish breast fluid called colostrum can be expressed by the third trimester. This fluid provides nourishment for the breastfeeding newborn during the first few days of life (see Chapters 15 and 16 for more information). Table 11.2 summarizes reproductive system adaptations.

General Body System Adaptations

In addition to changes in the reproductive system, the pregnant client also experiences changes in virtually every other body system in response to the growing fetus.

Gastrointestinal System

The gastrointestinal system begins in the oral cavity and ends at the rectum. During pregnancy, the gums become hyperemic, swollen, and friable and tend to bleed easily. This change is influenced by estrogen and increased proliferation of blood vessels and circulation to the mouth. In addition, the saliva produced in the mouth becomes more acidic. Some people complain about excessive salivation, termed *ptyalism,* which may be caused by the decrease in unconscious swallowing when nauseated. Ptyalism typically resolves spontaneously, although in some people it endures throughout the pregnancy. Some clients get temporary relief from gum chewing or sucking on hard candies (King et al., 2015). Dental plaque, calculus, and debris deposits increase during pregnancy and are all associated with gingivitis. An increased production of female hormones during pregnancy contributes to the development of gingivitis and periodontitis because vascular permeability and possible tissue edema are both increased. It is reported that as many as 50% to 70% of pregnant women will have some level of gingivitis during pregnancy as a result of hormonal changes that promote inflammation (Anil et al., 2015). Previous studies linked periodontal disease with preterm birth, preeclampsia, low–birth-weight risk, stillbirth, and early-onset neonatal sepsis, but more recent research findings indicated no reduction in preterm births with

TABLE 11.2	SUMMARY OF REPRODUCTIVE SYSTEM ADAPTATIONS
Reproductive Organ	**Adaptations**
Uterus	Size increases to 20 times that of nonpregnant size Capacity increases by 2,000 times to accommodate the developing fetus Weight increases from 2 oz to approximately 2 lb at term Uterine growth occurs as a result of both hyperplasia and hypertrophy of the myometrial cells Increased strength and elasticity allow uterus to contract and expel fetus during birth
Cervix	Increases in mass, water content, and vascularization Changes from a relatively rigid to a soft, distensible structure that allows the fetus to be expelled Under the influence of progesterone, a thick mucus plug is formed, which blocks the cervical os and protects the developing fetus from bacterial invasion
Vagina	Increased vascularity because of estrogen influences, resulting in pelvic congestion and hypertrophy Increased thickness of mucosa, along with an increase in vaginal secretions to prevent bacterial infections
Ovaries	Increased blood supply to the ovaries causes them to enlarge until approximately the 12–14th week of gestation. They actively produce hormones to support the pregnancy until weeks 6–7 when the placenta takes over the production of progesterone
Breasts	Breast changes begin soon after conception; they increase in size and areolar pigmentation The tubercles of Montgomery enlarge and become more prominent, and the nipples become more erect The blood vessels become more prominent, and blood flow to the breast doubles

the treatment of periodontal disease during pregnancy (Trivedi, Lal, & Singhal, 2015), and a recent Canadian study concluded that periodontal disease is associated with preeclampsia but not with spontaneous preterm birth (Soucy-Giguère et al., 2016).

Take Note!
Bleeding of gums during pregnancy results from increased estrogen levels that cause blood vessel proliferation. This then leads to increased blood vessels in the gums and an increased chance of bleeding.

Smooth muscle relaxation and decreased peristalsis occur related to the influence of progesterone. Elevated progesterone levels cause smooth muscle relaxation, which results in delayed gastric emptying and decreased peristalsis. Transition time of food throughout the gastrointestinal tract may be so much slower that more water than normal is reabsorbed, leading to bloating and constipation. Constipation can also result from low-fiber food choices, reduced fluid intake, use of iron supplements, decreased activity level, and intestinal displacement secondary to a growing uterus. Constipation, increased venous pressure, and the pressure of the gravid uterus contribute to the formation of hemorrhoids.

The slowed gastric emptying combined with relaxation of the cardiac sphincter allows reflux, which causes heartburn. Acid indigestion or heartburn (pyrosis) seems to be a universal problem for pregnant people. It is caused by regurgitation of the stomach contents into the upper esophagus and may be associated with the generalized relaxation of the entire digestive system. Over-the-counter antacids will usually relieve the symptoms, but they should be taken with the health care provider's knowledge and only as directed.

The emptying time of the gallbladder is prolonged secondary to the smooth muscle relaxation from progesterone. Hypercholesterolemia can follow, increasing the risk of gallstone formation. Other risk factors for gallbladder disease include obesity, Hispanic ethnicity, and increasing maternal age (Heuman, Mihas, & Allen, 2017).

Nausea and vomiting, better known as morning sickness, plague about 80% of pregnant people. This condition is usually self-limiting, but the symptoms can be distressing and interfere with work, social activities, and interrupt sleep. The Society of Obstetricians and Gynaecologists of Canada (SOGC) recommends that pyridoxine monotherapy or doxylamine/pyridoxine (Diclectin) combination therapy as first line in treating nausea and vomiting of pregnancy due to their efficacy and safety (Campbell, Rowe, Azzam, & Lane, 2016). Canada approved doxylamine succinate-pyridoxine HCl (Diclectin) in the late 1980s. Diclectin is currently the only prescription drug authorized in Canada for the treatment of nausea and vomiting in pregnancy (Health Canada, 2016a). In 2013, the United States FDA authorized Diclegis (the US equivalent to Diclectin) for the treatment of nausea and vomiting in pregnant clients as a "Category A drug" (the safest for use by pregnant people). This drug approval was supported by historical and recent data (Pope, Maltepe, & Koren, 2015). Although it occurs most often in the morning, the nauseated feeling can last all day in some people. The highest incidence of morning sickness occurs between 6 and 12 weeks. The physiologic basis for morning sickness is still debatable. It has been linked to the high levels of hCG, high levels of circulating estrogens, prostaglandins, reduced stomach acidity, advancing maternal age, slowed peristalsis, genetic factors, and the lowered tone and motility of the digestive tract (King et al., 2015).

The SOGC offers many suggestions for educating pregnant clients on ways to reduce nausea and vomiting in pregnancy, including (SOGC, 2012):

- Try eating crackers and resting for 15 minutes before getting up in the morning.
- Rise slowly and avoid lying down after eating.
- Eat small meals or snacks often (e.g., every 2 hours) to avoid an empty stomach. Try not to skip meals.
- Eat what you feel like and eat when you are hungry, although spicy, fatty, or fried foods may trigger or aggravate nausea.
- If the smell of food cooking is bothersome, open windows and turn on the stove fan. If possible, ask someone else to cook. Cold food may not smell as strongly.
- Sniffing lemons or ginger may help settle an upset stomach.
- A few salty potato chips can help settle the stomach enough to eat a meal.

Cardiovascular System

Cardiovascular changes occur early during pregnancy to meet the demands of the enlarging uterus and the placenta for more blood and more oxygen. The changes include an increase in heart rate (25%); cardiac output increases by 30% to 50% and peaks at 25 to 30 weeks of gestation; reduced total peripheral resistance; increased blood volume; increased plasma volume which leads to physiologic anemia. Perhaps the most striking cardiac alteration occurring during pregnancy is the increase in blood volume.

BLOOD VOLUME

Blood volume increases by approximately 1,500 mL, or up to 50% above nonpregnant levels, by the 32nd week of gestation, and remains more or less constant thereafter (Foo, Tay, Lees, McEniery, & Wilkinson, 2015). The increase is made up of 1,000 mL plasma plus 450 mL red blood cells. It begins at weeks 10 to 12, peaks at weeks 32 to 34, and decreases slightly by week 40.

Take Note!

The rise in blood volume correlates directly with fetal weight, supporting the concept of the placenta as an arteriovenous shunt in the maternal vascular compartment.

This increase in blood volume is needed to provide adequate hydration of fetal and maternal tissues, to supply blood flow to perfuse the enlarging uterus, and to provide a reserve to compensate for blood loss at birth and during postpartum. The maternal blood volume expansion occurs at a larger proportion than the increase in red blood cell mass, which results in physiologic anemia and hemodilution. Criteria of physiologic anemia include hemoglobin 10 g or less, red blood cells 3.5 million/mm^3, and normal morphology with central pallor (Sabina, Iftequar, Zaheer, Khan, & Khan, 2015). This increase is also necessary to meet the increased metabolic needs of the pregnant person and to meet the need for increased perfusion of other organs, especially the kidneys, because of the excretion of waste products for the fetus as well.

CARDIAC OUTPUT AND HEART RATE

Cardiac output, the product of stroke volume and heart rate, is a measure of the functional capacity of the heart. It increases from 30% to 50% over the nonpregnant rate by the 32nd week of pregnancy and declines to about a 20% increase at 40 weeks of gestation. The increase in cardiac output is associated with an increase in venous return and greater right ventricular output, especially in the left lateral position (Bope & Kellerman, 2015). Elevated cardiac output is also a result of increased stroke volume and heart rate and occurs in response to increased tissue demands for oxygen (Blackburn, 2013). Heart rate increases by 10 to 15 bpm between 14 and 20 weeks of gestation, and this persists to term. There is slight hypertrophy or enlargement of the heart during pregnancy. This is probably to accommodate the increase in blood volume and cardiac output. The heart works harder and pumps more blood to supply the oxygen needs of the fetus as well as those of the mother. Both heart rate and venous return are increased in pregnancy, contributing to the increase in cardiac output seen throughout gestation. A client with preexisting heart disease may become symptomatic and begin to decompensate during the time the blood volume peaks. Close monitoring is warranted during 28 to 35 weeks of gestation.

BLOOD PRESSURE

Blood pressure, especially the diastolic pressure, declines slightly during pregnancy as a result of peripheral vasodilation caused by progesterone. It usually reaches a low point at midpregnancy and thereafter increases to prepregnancy levels until term. During the first trimester, blood pressure typically remains at the prepregnancy level. During the second trimester, the blood pressure decreases 5 to 10 mm Hg and thereafter returns to first-trimester levels (Gaillard & Jaddoe, 2015). Any significant rise in blood pressure during pregnancy should be investigated to rule out gestational hypertension. Gestational hypertension is a clinical diagnosis defined by the new onset of hypertension (systolic of 140 mm Hg or higher and/or diastolic of 90 mm Hg or higher) after 20 weeks of gestation.

BLOOD COMPONENTS

The number of red blood cells also increases throughout pregnancy to a level 25% to 33% higher than nonpregnant values, depending on the amount of iron available. This increase is necessary to transport the additional oxygen required during pregnancy. Although there is an increase in red blood cells, there is a greater increase in the plasma volume as a result of hormonal factors and sodium and water retention. Because the plasma increase exceeds the increase of red blood cell production, normal hemoglobin and hematocrit values decrease. This state of hemodilution is referred to as **physiologic anemia of pregnancy**. Changes in red blood cell volume are due to increased circulating erythropoietin and accelerated red blood cell production. The rise in erythropoietin in the last two trimesters is stimulated by progesterone, prolactin, and human placental lactogen (hPL) (Jones & Lopez, 2014).

Iron requirements during pregnancy increase because of the demands of the growing fetus and the increase in maternal blood volume. The fetal tissues prevail over the mother's tissues with respect to use of iron stores. With the accelerated production of red blood cells, iron is necessary for hemoglobin formation, the oxygen-carrying component of red blood cells.

Take Note!

Because of the increased amounts of iron that is needed for a healthy pregnancy, pregnant clients are often encouraged to take prophylactic iron supplementation (Blackburn, 2013; Health Canada, 2016b). Teaching patients and families about adequate iron intake, either through diet or iron supplements, is an important role of the nurse.

Both fibrin and plasma fibrinogen levels increase, along with various blood-clotting factors. These factors make pregnancy a hypercoagulable state. These changes, coupled with venous stasis secondary to venous pooling, which occurs during late pregnancy after long periods of standing in the upright position with the pressure exerted by the uterus on the large pelvic veins, contribute to slowed venous return, pooling, and dependent edema. These factors also increase the client's risk for venous thrombosis (DeLoughery, 2015).

Respiratory System

The growing uterus and the increased production of the hormone progesterone cause the lungs to function differently during pregnancy. Oxygen consumption reflects the uptick of the pregnant client's metabolism by increasing between 20% and 30% by the time full term is reached. During pregnancy, the amount of space available to house the lungs decreases as the uterus puts pressure on the diaphragm and causes it to shift upward by 4 cm above its usual position. The growing uterus does change the size and shape of the thoracic cavity, but diaphragmatic excursion increases, chest circumference increases by 2 to 3 in, and the transverse diameter increases by an inch, allowing a larger tidal volume, as evidenced by deeper breathing (tidal volume, or the volume of air inhaled) increases by 30% to 40% (from 500 to 700 mL) as the pregnancy progresses. This increase results in hyperventilation and hypocapnia. As a result of these changes, the pregnant person's breathing becomes more diaphragmatic than abdominal. Concomitant with the increase in tidal volume is a 30% to 40% increase in oxygen consumption due to the increased oxygen requirements of the developing fetus, placenta, and the person's own organs.

Anatomic and physiologic changes of pregnancy predispose the mother to increased morbidity and mortality and increase the risks of a less than optimal outcome for the fetus. The frequency and significance of acute and chronic respiratory conditions in pregnant people have increased in recent years. Because of these various changes, pregnant people with asthma, pneumonia, or other respiratory pathology are more susceptible to early decompensation (Mehta, Chen, Hardy, & Powrie, 2015).

A pregnant person breathes faster and more deeply because of the need to supply the fetus with oxygen as well. Oxygen consumption increases during pregnancy even as airway resistance and lung compliance remain unchanged. Changes in the structures of the respiratory system take place to prepare the body for the enlarging uterus and increased lung volume (Alexander, LaRosa, Bader, & Garfield, 2014). As muscles and cartilage in the thoracic region relax, the chest broadens, with a conversion from abdominal breathing to thoracic breathing. This leads to a 50% increase in air volume per minute. All of these structural alterations are temporary and revert back to their prepregnant state at the end of the pregnancy.

Increased vascularity of the respiratory tract is influenced by increased estrogen levels, leading to congestion. Rising levels of sex hormones and heightened sensitivity to allergens may influence the nasal mucosa, precipitating epistaxis (nosebleed) and rhinitis. This congestion gives rise to nasal and sinus stuffiness and changes in the tone and quality of the pregnant client's voice (Jordan et al., 2014).

Renal/Urinary System

Hormonal changes during pregnancy allow for increased blood flow to the kidneys. The renal system must handle the effects of increased maternal intravascular and extracellular volume and metabolic waste products as well as excretion of fetal wastes. The predominant structural change in the renal system during pregnancy is dilation of the renal pelvis and uterus. Changes in renal structure occur as a result of the hormonal influences of estrogen and progesterone, pressure from an enlarging uterus, and an increase in maternal blood volume. Like the heart, the kidneys work harder throughout the pregnancy. Changes in kidney function occur to accommodate a heavier workload while maintaining a stable electrolyte balance and blood pressure. As more blood flows to the kidneys, the glomerular filtration rate (GFR) increases, leading to an increase in urine flow and volume, substances delivered to the kidneys, and filtration and excretion of urea, uric acid, creatinine, water, and solutes (Cox & Reid, 2015).

Anatomically, the kidneys enlarge during pregnancy. Each kidney increases in length by approximately 1 to 1.5 cm and weight as a result of hormonal effects that cause increased tone and decreased motility of the smooth muscle. The renal pelvis becomes dilated. The ureters (especially the right ureter) elongate, widen, and become more curved above the pelvic rim as early as the 10th gestational week (Thadhani & Maynard, 2018). Progesterone is thought to cause both of these changes because of its relaxing influence on smooth muscle.

Blood flow to the kidneys increases by 50% to 80% as a result of the increase in cardiac output and relaxin, which causes a decrease in both efferent and afferent resistance. This in turn leads to an increase in the GFR by as much as 40% to 60% starting during the second trimester, resulting in hyperfiltration. This elevation continues until birth. This change has important clinical implications for medication use because renally excreted drugs may require higher doses and more frequent administration for therapeutic blood levels during pregnancy (Larson, 2015).

The activity of the kidneys normally increases when a person lies down and decreases on standing. This difference is amplified during pregnancy, which is one reason a pregnant person feels the need to urinate frequently while trying to sleep. Late in the pregnancy, the increase in kidney activity is even greater when the client lies on one side rather than flat on their back. Lying on either side relieves the pressure that the enlarged uterus puts on the vena cava carrying blood from the legs. Subsequently, venous return to the heart increases, leading to increased cardiac output. Increased cardiac output results in increased renal perfusion and glomerular filtration. As a rule, all the physiologic changes maximize by the end of the second trimester and then start to return to the prepregnant level. However, changes in the anatomy take up to 3 months postpartum to subside (King et al., 2015).

Musculoskeletal System

Changes in the musculoskeletal system are progressive, resulting from the influence of hormones, fetal growth, and maternal weight gain. Pregnancy is characterized by changes in posture and gait. By the 10th to 12th week of pregnancy, the ligaments that hold the sacroiliac joints and the pubis symphysis in place begin to soften and stretch, and the articulations between the joints widen and become more movable (Bope & Kellerman, 2015). The relaxation of the joints peaks by the beginning of the third trimester. The purpose of these changes is to increase the size of the pelvic cavity and to make delivery easier.

The postural changes of pregnancy—an increased swayback and an upper spine extension to compensate for the enlarging abdomen—coupled with the loosening of the sacroiliac joints may result in lower back pain. The pregnant person's centre of gravity shifts forward, requiring a realignment of the spinal curvatures. Factors thought to contribute to these postural changes include the alteration to the centre of gravity that come with pregnancy, the influence of the pregnancy-related hormone relaxin on the pelvic joints, and the increasing weight and position of the growing fetus.

An increase in the normal lumbosacral curve (lordosis) occurs and a compensatory curvature in the cervicodorsal area develops to assist her in maintaining her balance (Fig. 11.3). In addition, relaxation and increased mobility of joints occur because of the hormones progesterone and relaxin, which lead to the characteristic "waddle" gait that pregnant people demonstrate toward term. Increased weight gain can add to this discomfort by accentuating the lumbar and dorsal curves (Kouhkan, Rahimi, Ghasemi, Naimi, & Baghban, 2015).

Integumentary System

There are a variety of skin changes that are associated with pregnancy. Increased activity of the maternal adrenal and pituitary glands, along with a contribution for the developing fetal endocrine glands, increasing cortisone levels, accelerated metabolism, and enhanced production of progesterone and estrogenic hormones are responsible for most skin changes in pregnancy (Tyler, 2015). Up to 90% of pregnant people will show signs of hyperpigmentation during pregnancy, and it is typically generalized and mild. The skin of pregnant people undergoes hyperpigmentation primarily as a result of estrogen, progesterone, and melanocyte-stimulating hormone (MSH) levels. These changes are mainly seen on the nipples, areola, umbilicus, perineum, and axilla. Although many integumentary changes disappear after giving birth,

FIGURE 11.3 Postural changes during (**A**) the first trimester and (**B**) the third trimester.

some only fade. Many pregnant people express concern about stretch marks, skin colour changes, and hair loss. Unfortunately, little is known about how to avoid these changes.

Complexion changes are not unusual. The increased pigmentation that occurs on the breasts and genitalia also develops on the face to form the "mask of pregnancy," which is also called facial melasma. It occurs in up to 70% of pregnant people. There is a genetic predisposition toward melasma, which is exacerbated by the sun, and it tends to recur in subsequent pregnancies. This blotchy, brownish pigment covers the forehead and cheeks in dark-haired people. Most facial pigmentation fades as the hormones subside at the end of the pregnancy, but some may linger. The skin in the middle of the abdomen may develop a pigmented line called **linea nigra,** which extends from the umbilicus to the pubic area (Fig. 11.4).

Striae gravidarum, or stretch marks, are irregular reddish streaks that appear on the abdomen, breasts, and buttocks in up to 90% of pregnant people. Striae are most prominent by 6 to 7 months. They result from genetics, reduced connective tissue strength resulting from the elevated adrenal steroid levels, and stretching of the structures secondary to growth (Tyler, 2015). They are more common in younger people, people with larger infants, and people with higher body mass indices. Non-Whites and people with a history of breast or thigh striae or a family history of striae gravidarum also are at higher risk. Several creams and lotions such as cocoa butter and olive oil have been touted as being able to prevent striae gravidarum, but research currently doesn't validate these claims. A study done by Tretti Clementoni and Lavagno

(2015) did find that laser treatments did improve pigmentation, volume, and textural appearance of striae gravidarum in >50% of the women enrolled in the study.

Vascular-Related Skin Changes

Vascular changes during pregnancy manifested in the integumentary system include varicosities of the legs, vulva, and perineum. Varicose veins commonly are the

FIGURE 11.4 Linea nigra.

result of distention, instability, and poor circulation secondary to prolonged standing or sitting and the heavy gravid uterus placing pressure on the pelvic veins, preventing complete venous return. Interventions to reduce the risk of developing varicosities include:

- Elevating both legs when sitting or lying down
- Avoiding prolonged standing or sitting; changing position frequently
- Resting in the left lateral position
- Walking daily for exercise
- Avoiding tight clothing or knee-high hosiery
- Wearing support hose if varicosities are a preexisting condition to pregnancy

Another skin manifestation, believed to be secondary to vascular changes and high estrogen levels, is the appearance of small blood vessels called vascular spiders. They may appear on the neck, thorax, face, and arms. They are especially obvious in White people and typically disappear after childbirth. Palmar erythema is a well-delineated pinkish area on the palmar surface of the hands. This integumentary change is also related to elevated estrogen levels (Rigby, 2016).

Hair and Nails

Some people also notice a decline in hair growth during pregnancy. The hair follicles normally undergo a growing and a resting phase. The resting phase is followed by a loss of hair; the hairs are then replaced by new ones. During pregnancy, fewer hair follicles go into the resting phase. After delivery, the body catches up with subsequent hair loss for several months. Nails typically grow faster during pregnancy. Pregnant people may experience increased brittleness, distal separation of the nail bed, whitish discolouration, and transverse grooves on the nails, but most of these conditions resolve in the postpartum period (King et al., 2015).

Endocrine System

The endocrine system undergoes many changes during pregnancy because hormonal changes are essential in meeting the needs of the growing fetus. Hormonal changes play a major role in controlling the supplies of maternal glucose, amino acids, and lipids to the fetus. Although estrogen and progesterone are the main hormones involved in pregnancy changes, other endocrine glands and hormones also change during pregnancy.

THYROID GLAND

The thyroid gland enlarges slightly and becomes more active during pregnancy as a result of increased vascularity and hyperplasia. Increased gland activity results in an increase in thyroid hormone secretion starting during the first trimester; levels taper off within a few weeks after birth and return to normal limits. Maternal thyroid

hormone is transferred to the fetus beginning soon after conception and is critical for fetal brain development, neurogenesis, and organizational processes prior to 20 weeks when fetal thyroid production is low. However, even after the fetal thyroid is producing increasing amounts of hormone, much of the thyroxin (T_4) needed for development continues to be provided by the mother. Low maternal thyroid levels with thyroid insufficiency, hypothyroidism, or low or inadequate iodine intake may compromise fetal neurologic development (Pearce, 2015). With an increase in the secretion of thyroid hormones, the basal metabolic rate (the amount of oxygen consumed by the body over a unit of time in milliliters per minute) progressively increases by 25%, along with heart rate and cardiac output (Medici, Korevaar, Visser, Visser, & Peeters, 2015).

PITUITARY GLAND

During pregnancy, major endocrine and metabolic alterations occur due to the physiologic hormonal secretion from the placenta. The pituitary gland adapts to these changes and all secretory axes are affected. During pregnancy, the pituitary gland enlarges; it returns to normal size after birth.

The anterior lobe of the pituitary is glandular tissue and produces multiple hormones. The release of these hormones is regulated by releasing and inhibiting hormones produced by the hypothalamus. Some of these anterior pituitary hormones induce other glands to secrete their hormones. The increase in blood levels of the hormones produced by the final target glands (e.g., the ovary or thyroid) inhibits the release of anterior pituitary hormones. Changes in levels of pituitary hormones are discussed in the following paragraphs.

FSH and LH secretion are inhibited during pregnancy, probably as a result of hCG produced by the placenta and corpus luteum, and the increased secretion of prolactin by the anterior pituitary gland. Levels remain decreased until after delivery.

Thyroid-stimulating hormone (TSH) is reduced during the first trimester but usually returns to normal for the remainder of the pregnancy. Decreased TSH is thought to be one of the factors, along with elevated hCG levels, associated with morning sickness, nausea, and vomiting during the first trimester.

Growth hormone (GH) is an anabolic hormone that promotes protein synthesis. It stimulates most body cells to grow in size and divide, facilitating the use of fats for fuel and conserving glucose. During pregnancy, there is a decrease in the number of GH-producing cells and a corresponding decrease in GH blood levels. The action of hPL is thought to decrease the need for and use of GH. During pregnancy, prolactin is secreted in pulses and increases 10-fold to promote breast development and the lactation process. High levels of progesterone secreted by the placenta inhibit the direct influence of

TABLE 11.3	PLACENTAL HORMONES
Hormone	**Description**
Human chorionic gonadotropin (hCG)	• Responsible for maintaining the maternal corpus luteum, which secretes progesterone and estrogens, with synthesis occurring before implantation • Production by fetal trophoblast cells until the placenta is developed sufficiently to take over that function • Basis for early pregnancy tests because it appears in the maternal bloodstream soon after implantation • Production peaks at 8 weeks and then gradually declines
hPL (also known as human chorionic somatomammotropin [hCS])	• Preparation of mammary glands for lactation and involved in the process of making glucose available for fetal growth by altering maternal carbohydrate, fat, and protein metabolism • Antagonist of insulin because it decreases tissue sensitivity or alters the ability to use insulin • Increase in the amount of circulating free fatty acids for maternal metabolic needs and decrease in maternal metabolism of glucose to facilitate fetal growth
Relaxin	• Secretion by the placenta as well as the corpus luteum during pregnancy • Thought to act synergistically with progesterone to maintain pregnancy • Increase in flexibility of the pubic symphysis, permitting the pelvis to expand during delivery • Dilation of the cervix, making it easier for the fetus to enter the vaginal canal; thought to suppress the release of oxytocin by the hypothalamus, thus delaying the onset of labour contractions
Progesterone	• Often called the "hormone of pregnancy" because of the critical role it plays in supporting the endometrium of the uterus • Supports the endometrium to provide an environment conducive to fetal survival • Produced by the corpus luteum during the first few weeks of pregnancy and then by the placenta until term • Initially, causes thickening of the uterine lining in anticipation of implantation of the fertilized ovum. From then on, it maintains the endometrium, inhibits uterine contractility, and assists in the development of the breasts for lactation
Estrogen	• Promotes enlargement of the genitals, uterus, and breasts, and increases vascularity, causing vasodilatation • Relaxation of pelvic ligaments and joints • Associated with hyperpigmentation, vascular changes in the skin, increased activity of the salivary glands, and hyperemia of the gums and nasal mucous membranes • Aids in developing the ductal system of the breasts in preparation for lactation

Adapted from Cunningham, F. G., Leveno, K. J., Bloom, S. L., Spong, C. Y., Dashe, J. S., Hoffman, B. L.,...Sheffield, J. S. (2014). *William's obstetrics* (24th ed.). New York: McGraw-Hill Education; Edelman, C. L., Kudzma, E. C., & *Mandle*, C. L. (2014). *Health promotion throughout the lifespan* (8th ed.). St. Louis, MO: Mosby Elsevier; Shields, A. D. (2017). Pregnancy diagnosis. *eMedicine*. Retrieved from http://emedicine.medscape.com/article/262591-overview

from foreign substances (antigens) that may cause tissue injury or disease. The mechanisms of innate and adaptive immunity work cooperatively to prevent, control, and eradicate foreign antigens in the body.

A general enhancement of innate immunity (inflammatory response and phagocytosis) and suppression of adaptive immunity (protective response to a specific foreign antigen) take place during pregnancy. These immunologic alterations help prevent the mother's immune system from rejecting the fetus (foreign body), increase her risk of developing certain infections such as urinary tract infections, and influence the course of chronic disorders such as autoimmune diseases. Some chronic conditions worsen (diabetes) while others seem to stabilize (asthma) during pregnancy, but this is individualized and

not predictable. In general, immune function in pregnant people is similar to immune function in nonpregnant people. Table 11.4 summarizes the general body systems' adaptations to pregnancy.

Marva **returns for her first prenatal appointment and tells the nurse that her whole body is "out of sorts." She is overwhelmed and feels poorly. Outline the bodily changes Marva can expect each trimester to help her understand the adaptations taking place. What guidance can the nurse give Marva to help her understand the changes of pregnancy?**

TABLE 11.4	SUMMARY OF GENERAL BODY SYSTEM ADAPTATIONS
System	**Adaptation**
Gastrointestinal system	*Mouth and pharynx:* Gums become hyperemic, swollen, and friable and tend to bleed easily. Saliva production increases. *Esophagus:* Decreased lower esophageal sphincter pressure and tone, which increases the risk of developing heartburn. *Stomach:* Decreased tone and mobility with delayed gastric emptying time, which increases the risk of gastroesophageal reflux and vomiting; decreased gastric acidity and histamine output, which improves symptoms of peptic ulcer disease. *Intestines:* Decreased intestinal tone motility with increased transit time, which increases risk of constipation and flatulence. *Gallbladder:* Decreased tone and motility, which may increase risk of gallstone formation.
Cardiovascular system	*Blood volume:* Marked increase in plasma (50%) and RBCs (25–33%) compared to nonpregnant values; causes hemodilution, which is reflected in a lower hematocrit and hemoglobin. *Cardiac output and heart rate:* CO increases from 30–50% over the nonpregnant rate by the 32nd week of pregnancy. The increase in CO is associated with an increase in venous return and greater right ventricular output, especially in the left lateral position. Heart rate increases by 10–15 bpm between 14 and 20 weeks of gestation, and this increase will persist to term. *Blood pressure:* Diastolic pressure decreases typically 10–15 mm Hg to reach its lowest point by midpregnancy; it then gradually returns to nonpregnant baseline values by term. *Blood components:* The number of RBCs increases throughout pregnancy to a level 25–33% higher than nonpregnant values. Both fibrin and plasma fibrinogen levels increase, along with various blood-clotting factors. These factors make pregnancy a hypercoagulable state.
Respiratory system	Enlargement of the uterus shifts the diaphragm up to 4 cm above its usual position. As muscles and cartilage in the thoracic region relax, the chest broadens, with conversion from abdominal breathing to thoracic breathing. This leads to a 50% increase in air volume per minute. Tidal volume, or the volume of air inhaled, increases gradually by 30–40% (from 500 to 700 mL) as the pregnancy progresses.
Renal/urinary system	The renal pelvis becomes dilated. The ureters (especially the right ureter) elongate, widen, and become more curved above the pelvic rim. Bladder tone decreases and bladder capacity doubles by term. GFR increases 40–60% during pregnancy. Blood flow to the kidneys increases by 50–80% as a result of the increase in cardiac output.
Musculoskeletal system	Distention of the abdomen with growth of the fetus tilts the pelvis forward, shifting the centre of gravity. The woman compensates by developing an increased curvature (lordosis) of the spine. Relaxation and increased mobility of joints occur because of the hormones progesterone and relaxin, which lead to the characteristic "waddle gait" that pregnant people demonstrate toward term.
Integumentary system	Hyperpigmentation of the skin is the most common alteration during pregnancy. The most common areas include the areola, genital skin, axilla, inner aspects of the thighs, and linea nigra. Striae gravidarum, or stretch marks, are irregular reddish streaks that may appear on the abdomen, breasts, and buttocks in about half of pregnant people. The skin in the middle of the abdomen may develop a pigmented line called linea nigra, which extends from the umbilicus to the pubic area. Melasma ("mask of pregnancy") occurs in up to 70% of pregnant people. It is characterized by irregular, blotchy areas of pigmentation on the face, most commonly on the cheeks, chin, and nose.
Endocrine system	Controls the integrity and duration of gestation by maintaining the corpus luteum via hCG secretion; production of estrogen, progesterone, hPL, and other hormones and growth factors via the placenta; release of oxytocin (by the posterior pituitary gland), prolactin (by the anterior pituitary), and relaxin (by the ovary, uterus, and placenta).
Immune system	A general enhancement of innate immunity (inflammatory response and phagocytosis) and suppression of adaptive immunity (protective response to a specific foreign antigen) take place during pregnancy. These immunologic alterations help prevent the mother's immune system from rejecting the fetus (foreign body), increase her risk of developing certain infections, and influence the course of chronic disorders such as autoimmune diseases.

CHANGING NUTRITIONAL NEEDS OF PREGNANCY

Maternal body weight and diet quality, even prepregnancy, can affect the uterine environment, birth weight, and the infant's subsequent health into adulthood. Healthy eating during pregnancy enables optimal gestational weight gain and reduces complications, both of which are associated with positive birth outcomes. During pregnancy, maternal nutritional needs change to meet the demands of the pregnancy. Healthy eating can help ensure that adequate nutrients are available for both mother and fetus.

Nutritional intake during pregnancy has a direct effect on fetal well-being and birth outcome. Inadequate nutritional intake, for example, is associated with preterm birth, low birth weight, and congenital anomalies. Excessive nutritional intake is connected with fetal macrosomia (>4,000 g), leading to a difficult birth, neonatal hypoglycemia, and continued obesity in the mother and the potential for childhood obesity and the components of metabolic syndrome (Ojha, Fainberg, Sebert, Budge, & Symonds, 2015).

Since the requirements for so many nutrients increase during pregnancy, pregnant clients should take a vitamin and mineral supplement daily. Prenatal vitamins are prescribed routinely as a safeguard against a less-than-optimal diet. In particular, iron and folic acid need to be supplemented because their increased requirements during pregnancy are usually too great to be met through diet alone. Iron and folic acid are needed to form new blood cells for the expanded maternal blood volume and to prevent anemia. Iron is essential for fetal growth and brain development and in the prevention of maternal anemia. An increase in folic acid is essential before pregnancy and in the early weeks of pregnancy to prevent neural tube defects in the fetus. In Canada, key messages on folic acid include eating according to Canada's Food Guide and taking a multivitamin that has 400 mcg (0.4 mg) of folic acid. Because many pregnancies are unplanned, all those of childbearing age (12–45 years of age) who could become pregnant should take a multivitamin with folic acid, three months prior to becoming pregnant (Society of Obstetricians and Gynaecologists of Canada [SOGC], 2015; Health Canada, 2009). People with a previous history of a fetus with a neural tube defect are often prescribed a higher dose of folic acid (SOGC, 2015).

There may be an abundance of conflicting advice about nutrition during pregnancy and what is good or bad to eat. Overall, the following guidelines are helpful:

- A person's nutritional and overall health, before and during pregnancy, influences the health of the developing baby.
- Eating well, combined with taking a daily multivitamin, will provide the nutrients needed to feel good, have energy, and support a healthy pregnancy.
- Follow Eating Well with Canada's Food Guide to eat the amount and type of food that is right for you and your baby.
- Include at least one dark green and orange vegetable each day and prepare vegetables with little or no added fat, sugar, and salt.
- Grain products are important: try to choose grain products that are lower in fat, sugar, and salt and look for whole grain varieties.
- Have milk and milk alternatives for healthy bones.
- Include meat and meat alternatives such as dried peas, beans, tofu, and lentils made with little or no added fat or salt.
- Have at least 150 g of cooked fish each week. Fish contains omega-3 fats and other important nutrients for pregnancy.
- All those who could become pregnant and those who are pregnant should take a multivitamin containing 0.4 mg of folic acid every day. Pregnant clients should also ensure that their multivitamin contains 16–20 mg of iron.
- Follow food safety advice and avoid eating foods that are a higher risk to you during your pregnancy.
- Gaining weight is a natural part of pregnancy. How much weight you should gain depends on your body mass index (BMI) before you became pregnant (Health Canada, 2019a).

In the months before conception, food choices are key. The foods and vitamins consumed can ensure that the pregnant person and the fetus will have the nutrients that are essential for the very start of pregnancy.

While most people recognize the importance of healthy eating during pregnancy, some may find it challenging to achieve. It is vital that nurses consider the determinants of health, including the social, structural, and individual factors that influence the health of Canadian people. Beyond a straightforward nutritional assessment, it is important that assessment of food security, including access and food skills is considered. Additional nutrition-related health problems must also be assessed for, such as diabetes, hypertension, and obesity. Many people also say they have little time and energy to devote to meal planning and preparation. Another barrier to healthy eating is conflicting messages from various sources, resulting in a lack of clear, reliable, and relevant information. It may be beneficial for people and families to be referred to a dietician for further supports and education on healthy meal planning and preparation. The federal government in Canada also supports the Canadian Prenatal Nutrition Program (CPNP) (Health Canada, 2015a). The CPNP is a community-based program that provides support to improve the health and well-being of pregnant clients, new mothers, and babies facing challenging life circumstances. The goals of CPNP are to improve maternal–infant health, increase the rates of healthy birth weights, and to promote and support breastfeeding. The program also aims to promote the creation of partnerships within communities and strengthen community capacity to increase support for pregnancy and for new mothers. The Public Health Agency of Canada (PHAC) currently funds hundreds of CPNP projects serving over 51,000 pregnant clients and parents and caregivers in over 2,000 communities across Canada each year. In addition, a separate stream of the program administered through Health Canada serves Indigenous people and their families living on-reserve (Health Canada, 2015a).

Nutritional Requirements During Pregnancy

Pregnancy is one of the most nutritionally demanding periods of a person's life. Gestation involves rapid cell division and organ development, and an adequate supply of nutrients is essential to support this tremendous fetal growth. Optimal maternal health via good nutritional practices during pregnancy reduces the risk of suboptimal fetal development.

In Canada, it is recommended that pregnant people follow the Canada's Food Guide (see Box 11.3). In the second and third trimester, pregnant clients should be encouraged to have two to three additional Canada Food Guide Servings each day. This may include having fruit and yogurt for a snack, or having an extra slice of toast at breakfast and an extra glass of milk at supper (Health Canada, 2012).

Most people are usually motivated to eat properly during pregnancy for the sake of the fetus. The Food and Nutrition Board of the National Research Council has made recommendations for nutrient intakes for people living in the United States, and the Institute of Medicine, in partnership with Health Canada publishes recommendations for **Dietary Reference Intakes** (DRIs) for people living in Canada and/or the United States. The DRIs include: Recommended Dietary Allowances (RDAs), Adequate Intakes (AIs), and Upper Limits (ULs). The DRIs are

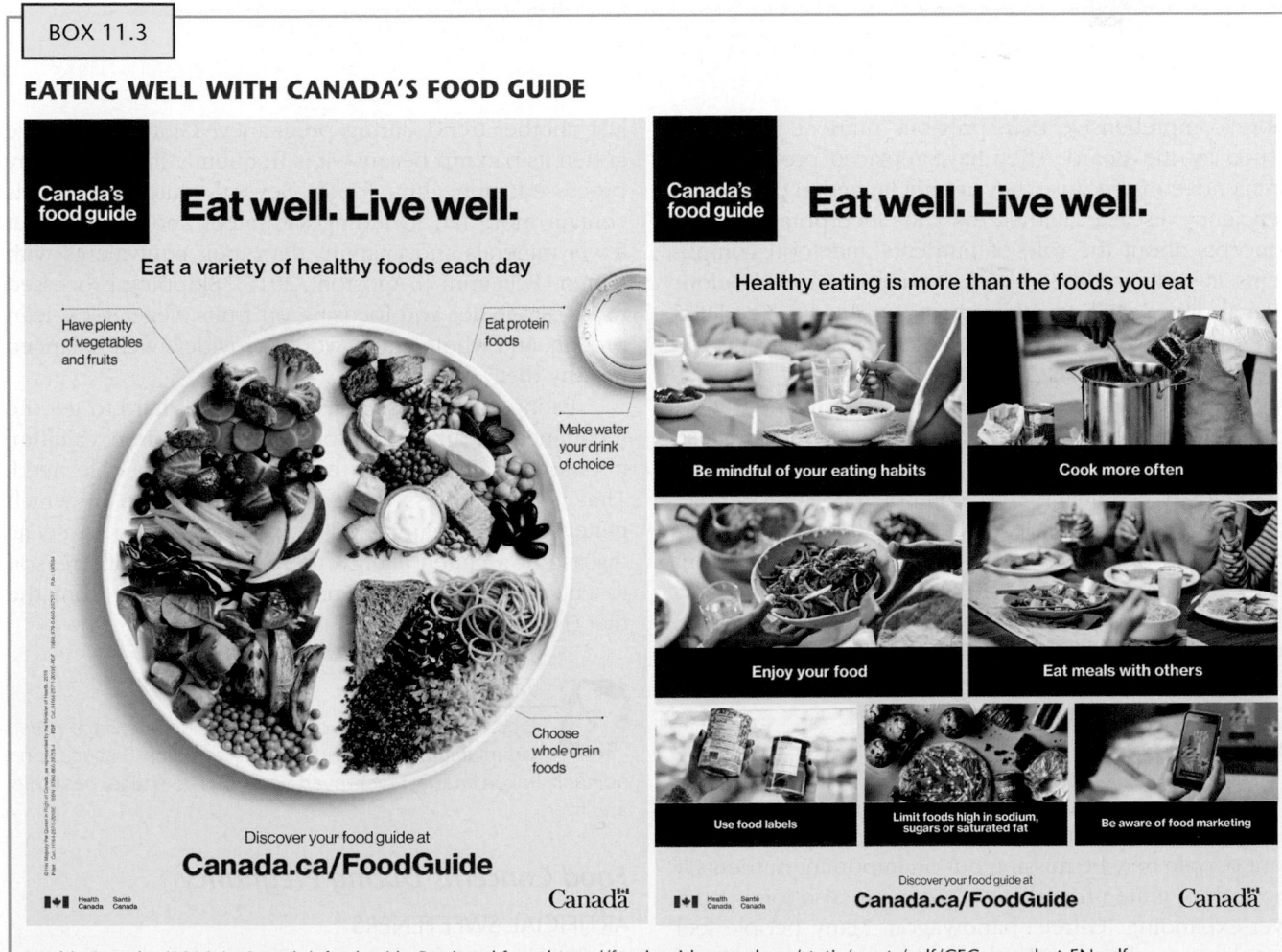

| BOX 11.3 |

EATING WELL WITH CANADA'S FOOD GUIDE

Health Canada. (2019c). *Canada's food guide.* Retrieved from https://food-guide.canada.ca/static/assets/pdf/CFG-snapshot-EN.pdf

| TABLE 11.5 | DIETARY RECOMMENDATIONS FOR PREGNANCY AND LACTATION |||

Recommended Dietary Allowance[a]	Women 19–50 years		
	Nonpregnant	Pregnant	Breastfeeding
Folate (mcg/day)	400	600	500
Iron (mg/day)	18	27	9
Vitamin A (mcg RAE[b]/day)	700	770	1,300
Vitamin C (mg/day)	75	85	120
Vitamin D (mcg/day)	**5**	**5**	**5**
Calcium (mg/day)	**1,000**	**1,000**	**1,000**
Zinc (mg/day)	8	11	12
Vitamin B$_6$ (mg/day)	1.3	1.9	2.0
Magnesium (mg/day)	310 *(19–30 years)* 320 *(31–50 years)*	350 *(19–30 years)* 360 *(31–50 years)*	310 *(19–30 years)* 320 *(31–50 years)*
Vitamin B$_{12}$ (mcg/day)	2.4	2.6	2.8

[a]Nutrient amounts in bold font indicate an Adequate Intake (AI).
[b]Retinol activity equivalent.
Health Canada. (2010). *Prenatal nutrition guidelines for health professionals: Background on Canada's Food Guide.* Retrieved from https://www.canada.ca/en/health-canada/services/publications/food-nutrition/prenatal-nutrition-guidelines-health-professionals-background-canada-food-guide-2009.html

more comprehensive than previous nutrient guidelines issued by the Board. They have replaced previous recommendations because they are not limited to preventing deficiency diseases. Rather, the DRIs incorporate current concepts about the role of nutrients and food components in reducing the risk of chronic disease, developmental disorders, and other related problems. The DRIs can be used to plan and assess diets for healthy people (Health Canada, 2010a; Kruger & Butte, 2015).

These dietary recommendations also include information for those who are pregnant or lactating, because growing fetal and maternal tissues require increased quantities of essential dietary components. For example, the current DRIs suggest an increase in the pregnant person's intake of protein from 60 to 80 g/day, iron from 18 to 27 g/day, and folic acid from 400 to 800 mcg/day, along with an increase of daily caloric intake (Jacobson, 2018; Walsh & McAuliffe, 2015) (Table 11.5).

Gluten-Free Diet During Pregnancy

In recent years, gluten-free foods have become popular, fueling a growing market for the Food Industry. Pregnant people may be missing out on important nutrients if they adopt gluten-free diets as many are also joining the ever-expanding "G-free" bandwagon. Many people feel that these products are healthier than their conventional counterparts. But is it really a health-promotion diet or just another trend during pregnancy? Gluten may have gotten its bad rap because it is frequently found in many processed, unhealthy foods. Several gluten-free foods contain more fat, including saturated, and sodium, but fewer minerals and vitamins than their equivalents with gluten (Pellegrini & Agostoni, 2015). Skipping processed foods altogether and focusing on fruits, vegetables, lean protein, and whole grains would provide a well-balanced healthy diet.

Eating a gluten-free diet can make it hard to get the recommended amount of folate, vitamin B, iron, calcium, fiber, and grain servings that all pregnant people need. That is why, unless there is medical reason in which gluten must be eliminated from the diet due to celiac disease or a gluten allergy, there isn't a scientific reason to cut out wholesome, nutrient-dense grains from the diet (Neifeld, 2018).

Take Note!

Good food sources of folic acid include dark green vegetables, such as broccoli, romaine lettuce, and spinach; baked beans; black-eyed peas; citrus fruits; peanuts; and liver.

Food Concerns During Pregnancy

ARTIFICIAL SWEETENERS

Artificial sweeteners or intense sweeteners are sugar substitutes that are used as an alternative to table sugar. They are many times sweeter than natural sugar and contain no calories. Extensive scientific research has demonstrated the safety of the six low-calorie sweeteners currently approved for use in foods in Canada, the United States, and Europe (stevia, acesulfame-K, aspartame, neotame, saccharin, and sucralose), if taken in acceptable quantities daily. For this reason, Health Canada has approved use of these sweeteners during pregnancy. There is an ongoing debate over whether artificial sweeteners pose a health threat (Qurrat-ul-Ain & Khan, 2015).

The safety of artificial sweeteners consumed during pregnancy remains controversial also. Some health care providers advise their pregnant clients to avoid all non-nutritive sweeteners during pregnancy, while others suggest they can be used in moderation (Hankey, 2015). The debate continues on this matter until additional research can be completed. Aspartame should be avoided by pregnant people with phenylketonuria (PKU).

FISH, SHELLFISH, AND LEVELS OF MERCURY

Fish and shellfish are an important part of a healthy diet because they contain high-quality protein, are low in saturated fat, and contain omega-3 fatty acids. However, nearly all fish and shellfish contain traces of mercury and some contain higher levels of mercury that may harm a developing fetus if ingested by pregnant people in large amounts. Human exposure to mercury occurs primarily through the consumption of fish contaminated through atmospheric mercury releases. The U.S. Environmental Protection Agency (EPA) and the United Nations Environment Program have identified coal-fired power plants as the source of 50% to 75% of the atmospheric mercury pollution worldwide. Once airborne, rainfall transfers mercury particles into waterways where it is converted to the neurotoxic methylmercury form through a microbial process. Plankton absorbs the methylmercury and as the smaller fish eat the plankton and the larger predatory fish consume the smaller fish, the methylmercury bioaccumulates up the food chain to humans. Mercury exposure in pregnancy has been associated with both pregnancy complications and developmental problems in infants. Apart from the environmental exposure, mercury is likely to arise from predatory fish consumption. It would be prudent to advise all pregnant people to avoid these potential problems and minimize any risk.

All fish contain methylmercury regardless of the size or the geographic location of the waters from which the fish is caught, although size and type of fish as well as the geographic location of waters can influence lower or higher amounts of methylmercury. In addition, because methylmercury resides in the tissue of the fish, no method of cleaning or cooking will reduce the amount of mercury in a meal of contaminated fish (Nelson, 2015).

Pregnant and breastfeeding clients should be especially careful when choosing fish and should be educated to select those that are low in mercury. As discussed earlier, it is recommended that pregnant people consume at least 150 g of cooked fish per week, as fish contributes to a healthy pregnancy, keeping in mind that larger fish which eat smaller fish are usually higher in mercury.

Clients who may become pregnant, those who are pregnant or nursing, and young children need to follow some precautions:

- Limit consumption of fresh or frozen tuna, shark, swordfish, escolar, marlin, and orange roughly to 150 g/month, and eat as much as 75 g/week of a variety of commercially caught fish and shellfish low in mercury such as shrimp, salmon, pollock, catfish, and canned light tuna (BC Health Link, 2016; Health Canada, 2019b).
- Canned tuna, especially canned light tuna, is one of the most popular types of fish for many Canadians. The fish used in canned tuna products are generally younger and smaller and have significantly less mercury than fresh or frozen tuna, so that most Canadians don't need to be concerned about consuming canned tuna (Health Canada, 2017).
- For those who consume large amounts of canned albacore tuna, there is some potential for exposure to higher levels of mercury than is considered acceptable. Because of this, Health Canada has issued advice for children and pregnant people on the consumption of canned albacore tuna. Canned albacore tuna is also often called canned white tuna, but it is not the same as canned light tuna. It should be limited to 300 g/week for pregnant clients (Health Canada, 2017).

LISTERIOSIS AND PREGNANCY

Another food issue concern for pregnant people is consumption of food contaminated with the gram-positive bacillus *Listeria*. *Listeria* is a type of bacteria found in soil, water, and sometimes on plants. *Listeria* is commonly found in processed and prepared foods and in raw or unpasteurized milk. Listeriosis is associated with high morbidity and mortality. Though *Listeria* is all around our environment, most *Listeria* infections in people result from eating contaminated foods. Listeriosis during pregnancy usually presents as an unremarkable febrile illness in the mother, but can be fatal for the fetus and newborn. Reliable laboratory testing for early diagnosis is lacking. Listeriosis can be passed to an unborn baby through the placenta even if the mother is not showing signs of illness. This can lead to preterm births, miscarriages, stillbirths, and high neonatal mortality rates (Allerberger & Huhulescu, 2015). Safe food alternatives for pregnant clients are provided in Table 11.6. Key points for pregnant clients and families include:

- Do not eat hot dogs, luncheon meats, or deli meats unless they are reheated until steaming hot.
- Avoid getting fluid from hot dog packages on other foods, utensils, and food preparation surfaces, and wash hands after handling hot dogs, luncheon meats, and deli meats.

TABLE 11.6	FOOD SAFETY FOR PREGNANT CLIENTS

Some types of food can be a higher risk for pregnant women because of how they are produced and stored. To lower your chances of getting food poisoning, you should avoid those foods. The following chart can help you make safer food choices

Type of Food	Food to Avoid	Safer Alternatives
Hot dogs	Hot dogs straight from the package, without further heating.	Hot dogs that are well cooked to a safe internal temperature. The middle of the hot dog should be steaming hot or 74°C (165°F). Tip: Avoid spreading juice from hot dog packages onto other food, or to cutting boards, utensils, dishes and counters. Wash your hands after touching hot dogs.
Deli meats	Nondried deli meats, such as bologna, roast beef, and turkey breast.	Dried and salted deli meats, such as salami and pepperoni. Nondried deli meats that are well heated and steaming hot.
Eggs and egg products	Raw or lightly cooked eggs, or egg products that contain raw eggs, including some salad dressings, cookie dough, cake batter, sauces, and drinks (like homemade eggnog).	Egg dishes that are well cooked to a safe internal temperature of 74°C (165°F). Cook eggs until the yolk is firm. Homemade eggnog heated to 71°C (160°F). Tip: Use pasteurized egg products when making uncooked food that calls for raw eggs.
Meat and poultry	Raw or undercooked meat or poultry, such as steak tartar.	Meat and poultry that are cooked to their safe internal temperature.
Seafood	Raw seafood, such as sushi. Raw oysters, clams, and mussels. Refrigerated smoked seafood.	Seafood cooked to a safe internal temperature of 74°C (165°F). Oysters, clams, and mussels that are cooked until the shell has opened. Smoked seafood in cans, or seafood that does not need to be refrigerated until it is opened.
Dairy products	Raw or unpasteurized dairy products. Unpasteurized and pasteurized soft cheeses, such as Brie and Camembert. Unpasteurized and pasteurized semisoft cheeses, such as Havarti. All unpasteurized and pasteurized blue-veined cheeses.	Pasteurized dairy products and any dairy products that are cooked, in a casserole or au gratin. Pasteurized cheeses such as cheese curds, cheddar, and cottage cheese. Pasteurized processed/spreadable cheeses such as cream cheese. Pasteurized and unpasteurized hard cheeses such as Romano and Parmesan.
Sprouts	Raw sprouts, such as alfalfa, clover, radish, and mung beans.	Thoroughly cooked sprouts.
Pâtés and meat spreads	Refrigerated pâtés and meat spreads.	Pâtés and meat spreads sold in cans, or that do not have to be refrigerated until they are opened.
Fruit juice and cider	Unpasteurized fruit juice and cider.	Unpasteurized fruit juice and cider that are brought to a rolling boil and cooled. Pasteurized fruit juice and cider.

Health Canada. (2015b). *Safe food handling for pregnant women.* Retrieved from https://www.canada.ca/en/health-canada/services/food-safety-vulnerable-populations/food-safety-pregnant-women.html

- Do not eat soft cheeses such as feta, Brie, Camembert, and blue-veined cheeses.
- It is safe to eat hard cheeses, semi-soft cheeses such as mozzarella, pasteurized processed cheese slices and spreads, cream cheese, and cottage cheese.
- Do not eat refrigerated pâté or meat spreads.
- It is safe to eat canned or shelf-stable pâté and meat spreads.
- Do not eat refrigerated smoked seafood unless it is an ingredient in a cooked dish such as a casserole. Examples of refrigerated smoked seafood include salmon, trout, whitefish, cod, tuna, and mackerel and are most often labeled as "nova-style," "lox," "kippered," "smoked," or "jerky." This fish is found in the refrigerated section or sold at deli counters of grocery stores and delicatessens.
- It is safe to eat canned fish such as salmon and tuna or shelf-stable smoked seafood.
- Do not drink raw (unpasteurized) milk or eat foods that contain unpasteurized milk.

- Use all refrigerated perishable items that are pre-cooked or ready-to-eat as soon as possible.
- Use a refrigerator thermometer to make sure that the refrigerator always stays at 5°C or below.
- Do not eat salads made in the store such as ham salad, chicken salad, egg salad, tuna salad, or seafood salad.
- Clean your refrigerator regularly.

(United States Department of Agriculture Food Safety and Inspection Service, 2017)

Maternal Weight Gain

The recommended weight gain during pregnancy varies from person to person. Pregnant people and their health care provider should set the goal for pregnancy weight gain based on their prepregnancy weight. See Table 11.7.

Weight gain should take place throughout the pregnancy. During the first and second trimesters, growth takes place primarily in maternal tissues whereas in the third trimester much of the growth occurs in the fetal tissues. Refer to Figure 11.5.

A client who is underweight before pregnancy or who has a low maternal weight gain pattern should be monitored carefully because of the risk of giving birth to a low–birth-weight infant (<2,500 g or 5.5 lb). Frequently these clients simply need advice on what to eat to add weight. Encourage the client to eat snacks that are high in calories such as nuts, peanut butter, milk shakes, cheese, fruit, yogurt, and ice cream. Any person who has a prepregnancy BMI of less than 18.5 is considered to be high risk and should be referred to a nutritionist (Sharma et al., 2015).

Conversely, people who start a pregnancy while overweight (BMI >25–29) run the risk of having a high-birth-weight infant, with resulting cephalopelvic disproportion and, potentially, a surgical birth. Two thirds of

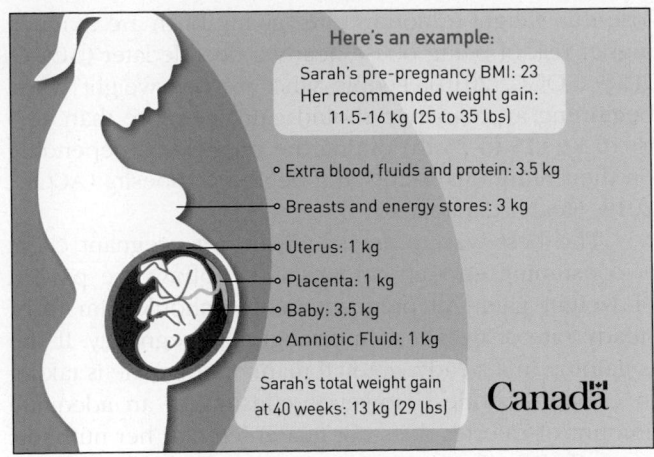

FIGURE 11.5 Where does the weight go? From Health Canada. (2010b). *Healthy weight gain during pregnancy.* Retrieved from https://www.canada.ca/content/dam/hc-sc/migration/hc-sc/fn-an/alt_formats/pdf/nutrition/prenatal/hwgdp-ppspg-eng.pdf

reproductive-age people in the United States are overweight or obese and at risk for numerous adverse pregnancy outcomes, in addition to a surgical birth. Some researchers have suggested that the uterine environment may influence the potential development of offspring obesity later in life. In a recent study, just a 10% weight loss before conception was associated with at least a 10% lower risk of preeclampsia, gestational diabetes, preterm birth, macrosomia, and stillbirth (Schummers, Hutcheon, Bodnar, Lieberman, & Himes, 2015). Dieting during pregnancy is never recommended, even for people who are obese. Severe restriction of caloric intake is associated with a decrease in birth weight. Because of the expansion of maternal blood volume and the development of fetal and placental tissues, some weight gain is essential for a healthy pregnancy. People who gain more than the recommended weight during pregnancy and who fail to

TABLE 11.7	RECOMMENDED WEIGHT GAIN FOR A SINGLETON PREGNANCY			
	Mean Rate of Weight Gain in the 2nd and 3rd Trimesters		Recommended Total Weight Gain	
Prepregnancy BMI	kg/wk	lb/wk	kg	lb
BMI < 18.5	0.5	1.0	12.5–18	28–40
BMI 18.5–24.9	0.4	1.0	11.5–16	25–35
BMI 25.0–29.9	0.3	0.6	7–11.5	15–25
BMI ≥ 30.0	0.2	0.5	5–9	11–20

Health Canada. (2010). *Prenatal nutrition guidelines for health professionals: Gestational weight gain.* Retrieved from https://www.canada.ca/content/dam/hc-sc/migration/hc-sc/fn-an/alt_formats/pdf/nutrition/prenatal/ewba-mbsa-eng.pdf lose this weight 6 months after giving birth are at much higher risk of being obese nearly a decade later (ACOG, 2018; SOGC, 2010). People who are overweight when beginning a pregnancy should gain no more than 11.5 to 16 kg (15 to 25 lb) during the pregnancy, depending on their nutritional status and degree of obesity (ACOG, 2018; Health Canada, 2014).

The best way to assess whether a pregnant client is consuming enough calories is to follow the pattern of weight gain. All pregnant people should aim for a steady rate of weight gain throughout pregnancy. If she is gaining in a steady, gradual manner, then she is taking in enough calories. However, consuming an adequate amount of calories does not guarantee that her nutrients are sufficient. It is critical to evaluate both the quantity and the quality of the foods eaten.

During the first trimester, for people whose prepregnancy weight is within the normal weight range, weight gain should be about 3.5 to 5 lb. For underweight people, weight gain should be at least 5 lb. For overweight people, weight gain should be about 2 lb. Much of the weight gained during the first trimester is caused by growth of the uterus and expansion of the blood volume.

During the second and third trimesters, the following pattern is recommended: for people whose prepregnancy weight is within the normal weight range, weight gain should be about 1 lb per week. For underweight people, weight gain should be slightly more than 1 lb per week. For overweight people, weight gain should be about two thirds of a pound per week (Hankey, 2015).

Nutrition Promotion

Through education, nurses can play an important role in ensuring adequate nutrition for pregnant people. During the initial prenatal visit, health care providers conduct a thorough assessment of a client's typical dietary practices and address any conditions that may cause inadequate nutrition, such as nausea and vomiting or lack of access to adequate food. Assess and reinforce dietary information at every prenatal visit to promote good nutrition. A normal pregnancy and a well-balanced diet generally provide most of the recommended nutrients except iron and folate, both of which must be supplemented in the form of prenatal vitamins. See Teaching Guidelines 11.1.

Teaching Guidelines 11.1
TEACHING TO PROMOTE OPTIMAL NUTRITION DURING PREGNANCY
- Follow Canada's Food Guide and select a variety of foods from each group
- Gain between 11.5 and 16 kg (25–35 lb) in a gradual and steady manner depending on prepregnancy weight as follows:

- Underweight (BMI > 18.5) total weight gain range = 12–18 kg
- Normal weight (BMI = 18.5–24.0) total weight gain range = 11.5–16 kg
- Overweight (BMI = 25–29) total weight gain range = 7–11.5 kg
- Obese (BMI = 30 or higher) total weight gain range = 7 kg (SOGC, 2010).
- Take your prenatal vitamin/mineral supplementation daily.
- Avoid weight-reduction diets during pregnancy.
- Do not skip meals; eat three meals with one or two snacks daily.
- Limit the intake of sodas and caffeine-rich drinks.
- Avoid the use of diuretics during pregnancy.
- Do not restrict the use of salt unless instructed to do so by your health care provider.
- Engage in reasonable physical activity daily.

Special Nutritional Considerations

Many factors play an important role in shaping a person's food habits, and these factors must be taken into account if nutritional counseling is to be realistic and appropriate. Nurses need to be aware of these factors to ensure individualized teaching and care.

Cultural Variations and Restrictions

Food is important to every cultural group. It is often part of celebrations and rituals. When working with people from various cultures, the nurse may need to adapt current Canadian nutritional guidelines to meet their nutritional needs. People in most cultures will be encouraged to eat a diet that is typical for them as an individual, while the nurse explores what each person's individual preferences are. Variations of food preferences, access, and availability may be different within a cultural or ethnic group and it is important that assumptions are not made about dietary preferences for a person or family. A relational approach and holistic assessment includes exploration of eating habits along with cultural preferences, celebrations, and rituals for that unique individual and family.

Lactose Intolerance

The best source of calcium is milk and dairy products, but for people with lactose intolerance, adaptations are necessary. People with lactose intolerance lack an enzyme (lactase) needed for the breakdown of lactose into its component simple sugars, glucose and galactose. Without adequate lactase, lactose passes through the small intestine undigested and causes abdominal discomfort, gas, and diarrhea. Lactose intolerance is especially common among women of African, Asian, and Middle Eastern descent (Szilagyi, 2015).

Additional or substitute sources of calcium may be necessary. These may include peanuts, almonds, sunflower seeds, broccoli, salmon, kale, and molasses (McIndoo, 2015). In addition, encourage the client to drink lactose-free dairy products or calcium-enriched orange juice or soy milk (Evidence-Based Practice 11.1).

Vegetarians

Vegetarian diets are becoming increasing prevalent in North America. People choose a vegetarian diet for various reasons including environmental, animal rights, philosophical, religious, and health beliefs (Dunlevy, 2015). Vegetarians choose not to eat meat, poultry, and fish. Their diets consist mostly of plant-based foods, such as legumes, vegetables, whole grains, nuts, and seeds.

Vegetarians fall into groups defined by the types of foods they eat. Lacto-ovo-vegetarians omit red meat, fish, and poultry, but eat eggs, milk, and dairy products in addition to plant-based foods. Lacto-vegetarians consume milk and dairy products along with plant-based foods; they omit eggs, meat, fish, and poultry. Vegans eliminate all foods from animals, including milk, eggs, and cheese, and eat only plant-based foods (Foster & Samman, 2015).

The concern with any form of vegetarianism, especially during pregnancy, is that the diet may be inadequate in nutrients. Other risks of vegetarian eating patterns during pregnancy may include low gestational weight gain, iron-deficiency anemia, compromised protein utilization, and decreased mineral absorption (Piccoli et al., 2015). A diet can become so restrictive that a person is not gaining weight or is consistently not eating enough from one or more of the food groups. Generally, the more restrictive the diet is, the greater the chance of nutrient deficiencies.

EVIDENCE-BASED PRACTICE 11.1 | **INTERVENTIONS FOR NAUSEA AND VOMITING IN EARLY PREGNANCY**

Nausea, retching or dry heaving, and vomiting in early pregnancy are very common and can be very distressing for people. Many treatments are available to people with "morning sickness," including drugs and complementary and alternative therapies. Because of concerns that taking medications may adversely affect the development of the fetus, this review aimed to examine if these treatments have been found to be effective and safe.

STUDY

The purpose of this study was to assess the effectiveness and safety of all interventions for nausea and vomiting in early pregnancy, up to 20 weeks of gestation. Thirty-seven trials involving 5,049 people met the inclusion criteria. These trials covered many interventions, including acupressure, acustimulation, acupuncture, ginger, chamomile, lemon oil, mint oil, vitamin B_6, and several antiemetic drugs.

Evidence regarding the effectiveness of P6 acupressure, auricular (ear) acupressure, and acustimulation of the P6 point was limited. Acupuncture (P6 or traditional) showed no significant benefit to people in pregnancy. The use of ginger products may be helpful to people, but the evidence of effectiveness was limited and not consistent, though two recent studies support ginger over placebo. There was only limited evidence from trials to support the use of pharmacologic agents including vitamin B_6, and antiemetic drugs to relieve mild or moderate nausea and vomiting. There was little information on maternal and fetal adverse outcomes and on psychological, social, or economic outcomes. The methodologic quality of the included studies was mixed.

Findings

This review found a lack of high-quality evidence to back up any advice on which interventions to use. Some of the studies showed a benefit in improving nausea and vomiting symptoms for people, but generally effects were inconsistent and limited. Studies were carried out in a way that meant they were at high risk of bias and, therefore, it was difficult to draw firm conclusions. Most studies had different ways of measuring the symptoms of nausea and vomiting and therefore, could not be looked at these findings together. Few studies reported maternal and fetal adverse outcomes and there was very little information on the effectiveness of treatments for improving people's quality of life.

Nursing Implications

Given the high prevalence of nausea and vomiting in early pregnancy, people and nurses caring for them need clear guidance about effective and safe interventions based on systematically reviewed evidence. Diclectin is the only approved medicine for treatment of morning sickness presently in Canada, but causes drowsiness, so people should avoid engaging in activities requiring complete mental alertness, such as driving. There is a lack of high-quality evidence to support any particular intervention at this time. This is not the same as saying that the interventions studied are ineffective, but that there is insufficient strong evidence for any one intervention. Advice provided by nurses to pregnant clients experiencing morning sickness should remain general and individualized, based on the findings of this study.

Adapted from Matthews, A., Haas, D. M., O'Mathúna, D. P., Dowswell, T., & Doyle, M. (2014). Interventions for nausea and vomiting in early pregnancy. *Cochrane Database of Systematic Reviews*, 2014, 3, CD007575.

Well-balanced vegetarian diets that include dairy products provide adequate caloric and nutrient intake and do not require special supplementation; however, vegan diets do not include any meat, eggs, or dairy products. Pregnant vegetarians must pay special attention to their intake of protein, iron, calcium, and vitamin B_{12}. Suggestions include:

- *For protein:* substitute soy foods, beans, lentils, nuts, grains, and seeds.
- *For iron:* eat a variety of meat alternatives, along with vitamin C–rich foods.
- *For calcium:* substitute soy, calcium-fortified orange juice, and tofu.
- *For vitamin B_{12}:* eat fortified soy foods and a B_{12} supplement.

Pica

Pica is a term used to describe the intense craving for and eating of nonfood items. Many people experience unusual food cravings during their pregnancy. Having cravings during pregnancy is perfectly normal. Sometimes, however, pregnant people crave substances that have no nutritional value and can even be dangerous to themselves and their fetus. Pica is the compulsive ingestion of nonfood substances. Pica is derived from the Latin term for magpie, a bird that is known to consume a variety of nonfood substances. Unlike the bird, however, pregnant people who develop a pica habit typically have one or two specific cravings.

The exact cause of pica is not known. Many theories have been advanced to explain it, but none has been proven scientifically. The incidence of pica is difficult to determine, since it is underreported. It is more common in the United States among African American people compared with other ethnicities, but the practice of pica is not limited to any one geographic area, race, creed, or culture. In North America, pica is also common in people from rural areas and people with a family history of it. Common substances ingested include dirt, clay, and laundry starch. Other pica cravings are burnt matches, stones, charcoal, mothballs, ice, cornstarch, toothpaste, soap, sand, plaster, coffee grounds, paint chips, coffee grounds, baking soda, and cigarette ashes (Jyothi, 2015).

The three main substances consumed by people with pica are soil or clay (geophagia), ice (pagophagia), and laundry starch (amylophagia). Nutritional implications include:

- *Soil:* replaces nutritive sources and causes iron-deficiency anemia
- *Clay:* produces constipation; can contain toxic substances and cause parasitic infection
- *Ice:* can cause iron-deficiency anemia, tooth fractures, freezer burn injuries
- *Laundry starch:* replaces iron-rich foods, leads to iron deficiencies, and replaces protein metabolism, thus depriving the fetus of amino acids needed for proper development (American Pregnancy Association, 2018)

Clinical manifestations of anemia often precede the identification of pica because the health care provider rarely addresses the behaviour and the client does not usually volunteer such information (King et al., 2015). Secrecy surrounding this habit makes research and diagnosis difficult because some people fail to view their behaviour as anything unusual, harmful, or worth reporting. Because of the clinical implications, pica should be discussed with all pregnant people as a preventive measure. The topic can be part of a general discussion of cravings, and the nurse should stress the harmful effects outlined above.

Suspect pica when the client exhibits anemia although the dietary intake seems appropriate. Ask about the client's usual dietary intake and include questions about the ingestion of nonfood substances. Consider the potential negative outcomes for the pregnant client and the fetus and take appropriate action.

PSYCHOSOCIAL ADAPTATIONS DURING PREGNANCY

Pregnancy is a unique time in a person's life. It is a time of dramatic alterations in the body and appearance, as well as a time of change in social status. All of these changes occur simultaneously. Concurrent with the physiologic changes within the body systems are psychosocial changes within the pregnant person and family members as they face significant role and lifestyle changes.

Maternal Emotional Responses

Motherhood, perhaps more than any role in society, has acquired a special significance for many people. Women are taught they should find fulfillment and satisfaction in the role of the "ever-bountiful, ever-giving, self-sacrificing mother." Pregnancy and transitioning to motherhood are critical experiences in a person's life, stirring a whole range of powerful emotions (Einstein, 2015). With such high expectations, many pregnant people experience various emotions throughout their pregnancy. The person's approach to these emotions is influenced by her emotional makeup, her sociologic and cultural background, her acceptance or rejection of the pregnancy, whether the pregnancy was planned, if the father is known, and her support network (Alexander et al., 2014).

Despite the wide-ranging emotions associated with the pregnancy, many people experience similar responses. These responses commonly include ambivalence, introversion, acceptance, mood swings, and changes in body image.

Ambivalence

The realization of a pregnancy can lead to fluctuating responses, possibly at the opposite ends of the spectrum. For example, regardless of whether the pregnancy was planned, the pregnant person may feel proud and excited by the news, while at the same time fearful and anxious of the implications. The reactions are influenced by several factors, including the way the client was raised, the current family situation, the quality of the relationship with the expectant father, and their hopes for the future. Some people express concern over the timing of the pregnancy, wishing that goals and life objectives had been met before becoming pregnant. Other people may question how a newborn or infant will affect their career or their relationships with friends and family. These feelings can cause conflict and confusion about the pregnancy.

Ambivalence, or having conflicting feelings at the same time, is a universal feeling and is considered normal when preparing for a lifestyle change and new role. Pregnant people commonly experience ambivalence during the first trimester. Usually ambivalence evolves into acceptance by the second trimester, after the first fetal movements (called **quickening**) are felt. The client's personality, ability to adapt to changing circumstances, and the reactions of the partner will affect a person's adjustment to being pregnant and the acceptance of impending motherhood.

Introversion

Introversion, or focusing on oneself, is common during the early part of pregnancy. The pregnant person may withdraw and become increasingly preoccupied with herself and the fetus. As a result, the client may participate less with the outside world, and may appear passive to family and friends.

This introspective behaviour is a normal psychological adaptation to motherhood for most people. Introversion seems to heighten during the first and third trimesters, when the pregnant person's focus is on behaviours that will ensure a safe and health pregnancy outcome. Couples need to be aware of this behaviour and should be informed about measures to maintain and support the focus on the family.

Acceptance

During the second trimester, the physical changes of the growing fetus, including an enlarging abdomen and fetal movement, bring reality and validity to the pregnancy. There are many tangible signs that someone separate from herself is present. The pregnant person feels fetal movement and may hear the heartbeat. Seeing the fetal image on an ultrasound screen and feeling distinct parts, as well as recognizing independent sleep and wake patterns, can help solidify the reality of growing fetus. The pregnant person becomes able to identify the fetus as a separate individual and accepts this.

Many people will verbalize positive feelings about the pregnancy and will conceptualize the fetus. The client may accept the new body image and talk about the new life within. Generating a discussion about the woman's feelings and offering support and validation at prenatal visits are important.

Mood Swings

Emotional lability is characteristic throughout most pregnancies. One moment a pregnant person can feel great joy, and within a short time can feel shock and disbelief. Frequently, pregnant people will start to cry without any apparent cause. Some people feel as though they are riding an emotional "roller-coaster." These extremes in emotion can make it difficult for partners and family members to communicate with the pregnant person without placing blame on themselves for their mood changes. Clear explanations about how common mood swings are during pregnancy are essential.

Change in Body Image

The way in which pregnancy affects a person's body image varies greatly. Some people feel as if they have never been more beautiful, whereas others spend their pregnancy feeling overweight and uncomfortable. For some clients, pregnancy is a relief from worrying about weight, whereas for others it only exacerbates their fears of weight gain. Changes in body image are normal but can be very stressful for the pregnant client. Offering a thorough explanation and initiating discussion of the expected bodily changes may help the family to cope with them.

Becoming a Mother

Reva Rubin (1984) identified maternal tasks that a woman must accomplish to incorporate the maternal role into her personality. Accomplishing these tasks helps the expectant mother to develop her self-concept as a mother and to form a mutually gratifying relationship with her infant. These tasks are listed in Box 11.4.

Pregnancy and Sexuality

Sexuality is an important part of health and well-being. Sexual behaviour modifies as pregnancy progresses, influenced by biologic, psychological, and social factors. The way a pregnant person feels and experiences their body during pregnancy can affect sexuality. The pregnant person's changing shape, emotional status, fetal activity, changes in breast size, pressure on the bladder, and other discomforts of pregnancy result in increased

RUBIN'S STAGES OF BECOMING A MOTHER

- **Ensuring safe passage throughout pregnancy and birth**
  - Primary focus of the woman's attention
  - First trimester: woman focuses on herself, not on the fetus
  - Second trimester: woman develops attachment of great value to her fetus
  - Third trimester: woman has concern for herself and her fetus as a unit
  - Participation in positive self-care activities related to diet, exercise, and overall well-being
- **Seeking acceptance of infant by others**
  - First trimester: acceptance of pregnancy by herself and others
  - Second trimester: family needs to relate to the fetus as member
  - Third trimester: unconditional acceptance without rejection
- **Seeking acceptance of self in maternal role to infant ("binding in")**
  - First trimester: mother accepts idea of pregnancy, but not of infant
  - Second trimester: with sensation of fetal movement (quickening), mother acknowledges fetus as a separate entity within her.
  - Third trimester: mother longs to hold infant and becomes tired of being pregnant.
- **Learning to give of oneself**
  - First trimester: identifies what must be given up to assume new role
  - Second trimester: identifies with infant, learns how to delay own desires
  - Third trimester: questions her ability to become a good mother to infant

Adapted from Rubin, R. (1984). *Maternal identity and the maternal experience*. New York: Springer.

recommended for clients who are at risk for preterm labour or for antepartum hemorrhage because of placenta previa (Boynton, 2015).

A person's sexual health is intimately linked to self-image. Sexual positions to increase comfort as the pregnancy progresses as well as alternative noncoital modes of sexual expression, such as cuddling, caressing, and holding, should be discussed. Giving permission to talk about and then normalizing sexuality can help enhance the sexual experience during pregnancy and, ultimately, the couple's relationship. If avenues of communication are open regarding sexuality during pregnancy, any fears and myths the couple may have can be dispelled.

Pregnancy and the Partner

Nursing care related to childbirth has expanded from a narrow emphasis on the physical health needs of the mother and infant to a broader focus on family-related social and emotional needs. One prominent feature of this family-centred approach is the recent movement toward promoting the mother–infant bond. To achieve a truly family-centred practice, nursing must make a comparable commitment to understanding and meeting the needs of the partner in the emerging family. Recent studies suggest that the partner's potential contribution to the infant's overall development has been misperceived or devalued and that the partner's ability and willingness to assume a more active role in the infant's care may have been underestimated.

Reactions to pregnancy and to the psychological and physical changes by the pregnant person's co-parent/partner vary greatly. Some enjoy the role of being the nurturer, whereas others experience alienation and may seek comfort or companionship elsewhere. Some expectant fathers may view pregnancy as proof of their masculinity and assume the dominant role, whereas others see their role as minimal, leaving the pregnancy up to the pregnant person entirely. Each expectant partner reacts uniquely.

Emotionally and psychologically, expectant partners may undergo fewer visible changes than the pregnant person, but most of these changes remain unexpressed and unappreciated (Davies, 2015). Expectant partners also experience a multitude of adjustments and concerns. Physically, they may gain weight around the middle and experience nausea and other GI disturbances—a reaction termed *couvade syndrome* that is a sympathetic response to their partner's pregnancy. They also experience ambivalence during early pregnancy, with extremes of emotions (e.g., pride and joy vs. an overwhelming sense of impending responsibility).

During the second trimester of pregnancy, partners go through acceptance of their role of breadwinner, caretaker, and support person. They come to accept the reality of the fetus when movement is felt, and they

physical and emotional demands. These can produce stress on the sexual relationship between the pregnant person and partner. As the changes of pregnancy ensue, many partners become confused, anxious, and fearful of how the relationship may be affected.

The sexual desire of pregnant people may change throughout the pregnancy. During the first trimester, the pregnant person may be less interested in sex because of fatigue, nausea, and fear of disturbing the early embryonic development. During the second trimester, sexual interest may increase because of the stability of the pregnancy. During the third trimester, the enlarging size may produce discomfort during sexual activity (Bope & Kellerman, 2015).

Potential complications of sex during pregnancy include preterm labour, pelvic inflammatory disease, antepartum hemorrhage in placenta previa, and venous air embolism. Generally, sexual relations are generally considered safe in pregnancy. Abstinence is usually only experience confusion when dealing with the pregnant partner's mood swings and introspection. During the third trimester, the partner prepares for the reality of this new role and negotiates what the role will be during the labour and birthing process. Many express concern about being the primary support person during labour and birth and worry how they will react when faced with their loved one in pain. Expectant partners share many of the same anxieties as their pregnant partners. However, it is uncommon for them to reveal these anxieties to the pregnant partner or health care providers. Often, how the expectant partner responds during the third trimester depends on the state of the marriage or partnership. When the marriage or partnership is struggling, the impending increase in responsibility toward the end of pregnancy acts to drive the expectant partner further away. Often it manifests as working late, staying out late with friends, or beginning new or superficial relationships. In the stable marriage or partnership, the expectant partner who may have been struggling to find his or her place in the pregnancy now finds concrete tasks to do—for example, painting the nursery, assembling the car seat, or attending Lamaze classes.

Pregnancy and Siblings

A sibling's reaction to pregnancy is age dependent. Some children might express excitement and anticipation, whereas others might have negative reactions. A young toddler might regress in toilet training or ask to drink from a bottle again. An older school-aged child may ignore the new addition to the family and engage in outside activities to avoid the new member. The introduction of an infant into the family is often the beginning of sibling rivalry, which results from the child's fear of change in the security of the relationship with his or her parents (Jordan et al., 2014). Preparation of the

FIGURE 11.6 Parents preparing sibling for the birth of a new baby.

siblings for the anticipated birth is imperative and must be designed according to the age and life experiences of the sibling at home. Constant reinforcement of love and caring will help to reduce the older child's fear of change and worry about being replaced by the new family member.

If possible, parents should include siblings in preparation for the birth of the new baby to help them feel as if they have an important role to play (Fig. 11.6). Parents must also continue to focus on the older sibling after the birth to reduce regressive or aggressive behaviour toward the newborn.

Pregnancy is an extremely busy time, not only in terms of the bodily changes taking place, but tasks that must be done such as choosing a provider to care for them, preparing for the new family member in a matter of months, and making lifestyle modifications to promote the best possible pregnancy outcome. We will explore this more in Chapter 12.

KEY CONCEPTS

- Pregnancy is a normal life event that involves considerable physical, psychosocial, emotional, and relationship adjustments.

- The signs and symptoms of pregnancy have been grouped into those that are subjective (presumptive) and experienced by the individual client, those that are objective (probable) and observed by the health care provider, and those that are the positive, certain signs.

- Physiologically, almost every system of a person's body changes during pregnancy with startling

rapidity to accommodate the needs of the growing fetus. A majority of the changes are influenced by hormonal changes.

- The placenta is a unique kind of endocrine gland; it has a feature possessed by no other endocrine organ—the ability to form protein and steroid hormones.

- Occurring in conjunction with the physiologic changes in the person's body systems are psychosocial changes occurring within the pregnant person and family members as they face significant role and lifestyle changes.

- Commonly experienced emotional responses to pregnancy include ambivalence, introversion, acceptance, mood swings, and changes in body image.

- Reactions of expectant partners to pregnancy and to the physical and psychological changes in the pregnant person vary greatly.

- A sibling's reaction to pregnancy is age dependent. The introduction of a new infant to the family is often the beginning of sibling rivalry, which results from the established child's fear of change in security of their relationships with their parents. Therefore, preparation of the siblings for the anticipated birth is imperative.

REFERENCES AND RECOMMENDED READINGS

Alexander, L. L., LaRosa, J. H., Bader, H., & Garfield, S. (2014). *New dimensions in women's health* (6th ed.). Sudbury, MA: Jones & Bartlett.

Allerberger, F., & Huhulescu, S. (2015). Pregnancy related listeriosis: Treatment and control. *Expert Review of Anti-infective Therapy, 13*(3), 395–403.

American College of Obstetricians and Gynaecologists (ACOG). (2018). *Nutrition during pregnancy.* Retrieved from https://www.acog.org/Patients/FAQs/Nutrition-During-Pregnancy

American Pregnancy Association. (2018). *Pregnancy and pica: Non-food cravings.* Retrieved from http://www.american-pregnancy.org/pregnancyhealth/unusualcravingspica.html

Anil, S., Alrowis, R. M., Chalisserry, E. P., Chalissery, V. P., AlMoharib, H. S., & Al-Sulaimani, A. F. (2015). Chapter 28: Oral health and adverse pregnancy outcomes. In M. Virdi (Ed.), *Emerging trends in oral health sciences and dentistry* (pp. 631–662). Retrieved from http://dx.doi.org/10.5772/59517

Banerjee, A., & Williamson, C. (2015). Chapter 5: Endocrine and metabolic emergencies in pregnancy. In G. Matfin (Ed.), *Endocrine and metabolic medical emergencies.* Retrieved from http://dx.doi.org/10.1210/EME.9781936704811.ch5

Blackburn, S. (2013). *Maternal, fetal, & neonatal physiology: A clinical perspective.* Maryland Heights, MO: Elsevier Saunders.

Bope, E. T., & Kellerman, R. D. (2015). *Conn's current therapy 2015.* Philadelphia, PA: Elsevier.

Boynton, P. M. (2015). Pregnancy: Relationships advice. In P. Whelehan, & A. Bolin (Eds.), *The international encyclopedia of human sexuality* (pp. 861–1042). Retrieved from http://dx.doi.org/10.1002/9781118896877.wbiehs372

Campbell, K., Rowe, H., Azzam, H., Lane, C. (2016). The management of nausea and vomiting of pregnancy. *Journal of Obstetrics and Gynaecology of Canada, 38*(12), 1127–1137.

Cheng, H. M. (2015). Water balance. In *Physiology question-based learning* (pp. 127–135). New York: Springer International Publishing.

Cox, S., & Reid, F. (2015). Urogynecological complications in pregnancy: An overview. *Obstetrics, Gynecology and Reproductive Medicine, 25*(5), 123–127.

Crowley, W. R. (2015). Neuroendocrine regulation of lactation and milk production. *Comprehensive Physiology, 5,* 255–291.

Cunningham, F. G., Leveno, K. J., Bloom, S. L., Spong, C. Y., Dashe, J. S., Hoffman, B. L., . . . Sheffield, J. S. (2014). *William's obstetrics* (24th ed.). New York: McGraw-Hill Education.

Davies, J. (2015). Fatherhood Institute: Supporting fathers to play their part. *Community Practitioner, 88*(1), 13–14.

DeLoughery, T. G. (2015). Bleeding and thrombosis: Women's issues. In *Hemostasis and thrombosis* (pp. 151–155). New York: Springer International Publishing.

Dunlevy, F. (2015). Nutritional assessment during pregnancy. *Topics in Clinical Nutrition, 30*(1), 71–79.

Edelman, C. L., Kudzma, E. C., & Mandle, C. L. (2014). *Health promotion throughout the lifespan* (8th ed.). St. Louis, MO: Mosby Elsevier.

Einstein, A. (2015). *Thinking about emotions. Thinking about thinking: Cognition, science, and psychotherapy* (pp. 68–85). New York: Routledge.

Foo, L., Tay, J., Lees, C. C., McEniery, C. M., & Wilkinson, I. B. (2015). Hypertension in pregnancy: Natural history and treatment options. *Current Hypertension Reports, 17*(5), 1–18.

Foster, M., & Samman, S. (2015). Vegetarian diets across the lifecycle: Impact on zinc intake and status. *Advances in Food and Nutrition Research, 74,* 93–131.

Gaillard, R., & Jaddoe, V. W. (2015). Assessment of maternal blood pressure development during pregnancy. *Journal of Hypertension, 33*(1), 61–62.

Hankey, C. R. (2015). Chapter 1: Importance of good health and nutrition before and during pregnancy. In L. Stewart, & J. Thompson (Eds.), *Early years nutrition and healthy weight* (pp. 1–13). Somerset, NJ: John Wiley & Sons.

Health Canada. (2009). *Prenatal nutrition guidelines for health professionals.* Retrieved from https://www.canada.ca/content/dam/hc-sc/migration/hc-sc/fn-an/alt_formats/hpfb-dgpsa/pdf/pubs/folate-eng.pdf

Health Canada. (2010a). *Dietary reference intakes definitions.* Retrieved from http://www.hc-sc.gc.ca/fn-an/alt_formats/hpfb-dgpsa/pdf/nutrition/dri_tables-eng.pdf

Health Canada. (2010b). *Healthy weight gain during pregnancy.* Retrieved from https://www.canada.ca/content/dam/hc-sc/migration/hc-sc/fn-an/alt_formats/pdf/nutrition/prenatal/hwgdp-ppspg-eng.pdf

Health Canada. (2014). *Prenatal nutrition guidelines for health professionals: Gestational weight gain.* Retrieved from https://www.canada.ca/en/health-canada/services/publications/food-nutrition/prenatal-nutrition-guidelines-health-professionals-background-canada-food-guide-2009.html

Health Canada. (2015a). *Canada prenatal nutrition program (CPNP).* Retrieved from https://www.canada.ca/en/public-health/services/health-promotion/childhood-adolescence/programs-initiatives/canada-prenatal-nutrition-program-cpnp.html

Health Canada. (2015b). *Safe food handling for pregnant women.* Retrieved from https://www.canada.ca/en/health-canada/services/food-safety-vulnerable-populations/food-safety-pregnant-women.html

Health Canada. (2016a). *Summary safety review: Diclectin (doxylamine and pyridoxine combination)—Assessing safety in pregnancy.* Retrieved from https://www.canada.

ca/en/health-canada/services/drugs-health-products/ medeffect-canada/safety-reviews/summary-safety-review- assessing-diclectin-doxylamine-pyridoxine-combination- safety-pregnancy.html

Health Canada. (2016b). *Iron and pregnancy.* Retrieved from https://www.canada.ca/en/public-health/services/preg- nancy/iron-pregnancy.html

Health Canada. (2017). *Mercury in fish.* Retrieved from https://www.canada.ca/en/health-canada/services/food- nutrition/food-safety/chemical-contaminants/environmental- contaminants/mercury/mercury-fish.html

Health Canada. (2019a). *Healthy eating and pregnancy.* Retrieved from https://www.canada.ca/en/public-health/ser- vices/pregnancy/healthy-eating-pregnancy.html

Health Canada. (2019b). *The sensible guide to a healthy pregnancy.* Retrieved from https://www.canada.ca/en/ public-health/services/health-promotion/healthy-pregnancy/ healthy-pregnancy-guide.html#a1

Health Canada. (2019c). *Canada's food guide.* Retrieved from https://food-guide.canada.ca/static/assets/pdf/CFG-snap- shot-EN.pdf

Health and Medicine Division [HMD]. (2009). *Weight gain during pregnancy: Reexamining the guidelines.* Retrieved from http://www.iom.edu/Reports/2009/Weight-Gain- During-Pregnancy-Reexamining-the-Guidelines.aspx

Health Link BC. (2016). *Food safety: Mercury in fish.* Retrieved from https://www.healthlinkbc.ca/healthlinkbc-files/ mercury-fish

Heffner, L. J., & Schust, D. J. (2014). *The reproductive system at a glance* (4th ed.). Somerset, NJ: Wiley Blackwell.

Heuman, D. M., Mihas, A. A., & Allen, J. (2017). Gallstones (cholelithiasis). *eMedicine.* Retrieved from http://emedicine. medscape.com/article/175667-overview

Jacobson, J. D. (2018). Eating right during pregnancy. *Medline- Plus.* Retrieved from http://www.nlm.nih.gov/medlineplus/ ency/patientinstructions/000584.htm

Jones, R. E., & Lopez, K. H. (2014). *Human reproductive biology* (4th ed.). Waltham, MA: Elsevier.

Jordan, R. G., Engstrom, J., Matrfell, J., & Farley, C. L. (2014). *Prenatal and postnatal care: A woman-centered approach.* Ames, IA: Wiley-Blackwell.

Jyothi, N. (2015). Case study on post pregnancy related com- plication of pica. *International Journal of Nursing Care,* *3*(1), 42–45.

Kim, S. H., Bennett, P. R., & Terzidou, V. (2015). Diverse roles of oxytocin. *Inflammation and Cell Signaling, 2*(1), 10–14.

King, T. L., Brucker, M. C., Kriebs, J. M., Fahey, J. O., Gegor, C. L., & Varney, H. (2015). *Varney's midwifery* (5th ed.). Burlington, MA: Jones & Bartlett Learning.

Kouhkan, S., Rahimi, A., Ghasemi, M., Naimi, S. S., & Bagh- ban, A. A. (2015). Postural changes during first pregnancy. *British Journal of Medicine and Medical Research, 7*(9), 744–753.

Krapf, J. M. (2018). Vulvovaginitis. *eMedicine.* Retrieved from http://emedicine.medscape.com/article/2188931-overview

Kruger, H. S., & Butte, N. F. (2015). Nutrition in pregnancy and lactation. In D. M. Bier, J. Mann, D. H. Alpers, H. E. Vorster, & M. J. Gibney (Eds.), *Nutrition for the primary care provider* (pp. 64–70). Basel: Karger.

Larson, L. (2015). Renal disease in pregnancy. In K. Rosene- Montella (Ed.), *Medical management of the pregnant patient* (pp. 261–272). New York: Springer Publishers.

Lutz, C. A., Mazur, E., & Litch, N. (2014). *Nutrition and diet therapy* (6th ed.). Philadelphia, PA: F. A. Davis.

Matthews, A., Haas, D. M., O'Mathúna, D. P., Dowswell, T., & Doyle, M. (2014). Interventions for nausea and vomiting in early pregnancy. *Cochrane Database of Systematic Reviews, 3,* CD007575.

McIndoo, H. (2015). The best plant-based milks. *Environmental Nutrition, 38*(1), 5–6.

Medici, M., Korevaar, T. I., Visser, W. E., Visser, T. J., & Peeters, R. P. (2015). Thyroid function in pregnancy: What is normal? *Clinical Chemistry, 61*(5), 704–713.

Mehta, N., Chen, K., Hardy, E., & Powrie, R. (2015). Respira- tory disease in pregnancy. *Best Practice & Research Clinical Obstetrics & Gynecology, 29*(5), 598–611.

Myers, K. M., Feltovich, H., Mazza, E., Vink, J., Bajka, M., Wapner, R. J., . . . House, M. (2015). The mechanical role of the cervix in pregnancy. *Journal of Biomechanics, 48*(9), 1511–1523.

Nas, K., Brcyer, H., & Tuu, L. (2015). The role of tailored treatment on conception and pregnancy at patients with insulin resistance. *Endocrine Abstracts, 37.* doi: 10.1530/ endoabs.37.EP189.

Neifeld, R. (2018). Gluten free for the gluten tolerant during pregnancy. *BabyMed.* Retrieved from http://www.babymed. com/food-and-nutrition/gluten-free-gluten-tolerant-during- pregnancy

Nelson, R. (2015). To eat fish or not to eat fish. *American Journal of Nursing, 115*(2), 18–19.

Ojha, S., Fainberg, H. P., Sebert, S., Budge, H., & Symonds, M. E. (2015). Maternal health and eating habits: Metabolic con sequences and impact on child health. *Trends in Molecular Medicine, 21*(2), 126–133.

Osol, G., & Moore, L. G. (2014). Maternal uterine vascular remodeling during pregnancy. *Microcirculation, 21*(1), 38–47.

Pearce, E. N. (2015). Thyroid disorders during pregnancy and postpartum. *Best Practice & Research Clinical Obstetrics & Gynecology, 29*(5), 700–706.

Pellegrini, N., & Agostoni, C. (2015). Nutritional aspects of gluten-free products. *Journal of the Science of Food and Agriculture, 95*(12), 2380–2385.

Piccoli, G., Clari, R., Vigotti, F., Leone, F., Attini, R., Cabiddu, G., . . . Avagnina, P. (2015). Vegan-vegetarian diets in preg- nancy: Danger or panacea? A systematic narrative review. *British Journal of Obstetrics and Gynaecology, 122*(5), 623–633.

Pope, E., Maltepe, C., & Koren, G. (2015). Comparing pyridox- ine and doxylamine succinate-pyridoxine HCl for nausea and vomiting of pregnancy: A matched, controlled cohort study. *Journal of Clinical Pharmacology, 55*(7), 809–814.

Qurrat-ul-Ain, & Khan, S. A. (2015). Artificial sweeteners: Safe or unsafe? *The Journal of the Pakistan Medical Association, 65*(2), 225–227.

Rigby, F. B. (2016). Common pregnancy complaints and ques- tions. *eMedicine.* Retrieved from http://emedicine.medscape. com/article/259724-overview

Rossier, B. C., Baker, M. E., & Studer, R. A. (2015). Epithelial sodium transport and its control by aldosterone: The story of our internal environment revisited. *Physiological Reviews, 95*(1), 297–340.

Rubin, R. (1984). *Maternal identity and the maternal experience.* New York: Springer.

Sabina, S., Iftequar, S., Zaheer, Z., Khan, M. M., & Khan, S. (2015). An overview of anemia in pregnancy. *Journal of Innovations in Pharmaceuticals and Biological Sciences, 2*(2), 144–151.

Schummers, L., Hutcheon, J. A., Bodnar, L. M., Lieberman, E., & Himes, K. P. (2015). Risk of adverse pregnancy outcomes by prepregnancy body mass index: A population-based study to inform prepregnancy weight loss counseling. *Obstetrics and Gynecology, 125*(1), 133–143.

Sharma, A. J., Vesco, K. K., Bulkley, J., Callaghan, W. M., Bruce, F. C., Staab, J., . . . Berg, C. J. (2015). Associations of gestational weight gain with preterm birth among underweight and normal weight women. *Maternal and Child Health Journal, 19*(9), 2066–2073.

Shields, A. D. (2017). Pregnancy diagnosis. *eMedicine.* Retrieved from http://emedicine.medscape.com/article/262591-overview

Soucy-Giguère, L., Tétu, A., Gauthier, S., Morand, M., Chandad, F., Giguère, Y., & Bujold, E. (2016). Periodontal disease and adverse pregnancy outcomes: A prospective study in a low-risk population. *Journal of Obstetrics and Gynaecology of Canada, 38* (4), 346–350.

Szilagyi, A. (2015). Adult lactose digestion status and effects on disease. *Canadian Journal of Gastroenterology and Hepatology, 29*(3), 149–156.

Thadhani, R. I., & Maynard, S. E. (2018). Renal and urinary physiology in normal pregnancy. *UpToDate.* Retrieved from http://www.uptodate.com/contents/renal-and-urinary-tract-physiology-in-normal-pregnancy

Tharpe, N. L., Farley, C. L., & Jordan, R. (2016). *Clinical practice guidelines for midwifery & women's health* (5th ed.). Sudbury, MA: Jones & Bartlett.

The Society of Obstetricians and Gynaecologists of Canada. (2010). Obesity in pregnancy. *Journal of Obstetrics and Gynaecology of Canada, 110*(2), 167–173.

The Society of Obstetricians and Gynaecologists of Canada. (2012). *Education: Nausea and vomiting in pregnancy.* Retrieved from http://pregnancy.sogc.org/wp-content/uploads/2014/05/PDF_nauseaandvomitinginpregnancy_ENG.pdf

The Society of Obstetricians and Gynaecologists of Canada. (2015). Pre-conception folic acid and multivitamin supplementation for the primary and secondary prevention of neural tube defects and other folic acid-sensitive congenital anomalies. *Journal of Obstetrics and Gynaecology of Canada, 37*(6), 534–549.

Tretti Clementoni, M., & Lavagno, R. (2015). A novel 1565 nm non-ablative fractional device for stretch marks: A preliminary report. *Journal of Cosmetic and Laser Therapy, 17*(3), 148–155.

Trivedi, S., Lal, N., & Singhal, R. (2015). Periodontal diseases and pregnancy. *Journal of Orofacial Sciences, 7*(1), 67–68.

Tyler, K. H. (2015). Physiological skin changes during pregnancy. *Clinical Obstetrics and Gynecology, 58*(1), 119–124.

United States Department of Agriculture Food Safety and Inspection Service. (2017). *Protect yourself and your baby from listeriosis.* Retrieved from https://www.fsis.usda.gov/wps/portal/fsis/topics/food-safety-education/get-answers/food-safety-fact-sheets/foodborne-illness-and-disease/protect-your-baby-and-yourself-from-listeriosis/ct_index

Walsh, J. M., & McAuliffe, F. M. (2015). Impact of maternal nutrition on pregnancy outcome—Does it matter what pregnant women eat? *Best Practice & Research Clinical Obstetrics & Gynecology, 29*(1), 63–78.

Zinaman, M. J., Johnson, S., & Marriott, L. (2015). Analysis of human chorionic gonadotropin levels in normal and failing pregnancies [40]. *Obstetrics and Gynecology, 125,* 21S–22S.

CHAPTER **WORKSHEET**

MULTIPLE CHOICE QUESTIONS

1. What factors would change during a pregnancy if the hormone progesterone were reduced or withdrawn?
   a. The pregnant person's gums would become red and swollen and would bleed easily.
   b. The uterus would contract more and peristalsis would increase.
   c. Morning sickness would increase and would be prolonged.
   d. The secretion of prolactin by the pituitary gland would be inhibited.

2. Which of the following is a presumptive sign or symptom of pregnancy?
   a. Restlessness
   b. Elevated mood
   c. Urinary frequency
   d. Low backache

3. When obtaining a blood test for pregnancy, which hormone would the nurse expect the test to measure?
   a. Human chorionic gonadotropin (hCG)
   b. Human placental lactogen (hPL)
   c. Follicle-stimulating hormone (FSH)
   d. Luteinizing hormone (LH)

4. During pregnancy, which of the following should the expectant person reduce or avoid?
   a. Raw meat or uncooked shellfish
   b. Fresh, washed fruits and vegetables
   c. Whole grains and cereals
   d. Protein and iron from meat sources

5. A feeling expressed by most people upon learning they are pregnant is:
   a. Acceptance
   b. Depression
   c. Jealousy
   d. Ambivalence

6. Reva Rubin identified four major tasks that the pregnant woman undertakes to form a mutually gratifying relationship with her infant. What is "binding in"?
   a. Ensuring safe passage through pregnancy, labour, and birth
   b. Seeking acceptance of this infant by others
   c. Seeking acceptance of self as mother to the infant
   d. Learning to give of oneself on behalf of the infant

7. A pregnant client close to term comes into the clinic for an exam. The client reports experiencing shortness of breath. The nurse knows that this symptom can be explained as the:
   a. Fetus is needing more oxygen now that his/her size is larger.
   b. Fundus of the uterus is high and pushing the diaphragm upward.
   c. Client is experiencing an allergic reaction because of high histamine levels.
   d. Oxygen partial pressure concentration is lower in the third trimester.

8. Which of the following fish should be limited in a pregnant person's diet because of the high mercury content?
   a. Salmon
   b. Cod
   c. Shrimp
   d. Sword fish

CRITICAL THINKING EXERCISES

1. When interviewing a woman at her first prenatal visit, the nurse asks about her feelings. The woman replies, "I'm frightened and confused. I don't know whether I want to be pregnant or not. Being pregnant means changing our whole life, and now having somebody to care for all the time. I'm not sure I would be a good mother. Plus I'm a bit afraid of all the changes that would happen to my body. Is this normal? Am I okay?"
   a. How should the nurse answer this question?
   b. What specific information is needed to support the client during this pregnancy?

2. Sally, age 23, is 9 weeks pregnant. At her clinic visit she says, "I'm so tired I can barely make it home from work. Then once I'm home, I don't have the energy to make dinner." She says she is so sick in the morning that she is frequently late to work and spends much of the day in the bathroom. Sally's current lab work is within normal limits.
   a. What explanation can the nurse offer Sally about her discomforts?
   b. What interventions can the nurse offer to Sally?

3. Bringing a new infant into the family affects the siblings. What strategies can a nurse discuss when a mother asks how to deal with this?

CHAPTER **WORKSHEET**

STUDY ACTIVITIES

1. Go to your local health department's maternity clinic and interview several people regarding their feelings and the bodily changes that have taken place since they became pregnant. Based on your findings, place them into appropriate trimesters of their pregnancy.

2. Search the Internet for information about the psychological changes that occur during pregnancy. Share information from the websites you found with your clinical group.

3. During pregnancy, the plasma volume increases by 50% but the RBC volume increases by only 25% to 33%. This disproportion is manifested as _____.

4. When a pregnant client in the third trimester lies on their back and experiences dizziness and light-headedness, the underlying cause of this is _____.

BRINGING IT ALL TOGETHER: A CASE STUDY

A 22-year-old pregnant client presents to the maternity clinic with a 4-day history of loss of appetite, constipation, and abdominal pain. She is in the first trimester of her first pregnancy and came to this country recently from India. Her mother accompanies her and answers most of the questions for her daughter. After much questioning, the mother reveals that her daughter frequently eats dirt, which was common practice in her country.

Go to thePoint **to find questions to consider about this case.**

12

Nursing Management During Pregnancy

Learning Objectives

Upon completion of the chapter, you will be able to:

1. Identify the information typically collected at the initial prenatal visit.

2. Determine an appropriate reproductive life plan based on a couple's risk profile.

3. Select the assessments completed at follow-up prenatal visits.

4. Evaluate the tests used to assess well-being of the childbearing person and fetus, including nursing management for each.

5. Outline appropriate nursing management to promote self-care during pregnancy and to minimize the common discomforts of pregnancy.

6. Examine the key components of perinatal education.

Linda and her partner, *Rob*, are eager to start a family within the next year. They are stable in their careers and financially secure. They decide to investigate a new midwifery practice associated with the local hospital, and they go for a preconception appointment. They leave their appointment overwhelmed with all the information they were given about having a healthy pregnancy.

INTRODUCTION

Pregnancy is a time of many physiologic and psychological changes that can positively or negatively affect the client, the fetus, and the family. Misconceptions, inadequate information, and unanswered questions about pregnancy, birth, and parenthood are common. The ultimate goal of any pregnancy is the birth of a healthy newborn, and nurses play a major role in helping the childbearing family achieve this goal. Ongoing assessment and education are essential.

This chapter describes the nursing management required during pregnancy. It begins with a brief discussion of preconception care and then describes the assessment of a childbearing person at the first prenatal visit and on follow-up visits. The chapter discusses tests commonly used to assess well-being of the client and fetus, including specific nursing management related to each test. The chapter also identifies important strategies to minimize the common discomforts of pregnancy and promote self-care. Finally, the chapter discusses perinatal education, including childbirth education, birthing options, health care provider options, preparation for breastfeeding or bottle feeding, and final preparation for labour and birth.

PRECONCEPTION CARE

Ideally, couples thinking about having a child should schedule a visit with their health care provider for preconception counselling to ensure that they are in the best possible state of health before pregnancy. **Preconception care** encompasses the interventions that identify and modify any medical, psychosocial, behavioural, or environmental risks to reproductive health and future pregnancies for the childbearing family (Public Health Agency of Canada [PHAC], 2017a). All persons of reproductive age are included in preconception care, and when based on the principles of Family-Centred Maternity and Newborn Care will empower individuals and families to actively participate in their care through informed decision making in practices that are safe and value the diversity of people's lives.

The Public Health Association of Canada (2017b), in partnership with maternal and newborn health experts, has outlined evidence-based guiding principles for Family-Centred Maternity and Newborn Care in Canada (Box 12.1).

Preconception care is advocated throughout the world as a tool for improving perinatal outcomes. Preconception care should occur any time a health care provider sees a client of reproductive age. Primary care for all clients of childbearing age by nurses should include a routine assessment of reproductive goals and planning. Those who could potentially become pregnant should

---

> **BOX 12.1**
>
> ### PRINCIPLES FOR FAMILY-CENTRED MATERNITY AND NEWBORN CARE IN CANADA
>
> 1. A family-centred approach to maternal and newborn care is optimal
> 2. Pregnancy and birth are normal, healthy processes
> 3. Early parent–infant attachment is critical for newborn and child development and the growth of healthy families
> 4. Family-centred maternal and newborn care applies to all care environments
> 5. Family-centred maternal and newborn care is informed by research evidence
> 6. Family-centred maternal and newborn care requires a holistic approach
> 7. Family-centred maternal and newborn care involves collaboration among care providers
> 8. Culturally appropriate care is important in a multicultural society
> 9. Indigenous people have distinctive needs during pregnancy and birth
> 10. Care as close to home as possible is ideal
> 11. Individualized maternal and newborn care is recommended
> 12. Childbearing families require knowledge about their care
> 13. Childbearing families play an integral role in decision making
> 14. The attitudes and language of health care providers have an impact on a family's experience of maternal and newborn care
> 15. Family-centred maternal and newborn care respects reproductive rights
> 16. Family-centred maternal and newborn care functions within a system that requires ongoing evaluation
> 17. Family-centred maternal and newborn care best practices for global settings may offer valuable options for Canadian consideration.
>
> Adapted from Public Health Agency of Canada. (2017a). Preconception care. Retrieved from https://www.canada.ca/content/dam/phac-aspc/documents/services/publications/healthy-living/maternity-newborn-care/maternity-newborn-care-guidelines-chapter-2-eng.pdf

---

be assessed for preconception risks and educated about the importance of individual health in ensuring healthy pregnancies. Clients may be motivated to address modifiable health risks by learning about the way their present health will affect a future pregnancy. For those not intending a pregnancy soon, preconception care should focus on contraception counselling (Callegari, Ma, & Schwartz, 2015). Personal and family history, physical examination, laboratory screening, reproductive plan, nutrition, supplements, weight, exercise, vaccinations, and injury prevention should be reviewed. Encourage folic acid 400 to 800 mcg per day depending on risk profile, as well as proper diet and exercise. Clients should receive the influenza vaccine if planning pregnancy during flu season; the rubella and varicella vaccines if there is no evidence of immunity to these viruses; and tetanus/diphtheria/pertussis if lacking adult vaccination. Offer specific interventions to reduce morbidity and mortality for both the individual who has been identified with chronic diseases or exposed to teratogens or illicit substances and their future baby. Several interventions have been proven to effectively improve pregnancy outcome when provided as preconception care. Recent research suggests that events that occur in the uterine decidua, even before an individual's awareness of being pregnant, may have a significant impact on fetal growth and the outcome of pregnancy. In addition, an intact immune system optimizes placental development and function and is essential for fetal survival (Regal, Gilbert, & Burwick, 2015). New insights reveal that the early embryo is extremely sensitive to signals from gametes, trophoblastic tissue, and periconception lifestyles. Also, environmental factors prior to and after conception have an enormous impact on the developing embryo and cause long-term health problems. There is a growing body of evidence that environmental factors during embryonic development can cause irreversible alteration in epigenetic markers and induce various adult diseases, such as cardiovascular, neurologic, and metabolic disorders later in life (Keytash, Jones, & Frances, 2015). With this in mind, shifting the focus on the periconception period and the very early stages of pregnancy should offer significant benefits to the health of both the client and the infant. The overall aim should be to effectively use every pregnancy as the health care opportunity of two lifetimes (Steeggers-Theunissen & Steegers, 2015).

Risk Factors for Adverse Pregnancy Outcomes

Preconception care is just as important as prenatal care to reduce adverse pregnancy outcomes such as perinatal mortality, preterm births, and low–birth-weight infants. Adverse pregnancy outcomes constitute a major public health challenge: 8.1% of infants are born preterm; 9.1% are born small for gestational age; 4.3% of infants are born with at least one congenital anomaly; and severe pregnancy complications are experienced at a rate of 14.2 per 1,000 deliveries (PHAC, 2017c). Risk factors for these adverse pregnancy outcomes are prevalent among the prepregnant population of reproductive age, as demonstrated by the following statistics:

- 23% who are aged 20 to 34 smoke tobacco.
- 16% who are aged 20 to 29 smoke marijuana.
- 73% who are aged 15 years and older consume alcohol, which can cause fetal alcohol spectrum disorder in children who are exposed to alcohol in utero.
- 42% do not take folic acid supplements prior to pregnancy, increasing the risk of neural tube defects in the newborn. Taking folic acid reduces the incidence of neural tube defects by two thirds.
- 16% aged 25 to 34 years are obese and another 22% are overweight, which may increase their risk of developing hypertension, diabetes, and thromboembolic disease and may increase the need for cesarean birth.
- Other individuals take prescription or over-the-counter medications that are known teratogens (substances harmful to the developing fetus), or have pre-existing medical conditions that can negatively affect pregnancy if unmanaged (PHAC, 2017a).

All of the preceding factors pose risks to pregnancy and could be addressed with early interventions if the individual or couple seeks preconception health care. Specific recognized risk factors for adverse pregnancy outcomes that fall into one or more of these categories are listed in Box 12.2.

The period of greatest environmental sensitivity and consequent risk for the developing embryo is between days 17 and 56 after conception. The first prenatal visit, which is usually a month or later after a missed menstrual period, may occur too late to affect reproductive outcomes associated with abnormal organogenesis secondary to risk exposure in the preconception period. In some cases, such as with unplanned pregnancies, individuals may delay seeking health care because they deny that they are pregnant or face barriers to access. Thus, commonly used prevention practices may begin too late to avert the morbidity and mortality associated with congenital anomalies and low birth weight. A large number of Canadian families continue to face multiple barriers to achieving optimal health. Those who experience poverty and associated food insecurity face higher rates of obesity, substance use, and exposure to environmental hazards and violence, leading to poor pregnancy outcomes. Indigenous families face higher than average rates of poverty, food insecurity, and underemployment, in addition to a lack of culturally relevant preconception services (PHAC, 2017a). A more global population health strategy is needed to improve pregnancy outcomes in the most vulnerable populations. Securing international level political priority for perinatal care remains critical to accomplish the goal of better health for all families. Ideally, all couples could take on the responsibility of developing their reproductive life plan and share it with their health care providers at office visits (Darmstadt, Shiffman, & Lawn, 2015).

What is the purpose of couples like Linda and Rob going for preconception counselling? What are the goals of preconception care for this couple? What psychological support can be offered by the nurse to this couple at this stage?

BOX 12.2

RISK FACTORS FOR ADVERSE PREGNANCY OUTCOMES

- **Isotretinoins.** Use of isotretinoins (e.g., Accutane®) in pregnancy to treat acne can result in high risk of congenital malformations which may include craniofacial, cardiac, and central nervous systems injuries. It is contraindicated in pregnancy.
- **Alcohol misuse.** No time during pregnancy is safe to drink alcohol, and harm can occur early, before a person even knows they are pregnant. Fetal alcohol syndrome and other alcohol-related birth defects can be prevented if intake of alcohol ceases before conception.
- **Antiepileptic drugs.** Certain antiepileptic drugs are known teratogens (e.g., valproic acid). Recommendations suggest that before conception, those who are on a regimen of these drugs and who are contemplating pregnancy should be prescribed a lower dosage of these drugs.
- **Diabetes (preconception).** The threefold increase in the prevalence of birth defects among infants born to individuals with type 1 and type 2 diabetes is substantially reduced through proper management of diabetes.
- **Folic acid deficiency.** Daily use of vitamin supplements containing folic acid (400 mcg) has been demonstrated to reduce the occurrence of neural tube defects by two thirds.
- **Hepatitis B.** Vaccination is recommended for anyone who may be at risk for acquiring hepatitis B virus (HBV) infection. Preventing HBV infection in people of childbearing age prevents transmission of infection to infants and eliminates the risk of HBV infection and

sequelae, including hepatic failure, liver carcinoma, cirrhosis, and death.
- **HIV/AIDS.** If HIV infection is identified before conception, timely antiretroviral treatment can be administered, and individuals (or couples) can be given additional information that can help prevent transmission to the child.
- **Rubella seronegativity.** Rubella vaccination provides protective seropositivity and prevents congenital rubella syndrome.
- **Obesity.** Adverse perinatal outcomes associated with obesity include neural tube defects, preterm delivery, diabetes, cesarean section, and hypertensive and thromboembolic disease. Appropriate weight loss and nutritional intake before pregnancy reduce these risks.
- **STIs.** *Chlamydia trachomatis* and *Neisseria gonorrhoeae* have been strongly associated with ectopic pregnancy, infertility, and chronic pelvic pain. STIs during pregnancy might result in fetal death or substantial physical and developmental disabilities, including intellectual disability and blindness. Early screening and treatment prevents these adverse outcomes.
- **Smoking.** Preterm birth, low birth weight, and other adverse perinatal outcomes associated with smoking in pregnancy can be prevented if smoking is stopped before or during early pregnancy. Because only 20% of individuals successfully control tobacco dependency during pregnancy, cessation of smoking is recommended before pregnancy.

Adapted from Centers for Disease Control and Prevention (CDC). (2015a). *Preconception care and health care*. Retrieved from http://www.cdc.gov/preconception/hcp/; March of Dimes. (2015a). *Pregnancy complications*. Retrieved from http://www.marchofdimes.com/pregnancy/pregnancy-complications.aspx; National Institutes of Health (NIH). (2015). *Health problems in pregnancy*. Retrieved from http://www.nlm.nih.gov/medlineplus/healthproblemsinpregnancy.html; and Senie, R. T. (2014). *Epidemiology of women's health*. Burlington, MA: Jones & Bartlett Learning.

Nursing Management

Traditionally, couples have thought that preconception care is a single visit made before getting pregnant; however, the maximum benefits are obtained when an individual and their partner receive care throughout the reproductive years. The nurse's role is vital in identifying risk factors and encouraging healthier behaviours that potentially improve perinatal outcomes. Preconception care involves obtaining a complete health history and physical examination of the individual and their partner. Key areas include:

- Immunization status
- Underlying medical conditions, such as cardiovascular and respiratory problems or genetic disorders
- Reproductive health data, such as pelvic examinations, use of contraceptives, and sexually transmitted infections (STIs)
- Sexuality and sexual practices, such as safer-sex practices and body image issues
- Nutrition history and present status

- Lifestyle practices, including occupation and recreational activities
- Psychosocial issues such as levels of stress and exposure to abuse and violence
- Medication and drug use, including use of tobacco, alcohol, over-the-counter and prescription medications, and illicit drugs
- Support system, including family, friends, and community

Figure 12.1 gives a sample preconception screening tool.

This information provides a foundation for planning health promotion activities and education. For example, to have a positive impact on the pregnancy:

- Ensure that immunizations are up to date.
- Create a reproductive life plan to address and outline their reproductive needs.
- Take a thorough history of both partners to identify any medical or genetic conditions that need treatment or a referral to specialists.

PRECONCEPTION SCREENING AND COUNSELING CHECKLIST

NAME	BIRTHPLACE	AGE

DATE: /   /   ARE YOU PLANNING TO GET PREGNANT IN THE NEXT SIX MONTHS? ___ Y ___N

IF YOUR ANSWER TO A QUESTION IS YES, PUT A CHECK MARK ON THE LINE IN FRONT OF THE QUESTION. FILL IN OTHER INFORMATION THAT APPLIES TO YOU.

DIET AND EXERCISE

What do you consider a healthy weight for you?_____
___Do you eat three meals a day?
___Do you follow a special diet (vegetarian, diabetic, other)?
___Which do you drink (__ coffee __ tea __ cola __ milk __ water __ soda/pop
   other_____)?
___Do you eat raw or undercooked food (meat, other)?
___Do you take folic acid?
___Do you take other vitamins daily (__ multivitamin __ vitamin A __ other)?
___Do you take dietary supplements (__ black cohosh __ pennyroyal __ other)?
___Do you have current/past problems with eating disorders?
___Do you exercise? Type/frequency:_____
Notes:

MEDICATION /DRUGS

___Are you taking prescribed drugs (Accutane, valproic acid, blood thinners)? List
   them_____
___Are you taking non-prescribed drugs?
   List them:_____
___Are you using birth control pills?
___Do you get injectable contraceptives or shots for birth control?
___Do you use any herbal remedies or alternative medicine?
   List:_____
NOTES:

WOMEN'S HEALTH

___Do you have any problems with your menstrual cycle?
___How many times have you been pregnant?
   What was/ were the outcomes(s)?_____
___Did you have difficulty getting pregnant last time?
___Have you been treated for infertility?
   Have you had surgery on your uterus, cervix, ovaries, or tubes?
___Did you mother take the hormone DES during pregnancy?
   Have you ever had HPV, genital warts or chlamydia?
___Have you ever been treated for a sexually transmitted infection (genital herpes,
   gonorrhea, syphilis, HIV/AIDS, other)? List:_____
NOTES:

HOME ENVIRONMENT

___Do you feel emotionally supported at home?
___Do you have help from relatives or friends if needed?
___Do you feel you have serious money/financial worries?
___Are you in a stable relationship?
___Do you feel safe at home?
___Does anyone threaten or physically hurt you?
___Do you have pets (cats, rodents, exotic animals)? List:_____
___Do have any contact with soil, cat litter, or sandboxes?

Baby preparation (if planning pregnancy):
___Do you have a place for a baby to sleep?
___Do you need any baby items?
Notes:

LIFESTYLE

___Do you smoke cigarettes or use other tobacco products?
   How many cigarettes/packs a day?_____
___Are you exposed to second-hand smoke?
___Do you drink alcohol?
   What kind?_____How often?_____How much?_____
___Do you use recreational drugs (cocaine, heroin, ecstasy, meth/ice, other?
   List:_____
___Do you see a dentist regularly?
   What kind of work do you do?_____
___Do you work or live near possible hazards (chemicals, x-ray or other radiation,
   lead)? List:_____
___Do you use saunas or hot tubs?
Notes:

MEDICAL/FAMILY HISTORY

Do you have or have you ever had:
___Epilepsy?
___Diabetes?
___Asthma?
___High blood pressure?
___Heart disease?
___Anemia?
___Kidney or bladder disorders?
___Thyroid disease?
___Chickenpox?
___Hepatitis C?
___Digestive problems?
___Depression or other mental health problem?
___Surgeries?
___Lupus?
___Scleroderma?
___Other conditions?
Have you ever been vaccinated for:
___Measles, mumps, rubella?
___Hepatitis B?
___Chickenpox?
NOTES:

GENETICS

Does your family have a history of   Or   Your partner's family
___Hemophilia?   ___
___Other bleeding disorders?   ___
___Tay-Sachs disease?   ___
___Blood diseases (sickle cell, thalassemia, other)?   ___
___Muscular dystrophy?   ___
___Down syndrome/mental retardation?   ___
___Cystic fibrosis?   ___
___Birth defects (spine/heart/kidney)?   ___
Your ethnic background is:_____
Your partner's ethnic background is: _____
NOTES:

OTHER

IS THERE ANYTHING ELSE YOU'D LIKE ME TO KNOW?

ARE THERE ANY QUESTIONS YOU'D LIKE TO ASK ME?

FIGURE 12.1 Sample preconception screening tool. (© 2019 March of Dimes.)

- Identify history of STIs and high-risk sexual practices so they can be modified.
- Complete a dietary history combined with nutritional counselling.
- Gather information regarding exercise and lifestyle practices to encourage daily exercise for well-being and weight maintenance.
- Stress the importance of taking folic acid to prevent neural tube defects.
- Inform of the benefit to achieving optimal weight before a pregnancy.
- Identify work environment and any needed changes to promote health.
- Address substance use issues, including smoking and drugs.
- Assess risk of intimate partner violence and assist with identifying help and supports if needed.
- Manage chronic conditions such as diabetes and asthma.
- Educate the couple about environmental hazards, including metals and herbs.
- Offer genetic counselling to identify carriers.
- Suggest the availability of support systems, if needed (Hurst & Linton, 2015; Templeton, 2015).

Nurses can act as advocates and educators, creating healthy, supportive communities for individuals and their partners in the childbearing phases of their lives. It is important to enter into a collaborative partnership with the client and their partner, enabling them to examine their own health and its influence on the health of their future baby. Provide information to allow clients to make an informed decision about having a baby, but keep in mind that this decision rests solely with the couple.

Take Note!

Because individuals of reproductive age, from menarche to menopause, benefit from preventive care, preconception care should be an integral part of that continuum (Boggess & Berggren, 2015).

Linda and *Rob* decide to change several aspects of their lifestyle and nutritional habits before conceiving a baby, based on advice from the nurse. They both want to lose weight, stop smoking, and increase their intake of fruits and vegetables. How will these lifestyle and dietary changes benefit the future pregnancy? What other areas might need to be brought up to date to prepare for a future pregnancy?

THE FIRST PRENATAL VISIT

Once a pregnancy is suspected and, in some cases, tentatively confirmed by a home pregnancy test, the individual should seek prenatal care to promote a healthy

outcome. Although the most opportune window (preconception) for improving pregnancy outcomes may be missed, appropriate nursing management starting at conception and continuing throughout the pregnancy can have a positive impact on the health of the patient and their unborn children.

The assessment process begins at this initial prenatal visit and continues throughout the pregnancy. The initial visit is an ideal time to screen for factors that might place the client and the fetus at risk for problems such as preterm delivery. The initial visit also is an optimal time to begin educating the client about expected changes that will affect daily life.

Prenatal care can be delivered in one of two methods: individually or in a group format termed *centering*. The first method is the traditional model whereby a pregnant client sees their health care provider at specified interims throughout the pregnancy and all visits occur on a one-to-one basis. The centering pregnancy model of group prenatal care involves groups of up to a dozen clients in similar gestational ages meeting with their health care provider for 10 sessions of approximately 1.5 to 2 hours each. The centering group method has been theorized to produce better birth outcomes than traditional individually delivered prenatal care due to increased client–provider interaction, increased social support, and greater perceived empowerment (Tracy, 2014). See Evidence-Based Practice 12.1.

The Canadian Diabetes Association recently released updated clinical practice guidelines for diabetes and pregnancy that reaffirmed their 2013 recommendations and continue to support universal screening for all pregnancies (Feig et al., 2018). While there remains a lack of international consensus on the approach to screening and diagnostic criteria for gestational diabetes, the Canadian Diabetes Association Expert Committee recommends the following:

- Clients at high risk of undiagnosed type 2 diabetes, should be screened early (at less than 20 weeks' gestation) to identify those with potentially overt diabetes.
- All pregnant clients without known pre-existing diabetes should be screened for gestational diabetes between 24 and 28 weeks' gestation.
- The preferred approach to screening is with a 2-step approach: with an initial 50-g glucose challenge test, followed by a 75-g oral glucose tolerance test if the results of the initial screening step are abnormal. An alternate 1-step approach could be offered, using just the 75-g oral glucose tolerance test with stricter diagnostic thresholds (Box 12.3) (Feig et al., 2018).

The incidence of gestational diabetes is increasing globally. The Society of Obstetricians and Gynecologists of Canada (SOGC) and the CDA recommend early screening in the first trimester for clients who are at higher risk for developing gestational diabetes, including those who

EVIDENCE-BASED PRACTICE 12.1   **THE EFFECTS OF CENTERING PREGNANCY GROUP PRENATAL CARE ON GESTATIONAL AGE, BIRTH WEIGHT, AND FETAL DEMISE**

STUDY

Although rates of infant mortality in the United States have declined over the last several decades, rates of preterm births (<37 weeks' gestation) and low birth weight (<2,500 g) have increased. Access to quality prenatal care has demonstrated improvement of perinatal outcomes, and may help reduce infant mortality, preterm birth, and low–birth-weight infants. The centering group prenatal care model has been theorized to produce better birth outcomes than traditional individually delivered prenatal care due to increased patient–provider interaction, increased social support, greater perceived empowerment, and increased exposure to useful skills and information about pregnancy, birthing, and childcare.

This study compared birth outcomes for childbearing clients who received two different forms of prenatal care. The objective of this study was to examine the effects of centering prenatal care versus individually delivered prenatal care on gestational age, birth weight, and fetal demise. Samples of 6,155 clients were divided into 2 groups—individual prenatal care and group prenatal care at 5 sites. The sample included clients who received prenatal care at one of five sites that offered both individual and group prenatal care.

Findings

Results indicated that clients in the centering pregnancy group prenatal care, compared with clients in traditional individually delivered prenatal care, had significantly longer gestational ages (b = 0.35, 95% CI [0.29, 0.41]) and higher overall birth weights (b = 28.6, 95% CI [4.8, 52.3]). Results also indicated that group delivered prenatal care was associated with significantly and substantially lower odds of very low birth weight and fetal demise.

Nursing Implications

At present there is support to provide centering group prenatal care where possible according to guidelines. The results indicated largely beneficial effects of group prenatal care on client's birth outcomes. Health policy reforms aimed at reducing adverse birth outcomes may consider group prenatal care a promising alternative format for delivering prenatal care. Nurses should continue to encourage all clients to obtain prenatal care (group or traditional) as part of their reproductive plan to enhance the outcomes of their pregnancy and all of their future children. Given the evidence of beneficial effects of centering group prenatal care and the cost implications of widespread implementation will be critical for informing state and local health policies aimed at improving perinatal health outcomes.

Adapted from Tanner-Smith, E., Steinka-Fry, K., & Lipsey, M. (2014). The effects of centering pregnancy group prenatal care on gestational age, birth weight, and fetal demise. *Maternal & Child Health Journal, 18*(4), 801–809.

are over 35 years old, are overweight (BMI ≥30 kg/m^2), have polycystic ovary syndrome, a history of a previous pregnancy with gestational diabetes, a first-degree relative with diabetes, or are a member of a high-risk population (African Canadian, Arab, Asian, Hispanic, Indigenous, or South Asian). Normoglycemia is the goal in all aspects of pregnancy and offers the benefits of decreased short- and long-term complications, and reduced incidence of diabetes related adverse pregnancy outcomes (Berger, Gagnon, & Dermer, 2016; Feig et al., 2018).

BOX 12.3

THRESHOLDS FOR DIAGNOSIS OF GESTATIONAL DIABETES

The thresholds for the diagnosis of gestational diabetes using the preferred 2-step screening approach are:
- 50-g glucose challenge test: 1-hour plasma glucose ≥ 11.1 mmol/L
- 75-g oral glucose tolerance test: Any one of the following:
  Fasting plasma glucose ≥5.3 mmol/L
  1-hour plasma glucose ≥10.6 mmol/L
  2-hour plasma glucose ≥9.0 mmol/L

Counselling and education of the pregnant client and their partner are critical to ensure healthy perinatal outcomes. Clients frequently have questions, misinformation, or misconceptions about what to eat, weight gain, physical discomforts, drug and alcohol use, sexuality, and the birthing process. The nurse needs to allow time to answer questions and provide anticipatory guidance during the pregnancy and to make appropriate community referrals to meet the individual needs of clients.

Comprehensive Health History

During the initial visit, a comprehensive health history is obtained, including age, menstrual history, prior obstetric history, past medical and surgical history, psychological screening, family history, genetic screening, dietary habits, lifestyle and health practices, medication or drug use, and history of exposure to STIs (Moses, 2015a). Often, use of a prenatal history form (Fig. 12.2) is the best way to document the data collected (Evidence-Based Practice 12.2.).

The initial health history typically includes questions about three major areas: the reason for seeking care; the client's past medical, surgical, and personal history, including that of the family and the partner; and the

(text continues on page 396)

Health History Summary
Maternal/Newborn Record System

Patient's name _____

ID. No. _____

_____

_____

Page 1 of 2

Demographic data

Date of birth _____ Age _____ ☐ N/A

Language ☐ English ☐ _____

Interpreter ☐ None ☐ _____

Religion ☐ _____ Race/ethnicity _____

Marital status S M SEP D W   Name of baby's father _____

Allergy/sensitivity

☐ **None** ☐ **Latex**

☐ Other _____

Primary/referring physician

Education	Occupation	Full	Part	Self	Unemp	Work Tel No	Home Tel No
Patient		☐	☐	☐	☐		
Father of baby		☐	☐	☐	☐		

Menstrual history

	Menarche yrs	Interval days	Length days	Abnormalities ☐ None

Certain ☐ Yes ☐ No

Normal ☐ Yes ☐ No

LMP ___/___/___

Positive pregnancy test ___/___/___

☐ Blood
☐ Urine

EDD

By dates ___/___/___

By ultrasound ___/___/___

Date of ultrasound ___/___/___

Pregnancy history

Gravida	Full term	Premature	Spontaneous Ab	Induced Ab	Ectopic	Multiple births	Live

No	Month/ year	Infant sex	Weight at birth	Wks gest	Hours in labor	Type of delivery	Anesthesia	Comments/complications
1								
2								
3								
4								
5								
6								
7								

Medical history

Check and detail positive findings below. Use reference numbers.

Obstetric   Patient
1. Anemia _____ ☐
2. Fetal/neonatal death or anomaly _____ ☐
3. Gestational diabetes _____ ☐
4. Hemorrhage _____ ☐
5. Hyperemesis _____ ☐
6. Incompetent cervix _____ ☐
7. Intrauterine growth retardation _____ ☐
8. Isoimmunization _____ ☐
9. Polyhydramnios _____ ☐
10. Postpartum depression _____ ☐
11. Pregnancy-induced hypertension _____ ☐
12. Preterm labor or birth _____ ☐
13. PROM-chorioamnionitis _____ ☐
14. Rhogam given _____ ☐
15. RH neg _____ ☐

Gynecologic
16. Contraceptive use _____ ☐
17. Abnormal PAP _____ ☐
18. Fibroids _____ ☐
19. Gyn· surgery _____ ☐

Gynecologic (cont'd.)   Patient
20. Infertility _____ ☐
21. In utero exposure to DES ___ ☐
22. Uterine/cervical anomaly _____ ☐

Sexually transmitted diseases
23. Chlamydia _____ ☐
24. Gonorrhea _____ ☐
25. Herpes (HSV) _____ ☐
26. Syphilis _____ ☐

Vaginal/genital infections
27. Trichomonas _____ ☐
28. Condylomata _____ ☐
29. Candidiasis _____ ☐

Other infections
30. Toxoplasmosis _____ ☐
31. Group B streptococcus _____ ☐
32. Rubella or immunization _____ ☐
33. Varicella or immunization _____ ☐
34. Cytomegalovirus (CMV) _____ ☐
35. AIDS (HIV) _____ ☐
36. Hepatitis (type ___) _____ ☐ or immunization (type ___)

FIGURE 12.2 Sample prenatal history form. (Used with permission. Copyright Briggs Corporation, 2001.)

Health History Summary
Maternal/newborn record system

Page 2 of 2

Patient's name _____

ID. No. _____

_____

_____

Check and detail positive findings below.
Use reference numbers.

Cardiovascular

	Patient	Family
37. Myocardial infarction	☐	☐
38. Heart disease	☐	☐
39. Rheumatic fever	☐	
40. Valve disease	☐	
41. Chronic hypertension	☐	☐
42. Disease of the aorta	☐	☐
43. Varicosities Thrombophlebitis	☐	☐
44. Previous pulmonary embolism	☐	
45. Blood disorders	☐	☐
46. Anemia/ hemoglobinopathy	☐	☐
47. Blood transfusions	☐	
48. Other	☐	

Pulmonary

	Patient	Family
49. Asthma	☐	
50. Tuberculosis	☐	☐
51. Chronic obstructive pulmonary disease	☐	☐

Endocrine

	Patient	Family
52. Diabetes	☐	☐
53. Thyroid dysfunction	☐	☐
54. Maternal PKU	☐	
55. Endocrinopathy	☐	☐
56. Gastrointestinal	☐	
57. Liver disease	☐	

Renal disease

	Patient	Family
58. Cystitis	☐	
59. Pyelonephritis	☐	
60. Asymptomatic bacteriuria	☐	
61. Chronic renal disease	☐	☐
62. Autoimmune disease	☐	☐
63. Cancer	☐	☐

Neurologic disease

	Patient	Family
64. Cerebrovascular accident	☐	☐
65. Seizure disorder	☐	☐
66. Migraine headaches	☐	☐
67. Degenerative disease	☐	☐
68. Other	☐	

Psychological/surgical

	Patient	Family
69. Psychiatric disease Mental illness	☐	☐
70. Physical abuse or neglect	☐	☐
71. Emotional abuse or neglect	☐	☐
72. Addiction (drug, alcohol, nicotine)	☐	☐
73. Major accidents	☐	
74. Surgery	☐	
75. Anesthetic complications	☐	
76. Non-surgical hospitalization	☐	
77. Other	☐	
78. **No known disease/problems**	☐	

Genetic history

	Patient	Father of baby	Family
79. Age 35 or older (female) 50 or older (male)	☐	☐	☐
80. Cerebral palsy	☐	☐	☐
81. Cleft lip/palate	☐	☐	☐
82. Congenital anomalies	☐	☐	☐
83. Congenital heart disease	☐	☐	☐
84. Consanguinity	☐	☐	☐
85. Cystic fibrosis	☐	☐	☐
86. Down's syndrome	☐	☐	☐
87. Hemophilia	☐	☐	☐
88. Huntington's chorea	☐	☐	☐

	Patient	Father of baby	Family
89. Mental retardation	☐	☐	☐
90. Muscular dystrophy	☐	☐	☐
91. Neural tube defect	☐	☐	☐
92. Sickle cell disease or trait	☐	☐	☐
93. Tay-Sachs disease	☐	☐	☐
94. Test for fragile X	☐	☐	☐
95. Thalassemia A or B	☐	☐	☐
96. Other	☐	☐	☐
97. Other	☐	☐	☐
98. Other	☐	☐	☐

Historical risk status   ☐ No risk factors noted
☐ **At risk (identify)**

Signature

FIGURE 12.2 (*continued*)

EVIDENCE-BASED PRACTICE 12.2   **ANTENATAL DIETARY EDUCATION AND SUPPLEMENTATION TO INCREASE ENERGY AND PROTEIN INTAKE**

STUDY

Gestational weight gain is positively associated with fetal growth, and observational studies of food supplementation in pregnancy have reported increases in gestational weight gain and fetal growth. During pregnancy, the fetus develops based on the nutrition of the childbearing person. Inadequate intake during pregnancy can lead to malnutrition and poor outcomes for the fetus. The objective of this study was to assess the effects of education during pregnancy to increase energy and protein intake, or of actual energy and protein supplementation, on energy and protein intake, and the effect on maternal and infant health outcomes.

Findings

The review included 17 randomized controlled trials, involving 9,030 clients. Four main findings included (1) providing nutritional advice resulted in an increase in the clients' protein intake with resulting fewer preterm births and low birth weights; (2) giving clients balanced energy and protein supplements was associated with fewer infants dying during labour and infants had an increase in birth weights; (3) high protein supplementation showed no benefit for childbearing persons and potential harm for the infant with more becoming small for gestational age at birth; and (4) isocaloric protein supplementations showed no benefit for higher birth weight in the infant and weekly gestational gain for the client.

Nursing Implications

This review provides encouraging evidence that prenatal nutritional education with the aim of increasing energy and protein intake in the childbearing population appears to be effective in reducing the risk of preterm birth, low birth weight, increasing head circumference at birth, increasing birth weight among undernourished clients, and increasing protein intake. There remains question about high protein supplementation being beneficial. Nurses can continue to provide good sound evidence-based nutritional education to their pregnant clients to bring about healthy outcomes.

Adapted from Ota, E., Hori, H., Mori, R., Tobe-Gai, R., & Farrar, D. (2015). Antenatal dietary education and supplementation to increase energy and protein intake. *Cochrane Database of Systematic Reviews, 6,* CD000032.

client's reproductive history. During the history-taking process, the nurse and client establish the foundation of a trusting relationship and jointly develop a plan of care for the pregnancy. They tailor this plan to the client's lifestyle as much as possible and focus primarily on education for overall wellness during the pregnancy. The ultimate goal for the first prenatal visit is to collect baseline data about the client and their partner and to detect any risk factors that need to be addressed to facilitate a healthy pregnancy (King et al., 2015).

Reason for Seeking Care

The client commonly comes for prenatal care based on the suspicion of being pregnant. The client may report a missed menstrual period or a positive result on a home pregnancy test. Ask for the date of the last normal menstrual period (LMP). Also ask about any presumptive or probable signs of pregnancy that the client might be experiencing. Typically a urine or blood test to check for evidence of human chorionic gonadotropin (hCG) is done to confirm the pregnancy.

Past History

Ask about past medical and surgical history. This information is important because conditions that the client experienced in the past (e.g., urinary tract infections) may recur or be exacerbated during pregnancy. Also, chronic illnesses, such as diabetes or heart disease, can increase the risk for complications during pregnancy for the individual and the fetus. Ask about any history of allergies to medications, foods, or environmental substances. Ask about any mental health problems, such as depression or anxiety. Gather similar information about the client's family and partner.

The client's personal history also is important. Ask about occupation, possible exposure to teratogens, exercise and activity level, recreational patterns (including the use of substances such as alcohol, tobacco, and drugs), use of alternative and complementary therapies, sleep patterns, nutritional habits, and general lifestyle. Each of these may have an impact on the outcome of the pregnancy. For example, if the client smokes during pregnancy, nicotine in the cigarettes causes vasoconstriction, leading to reduced placental perfusion. As a result, the newborn is at risk of being small for gestational age, and is at risk for nicotine withdrawal after birth. In addition, no safe level of alcohol ingestion in pregnancy has been determined. Many fetuses exposed to heavy alcohol levels during pregnancy develop fetal alcohol syndrome, a collection of deformities and disabilities.

Reproductive History

The client's reproductive history includes a menstrual, obstetric, and gynecologic history. Typically, this history begins with a description of the menstrual cycle, including age at menarche, number of days in the cycle, typical flow characteristics, and any discomfort experienced.

The use of contraception also is important, including when the client last used any contraception.

Establishing an accurate due date is one of the most important assessments, one that has both social and medical significance. For expectant families, this estimated due date (EDD) represents the long-awaited birthday of their child and is a time frame around which many economic and social activities are planned. This end point date provides guidance for the timing of specific prenatal testing, gauges fetal growth parameters, and provides well-established timelines for specific interventions in the management of prenatal complications. In fact, critical decisions, such as preterm labour management, timing of postdate induction of labour, and identification of fetal growth restriction (FGR), are all based on the presumed gestational age of the fetus, which is calculated backward from the EDD (Bond, 2015).

Ask the client the date of the LMP to determine the estimated due date or EDD. Several methods may be used to estimate the date of birth. Nagele's rule can be used to establish the EDD (Box 12.4). Using this rule, subtract 3 months from the month of the LMP and then add 7 days to the first day of the LMP. Then correct the year by adding 1 to it where necessary. An alternative way is to add 7 days and then add 9 months = year where needed. This date has a margin of error of plus or minus 2 weeks. For instance, if the client reports that the LMP was October 14, 2018, you would

---

BOX 12.4

NAGELE RULE FOR CALCULATING THE ESTIMATED DUE DATE (EDD)

1. Use the first day of the last normal menstrual period   10/14/18
2. Subtract 3 from the number of months   7/14/18
3. Add 7 to the number of days   7/21/18
4. Adjust the year by adding one year   7/21/19
5. Estimated due date (+ or – 2 weeks) = July 21st 2019

---

subtract 3 months (July) and add 7 days (21), then add 1 year (2016). The client's EDD is July 21, 2019.

Because of the normal variations in people's menstrual cycles, differences in the normal length of gestation among ethnic groups, and errors in dating methods, there is no such thing as an exact due date. In general, a birth 2 weeks before or 2 weeks after the EDD is considered normal. Nagele's rule is less accurate if the client's menstrual cycles are irregular, if the client conceives while breastfeeding or before the regular menstrual cycle is established after childbirth, if the client is ovulating although amenorrheic, or after discontinuing oral contraceptives (Schuiling & Likis, 2016).

A gestational or birth calculator or wheel can also be used to calculate the due date (Fig. 12.3). Some

FIGURE 12.3 EDD using a birth wheel. The first day of the client's last normal menstrual period was October 1. Using the birth wheel, the EDD would be approximately July 8 of the following year. (Used with permission. Copyright March of Dimes, 2015.)

practitioners use ultrasound to more accurately determine the gestational age and date the pregnancy. Ultrasound is typically the most accurate method of dating a pregnancy.

Typically, an obstetric history provides information about the client's past pregnancies, including any problems encountered during the pregnancy, labour, birth, and postpartum. Such information can provide clues to problems that might develop in the current pregnancy. Some common terms used to describe and document an obstetric history include gravid, gravida, gravida I (primigravida), gravida II (secundigravida), multigravida, and para (Table 12.1).

Other systems may be used to document a client's obstetric history. These systems often break down the category of para more specifically (Box 12.5).

Information about the client's gynecologic history is important. Ask about any reproductive tract surgeries

BOX 12.5

OBSTETRIC HISTORY TERMS: GTPAL OR TPAL

G = gravida, T = term births, P = preterm births, A = abortions, L = living children

- G—the current pregnancy to be included in count
- T—the number of term gestations delivering between 38 and 42 weeks
- P—the number of preterm pregnancies ending >20 weeks or viability but before completion of 37 weeks
- A—the number of pregnancies ending before 20 weeks or viability
- L—the number of children currently living

Consider this example:

Mary Johnson is pregnant for the fourth time. Mary had one abortion at 8 weeks' gestation.

She has a daughter who was born at 40 weeks' gestation and a son born at 34 weeks.

Mary's obstetric history would be documented as follows:

- Using the gravida/para method: gravida 4, para 2
- Using the TPAL method: 1112 (T = 1 [daughter born at 40 weeks]; P = 1 [son born at 34 weeks]; A = 1 [abortion at 8 weeks]; L = 2 [two living children])

TABLE 12.1	PREGNANCY TERMS

Term	Definition
Gravid	The state of being pregnant.
Gravida/ Gravidity	The total number of times a person has been pregnant, regardless of whether the pregnancy resulted in a termination or if multiple infants were born from a pregnancy.
Nulligravida	A person who has never experienced pregnancy.
Primigravida	A person pregnant for the first time.
Secundigravida	A person pregnant for the second time.
Multigravida	A person pregnant for at least the third time.
Para	The number of times a person has given birth to a fetus of at least 20 gestational weeks (viable or not), counting multiple births as one birth event.
Parity	Refers to the number of pregnancies, not the number of fetuses, carried to the point of viability, regardless of the outcome.
Nullipara (para 0)	A person who has not produced a viable offspring.
Primipara	A person who has given birth once after a pregnancy of at least 20 weeks, commonly referred to as a "primip" in clinical practice.
Multipara	A person who has had two or more pregnancies of at least 20 weeks' gestation resulting in viable offspring. Commonly referred to as a "multip."

the client has undergone. For example, surgery on the uterus may affect its ability to contract effectively during labour. A history of tubal pregnancy increases the risk for another tubal pregnancy. Also ask about safe-sex practices and any history of STIs.

Physical Examination

The next step in the assessment process is the physical examination. While not every aspect of the physical exam outlined is required specifically for the first prenatal visit, this provides an optimal opportunity for a thorough exam for the otherwise healthy childbearing person who may not commonly have reason to access health care, and to detect any unknown physical problems that have the potential to affect the pregnancy outcome. The initial physical examination also provides a baseline for evaluating changes during future visits.

Preparation

Instruct the client to undress and put on a gown. Transgendered people have all the same preventative health care needs as others and care that is congruent with the person's anatomy should be provided in a culturally safe way that is respectful of their gender identity (PHAC, 2017a). Ask the client to empty their bladder and, in doing so, to collect a urine specimen. Typically, this specimen is a clean-catch urine specimen that is sent to the laboratory for a urinalysis to detect a possible urinary tract infection. It is further recommended that all childbearing persons are screened for the presence of proteinuria and possible pre-existing renal disease in early pregnancy (Magee, Pels, Helewa, Rey, & von Dadelszen, 2014).

Begin the physical examination by obtaining vital signs, including blood pressure, respiratory rate, temperature, and pulse. Also measure the client's height and weight. Abnormalities such as an elevated blood pressure may suggest pregestational hypertension, requiring further evaluation. Abnormalities in pulse rate and respiration require further investigation for possible cardiac or respiratory disease. If the client weighs less than 100 lb or more than 200 lb or there has been a sudden weight gain, report these findings to the primary care provider; medical treatment or nutritional counselling may be necessary.

Head-to-Toe Assessment

A complete head-to-toe assessment is usually performed by the health care provider. Each body system is assessed. Some of the major areas are discussed here. Throughout the assessment, be sure to drape the client appropriately to ensure privacy and prevent chilling.

HEAD AND NECK

Assess the head and neck area for any previous injuries and sequelae. Evaluate for any limitations in range of motion. Palpate for any enlarged lymph nodes or swelling. Note any edema of the nasal mucosa or hypertrophy of gingival tissue in the mouth; these are typical responses to increased estrogen levels in pregnancy. Palpate the thyroid gland for enlargement. Slight enlargement is normal, but marked enlargement may indicate hyperthyroidism, requiring further investigation.

CHEST

Auscultate heart sounds, noting any abnormalities. A soft systolic murmur caused by the increase in blood volume may be noted. Anticipate an increase in heart rate by 10 to 15 beats per minute (bpm) (starting between 14 and 20 weeks of pregnancy) secondary to increases in cardiac output and blood volume. The body adapts to the increase in blood volume with peripheral dilation to maintain blood pressure. Progesterone causes peripheral dilation.

Auscultate the chest for breath sounds, which should be clear. Also note symmetry of chest movement and thoracic breathing patterns. Estrogen promotes relaxation of the ligaments and joints of the ribs, with a resulting increase in the anteroposterior chest diameter. Expect a slight increase in respiratory rate to accommodate the increase in tidal volume and oxygen consumption.

After obtaining the client's permission, inspect and palpate the breast tissue and nipples for symmetry and colour.

Increases in estrogen and progesterone and blood supply make the breasts feel full and more nodular, with increased sensitivity to touch. Blood vessels become more visible and there is an increase in breast size. Striae gravidarum (stretch marks) may be visible in a client with large breasts. Darker pigmentation of the nipple and areola is present, along with enlargement of Montgomery glands. Colostrum (yellowish secretion that precedes mature breast milk) is excreted typically in the third trimester.

 Take Note!

Use this opportunity to reinforce and teach breast self-examination if the client has a high-risk history.

ABDOMEN

The appearance of the abdomen depends on the number of weeks of gestation. The abdomen enlarges progressively as the fetus grows. Inspect the abdomen for striae, scars, shape, and size. Inspection may reveal striae gravidarum (stretch marks) and **linea nigra,** a thin brownish black pigmented line running from the umbilicus to the symphysis pubis, depending on the duration of the pregnancy. Palpate the abdomen, which should be rounded and nontender. A decrease in muscle tone may be noted due to the influence of progesterone.

Typically, the height of the fundus is measured when the uterus arises out of the pelvis to evaluate fetal growth. At 12 weeks' gestation the fundus can be palpated at the symphysis pubis. At 16 weeks' gestation the fundus is midway between the symphysis and the umbilicus. At 20 weeks the fundus can be palpated at the umbilicus and measures approximately 20 cm from the symphysis pubis. By 36 weeks the fundus is just below the xiphoid process and measures approximately 36 cm. The uterus maintains a globular/ovoid shape throughout pregnancy (Bope & Kellerman, 2015).

EXTREMITIES

Inspect and palpate both legs for dependent edema, pulses, and varicose veins. If edema is present in early pregnancy, further evaluation may be needed to rule out gestational hypertension. During the third trimester, dependent edema is a normal finding. Ask the client if they have any pain in the calves that increases when ambulating. This might indicate a deep vein thrombosis (DVT). High levels of estrogen during pregnancy increase the risk for DVT.

Pelvic Examination

The pelvic examination provides information about the internal and external reproductive organs. In addition, it aids in assessing some of the presumptive and probable signs of pregnancy and allows for determination of pelvic adequacy. Note that a pelvic examination can be both physically and emotionally uncomfortable for some clients, particularly those who have a history of sexual abuse, which may or may not have been revealed during the Past Health History data collection. After a client has consented to a pelvic examination, remain in the examining room to assist the health care provider with any specimen collection, fixation, and labelling. Also provide comfort and emotional support for the client, who might be anxious. Throughout the examination, offer anticipatory education, explaining what will happen and why, and answer any questions as necessary.

EXTERNAL GENITALIA

After the client settles in the lithotomy position and is draped appropriately, the external genitalia are inspected visually. They should be free from lesions, discharge, hematomas, varicosities, and inflammation upon inspection. A culture for STIs may be collected at this time.

INTERNAL GENITALIA

Next, the internal genitalia are examined via a speculum. The cervix should be smooth, long, thick, and closed. Because of increased pelvic congestion, the cervix will be softened (Goodell sign), the uterine isthmus will be softened (Hegar sign), and there will be a bluish colouration of the cervix and vaginal mucosa (Chadwick sign).

The uterus typically is pear shaped and mobile, with a smooth surface. It will undergo cell hypertrophy and hyperplasia so that it enlarges throughout the pregnancy to accommodate the growing fetus.

During the pelvic examination, a Papanicolaou (Pap) smear may be obtained. Additional cultures, such as for gonorrhea and chlamydia screening, also may be obtained. Ensure that all specimens obtained are labelled correctly and sent to the laboratory for evaluation. A

rectal examination is done last to assess for lesions, masses, prolapse, or hemorrhoids.

Once the examination of the internal genitalia is completed and the speculum is removed, a bimanual examination is performed to estimate the size of the uterus to confirm dates and to palpate the ovaries. The ovaries should be small and nontender, without masses. At the conclusion of the bimanual examination, the health care provider reinserts the index finger into the vagina and the middle finger into the rectum to assess the strength and regularity of the posterior vaginal wall.

PELVIC SIZE, SHAPE, AND MEASUREMENTS

The size and shape of the pelvis can affect the ability to give birth vaginally. Pelvic shape is typically classified as one of four types: gynecoid, android, anthropoid, and platypelloid. Refer to Chapter 13 for an in-depth discussion of pelvic size and shape.

Taking internal pelvic measurements determines the actual diameters of the inlet and outlet through which the fetus will pass. This is extremely important if the client has never given birth vaginally. Taking pelvic measurements is unnecessary for the client who has given birth vaginally before (unless they have experienced some type of trauma to the area) because vaginal delivery demonstrates that the pelvis is adequate for the passage of the fetus.

Three measurements are assessed: diagonal conjugate, true conjugate, and ischial tuberosity (Fig. 12.4). The diagonal conjugate is the distance between the anterior surface of the sacral prominence and the anterior surface of the inferior margin of the symphysis pubis (Bope & Kellerman, 2015). This measurement, usually 12.5 cm or greater, represents the anteroposterior diameter of the

A **B**

FIGURE 12.4 Pelvic measurements. **A.** Diagonal conjugate (*solid line*) and true conjugate (*dotted line*). **B.** Ischial tuberosity diameter.

pelvic inlet through which the fetal head passes first. The diagonal conjugate is the most useful measurement for estimating pelvic size because a misfit with the fetal head occurs if it is too small.

The true conjugate, also called the obstetric conjugate, is the measurement from the anterior surface of the sacral prominence to the posterior surface of the inferior margin of the symphysis pubis. This diameter cannot be measured directly; rather, it is estimated by subtracting 1 to 2 cm from the diagonal conjugate measurement. The average true conjugate diameter is at least 11.5 cm (Cunningham et al., 2014). This measurement is important because it is the smallest front-to-back diameter through which the fetal head must pass when moving through the pelvic inlet.

The ischial tuberosity diameter is the transverse diameter of the pelvic outlet. This measurement is made outside the pelvis at the lowest aspect of the ischial tuberosities. A diameter of 10.5 cm or more is considered adequate for passage of the fetal head (Tharpe, Farley, & Jordan, 2016).

Laboratory Tests

A series of tests is generally ordered during the initial visit so that baseline data can be obtained, allowing for early detection and prompt intervention if any problems occur. Tests that are generally conducted for all pregnancies include urinalysis and blood studies. The urine is analyzed for albumin, glucose, ketones, and bacteria casts. Blood studies usually include a complete blood count (hemoglobin, hematocrit, red and white blood cell counts, and platelets), blood typing and Rh factor, glucose screening for high-risk clients, a rubella titer, hepatitis B surface antibody antigen, HIV, venereal disease research laboratory (VDRL) or rapid plasma reagin (RPR) tests, and cervical smears to detect STIs (Common Laboratory and Diagnostic Tests 12.1).

The need for additional laboratory studies is determined by a client's history, physical examination findings, current health status, and risk factors identified in the initial interview. Additional tests can be offered (e.g., screening for genetic diseases, blood lead screening,

COMMON LABORATORY AND DIAGNOSTIC TESTS 12.1

Test	Explanation
Complete blood cell count (CBC)	Evaluates hemoglobin (120 to 160 g/L) and hematocrit (0.37 to 0.47) levels and red blood cell count (4.2 to 5.4 x 10^{12}/L) to detect presence of anemia; identifies white blood cell level (3.5 to 12.0 x 10^9/L), which if elevated may indicate an infection; determines platelet count (150 to 400 x 10^9/L) to assess clotting ability
Blood typing	Determines client's blood type and Rh status to rule out any blood incompatibility issues early; Rh-negative client would likely receive RhoGAM (at 28 weeks' gestation) and again within 72 hours after childbirth, if Rh sensitive
Rubella titer	Detects antibodies for the virus that causes German measles; if titer is 1:8 or less, the client is not immune; requires immunization after birth; and client is advised to avoid people with undiagnosed rashes
Hepatitis B	Determines if the client has hepatitis B by detecting presence of hepatitis antibody surface antigen (HbsAg) in the blood
HIV testing	Detects HIV antibodies and if positive requires more specific testing, counselling, and treatment during pregnancy with antiretroviral medications to prevent transmission to fetus
STI screening: Venereal Disease Research Laboratory (VDRL) or rapid plasma reagin (RPR) serologic tests or by cervical smears, cultures, or visual identification of suspicious lesions	Detects STIs (such as syphilis, herpes, HPV, gonorrhea) so that treatment can be initiated early to prevent transmission to fetus
Cervical smears	Detects abnormalities such as cervical cancer (Pap test) or infections such as gonorrhea, chlamydia, or group B streptococcus so that treatment can be initiated if positive

Adapted from Fischbach, F., & Dunning, M. B. (2014). *A manual of laboratory and diagnostic tests* (9th ed.). Philadelphia, PA: Lippincott Williams & Wilkins; Ferri, F. F. (2014). *Ferri's best test: A practical guide to laboratory medicine and diagnostic imaging* (3rd ed.). Philadelphia, PA: Elsevier Health Sciences; and Royal College of Physicians and Surgeons of Canada. (2015). *Clinical laboratory tests—Reference Values*. Retrieved from http://www.royalcollege.ca/portal/page/portal/rc/common/documents/exams/examiners/clinical_lab_tests_reference_values_e.pdf rubeola, and so on), but ultimately the client and their partner make the decision about undergoing them. Educate the client and partner about the tests, including the rationale. In addition, support the client and their partner in their decision-making process, regardless of whether you agree with the couple's decision. The couple's decisions about their health care are based on the ethical principle of autonomy, which allows an individual the right to make decisions about their own body.

> **Remember Linda and Rob, the couple who want to start a family? Ten months after the preconception appointment, Linda calls to make a first prenatal appointment. What key areas will be addressed at this first prenatal visit? What interventions might be suggested for Linda to implement in order to ensure a healthy newborn? What emotional support might be needed by Linda at this time in her first trimester of pregnancy?**

FOLLOW-UP VISITS

Continuous prenatal care is important for a successful pregnancy outcome. The recommended follow-up visit schedule for a healthy client who is pregnant is as follows:

- Every 4 weeks up to 28 weeks (7 months)
- Every 2 weeks from 29 to 36 weeks
- Every week from 37 weeks to birth

At each subsequent prenatal visit the following assessments are completed:

- Weight and blood pressure, which are compared with baseline values
- Urine testing for protein, glucose, ketones, and nitrites, if indicated
- Fundal height measurement to assess fetal growth
- Assessment for quickening/fetal movement to determine fetal well-being
- Assessment of fetal heart rate (should be 110 to 160 bpm)

At each follow-up visit answer questions, provide anticipatory guidance and education, review nutritional guidelines, and evaluate the client for adherence to prenatal vitamin therapy. Throughout the pregnancy, encourage the client's partner to participate if possible.

Follow-Up Visit Intervals and Assessments

Up to 28 weeks' gestation, follow-up visits involve assessment of the client's blood pressure and weight. The urine is tested for protein and glucose, if indicated based on existing diabetes or kidney disease, or the presence of

new concerning symptoms that may indicate the development of preeclampsia (Magee et al., 2014). Fundal height and fetal heart rate are assessed at every office visit.

The best procedure for screening and diagnosing gestational diabetes remains controversial. All strategies involve an oral glucose test, but there remains disagreement about how many grams of glucose (50, 75, or 100) the client ingests and how long afterward the blood sample is drawn. A recent *Cochrane Review* concluded that there was insufficient evidence to permit assessment of which is the best method to use to identify clients who have gestational diabetes (Farrar, Duley, Medley, & Lawlor, 2015). Screening for gestational diabetes is best done between 24 and 28 weeks' gestation, unless screening is warranted in the first trimester for those identified to be at high-risk. Using the CDA preferred screening method, a blood glucose level is obtained using an oral 50-g glucose control test followed by a 1-hour plasma glucose determination. If the result is ≥11.1 mmol/L, a diagnosis of gestational diabetes can be made. If the result is between 7.8 and 11.0 mmol/L, further testing with a 2-hour 75-g oral glucose tolerance test, is warranted to determine whether gestational diabetes is present (Feig et al., 2018). Because insulin resistance increases as pregnancy advances, testing at this gestational point yields a higher rate of abnormal test results.

During this time, review the common discomforts of pregnancy, evaluate any client complaints, and answer questions. Reinforce the importance of good nutrition and use of prenatal vitamins, along with daily exercise.

Between 29 and 36 weeks' gestation, all the assessments of previous visits are completed, along with assessment for edema. Special attention is focused on the presence and location of edema during the last trimester. Pregnant clients commonly experience dependent edema of the lower extremities from constriction of blood vessels secondary to the heavy gravid uterus. Periorbital edema around the eyes, edema of the hands, and pretibial edema (edema on the front, or shin part of the leg) are abnormal and could be signs of gestational hypertension. Inspecting and palpating both extremities, listening for complaints of tight rings on fingers, and observing for swelling around the eyes are important assessments. Abnormal findings in any of these areas need to be reported.

If the client is Rh negative, their antibody titer is evaluated. RhoGAM is given if indicated. RhoGAM is used to prevent development of antibodies to Rh-positive red cells whenever fetal cells are known or suspected of entering the maternal circulation such as after a spontaneous abortion or amniocentesis. It is also recommended for prophylaxis at 28 weeks' gestation and following birth if the infant is Rh positive (King et al., 2015). The client also is evaluated for risk of preterm labour. At each visit, ask if they are experiencing any common signs or symptoms of preterm labour (e.g., uterine contractions, dull backache, feeling of pressure in the pelvic area or thighs, increased vaginal discharge, menstrual-like cramps, vaginal bleeding). If the client has had a previous preterm birth, they are at risk for another and close monitoring is warranted. An initial preterm labour evaluation if the client reports signs and symptoms of preterm labour includes review of prenatal record for risk factors, evaluation of reported symptoms, physical examination (uterine contractions, vital signs, fetal heart rate, pelvic examination for cervical dilation and effacement assessment, and status of fetal membranes), and a urine culture to diagnose asymptomatic bacteriuria (Jordan, Engstrom, Marfell, & Farley, 2014). If positive for preterm labour, the client may require enhanced observation and monitoring and medications to stop contractions may be in order.

Counsel the client about choosing a health care provider for the newborn, if one has not yet been selected. The nurse should allow the opportunity to discuss the client's values and ideas about infant feeding, and provide education about the benefits of breastfeeding so that the client is able to make an informed decision for feeding their baby. The nurse can refer the client to *Nursing Mothers* and *La Leche League* websites for further information to assist in making that decision. Reinforce the importance of daily fetal movement monitoring as an indicator of fetal well-being. Reevaluate hemoglobin and hematocrit levels to assess for anemia.

Between 37 and 40 weeks' gestation, the same assessments are done as for the previous weeks. In addition, screening for group B streptococcus is required, and gonorrhea and chlamydia screening may be done or repeated at this time. Fetal presentation and position (via Leopold manoeuvres) are assessed. Review the signs and symptoms of labour and forward a copy of the prenatal record to the hospital labour and birthing unit for future reference. Review the client's desire for family planning after birth as well as their decision to breastfeed or bottle feed. Remind the client that an infant car seat is required by law and must be used to drive the newborn home from the hospital or birthing centre.

Fundal Height Measurement

Fundal height is the distance (in centimetres) measured with a tape measure from the top of the pubic bone to the top of the uterus (fundus) with the client lying on their back with knees slightly flexed (Fig. 12.5). Measurement in this way is termed the McDonald method. Fundal height typically increases as the pregnancy progresses; it reflects fetal growth and provides a gross estimate of the duration of the pregnancy.

Between 12 and 14 weeks' gestation, the fundus can be palpated above the symphysis pubis. The fundus reaches the level of the umbilicus at approximately

FIGURE 12.5 **Fundal height measurement.**

20 weeks and measures 20 cm. Fundal measurement should approximately equal the number of weeks of gestation until week 36. For example, a fundal height of 24 cm suggests a fetus at 24 weeks' gestation. After 36 weeks, the fundal height then drops due to lightening and may no longer correspond with the week of gestation.

It is expected that the fundal height will increase progressively throughout the pregnancy, reflecting fetal growth. However, if the growth curve flattens or stays stable, it may indicate the presence of FGR. If the fundal height measurement is greater than 4 cm from the estimated gestational age, further evaluation is warranted if a multifetal gestation has not been diagnosed or hydramnios has not been ruled out (Weber & Kelley, 2014).

Fetal Movement Determination

Perception of fetal movement typically begins in the second trimester, and occurs earlier in multiparous verses nulliparous clients. The client's first perception of fetal movement, termed "quickening," is commonly described as a gentle fluttering. This perceived fetal movement is most often related to trunk and limb motion and rollovers, or flips (Moses, 2015b). Perception of fetal movement is an important screening method for fetal well-being, because decreased fetal movement is associated with a range of pregnancy pathologies and poor pregnancy outcomes. Decreased fetal movement may indicate asphyxia and FGR. If compromised, the fetus decreases its oxygen requirements by decreasing activity. Reduced fetal movement is thought to represent fetal compensation in a chronic hypoxic environment due to inadequacies in the placental supply of oxygen and nutrients (Fretts, 2014). A decrease in fetal movement may also be related to other factors as well, such as client use of central nervous system depressants, fetal sleep cycles, hydrocephalus, bilateral renal agenesis, stillbirth, placental dysfunction, and bilateral hip dislocation (Heazell, 2015).

Fetal movement counting is a method used by the client to quantify the fetus's movement. However, the optimal number of movements and the ideal duration of counting them remain controversial. Many variations for determining fetal movement, also called fetal movement counts, have been developed, but the one most common method is described as follows. Determining fetal movement is a noninvasive method of screening and can be easily taught to all pregnant clients. Any technique used requires client participation and cooperation.

Instruct the client about how to count fetal movements, the reasons for doing so, and the significance of decreased fetal movements. Urge the client to perform the counts in a relaxed environment and a comfortable position, such as semi-Fowler's or side-lying. Provide the client with detailed information concerning fetal movement counts and stress the need for consistency in monitoring (at approximately the same time each day) and the importance of informing the health care provider promptly of any reduced movements. Providing clients with "fetal kick count" charts to record movement helps promote adherence to your instructions. No values for fetal movement have been established that indicate fetal well-being, so the client needs to be aware of a decrease in the number of movements when last assessed. The most common method used is "Count to 10," whereby the client focuses attention on the fetus's movement and records how long it takes to document 10 movements. If it takes longer than 2 hours, the client should contact their health care provider for further evaluation. Fetal kick counting in current prenatal care appears to be underutilized and nurses need to educate clients about this assessment in their pregnancy care.

Fetal Heart Rate Measurement

Fetal heart rate measurement is integral to fetal surveillance throughout the pregnancy. Auscultating the fetal heart rate with a handheld Doppler at each prenatal visit helps confirm that the intrauterine environment is still supportive to the growing fetus. The purpose of assessing fetal heart rate is to determine rate and rhythm. The normal fetal heart rate range is 110 to 160 bpm. Nursing Procedure 12.1 lists the steps in measuring fetal heart rate.

Teaching About the Danger Signs of Pregnancy

It is important to educate the client about danger signs during pregnancy that require further evaluation. Explain that they should contact their health care provider immediately if experiencing any of the following:
- *During the first trimester:* spotting or bleeding (miscarriage), painful urination (infection), severe persistent vomiting (hyperemesis gravidarum), fever >37.5°C (infection), and lower abdominal pain with dizziness

NURSING PROCEDURE 12.1

Measuring Fetal Heart Rate

Purpose: To assess fetal well-being

1. Assist the client onto the examining table and have them lie down.
2. Cover the client with a sheet to ensure privacy, and then expose the abdomen.
3. Palpate the abdomen to determine the fetal lie, position, and presentation.
4. Locate the back of the fetus (the ideal position to hear the heart rate).
5. Apply lubricant gel to abdomen in the area where the back has been located.
6. Turn on the handheld Doppler device and place it on the spot over the fetal back.
7. Listen for the sound of the amplified heart rate, moving the device slightly from side to side as necessary to obtain the loudest sound. Assess the client's pulse rate and compare it to the amplified sound. If the rates appear the same, reposition the Doppler device.
8. Once the fetal heart rate has been identified, count the number of beats in 1 minute and record the results.
9. Remove the Doppler device and wipe off any remaining gel from the client's abdomen and the device.
10. Record the heart rate on the client's medical record; normal range is 110 to 160 bpm.
11. Provide information to the client regarding fetal well-being based on findings.

and accompanied by shoulder pain (ruptured ectopic pregnancy).
- *During the second trimester:* regular uterine contractions (preterm labour); pain in calf, often increased with foot flexion (blood clot in deep vein); sudden gush or leakage of fluid from vagina (premature rupture of membranes); and absence of fetal movement for more than 12 hours (possible fetal distress or demise).
- *During the third trimester:* sudden weight gain; periorbital or facial edema, severe upper abdominal pain, or headache with visual changes (gestational hypertension and/or preeclampsia); and a decrease in fetal daily movement for more than 24 hours (possible demise). Any of the previous warning signs and symptoms can also be present in this last trimester (March of Dimes, 2015a).

Early Contractions

One of the warning signs that should be emphasized is early contractions, which can lead to preterm birth. The client should not confuse these early preterm contractions with Braxton Hicks contractions, which are not true labour pains because they go away when walking around or resting. They often go away when the client goes to sleep. Braxton Hicks contractions are usually felt in the abdomen versus in the lower back with true preterm labour contractions. Signs of preterm labour that a client may experience include contractions every 10 minutes or more frequently, change in vaginal discharge, pelvic pressure, low, dull backache, pelvic cramps, and diarrhea (Nagtalon-Ramos, 2014).

All childbearing clients need to be able to recognize early signs of contractions to prevent preterm labour. Worldwide, 15 million infants are born too soon each year (March of Dimes, 2015b). These preterm infants (born at less than 37 weeks' gestation) can suffer lifelong health consequences such as intellectual disability, chronic lung disease, cerebral palsy, seizure disorders, and blindness (March of Dimes, 2015c). Preterm labour can happen in any pregnancy, at any time. In many cases, it can be stopped with medications if it is recognized early, before significant cervical dilation has taken place. If the client experiences menstrual-like cramps occurring every 10 minutes accompanied by a low, dull backache, they should stop what they are doing and lie down on the left side for 1 hour and drink two or three glasses of water. If the symptoms worsen or do not subside after 1 hour, the client should contact their health care provider.

ASSESSMENT OF FETAL WELL-BEING

During the antepartum period, several tests are performed routinely to monitor fetal well-being and to detect possible problems. When a high-risk pregnancy is identified, additional antepartum testing can be initiated to promote positive perinatal outcomes. **High-risk pregnancies** include those that are complicated by maternal or fetal conditions (coincidental with or unique to pregnancy) that jeopardize the health status of the client and put the fetus at risk for uteroplacental insufficiency, hypoxia, and death (CDC, 2015d). However, additional antepartum fetal testing should take place only when the results obtained will guide future care, whether it is reassurance, more frequent testing, admission to the hospital, or the need for immediate delivery (Brown, 2015).

Ultrasonography

Since its introduction in the late 1950s, ultrasonography has become a very useful diagnostic tool in obstetrics. Real-time scanners can produce a continuous picture of the fetus on a monitor screen. A transducer that emits high-frequency sound waves is placed on the client's abdomen and moved to visualize the fetus (Fig. 12.6). The fetal heartbeat and any malformations in the fetus can be assessed and measurements can be made accurately from the picture on the monitor screen.

Obstetric ultrasound is a standard component of prenatal care used to identify pregnancy complications and to establish an accurate gestational age in order to improve pregnancy outcomes. Because the ultrasound procedure is noninvasive, it is a safe, but not evidence-based practice for low-risk clients, accurate, and cost-effective tool. It provides important information about fetal activity, growth, and gestational age; assesses fetal well-being; and determines the need for invasive intrauterine tests (Maeda, 2015).

There are no hard-and-fast rules as to the number of ultrasounds a client should have during pregnancy. A low-risk client does not necessarily require any, but most practices do them as part of their prenatal care routine. Currently, the SOGC recommends that all childbearing persons be offered a first trimester dating ultrasound

FIGURE 12.6 Ultrasound. **A.** Ultrasound device being applied to client's abdomen. **B.** View of monitor.

between 8 and 12 weeks' gestation (Butt & Lim, 2014). A transvaginal ultrasound may be performed in the first trimester to confirm pregnancy, exclude ectopic (in which a fertilized egg implants somewhere other than the main cavity of the uterus) or molar (hydatidiform mole, a benign tumour that develops in the uterus) pregnancies, and confirm cardiac pulsation. An anatomy scan is recommended at about 18 to 20 weeks to look for congenital malformations, exclude multifetal pregnancies, and verify dates and growth. Additional ultrasound scans may be indicated to further evaluate fetal growth, assess fetal positioning, and verify placental position (Everett & Peebles, 2015). An ultrasound is used to confirm placental location during amniocentesis and to provide visualization during chorionic villus sampling. An ultrasound is also ordered whenever an abnormality is suspected.

During the past several years, ultrasound technology has advanced significantly. Now available for expecting parents is 3D/4D ultrasound imaging. Unlike traditional 2D imaging, which takes a look at the developing fetus from one angle (thus creating the "flat" image), three-dimensional (3D) imaging takes a view of the fetus from three different angles. Software then takes these three images and merges them to produce a 3D image. Because the fourth dimension is time and movement, with 4D parents are able to watch the live movements of their fetus in 3D.

Nursing management during the ultrasound procedure focuses on educating the client about the ultrasound test and reassuring that there will not be any experience of sensation from the sound waves during the test. No special client preparation is needed before performing the ultrasound, although in early pregnancy the client may need to have a full bladder. Inform them that they may experience some discomfort from the pressure on the full bladder during the scan, but it will last only a short time. Tell the client that the conducting gel used on the abdomen during the scan may feel cold initially.

Doppler Flow Studies

Comprehensive assessment of fetal well-being involves monitoring of fetal growth, placental function, central venous pressure, and cardiac function. Ultrasound evaluation of the fetus using 2D, colour Doppler, and pulse-wave Doppler techniques forms the foundation of prenatal diagnosis of structural anomalies, rhythm abnormalities, and altered fetal circulation (Pruetz, Votava-Smith, & Miller, 2015). Doppler flow studies can be used to measure the velocity of blood flow via ultrasound. Doppler flow studies can detect fetal compromise in high-risk pregnancies. The test is noninvasive and has no contraindications. The colour images produced help to identify abnormalities in diastolic flow within the

umbilical vessels. The velocity of the fetal red blood cells can be determined by measuring the change in the frequency of the sound wave reflected off the cells. Thus, Doppler flow studies can detect the movement of red blood cells in vessels (Everett & Peebles, 2015). In pregnancies complicated by hypertension or FGRs diastolic blood flow may be absent or even reversed (Alfirevic, Stampalija, & Medley, 2015). Doppler flow studies also can be used to evaluate the blood flow through other fetal blood vessels, such as the aorta and those in the brain. Research continues to determine the indications for Doppler flow studies to improve pregnancy outcomes. Nursing management of the client undergoing Doppler flow studies is similar to that described for an ultrasound.

Alpha-Fetoprotein Analysis

Alpha-fetoprotein (AFP) is a glycoprotein produced initially by the yolk sac and fetal gut, and later predominantly by the fetal liver. In a fetus, the serum AFP level increases until approximately 14 to 15 weeks, and then falls progressively. In normal pregnancies, AFP from fetal serum enters the amniotic fluid (in microgram quantities) through fetal urination, fetal gastrointestinal secretions, and transudation across fetal membranes (amnion and placenta). About 30 years ago, elevated levels of maternal serum AFP (MSAFP) or amniotic fluid AFP were first linked to the occurrence of fetal neural tube defects. This biomarker screening test is now recommended for all pregnancies along with other prenatal screening tests depending on risk profile (Alexander, LaRosa, Bader, & Garfield, 2014; American College of Obstetricians and Gynecologists [ACOG], 2015b).

AFP is present in amniotic fluid in low concentrations between 10 and 14 weeks' gestation and can be detected in maternal serum beginning at approximately 12 to 14 weeks' gestation (Callahan, 2016). If a developmental defect is present, such as failure of the neural tube to close, more AFP escapes into amniotic fluid from the fetus. AFP then enters the client circulation by crossing the placenta, and the level in the client's serum can be measured. The optimal time for AFP screening is 16 to 18 weeks' gestation. Correct information about gestational dating, maternal weight, race, number of fetuses, and insulin dependency is necessary to ensure the accuracy of this screening test. If incorrect information is submitted or the blood specimen is not drawn during the appropriate time frame, false-positive results may occur, increasing the client's anxiety. Subsequently, further testing might be ordered based on an inaccurate interpretation, resulting in additional emotional stress to the client and family.

A variety of situations can lead to elevation of MSAFP, including open neural tube defect, underestimation of gestational age, the presence of multiple fetuses, gastrointestinal defects, low birth weight, oligohydramnios, maternal age, diabetes, and decreased maternal weight (King et al., 2015). Lower-than-expected MSAFP levels are seen when fetal gestational age is overestimated or in cases of fetal death, hydatidiform mole, increased maternal weight, maternal type 1 diabetes, and fetal trisomy 21 (Down syndrome) or trisomy 18 (Edwards syndrome) (Khalil & Coates, 2015).

Measurement of MSAFP is minimally invasive, requiring only a venipuncture for a blood sample. AFP has now been combined with other biomarker screening tests to determine the risk of neural tube defects and Down syndrome.

Nursing management for AFP testing consists of preparing the client for this screening test by gathering accurate information about the date of the LMP, weight, race, and gestational dating. Accurately determining the window of 16 to 18 weeks' gestation will help to ensure that the test results are correct. Also explain that the test involves obtaining a blood specimen.

Marker Screening Tests

Using maternal serum is an effective, noninvasive method for identifying fetal risk for aneuploidy (trisomies 13, 18, and 21) and neural tube defects. Prenatal screening for Down syndrome in the early second trimester with multiple maternal serum markers has been available for more than 15 years. Abnormalities in maternal serum marker levels and fetal measurements obtained during the first trimester screening can be markers for not only certain chromosomal disorders and anomalies in the fetus, but also for specific pregnancy complications. Pregnancy-associated plasma protein A (PAPP-A) is a key regulator of insulin-like growth factor essential for normal fetal development. In the client's blood, this protein increases with gestational age. It is routinely used for Down syndrome screening in the first trimester. A low maternal serum PAPP-A, at 11 to 13 weeks' gestation, is associated with stillbirth, infant death, preterm birth, preeclampsia, and chromosomal abnormalities (Kalousova, Muravska, & Zima, 2014; Patil, Panchanadikar, & Wagh, 2014). Multiple blood screening tests may be used to determine the risk of open neural tube defects and Down syndrome: the triple-marker screen (AFP, hCG, and unconjugated estriol) or the quad screen, which includes the triple screening tests with the addition of a fourth marker, inhibin A (glycoprotein secreted by the placenta). The quad screen is used to enhance the accuracy of screening for Down syndrome in clients younger than 35 years of age. Low inhibin A levels indicate the possibility of Down syndrome (ACOG, 2015b). These biomarkers are merely screening tests and identify clients who need further definitive procedures (i.e., ultrasound, amniocentesis, and genetic counselling) to make a diagnosis of neural tube defects (anencephaly,

spina bifida, and encephalocele) or Down syndrome in the fetus. Most screening tests are performed between 15 and 22 weeks' gestation (16 to 18 weeks is ideal), except for the cffDNA test which can be performed around 9 to 10 weeks' gestation (Dempsey & Overton, 2015).

With these multiple screening tests, low MSAFP, unconjugated estriol levels, and a high hCG level suggest the possibility of Down syndrome. Elevated levels of MSAFP are associated with open neural tube defects, ventral wall defects, some renal abnormalities, multiple gestation, certain skin disorders, fetal demise, and placental abnormality. The multiple marker combination with the highest screening performance currently available is AFP, unconjugated estriol (uE3), hCG, and inhibin A, together with the client's age (the so-called quad marker test). With this combination, a detection rate of 80% at a 5% false-positive rate is achieved (Hixson et al., 2015).

A number of factors influence the interpretation of an MSAFP value. The most important is the accuracy of the gestational age determination. A variation of 2 weeks can be misleading and lead to a wrong interpretation. Client's weight (>250 lb), ethnicity, tobacco smoking, fetal sex, gravidity, para status, and presence of insulin-dependent diabetes also may alter the levels of MSAFP and need to be taken into consideration when interpreting the results (Latendresse & Deneris, 2015). Recent research studies indicate prenatal testing with the use of cell free DNA (cfDNA) has significantly lower false positives and high positive predictive values for detection of trisomies than standard testing (Greeley, Kessler, & Vohra, 2015).

Nursing Management

Accurate test interpretation and risk determination are dependent on accurate pregnancy dating and reporting of relevant client characteristics. This is why it is so important for nurses, if an abnormal test result is reported, for them to confirm pregnancy dating and report any significant client factors relevant to test accuracy. In addition, nurses have a big role in providing education about the tests to the couples. Prenatal screening has become standard in prenatal care. However, for many couples it remains confusing, emotionally charged, and filled with uncertain risks. Offer a thorough explanation of the test, reinforcing the information given by the health care professional. Provide couples with a description of the risks and benefits of performing these screens, emphasizing that these tests are for screening purposes only. Remind the couple that a definitive diagnosis is not made without further tests such as an amniocentesis. Answer any questions about these prenatal screening tests and respect the couple's decision if they choose not to have them done. Many couples may choose not to know because they would not consider having an abortion regardless of the test results.

gender determination and to identify sex-linked disorders such as hemophilia, sickle cell anemia, and Tay–Sachs disease (Greeley et al., 2015). Chorionic villi are finger-like projections that cover the embryo and anchor it to the uterine lining before the placenta is developed. Because they are of embryonic origin, sampling provides information about the developing fetus. CVS can be used to detect numerous genetic disorders, with the exception of neural tube defects (Latendresse & Deneris, 2015).

There has been an impetus to develop earlier prenatal diagnostic procedures so that couples can make an early decision to terminate the pregnancy if an anomaly is confirmed. Early prenatal diagnosis by CVS has been proposed as an alternative to routine amniocentesis, which carries fewer risks if done later in the pregnancy. In addition, results of CVS testing are available sooner than those of amniocentesis, usually within 48 hours.

Procedure

CVS is generally performed 10 to 13 weeks after the LMP. Earlier, chorionic villi may not be sufficiently developed for adequate tissue sampling and the risk of limb defects is increased (Khalil & Coates, 2015). First, an ultrasound is done to confirm gestational age and viability. Then, under continuous ultrasound guidance, CVS is performed using either a transcervical or transabdominal approach. With the transcervical approach, the client is placed in the lithotomy position and a sterile catheter is introduced through the cervix and inserted in the placenta, where a sample of chorionic villi is aspirated. This approach requires the client to have a full bladder to push the uterus and placenta into a position that is more accessible to the catheter. A full bladder also helps in better visualization of the structures. With the transabdominal approach, an 18-gauge spinal needle is inserted through the abdominal wall into the placental tissue and a sample of chorionic villi is aspirated. Regardless of the approach used, the sample is sent to the cytogenetics laboratory for analysis.

Potential complications of CVS include postprocedure vaginal bleeding and cramping (most common), hematomas, spontaneous abortion, limb abnormalities, rupture of membranes, infection, chorioamnionitis, and fetal–maternal hemorrhage (March of Dimes, 2015e). The pregnancy loss rate or procedure-related miscarriage rate is approximately 0.5% to 1.0%, which is the same rate for amniocentesis. In addition, clients who are Rh negative should receive immune globulin (RhoGAM) to avoid isoimmunization (Jordan et al., 2014).

Nursing Management

Explain to the client that the procedure will last about 15 minutes. An ultrasound will be done first to locate the embryo, and a baseline set of vital signs will be taken before starting. Make sure the client is informed of the risks related to the procedure, including their incidence. If a transabdominal CVS procedure is planned, advise them to fill their bladder by drinking increased amounts of water. Inform them that a needle will be inserted through the abdominal wall and samples will be collected. Once the samples are collected, the needle will be withdrawn and the samples will be sent to the genetics laboratory for evaluation.

For transcervical CVS, inform the client that a speculum will be placed into the vagina under ultrasound guidance. Then the vagina is cleaned and a small catheter is inserted through the cervix. The samples obtained through the catheter are then sent to a laboratory.

After either procedure, assist the client to a position of comfort and clean any excess lubricant or secretions from the area. Instruct them about signs to watch for and report, such as fever, cramping, and vaginal bleeding. Urge the client not to engage in any strenuous activity for the next 48 hours. Assess the fetal heart rate for changes and administer RhoGAM to an unsensitized Rh-negative client after the procedure.

Nonstress Test

The nonstress test (NST) is the most common method of prenatal testing used in practice today. The NST provides an indirect measurement of uteroplacental function. Unlike the fetal movement counting done by the client alone, this procedure requires specialized equipment and trained personnel. The basis for the NST is that the normal fetus produces characteristic fetal heart rate patterns in response to fetal movements. In the healthy fetus there is an acceleration of the fetal heart rate with fetal movement. Currently, enhanced fetal surveillance with an NST is recommended for clients with diabetes and other high-risk conditions, such as IUGR, preeclampsia, post term pregnancy, renal disease, and multifetal pregnancies (Cunningham et al., 2014). NST is a noninvasive test that requires no initiation of contractions. It is quick to perform and there are no known side effects.

Procedure

The client is advised to empty their bladder, then is placed in the left lateral recumbent position to avoid supine hypotension syndrome. An external electronic fetal monitoring device is applied to the abdomen. The device consists of two belts, each with a sensor. One of the sensors records uterine activity, while the second sensor records fetal heart rate. The client is handed an "event marker" with a button that to push every time fetal movement is felt. When the button is pushed, the fetal monitor strip is marked to identify that fetal movement has occurred. The procedure usually lasts 20 to 30 minutes.

Nursing Management

Prior to the NST, explain the testing procedure, assist with positioning, and apply the two external monitor belts. Document the date and time the test is started, client information, the reason for the test, and the maternal vital signs. Obtain a baseline fetal monitor strip over 15 to 30 minutes.

During the test, observe for signs of fetal activity with a concurrent acceleration of the fetal heart rate. Interpret the NST as normal, atypical, or abnormal. A normal NST will have a baseline fetal heart rate in the normal range (110 to 160 bpm), moderate variability, includes at least two fetal heart rate accelerations from the baseline of at least 15 bpm for at least 15 seconds within the 20-minute recording period, and no decelerations. If the test does not meet these criteria after 40 minutes, it is considered either atypical or abnormal depending on the findings. Additional testing, such as a biophysical profile, should be considered (King et al., 2015).

After the NST procedure, assist the client off the table, provide them with fluids, and allow them to use the restroom. Typically, the health care provider discusses the results at this time. Provide teaching about signs and symptoms to report. If serial NSTs are being done, schedule the next testing session.

Biophysical Profile

A **biophysical profile (BPP)** uses a real-time ultrasound and NST to allow assessment of various parameters of fetal well-being. A BPP includes ultrasound monitoring of fetal movements, fetal tone, and fetal breathing and ultrasound assessment of amniotic fluid volume with or without assessment of the fetal heart rate. A BPP is performed in an effort to identify infants who may be at risk of poor pregnancy outcome, so that additional assessments of well-being may be performed, or labour may be induced or a cesarean section performed to expedite birth. The primary objectives of the BPP are to reduce stillbirth and to detect hypoxia early enough to allow delivery in time to avoid permanent fetal damage resulting from fetal asphyxia. These parameters, together with the NST, constitute the BPP. Each parameter is controlled by a different structure in the fetal brain: fetal tone by the cortex; fetal movements by the cortex and motor nuclei; fetal breathing movements by the centres close to the fourth ventricle; and the NST by the posterior hypothalamus and medulla. The amniotic fluid is the result of fetal urine volume. Some facilities do not perform an NST unless other parameters of the profile are abnormal (King et al., 2015).

The BPP is based on the concept that a fetus that experiences hypoxia loses certain behavioural parameters in the reverse order in which they were acquired during fetal development (normal order of development: tone at 8 weeks; movement at 9 weeks; breathing at 20 weeks; and fetal heart rate reactivity at 24 weeks).

Scoring and Interpretation

The BPP is a scored test with five components, each worth two points if present. A total score of 10 is possible if the NST is used. Thirty minutes are allotted for testing, although less than 10 minutes is usually needed. The following criteria must be met to obtain a score of 2; anything less is scored as 0 (Moses, 2015c):

- *Body movements:* three or more discrete limb or trunk movements
- *Fetal tone:* one or more instances of full extension and flexion of a limb or trunk
- *Fetal breathing:* one or more fetal breathing movements of more than 30 seconds
- *Amniotic fluid volume:* one or more pockets of fluid measuring 2 cm
- *NST:* normal NST = 2 points; abnormal NST = 0 points

Interpretation of the BPP score can be complicated, depending on several fetal and client variables. Because it is indicated as a result of atypical or abnormal findings from previous fetal surveillance tests, this test can be used to quantify the interpretation, and intervention can be initiated if appropriate. A maximum score of 10 can be achieved and the test is complete once all of the variables have been observed. For the test to be judged abnormal and a score of zero awarded for the absence of fetal movement, fetal tone, or fetal breathing movements, a period of not less than 30 minutes must have elapsed. Because of the excellent sensitivity of fetal NST for fetal acidemia, it has been proposed that this acute marker alone may be used for fetal assessment in combination with the amniotic fluid volume assessment, a chronic marker. This combination, also known as the modified BPP, has been shown to have excellent false-negative rates that compare with that of the complete BPP. In addition, a recent study reported that BPP scores correlate fairly closely with the APGAR scores obtained after birth (Nisa, Hamid, Nasreen, & Khanum, 2015).

One of the important factors is the amniotic fluid volume, taken in conjunction with the results of the NST. Amniotic fluid is largely composed of fetal urine. As placental function decreases, perfusion of fetal organs, such as kidneys, decreases, and this can lead to a reduction of amniotic fluid. If oligohydramnios or decreased amniotic fluid is present, the potential exists for antepartum or intrapartum fetal compromise (Lakshmi & Jyothsna, 2015).

Overall, a score of 8 to 10 is considered normal if the amniotic fluid volume is adequate. A score of 6 or below is suspicious, possibly indicating a compromised fetus; further investigation of fetal well-being is needed.

Because the BPP is an ultrasonographic assessment of fetal behaviour, it requires more extensive equipment and more highly trained personnel than other testing modalities. The cost is much greater than with less sophisticated tests. It permits conservative therapy and prevents premature or unnecessary intervention. There are fewer false-positive results than with the NST alone (Callahan, 2016).

Nursing Management

Nursing management focuses primarily on offering the client support and answering questions. Expect to complete the NST before scheduling the BPP, and explain why further testing might be needed. Tell the client that the ultrasound will be done in the diagnostic imaging department.

NURSING MANAGEMENT FOR THE COMMON DISCOMFORTS OF PREGNANCY

Most clients experience common discomforts during pregnancy and ask a nurse's advice about ways to minimize them. However, other clients will not bring up their concerns unless asked. Therefore, the nurse needs to address the common discomforts that occur in each trimester at each prenatal visit and provide realistic measures to help the client deal with them (Teaching Guidelines 12.1). Nursing Care Plan 12.1 (at the end of the chapter) applies the nursing process to the care of a client experiencing some discomforts of pregnancy.

 Teaching Guidelines 12.1
TEACHING TO MANAGE THE DISCOMFORTS OF PREGNANCY

Urinary Frequency or Incontinence
* Try pelvic floor exercises to increase control over leakage.
* Empty your bladder when you first feel a full sensation.
* Avoid caffeinated drinks, which stimulate voiding.
* Reduce your fluid intake after dinner to reduce night-time urination.

Fatigue
* Attempt to get a full night's sleep, without interruptions.
* Eat a healthy balanced diet.
* Schedule a nap in the early afternoon daily.
* When you are feeling tired, rest.

Nausea and Vomiting
* Avoid an empty stomach at all times.
* Eat dry crackers/toast in bed before arising.
* Eat several small meals throughout the day.
* Avoid brushing teeth immediately after eating to avoid gag reflex.
* Acupressure wristbands can be worn daily.
* Drink fluids between meals rather than with meals.
* Avoid greasy, fried foods or ones with a strong odour, such as cabbage or Brussels sprouts.

Backache
* Avoid standing or sitting in one position for long periods.
* Apply heating pad (low setting) to the small of your back.
* Support your lower back with pillows when sitting.
* Use proper body mechanics for lifting anything.
* Avoid excessive bending, lifting, or walking without rest periods.
* Wear supportive low-heeled shoes; avoid high heels.
* Stand with your shoulders back to maintain correct posture.

Leg Cramps
* Elevate legs above heart level frequently throughout the day.
* If you get a cramp, straighten both legs and flex your feet toward your body.
* Ask your health care provider about taking additional calcium supplements, which may reduce leg spasms.

Varicosities
* Walk daily to improve circulation to extremities.
* Elevate both legs above heart level while resting.
* Avoid standing in one position for long periods of time.
* Don't wear constrictive stockings and socks.
* Don't cross the legs when sitting for long periods.
* Wear support stockings to promote better circulation.

Hemorrhoids
* Establish a regular time for daily bowel elimination.
* Avoid constipation and straining during defecation.
* Prevent straining by drinking plenty of fluids and eating fibre-rich foods and exercising daily.
* Use warm sitz baths and cool witch hazel compresses for comfort.

Constipation
* Increase your intake of foods high in fibre and drink at least eight 8-oz glasses of fluid daily.
* Ingest prunes or prune juice which are natural laxatives.
* Consume warm liquids (tea) on rising, to stimulate peristalsis.
* Exercise each day (brisk walking) to promote movement through the intestine.
* Reduce the amount of cheese consumed.

Heartburn/Indigestion

- Avoid spicy or greasy foods and eat small frequent meals.
- Sleep on several pillows so that your head is elevated 30 degrees.
- Stop smoking and avoid caffeinated drinks to reduce stimulation.
- Avoid lying down for at least 3 hours after meals.
- Try drinking sips of water to reduce burning sensation.
- Avoid foods that trigger symptoms—fried foods, citrus, soda, chocolate.
- Take antacids sparingly if burning sensation is severe.

Braxton Hicks Contractions

- Keep in mind that these contractions are a normal sensation. Try changing your position or engaging in mild exercise to help reduce the sensation.
- Drink more fluids if possible.

First-Trimester Discomforts

During the first 3 months of pregnancy, the client's body is undergoing numerous changes. Some will experience many discomforts, but others have few. These discomforts are caused by the changes taking place within the body and they pass as the pregnancy progresses.

Urinary Frequency or Incontinence

Urinary frequency or incontinence is common in the first trimester because the growing uterus compresses the bladder. This also is a common complaint during the third trimester, especially when the fetal head settles into the pelvis. However, the discomfort tends to improve in the second trimester, when the uterus becomes an abdominal organ and moves away from the bladder region.

After infection and gestational diabetes have been ruled out as causative factors of increased urinary frequency, suggest that the client decrease their fluid intake 2 to 3 hours before bedtime and limit intake of caffeinated beverages. Increased voiding is normal, but encourage the client to report any pain or burning during urination. Also explain that increased urinary frequency may subside once in the second trimester, only to recur in the third trimester. Teach the client to perform pelvic floor muscle training exercises, formally termed Kegel exercises, to increase support of the uterus, bladder, small intestine, and rectum throughout the day to help strengthen perineal muscle tone, thereby enhancing urinary control and decreasing the possibility of incontinence.

Fatigue

Fatigue plagues all pregnant clients, primarily in the first and third trimesters (the highest-energy levels typically occur during the second trimester), even if they get their normal amount of sleep at night. First-trimester fatigue most often is related to the many physical changes (e.g., increased oxygen consumption, increased levels of progesterone and relaxin, increased metabolic demands) and psychosocial changes (e.g., mood swings, multiple role demands) of pregnancy. Third-trimester fatigue can be caused by sleep disturbances from increased weight (many cannot find a comfortable sleeping position due to the enlarging abdomen), physical discomforts such as heartburn, and insomnia due to mood swings, multiple role anxiety, and a decrease in exercise (Rigby, 2015).

Once anemia, infection, and blood dyscrasias have been ruled out as contributing to the client's fatigue, advise them to arrange work, child care, and other life demands to permit additional rest periods. Work with the client to devise a realistic schedule for rest. Using pillows for support in the left-side-lying position relieves pressure on major blood vessels that supply oxygen and nutrients to the fetus when resting (Fig. 12.8). Also recommend the use of relaxation techniques, providing instructions as necessary, and suggest increasing daily exercise level.

Nausea and Vomiting

It is estimated that somewhere between 70% and 80% of pregnant people experience nausea and vomiting. The problem is generally time limited, with the onset about the fifth week after the LMP, a peak at 8 to 12 weeks, and resolution by 16 to 18 weeks. Despite popular use of the term *morning sickness,* nausea and vomiting of pregnancy persists throughout the day in the majority of those affected, and has been found to be limited to the morning in less than 2% of clients (Tyler & Nagtalon-Ramos, 2015). The physiologic changes that cause nausea and vomiting

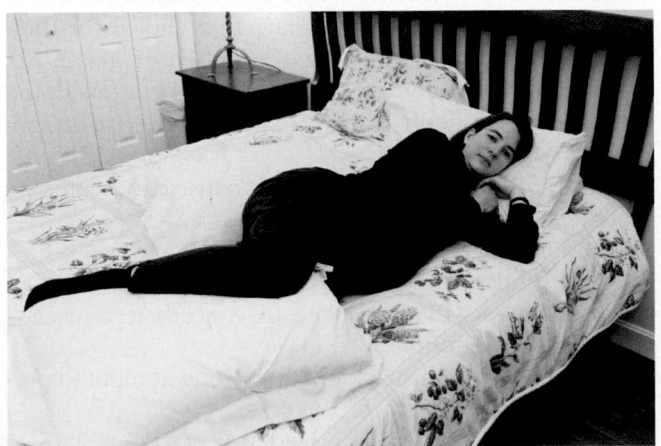

FIGURE 12.8 Using pillows for support in the side-lying position.

are unknown, but research suggests that unusually high levels of estrogen, progesterone, and hCG and a vitamin B_6 deficiency may be contributing factors. Symptoms generally last until the second trimester and are generally associated with a positive pregnancy outcome, in terms of lower rates of miscarriages, congenital malformations, and preterm births (Cunningham et al., 2014). In summary, the etiology of nausea and vomiting in pregnancy is physiologic, thus assessment of the condition focuses on severity, and the management is largely supportive.

Nausea and vomiting of pregnancy can take a physical and psychological toll on the pregnant client, and may have an adverse effect on their partner, family members, and even coworkers. The burden it places on the client is usually minimized, as it is considered a normal part of pregnancy, thus it may not be worthy of evaluation, diagnosis, management, and emotional support. As a result, it may not be taken seriously because it is so common and time-limited; leading some clients to feel frustrated and feel guilty that they are even complaining about their symptoms. Nurses need to pick up on this, address it and provide support.

The goal of treatment is to improve symptoms while minimizing risks to the client and fetus. Treatment management ranges from simple dietary modifications to drug therapy. To help alleviate nausea and vomiting, advise the client to eat small, frequent meals that are bland and low in fat (five or six a day) to prevent the stomach from becoming completely empty. Other helpful suggestions include eating dry crackers, Cheerios, or cheese or drinking lemonade before getting out of bed in the morning and increasing the intake of foods high in vitamin B_6, such as meat, poultry, bananas, fish, green leafy vegetables, peanuts, raisins, walnuts, and whole grains, or making sure to receive enough vitamin B_6 by taking prescribed prenatal vitamins.

Pharmacologic treatment of nausea and vomiting in pregnancy is limited. Doxylamine-pyridoxine (e.g., Diclectin) is shown to be a safe and effective for use in pregnancy, and is an appropriate first choice for therapy of nausea and vomiting (Campbell et al., 2016). Other pharmacotherapies that might be considered may include dimenhydrinate (e.g., Gravol), or ondansetron (e.g., Zofran).

Other helpful tips to deal with nausea and vomiting include:
- Get out of bed in the morning very slowly.
- Avoid sudden movements.
- Avoid triggers that stimulate or exacerbate nausea—strong food odours.
- Eat a high-protein snack before retiring at night to prevent an empty stomach.
- Take ginger (up to 1 g in divided doses daily; 250-mg capsules QID), which increases tone and peristalsis in the gastrointestinal tract.

- Open a window to remove odours of food being cooked.
- Eat more protein than carbohydrates and take in more liquids than solids.
- Limit intake of fluids or soups during meals (drink them between meals).
- Avoid fried foods and foods cooked with grease, oils, or fatty meats, because they tend to upset the stomach.
- Avoid highly seasoned foods such as those cooked with garlic, onions, peppers, and chili.
- Drink a small amount of caffeine-free carbonated beverage (ginger ale) if nauseated.
- Trying acupressure using a wristband has been FDA approved for nausea.
- Avoid wearing tight or restricting clothes, which might place increased pressure on the expanding abdomen.
- Avoid stress (Bope & Kellerman, 2015; Jordan et al., 2014; King et al., 2015).

Breast Tenderness

As a result of increased estrogen and progesterone levels, which cause the fat layer of the breast tissue to thicken and the number of milk ducts and glands to increase during the first trimester, many clients experience breast tenderness. Offering a thorough explanation about the reasons for the breast discomfort is important. Wearing a larger bra with good support can help alleviate this discomfort. Advise clients to wear a supportive bra, even while sleeping. As the breasts increase in size, advise clients to increase their bra size to ensure adequate support.

Constipation

Constipation affects up to 38% of pregnancies (Verghese, Futaba, & Latthe, 2015). Increasing levels of progesterone during pregnancy lead to decreased contractility of the gastrointestinal tract, slowed movement of substances through the colon, and a resulting increase in water absorption. All of these factors lead to constipation. Lack of exercise or too little fibre or fluids in the diet can also promote constipation. In addition, the large bowel is mechanically compressed by the enlarging uterus, adding to this discomfort. The iron and calcium in prenatal vitamins can also contribute to constipation during the first and third trimesters.

Explain how pregnancy exacerbates the symptoms of constipation and offer the following suggestions:
- Eat fresh or dried fruit daily.
- Eat more raw fruits and vegetables, including their skins.
- Eat whole-grain cereals and breads such as raisin bran or bran flakes.
- Participate in physical activity every day.
- Engage in pelvis floor exercises, stretching exercises, and yoga daily.

- Eat meals at regular intervals.
- Establish a time of day to defecate, and elevate feet on a stool to avoid straining.
- Drink six to eight glasses of water daily.
- Decrease intake of refined carbohydrates.
- Drink warm fluids on arising to stimulate bowel motility.
- Decrease consumption of sugary sodas.
- Avoid eating large amounts of cheese.

If the suggestions above are ineffective, suggest that the client use a bulk-forming laxative such as Metamucil®.

Nasal Stuffiness, Bleeding Gums, Epistaxis (Nosebleeds)

Increased levels of estrogen cause edema of the mucous membranes of the nasal and oral cavities. Advise clients to drink extra water for hydration of the mucous membranes or to use a cool mist humidifier in the bedroom at night. If they need to blow their nose to relieve nasal stuffiness, advise blowing gently, one nostril at a time. Advise clients to avoid the use of nasal decongestants and sprays.

If a nosebleed occurs, advise the client to loosen the clothing around the neck, sit with head tilted forward, pinch the nostrils with thumb and forefinger for 10 to 15 minutes, and apply an ice pack to the bridge of the nose.

If the client has bleeding gums, encourage the practice of good oral hygiene by using a soft toothbrush and flossing daily. Warm saline mouthwashes can relieve discomfort. If the gum problem persists, instruct the client to see a dentist.

Cravings

Food craving refers to an intense desire to consume a specific food. Desires for certain foods and beverages are likely to begin during the first trimester but do not appear to reflect any physiologic need. Foods with a high sodium or sugar content often are the ones craved. At times, some individuals crave nonfood substances such as clay, cornstarch, laundry detergent, baking soda, soap, paint chips, dirt, ice, or wax. As explained in Chapter 11, this craving for nonfood substances, termed *pica,* may indicate a severe dietary deficiency of minerals or vitamins, or it may have cultural roots (Jyothi, 2015).

Leukorrhea

Increased vaginal discharge begins during the first trimester and continues throughout pregnancy. The physiologic changes behind leukorrhea arise from the high levels of estrogen, which cause increased vascularity and hypertrophy of cervical glands as well as vaginal cells

(Cunningham et al., 2014). The result is progressively increasing vaginal secretions throughout pregnancy.

Advise the client to keep the perineal area clean and dry, washing the area with mild soap and water during a daily shower. Also recommend that clients avoid wearing pantyhose and other tight-fitting nylon clothes that prevent air from circulating to the genital area. Encourage the use of cotton underwear and suggest wearing a nightgown rather than pajamas to allow for increased airflow. Also instruct clients to avoid douching and tampon use.

Second-Trimester Discomforts

A sense of well-being typically characterizes the second trimester. By this time, the fatigue, nausea, and vomiting have subsided and the uncomfortable changes of the third trimester are a few months away. Not everyone experiences the same discomforts during this time, so nursing assessments and interventions must be individualized.

Backache

Musculoskeletal pain is a common occurrence in pregnancy and postpartum. Half of childbearing individuals report having back pain at some point during pregnancy. This can seriously impact the quality of life and have socioeconomic issues from loss days at work. The pain can be lumbar or sacroiliac. The pain may also be present only at night. Back pain is thought to be due to multiple factors, which include shifting of the centre of gravity caused by the enlarging uterus, increased joint laxity due to an increase in relaxin, stretching of the ligaments (which are pain-sensitive structures), and pregnancy-related circulatory changes.

Treatment is heat and ice, acetaminophen, massage, proper posturing, good support shoes, and a good exercise program for strength and conditioning. Pregnant clients may also relieve back pain by placing one foot on a stool when standing for long periods of time and placing a pillow between the legs when lying down (Plastaras & Appasamy, 2015). After exploring other reasons that might cause backache, such as uterine contractions, urinary tract infection, ulcers, or musculoskeletal back disorders, the following instructions may be helpful:

- Maintain correct posture, with head up and shoulders back.
- Wear low-heeled shoes with good arch support.
- When standing for long periods, place one foot on a stool or box.
- Use good body mechanics when lifting objects.
- When sitting, use foot supports and pillows behind the back.

• Try pelvic tilt or rocking exercises to strengthen the back (ACOG, 2015c).

The pelvic tilt or pelvic rock is used to alleviate pressure on the lower back during pregnancy by stretching the lower back muscles. It can be done sitting, standing, or on all fours. To do it on all fours, the hands are positioned directly under the shoulders and the knees under the hips. The back should be in a neutral position with the head and neck aligned with the straight back. The person then presses up with the lower back and holds this position for a few seconds, then relaxes to a neutral position. This action of pressing upward is repeated frequently throughout the day to prevent a sore back (Rigby, 2015).

Leg Cramps

Many clients experience leg cramps in pregnancy. They become more common as pregnancy progresses and are especially troublesome at night. They occur primarily in the second and third trimesters and could be related to the pressure of the gravid uterus on pelvic nerves and blood vessels. During pregnancy, up to 50% of clients can be affected by leg cramps, and up to 25% can be affected by restless legs syndrome (King et al., 2015). Along with lack of exercise, diet can also be a contributing factor if they are not consuming enough of certain minerals, such as calcium and magnesium. The sudden stretching of leg muscles may also play a role in causing leg cramps (Kondhare & Khodgire, 2015).

Encourage the client to gently stretch the muscle by dorsiflexing the foot up toward the body. Wrapping a warm, moist towel around the leg muscle can also help the muscle to relax. Advise the client to avoid stretching the legs, pointing the toes, and walking excessively. Stress the importance of wearing low-heeled shoes and support hose and arising slowly from a sitting position. If the leg cramps are due to deficiencies in minerals, the condition can be remedied by eating more foods rich in these nutrients. Also instruct the client on calf-stretching exercises: have them stand 3 ft from the wall and lean toward it, resting the lower arms against it, while keeping the heels on the floor. This may help reduce cramping if it is done before going to bed.

Elevating the legs throughout the day will help relieve pressure and minimize strain. Wearing support hose and avoiding curling the toes may help to relieve leg discomfort. Also instruct the client to avoid standing in one spot for a prolonged period or crossing the legs. If standing for prolonged periods is unavoidable, suggest a change in position at least every 2 hours by walking or sitting to reduce the risk of leg cramps. Encourage drinking eight 8-oz glasses of fluid throughout the day to ensure adequate hydration. Taking daily walks can also help reduce leg cramping because ambulation improves circulation to the muscles.

Varicosities of the Vulva and Legs

Varicosities of the vulva and legs are associated with the increased venous stasis caused by the pressure of the gravid uterus on pelvic vessels and the vasodilation resulting from increased progesterone levels. Progesterone relaxes the vein walls, making it difficult for blood to return to the heart from the extremities; pooling can result. Genetic predisposition, inactivity, obesity, and poor muscle tone are also contributing factors.

Encourage clients to wear support hose and teach proper application. Advise elevating the legs above the level of the heart while lying back for 10 minutes before getting out of bed in the morning, thus promoting venous return before applying the hose. Instruct clients to avoid crossing their legs and avoid wearing knee-high stockings. These can cause constriction of leg vessels and muscles and contribute to venous stasis. Also encourage clients to elevate both legs above the level of the heart for 5 to 10 minutes at least twice a day (Fig. 12.9); to wear low-heeled shoes; and to avoid long periods of standing or sitting, frequently changing position. If a client has vulvar varicosities, suggest applying ice packs to the area when lying down.

Hemorrhoids

Hemorrhoids are varicosities of the rectum and may be external (outside the anal sphincter) or internal (above the sphincter) (ACOG, 2015d). They occur as a result of progesterone-induced vasodilation and from pressure of the enlarged uterus on the lower intestine and rectum. Hemorrhoids are more common in people with constipation, poor fluid intake or poor dietary habits,

FIGURE 12.9 Childbearing person elevating legs while working.

smokers, or those with a previous history of hemorrhoids (Zielinski, Searing, & Deibel, 2015).

Instruct the client in measures to prevent constipation, including increasing fibre intake and drinking at least 2 L of fluid per day. Recommend the use of topical anesthetics (e.g., Preparation H®, Anusol, witch hazel compresses such as Tucks®) to reduce pain, itching, and swelling, if permitted by the health care provider. Teach the client about local comfort measures such as warm sitz baths, witch hazel compresses, or cold compresses. To minimize the risk of straining while defecating, suggest elevating the feet on a stool. Also encourage the client to avoid prolonged sitting or standing (ACOG, 2015d).

Flatulence With Bloating

Flatulence and gas pain are another result of decreased gastrointestinal motility. The physiologic changes that result in constipation (reduced gastrointestinal motility and dilation secondary to progesterone's influence) may also result in increased flatulence. As the enlarging uterus compresses the bowel, it delays the passage of food through the intestines, thus allowing more time for gas to be formed by bacteria in the colon. The client usually reports increased passage of rectal gas, abdominal bloating, or belching. Instruct them to avoid gas-forming foods, such as beans, cabbage, and onions, as well as foods that have a high content of white sugar. Adding more fibre to the diet, increasing fluid intake, and increasing physical exercise are also helpful in reducing flatus. In addition, reducing the amount of swallowed air, if chewing gum, will reduce gas build-up. The knee-chest position may also help with discomfort from unexpelled gas. Reducing the intake of carbonated beverages and cheese and eating mints can also help reduce flatulence during pregnancy (Almansa, De Vault, & Houghton, 2015).

Third-Trimester Discomforts

As clients enter their third trimester, many experience a return of the first-trimester discomforts of fatigue, urinary frequency, leukorrhea, and constipation. These discomforts are secondary to the ever-enlarging uterus compressing adjacent structures, increasing hormone levels, and the metabolic demands of the fetus. In addition to these discomforts, many individuals experience shortness of breath, heartburn and indigestion, swelling, and Braxton Hicks contractions.

Shortness of Breath and Dyspnea

Dyspnea is a common complaint in pregnancy. Physiologic and hemodynamic changes can result in a significant dyspnea in such cases. In some individuals, dyspnea in normal daily activities can be a sign of heart and lung disease and may be associated with poor perinatal and cardiac outcome in which early detection can prevent adverse events. The increasing growth of the uterus prevents complete lung expansion late in pregnancy. As the uterus enlarges upward in the second and third trimesters, the expansion of the diaphragm is limited. Dyspnea can occur when the individual lies on their back and the pressure of the gravid uterus against the vena cava reduces venous return to the heart (Tara, Vakilian, Moosavi-Baigy, Salehi, & Moghiman, 2015).

Explain to the client that dyspnea is normal and will improve when the fetus drops into the pelvis (lightening). Instruct them to adjust their body position to allow for maximum expansion of the chest and to avoid large meals, which increase abdominal pressure. Raising the head of the bed on blocks or placing pillows behind the back is helpful too. Under normal circumstances, resting with the head elevated while taking slow, deep breaths reduces shortness of breath symptoms. In addition, stress that lying on the left side will displace the uterus off the vena cava and improve breathing. Having the client periodically stand up to stretch the arms above the head and take a deep breath is helpful to relieve dyspnea. Also, advise them to avoid exercise that precipitates dyspnea, to rest after exercise, and to avoid overheating in warm climates. If the client still smokes, encourage them to stop.

Heartburn and Indigestion

Heartburn and indigestion result when high progesterone levels cause relaxation of the cardiac sphincter, allowing food and digestive juices to flow backward from the stomach into the esophagus. Irritation of the esophageal lining occurs, causing the burning sensation known as heartburn. It occurs in up to 70% of individuals at some point during pregnancy, with an increased frequency seen in the third trimester (King et al., 2015). The pain may radiate to the neck and throat. It worsens when the client lies down, bends over after eating, or wears tight clothes. Indigestion (vague abdominal discomfort after meals) results from eating too much or too fast; from eating when tense, tired, or emotionally upset; from eating food that is too fatty or spicy; and from eating heavy food or food that has been badly cooked or processed (Nagtalon-Ramos, 2014). In addition, the stomach is displaced upward and compressed by the large uterus in the third trimester, thus limiting the stomach's capacity to empty quickly. Food sits, causing heartburn and indigestion.

Review clients' usual dietary intake and suggest that they limit or avoid gas-producing or fatty foods and large meals. Instruct clients to pay attention to the timing of any discomfort. When the pain occurs 30 to 45 minutes after a meal, the cause may be heartburn. Encourage clients to maintain proper posture and remain in the sitting position for 1 to 3 hours after eating to prevent reflux of gastric acids into the esophagus by gravity. Urge clients to consume small, frequent meals, to eat slowly, chewing food thoroughly to prevent excessive swallowing of air, which can lead to increased gastric pressure. Instruct clients to avoid foods that act as triggers such as caffeinated drinks, greasy, gas-forming foods, citrus, spiced foods, chocolate, coffee, alcohol, and spearmint or peppermint. These items stimulate the release of gastric digestive acids, which may cause reflux into the esophagus. Avoid late-night or large meals and gum chewing. Avoid lying down within 3 hours after eating. Finally, elevate the head of the bed by 10 to 30 degrees.

Dependent Edema

Swelling is the result of increased capillary permeability caused by elevated hormone levels and increased blood volume. Sodium and water are retained and thirst increases. Edema occurs most often in dependent areas such as the legs and feet throughout the day due to gravity; it improves after a night's sleep. Warm weather or prolonged standing or sitting may increase edema. Generalized edema, appearing in the face, hands, and feet, can signal preeclampsia if accompanied by dizziness, blurred vision, headaches, upper quadrant pain, or nausea (Rigby, 2015). This edema should be reported to the health care provider. Appropriate suggestions to minimize dependent edema include:

- Elevate your feet and legs above the level of the heart periodically throughout the day.
- Wear support hose when standing or sitting for long periods.
- Change position frequently throughout the day.
- Walk at a sensible pace to help contract leg muscles to promote venous return.
- When taking a long car ride, stop to walk around every 2 hours.
- When standing, rock from the ball of the foot to the toes to stimulate circulation.
- Lie on your left side to keep the gravid uterus off the vena cava to return blood to the heart.
- Avoid foods high in sodium, such as lunch meats, potato chips, and bacon.
- Avoid wearing knee-high stockings.
- Drink six to eight glasses of water daily to replace fluids lost through perspiration.
- Avoid high intake of sugar and fats, because they cause water retention.

Braxton Hicks Contractions

Braxton Hicks contractions are irregular, painless contractions that occur without cervical dilation. Typically, they intensify in the third trimester in preparation for labour. In reality, they have been present since early in the pregnancy but may have gone unnoticed. They are thought to increase the tone of uterine muscles for labour purposes (Grant, Strevens, & Thornton, 2015).

Reassure the client that these contractions are normal. Instruct the client in how to differentiate between Braxton Hicks and labour contractions. Explain that true labour contractions usually grow longer, stronger, and closer together and occur at regular intervals. Walking usually strengthens true labour contractions, whereas Braxton Hicks contractions tend to decrease in intensity and taper off. Advise the client to keep well hydrated and to rest in a left-side-lying position to help relieve the discomfort. Suggest using breathing techniques such as Lamaze techniques to ease the discomfort.

Consider This

One has to wonder sometimes why people go through what they do. During my first pregnancy, I was sick for the first 2 months. I would experience waves of nausea from the moment I got out of bed until midmorning. Needless to say, I wasn't the happiest camper around. After the third month, my life seemed to settle down and I was beginning to think that being pregnant wasn't too bad after all. For the moment, I was fooled. Then, during my last 2 months, another wave of discomfort struck—heartburn and constipation—a double whammy! I now feared eating anything that might trigger acid indigestion and also might remain in my body too long. I literally had to become the "fibre queen" to combat these two challenges. Needless to say, my "suffering" was well worth our bright-eyed baby girl in the end.

Thoughts: *Despite the various discomforts associated with pregnancy, most individuals wouldn't change their end result. Do most clients experience these discomforts? What suggestions could be made to reduce them?*

NURSING MANAGEMENT TO PROMOTE SELF-CARE

Pregnancy is considered a time of health, not illness. Health promotion and maintenance activities are essential to promoting an optimal outcome for the client and the fetus. Pregnant clients commonly have many questions about the changes occurring during pregnancy: how these changes affect their usual routine, such as working, travelling, exercising, or engaging in sexual activity; how the changes influence their typical self-care activities, such as bathing, perineal care, or dental care; and whether these changes are signs of a problem.

Take Note!

Clients may have heard stories about or been told by others what to do and what not to do during pregnancy, leading to many misconceptions and much misinformation.

Nurses can play a major role in providing anticipatory guidance and teaching to foster the client's responsibility for self-care, helping to clarify misconceptions and correct any misinformation. Educating the client to identify threats to safety posed by their lifestyle or environment and proposing ways to modify them to avoid a negative outcome are important. Counselling should also include healthy ways to prepare food, advice to avoid medications unless they are prescribed, and advice on identifying teratogens within the environment or at work and how to reduce risk from exposure. The pregnant client can better care for themselves and the fetus if their concerns are anticipated and identified by the nurse and are incorporated into teaching sessions at each prenatal visit.

Personal Hygiene

Hygiene is a necessity for the maintenance of good health. Cleansing the skin removes dirt, bacteria, sweat, dead skin cells, and body secretions. Counsel clients to wash their hands and under their fingernails frequently throughout the day in order to lower the bacterial count on both. During pregnancy the sebaceous (sweat) glands become more active under the influence of hormones, and sweating is more profuse. This increase may make it necessary to use a stronger deodorant and shower more frequently. The cervical and vaginal glands also produce more secretions during pregnancy. Frequent showering helps to keep the area dry and promotes better hygiene. Encourage the use of cotton underwear to allow greater air circulation. Taking a tub bath throughout pregnancy is permitted, but closer to term, when the centre of gravity shifts, caution should be taken in tub and shower to prevent slipping.

Hot Tubs and Saunas

Caution pregnant clients to avoid using hot tubs, saunas, whirlpools, and tanning beds during pregnancy. The heat may cause fetal tachycardia as well as raise the individual's temperature. Exposure to bacteria in hot tubs that have not been cleaned sufficiently is another reason to avoid them during pregnancy.

Perineal Care

The glands in the cervical and vaginal areas become more active during pregnancy secondary to hormonal influences. This increase in activity will produce more vaginal secretions, especially in the last trimester. Advise clients to shower frequently and wear all-cotton underwear to minimize the effects of these secretions. Caution clients not to douche, because douching can increase the risk of infection, and not to wear panty liners, which block air circulation and promote moisture. Explain that they should also avoid perfumed soaps, lotions, perineal sprays, and harsh laundry detergents to help prevent irritation and potential infection.

Dental Care

Physiologic changes that occur in pregnancy can adversely affect oral health. Elevations in estrogen and progesterone enhance the inflammatory response and consequently alter gingival tissue. During pregnancy, the incidence of gingivitis and periodontitis increases (Anil et al., 2015). Pregnancy is a time when a person can be very receptive to health messaging. Pregnancy is no longer a contraindication for dental treatment; it is also a time when nurses can help clients understand that good oral health is important to a healthy pregnancy and can decrease the risk of dental caries in their children. When individuals see oral health as a priority for themselves, they are more likely to place a high priority on their children's oral health.

Periodontal disease is a contributing factor to systemic conditions, such as heart disease, respiratory diseases, diabetes mellitus, adverse pregnancy outcomes (preterm births, low–birth-weight infants, and small-for-gestational-age infants), anemia, and stroke (Trivedi, Lal, & Singhal, 2015). Research has established that the elevated levels of estrogen and progesterone during pregnancy cause individuals to be more sensitive to the effects of bacterial dental plaque, which can cause gingivitis, an oral infection characterized by swollen and bleeding gums (ACOG, 2013). Brushing and flossing teeth twice daily will help reduce bacteria in the mouth. Advise the client to visit a dentist early in the pregnancy to address any dental caries and have a thorough cleaning to prevent possible infection later in the pregnancy. Advise them to avoid exposure to x-rays by informing the hygienist of the pregnancy. If x-rays are necessary, the abdomen should be shielded with a lead apron.

Researchers have reported an association between prematurity and periodontitis, an oral infection that spreads beyond the gum tissues to invade the supporting structures of the teeth. Periodontitis is characterized by bleeding gums, loss of tooth attachment, loss of supporting bone, and bad breath due to pus formation. Unfortunately, because this infection is chronic and often painless, individuals frequently do not realize they have it and a preterm birth can result. During pregnancy, gingivitis occurs in 35% to 100% of clients, depending upon the study (Trivedi, Lal, & Singhal, 2015). Nurses should assess all clients' oral health status by taking an oral health history; checking their mouths for swollen or bleeding gums, untreated dental decay, mucosal lesions, and signs of infection; and document findings in the prenatal record.

Additional guidelines that the nurse should stress regarding maintaining dental health include:

- Seek professional dental care during the first trimester for assessment and care.
- Be reassured that oral health care is safe during pregnancy.
- Obtain treatment for dental pain and infection promptly during pregnancy.
- Brush twice daily for 2 minutes, especially before bed, with fluoridated toothpaste and rinse well. Use a soft-bristled toothbrush and be sure to brush at the gum line to remove food debris and plaque to keep gums healthy.
- Floss teeth daily with dental floss and rinse well afterward with plain water.
- Eat healthy foods, especially those high in vitamins A, C, and D and calcium.
- Avoid sugary snacks.
- Chew sugar-free gum for 10 minutes after a meal if brushing is not possible.
- After vomiting, rinse your mouth immediately with baking soda (¼ teaspoon) and warm water (1 cup) to neutralize the acid (National Maternal and Child Oral Health Resource Center, 2015).

Breast Care

Because the breasts enlarge significantly and become heavier throughout pregnancy, stress the need to wear a firm, supportive bra with wide straps to balance the weight of the breasts. Instruct the client to anticipate buying a larger-sized bra about halfway through the pregnancy because of the increasing size of the breasts. Advise them to avoid using soap on the nipple area because it can be very drying. Encourage rinsing the nipple area with plain water while bathing to keep it clean. The Montgomery glands (located in the areolar part of the nipple) secrete a lubricating substance that keeps the nipples moist and discourages growth of bacteria, so there is no need to use alcohol or other antiseptics on the nipples.

When a client plans to breastfeed, nipple preparation is unnecessary unless the nipples are inverted and do not become erect when stimulated. Breast shells can be worn during the last 2 months to address this issue (Alexander et al., 2014).

Around week 16 of pregnancy, colostrum secretion begins, which the client may notice as moisture in the bra. Advise them to place breast pads or a cotton cloth in the bra and change them frequently to prevent build-up, which may lead to excoriation.

Clothing

Many contemporary clothes are loose fitting and layered, so the client may not need to buy an entirely new wardrobe to accommodate the pregnancy. Some individuals may continue to wear tight clothes. Point out that loose clothing will be more comfortable for the client and their expanding waistline.

Advise clients to avoid wearing constricting clothes and girdles that compress the growing abdomen. Urge them to avoid knee-high hose, which might impede lower-extremity circulation and increase the risk of developing DVT. Low-heeled shoes will minimize pelvic tilt and possible backache. Wearing layered clothing that can be removed as the temperatures fluctuate may be more comfortable, especially toward term, when the client may feel overheated.

Exercise

A physically inactive lifestyle is associated with an increase in chronic diseases such as cardiovascular disease, type 2 diabetes, osteoporosis, and cancer. The proportion of the pregnant population who are overweight or obese is increasing globally, thus exercise is essential to reduce these risks and promote a healthy pregnancy. Exercise is well tolerated by a healthy individual during pregnancy. It promotes a feeling of well-being; improves circulation; helps reduce constipation, bloating, and swelling; may help prevent or treat gestational diabetes; promotes muscle tone, strength, and endurance; may improve the ability to cope with labour; increases energy levels; improves posture; helps sleep and promotes relaxation and rest; and relieves the lower back discomfort that often arises as the pregnancy progresses (Barakat, Lucia, & Ruiz, 2015). However, the duration and difficulty of exercise should be modified throughout pregnancy because of a decrease in performance efficiency with gestational age. Some individuals continue to push themselves to maintain their prior level of exercise, but most find that as their shape changes and their abdominal area enlarges, they must modify their exercise routines. Modification also helps to reduce the risk of injury caused by laxity of the joints and connective tissue due to the hormonal effects (Petrov Fieril, Glantz, & Fagevik Olsen, 2015).

Exercise during pregnancy is contraindicated in clients with preterm labour, poor weight gain, anemia, facial and hand edema, pain, hypertension, threatened abortion, dizziness, shortness of breath, multiple gestation, decreased fetal activity, cardiac disease, and palpitations (Rigby, 2015).

Federal physical activity guidelines recommend at least 150 minutes of moderate-intensity exercise per week during pregnancy (Dietz, 2015) (Fig. 12.10). It is believed that pregnancy is a unique time for behaviour modification

FIGURE 12.10 **Exercising during pregnancy.**

and that healthy behaviours maintained or adopted during pregnancy may improve the client's health for the rest of their life. The excess weight gained in pregnancy, which some never lose, is a major public health problem (Truong, Yee, Caughey, & Cheng, 2015). Exercise helps the client avoid gaining excess weight during pregnancy.

Exercise during pregnancy helps return a client's body to good health after the baby is born. The long-term benefits of exercise that begin in early pregnancy include improved posture, weight control, and improved muscle tone. Exercise also aids in the prevention of osteoporosis after menopause, reduces the risk of hypertension and diabetes, and assists in keeping the birth weight of the fetus within the normal range (Barakat et al., 2015). Teaching Guidelines 12.2 highlights recommendations for exercise during pregnancy.

Teaching Guidelines 12.2
TEACHING TO PROMOTE EXERCISE DURING PREGNANCY

- Consume liquids before, during, and after exercising.
  - Ask your health care provider before you start a new exercise routine.
- Avoid exercising in hot, humid weather or when you have a fever.
- Stop exercising if you experience vaginal bleeding, dizziness, chest pain, headache, muscle weakness, calf pain or swelling, uterine contractions, decreased fetal movement, or fluid leaking from the vagina.
- Exercise three or four times each week, not sporadically.
- Engage in brisk walking, swimming, biking, or low-impact aerobics; these are considered ideal activities.
- Avoid getting overheated during exercise.
- Wear comfortable exercise footwear that gives strong ankle and arch support.
- Contact sports should be avoided during pregnancy.
- Include relaxation and stretching before and after your exercise program.
- Reduce the intensity of workouts in late pregnancy.
- Avoid jerky, bouncy, or high-impact movements.
- Avoid lying flat (supine) after the fourth month because of hypotensive effect.
- Use pelvic tilt and pelvic rocking to relieve backache.
- Start with 5 to 10 minutes of stretching exercises.
- Rise slowly following an exercise session to avoid dizziness.
- Avoid activities such as skiing, surfing, scuba diving, and ice hockey.
- Never exercise to the point of exhaustion.

Adapted from Kader, M., & Naim-Shuchana, S. (2014). Physical activity and exercise during pregnancy. *European Journal of Physiotherapy, 16*(1), 2–9. doi: 10.3109/21679169.2013.861509; American College of Obstetricians & Gynecologists (ACOG). (2015e). *Exercise during pregnancy.* Retrieved from https://www.acog.org/Search?Keyword =exercise+guidelines; and American Pregnancy Association (APA). (2014b). Pregnancy exercise guidelines. Retrieved from http://americanpregnancy.org/pregnancyhealth/exerciseguidelines.html

Sleep and Rest

Getting enough sleep helps a person feel better and promotes optimal performance levels during the day. The body releases its greatest concentration of growth hormone during sleep, helping the body to repair damaged tissue and grow. Also, with the increased metabolic demands during pregnancy, fatigue is a constant challenge to many pregnant clients, especially during the first and third trimesters. The following tips can help promote adequate sleep:

- Stay on a regular schedule by going to bed and waking up at the same times.
- Eat regular meals at regular times to keep external body cues consistent.
- Take time to unwind and relax before bedtime.
- Establish a bedtime routine or pattern and follow it.
- Create a proper sleep environment by reducing the light and lowering the room temperature.
- Go to bed when you feel tired; if sleep does not occur, read a book until you are sleepy.
- Reduce caffeine intake later in the day.
- Limit fluid intake after dinner to minimize trips to the bathroom.
- Exercise daily to improve circulation and well-being.
- Use a modified Sims position to improve circulation in the lower extremities.
- Avoid lying on your back after the fourth month, which may compromise circulation to the uterus.
- Avoid sharply bending your knees, which promotes venous stasis below the knees.
- Keep anxieties and worries out of the bedroom. Set aside a specific area in the home or time of day for them.

Sexual Activity and Sexuality

Sexuality is an important part of health and well-being. Pregnancy is characterized by intense biologic, psychological, and social changes. These changes have direct and indirect, conscious and unconscious effects on an individual's sexuality. Pregnant people will experience dramatic alterations in their physiology, appearance, and body, as well as relationships. The sexual responses during pregnancy vary widely. Common symptoms such as fatigue, nausea, vomiting, breast tenderness, and urinary frequency may reduce the desire for sexual intimacy. However, many people report enhanced sexual desire due to increasing levels of estrogen. Usually sexual satisfaction does not change in pregnancy compared with the prepregnancy patterns despite a decline of sexual activity during the third trimester. A discussion of expected changes in sexuality should be routinely done in order to improve couples' perception of possible sexual modifications induced by pregnancy. It is clear that, despite some difficulties related to sexual activity during pregnancy, its need and importance are recognized for both participants.

 Take Note!

Fluctuations in sexual desire are normal and a highly individualized response throughout pregnancy.

The physical and emotional adjustments of pregnancy can cause changes in body image, fatigue, mood swings, and sexual activity. The client's changing shape, emotional status, fetal activity, changes in breast size, pressure on the bladder, and other common discomforts of pregnancy result in increased physical and emotional demands. These can produce stress on the sexual relationship of the pregnant individual and their partner. However, most will adjust well to the alterations and experience a satisfying sexual relationship. Research indicates that sexual intercourse is safe in the absence of ruptured membranes, bleeding, or placenta previa, but individuals engage in sex less often as the pregnancy progresses (ACOG, 2015f).

Often clients ask whether sexual intercourse is allowed during pregnancy or whether there are specific times when they should refrain from having sex. This is a good opportunity to educate clients about sexual behaviour during pregnancy and also to ask about their expectations and individual experience related to sexuality and possible changes. It is also a good time for nurses to address the impact of the changes associated with pregnancy on sexual desire and behaviour. Couples may enjoy sexual activity more because there is no fear of pregnancy and no need to disrupt spontaneity by using birth control. An increase in pelvic congestion and lubrication secondary to estrogen influence may heighten orgasm. Some individuals have a decrease in desire because of a negative body image, fear of harming the fetus by engaging in intercourse, and fatigue, nausea, and vomiting (Boynton, 2015). A couple may need assistance to adjust to the various changes brought about by pregnancy.

Reassure the client and partner that sexual activity is permissible during pregnancy unless there is a history of any of the following:

- Vaginal bleeding
- Placenta previa
- Risk of preterm labour
- Cervical insufficiency
- Premature rupture of membranes
- Presence of infection (Rigby, 2015)

Inform the couple that the fetus will not be injured by intercourse. Suggest that alternative positions may be more comfortable (e.g., side-lying), especially during the later stages of pregnancy. Some of the physical changes in pregnancy, which can affect a couple's relationship, for example, halitosis which can result from dehydration, but can be alleviated through extra fluids and better oral hygiene. Clients can have breast tissue tenderness and skin changes that can cause them feel unattractive to their partner during pregnancy. In addition, they can be worried about increases in vaginal discharge and need to know what is normal and what can be a sign of infection. Nurses should make clients feel comfortable talking about their fears, encouraging them to take pride in their changing bodies.

Many individuals feel a particular need for closeness during pregnancy, and they should communicate this need to their partner (Halford, Petch, & Creedy, 2015). Emphasize to the couple that closeness and cuddling need not culminate in intercourse, and that other forms of sexual expression, such as mutual masturbation, foot massage, holding hands, kissing, and hugging can be very satisfying (Halford et al., 2015).

Sex in pregnancy is normal. Research suggests that prepregnancy sexuality plays an important role in maintaining sexuality during pregnancy and postpartum (Yildiz, 2015). There are very few proven contraindications and risks to intercourse in low-risk pregnancies, and therefore these clients should be reassured. In pregnancies complicated by placenta previa or an increased risk of preterm labour, the evidence to support abstinence is lacking, but it is a reasonable benign recommendation given the theoretical catastrophic consequences (Yeniel & Petri, 2014).

Clients will experience a myriad of symptoms, feelings, and physical sensations during their pregnancy. Having a satisfying sexual relationship during pregnancy is certainly possible, but it requires honest communication between partners to determine what works best for them and a good relationship with their health care provider to ensure safety (March of Dimes, 2015f).

Employment

For the most part, clients can continue working until giving birth if they have no complications during their pregnancy and the workplace does not present any special hazards (Zolotor & Carlough, 2014). Hazardous occupations include health care workers, daycare providers, laboratory technicians, chemists, painters, hairstylists, veterinary workers, and carpenters (Guidotti, 2014). Jobs requiring strenuous work such as heavy lifting, climbing, carrying heavy objects, and standing for prolonged periods place a pregnant client at risk if modifications are not instituted.

Assess for environmental and occupational factors that place a pregnant client and the fetus at risk for injury. Interview the client about the employment environment. Ask about possible exposure to teratogens (substances with the potential to alter the fetus permanently in form or function) and the physical demands of employment: Are they exposed to temperature extremes? Do they need to stand for prolonged periods in a fixed position? A description of the work environment is important in providing anticipatory guidance to the client. Stress the importance of taking rest periods throughout the day, because constant physically intensive workloads

increase the likelihood of low birth weight and preterm labour and birth (Cunningham et al., 2014).

Because of the numerous physiologic and psychosocial changes that clients experience during their pregnancies, the employer may need to make special accommodations to reduce the risk of hazardous exposures and heavy workloads. The employer may need to provide adequate coverage so that the client can take rest breaks; be removed from any areas where they might be exposed to toxic substances; and avoid work assignments that require heavy lifting, hard physical labour, continuous standing, or constant moving. Some recommendations for working while pregnant are given in Teaching Guidelines 12.3.

Teaching Guidelines 12.3
TEACHING FOR THE CHILDBEARING CLIENT WHO IS WORKING

- Plan to take two 10- to 15-minute breaks within an 8-hour work day.
- Be sure there is a place available for you to rest, preferably in the side-lying position, with a restroom readily available.
- Avoid jobs that require strenuous workloads; if this is not possible, then request a modification of work duties (lighter tasks) to reduce your workload.
- Change your position from standing to sitting or vice versa at least every 2 hours.
- Ensure that you are allowed time off without penalty, if necessary, to ensure a healthy outcome for you and your fetus.
- Make sure the work environment is free of toxic substances.
- Ensure the work environment is smoke-free so passive smoking is not a concern.
- Minimize heavy lifting if associated with bending.

Travel

Pregnancy does not curtail the ability to travel in a car or in a plane. However, following a few safety guidelines can minimize the risk to themselves and their fetuses. According to SOGC (2019), individuals can travel safely throughout their pregnancy, although the second trimester is perhaps the best time to travel because there is the least chance of complications. Pregnant clients considering international travel should evaluate the problems that could occur during the journey as well as the quality of medical care available at the destination.

A client in the third trimester should be advised to defer overseas travel because of concerns about access to medical care in case of problems such as hypertension, phlebitis, or premature labour (CDC, 2015e). Individuals should be advised to consult with their health care providers before making any travel decisions.

Take Note!

Clinical manifestations that indicate the need for immediate medical attention while travelling are vaginal bleeding, passing tissue or clots, abdominal pain or cramps, contractions, ruptured membranes, excessive leg swelling or pain, headaches, or visual problems (Leggat & Zuckerman, 2015).

Advise clients to be aware of the potential for injuries and traumas related to travelling, and teach them ways to prevent injuries from occurring. Teaching Guidelines 12.4 offers tips for safe travel on planes and to foreign areas.

Teaching Guidelines 12.4
TEACHING TO PROMOTE SAFE TRAVEL ON PLANES AND IN FOREIGN COUNTRIES

- Bring along a copy of the prenatal record if your travel will be prolonged in case there is a medical emergency away from home.
- When travelling abroad, carry a foreign dictionary that includes words or phrases for the most common pregnancy emergencies.
- Travel with at least one companion at all times for personal safety.
- Check with your health care provider before receiving any immunizations necessary for foreign travel; some may be harmful to the fetus.
- When in a foreign country, avoid fresh fruit, vegetables, and local water.
- Avoid any milk that is not pasteurized.
- Eat only meat that is well cooked to avoid exposure to toxoplasmosis.
- Request an aisle seat and walk about the airplane every 2 hours.
- While sitting on long flights, practice calf-tensing exercises to improve circulation to the lower extremities.
- Be aware of typical problems encountered by pregnant travellers, such as fatigue, heartburn, indigestion, constipation, vaginal discharge, leg cramps, urinary frequency, and hemorrhoids.
- Always wear support hose while flying to prevent the development of blood clots.
- Drink plenty of water to keep well hydrated throughout the flight.
- Postpone travel if risks outweigh benefits.

Adapted from American College of Obstetricians and Gynecologists. (2015e). *Travel during pregnancy: FAQ 055*. Retrieved from http://www.acog.org/~/media/for%20patients/faq055.ashx; and Centers for Disease Control and Prevention (CDC). (2015g). *Pregnant travelers*. Retrieved from http://wwwnc.cdc.gov/travel/yellowbook/2014/chapter-8-advising-travelers-with-specific-needs/pregnant-travelers

---

When travelling by car, the major risk is a car accident. Motor vehicle accidents account for more than 50% of all traumas during pregnancy and 82% of fetal deaths occurring during these accidents (Eshaghabadi & Barati, 2015). The impact and momentum can lead to traumatic separation of the placenta from the wall of the uterus. Shock and massive hemorrhage might result. Tips that nurses can offer to promote safety during ground travel include:

- Always wear a three-point seat belt, no matter how short the trip, to prevent ejection or serious injury from collision.
- Apply a nonpadded shoulder strap properly; it should cross between the breasts and over the upper abdomen, above the uterus (Fig. 12.11).
- If no seat belts are available (buses or vans), ride in the back seat of the vehicle.
- Use a lap belt that crosses over the pelvis below the uterus.
- Deactivate the airbag if possible. If you can't, move the seat as far back from the dashboard as possible to minimize impact on the abdomen.
- Never use a cellular phone while driving to prevent distraction.
- Avoid driving when very fatigued in the first and third trimesters.
- Avoid late-night driving, when visibility might be compromised.
- Direct a tilting steering wheel away from the abdomen (CDC, 2015e).

FIGURE 12.11 Proper application of a seat belt during pregnancy.

Immunizations and Medications

Vaccines are among the greatest public health achievements of the 21st century, credited with significant reduction of morbidity and mortality from many diseases caused by bacteria and viruses (Senie, 2014). Ideally, clients should receive all childhood immunizations before conception to protect the fetus from any risk of congenital anomalies. If the client comes for a preconception visit, discuss immunizations such as measles, mumps, and rubella (MMR), hepatitis B, and diphtheria/tetanus (every 10 years); administer them at this time if needed.

The risk to a developing fetus from vaccination of the childbearing person during pregnancy is primarily theoretical. Routine immunizations are not usually indicated during pregnancy. However, no evidence exists of risk from vaccinating pregnant individuals with inactivated virus or bacterial vaccines or toxoids. A number of other vaccines have not been adequately studied, and thus theoretical risks of vaccination must be weighed against the risks of the disease to the client and the fetus (CDC, 2015f).

Take Note!

Advise pregnant clients to avoid live virus vaccines (MMR and varicella), and to avoid becoming pregnant within 1 month of having received one of these vaccines because of the theoretical risk of transmission to the fetus (CDC, 2015f).

The current PHAC guidelines for vaccine administration in pregnancy are highlighted in Box 12.6.

Little is known about the effects of taking most medications during pregnancy. Less than 10% of medications approved by the U.S. FDA since 1980 have enough information to determine their risk for birth defects (CDC, 2015g). Based on this lack of evidence, it is best for childbearing persons not to take any medications during their pregnancy. At the very least, encourage them to discuss with the health care provider their current medications and any herbal remedies they take so that they can learn about any potential risks should they continue to take them during pregnancy. Generally, if the client is taking medicine for seizures, high blood pressure, asthma, or depression, the benefits of continuing the medicine during pregnancy outweigh the risks to the fetus. The safety profile of some medications may change according to the gestational age of the fetus. Embryogenesis is completed by the end of the first trimester, when all fetal organs are complete. Thus, to cause a malformation, fetal drug exposure must occur in the first 12 weeks' gestation (Gadot & Koren, 2015).

The U.S. FDA has developed a system of ranking drugs that appears on drug labels and package inserts. These risk categories are summarized in Box 12.7. Always advise clients to check with the health care provider for guidance.

A common concern of many childbearing persons involves the use of over-the-counter medications and herbal

---

BOX 12.6

PHAC GUIDELINES FOR VACCINE ADMINISTRATION DURING PREGNANCY

Vaccines That Are Recommended in Pregnancy
- Inactivated Influenza Vaccine—in all pregnancies, at any gestation
- Tetanus/diphtheria/pertussis (Tdap)—in all pregnancies, between 27 and 32 weeks' gestation
- Hepatitis B—for those at high risk, as early as possible during the pregnancy

Vaccines That Should Be Considered if Otherwise Indicated, in High-Risk Situations if Potential Benefits Outweigh Risk
- Meningococcal conjugate
- Pneumococcal conjugate or polysaccharide—for post-exposure prophylaxis, delay pre-exposure prophylaxis unless substantial risk
- Inactivated Polio Vaccine (IPV)—if immediate protection is needed
- Hepatitis A
- Inactivated typhoid
- Cholera and traveller's diarrhea
- Japanese encephalitis

Vaccines Contraindicated During Pregnancy
- Influenza (live, attenuated vaccine) nasal spray
- Human papilloma virus (HPV) vaccine
- Measles
- Mumps
- Rubella
- Varicella
- BCG (tuberculosis)
- Oral Typhoid
- Small pox
- Yellow fever

Adapted from Public Health Agency of Canada. (2015). *Canadian immunization guide: Part 3—Vaccination of special populations.* Retrieved from https://www.canada.ca/en/public-health/services/publications/healthy-living/canadian-immunization-guide-part-3-vaccination-specific-populations/page-4-immunization-pregnancy-breastfeeding.html#p3c3t1; and Public Health Agency of Canada. (2018). An Advisory Committee Statement (ACS) National Advisory Committee of Immunization (NACI). *Update on immunization in pregnancy with tetanus toxoid, reduced diphtheria toxoid, and reduced acellular pertussis (Tdap) vaccine.* Retrieved from https://www.canada.ca/content/dam/phac-aspc/documents/services/publications/healthy-living/update-immunization-pregnancy-tdap-vaccine/update-immunization-pregnancy-tdap-vaccine-eng.pdf

---

agents. Many individuals consider these products benign simply because they are available without a prescription (King et al., 2015). Although herbal medications are commonly thought of as "natural" alternatives to other medicines, they can be just as potent as some prescription medications. A major concern about herbal medicine is the lack of consistent potency in the active ingredients in any given batch of product, making it difficult to know the exact strength by reading the label. Also, many herbs contain chemicals that cross the placenta and may cause harm to the fetus.

FDA PREGNANCY RISK CLASSIFICATION OF DRUGS

- *Category A:* These drugs have been tested and found safe during pregnancy. Examples: folic acid, vitamin B_6, and thyroid medicine.
- *Category B:* These drugs have been used frequently during pregnancy and do not appear to cause major birth defects or other fetal problems. Examples: antibiotics, acetamino phen (Tylenol), aspartame (artificial sweetener), famotidine (Pepcid), prednisone (cortisone), insulin, and ibuprofen. (Ibuprofen should not be used after 36 weeks of pregnancy to avoid increased blood loss during parturition and to avoid premature closure of the ductus arterious in the fetus.)
- *Category C:* These drugs are more likely to cause problems and safety studies have not been completed. Examples: prochlorperazine (Compazine), fluconazole (Diflucan), ciprofloxacin (Cipro), and some antidepressants.
- *Category D:* These drugs have clear health risks for the fetus. Examples: alcohol, lithium (treats bipolar disorders), phenytoin (Dilantin); all chemotherapeutic agents used to treat cancer.
- *Category X:* These drugs have demonstrated positive evidence of fetal abnormalities and are contraindicated in those who are or may become pregnant. Examples: Accutane (treats cystic acne), androgens (treat endometriosis), Coumadin (prevents blood clots), antithyroid medications for overactive thyroid; radiation therapy (cancer treatment), Tegison or Soriatane (treats psoriasis), streptomycin (treats tuberculosis); thalidomide (treats insomnia), diethylstilbestrol (DES) (treats menstrual disorders), and organic mercury from contaminated food.

Adapted from King, T. L., Brucker, M. C., Kriebs, J. M., Fahey, J. O., Gegor, C. L., & Varney, H. (2015). *Varney's midwifery* (5th ed.). Burlington, MA: Jones & Bartlett Learning; and Rigby, F. B. (2015). Common pregnancy complaints and questions. *eMedicine.* Retrieved from http://emedicine.medscape.com/article/259724-overview

Nurses are often asked about the safety of over-the-counter medicines and herbal agents. Unfortunately, many drugs have not been evaluated in controlled studies, and it is difficult to make general recommendations for these products. Therefore, encourage pregnant clients to check with their health care provider before taking anything. Questions about the use of over-the-counter and herbal products are part of the initial prenatal interview.

NURSING MANAGEMENT TO PREPARE THE CHILDBEARING PERSON AND THEIR PARTNER FOR LABOUR, BIRTH, AND PARENTHOOD

Pregnancy and birth are unique to every childbearing person. Clients and families hold different expectations during childbearing based on their knowledge, experiences, belief systems, culture, and social and family backgrounds. These differences should be understood and respected by the nurse, and care to them adapted to meet the individual needs of the clients and families. Understanding a person's needs, values, cultural background, preferences, and expectations during childbirth helps nurses to provide high-quality care to them. Childbirth today is a very different experience from childbirth in previous generations. In the past, clients were literally "put to sleep" with anesthetics, and they woke up with a baby. Most clients never remembered the details and had a passive role in childbirth as the physician delivered the newborn. In the 1950s, consumers began to insist on taking a more active role in their health care, and couples desired to be together during the extraordinary event of childbirth. Beginning in the 1970s, the partner or support person remained with the client throughout labour and birth. Partners today want to be seen as individuals who are part of the labouring couple. If the partners are left out, they tend to feel helpless; this can result in a feeling of panic and can put their support for their partner at risk (Schytt & Bergstrom, 2014).

Health beliefs related to pregnancy and childbirth exist in various cultures globally. A person's perception of their own status is critical to their decision-making process, because personal behaviours can significantly alter pregnancy-related risks. Childbearing people of diverse cultures hold a number of beliefs related to diet, behaviour related to prenatal care, and the use of herbs during pregnancy and postnatally. Nurses need to be aware of these cultural beliefs so as to incorporate those into their practices, while those posing a health risk should be discouraged respectfully (M'soka, Mabuza, & Pretorius, 2015).

Childbirth education began because the childbearing population demanded to become more involved in their birthing experience rather than simply turning control over to a health care provider. Nurses played a pivotal role in bringing about this change by providing information and supporting clients and their families, fostering a more active role in preparing for the upcoming birth.

Traditional childbirth education classes focused on developing and practicing techniques for use in managing pain and facilitating the progress of labour. Recently, the focus of this education has broadened: it now encompasses not only preparation for childbirth, but also preparation for breastfeeding, infant care, transition to new parenting roles, relationship skills, family health promotion, and sexuality (Varner, 2015). The term used to describe this broad range of topics is **perinatal education.** Subjects commonly addressed in perinatal education include:

- Anatomy and physiology of reproduction
- Fetal growth and development

- Prenatal exercise
- Physiologic and emotional changes during pregnancy
- Sex during pregnancy
- Infant growth and development
- Nutrition and healthy eating habits during pregnancy
- Teratogens and their impact on the fetus
- Signs and symptoms of labour
- Preparation for labour and birth (for parents, siblings, and other family members)
- Options for birth
- Infant nutrition, including preparation for breastfeeding
- Infant care, including safety, CPR, and first aid
- Family planning (March of Dimes, 2015g)

Childbirth Education Classes

Childbirth education classes teach the childbearing person and their supports about pregnancy, birth, and parenting. The classes are offered in local communities or online and are usually taught by certified childbirth educators. Most childbirth classes support the concept of **natural childbirth** (a birth without pain-relieving medications) so that the childbearing person can be in control throughout the experience as much as possible. The classes differ in their approach to specific comfort techniques and breathing patterns. The three most common childbirth methods are the Lamaze (psychoprophylactic) method, the Bradley (partner-coached childbirth) method, and the Dick-Read (natural childbirth) method.

Lamaze Method

Lamaze is a psychoprophylactic ("mind prevention") method of preparing for labour and birth that promotes the use of specific breathing and relaxation techniques. Dr. Fernand Lamaze, a French obstetrician, popularized this method of childbirth preparation in the 1960s. Lamaze believed that conquering fear through knowledge and support was important. He also believed that the childbearing person needed to alter the perception of suffering during childbirth. This perception change would come about by learning conditioned reflexes that, instead of signaling pain, would signal the work of producing a child, and thus would carry the person through labour awake, aware, and in control of their own body (Lamaze International, 2015). Lamaze felt strongly that all childbearing persons have the right to deliver their babies with minimal or no medication while maintaining their dignity, minimizing their pain, maximizing their self-esteem, and enjoying the miracle of birth.

Lamaze classes include information on toning exercises, relaxation exercises and techniques, and breathing methods for labour. The breathing techniques are used in labour to enhance relaxation and to reduce the client's perception of pain. The goal is for participants to become aware of their own comfortable rate of breathing in order to maintain relaxation and adequate oxygenation of the fetus. The following breathing techniques are an effective attention-focusing strategy to reduce pain:

- *Paced breathing* involves breathing techniques used to decrease stress responses and therefore decrease pain. This type of breathing implies self-regulation by the childbearing person. The person starts off by taking a cleansing breath at the onset and end of each contraction. This cleansing breath symbolizes freeing the mind from worries and concerns. This breath enhances oxygenation and puts them into a relaxed state.
- *Slow-paced breathing* is associated with relaxation and should be half the normal breathing rate (6 to 9 breaths/min). This type of breathing is the most relaxed pattern and is recommended throughout labour. Abdominal or chest breathing may be used. It is generally best to breathe in through the nose and breathe out either through the nose or mouth, whichever is more comfortable for the childbearing person.
- *Modified-paced breathing* can be used for increased work or stress during labour to increase alertness or focus attention or when slow-paced breathing is no longer effective in keeping the labouring person relaxed. The person's respiratory rate increases, but it does not exceed twice their normal rate. Modified-paced breathing is a quiet upper chest breath that is increased or decreased according to the intensity of the contraction. The inhalation and the exhalation are equal. This breathing technique should be practiced during pregnancy for optimal use during labour.
- *Patterned-paced breathing* is similar to modified-paced breathing but with a rhythmic pattern. It uses a variety of patterns, with an emphasis on the exhalation breath at regular intervals. Different patterns can be used, such as 4/1, 6/1, 4/1. A 4/1 rhythm is four upper chest breaths followed by an exhalation (a sighing out of air, like blowing out a candle). Random patterns can be chosen for use as long as the basic principles of rate and relaxation are met.

Couples practice these breathing patterns typically during the last few months of the pregnancy until they feel comfortable using them. Focal points (visual fixation on a designated object), effleurage (light abdominal massage by the client or partner), massage, and imagery (journey of the mind to a relaxing place) are also added to aid in relaxation. From the nurse's perspective, encourage the childbearing person to breathe at a level of comfort that allows them to cope. Always remain quiet during the client's periods of imagery and focal point visualization to avoid breaking their concentration.

Bradley (Partner-Coached) Method

The Bradley method uses various exercises and slow, controlled abdominal breathing to accomplish relaxation. Dr. Robert Bradley, a Denver-based obstetrician, advocated a completely unmedicated labour and birth experience. The Bradley method emphasizes the pleasurable sensations of childbirth, teaching clients to concentrate on these sensations while "turning on" to their own bodies (Bradley Method, 2014). In 1965, Bradley wrote *Husband-Coached Childbirth*, which advocated the active participation of the partner as labour coach.

A childbearing person is conditioned to work in harmony with the body using breath control and deep abdominopelvic breathing to promote general body relaxation during labour. This method stresses that childbirth is a joyful, natural process and emphasizes the partner's involvement during pregnancy, labour, birth, and the early newborn period. Thus, the training techniques are directed toward the coach, not the childbearing person. The coach is educated in massage/comfort techniques to use on the childbearing person throughout the labour and birth process.

Dick-Read Method

In 1944 Grantly Dick-Read, a British obstetrician, wrote *Childbirth Without Fear*. He believed that the attitude of a childbearing person toward the birthing process had a considerable influence on the ease of labour, and he believed that fear is the primary pain-producing agent in an otherwise normal labour. He felt that fear builds a state of tension, creating an antagonistic effect on the labouring muscles of the uterus, which results in pain. A private, undisturbed and dark environment, where client can feel safe can promote the release of oxytocin, the hormone responsible for uterine contractions and though to promote the release of the pain-relieving hormones endorphins. When this is not achieved, clients can experience fear–tension–pain syndrome, impeding labour progress and causing increased levels of pain (Westbury, 2015). Dick-Read sought to interrupt the circular pattern of fear, tension, and pain during the labour and birthing process. He promoted the belief that the degree of fear could be diminished with increased understanding of the normal physiologic response to labour (Alexander et al., 2014).

Dick-Read believed that prenatal instruction was essential for pain relief and that emotional factors during labour interfered with the normal labour progression. The childbearing person achieves relaxation and reduces pain by arming themselves with the knowledge of normal childbirth and using abdominal breathing during contractions.

Nursing Management and Childbirth Education

Childbirth education is less about methods than about mastery. The overall aim of any of the methods is to promote an internal locus of control that will enable each person to yield the body to the process of birth. As the childbearing person gains success and tangible benefits from the exercises taught, they begin to reframe their beliefs and gains practical knowledge, and the impetus will be there to engage in the conscious use of the techniques (Fig. 12.12). Nurses play a key role in supporting and encouraging each couple's use of the techniques taught in childbirth education classes.

Every childbearing person's labour is unique, and it is important for nurses not to generalize or stereotype clients. The most effective support a nurse can offer a couple using prepared childbirth methods is encouragement and presence. These nursing measures must be adapted to each individual throughout the labour process. Offering encouraging phrases such as "great job" or "you can do it" helps to reinforce their efforts and at the same time empowers them to continue. Using eye-to-eye contact to engage the client's total attention is important if they appear overwhelmed or appear to lose control during the transition phase of labour.

Nurses play a significant role in enhancing the couple's relationship by respecting the involvement of the partner and demonstrating concern for their needs throughout labour. Offering to stay with the childbearing

FIGURE 12.12 A couple practicing the techniques taught in a childbirth education class.

person to give the support person a break periodically allows them to meet their needs while at the same time still actively participating. Offer anticipatory guidance to the couple and assist during critical times in labour. Demonstrate many of the coping techniques to the partner and praise their successful use, which increases self-esteem. Focus on their strengths and the positive elements of the labour experience. Congratulating the couple for a job well done is paramount.

Throughout the labour experience, demonstrate personal warmth and project a friendly attitude. Frequently, a nurse's touch may help to prevent a crisis by reassuring the childbearing person that they are doing fine.

Options for Birth Settings and Care Providers

From the moment a person discovers they are pregnant, numerous decisions await them—where the infant will be born, what birth setting is best, and who will assist with the birth. The majority of childbearing persons are well and healthy and can consider the full range of birth settings—hospital, birth centre, or home setting—and care providers. They should be given information about each to ensure the most informed decision.

Birth Settings

HOSPITALS

Hospitals are the most common site for birth, and the only available option in some areas of the country. If the childbearing client has a serious medical condition or is at high risk for developing one, they will probably need to plan to give birth in a hospital setting under the care of an obstetrician. Giving birth in a hospital is advantageous for several reasons. Hospitals are best equipped to diagnose and treat clients and newborns with complications; trained personnel are available if necessary; and no transportation is needed if a complication should

arise during labour or birth. Disadvantages include the high-tech atmosphere; strict policies and restrictions that might limit who can be with the childbearing person; and the medical model of care.

Within the hospital setting, however, choices do exist regarding birth environments. The conventional delivery room resembles an operating room, where the health care professional delivers the newborn from the client, who may be positioned in stirrups. The client is then transferred to the recovery area on a stretcher and then again to the postpartum unit. The birthing suite is the other option within the hospital setting. In the birthing suite, the childbearing client and partner remain in one place for labour, birth, and recovery. The birthing suite is a private room decorated to look as homelike as possible. For example, the bed converts to allow for various birthing positions, and there may be a rocking chair or an easy chair for the support person. Despite the homey atmosphere, the room is still equipped with emergency resuscitative obstetric equipment and electronic fetal monitors in case they are needed quickly (Fig. 12.13A). Such settings provide a more personal childbirth experience in a less formal and intimidating atmosphere compared to the traditional delivery room.

FREESTANDING BIRTH CENTRE

A freestanding birth centre offers the childbearing person and family a comfortable setting where they can receive maternity care with appropriate levels of intervention. A freestanding birth centre (Fig. 12.13B) can be a good choice for a client who wants more personalized care than in a hospital but does not feel comfortable with a home birth. In contrast to the institutional environment in hospitals, most freestanding birth centres have a homelike atmosphere, and many are, in fact, located in converted homes. Some are located on hospital property and are affiliated with them. Birth centres are designed to provide maternity care to clients judged to be at low risk for

FIGURE 12.13 **A.** Birthing suite in hospital setting. **B.** Childbirth room in birthing centre.

obstetric complications. Clients are allowed and encouraged to give birth in the position most comfortable for them. Care in birth centres is often provided by midwives and is more relaxed, with no routine intravenous lines, fetal monitoring, and restrictive protocols. A disadvantage of the birth centre is the need to transport the client to a hospital quickly if an emergency arises, because emergency equipment is not readily available. In a research study comparing homelike to conventional institutional settings, the author concluded that there appeared to be some benefits from homelike settings for childbirth, although increased support from caregivers may be more important (Alliman, Jolles, & Summers, 2015).

HOME BIRTHS

A planned, midwife attended home birth for a healthy low risk childbearing person is a physically, culturally, spiritually, and emotionally safe option for childbearing families and is associated with fewer obstetrical interventions with no increase to perinatal mortality or morbidity compared to planned in hospital births (Canadian Association of Midwives, 2013). Most clients who choose a home birth believe that birth is a natural process that requires little medical intervention (Lewis, 2015). Research has shown that clients believe that planned home births increase privacy, comfort, and convenience; are associated with reduced rates of medical interventions; and facilitate family involvement in a relaxed, peaceful atmosphere (Budin, 2015).

Home births require qualified, experienced birth attendants and an emergency transfer system in place in case of serious complications. Many clients choose the home setting out of a strong desire to control their child's birth and to give birth surrounded by family members. Most home birth caregivers are midwives who have provided continuous care to the childbearing person throughout the pregnancy. Disadvantages include the need to transport the client to the hospital during or after labour if a problem arises, and the limited pain management available in the home setting.

Care Providers

The type of care provider available to the childbearing person and family varies across Canadian communities. Currently, the childbearing person may receive care during the prenatal, birth, and postpartum period from an obstetrician, a family practice physician, or a midwife. The difference is a matter of degrees and specialization. Obstetricians must finish a 4-year residency in obstetrics and gynecology in addition to medical school. Midwives must complete a 4-year baccalaureate midwifery education program, pass the national Canadian midwifery registration exam, and be registered with their respective provincial or territorial college (Canadian Association of Midwives, 2017b). Midwives usually care for low-risk

clients in a variety of settings. They are able to write prescriptions, provide prenatal care, childbirth care, postpartum care, and newborn care. Family practice physicians who maintain a practice in obstetrics also provide low risk prenatal, intrapartum, and well-baby care. Many deliver their clients' newborns in the hospital or birthing centres. Obstetricians can handle high-risk pregnancies and delivery emergencies; can administer or order pain-relief drugs; and are assisted by a support staff in the hospital setting. Midwives work in hospitals, birthing centres, and home settings to deliver care. They believe in the normalcy of birth and tolerate wide variations of what is considered normal during labour, which leads to fewer interventions applied during the childbirth process. Family physicians who maintain a practice in obstetrics are able to provide continuity of care throughout the life span, which includes the birth of newborns in hospital. They can attend to the full scope of needs within their family practice, and sometimes work in shared care arrangements for clients with additional risk factors or comorbidities.

In addition to the childbearing person's primary health care provider, some will hire a doula to be with them during the childbearing process. *Doula* is a Greek word that means "woman's servant." A doula is a layperson trained to provide childbearing families with encouragement, emotional and physical support, and information through late pregnancy, labour, birth, and postpartum. Doulas provide the client with continuous support throughout labour but do not perform any clinical procedures.

Preparation for Infant Feeding

Childbearing clients are faced with a decision about which method of feeding to choose. Educate the client about the advantages and disadvantages of each method, allowing the childbearing family to make an informed decision about the best method for their situation. Providing this information will increase the likelihood of a successful experience regardless of the method of feeding chosen. As part of health promotion/evidence-based interventions, nurses should be encouraging and educating all childbearing persons about the benefits associated with breastfeeding.

Breastfeeding

Substantial scientific evidence exists documenting the health benefits of breastfeeding for newborns. Current evidence cited by the Canadian Pediatric Society (CPS) reports that breastfeeding is protective against childhood obesity, gastrointestinal and respiratory infective illnesses, it reduces risk of breast and ovarian cancer among the breastfeeding individual (Critch, 2014). The American Academy of Pediatrics furthers that there are improved outcomes for breastfed infants with regard to otitis media, atopic dermatitis, childhood asthma, type 1 and type 2 diabetes, childhood leukemia, sudden infant death syndrome, and cognitive development (2012). The CPS recommends that infants be breastfed exclusively until the age 6 months, and continue to be breastfed for up to 2 years and beyond, with complimentary nutrition, as it is mutually desired (Critch, 2014). In addition, a lack of breastfeeding has a negative impact on the health care system by increasing the number of client visits, hospital admissions, rate of obesity, and health care costs. Most researchers agree that the duration of breastfeeding is inversely associated with overweight risk. Breastfeeding is a cost-effective, natural, and effective prevention strategy for reducing childhood obesity. A recent study from the United States estimates that $13 billion a year would be saved and 1,000 deaths prevented each year if 90% of infants in the United States were exclusively breastfed until 6 months (Office on Women's Health, 2014).

Human milk provides an ideal balance of nutrients for newborns (ACOG, 2015h). Breastfeeding is advantageous for the following reasons:

- Human milk is digestible and economical and requires no preparation.
- Infant bonding and attachment is promoted.
- Cost is less than purchasing formula.
- Ovulation is suppressed (however, this is not a reliable birth control method).
- The risk of ovarian cancer and the incidence of premenopausal breast cancer are reduced.
- Extra calories are used, which promotes weight loss gradually without dieting.
- Oxytocin is released to promote more rapid uterine involution with less bleeding.
- Sucking helps to develop the muscles in the infant's jaw.
- Absorption of lactose and minerals in the newborn is improved.
- The immunologic properties of breast milk help prevent infections in the baby.
- The composition of breast milk adapts to meet the infant's changing needs.
- Constipation in the baby is not a problem with adequate intake.
- Food allergies are less likely to develop in the breastfed baby.
- The incidence of otitis media and upper respiratory infections in the infant is reduced.
- Breastfed babies are less likely to be overfed, thus reducing the risk of adult obesity.
- Breastfed newborns are less prone to vomiting (American Academy of Family Physicians [2015]; AAP [2015]; ACOG [2015h]; Women, Infant, & Children [WIC], 2015).

One could say that lactation and breastfeeding are so natural that they should just happen on their own accord, but this is not the case. Learning to breastfeed takes practice, requires support from the partner, and requires dedication and patience; it may be necessary to work closely with a lactation consultant to be successful and comfortable when breastfeeding (Fig. 12.14 shows the different positions that may be used for breastfeeding). Nurses can encourage breastfeeding except for those who are HIV+, and are untreated, have active tuberculosis, use illicit drugs, or take prescribed cancer chemotherapeutic agents.

Breastfeeding also has some side effects. These include breast discomfort, sore nipples, mastitis, engorgement, milk stasis, vaginal dryness, and decreased libido (Alekseev, Vladimir, & Nadezhda, 2015). The most common cause of nipple pain is an improper latch and such discomfort is piercing, immediate and short lived, typically occurring as soon as the baby starts nursing and gradually subsiding during the feeding. Some individuals feel it is inconvenient or embarrassing, limits other activities, limits partner involvement, increases their dependency by being tied to the infant all the time, and restricts their use of alcohol or drugs. Nurses can help clients to cope with their fear of dependency and feelings of obligation by emphasizing the positive aspects of breastfeeding and encouraging bonding experiences. Nurses can be instrumental in helping clients prepare and continue to breastfeed after they return to work.

PREPARATION FOR BREASTFEEDING

Nipple preparation is not necessary during the prenatal period unless the nipples are inverted and do not become erect when stimulated. Assess for this by placing the forefinger and thumb above and below the areola and compressing behind the nipple. If it flattens or inverts, advise the client to wear breast shields during the last 2 months of pregnancy. Breast shields exert a continuous pressure around the areola, pushing the nipple through a central opening in the inner shield (La Leche League International, 2016). The shields are worn inside the bra. Initially the shields are worn for 1 hour, and then the client progressively increases the wearing time up to 8 hours daily. The client maintains this schedule until after childbirth, and then wears the shield 24 hours a day until the infant latches on easily (La Leche League International, 2016). In addition, suggest that the client wear a supportive nursing bra, 24 hours a day.

Encourage the client to request a certified lactation consultant (IBCLC) at the hospital, if giving birth there. Lactation consultants are health care providers who specialize in the clinical management of breastfeeding and lactation and are certified by the International Board of Lactation Consultant Examiners. Some run their own breastfeeding support groups as well. In addition, suggest that the client attend a breastfeeding support group (e.g., La Leche League), provide sources of information about infant feeding, and suggest reading a good reference book about lactation. All of these activities will help in the decision-making process and will be invaluable

FIGURE 12.14 Positions for breastfeeding: cradle (**A**), cross-cradle (**B**), clutch or football (**C**), side-lying (**D**), and laid-back (**E**). (From *Lippincott Procedures*.)

supports for breastfeeding success. Clients returning to work can pump their milk while working and store the milk in the refrigerator or freezer for future use.

Bottle Feeding

Recent research indicates that infants who are fed formula within the first 6 months do have an increased incidence of otitis media, diabetes, asthma, atopic dermatitis, reflux, diarrhea, colic, constipation, and lower respiratory infections (Schram, 2014). It is important to inform childbearing families of this.

Bottle feeding an infant is not just a matter of "open, pour, and feed." Families need information on types of formulas, preparation and storage of formula, equipment, and feeding positions. It is recommended that normal full-term infants receive conventional cow's milk-based formula; the physician should direct this choice. If the infant has a reaction (diarrhea, vomiting, abdominal pain, excessive gas) to the first formula, another formula should be tried. Sometimes a soy-based formula is substituted. In terms of preparation of formula and its use, the following guidelines should be stressed:

- Obtain adequate equipment (six 4-oz bottles, eight 8-oz bottles, and nipples).
- Consistency is important. Stay with a nipple that is comfortable to the infant.
- Frequently assess nipples for any loose pieces of rubber at the opening.
- Correct formula preparation is critical to the health and development of the infant. Formula is available in three forms: ready-to-feed, concentrate, and powder.
- Read the formula label thoroughly before mixing.
- Correct formula dilution is important to avoid fluid imbalances. For ready-to-use formula, use as is without dilution. For concentrated formulas, dilute with equal parts of water. For powdered formulas, mix one scoop of powder with 2 oz of water.
- If the water supply is safe, sterilization is not necessary.
- Bottles and nipples should be washed in hot, sudsy water using a bottle brush.
- Formula should be served at room temperature.
- If the water supply is questionable, water should be boiled for 5 minutes before use.
- Formula should not be heated in a microwave oven, because it is heated unevenly.
- Formula can be prepared 24 hours ahead of time and stored in the refrigerator.

Teach the family to feed the infant in a semi-upright position using the cradle hold in the arms. This position allows for face-to-face contact between the infant and caretaker. Advise the caretaker to hold the bottle so that the nipple is kept full of formula to prevent excessive air swallowing. Instruct the caretaker to feed the infant every 3 to 4 hours based on infant cues, and adapt the feeding times to the infant's needs. Frequent burping of the infant (every ounce) helps prevent gas from building up in the stomach. Caution the caretaker not to prop the bottle; propping the bottle can cause choking.

Bottle feeding should mirror breastfeeding as closely as possible. While nutrition is important, so are the emotional and interactive components of feeding. Encourage the caretaker to cuddle the infant closely and position the infant with the baby's head is in a comfortable position. Also encourage communication with the infant during feedings. Nurses should know the different types of formulas available to provide advice to mothers who have made the informed choice not to breastfeed or want to supplement or stop breastfeeding.

Take Note!

Warn the caretaker about the danger of putting the infant to bed with a bottle. This can lead to "baby bottle tooth decay" (nursing caries) because sugars in the formula stay in contact with the infant's developing teeth for prolonged periods.

Final Preparation for Labour and Birth

The nurse has played a supportive/education role for the childbearing family throughout the pregnancy and now needs to assist in preparing them for their "big event" by making sure they have made informed decisions and completed the following checklist:

- Attended childbirth preparation classes and practiced breathing techniques
- Selected a birth setting and made arrangements there
- Know what to expect during labour and birth
- Toured the birthing facility
- Packed a suitcase to take to the birthing facility when labour starts
- Made arrangements to have siblings and/or pets taken care of during labour
- Been instructed on signs and symptoms of labour and what to do
- Know what to do if membranes rupture prior to going into labour
- Know how to reach their health care provider when labour starts
- Communicated their needs and desires concerning pain management
- Discussed the possibility of a cesarean birth if complications occur
- Discussed possible names for the newborn
- Selected a feeding method (breast or bottle) with which they feel comfortable
- Have had the opportunity to discuss male infant circumcision
- Purchased an infant safety car seat in which to bring their newborn home

- Have items needed to prepare for the newborn's home-coming:
  - Infant clothes in several sizes
  - Nursing bras
  - Infant crib with spaces between the slats that are 2 in or less apart
  - Diapers (cloth or disposable)
  - Feeding supplies (bottles and nipples if bottle feeding)
  - Infant thermometer
- Selected a family planning method to use after the birth

At each prenatal visit the nurse has had the opportunity to discuss and reinforce the importance of being prepared for the birth of the child with the childbearing family. It is now up to the family to use the nurse's guidance and put it into action to be ready for the upcoming birth.

A recent national survey entitled *Listening to Mothers III: Pregnancy and Birth* revealed concerns about over-use of maternity care practices and women's readiness to make informed decisions. Key findings point to the need for quality improvement, consumer engagement, and shared decision making (Declercq, Sakala, Corry, Applebaum, & Herrlick, 2014). These findings present a challenge for all nurses caring for maternity clients to thoroughly explain all procedures, along with their rationales, and truly listen to what the client desires to make the childbirth experience outcome a positive one.

All nurses have the responsibility to impart their knowledge to all childbearing clients and their families—and that starts with teaching themselves first. The evidence is clear that clients have better outcomes when nurses intervene only when needed in the childbirth process. Nurses need to personalize their care to every childbearing person based on their needs, desires, and state of health. Nurses must focus on teaching clients and their families to understand the value of birth and its long-lasting effects on the family. In addition, women nurses must provide birth settings that are safe, whether in the hospital, birth centre, or at home. This includes, but is not limited to, providing continuous support in labour, allowing clients the freedom to move and assume positions of choice, offering nourishment of the client's body and spirit, using nonpharmacologic pain relief modalities whenever possible, and ensuring seamless, collaborative teamwork. Continuous labour support is a nonpharmacologic, evidence-based strategy associated with reduced cesarean rates (Baum, Crawford, & Humphrey-Shelton, 2015).

NURSING CARE PLAN 12.1

Overview of the Childbearing Person Experiencing Common Discomforts of Pregnancy

Alicia, a 32-year-old, G1 P0, at 10 weeks' gestation, comes to the clinic for a visit. During the interview Alicia tells you, "I'm running to the bathroom to urinate it seems like all the time, and I'm so nauseous that I'm having trouble eating." Alicia denies any burning or pain on urination. Vital signs are within acceptable limits.

NURSING DIAGNOSIS: Impaired urinary elimination related to frequency secondary to physiologic changes of pregnancy

Outcome Identification and Evaluation

The client will report a decrease in urinary complaints, as evidenced by a decrease in the number of times they use the bathroom to void, reports feeling that the bladder is empty after voiding, and use of Kegel exercises.

Interventions: *Promoting Normal Urinary Elimination Patterns*

- Assess client's usual bladder elimination patterns to establish a baseline for comparison.
- Obtain a urine specimen for analysis to rule out infection or glucosuria.
- Review with client the physiologic basis for the increased frequency during pregnancy; inform client that frequency should abate during the second trimester and that it most likely will return during the third trimester. This will promote understanding of the problem.
- Encourage the client to empty the bladder when first feeling a sensation of fullness to minimize risk of urinary retention.
- Suggest client avoid caffeinated drinks, which can stimulate the need to void.

NURSING CARE PLAN 12.1

Overview of the Childbearing Person Experiencing Common Discomforts of Pregnancy (continued)

- Encourage client to drink adequate amounts of fluid throughout the day; however, have client reduce fluid intake before bedtime to reduce nighttime urination.
- Urge client to keep perineal area clean and dry to prevent irritation and excoriation from any leakage.

- Instruct client in Kegel exercises to increase perineal muscle tone and control over leakage.
- Teach client about the signs and symptoms of urinary tract infection and encourage seeking medical assistance should they occur to ensure early detection and prompt intervention.

NURSING DIAGNOSIS: Imbalanced nutrition: less than body requirements, related to nausea and vomiting

Outcome Identification and Evaluation

The client will ingest adequate amounts of nutrients for both client and fetal well-being as evidenced by acceptable weight gain pattern and statements indicating an increase in food intake with a decrease in the number of episodes of nausea and vomiting.

Interventions: *Promoting Adequate Nutrition*

1. Obtain weight and compare to baseline to determine effects of nausea and vomiting on nutritional intake.
2. Review client's typical dietary intake over 24 hours to determine nutritional intake and patterns so that suggestions can be individualized.
3. Encourage client to eat five or six small frequent meals throughout the day to prevent the stomach from becoming empty.
4. Suggest that the client munch on dry crackers, toast, cereal, or cheese or drink a small amount of lemonade before arising to minimize nausea.
5. Encourage client to arise slowly from bed in the morning and avoid sudden movements to reduce stimulation of the vomiting centre.
6. Advise client to drink fluids between meals rather than with meals to avoid overdistention of the abdomen and subsequent increase in abdominal pressure.
7. Encourage the client to increase the intake of foods high in vitamin B_6 such as meat, poultry, bananas, fish, green leafy vegetables, peanuts, raisins, walnuts, and whole grains, as tolerated, to ensure adequate nutrient intake.
8. Advise the client to avoid greasy, fried, or highly spiced foods and to avoid strong odours, including foods such as cabbage, to minimize gastrointestinal upset.
9. Encourage the client to avoid wearing tight or restricting clothes to minimize pressure on the expanding abdomen.
10. Arrange for consultation with nutritionist as necessary to assist with diet planning.

KEY CONCEPTS

- Preconception care is the promotion of the health and well-being of a childbearing person and their family before pregnancy. The goal of preconception care is to identify any areas such as health problems, lifestyle behaviours, or social concerns that might unfavourably affect pregnancy.

- A thorough history and physical examination are performed on the initial prenatal visit.

- A primary aspect of nursing management during the antepartum period is counselling and educating the childbearing person and their partner to promote healthy outcomes for all involved.

- Nagele rule can be used to establish the estimated date of birth. Using this rule, subtract 3 months from the month of their last LMP, add 7 days to the first day of the last normal menstrual period, then correct the year by adding 1 to it. This date is within plus or minus 2 weeks (margin of error).

- Pelvic shape is typically classified as one of four types: gynecoid, android, anthropoid, and platypelloid. The gynecoid type is the most common and offers the best shape for a vaginal delivery.

- Continuous prenatal care is important for a successful outcome. The recommended schedule is every 4 weeks up to 28 weeks (7 months); every 2 weeks from 29 to 36 weeks; and every week from 37 weeks to birth.

- The height of the fundus is measured when the uterus arises out of the pelvis to evaluate fetal growth.

- The fundus reaches the level of the umbilicus at approximately 20 weeks and measures 20 cm. The fundal measurement should approximately equal the number of weeks of gestation until week 36.

- At each visit the childbearing person is asked whether they are having any common signs or symptoms of preterm labour, which might include uterine contractions, dull backache, pressure in the pelvic area or thighs, increased vaginal discharge, menstrual-like cramps, and vaginal bleeding.

- Prenatal screening has become standard in prenatal care to detect neural tube defects and genetic abnormalities.

- The nurse should address matter of factly common discomforts that occur in each trimester at all prenatal visits and should provide realistic measures to help the client deal with them effectively.

- The pregnant client can better care for themselves and the fetus if their concerns are anticipated by the nurse and incorporated into guidance sessions at each prenatal visit.

- Iron and folic acid need to be supplemented because their increased requirements during pregnancy are usually too great to be met through diet alone.

- Throughout pregnancy, a well-balanced diet is critical for a healthy baby.

- Perinatal education has broadened its focus to include preparation for pregnancy and family adaptation to the new parenting roles. Childbirth education began because of increasing pressure from consumers who wanted to become more involved in their birthing experience.

- Three common childbirth education methods are Lamaze (psychoprophylactic), Bradley (partner-coached childbirth), and Dick-Read (natural childbirth).

- The great majorities of childbearing persons are well and healthy and can consider the full range of birth settings: hospital, birth centre, or home setting.

- All pregnant clients need to be able to recognize early signs of contractions to prevent preterm labour.

REFERENCES AND RECOMMENDED READINGS

Akolekar, R., Beta, J., Picciarelli, G., Ogilvie, C., & D'Antonio, F. (2015). Procedure-related risk of miscarriage following amniocentesis and chorionic villus sampling: A systematic review and meta-analysis. *Ultrasound in Obstetrics & Gynecology, 45*(1), 16–26.

Alekseev, N. P., Vladimir, I. I., & Nadezhda, T. E. (2015). Pathological postpartum breast engorgement: Prediction, prevention, and resolution. *Breastfeeding Medicine, 10*(4), 203–208.

Alexander, L. L., LaRosa, J. H., Bader, H., & Garfield, S. (2014). *New dimensions in women's health* (6th ed.). Sudbury, MA: Jones & Bartlett.

Alfirevic, Z., Stampalija, T., & Medley N. (2015). Fetal and umbilical Doppler ultrasound in normal pregnancy. *Cochrane Database of Systematic Reviews,* (4), CD001450.

Alliman, J., Jolles, D., & Summers, L. (2015). The innovation imperative: Scaling freestanding birth centers, centering pregnancy, and midwifery-led maternity health homes. *Journal of Midwifery & Women's Health, 60*(3), 244–249.

Almansa, C., DeVault, K., & Houghton, L. A. (2015). Gas and bloating. In *Functional and motility disorders of the gastrointestinal tract* (pp. 113–123). New York: Springer Publishers.

American Academy of Family Physicians. (2015). *Summary of recommendations for clinical preventive services.* Retrieved from http://www.aafp.org/dam/AAFP/documents/patient_care/clinical_recommendations/cps-recommendations.pdf

American Academy of Pediatrics (AAP). (2012). Breastfeeding and the use of human milk. *Pediatrics, 129*(3), 827–841.

American Academy of Pediatrics. (2015). *Breastfeeding.* Retrieved from https://www2.aap.org/breastfeeding/index.html

American College of Nurse-Midwives. (2015). *About midwives.* Retrieved from http://www.midwife.org/About-Midwives

American College of Obstetricians & Gynecologists (ACOG). (2013). *Oral health care during pregnancy and through the lifespan.* Retrieved from http://www.acog.org/Resources-And-Publications/Committee-Opinions/Committee-on-Health-Care-for-Underserved-Women/Oral-Health-Care-During-Pregnancy-and-Through-the-Lifespan

American College of Obstetricians and Gynecologists (ACOG). (2015a). *Routine tests in pregnancy FAQ 133.* Retrieved from http://www.acog.org/For_Patients/Search_FAQs?Topics=906bff1e-0656-4579-a7df-4a22f9bce483&pipe;fb741a4b-41f7-4b37-8307-f4844738b26f

American College of Obstetricians and Gynecologists (ACOG). (2015b). *Screening tests for birth defects*. Retrieved from http://www.acog.org/~/media/For%20Patients/faq165.pdf?dmc=1&ts=20140517T0925037578

American College of Obstetricians and Gynecologists (ACOG). (2015c). *Easing back pain during pregnancy*. Retrieved from http://www.acog.org/~/media/For%20Patients/faq115.pdf?dmc=1&ts=20140517T1536210126

American College of Obstetricians and Gynecologists (ACOG). (2015d). *Problems of the digestive system*. Retrieved from http://www.acog.org/~/media/For%20Patients/faq120.pdf?dmc=1&ts=20140518T1321141397

American College of Obstetricians & Gynecologists (ACOG). (2015e). *Exercise during pregnancy*. Retrieved from https://www.acog.org/Search?Keyword=exercise+guidelines

American College of Obstetricians & Gynecologists (ACOG). (2015f). *Sexuality and sexual problems*. Retrieved from http://pause.acog.org/topics/sexuality-and-sexual-problems

American College of Obstetricians & Gynecologists (ACOG). (2015g). *Travel during pregnancy*. Retrieved from http://www.acog.org/~/media/For%20Patients/faq055.pdf?dmc=1&ts=20140519T1526511729

American College of Obstetricians & Gynecologists (ACOG). (2015h). *Breastfeeding your baby*. Retrieved from http://www.acog.org/~/media/For%20Patients/faq029.pdf?dmc=1&ts=20140520T0943394126

American Diabetes Association (ADA). (2015). Classification and diagnosis of diabetes. *Diabetes Care, 38*(Suppl 1), S8–S16.

American Pregnancy Association (APA). (2014a). *Maternal serum alpha-fetoprotein screening (MSAFP)*. Retrieved from http://americanpregnancy.org/prenataltesting/afp.html

American Pregnancy Association (APA). (2014b). *Pregnancy exercise guidelines*. Retrieved from http://americanpregnancy.org/pregnancyhealth/exerciseguidelines.html

Anil, S., Alrowis, R. M., Chalisserry, E. P., Chalissery, V. P., AlMoharib, H. S., & Al-Sulaimani, A. F. (2015). Oral health and adverse pregnancy outcomes. In *Emerging trends in oral health sciences and dentistry*. (pp. 631–662). Retrieved from http://dx.doi.org/10.5772/59517

Barakat, R., Lucía, A., & Ruiz, J. (2015). Exercise and pregnancy. In M. L. Mountjoy (Ed.). *Handbook of sports medicine and science: The female athlete*. Hoboken, NJ, USA: John Wiley & Sons, Inc.

Baum, A., Crawford, P., & Humphrey-Shelton, M. (2015). Clinical inquiry: Does the presence of a trained support person during labor decrease C-section rates? *The Journal of Family Practice, 64*(3), 192–193.

Berger, H., Gagnon, R., & Sermer, M. (2016). Diabetes in pregnancy. *Journal of Obstetrics and Gynecology Canada, 38*(7), 667–679.

Biswas, A., & Choolani, M. (2015). Prenatal diagnosis of chromosomal abnormalities—shifting paradigm. *Annals of the Academy of Medicine, Singapore, 44*(2), 40–42.

Boggess, K. A., & Berggren, E. K. (2015). Preconception care has the potential for a high return on investment. *American Journal of Obstetrics & Gynecology, 212*(1), A1–A20.

Bond, S. (2015). American College of Obstetricians and Gynecologists releases committee opinion on estimation of due date. *Journal of Midwifery & Women's Health, 60*(2), 220–224.

Bope, E. T., & Kellerman, R. D. (2015). *Conn's current therapy 2015*. Philadelphia, PA: Saunders Elsevier.

Boynton, P. M. (2015). Pregnancy: Relationships advice. *The International Encyclopedia of Human Sexuality*, 861–1042.

Bradley Method. (2014). *Introduction to the Bradley method*. Retrieved from http://www.bradleybirth.com

Brown, H. L. (2015). ACOG guidelines at a glance: Antepartum fetal surveillance. Contemporary OB/GYN. Retrieved from http://contemporaryobgyn.modernmedicine.com/contemporary-obgyn/news/acog-guidelines-glance-antepartum-fetal-surveillance?page = full

Budin, W. C. (2015). Choosing wisely for birth. *The Journal of Perinatal Education, 24*(1), 3–5.

Butt, K., & Lim, K. (2014). Determination of gestational age by ultrasound. *Journal of Obstetrics and Gynecology Canada, 36*(2), 171–181.

Callahan, T. L. (2016). *Tarascon Ob/Gyn Pocketbook*. Burlington, MA: Jones & Bartlett Learning.

Callegari, L. S., Ma, E. W., & Schwarz, E. B. (2015). Preconception care and reproductive planning in primary care. *Medical Clinics of North America, 99*(3), 663–682.

Campbell, K., Rowe, H., Azzam, H., & Lane, C.A. (2016). The management of nausea and vomiting of pregnancy. *Journal of Obstetrics and Gynaecology Canada, 38*(12), 1127–1137. doi: 10.1016/j.jogc.2016.08.009

Canadian Association of Midwives (2013). *Position statement on home birth*. Retrieved from https://canadianmidwives.org/wp-content/uploads/2016/06/CAMACSF-HomeBirthPS-FINAL-2013ENG.pdf

Canadian Association of Midwives (2017a). *Midwifery education*. Retrieved from https://canadianmidwives.org/education/

Canadian Association of Midwives (2017b). *Midwifery regulation*. Retrieved from https://canadianmidwives.org/midwifery-regulation/

Centers for Disease Control and Prevention (CDC). (2015a). *Preconception care and health care*. Retrieved from http://www.cdc.gov/preconception/hcp/

Centers for Disease Control and Prevention (CDC). (2015b). *Preconception care recommendations*. Retrieved from http://www.cdc.gov/preconception/hcp/recommendations.html

Centers for Disease Control and Prevention (CDC). (2015c). *Facts about birth defects*. Retrieved from http://www.cdc.gov/ncbddd/birthdefects/facts.html

Centers for Disease Control and Prevention (CDC). (2015d). *Pregnancy complications*. Retrieved from http://www.cdc.gov/reproductivehealth/MaternalInfantHealth/PregComplications.htm#n5

Centers for Disease Control and Prevention (CDC). (2015e). *Pregnant travelers*. Retrieved from http://wwwnc.cdc.gov/travel/yellowbook/2014/chapter-8-advising-travelers-with-specific-needs/pregnant-travelers

Centers for Disease Control and Prevention (CDC). (2015f). *Vaccines for pregnant women*. Retrieved from http://www.cdc.gov/vaccines/adults/rec-vac/pregnant.html

Centers for Disease Control and Prevention (CDC). (2015g). *Mediations and pregnancy*. Retrieved from http://www.cdc.gov/pregnancy/meds/

Critch, J. N. (2014). Nutrition for healthy term infants, six to 24 months: An overview. *Pediatrics & Child Health, 19*(10), 547–549. Retrieved from https://www.cps.ca/en/documents/position/nutrition-healthy-term-infants-6-to-24-months

Cunningham, F., Leveno, K., Bloom, S., Spong, K., Dashe, J. S., Hoffman, B. L., … Sheffield, J. S. (2014). *Williams obstetrics* (24th ed.). New York: McGraw-Hill Education.

Darmstadt, G. L., Shiffman, J., & Lawn, J. E. (2015). Advancing the newborn and stillbirth global agenda: Priorities for the next decade. *Archives of Disease in Childhood, 100*(Suppl 1), S13–S18.

Declercq, E. R., Sakala, C., Corry, M. P., Applebaum, S., & Herrlich, A. (2014). Major survey findings of listening to mothers (SM) III: New mothers speak out: Report of national surveys of women's childbearing experiences conducted October 2102 and January-April 2013. *Journal of Perinatal Education. Winter, 23*(1), 17–24. doi: 10.1891/1058-1243.23.1.17

Declercq, E., & Stotland, N. E. (2015). Planned home birth. *UpToDate.* Retrieved from http://www.uptodate.com. ksclib.keene.edu/contents/planned-homebirth?source = search_result&search = planned+home+birth&selectedTit le = 1~150

Dempsey, Á. C., & Overton, T. G. (2015). Advances in fetal therapy. *Obstetrics, Gynecology & Reproductive Medicine. 25*(7), 203–207.

Dietz, W. H. (2015). The response of the US Centers for Disease Control and Prevention to the obesity epidemic. *Annual Review of Public Health, 36,* 575–596.

Eshaghabadi, A., & Barati, P. (2015). P97: Motor vehicle accident during the pregnancy. *The Neuroscience Journal of Shefaye Khatam, 2*(4), 147–147.

Evans, M. I., Andriole, S., & Evans, S. M. (2015). Genetics: Update on prenatal screening and diagnosis. *Obstetrics and Gynecology Clinics of North America, 42*(2), 193–208.

Everett, T. R., & Peebles, D. M. (2015). Antenatal tests of fetal wellbeing. In *Seminars in fetal and neonatal medicine.* WB Saunders.

Farrar, D., Duley, L., Medley, N., & Lawlor D. A. (2015). Different strategies for diagnosing gestational diabetes to improve maternal and infant health. *Cochrane Database of Systematic Reviews, 1,* CD007122.

Feig, D. S., Berger, H., Donovan, L., Godbout, A., Kader, T., Keely, E., & Sanghera, R. (2018). 2018 Clinical practice guidelines. Diabetes and pregnancy. *Canadian Journal of Diabetes,42,* S255–S282.

Ferri, F. F. (2014). *Ferri's best test: A practical guide to laboratory medicine and diagnostic imaging* (3rd ed.). Philadelphia, PA: Elsevier Health Sciences.

Fischbach, F., & Dunning, M. B. (2014). *A manual of laboratory and diagnostic tests.* (9th ed.). Philadelphia, PA: Lippincott Williams & Wilkins.

Fretts, R. C. (2014). Evaluation of decreased fetal movements. *UpToDate.* Retrieved from http://www.uptodate.com/contents/evaluation-of-decreased-fetal-movements

Gadot, Y., & Koren, G. (2015). Medications in pregnancy: Can we treat the mother while protecting the unborn? In *Optimizing treatment for children in the developing world* (pp. 65–70). Springer International Publishing.

Grant, N., Strevens, H., & Thornton, J. (2015). Physiology of labor. In *Epidural labor analgesia* (pp. 1–10). Springer International Publishing.

Greeley, E. T., Kessler, K. A., & Vohra, N. (2015). Clinical applications of noninvasive prenatal testing. *Journal of Fetal Medicine, 2*(1):11–17.

Guidotti, T. L. (2014). Demystifying reproductive hazards in the workplace. *Archives of Environmental & Occupational Health, 69*(2), 125–126.

Halford, W. K., Petch, J., & Creedy, D. (2015). Caring and sexuality. In *Clinical guide to helping new parents* (pp. 131–150). New York: Springer Publishers.

Heazell, A. (2015). A kick in the right direction-reduced fetal movements and stillbirth prevention. *BMC Pregnancy and Childbirth, 15*(Suppl 1), A7.

Hehir, M. P., Dalrymple, J., & Malone, F. D. (2015). Decision-support guide and use of prenatal genetic testing. *JAMA, 313*(2), 199.

Hixson, L., Goel, S., Schuber, P., Faltas, V., Lee, J., Narayakkadan, A., … Osborne, J. (2015). An overview on prenatal screening for chromosomal aberrations. *Journal of Laboratory Automation, 20*(5), 562–573.

Hurst, H. M., & Linton, D. M. (2015). Preconception care: Planning for the future. *The Journal for Nurse Practitioners, 11*(3), 335–340.

Jordan, R. G., Engstrom, J., Marfell, J., & Farley, C. L. (2014). *Prenatal and postnatal care: A women-centered approach.* Ames, Iowa: John Wiley & Sons.

Jyothi, M. N. (2015). A case report on pica: A rare pregnancy related complication. *Asian Journal of Nursing Education and Research, 5*(1), 137–139.

Kader, M., & Naim-Shuchana, S. (2014). Physical activity and exercise during pregnancy. *European Journal of Physiotherapy, 16*(1), 2–9.

Kalousová, M., Muravská, A., & Zima, T. (2014). Pregnancy-associated plasma protein A (PAPP-A) and preeclampsia. *Advances in Clinical Chemistry, 63,* 169–209.

Keytash, A., Jones, L., & Frances, A. (2015). Strong healthy behavioral change program for women. *Australian Nursing and Midwifery Journal, 22*(9), 45–46.

Khalil, A., & Coates, A. (2015). *Prenatal diagnosis of chromosomal abnormalities. Arias' practical guide to high-risk pregnancy and delivery: A South Asian perspective* (4th ed., pp. 1–13). Elsevier Health Sciences.

King, T. L., Brucker, M. C., Kriebs, J. M., Fahey, J. O., Gcgor, C. L., & Varney, H. (2015). *Varney's midwifery* (5th ed.). Burlington, MA: Jones & Bartlett Learning.

Kondhare, M. M., & Khodgire, U. (2015). Benefits of exercises on selected physiological common complaints during pregnancy. *Journal of Physical Education Research, 1,* 13–26.

Lakshmi, G. R., & Jyothsna, D. (2015). Influence of amniotic fluid index on fetal outcome. *Journal of Evidence Based Medicine and Healthcare, 2*(10), 1455–1463.

La Leche League International. (2016). *Breastfeeding help.* Retrieved from http://www.llli.org/resources/assistance. html?m=0,0

Lamaze International. (2015). *Healthy birth practices.* Retrieved from http://www.lamaze.org

Latendresse, G., & Deneris, A. (2015). An update on current prenatal testing options: First trimester and noninvasive prenatal testing. *Journal of Midwifery & Women's Health, 60*(1), 24–36.

Leggat, P. A., & Zuckerman, J. N. (2015). *Pre-travel health risk assessment. Essential Travel Medicine* (pp. 23–34). West Sussex, UK: John Wiley & Sons.

Lewis, R. (2015). As home births increase, recent studies illuminate controversies and complexities. *JAMA, 313*(6), 553–555.

Maeda, K. (2015). Ultrasound diagnosis of the fetus in-utero. *Journal of Health Medical Informatics, 6*(174), 2.

Magee, L. A., Pels, A., Helewa, M., Rey, E., & von Dadelszen, P. (2014). Diagnosis, evaluation, and management of the hypertensive disorders of pregnancy. Pregnancy Hypertension. *An International Journal of Women's Cardiovascular Health, 4,* 105–145.

March of Dimes. (2015a). *Pregnancy complications.* Retrieved from http://www.marchofdimes.com/pregnancy/pregnancy-complications.aspx

March of Dimes. (2015b). *The serious problem of premature birth.* Retrieved from http://www.marchofdimes.com/mission/prematurity-campaign.aspx

March of Dimes. (2015c). *Preterm labor.* Retrieved from http://www.marchofdimes.com/pregnancy/preterm-labor-and-birth.aspx

March of Dimes. (2015d). *Aminocentesis.* Retrieved from http://www.marchofdimes.com/pregnancy/amniocentesis.aspx

March of Dimes. (2015e). *Chorionic villus sampling.* Retrieved from http://www.marchofdimes.com/pregnancy/chorionic-villus-sampling.aspx

March of Dimes. (2015f). *Sex during pregnancy.* Retrieved from http://www.marchofdimes.com/pregnancy/physicalactivity_sex.html

March of Dimes. (2015g). *Childbirth education classes.* Retrieved from http://www.marchofdimes.com/pregnancy/childbirth-education-classes.aspx

March of Dimes. (2015h). *Vaccinations during pregnancy.* Retrieved from http://www.marchofdimes.com/pregnancy/vaccinations-during-pregnancy.aspx

Moses, S. (2015a). *Routine obstetric visit—Family Practice Notebook.* Retrieved from http://www.fpnotebook.com/ob/Exam/RtnObstrcVst.htm

Moses, S. (2015b). *Fetal movement count—Family Practice Notebook.* Retrieved from http://www.fpnotebook.com/ob/fetus/FtlMvmntCnt.htm

Moses, S. (2015c). *Biophysical profile—Family Practice Notebook.* Retrieved from http://www.fpnotebook.com/ob/fetus/BphysclPrfl.htm

M'soka, N. C., Mabuza, L. H., & Pretorius, D. (2015). Cultural and health beliefs of pregnant women in Zambia regarding pregnancy and child birth. *Curationis, 38*(1), 1–7.

Nagtalon-Ramos, J. (2014). *Best evidence-based practices in maternal-newborn care.* Philadelphia, PA: F. A. Davis Company.

National Institutes of Health. (2015). *Health problems in pregnancy.* Retrieved from http://www.nlm.nih.gov/medlineplus/healthproblemsinpregnancy.html

National Maternal and Child Health Resource Center. (2015). *Oral health care during pregnancy: A national consensus statement.* Retrieved from http://www.mchoralhealth.org/materials/consensus_statement.html

Nisa, M. U., Hamid, N., Nasreen, F., & Khanum, F. (2015). Co-relation of biophysical profile with APGAR score. *Cell, 92.* doi: 321–9001662.

Office on Women's Health. (2014). Why breastfeeding is important. *Womenshealth.gov.* Retrieved from http://www.womenshealth.gov/breastfeeding/why-breastfeeding-is-important/

Ota, E., Hori, H., Mori, R., Tobe-Gai, R., & Farrar, D. (2015). Antenatal dietary education and supplementation to increase energy and protein intake. *Cochrane Database of Systematic Reviews,* (6), CD000032.

Patil, M., Panchanadikar, T., & Wagh, G. (2014). Variation of PAPP-A level in the first trimester of pregnancy and its clinical outcome. *Journal of Obstetrics and Gynecology of India, 64*(2), 116–119.

Petrov Fieril, K., Glantz, A., & Fagevik Olsen, M. (2015). The efficacy of moderate to vigorous resistance exercise during pregnancy: A randomized controlled trial. *Acta Obstetricia et Gynecologica Scandinavica, 94*(1), 35–42.

Plastaras, C. T., & Appasamy, M. (2015). Interventional procedures for musculoskeletal pain in pregnancy and postpartum: Efficacy and safety. In *Musculoskeletal health in pregnancy and postpartum* (pp. 115–133). Springer International Publishing.

Pruetz, J. D., Votava-Smith, J., & Miller, D. A. (2015). Clinical relevance of fetal hemodynamic monitoring: Perinatal implications. In *Seminars in fetal and neonatal medicine.* WB Saunders. doi:10.1016/j.siny.2015.03.007

Public Health Agency of Canada (2015). *Canadian immunization guide: Part 3—Vaccination of special populations.* Retrieved from https://www.canada.ca/en/public-health/services/publications/healthy-living/canadian-immunization-guide-part-3-vaccination-specific-populations/page-4-immunization-pregnancy-breastfeeding.html#p3c3t1

Public Health Agency of Canada (2017a). *Preconception care.* Retrieved from https://www.canada.ca/content/dam/phac-aspc/documents/services/publications/healthy-living/maternity-newborn-care/maternity-newborn-care-guidelines-chapter-2-eng.pdf

Public Health Agency of Canada (2017b). *Family-centred maternity and newborn care in Canada: Underlying philosophy and principles.* Retrieved from https://www.canada.ca/content/dam/phac-aspc/documents/services/publications/healthy-living/maternity-newborn-care/maternity-newborn-care-guidelines-chapter-1-eng.pdf

Public Health Agency of Canada (2017c). *Perinatal health indicators for Canada 2017. A report from the Canadian perinatal surveillance system.* Retrieved from http://publications.gc.ca/site/eng/9.506796/publication.html

Public Health Agency of Canada (2018). An Advisory Committee Statement (ACS) National Advisory Committee of Immunization (NACI). *Update on immunization in pregnancy with tetanus toxoid, reduced diphtheria toxoid, and reduced acellular pertussis (Tdap) vaccine.* Retrieved from https://www.canada.ca/content/dam/phac-aspc/documents/services/publications/healthy-living/update-immunization-pregnancy-tdap-vaccine/update-immunization-pregnancy-tdap-vaccine-eng.pdf

Rayburn, W. F., Jolley, J. A., Simpson, L. L. (2015). Advances in ultrasound imaging for congenital malformations during early gestation. *Birth Defects Research Part A: Clinical and Molecular Teratology, 103*(4), 260–268. doi: 10.1002/bdra.23353

Regal, J. F., Gilbert, J. S., & Burwick, R. M. (2015). The complement system and adverse pregnancy outcomes. *Molecular Immunology, 67*(1), 56–70.

Rigby, F. B. (2015). Common pregnancy complaints and questions. *eMedicine.* Retrieved from http://emedicine.medscape.com/article/259724-overview

Royal College of Physicians and Surgeons of Canada (2015). *Clinical laboratory tests—Reference Values.* Retrieved from http://www.royalcollege.ca/portal/page/portal/rc/common/

documents/exams/examiners/clinical_lab_tests_reference_values_e.pdf

Satyan, M. T., Grothusen, J., Drummond, K., Kennedy, B., Weiner, C., & Lee, G. (2015). 200: A retrospective review of the impact of HAPO based screening guidelines for gestational diabetes. *American Journal of Obstetrics & Gynecology, 212*(1), S113–S114.

Schram, J. (2014). Food for thought. *World of Irish Nursing & Midwifery, 22*(3), 46–47.

Schuiling, K. D., & Likis, F. E. (2016). *Women's gynecologic health* (3rd ed.). Burlington, MA: Jones & Bartlett Learning.

Schytt, E., & Bergström, M. (2014). First-time fathers' expectations and experiences of childbirth in relation to age. *Midwifery, 30*(1), 82–88.

Senie, R. T. (2014). *Epidemiology of women's health.* Burlington, MA: Jones & Bartlett Learning.

Slaughter, S., Hearns-Stokes, R., van der Vlugt, T., & Joffe, H. (2014). FDA approval of doxylamine-pyridoxine therapy for use in pregnancy. *New England Journal of Medicine, 370*(12), 1081–1083.

Society of Obstetricians and Gynaecologist of Canada. (2019). *Travel and Pregnancy.* Retrieved from https://www.pregnancyinfo.ca/your-pregnancy/special-consideration/travel-and-pregnancy/

Springer, S. C. (2018). Prenatal diagnosis and fetal therapy. *eMedicine.* Retrieved from https://emedicine.medscape.com/article/936318-overview

Steegers-Theunissen, R. P., & Steegers, E. A. (2015). Embryonic health: New insights, health and personalized patient care. *Reproduction, Fertility and Development, 27*(4), 712–715.

Tanner-Smith, E., Steinka-Fry, K., & Lipsey, M. (2014). The effects of centering pregnancy group prenatal care on gestational age, birth weight, and fetal demise. *Maternal & Child Health Journal, 18*(4), 801–809.

Tara, F., Vakilian, F., Moosavi-Baigy, F., Salehi, M., & Moghiman, T. (2015). Prenatal and cardiovascular outcome in pregnant patients with dyspnea. *Research in Cardiovascular Medicine, 4*(2), e20950. doi: 10.5812/cardiovascmed.20950

Templeton, A. (2015). The public health importance of antenatal care. *Facts, Views & Vision in ObGyn, 7*(1), 5–6.

Tharpe, N. L., Farley, C. L., & Jordan, R. (2016). *Clinical practice guidelines for midwifery & women's health* (5th ed.). Sudbury, MA: Jones & Bartlett.

Tracy, M. (2014). Centering pregnancy: An alternative model of prenatal care. *The Citizen.* Retrieved from http://www.auburnhospital.org/news-events/articles/centering-pregnancy-an-alternate-model-of-prenatal-care

Trivedi, S., Lal, N., & Singhal, R. (2015). Periodontal diseases and pregnancy. *Journal of Orofacial Sciences, 7*(1), 67–68.

Truong, Y. N., Yee, L. M., Caughey, A. B., & Cheng, Y. W. (2015). Weight gain in pregnancy: Does the Health and Medicine Division have it right? *American Journal of Obstetrics and Gynecology, 212*(3), 362–370.

Tyler, S., & Nagtalon-Ramos, J. (2015). Managing nausea and vomiting of pregnancy. *NP Women's Healthcare, 3*(2), 7–13.

U.S. Department of Health and Human Services. (2010). *Healthy People 2020.* Retrieved from http://www.healthypeople.gov/2020/topicsobjectives2020/objectiveslist.aspx?topicId = 26

U.S. Preventive Services Task Force (USPSTF). (2015). *Screening for gestational diabetes mellitus.* Retrieved from http://www.uspreventiveservicestaskforce.org/uspstf/uspsgdm.htm

Varner, C. A. (2015). Comparison of the Bradley method and HypnoBirthing childbirth education classes. *The Journal of Perinatal Education, 24*(2), 128–136.

Verghese, T. S., Futaba, K., & Latthe, P. (2015). Constipation in pregnancy. *The Obstetrician & Gynecologist, 17*(2), 111–115.

Weber, J., & Kelley, J. H. (2014). *Health assessment in nursing* (5th ed.). Philadelphia, PA: Lippincott Williams & Wilkins.

Westbury, B. (2015). The power of environment. *The Practicing Midwife, 18*(6), 24–26.

Women, Infants and Children (WIC). (2015). *Breastfeeding promotion and support in WIC.* Retrieved from http://www.fns.usda.gov/wic/breastfeeding-promotion-and-support-wic

Yeniel, A. A., & Petri, E. E. (2014). Pregnancy, childbirth, and sexual function: Perceptions and facts. *International Urogynecology Journal, 25*(1), 5–14.

Yildiz, H. (2015). The relation between prepregnancy sexuality and sexual function during pregnancy and the postpartum period: A prospective study. *Journal of Sex & Marital Therapy, 41*(1), 49–59.

Zelig, C. M., Knutzen, D. M., Ennen, C. S., Dolinsky, B. M., & Napolitano, P. G. (2016). Chorionic villus sampling, early amniocentesis, and termination of pregnancy without diagnostic testing: Comparison of fetal risk following positive non-invasive prenatal testing. *Journal of Obstetrics and Gynaecology Canada, 38*(5), 441–445. doi: 10.1016/j.jogc.2016.03.006

Zielinski, R., Ackerson, K., & Low, L. K. (2015). Planned home birth: Benefits, risks, and opportunities. *International Journal of Women's Health, 7*, 361–377.

Zielinski, R., Searing, K., & Deibel, M. (2015). Gastrointestinal distress in pregnancy: Prevalence, assessment, and treatment of 5 common minor discomforts. *The Journal of Perinatal & Neonatal Nursing, 29*(1), 23–31.

Zolotor, A., & Carlough, M. (2014). Update on prenatal care. *American Family Physician, 89*(3), 199–208.

MULTIPLE CHOICE QUESTIONS

1. Which of the following biophysical profile findings indicate poor oxygenation to the fetus?
   a. Two pockets of amniotic fluid
   b. Well-flexed arms and legs
   c. Abnormal fetal heart rate
   d. Fetal breathing movements noted

2. The nurse teaches the pregnant client how to perform Kegel exercises as a way to accomplish which of the following?
   a. Prevent perineal lacerations
   b. Stimulate labour contractions
   c. Increase pelvic muscle tone
   d. Lose pregnancy weight quickly

3. During a clinic visit, a pregnant client at 30 weeks' gestation tells the nurse, "I've had some mild cramps that are pretty irregular. What does this mean?" The cramps are probably:
   a. The beginning of labour in the very early stages
   b. An ominous finding indicating that the client is about to have a miscarriage
   c. Related to over hydration
   d. Braxton Hicks contractions, which occur throughout pregnancy

4. The nurse is preparing a teaching plan for a client who has just had a pregnancy confirmed. Which of the following should be included in it? Select all that apply.
   a. Prevent constipation by taking a daily laxative
   b. Balance your dietary intake by increasing your calories by 300 daily
   c. Continue your daily walking routine just as you did before this pregnancy
   d. Tetanus, measles, mumps, and rubella vaccines will be given to you now
   e. Avoid tub baths now that you are pregnant to prevent vaginal infections
   f. Sexual activity is permitted as long as your membranes are intact
   g. Increase your consumption of milk to meet your iron needs

5. A pregnant client's last normal menstrual period was on August 10. Using Nagele rule, the nurse calculates that the estimated due date (EDD) will be which of the following?
   a. June 23
   b. July 10
   c. July 30
   d. May 17

6. Which of the following is not true about breastfeeding?
   a. Breastfed infants experience more obesity and allergies
   b. Breast milk is perfectly suited to the infant's nutritional needs
   c. Breast milk contains maternal antibodies to stimulate infant's immunity
   d. Breastfeeding enhances maternal bonding and attachment

7. Practicing good oral hygiene is important for all childbearing persons throughout their pregnancy. As a nurse providing anticipatory guidance for pregnant client, what condition can result from periodontal disease if good dental care isn't practiced?
   a. Post-dates pregnancy
   b. Large for gestational age infant
   c. Advanced reproductive cancer
   d. Preterm or low–birth-weight infant

8. Anticipatory guidance regarding sexual activity during pregnancy includes which of the following? Select all that apply:
   a. Sexual activity is contraindicated throughout pregnancy
   b. Most childbearing persons don't desire intimacy after the first trimester
   c. Sexual activity may continue up until the end of the second trimester
   d. Sexual intercourse is prohibited if a history of preterm labour exists
   e. A childbearing person's sexual desire may change throughout the pregnancy
   f. Couples can try a variety of positions of comfort during pregnancy

9. Which of the following would be considered risk factors for psychological well-being in pregnancy? Select all that apply:
   a. Limited support system and network of friends and family
   b. Introverted personality at any point in the pregnancy
   c. Ambivalence any time during the pregnancy
   d. High levels of stress due to family discord
   e. History of previous high-risk pregnancy with complications
   f. Depression prior to pregnancy and on medication

CHAPTER **WORKSHEET**

CRITICAL THINKING EXERCISES

1. Mary Jones comes to the Women's Health Center, where you work as a nurse. Mary is in the first trimester of pregnancy and tells you that her main complaints are nausea and fatigue, to the point of wanting to sleep most of the time and eats one meal daily. She appears pale and tired. The mucous membranes are pale. Mary reports that getting 8 to 9 hours of sleep each night but still can't seem to stay awake and alert at work. Mary reports not eating well, due to not being hungry. On blood work, the hemoglobin and hematocrit are low.
   a. What subjective and objective data do you have to make your assessment?
   b. What is your impression of this client?
   c. What nursing interventions would be appropriate for this client?
   d. How will you evaluate the effectiveness of your interventions?

2. Monica, a 16-year-old African Canadian high school student, is here for the first prenatal visit. The last normal menstrual period was 2 months ago, and Monica states being "sick ever since." Monica is 5 ft, 6 in tall, and weighs 110 lb. In completing a dietary assessment, the nurse asks about intake of milk and dairy products. Monica reports not liking "that stuff" and doesn't want to put on too much weight because it "might ruin my figure."
   a. In addition to the routine obstetric assessments, which additional ones might be warranted for this client?
   b. What dietary instruction should be provided to this client based on the history?
   c. What follow-up monitoring should be included in subsequent prenatal visits?

3. Maria, a 27-year-old Hispanic childbearing client in the last trimester of pregnancy (34 weeks), complains to the clinic nurse of being constipated and feeling miserable most of the time. Maria reports having started taking laxatives, but they don't help much. When questioned about dietary habits, Maria reports eating beans and rice and drinking tea with most meals. Maria has tried to limit fluid intake to limit having to go to the bathroom so much because the supervisor at work does not approve of taking so many breaks.
   a. What additional information would the nurse need to assess the client's complaint?
   b. What interventions would be appropriate for Maria?
   c. What adaptations will Maria need to make to alleviate the constipation?

STUDY ACTIVITIES

1. Visit a freestanding birth centre and compare it to a traditional hospital setting in terms of restrictions, and type of pain management available.

2. Arrange to shadow a midwife for a day to see the role in working with the childbearing family.

3. Visit the student resources on and select two of the supplied websites that correspond to this chapter. Note their target audience, the validity of information offered, and their appeal to expectant couples. Present your findings.

4. Request permission to attend a childbirth education class in your local area and help a childbearing person and their partner practice the paced breathing exercises. Present the information you learned and think about how you can apply it while taking care of a client during labour.

5. A layperson with a specialized education and experience in assisting a childbearing person during labour is a _____.

BRINGING IT ALL TOGETHER: A CASE STUDY

A 19-year-old client came to the public health clinic. This was the first prenatal visit, despite being 8 months pregnant. The client's explanation for not coming there before was: "It was summer and everything had been going good until my back started hurting two days ago."

ASSESSMENT

Vital signs were within normal range. Weight was 175 lb. On physical examination, the back area was normal without tenderness when palpated. Fundal height was 36 cm; fetal heart rate was 150 bpm; urinalysis was negative for blood, glucose, or leukocytes. The pelvic examination showed the cervix to be long, thick, and closed. Missed routine prenatal lab work was done since this was the first visit. When questioned further about when the back seemed to cause the most discomfort, the client reported working as a waitress and when finished the shift, was barely able to walk home.

1. What additional information is needed to make a diagnosis?

2. Based on the assessment, what might be suspected as the cause of the back pain?

3. What lab work might be included in the routine prenatal assessment that was missed?

CHAPTER **WORKSHEET**

It would be important to know what the client's pre-pregnant weight was to compare it with the present weight. If the client has gained a large amount of weight during this pregnancy, it might be a contributing factor to the low back pain. Low back pain can also be a symptom of early labour, but in this case, the client hasn't noticed any contractions and no cervical changes have taken place based on the examination. Low back pain in the lumbosacral region generally occurs in the last trimester and increases in intensity as the pregnancy progresses secondary to the increasing weight of the enlarged uterus and relaxation of the sacroiliac ligaments. The normal lordosis of pregnancy strains the back muscles and causes pain. Routine lab work may include a complete blood count (CBC), blood type, Rh type, and antibody screen, hepatitis B surface antigen, HIV screening test, syphilis screening test, diabetic screening, and urinalysis or dipstick for protein.

PLAN

1. What health teaching by the nurse is needed for this client?

2. What specific relief measures are helpful to address the client's concern?

3. What changes in the work environment might be suggested?

4. How can the lack of prenatal care be addressed by the nurse?

Since this is the first prenatal visit, the client has not had the benefit of any health teaching throughout the pregnancy thus far. Since this is now the last trimester, focus should be on preparing for labour and birth, making arrangements for childbirth at a local hospital, and referring the client to any community resources available. Specific relief measures for low back pain would include instructing the client to rest in a side-lying position to take the weight off the back; use proper body mechanics for lifting, stooping rather than bending so that the legs, rather than the back bear the weight and strain; and wearing low-heeled shoes. Excessive standing for long periods of time can contribute to low back pain, so periodic rest periods may need to be instituted in the work environment to reduce the low back pain. Since this client is already in the 8th month of pregnancy, the nurse should encourage them to keep their weekly prenatal appointments without placing judgment on the previous behaviour. Making judgments and placing blame are not therapeutic interventions that provide an accepting environment to any client. Stressing the importance of prenatal care to the health of the baby and the client are important.

Unit 4

Labour and Birth

13

Labour and Birth Process

Learning Objectives

Upon completion of the chapter, you will be able to:

1. Relate premonitory signs of labour.
2. Compare and contrast true versus false labour.
3. Categorize the critical factors affecting labour and birth.
4. Analyze the cardinal movements of labour.
5. Evaluate the client and fetal responses to labour and birth.
6. Classify the stages of labour and the critical events in each stage.
7. Characterize the normal physiologic/psychological changes occurring during all four stages of labour.
8. Formulate the concept of pain as it relates to the client in labour.

Kathy and Chuck have been eagerly awaiting the birth of their first child for what seems to them an eternity. When Kathy finally feels contractions in her abdomen, she and Chuck rush to the birthing centre. After the OB nurse finishes a complete history and physical assessment, she informs Kathy and her husband that she must have experienced "false labour" and that they should return home until she starts true labour.

INTRODUCTION

The process of labour and birth involves more than the birth of a newborn. Numerous physiologic and psychological events occur that ultimately result in the birth of a newborn and the creation or expansion of the family. This chapter describes labour and birth as a process. It addresses initiation of labour, the premonitory signs of labour, including true and false labour, critical factors affecting labour and birth, client and fetal response to the labouring process, and the four stages of labour. The chapter also identifies critical factors related to each stage of labour: the "10 P's of labour."

INITIATION OF LABOUR

Labour is a physiologic event involving a sequential, integrated set of changes within the myometrium, decidua, and cervix that occurs gradually over a period of days to weeks in order to expel the fetus from the uterus. It is difficult to determine exactly why labour begins and what initiates it. Although several theories have been proposed to explain the onset and maintenance of labour, none of these have been proved scientifically. It is widely believed that labour is influenced by a cascade of events, including uterine stretch from the fetus and amniotic fluid volume, progesterone withdrawal to estrogen dominance, increased oxytocin sensitivity, and increased release of prostaglandins.

One theory suggests that labour is initiated by a change in the estrogen-to-progesterone ratio. During the last trimester of pregnancy, estrogen levels increase and progesterone levels decrease. This change leads to an increase in the number of myometrium gap junctions. Gap junctions are proteins that connect cell membranes and facilitate coordination of uterine contractions and myometrial stretching (Norwitz, 2018).

Although physiologic evidence for the role of oxytocin in the initiation of labour is inconclusive, the number of oxytocin receptors in the uterus increases at the end of pregnancy. This creates an increased sensitivity to oxytocin. Estrogen, the levels of which are also rising, increases myometrial sensitivity to oxytocin. With the increasing levels of oxytocin in the pregnant client's blood in conjunction with increasing fetal cortisol levels that synthesize prostaglandins, uterine contractions are initiated. Oxytocin also aids in stimulating prostaglandin synthesis through receptors in the decidua. Prostaglandins lead to additional contractions, cervical softening, gap junction induction, and myometrial sensitization, thereby leading to a progressive cervical **dilation** (the opening or enlargement of the external cervical os). Uterine contractions have two main functions: to dilate the cervix and to push the fetus through the birth canal (Funai & Norwitz, 2018).

PREMONITORY SIGNS OF LABOUR

Before the onset of labour, a pregnant client's body undergoes several changes in preparation for the birth of the newborn. The changes that occur often lead to characteristic signs and symptoms that suggest that labour is near. These premonitory signs and symptoms can vary, and each pregnant person may experience some, none, or all, and in different ways.

Cervical Changes

Before labour begins, cervical softening and possible cervical dilation with descent of the presenting part into the pelvis occur. These changes can occur 1 month to 1 hour before actual labour begins.

As labour approaches, the cervix changes from an elongated structure to a shortened, thinned segment. Cervical collagen fibres undergo enzymatic rearrangement into smaller, more flexible fibres that facilitate water absorption, leading to a softer, more stretchable cervix. These changes occur secondary to the effects of prostaglandins. The ripening and softening of the cervix are essential for effacement and dilation, which reflect the enhanced collagen breakdown that was previously inhibited by progesterone (Grant, Strevens, & Thornton, 2015).

Lightening

Lightening occurs when the fetal presenting part begins to descend into the true pelvis. The uterus depresses and moves into a more anterior position. The shape of the abdomen changes as a result of the change in the uterus. With this descent, the client usually notes that breathing is now much easier and that there is a decrease in gastric reflux. However, the client may simultaneously experience increased pelvic pressure, leg cramping, dependent edema in the lower legs, low back discomfort, and increased bladder pressure and urinary frequency. There may be an increase in vaginal discharge. In primiparas, lightening can occur 2 weeks or more before labour begins; among multiparas it may not occur until labour starts (Cheng & Caughey, 2017).

Increased Energy Level

Some clients report a sudden increase in energy before labour. This is sometimes referred to as nesting, because many people will focus this energy toward childbirth preparation by cleaning, cooking, preparing the home for the baby, and spending extra time with other children. The increased energy level usually occurs 24 to 48 hours before the onset of labour. It is thought to be the result of an increase in epinephrine release caused by a decrease in progesterone (Jordan, Engstrom, Marfell, & Farley, 2014).

Bloody Show

At the onset of labour or before, the mucous plug that fills the cervical canal during pregnancy is expelled as a result of cervical softening and increased pressure of the presenting part. These ruptured cervical capillaries release a small amount of blood that mixes with mucus, resulting in the pink-tinged secretions known as bloody show.

Braxton Hicks Contractions

Braxton Hicks contractions, which the client may have been experiencing throughout the pregnancy, may become stronger and more frequent. Braxton Hicks contractions are typically felt as a tightening or pulling sensation of the top of the uterus. They occur primarily in the abdomen and groin and gradually spread downward before relaxing. These contractions aid in moving the cervix from a posterior position to an anterior position. They also help in ripening and softening the cervix. However, the contractions are irregular and are not increased by activity. Clients may find they can be distracted from these contractions by eating, increasing fluid intake, or changing position.

Braxton Hicks contractions are irregular in duration: lasting as little as 30 seconds or persisting for as long as 2 minutes. As birth draws near and the uterus becomes more sensitive to oxytocin, the frequency and intensity of these contractions increase. However, if the contractions last longer than 30 seconds and occur more often than four to six times an hour, advise the client to contact their health care provider in order to be evaluated for possible preterm labour, especially prior to 37 weeks pregnant.

Take Note!

Infants born prior to 36 completed weeks are classified as preterm. An infant born between 34 0/7 and 36 6/7 weeks of gestation is identified as "late preterm" and may experience many of the same health issues as other preterm birth infants such as temperature instability, breathing issues, and feeding challenges (Horgan, 2015; Whyte & Canadian Pediatric Society Fetus and Newborn Committee, 2017).

Spontaneous Rupture of Membranes

Rupture of membranes with loss of amniotic fluid prior to the onset of labour is termed prelabour rupture of membranes. It occurs in 8% to 10% of term pregnancies, the majority of whom will begin labour spontaneously within 24 hours (King et al., 2015). The rupture of membranes can result in either a sudden gush or a steady leakage of amniotic fluid. Although much of the amniotic fluid is lost when the rupture occurs, a continuous

supply is produced to ensure protection of the fetus until birth.

After the amniotic sac has ruptured, the barrier to infection is gone and the client and fetus are more at risk for an ascending infection. In addition, there is a danger of cord prolapse if fetal engagement has not occurred with the sudden release of fluid and pressure with rupture. Due to the possibility of these complications occurring, clients should be advised to contact their health care provider and to go in for an evaluation after their water breaks.

Consider This

I always pictured myself a dignified woman and behaved in ways to demonstrate that, for that was the way I was raised. My mother and grandmother always stressed that you should look good, dress well, and do nothing to embarrass yourself in public. I did a fairly good job of living up to their expectations until an incident occurred at the end of my first pregnancy. I recall I was overdue according to my dates and was miserable in the summer heat. I decided to go to the store for some ice cream. As I waddled down the grocery aisles, all of a sudden, my water broke and came pouring down my legs all over the floor. Not wanting to make a spectacle of myself and remembering what my mother always said about being dignified at all times in public, I quickly reached up onto the grocery shelf and "accidentally" knocked off a large jar of pickles right where my puddle was. As I walked hurriedly away from that mess without my ice cream, I heard on the store loudspeaker, "Clean-up on aisle 13!"

Thoughts: We tend to live by what we are taught, and in this case, this woman needed to save face from her ruptured membranes. Many clients experience ruptured membranes before the onset of labour, so it is not out of the ordinary for this to happen in public. What risks can occur when membranes do rupture? What action should this individual take now to minimize these risks? How will the nurse confirm that the membranes have ruptured?

TRUE VERSUS FALSE LABOUR

False labour is a condition occurring during the latter weeks of some pregnancies in which irregular uterine contractions are felt, but the cervix is not affected. In contrast, true labour is characterized by contractions occurring at regular intervals that increase in frequency, duration, and intensity. True labour contractions bring about progressive cervical dilation and effacement. Table 13.1 summarizes the differences between true and false labour. False labour, prodromal labour, and Braxton Hicks contractions are all names for contractions that do not cause a measurable change in the cervix. Distinguishing between true

TABLE 13.1	DIFFERENCES BETWEEN TRUE AND FALSE LABOUR	
Parameters	**True Labour**	**False Labour**
Contraction timing	Regular, becoming closer together, usually 4–6 minutes apart, lasting 30–60 seconds	Irregular, not occurring close together
Contraction strength	Become stronger with time, vaginal pressure is usually felt	Frequently weak, not getting stronger with time or alternating (a strong one followed by weaker ones)
Contraction discomfort	Starts in the back and radiates around toward the front of the abdomen	Usually felt in the front of the abdomen
Any change in activity	Contractions continue no matter what positional change is made	Contractions may stop or slow down with walking or making a position change
Stay or go?	Stay home until contractions are 5 minutes apart, last 45–60 seconds, and are strong enough so that a conversation during one is not possible—then go to the hospital or birthing centre	Drink fluids and walk around to see if there is any change in the intensity of the contractions; if the contractions diminish in intensity after either or both—stay home

Adapted from Cunningham, F. G., Leveno, K. J., Bloom, S. L., Spong, C. Y., Dashe, J. S., Hoffman, B. L., . . . Sheffield, J. S. (2014). *Williams obstetrics* (24th ed.). New York: McGraw-Hill Education; King, T. L., Brucker, M. C., Kriebs, J. M., Fahey, J. O., Gegor, C. L., & Varney, H. (2015). *Varney's midwifery* (5th ed.). Burlington, MA: Jones & Bartlett Learning; and Tharpe, N. L., Farley, C. L., & Jordan, R. (2016). *Clinical practice guidelines for midwifery & women's health* (4th ed.). Sudbury, MA: Jones & Bartlett.

and false labour is an essential nursing assessment skill and one that develops with experience.

Many people fear being sent home from the hospital with false labour. All pregnant clients feel anxious when they feel contractions, but they should be informed that labour could be a long process, especially if it is their first pregnancy. Encourage the client to think of false labour as prelabour signs, and that this is a positive thing, because prelabour contractions are part of the labour continuum. With first pregnancies, the cervix can take up to 20 hours to dilate completely to 10 cm and be fully effaced (Cunningham et al., 2014).

Remember Kathy and Chuck, the anxious couple who came to the hospital too early? Kathy felt sure she was in labour and is now confused. What explanations and anticipatory guidance should be offered to this couple? What term would describe her earlier contractions?

FACTORS AFFECTING THE LABOUR PROCESS

Traditionally, the critical factors that affect the process of labour and birth are outlined as the "five P's":
1. **P**assageway (birth canal)
2. **P**assenger (fetus and placenta)
3. **P**owers (contractions)
4. **P**osition (of the labouring client)
5. **P**sychological response or **P**syche

These critical factors are commonly accepted and discussed by health care providers. However, five additional "P's" can also affect the labour process:
1. **P**hilosophy (low tech, high touch)
2. **P**artners (support caregivers)
3. **P**atience (natural timing)
4. **P**atient (client) preparation (childbirth knowledge base)
5. **P**ain management (comfort measures)

These five additional P's are helpful in planning care for the labouring family. These client-focused factors are an attempt to foster labour that can be managed through the use of high touch, patience, support, knowledge, and pain management.

Passageway

The birth passageway is the route through which the fetus must travel to be born vaginally. Compared to other primates, childbirth is remarkably difficult in humans because the head of the neonate is large relative to the birth-relevant dimensions of the birthing parent's pelvis. The passageway consists of the bony pelvis and soft tissues. Of the two, however, the bony pelvis is more important because it is relatively unyielding (except for the coccyx). Typically, the pelvis is assessed and measured during the first trimester, often at the first visit to the health care provider, to identify any abnormalities that might hinder a successful vaginal birth. As the pregnancy progresses, the hormones relaxin and estrogen cause the connective tissues to become more relaxed and elastic and this causes the joints to become more

False pelvis

Pelvic outlet

True pelvis   Linea terminalis   Pelvic inlet

Anterior view   Superior view   Inferior view

FIGURE 13.1 **The bony pelvis.**

flexible to prepare the client's pelvis for birth. Additionally, the soft tissues usually yield to the forces of labour.

Bony Pelvis

The bony pelvis can be divided into the true and false portions. The false (or greater) pelvis is composed of the upper flared parts of the two iliac bones with their concavities and the wings of the base of the sacrum. The false pelvis is divided from the true pelvis by an imaginary line drawn from the sacral prominence at the back to the superior aspect of the symphysis pubis at the front of the pelvis. This imaginary line is called the linea terminalis. The false pelvis lies above this imaginary line; the true pelvis lies below it (Fig. 13.1). The true pelvis is the bony passageway through which the fetus must travel. It is made up of three planes: the inlet, the mid-pelvis (cavity), and the outlet.

PELVIC INLET

The pelvic inlet allows entrance to the true pelvis. It is bounded by the sacral prominence in the back, the ilium on the sides, and the superior aspect of the symphysis pubis in the front (Jones & Lopez, 2014). The pelvic inlet is wider in the transverse aspect (sideways) than it is from front to back.

MID-PELVIS

The mid-pelvis (cavity) occupies the space between the inlet and outlet. It is through this snug, curved space that the fetus must travel to reach the outside. As the fetus passes through this small area its chest is compressed, causing lung fluid and mucus to be expelled. This expulsion removes the space-occupying fluid so that air can enter the lungs with the newborn's first breath.

PELVIC OUTLET

The pelvic outlet is bound by the ischial tuberosities, the lower rim of the symphysis pubis, and the tip of the

coccyx. In comparison with the pelvic inlet, the outlet is wider from front to back. For the fetus to pass through the pelvis, the outlet must be large enough. To ensure the adequacy of the pelvic outlet for vaginal birth, the following pelvic measurements are assessed:
- Diagonal conjugate of the inlet (distance between the anterior surface of the sacral prominence and the anterior surface of the inferior margin of the symphysis pubis)
- Transverse or ischial tuberosity diameter of the outlet (distance at the medial and lowest aspect of the ischial tuberosities, at the level of the anus; a known hand span or clenched-fist measurement is generally used to obtain this measurement)
- True or obstetric conjugate (distance estimated from the measurement of the diagonal conjugate; 1.5 cm is subtracted from the diagonal conjugate measurement)

For more information about pelvic measurements, see Chapter 12.

If the diagonal conjugate measures at least 11.5 cm and the true or obstetric conjugate measures 10 cm or more (1.5 cm less than the diagonal conjugate, or about 10 cm), then the pelvis is large enough for a vaginal birth of what would be considered a normal-size newborn.

Pelvic Shape

In addition to size, the shape of the pelvis is a determining factor for a vaginal birth. Each plane of the pelvis has a shape, which is defined by the anterior–posterior and transverse diameters. The pelvis is divided into four main shapes: gynecoid, anthropoid, android, and platypelloid (Fig. 13.2).

GYNECOID PELVIS

The gynecoid pelvis is considered the "true female pelvis," occurring in about 40% of all cis-gender women; it is less common in cis-gender men (Fischer & Mitteroecker, 2015).

FIGURE 13.2 Pelvic shapes. **A.** Gynecoid. **B.** Android. **C.** Anthropoid. **D.** Platypelloid.

A   Gynecoid

C   Anthropoid

B   Android

D   Platypelloid

Vaginal birth is most favourable with this type of pelvis because the inlet is round and the outlet is roomy. This shape offers the optimal diameters in all three planes of the pelvis. This type of pelvis allows early and complete fetal internal rotation during labour.

ANTHROPOID PELVIS

The anthropoid pelvis is common in cis-gender men and is most common in women of colour. It occurs in approximately 25% of cis-gender women (Marani & Koch, 2014). The pelvic inlet is oval and the sacrum is long, producing a deep pelvis (wider front to back [anterior to posterior] than side to side [transverse]). Vaginal birth is more favourable with this pelvic shape compared with the android or platypelloid shape (Tharpe, Farley, & Jordan, 2016).

ANDROID PELVIS

The android pelvis is considered the "male-shaped" pelvis and is characterized by a funnel shape. It occurs in approximately 20% of cis-gender women (Cunningham et al., 2014). The pelvic inlet is heart-shaped and the posterior segments are reduced in all pelvic planes. Descent of the fetal head into the pelvis is slow, and failure of the fetus to rotate is common. The prognosis for labour is poor, subsequently leading to cesarean birth.

PLATYPELLOID (FLAT) PELVIS

The platypelloid or flat pelvis is the least common type of pelvic structure, with an approximate incidence of 3% (King et al., 2015). The pelvic cavity is shallow but widens at the pelvic outlet, making it difficult for the fetus to descend through the mid-pelvis. Labour prognosis is poor with arrest at the inlet occurring frequently. It is not favourable for a vaginal birth unless the fetal head can pass through the inlet. Pregnant individuals with this type of pelvis usually require cesarean birth.

An important principle is that most pelvises are not purely defined but occur in nature as mixed types. Many people have a combination of these four basic pelvis types, with no two pelvises being exactly the same. Regardless of the shape, the newborn can be born vaginally if size and positioning remain compatible. The narrowest part of the fetus attempts to align itself with the narrowest pelvic dimension (e.g., biparietal to interspinous diameters, which means the fetus generally tends to rotate to the most ample portion of the pelvis).

Soft Tissues

The soft tissues of the passageway consist of the cervix, the pelvic floor muscles, and the vagina. Through **effacement,** the cervix effaces (thins) to allow the presenting fetal part to descend into the vagina.

The pelvic floor muscles help the fetus to rotate anteriorly as it passes through the birth canal. The soft tissues of the vagina expand to accommodate the fetus during birth.

Passenger

The fetus (with placenta) is the passenger. The fetal head (size and presence of moulding), fetal **attitude** (degree of body flexion), fetal **lie** (relationship of body parts), fetal **presentation** (first body part), fetal **position** (relationship to the client's pelvis), fetal station, and fetal engagement are all important factors that have an impact on the ultimate outcome in the birthing process.

Fetal Head

The fetal head is the largest fetal structure, making it an important factor in relation to labour and birth. Considerable variation in the size and diameter of the fetal skull is often seen.

Compared with an adult's head, the fetal head is large in proportion to the rest of the body, usually about one quarter of the body surface area (Martin, Fanaroff, & Walsh, 2014). The bones that make up the face and cranial base are fused and essentially fixed. However, the five bones that make up the rest of the cranium (two frontal bones, two parietal bones, and the occipital bone) are not fused; rather, they are soft and pliable, with gaps between the plates of bone. These gaps or membranous spaces between the cranial bones are called sutures, and the intersections of these sutures are called fontanelles. Sutures are important because they allow the cranial bones to overlap in order for the head to adjust in shape (elongate) when pressure is exerted on it by uterine contractions or the bony pelvis. Some diameters shorten, whereas others lengthen as the head is moulded during the labour and birthing process. This malleability of the fetal skull may decrease fetal skull dimensions by 0.5 to 1 cm (King et al., 2015). After birth, the fetal head will return to its pre-birth shape. Over the next few months the sutures close as the bones grow and the brain reaches its full growth.

The changed (elongated) shape of the fetal skull at birth as a result of overlapping of the cranial bones is known as **moulding.** Along with moulding, fluid can also collect in the scalp (caput succedaneum) or blood can collect beneath the scalp (cephalohematoma), further distorting the shape and appearance of the fetal head. Caput succedaneum can be described as edema

of the scalp at the presenting part. This swelling crosses suture lines and disappears within 3 to 4 days. Cephalohematoma is a collection of blood between the periosteum and the bone that occurs several hours after birth. It does not cross suture lines and is generally reabsorbed over the next 6 to 8 weeks (Collins & Reed, 2014). (See full discussion in Chapter 18.)

Sutures also play a role in helping to identify the position of the fetal head during a vaginal examination. Figure 13.3 shows a fetal skull. During a pelvic examination, palpation of these sutures by the examiner reveals the position of the fetal head and the degree of rotation that has occurred.

The anterior and posterior fontanelles are also useful in helping to identify the position of the fetal head. They allow for moulding and are important when evaluating the newborn. The anterior fontanelle is the famous "soft spot" of the newborn's head. It is a diamond-shaped space that measures from 1 to 4 cm. It remains open for 12 to 18 months after birth to allow for growth of the brain (Verklan & Walden, 2014). The posterior fontanelle corresponds to the anterior one but is located at the back of the fetal head; it is triangular. This one closes within 8 to 12 weeks after birth and measures, on average, 1 to 2 cm at its widest diameter (Weber & Kelley, 2014).

The diameter of the fetal skull is an important consideration during the labour and birth process. Fetal skull diameters are measured between the various landmarks of the skull. Diameters include occipitofrontal, occipitomental, suboccipitobregmatic, and biparietal (Fig. 13.4). The two most important diameters that can affect the birth process are the suboccipitobregmatic (approximately 9.5 cm

FIGURE 13.3 Fetal skull.

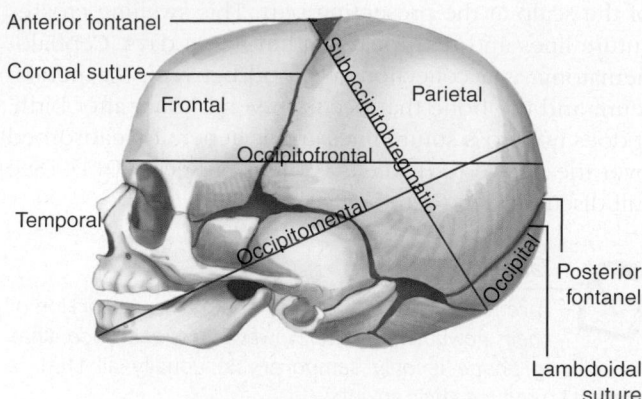

FIGURE 13.4 **Fetal skull diameters.**

at term) and the biparietal (approximately 9.25 cm at term) diameters. The suboccipitobregmatic diameter, measured from the base of the occiput to the centre of the anterior fontanelle, identifies the smallest anteroposterior diameter of the fetal skull. The biparietal diameter measures the largest transverse diameter of the fetal skull: the distance between the two parietal bones. In a cephalic (head first) presentation, which occurs in 95% of all term births, if the fetus presents in a flexed position in which the chin is resting on the chest, the optimal or smallest fetal skull dimensions for a vaginal birth are demonstrated. If the fetal head is not fully flexed at birth, the anteroposterior diameter increases. This increase in dimension might prevent the fetal skull from entering the client's pelvis.

Fetal Attitude

Fetal attitude is another important consideration related to the passenger. Fetal attitude refers to the posturing (flexion or extension) of the joints and the relationship of fetal parts to one another. The most common fetal attitude when labour begins is with all joints flexed—the fetal back is rounded, the chin is on the chest, the thighs are flexed on the abdomen, and the legs are flexed at the knees, and the head is presenting (Fig. 13.5). This

normal fetal position is most favourable for vaginal birth, presenting the smallest fetal skull diameters to the pelvis.

When the fetus presents to the pelvis with abnormal attitudes (no flexion or extension), their nonflexed position can increase the diameter of the presenting part as it passes through the pelvis, increasing the difficulty of birth. An attitude of extension tends to present larger fetal skull diameters, which may make birth difficult.

Fetal Lie

Fetal lie refers to the relationship of the long axis (spine) of the fetus to the long axis (spine) of the pregnant person. There are three possible lies: longitudinal (which is the most common), transverse (Fig. 13.6), and oblique.

A longitudinal lie occurs when the long axis of the fetus is parallel to that of the pregnant person (spines side-by-side). A transverse lie occurs when the long axis of the fetus is perpendicular to the long axis of the pregnant person (fetal spine lies horizontally across the abdomen, crossing the spine). In an oblique lie, the fetal long axis is at an angle to the bony inlet, and no palpable fetal part is presenting. This lie is usually transitory and occurs during fetal conversion between other lies. A fetus in a transverse or oblique lie position cannot be delivered vaginally (Cunningham et al., 2014).

Fetal Presentation

Fetal presentation refers to the body part of the fetus that enters the pelvic inlet first (the "presenting part"). This is the fetal part that lies over the inlet of the pelvis or

A. Longitudinal lie

B. Transverse lie

FIGURE 13.6 **Fetal lie.**

FIGURE 13.5 **Fetal attitude: full flexion.** Note that the smallest diameter presents to the pelvis.

FIGURE 13.7 Fetal presentation: cephalic presentations. **A.** Vertex. **B.** Military. **C.** Brow. **D.** Face.

the cervical os. Knowing which fetal part is coming first at birth is critical for planning and initiating appropriate interventions.

The three main fetal presentations are cephalic (head first), breech (pelvis or feet first), and shoulder (scapula first). The majority of term newborns (95%) enter this world in a cephalic presentation; breech presentations account for 3% of term births, and shoulder presentations for approximately 2% (Tharpe et al., 2016).

In a cephalic presentation, the presenting part is usually the occipital portion of the fetal head (Fig. 13.7). This presentation is also referred to as a vertex presentation. Variations in a vertex presentation include the brow and facial presentations.

BREECH PRESENTATION

By term, approximately 97% of infants actively turn to a cephalic presentation. It is determined by abdominal palpation (Hofmeyr, 2015) and ultrasound. Breech presentation occurs when the fetal buttocks or feet enter the

pelvis first and the fetal skull enters last. This abnormal presentation poses several challenges at birth. Primarily, the largest part of the fetus (skull) is born last and may become "hung up" or stuck in the pelvis. In addition, the umbilical cord can become compressed between the fetal skull and the pelvis after the fetal chest is born because the head is the last to exit. Moreover, unlike the hard fetal skull, the buttocks are soft and are not as effective as a cervical dilator during labour compared with a cephalic presentation. Finally, there is the possibility of trauma to the head as a result of the lack of opportunity for moulding.

The types of breech presentations are determined by the positioning of the fetal legs (Fig. 13.8). In a frank breech (50% to 70%), the buttocks present first with both legs extended up toward the face as in a pike position. In a full or complete breech (5% to 10%), the fetus sits crossed-legged above the cervix. In a footling or incomplete breech (10% to 30%), one or both legs are presenting. Breech presentations are associated with prematurity,

FIGURE 13.8 Breech presentations. **A.** Frank breech. **B.** Complete breech. **C.** Single footling breech. **D.** Double footling breech.

placenta previa, multiparity, uterine abnormalities (such as fibroids), and some congenital anomalies such as hydrocephaly (Hofmeyr, 2015). A frank breech can result in a vaginal birth, but complete, footling, and incomplete breech presentations generally necessitate a cesarean birth.

SHOULDER PRESENTATION

A shoulder presentation occurs when the fetal shoulders present first, with the head tucked inside. Odds of a shoulder presentation are 1 in 300 births (Cunningham et al., 2014). The fetus is in a transverse lie with the shoulder as the presenting part.

Conditions associated with shoulder or arm or compound presentation include placenta previa, prematurity, high parity, premature rupture of membranes, multiple gestation, or fetal anomalies. A cesarean birth will be necessary.

Fetal Position

Fetal position describes the relationship of a given point on the presenting part of the fetus to a designated point

of the pelvis (King et al., 2015). The landmark fetal presenting parts include the occipital bone (O), which designates a vertex presentation; the chin (mentum [M]), which designates a face presentation; the buttocks (sacrum [S]), which designate a breech presentation; and the scapula (acromion process [A]), which designates a shoulder presentation.

In addition, the pelvis is divided into four quadrants: right anterior, left anterior, right posterior, and left posterior. These quadrants designate whether the presenting part is directed toward the front, back, left, or right side of the pelvis. Fetal position is determined by identifying first the presenting part and then the quadrant of the bony pelvis that the presenting part is facing (Fig. 13.9). Position is indicated by a three-letter abbreviation as follows:

- The first letter defines whether the presenting part is tilted toward the left (L) or the right (R) side of the pelvis, from the client's (not the caregiver's) perspective.
- The second letter represents the particular presenting part of the fetus: O for occiput, S for sacrum (buttocks), M for mentum (chin), A for acromion process (shoulder) (Cheng & Caughey, 2017).

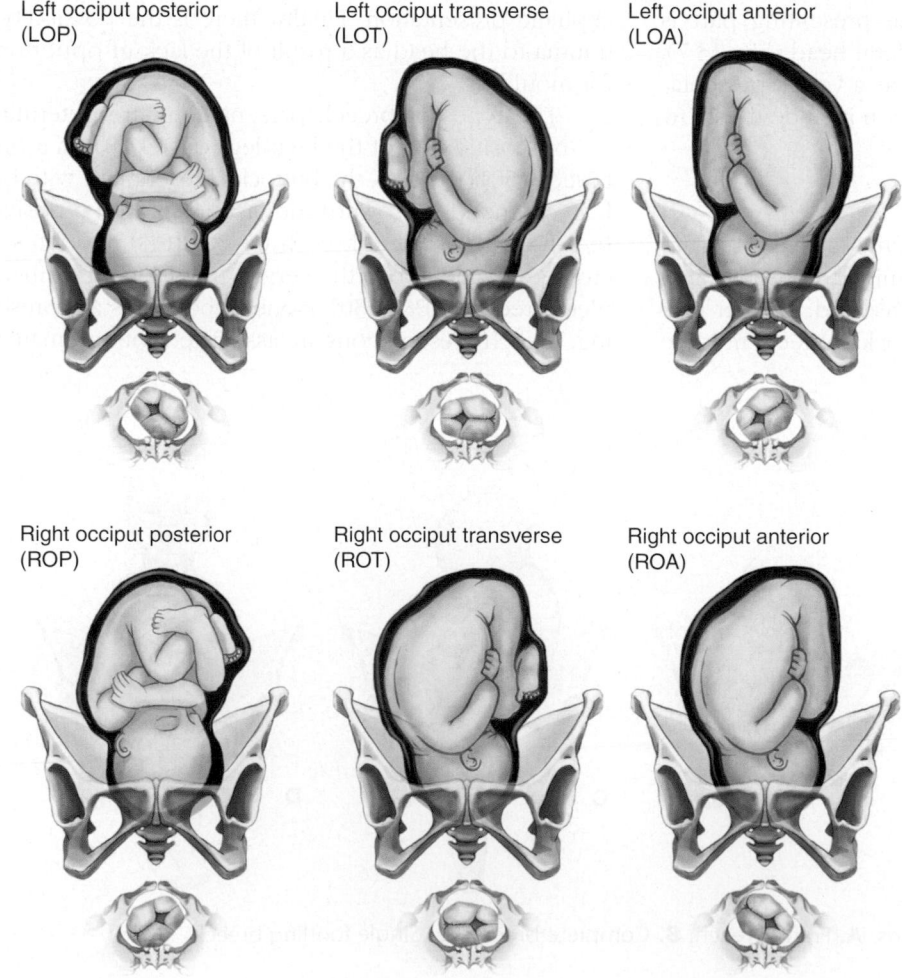

Left occiput posterior (LOP)

Left occiput transverse (LOT)

Left occiput anterior (LOA)

Right occiput posterior (ROP)

Right occiput transverse (ROT)

Right occiput anterior (ROA)

FIGURE 13.9 Examples of fetal positions in a vertex presentation. The lie is longitudinal for each illustration. The attitude is one of flexion. Notice that the view of the top illustration is seen when facing the pregnant client. The bottom view is that seen with the client in a dorsal recumbent position.

- The third letter defines the location of the presenting part in relation to the anterior (A) portion or the posterior (P) portion of the pelvis. If the presenting part is directed to the side of the pelvis, the fetal presentation is designated as transverse (T).

For example, if the occiput is facing the left anterior quadrant of the pelvis, then the position is termed left occiput anterior and is recorded as LOA.

> ### Take Note!
> LOA is the most common (and most favourable) fetal position for birthing, followed by right occiput anterior (ROA). The positioning of the fetus allows the fetal head to contour to the diameters of the bony pelvis. LOA and ROA are optimal positions for a vaginal birth.

An occiput posterior position may lead to a long and difficult birth, and other positions may or may not be compatible with vaginal birth.

Fetal Station

Fetal **station** refers to the relationship of the presenting part to the level of the pelvic ischial spines. Fetal station is measured in centimetres and is referred to as a minus or plus, depending on its location above or below the ischial spines. Typically, the ischial spines are the narrowest part of the pelvis and are the natural measuring point for the birth progress.

Zero (0) station is designated when the presenting part is at the level of the ischial spines. When the presenting part is above the ischial spines, the distance is recorded as minus stations. When the presenting part is below the ischial spines, the distance is recorded as plus stations. For instance, if the presenting part is above the ischial spines by 1 cm, it is documented as being a –1 station; if the presenting part is below the ischial spines by 1 cm, it is documented as being a +1 station.

An easy way to understand this concept is to think in terms of meeting the goal, which is the birth. If the fetus is descending downward (past the ischial spines) and moving toward meeting the goal of birth, then the station is positive and the centimetre numbers grow bigger from +1 to +4. If the fetus is not descending past the ischial spines, then the station is negative and the centimetre numbers grow bigger from –1 to –4. The farther away the presenting part from the outside, the larger the negative number (–4 cm). The closer the presenting part of the fetus is to the outside, the larger the positive number (+4 cm). Figure 13.10 shows stations of the presenting part.

Fetal Engagement

Fetal **engagement** signifies the entrance of the largest diameter of the fetal presenting part (usually the fetal

FIGURE 13.10 **Fetal stations.**

head) into the smallest diameter of the pelvis (Alexander, LaRosa, Bader, & Garfield, 2014). The fetus is said to be engaged in the pelvis when the widest diameter of the presenting part reaches 0 station. Engagement is determined by pelvic examination.

The largest diameter of the fetal head is the biparietal diameter. It extends from one parietal prominence to the other. It is an important factor in the navigation through the bony pelvis. Engagement typically occurs in primigravidas 2 weeks before term, whereas multiparas may experience engagement several weeks before the onset of labour or not until labour begins.

> ### Take Note!
> The term floating is used when engagement has not occurred, because the presenting part is freely movable above the pelvic inlet.

Cardinal Movements of Labour

The fetus goes through many positional changes as it travels through the passageway. These positional changes are known as the cardinal movements of labour. They are deliberate, specific, and very precise movements that allow the smallest diameter of the fetal head to pass through a corresponding diameter of the pelvic structure. Although cardinal movements are conceptualized as separate and sequential, the movements are typically concurrent (Fig. 13.11).

Engagement, Descent, Flexion

Internal Rotation

Extension Beginning (rotation complete)

Extension Complete

External Rotation (restitution)

External Rotation (shoulder rotation)

Expulsion

FIGURE 13.11 Cardinal movements of labour.

ENGAGEMENT

Engagement occurs when the greatest transverse diameter of the head in vertex (biparietal diameter) passes through the pelvic inlet (usually 0 station). The head usually enters the pelvis with the sagittal suture aligned in the transverse diameter.

DESCENT

Descent is the downward movement of the fetal head until it is within the pelvic inlet. Descent occurs intermittently with contractions and is brought about by one or more of the following forces:

• Pressure of the amniotic fluid

• Direct pressure of the fundus on the fetus's buttocks or head (depending on which part is located in the top of the uterus)

• Contractions of the abdominal muscles (second stage)

• Extension and straightening of the fetal body

Descent occurs throughout labour, ending with birth. During this time, the client experiences discomfort, and may or may not be able to isolate this particular fetal movement from the overall discomfort.

FLEXION

Flexion occurs as the vertex meets resistance from the cervix, the walls of the pelvis, or the pelvic floor. As a result, the chin is brought into contact with the fetal thorax and the presenting diameter is changed from occipitofrontal to suboccipitobregmatic (9.5 cm), which achieves the smallest fetal skull diameter presenting to the pelvic dimensions.

INTERNAL ROTATION

After engagement, as the head descends, the lower portion of the head (usually the occiput) meets resistance from one side of the pelvic floor. As a result, the head rotates about 45 degrees anteriorly to the midline under the symphysis. This movement is known as *internal rotation*. Internal rotation brings the anteroposterior diameter of the head in line with the anteroposterior diameter of the pelvic outlet. It aligns the long axis of the fetal head with the long axis of the pelvis. The widest portion of the pelvis is the anteroposterior diameter, and thus the fetus must rotate to accommodate the pelvis.

EXTENSION

With further descent and full flexion of the head, the nucha (the base of the occiput) becomes impinged under the symphysis. Resistance from the pelvic floor causes the fetal head to extend so that it can pass under the pubic arch. *Extension* occurs after internal rotation is complete. The head emerges through extension under the symphysis pubis along with the shoulders. The anterior fontanel, brow, nose, mouth, and chin are born successively.

EXTERNAL ROTATION (RESTITUTION)

After the head is born and is free of resistance, it untwists, causing the occiput to move about 45 degrees back to its original left or right position (restitution). The sagittal suture has now resumed its normal right-angle relationship to the transverse (bisacromial) diameter of the shoulders (i.e., the head realigns with the position of the back in the birth canal). *External rotation* of the fetal head allows the shoulders to rotate internally to fit the pelvis.

EXPULSION

Expulsion of the rest of the body occurs more smoothly after the birth of the head and the anterior and posterior shoulders (Cheng & Caughey, 2017). See Figure 13.3 for an image of a fetal skull.

Powers

The primary stimulus powering labour is uterine contraction. Contractions cause complete dilation and effacement of the cervix during the first stage of labour. The secondary powers in labour involve the use of intra-abdominal pressure (voluntary muscle contractions) exerted by the client when pushing and bearing down during the second stage of labour.

Uterine Contractions

Uterine contractions are involuntary and therefore cannot be controlled by the pregnant person, regardless of whether they are spontaneous, augmented, or induced. Uterine contractions are rhythmic and intermittent, with a period of relaxation between contractions. This pause allows the person and the uterine muscles to rest. In addition, this pause restores blood flow to the uterus and placenta, which is temporarily reduced during each uterine contraction.

Uterine contractions are responsible for thinning and dilating the cervix, then thrusting the presenting part toward the lower uterine segment. The cervical canal reduces in length from 2 cm to a paper-thin entity and is described in terms of percentages from 0% to 100%. In primigravidas, effacement typically starts before the onset of labour and usually begins before dilation; in multiparas, however, neither effacement nor dilation may start until labour is underway (Fig. 13.12). On clinical examination, the following may be assessed:

- Cervical canal 2 cm in length would be described as 0% effaced.
- Cervical canal 1 cm in length would be described as 50% effaced.
- Cervical canal 0 cm in length would be described as 100% effaced.

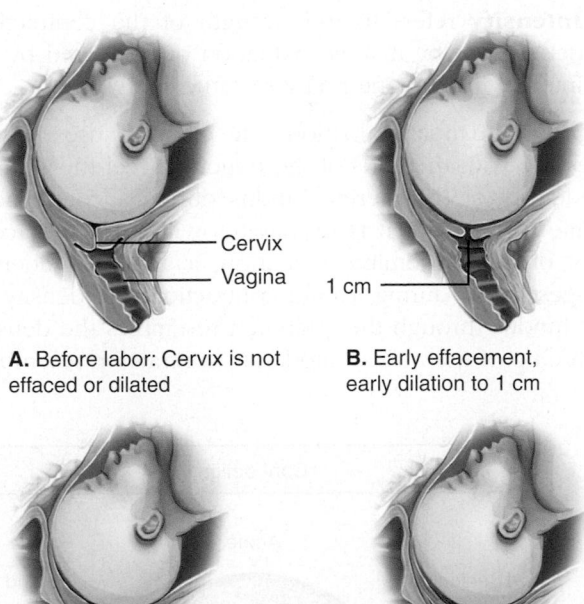

A. Before labor: Cervix is not effaced or dilated

B. Early effacement, early dilation to 1 cm

C. Complete effacement, mid-dilation to 5 cm

D. Full dilation to 10 cm

FIGURE 13.12 Cervical effacement and dilation. Cervical dilation is expressed in centimetres. **A.** Shows cervix not effaced or dilated. **B.** 50% effaced. **C.** 100% effaced. **D.** Fully dilated at 10 cm.

Dilation is dependent on the pressure of the presenting part and the contraction and retraction of the uterus. The diameter of the cervical os increases from less than 1 cm to approximately 10 cm to allow for birth. When the cervix is fully dilated, it is no longer palpable on vaginal examination. Descriptions may include the following:

- External cervical os closed: 0 cm dilated
- External cervical os half open: 5 cm dilated
- External cervical os fully open: 10 cm dilated

During early labour, uterine contractions are described as mild, they last about 30 seconds, and they occur about every 5 to 7 minutes. As labour progresses, contractions last longer (60 seconds), occur more frequently (2 to 3 minutes apart), and are described as being moderate to high in intensity. Each contraction has three phases: increment (buildup of the contraction), acme (peak or highest intensity), and decrement (descent or relaxation of the uterine muscle fibres; Fig. 13.13).

Uterine contractions are monitored and assessed according to three parameters: frequency, duration, and intensity.

1. **Frequency** refers to how often the contractions occur, and is measured from the beginning of one contraction to the beginning of the next contraction.
2. **Duration** refers to how long a contraction lasts, and is measured from the beginning of one contraction to the end of that same contraction.
3. **Intensity** refers to the strength of the contraction determined by manual palpation or measured by an internal intrauterine pressure catheter (IUPC).

With manual palpation, the clinician uses gentle pressure with the pads of the fingers to feel the change in density of the uterine fundus during a contraction. While the individual body habitus will affect the accuracy of this abdominal palpation, a general guideline suggests that: during a mild contraction, the density of the fundus through the abdomen resembles the density of the tip of the nose; a moderate contraction resembles the density felt by pressing a finger on the chin; and a strong contraction resembles the density of pressing on the forehead.

With an IUPC, the catheter is positioned in the uterine cavity through the cervix after the membranes have ruptured. It reports intensity by measuring the pressure of the amniotic fluid inside the uterus in millimetres of mercury. This is a more accurate, but invasive, method of assessing intensity of the contractions. It is not recommended for routine use in low-risk labouring clients due to the potential risk of infection and injury to the placenta or fetus. In a recent meta-analysis involving >2,000 labouring women, the researchers found an increase in surgical births and no advantages of using internal intrauterine pressure catheters over external monitoring during labour augmentation (Milton, Chelmow, & Ramus, 2015).

When an external fetal monitor is used for fetal health surveillance in labour, the tocodynamometer (often referred to as the "toco") attached to the machine will measure and record the frequency and duration of contractions, but does not accurately measure the intensity (Cohen, 2017).

Intra-Abdominal Pressure

Increased intra-abdominal pressure (voluntary muscle contractions) compresses the uterus and adds to the power of the expulsion forces of the uterine contractions (Grant et al., 2015). Coordination of these forces in unison promotes birth of the fetus and expulsion of the fetal membranes and placenta from the uterus. Interference with these forces (such as when a client is numb due to epidural anesthesia or extremely anxious) can compromise the effectiveness of these powers.

Position (of the Labouring Person)

Positioning for normal labour and birth has evolved. Until about 250 years ago, women were depicted in art and described in essays as sitting upright with flexed

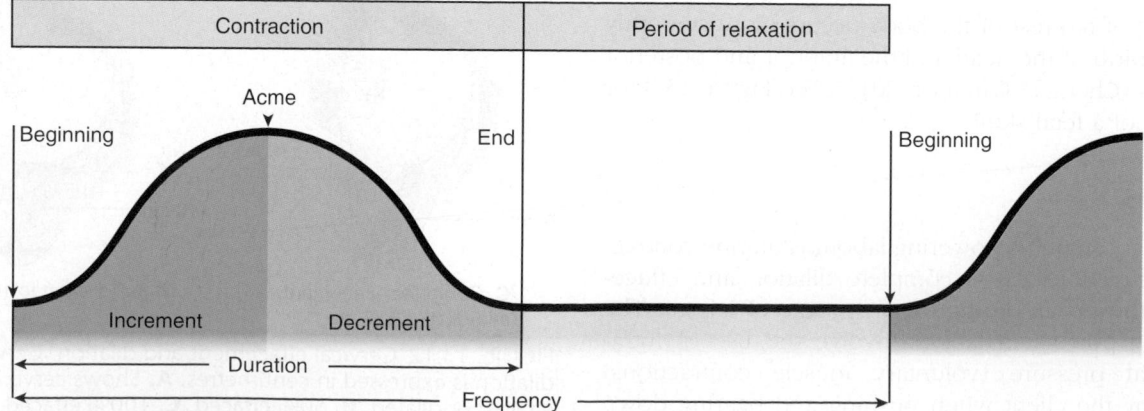

FIGURE 13.13 The three phases of a uterine contraction.

hips, squatting, or less commonly standing or kneeling during the childbirth process. These positions maintain flexion at the hip joint and somewhat straighten the pelvis (Nieuwenhuijze, Low, Korstjens, & Lagro-Janssen, 2014). In the past 250 years, dorsal and dorsal lithotomy positions evolved due to Western medicine practices. The medicalization of childbirth has reduced labouring clients' opportunity for a spontaneous position of choice to a recumbent one. Medical historians say the evolution was to facilitate forceps usage, to promote physicians' control over women, for better visualization of the birth for the physician, and for convenience after administration of anesthesia (Marani & Koch, 2014).

Positioning during labour has only recently been the subject of well-controlled research. Scientific evidence has shown that nonmoving, back-lying positions during labour are not healthy (Gizzo et al., 2014). However, despite this evidence to the contrary, many continue to be supine during labour. Some of the reasons why this practice continues include the beliefs that:

- labouring clients need to conserve their energy and not tire themselves
- nurses cannot keep track of the whereabouts of ambulating clients
- it is the preference of the health care provider
- the fetus can be better monitored in this position using an external fetal monitor
- the supine position facilitates vaginal examinations
- a bed is "where one is supposed to be" in a hospital setting
- the position is more convenient for the delivering health care provider
- labouring clients are "connected to things" that impede movement (Hanson & VandeVusse, 2014).

Labouring clients should be encouraged to assume any position of comfort for them. In a recent randomized, controlled study, the use of a peanut-shaped ball placed between the legs of the client in a side-lying position during labour decreased the length of labour and increased the rate of vaginal births. The use of the peanut ball was associated with a significantly lower incidence of cesarean births. The use and placement of the peanut ball can be a potentially successful nursing intervention to help progress labour and support vaginal birth for those labouring under epidural analgesia (Tussey et al., 2015).

Take Note!

If the only furniture provided is a bed, this is what the client will use. Furnishing rooms with comfortable chairs, beanbags, and other birth props allows a labouring client to choose from a variety of positions and to be free to move.

Changing positions and moving around during labour and birth offer several benefits. Position changes can influence pelvic size and contours. Changing position and walking affect the pelvis joints, which may facilitate fetal descent and rotation. Squatting enlarges the pelvic inlet and outlet diameters, whereas a kneeling position removes pressure on the client's vena cava and helps to rotate the fetus from a posterior position to an anterior one to facilitate birth (Budin, 2015). The use of any upright or lateral position, compared with supine or lithotomy positions, may:

- Reduce the length of the first stage of labour
- Reduce the duration of the second stage of labour
- Reduce the number of assisted deliveries (vacuum and forceps)
- Reduce the incidence of episiotomies and perineal tears
- Contribute to fewer abnormal fetal heart rate patterns
- Increase comfort/reduce requests for pain medication
- Enhance a sense of control by the mother
- Alter the shape and size of the pelvis, which assists in descent
- Assist gravity to move the fetus downward (Cox & King, 2015).

Using the research available can bring better outcomes, heightened professionalism, and evidence-based practice to childbearing practices. The National Institute for Health and Care Excellence (NICE) guidelines recommend discouraging labouring clients from lying supine or semi-supine and encourage them to adapt to any other position that they find comfortable since lying on their backs is associated with longer labours, an increase in surgical births, increased pain, and a higher incidence of FHR abnormalities. The Cochrane collaboration supports the current NICE guidance of positions (Camorcia, 2015).

Psychological Response

Childbearing can be one of the most life-altering experiences for a person. The experience of childbirth goes beyond the physiologic aspects: it influences a person's self-confidence, self-esteem, and view of life, relationships, and children. The state of mind (psyche) throughout the entire process is critical to bringing about a positive outcome. Factors promoting a positive birth experience include:

- Clear information about procedures
- Support, not being alone
- Sense of mastery, self-confidence
- Trust in the health care team
- Positive reaction to the pregnancy
- Personal control over breathing
- Preparation for the childbirth experience

Having a strong sense of self and meaningful support from others can often help clients manage labour well. Feeling safe and secure typically promotes a sense of control and ability to withstand the challenges of the childbearing experience. Anxiety and fear, however, decrease a person's ability to cope with the discomfort of labour. Catecholamines secreted in response to anxiety and fear can inhibit uterine blood flow and placental perfusion. In contrast, relaxation can augment the natural process of labour (Stoll, Swift, Fairbrother, Nethery, & Janssen, 2018). Preparing mentally for childbirth is important so that the client can work with, rather than against, the natural forces of labour.

Philosophy

Not everyone views childbirth in the same way. A philosophical continuum exists that extends from viewing labour as a disease process to a normal process. One philosophy assumes that individuals cannot manage the birth experience adequately and therefore need constant expert monitoring and management. The other philosophy assumes that every individual is capable of actively participating in their birth experience.

The health care systems in North America today appear to be leaning toward the former philosophy, applying technologic interventions to most people who enter the hospital system. Giving birth in a hospital in the 21st century has become "intervention intensive"—designed to start, continue, and end labour through medical management rather than allowing the normal process of birth to unfold. Advances in medical care have improved the safety for clients with high-risk pregnancies. However, the routine use of intravenous therapy, electronic fetal monitoring, labour augmentation, and epidural anesthesia has not necessarily improved birth outcomes for all pregnant people (Cook et al., 2017). A middle-of-the-road philosophy for intervening when circumstances dictate, along with weighing the risks and benefits before doing so, may be more appropriate for low-risk individuals.

During the 1970s, family-centred maternity care was developed in response to the consumer reaction to the depersonalization of birth. The hope was to shift the philosophy from "technologization" to personalization to humanize childbirth. The term *family-centred birthing* is more appropriate today to denote the low-tech, high-touch approach requested by many childbearing persons, who view childbirth as a normal process. Now the Society of Obstetricians and Gynecologists of Canada (SOGC) recommends continuous labour support for all clients in active labour, indicating that birthing units should provide 1-on-1 continuous support from an educated labour support person (Lee, Dy, & Azzam, 2016). The Association of Women's Health, Obstetric and Neonatal Nurses (AWHONN) specifies that continuous labour support be provided by a registered nurse (RN) to achieve improved birth outcomes through collaboration, assessments, and implementation of individualized care that supports the client's physical, psychological, and sociocultural needs (AWHONN, 2018).

Registered midwives have been champions of family-centred birthing, and their participation in the childbirth process is associated with fewer unnecessary interventions when compared with obstetricians. Registered midwives subscribe to a normal birth process where the labouring person uses their own instincts and bodily signs during labour. In short, midwives empower individuals within the birthing environment (Casey et al., 2015). In Canada, midwifery education consists of a 4-year baccalaureate degree, and to be eligible for professional practice, midwives must be registered and regulated through their provincial professional body (Canadian Association of Midwives, 2018). This differentiates **registered midwives** from *lay midwives*, who may have personal or lived experience with childbirth, but no formal education or professional oversight.

No matter what philosophy is held, it is ideal if everyone involved in the particular birth process—from the health care provider to the client—shares the same philosophy toward the birth process.

Partners

People desire support and attentive care during labour and birth. Caregivers can convey emotional support by offering their continued presence and words of encouragement. Throughout the world, few are left to labour totally alone: emotional, physical, or spiritual support during labour is the norm for most cultures. According to the Childbirth Connection's ongoing *Listening to Mothers Initiative III* Survey, 99% of women reported having received some type of supportive care during labour (Edmonds, Cwiertniewicz, & Stoll, 2015). A caring partner or health care professional such as a nurse or midwife can use massage, light touch, acupressure, hand-holding, stroking, and relaxation; can help the client communicate their wishes to the staff; and can provide a continuous, reassuring presence, all of which bring some degree of comfort to the labouring person (Capogna, 2015). Although the presence of the mother's significant other at the birth provides special emotional support, a partner can be anyone who is present to support the client throughout the experience. For many expectant parents, the essential ingredients for a safe and satisfying birth include a sense of empowerment and success in coping with or transcending the experience, in addition to having solid, positive encouragement from a support companion.

Doula is a Greek word meaning woman servant or caregiver. It now commonly refers to a person who offers emotional and practical support to an expectant client or couple before, during, and after childbirth. A doula believes in "mothering the mother," but clinical support remains the job of the nurse, midwife, or medical staff (Ahlemeyer & Mahon, 2015). The doula, who is an experienced labour companion, provides the labouring client and partner with emotional and physical support and information throughout the entire labour and birth experience. Research has shown that continuous presence of a trained support person throughout the process of labour reduces the need for medication for pain relief, the use of vacuum or forceps delivery, the need for cesarean births, and is associated with a reduction in the length of labour (Hodnett, Gates, Hofmeyr, & Sakala, 2017).

A recent study in the United States found that nursing care decreases the likelihood of negative evaluations of the childbirth experience, feelings of tenseness during labour, and finding labour worse than expected. Also reported were less perineal trauma, reduced difficulty in mothering, and reduced likelihood of early cessation of breastfeeding. Continuous support by nurses included reassurance, encouragement, praise, and explanation (Iravani, Zarean, Janghorbani, & Bahrami, 2015).

Given the many benefits of intrapartum support, labouring clients should always receive support, whether from nurses, doulas, significant others, or family. Whoever the labour support partner is, he or she should provide the labouring client with continuous presence, comfort, and encouragement. The overall objective of providing support during childbirth is to create a positive experience, while preserving physical and psychological health.

Patience

The birth process takes time. If more time were allowed for clients to labour naturally without intervention, the cesarean birth rate would most likely be reduced. In one study, continuous support provided by midwives during labour reduced the duration of labour and the number of cesarean births; this model of support should be available to all universally (Cox & King, 2015). The literature suggests that delaying interventions can give a labouring client enough time to progress in labour and reduce the need for surgical intervention (American College of Obstetricians and Gynecologists [ACOG], 2015).

We are a long way from achieving these goals—the current cesarean birth rate in Canada, at 28.2%, means that cesarean sections are the most commonly performed inpatient surgical procedure in Canada (Canadian Institute for Health Information [CIHI], 2018). Cesarean birth rate is associated with increased morbidity and mortality for both mother and infant as well as increased inpatient length of stay and health care costs (Centers for Disease Control and Prevention [CDC], 2014).

It is difficult to predict how a labour will progress and therefore equally difficult to determine how long a labour will last. There is no way to estimate the likely strength and frequency of uterine contractions, the extent to which the cervix will soften and dilate,

and how much the fetal head will mould to fit the birth canal. We cannot know beforehand whether the complex fetal rotations needed for an efficient labour will take place properly. All of these factors are unknowns when labour begins.

Induction of Labour

There is a trend in health care to attempt to manipulate the process of labour through medical means such as artificial rupture of membranes (amniotomy) and induction or augmentation of labour with oxytocin (Kriebs, 2015). The labour induction rate has doubled in North America since the 1990s (Leduc, Biringer, Lee, & Dy, 2013; Moses, 2018).

Approximately one in four pregnant clients are induced or have labour augmented with uterine-stimulating drugs or artificial rupture of membranes to accelerate the progress, and early term (in the 37th and 38th week) inductions have increased also. **Induction** of labour refers to medical interventions used to begin labour prior to its natural onset. **Augmentation** of labour means implementing a medical intervention to increase the frequency or efficacy of naturally occurring contractions. An amniotomy (artificial rupture of the fetal membranes) may be performed to induce or augment labour when the membranes have not ruptured spontaneously. Doing so allows the fetal head to have more direct contact with the cervix to dilate it. This procedure is performed with the fetal head at −2 station or lower, and with some degree of cervical dilation, usually 2 to 3 cm. Synthetic oxytocin (Pitocin) is also used to induce or augment labour by stimulating uterine contractions. It is administered piggybacked into the primary intravenous line with an infusion pump titrated to uterine activity.

Elective induction of labour is at an all-time high in North America despite known associated risks. It can lead to birth of an infant too early, a long labour, lengthy exposure to a high-alert medication with its potential side effects, unnecessary cesarean birth, and maternal and neonatal morbidity. Induction of labour brings a cascade of related interventions, such as an intravenous line, continuous electronic fetal monitoring, limitations in mobility with possible confinement to bed, amniotomy, pharmacologic labour-stimulating agents, parenteral pain medications, and regional anesthesia, each with its own set of potential complications and risks. These risks apply to all clients having the procedure; however, for nulliparous clients before 41 weeks of gestation with an unfavourable cervix, the main risk is cesarean birth after unsuccessful labour induction with the potential for maternal and neonatal morbidity and increased health care costs. When cesarean occurs, subsequent births are likely to be via cesarean as well (Caughey, 2014). Compelling evidence indicates that elective induction of labour may increase the risk of cesarean birth, especially for nulliparas (Le Ray et al., 2015). Elective induction of labour in nulliparas is also associated with postpartum hemorrhage, neonatal resuscitation, and longer hospitalizations without improvement in neonatal outcomes (Glavind & Uldbjerg, 2015). The belief is that many cesarean births could be avoided if labours were allowed more time, and if the natural labour process were allowed to complete the job. The longer wait (using the intervention of patience) usually results in less intervention. The ACOG attributes the dramatic increase in inductions in part to pressure from clients, convenience for health care providers, and liability concerns. Other reasons for the increase in inductions include the availability of better cervical ripening agents and a more relaxed attitude toward marginal indications for inductions. They recommend a cautious approach regarding elective induction until clinical trials can validate a more liberal use of labour inductions (ACOG, 2015). The SOGC's list of current medical indications for inducing labour includes:

- Preeclampsia ≥37 weeks
- Spontaneous rupture of membranes at term when GBS culture is positive
- Intra uterine growth restriction (IUGR)
- A pregnancy of more than 42 weeks of gestation
- Significant maternal disease not responding to treatment
- Significant but stable antepartum hemorrhage
- Oligohydramnios (Leduc et al., 2013)
- Chorioamnionitis

Note that suspected fetal macrosomia (estimated fetal weight >4,000 g) has previously been an identified indication for induction of labour, however the SOGC now advises against this (Leduc et al., 2013).

Augmentation of labour is initiated when labour began spontaneously, but progress becomes protracted (slowed) or arrested (stopped), which may occur in either the first stage or second stage of labour (Ehsanipoor & Satin, 2018). When the labouring client feels the urge to bear down and is fully dilated (to 10 cm), the second stage (or pushing phase) begins. Most people respond extremely well to messages from their body without requiring direction from their nurse or midwife, especially if they are not using analgesic or anesthetic medication. A more natural, undirected approach allows the client to wait and bear down only when the client feels the urge to push. Having patience and letting nature take its course will reduce the incidence of physiologic stress for the client, resulting in less trauma to perineal tissue.

Patient (Client) Preparation: Prenatal Education

Basic prenatal education can help clients manage their labour process and feel in control of their birthing experience. The literature indicates that if an individual is prepared before the labour and birth experience, the labour is more likely to remain normal or natural (without the need for medical intervention) (Byrne, Hauck, Fisher, Bayes, & Schutze, 2014). An increasing body of evidence also indicates that the well-prepared client, with good labour support, is less likely to need analgesia, anesthesia, or cesarean birth (Hoang, 2014).

Prenatal education teaches expectant parents about the childbirth experience and increases their sense of control. Clients and couples are then able to work as active participants during the labour and birth experience (Jordan et al., 2014). The research also suggests that prenatal preparation may affect intrapartum and postpartum psychosocial outcomes (Budin, 2014). For example, prenatal education covering parenting communication classes had a significant effect on postpartum anxiety and postpartum adjustment. In a recent study of Hispanic women attending a community prenatal education program, researchers found that many women experienced anguish from unknowns during their pregnancy, leading to a yearning to learn and understand more, but with a desire to do so without sacrificing their cultural identity (Fitzgerald, Cronin, & Boccella, 2016). In another study involving Somali couples, most did not attend prenatal classes because their religion doesn't allow women and men to learn in the same room, and the men are not allowed to look at naked figures displayed in photos and videos (Wojnar, 2015).

These findings have important implications for nurses teaching prenatal classes to diverse cultures. To be effective, the prenatal educational setting must be sensitive, inclusive, and respectful of people's beliefs. Prenatal education must be viewed as an opportunity to strengthen families by providing anticipatory guidance and improving family members' life skills. In short, prenatal education helps to promote healthy families during the transition to parenthood and beyond (Woods & Chesser, 2015).

There is evidence that some pregnant people use herbs to induce labour and also during labour for pain relief. Desire to have control over their health has been cited as the strongest motive for people to use herbal medicine. A few of the herbs used include *Caulophyllum*, made from the herb blue cohosh to induce labour contractions; blue and black cohosh, raspberry leaves, castor oil and evening primrose oil used for cervical ripening and induction of labour; and *Chanlibao* to shorten the second stage of labour by strengthening the contractions (Ramasubramaniam, Renganathan, Vijayalakshmi, & Mallo-Banatao, 2015). The use of herbs during labour have been found to benefit some individuals by easing the labour process without side effects, but clinical trials are lacking to prove the safety and effectiveness of them.

Pain Management

Labour and birth, although a normal physiologic process, can produce significant discomfort and pain. Pain during labour is a nearly universal experience. Controlling and reducing the uterine discomfort without harm to the fetus or labour process is the major focus of pain management during childbirth. Pain is a subjective experience involving a complex interaction of physiologic, spiritual, psychosocial, cultural, and environmental influences (Van der Gucht & Lewis, 2015). Cultural values and learned behaviours influence perception and response to pain, as do anxiety and fear, both of which tend to heighten the sense of pain (Jones, 2015). The challenge for care providers is to find the right combination of pain and coping management methods to keep the discomfort manageable while minimizing the negative effect on the fetus, the normal physiology of labour, bonding with the baby, breastfeeding, and a client's perception of the labour itself (King et al., 2015). Chapter 14 presents a full discussion of pain management during labour and birth.

PHYSIOLOGIC RESPONSES TO LABOUR

Labour is the process by which the birth canal is prepared to allow the fetus to pass from the uterine cavity to the outside world. During pregnancy, progesterone secreted from the placenta suppresses the spontaneous contractions of a typical uterus, keeping the fetus within the uterus. In addition, the cervix remains firm and noncompliant. At term, however, changes occur in the cervix that make it softer. In addition, uterine contractions become more frequent and regular, signaling the onset of labour.

The labour process involves a series of rhythmic, involuntary, usually quite uncomfortable uterine muscle contractions. The contractions bring about a shortening that causes effacement and dilation of the cervix and a bursting of the fetal membranes. Uterine contractions of an intensity of 30 mm Hg or greater promote cervical dilation. Then, accompanied by both reflex and voluntary contractions of the abdominal muscles (pushing), the uterine contractions result in the birth of the baby (Grant et al., 2015). During labour, the labouring client and the fetus make several physiologic adaptations.

Maternal Responses

As the client progresses through childbirth, numerous physiologic responses occur that assist the adaptation to the labour process. The labour process stresses several of the body systems, which react through numerous compensatory mechanisms. Anticipated physiologic responses include:

- Heart rate increases by 10 to 20 bpm.
- Cardiac output increases by 12% to 31% during the first stage of labour and by 50% during the second stage of labour.
- Blood pressure increases by up to 35 mm Hg during uterine contractions in all labour stages.
- The white blood cell count increases to 25,000 to 30,000 cells/mm^3, perhaps as a result of tissue trauma.
- Respiratory rate increases, and more oxygen is consumed related to the increase in metabolism.
- Gastric motility and food absorption decrease, which may increase the risk of nausea and vomiting during the transition stage of labour.
- Gastric emptying and gastric pH decrease, increasing the risk of vomiting.
- Temperature rises slightly, possibly due to an increase in muscle activity.
- Muscular aches/cramps occur as a result of the stressed musculoskeletal system.
- Basal metabolic rate increases, and blood glucose levels decrease because of the stress of labour (Cheng & Caughey, 2017).

A person's ability to adapt to the stress of labour is influenced by their psychological and physical state. Among the many factors that affect coping abilities are:

- Previous birth experiences and their outcomes (complications and previous birth outcomes)
- Current pregnancy experience (planned vs. unplanned, discomforts experienced, age, risk status of pregnancy, chronic illness, weight gain)
- Cultural considerations (values and beliefs about health status)
- Support system (presence and support of a valued partner during labour)
- Childbirth preparation (attended childbirth classes and has practiced paced breathing techniques)
- Exercise during pregnancy (muscle tone; ability to assist with intra-abdominal pushing)
- Expectations of the birthing experience (viewed as a meaningful or stressful event)
- Anxiety level (excessive anxiety may interfere with labour progress)
- Fear of labour and loss of control (fear may enhance pain perception, augmenting fear)
- Fatigue and weariness (King et al., 2015).

Fetal Responses

Although the focus during labour may be on assessing the client's adaptations, several physiologic adaptations occur in the fetus as well. The fetus is experiencing labour at the same time. If the fetus is healthy, the stress of labour usually has no adverse effects. The nurse needs to be alert to any abnormalities in the fetus's adaptation to labour. Fetal responses to labour include:

- Periodic fetal heart rate accelerations and possible slight decelerations related to fetal movement, fundal pressure, and uterine contractions
- Decrease in circulation and perfusion to the fetus secondary to uterine contractions (a healthy fetus is able to compensate for this drop)
- Increase in arterial carbon dioxide pressure (PCO_2)
- Decrease in fetal practice breathing movements throughout labour
- Decrease in fetal oxygen pressure with a decrease in the partial pressure of oxygen (PO_2) (Verklan & Walden, 2014).

Take Note!

Fetal respiratory changes during labour help to prepare the fetus for extrauterine respiration immediately after birth.

STAGES OF LABOUR

Labour is typically divided into four stages: dilation, expulsive, placental, and restorative. Table 13.2 summarizes the major events of each stage.

The first stage is the longest: it begins with the first true contraction and ends with full dilation (opening) of the cervix. Because this stage lasts so long, it is divided into three phases, each corresponding to the

TABLE 13.2	STAGES AND PHASES OF LABOUR			
	First Stage	**Second Stage**	**Third Stage**	**Fourth Stage**
Description	From 0 to 10 cm dilation; consists of three phases	From complete dilation (10 cm) to birth of the newborn; may last up to 3 hours or longer	Separation and delivery of the placenta; usually takes 5–10 minutes, but may take up to 30 minutes	1–4 hours after the birth of the newborn; time of significant physiologic adjustment
Phases	**Latent phase** (0–3 cm dilation) • Cervical dilation from 0 to 3 cm • Cervical effacement from 0% to 40% • Nullipara, lasts average of up to 9 hours; multipara, lasts average of up to 5–6 hours • Contraction frequency every 5–10 minutes • Contraction duration 30–45 seconds • Contraction intensity mild to palpation **Active phase** (4–7 cm dilation) • Cervical dilation from 4 to 7 cm • Cervical effacement from 40% to 80% • Nullipara, lasts up to 6 hours on average; multipara, lasts up to 4 hours on average • Contraction frequency every 2–5 minutes • Contraction duration 45–60 seconds • Contraction intensity moderate to palpation **Transition phase** (8–10 cm dilation) • Cervical dilation from 8 to 10 cm • Cervical effacement from 80% to 100% • Nullipara lasts up to 1 hour on average; multipara, lasts up to 30 minutes on average • Contraction frequency every 1–2 minutes • Contraction duration 60–90 seconds • Contraction intensity strong by palpation	**Pelvic phase** (period of fetal descent) **Perineal phase** (period of active pushing) • Nullipara, lasts up to 1 hour on average; multipara, lasts up to 30 minutes on average • Contraction frequency every 2–3 minutes or less • Contraction duration 60–90 seconds • Contraction intensity strong by palpation • Strong urge to push during the later perineal phase	**Placental separation:** detaching from uterine wall **Placental expulsion:** coming outside the vaginal opening	

Adapted from Cheng, Y. W., & Caughey, A. B. (2017). Normal labor and delivery. *eMedicine*. Retrieved from http://emedicine.medscape.com/article/260036-overview; Cunningham, F. G., Leveno, K. J., Bloom, S. L., Spong, C. Y., Dashe, J. S., Hoffman, B. L., . . . Sheffield, J. S. (2014). *Williams obstetrics* (24th ed.). New York: McGraw-Hill Education; and King, T. L., Brucker, M. C., Kriebs, J. M., Fahey, J. O., Gegor, C. L., & Varney, H. (2015). *Varney's midwifery* (5th ed.). Burlington, MA: Jones & Bartlett Learning.

progressive dilation of the cervix. The second stage of labour, or the expulsive stage, begins when the cervix is completely dilated and ends with the birth of the newborn. The expulsive stage can last from minutes to hours. The contractions typically occur every 2 to 3 minutes, lasting 60 to 90 seconds, and are strong by palpation. The labouring client is usually intent on the work of pushing during this stage. The third stage, or placental expulsion, starts after the newborn is born and ends with the separation and birth of the placenta. Continued uterine contractions typically cause the placenta to be expelled within 5 to 30 minutes. If the newborn is stable, bonding of infant and mother takes place during this stage through touching, holding, and skin-to-skin contact.

The fourth stage, or the restorative stage or immediate postpartum period, lasts from 1 to 4 hours after birth. This period is when the client's body begins to stabilize after the hard work of labour and the loss of the products of conception. The fourth stage is sometimes not recognized as a true stage of labour, but it is a critical period for physiologic transition as well as new family attachment. Close monitoring of both the client and newborn are essential during this stage (Green, 2015).

First Stage

During the first stage of labour, the fundamental change underlying the process is progressive dilation of the cervix. Cervical dilation is gauged subjectively by vaginal examination and is expressed in centimetres. The first stage ends when the cervix is dilated to 10 cm in diameter and is large enough to permit the passage of a fetal head of average size. The fetal membranes, or bag of waters, usually rupture during the first stage, but they may have burst earlier or may even remain intact until birth. For the primigravida, the first stage of labour lasts an average of 12 hours; however, this time can vary widely. For the multiparous client, the first stage often lasts approximately half that long.

During the first stage of labour, clients usually perceive the visceral pain of diffuse abdominal cramping and uterine contractions. Discomfort during the first stage of labour is primarily a result of the dilation of the cervix and lower uterine segment, and the distention (stretching) of these structures during contractions. The first stage is divided into three phases: latent or early phase, active phase, and transition phase.

Latent or Early Phase

The latent or early phase gives rise to the familiar signs and symptoms of labour. This phase begins with the start of regular contractions and ends when rapid cervical dilation begins. Cervical effacement occurs during this phase, and the cervix dilates from 0 to 3 cm.

Contractions usually occur every 5 to 10 minutes, last 30 to 45 seconds, and are mild by palpation. Assessment of intensity is evaluated by pressing down on the fundus during a contraction to see if it can be dented with the one's fingers. The ability to indent the fundus at the peak of the contraction would typically indicate a mild contraction. Effacement of the cervix is from 0% to 40%. Many clients will perceive their contractions to be similar to menstrual cramps.

For the nulliparous client, the latent phase lasts about 9 hours on average; in the multiparous client, it lasts about 6 hours on average (Cheng & Caughey, 2017). During this phase, labouring clients may be apprehensive but excited about the start of their labour after their long gestational period. The SOGC advises that health care providers encourage clients to remain home where they are comfortable during this phase, waiting until the onset of active labour before admission to birthing unit to reduce the number of unnecessary interventions in labour (Lee et al., 2016).

> Think back to the couple who were sent home from the hospital birthing centre. Three days later Kathy awoke with a wet sensation and intense discomfort in her back, spreading around to her abdomen. She decided to go for a walk, but her contractions didn't diminish. Instead, her contractions continued to occur every few minutes and grew stronger in intensity. She and Chuck decided to go back to the hospital birthing centre. Was there a difference in the location of Kathy's discomfort this time? What changes will the admission nurse find in Kathy if this is true labour?

Active Phase

The active phase of labour encompasses the time from an increase in the rate of cervical dilation (end of latent phase of labour) until completion of cervical dilation. Cervical dilation begins to occur more rapidly during the active phase. The cervix usually dilates from 4 to 7 cm, with 40% to 80% effacement taking place. This phase can last up to 6 hours for the nulliparous client and 4.5 hours for the multiparous client (Leap & Hunter, 2015). The fetus descends farther in the pelvis. Contractions become more frequent (every 2 to 5 minutes) and increase in duration (45 to 60 seconds). The client's discomfort intensifies as the efficacy of the contractions increases (moderate to strong by palpation). During this phase, labouring clients generally become more intense and inwardly focused, absorbed in the serious work of labour. The client may start to limit interactions with those in the room. Those who have attended childbirth education classes may begin to use the relaxation and paced breathing techniques that they learned to cope with the contractions. The expected dilation rate for the nulliparous client is at least 0.5 cm/hr (Lee et al., 2016); for the multiparous client, it is 1.5 cm/hr (Cunningham et al., 2014).

Transition Phase

The transition phase is the last phase of the first stage of labour. During this phase, dilation slows, progressing from 8 to 10 cm, with effacement from 80% to 100%. The transition phase can be the most uncomfortable and, fortunately, the shortest phase of the first stage, lasting approximately 1 hour in the first birth and perhaps 15 to 30 minutes in successive births (Tharpe et al., 2016). During transition, the contractions are stronger in intensity, more painful, more frequent (every 1 to 2 minutes), and they last longer (60 to 90 seconds). The average rate of fetal descent is 1 cm/hr in nulliparous clients and 2 cm/hr in multiparous clients. Pressure on the rectum is great, and there is a strong desire to contract the abdominal muscles and push.

Other symptoms labouring clients may experience during the transitional phase include nausea and vomiting, trembling extremities, backache, increased apprehension and irritability, restless movement, increased bloody show (a bloody mucous discharge from the vagina), inability to relax, diaphoresis, feelings of loss of control, and being overwhelmed (and may say, "I can't take it anymore") (Cunningham et al., 2014).

> In assessing Kathy, the nurse finds she is 4 cm dilated and 50% effaced with ruptured membranes. In what stage and phase of labour would this assessment finding place Kathy?

Second Stage

The second stage of labour begins with complete cervical dilation (10 cm) and effacement (100%) and ends with the birth of the newborn. Although the previous stage of labour primarily involved the thinning and opening of the cervix, this stage involves moving the fetus through the birth canal and out of the body. The cardinal movements of labour occur during the early phase of passive descent in the second stage of labour.

Contractions typically occur every 2 to 3 minutes, last 60 to 90 seconds, and are described as strong by palpation. The average length of the second stage of labour in a nullipara is approximately 1 to 2 hours and less than 30 minutes for a multipara. During this expulsive stage, the client usually feels more in control and

may feel less irritable and agitated, while focusing on the work of pushing. The urge to push is generally felt when there is direct contact of the fetus to the pelvic floor. Stretch receptors in the wall of the vagina, rectum, and perineum communicate the pressure of the fetus descending in the birth canal that, along with increased abdominal pressure, causes the overwhelming urge to push (Camorcia, 2015).

Pushing

The second stage of labour has two phases (pelvic and perineal) related to the existence and quality of the urge to push and to obstetric conditions related to fetal descent. The early phase of the second stage is called the pelvic phase, because it is during this phase that the fetal head is negotiating the pelvis, rotating, and advancing in descent. The later phase is called the perineal phase, because at this point the fetal head is lower in the pelvis and is distending the perineum. The occurrence of a strong urge to push characterizes the later phase of the second stage and has also been called the phase of active pushing (Cheng & Caughey, 2015).

The later perineal phase occurs when the client feels a tremendous urge to push as the fetal head is lowered and is distending the perineum. The perineum bulges and there is an increase in bloody show. The fetal head becomes apparent at the vaginal opening but disappears between contractions. When the top of the head no longer regresses between contractions, it is said to have crowned. The fetus rotates as it manoeuvres out. Evidence now shows that labour actually progresses slower than previously thought in the past. Many clients benefit from a little more time to labour and give birth vaginally instead of moving to a surgical birth (ACOG, 2014). The second stage commonly lasts up to 3 hours in a first labour and up to an hour in subsequent ones (Fig. 13.14).

SPONTANEOUS PUSHING VERSUS DIRECTED PUSHING

There are two ways of conducting the second stage of labour: *spontaneous* or *non-directed pushing* (following the client's spontaneous urge) and *directed pushing* (pushing directed by the caregiver). Spontaneous pushing represents a natural way of managing the second stage of labour. However, lately, and as a result of epidural analgesia, health care providers frequently resort to directed pushing without taking into account the potential negative repercussions this could have on the client and fetus.

Evidence is mounting that the management of the second stage, particularly pushing, is a modifiable risk factor in long-term perinatal outcomes (ACOG, 2015). Research supports spontaneous physiologic approaches to second-stage labour care; however, many labouring

FIGURE 13.14 Birth sequence from crowning through birth of the newborn. **A.** Early crowning of the fetal head. Notice the bulging of the perineum. **B.** Late crowning. Notice that the fetal head is appearing face down. This is the normal OA position. **C.** As the head extends, you can see that the occiput is to the client's right side—ROA position. **D.** The cardinal movement of extension. **E.** The shoulders are born. Notice how the head has turned to line up with the shoulders—the cardinal movement of external rotation. **F.** The body easily follows the shoulders. **G.** The newborn is held for the first time. (© B. Proud.)

clients in hospital settings continue to receive direction from health care providers to use prolonged Valsalva (holding breath) bearing-down efforts as soon as the cervix is completely dilated. Since the adoption of a medicalized approach to management of labour and birth in North America, labouring clients in the second stage have been taught to hold their breath to the count of 10, inhale again, push again, and repeat the process several times during a contraction. This sustained, strenuous style of pushing, that is, Valsalva bearing-down is linked to hemodynamic changes in the client and interferes with oxygen exchange between the pregnant individual and the fetus. In addition, it is associated with pelvic floor damage: the longer the push, the more damage to the pelvic floor. The SOGC recommends that the method of pushing (spontaneous or directed) should be based on the client's own preference (Lee et al., 2016).

In clinical practice, health care providers sometimes resist delaying the onset of pushing after the second stage of labour has begun because of a belief that it will increase labour time. Delaying bearing-down efforts during the second stage until the client feels the urge to push (labouring down) allows for optimal use of energy, has no detrimental effects, and results in improved fetal oxygenation (Osborne & Hanson, 2014). Research shows that delaying pushing for up to 90 minutes after complete cervical dilation resulted in a significant decrease in the time spent pushing without a significant increase in total time in second stage of labour (King et al., 2015). Because research does not support a policy of directed pushing, and some evidence suggests it may be harmful, the practice of directed pushing should be abandoned (Brodrick, 2014). The Association of Women's Health, Obstetric and Neonatal Nurses (AWHONN, 2014) recommends an open-glottis method in which air is released during pushing to prevent the buildup of intrathoracic pressure. Doing so also supports the client's involuntary bearing-down efforts (Holvey, 2014). The adoption of a physiologic, client-directed approach to bearing down is advocated (King et al., 2015).

Behaviours demonstrated by labouring clients during this time include pushing at the onset of the urge to bear down; using their own pattern and technique of bearing down in response to sensations they experience; using open-glottis bearing down with contractions; pushing with variations in strength and duration; pushing down with progressive intensity; and using multiple positions to increase progress and comfort. This approach is in stark contrast to management by arbitrary time limits and the directed bearing-down efforts seen in practice today. Labour nurses need to develop an evidence-based approach that acknowledges and reinforces clients' innate ability to birth and refrain from trying to direct clients' pushing behaviours (Reed, 2015). It is also important that labour nurses be able to advocate the need for the clients to push in this approach to other health care providers.

Labouring down (promotion of passive descent) is an alternative strategy for second-stage management in clients with epidurals. Using this approach, the fetus descends and is born without coached pushing.

Third Stage

The third stage of labour begins with the birth of the newborn and ends with the separation and birth of the placenta. It consists of two phases: placental separation and placental expulsion. Worldwide, approximately 800 individuals die each day from preventable causes related to giving birth. The single most common cause is severe bleeding, which can kill a person within hours if care is delayed. Prompt and effective management is paramount to saving these lives, and prevention measures can be initiated in the third stage of labour. Controversy continues about active versus expectant management of the third stage of labour. The SOGC recommends the routine use of oxytocic drugs in the third stage of labour to reduce the risk of hemorrhage (Lee et al., 2016). See Evidence-Based Practice 13.1.

Placental Separation

After the infant is born, the uterus continues to contract strongly and can now retract, decreasing markedly in size. These contractions cause the placenta to pull away from the uterine wall. The following signs of separation indicate that the placenta is ready to deliver:
- The uterus rises upward.
- The umbilical cord lengthens.
- A sudden trickle of blood is released from the vaginal opening.
- The uterus changes its shape to globular.

Spontaneous birth of the placenta occurs in one of two ways: the fetal side (shiny grey side) presenting first (called Schultz's mechanism or more commonly called "shiny Schultz's") or the uterine side (red raw side) presenting first (termed Duncan's mechanism or "dirty Duncan").

Placental Expulsion

After separation of the placenta from the uterine wall, continued uterine contractions cause the placenta to be expelled within 2 to 30 minutes unless there is gentle external traction to assist. After the placenta is expelled, the uterus is massaged briefly by the attending physician, nurse practitioner, or midwife until it is firm so that uterine blood vessels constrict, minimizing the possibility of

EVIDENCE-BASED PRACTICE 13.1   ACTIVE VERSUS EXPECTANT MANAGEMENT FOR CLIENTS IN LABOUR

STUDY

Once birth has taken place, the uterus continues to contract, causing the placenta to separate from the wall of the uterus. The client then delivers the placenta without outside intervention. This is termed expectant management of the third stage of labour. Active management of the third stage of labour involves giving a prophylactic uterotonic drug to contract the uterus, clamping the umbilical cord early before cord pulsations stops, and traction is applied to the cord with counter-pressure on the uterus to deliver the placenta. Active management was introduced to try to reduce postpartum hemorrhage, a major contributor to maternal mortality. The objective of this study was to compare the effectiveness of active versus expectant management of the third stage of labour.

Findings

Seven studies involving 8,247 women were analyzed. Because of the clinical heterogeneity of the sample,

random effects were used in the analysis. Active management showed a significant decrease in primary blood loss greater than 500 mL and subsequent anemia. However, it reduced the newborn's birthweight and increased the mother's blood pressure. Overall, the quality of the evidence was low and more data are needed to be confident in the findings.

Nursing Implications

Although there was lack of high-quality evidence in this review, active management of the third stage of labour reduced the risk of hemorrhage after childbirth, but adverse effects were identified. Pregnant clients should be provided information on the benefits and harms of both methods to support informed choice. Given the concerns about early cord clamping and the potential adverse effects of uterotonic drugs, it is important to look at the individual components of third-stage management and work toward modifications to bring about the best outcomes.

Adapted from Begley, C. M., Gyte, G. M. L., Devane, D., McGuire, W., & Weeks, A. (2015). Active versus expectant management for women in the third stage of labor. *Cochrane Database of Systematic Reviews*, (3), CD007412.

hemorrhage. Normal blood loss is approximately 500 mL for a vaginal birth and 1,000 mL for a cesarean birth. Blood loss of over 1,000 mL is considered severe (Pavord & Maybury, 2015).

If the placenta does not spontaneously deliver, the health care provider assists with its removal by manual extraction. On expulsion, the placenta is inspected for its intactness by the health care provider and the nurse to make sure all sections are present. If any piece is still attached to the uterine wall, the client is at risk for postpartum hemorrhage because it becomes a space-occupying object that interferes with the ability of the uterus to contract fully and effectively.

Fourth Stage

The fourth stage begins with completion of the expulsion of the placenta and membranes and ends with the initial physiologic adjustment and stabilization of the client (1 to 4 hours after birth). This stage initiates the postpartum period. The client usually feels a sense of peace and excitement, is wide awake, and may be very talkative initially. The attachment process begins with parents inspecting the

newborn and desiring to cuddle and breastfeed. The client's fundus should be firm and well contracted. Typically at this time, the fundus is located at the midline between the umbilicus and the symphysis, but it then slowly rises to the level of the umbilicus during the first hour after birth (Jordan et al., 2014). If the uterus becomes boggy, it is massaged to keep it firm. The lochia (vaginal discharge) is red, mixed with small clots, and of moderate flow. If the client has had a perineal tear or an episiotomy during the second stage of labour, it will be repaired at this point, and should then be intact, with the edges approximated and clean and no redness or edema present.

The focus during this stage is to monitor the client closely to prevent hemorrhage, bladder distention, and venous thrombosis. Usually the client is thirsty and hungry during this time and may request food and drink. The bladder is hypotonic and thus the client has limited sensation to acknowledge a full bladder or to void. Vital signs, the amount and consistency of the vaginal discharge (lochia), and the uterine fundus are typically monitored every 15 minutes for at least 1 hour. The client will be feeling cramp-like discomfort during this time due to the contracting uterus.

KEY CONCEPTS

- Labour is a complex, multifaceted interaction between the labouring individual and fetus. Thus, it is difficult to determine exactly why labour begins and what initiates it.

- Before the onset of labour, a pregnant person's body undergoes several changes in preparation for the birth of the newborn, often leading to characteristic signs and symptoms that suggest that labour is near. These changes include cervical changes, lightening, increased energy level, bloody show, Braxton Hicks contractions, and spontaneous rupture of membranes.

- False labour is a condition seen during the latter weeks of some pregnancies in which irregular uterine contractions are felt, but the cervix is not affected. This can be referred to as prelabour or practice labour.

- The critical factors in labour and birth are designated as the 10 P's: passageway (birth canal), passenger (fetus and placenta), powers (contractions), position (of the labouring client), psychological response, philosophy (low tech, high touch), partners (support caregivers), patience (natural timing), patient (client) preparation (childbirth knowledge base), and pain management (comfort measures).

- The size and shape of a pelvis are determining factors for a vaginal birth. The pelvis is classified according to four main shapes: gynecoid, anthropoid, android, and platypelloid.

- The labour process is comprised of a series of rhythmic, involuntary, usually quite uncomfortable uterine muscle contractions that bring about a shortening (effacement) and opening (dilation) of the cervix, and a bursting of the fetal membranes. Important parameters of uterine contractions are frequency, duration, and intensity.

- The diameters of the fetal skull vary considerably, with some diameters shortening and others lengthening as the head is moulded during the labour and birth process.

- Pain during labour is a nearly universal experience for childbearing individuals. Having a strong sense of self and meaningful support from others can often help clients manage labour well and reduce their sensation of pain.

- Preparing mentally for childbirth is important for clients to enable them to work with the natural forces of labour and not against them.

- As the client experiences and progresses through childbirth, numerous physiologic responses occur that assist in the adaptation to the labouring process.

- Labour is typically divided into four stages that are unequal in length.

- During the first stage, the fundamental change underlying the process is progressive dilation of the cervix. It is divided into three phases: latent phase, active phase, and transition.

- The second stage of labour is from complete cervical dilation (10 cm) and effacement (100%) through the birth of the infant.

- The third stage is that of separation and birth of the placenta. It consists of two phases: placental separation and placental expulsion.

- The fourth stage begins after the birth of the placenta and membranes and ends with the initial physiologic adjustment and stabilization of the postpartum client (1 to 4 hours).

REFERENCES AND RECOMMENDED READINGS

Ahlemeyer, J., & Mahon, S. (2015). Doulas for childbearing women. *MCN: The American Journal of Maternal/Child Nursing, 40*(2), 122–127.

Alexander, L. L., LaRosa, J. H., Bader, H., & Garfield, S. (2014). *New dimensions in women's health* (6th ed.). Sudbury, MA: Jones & Bartlett.

American College of Obstetricians & Gynecologists (ACOG). (2014). *Nation's OB/GYNs take aim at preventing cesareans: New guidelines recommends allowing women to labor longer to help avoid cesarean.* Retrieved from http://www.acog.org/About_ACOG/News_Room/News_Releases/2014/Nations_Ob-Gyns_Take_Aim_at_Preventing_Cesareans

American College of Obstetricians and Gynecologists (ACOG). (2015). Practice Bulletin 107 reaffirmed: Induction of labor. *Obstetrics and Gynecology, 113,* 386–397.

Association of Women's Health, Obstetric and Neonatal Nurses (AWHONN). (2014). *Nursing care and management of the 2nd stage of labor* (2nd ed.). Retrieved from https://www.awhonn.org/awhonn/content.do?name=08_Store/08_labormanagement.htm

Association of Women's Health, Obstetric and Neonatal Nurses. (2018). Continuous labor support for every woman. *Journal of Obstetric, Gynecologic, and Neonatal Nursing, 47*(1), 73–74.

Begley, C. M., Gyte, G. M., Devane, D., McGuire, W., & Weeks, A. (2015). Active versus expectant management for women in the third stage of labor. *Cochrane Database of Systematic Reviews,* (3), CD007412.

Brodrick, A. (2014). Too afraid to push: Dealing with fear of childbirth. *Practicing Midwife, 17*(3), 15–17.

Budin, W. C. (2014). What to teach?. *Journal of Perinatal Education, 23*(2), 59–61.

Budin, W. C. (2015). Choosing wisely for birth. *The Journal of Perinatal Education, 24*(1), 3–5.

Byrne, J., Hauck, Y., Fisher, C., Bayes, S., & Schutze, R. (2014). Effectiveness of a mindfulness-based childbirth education pilot study on maternal self-efficacy and fear of childbirth. *Journal of Midwifery & Women's Health, 59*(2), 192–197.

Camorcia, M. (2015). Chapter 9: The second and third stage of labor. In G. Capogna (Ed.), *Epidural labor analgesia* (pp. 103–119). New York: Springer International Publishing.

Canadian Association of Midwives. (2018). *Midwifery education*. Retrieved from https://canadianmidwives.org/education/

Canadian Institute for Health Information. (2018). *C-section rates continue to increase while birth rates decline*. Retrieved from https://www.cihi.ca/en/c-section-rates-continue-to-increase-while-birth-rates-decline

Capogna, G. (2015). Chapter 24: Humanization of childbirth and epidural analgesia. In G. Capogna (Ed.), *Epidural labor analgesia* (pp. 315–323). New York: Springer International Publishing.

Casey, M., Fealy, G., Kennedy, C., Hegarty, J., Prizeman, G., McNamara, M., . . . Rohde, D. (2015). Nurses', midwives' and key stakeholders' experiences and perceptions of a scope of nursing and midwifery practice framework. *Journal of Advanced Nursing, 71*(6), 1227–1237.

Caughey, A. (2014). Induction of labor: Does it increase the risk of cesarean delivery?. *BJOG: An International Journal of Obstetrics & Gynaecology, 121*(6), 658–661.

Centers for Disease Control and Prevention (CDC). (2014). Primary cesarean delivery rates, by state: Results from the revised birth certificate, 2006–2012. *National Vital Statistics Reports, 63*(1), 1–11.

Cheng, Y. W., & Caughey, A. B. (2015). Second stage of labor. *Clinical Obstetrics and Gynecology, 58*(2), 227–240.

Cheng, Y. W., & Caughey, A. B. (2017). Normal labor and delivery. *eMedicine*. Retrieved from http://emedicine.medscape.com/article/260036-overview

Cohen, W. R. (2017). Clinical assessment of uterine contractions. *International Journal of Gynaecology and Obstetrics, 139*(2), 137–142.

Collins, K. A., & Reed, R. C. (2014). Chapter 6: Birth trauma. In K. A. Collins, & R. W. Byard (Eds.), *Forensic pathology of infancy and childhood* (pp. 139–168). New York, NY: Springer International Publishing.

Cook, J. L., Majd, M., Blake, J., Barrett, J., Bouvet, S., Janssen, P., . . . Wong, T. (2017). Measuring maternal mortality and morbidity in Canada. *Journal of Obstetrics and Gynaecology Canada, 39*(11), 1028–1037.

Cox, K. J., & King, T. L. (2015). Preventing primary cesarean births: Midwifery care. *Clinical Obstetrics and Gynecology, 58*(2), 282–293.

Cunningham, F. G., Leveno, K. J., Bloom, S. L., Spong, C. Y., Dashe, J. S., Hoffman, B. L., . . . Sheffield, J. S. (2014). *Williams obstetrics* (24th ed.). New York: McGraw-Hill Education.

Edmonds, J. K., Cwiertniewicz, T., & Stoll, K. (2015). Childbirth education prior to pregnancy? Survey findings of childbirth preferences and attitudes among young women. *The Journal of Perinatal Education, 24*(2), 93–101.

Ehsanipoor, R. M., & Satin, A. J. (2018). Normal and abnormal labor progression. *UpToDate*, Topic 4464. Retrieved from https://www.uptodate.com/contents/normal-and-abnormal-labor-progression?search=abnormal%20labor&source=search_result&selectedTitle=1~150&usage_type=default&display_rank=1

Fischer, B., & Mitteroecker, P. (2015). Covariation between human pelvis shape, stature, and head size alleviates the obstetric dilemma. *Proceedings of the National Academy of Sciences, 112*(18), 5655–5660.

Fitzgerald, E. M., Cronin, S. N., & Boccella, S. H. (2016). Anguish, yearning, and identity: Toward a better understanding of the pregnant Hispanic woman's prenatal care experience. *Journal of Transcultural Nursing, 27,* 464–470.

Funai, E. F., & Norwitz, E. R. (2018). Mechanism of normal labor and delivery. *UpToDate*. Retrieved from http://www.uptodate.com/contents/mechanism-of-normal-labor-and-delivery

Gizzo, S., Di Gangi, S., Noventa, M., Bacile, V., Zambon, A., & Nardelli, G. B. (2014). Women's choice of positions during labour: Return to the past or a modern way to give birth?. *BioMed Research International, 2014.*

Glavind, J., & Uldbjerg, N. (2015). Elective cesarean delivery at 38 and 39 weeks: Neonatal and maternal risks. *Current Opinion in Obstetrics and Gynecology, 27*(2), 121–127.

Grant, N., Strevens, H., & Thornton, J. (2015). Chapter 1: Physiology of labor. In G. Capogna (Ed.), *Epidural labor analgesia* (pp. 1–10). New York: Springer International Publishing.

Green, C. J. (2015). *Maternal newborn nursing care plans.* (3rd ed.). Burlington, MA: Jones & Bartlett Learning.

Hanson, L., & VandeVusse, L. (2014). Supporting labor progress toward physiologic birth. *Journal of Perinatal & Neonatal Nursing, 28*(2), 101–107.

Hoang, S. (2014). Pregnancy and anxiety. *International Journal of Childbirth Education, 29*(1), 67–70.

Hodnett, E. D., Gates, S., Hofmeyr, G. J., & Sakala, C. (2017). Continuous support for women during childbirth. *Cochrane Database Systematic Reviews, 2017*(7).

Hofmeyr, G. J. (2015). Breech delivery. In *Protocols for high-risk pregnancies: An evidence-based approach* (6th ed., pp. 423–427). West Sussex, UK: John Wiley & Sons.

Holvey, N. (2014). Supporting women in the second stage of labor. *British Journal of Midwifery, 22*(3), 182–186.

Horgan, M. J. (2015). Management of the late preterm infant: Not quite ready for prime time. *Pediatric Clinics of North America, 62*(2), 439–451.

Iravani, M., Zarean, E., Janghorbani, M., & Bahrami, M. (2015). Women's needs and expectations during normal labor and delivery. *Journal of Education and Health Promotion, 4,* 6.

Jones, L. V. (2015). Non-pharmacological approaches for pain relief during labor can improve maternal satisfaction with childbirth and reduce obstetric interventions. *Evidence Based Nursing, 18*(3), 70.

Jones, R. E., & Lopez, K. H. (2014). *Human reproductive biology* (4th ed.). Waltham, MA: Elsevier Health Sciences.

Jordan, R. G., Engstrom, J., Marfell, J., & Farley, C. L. (2014). *Prenatal and postnatal care: A women-centered approach.* Ames, IA: John Wiley & Sons.

King, T. L., Brucker, M. C., Kriebs, J. M., Fahey, J. O., Gegor, C. L., & Varney, H. (2015). *Varney's midwifery* (5th ed.). Burlington, MA: Jones & Bartlett Learning.

Kriebs, J. M. (2015). Patient safety during induction of labor. *The Journal of Perinatal & Neonatal Nursing, 29*(2), 130–137.

Leap, N., & Hunter, B. (2015). *Supporting women for labor and birth: A companion.* Florence, KY: Routledge.

Leduc, D., Biringer, A., Lee, L., & Dy, J.; SOGC Clinical Practice Obstetrics Committee. (2013). SOGC clinical practice guideline: Induction of labour. *Journal of Obstetrics and Gynaecology Canada, 35*(9), S1–S18. Retrieved from https://sogc.org/wp-content/uploads/2013/08/September2013-CPG296-ENG-Online_REV-D.pdf

Lee, L., Dy, J., & Azzam, H. (2016). Management of spontaneous labour at term in healthy women. *Journal of Obstetrics and Gynaecology Canada, 38*(9), 843–865.

Le Ray, C., Blondel, B., Prunet, C., Khireddine, I., Deneux-Tharaux, C., & Goffinet, F. (2015). Stabilizing the caesarean rate: Which target population?. *British Journal of Obstetrics and Gynaecology, 122,* 690–699.

Marani, E., & Koch, W. (2014). *The pelvis: Structure, gender and society.* Philadelphia, PA: Springer Healthcare.

Martin, R. J., Fanaroff, A. A., & Walsh, M. C. (2014). *Neonatal-perinatal medicine* (10th ed.). St. Louis, MO: Elsevier Health Sciences.

Milton, S. K., Chelmow, D., & Ramus, R. M. (2015). Maternal and fetal outcomes with internal compared with external tocometry: A meta-analysis [218]. *Obstetrics & Gynecology, 125,* 71S.

Moses, S. (2018). Labor induction. *Family Practice Notebook.* Retrieved from http://www.fpnotebook.com/ob/ld/LbrIndctn.htm

Nieuwenhuijze, M., Low, L., Korstjens, I., & Lagro-Janssen, T. (2014). The role of maternity care providers in promoting shared decision making regarding birthing positions during the second stage of labor. *Journal of Midwifery & Women's Health, 59*(3), 277–285.

Norwitz, E. R. (2018). Physiology of parturition. *UpToDate.* Retrieved from http://www.uptodate.com/contents/physiology-of-parturition

Osborne, K., & Hanson, L. (2014). Labor down or bear down: A strategy to translate second-stage labor evidence to perinatal practice. *Journal of Perinatal & Neonatal Nursing, 28*(2), 117–126.

Pavord, S., & Maybury, H. (2015). How I treat postpartum hemorrhage. *Blood, 125*(18), 2759–2770.

Ramasubramaniam, S., Renganathan, L., Vijayalakshmi, G., & Mallo-Banatao, M. V. (2015). Use of herbal preparations among parturient women: Is there enough evidence—A review of literature. *International Journal of Herbal Medicine, 2*(5), 20–26.

Reed, R. (2015). Supporting women's instinctive pushing behavior during birth. *The Practising Midwife, 18*(6), 13–15.

Sharshiner, R., & Silver, R. M. (2015). Management of fetal malpresentation. *Clinical Obstetrics and Gynecology, 58*(2), 246–255.

Stoll, K., Swift, E. M., Fairbrother, N., Nethery, E., & Janssen, P. (2018). A systematic review of nonpharmacological prenatal interventions for pregnancy-specific anxiety and fear of childbirth. *Birth, 45*(1), 7–18.

Tharpe, N. L., Farley, C. L., & Jordan, R. (2016). *Clinical practice guidelines for midwifery & women's health* (5th ed.). Sudbury, MA: Jones & Bartlett.

Tussey, C. M., Botsios, E., Gerkin, R. D., Kelly, L. A., Gamez, J., & Mensik, J. (2015). Reducing length of labor and cesarean surgery rate using a peanut ball for women laboring with an epidural. *The Journal of Perinatal Education, 24*(1), 16–24.

Van der Gucht, N., & Lewis, K. (2015). Women's experiences of coping with pain during childbirth: A critical review of qualitative research. *Midwifery, 31*(3), 349–358.

Verklan, T., & Walden, M. (2014). *Core curriculum for neonatal intensive care nursing* (4th ed.). St. Louis, MO: Saunders Elsevier.

Weber, J., & Kelley, J. (2014). *Health assessment in nursing* (5th ed.). Philadelphia, PA: Lippincott Williams & Wilkins.

Whyte, R. K.; Canadian Pediatric Society Fetus and Newborn Committee. (2017). Position statement: Safe discharge of the late preterm infant. *Paediatric Child Health, 15*(10), 655–660. Retrieved from https://www.cps.ca/en/documents/position/safe-discharge-late-preterm-infant

Wojnar, D. M. (2015). Perinatal experiences of Somali couples in the United States. *Journal of Obstetric, Gynecologic and Neonatal Nursing, 44*(3), 358–369.

Woods, N. K., & Chesser, A. (2015). Becoming a mom: Improving birth outcomes through a community collaborative prenatal education model. *Journal of Family Medicine and Disease Prevention, 1*(002), 1–4.

CHAPTER **WORKSHEET**

MULTIPLE CHOICE QUESTIONS

1. When determining the frequency of contractions, the nurse would measure which of the following?
   a. Start of one contraction to the start of the next contraction
   b. Beginning of one contraction to the end of the same contraction
   c. Peak of one contraction to the peak of the next contraction
   d. End of one contraction to the beginning of the next contraction

2. Which fetal lie is most conducive to a spontaneous vaginal birth?
   a. Transverse
   b. Longitudinal
   c. Perpendicular
   d. Oblique

3. Which of the following observations would suggest that placental separation is occurring?
   a. Uterus stops contracting altogether.
   b. Umbilical cord pulsations stop.
   c. Uterine shape changes to globular.
   d. Client's blood pressure drops.

4. The nurse is explaining the difference between true versus false labour to a childbirth class, and states that the major difference between them is:
   a. Discomfort level is greater with false labour.
   b. Progressive cervical changes occur in true labour.
   c. There is a feeling of nausea with false labour.
   d. There is more fetal movement with true labour.

5. The shortest but most intense phase of labour is the:
   a. Latent phase
   b. Active phase
   c. Transition phase
   d. Placental expulsion phase

6. A labouring woman is admitted to the labour and birth suite at 6 cm dilation. She would be in which phase of the first stage of labour?
   a. Latent
   b. Active
   c. Transition
   d. Early

7. Which assessment would indicate that a client is in true labour?
   a. Membranes are ruptured and fluid is clear.
   b. Presenting part is engaged and not floating.
   c. Cervix is 4 cm dilated, 90% effaced.
   d. Contractions last 30 seconds, every 5 to 10 minutes.

8. Which of the following interventions are commonly underutilized in promoting a normal birth? Select all that apply.
   a. Oral nutrition and fluids in labour
   b. Open glottis pushing in the second stage of labour
   c. Skin-to-skin contact after birth for infant bonding
   d. Routine artificial rupture of membranes (amniotomy)
   e. Labour induction with Pitocin given intravenously
   f. Routine episiotomy to shorten labour length

9. Physiologic preparation for labour would be demonstrated by:
   a. Decrease in Braxton Hicks contractions
   b. Weight gain and increase in appetite
   c. Lightening, whereby the fetus drops into true pelvis
   d. Fetal heart rate accelerations and increased movements

CRITICAL THINKING EXERCISES

1. Cindy, a 20-year-old primipara, calls the birthing centre where you work as a nurse and reports that she thinks she is in labour because she feels labour pains. Her due date is this week. The midwives have been giving her prenatal care throughout this pregnancy.
   a. What additional information do you need to respond appropriately?
   b. What suggestions/recommendations would you make to her?
   c. What instructions need to be given to guide her decision making?
   d. What other premonitory signs of labour might the nurse ask about?
   e. What manifestations would be found if Cindy is experiencing true labour?

2. You are assigned to lead a community education class for women in their third trimester of pregnancy to prepare them for their upcoming birth. Prepare an outline of topics that should be addressed.

STUDY ACTIVITIES

1. During clinical post-conference, share with the other nursing students how the critical forces of labour influenced the length of labour and the birthing process for a labouring client assigned to you.

2. The cardinal movements of labour include which of the following? Select all that apply.
   a. Extension and rotation
   b. Descent and engagement
   c. Presentation and position
   d. Attitude and lie
   e. Flexion and expulsion

CHAPTER **WORKSHEET**

3. Interview a client on the postpartum unit who has given birth within the past few hours. Ask the client to describe the experience and examine psychological factors that may have influenced the labouring process.

4. On the following illustration, identify the parameters of uterine contractions by marking an "X" where the nurse would measure the duration of the contraction.

BRINGING IT ALL TOGETHER: A CASE STUDY

Moritza is a 20-year-old pregnant female who comes to the prenatal clinic with her boyfriend for her prenatal visit at 39 weeks of gestation. This is her first pregnancy and she has missed several of her previous prenatal office visits. Her pregnancy has been uneventful thus far, but she is concerned today about impending labour and how she will know when to go to the hospital. She feels unprepared for labour and admits she is very afraid of the pain since many of her friends and family members have shared their "horror" stories about their experiences. She admits she is scared about having an IV in her arm at the hospital. She wants a normal physiologic childbirth.

Go to thePoint **to find questions to consider about this case.**

14

Nursing Management During Labour and Birth

Learning Objectives

Upon completion of the chapter, you will be able to:

1. Examine the measures used to evaluate a client's status during labour and birth.

2. Differentiate the advantages and disadvantages of external and internal fetal monitoring, including the appropriate use for each.

3. Choose appropriate nursing interventions to address normal, atypical, and abnormal fetal heart tracings in accordance with the SOGC guidelines.

4. Outline the nurse's role in fetal assessment.

5. Appraise the various comfort promotion and pain relief strategies used during labour and birth.

6. Summarize the assessment data collected on admission to the perinatal unit.

7. Relate the ongoing assessments involved in each stage of labour and birth.

8. Analyze the nurse's role throughout the labour and birth process.

Sheila **was admitted in active labour to the labour and birth unit. She has progressed to the transition phase (dilated 8 cm) and is becoming increasingly more uncomfortable. She is using a patterned-paced breathing pattern now, but is thrashing around in the hospital bed.**

INTRODUCTION

The labouring and birthing process is a life-changing event for clients and families. Nurses need to be respectful, available, encouraging, supportive, and professional in dealing with all birthing families. Nursing management for labour and birth involves physical and emotional assessment of the birthing patient, and providing comfort measures, emotional support, information and instruction, advocacy, and support for the partner and family. Providing the highest quality in maternity care is dependent on nurses valuing the childbirth experience and recognizing it as a life-changing experience. Caring nursing practice encompasses technical skills and caring behaviours; giving care that protects, promotes, and supports physiologic childbirth; provides optimal, evidence-based care; and recognizes health disparity and cultural diversity in all patients in order to improve their childbirth experience across time, settings, and disciplines.

One of the components for care that is both evidence-based care and person-centred is to encourage and advocate for a patient's preferences to guide their own care during the birthing process. In a recent study, birthing parents' needs and expectations during labour and birth were assessed. Seven themes emerged—physiologic needs (nutrition, room environment, hygiene, comfort, and privacy); psychological needs (empathy and advocacy, constant emotional support and encouragement); informational needs (about labour process and hospital policies); communication needs (health care provider and familiar attendant); esteem needs (sense of value, confidence, involvement in decisions); security needs (calming fears); and medical needs (pain relief and prevention of unnecessary interventions during labour and birth) (Iravani, Zarean, Janghorbani, & Bahrami, 2015). It is important that nurses identify the expectations and needs of individuals in their care, so as to empower them to fully participate in their childbirth experience.

This chapter provides information about nursing management during labour and birth. First, the essentials for in-depth assessment of maternal/birthing parent status and fetal status during labour and birth are discussed. This is followed by a thorough description of the major methods of promoting comfort and providing pain management during the labour and birth process. The chapter concludes by combining the themes and the information with a discussion of the nursing care specific to each stage of labour, including the necessary data to be obtained with the admission assessment, methods to evaluate labour progress during the first stage of labour, and key nursing measures that focus on maternal/birthing parent assessment and fetal assessments and pain relief for all stages of labour.

ASSESSMENT OF THE CLIENT DURING LABOUR AND BIRTH

During labour and birth, various techniques are used to assess maternal/birthing parent status. These techniques provide an ongoing source of data to determine the client's response and progress in labour:

- Assessing vital signs, including temperature, blood pressure, pulse, respiration, and pain response, which are primary components of the physical examination and ongoing assessment.
- Reviewing the prenatal record to identify risk factors that may contribute to a decrease in uteroplacental circulation during labour. If these records are not available, taking a thorough obstetrical and health history.
- If there is no vaginal bleeding on admission and there are no risk factors present to preclude a vaginal exam (such as placenta praevia or prolonged rupture of membranes), performing a vaginal examination to assess cervical changes including consistency, effacement, position, and dilation, after which it is monitored periodically as necessary to identify progress.
- Evaluating pain and the effectiveness of pain management strategies at regular intervals during labour and birth.

Vaginal Examination

The World Health Organization (WHO) recommends digital vaginal examinations at intervals of 4 hours for routine assessment and identification of a delay in active labour (2015).

> **Take Note!**
> A vaginal examination is an assessment skill that takes time and experience to develop; only by doing it frequently in clinical practice can the practitioner's skill level improve.

The purpose of performing a vaginal examination is to assess cervical changes in regard to consistency (firm or soft), the percentage of cervical effacement, the extent of dilation, as well as the fetal membrane status, and to gather information on presentation, position, station, degree of fetal head flexion, and presence of fetal skull swelling or moulding (Fig. 14.1). The nurse should prepare the client by providing information about the procedure, what information will be obtained from it, how they can assist with the procedure, how it will be performed, and who will be performing it.

The client is typically supine with a slight left tilt during the vaginal examination. The vaginal examination is performed gently, with concern for the client's comfort.

After donning sterile gloves, the examiner inserts the index and middle fingers into the vaginal introitus. Next, the cervix is palpated to assess dilation, effacement, and

FIGURE 14.1 Vaginal examination to determine cervical dilation and effacement.

position (e.g., posterior or anterior). If the cervix is open to any degree, the presenting fetal part, fetal position, station, and presence of moulding can be assessed. In addition, the membranes can be evaluated and described as intact, bulging, or ruptured.

At the conclusion of the vaginal examination, the findings are discussed with the patient and family regarding the labour progress and any other findings. In addition, the findings are documented either electronically or in writing and reported to the primary health care provider in charge of the case. Assess the fetal heart after a vaginal examination and document this along with the other findings.

Cervical Dilation and Effacement

The amount of cervical dilation (opening) and the degree of cervical effacement (thinning) are key areas assessed during the vaginal examination. Although this finding is somewhat subjective, experienced examiners typically come up with similar findings. The width of the cervical opening determines dilation, and the length of the cervix assesses effacement. Effacement and dilation are used to assess cervical changes as follows:

- Effacement:
  - 0%: cervical canal is 2 cm long
  - 50%: cervical canal is 1 cm long
  - 100%: cervical canal is paper thin
- Dilation:
  - 0 cm: external cervical os is closed
  - 5 cm: external cervical os is halfway dilated
  - 10 cm: external os is fully dilated and ready for birth passage

The information yielded by this examination serves as a basis for determining which stage of labour the patient is in and how the ongoing care may be directed and given.

Fetal Descent and Presenting Part

In addition to cervical dilation and effacement findings, the vaginal examination can also determine fetal descent (station) and presenting part. During the vaginal examination, the gloved fingers palpate the fetal skull (if vertex presentation) through the opened cervix or the fetal buttocks in the case of a breech presentation. Station is assessed in relation to the patient's ischial spines and the presenting fetal part. These spines are not sharp protrusions but rather blunted prominences at the midpelvis. The ischial spines serve as landmarks and have been designated as zero station. If the presenting part is palpated higher than the ischial spines, a negative number is assigned; if the presenting fetal part is felt below the ischial spines, a plus number is assigned, denoting how many centimeters below the zero station (see Chapter 13 for a more detailed discussion).

Progressive fetal descent (−5 to +4) is the expected norm during labour; moving downward from the negative stations to zero station to the positive stations in a timely manner. If progressive fetal descent does not occur, there may be a disproportion between the client's pelvis and the fetus which will require investigation.

Rupture of Membranes

The integrity of the membranes can be determined during the vaginal examination. Typically, if intact, the membranes will be felt as a soft bulge that is more prominent during a contraction. If the membranes have ruptured, the client may have reported a sudden gush of fluid. Membrane rupture also may occur as a slow trickle of fluid. When membranes rupture, the priority focus should be on assessing fetal heart rate (FHR) first to identify a deceleration, which might indicate cord compression secondary to cord prolapse. If the membranes are ruptured when the client comes to the hospital, the health care provider should ascertain when it occurred. Prolonged ruptured membranes increase the risk of infection as a result of ascending vaginal pathologic organisms for both birthing client and fetus. Nurses must be alert for signs of intrauterine infection, which include fever and tachycardia, foul odour of vaginal discharge, and an increase in white blood cell count. Fetal tachycardia may also be present.

To confirm that membranes have ruptured, a sample of fluid is taken from the vagina via a nitrazine yellow dye swab to determine the fluid's pH. Vaginal fluid is acidic, whereas amniotic fluid is alkaline and turns a nitrazine swab blue. However, false-positive results can occur, especially in patients experiencing a large amount of bloody show, because blood is alkaline. The membranes are most likely intact if the nitrazine swab remains yellow to olive green, with pH between 5 and 6. The membranes are probably ruptured if the nitrazine swab turns a blue-green to deep blue, with pH ranging from 6.5 to 7.5 (Tharpe, Farley, & Jordan, 2016).

Because the nitrazine test can be inconclusive, an additional test, called the *fern test*, can be used to confirm rupture of membranes. With this test, a sample of vaginal fluid is obtained, applied to a microscope slide, and allowed to dry. Using a microscope, the slide is examined for a characteristic fern pattern that indicates the presence of amniotic fluid.

A more recent innovation in confirming ruptured membranes is the placental alpha-microglobulin-1 (PAMG-1) assay, under the trade name AmniSure. This point-of-care test is a rapid, noninvasive method which can detect PAMG-1 with as little as 0.25 µL of amniotic fluid in 1 mL of vaginal secretions. The care provider inserts a sterile swab into the vagina for 1 minute, then places the swab into a vial containing a solvent for 1 minute, and then an AmniSure test strip is dipped into that vial. The test result is revealed by the presence of one or two lines within the next 10 minutes. Many studies have demonstrated a high sensitivity (from 94.4% to 98.9%) and high specificity (from 87.5% to 100%). The test is quite costly and therefore is generally only used when the diagnosis remains uncertain after physical examination, nitrazine and fern tests, and ultrasound assessment (Duff, 2018).

Assessing Uterine Contractions

The primary power of labour is uterine contractions, which are involuntary. Uterine contractions increase intrauterine pressure, causing tension to be placed upon the cervix. This tension leads to cervical dilation and thinning, which in turn eventually forces the fetus through the birth canal. Normal uterine contractions have a contraction (systole) and a relaxation (diastole) phase. The contraction resembles a wave, moving downward to the cervix and upward to the fundus of the uterus. Each contraction starts with a building up (increment), gradually reaching an acme (peak intensity), and then a letting down (decrement). Each contraction is followed by an interval of rest, which ends when the next contraction begins. At the acme (peak) of the contraction, the entire uterus is contracting, with the greatest intensity in the fundal area. The relaxation phase follows and occurs simultaneously throughout the uterus.

Uterine contractions during labour are monitored by palpation and may also be monitored by electronic monitoring. Assessment of the contractions always includes frequency, duration, intensity, and uterine resting tone (see Chapter 13 for a more detailed discussion). It is important to note that if the nurse is doing abdominal palpation with an external tocodynamometer, subjective and objective assessment of the contractions are required.

To palpate the fundus for contraction intensity, place the pads of your fingers on the fundus and describe how it feels: like the tip of the nose (mild), like the chin (moderate), or like the forehead (strong). Palpation of intensity is a subjective judgment of the indentability of the

FIGURE 14.2 Nurse palpating the client's fundus during a contraction.

uterine wall; a descriptive term is assigned (mild, moderate, or strong) (Fig. 14.2).

Take Note!

Frequent clinical experience is needed to gain accuracy in assessing the intensity of uterine contractions. A well-trained nurse has proficient skills at palpating the intensity of contractions.

The second method used to assess the intensity of uterine contractions is electronic monitoring, either external or internal. Both methods provide a determination of frequency and duration of uterine contractions but only the internal method can accurately demonstrate the intensity of the contractions, if properly placed. This was discussed in detail in Chapter 13.

Performing Leopold Manoeuvres

Leopold manoeuvres are a method for determining the presentation, position, and lie of the fetus through the use of four specific steps. This method involves inspection and palpation of the client's abdomen as a screening assessment for malpresentation. A longitudinal lie is expected, and the presentation can be cephalic, breech, or shoulder. Each manoeuvre answers a question:

- *Manoeuvre 1*: What fetal part (head or buttocks) is located in the fundus (top of the uterus)?
- *Manoeuvre 2*: On which side is the fetal back located? (Fetal heart tones are best auscultated through the back of the fetus.)
- *Manoeuvre 3*: What is the presenting part?
- *Manoeuvre 4*: Is the fetal head flexed and engaged in the pelvis?

Leopold manoeuvres are described in Nursing Procedure 14.1.

NURSING PROCEDURE 14.1

Performing Leopold Manoeuvres

Purpose: To Determine Fetal Presentation, Position, and Lie

1. Place the client in the supine position and stand to the side of the bed/table.

2. Perform the first manoeuvre to determine presentation.

   a. Facing the client's head, place both hands on the abdomen to determine fetal position in the uterine fundus.

   b. Feel for the buttocks, which will feel soft and irregular (indicates vertex presentation); feel for the head, which will feel hard, smooth, and round (indicates a breech presentation).

3. Complete the second manoeuvre to determine position.

   a. While still facing the client's head, move hands down the lateral sides of the abdomen to palpate on which side the back is located (feels hard and smooth).

   b. Continue to palpate to determine on which side the limbs are located (irregular nodules with kicking and movement).

4. Perform the third manoeuvre to confirm presentation.

   a. Move hands down the sides of the abdomen to grasp the lower uterine segment and palpate the area just above the symphysis pubis.

   b. Place thumb and fingers of one hand apart and grasp the presenting part by bringing fingers together.

   c. Feel for the presenting part. If the presenting part is the head, it will be round, firm, and ballottable; if it is the buttocks, it will feel soft and irregular.

(continued)

fetal well-being is to start listening to the FHR immediately following the contraction to determine if there are decelerations after the contractions. Listening during contractions may be technically difficult and uncomfortable for the patient. The most important information will come from an assessment of the fetal heart after the contractions.

Intermittent FHR auscultation can be used to detect FHR baseline and rhythm and changes from baseline. However, unlike continuous electronic FHR monitoring, it cannot detect variability and types of decelerations (Wisner, 2015). Using intermittent auscultation to establish a baseline, the FHR is assessed for a full minute after a contraction and then if there are no problems detected, intermittent auscultation can continue in this fashion during the labour under the guidelines of the SOGC (Liston et al., 2018). If the client experiences a change in condition as labour progresses, auscultation assessments should be performed more frequently. Changes in condition include ruptured membranes or the onset of bleeding. In addition, more frequent assessments occur after periods of ambulation, a vaginal examination, administration of pain medications, or other clinically important events (King et al., 2019).

The FHR is heard most clearly at the fetal back. In a cephalic presentation, the FHR is best heard in the lower quadrant of the client's abdomen. In a breech presentation, it is heard at or above the level of the client's umbilicus (Fig. 14.4). As labour progresses, the FHR location will change accordingly as the fetus descends into the pelvis for the birthing process. To ensure that the client's heart rate is not confused with the FHR, palpate the patient's radial pulse simultaneously while the FHR is being auscultated through the abdomen.

For low-risk clients, the FHR and contraction characteristics should be assessed every 15 to 30 minutes in active labour and after every contraction while pushing, as well as before and after any digital vaginal examinations, membrane rupture, medication administered, and ambulation to the bathroom (Freeman, 2015).

Nursing Procedure 12.1 in Chapter 12 lists detailed steps for using a Doppler device to assess FHR. In brief, a small amount of water-soluble gel is applied to the client's abdomen or ultrasound device before auscultation with the Doppler to promote sound wave transmission. Usually the FHR is best heard in the client's lower abdominal quadrants; if the FHR is not found quickly, it may help to locate the fetal back by performing Leopold manoeuvres.

Although the intermittent method of FHR assessment allows the client to move about during labour, the information obtained fails to provide a complete picture of the well-being of the fetus from moment to moment. This leads to the question of what the fetal status is during the times that are not assessed, which is more concerning for client's at an increased risk for complications.

If a patient is at higher risk, having periods of time where the fetus is not being assessed might lead to health care team to miss indications of changes in the fetal status.

GUIDELINES FOR ASSESSING FETAL HEART RATE

National and international professional organizations have provided general guidelines for the frequency of assessments based on existing evidence. The American College of Obstetricians and Gynecologists (ACOG), the SOGC, the Royal College of Obstetricians, Institute for Clinical Systems Improvement (ICSI), and the Association of Women's Health, Obstetric and Neonatal Nurses (AWHONN) have published guidelines designed to assist clinicians in caring for labouring clients. Their recommendations are supported by large controlled studies. They recommend the following guidelines for assessing FHR:

- Completion of a prenatal and labour risk assessment on all patients
- Initial 10- to 20-minute continuous FHR assessment on entry into labour/birth area *only* if the client has risk factors for adverse perinatal outcomes. All healthy full-term pregnancies should be assessed by intermittent auscultation upon arrival to the birthing facility
- Intermittent auscultation every 30 minutes during active labour for a low-risk clients and every 15 minutes for a high-risk clients
- During the second stage of labour, every 5 to 15 minutes for the low-risk client and every 5 minutes for the high-risk client and during the pushing stage (Liston et al., 2018)

EVIDENCE-BASED RESULTS: INTERMITTENT VERSUS ELECTRONIC MONITORING

In several randomized controlled studies comparing intermittent auscultation with electronic monitoring in both low- and high-risk clients, no difference in intrapartum fetal death was found. However, in each study a nurse–client ratio of 1:1 was consistently maintained during labour (Liston et al., 2018). This suggests that adequate staffing is essential with intermittent FHR monitoring to ensure optimal outcomes for the client and fetus. There is insufficient evidence to indicate specific situations where continuous electronic FHR monitoring might result in better outcomes when compared to intermittent assessment. However, in pregnancies involving an increased risk of perinatal death, cerebral palsy, or neonatal encephalopathy and when oxytocin is used for induction or augmentation, it is recommended that continuous EFM be used rather than intermittent fetal auscultation (Liston et al., 2018).

Continuous Electronic Fetal Monitoring

Electronic fetal monitoring (EFM) detects the fetal pulse by sensing and analyzing tissue movements via Doppler ultrasound. The machine uses a transducer that is

FIGURE 14.4 Locations for auscultating fetal heart rate based on fetal position. **A.** Left occiput anterior (LOA). **B.** Right occiput anterior (ROA). **C.** Left occiput posterior (LOP). **D.** Right occiput posterior (ROP). **E.** Left sacral anterior (LSA).

capable of both sending and receiving ultrasound waves. The waves travel through the ultrasound gel, then body tissues, and are eventually reflected by any tissue. The fast reflections are analyzed and software in the machine determines the FHR. EFM is the recommended method of intrapartum fetal surveillance for high-risk pregnancies. Despite the questions about its efficacy and controversy regarding increased rates of surgical births

associated with its use, continuous cardiotocography (CTG) remains the predominant method of fetal monitoring today (Nageotte, 2015). The indications for offering birthing clients continuous fetal monitoring in labour include the following: clients whose labour is induced or augmented, who have had a previous cesarean section, are experiencing preterm labour, experience vaginal bleeding in labour, or have a condition which could compromise either fetal or the birthing client's health—prolonged rupture of membranes (>24 hours), hypertensive disorders of pregnancy, IUGR, or the presence of meconium in the amniotic fluid (Liston et al., 2018).

EFM uses a machine to produce a continuous tracing of the FHR. When the monitoring device is in place, a sound is produced with each heartbeat. In addition, a graphic record of the FHR pattern is produced. The primary objective of EFM is to provide information about fetal oxygenation and prevent fetal injury that could result from impaired fetal oxygenation during labour. The purpose of EFM is to detect FHR changes early before they are prolonged and profound. Fetal hypoxia is demonstrated in a heart rate pattern change and is by far the most common etiology of fetal injury and death that can be prevented with optimal fetal surveillance during labour and early interventions (Cox & King, 2015).

Current methods of continuous EFM were introduced during the 1970s, specifically for use in clients considered to be at high risk. However, the use of these methods gradually increased and they eventually came to be used for clients other than just those at high risk. This increased use has become controversial because it is suspected of being associated with the steadily increasing rates of cesarean births with no decrease in the rate of cerebral palsy (Omo-Aghoja, 2015). Many studies suggest that when compared with standardized intermittent auscultation, the use of intrapartum continuous EFM seems to increase the number of preterm and surgical births but has no significant effect on reducing the incidence of intrapartum death or long-term neurologic injury. An impetus for the overuse of EFM is the litigious nature of current society, but the benefits have not been proven scientifically. EFM has been given excessive importance in legal cases. Before assigning fault on events at birth, a better understanding of developmental neurobiology and limitations of the present biomarkers is warranted (Freeman, 2015). To date, continuous EFM is not evidence based for determining fetal health status, in spite of its widespread use in practice.

Concerns about the efficiency and safety of routine EFM in labour have led expert panels in Canada and the United States to recommend that such monitoring be limited to high-risk pregnancies. However, its use in low-risk pregnancies continues globally (Maso et al., 2015; Prior & Kumar, 2015). This remains an important research issue.

Continuous EFM can be performed externally (indirectly), with the equipment attached to the patient's abdominal wall, or internally (directly), with the equipment attached to the fetus. Both methods provide a continuous printout of the FHR, but they differ in their specificity. The efficacy of EFM depends on the accurate interpretation of the tracings, not necessarily which method (external vs. internal) is used.

CONTINUOUS EXTERNAL MONITORING

In external or indirect monitoring, two ultrasound transducers, each of which is attached to a belt, are applied around the client's abdomen. One transducer is called a tocotransducer, a pressure-sensitive device that is applied against the uterine fundus. It detects changes in uterine pressure and converts the pressure registered into an electronic signal that is recorded on graph paper (Farine, 2015). The tocotransducer is placed over the uterine fundus in the area of greatest contractility to monitor uterine contractions. The other ultrasound transducer records the baseline FHR, variability, accelerations, and decelerations. It is positioned on the client's abdomen in the midline between the umbilicus and the symphysis pubis. The diaphragm of the ultrasound transducer is moved to either side of the abdomen to obtain a stronger sound and is then attached to the second elastic belt. This transducer converts the fetal heart movements into beeping sounds and records them on a graph paper (Fig. 14.5).

Continuous data are provided on the FHR. External monitoring can be used while the membranes are still intact and the cervix is not yet dilated, but also can be used with ruptured membranes and a dilating cervix. It is noninvasive and can detect relative changes in abdominal pressure between uterine resting tone and contractions. External monitoring also records the duration and frequency of contractions, providing a permanent record with the FHR (Casanova, 2015).

However, the use of external monitoring can restrict the client's movements in labour. Signal disruptions can occur due to client size and obesity, positioning, fetal malpresentation, positioning, and fetal movement as well as by artefact. The term **artefact** is used to describe irregular variations or absence of the FHR on the fetal monitor record that result from mechanical limitations of the monitor or electrical interference. Additionally, gaps in the monitor strip can occur periodically without explanation.

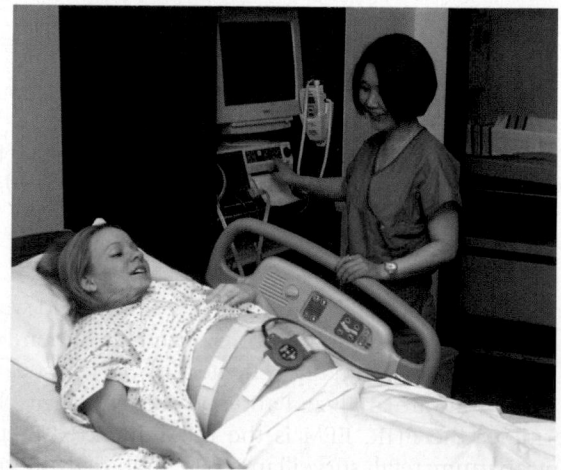

FIGURE 14.5 Continuous external electronic fetal monitoring device applied in labour.

Intrauterine pressure catheter

Internal fetal monitor
Electrode
Scalp

FIGURE 14.6 Continuous internal electronic fetal monitoring.

CONTINUOUS INTERNAL MONITORING

Continuous *internal* monitoring is usually indicated for clients considered to be at high risk. Possible conditions might include multiple gestation, decreased fetal movement, abnormal FHR on auscultation, IUGR, fever, preeclampsia, dysfunctional labour, preterm labour, or medical conditions such as diabetes or hypertension. It involves the placement of a spiral electrode into the fetal presenting part, usually the head, to assess FHR, with an option to continue with either external contraction monitoring or internal monitoring. The latter involves introducing a pressure transducer internally within the uterus to record uterine contractions (Fig. 14.6). The fetal spiral electrode is considered the most accurate method of detecting fetal heart characteristics and patterns because it involves receiving a signal directly from the fetus (Nageotte, 2015). Contraindications for internal fetal scalp monitoring include placenta previa, face presentation, human immunodeficiency virus (HIV)-positive status, or active genital herpes (Liston et al., 2018).

Both the FHR and the duration and interval of uterine contractions are recorded on the graph paper. This method permits evaluation of baseline heart rate and changes in rate and pattern.

Four specific criteria must be met for this type of monitoring to be used:
• Ruptured membranes
• Cervical dilation of at least 2 cm
• Presenting fetal part low enough to allow placement of the scalp electrode
• Skilled practitioner available to insert spiral electrode.

Compared with external monitoring, continuous internal monitoring can more accurately detect variability (normal fluctuations within the fetal heartbeats) and the changes in the amount of variability as well as FHR dysrhythmias. In addition, the client's position changes and movement do not interfere with the quality of the tracing. The client will be restricted to bed, unless the monitor used has wireless capabilities in which case the patient may be ambulating or even showering while still being monitored.

Determining FHR Patterns

Due to the rising costs of litigations related to birth asphyxia of the newborn and increasing complexity of obstetric populations, it has become absolutely mandatory that all nurses responsible for the care of labouring clients are trained adequately in interpretation and documentation of CTG tracings, as well as the guidelines for interventions based on the assessment of the tracing and overall clinical situation. Assessment parameters of the FHR include baseline FHR and variability, presence of accelerations, periodic or episodic decelerations, and changes or trends of FHR patterns over time. The nurse must be able to interpret the various parameters to determine if the FHR pattern is normal, which is strongly predictive of normal fetal acid–base status at the time of observation and needs no intervention; atypical which is not predictive of abnormal fetal acid–base status but does require evaluation and continued monitoring; or abnormal which is predictive of abnormal fetal acid–base status at the time of observation and requires prompt evaluation and interventions such as giving oxygen, changing patient position, discontinuing labour augmentation medication, and/or treating hypotension (Freeman, 2015). Table 14.1 summarizes these categories. Health care providers should be aware that terminology for fetal heart tracings may differ when used in other countries. For example, in the United States, normal, atypical, and abnormal are referred to as category I, category II, and category III (ACOG, 2010).

BASELINE FHR

Baseline FHR refers to the average FHR that occurs during a 10-minute segment that excludes periodic or episodic rate changes, such as tachycardia or bradycardia. It is assessed when the patient has no contractions and the fetus is not experiencing episodic FHR changes. The normal baseline FHR ranges between 110 and 160 beats per minute (bpm) (Liston, et al., 2018). The normal baseline FHR can be obtained by auscultation, ultrasound, or Doppler, or by a continuous internal direct fetal electrode.

Fetal bradycardia occurs when the FHR is below 110 bpm and lasts 10 minutes or longer (Maso et al., 2015). It can be the initial response of a healthy fetus to asphyxia. Causes of fetal bradycardia might include fetal

TABLE 14.1	INTERPRETING FHR PATTERNS
Normal	*Predictive of normal fetal acid–base status and do not require intervention* • Baseline rate (110–160 bpm) • Baseline variability moderate (6–25 bpm) • Accelerations present • Present or absent early decelerations • No late or occasional variable decelerations Can be monitored with intermittent auscultation during labour
Atypical	*Not predictive of abnormal fetal acid–base status, but require evaluation and continued surveillance* • Fetal tachycardia (>160 bpm) for <30 minutes • Bradycardia (100–110 bpm) • Variability absent or minimal (≤5 bpm) for 40–80 minutes • Variable decelerations, 30–60 seconds duration • Accelerations ≤2 in 40–80 minutes
Abnormal	*Predictive of abnormal fetus acid–base status and require intervention* • Fetal bradycardia (<110 bpm) • Fetal tachycardia (>160 pm) • Minimal or absent variability (≤5 bpm) for ≥80 minutes • Marked variability (>25 bpm) >10 minutes • Sinusoidal pattern (smooth, undulating baseline) • Recurrent late decelerations • Recurrent variable decelerations >60 seconds duration • Accelerations ≤2 in >80 minutes

Liston, R., Sawchuck, D., & Young, D. (2018). SOGC clinical practice guideline No. 197b, Fetal health surveillance: Intrapartum consensus guideline. *Journal of Obstetrics and Gynaecology Canada*. Retrieved from https://www.jogc.com/article/S1701-2163(18)30067-7/pdf

hypoxia, prolonged patient hypoglycemia, fetal acidosis, administration of analgesic drugs to the patient, hypothermia, anesthetic agents (epidural), patient hypotension, prolonged umbilical cord compression, and fetal congenital heart block (Nageotte, 2015). Bradycardia may be benign if it is an isolated event, but it is considered an ominous sign when accompanied by a decrease in baseline variability and late decelerations.

Fetal tachycardia is a baseline FHR greater than 160 bpm that lasts for 10 minutes or longer (Liston et al., 2018). It can represent an early compensatory response to asphyxia. Other causes of fetal tachycardia include fetal hypoxia, patient fever, patient dehydration, amnionitis, the presence of certain drugs such as cocaine, amphetamines, and nicotine, patients with hyperthyroidism, anxiety, fetal anemia, prematurity, fetal infection, chronic hypoxemia, congenital anomalies, fetal heart

failure, and fetal arrhythmias. Fetal tachycardia is considered an ominous sign if it is accompanied by a decrease in variability and late decelerations (Yuan, 2015).

BASELINE VARIABILITY

Baseline variability is defined as irregular fluctuations in the baseline FHR, which is measured as the amplitude of the peak to trough in bpm (Sholapurkar, 2015). It represents the interplay between the parasympathetic and sympathetic nervous systems. The constant interplay (push-and-pull effect) on the FHR from the parasympathetic and sympathetic systems produces a moment-to-moment change in the FHR. Because variability is in essence the combined result of autonomic nervous system branch function, its presence implies that both the branches are working and receiving adequate oxygen (Timmins & Clark, 2015). Thus, variability is one of the most important characteristics of the FHR. Variability is described in four categories as follows:
• fluctuation range undetectable: absent
• fluctuation range observed at less than 5 bpm: minimal
• fluctuation range from 6 to 25 bpm: moderate
• fluctuation range greater than 25 bpm: marked

Absent or minimal variability typically is caused by fetal acidemia secondary to uteroplacental insufficiency, cord compression, a preterm fetus, patients experiencing hypotension, uterine hyperstimulation, abruptio placenta, or a fetal dysrhythmia. Interventions to improve uteroplacental blood flow and perfusion through the umbilical cord include lateral positioning of the patient, increasing the IV fluid rate to improve the patient's circulation, administering oxygen at 8 to 10 L/min by mask, considering internal fetal monitoring, documenting findings, and reporting to the health care provider. Preparation for an imminent or surgical birth may be necessary if no changes occur after attempting the interventions.

Moderate viability indicates that the autonomic and central nervous systems (CNS) of the fetus are well developed and well oxygenated. It is considered a good sign of fetal well-being and correlates with the absence of significant metabolic acidosis (Fig. 14.7).

Marked variability occurs when there are more than 25 beats of fluctuation in the FHR baseline. Causes of this include cord prolapse or compression, patients with hypotension, uterine hyperstimulation, and abruptio placenta. It is abnormal if it lasts greater than 10 minutes and interventions necessary would be included determining the cause if possible, lateral positioning, increasing intravenous fluid rate, administering oxygen at 8 to 10 L/min by mask, discontinuing oxytocin infusion, observing for changes in tracing, considering internal fetal monitoring, communicating an abnormal pattern to the health care provider, and preparing for an expedient or surgical birth if no change in pattern is noted (Freeman, 2015).

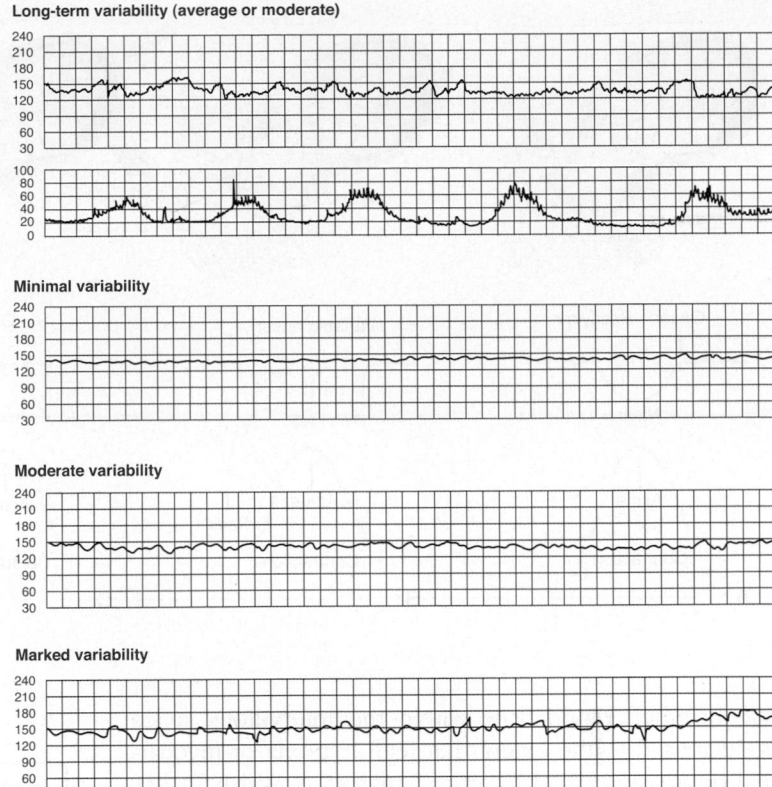

FIGURE 14.7 Examples of fetal monitoring strips.
A. Long-term variability (average or moderate).
B. Minimal variability. **C.** Moderate variability.
D. Marked variability.

FHR variability is an important clinical indicator that is predictive of fetal acid–base balance and cerebral tissue perfusion. It is influenced by fetal oxygenation status, cardiac output, and drug effects (King et al., 2019). As the CNS is desensitized by hypoxia and acidosis, FHR decreases until a smooth baseline pattern appears. Loss of variability may be associated with a poor outcome.

Take Note!

External EFM cannot assess variability accurately. Therefore, if external monitoring shows a baseline that is becoming smooth or losing variability, use of an internal spiral electrode should be considered to gain a more accurate picture of the fetal health status.

PERIODIC BASELINE CHANGES

Periodic baseline changes are temporary, recurrent changes made in response to a stimulus, such as a contraction. The FHR can demonstrate patterns of accelerations or decelerations in response to most stimuli. Fetal **accelerations** are transitory abrupt increases in the FHR above the baseline that last less than 30 seconds from onset to peak. They are associated with sympathetic nervous stimulation. They are visually apparent, with elevations of FHR of more than 15 bpm above the baseline, and their duration is greater than 15 seconds, but less than 2 minutes (Liston et al., 2018). They are generally considered reassuring and require no interventions.

Accelerations denote fetal movement and fetal well-being and are the basis for nonstress testing.

A **deceleration** is a transient fall in FHR caused by stimulation of the parasympathetic nervous system. Decelerations are described by their shape and often their timing in association to a uterine contraction. They are classified as early, late, and variable (Fig. 14.8).

Early decelerations are visually apparent, usually symmetrical, and characterized by a gradual decrease in the FHR with the nadir or lowest point being reached after or equal to 30 seconds and with peak of the contraction. They rarely decrease more than 30 to 40 bpm below the baseline. Typically, the onset, nadir, and recovery of the deceleration occur at the same time as the onset, peak, and recovery of the contraction. They are most often seen during the active stage of any normal labour, during pushing, crowning, or vacuum extraction. They are thought to be a result of fetal head compression that results in a reflex vagal response with a resultant slowing of the FHR during uterine contractions. Early decelerations are not indicative of fetal distress and do not require intervention.

Late decelerations are visually apparent, usually symmetrical, transitory decreases in FHR that occur after the peak of the contraction. They are also gradual in nature with the nadir being reached after or equal to 30 seconds, however the FHR does not return to baseline levels until well after the contraction has ended. Late decelerations are associated with uteroplacental insufficiency, which

Onset   Recovery

Nadir

Acme

Contraction

A

Variable onset

Acme

Nadir

Contraction

B

Onset   Recovery

Nadir

Acme

Contraction

C

FIGURE 14.8 Decelerations.
A. Early. **B.** Variable. **C.** Late.

occurs when blood flow within the intervillous space is decreased to the extent that fetal hypoxia or myocardial depression exists (Martin, Fanaroff, & Walsh, 2014). Conditions that may decrease uteroplacental perfusion with resultant decelerations include patients with hypotension, gestational hypertension, and placental aging secondary to diabetes and post maturity, hyperstimulation via oxytocin infusion, smoking, anemia, and cardiac disease. They imply some degree of fetal hypoxia. Recurrent or intermittent late decelerations are always atypical or abnormal regardless of depth of deceleration. Acute episodes with moderate variability are more likely to be correctable, whereas chronic episodes with loss of variability are less likely to be correctable (Sholapurkar, 2015). Box 14.1 highlights interventions for abnormal or category III decelerations.

Variable decelerations present as visually apparent abrupt decreases in FHR where the decreases occur in less than 30 seconds below baseline and have an unpredictable shape on the FHR baseline, possibly demonstrating no consistent relationship to uterine contractions. The shape of variable decelerations may be U, V, or W, or they may not resemble other patterns (Cahill & Spain, 2015). Variable decelerations usually occur abruptly with quick deceleration. They are the most common deceleration pattern found in the labouring patient and are usually transient and correctable (Ugwumadu, 2015). Variable decelerations are associated with cord compression. However, they are classified either as category atypical or abnormal depending on the accompanying change in baseline variability (Liston et al., 2018). The pattern of variable deceleration consistently related to the contractions with a slow return to FHR baseline warrants further monitoring and evaluation.

BOX 14.1

INTERVENTIONS FOR ABNORMAL FETAL HEART RATE PATTERNS

- Notify the health care provider about the pattern and obtain further orders, making sure to document all interventions and their effects on the FHR pattern.
- Discontinue any oxytocin or other uterotonic agents as dictated by the facility's protocol, if it is being administered.
- Turn the client on to the left or right lateral position, knee-chest, or hands and knees to increase placental perfusion or relieve cord compression.
- Administer oxygen via face mask to increase fetal oxygenation.
- Increase the intravenous fluid rate to improve intravascular volume and correct any hypotension.
- Assess the client for any underlying contributing causes.
- Reduce the client's anxiety by providing reassurance that interventions are to effect pattern change.
- Modify pushing in the second stage of labour to improve fetal oxygenation.
- Document any and all interventions and any changes in FHR patterns.
- Prepare for an expeditious surgical birth if the pattern is not corrected in 30 minutes.

Adapted from American College of Obstetricians and Gynecologists (ACOG). (2014). Safe prevention of the primary cesarean delivery. Obstetric Care Consensus 1. *Obstetrics & Gynecology, 123,* 693–711; Liston, R., Sawchuck, D., & Young, D. (2018). SOGC clinical practice guideline No. 197b, Fetal health surveillance: Intrapartum consensus guideline. *Journal of Obstetrics and Gynaecology Canada.* Retrieved from https://www.jogc.com/article/S1701-2163(18)30067-7/pdf

Prolonged decelerations are abrupt FHR declines of at least 15 bpm that last longer than 2 minutes, but less than 10 minutes (Liston et al., 2018). The rate usually drops to less than 90 bpm. Many factors are associated with this pattern, including prolonged cord compression, abruptio placenta, cord prolapse, supine patient position, vaginal examination, fetal blood sampling, patient seizures, regional anesthesia, or uterine rupture (Liston et al., 2018). Prolonged decelerations can be remedied by identifying the underlying cause and correcting it.

A *sinusoidal pattern* is described as having a visually apparent smooth, sinewave-like undulating pattern in the FHR baseline with a cycle frequency of 3 to 5 bpm that persists for >20 minutes. It is attributed to a derangement of CNS control of FHR and occurs when a severe degree of hypoxia secondary to fetal anemia and hypovolemia is present. It is always considered an abnormal, and to attempt to correct it, a fetal intrauterine transfusion would be needed (Nageotte, 2015) if delivery is not advised.

Combinations of FHR patterns obtained by EFM during labour are not infrequent. Atypical and abnormal patterns are more significant if they are mixed, persist for long periods, or have frequent prolonged late decelerations, absent or minimal variability, bradycardia or tachycardia, and prolonged variable decelerations lower than 60 bpm. The likelihood of fetal compromise is increased if atypical and abnormal patterns are associated with decreased baseline variability or abnormal contraction patterns (Liston et al., 2018).

Other Fetal Assessment Methods

In situations suggesting the possibility of fetal compromise, such as atypical or abnormal FHR patterns, further ancillary testing such as scalp pH blood analysis or scalp lactate and fetal scalp stimulation may be used to validate the FHR findings and assist in planning interventions.

Take Note!

In recent years, the use of fetal scalp sampling has decreased, being replaced by techniques that yield similar information. It has been shown to have a poor positive predictive value for intrapartum hypoxia and recent systematic reviews have reported no evidence of benefit in reducing cesarean section rates (Chandraharan, 2014).

Umbilical Cord Blood Analysis

Neonatal and childhood mortality and morbidity, including cerebral palsy, are often attributed to fetal acidosis, as defined by a low cord pH at birth. Umbilical cord blood acid–base analysis drawn at birth provides an objective method of evaluating a newborn's condition, identifying the presence of intrapartum hypoxia and acidemia. This test is considered a good indicator of fetal oxygenation and acid–base condition at birth (Martin et al., 2014). The normal mean pH value range is 7.2 to 7.3. The pH values are useful for planning interventions for the newborn born with low 5-minute Apgar scores, atypical and abnormal FHR patterns during labour, umbilical cord prolapse, uterine rupture, patient fever, placental abruption, meconium-stained amniotic fluid, and post-term births (Gujral & Nayar, 2015). The interventions needed for the compromised newborn might include providing an optimal extrauterine environment, fluids, oxygen, medications, and other treatments.

Fetal Scalp Stimulation

An indirect method used to evaluate fetal oxygenation and acid–base balance to identify fetal hypoxia is fetal scalp stimulation or vibroacoustic stimulation. If the fetus does not have adequate oxygen reserves, carbon dioxide builds up, leading to acidemia and hypoxemia. These metabolic states are reflected in abnormal FHR patterns as well as fetal inactivity. Fetal stimulation is performed to promote fetal movement with the hope that FHR accelerations will accompany the movement.

Fetal movement can be stimulated with a vibroacoustic stimulator (artificial larynx) applied to the woman's lower abdomen and turned on for 3 to 5 seconds to produce sound and vibration or by placing a gloved finger on the fetal scalp and applying firm pressure. A well-oxygenated fetus will respond when stimulated (tactile or by noise) by moving in conjunction with an acceleration of 15 bpm above the baseline heart rate that lasts at least 15 seconds. This FHR acceleration reflects a pH of more than 7 and a fetus with an intact CNS. Fetal scalp stimulation is not done during a contraction, if the fetus is preterm, or if the patient has an intrauterine infection, a diagnosis of placenta previa (which could lead to hemorrhage), or a fever (which increases the risk of an ascending infection) (King et al., 2019). If no acceleratory response by the fetus is exhibited with either scalp stimulation or vibroacoustic stimulation, further evaluation of the fetus is warranted.

Nurses play an essential role in the evaluation of labouring client and fetal status during labour, continued surveillance, initiation of corrective measures when indicated, and reevaluation. A vital attribute of nursing surveillance is that it is a systematic process for assessment, intervention, and evaluation.

PROMOTING COMFORT AND PROVIDING PAIN MANAGEMENT DURING LABOUR

Pain during labour is a universal experience, although the intensity of the pain may vary. Labour pain is unique to every person based on various contributing physiologic, emotional, social, and cultural factors. Although labour and childbirth are viewed as natural processes, both can produce significant pain and discomfort. The physical causes of pain during labour include cervical stretching, hypoxia of the uterine muscle due to a decrease in perfusion during contractions, pressure on the urethra, bladder, and rectum, and distention of the muscles of the pelvic floor (Leonard, 2018).

Pain during labour is a physiologic phenomenon. The etiology of pain during the first stage of labour is associated with ischemia of the uterus during contractions. In the second stage, pain is caused by the stretching of the vagina and perineum and compression of the pelvic structures. A patient's pain perception can be influenced by previous experiences with pain, fatigue, pain anticipation, genetics, positive or negative support system, health care provider's presence and encouragement, labour and birth environment, cultural expectations, and level of emotional stress and anxiety. Pain perception during labour changes in intensity and nature as labour progresses, and this is associated with, and can influence, behavioural changes in the labouring clients. Supporting clients to maintain a sense of control and empowerment during their labour process can help women to experience pain more as a physiological process, rather than as suffering (Bonapace et al., 2018).

The techniques used to manage the pain of labour vary according to geography and culture. For example, some Appalachians believe that placing a hatchet or knife under the bed of a labouring person may help "cut the pain of childbirth," and someone from this background may wish to do so in the hospital setting (Bowers, 2015). Asian, Latino, and Orthodox Jewish patients may request that their own mothers, not their partners, attend their births. In some cultures, the partners do not actively participate in the birthing process. People of Cherokee, Hmong, and Japanese backgrounds may remain quiet during labour and birth and not complain of pain because outwardly expressing pain is not appropriate in their cultures. Never interpret their quietness as the absence of pain. The concept of pain and pain expression during labour has different meanings for people of different cultures. Several points for the nurse to consider when caring for diverse cultural clients include using a qualified interpreter to communicate about pain as needed, offer and support culturally acceptable forms of pain relief, and assess for pain frequently (Wojnar & Narruhn, 2016).

Immigrating to a new country is a stressful process of readjustment and change. Effective verbal communication and understanding nonverbal social cues are invaluable when providing care to diverse cultures. Culturally diverse childbearing families present to the labour and birth suites with the same needs and desires of all families. Make sure they have a high-quality birth experience:

uphold their religious, ethnic, gender identities, gender expressions, and cultural values and integrate them into care

Today, clients have many safe nonpharmacologic and pharmacologic choices for the management of pain during labour and birth, which may be used separately or in combination with one another. Pharmacologic approaches are directed at eliminating the physical sensation of labour pain, whereas nonpharmacologic approaches are largely directed at prevention of suffering.

Nurses are in an ideal position to provide childbearing families with balanced, clear, concise information about effective nonpharmacologic and pharmacologic measures to relieve pain. Pain management standards issued by The Joint Commission mandate that pain be assessed in all clients admitted to a health care facility. Attention to the pain that occurs during labour and childbirth should be a priority of care for all nurses (Bonapace et al., 2018). A pain assessment tool named the *Coping with Labour Algorithm* uses the FOCUS format "Plan, Do, Check, and Act" cycle in labouring patients. This tool provides a mechanism for pain documentation and links it to nursing care interventions (Roberts, Gulliver, Fisher, & Cloyes, 2010). Thus, it is important for nurses to be knowledgeable about the most recent scientific research on labour pain relief modalities, to make sure that accurate and unbiased information about effective pain relief measures is available to labouring patients, to be sure that the person determines what is an acceptable labour pain level for them, and to allow for their choice of pain relief method to be honoured.

Nonpharmacologic Measures

Nonpharmacologic measures may include continuous labour support, hydrotherapy, hypnosis, ambulation and position changes, transcutaneous electrical nerve stimulation (TENS), acupuncture and acupressure, attention focusing and imagery, therapeutic touch and massage, breathing techniques, and effleurage. Most of these methods are based on the *gate control theory of pain*, which proposes that local physical stimulation can interfere with pain stimuli by closing a hypothetical gate in the spinal cord, thus blocking pain signals from reaching the brain (McGeary, Swanholm, & Gatchel, 2015). It has long been a standard of care for labour nurses to first provide or encourage a variety of nonpharmacologic measures before moving to the pharmacologic interventions.

Nonpharmacologic measures are usually simple, safe, and inexpensive to use. Many of these measures are taught in childbirth classes, and expectant patients should be encouraged to try a variety of methods prior to the real labour. Many of the measures need to be practiced for best results and coordinated with the partner/coach. The nurse can and should provide support and

EVIDENCE-BASED PRACTICE 14.2 — EFFECTIVENESS OF AROMATHERAPY AND BIOFEEDBACK IN PROMOTION OF LABOUR OUTCOME DURING CHILDBIRTH AMONG PRIMIGRAVIDAS

STUDY

Labour pain is described as the most severe form of pain that a person may experience during their lifetime. When considering labour analgesia, one is faced with a number of choices each with different advantages and disadvantages depending on the individual's expectations and preferences. Many clients would like to avoid taking medications or invasive methods for pain management because of the potential negative impact on their fetus during labour. Severe pain triggers a stress response which may lead to harmful effects on both labouring individual and fetus. The purpose of this study was to evaluate the effect of aromatherapy (essential oils from plants are massaged in the skin and inhaled) and biofeedback (mother was asked to experience both the fetal heart sound and variation in contractions and consciously regulate them) in promotion of labour outcome during childbirth.

Findings

Six hundred nulliparous women were selected randomly and assigned to an aromatherapy group (n = 200), a biofeedback group (n = 200), or a control group (n = 200). The researchers rated pain by using a visual pain analog scale during their labours. Sixty-nine percent of cases in the aromatherapy group expressed it was helpful, provided pain relief and emotional well-being during their labours. Biofeedback was also effective in reducing pain and duration of labour during childbirth compared with the control group.

Nursing Implications

The results of this study indicated that the use of aromatherapy and biofeedback, as nonpharmacologic methods were both effective methods of reducing pain perception and duration of labour among women during labour. As a nonpharmacologic nursing intervention, these are easy to administer, cost-effective, harmless, and appealing to the mother without any apparent maternal or neonatal adverse effects.

Adopted from Janula, R., & Mahipal, S. (2015). Effectiveness of aromatherapy and biofeedback in promotion of labour outcome during childbirth among primigravidas. *Health Science Journal, 9*(1), 1–5.

encouragement for the patient and their partner using nonpharmacologic methods. Although clients cannot consciously direct the labour contractions, they can control how they respond to them, thereby enhancing their feelings of control. See Evidence-Based Practice 14.2 for more information.

Continuous Labour Support

Continuous labour support involves offering a sustained presence to the labouring patient by providing emotional support, comfort measures, advocacy, information and advice, and support for the partner. Continuous labour support is a nonpharmacologic, evidence-based strategy associated with reduced cesarean rates (Bonapace et al., 2018). The client's family, a doula, or anyone else close to the client can provide this continuous presence, however, the labour nurse is ideally situated to provide this support, with a sound medical and physiologic base. A support person can assist the client to ambulate, reposition, and use breathing techniques. A support person can also aid with the use of acupressure, massage, music therapy, or therapeutic touch. During the natural course of childbirth, a labouring client's functional ability is limited secondary to pain, and clients often have trouble making decisions. The support person can help the client to make decisions based on their birth plan and personal wishes.

Research has validated the value of continuous labour support versus intermittent support in terms of fewer operative deliveries, cesarean births, and requests for pain medication. Continuous labour support has shown to have beneficial effects on the birthing parent and the newborn primarily due to the reduction in anxiety during the labouring experience. Most birthing parents expressed greater satisfaction with their childbirth experience (Bonapace et al., 2018; Simkin & Klein, 2018).

Take Note!

The human presence is of immeasurable value to help the labouring client feel secure.

Hydrotherapy

Hydrotherapy is a nonpharmacologic measure that may involve showering or soaking in a regular tub or whirlpool bath. When showering is the selected method of hydrotherapy, the patient stands or sits in a shower chair in a warm shower and allows the water to gently glide over the abdomen and back. If a tub or whirlpool is chosen, the patient is immersed in warm water for relaxation and relief of discomfort. The warmth and buoyancy of being in the water help to release muscle tension and can impart a sense of well-being (Taghavi, Barband, & Khaki, 2015) and contractions are usually less painful. Warm water provides soothing stimulation of nerves in the skin, promoting vasodilation, reversal of sympathetic nervous response, and a reduction in catecholamines (Dalal, 2015). Recent research findings reported that patients who used hydrotherapy had significantly reduced surgical birth rates, a shorter second stage of labour, reduced analgesic requirements, and a lower incidence of perineal trauma (Taghavi et al., 2015). The research concluded that hydrotherapy during labour significantly aids the labour process, minimizes the use of analgesic medications, offers fast- and short-acting pain and anxiety relief, and should be considered as a safe and effective birthing aid (Simkin & Klein, 2018).

A wide range of hydrotherapy options are available, from ordinary bathtubs to whirlpool baths and showers, combined with low lighting and music. Many hospitals provide showers and whirlpool baths for labouring patients for pain relief. However, hydrotherapy is more commonly practiced in birthing centres managed by midwives. The recommendation for initiating hydrotherapy is that the labouring patient be in active labour (more than 5 cm dilated) to prevent the slowing of labour contractions secondary to muscular relaxation. The membranes can be intact or ruptured. Clients are encouraged to stay in the bath or shower as long as they feel they are comfortable. The water temperature should not exceed body temperature.

Hydrotherapy is an effective pain management option for many people. Patients who are experiencing a healthy pregnancy can be offered this option. The potential risks associated with hydrotherapy include hyperthermia, hypothermia, changes in patient heart rate, fetal tachycardia, and unplanned underwater birth. The benefits include reducing pain, relieving anxiety, and promoting a sense of control during labour (Nutter, 2016).

Ambulation and Position Changes

Ambulation and position changes during labour are another extremely useful comfort measure. Historically, the person in labour adopted a variety of positions during labour, rarely using the recumbent position until during the first half of the 20th century. The medical profession has favoured recumbent positions during labour, but without evidence to demonstrate its appropriateness. A Cochrane database systematic review reported there is evidence that walking and upright positions in the first stage of labour reduce the length of labour and do not seem to be associated with increased intervention or negative effects on labouring patient's and fetal well-being. In an upright posture, gravity directs the weight of the fetus and amniotic fluid downward, successively dilating the cervix and the birth canal. Uterine contractions have been shown to be better spaced, stronger and more efficient in dilating the cervix when the patient is in an upright position when compared to being in the supine position (Cox & King, 2015). Patients should be encouraged to take up

whatever position they find most comfortable in the first stage of labour (Simkin & Klein, 2018).

Changing position frequently, at least every 30 minutes, such as sitting, walking, kneeling, standing, lying down, getting on hands and knees, and using a birthing ball, helps to relieve pain (Fig. 14.9). Position changes also may help to speed labour by adding the benefits of gravity and changing the shape of the pelvis. Research has found that the position that the patient assumes and the frequency of position changes have a profound effect on uterine activity and efficiency. Allowing the patient to obtain a position of comfort frequently facilitates a favourable fetal rotation by altering the alignment of the presenting part with the pelvis. As the patient continues to change position based on comfort, the optimal presentation is afforded (Simkin & Klein, 2018). Supine positions should be avoided, since they may interfere with labour progress and can cause compression of the vena cava and decrease blood return to the heart resulting in a profound hypotensive episode.

Swaying from side to side, rocking, or other rhythmic movements may also be comforting. If labour is progressing slowly, ambulating may speed it up again (Fig. 14.10). Upright positions such as walking, kneeling forward, or doing the lunge on the birthing ball give most patients a greater sense of control and active movement than just lying down. Table 14.2 highlights some of the more common positions that can be used during labour and birth.

Acupuncture and Acupressure

Acupuncture and acupressure can be used to relieve pain during labour. Although controlled research studies of these methods are limited, there is adequate evidence that both are useful in relieving pain associated with labour and birth. However, both methods require a trained, certified clinician, and such a person is not available in many birth facilities (Halpern & Garg, 2015).

Acupuncture involves stimulating key trigger points with needles. This form of Chinese medicine has been practiced for approximately 3,000 years. Classical Chinese teaching holds that throughout the body there are meridians or channels of energy (*qi*) that when in balance regulate body functions. Pain reflects an imbalance or obstruction of the flow of energy. The purpose of acupuncture is to restore thus diminishing pain (Adams, Frawley, Steel, Broom, & Sibbritt, 2015). Stimulating the trigger points causes the release of endorphins, reducing the perception of pain.

Acupressure involves the application of a firm finger or massage used in acupuncture to reduce the pain sensation. The amount of pressure is important. The intensity of the pressure is determined by the needs of the person. Holding and squeezing the hand of a patient in labour may trigger the point most commonly used for both techniques. Some acupressure points are

FIGURE 14.9 Various positions for use during labour. **A.** Ambulation. **B.** Leaning forward. **C.** Sitting in a chair. **D.** Using a birthing ball.

found along the spine, neck, shoulder, toes, and soles of the feet. Pressure along the side of the spine can help relieve back pain during labour (Mollart, Adam, & Foureur, 2015). A Cochrane collaboration review found that acupuncture may indeed reduce labour pain, increasing satisfaction with pain management and reduced use of pharmacologic management. However, there is a need for further research (Simkin & Klein, 2018).

Application of Heat and Cold

Superficial applications of heat and/or cold, in various forms, are popular with labouring clients. They are easy to use, inexpensive, require no prior practice, and have minimal negative side effects when used properly. Heat is typically applied to the person's back, lower abdomen, groin, and/or perineum. Heat sources include a hot water bottle, heated rice-filled sock, warm compress, electric heating pad, warm blanket, and warm bath or shower. In addition to being used for pain relief, heat is used to relieve chills or trembling, decrease joint stiffness, reduce muscle spasm, and increase connective tissue extensibility (Liu, Fernando, & Mon, 2015).

Cold therapy, or cryotherapy, is usually applied on the back, chest, and/or face during labour. Forms of cold include a bag or surgical glove filled with ice, a frozen

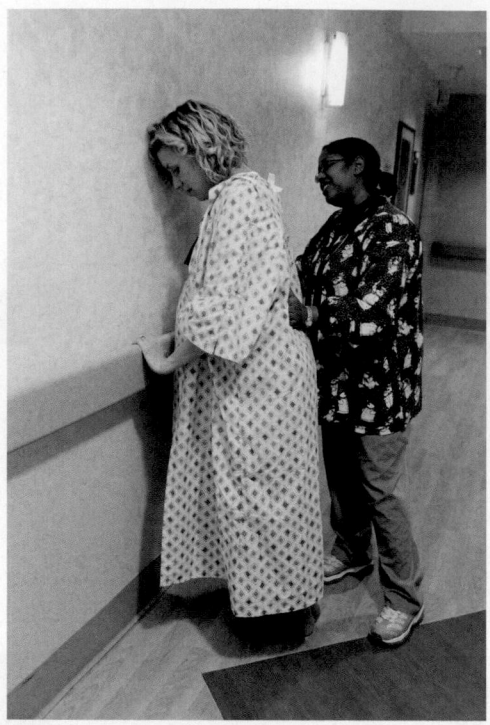

FIGURE 14.10 Nurse massaging the client's back during a contraction while she ambulates during labour.

gel pack, a hollow, plastic rolling pin or bottle filled with ice, a washcloth dipped in cold water, soda cans chilled in ice, and even a frozen bag of vegetables. Patients in labour who feel cold usually need to feel warm before they can comfortably tolerate using a cold pack. Chilled soda cans and rolling pins filled with ice give the added benefit of mechanical pressure when rolled on the low back. Cold has the additional effects of relieving muscle spasms and reducing inflammation and edema (Tharpe et al., 2016).

To date, no randomized controlled studies have evaluated the use of heat and cold, so further study is needed to determine if either approach is efficacious. With appropriate safety precautions, heat and cold offer comfort and relief, and their use should be dictated by the desires and responses of the labouring patient.

Attention Focusing and Imagery

Attention focusing and imagery use many of the senses and the mind to focus on stimuli. The person can focus on tactile stimuli such as touch, massage, or stroking. They may focus on auditory stimuli such as music, humming, or verbal encouragement. Visual stimuli might be any object in the room, or the person can imagine the beach, a mountaintop, a happy memory, or even the contractions of the uterine muscle pulling the cervix open and the fetus pressing downward to open the cervix. Some people focus on a particular mental activity such

as a song, a chant, counting backward, or a religious prayer or verse. Breathing, relaxation, positive thinking, and positive visualization work well for patients in labour. The use of these techniques keeps the sensory input perceived during the contraction from reaching the pain centre in the cortex of the brain (Capogna, 2015a).

Effleurage and Massage

Effleurage is a light, stroking, superficial touch of the abdomen, in rhythm with breathing during contractions. It is used as a relaxation and distraction technique from discomfort. External fetal monitor belts may interfere with the ability to accomplish this.

Effleurage and massage use the sense of touch to promote relaxation and pain relief. Massage works as a form of pain relief by increasing the production of endorphins in the body. Endorphins reduce the transmission of signals between nerve cells and thus lower the perception of pain. Because touch receptors go to the brain faster than pain receptors, massage—anywhere on the body—can block the pain message to the brain. In addition, light touch has been found to release endorphins and induce a relaxed state. In addition, touching and massage distract the person from discomfort. Massage involves manipulation of the body's soft tissues. It is commonly used to help relax tense muscles and to soothe and calm the individual. Massage may help to relieve pain by assisting with relaxation, inhibiting sensory transmission in the pain pathways, or improving blood flow and oxygenation of tissues (Neetu & Panchal, 2015).

Breathing Techniques

Conscious use of breath by the patient has the power to profoundly influence the labour and how the client manages it. The first action anyone takes in any situation is a breath. The breath affects the lungs, immediately cueing the nervous system. The nervous system responds by sending messages, which impact our entire psychophysiologic system. Messages sent from the nervous system affect us physically, emotionally, and mentally. If we alter how we breathe, we alter the constellation of messages and reactions in our entire mind–body experience (Cheng & Caughey, 2015).

Breathing techniques are effective in producing relaxation and pain relief through the use of distraction. If the client is concentrating on slow-paced rhythmic breathing, they are not likely to fully focus on contraction pain. Breathing techniques are often taught in childbirth education classes (see Chapter 12 for additional information).

Controlled breathing helps reduce the pain experienced by using stimulus–response conditioning. The client selects a focal point within the environment to

TABLE 14.2	COMMON POSITIONS FOR USE DURING LABOUR AND BIRTH
Standing	• Takes advantage of gravity during and between contractions • Makes contractions feel less painful and be more productive • Helps fetus line up with angle of maternal pelvis • Helps to increase urge to push in second stage of labour
Walking	• Has the same advantages as standing • Causes changes in the pelvic joints, helping the fetus move through the birth canal
Standing and leaning forward on partner, bed, birthing ball	• Has the same advantages as standing • Is a good position for a back massage • May feel more restful than standing • Can be used with electronic fetal monitor
Slow dancing (standing with client's arms around partner's neck, head resting on their chest or shoulder, sway to music and breathe in rhythm if it helps; partner can massage client's back)	• Has the same advantages as walking • Back pressure helps relieve back pain • Rhythm and music help clients relax and provide comfort
The lunge (standing facing a straight chair with one foot on the seat with knee and foot to the side; bending raised knee and hip, and lunging sideways repeatedly during a contraction, holding each lunge for 5 seconds; partner holds chair and helps with balance)	• Widens one side of the pelvis (the side toward lunge) • Encourages rotation of baby • Can also be done in a kneeling position
Sitting upright	• Helps promote rest • Has more gravity advantage than lying down • Can be used with electronic fetal monitor
Semi-sitting (setting the head of the bed at a 45-degree angle with pillows used for support)	• Has the same advantages as sitting upright • Is an easy position if on a bed
Sitting on toilet or commode	• Has the same advantages as sitting upright • May help relax the perineum for effective bearing down
Rocking in a chair	• Has the same advantages as sitting upright • May help speed labour (rocking movement)
Sitting, leaning forward with support	• Has the same advantages as sitting upright • Is a good position for a back massage
On all fours, on hands and knees	• Helps relieve backache • Assists rotation of baby in posterior position • Allows for pelvic rocking and body movement • Relieves pressure on hemorrhoids • Allows for vaginal examinations • Is sometimes preferred as a pushing position by clients with back labour
Kneeling, leaning forward with support on a chair seat, the raised head of the bed, or on a birthing ball	• Has the same advantages as all-fours position • Puts less strain on wrists and hands
Side-lying	• Is a very good position for resting and convenient for many kinds of medical interventions • Helps lower elevated blood pressure • May promote progress of labour when alternated with walking • Is useful to slow a very rapid second stage • Avoids vena cava syndrome • May offer increased control of pushing efforts • Takes pressure off hemorrhoids • Facilitates relaxation between contractions

(continued)

TABLE 14.2	**COMMON POSITIONS FOR USE DURING LABOUR AND BIRTH** (continued)
Squatting	• May relieve backache • Takes advantage of gravity • Requires less bearing-down effort • Widens pelvic outlet by approximately 28% • Pressure is evenly distributed to the perineum, reducing the need for episiotomy • May help fetus turn and move down in a difficult birth • Allows freedom to shift weight for comfort • Offers an advantage when pushing, since upper trunk presses on the top of the uterus
Supported squat (leaning back against partner, who provides supports under the arms; standing up between contractions)	• Requires great strength in partner • Lengthens trunk, allowing more room for fetus to manoeuvre into position • Lets gravity help
Dangle (partner sitting high on bed or counter with feet supported on chairs or footrests and thighs spread; client leaning back between partner's legs, placing flexed arms over partner's thighs; partner gripping sides with thighs; client lowers down and allows partner to support the full weight; standing up between contractions)	• Has the same advantages of a supported squat • Requires less physical strength from the partner

Adapted from Gizzo, S., Di Gangi, S., Noventa, M., Bacile, V., Zambon, A., & Nardelli, B. (2014). Women's choice of positions during labor: Return to the past or a modern way to give birth? A cohort study in Italy. *BioMed Research International.* Retrieved from http://dx.doi.org/10.1155/2014/638093; Hanson, L., & VandeVusse, L. (2014). Supporting labor progress toward physiologic birth. *Journal of Perinatal & Neonatal Nursing, 28*(2), 101–107; Magowan, B., Owen, P., & Thomson, A. (2014). *Clinical obstetrics & gynecology* (3rd ed.). St. Louis, MO: Saunders Elsevier; and Simkin, P., & Klein, M.C. (2018). Nonpharmacologic approaches to management of labor pain. *UpToDate.* Retrieved from http://www.uptodate.com/contents/nonpharmacological-approaches-to-management-of-labor-pain

stare at during the first sign of a contraction. This focus creates a visual stimulus that goes directly to the brain. The client takes a deep cleansing breath, which is followed by rhythmic breathing. Verbal commands from support people supply an ongoing auditory stimulus to the brain. Benefits of practicing patterned breathing include breathing that:

• becomes an automatic response to pain.
• increases relaxation and can be used to deal with life's everyday stresses.
• is calming during labour.
• provides a sense of well-being and a measure of control.
• brings purpose to each contraction, making them more productive.
• provides more oxygen for the client and the fetus (Bonapace et al., 2018).

Many people learn patterned-paced breathing during formal and informal education during the pregnancy. Three levels of breathing may be taught, each beginning and ending with a cleansing breath or sigh after each contraction. In the first pattern, also known as slow-paced breathing, the person inhales slowly through the nose and exhales through pursed lips. The breathing rate is typically 6 to 9 bpm. In the second pattern, the person inhales and exhales through the mouth at a rate of four breaths every 5 seconds. The rate can be accelerated to two breaths per second to assist in relaxation. The third

pattern, is similar to the second pattern except that the breathing is punctuated every few breaths by a forceful exhalation through pursed lips. All breaths are kept equal and rhythmic and can increase as contractions increase in intensity (Lindholm & Hildingsson, 2015).

Many childbirth educators do not recommend specific breathing techniques or try to teach parents to breathe the "right" way during labour and birth. People are encouraged to find breathing styles that enhance their relaxation and use them. There are numerous benefits to controlled and rhythmic breathing in childbirth (outlined previously), and many people will choose these techniques to manage their discomfort during labour.

Pharmacologic Measures

With varying degrees of success, generations of people have sought ways to relieve the pain of childbirth. Pharmacologic pain relief during labour includes systemic analgesia and regional or local anesthesia. Childbearing clients have seen dramatic changes in pharmacologic pain management options over the years. Methods have evolved from biting down on a stick to control their pain, experiencing "twilight sleep" during their labours and not remembering what happened, to a more complex pharmacologic approach such as epidural/intrathecal analgesia. Systemic analgesia and regional analgesia/anesthesia have become less common, while newer neuraxial analgesia/anesthesia techniques involving minimal motor blockade have become more effective and thus, more popular. **Neuraxial analgesia/anesthesia** is the administration of analgesic (opioids) or anesthetic (capable of producing a loss of sensation in an area of the body) agents, either continuously or intermittently, into the epidural or intrathecal space to relieve pain. Low-dose and ultra–low-dose epidural analgesia, spinal analgesia, and combined spinal–epidural (CSE) analgesia have replaced the traditional epidural for labour. Neuraxial analgesia does not interfere with the progress or outcome of labour. There is no need to withhold neuraxial analgesia until the active stage of labour (Grant, Tao, Craig, McIntire, & Leveno, 2015). This shift in pain management techniques allows a person to be an active participant in their own labour and determination of pain management.

Take Note!

Regardless of the approach used during labour, every person has the right to choose the methods of pain control and pain management that will best suit them and meet their needs.

Systemic Analgesia

Systemic analgesia involves the use of one or more drugs administered orally, intramuscularly, or intravenously and which become distributed throughout the body via the circulatory system. Depending on which administration method is used, the therapeutic effect of pain relief can occur within minutes and last up to several hours. The most important consideration is the associated with the use of this class of drugs is the complication of respiratory depression in both the patient and also in the newborn. Therefore, patients given these drugs require careful monitoring. Opioids given close to the time of birth can cause CNS depression in the newborn, necessitating assistance with effective respiratory ventilation after birth. These infants also need ongoing monitoring for risk of continued respiratory depression for several hours.

Several drug categories may be used for systemic analgesia:

- *Opioids*, such as butorphanol (Stadol), nalbuphine (Nubain), morphine, or fentanyl (Sublimaze)
- *Ataractics*, such as hydroxyzine (Vistaril), promethazine (Phenergan), or prochlorperazine (Compazine)
- *Benzodiazepines*, such as diazepam (Valium) or midazolam (Versed)

Drug Guide 14.1 highlights some of the major drugs used for systemic analgesia.

Systemic analgesics are typically administered parenterally, usually through an existing intravenous line. Nearly all medications given during labour cross the placenta and have a depressant effect on the fetus; therefore, it is important for the patient to receive the least amount of systemic medication that relieves the discomfort so that it does not cause any harm to the fetus (Cheng & Caughey, 2015). Historically opioids have been administered by nurses, but in the past decade there has been increasing use of client-controlled intravenous analgesia (patient-controlled analgesia or PCA). With this system, the patient is given a button connected to a computerized pump on the intravenous line. When analgesia is desired, the patient presses the button and the pump delivers a preset amount of medication. This system provides the patient with a sense of control over the pain management and be an active participation in the childbirth process.

OPIOIDS

Opioids are morphine-like medications that are most effective for the relief of moderate to severe pain and are typically administered intravenously. All opioids are lipophilic and cross the placental barrier, but do not affect labour progress in the active phase. Opioids are associated with newborn respiratory depression, newborn decreased alertness, inhibited sucking, and a delay in effective feeding (King et al., 2019).

Opioids decrease the transmission of pain impulses by binding to receptor site pathways that transmit the pain signals to the brain. The effect is increased tolerance to pain and respiratory depression related to a decrease in sensitivity to carbon dioxide (Skidmore-Roth, 2015). All opioids are considered good analgesics. However, respiratory depression can occur in the patient depending on the dose given. For the fetus, these medications may also cause a decrease in FHR variability identified on the fetal monitor strip. This FHR pattern change is usually transient. Other systemic side effects to the patient include nausea, vomiting, pruritus, delayed gastric emptying, drowsiness, hypoventilation, and in the newborn, there is a risk of respiratory depression. To reduce the incidence of newborn respiratory depression, birth should ideally occur within 1 hour or after 4 hours of administration to prevent the fetus from receiving the peak concentration (Cheng & Caughey, 2015). Staff trained in neonatal resuscitation should always be available to evaluate and treat the newborn for respiratory depression at birth.

A recent study reported that parenteral opioids provide some relief from pain in labour, but are associated with neonatal respiratory distress. Patient satisfaction with opioid analgesia appeared moderate at best (Kerr, Taylor, & Evans, 2015).

ANTIEMETICS

The antiemetic group of medications is used in combination with an opioid to decrease nausea and vomiting and lessen anxiety. These adjunct drugs potentiate the

DRUG GUIDE 14.1 COMMON AGENTS USED FOR SYSTEMIC ANALGESIA

Type	Drug	Comments
Opioids	Morphine 2–5 mg IV	May be given IV or epidurally Rapidly crosses the placenta, causes a decrease in FHR variability Can cause maternal and neonatal CNS depression Decreases uterine contractions
	Butorphanol (Stadol) 1–2 mg IV	Is given IV
	q2–4h	Is rapidly transferred across the placenta Causes neonatal respiratory depression
	Nalbuphine (Nubain) 10–20 mg IV	Is given IV Causes less maternal nausea and vomiting Causes decreased FHR variability, fetal bradycardia, and respiratory depression
	Fentanyl (Sublimaze) 50–100 mcg IV	Is given IV or epidurally Can cause hypotension, maternal and fetal respiratory depression Rapidly crosses placenta
Antiemetics	Hydroxyzine (Vistaril) 50–100 mg IM	Does not relieve pain but reduces anxiety and potentiates opioid analgesic effects; cannot be given IV Is used to decrease nausea and vomiting
	Promethazine (Phenergan) 25–50 mg IV or IM	Is used for antiemetic effect when combined with opioids Causes sedation and reduces apprehension May contribute to maternal hypotension and neonatal depression
	Prochlorperazine (Compazine) 5–10 mg IV or IM	Frequently given with morphine sulphate for sleep during prolonged latent phase; counteracts the nausea that opioids can produce
Benzodiazepines	Diazepam (Valium) 2–5 mg IV	Is given to enhance pain relief of opioid and cause sedation May be used to stop eclamptic seizures Decreases nausea and vomiting Can cause newborn depression; therefore, lowest possible dose should be used
	Midazolam (Versed) 1–5 mg IV	Is not used for analgesic but amnesia effect Is used as adjunct for anesthesia Is excreted in breastmilk

IV, intravenous; IM, intramuscular.
Adapted from Hagood Milton, S. (2017). Normal labor and delivery. Retrieved from http://emedicine.medscape.com/article/260036-overview#aw2aab6b2; King, T. L., Brucker, M. C., Osborne, K., & Jevitt, C. M. (2019). *Varney's midwifery* (6th ed.). Burlington, MA: Jones & Bartlett Learning.; and Skidmore-Roth, L. (2015). *Mosby's 2015 nursing drug reference* (28th ed.). St. Louis, MO: Mosby Elsevier.

effectiveness of the opioid so that a lesser dose of opioid can be given. They may also be used to increase sedation. Promethazine (Phenergan) can be given intravenously, but hydroxyzine (Vistaril) must be given by mouth or by intramuscular injection into a large muscle mass. Neither drug affects the progress of labour, but either one may cause a decrease in FHR variability and possible newborn respiratory depression (Skidmore-Roth, 2015). Prochlorperazine (Compazine) is typically given intravenously or intramuscularly with morphine sulphate for sleep during a prolonged latent phase. It counteracts the nausea associated with opioids (King et al., 2019).

BENZODIAZEPINES

Benzodiazepines are used for minor tranquilizing and sedative effects. Diazepam (Valium) also is given intravenously to stop seizures resulting from eclampsia. It can be administered to calm a patient feeling out of control, thereby enabling them to relax enough to participate effectively in the labour process. Lorazepam (Ativan) can also be used for its tranquilizing effect, but increased sedation is experienced with this medication (Skidmore-Roth, 2015). Midazolam (Versed), also given intravenously, produces good amnesia but no analgesia. It is most commonly used as an adjunct for anesthesia.

Diazepam and midazolam cause CNS depression for both the client and the newborn.

Inhaled Analgesics

Nitrous oxide is known by most people as "laughing gas." For labour pain, half nitrous oxide gas (50%) is mixed with half oxygen (50%) and breathed through a mask or mouthpiece. This has been recently introduced in the United States, but has been in widespread use in Europe and Canada for many years. Clients have generally reported satisfaction with the use of nitrous oxide for pain relief in labour. An additional factor that may contribute to the decreased perception of pain is that this is self-administered. Self-administration is not only empowering for patients, but it also acts as a safety mechanism because it is almost impossible to overdose when it is self-administered (Halpern & Garg, 2015). Potential side effects of nitrous oxide include nausea and vomiting, dizziness, and dysphoria, although these are rare. No FHR abnormalities have been attributed to its use (Badve & Vallejo, 2015).

Regional Analgesia/Anesthesia

Regional analgesia/anesthesia provides pain relief without loss of consciousness. It involves the use of local anesthetic agents, with or without added opioids, to bring about pain relief or numbness through the drug's effects on the spinal cord and nerve roots. Obstetric regional analgesia generally refers to a partial or complete loss of pain sensation below the T8 to T10 level of the spinal cord (Stocks & Griffiths, 2015).

The routes for regional pain relief include epidural block, CSE, local infiltration, pudendal block, and intrathecal (spinal) analgesia/anesthesia. Local and pudendal routes are used during birth for episiotomies (surgical incision into the perineum to facilitate birth); epidural and intrathecal routes are used for pain relief during active labour and birth. The major advantage of regional pain management techniques is that the patient can participate in the birthing process and still have good pain control (Lee, Dy, & Azzam, 2016).

EPIDURAL ANALGESIA

Patients requesting epidural analgesia in labour will do so when they feel they need pain relief, and for some it might be quite early in their labour. Epidural analgesia for labour and birth involves the injection of a local anesthetic agent (e.g., Lidocaine or Bupivacaine) and an opioid analgesic agent (e.g., Morphine or Fentanyl) into the lumbar epidural space. A small catheter is then passed through the epidural needle to provide continuous access to the epidural space for maintenance of analgesia throughout labour and birth (Fig. 14.11). Epidural analgesia may slightly increase the duration of the second stage of labour and may increase the rate of instrument-assisted vaginal deliveries as well as that of oxytocin administration (Camorcia, 2015). Approximately 58% of labouring clients in Canada, and 60%

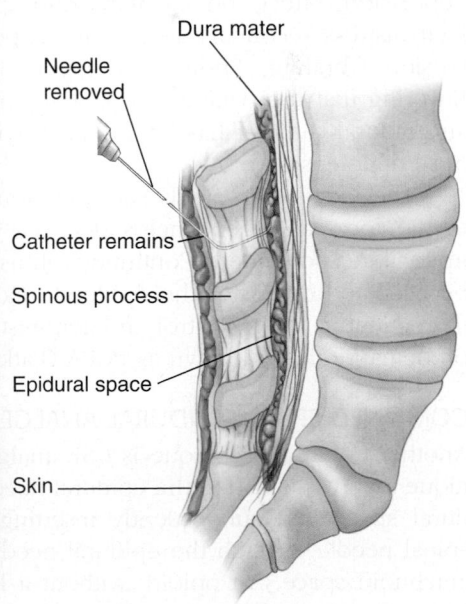

A   B

FIGURE 14.11 Epidural catheter insertion. **A.** A needle is inserted into the epidural space. **B.** A catheter is threaded into the epidural space; the needle is then removed. The catheter allows medication to be administered intermittently or continuously to relieve pain during labour and childbirth.

in the United States receive an epidural for pain relief during labour, but one in eight women who have an epidural during labour still need to use other methods of pain relief (Canadian Institute for Health Information, 2018). The frequency of epidural use varies across the country and may be dependent on the access and availability to the anesthesiologist.

An epidural involves the injection of a drug into the epidural space, which is located outside the dura mater between the dura and the spinal canal. The epidural space is typically entered through the third and fourth lumbar vertebrae with a needle, and a catheter is threaded into the epidural space. An epidural can be used for both vaginal and cesarean births. It has evolved from a regional block producing total loss of sensation to analgesia with minimal blockade. The effectiveness of epidural analgesia depends on the technique and medications used. Theoretically, epidural local anesthetics could block all labour pain if used in large volumes and high concentrations. However, pain relief is balanced against other goals such as walking during the first stage of labour, pushing effectively in the second stage, and minimizing patient and fetal side effects.

An epidural is contraindicated for people with a previous history of spinal surgery or spinal abnormalities, coagulation defects, cardiac disease, infections, and untreated hypovolemia. It also may be contraindicated for the patient who is receiving anticoagulation therapy.

Complications, from minor to major, include nausea and vomiting, hypotension, fever, pruritus, intravascular injection, patient fever, allergic reaction, and respiratory depression. Effects on the fetus during labour include fetal distress secondary to patients experiencing hypotension (Ibrahim, Fridman, Korst, & Gregory, 2015). Ensuring that the patient avoids a supine position after an epidural catheter has been placed will help to minimize hypotension.

The addition of opioids, such as Fentanyl or Morphine, to the local anesthetic helps decrease the amount of motor block obtained. Continuous infusion pumps can be used to administer the epidural analgesia, allowing the patient to be in control and administer a bolus dose on demand: this is known as PCEA (Patkar et al., 2015).

COMBINED SPINAL–EPIDURAL ANALGESIA

Another epidural technique is CSE analgesia. This technique involves inserting the epidural needle into the epidural space and subsequently inserting a small-gauge spinal needle through the epidural needle into the subarachnoid space. An opioid, without a local anesthetic, is injected into this space. The spinal needle is then removed and an epidural catheter is inserted for later use.

CSE is advantageous because of its rapid onset of pain relief (within 3 to 5 minutes) that can last up to 3 hours. It also allows the patient's motor function to remain active. The ability to bear down during the second stage

of labour is preserved because the pushing reflex is not lost, and the motor power remains intact. The CSE technique provides greater flexibility and reliability for labour than either spinal or epidural analgesia alone (Stocks & Griffiths, 2015). When compared with traditional epidural or spinal analgesia, which often keeps the patient lying in bed, CSE allows for patient ambulation ("walking epidural"). A recent Cochrane review contrasting the CSE analgesia approach with traditional and low-dose epidural analgesia in labour identified that CSE analgesia was associated with a greater incidence of pruritus, but a lower incidence of urinary retention and need for rescue analgesia, than epidural alone. In addition, CSE analgesia had a faster onset of pain relief, and there were no differences in labour outcomes (Heesen et al., 2015). Ambulating during labour provides several benefits: it may help control pain better, shorten the first stage of labour, increase the intensity of the contractions, and decrease the possibility of an operative vaginal or cesarean birth.

Consider This

When I was expecting my first child, I was determined to put my best foot forward and do everything right. I was an experienced OB nurse, and in my mind doing everything right was expected behaviour. I was already 2 weeks past my calculated due date and I was becoming increasingly worried. That particular day I went to work with a backache but felt no contractions.

I managed to finish my shift but felt completely wiped out. As I walked to my car outside the hospital, my water broke and I felt the warm fluid run down my legs. I went back inside to be admitted for this much-awaited event.

Although I had helped thousands of women go through their childbirth experience, I was now the one in the bed and not standing alongside it. My husband and I had practiced our breathing techniques to cope with the discomfort of labour, but this "discomfort" in my mind was more than I could tolerate. So, despite my best intentions of doing everything right, within an hour I begged for a painkiller to ease the pain. While the medication took the edge off my pain, I still felt every contraction and truly now appreciate the meaning of the word "labour." Although I wanted to use natural childbirth without any medication, I know that I was a full participant in my son's birthing experience, and that is what "doing everything right" was for me!

Thoughts: *Doing what is right varies for each individual, and as nurses we need to support whatever that is. Having a positive outcome from the childbirth experience is the goal; the means it takes to achieve it is less important. How can nurses support birthing patients in making their personal choices to achieve a healthy outcome? Are any people "failures" if they ask for pain medication to tolerate labour?*

Although clients can walk with CSE, they often choose not to because of fatigue. Often health care providers may not encourage or assist patients to ambulate for fear of injury. Nurses need to evaluate for ambulation safety that includes no postural hypotension and normal leg strength by the patient demonstrating a partial knee bend while standing; they also need to assist with ambulation at all times (Capogna, 2015b). Currently, anesthesiologists are performing walking epidurals using continuous infusion techniques as well as CSE and client-controlled epidural analgesia (Grant et al., 2015).

Complications for CSE include patient hypotension, intravascular injection, accidental intrathecal blockade, post-dural puncture headache, inadequate or failed block, fever, and pruritus. Hypotension and associated FHR changes are managed with patient positioning (semi-Fowler's position), intravenous hydration, and supplemental oxygen (Ibrahim et al., 2015).

PATIENT-CONTROLLED EPIDURAL ANALGESIA

Patient-controlled epidural analgesia (PCEA) involves the use of an indwelling epidural catheter with an infusion of medication and a programmed pump that allows the patient to control the dosing. This method allows the person to have a sense of control over their pain and reach their own individually acceptable analgesia level. When compared with traditional epidural analgesia, PCEA provides equivalent analgesia with lower anesthetic use, lower rates of supplementation, and higher client satisfaction (Van De Velde, 2015).

With PCEA, the client uses a handheld device connected to an analgesic agent that is attached to an epidural catheter. When they push the button, a set and timed bolus dose of agent is administered via the catheter to reduce the pain. This method allows one to manage the pain at will without having to ask a staff member to provide pain relief. Evidence supports the use of PCEA which appears to result in greater patient satisfaction and lower overall medication use (Sng, Kwok, & Sia, 2015).

LOCAL INFILTRATION

Local infiltration involves the injection of a local anesthetic, such as Lidocaine, into the superficial perineal nerves to numb the perineal area. This technique is done by the physician or midwife just before performing an episiotomy or before suturing a laceration. Local infiltration does not alter the pain of uterine contractions, but it does numb the immediate area of the episiotomy or laceration. Local infiltration does not cause side effects for the patient or the newborn.

PUDENDAL NERVE BLOCK

A pudendal nerve block refers to the injection of a local anesthetic agent (e.g., bupivacaine, ropivacaine) into

FIGURE 14.12 Pudendal nerve block.

the pudendal nerves near each ischial spine. It provides pain relief in the lower vagina, vulva, and perineum (Fig. 14.12).

A pudendal block is used for the second stage of labour, an episiotomy, or an operative vaginal birth with outlet forceps or vacuum extractor. It must be administered about 15 minutes before it would be needed to ensure its full effect. A transvaginal approach is generally used to inject an anesthetic agent at or near the pudendal nerve branch. Complications are uncommon, however there is a risk of transient fetal bradycardia from this procedure.

SPINAL (INTRATHECAL) ANALGESIA/ANESTHESIA

The spinal (intrathecal) pain management technique involves injection of an anesthetic "caine" agent, with or without opioids, into the subarachnoid space to provide pain relief during labour or cesarean birth. The subarachnoid space is a fluid-filled area located between the dura mater and the spinal cord. Spinal anesthesia is frequently used for elective and emergent cesarean births. The contraindications are similar to those for an epidural block. Adverse reactions for the patient include hypotension and spinal headache.

The subarachnoid injection of opioids alone, a technique termed intrathecal narcotics, has been gaining popularity since it was introduced in the 1980s. A narcotic is injected into the subarachnoid space, providing rapid pain relief while still maintaining motor function and sensation (Sng et al., 2015). An intrathecal narcotic is given during the active phase (more than 5 cm of dilation) of labour. Compared with epidural blocks, intrathecal narcotics are easy to administer, require a smaller volume of medication, produce excellent muscular relaxation, provide rapid-onset pain relief, are less likely to cause newborn respiratory depression, and do not cause motor blockade (Badve & Vallejo, 2015). Although pain relief is rapid with this technique, it is limited by the narcotic's duration of action, which may be only a few hours and not last through the labour. Additional pain measures may be needed to sustain pain management.

General Anesthesia

General anesthesia is typically reserved for emergency cesarean births when there is not enough time to provide spinal or epidural anesthesia or if the patient has a contraindication to the use of regional anesthesia. It can be started quickly and causes a rapid loss of consciousness. General anesthesia can be administered by intravenous injection, inhalation of anesthetic agents, or both. Commonly, Thiopental, a short-acting barbiturate, or propofol is given intravenously to produce unconsciousness. This is followed by administration of a muscle relaxant. After the patient is intubated, nitrous oxide and oxygen are administered. A volatile halogenated agent may also be administered to produce amnesia (Cheng & Caughey, 2015).

All anesthetic agents cross the placenta and affect the fetus. The primary complication with general anesthesia is fetal depression leading to newborn respiratory depression, along with uterine relaxation and potential maternal vomiting and aspiration. Complications relating to the inability to intubate the patient undergoing a general anesthesia complication are rare and the incidence of this complication has decreased greatly as a result of improved techniques (Hawkins, 2015).

Although the anesthesiologist or nurse anesthetist administers the various general anesthesia agents, the nurse needs to be knowledgeable about the pharmacologic aspects of the drugs used and must be aware of airway management. Ensure that the patient is not taking anything by mouth (NPO) and has a patent intravenous line. In addition, administer a nonparticulate (clear) oral antacid (e.g., Bicitra or sodium citrate) or a proton pump inhibitor (Protonix) as ordered to reduce gastric acidity. Assist with placement of a wedge under the patient's right hip to displace the gravid uterus and prevent vena cava compression in the supine position. Once the newborn has been removed from the uterus, assist the perinatal team in providing supportive care.

NURSING CARE DURING LABOUR AND BIRTH

Childbirth, a physiologic process that is fundamental to all human existence, is one of the most significant cultural, psychological, spiritual, and behavioural events in a person's life. Although the act of giving birth is a universal phenomenon, it is a unique experience for each individual. Continuous evaluation and appropriate intervention for patients and families during labour are essential to promoting a positive outcome for the family.

The nurse's role in childbirth is to ensure a safe environment for the labouring patient and the newborn. Nurses begin evaluating the patient and fetus during the admission procedures at the health care agency and continue to do so throughout labour. It is critical to provide anticipatory guidance and explain each procedure (fetal monitoring, intravenous therapy, medications given, and expected reactions) and what will happen next. This will prepare the patient and the family for the upcoming physical and emotional challenges, thereby helping to reduce anxiety. Acknowledging members of the support system helps allay their fears and concerns, thereby assisting them in carrying out their supportive role. Knowing how and when to evaluate a patient during the various stages of labour is essential for all labour and birth nurses to ensure a positive maternal experience and a healthy newborn.

A major focus of care for the woman during labour and birth is assisting one to maintain control over their pain, emotions, and actions while being an active participant. Nurses can help and support clients to be actively involved in their childbirth experience by allowing time for discussion, offering companionship, listening to worries and concerns, paying attention to the woman's emotional needs, and offering information to help her understand what is happening in each stage of labour. This is known as supportive care in labour.

Nursing Management During the First Stage of Labour

Depending on how far advanced the labour is when the client arrives at the facility; the nurse will determine assessment parameters of patient–fetal status and plan care accordingly. The nurse will provide supportive nursing care during the first stage of labour when admitting the client and family and orienting them to the labour and birth suite. The nurse is usually the primary gatekeeper of observations, interventions, treatments, and often the management of labour in the inpatient perinatal setting. Nursing care during this stage will include taking an admission history (reviewing the prenatal record); checking the results of routine laboratory tests and any special tests such as amniocentesis, genetic studies, and biophysical profile done during pregnancy; asking the client about any childbirth preparation (birth plan, classes taken, coping skills); and completing a physical assessment to establish baseline values for future comparison.

Key nursing interventions include:

- Identifying the estimated date of birth from the client and the prenatal chart
- Validating the client's prenatal history to determine fetal risk status
- Determining fundal height to validate dates and fetal growth
- Performing Leopold manoeuvres to determine fetal position, lie, and presentation
- Checking FHR
- Performing a vaginal examination (as appropriate) to evaluate effacement and dilation progress
- Instructing the client and partner about monitoring techniques and equipment
- Assessing fetal response and FHR if using intermittent auscultation. Interpreting fetal monitoring strips if continuous fetal monitoring is required
- Repositioning the client to obtain an optimal FHR pattern
- Recognizing FHR problems and initiating corrective measures
- Checking amniotic fluid for meconium staining, odour, and amount
- Comforting client throughout testing period and labour
- Documenting times of notification for team members if problems arise
- Supporting the client's decisions regarding intervention or avoidance of intervention
- Assessing the client's support system and coping status frequently

In addition to these interventions to promote optimal outcomes for the mother and fetus, the nurse must document care accurately and in a timely fashion. Accurate and timely documentation helps to decrease professional liability exposure, minimize the risk of preventable injuries to clients and infants during labour and birth, and preserve families (Simpson, 2015). Guidelines for recording care include documenting:

- All care given, to prove that standards were met
- Conversations with all providers, including notification times
- Nursing interventions before and after notifying provider
- Use of the chain of command and response at each level
- All flow sheets and forms, to validate care given
- All education given to client and response to it
- Facts, not personal opinions
- Detailed descriptions of any adverse outcome
- Initial nursing assessment, all encounters, and discharge plan
- All telephone conversations (Callahan, 2016)

This standard of documentation is needed to prevent or defend against litigation, which is prevalent in the childbirth arena.

Assessing the Client Upon Admission

The nurse usually first comes in contact with the client either by phone or in person. The nurse should ascertain whether the client is in true or prodromal phase of labour and whether they should be admitted or sent home. Upon admission to the labour and birth suite, the highest priorities include assessing FHR, determining whether membranes have ruptured or are intact, and assessing cervical dilation/effacement. These assessment data will guide the critical thinking in planning care for the client.

If the initial contact is by phone, establish a therapeutic relationship with the caller by using a calm, caring, and supportive tone of voice. Nurses providing a telephone triage service need to have sufficient clinical experience and have clear lines of responsibility to enable sound decision making. When completing a phone assessment, include questions about the following:

- Estimated date of birth, to determine if term or preterm
- Any significant medical history prior to or during the pregnancy
- Fetal movement (frequency in the past few days)
- Other premonitory signs of labour experienced
- Parity, gravida, and previous childbirth experiences
- Time from start of labour to birth in previous labours
- Characteristics of contractions, including frequency, duration, and intensity
- Appearance of any vaginal bloody show
- Membrane status (ruptured or intact)
- Presence of supportive adult in household or if she is alone

When speaking with the client over the telephone, review the signs and symptoms that denote true versus prodromal labour, and suggest various positions they can assume to provide comfort and increase placental perfusion. Also suggest walking, massage, and taking a warm shower to promote relaxation. Outline what foods and fluids are appropriate for oral intake in early labour. Throughout the phone call, listen to the labouring person's concerns and answer any questions clearly.

Reducing the risk of liability exposure and avoiding preventable injuries to clients and fetuses during labour and birth can be accomplished by adhering to two basic tenets of clinical practice: (1) use applicable evidence and/or published standards and guidelines as the foundation of care, and (2) whenever a clinical choice is presented, choose client safety (Miller, 2014). With these two tenets in mind, advise the client on the phone to contact her health care provider for further instructions or to come to the facility to be evaluated, since ruling out true labour and possible complications cannot be done accurately over the phone. Additional nursing responsibilities associated with a phone assessment include:

- Consulting the caller's prenatal record for parity status, estimated date of birth, and untoward events
- Calling the health care provider to inform them of the caller's status

- Preparing for admission to the perinatal unit to ensure adequate and safe staff assignment
- Documentation of the phone call and information received and given as per the institution's policy

If the nurse's first encounter with the client is in person, an assessment is completed to determine whether they should be admitted to the perinatal unit or sent home until the labour advances. Recent research findings suggest that patients admitted before active labour are approximately twice as likely to be augmented with oxytocin and give birth via cesarean when compared with women admitted in active labour (Lee et al., 2016). Nurses need to make careful assessment of labour progression *prior* to labour admission to decrease early admissions and to improve labour safety and birth outcomes.

Entering a facility is often an intimidating and stressful event for clients and families since it is an unfamiliar environment. Giving birth is a pivotal event in the lives of most people. Nurses must demonstrate respect and care when addressing the client, listening to the client, and expressing interest in their concerns. Nurses should ask clients and families how they would like to be addressed and what pronouns they, demonstrating awareness and acceptance of all gender identities. Nurses must value and respect clients and families and promote patient self-worth and sense of control by facilitating their involvement in making decisions. Allowing them a fair amount of autonomy in their childbirth decisions, supporting their personal worth, knowing them holistically, and using caring communication will increase client satisfaction (Bonapace et al., 2018).

An admission assessment includes the client's health history, physical assessment, laboratory studies, assessment of psychological status, and the fetal assessment. Usually the facility has a form that can be used throughout labour and birth to document assessment findings (Fig. 14.13).

HEALTH HISTORY AND CULTURAL ASSESSMENT

A client's health history should include typical biographical data such as the client's name and age and the name of the health care provider. Other information that is collected includes reason for admission, such as labour, cesarean birth, or observation for a complication; the prenatal record data, including the estimated date of birth, a history of the current pregnancy, and the results of any laboratory and diagnostic tests, such as blood type, Rh status, and group B streptococcal status; past pregnancy and obstetric history; past health history and family history; prenatal education; list of medications; allergies; risk factors such as diabetes, hypertension, and use of tobacco, alcohol, cannabis, or illicit drugs; pain management plan; history of domestic violence; time of last food ingestion; method chosen for infant feeding; name of birth attendant; primary care provider; and infant's health care provider.

Ascertaining this information is important so that an individualized plan of care can be developed for the client. If,

for example, the due date is still 2 months away, it is important to establish this information so interventions can be initiated to arrest the labour immediately or notify the intensive perinatal team to be available. In addition, if the patient has diabetes, it is critical to monitor their glucose levels during labour, to prepare for a surgical birth if dystocia of labour occurs, and to alert the newborn nursery of potential hypoglycemia in the newborn after birth. By collecting important information about each individual for whom they care, nurses can help improve the outcomes for all concerned.

Be sure to observe the client's emotions, support system, verbal interaction, cultural background and language spoken, body language and posture, perceptual acuity, and energy level. This psychosocial information provides cues about their emotional state, culture, and communication systems. For example, if the client arrives at the labour and birth suite extremely anxious, alone, and unable to communicate in English, how can the nurse meet their needs and plan care appropriately? It is only by assessing each person physically and psychosocially that the nurse can make astute decisions regarding proper care. In this case, an interpreter would be needed to assist in the communication process between the staff and the patient and family to initiate proper care.

It is important to acknowledge and try to understand the cultural differences in clients with cultural backgrounds different from that of the nurse. Attitudes toward childbirth are heavily influenced by the culture in which people have been raised. As a result, within every society, specific attitudes and values shape the patient's childbearing behaviours and it is important to be aware of what these may be. When carrying out a cultural assessment during the admission process, ask questions (Box 14.2) to help plan culturally competent care during labour and birth.

BOX 14.2

QUESTIONS FOR PROVIDING CULTURALLY COMPETENT CARE DURING LABOUR AND BIRTH

- Where were you born? How long have you lived in Canada?
- What languages do you speak and read?
- Who are your major support people?
- What are your religious practices?
- How do you view childbearing?
- Are there any special precautions or restrictions that are important?
- Is birth considered a private or a social experience?
- How would you like to manage your labour discomfort?
- Who will provide your labour support?

Adapted from Bowers, P. (2015). Cultural perspectives in childbearing. *Nursing spectrum.* Retrieved from http://ce.nurse.com/ce263-60/cultural-perspectives-in-childbearing; Canadian Nurses Association. (2010). Position statement: Promoting cultural competence in nursing. Retrieved from https://www.cna-aiic.ca/-/media/cna/page-content/pdf-en/6—ps114_cultural_competence_2010_e.pdf

ADMISSION ASSESSMENT OBSTETRICS

▲ PATIENT IDENTIFICATION ▲

ADMISSION DATA

Date		Time		Via		
				☐ Ambulatory ☐ Wheelchair ☐ Stretcher		

Grav.	Term	Pre-term	Ab.	Living	EDC	LMP	GA

Prev. adm. date _____ Reason _____
Obstetrician _____ Pediatrician _____
Ht.____ Wt.____ Wt. gain _____
Allergies (meds/food) ☐ None _____ ☐ Hx latex sensitivity
BP_____ T_____ P_____ R_____
FHR _____ Vag exam _____

Reason for Admission

☐ Labor / SROM   ☐ Induction _____
☐ Primary C/S _____ ☐ Repeat C/S
☐ Observation _____
☐ OB / Medical complication _____

Onset of labor: ☐ Not in labor
Date _____ Time _____
Membranes: ☐ Intact
☐ Ruptured / Date _____ Time _____
☐ Clear   ☐ Meconium   ☐ Bloody   ☐ Foul
Vaginal bleeding: ☐ None
☐ Normal show   ☐ _____

Current Pregnancy Labs   ☐ NPC

☐ POL   ☐ PPROM   ☐ Cerclage
☐ PIH   ☐ Chr. HTN   ☐ Other _____
☐ Diabetes _____ Diet _____
☐ Insulin _____
☐ Amniocentesis _____ Results _____
Bld type / RH____Date Rhogam____
Antibody screen☐Neg ☐Pos
Rubella ☐Non-immune ☐Immune
Diabetic screen☐ Normal ☐Abnormal
Recent exposure to chick pox☐
Current meds:_____
_____

	Pos	Neg	Tested
Hepatitis B	☐	☐	☐ No
HIV	☐	☐	☐ No
Group B strep	☐	☐	☐ No
GC	☐	☐	☐ No
Chlamydia	☐	☐	☐ No
RPR	☐	☐	☐ No

Previous OB History

☐POL   ☐ Multiple gestation
☐ Prev C/S type _____ Reason _____
☐PIH   ☐ Chronic HTN   ☐ Diabetes _____
☐ Stillbirth/demise   ☐ Neodeath   ☐ Anomalies
☐ Precipitous labor (<3 H)   ☐ Macrosomia
☐ PP Hemorrhage
☐ Hx Transfusion reaction   ☐Yes   ☐ No
☐ Other _____
Latest risk assessment   ☐ None
1. _____ 3. _____
2. _____ 4. _____

_____ Date _____
Signature _____ Time _____

NEUROLOGICAL
☐WNL
Variance: ☐HA
☐ Scotoma / visual changes
Reflexes   ☐ < 2 +   ☐ > 2 +
☐ Clonus____ bts
☐ Numbness   ☐ Tingling
☐ Hx Seizures
_____

RESPIRATORY
☐WNL
Variance: ☐ Hx Asthma ☐URI
Respirations: ☐ < 12 ☐ > 24
Effort: ☐ SOB
☐ Shallow ☐ Labored
Auscultation:
☐ Diminished ☐ Crackles
☐ Wheezes ☐ Rhonchi

	No	Yes
Cough for greater than 2 weeks?	☐	☐
Is the cough productive?	☐	☐
Blood in the sputum?	☐	☐
Experiencing any fever or night sweats?	☐	☐
Ever had TB in the past?	☐	☐
Recent exposure to TB?	☐	☐
Weight loss in last 3 weeks?	☐	☐

If the patient answers yes to any three of the above questions implement policy and procedure # 5725-0704.

GASTROINTESTINAL
☐WNL
Variance: ☐ Heartburn
☐ Epigastric pain   Nausea
☐ Vomiting   ☐ Diarrhea
☐ Constipation   ☐ Pain
☐ Wt. Gain < 2lbs / month**
☐ Recent change in appetite of < 50% of usual intake for > 5 days
☐ _____

INTEGUMENTARY
☐WNL
Variance: ☐ Rash ☐ Lacerations
☐ Abrasion ☐ Swelling
☐ Uticaria ☐ Bruising
☐ Diaphoretic/hot
☐ Clammy/cold
☐ Scars
☐ _____

FETAL ASSESSMENT
☐WNL
Variance:
☐NRFS
FHR ☐ < 110 ☐ > 160
LTV ☐ Absent ☐ Minimal
☐ Increased
STV Absent
Decelerations: _____
☐ Decreased fetal movement
☐ IUGR
☐ _____

Tobacco use	☐Denies ☐ Yes	Amt _____
Alcohol use	☐Denies ☐ Yes	Amt _____
Drug use	☐Denies ☐ Yes	Amt type____
Primary language	☐English ☐ Spanish	

CARDIOVASCULAR
☐WNL
Variance:
☐MVP
Heart rate: ☐< 60 ☐ > 100
B/P: Systolic: ☐ < 90 ☐ > 140
Diastolic: ☐< 50 ☐ > 90
☐ Edema
☐ Chest pain / palpitations
☐ _____

MUSCULOSKELETAL
☐WNL
Variance:
☐ Numbness   ☐ Tingling
☐ Paralysis   ☐ Deformity
☐ Scoliosis
☐ _____

GENITOURINARY
☐WNL
Variance: ☐ Albumin _____
Output:☐ < 30 cc/Hr.
☐ UTI   ☐ Rx   ☐ Frequency
☐ Dysuria   ☐ Hematuria
☐ CVA Tenderness
☐ Hx STD
☐ Vag. discharge _____
☐ Rash   ☐ Blisters
☐ Warts   ☐ Lesions
☐ _____

EARS, NOSE, THROAT, AND EYES
☐WNL
Variance:
☐ Sore throat   ☐ Eyeglasses
☐ Runny nose   ☐ Contact lenses
☐ Nasal congestion

PSYCHOSOCIAL
☐WNL
Variance: ☐ Hx depression
☐ Yes   ☐ No
☐ Emotional behavioral care
Affect: ☐ Flat   ☐ Anxious
☐ Uncooperative ☐ Combative
Living will   ☐ Yes   ☐ No
☐ On chart
Healthcare surrogate ☐ Yes ☐No
☐ On chart
Are you being hurt, hit, frightened by anyone at home or in your life? ☐ Yes ☐ No
Religious preference _____

PAIN ASSESSMENT
1. Do you have any ongoing pain problems? ☐ No ☐ Yes
2. Do you have any pain now? ☐ No ☐ Yes
3. If any of the above questions are answered yes, the patient has a positive pain screening.
4. Patient to be given pain management education material.
Complete pain / symptom assessment on flowsheet.
5. Please proceed to complete pain assessment.

FIGURE 14.13 Sample documentation form used for admission to the perinatal unit. (Used with permission. Briggs Corporation, 2001.)

PHYSICAL EXAMINATION

The physical examination typically includes a generalized assessment of the client's body systems, including hydration status, vital signs, auscultation of heart and lung sounds, and measurement of height and weight. The physical examination also includes the following assessments:

1. Pain level and coping behaviours demonstrated
2. Uterine activity, including contraction frequency, duration, and intensity
3. Fetal status, including heart rate, position, and station
4. Cervical dilation and degree of effacement
5. Status of membranes (intact or ruptured)
6. Vital signs: temperature, pulse, respirations, and blood pressure
7. Leopold manoeuvres to determine fetal lie
8. Fundal height measurement
9. Ability to ambulate safely

These assessment parameters form a baseline against which the nurse can compare all future values throughout labour. The findings should be similar to those of the patient's prepregnancy and pregnancy findings, with the exception of the pulse rate, which might be elevated secondary any anxiety that might be experienced in the labour.

LABORATORY STUDIES

On admission, laboratory studies typically are done to establish a baseline. Although the exact tests may vary among facilities, they may include a urinalysis via clean-catch urine specimen and complete blood count. Blood typing and Rh factor analysis may be necessary if the results of these are unknown or unavailable. In addition, if the following test results are not included in the prenatal history, it may be necessary to perform them at this time. They include syphilis screening, hepatitis B (HbsAg) screening, group B streptococcus (GBS), HIV testing (with consent), and possible drug screening if the history is positive.

GBS is a gram-positive organism that colonizes in the female genital tract and rectum and is present in 10% to 30% of all healthy females (King, Brucker, Osborne, & Jevitt, 2019). People with GBS are asymptomatic carriers but can cause GBS disease of the newborn through vertical transmission during labour and horizontal transmission after birth. The mortality rate of infected newborns varies according to time of onset (early or late). Risk factors for GBS include intrapartum fever, prolonged ruptured membranes (>12 to 18 hours), previous birth of an infected newborn, and GBS bacteriuria in the present pregnancy.

The SOGC and the Canadian Pediatric Society (CPS) in Canada, and the Centers for Disease Control and Prevention (CDC), ACOG, and the American Academy of Pediatrics in the United States have guidelines that advised universal screening of pregnant person at 35 to 37 weeks' gestation for GBS and intrapartum antibiotic therapy for GBS carriers. These new guidelines reaffirmed the major prevention strategy—universal antenatal GBS screening and intrapartum antibiotic prophylaxis for culture-positive and high-risk people. Also included are new recommendations for laboratory methods for identification of GBS colonization during pregnancy, algorithms for screening and intrapartum prophylaxis for people experiencing preterm labour and premature rupture of membranes, updated prophylaxis recommendations for those people with a penicillin allergy, and a revised algorithm for the care of newborn infants (CDC, 2016; CPS, 2017). Infections associated with GBS include acute chorioamnionitis, endometritis, and urinary tract infection. Neonatal clinical manifestations include pneumonia and sepsis. Identified GBS carriers receive intravenous antibiotic prophylaxis (Penicillin G or Ampicillin) at the onset of labour or ruptured membranes.

The SOGC, ACOG, and CDC each recommend that all pregnant clients be offered a screening test for HIV antibodies on their first prenatal visit, again during the third trimester if engaging in high-risk behaviours, and on admission to the labour and birth area. The CDC estimates that 50,000 individuals contract HIV in the United States each year, and 250,000 individuals have undiagnosed HIV infections (CDC, 2018).

If the HIV status is not documented, on admission to the labour and birth suite, the client can be asked if they consent to having rapid HIV testing done. To reduce perinatal transmission, patients who are HIV-positive are given zidovudine (2 mg/kg intravenously over an hour, and then a maintenance infusion of 1 mg/kg/hr until birth) or a single 200-mg oral dose of nevirapine at the onset of labour; the newborn is given zidovudine orally (2 mg/kg body weight every 6 hours) and should be continued for 6 weeks (Verklan & Walden, 2014). To further reduce the risk of perinatal transmission, SOGC and ACOG recommend that pregnant clients who are infected with HIV and have plasma viral loads of more than 1,000 copies/mL be counselled regarding the benefits of elective cesarean birth. In the absence of any medical intervention, the rate of vertical transmission of HIV to the fetus can range from 15% to 45% (Ashimi, Hoff, Sibai, & Hardwicke, 2015; Money, Tulloch, Boucoiran, & Caddy, 2014).

Additional interventions to reduce the transmission risk would include avoiding use of a scalp electrode for fetal monitoring or doing a scalp blood sampling for fetal pH, delaying amniotomy, advising for the use of formula for infant feeding, and avoiding invasive procedures such as forceps or vacuum-assisted devices. The nurse stresses the importance of all interventions and the goal to reduce transmission of HIV to the newborn.

Continuing Assessment During the First Stage of Labour

After the admission assessment is complete the client and the support people are oriented to the room, equipment, and procedures. Ongoing assessments continue for changes that would indicate that labour is progressing as expected and the nurse should assess the client's knowledge, experience, and expectations of labour. Typically, blood pressure, pulse, and respirations are assessed every hour during the latent phase of labour unless the clinical situation dictates that vital signs be taken more frequently. During the active and transition phases, they are assessed every 30 minutes. The temperature is taken every 4 hours throughout the first stage of labour and at least every 2 hours after membranes have ruptured to detect an elevation indicating an ascending infection.

Vaginal examinations are performed periodically to track labour progress. This assessment information is shared with the client to reinforce that they are making progress toward the goal of birth. Uterine contractions are monitored for frequency, duration, and intensity every 30 to 60 minutes during the latent phase, every 15 to 30 minutes during the active phase, and every 15 minutes during transition. Note the changes in the character of the contractions as labour progresses, and inform the client of the progress. Continually assess and determine the client's level of pain and ability to cope and use relaxation techniques effectively.

When the fetal membranes rupture, either spontaneously or artificially, assess the FHR and check the amniotic fluid for colour, odour, and amount. Assess the FHR intermittently or continuously via electronic monitoring. During the latent phase of labour, assess the FHR every 30 to 60 minutes; in the active phase, assess FHR at least every 15 to 30 minutes. Also, be sure to assess the FHR before ambulation, before any procedure, and before administering analgesia or anesthesia (Liston et al., 2018). Table 14.3 summarizes assessments for the first stage of labour.

Remember Sheila from the chapter-opening scenario? What is the nurse's role with Sheila in active labour? What additional comfort measures can the labour nurse offer Sheila?

Nursing Interventions

Nursing interventions during the admission process should include:

- Asking about the client's expectations of the birthing process
- Providing information about labour, birth, pain management options, and relaxation techniques
- Presenting information about fetal monitoring equipment and the procedures needed

TABLE 14.3	SUMMARY OF ASSESSMENTS DURING THE FIRST STAGE OF LABOUR		
Assessments[a]	Latent Phase (0–3 cm)	Active Phase (4–7 cm)	Transition (8–10 cm)
Vital signs (BP, pulse, respirations)	Every 30–60 minutes	Every 30 minutes	Every 15–30 minutes
Temperature	Every 4 hours; more frequently if membranes are ruptured	Every 4 hours; more frequently if membranes are ruptured	Every 4 hours; more frequently if membranes are ruptured
Contractions (frequency, duration, intensity)	Every 30–60 minutes by palpation or continuously if EFM	Every 15–30 minutes by palpation or continuously if EFM	Every 15 minutes by palpation or continuously if EFM
Fetal heart rate	Every hour by Doppler or continuously by EFM	Every 15–30 minutes by Doppler or continuously by EFM	Every 15–30 minutes by Doppler or continuously by EFM
Vaginal examination	Initially on admission to determine phase and as needed based on maternal cues to document labour progression	As needed to monitor labour progression	As needed to monitor labour progression
Behaviour/ psychosocial	With every client encounter: talkative, excited, anxious	With every client encounter: self-absorbed in labour; intense and quiet now	With every client encounter: discouraged, irritable, feels out of control, declining coping ability

[a]The frequency of assessments is dictated by the health status of the client and fetus and will be altered if either one of their conditions changes.
EFM, electronic fetal monitoring.
Adapted from Liston, R., Sawchuck, D., & Young, D. (2018). SOGC clinical practice guideline No. 197b, Fetal health surveillance: Intrapartum consensus guideline. *Journal of Obstetrics and Gynaecology Canada.* Retrieved from https://www.jogc.com/article/S1701-2163(18)30067-7/pdf

510 UNIT 4 Labour and Birth

- Monitoring FHR and identifying patterns that need further intervention
- Monitoring the patient's vital signs to obtain a baseline for later comparison
- Reassuring the client that the labour progress will be monitored closely and nursing care will focus on ensuring fetal and patient well-being throughout

As the client progresses through the first stage of labour, nursing interventions include:
- Encouraging the support people to participate as per the client's wishes
- Keeping the client and the support people up to date on the progress of the labour
- Orienting the client and the support people to the labour and birth unit and explaining all of the birthing procedures
- Providing clear fluids (e.g., ice chips, apple juice) as needed or requested
- If the client requires an IV line, maintaining parenteral fluid intake at the prescribed rate
- Encouraging use of comfort measures, such as back-rubs, cool cloths to the forehead, frequent position changes, ambulation, showers, leaning over a birthing ball, side-lying, or counterpressure on lower back (Teaching Guidelines 14.1)
- Encouraging the partner's involvement with supporting and encouraging breathing techniques
- Assisting the client and support people to focus on breathing techniques
- Informing the client that the discomfort will be intermittent and of limited duration; urging them to rest between contractions to preserve strength; and encouraging the use of distracting activities to lessen the focus on contractions
- Ensuring that the client takes deep cleansing breaths before and after each contraction to enhance gas exchange and oxygen to the fetus
- Changing bed linens and gown as needed
- Keeping the perineal area clean and dry
- Supporting the client's decisions about pain management
- Monitoring vital signs frequently and reporting any abnormal values to the health care providers
- Educating the client and the support people about the need for rest, and helping them plan strategies to conserve strength throughout the labour experience
- Monitoring FHR for baseline, accelerations, variability, and decelerations
- Checking bladder status and encouraging voiding at least every 2 hours to make room for birth or assessing need to empty bladder with intermittent straight in/out catheterization as required
- Assist the client to reposition as needed for optimal heart rate patterns
- Communicating requests from the client to appropriate personnel

- Respecting the patient's sense of privacy by using drapes and covers when performing invasive examinations
- Offering presence and remaining with the client, not leaving them alone for long periods
- Being patient with the natural labour pattern to allow time for change
- Encouraging movement throughout labour to increase the patient's level of comfort
- Dimming the lights in the room when appropriate and using softened voices be used to maintain a calm and centred ambiance
- Reporting any deviations from normal to the health care professional so that interventions can be initiated early to be effective (Green, 2016; Lucas, da Rocha, de Medonça Costa, de Oliveira, & Melo, 2015; Nagtalon-Ramos, 2014)

See Nursing Care Plan 14.1 (at the end of chapter).

 Teaching Guidelines 14.1

POSITIONING DURING THE FIRST STAGE OF LABOUR

- Walking with support from the partner (adds the force of gravity to contractions to promote fetal descent)
- Slow-dancing position with the partner supporting the client (adds the force of gravity to contractions and promotes support from and active participation of the partner)
- Side-lying with pillows between the knees for comfort (offers a restful position and improves oxygen flow to the uterus)
- Semi-sitting in bed or on a couch leaning against the partner (reduces back pain because fetus falls forward, away from the sacrum)
- Sitting in a chair with one foot on the floor and one on the chair (changes pelvic shape)
- Leaning forward by straddling a chair, a table, or a bed or kneeling over a birth ball (reduces back pain, adds the force of gravity to promote descent; possible pain relief if partner can apply sacral pressure)
- Sitting in a rocking chair or on a birth ball and shifting weight back and forth (provides comfort because rocking motion is soothing; uses the force of gravity to help fetal descent)
- Lunge by rocking weight back and forth with foot up on chair during contraction (uses force of gravity by being upright; enhances rotation of fetus through rocking)
- Open knee-chest position (helps to relieve back discomfort)
- Encourage any position of comfort for labour and birth (Simkin & Klein, 2018)

Nursing Management During the Second Stage of Labour

Management of the second stage of labour often follows tradition-based routines rather than evidence-based practices. Current evidence for management of the second stage of labour supports the practices of delayed pushing, spontaneous (nondirected) pushing, and client choice for positions (Cox & King, 2015). To be able to help patients through the second stage of labour requires the nurse to have a comprehensive understanding of physiology and be aware of the latest evidence-based research and apply it to practice (Green, 2016).

Nursing care during the second stage of labour focuses on supporting the client and the partner in making active decisions about care and labour management, implementing strategies to prolong the early passive phase of fetal descent, supporting involuntary bearing-down efforts, providing instruction and assistance, and using positions that can enhance descent and reduce pain (King et al., 2019). In the past, people gave birth unaided by following their bodies' signals to birth their babies, so the role of the nurse should be to support the client in their choice of pushing method and to encourage confidence in the natural instinct of when and how to push.

In the absence of any complications, nurses should not be attempting to control this stage of labour, but empowering patients to achieve a satisfying experience. The primary rationale for directing patients to push is to shorten the second stage of labour. Common practice in many labour units is still to coach clients to use closed glottis pushing with every contraction, starting when the cervix has reached 10 cm of dilation. This practice is not supported by research. Evidence suggests that directed pushing during the second stage may be accompanied by a significant decline in fetal pH and may cause patient muscle and nerve damage, as well as avoidable exhaustion, if done too early (Reed, 2015). Shortening the phase of active pushing and lengthening the early phase of passive descent can be achieved by encouraging the client not to push until there is a strong urge to do so and until the descent and rotation of the fetal head are well advanced. Effective pushing can be achieved by assisting the client to assume a more upright or squatting position. Supporting spontaneous pushing and encouraging patients to choose their own method of pushing should be accepted as best clinical practice (Cheng & Caughey, 2015).

Perineal lacerations or tears can occur during the second stage when the fetal head emerges through the vaginal introitus. The extent of the laceration is defined by depth: a first-degree laceration extends through the skin; a second-degree laceration extends through the muscles of the perineal body; a third-degree laceration continues through the anal sphincter muscle; and a fourth-degree laceration also involves the anterior rectal wall. Special attention needs to be paid to third- and fourth-degree lacerations to prevent fecal incontinence. Risks for third- or fourth-degree lacerations included nulliparity, being Asian or Pacific Islander, increased birth weight of newborn, operative vaginal birth, episiotomy, and longer second stage of labour. Increasing body mass index was associated with fewer lacerations (Sides et al., 2015). The primary care provider should repair any lacerations during the third stage of labour.

An **episiotomy** is an incision made in the perineum to enlarge the vaginal outlet, theoretically and historically used to shorten the second stage of labour. Alternative measures such as warm compresses and continual massage with oil have been successful in stretching the perineal area to prevent the need for cutting it.

Take Note!

Restrictive use of episiotomy has been recommended by the SOGC given the risks of the procedure and unclear benefits of routine use (Cargill & MacKinnon, 2018).

The application of warmed compresses and/or intrapartum perineal massage is associated with a decrease in trauma to the perineal area and reduced the need for an episiotomy (Green, 2016). Routine episiotomy has declined since liberal usage has been discouraged by the SOGC and ACOG, except to avoid several perineal lacerations, or to expedite difficult births. Anal sphincter laceration rates with spontaneous vaginal delivery have decreased, likely reflecting the decreased usage of episiotomy. The decline in operative vaginal delivery corresponds with a sharp increase in cesarean births, which may indicate that health care providers are favouring cesarean births for difficult births (Faisal-Cury, Menezes, Quayle, Matijasevich, & Diniz, 2015). Figure 14.14 shows episiotomy locations.

Continuous Assessment During the Second Stage of Labour

Assessment is continuous during the second stage of labour. Hospital policies dictate the specific type and timing of assessments, as well as the way in which they are documented. Assessment involves identifying the signs typical of the second stage of labour, including:

- Increase in apprehension or irritability
- Spontaneous rupture of membranes
- Increase in blood-tinged show
- Low grunting sounds from the client
- Reports of rectal and perineal pressure
- Beginning of involuntary bearing-down efforts

Other ongoing assessments include the contraction frequency, duration, and intensity; monitoring vital signs every 5 to 15 minutes; fetal response to labour

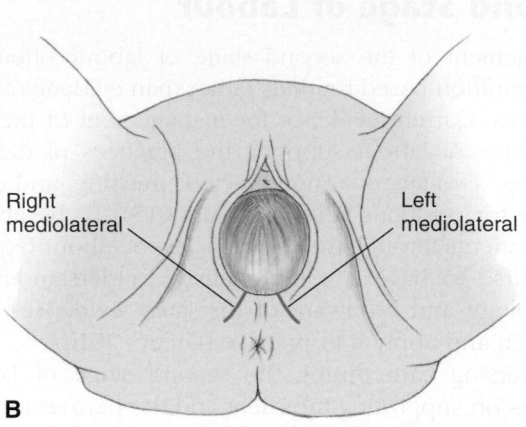

A

Right mediolateral

Left mediolateral

B

FIGURE 14.14 Location of an episiotomy. **A.** Midline episiotomy. **B.** Right and left mediolateral episiotomies.

as indicated by FHR patterns; amniotic fluid for colour, odour, and amount when membranes are ruptured; and the coping status of the client and any support people present (Table 14.4).

Assessment also focuses on determining the progress of labour. Associated signs include bulging of the perineum, labial separation, advancing and retreating of the newborn's head during and between bearing-down efforts, and **crowning** (fetal head is visible at vaginal opening; Fig. 14.15).

A vaginal examination is completed to determine if it is appropriate for the client to push. Pushing is appropriate if the cervix has fully dilated to 10 cm and the client feels the urge to do so.

TABLE 14.4	SUMMARY OF ASSESSMENTS DURING THE SECOND, THIRD, AND FOURTH STAGES OF LABOUR		
Assessments[a]	Second Stage of Labour (Birth of Neonate)	Third Stage of Labour (Placenta Expulsion)	Fourth Stage of Labour (Recovery)
Vital signs (BP, pulse, respirations)	Every 5–15 minutes	Every 15 minutes	Every 15 minutes
Fetal heart rate	Every 5 minutes by Doppler or continuously by EFM	Apgar scoring at 1 and 5 minutes	Newborn—complete head-to-toe assessment; vital signs every 15 minutes until stable
Contractions/uterus	Palpate every one	Observe for placental separation	Palpating for firmness and position every 15 minutes for first hour
Bearing down/pushing	Assist with every effort	None	None
Vaginal discharge	Observe for signs of descent—bulging of perineum, crowning	Assess bleeding after expulsion	Assess every 15 minutes with fundus firmness
Behaviour/psychosocial	Observe every 15 minutes: cooperative, focus is on work of pushing newborn out	Observe every 15 minutes: often feelings of relief after hearing newborn crying; calmer	Observe every 15 minutes: usually excited, talkative, awake; needs to hold newborn, be close, and inspect body
Hydration/urination	Ongoing	Ongoing	Ongoing

[a]The frequency of assessments is dictated by the health status of the client and fetus and will be altered if either one of their conditions changes.
EFM, electronic fetal monitoring.
Adapted from Holvey, N. (2014). Supporting women in the second stage of labor. *British Journal of Midwifery, 22*(3), 182–186; Werner, L. (2015). It's the little things. *Nursing for Women's Health, 19*(2), 203–204.

FIGURE 14.15 **Crowning.**

Nursing Interventions

Nursing interventions during this stage focus on motivating and supporting the client, assisting with positioning, encouraging the client to put all the effort to pushing this newborn to the outside world, and giving ongoing feedback about the progress. If the client is pushing without much progress, suggest the use of a mirror pointed toward the perineum to see the newborn's head emerge during pushing. Changing positions frequently will also help in making progress. During the second stage of labour, an ideal position would be one that opens the pelvic outlet as wide as possible, provides a smooth pathway for the fetus to descend through the birth canal, takes advantage of gravity to assist the fetus to descend, and gives the patient a sense of being safe and in control of the labour process (Capogna, 2015a). Some suggestions for positions in the second stage include:

- Semi-sitting with pillows underneath knees, arms, and back
- Lateral/side-lying with curved back and upper leg supported by partner or nurse
- Sitting on birthing stool: opens pelvis, enhances the pull of gravity and helps with pushing
- Squatting/supported squatting
- Kneeling with hands on bed and knees comfortably apart

The Lithotomy position, with feet up in stirrups and the patient supine, is the most convenient position for caregivers, although EBP findings do not support this position physiologically and it should be the last choice as a pushing position.

Other important nursing interventions during the second stage include:
- Providing continuous comfort measures such as mouth care, encouraging position changes, changing bed linen and underpads
- Providing a quiet, focused environment
- Instructing the client regarding bearing-down positions and techniques as required. These may include:
  - Pushing only when there is an urge to push
  - Delaying pushing for up to 90 minutes after complete dilation until there is an urge to push
  - Using abdominal muscles when bearing down
  - Using short pushes of 6 to 7 seconds
  - Focusing attention on the perineal area to visualize the newborn
  - Relaxing and conserving energy between contractions
  - Pushing several times with each contraction
  - Pushing with an open glottis and slight exhalation (Petrocnik & Marshall, 2015)
- Continuing to monitor contraction and FHR patterns to identify problems
- Providing brief, explicit directions throughout this stage
- Continuing to provide psychosocial support by reassuring and coaching
- Facilitating the upright position to encourage the fetus to descend
- Continuing to assess blood pressure, pulse, respirations, uterine contractions, bearing-down efforts, FHR, and coping status of the patient
- Providing pain management if needed
- Providing a continuous nursing presence
- Offering praise for the client's efforts
- Preparing for and assisting with delivery by:
  - Notifying the health care provider of the estimated time frame for birth
  - Preparing the birthing bed and positioning the client
  - Offering a mirror and adjusting it so the patient can see the birth
  - Explaining all procedures and equipment to the client and support person/people
  - Setting up delivery instruments needed while maintaining sterility
  - Assessing for need to empty bladder if indicated
  - Using standard precautions for personal protective devices during the birthing process to avoid body fluid splashes
  - Recording the time of birth, time of placenta, and type of birth
  - Assessing the newborn and placing the infant skin-to-skin on the patient's chest/abdomen while drying and covering with warm blankets, if stable
  - Or, ensuring that the infant has been moved to a resuscitation area for resuscitation efforts if needed
  - Providing initial care and assessment of the newborn (see the Birth section)

Sheila **is completely dilated now and experiencing the urge to push. How can the nurse help Sheila with her pushing efforts? What additional interventions can the labour nurse offer Sheila now? In addition to encouraging Sheila to rest between pushing and offering praise for her efforts, what is the nurse's role during the birthing process?**

BIRTH

The second stage of labour ends with the birth of the newborn. The client's position for birth varies from the standard lithotomy position to side-lying to squatting to standing or kneeling, depending on the birthing location, the client's preference, and the health care provider preference or needs. When the patient is positioned for birth the primary health care provider then takes charge after donning protective eyewear and gloves.

Once the fetal head has emerged, the primary care provider explores the fetal neck to see if the umbilical cord is wrapped around it. If it is, the cord is slipped over the head to facilitate delivery. As soon as the head emerges and restitution occurs, the shoulders are delivered and the umbilical cord may be cut or left to pulsate for delayed cord clamping, depending on patient wishes and newborn status. When ready to be cut, the umbilical cord is double-clamped and cut between the clamps by the birth attendant or the support person if desired. With the first cries of the newborn, the second stage of labour ends. For care of the client undergoing a surgical birth, refer to Chapter 21.

In addition to encouraging Sheila to rest between pushing and offering praise for her efforts, what is the nurse's role during the birthing process?

IMMEDIATE CARE OF THE NEWBORN

Once birth takes place, the newborn can be placed directly on the client's chest and covered with warm blankets. If the newborn requires any resuscitation, it would be placed under a radiant warmer, dried, assessed. The stable infant can then go to the parent and be placed on skin-to-skin, covered in warm blankets. In any situation, the stability of the newborn dictates the location of aftercare. The nurse will also assist the new parent with the first breastfeeding.

Assessment of the newborn begins at the moment of birth and continues until the newborn is discharged. Drying the newborn and providing warmth to prevent heat loss by evaporation is essential to help support thermoregulation and provide stimulation. Placing the newborn skin-to-skin with a stockinet/knitted cap will further reduce heat loss after drying. If the newborn is not able to be skin-to-skin with a parent, they should be placed under a radiant heat source during this time.

Assess the newborn by assigning an Apgar score at 1 and 5 minutes. The Apgar score assesses five parameters—(1) heart rate (absent, slow, or fast), (2) respiratory effort (absent, weak cry, or good strong yell), (3) muscle tone (limp, or lively and active), (4) response to irritation stimulus, and (5) colour—that evaluate a newborn's cardiorespiratory adaptation after birth. The parameters are arranged from the most important (heart rate) to the least important (colour). The newborn is assigned a score of 0 to 2 in each of the five parameters. The purpose of the Apgar assessment is to evaluate the physiologic status of the newborn; see Chapter 18 for additional information on Apgar scoring.

Secure two identification bands on the newborn's wrist and ankle that match the band on the birthing parent's wrist to ensure the newborn's identity. This identification process is completed in the birthing suite before anyone leaves the room.

Other types of newborn security systems can also be used to prevent abduction. Some systems have sensors that are attached to the newborn's identification bracelet or cord clamp. An alarm is set off if the bracelet or clamp activates receivers near exits. Others have an alarm that is activated when the sensor is removed from the newborn (Fig. 14.16). Even with the use of electronic sensors, the parents, nursing staff, and security personnel are responsible for prevention strategies and ensuring the safety and protection of all newborns (National Center for Missing and Exploited Children [NCMEC], 2015). Nurses can help in preventing newborn abduction by educating parents about abduction risks, using identically numbered bands on the baby and parents, by instructing parents to keep their newborn in their direct line of vision within their hospital room at all times, taking colour photographs of the infant, wearing colour photograph ID badges themselves, discouraging parents/families from

FIGURE 14.16 An example of a security sensor applied to a newborn's arm.

publishing birth notices in the public media with names and addresses, controlling access to nursery/postpartum unit with locked doors, and utilizing infant security tags or abduction alarm systems (NCMEC, 2015).

> ***Sheila*** **gave birth to a healthy 7-lb, 7-oz baby girl. She is eager to hold and nurse her newborn. What is the initial care of the newborn? How can the nurse meet the needs of both the newborn and Sheila, who is exhausted but eager to bond with her newborn?**

Nursing Management During the Third Stage of Labour

During the third stage of labour, strong uterine contractions continue at regular intervals under the continuing influence of oxytocin. The uterine muscle fibers shorten, or retract, with each contraction, leading to a gradual decrease in the size of the uterus, which helps shear the placenta away from its attachment site. The third stage is complete when the placenta is delivered. Nursing care during the third stage of labour primarily focuses on immediate newborn care and assessment and observing for signs of placental separation, being available to assist with the delivery of the placenta, recording the time of expulsion and inspecting it for intactness. The nurse should also be assessing by palpating the uterus before and after placental expulsion.

Three hormones play important roles in the third stage. During this stage, the client experiences peak levels of oxytocin and endorphins, while the high adrenaline levels that occurred during the second stage of labour to aid with pushing begin falling. The hormone oxytocin causes uterine contractions and helps foster instinctive bonding behaviours such as holding the newborn close to the body and cuddling the baby.

Skin-to-skin contact immediately after birth and the newborn's first attempt at breastfeeding further augment these oxytocin levels, strengthening the uterine contractions that will help the placenta to separate and the uterus to contract to prevent hemorrhage. Endorphins, the body's natural opiates, produce an altered state of consciousness and aid in blocking out pain. In addition, the drop in the adrenaline level from the second stage, which had kept the client and baby alert at first contact, causes most clients to shiver and feel cold shortly after giving birth.

Take Note!

A crucial role for nurses during this time is to protect the natural hormonal process by ensuring unhurried and uninterrupted contact between birthing parent and newborn after birth, providing warmed blankets to prevent shivering, and allowing skin-to-skin contact with early breastfeeding.

Continuing Assessment During the Third Stage of Labour

Assessment during the third stage of labour includes:
- Monitoring placental separation by looking for the following signs:
  - Firmly contracting uterus
  - Change in uterine shape from discoid to globular ovoid
  - Sudden gush of dark blood from vaginal opening
  - Lengthening of umbilical cord protruding from vagina
- Examining the placenta and fetal membranes for intactness the second time (the health care provider assesses the placenta for intactness the first time) (Fig. 14.17)
- Assessing for any perineal trauma, such as the following, before allowing the birth attendant to leave:
  - Firm fundus with bright-red blood trickling: laceration
  - Boggy fundus with red blood flowing: uterine atony
  - Boggy fundus with dark blood and clots: retained placenta

FIGURE 14.17 Placenta. **A.** Fetal side. **B.** Uterine side.

- Assessing for perineal lacerations and ensuring repair by birth attendant
- Inspecting the perineum for condition of episiotomy if performed

Nursing Interventions

Interventions during the third stage of labour include:
- Describing the process of placental separation to the client
- Instructing the client to push when signs of separation are apparent
- Administering an oxytocic agent if ordered and indicated after placental expulsion
- Providing support and information about episiotomy and/or laceration if applicable
- Cleaning and assisting the client into a comfortable position after birth
- If stirrups were used, ensure that both legs are lifted out simultaneously to prevent strain
- Repositioning the birthing bed to serve as a recovery bed if applicable
- Assisting with transfer to the recovery area if applicable
- Providing warmth by providing warmed blankets
- Applying an ice pack to the perineal area to provide comfort to perineal stitches if present
- Explaining what assessments will be carried out over the next hour and offering support
- Inquiring about any needs
- Monitoring physical status by assessing:
  - Vaginal bleeding: amount, consistency, and colour
  - Vital signs: blood pressure, pulse, and respirations taken every 15 minutes
  - Uterine fundus, which should be firm, in the midline, and at the level of the umbilicus
  - The client's knowledge of breastfeeding to determine educational needs and then provide assistance with infant positioning and latching on, while watching for infant sucking and swallowing
- Recording all birthing statistics and charting as appropriate

Nursing Management During the Fourth Stage of Labour

The fourth stage of labour begins after the placenta is expelled and lasts up to 4 hours after birth, during which time recovery takes place. This recovery period may take place in the same room where the patient gave birth, in a separate recovery area, or in the postpartum room. During this stage, the client's body is beginning to undergo the many physiologic and psychological changes that occur after birth. The focus of nursing management during the fourth stage of labour involves frequent close observation for hemorrhage, provision of comfort measures, and promotion of family attachment.

Assessment

Assessments during the fourth stage centre on the client's vital signs, status of the uterine fundus and perineal area, comfort level, lochia amount, and bladder status. During the first hour after birth, vital signs are taken every 15 minutes, then every 30 minutes for the next hour if needed. The client's blood pressure should remain stable and within normal range after giving birth. A decrease may indicate uterine hemorrhage; an elevation might suggest preeclampsia.

The pulse usually is typically slower (60 to 70 bpm) than during labour. This may be associated with a decrease in blood volume following placental separation. An elevated pulse rate may be an early sign of blood loss. The blood pressure usually returns to its prepregnancy level and therefore is not a reliable early indicator of shock. Fever is indicative of dehydration (less than 38°C or 100.4°F) or infection (above 38.5°C or 101°F), which may involve the genitourinary tract. Respiratory rate is usually between 16 and 24 breaths per minute and regular. Respirations should be unlaboured unless there is an underlying pre-existing respiratory condition.

Assess fundal height, position, and firmness every 15 minutes during the first hour following birth. The fundus needs to remain firm to prevent excessive postpartum bleeding. The fundus should be firm (feels like the size and consistency of a grapefruit), located in the midline and below the umbilicus. If it is not firm (boggy), gently massage it until it is firm (see Table 22.2 for more information). Once firmness is obtained, stop massaging.

 Take Note!

If the fundus is displaced to the right or the left of the midline, suspect a full bladder as the cause.

The vagina and perineal areas are quite stretched and edematous following a vaginal birth. Assess the perineum, including the episiotomy if present, for possible hematoma formation. Suspect a hematoma if the client reports excruciating pain or cannot void or if a mass is noted in the perineal area. Also assess for hemorrhoids, which can cause discomfort.

Assess the client's comfort level frequently to determine the need for analgesia. Ask the client to rate any pain on a scale of 0 to 10; it should be less than 3. If it is higher, further evaluation is needed to make sure that there are not any deviations contributing to the discomfort.

Assess vaginal discharge (lochia) every 15 minutes for the first hour and every 30 minutes for the next hour. Palpate the fundus at the same time to ascertain its firmness and help to estimate the amount of vaginal discharge. In addition, palpate the bladder for fullness, since many clients receiving an epidural block experience limited sensation in the bladder region. Voiding should produce large amounts of urine (diuresis) each time. Palpating the client's bladder after each voiding helps to assess for complete emptying. A full bladder will displace the uterus to either side of the midline and potentiate uterine hemorrhage secondary to bogginess.

Nursing Interventions

Nursing interventions during the fourth stage might include:

- Providing support and information to the client regarding episiotomy repair and related pain relief and self-care measures
- Applying an ice pack to the perineum to promote comfort and reduce swelling
- Assisting with hygiene and perineal care; teaching the client how to use the perineal bottle after each pad change and voiding; helping the client into a new gown
- Monitoring for return of sensation and ability to void (if regional anesthesia was used)
- Encouraging the client to void by ambulating to the bathroom, listening to running water, or pouring warm water over the perineal area with the peribottle
- Assessing for postpartum hemorrhage and urinary retention via uterine palpation
- If unable to void, emptying the bladder with a straight in/out catheterization
- Monitoring vital signs and fundal and lochia status every 15 minutes and documenting them
- Promoting comfort by offering analgesia for after pains and warm blankets to reduce chilling
- Offering fluids and nourishment if desired
- Encouraging parent–infant attachment by providing privacy for the family

- Being knowledgeable about, and sensitive to, typical cultural practices after birth
- Assisting and encouraging the client to breastfeed during the recovery period to promote uterine firmness (the release of oxytocin from the posterior pituitary gland stimulates uterine contractions)
- Teaching the client how to assess her fundus for firmness periodically and to massage it if it is boggy
- Describing the lochia flow and normal parameters to observe for postpartum
- Demonstrating the use of the portable sitz bath as a comfort measure for her perineum if the client had a laceration or episiotomy repair
- Explaining comfort/hygiene measures and when to use them
- Assisting with ambulation when getting out of bed for the first time
- Providing information about the routine on the postpartum unit for the family's stay
- Observing for signs of early parent–infant attachment: fingertip touch to palm touch to enfolding of the infant (Green, 2016; Leonard, 2018)
- Teaching safety techniques to prevent newborn abduction

The nurse's role in labour and birth is a privileged one, supporting new parents at one of their most vulnerable times—childbirth. The nurse's focus during this time should be on supporting, protecting, advocating, and empowering clients. The nurse should also provide informational support, which would allow the client to realize personal aspirations and goals by making decisions through informed choice. Nurses make a long-term difference in the lives of childbearing client with small things they do for their clients which make a big difference to them.

NURSING CARE PLAN 14.1

Overview of a Client in the Active Phase of the First Stage of Labour

Candice, a 23-year-old gravida 1, para 0 (G1, P0), is admitted to the labour and birth suite at 39 weeks' gestation having contractions of moderate intensity every 5 to 6 minutes. A vaginal examination reveals that her cervix is 80% effaced and 5 cm dilated. The presenting part (vertex) is at 0 station and her membranes ruptured spontaneously 4 hours ago at home. She is admitted. FHR is auscultated with a Doppler and found to be 140 bpm and regular. Her partner is present at her bedside. Candice is now in the active phase of the first stage of labour, and her assessment findings are as follows: cervix dilated 7 cm, 80% effaced; moderate to strong contractions occurring regularly, every 3 to 5 minutes, lasting 45 to 60 seconds; at 0 station on pelvic examination; FHR auscultated loudest below umbilicus at 140 bpm; vaginal show—pink or bloody vaginal mucus; currently apprehensive, inwardly focused, with increased dependency; voicing concern about ability to cope with pain; limited ability to follow directions.

(continued)

Overview of a Client in the Active Phase of the First Stage of Labour (continued)

NURSING DIAGNOSIS: Anxiety related to labour and birth process and fear of the unknown related to client's first experience

Outcome Identification and Evaluation

The client will remain calm and in control as evidenced by ability to make decisions and use positive coping strategies.

Interventions: *Promoting Positive Coping Strategies*

- Provide instruction regarding the labour process to allay anxiety.
- Orient the client to the physical environment and equipment as necessary to keep her informed of events.
- Encourage verbalization of feelings and concerns to reduce anxiety.
- Listen attentively to the client and partner to demonstrate interest and concern.
- Inform client and partner of standard procedures/processes to ensure adequate understanding of events and procedures.

- Frequently update client of progress and labour status to provide positive reinforcement for actions.
- Reinforce relaxation techniques and provide instruction if needed to aid in coping.
- Encourage participation of the partner in the coaching role; role-model to facilitate partner participation in labour process to provide support and encouragement to the client.
- Provide a presence and remain with the client as much as possible to provide comfort and support.

NURSING DIAGNOSIS: Acute pain related to uterine contractions and stretching of the cervix and birth canal

Outcome Identification and Evaluation

The client will maintain a tolerable level of pain and discomfort as evidenced by statements of pain relief, and absence of adverse effects in client and fetus from analgesia or anesthesia.

Interventions: *Providing Pain Relief*

- Monitor vital signs, observe for signs of pain, and have client rate pain on a scale of 0 to 10 to provide baseline for comparison.
- Encourage client to void every 1 to 2 hours to decrease pressure from a full bladder.
- Assist client to change positions frequently to increase comfort and promote labour progress.
- Encourage use of distraction to reduce focus on contraction pain.
- Suggest pelvic rocking, massage, or back counter pressure to reduce pain.
- Assist with use of relaxation and breathing techniques to promote relaxation.
- Use touch appropriately (backrub) when desired by the client to promote comfort.
- Integrate use of nonpharmacologic measures for pain relief, such as warm water, birthing ball, or other techniques to facilitate pain relief.
- Administer pharmacologic agents as ordered when requested to control pain.
- Provide reassurance and encouragement between contractions to foster self-esteem and continued participation in labour process.

NURSING CARE PLAN 14.1

Overview of a Client in the Active Phase of the First Stage
of Labour (continued)

NURSING DIAGNOSIS: Risk for infection related to multiple vaginal examinations following rupture of membranes and tissue trauma

Outcome Identification and Evaluation

The client will remain free of infection as evidenced by the absence of signs and symptoms of infection, vital signs and FHR within acceptable parameters, lab test results within normal limits, and clear amniotic fluid without odour.

Interventions: *Preventing Infection*

- Monitor vital signs (every 2 hours after rupture of membranes [ROM]) and FHR frequently as per protocol to allow for early detection of problems; report fetal tachycardia (early sign of maternal infection) to ensure prompt treatment.
- Provide frequent perineal care and pad changes to maintain good perineal hygiene.
- Change linens and client's gown as needed to maintain cleanliness.
- Ensure that vaginal examinations are performed only when needed to prevent introducing pathogens into the vaginal vault.

- Monitor lab test results such as white blood cell count to assess for elevations indicating infection.
- Use aseptic technique for all invasive procedures to prevent infection transmission.
- Carry out proper handwashing techniques before and after procedures and use standard precautions as appropriate to minimize risk of infection transmission.
- Document amniotic fluid characteristics—colour, odour—to establish baseline for comparison.

KEY CONCEPTS

- A nurse provides physical and emotional support during the labour and birth process to assist clients to achieve their own goals.

- When a client is admitted to the labour and birth area, the admitting nurse must assess and evaluate the risk status of the pregnancy and initiate appropriate interventions to provide optimal care for that client.

- Completing an admission assessment includes taking a health history; performing physical assessments on the client and fetus, which includes emotional and psychosocial status; and obtaining the necessary laboratory studies.

- The nurse's role in fetal assessment for labour and birth includes determining fetal well-being and interpreting signs and symptoms of possible compromise. Determining the fetal heart rate (FHR) pattern and assessing amniotic fluid characteristics are key.

- FHR can be assessed intermittently or continuously. The intermittent method allows the client to move about during labour and is the preferred method for healthy, low-risk, full-term births.

- Assessment parameters of the FHR are classified as baseline rate, baseline variability (with continuous EFM only), and periodic changes in the rate (accelerations and decelerations).

- The nurse monitoring the labouring client needs to be knowledgeable about which category the FHR pattern is in so that appropriate interventions can be instituted.

- For atypical or abnormal FHR patterns, the nurse should notify the health care provider about the pattern and obtain further orders, making sure to document all interventions and their effects on the FHR pattern.

- In addition to interpreting assessment findings and initiating appropriate inventions for the labouring client, accurate and timely documentation must be carried out continuously.

- Clients have many safe nonpharmacologic and pharmacologic choices for the management of pain during childbirth. They may be used individually or in combination to complement one another.

- Nursing management during labour and birth includes comfort measures, emotional support, information and instruction, advocacy, and support for the partner.

- Nursing care during the first stage of labour includes taking an admission history (reviewing the prenatal record), checking the results of routine laboratory work and special tests done during pregnancy, asking the client about childbirth preparation (birth plan, classes taken, coping skills), and completing a physical assessment to establish baseline values for future comparison.

- Nursing care during the second stage of labour focuses on supporting the client and partner in making decisions about their care and labour management, implementing strategies to prolong the early passive phase of fetal descent, supporting involuntary bearing-down efforts, providing support and assistance, and encouraging the use of position changes that can enhance descent and reduce the pain.

- Nursing care during the third stage of labour primarily focuses on immediate newborn care and assessment, and being available to assist with the delivery of the placenta and inspecting it for intactness.

- The focus of nursing management during the fourth stage of labour involves frequently observing the client for hemorrhage, providing comfort measures, assisting with the first feeding, and promoting family attachment.

REFERENCES AND RECOMMENDED READINGS

Adams, J., Frawley, J., Steel, A., Broom, A., & Sibbritt, D. (2015). Use of pharmacological and non-pharmacological labor pain management techniques and their relationship to maternal and infant birth outcomes: Examination of a nationally representative sample of 1835 pregnant women. *Midwifery, 31*(4), 458–463.

American College of Obstetricians and Gynecologists (ACOG). (2010). Practice bulletin No. 116: Management of intrapartum fetal heart rate tracings. Retrieved from http://simponline.it/wp-content/uploads/2014/11/pb116-PR-Bull-Intrapartuma-FHR.pdf

American College of Obstetricians and Gynecologists (ACOG), & Society for Maternal Fetal Medicine (SMFM). (2014). Safe prevention of the primary cesarean delivery. Obstetric Care Consensus 1. *Obstetrics & Gynecology, 123*(3), 693–711.

American College of Obstetricians and Gynecologists (ACOG). (2018 [reaffirmed]). Committee opinion: Amnioinfusion does not prevent meconium aspiration syndrome. Retrieved from https://www.acog.org/Clinical-Guidance-and-Publications/Committee-Opinions/Committee-on-Obstetric-Practice/Amnioinfusion-Does-Not-Prevent-Meconium-Aspiration-Syndrome

Ashimi, O., Hoff, E., Sibai, B., & Hardwicke, R. (2015). 212: Should the current DHHS recommendations for use of antiretroviral drugs in maternal HIV-1 RNA undergo a review? An urban academic experience. *American Journal of Obstetrics & Gynecology, 212*(1), S119–S120.

Association of Women's Health, Obstetric and Neonatal Nurses (AWHONN). (2015). *Fetal heart monitoring: Principles and practices* (5th ed.). Washington, DC: AWHONN.

Badve, M., & Vallejo, M. C. (2015). Obstetric anesthesia. In P. K. Sikka, S. T. Beaman, & J. A. Street (Eds.), *Basic clinical anesthesia* (pp. 501–527). New York: Springer Publishers.

Bonapace, J., Gagné, G. P., Chaillet, N., Gagnon, R., Hébert, E., & Buckley, S. (2018). SOGC clinical practice guideline No. 355-Physiologic basis of pain in labour and delivery: An evidence-based approach to its management. *Journal of Obstetrics and Gynaecology Canada, 40*(2), 227–245.

Bowers, P. (2015). Cultural perspectives in childbearing. *Nursing spectrum.* Retrieved from http://ce.nurse.com/ce263-60/cultural-perspectives-in-childbearing

Cahill, A. G., & Spain, J. (2015). Intrapartum fetal monitoring. *Clinical Obstetrics and Gynecology, 58*(2), 263–268.

Callahan, T. L. (2016). *Tarascon's OB/GYN pocketbook.* Burlington, MA: Jones & Bartlett Learning.

Camorcia, M. (2015). The second and third stage of labor. In *Epidural labor analgesia* (pp. 103–119). Switzerland: Springer International Publishing.

Canadian Institute for Health Information. (2018). Inpatient hospitalizations, surgeries, newborns and childbirth Indicators, 2016–2017. Retrieved from https://secure.cihi.ca/free_products/hospch-hosp-2016-2017-snapshot_en.pdf

Canadian Nurses Association. (2010). Position statement: Promoting cultural competence in nursing. Retrieved from https://www.cna-aiic.ca/-/media/cna/page-content/pdf-en/6—ps114_cultural_competence_2010_e.pdf

Canadian Pediatric Society (CPS). (2017). Position statement: Management of term infants at increased risk for early onset bacterial sepsis. Retrieved from https://www.cps.ca/en/documents/position/management-infant-sepsis

Capogna, G. (2015a). Humanization of childbirth and epidural analgesia. In G. Capogna (Ed.), *Epidural labor analgesia* (pp. 315–323). Switzerland: Springer International Publishing.

Capogna, G. (2015b). Maintenance of labor analgesia. In G. Capogna (Ed.), *Epidural labor analgesia* (pp. 89–101). Switzerland: Springer International Publishing.

Cargill, Y. M., & MacKinnon, C. J. (2018). SOGC Clinical practice guideline: No. 148-Guidelines for operative vaginal birth. *Journal of Obstetrics and Gynaecology Canada, 40*(2), e74–e80.

Casanova, R. (2015). *Shelf-life obstetrics and gynecology.* Philadelphia, PA: Lippincott Williams & Wilkins.

Centers for Disease Control and Prevention (CDC). (2016). *Group B strep (GBS) guidelines.* Retrieved from http://www.cdc.gov/groupbstrep/guidelines/new-differences.html

Centers for Disease Control and Prevention (CDC). (2018). *HIV/AIDS testing.* Retrieved from http://www.cdc.gov/hiv/basics/testing.html

Chandraharan, E. (2014). Fetal scalp sampling during labor: Is it a useful diagnostic test or a historical test that no longer has a place in modern obstetrics? *An International Journal of Obstetrics & Gynaecology, 121*(9), 1056–1060; discussion 1060–1062.

Cheng, Y. W., & Caughey, A. B. (2015). Second stage of labor. *Clinical Obstetrics and Gynecology, 58*(2), 227–240.

Cibils, L. A. (2014). *Electronic fetal-maternal monitoring: Antepartum/intrapartum* (2nd ed.). New York: Springer Publishers.

Cox, K. J., & King, T. L. (2015). Preventing primary cesarean births: Midwifery care. *Clinical Obstetrics and Gynecology, 58*(2), 282–293.

Dalal, S. M. (2015). Newer aspects in labor analgesia. *Research Chronicle in Health Sciences, 1*(2), 130–138.

Duff, P. (2018). Preterm prelabor rupture of membranes. *UpToDate.* Retrieved from https://www.uptodate.com/contents/preterm-prelabor-rupture-of-membranes

Faisal-Cury, A., Menezes, P. R., Quayle, J., Matijasevich, A., & Diniz, S. G. (2015). The relationship between mode of delivery and sexual health outcomes after childbirth. *The Journal of Sexual Medicine, 12*(5), 1212–1220.

Farine, D. (Ed.). (2015). *New technologies for managing labor.* Boston, MA: Walter de Gruyter GmbH & Co. KG.

Freeman, R. K. (2015). Intrapartum fetal heart rate monitoring. In J. T. Queenan, C. Y. Spong, & C. J. Lockwood (Eds.), *Protocols for high-risk pregnancies: An evidence-based approach.* Chichester, UK: John Wiley & Sons, Ltd.

Friedman, A. M., Ananth, C. V., Prendergast, E., D'Alton, M. E., & Wright, J. D. (2015). Variation in and factors associated with use of episiotomy. *Journal of the American Medical Association, 313*(2), 197–199.

Gizzo, S., Di Gangi, S., Noventa, M., Bacile, V., Zambon, A., & Nardelli, B. (2014). Women's choice of positions during labor: Return to the past or a modern way to give birth? A cohort study in Italy. *BioMed Research International, 2014,* 638093.

Grant, E. N., Tao, W., Craig, M., McIntire, D., & Leveno, K. (2015). Neuraxial analgesia effects on labor progression: Facts, fallacies, uncertainties and the future. *British Journal of Obstetrics and Gynaecology, 122*(3), 288–293.

Green, C. J. (2016). *Maternal newborn nursing care plans* (3rd ed.). Burlington, MA: Jones & Bartlett Learning.

Gujral, K., & Nayar, S. (2015). Current trends in management of fetal growth restriction. *Journal of Fetal Medicine, 1*(3), 125–129.

Hagood Milton, S. (2017). Normal labor and delivery. *eMedicine.* Retrieved from http://emedicine.medscape.com/article/260036-overview#aw2aab6b2

Halpern, S. H., & Garg, R. (2015). Evidence-based medicine and labor analgesia. In G. Capogna (Ed.), *Epidural labor analgesia* (pp. 285–295). Switzerland: Springer International Publishing.

Hanson, L., & VandeVusse, L. (2014). Supporting labor progress toward physiologic birth. *Journal of Perinatal & Neonatal Nursing, 28*(2), 101–107.

Hastings, C. (2015). The role of fetal monitoring in intrapartum care. *British Journal of Healthcare Management, [serial online], 21*(4), 166–170.

Hawkins, J. L. (2015). Excess in moderation: General anesthesia for cesarean delivery. *Anesthesia & Analgesia, 120*(6), 1175–1177.

Heesen, M., Van de Velde, M., Klöhr, S., Lehberger, J., Rossaint, R., & Straube, S. (2014). Meta-analysis of the success of block following combined spinal-epidural vs epidural analgesia during labor. *Anaesthesia, 69*(1), 64–71. doi: 10.1111/anae.12456.

Hersh, S., Megregian, M., & Emeis, C. (2014). Intermittent auscultation of the fetal heart rate during labor: An opportunity for shared decision making. *Journal of Midwifery & Women's Health, 59*(3), 344–349.

Hiersch, L., Rosen, H., Salzer, L., Aviram, A., Ben-Haroush, A., & Yogev, Y. (2015). Does artificial rupturing of membranes in the active phase of labor enhance myometrial electrical activity? *The Journal of Maternal-Fetal & Neonatal Medicine, 28*(5), 515–518.

Holvey, N. (2014). Supporting women in the second stage of labor. *British Journal of Midwifery, 22*(3), 182–186.

Ibrahim, S. E. H., Fridman, M., Korst, L. M., & Gregory, K. D. (2015). Anesthesia complications as a childbirth patient safety indicator. *Survey of Anesthesiology, 59*(3), 127–129.

Iravani, M., Zarean, E., Janghorbani, M., & Bahrami, M. (2015). Women's needs and expectations during normal labor and delivery. *Journal of Education and Health Promotion, 4,* 6.

Ivory, C. H. (2014). Standardizing the words nurses use to document elements of perinatal failure to rescue. *JOGNN: Journal of Obstetric, Gynecologic & Neonatal Nursing, 43*(1), 13–24.

Jackson, S., & Gregory, K. D. (2015). Management of the first stage of labor: Potential strategies to lower the cesarean delivery rate. *Clinical Obstetrics and Gynecology, 58*(2), 217–226.

Janula, R., & Mahipal, S. (2015). Effectiveness of aromatherapy and biofeedback in promotion of labor outcome during childbirth among primigravidas. *Health Science Journal, 9*(1), 1–5.

Jones, L. E., Whitburn, L. Y., Davey, M. A., & Small, R. (2015). Assessment of pain associated with childbirth: Women's perspectives, preferences and solutions. *Midwifery, 31*(7), 708–712.

Kerr, D., Taylor, D., & Evans, B. (2015). Patient-controlled intranasal fentanyl analgesia: A pilot study to assess practicality and tolerability during childbirth. *International Journal of Obstetric Anesthesia, 24*(2), 117–123.

King, T. L., Brucker, M. C., Osborne, K., & Jevitt, C. M. (2019). *Varney's midwifery* (6th ed.). Burlington, MA: Jones & Bartlett Learning.

Lee, L., Dy, J., & Azzam, H. (2016). SOGC clinical practice guideline: Management of spontaneous labour at term in healthy women. *Journal of Obstetrics and Gynaecology Canada, 38*(9), e843–e865.

Leonard, P. (2018). Support of the childbearing family through education. *Nursing spectrum.* Retrieved from https://www.nurse.com/ce/support-of-the-childbearing-family-through-education

Lindholm, A., & Hildingsson, I. (2015). Women's preferences and received pain relief in childbirth—a prospective longitudinal study in a northern region of Sweden. *Sexual & Reproductive Healthcare, 6*(2), 74–81.

Liston, R., Sawchuck, D., & Young, D. (2018). SOGC clinical practice guideline No. 197b, Fetal health surveillance: Intrapartum consensus guideline. *Journal of Obstetrics and Gynaecology Canada, 40*(4):e298–e322. Retrieved from https://www.jogc.com/article/S1701-2163(18)30067-7/pdf

Liu, Y. M., Fernando, R., & Mon, W. Y. (2015). Labor pain. In G. Capogna (Ed.), *Epidural labor analgesia* (pp. 21–37). Switzerland: Springer International Publishing.

Lucas, M. T. B., da Rocha, M. J. F., de Medonça Costa, K. M., de Oliveira, G. G., & Melo, J. O. (2015). Nursing care during labor in a model maternity unit: Cross-sectional study. *Online Brazilian Journal of Nursing, 14*(1), 32–40.

Macones, G. (2018). Management of intrapartum category I, II, and III fetal heart rate tracings. *UpToDate*. Retrieved from https://www.uptodate.com/contents/management-of-intrapartum-category-i-ii-and-iii-fetal-heart-rate-tracings

Magowan, B., Owen, P., & Thomson, A. (2014). *Clinical obstetrics & gynecology* (3rd ed.). St. Louis, MO: Saunders Elsevier.

Martin, R. J., Fanaroff, A. A., & Walsh, M. C. (2014). *Neonatal-perinatal medicine* (10th ed.). Philadelphia, PA: Elsevier Health Sciences.

Maso, G., Piccoli, M., De Seta, F., Parolin, S., Banco, R., Camacho, M. L., . . . Alberico S. (2015). Intrapartum fetal heart rate monitoring interpretation in labor: A critical appraisal. *Minerva Ginecologica, 67*(1), 65–79.

McGeary, C. A., Swanholm, E., & Gatchel, R. J. (2015). Pain management. *The Encyclopedia of Clinical Psychology,* 1–6. doi: 10.1002/9781118625392.wbecp144

Miller, L. A. (2014). Ask an expert: Frequently asked questions on nursing liability issues. *Journal of Perinatal & Neonatal Nursing, 28*(1), 9–11.

Mollart, L. J., Adam, J., & Foureur, M. (2015). Impact of acupressure on onset of labor and labor duration: A systematic review. *Women and Birth, 28*(3), 199–206.

Money, D., Tulloch, K., Boucoiran, I., & Caddy, S. (2014). SOGC Clinical practice guideline: Guidelines for the care of pregnant women living with HIV and interventions to reduce perinatal transmission. Retrieved from https://sogc.org/wp-content/uploads/2014/08/August2014-CPG310-ENG-online-Complete-REV.pdf

Nageotte, M. P. (2015). Fetal heart rate monitoring. *Seminars in Fetal and Neonatal Medicine, 20*(3), 144–148.

Nagtalon-Ramos, J. (2014). *Best evidence-based practices in maternal-newborn nursing care.* Philadelphia, PA: F. A. Davis Company.

National Center for Missing and Exploited Children (NCMEC). (2015). For health care professionals: Guidelines on prevention of and response to infant abductions. Retrieved from http://www.missingkids.com/content/dam/pdfs/publications/nc05.pdf

National Institute for Health and Care Excellence (NICE). (2014). *Intrapartum care: Care of healthy women and their babies during childbirth. CG190.* London, UK: NICE.

Neal, J. L., Lamp, J. M., Buck, J. S., Lowe, N. K., Gillespie, S. L., & Ryan, S. L. (2014). Outcomes of nulliparous women with spontaneous labor onset admitted to hospitals in preactive versus active labor. *Journal of Midwifery & Women's Health, 59*(1), 28–34.

Neetu, P. S., & Panchal, R. (2015). A study to assess the effectiveness of abdominal effleurage on labor pain intensity and labor outcomes among nullipara mothers during first stage of labor in selected Hospitals of District Ambala, Haryana. *International Journal of Science & Research, 4*(1), 1585–1590.

Nutter, E. (2016). *Decreasing vulnerability in childbirth: Waterbirth in military treatment facilities. Caring for the vulnerable* (4th ed., pp. 253–262). Burlington, MA: Jones & Bartlett Learning.

Omo-Aghoja, L. (2015). Maternal and fetal acid-base chemistry: A major determinant of perinatal outcome. *Annals of Medical and Health Sciences Research, 4*(1), 8–17.

Patkar, C. S., Vora, K., Patel, H., Shah, V., Modi, M. P., & Parikh, G. (2015). A comparison of continuous infusion and intermittent bolus administration of 0.1% ropivacaine with 0.0002% fentanyl for epidural labor analgesia. *Journal of Anesthesiology, Clinical Pharmacology, 31*(2), 234–238.

Petrocnik, P., & Marshall, J. E. (2015). Hands-poised technique: The future technique for perineal management of second stage of labor? A modified systematic literature review. *Midwifery, 31*(2), 274–279.

Prior, T., & Kumar, S. (2015). Expert review: Identification of intra-partum fetal compromise. *European Journal of Obstetrics & Gynecology and Reproductive Biology, 190,* 1–6.

Reed, R. (2015). Supporting women's instinctive pushing behaviour during birth. *The Practicing Midwife, 18*(6), 13–15.

Regi, A., Alexander, N., Jose, R., Lionel, J., Varghese, L., Peedicayil, A. (2009). Amnioinfusion for relief of recurrent severe and moderate variable decelerations in labor. *Journal of Reproductive Medicine, 54*(5), 295–302. Retrieved from https://www.ncbi.nlm.nih.gov/pubmed/19517694

Roberts, L., Gulliver, B., Fisher, J., & Cloyes, K. G. (2010). The coping with labor algorithm: An alternate pain assessment tool for the laboring woman. *Journal of Midwifery & Women's Health, 55*(2), 107–116.

Royal College of Midwives & Royal College of Obstetricians and Gynaecologists. (2017). RCM/RCOG consensus statement on electronic fetal monitoring (EFM). Retrieved from https://www.rcm.org.uk/sites/default/files/RCMRCOG%20Consensus%20Statement%20on%20EFM%20A4_3_0.pdf

Sholapurkar, M. S. L. (2015). Intrapartum fetal monitoring: Overview, controversies and pitfalls. *The Health Foundation,* 1–8.

Sholapurkar, S. (2014). Algorithm for management of category II fetal heart rate tracings: A standardization of right sort? *American Journal of Obstetrics and Gynecology, 210*(2), 175.

Sides, C., Rios, A. R., Lam, M. C., Ward, A. R., Stoltzfus, J., & Lucente, V. R. (2015). Above all, do no harm: Modifiable risk factors for high-risk perineal lacerations. *Obstetrics & Gynecology, 125,* 49S.

Simkin, P., & Klein, M. C. (2018). Nonpharmacologic approaches to management of labor pain. *UpToDate.* Retrieved from http://www.uptodate.com/contents/non-pharmacological-approaches-to-management-of-labor-pain

Simpson, K. R. (2015). Electronic health records. *MCN: The American Journal of Maternal/Child Nursing, 40*(1), 68.

Skidmore-Roth, L. (2015). *Mosby's 2015 nursing drug reference* (28th ed.). St. Louis, MO: Mosby Elsevier.

Sng, B. L., Kwok, S. C., & Sia, A. T. (2015). Modern neuraxial labor analgesia. *Current Opinion in Anesthesiology, 28*(3), 285–289.

Sng, B. L., Zhang, Q., Leong, W. L., Ocampo, C., Assam, P. N., & Sia, A. T. (2015). Incidence and characteristics of breakthrough pain in parturients using computer-integrated patient-controlled epidural analgesia. *Journal of Clinical Anesthesia, 27*(4), 277–284.

Stocks, G. M., & Griffiths, S. K. (2015). Initiation of labor analgesia: Epidural, CSE. In *Epidural labor analgesia* (pp. 73–88). Switzerland: Springer International Publishing.

Taghavi, S., Barband, S., & Khaki, A. (2015). Effect of hydrotherapy on pain of labor process. *BALTICA, 28*(1), 116–121.

Tharpe, N. L., Farley, C. L., & Jordan, R. (2016). *Clinical practice guidelines for midwifery & women's health* (5th ed.). Sudbury, MA: Jones & Bartlett.

Timmins, A. E., & Clark, S. L. (2015). How to approach intrapartum category II tracings. *Obstetrics and Gynecology Clinics of North America, 42*(2), 363–375.

Ugwumadu, A. (2015). Author's reply re: Are we (mis)guided by current guidelines on intrapartum fetal heart rate monitoring? Case for a more physiological approach to interpretation. *BJOG: An International Journal of Obstetrics & Gynecology, 122*(4), 589.

Van de Velde, M. (2015). Patient-controlled intravenous analgesia remifentanil for labor analgesia: Time to stop, think and reconsider. *Current Opinion in Anesthesiology, 28*(3), 237–239.

Verklan, T., & Walden, M. (2014). *Core curriculum for neonatal intensive care nursing* (4th ed.). St. Louis, MO: Saunders Elsevier.

Walker, S., & Sabrosa, R. (2014). Assessment of fetal presentation: Exploring a woman-centered approach. *British Journal of Midwifery, 22*(4), 240–244.

Wenner, L. (2015). It's the little things. *Nursing for Women's Health, 19*(2), 203–204.

Wisner, K. (2015). Intermittent auscultation in low-risk labor. *MCN: The American Journal of Maternal/Child Nursing, 40*(1), 58.

Wojnar, D. M., & Narruhn, R. A. (2016). *Transcultural aspects of perinatal health care of Somali women. Caring for the vulnerable* (4th ed., pp. 287–302). Burlington, MA: Jones & Bartlett Learning.

World Health Organization. (2015). Recommendations for augmentation of labour. Retrieved from http://apps.who.int/iris/bitstream/handle/10665/174001/WHO_RHR_15.05_eng.pdf?sequence = 1

Yuan, S. M. (2015). Fetal cardiac interventions. *Pediatrics & Neonatology, 56*(2), 81–87.

CHAPTER **WORKSHEET**

MULTIPLE CHOICE QUESTIONS

1. When a client in labour is fully dilated, which instruction would be most effective to assist and encourage effective pushing?
   a. Hold your breath and push through entire contraction.
   b. Use chest-breathing with the contraction.
   c. Pant and blow during each contraction.
   d. Wait until you feel the urge to push.

2. During the fourth stage of labour, the nurse assesses the client at frequent intervals after giving childbirth. What assessment data would cause the nurse the most concern?
   a. Moderate amount of dark red lochia drainage on peripad
   b. Uterine fundus palpated to the right of the umbilicus
   c. An oral temperature reading of 38.1°C (100.6°F)
   d. Perineal area bruised and edematous

3. When managing a client's pain during labour, nurses should:
   a. Make sure the agents given do not prolong labour.
   b. Know that all pain relief measures are similar.
   c. Support the client's decisions and requests.
   d. Not recommend nonpharmacologic methods.

4. When caring for a client during the active phase of labour without continuous electronic fetal monitoring, the nurse would intermittently assess FHR every:
   a. 15 to 30 minutes.
   b. 5 to 10 minutes.
   c. 45 to 60 minutes.
   d. 60 to 75 minutes.

5. The nurse notes the presence of transient fetal accelerations on the fetal monitoring strip. Which intervention would be most appropriate?
   a. Reposition the client on the left side.
   b. Begin 100% oxygen via face mask.
   c. Document this as indicating a normal pattern.
   d. Call the health care provider immediately.

6. By the end of the second stage of labour, the nurse would expect which of the following events?
   a. The cervix is fully dilated and effaced.
   b. The placenta is detached and expelled.
   c. The fetus is born and placed on the client's chest.
   d. The client to request pain medication.

7. Which of the following practices would not be included in a physiologic birth?
   a. Early induction of labour <39 weeks' gestation
   b. Freedom of movement for the labouring client
   c. Continuous presence and support throughout labour
   d. Encouraging spontaneous pushing when urge felt

CRITICAL THINKING EXERCISES

1. A 20-year-old primigravida at term, comes to the birthing center in active labour (dilation 5 cm and 80% effaced, −1 station) with ruptured membranes. She states she wants an "all-natural" birth without medication. Her partner is with her and appears anxious but supportive. On the admission assessment, this client's prenatal history is unremarkable; vital signs are within normal limits; FHR via Doppler ranges between 140 and 144 bpm and is regular.
   a. Based on your assessment data and the woman's request not to have medication, what nonpharmacologic interventions could you offer her?
   b. What positions might be suggested to facilitate fetal descent?

2. Several hours later, the client complains of nausea and turns to her partner and angrily tells him to not touch her and to go away.
   a. What assessment needs to be done to determine what is happening?
   b. What explanation can you offer this client's partner regarding her change in behaviour?

STUDY ACTIVITIES

1. Share experiences within a post clinical conference group regarding the pain management interventions of the clients to which you were assigned. Compare and evaluate the effectiveness of different methods used, maternal behaviour observed, and neonatal outcome in terms of Apgar scores.

2. On the fetal heart monitor, the nurse notices an elevation of the fetal baseline with the onset of contractions. This elevation would describe _____.

3. Compare and contrast a birthing centre to a community hospital's birthing suite in terms of the pain management techniques and fetal monitoring used.

4. Select a childbirth website for expectant parents and critique the information provided in terms of its educational level and amount of advertising.

BRINGING IT ALL TOGETHER: A CASE STUDY

A 30-year-old woman at term presents to the emergency room with abdominal pain. This is her first pregnancy and she is accompanied by her partner and her very anxious sister. She is 40 weeks and 6 days based on her last ultrasound. All pregnancy blood tests have been normal. Earlier in the day she had a mucus-like dark red discharge followed by the onset of irregular period-type cramps. Two hours ago, she felt a gush of clear fluid from her vagina and since then she has felt miserable. She took two Tylenol at home for the pain, but she is now in distress and came to the hospital for assessment.

Go to thePoint **to find questions to consider about this case.**

Postpartum
Period

15

Postpartum Adaptations

Learning Objectives

Upon completion of the chapter, you will be able to:

1. Examine the systemic physiologic changes occurring after childbirth.

2. Determine the psychological changes that occur in the postpartum period.

3. Relate effective self-care measures for clients to implement in the postpartum period.

4. Integrate dimensions of cultural safety into care of the family during the postpartum period.

5. Plan nursing interventions to support bonding in the postpartum period.

6. Assess the phases of parental role adjustment and accompanying behaviours.

7. Analyze new parents' psychological adaptations after childbirth.

Betsy had been home only 3 days when she called the maternity unit where she had given birth and asked to speak to the lactation consultant. She reported pain in both breasts. Her nipples were tender due to frequent breastfeeding and she described her breasts as heavy, hard, and swollen.

INTRODUCTION

The postpartum period is a critical transition time for a postpartum client, the newborn, and the family on physiologic and psychological levels. The **puerperium** period begins after the delivery of the placenta and lasts approximately 6 weeks. During this period the client's body begins to return to its prepregnant state, and these changes generally resolve by the 6th week after giving birth. The postpartum period can also be defined to include the changes in all aspects of the new parent's life that occur during the 1st year after a child is born. Some believe that the postpartum adjustment period lasts well into the 1st year, making the fourth phase of labour the longest. Keeping this in mind, the true postpartum period could last up to 12 months as the parent works to lose the weight gained during the pregnancy and adjusts psychologically to the changes of parenthood and infant feeding.

Nurses caring for childbearing families should consider all aspects of culture, including communication, space, and family roles. Communication encompasses an understanding of not only a person's language, and loudness of speech, but also the meaning of touch and gestures. The concept of personal space and the dimensions of comfort zones differ from culture to culture. Touching, placing clients in proximity to others, and taking away personal possessions can reduce a client's personal security and heighten her anxiety. Nurses must be sensitive to how people respond when being touched and should refrain from touching if the client's response indicates that it is unwelcome. Cultural norms also have an impact on family roles, expectations, and behaviours associated with a member's position in the family. For example, culture may influence whether a man actively participates in the pregnancy and childbirth. Maternity health care professionals in North America expect men to be involved, but this role expectation may conflict with that of many of the diverse groups now living in North America. Families from a variety of cultural backgrounds, including Mexican, Arab, Asian, and Orthodox Jewish families, for example, may view the birthing experience as a woman's affair (Purnell, 2014).

Our major role as nurses is to provide safe and evidence-based care to promote optimal birth outcomes for all women/clients and families, regardless of their cultural background. Nurses need to remember that there is more than one way to provide this care. Nurses are important cultural brokers as they welcome clients and their families into our obstetrical units, where nurses share with those families one of the most intimate experiences of their lives (Bowers & Ceballos, 2015).

This chapter describes the major physiologic and psychological changes that occur after childbirth. Various systemic adaptations take place throughout the client's body. In addition, the client and the family adjust to the new addition psychologically. The birth of a child changes the family structure and the roles of the family members. The adaptations are dynamic and continue to evolve as physical changes occur and new roles emerge.

PHYSIOLOGIC ADAPTATIONS

During pregnancy, the entire body changes to accommodate the needs of the growing fetus. After birth, the body once again undergoes significant changes in all systems to return to its prepregnant state.

Reproductive System Adaptations

The reproductive system goes through tremendous adaptations to return to the prepregnancy state. All organs and tissues of the reproductive system are involved. The female reproductive system is unique in its capacity to remodel itself throughout the reproductive life. The events after birth, with the shedding of the placenta and subsequent uterine involution, involve substantial tissue destruction and subsequent repair and remodeling. For example, if the client is not breastfeeding, the menstrual cycle will return several weeks after childbirth. Nurses must inform clients that ovulation will resume prior to the first menstrual period, thus the absences of menses should not be considered guaranteed protection against pregnancy. The uterus, which has undergone tremendous expansion during pregnancy to accommodate progressive fetal growth, will return to its prepregnant size over several weeks. The breasts have grown to prepare for lactation and do not return to their prepregnant size as the uterus does.

Uterine Involution

The uterus returns to its normal size through a gradual process of **involution,** which involves retrogressive changes that return it to its nonpregnant size and condition. Involution involves three retrogressive processes:

1. Contraction of muscle fibers to reduce those previously stretched during pregnancy
2. Catabolism, which shrinks enlarged, individual myometrial cells
3. Regeneration of uterine epithelium from the lower layer of the decidua after the upper layers have been sloughed off and shed during lochial discharge (Mattson & Smith, 2015).

The uterus, which weighs approximately 1,000 g (2.2 lb) soon after birth, undergoes physiologic involution as it returns to its nonpregnant state. Approximately 1 week after birth, the uterus shrinks in size by 50% and weighs about 500 g (1 lb); at the end of 6 weeks, it weighs approximately 60 g (2 oz), about the weight before the pregnancy (Jordan, Engstrom, Marfell, & Farley, 2014) (Fig. 15.1). During the first few days after

— Umbilicus

--- Postpartum day 1
--- Postpartum day 2
--- Postpartum day 3
--- Postpartum day 4
--- Postpartum day 5
--- Postpartum day 6
--- Postpartum day 7
--- Postpartum day 8
--- Postpartum day 9

FIGURE 15.1 Uterine involution.

birth, the uterus typically descends from the level of the umbilicus at a rate of 1 cm (1 fingerbreadth) per day. By 3 days, the fundus lies 2 to 3 cm below the umbilicus (or slightly higher in multiparous individuals). By the end of 10 days, the fundus usually cannot be palpated because it has descended into the true pelvis.

If these retrogressive changes do not occur as a result of retained placental fragments or infection, then subinvolution of the uterus typically results (delayed or absent involution). Subinvolution is generally responsive to early diagnosis and treatment. Factors that facilitate uterine involution include complete expulsion of amniotic membranes and placenta at birth, a complication-free labour and birth process, breastfeeding, and early ambulation. Factors that inhibit involution include a prolonged labour and difficult birth, incomplete expulsion of amniotic membranes and placenta, uterine infection, over-distention of uterine muscles (such as by multiple gestation, hydramnios, or a large singleton fetus), a full bladder (which displaces the uterus and interferes with contractions), anesthesia (which relaxes uterine muscles), and close childbirth spacing (frequent and repeated distention decreases tone and causes muscular relaxation).

LOCHIA

Lochia is the vaginal discharge that occurs after birth and continues for approximately 4 to 8 weeks. It results from involution, during which the superficial layer of the decidua basalis becomes necrotic and is sloughed off. Immediately after childbirth, lochia is bright red and consists mainly of blood, fibrinous products, decidual cells, and red and white blood cells. The lochia from the

uterus is alkaline but becomes acidic as it passes through the vagina. It is roughly equal to the amount occurring during a heavy menstrual period. The average amount of lochial discharge is 240 to 270 mL (8 to 9 oz) (Bope & Kellerman, 2015).

Clients who have had caesarean births tend to have less flow because the uterine debris is removed manually along with delivery of the placenta. Lochia is present for at least 3 weeks after childbirth but can persist for as long as 6 weeks.

Lochia passes through three stages:
- *Lochia rubra* is a deep-red mixture of mucus, tissue debris, and blood that occurs for the first 3 to 4 days after birth. As uterine bleeding subsides, it becomes paler and more serous.
- *Lochia serosa* is the second stage. It is pinkish brown and is expelled 3 to 10 days postpartum. Lochia serosa primarily contains leukocytes, decidual tissue, red blood cells, and serous fluid.
- *Lochia alba* is the final stage. The discharge is creamy white or light brown and consists of leukocytes, decidual tissue, and reduced fluid content. It occurs from days 10 to 14 but can last 3 to 6 weeks postpartum in some women and still be considered normal.

Lochia at any stage should have a fleshy smell; an offensive odour usually indicates an infection, such as endometritis.

Take Note!

A danger sign is the reappearance of bright-red blood after lochia rubra has stopped. Reevaluation by a health care provider is essential if this occurs.

AFTERPAINS

Part of the involution process involves uterine contractions. Subsequently, many clients are frequently bothered by painful uterine contractions termed *afterpains*. All postpartum clients experience afterpains, but they are more acute in those who are multiparous and breast-feeding, secondary to repeated stretching of the uterine muscles from multiple pregnancies or stimulation during breastfeeding with oxytocin released from the pituitary gland. Primiparous clients typically experience mild afterpains because their uterus is able to maintain a contracted state. Breastfeeding and administration of exogenous oxytocin both cause powerful and painful uterine contractions. Afterpains are usually relieved by oral analgesics.

Take Note!

Afterpains are usually stronger during breastfeeding because oxytocin released by the sucking reflex strengthens the contractions. Mild analgesics can reduce this discomfort.

FIGURE 15.2 Appearance of the cervical os, (**A**) before the first pregnancy, and (**B**) after pregnancy.

Cervix

The cervix typically returns to its prepregnant state by week 6 of the postpartum period. The cervix gradually closes but never regains its prepregnant appearance. Immediately after childbirth, the cervix is shapeless and edematous and is easily distensible for several days. The internal cervical os gradually closes and returns to normal by 2 weeks, whereas the external os widens and never appears the same after childbirth. The external cervical os is no longer shaped like a circle, but instead appears as a jagged slit-like opening, often described as a "fish mouth" (Fig. 15.2).

Vagina

Shortly after birth, the vaginal mucosa is edematous and thin, with few rugae. As ovarian function returns and estrogen production resumes, the mucosa thickens and rugae return in approximately 3 weeks. The vagina gapes at the opening and is generally lax. The vagina returns to its approximate prepregnant size by 6 to 8 weeks postpartum but will always remain a bit larger than it had been before pregnancy.

Normal mucus production and thickening of the vaginal mucosa usually return with ovulation. The vagina gradually decreases in size and regains tone over several weeks. By 3 to 4 weeks, the edema and vascularity have decreased. The vaginal epithelium is generally restored by 6 to 8 weeks postpartum (Mattson & Smith, 2015). Localized dryness and coital discomfort (dyspareunia) usually plague most women until menstruation returns. Water-soluble lubricants can reduce discomfort during intercourse.

Perineum

The perineum is often edematous and bruised for the first day or two after birth. If the birth involved an episiotomy or laceration, complete healing may take as long as 4 to 6 months in the absence of complications at the site, such as hematoma or infection. The muscle tone may or may not return to normal, depending on the extent of injury to muscle, nerve, and connecting tissues (Kansky & Isaacs, 2016). Perineal lacerations may extend into the anus and cause considerable discomfort when the client is attempting to defecate or ambulate. The presence of swollen hemorrhoids may also heighten discomfort. Local comfort measures such as ice packs, pouring warm water over the area via a peribottle, witch hazel pads, anesthetic sprays, and sitz baths can relieve pain.

Supportive tissues of the pelvic floor are stretched during the childbirth process and restoring their tone may take up to 6 months. Pelvic relaxation can occur in any client experiencing a vaginal birth. Nurses should encourage all clients to practice pelvic floor muscle training (PFMT) exercises to improve pelvic floor tone, strengthen the perineal muscles, and promote healing. See Evidence-Based Practice 15.1.

Take Note!

Failure to maintain and restore perineal muscular tone can lead to urinary incontinence later in life.

Cardiovascular System Adaptations

The cardiovascular system undergoes dramatic changes after birth. During pregnancy, the heart is displaced slightly upward and to the left. This reverses as the uterus undergoes involution. Cardiac output remains high for the first few days postpartum and then gradually declines to nonpregnant values within 3 months of birth.

Blood volume, which increases substantially during pregnancy, drops rapidly after birth and returns to normal within 4 weeks postpartum. The decrease in both cardiac output and blood volume reflects the birth-related blood loss (an average of 500 mL with a vaginal birth and 1,000 mL with a caesarean birth). The cardiac output deceases to prelabour values 24 to 72 hours postpartum, rapidly falls over the next 2 weeks and usually returns to nonpregnant levels within 6 to 8 weeks postpartum. Blood plasma volume is further reduced through diuresis, which occurs during the early postpartum period (Hagood Milton, 2017). Despite the decrease in blood volume, the hematocrit level remains relatively stable and may even increase, reflecting the predominant loss of plasma. Thus, an acute decrease in hematocrit is not an expected finding and may indicate hemorrhage.

Pulse and Blood Pressure

The increase in cardiac output and stroke volume during pregnancy begins to diminish after birth once the placenta has been delivered. This decrease in cardiac output is reflected in bradycardia (40 to 60 bpm) for up to the first 2 weeks postpartum. This slowing of the heart rate is related to the increased blood that flows back to the heart and to the central circulation after it is no longer

PELVIC FLOOR MUSCLE TRAINING VERSUS NO TREATMENT, OR INACTIVE CONTROL TREATMENTS, FOR URINARY INCONTINENCE IN WOMEN

Stress incontinence is the involuntary leakage of urine with a physical activity that increases intra-abdominal pressure such as coughing or sneezing. This incontinence can occur after childbirth secondary to perineal trauma. Pelvic floor muscle training (PFMT) is the most common intervention for women that experience stress urinary incontinence. The objective of this study was to determine the effects of PFMT for women with urinary incontinence when compared with no treatment, placebo, or other inactive control treatments.

STUDY

Randomized or quasi-randomized trials in women experiencing stress incontinence were reviewed. Twenty-one trials involving 1,281 women met the inclusion criteria. Women with stress urinary incontinence who were in the PFMT groups were 8 times more likely than the controls to report that they were cured (46/82 [56.1%] vs. 5/83 [6.0%], RR 8.38, 95% CI 3.68 to 19.07) and 17 times more likely to report cure or improvement (32/58 [55%] vs. 2/63 [3.2%], RR 17.33, 95% CI 4.31 to 69.64). In trials in women with any type of urinary incontinence, PFMT groups were also more likely to report cure, or more cure and improvement, than the women in the control groups, although the effect size was reduced. Women with stress urinary incontinence were also more satisfied with the active treatment, while women in the control groups were more likely to seek further treatment. Women treated with PFMT leaked urine less often, lost smaller amounts on the short office-based pad test, and emptied their bladders less often during the day.

Findings

The review of trials found that PFMT (muscle-clenching exercises) helps women cure and improve stress urinary incontinence in particular, and all types of incontinence.

Nursing Implications

The review provides support for the widespread recommendation that PFMT be included in first-line conservative management programs for women with stress and any type of urinary incontinence. Long-term effectiveness of PFMT needs to be further researched. The take-away message for nurses working with postpartum women should be to instruct them how to perform PFMT exercises at home to assist in restoring pelvic floor strength and tone. In addition to PFMT exercises, the promotion of healthy weight can also help prevent or reduce incontinence as a person ages.

Adapted from Dumoulin C., Hay-Smith, E. J. C., & Mac Habée-Séguin, G. (2014). Pelvic floor muscle training versus no treatment, or inactive control treatments, for urinary incontinence in women. *Cochrane Database of Systematic Reviews, 5*, CD005654.

---

perfusing the placenta. This increase in central circulation brings about an increased stroke volume and allows a slower heart rate to provide ample circulation. Gradually, cardiac output returns to prepregnant levels by 3 months after childbirth (Mahendru, Everett, Wilkinson, Lees, & McEniery, 2014).

Tachycardia (heart rate above 100 bpm) in the postpartum client warrants further investigation. It may indicate hypovolemia, dehydration, or hemorrhage. However, because of the increased blood volume during pregnancy, a considerable loss of blood may be well tolerated and not cause a compensatory cardiovascular response such as tachycardia. In most instances of postpartum hemorrhage, blood pressure and cardiac output remain increased because of the compensatory increase in heart rate. Thus, a decrease in blood pressure and cardiac output are not expected changes during the postpartum period. Early identification is essential to ensure prompt intervention.

Blood pressure falls mostly in the first 2 days and then increases 3 to 7 days after childbirth and returns to prepregnancy levels by 6 weeks (Parpaglioni, 2015). A significant increase accompanied by headache might indicate preeclampsia and requires further investigation. Decreased blood pressure may suggest an infection or a uterine hemorrhage.

Coagulation

Normal physiologic changes of pregnancy, including alterations in hemostasis that favour coagulation, reduced fibrinolysis, and pooling and stasis of blood in the lower limbs, place postpartum clients at risk for blood clots. These changes, which usually return to prepregnant levels 3 weeks postpartum, are important for minimizing blood loss at childbirth. Smoking, obesity, immobility, and postpartum factors such as infection, bleeding, and emergency surgery (including emergency caesarean section) also increase the risk of coagulation disorders (Creasy et al., 2014).

Clotting factors that increased during pregnancy tend to remain elevated during the early postpartum period. Giving birth stimulates this hypercoagulability state further. As a result, these coagulation factors remain elevated for 2 to 3 weeks postpartum (King et al., 2015). This hypercoagulable state, combined with vessel damage during birth and immobility, places the client at risk for thromboembolism (blood clots) in the lower extremities and the lungs.

Blood Cellular Components

Red blood cell production ceases early in the puerperium, causing mean hemoglobin and hematocrit levels to decrease slightly in the first 24 hours. During the next 2 weeks, both levels rise slowly. The white blood count, which increases in labour, remains elevated for first 4 to 6 days after birth but then falls to 6,000 to 10,000/mm³. This white blood cell elevation can complicate a diagnosis of infection in the immediate postpartum period.

Urinary System Adaptations

Pregnancy and birth can have profound effects on the urinary system. During pregnancy, the glomerular filtration rate and renal plasma flow increase significantly. Both usually return to normal by 6 weeks after birth. There is a gradual return of bladder tone and normal size and function of the bladder, ureters, and renal pelvis, all of which were dilated during pregnancy.

Many postpartum clients have difficulty feeling the sensation to void after giving birth if they received an anesthetic block during labour (which inhibits neural functioning of the bladder) or if they received oxytocin to induce or augment their labour (antidiuretic effect). These clients will be at risk for incomplete emptying, bladder distention, difficulty voiding, and urinary retention. In addition, urination may be impeded by:

- Perineal lacerations
- Generalized swelling and bruising of the perineum and tissues surrounding the urinary meatus
- Hematomas
- Decreased bladder tone as a result of regional anesthesia
- Diminished sensation of bladder pressure as a result of swelling, poor bladder tone, and numbing effects of regional anesthesia used during labour (Bope & Kellerman, 2015).

Difficulty voiding can lead to urinary retention, bladder distention, and ultimately urinary tract infection. Urinary retention and bladder distention can cause displacement of the uterus from the midline to the right and can inhibit the uterus from contracting properly, which increases the risk of postpartum hemorrhage. Urinary retention is a major cause of **uterine atony** (loss of uterine muscle tone), which allows excessive bleeding. Frequent voiding of small amounts (less than 150 mL) suggests urinary retention with overflow, and catheterization may be necessary to empty the bladder to restore tone.

Postpartum diuresis occurs as a result of several mechanisms: the large amounts of intravenous fluids given during labour, a decreasing antidiuretic effect of oxytocin as its level declines, the buildup and retention of extra fluids during pregnancy, and a decreasing production of aldosterone—the hormone that decreases sodium retention and increases urine production (Evans & De Franco, 2014). All of these factors contribute to rapid filling of the bladder within 12 hours of birth. Diuresis begins within 12 hours after childbirth and continues throughout the 1st week postpartum. Normal function returns within a month after birth (Cunningham et al., 2014).

Consider This

Have you ever felt foolish by not being able to complete a simple task in life? I had a beautiful baby boy after only 6 hours of labour. My epidural worked well, and I actually felt very little discomfort throughout my labour. Because it was in the middle of the night when they brought me to my postpartum room, I felt a few hours of sleep would be all I needed to be back to normal. During an assessment early the next morning, the nurse found my uterus had shifted to the right from my midline, and I was instructed to empty my bladder. I didn't understand why the nurse was concerned about where my uterus was located and, besides, I didn't feel any sensation of a full bladder. But I did get up anyway and tried to comply. Despite all the nurse's tricks of running the faucet for sound effects, in addition to having warm water poured over my thighs via the peribottle, I was unable to urinate. How could I not accomplish one of life's simplest tasks?

Thoughts: Clients who receive regional anesthesia frequently experience reduced sensation to their perineal area and do not feel a full bladder. The nursing assessment revealed a displaced uterus secondary to a full bladder. What additional "tricks" can be used to assist this woman to void? What explanation should be offered to her regarding why she is having difficulty urinating?

Gastrointestinal System Adaptations

The gastrointestinal system quickly returns to normal after birth because the gravid uterus is no longer filling the abdominal cavity and producing pressure on the abdominal organs. Progesterone levels, which caused relaxation of smooth muscle during pregnancy and diminished bowel tone, also are declining.

Regardless of the type of delivery, most postpartum clients experience decreased bowel tone and sluggish bowels for several days after birth. Decreased peristalsis occurs in response to analgesics, surgery, diminished intra-abdominal pressure, low fiber diet, insufficient fluid intake, and diminished muscle tone. In addition, clients with an episiotomy, perineal laceration, or hemorrhoids may fear pain or damage to the perineum with their first bowel movement and may attempt to delay it. Subsequently, constipation is a common problem during the postpartum period. A stool softener can be prescribed for this reason.

Most clients are hungry and thirsty after childbirth, commonly related to nothing-by-mouth (NPO) restrictions and the energy expended during labour. Their appetite returns to normal immediately after giving birth.

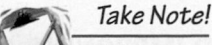 **Take Note!**

Anticipate the client's need to replenish the body with food and fluids and provide both soon after giving birth.

Musculoskeletal System Adaptations

The effects of pregnancy on the muscles and joints vary widely. Musculoskeletal changes associated with pregnancy, such as increased ligament laxity, weight gain, change in the centre of gravity, and carpal tunnel syndrome, revert back during the postpartum period. During pregnancy, the hormones relaxin, estrogen, and progesterone relax the joints. After birth, levels of these hormones decline, resulting in a return of all joints to their prepregnant state, with the exception of the feet. Parous clients may note a permanent increase in their shoe size (Jordan et al., 2014).

Postpartum clients commonly experience fatigue and activity intolerance and have a distorted body image for weeks after birth secondary to declining relaxin and progesterone levels, which cause hip and joint pain that interferes with ambulation and exercise. Good body mechanics and correct positioning are important during this time to prevent low back pain and injury to the joints. Within 6 to 8 weeks after delivery, joints are completely stabilized and return to normal.

During pregnancy, stretching of the abdominal wall muscles occurs to accommodate the enlarging uterus. This stretching leads to a loss in muscle tone and possibly separation of the longitudinal muscles (rectus abdominis muscles) of the abdomen. Separation of the rectus abdominis muscles, called diastasis recti, is more common in those who have poor abdominal muscle tone before pregnancy. After birth, muscle tone is diminished and the abdominal muscles are soft and flabby. Specific exercises are necessary to help the client regain muscle tone. Fortunately, diastasis responds well to exercise, and abdominal muscle tone can be improved. (See Chapter 16 for more information about exercises to improve muscle tone.)

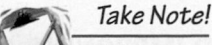 **Take Note!**

If rectus muscle tone is not regained through exercise, support may not be adequate during future pregnancies.

Integumentary System Adaptations

Another system that experiences lasting effects of pregnancy is the integumentary system. As estrogen and progesterone levels decrease, the darkened pigmentation on the abdomen (linea nigra), face (melasma), and nipples gradually fades. Some clients experience hair loss during pregnancy and the postpartum periods. Approximately 90% of hairs are growing at any one time, with the other 10% entering a resting phase. Because of the high estrogen levels present during pregnancy, an increased number of hairs go into the resting phase, which is part of the normal hair loss cycle. The most common period for hair loss is within 3 months after birth, when estrogen returns to normal levels and more hairs are allowed to fall out. This hair loss is temporary, and regrowth generally returns to normal levels in 4 to 6 months in two thirds of postpartum clients and by 15 months in the remainder, although hair may be less abundant than before pregnancy (King et al., 2015).

Striae gravidarum (stretch marks) that developed during pregnancy on the breasts, abdomen, and hips gradually fade to silvery lines. However, these lines do not disappear completely. Although many products on the market claim to make stretch marks disappear, their effectiveness is highly questionable.

The profuse diaphoresis (sweating) that is common during the early postpartum period is one of the most noticeable adaptations in the integumentary system. Many postpartum clients will wake up drenched with perspiration during this time. This postpartum diaphoresis is a mechanism to reduce the amount of fluids retained during pregnancy and restore prepregnant body fluid levels. It can be profuse at times. It is common, especially at night during the 1st week after birth. Reassure clients that this is normal and encourage them to change pyjamas to prevent chilling.

Respiratory System Adaptations

Respirations usually remain within the normal adult range of 16 to 24 breaths per minute. As the abdominal organs resume their nonpregnant position, the diaphragm returns to its usual position. Anatomic changes in the thoracic cavity and rib cage caused by increasing uterine growth resolve quickly. As a result, discomforts such as shortness of breath and rib aches are relieved. Tidal volume, minute volume, vital capacity, and functional residual capacity return to prepregnant values, typically within 1 to 3 weeks of birth (Mattson & Smith, 2015).

Endocrine System Adaptations

The endocrine system rapidly undergoes several changes after birth. Levels of circulating estrogen and progesterone drop quickly with delivery of the placenta. Decreased estrogen levels are associated with breast engorgement and with the diuresis of excess extracellular fluid accumulated during pregnancy (Creasy et al., 2014). Estrogen is at its lowest level a week after birth. While breastfeeding, estrogen levels remain low until the frequency baby

EVIDENCE-BASED PRACTICE 15.2

REDUCING POSTPARTUM WEIGHT RETENTION AND IMPROVING BREASTFEEDING OUTCOMES IN OVERWEIGHT WOMEN: A PILOT RANDOMIZED CONTROLLED TRIAL

Women naturally gain weight during pregnancy and many gradually lose it afterward. Some women, though, find it difficult to lose the pregnancy-related weight during the postpartum period and there is concern that this may be a health risk. The retention of weight gained during pregnancy may contribute to obesity. Obesity in the general population increases the risk of diabetes, heart disease, and high blood pressure. It is suggested that women who return to their prepregnancy weight by about 6 months after childbirth have a lower risk of being overweight 10 years later. Weight gain is also associated with lower rates of breastfeeding initiation and duration. The purpose of this randomized study was to help women reduce their postpartum weight retention and improve breastfeeding outcomes.

STUDY

Thirty-six women with a BMI of >25 were recruited, stratified by BMI and randomized to one of three groups with follow-up to 6 months postpartum. Women received a dietary intervention with or without breastfeeding support from a lactation consultant. All participants initiated breastfeeding, but the group that had lactation support had a longer duration of breastfeeding than the group without

the lactation support. In addition, the women with longer breastfeeding duration also lost the most weight during the 6-month period.

Findings

The study provided evidence to support the feasibility of providing overweight and obese women with targeted dietary advice and breastfeeding support to improve weight and breastfeeding outcomes.

Nursing Implications

Based on the findings of this study, nurses can recommend to their postpartum mothers desiring to lose their pregnancy weight should be encouraged to breastfeed and sustain it for at least six months to lose their pregnancy weight gained. Research findings associate breastfeeding with postpartum weight loss due to the increase in women's metabolic rates which burn calories. This information should be reported to postpartum mothers desiring to lose weight and breastfeed. Overall, if gained weight through the pregnancy isn't lost, their risk of cardiovascular diseases, diabetes, hypertension, and cancer will be increased as they age. The weight loss will help prevent these conditions or at the very least reduce their risks.

Adapted from Martin, J., MacDonald-Wicks, L., Hure, A., Smith, R., & Collins, C. E. (2015). Reducing postpartum weight retention and improving breastfeeding outcomes in overweight women: A pilot randomized controlled trial. *Nutrients, 7*(3), 1464–1479.

starts to wean If the client is not breastfeeding, estrogen levels begin to increase by 2 weeks after birth.

Other placental hormones (human chorionic gonadotropin [hCG], human placental lactogen [hPL], progesterone) decline rapidly after birth. The hCG levels are nonexistent at the end of the first postpartum week, and hPL is undetectable within 1 day after birth (Mattson & Smith, 2016). Progesterone levels are undetectable by 3 days after childbirth, and production is reestablished with the first menses. Prolactin is a hormone secreted by the anterior pituitary gland involved with lactation and reproduction. Prolactin levels remain elevated throughout lactation but decline within 2 weeks in clients who are not breastfeeding (Jin, Yu, Jin, Du, & Yang, 2015).

Weight Loss After Childbirth

Breastfeeding has many essential health implications for both mother and infant. Excessive weight gain in pregnancy and postpartum weight retention can increase the risk of obesity. Research has indicated that exclusive breastfeeding for a minimum of 3 months is associated with increased weight loss (Lopez-Olmedo et al., 2016).

The rate and amount of weight loss in the postpartum period seem to be determined by the same factors

that determine weight loss at any point in a person's life, including existing weight/body mass index (BMI), diet, age, and activity level (Nascimento, Pudwell, Surita, Adamo, & Smith, 2014). Thus, there is also benefit from overall lifestyle interventions on weight loss in postpartum clients which include exercise plus dietary changes to achieve their weight reduction goals. See Evidence-Based Practice 15.2.

> **Think back to Betsy, the woman experiencing painful changes in her breasts. What is Betsy describing to the lactation consultant? Why has the condition of her breasts changed compared with when she was in the hospital?**

Global Health of Childbearing Individuals

Globalization has changed our society in numerous ways, yet the health of women is remaining stagnant or growing worse in many parts of the world. Many women in developing counties are denied their fundamental right to enjoy a complete state of health as defined by the World Health Organization (Boyd-Judson & James, 2014). More than half a million women die each year from complications during and after childbirth (bleeding and infections), the vast majority of them in Africa and Asia (Webber & Chirangi, 2014).

Women throughout the world continue to face enormous obstacles in attempting to access obstetric care. Skilled attendance at childbirth is critical for decreasing postpartum and neonatal mortality, yet many women in developing countries give birth outside health facilities, without skilled help. Nurses throughout the world can help advocate for cost-effective, evidence-based interventions to prevent and battle complications from childbirth to save clients' lives. The challenge is to guarantee that every pregnant individual who needs care gets it. Nurses can make a difference outside their own country's borders by advocating for all international clients through their governmental political systems and encouraging those governments to offer help and save lives.

Lactation

Lactation is the secretion of milk by the breasts. It is thought to be brought about by the interaction of progesterone, estrogen, prolactin, and oxytocin. Breastmilk typically appears within 4 to 5 days after childbirth.

BREASTFEEDING

Breastfeeding is a dynamic process, which requires coupling between periodic motions of the infant's jaws, undulation of the tongue, and breastmilk ejection reflex. All mechanisms must be coordinated to be successful. All major health organizations recommend breastfeeding. The Canadian Pediatrics Society (CPS) recommends exclusive breastfeeding for 6 months (CPS, 2016), followed by the introduction of appropriate complementary foods and continued breastfeeding to 2 years and beyond (CPS, 2017). These recommendations are considered the standard of care today. Nurses have an important role in promoting, supporting, and protecting breastfeeding. Proper positioning, latching-on, sucking, and swallowing are the foundation for successful breastfeeding. Although breastfeeding is recommended by international and national organizations, the nurse must respect and support all mothers in either infant feeding method chosen.

During pregnancy, the breasts increase in size and functional ability in preparation for breastfeeding. Estrogen stimulates growth of the milk collection (ductal) system, whereas progesterone stimulates growth of the milk production system. Within the 1st month of gestation, the ducts of the mammary glands grow branches, forming more lobules and alveoli. These structural changes make the breasts larger, more tender, and heavy. Each breast gains nearly 1 pound in weight by term, the glandular cells fill with secretions, blood vessels increase in number, and the amounts of connective tissue and fat cells increase (Engel, Kon, Mawson, & Folley, 2015).

Prolactin from the anterior pituitary gland, secreted in increasing levels throughout pregnancy, triggers the synthesis and secretion of milk after giving birth. During pregnancy, prolactin, estrogen, and progesterone cause synthesis and secretion of *colostrum*, which contains protein and carbohydrate but no milk fat. It is only after birth takes place, when the high levels of estrogen and progesterone are abruptly withdrawn, that prolactin is able to stimulate the glandular cells to secrete milk instead of colostrum. This takes place within 3 to 5 days after giving birth.

Prolactin and oxytocin result in milk production if stimulated by sucking. The newborn's sucking will release milk by stimulating oxytocin which causes milk to be ejected from the alveoli down to the nipple. Prolactin levels also increase in response to nipple stimulation during feedings. Therefore, a decrease in the quality of stimulation causes a decrease in prolactin surges and thus a decrease in milk production (Stuebe, Meltzer-Brody, Pearson, Pedersen, & Grewen, 2015) (Fig. 15.3). If a postpartum client is not breastfeeding, breast engorgement and milk production will subside within days postpartum as the stimulus (sucking) is not present.

Skin-to-skin contact during the first 1 to 2 hours following birth is the gold standard to initiate breastfeeding. A newborn's instinct is to seek nourishment after birth. When placed on their mother's abdomen, they will move upward to the breast instinctively. This instinct arises when a newborn, left undisturbed and skin-to-skin on the mother's trunk following birth, moves toward her/his mother's breast for the purpose of locating and self-attaching for the first feeding. From there, the newborn uses leg and arm movements to propel her/himself toward the breast. Upon reaching the sternum, the newborn will bounce her/his head up and down and side to side. As the newborn approaches the nipple, his/her mouth opens and, after several attempts, latch-on and suckling take place. Newborns have senses and skills that enable early initiation of feeding at the breast. Researchers termed this movement the *breast crawl* that helps initiate breastfeeding immediately after childbirth. Nurses can help facilitate the breast crawl as a continuation of the birthing process. Nurses have a responsibility to promote the health of their childbearing families and provide evidence-based care. Encouraging use of the breast crawl can be the first step in health promotion for every newborn (Zanardo & Straface, 2015).

Breastmilk production can be summarized as follows:

- Prolactin levels increase at term with a decrease in estrogen and progesterone levels.
- Estrogen and progesterone levels decrease after the placenta is delivered.

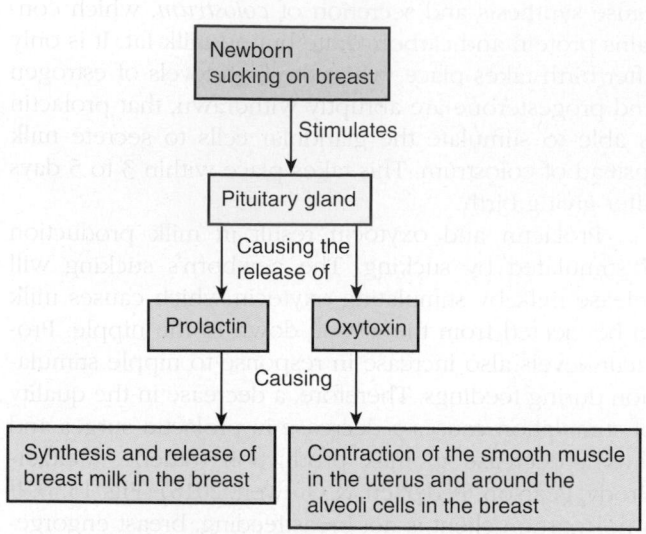

```
┌──────────────────────┐
│ Newborn              │
│ sucking on breast    │
└──────────────────────┘
           │
       Stimulates
           ↓
┌──────────────────────┐
│ Pituitary gland      │
└──────────────────────┘
     Causing the
     release of
           │
    ┌──────┴──────┐
    ↓             ↓
┌──────────┐  ┌──────────┐
│ Prolactin│  │ Oxytoxin │
└──────────┘  └──────────┘
         Causing
    │             │
    ↓             ↓
┌────────────────┐ ┌──────────────────────────┐
│ Synthesis and  │ │ Contraction of the smooth│
│ release of     │ │ muscle in the uterus and │
│ breast milk in │ │ around the alveoli cells │
│ the breast     │ │ in the breast            │
└────────────────┘ └──────────────────────────┘
```

FIGURE 15.3 Physiology of lactation.

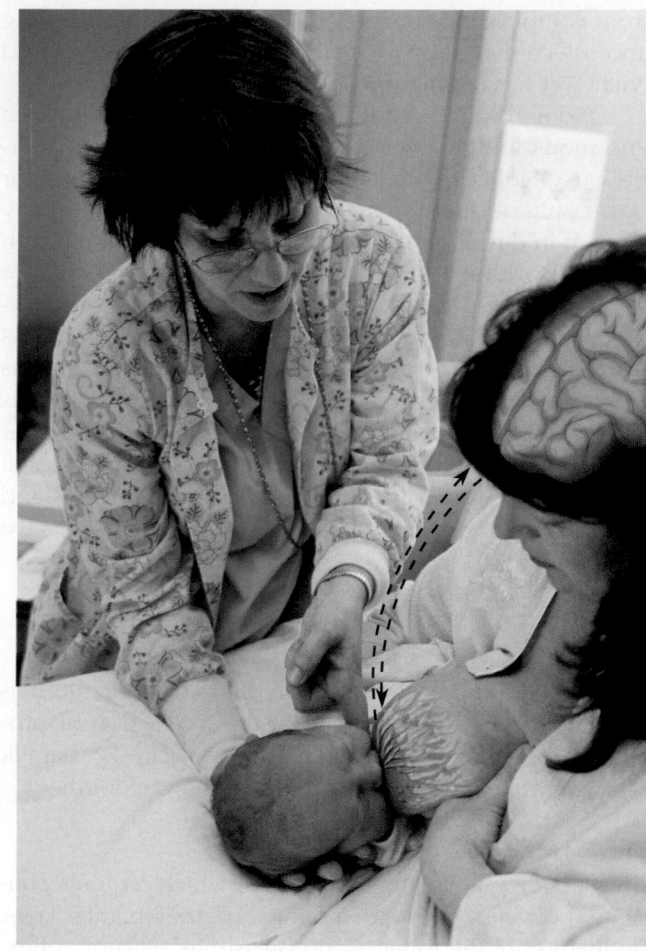

- Prolactin is released from the anterior pituitary gland and initiates milk production.
- Oxytocin is released from the posterior pituitary gland to promote milk let-down.
- Infant sucking at each feeding provides continuous stimulus for prolactin and oxytocin release (Wambach & Riordan, 2014).

Typically, during the first 2 days after birth, the breasts are soft and nontender. The postpartum client also may report a tingling sensation in the breasts, which is the "let-down reflex" that occurs immediately before or during breastfeeding. After this time, breast changes depend on whether the client is breastfeeding or taking measures to prevent lactation.

Engorgement is a physiologic painful condition during the postnatal period in which distention and swelling of the breast tissue occurs due to an increase in blood and lymph supply as a precursor to lactation (Fig. 15.4). Breast engorgement usually peaks in 3 to 5 days postpartum and usually subsides within the following 24 to 36 hours (Alekseev, Vladimir, & Nadezhda, 2015). Engorgement can occur from infrequent feeding

or ineffective emptying of the breasts and typically lasts about 24 hours. Breasts increase in vascularity and swell in response to prolactin 2 to 4 days after birth. If engorged, the breasts will be hard and tender to touch. They are temporarily full, tender, and very uncomfortable until the milk supply is ready. Frequent emptying of the breasts helps to minimize discomfort and resolve engorgement. Standing in a warm shower or applying warm compresses immediately before feedings will help to soften the breasts and nipples in order to allow the newborn to latch on more easily.

Treatments to reduce the pain of breast engorgement include heat or cold applications, cabbage leaf compresses, breast massage and milk expression, ultrasound, breast pumping, and anti-inflammatory agents (King et al., 2015). A nonprescription anti-inflammatory medication can also be taken for the breast discomfort and swelling resulting from engorgement. These measures will also enhance the let-down reflex. Between feedings, applying cold compresses to the breasts helps to reduce swelling. To maintain milk supply, the breasts need to be stimulated by a nursing infant, a breast pump, or manual expression of the milk (Fig. 15.5).

A **B1** **B2**

FIGURE 15.4 **A:** Image of engorged breasts. Note swelling and inflammation of both breasts. **B:** Breast engorgement can disrupt breastfeeding: (1) When sucking at a normal breast, the infant's lips compress the areola and fit neatly against the sides of the nipple. The infant also has adequate room to breathe. (2) When a breast is engorged, however, the infant has difficulty grasping the nipple and breathing ability is compromised. (From Pillitteri, A. [2014]. *Maternal and child nursing* [7th ed.]. Philadelphia, PA: Lippincott Williams & Wilkins.)

Remember Betsy, with the breast discomfort? The lactation consultant explained that she was experiencing normal breast engorgement and offered several suggestions to help her. What relief measures might she have suggested? What reassurance can be given to Betsy at this time?

SUPPRESSING LACTATION

While the vast majority of newborns are breastfed in Canada, approximately 11% of newborns are formula fed from birth (Gionet, 2015). Various pharmacologic and nonpharmacologic interventions have been used to suppress lactation after childbirth and relieve associated symptoms for those choosing not to breastfeed. Despite the large volume of literature on the subject, there is currently no universal guideline on the most appropriate

FIGURE 15.5 Nurse instructs the new breastfeeding mother about use of a breast pump. (Copyright B. Proud.)

approach for suppressing lactation in the postpartum period (Cunningham et al., 2014). Although physiologic cessation of lactation eventually occurs in the absence of physical stimulus such as infant suckling, a large number of clients experience moderate to severe milk leakage and discomfort before lactation ceases.

Up to two thirds of non–breastfeeding clients experience moderate to severe engorgement and breast pain when no treatment is applied (Spencer, 2015). If a client does not desire to breastfeed, some relief measures include wearing a firm, supportive bra 24 hours daily, applying ice to the breasts for approximately 15 to 20 minutes every other hour, avoiding sexual stimulation, and not stimulating the breasts by squeezing or manually expressing milk from the nipples. In addition, avoiding exposing the breasts to warmth (e.g., a hot shower) will help relieve breast engorgement. In those who are not breastfeeding, engorgement typically subsides within 2 to 3 days with application of these measures.

Ovulation and Return of Menstruation

Changing hormone levels constantly interact with one another to produce bodily changes. Four major hormones are influential during the postpartum period: estrogen, progesterone, prolactin, and oxytocin. Estrogen plays a major role during pregnancy, but levels drop profoundly at birth and reach their lowest level a week into the postpartum period. Progesterone quiets the uterus to prevent a preterm birth during pregnancy, and its increasing levels during pregnancy prevent lactation from starting before birth takes place. As with estrogen, progesterone levels decrease dramatically after birth and are undetectable 72 hours after birth. Progesterone levels are reestablished with the first menstrual cycle (Creasy et al., 2014).

During the postpartum period, oxytocin stimulates the uterus to contract during the breastfeeding session and for as long as 20 minutes after each feeding. Oxytocin also acts on the breast by eliciting the milk let-down reflex during breastfeeding. Prolactin is also associated with the breastfeeding process by stimulating milk production. In clients who breastfeed, prolactin levels remain elevated into the 6th week after birth (Bope & Kellerman, 2015). The levels of prolactin fluctuate in proportion to nipple stimulation. Prolactin levels decrease in nonlactating client, reaching prepregnant levels by the third postpartum week. High levels of prolactin have been found to delay ovulation by inhibiting ovarian response to follicle-stimulating hormone (Bernard, Young, Chanson, & Binart, 2015).

The timing of first menses and ovulation after birth differs between those who are breastfeeding and those who are not. For nonlactating clients, menstruation may resume as early as 7 to 9 weeks after giving birth, but the majority take up to 3 months (Barrett, Parlett, Windham, & Swan, 2014). The return of menses in the lactating client depends on breastfeeding frequency and duration. It can return any time after childbirth, depending on whether the client is exclusively breastfeeding or supplementing with formula.

Take Note!

Ovulation may occur before menstruation. Therefore, breastfeeding is not a totally reliable method of contraception unless the client exclusively breastfeeds, has had no menstrual period since giving birth, and whose infant is younger than 6 months old (Alexander, LaRosa, Bader, & Garfield, 2014).

Betsy tries several of the measures the lactation consultant suggested to relieve her breast discomfort, but is still having heaviness and pain. She feels discouraged and tells the nurse she is thinking of reducing her breastfeeding and using formula to feed her newborn. Is that a good choice? Why or why not? What interventions will help Betsy get through this difficult time?

CULTURAL CONSIDERATIONS FOR THE POSTPARTUM PERIOD

Cultures vary in their postpartum beliefs, practices, and customs. Nurses practice in an increasingly multicultural society. Therefore, they must be open, respectful, nonjudgmental, and willing to learn about ethnically diverse populations. Although childbirth and the postpartum period are unique experiences for each individual, how the client perceives and makes meaning of these is culturally defined. For example, Somali women are highly regarded in Somali society for their roles as mothers. Postpartum women stay at home and refrain from sexual activity for 40 days. At the end of 40 days, there is a celebration, and this typically marks the first time the mother and infant have left their home since childbirth. The majority of Somalian and Arab women breastfeed and do so for extended periods of time (Wojnar & Narruhn, 2016). Nurses need to offer early breastfeeding instruction to support their efforts while still in the hospital setting before discharge.

Balance of Hot and Cold

Two areas that are significantly different from Western culture involve beliefs about the balance of hot and cold and confinement after childbirth. Vietnamese clients view the postpartum period as a cold state (duong) and protect themselves through warmth. Cultural practices include warm water for hygiene and stimulation of lactation, consuming warm foods, and staying indoors. In Canada, childbearing and recovery are viewed as healthy states and clients receive little formal support for both their recovery and infant care. In China, childbearing and postpartum are viewed as states which disturb the normal health balance between yin and yang. In order to restore balance in health, postpartum clients engage in practices for a month related to physical activity, maintenance of body warmth, and certain food consumption that will restore their balance. Recent research findings in a small sample of Chinese women found that postpartum confinement negatively correlated with aerobic endurance and positively correlated with depression. These findings may challenge the assumption that practices of confinement are healthy for Chinese women's recovery after childbirth (Liu, Maloni, & Petrini, 2014).

For many cultures, good health requires the balancing of hot and cold substances. Because childbirth involves the loss of blood, which is considered hot, the postpartum period is considered cold, so the mother must balance that with the intake of hot food. Foods consumed should be hot in nature, and cold foods, such as fruits and vegetables, avoided. Western practices frequently use cold packs or sitz baths to reduce perineal swelling and discomfort. These practices are not acceptable to clients of many cultures and can be viewed as harmful. Hot–cold beliefs are common among Latin American, African, and Asian people (Purnell, 2014).

To reduce vulnerability and potential illness in the newborn/postpartum period, families may practice a month-long confinement period after childbirth. During this confinement period, new mothers rest and recuperate. The postpartum period is a time to avoid cold—both in temperature and foods. Women are kept warm, stay inside to prevent becoming chilled, bathe infrequently, and avoid exercise (Rice & Manderson, 2014).

Postpartum Cultural Beliefs

With increasing multiculturalism in Canada, understanding various cultures' views of the postnatal period as it relates to their recovery and well-being after childbirth is important for all nurses. Postpartum nurses need to understand these diverse cultural beliefs and provide creative strategies for encouraging hygiene (sponge baths, perineal care), exercise, and balanced nutrition, while remaining respectful of the cultural significance of these practices. The best approach is to ask all clients to describe what cultural practices are important to them and plan accordingly.

PSYCHOLOGICAL ADAPTATIONS

The process of becoming a mother (BAM) requires extensive psychological, social, and physical work. Women experience heightened vulnerability and face tremendous challenges as they make this transition. Nurses have a remarkable opportunity to help clients learn, gain confidence, and experience growth as they assume the parental identity.

The transition to parenthood, while an exciting time to celebrate the life of their child, causes parents to face new challenges such as physical exhaustion, role overload, and less time for themselves and their partners (Public Health Agency of Canada, 2019). Parents' experiences of pregnancy are necessarily different, and this difference continues after childbirth as they adjust to their new parenting roles. Many people and couples struggle to adapt to parenthood. Parenting involves caring for infants physically and emotionally to foster the growth and development of responsible, caring adults. A substantial body of research finds no biologically based differences between mothers and fathers in sensitivity to infants, capacity to provide care, or acquisition of parenting skills. Within 15 minutes of holding a newborn, men experience raised levels of oxytocin, cortisol, and prolactin. The increased levels of these nurturing hormones are the same in men and women exposed to infants (Davies, 2015). Other members of the newborn's family, such as siblings and grandparents, also experience changes related to the birth of the newborn (see Chapter 16). Early parent–infant contact after birth improves attachment behaviours.

Parental Attachment Behaviours

The postpartum period is a unique time distinguished by the inseparable relationship parents have with their newborn. To enable an attachment to be built, closeness of this family unit is essential. **Attachment** is the formation of a relationship between a parent and his or her newborn through a process of physical and emotional interactions. Attachment between a client and her newborn has lifelong implications (King et al., 2015). Attachment has the potential to affect both child development and parenting. The bond between a parent and their newborn is one of strength, power, and potential. Attachment begins before birth, during the prenatal period where acceptance and nurturing of the growing fetus takes place. It continues after giving birth as parents learn to recognize their newborn's cues, adapt to their newborn's behaviours and responses, and meet their newborn's needs.

Several factors take place during the early postpartum period that can have a large influence on the attachment/bonding that occurs during this time. Oxytocin plays an essential role in the chemistry aspect of bonding, and its effects can be enhanced by skin-to-skin contact, breastfeeding, eye contact, social vocalizations, and milk odours, which are soothing for the newborn, and newborn message during the first postpartum hour (Hutcheson & Cheeseman, 2015; Buckley, 2015).

Early and sustained contact between newborns and their parents is vital for initiating their relationship.

Nurses play a crucial role in assisting the attachment process by promoting early parent–newborn interactions. In addition, nurses can facilitate skin-to-skin contact (kangaroo care) by placing the infant onto the bare chests of mothers and fathers to enhance parent–newborn attachment. This activity will enable them to get close to their newborn and experience an intense feeling of connectedness and evoke feelings of being nurturing parents. Encouraging breastfeeding is another way to foster attachment between clients and their newborns. Finally, nurses can encourage nurturing activities and contact such as touching, talking, singing, comforting, changing diapers, feeding—in short, participating in routine newborn care.

The process of attachment is complex and is influenced by many factors including environmental circumstances, the newborn's health status, and the quality of nursing care (Buckley, 2015). Nurses need to minimize parent–newborn separation by promoting parent–newborn interactions through kangaroo care, breastfeeding, and participation in their newborn care. Nurses who provide positive psychosocial support and clear communication to parents will help support the attachment process within family units.

Psychological Adaptations

Childbirth is a joyous period in a client's life involving such spiritual experiences as giving birth and being able to give life to another being. For many, this can be a life-changing event. Childbirth and child rearing can also be very stressful, financially challenging, and emotionally demanding.

Mood Disorders

Although many people consider childbirth a time of happiness and well-being, it is common for new parents to experience changes in their mood during this time. These changes may include being fatigued, irritable, or worried, and frequently these mood symptoms become severe enough to seek intervention from health care professionals. In the postpartum period, mood disorders can be divided into three distinct entities in ascending order of severity: baby blues, postpartum depression, and psychosis. Differences between these have not been clearly demarcated and the severity of their effects is often variable and sometimes debated (Finley & Brizendine, 2015).

Up to 85% of new mothers suffer from the short-lived postpartum mood disorder termed "baby blues" which is characterized by mild depressive symptoms, anxiety, irritability, mood swings, loss of appetite, trouble with sleeping, unexplained tearfulness increased sensitivity, and fatigue (Flynn, 2015). The "blues" typically peak on postpartum days 4 and 5, may last hours to days, and usually resolve by day 10. Although these symptoms may be distressing, they do not reflect psychopathology, and they typically do not affect the mother's ability to function and care for her child. For additional information on perinatal mood disorders, see Chapter 22.

Phases of Adaptation to Parenthood

Parenthood is a highly anticipated and positive event for most clients. Society has constructed many ideal images of motherhood, in particular, giving standards for women to live up to, and frequently setting them up for disappointment. Most clients are able to experience this mismatch between their ideal and actual self and adapt with minimal discrepancy (Adams, 2015). The client experiences a variety of responses as she adjusts to a new family member and to postpartum discomforts, changes in her body image, and the reality of change in her life. In the early 1960s, Reva Rubin identified three phases that a mother goes through to adjust to her new role. Rubin's maternal role framework can be used to monitor the client's progress as she "tries on" her new role as a mother. The absence of these processes or inability to progress through the phases satisfactorily may impede the appropriate development of the role (Rubin, 1984). Although Rubin's maternal role development theories are of value, some of her observations regarding the length of each phase may not be completely relevant for the contemporary childbearing individuals of the 21st century. Today, many parents know their infant's sex, have "seen" their fetus in utero through four-dimensional ultrasound, and have a working knowledge of childbirth and child care. They are less passive than in years past and progress

through the phases of attaining the parental role at a much faster pace than Rubin would have imagined. Still, Rubin's framework is timeless for assessing and monitoring expected role behaviours when planning care and appropriate interventions.

TAKING-IN PHASE

The **taking-in phase** is the time immediately after birth when the client needs sleep, depends on others to meet her needs, and relives the events surrounding the birth process. This phase is characterized by dependent behaviour. During the first 24 to 48 hours after giving birth, clients often assume a very passive role in meeting their own basic needs for food, fluids, and rest, allowing the nurse to make decisions for them concerning activities and care. They spend time recounting their labour experience to anyone who will listen. Such actions help the client integrate the birth experience into reality—that is, the pregnancy is over, and the newborn is now a unique individual, separate from herself. When interacting with the newborn, new mothers spend time claiming the newborn and touching him or her, commonly identifying specific features in the newborn, such as "he has my nose" or "his fingers are long like his father's" (Fig. 15.6).

Take Note!
The taking-in phase typically lasts 1 to 2 days and may be the only phase observed by nurses in the hospital setting because of the shortened length of hospital stays postpartum.

TAKING-HOLD PHASE

The **taking-hold phase**, the second phase of adaptation, is characterized by dependent and independent

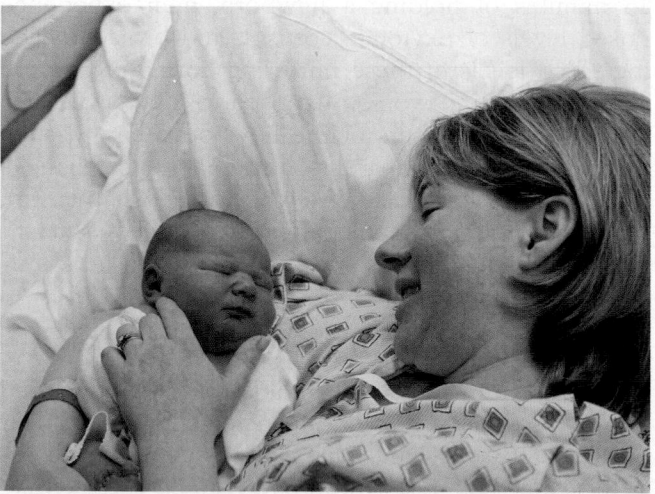

FIGURE 15.6 Mother bonding with newborn during the taking-in phase.

maternal behaviour. This phase typically starts on the 2nd to 3rd day postpartum and may last several weeks.

As the client regains control over her bodily functions during the next few days, she will be taking hold and becoming preoccupied with the present. She will be particularly concerned about her health, the infant's condition, and her ability to care for her or him. She demonstrates increased autonomy and mastery of her own body's functioning, and a desire to take charge with support and help from others. She will show independence by caring for herself and learning to care for her newborn, but she still requires assurance that she is doing well as a mother. She expresses a strong interest in caring for her newborn by herself.

LETTING-GO PHASE

In the **letting-go phase**, the third phase of maternal adaptation, the client reestablishes relationships with other people. She adapts to parenthood through her new role postpartum. She assumes the responsibility and care of the newborn with a bit more confidence now (Edelman, Kudzma, & Mandle, 2014). The focus of this phase is to move forward by assuming the parental role and to separate herself from the symbiotic relationship that she and her newborn had during pregnancy. She establishes a lifestyle that includes the infant. The client relinquishes the fantasy infant and accepts the real one.

Nurses have recognized the importance of the process of BAM to maternal–infant nursing since Rubin's report on maternal role attainment (MRA). Mothers' perceptions of their competence or confidence, or both, in mothering and their expressions of love for their newborns include age, relationship with the partner, socioeconomic status, birth experience, experienced stress, available support, personality traits, self-concept, child-rearing attitudes, role strain, health status, preparation during pregnancy, relationships with own mother, depression, and anxiety. Newborn variables identified as influencing MRA/BAM include appearance, responsiveness, temperament, and health status (DiPietro, Goldshore, Kivlighan, Pater, & Costigan, 2015). More current research has led to renaming the four stages a client progresses through in establishing a maternal identity in BAM:

1. Commitment, attachment to the unborn baby, and preparation for delivery and motherhood during pregnancy
2. Acquaintance/attachment to the infant, learning to care for the infant, and physical restoration during the first 2 to 6 weeks following birth
3. Moving toward a new normal
4. Achievement of a maternal identity through redefining self to incorporate motherhood (around 4 months). The mother feels self-confident and competent in her mothering and expresses love for and pleasure interacting with her infant (Mercer & Walker, 2006)

The client's work in the first stage is to make a commitment to the pregnancy and to the safe birth and care of her unborn child. This commitment is associated with a positive adaptation to motherhood. During the second stage while the client is placing the newborn in her family context and learning how to care for her newborn, her attachment and attitude toward her newborn, and her self-confidence or sense of competence in mothering, or both, consistently indicate an interdependence of these two variables. The nursing care provided during the first two stages is especially important in assisting clients as they begin to nurture. Follow-up by nurses is needed as clients move toward a new normal and recognize that a transformation of self in BAM. Nurses can continue to reinforce their new mothering capabilities (Mercer, 2006).

To foster MRA, three specific interventions for nurses were identified in a review of the literature (Ferrarello & Hatfield, 2014). First, instructions about newborn care and the newborn's capabilities are more effective if they are specifically focused on that particular client's newborn. Second, clients prefer live classes rather than videotapes so they can ask questions. In short, interactive nurse–client relationships are associated with positive maternal growth. Third, identifying barriers that reduce skin-to-skin periods of mother-to-infant during the postpartum hospital stay and intervening to reduce them have implications for both maternal role development and breastfeeding success. Providing times for skin-to-skin client and newborn contact has a positive impact on the long-term health of both. Nurses who interact with clients' long term during pregnancy, childbirth, and during well child care help build maternal competence. Pregnancy, birth, and becoming a parent collectively represent a critical period of physical and emotional upheaval in a person's life. The need for a holistic care approach that supports the emotional and physical health of the dyad is imperative (Spiteri, Borg Xuereb, Carrick-Sen, Kaner, & Martin, 2014).

Transition to motherhood theories (Rubin and Mercer) describe women in a prescribed role—that of being a mother and indeed a predetermined type of mother. In that sense transition to motherhood theory is baby-centred. New theories need to be developed that are person-centred and which conceptualize the parent as an embodied self who is powerful in their own life.

Partner Psychological Adaptations

For partners, whether they are husbands, wives, significant others, boyfriends, life partners, or just friends, becoming a parent or just sharing the childbirth experience can be a perplexing time as well as a time of great change. This transition is influenced by many factors, including participation in childbirth, relationships with significant others, competence in child care, the family role organization, the individual's cultural background, and the method of infant feeding.

The transition from being merely a partner to being a parent can propel many partners to reorganize their lifestyles. During the postpartum period, partners frequently find themselves struggling to balance personal and work needs with the new demands of parent status and their new self-image. The complexities of the transitional process involved in forging a parenthood identity can be viewed at three different levels: readjustment to a new self-image, formation of a triadic family relationship, and adaptation to redefining themselves and their relationship with their partner: the "more united tag team" (Halford, Petch, & Creedy, 2015).

Nurses can play a key role in supporting a partner's transition to parenthood by keeping partners informed about birth and postpartum routines, reporting on their newborn's health status, and reviewing infant development. They can also contribute by creating participative space for new partners during the postpartum period. This can be achieved, for example, by helping partners take on their new role by supporting and promoting their degree of involvement in the process. They can also be encouraged to actively participate in caring for, and maintaining contact with, their newborns.

Take Note!

Most research findings stress the importance of early contact between the partner or significant other and the newborn, as well as participation in infant care activities, to foster the relationship (Nolan, 2015).

Infants have a powerful effect on their parents and others, who become intensely involved with them (Fig. 15.7). The father's or partner's developing bond with the newborn—a time of intense absorption, preoccupation, and interest—is called **engrossment**.

Engrossment

Engrossment is characterized by seven behaviours:
1. Visual awareness of the newborn—the partner perceives the newborn as attractive, pretty, or beautiful.
2. Tactile awareness of the newborn—the partner has a desire to touch or hold the newborn and considers this activity to be pleasurable.
3. Perception of the newborn as perfect—the partner does not "see" any imperfections.
4. Strong attraction to the newborn—the partner focuses all attention on the newborn when they are in the room.
5. Awareness of distinct features of the newborn—the partner can distinguish his/her newborn from others in the nursery.

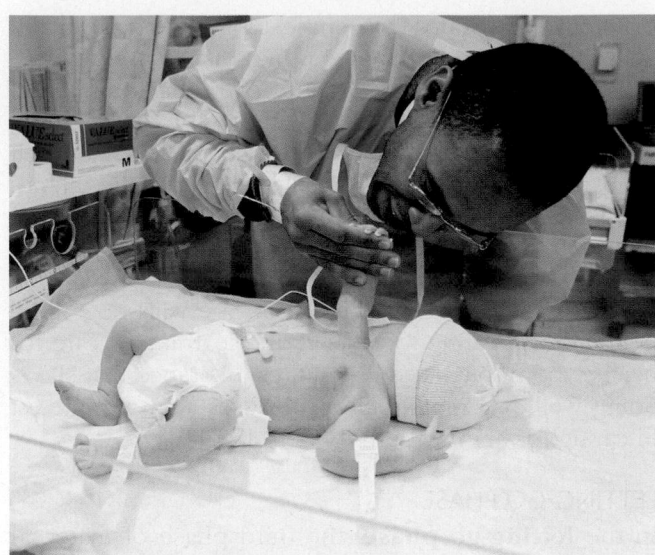

FIGURE 15.7 **Engrossment of the father and his newborn.**

6. Extreme elation—the partner feels a "high" after the birth of his/her child.
7. Increased sense of self-esteem—the partner feels proud, "bigger," more mature, and older after the birth of his/her child (Sears & Sears, 2018).

Frequently, partners are portrayed as well-meaning but bumbling when caring for newborns. However, they have their own unique way of relating to their newborns and can become as nurturing as mothers. A partner's nurturing responses may be less automatic and slower to unfold than a biologic mother's, but they are capable of a strong bonding attachment to their newborns (Sears & Sears, 2018). Encouraging partners to express their feelings by seeing, touching, and holding their son or daughter and by cuddling, talking to, and feeding him or her will help to cement this new relationship. Reinforcement of this engrossing behaviour helps partners to make a positive attachment during this critical period.

Three-Stage Role Development Process

Similar to mothers, partners also go through a predictable three-stage process during the first 3 weeks as they too "try on" their roles as parents. The three stages are expectations, reality, and transition to mastery (Sears & Sears, 2018).

STAGE 1: EXPECTATIONS
New partners pass through stage 1 (expectations) with preconceptions about what home life will be like with a newborn. Many partners may be unaware of the dramatic changes that can occur when this newborn comes home to live with them. For some, it is an eye-opening experience.

STAGE 2: REALITY

Stage 2 (reality) occurs when partners realize that their expectations in stage 1 are not realistic. Their feelings change from elation to sadness, ambivalence, jealousy, and frustration. Many wish to be more involved in the newborn's care and yet do not feel prepared to do so. Some find parenting fun but at the same time do not feel fully prepared to take on that role.

Partner's stress, irritability, and frustration in the days, weeks, and months after the birth of their child can turn into depression, just like new parental experience. Unfortunately, partners rarely discuss their feelings or ask for help, especially during a time when they are supposed to be the "strong one" for the new mother. Depression in partners can cause marital conflicts, reckless or violent behaviour, withdrawn parental interactions with the newborn, poor job performance, and substance abuse. In addition, paternal depression following childbirth can have a detrimental effect on a couple's relationship, on the parent–child relationship, and on their children's future development (Sethna, Murray, Netsi, Psychogiou, & Ramchandani, 2015).

Risk factors for partner postpartum depression include previous history of depression, financial problems, a poor relationship with his/her partner, and an unplanned pregnancy. Symptoms of depression appear 1 to 3 weeks after birth and can include feelings of being very stressed and anxious, being discouraged or fatigued, resentment toward the infant and the attention he or she is getting, and headaches. Partners experiencing these symptoms should understand that it is not a sign of weakness and professional help can be helpful for them.

STAGE 3: TRANSITION TO MASTERY

In stage 3 (transition to mastery), the partner makes a conscious decision to take control and be at the centre of his/her newborn's life regardless of his/her preparedness. This adjustment period is similar to that of the client's letting-go phase, when she incorporates the newest member into the family.

KEY CONCEPTS

- The puerperium period refers to the first 6 weeks after delivery. During this period, the postpartum client experiences many physiologic and psychological adaptations to return to the prepregnant state.

- Involution involves three processes: contraction of muscle fibers to reduce stretched ones, catabolism (which reduces enlarged, individual cells), and regeneration of uterine epithelium from the lower layer of the decidua after the upper layers have been sloughed off and shed in lochia.

- Lochia passes through three stages—lochia rubra, lochia serosa, and lochia alba—during the postpartum period.

- The postpartum client's blood plasma volume decreases rapidly after birth and returns to normal within 4 weeks postpartum.

- Reva Rubin (1984) identified three phases the mother goes through to adjust to her new maternal role: the taking-in, taking-hold, and letting-go phases.

- The transition to fatherhood/coparenthood is influenced by many factors, including participation in childbirth, relationships with significant others, competence in child care, the family role organization, the father's cultural background, and the method of infant feeding.

- Like mothers, partners go through a predictable three-stage process during the first 3 weeks as they too "try on" their roles as partners. The three stages include expectations, reality, and transition to mastery.

REFERENCES AND RECOMMENDED READING

Adams, M. (2015). Motherhood: A discrepancy theory. *Research and Theory for Nursing Practice, 29*(2), 143–157.

Alekseev, N. P., Vladimir, I. I., & Nadezhda, T. E. (2015). Pathological postpartum breast engorgement: Prediction, prevention, and resolution. *Breastfeeding Medicine, 10*(4), 203–208.

Alexander, L. L., LaRosa, J. H., Bader, H., & Garfield, S. (2014). *New dimensions in women's health* (6th ed.). Sudbury, MA: Jones & Bartlett.

American Academy of Pediatrics [AAP]. (2015). *Caring for your baby and young child: Birth to age 5* (6th ed.). Elk Grove Village, IL: AAP.

Barrett, E. S., Parlett, L. E., Windham, G. C., & Swan, S. H. (2014). Differences in ovarian hormones in relation to parity and time since last birth. *Fertility & Sterility, 101*(6), 1773–1780.

Bernard, V., Young, J., Chanson, P., & Binart, N. (2015). New insights in prolactin: Pathological implications. *Nature Reviews Endocrinology, 11*(5), 265–275.

Bope, E., & Kellerman, R. (2015). *Conn's current therapy 2015*. Philadelphia, PA: Saunders Elsevier.

Bowers, P., & Ceballos, K.. (2015). Cultural perspectives in childbearing. *Nurse.com*. Retrieved from http://ce.nurse.com/course/ce263-60/cultural-perspectives-in-childbearing.

Boyd-Judson, L., & James, P. (2014). *Women's global health: Norms and state policies*. Plymouth, UK: Lexington Books.

Buckley, S. (2015). *Hormonal physiology of childbearing: Evidence and implications for women, babies and maternity care*. Washington, DC: Childbirth Connection, National Partnership for Women & Families.

Canadian Pediatric Society. (2016). *Nutrition for healthy term infants, birth to six months: An overview*. Retrieved from https://www.cps.ca/en/documents/position/nutrition-healthy-term-infants-overview.

Canadian Pediatric Society. (2017). *Nutrition for healthy term infants, six to 24 months: An overview*. Retrieved from https://www.cps.ca/en/documents/position/nutrition-healthy-term-infants-6-to-24-months.

Creasy, R. K., Resnik, R., Iams, J. D., Lockwood, C. J., Moore, T. R., & Greene, M. F. (2014). *Creasy & Resnik's maternal-fetal medicine: Principles and practice* (7th ed.). Philadelphia, PA: Elsevier Saunders.

Cunningham, F. G., Leveno, K. J., Bloom, S. L., Spong, C., Dashe, J. S., Hoffman, B. L., … Sheffield, J. S. (2014). *Williams obstetrics* (24th ed.). New York: McGraw-Hill Publishers.

Davies, J. (2015). Fatherhood Institute: Supporting fathers to play their part. *Community Practitioner, 88*(1), 13–14.

DiPietro, J. A., Goldshore, M. A., Kivlighan, K. T., Pater, H. A., & Costigan, K. A. (2015). The ups and downs of early mothering. *Journal of Psychosomatic Obstetrics & Gynecology*, 1–9.

Dumoulin, C., Hay-Smith, E. J., & Mac Habée-Séguin, G. (2014). Pelvic floor muscle training versus no treatment, or inactive control treatments, for urinary incontinence in women. *Cochrane Database of Systematic Reviews, 5*, CD005654.

Edelman, C. L., Kudzma, E. C., & Mandle, C. L. (2014). *Health promotion throughout the lifespan* (8th ed.). St. Louis, MO: Mosby Elsevier.

Engel, S., Kon, S. K., Mawson, E. H., & Folley, S. J. (2015). Discussion of some recent developments in knowledge of the physiology of the breast. *Proceedings of the Royal Society of Medicine, 40*, 899–906.

Evans, A. T., & De Franco, E. (2014). *Manual of obstetrics* (8th ed.). Philadelphia, PA: Lippincott Williams & Wilkins.

Ferrarello, D., & Hatfield, L. (2014). Barriers to skin-to-skin care during the postpartum stay. *MCN. The American Journal of Maternal Child Nursing, 39*(1), 56–61.

Finley, P. R., & Brizendine, L. (2015). Enhancing our understanding of perinatal depression. *CNS Spectrums, 20*(1), 9–10.

Flynn, R. (2015). Mood disorders during and after pregnancy. *South African Journal of Diabetes, 8*(2), 27–33.

Gionet, L. (2015). *Breastfeeding trends in Canada. Statistics Canada catalogue no. 82-624-X*. Retrieved from https://www.statcan.gc.ca/pub/82-624-x/2013001/article/11879-eng.htm.

Hagood Milton, S. (2017). Normal labor and delivery. *eMedicine*. Retrieved from http://emedicine.medscape.com/article/260036-overview.

Halford, W. K., Petch, J., & Creedy, D. (2015). *Clinical guide to helping new parents: The couple CARE for parents program*. New York: Springer Publishers.

Hutcheson, J. L., & Cheeseman, S. E. (2015). An innovative strategy to improve family—infant bonding. *Neonatal Network, 34*(3), 189–191.

Jin, B., Yu, H., Jin, M., Du, X., & Yang, S. (2015). Measurement of prolactin and estradiol to estimate menses return of breastfeeding mothers. *Reproduction and Contraception, 14*(2), 111–117.

Jordan, R. G., Engstrom, J., Marfell, J., & Farley, C. L. (2014). *Prenatal & postnatal care: A women-centered approach*. Ames, IA: John Wiley & Sons.

Kansky, C., & Isaacs, C. (2016). Normal and abnormal puerperium. *eMedicine*. Retrieved from http://emedicine.medscape.com/article/260187-overview#a1.

King, T. L., Brucker, M. C., Kriebs, J. M., Fahey, J. O., Gegor, C. L., & Varney, H. (2015). *Varney's midwifery* (5th ed.). Burlington, MA: Jones & Bartlett Learning.

Liu, Y., Maloni, J. A., & Petrini, M. A. (2014). Effect of postpartum practices of doing the month on Chinese women's physical and psychological health. *Biological Research for Nursing, 16*(1), 55–63.

Lopez-Olmedo, N., Hernandez-Cordero, S., Neufeld, L. M., Garcia-Guerra, A., Mejia-Rodriguez, F., & Gomez-Humaran, I. M. (2016). The associations of maternal weight change with breastfeeding, diet and physical activity during the postpartum period. *Maternal Child Health Journal, 20*, 270–280.

Mahendru, A., Everett, T., Wilkinson, I., Lees, C., & McEniery, C. (2014). A longitudinal study of maternal cardiovascular function from preconception to the postpartum period. *Journal of Hypertension, 32*(4), 849–856.

Martin, J., MacDonald-Wicks, L., Hure, A., Smith, R., & Collins, C. E. (2015). Reducing postpartum weight retention and improving breastfeeding outcomes in overweight women: A pilot randomized controlled trial. *Nutrients, 7*(3), 1464–1479.

Mattson, S., & Smith, J. (2016). *Core Curriculum for maternal-newborn nursing* (5th ed.). St. Louis, MO: Elsevier Saunders.

Mercer, R. (2006). Nursing support of the process of becoming a mother. *Journal of Obstetric, Gynecologic & Neonatal Nursing, 35*(5), 649–651.

Mercer, R., & Walker, L. (2006). A review of nursing interventions to foster becoming a mother. *Journal of Obstetric, Gynecologic & Neonatal Nursing, 35*(5), 568–582.

Nascimento, S., Pudwell, J., Surita, F., Adamo, K., & Smith, G. (2014). The effect of physical exercise strategies on weight loss in postpartum women: A systematic review and meta-analysis. *International Journal of Obesity, 38*(5), 626–635.

Neville, C., McKinley, M., Holmes, V., Spence, D., & Woodside, J. (2014). The relationship between breastfeeding and postpartum weight change—A systematic review and critical evaluation. *International Journal of Obesity, 38*(4), 577–590.

Nolan, M. (2015). Why it is important to involve new fathers in the care of their child: Mary Nolan explores research into the often-neglected role of men and suggests how primary care nurses can develop services to increase their involvement. *Primary Health Care, 25*(3), 18–23.

Norwitz, E. R., & Schorge, J. O. (2015). *Obstetrics & gynecology at a glance* (5th ed.). Oxford, UK: Wiley-Blackwell.

Parpaglioni, R. (2015). Anatomo-physiological changes during labor and after delivery. In: G. Capogna (Ed.), *Epidural labor analgesia* (pp. 11–20). New York: Springer International Publishing.

Public Health Agency of Canada. (2019). *Nobody's perfect.* Retrieved from https://www.canada.ca/en/public-health/services/health-promotion/childhood-adolescence/parent/nobody-perfect.html

Purnell, L. D. (2014). *Guide to culturally competent health care* (3rd ed.). Philadelphia, PA: F. A. Davis.

Rice, P. L., & Manderson, L. (2014). *Maternity and reproductive health in Asian societies.* Abingdon, Oxon: Routledge.

Rubin, R. (1984). *Maternal identity and the maternal experience.* New York: Springer.

Sears, R. W., & Sears, J. M. (2018). Father–newborn bonding. Ask Dr. Sears. Retrieved from http://www.askdrsears.com/topics/pregnancy-childbirth/tenth-month-post-partum/bonding-with-your-newborn/father-newborn-bonding.

Senie, R. T. (2014). *Epidemiology of women's health.* Burlington, MA: Jones & Bartlett Learning.

Sethna, V., Murray, L., Netsi, E., Psychogiou, L., & Ramchandani, P. G. (2015). Paternal depression in the postnatal period and early father–infant interactions. *Parenting, 15*(1), 1–8.

Spencer, B. (2015). Medications and breastfeeding for mothers with chronic illness. *Journal of Obstetric, Gynecologic, & Neonatal Nursing, 44*(4), 543–552.

Spiteri, G., Borg Xuereb, R., Carrick-Sen, D., Kaner, E., & Martin, C. R. (2014). Preparation for parenthood: A concept analysis. *Journal of Reproductive & Infant Psychology, 32*(2), 148–165.

Stuebe, A. M., Meltzer-Brody, S., Pearson, B., Pedersen, C., & Grewen, K. (2015). Maternal neuroendocrine serum levels in exclusively breastfeeding mothers. *Breastfeeding Medicine, 10*(4), 197–202.

Wambach, K., & Riordan, J. (2014). *Breastfeeding and human lactation.* (5th ed.). Burlington, MA: Jones and Bartlett Learning.

Webber, G. C., & Chirangi, B. (2014). Women's health in women's hands: A pilot study assessing the feasibility of providing women with medications to reduce postpartum hemorrhage and sepsis in rural Tanzania. *Health Care for Women International, 35*(7–9), 758–770.

Wojnar, D. M., & Narruhn, R. A. (2015). Chapter 18: Transcultural aspects of perinatal health care of Somali women. In M. De Chesnay & B. A. Anderson (Eds.), *Caring for the vulnerable* (4th ed., pp. 287–302). Burlington, MA: Jones & Bartlett Learning.

Zanardo, V., & Straface, G. (2015). The higher temperature in the areola supports the natural progression of the birth to breastfeeding continuum. *PloS One, 10*(3), e0118774.

CHAPTER **WORKSHEET**

MULTIPLE CHOICE QUESTIONS

1. Postpartum breast engorgement occurs 48 to 72 hours after giving birth. What physiologic change influences breast engorgement?
   a. An increase in blood and lymph supply to the breasts
   b. An increase in estrogen and progesterone levels
   c. Colostrum production increases dramatically
   d. Fluid retention in the breasts due to the intravenous fluids given during labour

2. In the taking-in maternal role phase described by Rubin (1984), the nurse would expect the client's behaviour to be characterized as which of the following?
   a. Gaining self-confidence
   b. Adjusting to her new relationships
   c. Being passive and dependent
   d. Resuming control over her life

3. The nurse is explaining to a postpartum client 48 hours after her giving childbirth that afterpains can be the result of which of the following?
   a. Abdominal cramping as a sign of endometriosis
   b. A small infant weighing less than 8 pounds
   c. Pregnancies that were too closely spaced
   d. Contractions of the uterus after birth

4. The nurse would expect a postpartum client to demonstrate lochia in which sequence?
   a. Rubra, alba, serosa
   b. Rubra, serosa, alba
   c. Serosa, alba, rubra
   d. Alba, rubra, serosa

5. The nurse is assessing Ms. Smith, who gave birth to her first child 5 days ago. What findings by the nurse would be expected?
   a. Cream-coloured lochia; uterus above the umbilicus
   b. Bright-red lochia with clots; uterus 2 fingerbreadths below umbilicus
   c. Light pink or brown lochia; uterus 4 to 5 fingerbreadths below umbilicus
   d. Yellow, mucousy lochia; uterus at the level of the umbilicus

6. Prioritize the postpartum client's needs 4 hours after giving birth by placing a number 1, 2, 3, or 4 in the blank before each need.
   a. _____ Learn how to hold and cuddle the infant
   b. _____ Watch a baby bath demonstration given by the nurse
   c. _____ Sleep and rest without being disturbed for a few hours
   d. _____ Interaction time (first 30 minutes) with the infant to facilitate bonding

7. Immediately after childbirth in the recovery area, the nurse observes the client's partner's fascination and interest in their new son. This behaviour is often termed:
   a. Attachment
   b. Engrossment
   c. Bonding
   d. Temperament

8. After the nurse provides instructions to a postpartum client about postpartum blues, which statement would indicate understanding of it? "I will…
   a. "need to take medication daily to treat the anxiety and sadness"
   b. "call the support line only if I start to hear voices"
   c. "contact my doctor if I become dizzy and fell nauseated"
   d. "feel like laughing one minute and crying the next minute"

CRITICAL THINKING EXERCISES

1. A new nurse assigned to the postpartum unit makes a comment to the oncoming shift that, a 25-year-old primipara patient seems lazy and shows no initiative in taking care of herself or her baby. The nurse reported that this new mother talks excessively about her labour and birth experience and seems preoccupied with herself and her needs, not her newborn's care. She wonders if something is wrong with this mother because she seems so self-centred and has to be directed to do everything.
   a. Is there something "wrong" with this client's behaviour? Why or why not?
   b. What maternal role phase is being described by the new nurse?
   c. What role can the nurse play to support the mother through this phase?

2. Mrs. Lenhart, a primipara, gave birth to a healthy baby boy yesterday. Her partner seemed elated at the birth, calling their friends and family on his cell phone minutes after the birth. He passed out cigars and praised his wife for her efforts. Today, when the nurse walked into their room, her partner seemed very anxious around his new son and called for the nurse whenever the baby cried or needed a diaper change. He seemed standoffish when asked to hold his son, and he spent time talking to other fathers in the waiting room, leaving his wife alone in the room.

   a. Would you consider Mr. Lenhart's paternal behaviour to be normal at this time?

   b. What might Mr. Lenhart be feeling at this time?

   c. How can the nurse help this new father adjust to his new role?

STUDY ACTIVITIES

1. Find an Internet resource that discusses general postpartum care for new parents who might have questions after discharge. Evaluate the website's information as to how credible, accurate, and current the information is.

2. Prepare a teaching plan for new mothers, outlining the various physiologic changes that will take place after discharge.

3. The term that describes the return of the uterus to its prepregnant state is _____.

4. A deviated fundus to the right side of the abdomen would indicate a _____.

BRINGING IT ALL TOGETHER: A CASE STUDY

A 29-year-old married mother of four children lived with her migrant husband and his parents in a small rural border town. She had given birth to her fourth child 7 weeks ago. She now had four children in the past 4 years. Her pregnancy, labour, and birth had been uneventful, and an untrained neighbor woman helped conduct the home birth. Because pregnancy was viewed as a normal occurrence that did not require any medical attention, she did not receive any prenatal care for any of her four pregnancies. For the 1st month after birth, she felt normal, but then began to exhibit bizarre behaviours. She became isolated from her family, stopped speaking to them, and ceased to care for her newborn or other children. Her family wondered about her isolation, but seemed indifferent to her condition, as they were all busy with their own lives. One day when all of her family members and her children had gone to work in the fields, she ended her life.

Go to the Point to find questions to consider about this case.

16

Nursing Management During the Postpartum Period

Learning Objectives

Upon completion of the chapter, you will be able to:

1. Characterize the normal physiologic and psychological adaptations to the postpartum period.

2. Determine the parameters that need to be assessed during the postpartum period.

3. Compare and contrast bonding to the attachment process.

4. Select behaviours that enhance or inhibit the attachment process.

5. Outline nursing management for the client and family during the postpartum period.

6. Examine the role of the nurse in promoting successful breastfeeding.

7. Plan areas of health education needed for discharge planning, home care, and follow-up.

A 24-year-old Muslim primipara has just been admitted to the postpartum unit. Her husband sits at the bedside. Despite a lengthy labour and difficult birth, her husband does not appear to provide her with any physical or emotional support.

INTRODUCTION

The postpartum period is a time of major adjustments and adaptations not just for the client, but for all members of the family. It is during this time that parenting starts and a relationship with the newborn begins. A positive, loving relationship between a parent and the newborn promotes the emotional well-being of all. This relationship endures and has profound effects on the child's growth and development.

Take Note!

Parenting is a skill that is often learned by trial and error, with varying degrees of success. Successful parenting, a continuous and complex interactive process, requires the parents to learn new skills and to integrate the new member into the family.

FIGURE 16.1 **Parents and grandmother interacting with the newborn.**

After giving birth, each system in the client's body takes several weeks to return to its nonpregnant state. The physiologic changes in these clients during the postpartum period are dramatic. Nurses should be aware of these changes and should be able to make observations and assessments to validate normal occurrences and detect any deviations.

This chapter describes the nursing management of the client and family during the postpartum period. (See Chapter 21 for a detailed discussion of the postpartum care of the client undergoing a surgical birth.) Nursing management during the postpartum period focuses on assessing the client's ability to adapt to the physiologic and psychological changes occurring at this time (see Chapter 15 for a detailed discussion of these adaptations). This chapter outlines physical assessment parameters for postpartum clients and newborns. It also focuses on bonding and attachment behaviours; nurses need to be aware of these behaviours, so they can perform appropriate interventions. Family members are also assessed to determine how well they are making the transition to this new stage.

Based on assessment findings, the nurse plans and implements care to address the family's needs. Steps to address physiologic needs such as comfort, self-care, nutrition, and contraception are described. Ways to help the client and her family adapt to the birth of the newborn are also discussed (Fig. 16.1). Because of today's shortened lengths of stay, the nurse may need to prioritize her care and arrange for follow-up in the home to ensure that all the family's needs are met.

SOCIAL SUPPORT AND CULTURAL CONSIDERATIONS

In addition to physical assessment and care of the client in the postpartum period, strong social support is vital to help her integrate the baby into the family. A key to providing effective postpartum care is to understand the client in both social and cultural contexts, so that all care provided is culturally competent and sensitive. In today's mobile society, extended families may live far away and may be unable to help care for the new family. Many new parents turn to health care providers for information as well as physical and emotional support during this adjustment period. Nurses can be an invaluable resource by serving as mentors, teaching about self-care measures and baby care basics, and providing emotional support. The nurse's support and care through this critical time can increase the new parents' confidence, giving them a sense of accomplishment in their parenting skills. The United Nations International Children's Emergency Fund (UNICEF) and the World Health Organization (WHO) outline the promotion of breastfeeding as a responsibility of facilities providing maternity and newborn care (UNICEF & WHO, 2018).

As in all nursing care, nurses should provide culturally competent care during the postpartum period. The nurse should engage in ongoing cultural self-assessment and overcome any stereotypes that perpetuate prejudice or discrimination against any cultural group (Bowers & Ceballos, 2015). Providing culturally competent nursing care during the postpartum period requires time, open-mindedness, and patience. The global migration of diverse populations presents nurses with the challenge of providing care to unprecedented numbers of clients and their families with health care beliefs and practices that differ from their own. Sensitivity cannot be assumed; it needs to be nurtured and developed. The skill set needed by nurses to provide culturally competent care to postpartum clients and their families includes understanding their beliefs, experiences, and family environment; facilitating their language through appropriate use of interpreters so that the information provided can be understood; and compassionately respecting clients and their human rights. Nurses must explore a client and family's cultural beliefs, values, and practices in order to base nursing interventions on information provided by the client or members of the family, as opposed to making harmful assumptions which could be perceived as stereotyping (CAPWHN, 2017; CNA, 2010).

Remember the couple introduced at the beginning of the chapter? When the postpartum nurse comes to examine Raina, her husband quickly leaves the room and returns a short time later after the examination is complete. How do you interpret his behaviour in relation to his wife? What might you communicate to this couple?

NURSING ASSESSMENT IN THE POSTPARTUM PERIOD

Many adaptations and adjustments must be made to accommodate the new family member. The nurse's focus is on assistance for families to maximize their adjustment, surveillance for maladaptation, and education, consultation, collaboration as needed. Comprehensive nursing assessment begins immediately after the client gives birth and continues through discharge.

 Take Note!

Nurses need a firm grasp of normal findings to be able to recognize abnormal findings and intervene appropriately.

This postpartum assessment includes vital signs and physical and psychosocial assessments. It also includes assessing the parents and other family members, such as siblings and grandparents, for attachment and bonding with the newborn. Although the exact protocol may vary among facilities, postpartum assessment typically is performed as follows:

- During the first hour: every 15 minutes
- During the second hour: every 30 minutes
- During the first 24 hours: every 4 to 8 hours
- After 24 hours: every 8 hours (Jordan, Engstrom, Marfell, & Farley, 2014; Mattson & Smith, 2016).

During each assessment, keep in mind risk factors that may lead to complications, such as infection or hemorrhage, during the recovery period (Box 16.1). Early identification is critical to ensure prompt intervention.

The postpartum period is a time of transition. The end of the pregnancy and childbirth initiates physiologic changes as many body systems return to their nonpregnant state. Nurses need to be aware of the normal physiologic and psychological changes that take place in clients' bodies and minds in order to provide

---

BOX 16.1

FACTORS INCREASING THE RISK FOR POSTPARTUM COMPLICATIONS

Risk Factors for Postpartum Infection

- Operative procedure (forceps, cesarean birth, vacuum extraction)
- History of diabetes, including gestational diabetes
- Prolonged labour (more than 24 hours)
- Use of indwelling urinary catheter
- Anemia (hemoglobin <100 g/L)
- Multiple vaginal examinations during labour
- Prolonged rupture of membranes (>18 hours)
- Manual extraction of placenta
- Compromised immune system (HIV positive)

Risk Factors for Postpartum Hemorrhage

- Precipitous labour (less than 3 hours)
- Uterine atony
- Placenta previa or abruptio placenta
- Labour induction or augmentation
- Operative procedures (vacuum extraction, forceps, cesarean birth)
- Retained placental fragments
- Prolonged third stage of labour (more than 30 minutes)
- Multiparity, more than three births closely spaced
- Uterine overdistention (large infant, twins, polyhydramnios)

---

comprehensive care during the postpartum period. In addition to client and family teaching, one of the most significant responsibilities of the postpartum nurse is to recognize potential complications after childbirth.

As with any assessment, always review the client's medical record for information about the pregnancy, labour, and birth. Note any pre-existing conditions, any complications that occurred during pregnancy, labour, birth, and immediately afterward, and any treatments provided.

Postpartum assessment typically includes vital signs, pain level, epidural site inspection for infection, and a systematic head-to-toe review of body systems. The acronym **BUBBLE-EE**—**b**reasts, **u**terus, **b**ladder, **b**owels, **l**ochia, **e**pisiotomy/perineum/epidural site, **e**xtremities, and **e**motional status—can be used as a guide for this head-to-toe review (Cunningham et al., 2014).

While assessing the client and family during the postpartum period, be alert for danger signs (Box 16.2). Notify the primary health care provider immediately if any are noted.

Vital Signs Assessment

Obtain vital signs and compare them with the previous values, noting and reporting any deviations. Vital sign changes can be an early indicator of complications.

POSTPARTUM DANGER SIGNS

- Fever more than 38°C (100.4°F)
- Foul-smelling lochia or an unexpected change in colour or amount
- Large blood clots, or bleeding that saturates a peri-pad in 1 hour
- Severe headaches or blurred vision
- Visual changes, such as blurred vision or spots, or headaches
- Calf pain with dorsiflexion of the foot
- Swelling, redness, or discharge at the episiotomy, epidural, or abdominal sites
- Dysuria, burning, or incomplete emptying of the bladder
- Shortness of breath or difficulty breathing without exertion
- Depression or extreme mood swings

Temperature

Use a consistent measurement technique (oral, axillary, or tympanic) to get the most accurate readings. Typically, the client's temperature during the first 24 hours postpartum is within the normal range or a low-grade elevation. Some postpartum clients experience a slight fever, up to 38°C, during the first 24 hours. This elevation may be the result of dehydration because of fluid loss during labour. Temperature should be normal after 24 hours with replacement of fluids lost during labour and birth (Green, 2016).

A temperature above 38°C at any time or an abnormal temperature after the first 24 hours may indicate infection and must be reported. Abnormal temperature readings warrant continued monitoring until an infection can be ruled out through cultures or blood studies. An elevated temperature can identify sepsis, which results in significant morbidity and mortality worldwide. To improve the outcome, it is essential that nurses be vigilant in obtaining accurate values and monitoring their client's temperature.

Pulse

Pulse rates of 60 to 80 beats per minute (bpm) at rest are normal during the first week after birth. This pulse rate is called puerperal bradycardia. During pregnancy, the heavy gravid uterus causes a decreased flow of venous blood to the heart. After giving birth, there is an increase in intravascular volume. The cardiac output is most likely caused by an increased stroke volume from the venous return now. The elevated stroke volume leads to a decreased heart rate (Creasy et al., 2014). Tachycardia in the postpartum period can suggest anxiety, excitement, fatigue, pain, excessive blood loss or delayed

hemorrhage, infection, or underlying cardiac problems. Any pulse rate higher than 100 bpm warrants further investigation to rule out complications.

Respirations

Respiratory rates in the postpartum client should be within the normal range of 12 to 20 breaths per minute at rest. Pulmonary function typically returns to the prepregnant state after childbirth when the diaphragm descends, and the organs revert to their normal positions. Any change in respiratory rate out of the normal range might indicate pulmonary edema, atelectasis, a side effect of epidural anesthesia, or pulmonary embolism and must be reported. Lungs should be clear on auscultation.

Blood Pressure

Assess the client's blood pressure and compare it with the usual range. Report any deviation from this range. Immediately after childbirth, the blood pressure should remain the same as during labour. An increase in blood pressure could indicate gestational hypertension, whereas a decrease could indicate shock or orthostatic hypotension or dehydration, a side effect of epidural anesthesia. Blood pressure readings should not be higher than 140/90 mm Hg or lower than 85/60 mm Hg (King et al., 2015). Blood pressure also may vary based on the client's position, so assess blood pressure with the client in the same position every time. Be alert for orthostatic hypotension, which can occur when the client moves rapidly from a lying or sitting position to a standing one.

Pain

Pain, the fifth vital sign, is assessed along with the other four parameters. Pain assessment should include questions about the presence, quality, radiation, severity, and quality of pain. Severity is measured using a numeric scale from 0 to 10 points. Nursing care should focus on providing comfort measures to ease pain which might include perineal care, clean gown, mouth care, providing warm blankets, ensuring adequate fluid intake to facilitate healing, repositioning frequently, and encouraging rest between assessments (Nagtalon-Ramos, 2014).

The goal of pain management is to have the client's pain scale rating maintained between 0 and 2 points at all times, especially after breastfeeding. This can be accomplished by assessing the client's pain level frequently and preventing pain by administering analgesics. If the client has severe pain in the perineal region despite use of physical comfort measures, check for a hematoma by inspecting and palpating the area. If one is found, notify the health care provider immediately.

Physical Examination

Physical examination of the postpartum client focuses on assessing the breasts, uterus, bladder, bowels, lochia, episiotomy/perineum, epidural site, and extremities.

Breasts

Inspect the breasts for size, contour, asymmetry, fullness, or erythema. Check the nipples for cracks, redness, fissures, or bleeding, and note whether they are erect, flat, or inverted. Flat or inverted nipples can make breastfeeding challenging for both the client and the infant. Cracked, blistered, fissured, bruised, or bleeding nipples in a client who is breastfeeding are typically an indication that the baby is improperly positioned on the breast. With the client's permission, palpate the breasts lightly to ascertain if they are soft, filling, or engorged, and document your findings. A breast assessment also needs to be conducted on clients who choose not to breastfeed. Teaching for these clients should include avoidance of breast stimulation so as not to exacerbate engorgement.

Lactogenesis (the onset of milk production) is initially triggered by the delivery of the placenta, which results in falling levels of estrogen and progesterone, with the continued presence of prolactin. If the client has chosen not to breastfeed, the prolactin levels fall and return to normal levels within 2 to 3 weeks. As milk to the full milk supply comes in, the breasts become firmer; this is charted as "filling." Engorged breasts are hard, tender, and taut. Assess for any nipple discomfort. With the client's permission, palpate the breasts for any nodules, masses, or areas of warmth, which may indicate a plugged duct that may progress to mastitis if not treated promptly. Any discharge from the nipple should be described and documented if it is not colostrum (creamy yellow) or milk (bluish white). Over the first week, the breast milk matures and contains all necessary nutrients in the neonatal period. The breast milk continues to change as breastfeeding progresses to meet the changing demands of the growing infant.

Uterus

Assess the fundus (top portion of the uterus) to determine the degree of uterine involution. Make sure that the client's bladder is empty before assessing the fundus and auscultate for bowel sounds prior to uterine palpation. If the client has had a cesarean birth and has a patient-controlled anesthesia (PCA) pump, evaluate whether self-medication is needed prior to fundal assessment to decrease the discomfort.

Using a two-handed approach, with the client in the supine position with knees flexed slightly and the bed in a flat position or as low as possible, palpate the abdomen gently, feeling for the top of the uterus while the

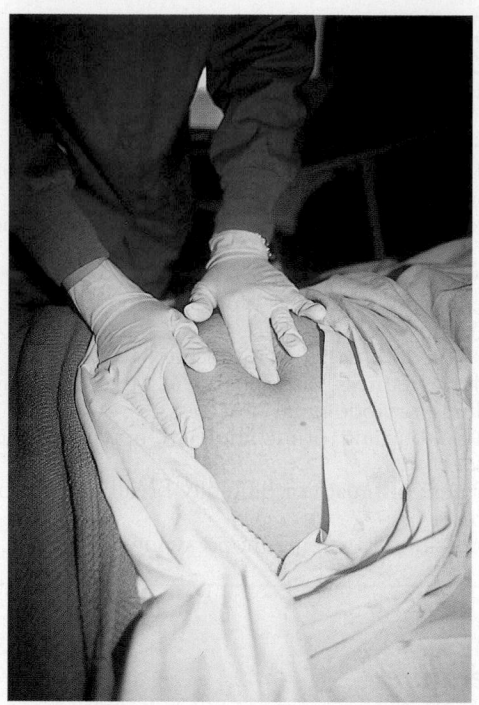

FIGURE 16.2 Palpating the fundus.

other hand is placed on the lower segment of the uterus to stabilize it (Fig. 16.2).

The fundus should be midline and should feel firm. A boggy or relaxed uterus is a sign of uterine atony (loss of muscle tone in the uterus). This can be the result of bladder distention, which displaces the uterus upward and to the right, or retained placental fragments. Either situation predisposes the client to hemorrhage.

Once the fundus is located, place your index finger on the fundus and count the number of fingerbreadths between the fundus and the umbilicus (1 fingerbreadth is approximately equal to 1 cm). One to 2 hours after birth, the fundus typically is between the umbilicus and the symphysis pubis. Approximately 6 to 12 hours after birth, the fundus usually is at the level of the umbilicus. If the fundal height is significantly above the umbilicus, investigate this immediately to prevent excessive bleeding. A full bladder will displace the uterus up and to either side of the midline. Assist the client to empty the bladder and then reassess the location of the fundus.

Normally, the fundus progresses downward at a rate of 1 fingerbreadth (or 1 cm) per day after childbirth and should be nonpalpable by 10 to 14 days postpartum. By day 14, the uterus has descended below the rim of the symphysis pubis and is no longer palpable (Cunningham et al., 2014). On the first postpartum day, the top of the fundus is located 1 cm below the umbilicus and is recorded as U/1. Similarly, on the second postpartum day, the fundus would be 2 cm below the umbilicus and should be recorded as U/2, and so on. Health care agencies differ according to how fundal heights are charted, so follow their protocols for this. If the fundus is not firm, gently massage the uterus using a circular motion until it becomes firm. If the fundus remains boggy despite fundal massage, inform the health care provider immediately. Uterine atony is the leading cause of postpartum hemorrhage worldwide, and postpartum hemorrhage is the third leading cause of perinatal mortality in Canada (Public Health Agency of Canada, 2014).

Bladder

Considerable diuresis—as much as 3,000 mL/day—begins within 12 hours after childbirth and continues for several days. A single voiding may be 500 mL or more. By 21 days postpartum, the diuresis is usually complete (Jordan et al., 2014). It is possible that the sensation to void, even if the bladder is full, will be diminished in the early postpartum days. In this situation the bladder can become distended and displace the uterus upward and to the side, preventing the uterine muscles from contracting properly and can lead to excessive bleeding. Urinary retention as a result of decreased bladder tone and emptying can lead to urinary tract infections. It is imperative that nurses monitor clients for signs of urinary tract infections, including fever, urinary frequency and/or urgency, difficult or painful urination, and tenderness over the costovertebral angle (Wilson, Passante, Rauschenbach, Yang, & Wong, 2015). Clients who received regional anesthesia during labour are at risk for urinary tract infections due to continuous urinary catheterization to prevent urinary retention during labour, which is thought to delay fetal descent. They also experience difficulty voiding and loss of sensation and must wait until it returns to feel a full bladder which might be several hours after childbirth.

Assess for voiding problems by asking the following questions:

- Have you (voided, urinated, gone to the bathroom) yet?
- Have you noticed any burning or discomfort with urination?
- Do you have any difficulty passing your urine?
- Do you feel that your bladder is empty when you finish urinating?
- Do you have any signs of infection such as urgency, frequency, or pain?
- Are you able to control the flow of urine by squeezing your muscles?
- Have you noticed any leakage of urine when you cough, laugh, or sneeze?

Assess the bladder for distention and adequate emptying after efforts to void. Palpate the area over the symphysis pubis. If empty, the bladder is not palpable. Palpation of a rounded mass suggests bladder distention. If you are unsure, percuss the area: a full bladder is dull to percussion. If the bladder is full, lochia drainage will be more than normal because the uterus cannot contract to suppress the bleeding.

Take Note!

Note the location and condition of the fundus; a full bladder tends to displace the uterus up and to the right.

After the client has voided, palpate and percuss the area again to determine adequate emptying of the bladder. If the bladder remains distended, there may be retained urine in the bladder, and measures to initiate voiding should be instituted. Be alert for signs of infection, including infrequent or insufficient voiding (less than 200 mL), discomfort, burning, urgency, or foul-smelling urine (Mattson & Smith, 2016). Document all urine output.

Bowels

Spontaneous bowel movements may not occur for 1 to 3 days after giving birth because of a decrease in muscle tone in the intestines as a result of elevated progesterone levels. Normal patterns of bowel elimination usually return within a week after birth (Verghese, Futaba, & Latthe, 2015). Often clients are hesitant to have a bowel movement due to pain in the perineal area resulting from an episiotomy, lacerations, or hemorrhoids. Some are fearful that they may "rip their stitches" should they strain. Nurses should reassure their clients that stool softeners and/or laxatives to treat constipation have been prescribed for them to reduce discomfort.

Inspect the abdomen for distention, auscultate for bowel sounds in all four quadrants prior to palpating the uterine fundus, and palpate for tenderness. The abdomen typically is soft, nontender, and nondistended. Bowel sounds are present in all four quadrants. Ask if the client has had a bowel movement or has passed gas since giving birth, because constipation is a common challenge during the postpartum period and many clients will not offer this information unless asked about it. Normal assessment findings are active bowel sounds, passing gas, and a nondistended abdomen.

Lochia

Assess lochia in terms of amount, colour, odour, and change with activity and time. To assess the extent of bleeding, ask the client how many perineal pads have been used in the past 1 to 2 hours and how much drainage was on each pad. For example, did the client saturate the pad completely, or was only half of the pad covered with drainage? Ask about the colour of the drainage, odour, and the presence of any clots. Lochia has a musky scent, with an odour similar to that of menstrual flow, and without large clots (fist size). Foul-smelling lochia suggests an infection, and large clots suggest poor uterine involution, necessitating additional intervention.

FIGURE 16.3 **Assessing lochia.**

To determine the amount of lochia, observe the amount of lochia saturation on the perineal pad and relate it to time (Fig. 16.3). Also, take into consideration the specific type of peripad used, because some are more absorbent than others. Lochia flow will increase when the client gets out of bed (lochia pools in the vagina and the uterus while lying down) and when breastfeeding (oxytocin release causes uterine contractions). A perineal pad being saturated within 30 to 60 minutes indicates a large amount of bleeding, compared to one pad being saturated in 2 hours (which is considered a moderate amount).

Typically, the amount of lochia is described as follows:

- *Scant:* a 2.5- to 5-cm lochia stain on the perineal pad or approximately a 10-mL loss
- *Light or small:* an approximately 10-cm stain or a 10- to 25-mL loss
- *Moderate:* a 10- to 15-cm stain with an estimated loss of 25 to 50 mL
- *Large or heavy:* a pad is saturated within 1 hour after changing it (Bope & Kellerman, 2015)

The total volume of lochial discharge varies based on parity, but the amount decreases daily. Check underneath the client, by positioning the client on either side, to make sure additional blood is not hidden and not being absorbed on the perineal pad. This also a good time to assess for the presence and condition of hemorrhoids since the nurse is visually inspecting the perineum.

Report any abnormal findings, such as heavy, bright-red lochia with large tissue fragments or a foul odour. If excessive bleeding occurs, the first step would be to massage the boggy fundus until it is firm to reduce the flow of blood. Document all findings.

Clients who had a cesarean birth will have less lochia discharge than those who had a vaginal birth, but stages and colour changes remain the same. Although the abdomen will be tender after surgery, the nurse must palpate the fundus and assess the lochia to make sure they are within the normal range and that there is no excessive bleeding.

Anticipatory guidance given at discharge should include information about lochia and the expected changes. Stress the importance of notifying the health care provider if lochia rubra returns after the serosa and alba transitions have taken place. This is abnormal and may indicate subinvolution or that the client is too active and needs to rest more. Lochia is an excellent medium for bacterial growth. Explain that frequent changing of perineal pads, continued use of the peribottle for rinsing the perineal area, and hand hygiene before and after pad changes are important infection control measures.

Episiotomy/Perineum and Epidural Site

If the client has an episiotomy, which is not routinely done, assess the episiotomy and perineal area. Position the client on one side with the top leg flexed upward at the knee and drawn up toward the waist. If necessary, use a penlight to provide adequate lighting during the assessment. Wearing gloves and standing at the client's back side, gently lift the upper buttock to expose the perineum and anus (Fig. 16.4). Inspect the episiotomy for irritation, ecchymosis, tenderness, or hematomas. Assess for hemorrhoids and their condition.

During the early postpartum period, the perineal tissue surrounding the episiotomy is typically edematous and slightly bruised. The normal episiotomy site should not have redness, discharge, or edema. The majority of healing takes place within the first 2 weeks, but it may take 4 to 6 months for the episiotomy to heal completely (King et al., 2015).

Lacerations to the perineal area sustained during the birthing process that were identified and repaired also need to be assessed to determine their healing status.

FIGURE 16.4 **Inspecting the perineum.**

Lacerations are classified based on their severity and tissue involvement:

- *First-degree laceration:* involves only skin and superficial structures above muscle
- *Second-degree laceration:* extends through perineal muscles
- *Third-degree laceration:* extends through the anal sphincter muscle
- *Fourth-degree laceration:* continues through anterior rectal wall

Assess the episiotomy and any lacerations at least every 8 hours to detect hematomas or signs of infection. Large areas of swollen, bluish skin with complaints of severe pain in the perineal area indicate pelvic or vulvar hematomas. Redness, swelling, increasing discomfort, or purulent drainage may indicate infection. Both findings need to be reported immediately.

A white line running the length of the episiotomy is a sign of infection, as well as swelling or discharge. Severe, intractable pain, perineal discolouration, and ecchymosis indicate a perineal hematoma, a potentially dangerous condition. Report any unusual findings to the health care provider. Ice can be applied to relieve discomfort and reduce edema; sitz baths also can promote comfort and perineal healing (see "Promoting Comfort" in the Nursing Interventions section).

If the client has had an epidural during labour, assessment of the epidural wound site is important as well as checking for any side effects of the medication injected such as itching, nausea and vomiting, or urinary retention. Visual inspection of the epidural site and an accurate documentation of intake and output are essential.

Extremities

Pregnancy is associated with an increased risk of venous thromboembolism (VTE), which includes pulmonary embolism and deep vein thrombosis. During pregnancy, the state of hypercoagulability protects the mother against excessive blood loss during childbirth and placental separation. However, this hypercoagulable state can increase the risk of thromboembolic disorders during pregnancy and postpartum. Three factors can predispose to thromboembolic disorders during pregnancy: stasis (compression of the large veins because of the gravid uterus), altered coagulation (state of pregnancy), and localized vascular damage (may occur during the birthing process). All these factors increase the risk of clot formation and having it travel to the lungs.

While inspecting the client's extremities, also determine the degree of sensory and motor function return (recovery from anesthesia) by asking if the client feels sensation at various areas the nurse touches, and by observing her ambulation stability.

Take Note!

Pulmonary embolism occurs in up to 3 per 1,000 births and is a major cause of maternal mortality (Kim, Kim, Kim, & Ha, 2015).

Pulmonary emboli typically result from dislodged deep vein thrombi in the lower extremities. Risk factors associated with thromboembolic conditions include:

- Anemia
- Diabetes mellitus
- Cigarette smoking
- Obesity
- Preeclampsia
- Hypertension
- Severe varicose veins
- Pregnancy
- Multiple pregnancies
- Cardiovascular disease
- Sickle cell disease
- Postpartum hemorrhage
- Oral contraceptive use
- Cesarean birth
- Severe infection
- Previous thromboembolic disease
- Multiparity
- Bed rest or immobility for 4 days or more
- Advanced maternal age >35 years (Kline & Kabrhel, 2015)

Because of the subtle presentation of thromboembolic disorders, the physical examination may not be enough to detect them. An accurate diagnosis of pulmonary embolism is needed because it requires (1) prolonged therapy ($\leq$9 months of heparin during pregnancy), (2) prophylaxis during future pregnancies, and (3) avoidance of oral contraceptive pills. The woman may report lower extremity tightness or aching when ambulating that is relieved with rest and elevation of the leg. Edema in the affected leg (typically the left), along with warmth and tenderness, and a low-grade fever may also be noted. A duplex ultrasound (two-dimensional ultrasound and Doppler ultrasound that compresses the vein to assess for changes in venous flow) in conjunction with the physical findings frequently is needed for a conclusive diagnosis (Sucker & Zotz, 2015).

Those with an increased risk for this condition during the postpartum period should wear anti-embolic stockings or use sequential compression devices to reduce the risk of venous stasis by preventing blood from pooling in the calves of the legs. Encouraging the client to ambulate after childbirth reduces the incidence of thrombophlebitis.

Psychosocial Assessment

Psychosocial assessment of the postpartum client focuses on emotional status as well as bonding and attachment.

Emotional Status

Assess new parents' emotional status by observing how they interact with their family, as well as their level of independence, energy levels, eye contact (within a cultural context), posture and comfort level while holding the newborn, and sleep and rest patterns. Be alert for mood swings, irritability, or crying episodes.

> Remember Raina and her "quiet" husband? The postpartum nurse informs Raina that her doctor, Nancy Schultz, has been called away for emergency surgery and won't be available the rest of the day. The nurse explains that Dr. Robert Nappo will be making rounds for her. Raina and her husband become upset. What could potentially have led to them being upset? How could the nurse frame her care for the client keeping cultural competency in mind?

Bonding and Attachment

Nurses can be instrumental in promoting attachment by assessing attachment behaviours (positive and negative) and intervening appropriately when needed. Nurses must be able to identify any family discord that might interfere with the attachment process. Remember, however, that a nurse must first consider their own cultural influences, values, and behaviours, and recognize the influence of culture on these for all new parents. For example, Indigenous parents may handle their newborns less often and use cradle boards to carry them. People from some cultures will delay breastfeeding until the full milk supply comes in, due to a belief that colostrum is harmful for the newborn (Bowers & Ceballos, 2015). A baseline knowledge of various customs and traditions is an important foundation for a culturally sensitive nursing practice, however, a nurse must never assume that every client/family will follow their traditional cultural beliefs and practices. Nurses can avoid stereotyping by assessing each client individually and basing nursing care on the information that is provided by the client or members of the client's support system.

Meeting the newborn for the first time after birth can be an exhilarating experience for parents. Although many hours have been spent dreaming of the unborn baby and how he or she will look, it is not until after birth that they meet face to face. They both need to get to know one another and to develop feelings for one another.

Bonding is the close emotional attraction to a newborn by the parents that develops during the first 30 to 60 minutes after birth. It is thought that optimal bonding of the parents to a newborn requires a period of close contact within the first few minutes to a few hours after

birth. Bonding is really a continuation of the relationship that began during pregnancy (Sears & Sears, 2015b). It is affected by a multitude of factors, including the parent's socioeconomic status, family history, role models, support systems, cultural factors, and birth experiences. Bonding is initiated when a new parent caresses the infant and exhibits certain behaviours typical of tending to a child. The infant's responses to this, such as body and eye movements, are a necessary part of the process. During this initial period immediately following birth, the infant is in a quiet, alert state, looking directly at the holder.

Take Note!

The length of time necessary for bonding depends on the health of the infant and parent, as well as the circumstances surrounding the labour and birth (Tester-Jones, O'Mahen, Watkins, & Karl, 2015).

Attachment is the development of strong affection between an infant and a significant other (parent, sibling, and caretaker). This attachment is reciprocal; both the significant other and the newborn exhibit attachment behaviours. The attachment relationship formed between the infant and primary caregiver influences the child's view of the world and future relationships (Sette, Coppola, & Cassibba, 2015). This tie between two people is psychological rather than biologic, and it does not occur overnight. The process of attachment follows a progressive or developmental course that changes over time. Attachment is an individualized and multifactorial process that differs based on the health of the infant, the parent, environmental circumstances, and the quality of care the infant receives. The newborn responds to the significant other by cooing, grasping, smiling, and crying. Nurses can assess for attachment behaviours by observing the interaction between the newborn and the person holding him or her (Mattson & Smith, 2016). It occurs through mutually satisfying experiences. Attachment begins during pregnancy as the result of fetal movement and the pregnant person's fantasies about the infant and continues through the birth and postpartum periods. Attachment behaviours include seeking, physical caretaking behaviours, emotional attentiveness to infant's needs, staying close to, touching, kissing, cuddling, choosing the *en face* (face-to-face) position while holding or feeding the newborn, expressing pride in the newborn and exchanging gratifying experiences with the infant (McComish, 2015). In a high-risk pregnancy, the attachment process may be complicated by premature birth (lack of time to develop a relationship with the unborn baby) and by parental stress due to the fetal and/or maternal vulnerability.

Bonding is a vital component of the attachment process and is necessary in establishing parent–infant attachment and a healthy, loving relationship. The infant may

FIGURE 16.5 *En face* position.

be visually and physically "explored," initially using fingertips on the infant's face and extremities and progressing to massaging and stroking the infant. This is followed by palm contact on the trunk. Eventually, the infant is drawn toward the parent and held (Fig. 16.5).

Generally, research on attachment has found that the process is similar for partners as for the birthing parent, but the pace may be different. Partners or co-parents also manifest attachment behaviours during pregnancy. Indeed, Baltes, Featherman, and Lerner (2014) found that the best predictors of early postnatal attachment for partners were those who viewed the supportive caregiving role as important and had greater marital quality. Higher levels of parental sensitivity were associated with better infant–parent attachment. Becoming a parent requires the person to build on the experiences he/she has had throughout childhood and adolescence. Co-parents develop an emotional tie with their infants in a variety of ways. They seek and maintain closeness with the infant and can recognize characteristics of the infant. Another study further described co-parent's attachment as a permanent, cyclical concept characterized by changes in response to the child's developmental stage. When children have a secure, supportive, and sensitive relationship with their non-birthing parent, they are generally better adjusted than those that have an unsupportive relationship (Lickenbrock & Braungart-Rieker, 2015).

Attachment is a process; it does not occur instantaneously, even though many parents believe in a romanticized version of attachment happening right after birth. A delay in the attachment process can occur if either the physical and emotional states are adversely affected by exhaustion, pain, or the absence of a support system; if the infant is in NICU and is separated from their parent(s); or had a traumatic birth experience, anesthesia, or an unwanted outcome, such as an ill infant (Lee, Carter, Stevenson, & Harrison, 2014).

Take Note!

Touch is a basic instinctual interaction between parents and their infants and has a vital role in infants' early development. Parents provide a variety of tactile stimulation while addressing their infant's daily care routines (Hugill, 2015).

The developmental task for the infant is learning to differentiate between trust and mistrust. If the primary parent is consistently responsive to the infant's care, meeting the baby's physical and psychological needs, the infant will likely learn to trust the caretaker, view the world as a safe place, and grow up to be secure, self-reliant, trusting, cooperative, and helpful. However, if the infant's needs are not met, the child is more likely to face developmental delays, neglect, and child abuse (Klebanov & Travis, 2015).

"Becoming" a parent may take 4 to 6 months. The transition to parenthood, according to Mercer (2006), involves four stages:
1. Commitment, attachment, and preparation for an infant during pregnancy
2. Acquaintance with and increasing attachment to the infant, learning how to care for the infant, and physical restoration during the first weeks after birth
3. Moving toward a new normal routine in the first 4 months after birth
4. Achievement of a parenthood role around 4 months

The stages overlap, and the timing of each is affected by variables such as the environment, family dynamics, and the partners (Mercer, 2006).

FACTORS AFFECTING ATTACHMENT

Attachment behaviours are influenced by three major factors:
1. Parents' background (includes the care that the parents received when growing up, cultural practices, relationship within the family, experience with previous pregnancies and planning and course of events during pregnancy, postpartum depression)
2. Infant (includes the infant's temperament and health at birth)
3. Care practices (the behaviours of physicians, nurse practitioners, midwives, nurses, and hospital personnel, care and support during labour, first day of life in separation from parent, and rules of the hospital or birthing centre) (Lewis & Rudolph, 2014).

Attachment occurs more readily with the infant whose temperament, health, appearance, and sex fit the parent's expectations. If the infant does not meet these expectations, attachment can be delayed (Lickenbrock & Braungart-Rieker, 2015).

Factors associated with the health care facility or birthing unit can also hinder attachment. These include:
- Separation of infant and parents immediately after birth and for long periods during the day

TABLE 16.1	POSITIVE AND NEGATIVE ATTACHMENT BEHAVIOURS	
	Positive Behaviours	**Negative Behaviours**
Infant	Is alert; demonstrates strong grasp reflex to hold parent's finger; sucks well, feeds easily; enjoys being held close; makes eye-to-eye contact; follows parent's face; appears facially appealing; smiles; is consolable when crying	Feeds poorly, regurgitates often; cries for long periods, colicky and inconsolable; shows flat affect, rarely smiles even when prompted; resists holding and closeness; sleeps with eyes closed most of time; stiffens body when held; is unresponsive to parents; doesn't pay attention to parents' faces
Parent	Makes direct eye contact; assumes *en face* position when holding infant; claims infant as family member, pointing out common features; expresses pride in infant; assigns meaning to infant's actions; smiles and gazes at infant; touches infant, progressing from fingertips to holding; names infant; requests to be close to infant as much as allowed; speaks positively about infant	Expresses disappointment or displeasure in infant; fails to "explore" infant visually or physically; fails to claim infant as part of family; avoids caring for infant; finds excuses not to hold infant close; has negative self-concept; appears uninterested in having infant in room; frequently asks the nurse to provide infant's care; assigns negative attributes to infant; and calls infant inappropriate, negative names

Adapted from Bope, E., & Kellerman, R. (2015). *Conn's current therapy 2015*. Philadelphia, PA: Saunders Elsevier; Park, S., Kim, S., & Kang, K. (2014). Integrative review of nursing intervention studies on mother-infant interactions. *Child Health Nursing Research, 20*(2), 75–86; and Barnes, D. L. (2014). *Women's reproductive mental health across the lifespan*. New York: Springer Publishers.

- Policies that discourage unwrapping and exploring the infant
- Intensive care environment, restrictive visiting policies
- Staff indifference or lack of support for parent's caretaking attempts and abilities

Take Note!

It is important for parents to visit their child in the special care nursery, but the priority of the nurse is to assist the postpartum client in dealing with the grief that accompanies giving birth to a child with special needs. The loss of the "perfect child" must first be mourned before a new parent may be ready to parent the child who has arrived.

CRITICAL ATTRIBUTES OF ATTACHMENT

The terms *bonding* and *attachment* are often used interchangeably, even though they involve different time frames and interactions. Attachment stages include proximity, reciprocity, and commitment.

Proximity refers to the physical and psychological experience of the parents being close to their infant. This attribute has three dimensions:
1. *Contact:* The sensory experiences of touching, holding, and gazing at the infant are part of proximity-seeking behaviour.
2. *Emotional state:* The emotional state emerges from the affective experience of the new parents toward their infant and their parental role.
3. *Individualization:* Parents are aware of the need to differentiate the infant's needs from themselves and to recognize and respond to them appropriately, making the attachment process also, in some way, one of detachment.

Reciprocity is the process by which the infant's abilities and behaviours elicit parental response. Reciprocity is described by two dimensions: complementary behaviour and sensitivity. Complementary behaviour involves taking turns and stopping when the other is not interested or becomes tired. An infant can coo and stare at the parent to elicit a similar parental response to complement his or her behaviour. Parents who are sensitive and responsive to their infant's cues will promote their development and growth. Parents who become skilled at recognizing the ways their infant communicates will respond appropriately by smiling, vocalizing, touching, and kissing.

Commitment refers to the enduring nature of the relationship. The components of this are twofold: centrality and parent role exploration. In centrality, parents place the infant at the centre of their lives. They acknowledge and accept their responsibility to promote the infant's safety, growth, and development. Parent role exploration is the parents' ability to find their own way and integrate the parental identity into themselves (Sears & Sears, 2015a).

POSITIVE AND NEGATIVE ATTACHMENT BEHAVIOURS

Positive bonding behaviours include maintaining close physical contact, making eye-to-eye contact, speaking in soft, high-pitched tones, and touching and exploring the infant. Table 16.1 highlights typical positive and negative attachment behaviours.

NURSING INTERVENTIONS

In terms of postpartum hospital stays today, "less is more." A client who had a vaginal birth may be discharged

EVIDENCE-BASED PRACTICE 16.1   ENHANCING NEONATAL WELLNESS WITH HOME VISITATION

STUDY

According to Health Canada and the CPS, there is substantial evidence that breastfeeding provides the optimal nutrition for newborns and should be continued for the first 6 months followed by continued breastfeeding during the 2 years or more, as solid foods are introduced. The purpose of this study was to measure the effectiveness of home visits by RNs on neonatal wellness as measured by the continuance of breastfeeding at 6 months, reduce readmissions for newborn jaundice and identify any maternal or newborn health issues. The home visits were made on days 3 and 7 after discharge from the hospital. A complete physical assessment on both mother and infant was performed at each home visit.

Findings

The study used a longitudinal, mixed method, within-subject design involving 1,705 participants. Quantitative data were compared to regional and national benchmarks. Qualitative data from study participant interviews were analyzed to identify common themes. The data indicated the home visits did help mothers to continue to breastfeed longer when compared to the regional and national statistics and the home visits also effectively identified newborn jaundice with a reduction in the average length of stay for infants readmitted in comparison to benchmarks.

Nursing Implications

The study's results reinforce the need for extended breastfeeding support beyond the hospital setting discharge for new mothers to continue to breastfeed longer. Clients need to have access to community-based interventions after discharge to reinforce their postpartum education. Nurses can be instrumental in making referrals for home visitations to promote the safe transition from the hospital to the home.

Adapted from Parker, C., Warmuskerken, G., & Sinclair, L. (2015). Enhancing neonatal wellness with home visitation. *Nursing for Women's Health*, *19*(1), 36–45.

within 48 hours or sooner. After a cesarean birth, the client may remain hospitalized for up to 72 hours. This shortened stay leaves little time for nurses to prepare the client and family for the many changes that will occur upon returning home. Research shows that many new parents feel unprepared, uninformed, and unsupported during the postpartum period as they struggle with physical and emotional issues, infant caregiving, breastfeeding concerns, and lifestyle adjustments (Walker, Murphey, & Nichols, 2015). Nurses need to focus on pain and discomfort, immunizations, nutrition, activity and exercise, infant care, lactation instruction, discharge teaching, sexuality and contraception, and follow-up with the limited time they have with their clients (see Nursing Care Plan 16.1, at the end of the chapter). Planning home visits to reinforce postpartum instructions may enhance maternal-infant wellness. (See Evidence-Based Practice 16.1.)

Take Note!

Always adhere to standard precautions when providing direct care to reduce the risk of disease transmission.

Providing Culturally Sensitive Care

As the face of Canada is becoming more diverse, nurses must be prepared to care for childbearing families from various cultures. In many cultures, the entire community will become involved in the caring and nurturing of a new family for weeks and even months after the birth. Overall, the culturally competent care for all childbearing families include understanding of traditional folk beliefs; involvement and support by family members; respect; presence of a significant other; breastfeeding and eating healthy; observing the principles of hot and cold; avoidance of sexual intercourse postnatally; encouragement; empowerment; their spiritual dimensions as important; avoidance of evil spirits; and the hope that nurses will anticipate the needs of the mother and infant (McFarland & Wehbe-Alamah, 2015). Box 16.3 highlights some of the major cultural variants during the postpartum period.

Nurses need to remember that childbearing practices and beliefs vary from culture to culture. To provide appropriate nursing care, the nurse should determine the client's preferences before intervening. Cultural practices may include dietary restrictions, certain clothes, taboos, activities for maintaining mental health, and the use of silence, prayer, or meditation. Restoring health may involve taking folk medicines or conferring with a tribal healer. A language barrier might interfere with communication between the client and health providers, followed by health care provider's lack of cultural sensitivity, leading to a new parent's reluctance in using health services (Santiago & Figueiredo, 2015). Providing culturally diverse care within our global community is challenging for all nurses, because they must remember that one's culture cannot be easily summarized in a reference book but must be viewed through one's own life experiences.

Raina and her husband divulge to the nurse that she would like to respect her Muslim cultural beliefs of modesty and would appreciate being cared for by a female doctor. What should the nurse do in this situation?

BOX 16.3

CULTURAL INFLUENCES DURING THE POSTPARTUM PERIOD

African Canadian Families

- Client may share care of the infant with extended family members.
- Experiences of older women within the family may influence infant care.
- Clients may protect their newborns from strangers for several weeks.
- Clients may choose not to bathe their newborns for the first week. Oils may be applied to skin and hair to prevent dryness and cradle cap.
- Silver dollars may be taped over the infant's umbilicus to flatten the slightly protruding umbilical stump.
- Parents may be inclined to have the baby sleep with them.

Amish Families

- Clients consider childbearing their primary role in society.
- They generally oppose birth control.
- Pregnancy and childbirth are considered a private matter; they may conceal it from public knowledge.
- Clients typically do not respond favourably when hurried to complete a self-care task. Nurses need to take cues from women indicating their readiness to complete morning self-care activities.

Filipino Families

- Grandparents often assist in the care of their grandchildren.
- Breastfeeding is encouraged, and breastfeeding for up to 2 years may be common.
- Clients may have difficulty discussing birth control and sexual matters.
- Families may have strong religious beliefs and bedside prayer may be practiced.
- Families may be very close-knit and numerous visitors may be expected at the hospital after childbirth.

Indigenous Families

- Women may keep pregnancies private and not reveal them until later in the gestation.
- Traditionally, touching was not a typical female behaviour, and eye contact may be brief.

- Clients may benefit from time to sit and talk without feeling hurried or rushed.
  Many Indigenous groups have traditionally considered the placenta as sacred. Families would save the placenta to later bury in the ground under a tree or bush. Some would also keep the umbilical cord remnant.

Japanese Families

- Cleanliness and protection from cold are traditional components of newborn care.
- Newborns might not be taken outside the home due to a traditional belief that they should not be exposed to outside or cold air. Families may prefer to keep infants should in a quiet, clean, warm place for the first month of life.
- Breastfeeding has traditionally been the primary method of feeding.
- Many women stay with their parents' for 1 to 2 months after birth.
- Bathing the infant can be the centre of family activity at home.

Muslim Families

- Modesty is a primary concern; nurses need to protect the client's modesty.
- Muslims are not permitted to eat pork; check all food items before serving.
- Muslims prefer a same-sex health care provider; male–female touching is prohibited except in an emergency.
- A Muslim woman traditionally stays in the house for 40 days after birth, being cared for by the female members of her family.
- Most women will breastfeed. Religious events call for periods of fasting, which may increase the risk of dehydration or malnutrition, however many groups recognize the need for pregnant or lactating women to break the fast.
- Women are exempt from obligatory five-times-daily prayers during the time when lochia is present.
- Extended family may be present throughout much of the woman's hospital stay. They will need an empty room to perform their prayers without having to leave the hospital.

Adapted from Bowers, P., & Ceballos, K. (2015). *Cultural perspectives in childbearing.* Retrieved from http://ce.nurse.com/ce263-60/Cultural-Perspectives-in-Childbearing; Dayer-Berenson, L. (2014). *Cultural competencies of nurses: Impact on health and illness* (2nd ed.). Burlington, MA: Jones & Bartlett Learning; Andrews, M. M., & Boyle, J. S. (2012). *Transcultural concepts in nursing care* (6th ed.). Philadelphia, PA: Wolters Kluwer Health; and O'Driscoll, T., Payne, L., Kelly, L., Cromarty, H., St. Pierre-Hansen, N., & Terry, C. (2011). Traditional First Nations birthing practices: Interviews with elders in northwestern Ontario. *Journal of Obstetrics and Gynecology Canada, 33*(1), 24–29.

Promoting Comfort

The postpartum client may have discomfort and pain from a variety of sources, such as an episiotomy, perineal lacerations, backache as a result of the epidural, pain from a full bladder, an edematous perineum, inflamed hemorrhoids, engorged breasts, afterbirth pains secondary to uterine contractions in breastfeeding and multiparity, and sore nipples if breastfeeding. Relieving the underlying problem is the first step in pain management. Most practices traditionally

employed for postpartum discomforts are not evidence based, so both nonpharmacologic and pharmacologic measures are often used in tandem (King et al., 2015).

Applications of Cold and Heat

COLD

Commonly, an ice pack is the first measure used after a vaginal birth to relieve perineal discomfort from edema, an episiotomy, or a laceration. An ice pack seems to minimize edema, reduce inflammation, decrease capillary permeability, and reduce nerve conduction to the site. It is applied during the fourth stage of labour and can be used for the first 24 hours to reduce perineal edema and to prevent hematoma formation, thus reducing pain and promoting healing. Ice packs are wrapped in a disposable covering or clean washcloth and are applied to the perineal area. Usually the ice pack is applied intermittently for 20 minutes and removed for 10 minutes. Many commercially prepared ice packs are available, but a clean disposable glove filled with crushed ice and covered can also be used. Ensure that the ice pack is changed frequently to promote good hygiene and to allow for periodic assessments.

HEAT

The **peribottle** is a plastic squeeze bottle filled with warm tap water that is sprayed over the perineal area during and after voiding, and before applying a new perineal pad. Usually the peribottle is introduced when the client is assisted to the bathroom to freshen up and void for the first time—in most instances, once vital signs are stable after the first hour. Provide instructions on how and when to use the peribottle. Reinforce this practice each time the client changes the perineal pad, voids, or defecates, making sure that the client understands to direct the flow of water from front to back. The peribottle can be taken home and used over the next several weeks until the lochia discharge stops. The peribottle can be used by clients who had either vaginal or cesarean births to provide comfort and hygiene to the perineal area.

After the first 24 hours, a **sitz bath** with room temperature water may be prescribed and substituted for the ice pack to reduce local swelling and promote comfort for an episiotomy, perineal trauma, or inflamed hemorrhoids. The change from cold to room temperature therapy enhances vascular circulation and healing. When compared with an infrared light to promote healing and reduce perineal pain, sitz baths were significantly more effective in promoting episiotomy wound healing (Sukhwinder, Poonam, Sulakshna, & Jodibala, 2014). Before using a sitz bath, the client should cleanse the perineum with a peribottle or shower.

Most health care agencies use plastic disposable sitz baths that clients can take home. The plastic sitz bath consists of a basin that fits on the commode; a bag filled with warm water is hung on a hook and connected via a tube onto the front of the basin (Fig. 16.6). Teaching Guidelines 16.1 highlights the steps in using a sitz bath.

Teaching Guidelines 16.1
USING A SITZ BATH

1. Close clamp on tubing before filling bag with water to prevent leakage.
2. Fill sitz bath basin and plastic bag with room-temperature water (comfortable to touch).

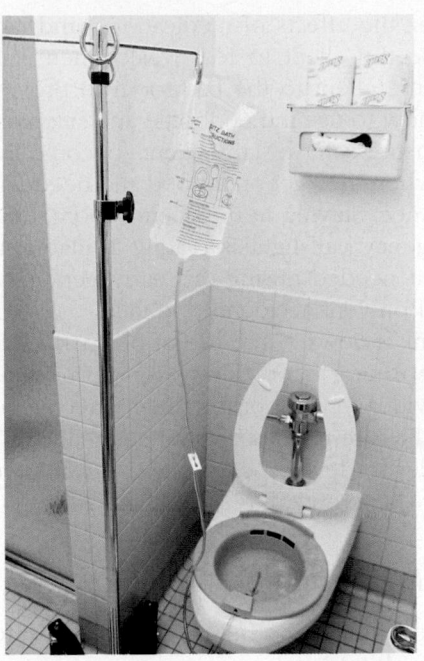

FIGURE 16.6 Sitz bath setup.

3. Place the filled basin on the toilet with the seat raised and the overflow opening facing toward the back of the toilet.
4. Hang the filled plastic bag on a hook close to the toilet or an IV pole.
5. Attach the tubing to the opening on the basin.
6. Sit on the basin positioned on the toilet seat and release the clamp to allow warm water to irrigate the perineum.
7. Remain sitting on the basin for approximately 15 to 20 minutes.
8. Stand up and pat the perineum dry. Apply a clean peripad.
9. Tip the basin to remove any remaining water and flush the toilet.
10. Wash the basin with warm water and soap and dry it in the sink.
11. Store basin and tubing in a clean, dry area until the next use.
12. Wash hands with soap and water.

Advise the client to use the sitz bath several times daily to provide hygiene and comfort to the perineal area. Encourage continuing this measure after discharge. Some facilities have hygienic sitz baths in the bathroom that spray an antiseptic, water, or both onto the perineum. The client sits on the toilet with legs apart so that the nozzle spray reaches her perineal area.

Keep in mind that tremendous hemodynamic changes are taking place during this early postpartum period, and the client's safety must be a priority. Fatigue, blood loss, the effects of medications, and lack of food may cause the client to feel weak when standing up. Assisting the client to the bathroom to provide instructions on how to use the peribottle and sitz bath is necessary to ensure safety. Many clients become lightheaded or dizzy when they get out of bed and need direct physical assistance. Staying in the client's room, ensuring that the emergency call light is readily available, and being available if needed during this early period will ensure safety and prevent accidents and falls.

Recent reviews of the use of postpartum local cooling and warming interventions for perineal pain found limited evidence supporting their effectiveness. Additional studies are needed around perineal pain and healing in order to develop evidence-based interventions in the future (Mooventhan & Nivethitha, 2014).

Topical Preparations

Several treatments may be applied topically for temporary relief of perineal pain and discomfort. One such treatment is a local anesthetic spray such as benzocaine topical. These agents numb the perineal area and are used after cleansing the area with water via the peribottle and/or a sitz bath.

Postpartum clients are predisposed to hemorrhoid development due to pressure during vaginal birth, constipation, relaxation of the smooth muscles in vein walls, and impaired blood return, all related to increased pressure from the heavy gravid uterus. Nonpharmacologic measures to reduce hemorrhoid discomfort include ice packs, ice sitz baths, and application of cool witch hazel pads, such as Tucks®. The pads are placed at the rectal area, between the hemorrhoids and the perineal pad. These pads cool the area, help relieve swelling, and minimize itching. Pharmacologic methods used to reduce hemorrhoid pain include local anesthetics (dibucaine) or steroids (hydrocortisone acetate). Prevention or correction of constipation, encouraging the use of the side-lying position, proper toileting habits, assuming positions that minimize putting pressure on the hemorrhoids, and not straining during defecation will be helpful in reducing discomfort (King et al., 2015).

Nipple pain is difficult to treat, although a wide variety of topical creams, ointments, and gels are available to do so. This group includes beeswax, glycerin-based products, petrolatum, lanolin, and hydrogel products. Many people find these products comforting. Beeswax, glycerin-based products, and petrolatum all need to be removed before breastfeeding. These products should be avoided in order to limit infant exposure because the process of removal may increase nipple irritation. All breastfeeding clients should be taught to apply expressed breast milk to nipples and allowing it to dry as a strategy to reduce nipple pain and promote healing. Usually the pain is due to incorrect latch-on and/or removal of

the nursing infant from the breast. Early assistance with breastfeeding to ensure correct positioning can help prevent nipple trauma.

Analgesics

Analgesics such as acetaminophen and oral nonsteroidal anti-inflammatory drugs (NSAIDs) such as ibuprofen or naproxen are prescribed to relieve mild postpartum discomfort. For moderate to severe pain, a narcotic analgesic such as codeine or oxycodone in conjunction with aspirin or acetaminophen may be prescribed. Instruct postpartum clients about adverse effects of any medication prescribed. Common adverse effects of oral analgesics include dizziness, lightheadedness, nausea and vomiting, constipation, and sedation (Skidmore-Roth, 2015).

Also inform the client that the drugs are secreted in breast milk. Nearly all medications that the client takes are passed into her breast milk; however, the mild analgesics (e.g., acetaminophen or ibuprofen) are considered relatively safe for breastfeeding (King et al., 2015). Administering a mild analgesic approximately an hour before breastfeeding will usually relieve afterpains and/or perineal discomfort.

Assisting With Elimination

The bladder is edematous, hypotonic, and congested immediately postpartum. Consequently, bladder distention, incomplete emptying, and inability to void are common. A full bladder interferes with uterine contraction and may lead to hemorrhage, because it will displace the uterus out of the midline. Encourage the client to void. Often, assisting the client into the normal voiding position on the commode facilitates this. If the client has difficulty voiding, strategies to attempt include: pouring warm water over the perineal area, hearing the sound of running tap water, blowing bubbles through a straw, taking a warm shower, drinking fluids, providing her with privacy, or placing her hand in a basin of warm water. If these actions do not stimulate urination within 4 to 6 hours after giving birth, catheterization may be needed. Palpate the bladder for distention and ask if the client is voiding in small amounts (less than 100 mL) frequently (retention with overflow). If catheterization is necessary, use sterile technique to reduce the risk of infection.

Decreased bowel motility during labour, high iron content in prenatal vitamins, postpartum fluid loss, and the adverse effects of pain medications and/or anesthesia may predispose the postpartum client to constipation. In addition, the client may fear that bowel movements will cause pain or injury, especially if she had an episiotomy or a laceration that was repaired with sutures.

Usually a stool softener, such as docusate, with or without a laxative might be helpful if the client has difficulty with bowel elimination. Other measures, such as ambulating and increasing fluid and fibre intake, may also help. Nutritional instruction might include increasing fruits and vegetables in the diet; drinking plenty of fluids (8 to 12 cups daily) to keep the stool soft; drinking small amounts of prune juice and/or hot liquids to stimulate peristalsis; eating high-fibre foods such as bran cereals, whole grains, dried fruits, fresh fruits, and raw vegetables; and walking daily.

Promoting Activity, Rest, and Exercise

The postpartum period is an ideal time for nurses to promote the importance of physical fitness, help clients incorporate exercise into their lifestyle, and encourage them to overcome barriers to exercise. The lifestyle changes that occur postpartum may affect a person's health for decades. Early ambulation is encouraged to reduce the risk of thromboembolism and to improve strengthening.

Many changes occur postpartum, and caring for a newborn alters the client's eating and sleeping habits, work schedules, and time allocation. Postpartum fatigue is common during the early days after childbirth, and it may continue for weeks or months. Having adequate sleep is critical because shorter sleep time, a high percentage of sleep disturbances, and greater fatigue are associated with depressive symptoms in the postpartum period (Bhati & Richards, 2015). Working partners with newborns experience fatigue during early parenthood and are unable to recover due to interrupted and poor sleep patterns. This sleep deficit can compromise their work safety (Parfitt & Ayers, 2014). It can also affect relationships with significant others as well as the ability to fulfill household and child care responsibilities. Be sure that the client recognizes the need for rest and sleep and has realistic expectations. Some suggestions include the following:

- Nap when the infant is sleeping, because getting uninterrupted sleep at night is difficult.
- Reduce participation in outside activities and limit the number of visitors.
- Determine the infant's sleep–wake cycles and attempt to increase wakeful periods during the day so the baby sleeps for longer periods at night.
- Eat a balanced diet to promote healing and to increase energy levels.
- Share household tasks to conserve your energy.
- Ask family members or other supports to assist in the care baby, allowing for more opportunities for rest.
- Review your family's daily routine and see if you can "cluster" activities to conserve energy and promote rest.

The demands of parenthood may reduce or prevent exercise in even the most committed person. A targeted exercise program and proper body mechanics can help the client to deal with the physical challenges of the postpartum period. Emphasize the benefits of a regular exercise program, which include:

- Helps to lose pregnancy weight
- Reduces the risk of obesity later in life
- Increases overall postpartum well-being
- Increases energy level so the woman can cope with her new responsibilities
- Speeds the return to prepregnant size and shape
- Reduces risk of postpartum depression
- Reduces risk of constipation
- Reduces mental fatigue
- Provides an outlet for stress (Covan, 2015)

Overweight and obesity are epidemic in Canada. Obesity is a risk factor for numerous conditions, including diabetes, hypertension, high cholesterol, stroke, heart disease, cancer, and arthritis. Approximately 6 per 1,000 pregnant women in Canada experience extreme obesity (Crane, Murphy, Burrage, & Hutchens, 2013). Although the average gestational weight gain is small (approximately 25 to 35 lb), excess weight gain and failure to lose weight after pregnancy are important predictors of long-term obesity. The postpartum period is a vulnerable time for excessive weight retention, particularly for the increasing number of clients who are overweight at the start of their pregnancy and subsequently find it difficult to lose the additional weight gained during pregnancy. Breastfeeding and exercise may help to control weight in the long term (Neville, McKinley, Holmes, Spence, & Woodside, 2014).

Take Note!

Clients who are unable to return to a healthy weight by 6 months postpartum increase their risk factors for the development of chronic diseases including metabolic syndrome, obesity, and cardiovascular disease (Brekke et al., 2014). Encourage the loss of pregnancy weight by 6 months postpartum, and refer those with difficulty to a dietician, nutritionist, or community weight-loss program.

The postpartum client may face some obstacles to exercising, including physical changes (ligament laxity), competing demands (newborn care), lack of information about weight retention (inactivity equates to weight gain), and stress incontinence (leaking of urine during activity).

A healthy client with an uncomplicated vaginal birth can resume exercise in the immediate postpartum period. Advise the client to start slowly and increase the level of exercise over a period of several weeks as tolerated. Infant strollers/carriers may be an option for some, allowing them to walk with their newborns for exercise. Jogging strollers can be used later when the infant is 6 to 12 months old and can hold his or her head up. Also, exercise videos and home exercise equipment allow new parents to work out while the newborn naps.

Exercising after giving birth promotes feelings of well-being and restores muscle tone lost during pregnancy. Routine exercise should be resumed gradually, beginning with pelvic floor exercises on the first postpartum day and, by the second week, progressing to abdominal, buttock, and thigh-toning exercises. Most postpartum clients fail to meet national guidelines for physical activity which may elevate their risk for morbidity and contribute to the intergenerational impact of obesity on their offspring (Downs, Evenson, & Chasan-Taber, 2014). Walking is an excellent form of early exercise as long as the individual avoids jarring and bouncing movements, because joints do not stabilize until 6 to 8 weeks postpartum. Exercising too much too soon can cause increased bleeding and lochia may return to bright red. If this occurs, instruct the client to stop exercising and rest lying down until the bleeding slows. This increase in bleeding should be a warning that the client is over doing it and needs to slow down the exercise routine.

Recommended exercises for the first few weeks postpartum include abdominal breathing, head lifts, modified sit-ups, double knee roll, and pelvic tilt (Teaching Guidelines 16.2). The number of exercises and their duration is gradually increased as the client gains strength.

Teaching Guidelines 16.2
POSTPARTUM EXERCISES

Abdominal Breathing
1. While lying on a flat surface (floor or bed), take a deep breath through your nose and expand your abdominal muscles (they will rise up from your midsection).
2. Slowly exhale and tighten your abdominal muscles for 3 to 5 seconds.
3. Repeat this several times.

Head Lift
1. Lie on a flat surface with knees flexed and feet flat on the surface.
2. Lift your head off the flat surface, tuck it onto your chest, and hold for 3 to 5 seconds.
3. Relax your head and return to the starting position.
4. Repeat this several times.

Modified Sit-Ups
1. Lie on a flat surface and raise your head and shoulders 15 to 20 cm so that your outstretched hands reach your knees.
2. Keep your waist on the flat surface.
3. Slowly return to the starting position.
4. Repeat, increasing in frequency as your comfort level allows.

Double Knee Roll
1. Lie on a flat surface with your knees bent.
2. While keeping your shoulders flat, slowly roll your knees to your right side to touch the flat surface (floor or bed).
3. Roll your knees back over your body to the left side until they touch the opposite side of the flat surface.
4. Return to the starting position on your back and rest.
5. Repeat this exercise several times.

Pelvic Tilt
1. Lie on your back on a flat surface with your knees bent and your arms at your side.
2. Slowly contract your abdominal muscles while lifting your pelvis up toward the ceiling.
3. Hold for 3 to 5 seconds and slowly return to your starting position.
4. Repeat several times.

Remember that cultures have different attitudes toward exercise. Some clients follow cultural beliefs that observe a specific period of bed rest or activity restriction; thus, recommending active exercise during the early postpartum period may not be appropriate (Bowers & Ceballos, 2015).

Preventing Stress Incontinence

Fifty percent of all parous clients develop some degree of pelvic prolapse in their lifetime that is associated with stress incontinence. Stress incontinence causes reduced quality of life and withdrawal from fitness and exercise activities typically. Research suggests that having a vaginal delivery results in direct pelvic muscle trauma and disruption of fascial supports, and also causes damage to the levator ani muscle and pudendal nerve injury. Offering pelvic floor muscle exercise instruction to all clients during their first pregnancy and again after having a vaginal birth is recommended by the National Institute for Health and Care Excellence (NICE) guidelines. Nurses can offer them as a first-line intervention in the prevention of urinary incontinence postpartum (Hall & Woodward, 2015). The more vaginal deliveries a person has had, the more likely stress incontinence becomes. Stress incontinence can occur with any activity that causes an increase in intra-abdominal pressure. Low-impact activities might be preferable, such as walking, biking, swimming, or low-impact aerobics so they can resume physical activity while strengthening the pelvic floor.

Suggestions to prevent stress incontinence are:
- Start a regular program of pelvic floor muscle exercises after childbirth.
- Lose weight if necessary; obesity is associated with stress incontinence.
- Avoid smoking; limit intake of alcohol and caffeinated beverages, which irritate the bladder.
- Adjust fluid intake to produce a 24-hourly urine output of 1,000 to 2,000 mL.
- Use either an intravaginal or intraurethral device that puts pressure onto the urethra so that urine will not leak when bladder pressure rises (Laliberte, 2015).

Pelvic floor exercises (Kegel exercises) help to strengthen the pelvic floor muscles if done properly and regularly (Ciaghi, Bianco, & Guarese, 2015). These pelvic floor strengthening exercises were originally developed by Dr. Arnold Kegel in the 1940s as a method of controlling incontinence after childbirth. The principle behind these exercises is that strengthening the muscles of the pelvic floor improves urethral sphincter function.

While providing postpartum care, instruct clients on primary prevention of stress incontinence by discussing the value and purpose of pelvic floor muscle exercises. Approach the subject sensitively, avoiding the term *incontinent*. The terms *leakage, loss of urine,* or *bladder control issues* are more acceptable.

Take Note!

When properly performed, pelvic floor exercises have been effective in preventing or improving urinary continence (Jones & Hawkes, 2015).

Pelvic floor exercises can be performed by doing ten 5-second contractions, whenever they change diapers, talk on the phone, or watch TV. Teach the client to perform pelvic floor exercises properly; help her to identify the correct muscles by trying to stop and start the flow of urine when sitting on the toilet (Teaching Guidelines 16.3). Pelvic floor exercises can be done without anyone knowing.

Teaching Guidelines 16.3
PERFORMING PELVIC FLOOR MUSCLE EXERCISES

1. Identify the correct pelvic floor muscles by contracting them to stop the flow of urine while sitting on the toilet.
2. Repeat this contraction several times to become familiar with it.
3. Start the exercises by emptying the bladder.
4. Tighten the pelvic floor muscles and hold for 10 seconds.
5. Relax the muscle completely for 10 seconds.
6. Perform 10 exercises at least three times daily. Progressively increase the number that you perform.
7. Perform the exercises in different positions, such as standing, lying, and sitting.
8. Keep breathing during the exercises.
9. Don't contract your abdominal, thigh, leg, or buttocks muscles during these exercises.
10. Relax while doing pelvic floor exercises and concentrate on isolating the right muscles.
11. Attempt to tighten your pelvic muscles before sneezing, jumping, or laughing.
12. Remember that you can perform these exercises anywhere without anyone noticing.

Assisting With Self-Care Measures

Demonstrate and discuss ways to prevent infection during the postpartum period. Because the client may experience lochia drainage for as long as a month after childbirth, describe practices to promote well-being and healing. These measures include:

- Frequently change perineal pads, applying and removing them from front to back to prevent spreading contamination from the rectal area to the genital area.
- Avoid using tampons after giving birth to decrease the risk of infection.
- Shower once or twice daily using a mild soap. Avoid using soap on nipples.
- Use a sitz bath after every bowel movement to cleanse the rectal area and relieve enlarged hemorrhoids.
- Use the peribottle filled with warm water after urinating and before applying a new perineal pad.
- Avoid tub baths for 4 to 6 weeks, until joints and balance are restored, to prevent falls.
- Wash your hands before changing perineal pads, after disposing of soiled pads, and after voiding (Mattson & Smith, 2016).

To reduce the risk of infection at the episiotomy site, reinforce proper perineal care with the client, showing the client how to rinse the perineum with the peribottle after voiding or defecation. Stress the importance of always patting gently from front to back and washing hands thoroughly before and after perineal care. For hemorrhoids, have the client apply witch hazel-soaked pads (Tucks®), ice packs to relieve swelling, or hemorrhoidal cream or ointment if ordered.

Ensuring Safety

One of the safety concerns during the postpartum period is orthostatic hypotension. When the client rapidly moves from a lying or sitting position to a standing one, blood pressure can suddenly drop, causing the pulse rate to increase. The client may become dizzy and faint. Be aware of this problem and initiate the following safeguards:

- Check blood pressure first before ambulation.
- Elevate the head of the bed for a few minutes before the client ambulates.
- Have the client sit on the side of the bed for a few moments before getting up.
- Help the client to stand up, and stay close.
- Ambulate alongside the client and provide support if needed.
- Frequently ask how the client is feeling.
- Stay close by to assist if the client reports feeling light-headed.

Additional topics to address orthostatic hypotension that may concern infant safety include instructing the client to place the newborn back in the crib on his or her back when feeling sleepy to prevent a fall. If a parent falls asleep while holding the newborn, the baby could fall. Also, instruct parents to keep the door to their room closed when their newborn is in their room with them, and to check the identification of anyone who enters their room or who wants to take the newborn out of the room. This will prevent infant abduction.

Counselling About Sexuality and Contraception

Pregnancy and childbirth are special periods in life that involve significant physical, hormonal, psychological, social, and cultural changes that may influence a person's sexuality as well as the health of a couple's sexual relationship. This is often a time period filled with excitement, changes, and challenges. Postpartum clients often face changes in their own sexuality in their adjustment to motherhood. Sexuality is an important part of every person's life. Clients may want to get back to "normal" as soon as possible after giving birth, but a couple's sexual relationship cannot be isolated from the psychological and psychosocial adjustments that both partners are going through.

Childbirth is a significant life transition that has a measurable impact on postpartum clients' sexual function. There are physical (perineal pain), psychological (depression), and contextual factors (parenthood) that contribute to the change in many people's sex lives after experiencing childbirth. They may experience hesitation to resume sexual relations for a number of reasons. During the postpartum period, new parents may deal with have fatigue, weakness, loss of sexual desire, perception of decreased attractiveness, change in body appearance, vaginal bleeding, perineal discomfort, hemorrhoids, sore breasts, decreased vaginal lubrication resulting from low estrogen levels, and dyspareunia. Fatigue, the physical demands made by the infant, and the stress of new roles and responsibilities may stress the emotional reserves of couples. New parents may not get much privacy or rest, both of which are necessary for sexual pleasure (Whittock, 2015).

Partners may feel they now have a secondary role within the family, and they may not understand their partner's daily routine. The delicate nature of postpartum sexuality makes it difficult for couples to discuss. These issues, combined with increased investment in the parenting role, can strain the couple's sexual relationship.

Although couples are reluctant to ask, they often want to know when they can safely resume sexual intercourse after childbirth. Typically, sexual intercourse can be resumed once the red bleeding has stopped and the perineum is healed from an episiotomy or lacerations. This is usually by the third to the sixth week postpartum. However, there is no prescribed time at which to resume sexual intercourse after childbirth. There is no scientific basis for the traditional recommendation to delay sexual

activity until the 6-week postpartum check-up. Each couple must set their own time frame when they feel it is appropriate to resume sexual intercourse. Despite fears and myths about sexual activity during pregnancy, maintaining a couple's sexual interactions throughout pregnancy and the postpartum period can promote sexual health and well-being and a greater depth of intimacy.

Postpartum sexual health and sexual problems are common, which receive little attention from health care providers during the postpartum period, need to be addressed (Halford, Petch, & Creedy, 2015). When counselling the couple about sexuality, determine what knowledge and concerns the couple have about their sexual relationship. Inform the couple that fluctuations in sexual interest are normal. Reassure the breastfeeding client that a let-down reflex may occur during orgasm and the breasts may be very sensitive when touched. Also inform the couple about how to prevent discomfort. Precoital vaginal lubrication may be impaired during the postpartum period, especially in those who are breastfeeding. Use of water-based gel lubricants (K-Y® jelly, Astroglide) can help. Pelvic floor exercises, in addition to preventing stress incontinence, can also enhance sensation.

Initiation of contraception during the postpartum period is important for heterosexual couples to prevent unintended pregnancy and short birth intervals, which can lead to negative health outcomes for both the client and infant. Contraceptive options should be included in the discussions with the couple so that they can make an informed decision before resuming sexual activity. Many couples are overwhelmed with the amount of new information given to them during their brief hospitalization, so many are not ready for a lengthy discussion about contraceptives. Presenting a brief overview of the options, along with literature, may be appropriate. It may be suitable to ask them to think about contraceptive needs and preferences and advise them to use a barrier method (condom with spermicidal gel or foam) until they choose another form of contraception. This advice is especially important if the follow-up appointment will not occur for 4 to 6 weeks after childbirth, because many couples will resume sexual activity before this time. Some postpartum clients ovulate before their menstrual period returns and thus need contraceptive protection to prevent another pregnancy.

Recently, the CDC assessed evidence regarding the safety of estrogen-containing contraceptive methods use during the postpartum period. They recommend that combined hormonal contraceptives not be used during the first 21 days after childbirth because of the high risk for VTE during this period. During days 21 to 42 postpartum, clients without risk factors for VTE generally can initiate estrogen-containing contraceptives, but those with risk factors for VTE (e.g., previous VTE or recent cesarean delivery) generally should not use these methods. After 42 days postpartum, no restrictions on the use of combined hormonal contraceptives based on postpartum status apply (Centers for Disease Control & Prevention [CDC], 2015a).

Open and effective communication is necessary for effective contraceptive counselling so that information is clearly understood. Provide clear, consistent information appropriate to the client and partner's language, culture, and educational level. This will help the couple select the best contraceptive method. Research supports that postpartum education about contraception leads to more contraception use and fewer unplanned pregnancies and that both short-term and multiple-contact interventions had effects. The use of contraceptives was highest when contraceptive counselling was provided prenatally and again in the postpartum period (Zapata et al., 2015).

Promoting Nutrition

The postpartum period can be a stressful one for myriad reasons, such as fatigue, the physical stress of pregnancy and birth, and the nonstop work required to take care of the newborn and to meet the needs of other family members. As a result, new parents may ignore their own nutrition needs. Whether breastfeeding or bottle-feeding, encourage the postpartum client to perform self-care and eat a healthy diet so that the nutrients lost during pregnancy can be replaced and to return to a healthy weight. In general, postpartum nutrition recommendations include the following:

- Eat a wide variety of foods with high nutrient density.
- Eat meals that require little or no preparation.
- Avoid high-fat fast foods.
- Drink plenty of fluids daily—at least 2,500 mL (approximately 84 oz).
- Avoid fad weight-reduction diets and harmful substances such as alcohol, tobacco, and drugs.
- Avoid excessive intake of fat, salt, sugar, and caffeine.
- Eat the recommended daily servings from each food group (Box 16.4).

Nutrition During Lactation

The breastfeeding client's nutritional needs are higher than they were during pregnancy. The client's diet and nutritional status influence the quantity and quality of breast milk. The Dieticians of Canada (2014) recommend that breastfeeding women consume foods that contain iodine, an element that is crucial to healthy brain development and may be lacking in their present diets. Iodine is necessary to produce thyroid hormone, which in turn helps brain development. To meet the needs for breast milk production, the client's nutritional needs increase as follows:

- *Calories:* + 500 cal/day for the first and second 6 months of lactation
- *Protein:* + 20 g/day, adding an extra 2 cups of skim milk
- *Calcium:* + 400 mg daily—consumption of four or more servings of milk

---

BOX 16.4

NUTRITIONAL RECOMMENDATIONS FOR NUTRITION DURING THE POSTPARTUM PERIOD

Recommendations for the Breastfeeding Client from the Canada's Food Guide for Health Eating (see Chapter 11)

- Fruits: 4 servings
- Vegetables: 4 servings
- Milk: 4 servings
- Bread, cereal, pasta: 6 to 7 servings
- Meat, poultry, fish, eggs: 3 servings
- Fats, oils: 30 to 45 mL (2 to 3 tbsp) of unsaturated fat per day.

General Dietary Guidelines from Eating Well with Canada's Food Guide (for the non–breast-feeding client)

- Eat at least one dark green and one orange vegetable each day.
- Choose vegetables and fruit prepared with little or no added fat, sugar or salt. Have vegetables and fruit more often than juice.
- Make at least half of your grain products whole grain each day.
- Choose grain products that are lower in fat, sugar or salt.
- Drink skim, 1%, or 2% milk each day.
- Select lower fat milk alternatives: Compare the Nutrition Facts table on yogurts or cheeses to make wise choices.
- Have meat alternatives such as beans, lentils, and tofu often.
- Eat at least two Food Guide Servings of fish each week. (*See Health Canada's recommendations for limiting exposure to mercury from certain fish.*)
- Select lean meat and alternatives prepared with little or no added fat or salt (Health Canada, 2011).

- *Iodine:* 290 mcg daily—dairy products, seafood, and iodized salt
- *Fluid:* + 2 to 3 quarts of fluids daily (milk, juice, or water); no sodas

Some foods eaten by the breastfeeding clients may affect the flavour of the breast milk or cause gastrointestinal problems for the infant. Not all infants are affected by the same foods. It is suggested that the food item that may be causing a problem for the infant be identified and its intake be reduced or eliminated completely.

Nutritional needs for breastfeeding clients are based on the nutritional content of breast milk and the energy expended to produce it. If intake of calories exceeds the energy expended, weight gain occurs. The highest incidence of obesity occurs during the childbearing years. Clients need to be made aware that weight gained during their reproductive years will have a negative impact on their health as they age. Nurses can support a postpartum weight management program by assessing the client's readiness to change to lose their pregnancy weight gain; assessing their breastfeeding status, dietary intake, and activity levels; and assessing them for stress and depressive symptoms, which might hinder their weight loss (Green, 2016).

Take Note!

During a client's brief stay in a health care facility, they may demonstrate healthy appetite and eat well. Nutritional problems usually start at home when people make their own food selections and prepare their own meals. This is a crucial area to address during follow-up.

Supporting Informed Decision Making for Infant Feeding

The WHO (2014b), Health Canada, Canadian Paediatric Society, Dietitians of Canada, and Breastfeeding Committee for Canada (2015), as well as the Canadian Nurses Association (CNA) and Canadian Association of Midwives (2014), have all released position statements in support of exclusive breastfeeding for the first 6 months of life, recognizing that breastfeeding is the "normal and unequalled method of feeding infants" (Health Canada, CPS, Dietitians of Canada, & Breastfeeding Committee for Canada, 2015, para 4) which nurses must encourage as part of evidence-based practice. There is extensive evidence that breastfeeding has numerous health benefits for both members of the breastfeeding dyad. However, some clients will choose to feed their infants with breast milk substitutes (formula) for the first year of life. Nurses must be able to deliver sound, evidence-based information to help new parents choose the best way to feed their infants and must support them in their decisions. Research findings indicate that parents do listen to nurses' instructions on feeding practices (Stagg & Ustianov, 2015). Many factors affect a client's choice of feeding method, such as culture, employment demands, support from significant others and family, and knowledge base. Breastfeeding is the optimal food for every baby and nurses must ensure that parents have the information they need to make an informed decision. Whether a parent chooses to breastfeed or formula-feed the newborn, nurses must then support and respect their choice.

Indications for Not Breastfeeding

While breastfeeding is generally the optimal choice for infant feeding, there are a few situations in which breastfeeding would not be safe. Drugs such as antithyroid drugs, antineoplastic drugs, or street drugs (methamphetamines, cocaine, PCP) enter the breast milk and would harm an infant, so clients who are not able to stop taking these substances should not breastfeed. With the legalization of cannabis in Canada, many clients and care providers have questions about the safety of cannabis use while breastfeeding. Research in this area in ongoing, however there is not adequate evidence at this time to indicate that cannabis

use is safe during lactation. Clients should be warned of potential risks, which early research indicates could include decreased attention span, memory function, and problem-solving abilities in growing children (Health Canada, 2018a).

To prevent HIV transmission to a newborn, clients who are HIV positive should be advised not to breastfeed. Those with active herpes infection on the breasts could pass the virus on to the baby and should not breastfeed from an affected breast. Other contraindications to breastfeeding include a newborn with an inborn error of metabolism such as galactosemia or phenylketonuria (PKU), or active tuberculosis (Denne, 2015).

Providing Assistance With Infant Feeding

First-time parents often have many questions about feeding, and even clients who have had experience with feeding may have questions. Regardless of whether new parents are breastfeeding or bottle-feeding, they will benefit from instruction.

SUPPORTING BREASTFEEDING

The CPS recommends breastfeeding for all full-term newborns. Exclusive breastfeeding is sufficient to support optimal growth and development for approximately the first 6 months of life. Breastfeeding should be continued for at least the first year of life and beyond for as long as mutually desired. Educating parents about breastfeeding will increase the likelihood of a successful breastfeeding experience.

At birth, all newborns should be quickly dried, assessed, and, if stable, placed immediately in uninterrupted skin-to-skin contact (kangaroo care) with their parent. This is good practice whether the client is going to breastfeed or bottle-feed. Numerous benefits of kangaroo care have been reported related to physiologic (thermoregulation, cardiorespiratory stability), behavioural (sleep, breastfeeding duration, and degree of exclusivity), domains, as an effective therapy to relieve procedural pain, and improve neurodevelopment. In addition, kangaroo care provides the newborn with optimal physiologic stability, warmth, and opportunities for the first feed (Campbell-Yeo, Disher, Benoit, & Johnston, 2015).

The benefits of breastfeeding for infants are clear (see Chapter 18). To promote breastfeeding, the Baby-Friendly Hospital Initiative (BFHI), an international program of the WHO and UNICEF, was started in 1991. This global health promotion initiative was put forth to improve maternal-infant health by improving rates of exclusive breastfeeding. In Canada, the Breastfeeding Committee for Canada (2017) revised the BFHI to implement the *Baby-Friendly Initiative*, which bridges both in-patient and community support for breastfeeding families. The following 10 steps to provide "an optimal environment for the promotion, protection, and support of breastfeeding:

1. Have a written infant feeding policy that is routinely communicated to all staff, health care providers, and volunteers.

2. Ensure all staff, health care providers, and volunteers have the knowledge and skills necessary to implement the infant feeding policy.

3. Inform pregnant women and their families about the importance and process of breastfeeding.

4. Place babies in uninterrupted skin-to-skin contact with their mothers immediately following birth for at least an hour or until completion of the first feeding or as long as the mother wishes. Encourage mothers to recognize when their babies are ready to feed, offering help as needed.

5. Assist mothers to breastfeed and maintain lactation should they face challenges including separation from their infants.

6. Support mothers to exclusively breastfeed for the first 6 months, unless supplements are medically indicated.

7. Facilitate 24-hour rooming-in for all mother–infant dyads: mothers and infants remain together.

8. Encourage responsive, cue-based feeding. Encourage sustained breastfeeding beyond 6 months with appropriate introduction of complementary foods.

9. Support mothers to feed and care for their breastfeeding babies without the use of artificial teats or pacifiers (dummies or soothers).

10. Provide a seamless transition between the services provided by the hospital, community health services, and peer support programs. Apply principles of Primary Health Care and Population Health to support the continuum of care and implement strategies that affect the broad determinants that will improve breastfeeding outcomes.

The nurse is responsible for protecting, promoting, and supporting breastfeeding. For the families who choose to breastfeed their infant, the nurse or lactation consultant will need to spend time providing instruction about how to do so successfully. Many new parents have the impression that breastfeeding is simple. Although it is a natural process, some may experience some difficulty in breastfeeding their newborns. Nurses can assist clients in smoothing out this transition. Assist and provide one-to-one instruction to breastfeeding parents, especially first-time breastfeeding parents, to ensure correct technique. Suggestions are highlighted in Teaching Guidelines 16.4. (See Evidence-Based Practice 16.2.)

Take Note!

Some newborns "latch on and catch on" right away, and others take more time and patience. Inform parents about this to reduce their frustration and uncertainty about their ability to breastfeed.

Clients need to believe in themselves and their ability to accomplish this task. They should not panic if breastfeeding does not go smoothly at first; it takes time and practice. Additional suggestions to help clients relax and feel more comfortable breastfeeding, especially when they return home, include the following:

• Select a quiet corner or room where you won't be disturbed.
• Use a rocking chair to soothe both you and your infant.
• Take long, slow deep breaths to relax before nursing.
• Drink noncaffeinated beverages while breastfeeding to replenish body fluids.

EVIDENCE-BASED PRACTICE 16.2 | **NURSES IMPROVING THE HEALTH OF MOTHERS AND INFANTS BY DANCING THE 10 STEPS TO SUCCESSFUL BREASTFEEDING**

STUDY

The Baby Friendly Hospital Initiative gained momentum around the world in recent years. The principles of it are evidence-based and indicate that promoting breastfeeding improves health outcomes and neurocognitive development in infants. The purpose of this study was to implement the Ten Steps to Successful Breastfeeding and see if the rates and duration of breastfeeding improved. The implementation strategies included assessment of current practices, identification of barriers and opportunities, and strategies to support changes in 89 hospitals that participated. The initiative was to increase the number of Baby Friendly designated hospitals in the United States over a 2-year process-improvement time frame.

Findings

Results included heightened professional environment of competence, enhanced delivery of client-centred care, improved health of mothers and infants, increased client satisfaction, and achievement of benchmarks. The implementation of the Ten Steps to Successful Breastfeeding resulted in improved rates of breastfeeding in all 89 hospitals.

Nursing Implications

This study demonstrated the positive effect of a nurse-led initiative that improved the continuum of care for mothers and infants from the prenatal period through post discharge community care. Nurses can be instrumental in breastfeeding success by applying principles of evidence-based practices and bring forth change within their health care agencies to improve the outcomes for mothers and their infants.

Adapted from Allen, M., & Schafer, D. J. (2015). Nurses improving the health of mothers and infants by dancing the 10 steps to successful breastfeeding. *Journal of Obstetric, Gynecologic, & Neonatal Nursing, 44,* S52.

Teaching Guidelines 16.4

EDUCATION FOR BREASTFEEDING PARENTS

1. Explain that breastfeeding is a learned skill for both parties.
2. Instruct the client to wash hands before starting.
3. Inform the client that afterpains will increase while breastfeeding.
4. Make sure the client is comfortable and not hungry.
5. Tell the client to identify early feeding cues, to respond to the baby during quiet and alert states, rather than waiting for late feeding cues (such as crying).
6. Assist the client to position herself correctly for comfort.
7. Facilitate the client's relaxation to encourage the let-down reflex.
8. Teach the client to form a "C" hold to support the breast with thumb on top and other four fingers under the breast.
9. Encourage the client lightly tickle the infant's upper lip with the nipple to stimulate the infant to open the mouth wide.
10. Teach the client to latch the baby on by bringing the infant rapidly to the breast when the baby opens the mouth wide.
11. Show the client and co-parent how to check that the newborn's mouth position is correct, and to listen for swallowing.
12. Demonstrate correct removal from the breast, using a finger to break the suction.
13. Instruct the client on how to burp the infant before changing from one breast to another.
14. Teach about different positions, such as cross-cradle and football holds and side-lying positions (see Chapter 18).
15. Reinforce and praise the client for the efforts and abilities demonstrated.
16. Allow ample time to answer questions and address concerns.
17. Refer the client to support groups and community resources for ongoing support and assistance.

- Listen to soothing music while breastfeeding.
- Cuddle and caress the infant while feeding.
- Set out extra cloths within reach to use as burping cloths.
- Allow sufficient time to enjoy each other in an unhurried atmosphere.
- Involve other family members in all aspects of the infant's care from the start.
- Contact a local La Leche League or Nursing Mother's group for continued guidance/support.

Because obesity in Canada is increasing in all walks of life, it is important for nurses to be knowledgeable about how it impacts breastfeeding and ways to support the obese client. Research shows that clients who are obese (BMI >30) are less likely to initiate lactation, have difficulties with latching on, have delayed lactogenesis, experience mechanical challenges, and are prone to early cessation of breastfeeding (Shannon, Chao, & Ramos, 2015). Clients who are overweight and obese have lowered prolactin responses to infant sucking, thus milk production may be inhibited. Lactation plays a significant role in preventing future obesity in both the client and the infant (Masho, Cha, & Morris, 2015).

Nurses can assist in managing obesity-related lactation challenges by encouraging rooming-in to facilitate early and frequent sucking to trigger prolactin and oxytocin production, which will help negate the obesity-related blunting of the prolactin response. Suggesting a sandwich technique to insert the breast into the newborn's mouth to elicit sucking might be helpful for the client with large breasts. In the sandwich technique, the client is taught to grasp the breast by making a "C" with the thumb and index finger. The thumb stabilizes the top of the breast while the remaining four fingers support the breast from below. Massage or pumping the breast may soften and extend the nipple for easier infant latch-on. In short, nurses can make a difference by observing lactation, assessing infant hydration and satisfaction, and reassuring the client about breastfeeding ability.

PROVIDING ASSISTANCE WITH FEEDING BREAST MILK SUBSTITUTES

If the couple has chosen to feed their newborn with infant formula, the nurse must respect and support their decision. Discuss with the parents what type of formula they will use. Commercial formulas are classified as cow's milk-based, soy protein-based, or specialized or therapeutic formulas for infants with protein allergies. Commercial formulas can also be purchased in various forms: powdered (must be mixed with water), condensed liquid (must be diluted with equal amounts of water), ready to use (poured directly into bottles), and prepackaged (ready to use in disposable bottles).

Breast milk is a dynamic fluid with compositional changes occurring throughout the period of lactation that reflects the growth rate and developmental needs of the infant. Infant formula, in contrast, has a static composition, intended to meet the nutritional requirements of infants from birth to 12 months of age (Lönnerdal & Hernell, 2015). Nurses need to bring this information to the attention of parents who choose to formula-feed their infants that changes may be needed in different stages of growth to meet the nutritional needs of their infant. Parents must be taught about safe preparation of infant formula and advised to avoid feeding their babies home-made formula recipes. Cow milk, evaporated milk, goat milk, soy beverage, rice beverage, or any other beverages should not be given to young infants as these will not have the appropriate nutritional contents which infants require (Health Canada et al., 2015).

Newborns who are older than 1 week need about 108 cal/kg or approximately 650 cal/day. Therefore, explain to parents that a newborn will need 60 to 120 mL to feel satisfied at each feeding. Until about age 4 months, most bottle-fed infants need six feedings a day. After this time, the number of feedings declines to accommodate other foods in the diet, such as fruits, cereals, and vegetables. For more information on newborn nutrition and bottle-feeding, see Chapter 18.

When providing individual education about bottle-feeding, provide the following guidelines:
- Wash hands with soap and water and dry using a clean or disposable cloth.
- Make sure all bottles, nipples, and other utensils are clean.
- Make feeding a relaxing time, a time to provide both food and comfort to your newborn.
- Use the feeding period to promote bonding by smiling, singing, making eye contact, and talking to the infant.
- Store any formula prepared in advance in the refrigerator to keep bacteria from growing. Use prepared bottles within 24 hours.
- Do not microwave formula; the microwave won't heat it evenly, causing hot spots.
- Always hold the newborn when feeding. Never prop the bottle.
- Use a comfortable position when feeding the newborn. Place the newborn in your dominant arm, which is supported by a pillow. Or have the newborn in a semi-upright position supported in the crook of your arm. (This position reduces choking and the flow of milk into the middle ear.)
- Tilt the bottle so that the nipple and the neck of the bottle are always filled with formula. This prevents the infant from taking in too much air.
- Stimulate the sucking reflex by touching the nipple to the infant's lips.
- Discard any formula not taken; do not keep it for future feedings.
- Burp the infant frequently and place the baby on his or her back for sleeping.
- Use only iron-fortified infant formula for the first year (Health Canada, 2012; Moses, 2014).

Teaching About Breast Care

Regardless of whether or not the client is breastfeeding, encourage the use of a supportive, snug-fitting bra 24 hours a day to support enlarged breasts and promote comfort. A client who is breastfeeding should wear a supportive bra throughout the lactation period. Those who are not nursing should wear it until engorgement ceases, and then should wear a less restrictive one. The bra should fit snugly while still allowing comfortable breathing without restriction. All postpartum clients should use plain water to clean their breasts, especially the nipple area; soap is drying and should be avoided.

Assessing the Breasts

Instruct client how to examine the breasts daily. Daily assessment includes the milk supply (breasts will feel full as they are filling), the condition of the nipples (red, bruised, fissured, or bleeding), and the success of breastfeeding. The fullness of the breasts may progress to engorgement in the breastfeeding client if feedings are delayed or breastfeeding is ineffective. Palpating both breasts will help identify whether the breasts are soft, filling, or engorged. A similar assessment of the breasts should be completed on the nonlactating client to identify any problems, such as engorgement or mastitis.

Alleviating Breast Engorgement

Breast engorgement can occur during the first week postpartum. It is a common response of the breasts to the sudden change in hormones and the presence of an increased amount of milk. Reassure the client that this condition is temporary and usually resolves within 72 hours.

ALLEVIATING BREAST ENGORGEMENT WHEN BREASTFEEDING

If the client is breastfeeding, encourage frequent feedings, at least 8 feeds per day, using manual expression just before feeding to soften the breast so the newborn can latch on more effectively. Advise the client to allow the newborn to feed on the first breast until it softens before switching to the other side. See Chapter 18 for more information on alleviating breast engorgement and other potential breastfeeding concerns.

ALLEVIATING BREAST ENGORGEMENT AND SUPPRESSING LACTATION IF NOT BREASTFEEDING

If the client decides to feed the baby with infant formula, explain that breast engorgement is a self-limiting phenomenon that disappears as increasing estrogen levels suppress milk formation (i.e., lactation suppression). If the client is not planning to express any breastmilk for feeding the baby (even by bottle), provide education about avoiding stimulation to the breasts that might foster milk production, such as warm showers or pumping or massaging the breasts. Encourage the client to use ice packs, to wear a snug, supportive bra 24 hours a day, and to take mild analgesics such as acetaminophen. Medication is no longer given to hasten lactation suppression because these agents had limited effectiveness and adverse side effects. Teaching Guidelines 16.5 provides tips on lactation suppression.

Teaching Guidelines 16.5
SUPPRESSING LACTATION

1. Wear a supportive, snugly fitting bra 24 hours daily, but not one that binds the breasts too tightly or interferes with your breathing.
2. Suppression may take 5 to 7 days to accomplish.
3. Take mild analgesics to reduce breast discomfort.

4. Let shower water flow over your back rather than your breasts.
5. Avoid any breast stimulation, including sucking or massage.
6. Drink to quench your thirst. Restricting your fluid intake will not dry up your milk.
7. Reduce your salt intake to decrease fluid retention.
8. Use ice packs or cool compresses (e.g., cool cabbage leaves) inside the bra to decrease local pain and swelling; change them every 30 minutes (King et al., 2015).

Promoting Family Adjustment and Well-Being

The postpartum period involves extraordinary physiologic, psychological, and sociocultural changes in the life of a postpartum person and family. Adapting to the role of a parent is not an easy process. The postpartum period is a "getting-to-know-you" time when parents begin to integrate the newborn into their lives as they reconcile the fantasy child with the real one. This can be a very challenging period for families. Nurses play a major role in assisting families to adapt to the changes, promoting a smooth transition into parenthood. Appropriate and timely interventions can help parents adjust to the role changes and promote attachment to the newborn (Fig. 16.7).

For couples who already have children, the addition of a new member may bring role conflict and challenges. The nurse should provide anticipatory guidance about siblings' responses to the new baby, increased emotional tension, child development, and meeting the multiple needs of the expanding family. Although the multiparous client has had experience with newborns, do not assume that their knowledge is current and accurate, especially if some time has elapsed since the previous child was born. Reinforcing information is important for all families.

Promoting Parental Roles

Parents' roles develop and grow when they interact with their newborn (see Chapter 15 for information on paternal adaptation). The pleasure they derive from this interaction stimulates and reinforces this behaviour. With repeated, continued contact with the newborn, parents learn to recognize cues and understand the newborn's behaviour. This positive interaction contributes to family harmony.

Nurses need to know the stages parents go through as they make their new parenting roles fit into their life experience. Assess the parents for attachment behaviours (normal and deviant), adjustment to the new parental role, family member adjustment, social support system, and educational needs. To promote parental role

A

B

C

FIGURE 16.7 Examples of family members carrying out roles to promote adjustment and well-being. **A.** An aunt admiring the newest member of the family. **B.** A father holding his newborn closely on his chest. **C.** Grandparents welcoming the newest little one to the family circle.

adaptation and parent–newborn attachment, provide the following nursing interventions:

- Provide as many opportunities as possible for parents to interact with their newborn. Encourage parents to explore, hold, and provide care for their newborn. Praise them for their efforts.
- Model behaviours by holding the newborn close, calling the newborn's name, and speaking positively.
- Speak directly to the newborn in a calm voice, while pointing out the newborn's positive features to the parents.
- Evaluate the family's strengths and weaknesses and readiness for parenting.
- Assess for risk factors such as lack of social support and the presence of stressors.
- Observe the effect of culture on the family interaction to determine healthy family dynamics.

- Monitor parental attachment behaviours to determine whether alterations require referral. Positive behaviours include holding the newborn closely or in an *en face* position, talking to or admiring the newborn, or demonstrating closeness. Negative behaviours include avoiding contact with the newborn, calling it names, or showing a lack of interest in caring for the newborn (see Table 16.1).
- Monitor the parents' coping behaviours to determine alterations that need intervention. Positive coping behaviours include positive conversations between the partners, both parents wanting to be involved with newborn care, and lack of arguments between the parents. Negative behaviours include not visiting, limited conversations or periods of silence, and heated arguments or conflict.
- Identify the support systems available to the new family and encourage them to ask for help. Ask direct

questions about home or community support. Make referrals to community resources to meet the family's needs.

- Arrange for community home visits in high-risk families to provide positive reinforcement of parenting skills and nurturing behaviours with the newborn.
- Provide anticipatory guidance about the following before discharge to reduce the new parents' frustration:
  - Newborn sleep–wake cycles (they may be reversed)
  - Variations in newborn appearance and developmental milestones (growth spurts)
  - How to interpret crying cues (hunger, wet, discomfort) and what to do about them
  - Sensory enrichment/stimulation (colourful images or toys)
  - Signs and symptoms of illness and how to assess for fever
  - Important phone numbers, follow-up care, and immunization schedule
  - Physical and emotional changes associated with the postpartum period
  - Need to integrate siblings into care of the newborn; stress that sibling rivalry is normal and offer ways to reduce it
  - Ways to make time together for the couple.

In addition, nurses can help fathers/co-parents to feel more competent in assuming their parental role by teaching and providing information (Fig. 16.8). Education can dispel any unrealistic expectations they may have, helping them to cope more successfully with the demands of fatherhood/parenthood and thereby fostering a nurturing family relationship.

Explaining Sibling Roles

It can be overwhelming to a young child to have another family member introduced into his or her small, stable world. Although most parents try to prepare siblings for the arrival of their new little brother or sister, many young children experience stress. They may view the new infant as competition, or fear that they will be replaced in the parents' affection. All siblings need extra attention from their parents and reassurance that they are loved and important. Many parents need reassurance that sibling rivalry is normal. Suggest the following to help parents minimize sibling rivalry:

- Expect and tolerate some regression (thumb sucking, bedwetting).
- Explain childbirth in an appropriate way for the child's age.
- Encourage discussion about the new infant during relaxed family times.
- Encourage the sibling(s) to participate in decisions, such as the baby's name, preparing the baby's room, and/or toys to buy.
- Take the sibling on a tour of the maternity suite.
- Make or buy a T-shirt that says "I'm the big [brother or sister]."
- Spend "special time" with the child.
- Read with the child.
- Plan time for each child throughout the day.
- Role-play safe handling of a newborn, using a doll. Give the preschooler or school-age child a doll to care for.
- Encourage older children to verbalize emotions about the newborn.
- Purchase a gift that the child can give to the newborn.
- Purchase a gift that can be given to the child by the newborn.
- Arrange for the child to come to the hospital to see the newborn (Fig. 16.9).

FIGURE 16.8 Father participating in newborn care.

FIGURE 16.9 Sibling visitation.

- Move the sibling from his or her crib to a youth bed months in advance of the birth of the newborn.
- Show the older sibling photos of the growing baby in the belly. Let them pat the baby beneath the bulge, talk to baby, and feel the baby kick.
- Make the older sibling feel important by giving them a title "mommy's/daddy's helper."
- Encourage grandparents to pay attention to the older child when visiting.
- Tell the older sibling that their friends may come and go, but siblings are forever.
- Encourage "Do unto others as you would have them do unto you" (Sears & Sears, 2015c).

Consider This

Katie and Molly have been excited about having a new baby sister ever since they were told about their mother's pregnancy. The 6-year-old twins are eagerly looking out the front window, waiting for their parents to bring their new sister, Jessica, home. The girls are big enough to help care for their new sibling, and for the past few months they have been fixing up the new nursery and selecting baby clothes. They practiced diapering their dolls— their mother was specific about not using any powder or lotion on Jessica's bottom—and holding them correctly to feed them bottles. Finally, their mother arrives home from the hospital with Jessica in her arms!

The girls notice that their mother is very protective of Jessica and watches them carefully when they care for her. They fight over the opportunity to hold her or feed her. What is special to both of them is the time they spend alone with their parents. Although a new family member has been added, the twins still feel special and loved by their parents.

Thoughts: *Bringing a new baby into an established family can cause conflict and jealousy. What preparation did the older siblings have before Jessica arrived? Why is it important for parents to spend time with each sibling separately?*

Discussing Grandparents' Role

Grandparents can be a source of support and comfort to the postpartum family if effective communication skills are used and roles are defined. The grandparents' role and involvement will depend on how close they live to the family, their willingness to become involved, and cultural expectations of their role. Just as parents and siblings go through developmental changes, so too do grandparents. These changes can have a positive or negative effect on the relationship.

Newborn care, feeding, and child-rearing practices have changed since the grandparents raised the parents. New parents may lack parenting skills but nonetheless want their parents' support without criticism. A grandparent's

"take-charge approach" may not be welcome by new parents who are testing their own parenting roles, and family conflict may ensue. However, many grandparents respect their adult children's wishes for autonomy and remain "resource people" for them when requested.

Take Note!

Grandparents' involvement can enrich the lives of the entire family if accepted in the right context and dose by the family.

Nurses can assist in the grandparents' role transition by assessing their communication skills, role expectations, and support skills during the prenatal period. Find out whether the grandparents are included in the couple's social support network and whether their support is wanted or helpful. If they are, and it is, then encourage the grandparents to learn about the parenting, feeding, and child-rearing skills their children have learned in childbirth classes. This information is commonly found in "grandparenting" classes, which introduce new parenting concepts and bring the grandparents up to date on today's childbirth practices. On the postpartum unit, nurses can facilitate grandparents' understanding of current evidence-based approaches to infant care by including them in the teaching provided to the new parents. This could include bathing, diapering, and feeding, when they are in visiting their new grandchild.

Teaching About Postpartum Blues

The postpartum period is typically a happy yet stressful time, because the birth of an infant is accompanied by enormous physical, social, and emotional changes. The postpartum client may report feelings of emotional lability, such as crying one minute and laughing the next. (See Chapter 15 for Postpartum Blues discussion.) Although **postpartum blues** is usually benign and self-limited, these mood changes can be frightening. It is prudent to ask two questions: about having pleasure and interest in things, or feeling predominately down, depressed, or hopeless. Once postpartum blues are determined to be the likely cause of the mood symptoms, the nurse can offer anticipatory guidance that these mood swings are commonly experienced by a majority of people in the postpartum period, usually resolve spontaneously within 2 weeks, and offer reassurance. Clients should also be counselled to seek further evaluation if these moods do not resolve within 2 weeks, as postpartum depression may be developing (King et al., 2015).

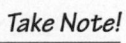

Take Note!

Postpartum blues have been regarded as brief, benign, and without clinical significance, but several studies have proposed a link between blues and subsequent depression in the 6 months following childbirth (Cristescu, Behrman, Jones, Chouliaras, & Ebmeier, 2015).

Postpartum blues require no formal treatment other than support and reassurance because they do not usually interfere with the person's ability to function and care for the infant. Nurses can ease a client's distress by encouraging venting of feelings and by demonstrating patience and understanding with the client and the family. Suggest that getting outside help with housework and infant care might help the client to feel less overwhelmed until the blues ease. Provide telephone numbers to call if feeling down during the day. Increasing awareness of this disorder during pregnancy will increase their knowledge about this mood disturbance, which may lessen their embarrassment and increase their willingness to ask for and accept help if it does occur.

The postpartum client is also at risk for postpartum depression and postpartum psychosis; these conditions are discussed in Chapter 22.

Preparing for Discharge

The WHO recommends that the length of stay in the health care facility should be individualized for each dyad, but should be at least 24 hours after birth (WHO, 2014b). A shortened hospital stay may be indicated if the following criteria are met:

- Client is afebrile and vital signs are within normal range.
- Lochia is appropriate amount and colour for stage of recovery.
- Hemoglobin and hematocrit values are within normal range.
- Uterine fundus is firm; urinary output is adequate.
- ABO blood groups and RhD status are known and, if indicated, anti-D immunoglobulin has been administered.
- Surgical wounds are healing and no signs of infection are present.
- Client is able to ambulate without difficulty.
- Food and fluids are taken without difficulty.
- Self-care and infant care are understood and demonstrated.
- Family or other support system is available to care for both.
- Client is aware of possible complications (WHO, 2014b).

Providing Immunizations

Prior to discharge, check the immunity status for rubella for all postpartum clients and give a subcutaneous injection of rubella vaccine if they are not immune. The benchmark for serologic immunity to rubella varies across countries; the WHO indicates that a laboratory result of ≥10 IU/mL rubella IgG antibodies is evidence of immunity (WHO, 2011). Obtain the client's informed consent to receive the vaccine. The rubella vaccine should not be given to any person who is immune compromised, and

the immune status of close contacts needs to be determined before any vaccine is administered to prevent a more virulent case of the vaccine-preventable illness or potential death. With the recent increase in the number of pertussis in infants younger than 3 months of age, Health Canada recommends vaccination with (Tdap) (combination of diphtheria, pertussis, and tetanus vaccines) for all pregnant clients at the beginning of the third trimester (between 27 and 32 weeks' gestation). Any client who did not receive the Tdap vaccination during the pregnancy should be encouraged to receive it during the postpartum stay (Health Canada, 2018b). Those who are breastfeeding can receive the Tdap vaccine because the live, attenuated rubella virus is not communicable via breastmilk. Inform all parents receiving immunization about adverse effects (rash, joint symptoms, and a low-grade fever 5 to 21 days later) and the need to avoid pregnancy for at least 28 days after being vaccinated because of the risk of teratogenic effects (CDC, 2015b; Health Canada, 2018b).

Rh Status

If the client is Rh-negative, check the Rh status of the newborn. Verify that the client is Rh-negative and has not been sensitized, that the indirect Coombs test (antibody screen) is negative, and that the newborn is Rh-positive. Those who are Rh-negative and have given birth to an infant who is Rh-positive should receive an injection of Rh immunoglobulin within 72 hours after birth to prevent a sensitization reaction in the Rh-negative client who was exposed to Rh-positive blood cells during the birthing process. Administering RhoGAM prevents initial isoimmunization in Rh-negative clients by destroying fetal erythrocytes in the maternal system before maternal antibodies can develop and maternal memory cells become sensitized. This is a classic passive immunization technique. The usual protocol for the Rh-negative client is to receive two doses of Rh immunoglobulin (RhoGAM), one at 28 weeks' gestation and the second dose within 72 hours after childbirth. The standard dose of Rho(D) immune globulin (RhoGAM) is 300 mcg given intramuscularly, which prevents the development of antibodies for an exposure of up to 15 mL of fetal red blood cells (King et al., 2015). A signed consent form is needed after a thorough explanation is provided about the procedure, including its purpose, possible adverse effects, and effect on future pregnancies.

RhoGAM contains actual Rh antibodies produced by people who have become sensitized. It is therefore, a blood product. Each dose contains enough anti-D to suppress the immune response of 15 mL of Rh-positive red blood cells (Jordan et al., 2014). Clients with religious beliefs prohibiting the use of blood products, such as Jehovah's Witness, may wish to consult their ecclesiastical leaders about the use of RhoGAM. Nurses are responsible for ensuring that clients understand all the information presented to them, and then must respect the client's decision, whether the nurse agrees with that decision or not.

Ensuring Follow-Up Care

New parents need to be attended to over an extended period of time by nurses knowledgeable about postpartum care, infant feeding (breastfeeding and formula-feeding), infant care, and nutrition. Although continuous nursing care stops on discharge from the hospital or birthing centre, extended episodic nursing care needs to be provided at home. Some of the challenges faced by families after discharge are described in Box 16.5.

Many clients are hesitant to leave the health care facility, and some will benefit from expanded community services. Being discharged too early from the hospital runs the risk of uterine subinvolution, discomfort at an episiotomy or cesarean site, infection, fatigue, and maladjustment to their new role. Postpartum nursing care should include a range of family-focused care, including telephone calls, outpatient clinics, and home visits. Typically, public health nurses, community and home health nurses, and the health care provider's office staff will provide postpartum care after hospital discharge.

PROVIDING TELEPHONE FOLLOW-UP

Telephone follow-up typically occurs during the first week after discharge to check on how things are going at home. Calls can be made by perinatal nurses within the

---

BOX 16.5

CHALLENGES IDENTIFIED BY FAMILIES AFTER DISCHARGE

- Lack of role models for breastfeeding and infant care
- Lack of support from the new parents' mothers if they did not breastfeed
- Increased mobility of society, which means that extended family may live far away and cannot help care for the newborn and support the new family
- Feelings of isolation and limited community ties for those who work full time
- Shortened hospital stays: parents may be overwhelmed by all the information they are given in the brief hospital stay
- Prenatal classes usually focus on the birth itself rather than on skills needed to care for themselves and the newborn during the postpartum period
- Limited access to education and support systems for families from diverse cultures

Adapted from Bope, E., & Kellerman, R. (2015). *Conn's current therapy 2015.* Philadelphia, PA: Saunders Elsevier; Bang, K., Huh, B., & Kwon, M. (2014). The effect of a postpartum nursing intervention program for immigrant mothers. *Child Health Nursing Research, 20*(1), 11–19.

---

agency as part of follow-up care or by the local health department nurses. One disadvantage of a phone call assessment is that the nurse cannot see the client and thus must rely on the client or the family's observations. The experienced nurse needs to be able to recognize distress and give appropriate advice and referral information if needed.

PROVIDING OUTPATIENT FOLLOW-UP

For clients with established health care providers such as a family physician, nurse practitioner, visits to the office are arranged soon after discharge. For the client with an uncomplicated vaginal birth, an office visit is usually scheduled for 4 to 6 weeks after childbirth with their primary care provider. A client who had a cesarean birth frequently is may have follow-up arranged with the obstetrician. Hospital discharge orders will specify when these visits should be made. Newborn examinations and further diagnostic laboratory studies are scheduled within the first week.

> **Take Note!**
>
> The hospital stay of the dyad should be long enough to allow identification of early problems and to ensure that the family is able and prepared to care for the infant at home (WHO, 2014b).

Outpatient clinics are available in many communities. If family members run into a problem, the local clinic is available to provide assessment and treatment. Clinic visits can replace or supplement home visits. Although these clinics are open during daytime hours only and the staff members are unfamiliar with the family, they can be a valuable resource for the new family with a problem or concern.

PROVIDING HOME VISIT FOLLOW-UP

Home visits are usually made within the first week after discharge to assess the dyad. During the home visit, the nurse assesses for and manages common physical and psychosocial problems. In addition, the home nurse can help the new parents adjust to the change in their lives. The postpartum home visit usually includes the following:

- *Postpartum client assessment:* general well-being, vital signs, breast health and care, abdominal and musculoskeletal status, voiding status, fundus and lochia status, psychological and coping status, family relationships, proper feeding technique, environmental safety check, newborn care knowledge, and health teaching needed (Fig. 16.10 shows sample assessment forms.)
- *Infant assessment:* physical examination, general appearance, vital signs, home safety check, child development status, any education needed to improve parents' skills

(text continues on page 583)

Maternal Assessment
Maternal/Newborn Record System

Page 1 of 2

Date __MO_ /_DAY_ /_YR_ Time begin: _____ Date of delivery __MO_ / _DAY_ / _YR_
Time end: _____

Medication allergy   ☐ None   Identify_____
Significant health history ☐ None   Identify_____

PHYSICAL

TEMP.	PULSE	RESP.	BP /

Breasts ☐ Nursing   ☐ Non-nursing
Color   ☐ Normal   ☐ Reddened
Condition ☐ Soft ☐ Firm ☐ Engorged ☐ Blocked ducts
Secretion ☐ Colostrum ☐ Milk ☐ Other_____
Support bra ☐ No ☐ Yes, fit ☐ Appropriate
☐ Inappropriate

Nipples (If nursing) ☐ Erect ☐ Flat ☐ Inverted
Condition ☐ Intact ☐ Bruised ☐ Blistered
☐ Fissured ☐ Bleeding ☐ Scabbed
Care ☐ Water only ☐ Soap ☐ Air dry
☐ Topical agent (type/frequency) _____

☐ Other _____
Self-exam ☐ Accurate ☐ Inaccurate/instructed

Abdomen

Diastasis recti ☐ Absent ☐ Present_____cm
☐ Exercise taught
Incision ☐ None
Type ☐ Transverse ☐ Vertical ☐ Umbilical
Closure ☐ Staples ☐ Sutures ☐ Steri-strips
Condition ☐ Approximated ☐ Open_____cm
☐ Redness _____
☐ Swelling _____
☐ Discharge _____
☐ Other_____

Reproductive Tract

Uterus ☐ Firm ☐ Firm with massage ☐ Boggy
Height_____ ☐ Midline ☐ Displaced L R
☐ Non tender ☐ Tender ☐ With touch ☐ Constant
Lochia ☐ Rubra ☐ Serosa ☐ Alba
☐ Clots (describe)_____
☐ Fleshy odor ☐ Foul odor
Pads Type_____ Number/day _____
Saturation %—+——+——+——+——
0 25 50 75 100

Perineum ☐ Intact ☐ Laceration
☐ Episiotomy Type_____ Extension_____
Condition ☐ Redness _____
☐ Edema _____
☐ Ecchymosis _____
☐ Discharge _____
☐ Approximation _____
Care ☐ Front-to-back cleansing ☐ Peri-bottle
☐ Soap/water
☐ Ice ☐ Sitz bath ☐ Warm ☐ Cool
☐ Topical agent (type/frequency) _____

☐ Other _____

Elimination

Urinary tract
Voiding pattern ☐ Normal ☐ Incontinence
☐ Bladder distention ☐ Catheter (type)
Signs of infection ☐ None/reviewed ☐ Urgency ☐ Frequency
☐ Dysuria ☐ CVA tenderness L R
Gastrointestinal tract
Bowel pattern ☐ Normal ☐ No BM
☐ Constipation ☐ Diarrhea
☐ Meds/treatments (type, frequency, effect)

Hemorrhoids ☐ No ☐ Yes (describe) _____
☐ Meds/treatments (type, frequency, effect) _____

Lower Extremities

Edema ☐ None ☐ Pedal ☐ Ankle ☐ Pretibial ☐ Thigh
☐ Pitting (describe) _____
Signs of thrombophlebitis ☐ None

	L	R		L	R
Homan's sign	☐	☐	Redness	☐	☐
Pain	☐	☐	Warmth	☐	☐
Swelling	☐	☐			

Pain

	No	Managed (Yes)	Problematic (Yes)
Abdominal incision	☐	☐	☐
Back	☐	☐	☐
Breasts	☐	☐	☐
Headache	☐	☐	☐
Hemorrhoid	☐	☐	☐
Nipple	☐	☐	☐
Perineum	☐	☐	☐
Uterine cramping	☐	☐	☐
Other ___	☐	☐	☐

Analgesic ☐ No
☐ Yes (type/dose/frequency) _____

Reportable danger signs ☐ Aware ☐ Unaware/instructed

TESTS ☐ None
☐ Urinalysis
☐ CBC
☐ _____

IDENTIFIED NEEDS

_____
_____
_____
_____
_____
_____
_____
_____

Signature _____

A

FIGURE 16.10 Sample postpartum home visit assessment form. **A.** Maternal assessment. **B.** Newborn assessment. (Used with permission: Copyright Briggs Corporation. Professional Nurse Associates.)

Maternal Assessment
Maternal/Newborn Record System

Page 2 of 2

PATIENT IDENTIFICATION
Record No. _____

Name _____
Home
address _____
STREET
CITY   STATE   ZIP

ACTIVITIES OF DAILY LIVING - 24 HOUR HISTORY

Date _MO_ / _DAY_ / _YR_

Nutrition

Appetite	☐ Good	☐ Fair	☐ Poor
Usual pattern	☐ Yes	☐ No _____
Special diet	☐ No	☐ Yes _____
Food intolerance/allergy	☐ No	☐ Yes _____
Vitamin/mineral supplement	☐ No	☐ Yes _____

Fluid intake (type/amount) _____

BREAKFAST	LUNCH	DINNER	SNACKS
_____	_____	_____	_____
_____	_____	_____	_____
_____	_____	_____	_____

General Hygiene   ☐ Adequate   ☐ Inadequate (describe) _____

Sleep/Activity

Amount of Activity
Night, uninterrupted _____ hrs

Naps ☐ No ☐ Yes _____ hrs

Fatigue ☐ None ☐ Minimal ☐ Moderate
☐ Exhausted

Activities
Limitations ☐ None   Identify _____

	Appropriate	Inappropriate/instructed
☐ Self-care	☐ Infant care	
Stair climbing	☐	☐
Lifting	☐	☐
Household tasks	☐	☐
Outside home	☐	☐
Other _____		

Exercise
☐ None

	Accurate	Inaccurate/instructed
Kegel	☐	☐
Postpartum	☐	☐
Other _____		

PSYCHOLOGICAL

Review of Labor and Birth

Missing pieces	☐ No	☐ Yes
Unmet expectations	☐ No	☐ Yes
Unresolved feelings	☐ No	☐ Yes

Pertinent data _____

Postpartum Timetable   (Key on reverse side)
☐ Taking in   ☐ Taking hold   ☐ Letting go

Emotional Status   ☐ Happy ☐ Ambivalent ☐ Anxious
☐ Sad ☐ Other _____
Postpartum-depression (Key on reverse side)
☐ 0 ☐ 1 ☐ 2 ☐ 3 ☐ 4
☐ Signs/Symptoms Reviewed

General Comments   (body image, role changes, concerns) _____
_____
_____

SEXUALITY

	Aware	Unaware/instructed
Relationship with partner		
Adjustment	☐	☐
Expressions of affection	☐	☐
Resuming Intercourse		
Timing (lack of lochia, comfort)	☐	☐
Vaginal dryness	☐	☐
Milk ejection (if lactating)	☐	☐
Position variation	☐	☐
Libidinal changes	☐	☐
Return of Menses	☐	☐

Contraceptive Method
☐ None   ☐ Undecided/aware of options
☐ Natural family planning
☐ Cervical cap
☐ Condom
☐ Diaphragm
☐ Hormones ☐ Pill ☐ Injection ☐ Implant
☐ IUD
☐ Spermicide
☐ Sterilization ☐ Female ☐ Male
☐ Other _____

Accurate use   ☐ Yes   ☐ No/instructed

IDENTIFIED NEEDS

_____
_____
_____

Signature _____

FIGURE 16.10 *(continued)*

Maternal Assessment
Maternal/Newborn Record System

PATIENT IDENTIFICATION

Record No. _____

Name _____

Home
address _____
                          STREET

CITY   STATE   ZIP

Date _MO_ / _DAY_ / _YR_ Time begin: _____ Date of Birth _MO_ / _DAY_ / _YR_
                          Time end: _____
Significant history ☐ None   Identify _____

PHYSICAL

Temp _____ Pulse (rate/rhythm) _____ Resp _____
Weight _____ Birth weight _____ % Change _____
Length _____ Head _____ Chest _____

HEAD/NECK

	Level	Bulging	Depressed
1. Fontanels			
Anterior	☐	☐	☐
Posterior	☐	☐	☐

Sutures ☐ Open ☐ Closed ☐ Overriding
2. Variations ☐ Molding ☐ Caput ☐ Cephalhematoma

	NORMAL	ABNORMAL	DETAIL VARIATIONS/ ABNORMAL FINDINGS
3. Face (symmetry)	☐	☐	
4. Eyes (symmetry, conjunctiva, sciera, eyelids, PERL)	☐	☐	
5. Ears (shape, position, auditory response)	☐	☐	
6. Nose (patency)	☐	☐	
7. Mouth (lip, mucous membranes, tongue, palate)	☐	☐	
8. Neck (ROM, symmetry)	☐	☐	

Chest

9. Appearance (shape, breasts, nipples)	☐	☐	
10. Breath sounds	☐	☐	
11. Clavicles	☐	☐	

Cardiovascular

12. Heart sounds	☐	☐	
13. Brachial/femoral pulses (compare strength, equality)	☐	☐	

Abdomen

14. Appearance (shape, size)	☐	☐	
15. Cord (condition)	☐	☐	
16. Liver (less than or equal to 3 cm ↓ ®costal margin)	☐	☐	

Genitalia

17. Female (labia, introitus, discharge)	☐	☐	
18. Male (meatus, scrotum, testes)	☐	☐	
19. Circumcision ☐ No ☐ Yes	☐	☐	

Musculoskeletal

20. Muscle tone	☐	☐	
21. Extremities (symmetry, digits, ROM)	☐	☐	
22. Hips (symmetry, ROM)	☐	☐	
23. Spine (alignment, integrity)	☐	☐	

Neurologic

24. Reflexes (presence, symmetry)

Moro	☐	☐	
Grasp	☐	☐	
Babinski	☐	☐	
25. Cry (presence, quality)	☐	☐	

PHYSICAL (CONT'D)
Skin
Turgor ☐ Good ☐ Poor
Condition ☐ Smooth ☐ Dry, cracked ☐ Peeling
Color ☐ Pink ☐ Ruddy ☐ Cyanotic ☐ Pale
☐ Jaundice (note levels)
  ☐ Head (3 mg/dl)
  ☐ Head and upper chest (6 mg/dl)
  ☐ Head and entire chest (9 mg/dl)
  ☐ Head, chest and abdomen to umbilicus (12 mg/dl)
  ☐ Head, chest and entire abdomen (15 mg/dl)
  ☐ Head, chest, abdomen, legs and feet (18 mg/dl)
Variations (Rashes, lesions, birthmarks). _____

NUTRITION
Feeding
Reflexes ☐ Root ☐ Suck ☐ Swallow
Hunger cues identified ☐ Yes ☐ No/instructed

BREAST	FORMULA
Frequency___times in _____ hours	Type _____
Time per breast_____ min _____min	Amount _____ oz.
Positioning ☐ Correct	Frequency _____
☐ Incorrect_____	Preparation ☐ Correct
Latch ☐ Correct	☐ Incorrect_____
☐ Incorrect_____	
Appropriate audible swallows	☐ Correct
☐ Yes ☐ No_____	☐ _____

Satiation demonstrated ☐ Yes
  ☐ No (describe)_____
Regurgitation ☐ No ☐ Yes (describe)_____
Pacifier use ☐ No ☐ Yes (type/pattern)_____

Stool (number/day, color, consistency)_____
Urine (number/day, color)_____

BEHAVIOR
Sleep/Activity Pattern (24 hours)
Sleep (16–20 hrs)   ☐ Yes ☐ No (describe)_____
_____

Awake-alert (2–3 hrs)   ☐ Yes ☐ No (describe)_____

Awake-crying (2–4 hrs)   ☐ Yes ☐ No (describe)_____
_____

Consolability (Key on reverse) ☐ 0 ☐ 1 ☐ 2 ☐ 3 ☐ 4

TESTS ☐ None   Time
☐ Metabolic screen kit no. _____ _____
☐ Bilirubin   _____
☐ Hematocrit   _____
☐ _____ _____
☐ _____ _____

IDENTIFIED NEEDS _____
_____
_____
_____
_____

Signature _____

B

FIGURE 16.10 *(continued)*

The home care nurse must be prepared to support and educate the client and family in the following areas:

- Breastfeeding or formula-feeding technique and procedures
- Appropriate parenting behaviour and problem solving
- Physical, psychosocial, cultural, and environmental needs of the dyad
- Emotional needs of the new family
- Warning signs of problems and how to prevent or eliminate them
- Sexuality issues, including contraceptive use
- Immunization needs for both client and infant
- Family dynamics for smooth transition
- Links to health care providers and community resources

NURSING CARE PLAN 16.1

Overview of the Postpartum Client

A 26-year-old G2P2, is a client on the postpartum unit after giving birth to a term 8-lb, 12-oz baby boy yesterday. The night nurse reports that she has an episiotomy, complains of a pain rating of 7 points on a scale of 1 to 10, is having difficulty breastfeeding, and had heavy lochia most of the night. The nurse also reports that the client seems focused on her own needs and not on those of her infant. Assessment this morning reveals the following:

B: **Breasts** are soft with colostrum leaking; nipples cracked
U: **Uterus** is 1 fingerbreadth below the umbilicus; deviated to right
B: **Bladder** is palpable; client states she hasn't been up to void yet
B: **Bowels** have not moved; bowel sounds present; passing flatus
L: **Lochia** is moderate; peripad soaked from night accumulation
E: **Episiotomy** site intact; swollen, bruised; hemorrhoids present
E: **Extremities**; no edema over tibia, no warmth or tenderness in calf
E: **Emotional status** is "distressed" because of discomfort and fatigue

---

NURSING DIAGNOSIS: Impaired tissue integrity related to episiotomy

Outcome Identification and Evaluation

The client will remain free of infection, without any signs and symptoms of infection, and exhibit evidence of progressive healing as demonstrated by clean, dry, decreased/absent edema, and an intact episiotomy site.

Interventions: *Promoting Tissue Integrity*

- Monitor episiotomy site for redness, edema, warmth, or discharge *to identify infection.*
- Assess vital signs at least every 4 hours *to identify changes suggesting infection.*
- Apply ice pack to episiotomy site *to reduce swelling.*
- Instruct client on use of sitz bath *to promote healing, hygiene, and comfort.*
- Encourage frequent perineal care and peripad changes *to prevent infection.*

- Recommend ambulation *to improve circulation and promote healing.*
- Instruct client on positioning *to relieve pressure on perineal area.*
- Demonstrate use of anesthetic sprays *to numb perineal area.*

NURSING DIAGNOSIS: Acute pain related to episiotomy, sore nipples, and hemorrhoids

Outcome Identification and Evaluation

The client will experience a decrease in pain as evidenced by reporting that her pain has diminished to a tolerable level and rating it as 2 points or less.

(continued)

NURSING CARE PLAN 16.1

Overview of the Postpartum Client (continued)

Interventions: *Providing Pain Relief*

- Thoroughly inspect perineum to rule out hematoma as cause of pain.
- Administer analgesic medication as ordered as needed to promote comfort.
- Carry out comfort measures to episiotomy as outlined earlier to reduce pain.
- Explain discomforts and reassure the client that they are time limited to assist in coping with pain.
- Apply Tucks® to swollen hemorrhoids to induce shrinkage and reduce pain.
- Suggest frequent use of sitz bath to reduce hemorrhoid pain.
- Administer stool softener and laxative to prevent straining with first bowel movement.
- Observe positioning and latching-on technique while breastfeeding. Offer suggestions based on observations to correct positioning/latching on to minimize trauma to the breast.
- Suggest expressing colostrum and rubbing it onto the nipples and allowing them to air-dry after breastfeeding to prevent nipple cracking.
- Teach relaxation techniques when breastfeeding to reduce anxiety and discomfort.

NURSING DIAGNOSIS: Ineffective coping related to mood alteration and pain

Outcome Identification and Evaluation

The client will cope with mood alterations, as evidenced by positive statements about newborn and participation in newborn care.

Interventions: *Promoting Effective Coping*

- Provide a supportive, nurturing environment and encourage the mother to vent her feelings and frustrations *to relieve anxiety.*
- Provide opportunities for the mother to rest and sleep *to combat fatigue.*
- Encourage the mother to eat a well-balanced diet *to increase her energy level.*
- Provide reassurance and explanations that mood alterations are common after birth secondary to waning hormones after pregnancy *to increase the mother's knowledge.*
- Allow the mother relief from newborn care *to afford opportunity for self-care.*
- Discuss with partner expected behaviour from mother and how additional support and help are needed during this stressful time *to promote partner's participation in care.*
- Make appropriate community referrals for mother–infant support *to ensure continuity of care.*
- Encourage frequent skin-to-skin contact and closeness between mother and infant *to facilitate bonding and attachment behaviours.*
- Encourage client to participate in infant care and provide instructions as needed *to foster a sense of independence and self-esteem.*
- Offer praise and reinforcement of positive mother–infant interactions *to enhance self-confidence in care.*

KEY CONCEPTS

- ○ The transitional adjustment period between birth and parenthood includes education about baby care basics, the roles of the new family, emotional support, breastfeeding or formula-feeding support, and parental mentoring.
- ○ Sensitivity to how childbearing practices and beliefs vary for diverse families and how best to

provide appropriate nursing care to meet their needs are essential nursing responsibilities during the postpartum period.

○ A thorough postpartum assessment is key to preventing complications as is frequent hand hygiene by the nurse, especially between handling clients and infants.

○ The postpartum assessment using the acronym BUBBLE-EE (breasts, uterus, bowel, bladder, lochia, episiotomy/perineum/epidural site, extremities, and emotions) is a helpful guide in performing a systematic head-to-toe postpartum assessment.

○ Lochia is assessed according to its amount, colour, and change with activity and time. It evolves from lochia rubra to serosa to alba.

○ Because of shortened agency stays, nurses must use this brief time with the client to address areas of comfort, elimination, activity, rest and exercise, self-care, sexuality and contraception, nutrition, family adaptation, discharge, and follow-up.

○ The CPS advocates breastfeeding for all full-term newborns, maintaining that, ideally, breast milk should be the sole nutrient for the first 6 months and continued with foods for 2 years or longer.

○ Successful parenting is a continuous and complex interactive process that requires the acquisition of new skills and the integration of the new member into the existing family unit.

○ Bonding is a vital component of the attachment process and is necessary in establishing parent–infant attachment and a healthy, loving relationship; attachment behaviours include seeking and maintaining proximity to, and exchanging gratifying experiences with, the infant.

○ Nurses can be instrumental in facilitating attachment by first understanding attachment behaviours (positive and negative) of newborns and parents, and intervening appropriately to promote and enhance attachment.

○ New families need to be attended to over an extended period of time by nurses knowledgeable about postpartum care, newborn feeding (breastfeeding or formula-feeding), newborn care, and nutrition.

REFERENCES AND RECOMMENDED READINGS

Allen, M., & Schafer, D. J. (2015). Nurses improving the health of mothers and infants by dancing the 10 steps to successful breastfeeding. *Journal of Obstetric, Gynecologic, & Neonatal Nursing, 44,* S52.

American Academy of Pediatrics (AAP). (2014a). *Iodine deficiency: Pregnant and breastfeeding women need supplementation.* AAP News. Retrieved from http://aapnews. aappublications.org/content/35/6/11.1.extract.

American Academy of Pediatrics (AAP). (2014b). *Ten steps to support parent's choice to breastfeed their baby.* Retrieved from http://www2.aap.org/breastfeeding/files/pdf/tensteps-poster.pdf.

American College of Obstetricians & Gynecologists (ACOG). (2014). Challenges for overweight and obese women. *Obstetrics & Gynecology, 1234*(3), 726–730.

Andrews, M. M., & Boyle, J. S. (2012). *Transcultural concepts in nursing care* (6th ed.). Philadelphia, PA: Wolters Kluwer Health.

Baltes, P. B., Featherman, D. L., & Lerner, R. M. (2014). *Life-span development and behavior* (10th ed.). New York: Psychology Press.

Bang, K., Huh, B., & Kwon, M. (2014). The effect of a postpartum nursing intervention program for immigrant mothers. *Child Health Nursing Research, 20*(1), 11–19.

Barnes, D. L. (2014). *Women's reproductive mental health across the lifespan.* New York: Springer Publishers.

Bhati, S., & Richards, K. (2015). A systematic review of the relationship between postpartum sleep disturbance and postpartum depression. *JOGNN: Journal of Obstetric, Gynecologic & Neonatal Nursing, 44*(3), 350–357.

Bope, E., & Kellerman, R. (2015). *Conn's current therapy 2015.* Philadelphia, PA: Saunders Elsevier.

Bowers, P., & Ceballos, K. (2015). *Cultural perspectives in childbearing.* Retrieved from http://ce.nurse.com/ce263-60/Cultural-Perspectives-in-Childbearing.

Breastfeeding Committee for Canada. (2017). *The BFI 10 steps and WHO Code outcome indicators for hospitals and community health services.* Retrieved from http://breastfeedingcanada.ca/documents/Indicators%20-%20complete%20June%202017.pdf.

Brekke, H. K., Bertz, F., Rasmussen, K. M., Bosaeus, I., Ellegård, L., & Winkvist, A. (2014). Diet and exercise interventions among overweight and obese lactating women: Randomized trial of effects on cardiovascular risk factors. *PLoS One, 9*(2), 1–8.

Campbell-Yeo, M. L., Disher, T. C., Benoit, B. L., & Johnston, C. C. (2015). Understanding kangaroo care and its benefits to preterm infants. *Pediatric Health, Medicine & Therapeutics, 6,* 15–33.

Canadian Association of Perinatal and Women's Health Nurses. (2017). *Position statement on cultural safety/humility.* Retrieved from http://www.capwhn.ca/uploads/documents//CAPWHN_Position_Statement_on_Cultural_Safety_Humility_Final.pdf.

Canadian Nurses Association. (2010). *Promoting cultural competence in nursing.* Retrieved from https://www.cna-aiic.ca/~/media/cna/page-content/pdf-en/ps114_cultural_competence_2010_e.pdf?la=en.

Canadian Nurses Association and Canadian Association of Midwives. (Reaffirmed 2014). *Joint statement on breastfeeding.* Retrieved from https://www.cna-aiic.ca/-/media/cna/page-content/pdf-en/jps94_breastfeeding_march_2008_e.pdf.

Centers for Disease Control and Prevention (CDC). (2015a). *Reproductive health.* Retrieved from http://www.cdc.gov/reproductivehealth/unintendedpregnancy/usmec.htm.

Centers for Disease Control and Prevention (CDC). (2015b). *Tdap for pregnant women: Information for providers.* Retrieved from http://www.cdc.gov/vaccines/vpd-vac/pertussis/tdap-pregnancy-hcp.htm.

Ciaghi, F., Bianco, A. D., & Guarese, O. (2015). Prevalence of pelvic floor disorders during the post-partum period. A prospective study and a proposal of a multidisciplinary prevention strategy. *Scienza Riabilitativa, 17*(1), 5–15.

Cleminson, J., Oddie, S., Renfrew, M. J., & McGuire, W. (2015). Being baby friendly: Evidence-based breastfeeding support. *Archives of Disease in Childhood-Fetal and Neonatal Edition, 100*(2), 173–178.

Covan, E. K. (2015). Benefits of exercise for body, mind, and spirit. *Health Care for Women International, 36*(3), 255.

Crane, J., Murphy, P., Burrage, L., & Hutchens, D. (2013). Maternal and perinatal outcomes of extreme obesity in pregnancy. *Journal of Obstetricians and Gynecologists of Canada, 35*(7), 606–611. Retrieved from https://doi.org/10.1016/S1701-2163(15)30879-3.

Creasy, R. K., Resnik, R., Iams, J. D., Lockwood, C. J., Moore, T. R., & Greene, M. F. (2014). *Creasy & Resnik's maternal-fetal medicine: Principles and practice* (7th ed.). Philadelphia, PA: Elsevier Saunders.

Cristescu, T., Behrman, S., Jones, S. V., Chouliaras, L., & Ebmeier, K. P. (2015). Be vigilant for perinatal mental health problems. *The Practitioner, 259*(1780), 19–23.

Critch, J., Canadian Paediatric Society, & Nutrition and Gastroenterology Committee. (2017). Nutrition for healthy term infants, birth to six months: And overview. *Pediatric Child Health,18*(4), 206–207.

Cunningham, F. G., Leveno, K. J., Bloom, S. L., Spong, C., Dashe, J. S., Hoffman, B. L., … Sheffield, J. S. (2014). *Williams' obstetrics* (24th ed.). New York: McGraw-Hill Publishers.

Dayer-Berenson, L. (2014). *Cultural competencies of nurses: Impact on health and illness* (2nd ed.). Burlington, MA: Jones & Bartlett Learning.

Dieticians of Canada. (2014). *Food sources of iodine.* Retrieved from https://www.dietitians.ca/getattachment/f92bb712-300a-44a0-a9ac-da7f4b19849e/FACTSHEET-Food-Sources-of-Iodine.pdf.aspx.

Denne, S. C. (2015). Neonatal nutrition. *Pediatric Clinics of North America, 62*(2), 427–438.

Downs, D. S., Evenson, K. R., & Chasan-Taber, L. (2014). Obesity and physical activity during pregnancy and postpartum: Evidence, guidelines, and recommendations. In *Obesity during pregnancy in clinical practice* (pp. 183–227). London, England: Springer.

Edelman, C. L., Kudzma, E. C., & Mandle, C. L. (2014). *Health promotion throughout the lifespan* (8th ed.). St. Louis, MO: Elsevier Mosby.

Green, C. J. (2016). *Maternal-newborn nursing care plans* (3rd ed.). Burlington, MA: Jones & Bartlett Learning.

Halford, W. K., Petch, J., & Creedy, D. (2015). Caring and sexuality. In *Clinical guide to helping new parents* (pp. 131–150). New York: Springer Publishers.

Hall, B., & Woodward, S. (2015). Pelvic floor muscle training for urinary incontinence postpartum. *British Journal of Nursing, 24*(11), 576–579.

Health Canada. (2011). *Eating well with Canada's food guide.* Retrieved from https://www.canada.ca/en/health-canada/services/food-nutrition/canada-food-guide/get-your-copy/eating-well-2007.html.

Health Canada. (2012). *Infant formula.* Retrieved from https://www.canada.ca/en/health-canada/services/infant-care/infant-formula.html.

Health Canada. (2018a). *Health effects of cannabis.* Retrieved from https://www.canada.ca/en/health-canada/services/drugs-medication/cannabis/health-effects/effects.html#a3.

Health Canada. (2018b). *Pertussis vaccine. Canadian immunization guide: Part 4—Active vaccines.* Retrieved from https://www.canada.ca/en/public-health/services/publications/healthy-living/canadian-immunization-guide-part-4-active-vaccines/page-15-pertussis-vaccine.html.

Health Canada, Canadian Paediatric Society, Dietitians of Canada, & Breastfeeding Committee for Canada. (2015). *Nutrition for healthy term infants: Recommendations from birth to six months.* Retrieved from https://www.canada.ca/en/health-canada/services/food-nutrition/healthy-eating/infant-feeding/nutrition-healthy-term-infants-recommendations-birth-six-months.html.

Hugill, K. (2015). The senses of touch and olfaction in early mother-infant interaction. *British Journal of Midwifery, 23*(4), 238–243.

Jones, C., & Hawkes, R. (2015). Managing pregnancy-related pelvic floor dysfunction. *Primary Health Care, 25*(1), 24–28.

Jordan, R. G., Engstrom, J., Marfell, J., & Farley, C. L. (2014). *Prenatal & postnatal care: A women-centered approach.* Ames, IA: John Wiley & Sons.

Kim, Y. K., Kim, K. B., Kim, C. H., & Ha, H. (2015). Pulmonary embolism and uterine venous plexus thrombosis in the postpartum period. *Korean Journal of Legal Medicine, 39*(2), 41–44.

King, T. L., Brucker, M. C., Kriebs, J. M., Fahey, J. O., Gegor, C. L., & Varney, H. (2015). *Varney's midwifery* (5th ed.). Burlington, MA: Jones & Bartlett Learning.

Klebanov, M. S., & Travis, A. D. (2015). *The critical role of parenting in human development.* New York: Routledge, Taylor & Francis Group.

Kline, J. A., & Kabrhel, C. (2015). Emergency evaluation for pulmonary embolism, Part 1: Clinical factors that increase risk. *The Journal of Emergency Medicine, 49*(1), 104–117.

Laliberte, R. (2015). Leaky bladder. *Prevention, 67*(7), 52–54.

Lee, A., & Brann, L. (2015). Influence of cultural beliefs on infant feeding, postpartum and childcare practices among Chinese-American mothers in New York City. *Journal of Community Health, 40*(3), 476–483.

Lee, L. A., Carter, M., Stevenson, S. B., & Harrison, H. (2014). Improving family-centered care practices in the NICU. *Neonatal Network, 33*(3), 125–132.

Lewis, M., & Rudolph, K. D. (2014). *Handbook of developmental psychopathology* (3rd ed.). New York: Springer Publishers.

Lickenbrock, D. M., & Braungart-Rieker, J. M. (2015). Examining antecedents of infant attachment security with mothers and fathers: An ecological systems perspective. *Infant Behavior & Development, 39*, 173–187.

Lönnerdal, B., & Hernell, O. (2015). An opinion on "staging" of infant formula: A developmental perspective on infant feeding. *Journal of Pediatric Gastroenterology and Nutrition, 62*(1), 9–21.

Masho, S. W., Cha, S., & Morris, M. R. (2015). Prepregnancy obesity and breastfeeding non-initiation in the United States: An examination of racial and ethnic differences. *Breastfeeding Medicine, 10*(5), 253–262.

Mattson, S., & Smith, J. E. (2016). *Core curriculum for maternal-newborn nursing* (5th ed.). St. Louis, MO: Saunders Elsevier.

McComish, J. F. (2015). Infant mental health and attachment. *Journal of Child & Adolescent Psychiatric Nursing, 28*(2), 63–64.

McFarland, M. R., & Wehbe-Alamah, H. B. (2015). *Leininger's cultural care and diversity and universality: A worldwide nursing theory* (3rd ed.). Burlington, MA: Jones & Bartlett Learning.

Mercer, R. T. (2006). Nursing support of the process of becoming a mother. *Journal of Obstetric, Gynecologic, and Neonatal Nursing, 35*(5), 649–651.

Mooventhan, A., & Nivethitha, L. (2014). Scientific evidence-based effects of hydrotherapy on various systems of the body. *North American Journal of Medical Sciences, 6*(5), 199–209.

Moses, S. (2014). *Formula feeding. Family Practice Notebook.* Retrieved from http://www.fpnotebook.com/pharm/NICU/FrmlFdng.htm.

Nagtalon-Ramos, J. (2014). *Best evidence-based practices in maternal-newborn nursing care.* Philadelphia, PA: F. A. Davis Company.

Neville, C., McKinley, M., Holmes, V., Spence, D., & Woodside, J. (2014). The effectiveness of weight management interventions in breastfeeding women—a systematic review and critical evaluation. *Birth, 41*(3), 223–236.

O'Driscoll, T., Payne, L., Kelly, L., Cromarty, H., St. Pierre-Hansen, N., & Terry, C. (2011). Traditional First Nations birthing practices: Interviews with elders in northwestern Ontario. *Journal of Obstetrics and Gynecology Canada, 33*(1), 24–29. Retrieved from https://www.jogc.com/article/S1701-2163(16)34768-5/pdf.

Parfitt, Y., & Ayers, S. (2014). Transition to parenthood and mental health in first-time parents. *Infant Mental Health Journal, 35*(3), 263–273.

Park, S., Kim, S., & Kang, K. (2014). Integrative review of nursing intervention studies on mother-infant interactions. *Child Health Nursing Research, 20*(2), 75–86.

Parker, C., Warmuskerken, G., & Sinclair, L. (2015). Enhancing neonatal wellness with home visitation. *Nursing for Women's Health, 19*(1), 36–45.

Public Health Agency of Canada. (2014). *Maternal mortality in Canada.* Retrieved from https://sogc.org/wp-content/uploads/2014/05/REVISEDMortality-EN-Final-PDF.pdf.

Purnell, L. D. (2014). *Guide to culturally competent health care* (3rd ed.). Philadelphia, PA: F. A. Davis.

Santiago, M., & Figueiredo, M. (2015). Immigrant women's perspective on prenatal and postpartum care: Systematic review. *Journal of Immigrant & Minority Health, 17*(1), 276–284.

Sears, R. W., & Sears, J. M. (2015a). *Attachment parenting.* Retrieved from http://www.askdrsears.com/topics/parenting/attachment-parenting.

Sears, R. W., & Sears, J. M. (2015b). *Bonding—What it means.* Retrieved from http://www.askdrsears.com/topics/pregnancy-childbirth/tenth-month-post-partum/bonding-with-your-newborn/bonding-what-it-means.

Sears, R. W., & Sears, J. M. (2015c). *Introducing a new baby: 11 smooth-entry tips.* Retrieved from http://www.askdrsears. com/topics/parenting/discipline-behavior/bothersome-behaviors/sibling-rivalry/introducing-new-baby-11.

Sette, G., Coppola, G., & Cassibba, R. (2015). The transmission of attachment across generations: The state of art and new theoretical perspectives. *Scandinavian Journal of Psychology, 56*(3), 315–326.

Shannon, C., Chao, M., & Ramos, D. E. (2015). A gap analysis of effective interventions for postpartum weight loss in obese new mothers. *Obstetrics & Gynecology, 125,* 56–59.

Skidmore-Roth, L. (2015). *Mosby's 2015 nursing drug reference* (28th ed.). St. Louis, MO: Mosby Elsevier.

Stagg, J., & Ustianov, J. (2015). Improving and sustaining breastfeeding practices through a statewide learning collaborative. *Journal of Obstetric, Gynecologic, & Neonatal Nursing, 44,* S55.

Sucker, C., & Zotz, R. B. (2015). Prophylaxis and treatment of venous thrombosis and pulmonary embolism in pregnancy. *Reviews in Vascular Medicine, 3*(2), 24–30.

Sukhwinder, K., Poonam, S., Sulakshna, C., & Jodibala, H. (2014). Comparison of infrared light therapy vs sitz bath on episiotomy in terms of wound healing and intensity of pain among postnatal mothers. *International Journal of Nursing Care, 2*(1), 37–41.

Tester-Jones, M., O'Mahen, H., Watkins, E., & Karl, A. (2015). The impact of maternal characteristics, infant temperament and contextual factors on maternal responsiveness to infant. *Infant Behavior & Development, 40,* 1–11.

UNICEF, & World Health Organization. (2018). *Protecting, promoting and supporting breastfeeding in facilities providing maternity and newborn services: The revised baby-friendly initiative.* Retrieved from http://www.who.int/nutrition/publications/infantfeeding/bfhi-implementation-2018.pdf?ua=1.

Verghese, T. S., Futaba, K., & Latthe, P. (2015). Constipation in pregnancy. *The Obstetrician & Gynecologist, 17*(2), 111–115.

Walker, L. O., Murphey, C. L., & Nichols, F. (2015). The broken thread of health promotion and disease prevention for women during the postpartum period. *Journal of Perinatal Education, 24*(2), 81–92.

Whittock, J. (2015). Promoting sexual health: Sex after childbirth. *MIDIRS Midwifery Digest, 25*(1), 77–80.

Wilson, B. L., Passante, T., Rauschenbach, D., Yang, R., & Wong, B. (2015). Bladder management with epidural anesthesia: A randomized controlled trial. *MCN: The American Journal of Maternal Child Nursing, 40*(4), 234–242.

World Health Organization (WHO). (2011). Rubella vaccines: WHO position paper. *Weekly Epidemiological Record, 86*(29), 301–316. Retrieved from http://www.who.int/wer/2011/wer8629.pdf?ua=1.

World Health Organization (WHO). (2014a). *Implementation of the baby-friendly hospital initiative.* Retrieved from http://www.who.int/elena/bbc/implementation_bfhi/en/.

World Health Organization (WHO). (2014b). *WHO recommendations on postnatal care of the mother and newborn.* Retrieved from http://apps.who.int/iris/bitstream/10665/97603/1/9789241506649_eng.pdf.

Zapata, L. B., Murtaza, S., Whiteman, M. K., Jamieson, D. J., Robbins, C. L., Marchbanks, P. A.,…Curtis, K. M. (2015). Contraceptive counseling and postpartum contraceptive use. *American Journal of Obstetrics and Gynecology, 212*(2), 171–179.

MULTIPLE CHOICE QUESTIONS

1. When assessing a postpartum client, which of the following would lead the nurse to suspect postpartum blues?
   a. Panic attacks and suicidal thoughts
   b. Anger toward self and infant
   c. Periodic crying and insomnia
   d. Obsessive thoughts and hallucinations

2. Which of these activities would best help the postpartum nurse to provide culturally sensitive care for the childbearing family?
   a. Taking a transcultural course
   b. Caring for only families of his or her cultural origin
   c. Teaching Western beliefs to culturally diverse families
   d. Seeking education regarding diverse cultural perinatal practices

3. Which of the following suggestions would be most appropriate to include in the teaching plan for a postpartum client who would benefit from losing weight?
   a. Increase fluid intake and acid-producing foods in her diet.
   b. Avoid empty-calorie foods, breastfeed, increase exercise.
   c. Start a high-protein, low carbohydrate diet and restrict fluids.
   d. Eat no snacks or carbohydrates after dinner.

4. After teaching a group of breastfeeding clients about nutritional needs, the nurse determines that the teaching was successful when the clients state that they need to increase their intake of which nutrients?
   a. Carbohydrates and fibre
   b. Fats and vitamins
   c. Calories and protein
   d. Iron-rich foods and minerals

5. Which of the following would lead the nurse to suspect that a postpartum client was developing a complication?
   a. Fatigue and irritability
   b. Perineal discomfort and pink discharge
   c. Pulse rate of 60 bpm
   d. Swollen, tender, hot area on breast

6. Which of the following would the nurse assess as indicating positive bonding between the parents and their newborn?
   a. Holding the infant close to the body
   b. Having visitors hold the infant
   c. Buying expensive infant clothes
   d. Requesting that the nurses care for the infant

7. Which activity would the nurse include in the teaching plan for parents with a newborn and an older child to reduce sibling rivalry when the newborn is brought home?
   a. Punishing the older child for bedwetting behaviour
   b. Sending the sibling to the grandparents' house
   c. Planning a daily "special time" for the older sibling
   d. Allowing the sibling to share a room with the infant

8. The major purpose of the first postpartum homecare visit is to:
   a. Identify complications that require interventions
   b. Obtain a blood specimen for PKU testing
   c. Complete the official birth certificate
   d. Support the new parents in their parenting roles

9. The nurse is instructing the postpartum client who plans to feed her newborn with infant formula about measures to prevent breast engorgement when she is discharged. Which of the following measures should the nurse include in the teaching plan?
   a. Decreasing her fluid intake for the first week at home
   b. Wearing a tight-fitting supportive bra 24 hours daily
   c. Take a diuretic to release the extra fluid in the breasts
   d. Manually express the milk that is accumulating

10. A client was brought to the postpartum unit who gave birth 12 hours ago. Because this is her first child, which of the following goals by the nurse is most appropriate?
    a. Early discharge for the dyad
    b. Rapid transition into her role of being a parent
    c. Minimal need for expression of her feelings now
    d. Effective education of both parents before discharge

CHAPTER **WORKSHEET**

CRITICAL THINKING EXERCISES

1. As a nurse working on a postpartum unit, you enter the room of, a 22-year-old primipara, and find her chatting on the phone while her newborn is crying loudly in the bassinette, which has been pushed into the bathroom. You pick up and comfort the newborn. While holding the baby, you ask the client if she was aware her newborn was crying. She replies, "That's about all that kid does since it was born!" You hand the newborn to her and she places the newborn on the bed away from her and continues her phone conversation.
   a. What is your nursing assessment of this encounter?
   b. What nursing interventions would be appropriate?
   c. What specific discharge interventions may be needed?

2. A 34-year-old single primipara, left the hospital after a 36-hour stay with her newborn son. She lives alone in a one-bedroom walk-up apartment. As the postpartum home health nurse visiting her 2 days later, you find the following:
   • Tearful client pacing the floor holding her crying son
   • Home cluttered and in disarray
   • Fundus firm and displaced to right of midline
   • Moderate lochia rubra; episiotomy site clean, dry, and intact
   • Vital signs within normal range; pain rating less than 3 on scale of 1 to 10
   • Breasts engorged slightly; supportive bra on
   • Newborn assessment within normal limits
   • Distended bladder upon palpation; reporting urinary frequency
   a. Which of these assessment findings warrants further investigation?
   b. What interventions are appropriate at this time, and why?
   c. What health teaching is needed before you leave this home?

3. The nurse walks into the room of a 24-year-old primigravida. The client asks the nurse to hand them the bottle sitting on the bedside table, stating, "I'm going to finish it off because my baby only ate half of it 3 hours ago when I fed him."
   a. What response by the nurse would be appropriate at this time?
   b. What action should the nurse take?
   c. What health teaching is needed for this new parent prior to discharge?

STUDY ACTIVITIES

1. Identify two questions that a nurse would ask a postpartum client to assess for postpartum blues.

2. Find a website that offers advice to new parents about breastfeeding. Critique the site, the author's credentials, and the accuracy of the content.

3. Outline instructions you would give to a postpartum client on how to use the peribottle.

4. Breast tissue swelling secondary to vascular congestion after childbirth and preceding lactation describes _____.

5. Listen to the postpartum story of one of your assigned clients and share it with your peers in class or as part of online discussion.

BRINGING IT ALL TOGETHER: A CASE STUDY

A 26-year-old client gave birth to a healthy term neonate yesterday and is preparing for discharge. The mother is illiterate and lives in a rural agricultural area outside of town. This is her fourth infant in 5 years. The postpartum nurse comes into the room and observes that this mother has wrapped a piece of unclean cloth tightly around the infant's abdomen with a quarter which covers the cord stump. The infant's outfit is not clean and not appropriate for the weather conditions outside. The mother is waiting for a ride home from a friend. The postpartum nurse is here to provide her with discharge instructions.

Go to thePoint **to find questions to consider about this case.**

The Newborn

Newborn Transitioning

Learning Objectives

Upon completion of the chapter, you will be able to:

1. Examine the major physiologic changes that occur as the newborn transitions to extrauterine life.

2. Determine the primary challenges faced by the newborn during the transition to extrauterine life.

3. Interpret the factors that influence the initiation of newborn respirations.

4. Compare and contrast the cardiovascular changes that take place from fetal circulation to extrauterine circulation after birth.

5. Relate three characteristics that predispose newborns to heat loss after birth.

6. Distinguish three primary immunoglobulins that help strengthen the newborn's immunologic system.

7. Differentiate the three behavioural patterns that newborns display after birth.

8. Assess the five typical behavioural responses triggered by external stimuli of the newborn.

The Public Health home care nurse reviewed the client's file in her car before she got out: 18-year-old primipara, 1 week postpartum with a term newborn girl weighing 7 lb. The new mother, Maria, greeted the nurse at the door and let her inside the house. After performing a postpartum assessment on Maria and an assessment of her newborn daughter, the nurse asked Maria if she had any questions or concerns. Maria's eyes welled up with tears: she is worried that her daughter can't see.

INTRODUCTION

When a child is born, the exhaustion and stress of labour are over for the parents, but now the newborn must begin the work of physiologically and behaviourally adapting to the new environment. The first 24 hours of life can be the most precarious (Swanson & Sinkin, 2015).

The **neonatal period** is defined as the first 28 days of life. It is a period of the most dramatic and rapid physiologic changes in humans. After birth, the newborn is exposed to a whole new world of sounds, colours, smells, and sensations. The newborn, previously confined to the warm, dark, wet intrauterine environment, is now thrust into an environment that is much brighter and cooler. As the newborn adapts to life after birth, numerous physiologic changes occur (Table 17.1).

Awareness of the adaptations that are occurring forms the foundation for providing support to the newborn during this crucial time. Physiologic and behavioural changes occur quickly during this transition period. Being aware of any deviations from the norm is crucial to ensure early identification and prompt intervention.

This chapter describes the physiologic changes of the newborn's major body systems. It also discusses the behavioural adaptations, including behavioural patterns and the newborn's behavioural responses, which occur during this transition period.

PHYSIOLOGIC TRANSITIONING

The adaptation from the intrauterine to extrauterine environment is complex and difficult, but required for all humans. Maternal medical and fetal conditions can have a profound effect on the successful transition. The mechanics of birth require a change in the newborn for survival outside the uterus. Immediately at birth, respiratory gas exchange, along with circulatory modifications, must occur to sustain extrauterine life. During this time, as newborns strive to attain homeostasis, they also experience complex changes in major organ systems. The newborn's most dramatic and most rapid extrauterine transitions occur in four interdependent areas: respiratory, circulatory, thermoregulation, and their ability to stabilize their blood glucose levels. All four areas must all make successful transitions for the newborn to adapt to extrauterine life. Although the transition usually takes place within the first 6 to 10 hours of life, many adaptations take weeks to attain full maturity.

Cardiovascular System Adaptations

During fetal life, the heart relies on certain unique structures that assist it in providing adequate perfusion of vital body parts. The umbilical vein carries oxygenated blood from the placenta to the fetus. The ductus venosus allows the majority of the umbilical vein blood to bypass the liver and merge with blood moving through the vena cava, bringing it to the heart sooner. The foramen ovale allows more than half the blood entering the right atrium to cross immediately to the left atrium, bypassing the pulmonary circulation. The ductus arteriosus connects the pulmonary artery to the aorta, which allows bypassing of the pulmonary circuit. Only a small portion of

TABLE 17.1	ANATOMIC AND PHYSIOLOGIC COMPARISON OF THE FETUS AND NEWBORN	
Topic of Comparison	**Fetus**	**Newborn**
Respiratory system	Fluid-filled, high-pressure system causes blood to be shunted from the lungs through the ductus arteriosus to the rest of the body.	Air-filled, low-pressure system encourages blood flow through the lungs for gas exchange; increased oxygen content of blood in the lungs contributes to the closing of the ductus arteriosus (becomes a ligament).
Site of gas exchange	Placenta	Lungs
Circulation through the heart	Pressures in the right atrium are greater than in the left, encouraging blood flow through the foramen ovale.	Pressures in the left atrium are greater than in the right, causing the foramen ovale to close.
Hepatic portal circulation	Ductus venosus bypasses; maternal liver performs filtering functions.	Ductus venosus closes (becomes a ligament); hepatic portal circulation begins.
Thermoregulation	Body temperature is maintained by maternal body temperature and the warmth of the intrauterine environment.	Body temperature is maintained through a flexed posture and brown fat.

Adapted from Sharma, A., Ford, S., & Calvert, J. (2014). Adaptation for life: A review of neonatal physiology. *Anesthesia & Intensive Care Medicine, 15*(3), 89–95; Stave, U. (2014). *Perinatal physiology.* New York: Springer Publishers; and King, T. L., Brucker, M. C., Kriebs, J. M., Fahey, J. O., Gegor, C. L., & Varney, H. (2015). *Varney's midwifery* (5th ed.). Burlington, MA: Jones & Bartlett Learning.

blood passes through the pulmonary circuit for the main purpose of perfusion of the structure, rather than for oxygenation. The fetus depends on the placenta to provide oxygen and nutrients and to remove waste products.

At birth, the circulatory system must switch from fetal to newborn circulation and from placental to pulmonary gas exchange. Successful transition from fetal to postnatal circulation requires increased pulmonary blood flow, removal of the placenta, and closure of the intracardiac (foramen ovale) and extracardiac shunts (ductus venosus and ductus arteriosus). These changes are needed to equalize the right ventricular output with that of the left (Steinhorn, 2015). The physical forces of the contractions of labour and birth, mild asphyxia, increased intracranial pressure as a result of cord compression and uterine contractions, and the cold stress experienced immediately after birth lead to an increased release of catecholamines that is critical for the changes involved in the transition to extrauterine life. The increased levels of epinephrine and norepinephrine stimulate increased cardiac output and contractility, surfactant release, and promotion of pulmonary fluid clearance (Sharma, Ford, & Calvert, 2014).

Fetal to Neonatal Circulation Changes

Changes in circulation occur immediately at birth as the fetus separates from the placenta (Fig. 17.1). When the umbilical cord is clamped, the first breath is taken and the lungs begin to function. As a result, systemic vascular resistance increases and blood return to the heart via the inferior vena cava decreases. Concurrently with these changes, there is a rapid decrease in pulmonary vascular resistance and an increase in pulmonary blood flow (Cuneo, 2014). The foramen ovale functionally closes with a decrease in pulmonary vascular resistance, which leads to a decrease in right-sided heart pressures. An increase in systemic pressure, after clamping of the cord, leads to an increase in left-sided heart pressures. The ductus arteriosus, ductus venosus, and umbilical vessels that were vital during fetal life are no longer needed. Over a period of months, these fetal vessels form nonfunctional ligaments.

Before birth, the foramen ovale allowed most of the oxygenated blood entering the right atrium from the inferior vena cava to pass into the left atrium of the heart. With the newborn's first breath, air pushes into the lungs, triggering an increase in pulmonary blood flow and pulmonary venous return to the left side of the heart. As a result, the pressure in the left atrium becomes higher than in the right atrium. The increased left atrial pressure causes the foramen ovale to close, thus allowing the output from the right ventricle to flow entirely to the lungs. With closure of this fetal shunt, oxygenated blood is now separated from nonoxygenated blood. The subsequent increase in tissue oxygenation further promotes the increase in systemic blood pressure and continuing blood flow to the lungs. The foramen ovale normally closes functionally at birth when left atrial pressure increases and right atrial pressure decreases. Permanent anatomic closure, though, really occurs throughout the next several weeks.

During fetal life, the ductus arteriosus, located between the aorta and the pulmonary artery, protected the lungs against circulatory overload by shunting blood (right to left) into the descending aorta, bypassing the pulmonary circulation. Its patency during fetal life is promoted by continual production of prostaglandin E2 (PGE2) by the ductus arteriosus (van Vonderen et al., 2014). The ductus arteriosus becomes functionally closed within the first few hours after birth. Oxygen is the most important factor in controlling its closure. Closure depends on the high oxygen content of the aortic blood that results from aeration of the lungs at birth. At birth, pulmonary vascular resistance decreases, allowing pulmonary blood flow to increase and oxygen exchange to occur in the lungs. It occurs secondary to an increase in PO_2 coincident with the first breath and umbilical cord occlusion when it is clamped.

The ductus venosus shunted blood from the left umbilical vein to the inferior vena cava during intrauterine life. It closes within a few days after birth, because this shunting is no longer needed as a result of activation of the liver. The activated liver now takes over the functions of the placenta (which was expelled at birth). The ductus venosus becomes a ligament in extrauterine life.

The two umbilical arteries and one umbilical vein begin to constrict at birth, because with placental expulsion, blood flow ceases. In addition, peripheral circulation increases. Thus, the vessels are no longer needed, and they too become ligaments. Successful transition and closure of the three fetal shunts creates a neonatal circulation where deoxygenated blood returns to the heart through the inferior and superior vena cava. It enters the right atrium to the right ventricle and travels through the pulmonary artery to the pulmonary vascular bed. Oxygenated blood returns through pulmonary veins to the left atrium, the left ventricle, and through the aorta to the systemic circulation (Stave, 2014). Box 17.1 provides a summary of fetal to neonatal circulation.

Heart Rate

During the first few minutes after birth, the newborn's heart rate is approximately 110 to 160 bpm. Thereafter, it begins to decrease to an average of 120 to 130 bpm (Creasy et al., 2014). The newborn is highly dependent on heart rate for maintenance of cardiac output and blood pressure. Although the blood pressure is not taken routinely in the healthy term newborn, it is usually highest after birth and reaches a plateau within a week after birth. Cardiac defects may be identified in the newborn nursery by conducting a thorough and systematic physical assessment, including inspection, palpation, auscultation, and measurement of blood pressure and oxygen

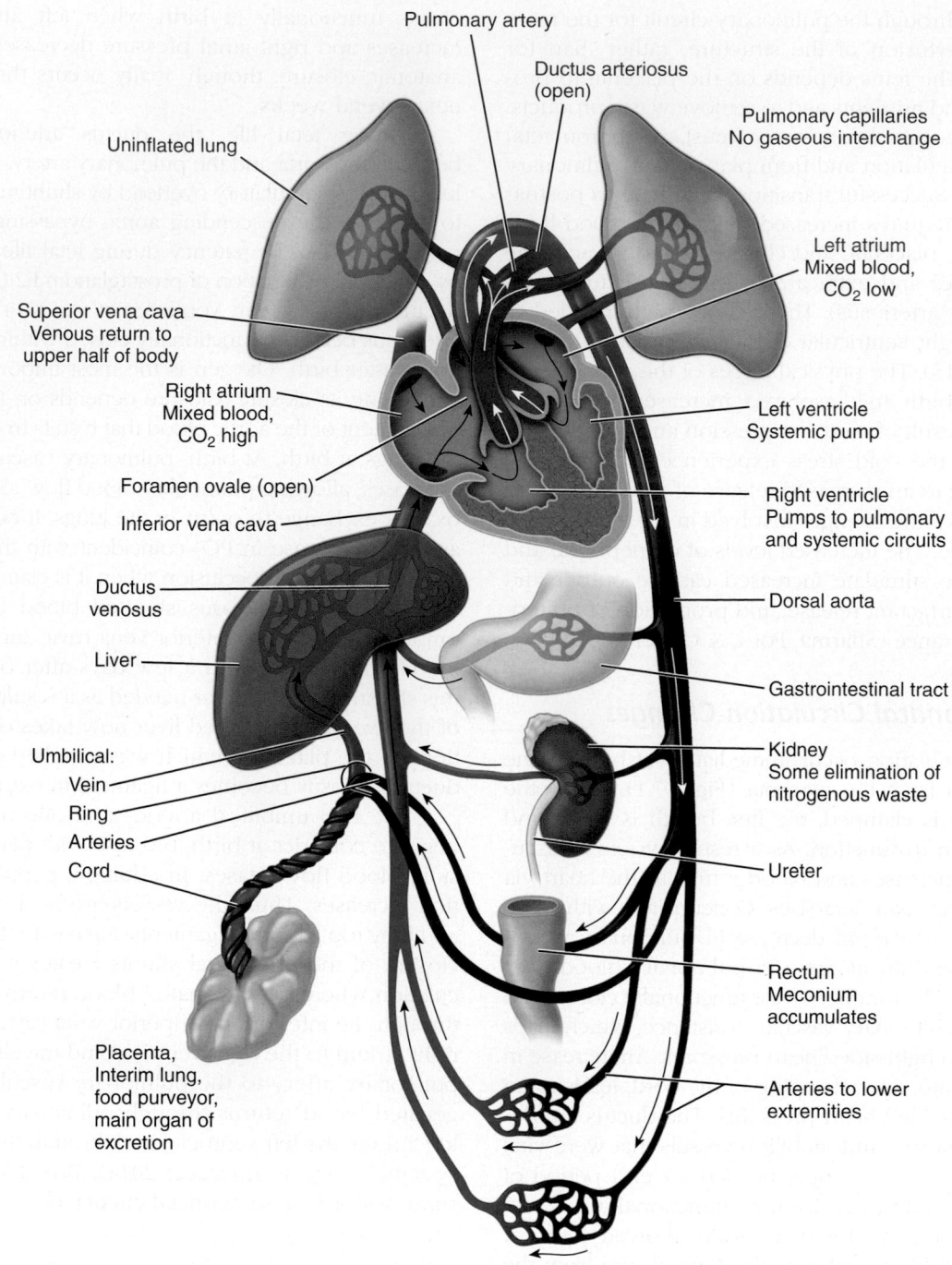

Pulmonary artery

Ductus arteriosus
(open)

Pulmonary capillaries
No gaseous interchange

Uninflated lung

Left atrium
Mixed blood,
CO_2 low

Superior vena cava
Venous return to
upper half of body

Right atrium
Mixed blood,
CO_2 high

Left ventricle
Systemic pump

Foramen ovale (open)

Inferior vena cava

Right ventricle
Pumps to pulmonary
and systemic circuits

Ductus
venosus

Dorsal aorta

Liver

Gastrointestinal tract

Umbilical:
Vein
Ring
Arteries
Cord

Kidney
Some elimination of
nitrogenous waste

Ureter

Rectum
Meconium
accumulates

Placenta,
Interim lung,
food purveyor,
main organ of
excretion

Arteries to lower
extremities

A

FIGURE 17.1 Cardiovascular adaptations of the newborn. Note the changes in oxygenation between (**A**) prenatal circulation and (**B**) postnatal (pulmonary) circulation.

saturations. The ability of the nurse to identify irregular findings during physical assessment aids rapid identification and treatment.

Take Note!

Transient functional cardiac murmurs may be heard during the neonatal period as a result of the changing dynamics of the cardiovascular system at birth (Fillipps & Bucciarelli, 2015).

The fluctuations in both the heart rate and blood pressure tend to follow the changes in the newborn's behavioural state. An increase in activity, such as wakefulness, movement, or crying, corresponds to an increase in heart rate and blood pressure. In contrast, the compromised newborn demonstrates markedly less physiologic variability overall. Tachycardia may be found with volume depletion, cardiorespiratory disease, drug withdrawal, and hyperthyroidism. Bradycardia

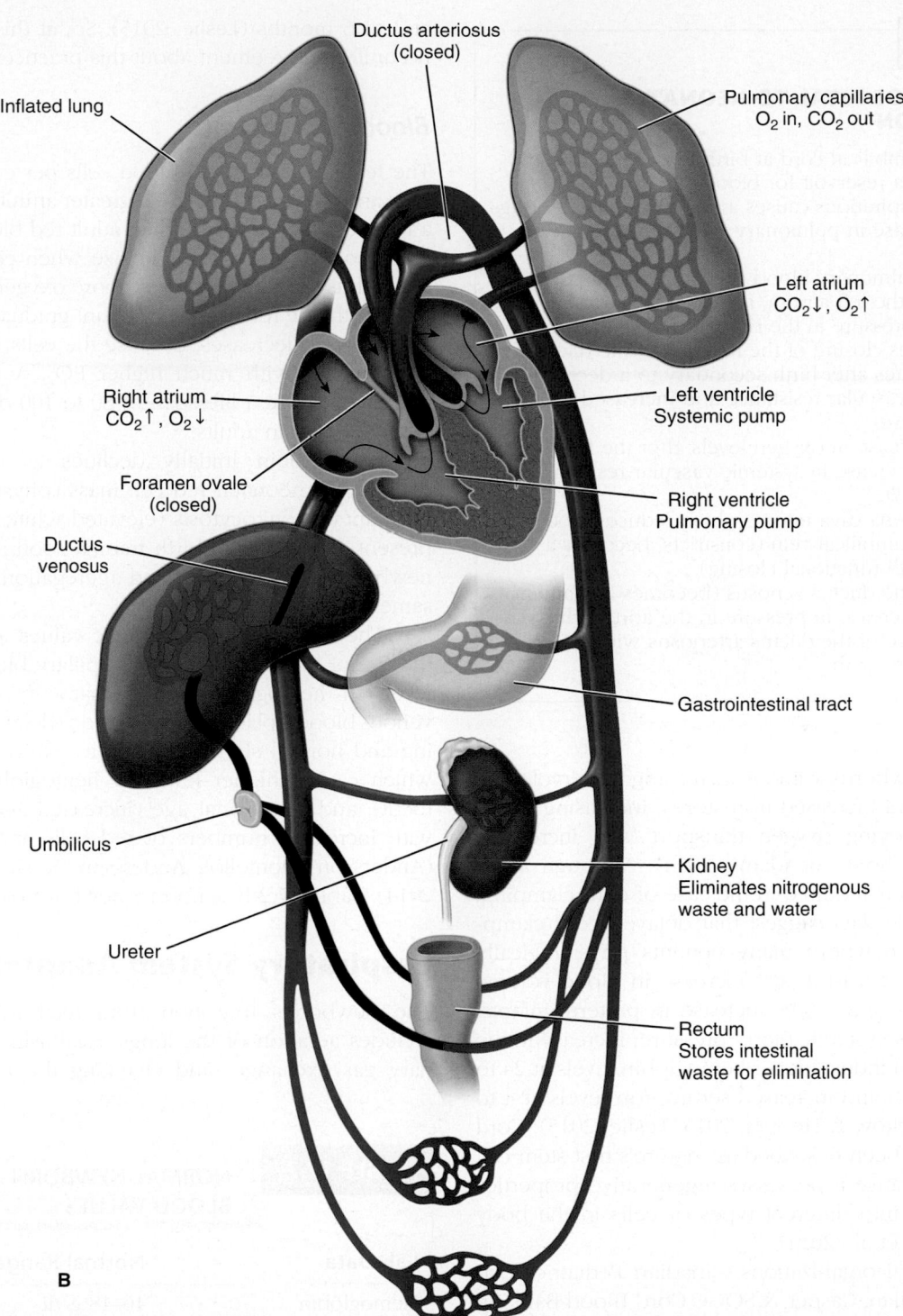

Ductus arteriosus
(closed)

Inflated lung

Pulmonary capillaries
O_2 in, CO_2 out

Left atrium
$CO_2\downarrow$, $O_2\uparrow$

Right atrium
$CO_2\uparrow$, $O_2\downarrow$

Left ventricle
Systemic pump

Foramen ovale
(closed)

Right ventricle
Pulmonary pump

Ductus
venosus

Gastrointestinal tract

Umbilicus

Kidney
Eliminates nitrogenous
waste and water

Ureter

Rectum
Stores intestinal
waste for elimination

B

FIGURE 17.1 *(continued)*

is often associated with apnea and is often seen with hypoxia.

Blood Volume

The blood volume of the newborn depends on the amount of blood transferred from the placenta at birth. It is usually estimated to be 80 to 85 mL/kg of body weight in the term infant (Stave, 2014). However, the volume may vary by as much as 25% to 40%, depending on when clamping of the umbilical cord occurs. Early (before 30 to 40 seconds) or late (after 3 minutes) clamping of the umbilical cord changes circulatory dynamics during transition. Recent studies indicate that the benefits of delayed cord clamping include improving the newborn's cardiopulmonary adaptation, preventing iron-deficient anemia

BOX 17.1

SUMMARY OF FETAL TO NEONATAL CIRCULATION

- Clamping umbilical cord at birth eliminates the placenta as a reservoir for blood.
- Onset of respirations causes a rise in PO_2 in the lungs and a decrease in pulmonary vascular resistance, *which...*
- Increases pulmonary blood flow and increases pressure in the left atrium, *which...*
- Decreases pressure in the right atrium of the heart, which causes closure of the foramen ovale (closes within minutes after birth secondary to a decreased pulmonary vascular resistance and increased left heart pressure).
- With an increase in oxygen levels after the first breath, an increase in systemic vascular resistance occurs, *which...*
- Decreases vena cava return, which reduces blood flow in the umbilical vein (constricts, becomes a ligament with functional closing).
- Closure of the ductus venosus (becomes a ligament) causes an increase in pressure in the aorta, which forces closure of the ductus arteriosus within 10 to 15 hours after birth.

in full-term newborns without increasing hypervolemia-related risks and increased iron stores, increasing blood pressure, improving oxygen transport, and increasing red blood cell flow (McAdams, 2014). Although a tailored approach is required in the case of cord clamping, current available data suggest that delayed cord clamping offers the newborn many benefits physiologically which include at least a 30% increase in blood volume for term infants and a 50% increase in preterm infants; improvement of systemic blood pressure; increase in the cerebral oxygen index; higher hemoglobin levels at 24 to 48 hours of age; and increased serum iron levels at 4 to 6 months (Kluckow & Hooper, 2015; Leslie, 2015). Cord blood has also been described as "nature's first stem cell transplant" because it possesses regenerative properties and can grow into different types of cells in the body (van Vonderen et al., 2014).

Professional organizations Canadian Pediatric Society (Armson, Allan, Casper, & SOGC Cord Blood Banking Working Group, 2015) and SOGC (2015) have released opinions that support delayed cord clamping for preterm infants but endorse continued research on this procedure for all infants. WHO (2014) released a report recommending delayed cord clamping for "all births" as a best practice. A recent Cochrane review on term infants and timing of umbilical cord clamping reported that those with delayed cord clamping had up to a 60% increase in red blood cells, high hemoglobin levels, and higher iron levels at 4 to 6 months. Infants whose cords were clamped early were twice as likely to be iron deficit

at 3 to 6 months (Leslie, 2015). So, at this time, there is no uniform agreement about this practice.

Blood Components

The fetus has more red blood cells per cubic millimetre than an adult and they have a greater affinity for oxygen at a lower oxygen pressure than adult red blood cells. Fetal red blood cells are larger in size when compared to an adult, thus each cell can carry more oxygen (Stave, 2014). After birth, the red blood cell count gradually increases as the cell size decreases, because the cells now live in an environment with much higher PO_2. A newborn's red blood cells have a life span of 80 to 100 days, compared with 120 days in adults.

Hemoglobin initially declines as a result of a decrease in neonatal red cell mass (physiologic anemia of infancy). Leukocytosis (elevated white blood cells) is present as a result of birth trauma soon after birth. The newborn's platelet count and aggregation ability are the same as those of adults.

The newborn's hematologic values are affected by the site of the blood sample (capillary blood has higher levels of hemoglobin and hematocrit compared with venous blood), placental transfusion (delayed cord clamping and normal shift of plasma to extravascular spaces, which causes higher levels of hemoglobin and hematocrit), and gestational age (increased age is associated with increased numbers of red cells and hemoglobin) (Andersson, Domellöf, Andersson, & Hellström-Westas, 2014). Table 17.2 lists normal newborn blood values.

Respiratory System Adaptations

The newborn's transition from fetal to neonatal life includes aeration of the lungs, establishment of pulmonary gas exchange, and changing the fetal circulation

TABLE 17.2	NORMAL NEWBORN BLOOD VALUES	
Lab Data	**Normal Range**	
Hemoglobin	16–18 g/dL	
Hematocrit	46–68%	
Platelets	150,000–350,000/µL	
Red blood cells	4.5–7.0 (1,000,000/µL)	
White blood cells	10–30,000/mm³	

Adapted from Fischbach, F., & Dunning, M. B. (2014). *Manual of laboratory and diagnostic tests* (9th ed.). Philadelphia, PA: Lippincott Williams & Wilkins; Verklan, T., & Walden, M. (2014). *Core curriculum for neonatal intensive care nursing* (4th ed.). St. Louis, MO: Elsevier; and Davidson, M. R. (2014). *Fast facts for the neonatal nurse: A nursing orientation and care guide in a nutshell.* New York: Springer.

into the adult type. Lung aeration leads to the establishment of functional residual capacity, allowing pulmonary gas exchange to start. The first breath of life is a gasp that generates an increase in transpulmonary pressure and results in diaphragmatic descent. Hypercapnia, hypoxia, and acidosis resulting from normal labour become stimuli for initiating respirations. Inspiration of air and expansion of the lungs allow for an increase in tidal volume (amount of air brought into the lungs). **Surfactant** is a surface tension–reducing lipoprotein found in the newborn's lungs that prevents alveolar collapse at the end of expiration and loss of lung volume. It lines the alveoli to enhance aeration of gas-free lungs, thus reducing surface tension and lowering the pressure required to open the alveoli. Healthy lung function depends on surfactant, which permits a decrease in surface tension at end expiration (to prevent atelectasis) and an increase in surface tension during lung expansion (to facilitate elastic recoil on inspiration). Surfactant provides the lung stability needed for gas exchange. The newborn's first breath, in conjunction with surfactant, overcomes the surface forces to permit aeration of the lungs. The chest wall of the newborn is floppy because of the high cartilage content and poorly developed musculature. Thus, accessory muscles to help in breathing are ineffective.

One of the most crucial adaptations that the newborn makes at birth is adjusting from a fluid-filled intrauterine environment to a gaseous extrauterine environment. During fetal life, the lungs are expanded with an ultrafiltrate of the amniotic fluid. During and after birth, this fluid must be removed and replaced with air. Passage through the birth canal allows intermittent compression of the thorax, which helps eliminate the fluid in the lungs. Pulmonary capillaries and the lymphatics remove the remaining fluid.

If fluid is removed too slowly or incompletely (e.g., with decreased thoracic squeezing during birth or diminished respiratory effort), transient tachypnea (respiratory rate above 60 breaths per minute) of the newborn occurs. Examples of situations involving decreased thoracic compression and diminished respiratory effort include cesarean birth and sedation in newborns. Research findings support the need for thoracic compression because the absence of the neonate's exposure to labour contractions, which may occur with cesarean births or heavy sedation during the labour process or general anesthesia administered during the surgical birth, is associated with an increased risk of transient tachypnea at term, with oxygen supplementation being needed for a longer duration (Hooper, Polglase, & Roehr, 2015).

Take Note!

A neonate born by cesarean section does not have the same benefit of the birth canal squeeze as does the newborn born by vaginal delivery. Closely observe the respirations of the newborn after cesarean delivery.

Lungs

Before the newborn's lungs can maintain respiratory function, the following events must occur:
- Initiation of respiratory movement
- Expansion of the lungs
- Establishing functional residual capacity (ability to retain some air in the lungs on expiration)
- Increased pulmonary blood flow
- Redistribution of cardiac output (Bope & Kellerman, 2015)

Initial breathing is probably the result of a reflex triggered by pressure changes, noise, light, temperature changes, touching, compression of the fetal chest during the birthing process, and high carbon dioxide and low oxygen concentrations of the newborn's blood. Central chemoreceptors stimulated by hypoxia and hypercapnia further increase the respiratory drive. Many theories address the initiation of respiration in the newborn, but most are based on speculation from observations rather than on empirical research (Sharma et al., 2014). Research continues to search for answers to these questions.

Respirations

After respirations are established in the newborn, they are shallow and irregular, ranging from 30 to 60 breaths per minute, with short periods of apnea (less than 15 seconds). The newborn's respiratory rate varies according to his or her activity; the more active the newborn, the higher the respiratory rate, on average. Signs of respiratory distress to observe for include cyanosis, tachypnea, expiratory grunting, sternal retractions, and nasal flaring. Respirations should not be laboured, and the chest movements should be symmetrical. In some cases, **periodic breathing** may occur, which is the cessation of breathing that lasts 5 to 10 seconds without changes in colour or heart rate (Davidson, 2014). Periodic breathing may be observed in newborns within the first few days of life and requires close monitoring.

Take Note!

Apneic periods lasting more than 15 seconds with cyanosis and heart rate changes require further evaluation (Mattson & Smith, 2015).

Body Temperature Regulation

Newborns are dependent on their environment for the maintenance of body temperature, much more so immediately after birth than later in life. One of the most important elements in a newborn's survival is obtaining a stable body temperature to promote an optimal transition to extrauterine life. On average, a newborn's temperature ranges from 36.6° to 37.6°C (97.9° to 99.7°F).

EVIDENCE-BASED PRACTICE 17.1

EFFECT OF EARLY MATERNAL/NEWBORN SKIN-TO-SKIN CONTACT AFTER BIRTH ON THE DURATION OF THIRD STAGE OF LABOUR AND INITIATION OF BREASTFEEDING

STUDY

The holding of a newborn with vertical skin-to-skin contact typically in an upright position with the swaddled newborn on the chest of the mother, is commonly referred to as kangaroo care. It has been recommended that this skin-to-skin contact is a feasible, natural, and cost-effective intervention for breastfeeding initiation, and thermoregulation. The aim of this study was to determine the effect of early maternal-newborn skin-to-skin contact after birth on the duration of the third stage of labour and initiation of breastfeeding.

Findings

A nonrandomized controlled clinical trial was conducted using a sample of 100 labouring women. The project included a study group (50) who had skin-to-skin contact and a control group (50) who received routine hospital care. Tools used to collect data included a structured interview, assessment of pregnant clients during the third stage of labour, and an outcome assessment of first breastfeeding. The results revealed that success in

first time breastfeeding during, complete separation of the placenta, and immediate contraction of the uterus was higher in the study group compared to the control group. There were statistically significant differences between the study and control groups in third stage of labour duration (9 minutes shorter), complete placental separation, and immediate contraction of the uterus or excessive bleeding. The study concluded that mothers who practice early mother/newborn skin-to-skin contact immediately after giving birth experienced a shorter third stage duration and early successful initiation of breastfeeding.

Nursing Implications

Based on these findings, it would make sense to incorporate early skin-to-skin contact immediate postbirth and delay routine infant care until the success of the first breastfeeding process for the benefits it provides to both mother and newborn. Nurses need to apply evidence-based research into their care since this application would improve maternal and child health outcomes.

Adapted from Essa, R. M., & Ismail, N. I. A. A. (2015). Effect of early maternal/newborn skin-to-skin contact after birth on the duration of third stage of labor and initiation of breastfeeding. *Journal of Nursing Education and Practice, 5*(4), 98–107.

Since newborns lose heat easily after birth, having uninterrupted skin-to-skin contact for 1 to 2 hours with their mothers/parent is recommended as the initial method for maintaining newborn body temperature. Safe skin-to-skin contact should be the first line of treatment for hypothermia and as a measure to reduce discomfort from painful procedures throughout the first days, weeks, and months of life. See Evidence-Based Practice 17.1.

Thermoregulation is the process of maintaining the balance between heat loss and heat production in order to maintain its core internal temperature. It is a critical physiologic function that is closely related to the transition and survival of the newborn. An appropriate thermal environment is essential for maintaining a normal body temperature. Compared with adults, newborns tolerate a narrower range of environmental temperatures and are extremely vulnerable to both under heating and overheating. Nurses play a key role in providing an appropriate environment to help newborns maintain thermal stability (Fig. 17.2).

Heat Loss

Newborns have several characteristics that predispose them to heat loss:

- Thin skin with blood vessels close to the surface
- Lack of shivering ability to produce heat until 3 months of age
- Limited stores of metabolic substrates (glucose, glycogen, fat)

- Limited use of voluntary muscle activity or movement to produce heat
- Large body surface area relative to body weight
- Lack of subcutaneous fat, which provides insulation
- Little ability to conserve heat by changing posture (fetal position)
- No ability to adjust their own clothing or blankets to achieve warmth
- Inability to communicate that they are too cold or too warm

FIGURE 17.2 Mother holding her newborn skin-to-skin after birth. Note the warm blanket to preserve body heat. A hat may also be placed on the baby's head.

Every newborn struggles to maintain body temperature from the moment of birth, when the newborn's wet body is exposed to the much cooler environment of the birthing room. The amniotic fluid covering the newborn cools as it evaporates rapidly in the low humidity and air conditioning of the room. The newborn's temperature may decrease several degrees within minutes after leaving the warmth of the pregnant client's uterus (37.5°C). The skin of newborns adjusts quickly to the challenging environmental conditions of extrauterine life. However, certain functions, for example, microcirculation,

continue to develop even beyond the neonatal period (McCall, Alderdice, Halliday, Johnston, & Vohra, 2014).

The transfer of heat depends on the temperature of the environment, air speed, and water vapour pressure or humidity. Heat exchange between the environment and the newborn involves the same mechanisms as those with any physical object and its environment. Heat can be lost by four mechanisms including conduction (3%), convection (34%), evaporation (24%), and radiation (39%) (Sharma et al., 2014). Prevention of heat loss is a key nursing intervention (Fig. 17.3).

A. Conduction

B. Convection

C. Evaporation

D. Radiation

FIGURE 17.3 The four mechanisms of heat loss in the newborn. **A.** Conduction. **B.** Convection. **C.** Evaporation. **D.** Radiation.

602 UNIT 6 The Newborn

CONDUCTION

Conduction involves the transfer of heat from one object to another when the two objects are in direct contact with each other. Conduction refers to heat fluctuation between the newborn's body surface when in contact with other solid surfaces, such as a cold mattress or scale. Heat loss by conduction can also occur when touching a newborn with cold hands or when the newborn has direct contact with a colder object such as a metal scale. Using a warmed cloth diaper or blanket to cover any cold surface touching a newborn directly helps to prevent heat loss through conduction. Keeping the newborn skin-to-skin with a parent also helps prevent heat loss through conduction.

CONVECTION

Convection involves the flow of heat from the body surface to cooler surrounding air or to air circulating over a body surface. An example of convection-related heat loss would be a cool breeze that flows over the newborn. To prevent heat loss by this mechanism, keep the newborn out of direct cool drafts (open doors, windows, fans, air conditioners) in the environment. If a newborn cannot be kept skin-to-skin (when resuscitation or advanced care measures are required), work inside an isolette as much as possible and minimize opening portholes that allow cold air to flow inside, and warm any oxygen or humidified air that comes in contact with the newborn. Using clothing and blankets in isolettes is an effective means of reducing the newborn's exposed surface area and providing external insulation. Also, if a baby must be transferred to a special care nursery, transporting the newborn in a warmed isolette, rather than carrying him or her, helps to maintain warmth and reduce exposure to the cool air.

EVAPORATION

Evaporation involves the loss of heat when a liquid is converted to a vapour. Evaporative loss may be insensible (such as from skin and respiration) or sensible (such as from sweating). Insensible loss occurs, but the individual is not aware of it. Sensible loss is objective and can be noticed. It depends on air speed and the absolute humidity of the air. For example, when the baby is born, the body is covered with amniotic fluid. The fluid evaporates into the air, leading to heat loss. Heat loss via evaporation also occurs when bathing a newborn. Drying newborns immediately after birth with warmed blankets and placing a hat on their dried head will help to prevent heat loss through evaporation. In addition, drying the newborn after bathing will help prevent heat loss through evaporation. Promptly changing wet linens, clothes, or diapers will also reduce heat loss and prevent chilling.

RADIATION

Radiation involves the loss of body heat to cooler, solid surfaces that are in proximity but not in direct contact with the newborn. The amount of heat loss depends on the size of the cold surface area, the surface temperature of the newborn's body, and the temperature of the receiving surface area. For example, when a newborn is placed in a single-wall isolette next to a cold window, heat loss from radiation occurs. A newborn will become cold even when in a heated isolette. To reduce heat loss by radiation, keep cribs and isolettes away from outside walls, cold windows, and air conditioners. Also, using radiant warmers for transporting newborns and when performing procedures that may expose the newborn to the cooler environment will help reduce heat loss.

A warmed transporter is an enclosed isolette on wheels. A radiant warmer is an open bed with a radiant heat source above. This type of environment allows health care providers to reach the newborn to carry out procedures and treatments.

Overheating

The newborn is also prone to overheating. Limited insulation and limited sweating ability can predispose any newborn to overheating. Control of body temperature is achieved via a complex negative feedback system that creates a balance between heat production, heat gain, and heat loss. The primary heat regulator is located in the hypothalamus and the central nervous system. The immaturity of the newborn's central nervous system makes it difficult to create and maintain this balance. Therefore, the newborn can become overheated easily. For example, an isolette that is too warm or one that is left too close to a sunny window may lead to hyperthermia. Although heat production can substantially increase in response to a cool environment, basal metabolic rate and the resultant heat produced cannot be reduced. Overheating increases fluid loss, the respiratory rate, and the metabolic rate considerably.

Thermoregulation

Humans have the ability to regulate their body temperature within a narrow range. Newborns have a decreased ability to regulate their body temperature, producing heat through nonshivering thermogenesis. **Thermoregulation**, the balance between heat loss and heat production, is related to the newborn's rate of metabolism and oxygen consumption. The newborn attempts to conserve heat and increase heat production by increasing the metabolic rate, increasing muscular activity through movement, increasing peripheral vasoconstriction, and assuming a fetal position to hold in heat and minimize exposed body surface area.

Take Note!

The newborn first experiences an increase in norepinephrine in response to a cold environment. This then influences the triglycerides to stimulate brown fat metabolism.

An environment in which body temperature is maintained without an increase in metabolic rate or oxygen use is called a **neutral thermal environment**. Within a neutral thermal environment, the rates of oxygen consumption and metabolism are minimal, and internal body temperature is maintained because of thermal balance. A neutral thermal environment promotes growth and stability, conserves energy for basic bodily functions, and minimizes heat (energy) and water loss (Knobel, 2014). Because newborns have difficulty maintaining their body heat through shivering or other mechanisms, they need a higher environmental temperature to maintain a neutral thermal environment. If the environmental temperature decreases, the newborn responds by consuming more oxygen. The respiratory rate increases (tachypnea) in response to the increased need for oxygen. As a result, the newborn's metabolic rate increases.

As noted earlier, the newborn's primary method of heat production is through nonshivering thermogenesis. This is a process in which brown fat (adipose tissue) is oxidized in response to cold exposure. Brown fat is a special kind of highly vascular fat found only in newborns. Brown adipose tissue is a unique tissue that is able to convert chemical energy directly into heat when activated by the sympathetic nervous system. It is produced during the third trimester; ordinarily disappears by 3 to 5 weeks after birth and is vital for thermogenesis. The brown colouring is derived from the fat's rich supply of blood vessels and nerve endings. These fat deposits, which are capable of intense metabolic activity—and thus can generate a great deal of heat—are found between the scapulae, axillae, at the nape of the neck, in the mediastinum, and in areas surrounding the kidneys and adrenal glands. Brown fat makes up about 6% of term body weight in the full-term newborn (Betz & Enerback, 2015). When the newborn experiences a cold environment, norepinephrine is released. This in turn stimulates brown fat metabolism by breaking down triglycerides. Cardiac output increases, increasing blood flow through the brown fat tissue. Subsequently, this blood becomes warmed as a result of the increased metabolic activity of the brown fat (Fig. 17.4).

Newborns can experience heat loss through all four mechanisms, ultimately resulting in cold stress. **Cold stress** is excessive heat loss that requires a newborn to use compensatory mechanisms (such as nonshivering thermogenesis and tachypnea) to maintain core body temperature (Davidson, 2014). The consequences of cold stress can be quite severe. As the body temperature decreases, the newborn becomes less active, lethargic, hypotonic, and weaker. All newborns are at risk for cold stress, particularly within the first 12 hours of life. However, preterm newborns are at the greatest risk for cold stress and experience more profound effects than full-term newborns because they have fewer fat stores,

FIGURE 17.4 Areas of brown fat in a newborn.

poorer vasomotor responses, and less insulation to cope with a hypothermic event.

Cold stress in the newborn can lead to the following problems if not reversed: depleted brown fat stores, increased oxygen needs, respiratory distress, increased glucose consumption leading to hypoglycemia, metabolic acidosis, jaundice, hypoxia, and decreased surfactant production (Mattson & Smith, 2015).

Take Note!

Nurses must be aware of the thermoregulatory needs of the newborn and must ensure that these needs are met to provide the newborn with the best start possible. Maintenance of temperature stability should be focused on preventative measures.

To minimize the effects of cold stress and maintain a neutral thermal environment, the following interventions are helpful:

- Prewarming blankets and hats to reduce heat loss through conduction
- Keeping the infant transporter (warmed isolette) fully charged and heated at all times
- Drying the newborn completely after birth to prevent heat loss from evaporation
- Facilitating early and continued skin-to-skin contact with the mother/parent for the stable newborn
- Promoting early breastfeeding to provide fuels for nonshivering thermogenesis
- Using heated and humidified oxygen
- Always using radiant warmers and double-wall isolettes to prevent heat loss from radiation
- Deferring bathing until the newborn is 12 to 24-hours old, and medically stable. Using a radiant heat source can minimize heat loss while bathing (Fig. 17.5)
- Avoiding the placement of a skin temperature probe over a bony area or one with brown fat, because it does

FIGURE 17.5 Bathing a newborn under a radiant warmer to prevent heat loss.

not give an accurate assessment of the whole body temperature (most temperature probes are placed over the liver when the newborn is supine or side-lying)

• Ensuring normal room temperature in order to promote neutral thermal environment and minimize heat loss

The preceding interventions allow the newborn to minimize his or her metabolic rate and oxygen consumption, thereby conserving vital energy stores required for optimum growth.

Hepatic System Function

The liver has an essential role in the synthesis, degradation, and regulation of pathways involved in the metabolism of carbohydrates, proteins, lipids, trace elements, and vitamins. At birth, the newborn's liver slowly assumes the functions that the placenta handled during fetal life. Most enzymatic pathways are present in the newborn, but are inactive at birth and generally become fully active at 3 months of age. These functions include blood coagulation, and also iron storage, carbohydrate metabolism, and conjugation of bilirubin, as discussed next. Glycogen reserves provide energy and may become depleted if the metabolic needs of the newborn increase, such as during respiratory distress or cold stress.

Iron Storage

As red blood cells are destroyed after birth, their iron is released and stored by the liver until new red cells need to be produced. Newborn iron stores are determined by total body hemoglobin content and length of gestation. If the pregnant person's iron intake was adequate during pregnancy, sufficient iron has been stored in the newborn's liver for use during the first 6 months of age.

Carbohydrate Metabolism

Glucose is an essential fuel for brain metabolism. When the placenta is lost at birth, the glucose supply is cut off. Initially, the newborn's serum glucose levels decline. Newborns must learn to regulate their blood glucose concentration and adjust to an intermittent feeding schedule. Usually, a term newborn's blood glucose level is 70% to 80% of the maternal blood glucose level at birth. Hypoglycemia is one of the most frequent problems encountered, and maintaining glucose homeostasis is one of the important physiologic events during the fetal-to-newborn transition. During the first 24 to 48 hours of life, as healthy neonates transition from intrauterine to extrauterine life, their plasma glucose levels are usually lower than later in life (Thornton et al., 2015).

Glucose is the main source of energy for the first several hours after birth. With the newborn's increased energy needs after birth, the liver releases glucose from glycogen stores for the first 24 hours. Initiating early breastfeeding, or feeding with formula, helps to stabilize the newborn's blood glucose levels. No evidence supports universal invasive routine measurement of glucose in healthy term newborns. Selective screening of at-risk newborns is more appropriate (Adamkin, 2015). Go to thePoint for the Canadian Pediatric Society's *Algorithm for the Screening and Immediate Management of Babies at Risk for Neonatal Hypoglycemia*.

Bilirubin Conjugation

The liver is also responsible for the conjugation of bilirubin—a yellow to orange bile pigment produced by the breakdown of red blood cells. In utero, elimination of bilirubin in the blood is handled by the placenta and the pregnant person's liver. However, once the cord is cut, the newborn must now assume this function.

Bilirubin normally circulates in plasma, is taken up by liver cells, and is changed to a water-soluble pigment that is excreted in the bile. This conjugated form of bilirubin is excreted from liver cells as a constituent of bile.

The principal source of bilirubin in the newborn is the hemolysis of erythrocytes. This is a normal occurrence after birth, when fewer red blood cells are needed to maintain extrauterine life. When red blood cells die after approximately 80 days of life, the heme in their hemoglobin is converted to bilirubin. Bilirubin is released in an unconjugated form called indirect bilirubin, which is fat soluble. Enzymes, proteins, and different cells in the reticuloendothelial system and liver process the unconjugated bilirubin into conjugated bilirubin or direct bilirubin. This form is water soluble and now enters the gastrointestinal system via the bile and is eventually excreted through feces. The kidneys also excrete a small amount.

Newborns produce bilirubin at a rate of approximately 6 to 8 mg/kg/day. This is more than twice the production rate in adults, primarily because of relative polycythemia and increased red blood cell turnover. Bilirubin production typically declines to the adult level within 10 to 14 days after birth (Bhutani, Wong, Vreman, & Stevenson, 2015). In addition, the metabolic pathways of the liver are relatively immature and thus cannot conjugate bilirubin as quickly as needed.

Failure of the liver cells to break down and excrete bilirubin can cause an increased amount of bilirubin in the bloodstream, leading to **jaundice** (Sharma et al., 2014). Bilirubin is toxic to the body and must be excreted. Blood tests ordered to determine bilirubin levels measure bilirubin in the serum. Total bilirubin is a combination of indirect (unconjugated) and direct (conjugated) bilirubin. When unconjugated bilirubin pigment is deposited in the skin and mucous membranes as a result of increased bilirubin levels, jaundice, also known as icterus, develops, with a yellowing of the skin, sclera, and mucous membranes. Visible jaundice as a result of increased blood bilirubin levels occurs in more than half of all healthy newborns. Even in healthy term newborns, extremely elevated blood levels of bilirubin during the first week of life can cause bilirubin encephalopathy, a permanent and devastating form of brain damage, called kernicterus (Wong & Bhutani, 2017).

Common risk factors for the development of jaundice include fetal–maternal blood group incompatibility, prematurity, asphyxia at birth, an insufficient intake of milk, drugs (such as diazepam [Valium], oxytocin [Pitocin], sulfisoxazole/erythromycin [Pediazole], and chloramphenicol [Chloromycetin]), maternal gestational diabetes, infrequent feedings, male sex, trauma during birth resulting in cephalohematoma, cutaneous bruising from birth trauma, polycythemia, previous sibling with hyperbilirubinemia, intrauterine infections such as TORCH (toxoplasmosis, other viruses, rubella, cytomegalovirus, herpes simplex viruses), sepsis, G6PD deficiency, and ethnicity such as Asian or Indigenous (Moses, 2018).

The causes of newborn jaundice can be classified into three groups based on the mechanism of accumulation:
1. Bilirubin overproduction, such as from blood incompatibility (Rh or ABO), drugs, trauma at birth, polycythemia, delayed cord clamping, and breastmilk jaundice
2. Decreased bilirubin conjugation, as seen in physiologic jaundice, hypothyroidism, and insufficient breastfeeding

3. Impaired bilirubin excretion, as seen in biliary obstruction (biliary atresia, gallstones, neoplasm), sepsis, hepatitis, chromosomal abnormality (Turner's syndrome, trisomies 18 and 21), and drugs (aspirin, acetaminophen, sulfa, alcohol, steroids, antibiotics) (Nagtalon-Ramos, 2014).

Jaundice in the newborn is discussed in more detail in Chapter 24.

Gastrointestinal System Adaptations

The full-term newborn has the capacity to swallow, digest, metabolize, and absorb food taken in soon after birth. At birth, the pH of the stomach contents is mildly acidic, reflecting the pH of the amniotic fluid. The once-sterile gut changes rapidly, depending on what feeding is received. Bowel sounds are normally heard shortly after birth, but may be hypoactive on the first day.

Mucosal Barrier Protection

Humans start their development in a sterile intrauterine environment, but from the very moment of birth all epithelial surfaces in direct contact with the environment (skin, respiratory, gastrointestinal, and urogenital tract) are colonized by microorganisms. An important adaptation of the gastrointestinal system is the development of a mucosal barrier to prevent the penetration of harmful substances (bacteria, toxins, and antigens) present within the intestinal lumen. At birth, the newborn must be prepared to deal with bacterial colonization of the gut. Colonization is dependent on oral intake. Nutrition plays a major role in early colonization patterns in the neonatal gut. It usually occurs within 24 hours of age and is required for the production of vitamin K (Gritz & Bhandari, 2015). After birth, environmental, oral, and cutaneous microbes from the parent(s) will be mechanically transferred to the newborn by several processes including suckling, kissing, and caressing. Thus, the proximity of the birth canal and the anus, as well as parental expression of neonatal care, is effective methods of ensuring transmission of microbes from one generation to the next. If harmful substances are allowed to penetrate the mucosal epithelial barrier under pathologic conditions, they can cause inflammatory and allergic reactions (Nylund, Satokari, Salminen, & de Vos, 2014).

Take Note!

Human breastmilk provides a passive mechanism to protect the newborn against the dangers of a deficient intestinal defense system. It contains antibodies, viable leukocytes, and many other substances that can interfere with bacterial colonization and prevent harmful penetration.

Stomach and Digestion

The newborn must rapidly adapt from receiving all nutrient and energy requirements via the placenta to obtaining them orally after birth. The physiologic capacity of the newborn stomach is considerably less than its anatomic capacity. There is a rapid gain in physiologic capacity during the first 4 days of life. After the first 4 days, the anatomic and physiologic capacities more closely approximate each other. Researchers have found that for the first 24 hours after birth, the newborn's small stomach does not stretch to hold more, as it will within a day or two later (Batchelor, 2014). This explains the experience of countless parents and nurses who have learned the hard way that if a newborn is bottle-fed an ounce or two during the first day of life, most of it tends to come right back up. The walls of the newborn stomach stay firm, expelling extra milk rather than stretching to hold it.

Breastfed newborns self-regulate how much they consume. For newborns who are bottle-fed, however, small, frequent feedings are important for setting up a healthy eating pattern right from the start. Experts now advise adults that it is healthier to eat smaller amounts more often and the same is true for babies and children. Coaxing an infant to take more milk leads to overfeeding. If feeling overfull at feedings becomes the norm for a young infant, this may lead to unhealthy eating habits that contribute to childhood and adult obesity later. This is believed to be one of the factors correlating breastfeeding with reduced rates of obesity later in life. Early-onset obesity is a precursor to a lifelong weight struggle and numerous comorbidities (Redsell et al., 2015; Reilly & Hughes, 2015).

The cardiac sphincter and nervous control of the stomach is immature, which may lead to uncoordinated peristaltic activity and frequent regurgitation. Immaturity of the pharyngoesophageal sphincter and absence of lower esophageal peristaltic waves also contribute to the reflux of gastric contents. Avoiding overfeeding and encouraging frequent burping may minimize regurgitation. Most digestive enzymes are available at birth, allowing newborns to digest simple carbohydrates and protein. However, they have limited ability to digest complex carbohydrates and fats, because amylase and lipase levels are low at birth. As a result, newborns excrete a fair amount of lipids, resulting in fatty stools.

Adequate digestion and absorption are essential for newborn growth and development. Normally, term newborns lose 5% to 10% of their birth weight as a result of shifting of intracellular water to extracellular space, insensible water loss, and potentially insufficient caloric intake within the first week after birth. To gain weight, the term newborn requires an intake of 108 kcal/kg/day from birth to 6 months of age. Understanding the role and importance of nutrition in early postnatal life on growth and development is vital, but how it links to later health has the potential of health benefits for all future generations (Robinson, 2015).

Bowel Elimination

The frequency, consistency, and type of stool passed by newborns vary widely. The evolution of a stool pattern begins with a newborn's first stool, which is **meconium**. Meconium is composed of amniotic fluid, shed mucosal cells, intestinal secretions, and blood. It is greenish black, has a tarry consistency, and is usually passed within 12 to 24 hours of birth. The first meconium stool passed is semisterile, but this changes rapidly with ingestion of bacteria through feedings. After feedings are initiated, a transitional stool develops, which is greenish brown to yellowish brown, thinner in consistency, and seedy in appearance. The stool of breastfed babies resembles light mustard with seed-like particles. If formula-fed, the stools will be tan or yellow in colour and firmer. The frequency of bowel movements varies widely from one infant to another.

Take Note!

Newborns who are fed early pass stools sooner, which helps to reduce bilirubin buildup (Mattson & Smith, 2015).

The last development in the stool pattern is the milk stool. Its characteristics differ in breastfed and formula-fed newborns. The stools of the breastfed newborn are yellow-gold, loose, and stringy to pasty in consistency, and typically have a mild odour. The stools of the formula-fed newborn vary depending on the type of formula ingested. They may be yellow, yellow-green, or greenish, and loose, pasty, or formed in consistency, and they have an unpleasant odour.

Renal System Changes

A full complement of one million nephrons is present by 34 weeks' gestation. The glomeruli and nephrons are functionally immature at birth, resulting in a reduced glomerular filtration rate (GFR) and limited concentrating ability. A limited ability to concentrate urine and the reduced GFR make the newborn susceptible to both dehydration and fluid overload (Sharma et al., 2014). Frequently the newborn's kidneys are described as immature, but they are able to carry out their usual responsibilities and can handle the challenge of excretion and maintaining acid–base balance. Only when the newborn is faced with unexpected imbalances of water, electrolytes, or a disruption of acid–base status secondary to a preterm birth or illness does it lack the ability to handle the body's fluid homeostasis. A newborn infant's body mass is 75% water, the highest proportion of body water at any stage of a person's life. The majority of term newborns void immediately after birth, indicating adequate renal function. Although the newborn's kidneys can produce urine, they are limited in their ability to concentrate it until about 3 months of age, when the kidneys become more mature. Until that time, a newborn voids frequently and the urine has a low specific gravity (1.001 to 1.020). About six to eight voids daily is expected for newborns past 4 days of age; this indicates adequate fluid intake (Harshman & Brophy, 2014).

The renal cortex is relatively underdeveloped at birth and does not reach maturity until 12 to 18 months of age. The GFR is the amount of fluid filtered each minute by all the glomeruli of both kidneys and is one index of kidney function. At birth, the newborn's GFR is approximately 30% of normal adult values, reaching approximately 50% of normal adult values by the tenth day of life and full adult values by the first year of life (Chishti, 2014). The low GFR and the limited excretion and conservation capability of the kidney affect the newborn's ability to excrete salt, water loads, and drugs.

Take Note!

The possibility of fluid overload is increased in newborns; keep this in mind when administering intravenous therapy to a newborn.

Immune System Adaptations

Essential to the newborn's survival is the ability to respond effectively to hostile environmental forces. The newborn's immune system begins working early in gestation, but many of the responses do not function adequately during the early neonatal period. The newborn is protected from certain infections, in part because of maternal antibodies circulating in their system until about 6 months of age. Immunoglobulin G (IgG) crosses the placenta to the fetus while in utero. Breastfed newborns receive antibodies from the breastmilk which includes IgE, IgA, IgM, and IgG (Nagtalon-Ramos, 2014). The risk of acquiring an infection is great because a newborn's immune system is immature and not able to respond for long periods of time to fight infections. The intrauterine environment usually protects the fetus from harmful microorganisms and the need for defensive immunologic responses. With exposure to a wide variety of microorganisms at birth, the newborn must develop a balance between its host defenses and the hostile environmental organisms to ensure a safe transition to the outside world. Healthy infants begin to produce their own antibodies, starting at 2 to 3 months of age.

Responses of the immune system serve three purposes: defense (protection from invading organisms), homeostasis (elimination of worn-out host cells), and surveillance (recognition and removal of enemy cells). The newborn's immune system response involves recognition of the pathogen or other foreign material, followed by activation of mechanisms to react against and eliminate it. All immune responses primarily involve leukocytes (white blood cells).

The immune system's responses can be divided into two categories: natural and acquired immunity. These mechanisms are interrelated and interdependent; both are required for immunocompetency.

Natural Immunity

Natural immunity includes responses or mechanisms that do not require previous exposure to the microorganism or antigen to operate efficiently. Physical barriers (such as intact skin and mucous membranes), chemical barriers (such as gastric acids and digestive enzymes), and resident nonpathologic organisms make up the newborn's natural immune system. Natural immunity involves the most basic host defense responses: ingestion and killing of microorganisms by phagocytic cells.

Acquired Immunity

Acquired immunity involves two primary processes: (1) the development of circulating antibodies or immunoglobulins capable of targeting specific invading agents (antigens) for destruction and (2) formation of activated lymphocytes designed to destroy foreign invaders. Acquired immunity is absent until after the first invasion by a foreign organism or toxin.

Immunologic ability depends heavily on immunoglobulins such as IgG, IgM, and IgA. The newborn depends largely on these three immunoglobulins for defense against microorganisms associated with illness. Newborns remain very susceptible to infections for months.

IgG is the major immunoglobulin and the most abundant, making up about 80% of all circulating antibodies (Martin, Fanaroff & Walsh, 2014). It is found in serum and interstitial fluid. It is the only class able to cross the placenta, with active placental transfer beginning at approximately 20 to 22 weeks' gestation. IgG produces antibodies against bacteria, bacterial toxins, and viral agents.

IgA is the second most abundant immunoglobulin in the serum. IgA does not cross the placenta, and maximum levels are reached during childhood. This immunoglobulin is believed to protect mucous membranes from viruses and bacteria. IgA is predominantly found in the gastrointestinal and respiratory tracts, tears, saliva, colostrum, and breastmilk.

Take Note!

A major source of IgA is human breastmilk, so breastfeeding has significant immunologic advantages over formula feeding (Walker, 2014).

IgM is found in blood and lymph fluid and is the first immunoglobulin to respond to infection. It does not cross the placenta, and levels are generally low at birth unless a congenital intrauterine infection is present. IgM offers a major source of protection from blood-borne infections. The predominant antibodies formed during neonatal or intrauterine infection are of this class.

Integumentary System Adaptations

The newborn skin is critical to its transition from intrauterine to extrauterine environments and to the journey to self-sufficiency. The newborn's skin is a large organ, making up approximately 13% of body weight in contrast to 3% of body weight in an adult. It is sensitive, fragile, with a neutral pH on the surface, lower lipid content and higher water content when compared with adults. Because of these characteristics, newborn skin is vulnerable to injury and infections (Visscher, Adam, Brink, & Odio, 2015). The most important function of the skin is to provide a protective barrier between the body and the environment. It limits the loss of water, prevents absorption of harmful agents, protects thermoregulation and fat storage, and protects against physical trauma. The epidermal barrier begins to develop during midgestation and is fully formed by about 32 weeks' gestation. Although the neonatal epidermis is similar to the adult epidermis in thickness and lipid composition, skin development is not complete at birth (King et al., 2015). Although the basic structure is the same as that of an adult, the less mature the newborn, the less mature the skin functions. Fewer fibrils connect the dermis and epidermis in the newborn compared with the adult. Also in a newborn, the risk of injury producing a break in the skin from the use of tapes and monitors and from handling is greater than for an adult. Improper handling of the newborn during daily skin care practices, such as bathing, can cause damage, prevent healing, and interfere with the normal maturation process.

Newborns vary greatly in appearance. Many of the variations are temporary and reflect the physiologic adaptations that the newborn is experiencing. Skin colouring varies, depending on the newborn's age, race or ethnic group, temperature, and whether he or she is crying. Skin colour changes with both the environment and health status. At birth, the newborn's skin is dark red to purple. As the newborn begins to breathe air his or her skin colour changes to red. This redness normally begins to fade the first day.

Neurologic System Adaptations

The nervous system is immature and continues to develop to achieve a full complement of cortical and brainstem cells by 1 year of age. The brain increases its size threefold during the first year of life. The nervous system consists of the brain, spinal cord, 12 cranial nerves, and a variety of spinal nerves that come from the spinal cord. Neurologic development follows cephalocaudal (head-to-toe) and proximal–distal (centre-to-outside) patterns. Myelin develops early on in sensory impulse transmitters. Thus, the newborn has an acute sense of hearing, smell, and taste. The newborn's sensory capabilities include the following:

- *Hearing*—well developed at birth, responds to noise by turning to sound
- *Taste*—ability to distinguish between sweet and sour by 72 hours old
- *Smell*—ability to distinguish between mother's breastmilk and breastmilk from others
- *Touch*—sensitivity to pain, responds to tactile stimuli
- *Vision*—is incomplete at birth. Maturation is dependent on nutrition and visual stimulation. Newborns have ability to focus only on close objects (20 to 25 cm away) with a visual acuity of 20/140; they can track objects in midline or beyond (230 cm). This is the least mature sense at birth. The ability to fix, follow, and be alert is indicative of an intact CNS (King et al., 2015).

Remember Maria, the new mother who is worried that her daughter can't see? What might the new mother notice about her daughter's behaviour? What might be the new mother's expectations?

Congenital Reflexes

Successful adaptations demonstrated by the respiratory, circulatory, thermoregulatory, and musculoskeletal systems indirectly indicate the central nervous system's successful transition from fetal to extrauterine life, because the central nervous system plays a major role in all these adaptations. In the newborn, congenital reflexes are the hallmarks of maturity of the central nervous system, viability, and adaptation to extrauterine life.

The presence and strength of a **reflex** is an important indication of neurologic development and function. A reflex is an involuntary muscular response to a sensory stimulus. It is built into the nervous system and does not need the intervention of conscious thought to take effect. The physical assessment of the neurologic system of the newborn includes evaluating the major reflexes (gag, Babinski, Moro, and Galant) and minor ones (finger grasp, toe grasp, rooting, sucking, head righting, stepping, and tonic neck).

To assess each reflex, the nurse progresses methodically, taking care to document each finding (Weber & Kelly, 2014). Many neonatal reflexes disappear with maturation, although some remain throughout adulthood.

The arcs of these reflexes end at different levels of the spine and brain stem, reflecting the function of the cranial nerves and motor systems. The ways newborns blink, move their limbs, focus on a caretaker's face, turn toward sound, suck, swallow, and respond to the environment are all indications of their neurologic abilities. Congenital defects within the central nervous system are frequently not overt but may be revealed in abnormalities in tone, posture, or behaviour (Davidson, 2014). Damage to the nervous system (birth trauma, perinatal hypoxia) during the birthing process can cause delays in the normal growth, development, and functioning of the newborn. Early identification may help to identify the cause and to start early intervention to decrease long-term complications or permanent sequelae.

Newborn reflexes are assessed to evaluate neurologic function and development. Absent or abnormal reflexes in a newborn, persistence of a reflex past the age when it is normally lost, or redevelopment of an infantile reflex in an older child or adult may indicate neurologic pathology. (See Chapter 18 for a description of newborn reflex assessment.)

> **The Public Health nurse explained to Maria that all newborns are born with some degree of myopia (near vision, or the inability to see distances) and that 20/20 vision is not generally achieved until 2 years of age. What developmental information should the nurse discuss with Maria?**

BEHAVIOURAL ADAPTATIONS

In addition to adapting physiologically, the newborn also adapts behaviourally. All newborns progress through a specific pattern of events after birth, regardless of their gestational age or the type of birth they experienced.

Behavioural Patterns

The newborn usually demonstrates a predictable pattern of behaviour during the first several hours after birth, characterized by two periods of reactivity separated by a sleep phase. Behavioural adaptation is a defined progression of events triggered by stimuli from the extrauterine environment after birth.

First Period of Reactivity

The first period of reactivity begins at birth and may last from 30 minutes up to 2 hours. The newborn is alert and moving and may appear hungry. This period is characterized by myoclonic movements of the eyes, spontaneous Moro reflexes, sucking motions, chewing, rooting, and

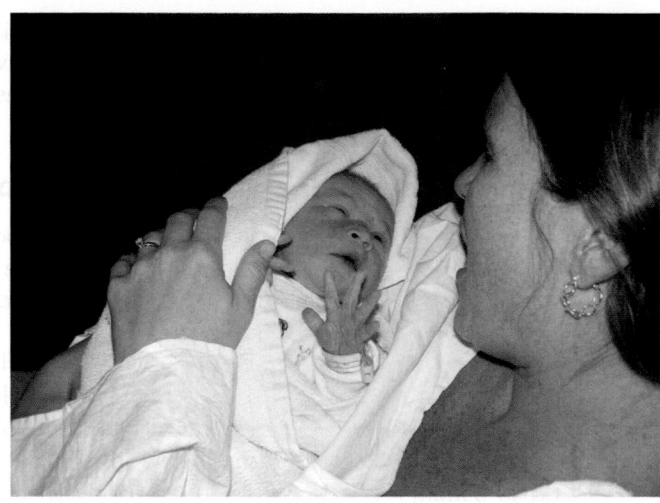

FIGURE 17.6 The first period of reactivity is an optimal time for interaction.

fine tremors of the extremities. Muscle tone and motor activity are increased (Healy & Fallon, 2014). Respiration and heart rate are elevated but gradually begin to slow as the next period begins.

This period of alertness allows parents to interact with their newborn and to enjoy close contact with their new baby (Fig. 17.6). The appearance of sucking and rooting behaviours provides a good opportunity for initiating breastfeeding. Many newborns latch on the nipple and suck well at this first experience.

Period of Decreased Responsiveness

At 30 to 120 minutes of age, the newborn enters the second stage of transition—that of the *sleep period* or a decrease in activity. This phase is referred to as a period of decreased responsiveness. Movements are less jerky and less frequent. Heart and respiratory rates decline as the newborn enters the sleep phase. The muscles become relaxed, and responsiveness to outside stimuli diminishes. During this phase, the newborn becomes difficult to arouse or stimulate. No interest in sucking is shown. This quiet time can be used for both the parent(s) and newborn to remain close and rest together after labour and the birthing experience.

Second Period of Reactivity

The second period of reactivity begins as the newborn awakens and shows an interest in environmental stimuli. This period lasts 2 to 8 hours in the healthy term newborn (Davidson, 2014). Heart and respiratory rates increase. Peristalsis also increases. Thus, it is common for the newborn to pass meconium or void during this period. In addition, motor activity and muscle tone increase in conjunction with an increase in muscular coordination (Fig. 17.7).

Andersson, O., Domellöf, M., Andersson, D., & Hellström-Westas, L. (2014). Effect of delayed vs early umbilical cord clamping on iron status and neurodevelopment at age 12 months: A randomized clinical trial. *JAMA Pediatrics, 168*(6), 547–554.

Armson, B. A., Allan, D., Casper, R., & SOGC Cord Blood Banking Working Group. (2015). Clinical practice guideline—Umbilical cord blood: Counselling, collection, and banking. *Journal of Obstetrics & Gynaecology Canada, 37*(9), 832–844. Retrieved from https://sogc.org/wp-content/uploads/2015/09/gui328CPG1509E.pdf

Batchelor, H. (2014). Pediatric development: Gastrointestinal. In *Pediatric formulations* (pp. 43–54). New York: Springer.

Betz, M. J., & Enerbäck, S. (2015). Human brown adipose tissue: What we have learned so far. *Diabetes, 64*(7), 2352–2360.

Bhutani, V. K., Wong, R. J., Vreman, H. J., & Stevenson, D. K. (2015). Bilirubin production and hour-specific bilirubin levels. *Journal of Perinatology, 35*(9), 735–738.

Bope, E. T., & Kellerman, R. D. (2015). *Conn's current therapy 2015.* Philadelphia, PA: Elsevier.

Canadian Pediatric Society. (2018). *Position statement: Minimizing blood loss and the need for transfusions in very premature infants.* Retrieved from https://www.cps.ca/en/documents/position/minimizing-blood-loss

Chishti, A. S. (2014). Assessment of renal function. In *Kidney and urinary tract diseases in the newborn* (pp. 117–126). Berlin, Heidelberg, Germany: Springer.

Creasy, R. K., Resnik, R., Iams, J. D., Lockwood, C. J., Moore, T. R., & Greene, M. F. (2014). *Creasy & Resnik's maternal-fetal medicine: Principles and practice* (7th ed.). St. Louis, MO: Elsevier.

Cuneo, B. (2014). Transition from fetal to neonatal circulation. In Da Cruz, E. M., Ivy, D., Jaggers, J. (Eds.), *Pediatric and congenital cardiology, cardiac surgery and intensive care* (pp. 179–199). London: Springer.

Davidson, M. R. (2014). *Fast facts for the neonatal nurse: A nursing orientation and care guide in a nutshell.* New York: Springer.

Essa, R. M., & Ismail, N. I. A. A. (2015). Effect of early maternal/newborn skin-to-skin contact after birth on the duration of third stage of labor and initiation of breastfeeding. *Journal of Nursing Education and Practice, 5*(4), 98–107.

Feldman-Winter, L., Goldsmith, J. P., & Committee on Fetus and Newborn Task Force on Sudden Infant Death Syndrome. (2016). Safe sleep and skin-to-skin care in the neonatal period for healthy term newborns. *Pediatrics, 138*(3), e20161889. Retrieved from http://pediatrics.aappublications.org/content/pediatrics/early/2016/08/18/peds.2016-1889.full.pdf

Fillipps, D. J., & Bucciarelli, R. L. (2015). Cardiac evaluation of the newborn. *Pediatric Clinics of North America, 62*(2), 471–489.

Fischbach, F., & Dunning, M. B. (2014). *Manual of laboratory and diagnostic tests* (9th ed.). Philadelphia, PA: Lippincott Williams & Wilkins.

Gritz, E. C., & Bhandari, V. (2015). The human neonatal gut microbiome: a brief review. *Frontiers in Pediatrics, 3*, 17–26.

Harshman, L. A., & Brophy, P. D. (2014). Development of renal function in the fetus and newborn. In *Kidney and urinary tract diseases in the newborn* (pp. 59–76). Berlin, Heidelberg, Germany: Springer.

Healy, P., & Fallon, A. (2014). Developments in neonatal care and nursing responses. *British Journal of Nursing, 23*(1), 21–24.

Hooper, S. B., Polglase, G. R., & Roehr, C. C. (2015). Cardiopulmonary changes with aeration of the newborn lung. *Pediatric Respiratory Reviews, 16*(3), 147–150.

Karp, H. (2014). *The happiest baby on the block.* New York: Bantam Dell.

King, T. L., Brucker, M. C., Kriebs, J. M., Fahey, J. O., Gegor, C. L., & Varney, H. (2015). *Varney's midwifery* (5th ed.). Burlington, MA: Jones & Bartlett Learning.

Kluckow, M., & Hooper, S. B. (2015). Using physiology to guide time to cord clamping. *Seminars in Fetal and Neonatal Medicine, 20*(4), 225–231.

Knobel, R. B. (2014). Fetal and neonatal thermal physiology. *Newborn and Infant Nursing Reviews, 14*(2), 45–49.

Leslie, M. S. (2015). Perspectives on implementing delayed cord clamping. *Nursing for Women's Health, 19*(2), 164–176.

Martin, R. J., Fanaroff, A. A., & Walsh, M. C. (2014). *Neonatal-perinatal medicine* (10th ed.). Philadelphia, PA: Elsevier.

Mattson, S., & Smith, J. (2015). *Core curriculum for maternal-newborn nursing* (5th ed.). Philadelphia, PA: Elsevier.

McAdams, R. M. (2014). Time to implement delayed cord clamping. *Obstetrics & Gynecology, 123*(3), 549–552.

McCall, E., Alderdice, F., Halliday, H., Johnston, L., & Vohra, S. (2014). Challenges of minimizing heat loss at birth: A narrative overview of evidence-based thermal care interventions. *Newborn and Infant Nursing Reviews, 14*(2), 56–63.

Moses, S. (2018). Jaundice in newborns. *Family Practice Notebook.* Retrieved from http://www.fpnotebook.com/NICU/GI/JndcInNwbrns.htm.

Nagtalon-Ramos, J. (2014). *Maternal-newborn nursing care: Best evidence-based practices.* Philadelphia, PA: F.A. Davis Company.

Nylund, L., Satokari, R., Salminen, S., & de Vos, W. M. (2014). Intestinal microbiota during early life—impact on health and disease. *Proceedings of the Nutrition Society, 73*(4), 457–469.

Public Health Agency of Canada. (2018). *Joint statement on safe sleep.* Retrieved from https://www.canada.ca/en/public-health/services/health-promotion/childhood-adolescence/stages-childhood/infancy-birth-two-years/safe-sleep/joint-statement-on-safe-sleep.html

Redsell, S. A., Edmonds, B., Swift, J. A., Siriwardena, A. N., Weng, S., Nathan, D., & Glazebrook, C. (2015). Systematic review of randomized controlled trials of interventions that aim to reduce the risk, either directly or indirectly, of overweight and obesity in infancy and early childhood. *Maternal & Child Nutrition, 12*(1), 24–38.

Reilly, J. J., & Hughes, A. R. (2015). Early life risk factors for childhood obesity. *Early Years Nutrition and Healthy Weight*, 40–45.

Robinson, S. M. (2015). Infant nutrition and lifelong health: Current perspectives and future challenges. *Journal of Developmental Origins of Health and Disease, 6*(5), 384–389.

Sharma, A., Ford, S., & Calvert, J. (2014). Adaptation for life: A review of neonatal physiology. *Anesthesia & Intensive Care Medicine, 15*(3), 89–95.

Stave, U. (2014). *Perinatal physiology.* New York: Springer.

Steinhorn, R. H. (2015). Persistent pulmonary hypertension of the newborn. *PanVascular Medicine*, 4135–4155.

Swanson, J. R., & Sinkin, R. A. (2015). Transition from fetus to newborn. *Pediatric Clinics of North America, 62*(2), 329–343.

Thornton, P. S., Stanley, C. A., De Leon, D. D., Harris, D., Haymond, M. W., Hussain, K., ... Wolfsdorf, J. I.; Pediatric Endocrine Society. (2015). Recommendations from the Pediatric Endocrine Society for evaluation and management of persistent hypoglycemia in neonates, infants, and children. *The Journal of Pediatrics, 167*(2), 238–245.

van Vonderen, J. J., Roest, A. A., Siew, M. L., Walther, F. J., Hooper, S. B., & te Pas, A. B. (2014). Measuring physiological changes during the transition to life after birth. *Neonatology, 105*(3), 230–242.

Verklan, T., & Walden, M. (2014). *Core curriculum for neonatal intensive care nursing* (4th ed.). St. Louis, MO: Elsevier.

Visscher, M. O., Adam, R., Brink, S., & Odio, M. (2015). Newborn infant skin: Physiology, development, and care. *Clinics in Dermatology, 33*(3), 271–280.

Walker, M. (2014). *Breastfeeding management for the clinician: Using the evidence* (3rd ed.). Burlington, MA: Jones & Bartlett Learning.

Weber, J., & Kelley, J. (2014). *Health assessment in nursing* (5th ed.). Philadelphia, PA: Lippincott Williams & Wilkins.

Wong, R. J., & Bhutani, V. K. (2017). Clinical manifestations of unconjugated hyperbilirubinemia in term and late preterm infants. *UpToDate.* Retrieved from http://www.uptodate.com/contents/clinical-manifestations-of-unconjugated-hyperbilirubinemia-in-term-and-late-preterm-infants

World Health Organization [WHO]. (2014). *Delayed clamping of the umbilical cord to reduce infant anemia* (Doc. No. WHO/RHR/14.19 ed.). Geneva, Switzerland: Author.

CHAPTER **WORKSHEET**

MULTIPLE CHOICE QUESTIONS

1. When assessing the term newborn, the following are observed: newborn is alert, heart and respiratory rates have stabilized, and meconium has been passed. The nurse determines that the newborn is exhibiting behaviours indicating:
   a. Initial period of reactivity
   b. Second period of reactivity
   c. Decreased responsiveness period
   d. Sleep period for newborns

2. A nurse observes a 3-day-old term newborn that is starting to appear mildly jaundiced. What might explain this condition?
   a. Physiologic jaundice
   b. Hemolytic disease of the newborn due to blood incompatibility
   c. Exposing the newborn to high levels of oxygen
   d. Overfeeding the newborn with too much glucose water

3. After teaching a group of nursing students about thermoregulation and appropriate measures to prevent heat loss by evaporation, which of the following student behaviours would indicate successful teaching?
   a. Transporting the newborn in an isolette
   b. Maintaining a warm room temperature
   c. Placing the newborn on a warmed surface
   d. Drying the newborn immediately after birth

4. After birth, the nurse would expect which fetal structure to close as a result of increases in the pressure gradients on the left side of the heart?
   a. Foramen ovale
   b. Ductus arteriosus
   c. Ductus venosus
   d. Umbilical vein

5. Which of the following newborns could be described as breathing normally?
   a. Newborn A is breathing deeply, with a regular rhythm, at a rate of 20 bpm.
   b. Newborn B is breathing diaphragmatically with sternal retractions, at a rate of 70 bpm.
   c. Newborn C is breathing shallowly, with 40-second periods of apnea and cyanosis.
   d. Newborn D is breathing shallowly, at a rate of 36 bpm, with short periods of apnea.

6. When assessing a term newborn (6 hours old), the nurse auscultates bowel sounds and documents recent passing of meconium. These findings would indicate:
   a. Abnormal gastrointestinal newborn transition and needs to be reported

   b. An intestinal anomaly that needs immediate surgery
   c. A patent anus with no bowel obstruction and normal peristalsis
   d. A malabsorption syndrome resulting in fatty stools

7. A nursing student questions the maternity nurse why they don't bathe the newborn immediately upon admission to the postpartum unit after birth. The nurse states that this would increase the risk of:
   a. Jaundice
   b. Infection
   c. Hypothermia
   d. Anemia

8. Because the newborn's red blood cells break down much sooner than those of an adult, what might result?
   a. Anemia
   b. Bruising
   c. Apnea
   d. Jaundice

9. The nurse performs a physical examination on a newborn 2 hours after birth. Which of the following findings indicate a need for a pediatric consultation? Select all that apply:
   a. Respiratory rate of 50 breaths per minute
   b. Intermittent episodes of apnea, lasting <10 seconds each
   c. Absent Moro reflex when startled
   d. Preauricular skin tag noted on left ear
   e. White raised bumps noted on nose and face
   f. Yellow blanching of the skin when pressure applied to the nose

CRITICAL THINKING EXERCISES

1. As the nurse manager, you have been orienting a new nurse in the maternity unit for the past few weeks. Although she has been demonstrating adequacy with most aspects of nursing care, today you observe her bathing several newborns without covering them, weighing them on the scale without a cover, leaving the storage door open with the transporter nearby, and leaving the newborns' laying in isolettes with head covers or blankets.
   a. What is your impression of this behaviour?
   b. What principles concerning thermoregulation need to be reinforced?
   c. How will you evaluate whether your instructions have been effective?

2. The most important adaptations for the newborn to make after birth are to establish respirations, make cardiovascular adjustments, and establish thermoregulation. Nursing care focuses on monitoring and supporting adjustments to extrauterine adaptation. Write appropriate nursing interventions to help achieve the following newborn adaptations:
   a. Respiratory adaptation
   b. Safety, including prevention of infection
   c. Thermoregulation

STUDY ACTIVITIES

1. While in the maternity clinical setting, identify the period of behavioural reactivity (first, inactivity, or second period) for two newborns born at different times. Share your findings during the post conference for that clinical day.

2. Dramatic changes occur in the cardiovascular system at birth. When the umbilical cord is clamped and the placenta is separated, there is a resultant increase in systemic blood pressure and changes to the three major fetal shunts (ductus venosus, foramen ovale, and ductus arteriosus) occur. Outline what happens to cause their functional closures during this period of transition.

3. Find two websites about the transition to extrauterine life that can be shared with other nursing students as well as nursery nurses. Critique the information presented in terms of how accurate and current it is.

4. The most common mechanism of heat loss in the newborn is _____.

5. The newborn creates heat in three ways—shivering, muscle activity, and through thermogenesis by the metabolism of brown adipose tissue. Which is the most effective?

BRINGING IT ALL TOGETHER: A CASE STUDY

An 18-year-old woman gave birth to her first infant 3 days ago, but she doesn't smile when the Public Health nurse greets her at a home visit. The nurse questions her about what has happened since she was discharged from the hospital 2 days ago. She tells the nurse that her breasts are swollen, hot, and very painful when touched. She states she knows that breastfeeding is best for her child, but she is not sure she wants to continue to breastfeed because of the pain. Her infant is lying on the bare kitchen table in only a diaper crying.

Go to thePoint **to find questions to consider about this case.**

TABLE 18.1	APGAR SCORING FOR NEWBORNS		
Parameter (Assessment Technique)	**0 Point**	**1 Point**	**2 Points**
Heart rate (auscultation of apical heart rate for one full minute)	Absent	Slow (<100 bpm)	>100 bpm
Respiratory effort (observation of the volume and vigour of the newborn's cry; auscultation of depth and rate of respirations)	Apneic	Slow, irregular, shallow	Regular respirations (usually 30–60 breaths/minute), strong, good cry
Muscle tone (observation of extent of flexion in the newborn's extremities and newborn's resistance when the extremities are pulled away from the body)	Limp, flaccid	Some flexion, limited resistance to extension	Tight flexion, good resistance to extension with quick return to flexed position after extension
Reflex irritability (stimulating the soles of the feet or suctioning of the nose with a bulb syringe)	No response	Grimace or frown when irritated	Sneeze, cough, or vigorous cry
Skin colour (inspection of trunk and extremities with the appropriate colour for ethnicity appearing within minutes after birth)	Cyanotic or pale	Appropriate body colour; blue extremities (acrocyanosis)	Completely appropriate colour (pink on both trunk and extremities)

Data from Cunningham, F. G., Leveno, K. J., Bloom, S. L., Spong, C. Y., Dashe, J. S., Hoffman, B. L., . . . Sheffield, J. S. (2018). *William's obstetrics* (25th ed.). New York: McGraw-Hill Medical; and Marcdante, K. J., & Kliegman, R. M. (2018). *Nelson essentials of pediatrics* (8th ed.). Philadelphia, PA: Elsevier Science Health.

Each parameter is assigned a score ranging from 0 to 2 points. A score of 0 points indicates an absent or poor response; a score of 2 points indicates a normal response (Table 18.1). A normal newborn's score should be 8 to 10 points. The higher the score, the better condition of the newborn. If the Apgar score is 8 points or higher, no intervention is needed other than supporting normal respiratory efforts and maintaining thermoregulation. Scores of 4 to 7 points signify moderate difficulty and scores of 0 to 3 points represent severe distress in adjusting to extrauterine life. The Apgar score is influenced by the presence of infection, newborn maturity, mother's age, congenital anomalies, physiologic immaturity, maternal sedation via medications, labour management, and neuromuscular disorders (Rüdiger & Konstantelos, 2015).

When the newborn experiences physiologic depression, the Apgar score characteristics disappear in a predictable manner: first the pink colouration is lost, next the respiratory effort, and then the tone, followed by reflex irritability and finally heart rate (Apgar, 2015).

Take Note!

Although Apgar scoring is done at 1 and 5 minutes, it also can be used as a guide during the immediate newborn period to evaluate the newborn's status for any changes because it focuses on critical parameters that must be assessed throughout the early transition period.

Length and Weight

Parents are eager to know their newborn's length and weight. These measurements are taken soon after birth. A disposable tape measure or a built-in measurement board located on the side of some scales can be used. Length is measured from the head of the newborn to the heel with the newborn unclothed (Fig. 18.1). Because of the flexed position of the newborn after birth, place the newborn in a supine position and extend the leg completely when measuring the length. The expected length range of a full-term newborn is usually 44 to 55 cm (17 to 22 in). **Moulding** can affect measurement (Weber & Kelley, 2017).

FIGURE 18.1 Measuring a newborn's length.

FIGURE 18.2 Weighing the newborn. Note how the nurse guards the newborn with one hand to prevent falling.

Most often, newborns are weighed using a digital scale that reads the weight in grams. Typically, the term newborn weighs 2,500 to 4,000 g (5 lb, 8 oz to 8 lb, 14 oz; Fig. 18.2). Birth weights less than 10% or more than 90% on a growth chart are outside the normal range and need further investigation (see Table 18.2). Weights taken at later times are compared with previous weights and are documented with regard to gain or loss on a nursing flow sheet. Newborns can lose up to 10% of their initial birth weight by 3 to 4 days of age secondary to loss of meconium, extracellular fluid, and limited food intake. This weight loss is usually regained by the 10th day of life (Fonseca, Severo, Barros, & Santos, 2014).

Newborns can be classified by their birth weight regardless of their gestational age (World Health Organization, 2006) as follows:

• Low birth weight: >2,500 g (>5.5 lb)
• Very low birth weight: >1,500 g (>3.5 lb)
• Extremely low birth weight: >1,000 g (>2.5 lb)

Vital Signs

Heart rate and respiratory rate are assessed immediately after birth with Apgar scoring. Heart rate, obtained by taking an apical pulse for one full minute, typically is 110 to 160 bpm. Newborns' respirations are assessed when they are quiet or sleeping. Place a stethoscope on the right side of the chest and count the breaths for one full minute to identify any irregularities. The newborn respiratory rate is 30 to 60 breaths/minute with symmetric chest movement. Heart and respiratory rates are usually assessed every 30 minutes until stable for 2 hours after birth. Once stable, the heart rate and respiratory rates are checked every 8 hours. These assessment time frames may vary per hospital protocols, so nurses should follow the facility's procedures (Nagtalon-Ramos, 2014).

Vital signs are assessed at birth, within 1 to 4 hours after birth according to hospital policy. Vital signs are used for identifying a variety of complications and for ensuring well-being of the newborn. In some health care agencies, temperatures are taken immediately after the Apgar score has been taken to allow for identification of hypothermia, which then requires a glucose check, but nurses need to follow their hospital protocols on this assessment timing. In term newborns, the normal axillary temperature range should be maintained at 36.5° to 37.5°C (97.7° to 99.5°F). The thermometer or temperature probe is held in the midaxillary space according to manufacturer's directions and hospital protocol. Blood pressure is not usually assessed as part of a normal newborn examination unless there is a clinical indication or low Apgar scores. If assessed, an oscillometer (Dinamap) is used. The typical range is 50 to 75 mm Hg (systolic) and 30 to 45 mm Hg (diastolic). Crying, moving, and late clamping of the umbilical cord will increase systolic pressure (Weber & Kelley, 2017). Typical values for newborn vital signs are provided in Table 18.3.

Gestational Age Assessment

To determine a newborn's gestational age (the stage of maturity), physical signs and neurologic characteristics are assessed. Typically, gestational age is determined by

TABLE 18.2	SMALL FOR GESTATIONAL AGE AND LARGE FOR GESTATIONAL AGE BIRTHWEIGHTS AT TERM

10th and 90th Percentile Birthweight at Term in Canadian Infants

Gestation (Completed Weeks)	Birthweight (g)			
	SGA: Under 10th Percentile		LGA: Over 90th Percentile	
	Male	Female	Male	Female
37	2,552	2,452	3,665	3,543
38	2,766	2,658	3,877	3,738
39	2,942	2,825	4,049	3,895
40	3,079	2,955	4,200	4,034
41	3,179	3,051	4,328	4,154
42	3,233	3,114	4,433	4,251

TABLE 18.3 NEWBORN VITAL SIGNS

Newborn Vital Signs	Ranges of Values
Temperature	36.5°–37.5°C (97.7°–99.5°F)
Heart rate (pulse) to 180 during crying	110–160 bpm; can increase
Respirations	30–60 breaths/minute at rest; will increase with crying
Blood pressure	50–75 mm Hg systolic, 30–45 mm Hg diastolic

From Moses, S. (2018). Pediatric vital signs. *Family practice notebook.* Retrieved from http://www.fpnotebook.com/cv/exam/pdtrcvtlsgns.htm; and Kliegman, R. M., Behrman, R. E., Jenson, H. B., & Stanton, B. F. (2016). *Nelson's textbook of pediatrics* (20th ed.). St. Louis, MO: Saunders Elsevier.

using a tool such as the Ballard gestational age assessment or Ballard scale. It determines a newborn's gestational age between 20 and 44 weeks. A score is assigned to the various parameters, and the total score corresponds to a maturity rating in weeks of gestation (Fig. 18.3). This scoring system provides an objective estimate of gestational age by scoring the specific parameters of physical and neuromuscular maturity. Points are given for each assessment parameter, with a low score of –1 point or –2 points for extreme immaturity to 4 or 5 points for postmaturity. The scores from each section are added to correspond to a specific gestational age in weeks.

The physical maturity section of the examination is done during the first 2 hours after birth. The physical maturity assessment section of the Ballard examination evaluates physical characteristics that appear different at different stages depending on a newborn's gestational maturity. Newborns that are physically mature have higher scores than those who are not. The areas assessed on the physical maturity examination include:

- *Skin texture*—typically ranges from sticky and transparent to smooth, with varying degrees of peeling and cracking, to parchment-like or leathery with significant cracking and wrinkling
- *Lanugo*—soft downy hair on the newborn's body, which is absent in preterm newborns, appears with maturity, and then disappears again with postmaturity
- *Plantar creases*—creases on the soles of the feet, which range from absent to covering the entire foot, depending on maturity (the greater the number of creases, the greater the newborn's maturity)
- *Breast tissue*—the thickness and size of breast tissue and areola (the darkened ring around each nipple), which range from being imperceptible to full and budding
- *Eyes and ears*—eyelids can be fused or open and ear cartilage and stiffness determine the degree of maturity

(the greater the amount of ear cartilage with stiffness, the greater the newborn's maturity)
- *Genitals*—in males, evidence of testicular descent and appearance of scrotum (which can range from smooth to covered with rugae) determine maturity; in females, appearance and size of clitoris and labia determine maturity (a prominent clitoris with flat labia suggests prematurity, whereas a clitoris covered by labia suggests greater maturity)

The neuromuscular maturity section typically is completed within 24 hours after birth. Six activities or manoeuvers that the newborn performs with various body parts are evaluated to determine the newborn's degree of maturity:

1. *Posture*—How does the newborn hold his or her extremities in relation to the trunk? The greater the degree of flexion, the greater the maturity. For example, extension of arms and legs is scored as 0 points and full flexion of arms and legs is scored as 4 points.
2. *Square window*—How far can the newborn's hands be flexed toward the wrist? The angle is measured and scored from more than 90 degrees to 0 degrees to determine the maturity rating. As the angle decreases, the newborn's maturity increases. For example, an angle of more than 90 degrees is scored as –1 point and an angle of 0 degrees is scored as 4 points.
3. *Arm recoil*—How far do the newborn's arms "spring back" to a flexed position? This measure evaluates the degree of arm flexion and the strength of recoil. The reaction of the arm is then scored from 0 to 4 points based on the degree of flexion as the arms are returned to their normal flexed position. The higher the points assigned, the greater the neuromuscular maturity (e.g., recoil less than a 90-degree angle is scored as 4 points).
4. *Popliteal angle*—How far will the newborn's knees extend? The angle created when the knee is extended is measured. An angle of less than 90 degrees indicates greater maturity. For example, an angle of 180 degrees is scored as –1 point and an angle of less than 90 degrees is scored as 5 points.
5. *Scarf sign*—How far can the elbows be moved across the newborn's chest? An elbow that does not reach midline indicates greater maturity. For example, if the elbow reaches or nears the level of the opposite shoulder, this is scored as –1 point; if the elbow does not cross the proximate axillary line, it is scored as 4 points.
6. *Heel to ear*—How close can the newborn's feet be moved to the ears? This manoeuver assesses hip flexibility: the lesser the flexibility, the greater the newborn's maturity. The heel-to-ear assessment is scored in the same manner as the scarf sign.

After the scoring is completed, the 12 scores are totalled and then compared with standardized values to determine the appropriate gestational age in weeks. Scores range from very low in preterm newborns to very high for mature and postmature newborns.

NEUROMUSCULAR MATURITY

NEUROMUSCULAR MATURITY SIGN	SCORE							RECORD SCORE HERE
	−1	0	1	2	3	4	5	
POSTURE								
SQUARE WINDOW (Wrist)	>90°	90°	60°	45°	30°	0°		
ARM RECOIL		180°	140°–180°	110°–140°	90°–110°	<90°		
POPLITEAL ANGLE	180°	160°	140°	120°	100°	90°	<90°	
SCARF SIGN								
HEEL TO EAR								
						TOTAL NEUROMUSCULAR MATURITY SCORE		

SCORE
Neuromuscular ——
Physical ——
Total ——

MATURITY RATING

Score	Weeks
−10	20
−5	22
0	24
5	26
10	28
15	30
20	32
25	34
30	36
35	38
40	40
45	42
50	44

PHYSICAL MATURITY

PHYSICAL MATURITY SIGN	SCORE							RECORD SCORE HERE
	−1	0	1	2	3	4	5	
SKIN	sticky, friable, transparent	gelatinous, red, translucent	smooth, pink, visible veins	superficial peeling and/or rash, few veins	cracking pale areas, rare veins	parchment, deep cracking, no vessels	leathery, cracked, wrinkled	
LANUGO	none	sparse	abundant	thinning	bald areas	mostly bald		
PLANTAR SURFACE	heel-toe 40–50 mm:−1 <40 mm:−2	>50 mm no crease	faint red marks	anterior transverse crease only	creases ant. 2/3	creases over entire sole		
BREAST	impercep-tible	barely perceptible	flat areola no bud	stippled areola 1–2 mm bud	raised areola 3–4 mm bud	full areola 5–10 mm bud		
EYE-EAR	lids fused loosely: −1 tightly: −2	lids open pinna flat stays folded	sl. curved pinna; soft; slow recoil	well-curved pinna; soft but ready recoil	formed and firm instant recoil	thick cartilage, ear stiff		
GENITALS (Male)	scrotum flat, smooth	scrotum empty, faint rugae	testes in upper canal, rare rugae	testes descending, few rugae	testes down, good rugae	testes pendulous, deep rugae		
GENITALS (Female)	clitoris prominent and labia flat	prominent clitoris and small labia minora	prominent clitoris and enlarging minora	majora and minora equally prominent	majora large, minora small	majora cover clitoris and minora		
						TOTAL PHYSICAL MATURITY SCORE		

FIGURE 18.3 Gestational age assessment tool. The New Ballard Score (2014). (Reprinted from Ballard, J. L., Khoury, J. C., Wedig, K., Wang, L., Eilers-Walsman, B. L., & Lipp R. [1991]. New Ballard Score, expanded to include extremely premature infants. *The Journal of Pediatrics, 119*(3), 417–423. Copyright © 1991 Elsevier. With permission.)

Typically newborns are also classified according to gestational age as:
- *Preterm or premature*—born prior to 37 completed weeks' gestation, regardless of birth weight
- *Term*—born between 38 and 42 weeks' gestation
- *Postterm or postdates*—born after completion of week 42 of gestation
- *Postmature*—born after 42 weeks and demonstrating signs of placental aging

Using the information about gestational age and then considering birth weight, newborns can also be classified as follows:
- ***Small for gestational age (SGA)***—weight less than the 10th percentile on standard growth charts (usually >5.5 lb)

- *Appropriate for gestational age (AGA)*—weight between 10th and 90th percentiles
- ***Large for gestational age (LGA)***—weight more than the 90th percentile on standard growth charts (Health Canada, 2004)

Chapter 23 describes these variations in birth weight and gestational age in greater detail.

> **Take Note!**
> Gestational age assessment is important because it allows the nurse to plot growth parameters and to anticipate problems related to prematurity, postmaturity, and growth abnormalities.

Nursing Interventions

During the immediate newborn period, care focuses on helping the newborn to make the transition to extrauterine life. The nursing interventions include maintaining airway patency, ensuring proper identification, administering prescribed medications, and maintaining thermoregulation.

Maintaining Airway Patency

Immediately after birth, a newborn's airway may be suctioned if needed to remove fluids and mucus from the mouth and nose (Fig. 18.4). Typically, the newborn's mouth is suctioned first using a bulb syringe to remove debris, and then the nose is suctioned. Suctioning in this manner helps to prevent aspiration of fluid into the lungs by an unexpected gasp. Recent studies, along with recommendations from leading maternal health experts and the WHO, support using a towel to wipe secretions from the mouth and nose of newborns for stable

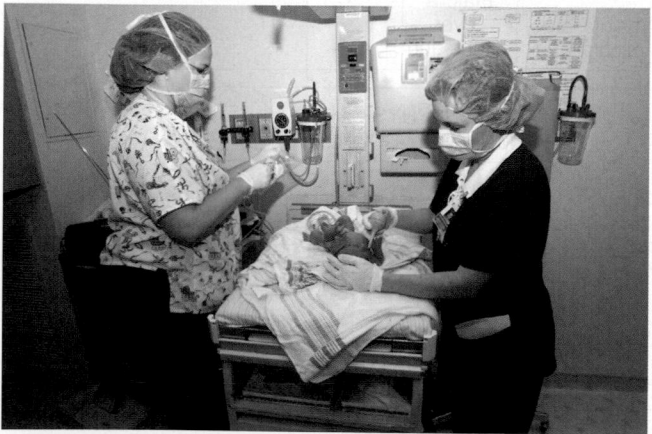

FIGURE 18.4 A newborn is suctioned by means of a bulb syringe to remove mucus from the mouth and nose. The head-down-and-to-the-side position facilitates drainage. Care is given with the infant under a radiant heat source.

newborns. Routine suctioning of the mouth and airways is not required. Despite evidence showing that the use of routine suctioning shows no benefit and may produce harm, the practice remains commonplace (Bond, 2015; Saugstad, 2015).

When suctioning a newborn with a bulb syringe, compress the bulb before placing it into the oral or nasal cavity. Release bulb compression slowly, making sure the tip is placed away from the mucous membranes to draw up the excess secretions. Remove the bulb syringe from the mouth or nose, and then, while holding the bulb syringe tip over an emesis basin lined with paper towel or tissue, compress the bulb to expel the secretions. Repeat the procedure several times until all secretions are removed or use a towel to wipe away secretions per hospital policy.

> **Take Note!**
> Always keep a bulb syringe near the newborn in case he or she develops sudden choking or a blockage in the nose. It may be lifesaving.

Ensuring Proper Identification

Infant abduction continues to be a threat in hospitals and health care organizations across North America. The abduction of newborns from health care facilities has clearly become a subject of concern for parents, perinatal nurses, health care security and risk management administrators, law enforcement officials, and the National Center for Missing and Exploited Children (NCMEC). Staff ID badges, training, video surveillance, access control, and tagging systems can help prevent a newborn from being abducted from the hospital. Proactive security measures must become everyone's responsibility to ensure the safety of all newborns and their families in all hospital settings.

Before the newborn and family leave the birthing area, be sure that agency policy about identification has been followed. Typically, the parent(s) and the newborn receive identification (ID) bracelets. The newborn commonly receives two ID bracelets, one on a wrist and one on an ankle. The mother receives a matching one, usually on her wrist. The ID bands usually state name, sex, date and time of birth, and identification number. The same identification number is on all matching bracelets.

These ID bracelets provide for the safety of the newborn and must be secured before the newborn is separated from their parents and/or the birthing area. The ID bracelets are checked by two nurses to validate that the correct newborn is brought to the right parent if they are separated for any period of time (Fig. 18.5). They also serve as the official newborn identification and should be checked before initiating any procedure on that newborn and on discharge from the unit (NCMEC, 2015). Taking the newborn's picture within 2 hours after birth

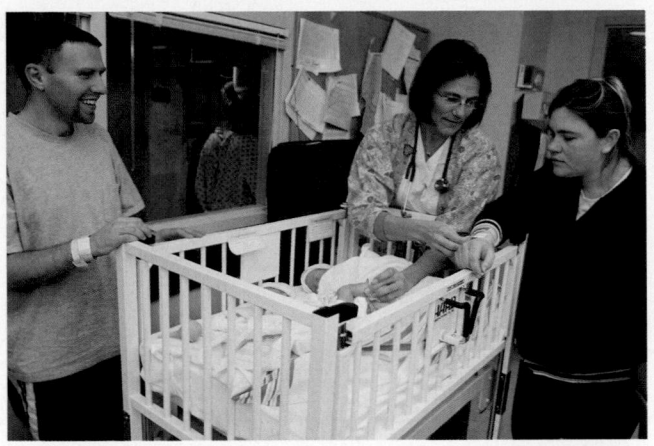

FIGURE 18.5 The nurse checks the newborn's identification band against the mother's.

with a colour camera or colour video/digital image also helps prevent mix-ups and abduction. Many facilities use electronic devices that sound an alarm if a newborn is taken beyond a certain point on the unit or removed from the area.

Prevention of infant abductions has been successful through a combination of increased security measures in hospitals, including video cameras and alarm devices, and education of staff and parents about precautions to

take while in the hospital. It is critical not to allow anyone without identification to take an infant for any reason and to keep the infant within sight of the parent or maternity staff at all times. These measures should be largely invisible and create a sense of security rather than increasing parental fears about abduction.

Although infant abduction rates are rare, the safety and security of infants and parents should remain a high priority for nurses. By being aware of physical security of maternity units, educating expectant parents on the methods used by potential abductors, and working with community resources, these tragic incidents can be prevented.

Administering Prescribed Medications

During the immediate newborn period, two medications are commonly ordered and administered with parents' consent: vitamin K and eye prophylaxis with either erythromycin or tetracycline ophthalmic ointment (Drug Guide 18.1).

VITAMIN K

Prophylactic treatment of newborns with intramuscular vitamin K has been the standard of care for decades in North America. Vitamin K, a fat-soluble vitamin, promotes

DRUG GUIDE 18.1   DRUGS FOR THE NEWBORN

Drug	Action/Indication	Nursing Implications
Phytonadione (vitamin K)	Provides the newborn with vitamin K (necessary for production of adequate clotting factors II, VII, IX, and X by the liver) during the 1st week of birth until newborn can manufacture it Prevents vitamin K deficiency bleeding (VKDB) of the newborn	Administer within 1–2 hours after birth Give as an IM injection at a 90-degree angle into the outer middle third of the vastus lateralis muscle Use a 25-gauge, 5/8-in needle for injection Hold the leg firmly and inject medication slowly Adhere to standard precautions Assess for bleeding at injection site after administration
Erythromycin ophthalmic ointment 0.5%	Provides bactericidal and bacteriostatic actions to prevent *Neisseria gonorrhea* and *Chlamydia trachomatis* conjunctivitis Prevents ophthalmia neonatorum	Be alert for chemical conjunctivitis for 1–2 days Wear gloves, and open eyes by placing thumb and finger above and below the eye Gently squeeze the tube or ampoule to apply medication into the conjunctival sac from the inner canthus to the outer canthus of each eye Do not touch the tip to the eye Close the eye to make sure the medication permeates Wipe off excess ointment after 1 minute

Adapted from King, T. L., Brucker, M. C., Osborne, K., & Jevitt, C. M. (2019). *Varney's midwifery* (6th ed.). Burlington, MA: Jones & Bartlett Learning; and Skidmore-Roth, L. (2018). *Mosby's 2018 nursing drug reference* (31st ed.). St. Louis, MO: Elsevier Health Sciences.

FIGURE 18.6 The nurse administers vitamin K IM to the newborn.

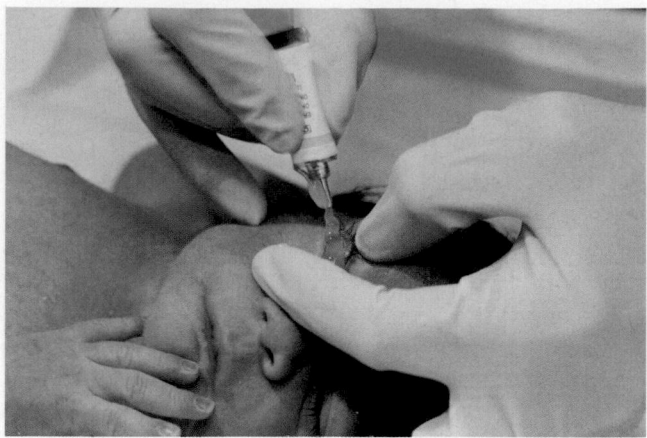

FIGURE 18.7 The nurse administers eye prophylaxis.

blood clotting by increasing the synthesis of prothrombin by the liver. A deficiency of this vitamin delays clotting and might lead to hemorrhage. Newborns are at risk for vitamin K deficiency and subsequent bleeding unless supplemented at birth. Vitamin K deficiency is an acquired coagulopathy in newborn infants because of an accumulation of inactive vitamin K coagulation factors, which leads to an increased bleeding tendency. Supplementation of vitamin K at birth has been recommended since 1961 and successfully reduces the risk of bleeding in newborns (Bellini, 2015).

In general, the bacteria of a mature intestine produce vitamin K in adequate quantities. However, the newborn's bowel is sterile, so vitamin K is not produced in the intestine until after microorganisms have been introduced, such as with the first feeding. Usually it takes about a week for the newborn to produce enough vitamin K to prevent vitamin K deficiency bleeding. Vitamin K may also be given orally to newborns outside North America, but at least three doses are needed over a 1-month period (Abrams & Savelli, 2014).

The efficacy of vitamin K in preventing early vitamin K deficiency bleeding is firmly established and has been the standard of care since the American Academy of Pediatrics (AAP) recommended it in the early 1960s. Both the AAP (2015) and the Canadian Paediatric Society (Ng, Loewy, & Fetus and Newborn Committee, 2018) recommend that vitamin K be administered to all newborns soon after birth in a single intramuscular dose of 0.5 to 1 mg (Fig. 18.6). The AAP also suggests that additional research is needed to validate the efficacy and safety of oral forms of vitamin K, which have been used in many parts of the world, but currently are not standard practice in North America.

EYE PROPHYLAXIS

Whether a baby is born vaginally or by cesarean birth, an installation of a prophylactic agent in their eyes within an hour or two of birth is recommended. This medical intervention dates back to the 1800s when silver nitrate was used to prevent vision loss due to neonatal ocular infection with *Neisseria gonorrhoeae*. Once a mandated practice in all Canadian provinces, this is now a recommended procedure, performed with parent's informed consent. **Ophthalmia neonatorum** is a hyperacute purulent conjunctivitis occurring during the first 10 days of life. It is usually contracted during birth when the baby comes in contact with vaginal discharge of the mother infected with gonorrhea. Historically it was believed that this antibiotic prophylaxis provided protection against chlamydia as well, however more recent studies have shown this intervention to be ineffective in preventing chlamydial conjunctivitis (Moore, MacDonald, & Canadian Paediatric Society Infectious Diseases and Immunization Committee, 2018).

Prophylactic agents that are currently recommended include erythromycin 0.5% ophthalmic ointment or tetracycline 1% ophthalmic ointment in a single application (Moore et al., 2018).

Regardless of which agent is used, instillation should be done within the first 1 to 2 hours after birth (Fig. 18.7). If instillation is delayed to allow visualization and bonding, the nursing staff should make sure the agent is administered by 2 hours of age.

Inform all parents about the eye treatment, including why it is recommended, what problems may arise if the treatment is not given, and possible adverse effects of the treatment.

> **Take Note!**
>
> Ophthalmia neonatorum is a severe form of conjunctivitis caused by chlamydia and/or gonococcal infections that is potentially a blinding condition in newborns.

Maintaining Thermoregulation

Newborns have trouble regulating their temperature; especially during the first few hours after birth (see

Chapter 17 for a complete discussion). Therefore, maintaining body temperature is crucial.

Take Note!

A 1-day-old infant should have adequate thermoregulation to remain out of the radiant heater. The best way to prevent heat loss is to ensure that the infant does not come in contact with cold surfaces.

Assess body temperature frequently during the immediate newborn period. The baby's temperature should be taken every 30 minutes for the first 2 hours or until the temperature has stabilized, and then every 8 hours until discharge or follow hospital protocols (King et al., 2019). In some health care facilities, a thermistor probe (automatic sensor) is attached to the newborn to record body temperature on a monitoring device. The probe is taped to the newborn's abdomen, usually in the right upper quadrant, which allows for position changes without having to readjust the probe. The other end of the thermistor probe is inserted into the radiant heat control panel. Temperature parameters are set on an alarm system connected to the heat panel that will sound if the newborn's temperature falls out of the set range. Check the probe connection periodically to make sure that it remains secure. Remember the potential for heat loss in newborns, and perform all nursing interventions in a way that minimizes heat loss and prevents hypothermia.

Axillary temperatures are also used to assess the newborn's body temperature. Place the thermometer under the newborn's axilla and place the arm over the chest to keep the thermometer in place and provide comfort to the newborn.

Nursing interventions to help maintain body temperature include:

- Dry the newborn immediately after birth to prevent heat loss through evaporation.
- Wrap the baby in warmed blankets to reduce heat loss via convection.
- Facilitate skin-to-skin contact with mother or parent immediately after birth (for all stable newborns).
- Use a warmed cover on the scale to weigh the unclothed newborn.
- Warm stethoscopes and hands before examining the baby or providing care.
- Avoid placing newborns in drafts or near air vents to prevent heat loss through convection.
- Delay the initial bath until the baby's temperature has stabilized to prevent heat loss through evaporation.
- Avoid placing cribs near cold outer walls to prevent heat loss through radiation.
- Put a cap on the newborn's head after it is thoroughly dried after birth.
- If the parents are unable to hold the baby skin-to-skin, place the newborn under a temperature-controlled radiant warmer (Fig. 18.8).

NURSING MANAGEMENT DURING THE EARLY NEWBORN PERIOD

The early newborn period is a time of great adjustment for both the newborn and parents, each of whom are adapting to many physiologic and psychological changes. In the past, mothers and newborns remained in the health care facility while these dramatic changes were taking place, with nurses and doctors readily available. However, today shorter hospital stays are the norm, and new parents can easily be overwhelmed by having to go through all of these changes in such a short time: the client gives birth, experiences marked physiologic and psychological changes, and must adapt to the newborn and learn the skills needed for self-care as well as care of the baby, all within 24 to 48 hours.

The nurse's role is to assist the parent(s) and newborn through this dramatic transition period. The newborn needs continued health assessment, and parents need to be taught to care for their new baby. At discharge, new parents may panic and feel insecure about their new roles as primary caretakers. Nurses play a major role in promoting the newborn's transition by providing ongoing assessment and care and in promoting the parents' confidence by serving as a role model and teaching about proper newborn care.

Assessment

The newborn requires ongoing assessment after leaving the birthing area to ensure that his or her transition to extrauterine life is progressing without problems. The nurse uses the data gathered during the initial assessment as a baseline for comparison.

Perinatal History

Pertinent maternal and fetal data are vital to formulate a plan of care for the parent(s) and newborn. Historical information is obtained from the medical record and from interviewing the pregnant client. Review the maternal history because it provides pertinent information, such as the presence of certain risk factors that could affect the newborn. Keep in mind that a comprehensive maternal history may not be available, especially if the mother has had limited or no prenatal care. Historical information usually includes the following:

- Mother's name, medical record number, blood type, serology result, rubella and hepatitis status
- Other maternal tests that are relevant to the newborn and care, such as human immunodeficiency virus (HIV) and group B streptococcus status
- Intrapartum maternal antibiotic therapy (type, dose, and duration)
- Maternal illness that can affect the pregnancy, evidence of chorioamnionitis, maternal use of medications such as steroids

FIGURE 18.8 Maintaining thermoregulation. **A.** Isolette. **B.** Radiant warmer. **C.** Plastic wrap. **D.** Combination unit: radiant warmer and isolette.

- Any history of substance abuse
- Prenatal care, including timing of first visit and subsequent visits
- Risk for blood group incompatibility, including Rh status and blood type
- Fetal heart rate patterns during labour
- Known inherited conditions such as sickle cell anemia and phenylketonuria (PKU)
- Birth weights of previous live-born children, along with identification of any newborn problems
- Social history, including tobacco, alcohol, and recreational drug use
- History of depression or domestic violence
- Cultural factors, including primary language and educational level
- Pregnancy complications associated with fetal growth, fetal anomalies, or abnormal results from tests of fetal well-being
- Information on the progress of labour, birth, labour complications, duration of ruptured membranes, and presence of meconium in the amniotic fluid
- Medications given during labour, at birth, and immediately after birth
- Time and method of delivery, including presentation and the use of forceps or a vacuum extractor
- Status of the newborn at birth, including Apgar scores at 1 and 5 minutes, the need for suctioning, weight, gestational age, vital signs, and umbilical cord status
- Medications administered to the newborn
- Postbirth maternal information, including placental findings, positive cultures, and presence of fever

Newborn Physical Examination

The initial newborn physical examination, which may demonstrate subtle differences related to the newborn's age, is carried out within the first 24 hours after birth. For example, a newborn who is 30 minutes old has not yet completed the normal transition from intrauterine to extrauterine life, and thus variability may exist in vital signs and in respiratory, neurologic, gastrointestinal, skin, and cardiovascular systems. Therefore, a comprehensive examination should be delayed until after the newborn has completed the transition.

The physical examination should not be initiated if the newborn is crying or appears to be upset. Instead, it is best to postpone the assessment until the newborn is calm. In a quiet newborn, begin the examination with the least invasive and noxious elements of the examination (auscultation of heart and lungs). Then examine the areas most likely to irritate the newborn (e.g., examining the hips and eliciting the Moro reflex). A general visual assessment provides an enormous amount of information about the well-being of a newborn. Initial observation gives an impression of a healthy (stable) versus an ill newborn and a term versus a preterm newborn.

A typical physical examination of a newborn includes a general survey of skin colour, posture, state of alertness, head size, overall behavioural state, respiratory status, sex, and any obvious congenital anomalies. Check the overall appearance for anything unusual. Then complete the examination in a systematic fashion.

> **Remember Kelly, who called the home health nurse and said her newborn son "looks like a canary"? What additional information is needed about the baby? What might be causing his yellow colour?**

ANTHROPOMETRIC MEASUREMENTS

Shortly after birth, after the sex of the child is revealed, most parents want to know the vital statistics of their newborn—length and weight—to report to their family and friends. Additional measurements, including head and chest circumference, are also taken and recorded. Abdominal measurements are not routinely obtained unless there is a suspicion of pathology that causes abdominal distention. The newborn's progress from that point on will be validated based on these early measurements. These measurements will be compared with future serial measurements to determine growth patterns, which are plotted on growth charts to evaluate normalcy. Therefore, accuracy is paramount.

Length. The average length of most newborns is 50 cm (20 in), but it can range from 44 to 55 cm (17 to 22 in). Measure length with the unclothed newborn lying on a warmed blanket placed on a flat surface with the knees held in an extended position. Then run a tape measure down the length of the newborn—from the head to the soles of the feet—and record this measurement in the newborn's record (Fig. 18.1).

Weight. At birth the average newborn weighs 3,400 g (7 lb, 7 oz), but normal birth weights can range from 2,500 to 4,000 g (5 lb, 8 oz to 8 lb, 13 oz). Newborns are

weighed immediately after birth and then daily. Newborns usually lose up to 7% of their birth weight within the first few days of life, but regain it in within 2 weeks.

Newborns are weighed within the first 2 hours of life, ideally with a digital portable scale in the presence of the parents. First, balance the scale if it is not balanced. Place a warmed protective cloth or paper as a barrier on the scale to prevent heat loss by conduction; recalibrate the scale to zero after applying the barrier. Next, place the unclothed newborn in the centre of the scale. Keep a hand above the newborn for safety (Fig. 18.2).

Weight is affected by racial origin, genetics, maternal age, size of the parents, maternal nutrition, maternal weight prenatally, and placental perfusion (Tawia & McGuire, 2014). Weight should be correlated with gestational age. A newborn who weighs more than normal might be LGA or an infant of a diabetic mother; a newborn who weighs less than normal might be SGA, preterm, or have a genetic syndrome. It is important to identify the cause for the deviation in size and to monitor the newborn for complications common to that etiology.

Head Circumference. The average newborn head circumference is 32 to 38 cm (13 to 15 in). Measure the circumference at the head's widest diameter (the occipitofrontal circumference). Wrap a flexible or paper measuring tape snugly around the newborn's head and record the measurement (Fig. 18.9A).

> **Take Note!**
> Head circumference will be remeasured if the shape of the head is altered from birth, if the baby had instrumental delivery, or if there is a suspected skull fracture or hematoma.

The head circumference should be approximately one fourth of the newborn's length or about half the infant's body length plus 10 cm. Expected head circumference for a term infant is between 32 and 37 cm (12.5 to 14.5 in) (Nagtalon-Ramos, 2014). A small head might indicate microcephaly caused by rubella, toxoplasmosis, or SGA status; an enlarged head might indicate hydrocephalus, intraventricular bleed, or increased intracranial pressure. Both need to be documented and reported for further investigation.

Chest Circumference. The average chest circumference is 30 to 36 cm (12 to 14 in). It is generally equal to or about 2 to 3 cm less than the head circumference (Weber & Kelley, 2017). Place a flexible or paper tape measure around the unclothed newborn's chest just below the nipple line without pulling it taut (Fig. 18.9B).

> **Take Note!**
> The head and chest circumferences are usually equal by about 1 year of age.

FIGURE 18.9 **A.** Measuring head circumference. **B.** Measuring chest circumference.

VITAL SIGNS

In the newborn, temperature, pulse, and respirations are monitored frequently and compared with baseline data obtained immediately after birth. In general, vital signs (excluding blood pressure) are taken:

- In the labour and birth room after the parent(s) hold and bond with the newborn
- Once every 30 minutes until the newborn has been stable for 2 hours
- Then once every 4 to 8 hours until discharge (Davidson, 2014)

Blood pressure is not routinely assessed in a healthy term newborn unless the baby's clinical condition warrants it. This schedule can change depending on the baby's health status.

Obtain a newborn's temperature by placing an electronic temperature probe in the midaxillary area or by monitoring the electronic thermistor probe that has been taped to the abdominal skin (applied when the newborn was placed under a radiant heat source). Monitor the newborn's temperature frequently per hospital protocol for changes until it stabilizes. If the temperature is higher, adjust the environment, such as removing some clothing

or blankets. If the temperature is lower, check the radiant warmer setting or add a warmed blanket. Report any abnormalities to the primary health care provider if simple adjustments to the environment do not change the baby's temperature as it may indicate condition such as sepsis.

Obtain an apical pulse by placing the stethoscope over the fourth left intercostal space on the chest. Listen for a full minute, noting rate, rhythm, and abnormal sounds such as murmurs. In the typical newborn, the heart rate is 110 to 160 bpm, with wide fluctuations with activity and sleep. Sinus arrhythmia is a normal finding. Murmurs detected during the newborn period do not necessarily indicate congenital heart disease, but they need to be evaluated further if they persist. Also palpate the apical, femoral, and brachial pulses for presence and equality (Fig. 18.10). Report any abnormalities to the primary health care provider for evaluation.

Assess respirations by observing the rise and fall of the chest for one full minute. Respirations should be symmetric, slightly irregular, shallow, and unlaboured at a rate of 30 to 60 breaths/minute. The newborn's respirations are predominantly diaphragmatic, but they are synchronous with abdominal movements. Also auscultate breath sounds. Note any abnormalities, such as tachypnea, bradypnea, grunting, gasping, periods of apnea lasting longer than 20 seconds, asymmetry or decreased chest expansion, abnormal breath sounds (rhonchi, crackles), or sternal retractions. Some variations might exist early after birth, but if the abnormal pattern persists, notify the primary health care provider.

SKIN

The newborn's skin is similar in structure to the adult's, but many of the functions are not fully developed. Observe the overall appearance of the skin, including colour, texture, turgor, and integrity. The newborn's skin should be smooth and flexible, and the colour should be consistent with genetic background.

Skin Condition and Colour. Check skin turgor by pinching a small area of skin over the chest or abdomen and note how quickly it returns to its original position. In a well-hydrated newborn, the skin should return to its normal position immediately. Skin that remains "tented" after being pinched may indicate dehydration. A small amount of lanugo (fine downy hair) may be observed over the shoulders and on the sides of the face and upper back. There may be some cracking and peeling of the skin, most commonly in babies born postdates (beyond their due date). The skin should be warm to the touch and intact.

The newborn's skin often appears blotchy or mottled, especially in the extremities. Persistent cyanosis of fingers, hands, toes, and feet with mottled blue or red discolouration and coldness is called **acrocyanosis**

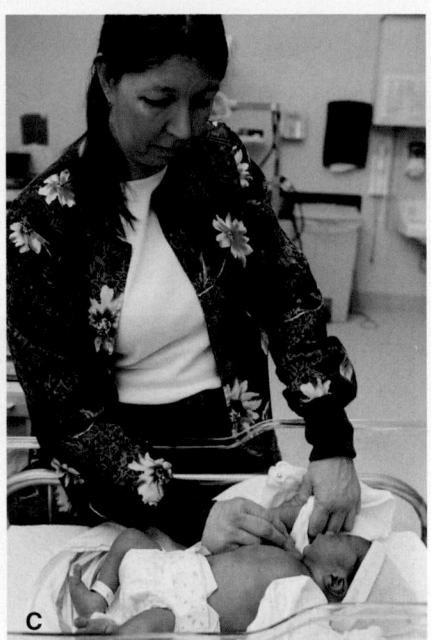

FIGURE 18.10 Assessing the newborn's vital signs. **A.** Assessing the apical pulse. **B.** Palpating the femoral pulse. **C.** Palpating the brachial pulse.

(Fig. 18.11). It may be seen in newborns during the first few weeks of life in response to exposure to cold. Acrocyanosis is normal and intermittent. Any change in colour of the newborn skin needs further investigation.

Newborn Skin Variations. While assessing the skin, make note of any rashes, ecchymoses or petechiae, nevi, or dark pigmentation. Skin lesions can be congenital or transient; they may be a result of infection or may result from the mode of birth. If any are present, observe the anatomic location, arrangement, type, and colour. Bruising may result from the use of devices such as a vacuum

FIGURE 18.11 Acrocyanosis. This commonly appears on the feet and hands of babies shortly after birth. This infant is a 32-week newborn. (From Fletcher, M. (1998). *Physical diagnosis in neonatology*. Philadelphia, PA: Lippincott-Raven Publishers.)

extractor during delivery. Petechiae may be the result of pressure on the skin during the birth process. Forceps marks may be observed over the cheeks and ears. A small puncture mark may be seen if internal fetal scalp electrode monitoring was used during labour.

Common skin variations include: **vernix caseosa**, **stork bites** or salmon patches, **milia**, **Mongolian spots**, **erythema toxicum**, **harlequin sign**, **nevus flammeus**, and **nevus vasculosus** (Fig. 18.12).

Vernix caseosa is a thick white substance that protects the skin of the fetus. It is formed by secretions from the fetus's oil glands and is found during the first 2 or 3 days after birth in body creases and the hair. It does not need to be removed because it acts as a protective moisturizer which will be absorbed into the skin.

Stork bites or salmon patches are superficial vascular areas found on the nape of the neck, on the eyelids, and between the eyes and upper lip (Fig. 18.12A). The name comes from the marks on the back of the neck where, as myth goes, a stork may have picked up the baby. They are caused by a concentration of immature blood vessels and are most visible when the newborn is crying. They are considered a normal variant, and most fade and disappear completely within the 1st year of life.

Milia are multiple pearly white or pale yellow unopened sebaceous glands frequently found on a newborn's nose. They may also appear on the chin and forehead (Fig. 18.12B). They form from oil glands and disappear on their own within 2 to 4 weeks. When they occur in a newborn's mouth and gums, they are termed **Epstein pearls**. They occur in approximately 80% of newborns. As most lesions break spontaneously within the first few

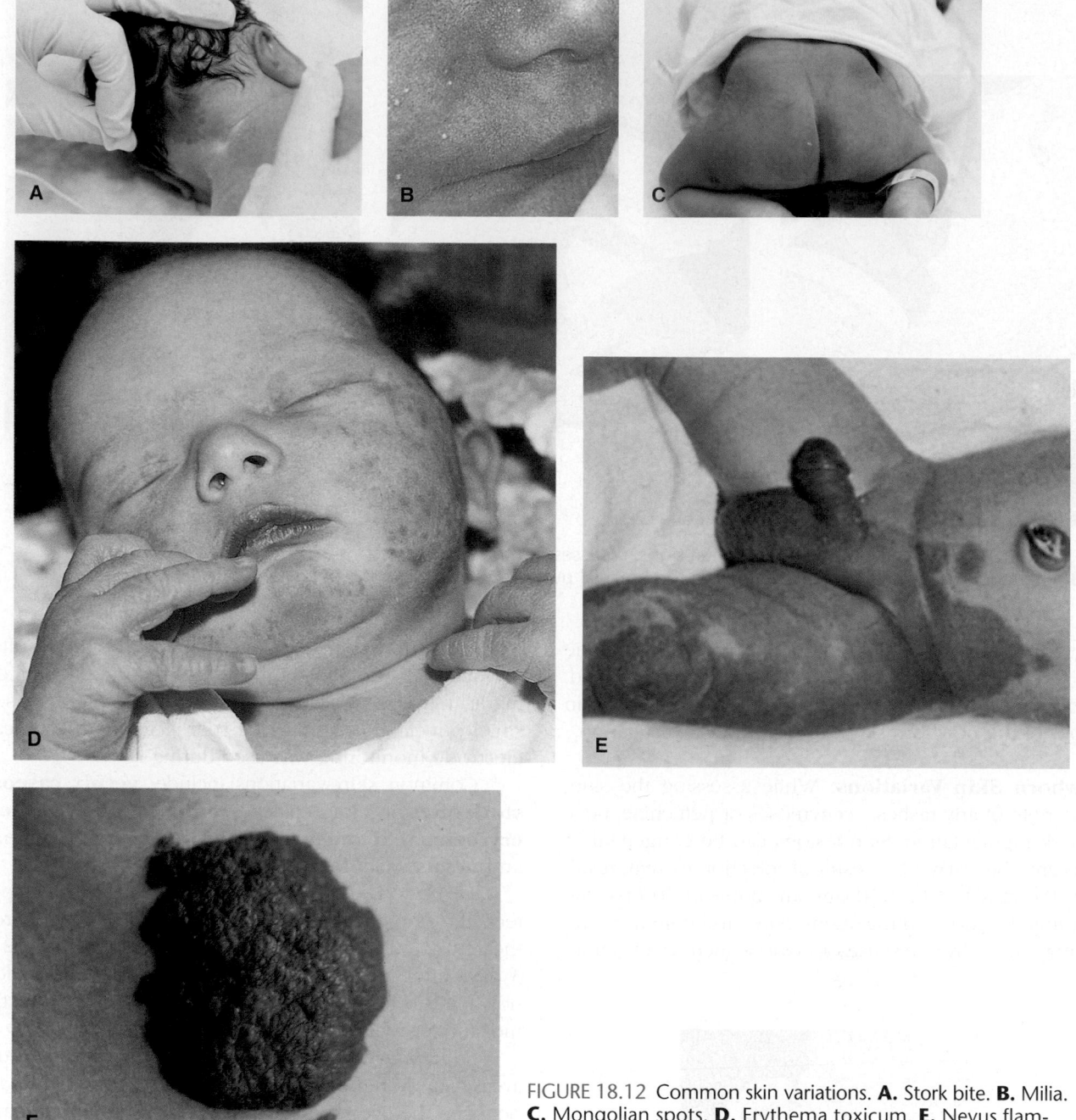

FIGURE 18.12 Common skin variations. **A.** Stork bite. **B.** Milia. **C.** Mongolian spots. **D.** Erythema toxicum. **E.** Nevus flammeus (port-wine stain). **F.** Strawberry hemangioma.

weeks of life, no therapy is indicated (El-Radhi, 2015). Parents should be taught that attempting to "pop" these spots can lead to permanent scarring on the baby's face.

Mongolian spots are benign blue or purple splotches that appear solitary on the lower back and buttocks of newborns, but may occur as multiple over the legs and shoulders (Fig. 18.12C). They tend to occur in African, Asian, Hispanic, and Indian newborns but can occur in dark-skinned newborns of all races. The spots are caused by a concentration of pigmented cells and usually disappear spontaneously within the first 4 years of life. They

should not be confused with bruises caused by trauma (Silverberg, 2015).

Erythema toxicum (newborn rash) is a benign, idiopathic, generalized, transient rash that occurs in up to 70% of all newborns during the 1st week of life. It consists of small papules or pustules on the skin resembling flea bites. It is often mistaken for staphylococcal pustules. The rash is common on the face, chest, and back (Fig. 18.12D). One of the chief characteristics of this rash is its lack of pattern. It is caused by the newborn's eosinophils reacting to the environment as the immune system matures. Histologically, erythema toxicum shows an abundance of eosinophils. Although it has been recognized and described for centuries, its etiology and pathogenesis remain unclear (Gloster, Gebauer, & Mistur, 2016a). It does not require any treatment and disappears in a few days.

Harlequin sign refers to the dilation of blood vessels on only one side of the body, giving the newborn the appearance of wearing a clown suit. It gives a distinct midline demarcation, which is described as pale on the nondependent side and red on the opposite, dependent side. It results from immature autoregulation of blood flow and is commonly seen in low–birth-weight newborns when there is a positional change (Lomax, 2015). It is transient, lasting as long as 20 minutes, and no intervention is needed.

Nevus flammeus, also called a port-wine stain, commonly appears on the newborn's face or other body areas (Fig. 18.12E). It is a capillary angioma located directly below the dermis. It is flat with sharp demarcations and is purple-red. This skin lesion is made up of mature capillaries that are congested and dilated. It ranges in size from a few millimeters to large, occasionally involving as much as half the body surface. Although it does not grow in area or size, it is permanent and will not fade. Although they may occur anywhere on the body, the majority are located in the head and neck areas. Port-wine stains may be associated with structural malformations, bony or muscular overgrowth, and certain cancers. Studies have noted an association between port-wine birthmarks and childhood cancer, so newborns with these lesions should be monitored with periodic eye examinations, neurologic imaging, and extremity measurements. Lasers and intense pulsed light have been used to remove larger lesions with some success. The optimal timing of treatment is before 1 year of age (Giese & Richter, 2015).

Nevus vasculosus, also called a strawberry mark or strawberry hemangioma, is a benign capillary hemangioma in the dermal and subdermal layers. It is raised, rough, dark red, and sharply demarcated (Fig. 18.12F). It is commonly found in the head region within a few weeks after birth and can increase in size or number. They are commonly found in about 10% of children. This type of hemangioma may be very subtle or even absent in the first few weeks of life, but they proliferate in the first few months of life. Commonly seen in premature infants weighing less than 1,500 g (El-Radhi, 2015), these hemangiomas tend to resolve by age 3 without any treatment.

The most important aspects of nursing management related to newborn skin variations include adequate recognition of the lesions and knowledge of their natural history so that accurate information can be offered to the parent(s). The majority of skin lesions do not require any therapeutic intervention, but referral is necessary if there is visual, airway or ear canal obstruction, extensive growth, severe facial disfigurement, recurrent bleeding, infection, ulceration, or excessive concerns of the parents.

HEAD

Head size varies with age, sex, and ethnicity and has a general correlation with body size. Inspect a newborn's head from all angles. The head should appear symmetric and round. As many as 90% of the congenital malformations present at birth are visible on the head and neck, so careful assessment is very important (Pfister & Ramel, 2014).

The newborn has two fontanels at the juncture of the cranial bones. The anterior fontanel is diamond shaped and closes by 18 to 24 months. Typically it measures 4 to 6 cm at the largest diameter (bone to bone). The posterior one is triangular, smaller than the anterior fontanel (usually fingertip size or 0.5 to 1 cm), and closes by 6 to 12 weeks. Palpate both fontanels, which should be soft, flat, and open. Then palpate the skull. It should feel somewhat smooth and fused, except at the area of the fontanels, over moulding areas, and sutures. Also assess the size of the head and the anterior and posterior fontanels, and compare them with appropriate standards.

Variations in Head Size and Appearance. During inspection and palpation, be alert for common variations that may cause asymmetry. These include moulding, **caput succedaneum**, and **cephalohematoma**.

Moulding is the elongated shaping of the fetal head to accommodate passage through the birth canal (Fig. 18.13). It occurs with a vaginal birth from a vertex position in which elongation of the fetal head occurs

FIGURE 18.13 Moulding in a newborn's head.

Scalp
Serum
Periosteum
Skull bone
Septal suture

A1

A2

Scalp
Periosteum
Skull bone

B1

B2

FIGURE 18.14 **A1** and **A2.** Caput succedaneum involves the collection of serous fluid and often crosses the suture line. **B1** and **B2.** Cephalohematoma involves the collection of blood and does not cross the suture line. (**A1, B1,** and **B2,** photos from O'Doherty, N. (1979). *Atlas of the newborn.* Philadelphia, PA: J B Lippincott, with permission. **A2,** photo from Chung, E. K., Atkinson-McEvoy, L. R., Boom, J. A., & Matz, P. S. (2010). *Visual diagnosis and treatment in pediatrics* (2nd ed.). Philadelphia, PA: LWW, Courtesy of the late Peter Sol, MD.)

with prominence of the occiput and overriding sagittal suture line. It typically resolves within a week after birth without intervention.

Caput succedaneum is the term for localized edema on the scalp that occurs from the pressure of the birth process. It is commonly observed after prolonged labour. Clinically, it appears as a poorly demarcated soft tissue swelling that crosses suture lines. Pitting

edema and overlying petechiae and ecchymosis are noted (Fig. 18.14A). The swelling will gradually dissipate in about 3 days without any treatment. Newborns who were born with the assistance of vacuum extraction usually have a caput in the area where the cup was used.

Cephalohematoma is a localized subperiosteal collection of blood of the skull which is always confined by one cranial bone. This condition is due to pressure on the head and disruption of the vessels during birth. It occurs after prolonged labour and use of obstetric interventions such as low forceps or vacuum extraction. The clinical features include a well-demarcated, often fluctuant swelling with no overlying skin discolouration. The swelling does not cross suture lines and is firmer to the touch than an edematous area (Fig. 18.14B). Aspiration is not required for resolution and is likely to increase the risk of infection. Hyperbilirubinemia occurs following the breakdown of the RBCs within the hematoma. This type of hyperbilirubinemia occurs later than classic physiologic hyperbilirubinemia. Cephalohematoma usually appears on the 2nd or 3rd day after birth and disappears within weeks or months. Large cephalohematomas can lead to increased bilirubin levels and subsequent jaundice (Lomax, 2015).

Common Abnormalities in Head or Fontanel Size.
Common abnormalities in head or fontanel size that may indicate a problem include:

- *Microcephaly*—a head circumference more than 2 standard deviations below average or less than 10% of normal parameters for gestational age, caused by inadequate brain development. There is a reduced production of neurons leading to a reduction of brain volume and as a consequence of that a reduced skull size. Microcephaly is fairly common; while the Canadian incidence is not currently known, more than 25,000 infants are born with microcephaly in the United States each year. Children with severe microcephaly, defined as more than 3 standard deviations below the mean for age and sex, are more likely to have imaging abnormalities and more severe developmental impairments than those with milder microcephaly. About 40% of children with microcephaly also have epilepsy, 20% have cerebral palsy, 50% have intellectual disability, and 20% to 50% have ophthalmologic and hearing disorders (Boom, 2018b). It can be familial, with autosomal dominant or recessive inheritance, and it may be associated with infections (cytomegalovirus), rubella, toxoplasmosis, and syndromes such as trisomy 13, 18, or 21 and fetal alcohol syndrome. In recent years, microcephaly has become a greater concern in pregnancy for Canadians travelling to warmer destinations where the Zika virus has been identified as a congenital risk factor (Nelson et al., 2017). Historically the incidence of microcephaly had not been tracked in Canada, however in 2016 the Canadian Paediatric Surveillance Program launched a multi-year study to track the incidence across the country (Nelson et al., 2017). In the United States, more than 25,000 infants are born with microcephaly each year. Genetic counselling and clinical management through carrier detection/prenatal diagnosis in families can help reduce the incidence of these disorders (Alcantara & O'Driscoll, 2014).
- *Macrocephaly*—a head circumference more than 90% of normal, typically related to hydrocephalus (Boom,

2018a). It is often familial (with autosomal dominant inheritance) and can be either an isolated anomaly or a manifestation of other anomalies, including hydrocephalus and skeletal disorders (achondroplasia).
- *Large fontanels*—more than 6 cm in the anterior diameter bone to bone or more than a 1-cm diameter in the posterior fontanel; possibly associated with malnutrition, hydrocephaly, congenital hypothyroidism, trisomies 13, 18, and 21, and various bone disorders such as osteogenesis imperfecta.
- *Small or closed fontanels*—smaller-than-normal anterior and posterior diameters or fontanels that are closed at birth. Craniosynostosis and abnormal brain development are associated with a small fontanel or early fontanel closure associated with microcephaly (Sheth, Ranalli, & Aldana, 2017).

FACE
Observe the newborn's face for fullness and symmetry. The face should have full cheeks and should be symmetric when the baby is resting and crying. If forceps were used during birth, the newborn may have bruising and reddened areas over both cheeks and parietal bones secondary to the pressure of the forceps blades. Reassure the parents that this resolves without treatment, and point out improvement each day.

Problems with the face can also involve facial nerve paralysis caused by trauma from the use of forceps. Paralysis is usually apparent on the 1st or 2nd day of life. Typically, the newborn will demonstrate asymmetry of the face with an inability to close the eye and move the lips on the affected side. Newborns with facial nerve paralysis have difficulty making a seal around the nipple, and consequently milk drools from the paralyzed side of the mouth. Most facial nerve palsies resolve spontaneously within days, although full recovery may require weeks to months. Attempt to determine the cause from the newborn's history.

Nose. Inspect the nose for size, symmetry, position, and lesions. The newborn's nose is small and narrow. The nose should have a midline placement, patent nares, and an intact septum. The nostrils should be of equal size and should be patent. A slight mucous discharge may be present, but there should be no actual drainage. The newborn is a preferential nose breather and will use sneezing to clear the nose if needed. The newborn can smell after the nasal passages are cleared of amniotic fluid and mucus (Clark-Gambelunghe & Clark, 2015).

Mouth. Inspect the newborn's mouth, lips, and interior structures. The lips should be intact with symmetric movement and positioned in the midline; there should be no lesions. Inspect the lips for pink colour, moisture, and cracking. The lips should encircle the examiner's finger to form a seal. Variations involving the lip might include

FIGURE 18.15 A natal tooth in a 16-day-old neonate. Natal teeth can be present at birth and are usually considered benign. No treatment is needed if they don't interfere with feeding.

cleft upper lip (separation extending up to the nose) or thin upper lip associated with fetal alcohol syndrome.

Assess the inside of the mouth for alignment of the mandible, intact soft and hard palate, sucking pads inside the cheeks, a midline uvula, a free-moving tongue, and working gag, swallow, and sucking reflexes. The mucous membranes lining the oral cavity should be pink and moist, with minimal saliva present.

Normal variations might include Epstein pearls (small, white epidermal cysts on the gums and hard palate that disappear in weeks), erupted natal teeth that may need to be removed to prevent aspiration (Fig. 18.15), and thrush (white plaque inside the mouth caused by exposure to *Candida albicans* during birth), which cannot be wiped away with a cotton-tipped applicator.

Eyes. Inspect the external eye structures, including the eyelids, lashes, conjunctiva, sclera, iris, and pupils, for position, colour, size, and movement. There may be marked edema of the eyelids and subconjunctival hemorrhages due to pressure during birth. The eyes should be clear and symmetrically placed. Test the blink reflex by bringing an object close to the eye; the newborn should respond quickly by blinking. Also test the newborn's pupillary reflex: pupils should be equal, round, and reactive to light bilaterally. Assess the newborn's gaze: he or she should be able to track objects to the midline. Movement may be uncoordinated during the first few weeks of life. Many newborns have transient strabismus (deviation or wandering of eyes independently) and searching nystagmus (involuntary repetitive eye movement), which is caused by immature muscular control. These are normal for the first 3 to 6 months of age.

Examine the internal eye structures. A red reflex (luminous red appearance seen on the retina) should be seen bilaterally on retinoscopy. The red reflex normally shows no dullness or irregularities.

Chemical conjunctivitis commonly occurs within 24 hours of instillation of eye prophylaxis after birth.

There is lid edema with sterile discharge from both eyes. Usually it resolves within 48 hours without treatment.

Ears. Inspect the ears for size, shape, skin condition, placement, amount of cartilage, and patency of the auditory canal. The ears should be soft and pliable and should recoil quickly and easily when folded and released. Ears should be aligned with the outer canthi of the eyes. Low-set ears and abnormally shaped ears are characteristic of many syndromes and genetic abnormalities, such as trisomy 13 or 18, and internal organ abnormalities involving the renal system. Findings of sinuses or preauricular skin tags should prompt further evaluation for possible renal abnormalities since both systems develop at the same time in utero.

An otoscopic examination is not typically done because the newborn's ear canals are filled with amniotic fluid and vernix caseosa, which would make visualization of the tympanic membrane difficult.

Newborn hearing screening is offered to families across Canada (discussed later in the chapter). Hearing loss is one of the most common birth defects, affecting nearly 2 in 1,000 newborns (Patel, Feldman, & Canadian Paediatric Society, Community Paediatrics Committee, 2018). Delays in identification and intervention may affect the child's cognitive, verbal, behavioural, and emotional development. Screening at birth has reduced the age at which newborns with hearing loss are identified and has improved early intervention rates dramatically. Available treatments include cochlear implantation, hearing augmentation, and follow-up by an audiologist, otolaryngologist, pediatrician, geneticist, and deaf education specialist (Nikolopoulos, 2015). Prior to universal newborn screening, children were usually older than 2 years before significant congenital hearing loss was detected; by this time it had already affected their speech and language skills (CDC, 2017).

Causes of hearing loss can be conductive, sensorineural, or central. Risk factors for congenital hearing loss include cytomegalovirus infection and preterm birth necessitating a stay in the neonatal intensive care unit.

To assess for hearing ability generally, observe the newborn's response to noises and conversations. The newborn typically turns toward these noises and startles with loud ones.

NECK

Inspect the newborn's neck for movement and ability to support the head. The newborn's neck will appear almost nonexistent because it is so short. Creases are usually noted. The neck should move freely in all directions and should be capable of holding the head in a midline position. The newborn should have enough head control to be able to hold it up briefly without support. Report any deviations such as restricted neck movement or absence of head control.

Also inspect the clavicles (collar bone), which should be straight and intact. The clavicles are the bones mostly commonly broken in infants, especially large babies experiencing difficult births, in operative vaginal births, abnormal fetal positions, and in maternal obesity. In most cases, the fractured clavicle is asymptomatic, but edema, crepitus, and decreased or absent movement and pain or tenderness on movement of the arm on the affected side may be noted. Major risk factors for clavicle fractures are typically vacuum births and large newborn birth weights (Ahn et al., 2015). If the newborn with clavicular fracture is in pain, the affected arm should be immobilized, with the arm abducted more than 60 degrees and the elbow flexed more than 90 degrees. In addition to immobilization, treatment involves minimizing pain overall.

CHEST

Inspect the newborn's chest for size, shape, and symmetry. The newborn's chest should be round, symmetric, and 2 to 3 cm smaller than the head circumference. The xiphoid process may be prominent at birth, but it usually becomes less apparent when adipose tissue accumulates. Nipples may be engorged and may secrete a white discharge. This discharge, which occurs in both boys and girls, is a result of exposure to high levels of maternal estrogen while in utero. Parents benefit from reassurance that this enlargement and milky discharge usually dissipates within a few weeks. Some newborns may have extra nipples, called supernumerary nipples. They are typically small, raised, pigmented areas vertical to the main nipple line, 5 to 6 cm below the normal nipple. Supernumerary nipples may be unilateral or bilateral, and they may include an areola, nipple, or both. They tend to be familial and do not contain glandular tissue. Supernumerary nipples are generally thought to be benign. Some studies have suggested an association with renal or urogenital anomalies, whereas other studies have failed to show this association. There is insufficient evidence to recommend imaging studies or removal in the absence of other clinical concerns or physical findings (Gloster, Gebauer, & Mistur, 2016b). Reassure parents that these extra small nipples are harmless.

The newborn chest is usually barrel shaped, with equal anteroposterior and lateral diameters, and symmetric. Auscultate the lungs bilaterally for equal breath sounds. Normal breath sounds should be heard, with little difference between inspiration and expiration. Fine crackles can be heard on inspiration soon after birth as a result of amniotic fluid being cleared from the lungs. Diminished breath sounds might indicate atelectasis or pneumonia (Weber & Kelley, 2017).

Listen to the heart when the newborn is quiet or sleeping. S1 and S2 heart sounds are accentuated at birth. The point of maximal impulse is a lateral to midclavicular line located at the fourth intercostal space. A displaced point of maximal impulse may indicate tension pneumothorax or cardiomegaly. Murmurs are common during the first few hours as the foramen ovale is closing. Although cardiac murmurs in the neonatal period do not necessarily indicate heart disease, they should be evaluated if they persist (Fillipps & Bucciarelli, 2015).

ABDOMEN

Inspect the abdomen for shape and movement. Typically the newborn's abdomen is protuberant but not distended. This contour is a result of the immaturity of the abdominal muscles. Abdominal movements are synchronous with respirations because newborns are, at times, abdominal breathers.

Auscultate bowel sounds in all four quadrants and then palpate the abdomen for consistency, masses, and tenderness. Perform auscultation and palpation systematically in a clockwise fashion until all four quadrants have been assessed. Palpate gently to feel the liver, the kidneys, and any masses. The liver is normally palpable 1 to 3 cm below the costal margin in the midclavicular line. The kidneys are 1 to 2 cm above and to both sides of the umbilicus. Normal findings would include bowel sounds in all four quadrants and no masses or tenderness on palpation. Absent or hyperactive bowel sounds might indicate an intestinal obstruction. Abdominal distention might indicate ascites, obstruction, infection, masses, or an enlarged abdominal organ. The newborn may also show signs of abdominal tenderness (Glasser & Springer, 2016). Imaging is a mainstay to diagnosis abdominal pathology and should be readily performed in a newborn with abdominal distention to determine the underlying etiology.

Inspect the umbilical cord area for the correct number of blood vessels (two arteries and one vein). The umbilical vein is larger than the two umbilical arteries. Evidence of only a single umbilical artery is associated with renal and gastrointestinal anomalies. Also inspect the umbilical area for signs of bleeding, infection, inflammation, redness, swelling, purulent drainage or bleeding, erythema around the umbilicus, granuloma, or abnormal communication with the intra-abdominal organs. Umbilical infections can occur because of an embryologic remnant or poor hygiene. Traditionally, gram-positive organisms, such as *Staphylococcus aureus* and *Streptococcus pyogens,* were most commonly identified, but gram-negative and polymicrobial infections are seen today. An umbilical cord infection (omphalitis) can spread to adjacent tissue, causing peritonitis, hepatic vein thrombosis, and hepatic abscess. Immediate evaluation and referral is needed (Lomax, 2015).

GENITALIA

Male. Inspect the penis and scrotum in the male. In the circumcised male newborn, the glans should be smooth, with the meatus centred at the tip of the penis. It will

FIGURE 18.16 Newborn genitalia. **A.** Male genitalia. Note the darkened colour of the scrotum. **B.** Female genitalia.

appear reddened until it heals. For the uncircumcised male, the foreskin should cover the glans. Check the position of the urinary meatus: it should be in the midline at the glans tip. If it is on the ventral surface of the penis, the condition is termed hypospadias; if it is on the dorsal surface of the penis, it is termed epispadias. In either case, **circumcision** should be avoided until further evaluation.

Inspect the scrotum for size, symmetry, colour, presence of rugae, and location of testes. The scrotum usually appears relatively large with well-formed rugae and that should cover the scrotal sac. There should not be bulging, edema, or discolouration (Fig. 18.16A).

Palpate the scrotum for evidence of the testes, which should be in the scrotal sac. The testes should feel firm and smooth and should be of equal size on both sides of the scrotal sac in the term newborn. Undescended testes (cryptorchidism) might be palpated in the inguinal canal in preterm infants; they can be unilateral or bilateral. If the testes are not palpable within the scrotal sac, further investigation is needed.

Female. In the female newborn, inspect the external genitalia. The urethral meatus is located below the clitoris in the midline (Mutter & Prat, 2014). In contrast to the male genitalia, the female genitalia will be engorged: the labia majora and minora may both be edematous. The labia majora is large and covers the labia minora. The clitoris is large and the hymen is thick. These findings are due to the maternal hormones estrogen and progesterone (Fig. 18.16B). A vaginal discharge composed of mucus mixed with blood may also be present during the first few weeks of life. This discharge, called **pseudomenstruation**, requires no treatment. Explain this phenomenon to the parents.

Variations in female newborns may include a labial bulge, which might indicate an inguinal hernia, ambiguous genitalia, a rectovaginal fistula with feces present in the vagina, and an imperforate hymen.

Male and Female. Inspect the anus in both male and female newborns for position and patency. Passage of meconium indicates patency. If meconium is not passed, a lubricated rectal thermometer can be inserted or a digital examination can be performed to determine patency. Abnormal findings would include anal fissures or fistulas and no meconium passed within 24 hours after birth.

EXTREMITIES AND BACK

Upper Extremities. Inspect the newborn's upper extremities for appearance and movement. Inspect the hands for shape, number, and position of fingers and presence of palmar creases. The newborn's arms and hands should be symmetric and should move through range of motion without hesitation. Observe for spontaneous movement of the extremities. Each hand should have five digits. Note any extra digits (polydactyly) or fusing of two or more digits (syndactyly). Most newborns have three palmar creases on the hand. A single palmar crease, called a simian line, is considered a soft marker (a possible association) for Down syndrome.

A brachial plexus injury can occur during a difficult birth involving shoulder dystocia. Erb palsy is an injury resulting from damage to the upper plexus, and palsies associated with the lower brachial plexus are termed Klumpke palsies. Factors associated with obstetric brachial plexus paralysis include large birth weight, breech delivery, labour anomalies, operative vaginal birth, and shoulder dystocia. Obstetric brachial plexus paralysis results from excessive lateral traction on the head away from the shoulder. This force on the brachial plexus can cause varying degrees of injury to the nerves. The affected arm hangs limp alongside the body, and the affected shoulder and arm are adducted, extended, and internally rotated with a pronated wrist. The Moro reflex is absent on the affected side in brachial palsy. Complete recovery may take 6 months or longer, and in some instances can lead to permanent functional impairment, including joint weakness, deformity, and limb length discrepancy. Current research studies support endogenous labour forces as the etiology

NURSING PROCEDURE 18.1

Performing Ortolani and Barlow Manoeuvers

Purpose: To Detect Congenital Developmental Dysplasia of the Hip

Ortolani Manoeuver

1. Place the newborn in the supine position and flex the hips and knees to 90 degrees at the hip.
2. Grasp the inner aspect of the thighs and abduct the hips (usually to approximately 180 degrees) while applying upward pressure.

3. Listen for any sounds during the manoeuver. There should be no "click" heard when the legs are abducted. Such a sound indicates the femoral head hitting the acetabulum as the head reenters the area. This suggests developmental hip dysplasia.

Barlow Manoeuver

1. With the newborn still lying supine and grasping the inner aspect of the thighs (as just mentioned), adduct the thighs while applying outward and downward pressure to the thighs.

2. Feel for the femoral head slipping out of the acetabulum; also listen for a click.

Adapted from Tamai, J., & McCarthy, J. J. (2018). Developmental dysplasia of the hip. *eMedicine*. Retrieved from http://emedicine.medscape.com/article/1248135-overview; and Weber, J., & Kelley, J. (2017). *Health assessment in nursing* (6th ed.). Philadelphia, PA: Lippincott Williams & Wilkins.

of this injury. Despite training in the management of shoulder dystocia and a rising institutional cesarean section rate, the incidence of brachial plexus injuries has remained unchanged compared with 10 years earlier (Coroneos et al., 2017; Tung & Moore, 2015).

Lower Extremities. Assess the lower extremities in the same manner. They should be of equal length, with symmetric skinfolds. Inspect the feet for clubfoot (a turning-inward position), which is secondary to intrauterine positioning. This may be positional or structural. Perform the Ortolani and Barlow manoeuvers to identify congenital hip dislocation, commonly termed developmental dysplasia of the hip (DDH). Nursing Procedure 18.1 highlights the steps for performing these manoeuvers. Table 18.4 summarizes the newborn assessment.

NEUROLOGIC STATUS

Assess the newborn's state of alertness, posture, muscle tone, and reflexes.

Newborn Alertness, Posture, and Muscle Tone. The newborn should be alert and not persistently lethargic. The normal posture is hips abducted and partially flexed, with knees flexed. Arms are adducted and flexed at the elbow. Fists are often clenched, with fingers covering the thumb.

To assess for muscle tone, support the newborn with one hand under the chest. Observe how the neck muscles hold the head. The neck extensors should be able to hold the head in line briefly. There should be only slight head lag when pulling the newborn from a supine position to a sitting one.

Newborn Reflexes. Assess the newborn's reflexes to evaluate neurologic function and development. Absent or abnormal reflexes in a newborn, persistence of a reflex past the age when the reflex is normally lost, or return of an infantile reflex in an older child or adult may indicate neurologic pathology (Table 18.5). Reflexes commonly assessed in the newborn include sucking,

TABLE 18.4	NEWBORN ASSESSMENT SUMMARY	
Assessment	Usual Findings	Variations and Common Problems
Anthropometric measurements	Head circumference: 33–37 cm (13–14 in) Chest circumference: 30–33 cm (12–13 in) Weight: 2,500–4,000 g (5.5–8.5 lb) Length: 45–55 cm (17–21 in)	SGA, LGA, preterm, postterm
Vital signs	Temperature: 36.5°–37.5°C (97°–99°F) Apical pulse: 110–160 bpm Respirations: 30–60 breaths/minute	
Skin	Expected: smooth, flexible, good skin turgor, well hydrated; warm	Jaundice, acrocyanosis, milia, Mongolian spots, stork bites
Head	Expected: varies with age, sex, ethnicity	Microcephaly, macrocephaly, enlarged fontanels
Face	Expected: full cheeks, facial features symmetric	Facial nerve paralysis, nevus flammeus, nevus vasculosus
Nose	Expected: small, placement in the midline and narrow, ability to smell	Malformation or blockage
Mouth	Expected: aligned in midline, symmetric, intact soft and hard palate	Epstein pearls, erupted precocious teeth, thrush
Neck	Expected: short, creased, moves freely, baby holds head in midline	Restricted movement, clavicular fractures
Eyes	Expected: clear and symmetrically placed on face; online with ears	Chemical conjunctivitis, subconjunctival hemorrhages
Ears	Expected: soft and pliable with quick recoil when folded and released	Low-set ears, hearing loss
Chest	Expected: round, symmetric, smaller than head	Nipple engorgement, whitish discharge
Abdomen	Expected: protuberant contour, soft, three vessels in umbilical cord	Distended, only two vessels in umbilical cord
Genitals	Expected in male: smooth glans, meatus centred at tip of penis Expected in female: swollen female genitals as a result of maternal estrogen	Edematous scrotum in males, vaginal discharge in females
Extremities and spine	Expected: extremities symmetric with free movement	Congenital hip dislocation; tuft or dimple on spine

Data from Davidson, M. R. (2014). *Fast facts for the neonatal nurse: A nursing orientation and care guide in a nutshell.* New York: Springer Publishing Company; and Weber, J., & Kelley, J. (2017). *Health assessment in nursing* (6th ed.). Philadelphia, PA: Lippincott Williams & Wilkins.

Moro, stepping, tonic neck, rooting, Babinski, palmar grasp, and plantar grasp reflexes. Spinal reflexes tested include truncal incurvation (Galant reflex) and anocutaneous reflex (anal wink).

The *sucking reflex* is elicited by gently stimulating the newborn's lips by touching them. The newborn will typically open the mouth and begin a sucking motion. Placing a gloved finger in the newborn's mouth will also elicit a sucking motion (Fig. 18.17A).

The *Moro reflex*, also called the embrace reflex, occurs when the neonate is startled. To elicit this reflex, place the newborn on his or her back. Support the upper body weight of the supine newborn by the arms, using a lifting motion, without lifting the newborn off the surface. Then release the arms suddenly. The newborn will throw the arms outward and flex the knees; the arms then return to the chest. The fingers also spread to form a C. The newborn initially appears startled and then relaxes to a normal resting position (Fig. 18.17B).

Assess the *stepping reflex* by holding the newborn upright and inclined forward with the soles of the feet touching a flat surface. The baby should make a stepping motion or walking, alternating flexion and extension with the soles of the feet (Fig. 18.17C).

The *tonic neck reflex* resembles the stance of a fencer and is often called the fencing reflex. Test this reflex by having the newborn lie on the back. Turn the baby's head to one side. The arm toward which the baby

TABLE 18.5	NEWBORN REFLEXES: APPEARANCE AND DISAPPEARANCE	
Reflex	**Appearance**	**Disappearance**
Blinking	Newborn	Persists into adulthood
Moro	Newborn	3–6 months
Grasp	Newborn	3–4 months
Stepping	Birth	1–2 months
Tonic neck	Newborn	3–4 months
Sneeze	Newborn	Persists into adulthood
Rooting	Birth	4–6 months
Gag reflex	Newborn	Persists into adulthood
Cough reflex	Newborn	Persists into adulthood
Babinski sign	Newborn	12 months

should fan out. A diminished response indicates a neurologic problem and requires follow-up (Fig. 18.17F).

The newborn exhibits two grasp reflexes: *palmar grasp* and *plantar grasp.* Elicit the palmar grasp reflex by placing a finger on the newborn's open palm. The baby's hand will close around the finger. Attempting to remove the finger causes the grip to tighten. Newborns have strong grasps and can almost be lifted from a flat surface if both hands are used. The grasp should be equal bilaterally (Fig. 18.17G). The plantar grasp is similar to the palmar grasp. Place a finger just below the newborn's toes. The toes typically curl over the finger (Fig. 18.17H).

Blinking, sneezing, gagging, and *coughing* are all protective reflexes and are elicited when an object or light is brought close to the eye (blinking), something irritating is swallowed or a bulb syringe is used for suctioning (gagging and coughing), or an irritant is brought close to the nose (sneezing).

The *truncal incurvation reflex (Galant reflex)* is present at birth and disappears in a few days to 4 weeks (Fig. 18.18). With the newborn in a prone position or held in ventral suspension, apply firm pressure and run a finger down either side of the spine. This stroking will cause the pelvis to flex toward the stimulated side. This indicates T2–S1 innervation. Lack of response indicates a neurologic or spinal cord problem.

The *anocutaneous reflex (anal wink)* is elicited by stimulating the perianal skin close to the anus. The external sphincter will constrict ("wink") immediately with stimulation. This indicates that innervation of the S4–S5 spinal nerves is intact (Marcdante & Kliegman, 2018).

is facing should extend straight away from the body with the hand partially open, whereas the arm on the side away from the face is flexed and the fist is clenched tightly. Reversing the direction to which the face is turned reverses the position (Fig. 18.17D).

Elicit the *rooting reflex* by stroking the newborn's cheek. The newborn will turn toward the side that was stroked and should begin to make sucking movements (Fig. 18.17E).

The *Babinski reflex* should be present at birth and disappears at approximately 1 year of age. It is elicited by stroking the lateral sole of the newborn's foot from the heel toward and across the ball of the foot. The toes

FIGURE 18.17 Newborn reflexes. **A.** Sucking reflex. **B.** Moro reflex. (*continued*)

FIGURE 18.17 (*continued*) **C.** Stepping reflex. **D.** Tonic neck reflex. **E.** Rooting reflex. **F.** Babinski reflex.

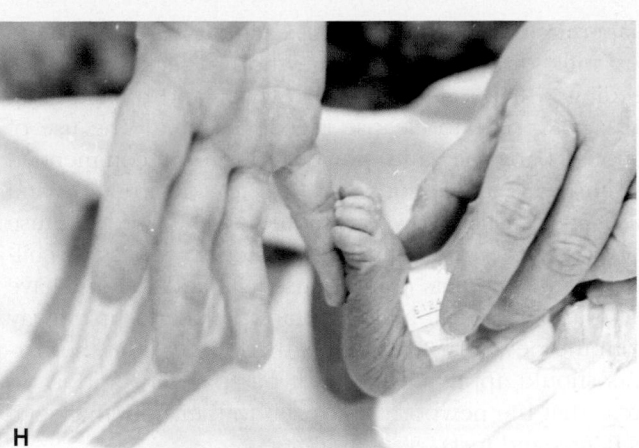

FIGURE 18.17 *(continued)* **G.** Palmar grasp. **H.** Plantar grasp.

Nursing Interventions

Developing confidence in caring for their newborn is challenging for most parents. It takes time and patience and a great deal of instruction provided by the nurse. "Showing and telling" parents about their newborn and all the procedures (e.g., feeding, bathing, changing, handling) involved in daily care are key nursing interventions.

Providing General Newborn Care

In general, newborn care involves bathing and hygiene, elimination and diaper area care, cord care, circumcision care, environmental safety measures, and prevention of infection. Nurses should teach these skills to parents and should serve as role models for appropriate and consistent interaction with newborns. Demonstrating respect for the newborn and family helps foster a

FIGURE 18.18 Trunk incurvation reflex. When the paravertebral area is stroked, the newborn flexes his or her trunk toward the direction of the stimulation.

positive atmosphere to promote the newborn's growth and development.

BATHING AND HYGIENE

Immediately after birth, drying the newborn and removing blood may minimize the risk of infection caused by hepatitis B, herpes simplex virus, and HIV, but the specific benefits of this practice remain unclear. Until the newborn has been thoroughly bathed, standard precautions should be used when handling the newborn. Nurses need to follow their hospital policies regarding the timing and procedures for newborn bathing and hygiene.

Newborns are bathed primarily for aesthetic reasons, and bathing is postponed until the newborn has established thermal and cardiorespiratory stability. Traditional reasons why nurses bathe the newborn are so they can conduct a physical assessment, reduce the effect of hypothermia, and allow the parent(s) to rest (Davidson, 2014). However, recent research suggests that nurses do not need to give the newborn an initial bath to reduce heat loss; rather, the parents could be given this opportunity, supported by nurses. A study found that the amount of heat loss was similar in newborns bathed by parents versus newborns who were bathed by nurses (Davidson, 2014). Current recommendations involve waiting at least 8 hours after birth until the first bath to allow vernix caseosa to moisturize the skin naturally, and allow the infant time to adjust to extrauterine life (Smith & Shell, 2017).

It is important for the nurse to assist the parent(s) to perform the bath efficiently, drying the baby thoroughly to prevent heat loss by evaporation. After bathing, place the newborn skin-to-skin with a parent, covered by a warm blanket, to prevent chilling. Check the baby's temperature within an hour to make sure it is within normal limits. If it is low, consider use of a radiant warmer.

After the initial bath, the newborn may not receive another full one during the stay in the birthing unit. The diaper area will be cleansed at each diaper change, and any milk dripped into the newborn's neck folds from feeding will be cleaned. Clear water and a mild soap are appropriate to cleanse the diaper area. The use of lotions, baby oil, and powders is not recommended because oils and lotions can lead to skin irritation and can cause rashes. Powders should not be used because they can be inhaled, causing respiratory illness in children. If the parents want to use oils and lotions, have them apply a small amount onto their hand first, away from the newborn; this warms the lotion. Then the parents should apply the lotion or oil sparingly, and avoid areas that the newborn can reach to their mouths (such as hands and feet).

Encourage the parent(s) to gather all items needed before starting the bath: one or two soft, clean washcloths; two cotton balls to clean the eyes; mild, unscented soap and shampoo; towels or blankets; a tub or basin with warm water; a clean diaper; and a change of clothes. Instruct parents that a frequency of two baths per week is sufficient for the 1st year; more frequent bathing may dry the skin. If the newborn has been circumcised, advise parents to wait until that area has also healed (usually 1 to 2 weeks) before submersing the baby in water; instead, teach them to perform a sponge bath. Parents should be taught to clean the circumcised penis with mild soap and water and apply a small amount of petroleum jelly to the tip to prevent the diaper from adhering to the penis. Instruct parents to apply the diaper loosely and place the newly circumcised male infant on his side or back to prevent pressure and irritation on the penis.

Other guidelines for bathing newborns are given in Teaching Guidelines 18.1.

Teaching Guidelines 18.1
BATHING A NEWBORN

- Select a warm room with a flat surface at a comfortable working height.
- Before the bath, gather all supplies needed so they will be within reach.
- Never leave the newborn alone or unattended at any time during the bath.
- Undress the newborn down to shirt and diaper.
- Always support the newborn's head and neck when moving or positioning him or her.
- Place a blanket or towel underneath the newborn for warmth and comfort.
- In this order, progressing from the cleanest to the dirtiest areas:
  - Wipe eyes with plain water, using either cotton balls or a washcloth. Wipe from the inner corner of the eyes to the outer with separate wipes.
  - Wash the rest of the face, including ears, with plain water.
  - Using baby shampoo, gently wash the hair and rinse with water.
  - Pay special attention to body creases, and dry thoroughly.
  - Wash extremities, trunk, and back. Wash, rinse, dry, cover.
  - Wash diaper area last, using soap and water, and dry; observe for rash.
- Put on a clean diaper and clean clothes after the bath.

ELIMINATION AND DIAPER AREA CARE

Newborn elimination patterns are highly individualized. Usually the urine is light amber in colour. Soaking at least six diapers a day indicates adequate hydration. Stools can change in colour, texture, and frequency without signalling a problem. Meconium is passed for the first 48 hours after birth; the stools appear thick, tarry, sticky, and dark green. Transitional stools (thin, brown to green, less sticky than meconium) typically appear by day 3. The stool characteristics after transitional stool depend on whether the newborn is breastfed or formula fed. Breast-fed newborns typically pass mustard-coloured, soft stool with a seedy consistency; formula-fed newborns pass yellow to brown, soft stools with a pasty consistency. As long as the newborn seems content, is eating normally, and shows no signs of illness, minor changes in bowel movements should not be a concern.

The newborn needs to be checked frequently to see whether a diaper change is needed, especially after feeding. Adhere to standard precautions when providing diaper area care. Instruct parents to keep the top edge of the diaper folded down below the umbilical cord area to prevent irritation and to allow air to help dry the cord. Teach all parents to wipe a female's diaper area from front to back, with a clean wipe, each time, to avoid urinary tract infections. For a male infant, instruct parents to point the penis down to prevent urine from wetting the top of the diaper where the umbilicus is located.

Meconium can be difficult to remove from the skin. Use plain water or special cleansing wipes if necessary to clean the area. Teach parents how to clean the diaper area properly and how to prevent skin irritation. Encourage them to avoid products such as powder and fragranced items, which could irritate the newborn's skin.

Discuss the pros and cons of using cloth diapers versus disposable diapers so that the parents can make informed decisions. Regardless of the type of diapers used, up to 10 diapers a day, or about 70 a week, will be needed.

Additional information about diapering might include:
- Before diapering, make sure all supplies are within reach, including clean diaper, cleaning agent or wipes, and ointment.
- Lay the newborn on a changing table and remove the dirty diaper.

- Use water and mild soap or wipes to gently wipe the genital area clean; wipe from front to back for girls.
- Wash your hands thoroughly before and after changing diapers.

While performing diaper area care, parents should observe the area closely for irritation or rash. Tips for preventing or healing a diaper rash include:

- Change diapers frequently, especially after bowel movements.
- Apply a "barrier" cream containing zinc after cleaning with mild soap and water.
- Use dye- and fragrance-free detergents to wash cloth diapers.
- Avoid the use of plastic pants, because they tend to hold in moisture.
- Expose the newborn's bottom to air several times a day.
- Place the newborn's buttocks in warm water after he or she has had a diaper on all night.

Take Note!

Advise parents that a rash that persists for more than 3 days may be fungal in origin and may require additional treatment. Encourage the parents to notify their health care provider.

CORD CARE

The umbilical cord begins drying within hours after birth and is shrivelled and darkened by the 2nd or 3rd day. Within 7 to 10 days, it sloughs off and the umbilicus heals. During this transition, frequent assessments of the area are necessary to detect any bleeding or signs of infection. Cord bleeding is abnormal and may occur if the cord clamp is loosened. Any cord drainage is also abnormal and is generally caused by infection, which requires immediate treatment.

Previously, health care practices concerning the umbilical cord included teaching parents to clean the stump with rubbing alcohol or an antimicrobial agent, however research over the years has demonstrated no apparent benefit to these practices compared to allow the cord to dry naturally (Dore et al., 1998; Zupan, Garner, & Omari, 2004).

Some facilities will remove the cord clamp approximately 24 hours after birth by using a cord-cutting clamp. However, if the cord is still moist, keep the clamp in place. Other facilities will leave the clamp in place, where it remains until the umbilical stump heals and falls off. Always adhere to agency policies regarding cord care; changes in policy may be necessary based on new research findings.

Many parents avoid contact with the cord site to make sure they don't "bother" it. Teach them how to care for the cord site when they go home to prevent complications (Teaching Guidelines 18.2).

Teaching Guidelines 18.2
UMBILICAL CORD CARE

- Observe for bleeding, redness, drainage, or foul odour from the cord stump and report it to your newborn's primary care provider immediately.
- Expose the cord stump to the air as much as possible throughout the day.
- Fold diapers below the level of the cord to prevent contamination of the site and to promote air-drying of the cord.
- Observe the cord stump, which will change colour from yellow to brown to black. This is normal.
- Never pull the cord or attempt to loosen it; it will fall off naturally.

CIRCUMCISION AND CARE OF THE PENIS

Circumcision is one of the oldest and most common surgical procedures performed worldwide, but the practice remains controversial. Over the past several decades, the number of circumcisions performed on newborn males has decreased in Canada and the United States. Both the Canadian Paediatric Society and the AAP have each published position statements indicating that circumcision is not medically indicated as a routine practice. It may still be performed for medical, religious, cultural, and social reasons. Circumcision is the surgical removal of all or part of the foreskin (prepuce) of the penis (Freedman & Hurwitz, 2015). This has been traditionally done for hygiene and medical reasons and is the oldest known religious rite. In the Jewish faith, circumcision is a ritual that is performed by a *mohel* (ordained circumciser) on the 8th day after birth if possible. The circumcision is followed by a *bris* (the Jewish religious ceremony), typically in the home, during which the newborn is named and symbolically enters the Jewish religious community.

The debate over routine newborn circumcision continues in the United States. For many years, the purported benefits and harms of circumcision have been debated in the medical literature and society at large, with no clear consensus to date. Despite the controversy, circumcision is the most common surgical procedure performed on newborns, and almost two thirds (61%) of American male newborns are circumcised (Owings, Uddin, & Williams, 2015).

Position Statement by Canadian Paediatric Society. The position statement by the CPS (Sorokan, Finlay, Jefferies, & Canadian Paediatric Society Fetus and Newborn Committee, 2018) indicates that newborn circumcision has potential disadvantages and risks as well as medical benefits and advantages. Risks to the newborn include infection, hemorrhage, skin dehiscence, adhesions, urethral fistula, and pain. Benefits to the newborn include the following:

- Urinary tract infections are slightly less common in circumcised boys. However, rates are low in both circumcised and uncircumcised boys and are easily treated without long-term sequelae.
- Sexually transmitted infections are less common in circumcised males, but the risk is believed to be related more to behavioural factors than to circumcision status. However, circumcised males have a 50% lower risk of acquiring HIV infection, herpes simplex virus, human papillomavirus (HPV), genital ulcer disease, bacterial vaginosis, and trichomoniasis (Tobian, Kacker, & Quinn, 2014).
- There appears to be a slightly lower rate of penile cancer in circumcised males. However, penile cancer is rare and risk factors such as genital warts, infection with HPV, multiple sex partners, and cigarette smoking seem to play a much larger role in causing penile cancer than circumcision status (Marcdante & Kliegman, 2018).

The CPS recommendations state that if parents decide to circumcise their newborn, pain relief must be provided. Research has found that newborns circumcised without analgesia experience pain and stress, indicated by changes in heart rate, blood pressure, oxygen saturation, and cortisol levels (Morrison, Herbst, Corbett, & Herndon, 2014). Analgesic methods may include EMLA® cream (a topical mixture of local anesthetics, lidocaine and prilocaine), a dorsal penile nerve block with buffered lidocaine, acetaminophen, skin-to-skin contact, a sucrose pacifier, and swaddling (Cunningham et al., 2018).

The CPS recommends that parents be given accurate and unbiased information about the risks and benefits of circumcision. As with other newborn procedures, research continues. Nurses must keep informed about current medical research to allow parents to make informed decisions. The absence of compelling medical evidence in favour of or against newborn circumcision makes informed consent of parents of paramount importance. The circumcision discussion involves cultural, religious, medical, and emotional considerations. Nurses may have difficulty remaining unbiased and unemotional as they present the facts to parents. Circumcision is a very personal decision for parents, and the nurse's major responsibility is to inform the parents of the risks and benefits of the procedure and to address concerns so that the parents can reach a fully informed decision.

Most circumcisions are performed in the hospital before the newborn is discharged as this is convenient for parents in facilities where the practice is offered. Circumcision may also be performed in a doctor's outpatient office after discharge. There are three commonly used methods of circumcision: the Gomco clamp, the Hollister Plastibell device, and the Mogen clamp. During the circumcision procedure, part of the foreskin is removed by clamping and cutting with a scalpel (Gomco or Mogen clamp) or by using a Plastibell. The Plastibell is fitted over the glans, and the excess foreskin is pulled over the plastic ring. A suture is tied around the rim to apply pressure to the blood vessels, creating hemostasis. The excess foreskin is cut away. The plastic rim remains in place until healing occurs. The plastic ring typically loosens and falls off in approximately 1 week. Petroleum jelly should be applied to the circumcised area after the procedure is done with the Gomco or Mogen clamp (Fig. 18.19) (Sinkey et al., 2015).

Take Note!

The decision to circumcise the male newborn is often a social one, with the strongest factor being whether the newborn's father is himself circumcised (Mielke, 2014).

Preoperative circumcision preparation should include confirmation of the following:

- Infant is at least 12 hours old or older
- Infant has received standard vitamin K prophylaxis

FIGURE 18.19 Circumcision. **A.** Before the procedure. **B.** Clamp applied and foreskin removed. **C.** Appearance after circumcision.

- Infant has voided normally at least once since birth
- Infant has not eaten for at least an hour prior to the procedure
- Written parental informed consent has been obtained
- Correct identification of the infant brought to procedure room

Immediately after circumcision, the tip of the penis is usually covered with petroleum jelly–coated gauze to keep the wound from sticking to the diaper. Continued care of this site includes:

- Assess for bleeding every 30 minutes for at least 2 hours.
- Document the first voiding to evaluate for urinary obstruction or edema.
- Squeeze soapy water over the area daily and then rinse with warm water. Pat dry.
- Apply a small amount of petroleum jelly with every diaper change if the Plastibell was used; clean with mild soap and water if other techniques were used.
- Fasten the diaper loosely over the penis and avoiding placing the newborn on his abdomen to prevent friction.

If a Plastibell has been used, it will fall off by itself in about a week. Inform parents of this and advise them not to pull it off sooner. Also instruct the parents to check daily for any foul-smelling drainage, bleeding, or unusual swelling.

For uncircumcised newborns, teach parents to wash the penis with mild soap and water after each diaper change and do not force the foreskin back; it will retract normally over time. Parents should be informed that forceful retraction of the foreskin prior to the natural release of adhesions can lead to cracking, bleeding, and scarring of the foreskin tissue (Canadian Urological Association, 2014).

SAFETY

Newborns are completely dependent on those around them for safety. Their safety must be ensured while in the health care facility and after they are discharged. Parental education is key, especially as the newborn grows and develops and begins to respond to and explore his or her surroundings (Teaching Guidelines 18.3).

 Teaching Guidelines 18.3
GENERAL NEWBORN SAFETY

- Have emergency telephone numbers readily available, such as those for emergency medical assistance and the poison control centre.
- Keep small or sharp objects out of reach to prevent them from being aspirated.
- Put safety plugs in wall sockets within the child's reach to prevent electrocution.

- Always supervise the newborn in the tub: a newborn can drown in 5 cm of water.
- Make sure the crib or changing table is sturdy, without any loose hardware, and is painted with lead-free paint.
- Avoid placing the crib or changing table near blinds or curtain cords.
- Provide a smoke-free environment for all infants.
- Place all infants on their backs to sleep to reduce the risk of sudden infant death syndrome.
- To prevent falls, do not leave the newborn alone on any elevated surface.
- Use sun shields on strollers and hats to avoid overexposing the newborn to the sun.
- To prevent infection, thoroughly wash your hands before preparing food, or handling the baby.
- Thoroughly investigate any infant care facility before using it (Health Canada, 2016).

Environmental Safety. People who enter a health care facility for treatment expect to be safe there until they return home, but ensuring a safe environment can be a daunting challenge to a health care facility.

Consider this scenario: A woman dressed in nurse's clothing entered the hospital room of a new mother soon after she had given birth. This "nurse" told the mother she needed to take her newborn to the nursery to have him weighed. Sometime later, a staff nurse making her routine rounds realized something was wrong when she saw that the newborn's bassinet in the mother's room was empty and the mother was sound asleep in her bed. The staff nurse called security immediately because she suspected that a newborn abduction had taken place.

This abduction scenario has, unfortunately, been repeated many times across North America in recent years. In infant abduction, someone who is not a family member takes a child less than 1 year old (NCMEC, 2015). Infant abductions are traumatic for the parents, the community, and the health care facility. The facility may also face huge financial liability if a lawsuit is filed by the parents.

Abductions typically occur during the day and are usually carried out by women who are not criminally sophisticated. Many of these women experienced a pregnancy loss in the past; they are often emotionally unstable and compulsive, with low self-esteem. Most female abductors can play the role of a hospital employee convincingly. Infants usually are abducted when taken for testing, during transport from one area to another, when left unattended, or while a parent was napping or showering (Joint Commission, 2018).

Health care agencies are challenged to prevent infant abduction by instituting sound security practices and systems (Joint Commission, 2018). Such measures include the following:

- All newborns must be transported in cribs and not carried.
- Nurses must respond immediately to any security alarm that sounds on the unit.
- Newborns must never be unattended at any time, especially in hallways.
- All staff must wear appropriate identification at all times.
- Encourage parents to keep their baby/bassinet on their far side, away from the door.
- Personnel should be wary of visitors who do not seem to be visiting a specific family.
- The electronic security system should be checked to make sure it is functional.
- Discontinue publication of birth notices in local newspapers.
- Develop and implement a proactive infant abduction prevention plan.
- Ensure the proper functioning and placement of any electronic sensors used on newborns.
- Parents should be taught what infant abduction is; why infant security is important; the schedule of nursery, feeding, and visiting hours; rules about visitor access; the facility's security policies and procedures; what parents can do to protect their infant in the hospital; which staff members are allowed to handle the newborn; and what a proper ID looks like.

Educating staff, educating parents, and access control are the three key steps to preventing abductions from any health care facility. Providing a safe and secure environment is a shared responsibility of the facility, staff, and parents. Preventing abductions requires everyone to learn and follow the rules and policies.

Car Safety. Every province requires the use of car seats for infants and children, because motor vehicle accidents are still the leading cause of unintentional injury and death in children under age 5. National Highway Traffic Safety Administration statistics show that nearly one half of deaths and injuries in infants occurred because they were not properly restrained. Child safety seats, when installed and used properly, can prevent injuries and save lives (AAP, 2015).

Despite evidence that the use of car seats can reduce the morbidity and mortality of motor vehicle crashes, parents who lack knowledge about them may underuse or misuse them (Hodges & Smith, 2014). Make sure that parents understand the importance of safely transporting their newborn in a federally approved safety car seat every time the infant rides in a car. Do not release any newborn unless the parents have a car seat in place for their newborn's ride home (Fig. 18.20). If they cannot afford one, many community organizations will provide one for them. According to the AAP's policy statement on child passenger safety

FIGURE 18.20 Newborn in a properly secured car seat.

(2015), no one car seat is considered to be the "safest" or the "best," but rather consistent and proper use is the key to preventing injuries and deaths. Instruct parents in the following:

- Select a car seat that is appropriate for the child's size and weight.
- Avoid cross-border shopping for a carseat: the Canadian safety standard is higher than in other countries. Use of a car seat without a National Safety Mark is illegal in Canada.
- Caution caregivers against the placement of car seats on elevated or soft surfaces outside the car to prevent falling.
- Use the car seat correctly, every time the child is in the car.
- Use rear-facing car safety seats for most infants up to 2 years of age or until they reach the highest weight or height allowed by the manufacturer of their CSS.
- Make sure the harness (most seats have a three- to five-point harness) is in the slots at or below the shoulders. Go to thePoint for Transport Canada's *Child Car Seat Safety* guidelines.

INFECTION PREVENTION

The nurse plays a major role in preventing infection in the newborn environment. Ways to control infection are as follows:

- Minimize exposure of newborns to organisms.
- Wash your hands before and after providing care, and insist that all personnel wash their hands before handling any newborn.
- Do not allow ill staff or visitors to visit or handle newborns.
- Avoid sharing any infant supplies with another infant.
- Monitor the umbilical cord stump and circumcision site for signs of infection.
- Provide eye prophylaxis by instilling erythromycin ointment soon after birth.

- Educate parents about appropriate home measures that will prevent infections, such as practicing good hand hygiene before and after diaper changes, keeping the newborn well hydrated, avoiding taking the infant into crowds (which may expose him or her to colds and flu viruses), observing for early signs of infection (fever, vomiting, loss of appetite, lethargy, laboured breathing, green watery stools, drainage from umbilical cord site or eyes), and keeping appointments for routine **immunizations**.

Promoting Sleep

Although many parents feel their newborns need them every minute of the day, babies actually need to sleep much of the day initially. Usually newborns sleep up to 15 hours daily. They sleep for 2 to 4 hours at a time but do not sleep through the night because their stomach capacity is too small to go long periods without nourishment.

Take Note!

All newborns develop their own sleep patterns and cycles, but it may take several months before the newborn sleeps through the night. Frequently, newborns have their day and night hours reversed and tend to sleep more during the daytime and less during the night.

Parents should place the newborn on his or her back to sleep. To prevent suffocation, all fluffy bedding, quilts, sheepskins, stuffed animals, and pillows should be removed from the sleep surface. Parents should be informed that the practice of "bed sharing" (having a baby sleep in the same bed as their parent[s]) is not safe. For example, infants who sleep in adult beds are more likely to suffocate than those who sleep in cribs (Task Force on Sudden Infant Death Syndrome, 2016). Suffocation can occur when the infant gets entangled in bedding or caught under pillows, or slips between the bed and the wall or the headboard and mattress. The parent may accidentally roll against or on top of the baby. The safest place for a newborn to sleep is in a crib or bassinette in their parents' room, without any movable objects close by. Benefits versus risks of a baby sleeping in the same bed with their parent(s) include:

- *Benefits*—Ease of breastfeeding; increases bonding time between infant and parent(s); promotes skin-to-skin contact; and may increase parental vigilance over infant.
- *Risks*—Increases risk for sudden infant death syndrome (SIDS), particularly for infants younger than 4 months; risk of death if parent rolls over the infant; interrupts infant sleeping patterns; risk of asphyxia due to entrapment or airway obstruction; and unsafe design of adult beds for infants (Health Canada, 2018).

Teach parents the safest sleep practices for their baby at home: Babies should be placed on their backs to sleep on a firm mattress, without the use of blankets, pillows, plush toys, or bumper pads, in their own crib/bassinet, ideally in the same room as their parent(s) for at least the first 4 months of life.

Parents should also be taught that exposure to tobacco smoke, alcohol, and illicit drugs or a high room temperature (causing overheating) are additional modifiable risk factors for SIDS; while breastfeeding offers protective benefits (Public Health Agency of Canada, Canadian Paediatric Society, Canadian Foundation for the Study of Infant Deaths, & Canadian Institute of Child Health, Health Canada, 2011). Recommendations for safe infant sleeping practices are an important aspect of education for new parents. It is important for nurses to assess families' cultural beliefs and their prior practices to fully understand how to make recommendations in a culturally sensitive manner. Health Canada's *Safe Sleep* campaign (2018) recommends that all parents receive the following information to reduce the risk of SIDS:

- Provide a smoke-free environment, before and after the baby is born.
- Breastfeeding provides protection against SIDS.
- Always place the baby on his or her back to sleep, at every naptime and night time.
- Provide the baby with a safe sleep environment that has a firm surface and no pillows, comforters, quilts, or bumper pads.
- Place the baby to sleep in a crib, cradle, or bassinet next to your bed.

Enhancing Bonding

Encourage and enhance parent—newborn interaction by involving parents with the baby and demonstrating appropriate nurturing behaviours:

- Say "hello" and introduce yourself to the newborn.
- Ask parents' permission to care for and hold their newborn. This helps parents to realize that they are responsible for their child and reminds nurses of their role.
- Show parents the power of a soothing voice to calm the newborn (Fig. 18.21).
- Provide care to the newborn in the least stressful way.
- Demonstrate ways to gently wake up the newborn for effective feeding.
- Tell parents what you are doing, why you are doing it, and how they can duplicate what you are doing at home.
- Offer the opportunity for parents to perform care while you observe them. Support their efforts to soothe the newborn throughout the care process.
- Help parents to interpret the communication cues the newborn uses.
- Point out the efforts the newborn is making to connect with the parents (e.g., alerting to the familiar voice,

FIGURE 18.21 **The father uses a soothing voice to calm the newborn.**

following the parents while they are speaking, quieting when held securely).

One of the most pleasurable aspects of newborn care is being close to them. Bonding begins soon after birth when parents cradle their newborn and gently stroke him or her with their fingers. Provide parents with opportunities for skin-to-skin contact with the newborn, holding the baby against their own skin with every feeding and at other times. Many newborns respond very positively to gentle massage. If necessary, recommend books and videos that cover the subject.

For newborns, crying is their only way to communicate that something is wrong. Try to find out the reason why: Is the diaper wet? Is the room too hot or too cold? Is the baby uncomfortable (e.g., diaper rash or tight clothing)? Suggest the following ways in which parents can soothe an upset newborn:

• Try feeding or burping to relieve air or stomach gas.
• Lightly rub the newborn's back and speak softly to him or her.
• Gently sway side to side, or rock back and forth in a rocking chair.
• Talk with the newborn while making eye contact.
• Take the newborn for a walk in a stroller or carriage to get fresh air.
• Change the (awake) baby's position from back to side or vice versa.
• Try singing, reciting poetry and nursery rhymes, or reading to the baby.
• Give more physical contact by walking, rocking, or patting the newborn.

Assisting With Screening Tests

Newborn screening has been among the most successful public health programs of the 21st century. Screening newborns for problems is important because some potentially life-threatening metabolic diseases may not be obvious at birth. Newborn screening tests that are routine before discharge are used to check for certain genetic and inborn errors of metabolism and hearing. Early identification and initiation of treatment can prevent significant complications and can minimize the negative effects of untreated disease.

GENETIC AND INBORN ERRORS OF METABOLISM SCREENING

Although each province and state mandates which conditions must be tested, the most common screening tests are for PKU, hypothyroidism, galactosemia, and sickle cell disease (Table 18.6).

The trend toward early discharge of newborns can affect the timing of screening and the accuracy of some test results. For example, the newborn needs to ingest enough milk to elevate phenylalanine levels for the screening test to identify PKU accurately, so newborn screening for PKU testing should not be performed before 24 hours of age.

Screening tests for genetic and inborn errors of metabolism require a few drops of blood taken from the newborn's heel (Fig. 18.22). These tests are usually performed shortly before discharge. Newborns who are discharged before 24 hours of age need to have repeat tests done within a week in an outpatient facility.

Be aware of which conditions your province regularly screens for at birth to ensure that the parents are taught about the tests and the importance of early treatment. Also be familiar with the optimal time frame for screening and conditions that could affect the results. Ensure that a satisfactory specimen has been obtained at the appropriate time and that circumstances that could cause false results have been minimized. Send out specimens and completed forms within 24 hours of collection to the appropriate laboratory (Nagtalon-Ramos, 2014).

HEARING SCREENING

Hearing loss is one of the most common birth disorders: approximately 3 to 5 newborns out of every 1,000 live births have some degree of hearing loss. Unlike a physical deformity, hearing loss is not clinically detectable at birth and thus remains difficult to assess (Patel et al., 2018). Factors associated with an increased risk of hearing loss include:

• Family history of hereditary childhood sensory hearing loss
• Congenital infections such as cytomegalovirus, rubella, toxoplasmosis, or herpes
• Craniofacial anomalies involving the pinna or ear canal

| TABLE 18.6 | SELECTED CONDITIONS SCREENED FOR IN THE NEWBORN |

Condition	Description	Clinical Picture/Effect If Not Treated	Treatment	Timing of Screening
PKU	Autosomal recessive inherited deficiency in one of the enzymes necessary for the metabolism of phenylalanine to tyrosine—essential amino acids found in most foods	Irritability, vomiting of protein feedings, and a musty odour to the skin or body secretions of the newborn; without early intervention: mental and motor retardation, seizures, microcephaly, and poor growth and development	Lifetime diet of foods low in phenylalanine (low protein) and monitoring of blood levels; special newborn formulas available	Universally screened for in Canada; testing is done 24–48 hours after protein feeding (PKU)
Congenital hypothyroidism	Deficiency of thyroid hormone necessary for healthy brain growth, calorie metabolism, and development; may result from maternal hypothyroidism	Increased risk in newborns with birth weight <2,000 g or >4,500 g, and those of Hispanic and Asian descent; feeding problems, growth and breathing problems; if not treated, irreversible brain damage and intellectual disability before age one	Lifelong thyroid replacement therapy	Testing (measures thyroxin [T_4] and TSH) is done between days 4 and 6 of life
Galactosemia	Absence of the enzyme needed for the conversion of the milk sugar galactose to glucose	Poor weight gain, vomiting, jaundice, mood changes, loss of eyesight, seizures, and intellectual disability; if untreated, galactose buildup causing permanent damage to the brain, eyes, and liver, and eventually death	Eliminate milk from diet; substitute soy milk	First test done on discharge from the hospital with a follow-up test within 1 month
Sickle cell anemia	Recessively inherited abnormality in hemoglobin structure, most commonly found in people of African descent	Anemia developing shortly after birth; increased risk for infection, growth restriction, vaso-occlusive crisis	Maintenance of hydration and hemodilution, rest, electrolyte replacement, pain management, blood replacement, and antibiotics	Bloodspot obtained at same time of other newborn screening tests or prior to 3 months of age

Adapted from Bhattacharya, K., Wotton, T., & Wiley, V. (2014). The evolution of blood-spot newborn screening. *Translational Pediatrics, 3*(2), 63–70; Boyle, C. A., Bocchini, J. A., & Kelly, J. (2014). Reflections on 50 years of newborn screening. *Pediatrics, 133*(6), 961 963; and Greene, C. L., & Matern, D. (2014). Newborn screening for inborn errors of metabolism. In N. Blau, M. Duran, K. M. Gibson, & C. Dionisi-Vici, (Eds.). *Physician's guide to the diagnosis, treatment, and follow-up of inherited metabolic diseases* (pp. 719–735). Berlin Heidelberg, Germany: Springer Publishers.

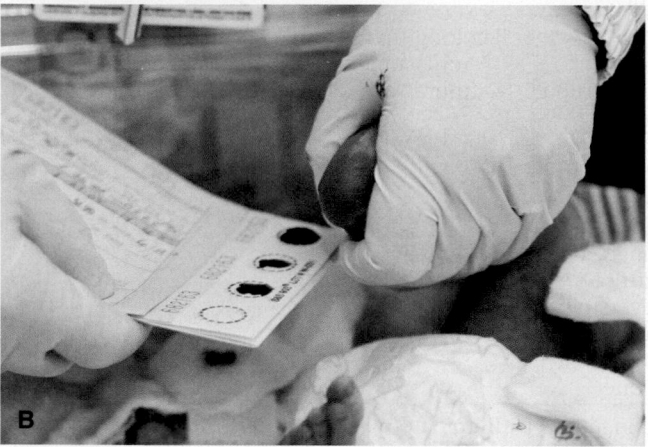

FIGURE 18.22 Screening for PKU. **A.** Performing a heel stick. **B.** Applying the blood specimen to the card for screening.

BOX 18.1

NEWBORN HEARING SCREENING METHODS

Newborn hearing screening is the standard of care in hospitals nationwide. The primary purpose of newborn hearing screening is to identify newborns who are likely to have a hearing loss and who require further evaluation. A newborn's hearing can be screened in one of two ways: otoacoustic emission (OAE) or automated auditory brain stem response (ABR).

In OAE, an earphone is placed in the infant's ear canal and the sounds produced by the newborn's inner ear are measured in response to certain tones or clicks presented through the earphone. Preset parameters in the equipment decide whether the OAEs are sufficient for the newborn to pass or whether a referral is necessary for further evaluation.

In ABR, an earphone is placed in the ear canal or an earmuff is placed over the newborn's ear, and a soft, rapid tapping noise is presented. Electrodes placed around the newborn's head, neck, and shoulders record neural activity from the infant's brain stem in response to the tapping noises. The ABR tests how well the ear and the nerves leading to the brain work. Like OAEs, automated ABR screening is sensitive to more than mild degrees of hearing loss, but a "pass" does not guarantee normal hearing.

Adapted from Patel, H., Feldman, M., & Canadian Paediatric Society, Community Paediatrics Committee. (2018). *Canadian Paediatric Society position statement: Universal newborn hearing screening*. Retrieved from https://www.cps.ca/en/documents/position/universal-hearing-screening-newborns; American Speech-Language-Hearing Association [ASHA]. (2018). *Newborn hearing screening*. Retrieved from https://www.asha.org/practice-portal/professional-issues/newborn-hearing-screening/

- Very low birth weight (less than 1,500 g)
- Postnatal infections such as bacterial meningitis
- Head trauma
- Hyperbilirubinemia requiring an exchange transfusion
- Exposure to ototoxic drugs, especially aminoglycosides
- Perinatal asphyxia (Nikolopoulos, 2015)

Delays in identification and intervention may affect the child's language development, academic performance, and cognitive development. Detection before 3 months greatly improves outcomes. Because of this, auditory screening programs for all newborns are recommended by the CPS (Patel et al., 2018). Screening only infants with risk factors is not enough, because as many as 50% of infants born with hearing loss have no known risk factors (CDC, 2017). Early identification and intervention can prevent severe psychosocial, educational, and language development delays.

The CPS recommends screening all infants by 1 month of age, confirming hearing loss with an audiologic examination by 3 months of age, and treat with comprehensive early intervention services before 6 months of age. All newborns should be screened prior to discharge to ensure that any newborn with a hearing loss is not missed. The methods of newborn hearing screening are described in Box 18.1. Those with suspected hearing loss should be referred for follow-up assessment. In addition, nurses should ensure that testing is accurate to facilitate early diagnosis and intervention services and to optimize the newborn's developmental potential. The implementation of newborn hearing screenings has lowered the mean age of hearing loss identification and many deaf children are now diagnosed in the early age of months old.

CCHD SCREEN

Most provinces and states are now doing critical congenital heart disease (CCHD) screen on all newborns after 24 hours of life before discharge.

CCHD refers to a group of serious heart defects that can affect the structure or vessels of the heart and are present from birth. CCHD prevents the heart from pumping blood effectively or reduces the amount of oxygen in the blood. Either can lead to organ damage and life-threatening complications. These conditions are called *critical* because they require surgery or intervention in the 1st year of life to ensure healthy outcomes for the baby.

Unfortunately, prenatal ultrasound detects only about half of CCHD. Changes in the structure and function of the newborn heart can lead to CCHD going unrecognized during the newborn hospital stay. Pulse oximetry newborn screening can identify some infants with CCHD before they show signs of the condition, resulting in better outcomes for the baby (Newborn Screening Ontario, 2018).

Common Concerns

During the newborn period of transition, certain conditions can develop that require intervention. These conditions, although not typically life-threatening, can be a source of anxiety for the parents. Common concerns include transient tachypnea of the newborn, physiologic jaundice, and hypoglycemia.

TRANSIENT TACHYPNEA OF THE NEWBORN

Transient tachypnea of the newborn appears soon after birth. It occurs when the fetal liquid in the lungs is removed slowly or incompletely. This can be due to the lack of thoracic squeezing that occurs during a cesarean birth or diminished respiratory effort if the baby was exposed to central nervous system depressant medication in utero, during labour. Prolonged labour, macrosomia of the fetus, and maternal asthma also have been associated with this condition. A vaginal birth appears to be protective against transient tachypnea of the newborn (Cunningham et al., 2018).

Transient tachypnea is accompanied by retractions, expiratory grunting, or cyanosis and is relieved by low-dose oxygen therapy. Mild or moderate respiratory distress typically is present at birth or within 6 hours of birth. Transient tachypnea of the newborn is generally a self-limited disorder without significant morbidity. Transient tachypnea of the newborn resolves over a 24-hour to 72-hour period.

Nursing interventions include providing supportive care: giving oxygen, ensuring warmth, observing respiratory status frequently, and allowing time for the pulmonary capillaries and the lymphatics to remove the remaining fluid. The clinical course is relatively benign, but any newborn respiratory issue can be very frightening to the parents. Provide a thorough explanation and reassure them that most often the condition will resolve over time Some newborns will require an admission into NICU for respiratory monitoring and support.

PHYSIOLOGIC JAUNDICE

Physiologic jaundice is very common in newborns, with the majority demonstrating yellowish skin, mucous membranes, and sclera within the first 3 days of life. In any given year, approximately 65% of the newborns will experience clinical jaundice (King et al., 2019). Jaundice is the visible manifestation of hyperbilirubinemia. It typically results from the deposition of unconjugated bilirubin pigment in the skin and mucous membranes.

Physiologic jaundice can be best understood as an imbalance between the production and elimination of bilirubin, with a multitude of factors and conditions affecting each of these processes. When an imbalance results because of an increase in circulating bilirubin (or the bilirubin load) to significantly high levels, it may go on to cause acute neurologic sequelae (acute bilirubin encephalopathy). In most infants, an increase in bilirubin production (e.g., due to hemolysis) is the primary cause of physiologic jaundice, and thus reducing bilirubin production is a rational approach for its management.

Factors that contribute to the development of physiologic jaundice in the newborn include an increased bilirubin load because of relative polycythemia, a shortened erythrocyte life span (80 days compared with the adult 120 days), and immature hepatic uptake and conjugation processes (Chu, 2014). Normally the liver removes bilirubin from the blood and changes it into a form that can be excreted. As the red blood cell breakdown continues at a fast pace, the newborn's liver cannot keep up with bilirubin removal. Thus, bilirubin accumulates in the blood, causing a yellowish discolouration on the skin.

CPS Guidelines for Prevention and Management of Hyperbilirubinemia in Newborns. The CPS *Guidelines for detection, management and prevention of hyperbilirubinemia in term and late-preterm newborn infants* (Barrington, Sankaran, Canadian Paediatric Society, & Fetus and Newborn Committee, 2018) provide the following recommendations for health care professionals:

- All pregnant clients should be tested for ABO and Rh(D) blood types and be screened for red cell antibodies during pregnancy.
- Selected at-risk infants (Mediterranean, Middle Eastern, African or Southeast Asian origin) should be screened for G6PD deficiency.
- A test for G6PD deficiency should be considered in all infants with severe hyperbilirubinemia.
- Either TSB or TcB concentration should be measured in all infants during the first 72 hours of life. If not required earlier because of clinical jaundice, a TSB measurement should be obtained at the same time as the metabolic screening test; alternatively, a TcB measurement should be obtained either at discharge or, if not yet discharged, at 72 hours of life.
- Any infant discharged before 24 hours of life should be reviewed within 24 hours by an individual with experience in the care of the newborn who has access to testing and treatment facilities.
- All newborns who are visibly jaundiced in the first 24 hours of life should have their bilirubin level determined.

- Intensive phototherapy will be required for infants with severe hyperbilirubinemia or those at greatly elevated risk of developing severe hyperbilirubinemia.
- A program for breastfeeding support should be instituted in every birthing facility.
- Routine supplementation of breastfed infants with water or dextrose water is not recommended.
- Breastfeeding should be continued during phototherapy.
- Infants with a TSB concentration above the thresholds should have immediate intensive phototherapy, and should be referred for further investigation and preparation for exchange transfusion.

Adequate follow-up should be ensured for all infants who are jaundiced. Infants requiring intensive phototherapy should be investigated for determination of the cause of jaundice.

In newborn infants, jaundice can be detected by blanching the skin with digital pressure on the bridge of the nose, sternum, or forehead, revealing the underlying colour of the skin and subcutaneous tissue. If jaundice is present, the blanched area will appear yellow before the capillary refill. The assessment of jaundice must be performed in a well-lit room or, preferably, in daylight at a window. Jaundice is usually seen first in the face and progresses caudally to the trunk and extremities (CPS, 2017).

Measures that parents can take to reduce the risk of jaundice include exposing the newborn to natural sunlight for short periods of time throughout the day to help oxidize the bilirubin deposits on the skin, breastfeeding on demand to promote elimination of bilirubin through urine and stooling, and avoiding glucose water supplementation, which hinders elimination.

If the levels of unconjugated serum bilirubin increase and do not return to normal levels with increased hydration, phototherapy is indicated. The serum level of bilirubin at which phototherapy is initiated is a matter of clinical judgment by the physician, but it is often begun when bilirubin levels reach 12 to 15 mg/dL in the first 48 hours of life in a term newborn (Davidson, 2014). **Phototherapy** involves exposing the newborn to ultraviolet light, which converts unconjugated bilirubin into products that can be excreted through feces and urine. Phototherapy is the most common treatment for hyperbilirubinemia and has significantly decreased the need for exchange transfusions in newborns now.

Take Note!

Exposure of newborns to sunlight represents the first documented use of phototherapy in the medical literature. Sister J. Ward, a charge nurse in Essex, England, recognized in 1956 that when jaundiced newborns were exposed to the sun they became less yellow. This observation changed the entire treatment of jaundice in newborns (Maisels, 2015).

Phototherapy reduces bilirubin levels in the blood by breaking down unconjugated bilirubin into colourless compounds. These compounds can then be excreted in the bile. Phototherapy aims to curtail the increase in bilirubin blood levels; thereby preventing kernicterus, a condition in which unconjugated bilirubin enters the brain. If not treated, kernicterus can lead to brain damage and death.

During the past several decades, phototherapy has generally been administered with either banks of fluorescent lights or spotlights. Factors that determine the dosage of phototherapy include spectrum of light emitted, irradiance of light source, design of light unit, surface area of newborn exposed to the light, and distance of the newborn from the light source (McDermott, 2015). For phototherapy to be effective, the rays must penetrate as much of the skin as possible. Thus, the newborn must be unclothed and turned frequently to ensure maximum exposure of the skin. Several side effects of standard phototherapy have been identified: frequent loose stools, increased insensible water loss, transient rash, and potential retinal damage if the newborn's eyes are not covered sufficiently.

Recently, fibreoptic pads (Biliblanket, Bilibed, or Bilivest) have been developed that can be wrapped around the newborn or on which the newborn can lie. The light is delivered from a tungsten–halogen bulb through a fiberoptic cable and is emitted from the sides and ends of the fibres inside a plastic pad (Barrington et al., 2018). These products work on the premise that phototherapy can be improved by delivering higher-intensity therapeutic light to decrease bilirubin levels. The pads do not produce appreciable heat like the banks of lights or spotlights do, so insensible water loss is not increased. Eye patches are still required to protect the baby's eyes. With fibreoptic pads, parents can feed and hold their newborns continuously to promote bonding.

When caring for newborns receiving phototherapy for jaundice, nurses must do the following:

- Closely monitor body temperature and fluid and electrolyte balance.
- Document frequency, character, and consistency of stools.
- Monitor hydration status (weight, specific gravity of urine, and urine output).
- Turn frequently to increase the infant's skin exposure to phototherapy.
- Observe skin integrity (as a result of exposure to diarrhea and phototherapy lights).
- Provide eye protection to prevent corneal injury related to phototherapy exposure.
- Encourage parents to participate in their newborn's care; prevent parent–infant separation.
- Provide eye care very time the nurse handles the baby, assess for eye discharge, adjust eye patches to ensure they fit well.

See Chapter 24 for a more detailed discussion of hyperbilirubinemia.

The home health nurse made a postpartum visit to Kelly to assess the situation. Kelly's son was slightly jaundiced when the home health nurse pressed gently over his sternum, but Kelly said he was nursing better compared with the previous 2 days. What home suggestions can the nurse make to Kelly to reduce the jaundice? What specific education about physiologic jaundice is needed?

HYPOGLYCEMIA

During the first 24 to 48 hours of life, as healthy newborns transition from intrauterine to extrauterine life, their plasma glucose levels are typically lower than later in life. Hypoglycemia affects as many as 40% of all full-term newborns. It is defined as a blood glucose level of less than 2.6 mmol/L (Aziz, Dancey, & Canadian Paediatric Society, Fetus and Newborn Committee, 2018). From a physiologic perspective, a newborn may be said to be hypoglycemic when glucose supply is inadequate to meet demand. In newborns, blood glucose levels fall to a low point during the first few hours of life because the source of glucose is removed when the placenta is expelled. This period of transition is usually smooth, but certain newborns are at greater risk for hypoglycemia: infants of those who have diabetes, preterm newborns, and newborns with intrauterine growth restriction (IUGR), small for gestation age (SGA), inadequate caloric intake, sepsis, asphyxia, hypothermia, polycythemia, glycogen storage disorders, and endocrine deficiencies (Adamkin, 2015).

Most newborns experience transient hypoglycemia and are asymptomatic. The symptoms, when present, are nonspecific and include jitteriness, lethargy, cyanosis, apnea, seizures, high-pitched or weak cry, hypothermia, and poor feeding. If hypoglycemia is prolonged or is left untreated, serious, long-term adverse neurologic sequelae such as learning disabilities and intellectual disabilities can occur (Stanley et al., 2015).

Treatment of hypoglycemia in the newborn includes administration of a rapid-acting source of glucose such as dextrose gel, expressed breastmilk and breastfeeding, or early formula feeding. In acute, severe cases, intravenous administration of IV dextrose solution may be required if oral feedings were not effective in rising blood sugar levels above 2.6 mmol/L. Continuous monitoring of glucose levels is not only prudent but mandatory in high-risk newborns. Although there is no specific means of preventing hypoglycemia in newborns, it is wise and cautious to monitor for symptoms and intervene as soon as symptoms are noted.

Subsequently, early diagnosis and appropriate intervention are essential for all newborns.

Nursing care of the hypoglycemic newborn includes monitoring for signs of hypoglycemia or identifying high-risk newborns prone to this disorder based on their perinatal history, physical examination, body measurements, and gestational age. Glucose screening should be performed only on at-risk infants and those with clinical symptoms compatible with hypoglycemia (Aziz et al., 2018).

Prevent hypoglycemia in newborns at risk by initiating feedings within the first 30 to 60 minutes after birth. If hypoglycemia persists despite feeding, notify the primary health care provider for orders such as intravenous therapy with dextrose solutions. Anticipate hypoglycemia in certain high-risk newborns and begin assessments immediately on nursery admission.

Promoting Nutrition

Several physiologic changes dictate the type and method of feeding throughout the newborn's 1st year. Some of these changes include the following:

- Stomach capacity is limited at birth. The emptying time is short (2 to 3 hours) and peristalsis is rapid. Therefore, small, frequent feedings are needed at first, with amounts progressively increasing as the baby grows.
- The immune system is immature at birth, so the baby is at a high risk for food allergies during the first 4 to 6 months of life. Introducing solid foods prior to this time increases the risk of developing food allergies.
- Pancreatic enzymes and bile, which assist in digestion of fat and starch, are in limited supply until about 3 to 6 months of age. Infants cannot digest cereal prior to this time.
- The kidneys are immature and unable to concentrate urine until about 4 to 6 weeks of age. Excess protein and mineral intake can place a strain on kidney function and can lead to dehydration.
- Immature muscular control at birth changes over time to assist in the feeding process by improving head and neck control, hand–eye coordination, swallowing, and ability to sit, grasp, and chew. By about 6 months, inborn reflexes disappear, head control develops, and the infant can sit to be fed, making spoon-feeding possible (Dudek, 2017).

NEWBORN NUTRITIONAL NEEDS

As newborns grow, their energy and nutrient requirements change to meet their body's changing needs. During infancy, energy, protein, vitamin, and mineral requirements per pound of body weight are higher than at any other time of life. These high levels are needed to fuel the rapid growth and development during this stage of life. In general, an infant's birth weight doubles by 6 months of life, and triples within the 1st year (Walker, 2017).

TABLE 18.7	COMPARISON OF HUMAN MILK WITH SELECTED FORMULA COMPOSITION				
Type	Brand Names	Calories/ Ounce	Carbohydrate Source	Protein Source	Indications
Human milk	None	20	Lactose	Human milk	Preferred for all infants
Term formula	Enfamil; Similac; Carnation Good Start	20	Lactose	Cow's milk	Appropriate for term infants
Term formula with DHA and ARA	Enfamil Lipil; Good Start DHA & ARA; Similac Advance	20	Lactose	Cow's milk	Appropriate for term infants
Preterm formula	Enfamil 24 Premature; Preemie SMA 24	24	Lactose	Cow's milk	Usually given to preterm infants <34 weeks' gestation
Soy formula	Enfamil Prosobee; Good Start Soy	20	Corn based	Soy	For infants with galactosemia
Hypoallergenic formula	Similac Alimentum; Enfamil Nutramigen; Enfamil Pregestimil	20	Corn or sucrose	Extensively hydrolyzed	For infants with a milk protein allergy
Nonallergenic formula	Neocate; Nutramigen AA	20	Corn or sucrose	Amino acids	For infants with a milk protein allergy
Antireflux formula	Enfamil AR; Similac Sensitive RS	20	Lactose thickened with rice starch	Cow's milk	For infants with gastric reflux disorder

Adapted from Lönnerdal, B. (2014). Infant formula and infant nutrition: Bioactive proteins of human milk and implications for composition of infant formulas. *The American Journal of Clinical Nutrition, 99*(3), 712S–717S; Kent, G. (2014). Regulating fatty acids in infant formula: Critical assessment of US policies and practices. *International Breastfeeding Journal, 9*(1), 2–10; and Abrams, S. A., & Schanler, R. J. (2014). Data do not support claims that "supplement formulas" are better than standard formulas for breastfed infants. *AAP News, 35*(6), 26–27.

A newborn's caloric needs range from 110 to 120 cal/kg body weight. Human milk and formulas contain approximately 20 cal/oz, so the caloric needs of young infants can be met if several feedings are given throughout the day. If a baby is fed with infant formula, there is no evidence to recommend one brand over the other since all commercially available brands are nutritionally similar. All formulas are classified based on three parameters: caloric density, carbohydrate source, and protein composition (Table 18.7).

Fluid requirements for the newborn and infant range from 100 to 150 mL/kg daily. This requirement can be met through breastfeeding or formula feeding. Additional water supplementation is not necessary. Adequate carbohydrates, fats, protein, and vitamins are achieved through consumption of breastmilk or formula. Health Canada (2014a) notes that commercially available infant formulas contain adequate iron for healthy term babies. The breastfed infant draws on iron reserves for the first 6 months and then needs iron-rich foods or supplementation added at 6 months of age. Health Canada (2014a) recommends that all breastfed infants receive a daily supplement of 400 IU of vitamin D starting within the first few days of life to prevent rickets and vitamin D deficiency. The AAP recommended that all pregnant and lactating individuals use iodized salt and take a supplement of 150 mcg of iodine daily. An iodine deficiency can affect fetal and early childhood neurocognitive development (AAP, 2014).

FACILITATING INFORMED DECISION MAKING REGARDING FEEDING METHOD

The importance of breastfeeding is significant and well documented. Numerous health-related professional organizations promote breastfeeding because of the health implications for both members of the breastfeeding dyad. Nurses should educate clients about breastfeeding and provide support for the family throughout their breastfeeding experiences. Parents typically decide about the method of feeding well before the infant is born. Prenatal and childbirth classes present information about infant feeding and allow the parents to decide which method is best for them. Various factors can influence their decision, including socioeconomic status, culture, sexual objectification, fear of a negative reaction, personal convenience, lack of social support, lack of self-efficacy, family violence, employment considerations, level of education, free formula provided by formula companies, range of care interventions provided during pregnancy, childbirth, and the early postpartum period, and especially partner support (Dunn, Kalich, Henning, & Fedrizzi, 2015). Nurses must provide evidence-based information to assist parents in making their decision. The nurse needs to ensure that the parent(s) are fully informed about feeding considerations. Regardless of which method is chosen, the nurse needs to respect and support the client/couple's decision.

FEEDING THE NEWBORN

The newborn can be fed at any time during the transition period if assessments are normal and a desire is demonstrated. Before the newborn can be fed, determine his or her ability to suck and swallow. Clear any mucus in the nares or mouth with a bulb syringe before initiating feeding if necessary. Auscultate bowel sounds, check for abdominal distention, and inspect the anus for patency. If these parameters are within normal limits, newborn feeding may be started. Parents often have many questions about feeding. In general, newborns should be fed on demand whenever they appear hungry. Most newborns will give clues about their hunger status by crying, placing their fingers or fist in their mouth, rooting around, and sucking. Parents are taught to recognize feeding cues so that they learn to feed their baby on demand, with at least eight or more feedings in 24 hours.

Newborns differ in their feeding needs and preferences, but most breastfed babies will want to be fed every 1½ to 3 hours. The length of feedings is up to the newborn. Parents should be taught to follow the baby's cues of hunger and fullness. Encourage parents to respond to the infant's cues and not feed according to a standard or preset schedule.

Formula-fed newborns usually feed every 3 to 4 hours, finishing a bottle in 30 minutes or less. After the first 2 weeks of life, daily formula intake for an infant should be 45 to 60 mL/lb of body weight divided in at least six feedings per day, but growth is a better measure of health than the amount of formula consumed (Schlenker & Gilbert, 2015). If the newborn seems satisfied, wets 6 to 10 diapers daily, produces several stools a day, sleeps well, and is gaining weight regularly, then he or she is probably receiving sufficient breastmilk or formula.

Newborns can swallow air during feedings, which causes discomfort and fussiness. Parents can prevent this by burping them frequently throughout the feeding. Tips about burping include:

- Hold the newborn upright with his or her head on the parent's shoulder (Fig. 18.23A).
- Support the head and neck while the parent gently pats or rubs the newborn's back (Fig. 18.23B).
- Have the newborn sit on the parent's lap, while supporting the baby's chest and head. Gently rub the newborn's back with the other hand.
- Lay the newborn on the parent's lap with the baby's back facing up.
- Support the newborn's head in the crook of the parent's arm and gently pat or rub the back.

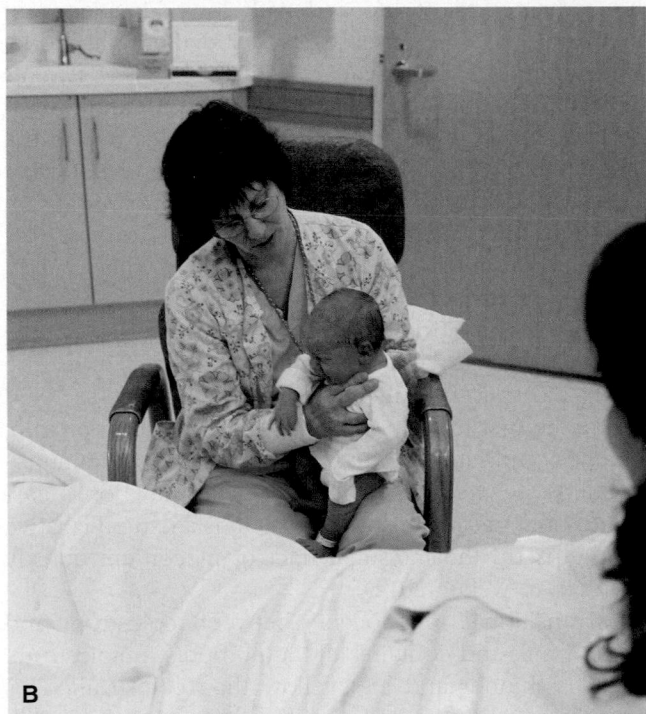

FIGURE 18.23 The nurse demonstrates (**A**) holding the newborn upright over the shoulder and (**B**) sitting the newborn upright, supporting the neck and chin.

Take Note!

It is the upright position, not the strength of the patting or rubbing that allows the newborn to release air accumulated in the stomach.

Stress to parents that feeding time is more than an opportunity to get nutrients into their newborn; it is also a time for closeness and sharing. Feedings are as much for the baby's emotional pleasure as his or her physical well-being. Encourage parents to maintain eye contact with the newborn during the feeding, hold him or her comfortably close to them, and talk softly during the feeding to promote closeness and security.

BREASTFEEDING

There is consensus in the medical community that breastfeeding is optimal for all newborns. The CPS, Health Canada, Public Health Agency of Canada, Dietitians of Canada, and the World Health Organization (WHO) all recommend breastfeeding exclusively for the first 6 months of life, continuing in conjunction with other food for 2 years or beyond. Data from 2010 indicated that over 87% of newborns in Canada initiated breastfeeding, however only 25.9% of babies were exclusively breastfed for the recommended 6 months (Health Canada, 2012a). Box 18.2 highlights the importance of breastfeeding. In addition, breastfeeding is associated with lower incidence of necrotizing enterocolitis and diarrhea during the early period of life and with lower incidence of inflammatory bowel diseases, type 2 diabetes, and obesity later in life (Martin, Fanaroff, & Welsh, 2014). Parents should be taught about the value of continuing breastfeeding during mild illnesses such as colds or the flu, as the baby will receive the maternal antibodies for that illness through the breastmilk, in essence providing an "immunization" against that illness. There are very few contraindications for breastfeeding. Those who are HIV positive are advised not to breastfeed.

The composition of human milk changes over time from colostrum, to transitional milk, and finally to mature milk. Colostrum is a thick, yellowish substance secreted during the first few days after birth. It is high in protein, minerals, and fat-soluble vitamins. It is rich in immunoglobulins (IgA), which help protect the newborn's gastrointestinal tract against infections. It is a natural laxative that helps rid the intestinal tract of meconium quickly (Gephart & Weller, 2014).

Transitional milk occurs between colostrum and mature milk and contains all the nutrients in colostrum, but it is thinner and less yellow than colostrum. This transitional milk is replaced by true or mature milk around day 10 after birth. Mature milk appears bluish and is not as thick as colostrum. It provides 20 cal/oz and contains:

- *Protein*—Although the content is lower than formula, it is ideal to support growth and development for the newborn. The majority of the protein is whey, which is easy to digest.
- *Fat*—Approximately 58% of total calories are fat, but they are easy to digest. Essential fatty acid content is high, as is the level of cholesterol, which helps develop

---

> ## BOX 18.2
>
> ## HEALTH IMPLICATIONS OF BREASTFEEDING
>
> ### Advantages for the Newborn
> - Contributes to the development of a strong immune system
> - Stimulates growth of positive bacteria in digestive tract
> - Reduces incidence of stomach upset, diarrhea, and colic
> - Begins the immunization process at birth by providing passive immunity
> - Promotes optimal bonding
> - Reduces risk of newborn constipation
> - Promotes greater developmental gains in preterm infants
> - Provides easily tolerated and digestible milk that is sterile, at proper temperature, and readily available with no artificial colourings, flavourings, or preservatives
> - Is less likely to result in overfeeding, leading to obesity
> - Promotes better tooth and jaw development as a result of sucking motions
> - Provides protection against food allergies
> - Lowers health care costs due to fewer illnesses
> - Is associated with reduced incidence of type 1 diabetes and heart disease later in life
>
> ### Advantages for the Breastfeeding Parent
> - Can facilitate postpartum weight loss by burning extra calories
> - Stimulates uterine contractions to control bleeding
> - Lowers risk for breast, ovarian, and endometrial cancers
> - Facilitates bonding with newborn infant
> - Lowers risk of type 2 diabetes
> - Breastmilk is free versus formula costs
> - Reduces risk of postpartum depression
> - Promotes uterine involution as a result of release of oxytocin
> - Lowers risk of osteoporosis
> - Affords some contraception effects
>
> Data from Schlenker, E., & Gilbert, J. A. (2015). *William's essentials of nutrition and diet therapy* (11th ed.). St. Louis, MO: Elsevier; Christopher, G. C., & Krell, J. K. (2014). Changing the breastfeeding conversation and our culture. *Breastfeeding Medicine, 9*(2), 53–55; and Walker, M. (2017). *Breastfeeding management for the clinician: Using the evidence* (4th ed.). Burlington, MA: Jones & Bartlett Learning.

enzyme systems capable of handling cholesterol later in life.

- *Carbohydrate*—Approximately 35% to 40% of total calories are in the form of lactose, which stimulates the growth of natural defense bacteria in the gastrointestinal system and promotes calcium absorption.
- *Water*—Water, the major nutrient in breastmilk, makes up 85% to 95% of the total volume. Total milk volume varies with the age of the infant and demand.
- *Minerals*—Breastmilk contains calcium, phosphorus, chlorine, potassium, and sodium, with trace amounts of iron, copper, and manganese. Iron absorption is about 50%, compared with about 4% for iron-fortified formulas.

- *Vitamins*—All vitamins are present in breastmilk; vitamin D is the lowest in amount. Vitamin D supplementation is recommended by Health Canada.
- *Enzymes*—Lipase and amylase are found in breastmilk to assist with digestion (Dudek, 2017).

Breastfeeding Support. Breastfeeding should be initiated immediately after birth. If the newborn is healthy and stable, wipe the newborn from head to toe with a dry cloth and place him or her skin-to-skin on the mother's abdomen. Then cover the mother-baby dyad with another warmed blanket to hold in the warmth. This immediate contact takes advantage of the newborn's natural alertness after a vaginal birth and fosters bonding. This immediate contact also reduces postpartum bleeding and stabilizes the newborn's temperature, blood glucose level, and respiratory rate (Khan, Vesel, Bahl, & Martines, 2014).

Left alone on the abdomen, a healthy full-term newborn scoots upward, pushing with the feet, pulling with the arms, and bobbing the head until finding and latching on to the nipple. A newborn's sense of smell is highly developed, which also helps in finding the nipple. As the newborn moves to the nipple, higher levels of oxytocin are stimulated and released, which contract the uterus, thereby minimizing bleeding. Oxytocin also causes the breasts to release colostrum when the newborn sucks on the nipple. Colostrum is rich in antibodies and thus provides the newborn with her "first immunization" against infection.

Keys to successful breastfeeding include:
- Initiating breastfeeding within the first hour of life
- Placing the newborn on the mother's chest/abdomen (skin-to-skin) immediately after birth
- Following the newborn's feeding schedule—8 to 12 or more times in 24 hours
- Providing unrestricted periods of breastfeeding
- Offering no supplement unless medically indicated
- Having a lactation consultant observe a feeding session
- Avoiding artificial nipples and pacifiers except during a painful procedure
- Increasing fluid intake to encourage greater milk production (Evidence-Based Practice Box 18.1)
- Offering both breasts at each feeding during the colostrum stage
- Watching for indicators of sufficient intake from infant:
  - 6 to 10 wet diapers daily
  - Waking up hungry 8 or more times in 24 hours
  - Acting content and falling asleep after feeding
- Keeping the newborn with the parent(s) throughout the hospital stay

EVIDENCE-BASED PRACTICE 18.1

PRIMARY CARE SETTING: A COMMUNITY PILOT PROJECT APPLYING THE TRI-CORE BREASTFEEDING MODEL: BEYOND THE BASICS

STUDY

Ongoing evidence-based practice findings strongly indicate that the lifelong health and economic benefits of breastfeeding contributes greatly to the health status of the infant, the mother, family, and society at large. Promotional lactation interventions are needed in the community to initiate and foster breastfeeding efforts beyond the hospital after discharge. The purpose of this study was to develop a primary care breastfeeding support program, bridging the gap from hospital discharge into primary care to improve breastfeeding rates. The study incorporated the three core interventions of the Tri-Core Model—(1) improving lactation support; (2) enhancing maternal and staff lactation education; and (3) fostering maternal confidence in their ability to breastfeed.

Findings

The study population (*N* = 50) included middle to low-income families that had recently given birth to a healthy full-term infant who desired to breastfeed within the early postpartum period. Outcomes were measured by the assessment of breastfeeding rates, durations, and reported maternal self-efficacy levels at 1-month, and a 2-month visit. Ongoing office support was provided with lactation visits and phone calls. Findings indicated significant gains in all three areas especially in overall breastfeeding rates when compared to previous rates, especially in rates of exclusive breastfeeding.

Nursing Implications

Based on the results of this study, nurses should remain instrumental in promoting successful breastfeeding practices by initiating breastfeeding as soon as possible after birth, assisting the mother to find a comfortable position for breastfeeding, assessing the infant's latch on to the breast, and reassuring her that the infant is getting adequate amount of breastmilk. In addition, utilizing multiprofessional community resources to encourage and support continued breastfeeding efforts is essential. Community referrals are important to help support the novice breastfeeding mother to reinforce breastfeeding instruction once she is discharged from the hospital. Nurses involved in improving breastfeeding rates benefit all ages and its greatest impact will be improving short- and long-term health care outcomes for all families.

Adapted from Busch, D., Nassar, L., & Silbert-Flagg, J. (2015). The necessity of breastfeeding—promoting breastfeeding in the primary care setting: A community pilot project applying the Tri-Core Breastfeeding Model: Beyond the basics. *Journal of Pregnancy & Child Health, 2*(3), 2–7.

- The nurse or lactation consultant should be available to guide and support breastfeeding while the family is on the postpartum unit
- Teaching every breastfeeding family about hand expressing breastmilk.

Help position the newborn so that latching-on is effective and is not painful. Placing pillows or a folded blanket under the client's head may help, or rolling on to one side and tucking the newborn in close. Assess both members of the dyad during this initial session to determine needs for assistance and education. One tool used frequently in this assessment is the LATCH scoring tool (Abbas & Hasan, 2015). The LATCH scoring tool is a breastfeeding charting system that provides a systematic method for gathering information about individual breastfeeding sessions. The system assigns a numerical score of 0, 1, or 2 to five key components of breastfeeding. Each letter of the acronym LATCH denotes an area of assessment: "L" is for how well the infant latches onto the breast; "A" is for the amount of audible swallowing noted; "T" is for the nipple type; "C" is for the level of comfort; and "H" is for the amount of help needed to hold the infant to the breast. The system is visually represented in the same form as the Apgar scoring grid, and the numbers are handled in the same way. With the LATCH system, the nurse can assess maternal and infant variables, define areas of needed intervention, and determine priorities in providing client care and teaching (Table 18.8). The higher the score, the less nursing intervention is needed. Higher LATCH scores have also been correlated with higher rates of breastfeeding exclusivity at six weeks postpartum (Sowjanya & Venugopalan, 2018).

Breastfeeding Positioning. Both members of the breastfeeding dyad must be in comfortable positions to ensure breastfeeding success. The four most common positions for breastfeeding are the football, cradle, cross-cradle, and side-lying holds. Each dyad should be assisted to try various positions and can decide which positions feel most comfortable for them (Fig. 18.24).

- In the football hold, the breastfeeding parent holds the infant's back and shoulders in their palm and tucks the infant under their arm. Remind the parent(s) to keep the infant's ears, shoulders, and hips in a straight line. The parent supports the breast with one hand and brings it to the infant's lips to latch on. The baby will benefit from the breast remaining supported until the infant is well established with breastfeeding. This position allows the parent to see the infant's mouth while guiding the infant to the nipple. This is a good choice for those who have had a cesarean birth because it avoids pressure on the incision.
- The cradling position is the one most commonly used. The parent holds the baby in the crook of the arm, with the infant facing belly-to-belly. The parent supports the breast with the opposite hand.
- In the cross-cradle position, the parent places a pillow across the lap, with the infant facing belly-to-belly. The parent supports the infant's back and shoulders with their palm and supports the breast from underneath. After the infant is in position, the infant is pulled forward to latch on.
- In the side-lying position, the parent lies on their side with a pillow supporting their back and another pillow supporting the newborn in the front. To start,

TABLE 18.8	THE LATCH SCORING TOOL		
Parameters	**0 Point**	**1 Point**	**2 Points**
L: latch	Sleepy infant, no sustained latch achieved	Must hold nipple in infant's mouth to sustain latch and suck; must stimulate infant to continue to suck	Grasps nipple; tongue down; rhythmic sucking
A: audible swallowing	None	A few observed with stimulation	Spontaneous and intermittent both <24-hours old and afterward
T: type of nipple	Inverted (drawn inward into breast tissue)	Flat (not protruding)	Everted or protruding out after stimulation
C: comfort of nipple	Engorged, cracked bleeding; severe discomfort	Filling; reddened, small blisters or bruises; mild to moderate discomfort	Soft, nontender
H: hold (positioning)	Nurse must hold infant to breast	Minimal assistance; help with positioning, then mother takes over	No assistance needed by nurse

Adapted from Walker, M. (2017). *Breastfeeding management for the clinician: Using the evidence* (4th ed.). Burlington, MA: Jones & Bartlett Learning; Altuntas, N., Turkyilmaz, C., Yildiz, H., Kulali, F., Hirfanoglu, I., Onal, E., . . . Atalay, Y. (2014). Validity and reliability of the infant breastfeeding assessment tool, the mother baby assessment tool, and the LATCH scoring system. *Breastfeeding Medicine, 9*(4), 191–195.

FIGURE 18.24 Breastfeeding positions. Cradling position (**A**), football hold position (**B**), and side-lying position (**C**).

the parent props up on an elbow and supports the newborn with that arm, while holding the breast with the opposite hand. Once nursing is started, the parent lies down in a comfortable position.

To promote latching-on, instruct parents to make a C or a V with their fingers. In the C hold, the thumb is placed well above the areola and the other four fingers below the areola and under the breast. In the V hold, the index finger is positioned above the areola and the other three fingers below the areola and under the breast. Either method can be used as long as the hand is well away from the nipple so the infant can easily latch on.

Breastfeeding Education. Breastfeeding is not an innate skill for everyone. Almost everyone who gives birth will have the potential to breastfeed successfully, but many do not achieve their personal breastfeeding goals because of inadequate knowledge. Nursing Care Plan 18.1 (at the end of the chapter) gives typical nursing diagnoses, outcomes, and interventions. For many breastfeeding dyads, feeding goes smoothly from the start, but for others it is a struggle. Nurses can help throughout the experience by being open, supportive, and avoiding making judgments, as well as by dem-

onstrating techniques and offering encouragement and praise for success. Correct positioning will enhance good attachment and will ensure effective milk transfer. Nurses should emphasize that the key to successful breastfeeding is correct positioning and latching-on.

Teaching by nurses has been shown to have a significant effect on both the ability to breastfeed successfully and the duration of lactation (Dudek, 2017). During the first few breastfeeding sessions, parents want to know how often the babies should be nursing, whether breastfeeding is going well, if the newborn is getting enough nourishment, and what problems may ensue and how to cope with them. Education for the breastfeeding family is highlighted in Teaching Guidelines 18.4.

Teaching Guidelines 18.4
BREASTFEEDING

• Set aside a quiet place where you can be relaxed and won't be disturbed. Relaxation promotes milk letdown.
• Sit in a comfortable chair or rocking chair or lie on a bed. Try to make each feeding calm, quiet, and leisurely. Avoid distractions.

- Listen to soothing music and sip a nutritious drink during feedings.
- Initially, nurse the newborn every few hours to stimulate milk production. Remember that the supply of milk is equal to the demand—the more sucking, the more milk.
- Watch for signals from the infant to indicate that he or she is hungry, such as:
  - Nuzzling against the breasts
  - Demonstrating the rooting reflex by making sucking motions
  - Placing fist or hands in mouth to suck on
  - Stretching and squirming
  - Smacking the lips
- Stimulate the rooting reflex by touching the newborn's cheek to initiate sucking.
- Look for signs indicating that the newborn has latched on correctly: wide-open mouth with the nipple and much of the areola in the mouth, lips rolled outward, and tongue over lower gum, visible jaw movement drawing milk out, rhythmic sucking with an audible swallowing (soft "ka" or "ah" sound indicates the infant is swallowing milk).
- Hold the newborn closely, facing the breast, with the newborn's ear, shoulder, and hip in direct alignment.
- Nurse the infant on demand, not on a rigid schedule. Feed every 2 to 3 hours within a 24-hour period for a total of 8 or more feedings.
- Alternate the breast you offer first; identify with a safety pin on bra.
- Vary your position for each feeding to empty breasts and reduce soreness.
- Look for signs that the newborn is getting enough milk:
  - At least six wet diapers and two to five loose yellow stools daily
  - Steady weight gain after the 1st week of age
  - Pale-yellow urine, not deep yellow or orange
  - Sleeping well, yet looks alert and healthy when awake
- Wake up the newborn if he or she has nursed less than 5 minutes by unwrapping him or her.
- Before removing the baby from the breast, break the infant's suction by inserting a finger.
- Burp the infant to release air when changing breasts and at the end of the breastfeeding session.
- Avoid supplemental formula feedings unless indicated for a medical reason. Do not take drugs or medications unless first discussed with the health care provider.
- Avoid drinking alcohol or caffeinated drinks because they pass through milk.
- Do not smoke; it increases the baby's risk of sudden infant death syndrome.

- Always wash your hands before expressing or handling milk to store.
- Wear nursing bras and clothes that are easy to undo (Dyson et al., 2014; Walker, 2017; La Leche League, 2018b).

Take Note!

Remember that the supply of milk is determined by the demand—the more sucking, the more milk.

Remember Kelly, who was concerned about jaundice in her newborn son? At her son's 2-week well-baby checkup at the clinic, his bilirubin level came back within normal limits. Kelly still felt he was not getting enough to eat and stated that she might switch to formula feeding her son. What information can the nurse present to promote and support breastfeeding? Should the nurse make a referral to the lactation consultant?

Breastmilk Storage and Expression. If a newborn must be separated from the parent(s) for any reason (e.g., illness, work, travel), the nurse must provide the parent(s) with instruction on how to express and store milk safely. Expressing milk can be done manually (hand compression of breast) or by using a breast pump. Handheld breast pumps are inexpensive and can be used by parents who occasionally need an extra bottle if they are going out (Fig. 18.25A). Electric breast pumps may be preferable for those who experience a lengthy separation from their infants and need to pump their breasts regularly, for example, those whose babies are premature or ill in NICU, or breastfeeding parents who must return to work shortly after birth (Fig. 18.25B).

To ensure the safety of expressed breastmilk, provide parents with the following instructions:
- Wash your hands before expressing milk or handling breastmilk.
- Find a quiet, clean place to express milk.
- Use clean containers to store expressed milk.
- Use fresh breastmilk stored in the refrigerator within 3 to 5 days.
- Use frozen expressed milk within 3 months.
- Use frozen expressed breastmilk that is stored in separate chest freezer within 6 to 12 months.
- Do not use microwave ovens to warm chilled milk.
- Discard any unused thawed milk; never refreeze it.
- Store milk in quantities to be used for each feeding (60 to 120 mL).

FIGURE 18.25 **A.** Handheld breast pump. **B.** Electric breast pump. (Part B from Lippincott's Nursing Procedures and Skills, 2007.)

- Thaw milk in warm water before using (CPS, 2018; La Leche League, 2018a).

Common Breastfeeding Concerns. Breastfeeding may present challenges for some, including cracked nipples, engorgement (the painful overfilling of the breasts with milk), or mastitis (inflammation of the breast). Breastfeeding should not be painful. If a breastfeeding client has sore, cracked nipples, the first step is to find the cause. Incorrect positioning or latching-on, removing the infant from the breast without first breaking the suction, or wearing a bra that is too tight can cause cracked or sore nipples. Cracked nipples can increase the risk of mastitis because a break in the skin may allow *S. aureus* or other organisms to enter the body.

Sore nipples usually are caused by improper infant attachment, which traumatizes the tissue. The nurse should review techniques for proper positioning and latching-on. It is important to get this correct from the first feed to assist in the prevention of incorrect attachment and associated nipple trauma. Recommend the following points:

- Use only warm water, not soap, to clean the nipples to prevent dryness.
- Express some milk before feeding to stimulate the milk ejection reflex.
- Avoid using breast pads with plastic liners, and change pads when they are wet.
- Wear a comfortable bra that is not too tight.
- Apply a few drops of breastmilk to the nipples after feeding.

- Leave the nursing bra flaps down after feeding to allow nipples to air-dry.
- Take systemic anti-inflammatory such as ibuprofen for discomfort.
- Rotate positions when feeding the infant to promote complete breast emptying.
- Inspect the nipples daily for redness or cracks (Walker, 2017).

To ease nipple pain and trauma, reinforce appropriate latching-on techniques and remind the parent(s) about the need to break the suction at the breast before removing the newborn from the breast. Additional measures may include applying cold compresses over the area and massaging breastmilk onto the nipple after feeding.

Engorgement may occur as the milk comes in around day 3 or 4 after birth of the newborn. Explain that engorgement, though uncomfortable, is self-limited and will resolve as the newborn continues to nurse. The parent should continue to nurse during engorgement to avoid a plugged milk duct, which could lead to mastitis. Provide the following tips for relieving engorgement:

- Take warm to hot showers to encourage milk release.
- Express some milk manually before breastfeeding.
- Wear a supportive nursing bra 24 hours a day to provide support.
- Feed the newborn in a variety of positions—sitting up and then lying down.
- Massage the breasts from under the axillary area down toward the nipple.

- Increase the frequency of feedings.
- Apply warm compresses to the breasts prior to nursing.
- Stay relaxed while breastfeeding.
- Use a breast pump if nursing or manual expression is not effective.
- Remember that this condition is temporary and resolves quickly.

Mastitis, or inflammation of the breast, causes flu-like symptoms, chills, fever, and malaise. These symptoms may occur before the development of soreness, aching, swelling, and redness in the breast (usually the upper outer quadrant). This condition usually occurs in just one breast when a milk duct becomes blocked, causing inflammation, or through a cracked or damaged nipple, allowing bacteria to infect a portion of the breast. Treatment consists of rest, warm compresses, antibiotics, breast support, and continued breastfeeding (the infection will not pass into the breastmilk). Explain that it is important to keep the milk flowing in the infected breast, whether it is through nursing or manual expression or with a breast pump.

FORMULA FEEDING

Despite the widespread acknowledgement that breastfeeding is the most desirable means of feeding infants, some parents choose formula feeding and will need as much education and support about this method of feeding as provided to parents who breastfeed.

Formula feeding requires more than just opening, pouring, and feeding. Parents need information about the types of formula available, safe preparation and storage of formula, equipment, feeding positions, and the amount to feed their newborn, as well as how to suppress lactation (see Chapter 16 for more information).

Commercially prepared formulas are regulated by the Food and Drug Administration (FDA), which sets minimum and maximum levels of nutrients. Formulas are manufactured by numerous manufacturers in Canada. Normal full-term infants usually receive conventional cow's milk–based formula. However, if an infant shows signs of a reaction or lactose intolerance, the health care provider will advise parents to switch to another formula type.

The general recommendation is for all infants to receive iron-fortified formula until the age of 1 year. The latest generation of infant formulas includes some fortification with docosahexaenoic acid (DHA) and arachidonic acid (ARA), two natural components of breastmilk. Many feel the FDA does not adequately regulate the use of fatty acid additives (DHA and ARA) to infant formula before they are marketed, and there is no systematic assessment after marketing is underway. Researchers are calling for more FDA regulation over additives in infant formulas (Kent, 2014). Commercial formulas come in three forms: powder, concentrate, and easy to feed or ready to use. All are similar in terms of nutritional content but differ in expense. Powdered formula is the least expensive, with concentrated formula the next most expensive. Both must be mixed with water before using. Ready-to-feed formula is the most expensive; once it is opened and poured into a bottle, it is fed directly to the infant.

Parents need information about the equipment needed for formula feeding. Basic supplies are four to six 120 mL bottles, eight to ten 240 mL bottles, eight to ten nipple units, a bottle brush, and a nipple brush. A key area of instruction is assessing for flow of formula through the nipple and checking for any nipple damage. When the bottle is filled and turned upside down, the flow from the nipple should be approximately one drop per second. If the parents are using bottles with disposable bags, instruct them to make sure they have a tight-fitting nipple to prevent leaks. Frequent observation of the flow rate from the nipple and the condition of the nipple will prevent choking and aspiration associated with the formula coming out too quickly or in too large an amount for the baby to swallow. Ask the parents to fill a bottle with formula and then turn it upside down and observe the rate at which the formula drips from the bottle. If it is too fast (more than one drop per second), then the nipple should be replaced.

Correct formula preparation is critical to the newborn's health and development. Improper dilution can cause severe illness and even death in newborns (Boué et al., 2018). Most errors in formula preparation result from a lack of education for the parents regarding how to prepare the formula and avoid measurement errors. The safety of the water supply should be considered. If well water is used, parents should have their well water tested regularly, and will need to sterilize the water by boiling it or should use bottled water. Many health care providers still recommend that all water used in formula preparation be brought to a rolling boil for 2 minutes and then cooled to no less than 70°C (158°F) before use mixing with powdered or liquid concentrate formula (Health Canada, 2012b).

Opened cans of readymade or concentrated formula should be covered and refrigerated after being prepared for the day (24 hours). Instruct parents to discard any unused portions after 48 hours.

Powdered infant formula (PIF) has been consumed by infants around the world for many years, and is considered to be a safe product. However, there have been a number of outbreaks among infants due to the consumption of PIF contaminated with harmful bacteria such as *Enterobacter sakazakii* (*Cronobacter* spp.) and *Salmonella enterica*. Proper preparation, handling and storage practices for PIF are recommended to reduce the risk of bacteria-related illness. Parents of infants under 2 months of age, or those who are premature, ill, or immunocompromised are encouraged to use liquid concentrate or ready-made formula, due to the sterility of these products. Parents are encouraged to speak with their primary care provider if they are considering using PIF (Health Canada, 2012b).

Take Note!

Any formula left in the bottle after feeding should be discarded after every feeding, because the infant's saliva has been mixed with it, causing the growth of bacteria within 1 to 2 hours.

To warm refrigerated formula, advise the parents to place the bottle in a pan of warm water or an electric bottle warmer and test the temperature by letting a few drops fall on the inside of the wrist. If it is comfortably warm on the inner arm, it is the correct temperature. Parents must be educated to never use the microwave to warm infant formula, as this causes hot spots within the milk which will burn the inside of the baby's mouth.

Formula-Feeding Assistance. The process of feeding a newborn formula from a bottle should mirror breastfeeding as closely as possible. Although nutrition is important, so are the emotional and interactive components of feeding. Encourage parents to cuddle their newborn closely and position him or her so that the head is in a comfortable position, not too far back or turned, which makes swallowing difficult (Fig. 18.26). Also urge parents to communicate with their newborn during the feedings by talking and singing to him or her.

Although it may seem that bottle feeding is not a difficult task, many new parents find it awkward or intimidating. At first glance, holding an infant and a bottle appears simple enough, but both the position of the baby and the angle of the bottle must be correct.

Formula-Feeding Positions. Advise parents to feed their newborns in a relaxed and quiet setting to create

FIGURE 18.26 Father holding his newborn securely while feeding.

a sense of calm for themselves and the baby. Make sure that comfort is a priority for both. The parent can sit in a comfortable chair, using a pillow to support the arm holding the baby. The parent can cradle the newborn in a semi-upright position, supporting the newborn's head in the crook of her arm. Holding the newborn close during feeding provides stimulation and helps prevent choking. Holding the newborn's head raised slightly will help prevent formula from washing backward into the eustachian tubes in the ears, which can lead to ear infections.

Formula-Feeding Education. Parents require teaching about the correct preparation and storage of formula as well as the techniques for feeding. Ensure that parents have an opportunity to perform a return demonstration of safe formula preparation education. See Teaching Guidelines 18.5.

 Teaching Guidelines 18.5
FORMULA FEEDING

- Wash your hands with soap and water before preparing formula.
- Mix the formula and water amounts exactly as the label specifies.
- Always hold the newborn and bottle during feedings; never prop the bottle.
- Never freeze formula.
- Never warm formula in the microwave.
- Place refrigerated formula in a pan of warm water for a few minutes to warm it.
- Test the temperature of the formula by shaking a few drops on the inside of the wrist.
- Hold the bottle like a pencil, keeping it tipped to prevent air from entering. Position the bottle so that the nipple remains filled with milk.
- Burp the infant after every few ounces to allow air swallowed to escape.
- Move the nipple around in the infant's mouth to stimulate sucking.
- Always keep a bulb syringe close by to use if choking occurs.
- Avoid putting the infant to bed with a bottle to prevent "baby bottle tooth decay."
- Feed the newborn approximately every 3 to 4 hours.
- Use an iron-fortified formula for the 1st year.
- Prepare enough formula for the next 24 hours. Store prepared bottles in the fridge for up to 24 hours.
- Check nipples regularly and discard any that are sticky, cracked, or leaking.
- Store unmixed, open liquid formula in the refrigerator for up to 48 hours.
- Throw away any formula left in the bottle after each feeding.

Proper positioning makes bottle feeding easier and more enjoyable for both the parent and the newborn. As in breastfeeding, frequent burping is key. Advise the parents to hold the bottle so that formula fills the nipple, thus allowing less air to enter. Infants get fussy from discomfort when they swallow air during feedings, and this need to be relieved every 60 to 90 mL.

Emphasize to parents that an electrolyte imbalance can occur in infants who are fed formula that has been incorrectly mixed. Mixing the formula with too *little* water (i.e., too thickly), can cause hypernatremia because the high concentration of sodium is too much for the baby's immature kidneys to handle. As a result, sodium is excreted along with water, leading to dehydration. Mixing the formula with too *much* water in an effort to save money can lead to failure to thrive, diminished nutrition, fluoride overdose, and lack of weight gain (Monahan, 2017).

WEANING AND INTRODUCTION OF SOLID FOODS

Weaning. Eventually, breastfeeding or formula feeding comes to an end. Weaning involves the transition from breast to bottle, from breast or bottle to cup, or from liquids to solids. Weaning from breastfeeding to cup has several advantages over weaning to a bottle because it eliminates the step of weaning first to a bottle and then to a cup. Another advantage is that the bottle does not become a security object for the infant.

Weaning can be done because the parent is returning to work and does not intend to keep breastfeeding, or because the infant is losing interest in breastfeeding and showing signs of independence. There is no "right" time to wean; it depends on the desires of each dyad. Weaning represents a significant change in the way the parent and infant interact, and each parent must decide when they are ready to take that step. Either one can start the weaning process, but usually it occurs between 6 months and 1 year of age.

To begin weaning from the breast, instruct parents to substitute one breastfeeding with a cup or bottle. Often the midday feeding is the easiest feeding to replace. A trainer cup with two handles and a snap-on lid with a spout is appropriate and minimizes spilling. Because weaning is a gradual process, it may take months. Instruct parents to proceed slowly and let the infant's willingness and interest guide them.

Weaning from the bottle to the cup also needs to be timed appropriately. Typically, the night bottle is the last to be given up, with cup drinking substituted throughout the day. After the child is at least 1 year old, slowly diluting the formula with water over a week can help in this process; the final result is an all-water bottle. To prevent the baby from sucking on the bottle during the night, remove it from the crib after the infant falls asleep.

Introduction of Solid Foods

When infants are 6 months old and have double their birth weight, it is time to consider introducing solid foods. Readiness cues include:

- Ability to sit up with minimal support and turn head away to indicate fullness
- Reduction of protrusion reflex so food can be propelled to back of throat
- Demonstration of interest in food others around them are eating
- Ability to open mouth automatically when food approaches it.

When introducing solid foods, certain principles apply:

- New foods should be introduced one at a time and several days apart so that if a problem develops, the responsible item can be identified; approximately every 3 to 5 days.
- Infants should be allowed to set the pace regarding how much they wish to eat.
- Iron-rich foods, such as meat and meat alternatives and iron-fortified cereals should be introduced first. Then vegetables, fruits, and milk products (such as cheese and yogurt) can be introduced between 6 and 9 months of age, along with the iron-rich foods.
- A relaxed, unhurried, calm atmosphere for meals is important.
- A variety of foods are provided to ensure a balanced diet.
- Infants should never be force fed (Health Canada, 2014b; Schlenker & Gilbert, 2015).

Nurses can promote good feeding practices by actively listening to new parents, helping them clarify their feelings, and discussing solutions. A warm, sincere manner and tone of voice will put an anxious parent at ease. Giving accurate information, making suggestions, and presenting options will enable parents to decide what is best for them and their infants. Nurses should be sensitive to the individual, family, and economic and cultural differences among parents before offering suggestions for feeding practices that may not be appropriate.

Preparing for Discharge

Preparing the parents for discharge is an essential task for the nurse. Because of today's shorter hospital stays, the nurse must identify the priority teaching topics that need to be covered. Nurses should assess the parents' baseline knowledge and learning needs and plan how to meet them. Using the following principles fosters a learner-centred approach:

- Make the environment conducive to learning. Encourage the parents to feel comfortable during this stressful time by using support and praise.
- Allow the parents to provide input about the content and the process of learning. What do they want and need to learn?

- Build the parents' self-esteem by confirming that their responses to the entire birthing process and aftercare are legitimate, and others have felt the same way.
- Ensure that what the parents learn is relevant to their day-to-day home situation.
- Encourage responsibility by reinforcing that their emotional and physical responses are within the normal range.
- Respect cultural beliefs and practices that are important to the family by taking into account their heritage and health beliefs regarding newborn care. Examples include placing a bellyband over the newborn's navel (as practiced by some Hispanic and African families), delaying naming the newborn (for some Asian and Haitian families), and delaying breastfeeding (some Asian families) (Bowers, 2015).

While in the hospital, parents have ready access to support and hands-on instruction regarding feeding and newborn care. When the family is discharged, this close supervision and support by nurses should not end abruptly. Providing the new parents with the phone number of the postpartum unit will help them through this stressful transitional period. Giving the new family information and offering backup support via the telephone will increase parenting success. (See Evidence-Based Practice 18.1.)

Consider This

I have always prided myself on being very organized and in control in most situations, but survival at home after childbirth wasn't one of them. I left the hospital 24 hours after giving birth to my son because my doctor said I could. The postpartum nurse encouraged me to stay longer, but wanting to be in control and sleeping in my own bed again won out. I thought my baby would be sleeping while I sent out birth announcements to my friends and family—wrong! What happened instead was my son didn't sleep as I imagined and my nipples became sore after breastfeeding every few hours. I was weary and tired and wanted to sleep, but I couldn't. Somehow I thought I would be getting a full night's sleep because I was up throughout the day, but that was a fantasy too. At 2 o'clock in the morning when you are up feeding your baby, you feel you are the only one in the world up at that time and feel very much alone. My feelings of being organized and in control all the time have changed dramatically since I left the hospital. I have learned to yield to the important needs of my son and derive satisfaction from being able to bring comfort to him and to let go of my control.

Thoughts: *It is interesting to see how a newborn changed this woman's need to organize and control her environment. What "tips of survival" could the nurse offer this woman to help in her transition to home with her newborn? How can friends and family help when women arrive home from the hospital with their newborns?*

ENSURING FOLLOW-UP CARE

Most newborns are scheduled for their first health follow-up appointment within 2 to 4 days after discharge so they can have additional laboratory work done as part of the newborn screening series, especially if they were discharged within 48 hours. After this first visit, the typical schedule of health care visits is as follows: 2 to 4 weeks of age; 2, 4, and 6 months of age for checkups and vaccines; 9 months of age for a checkup; 12 months for a checkup and vaccines; 15 and 18 months for checkups and vaccines; and 2 years of age for a checkup. These appointments provide an opportunity for parents to ask questions and receive anticipatory guidance as their child grows and develops.

In addition to encouraging parents to keep follow-up appointments, advise parents to call their health care provider if they notice signs of illness in their newborn. They should know which over-the-counter medicines should be kept on hand. Review the following warning signs of illness with parents:

- Temperature of 38.3°C (101°F) or higher
- Forceful, persistent vomiting; not just spitting up
- Refusal to take feedings
- Two or more green, watery diarrheal stools
- Infrequent wet diapers and change in bowel movements from normal pattern
- Lethargy or excessive sleepiness
- Inconsolable crying and extreme fussiness
- Abdominal distention
- Difficult or laboured breathing

PROVIDING IMMUNIZATION INFORMATION

In the last century, vaccinations have been the most effective medical intervention to reduce mortality and morbidity caused by communicable diseases. It is believed that vaccines save at least two to three million lives annually worldwide (Delany, Rappuoli, & De Gregorio, 2014). Parents also need instructions about immunizations for their newborn. Immunization is the process of rendering an individual immune or of becoming immune to certain communicable diseases (Verklan & Walden, 2015). The purpose of the immune system is to identify unknown (nonself) substances in the body and develop a defense against these invaders. Disease prevention by immunization is a public health priority. Despite many advances in vaccine delivery, the goal of universal immunization has not been reached (Davidson, 2014). Nurses can help to meet this goal by educating new parents about the importance of disease prevention through immunizations.

Immunity can be provided either passively or actively. Passive immunity is protection transferred via already formed antibodies from one person to another. Passive immunity includes the passage of antibodies through the placenta to the fetus, immunity passed through breastmilk, and immunity from immunoglobulins. Passive immunity provides limited protection and decreases over a period of weeks or months (Chu & Englund, 2014). Active immunity

TABLE 18.9   CANADA'S PROVINCIAL AND TERRITORIAL ROUTINE VACCINATION SCHEDULE

Canada's Provincial and Territorial Routine (and Catch-up) Vaccination Routine Schedule Programs for Infants and Children

This table summarizes the current routine vaccination schedule for infants and children in all provinces and territories across Canada. Changes to this schedule are updated regularly in collaboration with the Canadian Nursing Coalition for Immunization (CNCI) and the Canadian Immunization Committee (CIC). Additional information is available on Canada.ca\vaccines (last update: January 2019).

VACCINES — Provincial & Territorial Vaccination Schedules

Abbreviations	Description	BC	AB	SK	MB	ON	QC[6]	NB	NS	PE	NL	YT	NT	NU
DTaP-IPV-Hib	Diphtheria, tetanus, acellular pertussis, inactivated polio virus, *Haemophilus influenzae* type B vaccine	Age: 18 mos	Age: 18 mos	Age: 2, 4, 6, 18 mos	Age: 2, 4, 6, 18 mos	Age: 2, 4, 6, 18 mos	Age: 6 mos	Age: 2, 4, 6, 18 mos	Age: 2, 4, 6, 18 mos	Age: 18 mos	Age: 2, 4, 6, 18 mos	Age: 18 mos	Age: 2, 4, 6, 18 mos	Age: 2, 4, 6, 18 mos
DTaP-HB-IPV-Hib	Diphtheria, tetanus, acellular pertussis, hepatitis B, inactivated polio virus, *Haemophilus influenzae* type B vaccine	Age: 2, 4, 6 mos	Age: 2, 4, 6 mos				Age: 2, 4, 18 mos			Age: 2, 4, 6 mos		Age: 2, 4, 6 mos		
Tdap-IPV	Tetanus, diphtheria (reduced toxoid), acellular pertussis (reduced toxoid), inactivated polio virus vaccine	Age: 4–6 yrs	Age: 4–6 yrs	Age: 4–6 yrs	Age: 4–6 yrs	Age: 4–6 yrs	Age: 4–6 yrs	Age: 4 yrs	Age: 4–6 yrs	Age: 4–5 yrs	Age: 4–6 yrs[7]	Age: 4–6 yrs	Age: 4–6 yrs[7]	Age: 4–6 yrs
Tdap	Tetanus, diphtheria (reduced toxoid), acellular pertussis (reduced toxoid) vaccine	Grade 9	Grade 9	Grade 8	Age: 13–15 yrs	Age: 14–16 yrs	Grade: secondary III	Grade 7	Grade 7	Grade 9	Grade 9	Grade 9	Grade 7	Grade 6
HA	Hepatitis A vaccine	Greyed out	Greyed out	Greyed out	Greyed out	Greyed out	Grade 4							
HB	Hepatitis B vaccine	HB is provided in a three-dose combination vaccine (DTaP-HB-IPV-Hib) in infancy	(3-dose) Grade 6	(2-dose) Grade 6	(2-dose), Grade 6	(2-dose) Grade 7	HB is provided in a 3-dose combination vaccine (DTaP-HB-IPV-Hib) in infancy / (2-dose) Grade 4[3]	At birth, 2, 6 mos	(2-doses) Grade 7	HB is provided in a three-dose combination vaccine (DTaP-HB-IPV-Hib) in infancy	(2-dose) Grade 6	HB is provided in a three-dose combination vaccine (DTaP-HB-IPV-Hib) in infancy	At birth, 1, 6 mos	At birth, 1, 9 mos
MMR	Measles, mumps, rubella vaccine	Age: 12 mos				Age: 12 mos	Age: 12 mos					Age: 12 mos		
Var	Varicella vaccine	Age: 12 mos	Age: 12 mos	(2nd dose) Grade: 6		Age: 15 mos	Age: 4–6 yrs	(2nd dose) Grade 9				Age: 12 mos		Grade 6
MMRV	Measles, mumps, rubella, varicella vaccine	2nd dose Age: 4–6 yrs	Age: 12 mos, 4–6 yrs	Age: 12, 18 mos	Age: 12 mos, 4–6 yrs	2nd dose Age: 4–6 yrs	Age: 18 mos	Age: 12, 18 mos	Age: 12 mos, 18 mos–6 yrs	Age: 12, 18 mos	Age: 12, 18 mos	2nd dose Age: 4–6 yrs	Age: 12, 36 mos	Age: 12, 18 mos
Men-C-C	Meningococcal conjugate (strain C) vaccine	Age: 2, 12 mos	Age: 4, 12 mos	Age: 12 mos	Age: 12 mos[4]	Age: 12 mos	Age: 12 mos, Grade: secondary III	Age: 12 mos	Age: 12 mos	Age: 12 mos	Age: 12 mos	Age: 2, 12 mos	Age: 2, 12 mos	Age: 12 mos
Men-C-ACYW-135	Meningococcal conjugate (strains A, C, Y, W135) vaccine	Grade 9	Grade 9	Grade 6		Grade 7		Grade 9	Grade 7	Grade 9	Grade 4	Grade 9	Grade 12[1]	Grade 9
Pneu-C-13	Pneumococcal conjugate (13-valent) vaccine	Age: 2, 4, 12 mos	Age: 2, 4, 12 mos	Age: 2, 4, 12 mos	Age: 2, 4, 12 mos	Age: 2, 4, 12 mos	Age: 2, 4, 12 mos	Age: 2, 4, 12 mos	Age: 2, 4, 12 mos	Age: 2, 4, 12 mos	Age: 2, 4, 12 mos	Age: 2, 4, 12 mos	Age: 2, 4, 6, 18 mos	Age: 2, 4, 6, 18 mos
Pnue-C-10	Pneumococcal conjugate (10-valent) vaccine													
Rota	Rotavirus vaccine	Age: 2, 4, 6 mos	Age: 2, 4, 6 mos	Age: 2, 4, 6 mos	Age: 2, 4, 6 mos	Age: 2, 4, 6 mos	Age: 2, 4 mos	Age: 2, 4, 6 mos	Age: 2, 4, 6 mos	Age: 2, 4, 6 mos	Age: 2, 4, 6 mos	Age: 2, 4, 6 mos	Age: 2, 4, 6 mos	Age: 2, 4, 6 mos
HPV	Human papillomavirus vaccine	(2-dose) Grade: 6	(2-dose) Grade 5[5]	(2-dose) Grade 6	(2-dose) 2018/19 Grade: 8, 9[5]	(2 or 3-dose) Grade 8, to 12[2]	(2-dose) Grade 4	(2-dose) Grade 7	(2-dose) Grade 7	(2-dose) Grade 6	(2-dose) Grade 6	(2-dose) Grade 6	(9–14 yrs: 2-dose 15 yrs +: 3-dose) Grade 4-6	(2-dose) Grade 6

LEGEND

Abbreviation/footnote	Definition
yrs	Years (age).
mos	Months (age).
1	If attending post-secondary school out-of-territory.
2	Females only.
3	Males only.
4	Starting as early as September 2019, Manitoba's Meningococcal School-Based Immunization Program will be offered at a later grade; no child will miss the opportunity to be vaccinated
5	Students are provided with a combination vaccine that protects against hepatitis A and B
6	A catch-up program in the 3rd year of high-school evaluates student's vaccination history. Students will be provided any missed vaccination to protect against the following diseases: diphtheria, pertussis, tetanus, polio, measles, mumps, rubella, varicella, meningococcal serogroup C infections, hepatitis A and B, and human papilloma virus.
7	DTaP-IPV-Hib may be substituted for DTaP-IPV in times of shortage

Vaccine is not publicly funded in this province/territory.

A specific catch-up program is currently underway. A catch-up program is defined as a time-limited measure to implement a new vaccine program to a certain age cohort (e.g., an additional dose of a vaccine is recommended and a targeted program is put in place). It can also be used when a vaccine is added at a younger age (e.g., in infancy) and the existing program continues until that infancy age cohort "catches up" to the current age cohort (e.g., hepatitis B vaccine is added to the infancy program, but the school immunization program continues until those infants reach school-aged immunization). With that said, a province or territory can still provide catch-up vaccine at the individual level even if there's no specific program in place.

Health Canada. (2019). Canada's Provincial and Territorial Routine (and Catch-up) Vaccination Routine Schedule Programs for Infants and Children. Retrieved from https://www.canada.ca/content/dam/phac-aspc/documents/services/provincial-territorial-immunization-information/Childhood_Schedule_January2019.pdf is protection produced by an individual's own immune system. It can be obtained by having the actual disease or by receiving a vaccine that produces an immunologic response by that person's body. Active immunity may be lifelong either way. (See Chapter 17, for additional information.)

Young infants and children are susceptible to various illnesses because their immune systems are not yet mature. Many of these illnesses can be prevented by following the recommended schedule of childhood immunizations. Table 18.9 shows Health Canada's (2019) provincial and territorial routine vaccination routine schedule programs for infants and children. Refer to the**Point** for information about how to view the latest Health Canada immunization schedules, by province. The schedule for immunizations should be reviewed with parents, stressing the importance of continued follow-up health care to preserve their infant's health.

The newborn's first immunization (hepatitis B) is received in the hospital soon after birth. The first dose can also be given by age 2 months if the mother is HbsAg negative. If the mother is HbsAg positive, then the newborn should receive hepatitis B vaccine and hepatitis B immunoglobulin within 12 hours of birth (Cunningham et al., 2018).

Education for the parents should include the risks and benefits for each vaccine and possible adverse effects. Parents have the right to decline immunizations based on their religious or personal beliefs. When consent has been received, the nurse administering the vaccine must document the date and time it was given, name and manufacturer, lot number and expiration date of the vaccine given, site and route of administration, and the name and title of the nurse who administered the vaccine. Despite overwhelming evidence of vaccine safety, suspicion and misconception continues in small groups of hesitant or resistant parents/partners/significant others, often leading to outbreaks of vaccine-preventable infections. On the front lines of vaccinations, nurses can improve vaccination rates by developing trust with parents/partners/significant others and arming them with information based on sound evidence.

NURSING CARE PLAN 18.1

Overview of the Mother and Newborn Having Difficulty With Breastfeeding

Baby boy James, weight 7 lb, 4 oz, was born a few hours ago. His mother is a 19-year-old gravida 1, para 1. His Apgar scores were 9 points at both 1 and 5 minutes. Labour and birth were unremarkable. James' mother said she wished to breastfeed. The postpartum nurse assisted the new mother with positioning and latching-on and left the room for a few minutes. On returning, the mother was upset, James was crying, and she stated she wanted a bottle of formula to feed him since she didn't have milk and her nipples hurt.

Assessment reveals a young, inexperienced mother placed in an uncomfortable situation with limited knowledge of breastfeeding. Anxiety from the mother transferred to James, resulting in crying. The mother, apprehensive about breastfeeding, needs additional help.

NURSING DIAGNOSIS: Ineffective breastfeeding related to pain and limited skill

Outcome Identification and Evaluation

The mother will demonstrate understanding of breastfeeding skills as evidenced by use of correct positioning and technique, and verbalization of appropriate information related to breastfeeding.

Interventions: *Providing Education*

- Instruct mother on proper positioning for breastfeeding; suggest use of football hold, side-lying position, modified cradle, and across-the-lap position *to ensure comfort and to promote ease in breastfeeding.*
- Review breast anatomy and milk letdown reflex *to enhance mother's understanding of lactation.*
- Observe newborn's ability to suck and latch on to the nipple *to assess whether newborn has adequate ability.*

- Monitor sucking and newborn swallowing for several minutes *to ensure adequate latching on and to assess intake.*
- Reinforce nipple care with water and exposure to air *to maintain nipple integrity.*

(continued)

NURSING CARE PLAN 18.1

Overview of the Mother and Newborn Having Difficulty With Breastfeeding (continued)

NURSING DIAGNOSIS: Anxiety related to breastfeeding ability and irritable, crying newborn

Outcome Identification and Evaluation

The mother will verbalize increased comfort with breastfeeding as evidenced by positive statements related to breastfeeding and verbalization of desire to continue to breastfeed newborn.

Interventions: *Reducing Anxiety*

- Ensure that the environment is calm and soothing without distractions *to promote maternal and newborn relaxation.*
- Show mother correct latching-on technique *to promote breastfeeding.*
- Assist in calming newborn by holding and talking *to ensure that the newborn is relaxed prior to latching on.*
- Reassure mother she can be successful at breastfeeding *to enhance her self-esteem and confidence.*
- Encourage frequent trials and attempts *to enhance confidence.*
- Encourage the mother to verbalize her anxiety/fears *to reduce anxiety.*

NURSING DIAGNOSIS: Acute pain related to breastfeeding and incorrect latching-on technique

Outcome Identification and Evaluation

The mother will experience a decrease in pain during breastfeeding as evidenced by statements of less nipple pain.

Interventions: *Reducing Pain*

- Suggest several alternate positions for breastfeeding *to increase comfort.*
- Demonstrate how to break suction before removing infant from breast *to minimize trauma to nipple.*
- Inspect nipple area *to promote early identification of trauma.*
- Reinforce correct latching-on technique *to prevent nipple trauma.*
- Administer pain medication if indicated *to relieve pain.*
- Instruct about nipple care between feedings *to maintain nipple integrity.*

KEY CONCEPTS

- The period of transition from intrauterine to extrauterine life occurs during the first several hours after birth. It is a time of stabilization for the newborn's temperature, respiration, and cardiovascular dynamics.

- The newborn's bowel is sterile at birth. It usually takes about a week for the newborn to produce vitamin K in sufficient quantities to prevent VKDB.

- It is recommended that all newborns in Canada receive an installation of a prophylactic agent (erythromycin or tetracycline ophthalmic ointment) in their eyes within an hour or two of being born, with parents' consent.

- Nursing measures to maintain newborns' body temperature include drying them immediately with prewarmed blankets after birth to prevent heat loss through evaporation, putting a hat on their head, and placing them skin-to-skin on their parent's chest, or under a temperature-controlled radiant warmer.

○ The specific components of a typical newborn examination include a general survey of skin colour, posture, state of alertness, head size, overall behavioural state, respiratory status, sex, and any obvious congenital anomalies.

○ Gestational age assessment is pertinent because it allows the nurse to plot growth parameters and to anticipate potential problems related to prematurity/postmaturity and growth abnormalities such as SGA/LGA.

○ After the newborn has passed the transitional period and stabilized, the nurse needs to complete ongoing assessments, vital signs, weight and measurements, cord care, hygiene measures, newborn screening tests, and various other tasks until the newborn is discharged home from the birthing unit.

○ Important topics about which to educate parents include environmental safety, newborn characteristics, feeding and bathing, circumcision and cord care, sleep and elimination patterns of newborns, safe infant car seats, holding/positioning, and follow-up care.

○ Newborn screening tests consist of hearing and certain genetic and inborn errors of metabolism tests required in most states for newborns before discharge from the birth facility.

○ The World Health Organization (2018), Health Canada (2014a), and Canadian Paediatric Society (Critch, Canadian Paediatric Society, & Nutrition and Gastroenterology Committee, 2018) all recommend breastfeeding exclusively for the first 6 months of life and that it continue along with other food for 2 years or beyond, to the comfort of each breastfeeding dyad.

○ Parents who make the informed decision not to breastfeed need to know what types of formula are available, safe preparation and storage of formula, equipment, feeding positions, and how much to feed their infant.

○ Common problems associated with the newborn include transient tachypnea, physiologic jaundice, and hypoglycemia.

○ Transient tachypnea of the newborn appears soon after birth; is accompanied by retractions, expiratory grunting, or cyanosis. In many babies it resolves fairly quickly; some babies require additional respiratory support and admission into NICU.

○ Physiologic jaundice is a very common condition in newborns, with the majority demonstrating yellowish skin, mucous membranes, and sclera within the first 3 days of life. Newborns undergoing phototherapy in the treatment of jaundice require close monitoring of their body temperature and fluid and electrolyte balance; observation of skin integrity; eye protection; and parental participation in their care.

○ The newborn with hypoglycemia requires close monitoring for signs and symptoms of hypoglycemia if present. In addition, newborns at high risk need to be identified based on their perinatal history, physical examination, body measurements, and gestational age.

○ The schedule for immunizations should be reviewed with parents, stressing the importance of continual follow-up health care to safeguard their infant's health.

REFERENCES AND RECOMMENDED READINGS

Abbas, I. M., & Hasan, R. T. (2015). Assessment of LATCH tool regarding initiation of breastfeeding among women after childbirth. *Assessment, 5*(05), 38–44.

Abrams, S., & Savelli, S. L. (2014). Be prepared to address parents' concerns about vitamin K injection. *AAP News, 35*(5), 1–1.

Abrams, S. A., & Schanler, R. J. (2014). Data do not support claims that "supplement formulas" are better than standard formulas for breastfed infants. *AAP News, 35*(6), 26–27.

Adamkin, D. H. (2015). Metabolic screening and postnatal glucose homeostasis in the newborn. *Pediatric Clinics of North America, 62*(2), 385–409.

Ahn, E. S., Jung, M. S., Lee, Y. K., Ko, S. Y., Shin, S. M., & Hahn, M. H. (2015). Neonatal clavicular fracture: Recent 10 year study. *Pediatrics International, 57*(1), 60–63.

Alcantara, D., & O'Driscoll, M. (2014). Congenital microcephaly. *American Journal of Medical Genetics Part C: Seminars in Medical Genetics, 166C*, 124–139.

Altuntas, N., Turkyilmaz, C., Yildiz, H., Kulali, F., Hirfanoglu, I., Onal, E., . . . Atalay, Y. (2014). Validity and reliability of the infant breastfeeding assessment tool, the mother baby assessment tool, and the LATCH scoring system. *Breastfeeding Medicine, 9*(4), 191–195.

American Academy of Pediatrics (AAP). (2014). Iodine deficiency: Pregnant, breastfeeding women need supplementation, AAP says. *AAP News, 35*(6). Retrieved from http://aapnews.aappublications.org/content/35/6/11.1.extract.

American Academy of Pediatrics (AAP). (2015). *Where we stand: Administration of vitamin K*. Retrieved from http://www.healthychildren.org/English/ages-stages/prenatal/delivery-beyond/Pages/Where-We-Stand-Administration-of-Vitamin-K.aspx.

American Academy of Pediatrics (AAP). (2017). *Jaundice in newborns: Parent FAQs*. Retrieved from http://www.healthychildren.org/English/ages-stages/baby/Pages/Jaundice.aspx.

American Academy of Pediatrics (AAP). (2018a). *Car seats: Information for families.* Retrieved from http://www.healthychildren.org/English/safety-prevention/on-the-go/Pages/Car-Safety-Seats-Information-for-Families.aspx.

American Academy of Pediatrics (AAP). (2018b). *Purpose of newborn hearing screening.* Retrieved from http://www.healthychildren.org/English/ages-stages/baby/Pages/Purpose-of-Newborn-Hearing-Screening.aspx.

American Speech-Language-Hearing Association (ASHA). (2018). *Newborn hearing screening.* Retrieved from https://www.asha.org/practice-portal/professional-issues/newborn-hearing-screening/.

Apgar, V. (2015). A proposal for a new method of evaluation of the newborn infant. *Anesthesia & Analgesia, 120*(5), 1056–1059.

Aziz, K., Dancey, P., & Canadian Paediatric Society, Fetus and Newborn Committee. (2018). *Screening guidelines for newborns at risk for low blood glucose.* Retrieved from https://www.cps.ca/en/documents/position/newborns-low-blood-glucose.

Barrington, K. J., Sankaran, K., Canadian Paediatric Society, & Fetus and Newborn Committee. (2018). *Canadian Paediatric Society position statement: Guidelines for detection, management and prevention of hyperbilirubinemia in term and late preterm newborn infants.* Retrieved from https://www.cps.ca/en/documents/position/hyperbilirubinemia-newborn#ref7.

Bellini, S. (2015). What parents need to know about vitamin K administration at birth. *Nursing for Women's Health, 19*(3), 261–265.

Bhattacharya, K., Wotton, T., & Wiley, V. (2014). The evolution of blood-spot newborn screening. *Translational Pediatrics, 3*(2), 63–70.

Bond, S. (2015). Rethinking old practices: Evidence supports wiping, not suctioning, newborn secretions at birth. *Journal of Midwifery & Women's Health, 60*(2), 220–224.

Boom, J. A. (2018a). Macrocephaly in infants and children: Etiology and evaluation. *UpToDate.* Retrieved from http://www.uptodate.com/contents/macrocephaly-in-infants-and-children-etiology-and-evaluation.

Boom, J. A. (2018b). Microcephaly in infants and children: Etiology and evaluation. *UpToDate.* Retrieved from http://www.uptodate.com/contents/microcephaly-in-infants-and-children-etiology-and-evaluation.

Boué, G., Cummins, E., Guillou, S., Antignac, J. P., Le Bizec, B., & Membré, J. M. (2018). Public health risks and benefits associated with breast milk and infant formula consumption. *Critical Reviews in Food Science and Nutrition, 58*(1), 126–145.

Bowers, P. (2015). Cultural perspectives of childbearing. *Nursing Spectrum.* Retrieved from https://www.nurse.com/ce/cultural-perspectives-in-childbearing.

Boyle, C. A., Bocchini, J. A., & Kelly, J. (2014). Reflections on 50 years of newborn screening. *Pediatrics, 133*(6), 961–963.

Busch, D. W., Logan, K., & Wilkinson, A. (2014). Clinical practice breastfeeding recommendations for primary care: Applying a tri-core breastfeeding conceptual model. *Journal of Pediatric Health Care, 28*(6), 486–496.

Busch, D., Nassar, L., & Silbert-Flagg, J. (2015). The necessity of breastfeeding—promoting breastfeeding in the primary care setting: A community pilot project applying the Tri-Core Breastfeeding Model: Beyond the basics. *Journal of Pregnancy & Child Health, 2*(3), 2–7.

Canadian Paediatric Society. (2017). *Caring for kids: Jaundice.* Retrieved from https://www.caringforkids.cps.ca/handouts/jaundice_in_newborns.

Canadian Paediatric Society. (2018). *Breastfeeding.* Retrieved from https://www.caringforkids.cps.ca/handouts/breastfeeding.

Canadian Urological Association. (2014). *Urological health: Foreskin care for boys.* Retrieved from https://www.cua.org/themes/web/assets/files/patient_info/secured/en/15e-foreskin_boys_s.pdf.

Centers for Disease Control and Prevention (CDC). (2017). *Recommendations and guidelines: Newborn screening contingency plan, Version II, 2017.* Retrieved from http://www.cdc.gov/ncbddd/hearingloss/recommendations.html.

Christopher, G. C., & Krell, J. K. (2014). Changing the breastfeeding conversation and our culture. *Breastfeeding Medicine, 9*(2), 53–55.

Chu, J. (2014). Approach to jaundice in infancy. *Mount Sinai Expert Guides: Hepatology,* 374–381. doi: 10.1002/9781118748626.ch36

Chu, H. Y., & Englund, J. A. (2014). Maternal immunization. *Clinical Infectious Diseases, 59*(4), 560–568.

Clark-Gambelunghe, M. B., & Clark, D. A. (2015). Sensory development. *Pediatric Clinics of North America, 62*(2), 367–384.

Coroneos, C. J., Voineskos, S. H., Christakis, M. K., Thoma, A., Bain, J. R., & Brouwers, M. C. (2017). Obstetrical brachial plexus injury (OBPI): Canada's national clinical practice guideline. *BMJ Open, 7*(1), e014141. Retrieved from https://www.ncbi.nlm.nih.gov/pmc/articles/PMC5278272/.

Critch, J. N., Canadian Paediatric Society, & Nutrition and Gastroenterology Committee. (2018). *Nutrition for healthy term infants, birth to six months: An overview.* Retrieved from https://www.cps.ca/en/documents/position/nutrition-healthy-term-infants-overview.

Cunningham, F. G., Leveno, K. J., Bloom, S. L., Spong, C. Y., Dashe, J. S., Hoffman, B. L., . . . Sheffield, J. S. (2018). *William's obstetrics* (25th ed.). New York: McGraw-Hill Medical.

Davidson, M. R. (2014). *Fast facts for the neonatal nurse: A nursing orientation and care guide in a nutshell.* New York: Springer Publishing Company.

Delany, I., Rappuoli, R., & De Gregorio, E. (2014). Vaccines for the 21st century. *EMBO Molecular Medicine, 6*(6), 708–720.

Dore, S., Buchan, D., Coulas, S., Hamber, L., Stewart, M., Cowan, D., & Jamieson, L. (1998). Alcohol versus natural drying for newborn cord care. *Journal of Obstetric, Gynecologic & Neonatal Nursing, 27*(6), 621–627.

Dudek, S. G. (2017). *Nutrition essentials for nursing practice* (8th ed.). Philadelphia, PA: Lippincott Williams & Wilkins.

Dunn, R. L., Kalich, K. A., Henning, M. J., & Fedrizzi, R. (2015). Engaging field-based professionals in a qualitative assessment of barriers and positive contributors to breastfeeding using the social ecological model. *Maternal and Child Health Journal, 19*(1), 6–16.

Dyson, L., McCormick, F. M., & Renfrew, M. J. (2014). Interventions for promoting the initiation of breastfeeding. *Sao Paulo Medical Journal, 132*(1), 68–72.

El-Radhi, A. S. (2015). Management of common neonatal problems. *British Journal of Nursing, 24*(5), 258–266.

Fillipps, D. J., & Bucciarelli, R. L. (2015). Cardiac evaluation of the newborn. *Pediatric Clinics of North America, 62*(2), 471–489.

Fonseca, M. J., Severo, M., Barros, H., & Santos, A. C. (2014). Determinants of weight changes during the first 96 hours of life in full-term newborns. *Birth, 41*(2), 160–168.

Freedman, A. L., & Hurwitz, R. S. (2015). Complications of newborn circumcision: Prevention, diagnosis and treatment. In P. P. Godbole, M. A. Koyle, & D. T. Wilcox (Eds.). *Pediatric urology: Surgical complications and management* (2nd ed.). Hoboken, NJ: John Wiley & Sons.

Gephart, S. M., & Weller, M. (2014). Colostrum as oral immune therapy to promote neonatal health. *Advances in Neonatal Care, 14*(1), 44–51.

Giese, R. A., & Richter, G. T. (2015). *Capillary malformations. Head and neck vascular anomalies: A practical case-based approach* (pp. 127–128), San Diego, CA: Plural Publishing.

Glasser, J. G. & Springer, S. C. (2016). Intestinal obstruction in the newborn. *eMedicine.* Retrieved from http://emedicine.medscape.com/article/980360-overview.

Gloster, H. M. Jr, Gebauer, L. E., & Mistur, R. L. (2016a). Erythema toxicum neonatorum. In H. M. Gloster, L. E. Gebauer, & R. L. Mistur (Eds.). *Absolute dermatology review* (pp. 87–89). Cham, Switzerland: Springer International Publishing.

Gloster, H. M. Jr, Gebauer, L. E., & Mistur, R. L. (2016b). Supernumerary nipples. In H. M. Gloster, L. E. Gebauer, & R. L. Mistur (Eds.). *Absolute dermatology review* (pp. 355–356). Cham, Switzerland: Springer International Publishing.

Goyal, D., Nagar, S., & Kumar, B. (2014). An enhanced approach for face recognition of newborns using HMM and SVD coefficients. *International Journal of Computer Applications, 88*(14), 17–23.

Greene, C. L., & Matern, D. (2014). Newborn screening for inborn errors of metabolism. In N. Blau, M. Duran, K. M. Gibson, & C. Dionisi-Vici (Eds.). *Physician's guide to the diagnosis, treatment, and follow-up of inherited metabolic diseases* (pp. 719–735). Berlin Heidelberg, Germany: Springer Publishers.

Health Canada. (2004). *Canadian Perinatal Surveillance System: Birth weight for gestational age.* Retrieved from https://www.canada.ca/en/public-health/services/injury-prevention/health-surveillance-epidemiology-division/maternal-infant-health/birth-weight-gestational.html.

Health Canada. (2012a). *Breastfeeding initiation in Canada: Key statistics and graphics (2009–2010).* Retrieved from https://www.canada.ca/en/health-canada/services/food-nutrition/food-nutrition-surveillance/health-nutrition-surveys/canadian-community-health-survey-cchs/breastfeeding-initiation-canada-key-statistics-graphics-2009-2010-food-nutrition-surveillance-health-canada.html.

Health Canada. (2012b). *Infant formula.* Retrieved from https://www.canada.ca/en/health-canada/services/food-nutrition/food-nutrition-surveillance/health-nutrition-surveys/canadian-community-health-survey-cchs/breastfeeding-practices-canada-overview-food-nutrition-surveillance-health-canada.html.

Health Canada. (2014a). *Nutrition for healthy term infants: Recommendations from birth to six months.* Retrieved from https://www.canada.ca/en/health-canada/services/food-nutrition/healthy-eating/infant-feeding/nutrition-healthy-term-infants-recommendations-birth-six-months.html.

Health Canada. (2014b). *Nutrition for healthy term infants: Recommendations from six to 24 months.* Retrieved from https://www.canada.ca/en/health-canada/services/canada-food-guide/resources/infant-feeding/nutrition-healthy-term-infants-recommendations-birth-six-months/6-24-months.html.

Health Canada. (2016). *Safety around the house.* Retrieved from https://www.canada.ca/en/health-canada/services/home-safety/safety-around-house.html.

Health Canada. (2018). *Safe sleep.* Retrieved from https://www.canada.ca/en/public-health/services/health-promotion/childhood-adolescence/stages-childhood/infancy-birth-two-years/safe-sleep.html.

Health Canada. (2019). Canada's provincial and territorial routine (and catch-up) vaccination routine schedule programs for infants and children. Retrieved from https://www.canada.ca/content/dam/phac-aspc/documents/services/provincial-territorial-immunization-information/Childhood_Schedule_January2019.pdf.

Hodges, N. L., & Smith, G. A. (2014). Car safety. *Pediatrics in Review, 35*(4), 155–161.

Joint Commission. (2018). *Infant abductions: Preventing future occurrences.* Retrieved from http://www.jointcommission.org/SentinelEvents/SentinelEventAlert/sea_9.htm.

Kent, G. (2014). Regulating fatty acids in infant formula: Critical assessment of US policies and practices. *International Breastfeeding Journal, 9*(1), 2–10.

Khan, J., Vesel, L., Bahl, R., & Martines, J. C. (2014). Timing of breastfeeding initiation and exclusivity of breastfeeding during the first month of life: Effects on neonatal mortality and morbidity—a systematic review and meta-analysis. *Maternal and Child Health Journal, 19*(3), 468–479.

King, T. L., Brucker, M. C., Osborne, K., & Jevitt, C. M. (2019). *Varney's midwifery* (6th ed.). Burlington, MA: Jones & Bartlett Learning.

Kliegman, R. M., Behrman, R. E., Jenson, H. B., & Stanton, B. F. (2016). *Nelson's textbook of pediatrics* (20th ed.). St. Louis, MO: Elsevier.

La Leche League. (2018a). *Storing human milk.* Retrieved from https://www.llli.org/breastfeeding-info/storingmilk/.

La Leche League. (2018b). *The first week: Positioning and latch.* Retrieved from https://www.llli.org/breastfeeding-info/positioning/.

Lomax, A. (2015). *Examination of the newborn: An evidence-based guide* (2nd ed.). West Sussex, UK: John Wiley & Sons.

Lönnerdal, B. (2014). Infant formula and infant nutrition: Bioactive proteins of human milk and implications for composition of infant formulas. *The American Journal of Clinical Nutrition, 99*(3), 712S–717S.

Ludington-Hoe, S. M., & Morgan, K. (2014). Infant assessment and reduction of sudden unexpected postnatal collapse risk during skin-to-skin contact. *Newborn and Infant Nursing Reviews, 14*(1), 28–33.

Maisels, M. J. (2015). Sister Jean Ward, phototherapy, and jaundice: A unique human and photochemical interaction. *Journal of Perinatology, 35*(9), 671–675.

Marcdante, K. J., & Kliegman, R. M. (2018). *Nelson essentials of pediatrics* (8th ed.). Philadelphia, PA: Elsevier.

Martin, R. J., Fanaroff, A. A., & Walsh, M. C. (2014). *Fanaroff & Martin's neonatal-perinatal medicine* (10th ed.). Philadelphia, PA: Elsevier.

McDermott, J. L. (2015). G586 (P) Phototherapy management in jaundiced babies: Jaundice management tool. *Archives of Disease in Childhood, 100*(Suppl 3), A268–A269.

Mielke, R. T. (2014). Counseling parents who are considering newborn male circumcision. *Journal of Midwifery & Women's Health, 59*(2), 225.

Monahan, E. (2017). What are the dangers of diluted baby formula? *Livestrong.* Retrieved from http://www.livestrong.com/article/97662-dangers-diluted-baby-formula/.

Moore, D. L., MacDonald, N. E., & Canadian Paediatric Society Infectious Diseases and Immunization Committee. (2018). *Position statement: Preventing ophthalmia neonatorum. Pediatrics & child health.* Retrieved from https://www.cps.ca/en/documents/position/ophthalmia-neonatorum.

Morrison, K., Herbst, K., Corbett, S., & Herndon, C. D. (2014). Pain management practice patterns for common pediatric urology procedures. *Urology, 83*(1), 206–210.

Moses, S. (2018). *Pediatric vital signs. Family practice notebook.* Retrieved from http://www.fpnotebook.com/cv/exam/pdtrcvtlsgns.htm.

Mutter, G. L., & Prat, J. (2014). *Pathology of the female reproductive tract.* Philadelphia, PA: Elsevier Health Sciences.

Nagtalon-Ramos, J. (2014). *Maternal-newborn nursing care: Best evidence-based practices.* Philadelphia, PA: F.A. Davis Company.

National Center for Missing & Exploited Children (NCMEC). (2015). *For healthcare professionals: Guidelines on prevention of and response to infant abductions.* Retrieved from http://www.missingkids.com/content/dam/pdfs/publications/nc05.pdf.

National Institute of Child Health and Human Development (NICHD). (2018). *Safe to sleep public education campaign.* Retrieved from http://www.nichd.nih.gov/sts/news/downloadable/Pages/infographic_horizontal.aspx.

Nelson, C. R., Demarsh, A., Miller, S. P., Morris, S. K., Moore Hepburn, C., Bitnun, A., . . . Tataryn, J. (2017). Small bite, big problem: Understanding severe microcephaly in Canada. *Paediatrics & Child Health, 22*(8), 504–505.

Newborn Screening Ontario. (2018). *Health care providers: Education resources.* Retrieved from https://www.newbornscreening.on.ca/en/health-care-providers/submitters/cchd-screening-implementation/cchd-resources.

Ng, E., Loewy, A. D., & Fetus and Newborn Committee. (2018). *Canadian Paediatric Society position statement: Guidelines for vitamin K prophylaxis in newborns.* Retrieved from https://www.cps.ca/en/documents/position/vitamin-k-prophylaxis-in-newborns.

Nikolopoulos, T. P. (2015). Neonatal hearing screening: What we have achieved and what needs to be improved. *International Journal of Pediatric Otorhinolaryngology, 79*(5), 635–637.

Otsuka, Y. (2014). Face recognition in infants: A review of behavioral and near-infrared spectroscopic studies. *Japanese Psychological Research, 56*, 76–90.

Owings, M., Uddin, S., & Williams, S. (2015). *Trends in circumcision for male newborns in U.S. Hospitals: 1979–2010.* Retrieved from http://www.cdc.gov/nchs/data/hestat/circumcision_2013/circumcision_2013.htm.

Patel, H., Feldman, M., & Canadian Paediatric Society, Community Paediatrics Committee. (2018). *Canadian Paediatric Society position statement: Universal newborn hearing screening.* Retrieved from https://www.cps.ca/en/documents/position/universal-hearing-screening-newborns.

Pfister, K. M., & Ramel, S. E. (2014). Linear growth and neurodevelopmental outcomes. *Clinics in Perinatology, 41*(2), 309–321.

Public Health Agency of Canada, Canadian Paediatric Society, Canadian Foundation for the Study of Infant Deaths, & Canadian Institute of Child Health, Health Canada. (2011). *Joint statement on safe sleep: Preventing sudden infant deaths in Canada.* Retrieved from https://www.canada.ca/content/dam/phac-aspc/migration/phac-aspc/hp-ps/dca-dea/stages-etapes/childhood-enfance_0-2/sids/pdf/jsss-ecss2011-eng.pdf.

Rüdiger, M., & Konstantelos, D. (2015). Apgar score and risk of cause-specific infant mortality. *The Lancet, 385*(9967), 505–506.

Saugstad, O. D. (2015). Delivery room management of term and preterm newly born infants. *Neonatology, 107*(4), 365–371.

Schlenker, E., & Gilbert, J. A. (2015). *William's essentials of nutrition and diet therapy* (11th ed.). St. Louis, MO: Elsevier.

Sheth, R. D., Ranalli, N., & Aldana, P. (2017). Pediatric craniosynostosis. *eMedicine.* Retrieved from http://emedicine.medscape.com/article/1175957-overview.

Silverberg, N. B. (2015). Normal color variations in children of color. In N. B. Silverberg, C. Durán-McKinster, & Y-K. Tay (Eds.). *Pediatric skin of color* (pp. 63–68). New York: Springer.

Sinkey, R. G., Eschenbacher, M. A., Walsh, P. M., Doerger, R. G., Lambers, D. S., Sibai, B. M., & Habli, M. A. (2015). The GoMo study: A randomized clinical trial assessing neonatal pain with Gomco vs. Mogen clamp circumcision. *American Journal of Obstetrics and Gynecology, 212*(5), 664.e1–664.e8.

Skidmore-Roth, L. (2018). *Mosby's 2018 nursing drug reference* (31st ed.). St. Louis, MO: Elsevier.

Smith, E., & Shell, T. (2017). *ICEA position paper: Delayed bathing.* Retrieved from https://icea.org/wp-content/uploads/2018/02/ICEA-Position-Paper-Delayed-Bathing.pdf.

Sorokan, S. T., Finlay, J. C., Jefferies, A. L., & Canadian Paediatric Society Fetus And Newborn Committee. (2018). Position statement: Newborn circumcision. *Paediatrics & Child Health, 20*(6), 311–315. Retrieved from https://www.cps.ca/en/documents/position/circumcision.

Sowjanya, S. V. N. S. & Venugopalan, L. (2018). LATCH score as a predictor of exclusive breastfeeding at 6 weeks postpartum: A prospective cohort study. *Breastfeeding Medicine, 13*(6), 444--449. doi: 10.1089/bfm.2017.0142.

Stanley, C. A., Rozance, P. J., Thornton, P. S., De Leon, D. D., Harris, D., Haymond, M. W., . . . Wolfsdorf, J. I. (2015). Re-evaluating "transitional neonatal hypoglycemia": Mechanism and implications for management. *The Journal of Pediatrics, 166*(6), 1520–1525.e1.

Tamai, J., & McCarthy, J. J. (2018). Developmental dysplasia of the hip. *eMedicine.* Retrieved from http://emedicine.medscape.com/article/1248135-overview.

Task Force on Sudden Infant Death Syndrome. (2016). *SIDS and Other Sleep-Related Infant Deaths: Updated 2016 Recommendations for a Safe Infant Sleeping Environment.*

Pediatrics, 138(5), e20162938. Retrieved from http://pediatrics.aappublications.org/content/138/5/e20162938.

Tawia, S., & McGuire, L. (2014). Early weight loss and weight gain in healthy, full-term, exclusively-breastfed infants. *Breastfeeding Review, 22*(1), 31–42.

Thornton, P. S., Stanley, C. A., De Leon, D. D., Harris, D., Haymond, M. W., Hussain, K., . . . Wolfsdorf, J. I. (2015). Recommendations from the Pediatric Endocrine Society for evaluation and management of persistent hypoglycemia in neonates, infants, and children. *The Journal of Pediatrics, 167*(2), 238–245.

Tobian, A. A., Kacker, S., & Quinn, T. C. (2014). Male circumcision: A globally relevant but under-utilized method for the prevention of HIV and other sexually transmitted infections. *Annual Review of Medicine, 65,* 293–306.

Tung, T. H., & Moore, A. M. (2015). *14 brachial plexus injuries. Nerve surgery* (pp. 391–479). New York: Thieme Medical Publishers.

Verklan, M. T., & Walden, M. (2015). *Core curriculum for neonatal intensive care nursing* (5th ed.). St. Louis, MO: Elsevier.

Walker, M. (2017). *Breastfeeding management for the clinician: Using the evidence* (4th ed.). Burlington, MA: Jones & Bartlett Learning.

Weber, J., & Kelley, J. (2017). *Health assessment in nursing* (6th ed.). Philadelphia, PA: Lippincott Williams & Wilkins.

World Health Organization. (2006). *Newborns with low birth weight.* Retrieved from http://www.who.int/whosis/whostat-2006NewbornsLowBirthWeight.pdf.

World Health Organization. (2018). *Breastfeeding.* Retrieved from http://www.who.int/topics/breastfeeding/en/.

Zupan, J., Garner, P., & Omari, A. A. (2004). Topical umbilical cord care at birth. *Cochrane Database Systematic Reviews, 2004*(3), CD001057.

CHAPTER **WORKSHEET**

MULTIPLE-CHOICE QUESTIONS

1. At birth, a newborn's assessment reveals the following: heart rate of 140 bpm, loud crying, some flexion of extremities, crying when bulb syringe is introduced into the nares, and a pink body with blue extremities. The nurse would document the newborn's Apgar score as:
   a. 5 points
   b. 6 points
   c. 7 points
   d. 8 points

2. The nurse is explaining phototherapy to the parents of a newborn. The nurse would include which of the following as the purpose?
   a. Increase surfactant levels
   b. Stabilize the newborn's temperature
   c. Destroy Rh-negative antibodies
   d. Oxidize bilirubin on the skin

3. The nurse administers a single dose of vitamin K intramuscularly to a newborn after birth to promote:
   a. Conjugation of bilirubin
   b. Blood clotting
   c. Foreman ovale closure
   d. Digestion of complex proteins

4. A prophylactic agent is instilled in newborns' eyes to prevent which of the following conditions?
   a. Gonorrhea and chlamydia
   b. Thrush and enterobacter
   c. Staphylococcus and syphilis
   d. Hepatitis B and herpes

5. Health Canada and the Canadian Paediatric Society recommend that all newborns be placed on their backs to sleep to reduce the risk of:
   a. Respiratory distress syndrome
   b. Bottle mouth syndrome
   c. Sudden infant death syndrome
   d. GI regurgitation syndrome

6. Which one of the following immunizations is most commonly received by newborns before hospital discharge?
   a. Pneumococcus
   b. Varicella
   c. Hepatitis A
   d. Hepatitis B

7. Which condition would be missed if a newborn were screened before he had tolerated protein feedings for at least 24 hours?
   a. Hypothyroidism
   b. Cystic fibrosis
   c. Phenylketonuria
   d. Sickle cell disease

8. Which of the following findings in a newborn would the nurse document as abnormal when assessing the newborn head?
   a. Two soft spots palpated between the cranial bones
   b. A spongy area of edema outlined on the head
   c. Head circumference 32 cm, chest 34 cm
   d. Asymmetry of the head with overriding bones

9. Which of the following findings in a newborn would be considered normal?
   a. Passage of meconium within the first 24 hours
   b. Respiratory rate of 80 breaths per minute
   c. Yellow skin tones at 10 hours after birth
   d. Bleeding from the umbilicus area

CRITICAL THINKING EXERCISE

1. An African-born mother gave birth to her first baby and is on the postpartum unit. She calls the nurse into her room and expresses concern about how her daughter looks. The mother tells the nurse that her baby's head looks like a "banana" and is mushy to the touch, and she has "white spots" all over her nose. In addition, there appear to be "big bluish bruises" all over her baby's buttocks. She wants to know what is wrong with her baby and whether these problems will go away.
   a. How should the nurse respond to this mother's questions?
   b. What additional newborn instruction might be appropriate at this time?
   c. What reassurance can be given to this new mother regarding her daughter's appearance?

2. At approximately 12:30 AM on a Friday, a woman enters a hospital through a busy emergency department. She is wearing a white uniform and a lab coat with a stethoscope around her neck. She identifies herself as a new nurse coming back to check on something she had left on the unit on an earlier shift. She enters a postpartum client's room containing a newborn, and pushes the open crib down a hallway, escaping through an exit. The security cameras aren't working. The infant isn't discovered missing until the 2 AM check by the nurse.

   a. What impact does an infant abduction have on the family and the hospital?

   b. What security measure was the weak link in the chain of security?

   c. What can hospitals do to prevent infant abduction?

STUDY ACTIVITIES

1. Obtain a set of vital signs (temperature, pulse, respiration) of a newborn on admission to the postpartum unit. Repeat this procedure and compare changes in the values several hours later. Discuss what changes in the vital signs you would expect during this transitional period.

   The discussion of newborn changes noticed will vary from student to student, depending on the interview information obtained from the new parent(s).

2. Interview a new parent on the postpartum unit on their 2nd day about the changes noticed in the newborn's appearance and behaviour within the past 24 hours. Discuss your interview findings at postconference. This discussion will vary depending on questions asked during the bath demonstration as well as each individual client's response to it.

3. Demonstrate a newborn bath to a new parent in the room, using the principle of bathing from the cleanest to the dirtiest body part. Discuss the questions asked by the parent and their reaction to the demonstration in postconference.

4. Go to the La Leche League website (refer to thePoint). Review the information it provides on breastfeeding. How helpful would it be to new parents?

5. Debate the risks and benefits of neonatal circumcision within your nursing group at postconference. Did either side present a stronger position? What is your opinion, and why?

BRINGING IT ALL TOGETHER: A CASE STUDY

Two days after having a difficult birth of her first child at 37 weeks' gestation, 25-year-old Molly and her partner take their son home from the hospital. That evening while she is breastfeeding him, Molly notices that the whites of her son's eyes seem slightly yellow, a condition that worsens noticeably by the next day. Molly calls the Mother-Baby Clinic nurse and requests an appointment to evaluate her newborn.

Go to thePoint to find questions to consider about this case.

Childbearing at Risk

19

Nursing Management of Pregnancy at Risk: Pregnancy-Related Complications

Learning Objectives

Upon completion of the chapter, you will be able to:

1. Compare and contrast a normal pregnancy to a high risk one. Determine the common factors that might place a pregnancy at high risk.
2. Identify the causes of vaginal bleeding during early and late pregnancy.
3. Outline nursing assessment and management for the pregnant individual experiencing vaginal bleeding.
4. Develop a plan of care for the client experiencing preeclampsia, eclampsia, and HELLP syndrome.
5. Examine the pathophysiology of oligohydramnios and polyhydramnios and subsequent management.
6. Evaluate factors in a client's prenatal history that increase the risk for premature rupture of membranes (PROM).
7. Formulate a teaching plan for maintaining the health of pregnant clients experiencing a high-risk pregnancy.

Helen, **a 35-year-old G5 P4, presented to the labour and birth suite with severe abdominal pain, reporting that the pain began suddenly about an hour ago while resting. Helen has had two prior cesarean births and thus far has had an uneventful past 32 weeks. Helen appears distressed and is moaning. What additional assessments do you need to do to care for Helen? What might be your immediate nursing action?**

stillbirth refers to the loss of a fetus after the 20th week of gestation or after attaining a weight of 500 g (Statistics Canada, 2015), whereas abortion or miscarriage refers to a loss before the 20th week and less than 500 g. Nonmedical people often use the term *miscarriage* to denote an abortion that has occurred spontaneously. A miscarriage can occur during early pregnancy, and individuals who miscarry may not even be aware that they are pregnant. About 80% of spontaneous abortions occur within the first trimester. The terms *stillbirth* and *miscarriage* can sometimes be confusing. Both refer to the loss of an early pregnancy; however, stillbirth occurs later in pregnancy. Some stillbirths can occur right up to the time of labour and delivery at full term. Stillbirths are much less common than miscarriages, occurring in only 5 out of every 1,000 births (Statistics Canada, 2015).

The overall rate for spontaneous abortion is reported to be 15% to 20% of recognized pregnancies. The rate of spontaneous abortion however, varies greatly with age, with a rate of 10% at age 20, and a rate of 90% over age 45. At age 30, the spontaneous abortion rate is 15% (Heffner, 2004). However, with the development of highly sensitive assays for human chorionic gonadotropin (hCG) levels that detect pregnancies much earlier now, even prior to the expected next menses, the incidence of pregnancy loss increases significantly—to about 60% to 70% (King et al., 2015).

Pathophysiology

The causes of spontaneous abortion are varied and often unknown. The most common cause for first-trimester abortions is fetal genetic abnormalities, usually unrelated to the pregnant individual. Chromosomal abnormalities are more likely causes in the first trimester and maternal disease is more likely the cause in the second trimester. Those occurring during the second trimester are more likely related to maternal conditions, such as cervical insufficiency, congenital or acquired anomaly of the uterine cavity (uterine septum or fibroids), hypothyroidism, diabetes mellitus, chronic nephritis, use of crack cocaine, inherited and acquired thrombophilias, lupus, polycystic ovary syndrome, severe hypertension, and acute infection such as rubella virus, cytomegalovirus, herpes simplex virus, bacterial vaginosis, and toxoplasmosis (Jones & Lopez, 2014).

Individuals experiencing a spontaneous first-trimester abortion without a D&C require monitoring of hCG levels to validate that all the products of conception have been expelled. A D&C may not be necessary if the spontaneous abortion appears to be complete and hCG levels drop. Individuals going through a second-trimester abortion are admitted to the hospital to have an augmented labour and delivery. Nursing care would focus on care of the labouring individuals with careful attention paid to providing emotional support and pain management to the client and the family.

Nursing Assessment

When a pregnant individual calls and reports vaginal bleeding, the client should be seen as soon as possible by a health care professional to ascertain the etiology. Varying degrees of vaginal bleeding, low back pain, abdominal cramping, and passage of products of conception tissue may be reported. Ask the client about the colour of the vaginal bleeding (bright red is significant) and the amount—for example, ask questions about the number of peripads used in an hour and how full they are (saturation of one peripad hourly is significant) and enquire about the passage of any clots or tissue. Instruct the client to save any tissue or clots passed and bring them to the health care facility. Also, obtain a description of any other signs and symptoms the client may be experiencing, along with a description of their severity and duration. It is important to be attentive, calm, and listen to the client's description and voiced concerns.

When the client arrives at the health care facility, assess vital signs and observe the amount, colour, and characteristics of the bleeding. Obtain a current pain level rating, using an appropriate pain assessment tool. Also, evaluate the amount and intensity of abdominal cramping or contractions, and assess the client's level of understanding about what is happening. A thorough assessment helps in determining the type of spontaneous abortion, such as threatened abortion, inevitable abortion, incomplete or complete abortion, missed abortion, and any history of habitual or recurrent abortion (Table 19.1).

Nursing Management

Nursing management of the client with a spontaneous abortion focuses on providing continued monitoring and psychological support for the family that is experiencing acute loss and grief. An important component of this support is reassuring the client that spontaneous abortions usually result from an abnormality and that no individual actions would be likely to cause the abortion.

PROVIDING CONTINUED MONITORING

Continued monitoring and ongoing assessments are essential for the client experiencing a spontaneous abortion. Monitor the amount of vaginal bleeding through pad counts and observe for passage of products of conception tissue. Assess the client's pain level and provide appropriate pain management as needed for the discomfort.

Assist in preparing the client for procedures and treatments such as surgery to evacuate the uterus or medications such as misoprostol or PGE2. Provide teaching regarding expectant management when this route is an option so the client can make an informed decision regarding the plan of care. If the client is Rh negative and not sensitized,

TABLE 19.1	CATEGORIES OF ABORTION		
Category	**Assessment Findings**	**Diagnosis**	**Therapeutic Management**
Threatened abortion	Vaginal bleeding (often slight) early in a pregnancy No cervical dilation or change in cervical consistency Mild abdominal cramping Closed cervical os No passage of fetal tissue	Vaginal ultrasound to confirm if sac is empty Declining maternal serum hCG and progesterone levels to provide additional information about viability of pregnancy	Conservative supportive treatment Possible reduction in activity in conjunction with nutritious diet and adequate hydration
Inevitable abortion	Vaginal bleeding (greater than that associated with threatened abortion) Rupture of membranes Cervical dilation Strong abdominal cramping Possible passage of products of conception	Ultrasound and hCG levels to indicate pregnancy loss	Vacuum curettage if products of conception are not passed, to reduce risk of excessive bleeding and infection Prostaglandin analogues such as misoprostol to empty uterus of retained tissue (only used if fragments are not completely passed)
Incomplete abortion (passage of some of the products of conception)	Intense abdominal cramping Heavy vaginal bleeding Cervical dilation	Ultrasound confirmation that products of conception still in uterus	Client stabilization Evacuation of uterus via D&C or prostaglandin analogue
Complete abortion (passage of all products of conception)	History of vaginal bleeding and abdominal pain Passage of tissue with subsequent decrease in pain and significant decrease in vaginal bleeding	Ultrasound demonstrating an empty uterus	No medical or surgical intervention necessary Follow-up appointment to discuss family planning
Missed abortion (nonviable embryo retained in utero for at least 6 weeks)	Absent uterine contractions Irregular spotting Possible progression to inevitable abortion	Ultrasound to identify products of conception in uterus	Evacuation of uterus (if inevitable abortion does not occur): suction curettage during first trimester, dilation and evacuation during second trimester Induction of labour with intravaginal PGE2 suppository to empty uterus without surgical intervention
Habitual abortion	History of three or more consecutive spontaneous abortions Not carrying the pregnancy to viability or term	Validation via client's history	Identification and treatment of underlying cause (possible causes such as genetic or chromosomal abnormalities, reproductive tract abnormalities, chronic diseases, or immunologic problems) Cervical cerclage in second trimester if incompetent cervix is the cause

expect to administer Rh immune globulin within 72 hours after the onset of bleeding. Drug Guide 19.1 gives more information about these medications.

PROVIDING SUPPORT

A client's emotional reaction may vary depending on the desire for this pregnancy and the available support network. Provide both physical and emotional support. In addition, provide teaching, and the opportunity to ask questions as part of the informed decision-making process and to allow the client to have realistic expectations of next steps and possible outcomes. Explaining some of the causes of spontaneous abortions can help the client to understand what is happening and may allay fears and guilt that the client did something to cause the pregnancy loss. Most individuals experience an acute sense of loss

DRUG GUIDE 19.1 MEDICATIONS RELATED TO ABORTIONS

Medication	Action/Indications	Nursing Implications
Misoprostol (Cytotec)	Stimulates uterine contractions to terminate a pregnancy; to evacuate the uterus after abortion to ensure passage of all the products of conception	• Monitor for side effects such as diarrhea, abdominal pain, nausea, vomiting, dyspepsia. • Assess vaginal bleeding and report any increased bleeding, pain, or fever. • Monitor for signs and symptoms of shock, such as tachycardia, hypotension, and anxiety.
Mifepristone (RU-486)	Acts as progesterone antagonist, allowing prostaglandins to stimulate uterine contractions; causes the endometrium to slough; may be followed by administration of misoprostol within 48 hours	• Monitor for headache, vomiting, diarrhea, and heavy bleeding. • Anticipate administration of antiemetic prior to use to reduce nausea and vomiting. • Encourage client to use acetaminophen to reduce discomfort from cramping.
PGE2, dinoprostone (Cervidil, Prepidil Gel, Prostin E2)	Stimulates uterine contractions, causing expulsion of uterine contents; to expel uterine contents in fetal death or missed abortion during second trimester, or to efface and dilate the cervix in pregnancy at term	• Bring gel to room temperature before administering. • Avoid contact with skin. • Use sterile technique to administer. • Keep client supine for 30 minutes after administering. • Document time of insertion and dosing intervals. • Remove insert after 12 hours or at the onset of labour. • Explain purpose and expected response to client.
Rh(D) immune globulin WinRho	Suppresses immune response of nonsensitized Rh-negative clients who are exposed to Rh-positive blood; to prevent isoimmunization in Rh-negative women exposed to Rh-positive blood after abortions, miscarriages, and pregnancies	• Administer intramuscularly. • Educate client that Rh immune globulin will need after subsequent deliveries if newborns are Rh positive • Check lab study results to confirm Rh-negative status of client, and Rh-positive status of baby if available. Confirm antibody screen in negative prior to administering the drug.

Adapted from King, T. L., Brucker, M. C., Fahey, J. O., Kriebs, J. M., Gegor, C. L., & Varney, H. (2015). *Varney's midwifery* (5th ed.). Burlington, MA: Jones & Bartlett Learning; and Skidmore-Roth, L. (2015). *Mosby's 2015 nursing drug reference* (28th ed.). Philadelphia, PA: Elsevier.

and go through a grieving process with a spontaneous abortion. Providing sensitive listening, counselling, and anticipatory guidance to the client and family will allow them to verbalize their feelings and ask questions about future pregnancies.

The grieving period may last from weeks to years after a pregnancy loss, with each person grieving in a highly individual way. Encourage friends and family to be supportive but give the client and partner space and time to work through their feelings of loss. Referral to a community support group for parents who have experienced a miscarriage can be very helpful during this grief process.

Ectopic Pregnancy

An ectopic pregnancy is any pregnancy in which the fertilized ovum implants outside the uterine cavity. The term *ectopic* is derived from the Greek word *ektopos*,

meaning "out of place," and refers to the implantation of a fertilized egg in a location outside of the uterine cavity, including the fallopian tubes, cervix, ovary, and the abdominal cavity. This abnormally implanted embryo grows and draws its blood supply from the site of abnormal implantation. As the embryo enlarges, it creates the potential for organ rupture because only the uterine cavity is designed to expand and accommodate fetal development. Ectopic pregnancy can lead to massive hemorrhage, infertility, or death.

Ectopic pregnancies occur in approximately 1 in every 100 pregnancies in Canada, or roughly 1% of all pregnancies are diagnosed as ectopic; this rate has increased dramatically during the past 14 years (Hockin & Jessamine, 1984). It is a major health concern for individuals of reproductive age and is the primary cause of death during the first trimester of pregnancy in the United States (Szypulski, 2015). The discovery of ectopic pregnancies prior to rupture has increased dramatically in the past few decades as a result of improved diagnostic techniques such as the development of sensitive and specific radioimmunoassays for hCG, high-resolution ultrasonography, and the widespread availability of laparoscopy (Desai et al., 2014).

With an ectopic pregnancy, rupture and hemorrhage may occur due to the growth of the embryo. A ruptured ectopic pregnancy is a medical emergency; therefore, prediction of any tubal rupture before its occurrence is extremely important. It is a potentially life-threatening condition and involves pregnancy loss. Even in Canada, individuals may still die from ectopic pregnancy, although early diagnosis, advancements in treatment, and surgical techniques have helped manage ectopic pregnancy more safely and effectively.

Pathophysiology

Normally, the fertilized ovum implants in the uterus. In ectopic pregnancy, the journey along the fallopian tube is arrested or altered in some way. With an ectopic pregnancy, the ovum implants outside the uterus. The most common site for implantation is the fallopian tubes, but some ova may implant in the ovary, the intestine, the cervix, or the abdominal cavity (Fig. 19.1) (Sepilian & Wood, 2017). None of these anatomic sites can accommodate placental attachment or a growing embryo.

Risk Factors

Ectopic pregnancies usually result from conditions that obstruct or slow the passage of the fertilized ovum through the fallopian tube to the uterus. This may be a physical blockage in the tube, or failure of the tubal epithelium to move the zygote (the cell formed after the egg is fertilized) down the tube into the uterus. In the general population, most cases are the result of tubal scarring secondary to pelvic inflammatory disease (PID). Organisms such as *Neisseria gonorrhea* and *Chlamydia trachomatis* preferentially attack the fallopian tubes, producing silent infections. One study reported a twofold increased risk for ectopic pregnancy in individuals with a history of a chlamydia infection, secondary to tubal damage (Randall & LaMontagne, 2015). Other associated risk factors for ectopic pregnancy include previous tubal surgery, infertility, PID, previous pregnancy loss (induced or spontaneous), use of an intrauterine contraceptive system, previous ectopic pregnancy, uterine fibroids, sterilization, smoking (which alters tubal motility), history of multiple sexual partners, use of progestin-only oral contraceptives, douching, and exposure to diethylstilbestrol (DES) (Ardehali, Casikar, & Condous, 2015).

Therapeutic Management

The diagnosis of ectopic pregnancy can be challenging because many clients are asymptomatic before tubal rupture. The classic clinical triad of ectopic pregnancy includes abdominal pain, amenorrhea, and vaginal bleeding. Unfortunately, only about half of clients present with all three symptoms.

Diagnostic procedures used for a suspected ectopic pregnancy includes serum beta-hCG concentrations to determine a baseline and to assess pregnancy advancement, and a transvaginal ultrasound to visualize the size and location of the gestational sac (Bourne, 2015).

Historically, the treatment of ectopic pregnancy was limited to surgery. The therapeutic management of ectopic pregnancy depends on whether the tube is intact or has ruptured, creating a medical emergency. In the event of a surgical intervention, preservation of the affected fallopian tube is attempted (King et al., 2015).

MEDICAL INTERVENTION

With early diagnosis, most individuals with ectopic pregnancy could be treated with methotrexate. The overall success rate of medical treatment in properly selected individuals is nearly 90%. To be eligible for medical therapy, the client must be hemodynamically stable, with no signs of active bleeding in the peritoneal cavity, low beta-hCG levels (<5,000 mIU/mL) and the mass (which must measure less than 4 cm as determined by ultrasound) must be unruptured. Contraindications to medical treatment include an unstable client, severe persistent abdominal pain, renal or liver disease, immunodeficiency, active pulmonary disease, peptic ulcer, suspected intrauterine pregnancy, and poor client compliance (Tulandi, 2015). The potential advantages include avoidance of surgery, the preservation of tubal patency and function, and a lower cost.

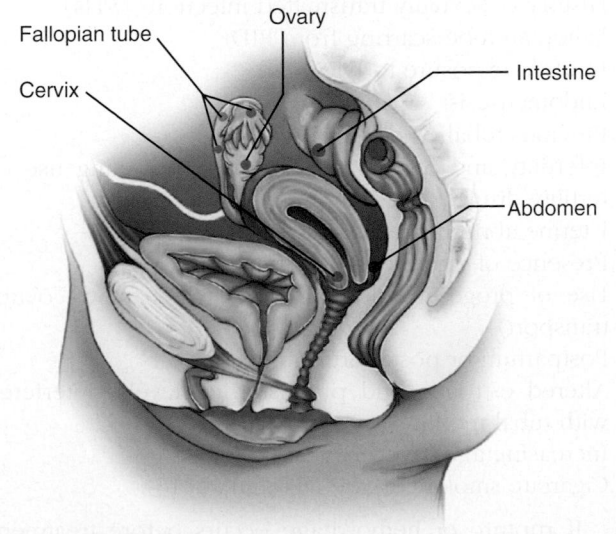

Fallopian tube
Ovary
Cervix
Intestine
Abdomen

FIGURE 19.1 **Possible sites for implantation with an ectopic pregnancy.**

The medical approach today for an unruptured tubal pregnancy most often consists of a single-dose intramuscular (IM) injection of methotrexate (Rheumatrex; Trexall) with outpatient follow-up. Medical management with methotrexate is widely used in areas where methotrexate is readily available and follow-up is easily arranged. Methotrexate is a folic acid antagonist that inhibits cell division in the developing embryo. It typically has been used as a chemotherapeutic agent in the treatment of leukemia, lymphomas, and carcinomas. It has been shown to produce results similar to that for surgical therapy in terms of high success rate, low complication rate, and good reproductive potential (Dalia, Price, Forsyth, Sokol, & Jaglal, 2015). Adverse effects associated with methotrexate include nausea, vomiting, stomatitis, diarrhea, gastric upset, increased abdominal pain, and dizziness. Methotrexate for an ectopic pregnancy is ordered based on the client's body surface area. The administration of methotrexate should be limited to people who have had education and training in the handling and administration of hazardous drugs. In some facilities, internal policies require that only nurses who have completed a chemotherapy certification and/or hazardous drug competency program can administer this product (Cohen et al., 2015).

Prior to receiving the single-dose intramuscular injection to treat unruptured ectopic pregnancies, the client needs to be counselled on the risks, benefits, adverse effects, and the possibility of failure of medical therapy, which could result in tubal rupture, necessitating surgery (Tulandi, 2015). After injection, the client is instructed to return, generally on days 2, 4, and 7 and then weekly for follow-up laboratory studies for the next several weeks until beta-hCG titers decrease. Beta-hCG level changes between days 0 and 4 after methotrexate therapy have clinical significance and predictive value. A decreasing beta-hCG level is highly predictive of treatment success (Agarwal & Odejinmi, 2014).

SURGICAL INTERVENTION

Surgical management for the unruptured fallopian tube might involve a linear salpingostomy to preserve the tube—an important consideration for the client wanting to preserve future fertility. It may also be considered when medical treatment is considered unsuitable.

With a ruptured ectopic pregnancy, surgery is necessary as a result of possible uncontrolled hemorrhage. A laparotomy with a removal of the tube (salpingectomy) may be necessary. With earlier diagnosis and medical management, the focus has changed from preventing maternal death to facilitating rapid recovery and preserving fertility.

Regardless of the treatment approach (medical or surgical), the client's beta-hCG level is monitored until it is undetectable to ensure that any residual trophoblastic tissue that forms the placenta is gone. Also, all Rh-negative unsensitized clients are given Rh immune globulin to prevent isoimmunization in future pregnancies.

Nursing Assessment

Nursing assessment focuses on determining the existence of an ectopic pregnancy and whether or not it has ruptured. A client with a suspected ectopic pregnancy may have to undergo several diagnostic tests, some of which are invasive. Using a patient-centred approach, consider the impact of the impending pregnancy loss, anticipated testing, fear of complications, and impact on usual routines and responsibilities; anticipate questions, and offer thorough explanations and reassurances. Ensure informed decision making has taken place considering the risks, benefits, and alternatives of management for ectopic pregnancy.

HEALTH HISTORY AND PHYSICAL EXAMINATION

Assess the client thoroughly for signs and symptoms that may suggest an ectopic pregnancy. The onset of signs and symptoms varies, but they usually begin at about the seventh or eighth week of gestation. A missed menstrual period, adnexal fullness, and tenderness may indicate an unruptured tubal pregnancy. As the tube stretches, the pain increases. Pain may be unilateral, bilateral, or diffuse over the abdomen.

Take Note!

The hallmark of ectopic pregnancy is abdominal pain with spotting within 6 to 8 weeks after a missed menstrual period. Although this is the classic triad, all three of these signs and symptoms occur in only about 50% of cases. Many clients will have symptoms typical of early pregnancy, such as breast tenderness, nausea, fatigue, and low back pain.

In addition, review the client's history for possible contributing factors. These may include:

- Previous ectopic pregnancy
- History of sexually transmitted infections (STIs)
- Fallopian tube scarring from PID
- In utero exposure to DES
- Endometriosis
- Previous tubal or pelvic surgery
- Infertility and infertility treatments, including use of fertility drugs
- Uterine abnormalities such as fibroids
- Presence of intrauterine contraception
- Use of progestin-only mini-pill (which slows ovum transport)
- Postpartum or postabortion infection
- Altered estrogen and progesterone levels (interferes with tubal motility)
- Increasing age (over 35 years)
- Cigarette smoking (Ardehali et al., 2015).

If rupture or hemorrhage occurs before treatment begins, symptoms may worsen and include severe, sharp, and sudden pain in the lower abdomen as the tube tears open and the embryo is expelled into the pelvic cavity;

feelings of faintness; referred pain to the shoulder area, indicating bleeding into the abdomen, caused by phrenic nerve irritation; hypotension; marked abdominal tenderness with distention; and hypovolemic shock (Cunningham et al., 2014).

LABORATORY AND DIAGNOSTIC TESTING

The use of transvaginal ultrasound to visualize the misplaced pregnancy and low levels of serum beta-hCG assist in diagnosing an ectopic pregnancy. The ultrasound determines whether the pregnancy is intrauterine, assesses the size of the pregnancy, and provides evidence of fetal viability. The visualization of an adnexal mass and the absence of an intrauterine gestational sac are diagnostic of ectopic pregnancy (Kao et al., 2014). In a normal intrauterine pregnancy, beta-hCG levels typically double every 2 to 4 days until peak values are reached 60 to 90 days after conception. Concentrations of hCG decrease after 10 to 11 weeks and reach a plateau at low levels by 100 to 130 days (Ko & Cheung, 2014). Therefore, low beta-hCG levels are suggestive of an ectopic pregnancy or impending abortion. Additional tests may be done to rule out other conditions such as spontaneous abortion, ruptured ovarian cyst, appendicitis, and salpingitis.

Nursing Management

Nursing management for the client with an ectopic pregnancy focuses on preparing the client for treatment and follow-up, providing support, and providing education about preventive measures.

PREPARING THE CLIENT FOR TREATMENT

Administer analgesics as ordered to promote comfort and relieve discomfort from abdominal pain. Although the intensity of the pain can vary, clients often report a great deal of pain. If the client is treated medically, explain the medication that will be used and what to expect. Also review signs and symptoms of possible adverse effects. If treatment will occur on an outpatient basis, outline the signs and symptoms of ectopic rupture (severe, sharp, stabbing, unilateral abdominal pain; vertigo/fainting; hypotension; and increased pulse) and advise the client to seek medical help immediately if any of these occur.

If surgery is needed, close assessment and monitoring of the client's vital signs, bleeding (peritoneal or vaginal), and pain status are critical to identify hypovolemic shock, which may occur with tubal rupture. Prepare the client physiologically and psychologically for surgery or any procedure. Provide a clear explanation of the expected outcome. Astute vigilance and early referral will help reduce short- and long-term morbidity.

PROVIDING EMOTIONAL SUPPORT

The client with an ectopic pregnancy requires support throughout diagnosis, treatment, and aftercare. A client's psychological reaction to an ectopic pregnancy is unpredictable. However, it is important to recognize that this person has experienced a pregnancy loss in addition to undergoing treatment for a potentially life-threatening condition. The client may find it difficult to comprehend what has happened because events occur so quickly. In the client's mind, a pregnancy has just begun and now it has ended abruptly. Bleeding during any pregnancy is traumatic because of the uncertainty of the outcome. Encourage the client and support network to express their feelings and concerns openly; validate that this is a loss of pregnancy and that it is okay to grieve over the loss. Although the client may have physically recovered following an ectopic pregnancy, the experience of significant grief and emotional distress may continue for a long time.

Provide emotional support, spiritual care, and information about community support groups as the client grieves for the loss of the unborn child and comes to terms with the medical complications of the situation. Acknowledge the client's pregnancy and allow for expression of feelings about what the pregnancy means. Also, stress the need for follow-up blood testing for several weeks to monitor hCG titers until they return to zero, indicating resolution of the ectopic pregnancy. Ask about feelings and concerns about future fertility, and provide teaching about the need to use contraceptives for at least three menstrual cycles to allow the reproductive tract to heal and the tissue to be repaired. Include the client's partner in this discussion to make sure both parties understand what has happened, what intervention is needed, and what the future holds regarding childbearing.

EDUCATING THE CLIENT

Preventing ectopic pregnancies through screening and client education is essential. Many can be prevented by avoiding conditions that might cause scarring of the fallopian tubes. In addition, a contributing factor to the development of ectopic pregnancy is a previous ectopic pregnancy. Therefore, educating the client is crucial. Prevention education may include the following:

- Reduce risk factors such as sexual intercourse with multiple partners or intercourse without a condom.
- Use safer sex practices to reduce the risk of contracting STIs that lead to PID.
- Obtain early diagnosis and adequate treatment of STIs.
- If an intrauterine contraceptive system is chosen, descriptions of the signs of PID should be included to reduce the risk of repeat ascending infections, which can be responsible for tubal scarring.
- Avoid smoking during childbearing years since a correlation and increase in risk exists.
- Seek prenatal care early to confirm the location of pregnancy.

Gestational Trophoblastic Disease (GTD)

GTD comprises a spectrum of neoplastic disorders that originate in the placenta. There is abnormal hyperproliferation of trophoblastic cells that normally would develop into the placenta during pregnancy. GTDs encompass hydatidiform mole (complete and partial), invasive mole, gestational choriocarcinoma, placental-site trophoblastic tumour, and epithelioid trophoblastic tumour (Nguyen & Slim, 2014). Gestational tissue is present, but the pregnancy is not viable. The incidence is hard to determine due to uncommon diagnosis and inaccuracy of documentation of pregnancy loss, but hydatidiform mole is thought to occur in about 1 to 2 in 1,000 pregnancies in the Canada (Colgan, Noor, Nanji, Chang, & Kolomietz, 2017); in Asian countries, the rate of GTD is 1 of every 120 pregnancies (American Cancer Society [ACS], 2017). The two most common types of GTD are hydatidiform mole (partial or complete) and choriocarcinoma.

Pathophysiology

The pathogenesis is unique because the tumour arises from gestational rather than maternal tissue. Hydatidiform mole is a benign neoplasm of the chorion in which the chorionic villi degenerate and become transparent vesicles containing clear, viscid fluid. Hydatidiform mole is classified as complete or partial, distinguished by differences in clinical presentation, pathology, genetics, and epidemiology (Strohl & Lurain, 2014). The complete mole contains no fetal tissue and develops from an "empty egg," which is fertilized by a normal sperm (the paternal chromosomes replicate, resulting in 46 all-paternal chromosomes) (Fig. 19.2). The embryo is not viable and dies. No

circulation is established, and no embryonic tissue is found. The complete mole is associated with the development of choriocarcinoma. Surgery can totally remove most complete moles, but as many as one in five affected persons will have some persistent molar tissue and require further treatment (ACS, 2017). Most individuals with a classic complete mole present with vaginal bleeding, anemia, excessively enlarged uterus, preeclampsia, and hyperemesis.

The partial mole has a triploid karyotype (69 chromosomes), because two sperm have provided a double contribution by fertilizing the ovum. Clients with a partial mole usually present with the clinical features of a missed or incomplete abortion, including vaginal bleeding and a small or normal size for date uterus (Dickson & Mullany, 2015).

The exact cause of molar pregnancy is unknown, but points to a genetic basis. Most complete molar pregnancies have a 46, XX karyotype, with all chromosomes coming from the sperm and none from the ovum (Baergan, 2019). Although the etiology remains uncertain, at some point in the pregnancy trophoblastic cells that normally would form the placenta proliferate and the chorionic villi become edematous. These swollen chorionic villi then become the grape-like clusters that characterize the molar pregnancy (King et al., 2015). Studies have revealed some remarkable features about molar pregnancies, including:

- Ability to invade into the wall of the uterus
- Tendency to recur in subsequent pregnancies
- Possible development into choriocarcinoma, a virulent cancer with metastasis to other organs
- Influence of nutritional factors, such as protein deficiency
- Tendency to affect older persons more often than younger persons

Having a molar pregnancy (partial or complete) results in the loss of the pregnancy and the possibility of developing choriocarcinoma, a chorionic malignancy from the trophoblastic tissue. Typically asymptomatic, the first symptoms of choriocarcinoma in 80% of cases are shortness of breath, indicative of metastasis to the lungs. Choriocarcinoma affects clients of all ages and can occur during pregnancy, after childbirth, or even years remote from the antecedent pregnancy. The most frequent sites of metastases are the lungs, lower genital tract, brain, and liver. Choriocarcinoma is highly responsive to chemotherapy, with an overall remission rate greater than 90% (Hensley & Shviraga, 2014). Partial moles rarely transform into choriocarcinoma.

Therapeutic Management

Treatment consists of immediate evacuation of the uterine contents as soon as the diagnosis is made and long-term follow-up of the client to detect any remaining trophoblastic tissue that might become malignant. D&C is used to empty the uterus. The tissue obtained is sent to the laboratory for analysis to evaluate for choriocarcinoma.

FIGURE 19.2 Complete hydatidiform mole as seen in a cutaway of a uterus. The chorionic villi degenerate and become filled with a viscid fluid, forming transparent vesicles. (From Reichert, R. A. [2011]. *Diagnostic gynecologic and obstetric pathology, Courtesy of Dr. Enrique Higa.* Philadelphia, PA: LWW.)

Serial levels of hCG are used to detect residual trophoblastic tissue for 1 year. If any tissue remains, hCG levels will not regress. In 80% of clients with a benign hydatidiform mole, serum hCG titers steadily drop to normal within 8 to 12 weeks after evacuation of the molar pregnancy. In the other 20% of pregnancies with a malignant hydatidiform mole, serum hCG levels begin to rise (Berkowitz, Goldstein, & Horowitz, 2014).

As a result of the increased risk for cancer, the client is advised to receive extensive follow-up therapy for the next 12 months. The follow-up protocol may include:

- Baseline hCG level, chest x-ray, and pelvic ultrasound
- Quantitative hCG levels every week until undetectable for 3 consecutive weeks; then serial hCG levels monthly for 1 year
- Chest x-ray every 6 months to detect pulmonary metastasis
- Regular pelvic examinations to assess uterine and ovarian regression
- Systemic assessments for symptoms indicative of lung, brain, liver, or vaginal metastasis
- Strong recommendation to avoid pregnancy for 1 year because the pregnancy can interfere with the monitoring of hCG levels
- Use of a reliable contraceptive for at least 1 year (Cunningham et al., 2014)

Nursing Assessment

The nurse plays an important role in identifying and bringing this condition to the attention of the health care provider based on sound knowledge of the typical clinical manifestations and through knowledge based antepartum assessments.

Clinical manifestations of GTD are very similar to those of spontaneous abortion at about 12 weeks of pregnancy. Assess the client for potential clinical manifestations at each antepartum visit. Be alert for the following:

- Report of early signs of pregnancy, such as amenorrhea, breast tenderness, fatigue
- Brownish vaginal bleeding/spotting
- Anemia
- Inability to detect a fetal heart rate after 10 to 12 weeks' gestation
- Fetal parts not evident with palpation
- Bilateral ovarian enlargement caused by cysts and elevated levels of hCG
- Persistent, often severe, nausea and vomiting (due to high hCG levels)
- Fluid retention and swelling
- Uterine size larger than expected for pregnancy dates
- Extremely high hCG levels present; no single value considered diagnostic
- Early development of preeclampsia (usually not present until after 24 weeks)
- Expulsion of grape-like vesicles

The diagnosis is made by very high hCG levels and the characteristic appearance of the vesicular molar pattern in the uterus via transvaginal ultrasound.

Nursing Management

Nursing management of the client with GTD focuses on preparing for a D&C, providing emotional support to deal with the loss and potential risks, and educating the client about the risk that cancer may develop after a molar pregnancy and the strict adherence needed with the follow-up program. The client must understand the need for the continued follow-up care regimen to improve chances of future pregnancies and to ensure continued quality of life.

PREPARING THE CLIENT
Upon diagnosis, the client will need an immediate evacuation of the uterus. Perform preoperative care, preparing the client physically and psychologically for the procedure.

PROVIDING EMOTIONAL SUPPORT
To aid the client and family in coping with the loss of the pregnancy and the possibility of a cancer diagnosis, use the following interventions:
- Listen to their concerns and fears.
- Allow them time to grieve for the pregnancy loss.
- Acknowledge their loss and sad feelings (tell them you are sorry for their loss).
- Encourage them to express their grief; allow them to cry.
- Provide them with as much factual information as possible to help them make sense of what is happening.
- Enlist support from additional family and friends as appropriate and with the client's permission.

EDUCATING THE CLIENT
After GTD is diagnosed, teach the client about the condition and appropriate interventions that may be necessary. Explain each phase of treatment accurately and provide support for the client and family as they go through the grieving process.

As with any facet of health care, be aware of the latest evidence-based practices, standards of care, and new therapies. Inform the client about follow-up care, which will probably involve close clinical surveillance for approximately 1 year, and reinforce its importance in monitoring the client's condition. Tell the client that serial serum beta-hCG levels are used to detect residual trophoblastic tissue. Continued high or increasing hCG titers are abnormal and need further evaluation.

Inform the client about the possible use of chemotherapy, such as methotrexate, which may be started prophylactically. Strongly urge the client to use a reliable contraceptive to prevent pregnancy for 1 year, because a pregnancy would interfere with tracking the serial beta-hCG levels used to identify a potential malignancy. Stress the need for the client to cooperate and adhere to the plan of therapy throughout this yearlong follow-up period.

Consider This

We had lived across the dorm hall from each other during nursing school but really didn't get to know each other except for a casual hello in passing. When we graduated, Rose went to work in the emergency room and I worked in OB. We saw each other occasionally in the cafeteria, but a quick hello was all that we usually exchanged. I heard she married one of the paramedics who worked in the ER and was soon pregnant. I finally got to say more than hello when she was admitted to the OB unit bleeding during her fourth month of pregnancy. GTD was discovered instead of a normal pregnancy. I remember holding her in my arms as she wept. She was told she had a complete molar pregnancy after surgery, and she would need extensive follow-up for the next year. I lost track of her that summer as my life became busier. Around Thanksgiving time, I heard she had died from choriocarcinoma. I attended her funeral, finally, to get the time to say a final hello and good-bye, but this time with sadness and tears.

Thoughts: Rose was only 26 years old when she succumbed to this very virulent cancer. I think back and realize I missed knowing this brave young woman and wished that I had taken the time to say more than hello. Could her outcome have been different? Why wasn't it recognized earlier? Did she not follow up after her diagnosis? I can only speculate regarding the whom, what, and where. She lived a short but purposeful life, and hopefully continued research will change outcomes in the future.

Cervical Insufficiency

Cervical insufficiency, also called premature dilation of the cervix, describes a weak, structurally and functionally defective cervix that spontaneously dilates in the absence of uterine contractions in the second trimester, or early third trimester, resulting in the loss or premature birth of the pregnancy. Since this often occurs in the fourth or fifth month of gestation before the point of fetal viability, the fetus dies unless the dilation can be arrested. The incidence of cervical insufficiency is about 1% in the obstetrical population in Canada and the United States (Agency for Healthcare Research and Quality [AHRQ], 2015; Brown, Gagnon, & Delisle, 2013).

Pathophysiology

The exact mechanism contributing to cervical insufficiency is not known. The cervix may have less elastin, less collagen, and greater amounts of smooth muscle than the normal cervix, and thus results in loss of sphincter tone (Magowan, Owen, & Thomson, 2014). Several theories have been proposed that focus on damage to the cervix as a key component of hormonal factors, such as increased amounts of relaxin. When the pressure of the expanding uterine contents becomes greater than the ability of the cervical sphincter to remain closed, the cervix suddenly relaxes, allowing effacement and dilation to proceed. The cervical dilation is typically rapid, relatively painless, and accompanied by minimal bleeding (Norwitz & Conroy, 2016).

Cervical insufficiency is likely to be the clinical end point of many pathologic processes, such as congenital cervical hypoplasia, in utero DES exposure that caused cervical hypoplasia, or trauma to the cervix (conization, amputation, obstetric laceration, or forced cervical dilatation). Other conditions such as previous precipitous birth, a prolonged second stage of labour, increased amounts of relaxin and progesterone, connective tissue disorders, or increased uterine volume (multiple gestation, hydramnios) are associated with cervical insufficiency (Berghella, 2018; Brown et al., 2013). However, the exact etiology of cervical insufficiency is not known.

Cervical length also has been associated with cervical insufficiency and, subsequently, preterm birth. Recent studies have examined the association between a short cervical length and the risk of preterm birth. Some have demonstrated a continuum of risk between a shorter cervix on ultrasound and a higher risk of preterm birth, leading to the hypothetical argument that clients with a short cervix on ultrasound might benefit from cervical cerclage (the sewing closed of the cervix). Both the Society of Obstetricians and Gynaecologists of Canada (SOGC) (Lim, Butt, & Crane, 2018) and the American Congress of Obstetricians and Gynecologists (American College of Obstetricians and Gynecologists [ACOG], 2014a) do not recommend cerclage placement for clients with a short cervix who do not have a history of preterm birth, as it has not been shown to be beneficial in this population. For clients with a history of preterm birth, ultrasound for cervical length may be beneficial.

Therapeutic Management

Cervical insufficiency may be treated in a variety of ways: bed rest; pelvic rest; avoidance of heavy lifting; progesterone supplementation in clients at risk for preterm birth; placement of a cervical pessary (a round, silicone device at the mouth of the cervix); or surgically, via a cervical cerclage procedure in the second trimester. Cerclage was devised more than 50 years ago based on the hypothesis that for some individuals, weakness or malfunction of the cervix has a causative role in the pathway to preterm birth. It can either be performed transvaginally

FIGURE 19.3 **A.** Cervical cerclage. **B.** Suturing the cervix for cervical insufficiency.

or transabdominally. Cervical cerclage involves using a heavy purse-string suture to secure and reinforce the internal os of the cervix (Fig. 19.3).

According to the SOGC clinical practice guideline, in asymptomatic individuals with a history of spontaneous preterm birth and an ultrasonographically diagnosed short cervical length (<25 mm) prior to 24 weeks' gestation, cervical cerclage should be considered to reduce the risk of preterm birth (Lim et al., 2018). Indications for cervical cerclage include: history of second-trimester pregnancy loss with painless dilatation; prior cerclage placement for cervical insufficiency; history of spontaneous preterm birth prior to 34 weeks' gestation; and painless cervical dilatation on physical examination in the second trimester (Brown et al., 2013). Complications associated with cerclage placement are suture displacement, rupture of membranes, and chorioamnionitis, and their incidence varies widely in relation to the timing and indications for the cerclage (Abu Hashim, Al-Inany, & Kilani, 2014). The optimal timing for cerclage removal is unclear, but the SOGC recommends removal at 36 to 38 weeks' gestation (Brown et al., 2013). A recent meta-analysis of randomized controlled trials concluded that either vaginal progesterone or cerclage are equally efficacious in the prevention of preterm birth in clients with a short cervix in the mid trimester, singleton gestation, and a previous preterm birth (Jena, Samal, & Behera, 2015; Lim et al., 2018).

Nursing Assessment

RISK FACTORS

Nursing assessment focuses on obtaining a thorough history to determine any risk factors that might be relevant to this pregnancy: previous cervical trauma, preterm labour, fetal loss in the second trimester, or previous surgeries or procedures involving the cervix. Also be alert for complaints of vaginal discharge or pelvic pressure. Commonly with cervical insufficiency the client will report a pink-tinged vaginal discharge or an increase in low pelvic pressure, mild cramping, minimal vaginal bleeding, or loss of amniotic fluid. As cervical dilation

continues, rupture of the membranes may occur, and uterine contractions will likely follow, resulting in delivery of the fetus, often before it is viable.

Take Note!

The diagnosis of cervical insufficiency remains difficult in many circumstances. The cornerstone of diagnosis is a history of a pregnancy loss during the second or early third trimester associated with painless cervical dilation without evidence of uterine activity.

DIAGNOSTIC TESTS

Transvaginal Ultrasound. For a client with a history of preterm birth or other risk factors, transvaginal ultrasound typically is done between 16 and 24 weeks' gestation to determine cervical length, evaluate for shortening, and attempt to predict an early preterm birth. Cervical shortening occurs from the internal os outward and can be viewed on ultrasound as funneling. The amount of funneling can be determined by dividing funnel length by cervical length. The most common time at which a short cervix or funneling develops is 16 to 24 weeks, so ultrasound screening should be performed during this interval (Herrera & Lewis, 2014). A cervical length of less than 25 mm is abnormal between 16 and 24 weeks and may increase the risk of preterm labour. Among clients with a short cervix, provide education concerning the signs and symptoms of preterm labour, especially as the pregnancy approaches potential viability. Prenatal visits/contacts may be scheduled at more frequent intervals to increase client interaction with the care provider, especially between 20 and 34 weeks' gestation. Although no specific randomized trials have been conducted to evaluate interventions in asymptomatic clients with history of preterm birth and with a shortened cervix teaching may include: reduction of activity level, work or travel, relocation if living far from a tertiary health care centre, increased surveillance, and administration of corticosteroids (Lim et al., 2018). Expect the client (particularly if pelvic pressure, backache, or increased mucoid discharge are present) to undergo serial transvaginal ultrasound evaluations every few days to avoid missing rapid changes in cervical dilation or until the trend in cervical length can be characterized (Cunningham et al., 2014; Lim et al., 2018).

Nursing Management

Nursing management focuses on monitoring the client very closely for signs of preterm labour: backache, increase in vaginal discharge, rupture of membranes, and uterine contractions. Provide emotional support and education to allay anxiety about the well-being of the fetus. Provide preoperative care and teaching as indicated if the client will be undergoing cerclage. Teach the client and family about the signs and symptoms of preterm labour and the need to report any changes immediately. Also reinforce the need for activity restrictions (if appropriate) and continued regular follow-up. Continuing surveillance throughout the pregnancy is important to promote a positive outcome for the family. The nurse can play a pivotal role in identifying preterm labour through risk assessment, physical examination, education and client advocacy.

Placenta Previa

Placenta previa is a placental condition that occurs during the last two trimesters of pregnancy which may be accompanied by mild to severe bleeding. In placenta previa (literally, "afterbirth first"), the placenta implants near or over the cervical os. It may cause serious morbidity and mortality to the fetus and client. The incidence of placenta previa in North America is about 2.9 per 1,000 pregnancies (Rowe, 2014). The risk of placenta previa rises to 1 in 160 after one cesarean section; 1 in 60 after two; 1 in 30 after three; and 1 in 10 after four cesarean sections and is associated with potentially serious consequences from hemorrhage, abruption (separation) of the placenta, or emergency cesarean birth (Bakker & Ramus, 2018). With the rising incidence of cesarean births combined with increasing maternal age and more infertility treatments, the number of cases of placenta previa is increasing dramatically. The cesarean section rate should continue to be an important quality measure and cesarean without obstetric indication should be avoided to decrease perinatal morbidity and mortality (Rowe, 2014). Comprehensive risk assessment, combined with advances in ultrasound, can provide earlier detection of this impaired placental implantation (Wiedaseck & Monchek, 2014).

Pathophysiology

The exact cause of placenta previa is unknown. It is initiated by implantation of the embryo in the lower uterus, perhaps due to uterine endometrial scarring or disturbance, the etiology of which is not clear. Fortunately, by a process called trophotropism, the placenta seeks an area of higher vascularity and often grows toward the upper segment of the uterus, away from the cervix as the pregnancy progresses, resolving up to 90% of low placentation in early pregnancy (Rowe, 2014). Uteroplacental underperfusion may also be present, which may increase the surface area required for placental attachment and may cause the placenta to encroach on the lower uterine segment. With placental attachment and growth, the cervical os may become covered by the developing placenta. Placenta previa is generally classified according to the degree of coverage or proximity to the internal os, as follows (Fig. 19.4):

- Total placenta previa: the internal cervical os is completely covered by the placenta
- Partial placenta previa: the internal os is partially covered by the placenta
- Marginal placenta previa: the placenta is at the margin or edge of the internal os
- Low-lying placenta previa: the placenta is implanted in the lower uterine segment and is near the internal os but does not reach it

Therapeutic Management

Therapeutic management depends on the extent of bleeding, the amount of placenta over the cervical os, whether the fetus is developed enough to survive outside the uterus, the position of the fetus, the client's parity, and the presence or absence of labour (Cunningham et al., 2014). Associated morbidity remains high due to the risk of hemorrhage. Prenatal care and timely diagnosis of placenta previa on ultrasound can decrease the associated morbidity.

If the client and fetus are both stable, therapeutic management may involve expectant management ("wait-and-see"). This care can be carried out at home or on an antepartum unit in the health care facility. There is no good evidence to recommend care at home versus hospital, and decisions should be made based on the individual (Rowe, 2014). If there is no active bleeding and the client has ready access to reliable transportation, can maintain bed rest at home, and can understand and follow instructions, expectant care at home is appropriate. However, if the client requires continuous care and monitoring and cannot meet the home care requirements, the antepartum unit is the best environment.

Nursing Assessment

Nursing assessment involves a thorough history, including possible risk factors, and physical examination. Evaluate the client closely for these risk factors:

- Advancing maternal age (more than 35 years)
- Previous cesarean birth
- Multiparity

FIGURE 19.4 **Classification of placenta previa. A.** Low-lying placenta. **B.** Marginal placenta previa.
C. Partial placental previa. **D.** Complete central placental previa. (From Stephenson, S. R. [2016].
Obstetrics and gynecology. Philadelphia, PA: Wolters Kluwer.)

- Uterine insult or injury
- Cocaine use
- Prior placenta previa
- Infertility treatment
- Multiple gestations
- Previous induced surgical abortion
- Smoking
- Previous myomectomy to remove fibroids
- Short interval between pregnancies
- Hypertension or diabetes (Archibong & Ahmed, 2015).

HEALTH HISTORY AND PHYSICAL EXAMINATION

Ask the client if there is any bleeding, now or in the recent past. The classical clinical presentation is painless, bright-red vaginal bleeding occurring during the second or third trimester. The initial bleeding usually is not profuse and it ceases spontaneously, but risk of recurrence is high. The first episode of bleeding occurs (on average) at 27 to 32 weeks' gestation. The bleeding is thought to arise secondary to the thinning of the lower uterine segment in preparation for the onset of labour. When the bleeding occurs at the implantation site in the lower uterus, the uterus cannot contract adequately to stop the flow of blood from the open vessels. Typically with normal placental implantation in the upper uterus, minor disruptive placental attachment is not a problem, because there is a larger volume of myometrial tissue able to contract and constrict bleeding vessels.

Assess the client for uterine contractions, which may or may not occur with the bleeding. Palpate the uterus;

typically it is soft and nontender on examination. Assess the fetal heart by continuous fetal monitoring; it commonly is within normal parameters. Fetal compromise is usually absent but may occur when cord problems arise, such as umbilical cord prolapse or cord compression, or when the client has experienced a chronic small blood loss or an acute episode to the extent that maternal shock or placental abruption has occurred (King et al., 2015).

LABORATORY AND DIAGNOSTIC TESTING

To validate the position of the placenta, a transvaginal ultrasound is done. In addition, magnetic resonance imaging (MRI) may be ordered when preparing for delivery because it allows identification of placenta **accreta** (placenta abnormally adherent to the myometrium), increta (placenta accreta with penetration of the myometrium), or percreta (placenta accreta with invasion of the myometrium to the peritoneal covering, causing rupture of the uterus) in addition to placenta previa. These placental abnormalities, although rare, carry a very high morbidity and mortality rate, possibly necessitating a hysterectomy at delivery.

Nursing Management

Whether the care setting is in the client's home or in the health care facility, the nurse focuses on monitoring the status of both the client and the fetus, including assessing for signs and symptoms of vaginal bleeding and fetal compromise, as well as providing support and education to the client and family, including providing information about the diagnostic studies and procedures that are performed. For the majority of clients, a cesarean birth will be planned, however, it is unclear how far the placenta should be from the internal os in order to proceed with vaginal birth, as the previous rule of 20 mm distance from the placental edge to the cervical os is being re-evaluated and for some clients, a distance of 11 to 20 mm may be safe for a vaginal birth (Rowe, 2014). Nursing Care Plan 19.1 (at the end of the chapter) discusses the nursing process for the client with placenta previa.

MONITORING THE CLIENT AND FETAL STATUS

Assess the degree of vaginal bleeding; inspect the perineal area for blood that may be pooled underneath the client. Estimate and document the amount of bleeding. Perform a peripad count on an ongoing basis. For heavy bleeding, weigh pads for more accurate blood loss, making sure to report any changes in amount or frequency to the health care provider. If the client is experiencing active bleeding, prepare for blood typing and cross-matching in the event a blood transfusion is needed.

Take Note!

Avoid doing vaginal examinations in the client with placenta previa because a digital exam may disrupt the placenta and cause hemorrhage.

Monitor vital signs and uterine contractility frequently for changes. Have the client rate their level of pain using an appropriate pain rating scale. Assess fetal heart rates via Doppler or electronic monitoring to detect fetal compromise. Monitor the client's cardiopulmonary status, reporting any abnormalities in blood pressure, heart rate, respirations, changes in skin colour, or difficulty breathing. Have oxygen equipment readily available should fetal or client distress develop. Encourage the client to lie on one side to enhance placental perfusion.

If the client has an intravenous (IV) line inserted, inspect the IV site frequently. Alternately, anticipate the insertion of an intermittent IV access device such as a saline lock, which can be used if quick access is needed for fluid restoration and infusion of blood products. Obtain laboratory tests as ordered, including complete blood count (CBC), coagulation studies, and Rh status if appropriate.

Administer pharmacologic agents as necessary. Give Rh immune globulin if the client is Rh negative at 28 weeks' gestation. Monitor tocolytic (anticontraction) medication if management of preterm labour is needed.

PROVIDING SUPPORT AND EDUCATION

Determine the client's level of understanding about placenta previa and the associated procedures and treatment plan. Explain all assessments and treatment measures before they occur. Doing so is important to prevent confusion and for the client to participate in informed decision making for treatments, procedures, and monitoring. Provide written information where available (after determining the client's literacy ability) and make sure that all information is consistent with information from the primary care provider. Act as a client advocate in obtaining information and care. Teach the client about monitoring blood loss, the contraindication to vaginal examination, how to perform and record daily fetal movement, and expected tests and monitoring. These actions serve two purposes: (1) Providing valuable information about the fetus and client and (2) Providing the client with the opportunity to participate, thereby fostering a sense of control, confidence, and competence. If the client will require prolonged hospitalization or home bed rest, assess the physical and emotional impact that this may have. Evaluate coping mechanisms to help determine the client's ability to adjust and adhere to the treatment plan. Allow the client to verbalize feelings and fears, and provide emotional support. Discuss personal preferences regarding opportunities for distraction. Provide teaching regarding the risk of anxiety, depression, and mood disorders related to prolonged antepartum bedrest, and evaluate the client's response,

In addition to the emotional impact of prolonged bed rest, thoroughly assess the client's skin to prevent skin breakdown and to help alleviate discomfort secondary to limited physical activity. Instruct the client in appropriate skin care measures. Encourage a balanced diet with adequate fluid intake to ensure adequate nutrition and hydration and prevent complications associated with urinary and bowel elimination secondary to bed rest. Teach the client and family about any signs and symptoms that should be reported immediately. In addition, prepare the client for the possibility of a cesarean birth. The client must notify the health care team about any bleeding episodes or backaches (may indicate preterm labour contractions) and must adhere to the prescribed bed rest regimen. To ensure adherence to the plan and a positive outcome, the client needs to be aware of and understand the rationales for the ongoing observations.

Abruptio Placentae

Abruptio placentae (or placental abruption) is the premature separation of a normally implanted placenta after the 20th week of gestation prior to birth, which leads to hemorrhage. It is a significant cause of third-trimester bleeding, with a high mortality rate. It occurs in about 1% of all pregnancies throughout the world, or approximately 1 in 100 pregnancies. There is a 10 to 20 times greater risk of reoccurrence in a subsequent pregnancy. It typically peaks between 24 and 26 weeks' gestation.

Potential risks include obstetric hemorrhage, need for blood transfusions, emergency hysterectomy, disseminated intravascular coagulopathy, and renal failure. Perinatal death is rare in developed countries, but seven times higher than the overall maternal mortality rate. Neonatal conditions associated with abruption include low birth weight, preterm delivery, asphyxia, stillbirth, and perinatal death. In developed countries, approximately 10% of all preterm births and 10% to 20% of all perinatal deaths are associated with placental abruption (Mukherjee, Bawa, Sharma, Nandanwar, & Gadam, 2014). The overall fetal mortality rate for placental abruption is up to 50%, depending on the extent of the abruption. Maternal mortality is approximately 6% in abruptio placentae and is related to cesarean birth and/or hemorrhage/coagulopathy (Jaju, Kulkarni, & Mundada, 2014).

Pathophysiology

The etiology of this condition is unknown; however, it has been proposed that abruption starts with degenerative changes in the small maternal blood vessels, resulting in blood clotting, degeneration of the decidua (uterine lining), and possible rupture of a vessel. Bleeding from the blood vessel forms a blood clot between the placenta and the uterine wall. The continued bleeding causes increased pressure behind the placenta and results in separation from the uterine wall (Moses, 2018a). Fetal blood supply is reduced and fetal compromise develops in proportion to the degree of placental separation. Poor neonatal outcomes are a result of the insult of the abruption and issues related to prematurity when early birth is required.

Abruptio placentae is classified according to the extent of separation and the amount of blood loss from the maternal circulation. Classifications include:
- *Mild (grade 1):* minimal bleeding (less than 500 mL), marginal separation (10% to 20%), tender uterus, no coagulopathy, no signs of shock, no fetal compromise
- *Moderate (grade 2):* moderate bleeding (1,000 to 1,500 mL), moderate separation (20% to 50%), continuous abdominal pain, mild shock, normal maternal blood pressure, maternal tachycardia
- *Severe (grade 3):* absent to moderate bleeding (more than 1,500 mL), severe separation (more than 50%), profound shock, dark vaginal bleeding, agonizing abdominal pain, decreased maternal blood pressure, significant maternal tachycardia, and development of disseminated intravascular coagulation (DIC) (Atkinson et al., 2015).

Abruptio placentae also may be classified as partial or complete, depending on the degree of separation. Alternately, it can be classified as concealed or apparent, by the type of bleeding (Fig. 19.5).

> **Remember Helen, the pregnant client with severe abdominal pain?** Electronic fetal monitoring revealed uterine hypertonicity with absent fetal heart sounds. Palpation of the abdomen revealed rigidity and extreme tenderness in all four quadrants. Vital signs were as follows: temperature, afebrile; pulse, 94; respirations, 22; blood pressure, 130/90 mm Hg. What might you suspect as the cause of Helen's abdominal pain? What course of action would you anticipate for Helen?

Therapeutic Management

Treatment of abruptio placentae is designed to assess, control, and restore the amount of blood lost; provide a positive outcome for both client and newborn; and prevent coagulation disorders, such as DIC (Box 19.2). Emergency measures include starting two large-bore IV lines with normal saline or lactated Ringer's solution to treat hypovolemia, obtaining blood specimens for evaluating hemodynamic status values and for typing and cross-matching, and frequently monitoring fetal and client well-being. After the severity of abruption is determined and appropriate blood and fluid replacement is given,

A Partial abruption, concealed hemorrhage

B Partial abruption, apparent hemorrhage

C Complete abruption, concealed hemorrhage

FIGURE 19.5 Classifications of abruptio placentae. **A.** Partial abruption with concealed hemorrhage. **B.** Partial abruption with apparent hemorrhage. **C.** Complete abruption with concealed hemorrhage.

BOX 19.2

DISSEMINATED INTRAVASCULAR COAGULATION

DIC is a bleeding disorder characterized by an abnormal reduction in the elements involved in blood clotting resulting from their widespread intravascular clotting (Davis & Kessler, 2014). This disorder can occur secondary to abruptio placentae, amniotic fluid embolism, endotoxin sepsis, retained dead fetus, posthemorrhagic shock, hydatidiform mole, and gynecologic malignancies.

The clinical and pathologic manifestations of DIC can be described as a loss of balance between the clot-forming activity of thrombin and the clot-lysing activity of plasmin. Therefore, too much thrombin tips the balance toward the prothrombic state and the client develops clots. Alternately, too much clot lysis (fibrinolysis) results from plasmin formation and the client hemorrhages. Small clots form throughout the body, and eventually the blood-clotting factors are used up, rendering them unavailable to form clots at sites of tissue injury. Clot-dissolving mechanisms are also increased, which results in bleeding (possibly severe).

DIC is usually associated with high mortality and morbidity rates. No single laboratory test is sensitive or specific enough to diagnose DIC definitively, but it can be diagnosed by using a combination of multiple clinical and laboratory tests that reflect the pathophysiology of the syndrome.

Laboratory studies that assist in the diagnosis include:
- Decreased fibrinogen and platelets
- Prolonged PT and aPTT
- Positive D-dimer tests and fibrin (split) degradation products (objective evidence of the simultaneous formation of thrombin and plasmin)

Adapted from Davis, S. J., & Kessler, C. M. (2014). Disseminated intravascular coagulation: Diagnosis and management. In *Hemostasis and thrombosis: Practical guidelines in clinical management* (pp. 151–168). Hoboken, NJ: Wiley Blackwell; and Kobayashi, T. (2014). Obstetrical disseminated intravascular coagulation score. *Journal of Obstetrics and Gynaecology Research*, 40(6), 1500–1506.

---

cesarean birth is facilitated immediately if fetal compromise is evident. If the fetal monitor tracing is normal, close monitoring continues, with delivery planned at the earliest signs of atypical or abnormal fetal heart rate tracing. Because of the possibility of fetal blood loss through the placenta, a neonatal resuscitation team should be present at the birth to assess and treat the newborn immediately for shock, blood loss, and hypoxia. Anticipate full resuscitation of the newborn including umbilical vein catheter and fluids or blood transfusion as needed.

If the client develops DIC, treatment focuses on determining the underlying cause of DIC and correcting it. Replacement therapy of the coagulation factors is achieved by transfusion of fresh-frozen plasma along with cryoprecipitate to maintain the circulating volume and provide oxygen to the cells of the body. Anticoagulant therapy (low–molecular-weight heparin), packed red cells, platelet concentrates, antithrombin concentrates, and nonclotting protein-containing volume expanders, such as plasma protein fraction or albumin, are also used to combat this serious condition. The use of blood products must be dictated by the clinical picture and not simply to normalize laboratory test results (Holt, 2015). Prompt identification and early intervention are essential for a client with acute DIC associated with abruptio placentae.

Nursing Assessment

Abruptio placentae is a medical emergency. The nurse plays a critical role in assessing the pregnant client presenting with abdominal pain and/or experiencing vaginal bleeding, especially in a concealed hemorrhage, in which the extent of bleeding is not recognized. Rapid assessment is essential to ensure prompt, effective interventions to prevent maternal and fetal morbidity and mortality. Comparison Chart 19.1 compares placenta previa with abruptio placentae.

COMPARISON CHART 19.1	PLACENTA PREVIA VERSUS ABRUPTIO PLACENTAE	
Manifestation	Placenta Previa	Abruptio Placentae
Onset	Insidious	Sudden
Type of bleeding	Always visible; slight, then more profuse	Can be concealed or visible
Blood description	Bright red	Dark
Discomfort/pain	None (painless)	Constant; uterine tenderness on palpation
Uterine tone	Soft and relaxed	Firm to rigid
Fetal heart rate	Usually in normal range	Fetal distress or absent
Fetal presentation	May be breech or transverse lie; engagement is absent	No relationship

HEALTH HISTORY AND PHYSICAL EXAMINATION

Abruptio placentae produces a wide range of clinical effects, depending on the extent of placental separation and the amount of maternal blood loss. Begin the health history by assessing the client for risk factors that may predispose her to abruptio placentae, such as advanced age (over 35 years old), poor nutrition, multiple gestation, excessive intrauterine pressure caused by polyhydramnios, chronic hypertension, cigarette smoking, severe trauma (e.g., auto accident, intimate partner violence), history of abruption in a previous pregnancy, placental abnormalities, cocaine or methamphetamine abuse, thrombophilia, alcohol ingestion, and multiparity (Deering, 2017). In addition, be alert for other notable risk factors, such as male fetal sex, chorioamnionitis, prolonged premature rupture of membranes (more than 18 hours), oligohydramnios, preeclampsia, and low socioeconomic status (Nagtalon-Ramos, 2014).

Assess the client for bleeding. As the placenta separates from the uterus, hemorrhage ensues. It can be apparent, appearing as vaginal bleeding, or it can be concealed. Vaginal bleeding is present in 80% of abruptio placentae cases and may be significant enough to jeopardize both the client and fetal health within a short time frame. The remaining 20% of abruptions are associated with a concealed hemorrhage and the absence of vaginal bleeding. Monitor the client's level of consciousness, noting any signs or symptoms that may suggest shock, including decreased level of consciousness, low blood pressure, and tachycardia.

Take Note!

Vital signs can be within normal range, even with significant blood loss, because a pregnant individual can lose up to 40% of the total blood volume without showing signs of shock (Schultz & McConachie, 2015).

Assess the client for reports of pain, including the type, onset, and location. Ask if there are any contractions

felt. Palpate the abdomen, noting any contractions, uterine tenderness, tenseness, or rigidity. Ask if the client has noticed any changes in fetal movement and activity. Decreased fetal movement may be the presenting complaint, resulting from fetal compromise or fetal death (Cunningham et al., 2014). Assess fetal heart rate and continue to monitor it electronically.

Take Note!

Classic manifestations of abruptio placentae include painful, dark-red vaginal bleeding (port-wine colour) because the bleeding comes from the clot that was formed behind the placenta; "knife-like" abdominal pain; uterine tenderness; contractions; and decreased fetal movement. Rapid assessment is essential to ensure prompt, effective interventions to prevent perinatal and fetal morbidity and mortality.

LABORATORY AND DIAGNOSTIC TESTING

Laboratory and diagnostic tests may be helpful in diagnosing the condition and guiding management. These studies may include:

- *Complete Blood Count (CBC)*—determines the current hemodynamic status; however, it is not reliable for estimating acute blood loss
- *Fibrinogen levels*—typically are increased in pregnancy (hyperfibrinogenemia); thus, a moderate dip in fibrinogen levels might suggest DIC and, if profuse bleeding occurs, the clotting cascade might be compromised
- *Prothrombin time (PT)/activated partial thromboplastin time (aPTT)*—determines the client's coagulation status, especially if surgery is planned
- *Type and cross-match*—determines blood type, Rh factor and antibody screen if a transfusion is needed
- *Nonstress test*—demonstrates findings of fetal compromise manifested by minimal variability, late decelerations, tachycardia, or bradycardia

• *Biophysical profile*—aids in evaluating clients with chronic abruption; a low score (less than 6 points) suggests possible fetal compromise (Resnik et al., 2014).

Ultrasound is not useful for making a definitive diagnosis because the clot is sonographically visible in less than 50% of the cases. A CT scan is a more reliable method for evaluation of placental abruption (Hosein, Abdel-Kariem, & Shriki, 2015).

Nursing Management

Nursing management of the client with abruptio placentae warrants immediate care to provide the best outcome for both the client and fetus.

ENSURING ADEQUATE TISSUE PERFUSION

When the client arrives at the facility, place them on strict bed rest and in a left lateral position to prevent pressure on the vena cava. This position provides uninterrupted perfusion to the fetus. Expect to administer oxygen therapy to ensure adequate tissue perfusion. Monitor oxygen saturation levels via pulse oximetry to evaluate the effectiveness of the interventions.

Obtain the client's vital signs frequently, as often as every 15 minutes as indicated, depending on the status and amount of blood loss. Observe for changes in vital signs suggesting hypovolemic shock and report them immediately. Also expect to insert an indwelling urinary (Foley) catheter to assess hourly urine output and initiate an IV infusion for fluid replacement using a large-bore catheter.

Assess fundal height for changes. An increase in size would indicate bleeding. Monitor the amount and characteristics of any vaginal bleeding as frequently as every 15 to 30 minutes. Be alert for signs and symptoms of DIC, such as bleeding gums, tachycardia, oozing from the IV insertion site, and petechiae, and administer blood products as ordered if DIC occurs.

Institute continuous electronic fetal monitoring. Assess uterine contractions and report any increased uterine tenseness or rigidity. Also observe the tracing for tetanic uterine contractions or changes in fetal heart rate patterns suggesting that the fetus has been compromised.

PROVIDING SUPPORT AND EDUCATION

A client diagnosed with abruptio placentae may be filled with a sense of heightened anxiety and apprehension regarding their own health as well as that of the fetus. Communicate empathy and understanding of the client's experience, and provide emotional support throughout this frightening time. Remain with the client and partner, acknowledge their emotions and fears, and address their spiritual and cultural needs. Answer their questions about the status of the fetus openly and honestly, being sure to explain indicators of fetal well-being. Provide information about the various diagnostic tests, treatments, and

procedures that may be done, including the possible need for a cesarean birth. Depending on the client's status, extent of bleeding, and length of gestation, the fetus may not survive. If the fetus does survive, the newborn will most likely require neonatal intensive care. Assist the client and family to deal with a loss or with the birth of a newborn in the neonatal intensive care unit.

Although abruptio placentae is not a preventable condition, client education is important to help reduce the risk for a recurrence of this condition. Encourage the client to avoid drinking, smoking, or using drugs during pregnancy. Urge the client to seek early and continuous prenatal care and to receive prompt health care if any signs and symptoms occur in future pregnancies.

> **Think back to Helen, the pregnant woman described at the beginning of the chapter. Helen was diagnosed with abruptio placentae and was prepared for an emergency cesarean birth. On exploration, there was almost a 75% abruption, with approximately 800 mL of concealed blood between the uterus and the placenta, with an additional 500 mL lost during surgery. What in Helen's history may have placed her at increased risk for abruption? What assessments and interventions would be essential during the postpartum recovery period secondary to the large blood loss? What psychosocial interventions would be necessary due to the fetal loss?**

Placenta Accreta

Placenta *accreta* is a potentially life-threatening obstetrical condition that can result in severe hemorrhage and requires a multidisciplinary approach to management. Abnormal placentation occurs when the placenta attaches unusually deep into the uterus and can be classified as placenta accreta, increta, or percreta. The incidence of abnormal placentation has increased 10- to 50-fold in the last 50 years and reportedly occurs in up to 1 in 530–550 pregnancies (Aitken et al., 2016). The increasing rate of placenta accreta has occurred alongside increasing rates of cesarean birth. A previous cesarean birth is the most easily identified risk factor for placenta accreta. Multiple previous cesarean births increases the risk exponentially. In addition, advanced age in pregnancy; multiparity; prior curettage procedures; and previous uterine surgery for Asherman's syndrome, embolization, or myomectomy increase the risk for invasive placentation (Aitken et al., 2016). Placenta accreta is a condition in which the placenta attaches itself too deeply, reaching beyond the decidua and into the surface of the myometrium. In *placenta increta*, the placenta invades more deeply into the myometrium, and with *placenta percreta*, the placenta extends through the myometrium and uterine serosa into adjacent tissue or organs. A common risk of placenta accreta during the birthing process is the possibility of hemorrhaging during manual attempts to detach the placenta.

According to ACOG (2014b), 90% of accretas have postpartum hemorrhage, and 50% of these will result in a hysterectomy (ACOG, 2014b). Clients at highest risk of emergency hysterectomy are those who are multiparous, had a cesarean birth in either a previous or the present pregnancy, or had abnormal placentation. The essential management issues are early detection and immediate and appropriate intervention. If a placenta accreta diagnosis is made, the client should be counselled that a cesarean section and possible hysterectomy may be necessary interventions (Resnik et al., 2014).

Placenta accreta is typically diagnosed after birth when the placenta fails to normally separate from the uterine wall. Diagnosis may be made prenatally via ultrasound and MRI, which can decrease maternal and fetal morbidities and mortalities through careful planning for the location of birth, readiness of an expert team, equipment, and blood products. A profuse hemorrhage may result because the uterus cannot contract to close off the open blood vessels. Management will depend on the severity of the bleeding and frequently necessitates a prompt hysterectomy (Humphrey, 2015). Nurses need to be prepared to assist in this emergency situation as dictated by the health care team.

HYPEREMESIS GRAVIDARUM

HG is a severe form of nausea and vomiting of pregnancy associated with significant costs and psychosocial impacts. At least 50% to 80% of individuals experience nausea and vomiting during their pregnancy (Campbell, Rowe, Azzam, & Lane, 2016). The term *morning sickness* is often used to describe this condition when symptoms are relatively mild. Such symptoms usually disappear after the first trimester. While mild nausea and vomiting mostly affects the quality of life of the pregnant client and family, severe hyperemesis or **hyperemesis gravidarum** can have a significant impact on the health, quality of life, and finances of the individual as well as financial impact on society (related to missed employment) and the health care system (Campbell et al., 2016). The physical effects of HG include dehydration, weight loss, electrolyte imbalance, and the need for hospitalization (Taylor, 2014). Possible effects on the fetus include low birth weight, preterm birth, small for gestational age, and lower Apgar scores (Campbell et al., 2016).

Unlike morning sickness, HG is a complication of pregnancy characterized by persistent, uncontrollable nausea and vomiting that begins in the first trimester and causes dehydration, ketosis, and weight loss of more than 5% of prepregnancy body weight (Campbell et al., 2016).

Risk factors for hyperemesis include previous pregnancy complicated by hyperemesis, molar pregnancies, history of helicobacter pylori infection, **multiple gestation**, prepregnancy history of genitourinary disorders, clinical hyperthyroid disorders, and prepregnancy psychiatric diagnosis (King et al., 2015), low body mass index, genetic predisposition, and female fetus (Campbell et al., 2016).

HG is estimated to occur in approximately 2% of pregnancies. The peak incidence is at 8 to 12 weeks of pregnancy, and symptoms usually resolve by week 20 (Maltepe et al., 2015).

Take Note!

Every pregnant client needs to be instructed to report any episodes of severe nausea and vomiting or episodes that extend beyond the first trimester.

Pathophysiology

Although the exact cause of hyperemesis is unknown, its effects—decreased placental blood flow, decreased maternal blood flow, and acidosis—can threaten the health of the pregnant client and fetus. Dehydration can also lead to preterm labour (Festin, 2014). Despite numerous theories, few studies have produced scientific evidence to identify the etiology of this condition. It is likely that multiple factors contribute to it.

Elevated levels of hCG are present in all pregnant individuals during early pregnancy, usually declining after 12 weeks. This corresponds to the usual duration of morning sickness. In HG, the hCG levels are often higher and extend beyond the first trimester. Symptoms exacerbate the disease. Decreased fluid intake and prolonged vomiting cause dehydration; dehydration increases the serum concentration of hCG, which in turn exacerbates the nausea and vomiting—a vicious cycle. A few other theories that have been proposed to explain its etiology include:

- *Endocrine theory*—high levels of hCG and estrogen during pregnancy
- *Metabolic theory*—vitamin B_6 deficiency
- *Genetic factors* that may predispose an individual to this condition
- *Psychological theory*—psychological stress increases the symptoms

Therapeutic Management

HG is a diagnosis of exclusion. Careful consideration of other conditions must be assessed when a client experiences severe and prolonged nausea and vomiting in pregnancy, not responsive to usual management strategies (Campbell, 2016).

Conservative management in the home is the first line of treatment for client HG. This usually focuses on dietary and lifestyle changes and medications for nausea and

If no improvement, proceed to next step

Give 10 mg of Pyridoxine 4 x a day po
The schedule and dose can be adjusted according to severity of symptoms

OR

Give 10 mg of doxylamine combined with 10 mg of pyridoxine po
Typical starting dose: one in the morning, one in the afternoon and 2 at bedtime. Titrate dose up to 8 tablets a day as needed. Adjust schedule dose according to severity of symptoms.

Add dimenhydrinate 50 mg q4–6h orally or rectally

No dehydration

Add any of the following:
• metoclopramide 5 to 10 mg q8h po or IM
• chlorpromazine 10 to 25 mg q4–6h po or 25 to 50 mg q4h IM
• prochlorperazine 5 to 10 mg q6–8h po or PR or IM
• promethazine 12.5 to 25 mg q4–6h po or IM

• Add ondansetron 8 mg q12h po or 4 mg q8h po prn

Notes:
• The use of this algorithm assumes that other causes of nausea and vomiting have been ruled out.

• At any time you may add any or all:
  - pyridoxine 25 mg q8h
  - ginger 250 mg q6h
  - P6 acupressure
  - Mindfulness-based cognitive behavioural therapy
  - In 1st trimester: substitute iron containing PV with folic acid

• At any step, when indicated, consider **parenteral nutrition.**

Dehydration

Start rehydration treatment:
• intravenous (IV) fluid replacement (per local protocol)
• multivitamin IV supplementation
• dimenhydrinate 50 mg q4–6h PR or IV

Add any of the following:
• metoclopramide 5 to 10 mg q8h IV
• chlorpromazine 12.5 to 50 mg q6–8h IM or IV
• prochlorperazine 5 to 10 mg q6–8h IV or IM
• promethazine 12.5 to 25 mg q4–6h IV

• Add ondansetron 8 mg q12h IV prn or 4 mg q8h IV prn

• Add methylprednisolone 15 to 20 mg q8h IV for up to 24 h

FIGURE 19.6 Treatment algorithm for nausea and vomiting of pregnancy. (From Campbell, K., Rowe, H., Azzam, H., & Lane, C. A. [2016]. The management of nausea and vomiting of pregnancy. *Journal of Obstetrics and Gynaecology Canada, 38*[12], 1127–1137.)

vomiting. Pharmacy grade ginger, acupressure, mindfulness-based cognitive therapy, and lifestyle changes such as increased rest and sleep are recommended as strategies with some evidence of effectiveness (Campbell et al., 2016). If conservative management fails to alleviate the client's symptoms, combinations of medications and fluid replacement may be effectively delivered in a home care setting. If severe dehydration occurs or HG is not responsive to home therapy, hospitalization may be necessary.

On admission to the hospital, blood tests are ordered to assess the severity of the client's dehydration, electrolyte imbalance, ketosis, and malnutrition. Parenteral fluids and drugs are ordered to rehydrate the client and reduce the symptoms. The first choice for fluid replacement is generally normal saline, which aids in preventing hyponatremia, with vitamins (pyridoxine [B₆]) and electrolytes added. There is no evidence to support dietary restrictions and clients should be encouraged to eat pregnancy safe foods in amounts and frequency that are tolerated (Campbell et al., 2016). Antiemetics and other therapies

are administered intravenously to control the nausea and vomiting and may include H1 antagonists (dimenhydrinate), metoclopramide, phenothiazines, and ondansetron. If the client does not improve after usual intravenous rehydration and medical therapy, total parenteral nutrition is instituted to prevent malnutrition (Fig. 19.6).

Take Note!

HG is nausea and vomiting in early pregnancy that prevents the pregnant individual from ingesting adequate nutrition. IV fluids, medication, cognitive and alternative therapies may be required for rehydration and stabilization of symptoms. In severe cases, total parenteral nutrition may be required. Dietary restrictions are not effective, and a diet-as-tolerated should be encouraged.

Nursing Assessment

Nursing assessment of the client with HG requires a thorough history and physical examination to identify signs and symptoms associated with this disorder. The client is extremely uncomfortable and may experience many hours of lost work productivity and sleep, adding to personal distress and potentially adversely affecting family relationships. If hyperemesis progresses untreated, it may cause neurologic disturbances, renal damage, dehydration, ketosis, alkalosis from loss of hydrochloric acid, hypokalemia, retinal hemorrhage, or death (Peled et al., 2014). Laboratory and diagnostic tests aid in determining the severity of the disorder.

Health History and Physical Examination

Begin the history by asking the client about the onset, duration, and course of nausea and vomiting. Ask about any medications or treatments already used and how effective they were in relieving the nausea and vomiting. Obtain a diet history from the client, including a dietary recall for the past week. Note the client's knowledge of nutrition and need for appropriate nutritional intake. Be alert for patterns that may contribute to or trigger distress. Also ask about any complaints of ptyalism (excessive salivation), anorexia, indigestion, abdominal pain or distention, or blood or mucus in the stool. Review the client's history for possible risk factors, such as young age, nausea and vomiting with previous pregnancy, nulliparity, trophoblastic disease, multiple gestation, emotional or psychological stress, genetic inheritance, previous affected pregnancies, lower body mass index, psychiatric or mood disorders, obesity, hyperthyroidism, and *Helicobacter pylori* seropositivity (Campbell et al., 2016; Ogunyemi, Fong, & Herrero, 2017). Weigh the client and compare this weight with the recorded weight before symptoms started and to the prepregnancy weight to estimate the degree of loss. With severe hyperemesis, weight loss usually exceeds 5% of body mass.

Inspect the mucous membranes for dryness and check skin turgor for evidence of fluid loss and dehydration. Assess blood pressure for changes, such as hypotension, that may suggest a fluid volume deficit. Also note any reports of weakness, fatigue, activity intolerance, dizziness, or sleep disturbances.

Assess the client's perception of the situation. Note any evidence of depression, anxiety, irritability, mood changes, and decreased ability to concentrate, which can add to emotional distress. Much of the psychological distress is self-limiting in this condition and may be part of the causal pathway (Tan, Zaidi, Azmi, Omar, & Khong, 2014). Determine the client's support systems available for help.

Laboratory and Diagnostic Testing

The results of laboratory and diagnostic tests may provide clues to the severity or etiology of the disorder. These may include:
- *Liver enzymes*—to rule out hepatitis, pancreatitis, and cholestasis; elevations of aspartate aminotransferase

(AST) and alanine aminotransferase (ALT) are usually present
- *CBC*—elevated levels of red blood cells and hematocrit, indicating dehydration
- *Urine ketones*—positive when the body breaks down fat to provide energy in the absence of adequate intake
- *TSH and T4* to rule out thyroid disease
- *Blood urea nitrogen*—increased in the presence of salt and water depletion
- *Urine specific gravity*—greater than 1.025, possibly indicating concentrated urine linked to inadequate fluid intake or excessive fluid loss
- *Serum electrolytes*—decreased levels of potassium, sodium, and chloride resulting from excessive vomiting and loss of hydrochloric acid in stomach
- *Ultrasound*—evaluation for molar pregnancy or multiple gestation (Cunningham et al., 2014).

Nursing Management

Nursing management for the client with HG focuses on promoting comfort by controlling the client's nausea and vomiting and promoting adequate nutrition. In addition, the nurse plays a major role in supporting and educating the client and family.

Promoting Comfort and Nutrition

During the initial period, expect to discuss current dietary patterns and strategies used by the client to maximize intake. Based on patterns of intake, encourage additional opportunities for nutritional intake, focusing on proteins and fluids, and avoidance of triggers. Administer prescribed antiemetics to relieve the nausea and vomiting and IV fluids to replace fluid losses. Monitor the rate of infusion to prevent overload and assess the IV insertion site to prevent infiltration or infection. Also administer electrolyte replacement therapy as ordered to correct any imbalances, and periodically check serum electrolyte levels to evaluate the effectiveness of therapy.

Provide physical comfort measures such as hygiene measures and oral care. Pay special attention to the environment, making sure to keep the area free of triggers such as odours or other stimulants. Monitor intake and output and assess the client's tolerance and any improvements.

Providing Support and Education

Pregnant individuals with HG commonly are fatigued physically and emotionally. Many are exhausted, frustrated, and anxious. Offer reassurance that all interventions are directed toward promoting positive pregnancy outcomes for both the client and fetus. Providing information about the expected plan of care may help to alleviate the client's anxiety. Listen to concerns and feelings, answering all questions honestly. Educate the client and family about the condition and its treatment options. Teach the client about therapeutic lifestyle changes, such as avoiding stressors and fatigue that may trigger nausea and vomiting. Offer ongoing support and encouragement and promote active participation in care decisions, thereby empowering the client and family. Attempting to provide the client with a sense of control may help mitigate the feelings of loss of control. Provide information for mindfulness cognitive-based therapy and other alternatives (acupressure or acupuncture). Suggest possible local or national support groups that the client may contact for additional information. Arrange for home care follow-up for the client, if available, and reinforce discharge instructions to promote understanding. Timely counselling, balanced nutrition, pharmacotherapy, and emotional support are associated with favourable outcomes for the client with this condition. Collaborate with community resources to ensure continuity of care.

HYPERTENSIVE DISORDERS OF PREGNANCY

Hypertensive disorders of pregnancy remain the leading cause of perinatal morbidity and mortality (Magee, Pels, Helewa, Rey, & von Dadelszen, 2014), complicating up to 15% of all pregnancies. These conditions result in frequent hospital admissions, maternal morbidity and mortality, and preterm births with concomitant neonatal morbidity and mortality. Hypertensive disorders of pregnancy comprise a spectrum of severity ranging from a mild elevation of blood pressure to severe preeclampsia, eclampsia and significant hematologic changes. Recent data show that hypertensive disorders of pregnancy are associated with long-term cardiovascular risks for the pregnant client (Miller & Carpenter, 2015).

Hypertensive disorders of pregnancy include chronic hypertension, gestational hypertension, preeclampsia, eclampsia, and chronic hypertension with superimposed preeclampsia (Magee et al., 2014). Preeclampsia complicates about 3% to 5% of pregnancies. Hypertensive disorders are associated with higher rates of maternal, fetal, and infant mortality and with severe morbidity, especially in cases of severe preeclampsia, eclampsia, and HELLP syndrome (ACOG, 2014c).

Hypertension may be a pre-existing condition (chronic hypertension) or it may present for the first time during pregnancy (gestational hypertension). Both chronic hypertension and gestational hypertension can be complicated by preeclampsia or eclampsia and can be subclassified as either mild or severe. Other definitions of hypertensive disorders include transient, white-coat, or masked hypertensive effects (Box 19.3). For hypertension, subclassification is dependent on systolic and diastolic values. For preeclampsia, subclassification

is dependent on the severity of end-organ involvement (Foley, Strong, & Garite, 2014; Magee et al., 2014).

The Society of Obstetricians and Gynecologist of Canada (SOGC) released a Clinical Practice Guideline (2014) for use in low- to high-risk settings to provide consistency in defining and approaching management, optimizing health outcomes with a consideration of cost-effectiveness. The classification of hypertensive disorders of pregnancy is outlined in Box 19.3.

Population-based data indicate that approximately 1% of pregnancies are complicated by chronic hypertension, 5% to 6% by gestational hypertension (without proteinuria), and 3% to 5% by preeclampsia (Carson & Gibson, 2018). Worldwide, 50,000 to 60,000 individuals die from preeclampsia each year, corresponding to 12% of all maternal deaths (Clausen & Bergholt, 2014).

Chronic Hypertension

Chronic hypertension is defined as blood pressure exceeding 140/90 mm Hg before pregnancy or before 20 weeks' gestation. When hypertension is first identified during pregnancy at less than 20 weeks' gestation, blood pressure elevations usually represent chronic hypertension. Chronic hypertension occurs in about 20% of individuals of childbearing age, with the prevalence varying according to age, race, and body mass index (BMI). As our nation's obesity rate rises, more individuals will start pregnancies with elevated blood pressures. About 25% of clients with chronic hypertension develop preeclampsia during pregnancy (Clausen & Bergholt, 2014). Clients with chronic hypertension in pregnancy should be monitored for the development of worsening hypertension and/or the development of superimposed preeclampsia.

Individuals with mild chronic hypertension often do not require antihypertensive therapy during most of the pregnancy. Pharmacologic treatment of mild hypertension does not reduce the likelihood of developing preeclampsia later in gestation and increases the likelihood of intrauterine growth restriction (IUGR). If maternal blood pressure exceeds 160/100 mm Hg, however, drug treatment is recommended (Magee et al., 2015). Nurses can play a large role in educating their hypertensive clients to help them understand potential complications and how simple changes in their lifestyles might be helpful in influencing the pregnancy outcome positively.

Gestational Hypertension

The gestational hypertension category is used for clients with nonproteinuric hypertension of pregnancy, in which the adverse conditions of preeclampsia are not present. Gestational hypertension is characterized by hypertension (>140/90) without proteinuria or other adverse conditions associated with preeclampsia (Box 19.3). It occurs after 20 weeks' gestation resolving by 12 weeks'

BOX 19.3

CLASSIFICATION OF THE HYPERTENSIVE DISORDERS OF PREGNANCY

Disorder	Comments
Pre-existing (chronic) hypertension	This is defined as hypertension that develops either prepregnancy or at <20+0 weeks' gestation
With comorbid condition(s)	Comorbid conditions (e.g., pregestational type I or II diabetes mellitus or kidney disease) warrant tighter BP control outside of pregnancy because of their association with heightened cardiovascular risk.
With evidence of preeclampsia	This is also known as superimposed preeclampsia, and is defined by the development of one or more of the following at ≥20 weeks: • resistant hypertension, *or* • new or worsening proteinuria, *or* • one or more adverse conditions,[a] *or* • one or more severe complications.[a] Severe preeclampsia is defined as preeclampsia with one or more severe complications.
Gestational hypertension	This is defined as hypertension that develops for the first time at ≥20+0 weeks' gestation.
With comorbid condition(s)	Comorbid conditions (e.g., pregestational type I or II diabetes mellitus or kidney disease) warrant tighter BP control outside of pregnancy because of their association with heightened cardiovascular risk.
With evidence of preeclampsia	Evidence of preeclampsia may appear only many weeks after the onset of gestational hypertension. Preeclampsia is defined as gestational hypertension with one or more of the following: • new proteinuria, *or* • one or more adverse conditions,[a] *or* • one or more severe complications.[a] Severe preeclampsia is defined as preeclampsia with one or more severe complications.
Preeclampsia	Preeclampsia may arise de novo. It is defined as gestational hypertension with one or more of the following: • new proteinuria, *or* • one or more adverse conditions,[a] *or* • one or more severe complications.[a] Severe preeclampsia is defined as preeclampsia with one or more severe complications.
Other hypertensive effects[b]	
Transient hypertensive effect	Elevated BP may be due to environmental stimuli, e.g., the pain of labour.
White-coat hypertensive effect	This is defined as BP that is elevated in the office (sBP ≥140 mm Hg or dBP ≥90 mm Hg), but consistently normal outside of the office (<135/85 mm Hg) by ABPM or HBPM
Masked hypertensive effect	This is defined as BP that is consistently normal in the office (sBP <140 mm Hg or dBP <90 mm Hg), but elevated outside of the office (≥135/85 mm Hg) by ABPM or repeated HBPM.

[a]Adverse conditions and severe complications of preeclampsia are defined in Comparison Chart 19.2.
[b]These may occur in women whose BP is elevated at <20+0 or ≥20+0 weeks who are suspected of having pre-existing or gestational hypertension/preeclampsia, respectively.
sBP, systolic BP; dBP, diastolic BP; ABPM, ambulatory BP monitoring; HBPM, home BP monitoring.
Adapted from Magee, L. A., Pels, A., Helewa, M., Rey, E., & von Dadelszen, P. (2014). SOGC Clinical practice guideline: Diagnosis, evaluation, and management of the hypertensive disorders of pregnancy: Executive summary. *Journal of Obstetrics and Gynaecology Canada, 36*(5), 416–438.

---

postpartum (Magowan et al., 2014). Previously, gestational hypertension was known as pregnancy-induced hypertension or toxemia of pregnancy, but these terms are no longer used. Gestational hypertension is defined as systolic blood pressure greater than 140 mm Hg and/or diastolic greater than 90 mm Hg on at least two occasions at least 15 minutes apart after the 20th week of gestation, in individuals known to be normotensive prior to this time and prior to pregnancy (Magee et al., 2014).

Preeclampsia and Eclampsia

Normal physiologic adaptations to pregnancy are altered in the individual who develops preeclampsia.

COMPARISON CHART 19.2 **ADVERSE CONDITIONS AND SEVERE COMPLICATIONS OF PREECLAMPSIA**

Organ System Affected	Adverse Conditions (That Increase the Risk of Severe Complications)	Severe Complications (That Warrant Delivery)
Central nervous system	Headache/visual symptoms	Eclampsia PRES Cortical blindness or retinal detachment Glasgow coma scale <13 Stroke, TIA, or RIND
Cardiorespiratory	Chest pain/dyspnea Oxygen saturation <97%	Uncontrolled severe hypertension (over a period of 12 hours despite use of three antihypertensive agents) Oxygen saturation <90%, need for ≥50% oxygen for >1 hour, intubation (other than for cesarean section), pulmonary edema Positive inotropic support Myocardial ischemia or infarction
Hematologic	Elevated WBC count Elevated INR or aPTT Low platelet count	Platelet count <50 × 109/L Transfusion of any blood product
Renal	Elevated serum creatinine Elevated serum uric acid	Acute kidney injury (creatinine >150 µM with no prior renal disease) New indication for dialysis
Hepatic	Nausea or vomiting RUQ or epigastric pain Elevated serum AST, ALT, LDH, or bilirubin Low plasma albumin	Hepatic dysfunction (INR >2 in absence of DIC or warfarin) Hepatic hematoma or rupture
Feto-placental	Abnormal FHR IUGR Oligohydramnios Absent or reversed end-diastolic flow by Doppler velocimetry	Abruption with evidence of maternal or fetal compromise Reverse ductus venosus A wave Stillbirth

PRES, posterior reversible leukoencephalopathy syndrome; TIA, transient ischemic attack; RIND, reversible ischemic neurologic deficit (<48 hours); WBC, white blood cell; INR, international normalized ratio; aPTT, activated partial thromboplastin time; RUQ, right upper quadrant; AST, aspartate aminotransferase; ALT, alanine aminotransferase; LDH, lactate dehydrogenase; DIC, disseminated intravascular coagulation; FHR, fetal heart rate.

Magee, L. A., Pels, A., Helewa, M., Rey, E., & von Dadelszen, P. (2014). SOGC Clinical practice guideline: Diagnosis, evaluation, and management of the hypertensive disorders of pregnancy: Executive summary. *Journal of Obstetrics and Gynaecology Canada, 36*(5), 416–438.

Preeclampsia can be described as a multisystem, vasopressive disorder that targets the cardiovascular, hepatic, renal, and central nervous systems (CNSs). Preeclampsia can be classified as mild or severe with a potential progression to eclampsia (severe preeclampsia with seizure). Comparison Chart 19.2 highlights adverse and severe complications of preeclampsia.

Pathophysiology

Preeclampsia remains an enigma. The condition can be devastating to both the client and fetus, yet the etiology remains a mystery to medical science despite decades of research. Many theories exist, but none has truly explained the widespread pathologic changes that result in pulmonary edema, oliguria, seizures, thrombocytopenia, and abnormal liver enzymes (Cunningham et al.,

2014). Despite the results of several research studies, the use of aspirin or supplementation with magnesium, zinc, or antioxidant therapy (vitamins C and E), salt restriction, diuretic therapy, or fish oils has not proved to prevent preeclampsia in low-risk individuals (Magee et al., 2014). According to recent studies, prevention of preeclampsia in clients at risk includes low-dose ASA daily, calcium supplementation where dietary intake in low, and low–molecular-weight heparin for clients with a history of placental pathology. Risk reduction for clients at low-risk includes calcium supplementation for those with a low dietary intake (less than 600 mg/day), as well as continuation of folate supplementation throughout pregnancy. L-arginine, increased rest and reduced stress may also be beneficial (Magee et al., 2014). Preeclampsia is a two-stage event; the underlying mechanisms involved are vasospasm and hypoperfusion. In the first stage, the key feature is widespread vasospasm. In addition, endothelial injury occurs, leading to platelet adherence, fibrin deposition, and the presence of schistocytes (fragment of an erythrocyte). The second stage of preeclampsia is the client's response to abnormal placentation, when symptoms of hypertension, proteinuria, and edema appear.

The first stage of generalized vasospasm results in elevation of blood pressure and reduced blood flow to the brain, liver, kidneys, placenta, and lungs. Decreased liver perfusion leads to impaired liver function and subcapsular hemorrhage. This is demonstrated by epigastric pain and elevated liver enzymes in the maternal serum. Decreased brain perfusion leads to small cerebral hemorrhages and symptoms of arterial vasospasm such as headaches, visual disturbances, blurred vision, and hyperactive deep tendon reflexes (DTRs). A thromboxane/prostacyclin imbalance leads to increased thromboxane (potent vasoconstrictor and stimulator of platelet aggregation) and decreased prostacyclin (potent vasodilator and inhibitor of platelet aggregation), which contribute to the hypertensive state. Decreased kidney perfusion reduces the glomerular filtration rate, resulting in decreased urine output and increased serum levels of sodium, BUN, uric acid, and creatinine, further increasing extracellular fluid and edema. Increased capillary permeability in the kidneys allows albumin to escape, which reduces plasma colloid osmotic pressure and moves more fluid into extracellular spaces; this leads to pulmonary edema and generalized edema. Poor placental perfusion resulting from prolonged vasoconstriction contributes to IUGR, premature separation of the placenta (abruptio placentae), persistent fetal hypoxia, and acidosis. In addition, hemoconcentration (resulting from decreased intravascular volume) causes increased blood viscosity and elevated hematocrit (ACOG, 2014c).

Therapeutic Management

Management of the client with preeclampsia varies depending on the severity of the condition and its effects on the fetus. Typically the client is managed conservatively if symptoms are mild. However, if the condition progresses, management becomes more aggressive. The "cure" for preeclampsia/eclampsia is always delivery of the placenta. The resolution following expulsion of the placenta supports theories related to the placental influence on the disease (Dekker, 2014).

MANAGEMENT FOR MILD PREECLAMPSIA

Conservative strategies for mild preeclampsia are used if the client exhibits no signs of renal or hepatic dysfunction or coagulopathy. The client will have increased antepartum visits for assessment of blood pressure and other monitoring, and increased diagnostic testing including CBC, clotting studies, liver enzymes, and platelet levels. The client will be asked to: monitor blood pressure daily (up to every 4 to 6 hours while awake) and report any increased readings; measure the amount of protein found in urine using a dipstick; and do daily weight checks to determine amount of weight gain. Daily fetal movement counting will be done to assess fetal well-being, and if there is any decrease in movement, the client needs to be instructed to seek assessment by the health care provider immediately. A balanced nutritional diet with no sodium restriction is advised. If home management fails to reduce the blood pressure, admission to the hospital is warranted and the treatment strategy is individualized based on the severity of the condition and the gestational age at the time of diagnosis.

During the hospitalization, the client with mild preeclampsia is monitored closely for signs and symptoms of severe preeclampsia or impending eclampsia (e.g., persistent headache, visual disturbances, hyperreflexia). Blood pressure measurements are frequently recorded along with daily weights to detect excessive weight gain resulting from edema. Fetal surveillance is instituted in the form of daily fetal movement counts, nonstress testing, and serial ultrasounds to evaluate fetal growth and amniotic fluid volume to confirm fetal well-being. Expectant management (watchful waiting) usually continues until the pregnancy reaches term, or complications develop that warrant immediate birth. Clients with mild preeclampsia are also at risk for postpartum hypertension (King et al., 2015).

Prevention of disease progression is the focus of treatment during labour. Blood pressure is monitored frequently and a quiet environment is important to minimize the risk of CNS stimulation and to promote rest. IV magnesium sulphate is infused to prevent seizure activity, along with antihypertensives if blood pressure values begin to rise. Calcium gluconate is kept at the bedside in case signs of magnesium toxicity become evident (including reduced respiratory rate or absent reflexes). Continued close monitoring of neurologic status is warranted to detect any signs or symptoms of hypoxemia, impending seizure activity, or increased intracranial pressure. An indwelling urinary (Foley) catheter is inserted to allow for accurate hourly measurement of urine output as adequate output required to clear the magnesium.

MANAGEMENT FOR SEVERE PREECLAMPSIA

Severe hypertension or preeclampsia may develop suddenly with high blood pressure of more than 160/110 mm Hg, proteinuria of more than 5 g in 24 hours, oliguria of less than 400 mL in 24 hours, cerebral and visual symptoms, and rapid weight gain and pulmonary edema. This clinical picture signals severe preeclampsia, and immediate hospitalization and expedited birth is needed.

Treatment is highly individualized and based on disease severity and fetal age. Birth of the infant and placenta is the only definitive relief, because preeclampsia depends on the presence of trophoblastic tissue. Therefore, the exact age of the fetus is assessed to determine viability.

Severe preeclampsia is treated aggressively because hypertension with adverse conditions, and risk of complications (proteinuria, low platelets, elevated liver enzymes, abnormal ultrasound findings), poses a serious threat to both the client and fetus. The goal of care is to stabilize the dyad and prepare for birth. Therapy focuses on controlling hypertension, preventing seizures, preventing long-term morbidity, and preventing client, fetal, or newborn death (Foo, Tay, Lees, McEniery, & Wilkinson, 2015).

The client in labour with severe preeclampsia typically receives oxytocin to stimulate uterine contractions and magnesium sulphate to prevent seizure activity. Oxytocin and magnesium sulphate is given simultaneously via infusion pumps through separate IV sites to ensure both are administered at the prescribed rate. A loading dose of 4 g of magnesium is given over 15 to 20 minutes. Then, a maintenance dose of 1 g/hr is given (Magee et al., 2014).

The client is evaluated closely for signs of magnesium toxicity including respiratory depression (less than 12 breaths/min) and absent DTRs. Serum magnesium levels are not recommended (Magee et al., 2014). If at all possible, a vaginal delivery is preferable to a cesarean birth for better client outcomes and less risk associated with a surgical birth. PGE2 gel may be used to ripen the cervix. A cesarean birth may be performed if the client is seriously ill. A full newborn resuscitation team including pediatrician/neonatologist or neonatal nurse practitioner should be available in the birthing room to care for the newborn. A newborn who was exposed to high doses of magnesium sulphate in utero needs to be monitored for respiratory depression, hypocalcemia, and hypotonia. Decreased fetal heart rate variability may occur but, in general, magnesium sulphate does not pose a risk to the fetus. The newborn may exhibit respiratory depression, loss of reflexes, muscle weakness, and neurologic depression (Martin, Fanaroff, & Walsh, 2014).

MANAGEMENT OF ECLAMPSIA

In the client who develops an eclamptic seizure, the convulsive activity begins with facial twitching, followed by generalized muscle rigidity. The client's face initially may become distorted, with protrusion of the eyes, and foaming at the mouth may occur. Respirations cease for the duration of the seizure, resulting from muscle spasms, thus compromising fetal oxygenation. Seizure complications can include tongue biting, head trauma, broken bones, and aspiration. Coma sometimes follows the seizure activity, with respiration resuming. Eclamptic seizures are life-threatening emergencies and require immediate treatment to decrease morbidity and mortality.

As with any seizure, the initial management is to clear the airway and administer adequate oxygen. Lateral positioning on the left side to protect the client from injury during the seizure is priority. Suction equipment must be readily available to remove secretions from the mouth

after the seizure is over. IV fluids are administered after the seizure at a rate to replace urine output and additional insensible losses. Fetal heart rate is monitored continuously. Magnesium sulphate is administered intravenously to prevent further seizures. Respiratory rate, reflexes, and urine output in clients receiving magnesium sulphate are closely monitored to avoid magnesium toxicity and prevent cardiac arrest. Serum magnesium levels are not recommended (Magee et al., 2014). Calcium gluconate (1 g intravenously) is typically ordered to counteract magnesium toxicity (respirations less than 12 per min, absent DTRs). Hypertension is controlled with antihypertensive medications. After the client's seizures are controlled, and if the client is stable, birth via induction or cesarean section is performed (Amorim et al., 2015). When the postpartum client's condition is stable, transfer to the postpartum unit for care may occur depending on unit protocols and based on available resources and expertise. If the client is unstable after giving birth, care may continue in the high-risk birthing unit or in a critical care unit for closer observation.

Nursing Assessment

Preventing complications related to preeclampsia requires the use of assessment, advocacy, and counselling skills. Assessment begins with the accurate measurement of the client's blood pressure at each encounter. In addition, nurses need to assess for subjective complaints that may indicate progression of the disease—visual changes, severe headaches, unusual bleeding or bruising, or epigastric pain (Nagtalon-Ramos, 2014). The significant signs of preeclampsia—proteinuria and hypertension occur without the client's awareness. By the time the client is experiencing symptoms, gestational hypertension and preeclampsia can be severe.

Take Note!

The absolute blood pressure (value that validates elevation) of 140/90 mm Hg should be obtained on two occasions 15 minutes apart to be diagnostic of hypertension. Proteinuria is defined as 300 mg or more of urinary protein. When urine dipstick is 1+ or greater, more definitive testing should be done for total protein and urine protein-creatinine ratio.

HEALTH HISTORY AND PHYSICAL EXAMINATION

Take a thorough history during the first antepartum visit to identify whether the client is at risk for preeclampsia. Risk factors include:

- Primigravida status
- Previous miscarriage at less than 10 weeks with same partner
- Assisted reproductive technologies
- Chromosomal abnormalities
- Structural congenital anomalies

- Multiple gestation
- Vaginal bleeding in early pregnancy
- Abnormal PAPP-A or free bHCG
- History of preeclampsia in a previous pregnancy
- Excessive placental tissue, as is seen in GTD
- Antiphospholipid antibody syndrome
- Infection during pregnancy (UTI, periodontal disease)
- IUGR
- Use of ovulation drugs
- Family history of preeclampsia (mother or sister) or early onset cardiovascular disease
- History of diabetes, hypertension, or renal disease
- Previous preterm birth
- Inherited thrombophilias
- Increased prepregnancy triglycerides
- Smoking
- Cocaine and methamphetamine use
- Poor nutrition
- Lower socioeconomic status
- African-Canadian ethnicity
- Age extremes (younger than 20 or older than 35)
- Obesity or excessive weight gain, low weight (Magee et al., 2014)

In addition, complete a nutritional assessment that includes the client's usual intake of protein, calcium, vitamin rich foods, folate, daily calories, and fluids.

Clients at risk for preeclampsia require more frequent prenatal visits throughout their pregnancy, and they require teaching about healthy lifestyles as well as signs and symptoms to watch for, so that they can report these promptly.

Blood pressure (BP) must be measured carefully and consistently. Obtain measurements with the client in the sitting position and arm at heart level. Use an appropriately sized cuff and if BP consistently higher in one arm, the arm with the higher measurements should be used. Automated and manual devices can be used but automated devices should be calibrated and validated. When the automated blood pressure is abnormal, confirm with a manual device (Magee et al., 2014). Obtain the client's weight (noting gain since last visit), and assess for amount and location of edema. Asking questions such as "Do your rings still fit on your fingers?" or "Is your face puffy when you get up in the morning?" will help to determine whether fluid retention is present or if the client's status has changed since her last visit.

Take Note!

Although edema is not a cardinal sign of preeclampsia, weight should be monitored frequently to identify sudden gains in a short time span. Current research relies less on the classic triad of symptoms (hypertension, proteinuria, and edema or weight gain) and more on decreased organ perfusion, endothelial dysfunction (capillary leaking and proteinuria), and elevated blood pressure as key indicators (Carson & Gibson, 2018).

If edema is present, assess the distribution, degree, and pitting. Document your findings and identify whether the edema is dependent or pitting. Dependent edema is present on the lower half of the body if the client is ambulatory, where hydrostatic pressure is greatest. It is usually observed in the feet and ankles or in the sacral area if the client is on bed rest. Pitting edema is edema that leaves a small depression or pit after finger pressure is applied to a swollen area (Carson & Gibson, 2018). Record the depth of pitting demonstrated when pressure is applied. Although subjective, the following is used to record relative degrees:

- 1+ pitting edema = 2-mm depression into skin; disappears rapidly
- 2+ pitting edema = 4-mm skin depression; disappears in 10 to 15 seconds
- 3+ pitting edema = 6-mm depression into skin; lasts more than 1 minute
- 4+ pitting edema = 8-mm depression into skin; lasts 2 to 3 minutes

At every antepartum visit, assess the fetal heart rate with a Doppler device. Also check a clean-catch urine specimen for protein using a dipstick and an analyser if available.

LABORATORY AND DIAGNOSTIC TESTING

Various laboratory tests may be performed to evaluate the client's status. Typically these include a CBC, serum electrolytes, BUN, creatinine, uric acid, and hepatic enzyme levels. Urine specimens are checked for protein; if levels are 1 to 2+ or greater, a 24-hour urine collection or a random urine protein/creatinine ratio is completed. The random urine protein/creatinine ratio is a single sample with immediate results so is advantageous over the 24-hour collection.

Nursing Management

Nursing management of the client with preeclampsia focuses on close monitoring of blood pressure and ongoing assessment for evidence of disease progression including adverse conditions outlined in Box 19.3. Throughout the client's pregnancy, fetal surveillance is essential.

INTERVENING FOR PREECLAMPSIA

The client with mild preeclampsia requires frequent monitoring to detect changes because preeclampsia can progress rapidly. Instruct all clients in the signs and symptoms of preeclampsia and urge them to contact their health care professional or birthing unit for immediate evaluation should any occur.

Typically, clients with mild preeclampsia can be managed at home if they have a good understanding of the disease process, blood pressure and vital signs are stable, there are no abnormal laboratory test results, and if good fetal movement is demonstrated (Teaching Guidelines 19.1). Continued assessments and monitoring remain essential. Ideally a home care nurse will make frequent visits and follow-up phone calls to assess the client's condition, to assist with scheduling periodic evaluations of the fetus (such as nonstress tests), and to evaluate any changes that might suggest a worsening of the client's condition.

Teaching Guidelines 19.1
TEACHING FOR THE CLIENT WITH MILD PREECLAMPSIA

- Rest in a quiet environment to prevent cerebral disturbances.
- Drink according to thirst.
- Consume a balanced, high-protein diet including high-fibre foods.
- Obtain intermittent bed rest to improve circulation to the heart and uterus.
- Limit your physical activity to promote urination and subsequent decrease in blood pressure.
- Enlist the aid of your family so that you can obtain appropriate rest time.
- Perform self-monitoring as instructed, including:
  - Taking your own blood pressure as directed
  - Checking and recording weight daily
  - Performing urine dipstick as directed
  - Recording the number of fetal movements daily and as needed
- Contact your health care provider if any of the following occurs:
  - Increase in blood pressure
  - Protein present in urine
  - Gain of more than 1 lb in 1 week
  - Burning or frequency when urinating
  - Decrease in fetal activity or movement
  - Headache (forehead or posterior neck region)
  - Dizziness or visual disturbances
  - Increase in swelling in hands, feet, legs, and face
  - Nausea and vomiting
  - Stomach pain, excessive heartburn, or upper abdominal pain
  - Decreased or infrequent urination
  - Contractions or low back pain
  - Easy or excessive bruising

Early detection and management of mild preeclampsia is associated with the greatest success in reducing progression of this condition. As long as the client carries out the guidelines of care as outlined by the health care provider and remains stable, home care can continue to maintain the pregnancy until the fetus is mature. If disease progression occurs, hospitalization is required.

INTERVENING FOR SEVERE PREECLAMPSIA

The client with severe preeclampsia requires hospitalization. Maintain the client on bed rest in the left lateral lying position. Ensure that the room is dark and quiet to reduce stimulation. Give sedatives as ordered to encourage quiet bed rest. The client is at risk for seizures if the condition progresses. Therefore, institute and maintain seizure precautions, such as having oxygen, suction equipment, and emergency call light for staff assistance readily available to protect the client from injury. Maintain emergency medications with doses, mixing and administration details in a kit or box. Review procedures and protocols and practice drills to maximize competence, confidence, and teamwork.

Take Note!

Preeclampsia increases the risk of placental abruption, preterm birth, intrauterine growth restriction, and fetal compromise during childbirth. Always be prepared if you see symptoms of preeclampsia!

Closely monitor the client's blood pressure. Administer antihypertensives as ordered to reduce blood pressure (Drug Guide 19.2). Assess the client's vision and level of consciousness. Report any changes and any complaints of headache or visual disturbances. Monitor the client's intake and output every hour and administer fluid and electrolyte replacements as ordered. Assess the client for signs and symptoms of pulmonary edema, such as crackles and wheezing heard on auscultation, dyspnea, decreased oxygen saturation levels, cough, neck vein distention, anxiety, and restlessness. The treatment of acute pulmonary edema is symptomatic and includes the administration of vasodilating agents and diuretics. The development of acute pulmonary edema in clients with hypertension during pregnancy is associated with high levels of IV fluid administration (Pauli & Repke, 2015).

Prepare the client for possible testing to evaluate fetal status as preeclampsia progresses. Testing may include the nonstress test, serial ultrasounds to track fetal growth, amniotic fluid levels and Doppler velocimetry to screen for fetal compromise, and biophysical profile to evaluate ongoing fetal well-being (Mattson & Smith, 2016).

Other laboratory tests may be performed to monitor the disease process and to determine if it is progressing into HELLP syndrome. These include liver enzymes such as lactic dehydrogenase (LDH), ALT, and AST; chemistry panel, such as creatinine, BUN, uric acid, and glucose; CBC, including platelet count; coagulation studies, such as PT, PTT, fibrinogen, and bleeding time; and a 24-hour urine or random urine sample collection for protein and creatinine clearance.

Administer parenteral magnesium sulphate as ordered to prevent seizures. Assess DTRs to evaluate

DRUG GUIDE 19.2 MEDICATIONS USED WITH PREECLAMPSIA AND ECLAMPSIA

Medication	Action/Indications	Nursing Implications
Magnesium sulphate	Blockage of neuromuscular transmission, vasodilation Prevention and treatment of eclamptic seizures	Loading dose of 4 g by IV in 100 mL of fluid administered over 15 to 20 minutes, followed by a maintenance dose of 1 to 2 g as a continuous intravenous infusion. Assess DTRs and check for ankle clonus. Monitor output hourly. Have calcium gluconate readily available in case of toxicity. Monitor for signs and symptoms of toxicity, such as flushing, sweating, hypotension, absent DTR, respirations less than 12/min, other signs of cardiac and central nervous system depression.
Hydralazine hydrochloride (Apresoline)	Vascular smooth muscle relaxant, thus improving perfusion to renal, uterine, and cerebral areas Reduction in blood pressure	Start with 5 mg IV; repeat 5 to 10 mg IV every 30 minutes, or 0.5 to 10 mg/hr IV, to a maximum of 20 mg IV (or 30 mg IM). Use parenteral form immediately after opening ampule. Withdraw drug slowly to prevent possible rebound hypertension. Monitor for adverse effects such as palpitations, headache, tachycardia, anorexia, nausea, vomiting, and diarrhea.
Labetalol hydrochloride (Trandate)	Alpha-1 and beta blocker Reduction in blood pressure	Be aware that drug lowers blood pressure without decreasing maternal heart rate or cardiac output. Start with 20 mg IV; repeat 20 to 80 mg IV q 30 min, or 1 to 2 mg/min, max 300 mg (then switch to oral). Monitor for possible adverse effects such as gastric pain, flatulence, constipation, dizziness, vertigo, and fatigue.
Nifedipine (Adalat)	Calcium channel blocker/dilation of coronary arteries, arterioles, and peripheral arterioles Reduction in blood pressure, potential reduction in uterine activity in preterm labour	5- to 10-mg capsule to be swallowed, or bitten then swallowed, every 30 minutes. Monitor for possible adverse effects such as dizziness, peripheral edema, angina, diarrhea, nasal congestions, cough. Staff should be aware of the distinction between short-acting nifedipine capsules used to treat severe hypertension and the slow-release tablets (XL) that are used for nonsevere hypertension.
Sodium nitroprusside For refractory hypertension only	Rapid vasodilation (arterial and venous) Severe hypertension requiring rapid reduction in blood pressure	Administer via continuous IV infusion with dose titrated according to blood pressure levels. Wrap intravenous infusion solution in foil or opaque material to protect from light. Monitor for possible adverse effects, such as apprehension, restlessness, retrosternal pressure, palpitations, diaphoresis, and abdominal pain.

Adapted from King, T. L., Brucker, M. C., Fahey, J. O., Kriebs, J. M., Gegor, C. L., & Varney, H. (2015). *Varney's midwifery* (5th ed.). Burlington, MA: Jones & Bartlett Learning; Skidmore-Roth, L. (2015). *Mosby's 2015 nursing drug reference* (28th ed.). Philadelphia, PA: Elsevier Health Science; and Magee, L. A., Pels, A., Helewa, M., Rey, E., & von Dadelszen, P. (2014). SOGC Clinical practice guideline: Diagnosis, evaluation, and management of the hypertensive disorders of pregnancy: Executive summary. *Journal of Obstetrics and Gynaecology Canada, 36*(5), 416–438.

the effectiveness of therapy and assess for toxicity. Clients with preeclampsia commonly present with hyperreflexia. Severe preeclampsia causes changes in the cortex, which disrupts the equilibrium of impulses between the cerebral cortex and the spinal cord. Brisk reflexes (hyperreflexia) are the result of an irritable cortex and indicate CNS involvement (Marik, 2015). Diminished or absent reflexes occur when the client develops magnesium toxicity. Because magnesium is a potent neuromuscular blockade, the afferent and efferent nerve pathways do not relay messages properly and hyporeflexia develops. Common sites used to assess DTRs are biceps reflex, triceps reflex, patellar reflex, Achilles reflex, and plantar reflex. Nursing Procedure 19.1 highlights the steps for assessing the patellar reflex.

NURSING PROCEDURE 19.1

Assessing the Patellar Reflex

Purpose: To Evaluate for Nervous System Irritability Related to Preeclampsia

- Place the client in the supine position (or sitting upright with the legs dangling freely over the side of the bed or examination table).
- If lying supine, have the client flex one knee slightly.
- Place a hand under the knee to support the leg and locate the patellar tendon. It should be midline just below the knee cap.
- Using a reflex hammer or the side of your hand, strike the area of the patellar tendon firmly and quickly.
- Note the movement of the leg and foot. A patellar reflex occurs when the leg and foot move (documented as 2+).
- Repeat the procedure on the opposite leg.

The National Institute of Neurological Disorders and Stroke, a division of the National Institutes of Health, published a scale in the early 1990s that, although subjective, is used widely today. It grades reflexes from 0 to 4+. Grades 2+ and 3+ are considered normal, whereas grades 0 and 4 may indicate pathology (Table 19.2). Because these are subjective assessments, to improve communication of reflex results, condensed descriptor categories such as absent, average, brisk, or clonus should be used rather than numeric codes (Magowan et al., 2014).

TABLE 19.2 GRADING DEEP TENDON REFLEXES

Description of Finding	Grade
Reflex absent, none elicited	0
Hypoactive response, sluggish	1
Reflex in lower half of normal range	2
Reflex in upper half of normal range	3
Hyperactive, brisk, clonus present	4

Adapted from King, T. L., Brucker, M. C., Fahey, J. O., Kriebs, J. M., Gegor, C. L., & Varney, H. (2015). *Varney's midwifery* (5th ed.). Burlington, MA: Jones & Bartlett Learning; and Nagtalon-Ramos, J. (2014). *Maternal-newborn nursing care: Best evidence-based practices.* Philadelphia, PA: F. A. Davis Company.

Clonus is the presence of rhythmic involuntary contractions, most often at the foot or ankle. Sustained clonus confirms CNS involvement. Nursing Procedure 19.2 highlights the steps when testing for ankle clonus.

With magnesium sulphate administration, the client is at risk for magnesium toxicity. Closely assess the client for signs of toxicity, which include a respiratory rate of less than 12 breaths/min, absence of DTRs, and a decrease in urinary output (<30 mL/hr). Urine output must remain adequate since magnesium is excreted through the kidneys and if output is low, magnesium toxicity is more likely. Low urine output is a contraindication to magnesium infusion. Although monitoring serum magnesium levels has been a practice in the past, evidence suggests that assessment of respiratory rate and DTRs provides best assessment of magnesium toxicity. Serum magnesium levels are not recommended (Magee et al., 2014). If signs and symptoms of magnesium toxicity develop, expect to administer calcium gluconate as the antidote.

Throughout the client's stay, monitor closely for signs and symptoms of labour. Perform continuous electronic fetal monitoring to assess fetal well-being. Note trends in baseline rate and variability and presence or absence of accelerations or decelerations. Observe for signs of fetal compromise and report them immediately. Administer glucocorticosteroids as ordered to enhance fetal lung maturity and prepare for labour induction if the client's condition warrants.

Keep the client and family informed of the individual's condition and educate them about the course of treatment. Provide emotional support for the client and family. Severe preeclampsia is very frightening for the client and family, and most expectant clients are very anxious about their own health as well as that of the fetus. To allay anxiety, use light touch to comfort and provide reassurance that the necessary actions are being taken. Actively listening to concerns and fears and communicating these to the health care provider are important to

NURSING PROCEDURE 19.2

Testing for Ankle Clonus

Purpose: To Evaluate for Nervous System Irritability Related to Preeclampsia

1. Place the client in the supine position.

2. Have the client slightly bend one knee and place a hand under the knee to support it.

3. Dorsiflex the foot briskly and then quickly release it.

4. Watch for the foot to rebound smoothly against your hand. If the movement is smooth without any rapid contractions of the ankle or calf muscle, then clonus is not present; if the movement is jerky and rapid, clonus is present.

5. Repeat on the opposite side.

keep open the lines of communication. Offering praise for small accomplishments can provide positive reinforcement for effective behaviours, enhancing self-efficacy and self-competence.

INTERVENING FOR ECLAMPSIA

The onset of seizure activity identifies **eclampsia**. Typically, eclamptic seizures are generalized and start with facial twitching. The body then becomes rigid, in a state of tonic muscular contraction. The clonic phase of the seizure involves alternating contraction and relaxation of all body muscles. Respirations stop during seizure activity and resume shortly after it ends. Client safety is the primary concern during eclamptic seizures. If possible, turn the client to lateral position and remain in attendance. Make sure that the bed is safe from points of injury. Dim the lights and keep the room quiet.

Document the time and sequence of events as soon as possible. After the seizure activity has ceased, suction the nasopharynx as necessary and administer oxygen. Continue the magnesium sulphate infusion to prevent further seizures. Ensure continuous electronic fetal monitoring, evaluating fetal status for changes. Also assess the client for uterine contractions. After the client is stabilized, prepare for the birthing process as soon as possible to reduce the risk of perinatal mortality.

PROVIDING FOLLOW-UP CARE

After delivery of the newborn, continue to monitor the client for signs and symptoms of preeclampsia/eclampsia for at least 48 hours. Expect to continue to administer magnesium sulphate infusion for 24 hours to prevent seizure activity, and monitor for signs of magnesium toxicity.

Assess vital signs at least every 4 hours, along with routine postpartum assessments: fundus, lochia, breasts, bladder, bowels, and the client's emotional state. Monitor urine output hourly. Diuresis is a positive sign that, along with a decrease in proteinuria, signals resolution of the disease.

HELLP SYNDROME

HELLP syndrome is an acronym for Hemolysis, Elevated Liver enzymes, and Low Platelet count. It is a variant of the preeclampsia/eclampsia syndrome that occurs in 10% to 20% of clients whose conditions are labelled as severe. Pregnant individuals with HELLP syndrome are at increased risk for complications such as cerebral hemorrhage, retinal detachment, hematoma/liver rupture, acute renal failure, DIC, placental abruption, and maternal death (Vigil-De Gracia, 2015). It is a life-threatening obstetric complication considered by many to be a severe form of preeclampsia involving hemolysis, thrombocytopenia, and liver dysfunction.

Both HELLP and preeclampsia occur during the later stages of pregnancy, and sometimes after childbirth. HELLP syndrome is a clinically progressive condition. Early diagnosis is critical to prevent liver distention, rupture, and hemorrhage, and the onset of DIC. If the condition presents prenatally, morbidity and mortality can affect both the client and the baby.

HELLP syndrome is unique, as it is a laboratory value–specific diagnosis. Clients with HELLP usually have fewer signs of abnormalities consistent with the metabolic syndrome and a lower prevalence of thrombophilia as compared with preeclamptic clients without HELLP (Sibai, 2018). Although it has been reported as early as 17 weeks' gestation, most of the time it is diagnosed between 22 and 36 weeks' gestation (Cunningham et al., 2014). It can present prior to the presence of an elevated blood pressure. HELLP syndrome leads to an increased risk for developing liver hematoma or rupture, stroke, cardiac arrest, seizure, pulmonary edema, DIC, subendocardial hemorrhage, adult respiratory distress syndrome, renal damage, sepsis, hypoxic encephalopathy, and client or fetal death (Moses, 2018b). The recognition of HELLP syndrome and an aggressive multidisciplinary approach and prompt transfer of these clients to obstetric centres with expertise in this field are required for the improvement of prognosis for both the client and fetus.

Pathophysiology

The hemolysis that occurs is termed microangiopathic hemolytic anemia. This cascade of events is thought to happen when red blood cells become fragmented as they pass through small, damaged blood vessels. Elevated liver enzymes are the result of reduced blood flow to the liver secondary to obstruction from fibrin deposits. At the same time, endothelial damage and fibrin deposition in the liver may lead to liver impairment and can result in hemorrhagic necrosis, indicated by right upper quadrant tenderness, nausea, and vomiting. Hyperbilirubinemia and jaundice result from liver impairment. Low platelets result from vascular damage, the result of vasospasm, and platelets aggregate at sites of damage, resulting in thrombocytopenia in multiple sites (Khan & Meirowitz, 2018).

Therapeutic Management

The treatment for HELLP syndrome is based on the severity of the disease, the gestational age of the fetus, and the condition of the client and fetus. The mainstay of treatment is lowering of high blood pressure with rapid-acting antihypertensive agents, prevention of seizures with magnesium sulphate, and use of steroids for fetal lung maturity if necessary, followed by the birth of the

infant and placenta (Foley et al., 2014). The client should be admitted or transferred to a tertiary centre with a neonatal intensive care unit. Additional treatment includes correction of the coagulopathies that accompany HELLP syndrome. After this syndrome is diagnosed and the client's condition is stable, birth of the infant is indicated.

Magnesium sulphate is used prophylactically to prevent seizures. Antihypertensives such as hydralazine or labetalol are given to control blood pressure. Blood component therapy—such as fresh-frozen plasma, packed red blood cells, or platelets—is transfused to address the microangiopathic hemolytic anemia. Birth may be delayed up to 96 hours so that betamethasone or dexamethasone can be given to stimulate lung maturation in the preterm fetus.

Nursing Assessment

Nursing assessment of the client with HELLP is similar to that for the client with severe preeclampsia. Be alert for reports of nausea (with or without vomiting), malaise, epigastric or right upper quadrant pain, and demonstrable edema. Perform systematic assessments frequently, as indicated by the client's condition and response to therapy.

A diagnosis of HELLP syndrome is made based on laboratory test results, including:
- Low hematocrit that is not explained by any blood loss
- Elevated LDH (liver impairment)
- Elevated AST (liver impairment)
- Elevated ALT (liver impairment)
- Elevated BUN
- Elevated bilirubin level
- Elevated uric acid and creatinine levels (renal involvement)
- Low platelet count (less than 100,000 cells/mm^3)

Nursing Management

Nursing management of the client diagnosed with HELLP syndrome is the same as that for the individual with severe preeclampsia. If possible, the client with HELLP syndrome should be transferred to a tertiary care centre once assessed and stabilized. Birthing units should be aware of the available resources and expertise when considering location of the antici pated birth. Consider any potential delay between ordering and receiving platelet units when planning care (Magee, 2014). Closely monitor the client for changes and provide ongoing support throughout this experience.

GESTATIONAL DIABETES

Gestational diabetes is a condition involving glucose intolerance that occurs during pregnancy. It is discussed in greater detail in Chapter 20.

BLOOD INCOMPATIBILITY

Blood incompatibility most commonly involves one of two issues: blood group or the Rh factor. *Blood group incompatibility*, also known as ABO incompatibility, may arise when an individual with blood group O becomes pregnant with a fetus with a different blood group (Group A, B, or AB). The pregnant individual with blood group O has serum which contains naturally occurring anti-A and anti-B antibodies, which can cross the placenta and hemolyze fetal red blood cells. It is usually less severe than Rh incompatibility. One reason is that fetal red blood cells express less of the ABO blood group antigens compared with adult levels. In addition, in contrast to the Rh antigens, the ABO blood group antigens are expressed by a variety of fetal (and adult) tissues, reducing the chances of anti-A and anti-B binding their target antigens on the fetal red blood cells. ABO incompatibility rarely causes significant hemolysis, and prenatal treatment is not warranted. Post-delivery, where the anti-A or anti-B has crossed the placenta and bound to the baby's blood, resultant ABO incompatibility can lead to significant hyperbilirubinemia in the newborn.

Rh isoimmunization occurs when a pregnant individual's immune system creates antibodies against fetal Rh blood factors. Although the client will exhibit no symptoms of Rh incompatibility, Rh antibodies adversely affect fetal health. Rh antibodies can cause fetal heart problems, breathing difficulties, jaundice, and a form of anemia known as hemolytic disease of the newborn. Rh sensitization occurs in approximately 1 in 1,000 births to Rh-negative pregnant individuals (March of Dimes, 2016). Today Rh isoimmunization in pregnant individuals and hemolytic disease of the newborn are rarely seen, primarily because clients who are Rh negative are given anti-D immune globulin prophylaxis (WinRho or Rho-GAM) in the third trimester of pregnancy, after childbirth (with Rh-positive baby) and with any identified antenatal risk of blood exchange (Fung & Eason, 2018).

Pathophysiology

ABO Incompatibility

Hemolysis associated with ABO incompatibility is limited to pregnant individual with type O blood with fetuses who have type A or B blood. In clients with type A and B blood, naturally occurring antibodies are of the IgM class, which do not cross the placenta, whereas in type O clients, the antibodies are predominantly IgG in nature. Because A and B antigens are widely expressed in a variety of tissues besides red blood cells, only a small portion of the antibodies crossing the placenta is available to bind to fetal red cells. In addition, fetal red cells appear to have less surface expression of A or B antigen,

resulting in few reactive sites—hence the low incidence of significant hemolysis in affected neonates.

Rh Incompatibility

Rh incompatibility is a condition that develops when an individual with Rh-negative blood type is exposed to Rh-positive blood cells and subsequently develops circulating titers of Rh antibodies. Individuals with Rh-positive blood type have the D antigen present on their red cells, whereas individuals with an Rh-negative blood type do not. The presence or absence of the Rh antigen on the RBC membrane is genetically controlled.

In Canada, about 16% of the population is Rh negative (Canadian Blood Services, 2018). There is a wide variation in blood Rh status based on ethnicity. In the United States, about 15% of the White population, 5% to 8% of the African-American and Hispanic populations, and 1% to 2% of the Asian and Indigenous populations are Rh negative. The vast majority (85%) of individuals is considered Rh positive (March of Dimes, 2016). Maternal isoimmunization still occurs in 0.4 per 1,000 births, or approximately 1% to 2% of D-negative women in Canada and the United Kingdom. This usually results from failure to administer anti-D immune globulin to eligible pregnant and postpartum clients or because of inadequate dosing (Fung & Eason, 2018).

Rh incompatibility most commonly arises with exposure of an Rh-negative client to Rh-positive fetal blood during pregnancy or birth, during which time erythrocytes from the fetal circulation leak into the maternal circulation. Isoimmunization can also occur during an amniocentesis, ectopic pregnancy, placenta previa, placenta abruption, in utero fetal death, spontaneous abortion, or abdominal/pelvic trauma. After a significant exposure, alloimmunization or sensitization occurs. As a result, maternal antibodies are produced against the foreign Rh antigen.

Theoretically, fetal blood and maternal blood do not mix during pregnancy. In reality, however, small placental accidents (transplacental bleeds secondary to minor separation), abortions, ectopic pregnancy, abdominal trauma, trophoblastic disease, amniocentesis, placenta previa, and abruptio placentae allow fetal blood to enter the maternal circulation and initiate the production of antibodies to destroy Rh-positive blood. The amount of fetal blood necessary to produce Rh incompatibility varies. In one study, less than 1 mL of Rh-positive blood was shown to result in sensitization of individuals who are Rh negative (Salem & Singer, 2017).

Once sensitized, it takes approximately a month for Rh antibodies in the maternal circulation to cross over into the fetal circulation. In 90% of cases, sensitization occurs during delivery (Cunningham et al., 2014). Thus, most firstborn infants with Rh-positive blood type are not affected because the short period from first exposure of

Rh-positive fetal erythrocytes to the birth of the infant is insufficient to produce a significant maternal IgG antibody response.

The risk and severity of alloimmune response increases with each subsequent pregnancy involving a fetus with Rh-positive blood. A second pregnancy with an Rh-positive fetus often produces a mildly anemic infant, whereas succeeding pregnancies produce infants with more serious hemolytic anemia.

Nursing Assessment

At the first prenatal visit, determine the client's blood group and Rh status. Obtain a thorough health history, noting any reports of previous events involving hemorrhage to delineate the risk for prior sensitization. All pregnant individuals (Rh negative or Rh positive) should be typed and screened for alloantibodies with an indirect antiglobulin test at the first prenatal visit and again at 28 weeks (Fung & Eason, 2018).

Nursing Management

If the prenatal antibody screen, or indirect Coombs test, is negative (meaning no antibodies are present), then the client is a candidate for Rh immune globulin. If the test is positive, the immune globulin is of no value because isoimmunization has already occurred. In this case, the fetus is carefully monitored for hemolytic disease.

The incidence of isoimmunization has declined dramatically as a result of administration of Rh immune globulin as prophylaxis (Fung & Eason, 2018). The standard dose is 300 mcg, which is effective for 15 mL of fetal blood cells. Pregnancy bleeding prior to 12 weeks' gestation requires 120 mcg. Rh immune globulin helps to destroy any fetal cells in the maternal circulation before sensitization occurs, thus inhibiting maternal antibody production. This provides temporary passive immunity, thereby preventing maternal sensitization.

The current recommendation is for every Rh-negative nonimmunized pregnant individual to receive Rh immune globulin at some point between 28 and 32 weeks' gestation, and again within 72 hours after giving birth if the baby is Rh positive. Other indications for Rh immune globulin include:

• Ectopic pregnancy
• Chorionic villus sampling
• Amniocentesis
• Cordocentesis
• Antepartum hemorrhage
• GTD
• Abdominal trauma
• External cephalic version
• Therapeutic or spontaneous abortion
• Fetal death
• Fetal surgery (Fung & Eason, 2018)

Despite the availability of Rh immune globulin and laboratory tests to identify clients and newborns at risk, isoimmunization remains a serious clinical reality that continues to contribute to perinatal and neonatal mortality. Nurses, as client advocates, are in a unique position to make sure test results are brought to the health care provider's attention so appropriate interventions can be initiated. In addition, nurses must stay informed of current literature, research, and best practices regarding isoimmunization and its management. Stress to all clients that early prenatal care can help identify and prevent this condition. Because Rh incompatibility is preventable with the use of Rh immune globulin, prevention remains the best treatment. Nurses can make a tremendous impact to ensure positive outcomes for the greatest possible number of pregnancies through education and advocacy.

AMNIOTIC FLUID IMBALANCES

Amniotic fluid develops from several maternal and fetal structures, including the amnion, chorion, maternal blood, fetal lungs, gastrointestinal tract, kidneys, and skin. Any alteration in one or more of the various sources will alter the amount of amniotic fluid. Polyhydramnios and oligohydramnios are two imbalances associated with amniotic fluid. Measurement of amniotic fluid continues to be a challenge technically and criteria for determining oligo- or polyhydramnios continue to be debated and studied. A technical bulletin from the SOGC recommends a single pocket measurement, with polyhydramnios defined as a single pocket greater than 8 cm × 1 cm and oligohydramnios as a single pocket of fluid less than 2 cm × 1 cm (Lim, Butt, Naud, & Smithies, 2017). Previously recommended, and still commonly used, is the amniotic fluid volume measurement which estimates amount of fluid in four quadrants of the abdomen and the sum is the Amniotic Fluid Index (AFI), with a normal range of 5 to 20 cm.

Polyhydramnios

Polyhydramnios is a condition in which there is too much amniotic fluid surrounding the fetus (single pocket greater than 8 cm × 1 cm, or AFI greater than 20 cm). It occurs in approximately 2% of all pregnancies and is associated with fetal anomalies of development such as upper gastrointestinal obstruction or atresias, neural tube defects, and anterior abdominal wall defects, together with impaired swallowing in fetuses with chromosomal anomalies, such as trisomies 13 and 18 (Carter & Boyd, 2015). Approximately 18% of all pregnant individuals with diabetes will develop polyhydramnios during their pregnancy. There is an increase in cesarean births for fetal labour intolerance, low 5-minute Apgar scores, increased neonatal birth weight, congenital anomalies, and newborn intensive care unit admissions for clients with too much amniotic fluid at term (Moore, 2015). Overall, it is associated with poorer fetal outcomes because of the increased incidence of preterm births, fetal malpresentation, and cord prolapse.

There are several causes of polyhydramnios. Generally, too much fluid is being produced, there is a problem with the fluid being taken up, or both. It can be associated with maternal disease and fetal anomalies, but it can also be idiopathic (of unknown cause) in nature.

Therapeutic Management

Treatment may include close monitoring and frequent follow-up visits with the health care provider if the polyhydramnios is mild to moderate. In severe cases in which the client is in pain and experiencing shortness of breath, an amniocentesis or artificial rupture of the membranes is done to reduce the fluid and the pressure. Removal of fluid by amniocentesis is only transiently effective. A noninvasive treatment may involve the use of a prostaglandin synthesis inhibitor (indomethacin) to decrease amniotic fluid volume by decreasing fetal urinary output, but this may cause premature closure of the fetal ductus arteriosus (King et al., 2015).

Nursing Assessment

Begin the assessment with a thorough history, being alert to risk factors such as diabetes or multiple gestations. Review the client history for information about possible fetal anomalies including fetal esophageal or intestinal atresia, neural tube defects, chromosomal deviations, fetal hydrops, CNS or cardiovascular anomalies, and hydrocephaly.

Determine the gestational age of the fetus and measure the client's fundal height. With polyhydramnios, there is a discrepancy between fundal height and gestational age, or a rapid growth of the uterus is noted. Note any reports of uterine contractions, which may result from overstretching of the uterus. Assess for shortness of breath resulting from pressure on the diaphragm and inspect the lower extremities for edema, which results from increased pressure on the vena cava. Palpate the abdomen and obtain the fetal heart rate. The fetal parts and heart rate may be more difficult to obtain because of the excess fluid present.

Prepare the client for possible diagnostic ultrasound testing to evaluate the amniotic fluid volume and possible causes of polyhydramnios, such as fetal structural anomaly.

Nursing Management

Nursing management of the client with polyhydramnios focuses on ongoing assessment and monitoring for symptoms of abdominal pain, dyspnea, uterine contractions, and edema of the lower extremities. Explain to the client and family that this condition can cause the uterus to become overdistended and may lead to preterm labour and preterm rupture of membranes. Outline the signs and symptoms of both conditions and instruct the client to contact the health care provider if they occur. If diabetes is present, assess the client's knowledge of diet and medications, and glycemic control. Review blood glucose records and refer for further diabetic education, support and follow-up as needed.

Oligohydramnios

Oligohydramnios is a decreased amount of amniotic fluid (single pocket less than 2 cm × 1 cm or AFI less than 5 cm). It occurs in approximately 4% of all pregnancies. Oligohydramnios may result from any condition that prevents the fetus from making urine or blocks it from going into the amniotic sac. It is most common in the last trimester of pregnancy, but it can develop at any time in the pregnancy. About one out of eight individuals whose pregnancies last 2 weeks past the due date develops oligohydramnios. This happens as amniotic fluid levels naturally decline. This condition puts the fetus at an increased risk of perinatal morbidity and mortality (March of Dimes, 2015). Reduction in amniotic fluid reduces the ability of the fetus to move freely without risk of cord compression, which increases the risk for fetal death and intrapartum hypoxia.

Therapeutic Management

The client with oligohydramnios can be managed on an outpatient basis with serial ultrasounds and fetal surveillance through nonstress testing. As long as fetal well-being is demonstrated with frequent testing, no intervention is necessary. If fetal well-being is compromised, however, birth is planned. If severe variable decelerations are present on electronic fetal monitoring, amnioinfusion may be used to introduce fluid into the uterus to relieve cord compression. The warmed fluid is introduced into the uterus through an intrauterine pressure catheter. The infusion is administered in a controlled fashion to prevent overdistention of the uterus and elevated uterine pressure. Amnioinfusion is thought to improve abnormal fetal heart rate patterns, thereby decreasing cesarean births (Carter & Boyd, 2017). Amnioinfusion has not been shown to improve outcomes related to meconium aspiration and is not indicated for meconium-stained fluid in labour.

Nursing Assessment

Review the client history for factors associated with oligohydramnios, including:

- Uteroplacental insufficiency
- Premature rupture of membranes (PROM) prior to labour onset
- Hypertension of pregnancy
- Diabetes

- Intrauterine growth restriction
- Postterm pregnancy
- Fetal renal agenesis
- Polycystic kidneys
- Urinary tract obstructions

Assess the client for complaints of fluid leaking from the vagina. Leaking of amniotic fluid from the vagina occurs with rupture of the amniotic sac. A uterus that is small for expected dates of gestation also suggests oligohydramnios. The client will usually not present with any symptoms. Typically, the reduced volume of amniotic fluid is identified on ultrasound.

Nursing Management

Nursing management of the client with oligohydramnios involves continuous monitoring of fetal well-being during nonstress testing or during labour and birth by identifying variable decelerations (complicated and uncomplicated) and determining if the fetal heart tracing is normal, atypical or abnormal). Variable decelerations indicating cord compression are common. Changing the client's position might be therapeutic in altering this fetal heart rate pattern. After the birth, evaluate the newborn for signs of postmaturity, congenital anomalies, and respiratory difficulty.

Assist with amnioinfusion where available and when indicated, and continue to assess the client's vital signs and contraction status and the fetal heart rate throughout the procedure. Provide comfort measures such as changing the bed linens and the client's bed clothes frequently because of the constant leakage of fluid from the vagina. Also provide frequent perineal care during the infusion.

MULTIPLE GESTATION

Multiple gestation is defined as a pregnancy with two or more fetuses. This includes twins, triplets, and higher-order multiples such as quadruplets. In the past two decades, the number of multiple gestations has jumped dramatically because of the widespread use of fertility drugs, older age of individuals having babies, and the development of assisted reproductive technologies to treat infertility. About one third of live births from assisted reproductive technology result in more than one infant, and twins represent 85% of those multiple-birth children (De Sutter, 2015).

The incidence of twins, triplets, and higher-order multiple gestations is approximately 3% in Canada and the United States (March of Dimes, 2017a; Statistics Canada, 2016). In 2013, 3.3% of all pregnancies were twins or higher multiples, up from 2.1% in 1991 (Statistics Canada, 2016). Two thirds of twins are dizygotic, meaning they are derived from two separate ova (March of Dimes, 2017b), while one in three are monozygotic. The increasing number of multiple gestations is a concern because clients who are expecting more than one infant are at high risk for preterm labour, polyhydramnios, HG, anemia, gestational diabetes, preeclampsia, and antepartum hemorrhage. Fetal/newborn risks or complications include prematurity, respiratory distress syndrome, birth asphyxia, congenital anomalies (CNS, cardiovascular, and gastrointestinal defects), twin-to-twin transfusion syndrome (transfusion of blood from one twin to the other twin), intrauterine growth restriction, and conjoined twins (Martin et al., 2014).

The two types of twins are monozygotic and dizygotic (Fig. 19.7). Monozygotic twins develop when a single, fertilized ovum splits during the first 2 weeks after conception. Monozygotic twins also are called identical twins. Two sperm fertilizing two ova produce dizygotic twins, which are called fraternal twins. Separate amnions, chorions, and placentas are formed in dizygotic twins. Triplets can be monozygotic, dizygotic, or trizygotic.

Therapeutic Management

When a multiple gestation is confirmed, the client is followed with serial ultrasounds to assess fetal growth patterns and development. Biophysical profiles along with

Placenta

Placenta
Chorion
Amnion

Placenta
Chorion
Amnion

Placenta

Chorion

Amnions

A

B

FIGURE 19.7 Multiple gestation with twins. **A.** Dizygotic twins, where each fetus has its own placenta, amnion, and chorion. **B.** Monozygotic twins, where the fetuses share one placenta, two amnions, and one chorion.

nonstress tests are ordered to determine fetal well-being. During the intrapartum period the client is closely monitored, with a perinatal team assigned to each newborn to assist after birth. Operative delivery is frequently indicated due to fetal malpresentation.

Nursing Assessment

Obtain a health history and perform a physical examination. Be alert for client reports of excessive fatigue and severe nausea and vomiting. Assess the client's abdomen and fundal height. Typically with a multiple gestation, the uterus is larger than expected based on the estimated date of birth. Laboratory test results may reveal anemia. Prepare the client for ultrasound, which typically confirms the diagnosis of a multiple gestation. Ultrasound in the first trimester is important to determine if the twins are monochorionic (sharing one placenta) or dichorionic (each have a separate placenta). Later ultrasounds cannot determine this with certainty since placentas can become fused and appear monochorionic).

Nursing Management

During the prenatal period, provide education and support for the client regarding nutrition, increased rest periods, and close observation for pregnancy complications such as anemia, excessive weight gain, proteinuria, edema, vaginal bleeding, and hypertension, and diabetes. Instruct the client to be alert for and report immediately any signs and symptoms of preterm labour: contractions, uterine cramping, low back ache, increase in vaginal discharge, loss of mucous plug, pelvic pain, and pressure.

With the onset of labour, expect to monitor fetal heart rates continuously. Prepare the client for an ultrasound to assess the presentation of each fetus to determine the best delivery approach. Ensure that extra nursing staff and the perinatal team are available for any birth or newborn complications.

After the babies are born, closely assess the client for hemorrhage by frequently assessing uterine involution. Palpate the uterine fundus and monitor the amount and characteristics of lochia. Distention of the uterine cavity in multiple gestation predisposes clients with multiple gestations to postpartum hemorrhage.

Throughout the entire pregnancy, birth, and hospital stay, inform and support the client and family. Encourage them to ask questions and verbalize any fears and concerns.

PREMATURE RUPTURE OF MEMBRANES

Premature rupture of membranes (**PROM**) is the rupture of the amniotic membrane (bag of waters) before the onset of labour. Prelabour rupture of membranes is another term also used for the same condition. There are a number of associated conditions and complications, such as infection, prolapsed cord, abruptio placentae, and preterm labour. High-risk factors associated with preterm PROM include low socioeconomic status, multiple gestation, low BMI, tobacco use, history of preterm labour, placenta previa, abruptio placentae, urinary tract infection, vaginal bleeding at any time in pregnancy, cerclage, and amniocentesis (Jazayeri, 2017).

If prolonged (greater than 18 hours), the client's risk for infection (chorioamnionitis, endometritis, sepsis, and neonatal infections) increases and continues to increase the longer the time since the membranes have ruptured (Jeffries & CPS, 2017). The time interval from rupture of membranes to the onset of regular contractions is termed the latent period.

Individuals with PROM present with leakage of fluid, vaginal discharge, vaginal bleeding, and pelvic pressure, but they are not having contractions. PROM is diagnosed by speculum vaginal examination of the cervix and vaginal cavity. Pooling of fluid in the vagina or leakage of fluid from the cervix, ferning of the dried fluid under microscopic examination, and alkalinity of the fluid as determined by nitrazine paper (pH indicator) are used for diagnosis. Ferning and pH testing have poor sensitivity and specificity, with detection rates in the 50% to 70% range. A more definitive test is available to detect PAMG, which is a molecule specific to the amniotic fluid. This test is performed by a simple vaginal swab and can be analyzed at point of care or by the lab with results in minutes. Although this test is more costly, the savings in unnecessary intervention (admission, antibiotics regimens) or missed diagnosis (perinatal morbidity and mortality) ultimately reduce costs to the health care system and psychosocial costs to families.

The terminology of PROM must be differentiated from PPROM. PROM is spontaneous rupture of the membranes prior to the onset of labour and is used appropriately when referring to a client who is at or beyond term (37 weeks' gestation) and is not in labour. A related term is ***preterm* premature rupture of membranes (PPROM)**, which is defined as rupture of membranes prior to the onset of labour in an individual who is *less* than 37 weeks' gestation. In Canada, preterm birth occurs in 7% to 8% of pregnancies (Yudin, van Schalkwyk, & Van Eyk, 2017) and preterm delivery is responsible for 60% to 80% of neonatal deaths, with PPROM occurring in close to one third of those preterm deliveries. Neonatal morbidity in a preterm birth can result from respiratory distress syndrome, intraventricular hemorrhage, necrotizing enterocolitis, sepsis, and retinopathy of prematurity (Catt, Chadha, Tang, Palmquist, & Lange, 2016).

The exact cause of PROM is not known, but may be associated with vaginal bleeding, placental abruption, microbial invasion of the amniotic cavity, and defective placentation. In many cases, PROM occurs spontaneously. Increasing evidence associates abnormalities in vaginal flora during pregnancy with preterm labour and birth with potential neonatal sequelae due to prematurity and poor perinatal outcome (Gilbert, 2014). Research has indicated that clients with previous PPROM are at increased risk for recurrence, and a short interval between pregnancies is associated with increased risk (Gibbins, Esplin, Varner, Eller, & Manuck, 2014).

Therapeutic Management

Treatment of PROM typically depends on the gestational age. To minimize risk of infection, vaginal examinations should be limited to active labour. Inspection of the cervix can be done initially by sterile speculum, and vaginal examination only if necessary. Induction of labour is initiated at 34 weeks and beyond. At less than 34 weeks, expectant management is reasonable if there are no signs of infection or maternal or fetal compromise. PROM is not a lone indicator for surgical birth. If less than 34 weeks, expectant management is carried out with adequate hydration, reduced physical activity, close observation for possible infection (vital signs and laboratory test results including white blood cell count). Management at 32 to 34 weeks is controversial. Recommendations include delivery if fetal lung maturity can be documented, since conservative management has been shown to prolong pregnancy only briefly with an increase the risk of amnionitis. If fetal lung maturity is uncertain, expectant management with antibiotics until 34 weeks is reasonable (Yudin et al., 2017). Corticosteroids may be given to enhance fetal lung maturity. Recent studies have shown clear benefits of antibiotics to decrease neonatal morbidity associated with PPROM, particularly at 32 weeks' gestation and earlier. Antibiotics may serve to reduce maternal infective responses, thereby prolonging the pregnancy, and reducing newborn morbidity by reducing infection in the fetus and complications of prematurity (Yudin et al., 2017).

Nursing Assessment

Nursing assessment focuses on obtaining a complete health history and performing a physical examination to determine maternal and fetal status. An accurate assessment of the gestational age and knowledge of the obstetrical, fetal, and neonatal risks are essential to appropriate evaluation, counselling, and management of clients with PROM and PPROM. Nurses need to be aware that the risk of infection increases with the duration of PPROM and that antibiotic therapy following a recommended regimen can reduce morbidity and mortality.

Health History and Physical Examination

Review the maternal history for risk factors such as infection, increased uterine size (polyhydramnios, macrosomia, multiple gestation), uterine and fetal anomalies, lower socioeconomic status, STIs, cervical insufficiency, vaginal bleeding, and cigarette smoking during pregnancy. Ask about any history or current symptoms of urinary tract infection (frequency, urgency, dysuria, or flank pain) or pelvic or vaginal infection (pain or vaginal discharge).

Assess for signs and symptoms of labour, such as cramping, pelvic pressure, or back pain. Also assess vital signs, noting any signs indicative of infection such as fever, tachycardia, hypotension. Note any elevation in white blood cell count (Nagtalon-Ramos, 2014).

Institute continuous electronic fetal heart rate monitoring to evaluate fetal well-being. When PROM is suspected, discuss plans for vaginal examination with the primary care provider to avoid multiple examinations. If PPROM exists, a sterile speculum examination (where the examiner inspects the cervix but does not palpate it) is done rather than a digital cervical examination because vaginal examination may diminish latency (period of time from rupture of membranes to birth), introduce infection, and increase newborn morbidity (Cunningham et al., 2014).

Observe the characteristics of the amniotic fluid. Note any evidence of meconium, or a foul odour. When meconium is present in the amniotic fluid, it typically indicates fetal compromise related to hypoxia. Meconium stains the fluid yellow to greenish brown, depending on the amount present. A foul odour of amniotic fluid indicates infection. Ultrasound will be useful to measure the amount of amniotic fluid. A decreased amount of amniotic fluid reduces the cushioning effect, thereby making cord compression a possibility. Some research shows that restoring the volume of lost amniotic fluid will help to reduce the risk of infection and reduce cord compression. See Evidence-Based Practice 19.1. Key assessments are summarized in Box 19.4.

Laboratory and Diagnostic Testing

To diagnose PROM or PPROM, several procedures may be used: the Nitrazine test and/or fern test, PAMG testing, or ultrasound. After the insertion of a sterile speculum, a sample of the fluid in the vaginal area is obtained. With a Nitrazine test, the pH of the fluid is tested; amniotic fluid is more basic (7.0) than normal vaginal secretions (4.5). Nitrazine paper turns blue in the presence of amniotic fluid. However, false-positive results can occur if blood, urine, semen, antiseptic chemicals, or infection are also present; all will increase the pH.

For the fern test, a sample of vaginal fluid is placed on a slide to be viewed directly under a microscope. Amniotic fluid will develop a fern-like pattern when it dries because of sodium chloride crystallization. If both of these tests are inconclusive, a transvaginal ultrasound can also be used to determine whether membranes have ruptured by demonstrating a decreased amount of amniotic fluid (oligohydramnios) in the uterus (Jazayeri,

EVIDENCE-BASED PRACTICE 19.1   A LOW-DOSE ASPIRIN FOR PREVENTING PREECLAMPSIA AND ITS COMPLICATIONS: A META-ANALYSIS

STUDY

Preeclampsia is a major cause of perinatal mortality and morbidity worldwide. The etiology of it remains unclear, but it is thought that the condition arises because of abnormal trophoblastic invasion of uterine vessels or endothelial cell activation and dysfunction. Low-dose aspirin is thought to prevent preeclampsia in high-risk pregnancy, but it is not universally used because of safety concerns. The World Health Organization (WHO), the Society of Obstetricians and Gynaecologists of Canada, and the US Preventive Services Task Force (USPSTF) recommend using low-dose aspirin in pregnant clients at high risk for preeclampsia. A systematic review and meta-analysis were analyzed using 29 studies involving 21,403 women.

Findings

The meta-analysis showed that low-dose aspirin significantly reduced the incidence of preeclampsia. Risk of preeclampsia was reduced when initiated before 16 weeks' gestation. Prophylactic low-dose aspirin, especially initiated before 16 weeks' gestation, is effective at preventing preeclampsia, preterm birth, and fetal growth restriction in high-risk pregnancies.

Nursing Implications

Based on the study's results, nurses can be involved in prenatal assessments of high-risk clients to identify them early so that prophylactic low-dose aspirin can be prescribed if deemed appropriate by the health care provider. The nurse can provide instruction and rationales for the use and timing of this therapy to the clients. Nurses can view this therapy as an evidence-based intervention to promote better outcomes for pregnant clients and infants.

Adapted from Xu, T. T., Zhou, F., Deng, C. Y., Huang, G. Q., Li, J. K., & Wang, X. D. (2015). Low-dose aspirin for preventing preeclampsia and its complications: A meta-analysis. *The Journal of Clinical Hypertension, 17*(7), 567–573.

BOX 19.4

KEY ASSESSMENT WITH PREMATURE RUPTURE OF MEMBRANES

For the client with PROM, the following assessments are essential:
- Determining the date, time, and duration of membrane rupture by client interview
- Ascertaining gestational age of the fetus based on date of client's last menstrual period, fundal height, and ultrasound dating
- Questioning the client about possible history of recent UTI or vaginal infection that might have contributed to PROM
- Assessing for any associated labour symptoms, such as back pain or pelvic pressure
- Assisting with or performing diagnostic tests to validate leakage of fluid, such as Nitrazine test, "ferning" on slide, PAMG swab, and ultrasound. Contamination of Nitrazine tape with lubricant or insufficient fluid will render the assessment unreliable.
- Continually assessing for signs of infection including:
  - Elevation of maternal temperature and pulse rate
  - Abdominal/uterine tenderness
  - Fetal tachycardia more than 160 bpm
  - Elevated white blood cell count and C-reactive protein
  - Cloudy, foul-smelling amniotic fluid

Adapted from Nagtalon-Ramos, J. (2014). *Maternal-newborn nursing care: Best evidence-based practices.* Philadelphia, PA: F. A. Davis Company; Cunningham, F. G., Leveno, K. J., Bloom, S. L., Spong, C. Y., Dashe, J. S., Hoffman, B. L., ... Sheffield, J. S. (2014). *Williams' obstetrics* (24th ed.). New York: McGraw-Hill Education; and Magowan, B. A., Owen, P., & Thomson, A. (2014). *Clinical obstetrics and gynecology* (3rd ed.). St. Louis, MO: Saunders Elsevier.

2017). This however, may not be helpful in the case where the fluid leak is slow and replaced over time.

To test for the presence of placental alpha microglobulin-1 (PAMG), a molecule specific to amniotic fluid, a swab is placed in the vagina, fluid allowed to soak in (1 minute) then the swab is placed in a small vial of liquid. That liquid is subsequently tested for the presence of PAMG. A brand of this test is AmniSure, which has demonstrated a positive predictive value of over 98% and a negative predictive value of over 97% (Abdelazim, Abdelrazak, Al-Kadi, Yehia, & Abdulkareem, 2014).

Other laboratory and diagnostic tests that may be used include:
- Urinalysis and urine culture for UTI or asymptomatic bacteriuria
- Cervical test or culture for chlamydia or gonorrhea
- Vaginal culture for bacterial vaginosis and trichomoniasis
- Vaginal introital/rectal culture for group B streptococcus

Nursing Management

Nursing management for the client with PROM or PPROM focuses on preventing infection and identifying uterine contractions. The risk for infection is great because of the break in the amniotic fluid membrane and its proximity to vaginal bacteria. Therefore, monitor vital signs closely. Be alert for a temperature elevation, an increase in pulse, or a reduction in blood pressure, which could indicate infection. Also monitor the fetal heart rate continuously, reporting any fetal tachycardia (which could indicate an infection) or variable decelerations (suggesting cord compression). If variable decelerations are present, anticipate amnioinfusion based on agency policy. Evaluate the results of laboratory tests such as a CBC. An elevation in white blood cells would suggest infection. Administer antibiotics if ordered.

Encourage the client and partner to verbalize their feelings and concerns. Educate them about the purpose of the protective membranes and the implications of early rupture. Keep them informed about planned interventions, including potential complications and required therapy. As appropriate, prepare the client for induction or augmentation of labour as appropriate if near term.

If labour does not start within 48 hours, the client with PPROM may be discharged home on expectant management, which may include:

- Antibiotics
- Activity restrictions
- Education about signs and symptoms of infection and when to call with problems or concerns (Teaching Guidelines 19.2)
- Frequent fetal testing for well-being
- Regular ultrasound examinations to assess amniotic fluid levels
- Possible corticosteroid treatment depending on gestational age
- Daily kick counts to assess fetal well-being

Ultimately, the decision whether to manage the case of a patient with PPROM on an outpatient basis needs to be individualized and made carefully after a thorough discussion of the risks and benefits of outpatient management (Yudin et al., 2017).

Teaching Guidelines 19.2
TEACHING FOR THE CLIENT WITH PPROM

- Monitor your baby's activity by performing fetal kick counts daily.
- Check your temperature twice daily or as directed and report any temperature increases to your health care provider.
- Watch for signs related to the beginning of labour. Report any tightening of the abdomen or contractions.
- Avoid any touching or manipulating of your breasts, which could stimulate labour.
- Do not insert anything into your vagina or vaginal area—no tampons, and avoid vaginal intercourse.
- Do not swim in pools or lakes/ocean or sit in a hot tub or Jacuzzi.
- Take showers for daily hygiene needs; avoid sitting in a tub bath.
- Maintain any specific activity restrictions as recommended.
- Wash your hands thoroughly after using the bathroom and make sure to wipe from front to back each time.
- Keep your perineal area clean and dry.
- Take your antibiotics as directed if your health care provider has prescribed them.
- Call your health care provider with changes in your condition, including fever, uterine tenderness, feeling like your heart is racing, and foul-smelling vaginal discharge.

NURSING CARE PLAN 19.1

Overview of the Client With Placenta Previa

A 39-year-old G5, P4, multigravida client at 32 weeks' gestation, was admitted to the labour and birth suite with sudden vaginal bleeding. There was no further active bleeding on arrival and no reports of any abdominal discomfort or tenderness. The client did complain of occasional "tightening" in the stomach. On palpation, the abdomen was soft. Fetal heart rates were in the 140s with accelerations with movement. The client was placed on bed rest with bathroom privileges. Ultrasound identified a low-lying placenta with a viable, normal-growth fetus. The client was diagnosed with placenta previa and admitted for observation and surveillance of fetal well-being. The obstetrical and medical history revealed two previous cesarean births, smoking half a pack of cigarettes per day, and postpartum endometritis with a previous pregnancy. Additional assessment findings included painless, bright-red vaginal bleeding with initial bleeding ceasing spontaneously; irregular, mild, and sporadic uterine contractions; vital signs and fetal heart rate within normal range; fetus in transverse lie; anxiety related to the outcome of pregnancy; and expression of feelings of helplessness.

NURSING DIAGNOSIS: Risk for injury (to client and fetus) related to threat to uteroplacental perfusion and hemorrhage

NURSING CARE PLAN 19.1

Overview of the Client With Placenta Previa (continued)

Outcome Identification and Evaluation

The client will maintain adequate tissue perfusion as evidenced by stable vital signs, decreased blood loss, few or no uterine contractions, normal fetal heart rate patterns and variability, and positive fetal movement.

Interventions: *Maintaining Adequate Tissue Perfusion*

- Establish intravenous access to allow for administration of fluids, blood, and medications as necessary.
- Obtain type and cross-match for at least 2 units blood products as ordered to ensure availability should bleeding continue.
- Obtain specimens as ordered for blood studies, such as CBC and clotting studies, to establish a baseline and use for future comparison.
- Monitor output to evaluate adequacy of renal perfusion.
- Administer intravenous fluid replacement therapy as ordered to maintain blood pressure and blood volume.
- Palpate for abdominal tenderness and rigidity to determine bleeding and evidence of uterine contractions.
- Institute bed rest, with limited activities when no bleeding.
- Assess for rupture of membranes to evaluate for possible onset of labour.
- Avoid vaginal examinations to prevent further bleeding episodes.
- Complete an Rh titer to identify need for Rh immunoglobulin.

- Avoid nipple stimulation to prevent uterine contractions.
- Continuously monitor for contractions or PROM to allow for prompt intervention.
- Administer tocolytic agents as ordered to stall preterm labour.
- Monitor vital signs frequently to identify possible hypovolemia and infection.
- Assess frequently for active vaginal bleeding to minimize risk of hemorrhage.
- Continuously monitor fetal heart rate with electronic fetal monitor to evaluate fetal status.
- Assist with fetal surveillance tests as ordered to aid in determining fetal well-being.
- Observe for abnormal fetal heart rate patterns, such as loss of variability, late decelerations, tachycardia, to identify fetal distress.
- Position client in side-lying position with wedge for support to maximize placental perfusion.
- Assess fetal movement to evaluate for possible fetal hypoxia.
- Teach client to monitor fetal movement to evaluate well-being.
- Administer oxygen as ordered to increase oxygenation to mother and fetus.

NURSING DIAGNOSIS: Anxiety related to threat to self and fetus, unknown future

Outcome Identification and Evaluation

The client will experience a decrease in anxiety as evidenced by verbal reports of less anxiety, use of effective coping measures, and calm demeanour.

Interventions: *Minimizing Anxiety*

- Provide factual information about diagnosis and treatment, and explain interventions and the rationale behind them *to provide client with understanding of the condition.*
- Answer questions about health status honestly *to establish a trusting relationship.*
- Speak calmly to client and family members *to minimize environmental stress.*
- Encourage the use of past effective techniques for coping *to promote relaxation and feelings of control.*

- Acknowledge and facilitate the client's spiritual needs *to promote effective coping.*
- Involve the client and family in the decision-making process *to foster self-confidence and control over situation.*
- Maintain a presence during stressful periods *to allay anxiety.*
- Use the sense of touch if appropriate *to convey caring and concern.*
- Encourage talking as a means *to release tension.*

KEY CONCEPTS

- Identifying risk factors early on and throughout the pregnancy is important to ensure the best outcome for every pregnancy. Risk assessment should start with the first prenatal visit and continue with subsequent visits.

- The three most common causes of hemorrhage early in pregnancy (first half of pregnancy) are spontaneous abortion, ectopic pregnancy, and GTD.

- Ectopic pregnancies occur in about 1 in 50 pregnancies and have increased dramatically during the past few decades.

- A molar pregnancy results is a nonviable pregnancy and could lead to the development of choriocarcinoma, a chronic malignancy from the trophoblastic tissue.

- The classic clinical picture presentation for placenta previa is painless, bright-red vaginal bleeding occurring during the third trimester.

- Treatment of abruptio placentae is designed to assess, control, and restore the amount of blood lost; to provide a positive outcome for both the pregnant client and infant; and to prevent coagulation disorders.

- DIC can be described in simplest terms as a loss of balance between the clot-forming activity of thrombin and the clot-lysing activity of plasmin.

- HG is a complication of pregnancy characterized by persistent, uncontrollable nausea and vomiting before the 20th week of gestation.

- Gestational hypertension is a leading cause of maternal death and the most common complication reported during pregnancy.

- HELLP is an acronym for a serious condition involving hemolysis, elevated liver enzymes, and low platelets.

- Rh incompatibility is a condition that develops when a client of Rh-negative blood type is exposed to Rh-positive fetal blood cells and subsequently develops circulating titers of Rh antibodies.

- Polyhydramnios occurs in approximately 3% to 4% of all pregnancies and is associated with fetal anomalies of development.

- Nursing care related to the client with oligohydramnios involves continuous monitoring of fetal well-being during nonstress testing or during labour and birth by identifying atypical and abnormal fetal heart rate patterns using a fetal monitor.

- The increasing number of multiple gestations is a concern because clients who are expecting more than one infant are at high risk for preterm labour, hydramnios, HG, anemia, preeclampsia, and antepartum hemorrhage.

- Nursing care related to PROM centres on preventing infection and identifying preterm labour contractions.

- PPROM requires monitoring of both vital signs and the fetal heart rate to increase the likelihood of a good outcome.

- It is essential that nurses educate all pregnant clients about how to detect the signs of PROM and what action is needed if it happens.

REFERENCES AND RECOMMENDED READINGS

Abdelazim, I. A., Abdelrazak, K. M., Al-Kadi, M., Yehia, A. H., & Abdulkareem, A. F. (2014). Fetal fibronectin (Quick Check fFN test) versus placental alpha microglobulin-1 (AmniSure test) for detection of premature rupture of fetal membranes. *Archives of Gynecology and Obstetrics, 290*(3), 457–464.

Abu Hashim, H., Al-Inany, H., & Kilani, Z. (2014). A review of the contemporary evidence on rescue cervical cerclage. *International Journal of Gynecology and Obstetrics, 124*(3), 198–203.

Agarwal, N., & Odejinmi, F. (2014). Early abdominal ectopic pregnancy: Challenges, update and review of current management. *Obstetrician and Gynaecologist, 16*(3), 193–198.

Agency for Healthcare Research and Quality (AHRQ). (2015). *Cerclage for the management of cervical insufficiency*. Retrieved from http://www.guideline.gov/content.aspx?id=47771

Aitken, K., Allen, L., Pantazi, S., Kingdom, J., Keating, S., Pollard, L., & Windrim, R. (2016). MRI significantly improves disease staging to direct surgical planning for abnormal invasive placentation: A single centre experience. *Journal of Obstetrics and Gynaecology Canada, 38*(3), 246–251

American Cancer Society (ACS). (2017). *Gestational trophoblastic disease*. Retrieved from http://www.cancer.org/cancer/gestationaltrophoblasticdisease/detailedguide/gestational-trophoblastic-disease-key-statistics

American College of Obstetricians and Gynecologists (ACOG). (2014a). ACOG Practice bulletin no. 142: Cerclage for the management of cervical insufficiency. *Obstetrics and Gynecology, 123*(2), 372–379.

American College of Obstetricians and Gynecologists (ACOG). (2014b). *Placenta accreta*. Retrieved from http://www.acog.org/Resources-And-Publications/Committee-Opinions/Committee-on-Obstetric-Practice/Placenta-Accreta

American College of Obstetricians and Gynecologists (ACOG). (2014c). ACOG task force on hypertension in pregnancy—A step forward in management. *Contemporary OB/GYN*. Retrieved from http://contemporaryobgyn.modernmedicine.

com/contemporary-obgyn/news/acog-task-force-hypertension-pregnancy-step-forward-management?page=full

Amorim, M. M., Katz, L., Barros, A. S., Almeida, T. S., Souza, A. S. R., & Faúndes, A. (2015). Maternal outcomes according to mode of delivery in women with severe preeclampsia: A cohort study. *The Journal of Maternal-Fetal and Neonatal Medicine, 28*(6), 654–660.

Ananth, C. V., & Kinzler, W. L. (2018). *Placental abruption: Pathophysiology, clinical features, diagnosis, and consequences. UpToDate.* Retrieved from http://www.uptodate.com/contents/placental-abruption-clinical-features-and-diagnosis

Archibong, E. I., & Ahmed, E. S. (2015). Risk factors maternal and neonatal outcome in major placenta previa: A prospective study. *Annals of Saudi Medicine, 21*(3–4), 245–247.

Ardehali, A., Casikar, I., & Condous, G. (2015). Identification of risk factors of ectopic pregnancy. In *Ectopic pregnancy* (pp. 1–10). Springer International Publishing.

Atkinson, A. L., Santolaya-Forgas, J., Blitzer, D. N., Santolaya, J. L., Matta, P., Canterino, J., & Oyelese, Y. (2015). Risk factors for perinatal mortality in patients admitted to the hospital with the diagnosis of placental abruption. *The Journal of Maternal-Fetal and Neonatal Medicine, 28*(5), 594–597.

Ayyavoo, A., Derraik, J. G., Hofman, P. L., & Cutfield, W. S. (2014). Hyperemesis gravidarum and long-term health of the offspring. *American Journal of Obstetrics and Gynecology, 210*(6), 521–525.

Baergan, R. (2019). Gestational trophoblastic disease: Pathology. *UpToDate.* Retrieved from https://www.uptodate.com/contents/gestational-trophoblastic-disease-pathology

Bakker, R., & Ramus, R. M. (2018). Placenta previa. *eMedicine.* Retrieved from http://emedicine.medscape.com/article/262063-overview

Berghella, V. (2018). Cervical insufficiency. *UpToDate.* Retrieved from http://www.uptodate.com/contents/cervical-insufficiency

Berkowitz, R. S., Goldstein, D. P., & Horowitz, N. S. (2014). Management options of gestational trophoblastic disease. *Current Obstetrics and Gynecology Reports, 3*(1), 76–83.

Boots, A. B., Sanchez-Ramos, L., Bowers, D. M., Kaunitz, A. M., Zamora, J., & Schlattmann, P. (2014). The short-term prediction of preterm birth: A systematic review and diagnostic metaanalysis. *American Journal of Obstetrics and Gynecology, 210*(1), 54. e1–e54.

Bourne, T. (2015). A missed opportunity for excellence: The NICE guideline on the diagnosis and initial management of ectopic pregnancy and miscarriage. *Journal of Family Planning and Reproductive Health Care, 41*(1), 13–19.

Brown, R., Gagnon, R., & Delisle, M. (2013). SOGC clinical practice guidelines: Cervical insufficiency and cervical cerclage. *Journal of Obstetrics and Gynaecology Canada, 35*(12), 1115–1127. Retrieved from https://sogc.org/wp-content/uploads/2013/11/December2013-CPG301-ENG-REV-Dec-13-13.pdf

Bujold, E. (2015). Low-dose aspirin reduces morbidity and mortality in pregnant women at high-risk for preeclampsia. *Evidence Based Nursing, 18*(3), 71.

Campbell, K., Rowe, H., Azzam, H., & Lane, C. A. (2016). The management of nausea and vomiting of pregnancy. *Journal of Obstetrics and Gynaecology Canada, 38*(12), 1127–1137.

Canadian Blood Services. (2018). *The facts about whole blood.* Retrieved from https://blood.ca/en/blood/facts-about-whole-blood

Carson, M. P., & Gibson, P. S. (2018). Hypertension and pregnancy. *eMedicine.* Retrieved from http://emedicine.medscape.com/article/261435-overview

Carter, B. S., & Boyd, R. L. (2017). Polyhydramnios and oligohydramnios. *eMedicine.* Retrieved from: http://reference.medscape.com/article/975821-overview

Castillo, M. J., & Phillippi, J. C. (2015). Hyperemesis gravidarum: A holistic overview and approach to clinical assessment and management. *The Journal of Perinatal and Neonatal Nursing, 29*(1), 12–22.

Catt, E., Chadha, R., Tang, S., Palmquist, E., & Lange, I. (2016). Management of preterm premature rupture of membranes: A comparison of inpatient and outpatient care. *Journal of Obstetrics and Gynaecology Canada, 38*(5), 433–440.

Clausen, T. D., & Bergholt, T. (2014). Chronic hypertension during pregnancy. *British Medical Journal, 348*, g2655.

Cohen, A., Zakar, L., Gil, Y., Amer-Alshick, J., Bibi, G., Almog, B., & Levin, I. (2015). Methotrexate success rates in progressing ectopic pregnancies: A reappraisal. *Obstetrical and Gynecological Survey, 70*(2), 88–89.

Colgan, T. J., Noor, A., Nanji, S., Chang, M. C., & Kolomietz, E. (2017). Molecular diagnosis of placental hydatidiform mole: Innovation and outcomes. *Journal of Obstetrics and Gynecology Canada, 39*(11), 1049–1052.

Cook, J. L., Majd, M., Blake, J., Barret, J., Bouvet, S., Janssen, P., … Wong, T. (2017). Measuring maternal mortality and morbidity in Canada. *Journal of Obstetrics and Gynaecology Canada, 9*(11), 1028–1037.

Creasy, R. K., Resnik, R., Iams, J. D., Lockwood, C. J., Moore, T. R., & Greene, M. F. (2014). *Creasy and Resnik's maternal-fetal medicine: Principles and practice* (7th ed.). Philadelphia, PA: Elsevier.

Cunningham, F. G., Leveno, K. J., Bloom, S. L., Spong, C. Y., Dashe, J. S., Hoffman, B. L., … Sheffield, J. S. (2014). *Williams' obstetrics* (24th ed.). New York: McGraw-Hill Education.

Dalia, S., Price, S., Forsyth, P., Sokol, L., & Jaglal, M. (2015). What is the optimal dose of high dose methotrexate in the initial treatment of primary Central Nervous System lymphoma?. *Leukemia and Lymphoma, 56*(2), 500–502.

Davidson, M. R. (2014). *Fast facts for the neonatal nurse: A nursing orientation and care guide in a nutshell.* New York: Springer Publishing Company.

Davis, S. J., & Kessler, C. M. (2014). Disseminated intravascular coagulation: Diagnosis and management. In *Hemostasis and thrombosis: Practical guidelines in clinical management* (pp. 151–168). Hoboken, NJ: Wiley Blackwell.

Deering, S. H. (2017). Abruptio placentae. *eMedicine.* Retrieved from http://emedicine.medscape.com/article/252810-overview

Dekker, G. A. (2014). Management of preeclampsia. *Pregnancy Hypertension, 4*(3), 246–247.

Desai, D., Lu, J., Wyness, S. P., Greene, D. N., Olson, K. N., Wiley, C. L., & Grenache, D. G. (2014). Human chorionic gonadotropin discriminatory zone in ectopic pregnancy: Does assay harmonization matter?. *Fertility and Sterility, 101*(6), 1671–1674.

De Sutter, P. (2015). The challenge of multiple pregnancies. In *Reducing risk in fertility treatment* (pp. 1–17). London, England: Springer Publishers.

Dickson, E. L., & Mullany, S. A. (2015). Gestational trophoblastic disease. In *Gynecologic oncology* (pp. 175–201). New York: Springer.

Festin, M. (2014). Nausea and vomiting in early pregnancy. *BMJ Clinical Evidence, 2014*, pii: 1405. Available from: MEDLINE, Ipswich, MA.

Foley, M., Strong, T. H., & Garite, T. (2014). *Obstetric intensive care manual* (4th ed.). New York: McGraw-Hill Publishers.

Foo, L., Tay, J., Lees, C. C., McEniery, C. M., & Wilkinson, I. B. (2015). Hypertension in pregnancy: Natural history and treatment options. *Current Hypertension Reports, 17*(5), 36.

Fung, K. F. K., & Eason, E. (2018). No. 133-Prevention of Rh alloimmunization. *Journal of Obstetrics and Gynaecology Canada, 40*(1), e1–e10.

Gaufberg, S. V. (2017). Early pregnancy loss in emergency medicine. *Drugs and Diseases: Emergency Medicine.* Retrieved from https://emedicine.medscape.com/article/795085-overview#a5

Gibbins, K., Esplin, M. S., Varner, M., Eller, A., & Manuck, T. (2014). 835: Subsequent pregnancy outcomes among women with a history of preterm premature rupture of membranes (PPROM) < 24.0 weeks gestation. *American Journal of Obstetrics and Gynecology, 210*(1), S405–S406.

Gilbert, R. (2014). Immediate delivery for group B streptococci-colonized women with preterm premature rupture of membranes. Don't forget the antibiotics. *BJOG: An International Journal of Obstetrics and Gynaecology, 121*, 1273.

Heffner, L. J. (2004). Advanced maternal age—how old is too old?. *New England Journal of Medicine, 351*(19), 1927–1929.

Hensley, J., & Shviraga, B. (2014). Metastatic choriocarcinoma in a term pregnancy: A case study. *MCN: The American Journal of Maternal Child Nursing, 39*(1), 8–15.

Herrera, K., & Lewis, D. (2014). Cervical insufficiency and cerclage. *Topics in Obstetrics and Gynecology, 34*(3), 1–5.

Hockin, J. C., & Jessamine, A. G. (1984). Trends in ectopic pregnancy in Canada. *CMAJ, 131*(7), 737–740.

Holt, J. L. (2015). Multidisciplinary care of a woman experiencing obstetric hemorrhage. *Journal of Obstetric, Gynecologic, and Neonatal Nursing, 44*, S85–S86.

Hosein, H., Abdel-Kariem, R., & Shriki, J. E. (2015). Placental abruption imaging. *eMedicine.* Retrieved from http://emedicine.medscape.com/article/402314-overview

Humphrey, J. (2015). Primary cesarean delivery results in emergency hysterectomy due to placenta accreta: A case study. *AANA Journal, 83*(1), 28–34.

Infante, F., Menakaya, U., & Condous, G. (2014). Medical treatment of ectopic pregnancy. *Fertility and Sterility, 101*(3), e16–e22. doi: http://dx.doi.org/10.1016/j.fertnstert.2013.12.013

Jaju, K. G., Kulkarni, A. P., & Mundada, S. K. (2014). Study of perinatal outcome in relation to abruptio placentae. *International Journal of Recent Trends in Science and Technology, 11*(3), 355–358.

Jazayeri, A. (2017). Premature rupture of membranes. *eMedicine.* Retrieved from http://emedicine.medscape.com/article/261137-overview

Jefferies, A. L.; Canadian Pediatric Society Fetus and Newborn Committee. (2017). Management of term infants at increased risk for early-onset bacterial sepsis. *Paediatrics and Child Health, 22*(4), 223–228.

Jena, S. K., Samal, S., & Behera, B. K. (2015). Cervical cerclage in modern obstetrics: A review. *The Health Agenda, 3*(1), 9–14.

Jones, R. E., & Lopez, K. H. (2014). *Human reproductive biology* (4th ed.). Waltham, MA: Academic Press/Elsevier.

Kao, L., Scheinfeld, M., Chernyak, V., Rozenblit, A., Oh, S., & Dym, R. (2014). Beyond ultrasound: CT and MRI of ectopic pregnancy. *American Journal of Roentgenology, 202*(4), 904–911.

Khan, H., & Meirowitz, N. B. (2018). HELLP syndrome. *eMedicine.* Retrieved from http://emedicine.medscape.com/article/1394126-overview

King, T. L., Brucker, M. C., Fahey, J. O., Kriebs, J. M., Gegor, C. L., & Varney, H. (2015). *Varney's midwifery* (5th ed.). Burlington, MA: Jones & Bartlett Learning.

Knez, J., Day, A., & Jurkovic, D. (2014). Ultrasound imaging in the management of bleeding and pain in early pregnancy. *Best Practice and Research Clinical Obstetrics and Gynaecology, 28*(5), 621–636.

Ko, J., & Cheung, V. (2014). Time to revisit the human chorionic gonadotropin discriminatory level in the management of pregnancy of unknown location. *Journal of Ultrasound in Medicine, 33*(3), 465–471.

Kobayashi, T. (2014). Obstetrical disseminated intravascular coagulation score. *Journal of Obstetrics and Gynaecology Research, 40*(6), 1500–1506.

Lim, K., Butt, K., & Crane, J. M. (2018). No. 257-Ultrasonographic cervical length assessment in predicting preterm birth in singleton pregnancies. *Journal of Obstetrics and Gynaecology Canada, 40*(2), 151–164.

Lim, K., Butt, K., Naud, K., & Smithies, M. (2017). Amniotic fluid: Technical update on physiology and measurement. *Journal of Obstetrics and Gynaecology Canada, 39*(1), 52–58.

Magee, L. A., Pels, A., Helewa, M., Rey, E., & von Dadelszen, P. (2014). SOGC Clinical practice guideline: Diagnosis, evaluation, and management of the hypertensive disorders of pregnancy: Executive summary. *Journal of Obstetrics and Gynaecology Canada, 36*(5), 416–438.

Magee, L. A., Pels, A., Helewa, M., Rey, E., von Dadelszen, P., Audibert, F., … Firoz, T. (2015). The hypertensive disorders of pregnancy (29.3). *Best Practice and Research Clinical Obstetrics and Gynaecology, 29*(5), 643–657.

Magowan, B. A., Owen, P., & Thomson, A. (2014). *Clinical obstetrics and gynecology* (3rd ed.). St. Louis, MO: Saunders Elsevier.

Maltepe, C., Popa, M. V., Bertucci, C., Farine, D., Koren, G., & Nulman, I. (2015). The effects of counseling and predictors of pregnancy outcomes in women with hyperemesis gravidarum [316]. *Obstetrics and Gynecology, 125*, 101S.

March of Dimes. (2015). *Oligohydramnios.* Retrieved from http://www.marchofdimes.com/pregnancy/oligohydramnios.aspx

March of Dimes. (2016). *Rh disease.* Retrieved from https://www.marchofdimes.org/baby/rh-disease.aspx

March of Dimes. (2017a). *Pregnancy loss.* Retrieved from http://www.marchofdimes.com/loss/stillbirth.aspx

March of Dimes. (2017b). *Multiples: Twins, triplets and beyond.* Retrieved from http://www.marchofdimes.com/pregnancy/multiples-twins-triplets-and-beyond.aspx

Marik, P. E. (2015). Pregnancy related disorders. In *Evidence-based critical care* (pp. 759–772). Springer International Publishing.

Martin, R. J., Fanaroff, A. A., & Walsh, M. C. (2014). *Fanaroff and Martin's neonatal-perinatal medicine* (10th ed.). Philadelphia, PA: Elsevier Health Sciences.

Matthews, A., Haas, D. M., O'Mathúna, D. P., Dowswell, T., & Doyle, M. (2014). Interventions for nausea and vomiting in early pregnancy. *Cochrane Database of Systematic Reviews, 3*, CD007575.

Mattson, S., & Smith, J. E. (2016). *Core curriculum for maternal-newborn nursing* (5th ed.). St. Louis, MO: Saunders Elsevier.

Miller, M. A., & Carpenter, M. (2015). Hypertensive disorders of pregnancy. In *Medical management of the pregnant patient* (pp. 177–193). New York: Springer Publishers.

Moore, T. R. (2015). Abnormal amniotic fluid. In J. T. Queenan, C. Y. Spong, C. J. Lockwood (Eds.). *Protocols for high-risk pregnancies: An evidence-based approach* (pp. 315–328). West Sussex, UK: John Wiley & Sons.

Moses, S. (2018a). Placental abruption. *Family Practice Notebook.* Retrieved from http://www.fpnotebook.com/ob/Bleed/PlcntlAbrptn.htm

Moses, S. (2018b). HELLP syndrome. *Family Practice Notebook.* Retrieved from http://www.fpnotebook.com/heme-onc/OB/HlpSyndrm.htm

Mukherjee, S., Bawa, A. K., Sharma, S., Nandanwar, Y. S., & Gadam, M. (2014). Retrospective study of risk factors and maternal and fetal outcome in patients with abruptio placentae. *Journal of Natural Science, Biology and Medicine, 5*(2), 425–428.

Nagtalon-Ramos, J. (2014). *Maternal-newborn nursing care: Best evidence-based practices.* Philadelphia, PA: F. A. Davis Company.

National High Blood Pressure Education Program Working Group on High Blood Pressure in Pregnancy. (2002). Working Group in High Blood Pressure in Pregnancy report. *American Journal of Obstetrics and Gynecology, 183,* S1–S22.

Nguyen, N., & Slim, R. (2014). Genetics and epigenetics of recurrent hydatidiform moles: Basic science and genetic counselling. *Current Obstetrics and Gynecology Reports, 3,* 55–64.

Norwitz, E. R., & Conroy, K. E. (2016). Cervical insufficiency. *eMedicine.* Retrieved from http://emedicine.medscape.com/article/1979914-overview

Ogunyemi, D. A., Fong, A., & Herrero, T. C. (2017). Hyperemesis gravidarum. *eMedicine.* Retrieved from http://emedicine.medscape.com/article/254751-overview

Pauli, J. M., & Repke, J. T. (2015). Preeclampsia: Short-term and long-term implications. *Obstetrics and Gynecology Clinics of North America, 42*(2), 299–313.

Peled, Y., Melamed, N., Hiersch, L., Pardo, J., Wiznitzer, A., & Yogev, Y. (2014). The impact of total parenteral nutrition support on pregnancy outcome in women with hyperemesis gravidarum. *Journal of Maternal-Fetal and Neonatal Medicine, 27*(11), 1146–1150.

Randall, S., & LaMontagne, D. S. (2015). Screening for chlamydia: Seize the day. *Journal of Family Planning and Reproductive Health Care, 31*(2), 98–100.

Rowe, T. (2014). Placenta Previa. *Journal of Obstetrics and Gynaecology Canada, 36,* 667–668. August, 2014 editorial.

Salem, L., & Singer, K. R. (2017). Rh incompatibility. *eMedicine.* Retrieved from http://emedicine.medscape.com/article/797150-overview

Schultz, W., & McConachie, I. (2015). Vital signs after hemorrhage—caution is appropriate. *Trends in Anesthesia and Critical Care, 5,* 89–92. doi: http://dx.doi.org/10.1016/j.tacc.2015.04.001

Sepilian, V., & Wood, E. (2017). Ectopic pregnancy. *eMedicine.* Retrieved from http://emedicine.medscape.com/article/2041923-overview

Sibai, B. M. (2018). HELLP syndrome. *UpToDate.* Retrieved from http://www.uptodate.com/contents/hellp-syndrome

Skidmore-Roth, L. (2015). *Mosby's 2015 nursing drug reference* (28th ed.). Philadelphia, PA: Elsevier Health Science.

Staneva, A., Bogossian, F., Pritchard, M., & Wittkowski, A. (2015). The effects of maternal depression, anxiety, and perceived stress during pregnancy on preterm birth: A systematic review. *Women and Birth, 28*(3), 179–193.

Statistics Canada. (2015). Fetal deaths (20 weeks or more of gestation) and late fetal deaths (28 weeks or more of gestation), Canada, provinces and territories. *Canadian Vital Statistics, Stillbirth Database.* Retrieved from http://www.statcan.gc.ca/pub/84f0210x/2009000/t024-eng.htm

Statistics Canada. (2016). Live births and fetal deaths (stillbirths), by type (single or multiple), Canada, provinces and territories. *CANSIM Table 102–4515.* Retrieved from http://bit.ly/1f3GCWu.

Strohl, A. E., & Lurain, J. R. (2014). Clinical epidemiology of gestational trophoblastic disease. *Current Obstetrics and Gynecology Reports, 3*(1), 40–43.

Szypulski, H. (2015). Practice guideline to prevent ectopic pregnancy rupture. *International Journal of Childbirth Education, 30*(1), 59–62.

Tan, P., Zaidi, S., Azmi, N., Omar, S., & Khong, S. (2014). Depression, anxiety, stress and hyperemesis gravidarum: Temporal and case controlled correlates. *PLoS One, 9*(3), e92036.

Taylor, T. (2014). Treatment of nausea and vomiting in pregnancy. *Australian Prescriber, 37*(2), 42–45.

Tulandi, T. (2015). Medical treatment of ectopic pregnancy. In *Ectopic pregnancy* (pp. 49–53). Springer International Publishing.

Tulandi, T., & Al-Fozan, H. M. (2018). Spontaneous abortion: Risk factors, etiology, clinical manifestations, and diagnostic evaluation. *UpToDate.* Retrieved from http://www.uptodate.com/contents/spontaneous-abortion-risk-factors-etiology-clinical-manifestations-and-diagnostic-evaluation

Urquhart, C., Currell, R., Harlow, F., & Callow, L. (2015). Home uterine monitoring for detecting preterm labor. *Cochrane Database of Systematic Reviews, 1,* CD006172.

Verklan, T., & Walden, M. (2014). *Core curriculum for neonatal intensive care nursing* (4th ed.). St. Louis, MO: Saunders Elsevier.

Vigil-De Gracia, P. (2015). HELLP syndrome. *Ginecología Y Obstetricia De México, 83*(1), 48–57.

Wiedaseck, S., & Monchek, R. (2014). Placental and cord insertion pathologies: Screening, diagnosis, and management. *Journal of Midwifery and Women's Health, 59*(3), 328–335.

World Health Organization (WHO). (2018). *Skilled birth attendants.* Retrieved from http://www.who.int/reproductivehealth/topics/mdgs/skilled_birth_attendant/en/

Xu, T. T., Zhou, F., Deng, C. Y., Huang, G. Q., Li, J. K., & Wang, X. D. (2015). Lowdose aspirin for preventing preeclampsia and its complications: A metaanalysis. *The Journal of Clinical Hypertension, 17*(7), 567–573.

Yudin, M. H., van Schalkwyk, J., & Van Eyk, N. (2017). SOGC Clinical practice guideline No. 233-Antibiotic therapy in preterm premature rupture of the membranes. *Journal of Obstetrics and Gynaecology Canada, 39*(9), e207–e212. doi: 10.1016/j.jogc.2017.06.003

Zainul Rashid, M. R., Lim, J., Nawawi, N. H., Luqman, M., Zolkeplai, M., Rangkuty, H., … Schindler, A. E. (2014). A pilot study to determine whether progestogen supplementation using dydrogesterone during the first trimester will reduce the incidence of gestational hypertension in primigravidae. *Gynecological Endocrinology, 30*(3), 217–220.

CHAPTER **WORKSHEET**

MULTIPLE CHOICE QUESTIONS

1. Which of the following clients should receive Rh immune globulin postpartum?
   a. Nonsensitized Rh-negative client with an Rh-negative newborn
   b. Nonsensitized Rh-negative client with an Rh-positive newborn
   c. Sensitized Rh-negative client with an Rh-positive newborn
   d. Sensitized Rh-negative client with an Rh-negative newborn

2. A pregnant client is suspected of having abruptio placentae. Which of the following would the nurse expect to assess as a classic symptom?
   a. Painless, bright-red bleeding
   b. "Knife-like" abdominal pain
   c. Excessive nausea and vomiting
   d. Hypertension and headache

3. Rh immune globulin is given to Rh-negative clients to prevent maternal sensitization. In addition to administration at 28 weeks' gestation, Rh-negative clients would also receive this medication after which of the following?
   a. Therapeutic or spontaneous abortion
   b. Head injury from a car accident
   c. Blood transfusion after a hemorrhage
   d. Unsuccessful artificial insemination procedure

4. After teaching a client about hyperemesis gravidarum and how it differs from the typical nausea and vomiting of pregnancy, which statement by the client indicates that the teaching was successful?
   a. "I can expect the nausea to last through my second trimester."
   b. "I should eat and drink whatever I feel I can tolerate that is safe for myself and baby."
   c. "I need to avoid strong odours, perfumes, or flavours."
   d. "I should lie down after I eat for about 2 hours."

5. A pregnant client, approximately 12 weeks' gestation, comes to the emergency department after calling the health care provider's office and reporting moderate vaginal bleeding. Assessment reveals cervical dilation and moderately strong abdominal cramps. The client reports that tissue has passed with the bleeding. The nurse interprets these findings to suggest which of the following?
   a. Threatened abortion
   b. Inevitable abortion
   c. Incomplete abortion
   d. Missed abortion

6. When administering magnesium sulphate to a client with preeclampsia, the nurse explains that this drug is given to:
   a. Reduce blood pressure
   b. Increase the progress of labour
   c. Prevent seizures
   d. Lower blood glucose levels

7. A client is being discharged after receiving treatment for a hydatidiform molar pregnancy. The nurse should include which of the following in the discharge teaching?
   a. Do not become pregnant for at least a year; use contraceptives to prevent it
   b. Have the client's blood pressure checked weekly in the clinic
   c. Rh immune globulin must be given within the next month
   d. An amniocentesis can detect a recurrence of this disorder in the future

CRITICAL THINKING EXERCISES

1. Suzanne is a 16-year-old primigravida, who presents to the perinatal clinic reporting continual nausea and vomiting for the past 3 days. The client states she is approximately 15 weeks pregnant and has been unable to hold anything down or take any fluids in without throwing up for the past 3 days. She reports she is dizzy and weak. On examination, Suzanne appears pale and anxious. Mucous membranes are dry, skin turgor is poor, and lips are dry and cracked.
   a. What is your impression of this condition?
   b. What risk factors does Suzanne have?
   c. What intervention is appropriate for this client?

2. An obese 39-year-old primigravida of African descent who is diagnosed with gestational hypertension presents to the prenatal clinic. History reveals that a sister developed preeclampsia during pregnancy. When describing her diet to the nurse, this client mentions that she tends to eat a lot of fast food.
   a. What risk factors does this client have that increase the risk for gestational hypertension?
   b. When assessing this client, what assessment findings would lead the nurse to suspect that this client has developed severe preeclampsia?

CHAPTER **WORKSHEET**

STUDY ACTIVITIES

1. Ask a community health maternity nurse how the signs and symptoms of gestational hypertension (including preeclampsia and eclampsia) are taught, and how effective efforts have been to reduce the incidence in the area.

2. Find a website designed to help parents who have suffered a pregnancy loss secondary to a spontaneous abortion. What is its audience level? Is the information up to date?

3. A pregnancy in which the blastocyst implants outside the uterus is a/an _____ pregnancy.

4. The most serious complication of hydatidiform mole is the development of _____ afterward.

5. Develop a teaching plan for a client with a multiple gestation. Discuss the increased risks associated with multiple gestation and signs and symptoms to monitor for those conditions.

BRINGING IT ALL TOGETHER: A CASE STUDY

A 21-year-old client presented to the local public health maternity clinic with a chief complaint of intermittent vaginal bleeding, abdominal cramping, and nausea. The stated last menstrual period was 8 weeks ago and a home pregnancy test prior to coming here was positive. The client was taking no medications and had no known drug allergies and admitted she was a half-pack a day smoker, but had been trying to quit.

Go to thePoint **to find questions to consider about this case.**

20

KEY TERMS

acquired immuno-
    deficiency
    syndrome (AIDS)
adolescence
anemia
fetal alcohol spectrum
    disorder (FASD)
gestational diabetes
    mellitus
glycosylated
    hemoglobin
    (HbA1C) level
human immuno-
    deficiency virus
    (HIV)
impaired fasting
    glucose
impaired glucose
    tolerance
multiple sclerosis (MS)
neonatal abstinence
    syndrome (NAS)
perinatal drug use
pica
rheumatoid arthritis
    (RA)
systemic lupus
    erythematosus (SLE)
teratogenicity
type 1 diabetes
type 2 diabetes

Nursing Management of the Pregnancy at Risk: Selected Health Conditions and Vulnerable Populations

Learning Objectives

Upon completion of the chapter, you will be able to:

1. Select at least two conditions present before pregnancy that can have a negative effect on a pregnancy.
2. Examine how a condition present before pregnancy can affect the client physiologically and psychologically during a pregnancy.
3. Evaluate the nursing assessment and management for a childbearing client with diabetes from that of a childbearing client without diabetes.
4. Explore how congenital and acquired heart conditions can affect a client's pregnancy.
5. Design the nursing assessment and management of a childbearing client with cardiovascular disorders and respiratory conditions.
6. Differentiate among the types of anemia affecting pregnant clients in terms of prevention and management.
7. Identify the nursing care needed for the childbearing client with an autoimmune disorder.
8. Compare the most common infections that can jeopardize a pregnancy and propose possible preventive strategies.
9. Develop a plan of care for the childbearing client who is HIV positive.
10. Outline the nurse's role in the prevention and management of adolescent pregnancy.
11. Determine the impact of pregnancy on a client over the age of 35.
12. Analyze the effects of substance abuse during pregnancy.

***Rose**, a thin 16-year-old who appears very pregnant, came into the clinic wheezing and having difficulty catching her breath. Rose had missed several previous prenatal visits but arrived at the clinic today in distress. Rose has a history of asthma since the age of 5. How might Rose's current condition affect the pregnancy? Is this picture typical of the pregnant client with asthma?*

INTRODUCTION

Pregnancy and childbirth are exciting yet complex facets within the continuum of health. Pregnancy is a special time in the lives of most childbearing people, but the 9-month waiting period can be very anxiety-producing if it is complicated by a medical condition which might jeopardize the fetal outcome. Ideally the childbearing person is free of any conditions that can affect a pregnancy, but in reality, many clients enter pregnancy with a multitude of health-related or psychosocial issues that can have a negative impact on the outcome. Currently, because of the obesity epidemic in the nation and people postponing pregnancies until later in their lives, nurses will increasingly see more clients with medical conditions that affect their pregnancies.

Many childbearing clients express the wish "I hope my baby is born healthy." Nurses can play a major role in helping this become a reality by educating clients before they become pregnant. Conditions such as diabetes, cardiac and respiratory disorders, **anemia**, autoimmune disorders, and specific infections frequently can be controlled through close prenatal management so that their impact on pregnancy is minimized. Nurses can provide pregnancy prevention strategies when counselling teenagers. Meeting the developmental needs of pregnant adolescents is a challenge. Finally, lifestyle factors can place many clients at risk during pregnancy, and nurses need to remain nonjudgmental when working with these special populations.

Chapter 19 described pregnancy-related conditions that place the client at risk. This chapter addresses common conditions that can have a negative impact on the pregnancy and special populations at risk, outlining appropriate nursing assessment and management for each condition or situation. The unique skills of nurses, in conjunction with the other members of the health care team, can increase the potential for a positive outcome in many high-risk pregnancies.

DIABETES MELLITUS

Diabetes mellitus is a chronic disease characterized by a relative lack of insulin or absence of the hormone that is necessary for glucose metabolism. The chronic hyperglycemia of diabetes is associated with long-term damage, dysfunction, and failure of the eyes, kidneys, nerves, heart, and blood vessels. Diabetes has been identified as a global health crisis by both the International Diabetes Federation and the World Health Organization. In Canada, 9.3% of the population are affected by diabetes, and the prevalence is estimated to increase to 12.1% by 2025. It was estimated that in 2015, prediabetes affected an additional 22.1% of the adult Canadian population (Houlden, 2018). Contributing factors to these increasing rates include inactive lifestyles, dietary changes, international migration of higher-risk populations, and the growing epidemic of childhood and adolescent obesity. We also know that the social determinants of health significantly influence the risk for developing diabetes, as persons with lower income are disproportionately affected. The rate of diabetes in Canada's Indigenous populations is three to five times higher than the general population; and Indigenous Canadians tend to be diagnosed at a younger age and experience higher rates of diabetes-related complications, which is compounded by the barriers they face to accessing culturally safe health care (Houlden, 2018).

The Diabetes Canada 2018 Clinical Practice Guidelines outline the classifications for diabetes, based on disease etiology (Punthakee, Goldenberg, & Katz, 2018). These groups include:

- **Type 1 diabetes:** absolute insulin deficiency resulting from pancreatic beta-cell destruction due to an autoimmune process or from unknown etiology; usually appears before the age of 30 years; approximately 5% of those diagnosed have type 1 diabetes.
- **Type 2 diabetes:** insulin resistance or deficiency (related to obesity, sedentary lifestyle); diagnosed primarily in adults older than 30 years of age but now being seen in children; the most common type of diabetes. It disproportionately affects persons from high-risk ethnic groups (African Canadian, Arab, Asian, Hispanic, Indigenous, and South Asian), as well as older adults.
- **Prediabetes:** characterized by hyperglycemia at a level lower than what qualifies as a diagnosis of diabetes; refers to **impaired fasting glucose** (fasting blood glucose level between 6.1 and 6.9 mmol/L), **impaired glucose tolerance** (blood glucose level between 7.8 and 11.0 mmol/L 2 hours following a 75-g oral glucose tolerance test), or altered glycated hemoglobin A1C levels (plasma A1C level between 6.0% and 6.4%); symptoms of diabetes are absent; newborns are at risk for being large for gestational age (LGA).
- **Gestational diabetes mellitus:** glucose intolerance with its onset, or recognition, during pregnancy, usually around the 24th week gestation. The prevalence of gestational diabetes has been increasing globally, along with increasing rates of obesity and increasing age of childbearing.

During pregnancy, diabetes typically is categorized into two groups: pre-existing diabetes (alteration in carbohydrate metabolism identified before conception), which includes individuals with type 1 or type 2 disease; and gestational diabetes, which develops during pregnancy.

The Diabetes Canada 2018 Clinical Practice Guidelines reaffirmed the recommendation for universal diabetes screening in all pregnancies (Feig et al., 2018). The Diabetes Canada Clinical Practice Guidelines Expert

TABLE 20.1	PREFERRED APPROACH FOR SCREENING AND DIAGNOSING HYPERGLYCEMIA IN PREGNANCY

Timing of screening:
- Early first trimester for individuals at high risk for developing gestational diabetes based on multiple clinical risk factors
- Between 24 and 28 weeks gestation for all childbearing persons

Test	Plasma Glucose Values	Interpretation
Step 1: 50-g glucose challenge test (GCT)	1-hour plasma glucose: • <7.8 mmol/L • 7.8–11.0 mmol/L • ≥11.1 mmol/L	• Normal • Elevated—further testing with 75-g oral glucose tolerance test (step 2) is required • Diagnostic—gestational diabetes
Step 2: 75-g oral glucose tolerance test (OGTT)	Fasting plasma glucose: • ≥5.3 mmol/L 1-hour plasma glucose: • ≥10.6 mmol/L 2-hour plasma glucose: • ≥9.0	One value met or exceeded for the fasting, 1-hour, or 2-hour plasma glucose, is diagnostic of gestational diabetes

Adapted from Feig, D. S., Berger, H., Donovan, L., Godbout, A., Kader, T., Keely, E., & Sanghera, R.; Diabetes Canada Clinical Practice Guidelines Expert Committee. (2018). 2018 Clinical practice guidelines. Diabetes and pregnancy. *Canadian Journal of Diabetes, 42,* S255–S282.

Committee has issued recommendations for the approach to screening and diagnosing hyperglycemia in pregnancy (see Table 20.1).

Gestational diabetes is associated with either neonatal complications such as macrosomia, hypoglycemia, and birth trauma or maternal complications such as preeclampsia and cesarean birth. All clients of childbearing age with diabetes should be counselled about the importance of strict glycemic control prior to conception. Observational studies show an increased risk of anencephaly, microcephaly, and congenital heart disease, which increases directly with elevations in A1C (Lapolla & Dalfrà, 2015).

Before the discovery of insulin in 1922, most clients with diabetes were infertile or experienced spontaneous abortion (March of Dimes, 2015a). During the past several decades, great strides have been made in improving the outcomes of childbearing persons with diabetes, but this chronic metabolic disorder remains a high-risk condition during pregnancy. A favourable outcome requires the client's commitment to adhere to frequent prenatal visits, dietary restrictions, self-monitoring of blood glucose (SMBG) levels, frequent laboratory tests, intensive fetal surveillance, and perhaps hospitalization.

Pathophysiology

Diabetes is a complex and progressive disease that has major societal and economic impact. It is a multifactorial disease, the pathophysiology of which involves not only the pancreas but also the liver, skeletal muscle, adipose tissue, gastrointestinal tract, brain, and kidney. Reduced sensitivity to insulin in the liver, muscle, and adipose tissue, and a progressive decline in pancreatic beta-cell function, leads to impaired insulin secretion, eventually resulting in hyperglycemia, the hallmark of diabetes (Cornell, 2015). Current understanding of the pathophysiology of gestational diabetes includes two key components. These are the existence of pancreatic beta-cell dysfunction prior to pregnancy and the unmasking of this problem by the development of insulin resistance during pregnancy, which requires enhanced insulin production to maintain normal blood glucose ranges.

Normal pregnancy is characterized by increasing peripheral resistance to insulin and a compensatory increase in insulin secretion. Therefore, pregnancy might be viewed as a stress test for the glucose homeostasis mechanisms. That is, clients who have some degree of chronic insulin resistance and compensatory increased insulin production resulting in beta-cell dysfunction before pregnancy may be unable to mount a sufficiently robust beta-cell response to pregnancy-mediated insulin resistance. Pregnancy is accompanied by insulin resistance, mediated by placental secretion of diabetogenic hormones. These and other metabolic changes that occur during pregnancy ensure that the fetus has an ample supply of nutrients.

With diabetes, there is a deficiency of or resistance to insulin. This alteration interferes with the body's ability to obtain essential nutrients for fuel and storage. If a pregnant client has pre-existing diabetes or develops gestational diabetes, the profound metabolic alterations that occur during pregnancy and that are necessary to support the growth and development of the fetus are greatly affected.

The pregnant client's metabolism is directed toward supplying adequate nutrition for the fetus. In pregnancy, placental hormones cause insulin resistance at a level that tends to parallel the growth of the fetoplacental unit. As the placenta grows, more placental hormones are

TABLE 20.2	DIABETES AND PREGNANCY: EFFECTS ON THE PREGNANT CLIENT AND FETUS

Effects on the Client	Effects on the Fetus/Neonate
• Hydramnios due to fetal diuresis caused by hyperglycemia • Gestational hypertension of unknown etiology • Ketoacidosis due to uncontrolled hyperglycemia • Preterm labour secondary to premature membrane rupture • Stillbirth in pregnancies complicated by ketoacidosis and poor glucose control • Hypoglycemia as glucose is diverted to the fetus (occurring in first trimester) • Urinary tract infections resulting from excess glucose in the urine (glucosuria), which promotes bacterial growth • Chronic monilial vaginitis due to glucosuria, which promotes growth of yeast • Difficult labour, cesarean birth, postpartum hemorrhage secondary to an overdistended uterus to accommodate a macrosomic infant	• Cord prolapse secondary to polyhydramnios and abnormal fetal presentation • Congenital anomaly due to hyperglycemia in the first trimester (cardiac problems, neural tube defects, skeletal deformities, and genitourinary problems) • Macrosomia resulting from hyperinsulinemia stimulated by fetal hyperglycemia • Birth trauma due to increased size of fetus, which complicates the birthing process (shoulder dystocia) • Preterm birth secondary to polyhydramnios and an aging placenta, which places the fetus in jeopardy if the pregnancy continues • Fetal asphyxia secondary to fetal hyperglycemia and hyperinsulinemia • Intrauterine growth restriction secondary to maternal vascular impairment and decreased placental perfusion, which restricts growth • Perinatal death due to poor placental perfusion and hypoxia • Respiratory distress syndrome resulting from poor surfactant production secondary to hyperinsulinemia inhibits the production of phospholipids that make up the surfactant • Polycythemia due to excessive red blood cell (RBC) production in response to hypoxia • Hyperbilirubinemia due to excessive RBC breakdown from hypoxia and an immature liver unable to break down bilirubin • Neonatal hypoglycemia resulting from ongoing hyperinsulinemia after the placenta is removed • Subsequent childhood obesity and carbohydrate intolerance

Adapted from Cunningham, F. G., Leveno, K. J., Bloom, S. L., Spong, C., Dashe, J., Hoffman, B. L., . . . Sheffield, J. S. (2014). *Williams' obstetrics* (24th ed.). New York: McGraw-Hill Professional Publishing; Moore, T. R. (2015). Diabetes mellitus and pregnancy. *eMedicine.* Retrieved from http://emedicine.medscape.com/article/127547; and March of Dimes. (2015a). *Gestational diabetes.* Retrieved from http://www.marchofdimes.com/pregnancy/gestational-diabetes.aspx.

secreted. Human placental lactogen (hPL) and growth hormone (somatotropin) increase in direct correlation with the growth of placental tissue, rising throughout the last 20 weeks of pregnancy and causing insulin resistance. Subsequently, insulin secretion increases to overcome the resistance of these two hormones. In the childbearing client without diabetes, the pancreas can respond to the demands for increased insulin production to maintain normal glucose levels throughout the pregnancy (Toledano, Hadar, & Hod, 2015). However, the client with diabetes during pregnancy cannot cope with changes in metabolism resulting from insufficient insulin to meet the needs during gestation.

Over the course of pregnancy, insulin resistance does change. It peaks in the last trimester to provide more nutrients to the fetus. The insulin resistance typically results in postprandial hyperglycemia, although some clients also have an elevated fasting blood glucose level (Aktas et al., 2014). With this increased demand on the pancreas in late pregnancy, clients with diabetes cannot accommodate the increased insulin demand; glucose levels rise as a result of insulin deficiency, leading to hyperglycemia. Subsequently, the childbearing person

and the fetus can experience major problems, as shown in Table 20.2.

Screening

Currently, there are inconsistent standards around the world for how childbearing clients are tested for gestational diabetes, as well cutoff values to diagnose it. The Society of Obstetricians and Gynecologists of Canada (SOGC) and Diabetes Canada currently recommend early screening in the first trimester for all pregnant clients who are at higher risk for developing gestational diabetes (Berger, Gagnon, & Sermer, 2016; Feig et al., 2018). This includes those who are over 35 years of age, are overweight (body mass index ≥ 30 kg/m²), have polycystic ovarian syndrome, a history of a previous pregnancy with gestational diabetes, a positive family history of diabetes, or are a member of a high-risk population (African Canadian, Arab, Asian, Hispanic, Indigenous, South Asian). All childbearing clients not known to have pre-existing diabetes, including those high-risk individuals who received a normal first trimester screen for diabetes, will be screened at 24 to 28 weeks of gestation. A client with abnormal plasma glucose results early in pregnancy may have had diabetes before the pregnancy, and the fetus is at great risk for congenital anomalies. For those individuals with the onset, or first recognition, of diabetes during pregnancy, testing with a 75-g oral glucose tolerance test should take place between 6 weeks and 6 months postpartum to detect diabetes and prediabetes.

The preferred approach to screening is with a 2-step approach (Berger et al., 2016; Feig et al., 2018). The initial step in screening is with a 50-g glucose challenge test, in which a 50-g oral glucose load is given, without regard to the timing or content of the last meal. Blood glucose is measured 1 hour later; a level of 11.1 mmol/L or greater is diagnostic of gestational diabetes, a level between 7.8 and 11.0 mmol/L is abnormal and requires further testing. At this time a 2-hour oral glucose tolerance test is done. One or more abnormal results on the 2-hour oral glucose tolerance test confirm a diagnosis of gestational diabetes:

- Fasting blood glucose level: greater than, or equal to 5.3 mmol/L
- At 1 hour: greater than, or equal to 10.6 mmol/L
- At 2 hours: greater than, or equal to 9.0 mmol/L

Therapeutic Management

Care for the Client With Pre-Existing Diabetes

Pre-existing diabetes is a significant public health problem that increases the risk for structural birth defects affecting perinatal outcomes. Clients who have pre-existing diabetes (the alteration in carbohydrate metabolism is identified before conception) need comprehensive prenatal care. Achieving good metabolic control during the period prior to conception is essential to reducing

congenital malformations that can occur in pregnancies complicated by diabetes. The primary goals of care are to maintain glycemic control and minimize the risks of the disease on the fetus. Key aspects of treatment include nutritional management, exercise, insulin regimens, and close surveillance of the client and the fetus (Fig. 20.1).

Preconception counselling is essential for the client with pre-existing diabetes to ensure that the disease state is stable. The challenge is that it is estimated that as many as half of all pregnancies are unplanned (Public Health Association of Canada, 2017). Thus, clients with chronic medical conditions such as diabetes might not have the opportunity to take steps to optimize management of their diabetes before becoming pregnant. When preconception care is possible, clients with pre-existing diabetes should be taught how to improve their metabolic control prior to conception to reduce the risk of birth defects. Nurses caring for clients of reproductive age can contribute to preconception care by helping to counsel someone who is prediabetic to avoid progression to diabetes and its attendant risks during pregnancy. The goals of preconception care are to:

- Provide counselling that includes the importance of glycemic control prior to pregnancy, the impact of body mass index (BMI) on pregnancy outcomes, and the importance of folic acid
- Strive to achieve a glycosylated hemoglobin A1C level of ≤7.0% (≤6.5% if this level can be reached safely)
- Offer counselling on using effective contraception until stable glycemic control is achieved
- Evaluate antihyperglycemic agents for their safety for use in pregnancy
- Identify and evaluate long-term diabetic complications such as retinopathy, nephropathy, neuropathy, cardiovascular disease (CVD), and hypertension (Feig et al., 2018; Gabbay-Benziv, Reece, Wang, & Yang, 2015).

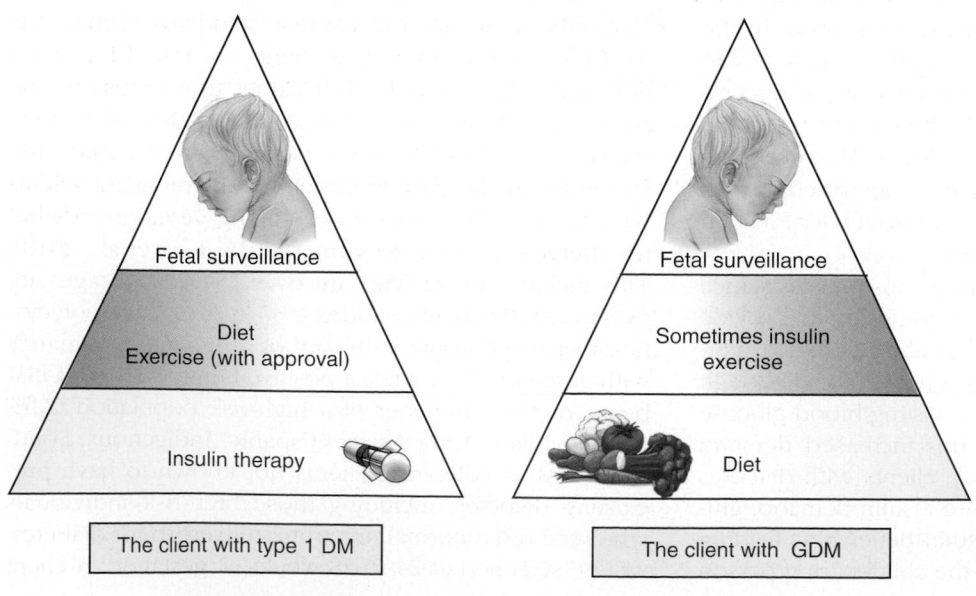

FIGURE 20.1 Treatment overview for diabetes in pregnancy. For clients with pregestational type 1 DM, the foundation of glycemic management is insulin therapy along with dietary management, exercise, and fetal surveillance. For the client who develops gestational diabetes, dietary modification is generally the foundation of treatment. Some clients may require insulin along with dietary modifications, whereas others will not require insulin therapy at all. Exercise and fetal surveillance are also important facets of care.

Fetal surveillance

Diet
Exercise (with approval)

Insulin therapy

The client with type 1 DM

Fetal surveillance

Sometimes insulin
exercise

Diet

The client with GDM

Excellent control of blood glucose, as evidenced by normal fasting blood glucose levels and **glycosylated hemoglobin (HbA1C) levels** (a measurement of the average glucose levels during the past 100 to 120 days), is crucial to achieve the best pregnancy outcome. A glycosylated hemoglobin level of less than 7% indicates good control. A childbearing client with pre-existing diabetes has up to a ninefold increase in birth defects, compared with the rate seen in nondiabetic pregnancies, if they do not have glycemic control (Mitanchez et al., 2015).

Preconception counselling is also important in helping to reduce the risk of congenital malformation. The most common malformations associated with diabetes occur in the renal, cardiac, skeletal, and central nervous systems. Since these defects occur by the eighth week of gestation, preconception counselling is critical. The rate of congenital anomalies in clients with pre-existing diabetes can be reduced if excellent glycemic control is achieved at the time of conception (Simeone et al., 2015). This information needs to be stressed with all clients with diabetes who are contemplating a pregnancy. In addition, the client with pre-existing diabetes needs to be evaluated for complications of diabetes. This evaluation should be part of baseline screening and continuing assessment during pregnancy.

Care During Pregnancy for the Client With Pre-Existing and Gestational Diabetes

Lifestyle modification, nutritional changes, and encouragement of physical activities form the primary mode of therapy for diabetes during pregnancy. Therapeutic management for the client with pre-existing and gestational diabetes mellitus focuses on tight glucose control. Diabetes Canada recommends maintaining a fasting blood glucose level below 5.3 mmol/L, with 1-hour postprandial levels below 7.8 mmol/L, and 2-hour postprandial levels below 6.7 mmol/L (Feig et al., 2018). In addition, clients with pre-existing diabetes would aim for a glycosylated hemoglobin A1C level of less than, or equal to 6.5%. Such tight control has been advocated because it is associated with a reduction in macrosomia and other perinatal complications. In addition, prepregnancy weight and weight gain during pregnancy appear to be significant and independent risk factors for macrosomia in clients with gestational diabetes (Grandy, Purnell, Thornburg, & Marshall, 2015).

Nutritional management focuses on maintaining balanced glucose levels and providing enough energy and nutrients for the childbearing person, while avoiding ketosis, and minimizing the risk of hypoglycemia in clients treated with insulin. Nutrition therapy is the cornerstone of therapy for clients with gestational diabetes. Clients should receive ethically appropriate nutritional advice on how to change their dietary habits from a dietitian. The diet counselling must be in keeping with their present cultural dietary patterns and not radically different

to become adopted and followed. If rice is a staple of a Chinese client's diet, then it must be incorporated into the diet counselling plan and not eliminated (He et al., 2015). A low-glycemic index diet is considered safe and has positive effects on the glycemic control and pregnancy outcomes for those with pre-existing type 2 diabetes and gestational diabetes. A moderately low carbohydrate diet with a carbohydrate content of 40% of the calories results in good glycemic control for most (Roskjær, Andersen, Ronneby, Damm, & Mathiesen, 2015). Eating for two during pregnancy for a client who has diabetes means eating not volume for two, but rather quality and timing to support both the client and the fetus. Childbearing clients who receive dietary instruction and follow it have been shown to have a better pregnancy outcome than those who do not receive dietary advice (Ma et al., 2015).

Exercise is another important component of comprehensive prenatal care for the childbearing client with diabetes. Regular exercise helps maintain glucose control by increasing the uptake of glucose into the cells and decreasing central obesity, hypertension, and dyslipidemia, which will ultimately decrease the client's insulin requirements (Jordan, Engstrom, Marfell, & Farley, 2014). Regular physical activity has been proven to result in marked benefits for the client and the fetus. Client benefits include improved cardiovascular function, limited pregnancy weight gain, decreased musculoskeletal discomfort, reduced incidence of muscle cramps and lower limb edema, mood stability, and reduction of gestational diabetes mellitus and gestational hypertension. Fetal benefits include decreased fat mass, improved stress tolerance, and advanced neurobehavioural maturation. Research also suggests the role of physical activity in prevention of gestational diabetes (Bain et al., 2015).

PHARMACOLOGIC THERAPY FOR GESTATIONAL DIABETES

For the client with gestational diabetes, nutritional management and exercise may be all that is necessary. Pharmacologic therapy is considered if nutrition and exercise fail to maintain target glucose levels. Blood glucose levels in the client can be controlled by nutritional therapy and exercise, but in uncontrolled cases, where target glycemic levels cannot be reached, insulin is also required. Insulin, which does not cross the placenta, historically has been the medication of choice for treating hyperglycemia in pregnancy and currently remains the first-line pharmacologic therapy. Insulin is calculated based on the client's weight. Combining intermediate and short-acting insulin yields the best result for most clients. Two insulin doses are given daily with two thirds of the total insulin in the morning to cover energy needs of the active day and one third at night.

Oral Medications for Management of Gestational Diabetes. Clients tend to manage oral medications better than insulin, so the standard of care may be moving toward the oral route (King et al., 2015). Some oral hypoglycemic medications are considered safe and may be used if nutrition and exercise are not adequate alone. Recent studies have examined the use of oral hypoglycemic medications in pregnancy with much success. Metformin can be used as an alternate to insulin, though information should be provided to the client that the medication does cross the placenta, and longer-term studies are not yet available (Feig et al., 2018). If clients do not tolerate or achieve adequate glycemic control with metformin, glyburide may be used. Perinatal outcomes are similar to those seen in clients who are treated with insulin. Oral hypoglycemic agents, however, must be further investigated to determine their safety with confidence and provide better treatment options for diabetes in pregnancy. Insulin, however, still has an important role to play in gestational diabetes (Buschur, Brown, & Wyckoff, 2015). Gestational diabetes offers a window of opportunity, which needs to be seized, for prevention of diabetes in future life (Nagtalon-Ramos, 2014).

The Society of Obstetricians and Gynecologists of Canada recommends that clients with pre-existing or gestational diabetes receive care by a multidisciplinary team (Berger et al., 2016). Diabetes Canada recommends that nutritional counselling be provided by a registered dietitian to include nutrition, weight, and blood glucose management (Feig et al., 2018). Diabetes Canada also recommends that if clients are unable to achieve glycemic targets within 2 weeks of initiating nutrition and physical activity therapy, then pharmacologic therapy is indicated.

Insulin for Management of Gestational Diabetes. Insulin remains the medication of choice for glycemic control if oral medications, diet, or exercise fail to yield results in pregnant and lactating clients with any type of diabetes (Moore, 2015). Generally, insulin doses are reduced in the first trimester to prevent hypoglycemia resulting from increased insulin sensitivity as well as from nausea and vomiting. Newer short-acting insulins such as lispro (Humalog) and aspart (NovoLog), which do not cross the placenta, may help reduce postprandial hyperglycemia, episodes of hypoglycemia between meals. Changes in diet and activity level add to the need for changes in insulin dosages throughout pregnancy.

Insulin regimens vary, and controversy remains over the best strategy for insulin delivery in pregnancy. Many health care providers use a split-dose therapy (two thirds of the daily dose in the morning and the remaining one third in the evening). Others advocate the use of an insulin pump to deliver a continuous subcutaneous insulin infusion. Regardless of which protocol is used, frequent blood glucose measurements are necessary, and the insulin dosage is adjusted on the basis of daily glucose levels. Insulin therapy or oral hypoglycemic agents, in addition to diet and exercise, are main elements of achieving glycemic control. See Evidence-Based Practice 20.1.

EVIDENCE-BASED PRACTICE 20.1   **PREVENTION OF GESTATIONAL DIABETES IN CHILDBEARING CLIENTS WITH RISK FACTORS FOR GESTATIONAL DIABETES: A SYSTEMATIC REVIEW AND META-ANALYSIS OF RANDOMIZED TRIALS**

STUDY

Gestational diabetes mellitus (GDM) is defined as the diabetes diagnosed during pregnancy that is not clearly overt diabetes. According to this definition, glycemic levels meeting the thresholds of overt diabetes are considered to have pre-existing diabetes and the rest are given diagnosis of GDM. The objective of the systematic review was to identify any intervention that could be used for primary prevention of gestational diabetes in those with risk factors for it.

A systematic review and meta-analysis was conducted by including randomized controlled trials comparing any form of therapeutic intervention in comparison to usual antenatal care. A literature search was conducted using electronic databases together with a hand search of relevant journals and conference proceedings.

Findings

A total of 2,422 clients from 14 randomized trials were included which compared diet, exercise, lifestyle changes, and metformin with standard care in clients with risk factors for gestational diabetes. Dietary intervention was associated with statistically significant lower incidence of gestational diabetes and gestational hypertension compared to standard of care. There was no statistically significant difference in the incidence of gestational diabetes with exercise, lifestyle changes, or metformin used compared to standard care.

Nursing Implications

Based on these findings, nurses can encourage healthy dietary changes as a primary prevention strategy to prevent gestational diabetes for high-risk clients, since this intervention was shown to be a statistically significant intervention over standard care. Instructing them on health dietary habits either preconceptually or at the first prenatal visit may help prevent gestational diabetes and turn the tide for better pregnancy outcomes for both the client and the infant.

Adapted from Madhuvrata, P., Govinden, G., Bustani, R., Song, S., & Farrell, T. A. (2015). Prevention of gestational diabetes in pregnant women with risk factors for gestational diabetes: A systematic review and meta-analysis of randomized trials. *Obstetric Medicine, 8*(2), 68–85.

Close surveillance of the client and the fetus is also essential. Frequent laboratory tests are done during pregnancy to monitor the client's status and glucose control. Fetal surveillance via diagnostic testing aids in evaluating fetal well-being and assisting in determining the best time for birth.

Care During and After Labour for the Client With Pre-Existing or Gestational Diabetes

For the labouring client with diabetes, intravenous saline or lactated Ringer's is given and blood glucose levels are monitored hourly. Glucose levels are maintained between 4.0 and 7.0 mmol/L throughout labour to reduce the likelihood of neonatal hypoglycemia. If necessary, an infusion of regular insulin and/or dextrose may be given to maintain this level (King et al., 2015). If the client was receiving insulin during the pregnancy, adjustments in dosage may be necessary after birth since glucose diversion across the placenta to supply the growing fetus is no longer present and insulin resistance is now removed. Frequently, the client with gestational diabetes can remain controlled through diet and weight management; the client with type 1 diabetes usually returns to prepregnant levels of insulin administration (Kim, 2014).

After giving birth, the overt glycemic abnormalities of gestational diabetes usually resolve. This phenomenon suggests that the diabetes is transient and that the consequences of gestational diabetes end with the birth of the infant. However, for the client, childbirth is not the end of the story. The diagnosis of gestational diabetes heralds future health risks. Knowledge of this "failed" stress test conveys new information about the future risk for type 2 diabetes, which warrants further screening and prevention efforts during the postpartum period and beyond.

Nursing Assessment

Nursing assessment begins at the first prenatal visit. A thorough history and physical examination in conjunction with specific laboratory and diagnostic testing aids in developing an individualized plan of care for the client with diabetes.

Health History and Physical Examination

For the client with pre-existing diabetes, obtain a thorough history of the pre-existing diabetic condition. Ask about the duration of disease, management of glucose levels (insulin injections, insulin pump, or oral hypoglycemic agents), dietary adjustments, presence of vascular complications and current vascular status, current insulin regimen, and technique used for glucose testing. Review any information that they may have received as part of preconception counselling and measures that were implemented during this time.

Be knowledgeable about the client's nutritional requirements and assess the adequacy and pattern of their dietary intake. Assess blood glucose self-monitoring in terms of technique, frequency, and their ability to adjust the insulin dose based on the changing patterns. Ask about the frequency of episodes of hypoglycemia or hyperglycemia to ascertain the client's ability to recognize and treat them. Continue to assess for signs and symptoms of hypo- and hyperglycemia.

During antepartum visits, assess the client's knowledge about the disease, including the signs and symptoms of hypoglycemia, hyperglycemia, and diabetic ketoacidosis, insulin administration techniques, and the impact of pregnancy on their chronic condition. If possible, have the client demonstrate their technique for blood glucose monitoring and insulin administration for correctness. It is essential that the nurse keeps in mind that there is a huge learning curve for clients with diabetes concerning the need for dietary changes, frequency of blood glucose monitoring, exercise, and insulin or oral medication administration. Suddenly, the client is expected to make rapid changes in their life, which can be overwhelming. The nurse can help facilitate these changes by exercising patience and understanding and reinforcing all verbal instructions with written material. Frequent encouragement is also needed to assist the client with their lifestyle changes. Although the client may have had diabetes for some time, do not assume that they have a firm knowledge base about the disease process or management of it (Fig. 20.2).

Assess the client's risk for gestational diabetes at the first prenatal visit. The clinical presentation of diabetes mellitus in pregnancy may be quite varied, but the classical triad of the symptoms of polydipsia, polyphagia, and polyuria may not be reported by most clients during pregnancy. Instead, the client may present with previous history

FIGURE 20.2 The nurse is demonstrating the technique for self-blood glucose monitoring with a pregnant client who has diabetes.

of medical complications of diabetes (chronic hypertension/chronic renal disease) and obesity. All of these conditions can influence pregnancy outcome. Diabetes Canada recommends early screening for any childbearing clients with multiple risk factors for developing gestational diabetes. Factors that place a client at high risk include:

- Previous infant with congenital anomaly (skeletal, renal, central nervous system, cardiac)
- History of gestational diabetes or polyhydramnios in a previous pregnancy
- History of prediabetes
- First-degree relative with diabetes
- Medications: corticosteroids or antipsychotics
- Age 35 years or older
- Polycystic ovarian syndrome
- Multiple pregnancy (twins, triplets)
- Previous delivery of a macrosomic infant (weighing more than 4,000 g)
- Previous unexplained fetal demise or neonatal death
- Obesity (body mass index [BMI] >30)
- Hypertension before pregnancy or in early pregnancy
- Member of a high-risk group (African Canadian, Arab, Asian, Hispanic, Indigenous, South Asian descent, or low socioeconomic status)
- Signs and symptoms of glucose intolerance (polyuria, polyphagia, polydipsia, fatigue)
- Presence of glycosuria (Ekoe, Goldenberg, & Katz, 2018; Gupta, Kalra, Baruah, Singla, & Kalra, 2015).

Clients with clinical characteristics consistent with a high risk for gestational diabetes should undergo glucose testing as soon as feasible.

Provide a close ongoing assessment throughout the antepartum period. Clients with gestational diabetes mellitus are at increased risk for preeclampsia and glucose control–related complications such as hypoglycemia, hyperglycemia, and ketoacidosis. Gestational diabetes of any severity increases the risk of fetal macrosomia, as noted earlier. It is also associated with an increased frequency of hypertensive disorders of pregnancy and operative births. This may be the result of fetal growth disorders (American Diabetes Association [ADA], 2015a). Even though gestational diabetes is diagnosed during pregnancy, it may have been present before the pregnancy. Therefore, monitor the client closely for signs and symptoms of possible complications.

Also assess the client's psychosocial adaptation to their condition. This assessment is critical to gauge their readiness for a change in regimen or the addition of a new regimen throughout pregnancy. Identify their support systems and note any financial constraints, because they will need intense monitoring and frequent fetal surveillance.

Laboratory and Diagnostic Testing

The results of laboratory and diagnostic tests provide valuable information about the well-being of the client and the fetus. Clients with pre-existing diabetes and those discovered to have gestational diabetes require ongoing surveillance during pregnancy to promote the best outcome.

SURVEILLANCE

Surveillance of the childbearing client may include the following:

- Urine check for protein (may indicate the need for further evaluation for preeclampsia) and for nitrates and leukocyte esterase (may indicate a urinary tract infection)
- Urine check for ketones (may indicate the need for evaluation of eating habits)
- Eye examination in the first trimester to evaluate the retina for vascular changes
- Monitor hemoglobin A1C levels in those with pre-existing diabetes (Jordan et al., 2014).

Fetal surveillance may include ultrasound to provide information about fetal growth, activity, and amniotic fluid volume and to validate gestational age. Alpha-fetoprotein levels may be obtained to detect congenital anomalies such as an open neural tube or ventral wall defects of omphalocele or gastroschisis, and a fetal echocardiogram may be necessary to rule out cardiac anomalies. Ultrasound assessments of fetal growth and amniotic fluid volume are recommended every 3 to 4 weeks beginning at 28 weeks' gestation (Berger et al., 2016). A biophysical profile helps to monitor fetal well-being and may be performed with or without a nonstress test weekly after 36 weeks' gestation. If the childbearing client has other coexisting comorbidities, poor glycemic control, or additional perinatal complications (such as a fetus that is small or large for gestational age, a previous stillbirth, or hypertension) additional surveillance with Doppler flow studies may be indicated.

Nursing Management

The ideal outcome of every pregnancy is a healthy newborn and client. Nurses can be pivotal in realizing this positive outcome for childbearing persons with pre-existing or gestational diabetes by implementing measures to minimize risks and complications. Since the client with diabetes is considered to be at high risk, antepartum visits may occur more frequently. This allows clients the opportunity to meet with a range of multidisciplinary providers who can support them in working through the various aspects of their diabetes management plan aimed at reducing risks for additional perinatal complications. This provides the nurse with numerous opportunities for ongoing assessment, education, and counselling (Nursing Care Plan 20.1, at the end of the chapter).

Promoting Optimal Glucose Control

At each visit, review the client's SMBG record, in addition to any laboratory test results. Reinforce the need to

FIGURE 20.3 **The pregnant client with diabetes eating a nutritious meal to ensure adequate glucose control.**

perform SMBG (usually four times a day but is individualized based on the type of management and stability of glycemic control, monitoring both pre and post meals) and to keep a record of the results. Also assess the client's techniques for SMBG and for administering insulin if ordered and offer support and guidance. If the client is receiving insulin therapy, assist with any changes needed if glucose levels are not controlled. Obtain a urine specimen and check for glucose, protein, and ketones. Ask the client if they have had any episodes of hypoglycemia and what was done to alleviate them. Discuss dietary measures related to blood glucose control (Fig. 20.3). In addition, recommend the following:

- Avoid weight loss and dieting during pregnancy.
- Ensure that food intake is adequate to prevent ketone formation and promote healthy gestational weight gain.
- Eat three meals a day plus three snacks to promote glycemic control:
  - 40% of calories from good-quality complex carbohydrates.
  - 35% of calories from protein sources.
  - 25% of calories from unsaturated fats.
  - Small frequent feedings throughout the day are recommended.
  - Bedtime snacks are recommended for all clients.
  - Include protein and fat at each meal (National Diabetes Information Clearing House, 2015).

Take Note!

Nutrient requirements and recommendations for weight gain for the childbearing client with diabetes are the same as those for the nondiabetic childbearing client.

If feasible, arrange for consultation with a registered dietitian to individualize the dietary plan. Also encourage the client to participate in an exercise program that includes at least three sessions lasting at least 30 minutes daily. Exercise may lessen the need for insulin or dosage adjustments.

When caring for the labouring clients with pre-existing or gestational diabetes, adjust the intravenous flow rate and the rate of supplemental regular insulin based on the blood glucose levels as ordered, to maintain plasma glucose levels between 4.0 and 7.0 mmol/L (Feig et al., 2018). Monitor blood glucose levels hourly, and intravenous dextrose solution should be available at the bedside to treat hypoglycemia below target levels. Monitor fetal heart rate patterns throughout labour to detect atypical or abnormal. Assess the client's vital signs every hour, in addition to assessing urinary output and urine ketone levels. If a cesarean birth is scheduled, monitor the client's blood glucose levels hourly and administer insulin or glucose based on the blood glucose levels, as ordered.

After birth, monitor blood glucose levels every 2 to 4 hours for the first 48 hours to determine the client's insulin need and continue intravenous fluid administration as ordered. Encourage breastfeeding to assist in maintaining good glucose control. For the client with pre-existing diabetes, expect insulin needs to decrease rapidly after birth: they may be reduced by half of the antepartum dose as meals are started (King et al., 2015). Some clients may return to their prepregnancy insulin dosage. In addition, the nurse must monitor the infant of the diabetic client for common problems seen in them, which include macrosomia, respiratory distress syndrome, hypoglycemia, polycythemia, hypocalcemia, hyperbilirubinemia, and a variety of congenital anomalies (Green, 2016).

The therapy plan after childbirth is individualized. If recommended dietary modifications are carried out along with weight loss, the client with gestational diabetes may return to their normal glucose levels. This is also true for the client with pre-existing diabetes, except that they will return to their prepregnancy insulin administration levels. This provides the nurse with a wonderful opportunity to reinforce healthy lifestyle interventions on the postpartum unit. Nurses can also become involved with community-based education to continue to offer their expertise.

Preventing Complications

Assess the client closely for signs and symptoms of complications at each visit. Anticipate possible complications and plan appropriate interventions or referrals. Check the client's blood pressure for changes and evaluate for proteinuria when obtaining a urine specimen. These might suggest the development of preeclampsia. Measure the fundal height and review gestational age. Note any discrepancies between the fundal height and gestational age or a sudden increase in uterine growth. These may suggest polyhydramnios.

Encourage the client to perform daily fetal movement counts to monitor fetal well-being. Tell them specifically when they should notify their health care provider. Also prepare the client if there is need for additional laboratory and diagnostic testing to evaluate fetal status. Assist with serial ultrasounds to monitor fetal growth and with nonstress tests and biophysical profiles to assess fetal well-being.

Consider This

Scott and I had been busy all day setting up the new crib in our nursery, and we finally sat down to rest. I was due any day, and we had been putting this off until we had a long weekend to complete the task. I was excited to think about all the cute things that decorated the room. I was sure that my new baby would love it as much as I loved them already. A few days later I barely noticed any fetal movement, but I thought that the baby must be as tired as I was by this point.

That night I went into labour and kept looking at the worried faces of the nurses and the midwife in attendance. I had been diagnosed with gestational diabetes a few months ago and had tried to follow the instructions regarding diet and exercise, but old habits are hard to change when you are 38 years old. I was finally told after a short time in the labour unit that they couldn't pick up a fetal heartbeat and an ultrasound was to be done—still no heartbeat was detected. Scott and I were finally told that our baby was a stillborn. All I could think about was that they would never get to see the beautiful nursery.

Providing Client Education and Counselling

The pregnant client with diabetes requires counselling and education about the need for strict glucose monitoring, diet and exercise, and signs and symptoms of complications. Encourage the client and their family to make any lifestyle changes needed to optimize the pregnancy outcome. Providing dietary education, weight control measures, and lifestyle advice that extends beyond pregnancy may lower the risk that the client will have gestational diabetes in subsequent pregnancies as well as type 2 diabetes (Hashemi-Beni et al., 2015). At each visit, stress the importance of performing blood glucose screening and documenting the results. With proper instruction, the client and their family will be able to cope with all the changes in their body during pregnancy (Teaching Guidelines 20.1).

Teaching Guidelines 20.1
TEACHING FOR THE PREGNANT CLIENT WITH DIABETES

- Be sure to keep your appointments for frequent prenatal visits and tests for fetal well-being.
- Perform blood glucose self-monitoring as directed, usually before each meal and at bedtime. Keep a record of your results and call your health care provider with any levels outside the established range. Bring your results to each prenatal visit.
- Perform daily "fetal kick counts." Document them and report any decrease in activity.
- Drink eight to ten 8-oz glasses of water each day to prevent bladder infections and maintain hydration.
- Wear proper, well-fitted footwear when walking to prevent injury.
- Engage in a regular exercise program such as walking to aid in glucose control, but avoid exercising in temperature extremes.
- Consider breastfeeding your infant to lower your blood glucose levels.
- If you are taking insulin:
  - Administer the correct dose of insulin at the correct time every day.
  - Eat breakfast within 30 minutes after injecting regular insulin to prevent a reaction.
  - Plan meals, as well as snacks, at a fixed time to prevent extremes in glucose levels.
- Avoid simple sugars (cake, candy, cookies), which raise blood glucose levels.
- Know the signs and symptoms of hypoglycemia and treatment needed:
  - Sweating, tremors, cold, clammy skin, headache
  - Feeling hungry, blurred vision, disorientation, irritability
  - Treatment: Drink 150 mL of juice or 15-g glucose in the form of tablets
- Carry "glucose boosters" (such as Life Savers) to treat hypoglycemia.
- Know the signs and symptoms of hyperglycemia and treatment needed:
  - Dry mouth, frequent urination, excessive thirst, rapid breathing
  - Feeling tired, flushed, hot skin, headache, drowsiness
  - Treatment: Notify health care provider, because hospitalization may be needed
- Wear a diabetic identification bracelet at all times.
- Wash your hands frequently to prevent infections.
- Report any signs and symptoms of illness, infection, and dehydration to your health care provider, because these can affect blood glucose control.

Review discussions about the timing of birth and the rationale. Counsel the client about the possibility for induction of labour between 38 and 40 weeks' gestation, based on glycemic control and other comorbid conditions, to reduce the risk of stillbirth (Feig et al., 2018). Also discuss the increased risk of cesarean birth and shoulder dystocia related to and having an infant that is large for gestational age.

Take Note!

In the client with well-controlled diabetes, birth is typically not induced before term unless complications arise, such as preeclampsia or fetal compromise. An early delivery date might be set for the client with poorly controlled diabetes or a large-sized fetus who is having complications.

Instruct the client about the benefits of breastfeeding related to blood glucose control. Breastfeeding helps to normalize blood glucose levels. Therefore, encourage the client to breastfeed their newborn. Also teach the client receiving insulin for diabetes that their insulin needs after birth will drastically decrease.

For the client with gestational diabetes, the focus is on lifestyle education. Clients with gestational diabetes have a greater than 50% increased risk of developing type 2 diabetes (ADA, 2015d). Inform the client that a repeat oral glucose tolerance test will need to be done between 6 weeks and 6 months postpartum. Clients with normal results at that visit typically are screened every 3 years thereafter, based on Diabetes Canada recommendations for diabetes screening (Ekoe et al., 2018). Teach the client how to maintain an optimal weight to reduce their risk of developing diabetes. If necessary, refer the client to a dietitian to help outline a balanced nutritious diet.

CARDIOVASCULAR DISORDERS

Despite an increase in awareness of a wide range of health concerns, the myth still exists that cardiovascular disease (CVD) primarily affects male-sexed persons. Heart disease is the leading cause for premature death in female-sexed persons in Canada, and affects those of Afro-Caribbean, Chinese, and South Asian decent as well as Canada's Indigenous peoples at much higher rates (Heart and Stroke Foundation, 2018). Risk factors such as hypertension, high blood cholesterol level, smoking, lack of physical activity, and obesity increase the probability of developing CVD. Menopause, gestational diabetes, oral contraceptive use, and bilateral oophorectomy in premenopausal clients also affect the risk of CVD (Chomistek et al., 2015).

Approximately 3% of childbearing persons have cardiac disease, which is responsible for 10% to 25%

of deaths in pregnancy (Cunningham et al., 2014). The prevalence of cardiac disease is increasing as a result of risk factors, including cigarette smoking, diabetes, and stress. As individuals are delaying childbearing, the incidence of cardiac disease in pregnancy will continue to increase. The cardiovascular adaptations during pregnancy are well tolerated by the normal heart, but may unveil undiagnosed underlying heart disease, or tip the hemodynamic balance and lead to decompensation in those with existing heart disease (Harvey, Coffman, & Miller, 2015).

Rheumatic heart disease used to represent the majority of cardiac conditions during pregnancy, but congenital heart disease now constitutes nearly half of all cases of heart disease encountered during pregnancy. Classic symptoms of heart disease mimic common symptoms of late pregnancy, such as palpitations, shortness of breath with exertion, and occasional chest pain. Few childbearing persons with heart disease die during pregnancy, but they are at risk for other complications, such as heart failure, arrhythmias, and stroke. Their offspring are also at risk for complications, such as premature birth, low birth weight for gestational age, respiratory distress syndrome, intraventricular hemorrhage, and death (Gilstrap & Wood, 2014).

Congenital and Acquired Heart Disease

Congenital heart disease often involves structural defects that are present at birth but may not be discovered at that time (Table 20.3). Until recently, individuals with congenital heart disease did not live long enough to bear children. Today, due to new surgical techniques to correct these defects, many of these clients can complete a successful pregnancy at relatively low risk when appropriate counselling and optimal care are provided. Increasing numbers of clients with complex congenital heart disease are reaching childbearing age. Complications such as growth restriction, preterm and premature birth, and fetal and neonatal mortality are more common among children of those with congenital heart disease. The risk of complications is determined by the severity of the cardiac lesion, the presence of cyanosis, the maternal functional class, and the use of anticoagulation therapy (Choreño-Machain, Barrios, & Reta, 2015).

Individuals with certain congenital conditions should avoid pregnancy. These include uncorrected tetralogy of Fallot or transposition of the great arteries, and Eisenmenger's syndrome, a defect with both cyanosis and pulmonary hypertension (Brickner, 2014).

Acquired heart diseases are conditions affecting the heart and its associated blood vessels that develop during a person's lifetime, in contrast with congenital heart diseases, which are present at birth. Acquired heart diseases include coronary artery disease, coronary heart

TABLE 20.3	SELECTED HEART CONDITIONS AFFECTING PREGNANCY	
Condition	**Description**	**Management**
Congenital		
Tetralogy of Fallot	Congenital defect involving four structural anomalies: obstruction to pulmonary flow; ventricular septal defect (abnormal opening between the right and left ventricles); dextroposition of the aorta (aortic opening overriding the septum and receiving blood from both ventricles); and right ventricular hypertrophy (increase in volume of the myocardium of the right ventricle)	Hospitalization and bed rest possible after the 20th week with hemodynamic monitoring via a pulmonary artery catheter to monitor volume status. Oxygen therapy may be necessary during labour and birth.
Atrial septal defect (ASD)	Congenital heart defect involving a communication or opening between the atria with left-to-right shunting due to greater left-sided pressure. Arrhythmias present in some.	Treatment with atrioventricular nodal blocking agents, and at times with electrical cardioversion.
Ventricular septal defect (VSD)	Congenital heart defect involving an opening in the ventricular septum, permitting blood flow from the left to the right ventricle. Complications include arrhythmias, heart failure, and pulmonary hypertension.	Rest with limited activity if symptomatic.
Patent ductus arteriosus	Abnormal persistence of an open lumen in the ductus arteriosus between the aorta and the pulmonary artery after birth; results in increased pulmonary blood flow and redistribution of flow to other organs.	Surgical ligation of the open ductus during infancy; subsequent problems minimal after surgical correction
Acquired		
Mitral valve prolapse	Very common in the general population, occurring most often in younger individuals. Leaflets of the mitral valve prolapse into the left atrium during ventricular contraction. The most common cause of mitral valve regurgitation if present during pregnancy. Usually improvements in mitral valve function due to increased blood volume and decreased systemic vascular resistance of pregnancy; most clients are able to tolerate pregnancy well.	Most clients are asymptomatic; diagnosis is made incidentally. Occasional palpations, chest pain, or arrhythmias in some clients, possibly requiring beta blockers. Usually no special precautions are necessary during pregnancy.
Mitral valve stenosis	Most common chronic rheumatic valvular lesion in pregnancy. Causes obstruction of blood flow from the atria to the ventricle, thereby decreasing ventricular filling and causing a fixed cardiac output. Resultant pulmonary edema, pulmonary hypertension, and right ventricular failure. Most childbearing clients with this condition can be managed medically.	General symptomatic improvement with medical management involving diuretics, beta blockers, and anticoagulant therapy. Activity restriction, reduction in sodium, and potentially bed rest if condition is severe.
Aortic stenosis	Narrowing of the opening of the aortic valve, leading to an obstruction to left ventricular ejection. Individuals with mild disease can tolerate hypervolemia of pregnancy; with progressive narrowing of the opening, cardiac output becomes fixed. Diagnosis can be confirmed with echocardiography. Most clients can be managed with medical therapy, bed rest, and close monitoring.	Diagnosis confirmed with echocardiography Pharmacologic treatment with beta blockers and/or antiarrhythmic agents to reduce risk of heart failure and/or dysrhythmias Bed rest/limited activity and close monitoring

TABLE 20.3	SELECTED HEART CONDITIONS AFFECTING PREGNANCY (continued)	
Condition	**Description**	**Management**
Peripartum cardiomyopathy	Rare congestive cardiomyopathy that may arise during pregnancy. Multiparity, age, multiple fetuses, hypertension, an infectious agent, autoimmune disease, or cocaine use may contribute to its presence. Development of heart failure in the last month of pregnancy or within 5 months of giving birth without any pre-existing heart disease or any identifiable cause.	Preload reduction with diuretic therapy Afterload reduction with vasodilators Improvement in contractility with inotropic agents Nonpharmacologic approaches include salt restriction and daily exercise such as walking or biking. The question of whether another pregnancy should be attempted is controversial due to the high risk of repeat complications.
Myocardial infarction (MI)	Rare during pregnancy but incidence is expected to increase as older individuals are becoming pregnant and the risk factors for coronary artery disease become more prevalent. Factors contributing to MI include family history, stress, smoking, age, obesity, multiple fetuses, hypercholesterolemia, and cocaine use. Increased plasma volume and cardiac output during pregnancy increase the cardiac workload as well as the myocardial oxygen demands; imbalance in supply and demand may contribute to myocardial ischemia.	Usual treatment modalities for any acute MI along with consideration for the fetus Anticoagulant therapy, rest, and lifestyle changes to preserve the health of both parties

Adapted from Brickner, M. E. (2014). Cardiovascular management in pregnancy: Congenital heart disease. *Circulation, 130*(3), 273–282; Gilstrap, L. G., & Wood, M. J. (2014). Cardiovascular disease in women and pregnancy. In *MGH cardiology board review* (pp. 205–223). London: Springer Publishers; Jordan, R. G., Engstrom, J. L., Marfell, J. A., & Farley, C. L. (2014). *Prenatal and postnatal care: A woman-centered approach.* Ames, IO: John Wiley & Sons, Inc.; and Mohamad, T. N., Fakhri, H. A., Bernal, J. M., Thatai, D., & Peterson, E. (2015). Cardiovascular disease and pregnancy. *eMedicine.* Retrieved from http://emedicine.medscape.com/article/162004-overview.

disease, rheumatic heart disease, diseases of the pulmonary vessels and the aorta, diseases of the tissues of the heart, and diseases of the heart valves. The incidence of rheumatic heart disease has declined dramatically in the past several decades because of prompt identification of streptococcal throat infections and treatment with antibiotics. When the heart is involved, valvular lesions, such as mitral stenosis, prolapse, or aortic stenosis, are common (see Table 20.3).

Many persons are postponing childbearing until their 30s and 40s. With advancing age at pregnancy, underlying medical conditions such as hypertension, diabetes, and hypercholesterolemia contributing to ischemic heart disease become more common and increase the incidence of acquired heart disease complicating pregnancy. Coronary artery disease and myocardial infarction may result.

A client's ability to function during the pregnancy is often more important than the actual diagnosis of the cardiac condition. The following is a functional classification system developed by the Criteria Committee of the New York Heart Association (1994) based on past and present disability and physical signs. It provides a simple way of classifying the extent of heart failure by placing people in one of four categories based on how much they are limited during physical activity, normal breathing, and varying degrees of shortness of breath and/or chest pain:

- *Class I:* asymptomatic with no limitation of physical activity; no objective evidence of cardiac disease. Ordinary physical activity does not cause undue fatigue, palpitation, dyspnea, or chest pain.
- *Class II:* symptomatic (dyspnea, chest pain) with increased activity resulting in slight limitation of physical activity. They are comfortable at rest. Ordinary physical activity results in fatigue, palpitation, dyspnea, or anginal pain. Minimal CVD present.
- *Class III:* symptomatic (fatigue, palpitations) with normal activity resulting in marked limitation of physical activity. They are comfortable at rest. Less than ordinary activity causes fatigue, palpitation, dyspnea, or anginal pain. Moderately severe CVD present.
- *Class IV:* symptomatic at rest or with any physical activity resulting in inability to carry on any physical activity without discomfort. Symptoms of heart failure or the anginal syndrome may be present even at rest. If any physical activity is undertaken, discomfort is increased. Severe CVD present.

BOX 20.1

CLASSIFICATION OF MATERNAL MORTALITY RISK

Group I (minimal risk) has a mortality rate of 1% and comprises clients with:
- Patent ductus arteriosus
- Tetralogy of Fallot, corrected
- Atrial septal defect
- Ventricular septal defect
- Mitral stenosis, class I and II

Group II (moderate risk) has a mortality rate of 5% to 15% and comprises clients with:
- Tetralogy of Fallot, uncorrected
- Mitral stenosis with atrial fibrillation
- Aortic stenosis, class III and IV
- Aortic coarctation without valvular involvement
- Artificial valve replacement

Group III (major risk) has a 25% to 50% mortality rate and comprises clients with:
- Pulmonary hypertension
- Complicated aortic coarctation
- Previous myocardial infarction

Adapted from American Heart Association (AHA). (2015). Women and heart disease. Retrieved from https://www.goredforwomen.org/about-heart-disease/facts_about_heart_disease_in_women-sub-category/statistics-at-a-glance/; Alonso-Gonzalez, R., & Swan, L. (2014). Treating cardiac disease in pregnancy. *Women's Health*, *10*(1), 79–90; and Mohamad, T. N., Fakhri, H. A., Bernal, J. M., Thatai, D., & Peterson, E. (2015). Cardiovascular disease and pregnancy. *eMedicine*. Retrieved from http://emedicine.medscape.com/article/162004-overview.

The classification may change as the pregnancy progresses and the client's body must cope with the increasing stress on the cardiovascular system resulting from the numerous physiologic changes taking place. The Canadian Cardiovascular Society recommends that childbearing persons with New York Heart Association (NYHA) class I or II cardiac disease can go through a pregnancy without major complications, and have a mortality rate of less than 1%, while those in class III or IV have a mortality rate of 5% to 15% (Howlett et al., 2010). A person with class III disease usually has to maintain bed rest during pregnancy. A person with class IV disease typically should be advised to avoid pregnancy (Grewal, Silversides, & Coleman, 2014). Clients with cardiac disease may benefit from preconception counselling so that they know the risks before deciding to become pregnant.

The American College of Obstetricians and Gynecologists (ACOG) has adopted a three-tiered classification according to the risk of death during pregnancy (Box 20.1).

Pathophysiology

Numerous hemodynamic changes occur in all childbearing persons. These normal physiologic changes can overstress the client's cardiovascular system, increasing her risk for problems. Increased cardiac workload and greater myocardial oxygen demand during pregnancy place the person's cardiovascular system at high risk for morbidity and mortality.

Pregnancy causes cardiac output to rise as early as the first trimester, reaching peak values at 20 to 24 weeks, and continues to increase until it plateaus between 28 and 34 weeks' gestation. This rise in cardiac output is due to a 30% to 50% increase in blood volume (stroke volume) and a 30% increase in heart rate. A normal resting heart rate for any pregnant person can be on average 20 beats per minute (bpm) above the normal values.

Take Note!

Uterine blood flow increases by at least 1 litre per minute, requiring the body to produce more blood during pregnancy. This results in a 25% increase in red blood cells, a 50% expansion of plasma volume during pregnancy, and an overall hemodilution. In addition, the increase in total red blood cellular volume includes an increase in clotting factors and platelets, defining the hypercoagulable state of pregnancy (Swan, 2014). These changes start as early as the second month of gestation.

Similarly, cardiac output increases steadily during pregnancy by 30% to 50% over prepregnancy levels. Stroke volume increases 20% to 30% from prepregnant levels, and the client's heart rate increases by 10 to 20 bpm. The increase is due to both the expansion in blood volume and the augmentation of stroke volume and heart rate. Other hemodynamic changes associated with pregnancy include a decrease in both the systemic vascular resistance and pulmonary vascular resistance, thereby lowering the systolic and diastolic blood pressure. In addition, the hypercoagulability associated with pregnancy might increase the risk of arterial thrombosis and embolization. These normal physiologic changes are important for a successful adaptation to pregnancy but create unique physiologic challenges for the clients with cardiac disease (Comparison Chart 20.1).

Therapeutic Management

Ideally, a client with a history of congenital or acquired heart disease should consult their health care provider and undergo a risk assessment before becoming pregnant. This risk assessment must consider the client's functional capacity, exercise tolerance, degree of cyanosis, medication needs, and history of arrhythmias. Data needed for risk assessment can be acquired from a thorough cardiovascular history and examination, a 12-lead electrocardiogram (ECG), and evaluation of oxygen saturation levels by pulse oximetry. The impact of heart disease on a client's childbearing potential needs to be clearly explained, and providing information on how pregnancy may affect the client and the fetus is important. This allows individuals to make an informed choice

COMPARISON CHART 20.1	CARDIOVASCULAR CHANGES: PREPREGNANCY VERSUS PREGNANCY	
Measurement	**Prepregnancy**	**Pregnancy**
Heart rate	72 (±10 bpm)	+10–20%
Cardiac output	4.3 (±0.9 L/min)	+30–50%
Blood volume	5 L	+20–50%
Stroke volume	73.3 (±9 mL)	+30%
Systemic vascular resistance	1,530 (±520 dyne/cm/sec)	−20%
Oxygen consumption	250 mL/min	+20–30%

Adapted from American Heart Association (AHA). (2015). Women and heart disease. Retrieved from https://www.goredforwomen.org/about-heart-disease/facts_about_heart_disease_in_women-sub-category/statistics-at-a-glance/; Mohamad, T. N., Fakhri, H. A., Bernal, J. M., Thatai, D., & Peterson, E. (2015). Cardiovascular disease and pregnancy. *eMedicine*. Retrieved from http://emedicine.medscape.com/article/162004-overview; and King, T. L., Brucker, M. C., Kriebs, J. M., Fahey, J. O., Gegor, C. L., & Varney, H. (2015). *Varney's midwifery* (5th ed.). Burlington, MA: Jones & Bartlett Learning.

about whether they wish to accept the risks associated with pregnancy. When possible, any surgical procedures, such as valve replacement, should be done before pregnancy to improve fetal and maternal outcomes (Sliwa, Johnson, Zilla, & Roos-Hesselink, 2015).

If the client presents for care after becoming pregnant, prenatal counselling focuses on the impact of the hemodynamic changes of pregnancy, the signs and symptoms of cardiac compromise, and dietary and lifestyle changes needed. More frequent prenatal visits (every 2 weeks until the last month and then weekly) are usually needed to ensure the health and safety of the client and fetus.

Nursing Assessment

Frequent and thorough assessments are crucial during the antepartum period to ensure early detection of and prompt intervention for problems. Assess the client's vital signs, noting any changes. Auscultate the apical heart rate and heart sounds, being especially alert for abnormalities, including irregularities in rhythm or murmurs. Check the client's weight and compare with baseline and weights obtained on previous visits. Report any weight gain outside recommended parameters. Inspect the extremities for edema and note any pitting.

Question the client about fetal activity, and ask if they have noticed any changes. Report any changes such as a decrease in fetal movements. Ask the client about any symptoms of preterm labour, such as low back pain, uterine contractions, and increased pelvic pressure and vaginal discharge, and report them immediately. Assess the fetal heart rate and review serial ultrasound results to monitor fetal growth.

Assess the client's lifestyle and ability to cope with the changes of pregnancy and its effect on cardiac status and ability to function. Evaluate the client's understanding of the condition and what restrictions and lifestyle changes may be needed to provide the best outcome for the client and the fetus. A healthy client and infant at the end of pregnancy is the ultimate goal. As the client's pregnancy advances, expect their functional class to be revised based on the level of disability. Suggest realistic modifications.

The nurse plays a major role in recognizing the signs and symptoms of cardiac decompensation. Decompensation refers to the heart's inability to maintain adequate circulation. As a result, tissue perfusion in the client and the fetus is impaired. Common complaints of normal pregnancy, such as dyspnea, fatigue, palpitations, orthopnea, and pedal edema, mimic symptoms of worsening cardiac disease and create challenges when trying to evaluate childbearing clients with cardiac disease. The pregnant client is most vulnerable for this complication from 28 to 32 weeks' gestation and in the first 48 hours postpartum (Gandhi & Martin, 2015). Assess the client for the following signs and symptoms:

- Shortness of breath on exertion, dyspnea
- Cyanosis of lips and nail beds
- Swelling of face, hands, and feet
- Jugular vein engorgement
- Rapid respirations
- Abnormal heartbeats, reports of heart racing or palpitations
- Chest pain with effort or emotion
- Syncope with exertion
- Increasing fatigue
- Moist, frequent cough

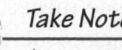 **Take Note!**

Assessing the childbearing client with heart disease for cardiac decompensation is vital because the client's hemodynamic status determines the health of the fetus.

Nursing Management

Nursing management of the childbearing client with heart disease focuses on assisting with measures to stabilize the client's hemodynamic status, because a decrease in blood pressure or volume will cause blood to be shunted away from the uterus, thus reducing placental perfusion. Pregnant clients with cardiac disease also need assistance in reducing risks that would lead to complications or further cardiac compromise; therefore, education and counselling are critical. Collaboration between the cardiologist, obstetrician, neonatologist, and nurse is needed to promote the best possible outcome.

Drug therapy may be indicated for the pregnant client with a cardiac disorder. Possible drugs include diuretics, such as Lasix, to prevent heart failure; digitalis to increase contractility and decrease heart rates; anti-arrhythmic agents (lidocaine); beta blockers (labetalol); calcium channel blockers (nifedipine) to treat hypertension; and anticoagulants (low–molecular-weight heparin). Warfarin (Coumadin) is not recommended because it crosses the placenta and may have teratogenic effects. It has been associated with spontaneous abortion, multiple birth defects, fetal growth restriction, and stillbirth (Lichtin & Philipson, 2014). The FDA's risk categories are as follows:

The FDA changed their drug risk categories in June of 2015. They are no longer using categories A, B, C, D, and X. The new rule requires removal of the previous letter pregnancy categories. The package inserts will now include three separate categories that provide information in a narrative format. The goal of the new labelling is to provide information about the drug to the consumer. They now use specific subheadings under each of the three categories: Pregnancy; lactation; and females and males of reproductive potential. For specific changes under each category, please access the FDA website via thePoint.

Encourage the client to continue taking any cardiac medications as prescribed. Review the indications, actions, and potential side effects of the medications. Reinforce the importance of frequent antepartum visits and close medical supervision throughout the pregnancy.

Discuss the need to conserve energy. Help the client to prioritize household chores and child care to allow rest periods. Encourage the client to rest in the side-lying position, which enhances placental perfusion.

Encourage the client to eat nutritious foods and consume a high-fibre diet to prevent straining and constipation. Discuss limiting sodium intake if indicated to reduce fluid retention. Contact a dietitian to assist the client in planning nutritionally appropriate meals.

Assist the client in preparing for diagnostic tests to evaluate fetal well-being. Describe the tests that may be done, such as ECG and echocardiogram, and explain the need for serial nonstress testing. Instruct the client in how to monitor fetal activity and movements. Urge them to do this daily and report any changes in activity immediately.

Although the morbidity and mortality rates of childbearing persons with cardiac disease have decreased greatly, hemodynamic changes during pregnancy (increased heart rate, stroke volume, cardiac output and blood volume) have a profound effect, which may increase cardiac work and might exceed the functional capacity of the diseased heart. These changes may result in pulmonary hypertension, pulmonary edema, heart failure, or death (Alonso-Gonzalez & Swan, 2014). Explain the signs and symptoms of these complications and review the sign and symptoms of cardiac decompensation, encouraging the client to notify their health care provider if any occur.

Provide support and encouragement throughout the antepartum period. Assess the support systems available to the client and their family and encourage use of them. If necessary, assist with referrals to community services for additional support.

During labour, anticipate the need for invasive hemodynamic monitoring, and make sure the client has been prepared for this beforehand. Monitor the fluid volume carefully to prevent overload. Anticipate the use of epidural anesthesia if a vaginal birth is planned. After birth, assess the client for fluid overload as peripheral fluids mobilize. This fluid shift from the periphery to the central circulation taxes the heart, and signs of heart failure such as cough, progressive dyspnea, edema, palpitations, and crackles in the lung bases may ensue before postpartum diuresis begins. Because hemodynamics do not return to baseline for several days after childbirth, clients at intermediate or high risk require monitoring for at least 48 hours postpartum (Cunningham et al., 2014).

Pregnancy offers a unique window through which clients at risk of future CVD may be identified. Nurses have the opportunity to implement health monitoring, lifestyle modifications, and other needed interventions to reduce the burden of future CVD in all of their pregnant clients. Dispelling the myths surrounding CVD and identifying risk factors would be huge in promoting awareness.

Hypertension in Pregnancy

The Society of Obstetricians and Gynecologists of Canada identify three classification categories for the hypertensive disorders of pregnancy: pre-existing hypertension, gestational hypertension, and preeclampsia (Magee, Pels, Helewa, Rey, & von Dadelszen, 2014). Both pre-existing hypertension and gestational hypertension have two subgroups: (1) with comorbid conditions requiring tighter blood pressure control, and (2) with preeclampsia. Preeclampsia is most commonly defined as new-onset proteinuria with hypertension, but can be diagnosed in the absence of proteinuria when one or more adverse conditions reflecting end-organ dysfunction (headache, visual symptoms, epigastric pain, and thrombocytopenia) are present. "Mild" is no longer used to categorize the severity of preeclampsia, though preeclampsia can be defined as severe when there is one or more severe complications present.

Pre-Existing Hypertension

Entering pregnancy with pre-existing hypertension is increasingly common. It is an important risk factor for pregnancy complications, including for the fetus or newborn, poor fetal growth, preterm birth, low birth weight, admission to the NICU and death, and for the client, superimposed preeclampsia/eclampsia, acute renal failure, pulmonary edema, surgical birth, placental abruption, stoke, postpartum cardiomyopathy, and mortality (Solomon & Greene, 2015). Pre-existing hypertension exists when the client has high blood pressure before pregnancy or before the 20th week of gestation, or when hypertension persists for more than 6 weeks postpartum.

Pre-existing hypertension occurs in up to 22% of clients of childbearing age, with the prevalence varying according to age, race, and BMI. It complicates at least 5% of pregnancies, with one in four clients developing preeclampsia during pregnancy (Sibai, 2015). Pre-existing hypertension is typically seen in older, obese persons with prediabetes or diabetes. The most common complication is preeclampsia, which is seen in approximately 25% of clients who enter the pregnancy with hypertension. Worldwide, about 60,000 clients die from preeclampsia each year, corresponding to 12% of all deaths in childbearing persons (Raio, Bolla, & Baumann, 2015). (See Chapter 19 for more information about preeclampsia.)

Therapeutic Management

Preconception counselling is important in fostering positive outcomes. Typically, it involves lifestyle changes such as diet, exercise, weight loss, and smoking cessation. Treatment for clients with pre-existing hypertension focuses on maintaining normal blood pressure, preventing superimposed preeclampsia/eclampsia, and ensuring normal fetal development.

Once the client is pregnant, antihypertensive agents may be considered, and are indicated with comorbid conditions, or in the presence of severe hypertension >160 mm Hg systolic and >110 mm Hg diastolic. Methyldopa is commonly prescribed because of its safety record during pregnancy. This slow-acting antihypertensive agent helps to improve uterine perfusion. Other antihypertensive agents that can be used include labetalol, and nifedipine XL preparation (Foo, Tay, Lees, McEniery, & Wilkinson, 2015; Magee et al., 2014). Intravenous labetalol or hydralazine, or short-acting nifedipine capsules are used with severe hypertension.

Daily aspirin given to those at high risk of developing preeclampsia from 14 weeks to 36 weeks' gestation has been shown to reduce the risk or preterm (but not term) preeclampsia, when administered as a 150-mg dose (Rolnik et al., 2017).

Lifestyle changes are needed and should continue throughout gestation. The client with pre-existing hypertension will be counselled about warning signs of preeclampsia, and will be monitored for proteinuria and other symptoms of preeclampsia. Additional ultrasound assessments of growth and amniotic fluid volume, Doppler flow studies, and biophysical profiles may be performed as the pregnancy progresses. Additional tests will be included if the client's status changes.

Nursing Assessment

Nursing assessment of the client with pre-existing hypertension involves a thorough history and physical examination. Review the client's history closely for risk factors. The pathogenesis of hypertension is multifactorial and includes many modifiable risk factors such as smoking, obesity, caffeine intake, excessive alcohol intake, excessive salt intake, and use of nonsteroidal anti-inflammatory drugs (NSAIDs). Also be alert for non-modifiable risk factors such as increasing age and high-risk groups, such as being African Canadian (Miller & Carpenter, 2015). Ask if the client has received any preconception counselling and what measures have been used to prevent or control hypertension.

Assess the client's vital signs, in particular the blood pressure. Evaluate blood pressure while sitting with feet flat on the floor. Assess for orthostatic hypertension when changing position from sitting to standing. Document your findings.

Ask if the client monitor their blood pressure at home; if so, inquire about the typical readings. Ask if the client use any medications for blood pressure control, including the drug, dosage, and frequency of administration, as well as any side effects. Ask the client about lifestyle modifications used to address any modifiable risk factors, and their effectiveness.

Hypertension during pregnancy decreases uteroplacental perfusion. Therefore, fetal well-being must be assessed and closely monitored. Anticipate serial ultrasounds to assess fetal growth and amniotic fluid volume. Question the client about fetal movement and evaluate the report of daily "kick counts." Assess fetal heart rate at every visit.

Nursing Management

Preconception counselling is the ideal time to discuss lifestyle changes to prevent or control hypertension. Areas to cover during this visit would be healthy nutrition, exercise, periconception folic acid, and calcium supplementation. Sodium restriction is not recommended (Magee et al., 2014). Encourage smoking cessation and avoidance of alcohol. If the client is overweight, encourage them to lose weight before becoming pregnant, not during the pregnancy (Killion, 2015). Stressing the positive benefits of a healthy lifestyle might help motivate the client to make the necessary modifications and change unhealthy habits.

Assist the client in scheduling appointments for antepartum visits and prepare the client for frequent fetal assessments. Explaining the rationale for the need to monitor fetal growth is important to gain the client's cooperation. Carefully monitor the client for signs and symptoms of abruptio placenta (abdominal pain, rigid abdomen, vaginal bleeding), as well as superimposed preeclampsia (new onset of proteinuria, headache, visual disturbances, epigastric pain). Alerting the client to these risks can mean early identification and prompt intervention.

Stress the importance of daily periods of rest (1 hour) in the left lateral recumbent position to maximize placental perfusion. Encourage client with pre-existing hypertension to use home blood pressure monitoring devices. Urge the client to report any elevations. As necessary, instruct the client and their family how to take and record a daily blood pressure, and reinforce the need for them to take their medications as prescribed to control blood pressure and to ensure the well-being of her unborn child. Providing praise for their efforts at each prenatal visit may motivate them to continue the regimen throughout the pregnancy.

The close monitoring of the client with pre-existing hypertension continues during labour and birth and during the postpartum period to prevent or identify the onset of preeclampsia. Accurate and frequent blood pressure readings and careful administration of antihypertensive medications, if prescribed, are essential components of care. Stressing the need for continued medical supervision after childbirth is vital to motivate the client to maintain or initiate lifestyle changes and dietary habits and stay compliant with their medication regimen.

RESPIRATORY CONDITIONS

During pregnancy, the respiratory system is affected by hormonal changes, mechanical changes, and prior respiratory conditions. These changes can cause a client with a history of compromised respiration to decompensate during pregnancy. Although upper respiratory infections are typically self-limiting, chronic respiratory conditions, such as asthma or tuberculosis (TB), can have a negative effect on the growing fetus when alterations in oxygenation occur in the client. The outcome of pregnancy in a client with a respiratory condition depends on the severity of the oxygen alteration as well as the degree and duration of hypoxia on the fetus.

Asthma

Worldwide, the prevalence of asthma among childbearing persons is on the rise; pregnancy leads to a worsening of asthma for many individuals (Nagtalon-Ramos, 2014). Asthma affects approximately up to 13% of pregnancies globally and is associated with an increased risk of infant death, preeclampsia, intrauterine growth restriction (IUGR), preterm birth, and low birth weight. These risks are linked to the severity of asthma: more severe asthma increases the risk (National Asthma Education and Prevention Program [NAEPP], 2015).

> **Remember Rose, the pregnant adolescent with asthma in acute distress described at the beginning of the chapter. What therapies might be offered to control the symptoms? Should Rose be treated differently than someone who is not pregnant? Why or why not?**

Pathophysiology

Asthma is an allergic-type inflammatory response of the respiratory tract to various stimuli such as allergens (pollen and animal dander), irritants (cigarette smoke and chemicals), stress, infections (colds or flu), and physical exertion. It is also known as reactive airway disease because the bronchioles constrict in response to these stimuli. Asthma is characterized by paroxysmal or persistent symptoms of bronchoconstriction including breathlessness, wheezing, chest tightness, cough, and sputum production. In addition to bronchoconstriction, inflammation of the airways produces thick mucus that further limits the movement of air and makes breathing difficult.

The normal physiologic changes of pregnancy affect the respiratory system. Although the respiratory rate does not change, hyperventilation increases at term by 48% due to high progesterone levels. Diaphragmatic elevation and a decrease in functional lung residual capacity occur late in pregnancy, which may reduce the ability to inspire deeply to take in more oxygen. Oxygen consumption and the metabolic rate both increase, placing additional stress on the respiratory system (American Academy of Allergy, Asthma, & Immunology [AAAAI], 2015).

Both the client and the fetus are at risk if asthma is not well managed during pregnancy. When a childbearing person has trouble breathing, the fetus also has trouble getting the oxygen it needs for adequate growth and development. Severe persistent asthma has been linked to the development of hypertension, low birth weight, preterm birth, preeclampsia, placenta previa, uterine hemorrhage, and oligohydramnios. Clients whose asthma is poorly controlled during pregnancy are at increased risk of preterm birth, low birth weight, and stillbirth (Vanders & Murphy, 2015).

The severity of the condition improves in one third of pregnant clients, remains unchanged in one third, and worsens in one third (Cunningham et al., 2014). However, the effect of pregnancy on asthma is unpredictable. The greatest increase in asthma attacks usually occurs between 24 and 36 weeks' gestation; flare-ups are rare during the last 4 weeks of pregnancy and during labour (AAAAI, 2015).

Therapeutic Management

Asthma should be treated as aggressively in pregnant clients as in nonpregnant clients because the benefits of averting an asthma attack outweigh the risks of medications. The ultimate goal of asthma therapy is to prevent hypoxic episodes to preserve continuous fetal oxygenation; improved perinatal outcomes are achieved with optimal control of asthma. One third of clients with asthma develop worsening of control during pregnancy; therefore, close monitoring and reevaluation are essential. Four important aspects of asthma treatment ensure optimal control: close monitoring, education of clients, avoidance of asthma triggers, and pharmacologic therapy.

Many clients with asthma have positive skin tests to allergens, the most common being animal dander, dust mites, cockroach antigens, pollens, and moulds. There are nonimmune triggers as well, including strong odours, tobacco smoke, air pollutants, and drugs such as aspirin and beta blockers. For exercise-triggered asthma, the use of a bronchodilator 5 to 60 minutes before exercise may reduce symptoms. Avoidance of these allergens and triggers can significantly reduce the need for medication and the occurrence of exacerbations during and after pregnancy. All clients should be strongly encouraged to stop smoking, but especially those with asthma because they are at increased risk for worsening chronic and acute asthma sequelae.

Allergy injections may benefit those with allergies and asthma, called allergic asthma. Also called immunotherapy, allergy shots do not "cure" asthma in the manner in which an injection of, say, antibiotics might cure an infection. Instead, allergy shots work a bit more like a vaccine. Allergy injections for asthma actually contain a very small amount of an allergen (substance causing allergy). Over time, the dosage is increased. Exposure to progressive amounts of the allergen is likely to help the body develop a tolerance to it. If the allergen buildup is effective, the allergic reaction will become much less severe. Allergy injections can reduce the symptoms of allergies and prevent the development of asthma.

Medical therapy includes a stepwise approach in an attempt to use the least amount of medication necessary to control a client's asthma and keep the severity in the mild range. Goals of therapy include having normal or near-normal pulmonary function and minimal or no chronic symptoms, exacerbations, or limitations on activities. The final goal is to minimize the adverse effects of treatment. Inhaled corticosteroids are preferred for the management of all levels of persistent asthma in pregnancy. Corticosteroids are the most effective treatment for the airway inflammation of asthma and reduce the hyperresponsiveness of airways to allergens and triggers.

NAEPP (2015) recommends three specific drugs to be used during pregnancy to control asthma:
- Budesonide (inhaled corticosteroid)
- Albuterol (short-acting beta2 agonist)
- Salmeterol (long-acting beta2 agonist)

Oral corticosteroids are not recommended for the long-term treatment of asthma during pregnancy, but they can be used to treat severe asthma attacks during pregnancy (AAAAI, 2015). In addition, hemabate, used for treating postpartum hemorrhage, is contraindicated for clients with asthma due to the risk of bronchial spasm and bronchoconstriction (King et al., 2015).

Nursing Assessment

Obtain a thorough history of the disease, including the client's usual therapy and control measures. Inquire about asthma triggers and strategies used to reduce exposure to them (Box 20.2). Review the client's medication therapy regimen.

Auscultate the lungs and assess respiratory and heart rates. Include the rate, rhythm, and depth of respirations;

BOX 20.2

COMMON ASTHMA TRIGGERS

- Smoke and chemical irritants
- Air pollution
- Dust mites
- Animal dander
- Seasonal changes with pollen, moulds, and spores
- Upper respiratory infections
- Esophageal reflux
- Medications, such as aspirin and nonsteroidal anti-inflammatory drugs (NSAIDs)
- Exercise
- Cold air
- Emotional stress

Adapted from American Academy of Allergy, Asthma & Immunology (AAAAI). (2015). *Asthma and pregnancy.* Retrieved from http://www.aaaai.org/conditions-and-treatments/library/asthma-library/asthma-and-pregnancy.aspx; March of Dimes. (2015l). *Asthma during pregnancy.* Retrieved from http://www.marchofdimes.org/pregnancy/asthma-during-pregnancy.aspx; and Cunningham, F. G., Leveno, K. J., Bloom, S. L., Spong, C., Dashe, J., Hoffman, B. L., . . . Sheffield, J. S. (2014). *Williams' obstetrics* (24th ed.). New York: McGraw-Hill Professional Publishing.

Nursing Management

Adherence to the multidrug therapy is critical to protect the client and the fetus from progression of TB. Provide education about the disease process, the mode of transmission, prevention, potential complications, and the importance of adhering to the treatment regimen.

Stressing the importance of health promotion activities throughout the pregnancy is important. Some suggestions might include avoiding crowded living conditions, avoiding sick people, maintaining adequate hydration, eating a nutritious, well-balanced diet, keeping all prenatal appointments to evaluate fetal growth and well-being, and getting plenty of fresh air outside. Determining the client's understanding of the condition and treatment plan is important for adherence. A language interpreter may be needed to validate and reinforce understanding if the client does not speak English.

Breastfeeding is not contraindicated during the time the client is on the medication regimen and should in fact be encouraged. If the client is untreated for TB at the time of childbirth, they should not breastfeed or be in direct contact with their newborn until at least 2 weeks after starting anti-tuberculin medications. Untreated clients can be encouraged to pump their milk to feed their newborns until they can breastfeed directly (AAP, 2015). Nurses should consult their hospital policies regarding mothers with TB for guidance. Management of the newborn of a parent with TB involves preventing transmission by teaching the parents not to cough, sneeze, or talk directly into the newborn's face. Nurses need to stay current about new therapies and screening techniques to treat this centuries-old disease.

HEMATOLOGIC CONDITIONS

Anemia, a reduction in red blood cell volume, is measured by hematocrit (Hct) or a decrease in the concentration of hemoglobin (Hgb) in the peripheral blood. This results in reduced capacity of the blood to carry oxygen to the vital organs of the client and the fetus. Anemia is a sign of an underlying problem but does not indicate its origin.

Iron-Deficiency Anemia

Iron deficiency is the most common pathologic cause of anemia in pregnancy. Increased risk during pregnancy is due to increased iron needs to support the pregnancy and demands from the growing fetus, increased erythrocyte mass; and, in the third trimester, expanded blood volume (Cantor, Bougatsos, Dana, Blazina, & McDonagh, 2015). Anemia affects one fourth of the world's population, and iron deficiency is the predominate cause. Iron-deficiency anemia mainly reflects poor nutrition, principally attributed to poor economic status

worldwide. A recent study supports that and found that iron-deficiency anemia is strongly associated with low socioeconomic status, which affects clients' knowledge and health-seeking behaviours. The study concludes that empowering clients in terms of education and economic status is the key factor in combating anemia in pregnancy to prevent the vicious cycle of associated problems (Friedman et al., 2015).

Iron-deficiency anemia accounts for 75% to 95% of the cases of anemia in childbearing client (affecting one in four pregnancies) and is usually related to an iron-deficient diet, gastrointestinal issues affecting absorption, or a short pregnancy interval (Jimenez, Kulnigg-Dabsch, & Gasche, 2015). A client who is pregnant often has insufficient iron stores to meet the demands of pregnancy.

The clinical consequences of iron-deficiency anemia include preterm delivery, perinatal mortality, and postpartum depression. Fetal and neonatal consequences include low birth weight and poor mental and psychomotor performance (Subramaniam & Girish, 2015). With significant maternal iron depletion, the fetus will attempt to store iron, but at a cost to the client. Anemia at term increases the perinatal risk for both the client and newborn. The risks of hemorrhage (impaired platelet function) and infection during and after birth also are increased. Clinical symptoms of iron-deficiency anemia include fatigue, diminished quality of life, impaired cognitive function, increased risk for thromboembolic events, headache, restless legs syndrome, and **pica** (consuming nonfood substances) eating behaviours (Camaschella, 2015).

Therapeutic Management

The goals of treatment for iron-deficiency anemia in pregnancy are to eliminate symptoms, correct the deficiency, and replenish iron stores. The Society of Obstetricians and Gynecologists recommend routine supplementation containing 16- to 20-mg elemental iron for all childbearing clients, and screening for iron deficiency in those at high risk (low meat intake, low socioeconomic status, or an immigrant from a developing country). Therapeutic doses of iron are indicated if clinical evidence of iron deficiency is present, as with low hemoglobin levels and serum ferritin less than 30 µg/L (O'Connor et al., 2016).

Nursing Assessment

Review the client's history for factors that may contribute to the development of iron-deficiency anemia, including poor nutrition, hemolysis, pica, multiple gestation, limited intervals between pregnancies, and blood loss. Assess the client's dietary intake as well as the quantity and timing of ingestion of substances that interfere with iron absorption, such as tea, coffee, chocolate, and high-fibre foods. Ask the client if they have fatigue, weakness, malaise, anorexia, or increased susceptibility to infection, such as frequent colds. Inspect the skin and mucous membranes, noting any pallor. Obtain vital signs and report any tachycardia.

Prepare the client for laboratory testing. Laboratory tests usually reveal low hemoglobin (<110 g/L), low hematocrit (<35%), low serum iron (<5 μmol/L), microcytic and hypochromic cells, and low serum ferritin (<30 μg/L).

> ### Take Note!
> Hemoglobin and hematocrit decrease normally during pregnancy in response to an increase in blood plasma in comparison to red blood cells. This hemodilution can lead to physiologic anemia of pregnancy, which does not indicate a decrease in oxygen-carrying capacity or true anemia.

Nursing Management

Nursing management of the client with iron-deficiency anemia focuses on encouraging adherence to drug therapy and providing dietary instruction about the intake of iron-rich foods. Although iron constitutes a minimal percentage of the body's total weight, it has several major roles: it assists in the transport of oxygen and carbon dioxide throughout the body, aids in the production of red blood cells, and plays a role in the body's immune response.

Stress the importance of taking the prenatal vitamin and iron supplement consistently. Encourage the client to take the iron supplement with vitamin C–containing fluids such as orange juice, which will promote absorption, rather than milk, which can inhibit iron absorption. Taking iron on an empty stomach improves its absorption, but many clients cannot tolerate the gastrointestinal discomfort it causes. In such cases, advise the client to take it with meals. Instruct the client about adverse effects, which are predominantly gastrointestinal and include gastric discomfort, nausea, vomiting, anorexia, diarrhea, metallic taste, and constipation. Suggest that the client take the iron supplement with meals and increase their intake of fibre and fluids to help overcome the most common side effects.

Provide dietary counselling. Recommend foods high in iron, such as dried fruits, whole grains, green leafy vegetables, meats, peanut butter, and iron-fortified cereals (Dudek, 2014). Anticipate the need for a referral to a dietitian. Teaching Guidelines 20.3 highlights instructions for the pregnant client with iron-deficiency anemia.

> ### Teaching Guidelines 20.3
> #### TEACHING FOR THE CLIENT WITH IRON-DEFICIENCY ANEMIA
> - Take your prenatal vitamin daily; if you miss a dose, take it as soon as you remember.
> - For best absorption, take iron supplements between meals.
> - Awareness of the side effects of iron supplementation
> - Avoid taking iron supplements with coffee, tea, chocolate, and high-fibre foods.
> - Eat foods rich in iron, such as:
>   - Meats, green leafy vegetables, legumes, dried fruits, whole grains
>   - Peanut butter, bean dip, whole-wheat fortified breads and cereals
> - For best iron absorption from foods, consume the food along with a food high in vitamin C.
> - Increase your exercise, fluids, and high-fibre foods to reduce constipation.
> - Plan frequent rest periods during the day.

Thalassemia

Thalassemia is a group of hereditary anemic disorders in which synthesis of one or both chains of hemoglobin molecules (alpha and beta) is defective. Inheritance is autosomal recessive. A low hemoglobin and a microcytic, hypochromic anemia results. The prevalence and severity of thalassemia depend on the client's racial background: persons of African, Asian, Mediterranean, Middle Eastern, or South Asian descent are most frequently affected.

Thalassemia occurs in two forms: alpha-thalassemia and beta-thalassemia. Alpha-thalassemia (minor), the heterozygous form, results from the inheritance of one abnormal gene from either parent, placing the offspring in a carrier trait state. These clients have little or no hematologic disease and are clinically asymptomatic (silent carrier state). Beta-thalassemia (major) is the form involving inheritance of the gene from both parents. Beta-thalassemia major can be very severe. Genetic counselling might be necessary when decisions about childbearing are being made.

Thalassemia minor has little effect on pregnancy, although the client will have mild, persistent anemia. This anemia does not respond to iron therapy, and iron supplements should not be prescribed. Several recent studies suggest that pregnancy appears safe for a client with well-treated beta-thalassemia major who does not have heart disease (Rigby, 2015).

Management of thalassemia during pregnancy depends on the severity of the disease. Apart from the routine prenatal visit schedule, childbearing clients with thalassemia need additional care which includes regular and periodic evaluation of cardiac function by a cardiologist to prevent fluid overload; and frequent hemoglobin and ferritin levels should be monitored to avoid iron overload. Identification and screening are important to plan care. The client's ethnic background, medical history, and blood studies are analyzed. If the client is determined to be a carrier, screening of the other parent of the child is indicated. Knowledge of the carrier state of each parent provides the genetic counsellor with knowledge about the risk that the fetus will be a carrier or will have the disease (Karimi, Cohan, & Parand, 2015). Mild anemia may be present, and instructions to rest and avoid infections are helpful. Nurses should provide supportive care and expectant management throughout the pregnancy.

Sickle Cell Anemia

Sickle cell anemia is an autosomal recessive inherited condition that results from a defective hemoglobin molecule (hemoglobin S). It is found most commonly in African Canadians, Southeast Asians, and Middle Eastern populations. Sickle cell disease affects millions of people across the globe.

Clients with sickle cell disease can have more adverse maternal outcomes such as preeclampsia, eclampsia, preterm labour, placental abruption, IUGR, low birth weight, and client mortality (Costa, Viana, & Aguiar, 2015). The gene offers protection against malaria, but can be a cause of chronic pain and early death. Life expectancy is shortened as a consequence of renal damage, cardiac damage, and infection (March of Dimes, 2015c). People with only one gene for the trait (heterozygous) will have sickle cell trait without obvious symptoms of the disease and with little effect on the pregnancy.

Pathophysiology

In the human body, the hemoglobin molecule serves as the oxygen-carrying component of the red blood cells. Most people have several types of circulating hemoglobin (HbA and HbA2) that make up the majority of their circulatory system. In sickle cell disease, the abnormal hemoglobin S (HbS) replaces HbA and HbA2. This abnormal hemoglobin (HbS) becomes "sickle" shaped as a result of any stress or trauma such as infection, fever, acidosis, dehydration, physical exertion, excessive cold exposure, or hypoxia. The sickle shape of the hemoglobin causes clumping together, which blocks the microvasculature. Significant anemia usually results.

Sickle cell anemia during pregnancy is associated with more severe anemia and frequent vaso-occlusive crises, with increased maternal and perinatal morbidity and mortality. In childbearing clients with sickle cell anemia, complications can occur at any time during gestation, labour and birth, or postpartum. This is believed to be secondary to hormonal modifications, hypercoagulable state, and increased susceptibility to infection. Microvascular sickling in the placental circulation is associated with miscarriages, placental abruption, preeclampsia, preterm labour, IUGR, fetal distress, and low birth weight (Vichinsky, 2018).

Therapeutic Management

Ideally, clients with hemoglobinopathies are screened before conception and are made aware of the risks of sickle cell anemia to themselves and to the fetus. A blood hemoglobin electrophoresis (lab study used for both DNA and RNA analyses) is done for all clients from high-risk ancestry at their first prenatal visit to determine the types and percentages of hemoglobin present. This information should help them in making reproductive decisions.

Treatment depends on the health status of the client. The effect of sickle cell disease on pregnancy depends on which manifestations the client is experiencing. For example, sickle cell anemia combined with the increased blood volume in pregnancy increases the risks for heart failure, should fluid overload occur in therapy for the anemia (Cunningham et al., 2014).

Early and continuous prenatal care is needed to safeguard the fetus/infant from potential complications during the antepartum, intrapartum, and postpartum periods. Toward this end, prenatal visits for the first and second trimesters should be scheduled more frequently. During pregnancy, only supportive therapy is used: blood transfusions for severe anemia, analgesics for pain, and antibiotics for infection.

Nursing Assessment

Assess the client for signs and symptoms of sickle cell anemia. Ask the client if they have anorexia, dyspnea, or malaise. Inspect the colour of the skin and mucous membranes, noting any pallor. Be alert for indicators of sickle cell crisis, including severe abdominal pain, muscle spasms, leg pains, joint pain, fever, stiff neck, nausea and vomiting, and seizures (Jordan et al., 2014).

Nursing Management

Clients require emotional support, education, and follow-up care to deal with this chronic condition, which can have a great impact on the client and family. Monitor vital signs, fetal heart rate, weight gain, and fetal growth. Assess hydration status at each visit and urge the client to drink 8 to 10 glasses of fluid daily to prevent dehydration. Teach the client about the need to avoid infections (including meticulous hand hygiene), cigarette smoking, alcohol consumption, and temperature extremes.

Assist the client in scheduling frequent fetal well-being assessments, such as biophysical profiles, nonstress tests, and monitor laboratory test results for changes. Throughout the antepartum period, be alert for early signs and symptoms of crisis.

During labour, encourage rest and provide pain management. Oxygen supplementation is typically used throughout labour, along with intravenous fluids to maintain hydration. The fetal heart rate is monitored closely.

After giving birth, the client is fitted with antiembolism stockings to prevent blood clot formation. Before discharge from the facility after birth of the newborn, discuss family planning options.

The ability to predict the clinical course of sickle cell anemia during pregnancy is difficult. Outcomes have improved for childbearing clients with the disease, and currently the majority can achieve a successful live birth. However, pregnancy is associated with an increased incidence of morbidity and mortality. Optimal management during pregnancy should be directed at preventing pain crises, chronic organ damage, and early mortality using a multidisciplinary team approach and prompt, effective, and safe relief of acute pain episodes. Although these measures do not remove the risk of perinatal complications, they are thought to minimize them, promoting a successful pregnancy outcome. As part of the obstetric health care team, the nurse provides nursing interventions for the labour and postpartum client aimed at pain management, safety for the client and the fetus, and education. The overall objective is a healthy outcome for the childbearing family. The nurse has a vital role in making this happen.

AUTOIMMUNE DISORDERS

Autoimmune disorders are a group of more than 80 distinct diseases that emerge when the immune system launches an immune response against its own cells and tissues. Two distinct types of autoimmune disease occur:

1. Localized disorders target-specific organs such as the thyroid gland in Hashimoto's thyroiditis and Graves' disease.
2. Systemic disorders affect multiple organs. For example, in **systemic lupus erythematosus (SLE)**, the immune system can target the lungs, hearts, joints, kidneys, brain, and red blood cells.

Autoimmune disorders may cause mild insidious symptoms that come and go or debilitating conditions with high mortality.

Autoimmune disease is more prevalent in female-sexed persons than in male-sexed individuals. Previously, the general advice to clients with autoimmune diseases, especially SLE, multiple sclerosis (MS), or rheumatoid syndromes, was to avoid pregnancy because there was a high risk of maternal and fetal morbidity and mortality. However, it is now clear that these risks can be reduced in general by avoiding pregnancy when the diseases are active and continuing appropriate medication to reduce the chances of disease flare during pregnancy.

Systemic Lupus Erythematosus

Lupus disease, also known as SLE, is diagnosed based on laboratory values, symptoms, and signs; SLE is a chronic, relapsing autoimmune disease of the connective tissues that can affect various organs, such as the skin, joints, kidneys, and serosal membranes. Lupus disease is of unknown etiology, but it is thought to be a failure of the regulatory mechanisms of the autoimmune system. It is usually managed with anti-inflammatory and anti-rheumatic medications. Several triggers that cause the disease to activate include estrogen; cigarette smoking; infections, especially Epstein–Barr virus; physical or psychological stress; exposure to ultraviolet light; and pregnancy. Lupus symptoms may include swollen joints, extreme fatigue, oral ulcers, skin rashes, and sensitivity to sunlight (Mohindra & Marwah, 2015). Lupus is a complex disorder characterized by periods of relative inactivity and periods of disease exacerbation (flare-ups). To be diagnosed with SLE, a client must have at least four out of eleven positive American College of Rheumatology Criteria which include red rash on face, photosensitivity, oral ulcers, arthritis, serositis, renal disease, seizures, fatigue, weight changes, anemia, and a positive antinuclear antibody test (Wasserman & Clowse, 2014).

The overall incidence of lupus in the United States is 150 per 100,000 people. The peak onset occurs between ages 15 and 45 with over 80% of the cases being diagnosed in clients who are in their childbearing years. SLE is more common among those of African Canadian, Caribbean, Asian, Indigenous, and Hispanic descent (Schur & Hahn, 2015).

Pathophysiology

The autoimmune responses in SLE prevent the body from recognizing "self" from "nonself," thus allowing antibodies to be formed that attack the body's own cells and proteins. This activity causes suppression of the body's normal immunity and damage to the body tissue. The autoimmune response may initially involve one organ or several. The most common organs/organ systems involved are the cardiovascular, integumentary, musculoskeletal, nervous systems, kidneys, and lungs. In pregnancy, inflammation of the connective tissue of the deciduas can result in placental implantation problems and poor functioning (Bartels & Muller, 2015).

Clients with SLE are at increased risk for adverse pregnancy outcomes and cardiovascular disease. A pregnancy with lupus is prone to complications, including flares of disease activity during pregnancy or in the postpartum period, preeclampsia, pregnancy loss, miscarriage, stillbirth, fetal growth restriction, and preterm birth. Active lupus nephritis poses the greatest risk. The recognition of a lupus flare during pregnancy may be difficult because the signs and symptoms may mimic those of normal pregnancy (Singh & Chowdhary, 2015).

Therapeutic Management

The focus of therapy is to control disease flare-ups, suppress symptoms, and prevent organ damage. Treatment decisions are based on severity of the condition and organ involvement. Treatment of SLE in pregnancy is generally limited to NSAIDs (e.g., ibuprofen), prednisone, and an antimalarial agent, hydroxychloroquine. During pregnancy in the person with SLE, the goal is to keep drug therapy to a minimum (King et al., 2015).

Nursing Assessment

The time at which the nurse comes in contact with the client in the childbearing life cycle will determine the focus of the assessment. If the client is considering pregnancy, it is recommended to postpone conception until the disease has been stable or in remission for 6 months. Active disease at time of conception and history of renal disease increase the likelihood of a poor pregnancy outcome (Cunningham et al., 2014). In particular, if pregnancy is planned during periods of inactive or stable disease, the result often is giving birth to healthy full-term babies without increased risks of pregnancy complications. Nonetheless, pregnancies in most autoimmune diseases are still classified as high risk because of the potential for major complications. Preconception counselling should include the medical and obstetric risks of spontaneous abortion, stillbirth, fetal death, fetal growth restriction, preeclampsia, preterm labour, and neonatal death and the need for more frequent visits for monitoring their condition (Hadar, Ashwal, & Hod, 2014).

If the client is already pregnant at the initial encounter with the nurse, the nurse will need to assess for the following:

• Duration and presence of SLE signs and symptoms (fatigue, fever, malaise, polyarthritis, skin rashes, and multiorgan involvement)
• Evidence of anemia, thrombocytopenia, and thrombophilias
• Underlying renal disease (check the urine for protein and specific gravity)
• Signs of flare-ups
• Abnormalities in laboratory tests
• Signs of infection (check at each prenatal visit especially urinary tract infections and upper respiratory infections, since prednisone can mask signs of infection and lower resistance)
• Fetal well-being and growth (check using ultrasound, fundal height measurements, nonstress tests, and biophysical profiles)

Nursing Management

The nurse should discuss with the client the importance of having good control over their SLE condition throughout the pregnancy. Discussions should focus on the effects of SLE during the pregnancy and possible risk for exacerbations. Emphasize the importance of frequent prenatal visits to detect early preeclampsia, preterm labour, or infections. Instruction should cover the implications and potential side effects of all drug therapies prescribed. Teach energy conservation techniques to prevent fatigue, signs and symptoms to report (extreme fatigue, edema, confusion, abdominal pain, weight loss, leg pain, anorexia), and the need for frequent and close monitoring for fetal well-being.

After childbirth, a discussion on birth control and the effects of the various methods on the disease is essential. Referral to self-help groups and local and national SLE organizations is important for further education of the client and their family.

SLE can greatly complicate a pregnancy if close supervision is not maintained. The keys to a successful outcome for the client and their infant include an accurate assessment of the disease and of the various systems involved, and vigilance during the pregnancy for disease progression, effects on the fetus, and development of complications. Nursing care should be directed at early detection of problematic signs and symptoms, education of the client and family, careful evaluation of the fetal status, and providing support to assist in strengthening coping strategies.

Multiple Sclerosis

Multiple sclerosis (MS) is a chronic inflammatory, demyelinating autoimmune disorder of the central nervous system. MS is more commonly seen in female-sexed persons than in male-sexed individuals, and the mean age of onset is 30 years. Globally, approximately 2.5 million are affected. There is no cure for the disease, and the disease usually becomes a chronic condition (2015).

In the early, inflammatory course of MS, autoreactive T cells cross the blood–brain barrier, attacking myelin proteins and leading to inflammation and demyelination. As the inflammatory process continues, repeated injury causes progressive neurodegeneration to the myelin membrane. The pathologic hallmark of MS can be described as multicentric, multiphasic central nervous system inflammation with resultant demyelination (Armon, Baquis, Howard, & Krupa, 2015).

Uncomplicated MS does not have adverse effects on fertility, labour, or birth. Rates of spontaneous abortion, congenital anomalies, and fetal mortality are no higher among clients with MS when compared with those in the general population (Vukusic & Marignier, 2015). There is no indication that clients with MS require different care or management during the labour and birth process. Childbearing clients with MS tend to have fewer relapses during gestation with a subsequent increase in disease activity in the first 3 months postpartum. Breastfeeding does not seem to have an influence on severity or frequency of exacerbations or the health of mothers and has been shown to decrease MS relapse rates during the first 6 months postpartum (Walker, 2014). Breastfeeding should be encouraged as long as the client is not being treated with disease-modifying agents.

The clinical presentation of MS can be similar to common pregnancy-related symptoms, especially fatigue, weakness, constipation, urinary frequency, balance problems, back pain, and visual changes. The similarity of the symptoms makes it difficult to attribute any symptoms that may develop during an established pregnancy to the disease process. These symptoms should be assessed carefully to assess MS exacerbations (Novotna & Ehler, 2014).

The focus of therapy for MS is to prevent clinical relapse and postpone neurodegeneration and the subsequent disability. Current medications include anti-inflammatories, immunosuppressants, immunomodulators/biologic agents, and a variety of complementary and alternative therapies such as vitamin/mineral supplementation, homeopathy, botanical products, and antioxidants. The complementary or alternative therapies have not been proven to reduce relapse rates or disease progression, but many MS sufferers turn to them (King et al., 2015). Most medications used in MS treatment during pregnancy are not FDA approved, but many have been used "off label" and have not shown to have any adverse effects.

Nursing care is similar to that outlined previously under SLE. The need for support at this life-changing time is crucial. Continuity of care, access to information tailored to their needs, when requested by the client or their family, and having a point of contact are all important aspects of nursing care.

Rheumatoid Arthritis

Rheumatoid arthritis (RA) is characterized by joint inflammation and progressive disability and is one of the most common chronic autoimmune disorders. It commonly affects persons of childbearing age and may complicate pregnancy. Approximately 1% of Canadian adults are affected by RA, but it occurs two times more frequently in female-sexed persons than in male-sexed individuals (Public Health Agency of Canada, 2010). RA is present in nearly all geographic areas and affects all ethnic groups. RA primarily affects synovial joints and tissues of the hands and feet, but any joint can be involved. Over time, bone and cartilage are damaged by the chronic inflammation process, resulting in joint deformity and loss of function. Progression of the disease and ensuing disability is unpredictable.

The course of RA during pregnancy is usually benign. In about three fourths of pregnancies, the symptoms of the disease lessen. In these cases, most clients experience relief in the first trimester that continues throughout the pregnancy. For many childbearing persons with RA, pregnancy can provide a reprieve from long-term joint pain and inflammation, but others will not experience remission and will continue to need medication. RA does not adversely affect pregnancy outcome. With occasional exceptions, RA returns after the third to fourth month postpartum (Strangfeld et al., 2015).

Individuals with RA typically present with pain, swelling, and tenderness in joints; decreased mobility; and stiffness after periods of inactivity. Treatment of RA focuses on reducing joint inflammation, managing pain, and preventing joint destruction. The categories of medications used to accomplish this are NSAIDs, glucocorticoids, hydroxychloroquine, methotrexate, immunomodulators/biologic agents and complementary alternative therapies such as physical therapy, exercise, acupuncture, and joint splinting for pain relief. During pregnancy, medications are limited to hydroxychloroquine, glucocorticoids, and NSAIDs. Methotrexate is contraindicated during pregnancy (Brucker & King, 2017). Careful preconception counselling and risk assessment is important in someone with RA. Antibody status and all medications need to be reviewed before pregnancy. Maintaining low disease activity before and during pregnancy is essential for optimal outcomes.

Nursing care should address the **teratogenicity** (the ability to cause birth defects) and adverse effects of some of the medications used to treat RA. Clients with RA must be monitored closely following childbirth because most are likely to have arthritis flare-ups during the postpartum period. The general nursing care is similar to that outlined for the low-risk pregnant client. Nurses caring for persons with any disability (physical or cognitive) in general need to provide level-appropriate education on all reproductive health issues and improved access to health care. The client's specific disability, resources, and approach to pregnancy and childbirth all help shape their experience. The nurse can play a role in making the experience a positive, memorable time in their life. Care for the client with a disability should be well planned and coordinated by ensuring all documentation of the client's needs and concerns is readily available to all personnel involved in their care. All members of the health care team should be involved in the plan of care and kept up to date of any changes. It is essential that the nurse facilitate care to ensure continuity of care throughout the client's pregnancy and childbirth experience (Ostensen, 2014).

INFECTIONS

A wide variety of infections can affect the progression of pregnancy, possibly having a negative impact on the outcome. The effect of the infection depends on the timing and severity of the infection and the body systems involved. Common viral infections include cytomegalovirus, rubella, herpes simplex, hepatitis B, varicella, parvovirus B19, and several sexually transmitted infections (STIs; Table 20.4). Toxoplasmosis and group B streptococcus are common nonviral infections. Only the most common infections will be discussed here.

TABLE 20.4	SEXUALLY TRANSMITTED INFECTIONS AFFECTING PREGNANCY	
Infection/Organism	Effect on Pregnancy and Fetus/Newborn	Implications
Syphilis (*Treponema pallidum*)	Client infection increases the risk of premature labour and birth. Newborn may be born with congenital syphilis—jaundice, rhinitis, anemia, IUGR, and CNS involvement.	All pregnant clients should be screened for this STI and treated with benzathine penicillin G 2.4 million units IM to prevent placental transmission.
Gonorrhea (*Neisseria gonorrhoeae*)	Majority of clients are asymptomatic. It causes ophthalmia neonatorum in the newborn from birth through infected birth canal.	All pregnant clients should be screened at first prenatal visit, with repeat screening in the third trimester, if indicated, and treated as necessary. The practice of administering erythromycin eye ointment to newborns, for prophylaxis within the first hour of life, continues in many Canadian jurisdictions.
Chlamydia (*Chlamydia trachomatis*)	Majority of clients are asymptomatic. Infection is associated with infertility and ectopic pregnancy, spontaneous abortions, preterm labour, premature rupture of membranes, low birth weight, stillbirth, and neonatal mortality. Infection is transmitted to newborn through vaginal birth. Neonate may develop conjunctivitis or pneumonia.	All pregnant clients should be screened at first prenatal visit and treated with erythromycin.
Human papillomavirus (HPV)	Infection causes warts in the anogenital area, known as condylomata acuminata. These warts may grow large enough to block a vaginal birth. Fetal exposure to HPV during birth is associated with laryngeal papillomas.	Warts are treated with trichloroacetic acid, liquid nitrogen, or laser therapy under colposcopy. Three HPV vaccines have been approved for use in Canada (Gardasil, Gardasil-9, and Cervarix) against the viral types most likely to cause cervical cancer (types 16 and 18) and genital warts (types 6 and 11). It is recommended for vaccination between ages 9 and 26 years old.
Trichomonas (*Trichomonas vaginalis*)	Infection produces itching and burning, dysuria, strawberry patches on cervix, and vaginal discharge. Infection is associated with premature rupture of membranes and preterm birth.	Treatment is with a single 2-g dose of metronidazole (Flagyl).

Adapted from King, T. L., Brucker, M. C., Kriebs, J. M., Fahey, J. O., Gegor, C. L., & Varney, H. (2015). *Varney's midwifery* (5th ed.). Burlington, MA: Jones & Bartlett Learning; Kumar, B., & Gupta, S. (2014). *Sexually transmitted infections* (2nd ed.). Philadelphia, PA: Elsevier Health Sciences; and Centers for Disease Control and Prevention (CDC). (2015r). *Sexually transmitted diseases*. Retrieved from http://www.cdc.gov/std/.

Cytomegalovirus

Human cytomegalovirus (CMV) infects greater than 50% of the human population. Humans are the only known hosts of CMV, which is transmitted via body fluids. Worldwide, the birth prevalence is estimated at 7 per 1,000 births with the highest rates seen in developing countries. It is typically asymptomatic in most individuals. CMV is the most common congenital and perinatal viral infection in the world (Fig. 20.4). CMV is the leading cause of congenital infection, with morbidity and

mortality at birth and sequelae. Each year approximately 1% to 7% of childbearing persons acquire a primary CMV infection (Kovacs & Briggs, 2015). Of these, about 30% to 40% transmit the infection to their fetuses. The risk of serious fetal injury is greatest when the client's infection develops in the first trimester or early in the second trimester. Between 10% and 15% of congenitally infected infants are acutely symptomatic at birth and most of the survivors have serious long-term complications (March of Dimes, 2015d). It is a leading cause of hearing loss and intellectual (Yinon, Farine, & Yudin, 2018). However,

FIGURE 20.4 Clinical appearance of infant with congenital CMV with stigmata of disease, including petechial rash, microcephaly, jaundice, and abnormal posture of upper extremities secondary to CNS damage.

there has been limited progress in developing interventions to prevent or treat CMV infection (Bialas, Swamy, & Permar, 2015). Pregnant persons acquire active disease primarily from sexual contact, blood transfusions, kissing, and contact with children in daycare centres. It can also be spread through vertical transmission from a childbearing person to their child in utero (causing congenital CMV), during birth, or through breastfeeding. The virus can be found in virtually all body fluids. CMV is not easily transmitted from host to recipient; the incidence of primary CMV infection occurs in 1% to 4% of pregnancies, and at higher rates among those of lower socioeconomic status (Yinon et al., 2018). CMV infection during pregnancy may result in abortion, stillbirth, low birth weight, IUGR, microcephaly, deafness, blindness, intellectual disability, jaundice, or congenital or neonatal infection. The first or primary infection, if it occurs during pregnancy, is the most dangerous to the fetus: the fetus has a 30% to 40% chance of being infected.

There are three time periods during which mother-to-child transmission can occur: in utero, during birth, and after birth. However, permanent disability only occurs in association with in utero infection. Such disability can result from infection of the childbearing person during any point in the pregnancy, but more severe disabilities are usually associated with infection during the first trimester.

Most clients are asymptomatic and do not know that they have been exposed to CMV. Symptoms of CMV in the fetus and newborn, known as CMV inclusion disease, include hepatomegaly, thrombocytopenia, IUGR, jaundice, microcephaly, hearing loss, chorioretinitis, and intellectual disability. Newborns that are asymptomatic at birth may go on to develop late neurodevelopmental sequelae, with sensorineural hearing loss being the most

common condition (Silasi et al., 2015). Prenatal screening for CMV infection is not routinely performed, and serologic testing should be used in clients who develop influenza-like illness (Yinon et al., 2018). Unfortunately, a preventive vaccine remains elusive. Since there is no therapy to prevent or treat CMV infections, nurses are responsible for educating and supporting childbearing-age clients at risk for CMV infection. Stressing the importance of good hand hygiene and the use of sound hygiene practices can help to reduce transmission of the virus. A few specific hygiene guidelines for pregnant clients include the following:

- Wash hands frequently with soap and water and wear gloves, especially after diaper changes, feeding, wiping nose or drool, and handling children's toys.
- Do not share cups, plates, utensils, food, or toothbrushes.
- Do not share towels or washcloths.
- Do not put a child's pacifier in your mouth.
- Clean toys, countertops, and other surfaces that come in contact with children's urine or saliva.
- Practice safe sex, including limiting sexual partners and use condoms consistently.

Rubella

Rubella, commonly called German measles, is spread by droplets or through direct contact with a contaminated object. The risk of a pregnant person transmitting this virus through the placenta to the fetus increases with earlier exposure to the virus. When infection occurs within the first month after conception, 50% of fetuses show signs of infection; in the second month following conception, 25% of fetuses will be infected; and in the third month, 10% of fetuses will be affected. Congenital rubella can manifest with a diverse range of symptoms in the newborn, including congenital cataracts, glaucoma, cardiac defects, microcephaly, as well as hearing and intellectual disabilities (Jyoti, Shirke, & Matalia, 2015).

Preconception care has been defined as a set of interventions designed to identify and modify risks to promote health and positive pregnancy outcomes through prevention and management. This care should be provided any time any health care provider sees a person of reproductive age. Personal and family history, physical exam, laboratory screening, reproductive plan, nutrition, supplements, weight, exercise, vaccinations, and injury prevention should be reviewed in all clients. Folic acid 400 mcg per day, as well as proper diet and exercise, should be encouraged. Clients should receive the influenza vaccine if planning pregnancy during flu season; the rubella and varicella vaccines if there is no evidence of immunity to these viruses; and tetanus/diphtheria/pertussis if lacking adult vaccination (Lambert, Strebel, Orenstein, Icenogle, & Poland, 2015).

Education for primary prevention is key. Ideally, all clients have been vaccinated and have adequate immunity against rubella. However, all childbearing persons are still screened at their first prenatal visit to determine their status. A rubella antibody titer of 1:8 or greater proves evidence of immunity. Clients who are not immune should be vaccinated during the immediate postpartum period so they will be immune before becoming pregnant again (Agent, 2015). Nurses need to check the rubella immune status of all new postpartum clients and should make sure those with a titer of less than 1:8 are immunized prior to discharge after birth of the newborn.

Herpes Simplex Virus

Genital herpes is an STI caused by the herpes simplex virus (HSV) type 1 or type 2. Both types can cause genital infections, and while HSV-2 has been more common with genital infections, primary HSV-1 genital infections are increasing in frequency (Money & Steben, 2017). HSV-2 is present in 17% of pregnancies, and neonates are affected at a rate of 1 per 17,000 live births in Canada. Untreated neonatal HSV infection is associated with a mortality rate of 60%, and survivors experience considerable disability (Ural, 2015). Despite strategies designed to prevent perinatal transmission, the number of cases of newborn HSV infection continues to rise, mirroring the rising prevalence of genital herpes infection in persons of childbearing age (Fig. 20.5) (James & Kimberlin, 2015).

HSV is a DNA virus with two subtypes: HSV-1 and HSV-2. HSV-1 infections were traditionally associated with oral lesions (fever blisters), whereas HSV-2 infections occurred in the genital region. Currently, either type can be found in either location (Ural, 2015).

FIGURE 20.5 Newborn with disseminated herpes simplex virus infection. Note the healing ulcerations on the abdomen of the infant. (From Sweet, R. L., Gibbs, R. S. [Eds.]. [2009]. *Infectious diseases of the female genital tract* [5th ed.]. Philadelphia, PA: Lippincott Williams & Wilkins.)

Infection occurs by direct contact of the skin or mucous membranes with an active lesion through such activities as kissing, sexual (vaginal, oral, anal) contact, or routine skin-to-skin contact. HSV is associated with infections of the genital tract that when acquired during pregnancy can result in severe systemic symptoms in the pregnant client and significant morbidity and mortality in the newborn. In addition, it may cause spontaneous abortion, birth anomalies, IUGR, or preterm labour. A 60% mortality rate may occur if the neonatal exposure is with an active primary infection (Silasi et al., 2015). Once the virus enters the body, it never leaves.

Infants born to clients with a primary HSV infection have a 30% to 50% risk of acquiring the infection via perinatal transmission near or during birth. Recurrent genital HSV infections carry a 1% to 3% risk of neonatal infection if the recurrence occurs around the time of vaginal birth (March of Dimes, 2015e). About one in four childbearing clients is infected with genital herpes, although most do not know it. Fortunately, only a small number pass the infection on to their newborns (March of Dimes, 2015e).

The greatest risk of transmission is when the pregnant person develops a primary infection near term and it is not recognized. Most neonatal infections are acquired at or around the time of birth through either ascending infection after ruptured membranes or contact with the virus at the time of birth. For clients with a primary infection identified in the third trimester, a cesarean birth is recommended (Money & Steben, 2017). For clients with recurrent genital HSV infection, in the absence of active lesions a vaginal birth is acceptable, but if the client has active herpetic lesions near or at term a cesarean birth should be offered. All invasive procedures that might cause a break in the infant's skin should be avoided, such as artificial rupture of membranes, fetal scalp electrode, or forceps and vacuum extraction (Jordan et al., 2014).

Management for the client with genital herpes during pregnancy involves caring for them as well as reducing the risk of newborn herpes. No therapy can eradicate HSV, and this chronic infection is noted for its frequent asymptomatic viral shedding. Because the majority of newborn herpes cases result from perinatal transmission of the virus during vaginal birth, and because transmission can result in severe neurologic impairment or death, treatment of the client with an antiviral agent such as acyclovir must be started as soon as the culture comes back positive with a primary infection, or in the presence of lesions with recurrent infection. The Society of Obstetricians and Gynecologists recommends offering all clients with chronic HSV infection antiviral treatment with acyclovir or valacyclovir, beginning at 36 weeks' gestation until the time of delivery, to reduce the risk of lesions and viral shedding at the time of delivery (Money & Steben, 2017). Use of condoms and antiviral medications assist in preventing transmission. Evidence does not support routine HSV serologic screening among asymptomatic pregnant clients currently (Workowski & Bolan, 2015), so nurses need to remain knowledgeable about current practice to provide accurate and sensitive care to all clients. Despite the surge in vaccine research, there is unfortunately no readily available or preventative or therapeutic vaccine for HSV to date.

Hepatitis B Virus

Hepatitis B is one of the most prevalent chronic diseases in the world. It is a serious global public health problem in Asia, Africa, Southern Europe, and Latin America, especially. Hepatitis B virus (HBV) has infected approximately 2 billion people worldwide, of whom more than 350 million are chronically infected. Life-threatening liver disease (cirrhosis, liver failure, and hepatocellular carcinoma) occurs in as many as 40% of people with hepatitis B. HBV can be transmitted through contaminated blood, illicit drug use, and sexual contact. The virus is 100 times more infectious than HIV and, unlike HIV, it can live outside the body in dried blood for more than a week (Salman, Priti, Molly, Kumar, & Zeenat, 2015).

Sexual transmission accounts for most adult HBV infections. Acutely infected clients develop hepatitis with anorexia, nausea, vomiting, fever, abdominal pain, and jaundice. In clients with acute hepatitis B, vertical transmission occurs in approximately 10% of newborns when infection occurs in the first trimester and in 80% to 90% of newborns when acute infection occurs in the third trimester. Without intervention, 40% of infants born to clients who are positive for hepatitis B will have chronic hepatitis B by 6 months of age (CDC, 2015g). In addition, hepatitis B infection during pregnancy is associated with an increased risk of preterm birth, fetal distress during labour, meconium peritonitis, low birth weight, and neonatal death. Newborns infected with HBV are likely to become chronic carriers of the virus, becoming reservoirs for continued infection in the population (CDC, 2015g). The fetus is at particular risk during birth because of the possible contact with contaminated blood at this time.

The CDC (2015g) recommends that all pregnant clients should be tested for hepatitis B surface antigen (HBsAg) regardless of previous HBV vaccine or screening. Infants born to HBsAg-positive person should receive single-antigen HBV vaccine and hepatitis B immunoglobulin (HBIG) within 12 hours of birth. Completion of the routine vaccine schedule is recommended, which in Canada includes HBV vaccination. There is a growing body of literature supporting the safety and efficacy of antiviral therapies administered in the third trimester of pregnancy to reduce the vertical transmission of the HBV from the childbearing person to the fetus, but to date there has not been any formal recommendations (Lamberth, Reddy, Pan, & Dasher, 2015).

Nursing Assessment

Review the client's history for factors placing them at high risk:
- History of STIs
- Household contacts with HBV-infected persons
- Employment as a health care provider
- Abuse of intravenous drugs
- Prostitution
- Foreign born
- Multiple sexual partners
- Chinese, Southeast Asian, or African heritage
- Sexual partners who are HBV infected (CDC, 2015g)

At the first prenatal visit, all pregnant clients should be screened for HbsAg via blood studies, even if they were previously vaccinated or tested. Expect to repeat this screening later in pregnancy for clients in high-risk groups (Park & Pan, 2014).

Nursing Management

If a client tests positive for HBV, expect to administer HBIG. The newborn will also receive HBV vaccine within 12 hours of birth. The timing of the second and third doses of the vaccine varies between provinces depending on the routine Provincial vaccine schedule (Castillo, Murphy, & Schalkwyk, 2017). The CDC recommends routine vaccination of all newborns.

Clients who are HbsAg negative may be vaccinated safely during pregnancy. No current research supports the use of surgical births to reduce vertical transmission of HBV. Breastfeeding by mothers with chronic HBV infection does not increase the risk of viral transmission to their newborns, nor is it a contraindication to breastfeeding, unless the client is taking antiviral medication or has bleeding nipples. Clients with bleeding nipples should abstain from breastfeeding until they are healed (Jhaveri, 2015).

Client education related to prevention of HBV is essential. Teach the client about safer sex practices, good hand hygiene techniques, and the use of standard precautions (Teaching Guidelines 20.4). Protection can be afforded with the highly effective hepatitis B vaccine.

Teaching Guidelines 20.4
TEACHING TO PREVENT HEPATITIS B VIRUS PROGRESSION
- Abstain from alcohol and potentially hepatotoxic medications.
- Avoid intravenous drug exposure or sharing of needles.
- Encourage all household contacts and sexual partners to be vaccinated.
- Receive immediate treatment for any STI.

- Know that your newborn will receive hepatitis B vaccine soon after birth.
- Use good hand hygiene techniques at all times.
- Avoid contact with blood or body fluids.
- Use barrier methods such as condoms during sexual intercourse.
- Avoid sharing any personal items, such as razors, toothbrushes, or eating utensils.
- Inform all health care providers of your HBV status.

Permanent remission of the disease even with treatment rarely occurs. Therefore, therapy is directed at long-term suppression of viral replication and prevention of end-stage liver disease. Urge the client to consume a high-protein diet and avoid fatigue. A healthy lifestyle can help delay disease progression. Initiate an open discussion about the modes of transmission and use of condoms to prevent spread.

Varicella Zoster Virus

Varicella zoster virus (VZV) is one of the eight herpes family viruses. It is the virus that causes both varicella (chickenpox) and herpes zoster (shingles). Primary VZV leads to varicella (chicken pox) and establishes latency in dorsal root ganglia. Reactivation of VZV causes herpes zoster, commonly called shingles. Herpes zoster can occur once immune response against the virus wanes, usually with advancing age.

Pregnant clients are at risk for developing varicella when they come in close contact with children who have active infection. Varicella occurs year round, but there is a higher incidence during winter and spring months. Varicella in the childbearing person can be transmitted to the fetus through the placenta, leading to congenital varicella syndrome, if the client is infected during the first half of pregnancy, via an ascending infection during birth, or by direct contact with infectious lesions, leading to infection after birth. Varicella occurs in approximately 1/1,000 pregnancies (Charlier et al., 2014).

Congenital varicella syndrome can occur in newborns of clients infected during early pregnancy. The vertical transmission rate is estimated to be between 2% and 10%. It is characterized by low birth weight, skin lesions in a dermatomal distribution, spontaneous abortion, chorioretinitis, cataracts, fetal growth restriction, delayed milestones, cutaneous scarring, limb hypoplasia, microcephaly, ocular abnormalities, intellectual disability, and early death (Swamy & Heine, 2015).

Preconception counselling is important for preventing this condition. A major component of counselling involves determining the client's varicella immunity. Vaccination is the cornerstone of prevention. The vaccine is administered if needed. Varicella vaccine is a live attenuated viral vaccine. It should be administered to all adolescents and adults 13 years of age and older who do not have evidence of varicella immunity (King et al., 2015). Provide education to clients who work in occupations that increase the risk of exposure to the virus, such as daycare workers, teachers of young children, and staff caring for children in institutional settings.

Varicella during pregnancy can be associated with severe illnesses for both the client and the newborn. If contracted in the first half of pregnancy, some childbearing clients are at risk for developing varicella pneumonia, which may put them at risk of life-threatening ventilatory compromise and death. Risk of varicella pneumonia appears to increase during pregnancy (Zhang, Patenaude, & Abenhaim, 2014). If the client develops varicella rashes close to the due date, generalized neonatal varicella leading to death in about 20% of cases can be expected (Jordan et al., 2014).

Parvovirus B19

Parvovirus B19 infection occurs worldwide with most infected persons asymptomatic. The incidence of acute B19 infection in pregnancy is about 3%. Approximately 30% to 50% of childbearing persons are not immune, and vertical transmission is common following maternal infection in pregnancy. Fetal infection may be associated with a normal outcome, but fetal death may also occur without ultrasound evidence of infectious sequelae (Desai & Brustman, 2014). Parvovirus B19 is a common, self-limiting, benign childhood virus that causes erythema infectiosum, also known as Fifth disease (referring to its fifth place in a list of common childhood infections). Approximately 65% of persons of reproductive age have developed immunity to parvovirus B19. Infection with parvovirus B19 affects 1 in 400 childbearing persons, but the majority has no adverse pregnancy outcome; those that do may experience spontaneous abortion and severe fetal anemia. There is no treatment for the pregnant client with parvovirus B19 infection (Malee, 2015).

Pathophysiology

The infection is spread transplacentally, by the oropharyngeal route in casual contact, and through infected blood. Infection of the fetus occurs through transplacental passage of the virus. Acute infection in pregnancy can cause B19 infection in the fetus, leading to nonimmune fetal hydrops (a serious abnormal accumulation of fluid in 2 or more fetal compartments, including ascites, pleural effusion, pericardial effusion, and skin edema), secondary to severe anemia or fetal loss, depending on the gestational age at the time of infection. The risk to the fetus is greatest when the pregnant person is exposed and infected within the first 20 weeks of gestation. In addition to hydrops, other fetal effects of parvovirus include spontaneous abortion, congenital anomalies (central nervous system, craniofacial, and eye), and long-term effects such as hepatic insufficiency, myocarditis, and learning disabilities (Edwards, 2014). Fetal infection with B19V is also associated with intrauterine fetal death, nonimmune hydrops fetalis, thrombocytopenia, myocarditis, and neurologic manifestations. Fetal infection can also remain clinically unrecognized (Suliman & Seopela, 2015).

Therapeutic Management

Generally, a diagnosis of parvovirus is based on clinical symptoms and serologic antibody testing for parvovirus immunoglobulin G (IgG) and parvovirus immunoglobulin M (IgM). Parvovirus B19 infection is followed by lifelong immunity, which is shown by positive serum B19 IgG. Childbearing clients who have been exposed to or who develop symptoms of parvovirus B19 require assessment to determine whether they are susceptible to infection (nonimmune). If the client is immune, they can be reassured that they will not develop infection and that the virus will not adversely affect the pregnancy. If the client is nonimmune, then referral to a maternal fetal medicine specialist is recommended and counselling regarding the risks of fetal transmission, fetal loss, and hydrops is necessary. Knowledge of how best to manage this infection during pregnancy lags behind our understanding of the potential adverse consequences.

Intrauterine B19 infection is a cause of fetal anemia, hydrops, and demise, and perhaps also of congenital anomalies. The best strategy for surveillance of the infected pregnant client is serial ultrasounds for detection of hydropic changes and fetal anemia, and treatment for severe fetal anemia. Serial ultrasounds are advocated because the rates of fetal death and complications peak 4 to 6 weeks after exposure, but they can occur as late as 3 months following onset of symptoms. The infected newborn is assessed for any anomaly and followed for up to 6 years to identify any sequelae (Smith, 2015).

Nursing Assessment

Review the client's history for any risk factors. School-teachers, daycare workers, and those living with school-aged children are at the highest risk for being seropositive for parvovirus B19, especially if a recent outbreak has occurred in those settings. Also assess the client for specific signs and symptoms. The characteristic rash starts on the face with a "slapped-cheeks" appearance and is followed by a generalized maculopapular rash. Fever, arthralgia, and generalized malaise are usually present in the client. Prepare the client for antibody testing.

Nursing Management

Prevention is the best strategy. Stress the need for hand hygiene after handling children; cleaning toys and surfaces that children have been in contact with; and avoiding the sharing of food and drinks. Screening for parvovirus B19 during early pregnancy may help in early diagnosis, but the cost-effectiveness of a national screening program has not been accepted to date. The nurse can provide information regarding risk factors and potential complications if exposed and support the parent's decision.

Group B Streptococcus

Group B streptococcus (GBS) is a naturally occurring bacterium found in approximately 50% of healthy adults. Clients who test positive for the GBS bacteria are considered carriers. Carrier status is transient and does not indicate illness. Approximately 25% of childbearing clients carry GBS in the rectum or vagina, thus introducing the risk of colonization of the fetus during birth. Approximately 1 out of every 100 to 200 newborns born to clients who carry GBS will develop signs and symptoms of GBS disease. Although GBS is rarely serious in adults, it can be life threatening to newborns. GBS is the most common cause of sepsis and meningitis in newborns and is a frequent cause of newborn pneumonia (Puopolo, Madoff, & Baker, 2015). Newborns with early-onset (within a week after birth) GBS infections may have pneumonia or sepsis, whereas late-onset (after the first week) infections often manifest with meningitis (CDC, 2015i).

Genital tract colonization poses the most serious threat to the newborn because of exposure during birth and to the client because of ascending infection after the membranes rupture. GBS colonization in the client is thought to cause chorioamnionitis, endometritis, and postpartum wound infection. Heavy colonization with GBS has also been associated with both preterm pre-labour rupture of membranes and preterm labour (Money & Allen, 2013).

Therapeutic Management

Antibiotic therapy usually is effective in treating clients with GBS infections of the urinary tract or uterus, or chorioamnionitis without any sequelae. Screening for asymptomatic bacteriuria is a standard component of prenatal care (Allen & Yudin, 2012). Childbearing clients who do not have a documented GBS bacteriuria at any point in the current pregnancy should be re-screened for GBS colonization with vaginal and rectal swabs at 35 to 37 weeks' gestation and treated in labour (Money & Allen, 2013). Clients with positive cultures are treated with a penicillin-based anti-infective agent during pregnancy for identified bacteriuria, and during labour if the positive detection with vaginal-rectal swabs.

Penicillin G is the treatment of choice for GBS infection because of its narrow spectrum. Alternative antibiotics can be prescribed for clients with a penicillin allergy. The drug is usually administered intravenously at least 4 hours before birth so that it can reach adequate levels in the serum and amniotic fluid to reduce the risk of newborn colonization. Close monitoring is required during the administration of intravenous antibiotics because severe allergic reactions can occur rapidly.

Nursing Assessment

Review the client's prenatal history and ask about any previous infection. Determine if the client's membranes have ruptured and the time of rupture. Rupture of amniotic membranes more than 18 hours increases the risk for infection. Monitor the client's vital signs, reporting any maternal fever greater than 38°C. Assess the client for other risk factors for perinatal transmission of GBS, including previous colonization with GBS, positive colonization at 35 to 37 weeks' gestation, GBS in urine sample at any time in the current pregnancy, previous birth of GBS-positive newborn (March of Dimes, 2015f). Document this information to help prevent vertical transmission to the newborn.

Many clients with GBS infection are asymptomatic, but they may have urinary tract infections, uterine infections, and chorioamnionitis.

Nursing Management

Nurses play major roles as educators and advocates for all clients and newborns to reduce the incidence of GBS infections. Ensure that pregnant clients between 35 and 37 weeks' gestation are screened for GBS infection during a prenatal visit. Record the results and notify the birth attendant if the client has tested positive for GBS. During labour, be prepared to administer intravenous antibiotics to all clients who are GBS positive.

Toxoplasmosis

Toxoplasmosis is a relatively widespread parasitic infection caused by a one-celled organism, *Toxoplasma gondii*. It is found all over the world, and can affect any warm-blooded animal, including humans, although the primary host is the cat. When a childbearing client is exposed to this protozoan, the infection can pose serious risks to the fetus through transplacental transfer from the client to the fetus. Cats are the definitive hosts of this parasite and shed it in their feces. It is transferred by hand to mouth after touching cat feces while changing the cat litter box or through gardening in contaminated soil. Consuming undercooked infected meat, such as pork, lamb, or venison drinking contaminated water, and eating unwashed fruits and vegetables can also transmit this organism.

A pregnant client that contracts toxoplasmosis for the first time has an approximately 40% chance of passing the infection to their fetus. Toxoplasmosis acquired during pregnancy means high risk of damage for the fetus (March of Dimes, 2015g). Although the client typically remains asymptomatic, transmission to the fetus can occur throughout pregnancy. A fetus that contracts congenital toxoplasmosis typically has a low birth weight, enlarged liver and spleen, chorioretinitis, jaundice, IUGR, hydrocephalus, microcephaly, neurologic damage, and anemia. Severity varies with gestational age; usually, the earlier the infection, the more severe the effects (Silasi et al., 2015).

Treatment of the client during pregnancy to reduce the risk of congenital infection is a combination of pyrimethamine, sulfadiazine, and folinic acid (Paquet & Yudin, 2013). Treatment with sulfonamides during pregnancy has been shown to reduce the risk of congenital infection.

Although there is much to learn about the best approach to the identification and treatment of toxoplasmosis, it is known that early treatment leads to the best neurodevelopmental outcomes in infants. Prevention is the key to managing this infection. Nurses play a key role in educating the client about measures to prevent toxoplasmosis (Teaching Guidelines 20.5).

Teaching Guidelines 20.5
TEACHING TO PREVENT TOXOPLASMOSIS

- Avoid eating raw or undercooked meat, especially lamb or pork. Cook all meat to an internal temperature of 160°F (71°C) throughout.
- Clean cutting boards, work surfaces, and utensils with hot soapy water after contact with raw meat or unwashed fruits and vegetables.
- Peel or thoroughly wash all raw fruits and vegetables before eating them.
- Wash hands thoroughly with warm water and soap after handling raw meat.
- Avoid feeding the cat raw or undercooked meats.
- Avoid emptying or cleaning the cat's litter box. Have someone else do it daily.
- Keep outdoor sandboxes covered to prevent cat feces contamination.
- Keep the cat indoors to prevent it from hunting and eating birds or rodents.
- Avoid uncooked eggs and unpasteurized milk.
- Wear gardening gloves when in contact with outdoor soil.
- Avoid contact with children's sandboxes, because cats can use them as litter boxes.

Clients Who Are HIV Positive

The **human immunodeficiency virus (HIV)** is a chronic infection caused by the retrovirus HIV, which infects T cells that causes immunodeficiency. Once the CD4-positive cell count falls below a certain level, HIV infection causes increased susceptibility to infections, cancers, and neurologic damage (Hardy, DegliEsposti, & Nee, 2015). HIV is transmitted by blood and body fluids. The number of people estimated to be living with HIV infection in Canada at the end of 2014 was 75,500 (Public Health Agency of Canada, 2015). There was a 9.7% increase from 2011 in the general population, but a 12.1% increase among Indigenous populations. Persons from countries where HIV is endemic are also over-represented in the proportion of those living with HIV.

Despite the revolutionary strides that have been made in treatment and detection and recent clinical advances and cautious optimism associated with combination therapies and vaccines, the number of individuals who are HIV positive continues to climb worldwide. Intensive efforts notwithstanding, no real "cure" can be seen on the horizon. To achieve a durable end to the HIV pandemic, a vaccine remains essential in the fight against this virus (Fauci, Folkers, & Marston, 2014). Also, despite dramatic reductions in perinatal transmission of HIV, barriers to prevention still exist and perinatal HIV infections continue.

The risk of acquiring HIV through heterosexual contact is greater for a person with vagina who has a sexual partner with a penis, due to exposure to the higher viral concentration in semen. In addition, sexual intercourse may cause breaks in the vaginal lining, increasing the chances that the virus will enter the body through the vaginal tissue. The same risk applies to individuals practicing anal intercourse. Recent data indicated that 78% of new HIV infections in Canadian individuals identified as female were attributed to heterosexual intercourse, and 22% of new infections were attributed to intravenous drug use (Challacombe, 2019).

Pathophysiology

The three recognized modes of HIV transmission are unprotected sexual intercourse with an infected partner, contact with infected blood or blood products, and perinatal transmission.

> **Take Note!**
>
> HIV is not transmitted by doorknobs, faucets, toilets, dirty dishes, mosquitoes, wet towels, coughing or sneezing, shaking hands, or being hugged or by any other indirect method.

The virus attacks the T4 cells, decreases the CD4 cell count, and disables the immune system. The HIV condition can progress to a severe immunosuppressed state termed **acquired immunodeficiency syndrome (AIDS)**. AIDS is a progressive, debilitating disease that suppresses cellular immunity, predisposing the infected person to opportunistic infections and malignancies. The CDC defines AIDS as an HIV-infected person with a specific opportunistic infection or a CD4 count of less than 200. Eventually, death occurs. The time from infection with HIV to development of AIDS is a median of 11 years but varies depending on whether the client is taking current antiretroviral therapy (ART) (Maartens, Celum, & Lewin, 2014). Research indicates that pregnancy does not accelerate the progression of HIV to AIDS or death (Calvert & Ronsmans, 2015).

Once infected with HIV, the client develops antibodies that can be detected with the enzyme-linked immunosorbent assay (ELISA) and confirmed with the Western blot test. Antibodies develop within 6 to 12 weeks after exposure, although this latent period is much longer in some female-sexed persons. Table 20.5

TABLE 20.5		STAGES OF HIV INFECTION OUTLINED BY THE CDC
Stages	**Description**	**Clinical Picture**
I	Acute infection	Early stage with pervasive viral production Flu-like symptoms 2–4 weeks after exposure Signs and symptoms: weight loss, low-grade fever, fatigue, sore throat, night sweats, and myalgia. Ability to spread HIV is highest during this stage because large amounts of HIV are being produced in the body and the CD4 count drops.
II	Asymptomatic infection or clinical latency	Viral replication continues within lymphatics, but slows down Usually free of symptoms; lymphadenopathy
III	Persistent generalized lymphadenopathy	Possibly remaining in this stage for years; AIDS develops in most within 7–10 years Opportunistic infections occur
IV	End-stage disease (AIDS)	Severe immune deficiency; very vulnerable to infections High viral load and low CD4 counts Signs and symptoms: bacterial, viral, or fungal opportunistic infections, fever, wasting syndrome, fatigue, neoplasms, and cognitive changes

Adapted from U.S. Centers of Disease Control and Prevention (CDC). (2015s). *About HIV/AIDS*. Retrieved from http://www.cdc.gov/hiv/basics/whatishiv.html.

highlights the four stages of HIV infection according to the CDC (2015l).

Impact of HIV on Pregnancy

When a person who is infected with HIV becomes pregnant, their personal risks, as well as the risk to the fetus and the newborn, are great. The risks are compounded by problems such as drug abuse, lack of access to prenatal care, poverty, poor nutrition, and high-risk behaviours such as unsafe sex practices and multiple sex partners, which can predispose the person to additional STIs including herpes, syphilis, or human papillomavirus (HPV). Additional risk factors to assess for include persons who exchange sex for money or drugs or have sex partners who do; a person whose past or present sex partners were HIV infected; and anyone who had a blood transfusion between 1978 and 1985. Early identification of HIV seropositivity allows early antiretroviral treatment to prevent client-to-child transmission, allows a provider to avoid obstetric practices that may increase the risk of transmission, and allows an opportunity to counsel the client against breastfeeding (also known to increase the risk of transmission) (U.S. Preventive Services Task Force [USPSTF], 2014). Subsequently, pregnant clients who are HIV positive are at risk for preterm delivery, fetal growth restriction, premature rupture of membranes, intrapartal or postpartum hemorrhage, postpartum infection, poor wound healing, and genitourinary tract infections (CDC, 2015m).

Perinatal transmission of HIV (from the pregnant person to the fetus or child) also can occur. However, such cases have decreased in the past several years, primarily due to the use of antiretroviral therapy in childbearing clients infected with HIV. This has not been the case in developing countries without similar resources. The Joint United Nations programs on HIV/AIDS (UNAIDS) estimate that over 2,000 new infections due to client-to-child transmission occur daily. This number is expected to increase rapidly as the prevalence rises in Southeast Asia (Rakhmanina & van den Anker, 2014). Perinatal transmission rates are as high as 35% when there is no intervention (ART) and below 1% when antiretroviral treatment and appropriate care are available. Lack of timely HIV testing during pregnancy is a major contributor to this outcome. Interventions are needed that will address knowledge barriers to HIV testing among persons identified as high risk. Research has found that clients who have information about methods to prevent perinatal HIV transmission and the importance of testing for the baby's or their own health are more likely to be HIV tested. Media campaigns addressing the benefits of HIV testing may be a significant intervention. Media campaigns are not only successful in promoting HIV testing but, in populations with high HIV prevalence, they also are cost-effective (International AIDS Society, 2015).

With perinatal transmission, approximately half of children manifest AIDS within the first year of life, and about 80% have clinical symptoms of the disease within 3 to 5 years (Rivera & Frye, 2014). Breastfeeding is a major contributing factor for client-to-child transmission, and the infected client must be informed about this (March of Dimes, 2015i). Breastfeeding is not recommended for persons who are HIV positive, and they should avoid breastfeeding to prevent HIV transmission to the newborn (Money, Tulloch, Boucoiran, & Caddy, 2014). Given the devastating effects of HIV infection on children, preventing its transmission is critical (National Institutes of Health [NIH], 2014).

In addition to perinatal transmission, the fetus and newborn also are at risk for prematurity, IUGR, low birth weight, and infection. Prompt treatment with antiretroviral medications for the infant with an HIV infection may slow the progression of the disease (Hughes & Cu-Uvin, 2019).

Therapeutic Management

Clients who are seropositive for HIV require counselling about the risk of perinatal transmission and the potential for obstetric complications. The risk of perinatal transmission directly correlates with the viral load (Drake, Wagner, Richardson, & John-Stewart, 2014). A discussion of the options on continuing the pregnancy, medication therapy, risks, perinatal outcomes, and treatment is warranted. Clients who elect to continue with the pregnancy should be treated with ART regardless of their CD4 count or viral load. Interventions to reduce HIV transmission include antiretroviral therapy to the client and the newborn, consideration of elective cesarean section in clients with elevated plasma viral load, and the avoidance of breastfeeding. With these interventions, the risk of HIV transmission is now less than 2% (Hughes & Cu-Uvin, 2019).

Drug therapy is the mainstay of treatment for childbearing clients infected with HIV. The standard treatment is oral antiretroviral drugs given twice daily until giving birth, intravenous administration during labour, and oral zidovudine (AZT) for the newborn within 6 to 12 hours of birth (Vogler, 2014). The goal of therapy is to reduce the viral load as much as possible, which reduces the risk of transmission to the fetus.

Decisions about the birthing method to be used are made on an individual basis based on several factors involving the client's health. Some reports suggest that cesarean birth may reduce the risk of HIV infection (King et al., 2015). Efforts to reduce instrumentation, such as avoiding the use of an episiotomy, fetal scalp electrodes, and fetal scalp sampling, will reduce the newborn's exposure to body fluids. The Society of Obstetricians and Gynecologists recommends discussing the preferred mode of delivery in detail with each client, and to base decisions on optimal antiretroviral therapy and plasma viral load in the 4 weeks prior to birth (Money et al., 2014).

With appropriate therapies, the prognosis for a childbearing person with an HIV infection has improved significantly. In addition, the newborns of clients with HIV infection who have received treatment usually do not become infected. Unfortunately, therapy is complicated, and medications are expensive. Moreover, the medications are associated with numerous adverse effects and possible toxic reactions. These therapies offer a dual purpose: reduce the likelihood of client-to-infant transmission and provide optimal suppression of the viral load in the client. The core goal of all medical therapy is to bring the client's viral load to an undetectable level, thus minimizing the risk of transmission to the fetus and newborn.

Nursing Assessment

Nursing assessment begins with a thorough history and physical examination. In addition, the client is offered screening for HIV antibodies. Screening and effective intervention for those who are HIV positive are essential components of prenatal services, which also include education, counselling, testing, treatment, and continued care.

HEALTH HISTORY AND PHYSICAL EXAMINATION

Review the client's history for risk factors, such as unsafe sex practices, multiple sex partners, and injectable drug use. Also have the client complete a risk assessment survey. In addition, question the person about any flu-like symptoms such as a low-grade fever, fatigue, sore throat, night sweats, diarrhea, cough, skin lesions, or muscle pain. Numerous factors influence perinatal transmission. Factors that increase risk of perinatal transmission include high viral load; immune depletion (low CD4 T cell counts); genital tract infections; nutritional deficiencies; drug abuse; cigarette smoking; unprotected sexual intercourse; other opportunistic and coexisting infections (TB, malaria); prolonged ruptured membranes; and breastfeeding. Nurses need to take a thorough history to identify risk factors present.

Perform a complete physical examination. Obtain the client's weight and determine if they have lost weight recently. Assess for signs and symptoms of STIs, such as vulvovaginal candidiasis, bacterial vaginosis, HSV, chancroid, CMV, or chlamydia because of the increased risk for STIs.

Take Note!

Clients who request an HIV test despite reporting no individual risk factors should be considered at risk, since many are not likely to disclose their high-risk behaviours.

LABORATORY AND DIAGNOSTIC TESTING

The Society of Obstetricians and Gynecologists of Canada recommends that all pregnant clients be offered HIV antibody testing, regardless of their risk of infection, and that testing be repeated each trimester for those at high risk (Money et al., 2014). Testing is essential because treatments are available that can reduce the likelihood of perinatal transmission and maintain the health of the client.

Take Note!

Screening only clients who are identified as high risk based on their histories is inadequate due to the prolonged latency period that can exist after exposure. Also, research indicating that treatment with antiretroviral agents could reduce vertical transmission from the infected pregnant client to the newborn has dramatically increased the importance of HIV antibody screening in pregnancy.

Offer all individuals who are pregnant or planning a pregnancy HIV testing using ELISA. Prepare the person with a reactive screening test for an additional test, such as the Western blot or an immunofluorescence assay. The Western blot is the confirmatory diagnostic test. A positive antibody test confirmed by a supplemental test indicates that the person has been infected with HIV and can pass it on to others. HIV antibodies are detectable in at least 95% of clients within 3 months after infection (Rayment, Asboe, & Sullivan, 2014).

In addition to the usual screening tests done in normal pregnancy, additional testing for STIs may be necessary. Clients infected with HIV have high rates of STIs, especially HPV, vulvovaginal candidiasis, bacterial vaginosis, syphilis, HSV, chancroid, CMV, gonorrhea, chlamydia, and hepatitis B (March of Dimes, 2015i).

Nursing Management

Clients infected with HIV should have comprehensive prenatal care, which starts with pre- and post-test counselling. In pretest counselling, the client completes a risk assessment survey and the nurse explains the meaning of positive versus negative test results, obtains informed consent for HIV testing, and educates the client on how to prevent HIV infection by changing lifestyle behaviours if needed. Post-test counselling includes informing the client of the test results, reviewing the meaning of the results again, and reinforcing safer sex guidelines. All pre- and post-test counselling should be documented in the client's chart.

EDUCATING THE CLIENT

Pregnant clients are dealing with many issues at their first prenatal visit. The confirmation of pregnancy may be accompanied by feelings of joy, anxiety, depression, or other emotions. Simultaneously, the client is given many pamphlets and receives advice and counselling about many important health issues (e.g., nutrition, prenatal development, appointment schedules). This health teaching may be done while the person feels excited, tired, and anxious. To expect everyone to understand detailed explanations of a complex disease entity (HIV/AIDS) too may be unrealistic. Determine the client's readiness for this discussion. Identify the client's individual needs for teaching, emotional support, and physical care. Nurses need to approach education and counselling of HIV-positive clients in a caring, sensitive manner. Address the following information:

- Infection control issues at home
- Safer sex precautions
- Stages of the HIV disease process and treatment for each stage
- Symptoms of opportunistic infections
- Preventive drug therapies for the unborn infant
- Avoidance of breastfeeding
- Referrals to community support, counselling, and financial aid
- Client's support system and potential caretaker
- Importance of continual prenatal care
- Need for a well-balanced diet
- Measures to reduce exposure to infections

Be knowledgeable about HIV infection and how HIV is transmitted and share this knowledge with all clients. Nurses also can work to influence legislators, public health officials, and the entire health establishment toward policies to address the HIV epidemic. Research toward treatment and cure is tremendously important, but the major key to prevention of the spread of the virus is education. Nurses play a major role in this education.

SUPPORTING THE CLIENT

Be aware of the psychosocial sequelae of HIV/AIDS. A diagnosis of HIV can put a client into an emotional tailspin, during which they are worried about their own health and that of their unborn infant. They may experience grief, fear, or anxiety about the future of their children. Along with the medications that are so important for health maintenance, address the client's mental health needs, family dynamics, capacity to work, and social concerns and provide appropriate support and guidance.

A stigma against both individuals and newborns who are HIV-exposed or infected persists as a challenge on many maternity care units. As nurses work to address this preventable disease, they should do so in a respectful conscientious manner. Beyond basic nursing care, nurses should strive to provide respectful care for all clients and their newborns together. To accomplish this, be aware of your personal beliefs and attitudes toward those who are HIV positive or have AIDS. Incorporate this awareness in your actions as you help the client face the reality of the diagnosis and treatment options. Empathy, understanding, caring, and assistance are key to helping the client and the family.

PREPARING FOR LABOUR, BIRTH, AND AFTERWARD

Prepare the client physically and emotionally for the possibility of cesarean birth and assist as necessary. Ensure that they understand the rationale for the surgical birth.

After the birth of the newborn, the motivation for taking antiretroviral medications may be lower, thus affecting the client's adherence to therapy. Encourage the client to continue therapy for their own sake as well as that of the newborn. Nurses can make a difference in helping clients to adhere to their complex drug regimens.

Reinforce family planning methods during this time, incorporating a realistic view of the disease status. It is clear that hormonal contraceptives are not protective against HIV infection and that dual protection with condoms should be the goal for individuals using hormonal contraception (U.S. Agency for International Development [USAID], 2014). Advise the client that breastfeeding is not recommended. Instruct the client who is HIV positive in self-care measures, including the proper method for disposing of perineal pads to reduce the risk of exposing others to infected body fluids. Finally, teach clients the signs and symptoms of infection in newborns and infants, encouraging them to report any to the health care provider.

The evolution of HIV infection into a chronic disease has implications across all clinical care settings. Every nurse should be knowledgeable about the prevention, testing, treatment, and chronicity of the disease in order to provide high-quality care to people with or at risk for HIV. Breakthroughs in the prevention of HIV important to public health include circumcision, antiretrovirals to prevent client-to-child transmission, ART in HIV+ people to prevent transmission, and antiretrovirals for pre-exposure prophylaxis. Nurses, therefore, need to have an understanding of the changing epidemiology of the disease, the most recent testing recommendations, the developments in screening technology, the implications of aging with HIV infection, and the nursing implications of this ongoing epidemic.

Take Note!

When providing direct care, **ALWAYS follow universal precautions.**

VULNERABLE POPULATIONS

Every year there are an estimated 208 million pregnancies worldwide. Each pregnancy runs the risk of an adverse outcome for the client and the baby, but risks are dramatically increased for certain vulnerable populations: adolescents, clients over the age of 35, those who are obese, and those who engage in substance abuse. Although risks cannot be totally eliminated once pregnancy has begun, they can be reduced through appropriate and timely interventions.

Every client's experience with pregnancy is unique and personal. The circumstances each one faces and what pregnancy means each person individually involve emotions and experiences that belong solely to them. Many clients in these special population groups go through this experience in confusion and isolation, feeling desperately in need of help but not knowing where to go. Although all pregnant clients experience these emotions to a certain extent, they are heightened in individuals who have numerous psychosocial issues. Pregnancy is a stressful time. Pregnant clients face wide-ranging changes in their lives, relationships, and bodies as they move toward parenthood. These changes can be challenging for a person without any additional stresses but are even more so in the face of age extremes, illness, or substance abuse.

Skilled nursing interventions are essential to promote the best outcome for the client and the baby. Timely support and appropriate interventions during the perinatal period can have long-standing implications for the client and the newborn, ultimately with the goal of stability and integration of the family as a unit.

Pregnant Adolescent

Adolescence lasts from the onset of puberty to the cessation of physical growth, roughly from 11 to 19 years of age. Adolescents vacillate between being children and being adults. They need to adjust to the physiologic changes their bodies are undergoing and establish a sexual identity during this time. They search for personal identity and desire freedom and independence of thought and action. However, they continue to have a strong dependence on their parents (Crockett & Crouter, 2014).

Adolescent pregnancy has emerged as one of the most significant social problems facing our society. Adolescent birth rates in Canada decreased between 2001 and 2010, with births to adolescents aged 10 to 17 accounting for less than 2% of all births, and less than 4% among those aged 18 to 19 (Public Health Agency of Canada, 2013). Rates of pregnancy among adolescents are highest in Nunavut and Northwest Territories (Fleming, O'Driscoll, Becker, & Spitzer, 2015). The birth rate is higher among older adolescents, whereas younger adolescents are more likely to have induced abortion, but the abortion rates have also decreased (Fleming et al., 2015). Among these approximately half will give birth, slightly over one third will opt for abortions, and the remaining 14% will have miscarriages or stillbirths. It is estimated that 11% of births worldwide are to adolescents 15 to 19 years old, but this age group accounts for 23% of perinatal morbidity and mortality (Fleming et al., 2015; Ganchimeg et al., 2014). In addition, about half of all teen pregnancies occur within 6 months of first having sexual intercourse. About one in four adolescent parents under age 18 have a second baby within

2 years after the birth of their first baby. Most of these teens are unmarried, and many are not ready for the emotional, psychological, and financial responsibilities of parenthood. Teens are least likely of all childbearing age groups to get early and regular prenatal care (March of Dimes, 2015j). Adolescent pregnancy is further complicated by the adolescent's lack of financial resources: their income is half that of childbearing persons who have given birth in their 20s (March of Dimes, 2015j).

Currently, fewer high school students are having sexual intercourse, and more sexually active students are using some method of contraception. However, many teens who have had sexual intercourse have not spoken with their parents about sex, and use of contraceptives remains rare (CDC, 2015a).

Impact of Pregnancy in Adolescence

The impact of adolescent pregnancy is evident in perinatal morbidity and mortality. Nonetheless, in addition to the age involved in precocious pregnancy, it also reflects previous conditions such as malnutrition, communicable diseases, and deficiencies in the health care given to pregnant adolescents. The most important impact lies in the psychosocial area: it contributes to a loss of self esteem, societal discrimination, a destruction of life projects, and the maintenance of the circle of poverty (WHO, 2015a).

Adolescents are a unique group with special needs related to their stage of development. Adolescent pregnancy can be an emotionally charged situation, laden with ethical dilemmas and decisions. Topics such as abstinence, safer sex, abortion, and the decision to have a child are sensitive issues.

A nurse's moral convictions may influence the care that they provide to pregnant adolescents depending on their beliefs. Nurses need to examine their own beliefs about teen sexuality to identify personal assumptions. Putting aside one's moral convictions may be difficult, but it is necessary when working with pregnant adolescents. To be effective, health care providers must be able to communicate with adolescents in a manner they can understand and respect them as individuals.

The evidence suggests that it's not enough to teach teens to "just say no," nor is it enough to give them information about contraceptive methods; teens need to be connected to their parents, their peers, and their community (Whitworth & Cockerill, 2014). Nurses should feel that there is always hope and the chance of positive outcomes; nurses see that every day, often in the faces of their youngest clients. Nurses have to believe in that and work toward *connecting* with their teen clients. Nurses are on the front line of health care and are often the first to interact and build rapport with teenagers. Teens who engage in risky sexual behaviour may seek out nurses first. Nurse's scope of practice includes providing

FIGURE 20.6 **Adolescents sharing time together.**

education and a source of comfort and support to all ages. It is therefore imperative for all nurses to be able to provide age-appropriate information about sexual health. In providing this care, the quality of life and outcome of both the client and the infant can be improved.

Developmental Issues

An adolescent must accomplish certain developmental tasks to advance to the next stage of maturity. These developmental tasks include:
- Seeking economic and social stability
- Adjusting to sexually maturing bodies and feelings
- Developing a personal value system
- Building meaningful relationships with others (Fig. 20.6)
- Becoming comfortable with their changing bodies
- Working to become independent from their parents
- Learning to verbalize conceptually (CDC, 2015n)

Adolescents have special needs when working to accomplish their developmental tasks and making a smooth transition to young adulthood. One of the biggest areas of need is sexual health. Adolescents commonly lack the information, skills, and services necessary to make informed choices related to their sexual and reproductive health. Developmentally, adolescents are trying to figure out who they are and how they fit into society. As adolescents mature, their parents become less influential and peers become more influential. Peer pressure can lead adolescents to participate in sexual activity, as can the typical adolescent's belief that "it won't happen to me" (Box 20.3). As a result, unplanned pregnancies occur. Work on the developmental tasks of adolescence, especially identity, can be interrupted as the adolescent attempts to integrate the tasks of pregnancy, bonding, and preparing to care for another with the tasks of developing self-identity and independence. A pregnant adolescent must try to meet their own needs along with those of their fetus. The process of learning how to separate from the parents while learning how to bond and attach

---

to a newborn brings conflict and stress. A pregnancy can exacerbate an adolescent's feeling of loss of control and helplessness (American Academy of Pediatrics, 2014).

Health and Social Issues

Adolescent pregnancy has a negative impact in terms of both health and social consequences. For example, 7 out of 10 adolescents will drop out of school. More than 75% will receive public assistance within 5 years of having their first child. In addition, children of adolescent parents are at greater risk of preterm birth, low birth weight, child abuse, neglect, poverty, and death. The younger the adolescent is at the time of the first pregnancy, the more likely it is that they will have another pregnancy during their teens (March of Dimes, 2015j). Adolescent pregnancy also places them at high risk for obstetric complications such as preterm labour and births, low–birth-weight infants, STIs, poor maternal weight gain, preeclampsia, iron-deficiency anemia, poor eating habits, and inadequate nutrition and postpartum depression (Rajoriya & Kalra, 2015).

The psychosocial risks associated with early childbearing often have an even greater impact on clients, families, and society than the obstetric or medical risks (Northridge & Coupey, 2015). Pregnant adolescents experience higher rates of domestic violence and substance abuse. Those experiencing abuse are more likely to abuse substances, receive inadequate prenatal care, and have lower pregnancy weight compared with those who are not (Smith et al., 2016). Moreover, substance abuse (cigarettes, alcohol, or illicit drugs) can contribute to low birth weight, fetal growth restriction, preterm births, newborn addiction, and sepsis (March of Dimes, 2015j).

Although early childbearing (12 to 19 years of age) occurs in all socioeconomic groups, it is more prevalent among poor individuals and those from minority backgrounds, who face more obstetric and newborn risks than their more affluent counterparts (March of Dimes, 2015j). Poverty often contributes to delayed prenatal care and medical complications related to poor nutrition, such as anemia.

There are social costs to society related to adolescent pregnancy in terms of the loss of human resources and the far-reaching intergenerational effects of adolescent parenting. For some adolescents, pregnancy may be seen as a hopeless situation: a grim story of poverty and lost dreams, of being trapped in a life that was never wanted. Health-related behaviours, such as smoking, diet, sexual behaviour, and help-seeking behaviours, which are developed during adolescence often, endure into later life (Fedorowicz, Hellerstedt, Schreiner, & Bolland, 2014). The consequences associated with an adolescent's less-than-optimal health status at this age due to pregnancy can ultimately affect their long-term health and that of their children. However, some adolescents can create a happy, stable life for themselves and their children by facing their challenges and working hard to beat the odds.

> **Recall Rose, the pregnant teenager with asthma. What issues would be important for the nurse to discuss related to the pregnancy, asthma, and her age?**

Nursing Assessment

Assessment of the pregnant adolescent is the same as that for any pregnant client. However, when dealing with pregnant teens, the nurse also needs to ask:

- How does the adolescent see themself in the future?
- Are realistic role models available?
- How much does the client know about child development?
- What financial resources are available?
- Does the client work? Does the client go to school?
- What emotional support is available?
- Can the client resolve conflicts and manage anger?
- What does the client know about health and nutrition for themselves and their child?
- Will the client need help dealing with the challenges of the new parenting role?
- Does the client need information about community resources?

Having an honest regard for adolescents requires getting to know them and being able to appreciate the important aspects of their life. Doing so forms a basis for the nurse's clinical judgment and promotes care that takes into account the concerns and practical circumstances of the teen and their family. Skillful practice includes knowing how and when to advise a teen and when to listen and refrain from giving advice. Giving advice can be misinterpreted as "preaching," and the adolescent will probably ignore the information. The nurse must be perceptive, flexible, and sensitive and must work to establish a therapeutic relationship.

Nursing Management

For adolescents, as for all clients, pregnancy can be a physically, emotionally, and socially stressful time. The pregnancy is often both the result of and cause of social problems and stressors that can be overwhelming to them. Nurses must support adolescents during the transition from childhood into adulthood, which is complicated by their emergence into parenthood. Assist the adolescent in identifying family and friends who want to be involved and provide support throughout the pregnancy.

Help the adolescent identify the options for this pregnancy, such as abortion, self-parenting of the child, temporary foster care for the baby or themself, or placement of the child for adoption. Explore with the adolescent if the pregnancy was planned or unintended. Becoming aware of why they decided to have a child is necessary to help with the development of the adolescent and their ability to parent. Identify barriers to seeking prenatal care, such as lack of transportation, too many problems at home, financial concerns, the long wait for an appointment, and lack of sensitivity on the part of the health care system. Encourage the client to set goals and work toward them. Assist them in returning to school and furthering their education. As appropriate, initiate a referral for career or job counselling.

Stress that the client's physical well-being is important for both themself and their developing fetus, which depends on them for its own health-related needs. Assist with arrangements for care, including stress management and self-care. Having a healthy newborn eases the transition to parenthood somewhat, rather than having to deal with the added stress of caring for an unhealthy baby (Rajoriya & Kalra, 2015). Monitor weight gain, sleep and rest patterns, and nutritional status to promote positive outcomes for both the client and the child. Stress the importance of attending prenatal education classes. Provide appropriate teaching based on the adolescent's developmental level and emphasize the importance of continued prenatal and follow-up care. Monitor well-being of the client and the fetus throughout pregnancy and labour (Fig. 20.7).

FIGURE 20.7 A pregnant adolescent receiving care during labour.

Nurses can also play a major role in preventing adolescent pregnancies, perhaps by volunteering to talk to teen groups. Teaching Guidelines 20.6 highlights the key areas for teaching adolescents about pregnancy prevention.

Teaching Guidelines 20.6

TOPICS FOR TEACHING ADOLESCENTS TO PREVENT PREGNANCY

- High-risk behaviours that lead to pregnancy
- Involvement in programs such as Free Teens, Teen Advisors, or Postponing Sexual Involvement
- Planning and goal setting to visualize their futures in terms of career, college, travel, and education
- Choice of abstinence or taking a step back to become a "second-time virgin"
- Discussions about sexuality with a wiser adult— someone they respect can help put things in perspective
- Protection against STIs and pregnancy if they choose to remain sexually active
- Critical observation and review of peers and friends to make sure they are creating the right atmosphere for friendship
- Empowerment to make choices that will shape their life for years to come, including getting control of their own lives now
- Appropriate use of recreational time, such as sports, drama, volunteer work, music, jobs, church activities, and school clubs

Adapted from Yoost, J. L., Hertweck, S. P., & Barnett, S. N. (2014). The effect of an educational approach to pregnancy prevention among high-risk early and late adolescents. *Journal of Adolescent Health, 55*(2), 222–227; Koh, H. (2014). The teen pregnancy prevention program: An evidence-based public health program model. *Journal of Adolescent Health, 54*(3), S1–S2; March of Dimes. (2015j). *Teenage pregnancy.* Retrieved from http://www.marchofdimes.com/professionals/14332_1159.asp.

Tackling the many issues surrounding adolescent pregnancy is difficult. Making connections with clients is crucial regardless of how complex their situation is. The future challenges nurses to find solutions to teenage pregnancies. Nurses must take proactive positions while working with adolescents, parents, schools, and communities to reduce the problems associated with early childbearing.

Nurses who provide care to adolescents have an opportunity to discuss future pregnancies and to use health care visits to teach about preconception health. Teaching adolescents who both express a desire for pregnancy and those who do not express such a desire is an important part of comprehensive nursing care. Teens require a thorough teaching about health care risks such as smoking cessation, body weight control, interpersonal violence, and the need for folic acid. Adolescents should be prime recipients of preconception education at every health care visit.

Teen childbearing is associated with adverse consequences for the parents and their children and imposes high public sector costs. Prevention of teen pregnancy requires evidence-based sex education, support for parents in talking with their children about pregnancy prevention and other aspects of sexual and reproductive health, and ready access to effective and affordable contraception for teens who are sexually active (CDC, 2015o).

Childbearing at Advanced Age

It is estimated that by the year 2025 about 25% of persons will begin their childbearing period at an "advanced age." Advanced age is a risk factor for infertility, pregnancy loss, fetal anomalies, stillbirth, and obstetric complications (Sauer, 2015). A few decades ago, a person having a baby after the age of 35 probably was giving birth to the last of several children, but today they may be having their first. With advances in technology and the tendency of individuals to seek career advancement prior to childbearing, the dramatic increase in having a first pregnancy after the age of 35 will likely continue.

Impact of Pregnancy on the Client of Advanced Age

Whether childbearing is delayed by choice or by chance, persons starting a family at age 35 or older are not doing so without risk. Clients in this age group may already have chronic health conditions that can put the pregnancy at risk. In addition, numerous studies have shown that increasing age is a risk factor for infertility and spontaneous abortions, gestational diabetes, chronic hypertension, postpartum hemorrhage, preeclampsia, preterm labour and birth, multiple pregnancy, genetic disorders and chromosomal abnormalities, placenta previa, fetal growth restriction, low Apgar scores, and surgical births

(Schimmel et al., 2015). However, even though increased age implies increased complications, most clients today who become pregnant after age 34 have healthy pregnancies and healthy newborns. The rate of first time births to persons over the age of 35 has been increasing, and the overall rate of live births occurring to persons aged 35 to 39 in 2010 was 49.3 per 1,000 (Public Health Agency of Canada, 2013).

Nursing Assessment

Nursing assessment of the pregnant client over age 34 is the same as that for any childbearing client. For a client of this age, a preconception visit is important to identify chronic health problems that might affect the pregnancy and also to address lifestyle issues that may take time to modify. Encourage the client of advanced maternal age to plan for the pregnancy by seeing their health care provider before getting pregnant to discuss pre-existing medical conditions, medications, and lifestyle choices. Assess the client for risk factors such as cigarette smoking, poor nutrition, overweight or underweight, alcohol use, or illicit drug use.

A preconception visit also provides the opportunity to educate the client about risk factors and provide information on how to modify their lifestyle habits to improve the pregnancy outcome. Assist the client with lifestyle changes so that they can begin pregnancy in an optimal state of health. For example, if the client is overweight, educate them about weight loss so that they can start the pregnancy at a healthy weight. If the client smokes, encourage smoking cessation to reduce the effects of nicotine on themself and their fetus.

Prepare the client for laboratory and diagnostic testing to establish a baseline for future comparisons. The risk of having a baby with Down syndrome increases with age, especially over age 34. Noninvasive screening, with a combination of serum and ultrasound markers, should be offered to all childbearing persons 35 years of age or older, and invasive diagnostic testing (amniocentesis, chorionic villus sampling) to any whose screening suggests high risk (Johnson & Tough, 2012). Advanced age is an independent risk factor for stillbirth; enhanced antepartum fetal surveillance with biophysical profiles and planned delivery by term for those in whom labour does not occur spontaneously can promote positive outcomes.

Nursing Management

During routine prenatal visits, the nurse can play a key role in promoting a healthy pregnancy. Consider social, genetic, and environmental factors that are unique to the childbearing client of advanced maternal age and prepare to address these factors when providing care. In a study by Mills and Lavender (2014), compared with the younger client, older clients had statistically similar rates of gestational hypertension, gestational diabetes, preterm premature rupture of membranes/preterm labour, and abnormal placentation. Cesarean birth was higher in older clients versus younger ones. Neonatal outcomes of gestational age and birth weight were excellent and similar between groups. Despite the increased risks, there are potential psychological and social advantages to delaying childbirth, and absolute numbers of complications are small.

Assess the client's knowledge about risk factors and measures to reduce them. Educate them about measures to promote a positive outcome. Encourage them to get early and regular prenatal care. Advise the client to eat a variety of nutritious foods, especially fortified cereals, enriched grain products, and fresh fruits and vegetables, and drink at least six to eight glasses of water daily and to take the prescribed vitamin containing 400 mcg of folic acid daily. Also stress the need for them to avoid alcohol intake during pregnancy, avoid exposure to secondhand smoke, and take no drugs unless they are prescribed. Provide continued surveillance of the pregnant client and fetus throughout the pregnancy.

The Obese Pregnant Client

Childbearing clients who are obese are a particularly vulnerable group because their disability (obesity) is highly visible. Excess weight and obesity have gained attention as serious health care threats globally. Obesity during pregnancy is defined as a BMI of 30 kg/m^2 or more calculated using the height and weight measured at the first prenatal visit. Compared to normal weight persons, overweight and obese persons tend to gain excessive weight in pregnancy and are at high risk for maternal and birth outcomes. Excessive gestational weight gain is strongly associated with postpartum weight retention which increases the risk of additional weight gains in subsequent pregnancies (Chang, Brown, Nitzke, Smith, & Eghtedary, 2015). Obesity contributes to social, psychological, and economic problems throughout a person's lifetime. Negative attitudes and discrimination by society can have negative consequences for the individual's quality of life. The number of clients who are overweight or obese during pregnancy has also increased. During pregnancy, excess weight increases both obstetric and neonatal risks, including:

- Gestational diabetes
- Hypertension
- Thromboembolism
- Preeclampsia
- Preterm labour and birth
- Congenital anomalies
- Childhood and adolescent obesity
- Fetal macrosomia (birth weight >4,000 g)
- Difficulty fighting postpartum infections
- Depression

- Tendency to remain overweight/obesity between pregnancies
- Prolongation of pregnancy/increased likelihood of post-term infant
- Increased risk of stillbirth
- Higher rate of cesarean births
- Increased risk of maternal mortality
- High risk for postpartum hemorrhage (American College of Obstetricians & Gynecologists [ACOG], 2014b)

Negative or judgmental attitudes toward overweight or obese individuals can be encountered within the health care community and its providers, including nurses. Nurses can find it difficult to discuss weight issues during prenatal visits with obese clients (Knight-Agarwal, Kaur, Williams, Davey, & Davis, 2014). Preconception assessment and counselling are needed for obese clients, which should include specific information about the perinatal risks linked to obesity in pregnancy, as well as encouragement to undertake a weight-reduction program, including diet, exercise, and behaviour modification, to achieve a healthy weight prior to conception.

Obese pregnant clients require individualized nursing care. Extra time may be needed to promote healthful practices, which should include dealing with issues of weight, diet, and exercise. Specialist dietary interventions and evidence-based guidelines for working with childbearing clients must be seen as a public health priority by all nurses. This care must be done with honesty and respect for all of the client's needs. There is an opportunity for health promotion aimed at disseminating information about the risks of obesity in pregnancy to overweight and obese clients of childbearing age.

The Pregnant Client and Substance Abuse

Substance abuse in pregnancy, or **perinatal substance use**, is a significant public health crisis causing increased morbidity in two individuals, the client and the fetus. The epidemic of substance abuse continues to pose a significant challenge to all nations. Although there is a tendency to simply associate drug abuse with poverty, the problem affects every social stratum, gender, and race; and pregnant persons are no exception. Substance use disorder involves cognitive, behavioural, and psychological symptoms indicating that a client continues to use harmful substances despite significant substance-related symptoms (Ordean, Wong, & Graves, 2017). The incidence of substance abuse during pregnancy is highly variable because most pregnant clients are reluctant to reveal the extent of their use. In Canada, 10.5% of childbearing persons report using tobacco, 10.5% report using alcohol, 2% use cannabis, and 1% use opioids in pregnancy (Cook et al., 2017; Ordean et al., 2017).

Impact of Substance Abuse on Pregnancy

Substance use can be viewed along a continuum between social recreational drug use and addiction. Substance abuse is very prevalent and continues to remain undetected and underdiagnosed in many pregnant persons. Substance abuse rarely starts during pregnancy. More often, a person enters pregnancy already abusing or dependent on drugs.

Prenatal education and counselling is essential to successfully impacting this high-risk population. The positive overall impact of adequate prenatal care on birth outcomes is well documented. For pregnant substance users, the receipt of adequate prenatal care is especially critical. Several studies have reported that increasing the adequacy of prenatal care utilization in pregnant substance users reduces risks for prematurity, low birth weight, and perinatal mortality. However, many childbearing clients who are substance users do not seek prenatal care for fear of being reported to Child Protective Services (Substance Abuse and Mental Health Services Administration [SAMHSA], 2015).

The use of drugs, legal or not, increases the risk of medical complications in the client and poor birth outcomes in the newborn. The placenta acts as an active transport mechanism, not as a barrier, and substances pass from a client to their fetus through the placenta. Thus, along with the client, the fetus experiences substance use, abuse, and addiction. Additionally, fetal vulnerability to drugs is much greater because the fetus has not developed the enzymatic system needed to metabolize drugs (Doulatram, Raj, & Govindaraj, 2015).

EFFECTS OF ADDICTION

Addiction is a multifaceted process that is affected by environmental, psychological, family, and physical factors. Clients who use drugs, alcohol, or tobacco come from all socioeconomic backgrounds, cultures, and lifestyles. Factors associated with substance abuse during a pregnancy may include low self-esteem, inadequate support systems, low self-expectations, high levels of anxiety, socioeconomic barriers, involvement in abusive relationships, chaotic familial and social systems, and a history of psychiatric illness or depression. Individuals often start using addictive substances to relieve their anxieties, previous physical, sexual, and emotional traumas in their life, depression, and feelings of worthlessness (Slater, 2015).

Societal attitudes regarding substance use may prohibit individuals from admitting the problem and seeking treatment. Society sanctions them for failing to live up to expectations of how a childbearing person "should" behave, thereby possibly driving them further away from the treatment they so desperately need. For many reasons, childbearing clients who abuse substances feel unwelcome in prenatal clinics or medical settings. Often they seek prenatal care late or not at all. They may fear being shamed or reported to legal or child protection authorities. A nonjudgmental atmosphere and unbiased teaching to all pregnant clients regardless of their lifestyle is crucial. A caring, concerned manner is critical to help these clients feel safe and respond honestly to assessment questions.

Pregnancy can be a motivator for some who want to try treatment. The goal of therapy is to help the client deal with pregnancy by developing a trusting relationship. Providing a full spectrum of medical, social, and emotional care is needed.

EFFECTS OF COMMONLY ABUSED SUBSTANCES

Routine screening and education of clients of childbearing age remain the most important ways to reduce addiction in pregnancy.

Substance abuse during pregnancy, particularly in the first trimester, has a negative effect on the health of the pregnant person and the growth and development of the fetus. The fetus experiences the same systemic effects as the client, but often more severely. The fetus cannot metabolize drugs as efficiently as the expectant person and will experience the effects long after the drugs have left the client's system. Substance abuse during pregnancy is associated with preterm labour, abortion, IUGR, abruptio placenta, depressed Apgar scores, third trimester bleeding, meconium staining at birth, fetal demise, low birth weight, neurobehavioural abnormalities, and long-term childhood developmental consequences (WHO, 2015c). Table 20.6 summarizes the effects of selected drugs during pregnancy.

Alcohol. Alcohol abuse is a major public health issue. Alcohol is a teratogen, a substance known to be toxic to human development. The true rate of prenatal alcohol consumption is unknown. It is recognized that **fetal alcohol spectrum disorder (FASD)** is entirely preventable through alcohol abstinence, but worldwide approximately 30% of pregnant individuals consume alcohol during pregnancy (Vall, Salat-Batlle, & Garcia-Algar, 2015). Theoretically, no client would give a glass of wine, beer, or hard liquor to their newborn, but when a pregnant person drinks, the embryo or fetus is exposed to the same blood alcohol concentration as the pregnant person is.

The teratogenic effects of heavy drinking have been recognized since 1973, when fetal alcohol syndrome was first described. Fetal alcohol syndrome is now a classification under the broader term of FASD; this disorder includes the full range of birth defects, such as structural anomalies and behavioural and neurocognitive disabilities caused by prenatal exposure to alcohol (Vaux & Chambers, 2015). FASD affects 1 in 100 infants each year, more than autism, Down syndrome, cerebral palsy, cystic fibrosis, spina bifida, and sudden infant death syndrome (SIDS) combined (National Organization on Fetal Alcohol

TABLE 20.6	EFFECTS OF SELECTED DRUGS ON PREGNANCY
Substance	**Effect on Pregnancy**
Alcohol	Spontaneous abortion, stillbirth, preterm birth, inadequate weight gain, intrauterine growth restriction (IUGR), fetal alcohol spectrum disorder, the leading cause of intellectual disability
Caffeine	Vasoconstriction and mild diuresis in mother; fetal stimulation, but teratogenic effects not documented via research
Nicotine	Vasoconstriction, reduced uteroplacental blood flow, decreased birth weight, abortion, prematurity, abruptio placentae, fetal demise
Cocaine	Vasoconstriction, gestational hypertension, abruptio placentae, premature rupture of membranes, preterm labour, uterine hypercontractility, spontaneous abortion, CNS defects, IUGR, SIDS
Cannabis	Long-term neurocognitive effects; hyperactive startle reflex, lower birth weight, increased incidence of tremors, and diminished crying in the neonate
Opiates and Narcotics	Maternal and fetal withdrawal symptoms (neonatal abstinence syndrome [NAS]), spontaneous abortion, stillbirth, abruptio placentae, preterm labour, premature rupture of membranes, perinatal asphyxia, newborn sepsis and death, intellectual impairment, malnutrition, IUGR
Sedatives	CNS depression, newborn withdrawal, maternal seizures in labour, newborn abstinence syndrome, delayed lung maturity
Amphetamines and Methamphetamines	IUGR, premature labour and delivery, low birth weight, neonatal withdrawal symptoms

Adapted from Centers for Disease Control and Prevention (CDC). (2015q). *Illegal drug use.* Retrieved from http://www.cdc.gov/nchs/fastats/drug-use-illegal.htm; March of Dimes. (2015k). *Smoking, alcohol, and drugs and pregnancy.* Retrieved from http://www.marchofdimes.org/pregnancy/illicit-drug-use-during-pregnancy.aspx; McKeever, A. E., Spaeth-Brayton, S., & Sheerin, S. (2014). The role of nurses in comprehensive care management of pregnant women with drug addiction. *Nursing for Women's Health, 18*(4), 284–293; and Cook, J. L., Green, C. R., de la Ronde, S., Dell, A. C., Graves, L., Ordean, A., . . . Wong, S. (2017). Epidemiology and effects of substance use in pregnancy. *Journal of Obstetrics and Gynaecology Canada, 39*(10), 906–915.

COMMON COGNITIVE AND BEHAVIOURAL PROBLEMS ASSOCIATED WITH FASD AND ATTENTION–DEFICIT/HYPERACTIVITY DISORDER

- Inability to foresee consequences
- Inability to learn from previous experience
- Lack of organization
- Intellectual disability or low IQ
- Difficulty in school, especially with math
- Learning difficulties
- Poor abstract thinking
- Poor reasoning and judgment skills
- Poor memory
- Poor impulse control
- Speech and language delays
- Poor judgment

Adapted from Centers for Disease Control and Prevention (CDC). (2015h). *Fetal alcohol spectrum disorders*. Retrieved from http://www.cdc.gov/ncbddd/fasd/alcohol-use.html

FIGURE 20.8 Typical facial characteristics of a newborn with FASD.

Syndrome [NOFAS], 2015). FASD is now recognized as a leading cause of nongenetic intellectual disability, possibly exceeding even Down syndrome. Alcohol consumption during pregnancy results in brain, craniofacial, and heart defects, neurotoxicity, and immune systems dysfunction.

Characteristics of FASD include craniofacial dysmorphia (thin upper lip, small head circumference, and small eyes), IUGR, microcephaly, and congenital anomalies such as limb abnormalities and cardiac defects. Long-term sequelae include postnatal growth restriction, attention deficits, delayed reaction time, and poor scholastic performance (NOFAS, 2015). The complex neurobehavioural problems typically manifest themselves insidiously. Children with prenatal alcohol exposure struggle with cognitive, academic, social, emotional, and behavioural challenges. These challenges reduce the child's ability to learn and function successfully in many structured environments (Mohammadzadeh & Farhat, 2014). Common cognitive and behavioural problems are listed in Box 20.4, and Figure 20.8 illustrates the characteristic facial features. See Chapter 24 for a more detailed discussion of the newborn with FASD.

The preferred action taken to prevent alcohol consumption during pregnancy is abstinence. However, the detection, diagnosis, and treatment of FASD remain major public health needs in this country and throughout the world. Not every client who drinks during pregnancy will give birth to an affected child. Based on the best research available, the following is known about alcohol consumption during pregnancy:

- Intake increases the risk of alcohol-related birth defects, including growth deficiencies, facial abnormalities, central nervous system impairment, behavioural disorders, and intellectual development.
- No amount of alcohol consumption is considered safe during pregnancy.
- Damage to the fetus can occur at any stage of pregnancy, even before a person knows they are pregnant.
- Cognitive defects and behavioural problems resulting from prenatal exposure are lifelong.
- Alcohol-related birth defects are completely preventable (ACOG, 2014c).

Risk factors for giving birth to an alcohol-affected newborn include client age, socioeconomic status, ethnicity, genetic factors, poor nutrition, depression, family disorganization, unplanned pregnancy, and late prenatal care (ACOG, 2014d). Identification of risk factors strongly associated with alcohol-related birth outcomes could help identify high-risk pregnancies requiring intervention.

One of the biggest challenges in determining the true prevalence of FASD is how to recognize the syndrome, which depends in part on the age and physical features of the person being assessed. Difficulty identifying alcohol abuse results from the client's denial of alcohol use, unwillingness to report alcohol consumption, underreporting, and limited ability to recollect the frequency, quantity, and type of alcohol consumed. This makes it difficult to identify clients who are drinking during pregnancy, institute preventive measures, or refer them for treatment.

Clients who drink excessively while pregnant are at high risk for giving birth to children with birth defects. To prevent these defects, someone should stop drinking during all phases of a pregnancy. Unfortunately, many people continue to drink during their pregnancy despite warnings from professionals.

Currently, it is not known whether there is a minimal amount of alcohol safe to drink during pregnancy; an occasional glass of wine might be harmless or might not be. Therefore, eliminating alcohol consumption during pregnancy is the ultimate goal to prevent FASD. Most individuals know they should not drink during pregnancy, but the window of vulnerability—that is, the time lag between conception and the discovery of pregnancy—may put substantial numbers of children at risk. Additionally, traditional alcohol-screening questionnaires, such as the Michigan Alcoholism Screening Test (MAST) and the CAGE Questionnaire, are not sensitive enough to detect low levels of alcohol consumption among clients.

Several challenges remain in preventing birth defects due to alcohol consumption:

- Ways to improve clinical recognition of high-risk clients who drink alcohol
- Ways to intervene more effectively to modify drinking behaviours
- In utero approaches to prevent or minimize fetal injury
- Strategies to address the neurodevelopmental problems of children affected by the client's alcohol ingestion

Sedatives. Sedatives relax the central nervous system and are used medically for inducing relaxation and sleep, relieving tension, and treating seizures. Sedatives easily cross the placenta and can cause birth defects and behavioural problems. Infants born to clients who abuse sedatives during pregnancy may be physically dependent on the drugs themselves and are more prone to respiratory problems, feeding difficulties, disturbed sleep, sweating, irritability, and fever (Alexander, LaRosa, Bader, & Garfield, 2014).

Nicotine. Cigarette smoking during pregnancy is the biggest preventable cause of death and illness in childbearing clients and infants and is associated with numerous obstetric, fetal, and developmental complications, as well as an increased risk of adverse health consequences in the adult offspring. Nicotine replacement therapy has been developed as a pharmacotherapy for smoking cessation and is considered to be a safer alternative for clients to smoking during pregnancy. The safety of nicotine replacement therapy (transdermal patches and bupropion) use during pregnancy has been evaluated in a limited number of short-term human trials, but there is currently no information on the long-term effects of developmental nicotine exposure in humans (Dhalwani, Szatkowski, Coleman, Fiaschi, & Tata, 2015).

Nicotine is found in cigarettes and is another substance that is harmful to the pregnant client and their fetus. Nicotine, which causes vasoconstriction, transfers across the placenta and reduces blood flow to the fetus, contributing to fetal hypoxia. When compared with alcohol, cannabis, and other illicit drug use, tobacco use is less likely to decline as the pregnancy progresses (Velez & Jansson, 2015). Smoking is associated with adverse pregnancy outcomes. However, these adverse outcomes can be avoided if the client stops smoking before becoming pregnant.

Smoking increases the risk of spontaneous abortion, tubal ectopic pregnancy, preterm labour and birth, fetal growth restriction, stillbirth, premature rupture of membranes, low fetal iron stores, maternal hypertension, placenta previa, and abruptio placentae. The perinatal death rate among infants of smoking clients is 20% to 35% higher than that of nonsmoking clients (Varner et al., 2014). Perinatal and childhood risks associated with smoking during their pregnancies include increased risk of cleft lip and palate, clubfoot, asthma, middle ear infections, SIDS, reduced head circumference, altered brainstem development, and cerebral palsy (Cunningham et al., 2014).

Smoking has also been considered an important risk factor for low birth weight, SIDS, and cognitive deficits, especially in language, reading, and vocabulary, as well as poorer performances on tests of reasoning and memory. Researchers have also reported behaviour problems, such as increased activity, inattention, impulsivity, opposition, and aggression (Skoglund, Chen, D'Onofrio, Lichtenstein, & Larsson, 2014). Clients who smoke during the pregnancy often continue to smoke after giving birth, and thus the infant will be exposed to nicotine after birth. This environmental or passive exposure affects the child's development and increases the risk of childhood respiratory disorders.

Caffeine. Caffeine is a widely used and accepted pharmacologically active substance. The socially sanctioned nature of caffeinated beverages promotes caffeine's popularity and at the same time obscures the fact that as a drug it can definitely be abused. The effect of caffeine intake during pregnancy on fetal growth and development is still unclear. A recent study found that caffeine intake of no more than 300 mg/day during pregnancy does not affect pregnancy duration and the condition of the newborn (Procter & Campbell, 2014). Caffeine, a stimulant of the central nervous system, is present in varying amounts in common products such as coffee, tea, colas, and chocolate. It is also in cold remedies and analgesics. Birth defects have not been linked to caffeine consumption, but coffee consumption decreases iron absorption and may increase the risk of anemia during pregnancy.

Moderate caffeine consumption (less than 300 mg/day) does not appear to be a major contributing factor in miscarriage or preterm birth. The relationship of caffeine to growth restriction remains undetermined. A final conclusion cannot be made at this time as to whether there is a correlation between high caffeine intake and miscarriage, due to lack of sufficient studies (Calhoun & Lewis, 2016).

Energy drinks represent a new class of caffeinated beverages that are marketed to improve energy, athletic performance, concentration, endurance, and weight loss, although the claims have not been supported by rigorous scientific evidence (Higgins, Yarlagadda, & Yang, 2015). All energy drinks surpass the FDA official soft drink concentration of caffeine limit, typically 2 to 4 times the amount seen in one serving of soda or tea. Adverse effects of energy drinks can occur in healthy people; however, pregnant clients would be considered in an at-risk group and should avoid excessive caffeine intake which has been linked to adverse reproductive outcomes, such as low birth weight. Consumption of energy drinks is associated with increased demand of the heart causing hypertension, tachycardia, dysrhythmias, coronary artery spasm, and sudden cardiac death (James, 2015). Given the rise in emergency room visits for complications of energy drink consumption, nurses should advise their pregnant clients to refrain from drinking them.

Cannabis. Cannabis is one of the most commonly used substances in pregnancy, with anywhere from 1.8% to 16.6% of childbearing persons in Canada using it during pregnancy (Cook et al., 2017). It is often called pot, reefer, herb, widow, hash, grass, weed, Mary Jane, or MJ (National Institute on Drug Abuse [NIDA], 2015c). Cannabis is a preparation of the leaves and flowering tops of *Cannabis sativa*, the hemp plant, which contains a number of pharmacologically active agents. Tetrahydrocannabinol (THC) is the most active ingredient of cannabis. With heavy smoking, THC narrows the bronchi and bronchioles and produces inflammation of the mucous membranes. Smoking cannabis causes tachycardia and a reduction in blood pressure, resulting in orthostatic hypotension. Cannabis is also currently used by some as a treatment for medical-specific conditions (chronic pain, chemotherapy related nausea and vomiting).

The effects of cannabis smoking on pregnancy are not yet fully understood because there are very few studies on its long-term effects on child development. Studies suggest that it is associated with neurocognitive and behavioural deficits, and deficits in executive functioning that are noted in older children and into adolescence (Cook et al., 2017). One can speculate that the effects of cannabis on the immature nervous system may be subtle and not detected until more complex functions are required, usually in a formal educational setting. There is some evidence that cannabis increases the risk of spontaneous abortion and preterm delivery (Desai, Mark, & Terplan, 2014). Although cannabis is not considered teratogenic, many newborns display altered responses to visual stimuli, increased tremulousness, and a high-pitched cry, which might indicate insults against the central nervous system (Volkow, Baler, Compton, & Weiss, 2014). A strong correlation exists between the use of cannabis and the use of alcohol and cigarettes.

Opiates and Narcotics. Opiates and narcotics include opium, heroin (known as horse, junk, smack, downtown), morphine, codeine, hydromorphone (Dilaudid; little D), oxycodone (Percodan, perkies), meperidine (Demerol, demise), and methadone (meth, dollies). Opiates can be inhaled, injected, snorted, ingested, or used subcutane-

ously. These drugs are central nervous system depressants that soothe and lull. They may be used medically for pain, but all have a high potential for abuse. Most cause an intense addiction in both the client and the newborn.

Narcotic dependence is particularly problematic in childbearing clients. It leads to medical, nutritional, and social neglect by the client due to the long-term risks of physical dependence, malnutrition, compromised immunity, hepatitis, and fatal overdose (Alexander et al., 2014). Taking opiates or narcotics during pregnancy places the client at increased risk for preterm labour, fetal growth restriction, abruptio placenta, perinatal mortality, preterm rupture of membranes, and preeclampsia (Prasad, 2014).

Heroin is the most common illicitly used opioid. It is derived from the seeds of the poppy plant and can be sniffed, smoked, or injected. It crosses the placenta via simple diffusion within 1 hour of maternal consumption (ACOG, 2014e). Use of heroin during pregnancy is believed to affect the developing brain of the fetus and may cause behavioural abnormalities in childhood. Risks of perinatal opiate exposure are not limited to the fetus. Opiate overdose deaths in the general population have increased dramatically.

The most common harmful effect of heroin and other narcotics on newborns is withdrawal, or **neonatal abstinence syndrome** (see Chapter 24). This collection of symptoms may include irritability, hypertonicity, jitteriness, fever, excessive and often high-pitched cry, vomiting, diarrhea, feeding disturbances, respiratory distress, disturbed sleeping, excessive sneezing and yawning, nasal stuffiness, diaphoresis, fever, poor sucking, tremors, and seizures (Slater, 2015).

Withdrawal from opiates during pregnancy is extremely dangerous for the fetus, so a prescribed oral methadone maintenance program combined with psychotherapy is recommended for the pregnant person. This closely supervised treatment program reduces withdrawal symptoms in the newborn, reduces drug cravings, and blocks the euphoric effects of narcotic drugs in order to reduce illicit drug use. Management of opioid addiction in pregnancy includes maintenance therapy with methadone or buprenorphine in addition to traditional prenatal care and psychosocial treatment of substance abuse, such as self-help, 12-step groups, individual and group substance abuse counselling, and psychotherapy. Maintenance therapy drugs provide a steady state of opiate levels, thus reducing the risk of withdrawal to the fetus and exposure to HIV and other STIs because the client is no longer injecting drugs. However, maintenance therapy drugs have the same withdrawal consequences for clients and their newborns as heroin does (McKeever, Spaeth-Brayton, & Sheerin, 2014).

Methamphetamines. Methamphetamine use is now more common than cocaine use in pregnancy, and its use by persons of childbearing age is. This highly addictive stimulant is commonly known as speed, meth, or chalk. In its smoked form, it is often referred to as ice, crystal, crank, and glass. Smoking or injecting the drug quickly delivers it to the brain for an immediate, intense euphoria. Because the pleasure also fades quickly, users often take repeated doses, in a "binge and crash" pattern. It is a white, odourless, bitter-tasting powder that was developed from its parent drug, amphetamine, and was used originally in nasal decongestants and bronchial inhalers. The maternal effects include increased energy and alertness, an intense rush, decreased appetite, tachycardia, and tachypnea. Chronic use can lead to psychosis, including paranoia, hallucinations, memory loss, and aggressive or violent behaviour. Signs of methamphetamine use include track marks from intravenous injection, malnutrition, severe dental decay (meth mouth), and skin abscesses from skin picking (ACOG, 2014f). Few studies have been done on the effects of methamphetamine abuse during pregnancy, but the few done indicate an increased risk for preterm births, low birth weight, placental abruption, fetal growth restriction, and congenital anomalies (NIDA, 2015d). These findings are hard to interpret, however, due to small sample size and polydrug use of the participants.

Cocaine. Cocaine use is second only to cannabis use in childbearing persons who use drugs during pregnancy. The incidence of cocaine exposure in utero is approximately 1 to 10 per 1,000 live births (Brandt, Leifheit, Finnegan, & Fischer, 2014). There is evidence that cocaine affects infant development both directly, via in utero exposure, and indirectly, via alterations in maternal care after birth.

Cocaine is a psychoactive drug derived from the leaves of the coca plant, which grows in the Andes Mountains of Peru, Ecuador, and Bolivia. The freebase form, called "crack" because of the cracking or popping noise made in its preparation, is less expensive, easily made, and smokable. Cocaine is a powerful vasoconstrictor. When sniffed into the mucous membranes of the nose, it produces an intense "rush" that some have compared to an orgasmic experience. Smoked crack is absorbed rapidly by the pulmonary vasculature and reaches the brain's circulation in 6 to 8 seconds (NIDA, 2015b).

Cocaine use produces vasoconstriction, dilates pupils, increases body temperature, tachycardia, and hypertension in both the client and the fetus (Kahn, Mikhael, & Vadivelu, 2015). Uteroplacental insufficiency may result from reduced blood flow and placental perfusion. Chronic use can result in low birth weight, the most common effect of cocaine use in pregnancy (NIDA, 2015b).

Studies suggest that perinatal cocaine use increases the risk of preterm labour, abortion, abruptio placentae, fetal growth restriction, intrauterine fetal distress and demise, seizures, withdrawal, and cerebral infarcts. Cocaine may increase the risk of uterine rupture and congenital anomalies (NIDA, 2015b). Fetal anomalies associated with cocaine use in early pregnancy involve neurologic problems such as neural tube defects and microcephaly; cardiovascular anomalies such as congenital heart defects; genitourinary conditions such as prune belly syndrome, hydronephrosis, and ambiguous genitalia; and gastrointestinal system problems such as necrotizing enterocolitis (Connery, 2014). Some infants exposed to cocaine in utero show increased irritability and are difficult to calm and soothe to sleep.

Nonmedical Use of Prescription Drugs. In addition to alcohol and illicit drug use, a new worldwide trend has emerged and may soon exceed illicit drug use; that is, the nonmedical use of prescription drugs found in many home medicine cabinets. Prescription drug abuse has reached epidemic levels. Common drugs of choice include analgesics, stimulants, sedatives, and tranquilizers. A frequent belief among abusers is that prescribed medications are less dangerous than street drugs and using a friend's medication is safe. Unfortunately, unintentional poisoning deaths occur frequently. In addition, the development of a counterfeit market has developed utilizing the Internet, thereby creating a global counterfeit drug market (McHugh, Nielsen, & Weiss, 2015).

Early detection through a comprehensive evaluation is essential to improve overall treatment outcomes. New research supports screening all childbearing clients for substance abuse. A major role of the nurse is to focus on prevention by educating all clients about the dangers associated with misuse of prescription medications. Community education is vital to manage risks to prevent problems from developing.

Nursing Assessment

Complete a thorough history and physical examination to evaluate a client for substance use and abuse. Substance abuse screening in pregnancy is done to detect the use of any substance known or suspected to exert a deleterious effect on the client or their fetus. Routinely ask about substance abuse with all clients of childbearing age, inform them of the risks involved, and advise them against continuing. Screening questionnaires are helpful in identifying potential users, may reduce the stigma of asking clients about substance abuse, and may result in a more accurate and consistent evaluation. The questions in Box 20.5 may be helpful in assessing a client who is at risk for substance abuse during pregnancy. Using "accepting" terminology may encourage the client to give honest answers without fear of reproach.

A client who reports taking no drugs while pregnant may be unaware that substances such as hair dye, diet cola, paint, or over-the-counter medications for colds or headaches are still considered drugs. Thus, it is very difficult to get a true picture of the real use of drugs by a childbearing person.

SAMPLE QUESTIONS FOR ASSESSING SUBSTANCE USE

- Have you ever used recreational drugs? If so, when and what?
- Have you ever taken a prescription drug other than as intended?
- What are your feelings about drug use during pregnancy?
- How often do you smoke cigarettes? How many per day?
- How often do you drink alcohol?
- Have you ever felt guilty about drinking or drug use?

If the assessment reveals substance use, obtain additional information by using the RAFFT questionnaire, which is a sensitive screening instrument for identifying substance abuse (Weekes & Lee, 2014):

R: Do you drink or take drugs to **R**elax, improve your self-image, or fit in?
A: Do you ever drink or take drugs while **A**lone?
F: Do you have any close **F**riends who drink or take drugs?
F: Does a close **F**amily member have a problem with alcohol or drugs?
T: Have you ever gotten in **T**rouble from drinking or taking drugs?

Many drugs are considered to have a teratogenic effect on growing fetuses. A teratogen is any environmental substance that can cause physical defects in the developing embryo and fetus. Pregnant clients with substance abuse commonly present with polysubstance abuse, which is likely to be more damaging than the use of any single substance. Thus, it is inherently difficult to ascribe a specific perinatal effect to any one substance (McKeever et al., 2014).

A urine toxicology screen may also be helpful in determining drug use, with consent of the client; although a urine screen identifies only recent or heavy use of drugs. The length of time a drug is present in urine is as follows:

- Cocaine: 24 to 48 hours in an adult, 72 to 96 hours in an infant
- Heroin: 24 hours in an adult, 24 to 48 hours in an infant
- Cannabis: 1 week to 1 month in an adult, up to a month or longer in an infant
- Methadone: up to 10 days in an infant (Wang, 2015).

Nursing Management

If the client's drug screen is positive, use this as an opportunity to discuss prenatal exposure to substances that may be harmful. The discussion may lead the nurse to refer the client for a diagnostic assessment or identify an intervention such as counselling that may be helpful. Being nonjudgmental is a key to success; a client is more apt to trust and reveal patterns of abuse if the nurse does not judge them and their lifestyle choices.

Be proactive, supportive, and accepting when caring for the client. Assure those with substance abuse challenges that sharing information of a confidential nature with health care providers will not render them liable to criminal prosecution. Provide counselling and education through brief interventions, which are short sessions incorporated into the routine prenatal care to provide the client with counselling, education, simple advice, and referrals as needed (Ordean et al., 2017). Brief interventions can emphasize the following:

- Effects of substance exposure on the fetus
- Interventions to improve client–child attachment and improve parenting
- Psychosocial support if treatment is needed to reduce substance abuse
- Referral to outreach programs to improve access to treatment facilities
- Hazardous legal substances to avoid during pregnancy
- Follow-up of children born to substance-dependent clients
- Dietary counselling to improve the pregnancy outcome for both client and child
- Drug screening to identify all drugs a client is using
- More frequent prenatal visits to monitor fetal well-being
- Client and fetal benefits of remaining drug free
- Cultural sensitivity
- Coping skills, support systems, and vocational assistance

There is nothing categorically different about addiction in pregnancy compared with addiction in general. Childbearing clients who use drugs are people who use drugs, get pregnant, and cannot stop using drugs. The fact that they are condemned in society leads to their further marginalization, which does nothing to improve their lives or the lives of their children.

Substance abuse is a complex problem that requires sensitivity to each client's unique situation and contributing factors. Be sure to address individual psychological and sociocultural factors to help the client regain control of their life. Nurses must be aware of these clients' unique needs and the related legal and ethical ramifications surrounding pregnancy. Treatment must combine different approaches and provide ongoing support for clients learning to live drug free. Developing personal strengths, such as communication skills, assertiveness, and self-confidence, will help the client to resist drug use. Encourage the use of healthy coping skills. Enhancing self-esteem also helps provide a foundation to avoid drugs. Through therapeutic communication, nursing interventions, clinical assessment, and building trusting relationships, nurses can have a significant impact in managing clients with substance abuse.

NURSING CARE PLAN 20.1

Overview of the Childbearing Client With Type 1 Diabetes

Donna, a 30-year-old client with type 1 diabetes, presents to the maternity clinic for pre-conception care. The client has had diabetes for 8 years and takes insulin twice daily by injection, and does blood glucose self-monitoring four times daily. The client reports that their disease is fairly well controlled, but "I'm worried about how my diabetes will affect a pregnancy and my baby. Will I need to make changes in my routine? Will my baby be normal?" The client reports that they recently had a foot infection and needed to go to the emergency department because it led to an episode of ketoacidosis. They state that their last glycosylated hemoglobin A1C test results were abnormal.

NURSING DIAGNOSIS: Ineffective health maintenance: related to deficient knowledge regarding care in diabetic condition in pregnancy as evidenced by questions about effect on pregnancy, possible changes in regimen, and pregnancy outcome.

Outcome Identification and Evaluation

The client will demonstrate increased knowledge of type 1 diabetes and effects on pregnancy as evidenced by proper techniques for blood glucose monitoring and insulin administration, ability to modify insulin doses and dietary intake to achieve control, and verbalization of need for glycemic control prior to pregnancy, with blood glucose levels remaining within normal range.

Interventions: *Providing Client Teaching*

- Assess client's knowledge of diabetes and pregnancy *to establish a baseline from which to develop an individualized teaching plan.*
- Review the underlying problems associated with diabetes and how pregnancy affects glucose control *to provide client with a firm knowledge base for decision-making.*
- Review signs and symptoms of hypoglycemia and hyperglycemia and prevention and management measures *to ensure client can deal with them should they occur.*
- Provide written materials describing diabetes and care needed for control *to provide opportunity for client's review and promote retention of learning.*
- Observe client administering insulin and self-glucose testing for technique and offer suggestions for improvement if needed *to ensure adequate self-care ability.*
- Discuss proper foot care to prevent future infections.
- Teach home treatment for symptomatic hypoglycemia to minimize risk to client and fetus.
- Outline acute and chronic diabetic complications to reinforce the importance of glucose control.

- Discuss use of contraceptives until blood glucose levels can be optimized before conception occurs *to promote the best possible health status before conception.*
- Explain the rationale for good glucose control and the importance of achieving excellent glycemic control before pregnancy to promote a positive pregnancy outcome.
- Review self-care practices (blood glucose monitoring and frequency of testing; insulin administration; adjustment of insulin dosages based on blood glucose levels) to foster independence in self-care and feelings of control over the situation.
- Refer client for dietary counselling to ensure optimal diet for glycemic control.
- Outline obstetric management and fetal surveillance needed for pregnancy to provide client with information on what to expect.
- Discuss strategies for maintaining optimal glycemic control during pregnancy to minimize risks to client and fetus.

(continued)

NURSING CARE PLAN 20.1

Overview of the Childbearing Client With Type 1 Diabetes (continued)

NURSING DIAGNOSIS: Anxiety related to threat to self and fetus as evidenced by questions about their condition's effect on the baby and baby being normal

Outcome Identification and Evaluation

The client will openly express their feelings related to diabetes and pregnancy as evidenced by statements of feeling better about the pre-existing condition and pregnancy outlook, and statements of understanding related to future childbearing by linking good glucose control with positive outcomes for both themself and their offspring.

Interventions: *Minimizing Anxiety*

- Review the need for a physical examination to evaluate for any effects of diabetes on the client's health status.
- Explain the rationale for assessing client's blood pressure, vision, and peripheral pulses at each visit to provide information related to possible effects of diabetes on health status.
- Identify any alterations in present diabetic condition that need intervention to aid in minimizing risks that may increase client's anxiety level.
- Review potential effects of diabetes on pregnancy to promote client understanding of risks and ways to control or minimize them.
- Encourage active participation in decision-making and planning pregnancy to promote

feelings of control over the situation and foster self-confidence.
- Discuss feelings about future childbearing and managing pregnancy to help reduce anxiety related to uncertainties.
- Encourage client to ask questions or voice concerns to help decrease anxiety related to the unknown.
- Emphasize the use of frequent and continued surveillance of client and fetal status during pregnancy to reduce the risk of complications and aid in alleviating anxieties related to the unknown.
- Provide positive reinforcement for healthy behaviours and actions to foster continued use and enhancement of self-esteem.

KEY CONCEPTS

- ○ Preconception counselling for the client with diabetes is helpful in promoting blood glucose control to prevent congenital anomalies.

- ○ The classification system for diabetes is based on disease etiology and not pharmacology; the classification includes type 1 diabetes, type 2 diabetes, gestational diabetes, and prediabetes.

- ○ A functional classification for heart disease during pregnancy is based on past and present disability: class I, asymptomatic with no limitation of physical activity; class II, symptomatic (dyspnea, chest pain) with increased activity; class III, symptomatic (fatigue, palpitation) with normal activity; and class IV, symptomatic at rest or with any physical activity.

- ○ Pre-existing hypertension exists when the client has a blood pressure of 140/90 mm Hg or higher

before pregnancy or before the 20th week of gestation or when hypertension persists for more than 12 weeks' postpartum.

- ○ Successful management of asthma in pregnancy involves elimination of environmental triggers, drug therapy, and client education.

- ○ Ideally, clients with hematologic conditions are screened before conception and are made aware of the risks to themselves and to a pregnancy.

- ○ A wide variety of infections, such as cytomegalovirus, rubella, herpes simplex, hepatitis B, varicella, parvovirus B19, and many sexually transmitted infections can affect a pregnancy, having a negative impact on its outcome.

- ○ There are only three recognized modes of HIV transmission: unprotected sexual intercourse with an infected partner, contact with infected blood or blood products, and perinatal transmission. Breast-feeding is a major contributing factor in client-to-child transmission of HIV.

○ Cases of perinatal AIDS have decreased in the past several years, primarily because of the use of anti-retroviral therapy in pregnant clients with HIV. All pregnant clients should be offered HIV antibody testing regardless of their risk of infection, and that testing should be done during the initial prenatal evaluation.

○ The younger an adolescent is at the time of their first pregnancy, the more likely it is that they will have another pregnancy during the teenage years.

○ The nurse's role in caring for the pregnant adolescent is to assist that client in identifying the options for this pregnancy, including abortion, self-parenting of the child, temporary foster care for the baby or the client, or placement for adoption.

○ Pregnant clients with substance abuse challenges commonly abuse several substances, making it difficult to ascribe a specific perinatal effect to any one substance. Societal attitudes regarding pregnant clients and substance abuse may prohibit them from admitting the problem and seeking treatment.

○ Substance abuse during pregnancy is associated with preterm labour, abortion, low birth weight, central nervous system and fetal anomalies, and long-term childhood developmental consequences.

○ Fetal alcohol spectrum disorder is a lifelong yet completely preventable set of physical, mental, and neurobehavioural birth defects; it is a leading cause of intellectual disability.

○ Nursing management for the client with substance abuse focuses on screening and preventing substance abuse to reduce the high incidence of obstetric and medical complications as well as the morbidity and mortality among newborns born substance dependent.

REFERENCES AND RECOMMENDED READINGS

Aberge, J. A. & Cespesdes, M. S. (2019). HIV and women. *UpToDate*. Retrieved from https://www.uptodate.com/contents/hiv-and-women

Agent, O. E. (2015). 19 Classic viral exanthems. In D. Schlossberg (Ed.). *Clinical infectious disease* (2nd ed., Chapter 19). Cambridge, MA: Cambridge University Press.

Aktas, G., Alcelik, A., Ozlu, T., Tosun, M., Tekce, B. K., Savli, H., . . . Dikbas, O. (2014). Association between omentin levels and insulin resistance in pregnancy. *Experimental and Clinical Endocrinology & Diabetes*, *122*(03), 163–166.

Alan Guttmacher Institute. (2015a). *Facts on American teens' sexual and reproductive health*. Retrieved from http://www.guttmacher.org/pubs/FB-ATSRH.html

Alan Guttmacher Institute. (2015b). *Pregnancy fact sheets*. Retrieved from http://www.guttmacher.org/in-the-know/pregnancy.html

Alexander, L. L., LaRosa, J. H., Bader, H., & Garfield, S. (2014). *New dimensions in women's health* (6th ed.). Sudbury, MA: Jones & Bartlett.

Allen, V. M., & Yudin, M. H. (2012). Management of group B streptococcal bacteriuria in pregnancy. *Journal of Obstetrics and Gynaecology Canada*, *34*(5), 482–486.

Alonso-Gonzalez, R., & Swan, L. (2014). Treating cardiac disease in pregnancy. *Women's Health*, *10*(1), 79–90.

American Academy of Allergy, Asthma & Immunology (AAAAI). (2015). *Asthma and pregnancy*. Retrieved from http://www.aaaai.org/conditions-and-treatments/library/asthma-library/asthma-and-pregnancy.aspx

American Academy of Pediatrics. (2014). Adolescent pregnancy: Current trends and issues. *AAP News*, *35*(5), 19–25.

American Academy of Pediatrics (AAP). (2015). *Serious illnesses and breastfeeding*. Retrieved from https://healthychildren.org/English/ages-stages/baby/breastfeeding/Pages/Serious-Illnesses-and-Breastfeeding.aspx

American College of Obstetricians & Gynecologists (ACOG). (2013). Hypertension in pregnancy. Report of the American College of Obstetricians and Gynecologists' Task Force on Hypertension in Pregnancy. *Obstetrics and Gynecology*, *122*, 1122–1131.

American College of Obstetricians & Gynecologists (ACOG). (2014a). ACOG guidelines at a glance: Gestational diabetes mellitus. *Contemporary OB/GYN*. Retrieved from http://contemporaryobgyn.modernmedicine.com/contemporary-obgyn/news/acog-guidelines-glance-gestational-diabetes-mellitus?page=full

American College of Obstetricians & Gynecologists (ACOG). (2014b). ACOG Committee opinion no. 549: Obesity in pregnancy. *Obstetrics and Gynecology*, *121*, 213–217.

American College of Obstetricians & Gynecologists (ACOG). (2014c). *Fetal alcohol spectrum disorders prevention handbook*. Retrieved from http://www.acog.org/About-ACOG/ACOG-Districts/District-II/Fetal-Alcohol-Spectrum-Disorders-Prevention-Handbook

American College of Obstetricians & Gynecologists (ACOG). (2014d). *Tobacco, alcohol, drugs, and pregnancy*. Retrieved from http://www.acog.org/Patients/FAQs/Tobacco-Alcohol-Drugs-and-Pregnancy

American College of Obstetricians & Gynecologists (ACOG). (2014e). *Opioid abuse, dependence, and addiction in pregnancy*. Retrieved from http://www.acog.org/Resources-And-Publications/Committee-Opinions/Committee-on-Health-Care-for-Underserved-Women/Opioid-Abuse-Dependence-and-Addiction-in-Pregnancy

American College of Obstetricians & Gynecologists (ACOG). (2014f). *Methamphetamine abuse in women of reproductive age*. Retrieved from http://www.acog.org/Resources-And-Publications/Committee-Opinions/Committee-on-Health-Care-for-Underserved-Women/Methamphetamine-Abuse-in-Women-of-Reproductive-Age

American College of Rheumatology. (2015). *Prevalence statistics*. Retrieved from http://www.rheumatology.org/Research/Prevalence_Statistics/

American Diabetes Association (ADA). (2015a). *Diabetes basics*. Retrieved from http://www.diabetes.org/diabetes-basics/

American Diabetes Association (ADA). (2015b). *What is gestational diabetes?* Retrieved from http://www.diabetes.org/diabetes-basics/gestational/what-is-gestational-diabetes.html

American Diabetes Association (ADA). (2015c). *How to treat gestational diabetes.* Retrieved from http://www.diabetes.org/diabetes-basics/gestational/how-to-treat-gestational.html

American Diabetes Association (ADA). (2015d). *Living with diabetes: After delivery.* Retrieved from http://www.diabetes.org/living-with-diabetes/

American Heart Association (AHA). (2015). *Women and heart disease.* Retrieved from https://www.goredforwomen.org/about-heart-disease/facts_about_heart_disease_in_women-sub-category/statistics-at-a-glance/

Armon, C., Baquis, G. D., Howard, G. F., & Krupa, M. J. (2015). Neurologic disease and pregnancy. *eMedicine.* Retrieved from http://emedicine.medscape.com/article/1149405-overview#a7

Bain, E., Crane, M., Tieu, J., Han, S., Crowther, C. A., & Middleton, P. (2015). Diet and exercise interventions for preventing gestational diabetes mellitus. *Cochrane Database of Systematic Reviews,* (4), CD010443.

Bartels, C. M., & Muller, D. (2015). Systemic lupus erythematosus. *eMedicine.* Retrieved from http://emedicine.medscape.com/article/332244-overview

Bates, M., Ahmed, Y., Kapata, N., Maeurer, M., Mwaba, P., & Zumla, A. (2015). Perspectives on tuberculosis in pregnancy. *International Journal of Infectious Diseases, 32,* 124–127.

Berger, H., Gagnon, R., & Sermer, W. (2016). Diabetes in Pregnancy. *Journal of Obstetrics and Gynecology Canada, 38*(7), 667–679.

Bialas, K. M., Swamy, G. K., & Permar, S. R. (2015). Perinatal cytomegalovirus and varicella zoster virus infections: Epidemiology, prevention, and treatment. *Clinics in Perinatology, 42*(1), 61–75.

Brandt, L., Leifheit, A. K., Finnegan, L. P., & Fischer, G. (2014). Management of substance abuse in pregnancy: Maternal and neonatal aspects. In M. Galbally, M. Snellen, & A. Lewis (Eds.). *Psychopharmacology and pregnancy* (pp. 169–195). Berlin: Springer Publishers.

Brickner, M. E. (2014). Cardiovascular management in pregnancy: Congenital heart disease. *Circulation, 130*(3), 273–282.

Brucker, M. C., & King, T. L. (2017). *Pharmacology for women's health* (2nd ed.). Burlington, MA: Jones & Bartlett Learning.

Buschur, E., Brown, F., & Wyckoff, J. (2015). Using oral agents to manage gestational diabetes: What have we learned?. *Current Diabetes Reports, 15*(2), 1–8.

Calhoun, B. C., & Lewis, T. (2016). *Tobacco cessation and substance abuse treatment in women's healthcare: A clinical guide.* Switzerland: Springer International Publishing.

Calvert, C., & Ronsmans, C. (2015). Pregnancy and HIV disease progression: A systematic review and meta-analysis. *Tropical Medicine & International Health, 20,* 122–145.

Camaschella, C. (2015). Iron-deficiency anemia. *New England Journal of Medicine, 372*(19), 1832–1843.

Cantor, A. G., Bougatsos, C., Dana, T., Blazina, I., & McDonagh, M. (2015). Routine iron supplementation and screening for iron deficiency anemia in pregnancy: A systematic review for the US Preventive Services Task Force. *Annals of Internal Medicine, 162*(8), 566–576.

Castillo, E., Murphy, K., & van Schalkwyk, J. (2017). Hepatitis B and pregnancy. *Journal of Obstetrics and Gynaecology Canada, 39*(3), 181–190.

Cennimo, D. J., & Dieudonne, A. (2015). Parvovirus B19 infection. *eMedicine.* Retrieved from http://emedicine.medscape.com/article/961063-overview

Centers for Disease Control and Prevention (CDC). (2015a). *Teen pregnancy in the United States.* Retrieved from http://www.cdc.gov/teenpregnancy/aboutteenpreg.htm

Centers for Disease Control and Prevention (CDC). (2015b). *Tuberculosis and pregnancy.* Retrieved from http://www.cdc.gov/tb/publications/factsheets/specpop/pregnancy.htm

Centers for Disease Control and Prevention (CDC). (2015c). *Fact sheet: Sickle cell disease.* Retrieved from http://www.cdc.gov/ncbddd/sicklecell/documents/scd-factsheet_what-is-scd.pdf

Centers for Disease Control and Prevention (CDC). (2015d). *Women and autoimmune diseases.* Retrieved from http://wwwnc.cdc.gov/eid/article/10/11/14-0367_article

Centers for Disease Control and Prevention (CDC). (2015e). *Cytomegalovirus and pregnant women.* Retrieved from http://www.cdc.gov/cmv/risk/preg-women.html

Centers for Disease Control and Prevention (CDC). (2015f). *Genital herpes—CDC fact sheet.* Retrieved from http://www.cdc.gov/std/herpes/stdfact-herpes.htm

Centers for Disease Control and Prevention (CDC). (2015g). *Hepatitis B information for health professionals: Perinatal transmission.* Retrieved from http://www.cdc.gov/hepatitis/HBV/PerinatalXmtn.htm

Centers for Disease Control and Prevention (CDC). (2015h). *Fetal alcohol spectrum disorders.* Retrieved from http://www.cdc.gov/ncbddd/fasd/alcohol-use.html

Centers for Disease Control and Prevention (CDC). (2015i). *Group B strep (GBS).* Retrieved from http://www.cdc.gov/groupbstrep/about/fast-facts.html

Centers for Disease Control and prevention (CDC). (2015j). *HIV in the United States: At a glance.* Retrieved from http://www.cdc.gov/hiv/statistics/basics/ataglance.html

Centers for Disease Control and Prevention (CDC). (2015k). *HIV among women.* Retrieved from http://www.cdc.gov/hiv/risk/gender/women/facts/index.html

Centers for Disease Control and Prevention (CDC). (2015l). *HIV transmission.* Retrieved from http://www.cdc.gov/hiv/basics/transmission.html

Centers for Disease Control and Prevention (CDC). (2015m). *HIV among pregnant women, infants, and children.* Retrieved from http://www.cdc.gov/hiv/risk/gender/pregnantwomen/facts/

Centers for Disease Control and Prevention (CDC). (2015n). *Child development: Teenagers (15–17 years old).* Retrieved from http://www.cdc.gov/ncbddd/childdevelopment/positiveparenting/adolescence2.html

Centers for Disease Control and Prevention (CDC). (2015o). *Health care providers and teen pregnancy prevention.* Retrieved from http://www.cdc.gov/teenpregnancy/healthcareproviders.htm

Centers for Disease Control and Prevention (CDC). (2015p). *Pregnancy complications: Obesity.* Retrieved from http://www.cdc.gov/reproductivehealth/maternalinfanthealth/pregcomplications.htm#n5

Centers for Disease Control and Prevention (CDC). (2015q). *Illegal drug use.* Retrieved from http://www.cdc.gov/nchs/fastats/drug-use-illegal.htm

Centers for Disease Control and Prevention (CDC). (2015r). *Sexually transmitted diseases.* Retrieved from http://www.cdc.gov/std/

Centers of Disease Control and Prevention (CDC). (2015s). *About HIV/AIDS.* Retrieved from http://www.cdc.gov/hiv/basics/whatishiv.html

Challacombe, L. (2019). The epidemiology of HIV in females. *CATIE.* Retrieved from https://www.catie.ca/en/fact-sheets/epidemiology/epidemiology-hiv-women

Chang, M. W., Brown, R., Nitzke, S., Smith, B., & Eghtedary, K. (2015). Stress, sleep, depression and dietary intakes among low-income overweight and obese pregnant women. *Maternal and Child Health Journal, 19*(5), 1047–1059.

Charlier, C., Le Mercier, D., Salomon, L. J., Ville, Y., Kermorvant-Duchemin, E., Frange, P., . . . Leruez-Ville, M. (2014). Varicella-zoster virus and pregnancy. *Presse Medicale, 43*(6), 665–675.

Cherry, A. L., & Dillon, M. E. (Eds.). (2014). *Adolescent pregnancy and mental health. International handbook of adolescent pregnancy* (pp. 79–102). New York: Springer Publishers.

Chomistek, A. K., Chiuve, S. E., Eliassen, A. H., Mukamal, K. J., Willett, W. C., & Rimm, E. B. (2015). Healthy lifestyle in young women greatly reduces CHD and development of CVD risk factors. *Journal of the American College of Cardiology, 65*(1), 43–51.

Choreño-Machain, T. C., Barrios, J., & Reta, E. B. (2015). Congenital and acquired heart disease in pregnancy. *Journal of the American College of Cardiology, 65*(Suppl 10), A548.

Connery, H. S. (2014). *Substance abuse during pregnancy, an issue of obstetrics and gynecology clinics.* Philadelphia, PA: Elsevier Health Sciences.

Contag, S. A., & Arrabal, P. P. (2015). Hepatitis in pregnancy. *eMedicine.* Retrieved from http://emedicine.medscape.com/article/1562368-overview#a1

Cook, J. L., Green, C. R., de la Ronde, S., Dell, C. A., Graves, L., Ordean, A., . . . Wong, S. (2017). Epidemiology and effects of substance use in pregnancy. *Journal of Obstetrics and Gynaecology Canada, 39*(10), 906–915.

Cornell, S. (2015). Continual evolution of type 2 diabetes: An update on pathophysiology and emerging treatment options. *Therapeutics and Clinical Risk Management, 11,* 621–632.

Costa, V. M., Viana, M. B., & Aguiar, R. A. (2015). Pregnancy in patients with sickle cell disease: Maternal and perinatal outcomes. *The Journal of Maternal-Fetal & Neonatal Medicine, 28*(6), 685–689.

Crockett, L. J., & Crouter, A. C. (Eds.). (2014). *Pathways through adolescence: Individual development in relation to social contexts.* New York: Psychology Press.

Cunningham, F. G., Leveno, K. J., Bloom, S. L., Spong, C., Dashe, J., Hoffman, B. L., . . . Sheffield, J. S. (2014). *Williams' obstetrics* (24th ed.). New York: McGraw-Hill Professional Publishing.

Desai, K. N., & Brustman, L. E. (2014). Parvovirus in pregnancy. *Postgraduate Obstetrics & Gynecology, 34*(8), 1–5.

Desai, A., Mark, K., & Terplan, M. (2014). Marijuana use and pregnancy: Prevalence, associated behaviors, and birth outcomes. *Obstetrics and Gynecology, 123,* 46S.

Dhalwani, N. N., Szatkowski, L., Coleman, T., Fiaschi, L., & Tata, L. J. (2015). Nicotine replacement therapy in pregnancy and major congenital anomalies in offspring. *Pediatrics, 135*(5), 859–867.

Doulatram, G., Raj, T. D., & Govindaraj, R. (2015). Pregnancy and substance abuse. In A. D. Kaye, N. Vadivelu, & R. D. Urman (Eds.). *Substance abuse* (pp. 453–494). New York: Springer Publishers.

Drake, A. L., Wagner, A., Richardson, B., & John-Stewart, G. (2014). Incident HIV during pregnancy and postpartum and risk of mother-to-child HIV transmission: A systematic review and meta-analysis. *PLoS Medicine, 11*(2), e1001608.

Dudek, S. G. (2014). *Nutrition essentials for nursing practice* (7th ed.). Philadelphia, PA: Lippincott Williams & Wilkins.

Edwards, M. S. (2014). Adverse fetal outcomes: Expanding the role of infection. *Journal of American Medical Association, 311*(11), 1115–1116.

Ekoe, J. M., Goldenberg, R., & Katz, P. (2018). 2018 Clinical Practice Guidelines. Screening for Diabetes in Adults. *Canadian Journal of Diabetes, 42,* S16–S19.

Farrar, D., Duley, L., Medley, N., & Lawlor, D. A. (2015). Different strategies for diagnosing gestational diabetes to improve maternal and infant health. *Cochrane Database of Systematic Reviews, 1,* CD007122.

Fauci, A. S., Folkers, G. K., & Marston, H. D. (2014). Ending the global HIV/AIDS pandemic: The critical role of an HIV vaccine. *Clinical Infectious Diseases, 59*(Suppl. 2), S80–S84.

Fedorowicz, A. R., Hellerstedt, W. L., Schreiner, P. J., & Bolland, J. M. (2014). Associations of adolescent hopelessness and self-worth with pregnancy attempts and pregnancy desire. *American Journal of Public Health, 104*(8), e133–e140.

Feig, D. S., Berger, H., Donovan, L., Godbout, A., Kader, T., Keely, E., & Sanghera, R.; Diabetes Canada Clinical Practice Guidelines Expert Committee. (2018). 2018 Clinical Practice Guidelines. Diabetes and pregnancy. *Canadian Journal of Diabetes, 42,* S255–S282.

Fleming, N., O'Driscoll, T., Becker, G., & Spitzer, R. F. (2015). Adolescent pregnancy guidelines. *Journal of Obstetrics and Gynaecology Canada, 37,* 740–756.

Foo, L., Tay, J., Lees, C. C., McEniery, C. M., & Wilkinson, I. B. (2015). Hypertension in pregnancy: Natural history and treatment options. *Current Hypertension Reports, 17*(5), 36.

Friedman, A. J., Shander, A., Martin, S. R., Calabrese, R. K., Ashton, M. E., Lew, I., . . . Goodnough, L. T. (2015). Iron deficiency anemia in women: A practical guide to detection, diagnosis, and treatment. *Obstetrical & Gynecological Survey, 70*(5), 342–353.

Gabbay-Benziv, R., Reece, E. A., Wang, F., & Yang, P. (2015). Birth defects in pregestational diabetes: Defect range, glycemic threshold and pathogenesis. *World Journal of Diabetes, 6*(3), 481–488.

Ganchimeg, T., Ota, E., Morisaki, N., Laopaiboon, M., Lumbiganon, P., Zhang, J., . . . Mori, R. (2014). Pregnancy and childbirth outcomes among adolescent mothers: A World Health Organization multicountry study. *BJOG: An International Journal of Obstetrics & Gynaecology, 121*(Suppl 1), 40–48.

Gandhi, M., & Martin, S. R. (2015). Cardiac disease in pregnancy. *Obstetrics and Gynecology Clinics of North America, 42*(2), 315–333.

Giles, M. L. (2015). HIV in pregnancy—Diagnosis, management and follow up of the neonate. *Pathology, 47,* S49.

Gilstrap, L. G., & Wood, M. J. (2014). Cardiovascular disease in women and pregnancy. In *MGH cardiology board review* (pp. 205–223). London: Springer Publishers.

Grandy, M., Purnell, J. Q., Thornburg, K. L., & Marshall, N. E. (2015). Gestational weight gain and maternal diet composition [272]. *Obstetrics & Gynecology, 125,* 87S–88S.

Green, C. J. (2016). *Maternal newborn nursing care plans* (3rd ed.). Burlington, MA: Jones & Bartlett Learning.

Grewal, J., Silversides, C. K., & Colman, J. M. (2014). Pregnancy in women with heart disease: Risk assessment and management of heart failure. *Heart Failure Clinics, 10*(1), 117–129.

Gupta, Y., Kalra, B., Baruah, M. P., Singla, R., & Kalra, S. (2015). Updated guidelines on screening for gestational diabetes. *International Journal of Women's Health, 7,* 539–550.

Hadar, E., Ashwal, E., & Hod, M. (2014). The preconceptional period as an opportunity for prediction and prevention of non-communicable disease. *Best Practice & Research Clinical Obstetrics & Gynaecology, 29*(1), 54–62.

Hamdan, A. H. (2015). Neonatal abstinence syndrome. *eMedicine.* Retrieved from http://emedicine.medscape.com/article/978763-overview

Hardy, E. J., DegliEsposti, S., & Nee, J. (2015). Viral infection in pregnancy: HIV and viral hepatitis. In *Medical management of the pregnant patient* (pp. 197–216). New York: Springer Publishers.

Harvey, R. E., Coffman, K. E., & Miller, V. M. (2015). Women-specific factors to consider in risk, diagnosis and treatment of cardiovascular disease. *Women's Health, 11*(2), 239–257.

Hashemi-Beni, M., Rahimi-Madiseh, M., Khosravi, A., Malekpur-Thehrani, A., Alijani, Z., & Ayazi, Z. (2015). Educational needs assessment of gestational diabetes in pregnant women for safe delivery and healthy baby birth. *Journal of Clinical Nursing and Midwifery, 4*(1), 59–67.

He, J. R., Yuan, M. Y., Chen, N. N., Lu, J. H., Hu, C. Y., Mai, W. B., . . . Qiu, X. (2015). Maternal dietary patterns and gestational diabetes mellitus: A large prospective cohort study in China. *British Journal of Nutrition, 113*(08), 1292–1300.

Heart and Stroke Foundation. (2018). *Heart and Stroke Foundation 2018 Heart Report.* Retrieved from http://www.heartandstroke.ca

Herchline, T. E., & Amorosa, J. K. (2015). Tuberculosis. *eMedicine.* Retrieved from http://emedicine.medscape.com/article/230802-overview

Higgins, J. P., Yarlagadda, S., & Yang, B. (2015). Cardiovascular complications of energy drinks. *Beverages, 1*(2), 104–126.

Hilfiker-Kleiner, D., & Arany, Z. (2014). Focus on pregnancy-mediated heart and vascular disease. *Cardiovascular Research, 101*(4), 543–544.

Hokelek, M. (2015). Toxoplasmosis. *eMedicine.* Retrieved from http://emedicine.medscape.com/article/229969-overview

Houlden, R. L. (2018). 2018 Clinical Practice Guidelines: Introduction. *Canadian Journal of Diabetes, 42,* S1–S5.

Howlett, J. G., McKelvie, R. S., Costigan, J., Ducharme, A., Estrella-Holder, E., Ezekowitz, J. A., . . . Zeiroth, S. (2010). The 2010 Canadian Cardiovascular Society guidelines for the diagnosis and management of heart failure update: Heart failure in ethnic minority populations, heart failure and pregnancy, disease management, and quality improvement/assurance programs. *Canadian Journal of Cardiology, 26*(4), 185–202.

Hughes, B. & Cu-Uvin, S. (2019). Antiretroviral and intrapartum management of pregnant HIV-infected women and their infants in resource-rich settings. *UpToDate.* Retrieved from https://www.uptodate.com/contents/antiretroviral-and-intrapartum-management-of-pregnant-hiv-infected-women-and-their-infants-in-resource-rich-settings

Institute for Alternative Futures. (2015). *Diabetes 2015—U.S., state, and metropolitan trends.* Retrieved from http://altfutures.org/diabetes2025/

International AIDS Society. (2015). Mass media campaigns effective for condom use and HIV knowledge. Retrieved from http://www.iasociety.org/Default.aspx?pageId = 5&elementId = 15969

James, J. E. (2015). Review: Higher caffeine intake during pregnancy increases risk of low birth weight. *Evidence Based Nursing, 18*(4), 111.

James, S. H., & Kimberlin, D. W. (2015). Neonatal herpes simplex virus infection: Epidemiology and treatment. *Clinics in Perinatology, 42*(1), 47–59.

James, P. A., Oparil, S., Carter, B. L., Cushman, W. C., Dennison-Himmelfarb, C., Handler, J., . . . Ortiz, E. (2014). 2014 evidence-based guideline for the management of high blood pressure in adults: Report from the panel members appointed to the Eighth Joint National Committee (JNC 8). *Journal of American Medical Association, 311*(5), 507–520.

Jhaveri, R. (2015). Prevention of hepatitis B virus vertical transmission: Time for the next step. *Pediatrics, 135*(5), e1286–e1287.

Jimenez, K., Kulnigg-Dabsch, S., & Gasche, C. (2015). Management of iron deficiency anemia. *Gastroenterology & Hepatology, 11*(4), 241–250.

Johnson, J. A., & Tough S. (2012). Delayed child-bearing. *Journal of Obstetrics and Gynaecology Canada, 34*(1), 80–93.

Joint National Committee. (2014). *Eighth report of the Joint National Committee on prevention, detection, evaluation, and treatment of high blood pressure (NIH Publication No. 035233).* Washington, DC: National Institutes of Health.

Jordan, R. G., Engstrom, J. L., Marfell, J. A., & Farley, C. L. (2014). *Prenatal and postnatal care: A woman-centered approach.* Ames, IO: John Wiley & Sons, Inc.

Jyoti, M., Shirke, S., & Matalia, H. (2015). Congenital rubella syndrome: Global issue. *Journal of Cataract & Refractive Surgery, 41*(5), 1127–1134.

Kahn, E., Mikhael, H., & Vadivelu, N. (2015). Cocaine abuse. In *Substance abuse* (pp. 143–154). New York: Springer Publishers.

Karimi, M., Cohan, N., & Parand, S. (2015). Thalassemia and women's health. *Women's Health Bulletin, 2*(3), E29440.

Kelly, W., Massoumi, A., & Lazarus, A. (2015). Asthma in pregnancy: Physiology, diagnosis, and management. *Postgraduate Medicine, 127*(4), 349–358.

Killion, M. (2015). New hypertension in pregnancy guidelines. *MCN: The American Journal of Maternal/Child Nursing, 40*(2), 128.

Kim, C. (2014). Maternal outcomes and follow-up after gestational diabetes mellitus. *Diabetic Medicine, 31*(3), 292–301.

King, T. L., Brucker, M. C., Kriebs, J. M., Fahey, J. O., Gegor, C. L., & Varney, H. (2015). *Varney's midwifery* (5th ed.), Burlington, MA: Jones & Bartlett Learning.

Knight-Agarwal, C. R., Kaur, M., Williams, L. T., Davey, R., & Davis, D. (2014). The views and attitudes of health professionals providing antenatal care to women with a high BMI: A qualitative research study. *Women and Birth, 27*(2), 138–144.

Knox, C. A., Delaney, J. A., & Winterstein, A. G. (2014). Antidiabetic drug utilization of pregnant diabetic women in us managed care. *BMC Pregnancy and Childbirth, 14*(1), 28–34.

Koh, H. (2014). The teen pregnancy prevention program: An evidence-based public health program model. *Journal of Adolescent Health, 54*(3), S1–S2.

Kovacs, G., & Briggs, P. (Eds.). (2015). Infections during pregnancy—Varicella, herpes, cytomegalovirus, toxoplasma, listeria, Group B Streptococcus. In *Lectures in obstetrics, gynecology and women's health* (pp. 133–137). Springer International Publishing.

Kumar, B., & Gupta, S. (2014). *Sexually transmitted infections* (2nd ed.). Philadelphia, PA: Elsevier Health Sciences.

Lambert, N., Strebel, P., Orenstein, W., Icenogle, J., & Poland, G. A. (2015). Rubella. *Lancet, 385*(9984), 2297–2307.

Lamberth, J. R., Reddy, S. C., Pan, J. J., & Dasher, K. J. (2015). Chronic hepatitis B infection in pregnancy. *World Journal of Hepatology, 7*(9), 1233–1237.

Lapolla, A., & Dalfrà, M. G. (2015). Pregnancy and diabetes. In D. Bruttomesso, & G. Grassi (Eds.). *Frontiers in diabetes* (Vol. *24*, pp. 11–22). Karger Medical & Scientific Publishers.

Lichtin, A., & Philipson, E. H. (2014). Pregnancy. In *The coagulation consult* (pp. 249–269). New York: Springer Publishers.

Ma, W. J., Huang, Z. H., Huang, B. X., Qi, B. H., Zhang, Y. J., Xiao, B. X., . . . Zhu, H. L. (2015). Intensive low-glycemic-load dietary intervention for the management of glycemia and serum lipids among women with gestational diabetes: A randomized control trial. *Public Health Nutrition, 18*(08), 1506–1513.

Maartens, G., Celum, C., & Lewin, S. R. (2014). HIV infection: Epidemiology, pathogeneses, treatment, and prevention. *Lancet, 384*(9939), 258–271.

Madhuvrata, P., Govinden, G., Bustani, R., Song, S., & Farrell, T. A. (2015). Prevention of gestational diabetes in pregnant women with risk factors for gestational diabetes: A systematic review and meta-analysis of randomized trials. *Obstetric Medicine, 8*(2), 68–85.

Magee, L. A., Pels, A., Helewa, M., Rey, E., & von Dadelszen, P. (2014). Diagnosis, evaluation, and management of the hypertensive disorders of pregnancy. *Pregnancy Hypertension, 4*, 105–145.

Malee, M. P. (2015). Protocol 30: Parvovirus B19 infection. In J. T. Queenan, C. Y. Spong, & C. J. Lockwood (Eds.). *Protocols for high-risk pregnancies: An evidence-based approach* (pp. 245–250). Chichester, UK: John Wiley & Sons.

March of Dimes. (2015a). *Gestational diabetes.* Retrieved from http://www.marchofdimes.com/pregnancy/gestational-diabetes.aspx

March of Dimes. (2015b). *Thalassemia.* Retrieved from http://www.marchofdimes.com/baby/thalassemia.aspx

March of Dimes. (2015c). *Sickle cell disease and pregnancy.* Retrieved from http://www.marchofdimes.com/pregnancy/sickle-cell-disease-and-pregnancy.aspx

March of Dimes. (2015d). *Cytomegalovirus and pregnancy.* Retrieved from http://www.marchofdimes.com/pregnancy/cytomegalovirus-and-pregnancy.aspx

March of Dimes. (2015e). *Genital herpes.* Retrieved from http://www.marchofdimes.com/pregnancy/genital-herpes.aspx

March of Dimes. (2015f). *Group B strep infection.* Retrieved from http://www.marchofdimes.com/pregnancy/group-b-strep-infection.aspx

March of Dimes. (2015g). *Toxoplasmosis.* Retrieved from http://www.marchofdimes.com/pregnancy/toxoplasmosis.aspx

March of Dimes. (2015h). *Keeping breastfeeding safe.* Retrieved from http://www.marchofdimes.org/baby/keeping-breastfeeding-safe.aspx

March of Dimes. (2015i). *Pregnancy complications: Sexually transmitted diseases.* Retrieved from http://www.marchofdimes.org/sexually-transmitted-diseases.aspx

March of Dimes. (2015j). *Teenage pregnancy.* Retrieved from http://www.marchofdimes.org/materials/teenage-pregnancy.pdf

March of Dimes. (2015k). *Smoking, alcohol, and drugs and pregnancy.* Retrieved from http://www.marchofdimes.org/pregnancy/illicit-drug-use-during-pregnancy.aspx

March of Dimes. (2015l). *Asthma during pregnancy.* Retrieved from http://www.marchofdimes.org/pregnancy/asthma-during-pregnancy.aspx

March of Dimes. (2015m). *A mommy after 35.* Retrieved from http://www.marchofdimes.org/pregnancy/a-mommy-after-35.aspx?gclid = CKqBr5zEwMACFWoR7AoddGQASQ

McHugh, R. K., Nielsen, S., & Weiss, R. D. (2015). Prescription drug abuse: From epidemiology to public policy. *Journal of Substance Abuse Treatment, 48*(1), 1–7.

McIntyre, H. D., Dyer, A. R., & Metzger, B. E. (2015). Odds, risks and appropriate diagnosis of gestational diabetes. *The Medical Journal of Australia, 202*(6), 309–311.

McKeever, A. E., Spaeth-Brayton, S., & Sheerin, S. (2014). The role of nurses in comprehensive care management of pregnant women with drug addiction. *Nursing for Women's Health, 18*(4), 284–293.

Mehta, N., Chen, K., Hardy, E., & Powrie, R. (2015). Respiratory disease in pregnancy. *Best Practice & Research Clinical Obstetrics & Gynaecology, 29*(5), 598–611.

Miller, M. A., & Carpenter, M. (2015). Hypertensive disorders of pregnancy. In K. R. Montella (Ed.). *Medical management of the pregnant patient* (pp. 177–193). New York: Springer Publishers.

Mills, T. A., & Lavender, T. (2014). Advanced maternal age. *Obstetrics, Gynaecology & Reproductive Medicine, 24*(3), 85–90.

Mitanchez, D., Yzydorczyk, C., Siddeek, B., Boubred, F., Benahmed, M., & Simeoni, U. (2015). The offspring of the diabetic mother—short-and long-term implications. *Best Practice & Research Clinical Obstetrics & Gynaecology, 29*(2), 256–269.

Mohamad, T. N., Fakhri, H. A., Bernal, J. M., Thatai, D., & Peterson, E. (2014). Cardiovascular disease and pregnancy. *eMedicine.* Retrieved from http://emedicine.medscape.com/article/162004-overview

Mohammadzadeh, A., & Farhat, A. (2014). Fetal alcohol syndrome. *Asia Pacific Journal of Medical Toxicology, 3*, 10.

Mohindra, R., & Marwah, S. (2015). Systemic lupus erythematosus in pregnancy-intricate, but wieldy. *International Journal of Reproduction, Contraception, Obstetrics and Gynecology, 4*(2), 295–300.

Money, D., & Allen, V. M. (2013). The prevention of early-onset neonatal group B streptococcal disease. *Journal of Obstetrics and Gynaecology Canada, 35*(10), 939–948.

Money, D. M., & Steben, M. (2017). No. 208-Guidelines for the management of herpes simplex virus in pregnancy. *Journal of Obstetrics and Gynaecology Canada, 39*(8), e199–e205.

Money, D., Tulloch, K., Boucoiran, I., & Caddy, S. (2014). Guidelines for the care of pregnant women living with HIV and interventions to reduce perinatal transmission: Executive summary. *Journal of Obstetrics and Gynaecology Canada, 36*(8), 721–734.

Moore, T. R. (2015). Diabetes mellitus and pregnancy. *eMedicine*. Retrieved from http://emedicine.medscape.com/article/127547-overview

Moses, S. (2015). Anemia in pregnancy. *Family Practice Notebook*. Retrieved from http://www.fpnotebook.com/heme-onc/OB/AnmInPrgncy.htm

Multiple Sclerosis Association of America (MSAA). (2015). *MS Overview*. Retrieved from http://mymsaa.org/about-ms/overview/

Nagtalon-Ramos, J. (2014). *Best evidence-based practices: Maternal-newborn nursing care*. Philadelphia, PA: F.A. Davis Company.

National Asthma Education and Prevention Program (NAEPP). (2015). *Guidelines for the diagnosis and management of asthma*. Retrieved from http://www.nhlbi.nih.gov/health-pro/guidelines/current/asthma-guidelines/index.htm

National Diabetes Information Clearing House. (2015). *What is gestational diabetes?*. Retrieved from http://www.diabetes.niddk.nih.gov/dm/pubs/pregnancy

National Institute on Drug Abuse (NIDA). (2015a). *What are the unique needs of pregnant women with substance abuse disorders?*. Retrieved from http://www.drugabuse.gov/publications/principles-drug-addiction-treatment-research-based-guide-second-edition/frequently-asked-questions/what-are-unique-needs-pregnant-women

National Institute on Drug Abuse (NIDA). (2015b). *Drug facts: Cocaine*. Retrieved from http://www.drugabuse.gov/publications/drugfacts/cocaine

National Institute on Drug Abuse (NIDA). (2015c). *Drug facts: Marijuana*. Retrieved from http://www.drugabuse.gov/publications/drugfacts/marijuana

National Institute on Drug Abuse (NIDA). (2015d). *Drug facts: Methamphetamine*. Retrieved from http://www.drugabuse.gov/publications/drugfacts/methamphetamine

National Institutes of Health (NIH). (2014). *Recommendations for use of antiretroviral drugs in pregnant HIV-infected women for maternal health and interventions to reduce perinatal transmission in the United States*. United Public Health Service. Retrieved from http://aidsinfo.nih.gov/contentfiles/lvguidelines/PerinatalGL.pdf

National Organization on Fetal Alcohol Syndrome (NOFAS). (2015). *What is fetal alcohol syndrome?*. Retrieved from http://www.nofas.org/main/what_is_FAS.htm.

New York Heart Association, Criteria Committee. (1994). *Nomenclature and criteria for diagnosis of diseases of the heart and great vessels* (9th ed., pp. 253–256). Boston, MA: Little, Brown.

Northridge, J. L., & Coupey, S. M. (2015). Realizing reproductive health equity for adolescents and young adults. *American Journal of Public Health, 105*(7), 1284.

Novotna, A., & Ehler, E. (2014). Multiple sclerosis and pregnancy. *Clinical Neurophysiology, 125*(5), e27.

O'Connor, D. L., Blake, J., Bell, R., Bowen, A., Callum, J., Fenton, S., . . . Cheung, A. (2016). Canadian consensus on female nutrition: Adolescence, reproduction, menopause, and beyond. *Journal of Obstetrics and Gynaecology Canada, 38*(6), 508–554.

Ordean, A., Wong, S., & Graves, L. (2017). Substance use in pregnancy. *Journal of Obstetrics and Gynaecology Canada, 39*(10), 922–937.

Ostensen, M. (2014). Contraception and pregnancy counseling in rheumatoid arthritis. *Current Opinion in Rheumatology, 26*(3), 302–307.

Paquet, C., & Yudin, M. H. (2013). Toxoplasmosis in pregnancy: Prevention, screening, and treatment. *Journal of Obstetrics and Gynaecology Canada, 35*(1), 78–81.

Park, J. S., & Pan, C. (2014). Current recommendations of managing HBV infection in preconception or pregnancy. *Frontiers of Medicine, 8*(2), 158–165.

Petry, C. J. (2014). Gestational diabetes: Origins, complications, and treatment. Boca Raton, FL: CRC Press Taylor & Francis Group.

Prasad, M. (2014). When opiate abuse complicates pregnancy. *Contemporary OB/GYN*. (Online, February 1, 2014).

Procter, S. B., & Campbell, C. G. (2014). Position of the Academy of Nutrition and Dietetics: Nutrition and lifestyle for a healthy pregnancy outcome. *Journal of the Academy of Nutrition and Dietetics, 114*(7), 1099–1103.

Public Health Agency of Canada. (2010). *Life with arthritis in Canada. A personal and public health challenge*. Retrieved from https://www.canada.ca/content/dam/phac-aspc/migration/phac-aspc/cd-mc/arthritis-arthrite/lwaic-vaaac-10/pdf/arthritis-2010-eng.pdf

Public Health Agency of Canada. (2013). *Perinatal health indicators for Canada, 2013. A report from the Canadian Perinatal Surveillance System*. Retrieved from https://sogc.org/wp-content/uploads/2014/05/REVISEDPerinatal_Health_Indicators_for_Canada_2013.pdf

Public Health Agency of Canada. (2015). *Summary: Estimates of HIV incidence, prevalence and proportion undiagnosed in Canada, 2014*. Retrieved from https://www.canada.ca/content/dam/canada/health-canada/migration/healthy-canadians/publications/diseases-conditions-maladies-affections/hiv-aids-estimates-2014-vih-sida-estimations/alt/hiv-aids-estimates-2014-vih-sida-estimations-eng.pdf

Public Health Agency of Canada. (2017). *Preconception care*. Retrieved from https://www.canada.ca/content/dam/phac-aspc/documents/services/publications/healthy-living/maternity-newborn-care/maternity-newborn-care-guidelines-chapter-2-eng.pdf

Punthakee, Z., Goldenberg, R., & Katz, P. (2018). Definition, classification, and diagnosis of diabetes, prediabetes, and metabolic syndrome. *Canadian Journal of Diabetes, 42*, S10–S15.

Puopolo, K. M., Madoff, L. C., & Baker, C. J. (2015). Group B streptococcal infection in pregnant women. *UpToDate*. Retrieved from http://www.uptodate.com/contents/group-b-streptococcal-infection-in-pregnant-women

Raio, L., Bolla, D., & Baumann, M. (2015). Hypertension in pregnancy. *Current Opinion in Cardiology, 30*(4), 411–415.

Rajoriya, M., & Kalra, R. (2015). Challenges of motherhood in adolescent girls. *International Journal of Reproduction, Contraception, Obstetrics and Gynecology, 4*(3), 696–700.

Rakhmanina, N. Y., & van den Anker, J. N. (2014). Pharmacologic prevention of perinatal HIV infection. *Early Human Development, 90*(1), S13–S15.

Rayment, M., Asboe, D., & Sullivan, A. K. (2014). HIV testing and management of newly diagnosed HIV. *British Medical Journal, 349*, g4275.

Rigby, F. B. (2015). Anemias in pregnancy. *eMedicine*. Retrieved from http://emedicine.medscape.com/article/261586-overview

Rivera, D. M., & Frye, R. E. (2014). Pediatric HIV infection. *eMedicine*. Retrieved from http://emedicine.medscape.com/article/965086-overview

Roglie, G., & Colagiuri, S. (2014). Gestational diabetes mellitus: Squaring the circle. *Diabetes Care, 37*(6), e143–e144.

Rolnik, D. L, Wright, D., Poon, L. C., O'Gorman, N., Syngelaki, A., de Paco Matallana, C., . . . Nicolaides, K. H. (2017). Aspirin versus placebo in pregnancies at high risk for preterm preeclampsia. *New England Journal of Medicine, 377*, 613–622.

Roskjær, A. B., Andersen, J. R., Ronneby, H., Damm, P., & Mathiesen, E. R. (2015). Dietary advices on carbohydrate intake for pregnant women with type 1 diabetes. *The Journal of Maternal-Fetal & Neonatal Medicine, 28*(2), 229–233; 1–15.

Ross, S., Baird, A. S., & Porter, C. C. (2014). Teenage pregnancy: Strategies for prevention. *Obstetrics, Gynaecology & Reproductive Medicine, 24*(9), 266–273.

Salman, K., Priti, S., Molly, M., Kumar, V. S., & Zeenat, S. (2015). Hepatitis B virus infection in pregnant women and transmission to newborns. *Asian Pacific Journal of Tropical Disease, 5*(6), 421–429.

Sauer, M. V. (2015). Reproduction at an advanced maternal age and maternal health. *Fertility and Sterility, 103*(5), 1136–1143.

Schimmel, M. S., Bromiker, R., Hammerman, C., Chertman, L., Ioscovich, A., Granovsky-Grisaru, S., . . . Elstein, D. (2015). The effects of maternal age and parity on maternal and neonatal outcome. *Archives of Gynecology and Obstetrics, 291*(4), 793–798.

Schur, P. H., & Hahn, B. H. (2015). Epidemiology and pathogenesis of systemic lupus erythematosus. *UpToDate*. Retrieved from http://www.uptodate.com/contents/epidemiology-and-pathogenesis-of-systemic-lupus-erythematosus

Sedgh, G., Finer, L. B., Bankole, A., Eilers, M. A., & Singh, S. (2015). Adolescent pregnancy, birth, and abortion rates across countries: Levels and recent trends. *Journal of Adolescent Health, 56*(2), 223–230.

Seely, E. W., & Ecker, J. (2014). Chronic hypertension in pregnancy. *Circulation, 129*(11), 1254–1261.

Sibai, B. M. (2015). Protocol 25: Chronic hypertension. In J. T. Queenan, C. Y. Spong, & C. J. Lockwood (Eds.). *Protocols for high-risk pregnancies: An evidence-based approach*. Chichester, UK: John Wiley & Sons, Ltd.

Silasi, M., Cardenas, I., Kwon, J. Y., Racicot, K., Aldo, P., & Mor, G. (2015). Viral infections during pregnancy. *American Journal of Reproductive Immunology, 73*(3), 199–213.

Simeone, R. M., Devine, O. J., Marcinkevage, J. A., Gilboa, S. M., Razzaghi, H., Bardenheier, B. H., . . . Honein, M. A.

(2015). Diabetes and congenital heart defects: A systematic review, meta-analysis, and modeling project. *American Journal of Preventive Medicine, 48*(2), 195–204.

Singh, A. G., & Chowdhary, V. R. (2015). Pregnancy-related issues in women with systemic lupus erythematosus. *International Journal of Rheumatic Diseases, 18*, 172–181.

Skoglund, C., Chen, Q., D'Onofrio, B. M., Lichtenstein, P., & Larsson, H. (2014). Familial confounding of the association between maternal smoking during pregnancy and ADHD in offspring. *Journal of Child Psychology and Psychiatry, 55*, 61–68.

Slater, L. (2015). Substance use in pregnancy. *The Practicing Midwife, 18*(1), 10–13.

Sliwa, K., Johnson, M. R., Zilla, P., & Roos-Hesselink, J. W. (2015). Management of valvular disease in pregnancy: A global perspective. *European Heart Journal, 36*(18), 1078–1089.

Smith, B. (2015). Neonatal-perinatal infections: An update. In *Clinics in Perinatology*, 42(1), 77–104. Philadelphia, PA: Elsevier Health Sciences.

Smith, M. V., Gotman, N., & Yonkers, K. A. (2016). Early childhood adversity and pregnancy outcomes. *Maternal and Child Health Journal, 20*(4), 790–798.

Solomon, C. G., & Greene, M. F. (2015). Control of hypertension in pregnancy—If some is good, Is more worse?. *The New England Journal of Medicine, 372*(5), 475–476.

Strangfeld, A., Pattloch, D., Spilka, M., Manger, B., Krummel-Lorenz, B., Gräßler, A., . . . Zink, A. (2015). Pregnancies in patients with rheumatoid arthritis: Treatment decisions, course of the disease, and pregnancy outcomes. *Annals of the Rheumatic Diseases, 74*(Suppl. 2), 70–71.

Subramaniam, G., & Girish, M. (2015). Iron deficiency anemia in children. *The Indian Journal of Pediatrics, 82*(6), 558–564.

Substance Abuse and Mental Health Services Administration (SAMHSA). (2015). *Pregnant women, new mothers, and substance abuse*. Retrieved from http://www.samhsa.gov/samhsaNewsLetter/Volume_17_Number_3/PregnancySubstanceAbuse.aspx

Suliman, S., & Seopela, L. (2015). Congenital and neonatal infections: Review. *Obstetrics and Gynecology Forum, 25*(2), 27–32.

Swamy, G. K., & Heine, R. (2015). Vaccinations for pregnant women. *Obstetrics and Gynecology, 125*(1), 212–226.

Swan, L. (2014). Congenital heart disease in pregnancy. *Best Practice & Research Clinical Obstetrics & Gynaecology, 28*(4), 495–506.

Toledano, Y., Hadar, E., & Hod, M. (2015). Diabetes in pregnancy. In R. A. DeFronzo, E. Ferrannini, P. Zimmet, & K. G. M. M. Alberti (Eds.). *International textbook of diabetes mellitus* (4th ed.). Chichester, UK: John Wiley & Sons.

Ural, S. H. (2015). Genital herpes in pregnancy. *eMedicine*. Retrieved from http://emedicine.medscape.com/article/274874-overview

U.S. Agency for International Development (USAID). (2014). *Contraceptives for clients with STIs, HIV, and AIDS*. Retrieved from https://www.fphandbook.org/contraceptives-clients-stis-hiv-and-aids

U.S. Department of Health and Human Services. (2010). *Healthy People 2020*. Retrieved from http://www.healthy-people.gov/2020/topicsobjectives2020

U.S. Preventive Services Task Force (USPSTF). (2014). *Screening for HIV*. Retrieved from http://www.uspreventiveservicestaskforce.org/uspstf13/hiv/hivfinalrs.htm#summary

U.S. Preventive Services Task Force (USPTF). (2015). *Low-dose aspirin use for the prevention of morbidity and mortality from preeclampsia: Preventive medication*. Retrieved from http://www.uspreventiveservicestaskforce.org/Page/Topic/recommendation-summary/low-dose-aspirin-use-for-the-prevention-of-morbidity-and-mortality-from-preeclampsia-preventive-medication

Vachon, J., Gallant, V., & Siu, W. (2018). Tuberculosis in Canada, 2016. *Canadian Communicable Disease Report*, *44*(3/4), 75–81. Retrieved from https://doi.org/10.14745/ccdr.v44i03a01

Vall, O., Salat-Batlle, J., & Garcia-Algar, O. (2015). Alcohol consumption during pregnancy and adverse neurodevelopmental outcomes. *Journal of Epidemiology and Community Health*, *69*(10), 927–929.

Vanders, R. L., & Murphy, V. E. (2015). Maternal complications and the management of asthma in pregnancy. *Women's Health*, *11*(2), 183–191.

Varner, M. W., Silver, R. M., Rowland Hogue, C. J., Willinger, M., Parker, C. B., Thorsten, V. R., . . . Reddy, U. M. (2014). Association between stillbirth and illicit drug use and smoking during pregnancy. *Obstetrics and Gynecology*, *123*(1), 113–125.

Vaux, K. K., & Chambers, C. (2015). Fetal alcohol syndrome. *eMedicine*. Retrieved from http://emedicine.medscape.com/article/974016-overview

Velez, M. L., & Jansson, L. M. (2015). Perinatal addictions: Intrauterine exposures. In *Textbook of addiction treatment: International perspectives* (pp. 2333–2363). Springer Publishers.

Vinchinski, E. P. (2018). Pregnancy in women with sickle cell disease. *UpToDate*. Retrieved from http://www.uptodate.com/contents/pregnancy-in-women-with-sickle-cell-disease

Vogler, M. A. (2014). HIV and pregnancy. *Current Treatment Options in Infectious Diseases*, *6*(2), 183–195.

Volkow, N. D., Baler, R. D., Compton, W. M., & Weiss, S. R. (2014). Adverse health effects of marijuana use. *New England Journal of Medicine*, *370*(23), 2219–2227.

Vukusic, S., & Marignier, R. (2015). Multiple sclerosis and pregnancy in the "treatment era". *Nature Reviews Neurology*, *11*, 280–289.

Walker, M. (2014). *Breastfeeding management for the clinician: Using the evidence* (3rd ed.). Burlington, MA: Jones & Bartlett Learning.

Wang, M. (2015). Perinatal drug abuse and neonatal withdrawal. *eMedicine*. Retrieved from http://emedicine.medscape.com/article/978492-overview

Wasserman, S., & Clowse, M. E. (2014). Systemic lupus erythematosus. In L. R. Sammaritano, & B. L. Bermas (Eds.). *Contraception and pregnancy in patients with rheumatic disease* (pp. 79–97). New York: Springer Publishers.

Weber, J. R., & Kelley, J. H. (2014). *Health assessment in nursing* (5th ed.). Philadelphia, PA: Lippincott Williams & Wilkins.

Weekes, A. J., & Lee, D. S. (2014). Pediatric cocaine abuse clinical presentation. *eMedicine*. Retrieved from http://emedicine.medscape.com/article/917385-clinical

Whitworth, M., & Cockerill, R. (2014). Antenatal management of teenage pregnancy. *Obstetrics, Gynaecology & Reproductive Medicine*, *24*(1), 23–28.

Worel, J. N., & Hayman, L. L. (2015). Cardiovascular disease prevention in women: Reducing the major threat to women's health. *Journal of Cardiovascular Nursing*, *30*(1), 5–7.

Workowski, K. A., & Bolan, G. A. (2015). Sexually transmitted diseases treatment guidelines, 2015. MMWR. Recommendations and Reports: Morbidity and Mortality Weekly Report. *Recommendations and Reports/Centers for Disease Control*, *64*(RR-03), 1–137.

World Health Organization (WHO). (2015a). *Health for the world's adolescents: A second chance in the second decade*. Geneva, Switzerland: Department of Maternal, Newborn, Child and Adolescent Health, WHO.

World Health Organization (WHO). (2015b). *Tuberculosis: Key facts*. Retrieved from http://www.who.int/mediacentre/factsheets/fs104/en/

World Health Organization (WHO). (2015c). *Guidelines for the identification and management of substance abuse use disorders in pregnancy*. Retrieved from http://www.cdc.gov/nchs/fastats/drug-use-illegal.htm

Worley, J. (2014). Identification and management of prescription drug abuse in pregnancy. *The Journal of Perinatal & Neonatal Nursing*, *28*(3), 196–203.

Yinon, Y., Farine, D., & Yudin, M. H. (2018). Cytomegalovirus infection in pregnancy. *Journal of Obstetrics and Gynaecology Canada*, *40*(2), e134–e141.

Yoost, J. L., Hertweck, S. P., & Barnett, S. N. (2014). The effect of an educational approach to pregnancy prevention among high-risk early and late adolescents. *Journal of Adolescent Health*, *55*(2), 222–227.

Zhang, H. J., Patenaude, V., & Abenhaim, H. (2014). Maternal outcomes in pregnancies affected by varicella zoster virus infections. *Obstetrics & Gynaecology*, *123*, 86S–87S.

CHAPTER **WORKSHEET**

MULTIPLE CHOICE QUESTIONS

1. Which of the following would the nurse include when teaching a pregnant client about the pathophysiologic mechanisms associated with gestational diabetes?
   a. Pregnancy fosters the development of carbohydrate cravings.
   b. There is progressive resistance to the effects of insulin.
   c. Hypoinsulinemia develops early in the first trimester.
   d. Glucose levels decrease to accommodate fetal growth.

2. When providing prenatal education to a pregnant client with asthma, which of the following would be important for the nurse to do?
   a. Explain that they should avoid steroids during the pregnancy.
   b. Demonstrate how to assess blood glucose levels.
   c. Teach correct administration of subcutaneous bronchodilators.
   d. Ensure they seek treatment for any acute exacerbation.

3. Which of the following conditions would most likely cause a pregnant client with type 1 diabetes the greatest difficulty during their pregnancy?
   a. Placenta previa
   b. Hyperemesis gravidarum
   c. Abruptio placentae
   d. Rh incompatibility

4. Childbearing clients who drink alcohol during pregnancy:
   a. Often produce more alcohol dehydrogenase
   b. Usually become intoxicated faster than before
   c. Can give birth to an infant with fetal alcohol spectrum disorder
   d. Gain fewer pounds throughout the gestation

5. When explaining to a pregnant client about HIV infection and transmission, which of the following would the nurse include?
   a. It primarily occurs when there is a large viral load in the blood.
   b. HIV is most commonly transmitted via sexual contact.
   c. It affects the majority of infants of persons with HIV infection.
   d. Nurses are most frequently affected due to needlesticks.

6. Clients who are obese have a greater risk of developing which of the following during pregnancy?
   a. Type 1 diabetes
   b. Hypotension
   c. Low–birth-weight infant
   d. Gestational hypertension

7. Maintenance on methadone or buprenorphine is the most common medical treatment for which of the following drug addictions?
   a. Alcohol
   b. Nicotine
   c. Opiates
   d. Marijuana

CRITICAL THINKING EXERCISES

1. A client at 26 weeks' gestation came to the clinic to follow up on their previous 1-hour glucose screening. The results had come back outside the accepted screening range, and a 2-hour oral glucose tolerance test (OGTT) had been ordered. It resulted in three abnormal values, confirming a diagnosis of gestational diabetes. As the nurse in the prenatal clinic you are seeing the client for the first time.
   a. What additional information will you need to provide care?
   b. What education will the client need to address this new diagnosis?
   c. How will you evaluate the effectiveness of your interventions?

2. A 14-year-old comes to the public health clinic with their parent. The parent tells you that their adolescent child has been "out messing around and has gotten themself pregnant." The young person is crying quietly in the corner and avoids eye contact with you. The parent reports that their child "must be following in my footsteps" because they had become pregnant when only 15 years old. The client's parent goes back out into the waiting room and leaves the client with you.
   a. What is your first approach with the client to gain their trust?
   b. List the client's educational needs during this pregnancy.
   c. What prevention strategies are needed to prevent a second pregnancy?

3. Della, a 27-year-old G3P2, is admitted to the labour and birth suite because of preterm rupture of membranes at an estimated 35 weeks' gestation. The client has received no prenatal care and reports this was an unplanned pregnancy. Della appears distracted and very thin. The client reports that their two previous children have been in foster care since birth because the child welfare authorities "didn't think I was an adequate parent." Della denies any recent use of alcohol or drugs, but you smell alcohol on their breath. Della has a spontaneous vaginal birth a few hours later, producing a 4-lb baby with Apgar scores of 8 at 1 minute and 9 at 5 minutes.

   a. What aspects of this client's history may lead the nurse to suspect that this infant may be at risk for fetal alcohol spectrum disorder?

   b. What additional screening or laboratory tests might validate your suspicion?

   c. What physical and neurodevelopmental deficits might present later in life if the infant has fetal alcohol spectrum disorder?

STUDY ACTIVITIES

1. In the maternity clinic or hospital setting, interview a pregnant client with a pre-existing medical condition (e.g., diabetes, asthma, sickle cell anemia) and find out how this condition affects their life and this pregnancy, especially their lifestyle choices.

2. You have a close friend who has a problem with alcohol but denies it. The friend now admits to you that they think they are pregnant because of a missed period. What specific information and advice should you give the friend concerning alcohol use during pregnancy?

3. Marijuana has been legalized in Canada for recreational use in addition to authorized medical use. What impact might your view (pro or con) have on childbearing clients and their offspring?

4. Outline a discussion you might have with an HIV-positive pregnant client who doesn't see the need to take antiretroviral agents to prevent perinatal transmission.

5. The nurse is preparing a teaching session about breastfeeding for a group of pregnant clients who have various infections listed below. The nurse would include persons with which of the following conditions? Select all that apply.

   a. Hepatitis B
   b. Parvovirus B19
   c. Herpesvirus type 2
   d. HIV-positive status
   e. Cytomegalovirus
   f. Varicella zoster virus

BRINGING IT ALL TOGETHER: A CASE STUDY

Linda is an 18-year-old, very thin client who has been abusing alcohol since the age of 12. The client has lived in foster care for much of their life and is recently on their own with a part-time job. Linda reports having experienced both emotional and sexual abuse during childhood. At 16, Linda was introduced to crack cocaine. So many friends and relatives were using, that it was impossible for the client to see any other lifestyle or want to seek help for the addiction. Linda states wanting to start a new life and get clean when they found out was about being pregnant, but admitted still ended up partying and using drugs for the past 4 months of this pregnancy. The client presents today for a first prenatal visit. The client claims that they are ready to commit to a positive change.

Go to thePoint **to find questions to consider about this case.**

21

Nursing Management of Labour and Birth at Risk

Learning Objectives

Upon completion of the chapter, you will be able to:

1. Propose at least five risk factors associated with dystocia.

2. Differentiate the four major abnormalities or problems associated with dysfunctional labour patterns, giving examples of each problem.

3. Examine the nursing management for the client with dysfunctional labour experiencing a problem with the powers, passenger, passageway, or psyche.

4. Devise a plan of care for the client experiencing preterm labour.

5. Relate the nursing assessment and management of the client experiencing a prolonged pregnancy.

6. Assess four obstetric emergencies that can complicate labour and birth, including appropriate management for each.

7. Compare and contrast the nursing management for the client undergoing labour induction or augmentation, and forceps or vacuum-assisted birth.

8. Summarize the plan of care for a client who is to undergo a caesarean birth.

9. Evaluate the key areas to be addressed when caring for a client who undergoes a vaginal birth after caesarean (VBAC).

Jennifer, a 29-year-old G1P0, is at 41 weeks' gestation. Her health care provider has recommended that she come in for induction. She is very anxious about doing this since she has heard "horror stories" about the "hard painful contractions" that can result. What can the nurse do to calm her fears?

TABLE 21.1 DIAGNOSIS AND MANAGEMENT OF COMMON PROBLEMS ASSOCIATED WITH DYSTOCIA

	Description	Diagnosis	Therapeutic Management	Nursing Management
Problems with the Powers				
Hypertonic uterine dysfunction	Occurring in the latent phase of the first stage of labour (cervical dilation of <4 cm); uncoordinated contractions. Force of contraction typically in the midsection of uterus at the junction of the active upper and passive lower segments of the uterus rather than in the fundus. Loss of downward pressure to push the presenting part against the cervix. Labouring client commonly becomes discouraged due to lack of progress; also has increased pain secondary to uterine anoxia.	Characteristic hypertonicity of the contractions that is frequent, often short in duration with moderate to strong intensity on palpation and short or no resting tone between contractions accompanied by lack of labour progress	Therapeutic rest with the use of hydration and sedatives to promote relaxation and stop the abnormal activity of the uterus. Identification and intervention of any contributing factors (use of prostaglandins). Ruling out abruptio placentae (also associated with high resting tone and persistent pain). Onset of a normal labour pattern often occurs after a 4- to 6-hour rest period.	Institute bed rest and sedation to promote relaxation and reduce pain. Assist with measures to rule out fetopelvic disproportion and fetal malpresentation. Evaluate fetal tolerance to labour pattern, such as monitoring of FHR patterns. Assess for signs of infection. Promote adequate hydration through IV therapy. Provide pain management via epidural or IV analgesics. Assist with amniotomy to augment labour. Explain to client and family about dysfunctional pattern. Plan for operative birth if normal labour pattern is not achieved.
Hypotonic uterine dysfunction	Often termed secondary uterine inertia because the labour begins normally and then the frequency and intensity of contractions decrease. Possible contributing factors: overdistended uterus with multifetal pregnancy, large single fetus, or polyhydramnios, too much pain medicine given too early in labour, fetal malposition, and regional anaesthesia	Evaluation of the client's labour to confirm that she is having hypotonic active labour rather than a long latent phase. Evaluation of the pelvis and fetal presentation and position to ensure that they are not contributing to the prolonged labour without noticeable progress.	Identification of possible cause of inefficient uterine action (a malpositioned fetus, pelvis that is too small, overdistention of the uterus with multiple fetuses, excess amniotic fluid or a macrosomic fetus). Rupture of amniotic sac (amniotomy) if all causes ruled out. Possible augmentation with oxytocin to stimulate effective uterine contractions. Caesarean birth if amniotomy and augmentation ineffective.	Administer oxytocin as ordered once fetopelvic disproportion is ruled out. Assist with amniotomy if membranes are intact. Provide continuous electronic fetal monitoring. Monitor vital signs, uterine activity, and cervix continually. Assess for signs of infection. Explain to client and family about dysfunctional pattern. Plan for surgical birth if normal labour pattern is not achieved or fetal compromise occurs.
Precipitate labour	Abrupt onset of high intensity contractions occurring in a shorter period of time instead of the more gradual increase in frequency, duration, and intensity resulting in rapid effacement and dilatation of the cervix and fetal descent and birth	Identification based on the rapid progress through the stages of labour	Vaginal delivery if pelvis is adequate	Closely monitor client with previous history. Anticipate use of scheduled induction to control labour rate and location. Administer pharmacologic agents, such as tocolytics, to slow labour if fetus compromised. Stay in constant attendance to monitor progress.

Problem	Description	Management	Nursing Interventions
Problems with the Passenger Persistent occiput posterior position	Engagement of fetal head in the left or right occipitotransverse position with the occiput rotating posteriorly rather than into the more favorable occiput anterior position (fetus born facing upward instead of the normal downward position) Labour usually much longer and more uncomfortable (causing increased back pain during labour) if fetus remains in this position. Possible extensive caput succedaneum and moulding from the sustained occiput posterior position.	Labour to proceed, preparing the client for a long labour (spontaneous resolution possible). Comfort measures and positioning to help promote fetal head rotation. Delayed pushing to allow fetal head to rotate with contractions.	Assess for complaints of intense back pain in first stage of labour. Anticipate possible use of forceps to rotate to anterior position at birth or manual rotation to anterior position at end of second stage. Assess for prolonged second stage of labour with arrest of descent (common with this malposition). Encourage position changes to promote fetal head rotation: hands and knees and rocking pelvis back and forth; side-lying position; side lunges during contractions; sitting, kneeling, or standing while leaning forward; squatting position to give birth and enlarge pelvic outlet. Prepare for possible caesarean birth if rotation is not achieved. Administer agents as ordered for pain relief (effective pain relief crucial to help the client to tolerate the back discomfort). Apply low back counter pressure during contractions to ease the discomfort. Provide measures to reduce anxiety. Continuously reinforce the client's progress. Teach client about possible interventions to facilitate fetal head rotation.
Face and brow presentation	Face presentation with complete extension of the fetal head. Brow presentation: fetal head between full extension and full flexion so that the largest fetal skull diameter presents to the pelvis.	Diagnosis only once labour is well established via vaginal examination; palpation of facial features as the presenting part rather than the fetal head	Vaginal birth possible with face presentation with an adequate pelvis and fetal head rotation; caesarean birth if head rotates backward. Caesarean birth for brow presentation unless head flexes.	Assist with evaluating for fetopelvic disproportion. Anticipate caesarean birth if vertex position is not achieved. Explain fetal malposition to the client and partner. Provide close observation for any signs of fetal hypoxia, as evidenced by late decelerations and minimal variability on the fetal monitor.

TABLE 21.1 DIAGNOSIS AND MANAGEMENT OF COMMON PROBLEMS ASSOCIATED WITH DYSTOCIA (continued)

	Description	Diagnosis	Therapeutic Management	Nursing Management
Breech presentation	Fetal buttocks, or breech, presenting first rather than the head. 1. Frank breech: buttock as the presenting part, with hips flexed and legs and knees extended upward 2. Complete breech (or full breech): buttock as presenting part, with hips flexed and knees flexed in a "cannonball" position 3. Footling or incomplete breech: one or two feet as the presenting part, with one or both hips extended	Vaginal examination to determine breech presentation. Ideally, ultrasound to confirm a clinically suspected presentation and to identify any fetal anomalies.	The optimal method of birth is controversial: caesarean birth by some providers unless the fetus is small and the client has a large pelvis; vaginal birth by others with each occurrence treated individually and labour monitored very closely. Regardless of the birth method selected, the risk for trauma is high. Vaginal delivery: fetus allowed to spontaneously deliver up to the umbilicus; then manoeuvres to assist in the delivery of the remainder of the body, arms, and head; fetal membranes left intact as long as possible to act as a dilating wedge and to prevent cord prolapse; anesthesiologist and neonatal resuscitation team present. Caesarean birth; use of external cephalic version to reduce the chance of breech presentation at birth; attempted after the 35th week of gestation but before the start of labour (some fetuses spontaneously turn to a cephalic presentation on their own) toward term, and some will return to the breech presentation if external cephalic version is attempted too early; variable success rates, with risk for fractured bones, ruptured viscera, abruptio placentae, fetomaternal hemorrhage, and umbilical cord entanglement. Tocolytic drugs may be used to relax the uterus, to facilitate external cephalic version at term. Individual evaluation of each client for all factors before any interventions is initiated.	Assess for associated conditions such as placenta praevia, hydramnios, fetal anomalies, and multifetal pregnancy. Arrange for ultrasound to confirm fetal presentation. Assist with external cephalic version possible after 36 weeks. Anticipate trial of labour for 4–6 hours to evaluate progress if version is successful and fetus is at term. Plan for caesarean birth if no progress is seen or fetal compromise occurs. After external cephalic version, administer RhoGAM to the Rh-negative client to prevent a sensitization reaction in case trauma has occurred and the potential for mixing of blood exists.

Shoulder dystocia	Delivery of fetal head with neck not appearing; retraction of chin against the perineum; shoulders remaining wedged behind the client's pubic bone, causing a difficult birth with potential for injury to both client and baby. If shoulders still above the brim at this stage, no advancement. Newborn's chest trapped within the vaginal vault; chest unable to expand with respiration (although nose and mouth are outside). Risk of umbilical cord compression between the fetal body and the pelvis.	Emergency, often unexpected complication. Diagnosis made when newborn's head delivers without delivery of neck and remaining body structures. Primary risk factors, include diabetes mellitus, obesity, excessive weight gain, abnormal pelvic anatomy, postdated pregnancy, short stature, a history of previous shoulder dystocia, use of epidural analgesia or operative vaginal birth, and suspected infant macrosomia (weight >4,500 g)	If anticipated, preparatory tasks instituted: alerting of key personnel; education of client and family regarding steps to be taken in the event of a difficult birth; emptying of client's bladder to allow additional room for possible manoeuvres needed for the birth. McRoberts manoeuvre. Suprapubic pressure (not fundal) (Fig. 21.1). Combination of manoeuvres effective in more than 50% of cases of shoulder dystocia Newborn resuscitation team readily available.	Intervene immediately due to cord compression. Perform McRoberts manoeuvre and application of suprapubic pressure. Assist with positioning the client in squatting position, hands-and-knees position, or lateral recumbent position for birth to free shoulder. After the birth, assess newborn for crepitus, deformity, Erb palsy, or bruising, which might suggest neurologic damage or a fracture.
Multiple pregnancy	More than one fetus, leading to uterine overdistention and possibly resulting in hypotonic contractions and abnormal presentations of the fetuses.	Nearly all multiples are now diagnosed early by ultrasound. The risk of preterm labour is high.	Admission to facility with equipment, resources and experience in care of twins. Spontaneous progression of labour if client has no complicating factors and first fetus is a cephalic presentation. Simultaneous monitoring of each FHR during labour and birth. Use of fetal scalp electrode on presenting twin recommended	Assess for hypotonic labour pattern due to overdistention. Evaluate for fetal presentation, and gestational age to determine mode of delivery. Vaginal birth to take place in presence of immediately avail caesarean (in operating room, room set and surgery can be immediate) Ensure presence of two neonatal teams for birth of multiples.

(continued)

TABLE 21.1 DIAGNOSIS AND MANAGEMENT OF COMMON PROBLEMS ASSOCIATED WITH DYSTOCIA (continued)

	Description	Diagnosis	Therapeutic Management	Nursing Management
	Fetal hypoxia during labour is a significant threat due to placenta variations (one shared placenta, or one placenta less efficient than other, risk of premature separation/abruption)		After birth of first fetus, clamping of cord and lie of the second twin assessed. Possible external cephalic version necessary to assist in providing a cephalic presentation or second fetus delivered breech. Second and subsequent fetuses at greater risk for birth-related complications, such as umbilical cord prolapse, malpresentation, and abruptio placentae. Caesarean birth if risk factors high.	Anticipate need for caesarean birth, which is common in multifetal pregnancy.
Excessive fetal size (greater than 4,500–5,000 g) and fetal anatomic abnormalities	Macrosomia leading to fetopelvic disproportion (fetus unable to fit through the pelvis to be born vaginally). Reduced contraction strength due to overdistention by a large fetus leading to a prolonged labour and the potential for birth injury and trauma. Fetal abnormalities possibly interfering with fetal descent, leading to prolonged labour and difficult birth.	A diagnosis of fetal macrosomia can be confirmed by measuring the birth weight after birth. Suspicion of macrosomia based on the findings of an ultrasound examination (large margin of inaccuracy) before onset of labour (if suspected due to conditions such as maternal diabetes or obesity, estimation of fetal weight via ultrasound). Leopold manoeuvres to estimate fetal weight and position on admission to labour and birth unit.	Scheduled caesarean birth if diagnosis is made before the onset of labour to reduce the risk of injury to both the newborn and the client. If identified by Leopold manoeuvres, possible trial of labour to evaluate progress; however, providers may opt to discuss the risks and benefits of a planned caesarean birth in a primigravida with a macrosomic fetus.	Anticipate need for vacuum and forceps-assisted births (common). Plan for caesarean birth if parameters are inadequate to give birth to large fetus.
Problems with the Passageway	Contraction of one or more of the three planes/diameters of the pelvis. Poorer prognosis for vaginal birth in clients with android and platypelloid types of pelvis.		Focus on allowing natural forces of labour contractions to push the largest diameter (biparietal) of the fetal head beyond the obstruction or narrow passage. Possible forceps and vacuum extraction to assist navigation through this passageway.	Assess for poor contractions, slow dilatation, prolonged labour. Evaluate bowel and bladder status to reduce soft tissue obstruction and allow increased pelvic space. Anticipate trial of labour; if no labour progression after an adequate trial, plan for caesarean birth.

	Obstruction in the birth canal, such as placenta praevia that partially or completely obstructs the internal os of the cervix, fibroids in the lower uterine segment, multiple or large human papilloma virus (HPV) warts in birth canal, or a full bladder or rectum, an edematous cervix caused by premature bearing-down efforts.	Diagnosis by ultrasound (praevia or fibroids), bladder, rectum and cervix palpated.	Caesarean birth for placenta praevia and lower segment fibroids HPV, assist with bladder and bowel emptying as needed.	Provide coaching, encouragement and support for client with involuntary pushing efforts. Anticipate caesarean birth for obstructions that cannot be relieved.
Problems with the Psyche	Release of stress-related hormones (catecholamines, cortisol, epinephrine, beta-endorphin), which act on smooth muscle (uterus) and reduce uterine contractility. Release also results in decreased uteroplacental perfusion and increased risk for poor newborn adjustment.	Ruling out of other possible causes of dystocia	Treatment dependent on client's responses such as anxiety, fear, anger, frustration, or denial (highly variable due to client's understanding of the condition itself, past experiences, previous coping mechanisms, and the amount of family and nursing support received). Appropriate medical or surgical interventions depending on the underlying condition.	Provide comfortable environment—dim lighting, music. Encourage partner to participate. Provide pain management to reduce anxiety and stress. Ensure continuous presence of nurse to provide support, encouragement and reassurance as well as strategies to reduce anxiety. Provide frequent updates concerning fetal status and progress. Offer anticipatory guidance and reassurance to increase self-efficacy and ability to cope.

Adapted from American Academy of Pediatrics. (2015). *Delivery by caesarean section.* Retrieved from https://www.healthychildren.org/English/ages-stages/prenatal/delivery-beyond/Pages/Delivery-by-Caesarean-Section.aspx; Caughey, A. B., & Butler, J. R. (2016). Postterm pregnancy. *eMedicine.* Retrieved from http://emedicine.medscape.com/article/261369-overview; Cunningham, F. G., Leveno, K. J., Bloom, S. L., Spong, C. Y., Dashe, J., Hoffman, B. L., ... Sheffield, J. S. (2014). *Williams' obstetrics* (24th ed.). New York: McGraw-Hill; Fischer, R. (2016). Breech presentation. *eMedicine.* Retrieved from http://emedicine.medscape.com/article/262159-overview; Olsen, N. S. & Karjane, N. W. (2017). Abnormal labour. *eMedicine.* Retrieved from http://emedicine.medscape.com/article/273053-overview; and King, T. L., Brucker, M. C., Osborne, K., & Jevitt, C. M. (2019). *Varney's midwifery* (6th ed.). Burlington, MA: Jones & Bartlett Learning.

contractions. Continuous monitoring, frequent updates on the progress of labour, pain management, and reassurance about the condition can assist in reducing the client's anxious state of mind. Management includes readiness of the health care team for this rapid birth.

Problems With the Passenger

Any presentation other than occiput anterior (head down and the occiput is anterior facing), or a slight variation of the fetal position or size, increases the probability of dystocia. These variations can affect the contractions or fetal descent through the pelvis. Common problems contributing to protracted labour and involving the fetus include occiput posterior position, breech presentation, multifetal pregnancy, excessive size (macrosomia), and fetal anomalies.

Persistent occiput posterior is the most common malposition, occurring in about 15% of labouring clients. The reasons for this malposition are often unclear. This position presents slightly larger diameters to the pelvis, thus slowing fetal descent. A fetal head that is poorly flexed may be responsible. In addition, poor uterine contractions may not push the fetal head down into the pelvic floor to the extent that the fetal occiput sinks into it rather than being pushed to rotate in an anterior direction.

Face and brow presentations are rare and are associated with fetal abnormalities (anencephaly), pelvic contractures, high parity, placenta praevia, hydramnios, low birth weight, or a large fetus (World Health Organization [WHO], 2014a).

By 35 to 36 weeks' gestation, the majority of fetuses will spontaneously settle into the vertex presentation (head down, toward the birth canal). In about 3% to 4% of cases, however, the fetus will remain in a breech presentation with the buttocks or feet presenting. There is less risk to the fetus and pregnant client when the head is down at the time of birth. Breech presentation is frequently associated with multifetal or multiple pregnancies, grand multiparity (more than five births), pregnancy over age 35 ("advanced maternal age"), placenta praevia, hydramnios, preterm births, uterine malformations or fibroids, a scarred uterus, a female infant, and fetal anomalies such as hydrocephaly (Sharshiner & Silver, 2015). In a persistent breech presentation, perinatal morbidity and mortality from a difficult birth may occur (Cunningham et al., 2014). A breech presentation may be an indicator for subtle fetal abnormalities, as apparently healthy breech infants have on average poorer long-term neurodevelopmental scores than cephalic infants (Hofmeyr, 2015). Perinatal mortality is increased two- to fourfold with a breech presentation, regardless of the mode of delivery.

External cephalic version refers to a procedure in which the fetus is rotated from the breech to the cephalic presentation by manipulation through the mother's abdominal wall at or near term. Several national organizations (ACOG, WHO, AFP) recommend that this manoeuvre be offered to clients between 36 and 38 weeks' gestation. It is performed only in a hospital setting under direct ultrasound guidance and fetal monitoring. External cephalic version is successful in approximately 50% of cases. Clients with a breech presentation today are often advised to have a surgical birth with no attempt to rotate the fetal position (Hofmeyr, Kulier, & West, 2015).

Shoulder dystocia is defined as the obstruction of fetal descent and birth by the axis of the fetal shoulders after the fetal head has been delivered. The incidence of shoulder dystocia is increasing due to increasing birth weight with a range of 0.7% to 2.0%. The rate of impacted shoulders in diabetics is higher (1.9%), newborns delivered by vacuum or forceps have a shoulder dystocia rate of 2.0% compared to 0.6%, for spontaneous birth (Hansen & Chauhan, 2014). It is an obstetric emergency with no reliable predictors that requires a coordinated team response to decrease the rate at which adverse outcomes occur (Gherman, 2015). It is one of the most anxiety-provoking emergencies encountered in labour. Failure of the shoulders to deliver spontaneously places both the birthing client and the fetus at risk for injury. Postpartum hemorrhage, secondary to uterine atony, vaginal lacerations, anal tears, and uterine rupture are major complications to the client. Transient Erb or Duchenne brachial plexus palsies and clavicular or humeral fractures are the most common fetal injuries encountered with shoulder dystocia. The occurrence of neonatal brachial plexus palsy is 1.5 per 1,000 live births, with about one third suffering permanent upper extremity functional insufficiencies (Mehlman, 2015). Newborns experiencing shoulder dystocia typically have greater shoulder-to-head and chest-to-head disproportions compared with those delivered without dystocia (Cunningham et al., 2014). Prompt recognition and appropriate management, such as with McRoberts manoeuvre or suprapubic pressure, can reduce the severity of injuries to the client and newborn (Fig. 21.1).

Take Note!

Prompt recognition and appropriate management of shoulder dystocia can reduce the severity of injuries to the birthing client and infant. Immediately assess the infant for signs of trauma such as a fractured clavicle, Erb palsy, or neonatal asphyxia. Assess the client for excessive vaginal bleeding (uterine atony or tissue trauma) and blood in the urine from bladder trauma.

Multiple or **multifetal gestation** refers to twins, triplets, or more infants within a single pregnancy (Box 21.1). The incidence is increasing, primarily as a result of infertility treatment (both ovarian stimulation and in vitro fertilization) and an increased number of clients giving birth at older ages. The incidence of twins, triplets, and higher-order multiple gestations is approximately 3% in Canada and the United States (March of Dimes, 2017;

FIGURE 21.1 Manoeuvres to relieve shoulder dystocia. **A.** McRoberts manoeuvre. The mother's thighs are flexed and abducted as much as possible to straighten the pelvic curve. **B.** Suprapubic pressure. Light pressure is applied just above the pubic bone, pushing the fetal anterior shoulder forward to displace it from above the mother's symphysis pubis.

Statistics Canada, 2018). In 2013, 3.3% of all pregnancies were twins or higher multiples, up from 2.1% in 1991 (Statistics Canada, 2018). The incidence of twins is approximately 1 in 30 conceptions, with about two thirds of them due to the fertilization of two ova (dizygotic or fraternal) and about one third occurring from the splitting of one fertilized ovum (monozygotic or identical twins). One in approximately 8,100 pregnancies results in triplets (March of Dimes, 2017). The most common complication for the childbearing person is postpartum hemorrhage resulting from uterine atony. Compared with singletons (one fetus), the risk of perinatal morbidity and mortality is markedly increased in multiple gestations. Based on recent level 1 evidence from a randomized controlled study, it was found that there was no difference in newborn outcomes between a planned surgical birth versus a planned vaginal birth for twins between 32 to 39 weeks' gestation. As long as the presenting twin is vertex, a vaginal birth should be considered (Bibbo & Robinson, 2015).

Excessive fetal size and abnormalities can also contribute to labour and birth dystocias. **Macrosomia,** in which a newborn weighs 4,000 to 4,500 g (8.81 to 9.92 lb) or more at birth, complicates approximately 10% of all pregnancies. It is the result of a change in body

---

BOX 21.1

MULTIPLE PREGNANCY

As the name implies, a multiple pregnancy or a multifetal pregnancy involves more than one fetus. These fetuses can result from fertilization of a single ovum or multiple ova. Monozygotic (identical) twins develop from one single ovum that divides into equal halves during early cleavage phase. Monozygotic twins are genetically identical; always the same gender, and look very similar in appearance. The number of amnions and chorions depends on the timing of division (cleavage). One fertilized ovum splitting into two separate individuals is termed *natural clones.* This type of twinning occurs in approximately 1 of 250 live births (March of Dimes, 2017).

Twin pregnancies that are multiple-ova conceptions (dizygotic twins) result from two ova fertilized by two sperm. They are referred to as fraternal twins. Genetically, dizygotic twins are as alike (or unlike) as any other pair or siblings. There are separate amnions and chorions although the chorions and placentas may be fused. The incidence of dizygotic twinning is approximately 1 in 500 Asians, 1 in 125 Whites, and as high as 1 in 20 in African populations (March of Dimes, 2017). Fraternal twins account for two thirds of all twins and there is a tendency to repeat within families. Currently the incidence of fraternal twins is increasing secondary to advancing childbearing age when pregnancy occurs and an increase in use of fertility drugs and procedures being done.

Multiple births other than twins can be of the identical type, the fraternal type, or combinations of the two. Triplets can occur from the division of one zygote into two, with one dividing again, producing identical triplets, or they can come from two zygotes, one dividing into a set of identical twins, and the second zygote developing as a single fraternal sibling, or from three separate zygotes. Triplets are said to occur once in 7,000 births and quadruplets once in 660,000 births (March of Dimes, 2017). In recent years, fertility drugs used to induce ovulation have resulted in a greater frequency of quadruplets, quintuplets, sextuplets, and even octuplets.

composition in the neonate with an increase in both percentage of fat and fat mass. Macrosomia is associated with later life obesity, diabetes, and cardiovascular disease (Bauer & Springel, 2017). Fetal abnormalities may include hydrocephalus, ascites, or a large mass on the neck or head. Complications associated with dystocia related to excessive fetal size and anomalies include an increased risk for postpartum hemorrhage, shoulder dystocia, low Apgar scores, dysfunctional labour, fetopelvic disproportion, soft tissue laceration during vaginal birth, fetal injuries or fractures, and perinatal asphyxia (Hobbins, 2015).

Problems With the Passage

Problems with the passage (pelvis and birth canal) are related to a contraction of one or more of the three planes of the pelvis: inlet, midpelvis, and outlet. The pelvis can be classified into four types based on the shape of the pelvic inlet, which is bounded anteriorly by the posterior border of the symphysis pubis, posteriorly by the sacral promontory, and laterally by the linea terminalis. The four basic types are gynecoid, anthropoid, android, and platypelloid (see Chapter 13 for additional information). Contraction of the midpelvis is more common than inlet contraction and typically causes an arrest of fetal descent. Obstructions in the birth canal, such as swelling of the soft tissue and cervix, termed soft tissue dystocia, can also hamper fetal descent and impede labour progression outside the bony pelvis.

Problems With the Psyche

Many clients experience an array of emotions during labour, which may include fear, anxiety, helplessness, isolation, and weariness. These emotions can lead to psychological stress, which indirectly can cause dystocia. Hormones released in response to anxiety can contribute to dystocia. Intense anxiety stimulates the sympathetic nervous system, which releases catecholamines that can lead to myometrial dysfunction. Norepinephrine and epinephrine then lead to uncoordinated or increased uterine activity (Hagood Milton, 2017).

Labour support describes the caring work, or social support provided to a labouring client. It consists of emotional support (continuous presence, reassurance, and praise), comfort measures (touch, massage, warm baths/showers, encouraging fluid intake and output), advocacy (communicating the client's wishes), and provision of information (coping methods, update on progress of labour). Continuous labour support was associated with reduced use of intrapartum pain medication, reduced use of regional analgesia/anaesthesia, decreased operative vaginal deliveries, decreased caesarean births, increased spontaneous vaginal births, and reduced likelihood of reports of negative experiences. On the basis of these findings, all clients should have support throughout labour and birth (Bohren, Hofmeyr, Sakala, Fukuzawa, & Cuthbert, 2017).

Nursing Assessment

Begin the assessment by reviewing the client's history to look for risk factors for dystocia which may include short stature, obesity, hydramnios, uterine abnormalities, fetal malpresentation, cephalopelvic disproportion, overstimulation with oxytocin, exhaustion, ineffective pushing, excessive fetal size, ineffective positioning in labour, and anxiety or fear (Green, 2016). Include in the assessment the client's frame of mind to identify fear, anxiety, stress, lack of support, and pain, which can interfere with uterine contractions and impede labour progress. Helping the client to relax will promote normal labour progress.

Assess the client's vital signs. Note any elevation in temperature (suggestive of an infection) or changes in heart rate or blood pressure (hypovolemia). Evaluate the uterine contractions for frequency and intensity. Question the client about any changes in the contraction pattern, such as a decrease or increase in frequency or intensity. Assess FHR and pattern, reporting any abnormal patterns immediately.

Assess fetal position via *Leopold manoeuvres* (see Chapter 14 for more information) to identify any deviations in presentation or position and report abnormal findings. Assist with or perform a vaginal examination to determine cervical dilation, effacement, and engagement of the fetal presenting part. Evaluate for evidence of membrane rupture. Report any malodorous, blood- or meconium-stained fluid.

Nursing Management

Nursing management of the client with dystocia, regardless of the etiology, requires a thorough and caring approach. The nurse should provide physical and emotional support to the client and family. The final outcome of any labour depends on the size and shape of the pelvis, the quality of the uterine contractions, and the size, presentation, and position of the fetus. Thus, dystocia is diagnosed after labour has progressed for a time, not at the beginning of labour.

PROMOTING THE PROGRESS OF LABOUR

The nurse plays a major role in determining the progress of labour. Continue to assess the client, frequently monitoring cervical dilation and effacement, uterine contractions, and fetal descent, and document that all assessed parameters are progressing. Evaluate progress in active labour by using the simple rule of 0.5 to 1 cm per hour for cervical dilation. When the client's membranes rupture, if they have not already ruptured, observe for colour of fluid and signs of cord prolapse (fetal heart changes, palpation of cord on vaginal examination or cord visible from vagina).

If a protracted labour occurs, contractions will slow or fail to advance in frequency, duration, or intensity; the cervix will fail to respond to uterine contractions by dilating and effacing; and the fetus will fail to descend.

Throughout labour, assess the client's fluid balance status. Check skin turgor and mucous membranes. Monitor intake and output. Also monitor the client's bladder for distention at least every 2 hours and encourage frequent emptying of the bladder. In addition, monitor bowel status. A full bladder or rectum can impede fetal descent.

Continue to monitor fetal well-being. If the fetus is in the breech position, be especially observant for visible cord prolapse and note any variable or prolonged decelerations in the heart rate. If either occurs, report it immediately.

Be prepared to administer a labour stimulant such as oxytocin if ordered to treat hypotonic labour contractions. Anticipate the need to assist with manipulations if shoulder dystocia is diagnosed. Prepare the client and family for the possibility of a caesarean birth if labour does not progress.

PROVIDING PHYSICAL AND EMOTIONAL COMFORT

Employ physical comfort measures to promote relaxation and reduce pain and stress. Offer blankets for warmth and a backrub, if the client wishes, to reduce muscle tension. Provide an environment conducive to rest so the client can conserve energy. Lower the lights and reduce external noise by closing the hallway door. Offer a warm shower or bath to promote relaxation (if not contraindicated). Use pillows to support the client in a comfortable position and encourage changing position every 30 minutes to reduce tension and to enhance uterine activity and efficiency. Offer fluids/food as appropriate to moisten the mouth and replenish energy (Fig. 21.2).

Assist with providing counter pressure in the lower back if the fetus is in the occiput posterior position. Encourage the client to assume different positions to promote fetal rotation. Upright positions are helpful in facilitating fetal rotation and descent. Also encourage the client to visualize the descent and birth of the fetus to promote focus and sense of self-efficacy.

Assess the client's level of pain and degree of distress. Administer analgesics as ordered after an informed decision-making discussion has occurred with the client. Evaluate the client's level of fatigue throughout labour, such as verbal expressions of feeling exhausted, inability to cope in early labour, or inability to rest between contractions. Praise the client and partner for their efforts. Provide empathetic listening to increase the client's coping ability and remain with the client to demonstrate caring and provide one-to-one professional support.

PROMOTING EMPOWERMENT

Educate the client and family about protracted labour and its causes and therapies. Explain therapeutic interventions

FIGURE 21.2 Continuous one-to-one labour support: The nurse provides support and comfort measures while monitoring the effects of dystocia on the labouring client and fetus.

that may be needed to assist with the labour process. Include the client and partner in the informed decision-making process about any proposed interventions.

Assist the client and partner in expressing their fears and anxieties. Provide encouragement to help them to maintain a sense of control and self-efficacy. Support the client and partner in their coping efforts. Keep the client and partner informed of progress and advocate for them. Provide continuous one-to-one professional supportive care to reduce interventions in labour and birth.

PRETERM LABOUR

Preterm labour is defined as the occurrence of regular uterine contractions accompanied by cervical effacement and dilation before the end of the 37th week of gestation. If not halted, it leads to preterm birth. Preterm births remain one of the biggest contributors to perinatal morbidity and mortality in the world and occur in approximately 8% of all births in Canada (Public Health Agency of Canada, 2013).

Preterm birth is one of the most common obstetric complications, and its sequelae have a profound effect on the survival and health of the newborn. Preterm births account for 75% of neurodevelopmental disorders and other serious morbidities, as well as behavioural and social problems. They account for 85% of all perinatal morbidity and mortality. In addition, up to $30 billion is spent on maternal and infant care related to prematurity annually in the United States (March of Dimes, 2018). Infants born prematurely also are at risk for serious sequelae such as respiratory distress syndrome, infections, congenital heart defects, thermoregulation problems that can lead to acidosis and weight loss, intraventricular hemorrhage, jaundice, hypoglycemia, feeding difficulties resulting from diminished stomach capacity and an underdeveloped suck reflex, and neurologic disorders related to hypoxia and trauma at birth. Many will face the prospect of numerous lifelong disabilities, such as cerebral palsy, intellectual impairment, vision defects, and hearing loss. A recent study's findings indicated that a single course of corticosteroids prenatally improved most neonates' neurodevelopmental outcomes if given before 34 weeks' gestation (Sotiriadis et al., 2015). Although great strides have been made in neonatal intensive care, prematurity remains the leading cause of death within the first month of life and is the second leading cause of all infant deaths (March of Dimes, 2018). The exact cause of preterm labour is not known. Currently, prevention is the goal.

Therapeutic Management

Predicting the likelihood of preterm birth is valuable to be able to use strategies that are likely to improve the situation. Many factors influence the decision to intervene when clients present with symptoms of preterm labour, including the probability of progressive labour, gestational age, and the risks of treatment. The Society of Obstetricians and Gynaecologist of Canada (SOGC) and ACOG recommends the following guidelines:

- There are no clear first-line **tocolytic** drugs (drugs that promote uterine relaxation by interfering with uterine contractions) to manage preterm labour, and the results of research on their efficacy are mixed. Clinical circumstances and the health care provider's preference should dictate treatment.
- Antibiotics do not appear to prolong gestation and should be reserved for group B streptococcal prophylaxis when birth is imminent.
- Tocolytic drugs may prolong pregnancy for 2 to 7 days; during this time, steroids can be given to improve fetal lung maturity and the client can be transported to a tertiary care centre.
- A single course of corticosteroids is recommended for all pregnant clients between 24 and 34 weeks of gestation who are at risk of preterm birth within 7 days. Prenatal corticosteroids significantly reduce the incidence and severity of neonatal respiratory distress syndrome.
- In 2011, intramuscular progesterone was approved for the prevention of preterm birth; however, more research is needed to provide evidence of the risks and benefits of this therapy (ACOG, 2014b; Skoll et al., 2018).

With these recommendations, health care providers continue to prescribe pharmacologic treatment for preterm labour. This treatment sometimes includes tocolytics and varying degrees of activity restriction. Antibiotics may also be prescribed to treat presumed or confirmed infections. Steroids may be given to enhance fetal lung maturity between 24 and 34 weeks' gestation. Magnesium sulphate may be given to minimize injury to the fetal brain. As evidence emerges, progesterone may be used to prevent preterm birth in clients identified as having risk factors (Jarde et al., 2017; Lim, Butt, & Crane, 2018).

Tocolytic Therapy

The decision to delay preterm birth is individualized based on risk factors, extent of cervical dilation, membrane status, fetal gestational age, and presence or absence of infection. Tocolytic therapy is most likely ordered if preterm labour occurs before the 34th week of gestation in an attempt to delay birth and thereby to reduce the severity of respiratory distress syndrome and other complications associated with prematurity. Tocolytic therapy does not typically prevent preterm birth, but it may delay it. It is contraindicated for abruptio placentae, acute fetal compromise or death, eclampsia or severe preeclampsia, active vaginal bleeding, dilation of more than 6 cm, chorioamnionitis, and hemodynamic instability (Locatelli, Consonni, & Ghidini, 2015).

Medications commonly used for tocolysis include indomethacin (a prostaglandin synthetase inhibitor), and nifedipine (a calcium channel blocker). (Evidence-Based Practice box 21.1). These drugs are used "off label," which means that they are effective for this purpose but have not been officially tested and developed for this purpose by Health Canada or the U.S. Food and Drug Administration (FDA) (Haas, Benjamin, Sawyer, & Quinney, 2014). In a Cochrane review study, calcium channel blockers were found to be better in preventing preterm labour when compared to beta-mimetics (Flenady et al., 2014). All of these medications have serious side effects, and the client requires close assessment and monitoring when they are being administered (Drug Guide 21.1).

Corticosteroids

Corticosteroids given to the client in preterm labour can help prevent or reduce the frequency and severity of respiratory distress syndrome in premature infants delivered between 24 and 34 weeks' gestation (Skoll et al., 2018). The beneficial effects of corticosteroids on fetal lung maturation have been reported within 48 hours of initial administration. A recent Cochrane review found that corticosteroids repeatedly administered to the client in preterm labour provided short-term benefits to the preterm infant of less respiratory distress and fewer serious health problems in the first few weeks after birth. They supported the use of repeat dose(s) of prenatal

EVIDENCE-BASED PRACTICE 21.1 BED REST IN SINGLETON PREGNANCIES FOR PREVENTING PRETERM BIRTH

STUDY

Preterm birth, defined a birth occurring prior to 37 weeks of gestation occurs in up to 10% of all pregnancies worldwide. Although there are many different therapies available for preventing preterm birth, very few are proven to be effective and recommended for clinical use. One therapy, bed rest, has been traditionally been recommended for preventing preterm birth as a first step in treatment. This therapy is based on the observation that hard work and hard physical activity during pregnancy could be associated with preterm birth, and with the idea that bed rest could reduce uterine activity. Bed rest does have adverse effects such as increasing the incidence of venous thrombosis, muscle atrophy, and cardiovascular deconditioning. The purpose of this study was to evaluate the effect of bed rest in the hospital or at home for preventing preterm birth.

Findings

Randomized, cluster-randomized and quasi-randomized control studies were sought. Two studies met the inclusion criteria with 1,266 women participating. There was no evidence found to support or refute the use of bed rest at home or in the hospital to prevent preterm birth. Due to the potential adverse effects that bed rest can have on women, it is suggested that health care providers discuss this intervention thoroughly with their clients. Additional research is needed.

Nursing Implications

Although the study did not reveal results that were statistically significant, nurses need to be aware of the potential benefits and limitations associated with bed rest employed to delay a preterm birth so that they can provide women and their families with the most appropriate information about options to prolonged pregnancy. Potential benefits and harms should be discussed with women facing an increased risk of preterm birth. Nurses can integrate evidence informed information from this study in their teaching about the risks associated with preterm labour and births. They can also use this information to help answer couple's questions about interventions currently used and their effectiveness as well as provide anticipatory guidance about the procedure. Doing so fosters empowerment of the client and family, promoting optimal informed decision making.

Adapted from Sosa, C. G., Althabe, F., Belizan, J. M., & Bergel, E. (2015). Bed rest in singleton pregnancies for preventing preterm birth. *Cochrane Database of Systematic Reviews, 30*(3), CD003581. doi: 10.1002/14651858.CD003581.pub3

corticosteroids for clients still at risk of preterm birth 7 days or more after an initial course. These benefits were associated with a small reduction in size at birth. The current available evidence reassuringly shows no significant harm in early childhood, although no benefit.

Further research is needed on the long-term benefits and risks for the client and baby (Cabbad, De Los Heros, Baltajian, & Robertazzi, 2015; Skoll et al., 2018). These drugs require at least 24 hours to become effective, so timely administration is crucial.

DRUG GUIDE 21.1 MEDICATIONS USED WITH PRETERM LABOUR

Drug	Action/Indication	Nursing Implications
Magnesium sulfate	Used for fetal neuroprotection, magnesium sulphate can reduce the risk of cerebral palsy in newborns delivered preterm and is recommended for labours less than 32 weeks Magnesium sulphate is also used in seizure prophylaxis and treatment of seizures in preeclamptic and eclamptic clients for almost 100 years	Administer IV with a loading dose of 4 g over 30 minutes initially, and then maintain infusion at 1 g/hr. Assess for signs for magnesium toxicity including vital signs and deep tendon reflexes (DTRs) hourly; report any hypotension or depressed or absent DTRs and reduced respiratory rate (<12/min). Monitor level of consciousness; report any headache, blurred vision, dizziness, or altered level of consciousness. Perform continuous electronic fetal monitoring; anticipate a reduction in FHR variability monitor for changes in baseline and presence of complicated variable or late decelerations. Monitor intake and output hourly; report any decrease in output (<30 mL/hr). Monitor for common side effects, including flushing, nausea and vomiting, dry mouth, lethargy, blurred vision, and headache. Have calcium gluconate readily available at the bedside to reverse magnesium toxicity.

(continued)

DRUG GUIDE 21.1 MEDICATIONS USED WITH PRETERM LABOUR (continued)

Drug	Action/Indication	Nursing Implications
Indomethacin (Indocin)	Inhibits prostaglandin synthesis (stimulates contractions), therefore reduces uterine activity to delay or arrest preterm labour	Continuously assess vital signs, uterine activity, and FHR. Administer oral form with food to reduce GI irritation. Do not give to individuals with peptic ulcer disease. Schedule ultrasound to assess amniotic fluid volume and function of ductus arteriosus before initiating therapy; monitor for signs of hemorrhage. Be alert for adverse effects such as nausea and vomiting, heartburn, rash, prolonged bleeding time, oligohydramnios, and hypertension. Monitor for neonatal adverse effects, including constriction of ductus arteriosus, premature ductus closure, necrotizing enterocolitis, oligohydramnios, and pulmonary hypertension. Contraindicated in >32 weeks' gestations, fetal growth restriction, history of asthma, urticaria, or allergic type reactions to aspirin or NSAIDs.
Nifedipine	Blocks calcium movement into muscle cells, inhibits uterine activity to reduce or arrest preterm labour	Use caution if giving this drug with magnesium sulphate because of increased risk for hypotension. Monitor blood pressure hourly if giving with magnesium sulphate; report a pulse rate >110 bpm. Monitor for fetal effects such as decreased uteroplacental blood flow manifested by fetal bradycardia, which can lead to fetal hypoxia. Monitor for adverse effects, such as flushing of the skin, headache, transient tachycardia, palpitations, postural hypotension, peripheral edema, and transient fetal tachycardia. Contraindicated in those with cardiovascular disease or hemodynamic instability.
Betamethasone (Celestone)	Promotes fetal lung maturity by stimulating surfactant production; prevents or reduces risk of respiratory distress syndrome and intraventricular hemorrhage in the preterm neonate less than 34 weeks' gestation	Administer two doses intramuscularly 24 hours apart. Monitor for signs of infection or pulmonary edema. Educate parents about potential benefits of drug to preterm infant. Counsel the diabetic patient that blood glucose levels may be transiently elevated.

Adapted from Chandrasekaran, S., & Srinivas, S. K. (2014). Antenatal corticosteroid administration: Understanding its use as an obstetric quality metric. *American Journal of Obstetrics and Gynecology, 210*(2), 143–150; Jørgensen, J. S., Weile, L. K. K., & Lamont, R. F. (2014). Preterm labour: Current tocolytic options for the treatment of preterm labour. *Expert Opinion on Pharmacotherapy, 15*(5), 585–588; King, T.L., Brucker, M.C., Osborne, K., & Jevitt, C.M. (2019). *Varney's midwifery* (6th ed.). Burlington, MA: Jones & Bartlett Learning. Magee, L., Sawchuk, D., Synnes, A. & von Dadelszen, P. (2011) SOGC Clinical practice guideline: Magnesium sulphate for fetal neuroprotection. *JOGC, 33*(5), 516–519.

Nursing Assessment

The preterm birth rate cannot be reduced until there are ways to predict the risk for preterm birth and impede the progress of preterm labour. Because the etiology is often multifactorial, an individualized approach is needed.

Health History and Physical Examination

The signs of preterm labour are subtle and may be overlooked by the client as well as the health care provider. Obtain a thorough health history and be alert for risk factors associated with preterm labour and birth (Box 21.2).

Frequently, clients are unaware that uterine contractions, effacement, and dilation are occurring, thus making early intervention ineffective in arresting preterm labour and preventing the birth of a premature newborn. Ask the client about any complaints, being alert for the subtle symptoms of preterm labour, which may include:

RISK FACTORS ASSOCIATED WITH PRETERM LABOUR AND BIRTH

- Childbearing in age extremes (<16 years and >40 years old)
- Low socioeconomic status
- Alcohol or other drug use, especially cocaine
- Poor nutrition
- Periodontal disease
- Cigarette smoking
- Low level of education
- History of prior preterm birth (triples the risk)
- Uterine abnormalities, such as fibroids
- Low pregnancy weight for height
- Pre-existing diabetes or hypertension
- Multiple pregnancy
- Premature rupture of membranes
- Late or no prenatal care
- Short cervical length
- Sexually transmitted infections: gonorrhea, chlamydia, trichomoniasis
- Bacterial vaginosis (50% increased risk)
- Chorioamnionitis
- Hydramnios
- Gestational hypertension
- Cervical insufficiency
- Short interpregnancy interval (<1 year between births)
- Placental problems, such as placenta praevia and abruption placenta
- Anemia
- Urinary tract infection
- Domestic violence
- Stress, acute and chronic

Adapted from March of Dimes. (2018). *Preterm labour and premature birth.* Retrieved from https://www.marchofdimes.org/complications/preterm-labor-and-premature-baby.aspx

- Change or increase in vaginal discharge with mucus, water, or blood in it
- Pelvic pressure (pushing-down sensation)
- Low, dull backache
- Menstrual-like cramps
- Urinary tract infection symptoms
- Feeling of pelvic pressure or fullness
- Gastrointestinal upset: nausea, vomiting, and diarrhea
- General sense of discomfort or unease
- Heaviness or aching in the thighs
- Uterine contractions, with or without pain
- More than six contractions per hour
- Intestinal cramping, with or without diarrhea (Jordan et al., 2014).

Assess the pattern of the contractions. Evaluate cervical dilation and effacement: cervical effacement is 80% or greater and cervical dilation is greater than 1 cm (ACOG, 2014b). On examination, engagement of the fetal presenting part will be noted.

Laboratory and Diagnostic Testing

Commonly used diagnostic testing for preterm labour risk assessment includes a complete blood count to detect infection, which may be a contributing factor to preterm labour, and urinalysis to detect bacteria and nitrites, which are indicative of a urinary tract infection. Other tests that may be used for preterm labour prediction include fetal fibronectin testing and cervical length evaluation by transvaginal ultrasound. Fetal fibronectin and cervical length examinations have a high negative predictive value and are thus better at predicting which pregnant clients are unlikely to have a preterm birth as opposed to predicting those who will (van Baaren et al., 2015). Ultrasonographic cervical length assessment and fetal fibronectin testing appear to be similar in predictive ability, and the combination of both is needed in this area (Lim et al., 2018).

FETAL FIBRONECTIN

Fetal fibronectin, a glycoprotein produced by the chorion, is found at the junction of the chorion and decidua (fetal membranes and uterus). It acts as biologic glue, attaching the fetal sac to the uterine lining. It normally is present in cervicovaginal secretions up to 22 weeks of pregnancy and again at the end of the last trimester (1 to 3 weeks before labour). It usually cannot be detected between 24 and 34 weeks of pregnancy (5½ to 8½ months) unless there has been a disruption between the chorion and deciduas. It is present in cervicovaginal fluid prior to delivery, regardless of gestational age.

The test is a useful marker for impending membrane rupture within 7 to 14 days if the level increases to greater than 0.05 mcg/mL. The accuracy of fetal fibronectin is decreased in the presence of lubricants, blood, recent intercourse, or cervical manipulation within the previous 24 hours. Conversely, a negative fetal fibronectin test is a strong predictor that preterm labour in the next 2 weeks is unlikely (Abbott et al., 2015).

A sterile applicator is used to collect a cervicovaginal sample during an examination by speculum. The result is either positive (fetal fibronectin is present) or negative (fetal fibronectin is not present). Interpretation of fetal fibronectin results must always be viewed in conjunction with the clinical findings; it is not used as a lone indicator for predicting preterm labour. The primary importance of cervicovaginal fetal fibronectin lies in the high negative predictive values of the test for reducing preterm birth risk. Fibronectin testing can be a useful tool in the triaging of clients symptomatic for preterm labour, particularly in low-risk level of care settings in remote areas.

CERVICAL LENGTH MEASUREMENT

Transvaginal ultrasound of the cervix has been used as a tool to predict preterm labour in high-risk pregnancies and to differentiate between true and false preterm labour. Three parameters are evaluated during the transvaginal ultrasound: cervical length and width and funnelling. Measurement of the closed portion of the cervix visualized during the transvaginal ultrasound is the single most reliable parameter for prediction of preterm delivery in high-risk clients (van Baaren et al., 2014).

Cervical length varies during pregnancy and can be measured fairly reliably after 16 weeks' gestation using an ultrasound probe inserted in the vagina. A cervical length of 3 cm or more indicates that birth within 14 days is unlikely. Clients with a short cervical length of 2.5 cm during the midtrimester have a substantially greater risk of preterm birth prior to 35 weeks' gestation. As with fetal fibronectin testing, negative results can be reassuring and prevent unnecessary interventions (Souka, Papastefanou, Papadopoulos, Chrelias, & Kassanos, 2015).

Nursing Management

Nurses play a key role in reducing preterm labour and births to improve pregnancy outcomes for both birthing parents and their infants. Early detection of preterm labour is currently the best strategy to improve outcomes. Because of the numerous factors associated with preterm labour, it is challenging to identify and address all of them, especially when clients experiencing contractions are frequently falsely reassured and not assessed thoroughly to determine the cause. This delay impedes initiation of interventions to reduce infant death and morbidity.

Preterm birth prevention programs for clients at high risk have used self-monitoring of symptoms and patterns, weekly cervical examinations, clinical markers, telephone monitoring, home visiting, alone or in combination, with disappointing results. Preterm labour is currently thought to be a chronic, long-term multifactorial process with a genetic component. A recent study found a multiple pregnancy, prior preterm birth, low socioeconomic status, medical disorders, and infections were statistically significant risk factors for predicting spontaneous preterm labour (Patel, Pitre, & Bhooker, 2015). Despite technologic and pharmacologic advances in the identification and treatment of preterm labour, the incidence remains high.

Supportive nursing care is needed for the client in preterm labour. Nursing care includes monitoring vital signs, measuring intake and output, encouraging bed rest on the client's left side to enhance placental perfusion, monitoring the FHR via an external monitor continuously, limiting vaginal examinations to prevent an ascending infection, and monitoring the client and fetus closely for any adverse effects from the tocolytic agents. Offering the couple ongoing explanations will help prepare them for the birth.

Administering Tocolytic Therapy

Tocolysis is the use of drugs to inhibit uterine contractions. The primary goals of tocolytic therapy are to arrest labour and delay birth long enough to initiate prophylactic corticosteroid therapy when indicated for stimulation of fetal lung maturity and to arrange for transfer to a perinatal tertiary care hospital. A firm diagnosis of preterm labour is necessary before treatment is considered. Diagnosis requires the presence of both uterine contractions and cervical change (or an initial cervical examination of more than 2 cm and/or more than 80% effacement in a nulliparous client). A cause for preterm labour should always be sought.

Absolute contraindications to administering tocolytic agents to stop labour include intrauterine infection, active hemorrhage, fetal compromise, fetus before viability, fetal abnormality incompatible with life, fetal growth restriction, severe preeclampsia, heart disease, prolonged premature rupture of the membranes (PPROM), and intrauterine demise (Callahan, 2016). Bed rest and hydration are commonly recommended, but without proven efficacy.

Magnesium sulphate has been used in the past as a tocolytic. In the absence of evidence that it is effective, this practice has been largely abandoned in Canada. More commonly, magnesium sulphate is administered in preterm labour to protect the fetal brain or in clients who develop preeclampsia or eclampsia. This agent acts as a physiologic calcium antagonist and a general inhibitor of neurotransmission. Expect to administer it intravenously. Monitor the client for nausea, vomiting, headache, weakness, hypotension, and respiratory depression. Frequent monitoring of respiratory effort and deep tendon reflexes is essential for early recognition of toxicity. Because magnesium is exclusively excreted by the kidneys, adequate renal function is essential for safe administration. Assess the fetus for decreased FHR variability, drowsiness, and hypotonia. Magnesium has a wide margin of safety but is not any more effective in delaying preterm birth than any other tocolytic agent.

Calcium channel blockers promote uterine relaxation by decreasing the influx of calcium ions into myometrium cells to inhibit contractions. Although calcium channel blockers may be prescribed to manage preterm labour, available literature provides little evidence that they have better efficacy in treating preterm labour than other tocolytic agents. Administer calcium channel blockers (nifedipine) orally or sublingually every 4 to 8 hours as ordered. Monitor the client for hypotension, reflex tachycardia, headache, nausea, and facial flushing.

Prostaglandin synthetase inhibitor (indomethacin) reduces prostaglandin synthesis from decidual macrophages. It readily crosses the placenta and can cause oligohydramnios due to a decrease in fetal renal blood flow if used for more than 48 hours. During treatment, urine output, temperature, and amniotic fluid index

(AFI) should be evaluated periodically. The initial recommended dose is 50 to 100 mg orally or per rectum followed by 25 to 50 mg every 6 hours for 8 doses. Indomethacin therapy is not recommended for gestations of 32 weeks or greater (Ross, 2018).

Educating the Client

Ensure that every pregnant client receives basic education about preterm labour, including information about harmful actions, the signs of genitourinary infections and preterm labour, and the appropriate response to these symptoms. Teach the client how to palpate for and time uterine contractions. Provide written materials to support this education at a level and in a language appropriate for the client. Also educate clients about the importance of prenatal care, risk reduction, and recognizing the signs and symptoms of preterm labour. Teaching Guidelines 21.1 highlights important instructions related to preventing preterm labour.

Teaching Guidelines 21.1
TEACHING TO PREVENT PRETERM LABOUR

We don't really know why some pregnancies are complicated by premature labour, and others are not. We do know that about half of all premature labours begin for unknown reasons, in pregnancies which were otherwise normal. However, we do know that some risks increase the chance of going into early labour.

Research has shown that the more people know about the signs and risks of premature labour, the lower the rate of premature births. Your choices and actions during the pregnancy can help you carry your baby longer, and give your baby the best start possible. The following are things which you can do in an effort to try to prevent your baby from being born too soon.

Quit smoking: Try to understand why you smoke, and seek help to learn other ways of dealing with these issues. Ask around in your community about "Quit Smoking" programs. Ask your care provider about programs to help you quit.

Eat properly: Talk to a registered dietitian about your eating habits. Plan your meals around the basic food groups and avoid junk food. Drink plenty of milk.

Get help if you need it: You have a right to feel safe. If you are being abused, call your local women's shelter and ask where you can go for help.

Get plenty of rest: Plan ahead to be sure a certain part of your day will be set aside for you to rest. Don't feel guilty for resting. It is very important during pregnancy.

Learn ways to reduce stress: Talk to people you trust about how you feel. Learn relaxation techniques such as meditation and self-massage to reduce your stress. Consider yoga.

Avoid strenuous work

Avoid overexertion when exercising during pregnancy: Even though you are physically fit, it is important not to increase your workout intensity during certain times of your pregnancy.

Learn to recognize the signs of premature labour: Prenatal classes through your hospital or community are an excellent way to learn. Talk to your primary care provider.

Learn the steps to take if you think you are in premature labour: Talk to your care provider about what you should do. Write down the phone numbers to call and what to do if you go into premature labour.

Visit your doctor or midwife regularly during pregnancy: This is one of the most important things you can do to prevent premature labour because it gives your care provider a chance to find or prevent problems, which may cause your baby to be born early.

Adapted from Society of Obstetricians and Gynaecologists of Canada (SOGC). (2018). *Preterm labour.* Retrieved from http://pregnancy.sogc.org/other-considerations/preterm-labour/

Explaining to the couple what is happening in terms of labour progress, the treatment regimen, and the status of the fetus is important to reduce the anxiety associated with the risk of giving birth to a preterm infant. Advocate for a consultation with a pediatrician or neonatologist prior to birth to discuss the developmental stage of the fetus and the expectation of needs and care post birth. Educate them about the importance of promotion of fetal lung maturity with corticosteroids. Include supportive family members in all education. Allow time for the client and family to express their concerns about the possible outcome for the infant. Encourage them to express any feelings of apprehension, fear, anxiety, uncertainty, and anger they may experience. Provide the client and family with an honest appraisal of the situation and plan of treatment throughout the birthing experience.

Providing Psychological Support

Preterm labour and birth present multifactorial challenges for everyone involved. If the client's activities are restricted, additional stresses may be placed on the family, contributing to the crisis. Assess the stress levels of the client and family, and make appropriate referrals. Emphasize the need for more frequent supervision and office visits, and encourage clients to talk to their health care provider for reassurance.

Every case of spontaneous preterm labour is unique. Care must take into account the clinical circumstances, and the full and informed consent of the client and partner is needed. Half of all those who ultimately give birth prematurely have no identifiable risk factors. Nurses should be sensitive to any complaint and should provide

TABLE 21.2	BISHOP SCORING SYSTEM		
		Score	
Factor	0	1	2
Dilatation (cm)	0	1–2	3–4
Effacement (%)	0–30	40–50	60–70
Length (cm)	>3	1–3	<1
Consistency	Firm	Medium	Soft
Position	Posterior	Mid	Anterior
Station	−3 or above	−2	−1 or 0

From Leduc, D., Biringer, A., Lee, L., & Dy, J. (2013). SOGC Clinical practice guideline No. 296, Induction of labour. *Journal of Obstetrics and Gynaecology Canada*. Retrieved from https://sogc.org/wp-content/uploads/2013/08/September2013-CPG296-ENG-Online_REV-D.pdf

fetal lie, prolapsed umbilical cord, a prior classic uterine incision that entered the uterine cavity, pelvic structure abnormality, previous myomectomy, vaginal bleeding with unknown cause, invasive cervical cancer, active genital herpes infection, and abnormal FHR patterns (Cunningham et al., 2014). In general, labour induction is indicated when the benefits of birth outweigh the risks to the pregnant client or fetus for continuing the pregnancy. However, the balance between risk and benefit remains controversial.

Take Note!

Before labour induction is started, fetal maturity (dating, ultrasound) and cervical readiness (vaginal examination, Bishop scoring; Table 21.2) must be assessed. Both need to be favourable for a successful induction.

Therapeutic Management

The decision to induce labour is based on a thorough evaluation of the client and fetal status. Typically, this includes an early ultrasound to confirm gestational age; ultrasound to evaluate fetal size, position, and to locate the placenta; engaged presenting fetal part; a nonstress test to evaluate fetal well-being; complete blood count and urinalysis to rule out infection; and a vaginal examination to evaluate the cervix for readiness (Kriebs, 2015).

Cervical Ripening

Cervical ripening is a process by which the cervix softens via the breakdown of collagen fibrils. It is the first step in the process of cervical effacement and dilation so that, on average, the cervix is approximately 50% effaced and 2 cm dilated at the onset of labour, although wide differences do exist. There has been increasing awareness that if the cervix is unfavourable or unripe, a successful vaginal birth is less likely. Cervical ripeness is

an important variable when labour induction is being considered. A ripe cervix is shortened, centred (anterior), softened, and partially dilated. An unripe cervix is long, closed, posterior, and firm. Cervical ripening usually begins prior to the onset of labour contractions and is necessary for cervical dilation.

Various scoring systems to assess cervical ripeness have been introduced, but the Bishop score is most commonly used today. The Bishop score helps identify clients who would be most likely to achieve a successful induction (Table 21.2). The duration of labour is inversely correlated with the Bishop score: a score over 8 indicates a successful vaginal birth. Bishop scores of less than 6 usually indicate that a cervical ripening method should be used prior to induction (Goldberg, 2018). Medical induction of labour has two components: cervical ripening and induction of contractions. When induction of labour is indicated, cervical readiness for labour is evaluated by pelvic examination and determination of a Bishop score is documented.

COMPLEMENTARY AND ALTERNATIVE MEDICINE METHODS

Alternative or complimentary methods for cervical ripening are less frequently used today, but nurses need to be aware of them and question clients about their use. Methods may include herbal agents such as evening primrose oil, black haw, black and blue cohosh, and red raspberry leaves. In addition, castor oil, hot baths, and enemas are used for cervical ripening and labour induction. The risks and benefits of these agents are unknown. Few have been evaluated scientifically, and thus, none can be recommended regarding their efficacy or safety.

Other nonpharmacologic methods suggested for labour induction include sexual intercourse or breast stimulation. Breast stimulation promotes the release of oxytocin, which stimulates uterine contractions. In addition, human semen is a biologic source of prostaglandins used for cervical ripening. According to a Cochrane review, sexual intercourse with breast stimulation would appear beneficial, but safety issues have not been fully evaluated, nor can this activity be standardized. It appears to shorten the latent phase of labour (King et al., 2019). Its use as a method for labour induction is not validated by research and if used should follow an established protocol for breast stimulation methods and assessment of fetal well-being.

MECHANICAL METHODS

Mechanical methods are used to open the cervix and stimulate the progression of labour. All share a similar mechanism of action: application of local pressure stimulates the release of prostaglandins to ripen the cervix. Potential advantages of mechanical methods, compared with pharmacologic methods, may include simplicity or preservation of the cervical tissue or structure, lower cost, and fewer side effects. The risks associated with these methods include infection, bleeding, membrane rupture, and placental disruption (Sciscione, 2014). For example, an indwelling (Foley) catheter (e.g., 26 French) can be inserted into the endocervical canal to ripen and dilate the cervix. The catheter is placed in the uterus, and the balloon is filled. Direct pressure is then applied to the lower segment of the uterus and the cervix. This direct pressure causes stress in the lower uterine segment and probably the local production of prostaglandins. The risks, benefits, and expected side effects should be explained to the client prior to the insertion of the balloon catheter (Fuks, Robinson, Rothschild, Akinnawonu, & Salafia, 2015).

Hygroscopic dilators absorb endocervical and local tissue fluids; as they enlarge, they expand the endocervix and provide controlled mechanical pressure. Laminaria, a type of dried seaweed, is an example of a hygroscopic dilator. Hygroscopic dilators are advantageous because they can be inserted on an outpatient basis and no fetal monitoring is needed. They are inserted in the cervix and expand over 12 to 24 hours as they absorb water. They are a reliable alternative when prostaglandins are contraindicated or unavailable (Goldberg, 2018). Recently there has been a reduction in the use of hygroscopic and osmotic dilators for the induction of labour in favour of pharmacologic agents. The increased risk of infections with hygroscopic and osmotic dilators when compared with that associated with the use of other pharmacologic agents and the ease of pharmacologic administration may be reasons for the decline. Placement of dilators also requires additional training and may be associated with rupture of membranes, vaginal bleeding, and client discomfort or pain (Drunecký et al., 2015).

SURGICAL METHODS

Surgical methods used to ripen the cervix and induce labour include stripping of the membranes and performing an amniotomy. Stripping of the membranes is accomplished by inserting a finger through the internal cervical os and moving it in a circular direction. This motion causes the membranes to detach. Manual separation of the amniotic membranes from the cervix is thought to induce cervical ripening and the onset of labour (Afzal, Asif, & Miraj, 2015). Stripping (or sweeping of the membranes is recommended beginning at 38 weeks to reduce the likelihood of induction of labour (Delaney & Roggensack, 2017). An amniotomy involves inserting a cervical hook (Amnihook) through the dilated cervical os to deliberately rupture the membranes. This promotes pressure of the presenting part on the cervix and stimulates an increase in the activity of prostaglandins locally. Risks associated with these procedures include umbilical cord prolapse or compression, infection, FHR deceleration, bleeding, and client discomfort (King et al., 2019).

When either of these techniques is used, amniotic fluid characteristics (such as whether it is clear or bloody, or meconium is present) and fetal status must be monitored closely.

PHARMACOLOGIC METHODS

The use of pharmacologic agents has revolutionized cervical ripening. The use of prostaglandins to attain cervical ripening has been found to be highly effective in producing cervical changes independent of uterine contractions (Grobman, 2015). In some cases, clients will go into labour and require no additional stimulants for induction. Induction of labour with prostaglandins offers the advantage of promoting both cervical ripening and uterine contractility. A drawback of prostaglandins is their ability to induce excessive uterine contractions, which can increase perinatal morbidity (Callahan, 2016). Prostaglandin analogues commonly used for cervical ripening include dinoprostone gel (Prepidil), dinoprostone inserts (Cervidil), and misoprostol (Cytotec). Misoprostol (Cytotec), a synthetic PGE1 analogue, is a gastric cytoprotective agent used in the treatment and prevention of peptic ulcers. It can be administered intravaginally or orally to ripen the cervix or induce labour. It is available in 100 mcg or 200 mcg tablets, but doses of 25 to 50 mcg are typically used. It is important to note that only dinoprostone is approved by Health Canada for use as a cervical ripening agent, although ACOG acknowledges the apparent safety and effectiveness of misoprostol for this purpose (King et al., 2019). Misoprostol is most commonly used in Canada for induction of labour in a fetal demise in early pregnancy, and management of postpartum hemorrhage since hyperstimulation of the uterus, with marked impairment of uteroplacental blood flow, uterine rupture, or amniotic fluid embolism are documented risks in full-term induction with misoprostol (Ahmed, Garba, Nafi'ah, & Yakasai, 2015). Furthermore, it is contraindicated for clients with prior uterine scars and therefore should not be used for cervical ripening in

DRUG GUIDE 21.2 DRUGS USED FOR CERVICAL RIPENING AND LABOUR INDUCTION

Drug	Action/Indication	Nursing Implications
Dinoprostone (Cervidil insert; Prepidil gel)	Directly softens and dilates the cervix/to ripen cervix and induce labour	Provide emotional support. Administer pain medications as needed. Frequently assess degree of effacement and dilation. Monitor uterine contractions for frequency, duration, intensity, and resting tone. Assess FHR pattern frequently. Monitor client for possible adverse effects such as headache, nausea and vomiting, and diarrhea.
Oxytocin	Acts on uterine myofibrils to contract/to initiate or augment labour	Administer as an IV infusion via pump, increasing dose based on protocol until adequate labour progress is achieved. Assess baseline vital signs and FHR and then frequently after initiating oxytocin infusion. Determine frequency, duration, intensity and resting tone of contractions frequently. Notify health care provider of any uterine hypertonicity or atypical or abnormal FHR patterns. Maintain I&O, being alert for water intoxication. Keep client informed of labour progress. Monitor for possible adverse effects such as hyperstimulation of the uterus, impaired uterine blood flow leading to fetal hypoxia, rapid labour leading to cervical lacerations or uterine rupture, water intoxication (if oxytocin is given in electrolyte-free solution or at a rate exceeding 20 mU/min), and hypotension.

Adapted from Goldberg, A. E. (2018). Cervical ripening. *eMedicine*. Retrieved from http://emedicine.medscape.com/article/263311-overview#aw2aab6b7; King, T. L., Brucker, M. C., Osborne, K., & Jevitt, C. M. (2019). *Varney's midwifery* (6th ed.). Burlington, MA: Jones & Bartlett Learning; and Goetzl, L. (2014). Methods of cervical ripening and labor induction: Pharmacologic. *Clinical Obstetrics and Gynecology, 57*(2), 377–390; Liston, R., Sawchuk, D. & Young, D. (2018). SOGC Clinical practice guideline: No. 197b-Fetal Health Surveillance: Intrapartum Consensus Guideline. *Journal of Obstetrics and Gynaecology Canada, 40*(4), e298–e322.

those attempting a vaginal birth after caesarean (VBAC). See Drug Guide 21.2 for additional information.

Oxytocin

Oxytocin is a potent endogenous uterotonic agent used for both induction and augmentation of labour. It is produced naturally by the posterior pituitary gland and stimulates contractions of the uterus. For clients with low Bishop scores, cervical ripening is typically initiated before oxytocin is used to increase the likelihood of successful induction. Once the cervix is ripe, oxytocin is the most popular pharmacologic agent used for inducing or augmenting labour.

Response to oxytocin varies widely: some people are very sensitive to even small amounts. The most common adverse effect of oxytocin is uterine hyperstimulation, leading to impaired oxygenation and fetal compromise (King et al., 2019). The response of the uterus to the drug is closely monitored throughout labour so that the oxytocin infusion can be titrated appropriately. In addition,

oxytocin has an antidiuretic effect, resulting in decreased urine flow that may lead to water intoxication. Symptoms to watch for include headache and vomiting.

Oxytocin is administered via an intravenous infusion pump piggybacked into the main intravenous line at the port most proximal to the insertion site. Typically, 10 or 20 units of oxytocin is added to 1 L of isotonic solution depending on unit protocols. The dose is titrated according to protocol to achieve stable contractions every 2 to 3 minutes lasting 60 seconds. Recent studies suggest that a conservative oxytocin protocol with lower doses reduces the number of neonatal intensive care unit admissions and lower caesarean sections (Lewis et al., 2014; Manjula, Bagga, Kalra, & Dutta, 2015).

The uterus should relax between contractions. If the resting uterine tone remains above 20 mm Hg, uteroplacental insufficiency and fetal hypoxia can result. This underscores the importance of continuous FHR monitoring. Unfortunately, neither the optimal oxytocin administration regimen nor the maximum oxytocin dose has been established or agreed upon through research or

FIGURE 21.3 The nurse monitors an intravenous infusion of oxytocin being administered to a woman in labour who is being induced. (From Lippincott Professional Development, September 2014.)

expert opinion. Nurses assisting with labour inductions need to become familiar with their hospital protocols concerning dosage, infusion rates, frequency of change, assessments, and processes related to decreasing or turning off the infusion in the presence of atypical or abnormal FHR monitoring.

Oxytocin has many advantages: it is potent and easy to titrate, it has a short half-life (1 to 5 minutes), and it is generally well tolerated. Induction using oxytocin has side effects (water intoxication, hypotension, and uterine hypertonicity), but because the drug does not cross the placental barrier, no direct fetal problems have been observed (Arrowsmith & Wray, 2014) (Fig. 21.3).

> **Remember Jennifer, the young woman described at the beginning of the chapter? After her cervix is ripened, an oxytocin infusion is started and her progress is slow. What encouragement can the nurse offer? After a few hours, her contractions begin to increase in intensity and frequency. What typical pain management measures can the nurse implement, and how would the nurse evaluate the effectiveness of these measures?**

Nursing Assessment

Nursing assessment of the client who is undergoing labour induction or augmentation involves a thorough history and physical examination. Review the client's history for relative indications for induction or augmentation, such as diabetes, hypertension, postterm status, dysfunctional labour pattern, prolonged ruptured

membranes, and infection, and for contraindications such as placenta praevia, overdistended uterus, active genital herpes, fetopelvic disproportion, fetal malposition, or fetal compromise.

Assist with determining the gestational age of the fetus to prevent a preterm birth. Assess fetal well-being to validate the client's and fetus' ability to withstand labour contractions. Evaluate the client's cervical status, including cervical dilation and effacement, and station via vaginal examination as appropriate before cervical ripening or induction is started. Determine the Bishop score to determine the probable success of induction.

 Take Note!

Nurses working with clients in labour play an important role acting as the eyes and ears for the birth attendant because they remain at the client's bedside throughout the entire experience. Close, frequent assessment and follow-up interventions are essential to ensure the safety of the client and the unborn child during cervical ripening and labour induction or augmentation.

Nursing Management

Explain to the client and partner about the induction or augmentation procedure clearly, using simple terms (Teaching Guidelines 21.2). Ensure that an informed consent has been obtained after the client and partner have received complete information about the procedure, including its advantages, disadvantages, alternatives, and potential risks. Ensure that the Bishop score has been determined before proceeding. Nursing Care Plan 21.1 (at the end of the chapter) presents an overview of the nursing care for a client undergoing labour induction.

> Teaching Guidelines 21.2
> ### TEACHING IN PREPARATION FOR LABOUR INDUCTION
> • Your health care provider may recommend that you have your labour induced. This may be necessary for a variety of reasons, such as elevated blood pressure, a medical condition, prolonged pregnancy over 41 weeks, or problems with fetal heart rate patterns or fetal growth.
> • Your health care provider may use one or more methods to induce labour, such as stripping the membranes, breaking the amniotic sac to release the fluid, administering medication close to or in the cervix to soften it, or administering a medication called oxytocin to stimulate contractions.
> • Labour induction is associated with some risks and disadvantages, such as overactivity of the uterus; nausea, vomiting, or diarrhea; and changes in fetal heart rate.

- Prior to inducing your labour, your health care provider may perform a procedure to ripen your cervix to increase the likelihood of a successful induction. Medication may be placed around your cervix to make it thinner and softer.
- During the induction, your contractions may feel stronger than normal. However, the length of your labour may be reduced with induction.
- Medications for pain relief and comfort measures will be readily available.
- Health care team members will be present throughout labour.

Administering Oxytocin

If not already done, prepare the oxytocin infusion by diluting 10 units of oxytocin in 1,000 mL of lactated Ringer solution or ordered isotonic solution (or per unit protocol). Use an infusion pump on a secondary line connected to the primary infusion at the most proximal site. Start the oxytocin infusion in mU/min as ordered. Each hospital has its own standards/protocols for oxytocin infusion and dilution. The nurse needs to follow that procedure when administering this medication. Maintain the rate once the desired contraction frequency has been reached. To ensure adequate surveillance and support during induction or augmentation, the nurse-to-client ratio should not exceed 1:1 (Liston et al., 2018).

During induction or augmentation, monitoring of the client and fetal status is essential. Apply an external electronic fetal monitor or assist with placement of an internal device. Obtain vital signs and assess the electronic FHR tracing every 15 to 30 minutes during the first stage. Evaluate the contractions (frequency, duration, and intensity) and resting tone, and adjust the oxytocin infusion rate accordingly. Monitor the FHR, including baseline rate, baseline variability, and accelerations and decelerations, to determine whether the oxytocin rate needs adjustment. Discontinue the oxytocin and notify the birth attendant if uterine hyperstimulation or atypical/abnormal FHR pattern occurs (Liston et al., 2018). Perform or assist with periodic vaginal examinations to determine cervical dilation and fetal descent: cervical dilation of 1 cm per hour typically indicates satisfactory progress. Continue to monitor the FHR continuously and document it every 15 to 30 minutes during the active phase of labour and every 5 minutes during the second stage. Assist with pushing efforts during the second stage. Measure and record intake and output to prevent excess fluid volume. Encourage the client to urinate every 2 hours to prevent soft tissue obstruction.

Providing Pain Relief and Support

As recommended by the SOGC Clinical Practice Guideline for intrapartum Fetal Surveillance, clients in active labour should receive continuous close support from an appropriately trained person. A systematic review of 15 randomized controlled trials found that continuous labour support was associated with reduced use of intrapartum pain medication, reduced use of regional analgesia/anaesthesia, decreased operative vaginal deliveries, decreased caesarean births, increased spontaneous vaginal births, and reduced likelihood of reports of negative experiences (Liston et al., 2018).

Ask the client frequently to rate any pain and provide pain management as needed. Offer position changes and other nonpharmacologic measures. Note the reaction to any medication given and document its effect. Monitor the need for comfort measures as contractions increase.

Throughout induction and augmentation, frequently reassure the client and partner about the fetal status and labour progress. Provide them with frequent updates on the condition of the client and the fetus. Assess the client's ability to cope with stronger contractions and follow protocols of the hospital about how frequent pain assessments are performed for each phase and stage of labour (Nagtalon-Ramos, 2014). Provide support and encouragement as indicated.

After a very long day, Jennifer gives birth to a healthy baby boy with Apgar scores of 9 at 1 minute and 10 at 5 minutes. When transferring her to the postpartum unit, what information is essential to include for the accepting nurse? What specific nursing information should be given to the nursery nurse regarding the labour experience? With such a lengthy labour, what assessments might the postpartum nurse need to focus on for the first few hours after birth?

VAGINAL BIRTH AFTER CAESAREAN

Vaginal birth after caesarean (VBAC) describes a client who gives birth vaginally after having at least one previous caesarean birth. Despite evidence that most clients who have had a caesarean birth are candidates for vaginal birth, many clients who have had a caesarean birth once undergo another for subsequent pregnancies. In Canada, the rate of repeat caesarean sections has risen significantly, from 64% in 1996, to 81% in 2016 (Public Health Agency of Canada, 2018).

The SOGC published clinical practice guidelines pertaining to VBAC in 1995 and reaffirmed those guidelines in 2018. The first recommendation is that: "Provided there are no contraindications, a woman with 1 previous transverse low-segment Caesarean section should be offered a TOL with appropriate discussion of maternal and perinatal risks and benefits. The process of informed consent with appropriate documentation should be an important part of the birth plan in a woman with a previous caesarean section" (Martel & MacKinnon, 2018, p. 3195).

Contraindications to VBAC include a prior classic uterine incision, prior transfundal uterine surgery (myomectomy), uterine scar other than low-transverse caesarean scar, contracted pelvis, previous uterine rupture, other contraindications to vaginal birth such as placenta praevia or malpresentation, inadequate staff or facility to provide an emergency caesarean if one is indicated, and consent not received for TOL with client requesting repeat caesarean birth (Caughey, 2018; Martel & MacKinnon, 2018). The use of cervical ripening agents increases the risk of uterine rupture and thus is contraindicated in VBAC clients. Oxytocin augmentation is not contraindicated in VBAC but oxytocin for induction increases the risk of uterine rupture and should be reserved for rare situations (Martel & MacKinnon, 2018). The client considering induction of labour after a previous caesarean birth needs to be informed of the risks versus benefits with an induction than with spontaneous labour (Scott, 2015).

Clients are the primary decision makers about the choice of birth method, but they need education about VBAC during their prenatal course. Management is similar for any clients experiencing labour, but certain areas require special focus:

- *Consent:* Fully informed consent is essential for the client who wants to have a TOL after caesarean birth. The client must be advised about the risks as well as the benefits. She must understand the ramifications of uterine rupture, even though the risk is small.
- *Documentation:* Record keeping is an important component of safe client care. If and when an emergency occurs, it is imperative to take care of the client, but also to keep track of the plan of care, interventions and their timing, and the client's response. Events and activities can be written right on the fetal monitoring tracing to correlate with the change in fetal status.
- *Surveillance:* An atypical or abnormal fetal monitor tracing in a client undergoing a TOL after a caesarean birth should alert the nurse to the possibility of uterine rupture and possible impending need for emergency caesarean delivery.
- *Readiness for emergency:* According to the SOGC and ACOG clinical practice guideline for VBAC, criteria for a safe TOL for a client who has had a previous caesarean birth includes the immediate availability of the multidisciplinary team including the nurse, obstetrician, anaesthesiologist, pediatrician, and operating room staff (ACOG, 2010; Martel & MacKinnon, 2018). Clients and their health care providers are advised to consider VBAC in the context of potential risk, available resources, and the health care system. VBACs are safe and appropriate for most people. Thorough counselling, shared decision making, and client autonomy are essential to the informed consent process. Nurses must act as advocates, giving input on the appropriate selection of those who

wish to undergo VBAC. Nurses also need to become experts at interpretation of fetal monitoring tracings to identify fetal compromise and resuscitative measures, and initiate an emergency birth if indicated. Including all of these nursing strategies will make VBAC safer for all.

INTRAUTERINE FETAL DEMISE

Pregnancy and childbirth are associated with hopes, expectations, joy, and happiness for the future. When an unborn life suddenly ends with fetal loss, the family members are profoundly affected. IUFD is fetal death that occurs after 20 weeks' gestation but before birth. The cause of IUFD is often unknown. The sudden loss of an expected child is tragic and the family's grief can be very intense: it can last for years and can cause extreme psychological stress and emotional problems (Sousou & Smart, 2015). The family's anticipation of a joyous birth is supplanted by despair, confusion, and loss. To clients and their families who have gone through this experience, culturally appropriate and sensitive care is crucial. Death of a fetus can occur at any gestation. Generally, fetal death and delivery after 20 weeks or after fetal weight of 500 g is attained, is termed a stillbirth, while fetal loss prior to 20 weeks and with a fetal weight of less than 500 g is defined as an abortion. These definitions vary slightly by jurisdiction and should be confirmed for your area.

Fetal demise in later pregnancy can be due to an extensive range of risk factors and possible causes, such as postterm pregnancy, renal disease, substance abuse, infection, hypertension, advanced childbearing age, multiple gestation, Rh disease, uterine rupture, diabetes, congenital anomalies, obesity, smoking, cord accident, abruption, blunt trauma (accidents, assault), premature rupture of membranes, or hemorrhage—or it may go unexplained (Mattingly & Joy, 2016). Early pregnancy loss may be through a spontaneous abortion (miscarriage), an induced abortion (therapeutic abortion), or a ruptured ectopic pregnancy. A wide spectrum of feelings may be expressed, from relief to sadness and despair. A fetal death can occur at any gestational age, and typically there is little or no warning other than reduced fetal movement. The effects of childbearing loss may affect clients and their families for a lifetime. The need to reflect, share, and regain strength is universal for all families dealing with loss. Grief, the typical response to the loss of a valued object, is not an intellectual response. Rather, it is personally experienced as a deep emotion of sadness and sorrow. Feelings such as helplessness, disbelief, unreality, and powerlessness are common. Emotional recovery from the pain of perinatal loss occurs with time, but it varies with each person.

The moment that fetal death is diagnosed can frequently be described very clearly and in detail by most who have experienced this tragic event. In many cases, the death was sudden, and expectant parents have no chance to prepare for the impending grief. Once IUFD is confirmed, most clients choose to immediately undergo induction of labour. Approximately 90% of clients will go into spontaneous labour within 2 weeks of fetal death (Green, 2016). With the death of a fetus or neonate, a couple's dreams and hopes for their expected child suddenly dissolve. To those who have experienced a sudden fetal death, the following processes may take place: experiencing a quiet birth without the infant, eclipsed by emptiness, anger, anxiety, loneliness, and sorrow; living without their infant, making it very difficult to see others with young infants; and experiencing differences with their partner over the loss (Callister, 2014). The process of grieving a death is not completed within a specific time frame, and for some, it is never complete. In general, the grief accompanying the loss of a fetus proceeds in the following order:

1. Accepting the reality of the loss
2. Getting over suffering from the loss
3. Adapting to the new environment without the deceased
4. Emotionally relocating the deceased and getting on with life (Grunebaum & Chervenak, 2018).

The period following a fetal death is extremely difficult for the family. The feelings of loss can be intense. The grief response in some parents may be so great that their relationships become strained, and healing can become hampered unless appropriate interventions and support are provided.

Fetal death also affects the health care staff. Despite the trauma that the loss of a fetus causes, some staff members avoid dealing with the bereaved family, never talking about or acknowledging their grief. This seems to imply that not discussing the problem will allow the grief to dissolve and vanish. As a result, the family's needs go unrecognized. Failing to keep the lines of communication open with a bereaved client and family closes off some of the channels to recovery and healing that may be desperately needed. Subsequently, the bereaved family members may feel isolated.

Nursing Assessment

An individual experiencing an IUFD is likely to seek care upon noticing that the fetus is not moving or when experiencing contractions, loss of fluid, or vaginal bleeding. History and physical examination frequently are of limited value in the diagnosis of fetal death, since many times the only history tends to be recent absence of fetal movement and no fetal heartbeat heard. An inability to obtain fetal heart sounds on examination suggests fetal demise, but an ultrasound is necessary to confirm the absence of fetal cardiac activity. Once fetal demise is confirmed, induction of labour or expectant management is offered.

Nursing Management

IUFD is associated with posttraumatic stress disorder (PTSD) and anxiety in a subsequent pregnancy (Robinson, 2014). The nurse can play a major role in assisting the grieving family. Nurses who can deal honestly with their own feelings regarding loss will be better able to help others cope with theirs. With skillful intervention, the bereaved family may be better prepared to resolve their grief and move forward.

To assist families in the grieving process, include the following measures:

- Provide accurate, understandable information to the family.
- Acknowledge that the client's feelings of loss are legitimate.
- Reassure parents that this outcome was beyond their control.
- Be knowledgeable about the grief process and comfortable in sharing another's grief.
- Utilize active listening to provide needed encouragement to the family members to open up to their feelings.
- Create a warm, receptive, accepting, and caring environment conducive to dialogue.
- Acknowledge grief, feelings of extreme sadness, anger and/or guilt.
- Recognize that each family member may express their grief differently.
- Provide reassurance about successful future pregnancies as appropriate.
- Encourage discussion of the loss and feelings of grief and guilt.
- Provide the family with baby mementos and pictures to validate the reality of death.
- Allow unlimited time with the stillborn infant after birth to validate the death; provide time for the family members to be together and grieve; offer the family the opportunity to see, touch, and hold the infant.
- Use appropriate touch, such as holding a hand or touching a shoulder.
- Offer and provide spiritual care support in the form requested by the family or modified as appropriate and agreed upon.
- Assist the parents with the funeral arrangements or disposition of the body.
- Provide the parents with brochures offering advice about how to talk to other siblings about the loss.
- Refer the family to a support group for pregnancy and infant loss which is designed for those who have lost an infant through abortion, miscarriage, fetal death, stillbirth, or other tragic circumstances.
- Make community referrals to promote a continuum of care after discharge.

Openness to talking with couples about their loss and grief is the basis for support provided by nurses,

FIGURE 21.4 Prolapsed cord.
A. Prolapse within the uterus (occult prolapse). **B.** Prolapse with the cord visible at the vulva.

which can have a positive influence on the long-term adjustment of couples and families coping with perinatal loss. An empathetic nurse who is comfortable talking about loss and is able to assist couples in navigating the process of grief provides a starting point for a healthy grieving process. Couples need to talk about their loss, its meaning, and the emotions that accompany it while the nurse listens. Nurses play a significant role in linking parents to appropriate professional support. As couples move through their grief and begin to consider another pregnancy, sensitive nursing care may mediate the understandable anxiety and concern that accompany this process. Nurses are a vital part of the interdisciplinary health care team caring for families with IUFD, who continue to require timely and sensitive care throughout the grieving process.

CLIENTS EXPERIENCING AN OBSTETRIC EMERGENCY

Obstetric emergencies are challenging to all labour and birth personnel because of the often-unpredictable nature of the event and increased risk of adverse outcomes for the client and fetus. Quick clinical judgment and good critical decision making will increase the likelihood of a positive outcome for both client and fetus. This section discusses a few of these emergencies: umbilical cord prolapse, placenta praevia, placental abruption, uterine rupture, and amniotic fluid embolism (AFE).

Umbilical Cord Prolapse

Umbilical cord prolapse is a rare obstetrical emergency that occurs when the cord precedes the fetal presenting part. An umbilical cord prolapse is the protrusion of the umbilical cord alongside (occult) or ahead of the presenting part of the fetus (Fig. 21.4). This condition occurs in 1 out of every 300 births and requires prompt recognition and intervention for a positive outcome (March of Dimes, 2016). Cord prolapse occurs in 3% of deliveries when the fetus is in the vertex position and in 3.7% of deliveries when the fetus is in the breech position. The risk is increased further when the presenting part does not fill the lower uterine segment, as is the case with incomplete breech presentations (5% to 10%), premature infants, and multiparous clients (Bush, Eddleman, & Belogolovkin, 2018). With a 50% perinatal mortality rate, it is one of the most catastrophic events in the intrapartum period (Beall & Ross, 2018).

Pathophysiology

Prolapse usually leads to total or partial occlusion of the cord. Since this is the fetus' only source of oxygen reception and waste removal, fetal perfusion deteriorates rapidly. Complete occlusion renders the fetus deprived of oxygen supply and unable to remove waste (carbon dioxide). The fetus will die if the cord compression is not relieved.

Nursing Assessment

Identification of clients at risk for cord prolapse can minimize the incidence of occurrence and reduce severity of outcome if anticipated. Carefully assess each client to help predict the risk status. Be aware that cord prolapse is more common in pregnancies involving malpresentation, growth restriction, prematurity, ruptured membranes with a fetus at a high station, polyhydramnios, grandmultiparity, and multiple gestation (Cunningham et al., 2014). Continuously assess the client and fetus to detect changes and to evaluate the effectiveness of any interventions performed.

Take Note!

When the presenting part does not fully occupy the pelvic inlet, prolapse is more likely to occur.

Nursing Management

Prompt recognition of a prolapsed cord is essential to reduce the risk of fetal hypoxia resulting from prolonged cord compression. Often the first sign of cord prolapse is a sudden fetal bradycardia or recurrent complicated variable decelerations that become progressively more severe. Call for help immediately and do not leave the client. Inform the client of what is happening and what options may be discussed by the health care provider. When membranes are artificially ruptured, assist with verifying that the presenting part is well applied to the cervix and engaged into the pelvis. If compression of the cord occurs, assist with measures to relieve the compression. Typically, the examiner places a sterile gloved hand into the vagina and holds the presenting part off the umbilical cord until delivery. Changing the client's position to a modified Sims, Trendelenburg, or knee-chest position also helps relieve cord pressure. Do not attempt to replace the cord in the uterus. Monitor FHR, maintain bed rest, and administer oxygen if ordered. Provide emotional support and explanations as to what is going on to allay the client's fears and anxiety. If the client's cervix is not fully dilated, prepare for an emergency caesarean birth as planned for by the health care provider.

Placenta Praevia

Placenta praevia is placental implantation in the lower uterine segment over or near the internal os of the cervix, typically during the second or third trimester of pregnancy. Placenta praevia has an overall prevalence in North America of 2.9 per 1,000 pregnancies (Rowe, 2014). With uterine segment formation and cervical dilation, placental implantation over or near the cervical os, instead of along the uterine wall inevitably results in trauma to the placenta and subsequent hemorrhage. This placenta over the cervix also creates a barrier for the fetus to pass into the vagina. As the cervix begins to thin and dilate (open up) in preparation for labour, blood vessels that connect the placenta to the uterus may tear and cause bleeding. It is the most common cause of significant bleeding in the second half of pregnancy and should be suspected in anyone beyond 24 weeks' gestation presenting with vaginal bleeding. Ultrasonography (transvaginal) is used to confirm diagnosis of placenta praevia. During labour and birth, bleeding can be severe, which can place both the client and fetus at risk. There is a direct relationship between the number of previous caesarean births and the risk of placenta praevia, probably due to uterine scarring. The degree of occlusion

of the internal cervical os may depend on the degree of cervical dilation, so what may appear to be a low-lying or marginal placenta praevia prior to the onset of labour can progress to become more serious as the cervix effaces and opens up (King et al., 2019).

The incidence of maternal mortality is less than 1%, but common morbidities include septicemia, renal failure, hemorrhage and hypovolemic shock, invasive placenta (accrete, increta, and percreta), and postpartum anemia. Risk factors for placenta praevia include previous caesarean section, advanced childbearing age >35, multiparity, multiple gestation, prior placenta praevia, and cigarette smoking. The risk for perinatal mortality is less than 10%, but common neonatal morbidities include stillbirth, prematurity, malpresentation, fetal growth restriction, and fetal anemia (Bakker & Ramus, 2018).

Signs and symptoms of placenta praevia include sudden, painless bleeding (scant to large volumes), anemia, pallor, hypoxia, low blood pressure, tachycardia, soft and nontender uterus, and rapid, weak pulse. Bleeding may be episodic, with spontaneous initiation and cessation. In some cases, it is asymptomatic because there is intrauterine bleeding only without external signs.

Management of placenta praevia varies by type and gestational age, and frequent medical surveillance may be sufficient in marginal cases; prompt treatment with bed rest, close monitoring, and control/replacement of blood loss greatly reduces risk for client and fetal complications and death. Vaginal delivery is possible when bleeding is minimal, placenta praevia is marginal, or labour is rapid. Pregnancy termination, early birth by caesarean section, or a hysterectomy may be necessary in order to control severe bleeding, especially for clients with complete placenta praevia. The overall prognosis is good if hemorrhage is controlled and sepsis or other complications are prevented. Fetal prognosis is directly related to the amount of blood loss. The United States perinatal mortality rate associated with placental praevia is 2% to 3%, and the maternal mortality rate is 0.03%. Risk for placenta praevia recurrence in subsequent pregnancies is 4% to 8% (Lal & Hibbard, 2015).

Nursing management within the acute care setting includes the following: monitor vital signs, intake and output, vaginal bleeding, and physiologic status for signs of hemorrhage, shock, or infection; closely monitor fetal heart rate for compromise (e.g., bradycardia, tachycardia, baseline changes, reduced variability); and treat fetus with resuscitative measures, as ordered. Administer prescribed intravenous fluids, packed red blood cells, platelets, and frozen plasma for transfusion. Administer Rho(D) immune globulin, if the client is Rh negative, and in cases of preterm labour, tocolytics if available to inhibit uterine contractions and corticosteroids (e.g., betamethasone) to enhance fetal lung maturity. Follow facility pre- and postsurgical protocols if the client becomes a surgical candidate (e.g., for caesarean section); reinforce pre- and postsurgical education and ensure completion of informed consent process. Closely monitor postsurgically for bleeding, infection, and other complications; assess client's anxiety level and coping ability; and provide emotional support and reassurance.

Frequently there is expectant management for the client after a first placenta praevia bleed if it isn't severe and fetal well-being is validated. After assessment and confirmation of client and fetal well-being, the client may be discharged home. It is common to experience an initial bleeding episode, which then subsides. These clients are monitored at home and instructed to report any additional bleeding episodes and come to hospital to be evaluated (King et al., 2019).

Placental Abruption

Placental abruption refers to premature separation of a normally implanted placenta from the myometrium. Placental abruption occurs in about 1% of all pregnancies throughout the world and is associated with significant perinatal mortality and morbidity (March of Dimes, 2015b). Risk factors include preeclampsia, gestational hypertension, seizure activity, advanced childbearing age >35, uterine rupture, trauma, smoking, cocaine use, coagulation defects, chorioamnionitis, premature rupture of membranes, oligohydramnios, uterine trauma, external cephalic version for breech presentation, previous history of abruption, domestic violence, and placental pathology. These conditions may force blood into the underlayer of the placenta and cause it to detach (Deering, 2018).

Management of placental abruption depends on the gestational age, the extent of the hemorrhage, and placental oxygenation perfusion/reserve status (see Chapter 19 for additional information on abruptio placentae). Treatment is based on the circumstances. Typically, once the diagnosis is established, the focus is on maintaining the cardiovascular status of the client and developing a plan to deliver the fetus quickly. A caesarean birth may take place quickly if the fetus is still alive with only a partial abruption. A vaginal birth may take place if delivery is imminent or fetal demise has occurred secondary to a complete abruption with a stable client and bleeding has subsided.

Uterine Rupture

Uterine rupture in pregnancy is a rare and often catastrophic complication with a high risk of morbidity for both the childbearing person and the fetus. Uterine rupture is a tearing of the uterus at the site of a previous scar into the abdominal cavity. Rarely it can occur in a nonscarred uterus and is related to overstimulation by oxytocin. Uterine rupture is often marked only by sudden fetal bradycardia, and treatment requires rapid surgery for good outcomes. From the time of diagnosis to delivery, only 10 to 30 minutes are available before clinically significant

fetal morbidity occurs. Fetal morbidity occurs secondary to catastrophic hemorrhage and subsequent fetal anoxia.

Nursing Assessment

Review the client's history for risk conditions such as uterine scars, prior caesarean births, prior rupture, trauma, prior invasive molar pregnancy, history of placenta percreta or increta, congenital uterine anomalies, multiparity, previous uterine myomectomy, malpresentation, labour induction with excessive uterine stimulation, and cocaine use (Nahum & Pham, 2018). Knowledge of a client's history for risk factors allows for increased surveillance and improved identification of abruption, allowing for more timely intervention.

Generally, the first and most reliable symptom of uterine rupture is sudden fetal compromise on the fetal tracing. Other signs may include acute and continuous abdominal pain with or without an epidural, vaginal bleeding, hematuria, irregular abdominal wall contour, loss of station in the fetal presenting part, and hypovolemic shock in the pregnant client, fetus, or both (Scott, 2015).

Timely management of uterine rupture depends on prompt detection. The nurse must be familiar with the signs and symptoms of uterine rupture when caring for a client with a previous caesarean birth. It is difficult to prevent uterine rupture or to predict who will experience rupture, so constant preparedness is necessary. Screening everyone with previous uterine surgical scars is important, and continuous electronic fetal monitoring should be used during labour because this may provide the only indication of an impending rupture.

Nursing Management

Because the presenting signs may be nonspecific, the initial management will be the same as that for any other cause of acute fetal distress. Urgent delivery by caesarean birth is usually indicated. Monitor vital signs and observe for hypotension and tachycardia, which might indicate hypovolemic shock. Assist in preparing for an emergency caesarean birth by alerting the operating room staff, anaesthesia provider, and neonatal team. Insert an indwelling urinary (Foley) catheter if one is not in place already. Inform the client of the seriousness of this event and state that the health care staff will be working quickly to ensure her health and that of her fetus. Remain calm and provide reassurance that everything is being done to ensure a safe outcome for both.

The life-threatening nature of uterine rupture is underscored by the fact that the pregnant person's circulatory system delivers approximately 500 mL of blood to the term uterus every minute (Cunningham et al., 2014). Maternal death is a possibility without rapid intervention. Newborn outcome after rupture depends largely on the speed with which surgical rescue is carried out. As in any case of acute obstetric emergency, preparation and timely mobilization of all necessary personnel including a newborn resuscitation team and lab and blood bank staff is essential to optimizing outcome.

> **Take Note!**
> When excessive bleeding occurs during the childbirth process and it persists or signs such as bruising or petechiae appear, disseminated intravascular coagulation (DIC) should be suspected.

Amniotic Fluid Embolism

Amniotic fluid embolism (AFE) is an unforeseeable, life-threatening complication of childbirth. AFE remains an enigmatic, but devastating obstetric condition associated with significant morbidity and mortality for both the client and newborn. It is a rare and often fatal event characterized by the sudden onset of hypotension, hypoxia, and coagulopathy. Amniotic fluid containing particles of debris (e.g., hair, skin, vernix, meconium) enters the pregnant client's circulation and obstructs the pulmonary vessels, causing respiratory distress and circulatory collapse (Sadera & Vasudevan, 2015). Prediction and diagnosis of the event are nearly impossible. However, timely recognition and response is critical in saving a client's life. Although estimates vary, AFE, also referred to as anaphylactoid syndrome of pregnancy, occurs in 1 in 15,000 births, with a reported mortality rate reaching 60% despite technologic advances in critical care life support (Moore, 2017).

Pathophysiology

The pathophysiology appears to involve an abnormal physiologic response to fetal tissue exposure. Normally, amniotic fluid does not enter the pregnant person's circulation because it is contained within the uterus, sealed off by the amniotic sac. An AFE occurs when the barrier between the pregnant client's circulation and the amniotic fluid is broken and amniotic fluid enters the client's venous system via the endocervical veins, the placental site (if the placenta is separated), or a site of uterine trauma. This condition has a high mortality rate: as many as 50% of people die within the first hour after the onset of symptoms, and about 85% of survivors have permanent hypoxia-induced neurologic damage (Sadera & Vasudevan, 2015).

Although medical science has supplied many answers to questions about this condition, health care providers remain largely unable to predict or prevent an AFE or to decrease its mortality rate.

Nursing Assessment

Predisposing factors associated with AFE include placental abruption, uterine over distention, fetal demise, uterine

trauma, oxytocin-stimulated labour, amnioinfusion, multiparity, advanced childbearing age, and ruptured membranes. However, many clients present without any of the risk factors.

Nurses should be prepared at all times in this obstetric emergency. A team response is essential because every person will be needed. No test can diagnose an AFE. Therefore, the nurse's assessment skills are critical. Immediate recognition and diagnosis of this condition are essential to improve client and fetal outcomes. Until recently, the diagnosis could be made only after an autopsy of the client revealed squamous cells, lanugo hair, or other fetal and amniotic material in the pulmonary arterial vasculature (Baldisseri, 2018).

The clinical appearance is varied, but most clients report difficulty breathing. Other symptoms include hypotension, cyanosis, hypoxemia, uterine atony, seizures, tachycardia, coagulation failure, disseminated intravascular coagulation (DIC), pulmonary edema, seizures, uterine atony with subsequent hemorrhage, adult respiratory distress syndrome, and cardiac arrest (Baldisseri, 2018).

> **Take Note!**
> Amniotic fluid embolism should be suspected in any pregnant clients with an acute onset of dyspnea, hypotension, and DIC. By knowing how to intervene, the nurse can promote a better chance of survival for both the client and newborn. Most clients are transferred to the intensive care unit.

Nursing Management

Upon recognizing the signs and symptoms of this life-threatening diagnosis, institute supportive measures: oxygenation (resuscitation and 100% oxygen), circulation (intravenous fluids, inotropic agents to maintain cardiac output and blood pressure), control of hemorrhage and coagulopathy (oxytocic agents to control uterine atony and bleeding), seizure precautions, and administration of steroids to control the inflammatory response. Monitor vital signs, pulse oximetry, skin colour, and temperature and observe for clinical signs of coagulopathy (vaginal bleeding, bleeding from intravenous site, bleeding from gums) (Moses, 2018).

Care is largely supportive and aimed at maintaining oxygenation and hemodynamic function and correcting coagulopathy. There is no specific therapy that is life-saving once this condition starts. Adequate oxygenation is necessary, with endotracheal intubation and mechanical ventilation for most clients. Vasopressors are used to maintain hemodynamic stability. Management of DIC may involve replacement with packed red blood cells or fresh frozen plasma as necessary. Oxytocin infusions and prostaglandin analogues can be used to address uterine atony.

Explain to the client and family what is happening and what therapies are being instituted. The client

FIGURE 21.5 Forceps delivery. **A.** Example of forceps. **B.** Forceps being applied to the fetus. **C.** Forceps marks are commonly found in newborns delivered by forceps. Such marks are transient and disappear in a day or two.

is usually transferred to a critical care unit for intensive observation and care. Assist the family to express their feelings and provide support as needed. Inform and reassure the client and family as much as possible during this crisis.

CLIENTS REQUIRING BIRTH-RELATED PROCEDURES

Many clients can give birth without the need for operative or medical obstetric interventions. However, in some situations interventions are necessary to safeguard the health of the client and fetus. The most common birth-related procedures are forceps-assisted or vacuum-assisted birth, caesarean birth, episiotomy (see Chapter 14), and vaginal birth following a previous caesarean birth (see section earlier in this chapter). Increasingly common in Canada is the use of amniofusion for atypical or abnormal fetal heart pattern. Nurses play a major role in helping couples to cope with any unanticipated procedures by offering thorough explanations of the procedure, its anticipated benefits and risks, and any other options available.

Forceps- or Vacuum-Assisted Birth

Forceps or a vacuum extractor may be used to apply traction to the fetal head or to provide a method of rotating the fetal head during birth. **Forceps** are stainless-steel instruments, similar to tongs, with rounded edges that fit around the fetus' head. Some forceps have open blades and some have solid blades. Outlet forceps are used when the fetal head is crowning and low forceps are used when the fetal head is at a +2 station or lower but not yet crowning. The forceps are applied to the sides of the fetal head. The type of forceps used is determined by the birth attendant. All forceps have a locking mechanism that prevents the blades from compressing

the fetal skull. Use of forceps has declined in popularity recently because many obstetricians are not trained to use them in their residency since they are rarely used in obstetrical practice today (Fig. 21.5).

A **vacuum extractor** is a cup-shaped instrument attached to a suction pump used for extraction of the fetal head (Fig. 21.6). The suction cup is placed against

FIGURE 21.6 Vacuum extractor for delivery. There are 2 common shapes with different uses. **A.** Typical bell-shaped cup with a hand pump. **B.** Disposable plastic version of the Bird cup with combined pump and traction bar. (From Ronald, S. G., Beth, Y. K., Arthur, F. H., & Ingrid, E. N. (2008). *Danforth's obstetrics and gynecology* (10th ed.). Philadelphia, PA: Wolters Kluwer.)

positioning in bed with the newborn, medications and other strategies for pain relief. Complete the preoperative procedures, which may include:

- Preparing the surgical site as ordered
- Starting an intravenous infusion for fluid replacement therapy as ordered
- Inserting an indwelling (Foley) catheter and informing the client about how long it will remain in place (usually 12 to 24 hours)
- Administering any preoperative medications as ordered; documenting the time administered and the client's reaction
- Completing a surgical safety checklist

PROVIDING POSTOPERATIVE CARE

Postoperative care for the client who has had a caesarean delivery is similar to that for one who has had a vaginal birth, with a few additional measures. Assess vital signs and lochia flow every 15 minutes for the first hour, then every 30 minutes for the next hour, and then every 4 hours if stable. Assist with perineal care and instruct the client in the same. Inspect the abdominal dressing and document description, including any evidence of drainage. Assess uterine tone to determine fundal firmness. Check the patency of the intravenous line, making sure the infusion is flowing at the correct rate. Inspect the infusion site frequently for redness.

Assess the client's level of consciousness if sedative drugs were administered. Institute safety precautions until the client is fully alert and responsive. If a regional anaesthetic was used, monitor for the return of sensation and motor control to the legs.

Assess for evidence of abdominal distention and auscultate bowel sounds. Assist with early ambulation to prevent respiratory and cardiovascular complications and to promote peristalsis. Monitor intake and output at least every 4 hours initially and then every 8 hours as indicated.

If the client has had a general anaesthetic, encourage coughing, performing deep-breathing exercises, and use the incentive spirometer every 2 hours. Enhance comfort and general well-being. Administer analgesics as ordered and provide comfort measures such as splinting the incision and pillows for positioning. Assist the client to move in bed and turn side to side to improve circulation. Also encourage the client to ambulate to promote venous return from the extremities. Prevent/minimize postoperative complications.

Encourage early touching and holding and skin-to-skin care of the newborn to promote bonding and physiologic transition. Assist with breastfeeding initiation and offer continued support. Suggest alternate positioning techniques to reduce incisional discomfort while breastfeeding. (See Chapter 18 for breastfeeding positions.)

Review with the couple their perception of the surgical birth experience. Allow them to verbalize their feelings and assist them in positive coping measures. Promote a positive emotional response to the birth experience and parenting role. Prior to discharge, teach the client about the need for adequate rest, activity restrictions such as lifting, incision care, pain management strategies including review of any prescriptions and signs and symptoms of infection and postpartum hemorrhage. Provide information about postpartum care at home and available community supports and services.

Amnioinfusion

Amnioinfusion is a technique in which a volume of warmed, sterile, normal saline or Ringer's lactate solution is introduced into the uterus transcervically through an intrauterine pressure catheter to increase the volume of fluid when oligohydramnios is present, during labour. It is used to change the relationship of the uterus, placenta, cord, and fetus to improve placental and fetal oxygenation. Instilling an isotonic glucose-free solution into the uterus helps to cushion the umbilical cord to prevent compression. Studies support the use of this procedure as safe and effective in resolving FHR decelerations (Liston et al., 2018).

This procedure is commonly indicated for severe variable decelerations due to cord compression, oligohydramnios due to placental insufficiency, postmaturity or rupture of membranes, preterm labour with premature rupture of membrane. However, it does not prevent meconium aspiration syndrome (Hofmeyr, Xu, & Eke, 2014). Contraindications to amnioinfusion include vaginal bleeding of unknown origin, umbilical cord prolapse, amnionitis, uterine hypertonicity, and severe fetal distress (Fong, Chau, Pan, & Ogunyemi, 2014).

There is no standard protocol for amnioinfusion; nurses should follow their own institution protocols. After obtaining informed consent, a vaginal examination is performed to evaluate for cord prolapse, establish dilatation, and confirm presentation. Next, 250 to 500 mL of warmed normal saline or lactated Ringer solution is administered using an infusion pump over 20 to 30 minutes. Overdistention of the uterus is a risk, so the amount of fluid infused must be monitored closely. In addition, the intrauterine pressure must be monitored using an intrauterine pressure catheter with pressure readings on the electronic fetal monitor. Amnioinfusion should reach therapeutic result or increase the amniotic fluid volume in approximately 30 minutes (Mattson & Smith, 2016).

When caring for the client who is receiving an amnioinfusion, include the following:
- Explain the need for the procedure, what it involves, and how it may solve the problem.
- Inform the client of the need to remain on bed rest during the procedure.
- Assess the client's vital signs and associated discomfort level.

- Maintain intake and output records.
- Assess the duration and intensity of uterine contractions frequently to identify overdistention or increased uterine tone. Monitor intrauterine pressures.
- Assess for fluid leakage by evaluating the pad under the client to determine that it is not being retained in

the uterus, which could lead to increased uterine pressure.
- Monitor the FHR pattern to determine whether the amnioinfusion is improving the fetal status.
- Prepare the client for a possible caesarean birth if the FHR does not improve after the amnioinfusion.

NURSING CARE PLAN 21.1

Overview of the Client Undergoing Labour Induction

Rose, a 29-year-old primipara, is admitted to the labour and birth suite at 41 weeks' gestation for induction of labour. Assessment reveals that the cervix is favourable at 80% effaced, and dilated to 2 cm. Rose says, "I'm a bit nervous about being induced. I've never been through labour before and I'm afraid that I'll have a lot of pain from the medicine used to start the contractions." She consents to being induced but wants reassurance that this procedure won't harm the baby. Upon examination, the fetus is engaged and in a cephalic presentation, with the vertex as the presenting part. Her partner is at her side. Induction is initiated with oxytocin. Rose reports that contractions have started and are beginning to get stronger.

NURSING DIAGNOSIS: Anxiety related to induction of labour and associated medical interventions needed as evidenced by statements about being nervous, not having gone through labour before, fear of pain and potential harm to fetus

Outcome Identification and Evaluation

The client will experience decrease in anxiety as evidenced by ability to verbalize understanding of procedures involved and use of positive coping skills to reduce anxious state.

Interventions: *Minimizing Anxiety*

- Provide a clear explanation of the labour induction process *to provide client and partner with a knowledge base.*
- Maintain continuous physical presence *to provide physical and emotional support and demonstrate concern for client and fetal well-being.*
- Explain each procedure before carrying it out and answer questions *to promote understanding of procedure and rationale for use and decrease fear of the unknown.*
- Review with client measures used in the past to deal with stressful situations *to determine effectiveness;*

encourage use of past effective coping strategies *to aid in controlling anxiety.*
- Instruct client's partner in helpful measures to assist client in coping and encourage their use *to foster joint participation in the process and feelings of being in control and to provide support to the client.*
- Offer frequent reassurance of fetal status and labour progress *to help alleviate client's concerns and foster continued participation in the labour process.*

NURSING DIAGNOSIS: Risk for injury related to induction procedure risk factors: hypertonic uterine contractions, fetal compromise related to potential decreased placental flow, cord compromise, placenta complications (abruption) or fetal birth trauma

Outcome Identification and Evaluation

The client will remain free of complications associated with induction as evidenced by progression of labour as expected, delivery of healthy newborn, and absence of signs and symptoms of adverse effects.

(continued)

NURSING CARE PLAN 21.1

Overview of the Client Undergoing Labour Induction (continued)

Interventions: *Promoting Client and Fetal Safety*

- Follow agency's protocol for medication use and infusion rate *to ensure accurate, safe drug administration.*
- Set up oxytocin IV infusion to piggyback into the primary IV infusion line at most proximal site *to allow for prompt discontinuation should adverse effects occur.*
- Use an infusion pump *to deliver accurate dose as ordered.*
- *Use independent double check to verify concentration and pump settings*
- Gradually increase oxytocin dose in increments based on assessment findings and protocol *to promote effective uterine contractions.*
- Maintain oxytocin rate once desired frequency of contractions has been reached *to ensure continued progress in labour.*
- Accurately monitor contractions for frequency, duration, and intensity and resting tone *to prevent development of hypertonic contractions.*
- Maintain a nurse-to-client ratio of 1:1 *to ensure client and fetal safety.*
- Monitor FHR via electronic fetal monitoring during induction and interpret the FHR response to titrated medication rate *to ensure fetal well-being and identify adverse effects immediately.*
- Obtain vital signs every 1 to 2 hours or as indicated by agency's protocol, reporting any deviations, *to promote client's well-being and allow for prompt identification of deviations from normal.*
- Communicate with birth attendant and health care team frequently concerning progress *to ensure continuity of care.*
- Discontinue oxytocin infusion if tetanic contractions (>90 seconds), uterine tachysystole (more than 5 contractions in 10 minutes), elevated uterine resting tone, or an atypical or abnormal FHR pattern occurs *to minimize risk of drug's adverse effects.*
- Provide client with frequent reassurance of current status *to minimize anxiety.*

NURSING DIAGNOSIS: Labor pain related to uterine contractions as evidenced by client's statements about contractions increasing in intensity and expected effect of oxytocin administration

Outcome Identification and Evaluation

The client will report a decrease in pain as evidenced by statements of increased comfort and pain rating of 3 or less on numeric pain rating scale.

Interventions: *Promoting Safety*

- Explain that the client will experience discomfort sooner than with naturally occurring labour *to promote client's awareness of events and prepare client for the experience.*
- Frequently assess client's pain using a pain rating scale *to quantify client's level of pain and evaluate effectiveness of pain relief measures.*
- Provide comfort measures, such as hygiene, backrubs, music, and distraction, and encourage the use of breathing and relaxation techniques *to help promote relaxation.*
- Provide support for the partner *to aid in alleviating stress and concerns.*
- Employ nonpharmacologic methods, such as position changes, birthing ball, hydrotherapy, visual imagery, and effleurage, *to help in managing pain and foster feelings of control over situation.*
- Administer pharmacologic agents such as analgesia or anaesthesia as appropriate and as ordered *to control pain.*
- Continuously reassess client's pain level *to evaluate effectiveness of pain management techniques used.*

KEY CONCEPTS

- Risk factors for dystocia include epidural analgesia, occiput posterior position, longer first stage of labour, nulliparity, short stature (<5 ft tall), high body mass index (BMI), age older than 35 years, gestational age more than 41 weeks, chorioamnionitis, pelvic contractions, macrosomia, and high station at complete cervical dilation.

- Dystocia may result from problems in the powers, passenger, passage, or psyche.

- Problems involving the powers that lead to dystocia include hypertonic uterine dysfunction, hypotonic uterine dysfunction, and precipitate labour.

- Management of hypertonic labour pattern involves therapeutic rest with the use of sedatives to promote relaxation and stop the abnormal activity of the uterus.

- Any presentation other than occiput or a slight variation of the fetal position or size increases the probability of dystocia.

- Multiple pregnancy may result in dysfunctional labour due to uterine overdistention, which may lead to hypotonic dystocia and abnormal presentation of the fetuses.

- During labour, evaluation of fetal descent, cervical effacement and dilation, and characteristics of uterine contractions are essential to determine progress or lack of progress.

- Antepartum assessment for a postterm pregnancy typically includes daily fetal movement counts done by the client, nonstress tests done twice weekly, amniotic fluid assessments as part of the biophysical profile, and weekly cervical examinations to check for ripening for induction. Membrane stripping can increase the likelihood of spontaneous labour.

- Once the cervix is ripe, oxytocin is the most commonly used pharmacologic agent used for inducing or augmenting labour.

- Generally, the first and most reliable symptom of uterine rupture is abnormal fetal tracing on electronic fetal monitoring.

- Amniotic fluid embolism is a rare but often fatal event characterized by the sudden onset of hypotension, hypoxia, and coagulopathy.

- Caesarean births have steadily risen in Canada; today, approximately one in three births occurs this way. Caesarean birth is a major surgical procedure and has increased risks over vaginal birth, which must be weighed against the benefits of surgical delivery to client and/or baby.

REFERENCES AND RECOMMENDED READINGS

Abbott, D. S., Hezelgrave, N. L., Seed, P. T., Norman, J. E., David, A. L., Bennett, P. R., … Shennan, A. H. (2015). Quantitative fetal fibronectin to predict preterm birth in asymptomatic women at high risk. *Obstetrics & Gynecology, 125*(5), 1168–1176.

Afzal, M., Asif, U., & Miraj, B. (2015). Induction of labor: Efficacy of sweeping of membranes at term in previous one C-section. *Professional Medical Journal, 22*(4), 385–389.

Ahmed, Z. D., Garba, I., Nafi'ah, T., & Yakasai, I. A. (2015). Misoprostol: An effective agent for cervical ripening and labor induction: A 2-year review in a tertiary center. *Open Journal of Obstetrics and Gynecology, 5*(05), 274–279.

American Academy of Pediatrics & American College of Obstetricians and Gynecologists. (2010). *Guidelines for perinatal care* (6th ed.). Washington, DC: Author.

American Academy of Pediatrics. (2015). *Delivery by cesarean section*. Retrieved from http://www.healthychildren.org/English/ages-stages/prenatal/delivery-beyond/pages/Delivery-by-Cesarean-Section.aspx

American College of Obstetricians and Gynecologists [ACOG]. (2010). ACOG practice bulletin no. 115: Vaginal birth after previous cesarean delivery. *Obstetrics and Gynecology, 116*, 450–463.

American College of Obstetricians & Gynecologists [ACOG]. (2014a). Safe prevention of primary cesarean delivery. *American Journal of Obstetrics & Gynecology, 123*, 693–711.

American College of Obstetricians & Gynecologists [ACOG]. (2014b). *Preterm labor practice guidelines*. Retrieved from http://www.acog.org/Womens-Health/Preterm-Premature-Labor-and-BirthAmerican

Arrowsmith, S., & Wray, S. (2014). Oxytocin: Its mechanism of action and receptor signaling in the myometrium. *Journal of Neuroendocrinology, 26*, 356–369.

Bakker, R., & Ramus, R. M. (2018). Placenta previa. *eMedicine*. Retrieved from http://emedicine.medscape.com/article/262063-overview

Baldisseri, M. R. (2018). Amniotic fluid embolism syndrome. *UpToDate*. Retrieved from http://www.uptodate.com/contents/amniotic-fluid-embolism-syndrome

Bauer, A. R., & Springel, E. H. (2017). Macrosomia. *eMedicine*. Retrieved from http://emedicine.medscape.com/article/262679-overview

Beall, M. H., & Ross, M. G. (2018). Umbilical cord complications. *eMedicine*. Retrieved from http://emedicine.medscape.com/article/262470-overview

Bibbo, C., & Robinson, J. N. (2015). Management of twins: Vaginal or cesarean delivery?. *Clinical Obstetrics & Gynecology, 58*(2), 294–308.

Bohren, M. A., Hofmeyr, G. J., Sakala, C., Fukuzawa, R. K., & Cuthbert, A. (2017). Continuous support for women during childbirth [Cochrane review]. *Cochrane Database of Systematic Reviews, 7,* CD003766.

Born, K., Konkin, J., Tepper, J., & Okun, N. (2014). *Healthy debate: Pulling back the curtain on Canada's rising C-section rate.* Retrieved from http://healthydebate.ca/2014/05/topic/quality/c-section-variation

Bush, M., Eddleman, K., & Belogolovkin, V. (2018). *Umbilical cord prolapse. UpToDate.* Retrieved from http://www.uptodate.com/contents/umbilical-cord-prolapse

Cabbad, M. F., De Los Heros, D., Baltajian, K. Z., & Robertazzi, R. R. (2015). Corticosteroid use in the face of threatened preterm labor [165]. *Obstetrics & Gynecology, 125,* 56S.

Callahan, T. L. (2016). *Tarascon Ob/Gyn Pocketbook.* Burlington, MA: Jones & Bartlett Publishers.

Callister, L. C. (2014). Global perspectives on perinatal loss. *MCN: The American Journal of Maternal/Child Nursing, 39*(3), 207.

Canadian Institute for Health Information. (2012). *Indicator Library: Caesarean section rate.* Retrieved from http://indicatorlibrary.cihi.ca/display/HSPIL/Caesarean±Section±Rate

Cargill, Y. M., & MacKinnon, C. J. (2018). Reaffirmed SOGC clinical practice guideline: No. 148, guidelines for operative vaginal birth. *Journal of Obstetrics and Gynaecology Canada, 40*(2), e74–e80.

Caughey, A. B. (2018). Vaginal birth after cesarean delivery. *eMedicine.* Retrieved from http://emedicine.medscape.com/article/272187-overview

Caughey, A. B., & Butler, J. R. (2016). Postterm pregnancy. *eMedicine.* Retrieved from http://emedicine.medscape.com/article/261369-overview

Centers for Disease Control and Prevention (CDC). (2018). Primary cesarean delivery rates, by State. *National Vital Statistics Reports, 67*(8). Retrieved from https://www.cdc.gov/nchs/data/nvsr/nvsr67/nvsr67_08_tables-508.pdf

Chandrasekaran, S., & Srinivas, S. K. (2014). Antenatal corticosteroid administration: Understanding its use as an obstetric quality metric. *American Journal of Obstetrics and Gynecology, 210*(2), 143–150.

Cunningham, F. G., Leveno, K. J., Bloom, S. L., Spong, C. Y., Dashe, J. S., Hoffman, B. L., ... Sheffield, J. S. (2014). *Williams' obstetrics* (24th ed.). New York: McGraw-Hill.

Deering, S. H. (2018). Abruptio placenta. *eMedicine.* Retrieved from http://emedicine.medscape.com/article/252810-overview

Delaney, M., & Roggensack, A. (2017). SOGC Clinical practice guideline No. 214--Guidelines for the management of pregnancy at 41D+0 to 42D+0 weeks. *Journal Obstetrics and Gynaecology Canada, 39*(8), e164–e174.

Drunecký, T., Reidingerová, M., Plisová, M., Dudič, M., Gdovinová, D., & Stoy, V. (2015). Experimental comparison of properties of natural and synthetic osmotic dilators. *Archives of Gynecology and Obstetrics, 292*(2), 349–354.

Fischer, R. (2016). Breech presentation. *eMedicine.* Retrieved from http://emedicine.medscape.com/article/262159-overview

Flenady, V., Wojcieszek, A. M., Papatsonis, D. N., Stock, O. M., Murray, L., Jardine, L. A., & Carbonne, B. (2014). Calcium channel blockers for inhibiting preterm labor and birth. *Cochrane Database of Systematic Reviews,* (6), CD002255.

Fong, A., Chau, C. T., Pan, D., & Ogunyemi, D. A. (2014). Amniotic fluid embolism: Antepartum, intrapartum and demographic factors. *The Journal of Maternal-Fetal & Neonatal Medicine, 28*(7), 793–798. (Online June 30, 2014), 1–6.

Fuks, A. M., Robinson, J. V., Rothschild, T. J., Akinnawonu, K. F., & Salafia, C. (2015). Mechanical labor induction using the Foley catheter balloon compared with the cook cervical balloon [96]. *Obstetrics & Gynecology, 125,* 37S.

Garrison, A. (2017). Vacuum extraction. *eMedicine.* Retrieved from http://emedicine.medscape.com/article/271175-overview#aw2aab6b4

Gherman, R. (2015). Shoulder dystocia. In J. T. Queenan, C. Y. Catherine, & C. J. Lockwood (Eds.). *Protocols for high-risk pregnancies: An evidence-based approach* (6th ed.). Hoboken, NJ: John Wiley & Sons.

Goetzl, L. (2014). Methods of cervical ripening and labor induction: Pharmacologic. *Clinical Obstetrics and Gynecology, 57*(2), 377–390.

Goldberg, A. E. (2018). Cervical ripening. *eMedicine.* Retrieved from http://emedicine.medscape.com/article/263311-overview

Green, C. J. (2016). *Maternal newborn nursing care plans* (3rd ed.). Burlington, MA: Jones & Bartlett Learning.

Grobman, W. A. (2015). Is it time for outpatient cervical ripening with prostaglandins?. *BJOG: An International Journal of Obstetrics & Gynecology, 122,* 105.

Grunebaum, A., & Chervenak, F. A. (2018). Counseling parents after fetal demise and stillbirth. *UpToDate.* Retrieved from http://www.uptodate.com/contents/counseling-parents-after-fetal-demise-and-stillbirth

Haas, D. M., Benjamin, T., Sawyer, R., & Quinney, S. K. (2014). Short-term tocolytics for preterm delivery—current perspectives. *International Journal of Women's Health, 6,* 343–349.

Hagood Milton, S. (2017). Normal labor and delivery. *eMedicine.* Retrieved from http://emedicine.medscape.com/article/260036-overview

Hansen, A. & Chauhan, S. P. (2014). Shoulder dystocia: Definitions and incidence. *Seminars in Perinatology, 38*(4), 184–188.

Hinshaw, K., & Kenyon, S. (2015). Abnormal labor. In F. Arias, A. G. Bhide, S. Arulkumaran, K. Damania, & S. N. Daftary (Eds.). *Arias' practical guide to high-risk pregnancy & delivery* (4th ed.). New Delhi, India: Elsevier.

Hobbins, J. C. (2015). Macrosomia. *OB/GYN Clinical Alert, 32*(2), 13–16.

Hofmeyr, G. J. (2015). Protocol 51: Breech delivery. In J. T. Queenan, C. Y. Spong, & C. J. Lockwood (Eds.). *Protocols for high-risk pregnancies: An evidence-based approach.* Chichester, UK: John Wiley & Sons.

Hofmeyr, G. J., Eke, A. C., & Lawrie, T. A. (2014). Amnioinfusion for third trimester preterm premature rupture of membranes. *Cochrane Database of Systematic Reviews, 3,* CD000942.

Hofmeyr G. J., Kulier, R., & West, H. M. (2015). External cephalic version for breech presentation at term. *Cochrane Database of Systematic Reviews, 4,* CD000083.

Hofmeyr, G. J., Xu, H., & Eke, A. C. (2014). Amnioinfusion for meconium-stained liquor in labor. *Cochrane Database of Systematic Reviews, 1,* CD000014.

Holley, S. R., & Pasch, L. A. (2015). Counseling lesbian, gay, bisexual, and transgender patients. *Fertility counseling* (pp. 180–194). Cambridge, UK: Cambridge University Press.

Iams, J. D. (2015). Clinical practice: Prevention of preterm parturition. *Obstetric Anesthesia Digest, 35*(1), 34–36.

International Childbirth Education Association [ICEA]. (2015). *ICEA position paper: Induction.* Retrieved from http://www. icea.org/sites/default/files/Induction%20PP-FINAL.pdf

Jarde, A., Lutsiv, O., Park, C. K., Beyene, J., Dodd, J. M., Barrett, J., ... McDonald, S. D. (2017). Effectiveness of progesterone, cerclage and pessary for preventing preterm birth in singleton pregnancies: A systematic review and network meta-analysis. *BJOG, 124*(8), 1176–1189.

Jordan, R. G., Engstrom, J. L., Marfell, J. A., & Farley, C. L. (2014). Prenatal and postnatal care: A woman-centered approach. Ames, Iowa: John Wiley & Sons, Inc.

Jørgensen, J. S., Weile, L. K. K., & Lamont, R. F. (2014). Preterm labor: Current tocolytic options for the treatment of preterm labor. *Expert Opinion on Pharmacotherapy, 15*(5), 585–588.

King, T. L., Brucker, M. C., Osborne, K., & Jevitt, C. M. (2019). *Varney's midwifery* (6th ed.). Burlington, MA: Jones & Bartlett Learning.

Kriebs, J. M. (2015). Patient safety during induction of labor. *The Journal of Perinatal & Neonatal Nursing, 29*(2), 130–137.

Lal, A. K., & Hibbard, J. U. (2015). Placenta previa: An outcome-based cohort study in a contemporary obstetric population. *Archives of Gynecology and Obstetrics, 292*(2), 299–305.

Leduc, D., Biringer, A., Lee, L., & Dy, J. (2013). SOGC Clinical practice guideline No. 296: Induction of labour. *Journal of Obstetrics and Gynaecology Canada.* Retrieved from https:// sogc.org/wp-content/uploads/2013/08/September2013-CPG296-ENG-Online_REV-D.pdf

Lee, L., Dy, J., & Azzam, H. (2016). Management of spontaneous labour at term in healthy women. *Journal of Obstetrics and Gynaecology Canada, 38*(9), 843–865.

Lewis, L. S., Pan, H. Y., Heine, R. P., Brown, H. L., Brancazio, L. R., & Grotegut, C. A. (2014). Labor and pregnancy outcomes after adoption of a more conservative oxytocin labor protocol. *Obstetrics & Gynecology, 123*, 66S.

Lim, K., Butt, K., & Crane, J. M. (2018). SOGC Clinical practice guideline No. 257, Ultrasonographic cervical length assessment in predicting preterm birth in singleton pregnancies. *Journal of Obstetrics and Gynaecology Canada, 40*(2), e151–e164.

Liston, R., Sawchuk, D., & Young, D. (2018). SOGC Clinical practice guideline: No. 197b—Fetal health surveillance: Intrapartum consensus guideline. *Journal of Obstetrics and Gynaecology Canada, 40*(4), e298–e322.

Locatelli, A., Consonni, S., & Ghidini, A. (2015). Preterm labor: Approach to decreasing complications of prematurity. *Obstetrics and Gynecology Clinics of North America, 42*(2), 255–274.

Manjula, B. G., Bagga, R., Kalra, J., & Dutta, S. (2015). Labor induction with an intermediate-dose oxytocin regimen has advantages over a high-dose regimen. *Journal of Obstetrics & Gynecology, 35*(4), 362–367.

March of Dimes. (2015a). *Placenta previa.* Retrieved from http:// www.marchofdimes.org/pregnancy/placenta-previa.aspx

March of Dimes. (2015b). *Placental abruption.* Retrieved from http://www.marchofdimes.org/pregnancy/placental-abruption.aspx

March of Dimes. (2016). *Umbilical cord conditions.* Retrieved from https://www.marchofdimes.org/complications/umbilical-cord-conditions.aspx

March of Dimes. (2017). *Being pregnant with twins, triplets and other multiples.* Retrieved from http://www.marchofdimes.com/professionals/14332_4545.asp

March of Dimes. (2018). *Preterm labor and premature birth.* Retrieved from https://www.marchofdimes.org/complications/preterm-labor-and-premature-baby.aspx

Martel, M. J., & MacKinnon, C. J. (2018). Reaffirmed SOGC clinical practice guideline: No. 155-Guidelines for vaginal birth after previous caesarean birth. *Journal of Obstetrics and Gynaecology Canada, 40*(3), e195–e207.

Mattingly, P. J., & Joy, S. (2016). Evaluation of fetal death. *eMedicine.* Retrieved from http://emedicine.medscape.com/article/259165-overview

Mattson, S., & Smith, J. E. (2016). *Core curriculum for maternal-newborn nursing* (5th ed.). Philadelphia, PA: Elsevier Health Sciences.

McCarthy, F. P., & Kenny, L. C. (2014). Induction of labor. *Obstetrics, Gynecology & Reproductive Medicine, 24*(1), 9–15.

Mehlman, C. T. (2015). Neonatal brachial plexus palsy. *The pediatric upper extremity* (pp. 589–605). New York: Springer Publishers.

Moore, L. E. (2017). Amniotic fluid embolism. *eMedicine.* Retrieved from http://emedicine.medscape.com/article/253068-overview#a5

Moses, S. (2018). *Amniotic fluid embolism. Family Practice Notebook.* Retrieved from http://www.fpnotebook.com/Lung/OB/AmntcFldEmblsm.htm

Nagtalon-Ramos, J. (2014). *Best evidence-based practices: Maternal-newborn nursing care.* Philadelphia, PA: F.A. Davis Company.

Nahum, G. G., & Pham, K. Q. (2018). Uterine rupture in pregnancy. *eMedicine.* Retrieved from http://emedicine.medscape.com/article/275854-overview

Nakazawa, H., Uchida, A., Minamitani, T., Makishi, A., Takamatsu, Y., Kiyoshi, K., ... Funakoshi, T. (2015). Factors affecting maternal serum magnesium levels during long-term magnesium sulfate tocolysis in singleton and twin pregnancy. *Journal of Obstetrics & Gynecology Research, 41*(8), 1178–1184.

Norwitz, E. R. (2018). Cesarean delivery on maternal request. *UpToDate.* Retrieved from http://www.uptodate.com/contents/cesarean-delivery-on-maternal-request

Olsen, N. S., & Karjane, N. W. (2017). Abnormal labor. *eMedicine.* Retrieved from http://emedicine.medscape.com/article/273053-overview

Optimal Birth BC. (2010). *Diagnosis of labour dystocia: Systematic review.* Retrieved from https://optimalbirthbc. ca/wp-content/uploads/2013/08/2-LabourDystocia_Sept28_2010.pdf

Patel, P. K., Pitre, D. S., & Bhooker, S. P. (2015). Predictive value of various risk factors for preterm labor. *Community Medicine, 6*(1), 121–125.

Public Health Agency of Canada. (2013). *Perinatal health indicators for Canada 2013: A report from the Canadian perinatal surveillance system.* Retrieved from http://publications.gc.ca/collections/collection_2014/aspc-phac/HP7-1-2013-eng.pdf

Public Health Agency of Canada (PHAC). (2018). Chapter 4: Care during labour and birth. In *Family-Centred Maternity and Newborn Care: National Guidelines.* Retrieved from https://www.canada.ca/en/public-health/services/publications/healthy-living/maternity-newborn-care-guidelines-chapter-4.html.

Robinson, G. E. (2014). Pregnancy loss. *Best Practice & Research Clinical Obstetrics & Gynecology, 28*(1), 169–178.

Ross, M. G. (2018). Preterm labor. *eMedicine.* Retrieved from https://emedicine.medscape.com/article/260998-overview#aw2aab6b7.

Rowe, T. (2014). Placenta previa. *Journal of Obstetrics and Gynaecology Canada, 36*(8), 667–668.

Sadera, G., & Vasudevan, B. (2015). Amniotic fluid embolism. *Journal of Obstetric Anesthesia and Critical Care, 5*(1), 3–8.

Saint Louis, H. (2017). Cesarean delivery. *eMedicine.* Retrieved from http://emedicine.medscape.com/article/263424-overview

Sciscione, A. C. (2014). Methods of cervical ripening and labor induction: Mechanical. *Clinical Obstetrics and Gynecology, 57*(2), 369–376.

Scott, J. R. (2015). Vaginal birth after cesarean. *Protocols for high-risk pregnancies: An evidence-based approach* (6th ed., pp. 428–432). Hoboken, NJ: John Wiley & Sons.

Sharshiner, R., & Silver, R. M. (2015). Management of fetal malpresentation. *Clinical Obstetrics and Gynecology, 58*(2), 246–255.

Skoll, A., Boutin, A., Bujold, E., Burrows, J., Crane, J., Geary M, ... Joseph, K. S. (2018). SOGC clinical practice guideline No. 364: Antenatal corticosteroid therapy for improving neonatal outcomes. *J Obstetrics & Gynaecology Canada, 40*(9), 1219–1239.

Soni, A., Vaishnav, G. D., & Gohil, J. (2015). Meconium and its significance and obstetric outcome. *Medicine Science International Medical Journal, 4*(1), 1861–1868.

Sosa, C. G., Althabe, F., Belizan, J. M., & Bergel, E. (2015). Bed rest in singleton pregnancies for preventing preterm birth. *Cochrane Database of Systematic Reviews, 30*(3), CD003581.

Sotiriadis, A., Tsiami, A., Papatheodorou, S., Baschat, A. A., Sarafidis, K., & Makrydimas, G. (2015). Neurodevelopmental outcome after a single course of antenatal steroids in children born preterm: A systematic review and meta-analysis. *Obstetrics & Gynecology, 125*(6), 1385–1396.

Souka, A. P., Papastefanou, I., Papadopoulos, G., Chrelias, C., & Kassanos, D. (2015). Cervical length in late second and third trimester: A mixture model for predicting delivery. *Ultrasound in Obstetrics & Gynecology, 45*(3), 308–312.

Sousou, J., & Smart, C. (2015). Care of the childbearing family with intrauterine fetal demise. *Nursing for Women's Health, 19*(3), 236–246.

Statistics Canada. (2018). *Live births and fetal deaths (stillbirths), by type (single or multiple), Canada, provinces and territories (CANSIM Table 102–4515).* Retrieved from https://www150.statcan.gc.ca/t1/tbl1/en/tv.action?pid=1310042801

Sue-A-Quan, A. K, Hannah, M. E., Cohen, M. M., Foster, G. A., & Liston, R. M. (1999). Effect of labour induction on rates of stillbirth and cesarean section in postterm pregnancies. *Canadian Medical Association Journal, 160*, 1145–1149.

Suzuki, S. (2015). Clinical significance of precipitous labor. *Journal of Clinical Medicine Research, 7*(3), 150–153.

van Baaren, G. J., Bruijn, M. M., Vis, J. Y., Wilms, F. F., Oudijk, M. A., Kwee, A., ... Mol, B. W. (2015). Risk factors for preterm delivery: Do they add to fetal fibronectin testing and cervical length measurement in the prediction of preterm delivery in symptomatic women?. *European Journal of Obstetrics & Gynecology and Reproductive Biology, 192*, 79–85.

van Baaren, G. J., Vis, J. Y., Wilms, F. F., Oudijk, M. A., Kwee, A., Porath, M. M., ... Mol, B. W. (2014). Predictive value of cervical length measurement and fibronectin testing in threatened preterm labor. *Obstetrics & Gynecology, 123*(6), 1185–1192.

van den Bosch, A. E., Ruys, T. P., & Roos-Hesselink, J. W. (2015). Use and impact of cardiac medication during pregnancy. *Future Cardiology, 11*(1), 89–100.

Viswanathan, M., Venkateswaran, V. K., & Daniel, S. (2014). Amniotic fluid embolism: A comprehensive review. *International Journal of Reproduction, Contraception, Obstetrics and Gynecology, 3*(2), 304–309.

Vogel, J. P., Gulmezoglu, A. M., Hofmeyr, G. J., & Temmerman, M. (2014). Global perspectives on elective induction of labor. *Clinical Obstetrics and Gynecology, 57*(2), 331–342.

Walker, N., & Gan, J. H. (2015). Prolonged pregnancy. *Obstetrics, Gynecology & Reproductive Medicine, 25*(3), 83–87.

Westwood, S., King, A., Almack, K., Suen, Y. T., & Bailey, L. (2015). Good practice in health and social care provision for LGBT older people in the UK. In J. Fish, & K. Karban (Eds.). *Lesbian, gay, bisexual and trans health inequalities: International perspectives in social work* (pp. 145–158). Chicago, IL: Policy Press.

World Health Organization. (2010). *International statistical classification of diseases and related health problems, 10th revision.* Retrieved from https://www.who.int/classifications/icd/ICD10Volume2_en_2010.pdf

World Health Organization [WHO]. (2014a). *Managing complications in pregnancy and childbirth: A guide for midwives and doctors.* Retrieved from http://www.who.int/maternal_child_adolescent/documents/9241545879/en/

World Health Organization [WHO]. (2014b). *WHO recommendations for augmentation of labor.* Retrieved from http://apps.who.int/iris/bitstream/10665/112825/1/9789241507363_eng.pdf

CHAPTER **WORKSHEET**

MULTIPLE-CHOICE QUESTIONS

1. When reviewing the medical record of a postpartum client, the nurse notes that the client has a condition in which the fetus could not physically pass through the pelvis. The nurse interprets this as:
   a. Cervical insufficiency
   b. Contracted pelvis
   c. Maternal disproportion
   d. Fetopelvic disproportion

2. The nurse would anticipate a caesarean birth for a client who has which active infection present at the onset of labour?
   a. Hepatitis
   b. Herpes simplex virus
   c. Toxoplasmosis
   d. Human papillomavirus

3. After a vaginal examination, the nurse determines that the fetus is in an occiput posterior position. The nurse would anticipate that the client will have:
   a. Intense back pain
   b. Frequent leg cramps
   c. Nausea and vomiting
   d. A precipitous birth

4. When assessing the following clients, which would the nurse identify as being at the greatest risk for preterm labour?
   a. Client who had twins in a previous pregnancy
   b. Client living in a large city close to the subway
   c. Client working full time as a computer programmer
   d. Client with a history of a previous preterm birth

5. The rationale for using a prostaglandin gel for a client prior to the induction of labour is to:
   a. Stimulate uterine contractions
   b. Numb cervical pain receptors
   c. Prevent cervical lacerations
   d. Soften and efface the cervix

6. A client who was in active labour and whose cervix had dilated to 4 cm experiences a weakening in the intensity and frequency of contractions and exhibits no further progress in labour. The nurse interprets this as a sign of:
   a. Hypertonic
   b. Precipitate labour
   c. Hypotonic
   d. Dysfunctional labour

7. The nurse is developing a plan of care for a client experiencing dystocia. Which of the following nursing interventions would be the nurse's high priority?
   a. Changing the client's position frequently
   b. Providing comfort measures to the client
   c. Monitoring the fetal heart rate patterns
   d. Keeping the couple informed of the labour progress

8. The nurse is caring for a client experiencing hypertonic uterine dystocia. The client's contractions are erratic in their frequency, duration, and of high intensity. The priority nursing interventions would be to:
   a. Encourage ambulation every 30 minutes
   b. Provide pain relief measures
   c. Monitor the oxytocin infusion rate closely
   d. Prepare the client for an amniotomy

CRITICAL THINKING EXERCISES

1. A 26-year-old multipara is admitted to the labour and birth suite in active labour. After a few hours, the nurse notices a change in the contraction pattern— poor contraction intensity and no progression of cervical dilatation beyond 5 cm. The client keeps asking about her labour progress and appears anxious about "how long this labour is taking."
   a. Based on the nurse's findings, what might you suspect is going on?
   b. How can the nurse address the client's anxiety?
   c. What are the appropriate interventions to change this labour pattern?

2. The client activates the call light and states, "I feel increased wetness down below."
   a. What might be occurring?
   b. How will the nurse confirm the suspicions?
   c. What interventions are appropriate for this finding?

STUDY ACTIVITIES

1. Visit the website of your local or regional perinatal bereavement support program and assess its helpfulness to parents. Is there anything you would add or change?

2. Outline the fetal and client risks of a forceps or vacuum-assisted birth.

3. Describe the risks and benefits to the client and fetus of a vaginal birth after caesarean (VBAC).

BRINGING IT ALL TOGETHER: A CASE STUDY

Tegan is a nulliparous client who is now at 41 3/7 weeks' gestation. Tegan presents for a routine prenatal visit. Fetal well-being is reassuring at this point with FHR 144, active fetal movement, no complaints voiced except for fatigue and a mild backache when standing for long periods of time. Tegan expresses concern about not having yet gone into labour.

Go to thePoint **to find questions to consider about this case.**

22

Nursing Management of the Postpartum Client at Risk

Learning Objectives

Upon completion of the chapter, you will be able to:

1. Examine the major conditions that place the postpartum client at risk.

2. Analyze the risk factors, assessment, preventive measures, and nursing management of common postpartum complications.

3. Differentiate the causes of postpartum hemorrhage based on the underlying pathophysiologic mechanisms.

4. Outline the nurse's role in assessing and managing the care of a client with a thromboembolic condition.

5. Characterize the nursing management of a client who develops a postpartum infection.

6. Compare and contrast at least two affective disorders that can occur after birth, describing specific therapeutic management for each.

Joan gave birth about an hour ago to her fifth baby boy, who weighed 4,536 g (10 lb), and she is resting in bed when the nurse comes in to assess her. She tells the nurse that she feels like there is "something really wet" between her legs. She also feels a bit light-headed. What would the nurse suspect is happening? What findings would support the nurse's suspicion? What should the nurse do first?

INTRODUCTION

The postpartum period is the culmination of the child-bearing experience. Numerous adaptations and adjustments must be made to assimilate the newborn into the established family unit. It is a time designed for recovery, family attachment, and new role development. Typically, recovery from childbirth progresses normally both physiologically and psychologically. Just like everything else in life, the body faces significant changes in the weeks and months following childbirth. It is a time filled with many changes and wide-ranging emotions, and the new parent commonly experiences a great sense of accomplishment. However, the person can experience deviations from the norm, developing a postpartum condition that increases risk.

This chapter addresses the nursing management of the most common conditions that place the postpartum client at risk: hemorrhage, thromboembolic disease, infections, and postpartum affective disorders.

POSTPARTUM HEMORRHAGE

Postpartum hemorrhage (PPH) is a potentially life-threatening complication that can occur after both vaginal and cesarean births. It is the leading cause of maternal death in both developed and developing countries, accounting for about 35% of all maternal deaths. Every year about 14 million individuals globally will experience a PPH or approximately 1 in 20 births (Agency for Healthcare Research and Quality [AHRQ], 2016). A hemorrhage occurs in 5% of all births and is responsible for a major part of maternal mortality. The majority of these deaths occur within 4 hours of childbirth, which indicates that they are a consequence of the third stage of labour management (Crowe & Faulkner, 2014; Ekin et al., 2015).

PPH is defined as a blood loss greater than 500 mL after vaginal birth or more than 1,000 mL after a cesarean birth. However, this definition is arbitrary, because estimates of blood loss at birth are subjective and generally inaccurate. Moreover, average blood loss from birth frequently exceeds 500 or 1,000 mL, and symptoms of hemorrhage or shock from blood loss may be hidden by normal plasma volume increases that occur during pregnancy. Morbidity from PPH can be severe, with sequelae including organ failure, shock, edema, thrombosis, acute respiratory distress, sepsis, anemia, intensive care admissions, and prolonged hospitalization (AHRQ, 2016). A major obstetric hemorrhage is defined as a blood loss of more than 1,500 mL to 2,500 mL or bleeding that requires more than 5 units of transfused blood (Pavord & Maybury, 2015). Hemorrhage is the most common reason postpartum clients are admitted to intensive care units and it is the most preventable cause of maternal death. Timely, accurate identification and initiation of appropriate interventions would improve outcomes (Clapp, 2015). Blood loss that occurs within 24 hours of birth is termed *primary (immediate or early) PPH;* blood loss that occurs 24 hours to 12 weeks after birth is termed *delayed (late) PPH.* A more objective definition of PPH would be any amount of bleeding that places the client in hemodynamic jeopardy.

Pathophysiology

Excessive bleeding can occur at any time between the separation of the placenta and its expulsion or removal. The most common cause of PPH is uterine atony, failure of the uterus to contract and retract after birth. The uterus must remain contracted after birth to control bleeding from the placental site. Uterine atony is responsible for 80% of primary or immediate PPH, while obstetric lacerations, uterine inversion, and rupture compromise about 20% of all primary or early PPHs (Kamel & Mastrogiannis, 2015). Any factor that causes the uterus to relax after birth will cause bleeding—even a full bladder that displaces the uterus.

During the third stage of labour the muscles of the uterus contract downward, causing constriction of the blood vessels that pass through the uterine wall to the placental surface and stopping the flow of blood. This action also causes the placenta to separate from the uterine wall. The absence of uterine contractions may result in excessive blood loss. Uterotonic medications promote uterine contractions to prevent atony and speed delivery of the placenta.

Over the course of pregnancy, maternal blood volume increases as much as 50% (from 4 to 6 L). The plasma volume increases twice as much in comparison to the total red blood cell volume. As a result, hemoglobin and hematocrit fall. The increase in blood volume meets the perfusion demands of the low-resistance uteroplacental unit and provides a reserve for the blood loss that occurs at delivery (Cunningham et al., 2014). Given this increase, the typical signs of hemorrhage (e.g., falling blood pressure, increasing pulse rate, and decreasing urinary output) do not appear until as much as 1,800 to 2,100 mL of blood has been lost. Current evidence on postpartum volume replacement suggests packed red blood cells, fresh frozen plasma, platelets, and recombinant factor VIIa be used for volume replacement (Nagtalon-Ramos, 2014). Clinical manifestations of shock resulting from blood loss are shown in Table 22.1.

In addition, accurate determination of actual blood loss is difficult because of blood pooling inside the uterus, on peripads, mattresses, and the floor. Because no universal clinical standard exists, nurses must remain vigilant, assessing for risk factors and checking clients carefully before the birth attendant leaves the birthing area.

TABLE 22.1	CLINICAL MANIFESTATIONS OF SHOCK DUE TO BLOOD LOSS		
Degree of Shock	Blood Loss (%)	Signs and Symptoms	
Mild	20	Diaphoresis Increased capillary refilling Cool extremities Maternal anxiety	
Moderate	20–40	Tachycardia Postural hypotension Oliguria	
Severe	>40	Hypotension Agitation/confusion Hemodynamic instability	

Adapted from Kolecki, P., & Menckhoff, C. R. (2016). *Hypovolemic shock. eMedicine.* Retrieved from http://emedicine.medscape.com/article/760145-overview; Belfort, M. A. (2018). *Overview of postpartum hemorrhage. UpToDate.* Retrieved from http://www.uptodate.com/contents/overview-of-postpartum-hemorrhage; and Cunningham, F. G., Leveno, K. J., Bloom, S. L., Spong, C., Dashe, J. S., Hoffman, B. L., . . . Sheffield, J. S. (2014). *Williams obstetrics* (24th ed.). New York: McGraw-Hill.

Other causes of PPH include lacerations of the genital tract, episiotomy, retained placental fragments, uterine inversion, coagulation disorders, large for gestational age newborn, failure to progress during the second stage of labour, placenta accreta, induction or augmentation of labour with oxytocin, surgical birth, and hematomas of the vulva, vagina, or subperitoneal areas (Moses, 2015). A helpful way to remember the causes of PPH is by using the 4 T's:

1. **T**one: uterine atony, distended bladder
2. **T**issue: retained placenta and clots; uterine subinvolution
3. **T**rauma: lacerations, hematoma, inversion, rupture
4. **T**hrombin: coagulopathy (pre-existing or acquired)

Tone

Altered uterine muscle tone most commonly results from overdistention of the uterus. Overdistention can be caused by multiple gestation, fetal macrosomia, hydramnios, fetal abnormality, placenta previa, precipitous birth, or retained placental fragments. Other causes might include prolonged or rapid, forceful labour, especially if stimulated by oxytocin; bacterial toxins (e.g., chorioamnionitis, endomyometritis, septicemia); use of anesthesia, especially halothane; and magnesium sulphate used in the treatment of preeclampsia (Jordan, Engstrom, Marfell, & Farley, 2014). Overdistention of the uterus is a major risk factor for **uterine atony,** the most common cause of early PPH, which can lead to hypovolemic shock. A distended bladder can also displace the uterus from the midline to either side, which impedes its ability to contract to reduce bleeding.

Tissue

Uterine contraction and retraction lead to detachment and expulsion of the placenta after birth. Classic signs of placental separation include a small gush of blood with lengthening of the umbilical cord and a slight rise of the uterus in the pelvis. Complete detachment and expulsion of the placenta permit continued contraction and optimal occlusion of blood vessels. Failure of complete placental separation and expulsion leads to retained fragments, which occupy space and prevent the uterus from contracting fully to clamp down on blood vessels; this can lead to hemorrhage. Clots can also occupy space, which inhibits uterine contractions.

After the placenta has been expelled, a thorough inspection is necessary to confirm its intactness; tears or fragments left inside may indicate an accessory lobe or placenta accreta (an uncommon condition in which the chorionic villi adhere to the myometrium, causing the placenta to adhere abnormally to the uterus and not separate and deliver spontaneously). Profuse hemorrhage results because the uterus cannot contract fully.

SUBINVOLUTION OF THE UTERUS

Subinvolution refers to incomplete involution of the uterus or failure to return to its normal size and condition after birth. Typically, subinvolution occurs when the myometrial fibres of the uterus do not contract effectively and causes relaxation. Complications of subinvolution include hemorrhage, pelvic peritonitis, salpingitis, and abscess formation (King et al., 2015). Causes of subinvolution include retained placental fragments, distended bladder, excessive maternal activity prohibiting proper recovery, uterine myoma, and infection. All of these conditions contribute to delayed postpartum bleeding. The clinical picture includes a postpartum fundal height that is higher than expected, with a boggy uterus; the lochia fails to change colours from red to serosa to alba within a few weeks. This condition is usually identified at the client's postpartum examination 4 to 6 weeks after birth with a bimanual vaginal examination or ultrasound. Treatment is directed toward stimulating the uterus to expel fragments with a uterine stimulant, and antibiotics are given to prevent infection.

Trauma

Damage to the genital tract may occur spontaneously or through the manipulations used during birth. Lacerations and hematomas resulting from birth trauma can cause significant blood loss. Hematomas can present as pain or as a change in vital signs disproportionate to the amount of blood loss. Most often, hematoma formation is associated with episiotomy, instrumental birth, or nulliparity. Many hematomas can be prevented with gentle, controlled birth, and appropriate inspection and repair of lacerations or episiotomy (Jordan et al., 2014). **Uterine**

inversion happens when the top of the uterus collapses into the inner cavity due to excessive fundal pressure or pulling on the umbilical cord when the placenta is still firmly attached to the fundus after the infant has been born. Treatment for uterine inversion includes giving uterine relaxants and immediate manual replacement by the health care provider. Additionally, uterine rupture can occur and cause damage to the genital tract and is more common in those with previous cesarean incisions or those who have undergone any procedure resulting in disruption of the uterine wall, including myomectomy, perforation of the uterus during a dilation and curettage (D&C), biopsy, or intrauterine system (IUS) insertion. Classically, its signs and symptoms combine pain, fetal heart rate abnormalities, and vaginal bleeding. Uterine rupture is a catastrophic complication that requires a rapid diagnosis and intervention, but initial clinical manifestations may be nonspecific (Nahum & Pham, 2018).

Trauma can also occur after prolonged or vigorous labour, especially if the uterus has been stimulated with oxytocin or prostaglandins. Trauma can also occur after extrauterine or intrauterine manipulation of the fetus.

Cervical lacerations commonly occur during a forceps delivery or in individuals who have not been able to resist bearing down before the cervix is fully dilated. Vaginal sidewall lacerations are associated with operative vaginal births but may occur spontaneously, especially if the fetal hand presents with the head. Lacerations can arise during manipulations to resolve shoulder dystocia. Lacerations should always be suspected in the face of a contracted uterus with bright-red blood continuing to trickle out of the vagina.

Thrombin

Thrombosis (formation of a blood clot) helps to prevent PPH immediately after birth by providing hemostasis. Fibrin deposits and clots in supplying vessels play a significant role in the hours and days after birth. Disorders that interfere with the clot formation can lead to PPH. Medication used to prevent hemorrhage by stimulating uterine contractions may delay the appearance of coagulation disorders. Coagulopathies should be suspected when postpartum bleeding persists without any identifiable cause (AHRQ, 2016).

Disorders of coagulation are relatively uncommon as a sole cause of PPH. Coagulation disturbances should be suspected in clients with a family history of such abnormalities and those with a history of menorrhagia. Clinical circumstances may also suggest coagulation defect as a cause of PPH. Diagnosis of a coagulation disorder often requires a high index of suspicion and should not be overlooked in the evaluation of obstetric hemorrhage (Yiadom & Carusi, 2015).

Ideally, the client's coagulation status is determined during pregnancy. However, if the client received no prenatal care, coagulation studies should be ordered immediately to determine the current status. Abnormal results typically include decreased platelet and fibrinogen levels; increased prothrombin time, partial thromboplastin time, and fibrin degradation products; and a prolonged bleeding time (Cunningham et al., 2014). Selected conditions associated with coagulopathies in the postpartum client include idiopathic thrombocytopenic purpura, von Willebrand disease (vWD), and disseminated intravascular coagulation (DIC).

IDIOPATHIC THROMBOCYTOPENIA PURPURA

Idiopathic thrombocytopenia purpura (ITP) is an autoimmune disorder of increased platelet destruction caused by autoantibodies, which can increase the risk of hemorrhaging. There is a decrease in the number of circulating platelets in the absence of toxic exposure or a disease associated with a low platelet count. It is most common in young people during childbearing age and may be associated with maternal and fetal complications. The incidence of ITP in adults is approximately 66 cases per 1,000,000 per year (Silverman, 2017). Glucocorticoids and immune globulin are the mainstays of medical therapy (Kessler, 2018).

VON WILLEBRAND DISEASE

vWD is a congenital bleeding disorder that is inherited as an autosomal dominant trait. It is characterized by a prolonged bleeding time, a deficiency of von Willebrand factor, and impairment of platelet adhesion (CDC, 2018c). It is the most common hereditary bleeding disorder, affecting approximately 1% of the general population (National Hemophilia Foundation, 2018). Although vWD is thought to affect men and women equally, it is diagnosed more frequently in women because of menorrhagia, and it is more common among White women than African-American women (American College of Obstetricians and Gynecologists [ACOG], 2017). Most cases remain undiagnosed due to lack of awareness, difficulty in diagnosis, a tendency to attribute bleeding to other causes, and variable symptoms.

The most common symptoms of vWD include bleeding gums, easy bruising, menorrhagia, blood in urine and stools, nosebleeds, and hematomas. Prolonged bleeding from trivial wounds, oral cavity bleeding, and excessive menstrual bleeding are common. Gastrointestinal bleeding is rare. During pregnancy, the von Willebrand factor level generally increases; thus, labour and birth usually proceed normally. However, all clients should be monitored for excessive bleeding, particularly during the first week postpartum (Pollak, 2018).

DISSEMINATED INTRAVASCULAR COAGULATION

DIC is a life-threatening, acquired coagulopathy in which the clotting system is abnormally activated, resulting in widespread clot formation in the small vessels throughout the body, which leads to the depletion of platelets and coagulation factors. This is why DIC is also known as consumption coagulopathy.

DIC is not itself a specific illness; rather it is always a secondary diagnosis that occurs as a complication of abruptio placentae, amniotic fluid embolism, intrauterine fetal death with prolonged retention of the fetus, acute fatty liver of pregnancy, severe preeclampsia, HELLP syndrome (hemolysis, i.e., the breakdown of red blood cells, elevated liver enzymes, and low platelet count), septicemia, and PPH. Clinical features include petechiae, ecchymoses, bleeding gums, fever, hypotension, acidosis, hematomas, tachycardia, proteinuria, uncontrolled bleeding during birth, and acute renal failure (Levi & Schmaier, 2018). Treatment goals are to maintain tissue perfusion through aggressive administration of fluid therapy, oxygen, heparin, and blood products. The most important treatment concept in DIC is that it is a secondary manifestation of an underlying disorder. The most important therapeutic manoeuvre is treating the initiating disorder. After treating the underlining cause, DIC will disappear, and the coagulation status will then become normalize. Without this, supportive measures ultimately fail (Erez, Mastrolia, & Thachil, 2015).

Therapeutic Management

Prompt diagnosis and understanding of the underlying triggers of this complication is essential for a favourable outcome. Team work and prompt treatment are essential for the successful management of a client with DIC. Therapeutic management focuses on the underlying cause of the hemorrhage. For example, uterine massage is used to treat uterine atony. If retained placental fragments are the cause, the fragments are usually manually separated and removed, and a uterine stimulant is given to promote the uterus to expel fragments. Antibiotics are administered to prevent infection. Lacerations are sutured or repaired. Glucocorticoids and intravenous immunoglobulin, intravenous anti-RhoD, and platelet transfusions may be given for ITP. Perinatal management of ITP should also include maintenance of maternal platelet count and regular monitoring of fetal growth along with prediction and prevention of fetal passive immune thrombocytopenia (Silverman, 2017).

The mainstays of therapy for vWD are desmopressin and plasma concentrates that contain von Willebrand factor. Delayed PPH may occur, despite adequate prophylaxis. Frequent monitoring and continued prophylaxis and/or treatment are recommended for at least 2 weeks after childbirth (Pollak, 2018).

Nursing Assessment

Most affected individuals will not have identifiable risk factors. Nonetheless, primary prevention of a PPH begins with an assessment of identifiable risk factors. Pregnancy and childbirth involve significant health risks, even for clients with no pre-existing health problems. In the Canada, where most births occur in hospitals and where resources are likely to be available as compared with developing countries, PPH still continues to be among the top causes of maternal deaths. Retrospective studies of these events suggest that some cases are preventable. As with many other sources of perinatal harm, delays in recognition, diagnosis, and treatment, problems with hierarchy and communication, and lack of knowledge, policies, and protocols were often cited as contributing factors (Shields, Wiesner, Fulton, & Pelletreau, 2015).

The period after the birth and the first hours postpartum are crucial times for the prevention, assessment, and management of bleeding. Compared with other maternal risks such as infection, bleeding can rapidly become life threatening, and nurses, along with other health care providers, need to identify this condition quickly and intervene appropriately.

Begin by reviewing the client's history, including labour and birth history, for risk factors associated with PPH (Table 22.2). The incidence of PPH has been rising, though the mortality has come down, suggesting improvement in the management of this condition. Although specific risk factors have been identified, PPH is often unanticipated and still occurs in approximately 5% of all births and increasing (Ekin et al., 2015).

Since the most common cause of immediate severe PPH is uterine atony (failure of the uterus to contract properly after birth), assess uterine tone after birth by palpating the fundus for firmness and location. A soft, boggy fundus indicates uterine atony.

Take Note!

A soft, boggy uterus that deviates from the midline suggests that a full bladder is interfering with uterine involution. If the uterus is not in correct position (midline), it will not be able to contract to control bleeding.

Assess the amount of bleeding. Visual estimation is the most frequently practiced method of determining blood loss during childbirth in the United States, and the results are usually included in the documentation of events pertaining to the birth. This method is used despite repeated studies showing its inaccuracy and underestimation. Weighing or counting peripads or using a Signaling a Postpartum Hemorrhage Emergency (SAPHE) mat would provide a more accurate estimate of blood loss. The mat was constructed so that each square on the mat would absorb up to 50 mL of blood. Blood loss is then calculated by multiplying the number of blood-saturated squares by 50 mL (Wilcox et al., 2015). In any method used, nurses should consult their hospital protocols and follow them. If bleeding continues even though there are no lacerations, suspect retained

TABLE 22.2	FACTORS PLACING A CLIENT AT RISK FOR POSTPARTUM HEMORRHAGE
Clinical Risk Factors	**Associated Clinical Conditions**
Tone (abnormalities of uterine contractions)	
Overdistention of uterus	Polyhydramnios Multifetal gestation Macrosomia
Uterine muscle exhaustion	Rapid labour Prolonged labour Oxytocin use
Uterine infection	Maternal fever Prolonged rupture of membranes
Tissue (retained in uterus)	
Products of conception	Incomplete placenta at birth
Retained blood clots	Atonic uterus
Trauma (of the genital tract)	
Lacerations anywhere	Precipitate birth or operative birth
Laceration extensions	Malposition of fetus Previous uterine surgery
Uterine inversion	Forceful pulling when placenta isn't separated yet; traction on the cord when uterus isn't contracted
Thrombin (coagulation abnormalities)	
Pre-existing conditions	Hereditary inheritance Hemophilia von Willebrand disease History of previous PPH Acquired in pregnancy Idiopathic thrombocytopenia purpura Bruising, elevated blood pressure Disseminated intravascular coagulation

Adapted from Centers for Disease Control and Prevention (CDC). (2018c). *Facts about von Willebrand Disease*. Retrieved from http://www.cdc.gov/ncbddd/vwd/facts.html; King, T. L., Brucker, M. C., Kriebs, J. M., Fahey, J. O., Gegor, C. L., & Varney, H. (2015). *Varney's midwifery* (5th ed.). Burlington, MA: Jones & Bartlett Learning; and Mattson, S., & Smith, J. E. (2015). *Core curriculum for maternal-newborn nursing* (5th ed.). St. Louis, MO: Saunders Elsevier.

placental fragments. The uterus remains large with painless, dark-red bleeding mixed with clots. This cause of hemorrhage can be prevented by carefully inspecting the placenta for intactness.

If trauma is suspected, attempt to identify the source and document it. Typically, the uterus will be firm with a steady stream or trickle of unclotted bright-red blood noted in the perineum. Most deaths from PPH are not due to gross bleeding, but rather to inadequate management of slow, steady blood loss (Clapp, 2015).

Assess for hematoma which may require surgical treatment. The uterus would be firm, with bright-red bleeding. Observe for a localized bluish bulging area just under the skin surface in the perineal area (Fig. 22.1). Often the client will report severe perineal or pelvic pain and will have difficulty voiding, and may exhibit

hypotension, tachycardia, and anemia. Frequently, the health care provider will incise the skin bulge to evacuate the hematoma of trapped blood. A pressure dressing is applied to this area to prevent further bleeding (Green, 2016).

Inspect the skin and mucous membranes for gingival bleeding or petechiae and ecchymoses. Check venipuncture sites for oozing or prolonged bleeding. These findings might suggest a coagulopathy as a cause of PPH. Also assess the amount of lochia, which would be much greater than usual. Urinary output would be diminished, with signs of acute renal failure. Vital signs would show an increased pulse rate and a decreased level of consciousness. However, signs of shock do not appear until hemorrhage is far advanced due to the increased fluid and blood volume of pregnancy.

FIGURE 22.1 Perineal hematoma. Note the bulging swollen mass.

Nursing Management

When excessive bleeding is encountered, initial management steps are aimed at improving uterine tone with immediate fundal massage, intravenous fluid resuscitation, and administration of uterotonic medications. If these methods fail to control bleeding, additional resources are mobilized and more aggressive interventions such as bimanual compression, internal uterine packing, and/or balloon tamponade techniques are employed by the health care provider. Other potential causes of bleeding should be thoroughly explored, and laboratory tests such as a complete blood count, type and cross-match, and coagulations studies should be obtained immediately. Transfusion of blood products should be instituted without hesitation once estimates of bleeding reach 1,500 mL (Nagtalon-Ramos, 2014).

Take Note!

Before initiating fundal massage, the nurse must first place a hand over the symphysis pubis to anchor the uterus and prevent possible uterine inversion.

Clearly, in all cases of unexpected hemorrhage, the interventions discussed as follows must be performed without delay. PPH is best managed by using a stepwise progressive approach. Manual message and pharmacologic therapies are first-line treatments. If the bleeding continues, second-line interventions might include the use of intrauterine balloon (or gauze) tamponade and uterine compression sutures. If these second-line therapies still don't stop the bleeding, the client may need to undergo radiologic embolization, pelvic

devascularization, or hysterectomy. Peripartum hysterectomy remains the last-resort lifesaving measure and carries with it a higher mortality rate compared with nonobstetric hysterectomy. It is a most demanding obstetric surgery performed under very trying circumstances of life-threatening hemorrhage (Van de Velde, Diez, & Varon, 2015). Moreover, high-volume transfusions are often required, and there are significant postsurgical morbidity risks such as renal failure, hepatic failure, respiratory distress syndrome, coagulopathies, septicemia, tissue hypoxia, and pituitary necrosis (Sheehan syndrome) (Rong, Yuna, & Yan, 2014). PPH outcomes can be improved by thorough preparation, anticipating the risks of PPH, and coordinating consultants for interventional procedures if warranted.

PPH is a serious complication of pregnancy that is often unanticipated. Even with prompt aggressive management, postpartum bleeding can quickly evolve into a life-threatening event. Perinatal nurses are often the first to observe significant postpartum bleeding and their prompt initial response and continued assessments are pivotal in the anticipation and coordination of necessary interventions. Multidisciplinary team support is critical because obstetric caregivers need a full array of medical and surgical strategies to manage intractable bleeding. Because all postpartum clients are at risk for hemorrhage, nurses need to possess the knowledge and skills to practice active management of the third stage of labour to prevent hemorrhage and to recognize, assess, and respond rapidly to excessive blood loss in their clients.

Massage the Uterus

Massage the uterus if uterine atony is noted. The uterine muscles are sensitive to touch; massage stimulates the muscle fibres to contract. Massage the boggy uterus to stimulate contractions and expression of any accumulated blood clots while supporting the lower uterine segment. As blood pools in the vagina, stasis of blood causes clots to form. These clots need to be expelled as pressure is placed on the fundus. Note, however, that overly forceful massage can tire the uterine muscles, resulting in further uterine atony and increased pain. See Nursing Procedure 22.1 for the steps in massaging the fundus.

Administer a Uterotonic Drug

Administer a uterotonic drug if repeated fundal massage and expression of clots fail, medication is probably needed to cause the uterus to contract in order to control bleeding from the placental site. The injection of a uterotonic drug immediately after birth is an important intervention used to prevent PPH. Oxytocin (Pitocin);

NURSING PROCEDURE 22.1

Massaging the Fundus

Purpose: To Promote Uterine Contraction

1. After explaining the procedure to the client, place one gloved hand on the area above the symphysis pubis (this helps to support the lower uterine segment).

2. Place the other gloved hand (usually the dominant hand) on the fundus.

3. With the hand on the fundus, gently massage the fundus in a circular manner. Be careful not to over massage the fundus, which could lead to muscle fatigue and uterine relaxation.

4. Assess for uterine firmness (uterine tissue responds quickly to touch).

5. If firm, apply gentle yet firm pressure in a downward motion toward the vagina to express any clots that may have accumulated.

6. Do not attempt to express clots until the fundus is firm because the application of firm pressure on an uncontracted uterus could cause uterine inversion, leading to massive hemorrhage.

7. Assist the client with perineal care and applying a new perineal pad.

8. Remove gloves and wash hands.

a synthetic analogue of prostaglandin E1, misoprostol (Cytotec) or dinoprostone (Prostin E2); methylergonovine maleate (Methergine); and a derivative of prostaglandin (PGF2α), carboprost (Hemabate), are drugs used to manage PPH (Drug Guide 22.1). However, misoprostol is not approved by Health Canada for this purpose. The choice of which uterotonic drug to use for management of bleeding depends on the judgment of the health care provider, the availability of drugs, and the risks and benefits of the drug.

All nurses need to be aware of the contraindications of administering each of the medications used to control PPH as follows:

- *Pitocin*—never give undiluted as a bolus injection intravenously
- *Cytotec*—allergy, active cardiovascular disease, pulmonary or hepatic disease
- *Prostin E2*—active cardiac, pulmonary, renal, or hepatic disease
- *Methergine*—if the client is hypertensive, do not administer.
- *Hemabate*—contraindicated with asthma due to risk of bronchial spasm

Remember Joan, the woman described at the beginning of the chapter? The nurse assesses her and finds that her uterus is boggy. What would the nurse do next? What additional nursing measures might be used if Joan's fundus remains boggy? When should the health care provider be notified?

Maintain the Primary Intravenous Infusion

Maintain the primary intravenous infusion and be prepared to start a second infusion at another site if blood transfusions are necessary. Draw blood for type and cross-match and send it to the laboratory. Administer oxytocics as ordered, correlating and titrating the infusion rate to assessment findings of uterine firmness and lochia. Assess for visible vaginal bleeding, and count or weigh perineal pads.

Take Note!

PPH outcomes can be improved by thorough preparation, anticipating the risks factors of PPH in every client admitted, and coordinating consultants for interventional procedures if warranted.

DRUG GUIDE 22.1 DRUGS USED TO CONTROL POSTPARTUM HEMORRHAGE

Drug	Action/Indication	Nursing Implications
Oxytocin (Pitocin) First-line therapy	Stimulates the uterus to contract to control bleeding from the placental site 20–40 units in a litre IV Or 10 units IM	Assess fundus for evidence of contraction and compare amount of bleeding every 15 minutes or according to orders. Monitor vital signs every 15 minutes. Monitor uterine tone to prevent hyperstimulation. Reassure client about the need for uterine contraction and administer analgesics for comfort. Offer explanation to client and family about what is happening and the purpose of the medication. Provide nonpharmacologic comfort measures to assist with pain management. Set up the IV infusion to be piggybacked into a primary IV line. This ensures that the medication can be discontinued readily if hyperstimulation or adverse effects occur while maintaining the IV site and primary infusion.
Misoprostol (Cytotec)	Stimulates the uterus to contract/ to reduce bleeding; a prosta- glandin analogue 800 mcg per rectum, one dose (range, 400–1,000 mcg)	Contraindications: never give undiluted as a bolus injection IV. As above. Not FDA approved for this indication, but a very effective drug therapy for acute postpartum hemorrhage. Contraindications: allergy, active CVD, pulmonary or hepatic disease; use with caution in individuals with asthma.
Dinoprostone (Prostin E2)	20 mg vaginal or rectal suppository May be repeated every 2 hours.	Monitor blood pressure frequently since hypotension is a frequent side effect along with vomiting and diarrhea, nausea, temperature elevation.
Methylergono- vine maleate (Methergine) Ergonovine Maleate	Stimulates the uterus/to prevent and treat postpartum hem- orrhage due to atony or subinvolution. 0.2 mg IM injection May be repeated in 5 minutes Thereafter every 2–4 hours	Assess baseline bleeding, uterine tone, and vital signs every 15 minutes or according to protocol. Offer explanation to client and family about what is happening and the purpose of the medication. Monitor for possible adverse effects, such as hypertension, seizures, uterine cramping, nausea, vomiting, and palpitations. Report any complaints of chest pain promptly. Contraindications: Hypertension, cardiovascular disease
Prostaglandin (PGF2α), Carboprost, (Hema- bate)	Stimulates uterine contractions/ to treat postpartum hemorrhage due to uterine atony when not controlled by other methods. 0.25 mg IM injection May be repeated every 15–90 minutes up to 8 doses. Stimulates uterine contractions to reduce bleeding when not controlled by the first-line therapy of oxytocin.	Assess vital signs, uterine contractions, client's comfort level, and bleeding status as per protocol. Offer explanation to client and family about what is happening and the purpose of the medication. Monitor for possible adverse effects, such as fever, chills, headache, nausea, vomiting, diarrhea, flushing, and bronchospasm. Contraindications: asthma or active cardiovascular disease Same as above Contraindications: active cardiac, pulmonary, renal, or hepatic disease
Tranexamic acid (Cyklokapron)	To stop prolonged bleeding and for blood clotting. Given to prevent PPH in someone with a known bleeding disorder. 10 mg/kg IV	Nausea, vomiting, diarrhea, dizziness. Contraindications: a history of blood clots or if taking anticoagulants

Adapted from Callahan, T. L. (2016). *Tarascon's OB/GYN pocketbook*. Burlington, MA: Jones & Bartlett Learning; Bohlmann, M., & Rath, W. (2014). Medical prevention and treatment of postpartum hemorrhage: A comparison of different guidelines. *Archives of Gynecology & Obstetrics, 289*(3), 555–567; Skidmore-Roth, L. (2015). *Mosby's 2015 nursing drug reference* (28th ed.). St. Louis, MO: Mosby Elsevier; and World Health Organization. (2017). *Updated WHO recommendation on tranexamic acid for the treatment of postpartum haemorrhage*. Retrieved from http://apps.who.int/iris/bitstream/handle/10665/259379/WHO-RHR-17.21-eng.pdf;jsessionid=6C1BBE9273754FFBA301457370D9E5B1?sequence=1; https://www.drugs.com/pro/cyklokapron.html

Check Vital Signs

Check vital signs every 15 to 30 minutes, depending on the acuity of the client's health status. Monitor the complete blood count to identify any deficit or assess the adequacy of replacement. Assess the client's level of consciousness to determine changes that may result from inadequate cerebral perfusion.

A Foley catheter is typically in place to keep the bladder empty to avoid displacement of the uterus. A fundus above the umbilicus and deviated laterally indicates a full bladder and interferes with uterine contractions to slow the bleeding.

Prepare the Client for Removal of Retained Placental Fragments

Prepare the client for removal of retained placental fragments. These fragments usually are manually separated and removed by the health care provider. Be sure that the health care provider remains long enough after birth to assess the bleeding status and determine the etiology. Assist the health care provider with suturing any lacerations immediately to control hemorrhage and repair the tissue.

Nurses should anticipate and prepare the client for transfer to the operating room for surgical intervention if tamponade techniques fail to achieve hemostasis. The blood bank should be notified that additional transfusions may be required and the client closely monitored for signs of hypovolemic shock.

Continually Assess the Client for Signs and Symptoms of Hemorrhagic Shock

Continually assess the woman for signs and symptoms of hemorrhagic shock, a condition in which inadequate perfusion of organs results in insufficient availability of oxygen to satisfy the metabolic needs of the tissues (Green, 2016). Hemorrhagic shock is the most common form of shock encountered in obstetric practice. Subsequently, a catabolic state develops, leading to inflammation, endothelial dysfunction, and disruption of normal metabolic processes in vital organs. Once these events become established, the process of shock is often irreversible, even if volume and red blood cell deficits are corrected. The main goals of treatment of hemorrhagic shock include fluid resuscitation, correction of the imbalance between oxygen delivery and consumption, and treating DIC (Tánczos, Németh, & Molnár, 2015).

A PPH is a traumatic experience because medical complications are unexpected during what is anticipated as a joyful time. Assess the client's anxiety level; the individual going into hypovolemic shock is highly anxious and may lose consciousness. The client's significant others experience a high level of anxiety as well and need a great deal of support.

Monitor blood pressure, pulse, capillary refill, mental status, and urinary output. These assessments allow estimation of the severity of blood loss and help direct treatment. If the client develops hemorrhagic shock, interventions focus on controlling the source of blood loss; restoring adequate oxygen-carrying capacity; and maintaining adequate tissue perfusion. Successful treatment depends on efficient collaboration among all health care team members to meet the client's specific needs.

For the client with ITP, expect to administer glucocorticoids, intravenous immunoglobulin, intravenous anti-RhoD, and platelet transfusions. Prepare the client for a splenectomy if the bleeding tissues do not respond to medical management. Be alert for abnormal bleeding tendencies, ensuring that they receive proper diagnosis and treatment. Teach them how to prevent severe hemorrhage by learning how to feel for and massage their fundus when boggy, assisting the nurse to keep track of the extent of bleeding on perineal pads, and avoiding any medications with antiplatelet activity such as aspirin, antihistamines, or nonsteroidal anti-inflammatory drugs (NSAIDs).

Institute Emergency Measures If DIC Develops

If the client develops DIC, institute emergency measures to control bleeding and impending shock and prepare for transfer to the intensive care unit. Identification of the underlying condition and elimination of the causative factor are essential to correct the coagulation problem. Be ready to replace fluid volume, administer blood component therapy, and optimize oxygenation and perfusion status to ensure adequate cardiac output and end-organ perfusion. Continually reassess the client's coagulation status via laboratory studies.

Monitor vital signs closely, being alert for changes that signal an increase in bleeding or impending shock. Observe for early signs of ecchymosis, including spontaneous bleeding from gums or nose, petechiae, excessive bleeding from the cesarean incision site or intravenous site, hematuria, and blood in the stool. Late signs include progressive changes in vital signs, skin colour, and reduction of urinary output. Collectively, these findings correlate with decreased blood volume, decreased organ and peripheral tissue perfusion, and clots in the microcirculation (Levi & Schmaier, 2018).

Take Note!

Always remember the five causes of PPH and the appropriate intervention for each: (1) uterine atony—massage and oxytocics; (2) retained placental tissue—evacuation and oxytocics; (3) lacerations or hematoma—surgical repair; (4) thrombin (bleeding disorders)—blood products; and (5) uterine inversion caused by too much cord traction—gentle replacement of uterus and oxytocics.

Institute measures to avoid tissue trauma or injury, such as giving injections and drawing blood. Also provide emotional support to the client and family throughout this critical time by being readily available and providing explanations and reassurance.

Preventing Postpartum Hemorrhage

Avoid an episiotomy unless an emergency birth is necessary and the perineum is a limiting factor. It is important to have the continuous intrapartum presence of an experienced labour and birth nurse. Provide active management of the third stage of labour, including administration of a uterotonic medication after birth of anterior shoulder, controlled and gentle cord traction to deliver the placenta, and uterine massage after the placenta is out. Authors of a Cochrane review concluded that active management of the third stage of labour is associated with reduced blood loss, reduced risk of PPH, and a reduced prolonged third stage of labour (Mousa, Blum, Abou El Senoun, Shakur, & Alfirevic, 2014).

Frequent staff education and PPH drills will help keep skills up to date. Nurses must identify and correct anemia and screen for coagulopathies before labour and birth. After birth, it is important to inspect the placenta (once it is delivered) for completeness. Assess the client for lower genital tract lacerations immediately after birth and reevaluate the vital signs and vaginal flow after childbirth. Finally, it is important to be aware of the client's beliefs about blood transfusions. Recently a workgroup representing all major perinatal health professional organizations developed an obstetric hemorrhage safety bundle for practice to improve PPH outcomes. Some of their selected readiness action domains include:

- Having a hemorrhage cart with supplies and instruction cards on every OB unit
- Having immediate access to medications used to treat a massive hemorrhage
- Establishing a response team within the hospital that can be called
- Developing emergency-release transfusion protocols in the blood bank
- Educating all staff on protocols and holding unit-based drills frequently (Main et al., 2015)

In summary, careful monitoring of the client's vital signs, laboratory tests (in particular, coagulation testing), and immediate diagnosis of the cause of PPH are important key factors to reduce maternal morbidity and mortality. Nurses must always be prepared to identify signs and symptoms of PPH, recognize maternal compromise and, deal with hemorrhage promptly. By identifying hemorrhage promptly and providing swift interventions, maternal mortality and morbidity can be reduced.

An intravenous oxytocin infusion is started for Joan. What assessments will need to be done frequently to make sure Joan is not losing too much blood? What discharge instructions need to be reinforced with Joan?

VENOUS THROMBOEMBOLIC CONDITIONS

Venous thromboembolism is one of the leading causes of maternal mortality and morbidity with an annual incidence of one per 1,000 pregnancies, a 10 times higher risk than the nonpregnant population (Testa et al., 2015). A thrombosis (blood clot within a blood vessel) can cause an inflammation of the blood vessel lining (thrombophlebitis), which in turn can lead to a thromboembolism (obstruction of a blood vessel by a blood clot carried by the circulation from the site of origin). Thrombi can involve the superficial or deep veins in the legs or pelvis. Superficial venous thrombosis usually involves the saphenous venous system and is confined to the lower leg. Superficial thrombophlebitis may be caused by the use of the lithotomy position during birth. Deep venous thrombosis (DVT) can involve deep veins from the foot to the calf, to the thighs, or pelvis. In both locations, thrombi can dislodge and migrate to the lungs, causing a pulmonary embolism (PE).

DVT is a common condition that can have serious complications. Deep venous thrombi have a high probability of propagating and leading to pulmonary emboli, which may cause chest pain, breathlessness, and sudden death. Thus, an accurate and timely diagnosis of DVT is imperative. Although DVT is often clinically silent, it may present with a number of signs, including calf pain, edema, and venous distention.

The three most common venous thromboembolic conditions occurring during the postpartum period are superficial venous thrombosis, DVT, and PE. Although venous thromboembolic disorders occur in less than 1% of all postpartum clients, pulmonary embolus can be fatal if a clot obstructs the lung circulation; thus, early identification and treatment are paramount. Risk for postpartum venous thromboembolism is highest during the first 3 weeks after childbirth. Individuals with obstetric complications are at highest risk for this, and this risk remains elevated throughout the first 12 weeks postpartum (Tepper et al., 2014).

Pathophysiology

Thrombus (blood clot) formation typically results from venous stasis, injury to the innermost layer of the blood vessel, and hypercoagulation. Venous stasis and hypercoagulation are both common in the postpartum period.

If a clot dislodges and travels to the pulmonary circulation, PE can occur. PE is a potentially fatal condition that occurs when the pulmonary artery is blocked by a blood clot that has travelled from another vein into the lungs, causing an obstruction and infarction. When the clot is large enough to block one or more of the pulmonary vessels that supply the lungs, it can result in sudden death. Approximately 600,000 PEs occur yearly in the United States, resulting in 60,000 to 100,000 deaths (CDC, 2018a). Only 25% of all clients with PE are actually diagnosed, indicating that thousands of PEs go undetected. Many deaths due to PE are unrecognized and the diagnosis is often made at autopsy. PE is the leading cause of pregnancy-related death in the United States, occurring in 2 out of 100,000 live births. It most commonly occurs up to 3 weeks postpartum and following a surgical birth (Conti et al., 2014). A national review of severe obstetric complications found a significant increase in the rate of PE associated with the increasing rate of cesarean births. Adequate treatment of thrombotic events in pregnancy is important to prevent progression of thrombosis to the development of PE (Sucker & Zotz, 2015).

Nursing Assessment

Assess the client closely for risk factors and signs and symptoms of thrombophlebitis. Look for risk factors in the client's history such as use of oral contraceptives before the pregnancy; smoking; employment that necessitates prolonged standing; history of thrombosis, thrombophlebitis, or endometritis; or evidence of current varicosities. Also look for other factors that can increase risk, such as prolonged bed rest, diabetes, obesity, cesarean birth, progesterone-induced distensibility of the veins of the lower legs during pregnancy, severe anemia, varicose veins, advanced maternal age (age 35 years or older), and multiparity. The likelihood of thrombophlebitis is increased through most of pregnancy and for approximately 12 weeks after childbirth. This is partly due to increased platelet stickiness and partly due to reduced fibrinolytic activity (Guimicheva, Czuprynska, & Arya, 2015).

Ask the client about pain or tenderness in the lower extremities. Suspect superficial venous thrombosis in a client with varicose veins who reports tenderness and discomfort over the site of the thrombosis, most commonly in the calf area. The area appears reddened along the vein and is warm to the touch. The client will report increased pain in the affected leg when ambulating and bearing weight.

Manifestations of DVT are often absent and diffuse. If present, they are caused by an inflammatory process and obstruction of venous return. Calf swelling, erythema, warmth, tenderness, and pedal edema may be noted. A positive Homans' sign (pain in the upper calf upon dorsiflexion) is not a definitive diagnostic sign as it is insensitive and nonspecific and is no longer recommended as an indicator of DVT. That is because calf pain can also be caused by a strained muscle, contusion, clients with herniated intervertebral discs, calf muscle spasm, neurogenic leg pain, ruptured Baker's cyst, and cellulitis (Heffline & Schmidt, 2014).

Be alert for signs and symptoms of PE, including unexplained sudden onset of shortness of breath and severe chest pain. The client may be apprehensive and diaphoretic. Additional manifestations may include tachypnea, tachycardia, hypotension, syncope, distention of the jugular vein, decreased oxygen saturation (shown by pulse oximetry), cardiac arrhythmias, hemoptysis, and a sudden change in mental status as a result of hypoxemia (Quellette, Harrington, & Kamangar, 2018). Prepare the client for a lung scan to confirm the diagnosis.

Nursing Management

Nursing management focuses on preventing thrombotic conditions, promoting adequate circulation if thrombosis occurs, and educating the client about preventive measures, anticoagulant therapy, and danger signs.

Preventing Thrombotic Conditions

Prevention of thrombotic conditions is an essential aspect of nursing management and can be achieved with the routine use of simple measures:

- Developing public awareness about risk factors, symptoms, and preventive measures
- Preventing venous stasis by encouraging activity that causes leg muscles to contract and promotes venous return (leg exercises and walking)
- Dorsi/plantar flexion of feet with prolonged sitting to promote venous return
- Using intermittent sequential compression devices to produce passive leg muscle contractions until the client is ambulatory
- Elevating the client legs above the heart level to promote venous return
- Stopping smoking to reduce or prevent vascular vasoconstriction
- Applying compression stockings and removing them daily for inspection of legs
- Using postoperative deep-breathing exercises to improve venous return by relieving the negative thoracic pressure on leg veins
- Reducing hypercoagulability with the use of aspirin or anticoagulation therapy
- Preventing venous pooling by avoiding pillows under knees, not crossing legs for long periods, and not leaving legs up in stirrups for long periods
- Padding stirrups to reduce pressure against the popliteal angle
- Avoiding sitting or standing in one position for prolonged periods

- Avoiding trauma to legs to prevent injury to the vein wall
- Increasing fluid intake to prevent dehydration
- Avoiding the use of oral contraceptives

In clients at risk, early ambulation is the easiest and most cost-effective method. Use of compression stockings decreases distal calf vein thrombosis by decreasing venous stasis and augmenting venous return (Wells, Forgie, & Rodger, 2014). Clients who are at a high risk for thromboembolic disease based on risk factors or a previous history of DVT or PE may be placed on prophylactic anticoagulation therapy during pregnancy. A low–molecular-weight heparin such as enoxaparin (Lovenox) can be given or rivaroxaban (Xarelto), apixaban (Eliquis), or dabigatran etexilate (Pradaxa) can be given (Middeldorp, 2015). It is typically discontinued during labour and birth and then restarted during the postpartum period.

Promoting Adequate Circulation

The mainstay of venous thromboembolic conditions is anticoagulation, while interventions such as thrombolysis and inferior vena cava filters are reserved for limited circumstances. For the client with superficial venous thrombosis, administer NSAIDs for analgesia, provide for rest and elevation of the affected leg, apply warm compresses to the affected area to promote healing, and use antiembolism stockings to promote circulation to the extremities.

Implement bed rest or limited ambulation if ordered and elevation of the affected extremity for the client with DVT. These actions help to reduce interstitial swelling and promote venous return from that leg. Apply antiembolism stockings to both extremities as ordered. Fit the stockings correctly to avoid excess pressure and constriction and urge the woman to wear them at all times. Sequential compression devices can also be used for clients with varicose veins, a history of thrombophlebitis, or a surgical birth.

Anticoagulant therapy using a continuous intravenous infusion of low–molecular-weight heparin along with vitamin K antagonists usually is initiated to prolong the clotting time and prevent extension of the thrombosis. Monitor the coagulation studies closely; these might include activated partial thromboplastin time (aPTT), whole-blood partial thromboplastin time, and platelet levels. A therapeutic aPTT value typically ranges from 35 to 45 seconds, depending on which standard values are used (Pagana, Pagana, & Pagana, 2014). Also apply warm moist compresses to the affected leg and administer analgesics as ordered to decrease the discomfort.

After several days of intravenous low–molecular-weight heparin therapy, expect to begin oral anticoagulant therapy as ordered. In most cases, the client will continue to take this medication for several months after discharge.

For the client who develops a PE, institute emergency measures immediately. The objectives of treatment are to prevent growth or multiplication of thrombi in the lower extremities, prevent more thrombi from travelling to the pulmonary vascular system, and provide cardiopulmonary support if needed. Administer oxygen via mask or cannula as ordered and initiate intravenous low–molecular-weight heparin therapy titrated according to the results of the coagulation studies. Maintain the client on bed rest, and administer analgesics as ordered for pain relief. Be prepared to assist with administering thrombolytic agents, such as alteplase (tPA), which might be used to dissolve pulmonary emboli and the source of the thrombus in the pelvis or deep leg veins, thus reducing the potential for a recurrence.

Educating the Client

Provide teaching about the use of anticoagulant therapy and danger signs that should be reported (Teaching Guidelines 22.1). Provide anticipatory guidance, support, and education about associated signs of complications and risks.

Teaching Guidelines 22.1

TEACHING TO PREVENT BLEEDING RELATED TO ANTICOAGULANT THERAPY

- Watch for possible signs of bleeding and notify your health care provider if any occur:
  - Nosebleeds
  - Bleeding from the gums or mouth
  - Black tarry stools
  - Brown "coffee grounds" vomitus
  - Red to brown speckled mucus from a cough
  - Oozing at incision, episiotomy site, cut, or scrape
  - Pink, red, or brown-tinged urine
  - Bruises, "black and blue marks"
  - Increased lochia discharge (from present level)
- Practice measures to reduce your risk of bleeding:
  - Brush your teeth gently using a soft toothbrush.
  - Use an electric razor for shaving.
  - Avoid activities that could lead to injury, scrapes, bruising, or cuts.
  - Do not use any over-the-counter products containing aspirin or aspirin-like derivatives.
  - Avoid consuming alcohol.
  - Inform other health care providers about the use of anticoagulants, especially dentists.
- Be sure to comply with follow-up laboratory testing as scheduled.
- If you accidentally cut or scrape yourself, apply firm direct pressure to the site for 5 to 10 minutes. Do the same after receiving any injections or having blood specimens drawn.

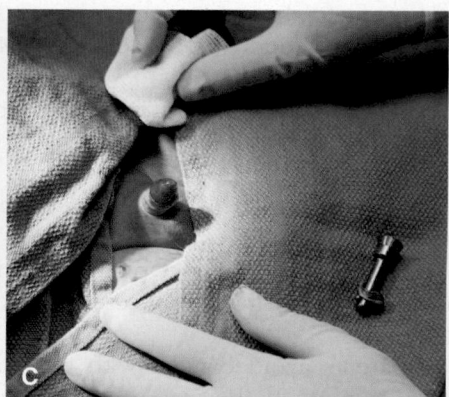

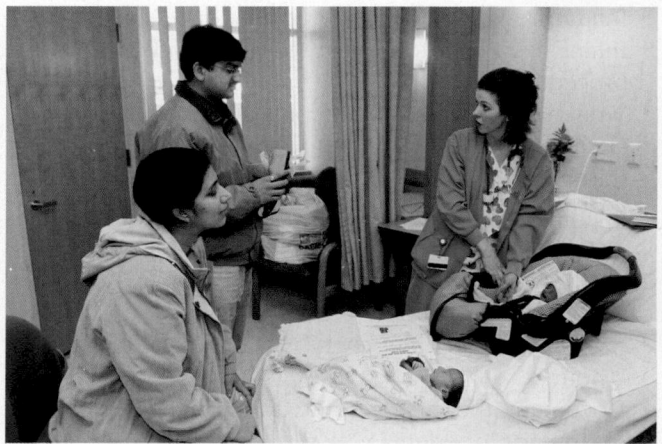

19

KEY TERMS

abortion
abruptio placentae
accreta
eclampsia
ectopic pregnancy
gestational
  hypertension
gestational
  trophoblastic
  disease (GTD)
high-risk pregnancy
hyperemesis
  gravidarum
multiple gestation
oligohydramnios
placenta accreta
placenta previa
polyhydramnios
preeclampsia
premature rupture
  of membranes
  (PROM)
preterm premature
  rupture of
  membranes
  (PPROM)

Nursing Management of Pregnancy at Risk: Pregnancy-Related Complications

Learning Objectives

Upon completion of the chapter, you will be able to:

1. Compare and contrast a normal pregnancy to a high risk one. Determine the common factors that might place a pregnancy at high risk.

2. Identify the causes of vaginal bleeding during early and late pregnancy.

3. Outline nursing assessment and management for the pregnant individual experiencing vaginal bleeding.

4. Develop a plan of care for the client experiencing preeclampsia, eclampsia, and HELLP syndrome.

5. Examine the pathophysiology of oligohydramnios and polyhydramnios and subsequent management.

6. Evaluate factors in a client's prenatal history that increase the risk for premature rupture of membranes (PROM).

7. Formulate a teaching plan for maintaining the health of pregnant clients experiencing a high-risk pregnancy.

Helen, a 35-year-old G5 P4, presented to the labour and birth suite with severe abdominal pain, reporting that the pain began suddenly about an hour ago while resting. Helen has had two prior cesarean births and thus far has had an uneventful past 32 weeks. Helen appears distressed and is moaning. What additional assessments do you need to do to care for Helen? What might be your immediate nursing action?

INTRODUCTION

Most people view pregnancy as a natural process with a positive outcome—the birth of a healthy newborn. Unfortunately, conditions can occur that may result in negative outcomes. A **high-risk pregnancy** is one in which a condition exists that jeopardizes the health of the pregnant client, the fetus, or both. The condition may result from the pregnancy, or it may be a condition that was present before the person became pregnant.

Approximately one in four pregnancies is considered to be at high risk or diagnosed with complications (Nagtalon-Ramos, 2014). Pregnancies that are considered to be at high risk have a higher morbidity and mortality compared with pregnant persons in the general population. The risk status of an individual and fetus can change during the pregnancy, with a number of problems occurring during labour, birth, or afterward, even in individuals without any known previous antepartum risk. Examples of high-risk conditions include **ectopic pregnancy** and gestational diabetes. Many obstetric complications and conditions are life-threatening emergencies with high morbidity and mortality rates. It is essential that these be identified early to ensure the best possible outcome for the client and infant. Early identification of the client at risk is essential to ensure that appropriate interventions are instituted promptly, increasing the opportunity to change the course of events and increase the likelihood of a positive outcome.

The term *risk* may have different meanings in the context of the care providers, the client, and the client's family and support network. Primary care providers may focus on the disease processes, diagnosis, and treatments to prevent complications. Nursing care will also focus on the psychosocial impact on the client and the family. The client's attention may be focused on their own needs, those of the family, and the impact of the risk on expectations and experiences both during the pregnancy and into the future. Together, working as a collaborative team, the ultimate goal of care is to ensure the best possible outcome for the client, fetus, family, and social support network.

Risk assessment begins at the first antenatal visit and continues with each subsequent visit because factors may be identified in later visits that were not apparent earlier in pregnancy. For example, as the nurse and client develop a trusting relationship, previously unidentified or unsuspected factors, such as substance abuse or intimate partner violence, may be revealed. Through education and support, the nurse can collaborate with the client, the primary health care provider, and the extended health care team to meet the physiologic and psychosocial needs of the client and family. Multiple factors are to be considered when determining a client's risk for adverse pregnancy outcomes, and a comprehensive approach to high-risk pregnancy is needed. For example,

prenatal stress and distress have been shown to have significant consequences for the client, child, and family. Pregnancy-specific stress such as depression, anxiety, and perceived stress may increase the risk for adverse birth outcomes and is associated with preterm births (Staneva, Bogossian, Pritchard, & Wittkowski, 2015). Risks are grouped into broad categories based on threats to health and pregnancy outcome. Current categories of risk are biophysical, psychosocial, sociodemographic, and environmental (Cunningham et al., 2014) (Box 19.1).

This chapter describes the major conditions directly related to pregnancy that can complicate a pregnancy, possibly affecting maternal and fetal outcomes. These include bleeding during pregnancy (threatened or spontaneous **abortion**, ectopic pregnancy, **gestational trophoblastic disease [GTD]**, cervical insufficiency, **placenta previa**, **abruptio placentae**, and **placenta accreta**), hyperemesis gravidarum (HG), **gestational hypertension**, HELLP syndrome, gestational diabetes, blood incompatibility, amniotic fluid imbalances (**polyhydramnios** and **oligohydramnios**), multiple gestation, and **premature rupture of membranes (PROM)**. Chapter 20 addresses pre-existing conditions that can complicate an individual's pregnancy as well as populations that are considered to be at high risk.

BLEEDING DURING PREGNANCY

Bleeding at any time during pregnancy is potentially life-threatening. Every minute of every day, an individual dies in pregnancy or childbirth. A major contributor to maternal death around the world is obstetric hemorrhage. In Canada, according to the 2014 Canadian Institute for Health Information's Discharge Abstract Database reports (excluding Québec) the most common severe maternal morbidity was blood transfusion (Cook et al., 2017). The successful treatment of obstetric hemorrhage is a challenge for both developed and developing countries. The presence of an attendant at every birth, and access to emergency obstetric care are strategic to reducing maternal morbidity and mortality (World Health Organization [WHO], 2018). Management of obstetric hemorrhage involves early recognition, assessment, and resuscitation. Various methods are available to try to stop the bleeding, ranging from pharmacologic methods to aid uterine contraction (e.g., oxytocin, ergometrine, and prostaglandins) to surgical methods to manage the bleeding (e.g., balloon tamponade, compression sutures, or arterial ligation). Bleeding can occur early or late in the pregnancy and may result from numerous conditions. Bleeding is experienced by approximately 20% of pregnant persons during the first trimester (Knez, Day, & Jurkovic, 2014). Conditions commonly associated with early bleeding (first half of pregnancy) include threatened or spontaneous abortion, uterine fibroids, ectopic pregnancy, GTD, and cervical insufficiency. Conditions

---

BOX 19.1

FACTORS PLACING A CLIENT AT RISK DURING PREGNANCY

Biophysical Factors

- Genetic conditions
- Chromosomal abnormalities
- Multiple pregnancy
- Defective genes
- Inherited disorders
- ABO incompatibility
- Large fetal size
- Medical and obstetric conditions
- Preterm labour and birth
- Cardiovascular disease
- Chronic hypertension
- Cervical insufficiency
- Placental abnormalities
- Infection
- Diabetes
- Maternal collagen diseases
- Thyroid disease
- Asthma
- Postterm pregnancy
- Hemoglobinopathies
- Nutritional status
- Inadequate dietary intake
- Food fads
- Excessive food intake
- Under- or overweight status
- Hematocrit value less than 33%
- Eating disorder
- Maternal Obesity

Psychosocial Factors

- Smoking
- Caffeine
- Alcohol and substance abuse
- Inadequate support system
- Situational crisis
- History of violence
- Emotional distress
- Unsafe cultural practices

Sociodemographic Factors

- Poverty
- Lack of prenatal care
- Age younger than 15 years or older than 35 years
- Parity—all first pregnancies and more than five pregnancies
- Marital status—increased risk for unmarried women
- Accessibility to health care
- Ethnicity—increased risk in individuals of colour

Environmental Factors

- Infections
- Radiation
- Pesticides
- Illicit drugs
- Industrial pollutants
- Second-hand cigarette smoke
- Personal stress
- Inadequate housing

Adapted from Martin, R. J., Fanaroff, A. A., & Walsh, M. C. (2014). *Fanaroff & Martin's neonatal-perinatal medicine* (10th ed.). Philadelphia, PA: Elsevier Health Sciences; Foley, M., Strong, T. M., & Garite, T. (2014). *Obstetric intensive care manual* (4th ed.). New York: McGraw-Hill Publishers; and Cunningham, F. G., Leveno, K. J., Bloom, S. L., Spong, C. Y., Dashe, J. S., Hoffman, B. L., . . . Sheffield, J. S. (2014). *Williams' obstetrics* (24th ed.). New York: McGraw-Hill Education.

---

associated with late bleeding include placenta previa, abruptio placentae, and placenta accreta, which usually occur after the 20th week of gestation.

Spontaneous Abortion

Abortion is considered not only a major reproductive health matter, but also a mental health risk factor for clients' well-being. Spontaneous abortion, also referred to as miscarriage, is the most common complication of early pregnancy (Tulandi & Al-Fozan, 2018). An abortion is the loss of an early pregnancy, before the 20th week of gestation and 500 g fetal weight. Abortion can be threatened, inevitable, incomplete or complete, or missed, and is either spontaneous or induced. A threatened abortion is when there is active bleeding and/or pelvic pain during a pregnancy, the cervix is closed, and there is no passage of tissue. About half of pregnancies at this stage of symptoms will continue as an ongoing pregnancy. The term "inevitable" abortion is used when there is active bleeding accompanied by severe cramping, the cervix

is open and the products of conception will certainly pass. An incomplete abortion describes the pregnancy in which the cervix is open, there is heavy bleeding, and products of conception are in the cervix or partially passed. In a complete abortion, the person may present with a history of bleeding, abdominal pain, and tissue passage. Bleeding and pain usually have subsided and ultrasound reveals a vacant uterus (Gaufberg, 2017). The term missed abortion is used when a pregnancy is not viable (when there is no fetal heart activity) but there are no symptoms of cramping or bleeding. Clients with a missed abortion may wait to start to cramp, may elect to have a dilation and curettage (D&C) procedure, or may choose a medical abortion. A habitual abortion refers to an abortion after three or more consecutive spontaneous abortions. A spontaneous abortion refers to the loss of a fetus resulting from natural causes, that is, not elective or therapeutically induced by a procedure. An induced abortion may also be called an elective or therapeutic abortion in which the abortion is achieved by surgical or medical means. In Canada (except in Quebec), a

21

Nursing Management of Labour and Birth at Risk

Learning Objectives

Upon completion of the chapter, you will be able to:

1. Propose at least five risk factors associated with dystocia.
2. Differentiate the four major abnormalities or problems associated with dysfunctional labour patterns, giving examples of each problem.
3. Examine the nursing management for the client with dysfunctional labour experiencing a problem with the powers, passenger, passageway, or psyche.
4. Devise a plan of care for the client experiencing preterm labour.
5. Relate the nursing assessment and management of the client experiencing a prolonged pregnancy.
6. Assess four obstetric emergencies that can complicate labour and birth, including appropriate management for each.
7. Compare and contrast the nursing management for the client undergoing labour induction or augmentation, and forceps or vacuum-assisted birth.
8. Summarize the plan of care for a client who is to undergo a caesarean birth.
9. Evaluate the key areas to be addressed when caring for a client who undergoes a vaginal birth after caesarean (VBAC).

KEY TERMS

amnioinfusion

arrest disorders

caesarean birth

dystocia

forceps

hypertonic uterine dysfunction

hypotonic uterine dysfunction

labour induction

macrosomia

multiple gestation

postterm pregnancy

precipitate labour

preterm labour

protracted disorders

shoulder dystocia

tocolytic

umbilical cord prolapse

vacuum extractor

vaginal birth after caesarean (VBAC)

Jennifer, **a 29-year-old G1P0, is at 41 weeks' gestation. Her health care provider has recommended that she come in for induction. She is very anxious about doing this since she has heard "horror stories" about the "hard painful contractions" that can result. What can the nurse do to calm her fears?**

Problems with the Passenger Persistent occiput posterior position	Engagement of fetal head in the left or right occipitotransverse position with the occiput rotating posteriorly rather than into the more favorable occiput anterior position (fetus born facing upward instead of the normal downward position) Labour usually much longer and more uncomfortable (causing increased back pain during labour) if fetus remains in this position. Possible extensive caput succedaneum and moulding from the sustained occiput posterior position.	Leopold manoeuvres and vaginal examination to determine position of fetal head in conjunction with the client's reports of severe back pain (back of fetal head pressing on the sacrum and coccyx).	Labour to proceed, preparing the client for a long labour (spontaneous resolution possible). Comfort measures and positioning to help promote fetal head rotation. Delayed pushing to allow fetal head to rotate with contractions.	Assess for complaints of intense back pain in first stage of labour. Anticipate possible use of forceps to rotate to anterior position at birth or manual rotation to anterior position at end of second stage. Assess for prolonged second stage of labour with arrest of descent (common with this malposition). Encourage position changes to promote fetal head rotation: hands and knees and rocking pelvis back and forth; side-lying position; side lunges during contractions; sitting, kneeling, or standing while leaning forward; squatting position to give birth and enlarge pelvic outlet. Prepare for possible caesarean birth if rotation is not achieved. Administer agents as ordered for pain relief (effective pain relief crucial to help the client to tolerate the back discomfort). Apply low back counter pressure during contractions to ease the discomfort. Provide measures to reduce anxiety. Continuously reinforce the client's progress. Teach client about possible interventions to facilitate fetal head rotation.
Face and brow presentation	Face presentation with complete extension of the fetal head. Brow presentation: fetal head between full extension and full flexion so that the largest fetal skull diameter presents to the pelvis.	Diagnosis only once labour is well established via vaginal examination; palpation of facial features as the presenting part rather than the fetal head	Vaginal birth possible with face presentation with an adequate pelvis and fetal head rotation; caesarean birth if head rotates backward. Caesarean birth for brow presentation unless head flexes.	Assist with evaluating for fetopelvic disproportion. Anticipate caesarean birth if vertex position is not achieved. Explain fetal malposition to the client and partner. Provide close observation for any signs of fetal hypoxia, as evidenced by late decelerations and minimal variability on the fetal monitor.

(continued)

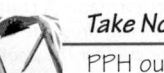

- Wear an identification bracelet or band that indicates that you are taking an anticoagulant.
- Elimination of modifiable risk factors for DVT (smoking, use of oral contraceptives, a sedentary lifestyle, and obesity)
- Importance of using compression stockings
- Avoidance of constrictive clothing and prolonged standing or sitting in a motionless, leg-dependent position
- Danger signs and symptoms (sudden onset of chest pain, dyspnea, and tachypnea) to report to the health care provider

POSTPARTUM INFECTION

Infection during the postpartum period is a common cause of maternal morbidity and mortality. Overall, postpartum infection (PPI) is estimated to occur in up to 8% of all births and accounts for 15% of global maternal mortality. There is a higher occurrence in cesarean births than in vaginal births (Mattson & Smith, 2015). PPI is defined as a fever of 38°C (100.4°F) or higher after the first 24 hours after childbirth, occurring on at least 2 of the first 10 days after birth, exclusive of the first 24 hours (Dalton & Castillo, 2014).

Risk factors include surgical birth, prolonged rupture of membranes, long labour with multiple vaginal examinations, inadequate hand hygiene, internal fetal monitoring, uterine manipulation, chorioamnionitis, instrumental birth, obesity, untreated infection prior to birth, retained placental fragments, obesity, gestational diabetes, extremes of client age, low socioeconomic status, and anemia during pregnancy (Jordan et al., 2014).

Infections can easily enter the female genital tract externally and ascend through the internal genital structures. Postpartum clients are at an increased risk for infection due to tissue trauma during birth, vulnerability from placenta separation site, and the incision from cesarean section. In addition, the normal physiologic changes of childbirth increase the risk of infection by decreasing the vaginal acidity due to the presence of amniotic fluid, blood, and lochia, all of which are alkaline. An alkaline environment encourages the growth of bacteria.

PPIs usually arise from organisms that constitute the normal vaginal flora, typically a mix of aerobic and anaerobic species. Generally, they are polymicrobial and involve the following microorganisms: *Staphylococcus aureus, Escherichia coli, Klebsiella, Gardnerella vaginalis,* gonococci, coliform bacteria, group A or B hemolytic streptococci, *Chlamydia trachomatis,* and the anaerobes that are common to bacterial vaginosis. Prevention can be achieved by screening and treating vaginal colonization during pregnancy (Callahan, 2016). Common PPIs include metritis, surgical site infections, urinary tract infections, and mastitis.

Metritis

Although usually referred to clinically as endometritis, postpartum uterine infections typically involve more than just the endometrial lining. **Metritis** is an infectious condition that involves the endometrium, decidua, and adjacent myometrium of the uterus. Extension of metritis can result in parametritis, which involves the broad ligament and possibly the ovaries and fallopian tubes, or septic pelvic thrombophlebitis, which results when the infection spreads along venous routes into the pelvis. It occurs within the first 2 days postpartum or as late as 2 to 6 weeks postpartum (King et al., 2015).

The uterine cavity is sterile until rupture of the amniotic sac. As a consequence of labour, birth, and associated manipulations, anaerobic and aerobic bacteria can contaminate the uterus. In most cases, the bacteria responsible for pelvic infections are those that normally reside in the bowel, vagina, perineum, and cervix, such as *E. coli, Klebsiella pneumoniae,* or *G. vaginalis.*

The risk of metritis increases dramatically after a cesarean birth; it complicates from 10% to 20% of cesarean births. This is typically an extension of chorioamnionitis that was present before birth (indeed, that may have been why the cesarean birth was performed). In addition, trauma to the tissues and a break in the skin (incision) provide entrances for bacteria to enter the body and multiply.

The Society of Obstetricians and Gynaecologists of Canada ([SOGC], 2015) and ACOG (2018) recommend use of one dose of prophylactic antibiotic therapy administered 1 hour before any cesarean section and this has become standard practice in Canada and the United States today. Once rupture of the amniotic membranes occurs during labour and birth, the uterus becomes more susceptible to colonization and infection, especially with a prolonged labour. Any area traumatized during childbirth is susceptible to infection.

Surgical Site Infections

Any break in the skin or mucous membranes provides a portal for bacteria. In the postpartum client, sites of wound infection include cesarean surgical incisions, the episiotomy site in the perineum, and genital tract lacerations (Fig. 22.2). Wound infections are usually not identified until the client has been discharged from the hospital because symptoms may not show up until 24 to 48 hours after birth.

Urinary Tract Infections

Urinary tract infections are most commonly caused by bacteria often found in bowel flora, including *E. coli, Klebsiella, Proteus,* and *Enterobacter* species. Invasive manipulation of the urethra (e.g., urinary catheterization),

A

B

FIGURE 22.2 Postpartum wound infections. **A.** Infected episiotomy site. **B.** Infected cesarean birth incision.

frequent vaginal examinations, and genital trauma increase the likelihood of a urinary tract infection. It is the most common cause of a fever in the postpartum person.

Mastitis

Mastitis is defined as inflammation of the mammary gland. A common problem that may occur within the first 2 days to 2 weeks postpartum. An estimated 5% of individuals who breastfeed will develop lactational mastitis (Kansky & Isaacs, 2016). Risk factors associated with mastitis include stasis of milk due to infrequent, inconsistent breastfeeding, and nipple trauma. As well as causing significant discomfort, it is a frequent reason identified for the cessation of breastfeeding. It can result from any event that creates milk stasis: insufficient drainage of the breast, rapid weaning, oversupply of milk, pressure on the breast from a poorly fitting bra, a blocked duct, missed feedings, and breakdown of the nipple via fissures, cracks, or blisters (Nagtalon-Ramos, 2014). The most common infecting organism is *S. aureus,* which comes from the breastfeeding infant's mouth or throat. *Staphylococcus albus, E. coli,* and streptococci are also causative agents, but found less frequently. Infection can be transmitted from the lactiferous ducts to a secreting lobule, from a nipple fissure to periductal lymphatics, or by circulation (Amir, 2014) (Fig. 22.3). A breast abscess may develop if mastitis is not treated adequately. Flu-like symptoms are often the first symptoms the client will experience. Breasts are red, tender, and hot to the touch. The upper, outer quadrant of the breast is the most common site for mastitis to occur because most of the breast tissue is located there with both the right and left breasts being equally affected. Effective milk removal, pain medication, and antibiotic therapy have been the mainstays of treatment.

Therapeutic Management

METRITIS

When metritis occurs, broad-spectrum antibiotics are used to treat the infection. Management also includes measures to restore and promote fluid and electrolyte balance, provide analgesia, and provide emotional support. Typically, after treatment, a fever will drop and symptoms cease within 48 to 72 hours after the start of antibiotic therapy.

SURGICAL SITE INFECTIONS

Management for surgical site infections involves recognition of the infection, followed by opening of the wound

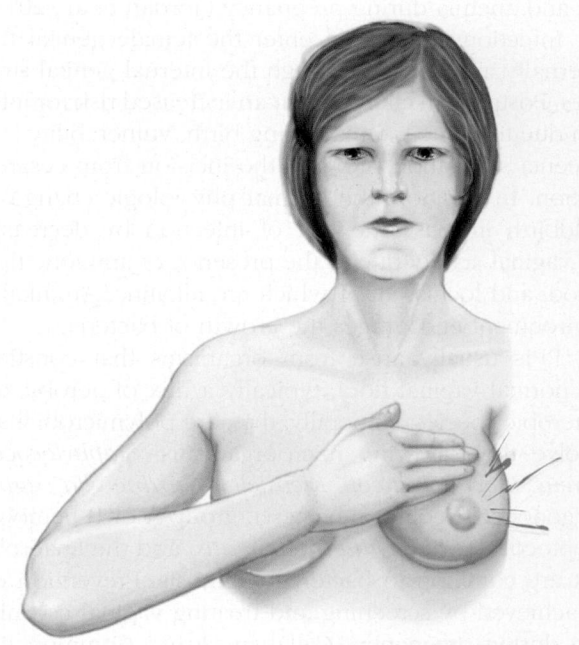

FIGURE 22.3 With mastitis, an area on one breast is tender, hot, red, and painful.

to allow drainage. Aseptic wound management with sterile gloves and frequent dressing changes if applicable, good hand hygiene, frequent perineal pad changes, hydration, and ambulation to prevent venous stasis and improve circulation are initiated to prevent development of a more serious infection or spread of the infection to adjacent structures. Parenteral antibiotics are the mainstay of treatment. Analgesics are also important, because clients often experience discomfort at the wound site.

URINARY TRACT INFECTIONS

Urinary tract infections are common during the postpartum period and could be prevented by timely removal of urinary catheters used during labour or surgical births. Risk factors include catheterization, epidural anesthesia, and vaginal procedures. If the client develops a urinary tract infection, fluids are used to treat dehydration. General nutrition measures include acidifying the urine by taking large doses of vitamin C or a regular intake of cranberry juice. Cranberry juice contains a substance with biologic activity that inhibits the growth of *E. coli* in the urinary tract (Wong & Rosh, 2017). Antibiotics may also be ordered if appropriate.

MASTITIS

Treatment of mastitis focuses on two areas: emptying the breasts and controlling the infection. Frequent breast emptying helps both infectious and noninfectious mastitis. The breast can be emptied either by the infant sucking or by manual expression. Increasing the frequency of nursing is advised. Lactation need not be suppressed. Control of infection is achieved with antibiotics. In addition, ice or warm packs and analgesics may be needed. In addition to antibiotics, management of lactational breast infections includes symptomatic treatment, assessment of the infant's attachment to the breast, and reassurance, emotional support, education, and support for ongoing breastfeeding.

Take Note!

Regardless of the etiology of mastitis, the focus is on reversing milk stasis, maintaining milk supply, and continuing breastfeeding, along with providing maternal comfort and preventing recurrence.

Nursing Assessment

Perinatal nurses are the primary caregivers for postpartum clients and have a unique opportunity to identify subtle changes that place individuals at risk for infection. Nurses play a key role in identifying signs and symptoms that suggest a PPI. Today families are commonly discharged 24 to 48 hours after giving birth. Therefore, nurses must assess for risk factors and identify early, subtle signs and symptoms of an infectious process. Factors that place an individual at risk for a PPI are highlighted in Box 22.1.

BOX 22.1

FACTORS PLACING A CLIENT AT RISK FOR POSTPARTUM INFECTION

- Prolonged (>18–24 hours) premature rupture of membranes (removes the barrier of amniotic fluid so bacteria can ascend)
- Cesarean birth (allows bacterial entry due to break in protective skin barrier)
- Urinary catheterization (could allow entry of bacteria into bladder due to break in aseptic technique)
- Regional anesthesia that decreases perception of need to void (causes urinary stasis and increases risk of urinary tract infection)
- Staff attending to the client are ill (promotes droplet infection from personnel)
- Compromised health status, such as anemia, obesity, smoking, drug abuse (reduces the body's immune system and decreases ability to fight infection)
- Pre-existing colonization of lower genital tract with bacterial vaginosis, *Chlamydia trachomatis,* group B streptococci, *S. aureus,* and *E. coli* (allows microbes to ascend)
- Retained placental fragments (provides medium for bacterial growth)
- Manual removal of a retained placenta (causes trauma to the lining of the uterus and thus opens up sites for bacterial invasion)
- Insertion of fetal scalp electrode or intrauterine pressure catheters for internal fetal monitoring during labour (provides entry into uterine cavity)
- Instrument-assisted childbirth, such as forceps or vacuum extraction (increases risk of trauma to genital tract, which provides bacteria access to grow)
- Trauma to the genital tract, such as episiotomy or lacerations (provides a portal of entry for bacteria)
- Prolonged labour with frequent vaginal examinations to check progress (allows time for bacteria to multiply and increases potential exposure to microorganisms or trauma)
- Poor nutritional status (reduces body's ability to repair tissue)
- Gestational diabetes (decreases body's healing ability and provides higher glucose levels on skin and in urine, which encourages bacterial growth)
- Break in aseptic technique during surgery or birthing process (allows entry of bacteria)

Adapted from Salam, R. A., Mansoor, T., Mallick, D., Lassi, Z. S., Das, J. K., & Bhutta, Z. A. (2014). Essential childbirth and postnatal interventions for improved maternal and neonatal health. *Reproductive Health, 11*(Suppl 1), S3–S20; Jordan, R. G., Engstrom, J. L., Marfell, J. A., & Farley, C. L. (2014). *Prenatal and postnatal care: A woman-centered approach.* Ames, Iowa: Wiley Blackwell; and Wong, A. W., & Rosh, A. J. (2017). Postpartum infections. *eMedicine.* Retrieved from http://emedicine.medscape.com/article/796892-overview

---

Review the client's history and physical examination and labour and birth record for factors that might increase the risk for developing an infection. Then complete the assessment (using the "BUBBLE-EE" parameters discussed in Chapter 16), paying particular attention to areas such as the abdomen and fundus, breasts, urinary

TABLE 22.3	SIGNS AND SYMPTOMS OF POSTPARTUM INFECTIONS
Postpartum Infection	**Signs and Symptoms**
Metritis	Lower abdominal tenderness or pain on one or both sides Temperature elevation (>38°C) Foul-smelling lochia Anorexia Nausea Fatigue and lethargy Leukocytosis and elevated sedimentation rate
Wound infection	Weeping serosanguineous or purulent drainage Separation of or unapproximated wound edges Edema Erythema Tenderness Discomfort at the site Maternal fever Elevated white blood cell count
Urinary tract infection	Urgency Frequency Dysuria Flank pain Low-grade fever Urinary retention Hematuria Urine positive for nitrates Cloudy urine with strong odour
Mastitis	Flu-like symptoms, including malaise, fever, and chills Tender, hot, red, painful area on one breast Inflammation of breast area Breast tenderness Cracking of skin around nipple or areola Breast distention with milk

Adapted from Dalton, E., & Castillo, E. (2014). Postpartum infections: A review for the non-OB/GYN. *Obstetric Medicine: The Medicine of Pregnancy, 7*(3), 98–102; Nagtalon-Ramos, J. (2014). *Maternal-newborn nursing care: Best evidence-based practices.* Philadelphia, PA: F.A. Davis Company; and Kansky, C., & Isaacs, C. (2016). Normal and abnormal puerperium. *eMedicine.* Retrieved from http://emedicine.medscape.com/article/260187-overview

tract, episiotomy, lacerations, or incisions and being alert for signs and symptoms of infection (Table 22.3).

Take Note!

A PPI is commonly associated with an elevated temperature, as mentioned previously. Other generalized signs and symptoms may include chills, foul-smelling vaginal discharge, headache, malaise, restlessness, anxiety, and tachycardia. In addition, the client may have specific signs and symptoms based on the type and location of the infection.

The acronym REEDA is frequently used for assessing a perineum after childbirth. It is derived from five components that have been identified to be associated with the healing process of the perineum. These include:
1. Redness—area may also feel warm to touch.
2. Edema—may indicate infection or a hematoma.
3. Ecchymosis—may indicate vaginal trauma.
4. Discharge—should follow the expected lochia pattern.
5. Approximation of skin edges—should be well aligned without gaps.

Each category is assessed, and a number assigned (0 to 3 points) for a total REEDA score ranging from 0 to 15. The higher scores indicate increased tissue trauma (Kaur, Sagar, Deol, & Kaur, 2015). See Figure 22.4 for the REEDA method for assessing perineum healing.

Monitor the vital signs, especially temperature. Changes may also signal an infection.

Nursing Management

Nursing management focuses on preventing PPIs. Use the following guidelines to reduce the incidence of PPIs:
- Maintain aseptic technique when performing invasive procedures such as urinary catheterization, when changing dressings, and during all surgical procedures.
- Use good hand hygiene technique before and after each client care activity.
- Reinforce measures for maintaining good perineal hygiene.
- Practice standard precautions whenever in contact with blood, body fluids, excretions.
- Use adequate lighting and turn the client to the side to assess the episiotomy site.
- Use extreme caution when handling sharp instruments, specimens, and waste disposal
- Screen all visitors for any signs of active infections to reduce the client's risk of exposure.
- Review the client's history for pre-existing infections or chronic conditions.
- Monitor vital signs and laboratory results for any abnormal values.
- Monitor the frequency of vaginal examinations and length of labour.
- Assess frequently for early signs of infection, especially fever and the appearance of lochia.
- Inspect wounds frequently for inflammation and drainage.
- Encourage rest, adequate hydration, and healthy eating habits.
- Reinforce preventive measures during any interaction with the client.

If the client develops an infection, review treatment measures, such as antibiotic therapy if ordered, and any special care measures, such as dressing changes, that might be needed (Nursing Care Plan 22.1, at the end of the chapter).

REEDA Method for Assessing Perineum Healing

➤ **R**edness

   o   none = 0 points

   o   Redness within .25 cm of incision bilaterally = 1

   o   Redness within .5 cm of incision bilaterally = 2

   o   Redness reaching beyond .5 cm of incision bilaterally = 3

➤ **E**dema – the more swelling present, the high the score

   o   None = 0 points

   o   <1 cm from incision = 1 point

   o   1–2 cm from incision = 2 points

   o   >2 cm from incision = 3 points

➤ **E**cchymosis – the more bruising observed, the higher the score

   o   None = 0 points

   o   1–2 cm from incision = 1 point

   o   .25–1 cm bilaterally or .5–2 cm unilaterally = 2 points

   o   >1 cm bilaterally or 2 cm unilaterally = 3 points

➤ **D**ischarge – range would be from none present to profuse

   o   None = 0 points

   o   Serum discharge present = 1 point

   o   Serosanguineous discharge present = 2 points

   o   Bloody, purulent discharge present = 3 points

➤ **A**pproximation of skin edges

   o   Closed, skin edges approximated well = 0 points

   o   Skin separated 3 cm or less = 1 point

   o   Skin and subcutaneous fat separated = 2 points

   o   Skin, subcutaneous fat and facial separation = 3 points

FIGURE 22.4 REEDA method for assessing perineum healing. (Adapted from Davidson, N. [1974]. REEDA: Evaluating postpartum healing. *Journal of Nurse Midwifery, 19*(2), 6–8; Nikpour, M., Shirvani, M. A., Azadbakht, M., Zanjani, R., & Mousavi, E. [2014]. The effect of honey gel on abdominal wound healing in caesarean section: A triple blind randomized clinical trial. *Oman Medical Journal, 29*(4), 255–259.)

Postpartum clients should be educated on the signs and symptoms of life-threatening conditions, including sepsis. Information should include the importance of good hand and perineal hygiene and of the need to seek immediate medical care if feeling unwell. Client teaching is a priority due to today's short lengths of stay after childbirth. Some infections may not manifest until after discharge. Review the signs and symptoms of infection, emphasizing the danger signs that need to be reported to the health care provider. Most importantly, stress proper hand hygiene, especially after perineal care and before and after breastfeeding. Also reinforce measures to promote breastfeeding, including proper breast care (see Chapter 16). Teaching Guidelines 22.2 highlights the major teaching points for a client with a PPI.

Teaching Guidelines 22.2
TEACHING FOR THE CLIENT WITH A POSTPARTUM INFECTION

- Continue your antibiotic therapy as prescribed.
- Take the medication exactly as ordered and continue with the medication until it is finished.
- Do not stop taking the medication even when you are feeling better.
- Check your temperature every day and call your health care provider if it is above 38°C (100.4°F).
- Watch for other signs and symptoms of infection, such as chills, increased abdominal pain, change in the colour or odour of your lochia, or increased redness, warmth, swelling, or drainage from a wound site such as your cesarean incision or episiotomy. Report any of these to your health care provider immediately.
- Practice good infection prevention:
- Always wash your hands thoroughly before and after eating, using the bathroom, touching your perineal area, or providing care for your newborn.
- Wipe from front to back after using the bathroom.
- Remove your perineal pad using a front-to-back motion. Fold the pad in half so that the inner sides of the pad that were touching your body are against each other. Wrap in toilet tissue or place in a plastic bag and discard.
- Wash your hands before applying a new pad.
- Apply a new perineal pad using a front-to-back motion. Handle the pad by the edges (top and bottom or sides) and avoid touching the inner aspect of the pad that will be against your body.
- When performing perineal care with a peribottle, angle the spray of water so that it flows from front to back.
- Drink plenty of fluids each day and eat a variety of foods that are high in vitamins, iron, and protein.
- Be sure to get adequate rest at night and periodically throughout the day.

POSTPARTUM AFFECTIVE DISORDERS

The postpartum period involves extraordinary physiologic, psychological, and sociocultural changes in the life of a person and family. It is an exhilarating time for most, but for others it may not be what they had expected. Individuals have varied reactions to their childbearing experiences, exhibiting a wide range of emotions. Typically, the delivery of a newborn is associated with positive feelings such as happiness, joy, and gratitude for the birth of a healthy infant. However, some will also feel weepy, overwhelmed, or unsure of what is happening to them. They may experience fear about loss of control; they may feel scared, alone, or guilty, or as if they have somehow failed. During the postpartum period, up to 85% of birthing parents experience some type of mood disorder (Joy, Mattingly, & Templeton, 2017).

Postpartum affective disorders have been documented for years, but only recently have they received medical attention. Plummeting levels of estrogen and progesterone immediately after birth can contribute to postpartum mood disorders. Reproductive hormones influence every biologic system and many individuals are particularly sensitive to the effects of perinatal changes in hormone levels after childbirth. It is believed that the greater the change in these hormone levels between pregnancy and postpartum, the greater the chance for developing a mood disorder (Schiller, Meltzer-Brody, & Rubinow, 2015).

Many types of affective disorders occur in the postpartum period. Although their description and classification may be controversial, the disorders are commonly classified on the basis of their severity as postpartum or baby blues, postpartum depression (PPD), and postpartum psychosis.

Postpartum Blues

Many postpartum individuals (approximately 80%) experience the "blues" (Callahan, 2016). The client experiences rapid cycling mood symptoms during the first postpartum week typically, and exhibits mild depressive symptoms of anxiety, irritability, mood swings, tearfulness, increased sensitivity, despondency, feelings of being overwhelmed, difficulty thinking clearly, and fatigue (Pop et al., 2015). Emotional lability is the most prominent symptom of the maternity blues. The "blues" typically peak on postpartum days 4 and 5 and usually resolve by postpartum day 10. Biologic, psychological, and social factors have been hypothesized as relevant to blues causation, but no studies have validated this. Although the symptoms may be distressing, they do not reflect psychopathology and usually do not affect the parent's ability to function and care for their infant.

Baby blues are usually self-limiting and require no formal treatment other than reassurance and validation of the experience, as well as assistance in self-care and caring for the newborn. However, follow-up of individuals with postpartum blues is important because up to 20% go on to develop PPD (Alexander, LaRosa, Bader, & Garfield, 2014).

Postpartum Depression

Depression is more prevalent in women than in men, which may be related to biologic, hormonal, and psychosocial factors. **Postpartum depression (PPD)** is a form of clinical depression that can affect women, and less frequently men, after childbirth. It affects 1 in 7 mothers and 1 in 10 fathers (CDC, 2018b; Joy et al., 2017). Unlike the postpartum blues, individuals with PPD feel worse over time, and changes in mood and behaviour do not go away on their own. PPD may persist for a minimum of 6 months if untreated. Different from the baby blues, the symptoms of PPD last longer, are more severe, and require intervention or treatment. Some signs and symptoms of PPD include feeling the following:

- Restless
- Worthless
- Guilty
- Hopeless
- Moody
- Sad
- Overwhelmed
- Loss of enjoyment
- Low energy level
- Loss of libido

The person may also:

- Cry a lot.
- Exhibit a lack of energy and motivation.
- Be unable to make decisions or focus.
- Have memory loss.
- Experience a lack of pleasure.
- Have changes in sleep or weight.
- Show a lack of concern for self.
- Withdraw from friends and family.
- Have pains that do not subside.
- Feel negatively toward the baby.
- Have appetite disturbances.
- Have feelings of isolation from others.
- Lack interest in the baby.
- Worry about hurting the baby.
- Act detached toward others and the infant.
- Have recurrent thoughts of suicide and death (Bobo & Yawn, 2014).

PPD affects not only the individual experiencing the symptoms but also the entire family. Identifying depression early can substantially improve the client and family outcomes. PPD usually has a gradual onset and becomes evident within the first 6 weeks postpartum.

The cause of PPD is not known, but research suggests that it is multifactorial, due to changes in the body with fluctuating hormone levels, social and familial roles, and lifestyle. The levels of estrogen, progesterone, serotonin, and thyroid hormone decrease sharply and return to normal during the immediate postpartum period, which can trigger depression and can change a person's mood and behaviour. Other aspects that can lead to PPD include:

- Unresolved feelings about the pregnancy
- Fatigue after delivery from lack of sleep or broken sleep
- Feelings of being less attractive
- Inadequate assistance from partner
- Lack of social support network
- History of sexual or physical abuse
- Unemployment or financial insecurity
- Doubts about the ability to be a good parent
- Stress from changes in work and home routines
- Loss of freedom and old identity (Finley & Brizendine, 2015)

PPD may lend itself to prophylactic intervention because its onset is predictable, the risk period for illness is well defined, and clients at high risk potentially could be identified using a screening tool. This is not the case for all, however (see Evidence-Based Practice 22.1). Prophylaxis starts with a prenatal risk assessment and education. Based on the client's history of prior depression, prophylactic antidepressant therapy may be needed during the third trimester or immediately after giving birth. Management mirrors that of any major depression: a combination of antidepressant medication, antianxiety medication, adequate sleep and rest, and psychotherapy in an outpatient or inpatient setting (Callahan, 2016). Marital counselling may be necessary if marital problems are contributing to the depressive symptoms.

The significant other's or partner's emotional health should not be overlooked during the pregnancy and throughout the first postpartum year. PPD, once expected only in new mothers, occurs in co-parents as well. Up to 50% of significant others or partners whose partners suffer from PPD also have depressive symptoms, and little is known about the impact of maternal PPD on them. Depressive symptoms are likely to decrease their ability to provide support. Partner's PPD can be difficult to identify. New co-parents may seem more angry and anxious than sad, yet depression is present. When left untreated, partner's PPD limits the significant other's or partner's capacity to provide emotional support to their partners and children. The highest rates of depression among fathers have been reported between 3 and 6 months postpartum. Factors that increase the risk of paternal PPD include a personal history of depression and/or anxiety, a low level

A SYSTEMATIC REVIEW OF THE RELATIONSHIP BETWEEN POSTPARTUM SLEEP DISTURBANCE AND POSTPARTUM DEPRESSION

STUDY

Sleep is closely associated with psychological well-being. Insufficient sleep leads to adverse medical and psychological consequences and a poorer quality of life. Despite commonly held beliefs of joy and happiness after childbirth, new parents are vulnerable to mood disorders during the postpartum period. Nighttime feedings and frequent nocturnal awakenings contribute to sleep maternal mood disturbances. Poor and fragmented sleep patterns are associated with a poor quality of life, a decrease in attentiveness and general well-being. More importantly, it may be a risk factor for postpartum depression. Postpartum depression has been linked with a series of psychosocial sequelae for mothers and their newborns. The purpose of this review was to analyze the relationship between postpartum sleep disturbance and postpartum depression.

Findings

A systematic review was conducted on 13 observational studies which included 3,793 women. The findings from all 13 studies revealed a consistent strong relationship between sleep disturbance and postpartum depression. Short sleep duration and insomnia are related to a range of impaired functional outcomes that may negatively impact the daily life of postpartum women and their newborns.

Nursing Implications

Based on this evidence, nurses can counsel postpartum clients about the importance of getting adequate sleep when they are discharged and the link between sleep disturbances and postpartum depression. Nurses can suggest several interventions to assist the new parent in obtaining adequate sleep such as bathing the newborn at night before bedtime, asking for help from family to assist in nighttime diaper changes, and taking naps throughout the day when the newborn sleeps. These simple helpful interventions may be a valuable prevention measure to assist in increasing the mother's wellness and reduce the risk of postpartum depression.

Adapted from Bhati, S., & Richards, K. (2015). A systematic review of the relationship between postpartum sleep disturbance and postpartum depression. *Journal of Obstetric, Gynecologic, & Neonatal Nursing, 44*(3), 350–357.

of marital satisfaction, excessive financial stressors, a lack of significant other or partner's parental leave, and the feeling that there is a great discrepancy between one's expectations of parenthood and its realities (Feeley, Bell, Hayton, Zelkowitz, & Carrier, 2016).

Assessing partner's PPD is not easy. Nevertheless, it is important for all nurses who have contact with new partners to remain open to the notion that new partners are predisposed to PPD, particularly if their partner is afflicted. Delving deeper into understanding behaviours of withdrawing, indecisiveness, cynicism, avoiding, drinking, using drugs, fighting, partner violence, extramarital affairs, and feelings of heightened irritation will reveal important insights. Asking new partners candidly if they are feeling depressed, anxious, or angry can open the door to further exploration of these emotions (Weissman, 2014).

Although partner depression is only now beginning to be defined and measured, sufficient evidence exists to warrant nurses' attention and concern. Nurses may be most able to help a new partner devastated by PPD when they plant seeds of awareness that the disorder exists, that they are not alone, and that help is available.

Despite the negative outcomes associated with PPD, rates of diagnosis and treatment are low mainly because of lack of recognition by the health care provider. In addition, PPD is the most misinterpreted, frequently dismissed, and most undiagnosed postpartum complication. Early recognition of PPD can eliminate the length of time that individuals have to suffer with this debilitating condition and can decrease the potentially harmful effects on the infants involved.

Screening for symptoms of PPD in all clients and partners is an important preliminary step to diagnosis and treatment, but the effectiveness of depression screening is dependent on the reliability and validity of the screening instruments in the population. Both the Edinburgh Postnatal Depression Scale (EPDS) and the Postpartum Depression Predictor Scale (PDSS) have been used to screen for PPD, but it is not clear which instrument best predicts a diagnosis of postpartum depression (Thombs et al., 2014).

The EPDS is a self-report, quick, and easy screening tool for PPD that consists of 10 questions with 4 possible responses. The individual or couple fill out the tool according to their symptoms during the past 7 days, with each response given a score of 0 to 3 points, creating a maximum score of 30. Using a cutoff score of 9 or 10, the sensitivity is 86%; the specificity, 78%; and positive predictive value, 73% (Zhao et al., 2015).

The PDSS is a self-report, 35-item Likert-type response scale divided into seven conceptual domains:

1. Anxiety/insecurity
2. Sleep/eating disturbance
3. Emotional liability
4. Loss of self-esteem
5. Guilt/shame
6. Cognitive impairment
7. Suicidal thoughts

The scores range from 35 to 175. The scale has five symptoms for each domain, and the client is asked to identify the degree of disagreement or agreement on the basis of their feelings over the past 2 weeks. The sensitivity of the PDSS is 91%; the specificity is 72% for detecting PPD. The PDSS takes 5 to 10 minutes to administer and is used during the postpartum period (King et al., 2015).

Early identification, screening, prevention, and treatment of PPD are crucial for improving overall outcomes for the parent and infant, as well as for decreasing mortality and morbidity. This is why it is crucial for nurses to understand and know about the risk factors, signs and symptoms, prevention, and use and interpretation of screening tools and to make appropriate referrals for treatment. Mass screening for PPD using a validated screening tool has been proven to improve the rates of detection and treatment of PPD and should be implemented in obstetricians' and pediatricians' offices and in primary care settings. The Edinburgh tool is shown in Figure 22.5.

Postpartum Psychosis

At the severe end of the continuum of postpartum emotional disorders is postpartum psychosis, which occurs in 1 in 1,000 live births (Doyle, Carballedo, & O'Keane, 2015). Postpartum psychosis, an emergency psychiatric condition, can result in a significant increased risk for suicide and infanticide. Symptoms of postpartum psychosis, such as mood lability, delusional beliefs, hallucinations, and disorganized thinking, can be frightening for those who are affected, and for their families. It generally surfaces within 3 months of giving birth and is manifested by sleep disturbances, fatigue, depression, and hypomania. The affected individual will be tearful, confused, and preoccupied with feelings of guilt and worthlessness. Early symptoms resemble those of depression, but they may escalate to delirium, hallucinations, extreme disorganization of thought, anger toward self and the infant, bizarre behaviour, delusions, disorientation, depersonalization, delirium-like appearance, manifestations of mania, and thoughts of hurting self and the infant. The individual frequently loses touch with reality and experiences a severe regressive breakdown, associated with a high risk of suicide or infanticide (del Corral Serrano, 2015). Individuals with postpartum psychosis should not be left alone with their infants. Most clients with postpartum psychosis are hospitalized for up to several months. Psychotropic drugs are almost always part of treatment, along with individual psychotherapy and support group therapy.

Take Note!

The greatest hazard of postpartum psychosis is suicide. Infanticide and child abuse are also risks if the individual is left alone with their infant. Early recognition and prompt treatment of this disorder are imperative.

Nursing Assessment

Postpartum affective disorders are often overlooked and go unrecognized despite the large percentage of individuals who experience them. The postpartum period is a time of increased vulnerability, but few receive education about the possibility of depression after birth. In addition, many new parents may feel ashamed of having negative emotions at a time when they "should" be happy; thus, they do not seek professional help. Nurses can play a major role in providing guidance about postpartum affective disorders, detecting manifestations, and assisting clients to obtain appropriate care.

Consider This

Even though I was an assertive practicing attorney in my thirties, my first pregnancy was filled with nagging feelings of doubt about this upcoming event in my life. Throughout my pregnancy I was so busy with trial work that I never had time to really evaluate my feelings. I was always reading about the bodily changes that were taking place, and on one level I was feeling excited, but on another level, I was emotionally drained. Shortly after the birth of my daughter, those suppressed nagging feelings of doubt surfaced big time and practically immobilized me. I felt exhausted all the time and was only too glad to have someone else care for my daughter. I didn't breastfeed because I thought it would tie me down too much. Although at the time I thought this "low mood" was normal for all new mothers, I have since found out it was postpartum depression. How could anyone be depressed about this wondrous event?

Thoughts: Now that postpartum depression has been "taken out of the closet" and recognized as a real emotional disorder, it can be treated. This woman showed tendencies during her pregnancy but was able to suppress the feelings and go forward. Her description of her depression is very typical of many who suffer in silence, hoping to get over these feelings in time. What can nurses do to promote awareness of this disorder? Can it be prevented?

Begin the assessment by reviewing the history to identify general risk factors that could predispose a person to depression:
- Poor coping skills
- First pregnancy
- Low self-esteem
- Numerous life stressors
- History of abuse
- Mood swings and emotional stress
- Previous psychological problems or a family history of psychiatric disorders
- Substance abuse
- Limited or lack of social support network

Edinburgh Postnatal Depression Scale

Name: _____   Address: _____

Your Date of Birth: _____   _____

Baby's Date of Birth: _____   Phone: _____

As you are pregnant or have recently had a baby, we would like to know how you are feeling. Please check the answer that comes closest to how you have felt **IN THE PAST 7 DAYS**, not just how you feel today.

Here is an example, already completed.

I have felt happy:
- ☐ Yes, all the time
- ☒ Yes, most of the time   This would mean: "I have felt happy most of the time" during the past week.
- ☐ No, not very often   Please complete the other questions in the same way.
- ☐ No, not at all

In the past 7 days:

1. I have been able to laugh and see the funny side of things
   - ☐ As much as I always could
   - ☐ Not quite so much now
   - ☐ Definitely not so much now
   - ☐ Not at all

2. I have looked forward with enjoyment to things
   - ☐ As much as I ever did
   - ☐ Rather less than I used to
   - ☐ Definitely less than I used to
   - ☐ Hardly at all

*3. I have blamed myself unnecessarily when things went wrong
   - ☐ Yes, most of the time
   - ☐ Yes, some of the time
   - ☐ Not very often
   - ☐ No, never

4. I have been anxious or worried for no good reason
   - ☐ No, not at all
   - ☐ Hardly ever
   - ☐ Yes, sometimes
   - ☐ Yes, very often

*5 I have felt scared or panicky for no very good reason
   - ☐ Yes, quite a lot
   - ☐ Yes, sometimes
   - ☐ No, not much
   - ☐ No, not at all

*6. Things have been getting on top of me
   - ☐ Yes, most of the time I haven't been able to cope at all
   - ☐ Yes, sometimes I haven't been coping as well as usual
   - ☐ No, most of the time I have copied quite well
   - ☐ No, I have been coping as well as ever

*7 I have been so unhappy that I have had difficulty sleeping
   - ☐ Yes, most of the time
   - ☐ Yes, sometimes
   - ☐ Not very often
   - ☐ No, not at all

*8 I have felt sad or miserable
   - ☐ Yes, most of the time
   - ☐ Yes, quite often
   - ☐ Not very often
   - ☐ No, not at all

*9 I have been so unhappy that I have been crying
   - ☐ Yes, most of the time
   - ☐ Yes, quite often
   - ☐ Only occasionally
   - ☐ No, never

*10 The thought of harming myself has occurred to me
   - ☐ Yes, quite often
   - ☐ Sometimes
   - ☐ Hardly ever
   - ☐ Never

Administered/Reviewed by _____   Date _____

FIGURE 22.5 Adapted Edinburgh Postnatal Depression Scale (EPDS). (From Cox, J. L., Holden, J. M., & Sagovsky, R. [1987]. Detection of postnatal depression: Development of the 10-item Edinburgh Postnatal Depression Scale. *British Journal of Psychiatry, 150,* 782–786.)

Also review the history for specific pregnancy and birth factors that may increase the client's risk for depression. These may include a history of PPD, evidence of depression during the pregnancy, prenatal anxiety, a difficult or complicated pregnancy, traumatic birth experience, or birth of a high-risk or special-needs infant (Callahan, 2016). The incidence of a major depressive disorder during pregnancy has been estimated at 5% to 16%, and up to 31% of postpartum individuals within the first year after birth. The incidence of anxiety disorders is also higher in the first year after giving birth (BC Reproductive Mental Health Program & Perinatal Services BC, 2014).

Be alert for physical findings. Assess the client's activity level, including level of fatigue. Ask about sleeping habits, noting any problems with insomnia. When interacting with the client, observe for verbal and nonverbal indicators of anxiety as well as any ability to concentrate during the interaction. Difficulty concentrating and anxious behaviours suggest a problem. Also assess nutritional intake: weight loss due to poor food intake may be seen. Assessment can identify clients with a high-risk profile for depression, and the nurse can educate them and make referrals for individual or family counselling if needed. Some common assessment findings associated with PPD are listed in Box 22.2.

Nursing Management

Nurses need to educate themselves about this disorder to facilitate early recognition of signs and symptoms of it, which, in turn, would make early treatment possible, thus supporting recovery. Furthermore, greater knowledge could contribute to providing more effective and compassionate care to these individuals and families. Nursing management focuses on assisting every postpartum person to cope with the changes of this period. Encourage clients to verbalize what they are going through and emphasize the importance of keeping their expectations realistic. Assist the client in structuring the day to regain a sense of control over the situation. Encourage clients to seek help if necessary, using available support systems. Also reinforce the need for good nutrition and adequate exercise and sleep (Bobo & Yawn, 2014).

The nurse can play an important role in assisting clients and their partners with postpartum adjustment. Providing facts about the enormous changes that occur during the postpartum period is critical. This information would include changes in the body. Review the signs and symptoms of all three affective disorders. This information is typically included as part of prenatal visits and childbirth education classes. Know the risk factors associated with these disorders and review the history of clients and their families. Use specific, nonthreatening questions to aid in early detection, such

---

| BOX 22.2 |

COMMON ASSESSMENT FINDINGS ASSOCIATED WITH POSTPARTUM DEPRESSION

- Loss of pleasure or interest in life
- Low mood, especially in the morning; sadness, tearfulness
- Exhaustion that is not relieved by sleep
- Feelings of guilt
- Weight loss
- Low energy
- Irritability
- Poor personal hygiene
- Constipation
- Being preoccupied and unfocused
- Indecisiveness
- Diminished concentration
- Anxiety
- Despair
- Compulsive thoughts
- Loss of libido
- Loss of confidence
- Sleep difficulties (insomnia)
- Loss of appetite
- Bleak and pessimistic view of the future
- Not responding to infant's cries or cues for attention
- Social isolation, not answering the door or the phone
- Feelings of failure as a mother

Adapted from Society of Obstetricians and Gynaecologist of Canada (SOGC). (2018). *Mental health and postpartum depression*. Retrieved from https://www.pregnancyinfo.ca/postpartum/postpartum/mental-health-and-postpartum-depression/; Centers for Disease Control and Prevention (CDC). (2018b). *Depression among women*. Retrieved from http://www.cdc.gov/reproductivehealth/depression/; and Joy, S., Mattingly, P. J., & Templeton, H. B. (2017). Postpartum depression. *eMedicine*. Retrieved from http://emedicine.medscape.com/article/271662-overview

---

as, "Have you felt down, depressed, or hopeless lately?" and, "Have you felt little interest or pleasure in doing things recently?"

Discuss factors that may increase a person's vulnerability to stress during the postpartum period, such as sleep deprivation and unrealistic expectations, so couples can understand and respond to those problems if they occur. Reinforce that many people need help after childbirth and that help is available from many sources, including people they already know. Assisting clients to learn how to ask for help is important so they can gain the support they need. Also provide educational materials about postpartum emotional disorders. Have available referral sources for psychotherapy and support groups appropriate for those experiencing postpartum adjustment difficulties, for example, Pacific Post Partum Support Society's *Postpartum Depression & Anxiety*. See Evidence-Based Practice 22.1.

NURSING CARE PLAN 22.1

Overview of the Client With a Postpartum Complication

Jennifer, a 16-year-old G1P1, gave birth to a boy 3 days ago. It was a cesarean birth due to cephalopelvic disproportion following 25 hours of labour with ruptured membranes. Her temperature is 39.2°C (102.6°F). She is complaining of chills and malaise and says, "My incision really hurts." Jennifer rates her pain as 7 to 8 out of 10. The incision site is red, swollen, and very warm to the touch. A 5-cm area of purulent drainage is noted on the dressing; a 3-cm area of the incision is slightly opened, with the wound edges separated. Jennifer's lochia is scant and dark red, with a strong odour. She asks the nurse to help take care of her baby because she doesn't feel well enough to care for him.

NURSING DIAGNOSIS: Ineffective thermoregulation related to bacterial invasion as evidenced by fever, complaints of chills and malaise, and statement of not feeling well

Outcome Identification and Evaluation

The client will exhibit a return to normothermia as evidenced by a body temperature being maintained below 37.2°C (99°F), reports of a decrease in chills and malaise, and statements of feeling better.

Interventions: *Promoting Fever Reduction*

- Assess vital signs every 2 to 4 hours and record results *to monitor progress of infection.*
- Administer antipyretics as ordered *to reduce temperature and help combat infection.*
- Encourage fluid intake *to promote fluid balance.*
- Document intake and output *to assess hydration status.*

- Offer cool bed bath or shower *to reduce temperature.*
- Place cool cloth on forehead and/or back of neck *to provide comfort.*
- Change bed linen and gown when damp from diaphoresis *to provide comfort and hygiene.*

NURSING DIAGNOSIS: Impaired skin integrity related to wound infection as evidenced by purulent drainage, redness, swelling, and separation of wound edges

Outcome Identification and Evaluation

The client will experience a resolution of wound infection as evidenced by a reduction in redness, swelling, and drainage from wound; absence of purulent drainage; and beginning signs and symptoms of wound healing.

Interventions: *Promoting Wound Healing*

- Administer antibiotic therapy as ordered *to treat infection.*
- Perform frequent dressing changes and wound care as ordered *to promote wound healing;* monitor dressing for drainage, including amount, colour, and characteristics, *to evaluate for resolution of infection.*

- Use aseptic technique *to prevent spread of infection.*
- Encourage fluid intake *to maintain fluid balance;* encourage adequate dietary intake, including protein, *to promote healing.*

NURSING CARE PLAN 22.1

Overview of the Client With a Postpartum Complication (continued)

NURSING DIAGNOSIS: Acute pain related to infectious process

Outcome Identification and Evaluation

The client will report a decrease in pain as evidenced by pain rating of 0 or 1 on pain scale, verbalization of relief with pain management, and statements of feeling better and ability to rest comfortably.

Interventions: *Relieving Pain*

- Place client in semi-Fowler's position to facilitate drainage and relieve pressure.
- Assess pain level on pain scale of 0 to 10 to quantify pain level; reassess pain level after intervening to determine effectiveness of intervention.
- Assess fundus gently to ensure appropriate involution.
- Administer analgesics as needed and on time as ordered to maintain pain relief.
- Provide for rest periods to allow for healing.
- Assist with positioning in bed with pillows to promote comfort.
- Offer nonpharmacologic pain measures such as a backrub to ease aches and discomfort if desired and enhance effectiveness of analgesics.

NURSING DIAGNOSIS: Risk for impaired attachment related to effects of postpartum infection as evidenced by mother's request to take baby back to the nursery

Outcome Identification and Evaluation

The client will begin to bond with newborn appropriately with each exposure as evidenced by desire to spend time with newborn, expression of positive feelings toward newborn when holding him, increasing participation in care of newborn as client's condition improves, and statements about help and support at home to care for self and newborn.

Interventions: *Promoting Parent–Infant Interaction*

- Promote adequate rest and sleep to ensure adequate energy for interaction and wound healing.
- Encourage self-care comfort and hygiene measures as well as analgesia to allow the client to focus energy on the child.
- Progressively encourage the client to care for and comfort the infant as energy level and pain level improve to promote self-confidence in caring for the newborn.
- Offer praise and positive reinforcement for caretaking tasks; stress positive attributes of newborn to the parent while caring for him to facilitate bonding and attachment.
- Contact family members to participate in care of the newborn to allow the client to rest and recover from infection.
- Encourage client to care for herself first and then the newborn to ensure adequate energy for newborn's care.
- Arrange for assistance and support after discharge from hospital to provide necessary backup.
- Refer to community health nurse for follow-up care of client and newborn at home to foster continued development of maternal–infant relationship.
- Discuss the community programs and services for support in development of parental–infant relationship as an adolescent parent.

KEY CONCEPTS

○ Postpartum hemorrhage is a potentially life-threatening complication of both vaginal and cesarean births. It is the leading cause of maternal mortality in the United States, and third leading cause in Canada.

○ A good way to remember the causes of postpartum hemorrhage is the "5 T's": tone, tissue, trauma, thrombin, and traction.

○ Uterine atony is the most common cause of early postpartum hemorrhage, which can lead to hypovolemic shock.

○ Oxytocin (Pitocin), misoprostol (Cytotec), dinoprostone (Prostin E2), methylergonovine maleate (Methergine), and prostaglandin PGF2α (carboprost [Hemabate]) are commonly used drugs used to manage postpartum hemorrhage.

○ Failure of the placenta to separate completely and be expelled interferes with the ability of the uterus to contract fully, thereby leading to hemorrhage.

○ Causes of subinvolution include retained placental fragments, distended bladder, uterine myoma, and infection.

○ Lacerations should always be suspected when the uterus is contracted, and bright-red blood continues to trickle out of the vagina.

○ Conditions that cause coagulopathies may include idiopathic thrombocytopenic purpura (ITP), von Willebrand disease (vWD), and disseminated intravascular coagulation (DIC).

○ Pulmonary embolism is a potentially fatal condition that occurs when the pulmonary artery is obstructed by a blood clot that has travelled from another vein into the lungs, causing obstruction and infarction.

○ The major causes of a thrombus formation (blood clot) are venous stasis and hypercoagulation, both of which are common in the postpartum period.

○ Postpartum infection is defined as a fever of 38°C (100.4°F) or higher after the first 24 hours after childbirth, occurring on at least 2 of the first 10 days exclusive of the first 24 hours.

○ Common postpartum infections include metritis, wound infections, urinary tract infections, and mastitis.

○ Postpartum emotional disorders are commonly classified on the basis of their severity: "baby blues," postpartum depression, and postpartum psychosis.

○ Management of postpartum depression mirrors the treatment of any major depression: a combination of antidepressant medication, antianxiety medication, and psychotherapy in an outpatient or inpatient setting.

REFERENCES AND RECOMMENDED READINGS

Agency for Healthcare Research and Quality (AHRQ). (2016). *Management of postpartum hemorrhage: Current state of the evidence*. Retrieved from https://effectivehealthcare.ahrq.gov/topics/hemorrhage-postpartum/clinician.

Alexander, L. L., LaRosa, J. H., Bader, H., & Garfield, S. (2014). *New dimensions in women's health* (6th ed.). Sudbury, MA: Jones & Bartlett.

American College of Obstetricians and Gynecologists (ACOG). (2017). *Von Willebrand Disease in women*. Retrieved from http://www.acog.org/Resources-And-Publications/Committee-Opinions/Committee-on-Adolescent-Health-Care/Von-Willebrand-Disease-in-Women.

American College of Obstetricians and Gynecologists (ACOG). (2018). *Use of prophylactic antibiotics in labor and delivery*. Retrieved from http://www.guideline.gov/content.aspx?id=34024.

Amir, L. H. (2014). The Academy of Breastfeeding Medicine Protocol Committee: Mastitis. *Breastfeeding Medicine, 9*(5): 239–243.

Anand, B., & Gujral, K. (2014). Monitoring of high-risk areas: Maternity wards. In C. Wattal, & N. Khardori (Eds.), *Hospital infection prevention* (pp. 133–136). New Delhi, India: Springer Publishers.

BC Reproductive Mental Health Program & Perinatal Services BC. (2014). *Best practice guidelines for mental health disorders in the perinatal period*. Retrieved from http://www.perinatalservicesbc.ca/Documents/Guidelines-Standards/Maternal/MentalHealthDisordersGuideline.pdf.

Belfort, M. A. (2018). Overview of postpartum hemorrhage. *UpToDate*. Retrieved from http://www.uptodate.com/contents/overview-of-postpartum-hemorrhage.

Bhati, S., & Richards, K. (2015). A systematic review of the relationship between postpartum sleep disturbance and postpartum depression. *Journal of Obstetric, Gynecologic, & Neonatal Nursing, 44*(3), 350–357.

Bobo, W. V., & Yawn, B. P. (2014). Concise review for physicians and other clinicians: Postpartum depression. *Mayo Clinic Proceedings, 89*(6), 835–844.

Bohlmann, M., & Rath, W. (2014). Medical prevention and treatment of postpartum hemorrhage: A comparison of different guidelines. *Archives of Gynecology & Obstetrics, 289*(3), 555–567.

Callahan, T. L. (2016). *Tarascon's OB/GYN pocketbook*. Burlington, MA: Jones & Bartlett Learning.

Centers for Disease Control and Prevention (CDC). (2018a). *Data and statistics on venous thromboembolism*. Retrieved from http://www.cdc.gov/ncbddd/dvt/data.html.

Centers for Disease Control and Prevention (CDC). (2018b). *Depression among women*. Retrieved from http://www.cdc.gov/reproductivehealth/depression/.

Centers for Disease Control and Prevention (CDC). (2018c). *Facts about von Willebrand Disease*. Retrieved from http://www.cdc.gov/ncbddd/vwd/facts.html.

Clapp, J. C. (2015). A multidisciplinary team approach to management of postpartum hemorrhage. *Journal of Obstetric, Gynecologic, & Neonatal Nursing, 44*, S22. doi: 10.1111/1552-6909.12693.

Conti, E., Zezza, L., Ralli, E., Comito, C., Sada, L., Passerini, J., . . . Volpe, M. (2014). Pulmonary embolism in pregnancy. *Journal of Thrombosis and Thrombolysis, 37*(3), 251–270.

Cox, J., Holden, J., & Henshaw, C. (2014). *Perinatal mental health: The Edinburgh Postnatal Depression Scale (EPDS) manual* (2nd ed.). London, England: RCPsych Publications.

Cox, J. L., Holden, J. M., & Sagovsky, R. (1987). Detection of postnatal depression: Development of the 10-item Edinburgh Postnatal Depression Scale. *British Journal of Psychiatry, 150*, 782–786.

Crowe, S. D., & Faulkner, B. (2014). Lean management system application in creation of a postpartum hemorrhage prevention bundle on postpartum units. *Obstetrics and Gynecology, 123*, 45S.

Cunningham, F. G., Leveno, K. J., Bloom, S. L., Spong, C., Dashe, J. S., Hoffman, B. L., . . . Sheffield, J. S. (2014). *Williams obstetrics* (24th ed.). New York: McGraw-Hill.

Dalton, E., & Castillo, E. (2014). Postpartum infections: A review for the non-OB/GYN. *Obstetric Medicine: The Medicine of Pregnancy, 7*(3), 98–102.

del Corral Serrano, J. (2015). Puerperal psychosis. In M. Sáenz-Herrero (Ed.), *Psychopathology in women* (pp. 497–510). New York: Springer International Publishing.

Doyle, M., Carballedo, A., & O'Keane, V. (2015). Perinatal depression and psychosis: an update. *Advances in Psychiatric Treatment, 21*(1), 5–14.

Ekin, A., Gezer, C., Solmaz, U., Taner, C. E., Dogan, A., & Ozeren, M. (2015). Predictors of severity in primary postpartum hemorrhage. *Archives of Gynecology and Obstetrics, 292*(6), 1247–154.

Erez, O., Mastrolia, S. A., & Thachil, J. (2015). Disseminated intravascular coagulation in pregnancy: Insights in pathophysiology, diagnosis and management. *American Journal of Obstetrics and Gynecology, 213*(4), 452–463.

Feeley, N., Bell, L., Hayton, B., Zelkowitz, P., & Carrier, M. E. (2016). Care for postpartum depression: What do women and their partners prefer? *Perspectives in Psychiatric Care, 52*(2):120–130.

Finley, P. R., & Brizendine, L. (2015). Enhancing our understanding of perinatal depression. *CNS Spectrums, 20*(1), 9–10.

Green, C. J. (2016). *Maternal newborn nursing care plans* (3rd ed.). Burlington, MA: Jones & Bartlett Learning.

Guimicheva, B., Czuprynska, J., & Arya, R. (2015). The prevention of pregnancy-related venous thromboembolism. *British Journal of Hematology, 168*(2), 163–174.

Heffline, M., & Schmidt, M. K. (2014). Chapter 19: Superficial thrombophlebitis and deep vein thrombosis. In C. R. Christensen, & P. A. Lewis (Eds.), *Core curriculum for vascular nursing* (pp. 370–399). Philadelphia, PA: Wolters Kluwer.

Jordan, R. G., Engstrom, J. L., Marfell, J. A., & Farley, C. L. (2014). *Prenatal and postnatal care: A woman-centered approach*. Ames, Iowa: Wiley Blackwell.

Joy, S., Mattingly, P. J., & Templeton, H. B. (2017). Postpartum depression. *eMedicine*. Retrieved from http://emedicine.medscape.com/article/271662-overview.

Kamel, I., & Mastrogiannis, D. S. (2015). The critically ill obstetric patient. Part 1: Epidemiology and pathophysiology. *Postgraduate Obstetrics & Gynecology, 35*(11), 1–7.

Kansky, C., & Isaacs, C. (2016). Normal and abnormal puerperium. *eMedicine*. Retrieved from https://emedicine.medscape.com/article/260187-overview.

Kaur, P., Sagar, N., Deol, R., & Kaur, J. (2015). Effectiveness of infra-red therapy upon level of episiotomy pain and wound healing among postnatal mothers. *International Journal of Nursing Education, 7*(2), 184–187.

Kessler, C. M. (2018). Immune thrombocytopenic purpura. *eMedicine*. Retrieved from http://emedicine.medscape.com/article/202158-overview.

King, T. L., Brucker, M. C., Kriebs, J. M., Fahey, J. O., Gegor, C. L., & Varney, H. (2015). *Varney's midwifery* (5th ed.). Burlington, MA: Jones & Bartlett Learning.

Kolecki, P., & Menckhoff, C. R. (2016). Hypovolemic shock. *eMedicine*. Retrieved from http://emedicine.medscape.com/article/760145-overview.

Levi, M. M., & Schmaier, A. H. (2018). Disseminated intravascular coagulation. *eMedicine*. Retrieved from http://emedicine.medscape.com/article/199627-overview.

Main, E. K., Goffman, D., Scavone, B. M., Low, L. K., Bingham, D., Fontaine, P. L., . . . Levy, B. S. (2015). National partnership for maternal safety: Consensus bundle on obstetric hemorrhage. *Journal of Obstetric, Gynecologic, & Neonatal Nursing, 121*(1), 142–148.

Mattson, S., & Smith, J. E. (2015). *Core curriculum for maternal-newborn nursing* (5th ed.). St. Louis, MO: Saunders Elsevier.

Middeldorp, S. (2015). New studies of low-molecular-weight heparin in pregnancy. *Thrombosis Research, 135*, S26–S29.

Moses, S. (2015). Postpartum hemorrhage. *Family practice notebook*. Retrieved from http://www.fpnotebook.com/ob/Bleed/PstprtmHmrhg.htm.

Mousa, H. A., Blum, J., Abou El Senoun, G., Shakur, H., Alfirevic, Z. (2014). Treatment for primary postpartum hemorrhage. *Cochrane Database of Systematic Reviews, 2*, CD003249. doi: 10.1002/14651858.CD003249.pub3.

Nagtalon-Ramos, J. (2014). *Maternal-newborn nursing care: Best evidence-based practices*. Philadelphia, PA: F.A. Davis Company.

Nahum, G. G., & Pham, K. Q. (2018). Uterine rupture in pregnancy. *eMedicine*. Retrieved from http://reference.medscape.com/article/275854-overview.

National Hemophilia Foundation. (2018). *Von Willebrand disease*. Retrieved from https://www.hemophilia.org/Bleeding-Disorders/Types-of-Bleeding-Disorders/Von-Willebrand-Disease.

Nikpour, M., Shirvani, M. A., Azadbakht, M., Zanjani, R., & Mousavi, E. (2014). The effect of honey gel on abdominal wound healing in caesarean section: A triple blind randomized clinical trial. *Oman Medical Journal, 29*(4), 255–259.

Pacific Post Partum Support Society (2014). *Postpartum depression & anxiety: A self-help guide for mothers.* (17th ed.). Burnaby, BC: Author.

Pagana, K. D., Pagana, T. J., & Pagana, T. N. (2014). *Mosby's diagnostic and laboratory test reference* (12th ed.). St. Louis, MO: Mosby Elsevier.

Pavord, S., & Maybury, H. (2015). How I treat postpartum hemorrhage. *Blood, 125*(18), 2759–2770.

Pollak, E. S. (2018). von Willebrand disease. *eMedicine.* Retrieved from http://emedicine.medscape.com/article/206996-overview.

Pop, V. J., Truijens, S. E., Spek, V., Wijnen, H. A., van Son, M. J., & Bergink, V. (2015). A new concept of maternity blues: Is there a subgroup of women with rapid cycling mood symptoms? *Journal of Affective Disorders, 177,* 74–79.

Quellette, D. R., Harrington, A., & Kamangar, N. (2018). Pulmonary embolism. *eMedicine.* Retrieved from http://emedicine.medscape.com/article/300901-overview.

Rong, J., Yuna, G., & Yan, C. (2014). Risk factors associated with emergency peripartum hysterectomy. *Chinese Medical Journal, 127*(5), 900–904.

Salam, R. A., Mansoor, T., Mallick, D., Lassi, Z. S., Das, J. K., & Bhutta, Z. A. (2014). Essential childbirth and postnatal interventions for improved maternal and neonatal health. *Reproductive Health, 11*(Suppl 1), S3–S20.

Schiller, C. E., Meltzer-Brody, S., & Rubinow, D. R. (2015). The role of reproductive hormones in postpartum depression. *CNS Spectrums, 20*(1), 48–59.

Shields, L. E., Wiesner, S., Fulton, J., & Pelletreau, B. (2015). Comprehensive maternal hemorrhage protocols reduce the use of blood products and improve patient safety. *American Journal of Obstetrics and Gynecology, 212*(3), 272–280.

Silverman, M. A. (2017). Idiopathic thrombocytopenic purpura. *eMedicine.* Retrieved from http://emedicine.medscape.com/article/779545-overview.

Skidmore-Roth, L. (2015). *Mosby's 2015 nursing drug reference* (28th ed.). St. Louis, MO: Mosby Elsevier.

Smithson, D.S., Twohey, R., Rice, T., Watts, N., Fernandes, C. M., & Gratton, R. (2013). Implementing an obstetric triage acuity scale: Interrater reliability and patient flow analysis. *American Journal Obstetrics and Gynecology, 209*(4), 287–293.

Society of Obstetricians and Gynaecologists of Canada. (2015). *Antibiotic prophylaxis in obstetric procedures.* Retrieved from https://sogc.org/wp-content/uploads/2013/01/gui247CPG1009ERe_Aff_Dis.pdf.

Sucker, C., & Zotz, R. B. (2015). Prophylaxis and treatment of venous thrombosis and pulmonary embolism in pregnancy. *Reviews in Vascular Medicine, 3*(2), 24–30.

Tánczos, K., Németh, M., & Molnár, Z. (2015). What's new in hemorrhagic shock? *Intensive Care Medicine, 41*(4), 712–714.

Tepper, N. K., Boulet, S. L., Whiteman, M. K., Monsour, M., Marchbanks, P. A., Hooper, W. C., & Curtis, K. M. (2014). Postpartum venous thromboembolism: Incidence and risk factors. *Obstetrics & Gynecology, 123*(5), 987–996.

Testa, S., Passamonti, S. M., Paoletti, O., Bucciarelli, P., Ronca, E., Riccardi, A., . . . Martinelli, I. (2015). The "Pregnancy Health-care Program" for the prevention of venous thromboembolism in pregnancy. *Internal and Emergency Medicine, 10*(2), 129–134.

Thombs, B. D., Arthurs, E., Coronado-Montoya, S., Roseman, M., Delisle, V. C., Leavens, A., . . . Zelkowitz, P. (2014). Depression screening and patient outcomes in pregnancy or postpartum: A systematic review. *Journal of Psychosomatic Research, 76*(6), 433–446.

Van de Velde, M., Diez, C., & Varon, A. J. (2015). Obstetric hemorrhage. *Current Opinion in Anesthesiology, 28*(2), 186–190.

Weissman, M. M. (2014). Treatment of depression: Men and women are different? *American Journal of Psychiatry, 171*(4), 384–387.

Wells, P. S., Forgie, M. A., & Rodger, M. A. (2014). Treatment of venous thromboembolism. *JAMA, 311*(7), 717–728.

Wilcox, L. L., Ramprasad, C., Gutierrez, A., Oden, M., Richards-Kortum, R., & Gandhi, M. (2015). Accuracy in estimation of blood loss using the SAPHE (Signaling a Postpartum Hemorrhage Emergency) Mat [51]. *Obstetrics & Gynecology, 125,* 25S. doi: 10.1097/AOG.0000000000000753.

Wong, A. W., & Rosh, A. J. (2017). Postpartum infections. *eMedicine.* Retrieved from http://emedicine.medscape.com/article/796892-overview.

World Health Organization. (2017). *Updated WHO recommendation on tranexamic acid for the treatment of postpartum haemorrhage.* Retrieved from http://apps.who.int/iris/bitstream/handle/10665/259379/WHO-RHR-17.21-eng.pdf;jsessionid=6C1BBE9273754FFBA301457370D9E5B1?sequence=1.

Yiadom, M. Y., & Carusi, D. (2015). Postpartum hemorrhage in emergency medicine. *eMedicine.* Retrieved from http://emedicine.medscape.com/article/796785-overview.

Zhao, Y., Kane, I., Wang, J., Shen, B., Luo, J., & Shi, S. (2015). Combined use of the postpartum depression screening scale (PDSS) and Edinburgh postnatal depression scale (EPDS) to identify antenatal depression among Chinese pregnant women with obstetric complications. *Psychiatry Research, 226*(1), 113–119.

CHAPTER **WORKSHEET**

MULTIPLE CHOICE QUESTIONS

1. A postpartum client appears very pale and states is bleeding heavily. The nurse should first:
   a. Call the client's health care provider immediately.
   b. Immediately set up an intravenous infusion of magnesium sulphate.
   c. Assess the fundus and ask about voiding status.
   d. Reassure the client that this is a normal finding after childbirth.

2. A postpartum client reports hearing voices and says, "The voices are telling me to do bad things to my baby." The clinic nurse interprets these findings as suggesting postpartum
   a. Psychosis.
   b. Anxiety disorder.
   c. Depression.
   d. Blues.

3. When implementing the plan of care for a multigravida postpartum client who gave birth just a few hours ago, the nurse vigilantly monitors the client for which complication?
   a. Deep venous thrombosis
   b. Postpartum psychosis
   c. Uterine infection
   d. Postpartum hemorrhage

4. Which of the following would the nurse expect to include in the plan of care for a client with mastitis who is receiving antibiotic therapy?
   a. Stop breastfeeding and apply lanolin.
   b. Administer analgesics and bind both breasts.
   c. Apply warm or cold compresses and administer analgesics.
   d. Remove the nursing bra and expose the breast to fresh air.

5. While assessing a postpartum multiparous client, the nurse detects a boggy uterus midline 2 cm above the umbilicus. Which intervention would be the priority?
   a. Assessing vital signs immediately
   b. Measuring the next urinary output
   c. Massaging the fundus
   d. Notifying the client's obstetrician

6. Methergine has been ordered for a postpartum client because of excessive bleeding. The nurse should question this order if which of the following is present?
   a. Mild abdominal cramping
   b. Tender inflamed breasts
   c. Pulse rate of 68 beats per minute
   d. Blood pressure of 158/96 mm Hg

7. Which of the following findings would lead the nurse to suspect that a client is developing a postpartum complication?
   a. Moderate lochia rubra for the first 24 hours
   b. Clear lung sounds upon auscultation
   c. Temperature of 38°C (100.4°F)
   d. Chest pain experienced when ambulating

8. Which of the following factors in a postpartum client's history would lead the nurse to monitor closely for an infection?
   a. Hemoglobin of 12 mg/dL
   b. Manually extracted placenta
   c. Labour of 10 hours length
   d. Multiparity of five pregnancies

CRITICAL THINKING EXERCISES

1. Mrs. Griffin had a 22-hour labour before a cesarean birth. Her membranes ruptured 20 hours before she came to the hospital. Her fetus showed signs of fetal distress, so internal electronic fetal monitoring was used. Her most recent test results indicate she is anemic.
   a. What postpartum complication is this client at highest risk for? Why?
   b. What assessments need to be done to detect this complication?
   c. What nursing measures will the nurse use to prevent this complication?

2. Tammy, a 32-year-old G9P9, had a spontaneous vaginal birth 2 hours ago. Tammy has been having a baby each year for the past 9 years. Her lochia has been heavy, with some clots. She hasn't been up to void since she had epidural anesthesia and has decreased sensation to her legs.
   a. What factors place Tammy at risk for postpartum hemorrhage?
   b. What assessments are needed before planning interventions?
   c. What nursing actions are needed to prevent a postpartum hemorrhage?

3. Lucy, a 25-year-old G2P2, gave birth 2 days ago and is expected to be discharged today. She had severe postpartum depression 2 years ago with her first child. Lucy has not been out of bed for the past 24 hours, is not eating, and provides no care for herself or her newborn. Lucy states she already has a boy at home and not having a girl this time is disappointing.
   a. What factors/behaviours place Lucy at risk for an affective disorder?
   b. Which interventions might be appropriate at this time?
   c. What education does the family need prior to discharge?

CHAPTER **WORKSHEET**

STUDY ACTIVITIES

1. Compare and contrast postpartum blues, postpartum depression, and postpartum psychosis in terms of their features and medical management.

2. Visit and select a website from the Student Resources for Chapter 22. Critique the website regarding its helpfulness to parents, the correctness of the information, and when it was last updated.

3. Interview an individual who has given birth and ask if there were any complications and what was most helpful during that experience.

4. The number one cause of postpartum hemorrhage is
_____.

5. When giving report to the nurse who will be caring for a client and newborn in the postpartum period, what information should the labour nurse convey?

BRINGING IT ALL TOGETHER: A CASE STUDY

Sheila is an 18-year-old G1P1 who had her first child 2 days ago via primary cesarean section. Her pregnancy was uneventful, but she didn't attend prenatal clinic very often. She presented to the hospital in labour at 39 weeks' gestation with ruptured membranes. The client reported that her membranes had been ruptured for a "couple of days," but she wasn't really sure. Upon admission, she was dilated 2 cm/40% effacement. She laboured for about 7 hours when the health care provider came in to check her. She was only 5 cm/completely effaced at that time. The health care provider inserted an internal fetal monitor with a scalp electrode and also an intrauterine pressure catheter because she was obese, and the nurse was having difficulty in picking up the FHR tracing. She had no progress for the next 4 hours and the fetus was noted to develop tachycardia with a baseline heart rate of 170 bpm. A primary cesarean section was performed, and she was given perioperative antibiotic prophylaxis at the time of surgery. Infant was LGA and Apgar scores were 9/9 at 1 minute and 5 minutes, respectively.

Go to thePoint **to find questions to consider about this case.**

Unit 8

The Newborn
at Risk

23

Nursing Care of the Newborn With Special Needs

Learning Objectives

Upon completion of the chapter, you will be able to:

1. Evaluate factors that assist in identifying a newborn at risk due to variations in birth weight and gestational age.

2. Select contributing factors and common complications associated with dysmature infants and their management.

3. Compare and contrast nursing assessment findings and nursing management of a small-for-gestational-age (SGA) newborn and a large-for-gestational-age (LGA) newborn; a postterm and a preterm newborn.

4. Analyze nursing assessment and management of newborn conditions associated with variations in birth weight and gestational ages.

5. Outline the nurse's role in helping parents experiencing perinatal grief or loss.

6. Integrate knowledge of the risks associated with late preterm births into nursing interventions, discharge planning, and parent education.

Anna and her husband were stunned when she went into labour at 7 months' gestation. They couldn't understand what would cause her to give birth early, but it happened. When they approached the NICU, Anna took a deep breath and looked down at her tiny baby with tubes coming from everywhere. What feelings might they be experiencing at this moment?

INTRODUCTION

All families look forward to the birth of a healthy newborn, but some pregnancy outcomes don't meet these expectations. Most newborns are born between 38 and 42 weeks' gestation and weigh 6 to 8 lb, but variations in birth weight or gestational age can occur, and newborns with these variations have special needs. Gestational age at birth is inversely correlated with the risk that the infant will experience physical, neurologic, or developmental challenges (March of Dimes, 2013). Some newborns are born very ill and require special advanced care to survive. Unexpected difficulties may occur during the pregnancy or childbirth, which change the whole course of events for the families. While reducing preterm births and **low birth weight (LBW)** remain important objectives, the fact remains that 9.8% of infants are born prematurely and 8% are of LBW (National Center for Health Statistics, 2017).

On giving birth to a newborn with problems involving immaturity or LBW, especially one who is considered high risk, parents may go through a grieving process in which they mourn the loss of the healthy full-term newborn they had expected. Through this process parents learn to come to terms with the experience they now face.

The key to identifying a newborn with special needs related to birth weight or gestational age variation is an awareness of the factors that could place a newborn at risk. These factors are similar to those that would suggest a high-risk pregnancy and include but not limited to:

- Maternal nutrition (malnutrition or overweight)
- Substandard living conditions or low socioeconomic status
- Maternal age of less than 20 or more than 35 years (advanced maternal age)
- Substance abuse
- Lack of prenatal care
- Smoking or exposure to passive smoke
- Periodontal disease
- Multiple gestation
- Iron deficiency anemia
- Maternal obesity
- Extreme maternal stress
- Abuse and violence
- History of mental health disorders
- Placental complications (placenta previa or abruptio placentae)
- History of previous preterm birth
- Maternal disease (e.g., hypertension, diabetes, HIV)
- Maternal infection (e.g., urinary tract infection, chorioamnionitis)
- Exposure to occupational hazards, working long hours, or very physical labour (Simpson, 2015)

The development of new technologies and regionalized care centres for the care of newborns with special needs has resulted in significant improvements in neonatal morbidity and mortality. Being able to anticipate the birth of a newborn at risk allows the birth to take place at a health care facility equipped with the resources to meet the newborn's needs. Nurses need to have a sound knowledge base to identify the newborn with special needs and to provide coordinated care.

This chapter discusses the nursing management of newborns with special needs related to variations in birth weight and gestational age. It also describes selected associated conditions affecting these newborns. Due to the frailty of these newborns, the care of the family experiencing perinatal loss and the role of the nurse in helping the family cope also are addressed.

BIRTH WEIGHT VARIATIONS

Fetal growth is influenced by maternal nutrition, genetics, placental function, environment, and a multitude of other factors. Assigning size to a newborn is a way to measure and monitor the growth and development of the newborn at birth. Newborns can be classified according to their birth weight and weeks of gestation. Knowing the group into which a newborn fits is important.

Appropriate for gestational age (AGA) describes a newborn with a weight that falls within the 10th to 90th percentile for that particular gestational age. This describes approximately 80% of all newborns (Mattson & Smith, 2015). Infants who are AGA have lower morbidity and mortality than other groups.

Small for gestational age (SGA) describes newborns that typically weigh less than 2,500 g (5 lb 8 oz) at term due to less growth than expected in utero. A newborn is also classified as SGA if his or her birth weight is at or below the 10th percentile as correlated with the number of weeks of gestation (Mandy, 2018a).

Large for gestational age (LGA) describes newborns whose birth weight is above the 90th percentile on a growth chart and who weigh more than 4,000 g (8 lb 13 oz) at term due to accelerated overgrowth for length of gestation (Mandy, 2018b).

The following terms describe other newborns with marginal weights at birth and of any gestational age:
- **Low birth weight:** less than 2,500 g (5.5 lb) (Fig. 23.1)
- **Very low birth weight:** less than 1,500 g (3 lb 5 oz)
- **Extremely low birth weight:** less than 1,000 g (2 lb 3 oz) (Cleary-Goldman & Robinson, 2018).

Small-for-Gestational-Age Newborns

Newborns are considered SGA when their weight falls below the 10th percentile for length, weight, or head circumference on a growth chart for gestational age. These infants can be preterm, term, or postterm. Some SGA newborns are constitutionally small; they are statistically small but otherwise healthy.

FIGURE 23.1 A low–birth-weight newborn in an isolette.

In some SGA newborns, the rate of growth does not meet the expected growth pattern. These infants are considered to have **fetal growth restriction** (FGR). FGR is the pathologic counterpart of SGA. Newborns with FGR are considered at risk, having increased morbidity and mortality rates as compared to those of AGA newborns. FGR can result from aneuploidy, congenital malformations, infections, or uteroplacental insufficiency (Resnik, 2018). The fetus is thought to have an inherent growth potential that, under normal circumstances, yields a healthy newborn of appropriate size. The maternal–placental–fetal units act in harmony to meet the needs of the fetus during gestation. However, growth potential in the fetus can be limited, and this is analogous to failure to thrive in the infant. The causes of both can be intrinsic or environmental. Factors that can contribute to the birth of an SGA newborn are highlighted in Box 23.1. FGR is usually categorized as symmetric or asymmetric. Symmetric FGR refers to fetuses with equally poor growth rates of the brain, the abdomen, and the long bones and is thought to result from an early global insult. All parameters of growth are affected. Asymmetric FGR refers to infants whose brain growth is spared compared to their abdomen and internal organs (Cunningham et al., 2018). Fetal growth is dependent on genetic, placental, and maternal factors. Cognitive and motor development during infancy forms the basis for children's subsequent development. Newborns that experience nutritional deficiencies in utero and are born with FGR are at risk for lifelong developmental deficits, and emotional and behavioural disorders (Verklan & Walden, 2015).

Nursing Assessment

Assessment of the SGA infant begins by reviewing the maternal history to identify risk factors such as smoking, drug abuse, alcohol consumption, preeclampsia, anemia, intrauterine viral infection, chronic maternal illness, hypertension, multiple gestation, or genetic disorders.

BOX 23.1

FACTORS CONTRIBUTING TO THE BIRTH OF SGA NEWBORNS

- Maternal causes
  - Chronic hypertension
  - Diabetes mellitus with vascular disease
  - Autoimmune diseases
  - Living at a high altitude (hypoxia)
  - Smoking or exposure to passive smoke
  - Periodontal disease of the mouth
  - Maternal age of 20 or 35 years
  - Failure to seek any prenatal care
  - Substandard living conditions
  - Low socioeconomic status
  - Abuse and violence
  - Substance abuse (heroin, cocaine, methamphetamines)
  - Hemoglobinopathies (sickle cell anemia)
  - Preeclampsia
  - Exposure to occupational hazards
  - Chronic renal disease
  - Maternal nutrition (malnutrition or obesity)
  - Extreme maternal stress
  - TORCH group infections
- Placental factors
  - Abnormal cord insertion
  - Chronic abruption
  - Decreased surface area, infarction
  - Decreased placental weight
  - Placenta previa
  - Placental insufficiency
- Fetal factors
  - Trisomy 13, 18, and 21
  - Turner syndrome
  - Chronic fetal infection (cytomegalovirus [CMV], rubella, syphilis, toxoplasmosis)
  - Congenital anomalies (heart, diaphragmatic hernia, tracheoesophageal fistula)
  - Radiation exposure
  - Multiple fetal gestation

Adapted from Cunningham, F. G., Leveno, K. J., Bloom, S. L., Spong, C. Y., Dashe, J. S., Hoffman, B. L., . . . Sheffield, J. S. (2018). *Williams obstetrics* (25th ed.). New York: McGraw-Hill; and Mandy, G. T. (2018a). Small for gestational age infant. *UpToDate*. Retrieved from http://www.uptodate.com/contents/small-for-gestational-age-infant

---

This information allows the nurse to anticipate a possible problem and to be prepared to intervene quickly should one occur. At birth, perform a thorough physical examination, closely observing the newborn for typical characteristics, including:

- Head disproportionately large compared with rest of body (asymmetric)
- Wasted appearance of extremities
- Reduced subcutaneous fat stores
- Jittery secondary to hypoglycemia
- Decreased amount of breast tissue
- Scaphoid abdomen (sunken appearance)
- Temperature instability
- Wide skull sutures secondary to inadequate bone growth

- Poor muscle tone over buttocks and cheeks
- Loose and dry skin that appears oversized
- Thin umbilical cord

Also assess the SGA newborn for any congenital malformations, neurologic insults, or indications of infection. SGA newborns commonly face problems after birth because of the decrease in placental function during gestation. Table 23.1 highlights some of the common problems associated with SGA newborns and others experiencing a variation in birth weight or gestational age. Anticipate the need for and provide resuscitation as indicated by the newborn's condition.

Nursing Management

Interventions for the SGA infant may include obtaining weight, length, and head circumference, comparing them with standards, and documenting the findings on a standardized growth chart. Perform frequent serial blood glucose measurements as ordered and monitor vital signs, being particularly alert for changes in respiratory status that might indicate respiratory distress. Institute measures to maintain a neutral thermal environment to prevent cold stress and acidosis.

Metabolic needs are increased for catch-up growth. Initiate early and frequent oral/enteral feedings unless contraindicated. At birth the newborn's glucose level is about 70% of the pregnant client's serum glucose. Neonatal hypoglycemia is a major cause of brain injury since the brain needs glucose continuously as a primary source of energy (Verklan & Walden, 2015). A newborn stressed at birth uses up available glucose stores quickly with resulting hypoglycemia, a plasma glucose concentration at or below 40 mg/dL (Nagtalon-Ramos, 2014). With the loss of the placenta at birth, the newborn now must assume control of glucose homeostasis through intermittent oral/enteral feedings. If oral feedings are not accepted, an intravenous infusion with 10% dextrose in water may be needed to maintain the glucose level above 40 mg/dL. Monitor feeding tolerance, sucking, and swallowing ability. Weigh the newborn daily and ensure that he or she has adequate rest periods to decrease metabolic requirements. Go to the Point for the Canadian Paediatric Society (CPS)'s *Algorithm for The Screening and Immediate Management of Babies at Risk for Neonatal Hypoglycemia*.

Polycythemia is not uncommon and is a potentially serious disorder of newborns. It is defined as a venous hematocrit above 65% and hemoglobin of more than 20 g. The hematocrit in a newborn peaks between 6 and 12 hours of age and decreases gradually after that. Polycythemia occurs in up to 12% of neonates, very commonly in SGA newborns 6 to 12 hours after birth (Kandasamy, 2017). The relationship between hematocrit and viscosity is almost linear until 65% and exponential thereafter. Increased viscosity of blood is associated with symptoms of hypoperfusion. Clinical features related to

hyperviscosity may affect all organ systems. Hyperviscosity of blood results in increased resistance to blood flow and decreased oxygen delivery. In the newborn, hyperviscosity can cause abnormalities of central nervous system (CNS) function, hypoglycemia, decreased renal function, cardiorespiratory distress, and coagulation disorders. Hyperviscosity has been reported to be associated with long-term motor and cognitive neurodevelopmental disorders (Fanaroff & Fanaroff, 2014). Newborns born SGA, infants of individuals with diabetes, and multiple births are at risk for polycythemia. They should therefore undergo screening at 2, 12, and 24 hours of age (Watchko, 2015). This treatment is performed in the NICU setting.

Observe for clinical signs of polycythemia (respiratory distress, cyanosis, jitteriness, jaundice, ruddy skin colour, and lethargy) and monitor blood results. Asymptomatic newborns with a hematocrit between 65% and 70% may simply be supported with fluids, close observation, and a repeat hematocrit level in 12 hours (Mahajan, Une, & Bansal, 2015). If the newborn is symptomatic, a partial exchange transfusion with replacement of removed red blood cell volume with volume expanders may be used, but this treatment is considered controversial and not validated by current evidence-based practice research.

Provide anticipatory guidance to parents about any treatments and procedures that are being done. Emphasize the need for close follow-up and careful monitoring of the infant's growth in length, weight, and head circumference and feeding patterns throughout the 1st year of life to confirm any "catch-up" growth taking place.

Large-for-Gestational-Age Newborns

A newborn whose weight is above the 90th percentile on growth charts or two standard deviations above the mean weight for gestational age is defined as LGA. LGA is also termed macrosomia. The infant's weight is over 4,000 g (>9 lb). LGA infants may be preterm, term, or postterm. Up to 10% of all infants are designated as LGA at birth. This large size can place both the labouring client and the newborn at risk for adverse outcomes (Baur, 2017).

Because of the newborn's large size, vaginal birth may be difficult and occasionally results in birth injury. In addition, shoulder dystocia, clavicular fractures, and facial palsies are common. The incidence of cesarean births is very high with LGA newborns to avoid arrested labour and birth trauma.

Take Note!

Maternal diabetes is commonly associated with LGA newborns. However, due to poor placental perfusion, the newborn may experience fetal growth restriction and be SGA (Potter & Kicklighter, 2016).

(text continues on page 876)

TABLE 23.1

COMMON PROBLEMS ASSOCIATED WITH NEWBORNS EXPERIENCING A VARIATION IN BIRTH WEIGHT OR GESTATIONAL AGE

Problem	Occurrence	Etiology/Pathophysiology	Assessment Findings	Nursing Implications
Perinatal asphyxia	SGA newborns (common)	Poor tolerance to stress of labour, frequently leading to acidosis and hypoxia Living in hypoxic environment prior to birth due to placental insufficiency, leaving little to no oxygen reserves available to withstand stress of labour: – Uterine contractions increase hypoxic stress – Possible depletion of glycogen stores due to chronic hypoxic state, leading to fetal distress – Impaired uteroplacental circulation due to maternal and uterine conditions predisposing to perinatal depression Compromised newborn at birth experiencing difficulty adjusting to extrauterine environment	Fetal distress (bradycardia, decelerations) during labour Low Apgar scores Potential meconium passage into amniotic fluid	Anticipate possible problem; assess for maternal risk factors Initiate resuscitation measures immediately at birth
	Postterm newborns	Placental deprivation or oligohydramnios, leading to cord compression and subsequent reduction in perfusion to fetus		
	Preterm newborns (common)	Surfactant deficiency Unstable chest wall Immaturity of respiratory control centres in the CNS Small respiratory passages, increasing risk for obstruction Inability to clear mucus from airways		
Difficulty with thermoregulation	SGA newborns (common)	Less muscle mass, less brown fat, less heat-preserving subcutaneous fat, and limited ability to control skin capillaries Associated with depleted glycogen stores, poor subcutaneous fat stores, and disturbances in CNS thermoregulation due to hypoxia Increased risk for acidosis and hypoglycemia secondary to metabolic stress	Temperature <36.4°C; temperature instability; skin cool to touch; cyanosis of hands and feet Bradypnea (<25 bpm) and tachypnea (>60 breaths/min) Tremors, irritability Wheezing, crackles, retractions Restlessness, lethargy Hypotonia Weak or high-pitched cry Seizures Poor feeding Grunting Acidosis	Maintain a neutral thermal environment to promote stabilization of newborn's temperature Assess skin temperature and respiration characteristics Monitor arterial blood gases and blood glucose levels Eliminate sources of heat loss: – Dry newborn thoroughly – Wrap in warmed blanket with stockinette cap on head – Use radiant heat source
	Postterm newborns	Loss of subcutaneous fat second to placental insufficiency Use of stored nutrients for nutrition due to lost ability of placenta to nourish fetus Subsequent wasting of subcutaneous fat, muscle, or both		

(continued)

TABLE 23.1 COMMON PROBLEMS ASSOCIATED WITH NEWBORNS EXPERIENCING A VARIATION IN BIRTH WEIGHT OR GESTATIONAL AGE (continued)

Problem	Occurrence	Etiology/Pathophysiology	Assessment Findings	Nursing Implications
	Preterm newborns (common)	Loss of natural insulation (subcutaneous fat) important in temperature regulation Immaturity of CNS (temperature-regulating centre) interferes with ability to regulate body temperature Inadequate amounts of subcutaneous fat Lack of muscle tone and flexion to conserve heat		
	Late preterm infant (common)	Inadequate brown fat to generate heat Limited muscle mass activity, reducing ability to produce own heat Inability to shiver to generate heat		
Hypoglycemia	SGA newborns (common)	Increased metabolic rate and lack of adequate glycogen stores to meet newborn's metabolic needs	Often subtle Lethargy, tachycardia Respiratory distress Jitteriness Drowsiness Poor feeding, feeble sucking Hypothermia, temperature instability Diaphoresis Weak cry Seizures Hypotonia Blood glucose levels <40 mg/dL for term newborns, <20 mg/dL for preterm newborns	Monitor blood glucose levels, initially on arrival to nursery and hourly thereafter Maintain fluid and electrolyte balance Watch for subtle changes. Initiate early oral feedings if possible; if not, administer IV infusion with 10% dextrose in water
	LGA newborns (common)	Commonly associated with infants of diabetic mothers Abrupt cessation of high-glucose maternal blood supply with birth and continued insulin production by the newborn Limited ability to release glucagons and catecholamines, which normally stimulate glucagon breakdown and glucose release		
	Postterm newborns	Hypoxia secondary to depleted glycogen reserves Placental insufficiency secondary to placental aging contributing to chronic fetal nutritional deficiency further depleting glycogen stores		
	Preterm newborns	Immature sucking and swallowing leading to insufficient intake Perinatal hypoxia Increased energy expenditure		
	Late preterm infants	Decreased subcutaneous and brown fat with little to no glycogen stores		

Condition	Newborn type	Pathophysiology	Signs and symptoms	Nursing interventions
Polycythemia	SGA newborns	Chronic mild hypoxia secondary to placental insufficiency; Stimulation of erythropoietin release, leading to increased RBC production	Venous hematocrit >65%; Plethora (ruddy appearance); Weak sucking reflex; Tachypnea; Jaundice; Lethargy; Jitteriness; Hypotonia; Irritability; Feeding difficulties; Difficulty in arousing; Seizures	Ensure adequate hydration (orally or IV); Monitor hematocrit levels (goal is ~60%); Administer partial exchange transfusion, albumin, or normal saline IV to reduce RBC volume and increase fluid volume (controversial)
	LGA newborns	Secondary to fetal hypoxia, trauma with bleeding, increased erythropoietin production, or delayed cord clamping		
	Postterm newborns	Intrauterine hypoxia triggers increased RBC cell production to compensate for lower oxygen levels.		
Meconium aspiration	SGA newborns	Release of meconium into amniotic fluid prior to birth; Inhalation of meconium-containing amniotic fluid by the newborn, leading to aspiration; Commonly associated with chronic intrauterine hypoxia	Green amniotic fluid with rupture of membranes during labour; Green staining of the umbilical cord or fingernails; Difficulty initiating respirations	Initiate resuscitation measures as necessary; Suction airways and support ventilation (see Chapter 24 for more information)
	Postterm newborns	Struggling by fetus making respiratory efforts and bearing down with abdominal muscles, leading to expulsion of meconium into amniotic fluid; Normal sucking and swallowing by fetus leads to meconium filling airways		
Hyperbilirubinemia	LGA newborns (common)	Associated with polycythemia and RBC breakdown; Inability to tolerate feedings in the first few days of life, leading to increased enterohepatic circulation of bilirubin	Elevated serum bilirubin levels; Jaundice; Tea-coloured urine; Clay-coloured stools	Ensure adequate hydration; Institute early feedings if possible; Administer phototherapy (see Chapter 24 for more information)
	Preterm newborns	Excessive bruising secondary to birth trauma, leading to higher-than-normal bilirubin levels		
	Late preterm infants	Increased breakdown of RBCs and immature liver function to handle excess load		
Birth trauma	LGA newborns	Large size requiring use of operative birth procedure	Obvious deformities; Bruising; Edema; Asymmetrical movement	Perform complete physical and neurologic assessment of the newborn; Note symmetry of structure and function; Assist parents in understanding situation (see Chapter 24 for more information)

Adapted from Fanaroff, A. A., & Fanaroff, J. M. (2014). *Klaus and Fanaroff's care of the high-risk neonate* (6th ed.). Philadelphia, PA: Elsevier Health Sciences; Green, C. J. (2016). *Maternal newborn nursing care plans* (3rd ed.). Burlington, MA: Jones & Bartlett Learning; Kandasamy, J. (2017). *Polycythemia of the newborn*. Retrieved from http://emedicine.medscape.com/article/976319-overview; and Verklan, M. T., & Walden, M. (2015). *Core curriculum for neonatal intensive care nursing* (5th ed.). St. Louis, MO: Saunders.

Nursing Assessment

Assessment of the LGA newborn begins with a review of the maternal history, which can provide clues as to whether the pregnant client has an increased risk of giving birth to an LGA newborn. Health factors that increase the chance of bearing an LGA newborn include diabetes mellitus or glucose intolerance, multiparity, prior history of a macrosomic infant, postterm gestation, maternal obesity, paternal height, gestational weight gain, male fetus, and genetics (Baur, 2017).

At birth, assess the newborn for common characteristics. The typical LGA newborn has a large body and appears plump and full-faced. The increase in body size is proportional. However, the head circumference and body length are in the upper limits of intrauterine growth. These newborns have poor motor skills and have difficulty in regulating behavioural states. LGA newborns are more difficult to arouse to a quiet alert state (Mandy, 2018b).

Thoroughly assess the LGA newborn at birth to identify traumatic birth injuries such as fractured clavicles, brachial palsy, facial paralysis, phrenic nerve palsy, skull fractures, or hematomas. Perform a neurologic examination to identify any nerve palsies, looking for abnormalities such as immobility of the upper arm. Observe and document any injuries discovered to allow for early intervention and improved outcomes.

LGA infants are at risk for hypoglycemia related to early depletion of glycogen stores in their liver. Obtain frequent blood glucose levels as ordered to evaluate for hypoglycemia. The clinical signs are often subtle and include lethargy, apathy, drowsiness, irritability, tachypnea, weak cry, temperature instability, jitteriness, seizures, apnea, bradycardia, cyanosis or pallor, feeble suck and poor feeding, hypotonia, and coma. Other disorders, including septicemia, severe respiratory distress, and congenital heart disease, may present with similar findings. In addition, be alert for other common problems, such as polycythemia and hyperbilirubinemia (see Table 23.1).

Nursing Management

Hypoglycemia in a neonate is defined as blood glucose value below 2.6 mmol/L (CPS, 2018). It is commonly associated with a variety of neonatal conditions like prematurity, FGR, and maternal diabetes. It may be asymptomatic in some newborns. Essential nursing care activities include early identification of clients at risk for diabetes, prevention of hypoglycemia, maintenance of fluid and electrolyte balance, and parental education and support. Screening for hypoglycemia in high-risk LGA infants is essential. Supervised breastfeeding or formula feeding may be initial treatment options in asymptomatic hypoglycemia. However, symptomatic hypoglycemia should always be treated with a continuous infusion of parenteral dextrose. LGA infants needing dextrose infusion rates above 12 mg/kg/min should be investigated for a definite cause of hypoglycemia. Hypoglycemia has been linked to poor neurodevelopmental outcome, and hence aggressive screening and treatment is recommended (Mattson & Smith, 2015).

Assist in stabilizing the LGA newborn. Monitor blood glucose levels at 2 hours of age. Recheck levels before feedings and also immediately in any infant suspected of having or showing clinical signs of hypoglycemia, regardless of age (CPS, 2018; Green, 2016). To help prevent hypoglycemia, initiate feedings, which can be formula or breast milk, with intravenous glucose supplementation as needed. Monitor and record intake and output and obtain daily weights to aid in evaluating nutritional intake.

Observe for signs of polycythemia and hyperbilirubinemia and report any, immediately to the health care provider so that early interventions can be taken to prevent poor long-term neurologic development outcomes. Polycythemia and hyperviscosity are associated with fine and gross motor delays, speech delays, and neurologic sequelae (Mandy, 2018b). Increasing fluid volume aids in decreasing blood viscosity. Partial exchange transfusion with plasma or normal saline may be used to lower hematocrit and decrease blood viscosity, but this treatment remains controversial (Kandasamy, 2017). Hydration, early feedings, and phototherapy are used to treat hyperbilirubinemia (see Chapter 24 for more information about hyperbilirubinemia). Provide parental guidance about the treatments and procedures being done and about the need for follow-up care for any abnormalities identified.

GESTATIONAL AGE VARIATIONS

The mean duration of pregnancy, calculated from the first day of the last normal menstrual period, is approximately 280 days, or 40 weeks. Gestational age is typically measured in weeks: a newborn born before completion of 37 weeks is classified as a **preterm newborn** and one born after completion of 42 weeks is classified as a **postterm newborn** (Cunningham et al., 2018). An infant born from the first day of the 38th week through 42 weeks is classified as a **full-term newborn**. A recent additional classification is that of the **late preterm newborn (near term)**—one that is born between 34 0/7 and 36 6/7 weeks' gestation. Late preterm births account for 72% of preterm births (Horgan, 2015).

- Preterm infant—born before 37 completed weeks of gestation
- Late preterm infant (near term)—34 0/7 to 36 6/7 weeks
- Full-term infant—37 through 41 completed weeks of gestation
- Postterm infant—42 weeks or more

Precise knowledge of a newborn's gestational age is imperative for effective postnatal management. Determination of gestational age by the nurse assists in planning appropriate care for the newborn and provides important information regarding potential problems that need interventions. See Chapter 18 for more information on assessing gestational age.

Take Note!

Although preterm and postterm newborns may appear to be at opposite ends of the gestational age spectrum and are very different in size and appearance, both are at high risk and need special care.

Postterm Newborn

A pregnancy that extends beyond 42 weeks' gestation (294 days) produces a postterm newborn. Other terms used to describe this late birth is a postmature infant. Postterm newborns may be LGA, SGA, or dysmature (newborn weighs less than established normal parameters for estimated gestational age [fetal growth restricted]), depending on placental function. A postmature infant's appearance typically shows the effects of progressive placental insufficiency.

The reason why some pregnancies last longer than others is not completely understood. What is known is that individuals who experience one postterm pregnancy are at increased risk in subsequent pregnancies. The incidence of prolonged pregnancy, beyond 42 weeks, is approximately 10% (Green, 2016).

The ability of the placenta to provide adequate oxygen and nutrients to the fetus after 42 weeks' gestation is thought to be compromised, leading to perinatal mortality and morbidity. After 42 weeks, the placenta begins aging. Deposits of fibrin and calcium, along with hemorrhagic infarcts, occur and the placental blood vessels begin to degenerate. All of these changes affect diffusion of oxygen to the fetus. As the placenta loses its ability to nourish the fetus, the fetus uses stored nutrients to stay alive, and wasting occurs. This wasted appearance at birth is secondary to the loss of muscle mass and subcutaneous fat. A recent study found that mortality in postterm infants was strongly related to FGR, not necessarily gestational age (Morken, Klungsoyr, & Skjaerven, 2014).

Nursing Assessment

Important nursing care activities include assessing neonate complications related to placental insufficiency, assessing for birth trauma, maintaining body temperature, and offering emotional support to the parent(s). A thorough assessment of the postterm newborn upon admission to the nursery provides a baseline from which to identify changes in clinical status. Review the maternal history for any risk factors associated with postterm birth.

Also be aware of the common physical characteristics and be able to identify any deviation from the expected. Postterm newborns typically exhibit the following characteristics:

- Dry, cracked, peeling, wrinkled skin
- Vernix caseosa and lanugo are absent.
- Long, thin extremities
- Creases that cover the entire soles of the feet
- Wide-eyed, alert expression
- Abundant hair on scalp
- Thin umbilical cord
- Long fingernails
- Limited vernix and lanugo
- Meconium-stained skin and fingernails (Mattson & Smith, 2015)

Assess the newborn's gestational age and complete a physical examination to identify any abnormalities. Review the medical record to determine the colour of the amniotic fluid when membranes ruptured and observe for a meconium-stained umbilical cord and fingernails to assess for possible meconium aspiration. Careful suctioning at the time of birth and afterward, if the condition dictates it, reduces the incidence of meconium aspiration (Verklan & Walden, 2015). Also be alert for other typical complications associated with a postterm newborn, such as perinatal asphyxia (caused by placental aging or oligohydramnios [decreased amniotic fluid]), hypoglycemia (caused by acute episodes of hypoxia related to cord compression which exhausts carbohydrate reserves), hypothermia (caused by loss of subcutaneous fat), and polycythemia (caused by an increased production of red blood cells to compensate for a reduced oxygen environment), and be prepared to initiate early interventions (see Table 23.1).

Nursing Management

The birth of a postterm newborn may create stress for the new parent(s) and their family. In most situations, birth of a newborn requiring special care was not anticipated. Postterm newborns are susceptible to several birth challenges secondary to placental dysfunction that place them at risk for asphyxia, hypoglycemia, and respiratory distress. The nurse must be vigilant for complications when managing these newborns.

The postterm newborn is at high risk for perinatal asphyxia, which is usually attributed to placental deprivation or oligohydramnios that leads to cord compression, thereby reducing perfusion to the fetus. Anticipating the need for newborn resuscitation is a priority. The newborn resuscitation team needs to be available in the birthing suite for immediate backup. The newborn may require transport to the neonatal intensive care unit (NICU) for continuous assessment, monitoring, and treatment, depending on his or her status after resuscitation.

Monitor and maintain the postterm newborn's blood glucose levels once stabilized. Intravenous dextrose 10%

and/or early initiation of feedings will help stabilize the blood glucose levels to prevent CNS sequelae.

Also monitor the postterm newborn's skin temperature; respiration characteristics; results of blood studies, such as arterial blood gases (ABGs) and serum bilirubin levels; and neurologic status. Institute measures to prevent or reduce the risk of hypothermia by eliminating sources of heat loss: thoroughly dry the newborn at birth, wrap him or her in a warmed blanket, and place a stockinette cap on the newborn's head. Providing environmental warmth via a radiant heat source will help stabilize the newborn's temperature. Holding the infant skin-to-skin on the parent's chest will also help to stabilize the temperature.

Closely assess all postterm newborns for polycythemia, which contributes to hyperbilirubinemia due to red blood cell destruction. Providing adequate hydration helps to reduce the viscosity of the newborn's blood to prevent thrombosis. Be alert to the early, often subtle signs to promote early identification and prompt treatment to prevent any neurodevelopmental delays (Green, 2016).

Consider This

I had been waiting for this baby since I can remember and now I was told to wait even longer. I was into my 3rd week past my due date and was just told that if I didn't go into labour on my own, the doctor would induce me on Monday. As I walked out of his office into the hot summer sun, I thought about all the comments that would await me at the office: "You're not still pregnant, are you?" "Weren't you due last month?" "You look as big as a house." "Are you sure you aren't expecting triplets?" I started to get into my car when I felt warm fluid slide down my legs. Although I was embarrassed at my wetness, I was thrilled I wouldn't have to go back to the office and drove myself to the hospital. Within hours my wait was finally over with the birth of my son, a postterm infant with peeling skin and a thick head of hair. He was certainly worth the wait!

Thoughts: Although most due dates are within plus or minus 2 weeks, we can't "go to the bank with it" because so many factors influence the start of labour. This woman was anxious about her overdue status, but nature prevailed. The old adage, "When the fruit is ripe, it will fall," doesn't always bring a good outcome: many clients need a little push to bring a healthy newborn forth. What happens when the fetus stays inside the uterus too long? What other features are typical of postterm infants?

Preterm Newborn

A preterm newborn is one who is born before the completion of 37 weeks' gestation. There has been an improved survival rate of preterm infants due to advancing technology and improved evidence-based perinatal care. Although the national birth rate has been declining since the 1990s, the preterm birth rate has been climbing rapidly. Approximately one in nine infants or nearly half a million infants are born before the 37th week of gestation (March of Dimes, 2018). Prematurity is now the leading cause of death worldwide within the 1st month of life and the second leading cause of all infant deaths.

The etiology of half of all preterm births is unknown (Cunningham et al., 2018). Preterm births take an enormous financial toll, estimated to be in the billions of dollars. They also take an emotional toll on those involved.

Changes in perinatal care practices, including regional care, have reduced newborn mortality rates. Transporting high-risk pregnant clients to a tertiary centre for birth rather than transferring the neonate after birth is associated with a reduction in neonatal mortality and morbidity (Kaneko et al., 2015). Despite increasing survival rates, preterm infants continue to be at high risk for neurodevelopmental disorders such as cerebral palsy or mental retardation, intraventricular hemorrhage, congenital anomalies, neurosensory impairment, behavioural problems, and chronic lung disease (Back, 2015). Making sure that all pregnant individuals receive quality prenatal care throughout pregnancy is a major method for preventing preterm births.

Preterm newborns face a myriad of possible complications as a result of their fragile health status or the procedures and treatments used. Some of the more common complications in preterm newborns include respiratory distress syndrome, periventricular–intraventricular hemorrhage, bronchopulmonary dysplasia, retinopathy of prematurity (ROP), hyperbilirubinemia, anemia, necrotizing enterocolitis, hypoglycemia, infection or septicemia, delayed growth and development, and mental or motor delays (Green, 2016). Several of these complications are described in Chapter 24.

Effects of Prematurity on Body Systems

Since the preterm newborn did not remain in utero long enough, every body system may be immature, affecting the newborn's transition from intrauterine to extrauterine life and placing him or her at risk for complications. Without full development, organ systems are not capable of functioning at the level needed to maintain extrauterine homeostasis (Carlo, 2015).

Recall Anna, who was described at the beginning of the chapter; she gave birth to a newborn at 7 months' gestation. What problems would you anticipate that her newborn might have?

RESPIRATORY SYSTEM

The respiratory system is one of the last body systems to mature. Therefore, the preterm newborn is at great risk for respiratory complications. A few of the problems that affect the preterm newborn's breathing ability and adjustment to extrauterine life include:

- Surfactant deficiency, leading to the development of respiratory distress syndrome
- Unstable chest wall, leading to atelectasis
- Immature respiratory control centres, leading to apnea
- Smaller respiratory passages, leading to an increased risk for obstruction
- Inability to clear fluid from passages, leading to transient tachypnea (Gardner, Carter, Hines, & Hernandez, 2016)

CARDIOVASCULAR SYSTEM

The preterm newborn has great difficulty in making the transition from intrauterine to extrauterine life in terms of changing from a fetal to a newborn circulation pattern. Higher oxygen levels in the circulation once air breathing begins spur this transition. If the oxygen levels remain low secondary to perinatal asphyxia, the fetal pattern of circulation may persist, causing blood flow to bypass the lungs. Another problem affecting the cardiovascular system is the increased incidence of congenital anomalies associated with continued fetal circulation—patent ductus arteriosus and an open foramen ovale. In addition, impaired regulation of blood pressure in preterm newborns may cause fluctuations throughout the circulatory system. One of special note is cerebral blood flow, which may predispose the fragile blood vessels in the brain to rupture, causing intracranial hemorrhage (Fanaroff & Fanaroff, 2014).

GASTROINTESTINAL SYSTEM

Preterm newborns usually lack the neuromuscular coordination required to maintain the sucking, swallowing, and breathing regimen necessary for sufficient calorie and fluid intake to support growth. Perinatal hypoxia causes shunting of blood from the gut to more important organs such as the heart and brain. Subsequently, ischemia and damage to the intestinal wall can occur. This combination of shunting, ischemia, damage to the intestinal wall, and poor sucking ability places the preterm infant at risk for malnutrition and weight loss.

In addition, preterm newborns have a small stomach capacity, weak abdominal muscles, compromised metabolic function, limited ability to digest proteins and absorb nutrients, and weak or absent suck and gag reflexes. All of these limitations place the preterm newborn at risk for nutritional deficiency and subsequent growth and development delays.

The preterm infant's ability to coordinate sucking, swallowing, and breathing is challenged. As a result, preterm infants often require enteral or parenteral nutrition.

Enteral tube feeding will help to conserve energy even in an infant who is able to suck. The exact nutritional needs of preterm infants depend on their gestational age, postnatal age, weight, route of nutritional intake, growth rate, activity, and thermal environment. Preterm infants that are ill or experiencing stressful situations have higher-energy requirements. Preterm infants take time to establish enteral intakes, and parenteral nutrition is typically an integral component of care, but safe amounts of macronutrients, and the optimal amino acid and lipid composition remains an uncertainty (Brennan, Murphy, & Kiely, 2015).

Currently, minimal enteral feeding is used to prepare the preterm newborn's gut to overcome the many feeding difficulties associated with gastrointestinal immaturity. It involves the introduction of small amounts, usually 0.5 to 1 mL/kg/h, of enteral feeding to induce surges in gut hormones that enhance maturation of the intestine. This minute amount of breastmilk or formula given via gavage (tube) feeding prepares the gut to absorb future introduction of nutrients. It builds mucosal bulk, stimulates development of enzymes, enhances pancreatic function, stimulates maturation of gastrointestinal hormones, reduces gastrointestinal distention and malabsorption, and enhances transition to oral feedings (Gardner et al., 2016).

RENAL SYSTEM

The renal system of the preterm newborn is immature, reducing the baby's ability to concentrate urine and slowing the glomerular filtration rate. As a result, the risk for fluid retention, with subsequent fluid and electrolyte disturbances, increases. In addition, preterm newborns have limited ability to clear drugs from their systems, thereby increasing the risk of drug toxicity. Close monitoring of the preterm newborn's acid–base and electrolyte balance is critical to identify metabolic inconsistencies. Prescribed medications require strict evaluation to prevent overwhelming the preterm baby's immature renal system (Mattson & Smith, 2015).

IMMUNE SYSTEM

The preterm newborn's immune system is very immature, increasing his or her susceptibility to infections. A deficiency of IgG may occur because transplacental transfer does not occur until after 34 weeks' gestation. This protection is lacking if the baby was born before this time. In addition, preterm newborns have an impaired ability to manufacture antibodies to fight infection if they were exposed to pathogens during the birth process. Moreover, the preterm newborn's thin skin and fragile blood vessels provide a limited protective barrier, adding to the increased risk for infection. Thus, anticipating and preventing infections is the goal; preventing infections has a better outcome than treating them (Gardner et al., 2016).

CENTRAL NERVOUS SYSTEM

The preterm newborn is susceptible to injury and insult to the CNS, increasing the potential for long-term disability into adulthood. Like all newborns, preterm newborns have difficulty in temperature regulation and maintaining stability. However, their risk for heat loss is compounded by inadequate amounts of insulating subcutaneous fat; lack of muscle tone and flexion to conserve heat; inadequate brown fat to generate heat; limited muscle mass activity, reducing the possibility of producing their own heat; inability to shiver to generate heat; and an immature temperature-regulating centre in the brain (Kenner & Lott, 2014). It is crucial to prevent cold stress, which would increase the newborn's metabolic and oxygen needs. The goal is to create a neutral thermal environment in which oxygen consumption is minimal, but body temperature is maintained (Fanaroff & Fanaroff, 2014).

In addition, the preterm newborn is especially susceptible to hypoglycemia due to immature glucose control mechanisms, decreased glucose stores, and a reduced availability of alternative fuels such as ketone bodies.

Take Note!

Glucose is needed by the brain and CNS to maintain and support numerous body system functions.

Nursing Assessment

Preterm newborns are at high risk for numerous problems and require special care. When preterm labour develops, and cannot be stopped by medical interventions, plans are necessary for appropriate management of the client and the preterm newborn, such as transporting them to a regional centre with facilities to care for preterm newborns or notifying the facility's NICU. Depending on the degree of prematurity, the preterm newborn may be kept in the NICU for months.

A thorough assessment of the preterm newborn upon admission to the nursery provides a baseline from which to identify changes in clinical status. Be aware of the common physical characteristics and be able to identify any deviation from the expected (Fig. 23.2). Common physical characteristics of preterm infants may include:

- Birth weight of less than 5.5 lb
- Scrawny appearance
- Head disproportionately larger than chest circumference
- Poor muscle tone and flexion
- Fontanels wide and soft with overriding sutures
- Minimal subcutaneous fat
- Undescended testes in males
- Plentiful lanugo (soft, downy hair), especially over the face and back
- Poorly formed ear pinna, with soft, pliable cartilage
- Fused eyelids
- Prominent clitoris and labia minora in females
- Soft and spongy skull bones, especially along suture lines
- Matted scalp hair, woolly in appearance
- Absent to a few creases in the soles and palms
- Minimal scrotal rugae in male infants
- Thin, transparent skin with visible veins
- Breast and nipples not clearly delineated
- Abundant vernix caseosa (Mattson & Smith, 2015)

Be alert for evidence that might suggest that the preterm newborn is developing a complication (see Table 23.1).

Review the maternal history to identify risk factors for preterm birth and check antepartum and intrapartum records for maternal infections to anticipate the need for treatment. Maternal risk factors associated with preterm birth include a previous preterm delivery, low socioeconomic status, preeclampsia, hypertension, poor maternal nutrition, smoking, multiple gestation, infection, advanced maternal age, and substance abuse.

Assess the newborn's gestational age and assess for FGR if appropriate. Inspect the newborn's skin closely, especially skin colour. Assess vital signs, including temperature via skin probe to identify hypothermia or fever, and heart rate for tachycardia or bradycardia. Evaluate the newborn's respiratory effort and respiratory rate. Observe for periods of apnea lasting longer than 20 seconds. Monitor oxygen saturation levels by pulse oximetry to validate perfusion status and capillary refill time. Note and report any signs of respiratory distress. Auscultate lung and heart sounds, being especially alert for possible murmur, which would indicate the presence of patent ductus arteriosus in a preterm newborn.

Assess neurologic status by observing the newborn's behaviour. Note any restlessness, hypotonia, or weak cry or sucking effort, and report unusual findings.

Monitor laboratory studies such as hemoglobin and hematocrit for signs of polycythemia. Screen for hypoglycemia upon admission and then hourly, while continuing to observe for nonspecific signs of hypoglycemia such as lethargy, poor feeding, and seizures. Evaluate serum bilirubin concentrations.

Finally, assess the parents and family members. Identify family strengths and coping mechanisms to establish a basis for intervention.

Nursing Management

The birth of a preterm newborn creates a crisis for the new parent(s) and family. Multiple studies have found that hospitalization for preterm newborns is often followed by negative mental health/behavioural outcomes, anxiety and depressive disorders, and long-term

FIGURE 23.2 Characteristics of a preterm newborn. **A:** Few plantar creases. **B:** Soft, pliable ear carti-lage, matted hair, and fused eyelids. **C:** Lax posture with poor muscle tone. **D:** Breast and nipple area barely visible. **E:** Male genitalia with minimal rugae on scrotum. **F:** Female genitalia with prominent labia and clitoris.

neurologic sequelae. Emerging evidence suggests that partners/significant others experience high rates of psy-chological stress in the first few months after a preterm birth (Feinberg, Roettger, Jones, Paul, & Kan, 2015). Pre-mature labour and birth are accompanied by feelings of helplessness, isolation, and loss of control (Gardner et al., 2016). Preterm newborns present with immaturity of all organ systems, abundant physiologic challenges, and significant morbidity and mortality globally (Verklan & Walden, 2015). The nurse must be vigilant for compli-cations when managing preterm newborns (Fig. 23.3) (Nursing Care Plan 23.1, at the end of the chapter).

FIGURE 23.3 The physical condition of a preterm newborn demands skilled assessment and nursing care.

PROMOTING OXYGENATION

Newborns normally start to breathe without assistance and often cry after birth, being stimulated by a change in pressure gradients and environmental temperature. The work of taking that first breath is primarily due to overcoming the surface tension of the walls of the terminal lung units at the gas–tissue interface. Subsequent breaths require less inspiratory pressure since there is an increase in functional capacity and air retained. By 1 minute of age, most newborns are breathing well. A newborn who fails to establish adequate, sustained respiration after birth is said to have **asphyxia** (perinatal acidosis), which is the deprivation of oxygen during the birth process, resulting in fetal hypoxia that can lead to organ damage and brain injury (Herrera-Marschitz et al., 2015).

The preterm infant lacks surfactant, which lowers surface tension in the alveoli and stabilizes them to prevent their collapse. Even if preterm newborns can initiate respirations, they have a limited ability to retain air due to insufficient surfactant. Therefore, preterm newborns develop atelectasis quickly without alveoli stabilization. The inability to initiate and establish respirations leads to hypoxemia and ultimately hypoxia (decreased oxygen), acidosis (decreased pH), and hypercarbia (increased carbon dioxide). This change in the newborn's biochemical environment may inhibit the transition to extrauterine circulation, thus allowing fetal circulation patterns to persist (Boxwell, 2010).

Failure to initiate extrauterine breathing or to breathe well after birth leads to hypoxia (too little oxygen in the cells of the body). As a result, the heart rate falls, cyanosis

develops, temperature decreases, blood pressure decreases, and respirations are altered (apnea, tachypnea, retractions, grunting, and nasal flaring) and the newborn becomes hypotonic and unresponsive. Although this can happen with any newborn, the risk is higher in preterm newborns.

Resuscitating the newborn. Approximately 10% of newborns require some assistance to begin breathing at birth. Nurses who provide care during labour and birth require certification in the Neonatal Resuscitation Program (NRP), through the CPS. The aim of neonatal resuscitation is to prevent neonatal death and adverse long-term neurodevelopmental sequelae associated with perinatal asphyxia (Yousaf, Hayat, & Afzal, 2015). For more information about NRP in Canada, go to thePoint to link to the CPS NRP site. Anticipation, adequate preparation, accurate evaluation, and prompt initiation of support are critical for successful newborn resuscitation. Have all basic equipment immediately available and in working order. Ensure that the equipment is evaluated daily, and document its condition and any needed repairs. Box 23.2 lists the equipment needed for basic newborn resuscitation.

Determine the need for resuscitation by performing a rapid assessment using the following questions:

- Is the newborn full term? Was the amniotic fluid clear of meconium?
- Is the newborn's heart rate greater than 100 bpm?
- Is the newborn breathing or crying now?
- Does the newborn have good muscle tone?

BOX 23.2

BASIC EQUIPMENT FOR NEWBORN RESUSCITATION

- A wall vacuum suction apparatus
- Infant-size stethoscopes
- Pulse oximeter
- Epinephrine 1:10,000 concentration
- Volume expander: 0.9% NaCl
- Intravenous fluids, IV insertion supplies, umbilical vein catheter insertion supplies, intraosseous needle,
- A wall source or tank source of 100% oxygen with a flow meter, blender
- A neonatal flow-inflating or self-inflating ventilation bag with correct-sized face masks
- A selection of endotracheal tubes (2.5, 3.0, or 3.5 mm) with introducers
- A laryngoscope with a small, straight blade and spare batteries and bulbs
- Ampules of naloxone (Narcan) with syringes and needles
- A wall clock to document timing of activities and events
- Hat, warm blanket, heat source
- A supply of disposable gloves in a variety of sizes for staff to use, gown, mask
- Documentation record

If the answers are "yes" to all questions, then routine care is initiated: provide warmth, clear the airway, dry the newborn. If the answer to any of these questions is "no," the newborn should receive one or more of the following actions, according to this sequence:

1. Stabilization—dry the newborn thoroughly with a warm towel; provide warmth by placing him or her under a radiant heater to prevent rapid heat loss through evaporation; position the head in a neutral position to open the airway; clear the airway with a bulb syringe or suction catheter if it is necessary; stimulate breathing. At times, handling and rubbing the newborn with a dry towel may be all that is needed to stimulate respirations.
2. Assess for breathing—bag the newborn if not breathing effectively or apneic.
3. Place pulse oximeter on the newborn's right hand or right wrist to determine oxygen saturation.
4. Continue positive pressure ventilation (PPV) if needed for 30 seconds.
5. Assess heart rate after 30 seconds of effective PPV.
6. Administer chest compressions if after 30 seconds of effective PPV the heart rate remains less than 60 beats per minute.
7. Administration of epinephrine and/or volume expansion (Vali, Matthew, & Lakshminrusimha, 2015).

The decision to progress from one set of actions to the next and the need for further resuscitative efforts is determined by the assessment of respirations, heart rate, and tone (CPS & Heart & Stroke Foundation, 2016). Nurses need to remember that preterm infants have immature lungs that may be more difficult to ventilate and are also more vulnerable to injury by PPV. They also have immature blood vessels in the brain that are prone to hemorrhage; thin skin and a large surface area, which contribute to rapid heat loss; increased susceptibility to infection; and increased risk of hypovolemic shock related to small blood volume. Anticipation, adequate preparation, accurate evaluation, and prompt initiation of support are critical for successful neonatal resuscitation.

When performing newborn resuscitation, use the mnemonic "ABCDs" (airway, breathing, circulation, and drugs) to remember the sequence of steps (Box 23.3).

Resuscitation measures are continued until the newborn has a pulse above 100 bpm, a good healthy cry or good breathing efforts, centrally pink, and oxygen saturation is within target range according to minutes of life. This last sign indicates a good oxygen supply to the brain. Effective ventilation is the key to successful resuscitation (Jaques & Kennea, 2015). Throughout the resuscitation period, keep the parents informed of what is happening to their newborn and what is being done and why. Provide support through this initial crisis. Once the newborn is stabilized, encourage bonding by having them stroke, touch, and when appropriate, hold the newborn.

BOX 23.3

ABCDs OF NEWBORN RESUSCITATION

- **A**irway
  - Place infant's head in "sniffing" position.
  - Suction mouth, then nose if required.
  - Suctioning of the trachea if meconium-stained and newborn is not vigorous (strong respiratory effort, good muscle tone, and heart rate >100 bpm) is no longer routinely indicated (CPS & Heart & Stroke Foundation, 2016). In a nonvigorous, meconium-stained newborn, suction the mouth and nose first and proceed with positive pressure ventilation (PPV). Utilize PPV corrective technique if the chest is not moving after 30 seconds of PPV.
- **B**reathing
  - Use PPV for apnea, grasping, or pulse <100 bpm.
  - Ventilate at a rate of 40 to 60 breaths/min.
  - Apply pulse oxymetry on right wrist or right hand.
  - Administer 21% oxygen (room air) to babies ≥35 weeks' gestation and 30% oxygen to babies ≤35 weeks' gestation. Titrate the oxygen based on the targeted saturation levels.
  - Listen for raising heart rate, audible breath sounds.
  - Look for slight chest movement with each breath.
  - Use carbon dioxide detector after intubation.
- **C**irculation
  - Start compressions if heart rate is <60 after 30 seconds of effective PPV.
  - Give three compressions: one breath, every 2 seconds (One-and-two-and-three-and-breath, and…).
  - Compress one third of the anterior–posterior diameter of the chest, ensure there is a full-chest recoil.
  - Place an advanced airway when chest compressions are initiated.
- **D**rugs
  - Give epinephrine if heart rate is <60 after 60 seconds of compressions and ventilation.
  - *Caution:* Epinephrine dosage is different for endotracheal and IV routes!
- **E**pinephrine: 1:10,000 concentration
  - 0.01 mg/kg IV (preferred method of administration)
  - 0.1 mg/kg via endotracheal tube, a maximum of 0.3 mg total

Adapted from Canadian Paediatric Society (CPS). (2017). *2016 medications for neonatal resuscitation program Canadian adaptation.* Retrieved from https://www.cps.ca/uploads/nrp/Medications_for_NRP_2016_v03_1.pdf.

Administering oxygen. Oxygen administration is a common therapy in the NICU, though the normal oxygen concentration for a preterm infant remains unknown. Use of large concentrations of oxygen and sustained oxygen saturations higher than 95% while on supplemental oxygen have been associated with the development of ROP as well as respiratory complications in the preterm newborn (Paul, 2015). For these reasons, oxygen should be administered judiciously to prevent the development of further complications. A guiding principle for oxygen therapy is it should be targeted to levels appropriate to the condition, gestational age, and postnatal age of the newborn. Current common practice is to maintain oxygen saturation levels in the high 80s to mid-90s, though a wide variation in practice may still occur. Room air is an emerging standard of care when initiating PPV during resuscitation (Ramji, Saugstad, & Jain, 2015). Refer to Chapter 39 for a more in-depth discussion of ROP.

Respiratory distress in preterm infants is commonly caused by a deficiency of surfactant, retained fluid in the lungs (wet lung syndrome), meconium aspiration, pneumonia, hypothermia, or anemia. The principles of care are the same regardless of the cause of respiratory distress.

- First, keep the newborn warm, preferably in a warmed isolette or with an overhead radiant warmer, to conserve the baby's energy and prevent cold stress.
- Handle the newborn as little as possible, because stimulation often increases the oxygen requirement.
- Provide energy through calories via intravenous dextrose or gavage or continuous tube feedings to prevent hypoglycemia. Be aware feeding newborn in respiratory distress via gavage feeding has a risk of aspiration and potentially worsening of the conditions.
- Treat cyanosis with an oxygen hood or blow-by oxygen placed near the newborn's face if respiratory distress is mild and short-term therapy is needed.
- Record the following important observations every hour or more frequently if indicated and document any deterioration in respiratory status:
  - Respiratory rate, quality of respirations, and respiratory effort
  - Airway patency, including removal of secretions per facility policy
  - Skin colour, including any changes to duskiness, blueness, or pallor
  - Lung sounds on auscultation to differentiate breath sounds in upper and lower fields, right and left side

- Equipment required for oxygen delivery, such as:
  - Blow-by oxygen delivered via mask or tube for short-term therapy
  - Oxygen hood (oxygen is delivered via a plastic hood placed over the newborn's head)
  - Nasal cannula (oxygen is delivered directly through the nares) (Fig. 23.4A)
  - Continuous positive airway pressure (CPAP), which prevents collapse of unstable alveoli and delivers high levels of inspired oxygen into the lungs
  - Humidified high flow nasal cannulae
  - Mechanical ventilation, which delivers consistent assisted ventilation and oxygen therapy, reducing the work of breathing for the fatigued infant (Fig. 23.4B)
- Correct placement of endotracheal tube (if present)
- Heart rate, including any changes
- Monitor the infant's respiratory status, clinically as well as by oxygen saturation, ABGs, and chest x-ray.
- Oxygen saturation levels via pulse oximetry to evaluate need for oxygen therapy modifications
- Suction as needed to remove secretions to maintain a patent airway and enhance oxygenation.
- Decrease stimulation; cluster all care to allow for rest.
- Maintain a neutral thermal environment.
- Administer medication, such as exogenous surfactant.
- Offer emotional support and progress reports on infant's condition to family.

If the newborn shows worsening cyanosis or if oxygen saturation levels fall below 90%, prepare to give additional oxygen as ordered. Evaluate ABG results periodically as ordered. Document any deterioration or changes in respiratory status. Administer exogenous surfactant as ordered. Throughout care, maintain strict asepsis and meticulous hand hygiene in order to reduce the risk of infection (Verklan & Walden, 2015).

FIGURE 23.4 **A:** A preterm newborn receiving oxygen therapy via a nasal cannula. The newborn also has an enteral feeding tube inserted for nutrition. **B:** A preterm newborn receiving mechanical ventilation.

MAINTAINING THERMAL REGULATION

Providing an optimal thermal environment is important. When a newborn becomes chilled, it attempts to conserve body heat by vasoconstriction and thermogenesis by metabolizing brown adipose tissue and increasing oxygen consumption. This increase in energy expenditure reduces the neonate's ability to gain weight. Immediately after birth, dry the newborn with a warmed towel and then place him or her in a second warm, dry towel before performing the assessment. This drying prevents rapid heat loss secondary to evaporation. Newborns that are active, breathing well, and crying are stable and can be placed on their parent's chest ("kangaroo care") to promote warmth and prevent hypothermia. Preterm newborns that are not considered stable may be placed under a radiant warmer or in a warmed isolette after they are dried with a warmed towel.

Typically, newborns use nonshivering thermogenesis for heat production by metabolizing their own brown adipose tissue. However, the preterm newborn has an inadequate supply of brown fat because he or she left the uterus early before the supply was adequate. The preterm newborn also has decreased muscle tone and thus cannot assume the flexed fetal position, which reduces the amount of skin exposed to a cooler environment. In addition, preterm newborns have large body surface areas compared to their weight. This allows an increased transfer of heat from their bodies to the environment.

Typically, a preterm newborn that is having problems with thermal regulation feels cold to the touch. The baby's hands, feet, and tongue may appear cyanotic. Respirations are shallow or slow, or signs of respiratory distress are present. The newborn is lethargic and hypotonic, feeds poorly, and has a feeble cry. Blood glucose levels are probably low, leading to hypoglycemia, due to the energy expended to keep warm.

When promoting thermal regulation for the preterm newborn:

- Remember the four mechanisms for heat transfer and ways to prevent loss:
  - Convection: heat loss through air currents (avoid drafts near the newborn)
  - Conduction: heat loss through direct contact (warm everything the newborn comes in contact with, such as blankets, mattress, stethoscope)
  - Radiation: heat loss without direct contact (keep isolettes away from cold sources and provide insulation to prevent heat transfer)
  - Evaporation: heat loss by conversion of liquid into vapor (keep the newborn dry and delay the first bath until the baby's temperature is stable)
- Frequently assess the temperature of the isolette or radiant warmer, adjusting the temperature as necessary to prevent hypo- or hyperthermia.
- Utilize plastic wraps and bags, skin-to-skin contact, or transwarmer mattresses if available to keep infants warmer and decrease the incidence of hypothermia.
- Assess the newborn's temperature every hour until stable.
- Observe for clinical signs of cold stress, such as respiratory distress, central cyanosis, hypoglycemia, lethargy, weak cry, abdominal distention, apnea, bradycardia, and acidosis.
- Remember the complications of hypothermia and frequently assess the newborn for signs:
  - Metabolic acidosis secondary to anaerobic metabolism used for heat production, which results in the production of lactic acid
  - Hypoglycemia due to depleted glycogen stores
  - Pulmonary hypertension secondary to pulmonary vasoconstriction
- Monitor the newborn for signs of hyperthermia such as tachycardia, tachypnea, apnea, warm to touch, flushed skin, lethargy, weak or absent cry, and CNS depression; adjust the environmental temperature appropriately.
- Explain to the parents the need to maintain the newborn's temperature, including the measures used; demonstrate ways to safeguard warmth and prevent heat loss (Gardner et al., 2016; Mattson & Smith, 2015).

PROMOTING NUTRITION AND FLUID BALANCE

Providing nutrition is challenging for preterm newborns because their needs are great but their ability to take in optimal amounts of energy/calories is reduced due to their compromised health status. Individual nutritional needs are highly variable.

Depending on their gestational age, preterm newborns receive nutrition orally, enterally, or parenterally via infusion. Several different methods can be used to provide nutrition: parenteral feedings administered through a percutaneous central venous catheter for long-term venous access with delivery of total parenteral nutrition (TPN); or enteral feedings, which can include oral feedings (formula or breastmilk), continuous nasogastric tube feedings, or intermittent gavage tube feedings. Gavage feedings are commonly used for compromised newborns to allow them to rest during the feeding process. Many have a weak suck and become fatigued and thus cannot consume enough calories to meet their needs.

Most newborns born after 34 weeks' gestation without significant complications can feed orally. Those born before 34 weeks' gestation typically start with parenteral nutrition within the first 24 hours of life. Then enteral nutrition is introduced and advanced based on the degree of maturity and clinical condition. Ultimately, enteral nutrition methods replace parenteral nutrition.

To promote nutrition and fluid balance in the preterm newborn:

- Measure daily weight and plot it on a growth curve.
- Monitor intake; calculate fluid and caloric intake daily.
- Assess fluid status by monitoring weight; urinary output; urine specific gravity; laboratory test results such as serum electrolyte levels, blood urea nitrogen,

creatinine, and hematocrit; skin turgor; and fontanels (Gardner et al., 2016). Be alert for signs of dehydration, such as a decrease in urinary output, sunken fontanels, temperature elevation, lethargy, and tachypnea.

- Continually assess for enteral feeding intolerance; measure abdominal girth, auscultate bowel sounds, and measure gastric residuals before the next tube feeding; monitor for vomiting.
- Encourage and support breastfeeding by facilitating maternal breast pumping, nonnutritive sucking, and skin-to-skin.
- Encourage nuzzling at the breast in conjunction with kangaroo care if the newborn is stable.

Take Note!

When assessing the fluid status of a preterm newborn, palpate the fontanels. Sunken fontanels suggest dehydration; bulging fontanels suggest overhydration.

PREVENTING INFECTION

Prevention of infection is critical when caring for preterm newborns. Infections are the most common cause of morbidity and mortality in the NICU population (Verklan & Walden, 2015). Sources of infection in a newborn can be divided into three categories: transplacental acquisition (intrauterine infection); perinatal acquisition during childbirth (intrapartum infection); and hospital acquisition in neonatal period (postnatal infection) from the parent(s), hospital environment, or staff (Gardner et al., 2016). Nursing assessment and early identification of infectious problems are imperative to improve outcomes.

Preterm newborns are at risk for infection because their early birth deprived them of maternal antibodies needed for passive protection. They are also susceptible to infection because of their limited ability to produce their own antibodies, asphyxia at birth, and thin, friable skin that is easily traumatized, providing an entry portal for microorganisms.

Early detection is crucial. The clinical manifestations can be nonspecific and subtle: apnea, diminished activity, poor feeding, temperature instability, respiratory distress, seizures, tachycardia, hypotonia, irritability, pallor, jaundice, hypoglycemia, and decreased oxygen saturations. Report any of these to the primary care provider immediately so that treatment can be instituted.

Include the following interventions when caring for a preterm or postterm newborn to prevent infection:

- Assess for risk factors in maternal history that place the newborn at increased risk.
- Monitor for changes in vital signs such as temperature instability, tachycardia, apnea, or tachypnea.
- Assess oxygen saturation levels and initiate oxygen therapy as ordered if oxygen saturation levels fall below acceptable parameters.

- Assess feeding tolerance, typically an early sign of infection.
- Monitor laboratory test results for changes.
- Avoid using tape on the newborn's skin to prevent tearing.
- Use equipment that can be thrown away after use.
- Adhere to standard precautions; use clean gloves to handle dirty diapers and dispose them of properly.
- Use sterile gloves when assisting with any invasive procedure; attempt to minimize the use of invasive procedures.
- Remove all jewelry on your hands prior to washing hands; wash hands upon entering the nursery and in between caring for newborns.
- Administer antibiotics as ordered and monitor for therapeutic and adverse effects.
- Avoid coming to work when ill, and screen all visitors for contagious infections.
- Follow isolation precautions as per organizational practice.

> Remember Anna, who was in a state of shock when she entered the NICU to see her preterm baby for the first time? How could the nurse have prepared her for this event? What information needs to be given at the isolette to reduce her anxiety and fear now?

PROVIDING APPROPRIATE STIMULATION

Newborn stimulation involves a series of activities to encourage normal development. Research on developmental interventions shows that when preterm newborns, in particular, receive sensorimotor interventions such as rocking, nonnutritive sucking with a pacifier, skin-to-skin contact with parents, containment (swaddling and surrounded by blanket rolls), music, nonnutritive sucking, breastfeeding, massage, holding, or sleeping on waterbeds, they gain weight faster, progress in feeding abilities more quickly, and show improved interactive behaviour compared to preterm newborns who were not stimulated (Verklan & Walden, 2015). Conversely, overstimulation may have negative effects by reducing oxygenation and causing stress. The NICU environment lends itself to persistent and unpredictable sounds that are in stark contrast to the protective sounds inside the womb. A newborn reacts to stress by flaying the hands or bringing an arm up to cover the face. When overstimulated, such as by noise, lights, excessive handling, alarms, and procedures, and stressed, heart and respiratory rates decrease, and periods of apnea or bradycardia may follow (Gardner et al., 2016).

Appropriate developmental stimulation that would not overtax the compromised newborn might include kangaroo (skin-to-skin) holding, rocking, soft singing

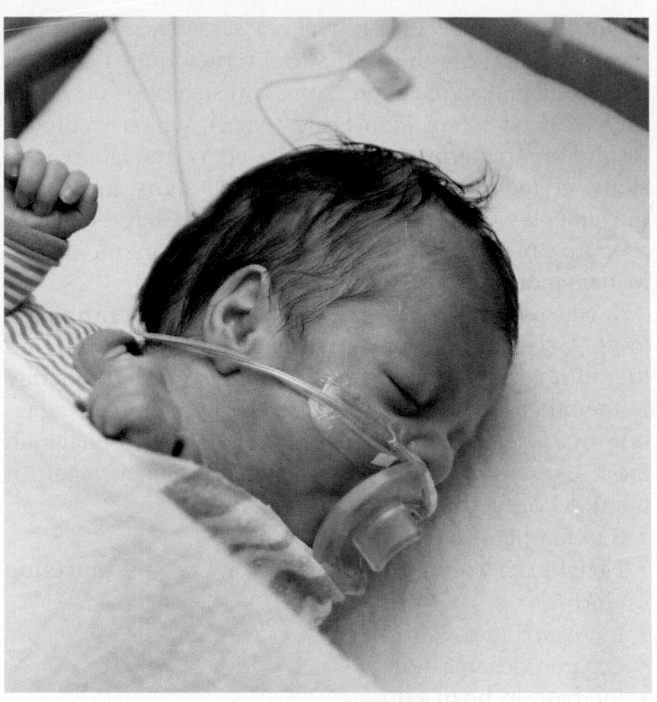

FIGURE 23.5 A preterm newborn receiving nonnutritive sucking.

FIGURE 23.6 A mother bonding with her preterm newborn.

or music, cuddling, gentle stroking of the infant's skin, colourful mobiles, gentle massage, waterbed mattresses, and nonnutritive sucking opportunities (Fig. 23.5) or providing 24% sucrose for painful procedures.

The NICU environment can be altered to provide periods of calm and rest for the newborn by dimming the lights, lowering the volume and tone of conversations, closing doors gently, setting the telephone ringer to the lowest volume possible, clustering nursing activities, and covering the isolette with a blanket to act as a light shield to promote rest at night (Verklan & Walden, 2015).

Encourage parents to hold and interact with their newborn. Doing so helps to acquaint the parents with their newborn, promotes self-confidence, and fosters parent–newborn attachment (Fig. 23.6).

> **Think back to Anna, the woman who gave birth to a preterm newborn at 7 months' gestation. Anna will be discharged but her newborn will be staying in the NICU for a while. What interventions would be appropriate to facilitate bonding despite their separation? What support can be provided specifically to her family?**

MANAGING PAIN

Effective pain control and prevention is imperative for ethical and clinical reasons and is required as a standard of excellence. Pain is an unpleasant sensory and emotional experience felt by all humans. Unlike adults, infants are incapable of rating their pain on a scale of 0 to 10, and yet from the moment they take their first breath, they are exposed to painful procedures. Newborns feel pain and require the same level of pain assessment and management as adults. Common indicators of pain in the newborn who is unable to vocalize include facial expressions, body movements, and physiologic changes such as oxygen saturation (Harrison, Bueno, & Reszel, 2015). Even though pain may not be expressed verbally in neonates, this does not negate their experiencing it. Untreated pain in newborns may result in increased morbidity and length of stay in the NICU, exaggerated responses to pain in later life, and altered psychosocial development (Valeri, Holsti, & Linhares, 2015). Parents commonly expect that health care providers will use appropriate measures to prevent pain in their newborns, but there are gaps in knowledge about the most effective way to accomplish this.

Recent research findings suggested that infants be given an appropriate-sized pacifier for comfort during painful procedures. Administration of oral sucrose with and without nonnutritive sucking and warmth is also frequently used as a nonpharmacologic intervention for procedural pain relief in neonates. The recommended sucrose concentration is a 24% solution (Gray, Garza, Zageris, Heilman, & Porges, 2015). Nurses need to be informed about the effectiveness of nonnutritive sucking, its analgesic mechanisms, and how to use and incorporate it into practice (Green, 2016).

Assessment of pain in the newborn remains a contentious and vexing problem. Newborns in the NICU are subjected to repeated procedures that cause them pain. Newborns, whether preterm, full term, or postterm, do experience pain, but the pain is difficult to validate with consistent behaviours. Considering that ill newborns undergo multiple noxious stimuli from invasive procedures, such as lumbar punctures, heel sticks, venipuncture, line insertions, chest tube placement, specimen collections, endotracheal intubation and suctioning, and mechanical ventilation, common sense would suggest that newborns experience pain from many of these activities and interventions. Historically, pain management in infants was not addressed formally but current guidelines address the nurse's role in assessing and managing neonatal pain (Yamada, Stevens, Sidani, & Watt-Watson, 2015). Refer to Box 23.4 for an overview of the principles of newborn pain prevention and management that all nurses should utilize.

Several psychometric tools are available to assess pain in the newborn. Examples include the Premature Infant Pain Profile (PIPP), which assesses heart rate and oxygen saturation; the CRIES tool (cry, requires oxygen, increased vital signs, expression, and sleeplessness); and the Neonatal Infant Pain Scale (NIPS), which evaluates respiratory patterns. Most are based on facial expressions, crying patterns, change in vital signs, and body movements (Gardner et al., 2016). See Chapter 36 for a more in-depth discussion of pain assessment and management.

Nurses play a key role in assessing a newborn's pain level. Assess the newborn frequently. Pain is considered the "fifth vital sign" and should be assessed as frequently as the other four vital signs. Differentiate pain from agitation by observing for changes in vital signs, behaviour, facial expression, and body movement. Suspect pain if the newborn exhibits the following:

- Sudden high-pitched cry
- Facial grimace with furrowing of brow and quivering chin
- Increased muscle tone
- Oxygen desaturation
- Increase in heart rate
- Body posturing, such as squirming, kicking, arching
- Limb withdrawal and thrashing movements
- Increased blood pressure, pulse, and respirations
- Fussiness and irritability (Verklan & Walden, 2015)

The goals of pain management are to minimize the amount, duration, and severity of pain and to assist the newborn in coping. It is essential that pain-related stress in preterm infants is accurately identified and appropriately managed, and that pain management strategies are evaluated for protective or adverse effects in the long term. Effective pain management strategies for newborns include preventing, limiting, or avoiding noxious stimuli; using nonpharmacologic techniques to reduce pain; and administering pharmacologic agents when appropriate. Box 23.5 lists some of the more commonly used nonpharmacologic pain management techniques for the preterm newborn.

Nonpharmacologic pain management strategies include nonnutritive sucking, breastfeeding, radiant heat to promote warmth, skin-to-skin contact, and sweetened solutions. Pharmacologic strategies include narcotic analgesics, but they are limited. Morphine and fentanyl, usually administered intravenously, are the most commonly used opioids for moderate to severe pain. Acetaminophen is effective for mild pain. Benzodiazepines are used as sedatives during painful procedures and can be combined with opioids for more effectiveness. Local or topical anesthetics (e.g., EMLA cream) also may be used before procedures such as venipuncture, lumbar puncture, and intravenous catheter insertion (Mattson & Smith, 2015). However, EMLA must be used cautiously in neonates and babies less than 3 months of age (Astra Pharmaceuticals, n.d.).

BOX 23.4

NEWBORN PAIN PREVENTION AND MANAGEMENT GUIDELINES

- Newborn pain frequently goes unrecognized and undertreated.
- Pain assessment is an essential activity prior to pain management.
- Newborns experience pain, and analgesics should be given.
- A procedure considered painful for an adult should also be considered painful for a newborn.
- Developmental maturity and health status must be considered when assessing for pain in newborns.
- Newborns may be more sensitive to pain than adults.
- Pain behaviour is frequently mistaken for irritability and agitation.
- Newborns are more susceptible to the long-term effects of pain.
- Adequate pain management may reduce complications and mortality.
- Nonpharmacologic measures can prevent, reduce, or eliminate newborn pain.
- Sedation does not provide pain relief and may mask pain responses.
- A newborn's response to both pharmacologic and nonpharmacologic pain therapy should be assessed within 30 minutes of administration or intervention.
- Health care professionals are responsible for pain assessment and treatment.
- Written guidelines are needed on each newborn unit.

Adapted from Kenner, C., & Lott, J. W. (2014). *Comprehensive neonatal care: An interdisciplinary approach* (5th ed.). St. Louis, MO: Saunders; Harrison, D., Bueno, M., & Reszel, J. (2015). Prevention and management of pain and stress in the neonate. *Research and Reports in Neonatology, 5*, 9–16; and Verklan, M. T., & Walden, M. (2015). *Core curriculum for neonatal intensive care nursing* (5th ed.). St. Louis, MO: Saunders.

BOX 23.5

NONPHARMACOLOGIC TECHNIQUES TO REDUCE PAIN IN THE PRETERM NEWBORN

- Gentle handling, rocking, caressing, cuddling, and massaging
- Rest periods before and after painful procedures
- Kangaroo care (skin-to-skin contact) during procedure
- Breastfeeding, if able, to reduce pain from minor procedures
- Use of a facilitated tuck (holding arms and legs in a flexed position)
- Application of topical anesthetics prior to venipuncture or lumbar puncture
  - EMLA topical anesthetic can be used 0 to 3 months but need to monitor methemoglobin levels
  - Ametop can be used in 1 month or older
- Swaddling and positioning to establish physical boundaries
- Nonnutritive sucking (pacifier dipped in sucrose) prior to procedure
- Minimal use of tape, with gentle removal to avoid skin tears
- Warm blankets for wrapping to facilitate relaxation
- Reduction of environmental stimuli by removing or turning down noxious stimuli such as noise from alarms, beepers, loud conversations, and bright lights
- Distraction, such as with coloured objects or mobiles

Adapted from Sabic, D., Blattner, C., & Metts, M. (2015). Newborn and infant pain control. *Clinical Pediatrics, 54*(7), 613–614; Nagtalon-Ramos, J. (2014). *Maternal-newborn nursing care: Best evidence-based practices.* Philadelphia, PA: F. A. Davis Company; and Verklan, M. T., & Walden, M. (2015). *Core curriculum for neonatal intensive care nursing* (5th ed.). St. Louis, MO: Saunders.

Be vigilant in assessing for adverse effects (respiratory depression or hypotension) when administering pharmacologic agents for pain management, especially in preterm newborns with neurologic impairment. These negative effects are usually dose and route related, so be knowledgeable about the pharmacokinetics and therapeutic dosing of any drug administered.

PROMOTING GROWTH AND DEVELOPMENT

In the late 1990s, researchers evaluated the NICU environment in terms of light and sound levels, caregiving activities, and handling of newborns. As a result of this research, many environmental modifications were made to reduce the stress and overstimulation of the NICU, and the concept of developmentally supportive care was introduced. Developmentally supportive care is defined as care of a newborn or infant to support positive growth and development. Developmental care focuses on what newborns or infants can do at that stage of development; it uses therapeutic interventions only to the point that they are beneficial; and it provides for the development of the newborn–family unit (White-Traut, 2015).

Family-centred developmental care is an essential element of neonatal intensive care. It is of particular importance when the infant is vulnerable and at greater risk for poor outcomes complicated by a family unit that is easily challenged by the unique needs of the infant; yet all newborns and their families deserve this philosophy of caregiving. Family-centred developmental care must continue to be tested through research to determine which interventions work, what does not work, and which interventions need further refinement (White & Wilson, 2015).

Developmental care is a philosophy of care that requires rethinking the relationships between newborns, families, and health care providers. It includes a variety of activities designed to manage the environment and individualize the care of the preterm or high-risk ill newborn based on behavioural observations (see Evidence-Based Practice 23.1).

Developmental care includes these strategies:

- Clustering care to promote rest and conserve the infant's energy
- Flexed positioning to simulate in utero positioning
- Environmental management to reduce noise and visual stimulation
- Kangaroo care to promote skin-to-skin sensation
- Placement of twins in the same isolette or open crib to reduce stress
- Activities to promote self-regulation and state regulation:
  - Surrounding the newborn with nesting rolls/devices
  - Swaddling with a blanket to maintain the flexed position
  - Providing sheepskin or a waterbed to simulate the uterine environment
  - Providing nonnutritive sucking (calms the infant)
  - Providing objects to grasp (comforts the newborn)
- Promotion of parent–infant bonding by making parents feel welcome in the NICU
- Open, honest communication with parents and staff
- Collaboration with the parents in planning the infant's care (Gardner et al., 2016; Verklan & Walden, 2015)

Developmental care can be fostered by clustering the lights in one area so that no lights are shining directly on newborns, installing visual alarm systems and limiting overhead pages to minimize noise, and monitoring continuous and peak noise levels. Nurses can play an active role by serving on committees that address these issues. In addition, nurses can provide direct developmentally supportive care. Doing so involves careful planning of nursing activities to provide the ideal environment for the newborn's development. For example:

- Dim the lights and cover isolettes at night to simulate nighttime.
- Support early extubation from mechanical ventilation.
- Encourage early and consistent feedings with breastmilk.
- Administer prescribed antibiotics judiciously.

EVIDENCE-BASED PRACTICE 23.1   **EFFECT OF DEVELOPMENTAL CARE FOR THE VERY PREMATURE INFANTS ON NEURODEVELOPMENTAL OUTCOME AT 2 YEARS OF AGE**

STUDY

Developmental care is a model for delivering individualized care to high-risk newborns within a family context that includes a developmentally supportive environment, flexible caregiving to meet the newborn's needs, parental involvement, and collaboration and communication with all individuals involved in the care. This study was done to determine the effect of developmental care on neurodevelopmental outcome in formerly preterm infants at the age of 2 years.

Findings

A prospective phase-lag study was performed which included 261 preterm infants divided into two groups. There were 124 placed in the conventional group and 137 placed in the developmental care group. It was found that the children in the developmental group showed less psychomotor delay than those in the control group. Not

smoking in pregnancy and higher gestational age were also significant predictors for a better psychomotor outcome at 2 years of age. The data implicated that developmental care may result in an improved 2-year psychomotor outcome in formerly preterm infants.

Nursing Implications

Based on the results of this study, nurses can feel confident in integrating the principles of developmental care into their practice to facilitate a positive impact on the infant's later neurodevelopmental outcome. Principles to incorporate into their nursing care would include clustering care to allow for rest periods, minimizing external stimuli (lights, noise, handling), respecting sleep states of the infant, utilizing comforting measures for painful procedures (swaddling, warmth, pacifiers, skin-to-skin), and engaging parents in their infant's care.

Source: Kiechl-Kohlendorfer, U., Merkle, U., Deufert, D., Neubauer, V., Peglow, U. P., & Griesmaier, E. (2015). Effect of developmental care for very premature infants on neurodevelopmental outcome at 2 years of age. *Infant Behavior and Development, 39*, 166–172.

- Position the newborn as if he or she was still in utero (a nesting fetal position).
- Promote kangaroo care by encouraging parents to hold the newborn against the chest for extended periods each day.
- Coordinate care to respect sleep and awake states.

Throughout the newborn's stay, work with the parents, developing a collaborative partnership so they feel comfortable caring for their newborn. Be prepared to make referrals to community support groups to enhance coping (Hall et al., 2015).

PROMOTING PARENTAL COPING

Generally, pregnancy and the birth of a newborn are exciting times, but when the newborn has serious, perhaps life-threatening problems, the exciting experience suddenly changes to one of anxiety, fear, guilt, loss, and grief.

Parents are typically unprepared for the birth of a preterm newborn and commonly experience an array of emotions, including disappointment, fear for the survival of the newborn, and anxiety due to the separation from their newborn immediately after birth. Gaining insight into the experience of parents of premature infants can help nurses ensure services more effectively meet the needs of these families (Discenza, 2015). Early interruptions in the bonding process and concern about the newborn's survival can create extreme anxiety and interfere with attachment (Mattson & Smith, 2015).

Nursing interventions aimed at reducing parental anxiety include:

- Reviewing with the parents the events that have occurred since birth

- Providing individualized support to parents while in NICU
- Providing simple relaxation and calming techniques (visual imagery, breathing)
- Exploring their perception of the newborn's condition and offering explanations
- Encouraging parental involvement with their newborn in NICU
- Validating their anxiety and behaviours as normal reactions to stress and trauma
- Providing a physical presence and support during emotional outbursts
- Providing anticipatory guidance about taking their infants home
- Exploring the coping strategies used successfully in the past and encouraging their use now
- Encouraging frequent visits to the NICU
- Addressing their reactions to the NICU environment and explaining all equipment used
- Identifying family and community resources available to them (Cano Gimenez & Sanchez-Luna, 2015; Rossman, Greene, & Meier, 2015)

Preparing for Discharge

Discharge planning typically begins with evidence that recovery of the newborn is certain. However, the exact date of discharge may not be predictable. The goal of the discharge plan is to make a successful transition to home care. Essential elements for discharge are a physiologically stable infant, a family who can provide the necessary care with appropriate support services in place in the community, and a pediatrician or primary care physician or nurse practitioner available for ongoing care (Krowchuk, 2015; Verklan & Walden, 2015).

The care of each high-risk newborn after discharge requires careful coordination to provide ongoing multidisciplinary support for the family. The discharge planning team typically includes the parents, primary care physician, neonatologists, neonatal nurses, and a social worker. Other professionals, such as surgical specialists and pediatric subspecialists, occupational, physical, speech, and respiratory therapists, nutritionists, home health care nurses, and a case manager, may be included as needed (Fanaroff & Fanaroff, 2014; Verklan & Walden, 2015). Critical components of discharge planning are summarized in Box 23.6.

Nurses involved in the discharge process are instrumental in bridging the gap between the hospital and home. When planning for discharge of the high-risk infant, the nurse should:

- Assess the physical status of the postpartum client and the newborn.
- Discuss the early signs of complications and what to do if they occur.
- Reinforce instructions for infant care and safety.
- Stress the importance of proper car seat use and reinforce instructions of car seat safety.
- Provide instructions for medication administration.
- Reinforce instructions for equipment operation, maintenance, and troubleshooting.
- Teach infant cardiopulmoary resuscitation and emergency care to the parent(s), including a return demonstration.

BOX 23.6

CRITICAL COMPONENTS OF DISCHARGE PLANNING

- Parental education—involvement and support in newborn care during NICU stay will ensure their readiness to care for the infant at home.
- Evaluation of unresolved medical problems—review of the active problem list and determination of what home care and follow-up is needed.
- Implementation of primary care—completion of newborn screening tests, immunizations, examinations such as funduscopic exam for ROP, and hematologic status evaluation
- Development of home care plan, including assessment of:
  - Equipment and supplies needed for care
  - In-home caregiver's preparation and ability to care for infant
  - Adequacy of the physical facilities in the home
  - An emergency care and transport plan if needed
  - Financial resources for home care costs
  - Family needs and coping skills
  - Community resources, including how they can be accessed
  - Support system available

- Demonstrate techniques for special care procedures such as dressings, ostomy care, artificial airway maintenance, chest physiotherapy, suctioning, and infant stimulation. Ensure parents are able to demonstrate these skills before discharge.
- Provide breastfeeding support or instruction on gavage feedings.
- Assist with defining roles in the adjustment period at home.
- Assess the parents' emotional stability and coping status.
- Provide support and reassurance to the family.
- Report abnormal findings to the health care team for intervention.
- Follow up with parents to ensure that they have connected with appropriate support systems in the community (Krowchuk, 2015; Verklan & Walden, 2015).

Take Note!

Infants born prematurely between 34 0/7 and 36 6/7 weeks are at higher risk for morbidity and mortality than those born after 37 weeks due to their physiologic and metabolic immunity (Boyle et al., 2015).

LATE PRETERM NEWBORN ("NEAR TERM")

The late preterm is a newborn that is born between 34 weeks and 36 6/7 weeks' gestation. Previously, infants born during this time frame were called "near term" or "slightly premature," which was a misnomer because the infants have special care needs. Some of the most common complications for late preterm infants are cold stress, respiratory distress, hypoglycemia, sepsis, cognitive delays, hyperbilirubinemia, and feeding difficulties (Barfield & Lee, 2019). In recent years, the subject of late preterm birth has received much attention, since this population of preterm newborns represents more than 70% of all preterm births in the United States and has increased by 30% in the past 20 years (CDC, 2017). With the sharp rise in the number of cesarean births performed, the incidence of late preterm newborns will also rise. Perinatal nurses need to understand the risks of late preterm births and the unique needs of this population in order to facilitate timely assessment and intervention to improve outcomes. Some of the challenges facing the late preterm newborn include:

- Respiratory distress (related to pulmonary immaturity, lack of adequate surfactant, retained lung fluid, cesarean section)
- Thermoregulation issues (less brown fat, limited ability to flex the trunk and extremities to decrease exposed surface area, less ability to shiver)
- Hypoglycemia related to the first two challenges (respiratory distress and cold stress)

- Apnea (related to poor respiratory control and immaturity)
- Jaundice and hyperbilirubinemia (related to immature bilirubin conjugation and excretion)
- Feeding challenges related to immature sucking and swallowing reflexes, GI system immaturity
- Sepsis because maternal antibodies are not fully transferred prior to the 37th week
- Neurodevelopmental delay (related to brain and CNS immaturity) (Gardner et al., 2016; Verklan & Walden, 2015)

These challenges are similar to those facing the preterm newborn and require similar management. Late preterm newborns have more clinical problems, longer lengths of stay, higher costs when compared with full-term newborns, and increased mortalities (Kenner & Lott, 2014). Anticipatory guidance for parents of late preterm infants should include recommending an infant cardiopulmonary resuscitation course, educating about sudden infant death syndrome prevention protocol (Back to Sleep), and advising the parents to avoid public places and limit visitors for the first few weeks after being discharged from the hospital. Consistent follow-up medical care, weekly weight checks, and up-to-date immunizations can help late preterm infants avoid complications (Baker, 2015). Nurses and parents must be aware of the risks associated with late preterm births to optimize care and outcomes for this group of newborns. For information related to discharge teaching for the family of the late preterm infant, refer to Teaching Guidelines 23.1.

Teaching Guidelines 23.1
DISCHARGING THE LATE PRETERM INFANT

When discharge planning for the late preterm infant, validate parents' understanding of:

- Dressing the infant appropriately in order to maintain appropriate temperature
- Practicing good handwashing and limiting contact with ill persons
- Maintaining adequate nutritional and fluid intake to promote growth and development; breastfeeding is preferred
- Avoiding secondhand smoke exposure
- Practicing safe sleep practices: avoid soft mattresses or blankets, place infant supine to sleep, light clothing, not too warm, no toys in the crib, no bed sharing
- Keeping appointments for health maintenance visits (checkups) as scheduled
- Notifying the pediatrician or nurse practitioner immediately if the infant:
  - Has difficulty breathing or turns blue (call for emergency services in this case)
  - Has a temperature below 36.1°C or above 38°C

- Displays a yellow colour to the skin (jaundice)
- Feeds poorly
- Vomits
- Fails to void for 12 hours, or to pass a bowel movement in 24 hours
- Acts lethargic, irritable or "just not right"

Adapted from Baker, B. (2015). Evidence-based practice to improve outcomes for late preterm infants. *Journal of Obstetric, Gynecologic, & Neonatal Nursing, 44,* 127–134.

Dealing With Perinatal Loss

It is estimated that over seven million perinatal losses occur globally each year. More than one million occur within the United States annually (Callister, 2014). Perinatal loss, defined as any pregnancy loss and/or neonatal death up to 1 month of age, continues to be a common occurrence even though major advances have taken place in perinatal health care. The prevalence of perinatal death reflects a very real possibility that all nurses will meet and care for a client who has experienced the death of a baby (Rondinelli, Long, Seelinger, Crawford, & Valdez, 2015).

Perinatal loss is a profound experience for the family. It engenders a unique kind of mourning since the infant is so much a part of the parents' identity. Instead of celebrating a new life as they expected, parents are mourning the loss of dreams and hopes and the loss of an extension of themselves. NICU nurses face a difficult situation when caring for newborns who may not survive. Newborn death is incomprehensible to most parents/partners/significant others. They are commonly offered time to see their infant, memory items, and support. This can make the grieving process more difficult because of the denial the parents commonly experience: what is happening "can't be real." Deciding whether to see, touch, or hold the dying newborn is extremely difficult for many parents. Nurses play a major role in assisting parents/partners/significant others to make their dying newborn "real" to them by providing them with as many memories as possible and encouraging them to see, hold, touch, dress, and take care of the infant and take photographs. These actions help to validate the partners'/significant others'/parents' sense of loss, relive the experience, and attach significance to the meaning of loss. A lock of hair, a name card, or an identification bracelet may serve as important mementos that can ease the grieving process. The memories created by these interventions can be useful allies in the grieving process and in resolving grief (Mattson & Smith, 2015; Verklan & Walden, 2015).

A nurse's willingness to sit quietly and observe, to remain open and nonjudgmental, and to explore what might be helpful are useful strategies to bridge cultural differences. Statements such as, "Help me understand how your family cares for someone who is dying," or, "What would be important for me to know about how best to care for your baby's body?" convey a nurse's willingness to learn what is most important to each family. Parents' answers may help guide nurses in providing culturally appropriate care for diverse populations. Nurses who are attentive to learning what is most important to parents, and subsequently work to incorporate such interventions into their care, foster relationships between parents and their infant (Steen, 2015).

Parent–newborn interaction is vital to the normal processes of attachment and bonding. The detachment process involved in a newborn's death is equally important for parents. Nurses can aid in this process by helping parents to see their newborn through the maze of equipment, explaining the various procedures and equipment, encouraging them to express their feelings about the newborn's status, and providing time for them to be with their dying newborn (Gardner et al., 2016; Steen, 2015).

A common reaction by many people when learning that a newborn is not going to survive is one of avoidance. Nurses are no exception. It is difficult to initiate a conversation about such a sensitive issue without knowing how the parents are going to react and cope with the impending loss. One way to begin a conversation with the parents is to convey concern and acknowledge their loss. Active listening can give parents a safe place to begin the healing process. The relationship that the nurse establishes with the parents is a unique one, providing an opportunity for both the nurse and the parents to share their feelings.

Be aware of personal feelings about loss and how these feelings are part of one's own life and personal belief system. Actively listen to the parents when they are talking about their experiences. Communicate empathy (understanding and feeling what another person is feeling), respect their feelings, and respond to them in helpful and supportive ways (Cunningham et al., 2018). Table 23.2 highlights appropriate interventions for a family experiencing a perinatal loss before and after a newborn dies.

TABLE 23.2	ASSISTING PARENTS TO COPE WITH PERINATAL LOSS
Before the newborn's death	Respect variations in the family's spiritual needs and readiness. Assess cultural beliefs and practices that may bring comfort; respect culturally appropriate requests for truth telling and informed refusal. Initiate spiritual comfort by calling the hospital clergy if appropriate; offer to pray with the family if appropriate. Encourage the parents to take photographs, make memory boxes, and record their thoughts in a journal. Explore with family members how they dealt with previous losses. Discuss techniques to reduce stress, such as meditation and relaxation. Recommend that family members maintain a healthy diet and get adequate rest and exercise to preserve their health. Participate in early and repeated care conferencing to reduce family stress. Allow family to be present at both medical rounds and resuscitation; provide explanations of all procedures, treatments, and findings; answer questions honestly and as completely as possible. Provide opportunities for the family to hold the newborn if they so choose. Assess the family's support network. Provide suggestions as to how friends can be helpful to the family.
After the newborn's death	Help the family to accept the reality of death by using the word "died." Acknowledge their grief and the fact that their newborn has died. Help the family to work through their grief by validating and listening. Provide the family with realistic information about the causes of death. Offer condolences to the family in a sincere manner. Encourage the father to cry and grieve with his partner. Provide opportunities for the family to hold the newborn if they desire.
At the time of the release of the newborn's body	Reassure the family that their feelings and grieving responses are normal. Encourage the parents to have a funeral or memorial service to bring closure. Suggest that the parents plant a tree or flowers to remember the infant. Address attachment issues concerning subsequent pregnancies. Provide information about local support groups. Provide anticipatory guidance regarding the grieving process. Present information about any impact on future childbearing, and refer the parents to appropriate specialists or genetic resources.

Adapted from Gardner, S. L., Carter, B. S., Hines, M. E., & Hernandez, J. A. (2016). *Merenstein & Gardner's handbook of neonatal intensive care* (8th ed.). St. Louis, MO: Mosby Elsevier; Steen, S. E. (2015). Perinatal death: Bereavement interventions used by US and Spanish nurses and midwives. *International Journal of Palliative Nursing, 21*(2), 79–86; and Fanaroff, A. A., & Fanaroff, J. M. (2014). *Klaus and Fanaroff's care of the high-risk neonate* (6th ed.). Philadelphia, PA: Elsevier Health Sciences.

In a time of crisis or loss, people are often more sensitive to other people's reactions. For example, the parents may be extremely aware of the nurse's facial expressions, choice of words, and tone of voice. Talking quickly, in a businesslike fashion, or ignoring the loss may inhibit parents from discussing their pain or how they are coping with it. Parents may need to vent their frustrations and anger, and the nurse may become the target. Validate their feelings and attempt to reframe or refocus the anger toward the real issue of loss. An example would be to say, "I understand your frustration and anger about this situation. You have experienced a tremendous loss and it must be difficult not to have an explanation for it at this time." Doing so helps to defuse the anger while allowing them to express their feelings.

The death of an infant will more than likely be one of the toughest moments in a family's life. Giving families some sense of control in an otherwise hopeless situation can provide some comfort. Some ideas to provide them a sense of control include:

- Ask the family who they wish to have present as the infant dies.
- Give the family a choice of rooms in which they can say good-bye to their infant.
- Provide privacy for the family during this time period by placing a sign on the door.
- Provide ideas for making or selecting memorial items for a memory box.
- The family should never be left to handle their emotions alone unless they request it.
- Respect a family's wishes if they refuse to be with their infant during the dying process or afterward. Everyone grieves differently.
- Accommodate cultural practices to the extent possible.

When assisting bereaved parents, start where the parents are in the grief process to avoid imposing your own agenda on them. You may feel uncomfortable at not being able to change the situation or take the pain away. The nurse's role is to provide immediate emotional support and facilitate the grieving process. Supporting and strengthening the family bond in the face of perinatal loss is essential.

Comforting the family after the infant's death is vital to give them a sense of closure and start the healing process. Some things the nurse can do to help the family during this time include:

- Sending the family a card from the nursing staff, signed by all who worked with their infant, within a week of leaving the hospital
- Attending the funeral to allow for a public good-bye and to support others in their time of loss
- Providing the family with a memory box, which might contain an outfit worn by their infant, a blanket used to cover their infant, a lock of hair, a card with hand and foot prints, and a photo with someone holding their infant
- Remembering their infant at various anniversaries by sending a card or calling the family to see how they are doing provides families much-needed comfort. Check with organizational privacy policy regarding regulations around contacting family after discharge
- Donating to a charity in memory of the infant, such as to March of Dimes
- Providing the family with resources that might help them. Information might include listings of local or online support groups as well as grief websites such as Share.org
- Referring the family to social work to help navigate the system of resources available

Being present during this traumatic event for families is tough. Serving infants and their families by bearing witness to their pain and grief is a special privilege. Being present for the family with compassion, comfort, support, and resources during their time of loss is truly an honourable gesture. Nurses are remembered years later for their kindness and guidance of the family members through this adverse event with dignity (Discenza, 2015).

NURSING CARE PLAN 23.1

Overview of the Care of a Preterm Newborn

Alice, an 18-year-old, felt she had done everything right during her first pregnancy and certainly didn't anticipate giving birth to a preterm newborn at 32 weeks' gestation. When Mary Kaye was born, she had respiratory distress and hypoglycemia and couldn't stabilize her temperature. Assessment revealed the following: newborn described as scrawny in appearance; skin thin and transparent with prominent veins over abdomen; hypotonia with lax, extended positioning; weak sucking reflex when nipple offered; respiratory distress with tachypnea (70 breaths/min), nasal flaring, and sternal retractions; low blood glucose level suggested by lethargy, tachycardia, jitteriness; axillary temperature of 36°C (96.8°F) despite warmed blanket; weight 2,146 g (4.73 lb); length 45 cm (17.72 in).

NURSING CARE PLAN 23.1

Overview of the Care of a Preterm Newborn (continued)

NURSING DIAGNOSIS: Ineffective breathing pattern related to immature respiratory system and respiratory distress as evidenced by tachypnea, nasal flaring, sternal retractions, and/or oxygen saturation <87%

Outcome Identification and Evaluation

Newborn's respiratory status returns to adequate level of functioning as evidenced by rate remaining within 30 to 60 breaths/min, maintenance of acceptable oxygen saturation levels, and minimal to absent signs of respiratory distress.

Interventions: *Promoting Optimal Breathing Pattern*

- Assess gestational age and risk factors for respiratory distress *to allow early detection.*
- Anticipate need for bag and mask setup and wall suction *to allow for prompt intervention should respiratory status continue to worsen.*
- Assess respiratory effort (rate, character, effort) *to identify changes.*
- Assess heart rate for tachycardia and auscultate heart sounds *to determine worsening of condition.*
- Observe for cues (grunting, shallow respirations, tachypnea, apnea, tachycardia, central cyanosis, hypotonia, increased effort) *to identify need for additional oxygen.*
- Maintain slight head elevation *to prevent upper airway obstruction (sniffing position).*
- Assess skin colour *to evaluate tissue perfusion.*
- Monitor oxygen saturation level via pulse oximetry *to provide objective indication of perfusion status and capillary refill.*

- Provide supplemental oxygen as indicated and ordered *to ensure adequate tissue oxygenation.*
- Assess blood gases to monitor blood pH, CO_2 clearance and oxygen levels.
- Assist with any ordered diagnostic tests, such as chest x-ray and arterial blood gases, *to determine effectiveness of treatments.*
- Cluster nursing activities *to reduce oxygen consumption.*
- Maintain a neutral thermal environment *to reduce oxygen consumption.*
- Monitor hydration status *to prevent fluid volume deficit or overload.*
- Explain all events and procedures to the parents *to help alleviate anxiety and promote understanding of the newborn's condition.*

NURSING DIAGNOSIS: Ineffective thermoregulation related to lack of fat stores and hypotonia as evidenced by extended positioning, low axillary temperature despite warmed blanket/radiant heat source/isolette, respiratory distress, and lethargy

Outcome Identification and Evaluation

Newborn will demonstrate ability to regulate temperature as evidenced by temperature remaining in normal range (36.5° to 37.5°C) and absent signs of cold stress.

Interventions: *Promoting Thermoregulation*

- Assess the axillary temperature every hour or use a thermistor probe *to monitor for changes.*
- Review maternal history *to identify risk factors contributing to problem.*
- Monitor vital signs, including heart rate and respiratory rate, every hour *to identify deviations.*
- Check radiant heat source or isolette *to ensure maintenance of appropriate temperature of the environment.*

- Assess environment for sources of heat loss or gain through evaporation, conduction, convection, or radiation *to minimize risk of heat loss.*
- Avoid bathing and exposing newborn *to prevent cold stress.*
- Warm all blankets and equipment that come in contact with newborn; place warmed cap on the newborn's head and keep it on *to minimize heat loss.*

(continued)

NURSING CARE PLAN 23.1

Overview of the Care of a Preterm Newborn (continued)

- Encourage kangaroo care (a parent holds preterm infant underneath clothing skin-to-skin and upright between breasts) *to provide warmth.*
- Educate parents on how to maintain a neutral thermal environment, including importance of keeping

the newborn warm with a cap and double-wrapping with blankets and changing them frequently to keep dry *to promote newborn's adjustment.*
- Demonstrate ways to safeguard warmth and prevent heat loss.

NURSING DIAGNOSIS: Imbalanced nutrition: less than body requirements to meet metabolic needs related to poor sucking and lack of glycogen stores necessary to meet the newborn's increased metabolic demands

Outcome Identification and Evaluation

Newborn will demonstrate adequate nutritional intake to progressively gain weight toward desired goal, remaining free of signs of hypoglycemia as evidenced by blood glucose levels being maintained above 45 mg/dL, enhanced sucking ability, and appropriate weight gain.

Interventions: *Promoting Optimal Nutrition*

- Identify newborn at risk based on behavioural characteristics, body measurements, and gestational age *to establish a baseline and allow for early detection.*
- Assess blood glucose levels as ordered *to determine status and establish a baseline for interventions.*
- Obtain blood glucose measurements upon admission to nursery and every 1 to 2 hours as indicated *to evaluate for changes.*
- Observe behaviour for signs of low blood glucose *to allow early identification.*
- Initiate early oral feedings or gavage feedings *to maintain blood glucose levels.*
- If oral or gavage feedings aren't tolerated, initiate an IV glucose infusion *to aid in stabilizing blood glucose levels.*
- Assess skin for pallor and sweating *to identify signs of hypoglycemia.*
- Assess neurologic status for tremors, seizures, jitteriness, and lethargy *to identify further drops in blood glucose levels.*

- Monitor weight daily for changes *to determine effectiveness of feedings.*
- Maintain temperature using warmed blankets, radiant warmer, or warmed isolette *to prevent heat loss and possible cold stress and reduce energy demands.*
- Monitor temperature *to prevent cold stress resulting in decreased blood glucose levels.*
- Offer opportunities for nonnutritive sucking on premature-size pacifier *to satisfy sucking needs.*
- Monitor for tolerance of oral feedings, including intake and output, *to determine effectiveness.*
- Administer IV dextrose if newborn is symptomatic *to raise blood glucose levels quickly.*
- Decrease energy requirements, including clustering care activities and providing rest periods, *to conserve glucose and glycogen stores.*
- Inform parents about procedures and treatments, including rationale for frequent blood glucose levels, *to help reduce their anxiety.*

KEY CONCEPTS

- Variations in birth weight and gestational age can place a newborn at risk for challenges that require special care.

- Variations in birth weight include the following categories: SGA, AGA, and LGA. Newborns who are SGA or LGA have special needs.

- The SGA newborn faces problems related to a decrease in placental function in utero; these problems may include perinatal asphyxia, hypothermia, hypoglycemia, polycythemia, and meconium aspiration.

- Risk factors for the birth of an LGA infant include maternal diabetes mellitus or glucose intolerance, multiparity, prior history of a macrosomic infant, postterm gestation, maternal obesity, male fetus, and genetics. LGA newborns face problems such as birth trauma due to cephalopelvic disproportion, hypoglycemia, and jaundice secondary to hyperbilirubinemia.

- Variations in gestational age include postterm and preterm newborns. Postterm newborns may be LGA or SGA, or dysmature, depending on placental function.

- The postterm newborn may develop complications after birth, including fetal hypoxia, hypoglycemia, hypothermia, polycythemia, and meconium aspiration.

- Preterm birth is the leading cause of death within the 1st month of life and the second leading cause of all infant deaths.

- The preterm newborn is at risk for complications because his or her organ systems are immature, thereby impeding the transition from intrauterine life to extrauterine life.

- Newborns can experience pain, but their pain is difficult to validate with consistent behaviours.

- Newborns with gestational age variations, primarily preterm newborns, benefit from developmental care, which includes a variety of activities designed to manage the environment and individualize the care based on behavioural observations.

- Nurses play a key role in assisting the parents and family of a newborn with special needs to cope with this crisis situation, including dealing with the possibility that the newborn may not survive. Nurses working with parents experiencing a perinatal loss can help by actively listening, understanding the parents' experiences, and communicating empathy.

- The goal of discharge planning is to make a successful transition to home care.

REFERENCES AND RECOMMENDED READINGS

Als, H. (2009). Newborn individualized developmental care and assessment program (NIDCAP): New frontier for neonatal and perinatal medicine. *Journal of Neonatal-Perinatal Medicine, 2,* 135–147.

American Academy of Pediatrics (AAP) and American Heart Association (AHA). (2014). *Documentation of neonatal resuscitation. 23*(1). Retrieved from https://www.aap.org/en-us/Documents/nrp_newsletter_2014_springsummer.pdf.

American College of Obstetrician and Gynecologist. (2013). *Definition of term pregnancy.* Retrieved from https://www.acog.org/Clinical-Guidance-and-Publications/Committee-Opinions/Committee-on-Obstetric-Practice/Definition-of-Term-Pregnancy.

Astra Pharmaceuticals. (n.d.). *EMLA cream [product monograph].* Retrieved from https://www.accessdata.fda.gov/drugsatfda_docs/label/2000/19941S11LBL.PDF.

Back, S. A. (2015). Brain injury in the preterm infant: New horizons for pathogenesis and prevention. *Pediatric Neurology, 53*(3), 185–192.

Baker, B. (2015). Evidence-based practice to improve outcomes for late preterm infants. *Journal of Obstetric, Gynecologic, & Neonatal Nursing, 44,* 127–134.

Barfield, W. D. & Lee, K. G. (2019). Late preterm infants. *UpToDate.* Retrieved from https://www.uptodate.com/contents/late-preterm-infants

Baur, A. R. (2017). Macrosomia. *eMedicine.* Retrieved from http://emedicine.medscape.com/article/262679-overview.

Boxwell, G. (Ed.). (2010). *Neonatal intensive care nursing* (2nd ed.). New York: Routledge.

Boyle, E. M., Johnson, S., Manktelow, B., Seaton, S. E., Draper, E. S., Smith, L. K., . . . Field, D. J. (2015). Neonatal outcomes and delivery of care for infants born late preterm or moderately preterm: A prospective population-based study. *Archives of Disease in Childhood: Fetal and Neonatal Edition, 100*(6), F479–F485.

Brennan, A. M., Murphy, B. P., & Kiely, M. (2015). Nutritional management and assessment of preterm infants: The Baby-Grow Longitudinal Nutrition and Growth study. *Topics in Clinical Nutrition, 30*(1), 80–93.

Callister, L. C. (2014). Global perspectives on perinatal loss. *MCN: The American Journal of Maternal/Child Nursing, 39*(3), 207–210.

Canadian Paediatric Society (CPS). (2017). *2016 medications for neonatal resuscitation program Canadian adaptation.* Retrieved from https://www.cps.ca/uploads/nrp/Medications_for_NRP_2016_v03_1.pdf.

Canadian Paediatric Society (CPS). (2018). *Screening guidelines for newborns at risk for low blood glucose.* Retrieved from https://www.cps.ca/en/documents/position/newborns-low-blood-glucose.

Canadian Paediatric Society (CPS) & Heart & Stroke Foundation. (2016). *Neonatal resuscitation program, 7th edition information.* Retrieved from https://www.cps.ca/en/nrp-prn/7th-edition-information.

Cano Giménez, E., & Sánchez-Luna, M. (2015). Providing parents with individualized support in a neonatal intensive care unit reduced stress, anxiety and depression. *Acta Paediatrica, 104*(7), e300–e305.

Carlo, W. A. (2015). Prematurity and intrauterine growth restriction. In R. M. Kliegman, B. R. Stanton, J. W. St. Geme, N. F. Schor, & R. E. Behrman (Eds.). *Nelson textbook of pediatrics* (20th ed.). Philadelphia, PA: Saunders.

Centers for Disease Control and Prevention (CDC). (2017). *Birthweight and gestation.* Retrieved from http://www.cdc.gov/nchs/fastats/birthweight.htm.

Cleary-Goldman, J., & Robinson, J. N. (2018). Delivery of the preterm low birth weight singleton fetus. *UpToDate.* Retrieved from http://www.uptodate.com/contents/delivery-of-the-preterm-low-birth-weight-singleton-fetus.

Cunningham, F. G., Leveno, K. J., Bloom, S. L., Dashe, J. S., Hoffman, B. L., Casey, B.M., & Spong, C. Y. (2014). *Williams obstetrics* (25th ed.). New York: McGraw-Hill.

Discenza, D. (2015). NICU helping hands: Supporting families through the whole journey. *Neonatal Network, 34*(1), 52–54.

Fanaroff, A. A., & Fanaroff, J. M. (2014). *Klaus and Fanaroff's care of the high-risk neonate* (6th ed.). Philadelphia, PA: Elsevier Health Sciences.

Feinberg, M. E., Roettger, M. E., Jones, D. E., Paul, I. M., & Kan, M. L. (2015). Effects of a psychosocial couple-based prevention program on adverse birth outcomes. *Maternal and Child Health Journal, 19*(1), 102–111.

Gardner, S. L., Carter, B. S., Hines, M. E., & Hernandez, J. A. (2016). *Merenstein & Gardner's handbook of neonatal intensive care* (8th ed.). St. Louis, MO: Mosby Elsevier.

Gray, L., Garza, E., Zageris, D., Heilman, K. J., & Porges, S. W. (2015). Sucrose and warmth for analgesia in healthy newborns: An RCT. *Pediatrics, 135*(3), e607–e614.

Green, C. J. (2016). *Maternal newborn nursing care plans* (3rd ed.). Burlington, MA: Jones & Bartlett Learning.

Hall, S., Hynan, M., Phillips, R., Press, J., Kenner, C., & Ryan, D. J. (2015). Development of program standards for psychosocial support of parents of infants admitted to a neonatal intensive care unit: A national interdisciplinary consensus model. *Newborn and Infant Nursing Reviews, 15*(1), 24–27.

Harrison, D., Bueno, M., & Reszel, J. (2015). Prevention and management of pain and stress in the neonate. *Research and Reports in Neonatology, 5*, 9–16.

Herrera-Marschitz, M., Neira-Peña, T., Leyton, L., Gebicke-Haerter, P., Rojas-Mancilla, E., Morales, P., & Bustamante, D. (2015). Short- and long-term consequences of perinatal asphyxia: Looking for neuroprotective strategies. In M. Antonelli (Ed.). *Perinatal programming of neurodevelopment* (pp. 169–198). New York: Springer Publishers.

Horgan, M. J. (2015). Management of the late preterm infant: Not quite ready for prime time. *Pediatric Clinics of North America, 62*(2), 439–451.

Jaques, S. C., & Kennea, N. (2015). Resuscitation of the newborn. *Obstetrics, Gynaecology & Reproductive Medicine, 25*(3), 61–67.

Kandasamy, J. (2017). *Polycythemia of the newborn*. Retrieved from http://emedicine.medscape.com/article/976319-overview.

Kaneko, M., Yamashita, R., Kai, K., Yamada, N., Sameshima, H., & Ikenoue, T. (2015). Perinatal morbidity and mortality for extremely low-birthweight infants: A population-based study of regionalized maternal and neonatal transport. *Journal of Obstetrics and Gynaecology Research, 41*(7), 1056–1066.

Kelly, M. M. (2010). Prematurity. In P. J. Allen, J. A. Vessey, & N. A. Schapiro (Eds.). *Primary care of the child with a chronic condition* (5th ed.). St. Louis, MO: Mosby.

Kenner, C., & Lott, J. W. (2014). *Comprehensive neonatal care: An interdisciplinary approach* (5th ed.). St. Louis, MO: Saunders.

Kiechl-Kohlendorfer, U., Merkle, U., Deufert, D., Neubauer, V., Peglow, U. P., & Griesmaier, E. (2015). Effect of developmental care for very premature infants on neurodevelopmental outcome at 2 years of age. *Infant Behavior and Development, 39*, 166–172.

Kliegman, R. M., Stanton, B., St. Geme, J., Schor, N., & Behrman, R. E. (Eds.). (2015). *Nelson textbook of pediatrics* (20th ed.). St. Louis, MO: Saunders Elsevier.

Krowchuk, H. (2015). Toward evidence-based practice: Paternal and maternal concerns for their very low-birth-weight infants transitioning from the NICU to home. *MCN:*

The American Journal of Maternal Child Nursing, 40(2), 134.

Mahajan, R. C., Une, L., & Bansal, S. (2015). Study of clinical features and in newborn with polycythemia: Antenatal and natal factors. *MedPulse—International Medical Journal, 2*(2), 66–71.

Mandy, G. T. (2018a). Small for gestational age infant. *UpToDate*. Retrieved from http://www.uptodate.com/contents/small-for-gestational-age-infant.

Mandy, G. T. (2018b). Large for gestational age newborn. *UpToDate*. Retrieved from http://www.uptodate.com/contents/large-for-gestational-age-newborn.

March of Dimes. (2013). *Premature babies*. Retrieved from http://www.marchofdimes.org/baby/premature-babies.aspx.

March of Dimes. (2018). *PeriStats*. Retrieved from http://www.marchofdimes.org/peristats/Peristats.aspx.

Mattson, S., & Smith, J. E. (2015). *Core curriculum for maternal–newborn nursing* (5th ed.). St. Louis, MO: Saunders Elsevier.

Morken, N. H., Klungsøyr, K., & Skjaerven, R. (2014). Perinatal mortality by gestational week and size at birth in singleton pregnancies at and beyond term: A nationwide population-based cohort study. *BMC Pregnancy and Childbirth, 14*(1), 172–175.

Nagtalon-Ramos, J. (2014). *Maternal-newborn nursing care: Best evidence-based practices*. Philadelphia, PA: F.A. Davis Company.

National Center for Health Statistics. (2017). *Birthweight and gestation*. Retrieved from http://www.cdc.gov/nchs/fastats/birthweight.htm.

Neonatal eHandbook. (2016a). *Diabetic mother–infant care*. Retrieved from https://www2.health.vic.gov.au/hospitals-and-health-services/patient-care/perinatal-reproductive/neonatal-ehandbook/conditions/diabetic-mother-infant-care.

Neonatal eHandbook. (2016b). *Polycythemia in neonates*. Retrieved from https://www2.health.vic.gov.au/hospitals-and-health-services/patient-care/perinatal-reproductive/neonatal-ehandbook/conditions/polycythaemia.

Neonatal eHandbook. (2016c). *Nutrition*. Retrieved from https://www2.health.vic.gov.au/hospitals-and-health-services/patient-care/perinatal-reproductive/neonatal-ehandbook/nutrition.

Paul, M. (2015). Oxygen administration to preterm neonates in the delivery room: Minimizing oxidative stress. *Advances in Neonatal Care, 15*(2), 94–103.

Potter, C. F., & Kicklighter, S. D. (2016) Infant of a diabetic mother. *eMedicine*. Retrieved from http://emedicine.medscape.com/article/974230-overview.

Ramji, S., Saugstad, O. D., & Jain, A. (2015). Current concepts of oxygen therapy in neonates. *The Indian Journal of Pediatrics, 82*(1), 46–52.

Resnik, R. (2018). Fetal growth restriction: Evaluation and management. *UpToDate*. Retrieved from https://www.uptodate.com/contents/fetal-growth-restriction-evaluation-and-management?search=fetal%20growth%20restriction&source=search_result&selectedTitle=1~150&usage_type=default&display_rank=1.

Rondinelli, J., Long, K., Seelinger, C., Crawford, C. L., & Valdez, R. (2015). Factors related to nurse comfort when caring for families experiencing perinatal loss: Evidence for bereavement program enhancement. *Journal for Nurses in Professional Development, 31*(3), 158–163.

Rossman, B., Greene, M. M., & Meier, P. P. (2015). The role of peer support in the development of maternal identity for 'NICU moms'. *JOGNN: Journal of Obstetric, Gynecologic & Neonatal Nursing, 44*(1), 3–16.

Sabic, D., Blattner, C., & Metts, M. (2015). Newborn and infant pain control. *Clinical Pediatrics, 54*(7), 613–614.

Simpson, L. (2015). *Best practices in high-risk pregnancy: An issue of obstetrics and gynecology clinics* (1st ed., Vol. 42-2). Philadelphia, PA: Elsevier Health Sciences.

Steen, S. E. (2015). Perinatal death: Bereavement interventions used by US and Spanish nurses and midwives. *International Journal of Palliative Nursing, 21*(2), 79–86.

Valeri, B. O., Holsti, L., & Linhares, M. B. (2015). Neonatal pain and developmental outcomes in children born preterm: A systematic review. *The Clinical Journal of Pain, 31*(4), 355–362.

Vali, P., Mathew, B., & Lakshminrusimha, S. (2015). Neonatal resuscitation: Evolving strategies. *Maternal Health, Neonatology and Perinatology, 1*(1), 4–23.

Verklan, M. T., & Walden, M. (2015). *Core curriculum for neonatal intensive care nursing* (5th ed.). St. Louis, MO: Saunders.

Watchko, J. F. (2015). Common hematologic problems in the newborn nursery. *Pediatric Clinics of North America, 62*(2), 509–524.

White, C., & Wilson, V. (2015). A longitudinal study of aspects of a hospital's family-centred nursing: Changing practice through data translation. *Journal of Advanced Nursing, 71*(1), 100–114.

White-Traut, R. (2015). Nurse management of the NICU environment is critical to optimal infant development. *Journal of Obstetric, Gynecologic, & Neonatal Nursing, 44*(2), 169–170.

Yamada, J., Stevens, B., Sidani, S., & Watt-Watson, J. (2015). Test of a process evaluation checklist to improve neonatal pain practices. *Western Journal of Nursing Research, 37*(5), 581–598.

Yousaf, U. F., Hayat, S., & Afzal, N. (2015). Resuscitation of newborn in high risk deliveries. *Journal of Ayub Medical College Abbottabad, 27*(2), 343–345.

CHAPTER **WORKSHEET**

MULTIPLE CHOICE QUESTIONS

1. The nurse documents that a newborn is postterm based on the understanding that he was born after:
   a. 38 weeks' gestation
   b. 40 weeks' gestation
   c. 42 weeks' gestation
   d. 44 weeks' gestation

2. SGA and LGA newborns have an excessive number of red blood cells related to:
   a. Hypoxia
   b. Hypoglycemia
   c. Hypocalcemia
   d. Hypothermia

3. Because subcutaneous and brown fat stores were used for survival in utero, the nurse would assess an SGA newborn for which of the following?
   a. Hyperbilirubinemia
   b. Hypothermia
   c. Polycythemia
   d. Hypoglycemia

4. In assessing a preterm newborn, which of the following findings would be of greatest concern?
   a. Milia over the bridge of the nose
   b. Thin transparent skin
   c. Poor muscle tone
   d. Heart murmur

5. In dealing with parents experiencing a perinatal loss, which of the following nursing interventions would be most appropriate?
   a. Sheltering the parents from the bad news
   b. Making all the decisions regarding care
   c. Encouraging them to participate in the newborn's care
   d. Leaving them by themselves to allow time to grieve

6. The nurse is providing care to several newborns with variations in gestational age and birth weight. When developing the plan of care for these newborns, the nurse focuses on energy conservation to promote growth and development. Which measures would the nurse include in the nursing plans of care? Select all that apply.
   a. Keeping the handling of the newborn to a minimum
   b. Maintaining a neutral thermal environment
   c. Decreasing environmental stimuli
   d. Initiating early oral feedings
   e. Using thermal warmers in all cribs

7. Which of the following concepts would the nurse incorporate into the plan of care when assessing pain in a newborn with special needs?
   a. Newborns experience pain primarily with surgical procedures.
   b. Preterm newborns in the NICU are at least risk for pain.
   c. Pain assessment needs to be comprehensive and frequent.
   d. A newborn's facial expression is the primary indicator of pain.

8. Evidence-based practice refers to the use of which of the following to validate your practice?
   a. Research findings
   b. Written guidelines
   c. Traditional practices
   d. Institutional policies

CRITICAL THINKING EXERCISES

1. After an abnormal fetal heart rate tracing was noted on the monitor, a postterm newborn was delivered via a difficult vacuum extraction. The newborn had low Apgar scores and had to be resuscitated before being transferred to the nursery. Once admitted, the nurse observed the following behaviours: jitteriness, tremors, hypotonia, lethargy, and rapid respirations.
   a. What might these behaviours indicate?
   b. For what other conditions might this newborn be at high risk?
   c. What intervention is needed to address this newborn's condition?

2. A preterm newborn was born at 35 weeks following an abruptio placenta due to a car accident. He was transported to the NICU at a nearby regional medical centre. After being stabilized, he was placed in an isolette close to the door and placed on a cardiac monitor. A short time later, the nurse notices that he is cool to the touch and lethargic, has a weak cry, and has an axillary temperature of 36°C.
   a. What might have contributed to this newborn's hypothermic condition?
   b. What transfer mechanism may have been a factor?
   c. What intervention would be appropriate for the nurse to initiate?

CHAPTER **WORKSHEET**

3. A term SGA newborn weighing 4 lb was brought to the nursery for admission a short time after birth. The labour and birth nurse reports the mother was a heavy smoker, used cocaine, and experienced physical abuse throughout her pregnancy. After stabilizing the newborn and correcting the hypoglycemia with oral feedings, the nurse observes the following: acrocyanosis, ruddy colour, poor circulation to the extremities, tachypnea, and irritability.

a. What complication might this SGA newborn be manifesting?

b. What factors may have contributed to this complication?

c. What would be an appropriate intervention to manage this condition?

STUDY ACTIVITIES

1. At a community health department maternity clinic, secure permission to interview the parents of a special needs child. Ask about their feelings throughout the experience. How are they managing and coping now?

2. Visit the March of Dimes website and review this group's national campaign to reduce the incidence of prematurity. Are their strategies workable or not? Explain your reasoning.

3. A common metabolic disorder present in both SGA and LGA newborns after birth is _____.

4. A 10-lb LGA newborn is brought to the nursery after a difficult vaginal birth. The nursery nurse should focus on detecting birth injuries such as _____.

BRINGING IT ALL TOGETHER: A CASE STUDY

Taylor was born at 29 weeks. Her premature birth has resulted in an increased risk both for respiratory distress and hypothermia. Her parents, Susan and Harvey, are interested and involved in Taylor's condition and care but are understandably anxious regarding their first child's health status. She is being cared for by nurses in the neonatal intensive care unit (NICU) of the university-affiliated medical centre where she was born.

Go to thePoint **to find questions to consider about this case.**

24

Nursing Management of the Newborn at Risk: Acquired and Congenital Newborn Conditions

Learning Objectives

Upon completion of the chapter, you will be able to:

1. Describe the most common acquired conditions affecting the newborn.
2. Characterize the nursing management of a newborn experiencing respiratory distress syndrome (RDS).
3. Outline the birthing room preparation and procedures necessary to prevent meconium aspiration syndrome (MAS) in the newborn at birth.
4. Differentiate risk factors for the development of necrotizing enterocolitis (NEC).
5. Analyze the impact of maternal diabetes on the newborn and the care needed.
6. Evaluate the assessment and intervention for a newborn experiencing substance withdrawal after birth.
7. Develop assessment and nursing management for newborns sustaining trauma and birth injuries.
8. Outline the assessment, interventions, prevention, and management of hyperbilirubinemia in newborns.
9. Summarize the interventions appropriate for a newborn with neonatal sepsis.
10. Research four gastrointestinal system congenital anomalies that can occur in a newborn.
11. Formulate a plan of care for a newborn with an acquired or congenital condition.
12. Relate the importance of parental participation in care of the newborn with a congenital or acquired condition, including the nurse's role in facilitating parental involvement.

***Kelly*, a 27-year-old G2P1, comes to the labour and birth area in active labour. She tells you she is overdue and relieved to finally be giving birth. Her membranes rupture on admission, revealing meconium-stained fluid. What additional nursing assessments need to be carried out now? What risk factors need to be considered when developing Kelly's plan of care?**

INTRODUCTION

Advances in pre- and neonatal medical and nursing care throughout the industrialized world have led to a marked increase in the number of newborns who have survived a high-risk pregnancy but experience acquired or congenital conditions. These newborns are considered one of our most vulnerable at-risk populations—that is, they are susceptible to morbidity and mortality because of the acquired or congenital disorder.

During the past several decades technologic and pharmacologic advances, genomic discoveries, and standardized policies and procedures have significantly improved survival rates for at-risk newborns. However, the risk of morbidity remains an important sequela. For example, some of these newborns are at risk for continuing health problems that require long-term technologic support. Other newborns remain at risk for physical and developmental problems into the school years and beyond. Although challenges exist in application of these advances to improve the newborn's health, the high-risk newborn will increasingly benefit from them in the future. Providing the complex care needed to maintain the child's health and well-being will have a tremendous emotional and economic impact on the family. Nurses are challenged to provide support to mothers and their families when neonatal well-being is threatened.

Acquired disorders typically occur at or soon after birth. They may result from problems or conditions experienced by the woman during her pregnancy or at birth, such as diabetes, maternal infection, or substance abuse, or conditions associated with labour and birth, such as prolonged rupture of membranes or fetal distress. However, there may be no identifiable cause for the disorder.

Congenital disorders can be defined as structural or functional or metabolic abnormalities at birth. According to the World Health Organization (WHO, 2016), an estimated 1 in 33 infants or over 3 million fetuses and infants globally are born each year with major congenital disorders. They are found in approximately 3% of all newborns (WHO, 2016). The most common serious defects are congenital heart defects, neural tube defects (NTDs), and Down syndrome (WHO, 2016). Congenital disorders, which often involve a problem with inheritance, include structural anomalies (commonly referred to as birth defects), chromosomal disorders, and inborn errors of metabolism. Most congenital disorders have a complex etiology, involving many interacting genes, gene products, and social and environmental factors during organogenesis (the origin and development of organs). Some alterations can be prevented or compensated for with pharmacologic, nutritional, or other types of interventions, while others cannot be changed. Only through a better understanding of the complex interplay of genetic, environmental, social, and cultural factors can these devastating and life-changing outcomes be prevented (March of Dimes, 2018b).

The field of genomics and genetic medicine has witnessed an explosion of new knowledge, much of it learned from the Human Genome Project. Advances in understanding of the genetic basis of development and function, as well as the interaction of genes and the environment, continue to foster new insights into human health. This chapter addresses selected acquired and congenital newborn conditions. In addition, it describes the nurse's role in assessment and management, emphasizing parental education and support. Nurses play a key role in helping the parents cope with the stress of having an ill newborn.

ACQUIRED DISORDERS

Acquired disorders are not passed genetically or caused by hereditary or developmental factors; they are obtained after birth by a reaction to environmental influences outside of the body. Examples of acquired disorders include perinatal asphyxia, respiratory distress syndrome (RDS), meconium aspiration syndrome (MAS), persistent pulmonary hypertension of the newborn (PPHN), intraventricular hemorrhage, necrotizing enterocolitis (NEC), retinopathy of prematurity, birth trauma, hyperbilirubinemia, and newborn infections.

Perinatal Asphyxia

At birth, the newborn's lungs are filled with fluid. This fluid must be cleared and replaced with air for successful respiration to begin after birth. As the newborn makes the transition to life outside the fluid-filled intrauterine environment, dramatic changes must occur to facilitate newborn respirations. Newborns normally start to breathe with routine warming, drying, airway suctioning, and mild stimulation. Most newborns make this transition such that by 1 minute of age, they are breathing well on their own. A newborn who fails to establish adequate, sustained respiration after birth is said to have **asphyxia**. Perinatal asphyxia, more appropriately known as hypoxic ischemic encephalopathy, is characterized by clinical and laboratory evidence of acute or subacute brain injury due to systemic hypoxemia or reduced cerebral blood flow (Zanelli, Stanley, & Kaufman, 2018). Physiologically, asphyxia can be defined as impairment in gas exchange resulting in a decrease in blood oxygen levels (hypoxemia) and an excess of carbon dioxide or hypercapnia that leads to acidosis. It occurs when pulmonary oxygenation is delayed or interrupted.

Asphyxia is the most common clinical insult in the perinatal period. As many as 10% of United States' newborns require some degree of active resuscitation to stimulate breathing with 1.5% requiring extensive resuscitation (Cunningham et al., 2014). More than a million newborns who survive asphyxia at birth develop long-term problems such as cerebral palsy, intellectual disability, speech disorders, hearing and/or visual impairment, and learning disabilities (Zanelli et al., 2018).

Pathophysiology

Asphyxia occurs when oxygen delivery is insufficient to meet metabolic demands, resulting in hypoxia, hypercarbia, and metabolic acidosis. Any condition that reduces oxygen delivery to the fetus can result in asphyxia. These conditions may include but are not limited to maternal hypoxia, such as from cardiac or respiratory disease, anemia, or postural hypotension; maternal vascular disease that leads to placental insufficiency, such as diabetes or hypertension; cord problems such as compression or prolapse; and postterm pregnancies, which may trigger meconium release into the amniotic fluid.

Initially, the newborn uses compensatory mechanisms including tachycardia and vasoconstriction to help bring oxygen to the vital organs for a time. However, without intervention, these mechanisms fail, leading to hypotension, bradycardia, and eventually cardiopulmonary arrest.

With failure to breathe well after birth, the newborn will develop hypoxia (too little oxygen in the cells of the body). As a result, the heart rate falls, cyanosis develops, and the newborn becomes hypotonic and unresponsive. Newborn resuscitation is needed to help initiate breathing in newborns that fail to breathe spontaneously at birth.

Nursing Assessment

The key to successful treatment of newborn asphyxia is early identification and recognition of newborns that may be at risk. Review the perinatal history for risk factors, including:

- Trauma: injury to the central or peripheral nervous system secondary to a long or difficult labour, a precipitous birth, multiple gestation, abnormal presentation, cephalopelvic disproportion, shoulder dystocia, or extraction by forceps or vacuum
- Intrauterine asphyxia: for example, fetal hypoxia secondary to maternal hypoxia, diabetes, hypertension, anemia, cord compression, or meconium aspiration
- Sepsis: acquired bacterial or viral organisms from infected amniotic fluid, maternal infection, or direct contact while passing through the birth canal
- Malformation: congenital anomalies including facial or upper airway deformities, renal anomalies, pulmonary hypoplasia, neuromuscular disorders, esophageal atresia, or NTDs
- Hypovolemic shock: secondary to abruptio placentae, placenta previa, or cord rupture resulting in blood loss to the fetus
- Medication: drugs given to mother during labour that can affect the fetus by causing placental hypoperfusion

and hypotension; use of hypnotics, analgesics, anesthetics, narcotics, oxytocin, and street drugs during pregnancy (Stark, 2018)

At birth, assess the newborn immediately. Observe the infant's colour, noting any pallor or cyanosis. Assess the work of breathing. Be alert for apnea, tachypnea, gasping respirations, grunting, nasal flaring, or retractions or other signs of respiratory distress. Evaluate heart rate and note bradycardia. Assess the newborn's temperature, noting hypothermia. Determine the Apgar score at 1 and 5 minutes. If the score is less than 7 at 5 minutes of age, Apgars should be repeated every 5 minutes for up to 20 minutes (Canadian Paediatric Society [CPS] & American Heart Association [AHA], 2016).

Laboratory or diagnostic testing may be used to identify etiologies for the newborn's asphyxia. For example, a chest x-ray may identify structural abnormalities that might interfere with respiration. A blood culture may identify an infectious process. A blood toxicology screen may detect any maternal drugs in the newborn (Verklan & Walden, 2015).

Methods of testing to identify the fetus at risk for developing perinatal asphyxia continue to be developed and refined. The perinatal nurse needs to be knowledgeable of each test's purpose, capabilities, limitations, and clinical issues. Appropriate nursing interventions based on this knowledge facilitate the testing process and promote the goal of improved perinatal outcome.

Nursing Management

Management of the newborn experiencing asphyxia includes immediate resuscitation. Ensure that the equipment needed for resuscitation is readily available and in working order. Essential equipment includes a wall suction apparatus, an oxygen source, a newborn ventilation bag, endotracheal tubes (2 to 3 mm), infant warmer, surgical blue towels, a laryngoscope and laryngoscope blade, pulse oximetry, suction catheters, IV insertion supplies, warm blankets, and hat. Effective ventilation is essential to successful newborn resuscitation. Ventilation is frequently initiated with a manual resuscitation bag and face mask followed by endotracheal intubation if respiratory depression continues (see Chapter 23 for a more detailed discussion of resuscitation).

Dry the newborn quickly with a warm towel and then place him or her under a radiant heater to prevent rapid heat loss through evaporation. Handling and rubbing the newborn with a dry towel may be all that is needed to stimulate the onset of breathing. If the newborn fails to respond to stimulation, then active resuscitation is needed.

The procedure for newborn resuscitation is easily remembered by the "ABCDs"—airway, breathing, circulation, and drugs (see Chapter 23, Box 23.3). Continue resuscitation until the newborn has a pulse above 100 bpm, a good healthy cry, or good breathing efforts, good tone, centrally pink, and has acceptable oxygen saturation levels. This last sign indicates a good oxygen supply to the brain (Jaques & Kennea, 2015).

Take Note!

According to the Canadian Paediatric Society and American Heart Association Guidelines for Neonatal Resuscitation, resuscitation efforts may be stopped if the newborn exhibits no detectable heart rate after 10 minutes of continuous and adequate resuscitation (CPS & AHA, 2016).

Provide continued observation and assessment of the newborn that has been successfully resuscitated. Monitor the newborn's vital signs and oxygen saturation levels closely for changes. Maintain a neutral thermal environment to prevent hypothermia, which would increase the newborn's metabolic and oxygen demands. Check the blood glucose level and observe for signs of hypoglycemia; if this develops, it can further stress the newborn.

The need for resuscitative measures can be extremely upsetting for the parents/partners/significant others. Explain to them the initial resuscitation activities being performed and offer ongoing explanations about any procedures being done, equipment being used, or medications given. Provide presence and support to them throughout the procedure and give frequent updates about procedures being used on their newborn.

Therapeutic hypothermia is a promising neuroprotective intervention for newborns with moderate to severe perinatal encephalopathy after perinatal asphyxia and has currently been incorporated in many neonatal intensive care units (NICUs). However, some infants with encephalopathy will benefit from hypothermia therapy though some will still develop significant adverse outcomes. Cooling the whole body to 33.5°C for 3 days has significant effects on normal physiology as well as pathologic processes. Some of these effects are desirable and neuroprotective, whereas others are not. To enhance the outcome, specific diagnostic predictors are needed to identify newborns likely to benefit from hypothermia treatment (Thoresen, 2015). This treatment decision must be made a collaborative one with the parents' full understanding of the risks involved. Nurses are in a unique position to detect parent anxiety and to maintain therapeutic communication that may help support them through this crisis.

Provide physical and emotional support to the parents through the initial crisis and throughout the newborn's stay. When the newborn is stable, allow parents to spend time with their newborn to promote bonding (Fig. 24.1). Point out the newborn's positive attributes (colour, activity, healthy cry) and give frequent updates on his or her status. Role model techniques for holding,

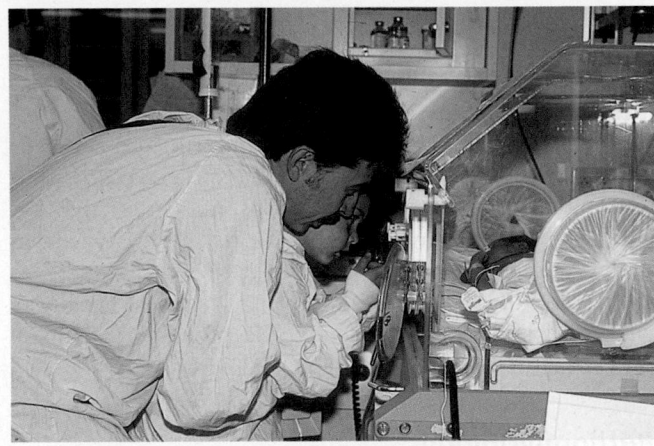

FIGURE 24.1 A father and sibling interacting with his newborn once the newborn's condition has stabilized.

interacting with, and caring for the newborn will assist to decrease the parents' anxiety.

Nurses need to remember developmental care practices for infants with perinatal asphyxia. A team approach incorporating developmental goals and intervention strategies into the nursing care of these infants is essential for optimal developmental outcome. Therapeutic management must always be appropriate for the infant's health status and gestational age. An understanding of the scientific basis for intervention and the therapeutic management techniques for newborns that are sick, recuperating, or convalescing will help the nurse to promote optimal development when caring for the asphyxiated infant (Smith et al., 2015).

Remember Kelly, the young woman described at the beginning of the chapter? Her son is intubated and tracheal suctioning is performed. Positive-pressure ventilation is also started with a self-inflating bag and 50% oxygen. Ventilation is continued for 1 minute and then gradually discontinued. The heart rate is now 120 bpm, and spontaneous respirations are noted. When free-flow oxygen is administered, the newborn begins to cry and turn pink. What continued care is needed in the special care nursery? What explanation should be offered to Kelly regarding her son?

Transient Tachypnea of the Newborn

Transient tachypnea of the newborn (TTN) is a self-limiting condition involving a mild degree of respiratory distress that requires minimal intervention, and resolves over 24 to 72 hours. It is described as the retention of lung fluid or transient pulmonary edema. It usually occurs within a few hours of birth and resolves by 72 hours of age. TTN occurs in approximately 1% to 2% of all live births and incidence is higher in males than females (Swanson & Sinkin, 2015).

Lower gestational age, caesarean birth, and male sex are independent risk factors for TTN (Lee, 2017). Performing elective caesarean sections no earlier than 39 weeks' gestation may decrease the risk of TTN. Labour before a caesarean section is not sufficient to decrease the frequency of TTN, even after 37 weeks of gestation, whereas vaginal birth appears to be protective against it (Pramanik, Rangaswamy, & Gates, 2015).

Pathophysiology

Most newborns make the transition from fetal to newborn life without incident. During fetal life, the lungs are filled with a serous fluid because the placenta, not the lungs, is used for nutrient and gas exchange. During and after birth, this fluid must be removed and replaced with air. An infant born by caesarean birth is at risk of having excessive pulmonary fluid as a result of not having experienced all the stages of labour. Passage through the birth canal during a vaginal birth compresses the thorax, which helps remove the majority of this fluid. Pulmonary circulation and the lymphatic drainage remove the remaining fluid shortly after birth. TTN occurs when the liquid in the lung is removed slowly or incompletely.

Nursing Assessment

Astutely observe the newborn with respiratory distress because TTN is a diagnosis of exclusion. Initially it might be difficult to distinguish this condition from RDS or group B streptococcal pneumonia, since the clinical picture is similar. However, the symptoms of transient tachypnea rarely last more than 72 hours and if they do, further investigation is warranted (Kim, Yang, & Kim, 2015).

HEALTH HISTORY AND PHYSICAL EXAMINATION

Review the perinatal history for risk factors related to TTN such as absence of labour, caesarean birth, precipitous delivery, prolonged labour, fetal macrosomia, infants born early, male gender, or maternal asthma and maternal smoking. Those factors are associated with a higher risk of TTN (Nagtalon-Ramos, 2014).

Closely assess the newborn for signs of TTN. Within the first few hours of birth, observe for tachypnea, expiratory grunting, retractions, laboured breathing, nasal flaring, and mild cyanosis. Mild to moderate respiratory distress is present by 6 hours of age; with respiratory rates as high as 100 to 140 breaths per minute. Also inspect the newborn's chest for hyperextension or a barrel shape. Auscultate breath sounds, which may be slightly diminished secondary to reduced air entry (Fanaroff & Fanaroff, 2014).

LABORATORY AND DIAGNOSTIC TESTING

To aid in the diagnosis, a chest x-ray may be done. It usually reveals mild symmetric lung overaeration and prominent perihilar interstitial markings and streaking. These findings correlate with lymphatic engorgement of retained fetal fluid. In addition, an arterial blood gas (ABG) assessment is important to ascertain the degree of gas exchange and acid–base balance. It typically demonstrates mild hypoxemia, mildly elevated CO_2, and a normal pH (Martin, 2018).

Nursing Management

Management of TTN is supportive. As the retained lung fluid is absorbed by the infant's lymphatic system, the pulmonary status improves. Nursing management focuses on providing adequate oxygenation and determining whether the newborn's respiratory manifestations appear to be resolving or persisting. Provide supportive care while the retained lung fluid is reabsorbed. Administer intravenous (IV) fluids and/or gavage feedings until the respiratory rate decreases enough to allow safe oral feeding. Provide supplemental oxygen via a nasal cannula or oxygen hood to maintain adequate oxygen saturation. Maintain a neutral thermal environment with minimal stimulation to minimize oxygen demand.

Provide ongoing assessment of the newborn's respiratory status. As TTN resolves, the newborn's respiratory rate declines to 60 breaths per minute or less, the oxygen requirement decreases, and the chest x-ray shows resolution of the perihilar streaking. Provide reassurance and progress reports to the parents to help them cope with this crisis.

Respiratory Distress Syndrome

Despite improved survival rates and advances in perinatal care, many high-risk newborns are at risk for respiratory problems, particularly **respiratory distress syndrome (RDS)**, a breathing disorder resulting from lung immaturity and lack of alveolar surfactant, which keeps the air sacs in the lungs from collapsing and allows them to inflate easily. Without surfactant, the alveoli collapse at the end of expiration. Since the link between RDS and surfactant deficiency was discovered more than 30 years ago, tremendous strides have been made in understanding the pathophysiology and treatment of this disorder. The introduction of prenatal steroids to accelerate lung maturity and the development of synthetic surfactant can be credited with the dramatic improvements in the outcome of newborns with RDS (CPS, 2017; Pramanik & Rosenkrantz, 2015).

The incidence of RDS declines with degree of maturity at birth. It occurs in 50% of preterm newborns born at 26 to 28 weeks' gestation, and in 30% of those born at 30 to 31 weeks (Pramanik & Rosenkrantz, 2015). Intensive respiratory care, usually with mechanical ventilation, is necessary.

Pathophysiology

Lung immaturity and surfactant deficiency contribute to the development of RDS. Surfactant is a complex mixture of phospholipids and proteins that adheres to the alveolar surface of the lungs. Anatomically, the immature lung cannot support oxygenation and ventilation, because the alveolar sacs are insufficiently developed, causing a deficient surface area for gas exchange. Physiologically, the amount of surfactant is insufficient to prevent collapse of unstable alveoli. Surfactant forms a coating over the inner surface of the alveoli, reducing the surface tension and preventing alveolar collapse at the end of expiration. In the affected newborn, surfactant is deficient or lacking, and this deficit results in stiff lungs and alveoli that tend to collapse, leading to diffuse atelectasis. The work of breathing is increased because increased pressure similar to that required to initiate the first breath is needed to inflate the lungs with each successive breath. Hypoxemia and acidemia result, leading to vasoconstriction of the pulmonary vasculature. Right-to-left shunting occurs and alveolar capillary circulation is limited, further inhibiting surfactant production. As the disease progresses, fluid and fibrin leak from the pulmonary capillaries, causing hyaline membranes to form in the bronchioles, alveolar ducts, and alveoli. Hyaline membranes produce a glassy appearance in the lung membranes that can be seen on x-rays. These membranes further decrease gas exchange. These factors decrease the total surface area of the gas exchange membrane. The end result is hypoxemia, academia, and a worsening respiratory distress. A vicious cycle is created, compounding the problem (Cunningham et al., 2014).

Nursing Assessment

Nursing assessment focuses on keen observation to identify the signs and symptoms of respiratory distress. In addition, assessment aids in differentiating RDS from other respiratory conditions, such as TTN or group B streptococcal pneumonia.

HISTORY AND PHYSICAL EXAMINATION

Review the history for risk factors associated with RDS. The most common risk factor for the development of RDS is premature birth. Additional risk factors particularly in the term infant include caesarean birth in the absence of preceding labour (related to the lack of thoracic squeezing), male gender, previous birth of an infant with RDS, perinatal asphyxia, cold stress, and maternal diabetes, which produces high levels of insulin which inhibit surfactant production (Rubarth & Quinn, 2015).

> **Take Note!**
> Prolonged rupture of membranes, gestational or chronic maternal hypertension, maternal narcotic addiction, and use of prenatal corticosteroids reduce the

newborn's risk for RDS because of the physiologic stress imposed on the fetus. Chronic stress experienced by the fetus in utero accelerates the production of surfactant before 35 weeks' gestation and thus reduces the incidence of RDS at birth (Pramanik & Rosenkrantz, 2015).

The newborn with RDS usually demonstrates signs at birth or within a few hours of birth. Observe the infant for expiratory grunting, shallow breathing, nasal flaring, chest wall retractions (Fig. 24.2), seesaw respirations, and generalized cyanosis. Auscultate the heart and lungs, noting tachycardia (rates above 150 to 180), fine inspiratory crackles, and tachypnea (rates above 60 breaths per minute).

The Silverman–Anderson Index is an assessment scoring system that can be used to evaluate five parameters of work of breathing as it assigns a numerical score for each parameter. Each category is scored as "0" for normal, "1" for moderate impairment, or "2" for severe impairment. Parameters assessed are retractions of the upper chest, lower chest, and xiphoid; nasal flaring; and expiratory grunt. Normally functioning infants should have a cumulative score of 0, whereas critically ill and severely depressed infants will have scores closer to 10 (Fig. 24.3).

LABORATORY AND DIAGNOSTIC TESTING

The diagnosis of RDS is based on the clinical picture, a lung ultrasound, or x-ray findings and ABGs that show hypoxemia and acidosis. A chest x-ray reveals hypoaeration, underexpansion, and a "ground-glass" pattern (Pramanik et al., 2015).

Nursing Management

If untreated, RDS will worsen. In many infants, respiratory symptoms decline after 72 hours, paralleling the

FIGURE 24.2 Sternal retractions are a sign of respiratory distress requiring immediate intervention, such as mechanical ventilation and other monitoring devices.

Suprasternal retractions

Intercostal retractions

Substernal retractions

Subcostal retractions

Score

FIGURE 24.3 **Assessing the degree of respiratory distress.** (Used with permission from Silverman, W. A., & Anderson, D. H. (1956). A controlled clinical trial of effects of water mist on obstructive respiratory signs, death rate, and necroscopy findings among premature infants. *Pediatrics, 17*(4), 1–10.)

production of surfactant in the alveoli (Gardner, Carter, Enzman-Hines, & Hernandez, 2016). The newborn needs supportive care until surfactant is produced. Effective therapies for established RDS include conventional mechanical ventilation, continuous positive airway pressure (CPAP), or positive end-expiratory pressure (PEEP) to prevent volume loss during expiration, and surfactant therapy. The use of exogenous surfactant replacement therapy to stabilize the newborn's lungs until postnatal surfactant synthesis matures has become a standard of care, but not necessarily evidence based. Knowledge of the surfactant proteins and lipids produced by the epithelial II cells was critical in the development of surfactant replacement preparations used to treat RDS. This preparation has dramatically improved morbidity and

mortality in preterm infants (Blennow & Bohlin, 2015; Whitsett, Wert, & Weaver, 2015).

Despite recent advances in the perinatal management of neonatal RDS, controversies still exist. Strong evidence exists for the role of a single course of prenatal steroids in RDS prevention, but the potential benefit and long-term safety of repeated courses are unclear. A Cochrane review concluded that the incidence of RDS was reduced in infants born before 48 hours and between 1 and 7 days of treatment of mothers with prenatal corticosteroids, but not those born <24 hours of administration (Gaur et al., 2015). Many practices involved in preterm neonatal stabilization at birth are not evidence based, including oxygen administration and positive-pressure lung inflation, and they may at times be harmful. Surfactant replacement therapy is crucial in the management of RDS, but the best preparation, optimal dose and timing of administration at different gestations has not been scientifically established. Respiratory support in the form of mechanical ventilation may also be lifesaving, but can cause lung injury, and protocols should be directed at avoiding mechanical ventilation where possible by using nasal CPAP or nasal ventilation. For newborns with RDS to have best outcomes, it is essential that they have optimal supportive care, including maintenance of a normal body temperature, proper fluid management, good nutritional support, and support of the circulation to maintain adequate tissue perfusion (Gardner et al., 2016).

As recommended, care of the newborn with RDS is primarily supportive and requires a multidisciplinary approach to obtain the best outcomes. Therapy focuses on improving oxygenation and maintaining optimal lung volumes. Expect to transfer the newborn to the NICU soon after birth. Apply the basic principles of newborn care, such as thermoregulation, cardiovascular and nutritional support, normal glucose level maintenance, and infection prevention, to achieve the therapeutic goals of reducing mortality and minimizing lung trauma.

Anticipate the administration of surfactant replacement therapy, prophylactically or as a rescue approach. With prophylactic administration, surfactant is given within minutes after birth, thus providing replacement surfactant before severe RDS develops. Rescue treatment is indicated for newborns with established RDS who require mechanical ventilation and supplemental oxygen. The earlier the surfactant is administered, the better the effect on gas exchange. Following surfactant administration, the newborn must be closely monitored, and preparation for reduced need for oxygen and ventilation should be anticipated (Mattson & Smith, 2015).

Administer the prescribed oxygen concentration via nasal cannula. Anticipate the need for ventilator therapy, which has greatly improved in the past several years, with significant advances in conventional and high-frequency ventilation therapies (Fig. 24.4). Recent studies show no difference in outcomes for newborns who received early treatment with high-frequency oscillatory ventilation compared with those receiving conventional mechanical ventilation. They are both equally effective (Jaecklin, Jarreau, & Kavanagh, 2015). Although mechanical ventilation has increased survival rates, it is also a contributing factor to bronchopulmonary dysplasia, pulmonary hypertension, and retinopathy of prematurity (Cunningham et al., 2014).

In addition, support the newborn with RDS using the following interventions:

- Continuously monitor the infant's cardiopulmonary status via invasive or noninvasive means (e.g., arterial lines or auscultation, respectively).
- Monitor oxygen saturation levels continuously; assess pulse oximeter values to determine oxygen saturation

FIGURE 24.4 **A newborn with RDS receiving mechanical ventilation.**

levels; avoid hyperoxygenation as it can be harmful to newborn's eyes and other organs.
- Closely monitor vital signs, acid–base status, and ABGs.
- Administer broad-spectrum antibiotics if blood cultures are positive.
- Administer sodium bicarbonate or acetate as ordered to correct metabolic acidosis.
- Provide fluids and vasopressor agents as needed to prevent or treat hypotension.
- Test blood glucose levels and administer dextrose as ordered for prevention or treatment of hypoglycemia.
- Cluster caretaking activities to avoid overtaxing and compromising the newborn.
- Place the newborn in the prone position to optimize respiratory status and reduce stress.
- Perform gentle suctioning to remove secretions and maintain a patent airway.
- Assess level of consciousness to identify intraventricular hemorrhage.
- Monitor x-ray studies to detect atelectasis or air leak.
- Maintain a neutral thermal environment to reduce metabolic and oxygen needs.
- Provide sufficient calories via gavage and IV feedings.
- Maintain adequate hydration and assess for signs of fluid overload.
- Provide information to the parents about treatment modalities; give thorough but simple explanations about the rationales for interventions.
- Encourage the parents to participate in care (Mattson & Smith, 2015; Verklan & Walden, 2015).

Provide ongoing assessment and be alert for complications. These may include air leak syndrome, bronchopulmonary dysplasia (chronic lung disease), patent ductus arteriosus, congestive heart failure, intraventricular hemorrhage, retinopathy of prematurity, NEC, complications resulting from IV catheter use (infection, thrombus formation), and developmental delay or disability (Kliegman, Stanton, St. Geme, Schor, & Behrman, 2015).

Meconium Aspiration Syndrome

Meconium is a viscous green substance composed primarily of water and other gastrointestinal secretions that can be noted in the fetal gastrointestinal tract as early as 10 to 16 weeks' gestation (Neonatal eHandbook, 2018). It is expelled as the newborn's first stool after birth. Meconium is sterile and does not contain bacteria, the primary factor that differentiates it from stool. Intrauterine distress can cause passage into the amniotic fluid. Factors that promote the passage in utero include placental insufficiency, maternal hypertension, preeclampsia, fetal hypoxia, transient umbilical compression, oligohydramnios, and maternal drug abuse, especially of tobacco and cocaine. Meconium can be aspirated before or during labour and after birth. Because meconium is rarely found in the amniotic fluid prior to 34 weeks' gestation, it mainly impacts infants born at term and postterm (Lindenskov, Castellheim, Saugstad, & Mollnes, 2015). It is usually expelled as the newborn's first stool after birth.

Meconium aspiration syndrome (MAS) occurs when the newborn inhales particulate meconium mixed with amniotic fluid into the lungs while still in utero or on taking the first breath after birth. It is a common cause of newborn respiratory distress and can lead to severe illness. MAS occurs in approximately 2% to 10% of infants born through meconium-stained amniotic fluid (Garcia-Prats, 2018). Aspiration induces airway obstruction, surfactant dysfunction, hypoxia, and chemical pneumonitis with inflammation of pulmonary tissues. Only 5% of infants with meconium-stained amniotic fluid actually progress to MAS (Geis & Clark, 2017). Severe MAS can lead to persistent pulmonary hypertension and death. The use of surfactant and inhaled nitric oxide has led to decreased mortality and the need for extracorporeal membrane oxygenation (ECMO).

Pathophysiology

The pathophysiology of MAS is complex, and the timing of the insult resulting in aspiration remains controversial. Meconium may be passed in utero secondary to hypoxic stress. Hypoxia induces the fetus to gasp or attempt to breathe. The fetus may bear down and pass meconium into the amniotic fluid or he or she may experience a vagal reflex that causes relaxation of the anal sphincter, allowing meconium to be passed into the amniotic fluid. The fetus then sucks or swallows this amniotic fluid in utero, or the infant may aspirate meconium with the first breath after birth as air rushes into the lungs.

Although the etiology is not well understood, the effects of meconium can be harmful to the fetus. Meconium alters the amniotic fluid by reducing antibacterial activity and subsequently increasing the risk of perinatal bacterial infection. Additionally, meconium is very irritating because it contains enzymes from the fetal pancreas.

When aspirated into the lungs, meconium blocks the bronchioles, causing an inflammatory reaction as well as a decrease in surfactant production. Gas exchange is impaired and atelectasis occurs. A ball valve effect occurs when air is inspired into the alveoli but cannot be fully expired secondary to reduced airway diameter. Significant respiratory distress is followed by persistent pulmonary hypertension, right-to-left shunting of blood, and patent ductus arteriosus. Conventional mechanical ventilation, ECMO, nitric oxide, high-frequency ventilation, or liquid ventilation may be necessary (Geis & Clark, 2017).

Nursing Assessment

Review prenatal and birth records to identify newborns that may be at high risk for meconium aspiration. Predisposing factors for MAS include postterm pregnancy; breech presentation, forceps, or vacuum extraction births; nulliparity; ethnicity (Pacific Islander, Indigenous Australian, African American); intrapartum fever; low Apgar score; prolonged or difficult labour associated with fetal distress in a term or postterm newborn; maternal drug abuse, especially of tobacco and cocaine; maternal infection/chorioamnionitis; maternal hypertension or diabetes; oligohydramnios; fetal growth restriction; prolapsed cord; or acute or chronic placental insufficiency (Choi et al., 2015).

Assess the amniotic fluid for meconium staining when the maternal membranes rupture. Green-stained amniotic fluid suggests the presence of meconium in the amniotic fluid and should be reported immediately. After birth, note any yellowish-green staining of the umbilical cord and nails and skin. This staining indicates that meconium has been present for some time.

> **Consider Kelly, the 27-year-old woman who gave birth to a son who required resuscitation. What findings would lead the nurse to suspect that her son aspirated meconium? What risk factors in Kelly's history would support the diagnosis of meconium aspiration syndrome?**

Take Note!

Standard prevention and treatment for meconium aspiration syndrome previously included suctioning the mouth and nares upon head delivery before body delivery. However, recent evidence suggests that aspiration occurs in utero, not at delivery; therefore, the infant's birth should not be impeded for suctioning. After full delivery, the infant should be handed to a neonatal team for evaluation and treatment. Although infants previously have been given intubation and airway suctioning, routine tracheal suction is no longer recommended for depressed infants (e.g., nonvigorous with depressed tone and respirations and/or heart rate

<100 bpm) and those with respiratory symptoms. Resuscitation of the nonvigorous infant starts with initial steps of positioning, drying, stimulation, and gentle oropharyngeal suction of the mouth and nose, as required. When the heart rate is <100 bpm or the infant has ineffective respirations, positive-pressure ventilation (PPV) should be provided. The efficacy of ventilation should be assessed after 15 seconds of PPV by evaluating heart rate and chest rise.

When ventilation is ineffective, corrective steps should be instituted. The MR.SOPA mnemonic—**M**ask adjustment, **R**eposition airway, **S**uction mouth and nose, **O**pen mouth, **P**ressure increase, and **A**lternative airway—summarizes the corrective actions. If thick meconium appears to be obstructing the infant's action airway, endotracheal intubation and suction are still indicated. Endotracheal tube placement to provide PPV may also be required if initial corrective steps do not result in effective ventilation (CPS & American Heart Association, 2016).

Observe the newborn for a barrel-shaped chest with an increased anterior–posterior (AP) chest diameter (similar to that found in a client with chronic obstructive pulmonary disease), prolonged tachypnea, progression from mild to severe respiratory distress, intercostal retractions, end-expiratory grunting, and cyanosis (Geis & Clark, 2017). Auscultate the lungs, noting coarse crackles and rhonchi.

Chest x-rays show patchy, fluffy infiltrates unevenly distributed throughout the lungs and marked hyperaeration mixed with areas of atelectasis. ABG analysis will indicate metabolic acidosis with a low blood pH, decreased PaO_2, and increased $PaCO_2$ (Gardner et al., 2016). Direct visualization of the vocal cords for meconium staining using an appropriate-size laryngoscope is needed to confirm the presence of meconium below the larynx.

Nursing Management

Nursing management focuses on ensuring adequate tissue perfusion and minimizing oxygen demand and energy expenditure. Caring for the newborn with meconium aspiration begins in the birthing unit when the birth attendant identifies meconium-stained amniotic fluid with membrane rupture during labour. The nonvigorous newborn is transferred to the NICU for close monitoring.

Maintain a neutral thermal environment, including placing the newborn under a radiant warmer or in a warmed isolette, to prevent hypothermia. In addition, minimize handling to reduce energy expenditure and oxygen consumption that could lead to further hypoxemia and acidosis.

Administer oxygen therapy as ordered via nasal cannula or with positive-pressure ventilation. Monitor oxygen saturation levels via pulse oximetry to evaluate the newborn's response to treatment and to detect changes. Increased pulmonary pressures associated with meconium aspiration may cause blood to be shunted away from the lungs. The newborn may exhibit uneven pulmonary ventilation, with hyperinflation in some areas and atelectasis in others. This leads to poor perfusion and subsequent hypoxemia, which in turn may increase pulmonary vasoconstriction, resulting in a worsening of hypoxemia and acidosis.

Expect to administer hyperoxygenation to dilate the pulmonary vasculature and close the ductus arteriosus or nitric oxide inhalation to decrease pulmonary vascular resistance, or to use high-frequency oscillatory ventilation to increase the chance of air trapping (Geis & Clark, 2017). In addition, administer vasopressors and pulmonary vasodilators as prescribed and administer surfactant as ordered to counteract inactivation by meconium. Monitor ABG results for changes and assist with measures to correct acid–base imbalances to facilitate perfusion of tissues and prevent pulmonary hypertension (Cunningham et al., 2014). If these measures are ineffective, be prepared to assist with the use of ECMO, a modified type of heart–lung machine.

In addition, perform the following interventions:

- Cluster newborn care to minimize oxygen demand.
- Maintain an optimal thermal environment to minimize oxygen consumption.
- Prevent and treat any complications such as hypotension, metabolic acidosis, or anemia.
- Incorporate developmental care practices when applicable.
- Pay special attention to systemic blood volume and blood pressure to reduce right-to-left shunting through the patent ductus.
- Administer broad-spectrum antibiotics to treat bacterial pneumonia.
- Administer sedation to reduce agitation and oxygen consumption.
- Continuously monitor the newborn's condition (cardiac and respiratory status, oximetry).
- Provide continuous reassurance and support to the parents throughout the experience (Gardner et al., 2016; Verklan & Walden, 2015).

Persistent Pulmonary Hypertension of the Newborn

PPHN, previously referred to as persistent fetal circulation, is a cardiopulmonary disorder characterized by marked pulmonary hypertension that causes right-to-left extrapulmonary shunting of blood and hypoxemia. It occurs when the newborn's circulatory system does not have normal transition after birth. PPHN can occur idiopathically or as a complication of perinatal asphyxia, MAS, maternal smoking, maternal obesity, hypocalcemia, maternal asthma, pneumonia, congenital heart defects, metabolic disorders such as hypoglycemia, hypothermia, hypovolemia, hyperviscosity, acute hypoxia with delayed resuscitation, sepsis, and RDS. It occurs in 2 to 6 newborns per 1,000 live births of term, near-term, or postterm infants. Current research findings link increased risk of developing PPHN to exposure to selective serotonin reuptake inhibitors (SSRIs) (antidepressants) in late pregnancy (Huybrechts, 2015). Treatment of depression with antidepressants is complicated by the mother's needs. Careful consideration must be given to the risks, benefits, and alternatives of utero medication exposure, and this should be discussed with the woman.

Pathophysiology

Normally, pulmonary artery pressure decreases when the newborn takes the first breath. However, interference with this ability to breathe allows pulmonary pressures to remain increased. Hypoxemia and acidosis also occur, leading to vasoconstriction of the pulmonary artery. These events cause an elevation in pulmonary vascular resistance. Normally, the decrease in pulmonary artery pressure and pulmonary vascular resistance with breathing leads to the closure of the ductus arteriosus and foramen ovale. However, with PPHN pulmonary vascular resistance is elevated to the point that venous blood is diverted to some degree through fetal shunts (i.e., the ductus arteriosus and foramen ovale) into the systemic circulation, bypasses the lungs, and results in systemic arterial hypoxemia.

Nursing Assessment

Assess the newborn's status closely. A newborn with persistent pulmonary hypertension demonstrates tachypnea within 12 hours after birth. Observe for marked cyanosis, grunting, respiratory distress with tachypnea, and retractions. Auscultate the heart, noting a systolic ejection harsh sound (tricuspid insufficiency murmur), and measure blood pressure for hypotension resulting from both heart failure and persistent hypoxemia (Kenner & Lott, 2014). Measure oxygen saturation via pulse oximetry and report low values. Prepare the newborn for an echocardiogram, which will reveal right-to-left shunting of blood that confirms the diagnosis.

Nursing Management

Nursing management focuses on ensuring adequate tissue profusion and minimizing oxygen demand and energy expenditure. When caring for the newborn with persistent pulmonary hypertension, pay meticulous attention to detail, with continuous monitoring of the newborn's oxygenation and perfusion status and blood pressure. The goals of therapy include improving alveolar oxygenation, correcting the acidosis, correcting hypovolemia and hypotension with the administration of volume replacement and vasopressors, and anticipating use of ECMO when support has failed to maintain acceptable oxygenation (Kim et al., 2015).

Provide immediate resuscitation after birth and administer oxygen therapy as ordered. Early and effective resuscitation and correction of acidosis and hypoxia are helpful in preventing persistent pulmonary hypertension. Monitor arterial blood gases frequently to evaluate the effectiveness of oxygen therapy. Provide respiratory support, which frequently necessitates the use of mechanical ventilation. Administer prescribed medications, monitor cardiopulmonary status, cluster care to reduce stimulation, and provide ongoing support and education to the parents.

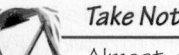

Take Note!

Almost any procedure, such as suctioning, weighing, changing diapers, or positioning, can precipitate severe hypoxemia due to the instability of the pulmonary vasculature. Therefore, minimize the newborn's exposure to stimulation as much as possible.

Periventricular–Intraventricular Hemorrhage

Periventricular–intraventricular hemorrhage (PVH–IVH) is defined as bleeding that usually originates in the subependymal germinal matrix region of the brain, often extending into the ventricular system (Annibale & Hill, 2018). IVH occurs in up to 50% of infants with birth weight less than 1,500 g and/or born at less than 35 weeks' gestation. It is uncommon in term neonates but may occur with birth trauma or asphyxia (Annibale & Hill, 2018). Complications resulting from IVH include hydrocephalus, seizure disorder, periventricular leukomalacia (an ischemic injury resulting from inadequate perfusion of the white matter adjacent to the ventricles), cerebral palsy, learning disabilities, vision or hearing deficits, and cognitive impairment (de Vries & Leijser, 2019).

Pathophysiology

The pathogenesis of PVH–IVH is attributed to the intrinsic weakness of germinal vasculature and to the fluctuation in the cerebral blood flow. Genetics appear to play a role in this condition (Szpecht, Szymankiewicz, Seremak-Mrozikiewicz, & Gadzinowski, 2015). The preterm newborn is at greatest risk for IVH because cerebral vascular development is immature, making it more vulnerable to injury. The earlier the newborn is, the greater the likelihood for brain damage. While all areas of the brain can be injured, the periventricular area is the most vulnerable (Gardner et al., 2016).

Each ventricular area contains a rich network of capillaries that are very thin, fragile, and easily ruptured. The causes of rupture vary and include fluctuations in systemic and cerebral blood flow, increases in cerebral blood flow from hypertension, IV infusions, seizure activity, increases in cerebral venous pressure due to vaginal delivery, hypoxia, and respiratory distress. With a preterm birth, the fetus is suddenly transported from a well-controlled uterine environment into a highly stimulating one. This tremendous physiologic stress and shock may contribute to the rupture of periventricular capillaries and subsequent hemorrhage. Most hemorrhages occur in the first 72 hours after birth (Annibale & Hill, 2018).

Nursing Assessment

The signs of intraventricular hemorrhage vary significantly, and some infants may display no clinical signs. Approximately 50% of PVH–IVH occurs by 24 hours of age, and 90% by 72 hours of age (Noori & Seri, 2015). Assess for risk factors such as:

- Preterm birth
- Low birth weight
- Acidosis
- Asphyxia
- Unstable blood pressure
- Seizures
- Acute blood loss or hypovolemia
- Respiratory distress with mechanical ventilation, intubation, apnea, hypoxia, or suctioning
- Use of hyperosmolar solutions or rapid volume expansion

Evaluate the newborn for an unexplained drop in hematocrit, pallor, and poor perfusion as evidenced by respiratory distress and oxygen desaturation. Note seizures, lethargy or other changes in level of consciousness, bulging fontanel, weak sucking, metabolic acidosis, high-pitched cry, or hypotonia. Palpate the anterior fontanel for tenseness. Assess vital signs, noting bradycardia and hypotension. Evaluate laboratory data for changes indicating metabolic acidosis or glucose instability. Frequently a bleed can progress rapidly and result in shock and death. Prepare the newborn for cranial ultrasonography, the diagnostic tool of choice to detect hemorrhage (Verklan & Walden, 2015).

Nursing Management

Prevention of preterm birth is essential in preventing IVH. Identify risk factors that can lead to hemorrhage, and focus care on interventions to decrease the risk of hemorrhage. For example, institute measures to prevent perinatal asphyxia and birth trauma and provide developmental care in the NICU. If a preterm birth is expected, having the mother deliver at a tertiary care facility with a NICU would be most appropriate.

Care of the newborn with IVH is primarily supportive. Correct anemia, acidosis, and hypotension with fluids and medications. Administer fluids slowly to prevent fluctuations in blood pressure. Avoid rapid volume expansion to minimize changes in cerebral blood flow. Keep the newborn in a flexed, contained position with the head elevated to prevent or minimize fluctuations in intracranial pressure. Continuously monitor the newborn for signs of hemorrhage, such as changes in the level of consciousness, bulging fontanel, seizures, apnea, and reduced activity level. Also, measuring head circumference daily to assess for expansion in size is essential in identifying complications early.

Minimize handling of the newborn by clustering nursing care, and limit stimulation in the newborn's environment to reduce stress. Also reduce the newborn's exposure to noxious stimuli to avoid a fluctuation in blood pressure and energy expenditure. Provide adequate oxygenation to promote tissue perfusion but controlled ventilation to decrease the risk of pneumothorax. Developmental care principles include avoiding lifting the lower extremities above the midline with diaper changes, giving rapid fluid boluses, and high oxygen and ventilation, as these can increase the chance of more cranial hemorrhage (Green, 2016).

Support for the parents to cope with the diagnosis and potential long-term sequelae is essential. The long-term neurodevelopmental outcome is determined by the severity of the bleed. Provide education and emotional support for the parents throughout the newborn's stay. Discuss expectations for short- and long-term care needs with the parents and assist them in obtaining the necessary support from appropriate community resources and Neonatal Follow-Up Clinic (Gardner et al., 2016).

Necrotizing Enterocolitis

NEC is an inflammatory disease of the bowel which can cause ischemic and necrotic injury in the gastrointestinal tract. It is the most common and most serious acquired gastrointestinal disorder among hospitalized preterm neonates and is associated with significant acute and chronic morbidity and mortality. NEC occurs in approximately 10% of infants who weigh less than 1,500 g, with mortality rates up to 50% (Johnson, Patel, Bigger, Engstrom, & Meier, 2015). Attempts to improve gastrointestinal function and reduce the risk of NEC include enteral antibiotics, judicious administration of parenteral fluids, monitoring tolerance of enteral feedings, oral immune therapy, human milk feedings, antenatal corticosteroids, enteral probiotics (*Lactobacillus acidophilus*), and slow continuous drip feedings (Springer & Annibale, 2017).

Pathophysiology

The pathophysiology of NEC is not clearly understood and is thought to be multifactorial in nature. Current research points to three major pathologic mechanisms that lead to NEC: bowel hypoxic ischemia events, perinatal stressors, an immature intestinal barrier, abnormal bacterial colonization, and formula feeding. The intestine of a preterm infant is characterized by underdeveloped immune defences and compromised mucosal barrier function. As a result, the immune intestine is susceptible to bacterial colonization by opportunistic pathogens, which follows oral feeding, which in turn incites an inflammatory response (Lim, Golden, & Ford, 2015).

During peri- or postnatal stress, oxygen is shunted away from the gut to more important organs such as the heart and brain. Ischemia and intestinal wall damage occur, allowing bacteria to invade. High-solute feedings allow bacteria to flourish. Mucosal or transmucosal necrosis of part of the intestine occurs. Although any region of the bowel can be affected, the distal ileum and proximal colon are the regions most commonly involved. NEC usually occurs between 3 and 12 days of life, but it can occur weeks later in some newborns (Springer & Annibale, 2017). See thePoint for links to websites that provide additional information.

Nursing Assessment

NEC can be devastating, and astute assessment is crucial. Assessing the newborn for the development of NEC includes the health history and physical examination as well as laboratory and diagnostic testing. The onset of NEC is heralded by the development of feeding intolerance, abdominal distention, and bloody stools in a preterm infant receiving enteral feedings. As the disease worsens, the infant develops signs and symptoms of septic shock (respiratory distress, temperature instability, lethargy, hypotension, and oliguria). Nurses need to be suspicious of this condition in caring for this preterm infant.

HEALTH HISTORY AND PHYSICAL EXAMINATION

Assess the newborn's history for risk factors associated with NEC. In addition to preterm birth, pre- and postnatal predisposing risk factors are highlighted in Box 24.1.

Also observe the newborn for common signs and symptoms, which may include:

- Cardiorespiratory baseline changes
- Feeding intolerance, bilious aspirates, vomiting
- Abdominal distention and tenderness, visible bowel loops, abdominal discolouration
- Bloody or hemoccult-positive stools
- Diarrhea
- Respiratory distress
- Metabolic acidosis
- Temperature instability
- Decreased or absent bowel sounds
- Signs of sepsis
- Lethargy
- Apnea, bradycardia, deceased oxygen saturations
- Hypoglycemia
- Shock (Fox, Thacker, & Hendricks-Muñoz, 2015)

Always keep the possibility of NEC in mind when dealing with preterm newborns, especially when enteral

---

BOX 24.1

PREDISPOSING FACTORS FOR THE DEVELOPMENT OF NECROTIZING ENTEROCOLITIS

Prenatal Factors
- Preterm labour
- Prolonged rupture of membranes
- Preeclampsia
- Maternal sepsis
- Amnionitis
- Uterine hypoxia

Postnatal Factors
- Respiratory distress syndrome
- Patent ductus arteriosus
- Congenital heart disease
- Exchange transfusion
- Low birth weight
- Low Apgar scores
- Umbilical catheterization
- Hypothermia
- Gastrointestinal infection
- Hypoglycemia
- Asphyxia

---

feedings are being administered. Note respiratory distress, cyanosis, lethargy, decreased activity level, temperature instability, feeding intolerance, diarrhea, bile-stained emesis, or grossly bloody stools. Assess blood pressure, noting hypotension. Evaluate the neonate's abdomen for distention, tenderness, and visible loops of bowel. Measure the abdominal circumference, noting an increase. Determine residual gastric volume prior to feeding; when it is elevated, be suspicious for NEC (Verklan & Walden, 2015).

LABORATORY AND DIAGNOSTIC TESTING

Common laboratory and diagnostic tests ordered for assessment of NEC include:

- Kidney, ureter, and bladder (KUB) of the abdomen x-ray: confirms the presence of pneumatosis intestinalis (air in the bowel wall) and persistently dilated loops of bowel
- An abdominal x-ray to demonstrate dilated bowel loops, abnormal gas patterns, air bubbles that occur from bacteria, and thickened bowel walls
- Blood values: may demonstrate metabolic acidosis, increased white blood cells, thrombocytopenia, neutropenia, electrolyte imbalance, or disseminated intravascular coagulation (DIC) (Springer & Annibale, 2017)

Nursing Management

Nursing management of the newborn with NEC focuses on maintaining fluid and nutritional status, providing supportive care, and teaching the family about the condition and prognosis. Therapeutic management initially consists of bowel rest and antibiotic therapy. Serial KUB x-rays and C-reactive protein levels are used to assess the resolution or progression of NEC. If medical treatment fails to stabilize the newborn or if free air is present on a left lateral decubitus film (where the infant is lying down on the left side), surgical intervention will be necessary to resect the portion of necrotic bowel while preserving as much of the intestinal length as possible. Surgery for NEC usually requires the placement of a proximal enterostomy until the anastomosis site is ready for reconnection. After surgery, post-op supportive care includes fluids, TPN, antibiotics, and bowel rest for 10 to 14 days.

MAINTAINING FLUID AND NUTRITIONAL STATUS

If NEC is suspected, immediately stop enteral feedings until a diagnosis is made. Administer IV fluids initially to restore proper fluid balance. If ordered, administer total parenteral nutrition (TPN) to keep the newborn supported nutritionally. Give prescribed IV antibiotics to prevent sepsis from the necrotic bowel (if surgery is required, antibiotics may be needed for an extended period of time). Institute gastric decompression as ordered with an orogastric tube attached to low intermittent suction. Carefully monitor intake and output. Restart enteral feedings once the disease has resolved (normal abdominal examination and KUB negative for pneumatosis) or as determined postoperatively by the surgeon.

PROVIDING SUPPORTIVE CARE

Manage pain by administering analgesics as ordered. Infection control is important, with an emphasis on careful handwashing. In addition, implement these interventions in an ongoing manner:

- Check stools for evidence of blood and report any positive findings.
- Measure the abdominal girth.
- Monitor blood pressure for hypotension.
- Palpate the abdomen for tenderness and rigidity.
- Auscultate for normal bowel sounds in all four quadrants.
- Monitor blood gases and oxygen saturation.
- Observe the abdomen for redness or shininess, which indicates peritonitis.
- Monitor feeding tolerance.
- Offer emotional support for parents/partners/significant others.

EDUCATING THE FAMILY

The diagnosis of NEC may cause significant family anxiety. Listen to the family's worries and fears. Answer their questions honestly. Inform the family that medically treated NEC is usually limited to a short period and resolves within 48 hours of stopping oral feedings, but

surgically treated NEC can be a much lengthier process. The amount of bowel that has necrosed, as determined during the bowel resection, significantly increases the likelihood of long-term medical problems. Short bowel syndrome may result from a large resection (short bowel syndrome is discussed in Chapter 42). Reassure the family that although some infants have more involved cases of NEC, the improved parenteral nutrition formulations have improved the outcomes for these infants. Provide education about ostomy care if surgery is required (refer to Chapter 42 for a discussion of ostomy care). Promote interaction with their newborn. Nursing actions of active engagement with parents and the sick infant (providing NICU orientation and physical care), providing cautious guidance (offering information and instruction on infant care), and their subtle presence (overseeing parent's interaction with their infant) all contribute to fostering a positive, trusting relationship with parents (Nagtalon-Ramos, 2014; Verklan & Walden, 2015).

Infants of Diabetic Mothers

An **infant of a diabetic mother** (IDM) is one born to a woman with pregestational or gestational diabetes (see Chapter 20 for additional information). The newborn of a diabetic woman is at high risk for numerous health-related complications, especially hypoglycemia. Gestational diabetes mellitus (GDM) from all causes of diabetes is the most common medical complication of pregnancy and is increasing in incidence, particularly as type 2 diabetes continues to increase worldwide. Despite advances in perinatal care, IDMs remain at risk for a multitude of physiologic, metabolic, and congenital complications such as preterm birth, macrosomia, asphyxia, respiratory distress, hypoglycemia, hypocalcemia, hyperbilirubinemia, polycythemia and hyperviscosity, hypertrophic cardiomyopathy, and congenital anomalies, particularly of the central nervous system. Overt type 1 diabetes around conception produces marked risk of NTDs, cardiac defects, and caudal regression syndrome; later in gestation, severe and unstable type 1 maternal diabetes carries a higher risk of intrauterine growth restriction, asphyxia, and fetal death. IDMs born to mothers with type 2 diabetes are more commonly obese (macrosomic) with milder conditions of the common problems found in IDMs. IDMs from all causes of GDM also are predisposed to later-life risk of obesity, diabetes, and cardiovascular disease (Mattson & Smith, 2015).

Impact of Diabetes on the Newborn

For more than a century, it has been known that diabetes during pregnancy can have severe adverse effects on fetal and newborn outcomes. Infants of diabetic mothers have increased morbidity and mortality in the perinatal period. The incidence of major congenital anomalies is much greater for these newborns than for other newborns (Potter & Kicklighter, 2016). Poor glycemic control in the first trimester, during organogenesis, is thought to be a major reason for congenital malformations. The most common types of malformations in infants of diabetic mothers involve the cardiovascular, skeletal, central nervous, gastrointestinal, and genitourinary systems. Cardiac anomalies are the most common (Gardner et al., 2016).

Infants of diabetic mothers can be large for gestational age (LGA) or small for gestational age (SGA), depending on the vascular impact of this chronic systemic disease on the mother prior to and during the pregnancy. Fetal macrosomia occurs in 25% to 42% of diabetic pregnancies because of hyperinsulinemia (Gardner et al., 2016). LGA infants (>90th percentile on growth chart) are longer and weigh more than 4,000 g with the majority of the excess weight composed of fat. They also have increased organ weights (organomegaly) and excessive fat deposits on their shoulders and trunk, contributing to the increased overall body weight and predisposing them to shoulder dystocia, brachial plexus injury, fracture, neonatal depression, or caesarean birth. These oversized newborns frequently require caesarean births for cephalopelvic disproportion and dysfunctional labour patterns. They are frequently hypoglycemic in the first few hours after birth (Korkmazer, Solak, & Tokgöz, 2015).

SGA infants (<10th percentile on growth chart) of diabetic mothers usually suffer from intrauterine malnutrition and have few glucose reserves to tolerate the rigours of labour and birth. Uteroplacental circulation is often impaired, leading to poor growth patterns and hypoxemia.

Despite their increased or decreased size and weight, they may be remarkably frail, showing behaviours similar to those of a preterm newborn. Thus, birth weight may not be a reliable criterion of maturity. Newborns of women with diabetes but without vascular complications often tend to be LGA, whereas those of women with diabetes and vascular disease are usually SGA (Green, 2016).

Pathophysiology

The large size of the IDM arises secondary to exposure to high levels of maternal glucose crossing the placenta into the fetal circulation. Maternal hyperglycemia acts as a fuel to stimulate increased production of fetal insulin, which in turn promotes somatic growth within the fetus. The fetus responds to these high levels by producing more insulin, which acts as a growth factor in the fetus (Kliegman et al., 2015). How the fetus will be affected and the problems that the newborn experiences depend on the severity, duration, and control of the diabetes in the mother during the pregnancy. Table 24.1 summarizes the common problems that may occur in infants of diabetic mothers.

Nursing Assessment

Assessment begins in the prenatal period by identifying women with diabetes and taking measures to control

TABLE 24.1	COMMON PROBLEMS OF INFANTS OF DIABETIC MOTHERS	
Condition	**Description**	**Effects**
Macrosomia	Newborn with an excessive birth weight; arbitrarily defined as a birth weight >4,000 g (8 lb 8 oz) to 4,500 g (9 lb 9 oz) or >90% for gestational age Complication in 10% of all pregnancies in the United States	• Increased risk for shoulder dystocia, traumatic birth injury, birth asphyxia • Risks for newborn hypoglycemia and hypomagnesemia, polycythemia, and electrolyte disturbances • Increased maternal risk for surgical birth, postpartum hemorrhage and infection, and birth canal lacerations • Increased risk of developing type 2 diabetes later in life for both • Higher weight and accumulation of fat in childhood and a higher rate of obesity in adults
Respiratory distress syndrome (RDS)	Cortisol-induced stimulation of lecithin/sphingomyelin (phospholipids) necessary for lung maturation is antagonized due to the high insulin environment within the fetus due to mother's hyperglycemia Less mature lung development than expected for gestational age Decrease in the phospholipid phosphatidylglycerol (PG), which stabilizes surfactant, compounding risk	• Most commonly, breathing normally at birth but developing laboured, grunting respiration with cough and a hoarse complaining cry within a few hours with chest retractions and varying degrees of cyanosis • IDMs with vascular disease seldom develop RDS because the chronic stress of poor intrauterine perfusion leads to increased production of steroids, which accelerates lung maturation

TABLE 24.1	**COMMON PROBLEMS OF INFANTS OF DIABETIC MOTHERS** (continued)	
Condition	**Description**	**Effects**
Hypoglycemia	Glucose is the major source of energy for organ function Typical characteristics: • Poor feedings • Jitteriness • Lethargy • High-pitched or weak cry • Apnea • Cyanosis and seizures Some newborns are asymptomatic	Low blood glucose levels are problematic during early postbirth period due to abrupt cessation of high-glucose maternal blood supply and the continuation of insulin production by the newborn Limited ability to release glucagon and catecholamines, which normally stimulate glucagon breakdown and glucose release Prolonged and untreated hypoglycemia leads to serious, long-term adverse neurologic sequelae such as learning disabilities and mental retardation
Hypocalcemia and hypomagnesemia	Hypocalcemia (drop in calcium levels) is manifested by tremors, hypotonia, apnea, high-pitched cry, and seizures due to abrupt cessation of maternal transfer of calcium to the fetus, primarily in the third trimester and experiencing birth asphyxia Associated hypomagnesemia is directly related to the maternal level before birth About half of IDMs affected	Newborn is at risk for a prolonged delay in parathyroid hormone production and cardiac dysrhythmias
Polycythemia	Venous hematocrit of >65% in the newborn Increased oxygen consumption by IDM secondary to fetal hyperglycemia and hyperinsulinemia Increased fetal erythropoiesis secondary to intrauterine hypoxia due to placental insufficiency from maternal diabetes Hypoxic stimulation of increased red blood cell (RBC) production as compensatory mechanism	Increased viscosity, resulting in poor blood flow predisposing newborn to decreased tissue oxygenation and development of microthrombi
Hyperbilirubinemia	Usually seen within the first few days after birth, manifested by a yellow appearance of the sclera and skin Excessive red cell hemolysis necessary to break down increased RBCs in circulation due to polycythemia Resultant elevated bilirubin levels Excessive bruising secondary to birth trauma of macrosomic infants, further adding to high bilirubin levels	If untreated, high levels of unconjugated bilirubin may lead to kernicterus (neurologic syndrome that results in irreversible damage) with long-term sequelae that include cerebral palsy, sensorineural hearing loss, and mental retardation
Congenital anomalies	Occur in up to 10% of infants of diabetic mothers, accounting for 30–50% of perinatal deaths Incidence is greatest among small-for-gestational-age newborns Overall, infants of diabetic mothers have three times the usual incidence of congenital anomalies compared to newborns from the nondiabetic general population	Most common anomalies: • Coarctation of the aorta • Atrial and ventricular septal defects • Transposition of the great vessels • Sacral agenesis • Hip and joint malformations • Anencephaly • Spina bifida • Caudal dysplasia • Hydrocephalus

Adapted from Green, C. J. (2016). *Maternal newborn nursing care plans* (3rd ed.). Burlington, MA: Jones & Bartlett Learning; Gardner, S. L., Carter, B. S., Enzman-Hines, M., & Hernandez, J. A. (2016). *Merenstein & Gardner's handbook of neonatal intensive care* (8th ed.). St. Louis, MO: Mosby Elsevier; and Verklan, M. T., & Walden, M. (2015). *Core curriculum for neonatal intensive care nursing* (5th ed.). St. Louis, MO: Saunders.

Wide shoulders

Rosy cheeks

Poor feeding

Distended abdomen

Excessive subcutaneous fat on extremities

FIGURE 24.5 Characteristics of an infant of a diabetic mother. A macrosomic infant of a diabetic mother (IDM) has head circumference and length that are at the 90th percentile; the IDM's body weight greatly exceeds the 90th percentile. The IDM has considerable fat deposition in the shoulder and intrascapular area. (McDonald, M. G., & Seshia, M. M. K. (2016). *Avery's neonatology: Pathophysiology & management of the newborn* (7th ed.). Philadelphia, PA: Wolters Kluwer.)

maternal glucose levels (see Chapter 20 for information on management of the pregnant client with diabetes).

PHYSICAL EXAMINATION

At birth, inspect the newborn for the following characteristic features. See also Figure 24.5.

- Full rosy cheeks with a ruddy skin colour
- Short neck (some describe "no-neck" appearance)
- Buffalo hump over the nape of the neck
- Massive shoulders with a full intrascapular area
- Distended upper abdomen due to organ overgrowth
- Excessive subcutaneous fat tissue, producing fat extremities

Be alert for hypoglycemia, which may occur immediately after birth or within an hour. Assess blood glucose levels, which should remain equal or above 2.6 mmol/L. Closely assess the newborn for signs of hypoglycemia, including listlessness, hypotonia, apathy, poor feeding, apneic episodes with a drop in oxygen saturation, cyanosis, temperature instability, pallor and sweating, tremors, irritability, and seizures.

Assess the newborn for signs of birth trauma involving the head (tense, bulging fontanels, cephalohematoma, skull fractures, and facial nerve paralysis), shoulders and extremities (posturing, paralysis), and skin (bruising). Inspect the newborn for compromised oxygenation by examining the skin for cyanosis, pallor, mottling, and sluggish capillary refill. Take the newborn's temperature frequently and provide a neutral thermal environment to prevent cold stress, which would increase the glucose utilization and contribute to the hypoglycemic state.

LABORATORY AND DIAGNOSTIC TESTING

Determine baseline serum calcium, magnesium, and bilirubin levels and monitor them frequently for changes (Table 24.2). Hypocalcemia is typically manifested in the first 2 to 3 days of life as a result of birth injury or a prolonged delay in parathyroid hormone production. Hypomagnesemia parallels calcium levels and is suspected only when hypocalcemia does not respond to calcium replacement therapy. Red blood cell (RBC) breakdown leads to increased hematocrit and polycythemia. In addition, hyperbilirubinemia may be caused by slightly decreased extracellular fluid volume, hepatic immaturity, and birth trauma forming enclosed hemorrhages. It can appear within the first 24 hours of life (pathologic) or after 24 hours of life (physiologic).

Nursing Management

The focus of care for these infants is early detection and initiation of therapy to address potential problems (Nursing Care Plan 24.1, at the end of the chapter). Perform a head-to-toe physical assessment to identify congenital anomalies. Institute measures to

TABLE 24.2	CRITICAL LABORATORY VALUES FOR INFANTS OF DIABETIC MOTHERS
Hypoglycemia	<40 mg/dL (2.6 mmol/L)
Hypocalcemia	<7 mg/dL
Hypomagnesemia	<1.5 mg/dL
Hyperbilirubinemia	>12 mg/dL (term infant)
Polycythemia	>65% (venous hematocrit)

Adapted from Fanaroff, A. A., & Fanaroff, J. M. (2014). *Klaus and Fanaroff's care of the high-risk neonate* (6th ed.). Philadelphia, PA: Elsevier Health Sciences; Kenner, C., & Lott, J. W. (2014). *Comprehensive neonatal nursing care* (5th ed.). New York: Springer Publishers; and Malcolm, W. (2015). *Beyond the NICU: Comprehensive care of the high risk infant.* New York: McGraw-Hill Education.

correct hypoglycemia, hypocalcemia, hypomagnesemia, dehydration, and jaundice. Provide oxygenation and ventilatory support as necessary. The focus of care includes correcting hypoglycemia and hypocalcemia, providing phototherapy for jaundice, administering fluid therapy, and maintaining oxygen and ventilation if needed.

PREVENTING HYPOGLYCEMIA

Prevent hypoglycemia by providing early oral feedings with breast milk or formula at frequent intervals (every 2 to 3 hours). Feedings help to control glucose levels, reduce hematocrit, and promote bilurubin excretion. Maintain a neutral thermal environment to avoid cold stress, which may stimulate the metabolic rate, thereby increasing the demand for glucose. Provide rest periods to decrease energy demand and expenditure.

Monitor blood glucose levels via heel stick at 2 hours of life and then every 3 to 6 hours before feeding according to CPS algorithm. Go to thePoint for the CPS newborn hypoglycemia screening guidelines. Document the results. Report unstable glucose values if oral feedings do not maintain and stabilize the newborn's blood glucose levels. If glucose levels are not stabilized, initiate IV glucose infusions as ordered and monitor that the infusions are flowing at the prescribed rate.

MAINTAINING FLUID AND ELECTROLYTE BALANCE

Monitor serum calcium levels for changes indicating the need for supplementation, such as with oral or IV calcium gluconate. Assess the newborn for signs of hypocalcemia, such as tremors, jitteriness, twitching, seizures, and high-pitched cry.

Also administer fluid therapy as ordered to maintain adequate hydration. Monitor serum bilirubin levels and institute phototherapy if the newborn is over 24 hours old.

PROVIDING PARENTAL SUPPORT

Good communication between the nurse and the family is essential. It should be supported by evidence-based, written information tailored to meet the woman's individual needs. Assist the parents and family in understanding the newborn's condition and need for frequent monitoring. Offer support and information to the parents and family about the benefits of breastfeeding for herself and the infant. They may erroneously interpret the newborn's large size as an indication that the newborn is free of problems. Encourage open communication and listen with empathy to the family's fears and concerns. Provide frequent opportunities for the parents to interact with their newborn. Make appropriate referrals to social services and community resources as necessary to help the family cope.

Birth Trauma

Injuries to the newborn from the forces of labour and birth are categorized as birth trauma. In the past, numerous injuries were associated with difficult births requiring external or internal version or mid or high forceps deliveries. Today, however, caesarean births have contributed to the decline in birth trauma. Damage occurs to the tissues and organs of the newborn caused by mechanical forces during childbirth often accompanied by impaired blood circulation and organ functioning. The most frequent and significant birth injuries are to the skull, brain, and spinal cord (Malcolm, 2015).

Significant birth trauma accounts for fewer than 3% of neonatal deaths and stillbirths in the United States (Loroia, 2015). They estimate that birth trauma in the United States occurs in approximately 29 per 1,000 births with the three most frequently diagnosed birth trauma conditions being injuries to the scalp, injuries to the skeleton, and fracture of the clavicle (Gardner et al., 2016). Improved prenatal diagnosis and monitoring during labour have helped to reduce the incidence of birth injuries today.

Pathophysiology

The process of birth is a blend of compression, contractions, torques, and traction. When fetal size, presentation, or neurologic immunity complicates this process, the forces of labour and birth may lead to tissue damage, edema, hemorrhages, or fractures in the newborn. For example, birth trauma may result from the pressure of birth, especially in a prolonged or abrupt labour, abnormal or difficult presentation, cephalopelvic disproportion, or mechanical forces, such as forceps or vacuum used during delivery. Table 24.3 summarizes the most common types of birth trauma.

Nursing Assessment

Recognition of trauma and birth injuries is imperative so that early treatment can be initiated. Review the labour and birth history for risk factors, such as a prolonged or abrupt labour, abnormal or difficult presentation, cephalopelvic disproportion, or mechanical forces, such as forceps or vacuum used during delivery. Also review the history for multiple fetus deliveries, large-for-date infants, extreme prematurity, large fetal head, or newborns with congenital anomalies.

Complete a careful physical and neurologic assessment of every newborn admitted to the nursery to establish whether injuries exist. Inspect the head for lumps, bumps, or bruises. Note if swelling or bruising crosses the suture line. Assess the eyes and face for facial paralysis, observing for asymmetry of the face with crying or appearance of the mouth being drawn

(text continues on page 922)

TABLE 24.3	COMMON TYPES OF BIRTH TRAUMA		
Type	**Description**	**Findings**	**Treatment**
Fractures	Most often occur during breech births or shoulder dystocia in newborns with macrosomia Midclavicular fractures are the most common type of fracture, secondary to shoulder dystocia Long bone fractures of the humerus or femur, usually midshaft, also can occur	Midclavicular fractures: The newborn is irritable and does not move the arm on the affected side either spontaneously or when the Moro reflex is elicited Femoral or humeral long bone fractures: The newborn shows loss of spontaneous leg or arm motion, respectively; usually swelling and pain accompany the limited movement X-rays confirm the fracture	Midclavicular fractures typically heal rapidly and uneventfully; arm motion may be limited by pinning the newborn's sleeve to the shirt Femoral and humeral shaft fractures are treated with splinting. Healing and complete recovery are expected within 2–4 wks without incident Explanation to the parents and reassurance are needed
Brachial plexus injury	Primarily in large babies, babies with shoulder dystocia, or breech delivery Results from stretching, hemorrhage within a nerve, or tearing of the nerve or the roots associated with cervical cord injury Associated traumatic injuries include fracture of the clavicle or humerus or subluxations of the shoulder or cervical spine Erb palsy is an upper brachial plexus injury Klumpke palsy is an injury to the lower brachial plexus (lower brachial injuries are less common)	In Erb palsy, the involved extremity usually presents adducted, prone, and internally rotated; shoulder movement is absent; Moro, bicep, and radial reflexes are absent, but the grasp reflex is usually present Klumpke palsy is manifested by weakness in the hand and wrist; grasp reflex is absent	Erb palsy usually involves immobilization of the upper arm across the upper abdomen/chest to protect the shoulder from excessive motion for the first week; then gentle passive range-of-motion exercises are performed daily to prevent contractures. There is usually no associated sensory loss, and this condition usually improves rapidly Treatment for Klumpke palsy involves placing the hand in a neutral position and using passive range-of-motion exercises In some cases deficits may persist, requiring continuing observation
Cranial nerve trauma	Most common is facial nerve palsy Frequently attributed to pressure resulting from forceps May also result from pressure on the nerve in utero, related to fetal positioning such as the head lying against the shoulder	Physical findings include asymmetry of the face when crying; mouth may be drawn toward the unaffected side; wrinkles are deeper on the unaffected side The paralyzed side may be smooth, with a swollen appearance. Eye is persistently open on the affected side	Most infants begin to recover in the first week, but full resolution may take up to several months; parents need reassurance about this In most cases, treatment is not necessary, only observation If the eye is affected and unable to close, protection with patches and synthetic tears may be necessary Parents need instruction about how to feed the newborn, since he or she cannot close the lips around the nipple without having milk seep out

TABLE 24.3	COMMON TYPES OF BIRTH TRAUMA (continued)		

Type	Description	Findings	Treatment
Head trauma	Mild trauma can cause soft tissue injuries such as cephalohematoma and caput succedaneum; greater trauma can cause depressed skull fractures **Cephalohematoma** (subperiosteal collection of blood secondary to the rupture of blood vessels between the skull and periosteum) occurs in 2.5% of all births and typically appears within hours after birth **Caput succedaneum** (soft tissue swelling) is caused by edema of the head against the dilating cervix during the birth process Subarachnoid hemorrhage (one of the most common types of intracranial trauma) may be due to hypoxia/ischemia, variations in blood pressure, and the pressure exerted on the head during labour. Bleeding is of venous origin, and underlying contusions also may occur Subdural hemorrhage (hematomas) occurs less often today because of improved obstetric techniques. Typically, tears of the major veins or venous sinuses overlying the cerebral hemispheres or cerebellum (most common in newborns of a primipara and large newborns, or after an instrumented birth) are the cause. Increased pressure on the blood vessels inside the skull leads to tears Depressed skull fractures (rare) may result from the pressure of a forceps delivery; can also occur during spontaneous or caesarean births and may be associated with other head trauma causing subdural bleeding, subarachnoid hemorrhage, or brain trauma	In cephalohematoma, suture lines delineate its extent; usually located on one side, over the parietal bone In caput succedaneum, swelling is not limited by suture lines: It extends across the midline and is associated with head moulding. It does not usually cause complications other than a misshapen head. Swelling is maximal at birth and then rapidly decreases in size In subarachnoid hemorrhage, some RBCs may appear in the CSF of full-term newborns. Newborns may present with apnea, seizures, lethargy, or abnormal findings on a neurologic examination Subdural hemorrhage can be asymptomatic, or the neonate can exhibit seizures, enlarging head size, decreased level of consciousness, or abnormal findings on a neurologic examination, with hypotonia, a poor Moro reflex, or extensive retinal hemorrhages Depressed skull fractures can be observed and palpated as depressions. Confirmation by x-ray is necessary	Cephalohematoma resolves gradually over 2–3 wks without treatment Caput succedaneum usually resolves over the first few days without treatment Subarachnoid hemorrhage requires minimal handling to reduce stress Subdural hematoma requires aspiration; can be life threatening if it is in an inaccessible location and cannot be aspirated Depressed skull fractures typically require a neurosurgical consultation

Adapted from Cunningham, F. G., Leveno, K. J., Bloom, S. L., Spong, C.Y., Dashe, J. S., Hoffman, B. L., . . . Sheffield, J. S. (2014). *Williams obstetrics* (24th ed.). New York: McGraw-Hill; Gardner, S. L., Carter, B. S., Enzman-Hines, M., & Hernandez, J. A. (2016). *Merenstein & Gardner's handbook of neonatal intensive care* (8th ed.). St. Louis, MO: Mosby Elsevier; and Loroia, N. (2015). Birth trauma. *eMedicine.* Retrieved from http://emedicine.medscape.com/article/980112-overview

to the unaffected side. Ensure that the newborn spontaneously moves all extremities. Note any absence of or decrease in deep tendon reflexes or abnormal positioning of extremities.

Assess and document symmetry of structure and function. Be prepared to assist with scheduling diagnostic studies to confirm trauma or injuries, which will be important in determining treatment modalities.

Nursing Management

Nursing management is primarily supportive and focuses on assessing for resolution of the trauma or any associated complications along with providing support and education to the parents. Provide the parents with explanations and reassurance that these injuries usually resolve with minimal or no treatment. Parents are alarmed when their newborn is unable to move an extremity or demonstrates asymmetric facial movements. Provide parents with a realistic picture of the situation to gain their understanding and trust. Be readily available to answer questions and teach them how to care for the newborn, including any modifications that might be necessary. Allow parents adequate time to understand the implications of the birth trauma or injury and what treatment modalities are needed, if any. Provide them with information about the length of time until the injury will resolve and when and if they need to seek further medical attention for the condition. Spending time with the parents and providing them with support, information, and teaching are important to allow them to make decisions and care for their newborn. Anticipate the need for community referral for ongoing follow-up and care, if necessary.

Newborns Exposed to Perinatal Substance Abuse

It is generally assumed that all parents want to provide a healthy environment for their unborn child and know how to avoid harm. However, pregnant individuals who use tobacco, alcohol, or illicit substances during pregnancy place themselves and their newborns at risk for numerous complications. Perinatal substance abuse is a persistent and significant public health issue, particularly affecting children, with high rates of reported abuse, neglect, and foster care placement. Substance use during pregnancy exposes the fetus to the possibility of fetal growth restriction, prematurity, neurobehavioural and neurophysiologic dysfunction, birth defects, infections, and long-term developmental sequelae (Wang, 2014). Infants exposed to perinatal substance abuse are more likely to suffer substantiated harm, enter foster care, and have more negative child protection outcomes. The effects of fetal alcohol syndrome (FAS) and spectrum disorders are well documented in the literature; studies attest to developmental delays, intellectual disabilities, attention disorders, and psychopathologies during the child's lifetime (Wang, 2014).

The full extent of the effects of prenatal drug exposure on a child is not known. However, studies show that various drugs of abuse may result in premature birth, miscarriage, low birth weight, and a variety of behavioural and cognitive problems.

It is difficult to establish the true prevalence of substance use in pregnancy; many people will deny taking any nonprescribed substance because of the associated social stigma and legal implications. The National Institute on Drug Abuse (NIDA) suggests that over 5% of pregnant individuals use alcohol or illicit drugs, thus exposing their fetuses to their effects (NIDA, 2018). Drug exposure may go unrecognized in these newborns, and they may be discharged from the newborn nursery at

Consider This

I admit, I had led a reckless life since I was a teen. I rebelled against my mother's authority and started smoking and doing drugs just to "check out" of my painful world. It was one big blast after another with a high and then a low. I never considered the consequences of my behaviour then and never thought it would hurt anyone until I learned I was about 4 months' pregnant. I convinced myself that if I cut back, everything would be fine.

Now, as I stand here in the NICU watching my tiny son struggle for air and tremble all over, I am not so convinced that I didn't hurt anyone except myself. As I witness my son fight against MY nicotine and drug addiction, my heart is heavy with guilt. I wonder how I could have thought that my troubles wouldn't become another's plight sooner or later. What must I have been thinking to isolate my addiction and not consider the impact that it would have on my mother and my son?

Thoughts: *This woman honestly regrets what her addiction has done to her son as she stands watching him go through withdrawal. Her lifestyle choices do affect others, despite her previous denial. One problem with addiction is the difficulty in getting help after deciding to finally quit. There are not enough rehab centres to deal with the large numbers needing their services and it can be difficult to get into one. What can be offered to pregnant women who abuse substances? How can nurses increase community awareness about the impact of this problem, especially during pregnancy?*

risk for medical and social problems, including abuse and neglect.

Tobacco, alcohol, and marijuana are the substances most commonly abused during pregnancy. Other drugs may include opioids such as morphine, codeine, methadone, meperidine, and heroin; CNS stimulants such as amphetamines and cocaine; CNS depressants such as barbiturates, diazepam (Valium), and sedative hypnotics; and hallucinogens such as LSD, inhalants, glue, paint thinner, nail polish remover, and nitrous oxide (NIDA, 2018). Table 24.4 highlights commonly used substances and their effects on the fetus and newborn.

Substance abuse during pregnancy is the subject of much controversy. The type of substance used and the timing of drug ingestion during pregnancy usually determines the type and severity of damage to the fetus. Frequently, the woman uses more than one substance, which compounds the problem. Nurses must be knowledgeable about the issues of substance abuse and must be alert for opportunities to identify, prevent, manage, and educate women and families about this key public health issue.

Fetal Alcohol Spectrum Disorders

Alcohol abuse during pregnancy is currently among the fastest-growing health care challenges in North America. Years ago, alcohol was not commonly recognized as a teratogen, an agent that can disrupt the development of a fetus. Today, it is known that prenatal alcohol exposure induces a variety of adverse effects on physical, neurologic, and behavioural development known as **fetal alcohol spectrum disorder (FASD)**. In Canada, over 3,000 babies are born with FASD each year, and over 30,000 Canadians are living with the effects (Health Canada, 2017). The adverse effects of alcohol consumption have been recognized for centuries, but the associated pattern of fetal anomalies was not labelled until the early 1970s. The distinctive pattern identified three specific findings: growth restriction (pre- and postnatal), craniofacial structural anomalies, and CNS dysfunction. These distinctive findings were called FAS, characterized by physical and mental disorders that appear at birth and remain problematic throughout the child's life. However, there are also circumstances in which the effects of prenatal alcohol exposure are apparent, but the newborn does not meet the entire criteria specific to FAS. Other disorders included in the grouping fetal alcohol spectrum disorders (FASDs) are alcohol-related neurodevelopmental disorder (ARND) and **alcohol-related birth defects** (ARBD). Children with ARND primarily display intellectual disabilities related to behaviour and learning while children with ARBD may have birth defects of the heart, kidneys, and/or bones. The

problems associated with any of the FASDs are lifelong and are entirely preventable by avoiding alcohol consumption during pregnancy (Centers for Disease Control and Prevention [CDC], 2018a). Box 24.2 summarizes the manifestations of FAS.

The exact prevalence of FASD in Canada is not known. Studies have demonstrated rates of 2.8 to 4.8 per 1,000 live births, with disproportionate higher rates among marginalized groups (CPS, 2018a). Heavy drinking and binge drinking place the fetus at highest risk (March of Dimes, 2016).

Decreasing or eliminating alcohol consumption during pregnancy is the only way to prevent FAS and fetal alcohol effects. Unfortunately, few treatment programs address the needs of pregnant women; so many newborns are exposed to alcohol in utero.

Neonatal Abstinence Syndrome

Neonatal abstinence syndrome (NAS) comprises a constellation of drug withdrawal symptoms that result from chronic intrauterine exposure to a variety of substances, including opioids, barbiturates, SSRIs, alcohol, benzodiazepines, caffeine, and nicotine. Newborns of women who abuse tobacco, illicit substances, caffeine, and alcohol can exhibit withdrawal behaviour. Withdrawal symptoms occur in 60% of all newborns exposed to drugs (March of Dimes, 2018a). Drug dependency acquired in utero is manifested by a constellation of neurologic and physical behaviours and is known as NAS. Although often treated as a single entity, NAS is not a single pathologic condition.

The manifestations of withdrawal are a function of the drug's half-life, the specific drug or combination of drugs used, dosage, route of administration, timing of drug exposure, and length of drug exposure (Hamdan, 2017). Typical newborn behaviours include CNS hypersensitivity, autonomic dysfunction, respiratory distress, temperature instability, hypoglycemia, tremors, seizures, abnormal cry patterns, feeding difficulties, and gastrointestinal disturbances (Gardner et al., 2016). NAS has both medical and developmental consequences for the newborn.

Nursing Assessment

A comprehensive prenatal medical and drug history, especially with respect to polydrug use, is vital. Fear of referral to child welfare agencies or the legal system has prompted women to conceal their drug abuse history. Frequently, the first inkling of drug use appears in the newborn when symptoms of withdrawal begin within 72 hours after birth. Typically the infant has been discharged by this time, unless the nurse has a high degree of suspicion that would prompt toxicology testing earlier.

(text continues on page 927)

TABLE 24.4	COMMON TYPES OF ABUSED SUBSTANCES		
Substance	**Description**	**Effects on Fetus and Newborn**	**Nursing Implications**
Alcohol	Consumption is pervasive and widely accepted, with use, abuse, and addiction affecting all levels of society It is a common misconception that a substance sold to the public without restriction is safe	Fetal alcohol syndrome (one of the most common known causes of mental retardation) Fetal alcohol spectrum disorders Alcohol-related birth defects	Provide education that decreasing or eliminating alcohol consumption during pregnancy is the only way to prevent fetal alcohol syndrome and fetal alcohol effects Assist pregnant clients in finding a treatment program if possible Inform all clients who are pregnant or planning to become pregnant about the detrimental effects of alcohol during pregnancy Educate clients using a nonjudgmental, culturally connected approach Warn clients that there is no safe time to drink or amount of alcohol they can consume
Tobacco/nicotine	Nicotine is an addictive substance. It causes epinephrine release from the adrenal cortex, leading to initial stimulation followed by depression and fatigue, causing the user to seek more nicotine Increased numbers of women are smoking (at least 11% smoke during pregnancy) Over 2,500 chemicals are found in cigarette smoke, including nicotine, tar, carbon monoxide, and cyanide. It is unknown which are harmful, but nicotine and carbon monoxide are believed to play a role in causing adverse pregnancy outcomes	Impaired oxygenation of mother and fetus due to nicotine crossing placenta and carbon monoxide combining with hemoglobin Increased risk for low birth weight (risk almost doubled), small for gestational age, and preterm birth Increased risk for sudden infant death syndrome (SIDS) and chronic respiratory illness	Provide support for smoking cessation Individualize counselling based on factors associated with the client's smoking and challenges faced (why woman smokes, stressors in life, and social support network) Suggest options such as group smoking cessation programs, relaxation techniques, individual counselling, hypnosis, and partner support counselling
Marijuana	Most widely used illicit psychoactive substance in the Western world Derived from *Cannabis sativa* plant	Not shown to have teratogenic effects on fetus; no consistent types of malformations identified Fetal growth restriction (FGR) is common due to delivery of carbon monoxide to fetus Increased risk for small for gestational age Altered responses to visual stimuli, sleep-pattern abnormalities, photophobia, lack of motor control, hyperirritability, increased tremulousness, and high-pitched cry noted in infants of mothers who smoked marijuana Research related to long-term effects is continuing	Provide teaching about healthy behaviours Provide support for cessation of marijuana use

TABLE 24.4	COMMON TYPES OF ABUSED SUBSTANCES (continued)		
Substance	**Description**	**Effects on Fetus and Newborn**	**Nursing Implications**
Methamphetamines	Addictive stimulant; use releases high levels of dopamine, which stimulates brain cells, enhancing mood and body movement High potential for abuse and addiction; can be inhaled, injected, smoked, or taken orally Many street names, such as speed, meth, ice, and chalk Primary effects include accelerated heart and respiratory rate, elevated blood pressure, papillary dilation; secondary effects include loss of appetite Used medically as treatment for obesity and narcolepsy in adults and hyperactivity in children	Little research on use during pregnancy because its use is less common than cocaine or narcotics Fetal effects similar to cocaine (suggesting vasoconstriction as possible underlying mechanism) Possible maternal malnutrition, leading to problems with fetal growth and development Increased risk for preterm birth and low–birth-weight newborns Infants may have withdrawal symptoms, including dysphoria, agitation, jitteriness, poor weight gain, abnormal sleep patterns, poor feeding, frantic fist sucking, high-pitched cry, respiratory distress soon after birth, frequent infections, and significant lassitude Long-term effects not known	Provide teaching about healthy behaviours Provide support for cessation of methamphetamine use Monitor the pregnant client for weight changes; emphasize the need for adequate nutritional intake to support fetal growth and development
Cocaine	Strong CNS stimulant that interferes with reabsorption of dopamine Physical effects: vasoconstriction; pupillary dilation; increased temperature, heart rate, and blood pressure Taken orally, sublingually, intranasally, intravenously, and via inhalation Estimated that 30–40% of cocaine addicts are female Maternal cocaine use during pregnancy is a significant health problem Increased potential for use of multiple drugs if mother using cocaine	Preterm birth and lower birth weight Unclear impact on later development Speculation that cocaine interferes with infant's cognitive development, leading to learning and memory difficulties later in life Associated congenital anomalies: GU, cardiac, and CNS defects, and prune belly syndrome Other typical newborn characteristics: smaller head circumference, piercing cry, limb defects, ambiguous genitalia, poor feeding, poor visual and auditory responses, poor sleep patterns, decreased impulse control, stiff, hyperextended positioning, irritability and hypersensitivity, inability to respond to caretaker. Elevated vital signs secondary to stimulating effect.	Educate the client about the effects of cocaine use on the fetus and newborn Assess for use of other substances Provide teaching about healthy behaviours Provide support and guidance for cessation of cocaine and other substance use

(continued)

TABLE 24.4	COMMON TYPES OF ABUSED SUBSTANCES (continued)		
Substance	**Description**	**Effects on Fetus and Newborn**	**Nursing Implications**
Heroin	Illegal, highly addictive opiate derived from morphine that can be sniffed, smoked, or injected Possible consequences include HIV infection, tuberculosis, crime, violence, and family disruption Severe physical addiction; CNS depressant producing mental dullness and drowsiness	Newborns of heroin-addicted mothers are born dependent on heroin Increased risk for transmission of hepatitis B and C and HIV to newborns when mothers share needles Significantly increased rates of stillbirth, FGR, preterm birth, and newborn mortality (three to seven times greater) Small-for-gestational-age newborns, meconium aspiration, high incidence of SIDS, and delayed effects from subacute withdrawal (restlessness, continual crying, agitation, sneezing, vomiting, fever, diarrhea, seizures, irritability, and poor socialization [possibly persisting for 4–6 months]); Intrauterine death or preterm birth is possible with abrupt cessation of heroin use	Educate the client about the effects of heroin use on the fetus and newborn Assess for use of other substances Provide teaching about healthy behaviours Warn the client not to abruptly stop heroin use. Encourage enrolment in a methadone maintenance program
Methadone	Synthetic opiate narcotic used, primarily as maintenance therapy for heroin addiction	Improvement in many of the detrimental fetal effects associated with heroin use Withdrawal symptoms are common in newborns. Possible low birth weight due to symmetric fetal growth restriction Increased severity and longer period of withdrawal (due to methadone's longer half-life) Seizures (commonly severe) do not usually occur until 2–3 wks of age, when the newborn is at home. Increased rate of SIDS (three to four times higher)	Methadone maintenance programs are the standard of care for pregnant clients with narcotic addiction Inform the client about the benefits and risks of methadone use versus heroin use. Advantages include improved fetal and newborn growth, reduced risk of fetal death, and reduced risk of HIV infections Advise the client that she will need to return consistently to receive the prescribed methadone dose Reinforce the need for continued prenatal care Inform the client that breastfeeding is encouraged while receiving methadone Teach parent(s) and caregivers about signs and symptoms of methadone withdrawal

BOX 24.2

CLINICAL PICTURE OF FETAL ALCOHOL SYNDROME

- Microcephaly (head circumference <10th percentile)[a]
- Small palpebral (eyelid) fissures[a]
- Abnormally small eyes
- Fetal growth restriction
- Maxillary hypoplasia (flattened or absent)
- Epicanthal folds (folds of skin of the upper eyelid over the eye)
- Thin upper lip[a]
- Missing vertical groove in median portion of upper lip[a]
- Short upturned nose
- Short birth length and low birth weight
- Joint and limb defects
- Small for gestational age
- Altered palmar crease pattern
- Pre- or postnatal growth ≤10th percentile[a]
- Congenital cardiac defects (septal defects)
- Delayed fine and gross motor development
- Poor eye–hand coordination
- Clinically significant brain abnormalities[a]
- Mental retardation
- Narrow forehead
- Performance substantially below expected level in cognitive or developmental functioning, executive or motor functioning, attention or hyperactivity, and social or language skills[a]
- Inadequate sucking reflex and poor appetite

[a]Diagnosis of fetal alcohol syndrome requires the presence of three findings:
1. Documentation of all three facial abnormalities
2. Documentation of growth deficits (height, weight, or both <10th percentile)
3. Documentation of CNS abnormalities (structural, neurologic, or functional)

Adapted from Centers for Disease Control and Prevention (CDC). (2018a). *Fetal alcohol spectrum disorders (FASDs)*. Retrieved from http://www.cdc.gov/ncbddd/fasd/facts.html; and Cook, J. L., Green, C. R., Lilley, C. M., Anderson, S. M., Baldwin, M. E., Chudley, A. E., ... Rosales, T. (2016). Fetal alcohol spectrum disorder: A guideline for diagnosis across the lifespan. *Canadian Medical Association Journal, 188*(3), 191–197. Retrieved from http://www.cmaj.ca/content/cmaj/188/3/191.full.pdf

Several assessment tools can be used to assess a drug-exposed newborn. Figure 24.6 shows an example. Regardless of the tool used for assessment, address these key areas:
- Maternal history to identify risk behaviours for substance abuse:
  - Previous unexplained fetal demise
  - Lack of prenatal care
  - Incarceration
  - Prostitution

- Cigarette smoking
- Fetal growth restriction
- Preterm birth
- History of STIs and/or HIV and/or HCV
- Mental health disorders
- History of intimate partner violence
- History of missed prenatal appointments
- Severe mood swings
- Precipitous labour
- Poor nutritional status
- Abruptio placentae
- Hypertensive episodes
- History of drug abuse
- Laboratory test results (toxicology) to identify substances in mother and newborn
- Signs of NAS (use the WITHDRAWAL acronym; see Box 24.3)
- Evidence of seizure activity and need for protective environment

The newborn's behaviour often prompts the health care provider or nurse to suspect intrauterine drug exposure. The newborn physical examination may also reveal low birth weight for gestational age or drug or ARBD and dysfunction. Assess the newborn for signs of NAS (Box 24.4).

Take Note!
Cocaine-exposed newborns are typically fussy, irritable, and inconsolable at times. Cocaine-exposed infants demonstrate poor coordination of sucking and swallowing, making feeding time frustrating for the newborn and caregiver alike.

Assist with obtaining diagnostic studies to identify the severity of withdrawal. Toxicology screening of the newborn's blood, urine, and meconium identifies the substances to which the newborn has been exposed. Urine drug screening identifies only recent substance exposure, whereas meconium samples may reveal exposure from the second trimester to the present (Hamdan, 2017). Take care to avoid contamination of meconium with urine, as this may affect the accuracy of the sample.

Nursing Management

The needs of the substance-exposed newborn are multiple, complex, and costly, both to the health care system and to society. Substance abuse takes place among people of all colours, sizes, shapes, incomes, types, and conditions. Most pregnant individuals are unaware of the adverse impact their substance abuse can have on the newborn. Pregnant clients dependent on opioids are maintained on methadone as the current standard of care,

CENTRAL NERVOUS SYSTEM DISTURBANCES

SIGNS AND SYMPTOMS	SCORE	AM							PM			
Excessive high-pitched cry	2											
Continuous high-pitched cry	3											
Sleeps <1 hour after feeding	3											
Sleeps <2 hours after feeding	2											
Sleeps <3 hours after feeding	1											
Hyperactive Moro reflex	2											
Markedly hyperactive Moro reflex	3											
Mild tremors disturbed	1											
Moderate–severe tremors disturbed	2											
Mild tremors undisturbed	1											
Moderate–severe tremors undisturbed	4											
Increased muscle tone	2											
Excoloration (specify area)	1											
Myoclonic jerks	3											
Generalized convulsions	5											

METABOLIC / VASOMOTOR/RESPIRATORY DISTURBANCES

Sweating												
Fever <101 (99–100.8°F/37.2–38.2°C)	1											
Fever >101 (38.2°C and higher)	2											
Frequent yawning (>3–4 times/interval)	1											
Mottling	1											
Nasal stuffiness	1											
Sneezing (>3–4 times/interval)	1											
Nasal flaring	2											
Respiratory rate >60 / min	1											
Respiratory rate >60 / min, with retractions	2											

GASTROINTESTINAL DISTURBANCES

Excessive sucking	1											
Poor feeding	2											
Regurgitation	2											
Projectile vomiting	3											
Loose stools	2											
Watery stools	3											
TOTAL SCORE												

FIGURE 24.6 Neonatal abstinence scoring system. (From Cloherty, J. P., Eichenwald, E. C., Hansen, A. R., & Stark, A. R. (2012). *Manual of neonatal care* (7th ed.). Philadelphia, PA: Lippincott Williams & Wilkins.)

BOX 24.3

WITHDRAWAL ACRONYM

Assess the newborn for signs of neonatal abstinence syndrome using the acronym WITHDRAWAL to focus the assessment:

W = **W**akefulness: sleep duration less than 3 hours after feeding
I = **I**rritability
T = **T**emperature variation, tachycardia, tremors
H = **H**yperactivity, high-pitched persistent cry, hyper-reflexia, hypertonus
D = **D**iarrhea, diaphoresis, disorganized suck
R = **R**espiratory distress, rub marks, rhinorrhea
A = **A**pneic attacks, autonomic dysfunction
W = **W**eight loss or failure to gain weight
A = **A**lkalosis (respiratory)
L = **L**acrimation (Hamdan, 2017)

---

which provides multiple benefits including improved prenatal care, reduced fetal mortality, and improved fetal growth (Jansson, 2018).

Nurses are in a unique position to help because they interact with high-risk parents and newborns in many settings, including the community, health care facilities,

and family agencies. It is the responsibility of all nurses to identify, educate, counsel, and refer pregnant clients with substance abusing challenges. For example, nurses can be instrumental in increasing the number of pregnant clients who make a serious attempt to quit smoking by using the "5 A's" approach:

- **A**sk: Ask all clients if they smoke and would like to quit.
- **A**dvise: Encourage the use of clinically proven treatment plans.
- **A**ssess: Provide motivation by discussing the "5 Rs":
  - **R**elevance of quitting to the client
  - **R**isk of continued smoking to the fetus
  - **R**ewards of quitting for both
  - **R**oadblocks to quitting
  - **R**epeat at every visit
- **A**ssist: Help the client to protect the fetus and newborn from the negative effects of smoking.
- **A**rrange: Schedule follow-up visits to reinforce the client's commitment to quit.

Although this approach is geared to smoking cessation, nurses can adapt it to focus on cessation for any substance use. Early, supportive, ongoing nursing care is critical to the well-being of the parent and newborn. Nurses have an ethical responsibility to provide

---

BOX 24.4

MANIFESTATIONS OF NEONATAL ABSTINENCE SYNDROME

CNS Dysfunction

- Tremors
- Generalized seizures
- Hyperactive reflexes
- Restlessness
- Hypertonic muscle tone, constant movement
- Shrill, high-pitched cry
- Disturbed sleep patterns

Metabolic, Vasomotor, and Respiratory Disturbances

- Fever
- Frequent yawning
- Mottling of the skin
- Sweating
- Frequent sneezing
- Nasal flaring
- Tachypnea >60 bpm
- Apnea

Gastrointestinal Dysfunction

- Poor feeding
- Frantic sucking or rooting
- Loose or watery stools
- Regurgitation or projectile vomiting

Adapted from Hamdan, A. H. (2016). Neonatal abstinence syndrome. *eMedicine*. Retrieved from http://emedicine.medscape.com/article/978763-overview; and Artigas, V. (2015). Management of neonatal abstinence syndrome in the newborn nursery. *Nursing for Women's Health, 18*(6), 509–514.

evidence-based and nonjudgmental care to this highly vulnerable population.

Caring for a substance-exposed newborn remains a major challenge to health care providers. The major goals include providing comfort to the newborn by relieving symptoms, improving feeding and weight gain, preventing seizures, promoting parent–newborn interactions, and reducing the incidence of newborn mortality and abnormal development (Mattson & Smith, 2015).

PROMOTING COMFORT

Supportive interventions to promote comfort include swaddling, low lighting, gentle handling, quiet environment with minimal stimulation, use of soft voices, pacifiers to promote "self-soothing," frequent small feedings, vertical rocking during infant disorganization periods, and rooming-in and positioning (Artigas, 2015). Keep environmental stimuli to a minimum. For example, decrease stimuli by dimming the lights in the nursery, and swaddle the newborn tightly to decrease irritability behaviours. Other techniques such as gentle rocking, using a flexed position, and offering a pacifier can help manage CNS irritability. A pacifier also helps satisfy the newborn's need for nonnutritive sucking. Swaddling, pacifiers, low lighting, oscillating cribs, and avoidance of abrupt changes in the infant's environment can be helpful. Use a calm, gentle approach when handling the newborn and plan activities to avoid overstimulating the newborn, allowing time for rest periods.

MEETING NUTRITIONAL NEEDS

Newborns suffering from NAS have impaired feeding behaviours, such as excessive sucking, poor feeding, regurgitation, and diarrhea, which may cause weight loss. To improve weight gain, they are supplemented with high-calorie formula. When feeding the newborn, use small amounts and position the newborn upright to prevent aspiration and to facilitate rhythmic sucking and swallowing. Frequent small feedings are preferable and should provide 150 to 250 kcal/kg per 24 hours for proper growth of the infant undergoing significant withdrawal (Gardner et al., 2016).

Breastfeeding is encouraged unless the mother is still using drugs. Monitor the newborn's weight daily to evaluate the success of food intake. Assess hydration; check skin turgor and fontanels. Assess the frequency and characteristics of bowel movements and monitor the newborn's fluid and electrolyte and acid–base status.

PREVENTING COMPLICATIONS

Pharmacologic treatment is warranted if conservative measures, such as swaddling and decreased environmental stimulation, are not adequate. The AAP recommends that for newborns with confirmed drug exposure, drug therapy is indicated if the newborn has seizures, diarrhea, and vomiting resulting in excessive weight loss and dehydration, poor feeding, inability to sleep, and fever unrelated to infection (Jones & Fielder, 2015). Common medications used in the management of newborn withdrawal include an opioid (morphine or methadone) and phenobarbital as a second drug if the opiate does not adequately control symptoms (Artigas, 2015). Administer the prescribed medications and document the newborn's behavioural responses.

The newborn is at risk for skin breakdown. Weight loss, diarrhea, dehydration, and irritability can contribute to this risk. Provide meticulous skin care and protect the newborn's elbows and knees against friction and abrasions.

PROMOTING PARENT–NEWBORN INTERACTION

For a parent who abuses substances, the birth of a drug-exposed newborn is both a crisis and an opportunity. The mother may feel guilty about the newborn's condition. Many of these newborns are unresponsive and have disorganized sleeping and feeding patterns. When awake, they can be easily overstimulated and irritated. Such characteristics make parent–newborn interactions difficult and frustrating, leading to possible detachment and avoidance. Nursing support, which includes a description of symptoms and their management, is vital if parental–infant attachment is to occur, and potential neglect or abuse is avoided (Gardner et al., 2016). Instruct the parent(s) or caretaker how to care for the newborn, including what to do after the newborn goes home (Teaching Guidelines 24.1).

 Teaching Guidelines 24.1
CARING FOR YOUR NEWBORN AT HOME

* Position your newborn with the head elevated to prevent choking.
* To aid your newborn's sucking and swallowing during feeding, position the chin downward and support it with your hand.
* Place your newborn on his or her back to sleep or nap, never on the stomach.
* Keep a bulb syringe close by to suction your newborn's mouth in case of choking.
* Cluster newborn care (bathing, feeding, dressing) to prevent overstimulation.
* If your newborn is fussy or crying, try these measures to help calm him or her:
  * Wrap your newborn snugly in a blanket and gently rock in rocking chair.
  * Take the baby for a ride in the car (using a newborn car seat).
  * Play soothing music and "dance" with the newborn.
  * Use a wind-up swing with music.

- To help your newborn get to sleep, try these measures:
  - Schedule a bath with a gentle massage prior to bedtime.
  - Change diaper and clothes to make the baby comfortable.
  - Feed the baby just prior to bedtime.
  - If the newborn cries when put in crib and all needs are met, allow him or her to cry.
  - Use a rocking chair to feed and sing a soft lullaby.
- Call your primary care provider if you observe withdrawal behaviours such as:
  - Slight tremors (shaking) of hands and legs
  - Stiff posture when held in your arms
  - Irritability and frequent fussiness
  - High-pitched cry, excessive sucking motions
  - Erratic sleep pattern
  - Frequent yawning, nasal stuffiness, sweating
  - Prolonged time needed to feed
  - Frequent vomiting after feeding

On the other hand, the newborn may be a powerful motivator for the parent(s) to undergo treatment and seek recovery. Offer referrals to community agencies to address addiction and the infant's developmental needs (Mattson & Smith, 2015). The nurse can play a pivotal role in assisting her to abstain from drug use and to promote effective parenting skills.

Hyperbilirubinemia

Hyperbilirubinemia is a total serum bilirubin level above 5 mg/dL resulting from unconjugated bilirubin being deposited in the skin and mucous membranes (Hansen, 2017). Hyperbilirubinemia is exhibited as jaundice (yellowing of the body tissues and fluids). Newborn jaundice is one of the most common reasons for hospital readmission. It occurs in 60% to 80% of term newborns in the first week of life and in virtually all preterm newborns (Fanaroff & Fanaroff, 2014).

Pathophysiology

Bilirubin has two forms—unconjugated or indirect, which is fat soluble and toxic to body tissues, and conjugated or direct, which is water soluble and nontoxic. Elevated serum bilirubin levels are manifested as jaundice in the newborn. Typically the total serum bilirubin level rises over the first 3 to 5 days and then declines.

Newborn jaundice results from an imbalance in the rate of bilirubin production and bilirubin elimination. This imbalance determines the pattern and degree of newborn hyperbilirubinemia (Hansen, 2017).

During the newborn period, a rapid transition from the intrauterine to the extrauterine pattern of bilirubin physiology occurs. Fetal unconjugated bilirubin is normally cleared by the placenta and the mother's liver in utero, so total bilirubin at birth is low. After the umbilical cord is cut, the newborn must conjugate bilirubin (convert a lipid-soluble pigment into a water-soluble pigment) in the liver on his or her own. The rate and amount of bilirubin conjugation depend on the rate of RBC breakdown, the bilirubin load, the maturity of the liver, and the number of albumin-binding sites. Bilirubin levels rise in newborns by three main mechanisms: increased production (accelerated RBC breakdown), decreased removal (transient liver enzyme insufficiency), and increased reabsorption (delay in bowel excretion) (Gardner et al., 2016). Bilirubin production increases after birth mainly because of a shortened RBC lifespan (70 days in the newborn vs. 90 days in the adult) combined with an increased RBC mass. Therefore, the amount of bilirubin the newborn must deal with is large compared to that of an adult.

PHYSIOLOGIC JAUNDICE
Physiologic jaundice is an unconjugated hyperbilirubinemia that occurs after the first postnatal day and can last up to 1 week. Total serum bilirubin concentrations peak in the first 3 to 5 postnatal days and decline to adult values over the next several weeks.

It occurs in 60% of term infants and up to 80% of preterm infants (Blackburn, 2012). Serum bilirubin levels reach up to 10 mg/dL and then decline rapidly over the first week after birth (Cunningham et al., 2014). Most newborns have been discharged by the time this jaundice peaks (at about 72 hours).

Physiologic jaundice may result from an increased bilirubin load because of relative polycythemia, a shortened RBC lifespan, immature hepatic uptake and conjugation process, and increased enterohepatic circulation (Hansen, 2017). Newborns with delayed passage of meconium are more likely to develop physiologic jaundice because meconium contains high levels of bilirubin (Kenner & Lott, 2014).

Physiologic jaundice differs between breastfed and bottle-fed newborns in relation to the onset of symptoms. Breastfed newborns typically have peak bilirubin levels on the fourth day of life; levels for bottle-fed newborns usually peak on the third day of life. The rate of bilirubin decline is less rapid in breastfed newborns compared to bottle-fed newborns because bottle-fed newborns tend to have more frequent bowel movements. Jaundice associated with breastfeeding presents in two distinct patterns: early-onset breastfeeding jaundice and late-onset breast milk jaundice.

Early-Onset Breastfeeding Jaundice. Early-onset breastfeeding jaundice is probably associated with ineffective breastfeeding practices because of relative caloric deprivation in the first few days of life. Decreased volume and frequency of feedings may result in mild dehydration and the delayed passage of meconium. This delayed defecation allows enterohepatic circulation reuptake of bilirubin and an increase in the serum level of unconjugated bilirubin. To prevent this, strategies to promote early effective breastfeeding are important. Health Canada and the CPS recommend early and frequent breastfeeding without supplemental water or dextrose water because they do not prevent hyperbilirubinemia and may lead to hyponatremia (Health Canada, 2015). Early frequent feedings can provide the newborn with adequate calories and fluid volume (via colostrum) to stimulate peristalsis and passage of meconium to eliminate bilirubin. Successful breastfeeding decreases the risk of hyperbilirubinemia. Infants need to be fed at least 8 to 12 times in the first few days after birth to help improve the mother's milk supply. The best way to judge successful breastfeeding is to monitor infant urine output, stool output, and weight. Newborns should have four to six wet diapers and three to four yellow, seedy stools per day by the fourth day after birth. Breastfeeding-associated jaundice is usually preventable through appropriate breastfeeding practices.

Late-Onset Breastfeeding Jaundice. Late-onset breastfeeding jaundice occurs later in the newborn period, with the bilirubin level usually peaking in the first 6 to 14 days of life. It typically occurs between the fourth and seventh days of life, when mature milk begins to replace colostrum. Total serum bilirubin levels may reach as high as 12 mg/dL, but the level is not considered pathologic (Lauwers & Swisher, 2016). The specific cause of late-onset breastfeeding jaundice is not entirely understood, but it may be related to a change in the milk composition resulting in enhanced enterohepatic circulation (Deshpande & Wagle, 2017). Additional research is needed to determine the cause. Interrupting breastfeeding is not recommended unless bilirubin levels reach dangerous levels; if this occurs, breastfeeding is stopped for only 1 or 2 days. Most cases require no interruption in breastfeeding. Frequent and effective breastfeeding soon after childbirth is associated with reducing the incidence and intensity of breastfeeding jaundice.

PATHOLOGIC JAUNDICE

Pathologic jaundice is manifested within the first 24 hours of life when total bilirubin levels increase by more than 5 mg/dL/day and the total serum bilirubin level is higher than 17 mg/dL in a full-term infant. This condition requires intervention (Ives, 2015). Conditions that alter the production, transport, uptake, metabolism, excretion, or reabsorption of bilirubin can cause pathologic jaundice in the newborn. A few conditions that contribute to RBC breakdown and thus higher bilirubin

levels include polycythemia, blood incompatibilities, and systemic acidosis. These altered conditions can lead to high levels of unconjugated bilirubin, possibly reaching toxic levels and resulting in a severe condition called **kernicterus** or bilirubin encephalopathy. It can be acute or chronic.

Hyperbilirubinemia is a great concern because of the potential for brain injury. The spectrum of bilirubin-induced neurologic dysfunction ranges from acute bilirubin encephalopathy to the devastating and irreversible chronic bilirubin encephalopathy or kernicterus.

Acute bilirubin encephalopathy describes the effects of hyperbilirubinemia in the first weeks of life. Clinical signs include lethargy, poor feeding, high-pitched cry, poor tone, a poor Moro reflex with incomplete flexion of the extremities, and a high-pitched cry. As symptoms of acute bilirubin encephalopathy worsen, the newborn progresses to apnea, seizures, coma, and death (Gardner et al., 2016).

Chronic bilirubin encephalopathy or kernicterus is characterized by four clinical manifestations: movement disorder (athetosis, dystonia, spasticity, hypotonia), auditory dysfunction (deafness), oculomotor impairment, and dental enamel hypoplasia of deciduous teeth (Springer & Annibale, 2014). Unconjugated bilirubin enters the brain and acts as a neurotoxin causing long-term neurologic sequelae. Cases of kernicterus should not be occurring today, but delays in diagnosing pathologic causes of prolonged jaundice are still being missed or overlooked (Ives, 2015).

The most common condition associated with pathologic jaundice is hemolytic disease of the newborn secondary to incompatibility of blood groups of the mother and the newborn. The most frequent conditions are Rh factor and ABO incompatibilities.

Take Note!

Significant jaundice in the newborn less than 24 hours of age should be immediately reported to the physician, as it may indicate a pathologic process.

Nursing Assessment

Neonatal jaundice first becomes visible in the face and forehead. Identification is aided by pressure on the skin, since blanching reveals the underlying colour. Jaundice then gradually becomes visible on the trunk and extremities. This cephalocaudal progression is well described. Jaundice disappears in the opposite direction. Nurses play an important role in early detection and identification of jaundice in the newborn. Keen observation skills are essential.

HEALTH HISTORY AND PHYSICAL EXAMINATION

Review the medical record for factors that might predispose the newborn to hyperbilirubinemia, such as:

- Polycythemia
- Significant bruising or cephalohematoma, which increases bilirubin production
- Infections such as TORCH (toxoplasmosis, hepatitis B, rubella, cytomegalovirus [CMV], herpes simplex virus)
- Use of drugs during labour and birth such as diazepam (Valium) or oxytocin (Pitocin)
- Prematurity
- Gestational age of 34 to 36 weeks
- Hemolysis due to ABO incompatibility or Rh isoimmunization
- Macrosomic IDM
- Delayed cord clamping, which increases the erythrocyte volume
- Decreased albumin-binding sites to transport unconjugated bilirubin to the liver because of acidosis
- Delayed meconium passage, which increases the amount of bilirubin that returns to the unconjugated state and can be absorbed by the intestinal mucosa
- Siblings who had significant jaundice
- Inadequate breastfeeding leading to dehydration, decreased caloric intake, weight loss, and delayed passage of meconium
- Ethnicity, such as Asian American, Mediterranean, or Indigenous
- Male gender
- Acidosis
- Sepsis
- Resuscitation at birth (CPS, 2018b; Gardner et al., 2016)

Perform a complete physical examination. Assess the skin, mucous membranes, sclerae, and bodily fluids (tears, urine) for a yellow colour. Detect jaundice by observing the infant in a well-lit room and blanching the skin with digital pressure over a bony prominence. Typically, jaundice begins on the head and gradually progresses to the abdomen and extremities. Also inspect for pallor (anemia), excessive bruising (bleeding), and

dehydration (sluggish circulation), which may contribute to the development of jaundice and the risk for kernicterus.

Assess the newborn for Rh incompatibility. Be alert for clinical manifestations such as ascites, anemia, congestive heart failure, edema, pallor, jaundice, hepatosplenomegaly, polyhydramnios, thick placenta, and dilation of the umbilical vein (Salem & Singer, 2017).

Hydropic newborns appear pale, edematous, and limp at birth and typically require resuscitation. The newborn with immune hydrops exhibits severe generalized edema, organ hypertrophy and enlargement, and effusion of fluid into body cavities.

LABORATORY AND DIAGNOSTIC TESTING

Determine maternal and fetal blood types, checking for incompatibilities (Comparison Chart 24.1). Assess laboratory values for bilirubin (both unconjugated and conjugated). Bilirubin levels establish the diagnosis of hyperbilirubinemia. The newborn with Rh incompatibility demonstrates a rapidly rising unconjugated bilirubin level at birth or in the first 24 hours. Also expect to obtain alkaline phosphatase, liver enzymes, and prothrombin time and partial thromboplastin time, as well as the following:

- Direct Coombs test—to identify hemolytic disease of the newborn; positive results indicate that the newborn's RBCs have been coated with antibodies and thus are sensitized
- Hemoglobin concentration—for evidence of anemia
- Blood type—to determine Rh status and any incompatibility of the newborn
- Total serum protein—to detect reduced binding capacity of albumin
- Reticulocyte count—to identify an elevated level indicating increased hemolysis

Assist with obtaining blood specimens. Use cord blood for hemoglobin concentration measurements and

COMPARISON CHART 24.1	RH VERSUS ABO INCOMPATIBILITY	
Clinical Picture	Rh Incompatibility	ABO Incompatibility
First born	Rare	Common
Later pregnancies	More severe	No increase in severity
Jaundice	Moderate to severe	Mild
Hydrops fetalis	Frequent	Rare
Anemia	Frequently severe	Rare
Ascites	Frequent	Rare
Hepatosplenomegaly	Frequent	Common

Coombs test. If cord blood is not available, use a heel stick for direct Coombs testing, hemoglobin concentration measurement, and bilirubin levels. Prepare the parents and newborn for radiologic evaluation if necessary to determine abnormalities that may be causing the jaundice.

Nursing Management

Nursing management of a newborn with hyperbilirubinemia requires a comprehensive approach. As members of the health care team, nurses share in the responsibility for early detection and identification, family education, management, and follow-up of the mother and newborn. Documentation of the timing of onset of jaundice is essential to differentiate between physiologic (>24 hours) and pathologic jaundice (<24 hours). Nurses can improve care by offering their presence and support and by following the AAP guidelines for preventing hyperbilirubinemia:

- Promote and support successful breastfeeding.
- Assess for risk factors that may increase bilirubin levels.
- Establish nursery protocols for identifying jaundice, including when a serum bilirubin can be ordered by a nurse.
- Measure total serum bilirubin on jaundiced infants in the first 24 hours.
- Interpret all bilirubin levels according to the infant's age in hours.
- Visual estimation of jaundice is inaccurate and shouldn't be used instead of labs.
- Infants <38 weeks, particularly if breastfed, should be considered high risk.
- Perform risk assessment on all newborns prior to discharge.
- Jaundiced newborns should be treated, if indicated, with phototherapy.
- Provide parents with written and oral information about jaundice at discharge.
- Follow-up care and referrals should be based on time of discharge and risk.
- Empower parents to make appropriate decisions once home (Green, 2016; Mattson & Smith, 2015).

REDUCING BILIRUBIN LEVELS

Encourage early initiation of feedings to prevent hypoglycemia and provide protein to maintain the albumin levels to transport bilirubin to the liver. Ensure newborn feedings (breast milk or formula) every 2 to 3 hours to promote prompt emptying of bilirubin from the bowel. Encourage the mother to breastfeed (8 to 12 or more feedings per day) to prevent inadequate intake and thus dehydration. Supplement breast milk with formula to supply protein if bilirubin levels continue

FIGURE 24.7 A newborn receiving phototherapy.

to increase with breastfeeding only. Monitor serum bilirubin levels frequently to reduce the risk of severe hyperbilirubinemia.

Phototherapy. For the newborn with jaundice, regardless of its etiology, phototherapy is used to convert unconjugated bilirubin to the less toxic water-soluble form that can be excreted. Phototherapy, via special lights placed above the newborn or a fibreoptic blanket placed under the newborn and wrapped around him or her, involves blue wavelengths of light to alter unconjugated bilirubin in the skin. For the newborn receiving phototherapy, place the newborn under the lights or on the fibreoptic blanket, exposing as much skin as possible. Cover the newborn's genitals and shield the eyes to protect these areas from becoming irritated or burned when using direct lights. Assess the intensity of the light source to prevent burns and excoriation (Fig. 24.7). Turn the newborn every 2 hours to maximize the area of exposure, removing the newborn from the lights only for feedings. Maintain a neutral thermal environment to decrease energy expenditure, and assess the newborn's neurologic status frequently. Research is finding that intermittent versus continuous phototherapy is as efficacious to lower bilirubin levels (Evidence-Based Practice 24.1).

Assess the newborn's temperature every 3 to 4 hours as indicated. Monitor fluid intake and output closely and assess daily weights for gains or losses. Check skin turgor for evidence of dehydration.

With feedings, remove the newborn from the lights and remove the eye shields to allow interaction with the newborn. Encourage breast- or bottle-feedings every 2 to 3 hours. Follow agency policy about removing the eye shields periodically to assess the eyes for discharge or corneal irritation secondary to eye shield pressure.

EVIDENCE-BASED PRACTICE 24.1   **INTERMITTENT VERSUS CONTINUOUS PHOTOTHERAPY FOR THE TREATMENT OF NEONATAL NONHEMOLYTIC MODERATE HYPERBILIRUBINEMIA IN INFANTS MORE THAN 34 WEEKS OF GESTATION: A RANDOMIZED CONTROL TRIAL**

STUDY

Neonatal hyperbilirubinemia is frequent reason for late preterm and full-term infants admitted to the NICU. Currently, phototherapy is the most effective therapy for management of neonatal hyperbilirubinemia. Phototherapy acts by three mechanisms to reduce the bilirubin level which include photooxidation, and photo and structural isomerization. The photochemical reaction requires a short period of time and the remaining time, the role of phototherapy is only minimal. With this process in mind, the purpose of this study was to compare intermittent phototherapy with 12 hours on and then 12 hours off with continuous phototherapy.

Findings

In this randomized control study, 75 healthy neonates >34 weeks' gestation were randomized either into intermittent or continuous phototherapy groups. The rate of fall of bilirubin was examined in each group. It was found that the rate of bilirubin fall was greater in the intermediate phototherapy group when compared to the continuous phototherapy group. This study concluded that intermittent phototherapy with 12-hour on and 12-hour off cycles is as efficacious as continuous phototherapy to reduce hyperbilirubinemia in neonates.

Nursing Implications

Nurses can begin the conversation within their clinical settings to bring about change in phototherapy protocols based on this study's findings. Although the sample size was small, it can be duplicated in larger clinical settings to demonstrate the effectiveness of intermittent phototherapy. This phototherapy protocol change could save costs and decrease the anxiety of parents/partners/significant others. Nurses can be instrumental in bringing evidence-based changes by serving on hospital policy and procedure committees.

Adapted from Sachdeva, M., Murki, S., Oleti, T. P., & Kandraju, H. (2015). Intermittent versus continuous phototherapy for the treatment of neonatal non-hemolytic moderate hyperbilirubinemia in infants more than 34 weeks of gestational age: A randomized controlled trial. *European Journal of Pediatrics, 174*(2), 177–181.

Typically, the eyes are assessed and eye shields removed once a shift.

Monitor stool for consistency and frequency. Unconjugated bilirubin excreted in the feces will produce a greenish appearance, and typically stools are loose. Lack of frequent green stools is a cause for concern.

Provide meticulous skin care. Assess skin surfaces frequently for dryness and irritation secondary to the dehydrating effects of phototherapy and irritation from highly acidic stool to prevent excoriation and skin breakdown (Green, 2016). Nursing responsibilities include ensuring effective irradiance delivery, maximizing skin exposure, providing eye protection and eye care, careful attention to thermoregulation, monitoring the newborn's skin turgor, maintaining adequate hydration, promoting elimination, and supporting parent–infant interaction (Nagtalon-Ramos, 2014).

A summary of the nursing care for the newborn undergoing phototherapy is as follows:

- Support parents, encouraging them to interact with their infant.
- Support breastfeeding with one-on-one instruction and patience.
- Place infants on their back to expose as much naked skin as possible.

- Provide eye care/protection every time the infant is exposed to the light.
- Check temperature and environment around infant to prevent overheating.
- Take daily weights to make sure the infant isn't becoming dehydrated.

Exchange Transfusion. If the total serum bilirubin level remains elevated after intensive phototherapy, an exchange transfusion with albumin administered before the transfusion, the quickest method for lowering serum bilirubin levels, may be necessary (Hansen, 2017). In the presence of hemolytic disease, severe anemia, or a rapid rise in the total serum bilirubin level, an exchange transfusion is recommended. An exchange transfusion removes the newborn's blood and replaces it with nonhemolyzed RBCs from a donor. During the transfusion, monitor the newborn's cardiovascular status continuously because serious complications can arise, such as acid–base imbalances, infection, hypovolemia, and fluid and electrolyte imbalances. Exchange transfusion is used only as a second-line therapy after phototherapy has failed to yield results. Intensive nursing care is needed.

Assist the physician or health care practitioner with an exchange transfusion if necessary. Exchange transfusion is done in intensive care setting with continuous monitoring. Monitor the newborn's status closely for changes, especially in vital signs and heart rate and rhythm, before, during, and after the procedure.

PROVIDING PARENT TEACHING AND SUPPORT

Nurses can help the parents to understand the diagnostic tests and treatment modalities by offering individualized teaching. Nurses are the ones who give discharge instructions to the family. Explore with the family their understanding of jaundice and treatment modalities to reduce anxiety and gain their cooperation in monitoring the infant. Teach the parents about jaundice and its potential risk using written and verbal material. Also show the parents how to identify newborn behaviours that might indicate rising bilirubin levels. Emphasize the need to seek treatment from their pediatrician should any of the following occur:

- Lethargy, sleepiness, poor muscle tone, floppiness
- Poor sucking, lack of interest in feeding
- High-pitched cry

Teach the parents how to assess their newborn for signs of jaundice because physiologic jaundice may not occur until after the newborn is discharged. After discharge is planned, parent education plays an important role in hyperbilirubinemia prevention, ensuring that the health care provider is contacted if concerning signs arise prior to the scheduled visit and also ensuring that the infant arrives at the scheduled visit. Frequency of breastfeeding, frequency of voiding and stooling, progression of jaundice, and signs of illness can all be monitored by the engaged parent and shared with the provider. Reinforce the need for appropriate follow-up with the primary care provider within 48 to 72 hours after discharge to assess jaundice status (Verklan & Walden, 2015).

The need for phototherapy can be anxiety producing for the parents. Explain the rationale for the procedure and demonstrate techniques that the parents can use to interact with their newborn. Additional education about phototherapy may be necessary when home phototherapy is used (Teaching Guidelines 24.2).

Teaching Guidelines 24.2

CARING FOR YOUR NEWBORN RECEIVING HOME PHOTOTHERAPY

- Inspect your newborn's skin, eyes, and mucous membranes for a yellow colour.
- Remember that a home health nurse will come to visit and help set up the light system.
- Keep the lights about 12 to 30 in above your newborn.
- Cover your newborn's eyes with patches or cotton balls and gauze to protect them.

- Keep the newborn undressed except for the diaper area; fold the diaper down below the newborn's navel in the front and as far as possible in the back to expose as much skin area as possible.
- Turn your newborn every 2 hours so that all areas of the body are exposed.
- Remove the newborn from the lights only for feeding.
- Remove the eye patches during feedings so that you can interact with your newborn.
- Record your newborn's temperature, weight, and fluid intake daily.
- Document the frequency, colour, and consistency of all stools; the stools should be loose and green as the bilirubin is broken down.
- Keep the skin clean and dry to prevent irritation.
- Feed your newborn frequently, including supplemental glucose water if allowed to provide added fluid, protein, and calories.
- Rock, cuddle, or hold the newborn to promote bonding when out of the lights.
- Contact your pediatrician or home health care agency with any questions or changes, including refusing feedings, fewer than five wet diapers in one day, vomiting of complete amounts of feeding, or elevated temperature.
- Keep appointments for follow-up laboratory testing to monitor bilirubin levels.

Neonatal Sepsis

Neonatal sepsis is defined as a clinical syndrome of bacteremia with systemic signs and symptoms of infection in the first month of life (Molyneux & Gest, 2015). Newborns have increased susceptibility to infections because their immune systems are immature and slow to react, and they have a poorly developed skin barrier. The antibodies that newborns received from their mother during pregnancy and from breast milk help protect them from invading organisms. However, these need time to reach optimal levels.

Bacterial infections of the newborn remain a major cause of illness and death in the neonatal period. The mortality rate from newborn sepsis may be as high as 50% if untreated. Infection is a major cause of death during the first month of life, contributing to 13% to 15% of all neonatal deaths (Anderson-Berry, Bellig, & Ohning, 2015).

Pathophysiology

When a pathologic organism overcomes the newborn's defences, infection and sepsis result. Neonatal sepsis is the presence of bacterial, fungal, or viral microorganisms or their toxins in blood or other tissues. Infections that have an onset within the first month of life are termed *newborn infections*. Exposure to a pathogenic organism, whether a virus, fungus, or bacteria, occurs, and it enters the newborn's body and begins to multiply.

Newborn infections are usually grouped into three classes according to their time of onset: congenital infection, acquired in utero (intrauterine infections) by vertical transmission with onset before birth; early-onset infections, acquired by vertical transmission in the perinatal period, either shortly before or during birth; and late-onset infections, acquired by horizontal transmission in the nursery. About 85% of neonatal infections have their onset in the first 2 days of life and usually are pneumonia and meningitis (Deleon, Shattuck, & Jain, 2015). Comparison Chart 24.2 compares the three classes of newborn infections.

Early-onset neonatal infections (<72 hours) are associated with acquisition of microorganisms from the mother. Transplacental infection or an ascending infection from the cervix may be caused by organisms that colonize in the mother's genitourinary tract, with acquisition of the microbe by passage through a colonized birth canal at delivery. The microorganisms most commonly associated with early-onset infection include group B *Streptococcus* (GBS), *Escherichia coli,* coagulase-negative *Staphylococcus, Haemophilus influenzae,* and *Listeria monocytogenes.*

Late-onset infections (>72 hours), acquired in the postpartum period, are primarily through horizontal transmission from family members or caregivers or through environmental exposures. Infections such as human immunodeficiency virus (HIV) and CMV can be acquired through breastfeeding (discussed in more

COMPARISON CHART 24.2	INTRAUTERINE VERSUS EARLY-ONSET VERSUS LATE-ONSET NEWBORN INFECTIONS		
	Intrauterine (Congenital)	**Early-Onset Infections**	**Late-Onset Infections**
Risk factors	• Immature immune system IgM, IgA, and T lymphocytes • Decreased gastric acid, which is needed to reduce organisms	• Prolonged rupture of membranes • Urinary tract infections • Preterm labour • Prolonged or difficult labour • Maternal fever • Colonization with group B streptococci • Maternal infections	• Low birth weight • Prematurity • Meconium staining • Need for resuscitation • Birth asphyxia • Improper handwashing
Common causative organisms	• Cytomegalovirus • Rubella • Toxoplasmosis • Syphilis	• *Escherichia coli* • Group B streptococci • *Klebsiella pneumoniae* • *Listeria monocytogenes* • Other enteric gram-negative bacilli	• *Candida albicans* • Coagulase-negative staphylococci • *Staphylococcus aureus* • *E. coli* • *Enterobacter* • *Klebsiella* • *Serratia* • *Pseudomonas* • Group B streptococci
Mechanism of infection	• Organism crossing placenta into fetal circulatory system; organism residing in amniotic fluid • Ascent of organism via the vagina, ultimately infecting membranes and causing rupture and leading to respiratory and gastrointestinal tract infections	• Most occur during birthing process when newborn comes into contact with infected birth canal (newborn cannot defend against host organisms) • Newborn susceptibility to infection by exogenous organisms possibly due to inadequacy of physical barriers (thin, friable skin with little subcutaneous tissue) • Lack of gastric acidity, possibly resulting in easy colonization by environmental organisms • Aspiration of microorganisms during birth with development of pneumonia	More common in newborns undergoing invasive procedures such as endotracheal intubation or catheter insertion; break in skin or mucosal protection barrier

Adapted from Anderson-Berry, A. L., Bellig, L. L., & Ohning, B. L. (2015). *Neonatal sepsis.* Retrieved from http://emedicine. medscape.com/article/978352-overview; Molyneux, E., & Gest, A. (2015). Neonatal sepsis: An old issue needing new answers. *The Lancet Infectious Diseases, 15*(5), 503–505; and Gardner, S. L., Carter, B. S., Enzman-Hines, M., & Hernandez, J. A. (2016). *Merenstein & Gardner's handbook of neonatal intensive care* (8th ed.). St. Louis, MO: Mosby Elsevier.

detail in Chapter 20) or by direct contact with family members or health care providers. These types of contacts and exposures are especially important in infants, primarily preterm, with prolonged hospital stays, where they are more likely to be exposed to multidrug-resistant hospital-associated organisms potentially from contact with caregivers or contaminated equipment. Organisms that cause late-onset sepsis include *Staphylococcus aureus, E. coli, Klebsiella, Pseudomonas, Enterobacter, Candida,* and *Anaerobes* (Mukhopadhyay & Puopolo, 2015).

Nursing Assessment

Diagnosis of neonatal infections is challenging. Most infants will have some risk factors and the presenting symptoms are many and nonspecific, including poor feeding, breathing difficulty, apneas and bradycardia, gastrointestinal problems, increased oxygen requirement, desaturations, hypoglycemia, or ventilator support needs, lethargy or hypotension, decreased or elevated temperature, unusual skin rash or colour change, persistent crying, or irritability, decreased muscle tone. Adding to the challenge of correctly identifying the infection, the list of conditions to consider in the differential diagnosis is extensive, including metabolic and congenital abnormalities (Bengtsson, van Houten, & Oster, 2015).

Nursing assessment focuses on early identification of a newborn at risk for infection to allow for prompt treatment, thus reducing mortality and morbidity. Be aware of the myriad risk factors associated with newborn sepsis. Among the factors that contribute to the newborn's overall vulnerability to infection are poor skin integrity, invasive procedures, exposure to numerous caregivers, and an environment conducive to bacterial colonization (Green, 2016).

Few newborn infections are easy to recognize because manifestations usually are nonspecific. Early symptoms can be vague because of the newborn's inability to mount an inflammatory response. Often, the observation is that the newborn does not "look right." Assess the newborn for common nonspecific signs of infection, including:

- Temperature instability
- Hypotension
- Tachycardia, bradycardia
- Pallor or duskiness, mottled skin colour
- Hypotonia
- Cyanosis
- Poor weight gain
- Irritability
- Seizures
- Rash
- Petechiae
- Jaundice

- Grunting
- Nasal flaring
- Increased oxygen demands and desaturations
- Apnea
- Lethargy
- Hypoglycemia
- Poor feeding (lack of interest in feeding)
- Abdominal distention (Gardner et al., 2016)

Since infection can be confused with other newborn conditions, laboratory and radiographic tests are needed to confirm the presence of infection. Be prepared to coordinate the timing of the various tests and assist as necessary.

Evaluate the complete blood count with a differential to identify anemia, leukocytosis, or leukopenia. Elevated C-reactive protein levels may indicate inflammation. As ordered, obtain x-rays of the chest and abdomen, which may reveal infectious processes located there. Blood, cerebrospinal fluid, and urine cultures are indicated to identify the location and type of infection present. Positive cultures confirm that the newborn has an infection. Initially, treatment is with ampicillin plus either gentamicin or cefotaxime, then narrowed down to organism-specific drugs as soon as the cultures identify the specific organism. This practice of empirically treating at-risk neonates leads to potentially harmful exposure for many uninfected infants, but in the absence of accurate rapid diagnostic tests, it is prudent to be safe (Oliver, Reagan, Slaughter, & Buhimschi, 2015).

Nursing Management

To enhance the newborn's chance of survival, early recognition and diagnosis are essential. Often the diagnosis of sepsis is based on a suspicious clinical picture. Antibiotic therapy is usually started before the laboratory results identify the infecting pathogen. Along with antibiotic therapy, circulatory, respiratory, nutritional, and developmental support is important. Antibiotic therapy is continued for 7 to 21 days if cultures are positive, or it is discontinued within 72 hours if cultures are negative. With the use of antibiotics along with early recognition and supportive care, mortality and morbidity rates have been reduced greatly.

Nurses possess the education and assessment tools to decrease the incidence of and reduce the impact of infections on affected individuals (see Chapter 20 for additional information) and their newborns. Implement measures for prevention and early recognition, including:

- Formulate a sepsis prevention plan that includes education of all members of the health care team on identification and treatment of sepsis.
- Maintain medical and surgical asepsis for all providing care.

- Screen all newborns daily for signs of sepsis.
- Monitor sepsis cases and outcomes to reinforce continued quality-improvement measures or to modify current practices.
- Outline and carry out measures to prevent hospital-acquired infections, such as:
  - Thorough handwashing hygiene for all staff
  - Monitor and support nutritional status
  - Frequent oral care and inspections of mucous membranes
  - Proper positioning and turning to prevent skin breakdown
  - Use of strict aseptic technique for all wound care, peripheral and central IV lines, blood work, and other invasive procedures
  - Frequent monitoring of invasive catheter sites for signs of infection
  - Follow infection control precautions and isolations as indicated
- Identify newborns at risk for sepsis by reviewing risk factors.
- Monitor vital sign changes and observe for subtle signs of infection.
- Monitor for signs of organ system dysfunction:
  - Cardiovascular compromise—tachycardia and hypotension
  - Respiratory compromise—respiratory distress and tachypnea
  - Renal compromise—oliguria or anuria
  - Systemic compromise—abnormal blood values
- Provide comprehensive sepsis treatment:
  - Circulatory support with fluids and vasopressors
  - Supplemental oxygen and invasive and noninvasive mechanical ventilation and other modalities of respiratory support
  - Obtaining culture samples, complete blood count, and CRP as requested
  - Antibiotic administration as ordered, observing for side effects
- Promote newborn comfort and pain management measures.
- Assess the family's educational needs and providing instructions as necessary.

Perinatal infections continue to be a public health problem, with severe consequences for those affected. By promoting a better understanding of newborn infections and appropriate use of therapies, nurses can lower the mortality rates associated with severe sepsis, especially with appropriate timing of interventions. The potential for nursing interventions to identify, prevent, and minimize the risk for sepsis is significant. Primary disease prevention must be a major focus for nurses. Family education plays a key role in the prevention of perinatal infections, in addition to following accepted practices in immunization.

CONGENITAL CONDITIONS

The human and economic toll of birth defects is significant and tragic. Each year an estimated 8 million children—6% of the total births globally—are born with a serious birth defect. Approximately 120,000 infants are born with a birth defect in the United States (March of Dimes, 2018b). Congenital conditions can arise from many etiologies, including single-gene disorders, chromosome aberrations, exposure to teratogens, and many sporadic conditions of unknown cause. Congenital conditions may be inherited or sporadic, isolated or multiple, apparent or hidden, gross or microscopic. They cause nearly half of all deaths in term newborns and cause long-term sequelae for many. The incidence varies according to the type of defect. When a serious anomaly is identified prenatally, the parents can decide whether or not to continue the pregnancy. When an anomaly is identified at or after birth, parents need to be informed promptly and given a realistic appraisal of the severity of the condition, the prognosis, and treatment options so that they can participate in all decisions pertaining to their child.

Congenital conditions can affect virtually any body system. This chapter describes common congenital conditions identified at or after birth. Some of these conditions warrant immediate treatment soon after birth. Other conditions, although identified in the newborn period, are long term with ongoing effects into childhood.

Ultimately, surveillance and research activities are translated into concrete strategies to prevent birth defects. Health Canada (2018) recommends that all women of childbearing age consume 400 micrograms (400 mcg or 0.4 mg) of folic acid daily to reduce the risk (up to 70%) of having a pregnancy affected by a **neural tube defect (NTD)** such as spina bifida and anencephaly. All women between 15 and 45 years of age should consume folic acid daily because half of pregnancies are unplanned and birth defects occur very early in pregnancy (3 to 4 weeks after conception), before most women know they are pregnant. This has spurred prevention activities at local and national levels to promote the folic acid message (CDC, 2018b).

Becoming a parent for most people implies a transition to something new and unknown in life. If the infant is born with a congenital defect, it is a very traumatic and challenging period for this overwhelmed family. In order to provide the best management for the infant and the family, guidelines based on scientific findings and recommendations should be followed. Nurses need to actively involve the parents/partners/significant others in the decision-making process, treatment options, and care of their infant in order to increase attachment and bonding.

Esophageal Atresia and Tracheoesophageal Fistula

Esophageal atresia and tracheoesophageal fistula are gastrointestinal anomalies in which the esophagus and trachea do not separate normally during embryonic development. Esophageal atresia refers to a congenitally interrupted esophagus where the proximal and distal ends do not communicate; the upper esophageal segment ends in a blind pouch and the lower segment ends a variable distance above the diaphragm (Fig. 24.8).

Tracheoesophageal fistula is an abnormal communication between the trachea and esophagus. When associated with esophageal atresia, the fistula most commonly occurs between the distal esophageal segment and the trachea. The incidence of esophageal atresia is 1 per 3,000 to 4,500 live births. The etiology has been attributed to genetic factors, infections, and teratogens, but in most cases, no cause is identifiable (Tewfik, Karsan, & Laberge, 2017).

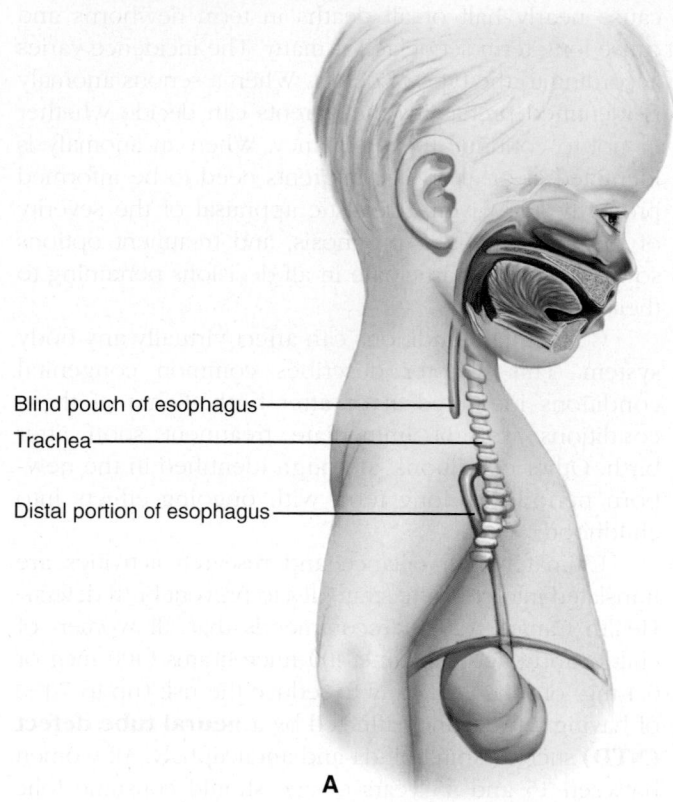

Blind pouch of esophagus ⎯⎯⎯

Trachea ⎯⎯⎯

Distal portion of esophagus ⎯⎯⎯

A

B   **C**   **D**

FIGURE 24.8 Esophageal atresia and tracheoesophageal fistula. **A.** The most common type of esophageal atresia, in which the esophagus ends in a blind pouch and a fistula connects the trachea with the distal portion of the esophagus. **B.** The upper and distal portions of the esophagus end in a blind pouch. **C.** The esophagus is one segment, but a portion of it is narrowed. **D.** The upper portion of the esophagus connects to the trachea.

Pathophysiology

Several types of esophageal atresia exist, but the most common anomaly is a fistula between the distal esophagus and the trachea, which occurs in 90% of newborns with an esophageal defect. Esophageal atresia and tracheoesophageal fistula are thought to be the result of incomplete separation of the lung bed from the foregut during early fetal development. A large percentage of these newborns have other congenital anomalies involving the vertebra, kidneys, heart, and musculoskeletal and gastrointestinal systems (Kliegman et al., 2015); most have several anomalies.

Nursing Assessment

Review the maternal history for polyhydramnios. Often this is the first sign of esophageal atresia because the fetus cannot swallow and absorb amniotic fluid in utero, leading to accumulation. Soon after birth, the newborn may exhibit copious, frothy bubbles of mucus in the mouth and nose, accompanied by drooling. Abdominal distention develops as air builds up in the stomach. In esophageal atresia, a gastric tube cannot be inserted beyond a certain point because the esophagus ends in a blind pouch. The newborn may have rattling respirations, excessive salivation, and drooling, and "the three Cs" (coughing, choking, and cyanosis) if feeding is attempted. The presence of a fistula increases the risk of respiratory complications such as pneumonitis and atelectasis due to aspiration of food and secretions (Gardner et al., 2016).

Take Note!

The "three Cs" of choking, coughing, and cyanosis in conjunction with feeding are considered the classic signs of tracheoesophageal fistula and atresia.

Prepare the newborn and parents for radiographic evaluation. Diagnosis is made by x-ray or an ultrasound or MRI, which will demonstrate a gastric tube coiled in the upper esophageal pouch, and air in the gastrointestinal tract indicates the presence of a fistula (Mattson & Smith, 2015). Once a diagnosis of esophageal atresia is established, begin preparations for surgery if the newborn is stable.

Nursing Management

Nursing management focuses on preparing the newborn and parents for surgery and providing meticulous postoperative care.

PROVIDING PREOPERATIVE CARE

Preoperative nursing interventions include the following measures:

- Initiate nothing by mouth (NPO) status.
- Elevate the head of the bed 30 to 45 degrees to prevent reflux and aspiration.
- Monitor hydration status and fluid and electrolyte balance; administer and monitor parenteral IV fluid infusions.
- Assess and maintain the patency of the orogastric tube; monitor the functioning of the tube, which is attached to low continuous suction; and avoid irrigation of the tube to prevent aspiration.
- Have oxygen and suctioning equipment readily available should the newborn experience respiratory distress.
- Assist with diagnostic studies to rule out other anomalies.
- Use comfort measures to minimize crying and prevent respiratory distress; provide nonnutritive sucking.
- Inform the parents about the rationales for the aspiration prevention measures.
- Document frequent observations of the newborn's condition (Kenner & Lott, 2014).

PROVIDING POSTOPERATIVE CARE

Surgery consists of closing the fistula and joining the two esophageal segments. Postoperative care involves closely observing all of the newborn's body systems to identify any complications. Expect to administer TPN and antibiotics until the esophageal anastomosis is proven intact and patent. Then begin oral feedings, usually within a week after surgery (Mahoney & Rosen, 2016). Keep the parents informed of their newborn's condition and progress. Closely assess the newborn during feeding and report any difficulty with swallowing. Provide parent teaching. Demonstrate and reinforce all teaching prior to discharge.

Omphalocele and Gastroschisis

Omphalocele and gastroschisis are congenital anomalies of the anterior abdominal wall at or near the umbilicus. Fetal abdominal wall defects result from disturbances in organogenesis during the early embryonic period. Gastroschisis occurs in 1 in 2,000 live births, while omphalocele occurs in 1 in 4,000 live births (Wagner & Lee, 2015). An **omphalocele** is a defect of the umbilical ring that allows evisceration of the abdominal contents into an external peritoneal sac. Defects vary in size; they may be limited to bowel loops or may include the entire gastrointestinal tract and liver (Fig. 24.9). Bowel malrotation is common, but the displaced organs are usually normal. Omphaloceles are associated with an abnormal karyotype or genetic syndrome in more than 50% of the cases (Stephenson, Lockwood, & MacKenzie, 2018). **Omphaloceles** are associated with other anomalies in more than 70% of the cases. This anomaly is usually detected during routine prenatal ultrasound of the fetus or during

FIGURE 24.9 Omphalocele in a newborn. Note the large, protruding sac.

investigation of an increased α-fetoprotein level (Glasser, 2017).

Gastroschisis is a herniation of the abdominal contents through an abdominal wall defect, at the umbilicus. Gastroschisis differs from omphalocele in that there is no peritoneal sac protecting the herniated organs, and thus exposure to amniotic fluid makes them thickened, edematous, and inflamed (Stephenson, Lockwood, & MacKenzie, 2019). Gastroschisis is associated with significant newborn mortality and morbidity rates. Despite surgical correction, feeding intolerance, failure to thrive, and prolonged hospital stays occur in nearly all newborns with this anomaly (Verklan & Walden, 2015).

Each of these diagnoses requires that a pediatric surgeon be available at delivery to determine the extent of the defect and complications.

Nursing Assessment

Abdominal wall defects are readily diagnosed by prenatal ultrasound, which is helpful in planning for the birth and needed therapy. An early birth may be planned if the ultrasound reveals evidence of progressive bowel distention and thickening. Review the gestational history for factors associated with high-risk pregnancies, such as illness and infection of the pregnant person, drug use, smoking, and genetic abnormalities. These factors are also associated with omphalocele and gastroschisis. They contribute to placental insufficiency and the birth of a small-for-gestational-age or preterm newborn, the populations in which both of these abdominal defects most commonly occur. The incidence of omphalocele is 1 case in 4,000 births and gastroschisis is 1 in 2,000 births (Glasser, 2017).

Omphalocele and gastroschisis are readily observed. Note the appearance of the protrusion on the abdomen and evidence of a sac. Inspect the sac closely for the presence of organs, most commonly the intestines but sometimes the liver. Also inspect the contents for any twisting of the intestines. Note the colour of the organs within the sac and measure the size of the omphalocele.

Also perform a complete physical examination of the newborn. Typically these congenital conditions are associated with other congenital anomalies, such as those involving the cardiovascular, genitourinary, and central nervous systems.

Assessment findings summary of omphalocele and gastroschisis:

- Usually detected on prenatal ultrasound examinations
- Eviscerated bowel without peritoneal covering—gastroschisis
- Eviscerated bowel with peritoneal covering—omphalocele
- Search for additional anomalies if omphalocele is diagnosed

Nursing Management

Nursing management of newborns with omphalocele or gastroschisis focuses on preventing hypothermia, maintaining perfusion to the eviscerated abdominal contents by minimizing fluid loss, and protecting the exposed abdominal contents from trauma and infection. These objectives can be accomplished by placing the infant in a sterile drawstring bowel bag that maintains a sterile environment for the exposed contents, allows visualization, reduces heat and moisture loss, and allows heat from radiant warmers to reach the infant. The infant is placed feet-first into the bag and the drawstring is secured around the torso (Mattson & Smith, 2015). Carefully handle the defect utilizing strict sterile technique to prevent contamination of the exposed abdominal contents as well as traumatic damage (Glasser, 2017).

An orogastric tube attached to low suction is used to prevent intestinal distention. IV therapy is administered to maintain fluid and electrolyte balance and provide a route for antibiotic therapy. Monitor the newborn's fluid status frequently. Closely observe the exposed bowel for vascular compromise, such as changes in colour or a decrease in temperature, and report these immediately.

PROVIDING POSTOPERATIVE CARE

Surgical repair of both defects occurs after initial stabilization and comprehensive evaluation for any other anomalies. It may have to occur in stages, depending on the defect (Box 24.5).

Postoperative care involves providing pain management, monitoring respiratory and cardiac status, monitoring intake and output, assessing for vascular

BOX 24.5

SURGERY TO REPAIR OMPHALOCELE AND GASTROSCHISIS

Surgical repair of gastroschisis is an emergency due to the high risk of intestinal atresia, resulting in obstruction. Primary repair of gastroschisis is usually performed without incident, unless the contents are unable to fit into the abdominal cavity. This occurs more often with a large omphalocele, requiring the surgeon to do a staged closure. This involves covering the defect with a synthetic material that is sequentially squeezed like toothpaste to reduce the defect into the abdominal cavity. After enough of the defect is in the abdominal cavity, a surgical repair is then performed (Glasser, 2017). If damage to the exposed organs occurs, such as necrosis, then the necrotic sections are removed during the repair. If a significant amount of small intestine is lost, then the complication of short bowel syndrome may occur.

compromise, maintaining the orogastric tube to suction, documenting the amount and colour of drainage, and administering ordered medications and treatments (Gardner et al., 2016). Also be alert for complications, such as short bowel syndrome (see Chapter 42 for additional information).

PROMOTING PARENT–NEWBORN INTERACTION

The parents need continued support and progress reports on their newborn. They may be distraught at the sight of the anomaly, and they may be frightened to touch their newborn. Encourage the parents to touch the newborn

and participate in care as much as possible. Because of the nature of this defect, bonding opportunities will be limited initially. However, strongly encourage frequent visiting. In addition, provide information to the parents about the defect, treatment modalities, and prognosis. After surgery, instruct the parents in care measures and provide them with home care instructions. Anticipate the need for a referral to a home health care agency and community resources for support.

Anorectal Malformations

An imperforate anus is a gastrointestinal system malformation of the anorectal opening and is identified in the newborn period. The rectum may end in a blind pouch that does not connect to the colon, or it may have fistulas (openings) between the rectum and the perineum (the vagina in girls or the urethra in boys) (Fig. 24.10). The malformations occur during early fetal development and may be associated with numerous other congenital anomalies (Rosen, 2016) in other body systems. Refer to Box 24.6 for anomalies associated with anorectal malformations.

Imperforate anus occurs in about 1 of every 3,500 live births (Malcolm, 2015). The defect can be further classified as a high or low type, depending on its level. The level significantly influences the outcome in terms of fecal continence as well as management (Fanaroff & Fanaroff, 2014).

Surgical intervention is needed for both high and low types of imperforate anus. Surgery for a high type of defect involves a colostomy in the newborn period,

FIGURE 24.10 Image **A** shows an imperforate anus, in which the rectum ends in a blind pouch. Image **B** shows an imperforate anus without fistula. The visible meconium streak along the raphe is consistent with a low imperforate anus. (Courtesy of Kevin P. Lally, MD.)

ANOMALIES ASSOCIATED WITH ANORECTAL MALFORMATIONS

VACTERL syndrome: vertebral, anorectal, cardiovascular, tracheoesophageal, renal, and limb
Esophageal atresia
Intestinal atresia
Bowel malrotation
Renal agenesis
Hypospadias
Vesicoureteral reflux
Bladder exstrophy
Cardiac anomalies
Skeletal anomalies

with corrective surgery performed in stages to allow for growth. Surgery for the low type of anomaly, which frequently includes a fistula, involves closure of the fistula, creation of an anal opening, and repositioning of the rectal pouch into the anal opening. A major challenge for either type of surgical repair is finding, using, or creating adequate nerve and muscle structures around the rectum to provide for normal evacuation (Malcolm, 2015).

Nursing Assessment

In the newborn, observe for an appropriate anal opening. If the anal opening exists, observe for passage of meconium stool within the first 24 hours of life. Assess urine output to identify genitourinary problems. For the newborn with an imperforate anus, inspection of the perineal area would reveal absence of the usual opening. In addition, meconium generally is not passed or present within 24 hours of birth.

In the infant with suspected imperforate anus, assess for common signs of intestinal obstruction, which may occur as a result of the malformation. These include abdominal distention and bilious vomiting.

Prepare the newborn and family for a perineal ultrasound and an abdominal x-ray that will be ordered to identify the level of defect in the absence of a perineal fistula and also to assess for complications associated with imperforate anus.

Nursing Management

Nursing management focuses on preparing the newborn and parent for surgery and providing postoperative care. Preoperatively, maintain the newborn's NPO status and provide gastric decompression. Administer IV therapy and antibiotic therapy as ordered and monitor the newborn's hydration status. Provide a full explanation of the defect, surgical options, potential complications, typical postoperative course, and long-term care needed to the parents. Make sure they are aware of the available treatment modalities. Prepare them for the possibility that the newborn may require an ostomy. Provide support to the parents and family.

Postoperative care includes ensuring adequate pain relief, maintaining NPO status and gastric decompression until normal bowel function is restored, and providing colostomy care if applicable. Refer to Chapter 42 for additional information related to ostomy care and postoperative care for children undergoing an intestinal pull-through procedure.

Bladder Exstrophy

In classic bladder exstrophy, a midline closure defect occurs during the embryonic period of gestation, leaving the bladder open and exposed outside of the abdomen. The incidence is 1 in 40,000 live births, and happens in males slightly more than females (Glasser, 2017). The bony pelvis may also be malformed, resulting in an opening in the pelvic arch. Bladder exstrophy may be diagnosed by prenatal ultrasound. Complications include UTI from ascending organisms. Treatment of bladder exstrophy involves surgical repair (Fig. 24.11).

FIGURE 24.11 Bladder exstrophy. **A.** Before surgical repair. **B.** After surgery.

Nursing Assessment

On physical examination of the infant or child, note the red appearance to the bladder seen on the abdominal wall. Draining urine will be visible. Note excoriation of abdominal skin around the bladder resulting from contact with urine. A malformed urethra may be present in females, whereas males may have an unformed or malformed penis or a normal penis with an epispadias.

Nursing Management

Nursing management consists of identifying the genitourinary defect at birth so immediate treatment can be initiated, preventing infection and skin breakdown, providing postoperative care, and catheterizing the stoma.

PREVENTING INFECTION AND SKIN BREAKDOWN

Bladder exstrophy requires surgical repair. In the preoperative period, care is focused on protecting the exstrophied bladder and preventing infection. Keep the infant in a supine position; keep the bladder moist and cover it with a sterile plastic bag. Change soiled diapers immediately to prevent contamination of the bladder with feces. Sponge-bathe the infant rather than immersing him or her in water to prevent pathogens in the bath water from entering the bladder. Prevent breakdown of the surrounding abdominal skin by applying protective barrier creams. In some instances it may be necessary to consult the ostomy nurse for further advice (see Chapter 43 for more information).

NURSING CARE PLAN 24.1

Overview of an Infant of a Diabetic Mother

Jamie, a 38-year-old Hispanic woman, gave birth to a term large-for-gestational-age newborn weighing 10 lb. She had a history of gestational diabetes but had not received any prenatal care. She arrived at the hospital in active labour. Despite macrosomia, the newborn's Apgar scores were 8 and 9 at 1 and 5 minutes, respectively. No resuscitative measures were needed.

One hour after birth, assessment revealed a pale, irritable newborn with sweating and several episodes of apnea. A glucose level obtained at this time via a heel stick was 1.7 mmol/L. Two hours later, the newborn begins exhibiting signs of respiratory distress—grunting, nasal flaring, retractions, tachypnea (respiratory rate 72 breaths/min), and tachycardia (heart rate 176 bpm).

NURSING DIAGNOSIS: Risk for unstable blood glucose level related to hypoglycemia secondary to intrauterine state of *hyperinsulinemia* resulting from maternal gestational diabetes as evidenced by low blood glucose level, irritability, pallor, sweating, and apnea.

Outcome Identification and Evaluation

The newborn will exhibit adequate glucose control as evidenced by maintaining blood glucose levels above 2.6 mmol/L and an absence of clinical signs of hypoglycemia.

Interventions: *Promoting Glucose Control*

- Monitor blood glucose levels at 2 hours of life and then every 3 to 6 hours before feeding or as necessary *to detect hypoglycemia, which would be <2.6 mmol/L.*
- Continue to observe for manifestations of hypoglycemia, such as pallor, tremors, jitteriness, lethargy, and poor feeding, *to allow for early detection and prompt intervention, thereby minimizing the risk of complications associated with hypoglycemia.*
- Monitor temperature frequently and institute measures to maintain a neutral thermal environment *to prevent cold stress, which would increase metabolic demands and further deplete glycogen stores.*
- Initiate early feedings every 2 to 3 hours or as appropriate or administer glucose supplements as ordered

to prevent hypoglycemia caused by the newborn's hyperinsulin state. Administer IV glucose infusions as ordered *to correct hypoglycemia if glucose levels do not stabilize with feeding.*
- Cluster infant care activities and provide for rest periods *to conserve the newborn's energy and reduce use of glucose and glycogen stores.*
- Reduce environmental stimuli by dimming lights and speaking softly *to reduce energy demands and further utilization of glucose.*
- Explain all events and procedures to the mother *to help alleviate anxiety and promote understanding of the newborn's condition.*

(continued)

NURSING CARE PLAN 24.1

Overview of an Infant of a Diabetic Mother (continued)

NURSING DIAGNOSIS: Impaired gas exchange related to respiratory distress secondary to delayed lung maturity resulting from inhibition of pulmonary surfactant production due to fetal hyperinsulinemia as evidenced by grunting, nasal flaring, retractions, tachypnea, and tachycardia.

Outcome Identification and Evaluation

Newborn will demonstrate signs of adequate oxygenation without respiratory distress as evidenced by respiratory rate and vital signs within acceptable parameters, absence of nasal flaring, retractions, and grunting, and oxygen saturation and arterial blood gas levels within acceptable parameters.

Interventions: *Promoting Oxygenation*

- Monitor newborn's vital signs to establish a baseline and evaluate for changes.
- Assess airway patency and perform gentle suctioning as ordered to ensure patency and allow for adequate oxygen intake.
- Position the newborn prone to optimize respiratory status and reduce stress.
- Assess lung sounds for changes to allow early detection of change in status.
- Continuously monitor oxygen saturation levels via pulse oximetry to determine adequacy of tissue perfusion.
- Assess arterial blood gas results to detect changes indicating acidosis, hypoxemia, or hypercarbia, which would suggest hypoxia. Administer medications as ordered to correct acidosis.
- Administer oxygen as ordered to promote adequate tissue perfusion.
- Assess newborn's skin to identify cyanosis, pallor, and mottling to detect changes indicating compromised oxygenation.
- Administer surfactant replacement therapy as ordered to aid in stabilizing the newborn's lungs until postnatal surfactant synthesis improves.
- Institute measures to maintain normal blood glucose levels and a neutral thermal environment, cluster care activities, and reduce excessive stimuli to reduce oxygen demand and consumption.

KEY CONCEPTS

- Asphyxia, the most common clinical insult in the perinatal period, results in brain injury and may lead to mental retardation, cerebral palsy, or seizures.

- TTN occurs when the liquid in the lung is removed slowly or incompletely.

- Common risk factors for respiratory distress syndrome (RDS) include young gestational age, perinatal asphyxia regardless of gestational age, caesarean birth in the absence of labour (related to the lack of thoracic squeeze), male gender, and maternal diabetes.

- Meconium aspiration has three major pulmonary effects: airway obstruction, surfactant dysfunction, and chemical pneumonitis.

- The management of PPHN requires meticulous attention to detail, with continuous monitoring of oxygenation, blood pressure, and perfusion.

- Intraventricular hemorrhage is bleeding that usually originates in the subependymal germinal matrix region of the brain with extension into the ventricular system.

- Necrotizing enterocolitis (NEC) is a serious gastrointestinal disease of unknown etiology in newborns that can result in necrosis of a segment of the bowel.

○ Infants born to a diabetic parent are at risk for malformations most frequently involving the cardiovascular, skeletal, central nervous, gastrointestinal, and genitourinary systems; cardiac anomalies are the most common.

○ Factors that place the newborn at risk for birth trauma include cephalopelvic disproportion, maternal pelvic anomalies, oligohydramnios, prolonged or rapid labour, abnormal presentation, fetal prematurity, fetal macrosomia, and fetal abnormalities.

○ Exposure to illicit or recreational drugs during pregnancy expose the fetus and newborn to the possibility of intrauterine growth restriction, prematurity, neurobehavioural and neurophysiologic dysfunction, birth defects, infections, and long-term developmental sequelae.

○ Newborns who were exposed to tobacco, illicit substances, caffeine, and alcohol in utero can exhibit withdrawal behaviour.

○ Physiologic jaundice is a common, normal newborn phenomenon that appears during the second or third day of life and then declines over the first week after birth. Pathologic jaundice is manifested within the first 24 hours of life when total bilirubin levels increase by more than 5 mg/dL/day and the total serum bilirubin level is higher than 17 mg/dL in a full-term infant.

○ Newborn infections are usually classified according to the time of onset and grouped into three categories: congenital infection, acquired in utero by vertical transmission with onset before birth; early-onset neonatal infections, acquired by vertical transmission in the perinatal period, either shortly before or during birth; and late-onset neonatal infections, acquired by horizontal transmission in the nursery.

○ Congenital conditions can arise from many etiologies including single-gene disorders, chromosome aberrations, exposure to teratogens, and many sporadic conditions of unknown cause. Congenital structural anomalies may be inherited or sporadic, isolated or multiple, apparent or hidden, and gross or microscopic.

○ Esophageal atresia refers to a congenitally interrupted esophagus where the proximal and distal ends do not communicate; the upper esophageal segment ends in a blind pouch and the lower segment ends a variable distance above the diaphragm. Tracheoesophageal fistula is an abnormal communication between the trachea and esophagus.

○ Omphalocele and gastroschisis are congenital anomalies of the anterior abdominal wall. An omphalocele is a defect of the umbilical ring that allows evisceration of abdominal contents into an external peritoneal sac. Gastroschisis is a herniation of abdominal contents through an abdominal wall defect, usually to the left or right of the umbilicus.

REFERENCES AND RECOMMENDED READINGS

American Academy of Pediatrics (AAP). (2012). Breastfeeding and the use of human milk. *Pediatrics, 129*(3), e827–e841.

Anderson-Berry, A. L., Bellig, L. L., & Ohning, B. L. (2015). *Neonatal sepsis.* Retrieved from http://emedicine.medscape.com/article/978352-overview

Annibale, D. J., & Hill, J. G. (2018). *Intraventricular hemorrhage in the preterm infant. eMedicine.* Retrieved from https://emedicine.medscape.com/article/976654-overview

Artigas, V. (2015). Management of neonatal abstinence syndrome in the newborn nursery. *Nursing for Women's Health, 18*(6), 509–514.

Aziz, K., Dancey, P., & Canadian Paediatric Society, Fetus and Newborn Committee. (2018). *Position statement: Screening guidelines for newborns at risk for low blood glucose.* Retrieved from https://www.cps.ca/en/documents/position/newborns-low-blood-glucose

Bengtsson, B. O. S., van Houten, J. P., & Oster, H. A. (2015). Index of suspicion in the nursery. *NeoReviews, 16*(2), e120–e122.

Blackburn, S. T. (2012). *Maternal, fetal and neonatal physiology: A clinical perspective* (4th ed.). St. Louis, MO: Saunders Elsevier.

Blennow, M., & Bohlin, K. (2015). Surfactant and noninvasive ventilation. *Neonatology, 107*(4), 330–336.

Canadian Paediatric Society (CPS) & American Heart Association (AHA). (2016). *Textbook of neonatal resuscitation* (7th ed.). Ottawa: Canadian Paediatric Society.

Canadian Paediatric Society (CPS). (2017). *Position statement: Recommendations for neonatal surfactant therapy.* Retrieved from https://www.cps.ca/en/documents/position/neonatal-surfactant-therapy

Canadian Paediatric Society (CPS). (2018a). *Position statement: Fetal alcohol syndrome.* Retrieved from https://www.cps.ca/en/documents/position/fetal-alcohol-syndrome

Canadian Paediatric Society (CPS). (2018b). *Position statement: Guidelines for detection, management and prevention of hyperbilirubinemia in term and late preterm newborn infants.* Retrieved from https://www.cps.ca/en/documents/position/hyperbilirubinemia-newborn

Centers for Disease Control and Prevention (CDC). (2018a). *Fetal alcohol spectrum disorders (FASDs).* Retrieved from http://www.cdc.gov/ncbddd/fasd/facts.html

Centers for Disease Control and Prevention (CDC). (2018b). *Recommendations: Women & folic acid.* Retrieved from http://www.cdc.gov/ncbddd/folicacid/recommendations.html

Choi, W., Jeong, H., Choi, S. J., Oh, S. Y., Kim, J. S., Roh, C. R., & Kim, J. H. (2015). Risk factors differentiating mild/moderate from severe meconium aspiration syndrome in meconium-stained neonates. *Obstetrics & Gynecology Science, 58*(1), 24–31.

Cook, J. L., Green, C. R., Lilley, C. M., Anderson, S. M., Baldwin, M. E., Chudley, A. E., ... Rosales, T. (2016). Fetal alcohol spectrum disorder: A guideline for diagnosis across the lifespan. *Canadian Medical Association Journal, 188*(3), 191–197. Retrieved from http://www.cmaj.ca/content/cmaj/188/3/191.full.pdf

Cunningham, F. G., Leveno, K. J., Bloom, S. L., Spong, C. Y., Dashe, J. S., Hoffman, B. L., . . . Sheffield, J. S. (2014). *Williams obstetrics* (24th ed.). New York: McGraw-Hill.

Deleon, C., Shattuck, K., & Jain, S. K. (2015). Biomarkers of neonatal sepsis. *NeoReviews, 16*(5), e297–e308.

Deshpande, P. G., & Wagle, S. (2017). Breast milk jaundice. *eMedicine.* Retrieved from http://emedicine.medscape.com/article/973629-overview

de Vries, L. S., & Leijser, L. M. (2019). Germinal matrix hemorrhage and intraventricular hemorrhage (GMH-IVH) in the newborn: Prevention, management, and complications. *UpToDate.* Retrieved from https://www.uptodate.com/contents/germinal-matrix-hemorrhage-and-intraventricular-hemorrhage-gmh-ivh-in-the-newborn-prevention-management-and-complications

Fanaroff, A. A., & Fanaroff, J. M. (2014). *Klaus and Fanaroff's care of the high-risk neonate* (6th ed.). Philadelphia, PA: Elsevier Health Sciences.

Fox, J. R., Thacker, L. R., & Hendricks-Muñoz, K. D. (2015). Early detection tool of intestinal dysfunction: Impact on necrotizing enterocolitis severity. *American Journal of Perinatology, 32*(10), 927–932.

Garcia-Prats, J. A. (2018). Clinical features and diagnosis of meconium aspiration syndrome. *UpToDate.* Retrieved from https://www-uptodate-com.proxy.hil.unb.ca/contents/clinical-features-and-diagnosis-of-meconium-aspiration-syndrome

Gardner, S. L., Carter, B. S., Enzman-Hines, M., & Hernandez, J. A. (2016). *Merenstein & Gardner's handbook of neonatal intensive care* (8th ed.). St. Louis, MO: Mosby Elsevier.

Gaur, K. V., Nimbalkar, S. M., Desai, R., & Ganguly, B. P. (2015). Effect of single dose antenatal steroid for pregnant mothers with high risk of preterm delivery on the respiratory outcome of neonates. *Journal of Clinical Neonatology, 4*(3), 217.

Geis, G. M., & Clark, D. A. (2017). Meconium aspiration syndrome. *eMedicine.* Retrieved from http://emedicine.medscape.com/article/974110-overview

Glasser, J. G. (2017). *Pediatric omphalocele and gastroschisis. eMedicine.* Retrieved from http://emedicine.medscape.com/article/975583-overview

Green, C. J. (2016). *Maternal newborn nursing care plans* (3rd ed.). Burlington, MA: Jones & Bartlett Learning.

Hamdan, A. H. (2017). Neonatal abstinence syndrome. *eMedicine.* Retrieved from http://emedicine.medscape.com/article/978763-overview

Hansen, T. W. (2017). Neonatal jaundice. *eMedicine.* Retrieved from http://emedicine.medscape.com/article/974786-overview

Health Canada. (2015). *Nutrition for healthy term infants: Recommendations from birth to six months.* Retrieved from https://www.canada.ca/en/health-canada/services/food-nutrition/healthy-eating/infant-feeding/nutrition-healthy-term-infants-recommendations-birth-six-months.html

Health Canada. (2017). *Fetal alcohol spectrum disorder.* Retrieved from https://www.canada.ca/en/health-canada/services/healthy-living/your-health/diseases/fetal-alcohol-spectrum-disorder.html

Health Canada. (2018). *Folic acid and neural tube defects.* Retrieved from https://www.canada.ca/en/public-health/services/pregnancy/folic-acid.html

Hudak, M. L., Tan, R. C.; Committee on Drugs, Committee on Fetus and Newborn, American Academy of Pediatrics (AAP). (2012). Neonatal drug withdrawal. *Pediatrics, 129*(2), e540–e560. [Erratum in *Pediatrics.* 2014, *133*(5), 937.]

Hudson, J. (2015). Facilitating normal physiology in the presence of meconium stained liquor. *The Practicing Midwife, 18*(6), 16–19.

Huybrechts, K. F. (2015). SSRI use in late pregnancy: Small risk of PPHN. *Reactions, 1556,* 11–20.

Ives, N. K. (2015). Management of neonatal jaundice. *Pediatrics and Child Health, 25*(6), 276–281.

Jaecklin, T., Jarreau, P. H., & Kavanagh, B. P. (2015). Ventilator-associated lung injury. In P. Rimensberger. *Pediatric and neonatal mechanical ventilation* (pp. 917–945). Berlin Heidelberg: Springer Publishers.

Jansson, L. M. (2018). Neonatal abstinence syndrome. *UpToDate.* Retrieved from http://www.uptodate.com/contents/neonatal-abstinence-syndrome

Jaques, S. C., & Kennea, N. (2015). Resuscitation of the newborn. Obstetrics. *Gynecology & Reproductive Medicine, 25*(3), 61–67.

Johnson, T. J., Patel, A. L., Bigger, H. R., Engstrom, J. L., & Meier, P. P. (2015). Cost savings of human milk as a strategy to reduce the incidence of necrotizing enterocolitis in very low birth weight infants. *Neonatology, 107*(4), 271–276.

Jones, H. E., & Fielder, A. (2015). Neonatal abstinence syndrome: Historical perspective, current focus, future directions. *Preventive Medicine, 80,* 12–17.

Kenner, C., & Lott, J. W. (2014). *Comprehensive neonatal nursing care* (5th ed.). New York: Springer Publishers.

Kim, H. A., Yang, G. E., & Kim, M. J. (2015). Early neonatal respiratory morbidities in term neonates. *Neonatal Medicine, 22*(1), 8–13.

Kliegman, R. M., Stanton, B., St. Geme, J., Schor, N., & Behrman, R. E. (2015). *Nelson's textbook of pediatrics* (20th ed.). St. Louis, MO: Saunders Elsevier.

Korkmazer, E., Solak, N., & Tokgöz, V. Y. (2015). Gestational diabetes: Screening, management, timing of delivery. *Current Obstetrics and Gynecology Reports, 4*(2), 132–138.

Lauwers, J., & Swisher, A. (2016). *Counseling the nursing mother: A lactation consultant's guide* (6th ed.). Burlington, MA: Jones & Bartlett Learning.

Lee, K. G. (2017). Transient tachypnea—newborn. *MedlinePlus.* Retrieved from http://www.nlm.nih.gov/medlineplus/ency/article/007233.htm

Lim, J. C., Golden, J. M., & Ford, H. R. (2015). Pathogenesis of neonatal necrotizing enterocolitis. *Pediatric Surgery International, 31*(6), 509–518.

Lindenskov, P. H., Castellheim, A., Saugstad, O. D., & Mollnes, T. E. (2015). Meconium aspiration syndrome: Possible pathophysiological mechanisms and future potential therapies. *Neonatology, 107*(3), 225–230.

Loroia, N. (2015). Birth trauma. *eMedicine.* Retrieved from http://emedicine.medscape.com/article/980112-overview

Mahoney, L., & Rosen, R. (2016). Feeding difficulties in children with esophageal atresia. *Pediatric Respiratory Reviews, 19.* 21-27. doi: 10.1016/j.prrv.2015.06.002.

Malcolm, W. (2015). *Beyond the NICU: Comprehensive care of the high risk infant.* New York: McGraw-Hill Education.

March of Dimes. (2016). *Alcohol during pregnancy.* Retrieved from http://www.marchofdimes.org/pregnancy/alcohol-during-pregnancy.aspx

March of Dimes. (2018a). *Neonatal abstinence syndrome (NAS)*. Retrieved from http://www.marchofdimes.org/baby/neonatal-abstinence-syndrome-(nas).aspx

March of Dimes. (2018b). *Birth defects and other health conditions*. Retrieved from http://www.marchofdimes.org/baby/birth-defects.aspx

March of Dimes. (2019). *Smoking during pregnancy*. Retrieved from http://www.marchofdimes.org/pregnancy/smoking-during-pregnancy.aspx

Martin, R. (2018). *Overview of neonatal respiratory distress: Disorders of transition. UpToDate*. Retrieved from http://www.uptodate.com/contents/overview-of-neonatal-respiratory-distress-disorders-of-transition

Mattson, S., & Smith, J. E. (2015). *Core curriculum for maternal-newborn nursing* (5th ed.). St. Louis, MO: Saunders Elsevier.

Molyneux, E., & Gest, A. (2015). Neonatal sepsis: An old issue needing new answers. *The Lancet Infectious Diseases, 15*(5), 503–505.

Mukhopadhyay, S., & Puopolo, K. M. (2015). Neonatal early-onset sepsis: Epidemiology and risk assessment. *NeoReviews, 16*(4), e221–e230.

Nagtalon-Ramos, J. (2014). *Maternal-newborn nursing care: Best evidence-based practices*. Philadelphia, PA: F. A. Davis Company.

National Institute for Health and Care Excellence (NICE). (2014). *Jaundice in newborn babies under 28 days*. Retrieved from http://www.nice.org.uk/guidance/qs57/chapter/introduction

National Institute on Drug Abuse (NIDA). (2018). *Substance use while pregnant and breastfeeding*. Retrieved from http://www.drugabuse.gov/publications/research-reports/substance-use-in-women/substance-use-while-pregnant-breastfeeding

Neonatal eHandbook. (2018). *Meconium aspiration syndrome*. Retrieved from https://www2.health.vic.gov.au/hospitals-and-health-services/patient-care/perinatal-reproductive/neonatal-ehandbook/conditions/meconium-aspiration-syndrome

Noori, S., & Seri, I. (2015). Hemodynamic antecedents of peri/intraventricular hemorrhage in very preterm neonates. *Seminars in Fetal and Neonatal Medicine, 20*(4), 232–237.

Oliver, E., Reagan, P., Slaughter, J., & Buhimschi, I. (2015). Patterns of empiric antibiotic use for presumed early onset neonatal sepsis (EONS). *American Journal of Obstetrics & Gynecology, 212*(1), S384. doi: http://dx.doi.org/10.1016/j.ajog.2014.10.999

Potter, C. F., & Kicklighter, S. D. (2016). Infant of a diabetic mother. *eMedicine*. Retrieved from http://emedicine.medscape.com/article/974230-overview

Pramanik, A. K., Rangaswamy, N., & Gates, T. (2015). Neonatal respiratory distress: A practical approach to its diagnosis and management. *Pediatric Clinics of North America, 62*(2), 453–469.

Pramanik, A. K., & Rosenkrantz, T. (2015). Respiratory distress syndrome. *eMedicine*. Retrieved from http://emedicine.medscape.com/article/976034-overview

Rosen, N. G. (2016). Pediatric imperforate anus. *eMedicine*. Retrieved from http://emedicine.medscape.com/article/929904-overview

Rubarth, L. B., & Quinn, J. (2015). Respiratory development and respiratory distress syndrome. *Neonatal Network, 34*(4), 231–238.

Sachdeva, M., Murki, S., Oleti, T. P., & Kandraju, H. (2015). Intermittent versus continuous phototherapy for the treatment of neonatal non-hemolytic moderate hyperbilirubinemia in infants more than 34 weeks of gestational age: A randomized controlled trial. *European Journal of Pediatrics, 174*(2), 177–181.

Salem, L., & Singer, K. R. (2017). Rh incompatibility. *eMedicine*. Retrieved from http://emedicine.medscape.com/article/797150-overview

Smith, J. R., Donze, A., Wolf, M., Smyser, C. D., Mathur, A., & Proctor, E. K. (2015). Ensuring quality in the NICU: Translating research into appropriate clinical care. *The Journal of Perinatal & Neonatal Nursing, 29*(3), 255–261.

Springer, S. C., & Annibale, D. J. (2014). Kernicterus. *eMedicine*. Retrieved from http://emedicine.medscape.com/article/975276-overview#a5

Springer, S. C., & Annibale, D. J. (2017). Necrotizing enterocolitis. *eMedicine*. Retrieved from http://emedicine.medscape.com/article/977956-overview

Stark, A. R. (2018). Systemic effects of perinatal asphyxia. Retrieved from http://www.uptodate.com/contents/systemic-effects-of-perinatal-asphyxia

Stephenson, C. D., Lockwood, C. J., & MacKenzie, A. P. (2018). Omphalocele. *UpToDate*. Retrieved from http://www.uptodate.com/contents/omphalocele

Stephenson, C. D., Lockwood, C. J., & MacKenzie, A. P. (2019). Gastroschisis. *UpToDate*. Retrieved from http://www.uptodate.com/contents/gastroschisis

Substance Abuse & Mental Health Services Administration (SAMHSA). (n.d.). *Fetal alcohol spectrum disorders (FASD)*. Retrieved from http://www.samhsa.gov/fetal-alcohol-spectrum-disorders-fasd-center

Swanson, J. R., & Sinkin, R. A. (2015). Transition from fetus to newborn. *Pediatric Clinics of North America, 62*(2), 329–343.

Szpecht, D., Szymankiewicz, M., Seremak-Mrozikiewicz, A., & Gadzinowski, J. (2015). Review paper: The role of genetic factors in the pathogenesis of neonatal intraventricular hemorrhage. *Folia Neuropathology, 53*(1), 1–7.

Tewfik, T. L., Karsan, N., & Laberge, J. M. (2017). Congenital malformations of the esophagus. *eMedicine*. Retrieved from http://emedicine.medscape.com/article/837879-overview#a3

Thoresen, M. (2015). Cooling after perinatal asphyxia. *Seminars in Fetal & Neonatal Medicine, 20*, 65–66.

Verklan, M. T., & Walden, M. (2015). *Core curriculum for neonatal intensive care nursing* (5th ed.). St. Louis, MO: Saunders.

Wagner, J. P., & Lee, S. L. (2015). Infant born with abdominal wall defect. In A. Grigorian & P. N. Frank (Eds.). *Surgery: A case based clinical review* (pp. 349–355). New York: Springer Publishers.

Wang, M. (2014). Perinatal drug abuse and neonatal drug withdrawal. *eMedicine*. Retrieved from http://emedicine.medscape.com/article/978492-overview

Whitsett, J. A., Wert, S. E., & Weaver, T. E. (2015). Diseases of pulmonary surfactant homeostasis. *Annual Review of Pathology, 10*, 371–393.

World Health Organization (WHO). (2016). *Congenital anomalies*. Retrieved from http://www.who.int/mediacentre/factsheets/fs370/en/

Zanelli, S. A., Stanley, D. P., & Kaufman, D. A. (2018). *Hypoxic-ischemic encephalopathy*. Retrieved from http://emedicine.medscape.com/article/973501-overview

CHAPTER **WORKSHEET**

MULTIPLE CHOICE QUESTIONS

1. Which finding would lead the nurse to suspect that a newborn is experiencing respiratory distress syndrome?
   a. Abdominal distention
   b. Acrocyanosis
   c. Depressed fontanels
   d. Nasal flaring

2. When assessing the substance-exposed newborn, which finding would the nurse expect?
   a. Calm facial appearance
   b. Daily weight gain
   c. Increasing irritability
   d. Feeding and sleeping well

3. A newborn with tracheoesophageal fistula is likely to present with which assessment finding?
   a. Subnormal temperature
   b. Absent Moro reflex
   c. Inability to swallow
   d. Drooling from mouth

4. In which of the following infants would the nurse would be most alert for the development of transient tachypnea?
   a. Infant born by caesarean section
   b. Neonate who received no sedation
   c. Newborn of a mother with heart disease
   d. Baby who is small for gestational age

5. The nurse is caring for a term neonate who was exposed to cocaine throughout the pregnancy. What effect would this exposure have on the neonate's vital signs?
   a. They would be lower than normal.
   b. They would be higher than normal.
   c. They would not be affected at all.
   d. BP would be lower, pulse would higher.

6. Characteristics of a newborn with fetal alcohol syndrome would include which of the following? Select all that apply:
   a. Hypocalcemia and hypokalemia
   b. Malformed ears and cataracts
   c. Microcephaly and thin upper lip
   d. Congenital cardiac defects and SGA
   e. Prominent cheekbones and LGA
   f. Hyperactive behaviour and feeding problems

CRITICAL THINKING EXERCISES

1. As the nursery nurse, you receive a newborn from the labour and birth suite and place him under the radiant warmer. The nurse who gives you the report states that the mother couldn't remember when her membranes broke before labour and that she ran a fever during labour for the past few hours. The Apgar scores were good, but the newborn seemed lethargic. As you begin your assessment, you note that he is pale and floppy and has a subnormal temperature; heart rate is 180 bpm and respiratory rate is 70 breaths per minute.
   a. What in the mother's history should raise a red flag to the nurse?
   b. For what condition is this newborn at high risk?
   c. What interventions are appropriate for this condition?

2. Terry, a-day-old baby girl, is very fretful, and calming measures don't seem to work. The nursery nurse notices that she is losing weight and her formula intake is poor, even though she is manifesting hungry behaviour. The mother received no prenatal care and denied drug use, but her drug screen was positive for heroin.
   a. What additional information does the nurse need to obtain from the mother?
   b. What additional laboratory work might be needed for Terry?
   c. What specific measures need to be made for her ongoing care?

3. Baby boy Sims, a term newborn, was brought to the nursery. His mother received no prenatal care, but the newborn's Apgar scores were fine. As the nurse carried out her newborn assessment, she noted an imperforate anus and palpated no testicles in the scrotal sac.
   a. What additional assessments should the nurse complete?
   b. Are anorectal agenesis and genitourinary tract anomalies common?
   c. What diagnostic tests might be ordered? What might be included in the treatment plan for this newborn?

STUDY ACTIVITIES

1. Arrange for a tour of a regional NICU to see the nurse's role in caring for sick neonates. Ask the nurse to give a quick history of each newborn's condition. Was the nurse's role like you imagined? What was your impression of the NICU, and how would you describe it to expectant parents?

2. Select a website from the list online at the Point. What kind of information is given? How helpful would it be for parents with an infant diagnosed with a specific condition?

3. A herniation of a newborn's abdominal contents present at birth describes _____.

BRINGING IT ALL TOGETHER: A CASE STUDY

Anna, a 17-year-old Indigenous client, was diagnosed with type 1 diabetes at the age of 5 years. She presented at the local clinic reporting that she has missed three periods and thinks she could be pregnant. A physical examination supports the possibility and a pregnancy test confirms that she is 12 weeks pregnant.

Go to the Point **to find questions to consider about this case.**

Health Promotion of the Growing Child and Family

Unit 9

Health Promotion of the Growing Child and Family

25

Growth and Development of the Newborn and Infant

Learning Objectives

Upon completion of the chapter, you will be able to:

1. Identify normal developmental changes occurring in the newborn and infant.
2. Identify the gross and fine motor milestones of the newborn and infant.
3. Express an understanding of language development in the first year of life.
4. Describe nutritional requirements of the newborn and infant.
5. Develop a nutritional plan for the first year of life.
6. Identify common issues related to growth and development in infancy.
7. Demonstrate knowledge of appropriate anticipatory guidance for common developmental issues.

Allison Johnson is a 6-month-old girl brought to the clinic by her mother and father for her 6-month checkup. As new parents, they have a list of questions and concerns. On assessment you find that Allison's weight is 7.26 kg (16 lb), length 65.41 cm (25¾ in), and head circumference 43.18 cm (17 in). As the nurse caring for her, assess Allison's growth and development, and then teach the parents what changes to expect in Allison over the next few months.

Infancy and early childhood is an extremely sensitive period in human development. Influences in the early years have a profound impact on health and well-being in adult life. The significance of biologic, environmental, community, spiritual, emotional, and psychosocial factors on infant development can inform future health outcomes (Boivin & Hertzman, 2012). The newborn or neonatal period of infancy is defined as the period from birth until 28 days of age. Infancy is defined as the period from birth to 12 months of age. Growth and development are interrelated, ongoing processes in infancy and childhood. **Growth** refers to an increase in physical size. **Development** is the sequential process by which infants and children gain various skills and functions. Heredity influences growth and development by determining the child's potential, while the environment contributes to the degree of achievement. **Maturation** refers to an increase in functionality of various body systems or developmental skills.

Growth and Development Overview

Growth and developmental changes in the first year of life are both numerous and dramatic. This period of rapid development is heavily influenced by the experiences and opportunities that infants are exposed to (Boivin & Hertzman, 2012). Physical growth, maturation of body systems, and gross and fine motor skills progress in an orderly and sequential fashion. Though timing may vary from infant to infant, the order in which developmental skills are acquired is consistent. Infants also exhibit vast areas of learning in the psychosocial and cognitive, language and communication, and social/emotional domains. Therefore, adequate growth and development depends on many factors including access to healthy families and resources, parenting or caregiver knowledge (health literacy) linked to infant development, social security needs being met—such as feelings of community connectedness, environmental safety being maintained (Takaro et al., 2015).

A recent study from Alberta has identified evidence of low parental knowledge in the areas of infant and child social and cognitive development, often as a result of factors such as parental stress, and limited availability of evidenced-based child development information and parent programs (Pujadas Botey et al., 2016). The nurse is well positioned to provide age-appropriate anticipatory guidance to parents or caregivers, and must endeavour to do so at any health encounter with the child and their family.

Early childhood experiences can become biologically embedded and influence outcomes in later life in either negative or positive ways. Disruptions in early life can impact behaviour, learning, emotional and cognitive development, and be a contributing burden to adult chronic disease. Adverse child experiences (ACEs), which include traumatic events such as sexual, emotional, or physical abuse, neglect, economic hardship, and family disruption (such as divorce), can have life-long health, social, and well-being impacts on the infant (HOPE, 2017). Early awareness of barriers that can prevent healthy infant development is critical since early intervention and building on encouraging aspects of the infant's life can have a tremendous positive influence on the future health of the infant and, as a result, society as a whole (The Royal College of Physicians and Surgeons of Canada [RCPSC], 2014). In addition, access to care must be equitable and timely, which is the underlying philosophy of Jordan's Principle. As such, Jordan's Principle is an important legislation that ensures First Nations children do not experience delays, disruptions, or denials of services ordinarily available to other Canadian children (Government of Canada, 2019).

Achievement of developmental milestones may be assessed in a variety of ways. While obtaining a health history, the nurse may ask the parent or caregiver if the skill is present and when it was attained. The infant may also demonstrate the skill during the interview or examination, or the nurse may elicit the skill from the infant. A number of screening tools are available to assess for developmental delay, such as the Rourke baby record; this example is used in some Canadian Provinces (Riverin, Li, Rourke, Leduc, & Rourke, 2015). The Denver II Development screening test and the Ages and Stages Questionnaire (ASQ) are other examples widely used in practice.

Infants that have experienced illness, congenital anomaly, or prematurity may exhibit delayed acquisition of physical growth and developmental skills. When assessing the growth and development of a premature infant, use the infant's corrected (adjusted) age to determine expected outcomes. To determine corrected age, subtract the number of weeks that the infant was premature from the infant's chronologic age. Plot growth parameters and assess developmental milestones based on corrected age. For example, a 6-month-old infant born at 28 weeks' gestation was born 12 weeks early (3 months). Subtract 12 weeks from chronologic age of 6 months to obtain the corrected age of 3 months. The infant's weight, length, and head circumference should closely match that of a healthy 3-month-old infant. Similarly, the infant would be expected to have the developmental skills typical of a 3- versus a 6-month-old infant. Growth parameters for premature infants smaller than 37 weeks' gestation (e.g., <37 weeks gestational age) should be corrected until at minimum, 24 months of chronologic age (Rourke Baby Record, 2014).

PHYSICAL GROWTH

Routine assessment of an infant's weight, length, and head circumference against expected norms is important so that excessive or inadequate growth can be identified early. Early diagnosis of any abnormalities in growth enables any possible causes to be corrected in order to achieve maximal growth potential.

Weight

The average newborn weighs 3.400 kg (7.5 lb) at birth, with boys being slightly heavier than girls (Olsson, 2011). Newborns may lose up to 10% of their body weight over the first week of life. The average newborn then gains about 30 g per day and regains his or her birth weight by 10 to 14 days of age. Most infants double their birth weight by 4 to 6 months of age and triple their birth weight by the time they are 1 year old (Feigelman, 2011).

Length

The average newborn is 50 cm (20 in) long at birth (Olsson, 2011). The infant grows quickly in length over the first 6 months, and by 12 months the infant's length has increased by 50% (Feigelman, 2011).

Head Circumference

The average head circumference of the full-term newborn is 35 cm (14 in). Similar to the weight and length, the head circumference increases rapidly during the first 6 months. Velocity slows slightly in the 6- to 12-month period, exhibiting an average 10-cm (4-in) gain from birth to 1 year of age (Feigelman, 2011).

ORGAN SYSTEM MATURATION

The newborn and infant organ systems undergo significant changes as the infant grows. Systems that undergo significant change include the neurologic system, the cardiovascular system, the respiratory system, the gastrointestinal (digestive) system, the renal system, the hematopoietic system, the immunologic system, and the integumentary system.

Neurologic System

The infant experiences tremendous maturation of the neurologic system over the first year of life. Critical brain growth and continued myelination of the spinal cord occur. Involuntary movement progresses to voluntary control, and immature vocalizations and cries evolve to purposeful vocalizations and language to communicate their needs. Recent advances in developmental neurobiology show a high level of plasticity in this early phase of brain organization which inform language development, cognitive skills, and emotional competencies (Boivin & Hertzman, 2012).

States of Consciousness

The normal-term newborn moves sequentially through states of consciousness reassure parents and health care providers (i.e., nurses, nurse practitioners, physicians) that the neurologic system, though immature, is intact. A normal newborn will ordinarily move through six states of consciousness:

1. Deep sleep: Sleeping with eyes closed and no movement.
2. Light sleep: Sleeping with eyes closed; rapid eye movements and irregular movements may be noticed.
3. Drowsiness: Eyes may close or be half-lidded; the infant may be dozing.
4. Quiet alert state: The infant's eyes are wide open and the body is calm.
5. Active alert state: The infant's eyes are open; body movements occur.
6. Crying: The infant cries or screams and it is difficult to gain the infant's attention (Brazelton & Nugent, 2011).

Newborns usually cycle through these states slowly, rather than going from deep sleep immediately into outright crying.

Brain Growth

The nervous system continues to mature throughout infancy, and the rapid increase in head circumference in the first 2 years of life reflects this period of tremendous brain growth. By 6 months of age the infant's brain weighs half that of the adult brain. At age 12 months, the brain has grown considerably, weighing 2½ times what it did at birth. The posterior fontanel normally closes by 4 months of age. Usually, the anterior fontanel remains open until 12 to 18 months of age to accommodate this rapid brain growth. However, the fontanel may close as early as 9 months of age, and this is not of concern in the infant with age-appropriate growth and development.

Myelination of the spinal cord and nerves continues over the first 2 years and is crucial to maturation of the nervous system.

Reflexes

Primitive reflexes are subcortical and involuntary, and are indicative of a healthy nervous system in the infant. Early primitive reflexes present at birth include Moro, rooting, sucking, asymmetric tonic neck, plantar and palmar grasp, step, and Babinski. These primitive reflexes disappear over the first few months of life following a clear sequence. This gives way to development of the protective reflexes (also termed postural responses or reflexes), which are useful in the maintenance of equilibrium. These protective reflexes, including the righting and parachute reflexes, are prerequisites for appropriate motor development and remain throughout life once they are established. Persistence of primitive reflexes beyond the usual age of disappearance may indicate an abnormality of the neurologic system and should be flagged and investigated.

Table 25.1 gives descriptions and pictures of several primitive and protective reflexes, as well as the timing of appearance and disappearance of these reflexes.

TABLE 25.1	SELECTED PRIMITIVE AND PROTECTIVE REFLEXES IN INFANCY		
	Description	Age Reflex Appears	Age Reflex Disappears
Primitive Reflexes			
Root	When infant's cheek is stroked, the infant turns to that side, searching with mouth.	Birth	3 months
Suck	Reflexive sucking when nipple or finger is placed in infant's mouth.	Birth	2–5 months
Moro	With sudden extension of the head, the arms abduct and move upward and the hands form a "C."	Birth	4 months

TABLE 25.1   SELECTED PRIMITIVE AND PROTECTIVE REFLEXES IN INFANCY (continued)

	Description	Age Reflex Appears	Age Reflex Disappears
Asymmetric tonic neck	While lying supine, extremities are extended on the side of the body to which the head is turned and opposite extremities are flexed (also called the "fencing" position).	Birth	4 months
Palmar grasp 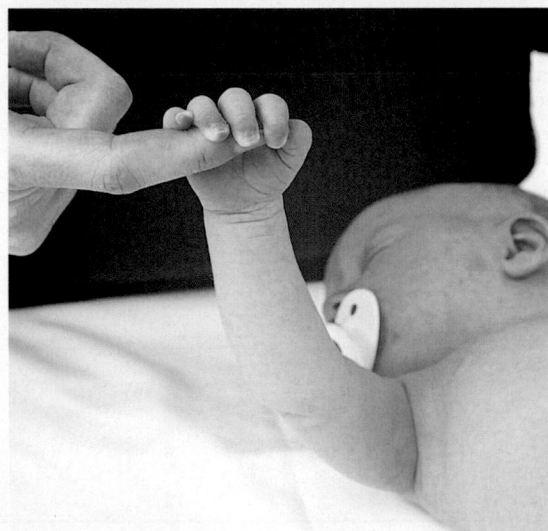	Infant reflexively grasps when palm is touched.	Birth	4–6 months
Plantar grasp 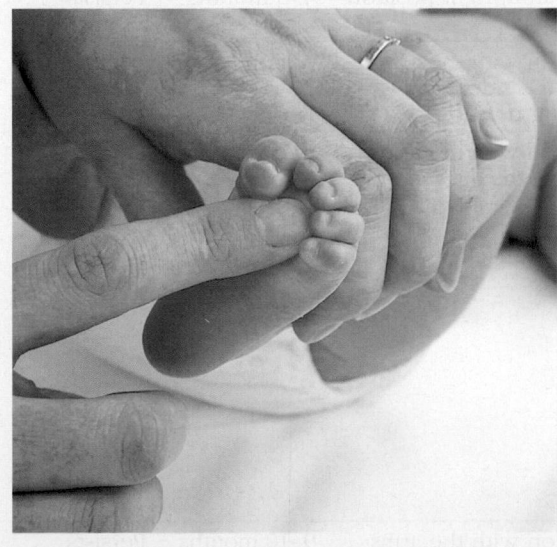	Infant reflexively grasps with bottom of foot when pressure is applied to plantar surface.	Birth	9 months

(continued)

TABLE 25.1	SELECTED PRIMITIVE AND PROTECTIVE REFLEXES IN INFANCY (continued)

	Description	Age Reflex Appears	Age Reflex Disappears
Babinski 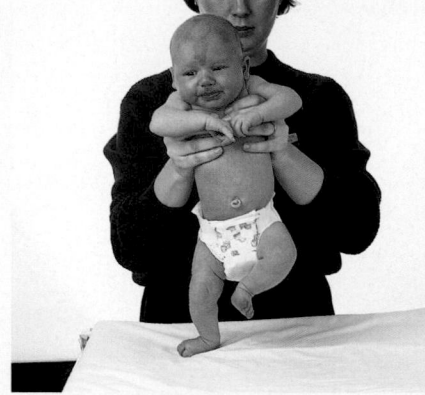	Stroking along the lateral aspect of the sole and across the plantar surface results in fanning and hyperextension of the toes.	Birth	12 months
Step	With one foot on a flat surface, the infant puts the other foot down as if to "step."	Birth	4–8 weeks

Protective Reflexes

	Description	Age Reflex Appears	Age Reflex Disappears
Neck righting	Neck keeps head in upright position when body is tilted.	4–6 months	Persists
Parachute (sideways)	Protective extension with the arms when tilted to the side in a supported sitting position.	6 months	Persists
Parachute (forward)	Protective extension with the arms when held up in the air and moved forward. The infant reflexively reaches forward to catch himself or herself.	6–7 months	Persists
Parachute (backward)	Protective extension with the arms when tilted backward.	9–10 months	Persists

Respiratory System

The respiratory system continues to mature over the first year of life. The respiratory rate slows from an average of 30 to 60 breaths in the newborn to about 24 to 40 in the 12 month old. The newborn breathes irregularly, with periodic pauses. As the infant matures, the respiratory pattern becomes more regular and rhythmic.

In comparison with the adult, in the infant:
- The nasal passages are narrower.
- The trachea and chest wall are more compliant.
- The bronchi and bronchioles are shorter and narrower.
- The larynx is more funnel shaped.
- The tongue is larger.
- There are significantly fewer alveoli.

These anatomic differences place the infant at higher risk for respiratory compromise. The respiratory system does not reach adult levels of maturity until about 7 years of age. The role of immunoglobulin A (IgA) in the mucosal lining of the upper respiratory tract may contribute to rates of infection in some children (Corthésy, 2013). Furthermore, breastfeeding can provide the infant with protection against various infections including pneumonia (Duijts, Jaddoe, Hofman, & Moll, 2010) and prevent *Haemophilus influenzae* from colonizing the nose and mouth.

Cardiovascular System

The heart doubles in size over the first year of life. As the cardiovascular system matures, the average pulse rate decreases from 120 to 160 in the newborn to about 100 in the 1 year old. Blood pressure steadily increases over the first 12 months of life, from an average of 60/40 in the newborn to 100/50 in the 12 month old. The peripheral capillaries are closer to the surface of the skin, thus making the newborn and young infant more susceptible to heat loss. Over the first year of life, thermoregulation (the body's ability to stabilize body temperature) becomes more effective: the peripheral capillaries constrict in response to a cold environment and dilate in response to heat.

Gastrointestinal System

Teeth

Occasionally, an infant is born with one or more teeth (termed natal teeth) or develops teeth in the first 28 days of life (termed neonatal teeth). The presence of natal or neonatal teeth may be associated with other birth anomalies. The vast majority of newborn do not have teeth at birth, nor do they develop them in the first month of life. On average, the first primary teeth begin to erupt between the ages of 6 and 8 months. The primary teeth (also termed deciduous teeth) are lost later in childhood and will be replaced by the permanent teeth. The gums

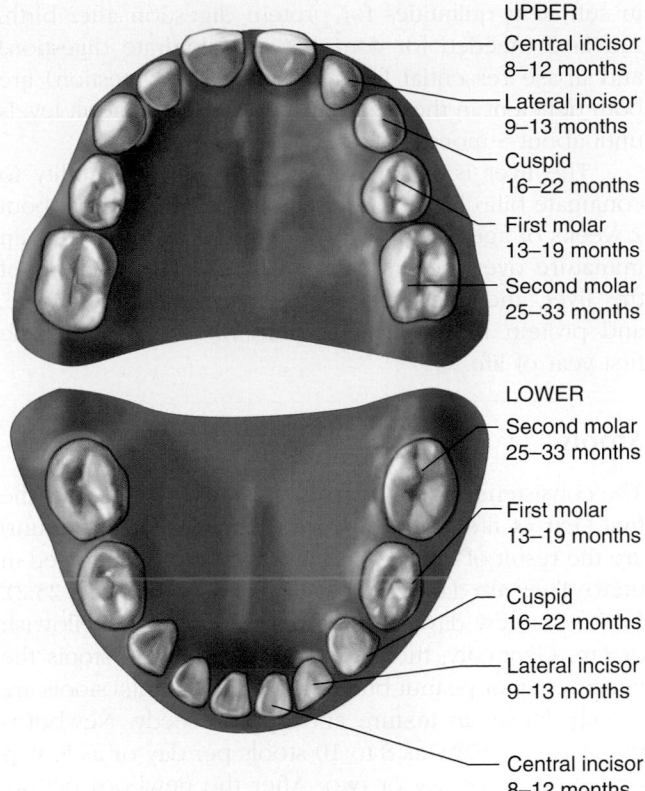

UPPER
- Central incisor 8–12 months
- Lateral incisor 9–13 months
- Cuspid 16–22 months
- First molar 13–19 months
- Second molar 25–33 months

LOWER
- Second molar 25–33 months
- First molar 13–19 months
- Cuspid 16–22 months
- Lateral incisor 9–13 months
- Central incisor 8–12 months

FIGURE 25.1 Sequence and average age of tooth eruption.

around the emerging tooth often swell, and can be associated with discomfort or pain. The lower central incisors are usually the first to appear, followed by the upper central incisors (Fig. 25.1). The average 12 month old has four to eight teeth. The Canadian Dental Association (CDA) recommends that infants receive their first dental visit by the age of 1 year or within 12 months of the eruption of their first tooth (CDA, 2010).

Digestion

The digestive system is not fully developed. Small amounts of saliva are present for the first 3 months of life and ptyalin is present only in small amounts in the saliva. Gastric digestion occurs as a result of the presence of hydrochloric acid and rennin. The stomach capacity is relatively small at birth and can hold up to 20 mL (Bergman, 2013), by a week 30 to 59 mL, and by 2 to 3 weeks 59 to 98 mL. Several factors influence stomach emptying including weight, time, and volume of feed as well as type and temperature. By 1 year of age the stomach can accommodate three full meals and several snacks per day. The small intestine is about 270 cm long and grows to the adult length over the first few years of life (Liacouras, 2011). In the duodenum, three enzymes in particular are important for digestion. Trypsin is available in sufficient quantities for protein digestion after birth. Amylase (needed for complex carbohydrate digestion) and lipase (essential for appropriate fat digestion) are both deficient in the infant and do not reach adult levels until about 5 months of age.

The liver is also immature at birth. The ability to conjugate bilirubin and secrete bile develops after about 2 weeks of age. Conjugation of medications may remain immature over the first year of life. Other functions of the liver, including gluconeogenesis, vitamin storage, and protein metabolism, remain immature during the first year of life.

Stools

The consistency and frequency of stools change over the first year of life. The newborn's first stools (meconium) are the result of digestion of amniotic fluid swallowed in utero. They are dark green to black and sticky (Fig. 25.2). In the first few days of life the stools become yellowish or tan. Generally, the formula-fed infant has stools the consistency of peanut butter. Breastfed infants' stools are usually looser in texture and appear seedy. Newborns may have as many as 8 to 10 stools per day or as few as one stool every day or two. After the newborn period, the number of stools may decrease, and some infants may not have a bowel movement every day. Infrequent stooling is considered normal if the bowel movement remains soft. Breastfed babies may go 8 to 10 days between stools, which is a normal variant. Due to the immaturity of the gastrointestinal system, newborns and young infants often grunt, strain, or cry while attempting to have a bowel movement. If the stool remains soft, there is no abdominal distention, and there is no vomiting, this is not concerning. Stool colour and texture may change depending on the foods that the infant has ingested. Iron

supplements may cause the stool to appear black or very dark green (Swanson, 2016).

Take Note!

Parents should call the primary care provider if the infant's stools are red, white, grey, or black; mucous-like; frequent and watery; frothy or foul-smelling; or hard, dry, formed, ribbon-like, or pellet-like; or if the baby is vomiting.

Genitourinary System

In the infant, extracellular fluid (lymph, interstitial fluid, and blood plasma) accounts for about 35% of body weight and intracellular fluid accounts for 40%, compared with the adult quantities of 20% and 40%, respectively (Greenbaum, 2011). Thus, the infant is more susceptible to dehydration. Infants urinate frequently and the urine has a relatively low specific gravity. The renal structures are immature and the glomerular filtration rate, tubular secretion, and reabsorption as well as renal perfusion are all reduced compared with the adult. The glomeruli reach full maturity by 2 years of age.

Integumentary System

In utero, the infant is covered with vernix caseosa, which protects the developing infant's skin. At birth, the infant may be covered with vernix (earlier gestational age) or vernix may be found in the folds of the skin, axilla, and groin areas (later gestational age). Production of vernix ceases at birth. Fine downy hair (lanugo) covers the body of many neonates. Often, this hair is lost over time and is not replaced. Darker-skinned infants tend to have more lanugo present at birth than those with light skin. Many newborns will develop tiny white bumps on their

A   B

FIGURE 25.2 **A**. Meconium stool. **B**. Typical stool after the first few days. Note the yellowish, seedy stool of a breastfed infant.

FIGURE 25.3 **A.** Acrocyanosis. Note blueness of the hands. **B.** Mottling of the skin in a young infant.

nose, cheeks, or chin, called Milia. Some will develop bright red raised bumps on their face, upper chest, or torso, often appearing with overheating or crying and then disappearing spontaneously. This is termed "baby acne," but is not the same as acne seen in adolescents. Both of these are benign and self-limiting skin conditions often seen in the newborn period.

Acrocyanosis (blueness of the hands and feet) is normal in the newborn; it decreases over the first few days of life (Fig. 25.3). Newborns often experience mottling of the skin (a pink-and-white marbled appearance) because of their immature circulatory system. Mottling decreases over the first few months of life.

The newborn and young infant's skin is significantly thinner than that of the adult, with the peripheral capillaries being closer to the surface. This, along with the absence of subcutaneous tissue predispose to increased absorption of topical medications.

Hematopoietic System

Significant changes in the hematopoietic system occur over the first year of life. At birth, fetal hemoglobin

(HgbF) is present in large amounts. After birth the production of HgbF nearly ceases, and adult hemoglobin (HgbA) is produced in steadily increasing amounts throughout the first 6 months. Since HgbF has a shorter lifespan than HgbA, infants may experience physiologic anemia at age 2 to 3 months (Lerner, 2011). During the last 3 months of gestation, maternal iron stores are transferred to the fetus. The newborn typically has 0.3 to 0.5 g of iron stores available. As the high concentrations of HgbF decrease over the first 2 to 3 months, iron is reclaimed and stored. However, the infant's stores of iron are largely depleted by 4 to 6 months of age. Exclusively breastfed infants, premature infants, and babies born to mothers with anemia or diabetes in pregnancy are at particularly high risk for iron deficiency (ID) and/or iron deficiency anemia (IDA). Infants with inadequate iron levels are at risk for significant conditions, including poor physiologic growth, slow brain development, cognitive delays, behavioural issues, and poorer developmental outcomes overall. IDA is more prevalent in Indigenous Canadian children (14% to 50%) as compared to non-Indigenous Canadian children (3.5% to 10.5%) (Abdullah, Zlotkin, Parkin, & Greiner, 2011), which is important to consider in the assessment of infants from a culturally diverse population.

Understanding parents' cultural beliefs and practices about feeding in infancy is an important step in supporting families who wish to feed their infants a culturally traditional healthy diet (Aboriginal Nurses Association of Canada, 2009; Canadian Nurses Association, 2010). Early and ongoing intake of iron-rich foods starting at 6 months of age will support the healthy growth and maturation of all body systems during first 2 years of life when iron needs are the greatest (Baker & Greer; The Committee on Nutrition, 2010).

Take Note!

Maternal iron stores are transferred to the fetus throughout the last trimester of pregnancy. Infants born prematurely miss all or at least a portion of this iron store transfer, placing them at increased risk for iron deficiency anemia compared with term infants.

Immunologic System

The newborns receive large amounts of IgG from their mother prior to birth since it is the only immunoglobulin small enough to pass through the placenta. Human milk will provide infants with IgG, IgA, IgM, and IgD, which confer passive immunity (short-term immunity passed from mother to infant) during the first 3 to 6 months of life. Infants then synthesize their own IgG, reaching approximately 60% of adult levels at age 12 months (Cherry, Demmler-Harrison, Kaplan, Steinbach, & Hotez, 2014). IgM is produced in significant amounts after birth, reaching adult levels by 9 months of age. IgA, IgD, and

IgE production increases very gradually, maturing in early childhood (Cherry et al., 2014).

PSYCHOSOCIAL DEVELOPMENT

Erikson (1963) identifies the psychosocial crisis of infancy as Trust versus Mistrust. Development of a sense of trust is crucial in the first year, as it serves as the foundation for later psychosocial tasks by providing the infant with feelings of physical comfort and security especially when in unfamiliar surrounds. The parent or primary caregiver can have a significant impact on the infant's development of a sense of trust. When the infant's needs are consistently met, the infant develops this sense of trust. But if the parent or caregiver is unavailable or inconsistent in meeting the infant's needs in a timely manner, then the infant develops a sense of mistrust. Table 25.2 lists activities that promote a sense of trust in infancy.

COGNITIVE DEVELOPMENT

The first stage of Jean Piaget's theory of cognitive development is referred to as the sensorimotor stage (birth to 2 years) (Piaget, 1969). Infants learn about themselves and the world through their developing sensory and motor capacities. Infants' development from birth to 1 year of age can be divided into four substages within the sensorimotor stage: reflexes, primary circular reaction, secondary circular reaction, and coordination of secondary schemes. Cause and effect guide most of the cognitive development seen in infancy (Table 25.2).

The concept of **object permanence** begins to develop between 4 and 7 months of age and is solidified by about 8 months of age (Piaget, 1969). If an object is hidden from the infant's sight, he or she will search for it in the last place it was seen, knowing it still exists. This development of object permanence is essential for the development of self-image. By age 12 months the infant knows he or she is separate from the parent or caregiver and can recognize themselves in the mirror. The 12 month old will explore objects in different ways, such as throwing, banging, dropping, and shaking. He or she may imitate gestures and knows how to use certain objects correctly (e.g., puts phone to ear, turns up cup to drink, attempts to comb hair) (Piaget, 1969).

MOTOR SKILL DEVELOPMENT

Infants exhibit phenomenal increases in their gross and fine motor skills over the first 12 months of life.

TABLE 25.2	DEVELOPMENTAL THEORIES	
Theorist	**Stage**	**Activities**
Erikson	Trust vs. mistrust (birth to 1 year)	Caregivers respond to the infant's basic needs by feeding, changing diapers, cleaning, touching, holding, and talking to the infant. This creates a sense of trust in the infant. As the nervous system matures, infants realize they are separate beings from their caregivers. Over time, the infant learns to tolerate small amounts of frustration and trusts that although gratification may be delayed, it will eventually be provided.
Piaget	Sensorimotor (birth to 2 years) Substage 1: use of reflexes (birth to 1 month) Substage 2: primary circular reactions (1 to 4 months) Substage 3: secondary circular reactions (4 to 8 months) Substage 4: coordination of secondary schemes (8 to 12 months)	Infant uses senses and motor skills to learn about the world. Reflexive sucking brings the pleasure of ingesting nutrition. Infant begins to gain control over reflexes and recognizes familiar objects, odours, and sounds. Thumb sucking may occur by chance; then the infant repeats it on purpose to bring pleasure. Imitation begins. Object permanence begins. Infant shows affect. Infant repeats actions to achieve wanted results (e.g., shakes rattle to hear the noise it makes). The infant's actions are purposeful but the infant does not always have an end goal in mind. Infants coordinate previously learned schemes with previously learned behaviours. They may grasp and shake a rattle intentionally or crawl across the room to reach a desired toy. Infant can anticipate events. Object permanence is fully present at about 8 months of age. The infant begins to associate symbols with events (e.g., waving goodbye means someone is leaving).
Freud	Oral stage (birth to 1 year)	Pleasure is focused on oral activities: feeding and sucking.

Adapted from Erikson, E. H. (1963). *Childhood and society* (2nd ed.). New York: W. W. Norton and Company; Goldson, E., & Reynolds, A. (2014). Child development and behavior. In W. W. Hay, Jr., M. J. Levin, R. R. Deterding, & M. J. Abzug (Eds.). *Current diagnosis and treatment: Pediatrics* (22nd ed.). New York: McGraw-Hill Education; and Piaget, J. (1969). *The theory of stages in cognitive development.* New York: McGraw-Hill.

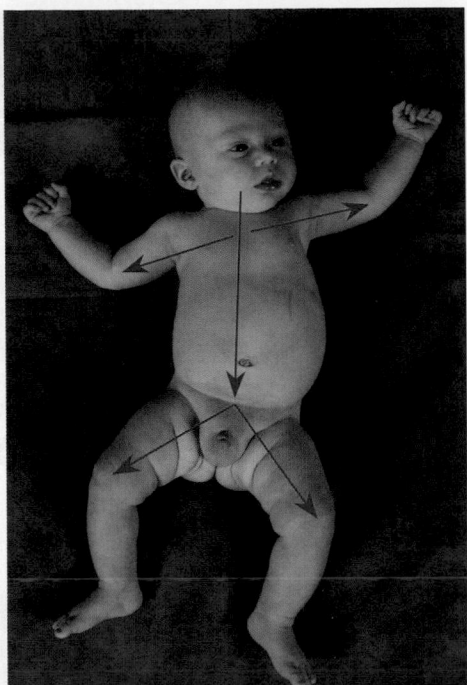

FIGURE 25.4 Gross motor skills develop in a cephalocaudal direction, fine motor skills in a proximodistal fashion.

Gross Motor Skills

The term "gross motor skills" refers to those that use the large muscles (e.g., head control, rolling, sitting, and walking). Gross motor skills develop in a **cephalocaudal** fashion (from the head to the tail) (Fig. 25.4). In other words, the baby learns to lift the head before learning to roll over and sit (Goldson & Reynolds, 2014). At birth, babies have poor head control and need to have their necks supported when being held. They can lift their heads only slightly while in a prone position. Over the next several months the infant's motor skills progress at a dramatic rate. First, the infant achieves head control, then the ability to roll over, sit, crawl, pull to stand, and, usually around 1 year of age, walk independently. Table 25.3 outlines when the infant typically develops each specific gross motor skill, as well as the typical sequence of acquisition. Diagnosing motor delays during the first year of life is important because these often indicate more generalized developmental delays or specific disabilities, such as cerebral palsy (Harris, 2016). Progression of gross motor skills is illustrated in Figures 25.5 through 25.7.

Take Note!

Warning signs that may indicate problems with motor development include the following: arms and legs are stiff or floppy; child cannot support head at 4 months of age; child reaches with one hand only; child cannot sit with assistance at 6 months of age; child does not crawl by 12 months of age; child cannot stand supported by 12 months of age. Of note, any infant that is experiencing

TABLE 25.3	DEVELOPMENT OF GROSS MOTOR SKILLS IN INFANCY
Age (months)	Gross Motor Skills
1	Lifts and turns head to side in prone position Head lag when pulled to sit Rounded back in sitting
2	Raises head and chest, holds position Improving head control
3	Raises head to 45 degrees in prone Slight head lag in pull to sit
4	Lifts head and looks around Rolls from prone to supine Head leads body when pulled to sit
5	Rolls from supine to prone and back again Sits with back upright when supported
6	Tripod sits
7	Sits alone with some use of hands for support
8	Sits unsupported
9	Crawls, abdomen off floor
10	Pulls to stand Cruises
12	Sits from standing position Walks independently

Adapted from Feigelman, S. (2011). The first year. In R. M. Kliegman, B. F. Stanton, J. W. St. Geme III, N. F. Schor, & R. E. Behrman (Eds.). *Nelson's textbook of pediatrics* (19th ed.). Philadelphia, PA: Elsevier, Saunders; Centers for Disease Control and Prevention. (2016). *Developmental milestones.* Retrieved from http://www.cdc.gov/ncbddd/actearly/milestones/index.html

a regression or loss of a specific motor skill that they had previously acquired, needs immediate evaluation by a health care provider to rule out an underlying cause.

Fine Motor Skills

Fine motor development includes the maturation of hand and finger use. Fine motor skills develop in a **proximodistal** fashion (from the centre to the periphery) (Fig. 25.4). In other words, the infant first bats with the whole hand, eventually progressing to grasping, before being capable of fine fingertip grasping (Fig. 25.8) (Goldson & Reynolds, 2014). The newborn's hand movements are involuntary in nature, whereas the 12 month old is capable of feeding himself or herself with a cup and spoon. By 12 months of age the infant should be able to eat with his or her fingers and assist with dressing (e.g., pushing an arm through the sleeve). Table 25.4 outlines the typical age and sequence of fine motor skill development.

FIGURE 25.5 When pulled to sit, an infant shows (**A**) significant head lag (newborn; 2 or 3 weeks old), (**B**) improving head control (2 months old), and (**C**) no head lag (4 months old).

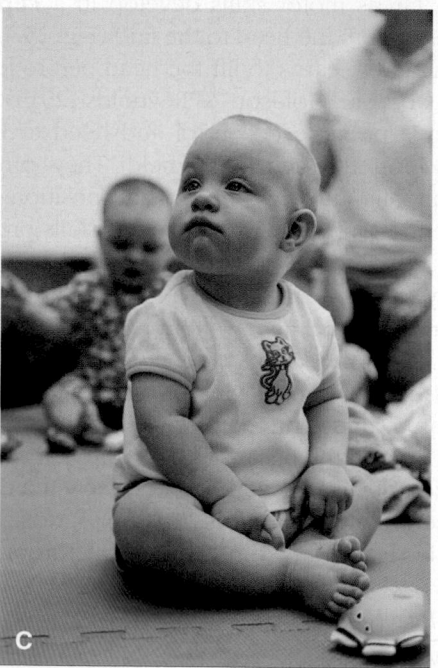

FIGURE 25.6 Development of sitting. **A**. At 4 months, the infant requires significant support. **B**. The 6-month-old infant sits in a tripod fashion. **C**. The 8 month old sits alone.

FIGURE 25.7 Development of locomotion. **A**. At 4 months the infant pushes up from a
prone position. **B**. At 8 months, the infant crawls with the abdomen off the floor. **C**. The
infant pulls to stand by 10 months of age. **D**. The infant cruises along furniture or (**E**) takes
steps with assistance at 10 to 11 months of age. **F**. The infant independently stands from a
crouched position and walks around at 12 months of age (plus or minus 3 months).

FIGURE 25.8 Development of the pincer grasp. Note the gross (whole-hand) approach to grasping a small object (**A**), compared with the fine (thumb-to-finger) ability (**B**).

SENSORY DEVELOPMENT

Sight

The newborn is near-sighted, preferring to view objects at a distance of 20 to 38 cm (8 to 15 in). Newborns prefer the human face to other objects and may even imitate the facial expressions made by those caring for them. In addition to human faces, newborns show a preference for certain objects, particularly those with contrasts such as black-and-white stripes. At 1 month of age the infant can recognize by sight the people he or she knows best. The infant will study objects within his or her visual range closely. The ability to fuse two ocular images into one cerebral picture (**binocularity**) begins to develop at 6 weeks of age and is well established by 4 months of age. The newborn's eyes may episodically wander or cross inward. The infant in whom this persists beyond 6 months of age should be assessed by a health care provider. Full colour vision develops by 7 months of age, as does distance vision and the ability to track objects.

Hearing

The newborn's hearing is intact at birth and as acute as that of an adult. Newborns prefer the sound of human voices to nonhuman sounds. By 1 month of age the infant can recognize the sounds of those he or she knows best.

Smell and Taste

The sense of smell develops rapidly: the 7-day-old infant can differentiate the smell of his or her mother's breast milk from that of another woman and will preferentially turn toward the mother's smell. Newborns prefer sweet tastes to all others. This persists for several months, and eventually the infant will accept non-sweet flavours.

Touch

The sense of touch is perhaps the most important of all the senses for newborn communication. Even the most immature infant responds to soothing stroking. The

TABLE 25.4	DEVELOPMENT OF FINE MOTOR SKILLS IN INFANCY
Age (months)	Fine Motor Skills
1	Fists mostly clenched Involuntary hand movements
3	Holds hand in front of face, hands open
4	Bats at objects
5	Grasps rattle
6	Releases object in hand to take another
7	Transfers object from one hand to the other
8	Gross pincer grasp (rakes)
9	Bangs objects together
10	Fine pincer grasp Puts objects into container and takes them out
11	Offers objects to others and releases them
12	Feeds self with cup and spoon Makes simple mark on paper Pokes with index finger

Adapted from Feigelman, S. (2011). The first year. In R. M. Kliegman, B. F. Stanton, J. W. St. Geme III, N. F. Schor, & R. E. Behrman (Eds.). *Nelson's textbook of pediatrics* (19th ed.). Philadelphia, PA: Elsevier, Saunders; Centers for Disease Control and Prevention. (2016). *Developmental milestones*. Retrieved from http://www.cdc.gov/ncbddd/actearly/milestones/index.html

infant prefers soft sensations to coarse sensations and dislikes rough handling which can provoke crying. Holding, stroking, rocking, or cuddling calms infants when they are upset. Infants learn to understand their caregiver's moods by the way they are touched and held by them.

Take Note!

Warning signs that may indicate an abnormality with sensory development that warrants evaluation include the following: young infant does not respond or startle to loud noises; does not follow a moving object by 2 to 3 months; does not focus on a near object; has persistent crossing or wandering of the eyes at any age; does not start to make sounds or babble by 4 months; does not turn to locate sound at age 4 months.

COMMUNICATION AND LANGUAGE DEVELOPMENT

The newborn and infant have many means of communication. The 1- to 3-month-old baby coos, makes other vocalizations, and demonstrates differentiated crying. At 4 to 5 months of age, the infant makes simple vowel sounds, laughs aloud, performs "raspberries," and vocalizes in response to voices. The infant also responds to his or her own name and begins to respond to "no." Between 4 and 7 months the infant begins to distinguish emotions based on the tone of voice. Squealing and yelling begin around 6 months of age; these may be used to express joy or displeasure. At age 7 to 10 months, babbling begins and progresses to strings (e.g., mamama, dadada) without meaning. The infant at this age is also able to respond to simple one-step commands. At 9 to 12 months of age the infant begins to attach meaning to "mama" and "dada" and starts to imitate other speech sounds. The average 12 month old uses two or three recognizable words with meaning, recognizes objects by name, and starts to imitate animal sounds. Pointing to specific objects to convey their wants is also typical. At this age, the infant pays increasing attention to speech and tries to imitate words; he or she may also say "uh-oh." The 12 month old also babbles with inflection (this babbling has the rhythm and timing of spoken language, but few of the "words" make sense) (Feigelman, 2011; Goldson & Reynolds, 2014).

It is important that parents and caregivers talk, read, and sing to their infant to promote the development of language and communication skills since receptive language skills develop much earlier than expressive language skills. Sometimes regression in language development occurs briefly when the child is focusing energy on other skills, such as crawling or walking. However, if hearing is normal, language acquisition should continue to progress. Infants in bilingual families may "language mix" (uses some words from each language). This is considered to be a normal progression in language development for these children (Lowry, 2011), but it makes it more difficult for the physician or nurse practitioner to determine delays in communication skills.

Language can be community and family specific with some parents needing to rebuild their confidence in speaking traditional dialects with their infants (Lyall & Ryan, 2015). As a result of historical legislation it is common for families who want to reconnect with their cultural history to have difficulty relearning traditional dialects. Language nests are approaches used by some communities to reconnect with their history and preserve stories and music for future generations (McIvor, 2006). Nurses can help families rebuild pride and confidence in their dialect and encourage elders, families, and communities to teach their infants and children (Indigenous and Northern Affairs Canada, 2017).

Take Note!

Warning signs that may indicate problems in language development are as follows: infant does not make sounds at 4 months of age; infant does not laugh or squeal by 6 months of age; infant does not babble by 8 months of age; infant does not point to desired objects at 12 months; infant does not use two to three single words with meaning at 12 months of age (mama, dada).

SOCIAL AND EMOTIONAL DEVELOPMENT

The newborn spends much of the time sleeping, but by 2 months of age the infant is ready to start socializing. The infant starts intentionally smiling at around 6 to 8 weeks of age. He or she spends a great deal of time while awake watching and observing what is going on around him or her. By about 3 months of age the infant will start an interaction with a caregiver by smiling widely and possibly gurgling. This prompts the caregiver to reciprocate, smile back, and talk to the infant. The infant responds with more smiling, cooing, and gurgles as well as moving the arms and legs. The 3 to 4 month old will also mimic the parent's facial movements, such as widening the eyes and sticking out the tongue. The baby may hesitate at first, but once the other person responds pleasantly to the infant, the infant engages and makes a reciprocal response within the interaction. The infant may cry when the pleasant interaction stops. At 6 to 8 months of age the infant may enjoy socially interactive games such as patty-cake and peek-a-boo (Feigelman, 2011; Goldson & Reynolds, 2014).

Stranger Anxiety

Around the age of 8 months the infant may develop **stranger anxiety**. The previously happy and very friendly infant may become clingy and cry when approached by strangers or unfamiliar people. Stranger anxiety is an indicator that the infant is recognizing himself or herself as separate from others and is an expected developmental phase. As the infant becomes more aware of new people and new places, he or she may view an interaction with a stranger as threatening and may start crying, even if the parent is right there. Family members, whom the child sees infrequently, as well as others the child does not spend a lot of time with, should approach the infant calmly and slowly, with the parent in sight. Sometimes this will prevent a sudden crying spell (Feigelman, 2011; Goldson & Reynolds, 2014).

Separation Anxiety

Separation anxiety may also start in the last few months of infancy. The infant becomes quite distressed when the parent leaves. The infant will eventually calm down and become engaged with the current caregiver. It is not until the infant is older that cognition and memory are sufficient for him or her to understand that the parent will come back (Feigelman, 2011; Goldson & Reynolds, 2014).

Take Note!

Warning signs of possible problems with social/emotional development include the following: infant does not offer a responsive smile at 3 months of age; infant refuses to cuddle or becomes irritable with close contact; infant makes little or no eye contact with others; shows no interest in peek-a-boo at 9 months of age.

Temperament

Temperament is an individual's nature; it is the child's inborn traits that determine how he or she interacts with the world (Child Development Institute [CDI], 2015). Temperament ranges from low or moderately active, regular, and predictable to highly active, more intense, and less adaptable. These are all considered normal along a continuum. An infant's innate temperament affects the way he or she responds to the environment. As parents take note of their infant's usual activity level, how intensely he or she reacts with others and the environment, and how stimulated he or she becomes with interactions, they start to learn about their infant's temperament. The parent should note how adaptable and flexible the infant is as well as how predictable and persistent the baby is.

When parents are familiar with how the baby approaches life on a routine basis, they will be better able to recognize when the baby is not acting like himself or herself. Nurses can help parents interpret observations about their infant's temperament and recommend ways to support the infant's individual behaviour. Some infants are slower to warm up than others; those infants should be approached slowly and calmly. Some infants

exhibit increased levels of activity compared to quieter, more passive babies; those infants generally require more direct play with the parent or caregiver and will be the type of older infant who is in constant motion. Some infants are loud and some are not. The quiet infant may become overwhelmed with excessive stimulation, whereas the very active baby may need additional stimulation to be satisfied. Becoming familiar with the infant's temperament also helps the parents describe the best approach to the infant by others (e.g., child care workers or health care professionals) (CDI, 2015).

CULTURAL INFLUENCES ON GROWTH AND DEVELOPMENT

Many culturally specific parenting practices have an impact on growth and development (International Council of Nurses, 2013). For example, some cultural groups carry their children well into the second year of life while other cultural groups expect the infant to learn to crawl and walk in the first year of life (Karasik, Adolph, Tamis-LeMonda, & Bornstein, 2010). Such practices affect the timing of the emergence of infants' motor skills. Parenting across different cultures needs to be respected and nurtured in light of the historical treatment of marginalized populations (Benzies, 2014). Furthermore, barriers can exist for immigrant parents seeking services for their children with various health care conditions (Khanlou, Haque, Mustafa, Vazquez, Mantini, & Weiss, 2017). The health needs of minority or marginalized populations, which include infants, can be linked to any race and ethnic group (Khan, Kobayashi, Vang, & Lee, 2017). Often mothers take a primary responsibility for caring for the child, but in some cultures, major health-related decisions may be deferred to the father or grandparents. Ethnicity influences some biologic variations such as stature; certain ethnic groups tend to be shorter than others because of their genetic makeup (Sinha, 2015). These children will not grow to be as tall as those from other ethnic backgrounds.

Suboptimal feeding practices, food insecurity (Roncarolo & Potvin, 2016), and lack of access to the traditional foods that are an important part of Indigenous peoples' diets can negatively impact infant health. This shift to a daily diet comprised of packaged market foods, many of which are nutrient poor and high in cost has resulted in poorer health outcomes such as obesity in some infants (Allison, 2016), and risk for hypertension and diabetes later in life. Children from families who follow a vegetarian diet need specific nutritional assessment to ensure their intake of protein and iron is adequate to maintain growth and healthy development.

Strengthening and improving the health and well-being of First Nations, Inuit, and Métis children, families, and communities is a key priority for nurses and other health professionals in Canada. Parenting approaches, lifestyle, and willingness to adopt evidence-based health practices such as infant immunization, can be significantly influenced by previous trauma (NCCAH, 2019). An understanding of the wider social determinants of health including poverty, lack of shelter, as well as cultural beliefs and practices are important in the provision of culturally competent health care to Canadian children (Benbow, Gorlick, Forchuk, Ward-Griffin, & Berman, 2016; Brittain & Blackstock, 2015). Health beliefs are influenced by an individual's religious or spiritual background. Sometimes this creates conflict in the health care setting when health providers have a different value system than that of the infant's family. Care should be taken by the nurse to provide an unbiased and judgment-free environment for each health encounter in order to develop a therapeutic family-centred care relationship with the family.

Take Note!

Many communities now include people from a variety of cultures, so it is important for nurses to practice transcultural nursing (nursing care that is directed by cultural aspects and that respects the individual's differences). Many nurse researchers are exploring the cultural aspects of health care and the impact that cultural diversity has upon health.

Refer back to Allison Johnson, who was introduced at the beginning of the chapter. What developmental milestones would you expect Allison to have reached by this age? How would this be different if Allison had been born 6 weeks premature?

The Nurse's Role in Newborn and Infant Growth and Development

Growth and developmental stages impact upon every aspect of the infant's life. As infants progress through various stages of development, they do so in a predictable fashion. It is important for the nurse to have a good understanding of expected growth and development at key stages which correspond to milestone health visits. Health care visits through infancy often focus primarily on **anticipatory guidance** (educating parents and caregivers about what to expect in the next phase of development). Therefore, nurses can be well placed to provide parents with resources and education to best support their infant's healthy development.

Hospital-based nurses also need to use their knowledge of growth and development when caring for infants that are unwell. Hospitalization often requires the infant to be confined to the crib or cot or the hospital room.

Nurses must support growth and development within the constraints imposed by the child's illness.

NURSING PROCESS OVERVIEW

After the infant's current growth and development status has been assessed against established expected norms, any abnormal findings may be identified. The nurse may then identify one or more nursing diagnoses, including:

- Ineffective breastfeeding
- Risk for disproportionate growth
- Imbalanced nutrition, less than body requirements
- Risk for impaired parent/infant attachment
- Delayed stages of development
- Risk for caregiver role strain

Nursing care planning for the infant with growth and development issues should be individualized based on the infant's and family's needs. Nursing Care Plan 25.1 (found at the end of the chapter) can be used as a guide in planning nursing care for the infant with a concern with growth and developmental progression. The nurse may choose the appropriate nursing diagnoses from the plan and individualize them as needed. The nursing care plan is intended to serve as a guide, not as an all-inclusive growth and development care plan.

PROMOTING HEALTHY GROWTH AND DEVELOPMENT

Adding a new person to the family produces both excitement and anxiety. Newborns are completely reliant upon their parents or caregivers to fill every need. It can be quite a burden and precious responsibility that new parents are taking on. Many parents read the latest books about caring for newborns, while others rely on information received from family and friends, health care professionals, or the Internet. Newborns and their mothers spend only a short time in the hospital after delivery, so it is very important that parents are provided with skills and information to safely care for their newborn, and know when to call the health care provider with concerns.

Periodic surveillance for adequate growth and development of the infant is recommended by the Canadian Paediatric Society (CPS) and the Canadian Task Force on Preventative Health Care (2016a). Routine health maintenance visits enable surveillance for high-risk situations, injury prevention, early identification of abnormalities, and are key to achieving optimal health outcomes in infants and children. The CPS and the National Advisory Committee on Immunization (NACI) make recommendations for immunization schedules. Immunizations are a very important part of the infant health maintenance visit.

Nurses caring for newborns and infants should be familiar with the recommended schedule for health visits as well as the current immunization schedule.

Promoting Growth and Development Through Play

Experts in child development and behaviour have said repeatedly that play is the work of children. Infants practice their gross and fine motor skills and language through play (Goldson & Reynolds, 2014). Play is a natural way for infants and children to learn. Play is critical to infant development, as it gives infants the opportunity to explore their environment, practice new skills, and solve problems. The newborn prefers interacting with the parent to toys. Parents can talk to and sing to their newborns while participating in the daily activities that infants need, such as feeding, bathing, and changing diapers. Newborns and young infants love to watch people's faces and often mimic the expressions they see.

As infants become older, toys may be geared toward the motor skills or language skills that the child is developing. Parents can promote fine motor development in infants by providing age-appropriate toys. For example, a rattle that a young infant can hold promotes reaching and attaining. The older infant builds fine motor skills by stacking cups or placing smaller toys inside larger ones. Gross motor skills are reinforced and practiced over and over again when the infant wants to reach something he or she is interested in.

When playing with toys, the infant usually engages in **solitary play**; he or she does not share with other infants or directly play with other infants (Feigelman, 2011; Goldson & Reynolds, 2014). A wide variety of toys are available for infants, but infants often enjoy the most basic ones, such as plastic containers of various shapes and sizes, soft balls, and wooden or plastic spoons.

Books are also very important toys for infants. Reading to all ages of infants is recommended, and the older infant develops fine motor skills by learning to turn book pages (Shaw, 2006). Table 25.5 lists age-appropriate toys.

Promoting Early Learning

Research has shown that reading aloud and sharing books during early infancy are critical to the development of neural networks that are important in the later tasks of reading and word recognition. Reading books increases listening comprehension, communication skills, and promotes learning (Shaw, 2006). Infants demonstrate their excitement about picture books by kicking and waving their arms and babbling when looking at them. At 6 to 12 months, the infant reaches for books and brings them to the mouth. Reading picture books and simple stories to infants starts a good habit that

TABLE 25.5	APPROPRIATE TOYS FOR NEWBORNS AND INFANTS
Age	**Appropriate Toys**
Newborn to 1 month	• Mobile with contrasting colours or patterns • Unbreakable mirror • Soft music via tape or music box • Soft, brightly coloured toys
1–4 months	• Bright mobile • Unbreakable mirror • Rattles • Singing by parent or caregiver, varied music • High-contrast patterns in books or images
4–7 months	• Fabric or board books • Different types of music • Easy-to-hold toys that do things or make noise (fancy rattles) • Floating, squirting bath toys • Soft dolls or animals
8–12 months	• Plastic cups, bowls, buckets • Unbreakable mirror • Large building blocks • Stacking toys • Busy boxes (with buttons or knobs that make things happen) • Balls • Dolls • Board books with large pictures • Toy telephone • Push–pull toys (older infants)

should be continued throughout childhood (Diener, Hobson-Rohrer, & Byington, 2012). Moreover, evidence shows that higher literacy skills are linked to positive health behaviours and better overall health through the lifespan (Canadian Public Health Association, 2003).

Promoting Safety and Injury Prevention

Hundreds of children younger than 1 year of age die each year as a result of injury (CPS, 2012). As infants become more mobile, they risk injury from falls down stairs, off chairs, tables, and other structures. Curiosity leads the infant to explore potentially dangerous items, such as electrical outlets and cords, computer cables, hot stove or furnace vents, mop buckets, and toilets. Since infants explore so much with their mouths, small objects or hard foods pose a choking hazard. The infant will invariably pick up any accessible object and bring it to the mouth. With increasing dexterity, poisoning from medications, household cleaning products, or other substances also becomes a problem.

Safety in the Car

Motor vehicle collisions are one source of injury, particularly if the infant is improperly restrained. It is against the law for any infant to be transported in a motor vehicle without proper restraint. Infant car seats should face the rear of the car until the infant exceeds the weight/height recommendations as per their specific car seat manufacturer. Infants and children should remain rear facing as long as possible for maximum safety (Transport Canada, 2016). The car seat should be secured tightly in the centre of the back seat. The infant should never be placed in a front seat that is equipped with an airbag.

Infants should never be left unattended in a motor vehicle. The temperature rises very quickly inside a closed vehicle, and an infant can suffocate from heat in a closed vehicle in the summer. Even during cooler weather, the heat generated within a closed vehicle can reach three to five times the exterior temperature. Kidnapping is also a concern if the baby is left unattended in a vehicle. Additional information on car safety can be found on thePoint.

Safety During Sleep

Important components of sleep safety include where the baby sleeps, his/her sleeping position, the type of crib, type of mattress and bedding, and the home environment. The safest sleep location for all babies is in a crib. Newborns and infants should always be placed to sleep on the back in order to reduce risk of sudden infant death syndrome (SIDS) and accidental suffocation (Public Health Agency of Canada, 2014). The baby's crib should have a firm mattress that fits snugly in the crib on a secure support. Loose blankets, stuffed animals, pillows, and bumper pads should be avoided. Also the sleeping environment should be smoke free, as exposure to smoke can raise the risk of SIDS and respiratory conditions later in life.

Safety in the Home

Even before the infant can roll over, he or she wiggles and pushes with the feet. The infant can easily fall from a changing table, sofa, or crib with the side rails down, so the infant should never be left unattended on any surface. If infant seats, bouncy seats, or swings are used, the infant should always be restrained in the seat with appropriate straps, and always supervised.

Health Canada (2013) discourages the use of infant walkers, because the walker may tip over and the baby may fall out of it or the infant may fall down the stairs in it. Walkers allow infants access to things they may not otherwise be capable of reaching until they are able to walk alone, such as hot stoves and items on the edge of the countertop.

As the infant learns to roll, crawl, and walk, new safety issues arise. Safety gates should be used at the tops and bottoms of stairways. Gates may also be used to block curious infants from rooms that may pose physical danger to them because of sharp-edged furniture or decorative objects. Electrical outlets should be covered with approved safety covers. Cabinets and drawers should be secured with child safety latches. Medications, household cleaning supplies, and other potentially hazardous substances should be stored completely out of reach of infants (Health Canada, 2012).

Choking is a risk because infants immediately bring small items to the mouth for exploration. To avoid choking, recommend the following to parents:

* Always supervise infants during feeding and meal times.
* Use only toys recommended for children 0 to 12 months of age.
* Avoid stuffed animals with eyes or buttons that can be dislodged by the persistent infant.
* Keep the floor free of small items (accidentally dropped coins, paper clips, straight pins).
* Avoid feeding popcorn, nuts, carrot slices, grapes, and hot dog pieces to infants.
* Keep plastic bags of any size away from infants.
* Avoid the risk of strangulation by keeping window blind and drapery cords out of the infant's reach.

Safety in the Water

Infants can drown in a very small amount of water. Never leave an infant unattended in the sink, a baby bathtub or standard bathtub, a swimming or wading pool, or any other body of water, even if it is quite shallow. The bathroom door should be kept closed and the toilet lid down. Water should be emptied from tubs, pails, or buckets immediately after use. If the family has a swimming pool, a locked fence or locked screen enclosure should surround it in compliance with local laws. Exterior doors should be kept locked to prevent the older infant from wandering out to the pool. Research has not sufficiently demonstrated that water survival skills taught to infants are effective (Hong Nguyen, 2003). Completing an aquatic program does not decrease the risk of drowning; vigilant supervision is still always required.

> Remember Allison Johnson, the infant described in the beginning of the chapter? What anticipatory guidance related to safety would you provide to Allison's parents?

Promoting Nutrition

Healthy eating can provide adequate nutrition which is essential for optimal growth and development. Parents or caregivers need to have access to information to be able to make informed decisions about infant feeding. The importance of breastfeeding is evidence based, but regardless of whether parents provide breast milk and/or human milk substitutes nurses need to have adequate knowledge to support the families feeding approach. Human milk or formula should provide the majority of the calories and nutrients to support optimal infant growth until 12 months of age (Dietitians of Canada, 2017; Health Canada, 2015). Solid foods are introduced at 6 months of age and should include iron-rich food sources, including meats, iron-fortified infant cereals, and non-meat iron-rich foods.

Cultural Factors

Many dietary practices are affected by culture, both in the types of traditional foods eaten and in the approach to progression of infant feeding. Access to food, concerns about food safety, and prevalence of allergies can influence various populations but have been shown to have a higher prevalence in various provinces in Canada (Ben-Shoshan et al., 2010; Bordeleau, Asselin, Mazerolle, & Imbeau, 2016; Gao, Rowe, Majaesic, O'Hara, & Senthilselvan, 2008). Therefore, the nurse must explore the cultural practices of the family related to infant feeding so that you can support the family's cultural values.

Nutritional Needs

Newborns and infants are experiencing tremendous growth and need diets that support these rapid changes. Table 25.6 compares fluid and caloric needs in the newborn and infant and further information can be found on thePoint.

Breastfeeding

Health Canada (2015) and CPS (2017) identify breastfeeding as a normal and unequalled method for infant feeding. Breastfeeding or feeding of expressed human milk is recommended for all infants, including sick or premature newborns (with rare exceptions). The exceptions include infants with galactosemia, maternal use of illicit drugs and a few prescription medications, maternal untreated active tuberculosis, and maternal HIV infection in developed countries.

Even partial breastfeeding is helpful and offers some of the health benefits of breastfeeding. Nurses in the community and the hospital are in an excellent position to promote and support breastfeeding, thereby contributing to the both provincial and federal direction to increase breastfeeding rates across Canada. Breastfeeding rates across Canada vary, with 7 out of 10 babies being breastfed exclusively when discharged from hospital (Perinatal Services BC, 2014). Rates for Indigenous mothers are comparable to non-Indigenous mothers. However, on average at 6 months only 1 in 4 babies is exclusively breastfed (Allison, 2016).

BREAST MILK COMPOSITION

Breast milk includes lactose, lipids, polyunsaturated fatty acids, and amino acids. The ratio of whey to casein protein in breast milk makes it readily digestible. The high concentration of fats and the balance of amino acids are believed to contribute to proper myelination of the nervous system. The concentration of iron in breast milk is less than that of formula, but the iron has increased bioavailability and is usually sufficient to meet the infant's requirements for the first 6 months of life.

In addition to complete nutrition, immunologic protection is transferred from mother to infant via breast milk and maternal–infant bonding is promoted. The benefits of breastfeeding are listed in Box 25.1.

BREAST MILK SUPPLY AND DEMAND

Frequent, on-demand breastfeeding of the newborn is necessary to establish an adequate milk supply. After delivery of the placenta, levels of progesterone drop dramatically, which stimulates the anterior pituitary to produce prolactin. Prolactin stimulates the production of milk in the acinar or alveolar cells of the breast. When the infant sucks at the breast, nervous impulses stimulate further production of breast milk.

TABLE 25.6	NUTRITIONAL REQUIREMENTS	
Nutritional Requirements	Newborn	Infant
Fluid	140–160 mL/kg/day	100 mL/kg/day for first 10 kg 50 mL/kg/day for next 10 kg
Calories	105–108 kcal/kg/day	1 to 6 months: 108 kcal/kg 6 to 12 months: 98 kcal/kg

Adapted from Engorn, B., & Flerlage, J. (Eds.). (2015). *The Harriett Lane handbook.* 20th ed. Philadelphia, PA: Saunders.

The first "milk" to be produced by the breasts is termed **colostrum**. It is produced in small amounts in the second and third trimester of pregnancy and increased amounts for the first 2 to 4 days after birth. Colostrum is a thin, watery, yellowish fluid that is easy to digest, as it is high in protein and low in sugar and fat. Colostrum is complete nutrition and all that is needed by the newborn for the first 2 to 4 days of life (La Leche League International [LLLI], 2013). Transitional breast milk replaces colostrum on days 2 to 4 after birth. By day 10 after birth, mature breast milk is produced. Mature breast milk has a slightly bluish colour and appears thin. The breastfeeding mother produces milk continually which is not stored in the breast but transported by ducts (Ramsay, Kent, Hartmann, & Hartmann, 2005). Ductal branches drain glandular tissue immediately below the nipple, often merging into the main collecting duct very close to the nipple, producing **foremilk**. This process is controlled by hormonal influences (Geddes, 2009). The **let-down reflex** is responsible for the release of further milk. When the baby sucks at the breast, oxytocin is released from the posterior pituitary which allows milk to "let down" into the nipples, and the infant then sucks the milk. The let-down reflex is triggered not only by suckling at the breast but also by thinking of the baby or by the sound of a baby crying. The foremilk let down also helps to wash down the fattier hindmilk (Mizuno et al., 2009). This **hindmilk** helps the breastfed infant to grow quickly since breast milk fat content is linked to

breast milk cell content and breast fullness prior to and 30 minutes after feeding (Hassiotou et al., 2013). Mothers should be informed that the production of oxytocin during suckling may also cause uterine contractions and may cause afterpains during breastfeeding.

BREASTFEEDING TECHNIQUE

Breastfeeding mothers may not have established adequate breastfeeding prior to leaving the hospital after birth of the newborn. The nurse may encounter an infant–mother dyad experiencing difficulty with breastfeeding for a variety of reasons. Thus, the nurse must be competent in counselling the breastfeeding mother. Before each breastfeeding session, mothers should wash their hands. It is not necessary to wash the breast in most cases. The mother should be positioned comfortably. A number of positions are possible, and they should be varied throughout the day (Fig. 25.9). The mother may hold the breast in a "C" position if that is helpful to her (Fig. 25.9C). Stroke the nipple against the baby's cheek (Fig. 25.10). This should stimulate the infant to open the mouth widely. Bring the baby's wide-open mouth to the breast to form a seal around all of the nipple and areola. When the infant is finished feeding they will generally release the nipple of their own accord since they are controlling their own appetite (Kakulas, 2013). Removing the infant from the breast prematurely can cause nipple soreness and cracking.

Watching and listening to the infant feed may help assess the adequacy of the baby's latch technique. The infant who is properly latched on to the breast will suck rhythmically, taking most or all of the areola into the mouth. Audible swallowing is a quiet sound but can be heard as milk is delivered into the infant's mouth. Alternatively, parents can observe the infant below the chin to watch for swallowing and note if the breast is softening once the milk comes in. The nurse should assess the mother for pain related to breastfeeding. She should not be in pain if the baby is latched on properly.

Establishment of breastfeeding is best achieved if the infant is allowed to feed on demand, whenever he or she is hungry. This may be as often as every 1 to 3 hours in the neonate. Infants may feed for 10 to 20 minutes on each breast at each feeding, or longer on just one breast, alternating the breast at each feeding. Both methods are acceptable.

The breastfeeding infant does not need supplementation with water or formula even in the first few days of life as long as the newborn continues to have wet and soiled diapers. After several days of age, the mother's milk supply should be well established. Adequate urine output and bowel movements, as well as continued weight gain in the infant, indicate the adequacy of breastfeeding. Working mothers in particular may need additional support from the nurse in order to continue breastfeeding if they desire to do so. Common problems occurring with breastfeeding are addressed in Teaching

FIGURE 25.9 Various positions may be used during breast-feeding: (**A**) cradle hold, (**B**) side-lying, (**C**) football hold (note the "C" position for holding the breast during latching on).

Guidelines 25.1. Additional reliable resources for mothers who desire to breastfeed may be found on the websites listed on thePoint.

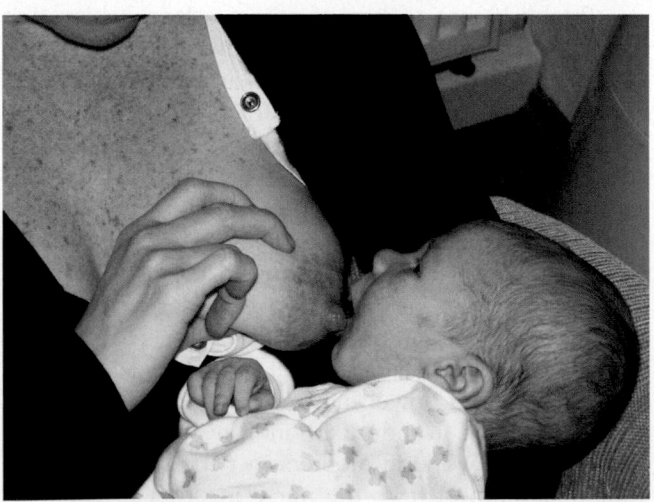

FIGURE 25.10 Stroking the infant's cheek with the nipple will elicit the rooting reflex.

Teaching Guidelines 25.1
PROMOTING BREASTFEEDING

Problem	Solutions
Sore nipples	Prevention: encourage appropriate latch on from the beginning
	Expose nipples to air between feedings
	Allow breast milk to dry on nipples
	Use aloe vera to help heal sore nipples. Vitamin E should not be used due to limited and conflicting evidence base.
	May use medical-grade lanolin or preservative-free lanolin product

Engagement	Apply warm compresses or encourage the mother to take a warm shower prior to having the baby latch on (warmth encourages some of the milk to be released, allowing the breast to soften and making it easier for the infant to latch on)
Poor sucking	Feed on cue, not on a schedule Encourage the sleepy infant by stroking the feet, undressing, and rubbing the head
Inadequate milk supply	Decrease maternal stress Encourage adequate maternal diet and fluid intake Instruct working mothers to pump in order to keep up milk supply when away from the infant
Father feels left out	Encourage father to participate in other aspects of care
Mother worries about adequacy of breast milk	If infant is voiding (and/or passing stool) per day and gaining weight, then he or she is receiving enough milk and appropriate nutrition

Bottle-Feeding

For the mother who makes a decision not to, or cannot, breastfeed, commercially prepared formulas are available for bottle-feeding. These formulas are designed to imitate human milk. Standard infant formulas based on cow's milk provide 20 kcal per 30 mL and use lactose as a source for carbohydrates (Stettler, Bhatia, Parish, & Stallings, 2011). Vegetable oil is used as the source of fat; whey or casein provides protein. Newer cow's milk–based formulas contain long-chain polyunsaturated fatty acids that are thought to improve brain development. Health Canada recommends that when making the transition to cow's milk as the child's main milk source, wait until the baby is between 9 and 12 months old. Start with homogenized cow's milk (3.25%); do not offer skim or partly skimmed milk (1% or 2%) before 2 years of age.

Take Note!

Cow's milk does not provide an adequate balance of nutrients for the growing infant, especially iron. It may also overload the infant's renal system with inappropriate amounts of protein, sodium, and minerals.

Only formulas that are fortified with iron should be used. Iron stores that the infant received prenatally are depleted by 4 to 6 months of age. To prevent IDA, poor growth patterns, and impaired development,

iron-fortified formulas must be used. The CPS recommends that commercial formulas provide 10 to 12 mg of iron per litre (Baker & Greer; The Committee on Nutrition, 2010). Commercial formulas also provide an adequate blend of essential vitamins and minerals.

FEEDING PATTERNS

Infant feeding is an opportune time to establish good eating behaviours. The infant should always be held while being bottle-fed. Cradling in a semi-upright position allows for additional bonding time, as the infant can see the caregiver's face while feeding (Fig. 25.11). Talking or singing during feeding time also increases bonding. As with breastfed infants, the bottle-fed infant should be fed on cue. Overfeeding with the bottle increases the incidence of spitting up and obesity, so families need to learn their baby's cues to hunger and satiety (Hill, 2015).

It is important to feed the baby when he or she displays signs of hunger. Crying is a late sign of hunger; earlier signs include making sucking motions, sucking on hands, or putting the fist to the chin. The infant should be burped two or three times per feeding, when he or she slows feeding or stops sucking. Newborns may only take 10 to 30 mL per feeding initially, working up to 60 to 90 mL in the first week to 10 days. They need to feed about 6 to 10 times per day. The infant will gradually be able to ingest more formula per feeding. By 6 months of age, babies feed 4 or 5 times per day and take 180 to 240 mL per feeding. Most infants

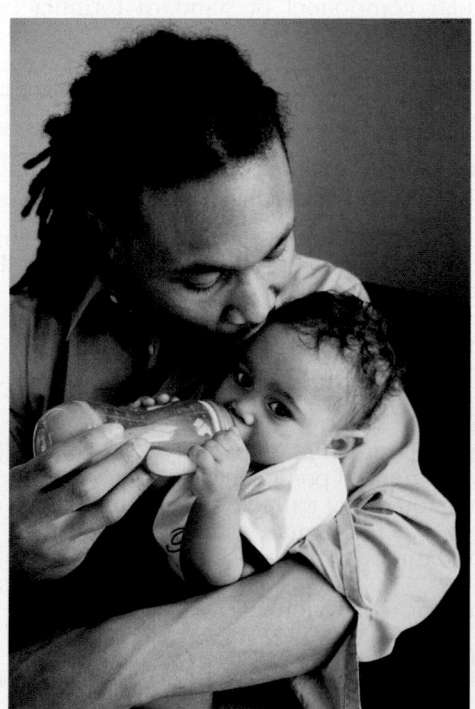

FIGURE 25.11 Technique for bottle-feeding the infant.

will not require specific amounts per feeding; the infant should be fed until full. To prevent overfeeding, healthy bottle-fed infants should be allowed to self-regulate the amount of formula ingested per feeding. When the baby is satiated, he or she might fall asleep, spit out the nipple or formula, play with the nipple, or lie quietly, only sucking once in a while (Hill, 2015).

TYPES OF FORMULAS AND BOTTLES

Parents may choose to use commercial formulas that are ready to feed or available as a concentrate or as a powder. Parents should follow the instructions for mixing the concentrate or powder to avoid dehydration or fluid and electrolyte imbalances. Purified or previously boiled room-temperature water should be used to mix formulas during the first 2 months of life. Bottles and nipples need to be properly sterilized between feedings for the first 4 months of life (HealthLinkBC, 2015a). Ready-to-feed formula should be used as is and never diluted (Stettler, et al., 2011).

A wide variety of baby bottles and nipple types are available for formula feeding, and the choice is purely individual. Few infants require special nipples or bottles. Box 25.2 gives guidelines on preparation and storage of formula and care of bottles.

SPECIAL FORMULAS

Cow's milk–based infant formulas are recommended for all healthy term infants as an alternative when breast-feeding is not possible (Dietitians of Canada, 2017; Health Canada, 2015). However, alternate formulas may be needed for the infant who may be allergic to a particular component of standard formula or has a renal, hepatic, metabolic, or intestinal disorder. Infants diagnosed with an intolerance to cow's milk may be recommended to consume a pre-digested or elemental formula. These special formulas should only be used under the recommendations of a health care provider who has diagnosed a specific condition which warrants their use. Infants who fail to gain weight may be placed on standard infant formula prepared to deliver a higher caloric density per ounce. Preterm infants (those born at less than 37 weeks' gestation) need nutrition and feeding reviews to monitor their growth and weight over the coming months (Stefanescu, Gillam-Krakauer, Stefanescu, Markham, & Kosinski, 2016). Evidence is starting to emerge that overfeeding small birth size babies after the age of 1 month to achieve a rapid postnatal growth increases the child's blood pressure (de Beer et al., 2016). Fortified human milk has been shown to have benefits to the preterm infant's long-term health outcome such as reduced infection rates and improved protein intake (Shah, Dereddy, Jones, Dhanireddy, & Talati, 2016).

Progressing to Solid Foods

After 6 months of age, infants require the nutrients available in solid foods in addition to their breast milk or formula. Progressing to feeding solid foods can be exciting and trying. Before solid foods are attempted, the infant should be assessed for readiness to progress. Parents need instruction and resources in choosing appropriate solid foods and support in the progression process.

ASSESSING INFANT READINESS

Several factors contribute to the appropriate timing of solid food introduction. The tongue extrusion reflex is necessary for sucking to be an automatic reaction—that is, when a nipple or other item is placed in the mouth, the tongue extrudes and sucking begins. This reflex disappears at about 4 to 6 months of age (Dietz & Stern, 2012). Introducing solid food with a spoon prior to 4 to 6 months of age will result in extrusion of the tongue. The parent may think that the infant does not want the food and is spitting it out intentionally, but this is not the case; the infant simply must be mature enough to eat with a spoon (absence of extrusion reflex).

> **Take Note!**
>
> **Infant Feeding**
>
> One percent to 2% cow's milk should never be given to an infant under 2 years since it is not nutritionally adequate to provide the calories, fats, and nutrients needed for healthy infant growth (Health Canada, 2015).

The ability to swallow solid food does not become completely functional until 4 to 6 months of age. Enzymes to appropriately digest food other than breast milk and

---

BOX 25.2

PREPARATION AND STORAGE OF BOTTLES AND FORMULA

- Wash nipples and bottles in hot soapy water and rinse well OR run nipples and bottles through the dishwasher.
- Store tightly covered ready-to-feed formula can after opening in refrigerator for up to 48 hours.
- After mixing concentrate or powdered formula, store tightly covered in refrigerator for up to 48 hours.
- Do not reheat and reuse partially used bottles. Throw away the unused portion after each feeding.
- Do not add cereal to the formula in the bottle.
- Do not sweeten formula with honey.
- Warm formula by placing bottle in a container of hot water.
- Do not microwave formula.

Adapted from Ben-Joseph, E. P. (2015). *Formula feeding FAQs: Preparation and storage.* Retrieved from kidshealth.org/parent/growth/feeding/formulafeed_storing.html#

formula are also not present in sufficient quantities until the age of 4 to 6 months.

Before the introduction of solid foods and the cup, the infant should be able to sit supported in a high chair. Solids should be fed with a spoon, with the infant in an upright position.

CHOOSING APPROPRIATE SOLID FOODS

Iron-fortified rice cereal mixed with a small amount of breast milk or formula is a good choice for the first solid food. The cereal is easily digested and its taste is generally well accepted. The cereal should be quite thin at first; it can be mixed to a thicker consistency as the infant gets older. Once the feeding of cereal with a spoon is successful, other single foods may be introduced. The foods should be soft and mashed or pureed to a smooth consistency, whether prepackaged "baby food" or foods prepared at home.

The introduction of one new food every 3 to 5 days is recommended (Stettler, et al., 2011). This allows for identification of food allergies (Box 25.3). No salt, sugar, or other seasoning should be added to these first foods.

Generally, by 6 to 8 months of age the infant is ready for more texture in his or her foods (see thePoint for additional links). Soft, smashed table food without large chunks is appropriate. Puree and food with meats can be given from 6 to 8 months as they are a source of zinc and iron (Government of Canada, 2017). The Government of Canada nutrition resource provides evidence of the nutritional needs for infants and offers menus for infants for a range of preferences including parents who advocate for a vegetarian diet in childhood. Finger foods such as cereals, soft green bean pieces, or soft peas may also be offered. Avoid hard foods that the infant may choke on, such as grapes, nuts, hot dogs, round berries.

The cup should be introduced at 6 to 8 months of age, 30 mL of breast milk or formula should be placed in the cup while the infant is learning. This will decrease the amount of mess should the cup be spilled. Old-fashioned sippy cups are generally acceptable for use, though older infants quickly learn to drink from an ordinary cup with assistance when they are thirsty. Older infants are also able to drink from a straw. Newer no-spill sippy cups are not recommended for general home use. They require sucking much like a bottle and do not really encourage the child to learn cup drinking. In addition, the no-spill sippy cup allows for juice or milk to be in constant contact with the baby's teeth increasing the risk of dental caries. Fruit juice and other sweetened drinks are never recommended for infants as they do not provide the nutritional requirements needed and they predispose to poor oral health and dental development (Stettler et al., 2011).

PROMOTING HEALTHY EATING HABITS

Infants and children learn about food within a social context, so the family plays an important role in creating healthy eating habits. Families "model" eating behaviours; infants and children learn about eating through watching others. Lifelong eating patterns are often established in childhood, so it is important to emphasize healthy eating practices beginning in infancy. Parents should not let infants eat whatever they want (permissive feeding style); this will lead to fights over eating in the future. Infants may require as many as 20 exposures to a new food before it is accepted. On the other hand, infants should not be coerced into eating all that is provided (authoritarian feeding style). Forcing an infant to eat when he or she is full sets the child up for overeating in the future and may lead to more power struggles (Dietz & Stern, 2012). Parents need to find a balance between the permissive and authoritarian feeding styles to establish lifelong healthy eating patterns in their children. By providing education about appropriate diet and feeding behaviours, the nurse can help the family accomplish this goal.

> **Think back to Allison Johnson. What questions should you ask Allison's parents related to her nutritional intake? What anticipatory guidance related to nutrition would be appropriate?**

Promoting Healthy Sleep and Rest

Newborns sleep about 20 hours a day, waking frequently to feed before quickly returning to sleep. By 3 months of age, some infants may sleep 6 hours per night without waking and they might be gaining weight well, so they

---

BOX 25.3

FOODS TO AVOID IN INFANCY
- Honey
- Excessive amounts of fruit juice
- Foods likely to cause choking
- Peanuts
- Popcorn
- Other small hard foods (e.g., raw carrot chunks)
- Grapes and hot dog slices (must be cut in smaller pieces)
- Foods likely to result in allergic reaction
- Citrus
- Strawberries
- Wheat
- Cow's milk (until 9 to 12 months)

Adapted from Brown, J. E. (2014). *Nutrition now* (7th ed.). Belmont, CA: Wadsworth, Cengage Learning.

do not need to feed as often during the night. They will continue to take about three naps a day. By 4 months of age the infant is more active and alert and may have more trouble going to sleep in the evening. Around 12 months of age infants sleep 8 to 12 hours per night and take two naps per day (Feigelman, 2011). There are wide variations of normal with regard to sleep routines in the first year of life, as each infant is individual. It is common for new parents to have concerns and questions about their baby's sleep duration and timing, especially if they have frequent night waking. The nurse can counsel parents about overall sleep requirements by referring to the CPS (2013b) guidelines on Healthy Sleep for your Baby and Child.

Take Note!

The Canadian Paediatric Society has determined that side sleeping is not as safe as supine sleeping.

In the newborn period, the primary caregiver should try to sleep when the baby is sleeping. Since newborns need to be fed every 1½ to 3 hours around the clock, parents may become exhausted quickly and are often eager for the infant to sleep through the night. Adding rice cereal to the evening bottle has not been proven to discourage night waking and is not recommended (Nevarez, Rifas-Shiman, Kleinman, Gillman, & Taveras, 2010). Provide support to parents of newborns and educate them on infant sleeping patterns.

It is important to establish a bedtime routine around 4 months of age due to the infant's increased alertness and activity level. The baby who is 4 months or older needs a time of calming and relaxation before going to sleep. A consistent bedtime routine should be established, perhaps a bath followed by rocking, singing, or reading to their child can be advocated. A variety of parenting strategies around sleep behaviours exist. Some parents believe that the infant should fall asleep in his or her own crib rather than being rocked to sleep while others may wish to cuddle their infant until he or she is relaxed, then put them in their crib. Occasionally, infants 12 to 24 months may exhibit head banging as a form of self-soothing and use this technique to fall asleep at night. When infants wake in the night, parents need to understand the cause which could be multifarious and include hunger, cold, or a need for comfort. Parents should minimize attention and stimulation when attending to the infant so as not to send mixed messages about sleeping patterns. Continued issues with night waking should be discussed with the infant's primary or other health care provider.

What anticipatory guidance should you provide to Allison's parents in relation to sleep?

Promoting Healthy Teeth and Gums

Healthy teeth and gums require proper oral hygiene practices and routine dental assessments by a qualified professional. The CDA recommends that infants receive their first dental visit by the age of 1 year or within 12 months of the eruption of their first tooth (CDA, 2010). Infants older than 6 months of age who are at risk for developing dental caries and whose drinking water source contains less than 0.3 parts per million may require fluoride supplementation (CDA, 2010). Variation in fluoride supplementation in water supplies exists across Canada and local information should be sought. Excess fluoride ingestion can result in discolouration of the teeth (fluorosis), thus should not be used unless specifically recommended by a health care provider. Early childhood dental caries can result from pooling of milk or juice around teeth and gums. Infants should not be allowed to take milk or juice bottles to bed, as the high sugar content of the fluid in contact with the teeth all night leads to dental caries.

Before tooth eruption, parents should clean the child's gums after feeding with a damp washcloth (teething is discussed below as a common developmental concern). After teeth have erupted, parents can continue to use a soft cloth for tooth cleaning and then eventually use a small soft-bristled toothbrush. Toothpaste is unnecessary in infancy. Weaning from the bottle at age 12 to 15 months may help prevent dental caries. No-spill sippy cups have also been implicated in the development of dental caries and should be avoided.

Promoting Secure Attachments and Setting Boundaries

Parenting requires ever-changing adaptations to the developing infant's needs. Unconditional love, patience, and compassion must be balanced with the parents' needs. Setting boundaries (which some may view as **discipline**) helps the child develop a positive behaviour and approach through instruction, practice, and consistency. The primary goal is to establish boundaries of acceptable and expected behaviour. Boundaries and predictable routines help build a sense of security in the infant. The infant's activities are based on the basic needs of food, security, warmth, love, and comfort. While crying may be as a result of an unmet need, infants who are ill, distressed, and afraid need comfort and reassurance from their caregivers (Cassidy & Shaver, 2016). Infant mental health promotion focuses on promoting early mental health and development and the importance this has on long-term outcome; for more information about infant mental health see thePoint.

As the infant is undergoing rapid changes in motor skills, safety needs increase. Nurses should encourage the parents to "childproof" their home so that the infant can develop physical skills without being at risk. Child-proofing involves removing or reducing hazards through means such as locking cupboards that contain cleaning products, covering electrical outlets, and moving items that may fall on or trip the infant as they learn to move around the home. In a childproof home, fewer restrictions need to be placed on the infant's behaviour, and he or she can explore.

Physical punishment or spanking should never be used with infants or children. The CPS (2013a) strongly discourages any use of physical punishment on children. It is normal for some infants to cry for a few hours per day, and this can be stressful and frustrating for parents. Parents have to learn strategies to cope with their infant that are not physically or emotionally punitive as infants are at increased risk for injury. Shaking or spanking an infant can cause significant head trauma which can lead to permanent disabling brain damage, blindness, seizures, paralysis, or even death (Government of Canada, 2013). Providing a safe environment, redirection away from undesirable behaviours, and saying "no" in appropriate instances are far more effective. For example, when the infant is in potential danger (e.g., inserting a key into an electrical outlet, attempting to ingest a poisonous substance, or reaching into the toilet), the parent must use a firm but calm and brisk approach. The nurse must be able to assess parental stress levels and ask about coping strategies used. Assessing for high-risk home situations and risk for infant injury is an essential component of the nurse's assessment in any health maintenance visit. The nurse can counsel parents about crying as a normal developmental stage in infancy, and provide education and resources on coping strategies as well as positive discipline approaches (CPS, 2013a).

Remaining calm, firm, and consistent is necessary. Immediacy is also an important component of appropriate discipline. The infant cannot make the connection between a subsequent punishment and discussion of behaviour with the earlier event itself. Positive reinforcement should be used to support good behaviour.

Addressing Child Care Needs

In Canada, many parents work outside the home, many households are single-parent families, and many families live a distance away from relatives. In all of these circumstances, infants may need to be cared for outside the home, often in child care settings or home day care centres. The number of children in paid child care in Canada has tripled from 357,000 to 1.36 million from 1967 to 1995 (Lang, 2008). The Canadian Child Care Federation offers a national statement focusing on assessing quality child care; see thePoint. The CPS offers recommendations for parents when making decisions around childcare; these include cost, quality, safety

levels. Parents need to carefully consider their options, and the nurse can be an important contact to discuss these at routine health review visits (Lang, 2008).

ADDRESSING COMMON DEVELOPMENTAL CONCERNS

Parents commonly have multiple concerns during normal infant growth and development. Although most of these issues are not actual disease states or behaviour problems, nurses must be aware of these issues to recognize them and to intervene appropriately.

Colic

Colic is defined as inconsolable crying that lasts 3 hours or longer per day and for which there is no physical cause. It may begin as early as 3 weeks of age, occur 3 to 7 days per week, especially in the evenings, and continue until around 3 months of age (HealthLinkBC, 2015b), coinciding with the age at which infants are better able to soothe themselves (e.g., by finger sucking). The cause of colic is not yet known, although possibly related to problems in the gastrointestinal or neurologic system (probably system immaturity), temperament, or parenting style of the mother or father. Some parents are overly anxious or overly attentive or, at the other extreme, may not give the infant the attention he or she needs. Any of these may contribute to a baby's fussing and crying.

Prolonged crying leads to increased stress among caregivers. Failure to stop the crying leads to frustration, and crying that prevents the parents from sleeping contributes to the exhaustion they are already experiencing.

Educate parents that normal crying increases by the time the infant is 6 weeks old and diminishes by about 12 weeks. When faced with a colicky baby, parents should develop a stepwise approach to checking that all of the infant's basic needs are met. When these needs are met, attempts at soothing the infant may be used. Reducing stimulation may decrease the length of crying. Carrying the infant more may also be helpful. Some infants respond to the motion of an infant swing or a car ride. Vibration, white noise, or gentle music may also help to decrease fussing in some infants. Pacifiers can be soothing to babies who need additional nonnutritive sucking. Parents should try one intervention at a time, taking care not to stimulate the infant excessively in the process of searching for solutions. Nurses should provide ongoing support to the parents of a colicky infant and reassure them that this is a temporary condition that will resolve in time (Ehrlich, 2014).

Spitting Up

Spitting up (regurgitating small amounts of stomach contents) occurs in all infants, and a significant number of normal infants spit up excessively. Although spitting up after feeding is normal, it can be a cause of great concern to parents. Overfed babies who feed based on a parent-designed schedule and those who burp poorly are more likely to spit up. For some infants, the amount and frequency of spitting up are significant, and those babies should be evaluated by the physician or nurse practitioner.

Teach parents that feeding smaller amounts on a more frequent basis may help to decrease spitting-up episodes. Always burp the baby at least two or three times per feeding. Keep the baby upright for 30 minutes after feeding and do not lay the infant prone after feeding. Avoid bouncing or excess activity immediately after feeding. Positioning in an infant seat compresses the stomach and is not recommended. Some parents report that their baby sleeps better "on their stomach," but the nurse should discourage this whenever possible. The safest sleep position for the infant is flat on their back in the crib. Reassure parents that if the infant is wetting diapers and gaining weight, the spitting up is normal. However, if the infant spits up most of his/her feedings, is very irritable during or after feeds, is not gaining weight appropriately, or has projectile emesis, then the primary care provider should be notified.

Thumb Sucking, Pacifiers, and Security Items

Infants demonstrate a clear need for nonnutritive sucking; even fetuses can be observed sucking their thumbs or fingers in utero. Thumb sucking is a healthy self-comforting activity. Infants who suck their thumbs or pacifiers often are better able to soothe themselves than those who do not. Studies have not shown that sucking either thumbs or pacifiers leads to the need for orthodontic braces unless the sucking continues well beyond the early school-age period, but it can lead to decreased breastfeeding in some infants. Pacifiers have also been shown to be protective against SIDS, however may be related to the development of ear infections (CPS, 2016b). Infants may also become attached to a doll, stuffed animal, or blanket. Just like thumb sucking, the attachment item gives the infant the security to self-soothe when he or she is uncomfortable.

Families need to explore their feelings and cultural preferences about sucking habits and security items. Parents should not try to break the habit during a stressful time for the infant. When the infant is intensely trying to master a new skill such as sitting or walking, he or she may need the sucking or security item to self-soothe. Pacifiers and security items can be physically taken away at some point, but the thumb is attached. The infant who has become attached to thumb sucking should not have additional attention drawn to the issue, as that may prolong thumb sucking.

Families of infants who use pacifiers may want to wean the infant from the pacifier when the child approaches 1 year of age, as this is the time when the need for additional sucking naturally decreases. Otherwise, weaning from the pacifier should occur by 2 to 3 years of age in order to limit adverse effects upon dentition (Nelson, 2012). Attempts to wean the child from a security blanket or toy should probably be reserved for after infancy (see Evidence-Based Practice 25.1).

Teething

Discomfort is common as the tooth breaks through the periodontal membrane. Infants may drool, bite on hard objects, or increase finger sucking. Some infants may become very irritable, refuse to eat, and not sleep well.

| EVIDENCE-BASED PRACTICE 25.1 | EVIDENCE AND RECOMMENDATIONS RELATED TO PACIFIER USE |

STUDY

The author performed a comprehensive review of research studies related to pacifier usage in order to provide nurses with the highest level of evidence to use when counselling parents about this topic. Studies reviewed included randomized controlled trials (RCTs), meta-analyses of RCTs, and critical literature reviews related to the risks and benefits of pacifier use. The author included only studies performed between 1990 and the present.

Findings

Upon analysis of the various research studies, the author reached several conclusions. Pacifier use has been shown to lower the risk of sudden infant death syndrome (SIDS) when used at the time of sleep. Additional benefits include the calming effect related to nonnutritive sucking and as an adjunct in pain relief. Potential disadvantages include negative effects on breastfeeding if pacifier is used early or extensively; increased incidence of otitis media; and the risks of injury, allergy, and dental malocclusion.

Nursing Implications

In light of the potential risks and benefits of pacifier use, nurses must be prepared to provide parents with accurate information related to the use of pacifiers. Educate parents to avoid introduction of the pacifier until breastfeeding is well established (4 to 6 weeks of age), to use pacifiers only during periods of sleep, and to never force a pacifier on an infant or replace a pacifier in a sleeping infant's mouth. In addition, parents should wean the child from the pacifier in late infancy so that it is not used by 2 to 3 years of age to avoid further dental issues.

Adapted from Nelson, A. M. (2012). A comprehensive review of evidence and current recommendations related to pacifier usage. *Journal of Pediatric Nursing, 27*, 690–699.

Fever, vomiting, and diarrhoea are generally not considered a sign of teething but rather of illness.

Teething pain results from inflammation. Teach parents that application of cold may be soothing to the gums. The infant may chew on a cold teething ring, or parents can rub an ice cube wrapped in a washcloth on the gums. Occasionally, oral acetaminophen or ibuprofen may be given to relieve pain (Tinanoff, 2011), but should be used under the recommendation of a health care provider and always follow the dosing instructions on the medication bottle.

> **Refer back to 6-month-old Allison Johnson. List some common developmental concerns of 6-month-old infants. What anticipatory guidance related to these concerns would you provide to her parents?**

NURSING CARE PLAN 25.1

Growth and Development Issues in the Newborn and Infant

NURSING DIAGNOSIS: Ineffective breastfeeding, related to lack of exposure, misconceptions, or knowledge deficit as evidenced by first baby, mother's verbalization, or nursing observations

Outcome Identification and Evaluation

Mother/infant dyad will experience successful breastfeeding: *infant will latch on, suck, and swallow at the breast; mother will not experience sore nipples.*

Interventions: *Promoting Effective Breastfeeding*

- Educate mother on recognition of and response to infant hunger cues *to promote on-cue breastfeeding, which will establish milk supply.*
- Mothers are encouraged to eat a healthy and well-balanced diet as they did during pregnancy and drink enough so that they are not thirsty.
- Demonstrate breastfeeding positions with infant at the breast *(appropriate positioning increases probability of successful latch).*
- Assess infant's latch technique, sucking motion, and audible swallowing *(an appropriately latched infant will take most of the areola in the mouth, suck in spurts, and demonstrate audible swallowing).*
- Assess infant voiding/stool patterns: *at least six voids per day and passage of stool ranging from one or more per day to one every several days is a normal pattern for breastfed infants.*
- Assess infant weight gain: *gain of 25 to 30 g per day after the second week of life indicates infant is receiving appropriate nutrition.*
- Assess mother's nipples for redness or soreness; *if infant appropriately latches on, nipples will not become sore.*

NURSING DIAGNOSIS: Risk for altered growth pattern* (risk factors: caregiver knowledge deficit, first infant, premature infant, or maladaptive feeding behaviours)

Outcome Identification and Evaluation

Infant will demonstrate adequate growth and appropriate feeding behaviours: *steady increases in weight, length, and head circumference; infant feeds appropriately for age.*

Interventions: *Promoting Adequate Growth*

- Observe mother/infant dyad breastfeeding or bottle-feeding to determine need for further education or identify infant difficulties with feeding.
- Educate mother about appropriate breastfeeding or bottle-feeding so that the mother is aware of what to expect in normal feeding pattern.
- When infant is old enough, provide education about addition of solid foods, spoon and cup feeding: after 6 months of age breast milk or formula needs to be supplemented with a variety of foods.

*Not on NANDA-I 2018-2020 list of nursing diagnoses.

(continued)

NURSING CARE PLAN 25.1

Growth and Development Issues in the Newborn and Infant (continued)

- Determine need for additional caloric intake, if necessary (premature infants and infants with chronic illnesses or metabolic disorders often need adjustments in caloric intake to demonstrate adequate or catch-up growth).
- Obtain daily weights if hospitalized (weekly if outpatient) and weekly length and head circumference to determine whether feeding pattern is sufficient to promote adequate growth in those infants there is concern around growth and development.

NURSING DIAGNOSIS: Imbalanced nutrition: less than body requirements, related to possible ineffective feeding pattern or inadequate caloric intake as evidenced by failure to gain weight or by inadequate increases in weight, length, and head circumference over time

Outcome Identification and Evaluation

Infant will take in adequate nutrients using effective feeding pattern: *infant will demonstrate adequate weight gain (25 to 30 g per day) and steady increases in length and head circumference.*

Interventions: *Promoting Adequate Nutritional Intake*

- Assess current feeding pattern and daily intake *to determine areas of concern.*
- Increase frequency of breastfeeding or volume of bottle-feeding, *if needed, to meet caloric needs.*
- Introduce solid foods on age-appropriate schedule: *introducing solids at the right time improves the chances that the child will learn to take solid foods.*
- Limit juice intake or discontinue altogether *(juice has little nutritive value and displaces nutrients from breast milk or formula).*

- Increase caloric density of formula (if ordered by a health care professional) by mixing to a more concentrated level or with additives (fats or carbohydrates) *to provide increased calories needed to support adequate growth.*
- If infant is taking solids already, choose higher calorie foods *to maximize nutrient intake.*

NURSING DIAGNOSIS: Risk for impaired parenting (risk factors: premature infant, parental knowledge deficit about normal newborn activity and care, infant with difficult temperament or medical problems).

Outcome Identification and Evaluation

Parent and infant will demonstrate appropriate attachment via *eye contact, parental response to infant cues, parental verbalization of caring for infant, infant response to parent's caretaking behaviours.*

Interventions: *Encouraging Appropriate Parent–Infant Attachment*

- Assess parent's response to infant cues to determine degree of attachment and level of parent's knowledge about infant care.
- Assess infant's response to parent's caretaking behaviours to determine degree of attachment.
- Determine infant's temperament to counsel parent effectively about responses appropriate for that type of temperament.

- Encourage face-to-face positioning for holding or feeding the young infant to encourage give-and-take response between infant and parent.
- Encourage parent to meet infant's needs promptly and with affection to promote sense of trust in the infant.
- Reinforce parent's attempts at improving attachment with infant (positive reinforcement naturally encourages appropriate behaviours).

NURSING CARE PLAN 25.1

Growth and Development Issues in the Newborn and Infant (continued)

NURSING DIAGNOSIS: Growth and development, altered*, related to speech, motor, psychosocial, or cognitive concerns as evidenced by delay in meeting expected milestones.

Outcome Identification and Evaluation

Development will be maximized: *infant will make continued progress toward attainment of developmental milestones.*

Interventions: *Maximizing Development*

- Use established developmental assessment tools to determine the infant's current level of functioning.
- Offer age-appropriate play, activities, and toys to encourage further development.
- Carry out interventions as prescribed by developmental specialist, physical therapist, occupational therapist, or speech therapist (repeated exposure to

the activities or exercises is needed to make developmental progress).
- Provide support to parents of infants with developmental concerns, as developmental progress can be slow and it is difficult for families to stay motivated and maintain hope.

NURSING DIAGNOSIS: Risk for caregiver role strain (risk factors: first baby, knowledge deficit about infant care, lack of prior exposure, fatigue if premature, ill, or developmentally delayed infant)

Outcome Identification and Evaluation

Parent will experience competence in role: *will demonstrate appropriate caretaking behaviours and verbalize comfort in new role.*

Interventions: *Preventing Caregiver Role Strain*

- Assess parent's knowledge of newborn/infant care and the issues that arise as a part of normal development *to determine parent's needs.*
- Provide education on normal newborn/infant care *so that parents have the knowledge they need to appropriately care for their new baby.*

- Provide anticipatory guidance related to normal infant development *to prepare parents for what to expect next and how to intervene.*
- Encourage respite for parents *(even a few hours away from the demands of attending to an infant's care can rejuvenate the parents. This can be someone coming in to the family home and allowing the parents time to rest but still be on hand if they were needed).*

NURSING DIAGNOSIS: Risk for injury (risk factors: developmental age, infant curiosity, rapidly progressing motor abilities)

Outcome Identification and Evaluation

Infant safety will be maintained: *infant will remain free from injury.*

Interventions: *Preventing Injury*

- Promote and educate about car seat safety to decrease risk of injury related to motor vehicles.
- Childproof home: as infant becomes more mobile, he or she will want to explore everything, increasing risk of injury.
- Parents should have the Poison Control Centre phone number available; should an accidental ingestion occur, Poison Control Centre can give parents the best advice for appropriate intervention.

- Never leave an infant unattended in the sink, bathtub, or swimming pool to prevent drowning.
- Teach parents first aid measures and infant CPR to minimize consequences of injury should it occur.
- Parents should watch the infant at all times (no amount of childproofing can replace the watchful eye of a caring parent) during feeding and meal time, when actively crawling or mobilizing, and during all awake hours.

---

*Not on NANDA-I 2018-2020 list of nursing diagnoses.

KEY CONCEPTS

- Infancy encompasses the period from birth to age 12 months.

- The infant exhibits tremendous growth, doubling the birth weight by 6 months of age and tripling it by 12 months of age.

- Most organ systems are immature at birth and develop and mature over the first year of life.

- Child development is orderly, sequential, and predictable, progressing in a cephalocaudal and proximodistal fashion.

- The infant is mastering the psychosocial task of Trust versus Mistrust.

- Cognitive development in infancy is sensorimotor; infants use their senses and progressing motor skills to master their environment.

- The 12 month old babbles expressively and uses two or three words with meaning.

- Promotion of safety is of key importance throughout infancy.

- Breastfeeding is the natural and preferred method for infant feeding.

- Breastfed and bottle-fed infants should both be fed on cue rather than on a parent-designed schedule.

- Solid foods should be introduced at age 6 months. A spoon should be used to feed the infant, and rice cereal should be the first food. New foods should be introduced no more frequently than every 3 to 5 days.

- The cup may be introduced at 6 months of age. No-spill sippy cups are generally not recommended.

- Spitting up and colic are parts of normal development in the otherwise thriving infant and do not require medical intervention.

REFERENCES AND RECOMMENDED READINGS

Abdullah, K., Zlotkin, S., Parkin, P., & Greiner, D. (2011). Iron-deficiency anemia in children. *Canadian Paediatric Surveillance Program*. Retrieved from http://www.cpsp.cps.ca/uploads/publications/RA-iron-deficiency-anemia.pdf

Aboriginal Nurses Association of Canada, Canadian Association of Schools of Nursing, & Canadian Nurses Association. (2009). *Cultural competence and cultural safety in nursing education*. Ottawa: Aboriginal Nurses Association of Canada. Retrieved from https://cna-aiic.ca/~/media/cna/page-content/pdf-en/first_nations_framework_e.pdf

Aguiar, W., & Halseth, R. (2015). *Addressing the healing of Aboriginal adults and families within a community model setting*. National Collaborating Centre for Aboriginal Health (NCCAH). Retrieved from http://www.nccah-ccnsa.ca/en/

Allison, S. (2016). *CMO child health status technical report, Northern BC*. Retrieved from https://www.northernhealth.ca/sites/northern_health/files/newsroom/documents/cmho-child-health-status-technical-report.pdf

Baker, R. D., & Greer, F. R., & The Committee on Nutrition. (2010). Diagnosis and prevention of iron deficiency and iron-deficiency anemia in infants and young children (0–3 years of age). *Pediatrics, 104*(1), 1040–1050. Retrieved from http://pediatrics.aappublications.org/content/pediatrics/126/5/1040.full.pdf

Benbow, S., Gorlick, C., Forchuk, C., Ward-Griffin, C., & Berman, H. (2016). Ontario's poverty reduction strategy: a critical discourse analysis. *Canadian Journal of Nursing Research, 48*(3-4), 100–109. Retrieved from https://doi.org/10.1177/0844562116684729

Ben-Joseph, E. P. (2015). *Formula feeding FAQs: Preparation and storage*. Retrieved from kidshealth.org/parent/growth/feeding/formulafeed_storing.html#

Ben-Shoshan, M., Harrington, D. W., Soller, L., Fragapane, J., Joseph, L., St Pierre, Y., … Clarke, A. E. (2010). A population-based study on peanut, tree nut, fish, shellfish, and sesame allergy prevalence in Canada. *Journal of Allergy and Clinical Immunology, 125*(6), 1327–1335. Retrieved from http://www.med.mcgill.ca/epidemiology/joseph/publications/medical/benshoshan2010.pdf

Benzies, K. M. (2014). Parenting in Canadian aboriginal cultures. In *Parenting across cultures* (pp. 379–392). Netherlands: Springer.

Bergman, N. J. (2013). Neonatal stomach volume and physiology suggest feeding at 1-h intervals. *Acta Paediatrica, 102*(8), 773–777. doi: 10.1111/apa.12291

Boivin, M., & Hertzman, C. (Eds.). (2012). *Early childhood development: adverse experiences and developmental health. Royal Society of Canada—Canadian Academy of Health Sciences Expert Panel (with Ronald Barr, Thomas Boyce, Alison Fleming, Harriet MacMillan, Candice Odgers, Marla Sokolowski, & Nico Trocmé)*. Ottawa, ON: Royal Society of Canada. Retrieved from https://rsc-src.ca/sites/default/files/pdf/ECD%20Report_0.pdf

Bordeleau, S., Asselin, H., Mazerolle, M. J., & Imbeau, L. (2016). Is it still safe to eat traditional food? Addressing traditional food safety concerns in aboriginal communities. *Science of the Total Environment, 565*, 529–538. Retrieved from https://www.researchgate.net/profile/Hugo_Asselin/publication/303248347_Is_it_still_safe_to_eat_traditional_food_Addressing_traditional_food_safety_concerns_in_aboriginal_communities/links/5739edb008ae298602e367b1.pdf?origin = publication_list

Brazelton, T. B., & Nugent, J. K. (2011). *Neonatal behavioral assessment scale* (4th ed.). London, UK: Mac Keith Press.

Brittain, M., & Blackstock, C. (2015). *First nations child poverty: A literature review and analysis*. Retrieved from https://fncaringsociety.com/sites/default/files/First%20

Nations%20Child%20Poverty%20-%20A%20Literature%20 Review%20and%20Analysis%202015-3.pdf

Brown, J. E. (2014). *Nutrition now* (7th ed.). Belmont, CA: Wadsworth, Cengage Learning.

Canadian Association of Poison Control Centres. (2017). Retrieved from http://www.capcc.ca/en

Canadian Dental Association. (2010). *Your child's first visit.* Retrieved from http://www.cda-adc.ca/en/oral_health/cfyt/ dental_care_children/first_visit.asp

Canadian Nurses Association. (2010). *Position statement. Promoting cultural competence in nursing.* Retrieved from https://www.cna-aiic.ca/~/media/cna/page-content/pdf-en/ps114_cultural_competence_2010_ e.pdf?la = en

Canadian Paediatric Society. (2003). *Swimming lessons for infants and toddlers.* Retrieved from http://www.cps.ca/ documents/position/swimming-lessons

Canadian Paediatric Society. (2008). *Transportation of infants and children in motor vehicles.* Retrieved from http://www. cps.ca/documents/position/car-seat-safety

Canadian Paediatric Society. (2012). *Child and youth injury prevention: A public health approach.* Retrieved from http:// www.cps.ca/documents/position/child-and-youth-injury-prevention

Canadian Paediatric Society. (2013a). *Caring for kids: guiding your young child with positive discipline.* Retrieved from http://www.caringforkids.cps.ca/handouts/guiding_with_ positive_discipline

Canadian Paediatric Society. (2013b). *Healthy sleep for your baby and child.* Retrieved from http://www.caringforkids. cps.ca/handouts/healthy_sleep_for_your_baby_and_child

Canadian Paediatric Society. (2016a). *Are we doing enough?* Retrieved from http://www.cps.ca/en/status-report

Canadian Paediatric Society. (2016b). *Management of acute otitis media in children six months of age and older.* Retrieved from https://www.cps.ca/en/documents/position/ acute-otitis-media

Canadian Paediatric Society. (2017). *Nutrition for healthy term infants, six to 24 months: An overview.* Retrieved from https://www.cps.ca/en/documents/position/nutrition-healthy-term-infants-6-to-24-months

Canadian Public Health Association. (2003). *Literacy and health in Canada.* Retrieved from http://www.cpha.ca/ uploads/portals/h-l/literacy_e.pdf

Canadian Task Force on Preventive Health Care. (2016). *Recommendations on screening for developmental delay (DD).* Retrieved from https://canadiantaskforce.ca/ updated-guideline-recommends-against-screening-with-stan-dardized-tools-to-detect-unrecognized-developmental-delay-in-primary-care/

Carpenito-Moyet, L. J. (2013). *Nursing diagnosis: Application to clinical practice* (14th ed.). Philadelphia, PA: Lippincott Williams & Wilkins.

Cassidy, J., & Shaver, P. R. (1999). *Handbook of attachment: Theory, research, and clinical applications.* New York: Guilford Press.

Cassidy, J., & Shaver, P. R. (2016). *Handbook of attachment third edition theory, research, and clinical applications.* New York, NY: Guildford Press.

Cherry, J., Demmler-Harrison, G. J., Kaplan, S. L., Steinbach, W. J., & Hotez, P. (2014). *Feigin and Cherry's textbook of pediatric infectious diseases* (7th ed.). Philadelphia, PA: Elsevier, Saunders.

Child Development Institute. (2015). *Temperament and your child's personality.* Retrieved from http://childdevelop-mentinfo.com/child-development/temperament_and_your_ child/

Corthésy, B. (2013). Role of secretory IgA in infection and maintenance of homeostasis. *Autoimmunity reviews, 12*(6), 661–665. Retrieved from http://dx.doi.org/10.1016/j.aut-rev.2012.10.012

de Beer, M., Vrijkotte, T. G., Fall, C. H., van Eijsden, M., Osmond, C., & Gemke, R. J. (2016). Associations of infant feeding and timing of weight gain and linear growth during early life with childhood blood pressure: findings from a prospective population based cohort study. *PloS One, 11*(11), e0166281. doi: 10.1371/journal.pone.0166281

Diener, M. L., Hobson-Rohrer, W., & Byington, C. L. (2012). Kindergarten readiness and performance of Latino children participating in Reach Out and Read. *Journal of Community Medicine & Health Education, 2*(3), 133. doi: 10.4172/ jcmhe.1000133

Dietitians of Canada. (2017). *Feeding infants and toddlers.* Retrieved from http://www.dietitians.ca/Dietitians-Views/ Prenatal-and-Infant/Infant-Feeding.aspx

Dietz, W. H., & Stern, L. (2012). *Nutrition: What every parent needs to know* (2nd ed.). Elk Grove Village, IL: American Academy of Pediatrics.

Douglas, M. K., Pierce, J. U., Rosenkoetter, M., Pacquiao, D., Callister, L. C., Hattar-Pollara, M., … Purnell, L. (2011). Standards of practice for culturally competent nursing care: 2011 update. *Journal of Transcultural Nursing, 22*(4), 317–333. Retrieved from https://doi. org/10.1177/1043659611412965

Duijts, L., Jaddoe, V. W., Hofman, A., & Moll, H. A. (2010). Prolonged and exclusive breastfeeding reduces the risk of infectious diseases in infancy. *Pediatrics, 126*(1), e18–e25. doi: 10.1542/peds.2008-3256

Ehrlich, S. D. (2014). *Infantile colic.* Retrieved from http:// umm.edu/health/medical/altmed/condition/infantile-colic

Engorn, B., & Flerlage, J. (Eds.). (2015). *The Harriett Lane handbook* (20th ed.). Philadelphia, PA: Saunders.

Erikson, E. H. (1963). *Childhood and society* (2nd ed.). New York: W. W. Norton and Company.

Feigelman, S. (2011). The first year. In R. M. Kliegman, B. F. Stanton, J. W. St. Geme III, N. F. Schor, & R. E. Behrman (Eds.). *Nelson's textbook of pediatrics* (19th ed.). Philadelphia, PA: Elsevier, Saunders.

Gao, Z., Rowe, B. H., Majaesic, C., O'Hara, C., & Senthilselvan, A. (2008). Prevalence of asthma and risk factors for asthma-like symptoms in Aboriginal and non-Aboriginal children in the northern territories of Canada. *Canadian Respiratory Journal, 15*(3), 139–145. Retrieved from https://www.ncbi. nlm.nih.gov/pmc/articles/PMC2677938/

Geddes, D. T. (2009). Ultrasound imaging of the lactating breast: methodology and application. *International Breast-feeding Journal, 4*(1), 4. Retrieved from https://www.ncbi. nlm.nih.gov/pmc/articles/PMC2687418/

Gionet, L. (2013). Breastfeeding trends in Canada. *Health at a Glance.* November. Statistics Canada Catalogue no. 82-624-X. Retrieved from http://www.statcan.gc.ca/pub/82-624-x/2013001/article/11879-eng.htm

Godel, J.; Canadian Paediatric Society, Nutrition and Gastroenterology Committee. (2002). The use of fluoride in infants and children. *Paediatrics & Child Health, 7*(8), 569–572. Retrieved from http://www.cps.ca/en/documents/position/fluoride-use

Goldson, E., & Reynolds, A. (2014). Child development and behavior. In W. W. Hay, Jr., M. J. Levin, R. R. Deterding, & M. J. Abzug (Eds.). *Current diagnosis and treatment: Pediatrics* (22nd ed.). New York: McGraw-Hill Education.

Government of Canada. (2013). Joint statement on shaken baby syndrome. Retrieved from http://publications.gc.ca/site/eng/9.663297/publication.html

Government of Canada. (2017). Infant nutrition. Retrieved from https://www.canada.ca/en/health-canada/services/infant-care/infant-nutrition.html

Government of Canada. (2019). Jordan's Principle. Retrieved from https://www.canada.ca/en/indigenous-services-canada/services/jordans-principle.html

Greenbaum, L. A. (2011). Electrolyte and acid-base disorders. In R. M. Kliegman, B. F. Stanton, J. W. St. Geme III, N. F. Schor, & R. E. Behrman (Eds.). *Nelson's textbook of pediatrics* (19th ed.). Philadelphia, PA: Elsevier, Saunders.

Grenier, D., & Leduc, D. (2008). Let's put a national childcare strategy back on the agenda. *Canadian Paediatric Society*. Retrieved from http://www.cps.ca/uploads/advocacy/Grenier.pdf

Harris, S. R. (2016). Early identification of motor delay. Family-centred screening tool. *Canadian Family Physician, 62*(8), 629–632. Retrieved from http://www.cfp.ca/content/62/8/629.long

Hassiotou, F., Hepworth, A. R., Williams, T. M., Twigger, A. J., Perrella, S., Lai, C. T., … Hartmann, P. E. (2013). Breastmilk cell and fat contents respond similarly to removal of breastmilk by the infant. *PloS One, 8*(11), e78232. Retrieved from http://journals.plos.org/plosone/article?id = 10.1371/journal.pone.0078232

Hay, W. W., & Hendrickson, K. C. (2016). Preterm formula use in the preterm very low birth weight infant. In *Seminars in Fetal and Neonatal Medicine*. WB Saunders. Retrieved from http://dx.doi.org/10.1016/j.siny.2016.08.005

Health Canada. (n.d.). *Nutrition for healthy term infants: Recommendations from birth to six months*. Retrieved from http://www.hc-sc.gc.ca/fn-an/nutrition/infant-nourisson/recom/index-eng.php#a4

Health Canada. *Children's Oral Health Initiative 2004*. Retrieved from http://www.hc-sc.gc.ca/ahc-asc/activit/strateg/fnih-spni-eng.php#cohi-isbde

Health Canada. (2012). *Is your child safe?* Retrieved from http://www.hc-sc.gc.ca/cps-spc/pubs/cons/child-enfant/play-jeu-eng.php

Health Canada (2013). Safety Brief—baby walkers. Retrieved from http://publications.gc.ca/site/eng/384190/publication.html

Health Canada. (2015). *Nutrition for healthy term infants: Recommendations for infants 6 to 24 months*. Retrieved from http://www.hc-sc.gc.ca/fn-an/nutrition/infant-nourisson/recom/recom-6-24-months-6-24-mois-eng.php#a19

Health Canada Joint Statement With Dieticians of Canada. (2015). Nutrition for healthy term infants: Recommendations from 6 to 24 months. Retrieved from http://www.hc-sc.gc.ca/fn-an/nutrition/infant-nourisson/recom/recom-6-24-months-6-24-mois-eng.php

HealthLinkBC. (2015a). Retrieved from https://www.healthlinkbc.ca/hlbc/files/documents/healthfiles/hfile69b.pdf

HealthLinkBC. (2015b). *Colic*. Retrieved from https://www.healthlinkbc.ca/health-topics/hw31504

Hill, D. L. (2015). *Bottle feeding basics*. Retrieved from https://www.healthychildren.org/English/ages-stages/baby/feeding-nutrition/Pages/Bottle-Feeding-How-Its-Done.aspx

Hong Nguyen, B. (2003). Swimming lessons for infants and toddlers. *Paediatrics & Child Health, 8*(2), 113–114. Retrieved from http://www.cps.ca/documents/position/swimming-lessons

HOPE. (2017). *Balancing adverse childhood experiences (ACEs) with HOPE. Casey Family Programs*. Retrieved from https://www.cssp.org/publications/documents/Balancing-ACEs-with-HOPE-FINAL.pdf

Indigenous and Northern Affairs Canada. (2017). *Truth and Reconciliation Commission of Canada*. Retrieved from https://www.aadnc-aandc.gc.ca/eng/1450124405592/1450124456123

Immunize Canada. (2016). Retrieved from http://www.immunize.ca/en/recommendations/schedules.aspx

International Council of Nurses. (2013). *Cultural and linguistic competence*. Retrieved from http://www.icn.ch/publications/position-statements/

Jordan's Principle Working Group. (2015). *Without denial, delay or disruption: ensuring first nations children's access to equitable services*. Ottawa, ON: Assembly of First Nations. Retrieved from http://cwrp.ca/publications/Jordans-Principle-Working-Group-Report

Kakulas, F. (2013). How breastfed babies control their own appetite. Retrieved from http://milkgenomics.org/article/how-breastfed-babies-control-their-own-appetite/

Karasik, L. B., Adolph, K. E., Tamis-LeMonda, C. S., & Bornstein, M. H. (2010). WEIRD walking: Cross-cultural research on motor development. *Behavioural and Brain Sciences, 33*(2/3), 35–36. doi: 10.1017/S0140525X10000117

Khan, M. M., Kobayashi, K., Vang, Z. M., & Lee, S. M. (2017). Are visible minorities' invisible' in Canadian health data and research? A scoping review. *International Journal of Migration, Health and Social Care, 13*(1), 126–143. Retrieved from http://dx.doi.org/10.1108/IJMHSC-10-2015-0036

Khanlou, N., Haque, N., Mustafa, N., Vazquez, L. M., Mantini, A., & Weiss, J. (2017). Access barriers to services by immigrant mothers of children with autism in Canada. *International Journal of Mental Health and Addiction, 15*(2), 239–259. Retrieved from http://link.springer.com/article/10.1007/s11469-017-9732-4

La Leche League International. (2013). *The early weeks*. Retrieved from http://www.llli.org/nb/nbearlyweeks.html

Lang, M.; Canadian Paediatric Society, Community Paediatrics Committee. (2008). Health implications of children in child care centres Part A: Canadian trends in child care, behaviour and developmental outcomes. *Paediatrics & Child Health, 13*(10), 863–867. Retrieved from http://www.cps.ca/documents/position/child-care-centres-trends-behaviour-development

Lawrence, R. (2011). *Breastfeeding: A guide for the medical professional* (7th ed.). Maryland Heights, MO: Mosby.

Lerner, N. B. (2011). Physiologic anemia of infancy. In R. M. Kliegman, B. F. Stanton, J. W. St. Geme III, N. F. Schor, & R.

E. Behrman (Eds.). *Nelson's textbook of pediatrics* (19th ed.). Philadelphia, PA: Elsevier, Saunders.

Liacouras, C. A. (2011). Normal development, structure, and function. In R. M. Kliegman, B. F. Stanton, J. W. St. Geme III, N. F. Schor, & R. E. Behrman (Eds.). *Nelson's textbook of pediatrics* (19th ed.). Philadelphia, PA: Elsevier, Saunders.

Lowry, L. (2011). *Bilingualism in young children: Separating fact from fiction.* Retrieved from http://www.hanen.org/Helpful-Info/Articles/Bilingualism-in-Young-Children–Separating-Fact-fr.aspx

Lyall, J., & Ryan, A. C. (2015). Inuit early childhood development: The foundation of optimal health and wellbeing. *International Meeting on Indigenous Child Health.* Retrieved from http://www.cps.ca/uploads/imich/imich-2015-program-downloads/imich15-b3-lyall.pdf

MacDonald, N. E. (2018). Maternal infectious diseases, antimicrobial therapy or immunizations: Very few contraindications to breastfeeding. *Canadian Journal of Infectious Diseases and Medical Microbiology, 17*(5), 270–272. Retrieved from https://www.cps.ca/en/documents/position/maternal-infectious-diseases-breastfeeding

Maqbool, A., Stettler, N., & Stallings, V. A. (2011). Nutritional requirements. In R. M. Kliegman, B. F. Stanton, J. W. St. Geme III, N. F. Schor, & R. E. Behrman (Eds.). *Nelson's textbook of pediatrics* (19th ed.). Philadelphia, PA: Elsevier, Saunders.

McIvor, O. (2006). *Language nest programs in BC. Early childhood immersion programs in two First Nations communities.* Retrieved from http://www.fpcc.ca/files/pdf/language-nest-programs_in_bc.pdf

Mizuno, K., Nishida, Y., Taki, M., Murase, M., Mukai, Y., Itabashi, K., … Iiyama, A. (2009). Is increased fat content of hindmilk due to the size or the number of milk fat globules?. *International Breastfeeding Journal, 4*(1), 7. Retrieved from https://internationalbreastfeedingjournal.biomedcentral.com/articles/10.1186/1746-4358-4-7

Moon, R. Y., & Fu, L. (2012). Sudden infant death syndrome: An update. *Pediatrics in Review, 33*(7), 314–320.

Multicultural Mental Health Resource Centre (MMHRC). (2016). Retrieved from http://www.multiculturalmentalhealth.ca

National Association for the Education of Young Children. (n.d.). *Good toys for young children by age and stage.* Retrieved from http://www.naeyc.org/toys

National Association of Pediatric Nurse Practitioners. (n.d.). *Infant and toddler discipline: Preventing bad behavior.* Retrieved from https://www.napnap.org/sites/default/files/userfiles/membership/No%20Hitting%20Infant%20Revised.pdf

National Association of Pediatric Nurse Practitioners. (2013). NAPNAP position statement on breastfeeding. *Journal of Pediatric Health Care, 27*(1), e13–e15.

National Collaborating Centre for Aboriginal Health (NCCAH). (2019). *Child health and wellness resource booklets.* Retrieved from https://www.nccah-ccnsa.ca/389/Childhood_Health_and_Wellness_Resource_Booklets.nccah

Nelson, A. M. (2012). A comprehensive review of evidence and current recommendations related to pacifier usage. *Journal of Pediatric Nursing, 27*, 690–699. Retrieved from https://www.mambaby.com/uploads/tx_dddownload/A_Comprehensive_Review_of_Evidence_and_Current_Recommendations_Related_to_Pacifier_Usage.pdf

Nevarez, M. D., Rifas-Shiman, S. L., Kleinman, K. P., Gillman, M. W., & Taveras, E. M. (2010). Associations of early life risk factors with infant sleep duration. *Academic Pediatrics, 10*(3), 187–193. doi: 10.1016/j.acap.2010.01.007.

Nieman, P., & Shea, S. (2004). Effective discipline for children. *Paediatrics & Child Health, 9*(1), 37–41. Retrieved from https://academic.oup.com/pch/article/9/1/37/2648475

Olsson, J. (2011). The newborn. In R. M. Kliegman, B. F. Stanton, J. W. St. Geme III, N. F. Schor, & R. E. Behrman (Eds.). *Nelson's textbook of pediatrics* (19th ed.). Philadelphia, PA: Elsevier, Saunders.

Organization for Economic Co-operation and Development Directorate for Education. (2008). *Early childhood education and care policy.* Retrieved from http://www.oecd.org/dataoecd/42/34/33850725.pdf

Perinatal Services BC. (2014). Fact sheet: Breastfeeding trends in British Columbia 2004/05 – 2012/13. Retrieved from http://www.perinatalservicesbc.ca/Documents/Data-Surveillance/Reports/BreastfeedingFactSheet_2014.pdf

Perniciaro, J. (2011). Development, behavior, and mental health. In R. M. Kliegman, B. F. Stanton, J. W. St. Geme III, N. F. Schor, & R. E. Behrman (Eds.). *Nelson's textbook of pediatrics* (19th ed.). Philadelphia, PA: Elsevier, Saunders.

Piaget, J. (1969). *The theory of stages in cognitive development.* New York: McGraw-Hill.

Public Health Agency of Canada. (2014). *Safe sleep.* Retrieved from http://www.phac-aspc.gc.ca/hp-ps/dca-dea/stages-etapes/childhood-enfance_0-2/sids/index-eng.php

Public Health Agency of Canada. (2017). *Canadian immunization guide.* Retrieved from http://www.phac-aspc.gc.ca/publicat/cig-gci/index-eng.php

Pujadas Botey, A., Vinturache, A., Bayrampour, H., Breitkreuz, R., Bukutu, C., Gibbard, B., & Tough, S. (2016). Adults' Knowledge of Child Development in Alberta, Canada: Comparing the Level of Knowledge of Adults in Two Samples in 2007 and 2013. *Child Care in Practice, 23*(4), 1–13.

Ramsay, D. T., Kent, J. C., Hartmann, R. A., & Hartmann, P. E. (2005). Anatomy of the lactating human breast redefined with ultrasound imaging. *Journal of Anatomy, 206*(6), 525–534. Retrieved from https://www.ncbi.nlm.nih.gov/pmc/articles/PMC1571528/

Riverin, B., Li, P., Rourke, L., Leduc, D., & Rourke, J. (2015). Rourke Baby Record 2014: Evidence-based tool for the health of infants and children from birth to age 5. *Canadian Family Physician, 61*, 949–955 (Clinical Review). Retrieved from http://www.cfp.ca/content/61/11/949.long

Roncarolo, F., & Potvin, L. (2016). Food insecurity as a symptom of a social disease. Analyzing a social problem from a medical perspective. *Canadian Family Physician, 62*(4), 291–292. Retrieved from https://www.ncbi.nlm.nih.gov/pmc/articles/PMC4830644/

Rourke Baby Record. (2014). Retrieved from http://www.rourkebabyrecord.ca

Royal College of Physicians and Surgeons of Canada. (2014). *Early childhood development. Position statement.* Retrieved from http://www.royalcollege.ca/portal/page/portal/rc/common/documents/advocacy/EBBDEL_statement_e.pdf

Safe Kids Worldwide. (2016). *Baby sleep safety and suffocation prevention*. Retrieved from http://www.safekids.org/safety-tips/field_age/babies-0%E2%80%9312-months/field_risks/sleep-safety

Shah, S. D., Dereddy, N., Jones, T. L., Dhanireddy, R., & Talati, A. J. (2016). Early versus delayed human milk fortification in very low birth weight infants—a randomized controlled trial. *The Journal of Pediatrics, 174*, 126–131. Retrieved from https://doi.org/10.1016/j.jpeds.2016.03.056

Shaw, A. (2006). Read, speak, sing: Promoting literacy in the physician's office. *Paediatrics & Child Health, 11*(9), 601–606. Retrieved from http://www.cps.ca/documents/position/read-speak-sing-promoting-literacy

Sinha, S. K. (2015). *Short stature*. Retrieved from http://emedicine.medscape.com/article/924411-overview

Statistics Canada. (2016a). *Children and youth*. Retrieved from http://www5.statcan.gc.ca/subject-sujet/index?lang=eng&MM=1

Statistics Canada. (2016b). *Immigrant children and youth*. Retrieved from http://www5.statcan.gc.ca/subject-sujet/subtheme-soustheme?pid=20000&id=20005&lang=eng&more=0

Stefanescu, B. M., Gillam-Krakauer, M., Stefanescu, A. R., Markham, M., & Kosinski, J. L. (2016). Very low birth weight infant care: adherence to a new nutrition protocol improves growth outcomes and reduces infectious risk. *Early Human Development, 94*, 25–30. Retrieved from http://dx.doi.org/10.1016/j.earlhumdev.2016.01.011

Stettler, N., Bhatia, J., Parish, A., & Stallings, V. A. (2011). Feeding healthy infants, children, and adolescents. In R. M. Kliegman, B. F. Stanton, J. W. St. Geme III, N. F. Schor, & R. E. Behrman (Eds.). *Nelson's textbook of pediatrics* (19th ed.). Philadelphia, PA: Elsevier, Saunders.

Swanson, W. S. (2016). *The scoop on poop: What's normal, what's not*. Retrieved from http://www.parents.com/baby/diapers/dirty/baby-bowel-movement/

Takaro, T. K., Scott, J. A., Allen, R. W., Anand, S. S., Becker, A. B., Befus, A. D., … Mandhane, P. J. (2015). The Canadian Healthy Infant Longitudinal Development (CHILD) birth cohort study: assessment of environmental exposures. *Journal of Exposure Science and Environmental Epidemiology, 25*(6), 580–592. doi: 10.1038/jes.2015.7

Tinanoff, N. (2011). The oral cavity. In R. M. Kliegman, B. F. Stanton, J. W. St. Geme III, N. F. Schor, & R. E. Behrman (Eds.). *Nelson's textbook of pediatrics* (19th ed.). Philadelphia, PA: Elsevier, Saunders.

Transport Canada. (2016). *Child car seat safety regulations*. Retrieved from http://www.tc.gc.ca/eng/motorvehicle-safety/safedrivers-childsafety-stage2-forward-facing-1085.htm

CHAPTER **WORKSHEET**

MULTIPLE CHOICE QUESTIONS

1. The mother of a 3-month-old boy asks the nurse about starting solid foods. What is the most appropriate response by the nurse?
   a. "It's okay to start puréed solids at this age if fed via the bottle."
   b. "Infants don't require solid food until 12 months of age."
   c. "Solid foods should be delayed until age 6 months, when the infant can handle a spoon on his own."
   d. "The tongue extrusion reflex disappears at age 4 to 6 months, making it a good time to start solid foods."

2. The father of a 2-month-old girl is expressing concern that his infant may be getting spoiled. The nurse's best response is:
   a. "She just needs love and attention. Don't worry; she's too young to spoil."
   b. "Consistently meeting the infant's needs helps promote a sense of trust."
   c. "Infants need to be fed and cleaned; if you're sure those needs are met, just let her cry."
   d. "Consistency in meeting needs is important, but you're right, holding her too much will spoil her."

3. Parents of an 8-month-old girl express concern that she cries when left with the babysitter. How does the nurse best explain this behaviour?
   a. Crying when left with the sitter may indicate difficulty with building trust.
   b. Stranger anxiety should not occur until toddlerhood; this concern should be investigated.
   c. Separation anxiety is normal at this age; the infant recognizes parents as separate beings.
   d. Perhaps the sitter doesn't meet the infant's needs; choose a different sitter.

4. The nurse is providing anticipatory guidance to the mother of a 6-month-old infant. What is the best instruction by the nurse in relation to the infant's oral health?
   a. "Start brushing her teeth after all the baby teeth come in."
   b. "Use a washcloth with toothpaste to clean her mouth."
   c. "Clean your baby's gums, then new teeth, with a washcloth."
   d. "Rinse your baby's mouth with water after every feeding."

5. A 9-month-old infant's mother is questioning why cow's milk is not recommended in the first year of life as it is much cheaper than formula. What rationale does the nurse include in her response?
   a. It is permissible to substitute cow's milk for formula at this age as he is so close to 1 year old.
   b. Cow's milk is poor in iron and does not provide the proper balance of nutrients for the infant.
   c. As long as the mother provides whole milk, rather than skim, she can start cow's milk in infancy.
   d. If the mother cannot afford the infant formula, she should dilute it to make it last longer.

CRITICAL THINKING EXERCISES

1. The mother of an 11-month-old boy who was born at 24 weeks' gestation is concerned about his size and motor skills. What information should the nurse provide?

2. An infant's mother thinks there may be something wrong with him because "he spits up so much." What further information should the nurse obtain?

3. If you determine that the infant in the question above is experiencing normal spitting up associated with his developmental age, develop a brief teaching plan to review with the mother.

STUDY ACTIVITIES

1. A mother brings her 9-month-old boy to the clinic for a well-child checkup. She has questions about feeding, speech, and walking. Develop a teaching plan of anticipatory guidance for the 9-month-old infant.

2. Develop a home and car safety plan for the 12-month-old infant.

3. In the clinical setting, observe two infants of the same age, one who is developing appropriately for his or her age and one who is delayed. Note the similarities and differences between the two infants.

BRINGING IT ALL TOGETHER: A CASE STUDY

Mario, a 9-month-old boy, is seen in the clinic for a well-child examination. He has been healthy since birth and now his mother is nervous, as she is considering putting him in day care so she can return to work. She is unsure how she will manage the return to work, as Mario is breastfeeding frequently throughout the day. Mario's grandmother has advised his mother that breast milk is better than baby food, so Mario's mom has not offered him baby food very much. His mother also expresses concern that Mario is not walking yet, because her cousin's baby walked at 9 months.

Go to thePoint **to find questions to consider about this case.**

26

KEY TERMS

animism

echolalia

egocentrism

expressive language

food jag

individuation

parallel play

receptive language

regression

separation

separation anxiety

sibling rivalry

telegraphic speech

Growth and Development of the Toddler

Learning Objectives

Upon completion of the chapter, you will be able to:

1. Explain normal physiologic, psychosocial, and cognitive changes occurring in the toddler.
2. Identify the gross and fine motor milestones of the toddler.
3. Demonstrate an understanding of language development in the toddler years.
4. Discuss sensory development of the toddler.
5. Demonstrate an understanding of emotional/social development and moral/spiritual development during toddlerhood.
6. Implement a nursing care plan to address common issues related to growth and development in toddlerhood.
7. Encourage growth and learning through play.
8. Develop a teaching plan for safety promotion in the toddler period.
9. Demonstrate an understanding of toddler needs related to sleep and rest, as well as dental health.
10. Develop a nutritional plan for the toddler based on average nutritional requirements.
11. Provide appropriate anticipatory guidance for common developmental issues that arise in the toddler period.
12. Demonstrate an understanding of appropriate methods of discipline for use during the toddler years.
13. Identify the role of the parent in the toddler's life and determine ways to support, encourage, and educate the parents about toddler growth, development, and concerns during this period.

Jose Gonzales **is a 2-year-old boy brought to the clinic by his mother and father for his planned check-up. During your assessment, you find that his weight is 13.6 kg (30 lb), height 83.82 cm (33 in), and head circumference 49.53 cm (19.5 in). As the nurse caring for him, assess Jose's growth and development, and then provide appropriate anticipatory guidance to the parents.**

A toddler is a child aged 12 to 36 months (1 to 3 years old). This developmental period is a time of significant advancement in growth and development for the child in addition to being a challenging time for many parents. The balance that children are trying to achieve during the toddler years is one of holding on and letting go. Having learned that parents are predictable and reliable, the toddler is now learning that his or her behaviour affects others. The challenge is to encourage independence and autonomy while keeping the curious toddler safe.

Take Note!

As more grandparents are assuming the primary caregiver role for their grandchildren, nurses should be alert to the possibility of increased stress that is placed upon the older caregiver, particularly during the active and sometimes trying years of toddlerhood (Smith & Segal, 2016).

GROWTH AND DEVELOPMENT OVERVIEW

While infancy was a time of intense growth and development, now the physical growth and acquisition of new motor skills is somewhat slower in toddlerhood. Refinement of motor skills, the acquisition of language, the development of problem-solving abilities, understanding of cause and effect, and the expansion of social-emotional skills need to mature. The nurse uses the knowledge of normal toddler development as a roadmap for assessment of the 1- to 3-year-old child.

PHYSICAL GROWTH

The toddler's increase in both height and weight tends to occur in spurts, rather than in a steady, linear fashion (Fig. 26.1). Height (length) increases by an average of 10 to 12 cm per year, generally reaching about half of their adult height by 2 years of age. The average toddler weight gain is 1.36 to 2.27 kg (3 to 6 lb) per year with boys being slightly heavier than girls. At 12 months, the brain has completed around half of its postnatal growth, and the head will be approaching 75% of its adult size (Merck manual, n.d.). Head circumference increases about 3.5 cm between 1 and 3 years of age. The anterior fontanel should be closed by the time the child is 18 months old. Head size becomes more proportional to the rest of the body around 3 years (Feigelman, 2011a, 2011b; Goldson & Reynolds, 2014).

ORGAN SYSTEM MATURATION

Though not as pronounced as the changes occurring during infancy, the toddler's organ systems continue to

FIGURE 26.1 The typical toddler appearance is that of a rounded abdomen, a slight swayback, and a wide-based stance.

grow and mature in their functioning. Significant functional changes occur within the neurologic, respiratory, cardiovascular, gastrointestinal, genitourinary, and musculoskeletal systems.

Neurologic System

Maturation of the brain and spinal cord continues to progress and is complete around 24 months of age. Myelination of the brain and cortical nerves results in improved coordination and equilibrium as well as the ability to exercise sphincter control, which is important for bowel and bladder mastery. Integration of the primitive reflexes in infancy allows for the emergence of the protective reflexes near the end of infancy or early in toddlerhood. The forward or downward parachute reflex is particularly helpful when the child starts to toddle and experiences frequent falls. Rapid increases in language skill and problem-solving ability are evidence of continued progression of cognitive development.

Respiratory System

The respiratory structures steadily grow in size and mature throughout toddlerhood. The alveoli continue to proliferate and reach maturity at about 7 years of age. The trachea and lower airways continue to grow but remain small compared with the adult. The tongue is relatively large in comparison to the size of the mouth, and similarly, the tonsils and adenoids are large relative to the size of the airway. The Eustachian tubes remain short and significantly straighter than those of the adult, which predisposes the toddler to poor drainage of nasal secretions and potential for middle ear infections.

Cardiovascular System

The heart rate decreases and blood pressure increases in toddlerhood. Blood vessels are close to the skin surface and so are compressed easily when palpated.

Gastrointestinal System

The stomach continues to increase in size to accommodate higher volumes, allowing the toddler to consume three regular meals per day. Pepsin production matures by 2 years of age. The small intestine continues to grow in length, though it does not reach the maximum length of 2 to 3 m until adulthood. Stool passage decreases in frequency to one or more per day. The colour of the stool may change (yellow, orange, brown, or green) depending on the toddler's diet. Since the toddler's intestines remain somewhat immature, the toddler may occasionally pass undigested food or have episodes of bloating when new foods or carbohydrate heavy foods are included in their diet. Many toddlers will achieve bowel control by age 3 years, but variation can exist with some children not being ready for toilet training until closer to 4 years of age.

Genitourinary System

Around 24 months of age, the kidneys reach adult functioning in their ability to filter blood and concentrate or dilute urine. Bladder capacity increases, allowing the toddler to retain urine for increased periods of times. Urine output should be about 1 mL/kg/hr, therefore a 2 year old could possibly excrete 500 to 600 mL of urine per day.

Musculoskeletal System

During toddlerhood, the bones increase in length and the ossification process continues. Connective tissues remain stronger than bone in this age, which predisposes toddlers to a higher risk of sustaining fractures due to falls and impact injuries. The abdominal musculature is weak in early toddlerhood, resulting in a pot-bellied appearance until around 3 years when increased strength results in a flatter abdominal appearance.

PSYCHOSOCIAL DEVELOPMENT

Erikson defines the toddler period as a time of autonomy versus shame and doubt. As compared with complete dependence in infancy, the toddler is ready to give up dependence and assert his or her sense of control and autonomy (Erikson, 1963). The toddler is struggling for self-mastery, to learn to do for himself or herself what others have been doing for him or her. Toddlers often flow between states of dependence and autonomy, resulting in emotional lability. The toddler may quickly change from happy and pleasant to crying and screaming. Exertion of independence also results in the toddler's favourite response "no." The toddler will often answer "no" even when he or she really means "yes." This negativism—always saying "no"—is a normal part of the healthy development of their understanding of self as separate from the parent. Table 26.1 gives further information related to developing a sense of autonomy.

COGNITIVE DEVELOPMENT

According to Jean Piaget (1969), toddlers move through the sensorimotor stage of cognitive development between 12 and 24 months of age. Young toddlers engage in tertiary circular reactions which is a period of trial-and-error experimentation whereby they use different sounds and behaviours to test out responses from others, thus adapting to a new situation. For example, restacking the blocks in a different way after knocking them down. Around 2 years of age, toddlers may demonstrate delayed imitation. For example, they may imitate a household task that they observed a parent doing several days ago.

Piaget identified the second stage of cognitive development as the preoperational stage. It occurs in children between ages 2 and 7 years. During this stage, toddlers begin to become more sophisticated with symbolic thought. The thinking patterns become more advanced than that of the infant or young toddler, who views the world as a series of objects. During the preoperational stage, objects begin to have characteristics that make them unique from one another. Objects are considered large or small, having a particular colour or shape, or having a unique texture. This moves beyond the connection of sensory information and physical action. Words and images allow the toddler to begin this process of developing symbolic thought by providing a label for the objects' characteristics (Piaget, 1969).

Toddlers also use symbols in dramatic play. First they imitate life with appropriate toy objects, and then they are able to substitute objects in their play. A bowl may be used to pretend to eat from, but then later it can be used upside down on the head as a hat (Fig. 26.2). Human feelings and characteristics may also be attributed to objects (**animism**) such as a doll or stuffed animal or an object causing an action, such as the "sofa made me fall over" (Papalia & Feldman,

TABLE 26.1	DEVELOPMENTAL THEORIES	
Theorist	**Stage**	**Activities**
Erikson	Autonomy vs. shame and doubt Age 1–3 years	Achieves autonomy and self-control Separates from parent/caregiver Withstands delayed gratification Negativism abounds Imitates adults and playmates Spontaneously shows affection Is increasingly enthusiastic about playmates Cannot take turns in games until age 3 years

Piaget	Sensorimotor
	Substage 5: tertiary circular
	  reactions
	Age: 12–18 months
	Substage 6: Mental combinations
	Age: 18–24 months
	Preoperational
	Age: 2–7 years
		Differentiates self from objects
		Increased object permanence (knows that objects that are out of
		  sight still exist [e.g., cookies in the cabinet])
		Uses ALL senses to explore environment
		Places items in and out of containers
		Imitates domestic chores (domestic mimicry)
		Imitation is more symbolic
		Starting to think before acting
		Understands requests and is capable of following simple
		  directions
		Has a sense of ownership (my, mine)
		Time, space, and causality understanding is increasing
		Uses mental trial and error rather than physical
		Makes mechanical toys work
		Plays make-believe with dolls, animals, and people
		Increased use of language for mental representation
		Understands concept of "two"
		Starting to make connections between an experience in the past
		  and a new one that is currently occurring
		Sorts objects by shape and colour
		Completes puzzles with four pieces
		Play becomes more complex

Freud	Anal stage
	Age: 1–3 years
		Focus is on achieving anal sphincter control. Satisfaction and/
		  or frustration may occur as the toddler learns to withhold and
		  expel stool.

Adapted from Erikson, E. H. (1963). *Childhood and society* (2nd ed.). New York: W.W. Norton and Company; Goldson, E., & Reynolds, A. (2014). Child development and behavior. In W. W. Hay Jr., M. J. Levin, R. R. Deterding, & M. J. Abzug (Eds.), *Current diagnosis and treatment: Pediatrics* (22nd ed.). New York: McGraw-Hill Education; Piaget, J. (1969). *The theory of stages in cognitive development.* New York: McGraw-Hill.

2011). See Table 26.1 for further explanation of cognitive development in toddlerhood.

Take Note!

Maternal depression is a risk factor for cognitive and socioemotional development of children. Mothers who are depressed may not be as sensitive or emotionally responsive to their child which has consequences on the toddler's development. An impaired maternal response to her child's attempts to interact or communicate, in order to elicit an emotional or reciprocal reaction, can result in dysregulated behaviour and interfere with the toddlers learning. Therefore, nursing assessment includes the mental health of the mother or primary caregiver so that appropriate interventions and necessary referrals can be made (Giles, Davies, Whitrow, Warin, & Moore, 2011).

MOTOR SKILL DEVELOPMENT

Toddlers continue to gain new motor skills as well as refine others. Walking progresses to running, climbing, and jumping. Pushing or pulling a toy, throwing a ball, and pedalling a tricycle are accomplished in toddlerhood. Fine motor skills progress from holding and pinching to the ability to manage utensils, hold a crayon, string a bead, and use a computer. Development of eye–hand coordination is necessary for the refinement of fine motor skills. These increased abilities of mobility and manipulation help the curious toddler explore and learn more about his or her environment (Fig. 26.3). As the toddler masters a new task, he or she has confidence to conquer the next challenge. Thus, mastery in motor skill development contributes to the toddler's growing sense of self-esteem. The toddler who is eager to face

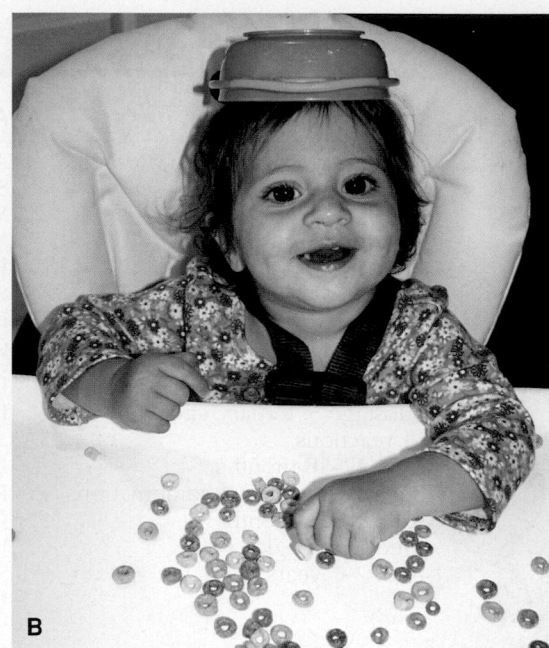

FIGURE 26.2 The toddler will (**A**) pretend with items in the way they are intended to be used as well as (**B**) find other creative uses for them.

challenges will likely develop more quickly than one who is reluctant. The senses of sight, hearing, and touch are useful in helping to coordinate gross and fine motor movement.

Gross Motor Skills

As gross motor skills are mastered and then used repeatedly, the large muscle groups in the toddler are strengthened. The "toddler gait" is characteristic of new walkers. The toddler does not walk smoothly and maturely. Instead, the legs are planted widely apart, toes are pointed forward, and the toddler seems to sway from side to side while moving forward (Fig. 26.4). Often, the toddler seems to speed along, be pitching forward, and may appear ready to topple over at any moment. The toddler may fall often, but will use outstretched arms to catch himself or herself (parachute reflex). After

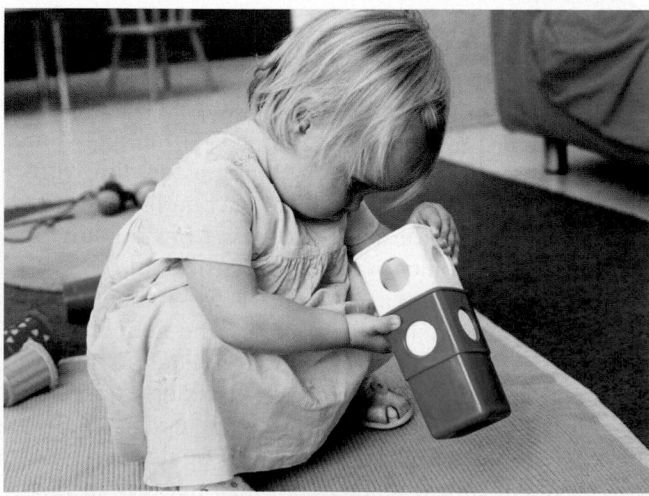

FIGURE 26.3 The toddler's curiosity about the world increases, as does her ability to explore it.

FIGURE 26.4 The young toddler (early walker) walks with a wide-based stance, feet pointing forward and arms akimbo.

TABLE 26.2	MOTOR SKILL DEVELOPMENT	
Age	**Expected Gross Motor Skill**	**Expected Fine Motor Skills**
12–15 months	Walks independently	Feeds self finger foods Uses index finger to point
18 months	Climbs stairs with assistance Pulls toys while walking	Masters reaching, grasping, and releasing: stacks blocks, puts things in slots Turns book pages (singly with board book, multiple if paper) Removes shoes and socks Stacks four cubes
24 months	Runs Kicks ball Can stand on tiptoe Carries several toys, or a large toy while walking Climbs onto and down from furniture without assistance	Builds tower of six or seven cubes Right- or left-handed Imitates circular and vertical strokes Scribbles and paints Starting to turn knobs Puts round pegs into holes
36 months	Climbs well Pedals tricycle Runs easily Walks up and down stairs with alternate feet Bends over easily without falling	Undresses self Copies circle Builds tower of nine or ten cubes Holds a pencil in writing position Screws/unscrews lids, nuts, bolts Turns book pages one at a time

Adapted from Feigelman, S. (2011a). Preschool years. In R. M. Kliegman, B. F. Stanton, J. W. St. Geme III, N. F. Schor, & R. E. Behrman (Eds.), *Nelson's textbook of pediatrics* (19th ed.). Philadelphia, PA: Elsevier, Saunders; Feigelman, S. (2011b). The second year. In R. M. Kliegman, B. F. Stanton, J. W. St. Geme III, N. F. Schor, & R. E. Behrman (Eds.), *Nelson's textbook of pediatrics* (19th ed.). Philadelphia, PA: Elsevier, Saunders; and Goldson, E., & Reynolds, A. (2014). Child development and behavior. In W. W. Hay Jr., M. J. Levin, R. R. Deterding, & M. J. Abzug (Eds.), *Current diagnosis and treatment: Pediatrics* (22nd ed.). New York, NY: McGraw-Hill Education.

about 6 months of practice walking, the toddler's gait is smoother, and the feet are closer together. By 3 years of age, the toddler walks in a heel-to-toe fashion similar to that of adults. Toddlers often use physical actions such as running, jumping, and hitting to express their emotions because they are only just learning to express their thoughts and feelings verbally. Table 26.2 lists motor skill expectations in relation to age.

Fine Motor Skills

Fine motor skills in the toddler period are improved and perfected. Holding utensils requires some control and agility, but greater dexterity is needed for buttoning and zipping. Adequate vision is necessary for the refinement of fine motor skills because eye–hand coordination is crucial for directing the fingers, hand, and wrist to accomplish small muscle tasks such as fitting a puzzle piece or stringing a bead. See Table 26.2 for age expectations for various motor skills.

SENSORY DEVELOPMENT

Toddlers use all of their senses to explore the world around them. Toddlers examine new items by feeling them, looking at them, shaking them to hear what sound they make, smelling them, and placing them in their mouths. Toddler vision continues to progress and should be 20/50 to 20/40 in both eyes. Depth perception also continues to mature. Hearing should be at the adult level, as infants are ordinarily born with hearing intact. The sense of smell continues to mature, and toddlers may comment if they do not care for the scent of something. Though taste discrimination is not completely developed, toddlers may exhibit preferences for certain flavours of foods. The toddler is more likely to try a new food if its appearance or smell is familiar. Lack of complete taste discrimination places the toddler at risk of accidental ingestion.

COMMUNICATION AND LANGUAGE DEVELOPMENT

Language usually develops rapidly during the toddler years. Cognitive development influences language development, which requires the toddler to have oral-motor ability, auditory perception, and understand syntax, semantics, and pragmatics (Murphy & Berry, 2013). The child's age, psychosocial, and cultural environment are important in motivating the toddler to listen to and engage with language. This is important in cultures where languages are undergoing a period of regeneration, for example in Indigenous Canadian communities (McIvor & Parker, 2016). **Receptive language** development (the ability to understand what is being said or asked) is typically far more advanced than **expressive language** development (the ability to communicate one's desires and feelings) (Goldson & Reynolds, 2014). In other words, the toddler understands language and is able to follow commands far sooner than he or she can actually use the words. Language is a very important part of the toddler's ability to organize his or her world and actually make sense of it. Thoughtfully planned use of language can provide behaviour guidance and contribute to the avoidance of power struggles. In regard to expressive language development, the young toddler begins to use short sentences and will progress to a vocabulary of 50 words by 2 years of age (Feigelman, 2011b). **Echolalia**

(repetition of words and phrases without understanding) normally occurs in toddlers younger than 30 months of age. "Why" and "what" questions dominate the older toddler's language. Telegraphic speech is common in the 3 year old. **Telegraphic speech** refers to speech that contains only the essential words to get the point across, much like a telegram. Rather than "I want a cookie and milk," the toddler might say, "want cookie milk." In telegraphic speech, the nouns and verbs are present and are verbalized in the appropriate order (Feigelman, 2011b). Table 26.3 gives an overview of receptive and expressive language development in the toddler.

Early identification and referral of children with potential speech delays is critical. If a delay is identified, intervention with a speech and language pathologist can support the child in acquiring age-appropriate expressive

TABLE 26.3	LANGUAGE DEVELOPMENT IN TODDLERS	
Age	**Receptive Language**	**Expressive Language**
12 months	Understands common words independent of context Follows a one-step command accompanied by gesture	Uses a finger to point to things Imitates or uses gestures such as waving goodbye Communicates desires with word and gesture combinations Vocal imitation First word
15 months	Looks at adult when communicating Follows a one-step command without gesture Understands 100–150 words	Repeats words that he or she hears Babbles in what sound like sentences
18 months	Understands the word "no" Comprehends 200 words Sometimes answers the question, "What's this?"	Uses at least 5–20 words Uses names of familiar objects
24 months	Points to named body parts Points to pictures in books Enjoys listening to simple stories Names a variety of objects in the environment Begins to use "my" or "mine"	Vocabulary of 40–50 words Sentences of two or three words ("me up," "want cookie") Asks questions ("what that?") Uses simple phrases Uses descriptive words (hungry, hot) Two thirds of what child says should be understandable by family members Repeats overheard words
30 months	Follows a series of two independent commands	Vocabulary of 150–300 words
36 months	Understands most sentences Understands physical relationships (on, in, under) Participates in short conversations May follow a three-part command	Speech usually understood by those who know the child, about half understood by those outside family Asks "why?" Three- to four-word sentences Talks about something that happened in the past Vocabulary of 1,000 words Can say name, age, and gender Uses pronouns and plurals

Adapted from Feigelman, S. (2011a). Preschool years. In R. M. Kliegman, B. F. Stanton, J. W. St. Geme III, N. F. Schor, & R. E. Behrman (Eds.), *Nelson's textbook of pediatrics* (19th ed.). Philadelphia, PA: Elsevier, Saunders; Feigelman, S. (2011b). The second year. In R. M. Kliegman, B. F. Stanton, J. W. St. Geme III, N. F. Schor, & R. E. Behrman (Eds.), *Nelson's textbook of pediatrics* (19th ed.). Philadelphia, PA: Elsevier, Saunders; and Goldson, E., & Reynolds, A. (2014). Child development and behavior. In W. W. Hay Jr., M. J. Levin, R. R. Deterding, & M. J. Abzug (Eds.), *Current diagnosis and treatment: Pediatrics* (22nd ed.). New York: McGraw-Hill Education.

language skills, thus reaching their full potential. Children with pre-existing conditions, such as genetic syndromes that are known to have an effect on language development, should be referred to a speech–language pathologist as soon as the condition is recognized rather than waiting until the child exhibits a delay.

Mild speech delay can be present in toddlers who are regularly exposed to two languages in the home (Murphy & Berry, 2013). In Canada, between 20% and 60% of Canadians speak two languages, depending on the region and proximity to an urban centre versus a more rural setting (Bialystok, 2012). In this bilingual context, a 1- to 2-year-old child may blend two languages—that is, parts of the word in both languages are blended into one word. Between age 2 and 3 years, mixing of words and phrases can be common. Despite blending and mixing languages, most bilingual children experience no delays in vocabulary development (Murphy & Berry, 2013). Current evidence suggests that bilingual children often have improved academic performance and potentially improved learning outcomes later in life (Bialystok, 2012). The nurse can provide resources and supports to parents with concerns about language development in the bilingual home. A list of websites that may be helpful is included on thePoint at http://thePoint.lww.com/EvansSanders2e.

EMOTIONAL AND SOCIAL DEVELOPMENT

Emotional development in the toddler years is focused on **separation** and **individuation** (Papalia & Feldman, 2011). For the toddler, learning that self is separate from the parent is accompanied by a sense of independence as demonstrated by exerting control over his or her environment. As this need to feel in control emerges, the toddler displays **egocentrism** (focus on self). The desire for independence results in emotional lability in the toddler. For example when boundaries are put in place: very happy and pleasant one moment, then intense emotional upset possibly escalating to a temper tantrum (Brazelton & Sparrow, 2006). As toddlers identify the boundaries between themselves and the parent or primary caregiver, they learn to negotiate a balance between attachment and independence. Toddlers initially rely on the parents' communication and signals in order to initiate appropriate behaviour or inhibit undesirable behaviour. They have a difficult time choosing between sets of behaviours as they occur in different situations. Power struggles often occur in this age group, and it is important for parents and caregivers to thoughtfully and intentionally develop the rituals and routines that will provide stability and security for the toddler (Feigelman, 2011b). Many toddlers rely on a security item (blanket, doll, or bear) to comfort themselves in stressful situations (Fig. 26.5). This ability to self-soothe is a function of autonomy and

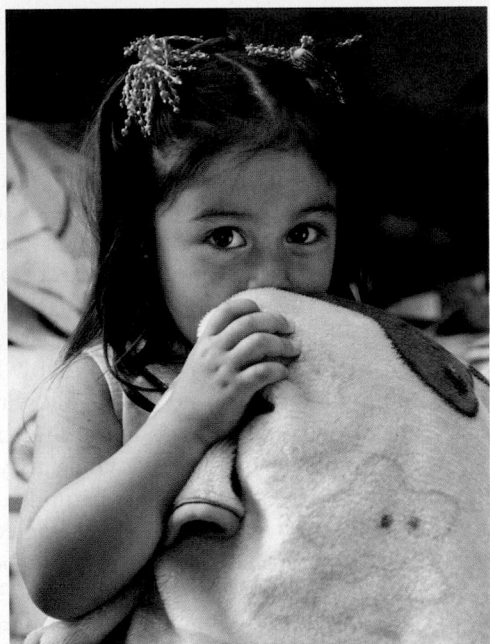

FIGURE 26.5 The toddler may be able to self-soothe and produce a sense of comfort during this stage of establishing autonomy by relying upon a security item such as a doll, bear, or blanket.

is viewed as a sign of a nurturing environment, rather than one of neglect.

Take Note!

Toddler Behaviour

When teaching parents about the stages of toddler emotional development, nurses can counsel parents to offer limited choices (usually two is sufficient) to assist with control over their environment. Nurses should advise parents that emotional lability and protest are typical in the toddler period, and these behaviours are not intentionally malicious or spiteful. In providing appropriate anticipatory guidance, the nurse may help parents understand what is motivating and driving their child's behaviour. This insight may enable parents to better cope with frequent emotional upset and tantrums, and lead to a more positive parent–child relationship. Additional access to parenting programs (Making Choices, n.d.), resources, and local community-based programs can support parents learning (Making Choices, n.d.). For example, First years First' (CPS, 2017) offers a link to education and various community resources and national directories that offer parenting resources.

Children also begin to learn about gender differences in the toddler years. They observe the differences between male and female anatomy. Toddlers may question parents about these differences and may begin to explore their own genitals. Toddlers also begin to understand and mimic social gender differences. They make observations about gender-specific behaviour dependent upon what they are exposed to.

Aggressive behaviours are typically displayed during the toddler years. Toddlers may hit, bite, or push other children and grab toys. Adults can assist the toddler in building empathy by pointing out when someone is hurt and explaining what happened. Toddlers should not be blamed for their impulsive behaviour; rather, they should be guided toward socially acceptable actions in order to foster development of appropriate social judgment. It is particularly important for the parent or caregiver to serve as a role model for appropriate behaviour, rather than losing his or her own temper, in order for the toddler to be able to learn how to acceptably handle frustrations. Limiting choices is one way of allowing toddlers some control over their environment and helping them to establish a sense of mastery which may minimize aggressive outburst. Since toddlers naturally have a short attention span, they become easily distracted from their present task, which enables their focus to be redirected away from the source of their frustration.

Though toddlers are becoming more self-aware, they still do not have clear body boundaries. They do not clearly understand the body's functions, though they are beginning to make appropriate connections. Feces may be viewed as a part of the child, and the toddler may become upset at seeing it disappear in the toilet. The toddler will protect his or her body by resisting intrusive procedures such as temperature or blood pressure measurement. In addition, injuries are a concern to the toddler, with minor cuts and abrasions, often generating lengthy or repeated discussion.

Separation Anxiety

As toddlers start to recognize that they can physically leave their parents and vice versa, some may become anxious about separation. As self-awareness develops and conflict over closeness versus exploration occurs, **separation anxiety** may re-emerge in the 18- to 24-month period (Brazelton & Sparrow, 2006). Power struggles may escalate and distress at separating from the parent may increase. Again, a predictable and consistent routine with appropriate limit setting may help toddlers to feel safe and secure during this period. For most toddlers between 24 and 36 months, separation anxiety eases. The older toddler begins to have a concept of object constancy: he or she has an internal representation of the parent or caregiver and is better able to tolerate separation, knowing that the parents will return.

Temperament

Temperament is the biologic basis for personality. It is our emotional and motivational core, around which the personality develops over time (Child Development Institute, 2015). Temperament affects how the toddler interacts with the environment. The "easygoing" toddler

may adapt more easily and not mind changes in routine as much as other toddlers. In addition, they often sleep and eat well and have more predictable and regular behaviours. However, the toddler may still express frustration by having a temper tantrum. The "difficult" toddler is more likely to have intense reactions, negative or positive, with temper tantrums being more likely, more frequent, and more intense than in other toddlers. The structure, routine, and boundaries that toddlers need to feel secure are essential for the difficult toddler; otherwise, the child feels insecure and as a result is more likely to behave inappropriately. The difficult toddler is also the most physically active of the three temperament types. The "slow-to-warm-up" toddler is more of a loner and may be very shy. He or she may experience more difficulty with separation anxiety. The behaviour of the slow-to-warm-up toddler is more passive; the toddler may be very watchful and withdrawn and may take longer to mature. Changes in routine usually do not result in as much upset, since the toddler's natural reaction is one of passivity (Brazelton & Sparrow, 2006).

Based on the toddler's temperament, make suggestions to the parents for interacting with the toddler in various situations. For example, to avoid temper tantrums in the difficult toddler, suggest that the parent should be especially diligent about maintaining structure and routine as well as avoiding tantrum triggers such as fatigue and hunger. Explain to parents that they may need to exercise additional patience with new activities to which the slow-to-warm-up toddler may need extra time becoming accustomed.

Fears

Common fears of toddlers include loss of parents (which contributes to separation anxiety) and fear of strangers. Some toddlers may be shy and actively avoid people they do not know. The nurse caring for a toddler in the clinic or hospital setting should take time to establish a relationship with the toddler in order to allay the toddler's fears. Toddlers may be afraid of loud noises and large or unfamiliar animals. Going to sleep may be a scary time for toddlers as they may be afraid of the dark. A nightlight in the toddler's room may be very helpful. Parents should avoid discussing scary or serious topics in the presence of the toddler, since the toddler is very adept at reading emotions which can heighten anxiety.

MORAL AND SPIRITUAL DEVELOPMENT

During the toddler years, parents are their children's first teachers on the importance of how to participate in family's spiritual or religious beliefs and practices (National Collaborating Centre for Aboriginal Health [NCCAH], 2013). For many Indigenous families teaching children how to be healthy in mind, body and spirit is an integral aspect of early learning (Smylie, 2011). However, toddlers have limited understanding of these beliefs because of their limited cognitive abilities. Kohlberg's (1984) description of moral development places the older toddler in the preconventional level. The toddler is only just beginning to learn right from wrong and does not understand the larger concept of morality. A capacity for empathy toward others with an ability to understand the emotional state of another is still undeveloped at this age.

CULTURAL INFLUENCES ON GROWTH AND DEVELOPMENT

Homelessness or poverty may directly influence the toddler's ability to grow adequately, as resources for the purchase and preparation of appropriate food may be lacking. Food customs and food insecurity can impact on the child's diet and ability to access the required nutrients for optimal growth (Allison, 2016). Toddlers from families who follow a vegetarian diet need specific nutritional assessment to ensure an adequate intake of iron, an essential nutrient for optimal growth and brain development.

Gendered family values may influence culture and toddler emotional development. For example, some families start at a very young age to discourage crying in boys, encouraging them to "act like a big boy" or "be a man." Ridicule for crying at this age may hurt the toddler's self-concept. Educating families about normal toddler growth and development while continuing to value and support cultural practices is important (Papalia & Feldman, 2011).

Remember Jose Gonzales, whom you met at the beginning of the chapter? What developmental milestones would you expect him to have reached at his age?

THE NURSE'S ROLE IN TODDLER GROWTH AND DEVELOPMENT

Though some toddlers may grow more quickly or reach developmental milestones sooner than others, growth and development remains orderly and sequential. The focus of any routine health monitoring visit is to assess for an adequate growth trajectory, and attainment and progression of all developmental skills. The nurse must have a good understanding of the changes that occur during the toddler years in order to provide appropriate anticipatory guidance and support to the family.

When the toddler is hospitalized, growth and development may be altered. The toddler's primary task is establishing autonomy, and the toddler's focus is mobility

FIGURE 26.6 **The hospitalized toddler continues to enjoy developmental tasks appropriate for his or her age, such as playing with manipulative toys.**

and language development. Hospitalization removes most opportunities for the toddler to learn through exploration of the environment. Isolation for contagious illness further constrains the toddler's ability to find some control over the environment. The nurse caring for the hospitalized toddler must use knowledge of normal growth and development to be successful in interactions with the toddler, promote continued development, and recognize delays (Fig. 26.6).

NURSING PROCESS OVERVIEW

Upon completion of assessment of a toddler's current growth and development status, problems or issues related to growth and development may be identified. The nurse may then identify one or more nursing diagnoses, including but not limited to:
- Delayed growth and development
- Imbalanced nutrition, less than body requirements
- Interrupted family processes
- Readiness for enhanced parenting
- Risk for caregiver role strain
- Risk for delayed development
- Risk for disproportionate growth
- Risk for injury

The nursing care plan for the toddler with growth and development issues should be individualized, strengths-based, and focused on meeting the specific needs of the child and family within a child and family-centred approach. Examples of a Nursing Care Plan can be found at the end of the chapter.

PROMOTING HEALTHY GROWTH AND DEVELOPMENT

Parents who show their toddler love and respect regardless of gender, temperament, behaviour, or capabilities are helping to lay the foundation for strong self-esteem. Self-esteem is also built through familiarity with the daily routine. Routine and ritual help toddlers develop a conscience. Making expectations known through everyday routines helps to reduce confrontations. If the toddler knows the routine, he or she knows what to expect and how he or she is expected to act. When routine and limits are absent, the toddler develops feelings of uncertainty and anxiety. Limit setting (and remaining consistent with those limits) helps toddlers master their behaviour, develop self-esteem, and become successful participants in the family. Children then are able to learn about cooperation throughout the predictable flow of daily life. Nurses need to be aware of normal developmental expectations in order to determine whether the toddler is progressing appropriately. Table 26.4 lists potential signs of developmental delay. Any toddler with one or more of these concerns should be referred for further developmental evaluation.

Promoting Growth and Development Through Play

Play is an essential component in toddlers' social, emotional, and physical development. Physical activity and outdoor unstructured play are key to fostering a child's well-being. Adequate physical activity is necessary for the development and refinement of gross motor skills, balance, and coordination. Recent guidelines from the Canadian Paediatric Society (CPS, 2012a) support the evidence by Tremblay et al. (2012), which suggests that toddlers and preschool children should engage in free play and movement, both structured and unstructured, for up to 180 minutes per day. Indoor and outdoor areas should encourage play activities that use the large muscle groups. Outdoor play structures should be positioned over surfaces that are soft enough to absorb a fall, such as sand, wood chips, or sawdust (Fig. 26.7). Box 26.1 lists recommended age-appropriate toys. Toddlers typically play alongside another child (**parallel play**) rather than cooperatively (Fig. 26.8). The short attention span of the toddler will make him or her often change toys and types of play. Toddlers do not need expensive toys and regular household items can make enjoyable toys. Toddlers are egocentric, a normal part of their development (Piaget, 1969) which makes it difficult for them to share. As they are developing a sense of self (who they are as a person), they may see their toys as an extension of themselves. Learning to share occurs in later toddlerhood. Toddlers also like dramatic play and play that

TABLE 26.4	SIGNS OF DEVELOPMENTAL DELAY
Age or Time Frame	**Concern**
After independent walking for several months	• Persistent tiptoe walking • Failure to develop a mature walking pattern (especially if older than 3 years)
By 18 months	• Not walking • Not speaking 15 words; persistent babbling • Poor eye contact with others, including parents • Does not understand function of common household items
By 2 years	• Does not use two-word sentences • Does not imitate actions • Cannot follow a 1-step command • Cannot push a toy with wheels
By 3 years	• Difficulty with stairs • Frequent falling • Cannot build tower of more than four blocks • Difficulty manipulating small objects • Extreme difficulty in separation from parent or caregiver • Cannot copy a circle • Does not engage in make-believe play • Cannot communicate in short 3-word phrases • Does not understand simple 2-step commands • Little interest in other children • Unclear speech, persistent drooling

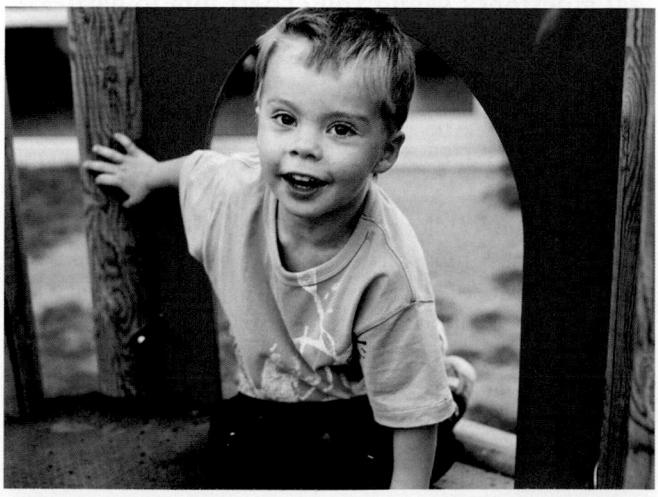

FIGURE 26.7 Toddlers love outdoor physical play, such as climbing on playground equipment. An adult should always supervise toddlers when they are playing outdoors.

Chapter 26 Growth and Development of the Toddler

BOX 26.1

APPROPRIATE TOYS FOR TODDLERS

- Familiar household items such as plastic bowls and cups of various sizes, large plastic serving utensils, pots and pans, wooden spoons, cardboard boxes and tubes (from paper towel rolls), old magazines, baskets, purses, hats. Avoid objects that are smaller in diameter than the inside of a toilet paper roll. Counsel parents to use this as a reference for judging whether an object is a choking hazard.
- Child-size household item toys (kitchen, broom, vacuum cleaner, lawnmower, telephone, and so on)
- Blocks, cars and trucks, plastic animals, trains, plastic figures (family, community helpers), simple dolls, stuffed animals, balls, doll beds, and carriages
- Manipulative toys with knobs, wind-ups, and buttons that make things happen; putting large pegs or shapes into matching holes; stringing large beads on shoelaces; blocks and containers that stack; jigsaw puzzles with large pieces; toys that can be taken apart and put back together again
- Gross motor toys: play gym, push and pull toys, wagons, tricycle or other ride-on toys, tunnels
- Sources of music (CD, radio), various musical instruments
- Chalk, large crayons, finger paint, Play-Doh, washable markers
- Bucket, plastic shovel, and other containers for sand and water play
- Squeaking, floating, and squirting toys for the bath

Adapted from National Association for the Education of Young Children. (n.d.). *Good toys for young children by age and stage.* Retrieved from http://www.naeyc.org/toys

recreates familiar activities in the home, such as caring for baby dolls or gardening. Toddlers like to listen to music of all kinds and will often dance to whatever they hear on the radio. Toddlers enjoy drums, xylophones, cymbals, and toy pianos. Musical instruments made at home are also enjoyed. A few pebbles or coins inside an empty water bottle with the top tightly secured are a great music maker; an empty yogurt container with a lid and a pair of wooden spoons makes a drum. All types of play, toys, and materials need to be safe for the toddler to interact with to minimize risk, for example from choking, or injury.

Interactive technology, screen time, and computer games should be used with caution in younger children. Toddlers should be limited to using less than one hour per day of screentime since it can limit language acquisition, social interactions, and gross motor play (CPS, 2012a). Such technologies can result in sedentary behaviour in the toddler which can limit the opportunity to maintain a healthy lifestyle and weight (CPS, 2012a).

Promoting Early Learning

The parent–child relationship and the interactions between parent and child form the context for the toddler's early learning.

Promoting Language Development

Toddlers learn and perfect language and communication skills through interactions with parents or caregivers. Talking and singing to the toddler during daily activities such as mealtimes and dressing provides an environment that encourages interactive conversation. Frequent, repetitive naming helps the toddler learn appropriate words for objects in their environment. The parent or caregiver should be attentive to what the toddler is saying as well as to his or her moods. Using clarification validates the toddler's emotions and ideas. Parents should listen to and answer the toddler's questions. They should sit down quietly with the toddler and gently repeat what the toddler is saying. Encouragement and elaboration convey confidence and interest to the toddler. The toddler needs time to complete his or her thoughts without being interrupted or rushed because he or she is just starting to be able to make the connections necessary to transfer thoughts and feelings into language.

Parents should not overreact to the child's use of the word "no." They can give the toddler opportunities to use the word "no" appropriately by asking silly questions such as, "Can a cat drive a car?" or "Is a banana purple?" When promoting language development, the parent or primary caregiver should teach the toddler appropriate words for body parts and objects and should help the toddler choose appropriate words to label feelings and emotions. Toddlers' receptive language and ability to interpret nonverbal cues from body language far surpass their expressive language, especially at a younger age (Goldson & Reynolds, 2014).

FIGURE 26.8 Parallel play. The toddler usually plays alongside another child rather than cooperatively.

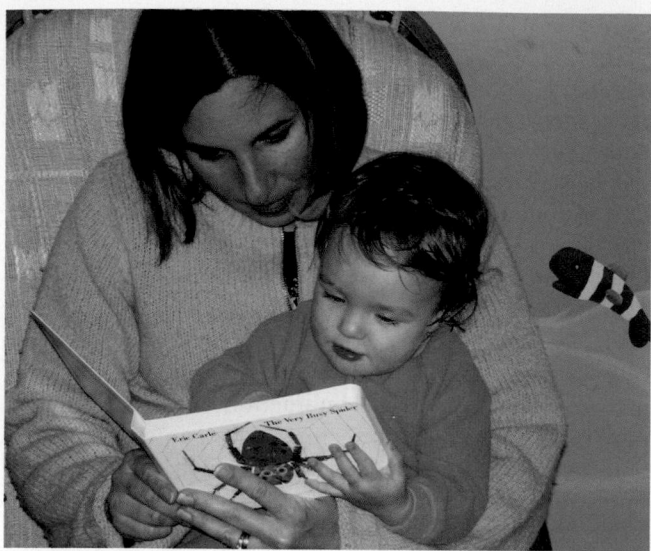

FIGURE 26.9 Reading to a toddler daily is one of the best ways to promote language development and school readiness.

Encouraging Reading

Reading to the toddler every day is the best way to promote language and cognitive development (Fig. 26.9). Toddlers particularly enjoy homemade or purchased books about feelings, family, friends, everyday life, animals and nature, and fun and fantasy. Board books have thick pages that are easier for young toddlers to turn; older toddlers can turn paper pages one at a time. The toddler may also enjoy "reading" the story to the parent. Reach Out and Read, a program designed to promote early literacy, offers tips for reading with young children (see Teaching Guidelines 26.1). Literacy is very closely related to major determinants of health, and is associated with school success, higher income, and overall better health outcomes (CPS, 2017a). As such, the nurse should ask about time spent reading and review its importance with parents at each health visit.

Teaching Guidelines 26.1
TIPS FOR READING WITH YOUNG CHILDREN
- Start at early age.
- Read at least a few minutes every day.
- Encourage your toddler to turn the pages.
- Read stories over and over to help the toddler learn.
- Ask the toddler questions about the book.
- Use voices for the story characters.
- Use body motions during the story.
- Ask questions about the story and about the pictures.
- Read anywhere, at any time.

Adapted from Reach Out and Read. (2013). *Reading tips for your young family.* Retrieved from http://www.reachoutandread.org/FileRepository/ReadingTips.pdf

Choosing a Preschool

Preschool readiness should be considered by the parents to allow them opportunity, if possible, to make decisions about their child's ability to cope with preschool, change in routine, and separation concerns (Murphy & Berry, 2013). The older toddler may benefit from the structure and socialization provided by attending preschool. Going to preschool can help the toddler become more mature and independent as well as provide a new setting in which to flourish. At this age, toddlers need supervised play with some direction that fosters their cognitive development. A strict curriculum is not necessary in this age group. When choosing a preschool, the parent needs to be able to evaluate the setting and feel confident their child is in a safe place. Parents can look for a preschool setting that has the following qualities:

- Goals and an overall philosophy with which the parents agree (promotion of independence and self-confidence through structured and free play)
- Teachers and assistants trained in early childhood development as well as child cardiopulmonary resuscitation (CPR)
- Small class sizes and an adult-to-child ratio with which the parent feels comfortable
- Disciplinary procedures consistent with the parents' values
- School is childproofed inside and out
- Appropriate hygiene procedures, including prohibiting sick children from attending

The nurse can educate parents about how to ease the toddler's transition to attending preschool. Encourage parents to talk about going to preschool and visit the preschool a couple of times. On the first day, parents should calmly and in a matter-of-fact tone tell the toddler that they will return to pick him or her up. The toddler may express some separation anxiety; however, the parent should remain calm and follow through with the plan for school attendance. It is helpful if parents emphasize to their child that they will return later to pick them up in order to build trust. Eventually, the child will feel secure that parents will return. Within a few days of this predictable routine, the child should have minimal crying when separating from parents.

Promoting Safety

Safety is of prime concern throughout the toddler period. Curiosity, mobility, and lack of impulse control all contribute to the incidence of unintentional injury in toddlerhood. Even when parents are vigilant, toddlers spontaneous actions can result in falls, accidents, and misadventure. Toddlers require direct observation and cannot be trusted to be left alone. A secure and childproof environment aims to provide a safe place for the toddler to explore and learn. Motor vehicle accidents, drowning, choking, burns, falls, and poisoning are the most common injuries suffered by toddlers. Safety and injury prevention focus on these categories.

Safety in the Car

In Canada, motor vehicle collisions are the leading cause of unintentional death to children aged 1 to 4 years (CPS, 2012a). The safest place for the toddler to ride is in the back seat of the car. Parents should use the appropriate size and style of car seat for the child's weight and age as required by local laws and safety recommendations outlined by Transport Canada (2014). The four stages of car seat use from Government Canada (2016) also suggest registering the product with the manufacturer and replacing out-of-date or damaged seats. A toddler riding in a pickup truck should never ride in the cargo area or truck bed. A full rear seat in the truck is the preferred placement for the toddler car seat. If an appropriate rear seat is unavailable, the air bag should be disarmed and the forward-facing car seat should be secured appropriately in the truck seat. The lower anchor and top tether are additionally required for all forward-facing car seats manufactured since 2002 and are accommodated by motor vehicles manufactured since that time. In older vehicles or car seats, seat belts are utilized for installation. Excellent resources about car seat safety appropriate for both parents and professionals can be found on thePoint https://www.canada.ca/en/services/transport/road/child-car-seat-safety.html.

Safety in the Home

Key areas of concern for keeping toddlers safe in the home include avoiding exposure to tobacco smoke, preventing injury, and preventing poisoning.

AVOIDING EXPOSURE TO TOBACCO SMOKE

Exposure to second-hand smoke has been associated with increased risk of respiratory disease and infection, decreased lung function, and increased incidence of middle ear effusion and recurrent otitis media. It may also hinder neurodevelopment and may be associated with behaviour problems (Health Canada, 2015). Parents should avoid cigarette smoking entirely to best protect their children. Even smoking outside of the home has risks to the child, as smoke lingers on parents' clothing and in the environment. This tobacco "dust" is a significant source of "third-hand smoke" which contains the same harmful chemicals as inhaled smoke. Toddlers are most vulnerable as they crawl on the floor, put objects in their mouths, and are often carried by parents where they inhale the chemicals in their clothing and hair. Studies show that children exposed to third-hand smoke have higher levels of the chemical by-products of nicotine in their blood and urine (American Thoracic Society, 2012). Counsel parents and provide resources to stop smoking as the best option for protecting their child's health. Harm may be reduced by never smoking inside the home or car, never smoking with the children present, and always changing their clothes after smoking and before hugging or holding their child (ATS, 2012).

PREVENTING INJURY

The focus of injury prevention is providing a safe environment coupled with active supervision (Murphy & Berry, 2013). The toddler is able to open drawers and doors, unlock deadbolts, and climb anywhere he or she wants to go. Toddlers have a limited concept of body boundaries and have not yet learnt safety rules. Toddlers may fall from any height to which they can climb (e.g., play structures, tables, counters). They may also fall from wheeled toys such as tricycles. As toddlers gain additional height and hand dexterity, they are able to reach potentially dangerous items on the counter or stove, leading to an accidental ingestion, burn, or cut. It is important to note that injury is the leading cause of death in Canadian Indigenous children and youth. As compared with 6% in the general Canadian population, 26% of all deaths among Indigenous people are caused by injuries (CPS, 2012b). Canadian federal gun control laws mandate that firearms be kept in a locked cabinet with the ammunition stored elsewhere (CPS, 2018).

To prevent injury in the home, stress the following to parents:

- Never leave a toddler unsupervised out of doors.
- Lock doors to dangerous rooms.
- Install safety gates at the top and bottom of staircases.
- Secure all open windows and locks safely. Windows left open, especially on upper floors of a home or apartment, post a significant risk of falls for young children.
- Keep pot handles on the stove turned inward, out of an inquisitive toddler's reach.
- Teach the toddler to avoid the oven, stove, fireplace, and iron.
- Keep electrical equipment, cords, and matches out of reach.
- Remove firearms from the home, or keep them in a locked cabinet out of the toddler's reach, as per Canadian laws and regulations.
- Always require the child to wear a helmet approved by the Consumer Products Safety Commission (CPSC) when riding a wheeled toy, bicycle, or scooter. This starts the habit of helmet wearing early, so it can be more easily carried over to the bicycle-riding years of the future.
- Begin teaching the toddler about watching for cars when crossing the street, but always carry or hold the hand of the toddler when crossing the street.
- Teach the toddler to avoid unknown animals.

Take Note!

Battery burns can cause significant health issues to toddlers in short periods of time. Often, children's toys contain small button batteries which can easily be ingested resulting in serious internal injury or death. Parents must act quickly if they think their child has swallowed a battery and seek medical advice (Government of Canada, 2014).

PREVENTING POISONING

As toddlers become more mobile, they are increasingly able to explore their environment and more easily gain access to materials that may be unsafe for them to handle. Their natural curiosity leads them into situations that may place them in danger. Poor taste discrimination in this age group allows for ingestion of chemicals or other materials that older children would find too unpleasant to swallow. Box 26.2 lists most potentially dangerous ingested poisons. Given poisoning is the second leading cause of accidental injury and hospitalization in toddlers 1 to 4 years of age (CPS, 2012a), the nurse should discuss poison prevention in the home at each well-child visit. Potentially poisonous substances (e.g., medications, cleaners, hair care products, car care products) should be stored out of the toddler's reach, out of the toddler's sight, and in a childproof, locked cabinet.

Encourage all families to take the following safety measures:

- Store all substances in original containers only.
- Never store any liquid other than soda in a soda pop bottle.
- Do not allow toddlers access to baby powder, lotion, cream, or other toddler hygiene products.
- Ensure all medications have child-safety caps.
- Do not leave within the toddler's reach medications such as lozenges or samples that are not packaged in safety bottles.
- Be very careful with medications that are provided in transdermal patch form.

BOX 26.2

MOST DANGEROUS POTENTIAL POISONS

- Medicines (especially iron)
- Cleaning products (especially bleach and solvents)
- Antifreeze, windshield washer solution
- Alcohol
- Pesticides
- Gasoline, kerosene, lamp oil, furniture polish, nail polish
- Wild mushrooms

Adapted from American Association of Poison Control Centers. (n.d.). *In the home.* Retrieved from http://www.aapcc.org/prevention/home/, and Canadian Association of Poison Control Centres. (n.d.). *Provincial centres.* Retrieved from http://www.capcc.ca/en/search/node/ipecac

---

- Do not refer to medicines as candy, as the toddler may mistake pills for candy and ingest them.
- Do not expose toddlers to hazardous vapours such as paints, cleaners, tobacco smoke, marijuana, e-cigarette smoke, and especially street drugs such as crack.
- Keep "button" batteries secured and away from a toddler's reach.
- Keep house plants off the floor, remove them from the home, or hang them or place them on a high shelf.

Take Note!

It is recommended that all families post the Poison Control Centre number in a readily accessible place in the home (Canadian Association of Poison Control Centres, n.d.). Since 2003, the American Thoracic Society (AAP, 2015) has discouraged the use of syrup of ipecac in the home to induce vomiting after an accidental ingestion. Instead, families should call their local provincial Poison Control Centre right away.

Safety in the Water

Drowning is the leading cause of unintentional injury and death in US and Canadian children, with nearly half of drowning victims being 4 years old and younger (Safe Kids, 2015). Drowning may occur in very small volumes of water such as a toilet, bucket, or bathtub, as well as the obvious sites such as swimming pools and other bodies of water. Toddlers' large heads in relation to their body size place them at risk for toppling over into a body of water that they are inquisitive about. Toddlers should be supervised at all times when in or around the water. In general, most children do not have the physical and cognitive capabilities necessary to become a true swimmer until 4 years of age. Parents who want to enrol a toddler in a swimming class should be aware that a water safety skills class would be most appropriate. However, even toddlers who have completed a swimming program still need *constant* supervision in the water (Safe Kids, 2016b). Box 26.3 gives recommendations for the prevention of drowning.

Remember Jose Gonzales, the 2 year old introduced at the beginning of the chapter? What anticipatory guidance related to safety should you provide to his parents?

Promoting Nutrition

The toddler's ability to chew and swallow is improving, and he or she learns to use utensils effectively to feed himself or herself. Forming healthy eating habits begins early in life, and diet has significant influence upon the child's future health status. By establishing healthier food choice patterns early in life, the child is better able to continue these healthy choices later in life. The child younger than 2 years of age should not have his or her fat intake restricted. A balanced diet high in nutrient-rich foods and low in refined sugars and prepackaged foods is endorsed by Health Canada and is reflected in the Canada Food Guide (2011). The culturally competent nurse should also be familiar with the Canada Food Guide (2007) for First Nations, Inuit, and Metis people, which incorporates traditional foods, values, and preparation methods.

Weaning

The timing of weaning from breastfeeding is influenced by a number of factors such as cultural beliefs, local and regional ethnic beliefs, the mother's work schedule, desired child spacing, or societal feelings about the nature of the mother–infant relationship. The CPS (2017b) recommends breastfeeding for the first 2 years of life, then for as long as is mutually agreeable to mother and child. Extending breastfeeding into toddlerhood is believed to be beneficial to the child. Extended breastfeeding provides nutritional, immunologic, and emotional benefits to the child. Note that breastfeeding does not offer contraception, it is biologically possible to become pregnant while breastfeeding. Breastfeeding a newborn appropriately can occur while continuing to nurse the older sibling.

Weaning from the breast is a highly individualized decision. Educate the mother about the benefits of extended breastfeeding and support her in her decision to wean at a given time.

Weaning from the bottle should occur by 12 to 15 months of age. Prolonged bottle-feeding is associated with the development of dental caries. No-spill "sippy cups" contain a valve that requires sucking by the toddler in order to obtain fluid, thus functioning similar to

a baby bottle. Hence, no-spill sippy cups can also be associated with dental caries and are not recommended (Canadian Dental Association, 2010). Cups with spouts that do not contain valves are acceptable. The 12 to 15 month old is developmentally capable of consuming adequate fluid amounts using a cup.

Teaching About Nutritional Needs

Adequate calcium and vitamin D intake, together with appropriate exercise, lays the foundation for proper bone mineralization. The toddler 1 to 4 years of age requires 700 mg of calcium per day, while the 4 to 8 year old requires 1,000 mg daily (National Institute of Health, 2016). Adequate vitamin D intake is essential as it works in synergy (aids in absorption) with calcium to support the development of strong bones. All children 1 year of age and older require 600 units of vitamin D per day (Health Canada, 2012). Dairy products were historically considered the primary sources of dietary calcium. However, because of ethnic and cultural diversity, many Canadians follow diets that do not include milk, such as those who follow a plant-based vegan diet, or those with a lactose intolerance, or a true allergy to cow milk. Children who follow one of these alternative diets require detailed nutritional assessment. Parents should be referred to nutrition guidelines published by Health Canada (2012) or the National Institute of Health (2016) for optimal recommended daily intakes for each age.

Iron-deficiency anemia in the first 2 years of life may be associated with developmental and psychomotor delays (Baker & Greer; Committee on Nutrition AAP, 2010). Although it is important for toddlers to consume adequate amounts of iron, they tend to have the lowest daily iron intake of any age group. When breastfeeding or formula-feeding ends (most often at 1 year of age), it is often replaced with iron-poor cow's milk. Limiting milk intake to approximately 470 mL (16 oz) per day can help reduce the risk of iron deficiency. Meats provide the most bioavailable source of iron, but non–meat-based iron-rich foods can also fulfil daily iron requirements. However, these are less bioavailable and require consumption of larger volumes which may be more challenging. Vitamin C rich foods should be consumed with iron to optimize its absorption. Likewise, calcium-rich foods should not be consumed with iron as it reduces its absorption by the gut.

Take Note!

Toddlers who consume a strictly vegan diet (no food from animal sources) are at risk for deficiencies in calcium, vitamin D, vitamin B_{12}, and iron. Supplementation with these nutrients should occur to promote adequate nutrition and growth (Stettler, Bhatia, Parish, & Stallings, 2011).

BOX 26.4

KEY NUTRIENTS PROVIDED BY FRUITS AND VEGETABLES

Dietary fibre: applesauce, carrots, corn, green beans, mangos, pears
Folate: avocados, broccoli, green peas, oranges, spinach and dark greens, strawberries
Vitamin A: apricots, cantaloupe, carrots, mangos, spinach and dark greens, sweet potatoes
Vitamin C: broccoli, cantaloupe, green peas, oranges, potatoes, strawberries, tomatoes

Adapted from Brown, J. (2011). *Nutrition now* (6th ed.). Florence, KY: Wadsworth Publishing.

Fat or cholesterol intake should not be restricted in children younger than age 2 years. The brain and body grow rapidly over the first 2 years of life. Toddlers are also constantly in motion, which raises their calorie requirements (metabolism) and thus their need for high-quality calories and fats. To promote healthy cholesterol levels, children older than age 2 years should consume a diet with a total fat content between 20% and 30% of total calories. Saturated fats should account for less than 10% of total calories (Stettler et al., 2011). Due to daily variations and the pickiness of the toddler, fat intake should be evaluated over a period of 1 week. The daily recommended intake of fibre for a 1 to 3 year old is 19 g. Generally, toddler serving sizes should be about two thirds that of an older child. Box 26.4 lists common sources of several nutrients.

Parents should encourage toddlers to drink water. Juice and other sweetened beverages are not recommended as they provide empty calories that take the place of nutritious foods. Maximal intake should be limited to 115 to 175 mL (4 to 6 oz) per day. Milk intake should be limited to approximately 470 to 700 mL (16 to 24 oz) per day. Juice and milk should be served along with meals or snacks. Water should be offered for between-meal drinking. Toddlers should drink from a cup.

Advancing Solid Foods

Parents should offer three full meals and two snacks daily. Portion sizes for toddlers are about one-quarter the size of adult portions. Large portions of a new or different food on the toddler's plate may intimidate the toddler. Normal toddler behaviours of mouthing, handling, tasting, extruding the food from the mouth, and then resampling the food often occur. These behaviours are distasteful to some parents but are a normal part of toddler development. Parents need to understand and tolerate these behaviours rather than scolding the toddler for them (Brazelton & Sparrow, 2006).

Toddlers are often afraid to try new things, so the parent or caregiver should be flexible with the toddler's acceptance or rejection of new foods. If the toddler refuses healthy food choices at meal or snack time, parents should not substitute high-fat, high-sugar, processed food just to make sure that the child eats something (Stettler et al., 2011). This sets the stage for future power struggles. The parent decides which foods will be served or offered. The toddler decides how much will be eaten. The toddler self-regulates the amount of food needed to sustain and allow further growth and development. The toddler may not eat well every day but, generally, over the course of several days, will consume the foods he or she needs (Zero to Three, 2016b).

Foods should be served near room temperature. Some of the food on the plate should be soft and moist. Food should always be cut into bite-size pieces. Teaching Guidelines 26.2 gives recommendations on ways to prevent choking.

 Teaching Guidelines 26.2
AVOIDING CHOKING

- Slowly add foods that are more difficult to chew as the toddler becomes more adept at chewing.
- Cut all foods into bite-sized pieces.
- Avoid foods that are hard to chew and may become lodged in the airway, such as:
  - Nuts
  - Gumdrops or other chewy candies
  - Raw carrots
  - Peanut butter (by itself)
  - Popcorn
- Cut hotdogs and grapes into quarters. Cook carrots until soft; if serving raw, then grate them.
- Always supervise the toddler while he or she is eating.

Adapted from Brown, J. (2011). *Nutrition now* (6th ed.). Florence, KY: Wadsworth Publishing.

Promoting Self-Feeding

Toddlers most often eat with their fingers, but they do need to learn to use utensils properly. The following are suggestions for parents:

- Use a child-sized spoon and fork with dull tines.
- Seat the toddler in a high chair or at a comfortable height in a secure chair. The toddler should have his or her feet supported rather than dangling (Fig. 26.10).
- Never leave the toddler unattended while eating.
- Minimize distractions during mealtime. Serve food to the toddler along with the other members of the family (Gavin, 2014b).

FIGURE 26.10 The toddler should be appropriately and safely seated in the high chair. The safety strap is secure, the toddler's feet are supported, and the tray table is locked in place.

Promoting Healthy Eating Habits

Since the toddler's rate of growth has slowed somewhat compared to that in infancy, their appetite may also slow. The toddler will also exhibit **food jags**, where he or she may prefer only one particular food for several days, then not want it for weeks. Again, it is important for the parent to continue to offer healthy food choices during a food jag and not give in by allowing the toddler to eat alternate sugary or processed foods (Gavin, 2014b).

The toddler may also engage in testing of limits during mealtime. Since toddlers still have reduced ability to express their emotions with words, they use nonverbal behaviours to do so. While eating, the toddler may dislike the taste of a particular food or experience a feeling of fullness but will communicate that feeling by screaming or throwing food. When the child exhibits these behaviours, the parent must remain calm and remove the toddler from the situation to avoid any negative reinforcement. Parents should strive for meal times to be calm and positive, as this can build positive mealtime rituals. Parents can model appropriate eating habits, but toddlers may also be willing to try more foods if they are exposed to other children who eat those foods. Praise the child for trying a new food, and never punish the toddler for refusing to try something

new. A new food may need to be offered upwards of 12 to 20 times before the toddler chooses to try it. Parents should be sure to include foods the child is familiar with and likes to eat at the same meal that the new food is being introduced (Zero to Three, 2016b). Teaching Guidelines 26.3 lists alternative foods that meet nutritional needs and a list of books for parents of the picky eater or alternatively encourage parents to check out their local library.

 Teaching Guidelines 26.3
MEETING NUTRITIONAL NEEDS OF THE PICKY EATER

Alternative Food Choices for the Picky Eater
- Won't drink milk? Obtain calcium through yogurt cheese, pudding, hot cocoa, and smoothies.
- Poor meat intake? Obtain iron through unsweetened iron-fortified cereals or breakfast bars, beans, tofu, pumpkin seeds, dried apricots or raisins; cook with an iron skillet.
- Loves processed white bread? Encourage fibre intake with fresh fruits and vegetables, bran muffins, beans, or peas (can be in soup).
- Refuses vegetables? Encourage vitamin A intake with apricots, sweet potatoes, and vegetable juices.

Books and resources for Parents of the Picky Eater
- The "Everything" Baby's First Food Book by J. Tarlou. Holbrook, MA: Adams Media Corp., 2001.
- Say goodbye to Picky Eating: https://www.eatright ontario.ca/en/Articles/Child-Toddler-Nutrition/Say-Goodbye-to-Picky-Eating!.aspx
- Government of Canada: Health Eating for Children. https://www.canada.ca/en/health-canada/services/tips-healthy-eating-tips-families/healthy-eating-children.html

Preventing Overweight and Obesity

In the child younger than 3 years of age, the greatest risk factor for the development of overweight or obesity is having a parent with a high body mass index (BMI) (Dev et al., 2013). The nurse can screen for overweight in the child older than 2 years of age by calculating the BMI and plotting the BMI on the standardized age- and gender-appropriate growth charts. Trends over time may be predictive of the development of overweight or obesity.

Another factor in development of obesity in young children is juice intake (Stettler et al., 2011). Toddlers who routinely drink excess fruit juice or eat high-calorie snacks are at high risk for becoming overweight or obesity because of the high sugar intake. Excess juice intake can also be associated with insufficient nutrient intake and malnutrition as juice occupies volume in the stomach and takes the place of nutrient-dense solid foods. Fruit juice intake should be limited to 115 to 175 mL (4 to 6 oz) per day. Internet links to feeding resources that can provide education to parents and professionals includes the Ellyn Satter Institute. This multipurpose educational evidence-based resource provides information and tools to help preventing child obesity by using the division of responsibility (sDOR) as a way in which to work toward restorative eating patterns.

> **Take Note!**
> Young children should consume only pasteurized juice, as unpasteurized juice consumption places the toddler at increased risk of *Escherichia coli*, *Salmonella*, and *Cryptosporidium* infection.

> Refer back to Jose Gonzales. What questions should you ask his parents related to his nutritional intake? What anticipatory guidance related to nutrition would be appropriate?

Promoting Healthy Sleep and Rest

The 18 month old generally requires 13.5 hours of sleep per day, the 24 month old 13 hours, and the 3 year old 12 hours (Feigelman, 2011a, 2011b). Every child is different however, and some require more or less sleep than another. A typical toddler should sleep through the night and take one daytime nap. Most children discontinue daytime napping at around 3 to 4 years of age. When the crib becomes unsafe (i.e., when the toddler becomes physically capable of climbing over the rails), then he or she must make the transition to a bed.

Consistent bedtime rituals help the toddler prepare for sleep. Choose a bedtime and stick to it as much as possible. The nightly routine might include a bath followed by reading a story. The routine should be a calm period with minimal outside distractions. Toddlers often require a security item to help them get to sleep. Older toddlers may be afraid of the dark, so a nightlight is often helpful.

Night waking is a fairly common occurrence for toddlers at some point. This may occur as a result of change in routine, getting over an illness, or as a desire for nighttime attention. Attention during night waking should be minimized so that the toddler receives no reward for being awake at night. For some toddlers, night waking is caused by nightmares. As the imagination and capacity for make-believe grow, the toddler may not be able to distinguish between reality and dream state. The parent should hold and comfort the toddler after a nightmare. Limiting television viewing (especially before bedtime; no TV or screen time 90 minutes before bed) may be helpful in limiting nightmares.

Some families practice "co-sleeping" (when children sleep in the parents' bed) based on preference or cultural norms. Although some professionals believe that co-sleeping may interfere with the toddler's struggle for independence, this theory has not been proven. The nurse should support the family's choice for sleep arrangements unless the co-sleeping is unsafe either physically or psychologically (SafeBedSharing.org, 2016). Refer to http://www.safebedsharing.org for bed-sharing safety guidelines.

> **Provide anticipatory guidance to Jose Gonzales' parents in relation to his sleep.**

Promoting Healthy Teeth and Gums

By around 3 years of age, most toddlers will have a full set of 20 primary ("baby") teeth. Parents may not appreciate the importance of preventing cavities in primary teeth since they will eventually be replaced by the permanent teeth. However, poor oral hygiene, prolonged use of a bottle or spill-proof sippy cup, lack of fluoride intake, and delayed or absent professional dental care may all contribute to the development of dental caries (CDA, 2010). Cleaning of the toddler's teeth should progress from brushing with simply water to using a very small amount (dry rice kernel) of fluoridated toothpaste with brushing beginning at 2 to 3 years of age, depending on local fluoride levels in the drinking water (Fig. 26.11).

FIGURE 26.11 The parent should brush the toddler's teeth to ensure proper cleaning of the teeth, gums, and tongue. Use only water for brushing before 2 years of age and a pea-sized amount of fluoride-containing toothpaste after age 2 years.

TABLE 26.5	RECOMMENDATIONS FOR FLUORIDE SUPPLEMENTATION		
	Fluoride Ion Level in Drinking Water (ppm)		
Age	*<0.3 ppm*	*0.3–0.6 ppm*	*>0.6 ppm*
Birth to 6 months	None	None	None
6 months to 3 years	0.25 mg/day	None	None
3–6 years	0.50 mg/day	0.25 mg/day	None
6–16 years	1.0 mg/day	0.50 mg/day	None

These recommendations are at public domain www.ada.org and were approved by the American Dental Association, the American Academy of Pediatrics, and the American Academy of Pediatric Dentistry. ppm, parts per million is equivalent to 1 mg/L.

At age 1 year, the toddler should have his or her first dentist visit to establish baseline health of the teeth and gums. Eating should be limited to meal and snack times, as "grazing" throughout the day exposes the teeth to food throughout the day. Sticky sugary or carbohydrate-containing foods such as raisins, dried mango or other fruits, fruit gummies, and goldfish crackers can be associated with dental decay, as these combine with oral bacteria to create a decreased oral pH level that is optimal for the development of dental caries (cavities).

Public water fluoridation is a public health initiative that ensures that most children receive adequate fluoride intake to prevent dental caries. Table 26.5 gives recommendations regarding fluoride supplementation. If the water supply contains adequate fluoride, no other supplementation is necessary other than brushing with a small amount of fluoride-containing toothpaste after age 2 years. Excess fluoride ingestion should be avoided, as it contributes to the development of fluorosis (mottling of the enamel). Fluorosis occurs most often in the toddler years (AAP, 2014). Risk factors for fluorosis development include:

- High fluoride levels in the local water supply
- Use of fluoride-containing toothpaste prior to age 2 years
- Excessive ingestion of fluoride either in toothpaste or foods
- Fluoride-containing foods: tea, ready-to-eat infant foods containing chicken, white or purple grape juice, and beverages, processed foods, and cereals that were manufactured with fluoride-containing water

Promoting Appropriate Discipline

Normal toddler development includes natural curiosity, and this curiosity often results in dangerous or problematic activities for the toddler (Lyness, 2013). Toddlers have a difficult time learning the rules and, in general, do not behave badly intentionally. Offering realistic choices helps give the toddler a sense of mastery. Rules should be simple and limited in number. Maintaining the toddler's schedule of meals and rest/sleep will help to prevent conflicts that occur as a result of hunger or fatigue. Toddlers should not be made to share, as this is a concept they do not understand. Parents should encourage simple activities enjoyed by the children involved and avoid confrontation over toys. Parents should offer toddlers appropriate choices to help them develop autonomy, but should not offer a choice when none exists.

Discipline is a common parental concern during toddlerhood. The toddler's intense personality and extreme emotional reactions can be difficult for parents to understand and cope with. The toddler needs firm, gentle, consistent guidance to learn what the expectations are and how to meet them. The parent's love and respect for the toddler teach the toddler to care about himself or herself and for others. Affection and praise is as important as the guidance aspect of discipline. Having realistic expectations of what the toddler is capable of learning and understanding can help the parent in the disciplinary process. The toddler's intense push for autonomy can often test a parent's limits. The easygoing infant usually becomes more challenging in toddlerhood. The toddler's continual quest for new experiences often places the toddler at risk, and his or her negativism very often taxes the parent's patience.

In an effort to prevent the toddler from experiencing harm and in response to his or her continual testing of limits, parents may resort to spanking. Physical punishment is not discipline. The Canadian Paediatric Society, and National Association Pediatric Nurse Practitioners recommend against corporal or physical punishment (CHEO, 2013). Recent research points out the dangers inherent in the use of corporal punishment as well as the possibilities for negative effects on the child's future behaviour (Box 26.5). Spanking or other forms of corporal punishment lead to a pro-violence attitude, create resentment and anger in some children, and contribute to the cycle of violence (NAPNAP, 2011). In Canada, forms of physical punishment are considered crimes, and

BOX 26.5

NEGATIVE IMPACT OF PHYSICAL PUNISHMENT

- Spanking and other forms of physical punishment are strongly discouraged by the Canadian Paediatric Society (2013), and play no role in the disciplining of a toddler or child. Most forms of physical punishment of children are considered crimes in Canada (Public Health Agency of Canada, 2016).
- The toddler lacks the cognitive ability to connect the spanking with the undesired behaviour.
- Physical punishment will create fear and mistrust of the parent, which is damaging to the parent–child relationship.
- May lead to a pro-violence attitude
- Is a poor model for learning effective problem solving
- May be correlated with antisocial and criminal behaviour later in life
- Leads to increased aggression in preschoolers, school-age children, and adults
- Childhood corporal punishment increases the probability of depression and substance abuse in adulthood.
- Spanking may escalate to more severe forms of punishment and to actual child abuse and maltreatment.
- The more frequently children are hit or spanked, the more likely they are to hit their own children and to be involved in spouse abuse as adults.

Adapted from Global Initiative to End All Corporal Punishment of Children. (n.d.). *Global initiative to end corporal punishment.* Retrieved from www.endcorporalpunishment.org; and National Association of Pediatric Nurse Practitioners. (2011). NAPNAP position statement on corporal punishment. *Journal of Pediatric Health Care, 25,* e31–e32.

all provinces and territories have laws in place to protect children from physical harm. It is against the law to "use force to punish a child under two" years of age (Department of Justice Canada, 2016).

Because their developmental stage is highly egocentric, toddlers lack the cognitive ability to understand broader consequences of their undesired behaviours on others or the environment around them. Verbal directions and explanations are often not effective at this age. Disciplinary approaches can include using consistent positive reinforcement actions from the parents or caregivers, physical removal and brief isolation "time out," or timely withdrawal of privileges (Murphy & Berry, 2013).

Positive reinforcement should be used as much as possible. When the toddler is displaying appropriate behaviour, the parent should offer specific label praise thereby reinforcing the good behaviour. "Extinction" is a particularly useful technique with 2 and 3 year olds. Extinction involves systematic ignoring of the undesired behaviour. Parents may unknowingly reinforce the unwanted behaviour by giving it negative attention. Parents who want to extinguish an annoying (nondangerous) behaviour should

resolve to ignore it every time it occurs. When the child withholds the undesired behaviour or performs the opposite (appropriate) behaviour, parents should provide specific labelled praise. It may be difficult to ignore a difficult behaviour, but the results are well worth the effort.

"Time-out" can be used effectively after 3 years of age. The young toddler is very susceptible to fears of abandonment and should not be kept in time-out away from the parent's line of sight. This is endorsed by the Canadian Paediatric Society (2016, 2018; Children's Hospital of Eastern Ontario, 2013). However, occasionally, a parent may become so frustrated with the child that it would be appropriate to ensure the toddler is in a safe contained place (e.g., crib or playpen) so the parent can take a break to calm and collect themselves. The nurse can screen for such higher risk situations by asking parents directly how they are coping with their toddler's challenging behaviour.

Teaching Guidelines 26.4 provides tips on avoiding power struggles and offering appropriate guidance to toddlers.

Teaching Guidelines 26.4
PROVIDING TODDLERS WITH GUIDANCE

- When giving the toddler instructions, tell the child what you would like them to do, NOT what not to do. This allows for a positive focus. If you must say "no," "don't," or "stop," then follow with a direction of what to do instead. For example, "legs are not for kicking others, you can kick a ball instead, feet are for the floor not for the furniture."
- Offer limited choices, when a choice is truly available. Say, "Do you want to wear your blue hat or your red hat?" NOT "Do you want to put on your hat?" This gives the toddler some, but not all, control.
- Role model appropriate communication, but don't feel like you have to speak nicely all the time. If the situation warrants, use a firm and even tone to get the point across. Avoid yelling as it is distressing for the child, and models an undesired response.
- Pay attention to the inflection in your voice. A statement or direction should not end in a questioning tone or with "Okay?" Be clear. Statements should sound like statements, and only questions should end in a questioning tone.
- When a toddler behaves aggressively, label the child's feelings calmly, but be firm and consistent with the expectation. For example, "I know you are mad that Johnny took the train. It is okay to be mad, but it is not okay to hit."

Adapted from Lyness, D. (2013). *Disciplining your toddler.* Retrieved from http://kidshealth.org/parent/positive/talk/toddler_tantrums.html# and Sears, W. & Sears, M. (2016b). 8 tools for toddler discipline. Retrieved from http://www.askdrsears.com/topics/parenting/discipline-behavior/8-tools-toddler-discipline

ADDRESSING COMMON DEVELOPMENTAL CONCERNS

Common developmental concerns of the toddler period are toilet teaching, temper tantrums, thumb sucking or pacifier use, sibling rivalry, and regression. An understanding of the normalcy of negativism, temper tantrums, and sibling rivalry will help the family cope with these issues. Prepare parents for these developmental events by giving appropriate anticipatory guidance.

Toilet Teaching

When myelination of the spinal cord is achieved around age 2 years, the toddler is capable of exercising voluntary control over the sphincters. Despite physiologic maturation, psychological and emotional readiness for toilet training may take time. Girls may be ready for toilet teaching earlier than boys. Toddlers are ready for toilet teaching when:

- Bowel movements occur on a fairly regular schedule.
- The toddler expresses knowledge of the need to defecate or urinate. This may be through verbalization, change in activity, or gestures such as:
  - Looks into or grabs diaper
  - Squats
  - Crosses legs
  - Grimaces and/or grunts
  - Hides behind a door or the couch when defecating
- The diaper is not always wet (this indicates the ability to hold the urine for a period of time).
- The toddler is willing to follow instructions.
- The toddler walks well alone and is able to pull down his or her pants.
- The toddler follows caregivers to the bathroom.
- The toddler climbs onto the potty chair or toilet.

Parents should approach toilet teaching with a calm, positive, and nonthreatening manner. Initially, it may be helpful to allow the toddler to observe a same-sex family member using the toilet. Start with the toddler fully clothed on the potty chair or toilet while the parent or caregiver talks about what the toilet is used for and when. The toddler will feel most comfortable with a toddler potty chair that sits on the floor (Fig. 26.12). If a potty chair is unavailable, facing toward the toilet tank may make the toddler feel more secure, as the buttocks remain on the front of the seat rather than sinking through the toilet seat opening. After a week or longer, remove a dirty diaper and place the contents in the toilet. Next, try having the toddler sit on the potty chair or toilet without pants or diaper on. The toddler may benefit from watching a caregiver or friend use the toilet. It may also be beneficial to demonstrate using the potty chair with a baby doll or with the use of a picture book.

Parents should always use gentle praise and no reproaches. Usually the best time to achieve success with

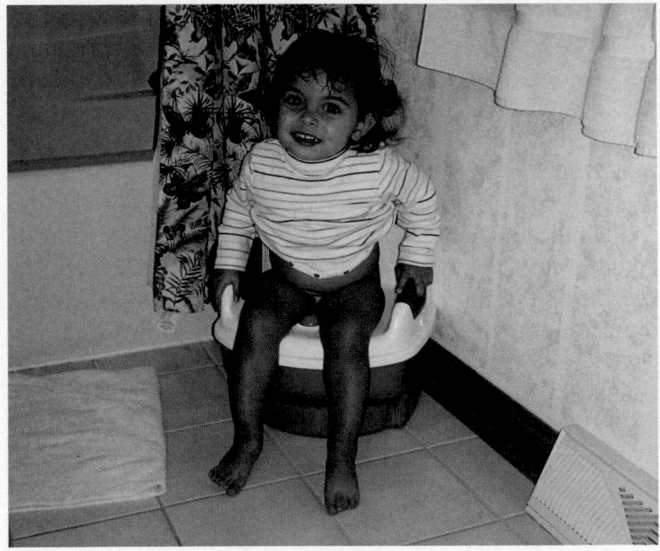

FIGURE 26.12 **The toddler will feel most comfortable with a potty chair that sits on the floor.**

defecation on the toilet is 20 minutes following a meal. When the toddler has achieved success with bowel control, bladder control will come next. It may be many months or several years before nighttime bladder control is achieved, and the toddler may still require a diaper at night. Parents should use appropriate words for body parts, urination, and defecation, and then use those words consistently so the toddler understands what to say and do.

After some success at toileting, the toddler may start wearing training pants. When toddlers have an accident and do not make it to the toilet, gently remind them about toileting and let them help clean up. Toddlers should never be punished for bowel or bladder "accidents."

With so much attention focused on the genitalia during toilet teaching and the frequency of being without a diaper, it is natural for toddlers to become more focused on their own genitalia. Boys and girls both will explore their genitalia and discover the resulting pleasurable sensation. Masturbation in the toddler often causes a great deal of discomfort in the parent. The parent should not draw attention to the activity, as that may increase its frequency. The parent should calmly explain to the toddler that this is an activity that may only be done in private (Feigelman, 2011b). If the toddler is masturbating excessively or refuses to stop when in public, then there may be additional stressors in the toddler's life that should be explored.

Negativism

Negativism is common in the toddler period (Brazelton & Sparrow, 2006). As the toddler separates from the parent, recognizes his or her own individuality, and exerts autonomy, negativism abounds. Parents should understand that this negativism is a normal developmental occurrence and not necessarily deliberate defiance. Avoid asking yes-or-no questions, as the toddler's usual response will be "no," whether he or she means it or not. Offering the child simple choices will give the toddler a sense of control. The parent should not ask the toddler if he or she "wants" to do something, if there is actually no choice. "Do you want to use the red cup or the blue cup?" is more appropriate than "Do you want your milk now?" When it is time to go outside, don't ask, "Do you want to put your shoes on?" Instead, state in a matter-of-fact tone that shoes must be worn outside, and give the toddler a choice of type of shoe or colour of socks. If the child continues with negative answers, then the parent should remain calm and make the decision for the child.

Temper Tantrums

Even children who displayed an easygoing personality as infants may lose their temper frequently during the toddler years (Fig. 26.13). A toddler who was more intense as an infant may have more temper tantrums. Temper tantrums are a natural result of the frustration that toddlers experience. Toddlers are eager to explore new things, but their efforts are often thwarted (usually for safety reasons). Toddlers do not behave badly on purpose. They need time and maturity to learn the rules and regulations. Some of their frustration may come from lack of language skills to express themselves. Toddlers are just starting to learn how to verbalize feelings and

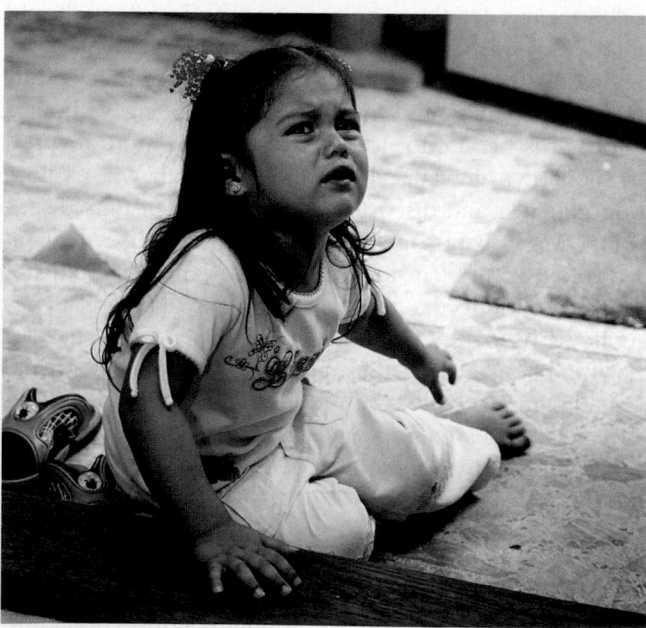

FIGURE 26.13 Tantrums are a normal component of toddler development.

to use alternative actions rather than just "pitching a fit." The temper tantrum may be manifested as a screaming and crying fit or a full-blown episode in which the toddler throws himself or herself on the floor kicking, screaming, and pounding, perhaps even holding their breath. Fatigue or hunger may limit the toddler's coping abilities and promote negative behaviour and temper tantrums (Lyness, 2013).

Although tantrums are annoying to parents and caregivers, they are a normal part of the toddler's quest for independence. As toddlers mature, they become better able to express themselves and to understand their environment, and tantrums should gradually abate.

Parents need to learn their toddler's behavioural cues in order to limit activity that is frustrating. When the parent notes the beginnings of frustration, a friendly warning might be given. Intervening early with an activity change might prevent a tantrum. Use distraction, refocusing, or removal from the situation.

When a temper tantrum does occur, the best course of action is to ignore the behaviour and ensure that the child is safe during the tantrum. If the tantrum occurs in public, it may be necessary for the parent to immobilize the child with a big bear hug and use a calm voice to soothe the toddler. It is very important for parents to model self-control. Since toddlers' tantrums most often result from frustration, the role-modelled behaviour of self-control helps to teach toddlers to control their temper when they can't get what they want (Lyness, 2013).

Thumb Sucking and Pacifiers

Infants bring their hands to their mouths and begin thumb sucking as a form of self-soothing (Sears & Sears, 2016c). This habit may continue into the toddler years and beyond. The pacifier is used for the same reason. Toddlers may calm themselves in a stressful situation by thumb sucking or sucking on a pacifier. Opinions about thumb and finger sucking and pacifier use are significantly affected by family history and culture. For most children, there is no need to worry about a sucking habit until it is time for the permanent teeth to erupt. Prolonged and frequent sucking in the withdrawn child is more likely to impact the tooth and jaw structure than sucking that is primarily used for self-soothing. Parents must clarify their own feelings about thumb sucking and pacifier use and then decide how they want to handle the habit.

To ensure safety with pacifier use:
• Use only one-piece pacifiers.
• Replace cracked and worn pacifiers with new ones.
• Never tie a pacifier around a toddler's neck.

Parents may want to limit thumb sucking and pacifier use to bedtime, in the car, and in stressful situations. The parent should calmly discuss these limits with the toddler and then remain consistent about enforcing them (Sears & Sears, 2016a, 2016c).

Sibling Rivalry

Many families have subsequent children when their first child is a toddler. The toddler has been accustomed to being the baby and receiving a great deal of attention, both at home and with the extended family. Since toddlers are normally egocentric, bringing a new baby into the home may be quite disruptive. To minimize issues with **sibling rivalry**, parents should attempt to keep the toddler's routine as close to normal as possible. Spend individual time with the toddler on a daily basis. Involve the toddler in the care of the baby. The toddler is capable of fetching a diaper or T-shirt, entertaining the baby with a toy, or helping sing a song to calm the baby (Hirsch, 2013). "Helping" the parent care for the baby gives the toddler a sense of importance (Fig. 26.14). The toddler will need significant support while holding the baby.

Regression

Some toddlers experience **regression** during a stressful event (e.g., the birth of a sibling, hospitalization). Stress in a toddler's life affects his or her ability to master new developmental tasks. During regression, the toddler may want to go back to an earlier stage. He or she may desire a bottle or pacifier forgotten long ago. The toddler may stop displaying previously achieved language or motor skills. A significant stress in the toddler's life may also disrupt the toilet teaching process (toilet teaching may not be achieved near the time a sibling is born). When regression occurs, parents should ignore the regressive behaviour and offer praise for age-appropriate behaviour or attainment of skills (Hirsch, 2013).

FIGURE 26.14 The toddler may be more likely to accept the new baby in a positive manner if she feels that this is "our baby," not just "mommy's baby." This toddler is meeting her new brother for the first time.

> Refer to Jose Gonzales, the 2 year old in the case study. List common developmental concerns of the toddler. What anticipatory guidance related to these concerns would the nurse provide to Jose's parents?

NURSING CARE PLAN 26.1

Growth and Development Issues in the Toddler

NURSING DIAGNOSIS: Risk for injury related to curiosity, increased mobility, and developmental immaturity

Outcome Identification and Evaluation

Toddler safety will be maintained: *Toddler will remain free from injury.*

Interventions: *Preventing Injury*

- Teach and encourage appropriate use of rear-facing car seat until 2 years of age and forward-facing car seat after 2 years of age *to decrease risk of toddler injury related to motor vehicles.*
- Teach toddlers to stay away from the street and provide constant supervision *to prevent pedestrian injury.*

- Require bicycle helmet use while riding any wheeled toy *to prevent head injury and form habit of helmet use.*
- Childproof the home *to provide a developmentally safe environment for the curious and increasingly mobile toddler.*
- Post poison control centre phone number *in case of accidental ingestion.*

(continued)

Growth and Development Issues in the Toddler (continued)

- Never leave a toddler unattended in a bath or pool or near any body of water *to prevent drowning.*
- Teach parents first-aid measures and child CPR *to minimize consequences of injury should it occur.*

- Provide close observation and keep side rails up on crib/bed in hospital *because toddlers are at particularly high risk for falling or becoming entangled in tubing as they attempt mobility.*

NURSING DIAGNOSIS: Imbalanced nutrition: less than body requirements, related to inappropriate nutritional intake to sustain growth needs (excess juice or milk intake, inadequate food variety intake) as evidenced by failure to attain adequate increases in height and weight over time

Outcome Identification and Evaluation

Toddler will consume adequate nutrients while using an appropriate feeding pattern: *Toddler will demonstrate weight gain and increases in height.*

Interventions: *Promoting Appropriate Nutrition*

- Assess current feeding schedule and usual intake, as well as methods used to feed, *to determine areas of adequacy versus inadequacy.*
- Determine toddler's ability to drink from cup, finger feed, swallow, and consume textures *to determine if additional exposure is needed or if further interventions such as speech or occupational therapy are required.*
- Weigh toddler daily on the same scale if hospitalized, weekly on the same scale if at home, and plot growth patterns weekly or monthly as appropriate on standardized growth charts *to determine if growth is increasing along a consistent curve.*
- Wean from bottle by 15 months of age *to discourage excess milk or juice intake in toddler who can carry bottle around.*

- Limit juice to 115 to 175 mL (4 to 6 oz) per day and milk to 470 to 700 mL (16 to 24 oz) per day *to discourage sense of fullness achieved with excess milk or juice intake, thereby increasing appetite for solid foods.*
- Provide three nutrient-dense meals and at least two healthy snacks per day *to encourage adequate nutrient consumption.*
- Feed toddler on a similar schedule daily, without distractions and with the family: *toddlers respond well to routine and structure and may eat better in the social context of meals, and they become distracted easily (TV should be off).*

NURSING DIAGNOSIS: Risk for delayed development related to motor, cognitive, language, or psychosocial concerns as evidenced by delay in meeting expected milestones

Outcome Identification and Evaluation

Development will be enhanced: *Toddler will make continued progress toward achievement of expected developmental milestones.*

Interventions: *Enhancing Growth and Development*

- Use a validated screening questionnaire to determine the toddler's present developmental ability.
- Offer age-appropriate toys, play, and activities (including gross motor) to encourage further development.
- Perform interventions as prescribed by physical, occupational, or speech pathologist: participation in those activities helps to promote function and accomplish acquisition of developmental skills.

- Provide support to families of toddlers with developmental delay (progress in achieving developmental milestones can be slow and ongoing motivation is needed).
- Reinforce positive attributes in the toddler to maintain motivation.
- Model age-appropriate communication skills to illustrate suitable means for parenting the toddler.

NURSING CARE PLAN 26.1

Growth and Development Issues in the Toddler (continued)

NURSING DIAGNOSIS: Risk for overweight related to excess milk or juice intake, late bottle weaning, and consumption of inappropriate foods or in excess amounts

Outcome Identification and Evaluation

Toddler will grow appropriately and not become overweight or obese: *Toddler will achieve and maintain a weight and height within the 5th to 95th percentiles on standardized World Health Organization growth chart*

Interventions: *Promoting Proportionate Growth*

- Wean from bottle and discourage use of no-spill sippy cups by 15 months of age (will keep mobile toddler from carrying around and continually drinking from cup or bottle).
- Discourage consumption of juice and other sweetened beverages altogether
- Provide a maximum intake of milk 470 to 700 mL (16 to 24 oz per day) from a cup at meal and snack time to encourage appropriate cup drinking.

- Provide only nutrient-rich foods without high sugar content for meals and snacks; even if the toddler won't eat, it is inappropriate to provide high-calorie junk food just so the toddler eats something.
- Ensure adequate physical activity to stimulate development of motor skills and provide appropriate caloric expenditure (approximately 180 minutes per day of active play/nonsedentary activity). This also sets the stage for forming lifelong habit of appropriate physical activity.

NURSING DIAGNOSIS: Interrupted family processes related to issues with toddler development, hospitalization, or situational crisis as evidenced by decreased parental visitation in hospital, parental verbalization of difficulty with current situation, possible crisis related to health of family member other than the toddler

Outcome Identification and Evaluation

Family will demonstrate adequate functioning: *Family will display coping and psychosocial adjustment.*

Interventions: *Enhancing Family Functioning*

- Assess the family's level of stress and ability to cope to determine family's ability to cope with multiple stressors.
- Engage in family-centred care to provide a holistic approach to care of the toddler and family.
- Encourage the family to verbalize feelings (verbalization is one method of decreasing anxiety levels), and acknowledge feelings and emotions.
- Encourage family visitation and provide for sleeping arrangements for a parent or caregiver to stay in the hospital with the toddler (contributes to family's sense of control of situation).
- Involve family members in toddler's care, giving them a feeling of control and connectedness.

NURSING DIAGNOSIS: Readiness for enhanced parenting related to parental desire for increased skills and success with toddler as evidenced by current healthy relationships and verbalization of desire for improved skills

Outcome Identification and Evaluation

Parent will provide safe and nurturing environment for the toddler.

(continued)

NURSING CARE PLAN 26.1

Growth and Development Issues in the Toddler (continued)

Interventions: *Increasing Parenting Skill Set*

- Use family-centred care to provide holistic approach.
- Educate parent about normal toddler development to provide basis for understanding the parenting skills needed in this time period.
- Acknowledge and encourage parent's verbalization of feelings related to chronic illness of child or difficulty with normal toddler behaviour to validate the normalcy of the parent's feelings.
- Encourage positive parenting with respect to toddlers and their normal development (helps parents develop approaches to toddlers that can be used in place of anger and frustration).
- Acknowledge and praise positive parenting skills already present to contribute to parents' confidence in their abilities to parent.
- Role model appropriate parenting behaviours related to communicating with and disciplining the toddler (role modelling actually shows rather than just telling the parent what to do).

KEY CONCEPTS

- The toddler's organ systems are continuing to mature, and growth slows during this period as compared with infancy.

- The psychosocial task of the toddler years is to attain a sense of autonomy and to experience separation and individuation from parents.

- Cognitive development in toddlerhood progresses from sensorimotor in nature to preoperational.

- The toddler refines gross motor skills after learning to walk and builds fine motor skills through the use of utensils and various manipulative toys.

- The toddler progresses from limited expressive language capabilities to a vocabulary of 900 words by age 3 years.

- Toddlers use all of their senses to explore and learn about their environment.

- Visual acuity progresses to at least 20/50 in the toddler period.

- Negativism abounds in toddlers as they attempt to exert their independence.

- Clear and predictable routines enhance feelings of security and safety.

- Toddler development may be promoted through active gross motor play, books, music, and block building.

- Safety is a primary concern in the toddler years as the child is more mobile, very curious, and experimenting with autonomy.

- Poisoning in the toddler period may be prevented through safe storage of medications and other potentially poisonous substances and appropriate supervision.

- Consistent bedtime rituals help ease the toddler's transition to sleep.

- All primary teeth generally erupt by 30 months of age; optimal oral hygiene includes twice daily brushing with very small amounts of fluorinated toothpaste. Fluoride supplementation may be required if drinking water is not fluoridated.

- The toddler may experience a decrease in appetite as growth slows, yet he or she still needs appropriate nutritional intake for continued development.

- Toilet teaching can be achieved after myelination of the spinal cord is complete, usually after 2 years of age but before 3 years.

- Thumb sucking, pacifier use, security items, and temper tantrums are normal expected issues in the toddler years.

- Toddler discipline should focus on clear limits and consistency. It should not involve spanking. It should be balanced with a caring and nurturing environment along with frequent praise for appropriate behaviour.

- Parental role modelling of appropriate behaviour, especially related to dealing with frustration, is beneficial to toddlers.

- Parents play an important role in toddler development, not only by providing a loving environment but also by role modelling appropriate behaviour in most areas of daily life.

REFERENCES AND RECOMMENDED READINGS

Allison, S. (2016). *Chief Medical Officer. Child health status report. Technical report.* Retrieved from https://northern health.ca/Portals/0/About/Community_Accountability/docu ments/CMHO-Child-Health-Status-Technical-Report.pdf

American Academy of Pediatric Dentistry. (2014). *Guideline on infant oral health care.* Retrieved from http://www. aapd.org/media/Policies_Guidelines/G_InfantOralHealth Care.pdf

American Academy of Pediatrics. (2015). *Poison prevention.* Retrieved from https://www.healthychildren.org/English/safety-prevention/all-around/Pages/Poison-Prevention.aspx

American Thoracic Society. (2012). Retrieved from http://www.thoracic.org/patients/patient-resources/resources/second-hand-smoke.pdf

Baker, R. D., & Greer, F. R.; Committee on Nutrition American Academy of Pediatrics. (2010). Diagnosis and prevention of iron deficiency and iron-deficiency anemia in infants and young children (0–3 years of age). *Pediatrics, 126*(5), 1040–1050.

Bialystok, E., Craik, F. I. M., Luk, G. (2012). *Bilingualism, consequences for mind and brain.* Retrieved from https://www.ncbi.nlm.nih.gov/pmc/articles/PMC3322418/

Brazelton, T. B., & Sparrow, J. D. (2006). *Touchpoints, birth to 3.* Cambridge, MA: Da Capo Press.

Brown, J. (2011). *Nutrition now* (6th ed.). Florence, KY: Wadsworth Publishing.

Canadian Association of Poison Control Centres. (n.d.). *Provincial centres.* Retrieved from http://www.capcc.ca/en

Canadian Dental Association. (2010). Report on early childhood caries. Retrieved from https://www.cda-adc.ca/_files/position_statements/earlyChildhoodCaries.pdf

Canadian Paediatric Society. (2012a). *Position statement. Health active living: Physical activity guidelines for children and adolescents.* Retrieved from https://www.cps.ca/en/documents/position/physical-activity-guidelines

Canadian Paediatric Society. (2012b). *Position statement. Child and youth injury prevention: A public health approach.* Retrieved from http://www.cps.ca/documents/position/child-and-youth-injury-prevention

Canadian Paediatric Society. (2016). *Community resources.* Retrieved from https://www.cps.ca/en/first-debut/community-resources

Canadian Paediatric Society. (2017). *Early Child Development: First years First.* Retrieved from https://www.cps.ca/en/first-debut

Canadian Paediatric Society. (2018). *The prevention of firearm injuries in Canadian youth.* Retrieved from https://www.cps.ca/en/documents/position/the-prevention-of-firearm-injuries-in-canadian-youth

Canadian Paediatric Society. (2017a). *Read, speak, sing: Promoting literacy in the physician's office.* Retrieved from http://www.cps.ca/documents/position/read-speak-sing-promoting-literacy

Canadian Paediatric Society. (2017b). *Nutrition for healthy term infants, six to 24 months: An overview.* Retrieved from http://www.cps.ca/en/documents/position/nutrition-healthy-term-infants-6-to-24-months

Child Development Institute. (2015). *Is your child easy or difficult to raise?* Retrieved from http://childdevelopmentinfo.com/child-development/temperament_and_your_child/

Children's Hospital of Eastern Ontario. (2013). *Joint Statement on Physical Punishment of Children and Youth.* Retrieved from http://www.cheo.on.ca/en/physicalpunishment

Dev, D. A., McBride, B. A., Fiese, B. H., Jones, B. L., Cho, H., & on Behalf of the Strong Kids Research Team. (2013). Risk factors for overweight/obesity in preschool children: An ecological approach. *Childhood Obesity, 9*(5), 399–408.

Erikson, E. H. (1963). *Childhood and society* (2nd ed.). New York: W.W. Norton and Company.

Feigelman, S. (2011a). Preschool years. In R. M. Kliegman, B. F. Stanton, J. W. St. Geme III, N. F. Schor, & R. E. Behrman (Eds.), *Nelson's textbook of pediatrics* (19th ed.). Philadelphia, PA: Elsevier, Saunders.

Feigelman, S. (2011b). The second year. In R. M. Kliegman, B. F. Stanton, J. W. St. Geme III, N. F. Schor, & R. E. Behrman (Eds.), *Nelson's textbook of pediatrics* (19th ed.). Philadelphia, PA: Elsevier, Saunders.

Flores, G., & Lin, H. (2013). Factors predicting overweight in U.S. kindergartners. *American Journal of Clinical Nutrition, 97*(6), 1178–1187.

Gavin, M. L. (2014a). *Fitness and your 2- to 3-year-old.* Retrieved from http://kidshealth.org/en/parents/fitness-2-3.html

Gavin, M. L. (2014b). *Toddlers at the table: Avoiding power struggles.* Retrieved from http://kidshealth.org/en/parents/toddler-meals.html#

Giles, L. C., Davies, M. J., Whitrow, M. J., Warin, M. J., & Moore, V. (2011). Maternal depressive symptoms and child care during toddlerhood relate to child behavior at age 5 years. *Pediatrics, 128*(1), e78–e84.

Global Initiative to End All Corporal Punishment of Children. (n.d.). *Global initiative to end corporal punishment.* Retrieved from www.endcorporalpunishment.org

Goldson, E., & Reynolds, A. (2014). Child development and behavior. In W. W. Hay Jr., M. J. Levin, R. R. Deterding, & M. J. Abzug (Eds.), *Current diagnosis and treatment: Pediatrics* (22nd ed.). New York: McGraw-Hill Education.

Government of Canada. (2014). *Battery safety.* Retrieved from https://www.canada.ca/en/health-canada/services/toy-safety/battery-safety.html?_ga=1.150134206.961975937.1400162627&wbdisable=true

Government of Canada. (2016). *Child car seat safety.* Retrieved from http://www.cps.ca/documents/position/child-and-youth-injury-prevention

Graber, E. (n.d.). *Physical growth of infants and children. Merck manual.* Retrieved from http://www.merckmanuals.com/en-ca/professional/pediatrics/growth-and-development/physical-growth-of-infants-and-children#v7821036

Health Canada. (2007). *Eating well with Canada's food guide – First nations, inuit and metis.* Retrieved from http://hc-sc.gc.ca/fn-an/food-guide-aliment/fnim-pnim/index-eng.php

Health Canada. (2012). *Vitamin D and calcium uptake.* Retrieved from http://www.hc-sc.gc.ca/fn-an/nutrition/vitamin/vita-d-eng.php#a10

Health Canada. (2015). *Second-hand smoke.* Retrieved from https://www.canada.ca/en/health-canada/services/smoking-tobacco/avoid-second-hand-smoke/second-hand-smoke.html

Hirsch, L. (2013). *Birth of a second child.* Retrieved from http://kidshealth.org/en/parents/second-child.html#

Kohlberg, L. (1984). *Moral development.* New York: Harper & Row.

Lowry, L. (2011). *Bilingualism in young children: Separating fact from fiction.* Retrieved from http://www.hanen.org/Helpful-Info/Articles/Bilingualism-in-Young-Children–Separating-Fact-fr.aspx

Lyness, D. (2013). *Disciplining your toddler.* Retrieved from http://kidshealth.org/parent/positive/talk/toddler_tantrums.html#

Making Choices. (n.d.). *Parenting program inventory.* Retrieved from http://www.parentsmatter.ca/index.cfm?fuseaction=page.viewpage&pageid=602&stopRedirect=1

McIvor, O., & Parker, A. (2016). Back to the future: Recreating natural Indigenous language learning environments through language nest early childhood immersion programs. *The International Journal of Holistic Early Learning and Development, 3,* 21–35. Retrieved from https://ijheld.lakeheadu.ca/article/view/1444/794

Murphy, M. A., & Berry, A. D. (2013). Developmental management of toddlers and pre-schoolers. In C. E. Burns, A. M. Dunn, M. A. Brady, N. B. Starr, & C. G. Blosser (Eds.), *Pediatric primary care* (5th ed.). Philadelphia, PA: Elsevier, Saunders.

National Association for the Education of Young Children. (n.d.). *Good toys for young children by age and stage.* Retrieved from http://www.naeyc.org/toys

National Association of Pediatric Nurse Practitioners. (2011). NAPNAP position statement on corporal punishment. *Journal of Pediatric Health Care, 25,* e31–e32.

National Collaborating Centre for Aboriginal Health. (2013). *Parents as first teachers.* Retrieved from http://www.nccah-ccnsa.ca/Publications/Lists/Publications/Attachments/90/parent_teacher_EN_web.pdf

National Institute Health. (2016). *Calcium.* Retrieved from https://ods.od.nih.gov/factsheets/Calcium-HealthProfessional/#h2

Papalia, D., & Feldman, R. (2011). *A child's world: Infancy through adolescence* (12th ed.). New York: McGraw-Hill.

Piaget, J. (1969). *The theory of stages in cognitive development.* New York: McGraw-Hill.

Public Health Agency of Canada and Department of Justice Canada. (2016). Retrieved from http://canada.justice.gc.ca/eng/rp-pr/cj-jp/fv-vf/mcb-cce/index.html

Reach Out and Read. (2013). Reading tips for your young family. Retrieved from http://www.reachoutandread.org/FileRepository/ReadingTips.pdf

Ross, C. A., Taylor, C. L., Yaktine, A. L., & Del Valle, H. B. (Eds.). (2014). *DRI dietary reference intakes calcium vitamin D.* Washington, DC: The National Academies Press.

Safe Kids. (2015). *Swimming and boating fact sheet (2015).* Retrieved from https://www.safekids.org/sites/default/files/documents/skw_swimming_fact_sheet_feb_2015.pdf

Safe Kids. (2016a). *Swimming.* Retrieved from https://www.safekids.org/poolsafety

Safe Kids. (2016b). *Water safety at home tips.* Retrieved from https://www.safekids.org/tip/water-safety-home-tips

SafeBedSharing.org. (2016). *Keep it safe.* Retrieved from http://www.safebedsharing.org/safetyguidelines.html

Sears, W., & Sears, M. (2016a). *Choosing and using a pacifier.* Retrieved from http://www.askdrsears.com/topics/parenting/child-rearing-and-development/bringing-baby-home/pacifiers-in-or-out/choosing-using

Sears, W., & Sears, M. (2016b). *8 tools for toddler discipline.* Retrieved from http://www.askdrsears.com/topics/parenting/discipline-behavior/8-tools-toddler-discipline

Sears, W., & Sears, M. (2016c). *Thumbsucking.* Retrieved from http://www.askdrsears.com/topics/parenting/discipline-behavior/bothersome-behaviors/thumbsucking

Smith, M. A., & Segal, J. (2016). *Grandparents as parents: The rewards & challenges of parenting the second time around.* Retrieved from http://www.helpguide.org/articles/grandparenting/grandparents-as-parents.htm

Smylie, J. (2011). *Honouring our children: Aboriginal children's health in British Columbia.* NCCAH. Retrieved from http://www.nccah-ccnsa.ca/docs/fact%20sheets/child%20and%20youth/Honouring%20Our%20Chilldren%20(English%20-%20Web).pdf

Stettler, N., Bhatia, J., Parish, A., & Stallings, V. A. (2011). Feeding healthy infants, children, and adolescents. In R. M. Kliegman, B. F. Stanton, J. W. St. Geme III, N. F. Schor, & R. E. Behrman (Eds.), *Nelson's textbook of pediatrics* (19th ed.). Philadelphia, PA: Elsevier, Saunders.

Transport Canada. (2014). *Motor Vehicle Safety Act.* Retrieved from http://www.tc.gc.ca/eng/acts-regulations/regulations-sor2010-90.htm

Tremblay, M. S., LeBlanc, A. G., Carson, V., Choquette, L., Connor Gorber, S., Dillman, C., … Timmons, B. W. (2012b). Canadian physical activity guidelines for the early years (aged 0–4 years). *Applied Physiology, Nutrition, and Metabolism, 37,* 345–356.

Zero to Three. (2016a). *Brain development.* Retrieved from https://www.zerotothree.org/early-development/brain-development

Zero to Three. (2016b). *How to handle picky eaters.* Retrieved from https://www.zerotothree.org/resources/1072-how-to-handle-picky-eaters

CHAPTER **WORKSHEET**

MULTIPLE CHOICE QUESTIONS

1. The nurse is caring for a hospitalized 30 month old who is resistant to care, is angry, and yells "no" all the time. The nurse identifies this toddler's behaviour as
   a. problematic, as it interferes with needed nursing care.
   b. normal for this stage of growth and development.
   c. normal because the child is hospitalized and out of his routine.

2. The mother of a 15 month old is concerned about a speech delay. She describes her toddler as being able to understand what she says, sometimes following commands, but using only one or two words with any consistency. What is the nurse's best response to this information?
   a. The toddler should have a developmental evaluation as soon as possible.
   b. If the mother would read to the child, then speech would develop faster.
   c. Receptive language normally develops earlier than expressive language.
   d. The mother should ask her child's physician for a speech pathologist assessment.

3. A 2 year old is having a temper tantrum. What advice should the nurse give the mother?
   a. For safety reasons, the toddler should be restrained during the tantrum.
   b. Punishment should be initiated, as tantrums should be controlled.
   c. The mother should promise the toddler a reward if the tantrum stops.
   d. The tantrum should be ignored as long as the toddler is safe.

4. What is the best advice about nutrition for the toddler?
   a. Encourage cup drinking and give water between meals and snacks.
   b. Encourage unlimited milk intake, because toddlers need the protein for growth.
   c. Avoid sugar-sweetened fruit drinks and allow as much natural fruit juice as desired.
   d. Allow the toddler unlimited access to the sippy cup to ensure adequate hydration.

5. To gain cooperation from a toddler, what is the best approach by the nurse?
   a. Immediately pick the toddler up from the mother's lap.
   b. Kneel in front of the toddler while he or she is on the mother's lap.
   c. Do the nursing tasks quickly so the toddler can play.
   d. Ask the toddler if it is okay if you begin the needed task.

CRITICAL THINKING EXERCISES

1. Develop a teaching plan about safety to present to a toddler-age preschool class.

2. Construct a 3-day menu for a 2 year old, one that is realistic and will provide the nutrients needed.

3. Develop a plan for educating the parent of a 34 month old who has been resistant to toilet teaching. Include assessments the nurse will make as well as the plan for teaching.

STUDY ACTIVITIES

1. Visit a preschool that provides care for special-needs toddlers as well as typical toddlers. Perform a developmental assessment on a typical toddler and one with special needs (both the same age). Compare and contrast your findings.

2. Care for two average 2 year olds in the clinical setting. Describe each toddler's behaviour, response to the parent, and response to the nurse and list strategies used to gain compliance and minimize stress to the toddler.

3. Observe in the toddler classroom of a typical preschool. Choose two toddlers of the same age with different temperaments. Record the toddlers' differences and similarities in response to structure and authority, interactions with classmates, attention levels, and language and activity levels.

BRINGING IT ALL TOGETHER: A CASE STUDY

Eva, an 18-month-old girl, comes to be seen in the pediatric office because her mother is concerned that she is not growing well. When Eva's growth measurements are plotted on the growth chart, they indicate she is at the 5th percentile for length and for weight, but at the 25th percentile for head circumference.

Go to the Point **to find questions to consider about this case.**

Growth and Development of the Preschooler

27

KEY TERMS

animism

empathy

imaginary friend

magical thinking

preoperational
    phase

school readiness

telegraphic speech

transduction

Learning Objectives

Upon completion of the chapter, you will be able to:

1. Identify normal physiologic, cognitive, and psychosocial changes occurring in the preschool-aged child.

2. Express an understanding of language development in the preschool years.

3. Implement a nursing care plan that addresses common concerns or delays in the preschooler's development.

4. Integrate knowledge of preschool growth and development with nursing care and health promotion of the preschool-aged child.

5. Develop a nutrition plan for the preschool-aged child.

6. Identify common issues and concerns related to growth and development during the preschool years.

7. Demonstrate knowledge of appropriate anticipatory guidance for common developmental issues that arise in the preschool period.

Nila Patel is a 4-year-old girl brought to the clinic by her mother and father for her school check-up. During your assessment you measure her weight to be 20 kg (44 lb) and her height 101.6 cm (40 in). As the nurse caring for her, assess Nila's growth and development, and then provide appropriate anticipatory guidance to her parents.

The preschool stage of development is often viewed as between 3 to 5 or 6 years of age depending on when children access formal education. This is a time of continued growth and development biologically, psychosocially, and spiritually. Physical growth continues at a much more subtle pace compared to earlier years. Achievements in cognitive, language, and psychosocial development are significant throughout the preschool period. Many tasks that are achieved in the toddler years are refined, mastered, and perfected during the preschool years. The child has learned to tolerate separation from parents, has a longer attention span, and continues to learn skills that will lead to later success in the school-age period. Preparation for success in school continues during this period with parents or caregivers playing an important role in facilitating the child's readiness for school life (Lukie, Skwarchuk, LeFevre, & Sowinski, 2014).

Growth and Development Overview

The healthy preschooler is slender and agile yet robust, with an upright posture. The formerly clumsy toddler becomes more graceful, demonstrating the ability to run more smoothly with control and speed; thereby athletic abilities may begin to develop. Major development occurs in the area of fine motor coordination. Psychosocial development is focused on the accomplishment of initiative. Preconceptual thought and intuitiveness dominate cognitive development. The preschooler is an inquisitive learner and absorbs new concepts with a level of curiosity and questioning.

PHYSICAL GROWTH

The average preschool-aged child will grow 6.5 to 7.8 cm (2.5 to 3 in) per year. The average 3 year old is 96.2-cm (37-in) tall, the average 4 year old is 103.7-cm (40.5-in) tall, and the average 5 year old is 118.5-cm (43-in) tall. Average weight gain during this time period is about 2.3 kg (4 to 5 lb) per year (Feigelman, 2011). The average weight of a 3 year old is 14.5 kg (32 lb), increasing to an average weight of 18.6 kg (41 lb) by age 5. A child should be weighed wearing light undergarments or lightweight outer clothing and always weighed using an accurate device, checking the measurements at least twice and precisely plotting on a validated growth chart, that is, WHO growth chart (Dietitians of Canada and Canadian Paediatric Society [DCCPS], 2014; Goldbloom, 2011). BMI-for-age is the recommended nutritional indicator for screening children 2 years and older to identify children who are potentially wasted, overweight, or obese (DCCPS, 2014). The loss of baby fat and the growth of muscle during the preschool years give the

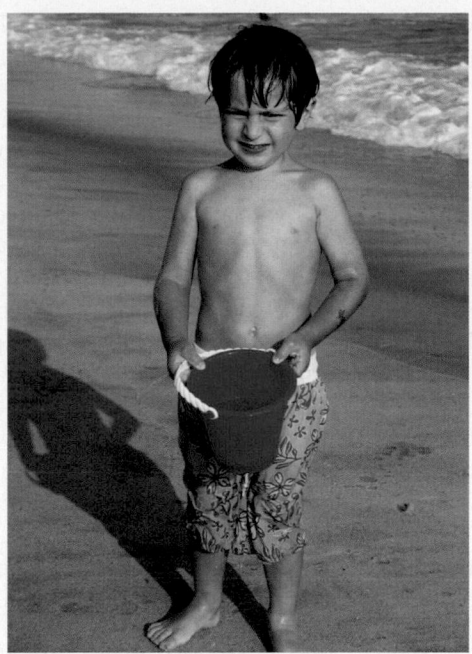

FIGURE 27.1 The preschool child has a more slender appearance and erect posture than the toddler.

child a stronger and more mature appearance (Fig. 27.1). If a child's head circumference is two standard deviations or more above the mean, it is helpful to check the parents' measurements to determine if having a larger head is a familial trait (Goldbloom, 2011). Occasionally below-expected head circumference can be benign or familial; however, more often it is associated with developmental delay (Goldbloom, 2011). The length of the skull also increases slightly, with the lower jaw becoming more pronounced. The upper jaw widens through the preschool years in preparation for the emergence of permanent teeth, usually starting around age 6.

ORGAN SYSTEM MATURATION

Most of the body systems have matured by the preschool years. Myelination of the spinal cord allows for bowel and bladder control to be complete in most children by age 3 years with some children taking up to the age of 5 to be dry at night (Canadian Paediatric Society [CPS], 2016c). The respiratory structures are continuing to grow in size, and the number of alveoli continues to increase, reaching the adult number at about 7 years of age. The normal respiratory rate in children aged 4 to 6 years is between 20 and 24 breaths/min. The eustachian tubes remain relatively short and straight. Heart rate decreases (beats per minute) when the child is resting, awake, and asleep with an increase during physical activity (PA). Blood pressure increases slightly during the preschool years. An innocent heart murmur may be heard upon auscultation, and splitting of the second heart sound may become evident. The preschooler should have 20 deciduous teeth present. Oral health is important as it can be an indicator of overall health status as well as affect functional, psychological, and social dimensions of a child's well-being (Rowan-Legg, 2013). Socioeconomic status has been reported as an indicator in early childhood caries (ECC) with new immigrants and Indigenous children at a greater risk and up to a 90% prevalence in their communities (Schroth, Harrison, & Moffatt, 2009). ECC is defined as the presence of one or more decayed, missing, or filled tooth surface in any primary tooth in a preschool-aged child (Canadian Dental Association, 2010). The small intestine is continuing to grow in length. Stool passage usually occurs once or twice per day in the average preschooler and appears similar to adult stool type. Child friendly stool charts can be a helpful way to gather information from the child and family with many resources found via the Internet. The 4 year old generally has adequate bowel control; any persistent or new episodes of soiling (encopresis) should be discussed with the health care provider. Functional bladder control is usually present in the 3 to 5 year olds, but an occasional accident may occur, particularly in stressful situations or when the child is absorbed in an interesting activity. Urinary tract infections can be more common in girls than boys due to their shorter urethra. Parents and caregivers can minimize risk by promoting good voiding routine and avoiding childhood constipation and irritants in the bath (such as bubble bath). The bones continue to increase in length and the muscles continue to strengthen and mature. However, the musculoskeletal (MSK) system is still not fully mature, making the preschooler susceptible to injury, particularly with overexertion or excess activity. Appropriate exercise, adequate nutrition, and rest and sleep are also important for MSK development.

PSYCHOSOCIAL DEVELOPMENT

According to Erik Erikson, the psychosocial task of the preschool years is establishing a sense of initiative versus guilt (Erikson, 1963). The preschooler is an inquisitive learner, very enthusiastic about discovering new phenomena, and will often fully engage in play, activities, and creative opportunities (such as story time). Preschoolers feel a sense of satisfaction when they succeed in activities (Fig. 27.2), and feeling pride in their accomplishments helps them to use their initiative. However, when the child oversteps the limits of their ability or extends himself or herself further than current capabilities allow, he or she may feel a sense of guilt in relation to their actions or feelings. The superego or conscience development is a significant task during the preschool period as this is the basis for moral development (understanding right and wrong) as well as an

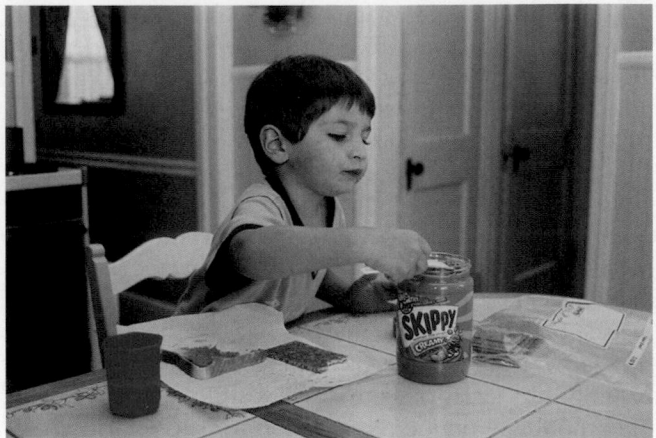

FIGURE 27.2 Allowing the preschooler to assist with simple household tasks such as preparing a sandwich encourages the development of initiative.

important stage in developing sociocultural awareness. Table 27.1 gives examples illustrating the stage of initiative versus guilt.

COGNITIVE DEVELOPMENT

According to Jean Piaget's theory (1969), the preschool-aged child continues in the preoperational stage. The **preoperational phase** dominates during this stage and is based on a self-centred understanding of the world. In the preconceptual phase of preoperational thought, the child remains egocentric and is able to approach a problem from a single point of view only. However, intuitive thinking starts developing around the age of 4 to 7 years. The transition between preconceptual toward intuitive thinking is the child's ability to shift from the egocentric thinking to an increased social awareness and the ability to consider other viewpoints. The younger preschooler is beginning to understand the concept of counting, therefore, exposing preschool children to numeracy activities during play at home can build future interest in the child (Lukie et al., 2014). The child in the intuitive phase can count 10 or more objects, correctly name at least 4 colours, and better understand the concept of time (although yesterday, tomorrow, and next week may hold little meaning for them) and he or she knows about things that are used in everyday life, such as appliances, money, and food. The preschooler uses **transduction** when reasoning: he or she extrapolates from a particular situation to another, even though the events may be unrelated. The preschooler also attributes life-like qualities to inanimate objects (**animism**) (Papalia & Feldman, 2011). Table 27.1 gives further examples illustrating this developmental stage.

Magical thinking is a normal part of preschool development. In magical thinking, the preschooler believes that his or her thoughts are all-powerful. The

TABLE 27.1	DEVELOPMENTAL THEORIES	
Theorist	**Stage**	**Activities**
Erikson	Initiative vs. guilt Age 3–6 years	Likes to please parents Begins to plan activities, make up games Initiates activities with others Acts out the roles of other people (real and imaginary) Develops sexual identity Develops conscience May take frustrations out on siblings Likes exploring new things Enjoys sports, shopping, cooking, working Feels remorse when makes wrong choice or behaves badly Cooperates with other children Negotiates solutions to conflicts
Piaget	Preoperational substage: Preconceptual phase Age 2–4 years	Exhibits egocentric thinking, which lessens as the child approaches age 4 Has short attention span Learns through observing and imitating Displays animism Forms concepts that are not as complete or as logical as the adult's Is able to make simple classifications By age 4 understands the concept of opposites (hot/cold, soft/hard) Reasoning is that of specific to specific Has an active imagination
	Preoperational substage: Intuitive phase Age 4–7 years	Is able to classify and relate objects Has intuitive thought processes; knows if something is right or wrong, though cannot state why Tolerates others' differences but doesn't understand them Is very curious about facts Knows acceptable cultural rules Uses words appropriately but often without true understanding of their meaning Has a more realistic sense of causality May begin to question parents' values
Kohlberg	Punishment–obedience orientation Age 2–7 years (preconventional morality)	Determines good vs. bad dependent upon associated punishment Children may learn inappropriate behaviour at this stage if parental intervention does not occur (if the child hits, bites, or is verbally disrespectful but is not punished for these activities, the child will view those behaviours as good and continue to participate in them)
Freud	Phallic stage Age 3–7 years	Child's pleasure centres on genitalia and masturbation. Superego is developing and conscience is emerging. Oedipal stage occurs: jealousy and rivalry toward same-sex parent, with love of the opposite-sex parent. This usually resolves by the end of the preschool years, when the child develops a strong identification with the same-sex parent.

Adapted from Erikson, E. H. (1963). *Childhood and society* (2nd ed.). New York: W. W. Norton and Company; Feigelman, S. (2011). Preschool years. In R. M. Kliegman, B. F. Stanton, J. W. St. Geme III, N. F. Schor, & R. E. Behrman (Eds.). *Nelson's textbook of pediatrics* (19th ed.). Philadelphia, PA: Elsevier, Saunders; Kohlberg, L. (1984). *Moral development*. New York: Harper & Row; and Piaget, J. (1969). *The theory of stages in cognitive development*. New York: McGraw-Hill.

fantasy experienced through magical thinking allows the preschooler to make room in his or her world for the actual or the real. Through make-believe and magical thinking, preschool-aged children satisfy their curiosity about differences in the world around them (Papalia & Feldman, 2011).

The preschooler often has an **imaginary friend** as well (Goldson & Reynolds, 2012). This friend serves as a creative way for the preschooler to sample different activities and behaviours and practice conversational skills. Despite this imagination, the preschooler is able to switch easily between fantasy and reality throughout the day.

The acquisition of language skills in the toddler period is enhanced in the preschool period. The expansion of vocabulary enables the preschooler to progress further with symbolic thought. At this age, children do not completely understand the concept of death or its permanence: they may ask when their grandparent or pet who died is returning. Preschoolers accept words "literally" and can misinterpret understanding or not associate an action with an outcome when parents or caregivers offer explanations or make requests without being specific. For example, positive label praise means telling the child exactly what it is they are doing right, that is, saying "thank you for picking up your toys" when the child has been asked to be tidy helps the child understand it was the action of putting toys away that was good. Since praise is a powerful reinforcer, this can promote social learning as well as strengthen the parent–child relationship.

DEVELOPMENT OF BODY IMAGE AND AWARENESS

During this phase, body image and gender identity start to develop. With developing language, cognition, and social awareness preschool children begin to recognise and ask about the differences between people such as variations in skin colour, bodily differences (i.e., wheel chair use), sexual orientation (i.e., same-sex parents). They can begin to question gender stereotype and present with gender (a)typical behaviour that parents may find confusing or worrying. Preschool-aged children are also becoming aware of social stereotypes and the meaning and association of words such as pretty or ugly, fat and skinny that may inform friendship preferences (Harrison, Rowlinson, & Hill, 2016). Increasingly 20% to 70% of children under the age of 6 years are experiencing body dissatisfaction (Tatangelo, McCabe, Mellor, & Mealey, 2016). During this time, curiosity around babies and body parts including the differences between boys and girls can arise. Parents or caregivers need to be mindful about how to have positive, simple, age-appropriate conversations with their child (AboutKidsHealth, n.d.). This curiosity is a normal function of the preschool years, and the curiosity may also involve playing with the genitals (see the section on masturbation later in this chapter).

MORAL AND SPIRITUAL DEVELOPMENT

The preschool-aged child is learning to understand the concepts of right and wrong and is beginning to develop a conscience. They may have little concern about why something is wrong and reason that an action is good or bad depending on whether it is rewarded or punished. Kohlberg identified this stage (between 2 and 7 years) as the preconventional stage, which is characterized by a punishment-and-obedience orientation (Kohlberg,

1984). Younger preschoolers have difficulty differentiating between reality and their imagination and fantasies, whereas older preschoolers are more aware of right and wrong. Preschool children see morality as external to themselves; they defer to power (that of the adult). The child's moral standards are those of their parents or other adults who influence them, not necessarily their own. Preschoolers adhere to those standards to gain rewards or avoid punishment. Since the preschool-aged child is facing the psychosocial task of initiative versus guilt, it is natural for the child to experience guilt when something goes wrong.

As the child's moral development progresses, he or she learns how to deal with angry feelings. Sometimes the way the child chooses to deal with those feelings may be inappropriate, such as fighting and biting. Lying, exaggeration, or fibbing often starts in the preschool period; reasons include forgetfulness, wishful thinking, active imagination, a desire to feel good, attention seeking, or a sense of control. Preschoolers also use their limited life experiences to make sense of and help them cope with crises. At times, when they may be frustrated, and as a result of limited life experience the preschool child can project feelings toward another object or person. For example, when a preschool child cannot get what they hoped for they may respond by being angry at their toy or shouting at a picture. They need to learn the socially acceptable limits of these behaviours that helps develop their wider social skills, such as being polite.

During the preoperational phase of cognitive development, the preschooler's concept of faith is intuitive and projective in nature (Keeley, 2010). The preschool-aged child's imagination allows for anything to be possible, so he or she does not have a logical view of the world (as adults do). They may use this projection to help them understand complex issues that are going on around them. Preschoolers may project their parents' or caregiver's feelings or characteristics onto "God": if mommy gets angry, then God also is probably angry.

The family's religious beliefs may affect the child's diet, the approaches to discipline that parents use, and even how they view their children. Knowing about a family's practices including prayer or meditation is helpful to the nurse so that he or she can help support beliefs and cultural practices when the child is ill or hospitalized or in need of ongoing health care (Fig. 27.3).

MOTOR SKILL DEVELOPMENT

As the preschooler's MSK system continues to mature, existing motor skills become refined and new ones develop. The preschooler has more voluntary control over his or her movements and is less clumsy than the toddler. Significant refinement in fine motor skills occurs during the preschool period (Table 27.2).

Gross Motor Skills

The preschooler is agile while standing, walking, running, and jumping (Fig. 27.4). He or she can go up and down stairs and walk forward and backward easily. Standing on tiptoes or on one foot still requires extra concentration. The preschooler seems to be in constant motion. He or she also uses the body to understand and describe new concepts (such as using the arms in a "chug-chug" motion when describing how the train wheels work). Often actions are incorporated into children's songs to help with memory and build learning capacity.

Fine Motor Skills

The 3 year old can move each finger independently and is capable of grasping utensils and crayons, with the thumb on one side and the fingers on the other. He or she can also scribble freely, copy a circle, trace a square, and feed himself or herself without spilling much. These skills are perfected over the next 2 years, and by 5 years of age the child can write letters, cut with scissors more accurately, and tie shoelaces (Fig. 27.5).

SENSORY DEVELOPMENT

Hearing is intact at birth and should remain so throughout the preschool years. The senses of smell and touch

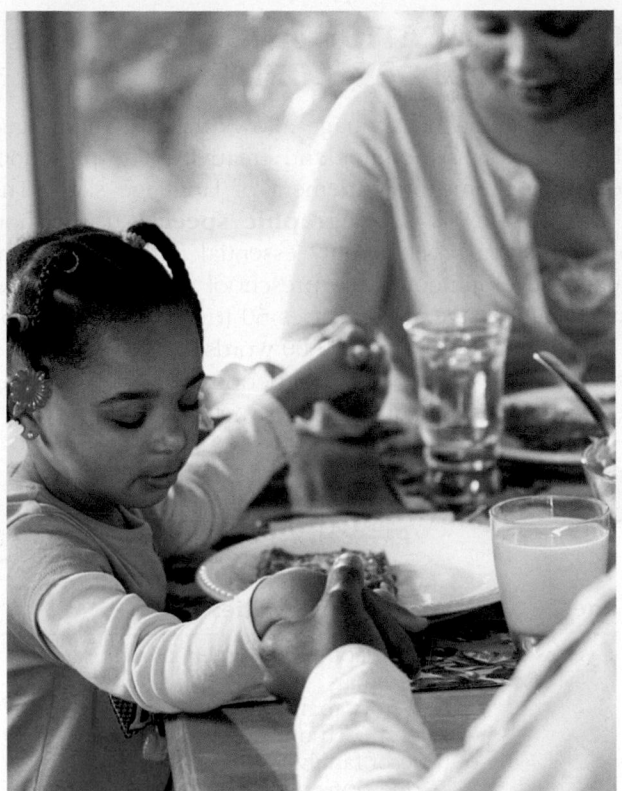

FIGURE 27.3 The preschool child may participate in religious rituals without having full understanding of their meaning.

TABLE 27.2	MOTOR SKILL DEVELOPMENT	
Age	Expected Gross Motor Skills	Expected Fine Motor Skills
3 years	• Climbs well • Pedals tricycle • Runs easily • Walks up and down stairs with alternate feet • Bends over easily without falling	• Undresses self • Copies circle • Builds tower of 9 or 10 cubes • Holds a pencil in writing position • Screws/unscrews lids, nuts, bolts • Turns book pages one at a time
4 years	• Throws ball overhand • Kicks ball forward • Catches bounced ball • Hops on one foot • Stands on one foot up to 5 seconds • Alternates feet going up and down steps • Moves backward and forward with agility	• Uses scissors successfully • Copies capital letters • Draws circles and squares • Traces a cross or diamond • Draws a person with two to four body parts • Laces shoes
5 years	• Stands on one foot for 10 seconds or longer • Swings and climbs well • May skip • Somersaults • May learn to skate and swim	• Prints some letters • Draws person with body and at least six parts • Dresses/undresses without assistance • Can learn to tie laces • Uses fork, spoon, and knife (supervised) well • Copies triangle and other geometric patterns • Mostly cares for own toileting needs

Adapted from Feigelman, S. (2011). Preschool years. In R. M. Kliegman, B. F. Stanton, J. W. St. Geme III, N. F. Schor, & R. E. Behrman, (Eds.). *Nelson's textbook of pediatrics* (19th ed.). Philadelphia, PA: Elsevier, Saunders; Goldson, E., & Reynolds, A. (2012). Child development & behaviour. In W. W. Hay, M. J. Levin, R. R., Deterding, & M. J. Abzug (Eds.). *Current diagnosis & treatment: Pediatrics* (21st ed.). New York: McGraw-Hill; and Papalia, D., & Feldman, R. (2011). *A child's world: Infancy through adolescence* (12th ed.). New York: McGraw-Hill.

FIGURE 27.4 The preschooler runs well, navigates stairs, and can balance on one foot.

continue to develop throughout the preschool years. The young preschooler may have a less discriminating sense of taste than the older child, putting him or her at increased risk for accidental ingestion. Visual acuity continues to progress and should be equal bilaterally. The typical 5 year old has visual acuity of 20/40 or 20/30. Colour vision is intact at this age.

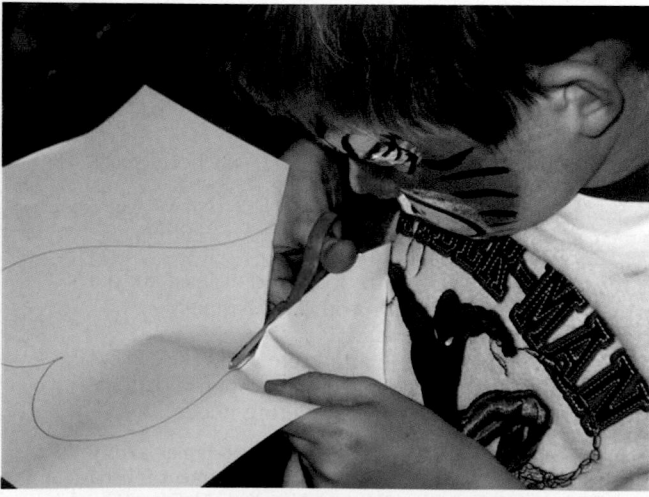

FIGURE 27.5 The 5 year old has the fine motor dexterity to cut well with scissors.

COMMUNICATION AND LANGUAGE DEVELOPMENT

The acquisition of language allows the preschool-aged child to express thoughts and creativity. The preschool years are a time of refinement of language skills. The 3 year old exhibits **telegraphic speech**, using short sentences that contain only essential information. Language development in the preschool years is extensive. At 2 years of age, a child uses 50 to 100 words and by 5 years of age uses about 2,000 words (Feigelman, 2011). By the end of the preschool period, the child is using sentences that are adult-like in structure (Table 27.3).

TABLE 27.3	COMMUNICATION SKILLS IN THE PRESCHOOL CHILD
Age	**Communication Abilities**
4 years	• Speaks in complete sentences using adult-like grammar • Tells a story that is easy to follow • 75% of speech understood by others outside of family • Asks questions with "who," "how," "how many" • Stays on topic in a conversation • Understands the concepts of "same" and "different" • Asks many questions • Knows names of familiar animals • Names common objects in books and magazines • Knows at least one colour • Uses language to engage in make-believe • Follows a three-part command • Can count a few numbers • Vocabulary of 1,500 words
5 years	• Persons outside of the family can understand most of the child's speech • Explains how an item is used • Participates in long, detailed conversations • Talks about past, future, and imaginary events • Answers questions that use "why" and "when" • Can count to 10 • Recalls part of a story • Speech should be completely intelligible, even if the child has articulation difficulties • Speech is generally grammatically correct • Vocabulary of 2,100 words • Says name and address

Adapted from Centers for Disease Control and Prevention. (2016). Developmental milestones. Retrieved from http://www.cdc.gov/ncbddd/actearly/milestones/index.html; Feigelman, S. (2011). Preschool years. In R. M. Kliegman, B. F. Stanton, J. W. St. Geme III, N. F. Schor, & R. E. Behrman, (Eds.). *Nelson's Textbook of Pediatrics* (19th ed.). Philadelphia, PA: Elsevier, Saunders; and Papalia, D., & Feldman, R. (2011). *A Child's World: Infancy through Adolescence* (12th ed.). New York: McGraw-Hill.

The 3 to 6 year old is starting to develop fluency (the ability to smoothly link sounds, syllables, and words when speaking). Initially, the child may exhibit dysfluency or stuttering. Speech may sound choppy, or the child may say repeated consonants or "um." Stuttering usually has its onset in the preschool years and will resolve in 80% of children by age 8 years (Feigelman, 2011). Parents should slow down their speech and should give the child time to speak without rushing or interrupting. Some sounds remain difficult for the preschooler to enunciate properly: "f," "v," "s," and "z" sounds are usually mastered by age 5 years, but some children do not master the sounds of "sh," "l," "th," and "r" until age 6 or later. The potentially bilingual child may lag slightly behind the single-language speaker, but will be able to differentiate and use both languages by the end of the preschool period (Lowry, 2011).

Communication in preschool children is concrete in nature, as they are not yet capable of abstract thought. Despite its concrete nature, the preschooler's communication can be quite elaborate and involved; he or she may talk about dreams and fantasies. In addition to acquiring a wider vocabulary they are becoming more sophisticated in how they use language.

The preschooler can be in tune with their parent's moods and picks up on negative or positive emotions in conversations. If the preschooler hears parents discussing things that are believed to be frightening their imagination may lead to worries, anxiety, or fears.

EMOTIONAL AND SOCIAL DEVELOPMENT

By the time a child enters kindergarten (unless they are home schooled), he or she should have developed a useful set of social skills that will help him or her have successful experiences in the school setting as well as in life in general. These skills include cooperation, sharing (of things and feelings), kindness, generosity, affection display, and conversation, expression of feelings, helping others, and making friends.

Preschoolers tend to have strong emotions. They can be very excited, happy, and giddy in one moment, then extremely disappointed in the next. The preschool-aged child has a vivid imagination, and fears are very real to preschoolers. Most children of this age have learned to control their behaviours. They should be able to name the feelings they are having rather than acting on them. Strong feelings may be expressed through outlets such as tactile materials like clay, water play, drawing, or painting, or dramatic play such as with puppets.

Preschoolers are developing a sense of identity. They recognize that they are boys or girls. They know that they belong to a particular family, community, or culture. They take pride in using self-control rather than

giving in to their impulses. The preschool-aged child is capable of helping others since they are sociable and willing to please.

Parents can encourage and assist preschool-aged children with developing the social and emotional skills that will be needed when the child enters school (Public Health Agency of Canada [PHAC], 2004). Preschool-aged children thrive on one-to-one communication with a parent. During interactive communication, children learn to express their feelings and ideas. Interactive communication fosters not only emotional and moral development but also self-esteem and cognitive development. Asking the preschool child questions requires the child to think out his or her own intention or motivation and encourages vocabulary development. Socioeconomic status may have an influence on vocabulary skills while general intelligence and speed of processing are not uniquely associated with disadvantage and school readiness (Fitzpatrick, McKinnon, Blair, & Willoughby, 2014). Parents may use individual communication as a time to explore beliefs about right and wrong, thus further contributing to moral development. Being listened to while answering parents' questions gives preschoolers a sense that they are valued, that what they think and have to say matters.

Establishing a few simple rules and enforcing them consistently give preschoolers the structure and security they need while promoting moral development. Parents or caregivers can help the child give a name to the emotion that is being experienced. Fears are very real to preschoolers because of their active imaginations and may result in a variety of emotions. Parents should validate the feeling or emotion, then discuss with the child alternatives for dealing with the emotion.

Preschoolers are developing their sense of identity, and parents should encourage preschoolers to do simple things for themselves, like dressing and washing their hands and face (Fig. 27.6). Parents should give the child the time he or she needs to complete the task. This helps to establish a sense of accomplishment.

Friendships

Preschoolers need interactions with friends as well as with adults. Learning how to make and keep a friend is an important part of social development. Friends may be other children in the neighbourhood or those at preschool or day care. A special friend is someone the preschooler can care about, talk to, and play with (Fig. 27.7). The preschooler is more likely to agree to rules and wants to please friends and be like them. The preschooler loves to sing, dance, and act and will enjoy these activities with friends. Disagreements may occur, but the parent can encourage the children to express their views, discuss and resolve conflicts, and continue being friends.

FIGURE 27.6 Encouraging the preschooler to complete simple tasks by himself or herself helps to build self-esteem.

Temperament

By the time children are 3 years old, they recognize that what they do actually matters. It is helpful for the parent to view the child as an active participant in the parent–child relationship. The child's temperament has become a reliable indicator of how a parent might expect the

FIGURE 27.7 The preschool child begins to develop friendships.

child to react in a certain situation. When the parent is in tune with the preschooler's temperament, it is easier to find ways to ease transitions and changes for that child. In the area of task orientation, temperament may range from the highly attentive and persistent to the more distractible and active.

A child's social flexibility is also evident by this age. A child who is quite adaptable will handle stimuli from the outside world in an approaching rather than a withdrawing manner. Temperament also determines the extent of reactivity (the child's sensory threshold of responsiveness, high vs. low). This determines the quality of the child's mood and the intensity of reactions to stimuli, change, or situations. When the parents are familiar with the child's task orientation, social flexibility, and reactivity, they can better structure activities and situations for the child. Furthermore, evidence suggests that children's personalities might influence their activity choices and levels of engagement (Tucker et al., 2013). Understanding how temperament and activity are linked may help ease tensions between the child's temperament–behaviour and the caregivers' reactions (Irwin, Johnson, Vanderloo, Burke, & Tucker, 2015). By the time a child is 4 years old he or she has learnt better self-control and can use experiences as ways to learn and grow. Temper tantrums should ease off by this age since they are better able to express themselves through language. The 5 year old who has a more vulnerable type of temperament, as opposed to a confident temperament, may be more apt to experience fears.

Fears

With their vivid imaginations, preschoolers experience a variety of fears. Preschoolers may be scared of loud noises such as fire engine sirens or barking dogs. Imaginary monsters may scare the child. Preschoolers are often afraid of people they do not know and of strange people (Santa Claus or people who look or dress very differently from what they are accustomed to). Many preschoolers are afraid of the dark. Preschoolers may also fear insects as well as animals they are not familiar with. The preschooler's memory is long enough that he or she may fear returning to the doctor's office when a painful procedure occurred during the prior visit.

Parents should acknowledge fears rather than minimizing them. They can then collaborate with the child on strategies for dealing with the fear.

CULTURAL AND FAMILY INFLUENCES ON GROWTH AND DEVELOPMENT

Children at this young age may learn prejudice or bias at home before entering school or day care (Bellini, Pereda, Cordero, & Suarez-Morales, 2016). The ways that families view other races or cultures may be subtly or overtly demonstrated in routine daily activities. The preschool-aged child is developing a conscience, so attitudes of tolerance or bias may influence the child's values (Bellini et al., 2016).

Some cultures value reading and education more than others. If reading is not valued or possible in the home, the preschool-aged child's first experience with books may not occur until he or she is in school. School readiness can vary as a result of geographical location. For children within both rural and urban landscapes the Aboriginal Head Start Program was a successful model, able to address cultural health concerns and well-being thereby enhancing school readiness of participating Aboriginal children (PHAC, 2016).

Food served in the home is often very specific to the family's ethnic background or limited by socioeconomic factors/food security, community sharing practices, or access to safe traditional food sources (Bhawra, Cooke, Guo, & Wilk, 2017; Collings et al., 2016). As the preschool-aged child is exposed to persons of other cultures in kindergarten, he or she may or may not like the food that is served. Exploring customs or cultural practices that the family participates in is important so that these practices may be safely incorporated into the child's plan of care.

Changes in the family composition, household characteristics, extended family networks, and family process have the capacity to influence the child's developing characteristics across a range of areas (i.e., physical, emotion development, impulsivity), which can influence their engagement and interactions with others (Gosselin et al., 2014).

> Refer back to Nila, who was introduced in the beginning of the chapter. What developmental milestones would you expect Nila to have reached at this age? Nila's mother expresses concerns about her child's imaginary friend, Sasha. How would you respond?

The Nurse's Role in Preschool Growth and Development

Growth and development in the preschool-aged child remain orderly and sequential. Some preschoolers grow faster than others or reach various developmental milestones sooner than others. Nurses must be aware of the usual growth and development patterns for this age group so that they can assess preschool-aged children appropriately and provide guidance to their families being mindful that screening for developmental delay in asymptomatic children (1 to 4 years) can be inconclusive (Warren et al., 2016). The changes that the preschool-aged child is experiencing affect not only the child but also the family. Health care visits throughout the preschool period continue to focus on expected growth and development and anticipatory guidance.

If the preschooler is hospitalized, growth and development may be altered. Hospitalization hinders the preschool-aged child's ability to explore the environment and engage in make-believe play and thus presents a challenge for the curious and inquisitive child. If the child must be isolated for an infectious illness, the opportunities for exploration and experimentation are further restricted. In addition, a preschooler who is unwell may feel a sense of guilt, worrying that maybe he or she caused the illness by negative thoughts or behaviours.

When caring for the hospitalized preschooler, the nurse must use knowledge of normal growth and development to recognize potential delays, promote continued appropriate growth and development, and interact successfully with the preschooler.

NURSING PROCESS OVERVIEW

Upon completion of assessment of the preschool-aged child's growth and development status, problems or issues related to growth and development may be identified. The nurse may then identify one or more nursing diagnoses, including but not limited to:
- Delayed growth and development
- Imbalanced nutrition, less than body requirements
- Interrupted family processes
- Readiness for enhanced parenting
- Risk for caregiver role strain
- Risk for delayed development
- Risk for disproportionate growth
- Risk for injury

Planning nursing care for the preschool child with growth and development issues should take into account the preschooler's and family's needs. The nursing care plan may be used as a guide in planning nursing care for the preschooler with a growth or developmental concern. The nurse may choose the appropriate nursing diagnoses from the Nursing Care Plan 27.1 (found at the end of the chapter) and individualize them as needed. The nursing care plan is intended to serve as a guide only and is not intended to be an inclusive growth and development plan.

PROMOTING HEALTHY GROWTH AND DEVELOPMENT

The building of self-esteem continues throughout the preschool period. It is of particular importance during these years, as the preschooler's developmental task is focused on the development of initiative rather than guilt (PHAC, 2004). A sense of guilt will contribute to low self-esteem, whereas a child who is rewarded for his or her initiative will have increased self-confidence. The parent who provides a loving and nurturing environment for the preschooler builds upon the earlier foundation.

Routine and ritual continue to be important throughout the preschool years, as they help the child to develop a sense of time as well as provide the structure for the child to feel safe and secure. Daily routine continues to assist with the development of conscience in the preschooler. As in toddlerhood, making expectations known through everyday routines helps to avoid confrontations. The preschooler is developing the maturity to know how to behave in various situations and is capable of learning manners.

Setting limits (and remaining consistent with those limits) continues to be important in the preschool period. Consistent limits provide the preschooler with expectation and guidance. As the preschooler increasingly participates in fantasy and imagination, the limits of routine and structure help guide his or her behaviour and ability to distinguish reality.

Nurses caring for preschoolers should have knowledge of normal developmental expectations so they can determine whether the preschool child is progressing appropriately. Table 27.4 lists potential signs of developmental delay. A preschool child with one or more of these concerns should be referred for further developmental evaluation.

Promoting Growth and Development Through Play

Play is important and should provide physical, social, and mental development opportunities for preschool children. Parents or caregivers are important partners in their child's play. By engaging in mutual play parents foster an ongoing reciprocal relationship with their child.

The preschool child will engage in various types of play including associative play; dramatic play is often imaginative and fantastical. Group play or associative play often entails children participating in identical activities with a level of freedom to allow for diversity and creativity. Giving children opportunities to decide how and with whom they want to play also helps them develop initiative. Preschool children like to write, colour, draw, paint with a brush or their fingers, and trace or copy patterns (Fig. 27.8). They may start small collections of toys or objects that may be sorted. They like using toys for their intended purpose as well as for whatever invented purpose they can imagine. Dramatic and fantasy play is imitative and imaginative, often it is cooperative (with other children). Children can enjoy dress-up, playing with toy versions of medical sets, using hand puppets, and interactions when they play with shared toys such as cars and

TABLE 27.4	SIGNS OF DEVELOPMENTAL DELAY
Age	**Concern**
4 years	• Cannot jump in place or ride a tricycle • Cannot stack four blocks • Cannot throw ball overhand • Does not grasp crayon with thumb and fingers • Has difficulty with scribbling • Cannot copy a circle • Does not use sentences with three or more words • Cannot use the words "me" and "you" appropriately • Ignores other children or does not show interest in interactive games • Will not respond to people outside the family; still clings or cries if parents leave • Resists using toilet, dressing, sleeping • Does not engage in fantasy play
5 years	• Is unhappy or sad often • Has little interest in playing with other children • Is unable to separate from parent without major protest • Is extremely aggressive • Is extremely fearful or timid, or unusually passive • Cannot build tower of six to eight blocks • Is easily distracted; cannot concentrate on single activity for 5 minutes • Rarely engages in fantasy play • Has trouble with eating, sleeping, or using the toilet • Cannot use plurals or past tense • Cannot brush teeth, wash and dry hands, or undress efficiently

a garage. Preschoolers have incredible imaginations and love to play fantasy and "make-believe" (Fig. 27.9).

Cooperative play encourages the preschool child to learn to share, take turns and compromise, listen to others' opinions, consider the feelings of others, and use self-control and overcome fears.

Furthermore, it encourages the preschooler to develop social skills such as taking turns, communication, paying attention, and responding to one another's words and actions. Fantasy play also allows preschoolers to explore complex social ideas such as power, compassion, and cruelty. Examples of dramatic play include the 3 year old who may mix the idea of reality and fantasy, running from scary creatures. Four year olds are more sophisticated with dramatic or pretend play: they know they are pretending, and they use dress-up clothes and props to act out more complex roles and scenarios (Fig. 27.10). Five year olds are capable of quite complex

FIGURE 27.9 Preschool children enjoy imitative play.

FIGURE 27.8 The preschool child loves to create things, so colouring and moulding clay are ideal activities for children of this age.

scenarios. They pretend they are real or fantasy characters. They often use dramatic play to express anxiety, try out negative feelings, or conquer their fears. Through role playing, children begin to develop their sexual identity as well. Play therapy can be a useful approach when working with children as they process experiences that may have been upsetting, painful, or frightening.

Since preschool children have vivid imaginations, it is important to be careful about what television they watch. The CPS recommends children ages 5 to 9 be limited to no more than 2 hours/day of recreational screen time (TV, tablet, computer, multimedia phones, video games) (CPS, 2012). For children ages 2 to 4, screen time should be limited to educational programming of less than 1 hour/day (CPS, 2012). Recent evidence has suggested that these targets for screen time were met by 22% of 3 to 4 year olds and 76% of 5 year olds (Garriguet et al., 2016). The violence in some television programs may scare the preschool child or inspire him or her to act out violent behaviour.

Physical activity for all Canadians is important as per the Pan-Canada sports, physical activity, and recreation programs (SPAR) (Pan-Canada Public Health Network, 2015). For preschool children, PA is important for long-term health as well as minimizing future obesity (Lipnowski & LeBlanc, 2012). Preschoolers should accumulate at least 180 minutes of PA spread throughout the day (Canadian Society for Exercise Physiology, 2012) with no more than 60 minutes of sedentary time between activity (Timmons, Naylor, & Pfeiffer, 2007). Currently, it is estimated that 73% of Canadian 3 to 4 year olds and 30% of 5 year olds meet their respective PA guidelines (Garriguet et al., 2016). Furthermore, PA should consider their natural activity patterns, gross motor play, and locomotor activities that children find fun and use both outdoor and inside activities. Outdoor play and nature-based

FIGURE 27.10 Preschool children love to dress up and pretend.

learning is a thoughtful Canada approach to both PA and learning; safe woodland play is worthy of consideration (Coe, 2016). Organized sports should be fun, affordable, and delivered in a safe environment.

Expensive toys that claim to teach the young child are not necessary (Pujadas Botey et al., 2016). Toys that require interactive rather than passive play, and that may include the involvement of the parent, are recommended. Box 27.1 lists appropriate playthings for the preschool child.

Promoting Early Learning

The family is the foundation for the child's early growth and development. Parents serve as role models for behaviour related to education and learning, as well as instilling values in their children. **School readiness** is a topic that has received a significant amount of national attention in recent years (Statistics Canada, 2006). Variation exists across Canada, and school readiness and success are influenced by sex, family characteristics, background, and home environment. Furthermore this report suggested that readiness to learn may already be

---

BOX 27.1

APPROPRIATE TOYS FOR PRESCHOOLERS

- Blocks, simple jigsaw puzzles (four to six large pieces), pegboards, wooden bead with string
- Supplies for creativity: chalk, large crayons, finger paint, Play-Doh or clay, washable markers, paper, paint and paintbrush, scissors, paste, or glue
- Puppets, dress-up clothes, and props for dramatic play
- Bucket, plastic shovel, and other containers for sand and water play
- Play kitchen with accessories and pretend food (empty food boxes can be recycled for kitchen play)
- Squeaking, floating, squirting toys for the bath
- Sandbox with shovel and various toys for building
- Dolls that can be dressed and undressed (large buttons, zippers, and snaps), doll care accessories (diapers, bottles, carriage, crib)
- Gross motor toys: tricycle or big wheel (with helmet), jungle gym or swing set (with supervision), hula hoop, tunnel, wagon
- Blocks, Legos, cars and trucks, plastic animals, trains, plastic figures (family, community helpers), stuffed animals, balls, sewing cards
- Tape or CD players for music, various musical instruments
- Simple card and board games (older preschooler)
- Dollhouse with furniture and accessories, people, and animals

Adapted from Dowshen, S. (2014). *Smart toys for every age.* Retrieved from http://kidshealth.org/en/parents/smart-toys.html#; National Association for the Education of Young Children. (n.d.). *Good toys for young children by age and stage.* Retrieved from http://www.naeyc.org/toys

---

evident 2 years earlier, when the children were 3 years old (Statistics Canada, 2006). Promoting language development, choosing a preschool, and making the transition to kindergarten are discussed in more detail below.

Promoting Language Development

The parent serves as the child's first teacher (National Reading Campaign, 2017). The interactions between parent and child in relation to books and other play activities model the types of interactions that the child will later have in school. Asking open-ended questions stimulates the development of thinking as well as language in the preschool child. The preschooler is a great imitator, so the parent should serve as a role model for appropriate language. Parents should avoid using language they would not want to hear their child use as the child is likely to repeat words even if he or she does not understand what they mean. Allowing children to pursue interests at their own pace will help them to develop the literacy and numeric skills that will enable them to later focus on academic skills. Preschoolers enjoy books with pictures that tell stories (Fig. 27.11). Stories with repeated phrases help to keep the child's attention. Children like stories that describe experiences similar to their own. The preschool child demonstrates early literacy skills by reciting stories or portions of books. He or she also may retell the story from the book, pretend to read books, and ask questions about the story. The preschool child has enough focus and expanded attention to notice when a page is skipped during reading and will call it

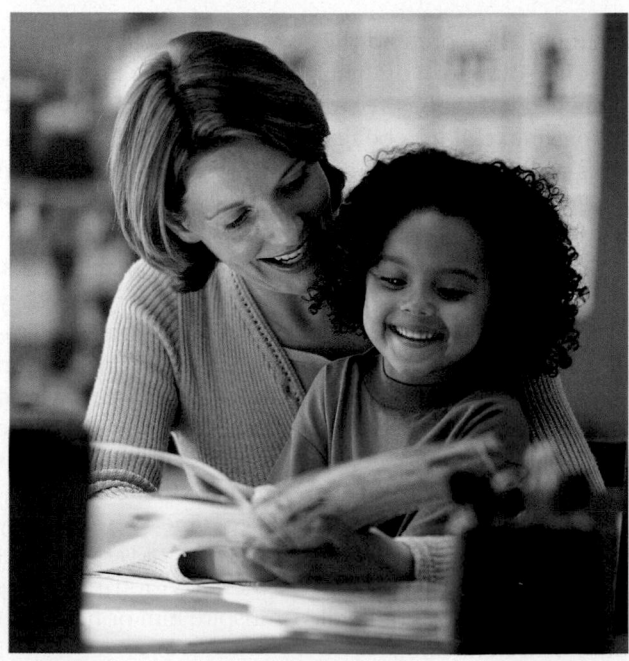

FIGURE 27.11 Preschool children enjoy being read to and looking at the pictures that go along with the story.

to the parent's attention. Literacy scores are generally good across Canada but are lower in some populations, therefore supporting parents who may struggle with literacy may help unlock potential for the child and parent (Gulati, 2013). When necessary the nurse can work with kindergarten teachers who are skilled using tools such as the Early Development Instrument to determine if the preschool child has areas of vulnerability around language and communication skills (Canadian Institute for Health Information, 2014).

> **Take Note!**
>
> Risk factors for lack of social and emotional readiness for school include insecure attachment in the early years, maternal depression, parental substance abuse, and low socioeconomic status. Nurses should screen for these factors, have knowledge about how to support families, and make referrals if appropriate.

Choosing a Preschool/ Starting Kindergarten

Licenced and early years programs are mandated to abide by provincial or territorial standards. The CPS can provide information on national directories for programs (CPS, n.d.). Many parents choose to enrol their child in preschool. Enrolment in such settings has shown that for some children (2 to 4 years) enhanced motor and social development are noted when mothers have chosen or needed to return to work (Lightbody & Williamson, 2017). Preschool should be used primarily as an opportunity to foster the child's social skills and accustom him or her to the group environment. When selecting a preschool, the parent may want to consider the accreditation of the school, the teachers' qualifications, and recommendations of other parents. The focus and philosophy of the school environment is also important since there can be wide variation in curriculum, teaching approach, and participation. Encourage the parent to visit or observe the classroom, evaluating the environment, noise level, and classroom routines as well as how the children interact with each other and how the teachers interact with the children.

The type of discipline and time-out for misbehaviour used in the school is also an important factor for parents to consider. The CPS discourages disciplinary spanking and all other forms of physical punishment (CPS, 2016).

Whether or not the child attended preschool, kindergarten will be the next big step. Kindergarten hours may be longer than preschool hours, and kindergarten is usually held 5 days/week. This may be a significant change for some children. For most children, the setting and personnel in kindergarten will be new. Rules and expectations are often very different from the home setting. When discussing starting kindergarten with the preschool child, parents should use an enthusiastic approach, keeping the conversation light and positive. Parents should meet with the child's teacher prior to the start of school, if possible, to discuss particular needs or concerns. Parents may want to schedule a tour of the school for the preschooler or attend the school's open house with the child to ease the transition. Practicing the new daily routine prior to the start of school will also be helpful.

It is important that the preschool child be up-to-date on immunizations and health screening before entering kindergarten. In Canada, Ontario and New Brunswick have mandatory immunizations that are required in order for the child to attend school. In these provinces parents must produce proof of the child's immunizations prior to school entry (Office of the Chief Medical Officer of Health, 2016; Ontario Ministry of Health and Long-Term Care, 2017).

Promoting Safety

In Canada, injury remains the leading cause of death not only for children, but also for adults between the ages of 1 and 44 years (CPS, 2012a). Various charitable, national, provincial, and territorial programs focus on this area including Parachute, Atlantic Collaborative on Injury Prevention (PHAC, n.d.; Yanchar, Warda, & Fuselli, 2012). Preschoolers are at an ideal age to be taught about safety and safe behaviours. They are cognitively able to absorb concrete information and they desire to master the situations they are in, but they continue to display poor judgment related to safety issues, that is, falls within the family home (Morrongiello & Corbett, 2016). The preschool child is capable of learning safe behaviours but may not always be able to transfer those behaviours to a different situation. Parents must continue to closely supervise preschool children to avoid accidental injury during this period.

Safety in the Car

Forward-facing car seats are for children with stronger back and neck muscles. The preschooler should use a forward-facing car seat until they grow out of it, or up until at least 18 kg (40 lb). Newer forward-facing car seats with a higher weight limits are also available up to 30 kg (65 lb) for preschoolers and large toddlers (Transport Canada, 2016a). Even if the preschooler weighs more than 18 kg (40 lb) and provincial/territorial law states you can use a booster seat, it is safer to continue to use the forward-facing car seat as long as the preschooler continues to be below the car seat's weight and height limits (Transport Canada, 2016b).

Once the preschooler has outgrown the forward-facing car seat, they should move to a booster seat. Booster seats are designed to position a child so the seat belt is correctly located on their lap and shoulder (Transport Canada, 2016c). Booster seats should continue to be used until at least 36 kg (80 lb), a height of 145 cm, and at least 8 years of age (CPS, 2008). Some booster seat models with higher weight limits are available up to 45 kg (100 lb). Once the child has reached these parameters, the child should be assessed whether the adult seatbelt fits appropriately before deciding a booster is no longer required (CPS, 2008).

The back seat of the car is always the safest place for a child to ride. If there is only a single occupant, the rear middle is considered the safest option as it is furthest away from side impacts and side air bags. Children should sit in the rear of the vehicle until at least 13 years of age as front passenger air bags can cause death or severely harm children (CPS, 2008).

Take Note!

Although motor vehicle accidents remain a major cause of injury and death in the preschool age group, many families do not use appropriate car seat/seat belt safety with their children. If you are unsure whether you have installed your car seat correctly, you may be able to attend a car seat clinic in your community. In addition the**Point** has links to Government of Canada's webpage, Child Car Safety, providing additional up-to-date information.

Safety in the Home

Injuries are the foremost cause of death in Canadian children (CPS, 2015). Firearms, matches, bodies of water, bicycle riding, and poisons continue to be sources of potential injury during the preschool years. Falls account for the highest percentage of nonfatal injuries among preschoolers and are the leading cause of hospitalization (Morrongiello & Corbett, 2016). In this age group, motor vehicle collisions are responsible for the most fatal injuries, followed by drowning (CPS, 2012a). In Aboriginal children, accidental injury occurs at disproportionality higher rates of three to four times the national average (CPS, 2015). In general, Indigenous communities are more at risk for accidental injury as they are far more likely to have substandard housing, poverty, and often experience difficulty accessing health care due to geographical constraints. In Indigenous children younger than 10 years of age, the most common causes of death due to injury are fires and motor vehicle collisions (CPS, 2015).

PREVENTING EXPOSURE TO TOBACCO SMOKE

Parents should protect their preschoolers from secondhand tobacco smoke. Exposure to tobacco smoke is associated with an increased incidence of otitis media and respiratory infections, as well as increased symptoms and medication use in children with asthma. Other effects include decreased lung function and behavioural difficulties. The preschool child should never be in an enclosed space (such as a car) where tobacco smoke is present.

PREVENTING INJURY

The preschool child who runs out into the street is at risk for being struck by a car. Teach preschoolers to stop at the road side and never go into the street without an adult or responsible person. The preschooler may learn to ride a bicycle (with or without training wheels). The child must be encouraged to wear an approved bicycle helmet any time he or she rides the bicycle, even if it is just in the driveway (CPS, 2016a). Requiring helmet use in the early years may lead to the habit of helmet use as the child gets older. Allowing the preschooler to choose his or her own helmet may encourage the child to use the helmet.

Bicycles should be safe for this age group. The size must be correct; the balls of the feet should reach both pedals while the child is sitting on the seat and has both hands on the handlebars. Children younger than 5 years of age have difficulty learning to use hand-operated brakes, so traditional pedal-back brakes are recommended in this age group. Preschoolers are not mature enough to ride a bicycle in the street even if they are riding with adults, so they should always ride on the sidewalk (Hagel & Yanchar, 2013).

It is important to make the inside of the home safe for the preschool child. Parents should install and maintain smoke alarms as well as carbon monoxide detectors in the home. Increased physical dexterity and refinement of motor skills enable the preschooler to strike matches or use a lighter and start a fire. The preschool child is capable of washing his or her hands independently, so the water heater should be set at 49°C (120°F) or below to prevent scalding (AAP, 2015).

The preschooler's active imagination and desire to play make-believe may result in a firearm injury. The average preschooler is physically capable of handling and firing a gun, particularly a handgun, which is smaller and lighter. If present in the home, Canadian federal gun control laws mandate that firearms be kept in a locked cabinet with the ammunition stored elsewhere (CPS, 2016d).

PREVENTING POISONING

Though it is continuing to develop, preschoolers still have unrefined taste discrimination, placing them at risk for accidental ingestion. Parents should never try to coax a child to take a vitamin supplement, tablet, or pill by calling it "candy." Dangerous fluids should be stored in their original containers and should be kept out of reach of preschoolers; they should not be poured into containers that look like ordinary drinking glasses or cups. Potentially dangerous cleaning or personal health and beauty products, gardening and pool chemicals, and automotive materials should be kept out of reach of preschoolers and in a locked cabinet if possible. Medications should have childproof caps and should be kept in a locked cabinet. The Poison Control Centre telephone number should be posted on or near the home phone. Please visit the Canadian Association of Poison Control

Centres at http://www.capcc.ca/en to determine your provincial telephone number (CAPCC, 2016).

Safety in the Water

A leading cause of unintentional injury resulting in death in preschool children (1 to 4 years) is drowning, 21% deaths (Yanchar, Warde, & Fuselli, 2012). Five years of age is an appropriate time for a child to learn to swim. Children at this age are physically capable of this activity and have the cognitive maturity to accomplish the task of swimming and basic water safety. Swimming programs should focus on appropriate swim techniques as well as safety measures. Parents and caregivers should be trained in infant/child cardiopulmonary resuscitation (CPR). Homes with swimming pools should have lifesaving devices readily accessible. Preschoolers should be taught never to dive into water until an adult has verified its depth. Preschoolers are still too young to be left unattended around any body of water, even if they know how to swim. Preschoolers should never be allowed to swim in a canal or any fast-moving water. Preschoolers who are riding in boats or fishing off riverbanks should wear a personal flotation device. Parents should also be cautioned about close supervision of young children walking, skating, or riding near thin or weak ice.

> **Recall Nila Patel, the 4 year old presented at the beginning of the chapter. What anticipatory guidance related to safety should you provide to her parents?**

Promoting Nutrition

The preschool child has a full set of primary teeth, is able to chew and swallow competently, and has learned to use utensils fairly effectively to feed himself or herself (Fig. 27.12). As in the toddler years, it is important for the preschool child to continue to learn and build upon healthy eating habits. These habits will last throughout the child's life. A diet high in nutrient-rich foods such as whole grains, vegetables, fruits, appropriate dairy foods, and lean meats is appropriate for the preschooler. Nutrient-poor, high-calorie foods such as sweets and typical fast foods should be offered only in limited amounts.

> **Take Note!**
> **Preschool Eating Habits**
> Preschoolers are erratic eaters and will eat very well one day and then may eat very little the next day. Food jags are not common in the preschooler, but are common in the toddler.

Nutritional Needs

Daily energy requirements for preschoolers are between 94 kcal/kg/day (2 to 3 years) and 100 kcal/kg/day (4 to 6 years) (Goldbloom, 2011). The 1 to 3 year old needs around 700-mg calcium daily while by 4 to 8 years it is 1,000 mg and 7- to 10-mg iron daily (Ross, Taylor, Yaktine, & Del Valle, 2011). Box 27.2 lists calcium and iron sources. Preschoolers should consume a minimum of 19-mg dietary fibre daily (Brown, 2011). Saturated fats should account for less than 10% of total calories. Preschool children's diets should include a daily total fat intake of no less than 20% and not more than 35% of total calories to promote and maintain healthy cholesterol levels (Haemer, Primark, & Krebs, 2012). A key resource is Canada's Food Guide; this provides information for professionals and parents including food tracker, recommended daily intake, choosing the right foods, understanding food labels, and maintaining healthy eating habits (Health Canada, 2016).

> **Take Note!**
> Drinking excess amounts of milk may lead to iron deficiency, as the calcium in milk blocks iron absorption.

Promoting Healthy Eating Habits

Preschool children may be picky eaters. They may eat only a limited variety of foods or foods prepared in certain ways and may not be very willing to try new things. The 3 or 4 year old may exhibit "food fads," eating only certain foods over a several-day period. As the child gets older, pickiness lessens. By 5 years of age the child is more focused on the social context of eating: table conversation and manners. The 5 year old is generally more willing to at least try new foods and may like to help with meal preparation and cleanup as appropriate.

FIGURE 27.12 The preschool child has the manual dexterity to handle utensils appropriately and feed himself or herself independently.

> BOX 27.2

DAILY CALCIUM AND IRON RECOMMENDATIONS FOR PRESCHOOL CHILDREN

Calcium: 700 mg (3 year old), 1,000 mg (4 to 8 year old)

Calcium in Foods
- 8-oz low-fat or whole milk: 275 to 300 mg
- 8-oz low-fat yogurt: 313 to 415 mg
- 1½-oz cheddar cheese: 307 mg
- 1-oz dried white beans (cooked): 75 mg
- ¼-cup tofu: 138 to 253 mg
- ½-cup raw broccoli: 21 mg

Iron: 7 mg (3 year old), 10 mg (4 to 8 year old)

Iron in Foods
- ¾-cup 100% fortified prepared cereal: 18 mg
- 3-oz beef: 3 mg
- 3-oz chicken (dark meat): 1.1 mg
- ½-cup cooked lentils: 3 mg
- 3-oz chicken (white meat): 0.9 mg
- 15.2-cm (6-in) slice watermelon: 0.7 mg
- ¼-cup fresh cooked spinach: 1.6 mg
- ¼-cup tofu: 1.7 mg
- ¼-cup raisins: 1 mg
- 1 slice enriched bread: 0.8 to 0.9 mg
- ¼-cup frozen spinach, cooked: 0.85 mg

Adapted from National Institutes of Health. (2016a). *Calcium dietary supplement fact sheet.* Retrieved from http://ods.od.nih.gov/factsheets/Calcium-HealthProfessional/#h3; National Institutes of Health. (2016b). *Iron dietary supplement fact sheet.* Retrieved from http://ods.od.nih.gov/factsheets/Iron-HealthProfessional/#h4

If the preschooler is growing well, then the pickiness is not a cause for worry. The concern may become the negative relationship that can develop between the parent and child relating to mealtime. The more the parent coaxes, cajoles, bribes, and threatens, the less likely the child is to try new foods or even eat the ones he or she likes that are served. The parent must maintain a positive and patient demeanour at mealtime. The child should be offered a healthy diet, with foods from all groups over the course of the day as recommended by Canada's Food Guide (Health Canada, 2016). Canada's Food Guide is available in 10 other languages. In addition, there is a separate Food Guide which reflects the values, traditions, and food choices of First Nations, Inuit, and Metis (Health Canada, 2016).

The parent should maintain a matter-of-fact approach, offer the meal or snack, and then allow the child to decide how much of the food, if any, he or she is going to eat. High-fat, nutrient-poor snacks should not be substituted for healthy foods just to coax the child to eat.

Preventing the Development of Overweight and Obesity

Worldwide, over 22 million children younger than 5 years old are obese. In Canada, over the past 25 years, the prevalence of obesity has nearly tripled with up to 26% of children aged 2 to 17 being overweight or obese (CPS, 2012b). This number jumps to 41% in Indigenous children aged 2 to 17 (CPS, 2012b). Overweight and obese children are at risk for hypertension, hyperlipidemia, and the development of insulin resistance. Having a high body mass index as a preschooler is consistently associated with adult and central obesity as well as early onset of metabolic syndrome (Graversen et al., 2014). The risk is increased if one or both parents are overweight.

Parents are in a strong position to be a positive influence on their preschooler's nutritional intake and activity level. The habits learned in early childhood will likely carry over into the school-age, adolescent, and adult years. Children whose parents take an authoritarian approach to mealtime may learn to overeat, as they are encouraged to finish the entire meal. If they are offered appropriate, healthy food choices, and access to high-calorie, nutrient-poor food is limited, preschoolers will learn to self-regulate (eat only until full). Food should not be used as either reward or punishment.

Parents should remain positive and patient at mealtime. Mealtimes should continue to be structured. Unstructured meals lead to an increase in fat and calorie consumption. Children who eat nutrient-dense and lower-fat foods are less likely to become overweight (Institute of Medicine, 2011). To limit the chance that overeating will occur, preschoolers should be offered a variety of healthy foods at each meal. The preschool child's serving size is usually one third to one half of the recommended size of an adult serving. The preschool child may imitate the other eaters at the table. Parents have a prime chance to be good role models, setting an example of eating vegetables and fruits.

Limiting television viewing and encouraging PA are also important strategies for the prevention of overweight and obesity. Canadian PA guidelines recommend that toddlers and preschoolers accumulate at least 180 minutes of PA a day at any intensity. This should include a variety of activities in different environments and activities that develop movement skills. By age 5, children should have progressed to at least 60 minutes of energetic play a day (Canadian Society for Exercise Physiology, 2012). The CPS suggests that screen time for children aged 2 to 4 should be limited to educational programing of less than 1 hour/day and for children aged 5 to 9 less than 2 hours/day as it is known that excessive screen time negatively impacts aspects of psychosocial and cognitive development and leads to obesity (see Evidence-Based Practice 27.1) (CPS, 2012b).

Promoting Healthy Sleep and Rest

Preschoolers should have access to a safe space to sleep as recommended by Health Canada (2012). Screen time before bed and access to televisions in the bedroom should be avoided since both have been found to be associated with excess body weight and short sleep duration in children (Chahal et al., 2013). The preschool child needs about 11 to 12 hours of sleep each day (Feigelman, 2011). Some preschool children continue to take a nap during the day. Unless very tired, many preschool children will resist going to bed from time to time. Bedtime routine is necessary; by having a time of relaxation with a decrease in stimulation allows the child to fall asleep more easily. Some children continue to need a security item at bedtime or naptime. A nightlight in the bedroom may be necessary, as many children of this age are afraid of the dark. Teaching Guidelines 27.1

gives information about assisting parents to establish a bedtime routine.

Teaching Guidelines 27.1
BEDTIME ROUTINES

- Establish a bedtime as well as morning wake-up time.
- Avoid sugar or caffeine consumption in the evening.
- Avoid stimulating activities such as roughhousing before bedtime.
- Do not allow television watching in bed or screen time 2 hours before bed.
- Make the child's bedroom a safe, inviting, and comfortable area of the home.
- Provide a nightlight in the child's bedroom if he or she is afraid of the dark.
- Promote and sustain a nightly routine.
- Turn television off at a certain time.
- Bath.
- Quiet game or story reading/telling.
- Bedtime song or prayer.
- Maintain quiet in the bedroom and nearby to increase the child's ability to fall asleep.

Adapted from Gupta, R. C. (2014). *Sleep and your preschooler.* Retrieved from http://kidshealth.org/parent/general/sleep/sleep_preschool.html; Goldson, E., & Reynolds, A. (2012). Child development & behaviour. In W. W. Hay, M. J. Levin, R. R. Deterding, M. J. Abzug (Eds.). *Current Diagnosis & Treatment: Pediatrics* (21st ed.). New York: McGraw-Hill.

EVIDENCE-BASED PRACTICE 27.1   PREVENTING PRESCHOOL OBESITY BY PROMOTING PHYSICAL ACTIVITY

STUDY

One of the most pressing public health issues is the continued rise in the childhood obesity epidemic. Early childhood obesity is associated with immediate health consequences as well as long-term issues such as adult obesity and early-onset metabolic syndrome.

The authors reviewed 14 recent US studies focusing on children aged 2 to 5 years, and measurement of physical activity as well as perceived factors related to physical activity. Independent reviews were undertaken followed by the authors reconvening and discussing the factors associated with physical activity among preschoolers.

Findings

The authors' literature review revealed discrepancies between parents' perceived notions about child physical activity and actual child physical activity. Families perceive their preschoolers to be active throughout the day, but studies show that much of this activity is sedentary in nature. The child's characteristics and personality traits

may have an influence on choice of play; children will be more active when engaged in a type of play that they personally enjoy. Parental involvement in physical activities also influences the preschooler's activity level. Perceived safety in the child care environment or home outdoor setting also affects children's physical activity levels.

Nursing Implications

Parents naturally want what is best for their children, but often need guidance from health care providers to encourage them to move toward healthy habits. Nurses are in a unique position to provide ongoing, repeated education about the importance of physical activity in preschoolers to families wherever they encounter them. Parents may be tired from their busy schedules, but nurses can provide positive reinforcement for even small steps (such as taking a brief walk after the evening meal, while the preschooler rides a bike or skates alongside). Encourage families to discover which physical activities their preschooler prefers, and encourage them to provide opportunities for participation in those activities.

Adapted from Hodges, E. A., Smith, C., Tidwell, S., & Berry, D. (2013). Promoting physical activity in preschoolers to prevent obesity: A review of the literature. *Journal of Pediatric Nursing, 28,* 3–19.

Nightmares often occur in preschool children as a result of the child's struggle to distinguish what is real from what is not. When a child awakens from a nightmare, he or she is often crying and may be able to recount what the dream was about. Parents should validate the child's fear rather than discounting it (Goldson & Reynolds, 2012). Saying, "Yes, I agree, monsters are scary; it's a good thing they aren't real" is more appropriate than, "Don't be silly: monsters aren't real." Sometimes children benefit from reading stories about dreams. Recommended books include:

- *Bedtime for Frances* by Russell Hoban
- *Ben's Dream* by Chris van Allsberg
- *In the Night Kitchen* by Maurice Sendak
- *There's a Nightmare in My Closet* by Mercer Mayer

Nightmares should not be confused with night terrors. After a nightmare, the child is aroused and interactive, but night terrors are different: a short time after falling asleep, the child seems to awaken and is screaming. The child usually does not respond much to the parent's soothing, but he or she eventually stops screaming and goes back to sleep. Night terrors are often frightening for parents because the child does not seem to be responding to them. One technique that may help to decrease the incidence of night terrors is to wake the child about 30 to 45 minutes into the sleep cycle. If continued nightly for about a week, the cycle of night terrors may be broken (Cavanaugh, 2011). See Comparison Chart 27.1.

> **Think back to Nila Patel. What anticipatory guidance would you provide to her parents in relation to sleep during the preschool years?**

Promoting Healthy Teeth and Gums

The Canadian Dental Association (2010) recognizes that ECC is a complex chronic disease influenced by biomedical factors (diet, bacteria, and host) and by social determinants of health. ECC has a lasting impact on both primary and permanent teeth and is the most common childhood disease. Dental caries prevention continues to be important and can be achieved through daily brushing and flossing, six monthly visits to the dentist, and early intervention including dietary supplements (Vitamin D as suggested by a health care provider). Parents should use only a pea-sized amount of toothpaste to prevent excess fluoride consumption, which can contribute to fluorosis (Clark & Krol, 2013). The preschooler may brush his or her own teeth, but the parent must continue to supervise to ensure adequate brushing. Parents must perform flossing because the preschool child cannot perform this task adequately. Oral health should be assessed regularly in high-risk groups such as immigration and refugee children (Reza et al., 2016) and First Nations children (Schroth et al., 2009).

Take Note!

Dental caries prevention is important in the primary teeth, because loss of these teeth to caries may affect the proper formation of permanent teeth as well as the width of the dental arch.

Promoting Appropriate Discipline

Successful discipline results from a loving and nurturing environment in which the preschooler's self-esteem is fostered and where limits are well chosen and enforced consistently. Spanking (striking with the open hand) is

COMPARISON CHART 27.1	NIGHTMARES VERSUS NIGHT TERRORS	
	Nightmare	**Night Terror**
Definition	Scary or bad dream followed by awakening	Partial arousal from deep sleep
When parents become aware	Child awakens parent after episode is over	Screaming and thrashing during the episode awakens the parent
Timing	Usually in the second half of the night	Usually about an hour after falling asleep
Behaviour	Crying, may be scared after awakening	Sits up, thrashes, cries, screams, talks, looks wild eyed. Sweats, may have racing heartbeat
Responsiveness	Responsive to parent's soothing and reassurances	Child unaware of parent's presence, may scream and thrash more if restrained
Return to sleep	Difficulty going back to sleep if afraid	Rapidly returns to sleep without full awakening
Memory of occurrence	May remember the dream and talk about it later	No memory of event

Adapted from Cavanaugh, K. (2011). Parasomnias. *Advance for NPs & Pas, 2*(2), 21–24.

the least effective discipline practice and is discouraged by the CPS (CPS, 2016). No item should be used to strike a child. The use of physical punishment has been associated with a number of additional problems in adulthood, such as antisocial and criminal behaviours.

If parents use consistent boundaries while encouraging the preschooler's normal growth and development of imagination and make-believe, the child will learn to accept that certain things are not allowed. The sense of initiative can be preserved and guilt avoided if the rules are clear and enforced consistently (Sears & Sears, 2015a).

Minimize the occurrence of misbehaviour by anticipating conditions likely to lead to the undesired or risky action. When the situation becomes difficult, parents should use distraction to change the preschooler's focus. When discussing the misbehaviour, be certain to label the behaviour and not the child (specific labelling). This helps to preserve the preschooler's self-esteem. When teaching preschoolers about undesired behaviour, be sure they also understand the reason why it is wrong or unacceptable to do it. This helps to encourage the child to use internal controls over behaviour. Parents should serve as role models for self-control, including choice of words, the tone they are delivered in, and the actions that accompany them.

Children work harder to obtain praise than to receive punishment, so always reward positive behaviours. Preschool children are becoming capable of understanding the concept of right and wrong. They start to understand each other's feelings (**empathy**) and are cognitively capable of remembering basic rules.

Time-out or time away from the situation can be very effective in this age group. The punishment should be used only for intentional misbehaviour (knowing something is forbidden but doing it anyway). It is particularly helpful with dangerous or destructive behaviour. The preschooler is given a warning that time-out will occur if the behaviour does not stop. The preschooler is removed from the situation and must stay in time-out for a specified (short) period of time. A particular time-out area is helpful; a boring corner of the room without distractions available is a good location. The generally recommended period of time is to require 1 minute of time-out per year of age; thus, a 4 year old would be in time-out for 4 minutes (Sears & Sears, 2015b). Set the timer so the child will know when the time-out is over. If the child gets up before the prescribed time, replace the child in time-out and restart the timer. Time-out works best if used each and every time the undesirable behaviour occurs. Also, praise the child when he or she follows the rules and behaves appropriately.

A simple and clear explanation of the misbehaviour should be given to the child; parents should also talk about acceptable alternative strategies that the child can use in the future instead of the undesired behaviour.

Removal of a privilege such as playing with a favourite toy can be as effective as time-out.

Books and other media that are available to help educate parents about appropriate discipline and to help the child learn self-control are listed in Box 27.3.

ADDRESSING COMMON DEVELOPMENTAL CONCERNS

Common developmental concerns of the preschool period include lying, how to address sex education, and masturbation. Parents often express difficulty in dealing with these issues with their preschool children. Offering appropriate anticipatory guidance may give the parents the support and confidence they need to deal with these issues.

Lying

Lying is common in preschool children. It may occur because the child fears punishment, has gotten carried away with imagination, or is imitating what he or she sees the parent do. The parent should ascertain the reason for the lie before punishing the child. If the child has broken a rule and fears punishment, then the parent must determine the truth. The child needs to learn that lying is usually far worse than the misbehaviour itself. The punishment for the misbehaviour should be lessened if the child admits the truth. The parent should remain calm and serve as a role model of an even temper. The next time the misbehaviour occurs, the child will be more apt to simply tell the truth.

If the child's lying is really just his or her imagination getting carried away, then the parent should guide the child in distinguishing between myth and reality (Sears & Sears, 2015c). The preschooler's imagination is very vivid, and the child needs direction in the use of that faculty. Parents should serve as role models of appropriate behaviour for their children to learn it.

Sex Education

Preschoolers are keen observers but are still not able to interpret all that they see correctly. The child may recognize, but not understand, sexual activity. Preschoolers are very inquisitive and want to learn about everything around them; therefore, they are very likely to ask questions about sex and where babies come from. Before attempting to answer questions, parents should try to find out first what the child is really asking and what the child already thinks about that subject. Then they should provide a short, simple, direct, and honest answer. The child needs only the information that he or she is requesting. Additional questions will occur in the future and should be addressed as they arise.

BOX 27.3

SELECTED RESOURCES FOR PARENTS AND PRESCHOOLERS

Books for Parents (about discipline)

- *How to Talk so Kids Will Listen and Listen so Kids Will Talk* by A. Faber & E. Mazlish (Harper Resource)
- *Kids Are Worth It: Giving Your Children the Gift of Inner Discipline* by B. Colorosos (Harper Collins Publishers)
- *Positive Discipline A to Z: 1001 Solutions to Everyday Parenting Problems* by J. Nelson, L. Lott, & S. G. Glenn (Three Rivers Press)
- *Setting Limits With Your Strong-Willed Child: Eliminating Conflict by Establishing Clear, Firm and Respectful Boundaries* by R. MacKenzie (Three Rivers Press)
- *The Case Against Spanking: How to Discipline Children Without Hitting* by I. A. Hyman (Jossey-Bass)
- *The Nurturing Parent: How to Raise Creative, Loving, Responsible Children* by J. S. Dacey & A. J. Packer (Fireside)
- *Without Spanking or Spoiling: A Practical Approach to Toddler and Preschool Guidance* by E. Crary (Parenting Press)

Books for Preschoolers (about dealing with feelings and learning how to behave)

- *Hands Are Not for Hitting* by M. Agassi (Free Spirit Publishing)
- *I Can't Wait* by E. Crary (Parenting Press)
- *I Want It* by E. Crary (Parenting Press)
- *I Want to Play* by E. Crary (Parenting Press)
- *I Was so Mad* by M. Mayer (Golden Books)
- *I Was so Mad* by N. Simon & D. Leder (Albert Whitman & Company)
- *I'm Excited* by E. Crary (Parenting Press)
- *I'm Frustrated* by E. Crary (Parenting Press)
- *I'm Mad* by E. Crary (Parenting Press)
- *I'm Scared* by E. Crary (Parenting Press)
- *Feet Are Not for Kicking* by E. Verdick (Free Spirit Publishing)
- *Teeth Are Not for Biting* by E. Verdick (Free Spirit Publishing)
- *When Sophie Gets Angry … Really, Really Angry* by M. Bang (Blue Sky Press)
- *Words Are Not for Hurting* by E. Verdick (Free Spirit Publishing)

Masturbation

The normal curiosity of the preschool years often leads children to explore their own genitals (Feigelman, 2011). This behaviour may be upsetting to some parents, but masturbation is a healthy and natural part of normal preschool development if it occurs in moderation. If the parent overreacts to this behaviour, then it may occur more frequently. Masturbation should be treated in a matter-of-fact way by the parent. The child needs to learn certain rules about this activity: nudity and masturbation are not acceptable in public. The child should also be taught safety: no other person can touch the private parts unless it is the parent, doctor, or nurse checking to see when something is wrong.

> **Think back to Nila Patel. What are some developmental concerns that are common during the preschool years? What anticipatory guidance related to these concerns would you provide to Nila's parents?**

NURSING CARE PLAN 27.1

Growth and Development Issues in the Preschool Child

NURSING DIAGNOSIS: Risk for injury (risk factors: developmental age, environment, and motor vehicle travel)

Outcome Identification and Evaluation

Child's safety will be maintained: *Child will remain free from injury.*

Interventions: *Preventing Injury*

- Teach and encourage appropriate use of forward-facing car seat or booster seat *to decrease risk of injury related to motor vehicles.*
- Teach preschoolers to stay away from street and to cross the street only when holding the hand of an adult *to prevent pedestrian injury.*

NURSING CARE PLAN 27.1

Growth and Development Issues in the Preschool Child (continued)

- Require bicycle helmet use while riding any wheeled toy *to prevent head injury and form habit of helmet use.*
- Teach the preschooler appropriate safety rules in the home (avoiding electric outlets, etc.): *the preschooler is able to follow simple directions and carry out directives. Limits help him or her to organize the environment.*
- Post Poison Control Centre phone number *(in case of accidental ingestion; the preschool child is very curious).*

- Never leave a preschool child unattended in a tub or pool or near any body of water *to prevent drowning.*
- Provide swimming lessons for children aged 4 or 5 *to encourage water safety, but not as a replacement for adult supervision.*
- Teach parents first-aid measures and child CPR *to minimize consequences of injury should it occur.*
- Provide close observation and keep side rails up on bed in hospital *because the preschool child continues to be at risk for falling or injuring self on equipment or tubing (because of curiosity).*

NURSING DIAGNOSIS: Imbalanced nutrition: less than body requirements, related to inappropriate nutritional intake to sustain growth needs (excess juice or milk intake, inadequate food variety intake) as evidenced by failure to attain adequate increases in height and weight over time

Outcome Identification and Evaluation

Child will consume adequate nutrients: Child will demonstrate weight gain and increases in height.

Interventions: *Promoting Appropriate Nutrition*

- Assess current feeding schedule and usual intake, as well as methods used to feed, *to determine areas of adequacy versus inadequacy.*
- Determine if the preschooler is unable to drink from a cup or does not finger feed or use utensils properly, or if the child has difficulty swallowing or tolerating certain textures of foods *to determine if further interventions such as speech or occupational therapy are required.*
- Weigh child daily on same scale if hospitalized, weekly on same scale if at home, and plot growth patterns weekly or monthly as appropriate on standardized growth charts *to determine if growth is improving.*
- Limit juice to 120 to 160 mL (4 to 6 oz) per day, milk to 480 to 720 mL (16 to 24 oz) per day, *to discourage sense of fullness achieved with excess milk or juice intake, thereby increasing appetite for appropriate solid foods. Remember milk on cereal counts.*
- Provide three nutrient-dense meals and at least two healthy snacks per day *to encourage adequate nutrient consumption.*
- Feed child on a similar schedule daily, without distractions and with the family: *preschool children continue to respond well to routine and structure. They are more interested in the social context of meals and are still apt to become distracted easily, so the TV should be off at mealtimes.*

NURSING DIAGNOSIS: Risk for delayed development related to motor, cognitive, language, or psychosocial concerns as evidenced by delay in meeting expected milestones

Outcome Identification and Evaluation

Development will be enhanced: Child will make continued progress toward realization of expected developmental milestones.

(continued)

NURSING CARE PLAN 27.1

Growth and Development Issues in the Preschool Child (continued)

Interventions *Enhancing Growth and Development*

- Screen for developmental capabilities to determine child's current level of functioning.
- Offer age-appropriate toys, play, and activities (including gross motor) to encourage further development.
- Perform interventions as prescribed by physical, occupational, or speech therapist: participation in those activities helps to promote function and accomplish acquisition of developmental skills.

- Provide support to families of preschoolers with developmental delay (progress in achieving developmental milestones can be slow and ongoing motivation is needed).
- Reinforce positive attributes in the child to maintain motivation.
- Model age-appropriate communication skills to illustrate suitable means for parenting the preschooler.

NURSING DIAGNOSIS: Risk for overweight (risk factors: excess milk or juice intake, consumption of inappropriate foods or in excess amounts)

Outcome Identification and Evaluation

Child will grow appropriately and not become overweight or obese: Child will achieve weight and height within the 5th to 85th percentiles on standardized growth charts.

Interventions: *Promoting Appropriate Growth*

- Discourage use of no-spill sippy cups (they contribute to dental caries and allow unlimited access to fluids, possibly decreasing appetite for appropriate solid foods).
- Provide juice (12 to 180 mL/day) and milk (480 to 720 mL/day) from a cup at meal and snack time and water in between to avoid having the child drink excessive juice or milk.
- Provide only nutrient-rich foods without high sugar content for meals and snacks; even if the preschooler is a picky eater, it is inappropriate to provide high-calorie junk food just so the child eats something.
- Teach parents to role model appropriate eating (nutrient-rich, varied diet) to encourage child to try/

accept new foods, as well as become familiar with a variety of foods.
- Severely limit the intake of fast foods and foods with high sugar and fat content to decrease intake of nutrient-poor, high-calorie foods.
- Ensure adequate physical activity to stimulate development of motor skills and provide appropriate caloric expenditure. This also sets the stage for forming life-long habit of appropriate physical activity.
- Teach parents to limit entertainment screen time to 1 to 2 hours/day to encourage participation in physical activities.

NURSING DIAGNOSIS: Interrupted family processes related to issues with preschool child's development, hospitalization, or situational crisis as evidenced by decreased parental visitation in hospital, parental verbalization of difficulty with current situation, possible crisis related to health of family member other than the preschool child

Outcome Identification and Evaluation

Family will demonstrate adequate functioning: Family will display coping and psychosocial adjustment.

NURSING CARE PLAN 27.1

Growth and Development Issues in the Preschool Child (continued)

Interventions: *Enhancing Family Functioning*

- Assess the family's level of stress and ability to cope to determine family's ability to cope with multiple stressors.
- Engage in family-centered care to provide a holistic approach to care of the preschooler and family.
- Encourage the family to verbalize feelings (verbalization is one method of decreasing anxiety levels) and acknowledge feelings and emotions.

- Use puppets or dramatic play with the child to elicit the preschooler's feelings about the current situation.
- Encourage family visitation and provide for sleeping arrangements for a parent or caregiver to stay in the hospital with the preschooler; this contributes to family's sense of control in situation.
- Involve family members in preschooler's care, giving them a feeling of control and connectedness.

NURSING DIAGNOSIS: Readiness for enhanced parenting related to parental desire for increased skill level and success with preschool child as evidenced by current healthy relationships and verbalization of desire for improved skills

---

Outcome Identification and Evaluation

Parent will provide safe and nurturing environment for the preschool child: *Parents will verbalize new skills they will employ in the family.*

Interventions: *Increasing Parenting Skill Set*

- Use family-centered care to provide holistic approach.
- Educate parent about normal preschool development to provide basis of understanding for parenting skills needed in this time period.
- Acknowledge and encourage parents' verbalization of feelings related to chronic illness of child or difficulty with normal preschool behaviour; this validates the normalcy of parents' feelings.
- Encourage positive parenting and respect for preschooler and his or her normal development (helps parents develop approaches to preschoolers that can be used in place of anger and frustration).
- Role model appropriate parenting behaviours related to communicating with and disciplining the child (role modelling actually demonstrates rather than just verbalizes what the parent should strive for).

KEY CONCEPTS

- The preschool child grows at a slower rate and takes on a more slender and upright appearance than the toddler.
- The primary psychosocial task of the preschool period is developing a sense of initiative.
- Cognitive development moves from an egocentric approach to the world toward a more empathetic understanding of what happens outside of the self.

- The preschooler gains additional motor skills and displays significant refinement of fine motor abilities.
- Cognitive and language skills that develop in the preschool years help prepare the child for success in school.
- Dysfluency or hesitancy in speech is a normal finding in the preschool period and occurs as a result of the fast pace with which the preschooler is gaining language skills and vocabulary.

- The vocabulary of a preschooler increases to about 2,100 words, and the child speaks in full sentences with appropriate use of tense and prepositions.

- Appropriate growth and development should be maintained in the ill or hospitalized child.

- Recognizing concerns or delays in growth and development is essential so that the appropriate referrals may be made and intervention can begin.

- The preschool child requires a well-balanced diet with fat content between 20% and 30% of calories consumed.

- Adequate physical activity and provision of a nutrient-dense diet (rather than foods high in fat and sugar) are the foundation for obesity prevention in the preschool child.

- Adequate dental care is important for the health of the primary teeth.

- Preschoolers need about 11 to 12 hours of sleep per day and benefit from a structured bedtime routine.

- Due to the active imagination of the preschooler, nightmares and night terrors may begin during this period.

- Safety and injury prevention remain a focus in the preschool years.

- Structure, appropriate limit setting, and consistency are the keys for effective discipline in the preschool period.

- Time-out is an effective disciplinary measure for preschoolers.

- Masturbation may occur as the preschooler discovers his or her body. If not excessive, it is considered a normal part of growth and development.

REFERENCES AND RECOMMENDED READINGS

AboutKidsHealth. (n.d). *Starting early with age-appropriate information about sex is a good idea*. Retrieved from http://www.aboutkidshealth.ca/En/HealthAZ/FamilyandPeerRelations/Sexuality/Pages/Sex-Education-for-Children-Why-Parents-Should-Talk-to-their-Kids-About-Sex.aspx.

American Academy of Pediatrics, The Injury Prevention Program. (2015). Safety for your child: 2 to 4 years. Retrieved from https://www.healthychildren.org/English/ages-stages/toddler/Pages/Safety-for-Your-Child-2-to-4-Years.aspx

Bellini, S., Pereda, V., Cordero, N., & Suarez-Morales, L. (2016). Developing multicultural awareness in preschool children: A pilot intervention. *Open Journal of Social Sciences, 4*(07), 182–189. Retrieved from http://dx.doi.org/10.4236/jss.2016.47028

Bhawra, J., Cooke, M. J., Guo, Y., & Wilk, P. (2017). The association of household food security, household characteristics and school environment with obesity status among off-reserve First Nations and Métis children and youth in Canada: results from the 2012 Aboriginal Peoples Survey. *Health Promotion and Chronic Disease Prevention in Canada: Research, Policy and Practice, 37*(3), 77–86. Retrieved from http://www.phac-aspc.gc.ca/publicat/hpcdp-pspmc/37-3/assets/pdf/ar-03-eng.pdf

Brown, J. (2011). *Nutrition now* (6th ed.). Florence, KY: Wadsworth Publishing.

Canadian Association of Poison Control Centre. (2016). *Provincial Centres*. Retrieved from http://www.capcc.ca/

Canadian Association of Poison Control Centres. (2017). Retrieved from http://www.capcc.ca/en

Canadian Dental Association. (2010). *Report on early childhood caries*. Retrieved from https://www.cda-adc.ca/_files/position_statements/earlyChildhoodCaries.pdf

Canadian Institute for Health Information (CIHI). (2014). *Children vulnerable in areas of early development: A determinant of child health*. Retrieved from https://secure.cihi.ca/free_products/Children_Vulnerable_in_Areas_of_Early_Development_EN.pdf

Canadian Paediatric Society. (n.d.). *Community resources*. Retrieved from http://www.cps.ca/en/first-debut/map/community-resources

Canadian Paediatric Society. (2008). Transportation of infants and children in motor vehicles. Retrieved from http://www.cps.ca/documents/position/car-seat-safety

Canadian Paediatric Society. (2012a). Child and youth injury prevention: A public health approach. Retrieved from http://www.cps.ca/documents/position/child-and-youth-injury-prevention

Canadian Paediatric Society. (2012b). Healthy active living: Physical activity guidelines for children and adolescents. Retrieved from http://www.cps.ca/documents/position/physical-activity-guidelines

Canadian Paediatric Society. (2015). Preventing unintentional injuries in Indigenous children and youth in Canada. Retrieved from http://www.cps.ca/en/documents/position/unintentional-injuries-indigenous-children-youth

Canadian Paediatric Society. (2016a). *Are we doing enough*. Retrieved from http://www.cps.ca/en/status-report

Canadian Paediatric Society. (2016b). Effective discipline for children. Retrieved from http://www.cps.ca/documents/position/discipline-for-children

Canadian Paediatric Society. (2016c). Position statement: Management of primary nocturnal enuresis by Feldman, M. Retrieved from http://www.cps.ca/en/documents/position/primary-nocturnal-enuresis

Canadian Paediatric Society. (2016d). Youth and firearms in Canada. Retrieved from http://www.cps.ca/documents/position/youth-and-firearms

Canadian Society for Exercise Physiology. (2012). Canadian physical activity guidelines for the early years: 0–4. Retrieved from http://www.csep.ca/CMFiles/Guidelines/CanadianPhysicalActivityGuidelinesStatements_E_5.pdf

Carpenito-Moyet, L. J. (2013). *Nursing diagnosis: Application to clinical practice* (14th ed.). Philadelphia, PA: Lippincott Williams & Wilkins.

Cavanaugh, K. (2011). Parasomnias. *Advance for NPs & Pas, 2*(2), 21–24.

Chahal, H., Fung, C., Kuhle, S., & Veugelers, P. J. (2013). Availability and night-time use of electronic entertainment and communication devices are associated with short sleep duration and obesity among Canadian children. *Pediatric Obesity, 8*(1), 42–51.

Clarke, M., & Krol, D. (2013). *Protecting all children's teeth (PACT): Oral health screening*. Retrieved from https://www.mededportal.org/publication/9462/ doi 10.15766/mep_2374-8265.9462

Coe, H. A. (2016). Embracing risk in the Canadian woodlands: Four children's risky play and risk-taking experiences in a Canadian Forest Kindergarten. *Journal of Early Childhood Research*. Retrieved from https://doi.org/10.1177/1476718X15614042

Collings, P., Marten, M. G., Pearce, T., & Young, A. G. (2016). Country food sharing networks, household structure, and implications for understanding food insecurity in Arctic Canada. *Ecology of food and nutrition, 55*(1), 30–49. Retrieved from http://dx.doi.org/10.1080/03670244.2015.1072812

Dietitians of Canada and Canadian Paediatric Society. (2014). A health professional's guide for using the WHO growth charts for Canada. Retrieved from http://www.dietitians.ca/Downloads/Public/DC_HealthProGrowthGuideE.aspx

Erikson, E. H. (1963). *Childhood and society* (2nd ed.). New York: W. W. Norton and Company.

Feigelman, S. (2011). Preschool years. In R. M. Kliegman, B. F. Stanton, J. W. St. Geme III, N. F. Schor, & R. E. Behrman (Eds.). *Nelson's textbook of pediatrics* (19th ed.). Philadelphia, PA: Elsevier, Saunders.

Fitzpatrick, C., McKinnon, R. D., Blair, C. B., & Willoughby, M. T. (2014). Do preschool executive function skills explain the school readiness gap between advantaged and disadvantaged children? *Learning and Instruction, 30*, 25–31. Retrieved from http://dx.doi.org/10.1016/j.learninstruc.2013.11.003

Garriguet, D., Carson, V., Colley, R. C., Janssen, I., Timmons, B. W., & Tremblay, M. S. (2016). Physical activity and sedentary behaviour of Canadian children aged 3 to 5. *Health Reports, 27*(9), 14–23.

Goldbloom, R. B. (2011). Assessing physical growth and nutrition. In R. B. Goldbloom (Ed.). *Paediatric Clinical Skills* (4th ed., pp. 22–37). Philadelphia, PA: Elsevier.

Goldson, E., & Reynolds, A. (2012). Child development & behaviour. In W. W. Hay, M. J. Levin, R. R. Deterding, & M. J. Abzug (Eds.). *Current diagnosis & treatment: Pediatrics* (21st ed.). New York: McGraw-Hill.

Gosselin, J., Romano, E., Bell, T., Babchishin, L., Buhs, I. H. V. D., Gagné, A., & Gosselin, N. (2014). Canadian portrait of changes in family structure and preschool children's behavioral outcomes. *International Journal of Behavioral Development, 38*(6), 518–528. Retrieved from https://doi.org/10.1177/0165025414535121

Graversen, L., Sørensen, T., Petersen, L., Sovio, U., Kaakinen, M., Sandbaek, A., ... Obel, C. (2014). Preschool weight and body mass index in relation to central obesity and metabolic syndrome in adulthood. *PLoS ONE, 9*(3), 1–9.

Guevremont, A., Bougie, E., & Kohen, D. (2016). Housing and Health among Young First Nations children living off reserve: Results from the 2006 Aboriginal Children's Survey. *Aboriginal Policy Studies, 5*(2). Retrieved from http://dx.doi.org/10.5663/aps.v5i2.24313

Gulati, S. (2013). *Literacy matters: Unlocking the literacy potential of Aboriginal peoples in Canada*. Retrieved from http://www.td.com/document/PDF/economics/special/LiteracyMattersUnlockingtheLiteracyPotentialofAboriginalPeoplesinCanada.pdf

Gupta, R. C. (2014). *Sleep and your preschooler*. Retrieved from http://kidshealth.org/parent/general/sleep/sleep_preschool.html

Haemer, M., Primark, L. E., & Krebs, N. R. (2012). Normal childhood nutrition and its disorders. In W. W. Hay, M. J. Levin, R. R. Deterding, & M. J. Abzug (Eds.). *Current Diagnosis & Treatment: Pediatrics* (21st ed.). New York: McGraw-Hill.

Hagel, B. E., & Yanchar, N. L. (2013). Bicycle helmet use in Canada: The need for legislation to reduce the risk of head injury. *Paediatric Child Health, 18*(9), 475–480. Retrieved from https://www.cps.ca/en/documents/position/bike-helmets-to-reduce-risk-of-head-injury

Hall, J. R. (2013). *Deaths and injuries due to non-fire exposure to gases*. Retrieved from http://www.nfpa.org/research/reports-and-statistics/non-fire-incidents/exposure-to-gases

Harrison, S., Rowlinson, M., & Hill, A. J. (2016). "No fat friend of mine": Young children's responses to overweight and disability. *Body Image, 18*, 65–73. Retrieved from http://dx.doi.org/10.1016/j.bodyim.2016.05.002

Health Canada. (2012). *Is your child safe? Sleep time*. Retrieved from http://www.hc-sc.gc.ca/cps-spc/pubs/cons/child-enfant/sleep-coucher-eng.php#a1

Health Canada. (2016). *Eating well with Canada's food guide*. Retrieved from http://www.hc-sc.gc.ca/fn-an/food-guide-aliment/index-eng.php

Hodges, E. A., Smith, C., Tidwell, S., & Berry, D. (2013). Promoting physical activity in preschoolers to prevent obesity: A review of the literature. *Journal of Pediatric Nursing, 28*, 3–19.

Institute of Medicine. (2011). *Early childhood obesity prevention policies*. Retrieved http://www.nationalacademies.org/hmd/Reports/2011/Early-Childhood-Obesity-Prevention-Policies.aspx

Irwin, J. D., Johnson, A. M., Vanderloo, L. M., Burke, S. M., & Tucker, P. (2015). Temperament and Objectively Measured Physical Activity and Sedentary Time among Canadian Preschoolers. *Preventive Medicine Reports, 2*, 598–601.

Keeley, R. J. (2010). Faith development and faith formation: More than just ages and stages. *Lifelong Faith, 4.3*, 20–27.

Kohlberg, L. (1984). *Moral development*. New York: Harper & Row.

Lightbody, T. K., & Williamson, D. L. (2017). The timing and intensity of maternal employment in early childhood: Implications for Canadian children. *Journal of Child and Family Studies, 26*, 1–13.

Lipnowski, S., & LeBlanc, C. M. A.; Canadian Paediatric Society; Healthy Active Living; Sports Medicine Committee. (2012). Healthy active living: Physical activity guidelines for children and adolescents. *Paediatrics & Child Health, 17*(4), 209–212. Retrieved from http://www.cps.ca/documents/position/physical-activity-guidelines

Lowry, L. (2011). Bilingualism in young children: Separating fact from fiction. Retrieved from http://www.hanen.org/Helpful-Info/Articles/Bilingualism-in-Young-Children–Separating-Fact-fr.aspx

Lukie, I. K., Skwarchuk, S. L., LeFevre, J. A., & Sowinski, C. (2014). The role of child interests and collaborative parent–child interactions in fostering numeracy and literacy development in Canadian homes. *Early Childhood Education Journal, 42*(4), 251–259.

Morrongiello, B. A., & Corbett, M. (2016). Parents' perspectives on preschool children's in-home falls: Implications for injury prevention. *Vulnerable Children and Youth Studies, 11*(2), 136–145. Retrieved from http://dx.doi.org/10.1080/17450128 .2016.1173754

National Institutes of Health. (2016). Iron dietary supplement fact sheet. Retrieved from http://ods.od.nih.gov/factsheets/ Iron-HealthProfessional/#h4

National Reading Campaign. (2017). Retrieved from http:// www.nationalreadingcampaign.ca

Office of the Chief Medical Officer of Health. (2016). Immunization program guide. Retrieved from http://www2.gnb.ca/ content/dam/gnb/Departments/h-s/pdf/en/CDC/Health Professionals/NBIPG-policy_2-9-e.pdf

Ontario Ministry of Health and Long-Term Care. (2017). Immunization. Retrieved from http://www.health.gov.on.ca/ en/pro/programs/immunization/ispa.aspx

Pan-Canadian Public Health Network. (2015). *Towards a healthier Canada—2015 progress report on advancing the federal/ provincial/territorial framework on healthy weights.* Retrieved from http://www.phn-rsp.ca/thcpr-vcpsre-2015/index-eng.php

Papalia, D., & Feldman, R. (2011). *A child's world: Infancy through adolescence* (12th ed.). New York: McGraw-Hill.

Piaget, J. (1969). *The theory of stages in cognitive development.* New York: McGraw-Hill.

Public Health Agency of Canada. (n.d.). *Injury prevention funding to promote active and safe play.* Retrieved from http://www.phac-aspc.gc.ca/inj-bles/fs-fr/2013_0121-eng.php

Public Health Agency of Canada. (2004). *Family front and centre.* Retrieved from http://www.phac-aspc.gc.ca/hp-ps/ dca-dea/publications/ffc-ief/assets/pdf/ffc_self_esteem.pdf

Public Health Agency of Canada. (2016). *To promote the health, well-being and school readiness of Aboriginal children.* Retrieved from http://www.phac-aspc.gc.ca/hp-ps/ dca-dea/prog-ini/fs-fr/2013_0114-eng.php

Pujadas Botey, A., Vinturache, A., Bayrampour, H., Breitkreuz, R., Bukutu, C., Gibbard, B., & Tough, S. (2016). Adults' knowledge of child development in Alberta, Canada: Comparing the level of knowledge of adults in two samples in 2007 and 2013. *Child Care in Practice, 23*(4), 1–13. Retrieved from http://dx.doi.org/10.1080/13575279.2016.1215292

Reza, M., Amin, M. S., Sgro, A., Abdelaziz, A., Ito, D., Main, P., & Azarpazhooh, A. (2016). Oral health status of immigrant and refugee children in North America: A scoping review. *Journal - Canadian Dental Association, 82*(g3), 1488–2159. Retrieved from http://www.jcda.ca/g3

Ross, C. A., Taylor, C. L., Yaktine, A. L., & Del Valle, H. B. (Eds.). (2011). *DRI dietary reference intakes calcium vitamin D.* Washington, DC: The National Academies Press.

Rowan-Legg, A. (2013). Oral health care for children—a call for action. *Paediatric Child Health, 18*(1), 37–43. Retrieved from http://www.cps.ca/documents/position/oral-health-care-for-children

Schroth, R. J., Harrison, R. L., & Moffatt, M. E. (2009). Oral health of indigenous children and the influence of early childhood caries on childhood health and well-being. *Pediatric Clinics of North America, 56*(6), 1481–1499. Retrieved from http://dx.doi.org/10.1016/j.pcl.2009.09.010

Sears, W., & Sears, M. (2015a). 10 techniques to shape children's behaviour. Retrieved from http://www.askdrsears. com/topics/parenting/discipline-behavior/shape-childrens-behavior

Sears, W., & Sears, M. (2015b). 10 time-out for children techniques. Retrieved from http://www.askdrsears.com/topics/ parenting/discipline-behavior/10-time-out-techniques

Sears, W., & Sears, M. (2015c). Why do kids lie—what to do. Retrieved from http://www.askdrsears.com/topics/parenting/ discipline-behavior/morals-manners/why-do-kids-lie

Statistics Canada. (2006). *Readiness to learn at school among 5 year old Canadians.* Retrieved from http://www.statcan. gc.ca/pub/89-599-m/2006004/4053157-eng.htm#1

Stettler, N., Bhatia, J., Parish, A., & Stallings, V. A. (2011). Feeding healthy infants, children, and adolescents. In R. M. Kliegman, B. F. Stanton, J. W. St. Geme III, N. F. Schor, & R. E. Behrman (Eds.). *Nelson's Textbook of Pediatrics* (19th ed.). Philadelphia, PA: Elsevier, Saunders.

Tatangelo, G., McCabe, M., Mellor, D., & Mealey, A. (2016). A systematic review of body dissatisfaction and sociocultural messages related to the body among preschool children. *Body Image, 18*, 86–95. Retrieved from http://dx.doi. org/10.1016/j.bodyim.2016.06.003

Timmons, B. W., Naylor, P. J., & Pfeiffer, K. A. (2007). Physical activity for preschool children—how much and how? This article is part of a supplement entitled Advancing physical activity measurement and guidelines in Canada: A scientific review and evidence-based foundation for the future of Canadian physical activity guidelines. *Can J Public Health* 98 (Suppl 2). *Applied Physiology, Nutrition, and Metabolism, 32*(S2E), S122–S134. Retrieved from http://www.nrcresearch-press.com/doi/pdf/10.1139/H07-112

Transport Canada. (2016a). Installing and using a child car seat, booster seat, or seat belt. Retrieved from https://www. canada.ca/en/services/transport/road/child-car-seat-safety/ installing-using-child-car-seat-booster-seat-seat-belt.html

Transport Canada. (2016b). Stage 2: Forward-facing car seats. Retrieved from https://www.tc.gc.ca/en/services/road/child-car-seat-safety/installing-child-car-seat-booster-seat/stage-2-forward-facing-seats.html

Transport Canada. (2016c). Stage 3: Booster seats. Retrieved from https://www.tc.gc.ca/en/services/road/child-car-seat-safety/installing-child-car-seat-booster-seat/stage-3-booster-seats.html

Tucker, P. (2008). The physical activity levels of preschool-aged children: A systematic review. *Early Childhood Research Quarterly, 23*, 547–558.

Tucker P., Vanderloo L. M., Newnham-Kanas C. (2013). Learning Environments' Activity Potential for Preschoolers (LEAPP): study rationale and design. *J Public Health Res, 2*(2), E19.

Warren, R., Kenny, M., Bennett, T., Fitzpatrick-Lewis, D., Ali, M. U., … Raina, P. (2016). Screening for developmental delay among children aged 1–4 years: A systematic review. *CMAJ Open, 4*(1), E20.

Yanchar, N. L., Warda, L. J., & Fuselli, P. (2012). Child and youth injury prevention: A public health approach. *Paediatrics & child health, 17*(9), 511–511.

CHAPTER **WORKSHEET**

MULTIPLE CHOICE QUESTIONS

1. The nurse is caring for a hospitalized 4 year old who insists on having the nurse perform every assessment and intervention on her imaginary friend first. She then agrees to have the assessment or intervention done to herself. The nurse identifies this preschooler's behaviour as:
   a. Problematic; the child is old enough to begin to have a basis in reality.
   b. Normal, because the child is hospitalized and out of her routine.
   c. Normal for this stage of growth and development.
   d. Problematic, as it interferes with needed nursing care.

2. The mother of a 3 year old is concerned about her child's speech. She describes her preschooler as hesitating at the beginning of sentences and repeating consonant sounds. What is the nurse's best response?
   a. Hesitancy and dysfluency are normal during this period of development.
   b. Reading to the child will help model appropriate speech.
   c. Expressive language concerns warrant a developmental evaluation.
   d. The mother should ask her child's physician for a speech therapy evaluation.

3. The mother of a 4 year old asks for advice on using time-out for discipline with her child. What advice should the nurse give the mother?
   a. If spanking is not working, then time-out is not likely to be helpful either.
   b. Place the child in time-out for 4 minutes.
   c. Use time-out only if removing privileges is unsuccessful.
   d. The child should stay in time-out until crying ceases.

4. A 5-year-old child is not gaining weight appropriately. Organic problems have been ruled out. What is the priority action by the nurse?
   a. Allow the child unlimited access to the sippy cup to ensure adequate hydration.
   b. Encourage sweets for the extra caloric content.
   c. Teach the mother about nutritional needs of the preschooler.
   d. Assess the child's usual intake pattern at home.

5. The nurse is providing teaching about accidental poisoning to the family of a 3 year old. The nurse understands that a child of this age is at increased risk of accidental ingestion due to which sensory alteration?
   a. A lack of fully developed hearing.
   b. A less discriminating sense of touch.
   c. Visual acuity that has not fully developed.
   d. A less discriminating sense of taste.

DOSAGE CALCULATION QUESTIONS

1. A child who weighs 33 kg has an order for acetaminophen 10 mg/kg/dose, every 4 hours prn pain or fever.
   a. How many milligrams will the child receive per dose?
   b. Acetaminophen elixir is provided as 160 mg/5 mL. How many milliliters will the nurse administer per dose?

CRITICAL THINKING EXERCISES

1. Teach a preschool class about bicycle and street safety. Be certain to design the content at an appropriate developmental level.

2. Construct a 3-day menu for a picky 4 year old. Include three daily meals and two snacks. Follow the nutritional guidelines recommended by the Canada Food Guide.

3. Colour or draw with a preschool child. Analyze the drawings and interactions or discussions you have with the child, relating them to psychosocial and cognitive development expected at this age.

STUDY ACTIVITIES

1. Care for two average 3-, 4-, or 5-year-old children in the clinical setting (make sure both are the same age). Describe each child's development level, response to hospitalization, and family dynamics.

2. Visit a preschool that provides care for special needs children as well as typically developing children. Perform a development assessment on a typical child and one with special needs (both the same age). Compare and contrast your findings.

3. Observe in a 3-, 4-, or 5-year-old classroom of a typical preschool. Choose two children who are the same age with different temperaments. Record the differences and similarities in their response to structure and authority, interactions with classmates, attention levels, and language and activity levels.

BRINGING IT ALL TOGETHER: A CASE STUDY

Steven, a 4-year-old boy, is seen in the paediatric office for a well-child examination. He is a healthy, active boy who attends extended-day preschool as his mother works long hours. His mother states she has some questions about Steven. She says she is concerned about Steven's growth, his language skills, and disciplining him. Steven's mother tells you that "he seems heavier than my other children did at his age." Upon measuring Steven you note his height to be 98 cm (38.5 in) and his weight to be 20.9 kg (46 lb). His calculated BMI of 21.76 plots well above the 95th percentile for age. After further discussion with Steven's mother, you determine that he has an excessive daily intake of fruit juice and whole milk, and eats numerous fast food meals weekly.

Go to thePoint **to find questions to consider about this case.**

Growth and Development of the School-Age Child

KEY TERMS

bruxism
caries
industry
inferiority
malocclusion
prepubescence
principle of
   conservation
school-age children
school refusal
self-esteem
temperament

Learning Objectives

Upon completion of the chapter, you will be able to:

1. Identify normal physiologic, cognitive, and moral changes occurring in the school-age child.

2. Describe the role of peers and schools in the development and socialization of the school-age child.

3. Identify the developmental milestones of the school-age child.

4. Identify the role of the nurse in promoting safety for the school-age child.

5. Demonstrate knowledge of the nutritional requirements of the school-age child.

6. Identify common developmental concerns in the school-age child.

7. Demonstrate knowledge of the appropriate nursing guidance for common developmental concerns.

Lawrence Jones **is a 10-year-old boy brought to the clinic by his mother for his annual school checkup. During your assessment, you measure his weight at 28.1 kg (62 lb) and his height at 137.2 cm (54 in). As the nurse caring for him, assess Lawrence's growth and development, and then provide appropriate anticipatory guidance to his mother.**

INTRODUCTION

School-age children, between the ages of 6 and 12 years, are experiencing a time of slow progressive physical growth, while their social and developmental growth accelerates and increases in complexity. The focus of their world expands from family to teachers, peers, and other outside influences (e.g., coaches, social media). The child at this stage becomes increasingly more independent while participating in activities outside the home.

 ## Growth and Development Overview

The school-age years are a time of continued maturation of the child's physical, social, and psychological characteristics. It is during this time that children move toward abstract thinking and seek approval of peers, teachers, and parents. Their eye–hand–muscle coordination allows them to participate in organized sports in school or the community. The school-age child typically values school attendance and school activities. The nurse uses knowledge of normal growth and development of the school-age child to assist the child with coping with disruptions and changes during this time period.

PHYSICAL GROWTH

From 6 to 12 years of age, children grow an average of 5 to 7 cm (2.5 in) per year, increasing their height by at least 30 to 60 cm. An increase of 3 to 3.5 kg (7 lb) per year in weight is expected (Feigelman, 2011a). In the early school-age years, girls and boys are similar in height and weight and appear thinner and more graceful than in previous years. In later school-age years, most girls begin to surpass boys in both height and weight. (See the Point for links to growth charts.) An example of comprehensive health assessment tools is the Greig Health Record. Both the Canadian Paediatric Society and the College of Family Physcians of Canada endorse the use of this record in clinical practice (CPS, 2016a).

Preadolescent boys and girls do not want to be different from peers of the same sex or the opposite sex, although there are differences in physical and physiologic growth during the school-age years. These differences, especially secondary sexual characteristics, are concerning and often a source of embarrassment for both sexes.

The differences between girls and boys are more apparent at the end of the middle-school years and may become extreme and a source of emotional problems. These differences in height and weight relationships, and changes in growth patterns, should be explained to parents and children (Fig. 28.1). Physical maturity is not necessarily associated with emotional and social maturity. An 8 year old who is the size of an 11 year old will think and act like an 8 year old. Many times, the expectations placed on these children are unrealistic and can impact the self-esteem and competence of the child. This can work in reverse, to similar effect, for an 11 year old who is the size of an 8 year old and is therefore treated as such.

ORGAN SYSTEMS MATURATION

Maturation of organs may differ with age or gender. Maturation of organs remains fairly consistent until late school age. In the late school-age years (10 to 12 year olds), boys experience a slowed growth in height and increased weight gain, which may lead to obesity. During this time, girls may begin to have changes in the body that soften body lines. Preadolescence is a period of rapid growth, especially for girls.

FIGURE 28.1 The different growth rates of school-age children are depicted by these same-age school-age children.

Neurologic System

The brain and skull grow very slowly during the school-age years. Brain growth is complete by the time the child is 10 years of age. The shape of the head is longer and the growth of the facial bones changes facial proportions.

Respiratory System

The respiratory system continues to mature with the development of the lungs and alveoli, resulting in fewer respiratory infections. Respiratory rates decrease, abdominal breathing disappears, and respirations become diaphragmatic in nature. The frontal sinuses are developed by 7 years of age. Tonsils decrease in size from the preschool years, but they remain larger than those of adolescents. The adenoids and tonsils may appear large normally, even in the absence of infection.

Cardiovascular System

The school-age child's blood pressure increases and the pulse rate decreases. The heart grows more slowly during the middle years and is smaller in size in relation to the rest of the body than at any other developmental stage.

Gastrointestinal System

During the school-age years, all 20 primary deciduous teeth are lost, replaced by 28 of 32 permanent teeth, with the exception of the third molars (commonly known as wisdom teeth). The school-age child experiences fewer gastrointestinal upsets compared with earlier years. Stomach capacity increases, which permits retention of food for longer periods of time. In addition, the caloric needs of the school-age child are lower than in the earlier years.

Genitourinary System

Bladder capacity increases, but varies among individual children. Girls generally have a greater bladder capacity than boys. Urination patterns vary with the amount of fluids ingested, the time they were ingested, and the stress level of the child. The formula for bladder capacity up to adult age can be estimated using the formula: age in years plus 2 × 30 mL. Therefore, the bladder capacity of the 7 year old would be 270 mL. Increased bladder capacity allows longer times between voiding.

Prepubescence

The late school-age years are also referred to as *preadolescence* (the time between middle childhood and the 13th birthday). During preadolescence, **prepubescence** occurs. Prepubescence typically occurs in the 2 years before the beginning of puberty and is characterized by the development of secondary sexual characteristics, a period of rapid growth for girls, and a period of continued growth for boys. There is approximately 2 years' difference in the onset of prepubescence between boys and girls. Sexual development in both boys and girls can lead to a negative perception of physical appearance and lowered self-esteem. Early development in girls can lead to embarrassment, concern over physical appearance, and lower self-esteem. Delayed development in boys can lead to a negative self-concept, increased risk-taking behaviours, and difficulties in relationships with peers and caregivers. It is important for the nurse and parents to educate the late school-age child about body changes, reframe thinking, be supportive and listen to any anxieties with a view to supporting the child learn about and adjust to their bodily changes, changing emotions and perhaps questions about sex and gender development, roles and orientation.

Musculoskeletal System

Musculoskeletal growth leads to greater coordination and strength, yet the muscles are still immature and can be injured easily. Bones continue to ossify throughout childhood, but mineralization is not complete until maturity.

Immune System

Lymphatic tissues continue to grow until the child is 9 years old; immunoglobulins A and G (IgA and IgG) reach adult levels at around 10 years of age. Due to the lymphatic system becoming more competent in localizing infections and producing antibody–antigen responses, school-age children may have fewer infections. They may experience more infections during the first 1 to 2 years of school due to exposure to other children who may have infections.

PSYCHOSOCIAL DEVELOPMENT

Erikson (1963) describes the task of the school-age years to be a sense of **industry** versus **inferiority** (Feigelman, 2011a). During this time, the child is developing his or her sense of self-worth by becoming involved in multiple activities at home, at school, and in the community, which develops his or her cognitive and social skills. The child is very interested in learning how things are made and work. The school-age child's satisfaction from achieving success in developing new skills, exploring his or her environment, and inclusion in peer activities supports him or her to increased sense of self-worth and level of competence. It is the role of the parents, teachers, coaches, and nurses of the school-age child to identify areas of competency and to build on the child's successful experiences to promote mastery, success, and self-esteem. If the expectations of adults are set too

TABLE 28.1		DEVELOPMENTAL THEORIES
Theorist	**Stage**	**Activities**
Erikson	Industry vs. inferiority	Interested in how things are made and run Success in personal and social tasks Increased activities outside home—clubs, sports Increased interactions with peers Increased interest in knowledge Needs support and encouragement from important people in child's life Needs support when child is not successful Inferiority occurs with repeated failures with little support or trust from those who are important to the child
Piaget	Concrete operational	Learns by manipulating concrete objects Lacks ability to think abstractly Learns that certain characteristics of objects remain constant Understands concepts of time Engages in serial ordering, addition, subtraction Classifies or groups objects by their common elements Understands relationships among objects Starts collections of items Can reverse thought process
Kohlberg	Conventional Stage 3: interpersonal conforming, "good child, bad child," age 7–10 years Stage 4: "law and order," age 10–12 years	An act is wrong because it brings punishment Behaviour is completely wrong or right Does not understand the reason behind rules If child and adult differ in opinions, the adult is right Can put self in another person's position Begins to exercise the "golden rule" Acts are judged in terms of intention, not just punishment
Freud	Latency	A time of tranquility between the Oedipal phase of early childhood and adolescence—focuses on activities that develop social and cognitive skills Develops social skills in relating to same-sex friends through joining clubs like Brownies, Girl Scouts, Boy Scouts

Adapted from Erikson, E. (1963). *Childhood and society* (2nd ed.). New York: Norton; Piaget, J. (1969). *The theory of stages in cognitive development.* New York: McGraw-Hill; Kohlberg, L. (1984). *Moral development.* New York: Harper & Row; and Feigelman, S. (2011b). Chapter 6: Overview and assessment variability. In R. M. Kleigman, B. F. Stanton, J. W. St. Geme III, N. F. Schor, & R. E. Behrman (Eds.). *Nelson textbook of pediatrics* (19th ed., p. 26). Philadelphia, PA: Saunders.

high, the child will develop a sense of inferiority and incompetence that can affect all aspects of his or her life. See Table 28.1 for a further explanation of psychosocial development in school-age children.

COGNITIVE DEVELOPMENT

Piaget's stage of cognitive development for the 7 to 11 year old is the period of concrete operational thoughts (Feigelman, 2011a). In developing concrete operations, the child is able to assimilate and coordinate information about his or her world from different dimensions. The child is able to see things from another person's point of view and think through an action, anticipating its consequences and the possibility of having to rethink the action. He or she is able to use stored memories of past experiences to evaluate and interpret present situations. The school-age child also develops the ability to classify or divide things into different sets and to identify their relationships to each other. The school-age child is able to classify members of four generations on a family tree vertically and horizontally, and at the same time see that one person can be a father, son, uncle, and grandson. It is at this time that the school-age child develops an interest in collecting objects. The child starts out collecting multiple objects and becomes more selective as he or she gets older. Also, during concrete operational thinking, the school-age child develops an understanding of the **principle of conservation**—that matter does not change when its form changes. For example, if the child pours a half cup of water into a short, wide glass and into a tall, thin glass, she still only has a half cup of water despite the fact that it looks like the tall, thin glass has more (Fig. 28.2). She learns about conserving matter in a sequence ranging from the simplest to the more complex. See Table 28.1 for further information about cognitive development of school-age children.

FIGURE 28.2 School-age children understand the theory of conservation (**A**). If you pour an equal amount of liquid into two glasses of unequal shape (**B**), the amount of water you have remains the same despite the unequal appearance in the two glasses (**C**).

MORAL AND SPIRITUAL DEVELOPMENT

During the school-age years, the child's sense of morality is constantly being developed. According to Kohlberg, the school-age child is at the conventional stage of moral development (Kohlberg, 1984). The 7 to 10 year old usually follows rules out of a sense of being a "good" person. He or she wants to be a good person to parents, friends, and teachers and to himself or herself. The adult is viewed as being right. This is stage 3: interpersonal conformity (good child, bad child), according to Kohlberg. The 10 to 12 year olds progress to stage 4: the "law and order" stage. At this stage, the child can determine if an action is good or bad based on the reason for the action, not just on the possible consequences of the action. The older school-age child's behaviour is guided by his or her desire to cooperate and by his or her respect for others. This leads to the school-age child's ability to understand and incorporate into his or her behaviour the concept of the "golden rule," to treat others how you would like to be treated (Feigelman, 2011a). See Table 28.1 for additional information about the moral development of school-age children.

During school age, children may develop a desire to understand more about their religion (CPS, 2016b) and should have the right to do so (Bennett & Auger, 2013). While they are still concrete thinkers guided by their family's religious and cultural beliefs, the opportunity to share and talk about spiritual beliefs is important (Smylie, 2011). They are comforted by the rituals of their religion and spirituality, but are just beginning to understand the differences between natural and supernatural. Incorporating religious practices in their lives can assist school-age children in coping with different stressors.

MOTOR SKILL DEVELOPMENT

Gross and fine motor skills continue to mature throughout the school-age years. Refinement of motor skills occurs, and speed and accuracy increase. To assess the motor skills of school-age children, ask questions about participation in sports and after-school activities, band membership, constructing models, and writing skills.

Gross Motor Skills

During the school-age years, coordination, balance, and rhythm improve, facilitating the opportunity to ride a two-wheel bike, jump rope, dance, and participate in a variety of other sports (Fig. 28.3). Older school-age children may become awkward due to their bodies growing faster than their ability to compensate.

School-age children between the ages of 6 and 8 enjoy gross motor activities such as bicycling, skating, and swimming. They are enthralled with the world and are in constant motion. Sometimes, fear is limited due to the strong impulses of exploration. Children between 8 and 10 years of age are less restless, but their energy level continues to be high with activities more subdued and directed. These children exhibit greater rhythm and gracefulness of muscular movements, allowing them to participate in physical activities that require longer and

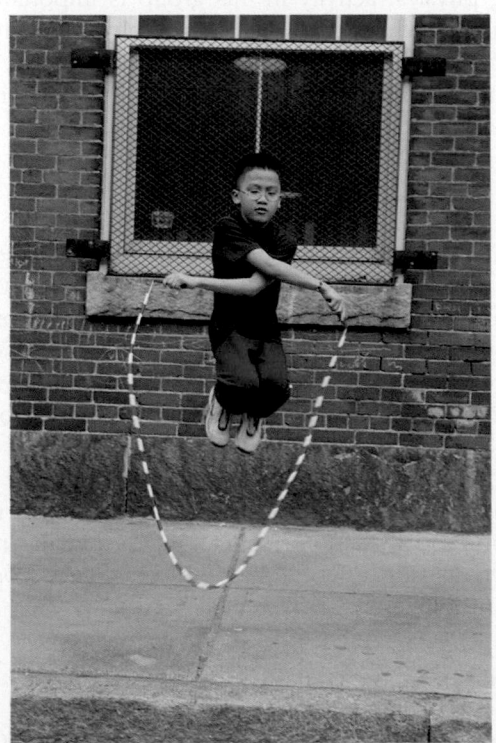

FIGURE 28.3 Jumping rope is an example of the increased development of gross motor skills of the school-age child.

FIGURE 28.4 School-age children improve their fine motor skills so they can play musical instruments well.

more concentrated attention and effort, such as baseball or soccer.

Between the ages of 10 and 12 years (the pubescent years for girls), energy levels remain high but are more controlled and focused. Physical skills in this age group are similar to those of adults, with strength and endurance increasing during adolescence.

All school-age children should be encouraged to engage in physical activities and learn physical skills that contribute to their health for the rest of their lives. Cardiovascular fitness, weight control, emotional tension release, and development of leadership and following skills are enhanced through physical activity and team sports. Promoting physical activity in this group is important, with >60 minutes of moderate to intensive physical daily activity that strengthens muscles and bone (CPS, 2015). Screen time should be limited to no more than 2 hours per day as well as sedentary time (such as sitting indoors).

Fine Motor Skills

Myelinization of the central nervous system is reflected by refinement of fine motor skills. Eye–hand coordination and balance improve with maturity and practice. Hand usage improves, becomes steadier and independent resulting in greater precision which allows the child to write, print words, sew, or build models or other crafts. The child between 10 and 12 years of age begins to exhibit manipulative skills comparable to adults. School-age children take pride in activities that require dexterity and fine motor skills such as playing musical instruments (Fig. 28.4). Talent and practice become the keys to proficiency.

SENSORY DEVELOPMENT

All senses are mature early in the school-age years. The typical school-age child has 20/20 visual acuity (Jarvis, 2012). Good vision is essential to the physical development

and educational progression of school-age children. Problems such as amblyopia (lazy eye), uncorrected refractive errors or other eye defects, and malalignment of the eyes (called *strabismus*) warrant referral if not noted at screening in preschool years (CPS, 2016c). Amblyopia is reduced vision in an eye that has not been adequately used during early development. Inadequate use can result from conditions such as strabismus, one eye being more nearsighted, farsighted, or astigmatic than the other eye. Amblyopia is the leading cause of visual impairment in children (CPS, 2016c). If untreated in childhood, it can persist into adulthood causing monocular visual impairments. This condition is correctable with glasses or patching which forces the child to use the weaker eye. Recent clinical trials have suggested that older children (7 to 17 years) may benefit from these treatments, which are more commonly used on younger children.

Hearing deficits that are severe are usually diagnosed in infancy, but the less severe may not be diagnosed until the child enters school and has difficulty learning or with speech. It is important to refer children to screen programs for problems with hearing and speech (CPS, 2016b) to ensure proper educational and social progression. Speech delay and language deficit can also be as a result of underlying conditions such as fetal alcohol syndrome promoting referral to appropriate local assessment and provider services (CPS, 2016d).

The sense of smell is mature and can be tested in the school-age child by using scents that children are familiar with, such as chocolate or other familiar odours. In addition, the school-age child may be tested for the sense of touch with objects to discriminate cold from hot, soft from hard, and blunt from sharp.

COMMUNICATION AND LANGUAGE DEVELOPMENT

Language skills continue to accelerate during the school-age years and vocabulary expands. Culturally specific words are used, with bilingual children speaking English in school and a second language at home. The school-age child learns to read and reading efficiency improves language skills. Reading skills are improved with increased reading exposure and early experiences helping set children up for success (CPS, 2017a). School-age children begin to use more complex grammatical forms such as plurals and pronouns. Also, they develop metalinguistic awareness—an ability to think about language and comment on its properties. This enables them to enjoy jokes and riddles due to their understanding of double meanings and play on words and sounds. They are also beginning to understand metaphors such as "a stitch in time saves nine." School-age children may experiment with profanity and dirty jokes if exposed. This age group tends to imitate parents, family members, or others. Therefore, role modelling is very important.

EMOTIONAL AND SOCIAL DEVELOPMENT

Patterns of temperamental traits identified in infancy may continue to influence behaviour in the school-age child. Analyzing past situations may provide clues to the way a child may react to new or different situations. Children may react differently over time due to their experiences and abilities. **Self-esteem** is the child's view of his or her individual worth. This view is impacted by feedback from family, teachers, and other authority figures.

Temperament

Temperament has been described as the way individuals behave. Three commonly grouped temperaments are the child that is easy and adaptable, the child that is slow to warm up, or the child that is difficult and easily frustrated (Feigelman, 2011b). Variations and combinations of these categories are seen. Not every child can be placed into one of these groups. Understanding a child's temperament can help care providers and parents to understand the child's behaviour, actions, and how the child relates to the world. For example, the child who is easy may adapt to school entry and other experiences smoothly and with little or no stress. The slow-to-warm child may be slow to adapt to changes. The slow-to-warm school-age child may exhibit discomfort when placed in different or new situations such as school. This child may need time to adjust to the new place or situation, and may demonstrate frustration with tears or somatic complaints. The slow-to-warm child should be allowed time to adjust to new situations and people (such as teachers) within his or her own time frame. All of these factors may impact the younger school-age child upon entering the school environment, with changes in authority and the introduction of many peers. The difficult or easily distracted child may benefit from an introduction to the new experience and people by role-playing, by visiting the site and being introduced to the teachers, and by hearing stories or participating in conversations about the upcoming school experience. These children require patience, firmness, and understanding to make the transition into a new situation or experience such as school. Assessment of temperament by a professional would include a combination of interview, observation, and a standardized questionnaire. Better understanding a child's temperament can assist parents with adjusting their parenting style to better fit their child and may help limit emotional and behavioural problems that occur when these areas are in conflict (Feigelman, 2011b).

Self-Esteem Development

Self-esteem mirrors the child's individual self-worth and consists of both positive and negative qualities. Children strive to achieve internalized goals of attainment, although they continually receive feedback from individuals they perceive as authorities (parent or teacher). By the school-age years, children have received feedback related to their performance or tasks. The direction of this feedback influences the child's opinion of self-worth, which influences self-esteem and self-evaluation.

Children face the process of self-evaluation from a framework of either self-confidence or self-doubt. Children who have mastered the earlier developmental task of autonomy and initiative face the world with feelings of pride rather than shame (Erikson, 1963).

If school-age children regard themselves as worthwhile, they have a positive self-concept and high self-esteem. Significant adults in school-age children's lives can manipulate the environment to facilitate success. This success impacts the self-esteem of the child.

Body Image

Body image is how the school-age child perceives his or her body. School-age children are knowledgeable about the human body but may have different perceptions about body parts. School-age children are very interested in peers' views and acceptances of their body, body changes, and clothing. This age group may model themselves after parents, peers, and persons in movies or on television. It is important for late school-agers to feel accepted by peers. If they feel different and are teased, there may be lifelong effects.

School-Age Fears

School-age children are less fearful of harm to their body than in their preschool years, but fear being kidnapped or undergoing surgery. They continue to fear the dark and worry about their past behaviours. They fear death and are fascinated by death and dying. They are less fearful of animals, such as dogs and noises. The school-age child needs reassurance that his or her fears are normal for this developmental age. Parents, teachers, and other caretakers should discuss the fears and answer questions posed by the child (Child Development Institute, 2013). Recognize the child's fears but do not cater to them. Teach the child coping strategies such as positive self-statements such as "I can do this" and relaxation techniques such as deep breathing and visualization (Lyness, 2013).

Peer Relationships

The school-age child's concept of self is shaped not only by his or her parents but also by relationships with others. Peer relationships influence children's independence from parents. Peers play an important role in the approval and critiquing of skills of school-age children. Previously, only adults such as parents and teachers have been authorities; now, peers influence school-age

FIGURE 28.5 School-age children like to join clubs. These children, in the acting club at school, are rehearsing for a play.

children's perceptions of themselves. Peer relationships help to support the school-age child by providing enough security to risk the parental conflict brought about when establishing independence. School-age children associate with peers of the same sex most of the time. Although games and other activities are shared by both boys and girls, the child's concept of the appropriate sex role is influenced by his or her relationship with peers.

Continuous peer relationships provide the most important social interaction for school-age children. Valuable lessons are learned from interactions with children of their own age. Children learn to respect differing points of view that are represented in their groups (Fig. 28.5). Peer groups establish norms and standards that signify acceptance or rejection. Children may modify behaviour to gain acceptance. A characteristic of school-age children is their formation of groups with rules and values. Peer and peer-group identification are important to the socialization of the school-age child (Feigelman, 2011a).

Teacher and School Influences

School serves as a means to transmit values of society and to establish peer relationships. Secondary only to the family, school exerts a profound influence on the social development of the child. Often, school requires changes for the child and parent. The child enters an environment that requires conforming to group activities that are structured and directed by an adult other than the parent. The parent's attitude and support influences the child's transition into the school setting. Parents who are positive and supportive promote a smooth entry into school. Parents who encourage clinging behaviours may delay a successful transition into school.

To facilitate the transition from home to school, the teacher must have the personality and knowledge of development that will allow him or her to meet the needs

of young children. Even though the teacher's responsibilities are primarily to stimulate and guide intellectual development, they must share in shaping the child's attitudes and values. The system of awards and punishment administered by teachers affects the self-concept of children and influences their response to school. Teachers and school are important in shaping the socialization, self-concept, and intellectual development of children.

Family Influences

The school-age years are a time for peer relationships, questioning of parents, and the potential for parental conflict but continued respect for family values. School-age years are the beginning of the time of peer-group influence, with testing of parental and family values. Although the peer group is influential, the family's values usually predominate when parental and peer-group values come into conflict. Even though the school-age child may question the parents' values, the child will usually incorporate the values from parents into his or her values.

Many times in the late school-age and preadolescent period, the child may prefer to be in the company of peers and show a decreased interest in family functions. This may require an adjustment for parents. Parents' awareness of this developmental trend and their continuing support for the child are important while they continue to enforce restrictions and take control of behaviours. The school-aged child is beginning to strive for independence, but parental authority and controls continue to impact choices and values.

Take Note!

School-age children continue to need parenting. They do not need parents as pals.

CULTURAL INFLUENCES ON GROWTH AND DEVELOPMENT

Culture influences habits, beliefs, language, and values. School-age children thrive on learning the music, language, traditions, holidays, games, values, gender roles, and other aspects of culture. Nurses must be aware of the effects on children of various groups' family structures and traditional values. The school-age child's cultural and ethnic backgrounds must be considered when assessing growth and development, including differences in growth in children of different racial and cultural backgrounds. Cultural implications must be considered for all children and families in order to provide appropriate care.

Refer back to Lawrence Jones, who was introduced at the beginning of this chapter. What developmental milestones would you expect him to have reached by this age?

The Nurse's Role in School-Age Growth and Development

Growth and development in the school-age child occurs in irregular spurts with a wide variation of sizes, shapes, and abilities seen. Nurses must be aware of the usual growth and development patterns for this age group so that they can assess school-age children appropriately and provide guidance to the child and his or her family. This is a time when children compare themselves to peers and self-esteem is a central issue. The school-age child is separating from his or her parents and seeks acceptance from peers and adults outside of his or her family. Health care visits throughout the school-age period continue to focus on expected growth and development and anticipatory guidance. Visits are more infrequent during the school-age years; therefore, the nurse needs to assess the child's functioning not only at home but also at school and within the community.

If the school-age child is hospitalized, growth and development may be altered. The school-age child is able to understand the reason for hospitalization and what will happen. He or she is often worried about pain or changes that may occur to his or her body. It is important for health care providers and family members to be honest and open with the school-age child. The school-age child may miss school and the interactions with his or her peers. As such, he or she may regress and exhibit behaviours of a younger child, such as needing special comfort toys or demanding attention from his or her parents. Hospitalization for the school-age child can bring with it a loss of control. The school-age child is used to controlling his or her self-care and making choices about his or her meals and activities.

When caring for the hospitalized school-age child, the nurse must use knowledge of normal growth and development to recognize potential delays, promote continued appropriate growth and development, and interact successfully with the school-age child. Provide opportunities for the school-age child to maintain independence, gain control, and increase self-esteem.

See the Nursing Care Plan at the end of the chapter.

NURSING PROCESS OVERVIEW

Upon completion of assessment of the school-age child's current growth and development status, problems or issues related to growth and development may be identified. The nurse may then identify one or more nursing diagnoses, including:
* Risk for disproportionate growth
* Imbalanced nutrition: more than body requirements
* Delayed growth and development
* Risk for caregiver role strain
* Risk for injury

Nursing care planning for the school-age child with growth and development issues should be individualized based on the school-age child's and family's needs. The nursing care plan can be used as a guide in planning nursing care for the school-age child with a growth and development concern. The nurse may choose the appropriate nursing diagnoses from Nursing Care Plan 28.1 and individualize them as needed. The nursing care plan is intended to serve as a guide, not to be an all-inclusive growth and development care plan.

PROMOTING HEALTHY GROWTH AND DEVELOPMENT

The family plays a critical role in promoting healthy growth and development of the school-age child. Respectful interchange of communication between the parent and child will foster self-esteem and self-confidence. This respect will give the child confidence in achieving personal, educational, and social goals appropriate for his or her age. The nurse should study interactions between parents and school-age children to observe for this respect or lack of respect ("putting the child down"). The nurse can model appropriate behaviours by listening to the child and making appropriate responses. The nurse can be a resource for parents and an advocate for the child in promoting healthy growth and development.

Promoting Growth and Development Through Play

Cooperative play is exhibited by the school-age child. Play for the school-age child includes both organized cooperative activities (such as team sports) and solitary activities. School-age children have the coordination and intellect to participate with other children of their age in sports such as soccer, baseball, football, and tennis. The school-age child comprehends that his or her cooperation with others will lead to a unified whole for the team. In addition, the child learns rules and the value of playing by the rules.

School-age children also enjoy solitary activities including board, card, video, and computer games, and dollhouse and other small-figure play (Fig. 28.6). Many school-agers start collections of stamps, cars, or other valuable or not-so-valuable items. During the school-age years, children may also begin a scrapbook or keep a diary. They may participate in activities such as dance or karate. Girls and boys may join clubs, organizations such as Brownies/Cub Scouts or Guides etc., or other special interest groups.

Active play has decreased in recent years as television viewing and computer games have increased. This trend has resulted in health risks such as obesity, type 2 diabetes, and cardiovascular problems.

FIGURE 28.6 This school-age girl enjoys solitary play with her dollhouse and dolls.

Promoting Learning

School attendance and learning are very important to the school-age child. Parent–child, child–teacher, and child–peer relationships and activities influence the school-age child's learning.

Formal Education

Most children are excited about starting school and making new friends. They like the notion of getting books, having book bags, and having homework assignments. The reality of the work involved with school and homework may decrease the enthusiasm about school.

Peers are very important within this age group. Both peers and teachers influence children. Attending school may be their first experience interacting with a large number of children of their own age. Through this interaction, children learn cooperation, competition, and the importance of following the rules. Peer approval and influences grow as the child matures. Teachers have significant influences on children. They help to guide the child's intellectual development by rewarding successes and helping the child deal with failures. The student–teacher relationship is a key to success. Teachers play a role in fostering feelings of industry and preventing feelings of inferiority (Fig. 28.7). School-age children also learn skills, rules, values, and other ways to work with peers and other authority figures.

Parental support is important for school adjustment and achievement. Parents must collaborate with teachers and school personnel to ensure that the child is fulfilling the expectations and requirements for this age group in school. Parents can monitor the child's homework assignments and friends, and observe for any changes in behaviour that would indicate school or behavioural problems.

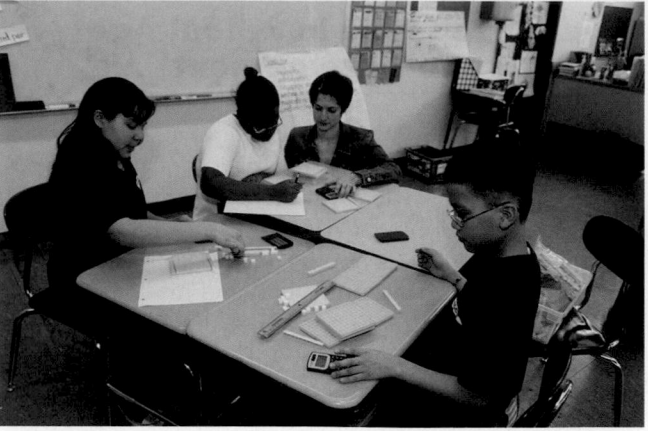

FIGURE 28.7 School is important to the school-age child.

Reading

Encouraging reading is an excellent way to promote learning in the school-age child. Trips to the library and purchasing books help to promote a love of reading. School-age children enjoy being read to as well as reading on their own. Younger school-age children (6 to 8 years) enjoy books that are simple to read with few words on a page (CPS, 2017a). They enjoy books about animals and trains and simple mysteries. Children 8 to 10 years of age have more advanced reading skills and enjoy those books from early childhood, plus more classic novels and adventures such as the Harry Potter series. Older children enjoy horror stories, mysteries, romances, and adventure stories as well as classic novels. School-age children of all ages benefit from books on topics related to things they may be experiencing, such as a visit to the hospital for a surgical procedure. See Box 28.1 for ideas for parents to promote reading in the school-age child.

BOX 28.1

PROMOTION OF READING IN SCHOOL-AGE CHILDREN

- Read to and with your children
- Ask teachers and librarians for advice on books appropriate for your child
- Choose stories that the child can relate to if the child has difficulty reading
- Choose books with movement if the child has a short attention span
- Take advantage of all reading opportunities (cereal boxes, road signs)
- Provide choices for the child to select a book of interest
- Talk about the text and ask questions to improve understanding
- Keep a record of what the child is reading
- Visit a library, get a library card, and check out books
- Demonstrate role modelling through reading books

Promoting Safety

School-age children become more independent with age. This independence leads to an increased self-confidence and decreased fears, which may contribute to accidents and injuries. School age is a time that the child may walk to school with peers who may influence his or her behaviour. Increased independence may also increase exposure to dangerous situations such as the approach of strangers or unsafe streets. Promotion of safe habits during the school-age years is important for parents and nurses. See Teaching Guidelines 28.1 for additional information on safety education for nurses and parents.

Teaching Guidelines 28.1
SAFETY ISSUES AND INTERVENTIONS OF THE SCHOOL-AGE CHILD

Safety Issue	Interventions
Car safety	• Seat belt or age- and weight-appropriate booster seat should be used at all times. The lap belt should lie low and flat on the hips and the shoulder belt should lie on the shoulder, not the neck or face (usually when the child is about 144.8 cm [57 in] tall) • Seat belts should be fastened before car is started • Children under 13 years must sit in back seat • Childproof locks should be used in back seat • Rules of conduct for car rides must be established
Pedestrian safety	• Child should be instructed to stop at the curb and look right, left, then right again before crossing the street; and crossing only at safe crossings • Older children and adults should provide supervision of younger children • Walking should only be done on sidewalks • In parking lots, children should know to watch for cars backing up and not dart out between parked cars • If children are playing outside, drivers should be aware of their presence before backing up
Bike safety: general	• Child should know to wear a properly fitted, CPSC (Consumer Product Safety Commission) or Snell-approved helmet every time he/she rides a bike • Proper fitting helmet should: sit level, not tilted, and firmly and comfortably on the head; have strong Y-shaped straps. These straps have limited movement i.e. when the child opens their mouth and stay in place when the child twists their head. Do not use a scarf under the helmet. • Bikes should be well maintained and appropriately sized • Child should be oriented to bike and demonstrate ability to ride bike safely before being allowed to ride on street • Safe areas for bike riding should be established as well as routes to and from area of activities • Riding bike barefoot, with someone else on bike, or with clothing that might get entangled in the bike should be prohibited • Child should know to wear sturdy, well-fitting shoes • Bike should be inspected often to ensure it is in proper working order • A basket should be used to carry heavy objects
Bike safety in traffic	• All traffic signs and signals must be observed • If riding at night, the bike should have lights and reflectors and the rider should wear light-coloured clothes • Child should know to ride on the side of the road travelling with traffic, and keep close to the side of the road in single file • Child should learn to watch and listen for cars • Headphones should not be used while riding a bike • Never hitch a ride on any vehicles
Sports safety	• Sports should be matched to child's ability and desire • Sports program should have warm up procedure • Coaches should be trained in CPR and first aid • Appropriate protection devices should be used for individual sport

Skateboarding and inline skating safety	• Child should wear helmet, and protective padding on knees, elbows, and wrists • Child should know not to skate in traffic or on streets or highways • Homemade ramps should be assessed for hazards before skating
All-terrain vehicle safety/ snowmobiles	• Child should be at least 16 years of age to operate vehicle • Helmets must be worn in addition to protective coverings • No nighttime riding • Use should be avoided on public roads • Never stand up in the vehicle or ride in a person's lap
Fire safety and burns	• All homes should have working smoke detectors, carbon monoxide detectors, and fire extinguishers. Change the batteries at least twice a year • Practice fire-escape plan regularly at home and school • Teach what to do in case of a fire: use fire extinguisher, call 911, and how to put out clothing fire • Use stove and other cooking facilities under adult supervision • All flammable materials and liquids should be stored safely • Fireplaces should have protective gratings • Teach children risk of wild fires, to raise an alarm, and to minimize risk • Teach children to avoid touching wires they might encounter while playing, hazard materials and structures (kites and high-tension wires, etc.) • Instruct child to cook safely (stove and microwave) and set water heater as 49°C to minimize scalds
Water safety	• Teach children how to swim and to never play around or in water without adult supervision • Child should know never swim alone—swim only where there is a lifeguard • Understand basic CPR • Teach child to never run or fool around at edge of pool • Drains in pool should be covered with appropriate cover • Life jackets should be worn when on boat • Make sure water is deep enough to support diving
Firearm safety	• Teach child never to play with guns; their lack of experience, development, and impulse control and understanding of consequences increases risk of accidental injury • If licenced guns (must be by law) are in household, they must be unloaded, secure, and in a safe place; use gun safety locks and store bullets in a separate place. (Regulations of Canada Firearms Act) • Inform parents that nonpowder guns and BB guns are dangerous weapons and should not be used without adult supervision
Toxin safety	• Teach child the hazards of accepting illegal drugs, alcohol, or dangerous drugs • Store potentially dangerous material in a safe place

Adapted from Canadian Paediatric Society (2012a, 2012b, 2017b).

Unintentional injuries are the leading cause of death in children between 1 and 19 years of age (CPS, 2012a). School-age children are very active at home, in the community, and at school. This increased mobility, activity, and time away from parents increase the risk for unintentional injuries. School-age children continue to need supervision and guidance. They need information and rules about car safety, pedestrian safety, bicycle and other sport safety, fire safety, and water safety.

Car Safety

Motor vehicle accidents are a common cause of injury in the school-age child. While travelling in the car, school-age children should always sit in the rear seat. The front seat is dangerous because of passenger-side airbags in most new-model cars. A school-age child over 18.1 kg (40 lb) (generally 4 to 8 years of age) should use a belt-positioning, forward-facing booster seat using both lap and shoulder belts. School-age children who outgrow the convertible restraint can sit in a booster seat until the vehicle seat belt restraint fits properly over the hips and shoulder, typically when they are 144.8 cm (4 ft 9 in) or taller, usually between 8 and 12 years of age (Transport Canada, 2017). The seat belt needs to lie low and flat over the hip bones and across the shoulder, not the neck or face. Children younger than 13 years of age should not ride in the front seat of a vehicle with an airbag.

Pedestrian Safety

Every year, children are injured or killed as pedestrians. Children younger than 10 years of age should not be unsupervised pedestrians (CPS, 2012b). Young school-age children therefore should walk to school or the bus with an older friend, sibling, or parent. Darting out into the street without looking both ways or from between cars is a common occurrence in the school-age years. Teach children safe street and pedestrian practices.

Bicycle and Sport Safety

Bicycling, riding scooters, skateboarding, and inline skating or roller skating are common activities of school-age children. Laws in some provinces require helmets for riding bicycles. In addition, when skating or skateboarding, school-age children should wear a helmet, kneepads, and elbow pads (CPS, 2012b).

Various studies have shown that head injuries due to bicycle accidents have reduced in the last 15 years in the region of 60% as a result of wearing a well-fitting helmet (Hagel & Yanchar, 2013). It is important for children to wear helmets that fit and that do not obstruct their vision or hearing. Because school-age children have completed most of their skull growth, a helmet can be worn into adolescence. It is important for the child to have a bicycle that is appropriate for his or her size and age. The child should be able to plant both feet on the ground when sitting on the seat of the bike (Fig. 28.8). It is important to stress to parents the importance of appropriate size and not to get a bike for the child to "grow into." If older school-agers are using the bike for transportation on busy streets, they should be taught to use bike lanes and to give appropriate hand signals for turning. Nonmotorized and motorized scooters also place children at risk for injury, so counsel families about the use of protective gear, including helmets, elbow pads, and kneepads.

Fire Safety

School-age children are eager to help parents with cooking and ironing. They are curious about fire and are drawn to play with fire, matches, and fireworks. Serious burns can occur from any exposure to fire. Educate children about the hazards of fire. In addition, teach children proper behaviour around fires at home and outdoors. Always supervise children in the use of matches. In the home setting, parents should develop a fire safety plan with their children, teach children what to do if their clothes catch on fire, and practice evacuating the house in the event of a fire. In the school setting, children should be aware of the appropriate response to fire drills and fire drills should be conducted on a regular basis.

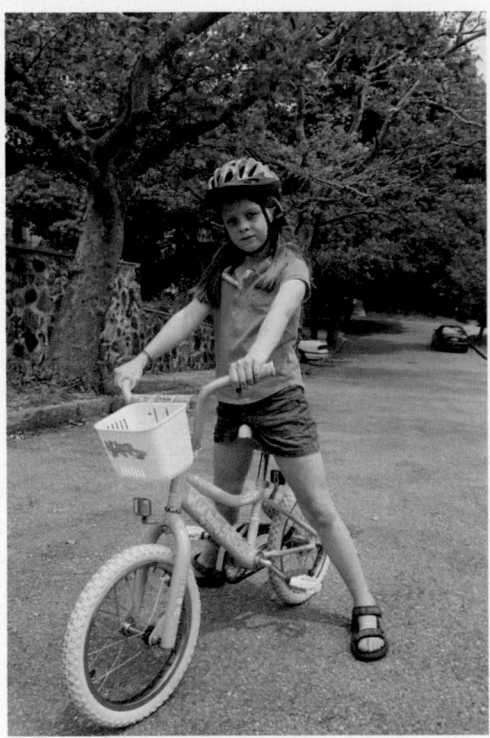

FIGURE 28.8 Wearing the appropriate safety equipment and having an appropriately sized bicycle are important to prevent injuries in school-age children.

Water Safety

Teach school-age children swim and water safety. An adult should always supervise children when they are swimming to prevent water-related accidents.

Abuse in Children

Child abuse, refers to the mistreatment, abuse or neglect of children (Ministry of Children and Families, BC, 2017). The abusers of children are often family, friends, or those in positions of power over a child but can also include strangers. It is important for parents to teach children the concept of "good touch" versus "bad touch" prior to school-age years; the underwear rule, for example, is one way to help parents talk about staying safely (National Society for the Prevention of Cruelty to Children, 2011). Whenever the school-age child's behaviour yields suspicion of physical or sexual abuse, the nurse should report to the appropriate authorities in his or her province.

Remember Lawrence Jones, the 10 year old presented in the case study? What anticipatory guidance related to safety should you provide to his mother?

Promoting Nutrition

Growth, body composition, and body shape remain constant during late school-age years. Needed calories decrease while the appetite increases. In preparation for adolescence, the body fat composition of school-age children increases. This tendency toward increased body fat occurs earlier in girls than in boys, with the amount of increase greater in girls. Boys have more lean body mass per inch of height than girls.

Diet preferences established in the preschool years continue during the school-age period. As the child grows older, influences of family, media, and peers can impact the eating habits of this age group. Some of these influences are parents' work schedule, outside activities, and exercise level of the child. Decreased exercise levels and poor nutritional choices lead to the mounting problem of obesity seen in this age group. See Box 28.2 for appropriate questions to ask the child and parent regarding nutritional status.

Nutritional Needs

The school-age child's calorie needs vary based on age, gender, and activity level with energy intake not exceeding energy need (Health Canada, 2012). In general, diet needs appear to be adequate for nutrients and vitamins, except lower Vitamin D and calcium between the ages of 4 and 8 years (Health Canada, 2012). In general, children with higher activity levels and male gender have higher calorie needs. Boys and girls 4 to 8 years old who are moderately active will need about 1,200 to 1,400 calories a day, but this depends on activity levels. Boys 9 to 13 years old who are moderately active need about 1,800 calories a day, while girls this age who are moderately active need about 1,600 calories a day. Of these calories, 45% to 65% should come from carbohydrates, 10% to 30% from protein, and 25% to 35% from fat (Health Canada, 2011). The 4- to 8-year-old child needs 800 to 1,000 mg of calcium, while the 9 to 13 year old needs 1,300 mg of calcium for maintenance of growth and good nutrition (Krebs, Primark, & Haemer, 2011). Calcium is needed for the development of strong bones and teeth. Milk, yogurt, and cheese provide protein, vitamins, and minerals and are an excellent source of calcium. Meats, poultry, fish, and eggs provide protein, vitamins, and minerals.

Promoting Healthy Eating Habits

The school-age child should be offered culturally appropriate foods from all groups over the course of the day as recommended by Canada's Food Guide (Health Canada, 2016). Parents may visit Health Canada's website (2016) or the Ellyn Satter website for additional information. Canada's Food Guide is available in 10 other languages. In addition, there is a separate Food Guide which reflects the values, traditions, and food choices of First Nations, Inuit and Métis (Health Canada, 2016). School-age children need to limit intake of fat and processed sugars. A prudent diet limits the use of fatty meats, high-fat dairy products, eggs, and hydrogenated shortenings and promotes the consumption of fish and the substitution of polyunsaturated vegetable oils and margarines.

Preventing the Development of Overweight and Obesity

In Canada, over the past 25 years, the prevalence of obesity has nearly tripled with up to 26% of children aged 2 to 17 reported as overweight or obese (CPS, 2012c). This number jumps to 41% in Indigenous children aged 2 to 17 (CPS, 2012c). Overweight is classified as a body mass index (BMI) greater than 85% and obese is classified as a BMI greater than 95% (Krebs et al., 2011) (see Healthy Promotion chapter 31). Obesity occurs when the intake of calories and food exceeds the expenditures. Some factors linked to causing obesity include family role modelling, lack of exercise, unstructured meals, consumption of sugar-sweetened beverages, large portion sizes, television viewing, and video gaming as well as cultural, genetic, environmental, and socioeconomic factors. Some factors that influence lack of exercise include the decreased number of days that school systems offer physical education programs and recess. Also, some children live in unsafe neighbourhoods or in a community

---

BOX 28.2

DIETARY QUESTIONS

Questions for the Child

- How often do you eat together as a family?
- What are the usual mealtimes?
- How often does the family eat out?
- Do you eat breakfast regularly?
- Where do you eat lunch?
- What do you drink/how much?
- What foods do you eat most often?
- What is your favourite food?
- How often do you eat fast foods?
- What type of exercise do you do?

Questions for the Parents

- How would you describe your child's usual appetite?
- Do you have any special cultural/religious practices regarding food?
- Has your child gained or lost weight recently?
- Do you have any concerns about his or her eating behaviours?
- How does your child exercise? Your family?
- Is there a family history of cancer, hypertension, diabetes, obesity, or heart disease?

that lacks sidewalks or parks and have no safe place to play outside; therefore, they spend time doing sedentary activities such as watching TV or playing video or computer games (CPS, 2015). Obese children are at risk for cardiovascular diseases such as high cholesterol and hypertension, type 2 (non–insulin-dependent) diabetes, respiratory complications such as obstructive sleep apnea, mental health issues such as depression, anxiety, decreased self-esteem, and eating disorders as well as orthopaedic problems.

Preventing obesity in childhood is important since the fat cells of childhood are carried into adulthood obesity which contributes to disease. Due to the risk of obesity, encourage parents to never use food as a reward. To prevent obesity, establish regular mealtimes and offer healthy foods and snacks. Encourage parents to praise their child's good food choices and to role model appropriate eating and exercise. The nurse also has to be mindful of food insecurity and the impact the social determinants of health have around food access and consumption (CPS, 2016b).

> **Regarding Lawrence Jones, what questions should you ask Lawrence's mother related to nutritional intake? What anticipatory guidance related to nutrition would be appropriate?**

Promoting Healthy Sleep and Rest

The number of hours of sleep required for growth and development decreases with age. Children between the ages of 6 and 8 years require about 12 hours of sleep per night, children between 8 and 10 years of age require at least 10 hours of sleep per night, and children between 10 and 12 years of age need 9 to 10 hours of sleep per night. Young school-age children may need an occasional brief nap for an energy boost after being in school for most of the day. Bedtime rituals and consistent schedules continue to be important throughout the school-age years. Parents must facilitate the bedtime schedule and quiet time before bed. Bedtime is a special time for parents and children to read together, listen to stories or soothing music, share events of the day, and exchange expressions of affection (CPS, 2016a). Children should have bedtime expectations as well as wake-up times and methods for waking up (alarm, calling by parent, and so forth).

Night terrors or sleepwalking may occur in 6 to 8 year olds, but should be resolved between the ages of 8 and 10 years. In the older school-age child (11 to 12 years), encourage parents to allow a variation in the sleep schedule on the weekends and a regular schedule on weekdays.

> **Provide anticipatory guidance to Lawrence Jones's mother in relation to proper sleep for her 10-year-old son.**

Promoting Healthy Teeth and Gums

Dental **caries** (tooth decay) remains a leading chronic disease and is an important public health issue. In Canada, it is estimated that 57% of children ages 6 to 11 have had a dental cavity (CPS, 2013). Unfortunately in Canada, dental care is not considered integral to health care and therefore is not subject to the tenets of the Canada Health Act, which ensures that health care is publicly administered, universal, portable, accessible, and comprehensive (CPS, 2013). Because of this, Canadians are largely responsible for financing their own dental care resulting in large disparities strongly linked to socioeconomic status (CPS, 2013). Dental care with emphasis on prevention of caries is important in this age group. School-age children need to brush their teeth two to three times per day for 2 to 3 minutes each time with fluoridated toothpaste (Fig. 28.9). Parents should replace the toothbrush (soft) every 3 to 4 months. Flossing the teeth at least once daily is recommended along with limiting the intake of sugar to aid in the prevention of cavities and improved oral health. Parents must

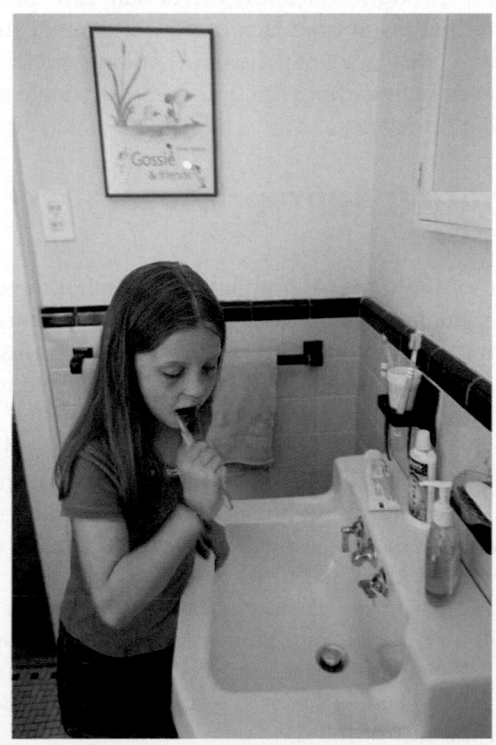

FIGURE 28.9 Using correct technique to brush the teeth is important in the prevention of cavities.

monitor teeth brushing, observe for abnormal alignment of their child's teeth, and schedule regular dental examinations every 6 months to ensure good dental health and prevent dental problems. Children will need help with brushing teeth until they are between 7 and 10 years of age.

Dental sealants are an easy way to protect a child's primary or permanent teeth as children with dental sealants have 60% less decay. The sealant is a plastic coating applied to biting surfaces to seal out tooth decay on back teeth and sometimes to cover deep pits or grooves. In addition, parents should give a fluoride supplement (as directed by the dentist) to their children if fluoride is not in the town's water supply. The school-age child should have an established dental home; if not, provide appropriate resources to establish one.

Proper alignment of teeth is important to tooth formation, speech development, and physical appearance. Many school-age children need braces or other orthodontic devices to correct **malocclusion**, a condition in which the teeth are crowded, crooked, or misaligned. **Bruxism** or teeth grinding while asleep may continue in the school-age years. Bruxism may result in grinding away of tooth enamel. Teeth grinding may be due to malalignment. A dental evaluation should be scheduled if consistent teeth grinding occurs.

Children wearing braces are more prone to cavities; encourage them to brush their teeth after meals and snacks. School personnel can assist these children with brushing after lunch. School nurses should promote dental health through education on dental care and gum problems that result from lack of proper dental care. Diet can play a part in dental health. Limiting sticky, high-sugar, and high-carbohydrate foods will decrease the possibility of cavities.

Promoting Appropriate Discipline

Because of the increasing ability of the school-age child to view situations from different angles, the school-age child should be able to see how his or her actions affect others. The school-age child is aware of the cause and effect of his or her behaviours and realizes that his or her behaviours have consequences. School-age children should be able to express emotions without using violence. Discipline techniques with consequences have both *natural* and *logical* consequences. Natural consequences allow the child to learn the results of his or her actions. For example, if the child throws a toy out of the window, then he or she cannot play with the toy anymore. In logical consequences, if the child does not put away his or her bike, he or she does not get to ride the bike for the rest of the day.

In disciplining children, parents should teach children the rules established by the family, values, and social rules of conduct. Rules should provide the school-age child with guidelines about behaviour that is acceptable and unacceptable. School-age children look to their parents for guidance and as role models. Parents should role model appropriate expressions of feelings and emotions and allow the child to express emotions and feelings. Discuss the effects of the child's temperament on his or her behaviour, as well as what constitutes age-appropriate behaviour. Include how the parents' temperament can influence the child's temperament.

Effective guidance, limit setting, and discipline focus on the development needs and level of the child. They can preserve the child's self-esteem and dignity. Discuss with parents, guidelines regarding discipline. Explain to parents that they should never belittle the child. Children may view parents and caretakers negatively if they are consistently belittled or insulted. These negative actions can inhibit learning and teach the child to react unkindly to others. Instead, parents should discipline with praise. Positive acknowledgements of progress are likely to encourage healthy development and appropriate behaviour. Discuss with parents how to be realistic when planning activities so as to not overwhelm the child, resulting in misbehaviour. Encourage parents to say "no" only when they mean it, to avoid a negative atmosphere in the home, and to avoid inconsistency.

When misbehaviours occur, the type and amount of discipline are based on different factors:
- Developmental level of both the child and the parents
- Severity of the misbehaviour
- Established rules of the family
- Temperament of the child
- Response of the child to rewards

Keep in mind that school-age children should participate in developing a plan of action for their misbehaviour. Whatever methods of discipline are chosen, it is important that parents are consistent in providing discipline in a nurturing environment.

ADDRESSING COMMON DEVELOPMENTAL CONCERNS

The developmental task (according to Erikson) of the school-age child is industry (Erikson, 1963; Feigelman, 2011a). The school-age child is busy learning, achieving, and exploring. As the school-age child becomes more independent, forces other than the family such as television, video games, and peers influence him or her. Some of these influences are positive and others are negative. Some of the common developmental concerns for the school-age child are discussed in the following sections. Guidelines to assist the parents and nurses when encountering these concerns are included in Teaching Guidelines 28.2.

Teaching Guidelines 28.2

ADDRESSING COMMON DEVELOPMENTAL CONCERNS

Television, Video Games, and the Internet
- Limit total screen time, which includes television watching, video game playing, and internet-connected devices to 1 to 2 hours per day, CPS (2015) recommends no more than 2 hours of any combination of these
- Monitor television programs and internet activity
- Prohibit television or video games with violence
- Do not put television, video games, or internet-connected devices in children's bedrooms. Place computers in an open area that allows easy monitoring by an adult
- Co-view television, video games, and internet content with the child
- Encourage sports, interactive play, and reading
- Teach your child internet safety, such as to never share personal information or meet a friend you have only met online without parental permission. Never share passwords. Never respond to a message that hurts your feelings or makes you uncomfortable. Never send mean messages over the internet

Obesity
- Provide healthy meals and snacks
- Schedule and encourage daily exercise
- Encourage involvement in sports
- Restrict sedentary behaviour, such as TV and computer game use
- Limit the amount of fast-food intake
- Provide education about healthy nutrition
- Never use food as a reward
- Be a good role model

School Refusal
- Return child to school
- Investigate cause of the fear
- Support child
- Collaborate with teachers
- Praise success in school attendance

Latchkey Kids
- Provide rules to follow and expectations, such as:
  - Not answering the door or phone
  - No friends in the house when parents are not home
  - No playing with fire
- Teach child to call a trusted neighbour when help is needed and 911 in the event of emergency
- Post all resource numbers (even numbers you think your child may have memorized), including after-school help lines if available, in a clearly viewable spot. Include physician's or nurse practitioner's number and preferred hospital
- Purchase caller ID for the phone system
- Enrol the child in an after-school program if available

- Discuss limitations of outside play
- Discuss limitations of television viewing and video game use
- Make sure the child knows how to contact the parent
- Set clear homework expectations
- DO NOT keep guns in the home
- Teach the child where first aid supplies are located
- Teach the child household emergency procedures such as circuit breakers and water shut-off valves
- Practice with your child. Have a trial run by leaving for a short time but staying close and role-playing situations that may occur
- Always check in with your child while you are away

Stealing and Dishonest Behaviour
- Educate parents about possibility of stealing
- Discuss ways to teach concept of ownership and property rights
- Handle situation openly and calmly
- Assist child in developing and enacting a plan to return what was stolen
- Make sure the punishment is appropriate for the action

Lying
- Help parents in understanding why the child is lying
- When the child lies, calmly confront the child and explain why the behaviour is not acceptable
- Educate parents that their behaviour should reflect what they teach and expect from their child
- Educate parents that too-rigid or severe punishments can decrease the child's sense of worth
- Seek professional help if lying persists in the older school-age child, to rule out underlying problems

Cheating
- Educate parents that the child must be mature enough to understand the concept of rules
- Handle cheating situations openly
- Help parents to understand why their child is cheating and to modify the trigger
- Develop appropriate punishment; inappropriate punishment could undermine the child
- Educate parents that their behaviour should reflect what they expect from their child
- Seek professional help if cheating persists in the older school-age child, to rule out underlying problems

Bullying
The Bullied Child
- Educate parents whose children are at risk for being bullied, such as:
  - Children who appear different from the majority
  - Children who act different from the majority
  - Children who have low self-esteem
  - Children with a mental or psychological problem

- Teach parents to role-play different scenarios the child may face at school; show the child different ways to react to being bullied
- Impress upon the child that he or she did not cause the bullying
- Develop ways to increase the child's self-esteem at home
- Discuss the situation with the teacher and develop a care plan

The Bullying Child

- Educate parents on reasons why it is important to correct the behaviour
- Discuss ways the child can appropriately show his or her anger and feelings
- Have parents help the child to see how it feels to be bullied
- Do not allow fighting at home
- Reward settling of conflicts without violence

Tobacco and Alcohol Education

- Inquire about tobacco and alcohol use. There may be locally adapted screening tools that can help guide questioning and risk
- Discuss the physical and social dangers of tobacco and alcohol use
- Urge parents to be good role models
- Provide age appropriate reading materials that provide education about substance use risks.
- Discuss the influences of tobacco and alcohol use by peers
- Educate the child on spit tobacco. Let them know it is just as dangerous as smoking tobacco
- Advocate for a smoke-free environment in the home and other places frequented
- Avoid having tobacco and alcohol products readily available in the home

Television, Video Games, and the Internet

The influence of television, video games, and the internet upon the school-age child is a growing concern for parents and child specialists. Children 8 to 10 years of age in the United States spend about 4 hours a day either watching TV or playing video games and another 2 hours on the computer outside of school work (CPC, 2017c). During that time, a child by the age of 18 will see 200,000 violent acts (CPC, 2017c). Although a school-age child can determine what is real from what is fantasy, research has shown that this amount of time in front of a screen—watching it or playing video games—can lead to aggressive behaviour, less physical activity, and obesity (CPC, 2017c).

Some television shows, video games, and internet activity can have positive influences on children, but parents should be taught guidelines on the use of TV, video games, and the internet. Parents should set limits on how much screen time the child can have. The CPS recommends 2 hours or less of screen time per day (CPS, 2017c). The parent should establish guidelines on when the child can watch TV, for example, after homework or when chores are completed (CPC, 2017c). Television watching, internet activity, or video gaming should not be used as a reward. The parents should be aware of what the child is watching and doing online. This can be accomplished by parents and children watching programs together and parents using that opportunity to discuss the subject matter with the child. There should be no TV during dinner and no TV or internet-connected devices in the child's room. The parents need to set an example for the child by reading instead of watching TV or by doing a physical activity together as a family. If the TV causes fights or arguments, it should be turned off for a period of time.

Take Note!

School-age children need supervision and monitoring when using the internet to ensure they are not exposed to inappropriate material or content (CPC, 2017c). Encourage parents of children in this age group to utilize internet safety tools that limit access to content and websites and that provide information on internet activities.

School Refusal

School refusal (also called *school phobia* or *school avoidance*) has been defined as a refusal to attend school or difficulty remaining in school for an entire day. Behaviours include frequent absences, skipping classes, chronically late for school, severe misbehaviour before school, or attending school with great fear. School phobia needs to be defined both symptomatically and operationally as the cause for the anxiety. School avoidance occurs in approximately 5% of children (AAP, 2013).

Some of the fears expressed by school-refusing children include separating from parents, riding the bus, tests, bullying, teacher reprimands, anxieties over toileting in a public bathroom, physical harm, or undressing in the locker room. Due to the emotional distress caused in these children when attending school, they are frequently classified as having school phobia. Young children may complain of stomachache or headache and older children may complain of palpitations or feeling faint.

It is important to investigate specific causes of school refusal/school phobia and take appropriate actions.

Many times, school phobia is a symptom of deeper problems. The physician or nurse practitioner should conduct a physical examination of the child to rule out any physical illness. After these measures are taken, the parent, teacher, school counsellor, and school administrator may devise a plan to assist the student to overcome a specific fear. In uncomplicated cases, parents must return the child to school as soon as possible. There may be altered schedules (partial days or decreased hours) to help promote a successful transition back to school. Another idea to help desensitize the child may be to have him or her spend part of the day in the counsellor's or school nurse's office.

Latchkey Children

With the increasing incidence of both parents in the workforce and many children living with just one parent, often times, children return home alone without adult supervision for a number of hours. Most young children are not capable of handling stress or making decisions on their own before 11 or 12 years of age. Parents not only need to consider their child's maturity and readiness to be home alone but also must comply with legal requirements in each province (Ruiz-Casares & Radic, 2015). Despite the level of maturity, children who are unsupervised are more likely to participate in risky behaviours such as smoking, drinking, and doing drugs. In addition, latchkey children may feel anxiety, stress, fear, boredom, loneliness; they miss more days of school, and have lower academic scores.

If children come home to no supervision, they should know the names, addresses, and phone numbers of parents and a neighbour, as well as emergency numbers. They should be given rules about answering the door and the phone. They should tell anyone who comes to the door or who calls that mom is home but busy at this time. Directions as to the handling of the house key and fire safety should be taught and demonstrated (see Teaching Guidelines 28.2).

Stealing, Lying, and Cheating

It is during the school-age years that antisocial behaviours can emerge. Children who were previously well behaved may now exhibit behaviours such as stealing, lying, and cheating (Mannheim, 2012). Parents are usually disturbed by this change in behaviour. In turn, they have difficulty in addressing these issues and need help in providing appropriate interventions.

Children between 6 and 8 years old do not fully understand the concept of ownership and property rights. These children may steal things because they like the look of the item. By the age of 9, the child should respect others' possessions and property and

understand that stealing is wrong (Roux, 2013). The school-age child may steal because he or she desires the item, feels peer pressure and is trying to impress his or her peers, or has a sense of low self-esteem (Roux, 2013). Stealing becomes a concern if the child steals and does not have remorse or steals continuously, or if stealing is accompanied by other behaviour problems (Roux, 2013).

Lying is more common in boys and in children between 5 and 8 years old (Roux, 2013). It is acceptable for these children to tell tall tales, but they should know what truth is and what make-believe is. These younger children typically lie to avoid punishment. However, they do not like others to lie and will tell on them if they lie. Children between 8 and 12 years old typically lie because they are unable to meet expectations of family and peers, they are testing the rules and limits placed on them, or they are unable to explain bad behaviour (Roux, 2013). If lying persists in older school-age children, if it is accompanied by other behaviour problems, or if the child does not show remorse with lying, parents should discuss the matter with a physician or nurse practitioner because the lying may be evidence of underlying problems.

The concept of cheating is not well understood until the child is 7 years old. Before this age, the desire to "win" is most important and rigid rules are hard to understand. In children between 8 and 12 years old, the concept of cheating is fully understood and following of rules becomes more important (Roux, 2013). Cheating is usually done because of competition and strong pressure placed on the child to succeed. If cheating persists in older school-age children, parents should discuss the matter with a physician or nurse practitioner because the behaviour may indicate underlying problems.

In dealing with children who exhibit stealing, lying, or cheating behaviours, parents must first realize the importance of their own behaviours in those areas. Parents are role models to the school-age child. Therefore, when the child sees or hears that parents lie, steal, or cheat (e.g., parents bragging about cheating on their taxes), they think it is all right to mimic those behaviours. Secondly, parents must directly confront any stealing, lying, or cheating behaviours and discuss (and follow through consistently with) the consequences of such behaviours (see Teaching Guidelines 28.2).

Bullying

Bullying, which is inflicting unwanted, repeated verbal, emotional, or physical abuse upon others, is on the rise (Schuster & Bogart, 2013). Utilizing email, text messages, social networking, and instant messaging, often referred to as cyberbullying, is a growing concern. Bullies often look for victims who appear shy, weak, and defenseless.

EVIDENCE-BASED PRACTICE 28.1 | **BENEFITS OF BULLYING-PREVENTION EDUCATION**

STUDY

Bullying and victimization continue to pose a problem in elementary schools. In addition to the behavioural disruption that occurs as a result of bullying and victimization, prior research has demonstrated that child bullies and victims are at increased risk for mental health problems, such as depression, anxiety, low self-esteem, and low social competence. Adverse consequences from bullying have led to prevention programs to decrease peer victimization. This study looked at the effectiveness of one such program, Youth Matters. It used a sample of 876 students in grades 4, 5, and 6. Children were placed in a control or experimental group and bullying and victimization were assessed at four different time points using surveys.

Findings

Upon analysis of the findings, the researchers reported in most cases children who participated in the bullying intervention program transitioned from being part of bullying, victim, or bullying–victim group to uninvolved group. The most positive effect was seen in children in the victim class. Findings support that bullying-prevention programs can help develop social and emotional skills and can assist in changing perceptions and attitudes to help prevent and help a child handle bullying incidents.

Nursing Implications

Nurses should continue to educate parents and teachers about bullying. Become actively involved in the local elementary school bullying prevention program and encourage school-wide interventions. When bullies are identified, refer them for education in bullying prevention programs that focus on skill building.

Adapted from Jenson, J. M., Brisson, D., Bender, K. A., & Williford, A. P. (2013). Effects of the Youth Matters Prevention Program on patterns of bullying and victimization in elementary and middle school. *Social Work Research, 37*(4), 361–372.

Children with health issues, such as disabilities, obesity, and food allergies, are at an increased risk of being bullied (Schuster & Bogart, 2013). Beginning in 2007, every February in Canada "Pink Shirt Day" occurs; a national anti-bullying campaign. On this day, children across Canada wear pink shirts to school to symbolize they do not tolerate bullying.

Take Note!

Bullying in School Children

Children who bully most often have low self-esteem, poor grades, and poor interpersonal skills. Both boys and girls are bullied, but boys tend to bully other boys and more often show force when bullying.

In general, about 10% of all children attending school are frightened and afraid most of the day (American Academy of Child and Adolescent Psychiatry, 2011). About 25% of children have been bullied (Robinson & Segal, 2014). Most of the bullying occurs at school (Augustyn & Zuckerman, 2011). Both boys and girls are bullied and can bully others; however, boys are twice as likely to be bullies and victims of bullying (Augustyn & Zuckerman, 2011). Being bullied can have negative results on children throughout life. These children often have increased episodes of headaches, stomachaches, sleep problems, anxiety, loneliness, depression, and suicidal tendencies (Schuster & Bogart, 2013). After the problem of either being bullied or being the bully has been identified, parents must work with the child, the school, and the physician or nurse practitioner to solve the problem (see Teaching Guidelines 28.2 and Evidence-Based Practice 28.1).

Tobacco and Alcohol Education

School-age children are eager to grow up and be independent. Peers and acceptance are very important at this time. School-age children may be exposed to messages that are in conflict with their parents' values regarding smoking and alcohol. Peers often exert pressure for children to experiment with tobacco and alcohol (see Health Promotion).

School-age children are ready to absorb information that deals with drugs and alcohol. Information from parents or other adults who are major influences in the child's life is essential at this time to set clear rules and model behaviours for children to embrace. Discussions with children need to be based on facts and focused on the present. Some topics for discussion include:

- What alcohol and drugs are like and how they harm you
- Differences in medical use versus illegal use of drugs
- How to think critically to interpret messages seen in advertising, media, sports, and entertainment personalities

Recall Lawrence Jones, the 10 year old presented at the beginning of the chapter. List potential developmental problems he may experience. What anticipatory guidance related to these concerns should you provide to his mother?

NURSING CARE PLAN 28.1

Growth and Development Issues of the School-Age Child

NURSING DIAGNOSIS: Risk for overweight (risk factors: caregiver knowledge deficit, frequent illnesses)

Outcome Identification and Evaluation

School-age child will demonstrate adequate growth: *appropriate weight gain and increases in height for age and gender*

Interventions: *Promoting Proportionate Growth*

* Assess parent's knowledge of nutritional needs of school-age children *to determine need for further education.*
* Plot out height, weight, and BMI *to detect possible pattern.*
* Determine need for additional caloric intake if necessary; *if very active in sports, if have a chronic illness, caloric needs may be altered.*
* Educate primary caregiver about appropriate serving sizes and foods *so that primary caregiver is aware of what to expect for school-age children.*

NURSING DIAGNOSIS: Ineffective health maintenance related to lack of exercise, increased caloric intake, poor food choices

Outcome Identification and Evaluation

School-age child will engage in health maintenance behaviours and lose weight at an appropriate rate: *increase amount of exercise, make appropriate eating choices, decrease caloric intake to appropriate amount for age and gender*

Interventions: *Promoting Appropriate Health Maintenance Behaviours*

* Assess knowledge of parents and child about nutritional needs of school-age children *to determine deficits in knowledge.*
* Plot out height, weight, and BMI *to detect weight loss or weight gain.*
* Have child keep food and exercise diary for 1 week *to determine current patterns of eating and exercise.*
* Interview parents in relationship to their eating habits and exercise habits *to determine where adjustments might need to be made.*
* Analyze preceding data, and base recommendations for changes on these data.
* Discuss ways to decrease temptation to overeat and to make good meal choices (see Teaching Guidelines 28.2).

* Have child assist in meal planning and grocery shopping *to allow him or her some sense of control in process.*
* Incorporate increase in daily exercise, which will stress sense of self-improvement, *to increase caloric expenditure and self-esteem.*
* Decrease TV/computer/device time *to increase caloric expenditure.*
* Develop reward system *to increase self-esteem.*
* Investigate joining weight-loss program for school-age children *to increase self-esteem and to increase awareness that other children have the same problem.*

NURSING DIAGNOSIS: Risk for delayed development related to speech, motor, psychosocial, or cognitive concerns as evidenced by delay in meeting expected school performances

Outcome Identification and Evaluation

Development will be maximized: *School-age child will make continued progress toward attainment of expected school performances.*

(continued)

development. The genital stage begins with the production of sex hormones and maturation of the reproductive system.

Girls reach physical maturity before boys and **menarche**, the first menstrual period, usually begins between the ages of 9 and 15 years (average 12.8 years). Breast budding (**thelarche**) occurs at approximately age 9 to 11 years and is followed by the growth of pubic hair.

The first sign of pubertal changes in boys is testicular enlargement in response to testosterone secretion, usually occurring in Tanner stage 2. As testosterone levels increase, the penis and scrotum enlarge, hair distribution increases, and scrotal skin texture changes. During late puberty, boys will typically experience their first ejaculation, which may occur while they are sleeping (nocturnal emissions). Nurses should provide anticipatory guidance to adolescent males regarding involuntary nocturnal emissions (wet dreams) to assure them that this is a normal occurrence.

Tanner stages 3 to 5 usually occur during adolescence. Refer to Figures 32.27, 32.33, and 32.35 for an illustration of the increase in breast tissue and pubic hair distribution in girls, and scrotal and penile changes as well as hair distribution changes in boys. The nurse should provide guidance to adolescents about the normalcy of the sexual feelings and evolving body changes that occur during puberty.

PHYSICAL GROWTH

Diet, exercise, and hereditary factors influence the height, weight, and body build of the adolescent. Over the past three decades, adolescents have become taller and heavier than their ancestors and the beginning of puberty is earlier. During the early adolescent period, there is an increase in the percentage of body fat and the head, neck, and hands reach adult proportions.

Both girls and boys experience changes in appearance and size. Height in girls increases rapidly after menarche and usually ceases 2 to 2½ years after menarche. Boys' growth spurt occurs later than girls' and usually begins between the ages of 10½ and 16 years and ends sometime between the ages of 13½ and 17½ years. Peak height velocity (PHV) occurs at approximately 12 years of age in girls or at about 6 to 12 months after menarche. Boys reach PHV at about 14 years of age. Peak weight velocity (PWV) occurs about 6 months after menarche in girls and at about 14 years of age in boys. Muscle mass increases in boys and fat deposits increase in girls (Fig. 29.1).

During early adolescence, growth is rapid, but it decreases in middle and late adolescence. Height for adolescent boys who are between the 50th and 95th percentile ranges from 132 cm (52½ in) to 176.8 cm (69½ in). Weight of boys in these percentiles ranges from 35.3 kg (77¼ lb) to 95.76 kg (211 lb). On average, boys will gain 10 to 30 cm (4 to 12 in) in height and 7 to 30 kg (15 to 65 lb) in weight.

Height for girls who are between the 50th and 95th percentile ranges from 144.8 cm (57 in) to 173.6 cm (68½ in), with weight ranging from 27.24 kg (60 lb) to 82.47 kg (181 lb). On average, girls will gain 5 to 20 cm (2 to 8 in) in height and 7 to 25 kg (15 to 55 lb) in weight during adolescence. See Appendix F WHO charts for this age group. Refer to Chapter 32, Box 32.1, for instructions for calculating body mass index (BMI).

FIGURE 29.1 These adolescents reflect the differences in sizes and shapes seen in adolescents of the same age.

ORGAN SYSTEM MATURATION

Adolescence is a time of metabolic slowing and of increasing size of some organs. The basal metabolic rate (BMR) reaches the adult level during late adolescence.

Neurologic System

During adolescence, there is continued brain growth, although the size of the brain does not increase significantly. Neurons do not increase in number, but growth of the myelin sheath enables faster neural processing.

Respiratory System

The adolescent years see an increase in diameter and length of the lungs. Respiratory rate decreases and reaches the adult rate of 15 to 20 breaths per minute. Respiratory volume and vital capacity increase. Volume and capacity are greater in boys than girls, which may be associated with increased chest and shoulder size in boys. The growth of the laryngeal cartilage, larynx, pharynx, vocal cords, and lungs produces the voice changes experienced in adolescence. These changes in the quality of the child's voice are often preceded with some voice instability where voice cracking is heard. Deepening of both male and female voices occurs but is more pronounced in boys.

Cardiovascular System

There is an increase in size and strength of the heart. Systolic blood pressure increases and heart rate decreases. Blood volume reaches higher levels in boys than girls, which may be due to boys' greater muscle mass.

Gastrointestinal System

The adolescent has a full set of permanent teeth with the exception of the last four molars (wisdom teeth), which may erupt between the ages of 17 and 20 years. The liver, spleen, kidneys, and digestive tract enlarge during the growth spurt in early adolescence, but do not change in function. These systems are mature in early school age.

Musculoskeletal System

The ossification of the skeletal system is incomplete until late adolescence in boys. Ossification is more advanced in girls and occurs at an earlier age. During the growth spurt, muscle mass and strength increase. At similar stages of development, muscle development is generally greater in boys. Estrogen, progesterone, and testosterone as well as other androgens are released from the gonads and affect changes in the muscles and bones. Low estrogen levels tend to stimulate skeletal growth, while higher levels inhibit growth. During middle adolescence, shoulder, chest, and hip breadth increase.

Integumentary System

During adolescence, the skin becomes thick and tough. Under the influence of androgens, the sebaceous glands become more active, particularly on the face, back, and genitals. Due to the increased levels of testosterone during Tanner stages 4 and 5 in both boys and girls, both sexes may have increased sebum production, which may lead to the development of acne and oily hair.

The exocrine and apocrine sweat glands function at adult levels during adolescence. The exocrine glands are all over the body and they produce sweat that helps to eliminate body heat through evaporation. The apocrine glands are found in the axillae, genital, and anal areas and around the breasts. The apocrine sweat glands produce sweat in response to hair follicles. This sweat is produced continuously and is stored and released in response to emotional stimuli.

PSYCHOSOCIAL DEVELOPMENT

According to Erikson (1963), it is during adolescence that teenagers achieve a sense of identity. As the adolescent is trying out many different roles in regard to his or her relationships with peers, family, community, and society, he or she is developing his or her own individual sense of self. If the adolescent is not successful in forming his or her own sense of self, he or she develops a sense of role confusion or diffusion. The adolescent culture becomes very important to the teenager. It is through his or her involvement with youth groups that the adolescent finds support and help with developing his or her own identity.

Erikson (1963) believed that during the task of developing his or her own sense of identity, the adolescent revisits each of the previous stages of development. The sense of trust is encountered as the adolescent strives to find out whom and what ideals he or she believes in. In revisiting the stage of autonomy, the adolescent is seeking out ways to express his or her individuality in an effective manner. The adolescent would avoid behaviours that would "shame" or ridicule him or her in front of his or her peers. The sense of initiative is revisited as the adolescent develops his or her vision for what he or she might become. And the sense of industry is again encountered as the adolescent makes his or her choice to participate in different activities at school, in the community, at church, and in the workforce.

The ability of the adolescent to successfully form a sense of self is dependent upon how well the adolescent

Foundations of Pediatric Nursing

Foundations of Pediatric Nursing

30

Atraumatic Care of Children and Families

Learning Objectives

Upon completion of the chapter, you will be able to:

1. Describe the major principles and concepts of atraumatic care.

2. Incorporate atraumatic care to prevent and minimize physical and emotional stress for children and families.

3. Discuss the major components and concepts of family-centred care.

4. Utilize excellent therapeutic communication and health teaching skills when interacting with children and their families.

5. Describe trauma-informed care and how you might incorporate this into pediatric nursing.

Emma Moore, 4 years old, is admitted to the pediatric unit with a suspected head injury from a fall. She was playing at a playground with her babysitter and fell from the top of the slide.

Atraumatic care is defined as therapeutic care that minimizes or eliminates the psychological and physical distress experienced by children and their families in the health care system (Wong, n.d.). This concept is based on the underlying premise of "do no harm." Box 30.1 highlights the major principles of atraumatic care.

Up to two thirds of children have been exposed to traumatic events, which may include abuse, neglect, witnessing death or violence, natural disasters, accidental injuries, or motor vehicle collisions. Children's exposure to traumatic events, often referred to as adverse childhood experiences (ACEs) may interrupt normal brain development and increase the risk of impairments in cognition and behavioural and psychological function (Gonzalez et al., 2018; Karatekin, 2018).

It is important to provide nursing care that decreases the child's exposure to stressful situations and prevents or minimizes pain and bodily injury. Pediatric nurses should be aware of situations that may cause distress, and should always consider how patients' and families' past experiences, such as trauma, may impact their current and future health care needs. Trauma is a threat to safety towards the child or someone close to them (Children's Health Policy Centre, 2011). Symptoms of trauma may include nightmares, repetitive play about the trauma, anger outbursts, self-injurious behaviour, and sexualized behaviour. Long-term consequences include increased risk of posttraumatic stress disorder, mood or anxiety disorders, and poor physical health (Marsac et al., 2016).

Nurses should incorporate trauma-informed approaches into their practices to ensure a safe and respectful care environment is fostered for the child and their family. **Trauma-informed care** refers to a way of delivering atraumatic health care that recognizes and responds to how individuals' past experiences of trauma can overlap and intersect to shape their interpretation of new events. It emphasizes minimizing the potential for medical care to trigger traumatic events, and it prioritizes individuals' safety, control, and choice (Arthur et al., 2013).

Atraumatic care also involves guiding children and their families through the health care experience using a family-centred approach by promoting family roles, fostering family support of the child, and providing age-appropriate information that is relevant to the child and the family's literacy levels and cultural context. Use of appropriate techniques for therapeutic communication (goal-directed, focused, purposeful communication), therapeutic play (type of play that provides an emotional outlet or improves the child's ability to cope with the stress of illness and hospitalization), and education can help the child and family understand the reason for the hospitalization and the necessary tests and procedures. In addition, the pediatric nurse can help the family and other health care personnel to obtain the resources and develop the relationships they need for optimal care. When combined with atraumatic and trauma-informed care, family-centred approaches enhance the health care experience for the child and family. Having an informed and educated family is key to providing optimal health care for children.

Table 30.1 gives suggestions for incorporating the principles of atraumatic care and trauma-informed care into nursing care for the child and family. Look for tips on atraumatic care as it relates to specific topics throughout the text.

BOX 30.1

Principles of Atraumatic Care

- Prevent or minimize physical stressors, including injections, urethral catheterization, sleep deprivation, inability to eat or drink, and changes in elimination.
- Avoid or reduce other kinds of physical distress, such as noise, smells, shivering, nausea and vomiting, sleeplessness, restraints, and skin trauma.
- Control pain via frequent assessments and use of pharmacologic and nonpharmacologic interventions.
- Promote family-centred care, treating the family as the patient.
- Prevent or minimize parent–child separation.

Principles of Trauma-Informed Care

- Trauma-informed care is a universal precaution; children and families should be provided care as if they have experienced trauma in the past or may currently be experiencing medically traumatic events.
- Consider all barriers to engagement in care that the child and family might be experiencing. This could include poverty, past emotional or physical abuse in an institutional setting such as a hospital or school, or parents' fear of losing their children based on past experience.
- Elicit the child's and family's priorities and hopes for care by finding out what is most worrisome for them and by clarifying their understanding of the care they are receiving.
- Elicit the family's knowledge about the child and his or her health condition, promoting partnerships, empowerment, and enabling.
- Reduce fear of the unknown through education, familiar articles, and decreasing the threat of the environment.
- Provide opportunities for control, such as participating in care, attempting to normalize daily schedule, and providing direct suggestions.

Adapted from Wong, D. L. (n.d.). *Innovative approaches for atraumatic cancer care.* Retrieved from http://www.authorstream.com/presentation/Carolina-48857-op077-INNOVATIVE-APPROACHES-ATRAUMATIC-CANCER-CARE-DEFINITION-SOURCES-PATIENT-FAMILY-STRESSORS-as-Entertainment-ppt-powerpoint/. Accessed August 25, 2013.

TABLE 30.1	SUGGESTIONS FOR ATRAUMATIC CARE
Principle	**Suggestions for Nursing Care**
Preventing or minimizing physical stressors	• For painful injections, blood draws, or IV insertion, use numbing techniques (see Chapter 36). • During painful or invasive procedures, avoid traditional restraint or "holding down" of the child. Use alternative positioning such as "therapeutic hugging." • If the above-mentioned positions are not an option, have the parent stand near the child's head to provide comfort. • Insert a saline lock if the child requires multiple doses of parenteral medications. • Advocate for minimal laboratory blood draws. • Minimize intramuscular or subcutaneous injections. • Provide appropriate pain management (refer to Chapter 36).
Preventing or minimizing child and family separation	• Promote family-centred care. • In the hospital, provide comfortable accommodations for the parent. • Allow the family the choice about whether to stay for an invasive procedure, and support them in their decision.
Promoting a sense of control	• Maintain the child's home routine related to activities of daily living. • Provide reassurance and realistic hope. • Encourage the child to have a security item present, if desired. • Involve the child and family in planning care from the moment of the first encounter. • Empower the family and child by providing knowledge. • Allow the child and family choices when they are available. • Make the environment more inviting and less intimidating.

PREVENTING/MINIMIZING PHYSICAL STRESSORS

The health care facility or hospital is an unfamiliar environment for children and parents and may upset or intimidate them. They may feel anxiety, fear, helplessness, anger, or loss of control. Even health care procedures performed in the home or school may be perceived as threatening to children. To prevent and minimize the stress experienced by children and their families in relation to health care, pediatric nurses and other health care professionals engage in atraumatic care.

Minimizing Stress During Procedures

Children undergo numerous diagnostic and therapeutic procedures in a wide range of settings during their development. These procedures may be performed in the community or outpatient setting or in a care facility. Regardless of the procedure and the setting, children need thorough preparation before the procedure and support during and after the procedure, to promote the best outcome and atraumatic care.

Using positions that are comforting to the child during painful procedures is an important aspect of atraumatic care (Fig. 30.1). **Therapeutic hugging** (a holding position that promotes close physical contact between the child and a parent or caregiver) may be used for certain procedures or treatments where the child must remain still. For example, the parent can hold the child in his or her lap snugly to prevent the child from moving during an injection or venepuncture. When using this technique, make sure the parent understands his or her role and knows which body parts to hold still in a safe manner. Alternatively, distraction or stimulation (such as with a toy) can help to gain the child's cooperation. Refer to Box 30.2 for distraction methods. See Figure 30.2.

Before the Procedure

Appropriate preparation for procedures helps to decrease the child's and family's anxiety level, promotes the child's

BOX 30.2

DISTRACTION METHODS

• Have the child point toes inward and wiggle them.
• Ask the child to squeeze your hand.
• Encourage the child to count aloud.
• Sing a song and have the child sing along.
• Point out the pictures on the ceiling.
• Have the child blow bubbles.
• Play music or read a book appealing to the child.

TABLE 30.2	ALTERNATIVES FOR CONFUSING OR MISUNDERSTOOD TERMS	
Term to Avoid	**How Children Might Interpret It**	**Use These Terms Instead**
Catheter	Too technical	Tube
Deaden	Kill	Make sleepy
Dye	"Die"	Special medicine to help the doctor see _____ (part of the body) better
Electrodes	Too technical	Stickers, ticklers, snaps
ICU	"I see you"	Special room with your own nurse
Incision, cut open, make a hole	Too explicit	Special or small opening
Monitor	Too technical	TV screen
Organ	Like a piano	Special place in the body
Pain	May be too explicit	Child's word for hurt; "boo-boo"
Put to sleep, anaesthesia	May confuse with putting a pet to sleep	Special kind of sleep
Shot	Children are scared of shots	Medication under the skin
Stool	Like you sit on	"Poop" or child's word for it
Stretcher or gurney	"Stretch her"	Rolling bed or special bed on wheels
Take your temperature/BP	Where are you going to "take" them	See how warm you are/hug your arm
Test	Like at school (the child will need to perform)	See how your heart is working
Tourniquet	Too technical	Special kind of rubber band
Urine	"You're in"	"Pee" or child's word for it
X-ray	Don't understand	Picture or big camera to take pictures of the inside of your body

Partially adapted from Florida Children's Hospital, Child Life Department. (n.d.). *Suggested vocabulary to use with children.* Orlando, FL: Author.

adults for assuming responsibility for their own health care needs.

The general principles of family-centred care include:
- Honest, objective, and unbiased exchange of information between families, children, and care providers
- Recognition of and respect for cultural, linguistic, and socioeconomic diversity and care preferences
- Collaboration and partnership between care providers and families that is supportive of the child and family's needs, strengths, and values
- Child and family care objectives are flexible
- Nursing and medical care decisions are made with consideration of the child's home and family life, school, daytime activities, and overall quality of life.

When children's health care is provided through a family-centred approach, many positive outcomes are possible, including the following:
- Anxiety is decreased.
- Children are calmer and pain management is enhanced.
- Recovery times are shortened.
- Families' confidence and problem-solving skills are improved.

- Communication between the health care team and the family is also improved, leading to greater satisfaction for both health care providers and health care consumers (families).
- A decrease in health care costs is seen and health care resources are used more effectively (Ontario Centre of Excellence for Child and Youth Mental Health, 2016).

Ways to increase collaboration between the family and the health care team may include a family advisory board, a newsletter, conferences, or parent resource notebooks. Methods for increasing communication between the health care team and the family may include the use of mailboxes or dry-erase boards for updating the daily plan of care, including the parents' participation in rounds, or through a daily assessment of health status by the child or family.

Nurses can offer support to parents through encouraging their participation and involvement in all aspects of their child's care. In particular, nurses should respect the parent's decision-making process regarding their child as well as be committed to advocating for parental presence during hospitalization and procedures. Address the family's emotional and spiritual needs, listen to their

FIGURE 30.3 Providing a comfortable area for the parent to rest is an important component of family-centred care.

concerns, and provide the best accommodations possible (when the child is hospitalized) (Fig. 30.3). This will empower the family and foster resilience, and allow the parents to develop a trusting relationship with the health care professionals caring for their child.

Take Note!

Some parents will not know how to advocate or speak up for their child; as a nurse, you must help open this door for them.

How could family-centred care help the Moore family described at the beginning of the chapter?

PROMOTING A SENSE OF CONTROL

During times of illness, hospitalization, or health-related interventions, the child and family can experience an extreme sense of loss of control. Promoting control in all health care interactions is crucial to atraumatic and trauma-informed practice because people who have experienced trauma have often experienced abuses of power in previous interactions. In addition, promoting control reduces the likelihood of making the current experience traumatizing for children or families. Providing communication and teaching that promotes a sense of safety and trustworthiness can help foster feelings of control and improve the child's and family's ability to understand, cope, and traverse the emotional upheaval of their child's illness. Assisting the family to obtain necessary information, resources, and relationships contributes to optimal health care for the child and family. Creating welcoming intake procedures, adapting the physical space to be less unfamiliar, ensuring informed consent and choice, and outlining realistic expectations

for procedures are key to promoting choice through a trauma-informed lens (Arthur et al., 2013).

Enhancing Communication

Clear and trustworthy communication with children and their parents is critical to providing atraumatic quality nursing care. Child- and parent-centred communication improves outcomes and satisfaction with nursing care. Effective communication is the foundation of the therapeutic relationship and leads to increased knowledge and health care behaviours on the part of the child and family (Levetown & American Academy of Paediatrics Committee on Bioethics, 2008). Nurses can support families and children in their communication with health care providers through advocating for the patient and family during health conversations, and clarifying misconceptions following medical encounters.

Children are often socialized to be passive participants in health care, doing as they are told, with or without protests. Yet, "as paediatric nurses, we have an obligation to listen, to hear, and to feel the voices of the children in our care" (McPherson & Thorne, 2000, p. 28). Children can inform nurses of their experiences and in turn nurses can respect, listen, and understand children's voices utilizing their innate wisdoms about their health to inform the clinical team and guide goal setting as well as health planning.

Nurses must become familiar with the unique communication patterns of their patients and their families. Some children are very talkative, while others are quiet. Children may be more apt to communicate if they are engaged in another activity or they may rely on nonverbal communication such as silence to communicate their needs. The pediatric nurse needs to consider the age of the child, and the child's cognitive and developmental level when communicating with patients. The nurse should also attune to the communication needs of the parents. Refer to Chapter 2 for information on verbal and nonverbal communication.

Developmental Techniques for Communicating With Children

Effective communication with children involves a variety of age-appropriate methods. With school-aged children and toddlers, give the child time to "warm up" to you. Speak to the parents first and follow their direction where possible in caring for their child. This therapeutic alliance is important in building strong trustworthy health care relationships. When the children are ready, use clear explanations in an unhurried and confident manner. Communicate at their eye level (Fig. 30.4A) using language that meets their developmental needs. Through the use of dolls, puppets, or stuffed animals, nurses can

Take Note!

There will always be some interest more immediate than protecting the well-being of children. There will never be one more important.

—UNICEF Report Card, 2016

Patient education occurs when nurses share information, knowledge, and skills with families, thus empowering them to take responsibility for their child's health care. Through patient education, families can overcome feelings of powerlessness and helplessness and gain the confidence and ability to step to the forefront of the health care team. Nurses spend innumerable hours teaching children and families; in fact, on some days in the hospital, more teaching than nursing care is provided. Given the importance of, and the amount of time spent on, child and family education, each nurse should become an expert at basic patient education principles.

Goals of Child and Family Education

The goals of child and family education are to:
- Improve the child's and family's health literacy
- Encourage communication with health care providers
- Improve health outcomes and promote healthy lifestyles
- Encourage involvement of the child and family in care and decision making about care
- Work with families to develop care plans that are culturally safe and relevant
- Promote a sense of autonomy and control

Overall goals for the child and family include the ability of children and families to make informed decisions, to perform basic health care skills, to recognize when the child has a problem and know how to respond to the problem, and to know how to get answers when questions arise.

Take Note!

Today health care consumers have information available at their fingertips. It is important to steer children and their families to reliable and credible health care resources. Refer to Chapter 2 for information on steps of client and family education.

Take Note!

Teaching Techniques

When given a diagnosis that will have a significant impact on a family's life, it is important for the nurse to allow the parents time to absorb the information about the disorder. The nurse should give parents only small amounts of information at a time to allow them time to absorb it.

Teaching Children and Adolescents

Teaching children and adolescents is a vital part of pediatric nursing practice. Children and adolescents have a great need for information about their illness as they attempt to master their anxiety and restore feelings of competency, self-confidence, and hope. As with adults, they learn best when their input is valued and they are actively involved in the learning process. The age and developmental level of the child will determine the amount, format, and timing of the information given. Before beginning to teach a child, it is important to establish rapport and lay the foundation for good communication. Refer to Developmental Techniques for Communicating With Children above and Table 30.3 for additional information related to communicating well with children and adolescents.

Teaching Preschool Children. When teaching young children, the nurse or family assumes part or all of the responsibility for what is learned, how it is learned, and when it is learned. Because they have vivid imaginations, young children often attempt to invent pieces of information, or they pick up bits and pieces of misinformation that can lead to false assumptions. Skilfully delivered and timed information can promote trust, calmness, and control in an otherwise apprehensive and uncooperative preschooler. Table 30.4 presents some general guidelines for teaching young children.

Teaching School-Aged Children. Unless they are quite ill, school-aged children usually want to participate in their care. They have a need to cooperate and achieve. When teaching, speak directly to them and include them in the education plan. Teach the school-aged child and parent together, as parents can often learn by observing the care being given and taught to their child. Table 30.5 provides some general guidelines to keep in mind when teaching school-aged children.

Teaching Adolescents. Adolescents are particularly sensitive about maintaining body image and feelings of control and autonomy. This is especially important with health care processes and decisions that affect them. Table 30.6 gives guidelines to use when teaching adolescents. Refer to Chapter 2 for information on evaluating learning and documenting education.

Consider This

Elsa is a 5-year-old girl on your unit who was recently diagnosed with diabetes. She is getting ready to be discharged home at the end of the week. Her grandparents are her primary caregivers.

What concerns regarding learning would you take into consideration during your assessment?

Describe different teaching strategies you would utilize with Elsa and her family.

How would you evaluate learning with Elsa and her family?

TABLE 30.4	GENERAL TEACHING TIPS FOR YOUNG CHILDREN

Teaching Tips	Practical Application
Offer simple, concise, concrete explanations based on the assessed needs, questions, and developmental level of the child.	Use a child's senses and relate what a procedure will look, sound, smell, taste, or feel like ("The MRI machine will sound very loud, like a big train").
Be honest, even when the information you need to convey is not positive. This helps the child to form a bond of trust and confidence with caregivers.	Use the family's words that the child understands; use "soft words" ("This will feel warm" instead of "This will burn").
Time explanations to decrease anxiety and excess worry before the event. Avoid telling unpleasant news close to bedtime.	As a general rule, give toddlers information about procedures, medicines, and other interventions immediately beforehand; give 4 to 7 year olds information 1 or 2 days in advance.
Parents know their child best. Eliciting information from them about their child's past behaviours and coping skills can often mean the difference between a positive and negative experience for their child.	Teach parents how to coach their child with pain management, visualization, or other methods of distraction when appropriate ("Remember when we went to the beach . . .").
Provide an active role for the child. This helps to foster a child's sense of self-confidence and control over the situation.	Allow the child to help with simple self-care activities such as holding a dressing or piece of tape. Provide props and dolls to touch and feel as much as possible ("Your job is to keep your hands still").
Children's wishes must be respected when they verbalize or demonstrate that they do not want more information.	Keep explanations short and simple; know when to stop teaching.
Praise the child and let him or her know how much you appreciate his or her help and cooperation.	Use "please" and "thank you" often ("Thank you. I like the way you held still for me").

TABLE 30.5	GENERAL GUIDELINES WHEN TEACHING SCHOOL-AGED CHILDREN

Teaching Tips	Practical Application
Allow the child some control and involvement in the decision-making process.	Offer choices whenever possible (taking the medicine with juice or milk), but don't offer choices when there are no alternatives (taking the medicine).
Children can relate present-day happenings to past experiences.	Use examples and past experiences that are familiar to the child ("Remember when you were first learning to swim . . .").
Achievement and accomplishment are very important to children at this age; so anything they can be actively involved in will help them adjust and learn.	Provide an active role and allow the child to do as much of his or her care as possible. Use props, dolls, games, and computers to enhance learning.
At this age, most children are able to sequence, understand cause and effect, and make sense of time.	Teach children the steps involved and how long it will take ("Today I'm going to teach you how to change your dressing. This will help keep your cut clean. First, wash your hands . . .").
Gaining control over the situation and preparing mentally are important for their self-confidence.	Provide information 3 to 7 days in advance, depending on the child's age and developmental level.
Praise the child and let him or her know how much you appreciate his or her help and cooperation.	Use "please" and "thank you" often ("Thanks! You did a great job using your inhaler").

TABLE 30.6	GENERAL GUIDELINES WHEN TEACHING ADOLESCENTS
Teaching Tips	**Practical Application**
Allow teens to be in control and involved in the decision-making process.	Speak directly to teens; consider their input in all decisions about their care and education.
Adolescents can process abstract information and understand how their actions affect long-term outcomes.	Provide reasons why something is important and discuss how their lives will be affected by their decision to take care of their health needs ("If you take your asthma medicine, you'll be better able to play tennis").
Adolescents are very concerned about how they look and how they fit in with peers.	Collaborate with the teen to develop acceptable solutions and strategies for dealing with health issues that affect personal appearance and peer acceptance (e.g., wig vs. head scarves for hair loss from chemotherapy).
Adolescents strive for independence and have personal values and ideologies that may conflict with those of parents and the medical community.	Expect some noncompliance with care, despite your best educational efforts. Work together to achieve win–win outcomes of educational goals.

KEY CONCEPTS

- Atraumatic care focuses on minimizing stressors and separation from the family and promoting a sense of control for the child and family.

- Children and families need appropriate explanation and education before a procedure is performed. Preparation may include explaining the procedure as well as physically preparing the child. Appropriate preparation helps to decrease the child's and family's anxiety, promote the child's cooperation, and support the child's and family's coping skills.

- A major aspect of preparation involves play.

- Include the child's parents in preparation because parents are usually the greatest source of comfort for the child.

- Be short, simple, and appropriate in explaining situations at the child's level of development. Explain what is to be done and what is expected of the child.

- Trauma-informed care encompasses how health care providers, organizations, and broader systems understand or respond to people who have experienced trauma or who are at risk for experiencing a traumatic event.

- Trauma-informed care places emphasis on reducing potentially traumatic medical events, providing patients with choice about their care, and emphasizes control in treatment options.

- Family-centred care is based on the concept that the family is the primary source of strength and support for the child.

- Family-centred care includes respect for the child and family, recognition of cultural diversity, identification of the family's strengths, assistance with emotional and other support of the family, providing honest and unbiased information, and collaborating and empowering families.

- Maintain open and honest lines of communication with children and their families.

- Therapeutic communication involves the use of open-ended questions, reflection, paraphrasing, acknowledgement of emotions, and active listening.

- To communicate effectively with children, provide information and support on the child's developmental level and utilize age-appropriate methods.

- When communicating with parents, be honest. Parents want to feel valued and should be equal partners in the health care team.

- It is vital for the family to have knowledge about their child's health.

- Patient education begins with the first patient encounter and proceeds through discharge and beyond. Reassessment after each step or change in the process is critical to success.

REFERENCES AND RECOMMENDED READINGS

Arthur, E., Seymour, A., Dartnall, M., Beltgens, P., Poole, N., Smylie, D., & Schmidt, R. (2013). *Trauma informed practice guide*. Retrieved from http://bccewh.bc.ca/wp-content/uploads/2012/05/2013_TIP-Guide.pdf

Bennett, C., & Pflaumer, D. (n.d.). *Positioning & comfort techniques*. Orlando, FL: Florida Children's Hospital.

Bray, L., Carter, B., & Snodin, J. (2016). Holding children for clinical procedures: Perseverance in spite of or persevering to be child-centered. *Research in nursing & health*, *39*(1), 30–41.

Canadian Paediatric Nursing Standards Advisory Group. (2017). *Canadian paediatric nursing standards: Standardizing high quality nursing care for Canada's children*. Retrieved from http://ken.caphc.org/xwiki/bin/download/Other+Resources/Canadian+Paediatric+Nursing+Standards/FINAL-Paediatric%20Nursing%20Standards.pdf

Children's Health Policy Centre. (2011). Helping children overcome trauma. *Children's mental health research quarterly*, *5*(3). Retrieved from http://childhealthpolicy.ca/wp-content/uploads/2012/12/RQ-3-11-Summer.pdf

Coyne, I. (2015). Families and health-care professionals' perspectives and expectations of family-centred care: Hidden expectations and unclear roles. *Health expectations 18*(5), 796–808.

Florida Children's Hospital, Child Life Department. (n.d.a). *Atraumatic care: An age specific approach*. Orlando, FL: Author.

Florida Children's Hospital, Child Life Department. (n.d.b). *Suggested vocabulary to use with children*. Orlando, FL: Author.

Gonzalez, A., Catherine, N., Boyle, M., Jack, S. M., Atkinson, L., Kobor, M., & MacMillan, H. L. (2018). Healthy Foundations Study: a randomised controlled trial to evaluate biological embedding of early-life experiences. *BMJ Open*, *8*(1), e018915.

Harrison, T. M. (2010). Family-centered pediatric nursing care: state of the science. *Journal of Pediatric Nursing, 25*(5), 335–343.

Karatekin, C. (2018). Adverse childhood experiences (ACEs), stress and mental health in college students. *Stress and Health, 34*(1), 36–45.

Koller, D. (2007). Child life council evidence-based practice statement: preparing children and adolescents for medical procedures. *Child Life Council*. Retrieved from http://www.childlife.org/files/ebppreparationstatement-complete.pdf

Kolucki, B., & Lemish, D. (2011). *Communicating with children: principles and practices to nurture, inspire, excite, educate and heal*. Retrieved from http://www.unicef.org/cwc/files/CwC_Web%282%29.pdf. AccessedAugust 29, 2013.

Leahy, S., Kennedy, R. M., Hesselgrave, J., Gurwitch, K., Barkey, M., & Millar, T. F. (2008). On the front lines: Lessons learned in implementing multidisciplinary peripheral venous access pain-management programs in pediatric hospitals. *Pediatrics, 122* Suppl 3, S161–S170. Retrieved from http://pediatrics.aappublications.org/cgi/reprint/122/Supplement_3/S161.pdf. Accessed March 31, 2011.

Levetown, M.; American Academy of Pediatrics Committee on Bioethics. (2008). Communicating with children and families: From everyday interactions to skill in conveying distressing information. *Pediatrics, 121*(5), e1441–e1460.

Manneheim, J. K. (2012). *Preschooler test or procedure preparation*. Retrieved from https://pediatrix.com/body.cfm?id=7&action=detail&AEArticleID=002057&AEProductID=Adam2004_1&AEProjectTypeIDURL=APT_1.

Marsac, M. L., Kassam-Adams, N., Hildenbrand, A. K., Nicholls, E., Winston, F. K., Leff, S. S., & Fein, J. (2016). Implementing a trauma-informed approach in pediatric health care networks. *JAMA Pediatrics, 170*(1), 70–77.

McPherson, G., & Thorne, S. (2000). Children's voices: can we hear them? *Journal of pediatric nursing, 15*(1), 22–29.

Ontario Centre of Excellence for Child and Youth Mental Health. (2016). *Evidence in-sight: best practices in engaging families in child and youth mental health*. Retrieved from http://www.excellenceforchildandyouth.ca/sites/default/files/eib_attach/FamilyEngagement_Final_Jan2016.pdf

UNICEF. (2016). *UNICEF report card 13: fairness for children*. Retrieved from http://www.unicef.ca/cn/unicef-report-card-13-fairness-children

Wong, D. L. (n.d.). *Innovative approaches to atraumatic cancer care*. Retrieved from http://www.authorstream.com/presentation/Carolina-48857-op077-INNOVATIVE-APPROACHES-ATRAUMATIC-CANCER-CARE-DEFINITION-SOURCES-PATIENT-FAMILY-STRESSORS-as-Entertainment-ppt-powerpoint/. Accessed August 25, 2013.

CHAPTER **WORKSHEET**

MULTIPLE CHOICE QUESTIONS

1. When providing atraumatic care to a child, which action would be the most appropriate?
   a. Applying restraints for any procedure that would be uncomfortable
   b. Keeping the lights on in the child's room throughout the day and night
   c. Limiting the use of topical anaesthetics for painful injections
   d. Allowing parents and children an informed choice about being together

2. A 2-year-old boy is scheduled to undergo an endoscopic procedure. His parents are asking when they should tell him about it. Based on the nurse's understanding of the child's developmental stage, when would be the most appropriate time to prepare the child for the procedure?
   a. About 1 week before the scheduled date
   b. A few days in advance of the scheduled date
   c. About 1 hour before the procedure is to occur
   d. Just before the procedure is to be performed

3. When working with children and families, which is a critical strategy for promoting therapeutic communication?
   a. Detailed explanations
   b. Attentive listening
   c. Comforting touch
   d. Closed-ended questions

4. The nurse is caring for a 2 year old in the hospital, and the mother expresses concern that the toddler will be scared. Which response by the nurse would be most appropriate?
   a. "Don't worry; we practice family-centred and atraumatic care here."
   b. "We will do our best to minimize the stress that your child experiences."
   c. "It will probably be upsetting for you as well, so you should stay home."
   d. "Our practice of atraumatic care will eliminate all pain and stress for your child."

5. When planning education for a child and parents, what is the first step the nurse should take?

   a. Decide which procedures and medications the child will be discharged on.
   b. Determine the child's and family's learning needs and styles.
   c. Ask the family if they have ever performed this type of procedure.
   d. Tell the child and family what the goals of the teaching session are.

CRITICAL THINKING EXERCISES

1. A 5-year-old boy is being admitted to your unit. The physician has ordered IV fluids along with laboratory work including a complete blood count, electrolytes, and a urine culture. As his nurse, how will you prepare him and his family before the procedure and support them during and after the procedure, to promote the best outcome and to ensure atraumatic care?

2. An 8 year old is admitted to your nursing unit. Please describe the steps the nurse should take to provide health care teaching to this child.

STUDY ACTIVITIES

1. Develop a teaching plan for one of the families that you care for in the clinical setting. Be sure to follow the appropriate steps for providing education.

2. Research the availability of language interpreters and translators in your local community, compiling a list of the available resources.

3. Describe health education topics that would be appropriate in a school setting for elementary students.

BRINGING IT ALL TOGETHER: A CASE STUDY

Mia, a 5-year-old girl, is admitted to your unit for pneumonia not improving at home on oral antibiotics. Orders for Mia include an IV insertion to begin IV antibiotics.

Go to thePoint **to find questions to consider about this case.**

31

KEY TERMS

capacity building
community health
 nurse (CHN)
comprehensive
 school health
determinants of
 health (DoH)
developmental
 screening
health promotion
health surveillance
home care
immunization
nursing process
partnership
prevention
primary care
primary health care
 (PHC)
priority populations
public health
school health
screening
social justice
strength-based
 approach
telehealth
vaccination
wellness

Health Promotion in the Community With Children and Families

Learning Objectives

Upon completion of the chapter, you will be able to:

1. Define child and family health concepts in community health nursing practice.
2. Describe principles of primary health care (PHC) in the community with children and families.
3. Define approaches to health surveillance and health promotion practices.
4. Describe practice and settings for nurses who work in the community.
5. Recognize priority populations of children.
6. Describe approaches to health promotion with priority populations.
7. Explain developmental surveillance and screening tools for healthy child development.
8. Describe approaches to prevention of disease and injury.
9. Demonstrate knowledge of an immunology and immunization.
10. Identify health promotion activities for different developmental stages and contexts.
11. Describe child health programs in the community.

Three-year-old Maya and 9-month-old Evan are brought to the clinic by their father. Maya was last seen in the clinic at 1 year of age, and Evan has never been seen. The father says that they have both been healthy, but now he is wondering about immunizations.

HEALTH IN THE COMMUNITY WITH CHILDREN AND FAMILIES

Our shared priority with children and families is optimal health. Health is a dynamic interplay of beliefs, context, and the influence of the determinants of health (DoH; Community Health Nurses of Canada [CHNC], 2011; Conference Board of Canada, 2015). Maintaining and improving health occurs where children and families live, play, and work within the community. This goal is supported by the community health nurse (CHN). The Community Health Nurses of Canada (CHNC, 2011) *Professional Practice Model and Standards of Practice* describes seven standards of practice, with respective focus priorities and implementation strategies. Community health nursing with children and families is guided by these standards, in conjunction with Canadian Paediatric Nursing Standards Advisory Group (CPNSAG, 2016), and professional nursing ethics of the Canadian Nursing Association (CNA, 2017a, 2017b). CHN practice priorities include health promotion, prevention, and health protection and health maintenance, restoration, and palliative care services (see Chapter 34). Recent approaches include access to care in early years (8 weeks to 5 years), universal access (for all children and families), and enhanced access (for vulnerable children and families). This chapter is organized around the components of health promotion within the community context, including developmental assessment, checks, and screening, prevention and health protection of injury and disease, recognition of priority populations, and providing strength-based care.

PRIMARY HEALTH CARE

Community health nursing encompasses primary health care (PHC) principles, with a focus on promoting health in the community. PHC is an overarching framework for optimizing health among individuals, families, and communities. This involves stakeholders working together in the health care system and with other sectors (e.g., education) to identify barriers to health, and create solutions, while being responsive, accountable, and collaborative (Canadian Nurses Association, 2015). By thinking about PHC, nurses can broaden their understanding of wider social, economic, physical, and political environments that influence child health and how to access related services (Allison, 2016).

PHC as an approach to health includes a spectrum of services beyond the traditional health care system. It includes all services that play a part in health, such as income, housing, education, and environment. Primary care is an element within PHC that focuses on health care services, including health promotion, illness and injury prevention, and the diagnosis and treatment of illness and injury.

Variation in the positioning and function of PHC and primary care exist and are summarized in Table 31.1.

In Canada, children and families continue to struggle with serious health issues, including poverty, chronic illness, disability, mental health, and obesity. DoH are major contributors to these serious health issues and require consideration at the broader societal level since this is where children and families are most affected (Raphael, 2014). Through PHC, CHNs focus on optimizing health for the child, family, and community. Health promotion visits with the family are viewed as part of a continuum of care, not as the accomplishment of isolated tasks. Therefore, nurses address issues beyond individual health encounters, and consider the influence of complex systemic factors influencing health within Canadian society. Through PHC, children and families have an opportunity to cocreate optimal wellness, and ultimately a healthier society.

TABLE 31.1	PRIMARY CARE AND PRIMARY HEALTH CARE	
Primary Health Care		**Primary Care**
Health for All based on 5 principles of Alma Ata Declaration (1978): accessibility, public participation, health promotion, appropriate technology, and intersectoral collaboration		Efficient, sustainable, comprehensive health care to optimize timely, seamless service delivery, and care coordination
Commitment to social justice, health equity, and community development to address the determinants of health		Commitment to accessible, integrated, and coordinated health care
Decentralized point of entry to the health care system led by interdisciplinary health care providers in collaboration with individuals, families, and community		Centralized point of entry to health care system led by physicians in collaboration with interdisciplinary health care teams
Comprehensive coordinated and integrated approach including health promotion and disease prevention, treatment, rehabilitation		Comprehensive coordinated and integrated approach including health promotion and disease prevention, treatment, rehabilitation
Population- (macro), community- (meso), and person-centred (micro) approach		Patient-centred approach with community care networks

HEALTH SURVEILLANCE

Health surveillance is an important concept within health, wellness, and prevention and is described by the Public Health Agency of Canada (PHAC, 2012) as the tracking and forecasting of events and determinants through the collection, analysis, and dissemination of data (para 1). As a result of this surveillance strategy, public health issues or outbreaks can be reported and managed quickly. In addition, evidenced-based, practical programs and policies are developed to meet the needs of Canadian children, families, and wider communities. Therefore, health surveillance has a broad reach into areas, including health promotion, routine assessment, chronic disease surveillance systems, and communicable disease (PHAC, 2012). Health surveillance will be discussed further in the upcoming section on Components of Health Care in the Community Screening and Surveillance.

Health Promotion

One key PHC principle is health promotion, which is a process that enables and empowers people to enhance their well-being at the individual, family, community, and population level (World Health Organization [WHO], 2017a). Health promotion supports optimal wellness through holistic growth and development (e.g., physical, social, mental), while preventing disease and injury (WHO, 1948/2017). The CHN facilitates health promotion–based strategies outlined in the Ottawa Charter by building healthy public policy, creating supportive environments, strengthening community action, and developing personal capacity (WHO, 1986). Five complex dimensions of child well-being are "material well-being, health and safety, education, behaviours and risks, and housing and environment" (UNICEF Office of Research-Innocenti, 2013, cited by Raphael, 2014) (Box 31.1). By recognizing the significance of five dimensions of child well-being from a community health perspective, the CHN promotes health through social justice, partnership, and strength-based approaches. Social justice is framed in how the CHN promotes health equity for children and families by acting on DoH at all levels (Commission on the Social Determinants of Health, 2008).

While health promotion is a distinct CHN standard (CHNC, 2011), in this chapter, health promotion is

---

BOX 31.1

FIVE COMPLEX DIMENSIONS OF CHILD WELL-BEING

Dimension	Key Components	Indicators
Economic and material well-being	Living in low-income households, financial deprivation, caregiver unemployment	Child poverty Increased level of vulnerability Poverty gap and rate—unmet food needs
Health and Safety– physical and social well-being	Prenatal care Health at birth Childhood mortality and morbidity	Infant mortality and morbidity rates, serious injury rates Birth weight and healthy eating in childhood Universal screening (i.e. vision, hearing, dental etc.) Rate of children in care Immunization rate Suicide rate Youth offending/conviction rates Incidence, reporting abuse—neglect
Education	Attendance Achievement and completion Employment and training (youth)	Readiness, engagement in pre-school and early years education Further education Child literacy, numeracy, exclusion
Behaviours and risk– including mental health	Health behaviours Risk taking Exposure to violence	Percentage children with healthy weight Youth physical activity levels Frequency tobacco, marijuana, alcohol use Prevalence asthma, chlamydia, teenage pregnancy Being bullied, gender(ed) discrimination
Environment, including housing	Housing Environmental safety	Living in poor housing conditions Youth not in employment or education Pollution (i.e. air, water etc.)

Adapted from UNCEF Office of Research-Innocenti (2013, pg 5) and Dimensions and Indicators of Children and Youth Health & Well-being in BC. Is "good" good enough (n.d.)

considered a broad term that encompasses optimizing wellness through all levels of prevention. Health promotion takes place in a variety of practice settings, including home, daycare, school, telehealth centres, ambulatory care centres, community health centres, and public health agencies (CHNC, 2011).

Partnerships

Developing partnerships involves working alongside children and families as well as the broader community to develop capacity, confidence, and capability (Shields, 2011). Shifting from a problem-based view does not mean that issues are overlooked. Rather, a strength-based approach supports resilience for children and families to face challenges, and be involved as active partners in health promotion (CPHA, 2010; CPNSAG, 2016). Strength-based CHN practice is focused on capacity building, and recognizes protective factors as assets. By focusing on strengths, rather than problems, the CHN supports families by generating solutions to challenges, and encourages self-determination through resourcefulness and resilience (Hammond, 2010).

Parental behaviours and life experiences can have a lasting impact on the child's health and development, and at times forecast child health outcomes (Donaldson, Handren, & Crano, 2016). For instance, if the family is in turmoil, the child may not receive the attention and energy they need to thrive. Furthermore, child health and social and emotional well-being are linked to the resources of his/her community. If the community has high levels of poverty, insufficient infrastructure, and lack of resources, children may not be able to access support services needed to reach their full potential. To be effective, the nurse must demonstrate commitment and develop ongoing partnerships with the child, family, and community whereby children and families are respected as partners in health promotion. This view is extended with the broader community to develop capacity and generate shared priorities and solutions. Community development is facilitated by building relationships and identifying community stakeholders working together towards positive change (CPHA, 2010).

Community Health Nursing: Practice With Children and Families

Community health nursing is a broad term that reflects a variety of practice settings where the CHN promotes health. Settings include home, clinics, school, and community-based services (CHNC, 2011). In addition, nurses can develop partnership models with the broader community such as city council, churches, and community agencies such as friendship centres and charitable organizations.

Take Note!

The main areas of practice where nurses work to promote the health with children and families are home health/care, telehealth, schools, primary care, and public health settings such as an immunization clinic.

Partnerships between the community and the CHN lead to greater awareness of available resources. With input from community partners, the nurse can perform an assessment of the community's assets and needs. The assessment then provides a foundation for the development of community-based health promotion programs. These programs expand the resources of the community, which in turn enhances the health of its members.

HOME CARE

Home care or home health care is nursing practice situated in the home or community environment, integrated within the child's context. Home care is supported by intersectoral programs, and builds long-term and comprehensive relationships with children, families, and interprofessional teams. Practices include health promotion, health teaching, disease prevention, and direct clinical care. The role of the nurse can vary from short focused intervention (i.e., wound care), teaching new skills to families and communities (i.e., diabetic management), and supportive care for children with complex or life-limiting health needs or working with children at end-of-life (Canadian Home Care Association, 2016). The home setting supports family-centred care that is highly accessible and collaboratively coordinated. Home care nursing is discussed further in Chapter 34.

TELEHEALTH

The CHN uses communication and information technology to provide care by distance (College of Registered Nurses of British Columbia, 2018). Canadian telehealth programs are offered in urban, rural, and remote areas, and include clinical services, remote monitoring, education, and videoconferencing (COACH, 2015). Such innovative distance care delivery is aligned with PHC to support community-based care with children, families, interprofessional providers, and agencies. Telehealth may optimize children's health by improving access, enhancing quality, and providing cost-effective health care within local settings (Canada Health Infoway, 2011). The nurse may be involved with health technologies that support the child or youth in a range of areas, including patient safety, promoting privacy, remote access, and health data updates (e.g., HbA1c mapping in youth is an example of this approach).

SCHOOLS

Children spend significant time at school, therefore the school becomes a priority setting for the CHN. Home care and public health nurses are often involved in school

CHILDREN AS PARTNERS IN HEALTH: COMPREHENSIVE SCHOOL HEALTH PILLARS

Pillars	Activity
Social and physical environments	Healthy relationships, healthy spaces, and places
Teaching and learning	Wellness resources, activities, and curriculum
Healthy school policy	Health-promoting policies and procedures
Partnerships and services	Collaboration with community stakeholders

Adapted from Pan-Canadian Joint Consortium for School Health (2017).

health promotion. Nurses support wellness of children and their school community in a collaborative, school-wide, holistic approach by providing direct or indirect education to children, youth, caregivers, and teachers. The Pan-Canadian joint consortium for school health (2017) advocates for a comprehensive school health framework built on four integrated pillars (Box 31.2). Further information can be found at thePoint.

PRIMARY CARE

CHNs also provide health promotion and disease prevention programs within primary care settings such as community health centres, primary care networks, and interprofessional health provider offices. CHNs working in primary care settings are called family practice nurses. They often are considered the first point of access to the health care system in urban, rural, and remote settings (Primary Care Initiative, 2017). Primary care nurses may be involved with general health promotion programs, developmental screening and surveillance programs, counselling, immunization, and referrals. Primary care settings are generally funded by health care or not-for-profit agencies such as the Alex Community Health outreach bus in Calgary, Alberta (The Alex, 2017) and community health centres for at-risk youth and families (Canadian Association of Community Health Centres, 2017).

PUBLIC HEALTH

Public health nursing is grounded in social sciences, behavioural theory, and public health sciences. The CHN in public health practice works in a variety of settings such as homes, clinics, community health centres, schools, and daycare centres. The CHN partners with communities and other systems, such as charitable organizations and local city councils, to meet the needs of children and families. The CHN links the health and illness experiences of individuals, families, and communities to population health promotion practice (CHNC, 2011). The key roles of public health nurses are health promotion, disease (e.g., immunization) and injury prevention (e.g., car seat safety), health protection (e.g., food safety), health surveillance (e.g., measles outbreak), population health assessment, and emergency preparedness and response (CPHA, 2010). Public health nursing practice focuses on health promotion by building healthy public policy, as well as prevention, surveillance, and control of injury and disease.

Nursing Process

The CHN promotes, protects, and preserves health of the child and family using the nursing process in an ongoing, dynamic, systematic, reciprocal, and purposeful manner (CHNC, 2011). This includes working with communities and populations to make substantive changes to health. The CHN *assessment* is ongoing and dynamic and requires feedback to be re-evaluated and reassessed in collaboration with the child, family, community, and population. The CHN conducts comprehensive assessments of needs and assets using multiple methods and sources. Methods of assessment include interviews, surveys, focus groups, and windshield surveys. A variety of data sources inform a comprehensive assessment such as relevant epidemiologic and health data; individual, family, community stakeholders; research; and nursing knowledge at local, provincial, and national levels.

Informed by theoretical knowledge such as developmental theory, family theory, DoH, behaviour change theory, population health, logic model, and ecological theory (CHNC, 2011), the CHN *diagnosis* identifies the key issue and underlying factors. Collaborative *planning and implementation* in partnership with the child and family determines actions required to promote health and reduce barriers to health and well-being. *Evaluation* of interventions within health promotion programs are ongoing, and measures outcomes, trends, and changes at the family and community over time. One such example is Early Development Instruments (EDI), a survey conducted with families to measure five domains of early child development which are known predictors of adult health, education, and social outcome (Human Early Years Partnership, 2016).

Priority Populations

The Canadian Pediatric Nursing Standards Advisory Group (2016) prioritized six population groups related to health inequities and disparities: *children living in poverty, Indigenous children, immigrant and refugee children, children experiencing mental health concerns, children living with chronic illness and disability,* and *children experiencing obesity.* It is important to understand the unique and overlapping experiences that determine health within these groups, while also considering health outcomes related to wellness and disease, function and disability, life expectancy, and mortality. Since community health nursing is based on social justice, strength-based approach, and partnership, it is crucial to address disparities by examining the opportunities for health equity.

HEALTH PROMOTION WITH CHILDREN AND FAMILIES EXPERIENCING POVERTY

Within Canadian society, poverty may be understood relatively, with multiple complex factors related to socioeconomic status, basic needs, life expectancy, literacy, and standard of living (Parliament of Canada, 2008). In Canada, over 1.3 million children live in poverty, with an increased rate among newcomers, Indigenous peoples, and those experiencing disability (Klein & Yalnizyan, 2016). Over the past two decades, child poverty rates have been relatively unchanged in Canada (Raphael, 2014). In 2015, the House of Commons passed a motion to eliminate child poverty (Government of Canada, 2017).

Critical aspects of poverty that impact child health include food and housing insecurity. In Canada, over 17% children experience food insecurity, and have greater risks associated with physical and mental health (PROOF, Food Insecurity Policy Research, 2017). The need to access food bank services is increasing in Canada, and it is estimated that 40% of food bank users are children (Raphael, 2014). While Canada is a highly developed country, many children and their families are struggling with homelessness and housing insecurity, including overcrowded and inadequate conditions. CNA (2010) prioritized poverty reduction as one of the defining attributes of social justice.

The CHN works in partnership with children and families experiencing poverty, noting strengths and capacities to leverage challenges (Hammond, 2010). Comprehensive care coordination requires trusting relationships, assessing situational barriers and facilitators, exploring reasonable strategies, identifying appropriate resources to address priorities, and integrating intersectoral programs and services (CNA, 2013). The CHN advocates at a broader societal level for poverty reduction through program and policy development for affordable housing, food security, healthy environments, and social inclusion (Fortier & Douglas, 2012).

HEALTH PROMOTION WITH INDIGENOUS CHILDREN AND FAMILIES

First Nations, Inuit, and Métis are the original peoples of Canada, and represent approximately 4% of the Canadian population (Statistics Canada, 2015, para 3). Indigenous peoples are the fastest growing and youngest population, with almost half under 25 years of age (Indigenous and Northern Affairs Canada, 2016, para 1–3). For centuries, Indigenous peoples lived in healthy societies on North American lands, respecting the interconnection of physical, social, emotional, and spiritual wellness (National Collaborating Centre for Aboriginal Health, 2013). European settlers devastated Indigenous peoples given dispossession of lands, resources, language, culture, social structures, and the spread of communicable diseases such as smallpox (United Nations, 2007). Indigenous peoples continue to experience marginalization, health inequity, and social disparities by dominant westernized systems, including interpersonal and structural racism (Loppie, Reading, & de Leeuw, 2014). Canadian history is tragically marked by the cultural genocide of over 150,000 Indigenous children who were separated from their families and communities to attend residential schools with the consequent loss of Indigenous culture, language, and family structure (Canadian Truth and Reconciliation Commission, 2015a). Currently, Canada's Indigenous children experience significant health disparities related to poverty, education, housing, safe drinking water, mental health, and suicide (Klein & Yalnizyan, 2016; Macdonald & Wilson, 2013).

The CHN may advance health equity through reconciliation efforts that address disparities while supporting Indigenous cultural strengths. The CHN role in reconciliation includes advocating for culturally safe care (CNA, 2014; Woods, 2010), parent participation, family unity, quality education (on and off reserve), and mental health (Truth and Reconciliation Commission of Canada, 2015b). The CHN has a responsibility to advance Indigenous child health equity by upholding the Canadian Truth and Reconciliation Commission (2015b) *Calls to Action* with a view to work towards improving many factors, including infant mortality rates, mental health, safety, and management of lifelong health conditions. From a social justice approach, the CHN is responsible to promote health holistically, respecting the complex intersection of Indigenous knowledge, spirituality, language, land, cultural practices, and social structures within the DoH. This includes partnering with Indigenous communities to create culturally safe health environments (Brown, McPherson, Peterson, Newman, & Cranmer, 2012) and advocating for Indigenous-directed health services (Allan & Smylie, 2015).

HEALTH PROMOTION WITH IMMIGRANT AND REFUGEE CHILDREN

Children new to Canada may have unique health challenges, including inadequate treatment for chronic conditions and experiences with illness not commonly seen in Canada. Health care practices considered routine in Canada, such as oral health and vision screening, may not have been conducted in countries of origin (Canadian Paediatric Society, 2017a). Also, attitudes and acceptance of developmental disabilities may vary, and families may avoid seeking treatment for conditions such as autism (Baxter & Mahoney, 2018). Since immunization history may be difficult to assess due to variations in practices and documentation, the National Advisory Committee on Immunization (PHAC, 2017a) established a catch-up schedule.

While many challenges are noted with children new to Canada, it is important for the CHN to recognize assets, and optimize health capacity within new communities. With a focus on social justice and cultural humility (Foronda, Baptiste, Reinholdt, & Ousman, 2015), the CHN considers how the dominant Canadian culture may influence health experiences of children and families new to Canada. The nurse works in partnership to promote health by supporting family and community strengths. Language, health practices, family dynamics, strengths, and spiritual beliefs provide effective family-centred, community-based care. While learning about various cultures is important, nurses must not assume that children from the same country of origin share similar health practices. Determining child and family's views on health and care will contribute towards a more successful partnership, leading to improved health outcomes.

HEALTH PROMOTION WITH CHILDREN EXPERIENCING MENTAL HEALTH CONCERNS
Mental health is important for all ages: infants, children, and youth. While over a million children in Canada experience mental illness, less than 20% will receive appropriate mental health care (Mental Health Commission of Canada, 2018, para 1). Priority fetal, infant, and child mental health concerns include brain health and neuroplasticity, reduction in stress and trauma from poverty and other challenges, neurodevelopmental disorders (i.e., autistic spectrum disorders/attention-deficit disorder), anxiety, bullying, intentional self-harm, mood disorders (e.g., depression and bipolar disorder), eating disorders, schizophrenia, and suicide (Butler & Pang, 2014; Freeman et al., 2012; Health Canada, 2007).

The CHN role includes advocacy, direct clinical care, counselling, and case management in a variety of settings, noting the importance of mental health promotion at home, school, and community (Association of Registered Nurses of Newfoundland and Labrador, 2008). CNA (2012b) endorsed the first national mental health strategy by the Mental Health Commission of Canada (2012). This national strategy has also been articulated from a youth perspective, outlining priorities for prevention, recovery, access, diversity, indigenous health, and care coordination (Mental Health Commission of Canada, 2016).

HEALTH PROMOTION WITH CHILDREN LIVING WITH CHRONIC CONDITIONS
Some health conditions for children are chronic, or lifelong, as a result of genetic (inherited) factors,

environment, or a combination of both (Torpy, Campbell, & Glass, 2010). Children living in the community with chronic conditions have a range of wellness and illness experiences. The three most common chronic conditions for children in Canada are asthma, diabetes, and cancer. See Chapter 34 for additional information.

The CHN works with children living with chronic conditions in the home, schools, and primary care clinics. Children with chronic conditions often need regular assessments to determine health maintenance needs. These assessments determine the frequency of health promotion visits and types of interventions needed. Effective partnerships shared between children, families, interprofessional health care team, and community are vital. Coordination of specialty services, parent and caregiver networks, and community-based care enhances the quality of life and health of children and families. Comprehensive care coordination includes frequent holistic health assessments of strengths and challenges.

HEALTH PROMOTION AND HEALTHY EATING
Healthy eating is fundamental to good health and wellbeing, supports growth, helps children develop a positive relationship with food and their bodies, and reduces the risk for chronic disease. Healthy eating is a complex process linked to food choices and security, nutrition, culture, and traditions (PROOF, 2017). A growing concern over recent decades has been a shift in children's weight and the impact of obesity in childhood on health outcomes. The incidence of obesity among children has risen significantly since the 1970s, now affecting almost one third of all 5- to 17-year-old children (Roberts, Shields, de Groh, Aziz, & Gilbert, 2011). Chronic conditions related to childhood obesity include type 2 diabetes, hypertension, social isolation, poverty, and impaired emotional health. Health behaviours that may contribute to obesity include poor eating habits and sedentary behaviours. Almost half of all children between 5 and 17 years spend at least 2 hours using screens such as television, computers, and gaming devices, and have a total estimated 8.5 hour of sedentary time each day (PHAC, 2016). Such behaviours are influenced by social, environmental, and biologic determinants (PHAC, 2011a).

Through a social justice lens, the CHN needs to assess the complex causes of obesity, which may include income, housing insecurity, education, transportation, and social exclusion (PROOF, 2017). The CHN designs, develops, and implements programs with children and families about healthy eating and physical activity within schools and other community settings. For example, the CHN collaborates with children and families to determine affordable food choices and fitness opportunities as reasonable interventions. In addition, the CHN advocates and lobbies for national health education programs and population-wide initiatives to reduce sedentary behaviour and encourage healthy food choices.

COMPONENTS OF HEALTH CARE IN THE COMMUNITY

Screening and surveillance, injury and disease prevention, and health promotion activities are the critical components of health care for children.

Screening and Surveillance

Screening is a secondary prevention intervention to identify risk factors in a client population (CPHA, 2010). Health surveillance, as mentioned earlier, is an epidemiologic practice for systematic, ongoing collection, comparison, and analysis of health-related information that is communicated on a regular and timely basis to inform decision-makers in health (PHAC, 2008). Developmental screening and surveillance monitors' child health related to growth and development. Universal screening is applied to an entire population without any qualifiers such as income, education, or place of origin. Targeted screening is applied to a subgroup of a defined population (e.g., children and families with risk for poor health outcomes) (National Collaborating Centre for Determinants of Health, 2013). Screening and surveillance tools are used to assess the five complex dimensions of child well-being (Raphael, 2014).

Screening Factors Influencing Children's Health

There are many internal and external factors influencing the health of infants and children that inform child health screening tools. Recognizing these factors is the first step in determining potential health concerns. Table 31.2 outlines infant/child development elements influencing biologic, behavioural, and environmental characteristics from a population health perspective.

There are several universal and targeted screening programs that exist in Canada, including maternal infant screening, developmental screening, metabolic screening, and vision and hearing screening. Screening is the first step in early identification and intervention to support children's optimal health.

Maternal Infant Screening

Maternal infant screening assesses health determinants, targeted for children and their families, to increase health and well-being. Screening may involve type of feeding (particularly breastfeeding), infant and maternal health, safety, housing, nutrition, health care access, attachment, social supports, developmental milestones, play and stimulation, and parenting skills (Ontario Ministry of Children and Youth Services, 2012). The CHN provides support to families and their newborn infants across Canada, including home visiting programs, outreach clinics, and community health nursing clinic visits (CHNC, 2011).

Table 31.3 describes the Ontario Ministry of Children and Youth Services (2012) *Healthy Babies Healthy Children* guidance document. Within the document is a screening tool for assessing families who may benefit from health programs. Data are collected from a provincial surveillance database to monitor children's health in the early years. Categories include pregnancy and birth, family, parenting supports, and the infant/child. Risk factors are provided under each category.

Developmental screening is a critical component in promoting children's health. The Canadian Paediatric Society recommended schedule for preventive health visits by the CHN are at birth, first week of life,

TABLE 31.2	POPULATION HEALTH FACTORS THAT INFLUENCE HEALTHY INFANT AND HEALTHY CHILD DEVELOPMENT
Infant/Child Development Elements	**Influencing Characteristics**
Physical health and well-being	Physical characteristics • Genetic makeup • Hearing, vision and speech abilities • Motor development • Growth (p. 67) Nutrition and food security (p. 67) Environmental conditions (p. 67)
Emotional well-being	Parenting and attachment (e.g., parenting practices/style) (p. 69)
Cognitive learning and language communication	Speech, language and communication development (p. 70)
Social knowledge and competence	Family structure and social relationships • Family income • Maternal education • Parental separation Socio-economic status (e.g., family income and parent education levels) • Neighbourhood socio-economic character • Access to quality child care and developmental opportunities (p. 70)

Adapted from the Ministry of Healthy Living and Sport (2009, pp. 67–70).

TABLE 31.3	HIGHLIGHTS OF HEALTHY BABIES HEALTHY CHILDREN SCREENING TOOL IN ONTARIO

Highlights of Screening Tool: Health Babies, Healthy Children

Pregnancy and birth	Lack of prenatal care Substance use during pregnancy Low birth weight Large for gestational age Multiple births Illness during pregnancy such as diabetes Complications during pregnancy and birth
Family	Age of mother Single status Less than high school education No health care insurance Previous pregnancy or loss of child Separation from infant for greater than 5 days
Parenting supports	Lack of identified parenting supports Concerns for housing, food, and basic financial needs Parental history of depression, anxiety, or other mental illness Parent expresses concerns about ability to parent baby/child Strain within parent relationship Parent involvement with child protection services Parental patterns are inconsistent or inappropriate in response to baby/child's cues
Infant and child characteristics	Hearing delays Speech and language delays Social and emotional developmental delays Motor delays Delays in self-help skills Cognitive delays

Adapted from the Ontario Ministry of Children and Youth Services (2012, p. 92).

2 months, 4 months, 6 months, 9 months, 12 months, 15 months, 18 months, 24 months, and 30 months (Rourke, Leduc, & Rourke, 2014), and then yearly until age 17 (Greig et al., 2016). Children with special needs or concerns have more frequent and intensive visits. However, the Canadian Task Force on Preventive Health Care (2016) recently recommended developmental check-in points to assess children without suspected delays, instead of standard screening between 1 and 4 years of age. The Task Force found no evidence that standardized screening increased the health outcomes of this age group.

The Rourke Baby Record (Rourke et al., 2014) is used for developmental screening from birth to 5 years of age. Embedded in the Rourke Baby Record is the NDDS (2017). Parents and caregivers are encouraged to complete the NDDS to guide discussion on strengths and concerns regarding children's development. This tool provides a checklist of milestones and corresponding activities to stimulate children's development. CHNs in several provinces promote NDDS to enable families to understand children's development, and how to seek help if needed.

For older children, The Greig Health Record (Greig et al., 2016) is an evidence-based clinical guideline recommended for ages 6 to 17, with similar developmental screening categories and education, with a psychosocial assessment and BMI. Additional information on either of these screening tools can be found on thePoint.

Development is the emergence of the child's abilities over a longitudinal process. Families, CHNs, and interprofessional health providers may share observations, concerns, accomplishments, and milestones over time. A population-based approach to developmental screening is the *Early Development Instrument* (McMaster University, 2016). At a local population level, data are collected by kindergarten teachers about physical, social, emotional, language/cognitive, and communication skills for each child, along with the data related to the DoH (Hertzman, Clinton, & Lynk, 2011). School records and test results provide academic performance data for school-aged children. Input from teachers, coaches, and other adults involved with the child give insight into the child's emotional and social development. When developmental delay is suspected, frequent developmental assessments are warranted. Enabling families to understand their children's development and learn strategies to manage developmental delays fosters caregiver involvement. A pattern of developmental delays warrants a formal evaluation.

Community health nursing with children requires knowledge of growth and development, screening proficiency for strengths and concerns, and community resources. Historical information obtained from families about developmental milestones provides insights about children's development and any red flags. Children with risk factors are screened carefully for developmental delays. This screening occurs in a prospective manner, with screenings occurring at frequent intervals for early identification of concerns.

Metabolic Screening

Provincial or territory health policy determines which metabolic screening tests are mandatory. For example, Saskatchewan is the only province in Canada where mandatory screening for congenital hypothyroid is legislated (Canadian Organization for Rare Diseases, 2015). The role of the CHN in neonatal metabolic screening also varies. All provinces and territories offer screening universally, to select populations or by request. In Table 31.4, the 11 core conditions, including hearing, and 20 core metabolic conditions are identified (Canadian Organization for Rare Diseases, 2015).

During the initial newborn visit in the community health clinic, home, or primary care setting, the CHN will confirm if newborn metabolic screening was performed prior to discharge from the birthing unit. If the test was not performed or was performed when the newborn was less than 24 hours of age, the screening is performed at that visit.

Hearing Screening

According to the Canadian Paediatric Society (Patel & Feldman, 2016), hearing loss is a common condition in newborns. Even mild hearing loss can cause delays in language acquisition, communication, social and emotional development, and cognitive function. In Canada, most universal newborn hearing programs aim for screening by 1 month of age, confirmation of the diagnosis by 3 months, with intervention by 6 months. If the CHN is aware of speech and language delays, referrals are coordinated in collaboration with the family and interprofessional providers, such as community audiologists who perform hearing screening.

Vision Screening

Vision screening including eye health and alignment is part of routine care from birth throughout childhood. Routine screening is inconsistent between jurisdictions in Canada. For example, a Canadian national survey found that seven provinces and territories conducted preschool vision screening, while six did not (Mema, McIntyre, & Musto, 2012). Jurisdictions with preschool vision screening programs were primarily administered by CHNs through community health programs. In jurisdictions without vision screening, the CHN often collaborates with local optometrists and schools to offer screening. Canadian Paediatric Society (2016b) recommendations for vision screening are outlined in Box 31.3.

Vision screening tests such as red reflex, corneal light reflex, or cover–uncover are included in the recommended schedule of routine health maintenance visits. Any infant or child unable to pass visual screening should be referred for further assessment. School-age children

TABLE 31.4	HIGHLIGHTS OF NEWBORN SCREENING IN CANADA

Core conditions (p. 1)
Hearing screening
    Endocrine conditions
Congenital hypothyroidism, congenital adrenal hyperplasia
    Hematologic conditions
Sickle cell anemia, S-βeta thalassemia, sickle cell disease
    Other genetic conditions
Biotinidase, cystic fibrosis, transferase-deficient galactosemia (classical), critical congenital heart disease, severe combined immunodeficiency
    Core metabolic conditions (p. 2)
    Fatty acid disorders
Not all provinces screen—presently medium-chain acyl-CoA dehydrogenase is universally screened while four other disorders may be screened for in various provinces
    Organic acid disorders—nine disorders are currently listed with isovaleric acidemia (isovaleryl-CoA dehydrogenase) universally screened across provinces
    Amino acid disorders—six disorders are currently listed with phenylketonuria
    Hyperphenylalaninemia universally screened across provinces

Adapted from Canadian Organization for Rare Diseases (2015, pp. 1–2; https://www.raredisorders.ca/content/uploads/Canada-NBS-status-updated-Sept.-3-2015.pdf).

VISION SCREENING

Newborn to 3 months of age (level of evidence rating BII):

A complete examination of the skin around and covering the eye, and external eye structures including the conjunctiva, cornea, iris, and pupils.

Check red reflex to exclude for eye disease.

Assess eye reflexes–one at a time–for slow or absent visualization.

High-risk newborns (e.g., prematurity and family histories of eye disease) should be examined by an ophthalmologist.

Six to twelve months of age (level of evidence rating BII):

A review examination of the skin around and covering the eye and structures.

Assess for strabismus.

Check for fixation and following of an object (the cover-uncover test).

Three to five years of age (level of evidence rating AII):

A review examination of the skin around and covering the eye and structures.

Visual acuity screening with an age-appropriate tool.

Based on Amit M; Canadian Paediatric Society, Community Paediatrics Committee. Vision screening in infants, children and youth, 2009 (reaffirmed 2018): https://www.cps.ca/en/documents/position/children-vision-screening.

who pass visual screening but have difficulties with reading should also be referred for further assessment.

Remember Maya and Evan, the children introduced at the beginning of the chapter? How would you assess their growth and development? Which screening tests are warranted for them, and why? What further information would you need to determine which tests should be performed?

INJURY AND DISEASE PREVENTION

The CHN works with children, families, and communities to promote health, and prevent injury and disease.

Prevention has three levels of intervention: primary, secondary, and tertiary (PHAC, 2013):

- Primary prevention requires an upstream approach with intervention prior to occurrence of injury or disease (e.g., vaccination).
- Secondary prevention involves early identification and treatment of injury or disease (e.g., vision screening).
- Tertiary prevention considers health maintenance and restoration of existing injury or disease (e.g., physical activity program with obese youth and families) (Association of Faculties of Medicine of Canada, n.d.).

The CHN addresses current and anticipated health needs among individuals, families, communities, and populations within diverse economic, geographic, and cultural settings. Emphasis on PHC and illness prevention within the Canadian health system has increased demand for local community-based services. Shifting from an illness-to-wellness perspective has expanded CHN roles. Ongoing changes require building healthy public policy that reflects the five complex dimensions of child well-being (Raphael, 2014). The CHN contributes to developing, analyzing, and advocating for healthy public policies that support children and families around income supports and benefits, housing and food security, employment and working conditions, and early child development and child care. These issues need to be at the forefront of public policy development, as they contribute to economic and social security necessary for children's health.

Injury Prevention

In Canada, injuries are the leading cause of death for children of all ages (Yanchar, Warda, & Fuselli, 2012). Adolescents have the highest rate of injury from all population age groups in Canada (Billette & Janz, 2015). Injuries can be unintentional (e.g., motor vehicle accidents, poisoning, falls, or drowning) or intentional (e.g., child abuse, homicide, or suicide) (Yanchar et al., 2012). The types of injuries a child is most likely to experience vary depending on age group. Therefore, a key mandate for the CHN is injury prevention, which is primarily accomplished through education, anticipatory guidance, and physical changes in the environment. Addressing injury prevention requires collaboration and interdisciplinary and intersectoral partnerships to reduce health inequities related to social exclusion and unaffordable recreation (CHNC, 2011). Good practices include engineering (e.g., modification of the product/environment); enforcement (e.g., policy/legislation and measures to ensure compliance) and education (e.g., behaviour change strategies) are critical strategies in injury prevention (MacKay, Vincenten, Brussoni, Towner, & Fuselli, 2011). When developing injury prevention programs, the CHN completes a situation assessment of the community. This includes identification of key community stakeholders (e.g., *SMARTRISK* program by Ontario Ministry of Health Promotion, 2012); protective factors among children (e.g., parental supervision, playground equipment meeting CSA standards); and risk factors (e.g., products such as trampolines).

The CHN broadly considers the effects of the DoH in the community, and lobbies for safe policies (e.g., equipment to decrease the risk of falling). The CHN also provides children and families with health education (e.g., bicycle helmet safety) and implements community education programs (e.g., *ThinkFirst Kids* in schools, Home Safety Checklist in homes) (Ontario Ministry of Health Promotion, 2010).

Although stringent public health initiatives have decreased mortality rates of childhood from unintentional injuries significantly in the past 50 years, rates remain high in some populations and continued vigilance and public health action remain necessary (PHAC, 2009). The CHN, in partnership with the family and the community, can have an enormous impact on child safety. Specific interventions are discussed in Chapters 25 through 29.

Disease Prevention

Another key mandate for the CHN is health protection through disease prevention. This includes communicable disease control, outbreak management, and maintenance of chronic disease (CHNC, 2011). Health promotion and disease prevention includes knowledge of normal childhood development, analysis of epidemiologic data to identify common risks, and addressing health issues within child and family populations. One of the main strategies for preventing disease is immunization programs. CHNs in primary care and public health assess and provide immunizations beginning in infancy to children across Canada (PHAC, 2017b).

Immunization

Immunization is a key disease prevention activity during childhood health visits. The development of effective vaccines, beginning in the 1940s, revolutionized children's health care. Immunization allowed the focus to shift from disease treatment to disease prevention. The CHN understands the principles of immunizations, the proper use of vaccines, and barriers to immunization. With this knowledge, the nurse partners with families to provide the highest level of disease protection to children. For information on vaccine-preventable communicable diseases, refer to Chapter 37.

PRINCIPLES OF IMMUNIZATION

The immune system has the ability to recognize materials present in the body as "self" or "nonself." Foreign materials (nonself) are called antigens. When an antigen is recognized by the immune system, the immune system responds by producing antibodies (immunoglobulins) or directing special cells to destroy and remove the antigen.

Immunity is the ability to destroy and remove a specific antigen from the body. The acquisition of immunity can be active or passive. Passive immunity

is produced when the immunoglobulins of one person are transferred to another. This immunity lasts only weeks or months. Passive immunity can be obtained by injection of exogenous immunoglobulins. It can also be transferred from mothers to infants via colostrum or the placenta. Active immunity is acquired when a person's own immune system generates the immune response. Active immunity lasts for many years or for a lifetime. This long-term protection is the result of immunologic memory. After the initial immune response, specialized cells for that antigen continue to exist. When an antigen returns, these memory cells rapidly produce a fresh supply of antibodies to re-establish protection. This immunity can occur after exposure to natural pathogens or after exposure to vaccines. Vaccines mimic the characteristics of the natural antigen. The immune system mounts a response and establishes an immunologic memory as it would for an infection (PHAC, 2016).

The classification of vaccines is based on the characteristics of the antigen present. The antigen may be viral or bacterial. It may be live attenuated (weakened) or killed. It may be the whole antigen or a portion of it (fractional).

- Live attenuated vaccines are modified living organisms that are weakened. The organism can produce an immune response but does not produce the complications of the illness.
- Killed vaccines contain whole dead organisms; they are incapable of reproducing but are capable of producing an immune response.
- Toxoid vaccines contain protein products produced by bacteria called toxins. The toxin is heat-treated to weaken its effect, but it retains its ability to produce an immune response.
- Conjugate vaccines are the result of chemically linking the bacterial cell wall polysaccharide (sugar-based) portions with proteins. This dramatically increases the immune response compared with presenting the polysaccharide portion alone.
- Recombinant vaccines use genetically engineered organisms. For example, the hepatitis B vaccine (HepB) is produced by splicing a gene portion of the virus into a gene of a yeast cell. The yeast cell is then able to produce hepatitis B surface antigen for vaccine production.

The safety and efficacy of existing vaccines are constantly reviewed, and research to improve vaccines is ongoing. The goal is to refine vaccines for a maximum immune response with the least amount of risk for the child.

IMMUNIZATION MANAGEMENT

The Public Health Agency of Canada is responsible for immunization programs in Canada and provides advice and recommendations for vaccines to the provinces and

BOX 31.4

VACCINATION AND IMMUNIZATION

Vaccination is when a vaccine is administered to protect a person from specific diseases. Most vaccines contain a small amount of a virus or bacteria (germs). These germs do not harm because they have been weakened, or made inactive, before being administered to the person (Government of Canada, 2014).

Immunization is when a person becomes protected against a disease through vaccination, which stimulates their own natural immune system (WHO, 2017c).

---

territories (see Box 31.4). The National Advisory Committee on Immunization (PHAC, 2018b) provides expertise and scientific evidence and publishes the Canadian Immunization Guide (PHAC, 2018a) as a comprehensive resource on immunization for health professionals. While immunizations are not mandatory in Canada, different jurisdictions determine immunization requirements for daycare and school admittance (Immunize Canada, 2018). Reference to the Canadian Immunization Guide (PHAC, 2018b) for recommendations for specific populations, including children who are immunosuppressed, or living with chronic disease, is advised. On an individualized basis, providers must weigh the benefits of immunization against the likelihood of an adverse event.

While Canada is working towards a coordinated national immunization registry (Government of Canada, 2016), each province and territory tracks immunization coverage, and determines their immunization schedule depending on resources and burden of illness. Table 31.5 is an example of a provincial routine immunization schedule for children in Alberta. The Canadian Immunization Guide (PHAC, 2018b) has routine immunization schedules for other provinces and territories. This guide also has additional immunization schedules for children not immunized in early infancy or during the school years. For additional information, see thePoint.

Prevention of disease is a core function and mandate of public health in Canada. As previously identified, community-based child health clinics are a common strategy to deliver publicly funded immunization programs. The impact of immunization is deemed an effective protective measure against many infectious diseases. Infectious diseases like smallpox and poliomyelitis have been eradicated through immunization programs. Vaccine-preventable diseases are identified in Table 31.5 with corresponding recommendation for immunization from 2 months of age to grade 9 in Alberta.

Vaccine storage and administration affect the efficacy of vaccines. Improperly stored or reconstituted vaccines can be ineffectual, leading to poor immunization conversion. Proper vaccine storage is critical to vaccine efficacy.

A vaccine that is not maintained at the proper storage temperature **should not be used** as it may be ineffective in preventing disease. A detailed discussion of storage and handling recommendations is beyond the scope of this chapter. Detailed information for vaccine providers and handlers is available by accessing thePoint. All vaccines must be given by the correct route Table 31.6. These are typically intradermal (ID), subcutaneous (SC), or intramuscular (IM) routes.

Any vaccine can have side effects, and the most common ones are mild, including redness, tenderness, and swelling at the site, low-grade fever, and fussiness. These symptoms usually resolve within a few days. CHNs provide information to parents to inform about

TABLE 31.5	ROUTINE IMMUNIZATION SCHEDULE (ALBERTA)
Age	**Vaccine**
2 months	• DTaP–IPV–Hib[a] • Pneumococcal conjugate (Pneu-CCV13) • Rotavirus
4 months	• DTaP–IPV–Hib • Pneumococcal conjugate (Pneu-C13) • Meningococcal conjugate (Mencon C) • Rotavirus
6 months	• DTaP–IPV–Hib • Pneumococcal conjugate (Pneu-C13) (for high-risk children only)
6 months and older	• Influenza[b] (annually)
12 months	• MMR-Var[c] • Meningococcal conjugate (Mencon C) • Pneumococcal conjugate (Pneu-CV13)
18 months	• DTaP–IPV–Hib
4–6 years	• dTap–DTaP–IPV[d] • MMR-Var[c] • Pneumococcal conjugate (Pneu-CV13) only for children up to 71 months (catchup program)
Grade 6	• Hepatitis B (3 doses) • HPV[e] (3 doses)
Grade 9	• DTaP[f] • MenC-ACYWCV4[g] • HPV (3 doses—catchup program for boys)

Each bullet represents one vaccine/injection unless otherwise noted.
[a]Diphtheria, tetanus, acellular pertussis, polio, Haemophilus influenzae type b.
[b]Annually, during influenza season.
[c]Measles, mumps, rubella, and varicella.
[d]Diphtheria, tetanus, acellular pertussis, polio.
[e]Human papillomavirus.
[f]Diphtheria, tetanus, acellular pertussis.
[g]Meningococcal conjugate vaccine (Groups A, C, W-135, and Y).
(Adapted from http://www.health.alberta.ca/health-info/imm-routine-schedule.html)

TABLE 31.6	VACCINATION ADMINISTRATION ROUTES	
Intramuscular	**Subcutaneous**	
DTaP, DT, dTap	IPV	
Hepatitis A, hepatitis B	MMR-VarR	
Hib	Varicella	
Influenza (quadrivalent)	MenC-ACYW	
Pneumococcal conjugate vaccine (PCV)		
HPV		
Mencon C		
IPV		

Adapted from Alberta Health Services. (2018). *Standard for the administration of immunization.* http://www.albertahealthservices. ca/assets/info/hp/cdc/if-hp-cdc-ipsm-standard-administrationimmunization-06-100.pdf

the benefits and risks, including potential side effects for each immunization. The CHN works in partnership with the family, using effective communication skills to encourage questions about immunization, explore misinformation, and offer reliable evidence-based information (PHAC, 2018b). The CHN will ask the parents about the child's reactions to previous immunizations, and screen for precautions and contraindications for each vaccine to be administered. Before the vaccine is given, the parents must provide their consent.

VACCINE HESITANCY

Immunization promotes optimal health by safely protecting children from preventable disease. However, some parents and caregivers may raise concerns about vaccines. It is important for the CHN to understand these concerns as a partner in care. Providing relevant facts to address concerns or myths is important. The nurse will share with parents how vaccines build immunity against harmful diseases, and there is no scientific evidence that vaccines cause autism (PHAC, 2018a). Another myth is that vaccines materials are not safe. In Canada, there are strict guidelines on vaccine development based on effective research testing. The vaccine process deactivates bacteria and makes vaccines safe and effective. As well, some parents think that multiple injections will overwhelm the baby's immune system. Vaccines are designed to protect infants soon after birth against more than one disease, and in fact strengthen the immune system. Viruses used in the development of vaccines are harmless, and act to stimulate the body's immune response to create that protection against the disease. An important example of vaccine-preventable disease is measles, which continues to be one of the leading causes of death in children globally, even though a safe and cost-effective vaccine is available (PHAC, 2018a).

Vaccine hesitancy may result with parents delaying or refusing immunization for their children. The World Health Organization (2017c) recognizes this as a serious issue and has established a Strategic Advisory Group of Experts (SAGE) Working Group on Vaccine Hesitancy. The nurse understands vaccine hesitancy from a broad perspective and considers the following three factors when addressing vaccine hesitancy as outlined in the Three Cs model:
- Confidence—trust in vaccine effectiveness and safety, health system, and policy
- Complacency—low perceived risk of vaccine-preventable disease
- Convenience—availability, affordability, and accessibility (Dubé et al., 2016)

The CHN will explore and address these complex factors in partnership with the family as it is important to understand the family's perspective. The nurse will share evidence-based information, including the risks of choosing to not vaccinate, and health benefits of vaccines (Canadian Paediatric Society, n.d.). Given the range of parent attitudes towards vaccination, there are several recommended approaches outlined in Table 31.7.

DOCUMENTATION

Documentation of vaccines in the child's permanent record includes the following:
- Date vaccines were administered
- Names of vaccine(s) (verify approved abbreviations)
- Lot number and expiration date of vaccine(s)
- Manufacturer's name
- Site and route by which vaccines were administered (e.g., left deltoid, intramuscularly)
- Name of the person administering the vaccine

Families should be provided with a copy of the child's immunizations. Any clinically significant adverse event that occurs after an immunization should be documented in the child's immunization record.

Vaccine Descriptions

This section reviews the most commonly used vaccines in Canada. Recommendations for administration site area identified in Table 31.7. These immunizations are recommended by the Public Health Agency of Canada (2018a).

Diphtheria, Tetanus, and Pertussis Vaccines. Immunization against diphtheria, tetanus, and pertussis diseases is given via a combination vaccine. The vaccine currently used for children younger than age 7 is diphtheria, tetanus, and acellular pertussis (DTaP). It contains diphtheria and tetanus toxoids and pertussis cell wall proteins. The older version of this vaccine—diphtheria, tetanus, pertussis (DPT)—contained killed whole cells of pertussis bacteria and caused more frequent and severe adverse reactions than DTaP. Diphtheria and

TABLE 31.7	COUNSELLING STRATEGIES TO ADDRESS PARENT/CAREGIVER ATTITUDES TOWARDS VACCINATION

Vaccine acceptors
- Recognize and acknowledge the parents'/caregivers' positive approach to immunization.
- Explain using evidence-based sources common side effects and rare adverse events with vaccines.
- Use both verbal and numeric descriptions of vaccine and disease risks.

Vaccine hesitant
- Build rapport, listen nonjudgmentally to questions and concerns.
- Establish honest, open dialogue, and provide information concerning risks and benefits about vaccines and impact of the diseases.
- Use decision aids and other quality information tools.
- Do not pressure the parent or caregiver to vaccinate; book another appointment to re-visit discussion, if needed.

Vaccine refusers
- Do not enter a debate/discussion about vaccination; remain impartial and approachable.
- Aim to share brief information on vaccines. Be open that you will have to document refusal to vaccinate in an open manner for future interactions with parents.
- Inform about risks of nonvaccination.

Adapted from Dubé, Bettinger, Fisher, Naus, Mahmud, and Hilderman (2016, p. 248).

tetanus (DT) vaccine is used for children younger than age 7 who have contraindications to pertussis immunization. Full-strength diphtheria toxoid causes significant adverse reactions in people older than age 7 years. For this group, the dTap adolescent preparation vaccine is used: it contains tetanus toxoid, reduced diphtheria toxoid, and acellular pertussis vaccine. The lowercase "d" is used to designate the lower dose of diphtheria toxoid. The Canadian Immunization Guide recommends that dTap be used for all tetanus boosters in adolescents (14 to 16 years) because dTap provides a boost to diphtheria and pertussis immunization (PHAC, 2018b).

Haemophilus Influenzae Type B Vaccines. *Haemophilus influenzae* type B is a bacterium that causes several life-threatening illnesses in children younger than 5 years of age. These infections include meningitis, epiglottitis, and septic arthritis. H. influenzae type B conjugate vaccines (Hib) have been extremely effective in reducing the rates of these diseases in children. A booster vaccine is needed at 12 months. Hib vaccine is not routinely given to children 5 years of age or older and is contraindicated in children younger than 6 weeks (PHAC, 2018b).

Polio Vaccine. Inactivated polio vaccine (IPV) is the only polio vaccine currently recommended in Canada (PHAC, 2018b). It is a killed virus vaccine that poses no risk for vaccine-acquired disease. Oral polio vaccine (OPV), a live attenuated virus vaccine, was the preferred polio vaccine until 2000. At that time, it became apparent that the only victims of poliomyelitis were people who had acquired it from OPV.

Measles, Mumps, and Rubella (MMR) Vaccines. MMR is a live attenuated virus combination vaccine. It is most commonly used in childhood immunizations. MMR can be given the same day as other live attenuated virus vaccines such as varicella vaccine (Var). However, if not given on the same day, the immunizations should be spaced at least 28 days apart (PHAC, 2018b). Anaphylactic reactions are believed to be associated with the neomycin or gelatin components of the vaccine rather than the egg component. The vaccine is not prepared from the allergenic albumen portion of the egg, so egg allergy is no longer a contraindication for measles vaccine (PHAC, 2018a). Pregnancy in a child's mother is also not a contraindication to the vaccination of the child (PHAC, 2018a).

Hepatitis A Vaccine. Hepatitis A vaccine (HepA) is an inactivated whole virus vaccine. Hepatitis A is spread through close physical contact and by eating or drinking contaminated food or water. It is one of the most frequently reported vaccine-preventable diseases in Canada. HepA is recommended for pre-exposure prevention for those who are most at risk for acquiring the disease (e.g., travellers to hepatitis A endemic countries, IV drug users, men who have sexual contact with men and outbreak control) (PHAC, 2018b).

Hepatitis B Vaccine. HepB is a recombinant vaccine. Hepatitis B virus can result in a serious infection that affects the liver. It is spread through contact with blood and body fluids and can be spread from an infected mother to a newborn at birth, unprotected sexual activity, and sharing injection drug equipment. Hepatitis B vaccination is recommended at birth for infants of infected mothers preferably within the first 12 hours, then at 1 to 2 months and 6 months (PHAC, 2018a). Hepatitis B is recommended for all children in Canada and is given at 10 to 12 years of age depending on the province and territory, for 2 or 3 doses (PHAC, 2018b).

Varicella (Chickenpox) Vaccine. Varicella vaccine (Var) is a live attenuated virus vaccine. All children aged 12 to 15 months who have not had varicella (chickenpox) should be immunized. A second dose is recommended starting at 18 months of age and no later than school entry. The vaccine provides effective postexposure prophylaxis if administered within 3 to 5 days after exposure. The Canadian Immunization Guide does recommend univalent vaccination for postexposure in children and adults without evidence of immunity and eligibility for the vaccination (not recommended for children younger than 12 months of age) (PHAC, 2018a). Varicella may be given the same day as other live attenuated virus vaccines. However, if not given on the same day, the immunizations should be spaced at least 28 days apart (PHAC, 2018a). Pregnancy of the child's mother is not a contraindication to the vaccination of the child.

Pneumococcal Vaccines. *Streptococcus pneumoniae* (pneumococcus) is the most common cause of pneumonia, sepsis, meningitis, and otitis media in young children (PHAC, 2018a). The two available pneumococcal vaccines are pneumococcal conjugate vaccine (Pneu-C-13) and pneumococcal polysaccharide vaccine (Pneu-P-23). Beginning in 2010, Pneu-C13, which contains 13 strains of *S. pneumoniae*, replaced PCV7, which contained only 7 strains, for use in routine vaccination for children (PHAC, 2018a). Pneu-C13 stimulates an immune response in infants and is given at 2 months of age as part of the initial immunization series but can be given as early as 6 weeks of age (PHAC, 2018a). PPSV contains 23 strains of *S. pneumoniae*. It does not provoke an immune response in children younger than 2 years of age. Pneu-P-23 is given to children older than 2 years of age who are at high risk for pneumococcal sepsis. This group includes children with anatomic/functional asplenia; sickle cell disease; chronic cardiac, pulmonary, or renal disease; diabetes mellitus; or HIV infection; children with cochlear implants; and children with immunosuppression (PHAC, 2018b).

Influenza Vaccines. Influenza immunization is recommended yearly for all persons 6 months of age or older. All children 6 months to 8 years of age who are receiving the influenza vaccination for the first time require two doses separated by 4 weeks. Only one dose is needed if the child has received two doses of seasonal influenza in previous years and at least one dose of 2009 H1N1–containing vaccine (Grohskopf et al., 2013). In 2009/2010, in addition to the seasonal influenza vaccinations, immunologists began recommending vaccination against H1N1 influenza due to the influenza pandemic that was occurring worldwide (PHAC, 2018b). There are two influenza vaccines available, the live attenuated influenza vaccine and the inactivated influenza vaccine. Canada's National Advisory Committee on Immunization (PHAC, 2018a) recommends inactivated vaccine in healthy children aged 2 years and older.

Take Note!

Quadrivalent seasonal influenza vaccine (QIV also known as Fluzone) is now available in Canada. This vaccine protects against four strains of influenza (quadrivalent) with an additional strain of influenza B to provide broader protection (PHAC, 2018b).

Human Papillomavirus Vaccine. Human papillomavirus (HPV) is a DNA tumour virus transmitted through direct skin-to-skin contact. HPV is contracted during vaginal, oral, or anal penetrative sexual acts as well as intimate skin-to-skin contact. HPV infection is the most common sexually transmitted infection in Canada (PHAC, 2018b). HPV causes genital warts and is linked to the future development of cancer. For these reasons, the Canadian Immunization Guide has recommended HPV vaccination in all preadolescent girls and boys and up to age 45 in females and age 26 in males (PHAC, 2018b). Three vaccines have been licensed: Cervarix®, Gardasil® and Gardasil®9. The two or three-vaccine series of either Cervarix®, Gardasil® or Gardasil®9 is recommended at 9 years of age over a 6-month period (NACI, 2017). Cervarix® is used for females, while Gardasil® and Gardasil®9 can be administered to males and females beginning at 9 years of age (NACI, 2017).

Meningococcal Vaccine. Meningococcal disease may manifest as meningitis, a deadly blood infection (meningococcemia), or bacteremic pneumonia. It is caused by the bacterium *Neisseria meningitidis*, which is spread through direct contact or by air droplets. It develops quickly, usually in healthy children and adolescents, and results in high rates of morbidity and mortality (PHAC, 2018b). For these reasons, the meningococcal vaccine is recommended for all previously unvaccinated children at 12 months of age (PHAC, 2018b). Routine vaccination is also recommended for children 2 months or older who are at an increased risk for the disease due to certain medical conditions such as anatomical or functional asplenia or complement component deficiency (PHAC, 2018b). Children 12 years of age and older up to the age of 24 years may be offered Mencon C (monovalent conjugate meningococcal vaccine) or Men C-ACYW (quadrivalent polysaccharide meningococcal vaccine) or MCV4 (meningococcal conjugate vaccine (Groups A, C, W-135, and Y) (PHAC, 2018b) even if previously vaccinated as infants or toddlers according to provincial and territorial schedules due to the potential spread of disease through sharing items such as water bottles during sports and activities. It can also be administered to certain at-risk groups to control an outbreak (PHAC, 2018b).

Recall the family, introduced at the beginning of the chapter. What vaccinations would be appropriate for the children to receive? Explain how you would administer the injections and discuss any contraindications or precautions.

HEALTH PROMOTION ACTIVITIES

The five complex dimensions of children's well-being are a key consideration when developing and implementing health promotion activities (Raphael, 2014). The CHN must consider the complex interplay of "material well-being, health and safety, education, behaviours and risks, and housing and environment" (p. 222). Health promotion activities by CHNs are delivered as population-based approaches to children and families to reflect all five dimensions. Each developmental childhood stage has unique opportunities to influence these dimensions through health promotion priorities. CHNs are mandated to provide health promotion activities to meet national public health goals in Canada. Key community health promotion activities for children and families are described next.

School-Age Health

The *Health Promoting School or Comprehensive School Health* framework (2017) described earlier guides CHN practice with school-aged children. Factors influencing the health of this population are different than children under 6 years of age. According to the following research finding, *Health behaviour in school-aged children in Canada: Focus on relationships* (Freeman, King, & Pickett, 2015), the social environment (e.g., family, friends, school, and community) makes an important difference in the health of school-aged children (ages 11 to 15). The information is based on a 4-year Canadian survey on health, well-being, and associated behavioural outcomes with school-aged children. There were 18 key findings described across three areas: relational supports, context, and health behaviours and outcomes.

Supports

1. *Family Support*—Related to having access to someone to talk with, someone who cared, spiritual health, and life satisfaction.
2. *School Climate*—School climate was important in preventing and reducing bullying and fighting among adolescents.
3. *Friend Support*—Healthy friend support was associated with positive behaviours, feeling good about oneself, and spiritual health.
4. *Community Support*—Community support had a weak association with positive health outcomes.

Contexts

1. *Home and Family*—Boys communicated more easily with parents than did girls; however, regardless of gender, grades 6 to 8 and grade 10 students preferred to communicate with their mothers rather than their fathers.
2. *School*—School can be positive experience offering academic support and positive supports from teachers.

3. *Peers*—Peers offer most of support through talking and sharing of highs and lows and being there during challenges and difficulties.
4. *Community*—Community is viewed as primarily with regard to neighbours as unsafe, unfriendly, and unsupportive compared with ratings from previous years.

Health Behaviours and Outcomes

1. *Physical Activity and Sedentary Behaviour*—1:5 children met the Canadian guidelines for physical activity. Only 1:10 children met the Canadian guidelines of less than 2 hours a day of screen time.
2. *Sleep Health*—Youth achieve the amount of sleep required which is generally 9 to 11 hours per night.
3. *Healthy Eating*—Almost half of boys (46%) and girls (37%) are eating neither fruits nor vegetables likely related to food insecurity issues. There is a reduction in junk food and sweet drink consumption over the years.
4. *Healthy Weights*—Unhealthy weights continue to be a concern with 1:3 boys and 1:4 girls who are identified as overweight or obese.
5. *Injury*—Almost half of children have at least one injury in 12 months. Sports related injuries are the most common with a high incidence of not wearing a helmet.
6. *Mental Health*—High school girls have issues related to self-confidence, psychosomatic symptoms, and emotional problems.
7. *Spiritual Health*—Spiritual health is more important for girls than boys and decreased with age. Youth with high spiritual health had also more positive health and education outcomes.
8. *Substance Use*—Cannabis use and smoking is declining in grades 9 to 10.
9. *Sexual Health*—Grade 10 students are waiting longer to become sexually active; however, those who are sexually active use safe sex practices only 20% of the time.
10. *Bullying and Fighting*—Bully and fighting behaviours are on the decline.

The complete report can be sources at the Point.

Promoting Healthy Eating

Healthy eating is considered one of the most important health promotion activities to increase energy levels, manage weight, enhance cognitive learning, and support children to access the activities they enjoy. Healthy eating requires access to appropriate foods which are nutritious and cost-effective. The focus of healthy eating should be health-centred, not weight-centred. Linking weight control to numbers on a scale increases the possibility of developing eating disorders, nutritional deficiencies, and negative body image. Instead, emphasizing the benefits of healthy eating focuses on incorporating nutritious food preferences and traditional food practices. Parents who have healthy eating patterns are likely to maintain and encourage those patterns in their children. The CHN provides parents with anticipatory guidance about age-related eating patterns. Parents with toddlers and pre-schoolers may have questions on coping with children's growing autonomy while providing a variety of nutritious options.

The CHN can begin by discussing healthy foods with families who have young children. Information and teaching modalities need to be age appropriate. Eating is a shared responsibility between the child and parent; it should be fun and engaging. Many provinces provide links to healthy eating via population health teams as well as wider organizations such as the Ellyn Satter Institute (additional information can be found at thePoint). With colourful posters and games, the nurse can teach the preschool child and families the difference between healthy and unhealthy food choices. As children enter school, group and peer-led activities can be very effective. Using the *Health Promoting School or Comprehensive School Health* framework (2017), nurses in school health promote change in food policies, provide resources on healthy eating to teachers to support the curriculum, and promote healthy eating events with appropriate food choice within the school. The nurse gears activities that develop children's' ability to make nutritious choices. Check the *Eat Well and Be Active Educational Toolkit* (Health Canada, 2014) for activity plans, poster, and presentations. See thePoint for further information. Detailed anticipatory guidance is provided in Chapters 25 through 29.

Promoting Physical Activity

Increasing physical activity and decreasing sedentary behaviour to reduce the risk for chronic conditions is critical. Healthy physical activity can take many forms and must be tailored to the developmental stage and abilities of the child (Lipnowski & LeBlanc, 2012b). During the preschool years, parents and caregivers are encouraged to provide a wide variety of physical activities. Exposure to multiple types of exercise increases the chances that children will enjoy exercise and maintain an active lifestyle. The focus should be on noncompetitive, fun activities. When children enter school, the lure of technology, social media, and computers can significantly diminish the amount of time spent in physical activity; therefore, the CHN and school community can promote physical activity by working towards a supportive social and physical environment. It is important to encourage children to limit the amount of time spent in sedentary activities, and to pursue enjoyable physical activities. In addition to verbal encouragement, families can promote exercise by participating in exercise with children. A family walk can increase physical fitness and interaction (Teaching Guideline 31.1).

Teaching Guidelines 31.1
HEALTHY ACTIVITY WITH CHILDREN AND FAMILIES

1. Plan physical activities that families can do as a group.
2. Incorporate exercise activities in daily schedules.
3. Look for activities that appeal to children's interests and abilities, such as dance, team sports, or swimming.
4. Place value on noncompetitive as well as competitive activities.
5. Demonstrate that exercise is important. Parents, caregivers, and families are encouraged to exercise daily.
6. Encourage the community to develop safe areas for spontaneous games and activities.

Adapted from the Canadian Society for Exercise Physiology (CSEP), 2016.

The *Canadian 24-Hour Movement Guidelines for Children and Youth* (ages 5 to 17 years) (Canadian Society for Exercise Physiology [CSEP], 2016) were released to address physical activity, sedentary behaviour, and sleep in a 24-hour period. These guidelines encourage children and youth to *sweat, step, sleep, and sit*. According to the guidelines, children should achieve high levels of physical activity, low levels of sedentary behaviour, and sufficient sleep each day.

Physical activity with children and youth is promoted in the *Health Promoting School and Comprehensive School Health* framework (2017). Promising evidence indicates that school-based curricular interventions have resulted in an increase in physical activity of most school-aged children. One example of implementing this evidence is an Ontario-based program called *Playground Activity Leaders in Schools* (Ghassemi, 2014). In this program, physical education focuses on skill development and noncompetitive sports, activity cards are used to support safe play equipment use during recess, and teachers are educated on increasing the physical activity in the classroom. Another health promotion approach is designing a community that supports physical activity outside of school using active transportation (CLASP, 2012) with programs such as *Active and Safe Routes to School* (Green Communities Canada, n.d.). The CHN partners with multiple stakeholders including parents to promote the use of active transportation for the daily trip to school, addressing health, physical activity, and traffic safety issues while taking action on air pollution and climate change.

Promoting Mental Well-Being

Mental health is linked to the capacity to feel, think, and act in ways that enhance our ability to enjoy life and deal with the challenges we face. It is a positive sense of emotional and spiritual well-being that respects the importance of culture, equity, social justice, interconnections, and personal dignity (PHAC, 2014). Promoting mental well-being from a CHN perspective considers upstream approaches, including mental health promotion and mental illness prevention. Mental health is positively correlated to healthy physical and emotional development, management of emotions, positive coping and problem-solving skills, and participation in recreational activities (Pan-Canadian Joint Consortium of School Health, 2017).

The school is identified as a critical environment to promote psychological resilience in children of primary school age (Stewart, Sun, Patterson, Lemerle, & Hardie, 2004). Mental health programs are often delivered within the school and community setting and create a positive culture of belonging for all students (Rowling, 2012, as cited in Mental Health Commission of Canada, 2012). The CHN delivers mental health programs with students to promote social skills and positive self-concept. Techniques include role playing, peer modeling, self-reflection, and skills training in social emotional learning, and cognitive behavioural training (Durlak et al., 2011, as cited in Mental Health Commission of Canada, 2012). These programs have been found to prevent mood disorders, anxiety disorders, and conduct disorders such as aggression. Such health promotion programs are most successful if started early within the school year and sustained for the entire year (Durlak et al., 2011, as cited in Mental Health Commission of Canada, 2012).

Promoting Oral Health Care

Effective oral health practices are essential to the overall health of children and adolescents. According to the Canadian Paediatric Society (Rowan-Legg, 2013), poor oral health contributes to pain, infection, and difficulties with learning, sleep, behaviour, self-esteem, socialization, and communication. The Oral Health Component of the Canadian Health Measures Survey (Health Canada, 2010) reports that tooth decay affects 57% of children aged 6 to 11 years. Early childhood caries affecting preschool children continue to be a concerning trend, and severe cases may require dental surgery (Rowan-Legg, 2013). The CHN provides anticipatory guidance with children and families to prevent factors affecting the incidence of early childhood caries such as poor eating habits, inappropriate infant feeding practices, and lack of professional dental care. Promoting fluoride is also important, and may be accessed in toothpaste, topical varnish dental treatments, or community drinking water (Rowan-Legg, 2013). The CHN promotes optimal children's oral health promotion through broad community and population health–related initiatives. Key recommendations by the Canadian Paediatric Society (Rowan-Legg, 2013) include support for publicly funded, affordable, accessible, and effective interdisciplinary oral health services for all children.

Promoting Sun Safety

Sun exposure and sunburns in childhood increase the risk of being diagnosed with skin cancer in adulthood. The incidence of cutaneous malignant melanoma in Canada has increased significantly since the 1970s (Taddeo & Stanwick, 2012). The CHN collaborates with parents, schools, community, interprofessional health providers, and policymakers to promote sun safety. Key messages include protecting children from hot surfaces such as pavement, car doors, or playground slides, limiting sun exposure during peak daylight hours, covering children with hats, loose clothing, the application of sunscreen prior to sun exposure, and highlighting the dangers of indoor tanning facilities for children and youth under 18 years of age due to the risk of skin cancer in adulthood (Canadian Paediatric Society, 2017b; Taddeo & Stanwick, 2012).

CHILD HEALTH PROGRAMS IN THE COMMUNITY

Across Canada, community health organizations provide various child health programs. One such program is *Healthy Babies Healthy Children*, which offers home visiting service to families at risk from birth to transition to school in Ontario. Many provinces/territories offer similar home visiting services. In addition, well-baby or child health clinics are provided to promote healthy child development and family health. Table 31.8 offers examples of community-based child health services that are funded nationally by the Public Health Agency of Canada (PHAC), Health Canada, or funded by public health organizations in distinct provinces and territories.

OVERALL CONCEPTS
- Health and wellness with children and families is a dynamic process.
- CHN practice is based on national standards by the Community Health Nurses of Canada (2011).
- The CHN implements health promotion using the strategies of the Ottawa Charter and principles of PHC.
- The CHN works in a variety of practice roles and settings, including home health, telehealth, schools, primary care, and public health, to promote health where children and families live, play, learn, and work.
- Wellness is optimized when the CHN considers social justice principles, and forms meaningful partnerships with children, families, and community using a strength-based approach.
- The CHN uses the nursing process to assess and manage the needs of children, families, communities, and populations. This process is client- and family-centred, relational, reciprocal, and dynamic.

TABLE 31.8	EXAMPLES OF COMMUNITY-BASED CHILD HEALTH SERVICES	
Child Health Service	**Service Description**	**Funding Level**
Canadian Prenatal Nutrition Program (CPNP) for pregnant to 6 months infant (PHAC, 2015a)	Supports the needs of pregnant women facing challenges that put their health and the health of their infants at risk including low-income women, Indigenous women, and recent immigrants. Challenges include poverty, teen pregnancy, social and geographic isolation, substance use, and family violence. Focus of CPNP includes community-based programs to strengthen and support women through partnerships, flexibility, and accessibility	Federal
Canadian Action Program for Children (CAPC) (PHAC, 2015b)	Offers a local service approach including family resource centres, parenting classes and drop-in groups, parent/child groups, home visiting, collective kitchens, and other specialized programs, such as support for mothers dealing with substance abuse	Federal
Aboriginal Head Start in Urban and Northern Communities for children 3–5 years (PHAC, 2017a)	Offers community-based children's program focused on early childhood development for First Nations, Inuit, and Métis children and their families living off-reserve (PHAC) and on reserve (Health Canada). It supports physical, intellectual, emotional, and spiritual development for children and their parents	Federal
Nobody's Perfect (PHAC, 2017b)	Provides a community-based parenting program for parents of preschool children. Parents who can participate in the program are young, physically or socially isolated, and/or have few financial or educational supports. Facilitators such as CHNs offer a strength-based approach in a group setting	Federal
Triple P-Positive Parenting Program® for birth to 12 years (Triple P International, n.d.)	Provides parenting and family evidence-based support that builds strong, nurturing relationships, good communication, and positive attention to children. Triple P aims to prevent behavioural, emotional, and developmental problems in children by enhancing the knowledge, skills, and confidence of parents	Ontario, Manitoba, Quebec, Nova Scotia, Prince Edward Island
Well Baby/Child Health Clinics	Supports families in the growth and development of their children, and prevents communicable disease outbreaks through drop in services, including weight and height assessments, developmental screening, parenting groups, immunization, oral health assessments, health education, and injury prevention	Most provinces and territories
Child protection prevention interventions	Provides a range of interventions within multiple settings such as teaching children and parents on healthy relationships and development, providing parenting resources, implementing positive parenting groups, supporting parents in their homes with resources and activities, reporting suspected child abuse to protective services, conducting home visiting, and collaborating with protective services and health care providers	All provinces and territories

- Anticipatory guidance involves knowledge of family strengths, healthy child development, parenting, and common childhood health issues.
- The CHN recognizes priority populations such as children who are living in poverty, indigenous children, refugees, children experiencing mental health issues, chronic illnesses, disability, and obesity.
- Screening and surveillance are part of monitoring child development, and prevention of injury and disease. The CHN uses risk assessments and screening tools to develop appropriate community health programs and services for children, families, and community.

- The principal components of injury and disease prevention are identifying risk factors, facilitating lifestyle changes to prevent, eliminate, or reduce those risk factors, and empowering children, families, and community to build capacity for optimizing health.
- Immunizations are a cornerstone of disease prevention for children and families. The CHN increases the effectiveness of immunization by understanding the principles of immunization and applying them to the child's context. Adhering to immunization practices and schedules, as outlined in the Canadian Immunization Guide (PHAC, 2018a), enhances health benefits and reduces risks.

- Barriers to full immunization include fragmented health care, concerns about vaccine safety, and lack of knowledge. The nurse can be pivotal in ensuring that children are fully immunized by serving as educator and advocate.

Health promotion activities based on PHC principles are designed, developed, and implemented with the community to optimize health through physical activity, healthy eating, injury prevention, mental well-being, oral care, and sun safety.

REFERENCES AND RECOMMENDED READINGS

Alberta Health. (2018). *Routine immunization schedule.* Retrieved from http://www.health.alberta.ca/health-info/imm-routine-schedule.html

Alberta Health Services. (2018). *Standard for the administration of immunizations.* Retrieved from https://www.albertahealthservices.ca/assets/info/hp/cdc/if-hp-cdc-ipsm-standard-administration-immunization-06-100.pdf

Alex Health Centre. (2017). *The Alex: Mobile health services, bringing good health to those in need.* Calgary, Alberta, Canada. Retrieved from http://www.thealex.ca/mobile/

Allan, B., & Smylie, J. (2015). *First peoples, second class treatment: The role of racism in the health and well-being of Indigenous peoples in Canada.* Toronto, ON: The Wellesley Institute. Retrieved from http://www.wellesleyinstitute.com/wp-content/uploads/2015/02/Report-First-Peoples-Second-Class-Treatment-Final.pdf

Allison, S. (2016). *Chief Medical Health Officer's health status report.* Retrieved from https://www.northernhealth.ca/Portals/0/About/Community_Accountability/documents/Northern-Health-CMHO.pdf

Amit, M.; Canadian Paediatric Society-Community Paediatrics Committee. (2016). Vision screening in infants, children and youth. Position statement. *Paediatric Child Health,14*(4), 246–248. Retrieved from http://www.cps.ca/documents/position/children-vision-screening

Association of Faculties of Medicine Canada (AFMC). (n.d.). The stages of prevention. Chapter 4: Basic concepts in prevention, surveillance and health promotion. AFMC primer on population health. Retrieved from http://phprimer.afmc.ca/Part1-TheoryThinkingAboutHealth/Chapter4BasicConceptsInPreventionSurveillanceAndHealthPromotion/Thestagesofprevention

Association of Registered Nurses of Newfoundland and Labrador. (2008). *Advancing the role of psychiatric-mental health nurse in the community.* St. John's, NL: Author. Retrieved from https://www.arnnl.ca/sites/default/files/documents/role_of_the_psychiatric_mental_health_nurse_working_in_the_comm_apr_08.pdf

Baxter, C., & Mahoney, W. (2018). Developmental disability across cultures. *Caring for Kids New to Canada.* Retrieved from https://www.kidsnewtocanada.ca/mental-health/developmental-disability

Billette, J. M., & Janz, T. (2015). *Injuries in Canada: Insights from the Canadian Community Health Survey. Health at a Glance. Statistics Canada.* Retrieved from http://www.statcan.gc.ca/pub/82-624-x/2011001/article/11506-eng.htm

Brown, H. J., McPherson, G., Peterson, R., Newman, V., & Cranmer, B. (2012). Our land, our language: Connecting dispossession and health equity in an indigenous context. *Canadian Journal of Nursing Research, 44*(92), 44–63.

Butler, M., & Pang, M. (2014). *Current issues in mental health in Canada: Child and youth mental health.* Ottawa, ON: Library of Parliament. Retrieved from http://www.lop.parl.gc.ca/Content/LOP/ResearchPublications/2014-13-e.pdf

Canada Health Infoway. (2011). *Telehealth benefits and adoption. Connecting people and providers across Canada.* Retrieved from https://www.infoway-inforoute.ca/en/component/edocman/334-telehealth-benefits-and-adoption-connecting-people-and-providers-summary/view-document?Itemid=101

Canadian Association of Community Health Centres. (2017). *About community health centres.* Retrieved from http://www.cachc.ca/about-chcs/

Canadian Home Care Association. (2016). *Home and community-based services and supports, children with complex needs.* Retrieved from http://www.cdnhomecare.ca/

Canadian Mental Health Association. (2016). *Your mental health.* Retrieved from http://www.cmha.ca/mental-health/your-mental-health/

Canadian Mental Health Association Ontario. (2017). *Social determinants of health.* Retrieved from http://ontario.cmha.ca/provincial-policy/social-determinants/

Canadian Nurses Association. (2010). *Social justice. A means to an end, an end in itself* (2nd ed.). Ottawa, ON: Author. Retrieved from https://www.cna-aiic.ca/~/media/cna/page-content/pdf-en/social_justice_2010_e.pdf

Canadian Nurses Association. (2012a). *Resolution 11. In support of Shannen's Dream and Jordan's principle.* Ottawa, ON: Author. Retrieved from https://cna-aiic.ca/~/media/cna/page-content/pdf-en/2012_resolution_11_e.pdf?la=en

Canadian Nurses Association. (2012b). *Position statement on mental health services.* Ottawa, ON: Author. Retrieved from https://www.cna-aiic.ca/~/media/cna/page-content/pdf-en/ps85_mental_health_e.pdf?la=en

Canadian Nurses Association. (2013). *Registered nurses: Stepping up to transform health care.* Ottawa, ON: Author. Retrieved from https://cna-aiic.ca/~/media/cna/files/en/registered_nurses_stepping_up_to_transform_health_care_e.pdf

Canadian Nurses Association. (2014). *Aboriginal health nursing and Aboriginal health: Charting policy direction for nursing in Canada.* Ottawa, ON: Author. Retrieved from https://cna-aiic.ca/~/media/cna/page-content/pdf-en/aboriginal-health-nursing-and-aboriginal-health_charting-policy-direction-for-nursing-in-canada.pdf?la=en

Canadian Nurses Association. (2015). *Primary health care.* Ottawa, ON: Author. Retrieved from http://www.cna-aiic.ca/~/media/cna/page-content/pdf-en/primary-health-care-position-statement.pdf?la=en

Canadian Nurses Association. (2017a). *Code of ethics for registered nurses*. Ottawa, ON: Author. Retrieved from https://www.cna-aiic.ca/en/nursing-practice/the-practice-of-nursing/nursing-ethics

Canadian Nurses Association. (2017b). *Social determinants of health*. Retrieved from https://cna-aiic.ca/en/on-the-issues/better-health/social-determinants-of-health

Canadian Organization for Rare Diseases. (2015). *Newborn screening in Canada status report*. Retrieved from https://www.raredisorders.ca/content/uploads/Canada-NBS-status-updated-Sept.-3-2015.pdf

Canadian Pediatric Nursing Standards Advisory Group. (2016). *Canadian pediatric nursing standards*. Retrieved from https://ken.childrenshealthcarecanada.ca/xwiki/bin/download/Other+Resources/Canadian+Paediatric+Nursing+Standards/FINAL-Paediatric%20Nursing%20Standards.pdf

Canadian Paediatric Society. (n.d.). *Choosing to not vaccinate your child?* Retrieved from http://www.caringforkids.cps.ca/uploads/handout_images/CFK_tearsheet-ENG(post).pdf

Canadian Pediatric Society. (2016). Behavioural and general developmental screening tools. Retrieved from http://www.cps.ca/en/tools-outils/behavioural-and-general-developmental-screening-tools

Canadian Paediatric Society. (2017a). *Caring for kids new to Canada. A guide for health professionals working with immigrant and refugee children and youth*. Retrieved from http://www.kidsnewtocanada.ca/

Canadian Paediatric Society. (2017b). *Sun safety. Caring for kids*. Retrieved from http://www.caringforkids.cps.ca/handouts/sun_safety

Canadian Public Health Association. (2010). *Public health. Community health nursing practice in Canada: Roles and activities*. (4th ed.). Retrieved from https://www.cpha.ca/sites/default/files/assets/pubs/3-1bk04214.pdf

Canadian Society for Exercise Physiology. (2016). Canadian 24-hour movement guidelines for children and youth: An integration of physical activity, sedentary behaviour, and sleep. Retrieved from http://www.csep.ca/CMFiles/Guidelines/24hrGlines/Canadian24HourMovementGuidelines2016.pdf

Canadian Task Force on Preventive Health Care. (2016). Recommendations on screening for developmental delay. *CMAJ, 188*(18), 579–587. Retrieved from http://www.cmaj.ca/content/188/8/579

Centre for Addictions and Mental Health. (2012). *Understanding resilience*. Retrieved from http://www.camh.ca/en/education/teachers_school_programs/resources_for_teachers_and_schools/growing_up_resilient_ways_to_build_resilience_in_children_and_youth/Pages/undertstanding_resilience.aspx

Child Health BC (n.d.) Is "Good" Good Enough? Dimensions of Health & Well-being. Retrieved from http://www.childhealthindicatorsbc.ca/overview/dimensions-health-well-being

Coalitions Linking Action and Science for Prevention (CLASP). (2012). *Active living, children and youth: What is the Canadian evidence saying?* Retrieved from http://cip-icu.ca/Files/Resources/FACTSHEETS-ChildrenYouth-FINALenglish.aspx

COACH. (2015). *Canadian telehealth report. Public version*. Toronto: ON: Author. Retrieved from https://www.lecsct.ca/wp-content/uploads/2012/10/2015-TeleHealth-Public-eBook-Final-10-9-15-secured.pdf

College of Registered Nurses of British Columbia. (2018). *Telehealth*. Retrieved from https://www.crnbc.ca/Standards/PracticeStandards/Pages/telehealth.aspx

Commission on the Social Determinants of Health. (2008). *Closing the gap in a generation: Health equity through action on the social determinants of health. Final Report of the Commission on Social Determinants of Health*. Geneva: World Health Organization. Retrieved from http://apps.who.int/iris/bitstream/10665/43943/1/9789241563703_eng.pdf

Community Health Nurses of Canada. (2011). *Canadian community health nursing: Professional practice model & standards of practice—revised March 2011*. Retrieved from https://www.chnc.ca/en/publications-resources

Conference Board of Canada. (2015). *How Canada performs. Provincial and territorial ranking: Health [Internet]*. Ottawa, ON: Author. Retrieved from http://www.conferenceboard.ca/hcp/provincial/health.aspx. Accessed February 26, 2016.

Donaldson, C. D., Handren, L. M., & Crano, W. D. (2016). The enduring impact of parents' monitoring, warmth, expectancies, and alcohol use on their children's future binge drinking and arrests: A longitudinal analysis. *Prevention Science, 17*(5), 606–614.

Dubé, E., Bettinger, J. A., Fisher, W. A., Naus, M., Mahmud, S. M., & Hilderman, T. (2016). Vaccine acceptance, hesitancy and refusal in Canada: Challenges and potential approaches. *Improving Vaccination Rates, Canada Communicable Disease Report, 42*(12), 246–251. Retrieved from http://www.phac-aspc.gc.ca/publicat/ccdr-rmtc/16vol42/dr-rm42-12/ar-02-eng.php

First Nations Child & Family Caring Society of Canada. (2016). 7 free ways to make a difference. Retrieved from https://fncaringsociety.com/7-free-ways-make-difference

Foronda, C., Baptiste, D. L., Reinholdt. M. M., & Ousman, K. (2015). Cultural humility: A concept analysis. *Journal of Transcultural Nursing, 27*(3), 201–217.

Fortier, J., & Douglas, J. (2012). Advocacy inside the maze. *Canadian Nurse, 108*(3), 22–27.

Freeman, J., King, M., & Pickett, W. (2015). Health behaviour in school-aged children in Canada: Focus on relationships. *Public Health Agency of Canada*. Retrieved from http://healthycanadians.gc.ca/publications/science-research-sciences-recherches/health-behaviour-children-canada-2015-comportements-sante-jeunes/alt/health-behaviour-children-canada-2015-comportements-sant%C3%A9-jeunes-eng.pdf

Freeman, J. G., King, M., Pickett, W., Craig, W., Elgar, F., Janssen, I., & Klinger, D. (2012). *The health of Canada's young people: A mental health focus*. Ottawa, ON: Public Health Agency of Canada. Retrieved from http://www.phac-aspc.gc.ca/hp-ps/dca-dea/publications/hbsc-mental-mentale/assets/pdf/hbsc-mental-mentale-eng.pdf

Ghassemi, M. (2014). *Effectiveness of school-based physical activity interventions in children and youth: Rapid review of evidence*. Region of Peel Public Health. Retrieved from https://www.peelregion.ca/health/library/pdf/school-pa-interventions.pdf

Green Communities Canada. (n.d.). *Active and safe routes to school*. Retrieved from http://www.saferoutestoschool.ca/about

Greig, A., Constantin, E., LeBlanc, C., Riverin, B., Tak-Sam Li, P., & Cummings, C. (2016). *An update to the Greig Health Record: Executive summary.* Retrieved from https://www.cps.ca/en/documents/position/greig-executive-summary

Government of Canada. (2012). What is primary health care? *About Primary Health Care.* Retrieved from https://www.canada.ca/en/health-canada/services/primary-health-care/about-primary-health-care.html

Government of Canada. (2014). *Get the facts about immunization.* Retrieved from https://www.canada.ca/en/public-health/services/vaccination-children/get-facts-about-immunization.html#s1

Government of Canada. (2016). *Immunization coverage and registries.* Retrieved from https://www.canada.ca/en/public-health/services/immunization-coverage-registries.html#a3

Government of Canada. (2017). *Poverty reduction strategy.* Retrieved from http://www.lop.parl.gc.ca/content/lop/researchpublications/prb0865-e.htm

Grohskopf, L. A., Shay, D. K., Shimabukuro, T. T., Sokolow, L. Z., Keitel, W. A., Bresee, J. S., & Cox, N. J. (2013). Prevention and control of seasonal influenza with vaccines: recommendations of the Advisory Committee on Immunization Practices—United States, 2013–2014. *Morbidity and Mortality Weekly Report: Recommendations and Reports, 62*(7), 1–43.

Hamilton, N., & Bhatti, T. (1995). Population health promotion: An integrated model of population health and health promotion. Working Paper. Health Promotion Development Division, Health Canada. Also reproduced by the Canadian Federal Government Health Promotion Development Division, February 1996. Retrieved from http://www.phac-aspc.gc.ca/ph-sp/php-psp/index-eng.php

Hammond, W. (2010). *Principles of strength-based practice.* Calgary, AB: Resiliency Initiatives. Retrieved from http://www.mentalhealth4kids.ca/healthlibrary_docs/principlesofstrength-basedpractice.p

Health Canada. (2007). *Reaching for the top: A report by the advisor on healthy children and youth.* Retrieved from http://www.hc-sc.gc.ca/hl-vs/pubs/child-enfant/advisor-conseillere/index-eng.php#a16

Health Canada. (2010). Report on the findings of the oral health component of the Canadian Health Measures Survey 2007–2009. Retrieved from http://publications.gc.ca/collections/collection_2010/sc-hc/H34-221-2010-eng.pdf

Hertzman, C., Clinton, J., & Lynk, A. (2011). Measuring in support of early childhood development. *Paediatrics & Child Health, 16*(10), 655–657.

Human Early Learning Partnership. *Early development instrument [Internet].* Vancouver, BC: University of British Columbia. Retrieved from http://earlylearning.ubc.ca/edi/. Accessed June 3, 2016.

Immunize Canada. (2018). *Is immunization mandatory in Canada?* Retrieved from https://immunize.ca/

Indigenous and Northern Affairs Canada. (2016). *Indigenous peoples and communities.* Retrieved from http://www.aadnc-aandc.gc.ca/eng/1100100013785/1304467449155

Institute for Patient and Family Centered Care. (2017). *Patient and family-centred care.* Retrieved from http://www.ipfcc.org/about/pfcc.html

Klein, S., & Yalnizyan, A. (2016). *Better is always possible: A federal plan to tackle poverty and inequality.* Ottawa, ON: Canadian Centre for Policy Alternatives. Retrieved from https://www.policyalternatives.ca/publications/reports/better-always-possible

Lipnowski, S., & LeBlanc, C. M. A.; Canadian Paediatric Society-Healthy Active Living and Sports Medicine Committee. (2012). Healthy active living: Physical activity guidelines for children and adolescents. Position statement. *Paediatric Child Health, 17*(4), 209–210. Retrieved from http://www.cps.ca/documents/position/physical-activity-guidelines

Loppie, S., Reading, C., & de Leeuw, S. (2014). *Aboriginal experiences with racism and its impacts. Social determinants of health.* Prince George, BC: National Collaborating Centre for Aboriginal Health. Retrieved from http://www.nccah-ccnsa.ca/Publications/Lists/Publications/Attachments/131/2014_07_09_FS_2426_RacismPart2_ExperiencesImpacts_EN_Web.pdf

Macdonald, D., & Wilson, D. (2013). *Poverty or prosperity. Indigenous children in Canada.* Ottawa, ON: Canadian Centre for Policy Alternatives. Retrieved from https://www.policyalternatives.ca/sites/default/files/uploads/publications/National%20Office/2013/06/Poverty_or_Prosperity_Indigenous_Children.pdf

MacKay, M., Vincenten, J., Brussoni, M., Towner, E., & Fuselli, P. (2011). *Child safety good practice guide: Good investments in unintentional child injury prevention and safety promotion—Canadian Edition.* Toronto, ON: The Hospital for Sick Children.

Marshall, M., Marshall, A., & Bartlett, C. (2015). Chapter 2. Two-eyed seeing in medicine. In M. Greenwood, S. de Leeuw, & C. Reading (Eds.), *Determinants of Indigenous peoples' health in Canada* (pp. 16–24). Toronto, ON: Canadian Scholar's Press.

McMaster University. (2016). *Early development instrument.* Retrieved from https://edi.offordcentre.com/

Mema, S. C., McIntyre, L., & Musto, R. (2012). Childhood vision screening in Canada: public health evidence and practice. *Canadian Journal of Public Health/Revue Canadienne de Sante'e Publique, 44–45*).

Mental Health Commission of Canada. (2012). *Changing directions changing lives. The mental health strategy for Canada.* Calgary, AB: Author. Retrieved from http://strategy.mentalhealthcommission.ca/pdf/strategy-images-en.pdf

Mental Health Commission of Canada. (2016). The mental health strategy for Canada: A youth perspective. Retrieved from http://www.mentalhealthcommission.ca/sites/default/files/2016-07/Youth_Strategy_Eng_2016.pdf

Mental Health Commission of Canada. (2018). *Children and youth.* Ottawa, ON: Mental Health Commission of Canada. Retrieved from https://www.mentalhealthcommission.ca/English/what-we-do/children-and-youth

Mikkonen, J., & Raphael, D. (2010). *Social determinants of health: The Canadian facts.* Toronto, ON: York University School of Health Policy and Management. Retrieved from http://www.thecanadianfacts.org/

Ministry of Children and Youth Services. (2012). *Healthy babies healthy children guidance document.* Retrieved from http://chd.region.waterloo.on.ca/en/partnersProfessionals/resources/HBHC_GuidanceDocument.pdf

Ministry of Healthy Living and Sport. (2009). *Core public health functions for BC: Model core program paper healthy infant and child development.* Retrieved from http://www2.gov.bc.ca/assets/gov/health/about-bc-s-health-care-system/

public-health/maternal-child-and-family-health/healthy_infant_and_child_development-model_core_program_paper.pdf

National Collaborating Centre for Aboriginal Health. (2013). *An overview of Aboriginal health in Canada.* Prince George, BC: Author. Retrieved from http://www.nccah-ccnsa.ca/Publications/Lists/Publications/Attachments/101/abororigi-nal_health_web.pdf

National Advisory Committee on Immunization (NACI). (2017). Updated Recommendations on Human Papilloma-virus (HPV) Vaccines: 9-valent HPV Vaccine and Clarifi-cation of Minimum Intervals Between Doses in the HPV immunization schedule. 2017. ON: Public Health Agency of Canada.

National Collaborating Centre for Determinants of Health. (2013). *Let's talk: Universal and targeted approaches to health equity.* Antigonish, NS: National Collaborating Centre for Determinants of Health, St. Francis Xavier University.

NDDS. (2017). NDDS checklist. Retrieved from http://www.ndds.ca/canada

Ontario Ministry of Children and Youth Services. (2012). *Healthy babies healthy children guidance document.* Retrieved from https://docplayer.net/52943408-Healthy-babies-healthy-children-guidance-document.html

Ontario Ministry of Health Promotion. (2010). *Prevention of injury: Guidance document.* Retrieved from http://www.health.gov.on.ca/en/pro/programs/publichealth/oph_standards/docs/mhp/PreventionofInjury.pdf

Pan-Canadian Joint Consortium for School Health. (2017). *Comprehensive school health.* Retrieved from http://www.jcsh-cces.ca/index.php/about/comprehensive-school-health

Parliament of Canada. (2008). *Measuring poverty: A challenge for Canada.* Retrieved from http://www.lop.parl.gc.ca/content/lop/researchpublications/prb0865-e.htm

Patel, H., & Feldman, M.; Canadian Pediatric Society. (2016). Universal newborn hearing screening. Position statement. *Paediatric Child Health, 16*(5), 301–305. Retrieved from http://www.cps.ca/documents/position/universal-hearing-screening-newborns

Primary Care Initiative. (2017). *What is the primary care ini-tiative?* Retrieved from https://www.scpcn.ca/primary-care-initiative

PROOF. Food Insecurity Policy Research. (2017). *Children in food insecure households.* Retrieved from http://proof.utoronto.ca/

Public Health Agency of Canada. (2008). *Core competen-cies for public health in Canada: Release 1.0.* Ottawa, ON: Author. Retrieved from http://www.phac-aspc.gc.ca/php-psp/ccph-cesp/pdfs/cc-manual-eng090407.pdf

Public Health Agency of Canada. (2009). *Chapter 3—The health of Canadian children. Report: The state of public health in Canada 2009.* Retrieved from http://www.phac-aspc.gc.ca/cphorsphc-respcacsp/2009/fr-rc/cphorsphc-respcacsp06-eng.php

Public Health Agency of Canada. (2011a). *What determines health?* Retrieved from http://www.phac-aspc.gc.ca/ph-sp/determinants/index-eng.php#key_determinants

Public Health Agency of Canada. (2012). *Curbing childhood obesity: A federal, provincial and territorial framework for action to promote healthy weights.* Retrieved from http://

www.phac-aspc.gc.ca/hp-ps/hl-mvs/framework-cadre/index-eng.php

Public Health Agency of Canada. (2013). *Implementing the population health approach.* Retrieved from http://www.phac-aspc.gc.ca/ph-sp/implement/index-eng.php

Public Health Agency of Canada. (2014). *Mental health pro-motion: Promoting mental health means promoting the best of ourselves.* Retrieved from http://www.phac-aspc.gc.ca/mh-sm/mhp-psm/index-eng.php

Public Health Agency of Canada. (2015a). *Canada prenatal nutrition program (CPNP).* Retrieved from http://www.phac-aspc.gc.ca/hp-ps/dca-dea/prog-ini/cpnp-pcnp/index-eng.php

Public Health Agency of Canada. (2015b). *Community action program for children (CAPC).* Retrieved from http://www.phac-aspc.gc.ca/hp-ps/dca-dea/prog-ini/capc-pace/index-eng.php

Public Health Agency of Canada. (2016). Chronic disease and injury indicator framework. Quick stats, 2016 edi-tion. *Health Promotion and Chronic Disease Prevention in Canada. Research, Policy and Practice, 36*(8), 171–171. Retrieved from http://www.phac-aspc.gc.ca/publicat/hpcdp-pspmc/36-8/assets/pdf/ar-04-eng.pdf

Public Health Agency of Canada. (2017a). *Aboriginal head start in urban and northern communities (AHSUNC).* Retrieved from http://www.phac-aspc.gc.ca/hp-ps/dca-dea/prog-ini/ahsunc-papacun/index-eng.php

Public Health Agency of Canada. (2017b). *Nobody's perfect.* Retrieved from http://www.phac-aspc.gc.ca/hp-ps/dca-dea/parent/nobody-personne/index-eng.php

Public Health Agency of Canada. (2018a). *National advisory committee on immunization (NACI).* Retrieved from http://www.phac-aspc.gc.ca/naci-ccni/

Public Health Agency of Canada. (2018b). *Canadian immu-nization guide.* Retrieved from https://www.canada.ca/en/public-health/services/canadian-immunization-guide.html

Raphael, D. (2014). Social determinants of children's health in Canada: Analysis and implications. *International Journal of Child, Youth and Family Studies, 5*(2), 220–239. Retrieved from https://journals.uvic.ca/index.php/ijcyfs/article/view/12899/3988

Roberts, K. C., Shields, M., de Groh, M., Aziz, A., & Gilbert, J. (2011). *Overweight and obesity in children and adolescents: Results from the 2009–2011 Canadian Health Measures Sur-vey. Statistics Canada.* Retrieved from http://www.statcan.gc.ca/pub/82-003-x/2012003/article/11706-eng.htm

Rourke, L., Leduc, D., & Rourke, J. (2014). *Rourke Baby Record: Evidence-based infant/child health maintenance guide.* Retrieved from http://www.rourkebabyrecord.ca

Rowan-Legg, A.; Canadian Paediatric Society-Community Pae-diatrics Committee. (2013). Oral health care for children—a call for action. Position statement. *Paediatric Child Health, 18*(1), 37–43. Retrieved from http://www.cps.ca/documents/position/oral-health-care-for-children

Shields, L., Mamun, A., Pereira, S., O'Nions, P., & Chaney, G. (2011). Measuring family centred care: working with chil-dren and their parents in a tertiary hospital. *The Interna-tional Journal of Person Centered Medicine, 1*(1), 155–160.

Statistics Canada. (2013). *Canadian survey on disability, 2012.* Retrieved from http://www.statcan.gc.ca/daily-quotidien/131203/dq131203a-eng.htm

Statistics Canada. (2015). *Aboriginal peoples: Fact sheet for Canada*. Retrieved from http://www.statcan.gc.ca/pub/89-656-x/89-656-x2015001-eng.htm

Stewart, D., Sun, J., Patterson, C., Lemerle, K., & Hardie, M. (2004). Promoting and building resilience in primary school communities: Evidence from a comprehensive "health promoting school" approach. *International Journal of Mental Health Promotion, 6*(3), 26–33.

Taddeo, D., & Stanwick, R.; Canadian Paediatric Society-Adolescent Health Committee. (2012). Banning children and youth under the age of 18 years from commercial tanning facilities. Position statement. *Paediatric Child Health, 17*(2), 89. Retrieved from http://www.cps.ca/documents/position/tanning-facilities

Torpy, J. M., Campbell, A., & Glass, R. M. (2010). Chronic diseases of children. *JAMA patient page. The Journal of the American Medical Association, 303*(7), 682. Retrieved from http://jamanetwork.com/journals/jama/fullarticle/185394

Triple P International. (n.d.). *Triple p-positive parenting program*®. Retrieved from http://www.triplep.net/glo-en/home/

Truth and Reconciliation Commission of Canada. (2015a). *Honoring the truth, reconciling for the future. Summary of the final report of the Truth and Reconciliation Commission of Canada*. Winnipeg, MB: Author. Retrieved from http://www.myrobust.com/websites/trcinstitution/File/Reports/Executive_Summary_English_Web.pdf

Truth and Reconciliation Commission of Canada. (2015b). *Truth and reconciliation commission of Canada: Calls to action*. Winnipeg, MB: Author. Retrieved from http://www.trc.ca/websites/trcinstitution/File/2015/Findings/Calls_to_Action_English2.pdfuture_July_23_2015.pdf

UNESCO. (2017). *Poverty*. Retrieved from http://www.unesco.org/new/en/social-and-human-sciences/themes/international-migration/glossary/poverty/

UNICEF. (2016). Fairness for children. Canada' challenge. *UNICEF Report Card 13*. Toronto, ON: Author. Retrieved from http://www.unicef.ca/sites/default/files/legacy/imce_uploads/images/advocacy/rc/irc13_canadian_companion_en_sp_new_.pdf

UNICEF Office of Research-Innocenti. (2013). *Child well-being in rich countries: A comparative overview,* Box 1, p. 5. Florence: Innocenti Research Centre. Retrieved from https://www.unicef-irc.org/publications/pdf/rc11_eng.pdf

United Nations. (2007). *United Nations declaration on the rights of Indigenous peoples*. Retrieved from https://www.un.org/development/desa/indigenouspeoples/declaration-on-the-rights-of-indigenous-peoples.html

Woods, M. (2010). Cultural safety and the socioethical nurse *Nursing ethics, 17*(6), 715–725.

World Health Organization. (1948/2017). *Constitution of the World Health Organization: Principles*. Retrieved from http://www.who.int/about/mission/en/

World Health Organization. (1986). *The Ottawa charter for health promotion*. Retrieved from http://www.who.int/healthpromotion/conferences/previous/ottawa/en/

World Health Organization. (2017a). *Health promotion*. Retrieved from http://www.who.int/topics/health_promotion/en/

World Health Organization. (2017b). *Patient safety. AAPS definition of partnership*. Retrieved from http://www.who.int/patientsafety/implementation/apps/definition/en/

World Health Organization. (2017c). *Immunization*. Retrieved from http://www.who.int/topics/immunization/en/

World Health Organization, Health and Welfare Canada, & Canadian Public Health Association. (1986). *Ottawa charter for health promotion*. Geneva: World Health Organization. Retrieved from http://www.who.int/healthpromotion/conferences/previous/ottawa/en/

Yanchar, N. L., Warda, L. W., & Fuselli, P.; Canadian Pediatric Society-Injury Prevention Committee. (2012). Child and youth injury prevention: A public health approach. *Paediatric Child Health, 17*(4), 511. Retrieved from http://www.cps.ca/documents/position/child-and-youth-injury-prevention

Assessment of the child's health status involves many components: the health interview and history; observation of the parent–child interaction; assessment of the child's emotional, physiologic, cognitive, and social development; and physical examination. The nurse's skills are vital to the success of the assessment process. The nurse must (Treitz, Bunik, & Fox, 2014):

- Establish rapport and trust
- Demonstrate respect for the child and the parent or caregiver
- Communicate effectively by listening actively, demonstrating empathy, and providing feedback
- Observe systematically (especially while the child is quiet)
- Obtain accurate data
- Validate and interpret data accurately

The focus of the assessment depends on the purpose of the visit and the needs of the child. Assessment should be thorough and is an ongoing process repeated to varying degrees at every encounter. The expert nurse uses thoughtful, direct, and indirect assessment techniques and strategies to evaluate each child's physiologic state, temperament, demeanour, and behaviour throughout the entire visit. Indeed, some of the most subtle developmental signs may express themselves only during relaxed and casual interaction such as child-centred play (Burns, Dunn, Brady, Starr, & Blosser, 2013). The nurse may observe gait while watching a child run down the hall, assess fine motor skills and social adaptation during collaborative play, or observe balance and coordination while the child is bouncing a ball. Playful activities such as tickling a child can give the nurse feedback related to upper body strength when the child attempts to push the nurse's arms away. The nurse must learn to perform a comprehensive and thorough examination in a timely way.

A systematic approach to the examination is the most effective manner in which to identify any potential concerns. A comprehensive history, a thorough examination, and review of developmental skills against expected age-based norms should be completed at every health visit. The Canadian Task Force on Preventive Health Care (2016) suggests **surveillance** as the "ongoing monitoring of development, identification of risk factors, and elicitation of parental concerns as part of standard clinical practice for children" (par1). Surveillance involves listening to parental concerns coupled with close observation during clinical assessment, thorough documentation of the child's developmental history, and early identification of potential risks. In contrast, developmental **screening** is the use of a validated screening tool at a specific time to measure specific developmental abilities against established norms per age. The Canadian Task Force on Preventive Health Care (2016) recommends against universal screening for developmental delay using standardized tools in children aged 1 to 4 years when there are

no parental concerns, children are identified as low risk with no apparent signs of developmental delay. If either developmental surveillance or case finding (e.g., infants with a history of low birth weight, prematurity, or risk linked to the social determinants of health) indicates the possibility of developmental delay then further specialist evaluation is clinically indicated. The history and physical examination also provide an opportunity for anticipatory health education, teaching about expected growth and development, and promotion of healthy lifestyle choices. The nurse uses critical thinking skills to analyze these data and establish priorities for nursing intervention or follow-up care (Burns et al., 2013).

The health assessment may be documented using a number of formats such as a written narrative, a written flow sheet, or an electronic health record. The information should be easily retrievable and available to all members of the child's health care team.

HEALTH HISTORY

The health history provides the nurse with an overall picture of what the child has experienced over a prescribed time period, highlighting areas of concern such as recurrent upper respiratory infections or headaches. This not only helps the nurse to assess those specific areas more comprehensively but also provides the opportunity to ask focused questions and identify areas where education may be needed. The time used to obtain the health history also gives the nurse an opportunity to interact with the child in a nonthreatening manner while the child watches the interactions between the nurse and the primary caregiver (Burns et al., 2013; Miller, n.d.).

Safety Check

GOAL: Improve the Safety of Medication Administration

Maintain and communicate accurate patient medication information.

Steps: When obtaining the health history, be sure to collect accurate information concerning the child's routine medications and supplements. Ask specific questions about the use of over-the-counter medications and vitamins.

Preparing for the Health History

Appropriate materials and a quiet, warm environment are needed when performing a thorough health history. Take into account family roles, values, and relevant cultural background. Consider the age and developmental stage of the child in order to approach the child appropriately and possibly involve him or her in the health history. Observe the child–parent interaction. Determine the extent of the health history that is needed in a given situation. Being well organized and staying flexible with the tone and pace of the interaction will help ensure success (Burns et al., 2013).

Gathering Materials

Before beginning, make sure the following are available: materials to record the history data (either a computer or chart paper and a pen), a private space with adequate lighting, chairs for adults and the nurse, and a bed or examination table for the child. The space should be safe for the child's developmental stage. Sit down for as much of the history taking as possible to demonstrate a relaxed and welcoming manner (Burns et al., 2013).

Approaching the Parent or Caregiver

Greet the parent or caregiver by name. While interviewing the parent, provide (cleaned) toys or books to occupy the child, allowing the parent to concentrate on the questions. Use open-ended questions and avoid making judgmental comments. Show respect by remaining approachable. Remember that the structure of the family and its roles and dynamic varies i.e., cultural traditions and practices can vary as a result of age, community, and history. For example, in Indigenous cultures it is seen as a sign of respect not to make eye contact with people older than you. This custom can often be misinterpreted as avoidance or lack of knowledge about the child. Attention to engagement with the child and family, respect of values, spirituality, and custom will affect how the family communicates and maybe how they make decisions about health care (CPS, 2014a). Demonstrate patience and be flexible to allow parents to fully express any concerns. Help the parent stay on track when there are several children present, which may be distracting. Refer to the child by name and ask the child direct questions, as appropriate to their age and developmental stage.

Take Note!

In some indigenous cultures, eye contact is considered disrespectful as the eyes are considered the "window to the soul." Nurses and other health professionals need to be cognizant and respectful of this custom.

Approaching the Child

Show a professional demeanour while still being warm and friendly to the caregivers and child. A white examination coat or all-white uniform may be frightening to children, who may associate the uniform with painful experiences or may associate it with negative emotions such as upset, nervousness, or worry (Albert et al., 2013). The nurse can wear a variety of professional-looking outfits, whether colourful uniform tops, aprons,

or smocks worn over white uniforms, or everyday clothing, depending on the setting of the nurse's practice. Ask the child or parent if they have a preferred name or how to pronounce the child's name correctly. Use slow deliberate gestures rather than very quick or grand ones, which may be frightening to shy children.

Some young children may want to be invisible in the room, such as hiding behind a parent before they tentatively appear. The nurse should give them time to become more familiar with the space. Utilize an approach that matches the child's developmental stage and corresponding skills for social–emotional interaction. For example, consider that babies often experience stranger anxiety from 9 to 15 months of age, and even longer for the particularly sensitive child. Direct eye contact, abrupt physical contact, and questions may overwhelm and upset them. The young child looks to their parent for cues on how to respond to an unfamiliar adult. When approaching the older infant or toddler, be sure to make eye contact and connect with the parent first. This will communicate safety and security to the child and help them warm up to the interaction with the nurse. Make physical contact with the child in a nonthreatening way at first. Briefly cuddling a newborn before returning him or her to the caregiver, laying a hand on the head or arm of toddlers and preschoolers, and warmly shaking the hand of older children and teens will convey a gentle demeanour. A joke, a puppet, a silly story, or even a simple magic trick may coax the child into warming up. Being at the same eye level as the child can also be more reassuring than standing over the child (Miller, n.d.). This may require having extra seating for the nurse at the same level as the child and parent/caregiver. Aim to be seen as a trustworthy adult who is the child's partner in feeling better and staying healthy.

Elicit the child's cooperation by allowing him or her control over the pace and order of the health history, or anything else that the child can control while still allowing the nurse to obtain the information needed. All of this establishes a personal relationship with the child and helps gain his or her cooperation (Miller, n.d.).

Communicating With the Child During the Health History

Give the child opportunities to actively participate in the health history and assessment process. For young children, such as toddlers and preschoolers, ask them to point to where it hurts and allow them to answer questions. Validation of the information by the parent/caregiver is essential because of the limited comprehension and language use of children at these ages. The school-aged child can answer more accurately because of his or her increased language skills and maturity.

Initially, address the child and obtain as much information from him or her as possible. School-aged children should be able to answer questions about interactions with friends and siblings and school and activities they enjoy or in which they are involved. Ask the parent/caregiver if any additional information or observations should be included.

Adolescents may not feel comfortable addressing health issues, answering questions, or being examined in the presence of the parent/caregiver. The nurse must establish a trusting relationship with the adolescent to provide him or her with optimal health care. Ask adolescents whether they would be more comfortable answering questions alone in the examination area or whether they prefer their parents to be present. Either way, the parent/caregiver will have an opportunity to talk with the nurse after the health history and assessment are completed (Burns et al., 2013).

Demonstrate an interest in the teen by asking questions about school, work, hobbies or activities, and friendships. Begin with these topics to make the teen feel comfortable in communicating with the nurse. Communicate honestly with the adolescent and explain the rationale for various aspects of the health history. Teens are very sensitive to nonverbal communication, so be very aware of gestures and expressions (Sass & Kaplan, 2014). Once a rapport has been established, move on to more emotionally charged questions that relate to sexuality, substance use, depression, and suicide.

Be honest with the child or teen about the limits of confidentiality and duty to report concerns about risk for neglect or abuse, imminent concerns of self-harm, danger to others, or medical emergency or information or records that maybe subpoenaed for legal proceedings (Burns et al., 2013). Remember the primary concern is maintaining the safety of the child or teen.

Take Note!

Do not try to become the adolescent's peer. Remain in the role of the nurse while demonstrating respect and acceptance toward the teen. Clarify the meaning of jargon or slang that the teen uses, but do not use these words yourself; the teen will simply not accept the nurse as a peer.

Observing the Parent–Child Interaction

Observation of the parent–child interaction begins during the focused conversation of the health interview and continues throughout the physical examination. Explore the family dynamics, not only through questions but also by observing the family for behavioural or nonverbal clues. Does the parent make eye contact with the infant and how does the infant or child respond to the parent? Does the parent anticipate and respond to the infant's needs? Is the infant soothed and comforted by the parent or do they flinch when the parent comes near them? Are

the parents ineffective when dealing with a toddler's temper tantrum? The plan of care may need to be adjusted to teach appropriate responses to the infant's needs or toddler's behaviour. Do the parents' comments increase the school-aged child's sense of self-worth or does the child display signs of anxiety, conflict, or withdrawal in response to the parents' comments? Behavioural observations are crucial to accurately assess the family's needs (Burns et al., 2013; Columbia University, College of Physicians and Surgeons, n.d.).

Observe and note if the parent appears to be overwhelmed and if his or her behaviour seems appropriate (Burns et al., 2013). Monitor the child's behavioural cues. Does the child look at the parent/caregiver before answering? Does the child seem relaxed and happy with the parent/caregiver, or is the child tense/anxious? The infant will appear calm and relaxed if his or her needs are generally met. Crying may occur when the baby is ill or frightened, but may also indicate discomfort with the parent or caregiver. Use a calm and comforting voice with the infant. When observing the relationship between the adolescent and the parent/caregiver, does the parent/caregiver allow the adolescent to speak, or does he or she frequently interrupt? Does the parent/caregiver contradict what is being said? Observe the body language of the adolescent: does the teen seem relaxed or tense? Since adolescents are between childhood and adulthood, they have unique needs. They are experiencing a time of multiple physical and emotional changes, many of which they cannot control. They need to know that the nurse is interested in what they have to say (Sass & Kaplan, 2014). The use of open-ended questions allows the adolescent to talk. "Tell me about your…." or "What have you noticed about…?" are comfortable phrases to use to elicit the information needed.

Be aware of your own reactions to the adolescent's questions or behaviours, such as nonverbal and facial expressions. Use accurate language and terminology when discussing topics such as sexuality, relationships, and puberty. Avoiding jargon and using anatomically appropriate terms when describing the body will convey professionalism and respect to the teen.

Determining the Type of History Needed

The purpose of the examination will determine how comprehensive the history must be. If the physician or nurse practitioner rarely sees the child or if the child is critically ill, a complete and detailed history is in order, no matter what the setting. The child who has received routine health care and presents with a mild illness may need only a problem-focused history. In critical situations, some of the history taking must be delayed until after the child's condition is stabilized. Evaluate the situation to determine the optimal timing and extent of the history required (Burns et al., 2013). Also, be sensitive to repetitive interviews in hospital situations, and collaborate with physicians or other members of the health care team to ensure that a family already under stress does not need to undergo prolonged or repetitive questioning.

Take Note!
Types of Health History

A child in an emergent situation should have a health history that is focused on the child's most immediate need. Conversely, a comprehensive health history is appropriate for the child who is having his first visit at a pediatrician's office, for example.

Remember Elliot, the 3 year old being seen for his annual examination? When you enter the room, he is hiding behind his mother's legs. Considering his age and developmental level, how will you proceed with obtaining a health history?

Performing a Health History

The health interview is the foundation of an accurate health assessment. A thorough and systematic interview with the child and/or the caregiver will reveal important information about the child's health (Burns et al., 2013). Depending on the objective of the health assessment, many of the questions will be direct, and many will require the caregiver or child to answer simply "yes" or "no." In nonemergent situations, asking open-ended questions offers an excellent opportunity to learn more about the patient's life. For example, "Are you happy at school?" may elicit a brief nod of the head, whereas "Tell me what it's like on your school playground" may result in a story about the child's friends, the kind of activities the child enjoys, any bullying that goes on, and so forth. These stories will provide the nurse with clues to the child's stage of physical, emotional, and moral development as well as his or her functional status (Burns et al., 2013; Columbia University, College of Physicians and Surgeons, n.d.).

Establish a therapeutic relationship with the child and family. A family-centred approach considers the child and family as a whole unit, where the health concerns of the child and the health of the family must be assessed together. A collaborative approach to the visit where the nurse involves the parent, and when possible the child, in the management plan will build respect and trust, thereby fostering a therapeutic environment. Without the trust that comes from this therapeutic relationship, the family may not reveal vital information due to fear, embarrassment, or mistrust (Treitz et al., 2014). Use therapeutic communication techniques such as active listening, open-ended questions, and eliminating barriers to communication. Establishing a "medical space" where ongoing health supervision occurs encourages trust through continuity of care and the family's continuing relationships with primary care providers.

The structure of the health interview is determined by the nature of the visit. At an initial visit, large amounts of historical data are collected. Having the family fill out a questionnaire can save time, but a questionnaire is not a substitute for the health interview. The questionnaire may serve as a springboard to begin structured conversations between the family and the nurse (be mindful that literacy levels can vary). At subsequent visits the health interview can focus on the pertinent issues of that visit as well as any specific health issues that are being monitored.

The health history includes demographics, chief complaint and history of present illness, past health history, review of systems, functional inquiry, social history (i.e., family genogram, resources, and home environment), family health history, and developmental history.

Take Note!

Any questionnaires used in the health care setting should be written at a fifth-grade reading level and be in the primary language of the person completing them (The Joint Commission, 2014). Assess and, where appropriate, inquire about literacy level; note if a child is the translator for the family. Perhaps consider helping the family complete the questionnaire.

Demographics

Initially, questions should be simple and nonintrusive; once a rapport between the nurse and patient has been achieved sensitive questions can be asked. First obtain data such as the child's name, preferred name, birth date, and gender they identify with. Determine the child's race or ethnicity, the language the child understands, and the language the child speaks. Record the child's address and home telephone number and the parent's or caregiver's work or alternative telephone number that a message can be left at if they do not have a telephone (i.e., extended family or Band representative). Some centres will ask for an email contact for the parent or caregiver. Identify who the historian is (the child or the parent or caregiver), and note how reliable this source of information is considered to be. Do not assume that an adult with the child is the child's parent or has guardianship of the child. Establish the relationship of the adult to the child, and ask who cares or has guardianship for the child if that person does not. Determine the composition of the household, including other children, other family members, or other persons who reside there.

Chief Complaint and History of Present Illness

Next, ask about the **chief complaint** (reason for the visit). The reason may not always be apparent to you.

- Routine health care and dental care (including frequency of dental visits, and whether any concerns were identified; ask about fluoride use and flossing)
- Nutrition, including a 24-hour dietary recall or week-long food diary, use of supplements and vitamins, feeding pattern and satisfaction with diet, amount of sugary drinks or sodas, caffeine, sweets, processed foods consumed, food likes and dislikes, food insecurity, and the parent's perception of the child's nutrition
- Physical activity, recreation, play, and organized sports
- Television and computer habits (amount of screen time per day)
- Sleep hygiene, location (bed sharing, room sharing), sleep hours, bedtime routines
- Elimination patterns (toilet training)
- Hearing or vision problems (dates of last screenings and results)
- Relationships with other family members and friends, coping and temperament, discipline strategies
- School environment (grade level, grades, supports, attention or behaviour problems)
- Religious involvement and other spiritual and cultural practices
- Use of adaptive and assistive devices such as eyeglasses or contact lenses, hearing aids, walker, braces, wheelchair

In the adolescent patient various assessment tools maybe helpful when raising difficult topics such as substance use or mental health. See thePoint for additional information:

- Sexual relationships, practices, use of barrier precautions and contraceptives (Burns et al., 2013)
- Substances (illicit drug or supplement use, alcohol, tobacco)
- Stress or mood disorders
- Suicide (active ideation or past attempts)

Social History (Family Composition, Resources, and Home Environment)

Determine the marital status of the parents. Does the child live with the parents, a stepparent, blended family, or other family member? Is the child adopted or in foster care? Are the parents the primary caretakers for the child? If not, who has guardianship of the child? This will be the individual who can consent to the child receiving medical treatment. Working parents may learn about a health or behaviour issue only after being alerted by the child's day care centre or babysitter. It may be helpful to expand the family history to include the grandparents and their interaction with the child.

Determine the employment status of the parents and their occupations, as this could affect the child's overall well-being; for example, the parents' work schedule may not allow them to spend much time with the child. Assess family income and financial resources, including health insurance, income assistance through the Ministry of Social Development and Social Innovation, or financial support through Aboriginal Affairs and Northern Development of Canada when families reside on reserve; or other governmental supplemental income. Major family changes, including separation or divorce, death of a family member, relocation to a new home or school, can stress family relationships and negatively impact the parent–child dynamic.

Ask about the family's home and its age and environment. Is there a safe outdoor play area? If there is a pool, are safety features in place? Determine whether the home has electricity and an indoor water supply. Also determine whether the home has heating and what kind, air conditioning, and refrigeration. What pets does the family have? How are they housed? Are there infestations of insects or rodents? Is there any dampness or mould in the home?

Take Note!

Homes or apartments built prior to 1978 may contain lead-based paint, and children who live there are at an increased risk for the development of lead poisoning (CDC, 2015b). Additionally, newcomers to Canada and international refugee children from developing nations, have much higher rates of lead exposure and lead poisoning. These children should be referred for baseline serum lead level testing, and be followed for ongoing monitoring depending on their risk profile.

PHYSICAL EXAMINATION

The next step after the health history is the physical examination. It should focus on the chief complaint and include any of the systems that were flagged by the nurse while obtaining the history. The examination will reflect the nurse's general practice style, the developmental stage and age of the child, the temperament of the child and caregiver, and the health status of the child. For example, a very ill child will not waste energy protesting the examination, so the nurse can move quickly in that situation. A healthy child, however, will express his or her normal developmental stage and show varying degrees of resistance to the examination (Columbia University, College of Physicians and Surgeons, n.d.; Miller, n.d.).

Preparing for the Physical Examination

When performing the physical examination, being prepared and organized ensures that the needed information will be obtained efficiently. The appropriate methods to use and ways to approach the child depend on the child's developmental stage.

Gathering Materials

The examination area should include an examination table or the child's hospital crib or bed. Appropriate lighting is necessary for adequate observation and inspection. Gather clean gloves and clean equipment necessary for the examination such as stethoscope, thermometer, sphygmomanometer, tape measure, reflex hammer, penlight, otoscope/ophthalmoscope, tongue depressor, and cotton ball. An infant or adult scale is needed, as well as a **stadiometer** for children capable of standing independently. Young children may be frightened by seeing a large amount of equipment, so take out one piece of equipment at a time. Some children can be very resistant to what they see as a threat or an invasion of their privacy, so it is helpful to have washable toys in the examination area to use as distractions during the assessment (Burns et al., 2013; Miller, n.d.).

Children and their parents may be able to sense any frustration or anxiety on the part of the examiner, so display a confident and matter-of-fact approach. If the child is not cooperative, use a game or a playful approach to the examination. Young children can be engaged with games and humour, which often helps them to be more receptive. It may be helpful to demonstrate the examination on a favourite doll or stuffed animal so that the child can participate as the "helper" and anticipate their turn. Regardless of the child's age, if the examination room is cold, the child will be uncomfortable and possibly less cooperative. Provide appropriate covers to ensure the child's comfort and dignity, or have the child remain dressed until the time of the examination (Miller, n.d.).

Approaching the Child

Approach the child according to his or her developmental age and stage. Table 32.2 outlines a general approach to the physical examination in each broad developmental category.

If several children are to be seen at the same time, begin with the child who will be most cooperative. If the other children do not see anything scary and realize that their sibling was examined without a problem, it sets the stage for better cooperation from the younger ones.

NEWBORNS AND INFANTS

If the infant is asleep, auscultate the heart, lungs, and abdomen first while the baby is quiet. Count the heart rate and respiratory rate for a full minute, before undressing the baby. Completely undress newborns and infants down to their diaper, removing it just at the end to examine the genitalia, anus, spine, and hips. It is best to examine the infant 1 to 2 hours before a feeding. Having the

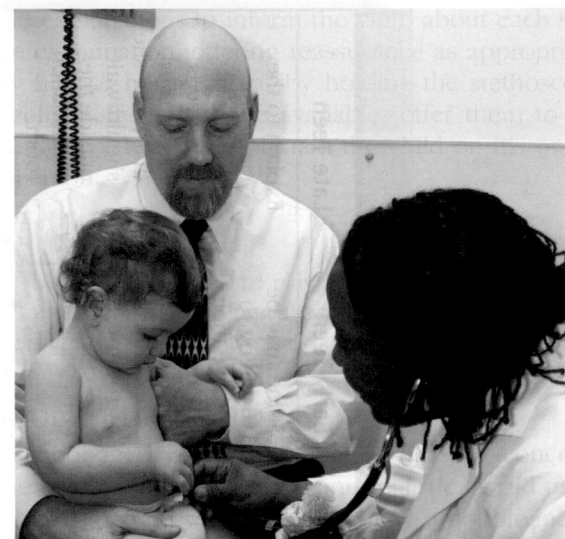

FIGURE 32.2 The infant or toddler may feel more comfortable and secure being examined while sitting in the parent or caregiver's lap.

parent or caregiver hold the child during the examination can help to alleviate fears and anxieties (Fig. 32.2). Allow the parent or caregiver to be a nurturer rather than assisting with painful procedures, unless there are no other choices available (Miller, n.d.).

Perform the assessment in a head-to-toe manner, leaving the most traumatic procedures, such as examination of the ears, nose, mouth, and throat, until last (Burns et al., 2013; Miller, n.d.). Also delay eliciting the Moro reflex until the end of the examination, as the startling sensation may make the infant cry. Use firm, gentle handling while examining the infant. Make sure your hands and the stethoscope are both clean and warm. Perform the assessment as quickly and completely as possible. Use a soft and crooning voice, smile, and engage the infant in eye contact. In addition, use brightly coloured sensory-based toys such as noisemakers or rattles to help assess vision, hearing, and attention skills. If the baby is crying, a pacifier may be useful.

Take Note!

Many older infants demonstrate stranger anxiety as a normal part of development. If the parent is not holding the infant, make sure the parent is within the infant's view; this will increase the baby's comfort and cooperation (Bickley, 2013; Burns et al., 2013).

TODDLERS

Toddlers usually prefer to remove their clothing one item at a time as needed for the examination. After one area is examined, the child may feel more comfortable replacing that item of clothing before removing another one (Treitz et al., 2014). An examination gown is usually

TABLE 32.3	HEART RATE AND RESPIRATORY RATE RANGES BY AGE GROUP				
	Infant	**Toddler**	**Preschooler**	**School Age**	**Adolescent**
Heart rate	80–150	70–120	65–110	60–100	55–95
Respiratory rate	25–55	20–30	20–25	14–22	12–18

Adapted from Kliegman, R. M., Stanton, B. F, St. Geme III, J. W., Schor, N. F., & Behrman, R. E. (Eds.). (2011). *Nelson textbook of pediatrics* (19th ed.). Philadelphia, PA: Saunders; and Marx, J., Hockberger, R., & Walls, R. (2014). *Rosen's emergency medicine—concepts and clinical practice* (8th ed.). Philadelphia, PA: Saunders.

ensure the child's mouth remains closed until the device registers the temperature. Oral intake, oxygen administration, and nebulized medications or treatments may affect oral temperature.

The axillary method may be used for children who are uncooperative, neurologically impaired, or immunosuppressed or have injuries or have had surgery to the oral cavity (Bowden & Greenberg, 2012). Place the tip of the electronic or digital thermometer in the axilla to obtain the reading. Make sure the tip is indeed in the axilla and not just between the arm and the child's side. Hold the thermometer parallel rather than perpendicular to the child's side to obtain the most accurate reading. Keep the child's arm pressed down to the side until the thermometer registers, which will be as little as 10 seconds with certain electronic models but 2 or 3 minutes with digital models commonly used at home.

Though long considered to reflect core temperature, the rectal route is invasive, not well accepted by children or parents, and probably unnecessary with the modern alternative methods now available (El Radhi, 2014). To take the rectal temperature, position the young infant supine with legs flexed. The older infant or child should be prone or side lying. Small children may lie across the parent's lap for additional comfort. Apply a water-soluble jelly to the covered probe, insert the thermometer past the anal sphincter no more than 1 in (2.5 cm), and hold it there until the temperature registers (as little as 15 seconds with certain electronic models but longer with digital models).

Take Note!

Avoid the rectal route of temperature measurement in the immunosuppressed child as well as the child who has diarrhoea, a bleeding disorder, or a history of rectal surgery (Asher & Northington, 2008).

PULSE

Assess the heart rate while the child is resting or sleeping. The heart rate in infants is much faster than in adults. It will be elevated in infants and children who are anxious, fearful, crying, or those who are febrile. As the child grows, the heart rate slows and the range of

normal values narrows. Table 32.3 lists heart rate ranges according to the child's age. The radial pulse is difficult to palpate accurately in children younger than 2 years of age because the blood vessels lie close to the skin surface and are easily obliterated (Bickley, 2013). For children younger than 10 years of age, auscultate the apical pulse with the stethoscope for a full minute (Jarvis, 2012). In older children, palpate the radial pulse for a full minute (Fig. 32.5). Note any irregularities in strength or rhythm. Finally, document the method used to obtain pulse measurement as well as any activity or crying during measurement.

Take Note!

In the infant and young child, the heart rate is often quite elevated due to fear or anxiety when the stethoscope is placed on the chest initially. For an accurate heart rate, wait several seconds until the rate slows, and then count for 1 full minute.

RESPIRATORY RATE

Assess respirations when the child is resting or sitting quietly, since respiratory rate often changes when infants or young children cry, feed, or become more active. They also tend to breathe faster when they are anxious or scared. The most accurate respiratory rate is obtained

FIGURE 32.5 Assessing the radial pulse of a young child.

before disturbing the infant or child (Bowden & Greenberg, 2012). This can often be done easily when the parent/caregiver is holding the child before any clothing is removed. Count the respiratory rate for a full minute to ensure accuracy. Infants' respirations are primarily diaphragmatic, so count the abdominal movements. After 1 year of age, count the thoracic movements. Table 32.3 lists ranges of respiratory rate according to the child's age. Document the rate, activity of the child, any deviations from normal, and any action taken.

> **Take Note!**
> Infants normally display an uneven or irregular breathing pattern, with short pauses between some breaths. This may be accentuated when they are ill (Bickley, 2013).

MEASURING OXYGEN SATURATION

Since the incidence of respiratory dysfunction is high in ill children, pulse oximetry is often routinely included in the vital signs assessment. This method is reliable and noninvasive. Pulse oximetry determines the oxygen saturation (SaO_2) in blood by using a sensor that measures the absorption of light waves as they pass through highly perfused areas of the body. The pulse rate on the oximeter should coincide with the apical pulse rate to ensure that the oxygen saturation reading is accurate. Nursing Procedure 32.2 details how to use the pulse oximeter.

A few guidelines to follow when using pulse oximetry are as follows:

- The probe may be placed on the finger, toe, ear, foot, or forehead. Avoid placing the probe on the same extremity with a blood pressure cuff or an intravenous or other type of line.
- Use the physician's or nurse practitioner's orders or health care agency guidelines to set parameters for high and low pulse rate as well as high and low oxygen saturation. Never turn off the alarm settings.
- Ensure that the probe is not applied too tightly, as this will prevent venous flow and cause inaccurate readings.
- It is helpful to use gauze dressing to shield the sensor from ambient light to prevent inaccurate results.

Potential sources of errors in pulse oximeter readings include abnormal haemoglobin value, poor perfusion, ambient light interference, motion artifact, and skin breakdown. Falsely low readings may be associated with a nonsecure connection (movement of child's foot or hand), and poor perfusion. Falsely high readings may be associated with carbon monoxide poisoning and severe anemia (Covidien, 2012).

BLOOD PRESSURE

At 3 years of age, children should have their blood pressure measured at every routine health maintenance visit (Harris et al., 2016). With the rising rates of early childhood obesity and sedentary behaviour in North American children, regular measurement of blood pressure allows health care providers to identify any changes from baseline and flag early signs of hypertension. Children younger than 2 to 3 years old should have blood pressure measured if they have one of the following risk factors:

- History of prematurity, very low birth weight, or other neonatal intensive care complication
- Congenital heart disease
- Recurrent urinary tract infections, hematuria, proteinuria, known renal disease or urologic malformations, family history of congenital renal disease
- Malignancy, bone marrow transplant, or solid organ transplant
- Treatment with medications that raise blood pressure
- Systemic illnesses associated with hypertension such as neurofibromatosis and tuberous sclerosis
- Increased intracranial pressure (U.S. Department of Health and Human Services, National Institutes of Health, National Heart, Lung, and Blood Institute, 2005)

In the hospital or outpatient setting when a child is ill or undergoing surgery or a procedure, the frequency of blood pressure measurement will depend on the child's physical status. Measurement of blood pressure can be frightening to a young child, so include an age-appropriate explanation and perform the procedure after obtaining the pulse rate and respirations (Fig. 32.6). Accuracy of blood pressure measurement depends on the cuff size, as well as the operator's skill and accurate calibration of an electronic device. The cuff bladder width should be at least 40% of the circumference of the upper arm at its midpoint (U.S. Department of Health and Human Services, National Institutes of Health, National Heart, Lung, and Blood Institute, 2005). The cuff bladder

FIGURE 32.6 Allowing children to handle the equipment gives them some control over the situation.

NURSING PROCEDURE 32.2

Pulse Oximetry Monitoring

1. Explain the procedure to the child and family (use a penlight to show how the sensor "looks through the skin")

2. Attach the probe to the child and connect to the monitor

3. Set the parameters for the alarm if monitoring pulse oximetry continuously

4. Observe and record pulse rate and oxygen saturation

5. Record the activity level of the child and the percentage of oxygen in use

6. Check skin condition and rotate sensor position every few hours if adhesive type used

Types of Sensors

a. Nonadhesive for infants (continuous use)

b. Finger adhesive (continuous use)

c. Finger reusable (intermittent use)

d. Forehead (can be used continuously for 2 days)—especially useful in instances of poor distal perfusion

Adapted from Covidien. (2012). *Covidien operator's manual: Nellcor™ bedside SpO$_2$ patient monitoring system.* Mansfield, MA: Author.

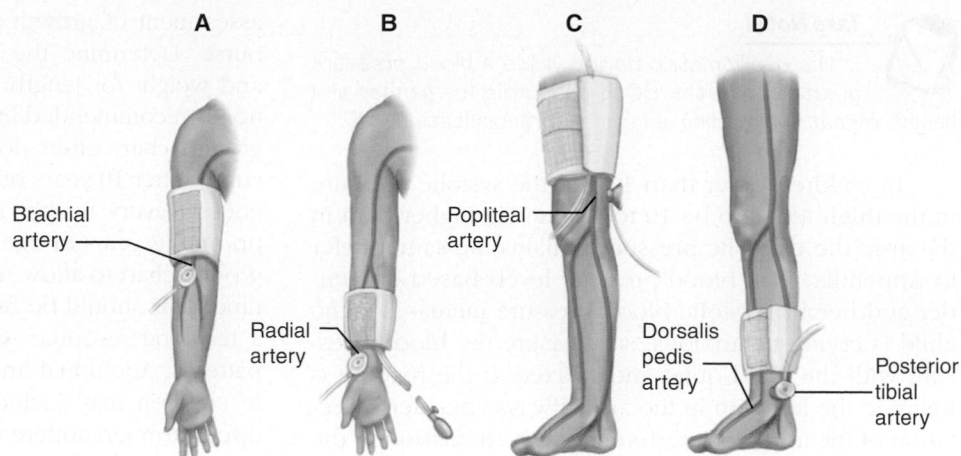

FIGURE 32.7 Various positions of cuff placement and auscultation area for obtaining blood pressure. **A.** Upper arm. **B.** Lower arm. **C.** Thigh. **D.** Calf/ankle.

length should cover 80% to 100% of the circumference of the upper arm. Various pediatric and infant cuffs are available, as well as larger thigh cuffs that may be used on an arm in an obese adolescent.

Take Note!

Using an accurate cuff size is important: a wider cuff yields a lower reading and a narrower cuff yields a higher reading.

Measure blood pressure in the upper arm, lower arm, thigh, or calf/ankle. The size of the cuff should match the extremity used. The measurement should be taken in the same limb, at the same place, and in the same position with each subsequent measurement to ensure consistency in tracking the blood pressure. To measure blood pressure using the upper arm, place the limb at the level of the heart, place the cuff around the upper arm, and auscultate at the brachial artery. When obtaining blood pressure in the lower arm, again, position the limb at the level of the heart, place the cuff above the wrist, and auscultate the radial artery. For measurement in the thigh, place the cuff above the knee and auscultate the popliteal artery. To obtain blood pressure on the calf or ankle, place the cuff above the malleolus or at the midcalf and auscultate the posterior tibial or dorsal pedal artery. Figure 32.7 shows appropriate cuff placement and auscultation points for the various sites.

Auscultation is the preferred method of obtaining blood pressure readings in children (Fig. 32.8). Systolic pressure in children is read at the moment the first Korotkoff sound is heard as the manometer pressure is lowered. The point at which the sound disappears is the diastolic pressure. In some children, the Korotkoff sounds can continue to zero, therefore record the diastolic pressure at the point at which the Korotkoff sounds first become muffled (Harris et al., 2016). Due to the small arm vessels in infants and young children, it may be very difficult to hear the Korotkoff sounds by auscultation (Jarvis, 2012). Alternative methods for obtaining blood pressure measurements in children include the use of Doppler or oscillometric (Dinamap) devices. The Doppler ultrasound method uses high-frequency sound waves that bounce off body parts to obtain blood pressure. Apply the gel to the Doppler end and listen with the Doppler device where Korotkoff sounds would normally be auscultated.

With either the Doppler method or auscultation, inflate the cuff 20 mm Hg past the point where the distal pulse disappears. Oscillometric equipment measures the mean arterial pulse and then calculates the systolic and diastolic readings. The accuracy of this method depends heavily on ongoing validation and calibration. Also, the cuff inflates to a preset value often far higher than the infant or child's blood pressure, resulting in a tight, uncomfortable cuff being in place for a longer period of time.

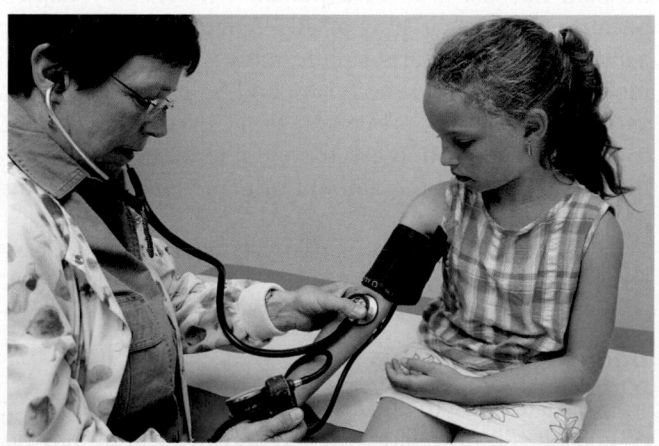

FIGURE 32.8 Auscultation is the preferred method for measuring blood pressure in children.

In children older than 1 year, the systolic pressure in the thigh tends to be 10 to 40 mm Hg higher than in the arm; the diastolic pressure remains the same. Refer to Appendix F for blood pressure levels based on gender and height. Systolic blood pressure increases if the child is crying or anxious, so measure the blood pressure with the child quiet and relaxed. If the reading is lower in the leg than in the arm, always consider coarctation of the aorta or interference with circulation to the lower extremities. Also pay attention to the pulse pressure (the difference between the systolic and diastolic readings): unusually wide (more than 50 mm Hg) or narrow (less than 10 mm Hg) pulse pressure readings suggest a congenital heart defect (Burns et al., 2013).

Pain Assessment

The symptoms of pain are considered to be important vital signs within the context of patient well-being (Levy, Sturgess, & Mills, 2018). However, caution around the use of language attributed to pain being the "5th vital sign" are shifting in light of patterns of medication prescribed in various countries (Levy, Sturgess, & Mills, 2018). In infants and young children, the FLACC pain scale can help to measure pain in those too young to verbally or conceptually quantify their pain, or when there is a language barrier (Manworren & Hynan, 2003). The FLACC pain scale consists of a possible 10 points, with 0, 1, or 2 points given for each of five clinical signs.

Children who are older and can express that pain is worsening or improving should use the Pain Faces Scale. Explain that each face represents a person who is happy or sad, depending on how much or how little pain he has: 0 is for a person who is "very happy because he doesn't hurt at all"; 1 means "it hurts just a little bit"; 2, "it hurts a little more"; 3, "it hurts even more"; 4, "it hurts a whole lot"; and 5, "it hurts as much as you can imagine—but you don't have to be crying to feel this bad." Then ask the child to point to the face that best describes the amount of pain being felt (Wong & Baker, 1988).

For additional information related to pain assessment, refer to Chapter 36.

Body Measurements

Appropriate growth in children is usually an indicator of good health. A child who is not growing well may be in poor health, have inappropriate or inadequate dietary intake, or have a chronic disease (Bickley, 2013). Accurate assessment of growth is a critical skill for the pediatric nurse. Determine the child's height or length, weight, and weight for length. Body mass index (BMI) calculation is recommended in children 2 to 19 years of age. The growth chart often does not include weight-for-height curves after 10 years of age. Measure the head circumference at every health office visit for all healthy children up until 2 years of age. Plot these measurements on the growth chart to allow monitoring of growth velocity over time. This should be reviewed with parents and used as a teaching resource when discussing expected growth patterns. Additional anthropometric measurements used in children may include the chest circumference, mid-upper arm circumference, and skinfold measurement at the triceps, abdomen, or subscapular regions, but these are not performed routinely and are usually used only when a nutritionist consultation is necessary.

The WHO Growth Chart for Canada is recommended for use with all Canadian infants and children as it reflects a broader ethnic population and includes both breastfed and formula fed infants in its subject groups (CPS, 2014C). This better represents the Canadian population of children and also allows the nurse to compare the child to other children of the same age and gender while allowing for normal genetic variation. Record each measurement in ink with a small dot at the correct location for the child's age and the date of the measurement written above it. Then use a straightedge to connect the previous measurement to the most current one. Children grow at variable rates; in infancy and prepuberty, the growth velocity is normally more rapid. When measurements follow a consistent percentile curve over time, it suggests the child is growing at an expected normal rate. Children whose measurements fall within the 5th and 95th percentiles are generally considered within the normal growth range (Reiter, 2011). Sudden increases or drops across percentile curves away from a period of consistent growth, may indicate a nutritional intake problem, or may reflect a chronic condition (Bickley, 2013). An abrupt upward increase or downward drop across two percentile curves between visits should be flagged by the nurse, and referred for further assessment by a provider with pediatric expertise.

The growth charts for boys and girls, ages birth to 24 months and 2 to 19 years used in Canada can be found at thePoint. It is recommended to use growth charts with all children, though special growth charts are also available for children with specific conditions such as the Fenton growth chart for preterm infants (Dieticians of Canada, 2014).

Take Note!

Please visit the Dieticians of Canada website for more information at http://www.dietitians.ca/Dietitians-Views/Prenatal-and-Infant/WHO-Growth-Charts.aspx.

FIGURE 32.9 The recumbent measuring board is the most accurate method for obtaining a length measurement in infants and very young children.

FIGURE 32.10 Standing height is most accurately measured with the stadiometer.

LENGTH OR HEIGHT

Calculate the length of the infant and toddler in a lying position until the age of 24 months. Use a measuring board (Fig. 32.9) or a cloth or paper measuring tape. Stretch out the legs to get a full extension of the body. Marking the examination paper at the child's head and extended foot is an option. When measuring horizontal length of a young child on an examination table with measuring tape, there may be excess movement which can lead to discrepancies in length by several centimetres. The use of a firm baby board provides the most accurate measure of length in the infant and young toddler. Make sure that the growth chart where the measurement is plotted is marked for length and not height, as the two measurements differ. Document the length in centimetres.

Once the child can cooperate and stand independently, begin measuring the standing height. Using a stadiometer is best (Fig. 32.10), but a cloth or paper tape can be used. Ask the child to remove his or her shoes and check that the back, shoulders, buttocks, and heels are against the wall, with the pelvis tucked as much as possible to correct for lordosis. The chin should be parallel to the floor. Plot this measurement on a growth chart marked for height rather than length. Record the height in centimetres as well as feet and inches.

Take Note!

Cloth and paper measuring tapes may stretch over time. Periodically replace or recalibrate all measuring tools.

WEIGHT

Measure weight on a scale that is calibrated between every measurement. Just before placing the child on the electronic scale, press the "zero" button and make sure

the reading is 0. Calibrate the balance-type scale by setting the weight at zero, observing the beam balance, and making adjustments as necessary. Infants and toddlers should be weighed on a platform-type electronic or balance scale, with an examination paper placed between the child and the scale surface. Calibrate the scale with the examination paper in place. Always remove the infant's diaper before placing him or her on the scale, as a soiled diaper can add significant weight and affect accuracy. Toddlers may sit on the scale with the nurse or caregiver nearby to avoid falls (Fig. 32.11). Weigh older children and adolescents on a standing scale (Fig. 32.12). They may keep their underpants on and wear a lightweight examination gown.

An alternate method for obtaining weight, though much less accurate, is to weigh the caregiver initially and then weigh the caregiver holding the child. The difference between the two weights is the child's weight. Regardless of the method used, weigh the infant to the nearest 10 g and the toddler and older child to the nearest 100 g. Record the weight in kilograms.

WEIGHT FOR LENGTH

For children between the ages of newborn and 24 months, plot weight on the growth chart in comparison to the child's length. This allows the nurse to determine whether the child is a healthy weight for how long he or she is. Children placing less than the 5th percentile on the weight-for-length chart are generally considered

FIGURE 32.11 A nurse or caregiver should remain nearby while weighing the infant or toddler.

FIGURE 32.12 Children who can stand independently can be weighed on a regular standing balance scale.

underweight. Those placing greater than the 95th percentile are considered to be overweight.

BODY MASS INDEX

With the recent increase in obesity in children, BMI is becoming an important measurement. **Body mass index (BMI)** is a measure of body fat and is determined by comparing the child's height and weight (see Evidence-Based Practice 32.1). Calculate the BMI using the child's weight and height by either the English or metric method. Box 32.1 provides BMI calculation formulas. BMI is included on the charts for children ages 2 to 19 years. Plot the BMI on the growth chart according to the child's age. A child whose BMI for age plots at less than the 3rd percentile is considered to be underweight. BMI between the 85th and 97th percentiles indicates risk for overweight (see Evidenced Based Practice 32.1). BMI greater than the 97th percentile indicates the child is overweight (Dieticians of Canada, 2014; CPS, 2014c).

The growth chart can indicate when a child is not growing adequately and can also be used to monitor for the development of overweight and obesity.

HEAD CIRCUMFERENCE

Healthy normal infants require head circumference measurement up until 24 months of age. Then measure it at the annual well-child visit until 6 years old if there are problems such as microcephaly or macrocephaly. Measure the largest point across the skull, not including the ears, with a nonstretching cloth or paper tape. Begin at the forehead just above the eyebrows and bring the tape around the head in a taut circle just above the occipital prominence at the back of the head (Fig. 32.13). Plot this measurement in relation to the child's age on the appropriate standardized growth chart, unless an alternate growth chart is being used for a chronic underlying condition (e.g., preterm infants).

Monitoring Equipment

Sometimes children in acute care settings require continuous monitoring of vital signs. This monitoring could be via an apnea monitor or a cardiopulmonary monitor. The

FIGURE 32.13 Measure occipitofrontal head circumference at the largest point.

FIGURE 32.14 Placement of cardiac apnea monitor leads: white on the right upper chest, black on the left upper chest, green or red on the abdomen (not over bone).

apnea monitor measures abnormal or irregular breathing in infants. The cardiopulmonary monitor generally measures heart rate and respiratory rate. Additional equipment on this monitor also allows for blood pressure and temperature monitoring. Set high and low alarm limits according to the health care facility's policies. Figure 32.14 indicates the placement of electrodes for the apnea and cardiopulmonary monitors. Assess the skin where the electrodes are placed to ensure there is no skin breakdown. If the alarm sounds, immediately check the child to ensure the leads are not disconnected or the child is not in distress.

Safety Check

GOAL: Reduce the Harm Associated With Clinical Alarm Systems

Improve the safety of clinical alarm systems.

Steps: Ensure alarms on biomedical equipment are properly set according to the child's age, clinical condition, prescribed orders, and facility policy. ALWAYS answer alarms promptly, checking the child first, then attending to the equipment.

Skin

The skin is the body's largest organ and reveals information about a child's nutrition, respiratory, cardiac, endocrine, and hydration status at a glance. A careful skin examination provides an invaluable understanding of a child's health (Jarvis, 2012).

EVIDENCE-BASED PRACTICE 32.1   PRESCHOOL BODY MASS INDEX ASSOCIATION WITH ADULT OBESITY

STUDY

Overweight and obesity have become significant public health concerns and are acknowledged to be responsible for a significant percentage of chronic disease in the adult population. In this study, a large cohort (4,111 children) was followed into adulthood. The researchers were able to include 2,120 children who had sufficient growth measurements throughout childhood. Preschool-age weight and body mass index, was compared to body mass index, metabolic syndrome, waist circumference, and other adult health markers at the adult age of 31 years.

Findings

Analysis of the preschool growth measurement data as compared to adult status revealed an important association. High preschool body mass index was consistently associated with adult obesity and early-onset metabolic

syndrome. Thus, routine growth measurements throughout the preschool years can help identify children who may benefit from intervention related to decreasing body mass index and preventing adult obesity.

Nursing Implications

Accurate growth measurements are critical for determining overall health in the growing child. Identifying children with slow or suboptimal growth is well known to be important for intervening early to ensure adequate growth. Pediatric nurses are also in the ideal position to identify preschoolers who demonstrate higher body mass indexes and heavier weight as noted on standardized growth charts. The nurse may then collaboratively develop a plan with the child and family to ensure healthy eating and exercise habits are instilled at this young age, in order to prevent adult obesity and its associated morbidities.

Adapted from Graversen, L., Sørensen, T., Petersen, L., Sovio, U., Kaakinen, M., Sandbaek, A., . . . Obel, C. (2014). Preschool weight and body mass index in relation to central obesity and metabolic syndrome in adulthood. *PLoS One, 9*(3), 19.

INSPECTION

Inspect the colour of the skin. The colour should be appropriate to the child's racial or ethnic background, with the nail beds, conjunctivae, soles of the feet, and palms of the hands appearing pink. Normal variations include the following:

- Blueness of the hands and feet, known as acrocyanosis, is normal in babies up to several days of age and results from an immature circulatory system completing the switch from fetal to extrauterine life (see Fig. 25.3A).
- Cooling or warming the newborn and young infant may produce a vasomotor response that causes a mottling of the skin over the trunk and extremities (see Fig. 25.3B).
- Babies of darkly pigmented First Nation, African, and Asian parents will be paler than their parents for many months until the melanocytes in the epidermis begin production.
- Dark-skinned infants commonly have hyperpigmented areolas, genitals, and linea nigra.

Other variations related to skin colour are discussed in Box 32.2.

Inspect the skin for the presence of **lanugo**. All infants display some degree of lanugo (soft, downy hair on the body, particularly the face and back). Lanugo is more abundant in infants of Hispanic descent and in premature infants and recedes over the first few weeks of life.

Inspect the entire body for nevi and vascular and other lesions or anomalies. Document carefully their location, size, distribution, characteristics, and colour,

FIGURE 32.15 Transient hyperpigmentation most often occurs in darker-skinned infants.

as this provides a baseline against which any new skin abnormalities may be compared and tracked. Pigmented nevi (also termed birthmarks) are indicated by a darker patch of skin and generally do not fade over time. Document the presence of hyperpigmented nevi (formerly called Mongolian spots). These are benign, flat, and irregularly shaped lesions, which appear as blue or grey (Fig. 32.15). These are a common finding in dark-skinned infants. These nevi fade over months to years as the child's skin pigment darkens. Do not mistake hyperpigmented nevi for bruises. Inspect the skin for the presence of any congenital vascular lesions. Some vascular lesions require ongoing monitoring, while some specific patterns of lesions are associated with underlying genetic conditions that require closer investigation. Here the nurse's role is to provide a thorough observation of the skin and carefully document the number, location, colour, and character of each lesion. Table 32.4 describes vascular lesions and their significance.

Rashes are common in children and are often associated with communicable diseases. Describe the rash in detail, noting types of lesions, distribution, drying, scabbing, scaling, and any drainage. The newborn and young infant may display milia (small white papules) on the forehead, chin, nose, and cheeks. These are of no concern and recede spontaneously. In adolescents, the skin examination may reveal open or closed comedones (pimples or blackheads) across the face, chest, and back. Teens may sport tattoos, brandings, or various body piercings; inspect these areas for signs of infection such as erythema or drainage (Fig. 32.16).

Document the presence of any lacerations, abrasions, or burns. Note the distribution of the injury and whether it seems consistent with the mechanism described in the health history. Be alert to the possibility of inflicted injury (or nonaccidental trauma) if the location, type or number of burns, lacerations, or bruises seems unusual for the situation or if the explanation

---

BOX 32.2

VARIATIONS IN SKIN COLOUR AND THEIR CAUSES

- **Pallor** (defined as decreased pinkness in light-skinned patients, ashy-grey in dark-skinned) is caused by anemia, shock, fever, or syncope.
- **Central cyanosis** (blueness of the lips, tongue, oral mucosa) is caused by hypoxia or circulatory collapse.
- Overall yellow colour (**jaundice**) may be physiologic in the newborn or related to liver or hematopoietic disease in any age child.
- **Yellowing** of nose, palms, and soles may result from excess intake of yellow vegetables.
- **Redness** of the skin results from blushing, exposure to cold, hyperthermia, inflammation (localized), or alcohol ingestion.
- **Lack of colour** in skin, hair, and eyes is related to albinism.

Adapted from Bickley, L. (2013). *Bates' guide to physical examination and history taking* (11th ed.). Philadelphia, PA: Lippincott Williams & Wilkins; Jarvis, C. (2012). *Physical examination and health assessment* (6th ed.). St. Louis, MO: Saunders.

TABLE 32.4	VASCULAR LESIONS AND THEIR SIGNIFICANCE
Description	**Significance**
Salmon nevi: light pink macule usually on eyelids, nasal bridge, back of neck ("stork bite")	Usually fade over time, but may never go away completely. No complications.
Strawberry nevus: raised reddish papule made of blood vessels (hemangiomas)	Present at or develop after birth; recede over time, usually by the age of 9 years. Usually no complications.
Nevus flammeus: dark purple-red flat patch, grows with the child ("port-wine stain")	May be associated with Sturge–Weber syndrome. May be disfiguring; may be removed with laser therapy.
Ecchymosis: purplish discoloration, changing to blue, brown, black (bruise)	Common on lower extremities in young children. Should correlate with the injury.
Petechiae: pinpoint reddish purple macules that do not blanch when pressed	Broken tiny blood vessels; occur with coughing, bleeding disorders, meningococcemia.
Purpura: larger purple macules that do not blanch when pressed	Bleeding under the skin; occur with bleeding disorders, meningococcemia.

Adapted from Bickley, L. (2013). *Bates' guide to physical examination and history taking* (11th ed.). Philadelphia, PA: Lippincott Williams & Wilkins; and Jarvis, C. (2012). *Physical examination and health assessment* (6th ed.). St. Louis, MO: Saunders.

for the injury is inconsistent with the type of injury or changes frequently.

Take Note!

Petechiae or ecchymosis may be found over areas traumatized by the birth process; these may take a few weeks to resolve. Certain cultures use "cupping" or "coining" when a child is ill, and these practices may yield bruises or mild burns (International Cupping Therapy Association, 2010).

PALPATION

Palpate the skin for temperature, moisture, texture, turgor, and edema. Use the back of your hand to assess the skin's temperature, comparing the right side of the body to the left and the upper body to the lower. The skin should feel uniformly warm. Cool extremities are associated with environmentally cool temperatures as well as impending circulatory collapse and shock. Newborn infants typically have cool and mottled peripheries, as they are extremely sensitive to any changes in temperature, especially when undressed for an examination. Warm skin may be associated with fever or sunburn, or locally a burn or infectious process. The skin should feel fairly dry, occasionally moister in the creases. Dry, flaking skin may occur in the young infant, particularly if born postmaturely. Overall skin dryness in the well-hydrated child may occur with excess sun exposure, poor nutrition, or overbathing. Moist skin occurs with perspiration, fever resolution, and shock. The infant's and young child's skin is usually very soft. Older children should continue to have a smooth and even skin texture. The preadolescent and adolescent may have oily feeling skin on the face, shoulders, or back.

Assess skin turgor by elevating the skin on the abdomen in the infant or on the back of the hand in the older child or teen. The "pinched-up" skin should quickly return to place. Skin that remains tented is strongly suggestive of moderate to severe dehydration. When edema is present, palpate the edematous area to determine its extent. Palpate any lumps or protrusions to determine firmness or tenderness. Palpate lesions or rashes with a gloved hand to document the size and extent of the lesions.

Hair and Nails

Inspect the hair and scalp, noting distribution of hair as well as colour, texture, amount, and quality. The young infant's hair may be absent entirely or quite thick; it will be replaced by hair that is of a texture and colour closer to what the child will have throughout childhood. Coarse, dry hair at any age may indicate a thyroid disorder or

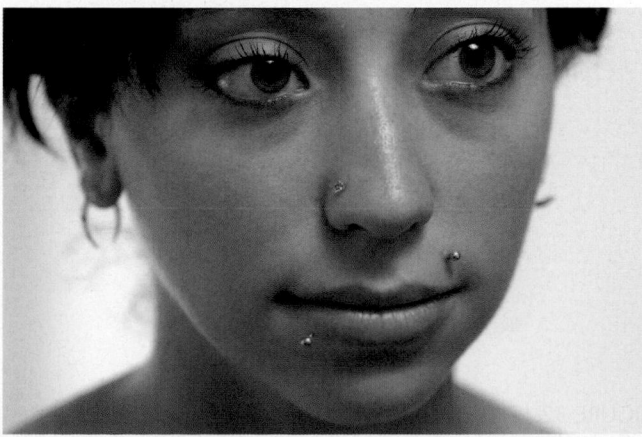

FIGURE 32.16 **Adolescent with multiple piercings.**

nutritional deficiency. Note the presence of a greasy, scaly plaque on the scalp of infants, termed seborrheic dermatitis or cradle cap; it is benign and easily treated.

Inspect the nails for colour, shape, and condition. Full-term infants may have long, papery fingernails that can scratch their skin if not trimmed. Children should have healthy nails. Dry, brittle nails may indicate a nutritional deficiency. Inspect the skin around the nails to ensure that it is intact and without signs of infection. Many children (especially school-aged children) have a nervous habit of nail biting or hangnail biting or pulling.

Inspect the school-aged child's or adolescent's toenails to ensure they are trimmed in a horizontal fashion. Self-trimming of toenails either too low or in a curved fashion places the child at risk for the development of ingrown nails. Clubbing of the nails indicates chronic hypoxemia related to respiratory or cardiac disease. Nails that curve inward or outward may be hereditary or linked with injury, infection, or iron-deficiency anemia.

Head

Examining the head is critical in the newborn and infant, but should not be overlooked in older children as an opportunity to check for diseases of the scalp, local infection, skin parasites (i.e., lice, noted as small greyish specks near the base of hair shafts, termed "nits"), and functional and developmental problems that are reflected in poor hygiene of the head and scalp. Note hair distribution and any bald or thinning areas. Use of gloves may be indicated, depending on the overall scalp cleanliness and chance of infestation.

INSPECTION

Examine the head and facial structures for shape and symmetry. In newborns, the head may be temporarily misshapen from uterine positioning or a lengthy vaginal delivery. If assistive devices such as forceps or vacuum were required for delivery, these infants may have prominent bruising or bossing of their scalp. Some infants have a slight flattening of the back of the head since the recommended sleeping position is supine. Note any irregularities or asymmetry. Observe the infant's head shape by looking down on it from above. Observe whether the head appears centred on the neck or tilts to one side. After 4 months of age, the infant should have achieved enough head control to hold the head erect and in midline when placed in a vertical position. Pull the infant from the supine position into sitting to determine the extent of head lag. To determine the extent of head control in older infants and children, ask the child to turn the head in different directions, either by simple commands or by following a colourful object.

Observe the infant's face when crying, smiling, or babbling for symmetry of muscle movement. In children who are old enough to follow directions, a game of

"Simon Says" is a playful way to determine facial symmetry and strength; ask them to puff out their cheeks, make kisses, look surprised, stick out their tongue, and so on (effectively testing function of cranial nerve VII [facial]) (Bickley, 2013).

Take Note!

When you note a flattened occiput in an infant, encourage the parent or caregiver to allow the infant "tummy time" for 3 to 5 minutes, several times per day. This helps strengthen the infant's head and neck control, while also taking the pressure off the back of the head. Parents should limit the infant's time in the car seat which can aggravate the flattening, and slow its improvement (Shah & Gupta, 2014).

PALPATION

Gently palpate the anterior and posterior **fontanels** (Fig. 32.17). The fontanels are the soft areas on the skull that remain open to allow for rapid brain growth in the first months of life. Note the size of the fontanels. The anterior fontanel's size is 1 to 4 cm in either direction until it can no longer be felt when it is closed by the age of 9 to 18 months (Rosenberg & Grover, 2014). If the anterior fontanel remains open beyond 24 months of age, the child needs prompt referral to a pediatrician for investigation. The posterior fontanel is much smaller and may close any time between shortly after birth and approximately 2 months of age. The posterior fontanel should close by 4 months of age. The fontanels should not be depressed or taut and bulging, though it is not uncommon to see them pulsate or briefly bulge if the baby cries. In an acutely ill infant, assess the fontanels while obtaining the vital signs. Dehydration can cause the fontanels to be sunken; increased intracranial pressure and overhydration can cause them to bulge. Palpate the skull for asymmetry, overriding or open sutures, and lumps or other deformities. A soft, swollen, or bruised area may be palpable to

FIGURE 32.17 Note location and size of the fontanels. The anterior fontanel is diamond shaped and closes between the ages of 9 and 18 months.

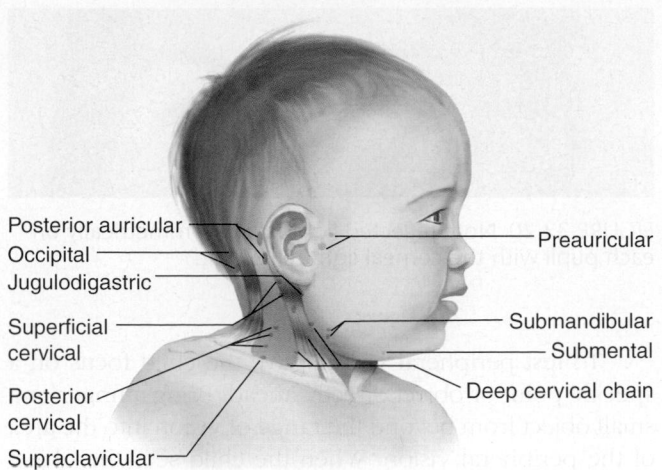

Posterior auricular
Occipital
Jugulodigastric
Superficial cervical
Posterior cervical
Supraclavicular

Preauricular
Submandibular
Submental
Deep cervical chain

FIGURE 32.18 Location of lymph nodes.

the upper back area of scalp of the newborn infant who required forceps or vacuum assist during birth. These are termed *caput succedaneum* or *cephalhematoma,* which should resolve within weeks of birth. However these can be associated with prolonged jaundice; thus should be monitored for resolution. Palpate the jaw joints as the child bites down to assess cranial nerve V (trigeminal). Use the fingertips to palpate for occipital, postauricular, preauricular, submental, and submandibular lymph nodes, noting their size, mobility, and consistency (Fig. 32.18).

Take Note!

Large fontanels may be associated with Down syndrome or congenital hypothyroidism. A fontanel that becomes larger over time rather than smaller may indicate the development of hydrocephalus, especially if accompanied by an accelerated increase in head circumference (Bickley, 2013). This child needs to be immediately evaluated, as this is a medical emergency.

Neck

Inspect the neck for symmetry. The infant's neck is short, but by 4 years of age the child's neck should be similar in appearance to the adult's. Webbing or excessive neck skin folds may be associated with Turner syndrome, and lax neck skin may occur with Down syndrome. Assess the flexibility of the neck through a full range of motion. Take younger children through a passive range of motion. Older children will be able to look in all directions on command and stretch their chins to their chests themselves. Test cranial nerve XI (accessory) in the older child by having the child attempt to turn the head against resistance. Assessment of neck mobility is particularly important when infections of the central nervous system are suspected. Pain or resistance to range of motion may indicate meningeal irritation. Do not assess neck mobility in the trauma victim.

Take Note!

The infant or child who has experienced a traumatic injury should have the cervical spine maintained completely immobile until a radiologist has determined that the spinal cord is not damaged.

Palpate the neck for masses and lymph nodes. Palpate the cervical and clavicular lymph nodes with the distal part of the fingers using gentle but firm pressure in a circular motion. Tilt the child's head upward slightly to allow better access. Assess the lymph nodes for swelling, mobility, temperature, and tenderness. In healthy infants and adolescents, the cervical lymph nodes are usually not palpable. In healthy children between 1 and 11 years, the cervical nodes are often found to be small, nontender, and mobile (see Fig. 32.18 for locations of lymph nodes). Typical benign lymph nodes are 1 cm in diameter or smaller. Enlarged cervical lymph nodes frequently occur in association with upper respiratory infections and otitis media. Report significant enlargement (>1.5 cm) to the physician or nurse practitioner. Palpate the trachea; the thyroid is usually palpable only in older children.

Eyes

Assessment of the eyes includes evaluation of the external and internal structures as well as screening for visual acuity. Any nurse caring for a child should be adept at examining the external structures. Assessment of the internal structures will also be covered below but is usually performed only by the advanced practitioner. Determination of visual acuity tests the function of cranial nerve II (optic).

EXTERNAL STRUCTURES

Observe the eyes for symmetry and spacing, presence and even distribution of eyelashes and eyelids, and presence of epicanthal folds. Note the child's ability to blink, and report an inability to do so. The pupils should be symmetric and in the midline when the child is looking directly ahead. The iris should be perfectly round and the sclerae should be clear. The cornea should be uniformly transparent. Inspect the corners of the eye (medial and lateral canthus) and the conjunctiva (lining of the eyelids). They should be free of discharge, inflammation, or swelling. Epicanthal folds may be present in children of Asian descent, children with genetic abnormalities, or those with fetal alcohol spectrum disorder. Using a small penlight or ophthalmoscope, inspect the function and clarity of the pupil by putting your nondominant hand on the child's forehead and moving the light toward and away from each eye. This will elicit the blink reflex. Next observe whether the pupil contracts with the light and expands when the light is removed. Make the same motion with a small toy or object and direct the child

FIGURE 32.19 The pupils should be equal, round, and reactive to light and accommodation (PERRLA).

FIGURE 32.20 Note reflected light falling symmetrically on each pupil with the corneal light reflex test.

to look at it. The eyes demonstrate **accommodation**, or focusing at different distances, if the pupil constricts as the object moves closer. If normal findings are present, report **PERRLA** (pupils are equal, round, reactive to light and accommodation) (Fig. 32.19). This is a particularly important assessment in head and eye injuries, as well as when other neurologic concerns are present. Absence of pupillary reflexive action after age 3 weeks may indicate blindness (Jarvis, 2012).

Take Note!

The normal infant may exhibit intermittent strabismus (crossing of the eyes) until about 4 months of age. However, persistent strabismus at any age or intermittent strabismus after 6 months of age should be evaluated promptly by a pediatric ophthalmologist (Burns et al., 2013).

Check extraocular muscle motility and function of cranial nerves III and IV (oculomotor and abducens) by instructing the child to follow the light through the six cardinal positions of gaze. Infants and very young children will follow an interesting object. Instruct the older child to look downward and inward (testing cranial nerve IV [trochlear]). Assess eye muscle strength using two tests. Using the corneal light reflex test, bring the penlight to the middle of your face and direct the child to look at it. The small dot of reflected light seen in the pupil should be placed symmetrically in each eye (Fig. 32.20). The cover test also assesses eye muscle strength. Cover one of the child's eyes and instruct the child to focus on an interesting object. The eye should not waver. While the child is still focusing with the first eye, remove the cover from the second. Observe the uncovered eye for movement. Any drift or movement is an abnormal finding and needs to be reported for further investigation.

To test peripheral vision, have the child focus on a specific point or object directly ahead. Bring a finger or a small object from beyond the range of vision into the area of the peripheral vision. When the child sees the object from the side, while still focusing on the object or point in front, the child should say "stop." This also tests cranial nerve II (optic). Visual acuity testing using a Snellen letter chart is generally not reliable in the preschool-aged child. The nurse can recommend parents seek vision testing from a community optometrist for best accuracy.

INTERNAL STRUCTURES

An advanced practitioner with experience in this type of assessment best accomplishes assessment of the internal structures of the eye. An adequate assessment requires that the child cooperate. Restraint for eye examination does not usually prove fruitful, as movement and tearing of the eyes interfere with the accuracy of the examination. Use the ophthalmoscope to inspect the internal eye structures. Observe the red reflex (creamy coloured in children with very dark eye colour). Inspect the optic disc, macula, fovea, and blood vessels. Refer any child with blurring or bulging of the optic disc or hemorrhage of vessels to a pediatric ophthalmologist for prompt evaluation.

Take Note!

Immediately report absence of the red reflex in one or both eyes, as this may indicate the presence of cataracts (Bickley, 2013) or retinoblastoma.

Ears

Assessment of the ears includes evaluation of the external and internal structures as well as screening for hearing. Any nurse caring for a child should be adept at examining the external structures. Assessment of the internal structures will also be covered below but is usually performed only by the advanced practitioner. Testing of hearing also tests the function of cranial nerve VIII (acoustic), although these may not be carried out by a nurse.

EXTERNAL STRUCTURES

Assess the placement of the external ears on the head. The top of the pinna should lie no lower than the eyes. The pinna should deviate no more than 10 degrees from an imaginary line that is perpendicular to a line drawn between the outer canthus of the eye and the top of the ear. Low-set ears may be associated with genetic abnormalities (i.e., kidney problems) or syndromes (Fig. 32.21). Note protrusion or flattening of the ears, which may be normal for that child or may indicate inflammation (protrusion) or persistent side-lying (flattening). Note the presence of pits or skin tags in the preauricular area. Observe the exterior ear canal. A waxy cerumen that is soft and in orangish-brown colour is normally found lubricating and protecting the external ear canal and should be left in place or washed gently away when bathing. Note drainage from the ear canal, which is always considered abnormal. Pull on the auricle and palpate the mastoid process, neither of which should result in pain in the healthy child.

Take Note!

Impacted and dry cerumen can be softened with a few drops of mineral oil once or twice daily for several days. This will lubricate the cerumen and allow passive drainage. **Never** irrigate the internal ear of a child with a syringe as this creates excessive pressure which may tear the tympanic membrane and damage the internal ear structures.

FIGURE 32.21 **Low-set ears may be associated with chromosomal or other genetic anomalies.**

Take Note!

Never attempt to flush a foreign object out with water until it has been identified, because small pieces of sponge, clay, or vegetative material like peas or beans swell with water, further obstructing the ear canal (Nettina, 2014).

Nose and Sinuses

The nose, as with all facial features in a child, should be symmetric, but it can be displaced temporarily by birth trauma in newborns. Children of Asian or African descent often display a flattened nasal bridge as a normal variation. Ensure that the nares provide unobstructed airflow by alternately occluding one nostril at a time and observing for air movement through the other nostril. If the child is breathing comfortably, there should be little nostril movement visible. Adolescents may have pierced their nose or nasal septum; ensure that the site is free from infection or loose jewellery that could migrate into the sinuses. Ideally the nose should not be draining, though clear mucus may be present if the child has been crying. Assess the amount, colour, thickness, and presence of any odour if drainage is present. Inspect the interior of the nose by tilting the child's head backward and pushing the tip of the nose upward. Direct the beam of a penlight in the nostril. The nasal mucosa should be uniformly firm, pink, and free from edema, excoriation, or masses. Test the older child's sense of smell by having the child close the eyes and identify a familiar scent such as peppermint or coffee (cranial nerve I [olfactory]). Palpate the sinuses for tenderness.

Take Note!

Infants up to 3 to 6 months of age have traditionally been thought to be **obligate nose breathers** because of their long soft palate and relatively large tongue, which allows for swallowing without aspiration during breast or artificial nipple feeding. This lessens with age and as the infant becomes better able to breathe through the mouth when necessary (Bickley, 2013).

Mouth and Throat

Wear a powder-free glove to examine the mouth, teeth, and throat. Inspection of the exterior of the mouth may be done at any point in the examination. Infants and young children may find assessment of the mouth and particularly the pharynx and uvula to be quite intrusive, so delay that part of the assessment until the end of the examination, after otoscopic evaluation. Assess the character and quality of the child's voice and the infant's cry. It should be neither too hoarse nor too shrill.

INSPECTION OF THE MOUTH

Observe the lips for colour, symmetry, and absence of inflammation or edema. Salivation in infants begins at

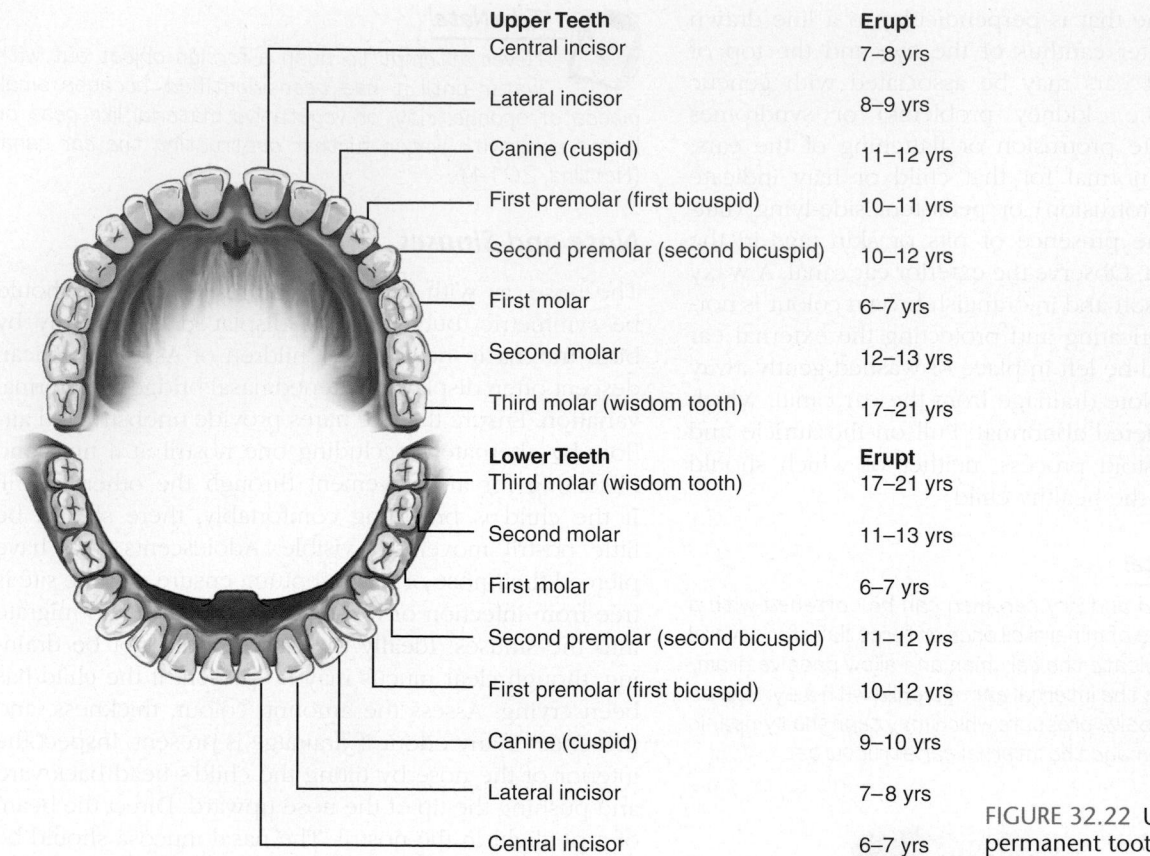

Upper Teeth	Erupt
Central incisor	7–8 yrs
Lateral incisor	8–9 yrs
Canine (cuspid)	11–12 yrs
First premolar (first bicuspid)	10–11 yrs
Second premolar (second bicuspid)	10–12 yrs
First molar	6–7 yrs
Second molar	12–13 yrs
Third molar (wisdom tooth)	17–21 yrs

Lower Teeth	Erupt
Third molar (wisdom tooth)	17–21 yrs
Second molar	11–13 yrs
First molar	6–7 yrs
Second premolar (second bicuspid)	11–12 yrs
First premolar (first bicuspid)	10–12 yrs
Canine (cuspid)	9–10 yrs
Lateral incisor	7–8 yrs
Central incisor	6–7 yrs

FIGURE 32.22 Usual sequence of permanent tooth eruption.

about 3 months of age; drooling occurs because the infant does not learn to swallow saliva until several months later. Next, inspect the interior of the mouth. The mouth is the first part of the digestive system, and a pink, moist, intact mucosal lining is indicative of a healthy gastrointestinal tract. In infants, the tongue should lie within the mouth at rest and should be capable of extending over the lower gum line to help the baby feed. The tongue extrusion reflex is normal in infants up until around the age of 6 months and allows the infant to suckle easily from birth. Observe movement of the tongue when the infant or young child babbles or cries. Ask the older child to touch the tongue to the roof of the mouth and then stick out the tongue and move it from side to side (testing cranial nerve XII [hypoglossal]). Full movement should be present and the tongue should be free from lesions or exudate. Visualize the hard and soft palate (which should be intact) or palpate with the gloved finger.

In infants, teeth may begin to erupt anywhere between 3 to 12 months of age. They may erupt one at a time, or have several teeth erupt simultaneously. Toddlers will have 20 teeth by 30 months of age. The infant may drool for several months before teething. During active teething the gums will be swollen at the location of the impending tooth, and parents may report increased fussiness, pain, and sleep disruption. Parents should be discouraged from applying any topical analgesics or

anaesthetics to their baby's gums, as these can anaesthetize the posterior pharynx and uvula and increase the risk of choking or aspiration. In older children, the secondary teeth replace the primary teeth much more slowly and with little discomfort from the 5th to the 20th year. Figure 32.22 shows the usual permanent tooth eruption pattern.

Look for dental caries or alignment problems and inspect the gums for signs of infection. Test cranial nerve IX (glossopharyngeal) by having the child identify taste with the posterior portion of the tongue.

Take Note!

Natal (present at birth) or neonatal (erupting by 30 days of age) teeth should be evaluated by a pediatric dentist for potential extraction, as they may pose an aspiration risk (Bickley, 2013).

INSPECTION OF THE THROAT

Inspect the tonsils, uvula, and oropharynx. Assess the infant's throat during a yawn or cry, as any forcible attempt to depress the tongue with a tongue depressor produces a strong reflex elevation of the base of the tongue that completely blocks the view of the pharynx. The young child will require restraint so that the nurse can depress the tongue and visualize the back of the mouth without injuring the child (Fig. 32.23). Asking the older child to open wide, stick out the tongue,

FIGURE 32.23 The young child may need to be restrained so that the throat examination can be done safely.

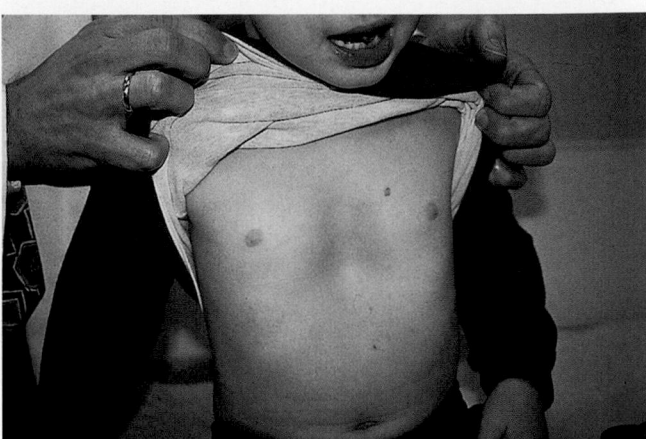

FIGURE 32.25 Pectus excavatum: note depression in xiphoid area.

and say "aaaah" simultaneously will allow for a quick look at the tonsils and pharynx without the need to use a tongue depressor, but the nurse must be very quick because the tongue rises rapidly after those manoeuvres are performed.

Tonsils usually cannot be seen in the infant. As the child becomes a toddler, the tonsils become dramatically larger and then begin to decrease in size again by the ninth year. The tonsils should be pink and may have crypts on their surfaces, which can sometimes be filled with debris or hard plaque-like stones. Ensure that the uvula is midline and rises if the gag reflex is elicited (cranial nerve X [vagus]). Inspect the oropharynx, which should be pink and free from exudate.

Thorax and Lungs

THORAX

Assessment of the thorax and lungs begins by observing the shape and contour of the thorax. Examine the chest with the head in a midline position to determine size and shape as well as symmetry, movement, and bony

landmarks. The newborn's chest should be smooth and round, with the transverse diameter nearly equal to the anterior–posterior diameter. The shape of the chest progresses to that of the adult by the age of 5 to 6 years. At that time the anterior–posterior diameter is about half the transverse diameter (Fig. 32.24). At the point where the xiphoid process and the right and left costal margins meet, the costal angle should measure 90 degrees or less. Inspect for structural deformity such as pectus excavatum (depressed sternum) or pectus carinatum (protuberant sternum) (Fig. 32.25). Note symmetric movement of the chest wall with respiration. Infants and younger children are primarily diaphragmatic breathers, so the abdomen and chest will rise and fall together. Older children, particularly adolescent females, demonstrate thoracic breathing, yet the abdomen and chest should continue to rise and fall together. Asymmetry of chest wall movement is an abnormal finding and should be flagged for further investigation.

Note the child's colour, which should be pink; cyanosis indicates hypoxia. Listen for audible stridor (inspiratory high-pitched sound), expiratory grunting or

A   B

FIGURE 32.24 **A.** The newborn's chest is round. **B.** The adult chest has an anterior–posterior diameter about half the transverse diameter.

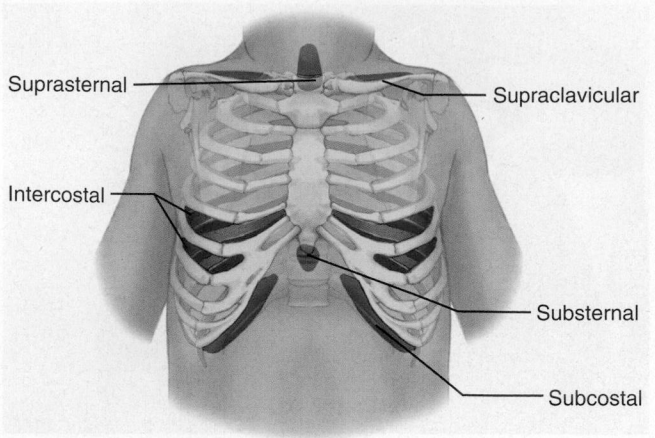

FIGURE 32.26 Location of retractions.

snoring, audible wheezing (heard with the naked ear), or cough. Document type and extent of cough. Observe the nail beds for clubbing, which occurs with diseases inducing chronic hypoxic states.

The nurse should assess the rate and quality of breathing at this stage, before physically touching or approaching the young child, which can trigger crying and make examination difficult. Observe the depth and regularity of respirations, noting the length of the inspiratory and expiratory phases in relation to each other. The newborn and young infant demonstrate an irregular respiratory pattern. Older infants and children should have a more regular respiratory pattern.

Assess the child's respiratory effort by first observing for nasal flaring, which indicates laboured breathing. Observe the chest wall and shoulders for accessory muscle use or heaving, which normally is not present. If retractions are present, note their location and severity. Typical locations for retractions include the intercostal, subcostal, substernal, suprasternal, and clavicular regions (Fig. 32.26). Pay attention to the position the child naturally assumes to breathe comfortably; children in respiratory distress often sit forward and are uncomfortable lying down or talking (Jarvis, 2012).

Observation must include assessment for signs of work of breathing, which may include an elevated respiratory rate, use of accessory chest muscles to ventilate, and any retractions between the intercostal vertebrae, at the trachea, or of the scalene muscles. An infant or young child showing signs of work of breathing must be immediately assessed by a physician or nurse practitioner, and transported to the emergency room setting as soon as possible if the signs suggest severe respiratory distress or failure.

LUNGS

Experienced examiners may palpate and percuss the lungs before using auscultation to evaluate the breath sounds.

Palpation and Percussion. Palpate for symmetric respiratory excursion by placing the thumbs and fingers together along the costal margin on the chest or back. Movement should be symmetric with each breath. Palpate for the normal presence of tactile fremitus with the palms or fingertips while the infant is crying or the older child says "99." Indirectly percuss the lungs of older children, noting resonance over lung fields. Hyperresonance may be present in conditions resulting in hyperaeration of the lungs, such as asthma.

Auscultation. Use the bell of the stethoscope or switch to a small diaphragm to auscultate lung sounds in the infant or child. The adult-sized diaphragm may be used for the adolescent. Auscultate the lung fields with the infant or child in a sitting position, even if that requires propping the infant in a parent's lap. Infants and young children have loud breath sounds because of their thin chest walls. Breath sounds should be clear with adequate aeration throughout all lung fields. Listen to a full inspiration and expiration at the apices of the lungs as well as symmetrically across the entire lung field, systematically comparing the right to the left side. Listen on the anterior chest, on the posterior chest, and in the axillary regions.

Playing games may encourage younger children to cooperate with deep breathing during lung assessment. The child can blow a cotton ball up in the air, blow a pinwheel, or "blow out" the light of the penlight (Miller, n.d.). Older children are capable of deep breathing when instructed to do so.

The child who has a respiratory disorder or who is experiencing respiratory distress may exhibit diminished breath sounds, most often in the lung bases. Diminished breath sounds are softer and quieter than lung sounds associated with adequate aeration. In the healthy infant or child, no adventitious sounds should be heard. If noisy breath sounds are heard in the infant or young child, particularly over all lung fields, compare the sound to the noises heard over the trachea or within the nose. Infants and young children with secretions in the nasopharyngeal area may have those sounds transmitted over the lung fields. These sounds usually clear with coughing or airway suctioning; they are not true adventitious sounds. Note adventitious breath sounds such as wheezes or crackles, documenting their location and whether they are present on inspiration, expiration, or both. It is most important to describe the abnormal breath sounds being heard rather than attempting to classify the sounds. Adventitious lung sounds are associated with a variety of disorders, and extensive experience is required to appropriately classify lung sounds. Adventitious breath sounds should be reported for further evaluation.

Breasts

Assess the breasts of children of all ages and both genders. Note the size of the breasts in relation to the age of the child. Palpate the axillary lymph nodes during the breast assessment.

INSPECTION

Observe the breasts for position, shape, size, symmetry, and colour. Newborns of both genders may have swollen nipples from the influence of maternal estrogen, but by several weeks of age the nipples should be flat and should continue to be so in all prepubertal children. In children the nipples are located lateral to the midclavicular line, usually between the fourth and fifth ribs. The areola becomes darker in colour as the child approaches puberty. Overweight children may appear to have enlarged breasts due to adipose tissue. Note the location of additional (supernumerary) nipples if present (usually located along the mammary ridge); they may appear as darkly pigmented, elevated, or nipple-like spots. These are usually of no concern as they do not change over time, but they may be associated with renal disorders.

Inspect the breasts for the current stage of development: widening of the areola, elevation of the nipple, and increase in breast size. Female breast development may begin as early as age 8, but starts by age 13 in most girls. Breast development then continues in a characteristic, but usually asymmetric, pattern, with one breast larger than the other throughout the lifespan. The sexual maturity rating scale developed by Tanner in 1962 is used to describe breast development (**Tanner stages**; Fig. 32.27). Adolescent boys may develop gynecomastia (enlargement of the breast tissue) due to hormonal

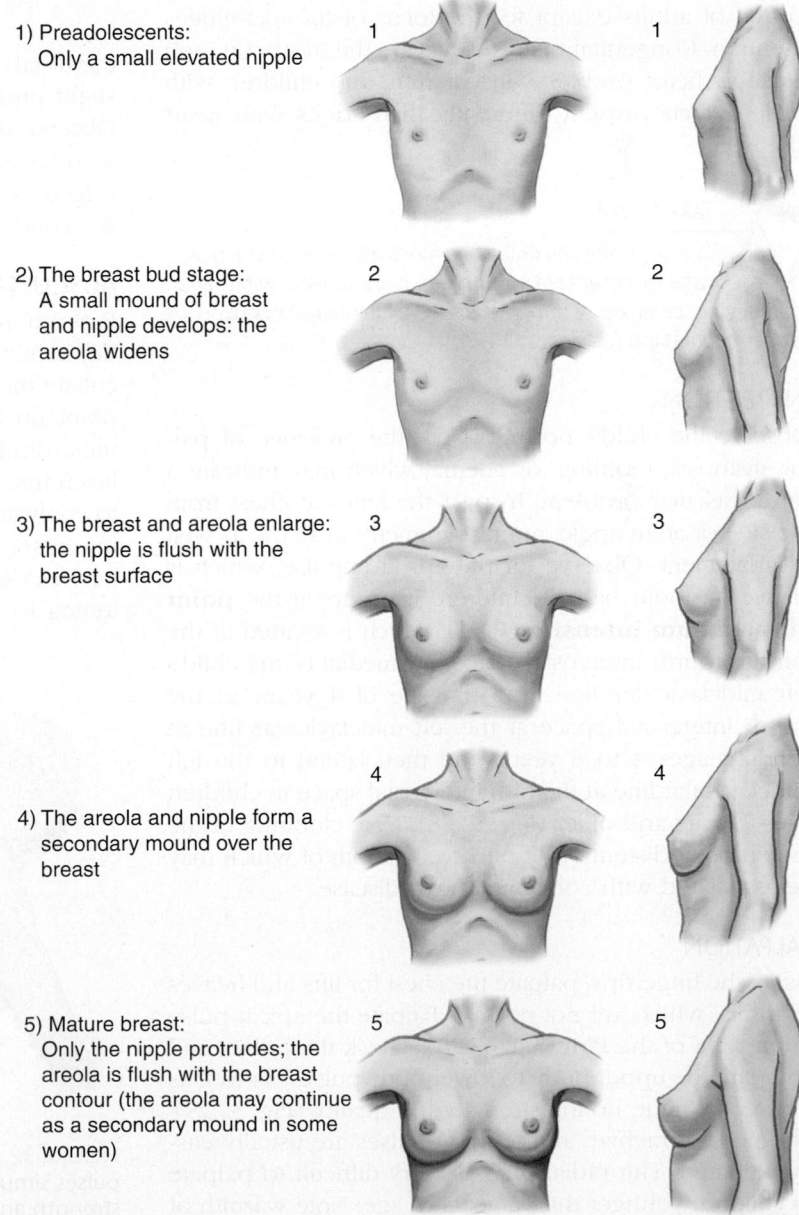

1) Preadolescents:
Only a small elevated nipple

2) The breast bud stage:
A small mound of breast and nipple develops: the areola widens

3) The breast and areola enlarge: the nipple is flush with the breast surface

4) The areola and nipple form a secondary mound over the breast

5) Mature breast:
Only the nipple protrudes; the areola is flush with the breast contour (the areola may continue as a secondary mound in some women)

FIGURE 32.27 Tanner sexual maturity rating for breast development. (Adapted from Tanner, J. M. [1962]. *Growth at adolescence*. Oxford, England: Blackwell Scientific Publications.)

pubertal changes. When the hormone levels stabilize, male adolescents then have flat nipples. Occasionally gynecomastia is caused by marijuana use, anabolic steroids, or hormonal dysfunction (Jarvis, 2012).

PALPATION

Palpate the breasts in a systematic fashion. A tender nodule palpated just under the nipple confirms pubertal changes. This change may be difficult to assess in girls with excessive adipose tissue. Normal breast tissue should feel smooth, firm, and elastic. Note masses or nodules if present. Palpate for axillary lymph nodes with the child's arms relaxed at the side but slightly abducted. Note size, number, and texture of nodes if present.

Heart and Peripheral Perfusion

The examination of the heart in children is identical to that of adults except for the focus of the examiner's attention. Congenital heart defects are the most common cause of heart problems in children, and children with these defects present differently than adults with heart disease.

Take Note!

The younger the child, the more responsive the heart rate is to activity changes. It increases with fever, fear, crying, or anxiety and decreases with sleep, sedation, or vagal stimulation (Jarvis, 2012).

INSPECTION

Observe the child's posture. Note the presence of pallor, cyanosis, mottling, or edema, which may indicate a cardiovascular problem. Inspect the anterior chest from the side or at an angle, noting symmetry in shape as well as movement. Observe for the apical impulse, which is visible in about half of children. It occurs at the **point of maximum intensity (PMI)**, which is located at the third to fourth intercostal space just medial of the child's left midclavicular line until the age of 4 years, at the fourth intercostal space at the left midclavicular line in children ages 4 to 6 years, and then lateral to the left midclavicular line at the fifth intercostal space in children ages 7 years and older (Fig. 32.28). Note clubbing of the fingertips or distention of neck veins, both of which may be associated with congenital heart disease.

PALPATION

Using the fingertips, palpate the chest for lifts and heaves or thrills, which are not normal. Palpate the apical pulse in the area of the PMI (Fig. 32.28). Check the pulses and compare the upper body to lower body pulses, as well as left versus right, noting strength and quality (Fig. 32.29). The pedal, brachial, and femoral pulses are usually easily palpated. The radial pulse is very difficult to palpate in children younger than 2 years of age. Note warmth of

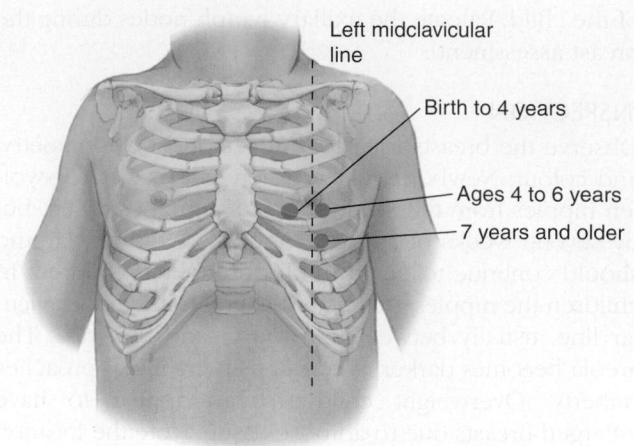

FIGURE 32.28 The point of maximum intensity (PMI) or apical impulse.

the distal extremities. To assess capillary refill time, place slight pressure on the nail beds and quickly release it. Observe the length of time required for refill and return to original colour. Compare capillary refill time of the fingers to the toes. A capillary refill time of less than 3 seconds indicates adequacy of perfusion.

AUSCULTATION

Perform auscultation of the heart with the child in two different positions, upright and reclined (Fig. 32.30). Auscultate the heart rate in the area of the PMI as this is the point on the chest wall where the heartbeat is heard most distinctly (Fig. 32.28). As you begin auscultation, listen first for respirations and note their timing so as not to confuse the heart sounds with the lung sounds. A crying infant may help by briefly holding his or her breath between cries. Once you are confident that you are listening to the heart, be sure to listen for 1 full minute

FIGURE 32.29 It is important to assess brachial and femoral pulses simultaneously to determine equality or differences in strength and intensity.

FIGURE 32.30 Auscultating the child's heart.

because of the irregularity of rhythms in some children. Count the heart rate, which should be consistent with the palpated pulse (either radial or brachial, depending on the child's age).

Develop a systematic approach to auscultation of the heart. Listen over all four valvular areas anteriorly (Fig. 32.31). In the infant or younger child, also auscultate the heart in the axillary region and posteriorly (certain murmurs radiate to these areas). Note S_1, S_2, extra heart sounds, or murmurs. S_1 is usually loudest at the mitral and tricuspid areas and increases in intensity with fever, exercise, and anemia. S_2 is usually most intense at the aortic and pulmonic areas. A split S_2 heard at the apex occurs in many infants and young children. S_3 may

be heard in many healthy children and is considered normal, though the child with a chronic cardiac condition may develop an S_3 when congestive heart failure is present. S_4 is usually considered abnormal, most often occurring with cardiac disease.

Sinus arrhythmia is a common and normal finding in children and adolescents. It results in an irregular heart rhythm: the heart rate increases with inhalation and decreases with exhalation. If the child holds his or her breath, the rhythm becomes regular.

Auscultate for murmurs. Note the location (where it is heard best or loudest) and timing of the murmur. A systolic murmur occurs in association with S_1 (closure of the atrioventricular valves), a diastolic murmur in association with S_2 (closure of the semilunar valves). Also note the duration of murmur. Does it occur early or late in diastole or systole? Does it occur all the way across systole (holosystolic, beginning at S_1 and continuing until S_2). Note the intensity of the murmur. Table 32.5 discusses grading of murmur intensity.

Innocent murmurs occur frequently in children because of the child's more dynamic circulation, thin chest wall, and angulated vessels (Darst, Collins, & Miyamoto, 2014). Innocent murmurs are also called functional murmurs or "Still's murmur." They are most common in children 3 to 8 years of age. They can spontaneously appear during period of increased blood flow such as during a febrile illness or with strenuous exercise. They are benign in nature, and do not reflect an underlying cardiac anomaly or condition. An innocent murmur is most often heard at the second or fourth intercostal space, and its timing is systolic. The innocent murmur is usually medium pitched and musical. Often

FIGURE 32.31 Areas where the sounds of heart valves radiate. A: Aortic valve—second intercostal space, just right of sternum. P: Pulmonic valve—second intercostal space, just left of sternum. T: Tricuspid valve—fourth intercostal space, just left of sternum. M: Mitral valve—fourth intercostal space at left midclavicular line.

TABLE 32.5	GRADING HEART MURMURS IN CHILDREN
Grade	Sound
1	Barely audible; sometimes heard, sometimes not. Usually heard only with intense concentration
2	Quiet, soft; heard each time the chest is auscultated
3	Audible, intermediate intensity
4	Audible, with a palpable thrill
5	Loud, audible with edge of the stethoscope lifted off the chest
6	Very loud, audible with the stethoscope placed near but not touching the chest

Adapted from Darst, J. R., Collins, K. K., & Miyamoto, S. D. (2014). Cardiovascular diseases. In W. W. Hay, Jr., M. J. Levin, R. R. Deterding, & M. J. Abzug (Eds.). *Current diagnosis and treatment: paediatrics* (22nd ed.). New York: McGraw-Hill.

an innocent murmur disappears when the child changes position. A venous hum that is heard in the supraclavicular area and possibly radiating down the chest is considered an innocent murmur. Refer any child with a murmur to an experienced practitioner for further evaluation.

Abdomen

The abdomen contains organs related to the genitourinary and lymphatic systems, in addition to the gastrointestinal system. These structures lie within the abdomen in approximately the same location as they do in adults. Dividing the abdomen into quadrants simplifies the description of normal organ location and the reporting of abnormalities. Draw an imaginary vertical line from the xiphoid process to the symphysis pubis. Cross this with an imaginary perpendicular line through the umbilicus. The sequence of physical examination is altered for the abdominal assessment: auscultation is done before percussion and palpation because manipulation of the lower abdomen may affect the bowel sounds (Bickley, 2013).

INSPECTION

Inspect the abdomen for size, shape, and symmetry. The abdomen in the infant and toddler is rounded and protuberant until the abdominal musculature becomes well developed. Though rounded, the abdomen should not be distended (at any age). By adolescence, the stature is more erect and the abdomen begins to appear flat when standing and concave when supine. The thin skin of a young child may allow the visualization of superficial venous circulation across the abdomen. Inspect the abdomen for movement. At eye level with the abdomen, note abdomen and thorax movement occurring simultaneously. Visible peristaltic waves are abnormal and should be reported immediately.

Inspect the newborn's umbilicus for colour, bleeding, odour, and drainage. The umbilical stump should slowly dry, become black and hard, and fall away from the cutaneous navel by the end of the second week of life. Note persistent drainage or granulation at the umbilical site indicating delayed drying of the umbilical stump. Report foul smelling drainage, inflammation, and signs of infection promptly, as this requires immediate assessment and intervention with antibiotics to avoid possible sepsis. Inspect the umbilicus in older infants and young children for the presence of umbilical hernia. Because the umbilicus divides the rectus abdominis muscle, it is not uncommon to see an umbilical hernia protrude through and become larger when the infant or toddler strains or cries. This is a benign finding and will usually disappear as the abdomen becomes stronger, generally around 3 to 4 years of age. The hernia is painless, and should be easily reducible back into

the abdominal cavity. If this cannot be done, the herniated tissues will have impaired blood flow, which is an emergency situation that requires immediate surgical intervention. Adolescents may have jewellery piercing the umbilicus.

AUSCULTATION

Auscultate the abdomen using the diaphragm or the bell of the stethoscope pressed firmly against the abdomen. Count the bowel sounds in each of the four quadrants for a full minute. Bowel sounds should be present by a few hours after birth and should remain active throughout life. Note whether bowel sounds are normally active, hyperactive, hypoactive, or absent. Normal bowel sounds can be described as growls, gurgles, and clicking sounds. Hypoactive bowel sounds may occur postoperatively. Hyperactive bowels sounds are common with diarrhoea. Classify bowel sounds as absent after listening for 5 full minutes in each area. Absent bowel sounds may indicate ileus or peritonitis.

PERCUSSION

Indirectly percuss all areas of the abdomen. Normal findings include dullness along the costal margins and tympany over the remainder of the abdomen. A full bladder may yield dullness to percussion.

PALPATION

Palpate the abdomen with the child in a supine position. If the child's legs are small enough, the knees may be brought up with the nondominant hand to flex the hips and relax the abdomen. Palpate all four quadrants of the abdomen in a systematic fashion, first lightly and then deeply. Apply light pressure with the fingertips to perform light palpation, assessing for tenderness and muscle tone (Fig. 32.32). Note skin turgor by gently elevating a piece of skin and allowing it to fall back into place. Perform deep palpation to assess the organs and any masses. Place one hand on top of the other and palpate from the lower quadrants to the upper (Fig. 32.32). The edge of the liver may be felt at the right costal margin, and the tip of the spleen can be felt at the left costal margin. The descending colon may be felt in the left lower quadrant as a small column and the bladder as a soft balloon below the umbilicus. The kidneys are rarely palpable. The abdomen should be soft and nontender to palpation. Report firmness, tenderness, distention, or masses. Palpate the inguinal area for the presence of hernia or enlarged lymph nodes.

Take Note!

To decrease ticklishness with abdominal palpation, place a flat, warm, still hand on the abdomen while distracting the child before palpation begins. An alternate technique is to first palpate with the child's hand over the examiner's hand.

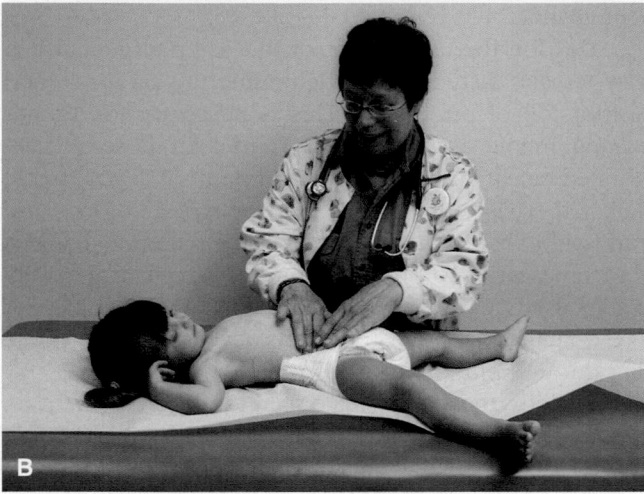

FIGURE 32.32 Light (**A**) and (**B**) deep palpation of the abdomen.

Genitalia and Anus

Examination of the genitals should immediately follow the abdominal assessment in the younger child and should be reserved for the end of the assessment in the adolescent. Though the anus is part of the gastrointestinal tract, it is best assessed during the genital examination. A parent should chaperone the genitalia and anus examination of the infant and child. In the case of the adolescent, a medical provider chaperone is recommended. Use of a chaperone should be recorded in nursing notes.

Ensure privacy for the older child and adolescent. Keep the child covered as much as possible. Use a casual, matter-of-fact approach to place the child or teen at ease. During the genital examination, teach the child or adolescent about normal variations and changes with puberty, as well as issues related to health promotion.

MALE

Inspect the penis and scrotum for size, colour, skin integrity, and obvious masses. The obese boy's penis may appear short because of additional fat pads at the pubis.

From top to bottom:

1) No pubic hair and scrotum size and proportion the same as during childhood

2) Few straight hairs at base of penis, little or no penis enlargement, testes/scrotum begin to enlarge

3) Sparse pubic hair growth over entire pubis, penis begins to lengthen, scrotum continues to enlarge

4) Thick pubic hair growth but not on thighs, penis grows in length and diameter, testes almost full grown

5) Pubic hair growth spread over medial thighs, penis and scrotum are adult size and shape

FIGURE 32.33 Tanner male sexual maturity rating for genitalia and pubic hair. (Adapted from Tanner, J. M. [1962]. *Growth at adolescence.* Oxford, England: Blackwell Scientific Publications.)

Penis size should correlate with pubertal stage (Fig. 32.33). The penis may have a foreskin that covers the glans, protecting and lubricating it. If present, never forcibly retract the foreskin. The foreskin typically retracts fully in older children (never in infants); note any scarring, lesions, or lichen sclerosis. In circumcised males, the urinary meatus is exposed and should be at the tip of the glans. Assess the meatus for absence of discharge. If possible, observe the stream of urine for strength of flow and patency of the urethral orifice. Skin lesions may indicate sexually transmitted infection. Report abnormal findings.

> ### Take Note!
> When you first remove a male infant's diaper, this is the ideal time to assess the force of the urine stream and the erection reflex, as the cool air may make the infant void and briefly experience an erection.

Assess the presence and distribution of pubic hair. Inspect the scrotum for size, slight asymmetry, colour, and absence of edema. The scrotum may initially be swollen from birth trauma or maternal hormones, but this swelling should decrease in the first few days of life. The scrotum is ordinarily more deeply pigmented than the rest of the boy's skin. Figure 32.33 illustrates scrotal changes that occur with puberty. Assess the testicles by placing one finger over the inguinal canal and palpating the scrotum with the other. This prevents the retractile testes in a young child from slipping back up the inguinal canal. The testicles should be smooth, of similar sizes, and freely moveable without any noted tenderness. The infant's testicles may be palpated in the scrotum or in the inguinal canal, where they can be easily moved into the scrotum with gentle pressure from the examiner's nondominant hand, called "milking" (Fig. 32.34). Beyond infancy, allow the boy to sit cross-legged to reduce the cremasteric reflex that retracts the testicles during palpation. An adolescent boy may need to stand for the nurse to fully palpate the scrotum. Document the presence of both testicles in the scrotal sac, if they are retractile, or if they are absent. If unable to locate and palpate the testes, promptly refer the child to another provider to repeat the assessment. Report an undescended testicle or testes or other abnormal findings.

FIGURE 32.34 Placing a digit over the inguinal canal during testicular palpation prevents retraction of the testis into the canal.

FEMALE

In most cases, the female genitalia examination is limited to assessment of the external genitalia. Internal examination is not routinely performed before maturity unless a pathology is suspected because of abnormal symptoms reported by the patient. If an internal examination is needed, refer the child or adolescent to the appropriate physician or nurse practitioner.

Position the infant in the parent's lap or on the examination table or crib. The toddler or preschooler should be examined in the parent's lap, in a frog-legged position. The school-aged or adolescent girl should lie on the examination table or bed. Provide for privacy by keeping the genital area covered until it is time for the examination.

Perform the assessment of the external genitalia in a systematic fashion. First, determine the presence and distribution of pubic hair. This is necessary for Tanner staging. Infants and young girls (particular those of dark-skinned races) may have a small amount of downy pubic hair. Otherwise, the appearance of typical coarse and curly pubic hair indicates the onset of pubertal changes, sometimes prior to breast changes. Pubic hair generally begins to appear by age 11 years, with age 13 being the latest. Figure 32.35 illustrates the development of pubic hair through puberty in girls.

Inspect the labia majora and minora for size, colour, and skin integrity. The newborn's labia minora are swollen from the effects of maternal estrogen but will decrease in size and be hidden by the labia majora within the first weeks of life. Redness or swelling of the labia may occur with infection, sexual abuse, or masturbation. Lesions on the external genitalia may indicate sexually transmitted infection. Gently spread the labia to inspect the clitoris, urethral meatus, and vaginal opening. Labial adhesions can occur in younger children and do not routinely need treatment unless problematic with vulvar soreness or dribbling urine. These should resolve in childhood. Some girls may prefer to spread the labia themselves. The urinary meatus and vaginal orifice should be visible and not occluded by the hymen. It is not uncommon to see a hymenal tag. Tears to the hymen should be noted and in cases of suspected sexual abuse follow duty to report as informed by local policy. Note any areas of lichen sclerosis in younger children who have a history of vulvar itching. Inspect the urinary meatus and vaginal opening for edema or redness, which should not be present. A small amount of blood-tinged or mucoid discharge may be noted in the first few weeks of life as a result of maternal hormone exposure. A small amount of clear mucous-like discharge is normal in all females. Discharge that is yellow/green or blood tinged, frothy or curdy, or accompanied by redness or excoriation of the vulva, are all considered abnormal findings and should be reported for further assessment.

Stage 1 Preadolescents. No pubic hair. Mons and labia covered with fine vellus hair as on abdomen.

Stage 2 Growth sparse and mostly on labia. Long, downy hair, slightly pigmented, straight or only slightly curly.

Stage 3 Growth sparse and spreading over mons pubis. Hair darker, coarser, curlier.

Stage 4 Hair is adult in type but over smaller area; none on medial thigh.

Stage 5 Adult in type and pattern; inverse triangle. Also on medial thigh surface.

FIGURE 32.35 Tanner female sexual maturity rating for pubic hair. (Adapted from Tanner, J. M. [1962]. *Growth at adolescence.* Oxford, England: Blackwell Scientific Publications.)

ANUS

Inspect the anal area for fissures, rash, prolapse, or skin tags. Examine the infant's anal area while examining the genitalia. The younger child may lie back in the parent's lap and flex the knees to the chest. The older child or adolescent may be prone or in a side-lying position. If the adolescent boy is already standing for the scrotal assessment, have him bend forward so that you can assess the anal area. The anus should appear moist and hairless and have tone. If it is relaxed and open refer for assessment to the physician or nurse practitioner.

Musculoskeletal

Assessment of the musculoskeletal system includes examination of the clavicles and shoulders, neck and spine, extremities, joints, and hips (CPS, 2014b). Determining the child's ability to move all extremities through the full range of motion is essential.

CLAVICLES AND SHOULDERS

Palpate the clavicles. In the newborn, tenderness or crepitus reveals a fracture sustained at birth. In the older infant or child, a bump indicates callus formation secondary to clavicle fracture. Test shoulder strength and the function of cranial nerve XI in the older child by requesting that the child shrug the shoulders while you apply downward pressure.

NECK AND SPINE

Observe the child's resting posture and alignment of the trunk. The newborn's position will look like the position the baby preferred in utero and is one of general flexion. The older infant moves more and can sit unassisted in the second half of the first year. Toddlers stand with a wide-based gait, a slightly swayed back, and the abdomen slightly protruding. The posture straightens in the preschool- and school-age years. Adolescents often demonstrate kyphosis as the skeleton and muscles are both growing rapidly (Fig. 32.36).

Inspect the child's spine. The newborn's spine has a single C-shaped curve and remains rounded for the first 3 months of life. The cervical curve begins to develop around 3 to 4 months of age as the baby gains head control. By 12 to 18 months of age, the lumbar curve develops, which corresponds to the onset of walking. The S-shaped spine in older children and adolescents is similar to that of the adult's. Inspect the newborn's spinal

FIGURE 32.36 The teen's posture often demonstrates kyphosis.

column for any discoloration, tufts of hair, or dimples. A pilonidal dimple is commonly seen at the base of the spine, but there should be no hair tufts, midline moles, or nevi along the spine. Should any of these be noted, the infant needs to be promptly assessed by a physician or nurse practitioner for further investigation for potential spinal cord malformation.

The spine should be flexible, with good muscle tone and no rigidity. Assess the back, and hip and shoulder heights for symmetry in the standing child. Examine the preadolescent and adolescent for the development of scoliosis. Scoliosis screening is generally performed during well-child examinations by the physician or nurse practitioner.

Note mobility of the vertebral column by having the child bend forward and side to side. Flex the neck and move it from side to side. No resistance or pain should occur.

JOINTS AND HIPS

Hip assessment for identification of developmental hip dysplasia should take place at every routine health maintenance visit for all Canadian infants up until the age of at least 12 months, or when the child can walk (Canadian Paediatric Society, 2014b; Rourke, Leduc, & Rourke, 2014). This is done by performing the Ortolani–Barlow test which is a manoeuver best performed by a proficient examiner. The hip assessment of the walking child and adolescent includes inspection and palpation for symmetry, strength, and range of motion. In the standing position, hip height should be symmetrical between sides, and there should be no redness, warmth, or tenderness noted. The older preschooler should be able to easily stand on one foot without dropping either hip. Observe the child squat down and then stand back up, taking note if the child needs to push up against the thighs to return to the upright position. This is an abnormal finding that reflects weakness in the hips and core, which should be reported for further evaluation.

EXTREMITIES

All children, even newborns, should be able to move all extremities spontaneously. Examination of the extremities includes inspection of size, symmetry, colour, and contour. This should be followed by palpation of upper and lower extremities for temperature, muscle tone, power, and range of motion. The infant's feet and legs appear bowed secondary to in utero positioning but can be straightened through passive range of motion. Observe the child in a standing position. Bowing of the lower legs (internal tibial torsion) lessens as the toddler begins to bear weight and usually resolves in the second or third year of life as the strength of the muscles and bones increases. When it persists past that time, it is termed genu varum (bowlegs). Genu valgum (knock knee) usually resolves around 7 years of age or beyond.

It is important to note that both of these are benign and developmentally normal features of gait progression in children. The nurse should provide ample reassurance to parents who articulate worries about the appearance of their young child's in-toeing or out-toeing position or gait. For the majority of children, all of these benign "deformities" will resolve spontaneously and not require any intervention. However, should a parent report any frequent tripping, clumsiness, or difficulty maintaining balance with running, the nurse should promptly refer this child for detailed assessment with their nurse practitioner or physician. If there is functional impairment, occasionally these may represent significant deformities that require surgical intervention or subspecialty management.

Observe the child walking, noting any asymmetry in strength, tone, or positioning of each limb between sides. Document any balance or coordination difficulties with walking, running, or squatting down to the ground, based on the child's age and developmental ability. Note the normal flat foot in the toddler and young child. The arch develops as the child grows, and the muscles and connective tissues become stronger and more well developed as the child's mobility progresses. Some children, however, may continue with flexible flat feet, which is considered a normal variation.

Perform passive range of motion of the young infant's extremities. Observe for any fixed extension of the foot and rigidity with flexion, as this indicates club-foot which is a congenital anomaly that requires immediate correction to allow achievement of normal gait and stance. Count the fingers and toes, noting abnormalities such as polydactyly (increased number of digits) or syndactyly (webbing of the digits). Palpate the infant's joints for warmth or tenderness, or crepitus. Check the mobility of the joints of the upper and lower extremities by performing passive range of motion through flexion, extension, adduction, abduction, and rotation. The nurse should note any asymmetry between sides or differences in the "end feel" of each movement.

Neurologic

The neurologic examination of the child should include level of consciousness, balance and coordination, sensory function, and reflexes. A developmental screening can be performed after completion of the neurologic assessment. Motor function is assessed within the musculoskeletal section. Cranial nerve function is generally tested within other portions of the physical assessment as it applies to that section.

LEVEL OF CONSCIOUSNESS

Note the general state of alertness and attentiveness to parents and the environment in the newborn and infant. Document if the infant is asleep, awake and alert, or alert and crying or distressed. Older infants become socially interactive as do toddlers and preschoolers. Younger children demonstrate healthy orientation and attachment to their caregivers by crying or fussing when they are separated from the parent, and conversely are easily comforted when returned to them. By school age, the child should be oriented to name and place and a few years later should be able to state the date as well (even if only the day of the week).

BALANCE AND COORDINATION

The cerebellum is involved in balance and coordination. Observe the child's gait while walking and running, noting any asymmetry, tripping, or clumsiness. Observe toddlers and older children rising and walking from a seated and supine position. They should be able to stand and balance without straining or holding on to objects. Continue to test cerebellar function by having the younger child skip or hop and requesting that the older child or adolescent walk heel to toe with one foot placed in front of the other "like walking on a tightrope." Further tests of cerebellar function responsible for balance and coordination are discussed in Box 32.3. Demonstrate each test and make sure the child understands your instructions.

BOX 32.3

CEREBELLAR FUNCTION TESTING

- Balance: Observe the child while standing. Look for any swaying from side to side. Note: this is NOT the Romberg test.

For the following tests, the child should demonstrate accuracy and smoothness:
- **Heel-to-shin:** Have the child lie in a supine position, place one heel on the opposite knee, and run it down the shin. Note any wobbling of the heel from side to side.
- **Rapid alternating movements:** The child pronates and supinates each hand quickly while patting the thighs with the hands. An alternate test is for the child to touch their thumb to each finger of the same hand starting at the index finger, then reverse the direction and repeat.
- **Finger-to-nose test:** The child's eyes are open. Ask child to alternate touching the examiner's finger with the index finger, and then touch his or her own nose. The examiner moves the finger to a different spot and the child repeats this process several times. Note any tremoring or overshooting where the child persistently reaches past the target.
- **Finger-to-nose:** The child's eyes are closed. The child stretches the arm with the index finger extended, then touches his or her nose with that finger, keeping the eyes closed.

Adapted from Bickley, L. (2013). *Bates' guide to physical examination and history taking* (11th ed.). Philadelphia, PA: Lippincott Williams & Wilkins; Jarvis, C. (2012). *Physical examination and health assessment* (6th ed.). St. Louis, MO: Saunders.

SENSORY TESTING

Portions of sensory testing related to most of the cranial nerves, vision, hearing, taste, and smell have already been incorporated into other sections as appropriate within the physical assessment. Take note that the sensory examination in young children (under the age of 5 to 6 years) is fairly imprecise and only gross neurologic deficits can be detected. Test cranial nerve V (trigeminal) by lightly touching the child's cheek with a cotton ball. The young infant will root toward the side that is touched. With the child's eyes closed, ask the child to identify other locations where he or she is lightly touched (several different ones) to assess sensation. Ask the child to tell you when he or she is touched. Make a game of this activity to encourage cooperation in younger children. Use the rounded end of a tongue blade for dull and the broken edge of a tongue blade for the sharp sensation. Do NOT use pinprick with children. In the older, school-aged child who knows the definition of sharp and dull, test for these sensations with the child's eyes closed. The child should be able to discriminate the sensations of sharp and dull.

REFLEXES

Assess the infant's primitive and protective reflexes. The primitive reflexes involve a whole-body response and are subcortical in origin. The primitive reflexes present at birth include Moro or "startle," root, suck, asymmetric tonic neck, plantar and palmar grasp, step, and Babinski. The primitive reflexes gradually disappear over the first few months of life, giving way to protective or postural reflexes. Protective reflexes are motor responses related to maintenance of equilibrium. They are necessary for appropriate motor development such as sitting, crawling, and walking and remain throughout life once they are established. The protective reflexes include the righting and parachute reactions.

Place one finger in each of the infant's hands to elicit the palmar grasp reflex (usually disappears by the age of 3 to 5 months). Touch the thumb to the ball of the infant's foot to elicit the plantar grasp reflex. The infant's toes will curl down (this reflex disappears by the age of 6 to 9 months). Refer to Table 25.1 for illustrations and additional explanation of the other reflexes. Appropriate presence and disappearance of primitive reflexes, as well as development of protective reflexes, is indicative of a healthy neurologic system. Primitive reflexes that persist beyond the usual age of disappearance may indicate an abnormality of the neurologic system and should be further investigated (Bickley, 2013).

Assess deep tendon reflexes in all infants and children. Appropriate responses indicate that the reflex arc is intact. Use the reflex hammer in all ages or the curved tips of the two first fingers to elicit the responses in infants. The limb must be relaxed and the muscle partly stretched. Use a snapping motion of the wrist to tap with the fingertips or the reflex hammer. Test the biceps, triceps, patellar, and Achilles reflexes as you would in the adult. It may help to place a finger under the infant's knee to encourage relaxation. Young children who tense up when their reflexes are being tested may relax the area if you have them focus on another area, so have the child clasp the hands while testing the Achilles and patellar reflexes. As the child focuses on the hands, the lower extremities relax (Jarvis, 2012). Distraction may also be helpful.

Grade the strength of the response using the standard scale from 0 to 4+:

- 0: no response
- 1+: diminished or sluggish
- 2+: average or *normal*
- 3+: brisker than average
- 4+: very brisk, may involve clonus

The newborn's deep tendon reflexes are normally brisk (3+). They decrease to average (2+) usually by 4 months of age. Healthy children should have reflexes of 2+ if the reflex has been elicited properly. Absent, sluggish, or hyperreactive responses usually indicate disease (Bickley, 2013).

DEVELOPMENTAL SCREENING

An important component of the neurologic assessment and following concerns or risks noted at developmental surveillance or checks is developmental screening. Developmental screening is used to focus assessment in children whose developmental status is delayed or if the child has increased risk of delay, for example prematurity. Developmental screening is often performed separately from the physical examination.

> **Refer back to Elliot, the 3 year old from the beginning of the chapter. What are some important considerations when performing his physical examination?**

KEY CONCEPTS

- The health history in children includes more than just the chief complaint, history of present illness, and past medical history; it is important to include the perinatal history and developmental milestones.

- Allow the chief complaint to determine which parts of the history and review of systems require a more detailed investigation.

- The developmental history and screening will consume a greater proportion of the health visit in the younger child, while school performance and adjustment will be more important in the school-aged child and adolescent.

- Though the parent will provide most of the health history for the infant and young child, allow the young verbal child to answer questions during the health history as appropriate.

- Direct health history questions to the school-aged child and adolescent, seeking clarification from the parents as needed.

- Provide confidentiality and privacy for the adolescent during the health history.

- Weight and length or height should be assessed at each well-child visit to determine adequacy of growth.

- Measure head circumference until age 2 years to monitor brain growth.

- Measure blood pressure in all children 3 years and older.

- Perform hearing and vision screenings for children of all ages.

- BMI can be used to identify children who are overweight or at risk for being overweight.

- The normal range of vital signs varies based on the child's age.

- The sequence of the physical examination in children should be based on the child's developmental age, his or her level of cooperation, and the severity of the illness.

- Obtain heart rate and respiratory rate and auscultate the heart and lungs while the infant or young child is quiet.

- Perform intrusive procedures such as examination of the ears, mouth, and throat last in the infant or young child.

- Perform the health assessment in a head-to-toe fashion in the school-aged child or adolescent, reserving the genitalia and anus examination for last.

- Plan the health assessment in such a way as to minimize trauma to the child or adolescent.

- Use age-appropriate measurement tools to assess pain in children.

- Allow the infant or young child to remain in the parent's lap for as much of the assessment as possible so that the child feels secure.

- Use age-appropriate games during the health assessment to gain cooperation in the younger child.

- Having the young boy sit cross-legged for a testicular examination may reduce the cremasteric reflex.

- The newborn may exhibit a wide variety of normal skin variations. Document all variations carefully to establish a baseline.

- The infant's fontanels should be soft and flat; report a bulging fontanel immediately, as this is a health emergency.

- Jaundice (outside of the newborn period), pallor, cyanosis, and poor skin turgor indicate illness and may need immediate intervention.

- Heart murmurs should be assessed for intensity, location, and duration. They may be innocent or may indicate a congenital heart defect.

- The infant's chest wall is relatively thin, allowing upper airway sounds to be transmitted throughout the lung fields.

- Any retractions of the chest wall in the subcostal, intercostal, suprasternal, supraclavicular, trachea, or scalene regions indicate that the child is labouring to breathe. Prominent retractions of more than one muscle group indicate significant distress. A fixed, depressed sternum (pectus excavatum) is a structural abnormality.

- The Tanner stages of sexual maturity provide a basis for assessing pubertal development in boys and girls. Use the breast and pubic hair charts for girls and the pubic hair and penis and scrotum size chart for boys.

REFERENCES AND RECOMMENDED READINGS

Albert, N. M., Burke, J., Bena, J. F., Morrison, S. M., Forney, J., & Krajewski, S. (2013). Nurses' uniform colour and feelings/emotions in school-aged children receiving health care. *Journal of Paediatric Nursing, 28*(2), 141–149.

American Academy of Pediatrics. (2011). Use of chaperones during the physical examination of the paediatric patient. *Pediatrics, 127*(5), 991–993.

Asher, C., & Northington, L. K. (2008). Position statement for measurement of temperature/fever in children. *Journal of Paediatric Nursing, 23*(3), 234–236.

Bickley, L. (2013). *Bates' guide to physical examination and history taking* (11th ed.). Philadelphia, PA: Lippincott Williams & Wilkins.

Bowden, V. R., & Greenberg, C. S. (2012). *Paediatric nursing procedures* (3rd ed.). Philadelphia, PA: Lippincott Williams & Wilkins.

Burns, C. E., Dunn, A. M., Brady, M. A., Starr, N. B., & Blosser, C. G. (2013). *Paediatric primary care* (5th ed.). Philadelphia, PA: Saunders.

Canadian Paediatric Society. (2014a). *Caring for kids new to Canada.* Retrieved from http://www.kidsnewtocanada.ca/screening/lead#screening

Canadian Paediatric Society. (2014b). *Guidelines hip screening.* Retrieved from https://www.cps.ca/en/tools-outils/rourke-baby-record

Canadian Paediatric Society. (2014c). *WHO growth charts.* Retrieved from http://www.cps.ca/tools-outils/who-growth-charts

Canadian Task Force on Preventive Health Care. (2016). *Recommendations on screening for developmental delay.* Retrieved from https://canadiantaskforce.ca/guidelines/published-guidelines/developmental-delay/

Centers for Disease Control and Prevention. (2010). *CDC growth charts.* Retrieved from http://www.cdc.gov/growth-charts/cdc_charts.htm

Centers for Disease Control and Prevention. (2015a). *Body mass index (BMI).* Retrieved from http://www.cdc.gov/healthyweight/assessing/bmi/index.html

Centers for Disease Control and Prevention. (2015b). *WHO growth chart training: Using the WHO growth charts to assess growth in the United States among children ages birth to 2 years.* Retrieved from http://www.cdc.gov/nccdphp/dnpao/growthcharts/who/index.htm

Centers for Disease Control and Prevention. (2016). *Lead.* Retrieved from http://www.cdc.gov/nceh/lead/

Columbia University, College of Physicians and Surgeons. (n.d.). *Points on the pediatric physical exam.* Retrieved from http://www.columbia.edu/itc/hs/medical/clerkships/peds/Student_Information/Reference_Materials/Pediatric_PE.html

Covidien. (2012). *Covidien operator's manual: Nellcor™ bedside spO2 patient monitoring system.* Mansfield, MA: Author.

Darst, J. R., Collins, K. K., & Miyamoto, S. D. (2014). Cardiovascular diseases. In W. W. Hay, Jr., M. J. Levin, R. R. Deterding, & M. J. Abzug (Eds.). *Current diagnosis and treatment: paediatrics* (22nd ed.). New York: McGraw-Hill.

Dieticians of Canada. (2014). *WHO growth charts.* Retrieved from https://www.dietitians.ca/Learn/Distance-Learning/Online-Courses/WHO-Growth-Chart-Training.aspx

El Radhi, A. S. (2014). Determining fever in children: The search for an ideal thermometer. *British Journal of Nursing, 23*(2), 91–94.

Exergen Corporation. (2014). Exergen temporal artery thermometer: instructions for use. Retrieved from http://www.exergen.com//medical/PDFs/tat2000c%20manual%20818621r5%20artwork.pdf

Gillespie, G. L., Gates, D. M., & Berry, P. (2013). Stressful incidents of physical violence against emergency nurses. *The Online Journal of Issues in Nursing, 18*(1), 2.

Graversen, L., Sørensen, T. I., Petersen, L., Sovio, U., Kaakinen, M., Sandbaek, A., . . . Obel, C. (2014). Preschool weight and body mass index in relation to central obesity and metabolic syndrome in adulthood. *PLoS One, 9*(3), 1–9.

Harris, K. C., Benoit, G., Dionne, J., Feber, J., Cloutier, L., Zarnke, K. B., . . . Fournier, A. (2016). *Canadian Hypertension Education Program guidelines for blood pressure measurement, diagnosis, and assessment of risk of pediatric hypertension.* Retrieved from http://www.onlinecjc.ca/article/S0828-282X(16)00221-X/pdf

International Cupping Therapy Association. (2010). A word on Cupping marks. Retrieved from https://www.cupping-therapy.org/pages/discolorations.htm

Jarvis, C. (2012). *Physical examination and health assessment* (6th ed.). St. Louis, MO: Saunders.

The Joint Commission. (2014). *Advancing effective communication, cultural competence, and patient- and family-centred care.* Retrieved from http://www.jointcommission.org/Advancing_Effective_Communication/

Kliegman, R. M., Stanton, B. F., St. Geme III, J. W., Schor, N. F., & Behrman, R. E. (Eds.). (2011). *Nelson textbook of pediatrics* (19th ed.). Philadelphia, PA: Saunders.

Levy, N., Sturgess, J., & Mills, P. (2018). *"Pain as the fifth vital sign" and dependence on the "numerical pain scale" is being abandoned in the US: Why?.* Retrieved from http://bjanaesthesia.org/article/S0007-0912(17)54182-3/fulltext

Manworren, R., & Hynan, L. (2003). Clinical validation of FLACC: Preverbal patient pain scale. *Paediatric Nursing, 29*(2), 140–146.

Marx, J., Hockberger, R., & Walls, R. (2014). *Rosen's emergency medicine—concepts and clinical practice* (8th ed.). Philadelphia, PA: Saunders.

Miller, S. (n.d.). *Paediatric physical exam video.* Retrieved from http://www.columbia.edu/itc/hs/medical/clerkships/peds/Student_Information/Reference_Materials/PE_Video.html

Nettina, M. S. (Ed.). (2014). *Lippincott manual of nursing practice* (10th ed.). Philadelphia, PA: Lippincott Williams & Wilkins.

Reiter, E. O. (2011). Growth and growth impairment. In C. D. Rudolph, A. M. Rudolph, G. E. Lister, L. First, & A. A. Gershon (Eds.). *Rudolph's pediatrics* (22nd ed.). New York: McGraw-Hill.

Rosenberg, A. A., & Grover, T. (2014). The newborn infant. In W. W. Hay, Jr., M. J. Levin, R. R. Deterding, & M. J. Abzug (Eds.). *Current diagnosis and treatment: pediatrics* (22nd ed.). New York: McGraw-Hill.

Rourke, L., Leduc, D., & Rourke, J. (2014). *Rourke baby record: evidence-based infant/child health maintenance guide.* Retrieved from http://www.rourkebabyrecord.ca/pdf/RBR2014Nat_Eng.pdf

Sass, A. E., & Kaplan, D. W. (2014). Adolescence. In W. W. Hay, Jr., M. J. Levin, R. R. Deterding, & M. J. Abzug (Eds.). *Current diagnosis and treatment: pediatrics* (22nd ed.). New York: McGraw-Hill.

Shah, M. N., & Gupta, R. C. (2014). *Flat head syndrome (positional plagiocephaly).* Retrieved from http://kidshealth.org/parent/growth/sleep/positional_plagiocephaly.html#

Supplementary Nutrition Assistance Program (SNAP-formerly food stamps). *Aid for women, infant and children (WIC).* Retrieved from http://www.wicprograms.org/ci/or-ontario

Tanner, J. M. (1962). *Growth at adolescence.* Oxford, England: Blackwell Scientific Publications.

Treitz, M., Bunik, M., & Fox, D. (2014). Ambulatory & office pediatrics. In W. W. Hay, Jr., M. J. Levin, R. R. Deterding, & M. J. Abzug (Eds.). *Current diagnosis and treatment: paediatrics* (22nd ed.). New York: McGraw-Hill.

U.S. Department of Health and Human Services. (2016). *Healthy People 2020.* Retrieved from http://www.healthypeople.gov/2020/default.aspx

U.S. Department of Health and Human Services; National Institutes of Health; National Heart, Lung, and Blood Institute. (2005). *The fourth report on the diagnosis, evaluation, and treatment of high blood pressure in children and adolescents. (NIH Publication No. 05–5267).* Washington, DC: U.S. Department of Health and Human Services.

Willis, M., Merkel, S., Voepel-Lewis, T., & Malviya, S. (2003). FLACC behavioural pain assessment scale: A comparison with the child's self-report. *Paediatric Nursing, 29*(3), 95–198.

Wong, D., & Baker, C. (1988). Pain in children: Comparison of assessment scales. *Paediatric Nursing, 14,* 9–17.

CHAPTER **WORKSHEET**

MULTIPLE CHOICE QUESTIONS

1. A 5-year-old boy visits the pediatric office with an upper respiratory infection. Which approach would give the nurse the most information about the child's developmental level?
   a. Playing a game with the child.
   b. Talking with the child about the teddy bear next to him.
   c. Using a screening tool during a follow-up office visit.
   d. Asking the 10-year-old sibling about the child.

2. Which statement indicates the best sequence for the nurse to conduct an assessment in a nonemergency situation?
   a. Introduce yourself, ask about any problems, take a history, and do the physical examination.
   b. Perform the physical examination and then ask the family if there are any problems in the child's life.
   c. Do the physical examination while at the same time asking about the child's previous illnesses; then talk about the family's concerns.
   d. Get a complete history of the family's health beliefs and practices, and then assess the child.

3. What approach by the nurse would most likely encourage a child to cooperate with an assessment of physical and developmental health?
   a. Explain to the child what's going to happen when the child asks questions.
   b. Explain what is going to happen in words the child can understand.
   c. Force the child to cooperate by having a parent hold him or her down.
   d. Give the child a sticker before beginning the examination.

4. A sleeping 5-month-old girl is being held by the mother when the nurse comes in to do a physical examination. What assessment should be done initially?
   a. Listening to the bowel sounds
   b. Counting the heart rate
   c. Checking the temperature
   d. Looking in the ears

5. Which assessment finding is considered normal in children?
   a. Irregular respiratory rate and rhythm
   b. Split S_2 and sinus arrhythmia
   c. Decreased heart rate with crying
   d. Genu varum past the age of 5 years

6. A child's weight is 35 lb, 7 oz. Convert the weight to kilograms.

7. A child's height is 41 in. Convert the height to centimetres.

CRITICAL THINKING EXERCISES

1. A soft and muffled heart murmur is heard in a 4-year-old patient. The mother states that she has never heard that the child has a murmur. What should the nurse do?

2. A nurse is helping a new mother breastfeed her 4-day-old baby. The mother notices that the baby has a bluish cast to the skin on his hands and that sometimes the infant has a tremor. She asks the nurse if the baby is cold, though the baby is swaddled and comfortably resting against the mother's skin. How might the nurse help teach this mother?

3. Devise a plan for encouraging cooperation of the toddler or preschooler during various parts of the physical examination.

STUDY ACTIVITIES

1. In the clinical setting, obtain a health history on an infant, child, or adolescent.

2. In the clinical setting, compare the approach you use for the physical examination of a toddler versus a school-aged child or adolescent.

3. No matter how thoughtfully and appropriately you plan your assessment, odds are good that you will have difficulty assessing a 2 year old. Discuss with your classmates the strategies that you have used for success and brainstorm with them about their ideas for assessing a crying or resistant young child.

BRINGING IT ALL TOGETHER: A CASE STUDY

Isabella is a 6-year-old, typically developing child. She has presented with her mother for an annual well-child check. Though appearing well developed, well nourished, and generally healthy, Isabella has been resistant to the examination. She refuses to hold the thermometer under her tongue appropriately for accurate temperature measurement. In fact, her distress with the thermometer seems to have set the tone for the entire visit.

Go to thePoint **to find questions to consider about this case.**

childhood and into adult life (Canadian Institutes of Health Research, 2013). Specific genetic factors, emotional or environmental influences, childhood trauma, and experiences of adversity can lead to chronic health conditions, especially when linked to the social determinants of health (Reuben et al., 2016). A recent UNICEF report identified Canadian children as below average when compared to other developed countries in relation to child poverty, infant mortality, general child health, and safety (Adamson, 2013; First Call BC Child Poverty Report Card, 2017). Furthermore, such reports suggest that the well-being of children living in Canada has not improved since 2001. Disparity across provinces, variations in access to health care, as well as barriers linked to rurality or chronic health care costs, and human resource shortages are key factors influencing service provision and children's access to health care (Allison, 2016; Minore, Boone, Arthur, & Sullivan, 2005). In Canada, a growing divide between rural and urban, Indigenous Canadians, immigrants, refugees, and marginalized populations is an ongoing cause for concern (Adelson, 2005; Canadian Paediatric Society, 2018; Gushulak, Pottie, Roberts, Torres, & DesMeules, 2011; Nakeyar, Esses, & Reid, 2017; Reading & Wien, 2009). All of these factors can place the child with acute or ongoing health needs at greater risk in relation to long-term outcomes for health and well-being (Ford-Jones, Williams, & Bertrand, 2008).

Hospitalization is typically a stressful and overwhelming time for children and their families (Coyne & Kirwan, 2012). Children react to the experience of hospitalization in various ways and respond in accordance with their development age and understanding of their health condition. Furthermore, an individual child's strengths and capabilities to cope with a hospital experience depend on other factors including; social and emotional capacity, parent coping skills before and after the child's illness or admission experience, family cultural beliefs, and the severity of the reason for hospitalization (Franck, Ferguson, Fryda, & Rubin, 2015). Nurses can prepare children and their families by assessing their individual needs, capacities, and plan interventions based on care that reflects the needs of each child and their family. Although a nurse may plan individualized care throughout their interactions with the child and family, a critical time to ensure the best outcome for the child and family is during the admission process. The nurse then continues to assess both the parents' and child's learning needs, health literacy capacity, and must consider ethics linked health management abilities during their stay and prior to discharge (Carnevale, Teachman, & Bogossian, 2017; Jacob, Ford-Jones, Wong, Warman, & Lovett, 2018). For the agreed interventions to be successful, the nurse must effectively communicate, support, and teach the individual child and their family at each stage of hospitalization.

Children's Reactions to Hospitalization

In general, children are more vulnerable to the effects of illness and hospitalization because of the change from their usual state of health and routine (Shields, 2015). They may also have limited understanding and coping mechanisms to assist them in resolving the stressors that might occur during this time. Hospitalization can create a series of traumatic and stressful events in a climate of uncertainty for children and their families, whether it is an elective procedure that is planned in advance or an emergency situation resulting from injury or illness. The stressors that children experience in relation to hospitalization may result in physical and emotional reactions at different times, including before admission, during hospitalization, and after discharge.

The effects of the health problem may go beyond the physiologic ones alone. The psychological, emotional, and social impact of having a chronic disease, acute illness, or hospitalization experience on a child, youth, and family can result in ongoing anxiety and fear related to the overall process and the potential (real or perceived) for bodily injury, physical harm, and pain. In addition, admission to hospital means that children are separated from their homes, families, and friends and what is familiar to them, which may result in **separation anxiety** (distress related to removal from family and familiar surroundings). There is diminished childhood agency which in real term means a general loss of control over their lives and sometimes their emotions and behaviours (Shields, 2015). The result may be feelings of anger and guilt, **regression** (return to a previous stage of development), acting out, and other types of defence mechanisms to cope with these effects. The typical coping strategies of both children and adolescents may be absent or changed during their experience of hospital admission or community health care interventions (Smyth, Kruze, Al Mamun, White, & Shields, 2016).

Anxiety and Fear

Levels of anxiety will be influenced by the uniqueness of the experience and/or the rapid onset of the illness or injury, particularly when the child has limited experiences with disease or injury. Normal fears may include the fear of separation from their parents (which includes other caregivers and guardians), family, or community; loss of control; and bodily injury, mutilation, or harm. Therefore, when the child is in the hospital, he or she may become distressed as a result of the unfamiliar environment (as well as its wider environmental effect [de Leeuw, 2017]) or medical equipment, unusual or frightening noises and smells (e.g., the sound of other children crying), health care procedures (e.g., the use of

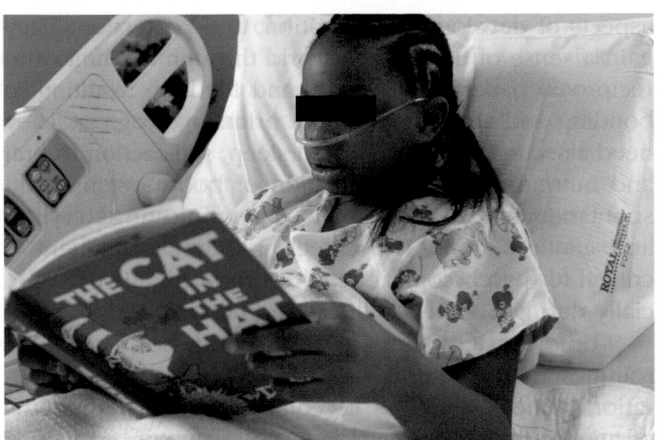

FIGURE 33.1 The presence of familiar objects and home routines normalizes the environment and helps the child cope with hospitalization. Reading a favourite bedtime story can be comforting.

needles), and the presence of large numbers of strangers and those dressed in medical attire (e.g., surgical caps, masks, gowns). This exposure to people, situations, and procedures that are unfamiliar or may result in pain leads to increased anxiety and fear (Fig. 33.1). Overall, hospitalization is a stressful experience for children that at times is also difficult for professionals as they navigate how to work with the child and also their family in a child- and/or family-centred way (Shields, Mamun, Flood, & Combs, 2014).

Separation Anxiety

Separation anxiety is a major stressor for children of certain ages. Timing of separation anxiety varies among children and can be linked to the role of the caregiver as well as the child's experiences over time. It typically begins once a child has developed object permanence (an understanding that things exist even when they are out of sight) which is usually around 4 to 9 months (Swanson, 2014). A central idea in Bowlby's attachment theory is concerned with the well-being of children who experience separations from their mothers (Kobak & Madsen, 2008). A secure attachment is derived from the child's appraisal of his/her mother's (or caregiver's) availability (Bowlby, 1973). Therefore, being resident with the child in hospital is important to the child. While Bowlby considered the separation or loss of a mother (temporary or permanent), Ainsworth (1990) expanded this idea further including the child's communication with their mother and the child's belief his/her mother will respond when called. Separation anxiety comprises three phases: protest, despair, and detachment (Hart & Rollins, 2011). While less commonplace within children's hospitals, as a consequence of family-centred models of care (Shields, 2015), nurses need to watch for signs of separation anxiety, particularly in younger children when their parents or caregivers cannot be present.

Loss of Control

When hospitalized, children and adolescents can be viewed as an extension of their parents which can result in limited inclusion in decision making and can give rise to conflict when there are differences in opinion between the child, youth, and parents or confrontation between professionals, parents, and youth (Ford et al., 2018). This loss of control can increase a child's perception of threat related to their hospitalization or health condition and may subsequently affect their coping skills as a result of feeling excluded (CAPHC, 2016; Carnevale et al., 2017). During hospitalization, children may lose control over routine self-care behaviours, favourite toys and play, as well as some decisions related to the care of their own bodies (Rasmussen, Water, & Dickinson, 2017). For example, if connected to tubes or IV lines, the child may not be able to visit the bathroom without additional help. The child has limited choices, for example, food choices, mealtimes, and may no longer be able to accomplish simple tasks independently as he or she does at home or school. Confinement to a cubicle room, bed, or cot can further heighten their feelings of having no control. As nurses, it is vital that children's interests and where possible independence, and choice remain central to practice.

Hospitalization also affects the child's and adolescent's control over decisions related to his or her own body. Many of the procedures and treatments that occur in the hospital are invasive or are at least disturbing to children. While distraction, play therapy, and inclusion in the decision-making process are advocated, often procedures are experienced as unpleasant and distressing. However, all children and adolescents should be provided with simple explanations of all procedures, with time for questions, to ensure they understand what will be happening to them. Until the child is competent to do so, parents or guardians have the legal responsibility to make decisions and provide informed consent for all interventions and procedures (e.g., Section 17, British Columbia Infants Act, 1996). Though the parents and nurses of hospitalized children have the children's best interest in mind, children may feel powerless when in the hospital. The nurse has a key role in facilitating communication and educating children, youth, and their families as well as ensuring that care is planned with the child and around the family (Shields, 2015), in order to limit power imbalances and respectfully promote their feelings and wishes.

Take Note!

When advocating for a child or adolescent, make sure to include the child's voice. Do not assume what his or her wishes may be; ask about them directly.

experience with hospitalization, and other health-related experiences, can facilitate children's coping or be a barrier to engaging with care providers if prior experiences were perceived as negative. For example, the child who associates the hospital with the opportunity to play with new toys while visiting an ill relative may view this experience as positive. However, the child who associates the hospital with the serious illness or death of a relative or close friend is likely to view the experience as negative.

The type of experience may contribute to increased anxiety and fear if the child is to be admitted to the hospital. If children have had previous experiences, how the experience unfolded and their response to it is likely to inform their emotional and even physical reaction to hospitalization. Older children may cling to their parents, kick, or create a scene because of their previous experience.

Recent Stresses and Changes and Individual Coping Skills

The effects of hospitalization on children are influenced by the nature and severity of the health problem, the condition of the child, and the degree to which activities and routines differ from those of everyday life. A lack of sensory stimulation in the hospital environment can lead to listlessness, indifference, unhappiness, and even appetite changes. When the child's motor activity is restricted, anger and hyperactivity may result. Play, recreation, and educational opportunities can provide an outlet to distract the child from the illness, provide pleasant experiences, and help the child understand his or her condition.

The child's ability to work through a situation will also affect his or her responses to illness and hospitalization. This ability depends on the age of the child, his or her perceptions of the event, previous encounters with health care personnel, and support from significant others. Box 33.2 lists various coping skills used by children and suggestions for promoting positive coping.

BOX 33.2

CHILDREN AND COPING

Behaviour/Methods for Coping	Suggestions to Promote Coping
Ignore or negate the problem	Breathing techniques such as blowing bubbles, pinwheels, or party noisemakers
Stoicism, passive acceptance	Distraction with books or games
Acting out—yelling, kicking, screaming, crying	Imagery with music, recordings, or scenarios
Anger, withdrawal, rejection	Music
Intellectualizing	Teaching before events or procedures

Parents' Response to Child's Hospitalization

Children can mirror their parents' anxiety and concern. For example, preschoolers may invent elaborate stories to explain what is happening to them. If parents do not tell children the truth or do not answer their questions (in ways that are developmentally appropriate), they may become confused and frightened, which can result in weakening of the child's trust in their parents. It is important for children to believe that someone is in control and that the person can be trusted. Some parents, however, have their own fears and insecurities which can transfer across to their child. Thus, a child's reaction can be influenced by their parents' reaction to the illness and hospitalization.

The relationship between the family and health care providers is important, since this dynamic is a core concept in the model of patient (person)- and family-centred care (PFCC/FCC) or child-centred care (CCC) (Ford et al., 2018; Kitson, Marshall, Bassett, & Zeitz, 2013; Shields, 2015). Using the framework of FCC, family strengths, respect and choice, information sharing, support, flexibility, collaboration, and empowerment are key concepts that professionals must pay attention to when working with families to build trust and foster open communication. An example of collaboration and relationship building is evidenced through development of a family-integrated care model in a Canadian neonatal intensive care unit. This approach was shown to support preterm babies, as well as support parent skill acquisition and build confidence (O'Brien et al., 2013). Additional information to research networks linked to child health can be found in thePoint.

> **Remember Jake, the 8-year-old with a suspected brain tumour? What responses to hospitalization might you see in him and his family?**

Family's Reactions to the Child's Hospitalization

Whether planned or unplanned, hospitalization increases the family's stress and anxiety level. The illness or serious injury of one family member affects all members of the family, since the process disrupts the family's usual routines and may alter family roles. Parents and siblings have their own reactions to this experience.

Reactions of Parents

Thinking that a child is in pain or watching a child in pain is difficult, especially when the parent is assisting with the procedure or trying to comfort their child. At these emotionally charged times, parents may feel guilty for not seeking care sooner. Parents will often have complex information needs, which at times professionals can fail to appreciate (Hummelinck & Pollack, 2006). Parents may also exhibit other feelings such as denial, anger, depression, and confusion (Gravdal Kvarme et al., 2016). On occasions, parents may deny that the child is unwell or wish to seek alternative treatments. They may express anger, especially directed at the nursing staff, another family member, or may question their spirituality or beliefs because of their loss of control in caring for the child. All of these emotions, coupled with the physiology of stress, can influence parents' coping at any stage of the hospital experience or when caring for a child with a chronic, life-limiting or life-altering condition. When there is uncertainty linked to diagnosis, or the understanding of their child's prognosis or illness trajectory, parents need to adapt. Family life changes to accommodate the child's altering needs (Somanadhan & Larkin, 2016). As a result of sleep deprivation, exhaustion, and the psychological and physical requirements of spending long hours in a hospital caring for their child, parents may be at risk of low mood, depression, and increased anxiety. Recounting the story around the child's health condition, having and recalling conversations with professionals, and learning how to communicate with their child about injury, health choices (including trans-gender treatment choices), or illness can also be stressful for parents or caregivers (Sanders, Edwards, & Keegan, 2017). Over time, the parents' marriage may become strained because of dual roles, long separation, and increased stress of caring for a child or adolescent with a chronic condition that requires ongoing health care support.

Reactions of Siblings

Siblings of children who are hospitalized may experience fear, confusion, anxiety, insecurity, and possibly even jealousy and resentment for the change in the parents' attention. They may wonder if their sibling is going to die or ever return home. Further, they may worry that their sibling's illness is going to happen to them. Certain age groups, such as preschoolers, may feel that they caused the illness. Little information or understanding about what is happening, combined with their magical and egocentric thinking, contributes to their fears that they may have caused the illness or injury by their thoughts, wishes, or behaviours. If the family roles or routines change significantly, the siblings may too feel insecure or anxious. They may develop changes in behaviour or in school performance. See Evidence-Based Practice 33.1.

Take Note!

Research supports the need to provide support and information to the siblings to decrease their stress, anxiety, and confusion and to promote psychological adjustment (Prchal, Graf, Bergstraesser, & Landolt, 2012).

Factors Influencing Family Reactions

The parenting style, along with the family–child relationship, can influence the hospital experience as well as

---

| EVIDENCE-BASED PRACTICE 33.1 | WHAT IS THE EFFECTIVENESS OF A TWO-SESSION PSYCHOLOGICAL INTERVENTION ON THE SIBLINGS OF A NEWLY DIAGNOSED CHILD WITH CANCER? |

Studies show that most siblings of a child with cancer adjust well but some suffer from cancer-related posttraumatic stress symptoms (PTSS) and have a poorer health-related quality of life. Siblings of a child with cancer are at risk for behavioural, emotional, and social problems.

STUDY

In order to test the effectiveness of the psychological interventions on siblings of children with cancer, a randomized control pilot trial was performed. Thirty siblings of a child recently diagnosed with cancer, ages 6 to 17 years, were recruited from two children's hospitals. Siblings assigned to the experimental group received two 50-minute sessions (2 weeks apart) within the first 2 months of diagnosis. Each session had three steps, including the provision of medical information, ways to cope with stressful situations, and information for parents. Siblings in the control group received standard psychosocial care.

Findings

The authors found that the psychological intervention had a positive affect on the sibling's psychological well-being, social support, and medical knowledge, but did not affect PTSS or anxiety.

Nursing Considerations

Recognize that siblings of an ill child often experience stress and anxiety. Provide education to the sibling of the ill child. Address the psychosocial and emotional needs of siblings of an ill child. Enlist CLSs to assist with the sibling of an ill child. Educate parents about the needs of siblings of an ill child.

Adapted from Prchal, A., Graf, A., Bergstraesser, E., & Landolt, M. A. (2012). A two-session psychological intervention for siblings of pediatric cancer patients: a randomized controlled pilot trial. *Child and Adolescent Psychiatry and Mental Health, 6*, 3.

each family member's coping skills. Cultural, ethnic, and religious variations, values, and practices related to illness, general response to stress, and attitudes about the care of a sick child have a significant influence on the family's response. For example, religious beliefs can raise problems or be a source of strength to the family and child. Families already in crisis or without support systems can experience increasing difficulty dealing with the added stress of hospitalization. Geography between the hospital and the family home can be a further barrier to visiting and may affect the family's reactions to the admission and the burden and impact of the child's or adolescent's illness. Furthermore, low-income populations are more likely to live in rural communities, find transport and access inhibitive, and in some areas are known to have a higher prevalence of children with complex chronic conditions necessitating hospitalization (Peltz et al., 2016). Chapter 1 gives further explanations of some of these influences on children and their families.

> Jake's parents are very upset that he has to be hospitalized. His mother says to you, "I'm worried how Jake is going to react to all of this. What can we do to help him?" How would you address his mother's concerns?

The Nurse's Role in Caring for the Hospitalized Child

The nurse is often central to supporting the child and their family during a time of hospital admission. The nurse is usually the first person to see the child and family and will spend more time with them when compared to other health care professionals. Nurses are part of a medical community that can help support decisions in the child's best interest, but the nurse needs to consider the child's rights and preferences (Ford et al., 2018). Furthermore, nurses should aim to minimize the child's (and parents') distress through atraumatic care and work with other professionals (e.g., child life specialists [CLSs]) to ensure that that the hospital stay is as positive an experience as possible. When establishing strategies to care for children in the hospital setting, nurses should examine the general effects of hospitalization on children in each developmental stage and should strive to understand both the reactions of the child and family to hospitalization and the factors affecting these reactions. Nursing Care Plan 33.1 summarizes the nursing care associated with a hospitalized child.

An Australian study that still has resonance with hospital care today; Crole and Smith (2002) found that the nursing care for a hospitalized child occurs in four phases: introduction, building a trusting relationship,

decision-making phase, and providing comfort and reassurance. All of these phases are interconnected. For example, if trust is not established, it becomes difficult to move to the next phase. Likewise, the introduction phase encompasses the initial contact with children and their families and establishes the foundation for a trusting relationship. During such situations, the use of favourite toys or talk about popular television shows, films, music or electronic games can help establish rapport and relationship building. Allowing the child to participate in the conversation, without the pressure of having to comply with requests or undergo any procedures, can also be helpful. Building a trusting relationship takes time but can start with using appropriate language, games, and play, such as singing a song during a procedure, preparing the child adequately for procedures, and providing explanations and encouragement. A key way in which nurses often demonstrate this, often intuitively, is when they will sit or play at the child's eye level, letting them take the lead in the game or story. In the decision-making phase, the nurse gives some control over to the child by allowing him or her to participate. This phase is critical to maintaining the trust the child has developed. For example, it is imperative to decide how much control the child will have during treatment, how much information to share with the child about upcoming events, and how parents should participate. Reinforce the child's use of coping strategies that lead to healthy outcomes by providing options whenever it is safe to do so. Finally, the comfort and reassurance phase uses techniques such as positive reinforcement, providing opportunities to cuddle with a favourite toy. This phase helps the nurse reestablish trust and provide comfort to the child to increase positive outcomes.

Preparing Children and Families for Hospitalization

When preparing children for hospitalization, be aware of the situations that may create distress in a child and try to minimize or eliminate them. Even the most minor situations may be frightening to young children. Remember, new experiences, unfamiliar sights and sounds, disruption of sleep patterns, and pain associated with procedures and treatments are major causes of stress for the hospitalized child and family. Table 33.1 presents some hospital activities that may seem scary or stressful to a child and gives suggestions for preparing the child and family. Thoughtful preparation for these situations may help relieve stress. Educate children about what to expect so they can cope with their imagination and distinguish reality from fantasy. Describe the intervention and the sequence of steps that will occur, and include sensory information such as how the child will feel.

TABLE 33.1	STRATEGIES TO REDUCE FEAR OF COMMON HOSPITALIZATION SITUATIONS
Situation	**Strategies to Reduce Fear**
Procedure involving intrusion into the body or use of equipment or technology	Describe the procedure and equipment in terms the child can understand Review the steps of the procedure or steps involved with the use of the equipment Explain what the child's role will be and what is or isn't allowed If appropriate, have the child rehearse with the equipment or role-play
Darkness, such as with radiologic examinations or at night	Keep a light on in the examination area Use a night light in the child's room If possible, allow the child to hold the caregiver's or nurse's hand or a favourite toy
Transport to other areas of the hospital	Allow caregiver to accompany child if possible Inform the child of where he or she is going, about how long he or she will be there, and approximately when he or she will return Introduce the child to the person who will be transporting the child
Numerous personnel in and out of child's room	Identify all staff members working with the child (each shift and each day) Place a small board in the child's room with the name of the nurse caring for the child that shift or day Inform the child how long the nurse will be caring for the child (adapt this information according to the child's cognitive level; e.g., instead of saying that you'll be there for 8 hours, say, "I'll be your nurse until just before dinner time" or "I'll be your nurse until you go for your test") Say good-bye to the child when leaving for the day; tell the child about his or her new nurse; inform the child of when you will return

Take Note!

Preparing the Child for Hospitalization

To help reduce the stress and trauma of hospitalization in a child, encourage the parents and child to work with a child life specialist (CLS) at the hospital who can give the child a comprehensive support through the transitions of illness and hospitalization. CLSs are often found in specialist children's hospitals or work in other children's settings (see Box 33.3).

BOX 33.3

EXAMPLES OF ACTIVITIES OF THE CHILD LIFE SPECIALIST

The **child life specialist** (CLS, or sometimes called play specialist in EU countries) is a specially trained individual who provides programs that prepare children for hospitalization, surgery, and other procedures that could be painful (Child Life Council, 2018). The CLS is a member of the multidisciplinary team and works in conjunction with the health care provider and parents to foster an atmosphere that promotes the child's well-being. Services provided by a CLS include:
• Nonmedical preparation for tests, surgeries, and other medical procedures
• Support during medical procedures
• Therapeutic and recreational play
• Activities to support normal growth and development
• Sibling support
• Advocacy for the child and family
• Grief and bereavement support
• Emergency room interventions for children and families
• Hospital preadmission tours and information programs
• Outpatient consultation with families

Good preparation can reduce the child's fears and increase his or her ability to cope with the hospital experience. Preparation should include exploring the child's perceptions, reviewing previous experiences, and identifying coping strategies. The goal should be to decrease fear and anxiety by allowing the child to better understand what is happening. Useful techniques include the following:
• Perform nursing care on stuffed animals or dolls and allow the child to do the same.
• Avoid the use of medical terms.
• Allow the child to handle some equipment.
• Teach the child the steps of the procedure or inform him or her exactly what will happen during the hospital stay.
• Show the child the room where he or she will be staying.
• Introduce the child to the health care personnel with whom he or she will come in contact.
• Explain the sounds the child may hear.

All techniques used to prepare the child for hospitalization should emphasize the philosophy of atraumatic care. Adapt all information to the cognitive and developmental level of the child. Identify what role the child will play in the situation: it is always helpful for children to have something to do, since it shows them that they are included. A rehearsal of what will occur in the hospital allows the child to become comfortable with the situation. If time permits, provide pamphlets that describe the procedure and suggest preparation activities for the child at home before admission.

FIGURE 33.2 A child is being prepared for hospitalization by becoming familiar with some of the equipment that might be used.

The child and family may be able to take a tour of the hospital unit or the surgical setting. Multimedia resources and books on hospitalization and surgery can serve as resources for the family and child. Some popular children's books are available that focus on hospital stays and procedures, such as *My Trip to the Hospital* in the Little Critter Series by Mercer Mayer and *Clifford Visits the Hospital* by Norman Bridwell. A list may be available at the hospital from the child life department or the patient education centre of the ward/unit or floor to which the child is being admitted. Many hospitals offer programs to familiarize children and families with the setting and may offer a guided tour of specific units, such as the day surgery unit. During the tour, opportunities are provided for role-playing, and during stops along the way, the child can see, touch, and feel the equipment that may be used (Fig. 33.2). If the tour guide notes a child or family member is really scared or concerned about something, the pediatric staff can be alerted and therefore address this issue, further leading to improved FCC. Nurses may support parents in preparing their children by reviewing the materials provided, answering questions, and being truthful and supportive. Teaching Guidelines 33.1 provides suggestions for parents in preparing their child for hospitalization.

Teaching Guidelines 33.1

PREPARING YOUR CHILD FOR HOSPITALIZATION

• Read stories about experiences with hospitals or surgery.
• Talk about going to the hospital and what it will be like coming home.
• Be honest and encourage the child to ask questions.
• Provide support to the child via your presence, telephone calls, and special items brought from home.

• Encourage the child to draw pictures to express how he or she is feeling.
• Include siblings in the preparation.

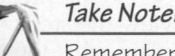

Take Note!

Remember to enlist the assistance of the child life specialist (CLS), if possible, to assist with preparing children and families for hospitalization. The CLS programs focus on the social and emotional impact of illness and hospitalization. www.sickkids.ca/patient-familyresources?Child-Life/index.html

Admitting the Child to the Health Care Setting

Admitting the child to the hospital involves preparing him or her for admission and introducing the child to the unit where he or she will be staying. Chapter 30 gives general information about communicating with and teaching children and families.

In today's health care environment, the admission process occurs quickly, with little time for extensive preparation; this is why preparation before admission is important. Of course, the urgency of the child's medical condition may also limit the amount of preparation that can be undertaken in advance.

Safety Check

GOAL: Improve the Safety of Using Medications

Maintain and communicate accurate patient medication information.

Steps: When admitting a child to the setting, be sure to collect accurate information concerning the child's usual medications. Compare this information with ordered medications to check for inconsistencies.

Canadian Patient Safety Institute and Health Canada can provide guidance around medication management with children http://www.patientsafetyinstitute.ca/en/Topic/Pages/Medication-Management.aspx & http://www.hc-sc.gc.ca/dhp-mps/index-eng.php as well as the Evidence Network Pharmaceutical Policy http://evidencenetwork.ca/pharmaceutical-policy

TYPES OF ADMISSIONS AND NURSING CARE

The hospital units to which a child may be admitted include:
• General inpatient unit
• Emergency and urgent care department
• Pediatric intensive care unit (PICU)
• Outpatient or special procedures unit
• Rehabilitation unit or hospital

Regardless of the site of care, nursing care must begin by establishing a trusting, caring relationship with the child and family. Smile, introduce yourself, and give your title; not only is this kind when the child and family may be feeling vulnerable, it is also a patient safety issue. Let the child and family know what will happen and what is expected of them. Ask the family and child what names they prefer to be called by. When talking with a younger child, start the conversation with the family first so the child can see that they trust you.

The next step, as the child's medical condition allows, involves an orientation to the hospital unit. Briefly explain policies and routines and the personnel who will be involved in the care of the child.

During the nursing interview that follows, obtain information about the child's history, routines, and reason for admission. Obtain baseline vital signs and height and weight, perform a physical assessment, and ensure that the child wears a patient identity band and allergy band where appropriate. Each health care setting has its own policies and procedures for this. Recognize the needs of the family and child during this process. If some of this information already exists, aim not ask for it again, except to confirm vital information such as allergies, medications taken at home, and history of the illness. Typically, the information is collected immediately if the child's condition is urgent; otherwise, the information is collected within the initial shift, except for the information that is required for safe care. Document nursing interventions in accordance with local pathways, policies, and data standard requirements to meet both regulatory standards as well as any health informatic measures (Nagle & White, 2016).

General Inpatient Unit Stays. Today, general inpatient unit stays for children are shorter and involve more acute conditions, resulting in little time for admission preparation. Many times, the admission procedure and treatment actually occur simultaneously. Sometimes, the stay is in a special 23-hour observation unit so the child is in the setting for less than 24 hours. General hospital stays may be in a pediatric hospital, a pediatric unit in a general hospital, or a general unit that occasionally admits children. General units often lack child-oriented services, such as play areas, child-size equipment, and staff familiar with caring for children.

Take Note!

When a child is admitted to a general unit, take extra time to orient and explain the routines and procedures to the child and family. Emphasize that the parents can stay with the child. If possible, place the child in a room close to the nurses' station and order food appropriate for the child's age and developmental level if the child is allowed to eat and drink (i.e., not listed for surgery). It is also important to recognize that information needs will continue during the time the child is an inpatient. While the provision of information is an individual right and important in enabling children to understand their illness and participate in decision making, the nurse should recognize that their needs may change as they develop understanding about their hospital experience and illness (Lambert, Glacken, & McCarron, 2013). It is important for the nurse to revisit key information over the course of the child's hospital admission.

Emergency and Urgent Care Departments. A major cause for illness and hospitalization in children is injuries from accidents (Yanchar, Warda, & Fuselli, 2012). Often, the ED is the first point of care for a child and their family. Due to the situation, the child and family may experience increased anxiety and may become overwhelmed as uncertainties develop and critical decisions must be made. The family may be frightened, insecure, and in a state of shock. Children in the ED setting have been found to adapt quickly and can use the language of professionals; however, this may not confer understanding. Furthermore, it can be difficult for children in this setting to differentiate between professionals and they may need extra reassurance about treatments and procedures (Jensen, Jackson, Kolbæk, & Glasdam, 2012), particularly if these are performed quickly with minimal time for preparation. The family is often not prepared for the visit, having little money or clothing with them. Siblings may be present if the parents did not have time to arrange other child care.

Due to the fast pace of the ED, professionals need to ensure the child safety and attend to the high emotions from children, youth, and parents (Ali, Thomson, Graham, Rickard, & Stang, 2017). Furthermore, the family may be hesitant to ask questions. Nurses should assess the understanding of the child and family and communicate effectively to keep the family and child well informed. Allowing the family to stay with the child, providing support, and facilitating participation in decision making are similarly important during these situations. Families may have a strong fear of the unknown and may be terrified that the child will die or be permanently disabled. Help the family to identify their concerns and support systems (do they need to call a friend or relative?) and prepare them for what they will experience. Provide comfort to the child and their family, such as holding their hand, therapeutic touch, talking softly, and other appropriate interventions according to age and developmental level.

Pediatric Intensive Care Units. The PICU specializes in caring for children in crisis. The same principles and concepts of general care of children apply to this setting, but everything is intensified. Families will be faced with an unfamiliar, high-tech environment and a large number of staff. Families may find it challenging to be involved in their child's care and communicate with professionals (Carnevale et al., 2007; Carnevale et al., 2016).

Families must deal with the critical situation that brought them to the PICU. The child will likely experience pain, unusual noises, and increased stimulation, and will probably undergo uncomfortable procedures that need to be managed appropriately (Stevens et al., 2011). Parents may be facing the possibility of losing their child. Sometimes the child cannot talk, eat, or display other appropriate developmental behaviours. Sensory overload (increased stimulation) or sensory deprivation (lack of stimulation) can affect both child and family in the short and longer term. Up to 25% of children have been reported to experience negative psychological and behavioural outcomes within the first year post discharge from PICU (Rennick et al., 2014).

Welcome families (if facility policy permits) and encourage them to stay with the child and participate in care. Explain everything to the parents and, when appropriate, to the child. Frequently use therapeutic touch with the child and encourage the parents to comfort him or her in the same way. Listen for clues about what the child and family need during the PICU stay and connect them with additional supports, such as religious connections, Elders, or others to provide emotional and spiritual support at this time.

Isolation Rooms. Isolation rooms are used for situations involving the risk for infection. When a child is admitted with an infectious disease, or there is a need to exclude an infectious disease or prevent infection due to impaired immune function, isolation will be necessary. Children in this setting may experience sensory deprivation due to the limited contact with others and the use of personal protective equipment such as gloves, masks, and gowns. Encourage the family to visit often, and help them to understand the reason for the isolation precautions; teaching and guiding them as to how to wash hands, use personal protective equipment, or complete any special procedures that are required. Introduce yourself before entering the room and allow the child to view your face before applying a mask, if possible. Continue to have contact with the child and hold and use therapeutic touch with the child as often as it is acceptable to the child or young person.

Rehabilitation Units. The rehabilitation unit provides care for children beyond the initial period of illness or injury. The care involves an interdisciplinary approach that assists the child to reach his or her potential and achieve developmental skills. For example, rehabilitation units help children regain abilities lost due to neurologic injuries or serious burns. The facilities often resemble a home environment, with special services to help children to relearn activities of daily living and to help them deal with the physical or mental challenges associated with the original illness or injury. Typically, families are encouraged to participate and are given support for their child's eventual return home.

Addressing the Effects of Hospitalization Developmentally

When addressing the fears, separation anxiety, and loss of control that occur in hospitalized children, the nurse should consider the child's age and cognitive or developmental level. Interventions are then based on how the child experiences these stressors at that age or developmental level. The content, timing, setting, and method of preparation are also based on the child's age and cognitive or developmental level. General guidelines for addressing fear and anxiety, separation anxiety, and loss of control are provided in Box 33.4.

NEWBORNS AND INFANTS

Assess the development, or lack of development, that is occurring in the infant and assess his or her attachment to the parents or primary caregivers. The infant's facial expression is the most consistent indicator of pain or bodily injury. To decrease fear and minimize separation anxiety, avoid separation from the primary caregiver if possible; this will also promote healthy attachment. If the

---

BOX 33.4

GUIDELINES TO ADDRESS THE GENERAL EFFECTS OF HOSPITALIZATION

Minimizing Fear and Anxiety
- Prepare the child and family for hospitalization and procedures.
- Explain everything to the child and their family before it occurs (see Chapter 30).
- Use age-appropriate communication techniques. Include the family in this process so they can help the child cope with fears.
- Allow time for children to play out their fears and concerns.
- Talk to the child and parents using a soft, friendly, comforting tone of voice.
- Have a calm, empathetic approach when caring for the child.

Addressing/Minimizing Separation Anxiety
- Know the stages of separation anxiety and be able to recognize them.
- Remember that behaviours demonstrated during the first stage do not indicate that the child is "bad."
- Encourage the family to stay with the child and always use a family-centred approach to care.
- Help the child cope, and intervene before the behaviours of detachment occur.

Addressing Loss of Control
- Minimize physical restrictions, altered routines and rituals, and dependency issues, because they produce loss of control.
- Allow as much independence as possible within the constraints of the diagnosis.
- Allow the child to participate in care and decisions regarding care whenever possible.

parent or primary caregiver cannot stay with the infant, arrange for volunteers to provide consistent comfort to the infant. Maintaining the infant's home routine with respect to sleep and feeding can help decrease feelings of loss of control. Weigh the infant daily, at the same time, on the same scale. Monitor intake and output closely. Be alert to signs of discomfort other than crying, such as a furrowed brow or tense body posture. Additional nursing goals related to ensuring safety and promoting growth and development of the infant are presented in Table 33.2.

TODDLERS

Key nursing concerns when caring for toddlers are separation anxiety, growth and development, and autonomy. Establishing a trusting relationship with the toddler through nonthreatening play may decrease the amount

of fear the toddler feels. Be alert to subtle, nonverbal indicators of grief or discontent.

Encourage the parent or primary caregiver to stay with the toddler in the hospital to decrease separation anxiety. Maintain the home routine related to meals and sleep where possible, since these provide structure and may help decrease the toddler's feelings of loss of control. If indicated, weigh the toddler daily. Closely monitor intake and output. Refer to Table 33.2 for additional nursing considerations related to ensuring safety and promoting growth and development in the hospitalized toddler.

PRESCHOOLERS

Nursing care for hospitalized preschoolers focuses on their special needs, fears, and fantasies. When working with preschoolers, remember that they use magical

TABLE 33.2	NURSING CONSIDERATIONS FOR PROVIDING SAFE, DEVELOPMENTALLY APPROPRIATE CARE	
	Ensuring Safety	**Promoting Healthy Growth and Development**
Infants	• Maintain close supervision of the infant. • Keep one hand on the infant when crib sides are down. • Keep crib rails up all the way when the infant is in the crib. • Avoid leaving small objects that are harmful or that can be swallowed in the crib. • Provide safe and appropriate toys for the infant. Clean as per infection control policies. • Place infants in rooms close to the nurses' station. • Encourage a family member to stay with the infant at all times.	• Use the face-to-face position when holding newborns. • Smile and talk to the infant during bathing, feeding, and other interactions. • Minimize the number of painful or uncomfortable procedures. • Provide comfort during and after procedures by holding or talking, using soothing tones and movements. • When handling the infant, use smooth, continuous movements. • Use gentle stroking and holding, which may reduce stress. • Serve as a role model for first-time parents. • Encourage the family to maintain home routines while in the hospital, planning nursing care around the usual feeding and sleep times. • Discuss the pacifier between feedings; being mindful may reduce breastfeeding in infants but in NPO may be a short-term soothing approach.
Toddlers	• Keep cot side rails up. • Never leave a toddler alone in the room unless secured in the crib. • Use a bed only for the older toddler who has an adult present in the room at all times. • Avoid leaving small objects that can be swallowed or are harmful in the crib or bed. • Place cot out of reach of cords, equipment, and electrical outlets. • Provide safe and appropriate toys for the toddler. • Place toddlers in rooms close to the nurses' station. • Always have someone with the toddler when ambulating.	• Encourage the parent to stay with the toddler to decrease separation anxiety. • To promote autonomy, allow the toddler to make appropriate choices, such as which juice to take the medicine with. • Encourage active play in the playroom or with push/pull toys in the hallway (accompanied by an adult). • Expect and plan for regression in areas of toilet training, eating, and other behaviours. • Expect increased temper tantrums in general and intense reactions to intrusive procedures. • Maintain home routine while in the hospital, planning nursing care around the usual feeding and sleep times. • Give simple directions with choices appropriate to the hospital situation. • Provide close supervision while encouraging independence.

(continued)

TABLE 33.2	NURSING CONSIDERATIONS FOR PROVIDING SAFE, DEVELOPMENTALLY APPROPRIATE CARE (continued)	
	Ensuring Safety	**Promoting Healthy Growth and Development**
Preschoolers	• Keep bed in low position with the side rails up when the preschooler is in the bed. • Instruct the child to call the nurse or caregiver for help getting out of bed. • Keep harmful objects out of reach of the child.	• Encourage parents to stay with the preschooler in the room as well as other areas of the hospital. • Encourage the preschooler to be involved in care by providing choices and opportunities for the child to help. • Use play as an opportunity to work through the preschooler's fears. • Explain activities in simple, concrete terms, being cautious with the words you use because of the preschooler's fantasies and magical thinking. • Expect reactions to pain and bodily injury to be verbally aggressive and specific. • Try to maintain home routines while the child is in the hospital, working them into the plan of care when possible.
School-Age Children	• Keep the bed in the low position with the side rails up while the child is in the bed, explaining that this is a hospital rule, not a punishment.	• Provide opportunities for the child to be involved in care. • Allow children to select their meals, assist with treatments, and keep their rooms neat. • Allow visits with other children if the condition allows. • Encourage parents to tell the child when they will return. • Plan care around the child's usual home routines (meals, sleep). • Encourage the child to do schoolwork.
Adolescents	• Be aware of the adolescent's whereabouts. The teen may not wish to stay in the room but may become confused about where the room or unit is located in the hospital.	• Allow teens to interact with others. • Alter hospital routines as possible to allow the teen to sleep in or stay up later at night. • Provide others close to their age as roommates. • Encourage visits from friends. • Provide emotional support for feelings of being alone or away from friends; be alert for regression, which may result in the teen becoming emotional. • Answer questions honestly and with appropriate information. • Give the teen a sense of control by allowing choices. • Be sensitive to concerns about being "different."

thinking and fantasy. Be honest and specific, providing information just prior to the intervention to allay the child's fears. As with toddlers, encouraging parental involvement may decrease the amount of separation anxiety the preschooler experiences while in the hospital. Allowing the preschooler to make simple decisions, such as which colour bandage to use or whether to take medicine from a cup or syringe, helps the child to feel some sense of control. Table 33.2 gives specific nursing considerations related to ensuring safety and promoting growth and development for the preschooler in the hospital.

SCHOOL-AGE CHILDREN

Provide honest information using concrete, meaningful words to the school-age child to minimize fear of the unknown. School-age children are still very attached to their parents, so encouraging parental involvement or rooming-in decreases separation anxiety. Involve the child in making simple decisions and planning the schedule as appropriate to give him or her a sense of control. Nursing considerations when caring for hospitalized school-age children include ensuring safety and promoting growth and development (Table 33.2).

ADOLESCENTS

Each adolescent who is hospitalized will have a different experience. Development, experience, and culture will all affect how an adolescent responds to each hospitalization. Youth with chronic conditions, who have had previous hospitalizations, will also have different expectations—impacted by the severity of their condition. Individualized care is the best approach, providing opportunities for questions, explanations, and decision making. Encourage visits from the adolescent's friends to minimize anxiety related to separation. Prepare a mutually agreeable schedule with the adolescent, as appropriate, that includes preferences while incorporating the required nursing care. Collaborating with the adolescent will support the young person in having some control. Refer to Table 33.2 for additional nursing considerations related to care of the adolescent in the hospital.

> **Think back to Jake, the 8-year-old from the beginning of the chapter. Discuss nursing care you could provide that will help minimize stressors.**

Preparing the Child and Family for Surgery

If the child is to undergo a surgical procedure, whether in the hospital or an outpatient setting, special interventions are necessary. The parents should be allowed to stay with the child until surgery begins. Parents should also be allowed to be with the child when he or she wakes up in the postanaesthesia recovery area. Good preparation provides reassurance and comfort to the child and allows him or her to know what will happen and what is expected of him or her.

Preoperative care for the child who is to undergo surgery is similar to that for an adult. The major difference is that the preparation and teaching must be geared to the child's age and developmental level. Table 33.3 discusses strategies for preoperative teaching. Many facilities offer special programs and supports to help prepare children and families for the surgical experience, such as CLSs. Preoperative preparation programs allow children and their families to experience a "trial run" in a supportive environment to help reduce anxiety, increase knowledge,

increase comfort level, and enhance coping skills. As mentioned earlier, books and tours can be helpful in preparing the child and family for an impending surgery.

Child and family teaching is essential. All teaching needs to be modified to meet the needs of the child and family. Like any intervention, all teaching should be adapted to the cognitive ability of those being taught and their desire to be engaged. Special attention should also be given to the parents' and/or caregivers' level of communication and capacity to understand the teaching. Games can be helpful with younger children; for example, when teaching a toddler or preschooler about breathing exercises, have the child blow a pinwheel or cotton balls across the table through a straw.

In preparation for surgery, use items such as stuffed animals or dolls to help children understand what is going to happen to them (Fig. 33.3). Allow the child to role-play various experiences with dolls. Dolls designed to simulate surgical experiences are available. For example, in the United States, Shadow Buddies are custom-made dolls that have the same illness or surgery as the child; the doll may have an ostomy, a scar, or a catheter (Shadow Buddies Foundation, 2014). Dolls have been made by families and many other countries have developed similar local resources working with specialist nurses or national charitable organizations. The aim behind these dolls or toys is to help the children explore difference and learn to talk about themselves by projecting their story onto another object. These dolls also provide the child with a companion to talk to.

Maintaining Safety During Hospitalization

Safety is a critical aspect of care of the child in the hospital. Due to their age and developmental level, children are vulnerable to harm. Ensure the child has an identification band in place at all times. Sometimes when

TABLE 33.3	STRATEGIES FOR PREOPERATIVE TEACHING
Developmental Level	**Implications for Teaching**
Infants and toddlers	Encourage parents to use a soft tone of voice and stroking, and secure, comfortable holding positions to promote calm Remind parents to use positive facial expressions Encourage the parent or caregiver to stay with the child as much as possible Use terms that the child and parents can understand For toddlers, provide information as close to the day of surgery as possible to prevent undue anxiety
Preschoolers and school-age children	Provide factual explanations using terms the child and parents can understand Incorporate pictures and other visual aids in explanation Tailor the timing of education to meet the child's learning needs, allowing enough time for the child to ask questions. For preschoolers, provide information 1 to 2 days before surgery. For school-age children, provide information 3 to 5 days before surgery
Adolescents	Provide detailed explanations of the procedure at least 7 to 10 days beforehand Answer questions honestly, ensuring privacy at all times Remain available for questions or concerns arising before or after surgery

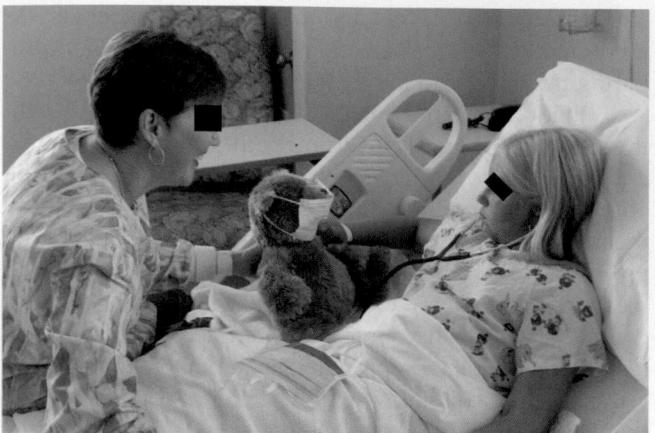

FIGURE 33.3 Using a stuffed animal to explain a surgical procedure to the child.

implementing an intervention, a name band is removed. In such circumstances, it is critical to ensure that the band is replaced or attached to another extremity. Monitor children closely to avoid accidents such as a child picking up a piece of equipment or supplies left in the bed or room, or climbing out of bed (Fig. 33.4). See Table 33.2, which highlights nursing goals for ensuring safe, developmentally appropriate care for the hospitalized child.

USE OF SECLUSION AND RESTRAINTS

When caring for children, some type of restriction may be necessary but should be considered a last resort when providing care (Kirwan & Coyne, 2016). The restriction, often referred to as a restraint, may be needed to ensure the child's safety, allow a therapeutic or diagnostic procedure to be completed safely and with the child's permission, immobilize a body part, or prevent disruption of prescribed therapy. Restraint can happen in various contexts and can be distressing for the nurse (Kangasniemi, Papinaho, & Korhonen, 2014), child, and family

FIGURE 33.4 Safety is an essential aspect of pediatric nursing. A clear plastic cover over the crib prevents the older infant or toddler from climbing out and falling.

members. An increasing number of studies have identified that children held for procedures are often younger and receiving urgent care (Bray, Snodin, & Carter, 2015). Nurses need to be clear about their boundaries when starting or continuing with a procedure when a child is distressed. Before, during, and after clinical procedures, the nurse should undertake procedural preparation and facilitate engagement activities with children and their parents. Working with other professionals skilled in child preparation, such as CLS (Bray, Carter, & Snodin, 2016), can also be helpful in such situations. Restraints can be overused and are not without risks to the safety (Emanuel, et al., 2017). Furthermore, emotional consequences may arise for the child, parent, and nurse (Bray et al., 2015). As a result, each setting will have specific procedures and policies in place related to the use of restraints based on local and provincial standards. Seclusion has historically been used within mental health settings, while its use in a pediatric setting is limited with one-to-one nursing should risk be identified. However, this may need to be discussed when a child or adolescent is presenting with disruptive, self-harming, aggressive, or violent behaviour (Ministry of Health, 2012; Timbo et al., 2016). Advice and direction should be sought from senior nursing and medical staff when caring for a child that may need to be restrained or secluded.

Atraumatic Care

Therapeutic hugging should be used for procedures and treatments, such as IV line insertion, for which the child needs to remain still. Refer to Chapter 30 for further information.

TRANSPORT OF THE CHILD

Children may need to move around the hospital for diagnostic tests or surgery, or move within the nursing unit to access a playroom or treatment area. When the child is transported to other areas, the nurse should consider potential safety issues, including the age and developmental level of the child, the child's physical condition, and the destination. This can ensure that an appropriate method of transport is utilized with the least amount of risk for the child. Various methods to transport children may be used, including carrying the infant or using strollers, wheel chairs, trollies, or rolling beds (Fig. 33.5). When using any equipment, this should always be clean, regularly inspected, and equipped with the necessary safety belts or harnesses (e.g., in strollers or wheelchair). Refer to local policies to ensure that you are up to date and compliant with patient moving and handling procedures to minimize risk to the child and staff. If possible, the parents should accompany the child to offer support and comfort.

A   B   C

D

FIGURE 33.5 Methods for transporting the infant or child. **A.** Cradle method for carrying infants up to 3 months of age. One hand grasps the infant's thighs; the other arm supports the infant's head and back. **B.** The "over-the-shoulder" method for carrying infants up to 7 months of age. Support the head if the infant does not have head control. **C.** Football method for carrying infants up to 2 months of age. The forearm and hand support the body and head of the infant. **D.** A wagon with rails and padding is used to transport small children.

Take Note!

Never leave a child unattended during transport. Keep the child visible at all times during the transport.

Providing Basic Care for the Hospitalized Child

Basic care involves general hygiene measures, including bathing, hair care, oral care, and nutritional care. Young children are dependent on an adult for most, if not all, of their self-care needs. If parents are present, allow them to provide care for the child to decrease the child's stress. Older children may perform hygiene measures themselves but may need some assistance from the nurse.

GENERAL HYGIENE MEASURES

General hygiene measures help to maintain healthy skin, hair, and teeth. Skin is a complex structure; its primary function is to protect the tissues that it encloses and to protect itself. Injury to the child's skin may occur when inserting and maintaining an IV line, removing a dressing, positioning a child in bed, changing a diaper, using and removing electrode patches, and maintaining restraints. Risk factors that can affect skin integrity include impaired mobility, protein malnutrition, edema, incontinence, sensory loss, anemia, and infection. A

TABLE 33.4	DEVELOPMENTAL CONSIDERATIONS FOR BATHING
Age of Child	**Special Considerations**
Infants	Use a sponge bath or tub bath to bathe young infants who cannot sit unaided. Support the infant's body at all times. Ensure appropriate water temperature. Avoid use of talcum powder.
Toddlers	Bathe older infants and toddlers at the bedside or in a regular bathtub, depending on their health condition.
School-age children and adolescents	Older children may prefer a shower if available and acceptable for their health condition. Assess whether a shower would be safe. Provide privacy.

good time to assess the child's skin is during bath or shower time.

Bathing. Bathing infants and children is a common daily hygiene measure in the health care environment. Although the parents or primary caregiver often does this in today's family-centred environment, the nurse is still responsible for ensuring that bathing is done safely and hygienically. Adhere to safety principles to prevent falls, burns, and aspiration of water. Never leave a child alone in a bathtub. Use a gentle, pH-balanced soap with moisturizer if there is a need to rehydrate the skin. Note any condition that might require special considerations or further assessment, such as paralysis, loss of sensation, surgical incisions, skin traction/cast, external lines (IV lines, urinary catheters, or feeding tubes), or other alterations in skin integrity. Pay close attention to the ears, between skin folds, the neck, the back, and the genital area for alterations in skin integrity. Table 33.4 highlights specific developmental considerations for bathing.

Before using the bath or shower or attending to the infant's or child's other hygiene measures, assess the family's preferences and home practices such as time of day the child has a bath, special equipment, or allergies to products. This is a good time to assess the amount of assistance that might be required by the parents and to address learning needs related to hygiene, such as not using narrow cotton tips to clean ears. Follow general guidelines that focus on bathing such as using equipment safely; attention to the temperature of the room and the water; need for privacy; and access to products and supplies such as deodorant, lotion, and clean clothing. For the adolescent patient, provide ample time for planning and preparation for washing and personal hygiene. Be mindful to ensure that adolescent girls who have started their periods have access to the products they may need. With physical changes as a result of illness, disease, or injury, refusal to take a bath or shower and attend to personal care can happen. Young people will need time, support, and opportunity to share their worries and concerns about any altered body image, how this makes them feel and how they believe others may perceive them. It is important to ensure they have privacy and the level of support necessary to ensure patient safety and respect their dignity.

Hair Care. Lying in bed can make the hair matted and tangled. Avoid pulling on the child's hair when combing or brushing it. If necessary, use commercial detangling solutions to ease combing.

If the hair requires washing, this is often done during the daily bath for infants. Typically, shampooing once or twice a week is sufficient for younger children. Adolescents may need more frequent shampooing due to the increase in sebaceous gland secretion. The frequency of shampooing also varies based on the child's condition; for example, if the child has experienced diaphoresis, more frequent shampooing may be indicated.

Shampooing may be done at the bedside with specially adapted equipment, at a readily accessible sink while the child is sitting in a chair or lying on a stretcher, or in a tub or shower. Commercial no-rinse shampoos may be available for use. With these products, the shampoo is applied to the hair and then brushed or combed out.

If the child uses the bath or shower for hair care, monitor the child's safety throughout to ensure that the child does not slip and fall due to the slippery surface. Check the temperature of the water to prevent scald injuries.

The child's ethnicity or religious beliefs may require special measures for hair care; discuss this with the child and family and ask if they can provide any specialist products, combs, or garments that may wish to be used.

Oral Hygiene. Oral hygiene is an important part of basic care. Wipe the infant's gums with a wet cloth after each feeding. Assist children in brushing and flossing their teeth after eating and before bedtime. The child who is immunosuppressed needs special attention to oral hygiene, such as using soft toothbrushes and moistened gauze sponges to prevent bleeding and careful inspection of the oral cavity for areas of breakdown.

NUTRITIONAL CARE

Adequate nutrition is necessary for growth, development, and tissue repair and is an essential component of optimal development of the child. If a CLS i[s avail]able, the nurse provides this type of activity[...] greater emphasis on the developmental and [so]cial implications of illness and hospitalizatio[n...] dation of the child's voice.

In emotional outlet play or traumatic pla[y...] acts out or dramatizes real-life stressors. Fo[r...] using a wooden hammer and pegs, a soft s[...] or boxing gloves can allow the child to exp[...] over separation from family and friends. [...] toys such as anatomically correct dolls and pu[...] removable parts so children can see variou[s...] the body. Sometimes, younger children "tal[k...] pets and dolls, allowing them to express their[...] a nonthreatening "person" about a specific [...] what they want from the health care provide[r...]

Other types of therapeutic play inclu[de...] and supervised "needle play." Drawing is a [way...] child to express his or her thoughts and feeli[ngs...] vised "needle play" assists children who mu[st...] frequent blood work, injections, or IV proced[ures...] can receive an injection as the child works o[ut...] anger and anxiety. Keep in mind safety and [...] growth and development level before plannir[g...] of directed play; an adult must always be pre[sent...]

Promoting Schoolwork and Educatio[n] During Hospitalization

Promote schoolwork while the child is in t[he...] Determine the amount of schoolwork that c[an...] by assessing the child's condition, the av[...] teachers, and the family situation. Many chi[l...] pitals have teachers at the hospitals; there m[ay...] rooms too. These teachers work closely wit[h...] school to continue schoolwork as the child[...] permits. Hospitals without an educational st[...] on parents to coordinate with the child's sch[...] may bring in schoolbooks and the child's ho[...] completion while in the hospital. This conne[...] child's school helps maintain normalcy for th[...] minimizes the disruption of everyday life.

Addressing the Needs of Family Mem[bers]

Assess the factors that may influence the fa[...] tion to the child's hospitalization and plan the[...] child to accommodate some of these issues [...] families to have support systems in place be[...] and after hospitalization. The practice of F[...] good communication and ensures that nur[...] address the needs and preferences of the chi[...] ily, and promote their satisfaction with the [...] setting (Best Practices in Engaging Families i[n...] Youth Mental Health, Ontario Centre of Ex[...] Child and Youth Mental Health, 2016).

care for the child that is unwell or in hospital. Often children and adolescents in hospital will have a change in their appetite. This may be compounded by other problems such as nausea and vomiting and taking nothing by mouth (NPO) due to restrictions for tests or surgery. The hospitalized child may adopt feeding habits that do not fit his or her age or stage of development, such as use of a bottle in an older infant/child or a child capable of self-feeding wanting to be fed. Support their return to independence as their condition improves. Food allergy and safety is important in the hospital setting (Watson, Kingon, Muston, Collins, & Sayers, 2016) and medical diets, restrictions, and additives can further disrupt the child's or adolescent's appetite. The appearance, temperature, taste, and consistency of food are important, as well as the social aspect of eating meals. Where possible, try to be creative at mealtimes, explore barriers to eating, and work with the catering staff and dieticians to explore alternatives if required.

Take Note!
Relieve pain and nausea at least 30 minutes before meals are served; if a child is in pain, they are less likely to eat, even if hungry.

If possible, schedule procedures or treatments away from mealtimes. In younger children, refusing to eat may be related to the child's feeling of separation; in others, refusing to eat may reflect the child's attempt to control the situation. Encourage parents to use gentle persuasion instead of force to assist with intake. The use of force can lead to an aversion for food that carries beyond the hospital stay into the home environment. They should give the child choices about what to eat; this reinforces the child's sense of control. Remind parents that the child's appetite will probably improve as his or her condition improves. Teaching Guidelines 33.2 provides tips for promoting nutrition in the hospitalized child. Although geared to parents, nurses can also incorporate these guidelines into the child's plan of care.

Teaching Guidelines 33.2
PROMOTING NUTRITION FOR YOUR HOSPITALIZED CHILD

- Check with the nurse about any restrictions related to your child's diet. Find out if intake and output are being monitored.
- Encourage your child to eat his or her favourite foods.
- Assist your child with eating or drinking as necessary; be present at mealtimes to promote socialization.
- Frequently offer small cups of fluid and finger foods; avoid giving large quantities at one time.

- Try offering fluids at different temperatures at different times for variety.
- Remember that children can ingest greater amounts of thin liquids (e.g., juice or water) than thicker liquids (e.g., cream soups or milkshakes).
- Include ice chips as fluid intake. Ice is approximately equivalent to half the same amount of water (e.g., 1 cup of ice equals a half cup of water).
- Use straws (unless not allowed) and brightly coloured utensils, cups, or dishes to provide contrast and stimulation.
- Offer the child choices; allow the child to choose what he or she wants from the menu.
- Talk with the dietitian to see if any special preferences can be addressed.
- Offer praise to your child for what he or she eats or drinks.
- Never punish the child for not eating or drinking.
- Encourage the older child to help keep track of what he or she eats and drinks.

Providing Play, Activities, and Recreation for the Hospitalized Child

Play is an important component in the child's plan of care. Today, many health care settings providing care for children have playrooms with age-appropriate toys, equipment, and other creative activities (Fig. 33.6). If the environment or unit setting is large enough, there may even be a separate area for teens where they can listen to music, play video games, and visit with peers.

Take Note!
Avoid using the term "playroom" when caring for older school-age children and adolescents. Instead, call it the "activity room" or "social room." Doing so promotes a greater feeling of maturity and makes it more likely that they will use the area.

Obviously, some children will not be able to use these facilities if their activity level is restricted or if isolation is necessary. Children may also play in their rooms. Ensure that opportunities for unstructured play are provided to all children who can engage in play. Therapeutic play may be used to teach children about their health status or to allow them to work through issues in their lives.

Take Note!
Keep the bed, cot, and playroom as "safe" places. Perform invasive procedures such as venipunctures in the treatment room if possible. Never perform any nursing interventions in the playroom, no matter how nonthreatening they may appear to the nurse.

FIGURE 33.6 Children occupied in a hospital pl
important to provide age-appropriate activities
and older children alike.

The nurse's greatest ally in the hospita
to atraumatic care, is the CLS. They not only
child for procedures but also provide activitie
to encourage play and normal growth and c

UNSTRUCTURED PLAY

Unstructured play allows children to co
ideas, and relationships. Encourage pare
small toys and favourite stuffed animals fr
make the child feel more comfortable in
environment of the hospital. Children also
ing small rewards such as new toys as sur
they are hospitalized. Many children enjoy
activities such as playing board games c
games, reading books, and watching TV, DV
their mobile devices. Quiet activities appro
child's developmental level provide the op
play and encourage the use and developr
motor skills, even if the child is confined to
and toddlers enjoy manipulating blocks
with stacking toys. The preschooler may e
ing, dollhouses, or playing with plastic buil
School-age children and adolescents may e

photographs back and forth between siblings, and allow siblings to talk on the phone.

Providing Child and Family Teaching

Not all experiences with hospitalization are negative; in fact, the experience may enhance the child's and family's coping skills, bolster self-esteem, and provide new socialization experiences. It may allow the child to master self-care skills and provide an opportunity for the child and family to learn new information. Parents may learn more about their child's growth and development skills, as well as additional parenting or caregiving skills, resulting in improved parenting abilities. In addition, the child's overall health may be improved because of the hospital stay and any new or associated learning.

The overall goals of child and family teaching are to minimize the child's and family's stress; educate them about treatment, nursing care, or medication management in the hospital; and ensure the family can provide appropriate care at home upon discharge. Assessing the child's and family's knowledge about the illness/disease or injury and taking time to listen to their hospital experiences are key in FCC. Providing support before, during, and after hospitalization may minimize stress and allow time for consolidated learning, relationship building, and meeting discharge needs. Using the time before discharge, the nurse can offer anticipatory guidance to focus on managing boundaries when the child is at home, recovering, and accessing support as needed for ongoing emotional issues as a result of hospital experiences. Therefore, every interaction with the child and family could provide an opportunity for teaching. Explaining, reinforcing, and revisiting information about the child's illness and treatment plan, as well as demonstrating and watching parents and children perform health care skills (i.e., measuring medications or catheterizing), can help them become confident in care at home.

Preparing the Child and Family for Discharge

Discharge planning actually begins upon admission. The goal of most hospital admissions is for the child or adolescent to return home, thus preparation for the discharge home should begin as soon as possible. The nurse and medical team assess the family's resources and knowledge level to determine what education and referrals they may need. Information, such as a discharge summary, is shared with the local primary care provider and any community team involved in the child's care. Upon discharge, children and their parents or caregivers receive written instructions about home care and a copy is retained in the medical record. These instructions are individualized for the child and may include links to

websites, support groups, and other resources. Generally, discharge instructions should include:

- Follow-up appointment information with family physician, pediatrician, specialists, and/or other providers, such as a dietician
- Guidelines about when to contact the physician or nurse practitioner (e.g., new or worsening symptoms or indications that the child is not improving) or seek emergency help
- Information about any new or altered diet
- Levels of activity level allowed over the next few weeks until a return to normal or agreed schedule is determined
- Medication prescriptions or supplies along with explicit instructions on dose, times to be given, route, adverse effects, special instructions, and storage
- Information on additional treatments the child requires at home. This may include where to obtain medical supplies (e.g., catheters) or application forms for relevant programs, such as the At Home Program; see thePoint for additional resource links
- Names and phone numbers of agencies to which the family has been referred
- Specific dates for when the child may return to school or day care, or instructions on how to apply for extended therapy to help children and youth be independent and reach educational goals

Provide and review educational booklets that give basic health information or general care for a child with a particular disease (Fig. 33.8). Online or digital resources, such as links to helpful organizations, support groups, or DVDs, may also be used if available.

Provide a written schedule or series of pictures, diagrams, or audio recordings for the family with limited or poor health literacy, especially if the child is to receive multiple medications, tube feedings, or other medical treatments. A teaching plan and record sheet may be used

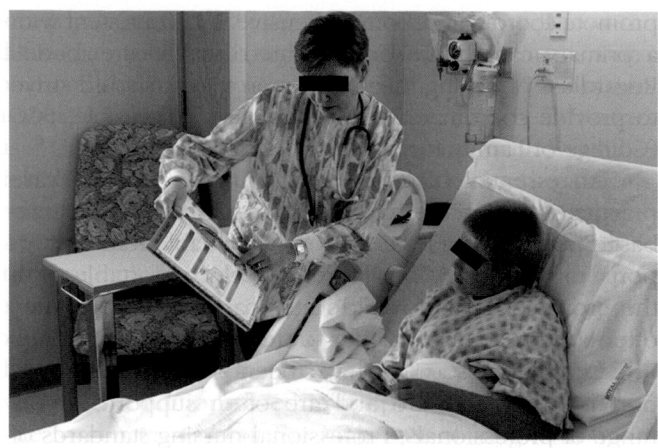

FIGURE 33.8 The nurse uses charts with pictures to perform client teaching before the child goes home.

to provide continuity of child/family education between various nurses. As the family attempts to perform each task, document whether the caregiver continues to require assistance or prompting with the task or whether he or she can perform the task independently.

Parents of children with multiple medical needs may benefit from a trial period of home care. This occurs while the child is still in the hospital, but the parents or caregivers provide all of the care that the child requires. Support the family and provide positive reinforcement in their accomplishments during this trial period.

COMMUNITY CARE IN CHILDHOOD

Remember Jake Jorgenson, the boy with suspected brain tumour from the beginning of the chapter? After a long hospital stay and complications resulting from his brain tumour, Jake requires intermittent gastrostomy feedings and has frequent respiratory infections. He has been receiving nursing care at home along with therapies, but is now ready to make the transition to the local elementary school.

Children receive most of their health care, in the community setting. Nurses play an important role in the health and wellness of a community. They not only meet the health care needs of individuals but also go beyond to create interventions that affect the community as a whole. Community health nursing refers to nursing care that strives to improve the health of a specific community as a whole (terms may vary in different settings and may include public health, primary health care, or home care nurses). Community-based nursing focuses more on providing care to the individual or family (which, of course, impacts the community) in settings outside of an acute care facility. Nurses practicing in the community promote the health of individuals, families, groups, communities, and populations, and promote an environment that supports health. See Chapter 2 for more information on Community Health and Community-Based Nursing. The following section focuses on community-based settings where nurses commonly care for children.

Community-Based Nursing Settings

Community-based nursing takes place in a variety of settings, including outpatient and ambulatory care settings, physicians' offices, clinics, health centres and nursing stations, urgent care centres, schools, camps, churches, shelters, and children's homes. Community-based nurses provide care during episodic conditions or long term for those with chronic illness or life-limiting conditions. They work to promote, preserve, and improve the health of children and families in these settings.

Outpatient and Ambulatory Care

Outpatient and ambulatory care is health care provided to individuals who do not require admission to the hospital as an inpatient. Due to advances in medical technology, more medical procedures, such as diagnostic tests, treatments, and surgeries, can be administered on an outpatient basis and do not require clients to be hospitalized. Outpatient and ambulatory care delivers convenient and cost-effective health care to children and their families, many times right within their own community. For children and youth with chronic conditions, such as diabetes, cystic fibrosis, heart conditions, and neuromuscular conditions, the majority of their care may be delivered in ambulatory settings, with hospitalizations only occurring to manage acute episodic conditions, complications, or surgery. Through these clinic visits, the pediatric patient receives surveillance of their condition, testing, teaching, and support. This can further reduce the need for hospitalization and allows the child and family to maintain a greater amount of normality in their lives. The clinic nurse may also provide phone advice and support to these families as needed.

Outpatient surgical units may be a part of the hospital or a freestanding unit. The child and family arrive in the morning; the child undergoes the procedure, test, or surgery, and then goes home in the evening. Examples of surgeries and procedures performed in outpatient settings include tympanostomy tube placement, adenoidectomy, arthroscopy of the knee, blood transfusions, dialysis, and chemotherapy. The advantages of this environment include minimal separation of the child from the family, minimal disruption of the family pattern, decreased risk of infection, and decreased cost. A and is considered an "extended service," so while there is no obligation, provinces and territories have implemented standards to address quantity and types of services provided (CHA, 2009; CHCA, 2016). The CHCA offers an inclusive definition of home care as "an array of services, provided in the home and community setting, that encompass health promotion and teaching, curative intervention, end-of-life care, rehabilitation, support and maintenance, social adaptation and integration and support for the informal (family) caregiver" (pages 21 and 22). Both the Kirby and the Romanow reports emphasized the need for an acute aspect to home care provision as well as the need to focus on priority areas including those who need ongoing care or are physically and/or mentally disabled (CHA, 2009; CHCA, 2016; Kirby & LeBreton, 2002; Romanow, 2002). Means testing within six provinces or territories informs home care access, with four provinces requiring a physician order if children are to access home care (CHA, 2009). Therefore, home care nursing access across Canada is variable for children and adolescents (up to 18 or 19 years of age). Access to home care in the acute phase of illness, for conditions and certain treatments such as IV antibiotics, may be limited by service availability, staffing, and geography.

Home care is geared toward the needs of the child and family and involves various team members working together. Provincial aid is often available to support families with the cost of caring for children with chronic medical conditions, though such financial and charitable support differs greatly across provinces. Nurses should connect with social workers to ensure that families are able to access the resources they need.

Home nursing care is used when more extensive care is needed; it may be delivered hourly (several hours per day) or on a full-time, live-in basis. Periodic visiting nursing care is used when the child needs intermittent interventions, such as IV antibiotic administration, follow-up with child and family teaching, and periodic monitoring, such as weight gain. The goals of nursing care in the home setting include promoting, restoring, and maintaining the health of the child. Home care focuses on minimizing the effects of the illness or disability, along with providing the family with support. In some cases, nurses train others and delegate components of the care to others. Nurses in the home care setting may be direct providers of care, child and family educators, advocates, or case managers. In some cases, home care nurses will provide palliative support to the child and family in the last stages of their lives.

There are added pressures on the patient and family when home care services are required. The presence of health care professionals in the home can be an intrusion on family privacy. Also, caring for children with complex medical needs can be overwhelming for some families.

FAMILY-CENTRED HOME CARE

FCC is a mainstay of pediatric nursing philosophy and is driven by evidence that a nurturing environment improves the chances of positive outcomes for the child. It places the family in a central position relative to the child and to the child's plan of care. This may include grandparents, extended family members, neighbours, and friends.

Family-centred home care focuses on increasing support for the emotional and developmental needs of the child. It encourages and supports families to confidently care for their children at home by providing advice, direction, support, empowerment, education, and expertise. In family-centred home care, the family and health care professionals build a partnership of trust to meet the needs of the child. The nurse must value the role and individuality of the child in the context of their family, while recognizing that the family members are ultimately the experts in caring for their child. In home care, the family is extensively involved in the child's care, and the home care nurse is there to facilitate and support this.

Any illness, especially a chronic illness, affects the entire family and can disrupt family structure. There is a change in the role of the parent when he or she has to care for an ill child. These role changes can result in stress for the family members and can affect their participation in the child's care. It is important for home care nurses to seek a partnership role with the family regarding care of the child. This can be difficult for both parties. Many times, nurses set limits on parental involvement and do not consider the parents' perspective, which is not consistent with an FCC approach. Many nurses are concerned that the parents may not be able to care for the child safely or may be concerned about the child's abilities to participate in decision making (Coyne, 2006). Therefore, it is important for nurses to use self-awareness and reflective practice to help them explore their reservations and perhaps reformulate this in ways that empower families and children. However, if there are child protection concerns, these need to be addressed through the appropriate child protection processes.

THE NURSE'S ROLE IN HOME CARE

Early discharge planning, teaching, and case management are key to promoting a successful transition from the hospital setting to home as the environments differ greatly. In the acute setting, the nurse is in control of the environment; in the home setting, the nurse is a guest in the home.

Nursing in the home care setting can be challenging. The focus is on meeting the child's physical, emotional, medical, and psychological needs while involving the family as active participants. Assessment in the home is similar to that in the acute care setting but involves obtaining first-hand data about the family and the way it functions. The nurse needs to assess the child's growth and development, as well as ensure the home environment offers a safe and nurturing setting for the child. In some cases, pediatric home support nursing is required postsurgery, or following discharge from a neonatal or PICU. Parents and families may be overwhelmed by the required care and technology for the child and initially need an increased level of support. Nursing support services will also provide coordination of other community-based services, locating required equipment, educating and training family members, and documenting the progress of the discharge home.

The home care nurse will also be required to assess the psychological impact on the family and their capacity to cope with the needs of their child. This includes the family's capacity to deal with the stress of the situation, follow-through on the child's care requirements, and ability to assess and contact emergency services as needed.

During the assessment phase, the nurse identifies the person who is the primary caregiver; this may be the mother, father, grandparent, or older sibling. It is essential to include this person when developing the plan of care, as he or she is the expert on the child and family. The primary caregiver can provide insight into direct care and which strategies will be most effective with this child, taking into account the physical layout of the home, the financial resources available, and the way the family functions. The home care nurse must also assess the family's learning needs in order to provide teaching that is appropriate to the educational and developmental levels of the child and family, as well as to make appropriate referrals to resources.

After the assessment is complete, the nurse develops appropriate nursing diagnoses and goals, and implements the plan of care. This will include the frequency and duration of the home visits, as well as the key nursing interventions that may be required. This nursing assessment, as well as letters from the physicians responsible for the child's care, will help to determine the number of nursing hours dedicated to the child and family. These hours are reassessed as needed to best meet the needs of the children and adolescents with complex chronic health conditions. The nurse may be the provider of

direct care to the child, or the care may be indirect, in which case the nurse plans and supervises the care that is given by others.

Nursing care in the home requires excellent critical thinking skills. The nurse has a great deal of independence, since there are no other nurses, supervisors, or physicians on site. When complex care is provided in the home, the nurse may need to adjust procedures to fit the setting. For example, feeding schedules may be adjusted to fit a child's school schedule or equipment may be adjusted to allow a child to receive feedings continuously while at school.

An important role of the home care nurse is to identify goals of home care and to empower children and their families to participate in as much of the child's care as possible. In many situations, parents or caregivers must learn all aspects of care very quickly in order to ensure the child's safety in the home setting. While there may be a steep learning curve for the patient and family, as the child grows and his or her condition stabilizes, the learning needs will change. For example, in a child with newly diagnosed diabetes, the initial learning needs will focus on monitoring and stabilization of blood glucose levels and adaptation to an altered health status. Over time, these learning needs may transition to supporting self-management in the older child or youth (Karlsson, Arman, & Wikblad, 2008). The home care nurse will have a role educating the child while supporting the parents to relinquish their control over the child's health care. As with any nursing care, the effectiveness of nursing interventions along with changes in the child's or family's status needs to be continuously evaluated and the plan of care altered as necessary.

As the home care nurse, what can you do to help with Jake's transition to school? On your last visit, Jake's parents expressed concerns about this transition and the added stress it is causing to the family. They appear tired from the round-the-clock care that Jake requires. What suggestions can you make to help ease their stress and fatigue?

NURSING CARE PLAN 33.1

Overview for the Hospitalized Child and Family

NURSING DIAGNOSIS: Anxiety related to hospital situation, fear of injury or bodily mutilation, separation from family or friends, changes in routine, painful procedures and treatments, and unfamiliar events and surroundings as evidenced by crying, fussing, withdrawal, or resistance

Outcome Identification and Evaluation

Child and family will exhibit a decrease in anxiety level as evidenced by positive coping strategies, verbalization or playing out of feelings, appropriate behaviours, positive interactions with staff, child and parent cooperation and participation, and absence of signs and symptoms of increasing anxiety and fear.

Interventions: *Minimizing Anxiety*

- Orient child and family to the unit and the child's room *to familiarize them with the setting.*
- Assess for signs and symptoms of anxiety and fear *to establish a baseline and assess effectiveness of interventions.*
- Place the child in a room with another child of a similar age, developmental level, and condition severity *to promote sharing.*
- Provide atraumatic care *to minimize exposure to distress, which would increase anxiety.*
- Explain all events, treatments, procedures, and activities to the parents and child (at a level the child can understand) in a calm, relaxed manner *to help the child prepare for what is to come and decrease fear of the unknown. A calm, relaxed manner helps to establish rapport and trust.*
- Enlist the aid of a CLS *to assist in age-appropriate preparation for all events, treatments, and procedures.*
- Encourage parents to room-in if possible *to provide the child with support;* if parents cannot stay, encourage them to call *to reduce child's fear of being alone.*

- Urge parents to inform the child when they will be leaving and when they are expected to return *to help child cope with their absence and promote trust.*
- Assess child's usual routine at home and attempt to incorporate aspects of usual routine into hospital routine *to ease the transition to the hospital and promote the child's participation in routine.*
- Offer comfort measures such as holding, stroking, and rocking *to relieve distress.*
- Encourage the child to play (unstructured and therapeutic play as necessary) *to allow for expression of feelings and fears and promote energy expenditure.*
- Suggest that parents bring in a special toy or object from home *to promote feelings of security.*
- Provide positive reinforcement for participation in care activities *to foster self-esteem.*
- Assess for regression behaviours and inform parents that such behaviours are common *to alleviate their concerns about this behaviour.*
- Provide consistency with care measures *to facilitate trust and acceptance.*

NURSING DIAGNOSIS: Risk for powerlessness (risk factors: lack of control over procedures, treatments and care, changes in usual routine, and continual hospital readmissions)

Outcome Identification and Evaluation

Child and family will demonstrate an increase in control over the situation as evidenced by participation in care activities, identification of needs and choices, and incorporation of appropriate aspects of child's usual routine with that of the hospital routine.

Interventions: *Promoting Control*

- Encourage child and parents to identify areas of concern *to help determine priority needs.*
- Encourage parent and child to participate in care activities *to promote feelings of control.*
- Incorporate aspects of child's routine at home and use terms similar to those used at home *to foster a sense of normality.*

NURSING CARE PLAN 33.1

Overview for the Hospitalized Child and Family (continued)

- Offer child choices as much as possible, such as options for foods, drinks, hygiene, activities, or clothing (if appropriate) *to promote feelings of individuality and control.*
- Allow child opportunities for being out of bed or room within limitations as appropriate *to foster independence.*
- Work with child, as age and development allow, and family to set up a schedule *to promote structure and routine.*

NURSING DIAGNOSIS: Decreased diversional activity engagement related to confinement in bed or health care setting, lack of appropriate stimulation from toys or peers, limited mobility, activity restrictions, or equipment as evidenced by verbalization of boredom or lack of participation in play, reading, or schoolwork

Outcome Identification and Evaluation

Child will participate in diversional activities, as evidenced by engagement in unstructured and therapeutic play that is developmentally appropriate and through interaction with family, staff, and other children.

Interventions: *Promoting Adequate Diversional Activities*

- Question child and family about favourite types of activities *to establish a baseline for developing appropriate choices during hospitalization.*
- Assist with planning activities within the limits of the child's condition *to maintain muscle tone and strength without overexerting the child.*
- Spend time with the child *to provide stimulation and foster trust.*
- Enlist the aid of a CLS *to provide suggestions for appropriate activities.*

- Encourage interaction with other children *to promote sharing and avoid loneliness.*
- Provide developmentally appropriate opportunities for unstructured and therapeutic play *to facilitate expression of feelings.*
- Encourage short trips to the playroom or activity room *to provide a change of scenery and sensory stimulation.*
- Integrate play activities with nursing care *to achieve therapeutic effect.*

NURSING DIAGNOSIS: Interrupted family processes related to separation from child due to hospitalization, increased demands of caring for an ill child, changes in role function and routine, and effect of hospitalization on other family members such as siblings, as evidenced by parental verbalization of issues, parental presence in hospital, or child's hospitalization requiring parent to miss work

Outcome Identification and Evaluation

Family will demonstrate positive coping strategies and mutual support for one another as evidenced by visiting frequently and staying with the child as necessary, sharing of family responsibilities, obtaining assistance for relief or respite, and visiting by other members of the child's family and friends.

Interventions: *Maximizing Family Functioning*

- Encourage parents and family members to verbalize concerns about child's illness, diagnosis, and prognosis *to promote family-centred care and identify areas where intervention may be needed.*
- Explain therapies, procedures, child's behaviours, and plan of care to parents *to promote understanding of*

the child's status and plan of care, and to decrease anxiety.
- Encourage parental involvement in care *to promote feelings of the parents being needed and valued, providing them with a sense of control over their child's health.*

(continued)

NURSING CARE PLAN 33.1

Overview for the Hospitalized Child and Family (continued)

- Identify support system for family and child *to identify resources available for coping.*
- Educate family and child on additional resources available *to promote a wider base of support to deal with the situation.*
- Suggest ways that parents can divide time between child and other siblings *to prevent feelings of guilt.*
- Provide support and positive reinforcement *to promote family coping and foster family strength.*
- Encourage frequent visits by family members, including siblings as appropriate, *to promote ongoing family functioning.*

- Stress the need for adequate rest, sleep, exercise, and nutrition for family members *to promote family health and minimize stress of hospitalization on family.*
- Assist with referrals for resources and help from additional family members and friends as necessary *to allow for respite or relief of care responsibilities.*
- Encourage family to maintain usual routine as much as possible *to minimize the effects of hospitalization on family functioning.*
- Enlist the aid of a CLS to work with any siblings *to provide support and education and to address the needs of a sibling of a hospitalized child.*

NURSING DIAGNOSIS: Bathing self-care deficit, dressing self-care deficit, feeding self-care deficit related to immobility, activity restrictions, regression, or use of equipment, devices, or prescribed treatments as evidenced by inability to feed, bathe, or dress self or accomplish other activities of daily living

Outcome Identification and Evaluation

Child will participate in self-care within limitations of condition as evidenced by assisting with bathing and hygiene, feeding, toileting, and dressing and grooming.

Interventions: *Promoting Self-Care*

- Assess child's usual routine for self-care and self-care abilities *to provide a baseline for individualizing interventions.*
- Provide child-sized equipment and devices *to promote child's ability to complete the self-care task.*
- Encourage parents and child to do as much self-care as possible, within limitations of the child's condi-

tion and developmental level, *to promote feelings of independence and foster growth and development.*
- Offer praise and encouragement for activities performed *to foster self-esteem, confidence, and competence.*
- Ensure adequate rest periods *to minimize energy expenditure associated with self-care activities.*

NURSING DIAGNOSIS: Risk for delayed development (risk factors: stressors associated with hospitalization, current condition or illness, separation from family, and sensory overload or sensory deprivation)

Outcome Identification and Evaluation

Child will demonstrate developmentally appropriate milestones as evidenced by age-appropriate behaviours and activities.

Interventions: *Promoting Growth and Development*

- Assess child's developmental stage *to establish a baseline and determine appropriate strategies.*
- Use unstructured and therapeutic play and adaptive toys *to promote developmental functioning.*
- Provide stimulating environment when possible *to maximize potential for growth and development.*
- Praise accomplishments and emphasize child's abilities *to foster self-esteem and encourage feelings of confidence and competence.*
- Include parents in techniques to foster growth and development *to promote feelings of control in their child's care.*

NURSING CARE PLAN 33.1

Overview for the Hospitalized Child and Family (continued)

NURSING DIAGNOSIS: Deficient knowledge related to hospitalization, surgery, treatments, procedures, required care, and follow-up as evidenced by questioning and verbalization, lack of prior exposure

Outcome Identification and Evaluation

Child and family will demonstrate understanding of all aspects of child's current situation as evidenced by identification of child's and family's needs, verbal statements of understanding and/or need for additional information, return demonstration of procedures and treatments, and verbalization of instructions for follow-up and continued care.

Interventions: *Providing Child and Family Teaching*

- Assess child's and family's willingness to learn *to ensure effective teaching.*
- Provide family with time to adjust to diagnosis *to facilitate their ability to learn and participate in the child's care.*
- Repeat information *to promote multiple opportunities for child and family to learn.*
- Teach in short sessions *to prevent overloading the child and parents with information.*
- Gear teaching to appropriate level of understanding for the child and the family (depends on age of child, physical condition, memory) *to promote learning.*
- Provide reinforcement and rewards *to facilitate the teaching/learning process.*

- Use multiple modes of learning, such as written information, verbal instruction, demonstrations, and media, when possible *to facilitate learning and retention of information.*
- Provide the child and family with written step-by-step instructions for procedures or care *to provide a reference, if needed, at a later date.*
- Have child and family provide return demonstrations of care procedures *to ensure effectiveness of teaching.*
- Arrange for trial home care during hospitalization and after discharge as appropriate *to ensure understanding and provide opportunities for additional teaching and learning.*

KEY CONCEPTS

- Stressors associated with hospitalization include separation from family and routines; fear of an unknown environment; potential for pain, bodily injury, or mutilation; and loss of control.

- Responses of children to the general stressors of hospitalization include anxiety, fear, anger, guilt, and regression.

- Parents may experience anger or guilt related to the hospitalization of their child.

- The responses of children and families to hospitalization can be influenced by the age and developmental level of the child, their perceptions of the situation, previous experiences, separation from family and peers, coping skills, and the preparation and support provided by the family, health care providers, and the nature of

the setting in which children access healthcare services.

- Play, including therapeutic play, is an important strategy to prepare children for hospitalization and to help them adapt to the effects of illness and hospitalization. It provides an emotional outlet, opportunities for teaching and learning, and the ability to become familiar with a situation and improve physiologic abilities. A CLS is a specially trained individual who is a member of the child's multidisciplinary team. He or she works in conjunction with the child's health care providers and parents to foster an atmosphere that promotes the child's well-being.

- FCC and atraumatic care are philosophies that pay special attention to the concerns of the family and child during hospitalization.

- Providing support to hospitalized children and their families is critical for minimizing stress.

- Whatever the reason for admission, preparation for admission is vital.

- Upon admission to the hospital or outpatient unit, orient the child and family to the unit, discuss unit policies and routines and the personnel who will be involved in the care of the child, and begin child/family teaching.

- Establish a trusting, caring relationship with the child and family. Let the child and family know what will happen and what is expected of them. Obtain information about the child's history, routines, and reason for admission. Obtain baseline vital signs and height and weight, and perform a physical assessment. Each health care setting has its own policies and procedures for this.

- Due to their age and developmental level, children may be vulnerable to harm, and the nurse must use appropriate safety measures in caring for children (e.g., identification of children, use of restraints and transportation, basic hygiene measures). These measures need to address developmental risks, such as that the infants, toddlers, and preschoolers require close supervision and the nurse must avoid leaving small objects within reach.

- Discharge planning begins upon admission. Each interaction with the family is an opportunity for child and family teaching.

- Provide and review discharge instructions with the child and primary caregiver. Use educational booklets or media such as videos or DVDs that give basic health information or general care for a child with a particular disease or health issue.

- Explain, demonstrate, and request a return demonstration of any treatments or procedures to be done at home. Provide a written schedule if the child is to receive multiple medications, tube feedings, or other medical treatments.

- Community-based nurses focus on the practice of nursing that provides personal care to children and families in the community. These nurses focus on promoting and preserving health as well as preventing disease or injury. They help children and their families cope with illness and disease. They are direct providers of care as well as advocates and educators working to minimize and remove barriers to allow the child to develop to his or her full potential.

- Due to the short lengths of stay in acute settings and the shift to home care for children with complex health needs, discharge planning and case management have become important nursing roles. Discharge planning provides a comprehensive plan for the safe discharge of a child from a health care setting and for continuing safe and effective care at home. Case management focuses on coordinating health care services while balancing quality and cost outcomes. Both contribute to improved transitions from hospital to home for children, their families, and the health care team.

- Nursing in the home care setting can be challenging. The focus is on meeting the child's physical and psychological needs while involving the family. Health care professionals provide the support, empowerment, education, and expertise in caring for the child that families need.

- Goals of the nurse in the home care setting include promoting, restoring, and maintaining the health of the child. Home care focuses on minimizing the effects of the illness or disability and providing the child or family with the means to care for the illness or disability at home. Nurses in the home care setting are direct providers of care, child and family educators, child and family advocates, and case managers.

- Community-based nursing takes place in a variety of settings, including physicians' offices, clinics, health centres and nursing stations, urgent care centres, clients' homes, schools, camps, churches, and shelters (such as shelters for abused women, homeless shelters, and disaster shelters). Nurses provide wellness care to enhance well-being (i.e. health promotion and prevention), episodic ill care, and chronic care to children and their families in these various settings.

- Advantages of home care include shorter hospital stays and decreased health care costs, but the major advantage of home care is the comfort and family support it provides, promoting an improved quality of life for these children. Caring for children at home not only improves their physical health but also allows for adequate growth and development while keeping them within their family.

- Disadvantages to home care include intrusion on family privacy. Caring for children with complex medical needs can be overwhelming for some families, and financial issues related to home care can become a large burden to families.

REFERENCES AND RECOMMENDED READINGS

Adamson, P. (2013). *UNICEF Office of Research. Innocenti Report Card 11*. Retrieved from https://www.unicef-irc.org/publications/series/16

Adelson, N. (2005). The embodiment of inequity: Health disparities in Aboriginal Canada. *Canadian Journal of Public Health/Revue Canadienne de Santé Publique, 96*(Suppl. 2), S45–S61.

Ainsworth, M. D. S. (1990). Some considerations regarding theory and assessment relevant to attachments beyond infancy. In M. T. Greenberg, D. Cicchetti, & E. M. Cummings (Eds.). *Attachment in preschool years: Theory, research, and interventions* (pp. 463–488). Chicago, IL: University of Chicago Press.

Ali, S., Thomson, D., Graham, T. A., Rickard, S. E., & Stang, A. S. (2017). High stakes and high emotions: Providing safe care in Canadian emergency departments. *Open Access Emergency Medicine: OAEM, 9,* 23–26.

Allison, S. (2016). *Chief Medical Health Officer child health status report (technical report).* Retrieved from https://northernhealth.ca/Portals/0/About/Community_Accountability/documents/CMHO-Child-Health-Status-Technical-Report.pdf

Amin, R., Sayal, P., Syed, F., Chaves, A., Moraes, T. J., & MacLusky, I. (2014). Pediatric long-term home mechanical ventilation: Twenty years of follow-up from one Canadian center. *Pediatric Pulmonology, 49*(8), 816–824.

Amin, R., Sayal, A., Syed, F., Daniels, C., Hoffman, A., Moraes, T. J., & Cox, P. (2015). How long does it take to initiate a child on long-term invasive ventilation? Results from a Canadian pediatric home ventilation program. *Canadian Respiratory Journal, 22*(2), 103–108.

Banerji, A., Panzov, V., Young, M., Robinson, J., Lee, B., Moraes, T., . . . Mahony, J. B. (2016). Hospital admissions for lower respiratory tract infections among infants in the Canadian Arctic: A cohort study. *CMAJ Open, 4*(4), E615–E622.

Berlin, E. A., & Fowkes, W. C., Jr. (1983). A teaching framework for cross-cultural health care. Application in family practice. *The Western Journal of Medicine, 139*(6), 934–938.

Bowden, V. R., & Greenberg, C. S. (2011). *Pediatric nursing procedures* (3rd ed.). Philadelphia, PA: Lippincott Williams & Wilkins.

Bowlby, J. (1973). *Attachment and loss: Vol II.* New York: Basic Books.

Bray, L., Carter, B., & Snodin, J. (2016). Holding children for clinical procedures: Perseverance in spite of or persevering to be child-centered. *Research in Nursing & Health, 39*(1), 30–41.

Bray, L., Snodin, J., & Carter, B. (2015). Holding and restraining children for clinical procedures within an acute care setting: An ethical consideration of the evidence. *Nursing Inquiry, 22*(2), 157–167.

Bretherton, I. (1992). The origins of attachment theory: John Bowlby and Mary Ainsworth. *Developmental Psychology, 28,* 759–775.

Browne, G., Birch, S., & Thabane, L. (2012). Better care: An analysis of nursing and healthcare system outcome. *CAN/CHSRF Report.* Retrieved from http://www.cfhi-fcass.ca/Libraries/Commissioned_Research_Reports/Browne-BetterCare-EN.sflb.ashx

Canadian Association of Paediatric Health Centres. (2016). *Listening to the voice of the child: An inclusive approach to ethical problems in paediatrics.* Retrieved from http://us1.campaign-archive1.com/?u=a34911d22f75af15c621abd3b&id=0463e347ab

Canadian Healthcare Association. (2009). *Home care in Canada: From the margins to the mainstream.* Retrieved from http://www.healthcarecan.ca/wp-content/uploads/2012/11/Home_Care_in_Canada_From_the_Margins_to_the_Mainstream_web.pdf

Canadian Home Care Association. (2016). *Home and community-based services and supports. Children with complex care needs.* Retrieved from http://www.cdnhomecare.ca/media.php?mid=4684Canadian Institute for Health Information

Canadian Institute for Health Information (CIHI). (2005). *Hospital trends in Canada. Results of a project to create a historical series of statistical and financial data for Canadian hospitals over twenty-seven years.* Retrieved from https://secure.cihi.ca/free_products/Hospital_Trends_in_Canada_e.pdf

Canadian Institutes of Health Research. (2013). *IHDCYH strategic plan 2013-2017: Healthy foundations of life.* Retrieved from http://www.cihr-irsc.gc.ca/e/47570.html

Canadian Nurses Association. (2013). *Optimizing the role of nursing in home health.* Retrieved from https://www.cna-aiic.ca/en

Canadian Paediatric Society. (2018). *Caring for kids new to Canada.* Retrieved from https://www.kidsnewtocanada.ca

Canadian Research Network for Care in the Community & the Children and Youth Home Care Network. (n.d.). *Caring for children, youth and families in home and community: Innovations and best practices from across Canada.* Retrieved from http://www.ryerson.ca/crncc/events-alphabetical-sort/caringforchildren

Carnevale, F. A., Canoui, P., Cremer, R., Farrell, C., Doussau, A., Seguin, M. J., . . . Larcroix, J. (2007). Parental involvement in treatment decisions regarding their critically ill child: A comparative study of France and Quebec. *Pediatric Critical Care Medicine, 8*(4), 337–342.

Carnevale, F. A., Farrell, C., Cremer, R., Séguret, S., Canouï, P., Leclerc, F., . . . Hubert, P. (2016). Communication in pediatric critical care: A proposal for an evidence-informed framework. *Journal of Child Health Care, 20*(1), 27–36.

Carnevale, F. A., Teachman, G., & Bogossian, A. (2017). A relational ethics framework for advancing practice with children with complex health care needs and their parents. *Comprehensive Child and Adolescent Nursing, 40*(4), 268–284.

Carpenito, L. J. (2013). *Nursing diagnosis: Application to clinical practice* (14th ed.). Philadelphia, PA: Lippincott Williams & Wilkins.

Carter, B., Bray, L., Dickinson, A., Edwards, M., & Ford, K. (2014). *Child-centred nursing: Promoting critical thinking.* Thousand Oaks, CA: Sage Publications Ltd.

Centers for Medicare & Medicaid Services (CMS). (2014). *State operations manual appendix A—survey protocol, regulations and interpretive guidelines for hospitals.* Retrieved from http://www.cms.gov/Regulations-and-Guidance/Guidance/Manuals/downloads/som107ap_a_hospitals.pdf

Child Life Council. (2018). *How do certified child life specialists help?* Retrieved from https://www.childlife.org/resources/for-parents-and-caregivers

Chundamala, J., Wright, J. G., & Kemp, S. M. (2009). An evidence-based review of parental presence during anaesthesia induction and parent/child anxiety. *Canadian Journal of Anaesthesia, 56*(1), 57–70.

Cohen, E., Kuo, D. Z., Agrawal, R., Berry, J. G., Bhagat, S. K., Simon, T. D., & Srivastava, R. (2011). Children with medical complexity: An emerging population for clinical and research initiatives. *Pediatrics, 127*(3), 529–538.

College of Family Physicians of Canada. (2011). *A vision for Canada. Family practice: The patient's medical home.* Retrieved from https://www.cfpc.ca/A_Vision_for_Canada/

Connors, C., & Millar, W. J. (1999). Changes in children's hospital use. *Health Reports, 11*(2), 9–19. Statistics Canada Catalogue 82-003. Retrieved from http://www.statcan.gc.ca/pub/82-003-x/1999002/article/4732-eng.pdf

Coyne, I. (2006). Consultation with children in hospital: Children, parents' and nurses' perspectives. *Journal of Clinical Nursing, 15*(1), 61–71.

Coyne, I., & Kirwan, L. (2012). Ascertaining children's wishes and feelings about hospital life. *Journal of Child Health Care, 16*(3), 293–304.

Crole, N., & Smith, L. (2002). Examining the phases of nursing care of the hospitalized child. *Australian Nursing Journal, 9*(8), 30–31.

de Leeuw, S. (2017). Honesty, not forgetting, and our fragile world: Linking ecological action and clinical encounters. *Canadian Family Physician, 63*(4), 308–311.

DesMeules, M., Pong, R., Lagace, C., Heng, D., Manuel, D., Pitblado, R., . . . Koren, I. (2006). How healthy are rural Canadians? An assessment of their health status and health determinants. *Canadian Institute for Health Information.* Retrieved from https://secure.cihi.ca/free_products/summary_rural_canadians_2006_e.pdf

Dowshen, S. (2014). Preparing Your Child for Surgery. *Kids Health.* Retrieved from https://kidshealth.org/en/parents/hosp-surgery.html

Elias, E. R., Murphy, N. A.; Council on Children with Disabilities. (2012). Home care of children and youth with complex health care needs and technology dependencies. *Pediatrics, 129*(5), 996–1005.

Emanuel, L. L., Taylor L., Hain, A., Combes, J. R., Hatlie, M. J., Karsh, B., … Walton, M, eds. (2017). The Patient Safety Education Program. Module 13d: Mental Health Care: Seclusion and Restraint: When All Else Fails. Ontario, Canada: The Patient saftey Education Program (TM). Retrieved from https://www.patientsafetyinstitute.ca/en/education/PatientSafetyEducationProgram/PatientSafetyEducationCurriculum/Documents/Module%2013d%20Seclusion%20and%20Restraint.pdf

Findlay, S., Pinzon, J., Goldberg, E., & Frappier, J. Y. (2008). Issues of care for hospitalized youth. *Paediatrics & Child Health, 13*(1), 61–64.

First Call BC Child Poverty Report Card. (2018). *1 out of 5 BC children are poor.* Retrieved from https://still1in5.ca

Ford, K., Dickinson, A., Water, T., Campbell, S., Bray, L. & Carter, B. (2018). Child-centred care: Challenging assumptions and repositioning children and young people. *Journal of Pediatric Nursing.* 43, e39–e43. Retrieved from https://www.sciencedirect.com/science/article/pii/S0882596318301660

Ford-Jones, E. L., Williams, R., & Bertrand, J. (2008). Social paediatrics and early child development: Part 1. *Paediatrics & Child Health, 13*(9), 755–758.

Forsner, M., Jansson, L., & Soderberg, A. (2009). Afraid of medical care school-aged children's narratives about medical fear. *Journal of Pediatric Nursing, 24*(6), 519–528.

Franck, L. S., Ferguson, D., Fryda, S., & Rubin, N. (2015). The child and family hospital experience: Is it influenced by family accommodation? *Medical Care Research and Review, 72*(4), 419–437.

Franck, L. S., Gay, C. L., & Rubin, N. (2013). Accommodating families during a child's hospital stay: Implications for family experience and perceptions of outcomes. *Families, Systems, & Health, 31*(3), 294–306.

Franck, L. S., Wray, J., Gay, C., Dearmun, A. K., Lee, K., & Cooper, B. A. (2015). Predictors of parent post-traumatic stress symptoms after child hospitalization on general pediatric wards: A prospective cohort study. *International Journal of Nursing Studies, 52*(1), 10–21.

Government of Canada. (2018). *Nursing.* Retrieved from https://www.canada.ca/en/services/health.html

Gravdal Kvarme, L., Albertini-Früh, E., Brekke, I., Gardsjord, R., Halvorsrud, L., & Liden, H. (2016). On duty all the time: Health and quality of life among immigrant parents caring for a child with complex health needs. *Journal of Clinical Nursing, 25*(3-4), 362–371.

Gushulak, B. D., Pottie, K., Roberts, J. H., Torres, S., & DesMeules, M. (2011). Migration and health in Canada: Health in the global village. *Canadian Medical Association Journal, 183*(12), E952–E958.

Hart, R., & Rollins, J. (2011). Chapter 1: Separation & stranger anxiety. In *Therapeutic activities for children and teens coping with health issues* (pp. 1–22). Hoboken, NJ: John Wiley & Sons, Inc.

Hummelinck, A., & Pollock, K. (2006). Parents' information needs about the treatment of their chronically ill child: A qualitative study. *Patient Education and Counseling, 62*(2), 228–234.

Infants Act. (1996). *Section 17 Children and Consent to Medical Treatment.* Retrieved from www.cbabc.org

Jacob, G., Ford-Jones, L., Wong, P. D., Warman, D., & Lovett, M. W. (2018). Literacy promotion by health care professionals: A comprehensive biomedical and psychosocial approach. *Paediatrics & Child Health, 23*, 6–11.

Jensen, C. S., Jackson, K., Kolbæk, R., & Glasdam, S. (2012). Children's experiences of acute hospitalization to a paediatric emergency and assessment unit—A qualitative study. *Journal of Child Health Care, 16*(3), 263–273.

Kangasniemi, M., Papinaho, O., & Korhonen, A. (2014). Nurses' perceptions of the use of restraint in pediatric somatic care. *Nursing Ethics, 21*(5), 608–620.

Karlsson, A., Arman, M., & Wikblad, K. (2008). Teenagers with type 1 diabetes—a phenomenological study of the transition towards autonomy in self-management. *International Journal of Nursing Studies, 45*(4), 562–570.

Kirby, M., & LeBreton, M. (2002). The health of Canadians—The federal role. Final report. Volume six: Recommendations for reform. *Ottawa: Government of Canada.* Retrieved from https://sencanada.ca/content/sen/committee/372/soci/rep/repoct02vol6part1-e.htm

Kirwan, L., & Coyne, I. (2016). Use of restraint with hospitalized children: A survey of nurses' perceptions of practices. *Journal of Child Health Care.* doi: https://doi.org/10.1177/1367493516666730

Kitson, A., Marshall, A., Bassett, K., & Zeitz, K. (2013). What are the core elements of patient-centered care? A narrative review and synthesis of the literature from health policy, medicine and nursing. *Journal of Advanced Nursing, 69*(1), 4–15.

Knight, K., Kenny, A., & Endacott, R. (2015). Assessing clinical urgency via telephone in rural Australia. *Nursing & Health Sciences, 17*(2), 201–207.

Kobak, R., & Madsen, S. D. (2008). The emotional dynamic of disruptions in attachment relationships: Implications for theory, research and clinical interventions. In J. Cassidy & P. R. Shaver (Eds.). *Handbook of attachment,* 1st ed. New York. Guilford Press. pp. 23–47.

Lambert, V., Glacken, M., & McCarron, M. (2013). Meeting the information needs of children in hospital. *Journal of Child Health Care, 17*(4), 338–353.

McNeil, S. A., Qizilbash, N., Ye, J., Gray, S., Zanotti, G., Munson, S., . . . Laferriere, C. (2016). A retrospective study of the clinical burden of hospitalized all-cause and pneumococcal pneumonia in Canada. *Canadian Respiratory Journal.* Retrieved from https://www.hindawi.com/journals/crj/2016/3605834/abs

Ministry of Health. (2012). *Secure rooms and seclusion standards and guidelines: A literature and evidence review.* Retrieved from http://www.health.gov.bc.ca/library/publications/year/2012/secure-rooms-seclusion-guidelines-lit-review.pdf

Minore, B., Boone, M., Arthur, A., & Sullivan, J. (2005). *Managing continuity of care for children with special needs in rural and remote parts of Northern Ontario.* Canadian Health Services Foundation (CHSF). Retrieved from http://www.cfhi-fcass.ca/Migrated/PDF/ResearchReports/OGC/minore2_final.pdf

Murphy, N. A., Carbone, P. S.; Council on Children with Disabilities. (2011). Parent-provider-community partnerships: Optimizing outcomes for children with disabilities. *Pediatrics, 128*(4), 795–802.

Nagle, L. M., & White, P. (2016). *National Nursing Data Standards Symposium Proceedings.* Retrieved from https://www.cna-aiic.ca/~/media/cna/page-content/pdf-en/national-nursing-data-standards-symposium-proceedings-report.pdf?la=en

Nakeyar, C., Esses, V., & Reid, G. J. (2017). The psychosocial needs of refugee children and youth and best practices for filling these needs: A systematic review. *Clinical Child Psychology and Psychiatry, 23*(2), 186–208.

O'Brien, K., Bracht, M., Macdonell, K., McBride, T., Robson, K., O'Leary, L., . . . Lee, S. K. (2013). A pilot cohort analytic study of family integrated care in a Canadian neonatal intensive care unit. *BMC Pregnancy and Childbirth, 13*(1), S12.

Open Minds, Healthy Minds: Ontario's Comprehensive Mental Health and Addictions Strategy. (2011). Retrieved from http://www.health.gov.on.ca/en/common/ministry/publications/reports/mental_health2011/mentalhealth_rep2011.pdf

Peltz, A., Wu, C. L., White, M. L., Wilson, K. M., Lorch, S. A., Thurm, C., . . . Berry, J. G. (2016). Characteristics of rural children admitted to pediatric hospitals. *Pediatrics, 137*(5), e20153156. Retrieved from http://pediatrics.aappublications.org/content/early/2016/04/07/peds

Prchal, A., Graf, A., Bergstraesser, E., & Landolt, M. A. (2012). A two-session psychological intervention for siblings of pediatric cancer patients: A randomized controlled pilot trial. *Child and Adolescent Psychiatry and Mental Health, 6,* 3. doi:10.1186/1753–2000–6–3

Public Health Agency of Canada. (2005). *The Rural Think Tank 2005—Understanding issues families face living in rural and remote communities.* Retrieved from http://www.phac-aspc.gc.ca/hp-ps/dca-dea/publications/rtt-grr-2005/2-eng.php#jmp-lan1

Ralph, S. S., & Taylor, C. M. (2011). *Nursing diagnosis pocket guide.* Philadelphia, PA: Wolters Kluwer/Lippincott Williams & Wilkins.

Randall, D., & Hill, A. (2012). Consulting children and young people on what makes a good nurse. *Nursing Children & Young People, 24,* 14–19.

Rasmussen, S., Water, T., & Dickinson, A. (2017). Children's perspectives in family-centred hospital care. *Contemporary Nurse,* 1–11. https://doi.org/10.1080/10376178.2017.1315829

Reading, C. L., & Wien, F. (2009). *Health inequalities and the social determinants of Aboriginal peoples' health.* Prince George, BC: National Collaborating Centre for Aboriginal Health. Retrieved from http://www.nccah-ccnsa.ca/docs/social%20determinates/nccah-loppie-wien_report.pdf

Rennick, J. E., Dougherty, G., Chambers, C., Stremler, R., Childerhose, J. E., Stack, D. M., . . . Hutchison, J. (2014). Children's psychological and behavioral responses following pediatric intensive care unit hospitalization: The caring intensively study. *BMC Pediatrics, 14*(1), 276.

Reuben, A., Moffitt, T. E., Caspi, A., Belsky, D. W., Harrington, H., Schroeder, F., . . . Danese, A. (2016). Lest we forget: Comparing retrospective and prospective assessments of adverse childhood experiences in the prediction of adult health. *Journal of Child Psychology and Psychiatry, and Allied Disciplines, 57*(10), 1103–1112.

Romanow, R. (2002). *Building on values: Report of the commission on the future of health care in Canada [Discussion Papers].*

Salmela, M., Salanterä, S., & Aronen, E. (2009). Child-reported hospital fears in 4 to 6 year-old-children. *Pediatric Nursing, 35*(5), 269–278.

Sanders, C., Edwards, Z., & Keegan, K. (2017). Exploring stakeholder experiences of interprofessional teamwork in sex development outpatient clinics. *Journal of Interprofessional Care, 31,* 376–385.

Shadow Buddies Foundation. (2014). *Shadow buddies foundation.* Retrieved from http://www.shadowbuddies.org

Shamian, J., & Lightstone, E. Y. (1997). Hospital restructuring initiatives in Canada. *Medical Care, 35*(10), OS62–OS69.

Shields, L. (2015). What is "family-centred care"? *European Journal for Person Centered Healthcare, 3*(2), 139–144.

Shields, L., Mamun, A. A., Flood, K., & Combs, S. (2014). Measuring family-centred care: working with children and their parents in two second level hospitals in Australia. *European Journal for Person Centered Healthcare, 2*(2), 206–211.

Smith, N. M., & Satyshur, R. D. (2016). Pediatric diabetes telemedicine program improves access to care for rural families: Role of APRNs. *Pediatric Nursing, 42*(6), 294–299.

Smyth, W., Kruze, R., Al Mamun, A., White, A., & Shields, L. (2016). Working with families in community services: Multidisciplinary perceptions of working with children and their parents. *Neonatal, Paediatric & Child Health Nursing, 19*(1), 18–23.

Somanadhan, S., & Larkin, P. J. (2016). Parents' experiences of living with, and caring for children, adolescents and young adults with mucopolysaccharidosis (MPS). *Orphanet Journal of Rare Diseases, 11*(1), 138.

Spalding, K., Watkins, J. R., & Williams, A. P. (2006). *Self managed care programs in Canada: A report to Health Canada.* Retrieved from https://www.canada.ca/content/dam/canada/health-canada/migration/healthy-canadians/publications/health-system-systeme-sante/2006-self-managed-soins-autogeres/alt/2006-self-managed-soins-autogeres-eng.pdf

Globally and within Canada children and youth with special, additional, or ongoing health care needs or disability can often be a marginalized group (UNICEF, 2013). The term "children with special health care needs" (SHCN) describes a broad range of behavioural, learning, emotional, developmental, medical, or psychiatric conditions (Dewan & Cohen, 2013). As such there are a growing number of terms used to describe the characteristics of **chronic illness**/disease and disability in children and youth (Box 34.1).

Children with SHCN may include those born with congenital anomalies and/or prematurity. These families experience a rapid learning trajectory that includes acquiring nursing and medical skills, possibly involving technologic devices required to support their child's well-being. In reality, families have to learn to care for their child with SHCN (Fig. 34.1). Gaining access to medication and equipment; education on the child's condition; and navigating the enhanced health resources such as speech therapy, occupational therapy, play therapy, physiotherapy, and mental health services all pose new social challenges that the family must navigate (Pearson & Li, 2015). Indigenous children and youth must have equal access to care without delay or disruption (Canadian Paediatric Society [CPS], 2016).

Nurses are in unique positions to have a significant and positive influence on the lives of these children and

FIGURE 34.1 **The special needs child often requires a significant amount of care at home throughout his life.**

BOX 34.1

TERMS ASSOCIATED WITH CHRONIC ILLNESS, DISEASE, AND DISABILITY

More common terms linked to children with special needs are those with physical disability, chronic conditions, intellectual disabilities, emotional problems, activity limitations, or learning disabilities (**https://www.ccsd.ca/index.php/evidence/research**).

Chronic condition—A condition that interferes with daily functioning for more than 3 months or results in hospitalization for more than 1 month per year or is likely to. Examples include diabetes, asthma, allergy, kidney disease.

Congenital disability—A disability that has existed from birth but not necessarily hereditary.

Acquired disability—These often stem from either an accident-related injury (head injury, spinal injury), an illness, or a health-related event (mental illness, stroke).

Developmental disability—Any mental or physical disability apparent before 22 years of age likely to continue in to adult life.

Developmental delay—Can be associated with prematurity, illness, or of unknown cause; described as an abnormal or slower rate of development than expected for age.

Disability—A temporary, prolonged, or permanent reduction or absence of the ability to perform certain common activities or roles. Examples include loss or reduction of hearing, vision, language, mobility, cognition, and recall.

Impairment—Is an abnormality in an organ or in a physical or mental function of the body that results in disability. Examples include partial or complete loss of a limb, cerebral palsy, neurologic disease or injury.

Learning difficulty—CICH reports this as the most common type of long-term condition in young Canadian children (0 to 14 years). Learning disabilities refer to a number of disorders which may affect the acquisition, organization, retention, understanding, or use of verbal or nonverbal information; these are distinct from global intellectual deficiency.

Life-limiting illness—Any birth condition, illness, or condition developed in childhood whereby the child's life expectancy is limited.

Technology-dependent child—A child from birth to 21 years of age with a chronic disability that requires the routine use of a medical device, that is, hearing aid, respiratory support.

Children with medical complexity—Presence of one or more complex chronic diseases often multisystem and severe necessitating specialized care; functional disability; and high health care utilization.

From The Canadian Encyclopedia. Retrieved from http://www.thecanadianencyclopedia.ca/en/article/disability/; The Canadian Council on Social Development (CCSD) Disability Research. Retrieved from http://www.ccsd.ca/index.php/about/24-site-pages/evidence/disability-research/47-disability-research; Children and Youth With Special Needs. Retrieved from http://www.ccsd.ca/images/research/DisabilityResearch/PDF/ChildrenYouthSpecialNeeds_2001.pdf; National Children's Alliance. Retrieved from https://www.nationalchildrensalliance.org/; Learning Disabilities Association of Canada. Retrieved from http://www.ldac-acta.ca/learn-more/ld-defined/official-definition-of-learning-disabilities; Centre for Excellence for Children & Adolescents With Special Needs. Retrieved from http://specialneedsproject.ca/resources/publications/resource-guide; and Dewan, T., & Cohen, E. (2013). Children with medical complexity in Canada. *Paediatrics & Child Health, 18*(10), 518–522. Retrieved from http://europepmc.org/articles/pmc3907346

their families, whether in the inpatient, outpatient, ambulatory clinic, community care, home, or school settings, as well as within any community context working with children and youth. For children with SHCN in addition to providing direct care, the nurse fills the critical role of child and family advocate and case manager throughout the trajectory of the child's condition. The role of the nurse extends from physical care into supporting families' access to spiritual care, as they meet the emotional needs of the child and family during diagnosis, care, treatment, and in some cases through palliation and death.

SCOPE

The participation and activities limitation surveys (Statistics Canada, 2006) estimated that 202,350 children between the ages of 4 and 14 years had activity limitations, for example, musculoskeletal impairments, speech defects, hearing loss, blindness, or visual impairment (Early Childhood Development, 2011; Pinzon & Harvey, 2006). However, when including all ages of Canadian children with SHCN prevalence is suggested as around 500,000 (SandBox Project, 2011). The most common chronic health conditions include respiratory conditions (e.g., asthma) and diabetes, often resulting in increased morbidity and mortality (Shooshtari et al., 2016). Improved medical technology and access to pediatric care has decreased the morbidity of children with chronic complex medical conditions with over 98% surviving to transfer to the adult health care system (Cohen et al., 2016). This group of youth and young adults includes young adults living with cerebral palsy and spina bifida (Metcalfe, 2017; Wajchendler, Anderson, & Koyle, 2017); young men living with muscular dystrophy beyond 25 years of age (Eagle et al., 2002); and individuals with cystic fibrosis in Canada (Cystic Fibrosis Canada, 2018). Childhood obesity is an increasing chronic health problem with recent statistics indicating that 13% of children and adolescents aged 3 to 19 years in Canada are classified as obese (Statistics Canada, 2015a).

The effects of illness such as childhood cancer can result in disability, chronic disease, or the need for end-of-life care. Between 2006 and 2010, an average of 905 new cases of cancer were diagnosed each year in children under the age of 15 years, while an average of 129 children in the same age group died annually from the disease (Statistics Canada, 2015b).

In Canada, it is estimated that 20% to 25% of children and youth are affected by mental health difficulties (Chief Public Health Officer Report on State of Public Health in Canada, 2011). For those youth who identify as two spirited, lesbian, gay, bisexual, transgender, or questioning (LGBTQ2S), mental and emotional well-being can be influenced by many factors including feelings of belonging to their school community (Burk, Park, & Saewyc, 2018).

Within Canada data from the National Longitudinal Survey of Children and Youth (NLSCY) have helped researchers better understand the needs and assess outcomes for children with SHCN. Many children with SHCN will require additional support in order to meet their developmental potential often from health care and social care providers (e.g., social workers, family support, and liaison), educational teams, and local community providers. In addition, charitable organizations and support groups can help the children and their families in their day-to-day lives, provide specific education resources, and connect families that may share similar experiences (Martinez & Ercikan, 2009).

Furthermore, studies have identified that children and youth, with or without SHCN, are living in Canadian households where their parents or caregivers have a chronic disease or a health condition (Leitch, 2007; Broemeling, Watson, & Prebtani, 2008). These children and youth will need additional support as they may be caregivers themselves. Numerous organizations exist across Canada that provide access to resources and advice or have co-created supportive research programs with families (e.g., Centre of Excellence for Early Childhood Development, the SandBox Project, CHILD-BRIGHT Network, and Canadian Institute for Health Research).

Impact of the Problem

Parents and families go through a wide range of feelings and emotions when an infant is born very prematurely, a child is injured and requires long-term special care and/or rehabilitation, or a child is diagnosed with a chronic health condition. While the infant or child is still in the hospital, nurses can help parents build on their strengths, empowering them to care for their child through building educational partnerships within a family-centred care (FCC) model (Hewitt-Taylor, 2012). Early discharge planning can help the child and family with transition into the community. Nurses should provide anticipatory guidance around nursing support needed in the community as well as identify ongoing learning requirements for family members.

Many children with SHCN progress through the stages of growth and development just as typical children do, though possibly at a slower pace. Exceptions will depend on the child's physical and cognitive abilities and capacity to learn. For example, interventions, parent teaching, and physical and occupational therapies will be focused on approaches that aim to maximize the child's psychomotor development. Children with SHCN desire to be treated in line with their peers and want to experience the same events that other children do.

Of particular concern is a growing subset of children with emotional, behavioural, and developmental special needs and/or chronic health problems. Special funds and programs, although limited, are being provided across Canada for children and youth who have been affected by some conditions including autism and fetal alcohol spectrum disorder (FASD) (PHAC, 2008). Many children with emotional, behavioural, or developmental problems also have chronic health problems. Often, these children's problems are not diagnosed early and treatment is difficult (Shepherd & Waddell, 2015). Ongoing provincial access to counselling, retesting for educational ability, and therapy can be very difficult for some families to obtain.

Effects of Special Needs on the Child

When a child has a special heath care need or disability, the child's coping ability may be affected as a result of biologic, social, and environmental context (Allison, 2016). In addition, the child's ability to cope is significantly affected by the family's response to stressors. There is a strong association between the child's disability status and the subjective well-being of those who have low social support and financial hardship (Savage, 2012).

Children with SHCN experience differing effects of the chronic illness or disability based on their developmental level, which naturally changes over time for most children.

Infants may fail to develop a sense of trust, attachment, or bonding with their parents because of frequent hospitalizations. Interactions with multiple caregivers, a lack of consistency in nurturing, or parental detachment or grieving over the child's condition can also influence the development of secure attachments. The infant's ability to learn through sensorimotor exploration may be impaired due to lack of appropriate stimulation, confinement to a crib or cot, or increased painful experiences (Vessey & Sullivan, 2010).

The toddler may experience difficulty developing autonomy because of increased dependency on the parent or parental overinvolvement. Motor and language skill development may be delayed if the toddler is not given adequate opportunities to test his or her limits and abilities (Vessey & Sullivan, 2010).

Limited opportunities also reduce the preschooler's development of a sense of initiative. The preschooler may experience limited opportunities for socialization, causing him or her to withdraw or to feel criticized. Body image development may be hindered due to painful exposures and anxiety. In preschoolers, magical thinking may lead to feelings of guilt for having caused their own disease or condition (Vessey & Sullivan, 2010).

The school-age child may have limited opportunities to achieve a sense of industry because of school absence and inability to participate in activities or competitive events. Lack of socialization limits the school-age child's ability to form peer relationships. The ability to learn via concrete operations is affected by the child's physical limitations or possibly the treatments he/she requires (Vessey & Sullivan, 2010).

Adolescents may feel as though they are different from their peers because of their lack of skills/abilities or their appearance. This may hinder the young person's ability to form a sense of personal identity. Since the young person with SHCN or disability often requires significant amounts of support from parents, it may be difficult for the adolescent to achieve independence. If the earlier stages of cognitive development have been delayed, then reaching the level of abstract thinking may be hindered (Vessey & Sullivan, 2010).

The child with SHCN may be able to focus on the positive experiences in his or her life as a method of coping, leading to as much independence as possible. However, some children may always feel different from their peers (in a negative sense) and may be withdrawn or quieter than their friends. The child's coping pattern may change over time or with certain situations, such as relapse or worsening of the condition. Children with overprotective parents may display ongoing dependence and may have a heightened sense of fear and worry in health, social, and educational settings. The nurse must assess the child's individual response to the current health care status and intervene as appropriate (Vessey & Sullivan, 2010).

Effects on the Family

Each member of the family experiences effects related to the child's special needs. Family members' experiences and their responses to the child's illness influence each other directly (Fig. 34.2).

Effects on Parents

Raising a child with special needs is generally not the life parents expected to have. Parents often need time (this can be brief or for some longer) to adapt to their child's illness or disability. Others may adapt but do not accept the child's condition and experience diminished then reemergence of chronic sorrow. Denial of their child's problem may prevent parents from processing grief, while for others it allows them to have a level of hope that they are comfortable with (Knafl & Santacroce, 2010). Often families may develop a level of resilience when raising children with special needs or disability (McConnell, Savage, & Breitkreuz, 2014).

However, caring for the child with special needs at home (rather than having the child in a facility) may decrease the parents' feelings of anxiety and helplessness. As with typically developing children, parents

FIGURE 34.2 A wheelchair-bound boy with his younger brother and older sister.

enjoy witnessing the emotional and social growth of the child. All parents experience a multitude of emotions and changes to their lives as a result of having children in their lives. They worry about their child's and family's well-being, and as experts in their child's care may feel burdened with continual care. They often feel helpless and overwhelmed when their child is discharged from the hospital. Though willing to carry the burden, they may experience fear, anger, sadness, guilt, frustration, or resentment. Many parents experience grief as a result of losing the perfect child of which they dreamed (Knafl & Santacroce, 2010).

Effects on Siblings

The brothers and sisters of children with SHCN can also be affected by their sibling's difficulties and the changes in the family dynamic. The siblings' relationship with their parents is frequently different from what it would have been if they had a typical brother or sister. Parents often need to spend more time with the child with SHCN and have less time with their healthy children. Children exhibit emotional and psychological responses to their sibling's long-term needs (Lane & Mason, 2014). The sibling's knowledge about the illness, the sibling's attitude toward and adjustment to it, the sibling's own

self-esteem, how socially supported the sibling is, and the parents' awareness of the sibling's feelings are all related to how well the sibling adjusts.

The Fabric of Everyday Life

Families with a child who has SHCN experience life differently from other families as highlighted in the in-depth report by McConnell et al. (2013). Families may have to change their housing situation to accommodate the child's needs. Sleep for parents, the affected child, and siblings can be altered, all of which has an influence on the day-to-day individual and family functioning (McConnell et al., 2013). Constant supervision of the technology-dependent child makes it difficult to carry out other basic household activities or results in carers being always present in the family home. In addition to providing basic child care and running the home, facilitating school life, preserving the emotional integrity of the family, and performing medical and technical care must be incorporated into daily life. Nursing and other health care professional visits are often disruptive to family life. The family's identity and the parents' employment may be altered temporarily or permanently. Holidays and vacations are also potentially affected, as it can be difficult to plan activities, buy adequate travel insurance, and find accommodation that can allow the child and family to travel safely. While mothers appear to carry the larger burden of care, fathers are not unaffected. Somehow, parents eventually take charge and though they may fear failure, they display vigilance, can negotiate and seek information, and become advocates for their child and experts on his or her care. Though parents may feel trapped and isolated and experience a loss of freedom, their need to survive as a family continues to motivate them. Parents may feel a need to be with their child at all times and experience stress related to coping with the heavy load of caregiving.

The extended burden of caregiving can also have adverse health effects on caregivers; only a small percentage of parents of children with SHCN report that they routinely participate in health-promoting activities for themselves. Parents of children with SHCN are at increased risk for the development of depression (Knafl & Santacroce, 2010). In addition to the caregiving burden, parents experience role conflicts, financial burdens, and the struggle between independence in providing care and the isolation associated with it. It is very difficult to enjoy spontaneous events outside the home because so much planning is necessary.

The possibility of independence revolves around mobility issues, education, and assistive technology. Though education for all children is federally mandated, parents have anxiety about educational decisions and also find it difficult to obtain the support and educational services the child needs.

Additional stress is associated with transition times in the care of a special needs child. These **transition** times include:

- Initial diagnosis or change in prognosis
- Increased symptoms
- When the child moves to a new setting (hospital, school)
- Parental absence
- During periods of developmental change (Caley, 2012; Knafl & Santacroce, 2010)

Nursing Care of the Child/Youth With SHCN and Their Family

FCC provides the optimal framework for caring for children with SHCN and their families. FCC aims to minimize the impact of chronic illness and maximize the degree of child and family inclusion in their care, decision making, and outcomes (Hodgetts, Nicholas, Zwaigenbaum, & McConnell, 2013). To provide opportunity for FCC the nurse must recognize the needs of the child and their family and work with them in order to address the nursing and wider issues. This reciprocal relationship builds safety, trust, and inclusion for the child and their family.

To ensure optimal functioning, children with SHCN require comprehensive and coordinated services from multiple professionals. In an ideal situation, these professionals should work collaboratively to address the child's health, educational, psychological, and social service needs. In addition to case management and advocacy, nursing management focuses on screening and ongoing assessment of the child, provision of home care, care of the technology-dependent child, education and support of the child and family, and referral for resources.

Developing a Therapeutic Relationship

Raising children is always challenging, but for the parent of a special needs child it is often overwhelming and exhausting. The parents' needs change continuously, therefore building and sustaining trusting relationships with professionals can be helpful for the child and their family. This also promotes trust and a more efficient two-way flow of information and inclusion in FCC (Sanders, Edwards, & Keegan, 2017). It is important to respect the parents' range of emotions and work with them as a team to manage the child's care. Parents are team members in developing the treatment plan and need to be recognized for their efforts and work to meet their child's daily needs.

Listening to, responding to, and empowering family members give them strength, energy, and hope. Furthermore, the need to respect the child's privacy and confidentiality is an important aspect of the nurse's role when navigating care (Noiseux, Rich, Bouchard, Noronha, & Carnevale, 2019). Box 34.2 lists principles related to family involvement.

BOX 34.2

PRINCIPLES RELATED TO FAMILY INVOLVEMENT

Families
- Are the constant in a child's life
- Need to have access to information and training
- Deserve to receive culturally competent care
- Know their strengths, limitations, and fears
- Merit mutual respect and responsibility for outcomes

Adapted from Goode, T. D., Haywood, S. H., Wells, N., & Rhee, K. (2009). Family-centred, culturally, and linguistically competent care: Essential components of the medical home. *Paediatric Annals, 38*(9), 505–512.

Screening and Ongoing Assessment

Nurses involved in the care of children with SHCN and their families should perform ongoing assessments to identify changes in the child's health, new safety concerns, changes in the families ability to cope, equipment and technology needs, and additional resources and services required. Children with SHCN may attain developmental milestones more slowly than typically developing children. When using any assessment screening tools be mindful to use the same tool when retesting. Screening tools are available and web links for additional information related to the screening tool can be found on thePoint.

Promoting Home Care

Home is the most developmentally appropriate environment for all children, even those who are technologically dependent (Hewitt-Taylor, 2012). The child's home provides an emotionally nurturing and socially stimulating environment. Children desire to be cared for at home, and those who are, often display an improved physical, emotional, psychological, spiritual, and social status (Canadian Home Care Association [CHCA], 2016). Challenges may exist for when nursing children in rural or remote settings. However, the CHCA (2008) offers that health care delivery in such context can be successful "through a mix of client resiliency, provider creativity and initiative, and system flexibility" (p. 3). In addition, Jordan's Principle is a legal ruling to ensure that all First Nation children can access the services and support needed, for example, respite care, therapy, school support, medical equipment, etc., in a timely fashion (Government of Canada, 2018).

Technology-dependent children may require supplemental oxygen, assisted ventilation, tracheostomy care, assisted enteral or parenteral feeding, or parenteral medication administration. Early discharge planning is important, and parents will need detailed instructions and support in caring for the technology-dependent child at home (see Chapter 33) (Hewitt-Taylor, 2012).

BOX 34.3

PREPARING FOR HOME CARE BEFORE DISCHARGE

- Promote liaison with community resources. Develop communication between various services. Plan appointments. Set up home nursing care (either private duty or visits).
- Teach skills, encouraging active caregiving in the hospital setting to increase the parents' self-confidence.
- Discuss psychological and emotional issues with parents.
- Obtain/organize equipment and supplies (running out of supplies may cause significant stress on families).
- Refer the family for necessary financial resources.
- Ensure the family's home environment is adequate (enough room for equipment, electricity on, air conditioner for warm weather, heater for cold weather, and refrigeration for food).
- For the baby being discharged from the neonatal intensive care unit (NICU):
  - Teach the parents about the infant's cues and behaviours and the preemie's different sleep–wake patterns.
  - Encourage kangaroo care and infant massage while in the NICU (as the infant's condition allows).
  - Educate the parents about possible effects on short- and long-term neurodevelopment.
  - Refer to local early intervention program.
  - Assist the family with finding a primary care provider who is experienced in the ongoing follow-up of high-risk infants.

Adapted from Smith, V. C., & Stewart, J. (2015). *Discharge planning for high-risk newborns*. Retrieved from http://www.uptodate.com/contents/discharge-planning-for-high-risk-newborns

EARLY DISCHARGE PLANNING

Early discharge planning and ongoing inclusion and education of the family facilitate continuity of care. Box 34.3 provides information about preparing the medically fragile child for discharge.

CARING FOR THE TECHNOLOGY-DEPENDENT CHILD AT HOME

Home care nurses are often involved in the care of technology-dependent children. Caring for a technology-dependent child at home is a complex process, yet children thrive in the home care setting with appropriate intervention and care. Many parents feel that rearing a technology-dependent child is different only because of the presence of the equipment (Carnevale, Teachman, & Bogossian, 2017). Most parents value normalization for their child, and strive to raise and provide discipline to all of their children in the same manner. Nurses should support this approach but above all, listen to parents' expectations for childrearing and respect parents' wishes.

Improved collaboration between parents and home care nurses may decrease the parents' stress and maximize opportunities for appropriate growth and development in the technology-dependent child. Thus, a strong

relationship, good communication, and good negotiation skills are assets to the family and child.

It may be the nurse's role to help the family to incorporate the medical regimen into daily life to minimize the child's self-perception of being different from other children. Teach families about the technical issues, such as home and travel oxygen therapy, use of the ventilator, suctioning, tube feedings and care of the feeding tube, and medications. Assist parents with the planning and management of routine care, respiratory treatments, nutritional support, and developmental interventions. Reinforce exercises and techniques as prescribed by developmental therapists. Refer to Chapter 33 for additional information about home care nursing.

Providing Care Coordination

Once a child with SHCN has been identified and discharged to the home setting, the nurse plays a vital role in care coordination. Any child with SHCN benefits from accessing care as framed within a patient medical home (PMH) model (Katz et al., 2017). As such the nurse in PMH is situated within primary care practice and is a critical team member, providing ongoing care coordination and follow-up. If such services are available in the local area, refer the family and child with special needs to an integrated health program that provides interdisciplinary, collaborative care for children requiring complex, coordinated care. Box 34.4 lists some suggested nursing interventions for families of children with SHCN.

BOX 34.4

NURSING INTERVENTIONS FOR FAMILIES OF CHILDREN WITH SPECIAL HEALTH CARE NEEDS

- Develop written health plans.
- Provide care coordination and collaboration with specialists in other disciplines, early intervention, schools, and public agencies.
- Address needs for prior authorization for treatments, medications, or specialist referrals; retain copies in the child's chart of authorization forms and approvals.
- Modify office routines to promote family and child comfort.
- Assist parents with child care decisions.
- Know community resources available to children with special health care needs.
- When the child is hospitalized, encourage high levels of parental participation.
- Provide care coordination across multiple health settings.
- Educate child care providers on child health needs.
- Help parents get involved with parent support networks.

Adapted from Looman, W. S., O'Conner-Von, S., & Lindeke, L. L. (2008). Caring for children with special health care needs and their families: What advanced practice nurses need to know. *Journal for Nurse Practitioners, 4*(7), 512–518; and McAllister, J. W., Presler, E., Turchi, R., & Antonelli, R. C. (2009). Achieving effective care coordination in the medical home. *Paediatric Annals, 38*(9), 491–497.

Providing Ongoing Follow-Up of the Former Premature Infant

Many former premature infants experience myriad medical and developmental problems throughout infancy, early childhood, and beyond. This group is at risk for one or more of the following medical or developmental problems:

- Chronic lung disease (bronchopulmonary dysplasia), increased rates of asthma
- Cardiac changes such as right ventricular hypertrophy and pulmonary artery hypertension
- Growth retardation, poor feeding, anemia of prematurity, other nutrient deficiencies
- Apnea of prematurity, gastroesophageal reflux disease, bradycardia
- Sudden infant death syndrome (SIDS)
- Rickets (osteopenia) of prematurity
- Hydrocephalus, ventriculomegaly, abnormal head magnetic resonance imaging results, ventriculoperitoneal shunt
- Inguinal or umbilical hernias
- Vision issues: retinopathy of prematurity, strabismus, decreased visual acuity
- Hearing deficits
- Delayed dentition
- Gross motor, fine motor, and language delay; sensory integration issues (Billimoria & Kamat, 2014; Kelly, 2010; Sullivan, Msall, & Miller, 2012)

Over the long term, former premature infants are at higher risk than typical infants of developing global developmental delay, cerebral palsy, poor motor abilities, attention deficit/hyperactivity disorder, increased anxiety, depression, learning disabilities, difficulties with socialization, and vulnerable child syndrome (Day et al., 2016; Poole et al., 2015; Sullivan et al., 2012).

For these reasons, high-risk infants require special attention and thorough, appropriate assessment to discern subtle changes that may affect their long-term physical, cognitive, emotional, spiritual, and social outcome. The pediatric nurse should have an understanding of the special concerns that former premature infants and children as well as their families may face (Fig. 34.3).

From the beginning, encourage families to keep a binder that includes all of the infant's pertinent checkup, insurance, and medical and developmental information; this will serve as a resource for the parents, and they will be able to supply complete information when visiting various providers.

PROVIDING ROUTINE WELL-CHILD CARE OF THE FORMER PREMATURE INFANT

Former premature infants require similar well-child care as typical infants do, with additional visits for management of multiple complex medical issues and developmental screening/intervention. Teach families routine

FIGURE 34.3 Parents of an infant discharged from the NICU may need to administer special care, such as feeding.

newborn care, including bathing, dressing, and avoidance of passive cigarette smoke. All visits for primary care follow-up will be scheduled based on the infant's chronologic age.

A common practice introduced in the 1990s was car seat tolerance screening (CSTS) in infants less than 37 weeks' gestational age or those leaving NICU, or with low term birth weight (Davis, 2015). Uncertainty, failure rates, risk factors, and adverse outcome data have resulted in the need for further studies (Jensen et al., 2018). However, as new data and recommendations are implemented parents should continue to be taught safe car seat use and be able to demonstrate the ability to ensure their infant is appropriately seated in their own car seat prior to discharge from hospital (Narvey, CPS, Fetus & Newborn Committee, 2016). It is recommended that children should only be seated in a car seat for travelling, and removed from the seat once the destination has been reached. Former premature infants require car seat use just as other infants do. Help the parents to find methods of padding the car seat to maintain an upright head position to ensure a patent airway. Some infants may need to continue cardiac/apnea monitoring while in the car seat if they have been found to have prolonged periods of apnea, bradycardia, or hypoxia necessitating continued monitoring.

Since the former premature infant is at increased risk for SIDS compared to the general population, it is critical to teach parents to put the infant on his or her back to sleep (Duncan & Byard, 2018). Parents are also highly encouraged to complete CPR training prior to the discharge of their infant home.

Give immunizations according to the current Centres for Disease Control and Prevention (CDC)–recommended immunization schedule, based on the infant's chronologic age. All former premature infants receive an annual influenza vaccine as recommended after 6 months of chronologic age. Respiratory syncytial virus (RSV) prophylaxis is critical for certain groups of premature infants (Billimoria & Kamat, 2014; Kelly, 2010). If indicated/prescribed, administer palivizumab (Synagis) vaccine according to the recommended schedule (refer to Chapter 40 for additional information about RSV prophylaxis).

ASSESSING GROWTH AND DEVELOPMENT OF THE FORMER PREMATURE INFANT

When assessing growth and development of the infant or child who was born prematurely, determine the child's adjusted or corrected age so that you can perform an accurate assessment. The corrected or adjusted age should be used for evaluating progression in growth as well as development. For example, if a 6-month-old infant was born at 28 weeks' gestation (12 weeks or 3 months early), his growth and development expectations are those of a 3-month-old (corrected age). Continue to correct age for growth and development until the child is 3 years old.

Breastfeeding the preterm infant can be challenging due to the infant's immaturity, which impacts his or her ability to suck, swallow, and draw in enough milk to provide an adequate caloric intake. In addition, mothers of preterm infants often need to establish a milk supply with the use of a breast pump, as their infant may not be able to orally feed for many weeks (Niela-Wilen, Melender, Axelin, Loyttyniemi, & Salantera, 2016). Breast milk is particularly important for the infant born prematurely, as it has been shown to benefit the infant's immune system, gastrointestinal mucosa, lowering their risk of sepsis and bowel infection, and provides important developmental stimulation through skin-to-skin interaction (Callen & Pinelli, 2005).

Many former premature infants require special diets to foster catch-up growth (Billimoria & Kamat, 2014; Carey, Russek, & Esposito, 2013). Extra calories are needed for increased growth needs. Additional calcium and phosphorus are required for bone mineralization. For these reasons, breastfed preterm infants may require expressed breast milk fortified with formula powder to provide additional nutrients and calories. These can be weaned off as the infant begins to demonstrate adequate growth and nutrition. Formula-fed preterm infants will require commercially prepared formula specific for premature infants. When formula-fed preterm infants demonstrate consistent and adequate growth prior to term corrected age, they may be switched to a specialized formula for preterm infants. Such formula has a higher calorie content than regular term infant formula, as well as more protein and vitamins and minerals to promote growth. If there are any concerns about the need for catch-up growth to reach normative growth curves or concerns for bone mineralization, preterm infants can be maintained on the specialized formula until as late as one year corrected age. When a preterm infant's growth is adequate, which most nutritionists define as tracking along what would be the normal growth pattern for a health unborn fetus of the same gestational age, they can be switched to a regular term formula like Similac or Enfamil. There is little evidence to suggest a benefit of continued use of a specialized preterm formula after term corrected age, unless for the aforementioned reasons (Fenton et al., 2013). Whether the infant is fed breast milk or formula, assess the infant's ability to latch and suck efficiently and refer him or her to a lactation consultant if breast-fed, or occupational or speech therapy if bottle-fed, if the infant demonstrates any of the following: slow feeder; uncoordinated suck and swallow; choking; or has any other difficulty feeding.

Premature infants commonly require iron-fortified formula, or iron supplementation due to anemia of prematurity. Some premature infants will experience constipation, and may require laxatives in the form of PEG or glycerine suppositories to maintain a normal stooling pattern.

All anticipatory guidance related to nutrition is based on the child's corrected age (D'Agostino et al., 2013). In other words, begin solids at 6 months corrected age, not chronologic age, and delay the addition of whole milk until 12 months corrected age, rather than 1 year chronologic age. Signs that the former premature infant may be ready to attempt spoon feeding include interest in feeding, decrease in tongue thrust, and adequate head control.

Early screening and intervention for issues related to development are critical to the attainment of optimal development in the former preemie. The comorbidities that preterm graduates exhibit in the form of prior and current medical problems place these infants at high risk for **developmental delay** (lag in meeting developmental milestones). Even mild developmental delays warrant evaluation and intervention. Parent-report questionnaires demonstrate fairly accurate estimations of developmental problems, and are simple to use. Most importantly, assess the child's development based on corrected age until the child is 3 years old. Refer infants and children early if developmental concerns are suspected.

Identifying and Managing Failure to Thrive and Feeding Disorders in Children With Special Needs

Failure to thrive (FTT) is a term used to describe inadequate growth in infants and children. The child fails to demonstrate appropriate weight gain over a prolonged period of time. Length or height velocity and head circumference growth may also be affected. Typical children may experience FTT, but it is much more common in the child with special needs. Adequate nutrition is critical for appropriate brain growth in the first 2 years of life and obviously for growth in general throughout childhood and adolescence (Starr et al., 2013). FTT is a multifactorial problem. **Developmental disability** (mental or physical or combination impairment resulting in lifelong disability) may contribute to FTT, as the child's ability to consume adequate nutrition is impaired because of sensory or motor delays, such as with cerebral palsy. Other organic causes of FTT include inability to suck and/or swallow correctly, malabsorption, diarrhoea, vomiting, or alterations in metabolism and caloric/nutrient needs associated with a variety of chronic illnesses. Infants and children with cardiac or metabolic disease, chronic lung disease (bronchopulmonary dysplasia), cleft palate, cystic fibrosis, or gastroesophageal reflux disease are at particular risk. Feeding disorders or food refusal may occur in infants or children who experienced delayed oral feeding as a result of prolonged mechanical ventilation, long-term enteral tube feedings, or an unpleasant event such as a choking episode. Additional causes of FTT include neglect, abuse, behavioural problems, lack of appropriate maternal interaction, poor feeding techniques, lack of parental knowledge, or parental mental illness. Poverty is the single greatest contributing risk factor (Kirkland, Motil, & Duryea, 2015a; Starr et al., 2013).

Screen all children for FTT to identify them early. In addition to poor growth, the infant or child with FTT may present with a history of developmental delay or loss of acquired milestones. Infants or children with feeding problems may display nipple, spoon, or food refusal; difficulty sucking; disinterest in feeding; or difficulty progressing from liquid to puréed to textured food. Perform a detailed dietary history and instruct the parents to complete a 3-day food diary to identify what the child actually eats and drinks. Assess the parent–child interaction, with particular attention to the parent's ability to read and respond to the infant's or child's cues. Observe feeding, noting the child's oral interest or aversion, oral–motor coordination, and swallowing ability, as well as parent–child interactions before, during, and after the feeding (Kirkland, Motil, & Duryea, 2015b).

Significant FTT may require hospitalization for evaluation and management. Sometimes, enteral tube feedings are necessary in order for children with FTT or feeding disorders to demonstrate adequate growth. Box 34.5 lists nursing interventions for the hospitalized child with FTT.

Take Note!

Infants and children who have experienced maternal neglect may not interact appropriately with their environment or caretaker (lack of eye contact) (Kirkland et al., 2015a).

Promoting Growth and Development

When caring for the infant with SHCN in the hospital, provide consistent care to encourage the infant to develop a sense of trust. Allow and encourage the parent to stay with the infant, providing a comfortable place for the parent

---

BOX 34.5

NURSING INTERVENTIONS DURING THE CHILD'S HOSPITALIZATION FOR FAILURE TO THRIVE

- Observe parent–child interactions, especially during feedings.
- Develop an appropriate feeding schedule.
- Provide feedings as prescribed (usually 120 kcal/kg/day is needed to demonstrate proper weight gain).
- Weigh the child daily and maintain strict records of intake and output.
- Educate parents about proper feeding techniques and volumes.
- Provide extensive support to alleviate parental anxiety related to the child's inability to gain weight.

Adapted from Kirkland, R. T., Motil, K. J., & Duryea, T. K. (2015b). *Failure to thrive (undernutrition) in children younger than two years: Management.* Retrieved from http://www.uptodate.com/contents/failure-to-thrive-undernutrition-in-children-younger-than-two-years-management

---

to sleep. To promote attachment, emphasize the baby's positive qualities. Encourage developmentally appropriate skills and allow the infant to have pleasurable experiences through all of the senses (Vessey & Sullivan, 2010).

For the toddler, begin developmentally appropriate limit setting and discipline. Encourage independence as the toddler is able. Modify gross motor and sensory activities to accommodate the toddler's limitations. To encourage a sense of control, offer the toddler simple choices. As the preschooler develops, encourage mastery of self-help skills as the child is able. Encourage socialization with same-age peers to develop a sense of friendship. Reinforce to the child that the illness or disability is not a punishment for wrongdoing or the child's fault in any way (Vessey & Sullivan, 2010).

Encourage the school-age child to attend school and make up work that must be missed for medical treatments or appointments. Provide education to the school staff and other students about the child's special needs. Promote involvement in appropriate sports activities; music, drama, or art activities; and clubs such as Scouts Canada. Educate the child about the illness or disability and the course of treatment (Vessey & Sullivan, 2010).

Inform parents of teens that those with chronic illness often participate in the same actions as typical teens, such as risk taking, rebelling, and trying out different identities. Assist the young person with coping and interpersonal skills. Promote involvement in activities with other teens with special needs as well as typical adolescents. Ensure that the teen participates in rites of passage as able, such as attending the prom or obtaining a driver's licence. Discuss future plans with the teen, such as college or vocation, as well as transition to adult-based health care services (Vessey & Sullivan, 2010).

Providing Resources to the Child and Family

Nurses should be familiar with community resources available to children with SHCN. Educational opportunities for children with SHCN include early intervention programs and programs offered through the public school system. Financial resources, respite care, and complementary therapies are other areas the nurse should become familiar with.

EDUCATIONAL OPPORTUNITIES FOR THE SPECIAL NEEDS CHILD

Early intervention programs are intended to enhance the development of infants and toddlers with, or at risk for, disabilities, thereby minimizing educational costs and special education. Early intervention is also directed toward enhancing the capacity of families to meet their child's needs as well as to maximize the likelihood of independent living (Berry, Garzon, & Deloian, 2012). Refer children suspected of developmental delay to the local early intervention program. For children receiving these services, collaborate with the service coordinator on an ongoing basis, with particular involvement at hospital discharge and when transition of services occurs at age 3 years.

> **Think back to Preet, the 2-year-old boy with a history of hydrocephalus and developmental delay, from the beginning of the chapter. Discuss with his mother the educational opportunities that are available for Preet. Explain what early intervention is and why it is important for Preet.**

Schools may have a profound impact on the child's overall health and development. Some children with special needs do not require additional services to succeed in school. For these children, the nurse's role is to assess for school success or failure and determine the effect of the school environment on the child's health. In 2014, the Council of Ministers of Education, Canada (CMEC), released the CMEC Early Learning and Development Framework. The framework presents a pan-Canadian vision for early learning and inclusion to be adapted to the needs of each province and territory. It is designed to serve as a resource to support the development of policies and initiatives by ministries and departments of education and their partners to enhance the quality and continuity of the learning experience in the early years and beyond.

According to the framework, each special needs student is entitled to an individualized education plan (IEP), which is a written plan designed to meet the preschool, primary, or secondary school student's individual needs. A committee consisting of the child's parent, a regular teacher, a special education teacher, and various other specialists develops the IEP. Nurses may be called to serve upon this committee. The IEP must include measurable short- and long-term goals. Parents are to be informed of the student's progress routinely and the IEP is reviewed at least annually.

Preschool special education through the local public school system is provided from age 3 to 5 years. A child is eligible for special needs preschool when a significant delay is present in the cognitive, language, adaptive, social-emotional, or motor development domains to the extent that it adversely affects the child's learning ability. The child receives (in the school setting) developmental therapy as needed to augment his or her ability to participate in the education process. The least restrictive environment is preferred, with special needs children participating in classes containing age-appropriate typical peers whenever possible. Special needs services are offered in the elementary school setting depending on specific diagnosed conditions, psychoeducational testing, and the resources of the school and region.

FINANCIAL AND INSURANCE RESOURCES

Many special needs children whose families demonstrate financial need may be eligible for different kinds of financial support. The amount and level of support will depend on the assessed need, other funds and services available to the child and/or family, and location (may differ even within provinces and territories). Financial aid also may be available from different sources—government agencies, charitable organizations, condition-specific groups, and local community or church groups. The role of the nurse working with children with SHCN and their families is to have knowledge of local resources, and/or programs, or websites that provide up-to-date quality, evidenced-based information. In addition, it may be the role of the nurse to help families complete assessment forms to ensure all the health care needs of the child are correctly explained, such as child disability benefit. Links to resources for special needs children are included on thePoint.

RESPITE CARE

Primary caregivers of children with SHCN must be dedicated, skilful, vigilant, and knowledgeable. Constant care is a stress on the primary caregiver, who needs temporary relief from the daily caregiving demands. **Respite care** provides an opportunity for families to take a break from the daily intensive caregiving responsibilities. Respite care should meet the child's health care needs and offer the child developmental opportunities. Finding and using respite care that the family is comfortable with and trusts may decrease the family's stress and lead to an enhanced quality of life for special needs children and their families. Nurses can facilitate access to respite care, educate respite providers, and ensure quality respite care practices through involvement in community agencies.

COMPLEMENTARY THERAPIES

Families of children with SHCN often use adjuvant therapies. These may include, among others, homeopathic and herbal medicine, traditional Indigenous medicine or ceremonies, pet therapy, hypnotherapy, music, and massage. Many families desire to blend natural, Eastern, or traditional Indigenous medicine with traditional allopathic medicine for their special needs child in search of palliation or a cure. When obtaining the health history, ask specifically about homeopathy or herbal medications the child may be taking. Pet therapy may be used to decrease stress or as a component of psychotherapy.

Hippotherapy is also referred to as horseback riding for the handicapped, therapeutic horseback riding, or equine-facilitated psychotherapy. Individuals with almost any cognitive, physical, or emotional disability may benefit from therapeutic riding or other supervised interaction with horses. The unique movement of the horse under the child helps the child with physical disabilities to achieve increased flexibility, balance, and muscle strength. Children with mental or emotional disabilities may experience increased self-esteem, confidence, and patience as a result of the unique relationship with the horse. A physical therapist or psychotherapist (depending on the situation) generally works very closely with specially trained equine staff (Granados & Agis, 2011). Box 34.6 lists chronic medical conditions for which hippotherapy may be beneficial. Additional information may be obtained through the Canadian Therapeutic Riding Association.

Music may be used to induce positive behavioural changes, reduce pain or stress, or various other positive effects. Massage therapy may be beneficial to a wide variety of children. It may be used to reduce pain, promote relaxation, or demonstrate a specific positive effect related to the child's particular medical condition (Cotton, Luberto, Bogenschutz, Pelley, & Dusek, 2014).

 Take Note!

Become familiar with the risks and benefits of homeopathic and herbal medications, as many families use these treatments in an effort to improve their child's quality of life or outcome.

Providing Support and Education

At the time of initial diagnosis, allow and encourage the family to express their feelings. Parents of children with SHCN require emotional, practical, economic, and social support. Encourage parents to obtain help with daily routines. Encourage stress reduction for the parents through exercise and allowing time for themselves. Be a supportive and encouraging listener, making sure to nurture the whole child, not just his or her special condition.

Parents value peer support groups, sometimes feeling that only other parents of disabled or chronically ill children could understand the heartache, fear, and other emotions they often experience. Pediatric nurses should be proactive in helping families find support systems.

Fathers have the same concerns about their children as mothers do, but they may show these concerns differently. It is important for nurses to involve them in the child's care. Teach skills to both parents, and actively involve fathers by asking about their observations and opinions.

Parents over time will become the experts on their child's needs and care, and they should be recognized as such. Parents need to be listened to and have their observations, needs, and concerns valued. As experts in their child's care, they should be viewed as having reliable and valuable information about their children. By being an active and reflective listener, the nurse can demonstrate to the parents that their opinion is valued, in addition to finding out what the child really needs. Some parents may hesitate to volunteer information, unsure about which information the nurse needs. Show respect for the parents' knowledge of their child's needs by seeking advice on the child's daily care, medical/physical needs, and current developmental level, no matter what the site of care is.

Families may need additional support from the nurse at times of transition—inpatient stays at a hospital, discharge home, changes in regular care providers, or the transfer of care to adult services. As the equipment or treatment needs change, adjust the teaching plan. Educate the child and family about the use of adaptive

---

BOX 34.6

CONDITIONS BENEFITING FROM HIPPOTHERAPY

- Muscular dystrophy
- Cerebral palsy
- Visual impairment
- Down syndrome
- Intellectual disability
- Autism
- Multiple sclerosis
- Brain injury
- Myelomeningocele
- Spinal cord injury
- Amputation
- Attention deficit disorder
- Learning disabilities
- Deafness
- Cerebrovascular accident (stroke)

Adapted from The Children's TherAplay Foundation, Inc. (2016). *Hippotherapy.* Retrieved from http://www.childrenstheraplay.org/hippotherapy

equipment. Ensure that families understand how specific activities must be modified to accommodate the child's needs. Provide anticipatory guidance related to expected developmental changes, including increasing autonomy, promoting independence and decision making as the child matures.

Assisting the Adolescent With Special Health Needs Making the Transition to Adulthood

Adolescence is a period of change involving extensive biologic, cognitive, emotional, and social changes. The CPS (2019) provides a functional, rather than chronologic definition of adolescence, stating "adolescence begins with the onset of physiologically normal puberty and ends when an adult identity and behaviours are accepted" (p. 577). This concept corresponds chronologically with ages 10 to 18 or 19 years of age, the legal voting and drinking age. Each person, despite their unique personal situation, is confronted with similar developmental tasks. For youth with SHCN, the opportunity and ability to meet their own needs, and formation of personal identity and psychological stability might be significantly altered by their health condition, family environment, health care providers, and the availability of services.

Adolescence is a time of physical changes, psychosocial challenges, and initiation of independence and emancipation from parents and family members. A chronic health condition and/or disability can impact an adolescent's life and development by limiting socialization with peers, altering sexual development, and limiting opportunities for independence. This may be due to the condition itself, effects of treatments or medications, and/or dependency on technology or personal care. Youth may struggle to fit in with their peers by hiding their illness or health care needs (ignoring them), complying poorly with treatment regimens, or participating in risky behaviours. At a time when the adolescent should be developing independence from parents, he or she may be experiencing significant dependence. For these reasons, the adolescent with SHCN and their parents may require increased amounts of support, teaching, and guidance from a nurse.

The transition to adult health care is not a single event but rather a complex process that occurs over time. During the transition process, health care is transferred from one organization to another (pediatric to adult services), with the understanding that it requires planning, therapeutic interactions, and flexibility. Transition programs, strategies, or interventions are developed to encompass the preparation, planning, and transfer of youth with SHCN from pediatric care until they are securely integrated and attached to the adult health care system (Canadian Association of Paediatric Health

Centres [CAPHC] & National Transitions Community of Practice, 2016). The process is complete once the young adult not only transfers to the adult system but is actively participating in activities of self-management and decision making.

Best practice for this population requires a combined holistic, medical, psychosocial, developmental, lifespan approach to transition (CPS, 2018). Making the transition to adult care for a child with SHCN can be difficult, and advance planning may lead to a smoother transition. Transition planning involves multidisciplinary care coordination; acknowledgement of the changing roles among the youth, family, and health care professionals; and fostering of the youth's self-management skills. A written plan for transition to adult care should be initiated in mid-adolescence. The youth and parents require ongoing conversations and skill building prior to the transfer to adult services. Many wider social, financial, and employment issues as well as housing and medical care needs when living independently will need to be considered in the transition phase (CAPHC & National Transitions Community of Practice, 2016).

The timeline for transition suggested by the CPS (2018) and supported by many consensus statements follows normal adolescent development categorized into content areas for early, middle, and late adolescence with counselling and teaching starting at or around 12 to 14 years of age. Care should be developmentally appropriate, flexible, and responsive to the cognitive abilities of the youth.

Nursing Role in Transition for Adolescents With SHCN

The nurse has a unique role in supporting the transition of adolescents with SHCN to adult care. Before moving to adult care (with an adult medical provider), ensure that the adolescent understands their treatment rationale, symptoms of worsening condition, and especially, danger signs. Teach the adolescent about when to seek help from a health professional. Taking a developmental approach, focus on the skills required by young adults engaging in care in adult setting. Skills will include self-advocacy, self-management, and independent health care behaviours. For young adults with cognitive injury or developmental delay—they may always require supported management by a guardian or support worker. Readiness checklists and clinical pathways are available to guide transition assessments for nursing (see thePoint for addition tools, checklists, and resources). Key to transition is that the youth is the central focus supported by the family. On transfer, the youth, family, and all health care providers should receive an updated health care record, transition plan, and current health tests and treatment plans.

THE DYING CHILD

The idea that a child may die is simply unimaginable to most people, yet children die daily. Each year, about 3,500 children die in Canada; approximately 1,200 of those deaths occur in infants before their first birthday (Statistics Canada, 2015a). The leading causes of death for infants are congenital abnormalities and problems of prematurity (Statistics Canada, 2011). For children aged 1 to 14 years, the leading causes of death were accidental injury followed by cancer (Statistics Canada, 2011). A child's chronic illness may progress to the point of becoming a life-threatening or life-limiting illness. A life-threatening condition is defined as a disease for which curative treatment may exist but may fail, such as cancer (Wolfe, Hinds, & Sourkes, 2011). A life-limiting condition has no reasonable hope for cure and the child will die from the condition, such as a degenerative neuromuscular disease (Wolfe et al., 2011). Pediatric nurses will inevitably encounter situations in which a child dies. These situations are extremely difficult for all persons involved and the nurse plays a key role in caring for the dying child and his or her family. Caring for the dying child is a family-centred, multidisciplinary process. Nurses must respond to the child's and family's physiologic, emotional, and spiritual needs during this difficult time. Children display differing responses to the dying process and impending death depending on their developmental level. Children and their families need significant amounts of support throughout the process of dying.

Palliative and Hospice Care of the Dying Child

Palliative care is an approach to care that seeks to ease pain and suffering caused by life-limiting or life-threatening conditions and support patients and their families to live as normally as possible, for as long as possible (Field & Behrman, 2003). The WHO's definition of pediatric palliative care (PPC) states that: "Palliative care for children is the active total care of the child's body, mind and spirit, and also involves giving support to the family" (WHO, n.d. a, para. 1). Palliative care should be initiated at the time of diagnosis, continuing while the child is in active stages of management. Effective palliative care requires a broad multidisciplinary approach that includes the family and makes use of available community resources; it can be successfully implemented even if resources are limited. Attention must be paid to the child's and family's physiologic, psychological, emotional, and spiritual needs as well as the child's developmental stage (Wolfe et al., 2011). Such care can be provided in tertiary care facilities, hospice settings, community health centres, and the child's home. Involving the family and

---

> **BOX 34.7**
>
> ### FIVE KEY COMPONENTS OF FAMILY-CENTRED CARE IN THE CONTEXT OF ALL ASPECTS OF CARE INCLUDING CARE OF THE DYING CHILD
>
> 1. Recognizing and respecting the pivotal role of the family in the lives of children;
> 2. Striving to support families in their caregiving roles by building upon their unique strengths as individuals and as families;
> 3. Respecting and encouraging the choices families make for their children;
> 4. Promoting normal patterns of living in the hospital, at home, and in the community; and
> 5. Promoting partnerships between families and professionals to ensure excellence at all levels of health care. (Jones et al., 2011, p. 135)

wider community in thoughtful and culturally sensitive ways can promote FCC (Box 34.7) (BCCH, 2013). When caring for a child, the nurse acknowledges the strengths of the family and employs the concepts of respect, choice, information sharing, support, collaboration, flexibility, and empowerment (BCCH, 2013).

Appropriate palliative care is essential for any child with a life-threatening or progressive incurable condition (Crozier & Hancock, 2012). Current recommended standards for pediatric palliative and hospice care are for palliative care to be given concurrently with potentially curative treatments (Canadian Hospice Palliative Care Association, 2006; Klein & Saroyan, 2011).

Whether palliative care is provided in the home, hospital, or hospice setting, the goal is to provide the best quality of life possible at the end of life while alleviating physical, psychological, emotional, and spiritual suffering (Crozier & Hancock, 2012). Hospice care allows for FCC in the child's home or a hospice facility. As with adult hospice care, the comfort of the entire family is important. The goal of pediatric hospice care is enhancement of quality of life for the child and family through an individualized plan of care. The first Canadian PPC program was created at Toronto's Hospital for Sick Children in 1986, followed by the establishment of North America's first free-standing children's hospice, Canuck Place Children's Hospice in Vancouver, British Columbia in 1995 (Widger, Cadell, Davies, Siden, & Steele, 2012). Among Canada's 12 specialized children's hospitals, there are 8 hospital-based PPC programs. There are now 7 freestanding children's hospices in Canada.

End-of-Life Decision Making

As medical technology advances and children with life-limiting and life-threatening conditions are living longer, advanced care planning, including code status, has gained more importance. It is essential that evidenced-informed, clear communication approaches are used to help prepare parents that their child might die, while still allowing for some hope. While curative treatments may continue to be the focus, as time progresses, and the child's condition deteriorates, a shift on the continuum from curative to palliative care occurs. All children, including those with intellectual disabilities, need to be informed and included in developmentally appropriate dialogues about their illness trajectory (Tuffrey-Wijne, 2013). Early conversations assure parents that many options are available to keep their child as comfortable as possible for as long as possible. Parents are obligated not only to protect their children from harm but also to do as much good for them as possible, both from an ethical and a legal standpoint. When the time comes for **end-of-life** decision making, parents are often torn about the "right" course of action. Parents may be asked to make decisions about stopping treatment, withdrawing treatment, providing palliative care, or consenting to "do not resuscitate" (DNR) orders. Meyer et al. (2006) found that parents want to have a voice in decision making, but not complete control over each life-sustaining decision. It is important for parents to feel supported, empowered, and respected for the decisions they make about their child's care as well as for maintaining their parental role throughout their child's illness. Nurses can work with families to involve them as much as possible or as the parent's desire. Emphasize that no matter what their decision is, the health care team is dedicated to the comfort and expert care of their child (Rushton, 2004).

Nurses involved in this process must examine their own values related to dying and consider the Canadian Nurses Association's code of ethics for nurses as well (CNA, 2008). Ensure that communication is family centred. Quality of life must be taken into consideration when making decisions to continue or withhold treatment. Provide parents facing end-of-life decisions with honest information and education from the time of the diagnosis/prognosis forward. Anticipate that parents may vacillate in the decision-making process. Clarify information for them and allow them private time to discuss the options. Do not make judgments about or question the parents' decision. Be sensitive to any ethnic, spiritual, or cultural preferences during the **terminal** stage of the illness. Encourage parents to interact with other parents who have a child with a terminal illness (Carter, Levetown, & Friebert, 2013).

Allowing Natural Death

The decision to institute a DNR order is one of the most difficult decisions a family and health care team may ever have to make. For many families, "DNR" is synonymous with "do nothing" and this can be a major cause of distress for them and make decision making very difficult. Parents may initially feel like this means they are giving up on their child. Nurses must educate families that full cardiopulmonary resuscitation may be inappropriate and lead to more suffering than if death were allowed to occur naturally. Language around resuscitation and code status is changing to more acceptable terminology including "do not attempt resuscitation," "allow natural death," and "levels of intervention." Goals of care decisions made by the health care team, family, and if developmentally appropriate, the child, can be clearly communicated with tools that document specific interventions that are appropriate for a child. Levels of intervention encompass limited interventions, when curative therapies are deemed no longer effective and the focus is on comfort; intermediate interventions that are focused on curing or controlling the child's condition, but usually do not include interventions that require care in a critical care unit; and advanced interventions that may also be focused on curing or controlling the child's condition and may include many aspects of resuscitation (BCCH DNAR form, 2012).

Organ or Tissue Donation

With large numbers of organ transplant candidates on waiting lists and the shortage of viable organs, pediatric organ and tissue donation is a priority (Cowl, Cummings, Yager, Miller, & Noviski, 2012). For many families, knowing that a child's organs or tissues may save another child's life provides a way to help others despite their own loss. A healthy child who dies unexpectedly is an excellent candidate for organ donation. Many chronic illnesses in children preclude the option of organ or tissue donation, though individual determinations of eligibility should be made.

The discussion of organ donation should be separated from the discussion of impending death or brain death notification. Written consent is necessary for organ donation, so the family must be appropriately informed and educated. Many families who never thought about it before may consider the option of donation if adequately educated about the process. Ask whether the dying child ever expressed a wish to donate organs and whether the parents have considered this.

Families need to know that procurement of the organs does not mar the child's appearance, so that an open casket at the child's funeral is still possible if the family desires. The donating child will not suffer further because of organ donation. The organs or tissues will be harvested in a timely fashion after the declaration of death, so the family need not worry about delay of the wake or funeral. The family's cultural and religious beliefs must be considered, and the team discussing organ donation with the family must do so in a sensitive and ethical manner (Cowl et al., 2012).

Nursing Management of the Dying Child

Though multidisciplinary care is essential for quality care at the end of life, it is the nurse who plays the key role of child/family advocate and who is usually the constant presence throughout the dying process. Nursing management of the dying child focuses on managing pain and discomfort, providing nutrition, providing emotional support to the dying child and family, and assisting the family through the grief process. Throughout the process, it is important to focus on the family as the unit of care.

Managing Pain and Discomfort

Pain management is an essential component of care for the child with a terminal illness. Adequately managing pain may enhance the child's quality of life and minimize suffering (Crozier & Hancock, 2012). Assess pain using a developmentally appropriate tool (see Chapter 36 for further information). Provide pain medication around the clock rather than on an "as needed" basis to prevent recurrence or escalation of pain. Determine the child's preferred comfort measures and use them to provide additional relief. Change the child's position frequently but gently to minimize discomfort. Limit nursing care to comfort measures that ease the child's discomfort. Maintain a calm environment, minimizing noise and light. Include integrative care interventions such as massage or healing touch as requested and/or tolerated. See Evidence-Based Practice 34.1.

Providing Nutrition

Since the body naturally requires less nutrition as the child is dying, do not excessively coax the child to eat or drink. Offer frequent small meals or a snack of the child's choosing. Soups and shakes require less energy to eat and so may be desirable. If the child desires a different food, where possible aim to provide this. Keep strong odours away from the child to decrease nausea. Administer antiemetics as needed. Provide mouth care and keep the lips lubricated to keep the mouth feeling clean and prevent the discomfort associated with chapped lips. Make sure the environment is a pleasant one for eating.

Providing Emotional Support to the Dying Child and Family

Be attuned to the entire family's needs and emotions in order to foster a holistic connection with the child and family. Nurses provide physical care through specific tasks and interventions for the dying child, but they also need to be fully present emotionally with the child and family. In general, people are uncomfortable with the concept of a dying child. Nurses should work through their own feelings about the situation in order to stay fully present with the child and family, attending to their individualized needs. Ask yourself how you can change in order to be fully present with the child and family (Carter et al., 2013).

Families and dying children benefit from the presence of the nurse, not just the interventions he or she performs. Families report that the simple act of being present with the family is very healing (Carter et al., 2013). Listen to the child and family; be still and silent for a time to accomplish this. Foster respect for the whole child by attending to him or her as such.

Respect the parents of the dying child by helping them honour the commitments they have made to their child. Acknowledge that parents have diverse needs for information and participation in decision making.

EVIDENCE-BASED PRACTICE 34.1 | **INTEGRATIVE THERAPIES FOR PAIN MANAGEMENT IN CHILDREN**

STUDY

Integrative care providers recorded data from 4,749 care visits to 2,404 children. The authors eliminated data from children whose records were incomplete or who were seen as outpatients. The remaining 519 children were included in the study data. Standard pain rating scales (based on developmental age and unit policy) were used to assess pain before and after the integrative treatment.

Findings

Mean pain scores decreased significantly following integrative care interventions. The data demonstrate that integrative care interventions (especially massage and healing touch) contribute to improvement in pain scores and relaxation in pediatric clients.

Nursing Implications

The results suggest that integrative care therapies may improve pain management and relaxation in children. Integrative care therapies continue to be primarily requested by the child or parent, rather than initiating from the health care provider. While the authors concede that additional rigorous studies are needed on this topic, integrative care interventions are not harmful to children and may help with decreasing pain.

Adapted from Cotton, S., Luberto, C. M., Bogenschutz, L. H., Pelley, T. J., & Dusek, J. (2014). Integrative care therapies and pain in hospitalized children and adolescents: A retrospective database review. *The Journal of Alternative and Complementary Medicine, 20*(2), 98–102.

Allow and encourage family customs or rituals in relation to death and dying. Families may desire the pastor, priest, or other spiritual leader to be present when the child's death is imminent. Certain rituals may be desired, depending on the family's religious or spiritual background. Ensure that these important events occur, and alter nursing care routines as needed to accommodate them. Respect the family's need to participate in these rituals and customs (Carter et al., 2013).

Work collaboratively with the family and health care team to provide for the needs of the child and family. Resources for families of a dying child are listed in Box 34.8. The Make-a-Wish Foundation works to grant the wishes of terminally ill children, giving the child and family an experience of hope, strength, and love. A link to the Canadian Children's Make-a-Wish Foundation is included on thePoint.

EASING ANXIETY OR FEARS

Parents may be afraid of their child dying alone or not know what to expect in the death process. This fear may contribute to increased anxiety, which the child may sense. Younger children may fear separation from their parents and older children may not want to die alone or experience pain or discomfort associated with dying. Each child and family is individual; discuss their particular fears and anxieties in order to determine the child's and family's needs for education and support (Carter et al., 2013).

Involve the parents and other family members in all phases of the child's care. Explain all aspects of care to the child to minimize anxiety related to nursing interventions. Answer the child's questions honestly. Involve the child in decision making whenever possible. Limit interventions to those related to palliation, rather than treatment, advocating for the child as needed. Remain

---

BOX 34.8

RESOURCES FOR FAMILIES OF A DYING CHILD

Websites
• Canadian Virtual Hospice has resources in English and French http://www.virtualhospice.ca/en_US/Main±Site±Navigation/Home/Support/Resources/Books_±Links_±and±More.aspx
• Canadian Paediatric Society (CPS). (2018). *Medical Assistance in Dying: A Paediatric Perspective*. https://www.cps.ca/en/documents/position/medical-assistance-in-dying
• SickKids. Grief Support Centres and Resources. http://www.sickkids.ca/patient-family-resources/paediatric-advance-care-team/Grief%20and%20bereavement%20resources/Grief-Support-Centres-%20Counselling-Resources/Grief-Support-Centres-PACT.html

---

with the child when a parent or family member is not in the room so the child will not fear dying alone.

MEETING THE DYING CHILD'S NEEDS ACCORDING TO DEVELOPMENTAL STAGE

It is important to provide the type of support and education that the dying child needs according to his or her developmental stage. For the infant, unconditional love and trust are of utmost importance. Ensure that the infant's family is available to the child. The toddler, 1 to 3 years old, thrives on familiarity and routine. Maximize the toddler's time with parents, be consistent, provide favourite toys, and ensure physical comfort. Spirituality in the preschool years focuses on the concept of right versus wrong. The 3 to 5 year old may see death as punishment for wrongdoing; correct this misunderstanding. Use honest and precise language. Help the parents to teach the child that though the family will miss the child, it will continue to function without him or her (Ethier, 2010).

The school-age child has a concrete understanding of death. Children who are 5 to 10 years old need specific, honest details (as desired). Encourage the child to help make decisions, and help the child to establish a sense of control (Ethier, 2010).

The young adolescent (10 to 14 years old) will benefit from reinforcement of self-esteem, self-respect, and a sense of worth. Respect the child's need for privacy and time alone as well as time requested with peers. Support the need for independence and encourage the child to participate in decision making. The older teen (14 to 18 years of age) has a more adult-like understanding of death and will need further support through honest, detailed explanations and will want to feel truly involved and listened to (Ethier, 2010).

Assisting the Family Through the Grief Process

The family may experience anticipatory grief when the diagnosis of terminal illness is made. Families may deny the prognosis, become angry at the health care system or a higher power, or experience depression. Acute grief is an intense process that occurs around the time of the actual death. Family members may feel short of breath or as though the throat is tight. They may verbalize that the situation is unreal to them or search for reasons why the death was not prevented. Families may also display hostility or restlessness, while others may display relief that their child is no longer suffering. Each individual will express grief in his or her own manner. Mourning the death of a loved one takes a long time, and families should be supported throughout the process (Carter et al., 2013; Ethier, 2010). Local and national resources are available for grieving parents. Several resources for grieving parents are listed on thePoint. Refer parents to bereavement resources as appropriate.

KEY CONCEPTS

- Children with special health care needs (SHCN) are those who have, or are at risk for, a chronic physical, developmental, behavioural, or emotional condition that generally requires more intensive and diverse health services, as well as coordination of those services, than do typical children.

- Most children with chronic illnesses or who are dependent on technology progress through stages of growth and development just as typical children do, though possibly at a slower pace.

- Parents of special needs children experience a multitude of emotions and changes in their lives, often carrying a heavy caregiving burden. They become the experts on their child's care and should be empowered and supported in their efforts.

- The child and family with special health care needs may require additional support during times of transition, such as at initial diagnosis or change in prognosis, when symptoms increase, when the child moves to a new setting (hospital, school), during periods of developmental change, or during a parent's absence.

- Children with SHCN are at increased risk for the development of vulnerable child syndrome, which may have psychologically harmful effects on the child and parents for many years.

- Home is the most developmentally appropriate environment for children with SHCN and those who are technology dependent. Children display an improved physical, emotional, psychological, and social status when they are cared for at home.

- Family-centred care provides the optimal framework for caring for children and families with special needs. Empowering the family strengthens them. A medical home or a permanent relationship with the physician or nurse practitioner benefits the family, as care coordination and advocacy are provided.

- Use adjusted (or corrected) age when assessing growth and development of the infant or child who was born prematurely. Provide early screening and intervention for issues related to development to maximize the former preemie's potential for growth and development.

- Become familiar with the risks and benefits of adjuvant therapies used by some families of children with SHCN.

- Screen children with SHCN for failure to thrive (FTT) or a feeding disorder.

- Screening helps to identify children with unmet health needs so that intervention may begin.

- Early intervention provides care coordination (developmental services and special education), as well as an individualized family service plan for qualifying children and their families.

- Each special needs student is entitled to an IEP, which is a written plan that is designed to meet the preschool, primary, or secondary school student's needs.

- Early discharge planning and ongoing inclusion and education of the family facilitate continuity of care. During mid-adolescence, initiate a written plan to help the special needs child make the transition to adult care.

- Support the dying child and the family throughout the end-of-life decision-making process, providing facts as desired about palliative care, hospice, and organ donation.

- Younger children who are dying generally need for their families to be close and to trust their needs will be provided for. Older children require honest explanations given at a level appropriate for the child's age or developmental stage.

REFERENCES AND RECOMMENDED READINGS

Allison, S. (2016). *Chief Medical Health Officer Child Health Status report (technical report)*. Retrieved from https://northernhealth.ca/Portals/0/About/Community_Accountability/documents/CMHO-Child-Health-Status-Technical-Report.pdf

Association of Paediatric Hematology/Oncology Nurses (APHON). (2003). *Precepts of palliative care for children, adolescents and their families*. Retrieved from http://www.apon.org/files/public/last_acts_precepts.pdf

Berry, A. D., Garzon, D. L., & Deloian, B. J. (2012). Developmental management in paediatric primary care. In C. E. Burns, A. M. Dunn, M. A. Brady, N. B. Starr, & C. G. Blosser (Eds.). *Paediatric primary care* (5th ed.). Philadelphia, PA: Elsevier Saunders.

Billimoria, Z. C., & Kamat, D. (2014). A pediatrician's guide to caring for the complex neonatal intensive care unit graduate. *Paediatric Annals, 43*(9), 369–372.

British Columbia Children's Hospital (BCCH). (2012). *Do Not Attempt Resuscitation Physician Order Form,* Vancouver, BC: Author.

British Columbia's Children's Hospital (BCCH). (2013). *Family-centred care*. Retrieved from http://www.bcchildrens.ca/YourVisit/Family-centredcare/default.htm

Broemeling, A. M., Watson, D. E., & Prebtani, F. (2008). Population patterns of chronic health conditions, co-morbidity and healthcare use in Canada: implications for policy and practice. *Healthcare Quarterly (Toronto, Ont.), 11*(3), 70–76.

Burk, J., Park, M., & Saewyc, E. (2018). A media-based school intervention to reduce sexual orientation prejudice and its relationship to discrimination, bullying, and the mental health of lesbian, gay, and bisexual adolescents in western Canada:

A population-based evaluation. *International Journal of Environmental Research and Public Health, 15*(11), 2447.

Caley, L. M. (2012). Risk and protective factors associated with stress in mothers whose children are enrolled in early intervention services. *Journal of Paediatric Health Care, 26*(5), 346–355.

Callen, J., & Pinelli, J. (2005). A review of the literature examining the benefits and challenges, incidence and duration, and barriers to breastfeeding in preterm infants. *Advances in Neonatal Care, 5*(2), 72–88.

Canadian Association of Paediatric Health Centres (CAPHC), National Transitions Community of Practice. (2016). *A guideline for transition from paediatric to adult health care for youth with special health care needs: A national approach.* Retrieved from https://ken.childrenshealthcarecanada.ca/xwiki/bin/view/Transitioning+from+Paediatric+to+Adult+Care/A+Guideline+for+Transition+from+Paediatric+to+Adult+Care.

Canadian Home Care Association (CHCA). (2008). *A scan of options for delivering home care in rural, remote and northern regions of Canada.* Retrieved from http://www.cdnhomecare.ca/content.php?doc=220

Canadian Home Care Association (CHCA). (2016). *Home and community-based services and supports. Children with complex needs.* Retrieved from http://www.cdnhomecare.ca

Canadian Hospice Palliative Care Association. (2006). Figure 1. The Role of Pediatric Hospice Palliative Care. In *Pediatric hospice palliative care: Guiding principles and norms of practice.* Ottawa, Ontario, Canada: Author. Retrieved from http://www.chpca.net/media/7841/Pediatric_Norms_of_Practice_March_31_2006_English.pdf

Canadian Institute of Child Health (CICH). (2000). *The health of Canada's children: A CICH profile, 3rd edition.* Retrieved from http://www.cich.ca/PDFFiles/ProfilePocketGuide.pdf

Canadian Nurses Association (CNA). (2008). *Code of ethics for registered nurses.* Retrieved from http://www.cna-aiic.ca

Canadian Paediatric Society (CPS). (2016). *Are we doing enough?* Retrieved from http://www.cps.ca/en/status-report/jordans-principle-2016-report

Canadian Paediatric Society. (2018). *Position statement: Transition to adult care for youth with special health care needs.* Retrieved from https://www.cps.ca/en/documents/position/transition-youth-special-needs

Canadian Paediatric Society. (2019). *Position statement: Age limits and adolescents.* Retrieved from https://www.cps.ca/en/documents/position/age-limits-and-adolescents

Carey, D., Russek, M., & Esposito, P. (2013). Supplementation in preterm and later preterm infants after discharge. *ICAN: Infant, Child, & Adolescent Nutrition, 5*(1), 26–28.

Carnevale, F. A., Teachman, G., & Bogossian, A. (2017). A relational ethics framework for advancing practice with children with complex health care needs and their parents. *Comprehensive Child and Adolescent Nursing, 40*(4), 268–284. https://doi.org/10.1080/24694193.2017.1373162

Carter, B. S., Levetown, M., & Friebert, S. E. (2013). *Palliative care for infants, children, and adolescents: A practical handbook* (2nd ed.). Baltimore, MD: Johns Hopkins University Press.

Chambers, P. L., Mahabee-Gittens, E. M., & Leonard, A. C. (2011). Vulnerable child syndrome, parental perception of child vulnerability, and emergency department usage. *Paediatric Emergency Care, 27*(11), 1009–1013.

Chief Public Health Officer's Report on the State of Public Health in Canada. (2011). *Chapter 3. The health and well-being of Canadian youth and young adults.* Retrieved from http://www.phac-aspc.gc.ca/cphorsphc-respcacsp/2011/cphorsphc-respcacsp-06-eng.php

Cohen, E., Gandhi, S., Toulany, A., Moore, C., Fu, L., Orkin, J., . . . Guttmann, A. (2016). Health care use during transfer to adult care among youth with chronic conditions. *Pediatrics, 137*(3), e20152734.

Cotton, S., Luberto, C. M., Bogenschutz, L. H., Pelley, T. J., & Dusek, J. (2014). Integrative care therapies and pain in hospitalized children and adolescents: A retrospective database review. *The Journal of Alternative and Complementary Medicine, 20*(2), 98–102.

Cowl, A. S., Cummings, B. M., Yager, P. H., Miller, B., & Noviski, N. (2012). Organ donation after cardiac death in children: Acceptance of a protocol by multidisciplinary staff. *American Journal of Critical Care, 21*(5), 322–327.

Crozier, F., & Hancock, L. E. (2012). Paediatric palliative care. *Paediatric Nursing, 38*(4), 198–203.

Cystic Fibrosis Canada. (2018). *The Canadian Cystic Fibrosis Registry.* Retrieved from https://www.cysticfibrosis.ca/our-programs/cf-registry.

D'Agostino, J. A., Gerdes, M., Hoffman, C., Manning, M. L., Phalen, A., & Bernbaum, J. (2013). Provider use of corrected age during health supervision visits for premature infants. *Journal of Paediatric Health Care, 27*(3), 172–179.

Davis, N. L. (2015). Car seat screening for low birth weight term neonates. *Pediatrics,* peds-2014. Retrieved from http://pediatrics.aappublications.org/content/pediatrics/136/1/89.full.pdf

Day, K. L., Schmidt, L. A., Vaillancourt, T., Saigal, S., Boyle, M. H., & Van Lieshout, R. J. (2016). Long-term psychiatric impact of peer victimization in adults born at extremely low birth weight. *Pediatrics, 137*(3), e20153383.

Dewan, T., & Cohen, E. (2013). Children with medical complexity in Canada. *Paediatrics & Child Health, 18*(10), 518–522.

Duncan, J. R., & Byard, R. W. (Eds.). (2018). *SIDS Sudden infant and early childhood death: The past, the present and the future.* South Australia: University of Adelaide Press. Retrieved from http://www.jstor.org/stable/10.20851/j.ctv2n7f0v.

Eagle, M., Baudouin, S. V., Chandler, C., Giddings, D. R., Bullock, R., & Bushby, K. (2002). Survival in Duchenne muscular dystrophy: improvements in life expectancy since 1967 and the impact of home nocturnal ventilation. *Neuromuscular Disorders, 12*(10), 926–929.

Early Childhood Development. (2011). *The well-being of Canada's young children: Government of Canada report.* Retrieved from http://www.dpe-agje-ecd-elcc.ca/eng/ecd/well-being/page11.shtml

Ethier, A. M. (2010). Care of the dying child and the family. In D. Tomlinson & N. E. Kline (Eds.). *Paediatric oncology nursing.* New York: Springer.

Fenton, T. R., Nasser, R., Eliasziw, M., Kim, J. H., Bilan, D., & Sauve, R. (2013). Validating the weight gain of preterm infants between the reference growth curve of the fetus and the term infant. *BMC Pediatrics, 13*, 92.

Field, M. J., & Behrman, R. E. (Eds.). (2003). *When children die: Improving palliative and end-of-life care for children and their families.* Washington, DC: Institute of Medicine, National Academies Press.

Goode, T. D., Haywood, S. H., Wells, N., & Rhee, K. (2009). Family-centered, culturally, and linguistically competent care: Essential components of the medical home. *Paediatric Annals, 38*(9), 505–512.

Government of Canada. (2018). *Jordan's principle*. Retrieved from https://www.canada.ca/en/indigenous-services-canada/services/jordans-principle.html

Granados, A. C., & Agis, I. F. (2011). Why children with special needs feel better with hippotherapy sessions: A conceptual review. *The Journal of Alternative and Complementary Medicine, 17*(3), 191–197.

Hasanbegovic, E., Cengic, N., Hasanbegovic, S., Heljic, J., Lutolli, I., & Begic, E. (2016). Evaluation and treatment of anemia in premature infants. *Medical Archives, 70*(6), 408–412.

Hewitt-Taylor, J. (2012). Planning the transition of children with complex needs from hospital to home. *Nursing Children and Young People, 24*(10), 28–36.

Hodgetts, S., Nicholas, D., Zwaigenbaum, L., & McConnell, D. (2013). Parents' and professionals' perceptions of family-centered care for children with autism spectrum disorder across service sectors. *Social Science & Medicine, 96*, 138–146.

Horowitz, J. A., & Marchetti, C. M. (2010). Mood disorders. In P. J. Allen, J. A. Vessey, & N. A. Schapiro (Eds.). *Primary care of the child with a chronic condition* (5th ed.). St. Louis, MO: Mosby. https://doi-org.prxy.lib.unbc.ca/10.1093/pch/pxy047

Jensen, E. A., Foglia, E. E., Dysart, K. C., Aghai, Z. H., Cook, A., Greenspan, J. S., & DeMauro, S. B. (2018). Car seat tolerance screening in the neonatal intensive care unit: Failure rates, risk factors, and adverse outcomes. *The Journal of Pediatrics, 194*, 60–66.

Jones, B. L., Gilmer, M. J., Parker-Raley, J., Dokken, D. L., Freyer, D. R., & Sydnor-Greenberg, N. (2011). Parent and sibling relationships and the family experience. In J. Wolfe, P. S. Hinds, & B. M. Sourkes (Eds.). *Textbook of interdisciplinary paediatric palliative care* (pp. 135–147). Philadelphia, PA: Saunders, Elsevier Inc.

Katz, A., Herpai, N., Smith, G., Aubrey-Bassler, K., Breton, M., Boivin, A., . . . Wong, S. T. (2017). Alignment of Canadian primary care with the patient medical home model: a QUALICO-PC study. *The Annals of Family Medicine, 15*(3), 230–236. Retrieved from http://www.annfammed.org/content/15/3/230.short

Kelly, M. M. (2010). Prematurity. In P. J. Allen, J. A. Vessey, & N. A. Schapiro (Eds.). *Primary care of the child with a chronic condition* (5th ed.). St. Louis, MO: Mosby.

Kirkland, R. T., Motil, K. J., & Duryea, T. K. (2015a). *Failure to thrive (undernutrition) in children younger than two years: Etiology and evaluation*. Retrieved from http://www.uptodate.com/contents/failure-to-thrive-undernutrition-in-children-younger-than-two-years-etiology-and-evaluation

Kirkland, R. T., Motil, K. J., & Duryea, T. K. (2015b). *Failure to thrive (undernutrition) in children younger than two years: Management*. Retrieved from http://www.uptodate.com/contents/failure-to-thrive-undernutrition-in-children-younger-than-two-years-management

Kirkland, R. T., Motil, K. J., & Duryea, T. K. (2016). Failure to thrive (undernutrition) in children younger than two years: Etiology and evaluation. *UpToDate. Waltham, MA: UpToDate*.

Klein, S. M., & Saroyan, J. M. (2011). Treating a child with a life-threatening condition. *Paediatric Annals, 40*(5), 259–265.

Knafl, K. A., & Santacroce, S. J. (2010). Chronic conditions & the family. In P. J. Allen, J. A. Vessey, & N. A. Schapiro (Eds.). *Primary care of the child with a chronic condition* (5th ed.). St. Louis, MO: Mosby.

Lane, C., & Mason, C. (2014). Meeting the needs of siblings of children with life-limiting illnesses. *Nursing Children & Young People, 26*(3), 16–20.

Leitch, K. K. (2007). *Reaching for the top. A report by the advisor on healthy children & youth*. Retrieved from https://static1.squarespace.com/static/575c7d10044262e4c49720f7/t/57e144023e00beb79cb78e3e/1474380812809/2007-reaching-for-the-top-english.pdf

Looman, W. S., O'Conner-Von, S., & Lindeke, L. L. (2008). Caring for children with special health care needs and their families: What advanced practice nurses need to know. *Journal for Nurse Practitioners, 4*(7), 512–517.

MacKenzie, T., Gifford, A. H., Sabadosa, K. A., Quinton, H. B., Knapp, E. A., Goss, C. H., & Marshall, B. C. (2014). Longevity of patients with cystic fibrosis in 2000 to 2010 and beyond: survival analysis of the cystic fibrosis foundation patient registry. *Annals of Internal Medicine, 161*(4), 233–241.

Martinez, Y. J., & Ercikan, K. (2009). Chronic illnesses in Canadian children: What is the effect of illness on academic achievement, and anxiety and emotional disorders? *Child: Care, Health and Development, 35*(3), 391–401.

McAllister, J. W., Presler, E., Turchi, R., & Antonelli, R. C. (2009). Achieving effective care coordination in the medical home. *Paediatric Annals, 38*(9), 491–497.

McConnell, D., Breitkreuz, R., Uditsky, B., Sobsey, R., Savage, A., & Parakkal, M. (2013). *Family life. Children with disabilities and the fabric of everyday family life*. Retrieved from https://cloudfront.ualberta.ca/-/media/rehabilitation/faculty-site/research/fdsi/documents/fdsi-reports/family-life-report.pdf

McConnell, D., Savage, A., & Breitkreuz, R. (2014). Resilience in families raising children with disabilities and behavior problems. *Research in Developmental Disabilities, 35*(4), 833–848. http://dx.doi.org/10.1016/j.ridd.2014.01.015

McDougall, J., King, G., De Wit, D. J., Miller, L. T., Hong, S., Offord, D. R., . . . Meyer, K. (2004). Chronic physical health conditions and disability among Canadian school-aged children: a national profile. *Disability and Rehabilitation, 26*(1), 35–45.

Mendes, M. A. (2013). Parents' descriptions of ideal home nursing care for their technology-dependent children. *Paediatric Nursing, 39*(2), 91–96.

Metcalfe, P. D. (2017). Neuropathic bladders: Investigation and treatment through their lifetime. *Canadian Urological Association Journal, 11*(1-2S), S81–S86.

Meyer, E. C., Ritholz, M. D., Burns, J. P., & Truog, R. D. (2006). Improving the quality of end-of-life care in the pediatric intensive care unit: Parents' priorities and recommendations. *Pediatrics, 117*(3), 649–657. doi:10.1542/peds.2005-0144.

Murphy, S. L., Xu, J., & Kochanek, K. D. (2013). Deaths: Final data for 2010. *National Vital Statistics Reports, 61*(4), 1–117.

Narvey, M. R.; Canadian Paediatric Society, Fetus and Newborn Committee. (2016). Assessment of cardiorespiratory stability using the infant car seat challenge before discharge in preterm infants (<37 weeks' gestational age). *Paediatrics & Child Health, 21*(3), 155–158.

National Association of Paediatric Nurse Practitioners. (2015). NAPNAP position statement on protection of children involved in research studies. *Journal of Paediatric Health Care, 29*(2), A13–A15.

Niela-Wilen, H., Melender, H. L., Axelin, A., Loyttyniemi, E., & Salantera, S. (2016). Predictors of breastfeeding initiation and frequency for preterm infants in the NICU. *Journal of Obstetric, Gynecologic & Neonatal Nursing, 45*(3), 346–358.

Noiseux, J., Rich, H., Bouchard, N., Noronha, C., & Carnevale, F. A. (2019). Children need privacy too: Respecting confidentiality in paediatric practice. *Paediatrics & Child Health, 24*(1):e8–e12. doi: 10.1093/pch/pxy047.

Pearson, L., & Li, L. (2015). *A Canada fit for children 2015: Identity, rights and belonging.* Retrieved from http://www.landonpearson. ca/uploads/6/0/1/4/6014680/a_canada_fit_for_children_2015.pdf

Pinzon, J., & Harvey, J. (2006). Care of the adolescents with chronic conditions. *Paediatric Child Health, 11*(1), 43–48. Retrieved from http://www.cps.ca//documents/position/ care-of-youth-chronic-conditions

Poole, K. L., Schmidt, L. A., Missiuna, C., Saigal, S., Boyle, M. H., & Van Lieshout, R. J. (2015). Motor coordination and mental health in extremely low birth weight survivors during the first four decades of life. *Research in Developmental Disabilities, 43–44,* 87–96.

Public Health Agency of Canada (PHAC). (2008). *Fetal alcohol spectrum disorder (FASD) prevention: Canadian perspectives.* Retrieved from http://www.phac-aspc.gc.ca/hp-ps/dca-dea/prog-ini/fasd-etcaf/publications/cp-pc/index-eng.php

Rushton, C. H. (2004). Ethics and palliative care in pediatrics: When should parents agree to withdraw life-sustaining therapy for children? *The American Journal of Nursing, 104*(4), 54–63.

SandBox Project. (2011). *Strategic action plan to improve the well-being of Canadian children & youth.* Retrieved from https:// static1.squarespace.com/static/575c7d10044262e4c49720f7/t/57 966ff6197aea8b4cf96228/1469476854935/Sandbox±Project±Wh ite±Paper±2012.pdf

Sanders, C., Edwards, Z., & Keegan, K. (2017). Exploring stakeholder experiences of interprofessional teamwork in sex development outpatient clinics. *Journal of Interprofessional Care, 31*(3), 376–385. Retrieved from http://www. tandfonline.com/doi/abs/10.1080/13561820.2016.1272559

Savage, A. (2012). *The well-being of Canadian youth with disability: A rights based perspective.* Retrieved from https:// cloudfront.ualberta.ca/-/media/rehabilitation/faculty-site/ research/fdsi/documents/presentations/amberiassid.pdf

Schulman, L. H., Meringolo, D., & Scott, G. (2007). Early intervention: A crash course for pediatricians. *Paediatric Annals, 36*(8), 463–469.

Shaw, T. M. (2012). Paediatric palliative pain and symptom management. *Paediatric Annals, 41*(8), 329–334.

Shepherd, C. A., & Waddell, C. (2015). A qualitative study of autism policy in Canada: Seeking consensus on children's services. *Journal of Autism and Developmental Disorders, 45*(11), 3550–3564. Retrieved from https://www.ncbi.nlm. nih.gov/pmc/articles/PMC4608990/

Shooshtari, S., Brownell, M., Mills, R. S. L., Dik, N., Yu, D. C., Chateau, D., . . . Wetzel, M. (2016). Comparing health status, health trajectories and use of health and social services between children with and without developmental disabilities: A population-based longitudinal study in manitoba. *Journal of Applied Research in Intellectual Disabilities, 30*(4), 584–601.

Smith, V. C., & Stewart, J. (2015). Discharge planning for high-risk newborns. Retrieved from http://www.uptodate.com/ contents/discharge-planning-for-high-risk-newborns

Social Security Administration. (n.d.). Title V–maternal and child health services block grant. Retrieved from http:// www.ssa.gov/OP_Home/ssact/title05/0500.htm

Starr, N. B., Blosser, C. G., Brady, M. A., Burns, C. E., Dunn, A. M., & Petersen-Smith, A. M. (2013). Gastrointestinal disorders. In C. E. Burns, A. M. Dunn, M. A. Brady, N. B. Starr, & C. G. Blosser (Eds.). *Paediatric primary care* (5th ed.). Philadelphia, PA: Elsevier Saunders.

Statistics Canada. (2006). *Participation and activity limitation survey. Children with disabilities and their families.* Retrieved from https://www.statcan.gc.ca/eng/survey/ household/participation/participation

Statistics Canada. (2015a). *Prevalence of obesity among children and adolescents in the United States and Canada, 1976 to 2013.* Retrieved from http://www.statcan.gc.ca/ daily-quotidien/150826/dq150826a-eng.htm

Statistics Canada. (2015b). *Study: Childhood cancer incidence and mortality in Canada, 1992 to 2010.* Retrieved from http:// www.statcan.gc.ca/daily-quotidien/150922/dq150922a-eng.htm

Sullivan, M. C., Msall, M. E., & Miller, R. J. (2012). 17-year outcome of preterm infants with diverse neonatal morbidities: Part 1—impact on physical, neurological, and psychological health status. *Journal for Specialists in Paediatric Nursing, 17*(3), 226–241.

Tabbers, M., DiLorenzo, M., Berger, M., Faure, C., Langendam, M., Nurko, S., . . . Benninga, M. (2014). Evaluation and treatment of functional constipation in infants and children: Evidence-based recommendations from ESPGHAN and NASPGHAN. *Journal of Pediatric Gastroenterology and Nutrition, 58*(2), 258–274.

The Canadian Encyclopedia. (2006). *Disability.* Retrieved from http://www.thecanadianencyclopedia.ca/en/article/ disability/#top

Tuffrey-Wijne, I. (2013). A new model for breaking bad news to people with intellectual disabilities. *Palliative Medicine, 27*(1), 5–12. DOI: 10.1177/0269216311433476

UNICEF. (2013). *Children and young people with disability. Fact sheet.* Retrieved from https://www.unicef.org/disabili-ties/files/Factsheet_A5__Web_NEW.pdf

Vessey, J. A., & Brown, S. S. (2010). Financing health care for children with chronic conditions. In P. J. Allen, J. A. Vessey, & N. A. Schapiro (Eds.). *Primary care of the child with a chronic condition* (5th ed.). St. Louis, MO: Mosby.

Vessey, J. A., & Sullivan, B. J. (2010). Chronic conditions and child development. In P. J. Allen, J. A. Vessey, & N. A. Schapiro (Eds.). *Primary care of the child with a chronic condition* (5th ed.). St. Louis, MO: Mosby.

Wajchendler, A., Anderson, P., & Koyle, M. A. (2017). The transition process of spina bifida patients to adult-centred care: An assessment of the Canadian urology landscape. *Canadian Urological Association Journal, 11*(1-2S), S88–S91.

Werner, S., & Shulman, C. (2013). Subjective well-being among family caregivers of individuals with developmental disabilities: the role of affiliate stigma and psychosocial moderating variables. *Research in Developmental Disabilities, 34*(11), 4103–4114.

Widger, K., Cadell., S., Davies, B., Siden, Hl., & Steele, R. (2012). Pediatric palliative care in Canada. In C. Knapp, V. Madden, & S. Fowler-Kerry (Eds.). *Pediatric palliative care: Global perspectives* (pp. 301–321). New York, NY: Springer.

Wolfe, J., Hinds, P. S., & Sourkes, B. M. (2011). The language of pediatric palliative care. In J. Wolfe, P. S. Hinds, & B. M. Sourkes (Eds.). *Textbook of interdisciplinary pediatric palliative care* (pp. 3-6). Philadelphia, PA: Elsevier/Saunders.

World Health Organization (WHO) (n.d. a). *Effective palliative care for children.* Retrieved from http://www.who.int/can-cer/palliative/en/

World Health Organization (WHO) (n.d. b). *WHO definition of palliative care.* Retrieved from http://www.who.int/cancer/ palliative/definition/en/

MULTIPLE CHOICE QUESTIONS

1. The parents of a 5-year-old with special health care needs talk to the parents of a 10-year-old with a similar condition for quite a while each day. What is the nurse's interpretation of this behaviour?
   a. The nurse has not provided enough emotional support for the parents.
   b. This relationship between the children's parents is potentially unhealthy.
   c. Support between parents of special children is extremely valuable.
   d. Confidentiality is a pressing issue in this particular situation.

2. The nurse is caring for a child who has received all possible medical care for cancer, yet continues to experience relapse and metastasis. It is time to make the transition from curative care attempts to palliative care. What is the most important nursing consideration at this time?
   a. The health care professionals should make the decision about the child's care.
   b. The family may lose a sense of hope, so cancer treatments should continue.
   c. Involve the family in the decision-making process about the shift to palliative care.
   d. Palliative care can take place only at home, so the child should be discharged.

3. The nurse is caring for a 3-year-old with a gastrostomy tube and tracheostomy who is on supplemental oxygen and multiple medications. The mother is rooming in during this hospitalization. What is the priority nursing action?
   a. Incorporate the mother's assistance in care when convenient.
   b. Recognize the mother as the expert on her child's needs and care.
   c. Recommend that the mother go home to get some rest.
   d. Provide family-centred care since the mother is there.

4. The nurse is caring for a child with a developmental disability who is starting kindergarten this year. The mother is tearful and doesn't want the child to go to school. What is the best response by the nurse?
   a. "Do you need some time alone to collect yourself?"
   b. "You've known for a while this time would come."
   c. "Can I call your husband or a friend for you?"
   e. "It is normal to feel stressed or sad at this time."

5. The parents of a child with a developmental disability ask the nurse for advice about disciplining their child. What is the best response by the nurse?
   a. "You should choose methods that are most congruent with your values about discipline."
   b. "Children like this really can't follow directions, so they may be very hard to discipline."
   c. "Punish your child only for socially unacceptable or offending behaviours."
   d. "Spanking works well for this type of child, as they really don't like pain."

CRITICAL THINKING EXERCISES

1. A 15-year-old boy is dying of cancer after all medical care options have been exhausted. Describe the plan of care for this child and his family. What strategies should the nurse use to support the child and his family through this difficult process?

2. A 5-month-old infant who was born at 24 weeks' gestation is ready to be discharged from the NICU. She will be going home on oxygen, gastrostomy tube feedings, and eight medications. Develop a teaching plan for the family.

STUDY ACTIVITIES

1. In the clinical setting, care for a child with a terminal illness. Reflect in your clinical journal about the feelings you had during the care of the child, as well as the feelings and behaviours that you noticed in the child, siblings, parents, and nursing staff.

2. Visit a preschool that provides care for developmentally delayed and typical children. Choose two same-age children, one with a disability or impairment and the other a typical healthy child. Perform a Denver developmental screening or developmental assessment on each of the two children. Compare and contrast your findings.

3. Spend the day with a home care nurse providing care for a technology-dependent child. What obstacles has the family overcome to have this child at home? What adjustments does the nurse make to provide family-centred care in the home (as compared to the hospital setting)?

BRINGING IT ALL TOGETHER: A CASE STUDY

Trey, a 7-month-old boy, will be receiving private duty nursing 8 hours per day upon his discharge from the NICU. He was born at 24 weeks' gestation and was discharged on oxygen via nasal cannula, a cardiac/apnea monitor, and oral feeding during the day with supplemental gastrostomy tube feedings overnight. In addition to twice-daily nebulized medications, he usually requires additional treatments throughout the day and is also on four additional oral/G-tube medications. His mother has verbalized being overwhelmed by the thought of caring for Trey at home.

Go to thePoint **to find questions to consider about this case.**

35

Medication Administration and Provision of Nutritional Support

Learning Objectives

Upon completion of this chapter, you will be able to:

1. Describe the "rights" of pediatric medication administration.

2. Explain the physiologic differences in children that can affect a medication's pharmacodynamic and pharmacokinetic properties.

3. Accurately determine recommended pediatric medication doses.

4. Demonstrate the proper technique for administering medication to children via oral, rectal, ophthalmic, optic, intravenous, intramuscular, and subcutaneous routes.

5. Integrate the concepts of atraumatic care in medication administration for children.

6. Identify the preferred sites for peripheral and central intravenous medication administration.

7. Describe nursing management related to maintenance of intravenous infusions in children, as well as prevention of complications.

8. Explain nursing care related to enteral tube feedings.

9. Describe nursing management of the child receiving total parenteral nutrition.

Lily Kline, a 9-month old, is admitted to your unit for failure to thrive. The physician has ordered insertion of a nasogastric tube to begin gavage feedings. The parents are very nervous and upset about this. They ask, "What will this tube do for Lily? It sounds very uncomfortable. What do you have to do to insert it? Will it have to stay in all the time? Won't it move?" How would you address their concerns?

The ill child often requires medications, intravenous (IV) therapy, or enteral nutrition to restore health. Such interventions occur most often in the inpatient setting, but with today's advanced technology, many children may receive treatment in the home, day care centre, school, healthcare provider office, healthcare facility, or other community setting.

This chapter will discuss the key elements of and guidelines for care related to medication administration, IV therapy, and nutritional support in children. Child and parent education is emphasized. The chapter will focus on adapting and modifying medication administration and nursing procedures based on the child's growth and development and providing these treatments using a family-centred, atraumatic approach.

MEDICATION ADMINISTRATION

At one time or another, every child is likely to require medication. As with adults, pediatric medication administration is a critical component of safe and effective nursing care. The pediatric nurse must adapt administration principles and techniques to meet the child's needs. Medication administration, regardless of the route, requires a solid knowledge base about the drug and its action. As with medication administration to any person, the nurse must adhere to the required "rights" of medication administration (Box 35.1). These rights

Safety Check

GOAL: Improve the Accuracy of Patient identification

Use at least two patient identifiers when providing care, treatment, and services.

Steps: When administering medications to a child, be sure to use a minimum of two patient identifiers that are directly associated with the patient and the medication to be given, such as full name, patient identification number, and birth date.

Accreditation Canada. (2015). *Required organizational practices: Handbook 2016.* Retrieved from https://accreditation.ca/sites/default/files/rop-handbook-2016-en.pdf

---

BOX 35.1

SEVEN RIGHTS OF PEDIATRIC MEDICATION ADMINISTRATION

Right Patient

- Confirm child identity by using two separate methods. Keep in mind that children may deny their identity or remove their ID bracelet in an attempt to avoid an unpleasant situation. They may also play in another child's room, which can lead to mistaken visual identification of the child.
- Confirm identity every time that medication is given.
- Verify child's name with caregiver to provide additional verification.
- Use technology when available (such as a bar code system).

Right Medication

- Check order and expiration dates of all medication.
- Know action of medication, potential side effects (use pharmacy, drug formulary), and what actions need to be taken in the event that a side effect occurs.
- Ensure that the medication provided is the medication that was actually ordered.

Right Time/Frequency

- Give medication within 20 to 30 minutes of the ordered time.
- For a medication given on an as-needed (PRN) basis, confirm when it was last given and how much has already been administered to the child over the past 24 hours.

Right Route

- Check ordered route and ensure this is the most effective, appropriate and safest route for this child; clarify any order that is confusing or unclear.

- Give the medication by the route ordered. If there is a need to change route, always check with prescriber (e.g., if a child is vomiting and has an order for an oral medication to be administered, the medication may need to be given via the IV or rectal route).

Right Dose

- Calculate the recommended dose according to child's weight and double-check your calculations. If you have any concerns, or if you do not have experience with the required type of calculation, ask a colleague to double-check it for you before you administer the medication to the child.
- Always question the pharmacist and/or prescriber if the ordered dose falls outside the recommended dose range.

Right Reason/Assessment

- Confirm the rationale for the medication that has been ordered. Understand the patient's medical history that precipitated the order.

Right Documentation

- Document administration of the medication only AFTER it has been given to the patient, never before.
- Appropriately chart all necessary information about the medication administration, including any laboratory values or vital signs that needed to be checked before the drug was administered to the patient.

were developed to ensure patient safety by decreasing the occurrence of medication errors. Some experts have added additional rights, such as right documentation, right to be educated, right to refuse, right form, and right approach. These additional rights are important considerations aimed at increasing patient safety and satisfaction.

Differences in Pharmacodynamics and Pharmacokinetics

Although a drug's mechanism of action is the same in any individual, the physiologic immaturity in some of the child's body systems can affect a drug's **pharmacodynamics** (behaviour of the medication at the cellular level). As a result, the body may not respond to the drug as intended, or as is expected. The effect may be erratic, enhanced, or diminished, necessitating a change in the dosage to ensure optimal effectiveness without increasing the child's risk for toxicity.

The child's age, weight, body surface area (BSA), and body composition also can affect the drug's **pharmacokinetics** (movement of drugs throughout the body via absorption, distribution, metabolism, and excretion). Drugs are administered to children via the same routes that are used for adults. However, this similarity ends once the drug has been administered. During the absorption process, drugs move from the administration site into the bloodstream. In infants and young children, the absorption of orally administered medications is affected by slower gastric emptying, increased intestinal motility, a proportionately larger small intestine surface area, higher gastric pH, and decreased lipase and amylase secretion compared with adults. Intramuscular (IM) absorption in infants and young children is affected by the amount of muscle mass, muscle tone and perfusion, and vasomotor instability. Similarly, decreased perfusion alters subcutaneous (SQ) absorption. In contrast, topical absorption of medications is increased in infants and young children as a result of greater BSA and skin permeability, which can result in adverse events (AEs) not seen in adults. The distribution of any administered medication (movement of a drug from the blood to interstitial spaces and then into cells) is also altered in infants and young children. Medication distribution in children is affected by:

- Higher percentage of body water than adults
- More rapid extracellular fluid exchange
- Decreased body fat
- Liver immaturity, altering first-pass elimination
- Decreased amounts of plasma proteins available for drug binding
- Immature blood–brain barrier, especially in neonates, allowing permeation by certain medications

The metabolism of medications in children is altered because of differences in hepatic enzyme production and the child's increased metabolic rate. Biotransformation (the alteration of chemical structures from their original form, which allows for eventual excretion of the substance) is affected by the same variations affecting distribution in children. In addition, immaturity of the kidneys until the age of 1 to 2 years affects renal blood flow, glomerular filtration, and active tubular secretion. This results in a longer half-life and increases the potential for toxicity of those drugs that are primarily excreted by the kidneys.

Developmental Issues and Concerns

Children are constantly growing and developing. The specific psychosocial, cognitive, physical, and motor development levels of children are important. Nurses need a solid understanding of growth and development to facilitate safe administration of medications to children. Table 35.1 details some growth and development issues related to administering medications to children. Always give developmentally appropriate, truthful explanations before administering medications to children, including:

- Why the drug is needed
- What the child may experience
- What is expected of the child
- Ways the parents can participate and support their child

The child's past experiences with taking medications, and the approaches that may have been used on those occasions, will often affect how the child reacts. Always approach children positively; let your manner convey the belief that they can accomplish this needed behaviour. Never label the child as "bad," even if he or she did not fully cooperate in taking medication. When medications must be administered with a needle (IM or SQ), assure the child that this method is not a consequence of the child's behaviour. Help parents to work through any feelings of frustration they may experience from the child's refusal to cooperate with medication administration. Provide parents with facts about growth and development issues and children's fears and anxieties related to medication administration. Always model appropriate ways of dealing with undesirable behaviour.

Take Note!

Always administer medications promptly, assist the child in holding still by using a comforting position for the child, and reward any positive behaviour. Remember that medication administration can be frightening for many children and they need your understanding and support.

Determination of Correct Dose

Administering the correct dose is a key component of medication administration and can obviously have significant safety implications. Children are more vulnerable

TABLE 35.1	GROWTH AND DEVELOPMENT ISSUES RELATED TO PEDIATRIC MEDICATION ADMINISTRATION	
Stage of Development	**Issue/Concern**	**Nursing Interventions**
Infant	Development of trust, which is fostered by consistent care; development of stranger anxiety later in infancy	Involve parents in medication administration to reduce stress for infant Ensure that parents hold and comfort infant during intervention
Toddler	Development of autonomy with displays of negativism; rituals, routines, and choices necessary to maintain some sense of control	Follow routines and rituals from home in giving medications if these are safe and positive approaches Involve parents in medication administration Offer simple choices (e.g., "Do you want Mom or me to give you your medicine?") Allow child to touch or handle equipment as appropriate
Preschooler	Development of initiative, which is fostered when they sense they are helping	Provide an opportunity to play with the equipment and respond positively to explanations and comforting Provide choices that are possible and keep them simple (e.g., "Do you want juice or water with your medication?" or "Which medication do you want to take first?") Do not ask, "Will you take your medicine now?" Involve parents in medication administration Be aware that giving suppositories is particularly upsetting to this age group because of their fears of bodily intrusion and mutilation
School-aged child	Development of industry, benefiting from being a part of their care; generally very cooperative	Explain to child in simple terms the purpose of the medication Seek their assistance, such as putting pills in cup or opening the packet, and allow a broader range of choices Establish a reward system to enhance their cooperation, if necessary
Adolescent	Development of identity, benefiting from much more control over their care	Approach in the same manner as adults, with respect and sensitivity to their needs Maintain the adolescent's privacy as much as possible

to even slight medication errors due to the individual dosing necessary for proper medication administration. Incorrect dosing or quantity has been found to be the most commonly reported medication error in the pediatric population (Manias, Kinney, Cranswick, & Williams, 2014). Many drug references list recommended pediatric dosages, and nurses are responsible for checking doses to ensure that they are appropriate for each child. Two common methods for determining pediatric doses are based on the unit of drug per kilogram of body weight or BSA.

Dose Determination by Body Weight

The most common method for calculating pediatric medication doses is based on body weight. The recommended dosage is usually expressed as the amount of drug to be given over a 24-hour period (mg/kg/day) or

as a single dose (mg/kg/dose). It is important to differentiate between the 24-hour dosage and the single dose. Use these guidelines to determine the correct dose by body weight:

1. Weigh the child.
2. If the child's weight is in pounds, convert it to kilograms by dividing the child's weight in pounds by 2.2.
3. Check a drug reference for the safe dose range (e.g., 10 to 20 mg/kg of body weight).
4. Calculate the low safe dose (Box 35.2).
5. Calculate the high safe dose (Box 35.2).
6. Determine if the ordered dose is within this safe range.

Take Note!

Pay close attention to whether the safe dose range has been given for 24 hours (mg/day) or is a single-dose period (mg/dose).

BOX 35.2

DOSAGE CALCULATION USING BODY WEIGHT

After converting the child's weight in pounds to kilograms and checking the safe dose range:
- Calculate the low safe dose range (e.g., 10 to 20 mg/kg and the child weighs 30 kg):
  - Set up a proportion using the low safe dose range
    10 mg/1 kg = x mg/30 kg
  - Solve for x by cross-multiplying:
    $1 \times x = 10 \times 30$
    $x = 300$ mg
- Calculate the high safe dose range:
  - Set up a proportion using the high safe dose range
    20 mg/1 kg = x mg/30 kg
  - Solve for x by cross-multiplying:
    $1 \times x = 20 \times 30$
    $x = 600$
- Compare the safe dose range (for this example, 300 to 600 mg) with the ordered dose. If the dose falls within the range, the dose is safe. If the dose falls outside the range, notify the prescriber *before* the medication is administered.

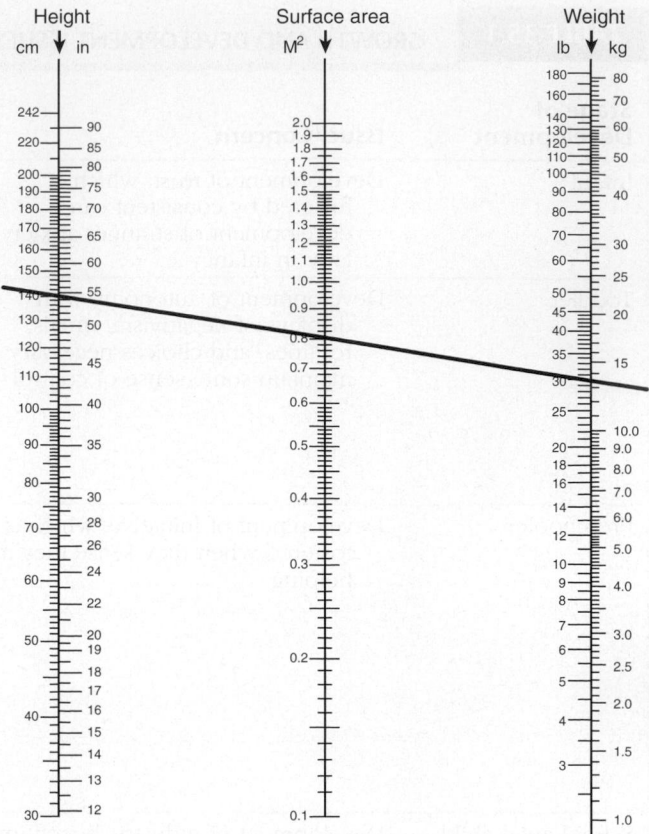

FIGURE 35.1 A nomogram to determine body surface area.

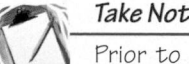

Take Note!

Prior to administering any medication to anyone, always remember to wash your hands. Also, don gloves if necessary. Adhere to the rights of medication administration.

The pediatric dosage should usually not exceed the minimum recommended adult dosage. Generally, once a child or adolescent weighs 40 to 50 kg or greater, the adult dose will frequently be prescribed (Bowden & Greenberg, 2011). However, it remains important to always verify that the prescribed dose does not exceed the maximum adult dose.

Dose Determination by Body Surface Area

Calculating the dosage based on BSA takes into account the child's metabolic rate and growth. It is commonly used for chemotherapeutic agents. Some recommended medication doses may read "mg/BSA/dose." To determine the dose using BSA, you will need to know the child's height and weight, which will be plotted on a nomogram (Fig. 35.1). A nomogram is a graph divided into three columns: height (left column), surface area (middle column), and weight (right column).

Use these guidelines to determine BSA:
1. Measure the child's height.
2. Determine the child's weight.
3. Using the nomogram, draw a line to connect the height measurement in the left column and the weight measurement in the right column.
4. Determine the point where this line intersects the line in the surface area column. This is the BSA, expressed in meters squared (m^2).

Once you have determined the BSA, use the recommended dosage range to calculate the safe dosage.

Oral Administration

Medications to be given via the oral route are supplied in many forms, including liquids (elixirs, syrups, or suspensions), powders, tablets, and capsules. Generally, children younger than the age of 5 to 6 are at higher risk for aspiration because they have difficulty swallowing tablets or capsules. Therefore, if a tablet or capsule is the only oral form available, it needs to be crushed or opened and mixed with a pleasant-tasting liquid or a small amount (generally no more than a tablespoon) of a nonessential food such as apple sauce. However, never crush or open an enteric-coated or time-release tablet or capsule without first discussing this option with a pharmacist or checking a trusted drug information resource. Elements of a crushed tablet or the insides of a capsule may taste bitter, so never mix it with formula or other essential foods; otherwise, the child may come to associate the bitter taste with the food and later refuse to eat it.

FIGURE 35.2 Devices used to administer oral medications to children.

> **Take Note!**
> Certain drug formulations should not be crushed. Before crushing a pill or opening a capsule, always check that this will not alter the intended effects of the drug. Crushing a time-release medication may result in immediate absorption of the entire dose of the medication; this can have lethal consequences.

Liquid medications, primarily suspensions, may separate over time. Always shake the liquid container gently before administration to ensure even drug distribution. The key to administering liquid forms of oral medications is to use calibrated equipment such as a medicine cup, spoon, plastic oral syringe, or dropper (Fig. 35.2).

> **Take Note!**
> Use a medicine cup or syringe with proper calibration instead of household cups or measuring spoons; the latter are not calibrated and may deliver an incorrect dose of medication.

If a dropper is packaged with a certain medication, never use it to administer another medication, since the drop size may vary from one dropper to another. If using a syringe for oral administration, only use the type intended for oral medications, not the one designed for parenteral administration. When using a dropper or oral syringe (without a needle) for infants or young children, direct the liquid toward the posterior portion of the mouth. Give the drug slowly in small amounts (0.2 to 0.5 mL at a time) and allow the child to swallow before more medication is placed in the mouth (Fig. 35.3). A nipple without the bottle attached is sometimes used to administer medication to infants. Place the medication directly in the nipple and keep the nipple filled with medication as the infant sucks so no air is taken in while the infant

FIGURE 35.3 Position the infant or young child with head elevated for safe medication administration. Holding the child or having a parent hold the child is preferred unless contraindicated.

takes the medication. Always place the infant or young child upright (at least a 45-degree angle) to avoid aspiration. The toddler or young preschooler may enjoy using the oral syringe to squirt the medicine slowly, into his or her own mouth. Older children can take oral medication from a medicine cup or measured medicine spoon.

> **Take Note!**
> Never force an oral medication into a child's mouth or pinch the child's nose. Doing so not only increases the risk for aspiration but also can interfere with the development of a trusting relationship.

As children adapt to swallowing tablets or capsules, administration is similar to that for adults. When helping the younger child learn how to swallow medication, the tablet or capsule can be placed at the back of the tongue or in a small amount of food, such as ice cream or apple sauce. Always tell children if there is medicine in the food; otherwise, they may learn not to trust you.

When the child has a nasogastric, orogastric, nasojejunal, nasoduodenal, **gastrostomy** (opening into the

- After administration of eye drops, gently press your finger for about 5 to 10 seconds against the inside corner where the eye meets the nose, blocking the tears and medication from exiting through the tear duct. This will help the eye to retain more of the medication. If the child is old enough, he or she may be able to do this unassisted.
- After administration of ointment, have the child close his or her eye and not rub the area.
- Ask the child not to blink or squeeze the eye shut more than normal, as this may wash away the medication prematurely.
- Using a clean tissue, gently dab away any tears or excess mediation that remains on the face.
- Wash your hands again and dry them thoroughly.

Adapted from The Hospital for Sick Children. (2017a). *Eye ointment: How to apply.* Retrieved from http://www.aboutkidshealth.ca/En/ HealthAZ/TestsAndTreatments/GivingMedication/Pages/ Eye-Ointment-How-to-Apply.aspx
Adapted from The Hospital for Sick Children. (2017b). *Eye drops: How to put in.* Retrieved from http://www.aboutkidshealth.ca/En/ HealthAZ/TestsAndTreatments/GivingMedication/Pages/Eye-Drops- How-to-Put-In.aspx

Otic Administration

Medications for otic administration are typically in the form of ear drops. This route of administration can be upsetting to the child because he or she will not be able to see what is happening. The child often receives otic drugs for an earache, and he or she may fear that the ear drops will increase the pain. To help allay such fears, explain to the child the purpose of the medication and the procedure for administration, using words and terms that he or she will be able to understand.

> ### Take Note!
> #### Administering Pediatric Ear Drops
> When administering pediatric ear drops, pulling the auricle down and back is correct if the child is younger than 3 years of age. To administer ear drops to a child who is 4 years old and above, the nurse should pull the auricle up and back.

Reinforce the need for the child to keep his or her head still. Younger children may require assistance to do so. Be sure that the ear drops are at room temperature. If necessary, roll the container between the palms of your hands to help warm the drops. Using cold ear drops can cause pain and possibly vertigo or vomiting when they reach the eardrum (Bowden & Greenberg, 2011).

Place the child in a supine or side-lying position with the affected ear exposed (Fig. 35.5). Pull the auricle downward and back in children younger than age 3 years; pull the auricle upward and back in older children. Instill the prescribed amount of medication using

FIGURE 35.5 Administering ear drops. (**A**) For the child younger than 3 years of age, the nurse pulls the pinna of the ear down and back. (**B**) For a child older than age 3 years, the nurse pulls the pinna of the affected ear up and back.

a dropper, being careful not to contaminate the tip of the dropper. Then, have the child remain in the same position for several minutes to ensure that the medication stays in the ear canal. Soothe, comfort, and distract the child to allow medication sufficient time to instill. Massage the area anterior to the affected ear to promote passage of the medication deeper into the ear canal. If necessary, place a piece of cotton or a cotton ball loosely in the ear canal to prevent the medication from leaking out as the child begins to move.

Nasal Administration

Nasally administered medications are typically in the form of drops and sprays. Administering nose drops to infants and young children may be difficult and additional help may be needed to help maintain the child's position. Ensure medication is at room temperature. Before medication is administered, have the child blow his nose or use a bulb syringe to clear nasal passage of secretions. For nose drops, position the child supine with the head hyperextended to ensure that the drops will

FIGURE 35.6 Administering nose drops. Tilt the head down and back to instill nose drops.

flow back into the nares. A pillow or folded towel can be used to facilitate this hyperextension. Place the tip of the dropper just at or inside the nasal opening, taking care not to touch the nares with the dropper (Fig. 35.6) since doing so might stimulate the child to sneeze. Although the nasal membranes are not sterile, the drop solution is; sneezing will contaminate the dropper, leading to contamination of the entire remaining drop solution when the dropper is returned back into the bottle. Once the drops have been instilled, maintain the child's head in hyperextension for at least 1 minute to ensure that the drops have come in contact with the nasal membranes.

For nasal sprays, position the child upright with head tilted slightly back. Place the tip of the spray bottle just inside the nasal opening and tilted toward the back. Hold one nostril closed (or have the child do this, if appropriate) and instruct the child to take a deep breath through the nostril while the medication is being administered. Squeeze the container, providing just enough force for the spray to be expelled from the container. Using too great a force can push the spray solution and secretions into the sinuses or eustachian tube. Repeat the same procedure with the other nostril if indicated. Small amounts of intranasal medication can be administered, as prescribed, during an acute event such as seizure (Zelcer & Goldman, 2016).

 Take Note!

In young infants, instill the medication in one naris at a time, since they are obligate nose breathers.

Intramuscular Administration

IM administration delivers medication to the muscle. In children, this method of medication administration is used as infrequently as possible, not only because it is painful but also because children often lack adequate muscle mass for medication absorption. However, IM administration is used to administer certain medications, such as immunizations.

Muscle development and the amount of fluid to be injected determine the IM injection site selected for use in children. Needle size (gauge and length) is determined by the size of the muscle and the viscosity of the medication. For example, more viscous medications often require a larger-gauge needle. In addition, the needle must be long enough to ensure that the medication actually reaches the muscle.

The preferred injection site for children less than 12 months of age is the vastus lateralis muscle in the anterolateral thigh (Centers for Disease Control and Prevention [CDC], 2016; Government of Canada, 2016). In children greater than 12 months of age, the deltoid muscle in the upper arm should be used (unless the muscle mass is not adequate, in which case the anterolateral thigh may be used instead) (CDC, 2016; Government of Canada, 2016). For children and adolescents between 3 years and 18 years of age, the deltoid muscle is preferred (CDC, 2016). The dorsogluteal site, often used in adults, is not recommended in children younger than 5 years of age. The muscle has not yet fully developed and, because the sciatic nerve occupies a larger portion of this area in the young child, the potential for development of sciatica is increased (BC Centre for Disease Control, 2010).

Take Note!

Many experts no longer recommend use of the dorsogluteal site at any age due to the risk of damaging the sciatic nerve (Aschenbrenner & Venable, 2012; Doyle & McCutcheon, 2015).

Figure 35.7 illustrates IM injection sites.

Select the needle size and gauge based on the size of the child's muscle. The goal is to use the smallest length and gauge that will deposit the medication into the muscle. Table 35.2 provides general guidelines for solution amount, needle size, and needle gauge when administering IM medications.

Insert the needle into the skin at a 90-degree angle. It is important to note that aspiration of blood used to be considered a part of IM injection procedure to ensure that the nurse had not inadvertently penetrated an artery or vein. However, critics of aspiration practice state it is nearly impossible for this to occur if the nurse is using proper technique and proper site selection; there are no large blood vessels present in the currently recommended injection sites, the vastus

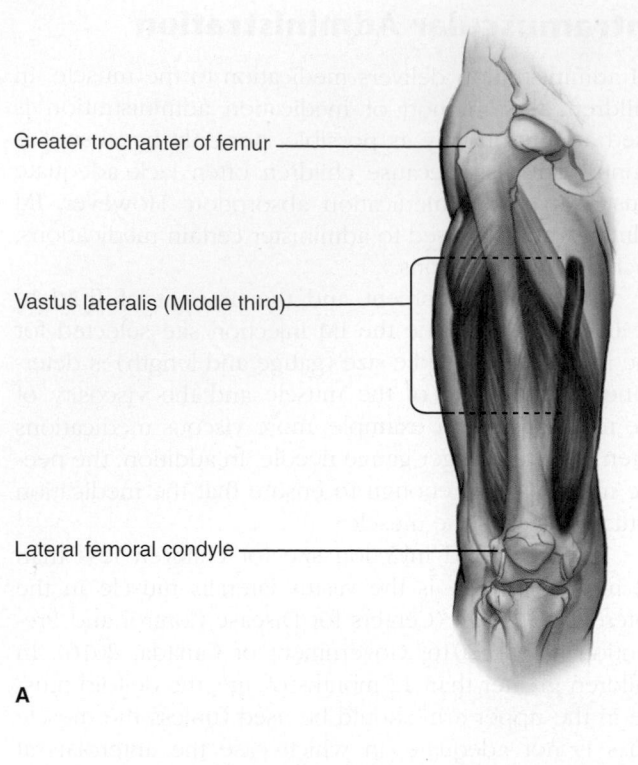

Greater trochanter of femur

Vastus lateralis (Middle third)

Lateral femoral condyle

A

Clavicle

Acromion process

Scapula

Deltoid muscle

Axilla

Humerus

Deep brachial artery

Radial nerve

B

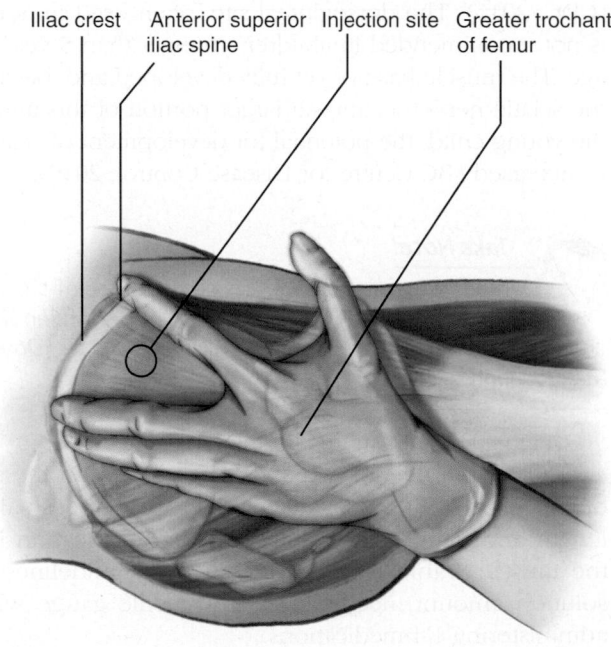

Iliac crest   Anterior superior   Injection site   Greater trochanter
                 iliac spine   of femur

C

FIGURE 35.7 Locating intramuscular injection sites. (**A**) Vastus lateralis: identify the greater trochanter and the lateral femoral condyle; inject in middle third and anterior lateral aspect. (**B**) Deltoid: locate the lateral side of the humerus, one to two finger widths below the acromion process. Inject into upper third of muscle. (**C**) Ventrogluteal: place palm of left hand on right greater trochanter so index finger points toward antero-superior iliac spine, spread middle finger to form a V, and inject in the middle of the V.

lateralis and deltoid muscles, so the risk of inadvertently hitting a blood vessel would be extremely slight (CDC, 2016; Davidson & Rourke, 2013; Taddio et al., 2010). Recent research has also shown decreased discomfort and no associated complications when IM immunizations are given using a rapid injection technique without

aspiration (BC Centre for Disease Control, 2009; CDC, 2016; Davidson & Rourke, 2013; Government of Canada, 2016). Therefore, the Government of Canada (2016) **no longer recommends aspiration** before injection of vaccines. In addition, a clinical practice guideline based on a systemic review of the literature, and developed by

TABLE 35.2	GUIDELINES FOR SOLUTION AMOUNT, NEEDLE LENGTH, AND NEEDLE GAUGE FOR IM INJECTIONS[a]				
	Solution Amount				
	Vastus Lateralis	*Deltoid*	*Ventrogluteal*	*Length*	*Gauge*
Infant	Preferred site; 0.5 mL	Not recommended	Not recommended until 12 months; then 0.5 mL	2.2–2.5 cm (7/8–1 in)	22–25
Toddler	0.5–1 mL	Preferred site; 0.5 mL	1 mL	2.2–2.5 cm (7/8–1 in)	22–25
Preschooler	1 mL	Preferred site; 0.5 mL	1.5 mL	2.2–2.5 cm (7/8–1 in)	22–25
School age	1.5–2 mL	Preferred site; 0.5–1 mL	1.5–2 mL	2.2–2.5 cm (7/8–1 in)	22–25
Adolescents		Preferred site; 0.5–1 mL		2.5–3.8 cm (1–1.5 in)	22–25

[a]Needle size and site need to be individualized based on the size of the muscle, amount of adipose tissue, amount of solution, and viscosity of solution to be administered.

Adapted from Government of Canada (2016) and BC Centre for Disease Control (2008).

representatives of many Canadian healthcare organizations, explicitly recommends that IM vaccines should be administered to children using a rapid injection technique *without* aspiration (Taddio et al., 2010).

Subcutaneous and Intradermal Administration

SQ administration distributes medication into the fatty layers of the body. It is used primarily for insulin administration, heparin, and certain immunizations, such as the measles, mumps, and rubella (MMR) vaccine. The amount of SQ tissue present differs between individuals. Therefore, when selecting a site and needle size, choose the most appropriate one based on adequacy and condition of the SQ tissue and the intended frequency and duration of the therapy. The preferred sites for SQ administration include the anterolateral thigh for infants less than 12 months of age and the upper triceps or anterolateral thigh for children older than 12 months (Government of Canada, 2016; Habib, Graydon, & Menezes, 2010). For all ages, a 1.6-cm (5/8 in), 25-gauge needle should be used (Government of Canada, 2016). Pinch up the skin to isolate the tissue from the muscle or pull it taut depending on the amount of adipose tissue present and length of needle, with the nondominant hand. Insert the needle at a 45-degree angle (Government of Canada, 2016), release the skin if pinched, and inject the medication. Remove the needle at the same angle it was inserted (Habib et al., 2010).

Intradermal (ID) administration deposits medication just under the epidermis. The forearm is the usual site for administration. ID administration is used primarily for tuberculosis screening and allergy testing. A 1-mL syringe with a 1.0-cm, 26- or 27-gauge needle is commonly used to administer the medication (Doyle & McCutcheon, 2015; Government of Canada, 2016). Insert the needle, with the bevel up, beneath the skin at a 5- to 15-degree angle (Doyle & McCutcheon, 2015). Keep the fingers and thumb resting on the sides of the syringe to ensure the proper angle.

Intravenous Administration

IV medication administration is commonly used with children, especially when a rapid response to a drug is desired or when absorption via other routes is difficult due to the child's illness or condition. In some cases, the IV route is the only effective method for administering a medication. Use of the IV route requires that the child have an IV device inserted, peripherally or centrally. Although insertion of this device is invasive and traumatic for the child, IV medication administration is considered to be less traumatic when compared with the trauma associated with multiple injections. Unfortunately, the veins of a child are small and easily irritated.

Most medications given by the IV route must be given at a specified rate and diluted properly to prevent overdose or toxicity due to the rapid onset of action that occurs with this route. Therefore, when administering medications via the IV route, knowledge of the drug, the amount of drug to be administered, the minimum dilution of the drug, the type of solution for dilution or infusion, the compatibility or various solutions and medications, the length of time for infusion, and the rate of

NURSING PROCEDURE 35.1

Administering Medication Via a Syringe Pump

Purpose: To Provide Accurate and Safe Administration of IV Medication

1. Verify the medication order.

2. Gather the medication and necessary equipment and supplies.

3. Wash hands and put on gloves.

4. Attach the syringe pump tubing to the medication syringe and purge air from the tubing by gently filling the tubing with medication from the syringe.

5. Insert the syringe into the pump according to the manufacturer's directions.

6. Clean the appropriate port on the child's IV access device or tubing, flush the device or tubing if appropriate (e.g., an intermittent infusion device [saline lock or heparin lock]), and attach the syringe tubing to the IV tubing or device.

7. Set the infusion rate on the pump as ordered.

8. When the medication infusion is completed, flush the syringe pump tubing to deliver any medication remaining in the tubing, according to institution protocol.

9. Document the procedure and the child's response to it.

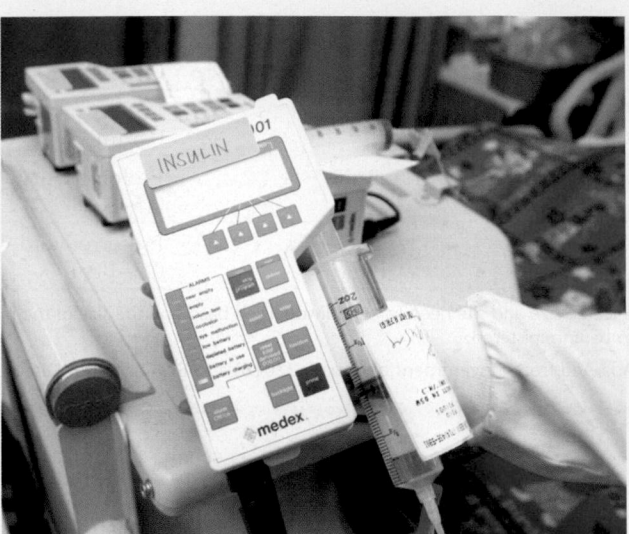

Adapted from Bowden, V. R., & Greenberg, C. S. (2011). *Pediatric nursing procedures* (3rd ed.). Philadelphia, PA: Lippincott Williams & Wilkins.

infusion are all required. Likewise, careful maintenance of the IV site is required to prevent complications.

The primary method for IV medication administration is a syringe pump. This method provides a high-precision rate of infusion. Nursing Procedure 35.1 gives the steps for administering medication via a syringe pump.

If a syringe pump is unavailable, the medication may be administered via a volume control device. The medication is added to this device with a specified amount of compatible fluid and is then infused at the ordered rate.

Take Note!

Some facilities have reduced or eliminated the use of volume control devices, especially for medication administration. Concerns include lack of identifying the medication in the volume control device and the potential for interaction or precipitation that may occur when multiple medications are administered using the same volume control device (ISMP, 2009). Be familiar with your facility's policies and procedures, and when using a volume control device, ensure that you label the chamber when medications are added and check for incompatibilities and potential interaction when multiple medications are given (ISMP, 2009).

Direct IV push medication is typically reserved for emergency situations and when therapeutic blood levels must be reached quickly to achieve the desired effect. Direct IV push administration requires that the drug be diluted appropriately and given at a specified rate, such as over 2 to 3 minutes. Care must be taken to prevent fluid overload, which may occur due to flushing needed to maintain IV patency and prevent drug incompatibilities, and from the administration of multiple drug therapies.

Providing Atraumatic Care

When administering any medication, including oral medications, use the principles of atraumatic care. Children can experience stress and fear or upset when they must take medications. The child may become upset or stressed when he or she must be secured snugly or positioned to minimize movement. The child may experience further discomfort if the medication has an unpleasant taste or results in pain, such as with an injection.

Atraumatic Care

Encourage the child to participate in care and provide the child with developmentally appropriate options, such as which fluid to drink with the medication or which flavour of ice pop to suck on before or after the administration (see Table 35.1).

To decrease discomfort and pain for the child who is to receive an injection, apply a topical anesthetic to the site before injection, when possible (Kroger et al., 2011), and inject the most painful medication last. Also, utilize developmentally appropriate distraction techniques, such as breastfeeding, music, books, blowing bubbles or a pinwheel, and deep breathing exercises.

Ensuring that the child will not move is essential to prevent injury when administering an injection. If the child is old enough to understand, taking the time to explain why he or she will be asked to remain still is an important first step toward gaining their cooperation and trust. Parents or caregivers can also be a significant source of support in effectively distracting the child during the injection. While it may ultimately be necessary to restrain the child to prevent injury, the least amount of restraint required should be used to keep the child still.

Take Note!

Research supports that children experience less pain and decreased fear if they are sitting versus lying down when receiving an injection (Eden et al., 2014).

Atraumatic Care

Use positions that are comforting to the child, such as therapeutic hugging, during injections. Have the child sit on the caregiver's lap with the caregiver holding the child's arms and legs to his or her body. After administration, encourage the parents or caregivers to hold and cuddle the child and offer praise.

Educating the Child and Parents

Teaching the child and parents or caregivers about medication administration is key. Many medications are given in the home, making the parents or caregivers the persons responsible for administration. They need to know what medications they are giving and why, how to give them, and what to expect from the drug. Since parents or caregivers often cite that AEs or side effects result in decisions to withhold medication, teaching

should include what AEs could occur (Hartling et al., 2016). Caregivers and parents often incorrectly dose medications or fail to follow prescribed orders, such as missing doses of medications or not completing the full course of medication (Yin et al., 2010; Walsh et al., 2013). Therefore, thorough instruction should be ensured, including frequency of administration, when the next dose is due, and length of time the medication is to be given. Emphasize the importance of completing the prescribed dose. Demonstrate use with an actual syringe if possible, encourage demonstration of correct medication administration procedures by the parent or caregiver (also known as "teach back"), advise against the use of home-measuring devices (such as a spoon, which can result in inaccurate medication measurement), and emphasize the importance of always using the calibrated dispensing device that was given with the medication. If the medication is to be given via injection, parents and caregivers need to learn how to administer the injection properly. Encourage questions or concerns from parents or caregivers.

Parents and caregivers commonly need suggestions about the best ways to administer the medication to their child. Provide them with tips for administration, such as mixing unpleasant-tasting medications with apple sauce or yogurt or offering a favourite liquid as a chaser. Pharmacies may be able to flavour medications to the child's preference. Also, teach the parents how to properly measure the amount of drug to be given. Teaching Guidelines 35.2 gives pointers about oral medication administration.

Teaching Guidelines 35.2
ADMINISTERING ORAL MEDICATIONS

- Be firm when telling the child that it is time for his or her medication. State, "It's time for your medicine" instead of asking, "Will you take your medicine?" or "Can you take your medicine for me?"
- Allow the child to choose an appropriate liquid to help swallow the medication or drink after taking it. Limit the choices to two or three.
- Never bribe or threaten the child to take his or her medication.
- Never refer to the medication as "candy."
- Be honest about the taste of the medication. If necessary, mix it with another food such as apple sauce, yogurt, or syrup to help mask the taste.
- Do not mix the medication with formula or baby food.
- Always check with your physician, nurse practitioner, or pharmacy about opening capsules or crushing tablets and mixing them with food. Some medications should not be opened or crushed.

- If you are giving a liquid using an oral syringe or dropper, place the medication slowly along the inside of the cheek. Never squirt the medication forcibly to the back of the child's throat. It may cause the child to gag and spit out the medication or aspirate it into his or her lungs.
- Always praise the child after taking the medication and provide comfort and cuddling.

Preventing Medication Errors

While medication delivery in virtually every area of health care can be highly complex, ensuring safe delivery to the pediatric population presents particular challenges and risk for errors to occur (ISMP Canada, 2009; Sears, Ross-White, & Godfrey, 2012). In one recent, large-scale medical review of pediatric admissions in the Canadian context, drug-related AEs accounted for 13.5% of all AEs identified in the study (Matlow et al., 2012). However, some estimates of the incidence of potentially harmful medication errors may be three times as high in pediatrics compared with adults (ISMP, 2015; Steering Committee on Quality Improvement and Management and Committee on Hospital Care, 2011). Many of these errors can be traced back to the need for weight-based dosing calculations, fractional dosing, the need for the use of decimal points, and a distinct lack of standardized, rigorous, easy-to-use dosage formulations and guidelines specifically created for the pediatric patient (Sears et al., 2012). Children are also more susceptible to medication harm because many drugs used in pediatrics have been formulated and packaged for adults, then provided to children without complete consideration and testing based on a child's younger age, stage of growth and development, lower body weight, and smaller BSA (Sears et al., 2012). It is important to remember that the pharmacokinetics and pharmacodynamics of a given drug "cannot simply be extrapolated to the pediatric population. For example, neonates have less physiologic reserve (i.e. volume of distribution) with which to buffer an overdose. These unique features of the pediatric population may put them at distinguishing risks for medication incidents when compared to adults" (Poon & Ho, 2011, p. 15). The variations in weight, BSA, and organ maturity significantly affect their ability to metabolize and excrete medications. Finally, infants and young children may be at significantly higher risk for medication errors because they are highly dependent on others for medication administration but may not yet have the ability to verbalize their subjective responses or adverse reactions to a medication dose or type (Sears et al., 2012). We continue to learn about various biological, developmental, and behavioural factors particular to children that can affect the safety and efficacy of the pharmaceuticals chosen for use in their treatment plans.

Confirming the child's identity and double-checking the dosage before administration of any medication are two critical safeguards that can play a major role in preventing medication errors. Other ways to prevent medication errors include the following:

- Always confirm that a child's listed weight is current.
- Always weigh children in kilograms.
- Double-check medication calculations; utilize another healthcare provider when possible, especially for high-risk medications.
- Utilize medication ordering and dispensing systems, if available.
- Always report medication errors or near-miss errors to help prevent future mistakes.
- Utilize the Institute for Safe Medication Practices ISMP Canada (2006), "Do not use: Dangerous abbreviations, symbols and dose designations."

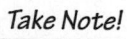 **Take Note!**

If any parent, caregiver, or child questions whether a medication should be given, listen attentively, answer their questions, and always double-check the order.

INTRAVENOUS THERAPY

IV access provides a route for the administration of medications and fluids. It is commonly used for children because it is the quickest, and often the most effective, method of administration. As with adults, numerous sites and various devices and equipment may be used to provide IV therapy over a short or long period of time. When administering IV therapy, safety is crucial. The nurse must have a solid knowledge base about the fluids or medications to be given as well as a thorough understanding of the child's physical and emotional development. Venipuncture can be a terrifying and painful experience for children and their families. Nurses play a crucial role in providing support and education to the child and family before, during, and after the procedure.

Sites

IV therapy may be administered via a peripheral vein or a central vein. Peripheral IV therapy sites commonly include the hands, feet, and forearms (Fig. 35.8). In neonates and young infants, the scalp veins may be used (O'Grady et al., 2011). The scalp veins are easily visualized, being covered by only a thin layer of SQ tissue. These veins do not have valves, so the device may be inserted in either direction, although the preference would be in the direction of blood flow. However, use of a scalp vein requires that the area of the infant's head be cleared of hair to enhance visualization. In addition, use of the scalp veins can be frightening to parents, who may think the fluid is infusing into the infant's brain. Thus, scalp veins are usually used only if attempts at other sites have been unsuccessful (Bergvall & Sawyer, 2012). When used, ensure appropriate education of the parents prior to insertion

and, if shaving the child's hair is needed, inquire whether parents would like to keep the child's hair.

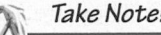
Take Note!

When selecting an IV site in an extremity, always choose the most distal site. Doing so prevents injury to the veins superior to the site and allows additional access sites should complications develop in the most distal site.

Central IV therapy usually is administered through a large vein, such as the subclavian, femoral, or jugular vein or the vena cava. The tip of the device lies in the superior vena cava just at the entrance to the right atrium. The device is inserted surgically or percutaneously and exits the body typically in the chest area, just below the clavicle. A device can be inserted via a peripheral vein, such as the median, cephalic, or basilic vein, and then threaded into the superior vena cava.

Equipment

The choice of equipment is determined by the solution or medication to be administered, the duration of the therapy, the age and developmental level of the child, the child's status, and the condition of his or her veins. Various types of IV devices are commercially available. In addition, different types of tubing and infusion control devices may be necessary, depending on the clinical circumstances.

Peripheral Access Devices

Devices used for peripheral venous access in a child include over-the-needle catheters or winged-infusion sets, commonly referred to as "butterflies" or scalp vein needles. These devices are inserted into the vein and then connected to the IV solution via tubing to provide a continuous infusion of fluid. These devices can also be inserted for intermittent use if the child does not require a continuous fluid infusion. Typically, the hub of the device is capped or plugged to allow intermittent access, such as for administering medications or obtaining blood specimens. When used in this manner, these devices are termed peripheral intermittent infusion devices or saline or heparin locks.

Needle size on the device also varies. Typically, the needle ranges from 21- to 25-gauge, depending on the child's size. The rule of thumb is to use the smallest-gauge catheter with the shortest length possible to prevent traumatizing the child's fragile veins. Typically, peripheral IV devices are used for short-term therapy lasting up to 1 week in duration (Moore, Bortolussi, & Canadian Paediatric Society, 2016). Midline catheters are also available and may be used if therapy is to exceed 1 week, although the Canadian Paediatric Society does note there is little data available on its duration of use in

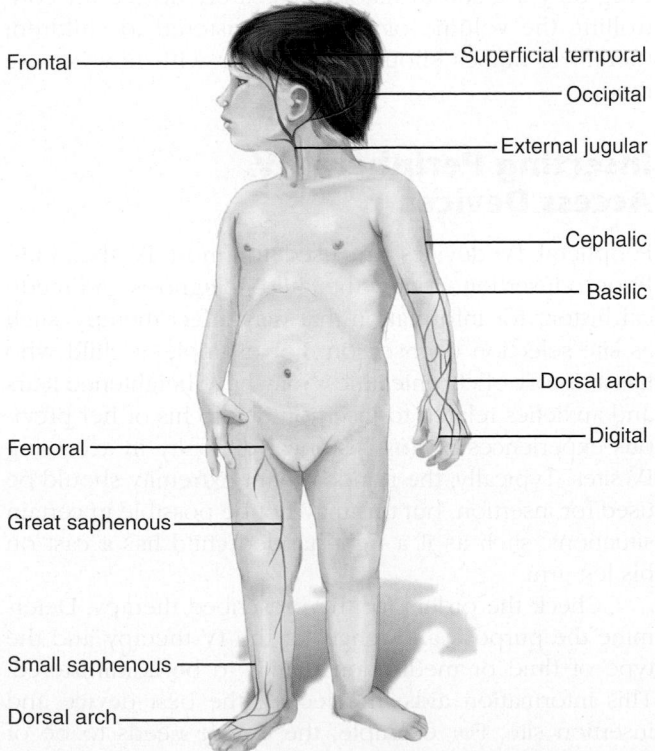

FIGURE 35.8 Preferred peripheral sites for IV insertion.

pediatric patients (Moore et al., 2016). These catheters are longer than peripheral catheters but still remain outside the central veins and can remain in place for up to 2 months (Bowden & Greenberg, 2011). They are seated deep in the cephalic or basilic veins, but the tip does not extend past the axilla.

Central Access Devices

Numerous devices for central venous access are available. The type chosen depends on several factors, including the duration of the therapy, the child's diagnosis, the risks to the child from insertion, and the ability of the child and family to care for the device. The device may have one or multiple lumens. Although central venous access devices can be used short term, the majority are used for moderate- to long-term therapy.

Safety Check

GOAL: Reduce the Risk of Health Care–Associated Infections

Implement evidence-based practices to prevent central line–associated bloodstream infections. Note: This requirement covers short- and long-term central venous catheters and peripherally inserted central catheter (PICC) lines.

Steps: When caring for a child with a central line, ensure to follow evidence-based policies and procedures strictly. Adhere to proper handwashing and aseptic techniques.

Public Health Agency of Canada. (2013); Safer Healthcare Now. (2012, June).

Central venous access devices are indicated when the child lacks suitable peripheral access, requires IV fluid or medication for a prolonged period of time, or is to receive specific treatments, such as the administration of highly concentrated solutions or irritating drugs like chemotherapeutic agents, parenteral nutrition or blood and blood products. Child preference is also a consideration. Central venous access is advantageous because it provides vascular access without the need for multiple IV starts, thus decreasing discomfort and fear. However, central venous access devices are also associated with complications such as infection at the site, sepsis due to the direct access to the central circulation, and thrombosis due to partial occlusion of the vessel. Typically, a chest x-ray is performed after a central venous access device is inserted to verify proper placement. No fluids are administered until correct placement is confirmed. Table 35.3 describes the major types of central venous access devices.

Infusion Control Devices

Infants and young children are at increased risk for fluid volume overload compared with adults. Also, malfunction at the IV insertion site, such as infiltration, may result in much greater injury than a similar incident would cause in an adult. Therefore, IV fluids must be carefully administered and monitored. To ensure accurate fluid administration, infusion control devices such as infusion pumps, syringe pumps, and volume control sets may be used.

Infusion pumps used for children are similar to those used for adults. In addition, syringe pumps are often used to deliver fluid and medications to children. These pumps can be programmed to deliver small amounts of fluid over controlled periods of time (see discussion on syringe pumps in the previous section).

An IV solution bag may be attached to a calibrated volume control set that has been filled with a specified amount of IV solution (Fig. 35.9). The fluid chamber holds a maximum of 100 to 150 mL of fluid that can be infused over a specified period of time as ordered. Usually, a maximum of a 2-hour infusion amount in the chamber avoids accidental fluid overload in the pediatric population. This chamber can be filled every 1 to 2 hours so that only small amounts of ordered quantities of fluid will be able to infuse and the child is protected from receiving too much fluid volume. Due to the advances in pump technology and the introduction of "smart pumps" which include dose error reduction systems such as hospital-defined drug libraries (drug lists) with standard drug concentrations, and dose limits, to potentially improve the safety of IV medication administration, the use of volume control devices is less common in practice (Loorand-Stiver, 2011). However, they are still available as a safety device for controlling the volume of fluid administered to children; therefore, nurses should be familiar with how to use them.

Inserting Peripheral IV Access Devices

Peripheral IV devices are used for most IV therapies. Prior to insertion, review the child's diagnosis and medical history for information that may affect therapy, such as site selection or insertion. For example, a child who has a history of chronic illness may have heightened fears and anxieties related to insertion due to his or her previous experiences or any historical difficulty in accessing IV sites. Typically, the nondominant extremity should be used for insertion, but this may not be possible in certain situations, such as if a right-handed child has a cast on his left arm.

Check the orders for the prescribed therapy. Determine the purpose and length of the IV therapy and the type of fluid or medication that is to be administered. This information aids in selecting the best device and insertion site. For example, the device needs to be of an adequate gauge to allow the solution or medication to infuse into the vein while at the same time allowing

TABLE 35.3	TYPES OF CENTRAL VENOUS ACCESS DEVICES

Device	Description
Peripherally inserted central catheter (PICC)	Short- to moderate-term therapy Insertion via a peripheral vein such as basilic, cephalic, or brachial vein Catheter typically threaded into superior vena cava; distal tip terminates in the superior vena cava, inferior vena cava, or proximal right atrium Insertion via saphenous vein with tip terminating in inferior vena cava above the diaphragm for infants Single or multiple lumens Can be inserted at the bedside; requires additional training and advanced skill
Nontunnelled central venous catheter (CVC)	Usually used short term One or more lumens Percutaneous insertion most commonly via the subclavian, internal jugular, or femoral vein with the tip of the catheter at the top of the superior vena cava just above the right atrium Useful for emergency situations Catheter sutured in place at the exit site Increased rate of central line–associated blood stream infection than tunnelled CVC
Tunnelled central venous catheter (e.g., Groshong, Hickman/Broviac)	Usually for long-term use Catheter inserted by a physician via small incision in jugular, femoral, or subclavian vein, and tunnelled in the subcutaneous tissue under the skin Initially sutured in place to stabilize position; sutures removed after approximately 1 to 2 weeks when cuff on catheter attaches to subcutaneous tissue Single or multiple lumens Some have valves that prevent backflow of blood and air entrance
Implanted ports (e.g., Port-a-Cath, Infus-a-Port, Mediport)	Surgically inserted by a physician Stainless steel port with a polyurethane or silicone catheter attached Catheter tip lying in subclavian or jugular vein; port implanted under skin in a subcutaneous pocket, usually on the upper chest wall Port covered completely by skin and visible only as a slight bulging on the chest; possibly more appealing to the older child and adolescent because there are no visible parts or dressings Access to port via a specially angled, noncoring needle (Huber needle) Site preparation and pain relief measures necessary before accessing the port Lowest risk for central line–associated blood stream infection

Adapted from The Joint Commission (2013). *Preventing central line–associated bloodstream infections: Useful tools, an international perspective.* Retrieved from http://www.jointcommission.org/Topics/Clabsi_toolkit.aspx; and Bowden, V. R., & Greenberg, C. S. (2011). *Pediatric nursing procedures* (3rd ed.). Philadelphia, PA: Lippincott Williams & Wilkins.

enough blood flow around the device to promote dilution of the infusion.

Establish rapport with the child and parents. Inform them about IV therapy and what to expect. Be honest with the child. Explain that the venipuncture will hurt but only for a short time. Provide the child with a time frame that he or she can understand, such as the time it takes to brush his or her teeth or eat a snack.

Atraumatic Care

Use therapeutic play to assist the child in preparation and coping for the procedure.

Insertion of an IV therapy device is traumatic. Follow the principles of atraumatic care, including the following:

• Gather all equipment needed before approaching the child.
• If possible, select a site using hand veins rather than wrist or upper arm veins to reduce the risk of phlebitis. Avoid using lower extremity veins and areas of joint flexion if possible because these are associated with an increased risk of thrombophlebitis and other complications (Bowden & Greenberg, 2011).
• Ensure adequate pain relief using pharmacologic and nonpharmacologic methods prior to insertion of the device.
• Allow the antiseptic used to prepare the site to dry completely before attempting insertion.

FIGURE 35.10 (**A**) IV house over the IV site on a child's hand. (**B**) IV house over the site on an infant's foot.

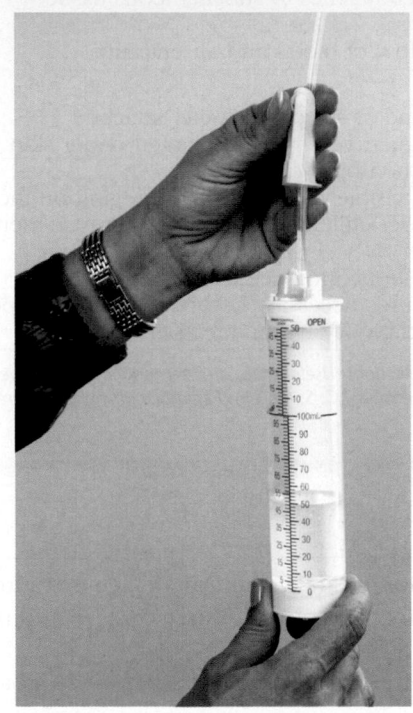

FIGURE 35.9 Volume control infusion device.

- Use a barrier such as gauze or a washcloth, or the sleeve of the child's gown, under the tourniquet to avoid pinching or damaging the skin.
- If the child's veins are difficult to locate, use a device to transilluminate the vein (utilizes a bright light, which illuminates the vein's size and direction of travel).
- Most facilities will have a policy that only allows a certain number of unsuccessful attempted IV starts by

an individual healthcare provider. Ensure that you are familiar with any such policy and, if you have reached that number of unsuccessful attempts, abide by policy directions regarding next steps. This may involve evaluating the need for insertion of a different type of access device.
- Encourage parental participation, as appropriate, in helping to position the child or to provide comfort positioning, such as therapeutic hugging.
- Coordinate care with other departments, such as the laboratory for blood specimen collection, to minimize the number of venipunctures required for a child.
- Secure the IV line using a minimal amount of tape or transparent dressing.
- Protect the site from bumping by using a security device such as the IV house dressing (Fig. 35.10).

IV Fluid Administration

Administering IV fluids to an infant or child requires close attention to the child's fluid status. Typically, the

TABLE 35.4	INTRAVENOUS MAINTENANCE FLUID CALCULATIONS BY BODY WEIGHT
<10 kg in weight	100 mL per kg of weight = # mL for 24 hours Example: A child weighs 7.4 kg 7.4 × 100 = 740 mL (daily requirement) 740/24 = 30.8 or 31 mL/hour
11–20 kg in weight	100 mL per kg of weight for the first 10 kg + 50 mL/kg for the next 10 kg = # mL for 24 hours Example: A child weighs 16 kg (10 × 100 = 1,000) plus (6 × 50 = 300) Total = 1,300 mL (daily requirement) 1,300/24 = 54 mL/hour
>20 kg in weight	100 mL/kg for the first 10 kg + 50 mL/kg for the next 10 kg + 20 mL/kg for each kg >20 kg = # mL for 24 hours Example: A child weighs 30 kg (10 × 100 = 1,000) plus (10 × 50 = 500) plus (10 × 20 = 200) Total = 1,700 mL (daily requirement) 1,700/24 = 70.8 or 71 mL/hour

amount of fluid to be administered within a 24-hour period is determined by the child's weight (in kilograms) and using the following formula:

100 mL per kg of body weight for the first 10 kg
50 mL per kg of body weight for the next 10 kg
20 mL per kg of body weight for the remainder of body weight in kilograms

Table 35.4 gives examples of calculating a child's fluid requirements using body weight. Once the 24-hour total fluid requirement is determined, this amount is then divided by 24 hours to arrive at the correct hourly rate of infusion.

Maintaining IV Fluid Therapy

Throughout the course of therapy, monitor the fluid infusion rate and volume closely, as often as every hour. If a volume control set is used to administer the IV infusion, fill the device with the allotted amount of fluid that the child is to receive in 1 hour. Doing so prevents inadvertent administration of too much fluid. Never assume that, just because an infusion pump is in use, the infusion is being administered without problems. Pumps can malfunction. The tubing can become blocked, or the IV device can move out of the vein lumen. Not enough fluid, fluid overload, or infiltration of the solution into the tissues can occur and cause significant complications for the child.

In addition to monitoring the fluid infusion, closely monitor the child's output. Expected urine output for children and adolescents is 1 to 2 mL/kg/hour.

Take Note!
When measuring the output of an infant or child who is not toilet trained or who is incontinent, weigh the diaper to determine the output. Remember that 1 g of weight is essentially equal to 1 mL of urine.

Flushing the IV line when the device is used intermittently may be necessary to maintain patency, such as before and/or after medication is administered and after obtaining blood specimens. However, there is much debate as to how often flushing should be done and the best flush solution to use: heparin or saline. Saline has been found to be more compatible with the numerous solutions and medications administered intravenously, and is less expensive and less irritating to the vein. In addition, using saline lessens the incidence of pain and phlebitis. Heparin is expensive and incompatible with numerous medications and solutions, and it can affect clotting time. A clinical trial is currently underway that is investigating normal saline versus heparinized solution flush for maintaining patency of peripheral venous catheters in children. Preliminary results favour the heparinized solution but the study is still in progress (Festini, Giusti, Ciofi, Olivini, & Bisogni, 2014). A recent systematic review of randomized control studies did show that continuous infusion of low-dose heparin resulted in increased catheter patency and decreased infusion failures while intermittent heparin flushing showed minimal benefits (Kumar, Vandermeer, Bassler, & Mansoor, 2013). Evidence appears to support that both heparin and normal saline are effective for maintaining patency of peripheral IV catheters. Additional research is needed to determine the best solution, volume and concentration of the flush solution, and interval for flushing. Flushing solutions and procedure will vary; therefore, it is important to always follow your agency's policy or provider order for flushing IV lines. Accreditation Canada (2015) currently advises that, for the flushing of intravenous lines, providers and facilities are encouraged to consult best practice guidelines to explore options other than heparin; heparin is considered to be a high-alert medication and may require additional strategies to ensure its safe use in this context.

If the child is receiving IV therapy via a central venous access device, provide site care using sterile technique and flush the device according to agency policy. Note the exit site for the device and inspect it frequently for signs of infection. If the device has multiple lumens, label each lumen with its use (i.e. blood specimen, medication, or fluid). Always check the compatibilities of any solutions and medications that are being given simultaneously.

Take Note!

When flushing or administering medications through a PICC line, follow the manufacturer's recommended syringe size because PICC lines are fragile. Using a larger volume syringe (i.e., 5 mL or larger) exerts less pressure on the PICC, thus reducing the risk of rupture (Bowden & Greenberg, 2011).

Preventing Complications

IV therapy is an invasive procedure that is associated with numerous complications. Strict aseptic technique is necessary when inserting the device and caring for the site. Ensure proper disinfecting of all catheter hubs, needleless connectors, and injection ports before accessing them or disconnecting/reconnecting tubing to minimize contamination. Adherence to standard infection control precautions is key to maximizing patient safety and minimizing risk.

Inspect the insertion site at least every 1 hour for **inflammation** (phlebitis) or **infiltration** (inadvertent infusion of a nonirritant solution or medication into the surrounding tissue). Note signs of inflammation such as warmth, redness, induration, or tender skin. Check closely for signs of infiltration such as cool, blanched, or puffy skin and compare limbs for any generalized edema. Use of a transparent dressing or IV house dressing provides easy access for assessing the IV insertion site. These types of dressings should be changed as necessary based on assessment. Dressings help to prevent movement of the catheter hub, thus minimizing the risk of mechanical irritation, dislodgement, and complications such as phlebitis or infection (Fig. 35.10). Never reinforce wet, stained, or damp dressing covering the IV site; rather, change the dressing and check the site.

Typically, in adults, an IV site is changed every 72 to 96 hours and at any time when the integrity of the system has been compromised or contamination is suspected (O'Grady et al., 2011). However, with children, the 72- to 96-hour time frame may need to be adjusted to minimize the child's exposure to the repeated trauma of insertion. Current recommendations include replacement in children only when clinically indicated (O'Grady et al., 2011). Follow local policies and procedures related to site changes. Replace IV administration tubing per agency

policy following a standardized protocol; SickKids (n.d.) suggest IV solution bags and syringes are replaced every 24 hours, tubing a minimum of every 72 hours.

Consider an alternative route for fluid and medication administration or the insertion of an alternative IV device, such as a PICC line. Catheter-related bloodstream infections often can occur with the use of central venous lines. These infections result in increased morbidity and healthcare costs, therefore prevention is paramount (O'Grady et al., 2011). Nurses need to practice proper hand hygiene, use maximal barrier protection during insertion, assess the site frequently, provide proper site care using strict sterile technique, and ensure that the child's central venous catheter is removed as soon as it is no longer needed. In children, it is important also to prevent the child from touching and playing with the central venous line site or dressing.

Take Note!

Chlorhexidine-impregnated sponge (Biopatch) dressings may be used to help prevent infection in children older than 2 months of age (O'Grady et al., 2011). Always follow institutional policies and procedures regarding site care.

Discontinuing the IV Device

Prepare the child for removal of the IV device in much the same manner as for insertion. Many children may fear the removal of the device to the same extent that they feared its insertion. Explain what is to occur and, where possible and appropriate, enlist the child's help in the removal so that they feel some degree of control over the procedure.

Atraumatic Care

If appropriate, allow the child to assist in removing the tape or dressing. This gives the child a sense of control over the situation and also encourages his or her cooperation.

In addition, practice atraumatic care by doing the following:
- Use water or adhesive remover to help loosen the tape.
- If a transparent dressing is in place, gently lift off the dressing by pulling up opposite corners using a motion parallel to the skin surface.
- Avoid using scissors to cut the tape, but if cutting the tape is necessary, be sure that the child's fingers are clear of the tape and scissors.
- Turn off the infusion solution and pump.
- Once all tape and dressings are removed, gently slide the IV device out using a motion opposite to that used for the insertion.

- Apply pressure to the site with a dry gauze dressing and then cover with a small adhesive bandage. If possible, allow the child to choose the bandage.

> ### Take Note!
>
> If the IV site was in the arm at or near the antecubital space, apply pressure until the bleeding stops. Do not have the child bend his or her arm after removal of the device as this is not sufficient pressure to prevent hematoma formation.

PROVIDING NUTRITIONAL SUPPORT

Adequate nutrition is important for all individuals but especially for children. During the growing years, the quality of a child's nutrition can have a significant effect on his or her overall health and development. The presence of a chronic illness, disease, or trauma can increase the child's nutritional demands; if the child cannot meet these even with oral supplementation, other measures may be necessary to provide adequate nutritional support. Such measures may include **enteral nutrition** (delivery of nutrition into the gastrointestinal tract via a tube) and **parenteral nutrition** (IV delivery of nutritional substances). The nutritional plan for any particular child will be determined by that child's age, developmental level, and health status.

Enteral Nutrition

Enteral nutrition, commonly called tube feedings, involves the insertion of a tube so that feedings can be delivered directly into the child's gastrointestinal tract. The tube may be inserted via the nose or mouth or through an opening in the abdominal area, with the tube ending in the stomach or small intestine. Nasogastric or orogastric tube feedings, a tube from the nose to the stomach or from the mouth to the stomach, respectively, are commonly referred to as **gavage feedings**. Nasoduodenal or nasojejunal feedings involve a tube that is inserted through the nose and ends in either the duodenum or jejunum. Gastrostomy feedings involve the insertion of a gastrostomy tube through an opening in the abdominal wall and into the stomach. Jejunostomy feedings are similar to gastrostomy feedings except that the tube lies in the jejunum.

Enteral nutrition is indicated for children who have a functioning gastrointestinal tract but cannot ingest sufficient nutrients orally to satisfy his or her needs. The child may be unconscious or have a severely debilitating condition that interferes with his or her ability to consume adequate food and fluids. Other conditions that may warrant the use of enteral nutrition include:
- Failure to thrive
- Inability to suck or tiring easily during sucking

FIGURE 35.11 **(A)** Gastrostomy tube. **(B)** Low-profile (button) gastrostomy tube. The filled balloon keeps the tube in place inside the stomach.

- Abnormalities of the throat or esophagus
- Swallowing difficulties or high risk for aspiration
- Respiratory distress
- Metabolic conditions
- Severe gastroesophageal reflux disease (GERD)
- Surgery
- Severe trauma

Enteral feedings may be given via nasogastric, orogastric, nasojejunal, nasoduodenal, gastrostomy, or jejunostomy tubes (Fig. 35.11). Table 35.5 provides additional information about these types of feeding tubes. Enteral feeding incurs lower costs and is associated with fewer complications, and is considered safer than parenteral feedings. However, tube misplacement is a serious complication of enteral feeding. Children considered to be at particularly high risk for misplaced or dislodged gastric enteral tubes include neonates, children with various neurological impairments, children who have a decreased gag reflex, and children who are sedated or critically ill (Irving et al., 2014).

Inserting a Nasogastric or Orogastric Feeding Tube (Gavage Feeding)

Tubes for gavage feeding can be inserted via the nose or mouth. For infants, who are obligate nose breathers, insertion via the mouth may be appropriate. Oral insertion also promotes sucking in the infant. For the older child, nasal insertion is usually the preferred method. If the tube is to remain in place, the nose also is considered to be more comfortable. Nursing Procedure 35.2 gives the steps for inserting a gavage feeding tube.

TABLE 35.5	TYPES OF ENTERAL FEEDING TUBES	
Type of Tube	**Indication**	**Nursing Implications**
Nasogastric (inserted via the nose into the stomach) Orogastric (inserted via the mouth into the stomach)	Short-term enteral feeding Orogastric usually limited to young infants only	• Long-term use or repeated insertion causes irritation and discomfort • Silicone and polyurethane tubes are very flexible and more comfortable; they require a stylet or guidewire for insertion • Length of long-term use varies according to the type of tube used and the institution protocol. Periodically, a nasogastric tube is removed and reinserted via the opposite nostril to prevent pressure on the nasal mucosa • Maintaining orogastric placement between feedings can be difficult due to oral secretions
Nasoduodenal (inserted via the nose to the duodenum) or nasojejunal (inserted via the nose to the jejunum)	Short-term enteral feeding. Indicated if child has trouble digesting food, cannot use his or her gastrointestinal tract secondary to congenital anomalies or surgery, or is at risk for or has a history of severe reflux or aspiration	• Silicone and polyurethane tubes with weighted tip allow tube to pass from pylorus into small intestines • Agency may require special training in order to place at bedside; may also be performed in radiology • Length of use same as nasogastric or orogastric tubes
Gastrostomy (surgically inserted through the abdominal wall into the stomach) Jejunostomy (surgically inserted through the abdominal wall into the jejunum)	Long-term enteral feeding or when esophageal atresia or stricture is present Jejunostomy tubes are indicated when gastric feeding is not tolerated	• The inner section of the tube is below the skin surface with the tip located in the stomach or jejunum (may be balloon, winged, or mushroom shaped). The outer section appears above the skin surface at the insertion site and has an opening or feeding port to which the feeding solution is attached • Low-profile gastrostomy device (gastrostomy button) is flush with the abdominal surface. The flip-top opening is anchored by a dome that fits against the stomach wall. Less conspicuous, it allows the child to be more active and mobile • After initial insertion, the tube length is measured from the insertion site to the far end of the tube and recorded. This measurement is checked at least daily to ensure that the tube has not moved • There are many different devices available. For any gastrostomy or jejunostomy tube, the type and size of tube inserted as well as the amount required to fill the balloon, if present, should be known

DETERMINING TUBING LENGTH FOR INSERTION

Improving the accuracy of predicting tube length will lead to an increase in successful nasogastric tube placements, and therefore, improved outcomes and decreased healthcare costs.

According to the Agency for Healthcare Research and Quality's National Guideline Clearinghouse (2012), determining tubing length for insertion of a nasogastric tube using age-related height-based (ARHB) methods versus the traditional morphologic method is more accurate for children greater than 2 weeks of age (National Guideline Clearinghouse, 2012). Refer to Table 35.6 for ARHB equations.

Continue to use traditional morphologic methods in neonates less than 2 weeks, children with short stature, or if unable to obtain an accurate height (Cincinnati Children's Hospital Medical Center, 2011; National Guideline Clearinghouse, 2012).

CHECKING TUBE PLACEMENT

Once the gavage feeding tube is inserted, checking for placement is an essential step. Tube placement must be confirmed each time the tube is inserted and before each use of the tube (including any use of the tube to administer medication). Radiologic confirmation of tube placement is considered the most accurate method (Irving et al., 2014;

NURSING PROCEDURE 35.2

Inserting a Gavage Feeding Tube

Purpose: To Provide a Means for Delivering Nutrition to the Child's Functioning Gastrointestinal Tract

1. Verify the order for gavage feeding.

2. Explain the procedure to the child and parents using appropriate language geared to the child's development level.

3. Gather the necessary equipment; remove formula for feeding from refrigerator if appropriate and allow it to come to room temperature.

4. Wash hands and put on gloves.

5. Inspect the child's nose and mouth for deformities that may interfere with passage of the tube.

6. Position an infant supine with the chin slightly raised and with the neck slightly hyperextended so that the nose is pointed upward. If necessary, place a rolled towel or blanket under the neck to help in maintaining this position. Assist an older child to a straight sitting position, if appropriate. Alternatively, have the parent or another person hold the child to promote comfort and reassurance. If needed, enlist the aid of additional persons, such as a parent or other healthcare team member, to assist in maintaining the child's position.

7. Determine the tubing length required for insertion: Use age-related height-based method (see Table 35.6) if possible, or the "NEMU" (**N**ose, **E**ar, **M**id-**U**mbilicus) measurement. For the latter, measure the tube from the tip of the child's nose to the base of the earlobe and then from the earlobe to the point midway between the xiphoid process and umbilicus. Mark this measurement on the tube with a permanent marker or with a piece of tape.

8. Lubricate the first 5 to 10 cm (2 to 4 in) of the tube with a generous amount of sterile water (many small-bore feeding tubes have a water-activated lubricant) or water-soluble lubricant to promote passage of the tube and minimize trauma to the child's mucosa.

9. Insert the tube into one of the nares or the mouth (if the child has already had a nasogastric tube inserted recently, try to alternate the nostril used with each change). Direct a nasally inserted tube straight back toward the occiput; direct an orally inserted tube toward the back of the throat.

10. Advance the tube slowly to the designated length; encourage the child (if capable) to swallow frequently to assist with advancing the tube.

11. Watch for signs of distress, such as gasping, coughing, or cyanosis, indicating that the tube is in the airway. If these signs develop, withdraw the tube and allow the child to rest before attempting reinsertion.

12. Temporarily secure tube to child's face with a small piece of tape (check the child has no allergy to tape/dressing to be used), remove stylet if applicable, and check for proper placement of the tube. Refer to Box 35.4.

13. Document the type of tube inserted; mark and record the length of tubing inserted; measurement of external tubing length, from nares to end of tube, after insertion; and confirmation of placement (see Box 35.4).

Adapted from Lyman, B., Yaworski, J. A., Duesing, L., & Moore, C. (2016). Verifying NG feeding tube placement in pediatric patients. *American Nurse Today, 11*(1), 1–3.

TABLE 35.6	AGE-RELATED HEIGHT-BASED (ARHB) EQUATIONS FOR PREDICTING OG/NG TUBE INSERTION LENGTHS	
Route	Age Group	Predicted Internal Distance to the Body of the Stomach Determined by:
Oral	Age ≤ 28 months	16.6 + 0.183 (height cm)
	Between ages 28 months and 100 months (8 years 4 months)	20.1 + 0.183 (height cm)
	Between ages 100 months (8 years 4 months) and 121 months (approx. 10 years)	17 + 0.218 (height cm)
	Greater than 121 months (approx. 10 years)	18.5 + 0.218 (height cm)
Nasal	Age < 28 months	17.6 + 0.197 (height cm)
	Between ages 28 months and 100 months (8 years 4 months)	21.1 + 0.197 (height cm)
	Between ages 100 months (8 years 4 months) and 121 months (approx. 10 years)	18.7 + 0.218 (height cm)
	Greater than 121 months (approx. 10 years)	21.2 + 0.218 (height cm)

Adapted from Cincinnati Children's Hospital Medical Center (2011). *Best evidence statement (BESt). Confirmation of nasogastric/orogastric tube (NGT/OGT) placement.* Cincinnati, OH: Cincinnati Children's Hospital Medical Center. Retrieved from http://www.cincinnatichildrens.org/assets/0/78/1067/2709/2777/2793/9198/ad67ab29–2a71–42a4-b78e-3d0e9710adac.pdf

Itkin et al., 2011), but the risks associated with repeated radiation exposure, high costs, and the impractical nature of obtaining a x-ray before feeding tube use can render it impractical (Cincinnati Children's Hospital Medical Center, 2011; Farrington, Lang, Cullen, & Stewart, 2009).

Take Note!

Instilling air into the tube and then auscultating for the sound is no longer considered a viable, single verification method for checking tube placement and is no longer recommended (Irving et al., 2014; Itkin et al., 2011; Lemyze, 2010; Lyman et al., 2016).

Research has suggested alternative methods such as using measurements of bilirubin, trypsin, and pepsin levels, CO_2 monitoring, transillumination and magnetic detection to enhance assessment of tube placement, but insufficient evidence is available to support these methods. Also, these methods have other limitations such as the cost, the availability of equipment, and the limited availability for bedside testing of these levels.

Refer to Box 35.4 for methods to verify feeding tube placement. However, keep in mind that even with these methods, tube malpositioning can occur. Therefore, nurses need to be vigilant in checking for tube placement using the recommended methods and be cautious and proactive if there is any suspicion that the tube may be misplaced.

Take Note!

If bedside methods of verifying tube placement are conflicting, or if the child is at high risk, such as children with swallowing problems, children with altered levels of consciousness, or children in the intensive care unit, radiologic verification is recommended as the "gold standard" confirmation method.

If the gavage feeding tube is to remain in place, secure it to the child's cheek. Do not tape the tube to the child's forehead, because this could lead to irritation and pressure on, and possible breakdown of, the nasal mucosa. Also, measure the length of the tube extending from the nose or mouth to the end and record this information. Double-check this measurement before administering each intermittent tube feeding, or administering medication through the tube, to verify that the feeding tube is in the proper position. Once the position of the gavage feeding tube is confirmed, the feeding solution or medication can be administered.

Knotting of a nasogastric tube, while rare, has been reported in the literature as case studies. Therefore, nurses need to be vigilant if any feeding, respiratory (stridor), or removal difficulties are noted and raise concerns with the physician.

Remember Lily, the 9-month-old infant, diagnosed with failure to thrive who is to receive gavage feedings with a nasogastric tube? What equipment will be needed, and what steps will you take to complete the procedure?

Administering Enteral Feedings

Enteral feedings can be given continuously or intermittently, regardless of the type of tube used. Intermittent feedings are commonly called **bolus feedings**. With a

BOX 35.4

METHODS FOR VERIFICATION OF FEEDING TUBE PLACEMENT

- Obtain radiographic confirmation of proper tube placement in children who are considered high risk for aspiration, such as children with neurologic impairment, children who are not fully alert, sedated, unconscious, critically ill, reduced gag reflex, or static encephalopathy, or when nonradiologic methods are not feasible or bedside results are conflicting.
- Nonradiologic verification is used in children who are not considered high risk for aspiration; document pH of aspirate; document insertion distance and external length of tube in the chart. Mark and document the tube's exit site from the nose or mouth.
- Use bedside techniques at regular intervals to determine proper tube positioning.
  - Measuring and recording pH.
    - Gastric secretions have a pH less than 5. Small intestine secretions will usually have a pH greater than 6, but this does not reliably predict proper tube placement. A pH greater than 6 can occur with respiratory or esophageal placement, with proper tube placement (gastric or intestinal) when feedings are given continuously, or if the child is receiving acid-inhibiting medications. Therefore, if the pH is greater than 5, additional assessment is warranted. Also check with local agency policy, for example clinical practice standards.
  - Observing appearance of fluid aspirated from tube (can be used in conjunction with pH testing but is not a reliable single verification method).
    - Gastric secretions are usually grassy green or clear and colourless and can have off-white or tan mucous shreds. It may also be brown tinged if blood is present.
    - Intestinal secretions are often bile stained, light golden yellow to brownish green. They tend to be thicker and more translucent than gastric secretions.
    - Respiratory secretions can be white, yellow, straw coloured, or clear.
  - Instill air into the tube and then auscultate for the sound (gastric auscultation) (can be used in conjunction with other assessment methods).
  - Check external markings on tube and external tube length (tube remaining from nares to end of tube) to determine if the tube seems to have migrated or been misplaced.
- Continually assess for signs indicative of feeding tube misplacement, such as unexplained gagging, vomiting, or coughing; signs and symptoms of respiratory distress; and decreased oxygen saturations.
- If bedside techniques reveal conflicting results or the child is at high risk, radiologic confirmation is recommended.
- Review routine chest and abdominal x-rays (if obtained) to double-check correct tube position.

Always follow agencies' policy and procedures.

Adapted from Cincinnati Children's Hospital Medical Center. (2011). *Best evidence statement (BESt). Confirmation of nasogastric/orogastric tube (NGT/OGT) placement.* Cincinnati, OH: Cincinnati Children's Hospital Medical Center. Retrieved from http://www.cincinnatichildrens.org/assets/0/78/1067/2709/2777/2793/9198/ad67ab29–2a71–42a4-b78e-3d0e9710adac.pdf

bolus feeding, a specified amount of feeding solution is given at specific intervals, usually over a short period of time such as 15 to 30 minutes. Given via a syringe, feeding bag, or infusion pump, bolus feedings most closely resemble regular meals. Continuous feedings are given at a slower rate over a longer period of time. In some cases, the feeding may be given during the night so that the child can be free to move about and participate in activities during the day. For continuous feedings, an enteral feeding pump is used to administer the solution at a prescribed rate.

Checking for tube placement is a priority before administering any intermittent tube feeding for the first time and periodic re-checking should also occur during continuous tube feedings, regardless of the type of tube being used (refer to Box 35.4). For gastrostomy and jejunostomy tubes, ensure that the calibration, if present, has not changed. Measure the length of the tube daily from the exit site on the stomach to the end of the tube. Assess the abdomen for distension and bowel sounds. Also, as directed, measure the **gastric residual** (the amount remaining in the stomach; indicates gastric emptying time) by aspirating the gastric contents with a syringe, measuring it, and then replacing the contents. Check the residuals periodically, according to the facility's policy, such as every 4 to 6 hours, and before each intermittent feeding. If the residual volume exceeds the amount specified by the physician's order, hold the feeding and notify the physician or nurse practitioner.

Begin the feeding by placing the child in a supine position with the head and shoulders elevated approximately 30 degrees so that the feeding will remain in the stomach area (Bowden & Greenberg, 2011). Flush the tube with a small amount of water to clear it and prevent occlusion. This is not necessary for a gavage feeding if the tube is being inserted each time a feeding is given. Ensure that the feeding solution is at room temperature. Administer the feed per the facility's policy.

Feeding solutions may be placed into the barrel of a syringe or into a feeding bag attached to the feeding tube and allowed to flow by gravity. The rate of flow for gravity-assisted feedings can be increased or decreased by raising or lowering the feeding solution container, respectively. Typically, intermittent feedings last from 15 to 30 minutes. A feeding bag also may be attached to a pump to control the rate of flow. Monitor the child's tolerance to the feeding.

Once the feeding is complete, but before the formula completely empties from the container, flush the tube with water. As the water leaves the syringe or tubing, clamp the tube to prevent air from entering the stomach. Then, disconnect the syringe or tube-feeding bag from the tube.

Take Note!

If the child vomits during the feeding, stop the feeding immediately and turn the child onto his or her side or sit him/her up.

If the child has a gastrostomy button, open the cap and connect an adaptor or insert extension tubing through the one-way valve. This allows access to the gastric conduit. The feeding solution container is connected to the extension tubing or adaptor and the feeding is given as described previously. After the feeding is completed, the extension tubing or adaptor is flushed with water, disconnected, and the flip-top opening is closed.

Burp the infant during and after any type of tube feeding in the same manner as for an infant who is bottle- or breast-fed. Also, position the child on his or her right side with the head slightly elevated, approximately 30 degrees, for about 1 hour after the feeding to facilitate gastric emptying and reduce the risk of aspiration and regurgitation. Some children have a difficult time with gas and burping on their own after tube placement. Venting, which helps relieve gas, may be ordered by the physician or nurse practitioner. It removes excess air and can be helpful if the child is bloated or the abdomen is distended. Use a catheter-tip syringe with the plunger removed and attach to the end of the tube. Hold the syringe above the child's stomach for a few minutes. Once the air or gas is removed, allow any stomach contents or formula to flow back into the stomach.

Weigh the child daily throughout enteral nutrition therapy to determine the effectiveness of the therapy.

Providing Skin and Insertion Site Care

Skin around the gastrostomy or jejunostomy insertion site may become irritated from movement of the tube, moisture, leakage of stomach or intestinal contents, or the adhesive device holding the tube in place. Keeping the skin clean and dry is important and will help prevent most of these problems.

The skin around a gastrostomy or jejunostomy tube requires cleaning at least once a day. Routine site care includes gentle cleansing with sterile water or saline for newly placed tubes, or for established tubes, soap, and water followed by rinsing or cleaning with water alone. To clean under an external disc or bumper, a cotton-tipped applicator may be used. Rotate the gastrostomy tube or button a quarter-turn to prevent skin adherence and irritation. Granulation tissue may form around the gastrostomy site which may result in a small amount of bleeding when cleaning. Always follow agency or institution policies and procedures when teaching parents or caregivers, and provide written advice and links to local and national support groups.

Take Note!

Do not rotate a jejunal or gastrojejunal tube because it can cause kinking (Bowden & Greenberg, 2011).

Assess the insertion site and condition of the surrounding skin for signs and symptoms of infection, such as erythema, induration, foul drainage, or pain. A small amount of clear or tan drainage is normal. If any drainage is present, a dressing can be placed. Use presplit 2 × 2 gauze and place it loosely around the site. Change this dressing when it is soiled. If no drainage is present, do not place a dressing as it can cause undue pressure and trap moisture, leading to skin irritation.

Preventing movement of the tube also helps reduce skin irritation. Check the volume of the balloon with a balloon-tipped device as per local policy and reinflate the balloon to the initial volume if needed. The tube should be able to move slightly in and out of the child's stomach. The plastic disc should be snug against the skin but not tight enough to cause pressure. Tube stabilization methods help prevent the tube from moving around and sliding further into the stomach or jejunum. Stabilize the tube by pulling gently on the tubing and sliding the stabilizer bar or disc snugly against the abdomen.

Take Note!

Rotate sites where the tube is secured to the abdomen to prevent tension on the stoma or skin breakdown.

Measure and record the length of the tube from the exit site of the abdominal wall to the end of the tube. All future measurements should be the same unless the tube length is changed. For tubes without a stabilizer bar or disc or for additional stabilization needs, several other methods may be used, including cut baby bottle nipples, taping methods, and commercially available stabilizers (Fig. 35.12). It is always important to follow agency policy.

Take Note!

When using the nipple method, make sure to cut several holes in the base of the nipple to allow air circulation and site assessment.

Promoting Growth and Development

Some children receive all of their nutritional needs through tube feedings, whereas other children use tube feedings as a supplement to eating by mouth. Feeding time is a special time for infants and children. Occasionally, babies who are fed solely through an enteral feeding tube may forget or lose the desire to eat by mouth. Use a pacifier to help avoid this, allowing the infant to associate the nipple in his or her mouth with a feeding (Children's Hospitals and Clinics of Minnesota, 2013). The sucking motion will also exercise the jaw and promote the flow of the feedings. The saliva produced during sucking aids in digestion. Combined with holding the infant and cuddling, rocking, and talking to him/her, this promotes a more normal feeding time.

FIGURE 35.12 Methods to stabilize a gastrostomy tube include (**A**) the nipple method, (**B**) taping methods, (**C**) the tension loop method, and (**D**) commercially available stabilizing devices (GripLok®; pictured here).

Talking with children, playing music, or reading a story promotes an active feeding time. At home, encourage parents to include the feeding as a part of regular family mealtime together to provide socialization for the child. Allow the child to participate in the feedings by gathering supplies and administering the actual feeding so that the child may experience independence and adaptation. If the child also eats food by mouth, feed him/her by mouth first and then administer the tube feeding. Children with feeding tubes should be allowed as normal a routine as possible. For example, they can crawl, walk, and jump just like children of the same age and developmental level. However, in some cases, contact sports such as football, hockey, and wrestling should be avoided because of the higher risk of injury. Securing the tubing under the child's clothing will prevent it from becoming accidentally dislodged and prevent the child from pulling and playing with it. Using one-piece outfits, an Ace wrap, or stretchy gauze to cover the tube can help protect it.

Educating the Child and Family

Educate children receiving enteral feedings and their parents thoroughly about this method of nutritional support. Reinforce the reason for the therapy and provide the child and parents with opportunities to verbalize their concerns and ask questions. Ensure that the parents understand the risks and benefits of the therapy and the expected duration.

Provide the child, if developmentally appropriate, and parents with opportunities to participate in the feeding sessions. This helps allay some of their fears and anxieties and promotes a sense of control over the situation. They will also gain valuable practice in learning the skill should the feedings be required at home. Teaching

Guidelines 35.3 identifies important topics to include in the teaching plan for a child receiving enteral nutrition at home. Troubleshooting problems at home is an important topic to cover. Refer to Teaching Guidelines 35.4. Education also involves helping the family develop appropriate coping strategies to adapt, solve problems, and access the support and services they will need after discharge.

Teaching Guidelines 35.3

TOPICS TO BE COVERED FOR HOME ENTERAL NUTRITION

- Type and size of tube
- Type of nutritional support
- Rationale for therapy
- Expected results from therapy
- Duration of therapy
- Frequency of feedings
- Feeding solution and equipment
- Tube insertion technique (if appropriate)
- Methods to check for correct placement
- Steps for administering the feeding (and medication, if ordered)
- Procedure for flushing tube
- Procedure for venting the tube, if appropriate
- Frequency of weighing the child
- Signs and symptoms of complications and when to notify physician or nurse practitioner
- Troubleshooting problems, such as clogging of the tube or dislodgement (see Teaching Guidelines 35.4)
- Daily tube care (e.g., cleaning the site, rotating tube)
- Site assessment
- Technique for reinsertion/replacement of tube as appropriate

• Equipment suppliers
• Resources for support
• Follow-up visits and referrals

 Teaching Guidelines 35.4
TROUBLESHOOTING COMPLICATIONS AT HOME

• If a tube appears clogged, instruct caregivers to first look for any kinks that may be preventing free flow of tube contents (e.g., has a clamp on the tube been closed accidently). If no reason for the clog can be seen, slowly push warm water (body temperature) into the tube. Amount and size of syringe will vary based on child's size and facility policy. Repeat if necessary. Instruct caregivers to never use an object or put anything into the tube. They should call the doctor or nurse if they are unable to unclog the tube. Declogging medications may be prescribed.

• If a tube is inadvertently removed, instruct the caregiver to cover the site with a small clean dressing tape, and then to call the physician or nurse immediately; the tube needs to be replaced as soon as possible or the tract will close. Some providers may have instructed and assessed parents' or caregivers' ability to replace G-Tubes at home. In this instance, local guidelines should be followed.

• If the site is red or irritated, instruct caregivers to continue with routine cleaning and call the physician or nurse practitioner. An antibiotic or skin barrier cream may be ordered. Assess for leakage and try to minimize, if possible. Check the tube's position and ensure tube is stabilized and secure and not dangling.

• If the tube is leaking, the caregiver needs to keep the dressing clean and dry. Assess tube position and secure the tube to avoid dangling. Assess if leaking is from stoma area or tube valve, if applicable. More frequent venting may help or the tube may need to be replaced; the physician or nurse practitioner should be notified.

• The caregiver should be made aware of the length of time that a gastrostomy tube can typically last before a replacement will be required. This length of time will depend on several factors, including the type of gastrostomy used for the child, any complications that have arisen during its placement (e.g., repeat occlusions or dislodgments), and adherence to preventative maintenance regimens (Itkin et al., 2011).

Always teach following the instructions per agency policy and procedure regarding home care.

Adapted from Sick Kids Nutrition Team. (2007). Guidelines for the administration of enteral and parenteral nutrition in paediatrics. Retrieved from https://www.sickkids.ca/pdfs/Clinical-Dietitians/19499-Enteral_Parenteral_Nutrition.pdf; and Ladhani, M. B. (Ed.). (2015–2016). *MacPeds pediatric survival guide.* Retrieved from https://www.macpeds.com/documents/Securedforwebsite-Final-MacPedsPediatricSurvivalGuide-.pdf

> **Remember Lily from the beginning of the chapter? She is to be discharged home after having a gastrostomy tube inserted to continue feedings at home.**
>
> **What teaching is needed for her family prior to discharge?**

Parenteral Nutrition

Nutritional support can be administered IV through a peripheral or central venous catheter. The concentration and components of the solution determine the type of parenteral nutrition. Parenteral nutrition given via a central venous access device is termed **total parenteral nutrition (TPN)**. Comparison Chart 35.1 gives information about peripheral and central parenteral nutrition.

Administering TPN

The physician or nurse practitioner, often in consultation with the pharmacy department, typically determines the concentration and components of the TPN solution based on a thorough assessment of the child's status, including the results of laboratory testing. This information is used as a baseline for evaluating the effectiveness of therapy.

The solution is prepared under sterile conditions in the pharmacy. For TPN, a central venous access device is inserted and secured, if one is not already in place. Specialized tubing with an in-line filter is used (the filter can prevent small microparticles from entering the circulation).

TPN solutions may be refrigerated until they are to be used. Once started, a single solution of TPN should hang for no longer than 24 hours (Doyle & McCutcheon, 2015; Weinstein & Hagle, 2014). The infusion of the solution is initiated at a slow rate that is gradually increased as ordered based on how the child tolerates the therapy. TPN solutions are highly concentrated glucose solutions that can cause hyperglycemia if given too rapidly. Use of an infusion pump is essential to control the rate of infusion. Fat emulsions are administered periodically to meet the child's need for essential fatty acids. These solutions are given as a piggyback solution into the TPN line, but below the in-line filter.

Throughout TPN therapy, be vigilant in monitoring the infusion rate, and report any changes in the infusion rate to the physician or nurse practitioner immediately. Gradual adjustments may be made to the rate, but only as ordered by the physician or nurse practitioner.

Initially, check blood glucose levels frequently, such as every 4 to 6 hours, to evaluate for hyperglycemia. These levels can be obtained with a bedside glucose meter. Minimize the trauma and discomfort associated with frequent invasive procedures by using the principles of atraumatic care. If blood glucose levels are

COMPARISON CHART 35.1	PERIPHERAL PARENTERAL NUTRITION VERSUS TOTAL PARENTERAL NUTRITION	

	Peripheral Parenteral Nutrition	**Total Parenteral Nutrition**
Indications/use	Primarily supplemental Short-term use to supply additional calories and nutrients	Provides all nutrients to meet child's needs Enough calories supplied to maintain a positive nitrogen balance[a]
Route	Peripheral vein	Central venous access to allow rapid dilution of hypertonic solution
Child's status	Nutritional status usually within acceptable parameters Oral intake decreased or absent	Child with a nonfunctioning gastrointestinal (GI) tract, such as a congenital or acquired GI disorder Severe failure to thrive Multisystem trauma or organ involvement Preterm newborns
Components	Fluid, electrolytes, and carbohydrates (dextrose); usually no protein or fats Carbohydrate concentration usually limited to 10% or less and osmolarity of <600 mOsm[a]	Highly concentrated solution of carbohydrates, electrolytes, vitamins, and minerals Lipid emulsion to supply the need for essential fatty acids Total nutrient admixture (TNA) with components of TPN plus lipids and other additives in one container

[a]Weinstein, S. M., & Hagle, M. E. (2014). *Plumer's principles & practice of infusion therapy* (9th ed.). Philadelphia, PA: Lippincott Williams & Wilkins.

elevated, SQ administration of insulin may be needed. Once the child's glucose levels stabilize, the frequency of blood glucose level testing decreases, such as every 8 to 12 hours, based on the facility's policy.

Take Note!
If for any reason the TPN infusion is interrupted or stops, be prepared to begin an infusion of a 5% to 10% dextrose solution at the same infusion rate as the TPN (Bowden & Greenberg, 2011). This helps to prevent rebound hypoglycemia that may occur due to the increased insulin secretion by the child's body in response to the use of the highly concentrated TPN solution.

Perform catheter site care, tubing and filter changes, and dressing changes according to the facility's policy. Inspect the insertion site closely for signs of infection. Also, monitor the child's vital signs, daily weights, and intake and output closely for changes. In addition, review laboratory test results, which can aid in early detection of problems, such as infection or electrolyte excesses or deficits.

TPN can be administered continuously over a 24-hour period, or after initiation it may be given on a cyclic basis, such as over a 12-hour period during the night. When administering cycled TPN, the solution is infused at half the prescribed rate for the first and last hour to prevent hyperglycemia and hypoglycemia.

Preventing Complications

Nurses play a key role in minimizing the risk for complications related to use of central venous access devices and

TPN. Box 35.5 describes these complications. Key measures to reduce the risk of complications include the following:

Take Note!
Never administer any medication, blood, or other solution through the TPN lumen (Weinstein & Hagle, 2014). Doing so increases the risk for contamination of the system and subsequent infection.

Promoting Growth and Development

Meals are a time for meeting nutritional needs as well as a time for love, comfort, support, and socialization. TPN meets the child's nutritional needs, but the child's need for love and support also must be met. Implement measures similar to those for children receiving enteral nutrition (see discussion earlier in this chapter). Also, provide opportunities for holding and cuddling the child. Allow the older child to participate in activities that can help to occupy the time associated with meals. When administering cyclic TPN, run the TPN over the night time hours, whenever possible, to allow the child to participate in developmentally appropriate activities during the day. Encourage the child and parents to participate in the care to promote a sense of independence as well as a sense of control over the situation.

Educating the Child and Family

Children who require long-term TPN therapy may receive TPN in the home. Administering TPN at home requires

BOX 35.5

COMPLICATIONS THAT CAN OCCUR WITH CENTRAL VENOUS ACCESS DEVICES AND TOTAL PARENTERAL NUTRITION (TPN)

- Air embolism from inadvertent entry of air into the system during tubing or cap changes or accidental disconnection.
- Cardiac tamponade due to catheter advancement with movement of the arm, neck, or shoulder.
- Catheter occlusion from the development of a fibrin sheath or thrombus at the catheter tip, malpositioning or kinking, or the deposition of precipitates or a blood clot.
- Venous thrombosis from injury to the vessel wall during insertion or movement of the catheter after insertion or from chemical irritation due to administration of concentrated solutions, vesicants, and other medications through the catheter.
- Hyperglycemia, typically with too rapid infusion of TPN.
- Hypoglycemia, which may occur with rapid cessation.
- Dehydration as the child's body attempts to rid itself of excess glucose through renal excretion.
- Electrolyte imbalance (particularly potassium, sodium, calcium, magnesium, and phosphorus).
- Infection at the skin insertion site, along the catheter pathway, or in the bloodstream. Organisms can arise from the skin, hands of caregivers, or other areas such as wound drainage, droplets from the lungs, or urine. For example, connection sites can be contaminated during tubing or dressing changes.
- Monitor the child's vital signs closely for changes.
- Adhere to strict aseptic technique when caring for the catheter and administering TPN.
- Ensure that the system remains a closed system at all times. Secure all connections and clamp the catheter or have the child perform the Valsalva maneuver during tubing and cap changes.
- Use occlusive dressings. Chlorhexidine-impregnated sponge (Biopatch) dressings may be used to help prevent infection. Always follow agency or institution policy and procedures.
- Adhere to agency policy for flushing of the catheter and maintaining catheter patency.
- Assess intake and output levels frequently.
- Monitor blood glucose levels and obtain laboratory tests as ordered to evaluate for changes in fluid and electrolytes.

thorough education of the child and parents. This teaching can occur in the healthcare agency or in the child's home. The amount of information to be taught can be overwhelming, so ensure that ample time is made available to give both caregivers and children the opportunity to ask questions and express concerns. Offer emotional support and guidance whenever necessary.

Provide written and verbal instructions about the care involved. Have the child (if appropriate) and parents demonstrate the care needed, including care of the central venous access device. Review with them the measures for obtaining, storing, and handling the solutions and supplies.

Develop plans for troubleshooting problems with devices and equipment, and give instructions on how to recognize and treat complications. Also, teach them about danger signs and symptoms that require immediate notification. Be sure they have the name and number of a contact person in case of emergency situations.

Initiate the appropriate referrals for support. Specialized home care infusion services may be available for follow-up in the home. In addition, social services can be helpful in providing assistance with finances, health insurance reimbursement, scheduling, transportation, emotional support, and community resources.

KEY CONCEPTS

○ The seven "rights" of pediatric medication administration are the right patient, right medication, right dose, right route, right time/frequency, right reason/assessment, and right documentation (Canadian references, see: College & Association of Registered Nurses of Alberta, 2015; College of Registered Nurses of British Columbia, 2017; College of Registered Nurses of Nova Scotia, 2017; Doyle & McCutcheon, 2015).

○ The physiologic immaturity of some body systems in children can affect a drug's pharmacodynamics, leading to differences in the body's response to the drug and thus enhancing or diminishing the drug's effects. The child's age, weight, BSA, and body composition can affect a drug's pharmacokinetics.

○ The two most common methods for determining pediatric drug doses involve the use of the child's body weight and BSA.

- Children younger than the age of 5 to 6 are at risk for aspiration when receiving tablets or capsules because they have difficulty swallowing them; liquids may be more appropriate. When administering oral medications to children, always tell them whether a medication is being mixed with food.

- Medication administration via the rectal route is not preferred because the drug's absorption may be erratic and unpredictable and children find this route extremely upsetting or embarrassing.

- When administering optic medications, pull the pinna downward and back if the child is younger than age 3, and up and back for older children.

- IM administration is used infrequently in children because it is painful and children often lack the adequate muscle mass. When used with infants less than 7 months, the preferred site is the vastus lateralis muscle.

- Administration of medication via the IV route is common with children, especially when a rapid response to the drug is desired or when absorption via other routes is difficult or impossible. The primary method for IV medication administration is via a syringe pump.

- Preferred sites for peripheral IV therapy include the veins of the hands, feet, and forearms. The scalp vein may be used in infants, but only if attempts at other sites have been unsuccessful. The rule of thumb for insertion of any peripheral devices is to use the smallest gauge catheter for the shortest length of time possible to prevent trauma to the child's fragile veins.

- Central venous therapy usually is administered through a large vein, such as the subclavian, femoral, or jugular vein or vena cava. The tip of the device lies in the superior vena cava just at the entrance to the right atrium. Devices include single- or multiple-lumen short- and long-term catheters, peripherally inserted central catheters, tunnelled catheters, and vascular access ports.

- Monitoring intake and output is important when a child is receiving IV therapy. Site inspection, proper care of the site, and proper dressing changes are key to preventing complications.

- Nutritional support can be administered enterally via a nasogastric or orogastric tube (gavage feeding) or via a gastrostomy or jejunostomy device or administered parenterally through a peripheral or central venous access device.

- Enteral nutrition is indicated for children who have a functioning gastrointestinal tract but cannot consume adequate amounts of nutrients orally.

- Prior to any enteral feeding, placement of the feeding tube must be confirmed. The gold standard for confirming placement is with an x-ray. At the bedside, nonradiologic methods are used to confirm placement including checking the colour and pH of the aspirate, checking external markings on the tube, verifying external tube length, and continually assessing for signs indicative of feeding tube misplacement, such as unexplained gagging, vomiting, or coughing; signs and symptoms of respiratory distress; and decreased oxygen saturations.

- Children receiving TPN require close monitoring of the infusion rate and volume, intake and output, vital signs, and blood glucose levels. Strict aseptic technique is necessary when caring for the central venous access site and TPN infusion.

REFERENCES AND RECOMMENDED READINGS

Accreditation Canada. (2015). *Required organizational practices: Handbook 2016*. Retrieved from https://accreditation.ca/sites/default/files/rop-handbook-2016-en.pdf

Aschenbrenner, D. S., & Venable, S. J. (2012). *Drug therapy in nursing* (4th ed.). Philadelphia, PA: Lippincott Williams & Wilkins.

BC Centre for Disease Control. (2008). *Communicable disease control: Immunization program. Section IV – Administration of biological products. 8.2: Needle size and sites for intramuscular (IM) injection*. Retrieved from http://www.bccdc.ca/resource-gallery/Documents/Guidelines%20and%20Forms/Guidelines%20and%20Manuals/Epid/CD%20Manual/Chapter%202%20-%20Imms/SectionIV_AdministrationofBiologicalProducts.pdf

BC Centre for Disease Control. (2009). *Communicable disease control: Immunization program. Section IV – Administration of biological products. 9.3: Intramuscular (IM) injection route*. Retrieved from http://www.bccdc.ca/resource-gallery/Documents/Guidelines%20and%20Forms/Guidelines%20and%20Manuals/Epid/CD%20Manual/Chapter%202%20-%20Imms/SectionIV_AdministrationofBiologicalProducts.pdf

BC Centre for Disease Control. (2010). *Communicable disease control: Immunization program. Section IV – Administration of biological products. 8.2.4: Dorsogluteal site*. Retrieved from http://www.bccdc.ca/resource-gallery/Documents/Guidelines%20and%20Forms/Guidelines%20and%20Manuals/Epid/CD%20Manual/Chapter%202%20-%20Imms/SectionIV_AdministrationofBiologicalProducts.pdf

Bergvall, E., & Sawyer, T. L. (2012). *Scalp vein catheterization*. Retrieved from http://emedicine.medscape.com/article/1348863-overview#a16

Bowden, V. R., & Greenberg, C. S. (2011). *Pediatric nursing procedures* (3rd ed.). Philadelphia, PA: Lippincott Williams & Wilkins.

British Columbia College of Nursing Professionals. (2018). *Practice standards: Medication administration*. Retrieved from https://www.bccnp.ca/Standards/RN_NP/PracticeStandards/Pages/medicationadmin.aspx

Canadian Nurses Protective Society. (2007). *Medication errors*. Retrieved from http://www.cnps.ca/index.php?page=97

Centers for Disease Control and Prevention. (2016). *Vaccine administration*. Retrieved from https://www.cdc.gov/vaccines/pubs/pinkbook/vac-admin.html

Cincinnati Children's Hospital Medical Center. (2011). *Best evidence statement (BESt). Confirmation of naso-gastric/orogastric tube (NGT/OGT) placement*. Cincinnati, OH: Cincinnati Children's Hospital Medical Center. Retrieved from http://www.cincinnatichildrens.org/assets/0/78/1067/2709/2777/2793/9198/ad67ab29-2a71-42a4-b78e-3d0e9710adac.pdf

Cincinnati Children's Hospital Medical Center. (2012). *Gastrostomy Tube (G-tube) home care*. Retrieved from http://www.cincinnatichildrens.org/health/info/abdomen/home/g-tube-care.htm

Children's Hospitals and Clinics of Minnesota. (2013). *Patient/family education: Nasogastric tube feeding*. Retrieved from http://www.childrensmn.org/manuals/pfs/homecare/018701.pdf

College & Association of Registered Nurses of Alberta. (2015). *Medication guidelines*. Retrieved from http://www.nurses.ab.ca/content/dam/carna/pdfs/DocumentList/Guidelines/MedicationGuidelines_Mar2015.pdf

College of Nurses of Ontario. (2015). *Medication*. Retrieved from http://www.cno.org/

College of Registered Nurses of Nova Scotia. (2017). *Medication guidelines for Registered Nurses*. Retrieved from http://crnns.ca/wp-content/uploads/2015/05/Medication-Guidelines.pdf

Davidson, K. M., & Rourke, L. (2013). Teaching best-evidence: Deltoid intramuscular injection technique. *Journal of Nursing Education and Practice, 3*(7), 120–128.

Doyle, G. R., & McCutcheon, J. A. (2015). *Clinical procedures for safer clinical care*. Retrieved from https://opentextbc.ca/clinicalskills/chapter/6-8-iv-push-medications-and-saline-lock-flush/

Eden, L. M., Macintosh, J. L., Luthy, K. E., & Beckstrand, R. L. (2014). Minimizing pain during childhood vaccination injections: Improving adherence to vaccination schedules. *Pediatrics Health, Medicines and Therapeutics*, 127–140.

Farrington, M., Lang, S., Cullen, L., & Stewart, S. (2009). Nasogastric tube placement verification in pediatric and neonatal patients. *Pediatric Nursing, 35*(1), 17–24.

Festini, F., Giusti, F., Ciofi, D., Olivini, N., & Bisogni, S. (2014). O-152 heparin solution vs normal saline for flushing peripheral venous catheters in children. Preliminary results of a RCT. *Archives of Disease in Childhood, 99*(Suppl 2), A82.

Government of Canada. (2016). *Canadian immunization guide: Part 1 – Key immunization information*. Retrieved from https://www.canada.ca/en/public-health/services/publications/healthy-living/canadian-immunization-guide-part-1-key-immunization-information/page-8-vaccine-administration-practices.html

Habib, S., Graydon, B., & Menezes, C. (2010). *Subcutaneous injections: Injecting at home*. Retrieved from http://www.aboutkidshealth.ca/En/HealthAZ/TestsAndTreatments/GivingMedication/Pages/Subcutaneous-Injections-Injecting-At-Home.aspx

Hartling, L., Ali, S., Dryden, D. M., Chordiya, P., Johnson, D. W., Plint, A. C., … Drendel, A. L. (2016). How safe are common analgesics for the treatment of acute pain for children? A systematic review. *Pain Research and Management, 2016*, 5346819.

Irving, S. Y., Lyman, B., Northington, L., Bartlett, J. A., Kemper, C., & NOVEL Project Work Group. (2014). Nasogastric tube placement and verification in children: Review of the current literature. *Nutrition in Clinical Practice, 29*(3), 267–276.

ISMP. (2009). *Medication safety alert! Safety briefs. 14(11)*. Retrieved from file:///C:/Users/Susan/Downloads/ISMP%20Newsletter%20Acute%20Care%206–4–09.pdf

ISMP. (2015). *Results of pediatric medication safety survey (part 2): Comparing data subsets points out areas for improvement*. Retrieved from https://www.ismp.org/newsletters/acutecare/showarticle.aspx?id=112

ISMP Canada. (2006). *Do not use: Dangerous abbreviations, symbols and dose designations*. Retrieved from https://www.ismp-canada.org/download/ISMPCanadaListOfDangerousAbbreviations.pdf

ISMP Canada. (2009). *ISMP Canada safety bulletin. National collaborative: Top 5 drugs reported as causing harm through medication error in paediatrics*. Retrieved from https://www.ismp-canada.org/download/safetyBulletins/ISMPCSB2009-6-NationalCollaborative-Top5DrugsReported.pdf

The Hospital for Sick Children. (2017a). *Eye ointment: How to apply*. Retrieved from http://www.aboutkidshealth.ca/En/HealthAZ/TestsAndTreatments/GivingMedication/Pages/Eye-Ointment-How-to-Apply.aspx

The Hospital for Sick Children. (2017b). *Eye drops: How to put in*. Retrieved from http://www.aboutkidshealth.ca/En/HealthAZ/TestsAndTreatments/GivingMedication/Pages/Eye-Drops-How-to-Put-In.aspx

Itkin, M., DeLegge, M. H., Fang, J. C., McClave, S. A., Kundu, S., d'Othee, B. J., … Cardella, J. F. (2011). Multidisciplinary practical guidelines for gastrointestinal access for enteral nutrition and decompression from the Society of Interventional Radiology and American Gastroenterological Association (AGA) Institute, with endorsement by Canadian Interventional Radiological Association (CIRA) and Cardiovascular and Interventional Radiological Society of Europe (CIRSE). *Journal of Vascular and Interventional Radiology, 22*(8), 1089–1106.

The Joint Commission. (2013). *Preventing central line–associated bloodstream infections: Useful tools, an international perspective*. Retrieved from http://www.jointcommission.org/Topics/Clabsi_toolkit.aspx

Kroger, A. T., Sumaya, C. V., Pickering, L. K., & Atkinson, W. L. (2011). General recommendations on immunization recommendations of the Advisory Committee on Immunization Practices (ACIP). *Morbidity and Mortality Weekly Report (MMWR), 60*(RR02), 1–60. Retrieved from http://www.cdc.gov/mmwr/preview/mmwrhtml/rr6002a1.htm?s_cid=rr6002a1_e

Kumar, M., Vandermeer, B., Bassler, D., & Mansoor, N. (2013). Low-dose heparin use and the patency of peripheral IV catheters in children: A systematic review. *Pediatrics, 131*, e864–e872.

Ladhani, M. B. (Ed.). (2015–2016). *MacPeds pediatric survival guide*. Retrieved from https://www.macpeds.com/documents/Securedforwebsite-Final-MacPedsPediatricSurvival-Guide-.pdf

Lemyze, M. (2010). Five things to know about the placement of nasogastric tubes. *Canadian Medical Association Journal*, *182*(8), 802.

Loorand-Stiver, L. (2011). *Pediatric intravenous administration of drugs and fluids. Environmental scan, 21*. Ottawa, ON: Canadian Agency for Drugs and Technologies in Health. Retrieved from http://www.cadth.ca/media/pdf/ES_Ped_IV_Admin_es21_e.pdf

Lyman, B., Yaworski, J. A., Duesing, L., & Moore, C. (2016). Verifying NG feeding tube placement in pediatric patients. *American Nurse Today*, *11*(1), 1–3.

Manias, E., Kinney, S., Cranswick, N., & Williams, A. (2014). Medication errors in hospitalised children. *Journal of Paediatrics and Child Health*, *50*(2014), 71–77.

Matlow, A. G., Baker, G. R., Flintoft, V., Cochrane, D., Coffey, M., Cohen, E., … Nijssen-Jordan, C. (2012). Adverse events among children in Canadian hospitals: The Canadian Paediatric Adverse Events study. *Canadian Medical Association Journal*, *184*(13), E709–E718.

Moore, D. L., Bortolussi, R., & Canadian Paediatric Society. (2016). *Home intravenous therapy: Accessibility for Canadian children and youth*. Retrieved from http://www.cps.ca/documents/position/home-intravenous-therapy

National Guideline Clearinghouse. (2012). *Best evidence statement (BESt). Confirmation of nasogastric tube placement in pediatric patients*. Retrieved from http://www.guideline.gov/content.aspx?id=35117

O'Grady, N. P., Alexander, M., Burns, L. A., Dellinger, E. P., Garland, J., Heard, S. O., … Saint, S. (2011, May). Guidelines for the prevention of intravascular catheter-related infections. *Clinical Infectious Diseases*, *52*, e1–e32.

Poon, C., & Ho, C. (2011, Fall). Medication safety in pediatrics. Retrieved from http://www.ocpinfo.com/library/PC/download/PC%20Fall%202011.pdf

Public Health Agency of Canada. (2013). *The Chief Public Health Officer's report on the state of public health in Canada, 2013: Infectious disease – The never-ending threat*. Retrieved from http://www.phac-aspc.gc.ca/cphorsphc-respcacsp/2013/infections-eng.php

Safer Healthcare Now. (2012). *Prevent central line infections: Getting started kit*. Retrieved from http://www.patientsafetyinstitute.ca/en/toolsResources/Documents/Interventions/Central%20Line-Associated%20Bloodstream%20Infection/CLI%20Getting%20Started%20Kit.pdf

Sears, K., Ross-White, A., & Godfrey, C. M. (2012). The incidence, prevalence and contributing factors associated with the occurrence of medication errors for children and adults in the community setting: A systematic review. *JBI Library of Systematic Reviews*, *10*(35), 2350–2464.

Shaw, M. (2016). How to administer eye drops and eye ointment. *Nursing Standard*, *30*(39), 34–36. Retrieved from https://rcni.com/sites/rcn_nspace/files/ns.30.39.34.s42.pdf

Sick Kids Nutrition Team. (2007). *Guidelines for the administration of enteral and parenteral nutrition in paediatrics*. Retrieved from https://www.sickkids.ca/pdfs/Clinical-Dietitians/19499-Enteral_Parenteral_Nutrition.pdf

SickKids (n.d.) *Paediatric IV therapy*. Retrieved from http://www.sickkids.ca/Nursing/Education-and-learning/Nursing-Student-Orientation/module-two-clinical-care/paediatric-iv-therapy/index.html

Steering Committee on Quality Improvement and Management and Committee on Hospital Care. (2011). Policy statement: Principles of pediatric patient safety: Reducing harm due to medical care. *Pediatrics*, *127*(6), 1199–1210. doi: 10.1542/peds.2011–0967

Taddio, A., Appleton, A., Bortolussi, R., Chambers, C., Dubey, V., Halperin, S., … Shah, V. (2010). Reducing the pain of childhood vaccination: An evidence-based clinical practice guideline. *Canadian Medical Association Journal*, *182*(18), E843–E855.

Walsh, K. E., Roblin, D. W., Weingart, S. N., Houlahan, K. E., Degar, B., Billett, A., … Mazor, K. M. (2013). Medication errors in the home: A multisite study of children with cancer. *Pediatrics*, *131*(5), e1405–e1414.

Weinstein, S. M., & Hagle, M. E. (2014). *Plumer's principles & practice of infusion therapy* (9th ed.). Philadelphia, PA: Lippincott Williams & Wilkins.

Yin, H. S., Mendelsohn, A. L., Wolf, M. S., Parker, R. M., Fierman, A., van Schaick, L., Dreyer, B. P. (2010). Parents' medication administration errors role of dosing instruments and health literacy. *Archives of Pediatrics & Adolescent Medicine*, *164*(2), 181–186.

Zelcer, M., & Goldman, R. D. (2016). Intranasal midazolam for seizure cessation in the community setting. *Canadian Family Physician*, *62*(7), 559–561. Retrieved from http://www.cfp.ca/content/cfp/62/7/559.full.pdf.1001/archpediatrics.2009.269

CHAPTER **WORKSHEET**

MULTIPLE CHOICE QUESTIONS

1. A 3-year-old child is to receive a medication that is supplied as an enteric-coated tablet. What is the best nursing action?
   a. Crush the tablet and mix it with apple sauce.
   b. Dissolve the medication in the child's milk.
   c. Place a pill in the posterior part of the pharynx and tell the child to swallow.
   d. Check with the prescriber to see if an alternative form can be used.

2. The nurse is caring for an infant who weighs 8.2 kg and is NPO and receiving IV fluid therapy. What rate does the nurse calculate as meeting the child's daily fluid requirements?
   a. 82 mL per hour
   b. 41 mL per hour
   c. 34 mL per hour
   d. 22 mL per hour

3. When administering ear drops to a 2-year old, which action would be most appropriate?
   a. Tell the child that the drops are to treat his infection.
   b. Pull the pinna of the child's ear down and back.
   c. Have the child turn his head to the opposite side after giving the drops.
   d. Massage the child's forehead to facilitate absorption of the medication.

4. An infant is to receive intermittent gavage feedings via a nasogastric tube every 6 hours. The feeding tube was inserted with a previous feeding and remains in place. The nurse is preparing to administer the next scheduled feeding. Place the events in the proper sequence.
   a. Check the placement of the feeding tube.
   b. Position the infant on his right side with the head of the bed slightly elevated.
   c. Allow the feeding to come to room temperature.
   d. Flush the tube with water.
   e. Clamp the tube to prevent air from entering the stomach.
   f. Pour the solution into the barrel of the syringe.

CRITICAL THINKING EXERCISES

1. When reviewing the medical record of a child, the nurse notes that the ordered dose of medication is different from the recommended dose. How should the nurse proceed?

2. While caring for a 5-year-old child who is receiving IV fluid therapy at a rate of 100 mL per hour, the nurse notes that the infusion is running slowly. The insertion site appears slightly reddened and swollen. What should the nurse do next?

3. A school-aged child is to be discharged, continuing TPN therapy at home. The child lives with his parents and two younger siblings. How would the nurse prepare this child and family for discharge? How could the nurse promote growth and development for this child during TPN therapy?

STUDY ACTIVITIES

1. Review the medical records of several children who are on a pediatric unit in your agency. Note the type of medication, route ordered, and what specific interventions are needed for each child related to the medication administration and developmental age of the child include atraumatic care interventions. Compile a list of the most commonly used routes.

2. Interview several parents about their experiences in giving medications to their children. From these interviews, develop a teaching sheet that provides tips to facilitate oral medication administration to children.

3. Create a chart that compares and contrasts the SQ, intramuscular, and IV methods of medication administration. Include examples of medications given via these routes, onset of action, appropriate sites, and necessary safety measures for each.

BRINGING IT ALL TOGETHER: A CASE STUDY

Fillipia, a 3-year old, is admitted to your unit with fever and lethargy. She is 36 lb and 101.6 cm (40 in) tall. Her current temperature is 38.8°C (101.8°F), HR 110, RR 22. Her orders include ceftriaxone 525 mg IM every 12 hours and acetaminophen 2 teaspoons PO every 4 hours as needed for temperature greater than 38.6°C (101.5°F). The safe dose range for ceftriaxone is 50 to 75 mg/kg/day for mild-to-moderate infections and acetaminophen is 10 to 15 mg/kg/dose (to a maximum of 5 doses per 24 hours). The concentration for ceftriaxone is 350 mg/mL and acetaminophen is 160 mg/5 mL.

Go to thePoint **to find questions to consider about this case.**

36

Pain Management in Children

Learning Objectives

Upon completion of the chapter, you will be able to:

1. Identify the major physiologic events associated with the perception of pain.

2. Discuss the factors that influence the pain response.

3. Identify the developmental considerations of the effects and management of pain in the infant, toddler, preschooler, school-age child, and adolescent.

4. Explain the principles of pain assessment as they relate to children.

5. Understand the use of the various pain-rating scales and physiologic monitoring for children.

6. Establish a nursing care plan for children related to management of pain, including pharmacologic and nonpharmacologic techniques and strategies.

Aiden Russell **is a 6-year-old on the pediatric unit admitted for a wound infection. He requires BID dressing changes. In report, you are told that Aiden cries and fights during the dressing change but otherwise seems to be playing and not experiencing much pain. The nurse reporting off duty states, "Aiden's mother keeps requesting pain medication for Aiden. She states he is complaining of pain most of the time. I'm not sure if I believe her: when I see Aiden, he's playing Nintendo games or watching television and seems to be fine. I've tried to hold off on his pain medication as long as I can."**

Pain is a highly individualized, subjective experience that can affect any person of any age. It is a complex phenomenon that involves multiple components and is influenced by a myriad of factors. **Pain** is defined by the International Association for the Study of Pain as "an unpleasant sensory and emotional experience that is associated with actual or potential tissue damage or described in terms of such damage" (International Association for the Study of Pain, 2012; WHO, 2012). Another definition of pain that is commonly used defines pain as whatever the person says it is, existing whenever the person says it does—that is, pain is present when the person says that it is (McCaffery, 1968; McCaffery & Pasero, 2011). The person experiencing the pain is the only one who can identify pain and know what the pain is like.

Pain is a universal experience, affecting adults and children of all ages, even preterm infants. Pain can result from numerous causes, including disease processes, injuries, procedures, and surgical interventions. The Canadian Pain Society supports the treatment of pain as a basic human right. Unlike adults, however, children may lack the verbal capacity to describe their pain accurately. In addition, many caregivers and health care providers have misconceptions about pain in children, it is difficult to assess the complex nature of the pain experience, and limited resources and research are available related to pain relief strategies for children. Therefore, pain is a major source of distress for children and their families as well as for health care providers.

If left unmanaged, pain in children can lead to serious physical and emotional consequences, such as increased oxygen consumption and alterations in blood glucose metabolism. In addition, the experience of untreated pain early in life may lead to long-term physiologic and psychological consequences for the child (Bowden & Greenberg, 2011). For example, inadequately controlled pain can have long-lasting negative outcomes such as increased distress during later procedures, non-adherence to treatment regimens, inactivity, prolonged bed rest, and the development of chronic pain. Detrimental effects on the course of the disease itself may also be seen with untreated pain. Preterm infants, due to long hospitalizations and numerous painful and invasive procedures, are often at greater risk for experiencing memories of pain (American Academy of Pediatrics, 2010).

All these factors make pain management a critical element in the plan of care for children. Treating pain reduces anxiety during procedures and decreases the need for physical restraints, reduces anxiety regarding subsequent procedures, and prevents short- and long-term consequences of inadequately treated pain, particularly in newborns (Cohen & Baxter, 2008; Kennedy, Luhmann, & Zempsky, 2008; Oakes & D'Arcy, 2011). Pain management in children has improved, but underestimation and inadequate management still remain a problem (Bowden & Greenberg, 2011). Various national health associations have issued position papers and guidelines related to the need to treat pain and suffering in children. Effective pain management involves initial pain assessment, therapeutic interventions, and reassessment for all children in any health care setting.

This chapter describes the pain experience in children, including the types of pain, factors influencing pain, and common fallacies and myths associated with pain in children. The nursing process is applied to provide an overview of the care for a child in pain. Various pain management strategies are described, including nonpharmacologic and pharmacologic interventions and measures to address procedure-related and chronic pain.

PHYSIOLOGY OF PAIN

The sensation of pain is a complex phenomenon that involves a sequence of physiologic events in the nervous system. These events are transduction, transmission, perception, and modulation.

Transduction

Peripheral nerve fibres extend from the spinal cord to various locations in and throughout the body's tissues, such as skin, joints, bones, and membranes covering the internal organs. At the end of these fibres are specialized receptors, called **nociceptors**, which become activated when they are exposed to noxious stimuli. The noxious stimuli can be mechanical, chemical, or thermal. Mechanical stimuli may include intense pressure to an area, a strong muscular contraction, or extensive pressure due to muscular overstretching. Chemical stimulation may involve the release of mediators, such as histamine, prostaglandins, leukotrienes, or bradykinin, as a response to tissue trauma, ischemia, or inflammation. Thermal stimuli typically involve extremes of heat and cold. This process of nociceptor activation is called **transduction**.

Transmission

When nociceptors are activated by noxious stimuli, the stimuli are converted to electrical impulses that are relayed along the peripheral nerves to the spinal cord and brain. Specialized afferent nerve fibres are responsible for moving the electrical impulse along. Myelinated A-delta fibres are large fibres that conduct the impulse at very rapid rates. The pain transmitted by these fibres is often referred to as fast pain, most commonly associated with mechanical or thermal stimuli (Bautista & Grossman, 2014). Pain also is transmitted by unmyelinated small C fibres. These fibres transmit the impulse slowly and are often activated by chemical stimuli or continued mechanical or thermal stimuli (Bautista & Grossman,

2014). These fibres carry the impulse to the spinal cord via the dorsal horn. Neurotransmitters are released to facilitate the transmission process to the brain.

Several theories have been proposed in an attempt to explain the process of pain transmission. The best known of these is the gate-control theory. According to this theory, the dorsal horn of the spinal cord contains interneuronal or interconnecting fibres. Large-diameter faster fibres carry nonnociceptive, tactile information, while small nerve fibres carry nociceptive or pain signals. Large fibres, when stimulated, close the gate or pathway to the brain, thereby inhibiting or blocking the transmission of the pain impulse. Subsequently, the impulse does not reach the brain, where it would be interpreted as pain. It is now known that pain modulation is a more complex process but this theory helps explain why some nonpharmacologic therapies, such as massage and pressure, are effective in reducing pain (Bautista & Grossman, 2014).

Perception

Once in the dorsal horn of the spinal cord, the nerve fibres divide and then cross to the opposite side and rise upward to the thalamus. The thalamus responds quickly and sends a message to the somatosensory cortex of the brain, where the impulse is interpreted as the physical sensation of pain. The impulses carried by the fast A-delta fibres lead to the perception of sharp, stabbing localized pain that also commonly involves a reflex response to withdraw from the stimulus. The impulses carried by the slow C fibres lead to the perception of diffuse, dull, burning, or aching pain. The point at which the person first feels the lowest intensity of the painful stimulus is termed the **pain threshold**. In addition to sending a message to the cerebral cortex, the thalamus also sends a message to the limbic system, where the sensation is interpreted emotionally, and to the brain stem centres, where autonomic nervous system responses begin.

Modulation

Research has identified substances called **neuromodulators** that appear to modify the pain sensation. These substances have been found to change a person's perception of pain. Examples of these neuromodulators include serotonin, endorphins, enkephalins, and dynorphins.

Pain perception can be modified peripherally or centrally. In the peripheral nerve fibres, chemical substances are released that either stimulate the nerve fibres or sensitize them. Peripheral sensitization allows the nerve fibres to react to a stimulus that is of lower intensity than would be needed to cause pain. As a result, the person perceives more pain. Actions that block or inhibit the release of these substances can lead to a decrease in pain perception.

FIGURE 36.1 Physiology of pain. (*1*) Exposure to thermal noxious stimuli results in activation of nociception (transduction). (*2*) Impulses are relayed along the peripheral nerves to the spinal cord through the dorsal horn (transmission). (*3, 4*) This results in the individual feeling the sensation of pain (perception). (*5*) Neurons in the brain stem send signals back down to the dorsal horn, and these fibres release substances such as endorphins, which can inhibit painful impulses in the dorsal horn (modulation). These neurotransmitters are taken back by the body, therefore limiting the analgesic value.

Modification of pain perception can occur centrally in the spinal cord at the dorsal horn. Substances released by the excited interneurons can potentiate the pain sensation. Other neurochemicals, through their binding to specific receptors, can inhibit the perception of pain. Figure 36.1 illustrates the physiology of pain.

TYPES OF PAIN

Many different systems can be used to classify pain. Most commonly, pain is classified based on its duration, etiology, or source or location.

Classification by Duration

Pain is classified by duration as acute or chronic.

Acute Pain

Acute pain is defined as pain that is associated with a rapid onset of varying intensity. It usually indicates tissue damage and resolves with healing of the injury. Acute pain reflects stimulation of nociceptors and serves a protective function (i.e., alerting the person to a problem). Examples of causes of acute pain include trauma, invasive procedures, acute illnesses such as sore throat or appendicitis, and surgery. This type of pain generally lasts a few days.

> **Take Note!**
> Children often experience pain associated with various procedures done in health care settings. This type of pain is usually short in duration. Preparation of the child and family will help to decrease fears or anxiety. Depending on the type of procedure and the child's age, cognitive level, and temperament, various techniques and methods can be used. Advocating for atraumatic care and adhering to its guidelines will help to minimize procedure-related pain.

Chronic Pain

Chronic pain is defined as pain that continues past the expected point of healing for injured tissue. It provides no protective function. It may be continuous or intermittent, with and without periods of exacerbation or remission. It often interferes with sleep and performance of activities of daily living. It can result in loss of appetite and depression. Thus, chronic pain impairs a person's ability to function. In contrast to acute pain, environmental and psychological factors influence behaviours associated with chronic pain. In children, chronic, recurrent pain is most commonly associated with abdominal pain, nonspecific headache, limb pain, or chest pain. Some conditions, such as sickle cell disease and migraines, have characteristics of both acute and chronic pain (Bautista & Grossman, 2014). Children with chronic pain may not exhibit the same physical or emotional responses as seen with acute pain. As pain becomes prolonged and continuous, the autonomic nervous system response tends to diminish.

Classification by Etiology

Pain can be classified by etiology as nociceptive or neuropathic.

Nociceptive Pain

Nociceptive pain reflects pain due to noxious stimuli that damages normal tissues or has the potential to do

so if the pain is prolonged. The pain perceived often correlates closely with the degree or intensity of the stimulus and the extent of real or possible tissue damage. With nociceptive pain, nervous system functioning is intact. Reports of nociceptive pain vary depending on the location of the nociceptors being stimulated. Nociceptive pain ranges from sharp or burning, to dull, aching, or cramping, and to deep aching or sharp stabbing. Examples of conditions that result in nociceptive pain include chemical burns, sunburn, cuts, appendicitis, and bladder distention.

Neuropathic Pain

Neuropathic pain is pain due to malfunctioning of the peripheral or central nervous system. It may be continuous or intermittent and is commonly described as burning, tingling, shooting, squeezing, or spasm-like pain. Examples of neuropathic pain include posttraumatic and postsurgical peripheral nerve injuries, pain after spinal cord injury, metabolic neuropathies, phantom limb pain after amputation, and post-stroke pain.

Classification by Source or Location

Pain also may be classified by the source or location of the area involved. It can be somatic pain (superficial and deep) or visceral pain. These classifications typically indicate nociceptive pain.

Somatic Pain

Somatic pain refers to pain that develops in the tissues. It can be further divided into two groups—superficial and deep. Superficial somatic pain, often called cutaneous pain, involves stimulation of nociceptors in the skin, subcutaneous tissue, or mucous membranes. Typically, the pain is well localized and described as a sharp, pricking, or burning sensation. Superficial somatic pain may be due to external mechanical, chemical, or thermal injury or skin disorders. Tenderness commonly is present.

Deep somatic pain typically involves the muscles, tendons, joints, fasciae, and bones. It can be localized or diffuse and is usually described as dull, aching, or cramping. Deep somatic pain may be due to strain from overuse or direct injury, ischemia, and inflammation. Tenderness and reflex spasm may be present. In addition, the person may exhibit sympathetic nervous system activation such as tachycardia, hypertension, tachypnea, diaphoresis, pallor, and pupillary dilation.

Visceral Pain

Visceral pain is pain that develops within organs such as the heart, lungs, gastrointestinal tract, pancreas, liver, gallbladder, kidneys, or bladder. It is often produced by disease. It usually is diffuse and poorly localized and is described as a deep ache or sharp stabbing sensation that may be referred to other areas. Visceral pain may be due to distention of the organ, organ muscular spasm, contraction, pulling, ischemia, or inflammation. Tenderness, nausea, vomiting, and diaphoresis may be present.

FACTORS INFLUENCING PAIN

Children, like adults, experience neurologic events that result in the perception of pain. However, research has found that environmental and psychological factors may exert a greater influence on the child's perception of pain (McGrath, 2005). Certain factors such as age, gender, cognitive level, temperament, previous pain experiences, and family and cultural background cannot be changed. However, situational factors involving behavioural, cognitive, and emotional aspects can be modified. These situation-specific factors that affect the child's pain experience include "what the child and parents understand, what they and the health care staff do, and how the child and parents feel. Certain situational factors can intensify pain and distress, whereas others can eventually trigger pain episodes, prolong pain-related disability or maintain the repeated pain episodes in recurrent pain syndrome" (McGrath, 2005, p. 437).

Age and Gender

Research has demonstrated that the nervous system structures needed for pain impulse transmission and perception are present before birth (American Medical Association, 2013). Therefore, children of any age, including preterm newborns, are capable of experiencing pain. Early on, children can interpret pain as an unpleasant sensation, but this interpretation is based on their comparison with other sensations. As they get older, they learn to use words to describe their pain more fully.

Gender and sex also may play a role in a child's perception of pain, but most of the research has been performed on adults, and therefore whether it holds true for children is unclear (Oakes & D'Arcy, 2011). It has been suggested that boys and girls differ in how they perceive, experience, express, and cope with pain and respond to analgesics. This may be influenced by various factors including genetics, hormones, family, and culture. Further research is warranted in this area to allow for more focused care in pain management.

Cognitive Level

Cognitive level is a key factor affecting a child's pain perception and response and usually goes hand in hand with the child's age. Cognitive level typically increases with age, thereby influencing the child's understanding of the pain and its impact and his or her choices for

coping strategies. In addition, as the child's cognitive level increases, his or her ability to communicate information about pain increases. However, this increased understanding and ability to communicate with advancing age may not apply to the child experiencing developmental delays. For example, a developmentally delayed school-age child or adolescent may have the cognitive level of a toddler or preschooler. Health care providers need to be cognizant of this difference when caring for the child in pain. Numerous research studies have revealed that young children often describe pain in concrete terms, whereas older children use more abstract terms that involve both physical and psychological components (McGrath, 2005).

Temperament

Literature suggests that temperament plays a role in predicting distress and pain levels in a child during painful events (Martin & Cohen, 2012). For example, a child with a "difficult temperament" is more likely to have an increased distress response to pain. Nurses can personalize interventions in the clinical environment and during the pain experience to better fit the child's temperament and other personality traits of the child and family.

Previous Pain Experiences

A child identifies pain based on his or her experiences with pain in the past. The number of episodes of pain, the type of pain, the severity or intensity of the previous pain experience, the effectiveness of treatment of pain, and how the child responded all affect how the child will perceive and respond to the current experience. Research suggests that severe pain experiences in the neonate or young infant can lead to sensory disturbances and altered pain responses lasting into adulthood (Hatfield, Chang, Bittle, Deluca, & Polomano, 2011). Previous pain experiences with inadequate pain control may lead to increased distress during future painful procedures. For example, research studies have demonstrated that neonates who had undergone painful procedures such as circumcision and heel lancing showed a stronger negative response to routine immunizations and venipuncture weeks to months later (Oakes & D'Arcy, 2011).

Family and Culture

The child's cultural and family background will influence how he or she will express and manage pain. Some cultures transmit the standard of accepting pain stoically; others allow outward expression. The parents have a strong influence on the child's ability to cope. For example, if a parent reacts to the child's pain in a positive manner and offers comfort measures, the child may have an easier time coping. If the parent shows anger or disapproval, the pain experience may be intensified for the child. Pain might be difficult for the youth to describe and they may want others to speak for them. Pain scales may not always be useful and storytelling can be an alternative (Latimer et al., 2015). *Two-eyes seeing*—as an embedded essential aspect of managing pain within the physical, psychosocial and historical context—is a growing area of study (CPS, 2017). The nurse must be sensitive to their own and the child's cultural background since culture, religion, and ethnicity can influence values and beliefs about health and pain. Resources linked via the Canadian Paediatric Society (2018), for example, Caring for Kids New to Canada, can offer additional information to guide nurses and other health professionals.

Situational Factors

Situational factors involve factors or elements that interact with the child and his or her current situation involving the experience of pain. These factors are highly variable and dependent on the specific situation. Situational factors result from the context in which the child is experiencing pain and include cognitive, which is what the child understands and believes about the pain experience; behavioural, which is how the child and family react and what they do about the pain experience; and emotional, which is how the child and family feel about the pain experience (Oakes & D'Arcy, 2011). Due to children's limited experience with pain, situational factors may affect them more than adults (McGrath, 2005). A thorough pain assessment must include assessment for situational factors that may exacerbate pain. Examples of situational factors include:

- Child's lack of understanding of the source of pain
- Child's lack of ability to use coping mechanisms or pain-relieving strategies to decrease pain
- Stress and anxiety in anticipation of pain
- Child's lack of control of cause of pain
- Child's lack of ability to understand what to expect from potentially painful experiences
- Increased anxiety exhibited by the family
- Overly protective behaviours exhibited by the family
- Presence of emotions such as fear, anxiety, frustration, distress, underlying anxiety, and depression (McGrath, 2005; Oakes & D'Arcy, 2011)

DEVELOPMENTAL CONSIDERATIONS

Since children of various developmental ages respond differently to pain and perceive pain in different ways, it is important to review developmental considerations. Refer to Chapters 25 through 29 for a more complete understanding of childhood development. Nurses must understand how children of various ages respond to painful stimuli and what behaviours may be expected on the basis of their developmental level. By understanding

these developmental considerations, the nurse can appropriately assess the child's pain and provide effective interventions.

Infants

Research has demonstrated that infants, including preterm infants, experience pain and can distinguish pain from other tactile experiences (American Medical Association, 2013). Much of this research focuses on pain related to invasive procedures, such as heel sticks and intravenous catheter insertion. Research suggests that neonates, especially preterm infants, actually experience pain at a greater intensity than older age children and adults (American Medical Association, 2013). The belief is related to the immaturity of the inhibitory mechanisms that develop higher in the central nervous system at a later time during fetal development. These mechanisms are more complex and do not become functional until later in gestation.

> **Take Note!**
> **Levels of Pain**
> When obtaining a blood sample with a heel stick, the nurse should remember that neonates, and in particular preterm infants, feel pain and feel it with greater intensity than older infants.

In preterm and term newborns, behavioural and physiologic indicators are used for determining pain. Behavioural indicators include facial expression, such as brow contracting and chin quivering; body movements; and crying (American Academy of Pediatrics, 2010). Physiologic signs include changes in heart rate, respiratory rate, blood pressure, oxygen saturation levels, intracranial pressure, vagal tone, palmar sweating, and an increase in plasma cortisol or catecholamine levels (American Academy of Pediatrics, 2010; Naughton & Ikuta, 2013).

In the younger infant, facial expression is the most common response to pain (Fig. 36.2). The brows may be lowered and drawn together, with the eyes tightly closed. The mouth is open, often forming a square. The body may be stiff, and thrashing may be seen. When the area is stimulated, the infant may demonstrate a generalized reflex withdrawal but will have no association between the approaching stimulus and the subsequent pain. The infant may exhibit a high-pitched, shrill cry. The older infant often displays similar behavioural manifestations of pain. The older infant may display an angry facial expression, but the eyes are open. He or she often demonstrates a definite withdrawal response when the area is stimulated. The older infant cries loudly and tries to push away the stimulus that is causing the pain. Other manifestations include irritability, restless sleeping, and poor feeding.

FIGURE 36.2 In the younger infant, facial expression is the most common response to pain.

![Take Note icon] **Take Note!**

Although an infant usually exhibits typical behaviours indicating pain, absence of these manifestations does not indicate a lack of pain; the response to pain is highly variable (Weissman, Aranovitch, Blazer, & Zimmer, 2009).

Infants also demonstrate physiologic responses to pain. These may include:

- Increased heart rate, usually averaging approximately 10 beats per minute; possibly bradycardia in preterm newborns
- Decreased vagal tone
- Decreased oxygen saturation
- Palmar or plantar sweating (as measured by skin conductivity testing); not reliable in infants before 37 weeks' gestation

Toddlers

Toddlers can react to painless procedures as intensely as painful ones, with intense emotional upset and physical resistance or aggression. They may bite, hit, scream, or kick and thrash their arms and legs. Other behaviours may include being very quiet, pointing to where it hurts, or saying such words as "oww," or "it hurts." Facial grimacing and teeth clenching may be noted. They may also react with fear and try to hide or leave the room. They often have limited vocabularies, so it may be difficult for them to express pain. It is important to ask about and encourage the child to verbalize his or her

pain. Ensure the use of words the toddler understands, such as "owie" or "boo-boo." Toddlers may demonstrate regressive behaviours, such as clinging to the parent or crying loudly.

![Take Note icon] **Take Note!**

Young children express pain by using simple words such as "hurt" or "ouchie" or by pointing to the area that hurts. By the age of 2 to 4 years, they can express the presence of pain and, by 5 years, they can usually describe pain and its intensity (WHO, 2012).

Preschoolers

Preschoolers may become quiet or try to withdraw and hide in response to actual or perceived pain. For example, the child may say he or she needs to go to the bathroom or needs to get something from another room. Linked to their magical type of thinking, preschoolers may believe pain is a punishment for misbehaving or having bad thoughts. Preschoolers may not verbally report their pain, thinking that pain is something to be expected or that the adults are aware of their pain. They can tell someone where it hurts and can use various tools to describe the severity of pain. However, because they may have limited experience with pain, they may have difficulty distinguishing between types of pain (sharp or dull), describing the intensity of the pain, and determining whether the pain is worse or better.

School-Age Children

School-age children can usually communicate the type, location, and severity of pain. Children older than the age of 8 years can use specific words, such as "sharp as a knife," "burning," or "pulling" to describe their pain. However, they may deny pain in an attempt to appear brave or to avoid further pain related to a procedure or intervention. They may be more concerned with their fear about the illness and its effects rather than the pain. They also may fear being embarrassed by acting-out behaviours in response to pain, such as screaming or thrashing. Thus, a typical response might be to withdraw by staring at the television. Other behaviours that may indicate pain in a school-age child include muscular rigidity, such as clenching the fists, stiffening the body, closing the eyes, wrinkling the forehead, or gritting the teeth. They may use stalling behaviours such as saying "wait a minute."

Adolescents

Adolescents may be concerned primarily about body image and fear losing control over their behaviour. This may result in denial or refusal of medications. Their mood and what they think is expected of them will also affect their response to pain. Adolescents often ask numerous questions and pay close attention to how others respond to them. Fearing that their behaviour may be viewed as juvenile, they may attempt to remain stoic and not exhibit any emotion. Subtle changes such as increased muscle tension with clenched fists and teeth, rapid breathing, and guarding the affected body part may occur. They may also show lack of interest in everyday activities or a decreased ability to concentrate. They exhibit more verbal expressions, such as "you're hurting me."

COMMON FALLACIES AND MYTHS ABOUT PAIN IN CHILDREN

In general, children respond to pain based on the type of pain, the extent of pain, and their age and developmental level. Table 36.1 highlights some common myths and misconceptions related to pain in children. Because

of these myths, children have been medicated less than adults with a similar diagnosis, leading to inadequate pain management.

NURSING PROCESS OVERVIEW FOR THE CHILD IN PAIN

Nursing care of the child with pain includes nursing assessment, nursing diagnosis, planning, interventions, and evaluation. Each step of this process must be individualized for each child. A general understanding of the physiology of pain, factors that influence pain, and effective pain management techniques can help to individualize the child's plan of care.

Assessment

Assessment of pain in children consists of both subjective and objective data collection. The acronym

TABLE 36.1	MYTHS AND MISCONCEPTIONS ABOUT CHILDREN AND PAIN
Myth or Misconception	**Fact**
Newborns do not feel pain	Newborns, including preterm newborns, do feel pain. The neurologic and hormonal systems needed for the transmission of painful stimuli are sufficiently developed
Exposure to pain at an early age has little to no effect on the child	Prolonged or severe pain can lead to increased newborn morbidity. Infants who have experienced pain during the neonatal period respond differently to subsequent painful events[a]
Infants and small children have little memory of pain	Repeated exposure to painful procedures and events can have long-term consequences. Memories of pain may be stored in the child's nervous system, influencing later reactions to painful stimuli[a]
The intensity of a child's behavioural reaction indicates the intensity of the child's pain	Numerous factors affect a child's response to pain. Each child is an individual, with his or her own set of responses
A child who is sleeping or playing is not in pain	Sleep or play may be a coping strategy for the child in pain. Sleep may reflect exhaustion of the child who is coping with pain
Children are truthful when they are asked if they are experiencing pain	Often children deny pain to avoid a painful situation or procedure, embarrassment, or loss of control. Children may assume that others know how they are feeling and thus will not verbalize their complaints
Children learn to adapt to pain and painful procedures	Repeated exposure to pain or painful procedures can result in an increase in behavioural manifestations
Children experience more adverse effects of narcotic analgesics than adults do	The risk of adverse effects of narcotic analgesics is the same for children as for adults
Children are more prone to addiction to narcotic analgesics	Addiction to narcotics when used appropriately to treat children's pain is very rare and no more common than in adults[b]

[a]Anand, K. J. S. (2013). Assessment of neonatal pain. UpToDate. Retrieved from http://www.uptodate.com/contents/assessment-of-neonatal-pain?source=search_result&search=neonatal+pain&selectedTitle=2~5#H12.

[b]Finley, G. A., Franck, L. S., Grunau, R. E., & von Baeyer, C. L. (2005). Why children's pain matters. *International Association for the Study of Pain. Pain: Clinical updates, XIII*(4), 1–6. Retrieved from http://iasp.files.cms-plus.com/Content/ContentFolders/Publications2/PainClinicalUpdates/Archives/PCU05-4_1390264071339_24.pdf.

Adapted from The Hospital for Sick Children. (2005). *Myths vs facts of children's pain.* Retrieved from http://www.iasp-pain.org/files/Content/ContentFolders/GlobalYearAgainstPain2/20052006PaininChildren/pdfist.pdf; Pawar, D., & Garten, L. (2010). Chapter 34: Pain management in children. In A. Kopf & N. B. Patel (Eds.), *Guide to pain management in low-resource settings* (pp. 255–268). Seattle, WA: International Association for the Study of Pain.

QUESTT is an excellent way to remember the key principles of pain assessment (Baker & Wong, 1987):

- **Q**uestion the child.
- **U**se a reliable and valid pain scale.
- **E**valuate the child's behaviour and physiologic changes to establish a baseline and determine the effectiveness of the intervention. The child's behaviour and motor activity may include irritability and protection as well as withdrawal of the affected painful area.
- **S**ecure the parent's involvement.
- **T**ake the cause of pain into account when intervening.
- **T**ake action.

 Take Note!

Children do experience pain! Pain management techniques work just as well with children as they do with adults.

Health History

When assessing pain in children, tailor the assessment to the child's developmental level and ask questions geared to the child's cognitive ability. During the health history, determine the child's previous exposure to pain, if any, and how the child responded. This information will provide clues about how the child copes and his or her current response. Attempt to determine what word the child uses to denote pain. Some children may not understand the term "pain" but do understand terms such as "ouchie" or "boo-boo."

The health history also includes questioning the parents about their cultural beliefs related to pain and their child's usual responses. This information aids in planning developmentally and culturally appropriate family-centred care.

QUESTIONING THE CHILD

When questioning the child, phrase the questions in a manner that the child will be able to understand based on his or her developmental level. Some input from the child's family may be helpful in determining where best to focus the questions.

Ask the child what pain means to him or her. Use words that the child may comprehend more easily, such as "hurt," "boo-boo," or "ouch," as appropriate. Inquire about similar experiences in the past and how he or she responded. Determine whether the child let others know that he or she was hurting and how this message was conveyed (e.g., crying, acting out, or pointing to the hurting area).

Review the history of the pain and various influences such as cultural aspects, caregiver attitudes or expectations, previous experiences, and any education or teaching related to pain management. Continue to formulate questions to ascertain the following:

- Location, quality, severity, and onset of the pain, as well as the circumstances in which the child experiences the pain. Have the child point to the area where it hurts or identify the location on a diagram or doll.
- Conditions, if any, that preceded the onset of pain and the conditions that followed the onset of pain.
- Any associated symptoms, such as weight loss, fever, vomiting, or diarrhea, which may indicate a current illness.
- Any recent trauma, including any interventions that were used in an attempt to relieve the pain.

Continue the health history by inquiring about what the child wants others, including the nurse, to do when they have pain (or something hurts). Conversely, ask the child what he or she does not want others to do. Finally, question the child about measures that seem to be most effective in relieving the pain. Ask if there is anything special the child wants to tell the nurse, such as a special pain relief technique or a specific comfort object.

If the child is experiencing chronic or recurrent pain, suggest the child and family record information in a symptom diary. Explain that this will be helpful in identifying the best ways to manage the pain.

QUESTIONING THE PARENTS

Parents play a key role in assessing pain in children. Often it is the parents who provide information about the child's current and past experiences with pain. In addition, parents can provide information about how the child exhibits and responds to pain. Parents may be aware of subtle changes in the child's behaviour that may precede the pain, occur with the pain, or indicate relief of pain. Including the parents in this process helps create a positive experience for all involved and promotes feelings of control over the situation.

The questions posed to the parents are similar in focus to those posed to the child. However, more detailed information may be obtained from the parents because they are usually able to describe events more fully or in greater detail due to their higher cognitive level. Parents typically know their child best.

 Take Note!

Parents may assume that nurses have greater expertise when it comes to assessing their child's pain and taking appropriate action. Thus, they may not always report when they notice changes suggesting that their child is uncomfortable. Emphasize the important role that parents play in reporting any changes in their child so that pain relief measures can be instituted as soon as possible.

When questioning the parents, use the following examples as a guide for assessing the child's pain:

- Has your child ever been in pain before? If so, what was the cause of the pain? How long did he or she have the pain? Where was the pain located?

- How did your child react to the pain? What did you do to lessen the pain?
- Did your child let you know that he or she was in pain? Did he or she tell you or did you notice something?
- Are there any special signs that let you know that your child is hurting? If so, what are they?
- Is there anything that your child does or that you do when he or she is hurting that helps relieve the pain?
- Does one thing work better than another when your child is hurting?
- Is there any special information that you want to tell me about your child?

USING PAIN RATING SCALES

Various pain assessment, or pain rating, scales are available. These scales allow the child to report his or her pain, and the pain level is quantified. These standardized rating scales provide a greater alignment between the child's pain and the nurse's assessment of the severity of the pain. Self-report is the primary source for the measurement of pain in children (von Baeyer, 2014). Self-report measures should be used in conjunction with observation and discussion with the child and family, especially in children younger than age 5 or in children with cognitive impairments (American Academy of Pediatrics and the American Pain Society, 2001; von Baeyer, 2014). Some studies have found validity in self-report tools used in children as young as 3 years of age, while others have found inconsistent findings when they are used in children younger than 5 years of age (Besenski, Forsyth, & von Baeyer, 2007; Oakes & D'Arcy, 2011). Therefore, it is important to assess young children's ability to perform self-report tasks rather than rely solely on their chronologic age (Besenski et al., 2007).

Many health care settings have specific policies and procedures related to pain assessment, including the frequency of assessment, the rating tool to use, and nursing interventions to be instituted on the basis of the rating. For example, acute care settings may require assessment of the child using a specific tool with each episode of documentation or at least once a shift and 30 minutes to 1 hour after a nonpharmacologic or pharmacologic pain relief intervention. This process provides a more objective method to determine whether the pain is increasing or decreasing and whether pain relief methods are effective.

Take Note!

Typically, different pain rating scales are appropriate for different developmental levels. However, children may regress when in pain, so a simpler tool may be needed to make sure that the child understands what is being asked. Regardless of the tool used, nurses need to be consistent in using the same tool so that appropriate comparisons can be made and effective interventions can

Wong-Baker FACES Pain Rating Scale

0	1	2	3	4	5
NO HURT	HURTS LITTLE BIT	HURTS LITTLE MORE	HURTS EVEN MORE	HURTS WHOLE LOT	HURTS WORST

Alternate coding: 0 2 4 6 8 10

Instructions: Explain to the person that each face is for a person who feels happy because he has no pain (hurt) or sad because he has some or a lot of pain. **Face 0** is very happy because he doesn't hurt at all. **Face 1** hurts just a little bit. **Face 2** hurts a little more. **Face 3** hurts even more. **Face 4** hurts a whole lot. **Face 5** hurts as much as you can imagine, although you don't have to be crying to feel this bad. Ask the person to choose the face that best describes how he is feeling.

FIGURE 36.3 FACES pain rating scale. (© 1983 Wong-Baker FACES Foundation. www.WongBakerFACES.org. Used with permission. Originally published in Whaley & Wong's Nursing Care of Infants and Children. © Elsevier Inc.)

be planned and implemented. Using the most appropriate tool consistently allows the most accurate assessment of the child's pain.

FACES Pain Rating Scale. The FACES pain rating scale-revised (Fig. 36.3) is a self-report tool that can be used by children as young as 3 (Oakes & D'Arcy, 2011). The scale consists of six illustrations of faces arranged horizontally; the faces show how much something can hurt. The face furthest to the left shows no pain, while the faces show more pain from left to right, till the last face hat shows the most pain. Under each face is a number ranging from 0+ no pain to 10 = most pain possible (International Association for the Study of Pain, 2012). The number scale can be 0, 1, 2, 3, 4, and 5 or 0, 2, 4, 6, 8, and 10. The nurse explains the words associated with each face to the child. Then, the nurse asks the child to select the facial expression that best describes the level of pain he or she is feeling. The nurse then documents the number corresponding to the word description and face. Facial coding systems can also be used with children with cerebral palsy when delivering treatments and interventions (Hadden, LeFort, O'Brien, Coyte, & Guerriere, 2016).

Oucher Pain Rating Scale. The Oucher pain rating scale is similar to the FACES scale in that it uses facial expressions to indicate increasing degrees of hurt. However, instead of illustrations, six photographs are used: "no hurt" is placed at the bottom of the arrangement and "most hurt" at the top. Alongside the photos is a scale ranging from 0 to 10 that corresponds to the facial expressions in the photographs (Fig. 36.4). After explaining the photos and numeric scale, the child is

OUCHER!

10 —
9 —
8 —
7 —
6 —
5 —
4 —
3 —
2 —
1 —
0 —

FIGURE 36.4 Oucher pain rating scale. (Used with permission from Beyer, J. E., Denyes, M. J., & Villarruel, A. M. (1992). The creation, validation, and continuing development of the Oucher: A measure of pain intensity in children. *Journal of Pediatric Nursing, 7*(5), 335–346.)

FIGURE 36.5 The poker chip tool. Here the nurse asks the child to identify the number of chips that indicate his degree of "hurt."

asked to point to the number that best describes his or her level of pain (Beyer, Denyes, & Villarruel, 1992).

This scale is useful for self-reporting of pain in children between 3 and 12 years of age (Oakes & D'Arcy, 2011). Different ethnicity versions have been developed for use with Caucasian, Hispanic, Asian, and African American children (Oakes & D'Arcy, 2011).

Poker Chip Tool. The poker chip tool, also known as the pieces of hurt tool, is a self-reporting pain assessment tool that uses four red poker chips to quantify the child's level of pain (American Medical Association, 2013). The chips are arranged in a horizontal line on a surface in front of the child. Starting with the chip closest to the child's left side, the nurse points to the chip and explains that the first chip means a little hurt, the next chip means more hurt, the third chip means more hurt, and the fourth chip means the worst hurt ever. Then, the nurse asks the child how many "pieces of hurt" he or she is having (Fig. 36.5). If the child is not experiencing any pain, typically the child will state that he or she isn't having any. When the child identifies the number of "pieces of hurt," the nurse follows up by asking the child to tell the nurse more about his or her hurt (Hester, 1979).

The poker chip tool is useful for assessing pain in children 4 to 7 years of age. Children may view this assessment tool as a game since it involves poker chips. However, the nurse needs to ensure that the child has the cognitive ability to distinguish the numbers.

Take Note!

Toddlers and preschoolers may not be used to being asked questions by strangers, and may not understand quantitative ratings or estimation. Preschoolers will often construct an answer even if they do not understand the question. They also will often use extremes of scales, such as no pain or the worst pain (von Baeyer, 2006).

Visual Analogue and Numeric Scales. Visual analogue and numeric scales involve a horizontal or vertical line with marked endpoints. With a visual analogue scale, the endpoints are identified as no pain and worst pain. A numeric scale typically has endpoints of 0 and 10, reflecting no pain and worst pain, respectively (Fig. 36.6). The nurse explains the scale to the child. With the visual analogue scale, the child makes a line that best describes the level of pain. The nurse then measures the distance from the "no pain" endpoint to the child's mark and records this as the pain score. With

Visual Analog Scale (VAS)

No pain

Pain as bad as it could possibly be

A

0 – 10 Numeric Pain Intensity Scale

0   1   2   3   4   5   6   7   8   9   10
No pain   Moderate   Worst
                         pain   possible
                                          pain

B

FIGURE 36.6 **A.** Visual analogue scale. **B.** Numeric scale.

the numeric scale, the nurse asks the child to pick the number that best describes his or her level of pain.

The visual analogue scale can be used in children 8 years or older but some studies report effectiveness in children 5 to 7 years of age (von Baeyer, 2014). The numeric scale can be used with children 8 years or older (von Baeyer, 2014). Even though a younger child may be able to count and give numbers on the scale, they have not yet developed an understanding of the quantitative significance of the numbers.

Adolescent Pediatric Pain Tool. The Adolescent Pediatric Pain Tool is a multidimensional self-report type of tool useful for older children, usually between 8 and 17 years of age (Oakes & D'Arcy, 2011). The tool involves three aspects of assessment. In the first assessment, the child identifies the location of the pain on two illustrations of the body—front and back views (Fig. 36.7).

The child is instructed to colour the areas where he or she is hurting. The child is also instructed to colour the area as big or as small as how much he or she is hurting. For example, if the hurt is mild or moderate, the child would colour a moderate area of the location; if the pain is severe, he or she would colour a much larger area. The second portion of the tool involves a scale that ranges from "no pain" to "worst possible pain." The nurse instructs the child to identify the severity of his or her pain. The third assessment is a list of words that may be used to describe pain, such as throbbing, pounding, stabbing, or sharp. The nurse asks the child to point to or circle the words that describe the current pain. Children with limited reading skills or vocabulary may have difficulty with some of the words listed to describe pain. Work with the child and encourage the parents to help the child understand the various descriptive words. Parental participation fosters control over the situation and gives the parents some insight into what their child is experiencing (Crandall & Savedra, 2005).

Thinking About Development

Kaylee Cooper is a 4-year-old female with a fractured femur. She has been in traction since arriving in the emergency room last night. When you enter her room at the beginning of your shift, you note she is quiet and withdrawn. How will Kaylee's developmental stage affect the use of self-report? What special considerations must the nurse think about when using self-report of pain with Kaylee? What is the most appropriate pain rating scale to be used for Kaylee?

Physical Examination

Physical examination of the child for pain primarily involves the skills of observation and inspection.

These skills are used to assess for physiologic and behavioural changes that indicate pain. Auscultation also may be used to assess for changes in vital signs, specifically heart rate and blood pressure.

OBSERVE FOR MANIFESTATIONS OF PAIN

Observe for physical signs and symptoms of pain, keeping in mind the child's developmental level. Look for facial expressions of discomfort, grimacing, or crying. Be alert for movements that may suggest pain. For example, an infant or toddler may pull on the ear when experiencing ear pain. The child may move the head from side to side, suggesting head pain. Typically, children with abdominal pain will lie on one side and draw their knees up to the abdomen. Inspect the child's gait: a limp or avoidance of weight bearing may suggest leg pain. Immobility, guarding of a particular body area, or refusal to move an area may be observed. Inspect the skin for flushing or diaphoresis, possible indicators of pain. Also monitor vital signs for changes. Pulse or heart rate, respiratory rate, and blood pressure may increase. Other physiologic parameters that suggest pain may include elevated intracranial pressure and pulmonary vascular resistance and decreased oxygen saturation levels.

Take Note!

The body responds to acute pain via the sympathetic nervous system, leading to stimulation and a subsequent increase in vital signs. However, if the child has persistent or chronic pain, the body adapts and these changes may be less noticeable (Oakes & D'Arcy, 2011).

The child also may exhibit behavioural changes indicating pain. Be alert for irritability and restlessness. Watch for clenching of teeth or fists, body stiffening, or increased muscle tension. Note any changes in the child's behaviour. For example, a child who previously was talkative and playful may become quiet and almost withdrawn in response to pain. Remember, a child in pain may sleep or play in order to cope with the pain. In addition, pay close attention to the child's cultural background and how these beliefs may be affecting the behavioural response to pain.

Each child is an individual with unique responses to pain, so the nurse must ensure that observations of behaviour do indeed reflect the child's pain level. To help ensure the accuracy of observations, several physiologic and behavioural assessment tools have been developed to help quantify the observations.

USING PHYSIOLOGIC AND BEHAVIOURAL PAIN ASSESSMENT TOOLS

Use of physiologic and behavioural pain assessment tools allows measurement of specific parameters and changes that would indicate that the child is experiencing

Right   Left Left   Right

Sensory

Aching ("pain all over")

Hurting ("pain all over")

Sore ("like a cut")

Beating (procedural pain "spots")

Pounding ("gets on your nerves")

Cutting ("hurts more than a cut")

Like a sharp knife ("stabbing and sharp")
Sharp (no meaning)

Stabbing (no meaning)

Cramping ("everywhere like a plane crash")
Crushing (no meaning)
Pressure ("pushing all over")
Itching ("all over")
Scratching ("helps sometimes")
Shocking (pain "surprises" her)
Splitting ("splitting in half" her body)
Numb ("knows pain is there"/ procedural pain)
Stiff ("cannot move")
Swollen ("meds do not help")
Tight ("cannot move")

Affective

Awful ("cannot do anything")

Crying ("hurts so bad")

Frightening ("scared it won't stop")

Screaming (afraid of "going to the hospital")

Terrifying ("cannot sleep," "really tired," "not going to live")

Dizzy ("don't know where I am")

Evaluative

Annoying ("cannot sleep")

Bad ("cannot stop the hurting")

Miserable ("cannot sleep or do stuff")

Terrible ("don't like it")

Uncomfortable ("can't stay in one spot")

Uncontrollable ("cannot stop it")

Temporal

Always ("pain always there")

Comes and goes ("always pain")

Comes on all of a sudden ("no warning")

Constant ("never goes away")

Continuous ("pain not going away")

Forever ("never will go away")

Once in a while ("in a month sometimes pain; sometimes not")
Sneaks up ("don't know when the pain will happen")
Sometimes ("goes away sometimes; sometimes not")

FIGURE 36.7 Adolescent Pediatric Assessment Tool. (**Top**) Adolescent Pediatric Pain Tool (APPT): body outline. (**Bottom**) Pain Quality: Words chosen and meaning of words. (Used with permission from Crandall, M., & Savedra, M. (2005). Multidimensional assessment using the adolescent pediatric pain tool: A case report. *Journal for Specialists in Pediatric Nursing, 10*(3), 115–123.)

TABLE 36.2	THE NEONATAL INFANT PAIN SCALE (NIPS)	
Parameter	**Finding**	**Score**
Facial expression	Relaxed (restful face; neutral expression)	0
	Grimace (tight facial muscles; furrowed brow, chin, or jaw; negative facial expression)	1
Cry	No cry (quiet; not crying)	0
	Whimper (mild intermittent moaning)	1
	Vigorous crying (loud screaming, shrill, continuous)	2
Breathing patterns	Relaxed	0
	Change in breathing (irregular; faster than usual; gagging; breath holding)	1
Arms	Relaxed (no muscular rigidity; occasional random movements of arm)	0
	Flexed/extended (tense, straight, rigid, or rapid flexion or extension)	1
Legs	Relaxed (no muscular rigidity; occasional random movements of leg)	0
	Flexed/extended (tense, straight, rigid, or rapid flexion or extension)	1
State of arousal	Sleeping/awake (quiet, peaceful, settled)	0
	Fussy (alert, restless, thrashing)	1

Reproduced with permission from Lawrence, J., Alcock, D., MacGrath, P., Kay, J., MacMurray, S. B., & Dulberg, C. (1993). The development of a tool to assess neonatal pain. *Neonatal Network*, *12*(6), 59–66. Copyright © 1993 Springer Publishing Company, LLC.

pain. These measurements aid in determining the intensity of the pain experience. Along with the self-report pain rating scales, measurement of these changes allows the nurse to objectively assess pain and the effectiveness of pain management measures.

Neonatal Infant Pain Scale. The Neonatal Infant Pain Scale (NIPS) is a behavioural assessment tool that is useful for measuring pain in preterm and full-term neonates (Lawrence et al., 1993). Six parameters are measured: facial expression, cry, breathing patterns, arms, legs, and state of arousal (Table 36.2). Each parameter except for cry is scored as 0 or 1; cry is scored as 0, 1, or 2. The scores are then totalled and the maximum score that can be achieved is 7. A higher score indicates increased pain. This scale does not include any physiologic parameters; therefore, it may not detect early pain in neonates who are too ill to respond, who are receiving paralyzing agents, or who are premature (Anand, 2013). In these cases, a falsely low score may be produced.

Riley Infant Pain Scale. The Riley Infant Pain Scale (RIPS) is a behavioural assessment tool useful for infants who lack verbal ability (Schade, Joyce, Gerkensmeyer, & Keck, 1996). Like NIPS, RIPS measures six parameters: facial expression, body movement, sleep, verbal or vocal ability, consolability, and response to movements and touch (Table 36.3). Each parameter is scored as 0, 1, 2, or 3. The score is then totalled and the maximum score that can be achieved is 18. The higher the total score, the more intense the pain.

Pain Observation Scale for Young Children. The Pain Observation Scale for Young Children (POCIS) is a behavioural assessment tool designed for use in children between 1 and 4 years of age (Boelen-van der Loo, Scheffer, de Haan, & de Groot, 1999). This tool measures seven parameters: facial expression, cry, breathing, torso, arms and fingers, legs and toes, and state of arousal (Table 36.4). Each parameter is scored as 0 or 1; the maximum score achievable is 7. The higher the score, the greater the pain being experienced by the child.

CRIES Scale for Neonatal Postoperative Pain Assessment. The CRIES scale is a behavioural assessment tool that also includes measures of physiologic parameters (Krechel & Bildner, 1995). It was developed to quantify postoperative pain in the newborn. The tool also may be used to monitor the infant's progress over time during recovery or after interventions. The tool assesses five parameters: cry, oxygen required for saturation levels less than 95%, increased vital signs, facial expression, and sleeplessness (Table 36.5). Each parameter is scored as 0, 1, or 2 and then totalled. As with other assessment tools, the higher the score, the greater the infant's pain.

r-FLACC Behavioural Scale for Pain in Nonverbal Young Children and Children With Cognitive Impairment. The original FLACC behavioural scale is a behavioural assessment tool that is useful in assessing a child's pain when the child cannot report accurately his or her level of pain (Merkel, Voepel-Lewis, Shayevitz, & Malviya, 1997). It has been demonstrated to be a reliable tool for children from age 2 months to 7 years of age (Oakes & D'Arcy, 2011). This tool measures five parameters: facial expression, legs, activity, cry, and

TABLE 36.3	THE RILEY INFANT PAIN SCALE	
Parameter		**Score**
• Facial expression		
• Neutral/smiling		0
• Frowning/grimacing		1
• Clenched teeth		2
• Full cry expression		3
• Body movement		
• Calm, relaxed		0
• Restless, fidgeting		1
• Moderate agitation or mobility; thrashing, flailing, incessant agitation or strong voluntary mobility		2
• Voluntary immobility		3
• Sleep		
• Sleeping quietly with easy respirations		0
• Restless while asleep		1
• Sleeping intermittently (sleep/awake)		2
• Sleeping for prolonged periods of time interrupted by jerky movements or inability to sleep		3
• Verbal/vocal		
• No cry		0
• Whimpering, complaining		1
• Pain crying		2
• Screaming, high-pitched cry		3
• Consolability		
• Neutral		0
• Easy to console		1
• Not easy to console		2
• Inconsolable		3
• Response to movement/touch		
• Moves easily		0
• Winces when touched or moved		1
• Cries out when moved or touched		2
• High-pitched cry or scream when touched or moved		3

Used with permission from Schade, J. G., Joyce, B. A., Gerkensmeyer, J., & Keck, J. F. (1996). Comparison of three preverbal scales for postoperative pain assessment in a diverse pediatric sample. *Journal of Pain and Symptom Management, 12*(6), 348–359.

TABLE 36.4	THE PAIN OBSERVATION SCALE FOR YOUNG CHILDREN (POCIS)	
Parameter	**Finding**	**Score**
Facial expression	Neutral	0
	Grimace (negative)	1
Cry	No cry	0
	Moan, scream	1
Breathing	Relaxed and regular	0
	Irregular and indrawn	1
Torso	At rest, inactive	0
	Tense, shivering	1
Arms and fingers	At rest, inactive	0
	Tense, restless	1
Legs and toes	At rest, inactive	0
	Tense, restless	1
State of arousal	Calm, sleepy	0
	Fussy	1

Used with permission from Boelen-van der Loo, W. J. C., Scheffer, E., de Haan, R. J., & de Groot, C. J. (1999). Clinimetric evaluation of the pain observation scale for young children in children aged between 1 and 4 years after ear, nose, and throat surgery. *Developmental and Behavioral Pediatrics, 20*(4), 222–227.

consolability (Table 36.6). Observe the child with the legs and body uncovered. If the child is awake, observe him or her for 1 to 2 minutes; if sleeping, observe the child for 2 minutes or longer. Each parameter is scored as 0, 1, or 2. The scores are totalled, with a maximum achievable score of 10. As with other assessment tools, the higher the score, the greater the pain.

The revised FLACC (r-FLACC) is used in the same manner as the original FLACC but it includes additional descriptors of behaviours most commonly associated with pain that have been validated in children with cognitive impairment (Hauer & Jones, 2014). Refer to Table 36.6. Pain assessment tools are a supplement to pain assessment and are not meant to replace caregiver/parent input. Review the descriptor terms with parents/caregivers and individualize the scale by adding pain-related behaviours that are specific indicators of pain observed in their child in the appropriate categories (Hauer & Jones, 2014).

Nursing Diagnoses, Goals, Interventions, and Evaluation

After assessing the child, the nurse identifies appropriate nursing diagnoses. The most commonly identified nursing diagnosis would be acute or chronic pain. However, the related factors and defining characteristics can vary widely. Nursing diagnoses will focus on the effects of pain on the child, for example, the stress incurred as a result of the pain or the fear or anxiety associated with the pain or events causing the pain. Moreover, pain can affect physiologic functions, such as sleep, nutrition, mobility, and elimination. Examples of common nursing diagnoses may include:

- Acute pain related to repeated need for invasive procedures, surgical experience, recent trauma, or infection
- Chronic pain related to prolonged illness or injury, effects of cancer on surrounding tissues, or treatment-related effects
- Fear related to the unknown, separation from family, anticipation of invasive procedures, or effects of treatment

TABLE 36.5	THE CRIES SCALE FOR NEONATAL POSTOPERATIVE PAIN ASSESSMENT		
Assessment	0	1	2
Crying	No	High-pitched, but consolable	High-pitched, inconsolable
Oxygen required for saturation above 95%	No	<30%	>30%
Increased vital signs	Heart rate and blood pressure within 10% of preoperative values	Heart rate or blood pressure 11–20% higher than preoperative values	Heart rate or blood pressure 21% or more above preoperative values
Expression	No grimace	Grimace	Grimace with grunt
Sleepless	No	Waking at frequent intervals	Constantly awake
Total infant score			

Used with permission from Krechel, S. W., & Bildner, J. (1995). CRIES: A new neonatal postoperative pain measurement score. Initial testing of validity and reliability. *Paediatric Anaesthesia, 5,* 53–61.

- Anxiety related to the stress and uncertainty of the situation
- Deficient knowledge related to current condition and appropriate methods for managing pain
- Sleep deprivation related to inability to manage pain effectively
- Impaired mobility related to increased episodes of pain
- Risk for constipation related to potential adverse effects of narcotic analgesic agents

When caring for a child experiencing pain, the ultimate goal is that the child will be free of pain as evidenced participation in age-appropriate activities of daily living and vital signs within age-appropriate parameters. However, at times, this may be unrealistic, especially if the child is experiencing chronic pain. Therefore, a more appropriate goal would be that the child reports that his or her pain has decreased to a tolerable level. Pain assessment tools can be used to quantify the amount by which the child's pain has decreased. For example, if the

TABLE 36.6	FLACC BEHAVIOURAL SCALE		
		Scoring	
Category	0	1	2
Face	No particular expression or smile	Occasional grimace or frown, withdrawn, disinterested; **appears sad or worried**[a]	Frequent to constant frown, clenched jaw, quivering chin; **distress-looking face: expression of fright or panic**[a]
Legs	Normal position or relaxed	Uneasy, restless, tense; **occasional tremors**[a]	Kicking, or legs drawn up; **marked increase in spasticity, constant tremors, or jerking**[a]
Activity	Lying quietly, normal position, moves easily	Squirming, shifting back and forth, tense; **mildly agitated (e.g., head back and forth, aggression); shallow, splinting respirations, intermittent sighs**[a]	Arched, rigid, or jerking; **severe agitation, head banging, shivering (not rigors); breath-holding, gasping, or sharp intake of breath; severe splinting**[a]
Cry	No cry (awake or asleep)	Moans or whimpers, occasional complaint; **occasional verbal outburst or grunt**[a]	Crying steadily, screams or sobs, frequent complaints; **repeated outbursts, constant grunting**[a]
Consolability	Content, relaxed	Reassured by occasional touching, hugging, or being talked to, distractible	Difficult to console or comfort; **pushing away caregiver, resisting care, or comfort measures**[a]

Each of the five categories is scored from 0 to 2, which results in a total score between 0 and 10. © 2002, The Regents of the University of Michigan. All rights reserved.
[a]Revised descriptors shown in bold.

child has rated the pain as 7 out of 10, a realistic goal might be that the child reports a pain rating of no more than 4 out of 10. Additional goals would reflect improvement or resolution of the identified problem. For example, a short-term goal for a child experiencing disturbed sleep due to the pain might be that the child sleeps for a minimum of 4 consecutive hours through the night. A long-term goal might be that the child sleeps for 7 to 8 hours undisturbed through the night.

Various interventions can be used for pain management. These interventions include nonpharmacologic and pharmacologic measures. A guiding principle when caring for the child experiencing pain is the provision of atraumatic care. For example, cognitive and behavioural approaches are appropriate for pain management, including pain management related to procedures. In addition to nonpharmacologic measures, pharmacologic measures are appropriate for pain management. For example, apply a topical anaesthetic cream to a site early enough before a venipuncture that it becomes effective. Another idea is to use an intermittent infusion device to obtain multiple blood specimen samples rather than performing repeated venipunctures. In addition, it is a good idea to consider the use of sedation for procedures that are or are perceived to be painful.

Throughout the child's care, be sure to discuss specific goals and interventions with the child and family as appropriate. Include the family in developing appropriate interventions so they can continue to support the child. Education of the child and family about interventions, including various therapies, is key. Ongoing pain assessment is crucial to determine the effectiveness of the pain relief measures with a view to achieving optimal pain management (Panjganj & Bevan, 2016).

Take Note!

The Registered Nurses' Association of Ontario (2013) provides evidence-informed clinical best practice guidelines in assessment and management of pain, across the life course. In addition, the centre for Pediatric Pain Research offers evidence-informed resources, research, and programs. Additional information can be found at thePoint.

Atraumatic Care

Play therapy may be helpful in allowing the child to express his or her feelings and adapt to the stressors of the current situation.

Nursing Care Plan 36.1 (at the end of the chapter) can be used as a guide in planning nursing care for the child experiencing pain. The nursing care plan should be individualized based on the child's symptoms and needs. Specific information related to pain management and the nurse's role will be discussed later in the chapter.

When you enter Aiden's room, he is crying and says his leg hurts. What will be your initial action? What will be your plan of care to manage Aiden's pain (refer to QUESTT assessment)? How would you address the statements made by the nurse in report? What approaches can you use to change staff behaviour about pain management?

MANAGEMENT OF PAIN

Management of pain begins with assessment of the child's comfort level. If pain or the potential for pain, such as during an invasive procedure, is identified, steps must be taken to minimize or treat the pain. Three general principles guide pain management in children:

1. Individualize interventions based on the amount of pain experienced and the child's characteristics, such as developmental level, temperament, previous pain experience, and coping strategies.
2. Use nonpharmacologic and pharmacologic approaches to ease or eliminate the pain.
3. Teach the child and family about pain relief interventions and techniques and discuss with the child and family expectations of pain management.

Specific strategies for pain management include nonpharmacologic interventions such as relaxation, distraction, and guided imagery and pharmacologic interventions such as analgesics, patient-controlled analgesia (PCA), local analgesia, epidural analgesia, and moderate sedation.

Nonpharmacologic Management

Various techniques may be available to assist in managing mild pain in children or to augment the effectiveness of medications for moderate or severe pain. Many of these nonpharmacologic techniques assist children in coping with pain and give them an opportunity to feel a sense of mastery or control over the situation. Two types of techniques are behavioural-cognitive strategies and biophysical strategies. It is important to involve the parents in the process when using these techniques.

Behavioural-Cognitive Strategies

Behavioural-cognitive strategies for pain management involve measures that require the child to focus on a specific area rather than the pain. These strategies help to change the interpretation of the painful stimuli, reducing pain perception or making pain more tolerable. In addition, these strategies help to decrease negative attitudes, thoughts, and anxieties, thereby improving the child's coping mechanisms. Research has shown strong evidence that these strategies reduce pain and distress with needle-related procedures in children (Hsu & Cravero, 2014). Typically, these interventions work well with older children, but younger children also benefit from these techniques if they are adapted to the child's age and developmental level. Common behavioural-cognitive strategies include relaxation, distraction, imagery, biofeedback, thought stopping, and positive self-talk.

RELAXATION

Relaxation aids in reducing muscle tension and anxiety. A wide variety of techniques can be used. Relaxation can be as simple as holding an infant or young child closely while stroking the child or speaking in a soft soothing manner, or having the child inhale and exhale slowly using rhythmically controlled deep breathing. It also can involve more sophisticated techniques such as progressive relaxation. With this technique, the child is asked to focus on one area of the body and let that body part go limp. Then, in an organized fashion, usually working from the toes to the head or vice versa, the child is asked to focus on another body part, making it go limp. Eventually, the exercises work through all body areas, leading to relaxation of the entire body.

DISTRACTION

Distraction involves having the child focus on another stimulus, thereby attempting to shield him or her from pain. Research has shown distraction to be associated with lower parental perception of pain and distress in younger children and decreased situational anxiety in older children (Hsu & Cravero, 2014).

This technique does not eliminate the pain but does help to make it more tolerable. Various methods can be used for distraction, including:

- Counting
- Repeating specific phrases or words, such as "ouch"
- Listening to music or singing
- Playing games, including computer and video games
- Blowing bubbles or blowing pinwheels or party favours
- Listening to favourite stories (Fig. 36.8)
- Watching cartoons, television shows, or movies
- Visiting with friends
- Humour

Humour has been demonstrated to be an effective distracting technique for pain management. However, make sure that the technique is age appropriate and be sure to determine what or who will make the child laugh. If possible, allow the child and his or her family to choose the materials that they consider humorous.

The type of distraction used depends on the age of the child. For example, a younger child may enjoy blowing pinwheels and blowing bubbles. He or she also will enjoy listening to favourite stories or books. Older

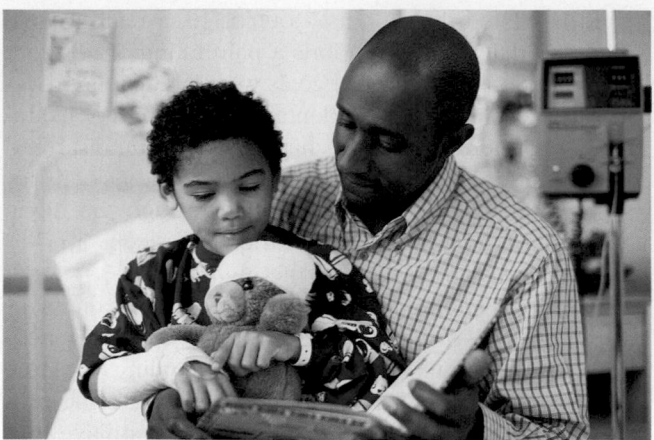

FIGURE 36.8 A child using distraction for pain management.

children may enjoy computer or video games, listening to favourite music, or visiting with friends.

IMAGERY

Imagery involves the use of the imagination to create a mental image. This mental image usually is a positive, pleasurable image, but it need not be real. The child is encouraged to include details and sensations that are associated with the image, such as specific descriptions of the image, colours, sounds, feelings, and smells. In some instances, the child may write down or record the image. When pain occurs, the child is encouraged to create the mental image or read or listen to the description.

BIOFEEDBACK

Biofeedback involves having the child gain an awareness of his or her body functions and learn ways to modify them voluntarily. The child usually is taught specific skills about how to modify body functions using an apparatus that measures pain-related changes in muscle tone or physiologic data, such as blood pressure or pulse rate. This teaching usually is performed by a specialized health care provider and occurs over several sessions, in advance of the pain experience. With practice, the child learns to control the changes without the apparatus. This technique can be used by older children, such as adolescents, who can concentrate for longer periods of time.

THOUGHT STOPPING

Thought stopping involves substituting a pleasurable or positive thought for the painful experience. Examples of positive thoughts might be, "It's only for a short time" or "It's important so I get better." The negative component of the pain is not ignored or suppressed; rather, it is transformed into something positive. Thought stopping also can involve the use of short, positive phrases. For example, the child may repeat "quick stick, feel better go

---

EVIDENCE-BASED PRACTICE 36.1

IS COMBINING NONNUTRITIVE SUCKING (NNS) WITH SUCROSE MORE EFFECTIVE AT REDUCING PROCEDURAL PAIN IN NEONATES THAN EITHER INTERVENTION ALONE?

Neonates who are hospitalized undergo numerous painful experiences. It is well established that neonates feel pain, with some research suggesting they have an increased sensitivity to pain. Pain in neonates has been found to have short- and long-term effects on the neonates' physical and developmental outcomes. Two common nonpharmacologic interventions used to decrease neonatal procedural pain are nonnutritive sucking (NNS) and sucrose.

STUDY

This study was an integrative review of the literature. Ten studies were included to determine if a synergistic effect exists when using NNS and sucrose before and during painful procedures to decrease procedural pain in the neonates.

Findings

The literature review found sufficient evidence to support the effectiveness of combining the use of NNS and sucrose to decrease procedural pain in the neonates.

Nursing Implications

The use of NNS and sucrose together is a safe and effective way to decrease procedural pain in neonates. Nurses should consider making it a standard of care policy in neonatal units. Further research is warranted to determine safe and effective concentration, dosing, and dosing intervals of sucrose in the neonatal population.

Adapted from Naughton K. A., & Ikuta, L. (2013). The combined use of sucrose and non-nutritive sucking for procedural pain in both term and preterm neonates: An integrative review of the literature. *Advances in Neonatal Care*, *13*(1), 9–19.

---

home soon" when he or she anticipates pain or experiences pain.

Thought stopping is a useful method for reducing anxiety before and during events associated with pain. Children can be taught to use this technique any time they experience anxiety related to a painful experience. Doing so helps to promote the child's sense of control over the situation.

POSITIVE SELF-TALK

Positive self-talk is similar to thought stopping in that it involves the use of positive statements. With positive self-talk, the child is taught to say positive statements when he or she is experiencing pain. For example, the child may be taught to say, "I will feel better and be able to go home and play with my friends."

Biophysical Interventions

Biophysical interventions focus on interfering with the transmission of pain impulses reaching the brain. The interventions involve some type of cutaneous stimulation near the site of the pain. This stimulation decreases the ability of the A-delta and C fibres to transmit pain impulses. Examples of biophysical interventions include the use of sucking and sucrose, application of heat and cold, massage and pressure, and transcutaneous electrical nerve stimulation (TENS).

SUCKING AND SUCROSE

Sucking is a behaviour from which infants derive satisfaction. Therefore, nonnutritive sucking (e.g., sucking a pacifier) can be used to reduce pain behaviours in

neonates undergoing painful procedures. In addition, infants show reduced pain behaviours after ingestion of sucrose or other sweet-tasting solutions such as glucose during single-event procedures, such as heel lancing (Anand, 2013). See Evidence-Based Practice 36.1. Optimal dosing for sucrose needs further research and caution must be used in extremely low–birth-weight infants and infants with unstable blood glucose levels.

Atraumatic Care

Breastfeeding is also a non-invasive, natural, and feasible way to use sucking to reduce pain in infants.

HEAT AND COLD APPLICATIONS

Heat and cold applications alter physiologic mechanisms associated with pain. Cold results in vasoconstriction and alters capillary permeability, leading to a decrease in edema at the site of injury. Due to vasoconstriction, blood flow is reduced and the release of pain-producing substances such as histamine and serotonin also is decreased. Moreover, transmission of painful stimuli via peripheral nerve fibres is decreased.

Heat results in vasodilation and increases blood flow to the area. It also leads to a decrease in nociceptive stimulation and removal of chemical substances that can stimulate nociceptive fibres. The increase in blood flow alters capillary permeability, leading to a reduction in swelling and pressure on nociceptive nerve fibres. Heat may also trigger the release of endogenous opioids, which mediate the pain response.

MASSAGE AND PRESSURE

Massage and pressure, like other biophysical interventions, are believed to inhibit stimulation of the A-delta and C fibres. These methods are helpful in relaxing muscles and reducing tension. In addition, these techniques can aid in distracting the child. Massage can be as simple as rubbing a body part or pressing on an area such as an injection site for about 10 seconds. It can also be more involved, requiring the use of another person to perform the massage. Lotion or ointment can be used during the massage and may provide a comforting effect. Contralateral pressure or massage of the opposite area may be used, especially if the area of pain cannot be accessed or if the affected area is too painful to touch.

A more formal method of pressure application is acupressure. In acupressure, the fingertip, the thumb, or a blunt instrument is used to apply gentle, firm pressure to specifically designated sites to control pain. The pressure may be applied in one motion followed by releasing, in a circular motion for several minutes and then releasing or with a vibrating motion using the fingertips. The motion of applying and then releasing pressure is thought to facilitate the release of endogenous endorphins and enkephalins. The techniques of pressure and massage are easy to learn and use and can be taught to children and parents.

The Nurse's Role in Nonpharmacologic Pain Intervention

The nurse plays a major role in teaching the child and family about nonpharmacologic pain interventions. Help the child and family choose the most appropriate and most effective methods and ensure that the child and parents use the method before pain occurs as well as before the pain increases. Teaching Guidelines 36.1 lists some helpful instructions for the parents and child about nonpharmacologic pain management.

Teaching Guidelines 36.1
TEACHING TO MANAGE PAIN WITHOUT DRUGS

- Review the methods available and choose the method(s) that your child and you find best for your situation.
- Learn to identify the ways in which your child shows pain or demonstrates he or she is anxious about the possibility of pain. For example, does he or she get restless, make a face, or get flushed in the face?
- Begin using the technique chosen before your child experiences pain or when your child first indicates he or she is anxious about, or beginning to experience, pain.
- Practice the technique with your child and encourage the child to use the technique when he or she

---

feels anxious about pain or anticipates that a procedure or experience will be painful.
- Perform the technique with your child. For example, take the deep breath in and out or blow bubbles with him or her; listen to the music or play the computer game with your child.
- Avoid using terms such as "hurt" or "pain" that suggest or cause your child to expect pain.
- Use descriptive terms like "pushing," "pulling," "pinching," or "heat."
- Avoid overly descriptive or judgmental statements such as, "This will really hurt a lot" or "This will be terrible."
- Stay with your child as much as possible; speak softly and gently stroke or cuddle your child.
- Offer praise, positive reinforcement, hugs, and support for using the technique even when it was not effective.

It is also important to assist the child and parents when using the technique in order to make sure that they are using the technique correctly. Offer suggestions for modifications or adaptations as necessary.

Parents are important components of the pain management program. Give them the option to stay with the child, or let them know that someone else will support the child if they opt not to stay. Offer simple, concrete ways to assist and help the child to manage pain. Many of the nonpharmacologic techniques can be done by parents, and children may respond better if their parents demonstrate the technique and encourage them to use it. Invite parents to participate in decisions as well as act as a coach to their child during procedures. Prepare the parents and explain the most appropriate pain management approaches and strategies. Discuss the type and amount of pain expected as well as the potential complications associated with pain management approaches. Ask how the parent predicts the child will react to a painful situation. Finally, offer techniques and strategies to the parents as they act as the coach during these situations.

Take Note!

Although parents want to help their children and some are able to act as coaches, the response of the child to pain and stress and to their parents' distraction interventions is highly variable. Some children appear to be soothed by their parents' distraction actions; others appear to become distressed. Be alert to factors that may influence the child's response, including age, sex, diagnosis, ethnicity, previous experience, temperament, anxiety, and coping style. Also be aware of parental factors, including ethnicity, sex, previous experience, belief in the helpfulness of the intervention, parenting style, and parental anxiety (McCarthy & Kleiber, 2006; McCarthy et al., 2010).

Pharmacologic Management

Pharmacologic interventions involve the administration of drugs for pain relief. Administration may occur using a wide variety of methods. The selection of the method is determined by the drug being administered; the child's status; the type, intensity, and location of the pain; and any factors that may be influencing the child's pain. Research overwhelmingly supports the appropriate use of analgesics to reduce pain perception in children.

Medications Used for Pain Management

Analgesics (medications for pain relief) typically fall into one of two categories—nonopioid analgesics and opioid analgesics. Anaesthetics also may be used. Drugs such as sedatives and hypnotics may be used as adjuvant medications to help minimize anxiety or provide or assist with pain relief when typical analgesics are ineffective.

NONOPIOID ANALGESICS

Nonopioid analgesics include acetaminophen and nonsteroidal anti-inflammatory drugs (NSAIDs) such as ibuprofen, ketorolac, naproxen, indomethacin, diclofenac, and piroxicam (Drug Guide 36.1). These agents may be used to treat mild-to-moderate pain, often for conditions such as arthritis; joint, bone, and muscle pain; headache; dental pain; and menstrual pain. Acetaminophen, probably the most widely known nonopioid analgesic, and ibuprofen are also commonly used to treat fever in children.

> **Take Note!**
>
> Aspirin should not be used in infants or children for analgesic or antipyretic purposes because of the high risk of Reye syndrome.

According to the World Health Organization's (WHO's) recommended two-step strategy, acetaminophen and NSAIDs are first-line agents for the treatment of pain (WHO, 2012). Nonopioid agents are typically administered orally or rectally. In some cases, such as with postoperative pain, they may be administered intravenously as a continuous infusion or as bolus doses. Administration via intramuscular injection is not recommended because the injection can cause significant pain and the onset of pain relief is not increased.

Acetaminophen is a relatively safe medication and it does not have the same GI or antiplatelet effects of NSAIDs; therefore, it is useful in children with cancer, with bleeding or clotting disorders, or children on anticoagulants. Acetaminophen toxicity and resulting hepatotoxicity can occur with misuse and overdosing. Adverse effects associated with NSAIDs are uncommon but include gastrointestinal irritation, blood clotting problems, and renal dysfunction (occasionally acute renal

failure). Nonopioids are relatively safe, have few incompatibilities with other medications, and do not depress the central nervous system. Unfortunately, they exhibit a ceiling effect for analgesia. That is, after a certain level, they do not provide increasing pain relief even when administered at increased doses. As a result, they may be combined with opioids for more effective pain relief.

OPIOID ANALGESICS

Opioid analgesics are typically used for moderate-to-severe pain. They are classified as either agonists (when they act as the neurotransmitter at the receptor site) or antagonists (when they block the action at the receptor site). Opioid agents that act as agonists include morphine, fentanyl, meperidine, hydromorphone, oxycodone, and hydrocodone. Opioids that act as mixed agonists–antagonists include pentazocine, butorphanol, and nalbuphine (see Drug Guide 36.1). Opioids can be administered orally, rectally, intramuscularly, or intravenously. In addition, some agents such as fentanyl can be administered transdermally or transmucosally. Morphine is considered the "gold standard" for all opioid agonists; it is the drug to which all other opioids are compared and is the drug of choice for severe pain (Oakes & D'Arcy, 2011; WHO, 2012). Tramadol is an opioid that has been considered for use in treating moderate pain and is associated with a lower risk of respiratory depression and constipation (Oakes & D'Arcy, 2011). Currently, the WHO states there is insufficient data to support its effectiveness and safety in children, and therefore more research is needed (WHO, 2012).

> **Take Note!**
>
> International and national guidelines recommend against the use of codeine in children due to serious safety concerns related to the genetic variability in its metabolism in children (some children are poor metabolizers while others are ultrametabolizers) (Kaiser et al., 2014; WHO, 2012).

Opioid agonists, such as morphine, are associated with numerous adverse effects, resulting primarily from their depressant action on the central nervous system.

> **Take Note!**
>
> When administering parenteral or epidural opioids, always have naloxone (Narcan) readily available to reverse the opioid's effects should respiratory depression occur.

Opioids stimulate the chemoreceptor trigger zone (CTZ), leading to nausea and vomiting. Moreover, **drug tolerance** (increased dosage required for the same pain relief previously achieved with a lower dose) and **physical dependence** (need for continued administration of the drug to prevent withdrawal symptoms) are

DRUG GUIDE 36.1 COMMON DRUGS FOR PAIN MANAGEMENT

Drug	Actions/Indications	Nursing Implications
Acetaminophen (Tylenol)	Possible inhibition of cyclooxygenase in the central nervous system Direct action on hypothalamic heat-regulating centre Mild-to-moderate pain, fever; arthritis, musculoskeletal pain, headache	• Administer orally, rectally, or intravenous. Do not exceed five doses or 60 mg/kg/day intravenous of drug in 24 hours • Caution parents to read labels of other over-the-counter (OTC) drugs carefully; some may contain acetaminophen and if given in conjunction may lead to overdose and toxicity
Ibuprofen (Motrin, Advil)	Inhibition of prostaglandin synthesis Mild-to-moderate pain, fever, treatment of inflammatory diseases	• Administer orally • Give with food or after meals if GI upset occurs • Assess for easy bruising, bleeding gums, or frank or occult blood in urine or stool • Monitor for nausea, vomiting, GI upset, diarrhea or constipation, dizziness, or drowsiness • Caution parents to read labels of OTC medications closely; some may contain ibuprofen or other NSAIDs and if given in conjunction may lead to overdose
Other NSAIDs: ketorolac (Toradol), diclofenac (Voltaren), indomethacin (Indocin), naproxen (Naprosyn, Aleve)	Inhibition of prostaglandin synthesis Moderate-to-severe pain	• Administer oral form with food or after meals if GI upset occurs • Monitor for headache, dizziness, nausea, vomiting, constipation, or diarrhea • Assess for signs and symptoms of bleeding, such as bruising, epistaxis, gingival bleeding, or frank or occult blood in urine or stool • Ketorolac: may also be given IV or IM. In children ages 2–16 years, recommended as single dose only • Naproxen: also available in combination products (caution parents to read OTC labels carefully) • Indomethacin: when administering IV, report oliguria or anuria • Diclofenac: may also be given rectally
Opioid agents: morphine, fentanyl (Sublimaze, Duragesic), hydromorphone (Dilaudid), oxycodone (OxyContin), methadone	Opioid agonist acting primarily at μ-receptor sites (morphine, fentanyl, hydromorphone, oxycodone, methadone) Moderate-to-severe acute and chronic pain Morphine: intractable pain, preoperative sedation Fentanyl: pain associated with short procedures such as bone marrow aspiration, fracture reductions, suturing	• Assess respiratory status frequently, noting any decrease in ventilatory rate or changes in breathing patterns; have naloxone readily available in case of respiratory depression (particularly morphine, fentanyl, hydromorphone) • Monitor for sedation dizziness, lethargy, or confusion • Educate parents and child that the drug may make the child sleepy, drowsy, or lightheaded • Institute safety measures to prevent injury to the child • Assess bowel sounds for decreased peristalsis; observe for abdominal distention • Ensure adequate fibre intake and administer stool softeners as prescribed to minimize risk for constipation • Monitor urine output for changes and report • Morphine: may cause itching, particularly facial • Fentanyl: observe for chest wall rigidity, which can occur with rapid IV infusion • Oxycodone is the opioid component of brand names products such as Tylox, Roxicet, and Percocet

DRUG GUIDE 36.1 COMMON DRUGS FOR PAIN MANAGEMENT (continued)

Drug	Actions/Indications	Nursing Implications
Mixed opioid agonist–antagonist: pentazocine (Talwin), butorphanol (Stadol), nalbuphine (Nubain)	Pentazocine: antagonist at μ-receptor sites, agonist at κ-receptor sites. Butorphanol: high affinity for κ-receptor sites, minimal affinity for κ-receptor sites. Nalbuphine: partial agonist at κ-receptor sites, antagonist at μ-receptor sites Moderate-to-severe pain Relief of migraine headache (butorphanol) Preoperative analgesia (nalbuphine)	• Monitor the child for sedation. Educate child and parents that the drug may make the child sleepy, drowsy, or lightheaded • Institute safety measures to prevent injury to the child • Pentazocine, butorphanol: monitor for diaphoresis, dizziness. Assess for tachycardia and hypertension • Butorphanol is given intranasally for migraine headaches

GI, gastrointestinal.

Adapted from Taketomo, C. K., Hodding, J. H., & Kraus, D. M. (2013). *Lexi-comp's drug reference handbook: Pediatric & neonatal dosage handbook* (20th ed.). Hudson, OH: Lexi-comp, Inc.

commonly noted when opioids are given repeatedly. Drug Guide 36.1 gives additional information related to the opioid analgesics.

Take Note!

Drug tolerance occurs when increasing doses are required to manage the pain. Physical dependence can occur after as few as 5 days of continuous use of the drug; symptoms of withdrawal begin if it is suddenly stopped (Oakes & D'Arcy, 2011).

Mixed agonist–antagonists are associated with less respiratory depression than agonists. Unfortunately, like NSAIDs, this group also has a ceiling effect, leading to inadequate pain relief even with increased dosages, and therefore limiting their use in treating severe pain (Oakes & D'Arcy, 2011).

Take Note!

Meperidine (Demerol), an opioid agonist, is not recommended as a first-choice agent for pain relief in children due to its toxicity on the central nervous system (WHO, 2012).

ADJUVANT DRUGS

Adjuvant drugs are drugs that are used to promote more effective pain relief, either alone or in combination with nonopioids or opioids. Their primary indication is for diagnoses other than pain. These agents are not classified as analgesics but may provide a coanalgesic effect or may treat side effects. Benzodiazepines, such as diazepam and midazolam, help to relieve anxiety. Midazolam also produces amnesia. Anticonvulsants, such as gabapentin, and tricyclic antidepressants, such as amitriptyline and nortriptyline, are used to treat neuropathic pain.

More recently, N-methyl-D-aspartate receptor antagonist, i.e., ketamine use is being explored for use within hospital settings as an adjunct to opioid management for children with acute and chronic pain (Sheehy et al., 2017).

LOCAL ANAESTHETICS

Local anaesthetics are commonly used to provide analgesia for procedures. They are effective in providing successful pain relief with only minimal risk of systemic adverse effects. However, local anaesthetics such as lidocaine historically were not used in children because these drugs need to be injected. The belief was that children feared needles and use of a local anaesthetic subjected the child to two needlesticks instead of one. Advances in technology have led to the development of improved methods of delivery such as topical ointments and iontophoresis for administration of local anaesthetics, thereby promoting atraumatic care. (For a more detailed discussion, see the next section on drug administration methods and later in the chapter on the nurse's role in managing procedure-related pain.)

Drug Administration Methods

With any medication administered for pain management, the timing of administration is vital. Timing depends on the type of pain. For continuous pain, the current recommendation is to administer analgesia around the clock at scheduled intervals to achieve the necessary effect (Oakes & D'Arcy, 2011; WHO, 2012). Scheduled dosing has been associated with decreased pain intensity ratings for children (Sutters et al., 2010). As-needed (PRN) dosing is not recommended for continuous pain. This method can lead to inadequate pain relief because of the delay before the drug reaches its peak effectiveness, and as a result, the child continues to experience pain, possibly necessitating a higher dose of analgesic to achieve relief. This then places the child at risk for over-medication and toxic effects.

For pain that can be predicted or considered tempo-rary, such as with a procedure, analgesia is administered so that the peak action of the drug matches the time of the painful event.

There are various methods for administering pain medications to children. The preferred methods are the oral, rectal, intravenous, topical, or local nerve block routes. Epidural administration and moderate sedation also can be used.

ORAL METHOD
The oral method is often preferred because it is sim-ple, easy, and convenient. The medication may be in the form of a pill, capsule, tablet, syrup, or elixir. Oral administration provides relatively steady blood levels of the drug when administered as a scheduled dose. Effec-tiveness typically occurs 1 to 2 hours after administration. As soon as possible, switch the child to oral dosing from parenteral dosing. However, keep in mind that higher doses of the oral medication may be needed to achieve the same effect.

RECTAL METHOD
The rectal method may be used when the child can-not take the medication orally, such as when he or she has difficulty swallowing or is experiencing nausea and vomiting. It is a viable alternative for drug administra-tion. Some analgesics are available in suppository form. For others that are not, the drug can be compounded into a suppository form. The absorption rate varies with rectal administration, and children may find insertion of a suppository uncomfortable and embarrassing (Bowden & Greenberg, 2011).

INTRAVENOUS METHOD
Intravenous analgesia administration is the method of choice in emergency situations and when pain is severe and quick relief is needed. With intravenous administra-tion, the drug usually takes effect within 5 minutes. Intra-venous administration can be accomplished with bolus injections or continuous infusions. Continuous infusions may be preferred over bolus doses because steady blood levels are more easily maintained, thereby enhancing the drug's effect in relieving pain. Typically, opioids such as morphine, hydromorphone, and fentanyl are used due to their short half-life and decreased risk for toxicity.

PATIENT-CONTROLLED ANALGESIA
In **patient-controlled analgesia (PCA)**, a computer-ized pump is programmed to deliver an infusion of anal-gesics via a catheter inserted intravenously, epidurally, or subcutaneously. The analgesic may be given as a continu-ous infusion, as a continuous infusion supplemented by

patient-delivered bolus doses, or as patient-delivered bolus doses only. Typically, the child presses a button to admin-ister a bolus dose. The pump has a lockout function that is preset with the dose and time interval. If the child presses the button before the preset time, he or she will not receive an overdose of medication. By delivering small, frequent doses of opioids, the child can experience pain relief with-out the effects of oversedation. The child also experiences a sense of control over the pain experience.

Both the Institute for Safe Medical Practices (ISMP) and The Joint Commission have identified infants and young children as not being good candidates for PCA usage (D'Arcy, 2011; Mann, 2014). However, PCA has been used successfully in children as young as 5 or 6 years old (Oakes & D'Arcy, 2011). It is essential to assess each child individually and consider his or her developmental level and psychosocial factors in determining appropriate PCA use. The child must have the necessary intellect, manual dexterity, and strength to operate the device.

PCA has been used to control postoperative pain and the pain associated with trauma, cancer, and sickle cell crisis. It can be used in acute care settings or in the home. Most commonly, morphine, hydromorphone, and fentanyl are the drugs used with PCA. The dosage is based on the child's response. Dosages for infusions depend on the child's age, the opioid used, and the type of pain. A commonly used range for morphine infusion to treat postoperative pain ranges from 0.01 to 0.04 mg/kg/hr. Higher dosage ranges have been used to treat the pain associated with sickle cell crisis and cancer.

Serious adverse events, such as oversedation, respira-tory depression, and even death, can occur when family members, caregivers, or clinicians who are not authorized administer PCA doses "by proxy" (Cooney et al., 2013; The Joint Commission, 2004). The ISMP recommends devel-oping specific criteria in any situation where authorized agent–activated PCA is being used (Cooney et al., 2013; D'Arcy, 2011). Proper education and instruction are crucial in any situation where someone other than the child may be administering PCA doses. Thorough assessment is nec-essary to ensure the child's pain is neither undertreated nor overtreated. To ensure safety with PCA use, each institution must have policies and procedures in place, appropriate education of health care staff, quality control measures, and quality machines.

LOCAL ANAESTHETIC APPLICATION
A local anaesthetic may sometimes be used to allevi-ate the pain associated with procedures such as veni-puncture, injections, wound repair, lumbar puncture, or accessing of implanted ports. Local anaesthesia is a type of regional analgesia that blocks or numbs spe-cific nerves in a region of the body. Medications called local anaesthetics include topical forms, such as creams, agents delivered by iontophoresis, vapocoolants, and skin refrigerants, and injectable forms.

Topical Forms. A common choice for effective, painless local anaesthesia is EMLA (eutectic mixture of local anaesthetics [lidocaine and prilocaine]). It achieves anaesthesia to a depth of 2 to 4 mm, so it reduces pain of phlebotomy, venous cannulation, and intramuscular injections for up to 24 hours after the injection. However, it requires a 60- to 90-minute application time to intact skin using an occlusive dressing for superficial procedures and up to 2 to 3 hours for deeper, more invasive procedures (Box 36.1). EMLA is approved for use in infants 37 weeks' gestation or older (Walden, 2014). Maximum dosage and maximum area of application are based on the child's weight. Parents can be taught how to apply the EMLA at home in preparation for a procedure (Fig. 36.9). Sometimes EMLA is not used due to the expense and the time needed to allow the drug to act. New approaches to EMLA delivery have been developed. Examples include other drug formulations and a patch delivery with a heat-activated system (Synera) that enhances the delivery of lidocaine and prilocaine. Synera

FIGURE 36.9 A parent applies EMLA cream to the child at home in preparation for a procedure.

is labelled for children older than 3 years of age and needs to be applied only 20 to 30 minutes before the procedure (Taketomo, Hodding, & Kraus, 2013).

Take Note!

EMLA is used with caution in children younger than 3 months and other susceptible persons because it may be associated with methemoglobinemia caused by prilocaine toxicity (Oakes & D'Arcy, 2011; Taketomo et al., 2013). It is contraindicated in children who have congenital or idiopathic methemoglobinemia (Taketomo et al., 2013). It must be used cautiously in those younger than age 12 months who are receiving methemoglobin-inducing agents, such as sulfonamides, phenytoin, phenobarbital, and acetaminophen (Taketomo et al., 2013). Use of these agents in combination with EMLA increases the child's risk for methemoglobinemia, a condition that could lead to cyanosis and hypoxemia.

Ametop (topical amethocaine) is a commonly used topical anaesthetic for venous cannulation. It has been shown to have a faster rate of onset than EMLA and has a similar action (Brown, Awad, Plant, McAdoo, & Shorten, 1999). It should be used cautiously in infants under 6 months. It may cause vasoconstriction, and therefore it is not always the best choice in situations where cannulation might be difficult.

Other examples of topical anaesthetics are TAC (tetracaine, epinephrine, cocaine) and LET (lidocaine, epinephrine, tetracaine). These are commonly used for lacerations that require suturing. The agent is applied directly to the wound with a cotton ball or swab for 20 to 30 minutes until the area is numb. These methods are not used in children with known sensitivity to any of these medications.

BOX 36.1

APPLYING EMLA

Follow these guidelines when applying EMLA:
- Explain the purpose of the medication to the child and parents, reinforcing that it will help the pain go away.
- Check the scheduled time for the procedure; plan to apply the cream 60 minutes before a superficial procedure such as an intramuscular injection or a venipuncture or 2 to 3 hours before a deeper procedure such as a lumbar puncture or bone marrow aspiration.
- Place a thick layer of the cream on the skin at the intended site of the procedure, making sure that the area where the cream is being applied is free of any breaks. Do not rub the cream in once it is applied to the skin.
- Cover the site with a transparent dressing such as Tegaderm or Op-site and secure it so that the dressing is occlusive. Alternatively, use plastic film wrap and tape the edges to secure the dressing.
- Instruct the child not to touch the dressing once it is secured. If necessary, cover the occlusive dressing with a protection device or a loosely applied gauze or elastic bandage.
- After the allotted time, remove the occlusive dressing and wipe the cream from the skin. Inspect the skin for a change in colour (blanching or redness), which indicates that the medication has penetrated the skin adequately.
- Verify that sensation is absent by lightly tapping or scratching the area. Use this technique also to demonstrate to the child that the anaesthetic is effective. If sensation is present, reapply the cream.
- Prepare the child for the procedure. Assess the child's pain after the procedure to evaluate for pain and to differentiate pain from fear and anxiety.

Lidocaine can also be dispersed in liposomes to allow for transcutaneous delivery (liposomal lidocaine). Over-the-counter LMX4 (lidocaine 4%), formerly called ELA-Max, is massaged into the skin without the use of an occlusive dressing. Anaesthesia to the area is reached in 15 to 30 minutes and lasts about 60 minutes. Recent studies suggest that the analgesic effect may be equal to that of EMLA with the advantage of a shorter onset (American Medical Association, 2013). Research has shown that liposomal lidocaine 4% cream was highly effective in reducing the pain associated with intravenous cannulation (Hsu, 2014; Zempsky, 2008). The researchers cited a short onset of action (30 minutes) and minimal vascular effects as benefits. They found that the liposomal encapsulation protects the anaesthetic from being metabolized too quickly (Zempsky, 2008). Study results have shown higher intravenous cannulation success rates, less pain, shorter total procedure time, and minor dermal changes among children (Hsu, 2014; Taddio, Soin, Schuh, Koren, & Scolnik, 2005).

Needle-free powder lidocaine (Zingo or J-tip) is another topical analgesic. It is labelled for use in children 3 to 18 years of age. It is a single-use, prefilled disposable system that provides analgesia in 1 to 3 minutes. Studies have shown it to be safe and well tolerated with a rapid onset and significant reduction in needlestick pain although the degree of relief varied (Hsu, 2014).

Another choice for local anaesthesia is iontophoresis. Iontophoretic lidocaine (Numby Stuff) provides a deeper analgesia in a shorter duration (approximately 10 to 25 minutes) and is used over intact skin. A mild electrical current from a small battery-powered generator and two iontophoretic drug-delivery electrodes push drug molecules (lidocaine HCl 2% with epinephrine 1:100,000) into the skin. A mild tingling sensation may be felt during drug delivery, with an increase in tingling noted with higher currents. This type of local anaesthesia is not recommended for use in children who have a history of allergy or sensitivity to these drugs, in children who have electrically sensitive equipment such as a pacemaker, or in children who have damaged skin or scar tissue.

Vapocoolant spray, another type of local analgesia, can be sprayed onto the skin or administered using a cotton ball soaked in liquid. The depth of anaesthesia is not known, but it appears to provide immediate pain control. It is inexpensive and requires no waiting time. The effect lasts for approximately 1 to 2 minutes. Studies have found it to be an effective analgesic for short-duration procedures (American Medical Association, 2013).

Injectable Forms. Injectable forms of lidocaine or procaine can be administered subcutaneously or intradermally around the procedural area approximately 5 to 10 minutes before the procedure. Common problems with this form of anaesthetic include the pain associated with the subcutaneous injection and some burning associated with lidocaine administration, as well as blanching of the skin.

Take Note!

The burning that lidocaine causes on injection may be diminished by buffering lidocaine with sodium bicarbonate, using 10 parts lidocaine and 1 part sodium bicarbonate (1 mL of 1% to 2% lidocaine and 0.1 mL of 8.4% sodium bicarbonate). Then, inject 0.1 mL or less of the solution intradermally at the site of venipuncture. Anaesthetic action is almost immediate. The solution is stable for only approximately 1 week if not refrigerated.

EPIDURAL ANALGESIA

For **epidural analgesia**, a catheter is inserted in the epidural space usually between the lumbar (L3) and the thoracic (T3) area. The drug, usually fentanyl or morphine, diffuses into the cerebrospinal fluid and crosses the dura mater to the spinal cord. Then, it binds with the opioid receptors located at the dorsal horn. The drugs can be administered as bolus injections (a one-time bolus or on an intermittent schedule), a continuous infusion, or PCA. Usually an opioid, such as morphine, fentanyl, or hydromorphone, is given in conjunction with a long-acting local anaesthetic such as bupivacaine.

Epidural analgesia is typically used postoperatively, providing analgesia to the lower body for approximately 12 to 14 hours. The small amount of medication used with this type of analgesia causes less sedation, thereby allowing the child to participate more actively in postoperative care activities. This type of analgesia also is effective for children undergoing upper or lower abdominal surgeries because it controls localized intense pain, somatic pain, and visceral pain.

When epidural analgesia is being administered, additional narcotic analgesics are not given in order to prevent complications such as respiratory depression, pruritus, nausea, vomiting, and urinary retention.

Take Note!

Respiratory depression, although rare when epidural analgesia is used, is always a possibility. When it does occur, it usually occurs gradually over a period of several hours after the medication is initiated. This allows adequate time for early detection and prompt intervention.

Constant assessment is essential because insertion of an epidural catheter and epidural analgesia can lead to infection at the site of the insertion, epidural hematoma, arachnoiditis, neuritis, spinal headache (rare) due to a cerebrospinal fluid leak, and respiratory depression. Frequent assessment, typically every 1 to 2 hours, of heart rate, respiratory rate, and depth of sedation, and every 2 to 4 hours of blood pressure, pain level, and motor function is imperative (Oakes & D'Arcy, 2011). Assessing for adverse reactions such as nausea and vomiting and pruritus, checking the tubing and catheter site, and ensuring the occlusive dressing is intact are all important nursing interventions. The dermatome, which is the

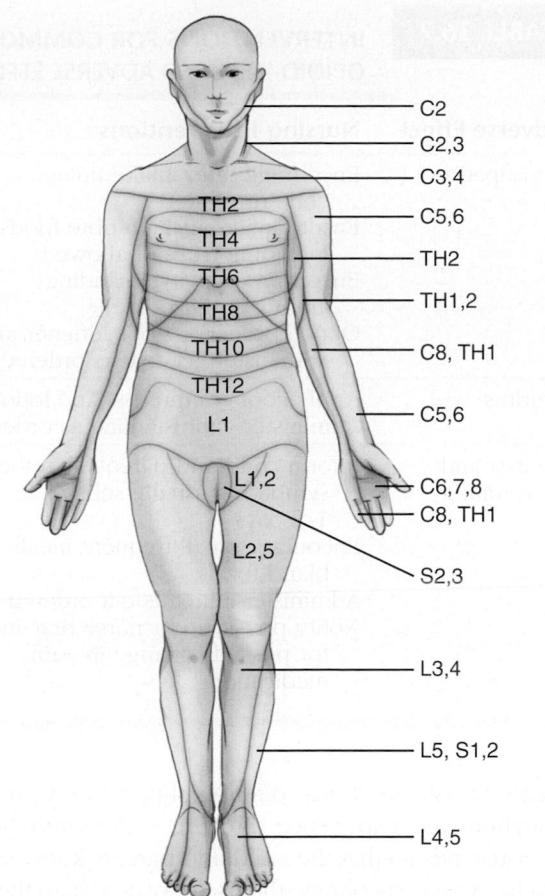

FIGURE 36.10 **The level of anaesthesia should not go higher than T4, the nipple line, in children.**

area of the body associated with supply by a particular nerve, that innervates the diaphragm can become suppressed during continuous epidural analgesia, resulting in respiratory depression. It is important to assess the child's sensory level frequently. Using cool water or an alcohol pad, bilaterally touch the child's body every 2 to 3 cm. The level where the child states he or she feels the temperature change is the level of anaesthesia. (Refer to Fig. 36.10 for dermatome levels.)

MODERATE (CONSCIOUS) SEDATION

Moderate sedation is used to be labelled conscious sedation, but the term "conscious" has been replaced since it can be misleading (Coté, Wilson, & The Work Group on Sedation, 2011). It is a medically controlled state of depressed consciousness that allows protective reflexes to be maintained so the child has the ability to maintain a patent airway and respond to physical or verbal stimulation. Sedation in children is different than in adults as it is often administered to help control behaviour in order to complete procedures or diagnostics studies (Coté et al., 2011). Moderate sedation requires adherence to specific protocols, and many regulatory bodies, such as the Joint Commission, and societies,

including the American Academy of Pediatrics, American Academy of Pediatric Dentistry, American Society of Anaesthesiologists, and American College of Emergency Physicians, have published standards and guidelines to improve patient safety and outcomes. The depressed state is obtained by using various agents such as morphine, fentanyl, midazolam, ketamine, chloral hydrate, diazepam, pentobarbital, nitrous oxide, or propofol. The medication used will depend on the expected degree of pain and discomfort, amount of motion restriction needed, and individual factors such as age, ability to cooperate, and medical history.

Moderate sedation is used for procedures that are painful and stressful. For example, moderate sedation is suggested instead of restraints, especially for toddlers and preschool children who are undergoing frightening or invasive procedures and who are manifesting extreme anxiety and behavioural upset. Other indications include situations involving:

- Evidence that the child is experiencing a heightened stress reaction (e.g., attempting to flee, crying inconsolably, or flailing)
- Verbalization by the child that he or she is frightened and does not want to be touched
- Inability to remain immobilized, such as during laceration repair or computed tomography
- Any procedure that is painful and fear-provoking

The route of administering the medications for sedation should follow the guidelines of atraumatic care. Oral, topical, or an existing intravenous route should be used. Studies have shown that pediatric clients often pass from the intended level of sedation to a deeper unintended level of sedation; therefore, personnel administering moderate sedation must be specially trained, with strong resuscitation and advanced pediatric life support skills, and emergency equipment and medications must be readily available (Coté et al., 2011).

The Nurse's Role in Pharmacologic Pain Management

The nurse plays a major role in providing pharmacologic pain relief. As with any medication, the nurse is responsible for adhering to the rights of medication administration—right drug, right dose, right route, right time, and right patient. In addition, the nurse also adheres to additional rights, such as the right of the child and parents to be educated, the right of the child to refuse the medication, the right documentation, the right form, and the right approach. The nurse also must have a solid knowledge base about the medications used for pain relief. This knowledge includes information about the drug's pharmacokinetics (absorption, distribution, metabolism, and excretion) and pharmacodynamics (mechanism of action, including adverse effects). Many factors can lead to children experiencing suboptimal pain management as noted in some Canadian EDs when children present with appendicitis (Robb, Ali, Poonai, & Thompson, 2016). The use of pain assessment tools; behavioural cues; communication between the nurse, parent, and patient; as well as clear and timely documentation and escalation of poor pain control are vital (Panjganj & Bevan, 2016).

Assessment is crucial when pharmacologic pain interventions are used. An initial assessment of pain provides a baseline from which options for relief can be chosen. Factors that can affect the choice of analgesic, such as the child's age, pain intensity, physiologic status, or previous experiences with pain, also need to be considered. The nurse acts as an advocate for the child and the family to ensure that the most appropriate pharmacologic agent is chosen for the situation.

Assessment is ongoing once the agent is administered. Monitor physiologic parameters such as level of consciousness, vital signs, oxygen saturation levels, and urinary output for changes that might indicate an adverse reaction to the agent. More intensive monitoring is needed when agents are administered intravenously or epidurally or by moderate sedation. For example, if the child is receiving moderate sedation, interventions include:

- Ensuring that emergency equipment is readily available
- Maintaining a patent airway
- Monitoring the child's level of consciousness and responsiveness
- Assessing the child's vital signs (especially heart rate, blood pressure, and respiratory rate)
- Monitoring oxygen saturation levels

Typically, a specially trained health care provider is specifically designated to perform these activities during the administration of the sedation. Afterward, the nurse is responsible for ongoing monitoring of the child's status.

Monitor the child closely for evidence of adverse effects. Table 36.7 describes the interventions useful for responding to these adverse effects. Be alert for signs and symptoms of respiratory depression secondary to opioid administration. Have an opioid antagonist such as naloxone (Narcan) and the benzodiazepine antagonist flumazenil (Romazicon) readily available should the child experience respiratory depression.

In addition to assessing physiologic parameters, assess the child's and parents' emotional status before and after the agent is administered. For example, increased anxiety and fear may necessitate a change in method of administration, such as topical application instead of an intradermal injection of a local anaesthetic. Use nonpharmacologic methods to help lessen anxiety, thereby promoting more effective relief from the drug.

Nurses also are responsible for ensuring that the child and parents are adequately prepared for the use of the pharmacologic agent. Teach the child and parents about the drug, why it is being used, its intended effects, and possible adverse effects, tailoring the teaching to the child's cognitive level. Provide opportunities for the child and

TABLE 36.7	INTERVENTIONS FOR COMMON OPIOID-INDUCED ADVERSE EFFECTS
Adverse Effect	**Nursing Interventions**
Constipation	Encourage fluid intake unless contraindicated Ensure intake of high-fibre foods, including fruits, if allowed Encourage activity, including ambulation if possible Obtain order for stool softener and administer laxative as ordered
Pruritus	Apply cool compresses and lotions Administer antihistamine as ordered
Nausea and vomiting	Inform child and parents that these symptoms usually subside in 1–2 days Encourage small frequent meals with bland foods Administer antiemetic if ordered Notify physician or nurse practitioner for possible change in pain medication

parents to ask questions, offering support and guidance throughout the experience. Provide a demonstration or use visual aids so that the child and parents know exactly what to expect. Encourage the use of play to help the child express fears and anxieties related to the administration.

Management of Procedure-Related Pain

One of the most common causes of pain in children is procedure-related pain. The procedure may be minor, such as an intramuscular injection, heel stick, or venipuncture, or it may be more involved, such as lumbar puncture, bone marrow aspiration, or wound care. Regardless, pain is real for children and painful procedures are often extremely distressing to them. Variables that affect pain include the intensity or length of the procedure and the skill of the health care provider performing the procedure.

The Nurse's Role in Managing Procedure-Related Pain

Through the use of behavioural and pharmacologic approaches, nurses can significantly reduce the pain and distress of procedures. Use the guiding principles of atraumatic care, which include the following:

- Use topical anesthetic, iontophoretic lidocaine, vapo-coolant spray, or buffered lidocaine at the intended site of a skin or vessel puncture. Inhalation approaches (i.e., nitrous oxide) may be used in some settings in line with local policies.
- Incorporate the use of nonpharmacologic strategies for pain relief in conjunction with pharmacologic methods.

- Prepare the child and parents ahead of time about the procedure and then keep all equipment out of sight until it is ready to be used.
- Use therapeutic hugging to secure the child.
- Use the smallest gauge needle possible or an automated lancet device to puncture the skin.
- Use an intermittent infusion device or peripherally inserted central catheter (PICC) if multiple or repeated blood samples are necessary. Coordinate care so that several tests can be performed from one sample if possible.
- Opt for venipuncture in newborns instead of heel sticks if the amount of blood needed would require much squeezing.
- Use kangaroo care (skin-to-skin contact) for newborns before and after heel stick.
- Provide nonnutritive sucking, with sucrose solution, if appropriate; pacifier; or breastfeeding for newborns several minutes before the procedure.

Take Note!

Individualize interventions based on the painfulness of the procedure and the child's developmental age and personality. Use behavioural-cognitive approaches and pharmacologic interventions. For example, encouraging the school-age child to assist during painful procedures in age-appropriate ways may actually help ease some of the pain related to a heightened state of anxiety, or at least assist the child in coping with the situation. Always use appropriate pharmacologic treatment especially for the first procedure to provide as painless an experience as possible for the child.

Nursing care for the child with procedure-related pain includes the child as well as the parents. Be sure to prepare them for the procedure using an appropriate developmental approach. Promote environmental comfort, too. Ensure that the child's privacy is maintained and that the lighting is adequate for the procedure but not so bright as to cause the child discomfort.

Painful procedures performed in the child's room can lead to an association of pain or fear with the room or bed. Many hospitals have a special treatment room where procedures can be performed. These rooms are usually equipped with many activities, toys, and decorations to help distract the child. The use of a treatment room may not be feasible or desirable in all situations or for all procedures. The ultimate goal is to do what is best for the child; therefore, the nurse needs to consider the needs of the child, the demands of the procedures, and the conditions that would facilitate the best outcome.

Unless contraindicated, encourage the parents to be present before, during, and after the procedure to provide comforting support to the child. Also, encourage the child and parents to use nonpharmacologic methods to help maximize pain relief and reduce anxiety. For example, nonpharmacologic methods that are helpful

for the toddler and preschooler may include positioning the child on the lap and hugging the child, distracting the child with toys or interactive books, and blowing bubbles.

Play therapy can be useful when preparing children for painful procedures, where possible engage a child life specialist (CLS) in the child's care. Encourage children to make decisions about their care related to pain management if their condition or procedure allows. It is also helpful to anticipate and recognize painful situations and provide pain medication before the actual procedure to ensure comfort. Many nonpharmacologic strategies can be enhanced and better implemented with the help of the CLS or play therapist, who have specialized training in these techniques.

Recall Aiden from the beginning of the chapter. What are some interventions that may be helpful prior to, during, and after his dressing change?

Management of Chronic Pain

Typically, pain in children is acute, but chronic pain is a significant problem in the pediatric population. Chronic pain is ongoing and recurrent pain that persists beyond the expected healing time, which has been typically defined as 3 to 6 months (Canadian Pain Society, n.d.). Chronic pain is the result of a complex interplay of biologic, psychological, and socio-cultural factors (Canadian Pain Society, n.d.). Children with chronic pain and their families experience significant emotional and social consequences from the pain and disability; also, the experience of chronic pain in childhood may predispose the individual to chronic pain in adulthood.

The Nurse's Role in Managing Chronic Pain

The nurse's role in managing chronic pain in children is similar to that for the child experiencing acute pain or procedure-related pain. Assessment of the child's pain is key and should include a history of the present problem. Questions should focus on the onset of the pain; its intensity, duration, and location; and any factors that alleviate or exacerbate it. In addition, it is important to question the child and parents about the impact of the pain on the child's daily life, such as sleep, play, eating, school, and interactions with peers, other family members, and friends. Also, address the impact of the child's chronic pain on the family's life.

Another key area of assessment is determining how the pain affects the child's and family's level of stress. Areas to address include the child's and parents' feelings of hopelessness, anxiety, and depression. Also, question the child and parents about what they think has caused the pain and how they have coped with it. In addition, ascertain what methods the child and parents have used to alleviate the pain and the success of these methods. Inquire about any home remedies or alternative therapies that may have been used.

Review past physical examination findings for clues to the underlying problem. Observe the child's overall appearance, gait, and posture. Assess the child's cognitive level and emotional response, especially related to the experience of pain. Expect to complete a neurologic examination and observe for muscle spasms, trigger points, and increased sensitivity to light touch. Abnormal body postures assumed by the child due to chronic pain

may result in the development of secondary pain in the muscles and fascia. When children tense their muscles due to fear of examination, somatic pain may occur.

Various nonpharmacologic and pharmacologic strategies are used to manage chronic pain. Often multiple strategies are combined to address pain relief as well as the pain's impact on other areas, such as sleep or school functioning. When pharmacologic agents are used, the oral form is the method of choice. As with any pain management strategy, education of the child and family is paramount. A referral to a pediatric pain specialist may be needed if the child's pain is not controlled effectively.

NURSING CARE PLAN 36.1

Overview for the Child in Pain

NURSING DIAGNOSIS: Acute pain related to need for invasive procedures, surgery, recent trauma, or infection as evidenced by pain rating scale, facial grimacing, crying, irritability, withdrawal activity, or changes in vital signs

Outcome Identification and Evaluation

Child will achieve adequate comfort level as evidenced by a decrease in rating number on a pain rating scale, quietness, calm resting behaviours, decrease in crying and irritability, and vital signs within acceptable parameters.

Interventions: *Promoting Pain Relief*

- Assess pain level using a developmentally appropriate pain rating tool *to establish a baseline.*
- Assess for verbal and nonverbal indicators of pain *to help determine child's pain level;* question parents about child's typical behaviours and previous experiences with pain *to determine factors that may be influencing child's response to pain.*
- Institute nonpharmacologic methods for pain control based on the child's age and cognitive level *to help decrease pain;* encourage parental participation in use of methods *to provide additional support and pain relief for the child.*
- Administer pharmacologic agents as ordered using the least traumatic route possible *to alter pain impulse transmission and minimize distress while promoting effective pain relief.*
- Explain the action of the drug and what the child should expect from the medication at a level that the child can understand *to promote trust and reduce fear while providing effective pain relief.*
- Give analgesics around the clock if pain is continuous and can be predicted *to maintain steady blood levels of the drug, thereby maximizing the drug's effect.*
- Perform atraumatic care at all times *to minimize the child's exposure to physical and psychological distress and pain.*

- Anticipate timing of procedures or situations that may lead to pain and provide appropriate analgesic therapy as ordered *to ensure that therapy is most effective at the time of the procedure.*
- Ensure that the child's environment is quiet and conducive to rest, dim the lights, and close the door or curtain *to reduce sensory overload that would increase the child's pain sensation.*
- Encourage the parents to stroke, touch, caress, and hold the child *to reduce discomfort and promote feelings of security.* The power of a parents' touch is an important management as well as calming technique (Campbell-Yeo, n.d.).
- Reassess the child's pain level after use of nonpharmacologic and pharmacologic methods *to determine effectiveness;* anticipate the need to modify or adapt nonpharmacologic methods or adjust analgesic dosage, route, or frequency *to promote maximum pain relief.*
- Perform nursing care activities after administering analgesic *to prevent exacerbating the child's pain.*
- Use diversional activities, distraction, and play appropriate to the child's age and cognitive level *to promote additional pain relief.*

NURSING CARE PLAN 36.1

Overview for the Child in Pain (continued)

NURSING DIAGNOSIS: Anxiety related to stress and uncertainty of the situation, unknown cause of pain, lack of familiarity with procedures, testing, and health care facility, and painful procedures, as evidenced by crying, irritability, withdrawal, stoic, or aggressive behaviours.

Outcome Identification and Evaluation

Child and family will demonstrate a decrease in anxiety level as evidenced by age-appropriate positive coping behaviours, verbalization of feelings, playing out of feelings, child and family cooperation with plan of care, and absence of signs and symptoms associated with escalating anxiety.

Interventions: *Minimizing Anxiety*

- Assess child's and parents' understanding of the situation, including their understanding of what may be causing the pain and the reasons for the procedures and testing, *to provide baseline information about the child's and parents' knowledge and possible clues to anxiety.*
- Spend time with the child and parents discussing what they think might be happening, encouraging the child and parents to talk openly about their feelings, *to facilitate continued expressions and communication.* Allow time for questions and answer questions honestly *to establish rapport and build trust.*
- Approach the child and family in a calm, relaxed manner *to foster trust and communication and decrease anxiety.*
- Allow the child options related to interventions as much as possible, such as fluid to drink or snack to eat, extremity to use for venipuncture (right or left), colour of bandage, or holding tape or dressing, *to foster feelings of control.*

- Provide atraumatic care *to reduce exposure to distress, which would exacerbate the child's anxiety level.*
- Explain any procedures, tests, or activities at a level the child can understand *to reduce fear of the unknown.*
- Incorporate aspects of the child's routine at home as much as possible *to reduce feelings of separation and promote feelings of normalcy.*
- Ensure consistency in care *to facilitate trust and acceptance.*
- Encourage parents in the use of comfort measures such as stroking, cuddling, holding, and rocking *to promote feelings of security and minimize stress.*
- Provide positive reinforcement for choices, participation in activities, and use of appropriate coping methods *to foster self-esteem.*
- Encourage the child's participation in play (unstructured and therapeutic play as needed) *to promote expression of feelings and fears.*

NURSING DIAGNOSIS: Deficient knowledge related to current condition and appropriate methods for managing pain as evidenced by crying, irritability, pushing away, and questions and verbalizations about pain and relief methods

Outcome Identification and Evaluation

Child and parents will demonstrate adequate knowledge about the child's current condition and use of pain relief methods as evidenced by statements about the cause of the child's pain, demonstration of chosen nonpharmacologic relief methods, use of pharmacologic agents, and statements related to signs and symptoms of increased and decreased pain.

Intervention: *Providing Child and Family Teaching*

- Assess the child's and parents' knowledge and understanding of the child's current condition and current pain level *to establish a baseline for teaching.*
- Provide time for the child and parents to ask questions; answer questions honestly and in terms they can understand *to promote learning.*

- Explain in simplified terms how the child's condition is associated with pain or the rationale for procedures needed that may contribute to pain *to promote understanding and foster trust.*
- Teach in short sessions *to prevent overloading the child and parents with information.*

(continued)

Overview for the Child in Pain (continued)

- Provide reinforcement and rewards *to help facilitate the teaching/learning process.*
- Use multiple modes of learning, such as written information, verbal instruction, demonstrations, and media when possible, *to facilitate learning and retention of information.*
- Instruct the parents and child as appropriate in non-pharmacologic methods for pain relief; encourage practice and participation by parents in methods chosen *to foster independence and use of method when necessary.*

- Teach the child as appropriate and parents about pharmacologic methods for pain relief; review specific information about the drug to be used, including action, duration, administration, possible adverse effects, and care necessary when the drug is used, *to promote learning;* have the child and parents report back information or demonstrate administration *to evaluate effectiveness of teaching.*
- Provide parents with written information about pain relief methods for use at home if indicated *to allow for reference at a later date.*

NURSING DIAGNOSIS: Sleep deprivation related to inability to manage pain effectively as evidenced by frequent waking by child during night, signs and symptoms of pain including irritability and restlessness, statements about being tired, pain rating scale remaining the same

Outcome Identification and Evaluation

Child will exhibit increased ability to sleep during the night as evidenced by increasing periods of calm and restfulness (initially starting at 2 hours and gradually increasing to 7 to 8 hours), decreased pain level on pain rating scale, and statements of decreased fatigue.

Intervention: *Promoting Sleep and Rest*

- Assist the child in using nonpharmacologic methods of pain relief, such as imagery, distraction, and muscle relaxation, *to promote relaxation.*
- Administer pharmacologic pain relief as ordered *to minimize pain interfering with sleep;* anticipate a change in drug therapy if pain relief is inadequate.
- Cluster nursing care activities *to minimize energy expenditure and disruptions in the child's ability to rest.*
- Help the child with a night-time routine similar to one he or she uses at home *to promote feelings of security.*
- Offer the child a back rub, warm bath, or warm liquids; reading a story; or listening to music *to facilitate relaxation;* provide stroking, hugging, cuddling, rocking, and light touch *to promote a sense of security and calm.*
- Dim the lights and close the curtain or door to the room *to provide a quiet, restful environment.*
- Ensure round-the-clock pain relief for the child through the night *to minimize the risk of pain.*

NURSING DIAGNOSIS: Risk for injury related to possible adverse effects of analgesics

Outcome Identification and Evaluation

Child will remain free of any injury related to signs and symptoms of adverse effects of analgesic therapy as evidenced by respiratory rate appropriate for age and no complaints of gastrointestinal (GI) upset, dizziness, or sedation, or episodes of constipation, nausea, vomiting, or pruritus.

NURSING CARE PLAN 36.1

Overview for the Child in Pain (continued)

Intervention: *Promoting Safety*

- Ensure that the child's call light is within reach *to allow for notification of health care personnel should problems arise.*
- Administer analgesic exactly as prescribed *to reduce the risk of error and development of adverse effects.*
- Assess the child's respiratory status closely for changes *to allow for early detection of respiratory depression.*
- If an opioid analgesic is being given, have naloxone readily available *to reverse the action of the narcotic if respiratory depression occurs.*
- Monitor appetite and assess bowel sounds for changes; note any abdominal distention or decreased bowel sounds, which would suggest decreased peristalsis, *to allow for early detection of constipation.*
- Ensure adequate fluid and fibre intake *to reduce risk of constipation.*
- Offer small frequent meals and give medication with food *to minimize risk of GI upset.*
- Assess for nausea and vomiting; if necessary, withhold food and fluids *to rest the GI tract* and administer antiemetics until nausea and vomiting resolve *to decrease nausea and vomiting.*
- Instruct the child to remain in bed after receiving analgesic, raise crib or side rails as appropriate, and instruct the child and parents to have someone accompany the child to the bathroom if allowed *to reduce the risk of falls from sedation.*
- Assess for complaints of itching and observe for rash or reddened areas; if pruritus occurs, urge the child not to scratch and expect to administer antihistamine as ordered *to reduce pruritus.*
- Provide the child with distraction *to assist in helping to reduce effects of pruritus.*

KEY CONCEPTS

- ○ Pain is a highly individualized subjective experience affecting persons of any age. It is a universal experience and is considered the fifth vital sign.

- ○ Pain management is a critical element in a child's plan of care because children may lack the verbal capacity to describe their pain experience; caregivers and health care providers often have misconceptions about pain; assessment of the complex nature of the pain experience is difficult; if left unmanaged, pain in children can lead to serious physical and emotional consequences; and available resources and research related to pain relief strategies in children are limited.

- ○ The sensation of pain involves a sequence of physiologic events: transduction, transmission, perception, and modulation.

- ○ Pain can be classified by duration as acute or chronic, by etiology as nociceptive or neuropathic, or by source or location as somatic or visceral.

- ○ Factors influencing a child's perception of pain include age and gender, cognitive level, temperament, previous pain experiences, and family and cultural background, all of which cannot be changed. Situational factors involve behavioural, cognitive, and emotional aspects and can be changed.

- ○ Infants, including preterm infants, experience pain. Behavioural and physiologic indicators are used to assess pain. Toddlers commonly react with intense emotional upset and physical resistance or aggression. Preschoolers may feel that pain is a punishment for misbehaving or having bad thoughts. School-age children can communicate the type, location, and severity of pain but may deny having pain to appear brave or avoid further pain. Adolescents, with their focus on body image and fear of loss of control, often ask numerous questions and may attempt to remain stoic to avoid being viewed as childish.

- ○ Assessment of pain in children includes both subjective and objective data. Nurses need to tailor the assessment to the child's developmental level and ask appropriate questions geared to the child's cognitive level. Parental questioning during the health history also is important.

- Self-report pain rating scales are valuable assessment tools that allow the child's level of pain to be quantified. Examples include the FACES pain scale-revised, the Oucher pain rating scale, the poker chip tool, the visual analogue and numeric scales, and the Adolescent Pediatric Pain Tool.

- Different pain rating scales are appropriate for different developmental levels. However, children may regress when in pain, so a simpler tool may be needed to make sure that the child understands what is being asked. Consistency in using the same tool is essential so that appropriate comparisons can be made and effective interventions can be planned and implemented. Furthermore, it may be more difficult to assess pain for an indigenous child. They may be more stoic and express pain through drawings or storytelling (Latimer et al., 2014).

- Physical examination of the child for pain primarily involves the skills of observation and inspection. These skills are used to assess for physiologic and behavioural changes that indicate pain. Auscultation also may be used to assess for changes in vital signs, specifically heart rate and blood pressure. Physiologic and behavioural pain assessment tools, such as the Neonatal Infant Pain Scale, Riley Infant Pain Scale, Pain Observation Scale for Young Children, CRIES Scale for Neonatal Postoperative Pain Assessment, and r-FLACC Behavioural Scale, measure specific parameters and changes that would indicate that the child is in pain.

- Nonpharmacologic pain management strategies aim to assist children in coping with pain and to give them a sense of mastery or control over the situation. These strategies may be categorized as behavioural-cognitive, in which the child focuses on a specific area or aspect rather than the pain (e.g., relaxation, distraction, imagery, biofeedback, thought stopping, and positive self-talk), or biophysical, in which the focus is on interfering with the transmission of pain impulses reaching the brain (e.g., heat and cold applications, massage, and pressure).

- The nurse plays a major role in teaching the child and family about available nonpharmacologic pain interventions, helping them choose the most appropriate and most effective methods, and ensuring that the child and parents use the method before the pain occurs as well as before it increases.

- Pharmacologic interventions involve the administration of drugs for pain relief, most commonly nonopioids and opioid analgesics. The selection of the method is determined by the drug being administered; the child's status; the type, intensity, and location of the pain; and any factors that may be influencing the child's pain. The preferred methods for administering analgesics include the oral, rectal, intravenous, or local nerve block routes; epidural administration; and moderate sedation.

- Nonopioid analgesics used to treat mild-to-moderate pain include acetaminophen and NSAIDs such as ibuprofen, ketorolac, naproxen, and, less commonly, indomethacin, diclofenac, and piroxicam.

- Morphine is considered the "gold standard" for all opioid agonists; it is the drug to which all other opioids are compared and is usually the drug of choice for severe pain (Oakes & D'Arcy, 2011).

- Local anaesthetics (vapocoolants) are commonly used to provide analgesia for procedures. They are effective in providing successful pain relief with only minimal risk of systemic adverse effects. The first choice for the most effective, painless local anaesthesia can be EMLA (eutectic mixture of local anaesthetics [lidocaine and prilocaine]) while other centres may use Ametop based on trends in the evidence literature or patient reaction to previous use. It achieves anaesthesia to a depth of 2 to 4 mm, so it reduces pain of phlebotomy, venous cannulation, and intramuscular injections up to 24 hours after injection.

- Epidural analgesia involves the insertion of a catheter into the epidural space through which drugs can be administered as bolus injections (a one-time bolus or on an intermittent schedule), as a continuous infusion, or as PCA. Usually an opioid, such as morphine, fentanyl, or hydromorphone, is given in conjunction with a long-acting local anaesthetic, such as bupivacaine.

- Moderate sedation is a medically controlled state of depressed consciousness that allows protective reflexes to be maintained so the child has the ability to maintain a patent airway and respond to physical or verbal stimulation.

- When providing pharmacologic pain relief, the nurse must adhere to the rights of medication administration and have a solid knowledge base about the medications used for pain relief and the drug's pharmacokinetics (absorption, distribution, metabolism, and excretion) and pharmacodynamics (mechanism of action, including adverse effects). Initial and ongoing assessment is crucial.

- The principles of atraumatic care guide nursing interventions for providing pain relief, especially for procedure-related pain.

- Chronic pain in children can significantly affect the child's daily life and activities as well as the family's life.

REFERENCES AND RECOMMENDED READINGS

American Academy of Pediatrics and the American Pain Society. (2001). Policy statement: The assessment and management of acute pain in infants, children, and adolescents. *Pediatrics, 108*(3), 793–797. Retrieved from http://pediatrics.aappublications.org/content/108/3/793.full

American Academy of Pediatrics, Committee on Fetus and Newborn and Section on Surgery, Section on Anesthesiology and Pain Medicine, Canadian Paediatric Society, Fetus and Newborn Committee. (2010). Policy statement. Prevention and management of pain in the Neonate: An update. *Pediatrics, 118*(5), 2231–2240. Retrieved from http://pediatrics.aappublications.org/content/118/5/2231.full.html

American Medical Association. (2013). *AMA pain management: Module 6 pain management: Pediatric pain management (continuing medical education).* Retrieved from https://cme.ama-assn.org/activity/1729042/detail.aspx

American Nurses Association (ANA). (2015). *Nursing-sensitive indicators.* Retrieved from http://nursingworld.org/MainMenu-Categories/ThePracticeofProfessionalNursing/PatientSafety-Quality/Research-Measurement/The-National-Database/Nursing-Sensitive-Indicators_1

American Pain Society. (1995). *Pain: The fifth vital sign.* Los Angeles, CA: Author.

Anand, K. J. S. (2013). *Assessment of neonatal pain.* UpToDate. Retrieved from http://www.uptodate.com/contents/assessment-of-neonatal-pain?source=search_result&search=neonatal+pain&selectedTitle=2~5#H12

Anand, K. J. S. (2014). *Prevention and treatment of neonatal pain.* UpToDate. Retrieved from http://www.uptodate.com/contents/prevention-and-treatment-of-neonatal-pain

Baker, C. M., & Wong, D. L. (1987). Q.U.E.S.T.: A process of pain assessment in children. *Orthopaedic Nursing, 6*(1), 11–21.

Bautista, C., & Grossman, S. (2014). Chapter 18: Somatosensory function, pain and headache. In S. C. Grossman & C. M. Porth (Eds.), *Porth's pathophysiology: Concepts of altered health states* (9th ed., pp. 422–451). Philadelphia, PA: Wolters Kluwer Health/Lippincott Williams & Wilkins.

Besenski, L. J., Forsyth, S. J., & von Baeyer, C. L. (2007). Commentary: Screening young children for their ability to use self-report pain scales. *Pediatric Pain Letter. Commentaries on Pain in Infants, Children and Adolescents, 9*(1), 1–7. Retrieved from http://childpain.org/ppl/issues/v9n1_2007/v9n1_besenski.pdf

Beyer, J. E., Denyes, M. J., & Villarruel, A. M. (1992). The creation, validation, and continuing development of the Oucher: A measure of pain intensity in children. *Journal of Pediatric Nursing, 7*(5), 335–346.

Boelen-van der Loo, W. J., Scheffer, E., de Haan, R. J., & de Groot, C. J. (1999). Clinimetric evaluation of the pain observation scale for young children in children aged between 1 and 4 years after ear, nose, and throat surgery. *Journal of Developmental and Behavioral Pediatrics, 20*(4), 222–227.

Bowden, V. R., & Greenberg, C. S. (2011). *Pediatric nursing procedures* (3rd ed.). Philadelphia, PA: Lippincott Williams & Wilkins.

Brown, J., Awad, I., Plant, R., McAdoo, J., & Shorten G. (1999). Topical amethocaine (Ametop) is superior to EMLA for intravenous cannulation. Eutectic Mixture Local Anaesthetics. Randomized controlled trial. *Canadian Journal of Anaesthesiology, 46*(11), 1014–1018.

Buck, M. L. (2010). Promethazine: Recommendations for safe use in children. *Pediatric Pharmacotherapy, 16*(3). Retrieved from http://www.medscape.com/viewarticle/720608

Campbell-Yeo, M (n.d.). The power of a parent's touch. Retrieved from http://itdoesnthavetohurt.ca

Canadian Paediatric Society. (2017). Aboriginal child's hurt & healing initiative: Art from the heart. Retrieved from https://www.cps.ca/uploads/imich/E41Latimer.pdf

Canadian Paediatric Society. (2018). *Caring for kids new to Canada.* Retrieved from https://www.kidsnewtocanada.ca

The Canadian Pain Society. (2014). *Pain in Canada fact sheet.* Retrieved from http://www.chronicpaintoronto.com/wp-content/uploads/2016/06/pain_fact_sheet_en.pdf

Canadian Pain Society. (n.d). CPS Position Statement. Retrieved from https://www.canadianpainsociety.ca/page/PositionStatement

Carpenito, L. J. (2013). *Nursing diagnosis: Application to clinical practice* (14th ed.). Philadelphia, PA: Lippincott Williams & Wilkins.

Cohen, M. R. (2009). *Patient-controlled analgesia: Making it safer for patients.* Retrieved from http://www.ismp.org/profdevelopment/PCAMonograph.pdf

Cohen, L. L., & Baxter, A. L. (2008). *Distraction techniques for procedural pain in children.* Retrieved from http://www.medscape.org/viewarticle/583976

Cooney, M. F., Czarnecki, M., Dunwoody, C., Eksterowicz, N., Merkel, S., Oakes, L., & Wuhrman, E. (2013). American Society for Pain Management Nursing position statement with clinical practice guidelines: Authorized agent controlled analgesia. *Pain Management Nursing, 14*(3), 176–181.

Coté, C. J., Wilson, S., & The Work Group on Sedation. (2011). *Guidelines for monitoring and management of pediatric patients during and after sedation for diagnostic and therapeutic procedures: An update.* Retrieved from http://pediatrics.aappublications.org/content/118/6/2587.long

Crandall, M., & Savedra, M. (2005). Multidimensional assessment using the adolescent pediatric pain tool: A case report. *Journal for Specialists in Pediatric Nursing, 10*(3), 115–123.

D'Arcy, Y. (2007). Patient safety issues with patient-controlled analgesia. *Topics in Advanced Practice Nursing eJournal, 7*(1). Retrieved from http://www.medscape.com/viewarticle/557394

D'Arcy, Y. (2011). New thinking about postoperative pain management. *OR Nurse, 5*(6), 28–36.

Fernandes, A. M., De Campos, C., Batalha, L., Perdigão, A., & Jacob, E. (2014). Pain assessment using the adolescent pediatric pain tool: A systematic review. *Pain Research & Management, 19*(4), 212–218.

Finley, G. A., Franck, L. S., Grunau, R. E., & von Baeyer, C. L. (2005). Why children's pain matters. *Pain: Clinician Updates, 13*(5), 1–6.

Hadden, K. L., LeFort, S., O'Brien, M., Coyte, P. C., & Guerriere, D. N. (2016). Validity of the child facial coding system for the assessment of acute pain in children with cerebral palsy. *Journal of Child Neurology, 31*(5), 597–602.

Hand, I. L., Noble, L., Geiss, D., Wozniak, L., & Hall, C. (2010). COVERS neonatal pain scale: Development and validation. *International Journal of Pediatrics, 2010*, 1–5.

Hatfield, L. A., Chang, K., Bittle, M., Deluca, J., & Polomano, R. C. (2011). The analgesic properties of intraoral sucrose: An integrative review. *Advances in Neonatal Care, 11*(2), 83–92.

Hauer, J., & Jones, B. L. (2014). *Evaluation and management of pain in children.* Retrieved from http://www.uptodate.com/contents/evaluation-and-management-of-pain-in-children?source=search_result&search=r+flacc&selectedTitle=1~2

Hester, N. K. (1979). The preoperational child's reaction to immunization. *Nursing Research, 28*(4), 250–255.

Hockenberry, M. J., & Wilson, D. (2009). *Wong's essentials of pediatric nursing* (8th ed., p. 162). St. Louis, MO: Elsevier Mosby.

The Hospital for Sick Children. (2005). *Myths vs facts of children's pain.* Retrieved from http://www.iasp-pain.org/files/Content/ContentFolders/GlobalYearAgainstPain2/20052006PaininChildren/pdfist.pdf

Hsu, D. C. (2014). *Topical anesthetics in children.* UpToDate. Retrieved from http://www.uptodate.com/contents/topical-anesthetics-in-children?source=machineLearning&search=EMLA&selectedTitle=5~49&sectionRank=2&anchor=H11#H11

Hsu, D. C., & Cravero, J. P. (2014). Procedural sedation in children outside of the operating room. Retrieved from http://www.uptodate.com/contents/procedural-sedation-in-children-outside-of-the-operating-room?source=see_link&anchor=H1684879#H1684879

International Association for the Study of Pain. (2012). *IASP taxonomy.* Retrieved from http://www.iasp-pain.org/Education/Content.aspx?ItemNumber=1698#Pain

The Joint Commission. (2004). Sentinel event alert. Patient controlled analgesia by proxy. Retrieved from https://psnet.ahrq.gov/resources/resource/1354/patient-controlled-analgesia-by-proxy

Kaiser, S. V., Asteria-Penaloza, R., Vittinghoff, E., Rosenbluth, G., Cabana, M. D., & Bardach, N. S. (2014). National patterns of codeine prescriptions for children in the emergency department. *Pediatrics, 133*(5), e1139–e1147.

Kennedy, R. M., Luhmann, J., & Zempsky, W. T. (2008). Clinical implications of unmanaged needle-insertion pain and distress in children. *Pediatrics, 122*(Suppl 3), S130–S133.

Krechel, S. W., & Bildner, J. (1995). CRIES: A new neonatal postoperative pain measurement score. Initial testing of validity and reliability. *Paediatric Anaesthesia, 5*, 53–61.

Latimer, M., & Paul, K. (2015). Understanding aboriginal children's pain from a two-eyed seeing perspective. *International Meeting of Indigenous Child Health.* Retrieved from https://www.cps.ca/uploads/imich/imich-2015-program-downloads/imich15-d3-latimer.pdf

Lawrence, J., Alcock, D., McGrath, P., Kay, J., MacMurray, S. B., & Dulberg, C. (1993). The development of a tool to assess neonatal pain. *Neonatal Network, 12*(6), 59–66.

Mann, A. (2014). *Patient-controlled analgesia: This mode of pain control involves careful selection, appropriate dosing and education. ADVANCE for Nurses.* Retrieved from http://nursing.advanceweb.com/article/patient-controlled-analgesia.aspx

Manworren, R. C., & Hynan, L. S. (2003). Clinical validation of FLACC: Preverbal patient pain scale. *Pediatric Nursing, 29*(2), 140–146.

Martin, S., & Cohen, L. L. (2012). Psychological approaches to pediatric pain relief. In A. M. Columbus (Ed.), *Advances in psychology research* (Vol. 89, pp. 115–130). New York: Nova Science Publishers.

McCaffery, M. (1968). *Nursing practice theories related to cognition, bodily pain and main environment interactions.* Los Angeles, CA: University of California Los Angeles.

McCaffery, M., & Pasero, C. (2011). *Pain assessment and pharmacologic management.* St. Louis, MO: Mosby.

McCarthy, A. M., & Kleiber, C. (2006). A conceptual model of factors influencing children's responses to a painful procedure when parents are distraction coaches. *Journal of Pediatric Nursing, 21*(2), 88–98.

McCarthy A. M., Kleiber, C., Hanrahan, K., Zimmerman, M. B., Westhus, N., & Allen, S. (2010). Factors explaining children's responses to intravenous needle insertions. *Nursing Research, 59*(6), 407–416.

McGrath, P. A. (2005). Children—not simply "little adults." In H. Merskey, J. D. Loeser, & R. Dubner (Eds.), *The paths of pain 1975–2005* (pp. 433–446). Seattle, WA: IASP Press.

Merkel, S. I., Voepel-Lewis, T., Shayevitz, J. R., & Malviya, S. (1997). The FLACC: A behavioural scale for scoring postoperative pain in young children. *Pediatric Nursing, 23*(3), 293–297.

Naughton, K. A., & Ikuta, L. (2013). The combined use of sucrose and non-nutritive sucking for procedural pain in both term and preterm neonates: An integrative review of the literature. *Advances in Neonatal Care, 13*(1), 9–19.

Oakes, L., & D'Arcy, Y. (2011). *Compact clinical guide to infant and child pain management. An evidence-based approach for nurses.* New York: Springer Publishing Company, LLC.

Panjganj, D., & Bevan, A. (2016). Children's nurses' postoperative pain assessment practices. *Nursing Children and Young People (2014+), 28*(5), 29–33.

Pawar, D., & Garten, L. (2010). Chapter 34: Pain management in children. In A. Kopf & N. B. Patel (Eds.), *Guide to pain management in low-resource settings* (pp. 255–268). Seattle, WA: International Association for the Study of Pain.

Registered Nurses' Association of Ontario. (2013). *Clinical Best Practice Guidelines. Assessment and Management of Pain* (3rd ed.). Retrieved from http://rnao.ca/sites/rnao-ca/files/AssessAndManagementOfPain2014.pdf

Robb, A. L., Ali, S., Poonai, N., & Thompson, G. C. (2016). Pain management of acute appendicitis in Canadian pediatric emergency departments. *Canadian Journal of Emergency Medicine*, 1–7.

Schade, J. G., Joyce, B. A., Gerkensmeyer, J., & Keck, J. F. (1996). Comparison of three preverbal scales for postoperative pain assessment in a diverse pediatric sample. *Journal of Pain and Symptom Management, 12*(6), 348–359.

Sheehy, K. A., Lippold, C., Rice, A. L., Nobrega, R., Finkel, J. C., & Quezado, Z. M. (2017). Subanesthetic ketamine for pain management in hospitalized children, adolescents, and young adults: A single-center cohort study. *Journal of Pain Research, 10,* 787.

Sutters, K. A., Miaskowski, C., Holdridge-Zeuner, D., Waite, S., Paul, S. M., Savedra, M. C., … Mahoney, K. (2010). A randomized clinical trial of the efficacy of scheduled dosing of acetaminophen and hydrocodone for the management of postoperative pain in children after tonsillectomy. *Clinical Journal of Pain, 26*(2), 95–103.

Taddio, A., Soin, H. K., Schuh, S., Koren, G., & Scolnik, D. (2005). Liposomal lidocaine to improve procedural success rates and reduce procedural pain among children: A randomized controlled trial. *Canadian Medical Association Journal, 172*(13), 1691–1695.

Taketomo, C. K., Hodding, J. H., & Kraus, D. M. (2013). *Lexicomp's drug reference handbook: Pediatric & neonatal dosage handbook* (20th ed.). Hudson, OH: Lexi-comp, Inc.

Vargas Schaffer, G. (2010). Is the WHO analgesic ladder still valid? Twenty-four years of experience. *Canadian Family Physician, 56*(6), 514–517. Retrieved from http://www.ncbi.nlm.nih.gov/pmc/articles/PMC2902929/

von Baeyer, C. L. (2006). Children's self-reports of pain intensity: Scale selection, limitations, and interpretation. *Pain Research and Management, 11*(3), 157–162.

von Baeyer, C. L. (2014). Chapter 36: Self report: The primary source of assessment after infancy. In P. J. McGrath, B. J. Stevens, S. M. Walker, & W. T. Zempsky (Eds.), *Oxford textbook of paediatric pain* (pp. 370–378). United Kingdom: Oxford University Press.

Walden, M. (2014). Chapter 23: Pain in the newborn and infant. In C. Kenner & J. W. Lott (Eds.), *Comprehensive neonatal nursing care* (5th ed., pp. 571–586). New York: Springer Publishing Company.

Weissman, A., Aranovitch, M., Blazer, S., & Zimmer, E. Z. (2009). Heel-lancing in newborns: Behavioural and spectral analysis assessment of pain control methods. *Pediatrics, 124*(5), e921–e926.

World Health Organization. (2012). *WHO guidelines on the pharmacological treatment of persisting pain in children with medical illnesses.* Retrieved from http://whqlibdoc.who.int/publications/2012/9789241548120_Guidelines.pdf?ua=1

Zeltzer, L. K., & Krane, E. J. (2011). Chapter 71: Pediatric pain management. In R. M. Kleigman, B. F. Stanton, J. W. St. Geme III, N. F. Schor, & R. E. Behrman (Eds.), *Nelson textbook of pediatrics* (19th ed., pp. 360–375). Philadelphia, PA: Saunders.

Zempsky, W. T. (2008). Pharmacologic approaches for reducing venous access pain in children. *Pediatrics, 122,* S140–S153. Retrieved from http://pediatrics.aappublications.org/cgi/content/full/122/Supplement_3/S140

Zempsky, W. T., Bean-Lijewski, J., Kauffman, R. E., Koh, J. L., Malviya, S. V., Rose, J. B., … Gennevois, D. J. (2008). Needle-free powder lidocaine delivery system provides rapid effective analgesia for venipuncture or cannulation pain in children: Randomized, double-blind comparison of venipuncture and venous cannulation pain after fast-onset needle-free powder lidocaine or placebo treatment trial. *Pediatrics, 121*(5), 979–987. Retrieved from http://pediatrics.aappublications.org/cgi/content/abstract/121/5/979

CHAPTER **WORKSHEET**

MULTIPLE-CHOICE QUESTIONS

1. The nurse is preparing to assess the pain of a 3-year-old child who had surgery the day before. Which pain assessment method would be most appropriate for the nurse to use?
   a. FACES pain rating scale and poker chip tool
   b. FACES pain rating scale, observation of the child, and parent report
   c. Asking the parents to rate their child's pain using the word-graphic rating scale
   d. Visual analogue scale

2. When developing the plan of care for a child in pain, the nurse identifies appropriate strategies aimed at modifying which factor influencing pain?
   a. Gender
   b. Cognitive level
   c. Previous pain experiences
   d. Anticipatory anxiety

3. An adolescent who is a competitive swimmer comes to the emergency department complaining of localized aching pain in his shoulder. He states, "I've been practicing really hard and long to get myself ready for my meet this weekend." The area is tender to the touch. The nurse determines that the adolescent is most likely experiencing which type of pain?
   a. Cutaneous pain
   b. Deep somatic pain
   c. Visceral pain
   d. Neuropathic pain

4. After teaching a child's parents about the different methods of distraction that can be used for pain management, which statement by the parents indicates a need for additional teaching?
   a. "We'll have her focus on her hand and count each finger slowly."
   b. "We'll read some of her favourite stories to her."
   c. "We'll have her imagine that she's at the beach this summer."
   d. "She likes to play video games, so we'll bring in some from home."

5. A child is scheduled for a bone marrow aspiration at 4 PM. The nurse would plan to apply EMLA cream to the intended site at which time?
   a. 1:30 PM
   b. 3:00 PM
   c. 3:30 PM
   d. 4:00 PM

CRITICAL THINKING EXERCISES

1. The nurse asks a 12-year-old girl if she is having pain. She denies pain, even though she is lying on her left side holding her abdomen with her knees flexed up to it. What might be some underlying factors leading the child to deny her pain? How would the nurse go about assessing this child's pain?

2. The nurse comes into the room of a 6-year-old who is sleeping. His mother states, "He's asleep, so he's not in pain." How should the nurse respond?

3. A child who is receiving ibuprofen is experiencing increased pain. The dosage of ibuprofen is increased but is no longer effective in providing adequate pain relief. What is occurring? What would be most likely to happen next?

STUDY ACTIVITIES

1. Interview nurses who work on a pediatric unit about their experiences with managing pain in children. Ask them how they assess pain in children and the major methods they use to assist the children in managing their pain.

2. Interview families of children with chronic illnesses who deal with pain. Ask the parents how they assess their children's pain level and what methods they have used in assisting their children in managing pain.

3. Compare and contrast the drugs fentanyl and midazolam when used for moderate sedation in terms of onset of action, duration, primary effects, and antidotes.

4. A child is receiving epidural analgesia with morphine. The nurse would be alert for which of the following adverse effects? (Select all that apply.)
   _____a. Respiratory depression
   _____b. Pruritus
   _____c. Constipation
   _____d. Vomiting
   _____e. Amnesia
   _____f. Hematoma

DOSAGE CALCULATION

After you have performed your nonpharmacologic interventions, your patient, who is an infant, is exhibiting kicking, is not reaching for toys, and is occasionally crying. There is an order for morphine sulfate 1 mg IV every 3 to 4 hours. The safe dose range for morphine sulfate is 0.1 to 0.2 mg/kg/dose every 3 to 4 hours. Morphine sulfate is supplied as 1 mg/mL.

1. Is this a safe dose?
2. Describe how you will administer this medication and what would you assess for after giving it.

BRINGING IT ALL TOGETHER: A CASE STUDY

You are caring for Chantal, a 7-month-old infant, during the postoperative period. She weighs 17 lb and is 26.5 in long. During your assessment, you find her current vital signs are as follows: temperature 37.1°C, heart rate 150, respiratory rate 32. Her behaviours include restlessness, moving a lot around the crib, and looking at her mother when the mother sings to her.

Go to thePoint **to find questions to consider about this case.**

Unit 11

Nursing Care of the Child With a Health Disorder

37

Nursing Care of the Child With an Infectious or Communicable Disorder

KEY TERMS

antibodies
antigen
chain of infection
communicability
endogenous
  pyrogens
exanthem
phagocytosis
vector-borne
zoonotic

Learning Objectives

Upon completion of the chapter, you will be able to:

1. Discuss anatomic and physiologic differences in children versus adults in relation to the infectious process.

2. Identify nursing interventions related to common laboratory and diagnostic tests used in the diagnosis and management of infectious conditions.

3. Identify appropriate nursing assessments and interventions related to medications and treatments for childhood infectious and communicable disorders.

4. Distinguish various infectious illnesses occurring in childhood.

5. Devise an individualized nursing care plan for the child with an infectious or communicable disorder.

6. Develop child/family teaching plans for the child with an infectious or communicable disorder.

Mrs. Goldberg brings her son Samuel, 3 months old, to the clinic. He presents with a history of fever and nasal congestion. His mother tells you, "He's been very irritable and crying more than usual."

Infection refers to the invasion of body tissue by microorganisms with the potential to cause illness or disease (Butler-Jones, 2013). Nurses encounter potential or actual infections in all types of clients and must detect problems and intervene early to prevent life-threatening complications. Infections (infectious and communicable diseases) are one of the leading causes of death worldwide. As the world has become increasingly connected, infectious diseases have presented new challenges with changes in microbial resistance, limitations in vaccine, and pharmacology developments influencing outcomes (Canadian Healthy Infant Longitudinal Development Study, n.d.). Children are particularly vulnerable to infectious disease. Their immune systems are still developing and their natural curiosity, especially in infants and toddlers, leads to wide-range handling of objects and surfaces coupled with a tendency to place their hands and objects in their mouths without washing first. However, infection risk is also linked to wider variables. For example, the determinants of health such as the social, physical, and economic environments that children live in can increase risk as a result of various factors such as poverty, poor parent health literacy linked to infection prevention, and management of infectious illness (see thePoint for further information). Infectious diseases in children can range in severity from mild with few symptoms to serious illness, resulting in damage to organs, and even death. Infectious and communicable diseases include bacterial infections (e.g., sepsis), viral infections (e.g., viral exanthems), zoonotic infections, vector-borne infections, parasitic and helminthic infections (e.g., roundworm [i.e., Ascariasis] and pediculosis capitis [head lice]), and sexually transmitted infections (e.g., chlamydia and gonorrhea).

There has been a dramatic decrease in the incidence and severity of infectious and communicable diseases since the advent of vaccines, antibiotics, antiviral drugs, and antitoxins (InterAction, 2013). Some diseases have been effectively controlled, but the vast majority will not be eliminated. New diseases emerge and old diseases are reappearing, sometimes in a drug-resistant form. The Public Health Agency of Canada (PHAC) tracks certain infectious diseases (Government of Canada, n.d.). This list of nationally reportable diseases is revised periodically to add new pathogens or remove diseases as their incidence declines. Box 37.1 lists nationally notifiable diseases in Canada.

Nurses, particularly those working in schools, primary care settings, child care centres, and clinics or outpatient settings, are often the first to see the signs of infectious or communicable diseases in children. These signs are often vague at first (e.g., a sore throat or rash). Therefore, nurses must have accurate assessment skills and be familiar with the signs and symptoms of common childhood infectious diseases so that they can provide prompt recognition, treatment, guidance, and support to

---

| BOX 37.1 |

NATIONALLY NOTIFIABLE DISEASES (INCLUDING DATES OF MANDATORY REPORTING)

- Anthrax 2002–present
- Botulism 1933–Present
- Chickenpox (Varicella) 1986–Present
- Chlamydia 1991–Present
- *Clostridium difficile* Associated Diarrhea (CDI) 2009–Present
- Congenital Syphilis 1993–Present
- Giardiasis 1983–Present
- Gonorrhea 1924–Present
- Group B Streptococcal Disease of the Newborn (GBS) 2000–Present
- Hanta Pulmonary Syndrome 2000–Present
- Hepatitis C 1991–Present
- HIV Infection 2000–Present
- Influenza, Laboratory confirmed 2000–Present
- Meningococcal Disease 1924–Present
- Pneumococcal Disease 2000–Present
- Lyme Disease 2009–Present
- Malaria 1983–Present
- Measles 1969–Present
- Mumps 1986–Present
- Norovirus Infection 2007–Present
- Pertussis 1924–Present
- Rubella 1969–Present
- Rabies 1927–Present
- SARS 2004–Present
- Tuberculosis 1924–Present
- West Nile Virus Infection 2003–Present

For a complete list of nationally notifiable disease in Canada, go to http://diseases.canada.ca/notifiable/diseases-list.

---

families. Identifying the infectious agent is of primary importance to prevent further spread.

Many infectious diseases can be prevented through simple and inexpensive methods such as handwashing, adequate immunization, proper handling and preparation of food, and judicious antibiotic use. Nurses play a key role in educating parents and the community on ways to prevent infectious and communicable diseases.

INFECTIOUS PROCESS

Infection occurs when an organism (viral, bacterial, fungal [parasite such as helminths or Protozoa can cause infection]) enters the body, invades and attacks host cells, and multiplies, thereby colonizing host tissue resulting in damage to cells, tissues, and organs. As a result of the infection, the body responds by triggering the immune system, thus prompting an inflammatory response. The body delivers fluid, blood, and nutrients to the area of infection or injury and attempts to eliminate the pathogens and repair the

TABLE 37.1	FUNCTION OF WHITE BLOOD CELLS BY LEUKOCYTE TYPE
Type of White Blood Cell	**Function**
Granulocytes • Neutrophils (polymorphonuclear leukocytes or PMNs, segs) • Eosinophils • Basophils	Phagocytic cells • First line of defence upon invasion of bacteria, fungus, cell debris, and other foreign substances • Respond to allergic disorders and parasitic infections • Respond to allergic disorders and hypersensitivity reactions; used to study chronic inflammation
Lymphocytes (B lymphocytes, T lymphocytes, and natural killer cells)	Main source of producing an immune response; respond to viral infections (measles, rubella, chickenpox, infectious mononucleosis); tumors
Monocytes	Second line of defence; respond to larger and more severe infections than neutrophils by phagocytosis; leukemias and lymphomas; chronic inflammation

Adapted from Fischbach, F. T., & Dunning, M. B, III. (2015). *A manual of laboratory and diagnostic tests* (9th ed., pp. 67–88). Philadelphia, PA: Wolters Kluwer/Lippincott Williams & Wilkins; and Grossman, S. (2014). Chapter 25: Blood cells and the hematopoietic system. In S. Grossman & C. M. Porth (Eds.). *Porth's pathophysiology: Concepts of altered health states* (9th ed., pp. 638–664). Philadelphia, PA: Wolters Kluwer Health/Lippincott Williams & Wilkins.

tissues. The body does this through vascular and cellular reactions. The vascular response is an initial period of vasoconstriction followed by vasodilatation. This vasodilatation allows for the increase of fluids, blood, and nutrients to the target area.

The cellular response involves the arrival of white blood cells (WBCs) to the area. WBCs are the body's defence against infection or injury. The types of WBCs are neutrophils, basophils, eosinophils, lymphocytes, and monocytes. Elevations in certain portions of the WBC count reflect different processes occurring in the body, such as infection, allergic reaction, or leukemia. Table 37.1 explains the function of each type of WBC. Each type is generally present in a balanced state; the types are reported as a percentage of the total WBC count or as the number per certain volume of blood.

WBCs use **phagocytosis** to ingest and destroy the pathogen. If bacteria escape the action of phagocytosis, they enter the bloodstream and lymph system and the immune system is activated. With activation of the immune system, B lymphocytes (humoral immunity) and T lymphocytes (cell-mediated immunity) are matured and activated. B and T cells recognize and attack infectious pathogens. B cells, which mature in the bone marrow, produce specific **antibodies** (specialized immune proteins) that bind to and neutralize a specific offending **antigen** (a substance that the body recognizes as foreign). T cells, which mature in the thymus, attack the antigen directly. Once B and T cells have been exposed to an antigen, some cells will remember the antigen. Therefore, if a particular antigen invades again, the body will act more quickly. A third type of lymphocyte, natural killer cells, is a part of the innate immune system and function to destroy foreign material present.

Fever

Infection or inflammation caused by bacteria, viruses, or other pathogens stimulates the release of **endogenous pyrogens** (interleukins, tumor necrosis factor, and interferon). The pyrogens act on the hypothalamus, where they trigger prostaglandin production and increase the body's temperature set point. This triggers the cold response, resulting in shivering, vasoconstriction, and a decrease in peripheral perfusion to help decrease heat loss and allow the body's temperature to rise to the new set point therefore resulting in fever. The definition of fever varies based on the age of the child, the method of temperature measurement, and the presence of any underlying conditions. There is no single value defined for fever due to individual variations but Box 37.2 shows generally accepted guidelines based on measurement route in an otherwise healthy child.

BOX 37.2

GENERAL GUIDELINE OF FEVER BASED ON MEASUREMENT ROUTE

• Oral: >37.8°C (100°F): normal range 36.5° to 37.5°C (95.9° to 99.5°F)
• Rectal: >38°C (100.4°F): normal range 36.6° to 38°C (97.9° to 100.4°F)
• Axillary: >37.2°C (99°F): normal range 36.5° to 37.5°C (97.8° to 99.5°F)
• Tympanic: >38°C (100.4°F): normal range 35.8° to 38°C (96.4° to 100.4°F)
• Temporal: >38°C (100.4°F)

Antipyretics are often used to lower fever and increase comfort. They decrease the temperature set point by inhibiting the production of prostaglandins. As a result, sweating and vasodilation occur and there is heat loss and a drop in temperature.

It is important to distinguish between fever and hyperthermia. Hyperthermia occurs when normal thermoregulation fails, resulting in an unregulated rise in core temperature. Hyperthermia may occur if the central nervous system of the child becomes impaired by disease, drugs, and abnormalities of heat production or thermal stressors, such as being left in a hot automobile or exertional heat stroke. In the absence of hyperthermia and in the neurologically intact child, the body does not allow fever to rise to lethal levels. The body actually produces a natural antipyretic, called cryogen. If there is no hyperthermic insult, it is rare to see a child's temperature rise above 41°C (105.8°F) (Ward, 2015a). Fever is a natural aspect of the body's defence system and a common symptom in young children (Kelly et al., 2017). Parents or caregivers may benefit from supportive education to minimize what is described as "fever phobia" (Purssell & Collin, 2016) which may improve parents misuse of antipyretics (either underdosing or overdosing) (Kelly et al., 2017).

Stages of Infectious Disease

Infectious diseases follow a similar pattern. They progress through certain stages (Table 37.2) in which **communicability** (ability to spread to others) can be predicted. It is important for nurses to understand these stages to help control and manage infectious diseases.

Chain of Infection

The **chain of infection** is the process by which an organism is spread. Behaviours of infants and young children,

mainly pertaining to hygiene, increase their exposure risk by promoting the chain of infection. Poor hygiene habits, including lack of handwashing, placing toys and hands in the mouth, can contribute to the spread of infection and communicable diseases. Table 37.3 reviews the chain of infection and nursing practice implications related to it.

Safety Check

GOAL: Reduce the Risk of Healthcare-Associated Infections

Implement evidence-based practices to prevent healthcare-associated infections due to multidrug-resistant organisms in acute care hospitals. Note: This requirement applies to, but is not limited to, epidemiologically important organisms such as methicillin-resistant *Staphylococcus aureus* (MRSA), *Clostridium difficile* (CDI), vancomycin-resistant enterococci (VRE), and multidrug-resistant Gram-negative bacteria

Steps: Follow strategies to break the chain of infection and prevent the spread of infection among hospitalized children

Public Health Agency of Canada. (2013). *The chief public health officer's report on the state of public health in Canada, 2013: Infectious disease-the never-ending threat.* Retrieved from http://www.phac-aspc.gc.ca/cphorsphc-respcacsp/2013/index-eng.php.

Preventing the Spread of Infection

Nurses play a key role in breaking the chain of infection and preventing the spread of diseases (see Box 37.3). It is important to follow infection control and prevention practices. It is also very important to educate parents and children on the measures they can take to prevent the spread of infection.

Take Note!

Frequent handwashing is the most important way to prevent the spread of infection.

TABLE 37.2	STAGES OF INFECTIOUS DISEASE
Stage	**Explanation**
Incubation	Time from entrance of pathogen into the body to appearance of first symptoms; during this time, pathogens grow and multiply
Prodrome	Time from onset of nonspecific symptoms such as fever, malaise, and fatigue to more specific symptoms
Illness	Time during which child demonstrates signs and symptoms specific to an infection type
Convalescence	Time when acute symptoms of illness disappear

Safety Check

GOAL: Reduce the Risk of Healthcare-Associated Infections

Comply with Infection Prevention and Control Canada (IPAC) guidelines information about hand hygiene guidelines or the current World Health Organization (WHO) hand hygiene guidelines

Steps: When caring for a child, perform proper handwashing before and after all care

IPAC. Information about Hand Hygiene. Retrieved both IPAC and PHAC from https://ipac-canada.org/hand-hygiene.php

https://ipac-canada.org/photos/custom/OldSite/pdf/2013_PHAC_Hand%20Hygiene-EN.pdf

http://www.publications.gc.ca/site/eng/440707/publication.html

TABLE 37.3	CHAIN OF INFECTION	
Chain Link	**Explanation**	**Nursing Implications**
Infectious agent	Any agent capable of causing infection; examples: bacteria, viruses, rickettsiae, protozoa, and fungi	Control or eliminate infectious agents through: • Handwashing • Wearing gloves • Cleaning, disinfecting, or sterilizing equipment
Reservoir	A place where the pathogen can thrive and reproduce; examples: human body, animals, insects, food, water, inanimate objects (e.g., stethoscopes)	• Control or eliminate reservoirs • Control sources of body fluids, drainage, or solutions that may harbour pathogens • Follow institutional guidelines for disposing of infectious wastes • Provide proper wound care; change dressings or bandages when soiled • Assist children to carry out appropriate skin and oral care • Keep linens clean and dry
Portal of exit	A way for the pathogen to exit the reservoir; examples: skin and mucous membranes, respiratory tract, urinary tract, gastrointestinal tract, reproductive tract	• Control portals of exit and educate children and families • Cover mouth and nose when sneezing or coughing • Avoid talking, coughing, or sneezing over open wounds or sterile fields • Use personal protective equipment
Modes of transmission	Direct transmission: body-to-body contact Indirect transmission: transferred by fomite or vector; spread by droplet or airborne transmission	• Wash hands before and after child contact, invasive procedures, or touching open wounds • Use personal protective equipment when necessary • Urge children and family to wash hands frequently, especially before eating or handling food, after eliminating, and after touching infectious material
Portal of entry	A way for the pathogen to enter the host; examples: skin and mucous membranes, respiratory tract, urinary tract, gastrointestinal tract, reproductive tract	• Use proper sterile technique during invasive procedures • Provide appropriate wound care • Dispose of needles and sharps in puncture-resistant containers • Provide all children with their own personal care items
Susceptible host	Any person who cannot resist the pathogen	• Protect susceptible host by promoting normal body defences against infection • Maintain integrity of the child's skin and mucous membranes • Protect normal defences by regular bathing and oral care, adequate fluid intake and nutrition, and proper immunization

Isolation precautions help nurses break the chain of infection and provide strategies to prevent the spread of pathogens among hospitalized children. Public Health Agency of Canada has developed guidelines that all health professionals need to be familiar with. The Centre for Communicable Diseases and Infection Control has presented two-tier guidelines for hospitalized children (Centre for Communicable Diseases and Infection Control, 2012). Tier 1 is standard precautions, which are designed for the care of all hospitalized children regardless of their diagnosis. Tier 2 is transmission-based precautions, designed for pediatric patients who are known, or suspected, to be infected with epidemiologically important pathogens. These pathogens can be spread by airborne, droplet, or contact transmission. Box 37.3 gives an overview of standard and transmission-based precautions.

Take Note!

Hand hygiene includes both handwashing with soap and water and the use of alcohol-based products (gels, rinses, foams) that do not require water. If there is no visible soiling of the hands, approved alcohol-based products are preferred because of their superior microbicidal activity, reduced drying of the skin, and convenience (Centre for Communicable Diseases and Infection Control, 2012).

When caring for children, these guidelines may need to be modified. For instance, diaper changing is routine in the pediatric setting. Handwashing before and after diaper change is acceptable, unless there are known infections or risk to patient or staff in which case additional precautions will be necessary. Pediatric units often have common rooms, such as playrooms and schoolrooms. Children placed on transmission-based

BOX 37.3

STANDARD PRECAUTIONS AND ISOLATION PRECAUTIONS

Standard Precautions or Routine Practices (Tier 1)

These are designed for the care of all patients in a hospital setting regardless of infection/illness status.

- Apply to all body fluids, secretions and excretions (except sweat), breast-milk, nonintact skin, and mucous membranes, and undiagnosed skin rashes
- Designed to reduce the risk of transmission of microorganisms from recognized and unrecognized sources including environmental surfaces
- Techniques include:
  - Proper hand hygiene (entering the room or attending to patient, before any aseptic intervention, after body fluid exposure and after patient–environment contact before leaving room or patient area)
  - Use of gloves (clean or sterile) when touching blood, body fluids, secretions or excretions, and contaminated items
  - Masks, eye protection, and face shields when patient care may include splashing or sprays of blood, body fluid secretions, or excretions, and during bronchoscopy, endotracheal intubation, and open suctioning of the respiratory tract
  - Fluid-resistant nonsterile gowns, to protect skin and clothing, when patient care may include splashing or sprays of blood, body fluid secretions, or excretions
  - Patient care equipment handled in a manner that prevents skin or mucous membrane exposure and contamination of clothing
  - All used linen is considered contaminated and needs to be handled and disposed of appropriately
  - Mouthpieces, resuscitation bags with one-way valves, and other ventilation devices should be readily available, with regular changing of such systems as per local policy
  - Cleaning and disinfecting noncritical surfaces in patient care areas, as per local policy
  - Respiratory hygiene/cough etiquette: applies to any person with signs of illness including cough, congestion, rhinorrhea, or increased respiratory secretions who is entering a healthcare facility. It includes education regarding covering the mouth/nose with a tissue; prompt disposal of used tissues, along with surgical masks used by a person who is coughing when appropriate; hand hygiene after contact with respiratory secretions; and separation, ideally greater than 3 ft, of persons with respiratory infections in common waiting areas when possible
  - Safe injection practices: use of sterile single-use disposable needle. When possible, use of single-dose vials; precautions used to prevent injury when using, cleaning, or disposing of needles and sharps
  - Use of masks for insertion of catheters or injection into the spinal or epidural space via lumbar puncture procedures

Transmission-Based Precautions or Additional Precautions (Tier 2)

Required to interrupt transmission of infectious agents which are known or suspected to be transmitted via airborne route, droplet, or contact

Airborne *(signs should be posted on the patients cubicle door to promote concordance with infection control practice; mask N95 and closed doors)*

- Designed to reduce the risk of infectious agents transmitted by airborne droplet nuclei or dust particles suspended in the air that may contain the infectious agent (<5 μm in diameter). These microorganisms are widely dispersed and inhaled by others. Examples of such illnesses include measles, varicella, pulmonary tuberculosis, and shingles
- Techniques include standard precautions as well as
  - Room with negative air pressure ventilation, with air externally exhausted or high-efficiency particulate air filtered if recirculated; if unavailable, mask the child and place in private room with the door closed
  - Wear a mask or respirator depending on specific recommendations based on disease, such as if infectious pulmonary tuberculosis is suspected or proven, wear a respiratory protective device, such as an N95 respirator, while in the child's room
  - Susceptible healthcare personnel should not enter the room of children with measles or varicella zoster infections

Droplet *(signs should be posted on the patients cubicle door to promote concordance with infection control practice; gloves, gown, eye protection, and mask)*

- Intended to prevent transmission of pathogens spread through close respiratory or mucous membrane contact with respiratory secretions. Designed to reduce the risk of infectious agents transmitted by contact of the conjunctivae or the mucous membranes of the nose or mouth of a susceptible person with large-particle droplets containing pathogens generated from a person (generally through coughing, sneezing, talking, or procedures such as suctioning) who has a clinical disease or who is a carrier of the disease. Note organisms can settle on objects in the patient's room and environment (travel distance is <2 m), and patient's unwashed hands. Since these droplets are large (5 microns in diameter), they do not remain in the air. Examples of such illnesses include respiratory infections (Influenza RSV, adenovirus), pertussis, mumps, rubella, and scarlet fever
- Enhanced Droplet Precautions are indicated when there is an international, regional, or local alert of an epidemiologically significant respiratory pathogen. Infection control advice should be sought, like the use of an N95 mask (regular FIT testing is mandatory). Examples include SARS, Pandemic influenza strains
- Techniques include standard precautions as well as:
  - Private room, single–use-only equipment, attention to hand hygiene, and disposal of gown/mask/eye gloves as per local guidelines

Contact *(signs should be posted on the patient's cubicle door to promote concordance with infection control practice; gloves and gown)*

- Includes direct and indirect transmission
- Direct-contact transmission involves skin-to-skin contact and physical transfer of pathogens between a susceptible host and an infected or colonized person. Examples include patient care activities that involve physical contact such as turning and bathing. Direct-contact

transmission also can occur between two children, where one serves as the source of infectious pathogen and the other as a susceptible host. Indirect-contact transmission involves contact of a susceptible host with a contaminated intermediate object, usually inanimate, in the child's environment
- Examples of such illnesses include gastroenteritis (i.e., Salmonellosis, Rotavirus), Enteroviral infections (i.e., hand-to-foot-and-mouth disease), Hepatitis A, Herpes Simplex (contained), Scabies
- Contact Precautions "R" are initiated for *Clostridium difficile* infection, which also include cleaning of the patient room with sporicidal agent and no sharing of equipment

- Contact Precautions "Mask" are initiated when patients have methicillin-resistant *Staphylococcus aureus* (MRSA)
- Techniques include standard precautions as well as:
  - Private room (if unavailable, consultation with infection control personnel is recommended)
  - Gloves (clean or sterile) should be used at all times
  - Proper hand hygiene after glove removal
  - Use gloves and gowns for all interactions that involve contact with the child or potentially contaminated areas. Don before entering and remove before leaving the child's room

Healthcare workers must practice within the specific institution's guidelines

Adapted from Siegel, J. D., Rhinehart, E., Jackson, M., Chiarello, L.; the Healthcare Infection Control Practices Advisory Committee. (2007). Guideline for isolation precautions: Preventing transmission of infectious agents in healthcare settings. Retrieved from http://www.cdc.gov/hicpac/pdf/isolation/Isolation2007.pdf and http://www.sickkids.ca/nursing/education-and-learning/nursing-student-orientation/module-one-safety/infection-control-at-sickkids/index.html

isolation are not allowed to leave their rooms and therefore are not allowed to use these common rooms.

VARIATIONS IN PEDIATRIC ANATOMY AND PHYSIOLOGY

Normal immune function is a complex protective response by the body. It involves various responses including humoral and cell-mediated immunity, phagocytosis, natural killer (NK) cells, and activation of the complement system (a system of plasma proteins usually activated by pathogens entering the body or pathogen-bound antibodies) (Merle, Noe, Halbwachs-Mccarclli, Frcmcaux-Bacchi, & Roumenina, 2015). Blood and lymph circulatory systems are responsible for transporting the agents of the immune system. Due to the immature responses of the immune system, infants and young children are more susceptible to infection. The newborn does not have a mature innate or adaptive immune (B and T lymphocytes) system (Simon, Hollander, & McMichael, 2015) which results in a decreased inflammatory response to pathogens (invading organisms) which in turn increases the infection risk. During the first few days and weeks of life, infant innate immunity capacity, a first line of defence present at birth, increases (Simon et al., 2015). The infants' blunted adaptive immune system strengthens overtime as antibody response process matures resulting in adaptive immunity (Simon et al., 2015). Since the infant has had limited exposure to disease and is losing the passive immunity acquired from maternal antibodies, the risk of infection is higher. Young children continue to have an increased risk for infection and communicable disorders because disease protection from immunizations is not complete.

COMMON MEDICAL TREATMENTS

A variety of medications and other medical treatments are used to treat infectious disorders in children. Most of these treatments will require a physician's or nurse practitioner's order when the child is in the hospital. The most common treatments and medications are listed in Common Medical Treatments 37.1 and Drug Guide 37.1. The nurse caring for the child with an infectious disorder should be familiar with what the procedures are, how they work, and common nursing implications related to use of these modalities.

NURSING PROCESS OVERVIEW FOR THE CHILD WITH AN INFECTIOUS OR COMMUNICABLE DISORDER

Care of the child with an infectious or communicable disorder includes assessment, nursing diagnosis, planning, interventions, and evaluation. There are a number of general concepts related to the nursing process that may be applied to the care of children with infectious disorders. From a general understanding of the care involved for a child with an infectious disorder, the nurse can then individualize the care based on the child's specifics.

Remember Samuel, the 3-month-old with fever, congestion, and irritability? What additional health history and physical examination assessment information should you obtain?

COMMON MEDICAL TREATMENTS 37.1

Treatment	Explanation	Indications	Nursing Implications
Hydration	Promoting proper fluid balance either orally or intravenously	Child who can't replace insensible loss due to fever, child who is vomiting or has diarrhea	• Encourage oral fluids, including breastfeeding • Offer child-preferred fluid; try popsicles or games to promote fluid intake • If administering IV fluids, ensure correct fluid and rate per order and assess IV site and fluid intake, minimally every hour • Maintain strict record of intake and output
Fever reduction	Reducing temperature by use of antipyretics or nonpharmacologic interventions	Febrile child who is uncomfortable or who can't keep up with the increased metabolic demands associated with fever	• Administer antipyretics, such as ibuprofen and acetaminophen • Avoid aspirin use in children and adolescents • Use nonpharmacologic interventions such as dressing lightly, removing blankets, use of a fan, tepid bath, and cooling blanket. Make sure that nonpharmacologic measures do not induce shivering or discomfort. If they do, they should be stopped immediately
IV, intravenous	Acts as a route for hydration if oral intake reduced and IV medication as prescribed	IV antipyretic use for fever >24 hours due to infection as a single dose, when oral medication is not possible or rapid reduction of temperature is required	• Observe for allergic reaction • Effectiveness dependent on child hepatic metabolism • Monitor vital signs as per local protocol, for example, Paediatric Early Warning Scores (PEWS)

DRUG GUIDE 37.1 COMMON DRUGS FOR COMMUNICABLE DISORDERS

Medication	Actions/Indications	Nursing Implications
Antibiotics	Kill and prevent the growth of bacteria Used for treatment of bacterial infections such as sepsis	• Check for antibiotic allergies • Give as prescribed for the length of time prescribed
Antivirals (e.g., acyclovir)	Kill and prevent the growth of viruses Used for treatment of viral infections such as herpes simplex type 2	• Observe infusion site for signs of tissue damage • If administering topically, clean and dry area before application and wear gloves • Give as prescribed for the length of time prescribed
Antipyretics (acetaminophen, ibuprofen)	Decrease the temperature set point (only in a child with a raised temperature) by inhibiting the production of prostaglandins, leading to heat loss (through vasodilation and sweating) and resulting in a reduction in fever Used to decrease temperature in the febrile child who is uncomfortable or who can't keep up with the increased metabolic demands associated with fever	• Ensure proper dosing, concentration, and dosing interval • Avoid aspirin use in children and adolescents • Avoid ibuprofen use in children with a bleeding disorder • Assess fever and any related symptoms such as tachycardia, shivering, or diaphoresis • Properly educate caregivers on appropriate dosing, concentration, dosing interval, and use of accurate measuring device
Antipruritics (usually antihistamines)	Given orally or topically to block the histamine reaction Used to relieve discomfort associated with itching	• When applying topically, wear gloves • Do not apply to open wounds • Oral antihistamines may cause drowsiness

Adapted from Taketokmo, C. K., Hodding, J. H., & Kraus, D. M. (2013). *Lexi-comp's drug reference handbook: Pediatric & neonatal dosage handbook* (20th ed.). Hudson, OH: Lexi-comp, Inc.

Assessment

Assessment of the child with a communicable or infectious disorder includes health history, physical examination, and laboratory and diagnostic testing.

Health History

The health history consists of the past medical history, including the mother's pregnancy history; family history; and history of present illness (when the symptoms started and how they have progressed), as well as treatments used at home. The pregnancy and birth history may highlight incomplete maternal immunizations, maternal infection during pregnancy or labour, prolonged difficult delivery, immunocompromise, and prematurity. Family history might be significant for lack of immunization or recent contact with others who have infectious or communicable disease. When eliciting the history of the present illness, inquire about the following:

- Any known exposure to infectious or communicable disease
- Immunization history
- History of having any common childhood communicable diseases
- Fever
- Sore throat
- Lethargy
- Malaise
- Poor feeding or decreased appetite
- Vomiting
- Diarrhea
- Cough
- Rash (in the older child, ask for a description [i.e., Is it painful? Does it itch?])

Take Note!

Many childhood infections and communicable diseases involve a rash. Rashes can be difficult to identify. Therefore, it is important to obtain a thorough description and history from the caregiver.

Physical Examination

Physical examination of the child with an infectious disorder includes inspection, observation, and palpation.

INSPECTION AND OBSERVATION

Begin the physical examination with inspection and observation. Assess the child's skin, mouth, throat, and hair for lesions or wounds. Note the colour, shape, size, and distribution of any lesions or wounds. Assess whether there is any exudate from the lesions or wounds. A thorough and accurate description is important to assist in identifying the rash and causative organism. Observe for scratching, restlessness, avoidance of the use of a body part, or guarding of a body part.

Observe the child's affect, energy level, and interaction with caregivers. Lethargy can indicate serious infection or sepsis. Observe if there is any discharge from the nose, cough, or respiratory difficulty.

Assess hydration status. Inspect the oral mucosa; dry and pale mucous membranes can indicate dehydration. Observe for other signs of dehydration, such as sunken eyes, reduced urine output, and no tears with crying.

Assessment of vital signs can provide more information about the child's condition. Elevated temperature can indicate infection. Often tachypnea and tachycardia accompany fever. Hypotension may also occur, but it is usually a late sign with sepsis.

Take Note!

Neonates may not present with fever; some may be hypothermic (Smitherman & Macias, 2015).

PALPATION

Palpate the skin to assess temperature, moisture, texture, and turgor. In a child with an infectious or communicable disease, the skin may be warm and moist due to fever. Turgor may be decreased secondary to dehydration. In infants, palpate the fontanels; if they are sunken, the infant may be dehydrated. Palpate the rash to determine if it is raised or flat. A thorough picture of the presenting rash can help identify the child's illness. Palpate the lymph nodes and note any that are swollen and tender.

Laboratory and Diagnostic Testing

Common Laboratory and Diagnostic Tests 37.1 discusses the tests used most commonly when communicable disorders are suspected. The tests can assist the physician or nurse practitioner in diagnosing the disorder and/or be used as guidelines in determining ongoing treatment. Laboratory or nonnursing personnel obtain some of the tests, while the nurse might obtain others. In either instance, the nurse should be familiar with how the tests are obtained, what they are used for, and normal versus abnormal results. This knowledge will also be necessary when providing child and family education related to the testing.

Safety Check

GOAL: Improve the Effectiveness of Communication Among Caregivers

Report critical results of tests and diagnostic procedures on a timely basis

Steps: When caring for a child with a potential or actual infectious or communicable disorder, notify appropriate healthcare provider with positive culture results, and critical changes to other laboratory values and diagnostic test results

(text continues on page 1342)

COMMON LABORATORY AND DIAGNOSTIC TESTS 37.1

(REFER TO LOCAL REFERENCE RANGES)

Test	Explanation	Indications	Nursing Implications
Complete blood count (CBC)	Evaluate white blood cell count (particularly the percentage of individual white blood cells)	Detect the presence of inflammation, infection	Normal values vary according to age and gender • White blood cell count differential is helpful in differentiating source of infection • May be affected by myelosuppressive drugs
Erythrocyte sedimentation rate (ESR)	Nonspecific test used in conjunction with other tests to determine presence of infection or inflammation	Detect the presence of inflammation, infection	• Send to laboratory immediately; specimens allowed to stand for longer than 3 hours may produce a falsely low result
C-reactive protein (CRP)	Nonspecific test that measures a type of protein produced in the liver that is present during episodes of acute inflammation or infection Usually used to diagnose bacterial infections; does not consistently rise with viral infections	To detect the presence of infection, CRP is a more sensitive and rapidly responding indicator than ESR	• Presence of an intrauterine device may cause positive test results because of tissue inflammation • Exogenous hormones, such as oral contraceptives, may cause increased levels • Nonsteroidal anti-inflammatories, salicylates, and steroids may cause decreased levels • Fasting may be required
Blood culture and sensitivity	Deliberate growing of microorganism in a solid or liquid medium. Once it has grown, it is tested against various antibiotics to determine which antibiotics will kill it	Detect the presence of bacteria or yeast, which may have spread from a certain site in the body into the bloodstream Determine which antibiotics the bacteria or yeast is sensitive to	• Follow aseptic technique and hospital protocol to prevent contamination • Two cultures obtained from two different sites are preferred • Ideally obtain before administering antibiotics; if child is taking antibiotics, notify laboratory and draw specimen shortly before next dose • Draw below IV line, if possible, to prevent dilution of sample • Deliver specimen to laboratory immediately (within 30 minutes)
Stool culture (including stool for ova and parasites [O&P])	To determine if bacteria or parasite has infected the intestines	Detect pathogens, including parasites or overgrowth of normal flora in the bowel. Indicated for children with diarrhea, fever, or abdominal pain	• Stool must be free of urine, water, and toilet paper • Do not retrieve out of toilet water • Deliver to laboratory immediately • Mineral oil, barium, and bismuth interfere with the detection of parasites; specimen collection should be delayed for 7–10 days • Often a minimum of three specimens on 3 separate days are required for adequate examination, since many parasites and worm eggs are shed intermittently

COMMON LABORATORY AND DIAGNOSTIC TESTS 37.1 (continued)

Test	Explanation	Indications	Nursing Implications
Urine culture	Collection of urine to detect the presence of bacteria in the urine	Detect the presence of bacteria in the urinary tract. Indicated for children with fever of unknown origin, dysuria, frequency, or urgency, or if urinalysis suggests infection	• Should be obtained by midstream clean-catch, catheterization, or suprapubic aspiration. Avoid contamination with stool, vaginal secretions, hands, or clothing • Placing bags on the perineum is less acceptable due to high chance of contamination • Obtain before antibiotics are administered • Deliver to laboratory immediately (preferable) or refrigerate
Wound culture	Allows for microbial growth and identification of specific organism	Identification of specific organism	• Do not take from exudate or eschar • If moderate-to-heavy drainage present, irrigate the wound with sterile saline • Specimens taken from wounds can harbour a variety of organisms. Pathogenicity depends of the quantity of organisms present • Avoid touching intact skin at the wound edges • Culture highly vascular granulation tissue
Throat culture	Vigorous swabbing of the tonsillar area and posterior pharynx to detect the presence of invasive organisms	Most reliable method of detecting group A streptococcal pharyngitis Will also detect *Bordetella pertussis, Corynebacterium diphtheriae* May be performed in those with fever of unknown origin	• Ensure specimen is of secretions in the pharyngeal or tonsillar area. Avoid touching tongue or lips with swab • When performing on young children, have adult hold child in lap • Healthcare worker needs to stabilize head by placing hand on the child's forehead
Nasal swabs (nasopharyngeal)	Insertion of swabs into the nose until reaching the nasopharynx to detect the presence of invasive organisms	Optimal method for detecting *Bordetella pertussis*. Also used to detect *Corynebacterium diphtheria* and viral illnesses such as *respiratory syncytial virus (RSV)*, parainfluenza	• The distance from the child's nose to ear gives an estimate of how far to insert the swab into the nostril to reach the nasopharynx • Insert swab straight back, not up, and leave in nasopharynx for several seconds • When performing on young children, have adult hold child in lap • Healthcare worker needs to stabilize head as child will likely try to pull away

Adapted from Fischbach, F. T., & Dunning, M. B, III. (2015). *A manual of laboratory and diagnostic tests* (9th ed.). Philadelphia, PA: Wolters Kluwer Health/Lippincott Williams & Wilkins.

Clinical Laboratory test reference ranges comparing SI units to Traditional Units can be found at http://www.royalcollege.ca/portal/page/portal/rc/common/documents/exams/normal_values_e.pdf.

OBTAINING BLOOD SPECIMENS

Giving a blood specimen may be very frightening to children because of the fear of needles, pain, and blood loss. Provide atraumatic care when collecting blood samples from children. Whether the laboratory technician or the nurse is drawing the blood, the procedure should be performed in an area other than the child's bed, such as the treatment room; the child's bed should be kept as a "safe" area. Provide teaching about the procedure based on the child's developmental level and readiness to learn. In infants and younger children, additional assistance with positioning and safe holding will be needed to perform the procedure safely and to ensure proper collection. Use a topical anesthetic cream or gel, refrigerant spray, or iontophoresis before venipuncture.

The usual sites for obtaining blood specimens via venipuncture are the superficial veins of the dorsal surface of the hand or the antecubital fossa, although other locations may also be used. In specific situations, the jugular or femoral vein may be used; in this case, either the physician or nurse practitioner will perform the venipuncture.

Capillary puncture of the child's fingertip, the great toe, or the infant's heel may also be used to obtain blood specimens. Fingertip puncture is similar to that in the adult, directed to the sides of the fingertip. Great toe puncture is performed in the same way. Capillary heel puncture must be performed in the proper location to avoid striking the medial plantar artery or periosteum (see Nursing Procedure 37.1). Automatic lancet devices can be used to deliver a more precise puncture depth.

Atraumatic Care

The young infant will benefit from the use of oral sucrose and nonnutritive sucking before and during the capillary puncture (Naughton & Ikuta, 2013).

Occasionally, blood samples may be obtained from an artery rather than a vein or capillary. Blood gases in particular are usually obtained by arterial puncture. Arterial puncture requires additional training and, in many institutions, is performed only by the respiratory therapist, physician, or nurse practitioner.

NURSING PROCEDURE 37.1

Capillary Heel Puncture

1. Choose the collection site and apply a commercial heel warmer or warm pack for several minutes prior to specimen collection
2. Assemble equipment:
   - Gloves
   - Automatic lancet
   - Antiseptic wipe
   - Cotton ball or dry gauze
   - Capillary blood collection tube
   - Band-aid (ensure child has no allergy to adhesive plasters and any local policy regarding band-aid use in infants)
3. Perform hand hygiene and don gloves. Remove the warm pack
4. Cleanse the site with antiseptic prep pad and allow to dry
5. Hold the dorsum of the foot with the nondominant hand; with the dominant hand, pierce the heel with the lancet. Place the extremity in the dependent position
6. Wipe away the first drop of blood with the cotton ball or dry gauze
7. Collect the blood specimen with a capillary specimen collection tube. Avoid squeezing the foot during specimen collection if possible, as it may contribute to hemolysis of the specimen
8. Hold dry gauze over the site until bleeding stops, elevate extremity above the level of the heart, and then apply appropriate pressure or a band-aid

Children with indwelling venous access devices may be spared the trauma of puncture for blood specimens. Follow your institution's guidelines for withdrawing blood from peripherally inserted venous catheters or central venous catheters. The initial blood will be discarded to prevent contamination with intravenous fluids or medications. The amount discarded depends on the size of the catheter, the weight of the child, and the institution's guidelines. After aspirating the specimen, flush the venous access device with normal saline to prevent clogging. The device may then be reconnected to the intravenous fluid or flushed according to the institution's protocol.

Nursing Diagnoses, Goals, Interventions, and Evaluations

After completing a thorough assessment, the nurse might identify several nursing diagnoses, including:

- Risk for ineffective thermoregulation
- Impaired comfort
- Impaired skin integrity
- Risk for infection
- Deficient fluid volume
- Social isolation
- Deficient knowledge (specify)

> **After completing an assessment of Samuel, you note the following: rectal temperature of 39°C, poor sucking, and lethargy. Based on these assessment findings, what would your top three nursing diagnoses be for Samuel?**

Nursing goals, interventions, and evaluation for the child with a communicable or infectious disorder are based on the nursing diagnoses. Nursing Care Plan 37.1 (at the end of the chapter) provides a general guide for planning care for a child with an infectious or communicable disorder. Additional information about nursing management will be included later in the chapter as it relates to specific disorders.

Managing Fever

Fever in their children is one of the most common reasons parents seek medical attention (Enarson et al., 2012). Most infections or communicable diseases are accompanied by fever. Many parents have great concerns about fever often labelled as "fever phobia" (Kelly et al., 2017). For example, they fear febrile seizures, neurologic complications, and a potential serious underlying disease. Many healthcare providers may share these fears, highlighting the need for supportive education for both professionals and parents (Elkon-Tamir, Rimon, Scolnik, & Glatstein, 2017). Failure to

advise and/or recognize the fever cycle can result in overtreatment or use of inappropriate treatments, such as inappropriate dosing of antipyretics, awakening the child during sleep to give antipyretics, or inappropriate use of nonpharmacologic treatments such as sponging the child with alcohol or cold water (Ward, 2015b).

It is important to educate parents that fever is a protective mechanism the body uses to fight infection. Evidence exists that an elevated body temperature actually enhances various components of the immune response (Sullivan & Farrar, 2011). Fever can slow the growth of bacteria and viruses and increase neutrophil production and T-cell proliferation (Sullivan & Farrar, 2011). Another concern is that reducing fever may hide signs of serious bacterial illness (Sullivan & Farrar, 2011; Ward, 2015a).

Take Note!

Infants younger than 3 months of age with a rectal temperature greater than 38°C should be seen by a physician or nurse practitioner. They are considered at risk for sepsis until proven otherwise due to their immature immune system and inability to localize or handle infection very well (Nield & Kamat, 2011).

In infants older than 3 months of age, fever less than 39°C usually does not require treatment (Nield & Kamat, 2011). Antipyretics provide symptomatic relief but do not change the course of the infection. The major benefits of decreasing fever are increasing comfort in the child and decreasing fluid requirements, which helps to prevent dehydration. Children with certain underlying conditions, such as cardiovascular disease or pulmonary disease, also benefit from treating fever because such treatment decreases demands on the body.

Home Management of Fever

Fever is typically managed at home, so it is important to give guidance and instruction at well-child visits and review this information at subsequent visits. Written and video materials about fever management may be effective in increasing caregivers' knowledge. Parents can refer to the written instructions when needed (see Teaching Guidelines 37.1).

Teaching Guidelines 37.1
FEVER MANAGEMENT

- Fever is a sign of illness, not a disease; it is the body's weapon to fight infection.
- Diurnal variation may allow temperature changes as much as 1°C (1.8°F) over a 24-hour period, peaking in the evening.

• Antipyretics are used if the child demonstrates discomfort or pain, for example, with swallowing. Always check correct doses before administration. Be aware that over-the-counter medications often contain acetaminophen which puts the child at risk of receiving additional doses. Never give aspirin or aspirin-containing products to a child younger than 19 years with a fever due to the risk of Reye syndrome.

• In some children, fever can be associated with a seizure or dehydration, but this will not lead to brain damage or death. Discuss the facts about febrile seizures.

• Watch for the signs and symptoms of dehydration; it is important to provide oral rehydration by increasing fluid intake.

• Dress the child lightly and avoid warm, binding clothing or blankets.

• The use of sponging with tepid water is controversial; if used, encourage the parent to give an antipyretic prior to sponging. Ensure the sponging does not produce shivering (which causes the body to produce heat and maintain the elevated set point), and reinforce the importance of using tepid water, not cold water or alcohol. Instruct the parent to stop if the child experiences discomfort.

• Call the provider for:
  • Any child younger than 3 months of age who has a rectal temperature above 38°C (100.4°F).
  • Any child who is lethargic or listless, regardless of temperature.
  • Fever lasting more than 3–5 days.
  • Fever greater than 40.6°C (105°F).
  • Any child who is immunocompromised by illness, such as cancer or HIV, will need further evaluation and treatment.

The use of acetaminophen or ibuprofen to reduce fever in children has been shown to be safe and effective when the appropriate dose is administered at the appropriate interval (Ward, 2015b). However, some studies have shown that ibuprofen is superior in reducing fever and lasts longer than acetaminophen (Ward, 2015b).

Box 37.4 gives dosing recommendations for both medications.

Take Note!

Never give aspirin to children to reduce fever, due to the risk of Reye syndrome.

Acetaminophen is widely used and accepted, with a long track record of safety and efficacy when used according to the label directions, but overdose can lead

---

BOX 37.4

DOSE RECOMMENDATIONS FOR ORAL ACETAMINOPHEN AND IBUPROFEN

Acetaminophen, 10–15 mg/kg/dose
• No more than every 4 hours
• No more than five doses in a 24-hour period

Ibuprofen, 4–10 mg/kg/dose
• Only children older than 6 months of age
• No more than four doses in a 24-hour period

Adapted from Taketomo, C. K., Hodding, J. H., & Kraus, D. M. (2013). *Lexi-comp's drug reference handbook: Pediatric & neonatal dosage handbook* (20th ed.). Hudson, OH: Lexi-comp, Inc.

---

to toxic reactions (Ward, 2015b). Causes of acetaminophen toxicity include overdosing or incorrect dosing due to failure to read and understand the label instructions, use of an incorrect measuring device or concentration, and coadministration with an over-the-counter fixed-dose combination medication (the parent may not recognize that it has acetaminophen in it).

Another factor that may cause acetaminophen toxicity is the controversial, but common, practice of alternating acetaminophen and ibuprofen to help reduce fever. Studies of the use of alternating acetaminophen with ibuprofen have had conflicting results (Ward, 2015b). This practice can result in overdose or improper administration. It can be hard for parents to keep track of the time each medication is due. Parents may confuse which medication is given every 4 hours and which is given every 6 hours. They may exceed the recommended daily doses or may confuse the strength or dosage of the medicines. See Evidence-Based Practice 37.1.

Rx **Dosage Calculation**

The nurse is caring for a toddler who is 2 years old and 13 kg. The order reads Ibuprofen 100 mg PO every 6 hours as needed for temperature greater than 38°C. Dosing range 6 months to 12 years, 5–10 mg/kg/dose PO q6–8h. Is this a safe and effective dose?

Managing Skin Rashes

Skin rashes accompany many infectious or communicable diseases. These rashes can be very uncomfortable and irritating for the child. Management often occurs at home, so it is important to educate parents on ways to relieve the discomfort and protect and maintain skin integrity. The physician may prescribe antipruritics, including oral medications or topical creams or ointments (see Drug Guide 37.1). Instruct parents on the importance of maintaining skin integrity to prevent infection or scarring. Teach parents to keep their

EVIDENCE-BASED PRACTICE 37.1   IS ALTERNATING ACETAMINOPHEN WITH IBUPROFEN MORE EFFECTIVE THAN EITHER ONE ALONE?

Fever is one of the most common health concerns seen in pediatrics. Alternating paracetamol, also known as acetaminophen, and ibuprofen for fever reduction is a common practice, but there has been limited evidence on its safety or efficacy. It may be a harmful practice due to combined toxicity and potential parental confusion in timing and dosing.

STUDY

This study performed a meta-analysis of randomized controlled trials. A total of six studies were included resulting in 915 enrolled participants. It evaluated the effects and side effects of combining paracetamol (acetaminophen) and ibuprofen or alternating them compared with single antipyretic therapy in treating fever in children.

Findings

Review of the studies suggested that some evidence exists that combining or alternating antipyretics may be more effective at reducing temperature for up to 4 hours than single antipyretic therapy. Evidence supporting whether these practices improve a febrile child's discomfort were inconclusive. No serious side effects were attributed to these practices in these studies.

Nursing Implications

Although this study suggests improved fever reduction with alternating of acetaminophen and ibuprofen, safety concerns appear to remain. Further research with larger sample sizes, longer follow-up, and a focus on measuring child's discomfort and safety of combining or alternating antipyretic regimens is warranted. To alleviate some of the concerns that parents have with fever, nurses should consistently educate parents about why fever occurs and fever facts and myths as well as encourage recording of when medication is administered to minimize the risk of medication misuse or inadvertent overdose.

Adapted from Wong, T., Stang, A. S., Ganshorn, H., Hartling, L., Maconochie, I. K., Thomsen, A. M., & Johnson, D. W. (2013). Combined and alternating paracetamol and ibuprofen therapy for febrile children. *Cochrane Database of Systematic Reviews*, (10), CD009572. doi: 10.1002/14651858. CD009572.pub2. Retrieved from http://www.aub.edu.lb/fm/cri/Documents/Cochrane%20review-Alternating%20antipyretic.pdf.

child's fingernails short and hands clean. Explain the importance of discouraging scratching, and discuss distraction techniques they can use with the child. Cool compresses or cool baths can relieve itching. Encourage the child to press on rather than scratch the itchy area; this can relieve discomfort while maintaining skin integrity.

Thinking About Development

Lisa Hernandez is a 4-year-old with a history of fever, cold-like symptoms, and presents currently with an itchy rash. Based on her developmental stage, how will you instruct her and her caregiver on managing her rash at home? How would your instructions change if the child was 12 years old?

Based on your top three nursing diagnoses for Samuel, describe appropriate nursing interventions.

SEPSIS

Sepsis is a systemic overresponse to infection resulting from bacteria and viruses, which are the most common, fungi, viruses, rickettsia, or parasites (Thompson & Kissoon, 2014). It can lead to septic shock, which results in hypotension, low blood flow, and multisystem organ failure. Septic shock is a medical emergency and children are usually admitted to an intensive care unit. Sepsis alert tools, awareness campaigns, guidelines, screening, and management bundles link to national standards, provincial groups, and health authorities. The cause of sepsis may not be known, but common causative organisms in infants less than 3 months include *Escherichia coli*, group B *Streptococcus*, *Staphylococcus aureus*, enteroviruses, and herpes simplex virus, and in older children include *Neisseria meningitidis*, *Streptococcus pneumoniae*, and *S. aureus* (Pomerantz & Weiss, 2015). Sepsis can affect any age group but infants less than 3 months of age, immunocompromised children, and children with an indwelling vascular catheter are at higher risk (Pomerantz & Weiss, 2015). Neonates and young infants have a higher susceptibility due to their immature immune system, inability to localize infections, and lack of immunoglobulin M (IgM), which is necessary to protect against bacterial infections.

The prognosis for sepsis is variable and depends on the child's age and the cause of the sepsis. The mortality rate ranges from 9% to 35% (Santhanam, 2015). Neonates are at the highest risk for a poor outcome. Due to this high mortality rate, when an ill-appearing febrile neonate presents, a full workup is indicated (Nield & Kamat, 2011b). Usually, admission to the hospital to rule out sepsis is standard practice.

Pathophysiology

Sepsis results in the systemic inflammatory response syndrome (SIRS) due to infection. The pathophysiology of sepsis is complex. It results from the effects of circulating bacterial products or toxins, mediated by cytokine release, occurring as a result of sustained bacteremia. The pathogens cause an overproduction of proinflammatory cytokines, previously termed endotoxins. These cytokines are responsible for the clinically observable effects of the sepsis. Impaired pulmonary, hepatic, or renal function may result from excessive cytokine release during the septic process.

Therapeutic Management

Therapeutic management of sepsis in infants, especially neonates, is more aggressive than for older children. Neonates and infants with sepsis or even suspected sepsis are treated in the hospital. The infant is admitted for close monitoring along with antibiotic therapy. Intravenous antibiotics are started immediately after the blood, urine, and cerebrospinal fluid cultures have been obtained. The length of therapy and the specific antibiotic used will be determined based on the source of the positive culture and the results of the culture and sensitivity. If final culture reports are negative and symptoms have subsided, antibiotics may be discontinued (usually after 72 hours of treatment). If the child is not responding to therapy and symptoms worsen, sepsis may be progressing to shock. Management of the child with septic shock requires intensive treatment, most commonly in an ICU, or if in rural settings, a specialty trained care team follows intensive care protocols to stabilize the child before transfer.

Nursing Assessment

For a full description of the assessment phase of the nursing process, refer to the assessment section of the Nursing Process Overview earlier in this chapter. Patient Early Warning Screening (PEWS) tools have been developed as screening approaches to aid in recognitions of sepsis (e.g., Child Health BC, 2015). Local providers and children's hospitals across Canada are likely to use PEWS as decision support aids. Assessment findings pertinent to sepsis are discussed below.

HEALTH HISTORY

Elicit a description of the present illness and chief complaint. Signs of sepsis can vary with each child. Some common signs and symptoms reported during the health history might include:

- Child just does not look or act right
- Crying more than usual, inconsolable
- Fever

- Hypothermia (in neonates and those with severe disease)
- Lethargic and less interactive or playful
- Increased irritability
- Poor feeding or poor suck
- Rash (e.g., petechiae, ecchymosis, diffuse erythema)
- Difficulty breathing
- Nasal congestion
- Diarrhea
- Vomiting
- Decreased urine output
- Hypotonia
- Changes in mental status (confused, anxious, excited)
- Seizures
- Older child may complain of heart racing

Explore the child's current and past medical history for risk factors such as:
- Prematurity
- Lack of immunizations
- Immunocompromise
- Exposure to communicable pathogens

In neonates and young infants, seek pregnancy and labour risk factors such as:
- Premature rupture of membranes or prolonged rupture
- Difficult delivery
- Maternal infection or fever, including sexually transmitted infections
- Resuscitation and other invasive procedures
- Positive maternal group β-streptococcal vaginosis

Sepsis may occur in the hospitalized child. Assess for risk factors such as:
- ICU stay
- Presence of central line or other invasive lines or tubes
- Immunosuppression

Take Note!

Listen to the parents' descriptions of the neonate's or infant's behaviour and appearance, as well as changes they have observed. Many times they are the first to notice when their child is not acting right, even before clinical signs of infection are seen.

PHYSICAL EXAMINATION

Perform a thorough physical examination of the infant or child with proven or suspected sepsis. Specific findings related to inspection and observation are noted below.

Inspection and Observation. Observe the child's general appearance, colour, level of arousal, and hydration status. The child with sepsis may appear lethargic and pale and show signs of dehydration. In neonates and infants, observe the quality of their cry and reaction to parental stimulation, noting weak cry, lack of smile or facial expression, or lack of responsiveness. Inspect the skin for petechiae or other skin lesions. Petechiae may indicate a serious bacterial infection (often *N. meningitidis*), and other skin lesion patterns may help identify the cause of the fever. Observe respiratory effort and rate. The infant or child with sepsis may demonstrate tachypnea and increased work of breathing, such as nasal flaring, grunting, and retractions.

Assess and report vital signs, noting abnormalities. Note elevation in temperature or hypothermia in the young infant. Note tachypnea or tachycardia in the child or apnea or bradycardia in the infant. Document blood pressure. Hypotension, especially when accompanied by signs of poor perfusion, can be a sign of worsening sepsis with progression to shock.

LABORATORY AND DIAGNOSTIC TESTS

Symptoms of sepsis can be vague in infants. Therefore, laboratory tests play a crucial role in confirming or ruling out sepsis. Common laboratory and diagnostic studies ordered for the assessment of sepsis include:

- Complete blood count: WBC levels will be elevated; in severe cases, they may be decreased (this is an ominous sign).
- C-reactive protein: elevated
- Blood culture: positive in septicemia, indicating bacteria is present in the blood
- Urine culture: may be positive, indicating presence of bacteria in the urine
- Cerebrospinal fluid analysis: may reveal increased WBCs and protein and low glucose
- Stool culture: may be positive for bacteria or other infectious organisms
- Culture of tubes, catheters, or shunts suspected to be infected: the fluid inside these tubes may be tested for bacteria.
- Chest x-ray: may reveal signs of pneumonia such as hyperinflation and patchy areas of atelectasis or infiltration

Nursing Management

Monitor the infant or child closely for changes in condition, especially the development of shock. Administer antibiotics as ordered. Refer to Nursing Care Plan 37.1 at the end of the chapter for nursing diagnoses and related interventions. In addition to these interventions, it is important to prevent infection and provide education to the child and family.

PREVENTING INFECTION

Sepsis is a potentially life-threatening illness, and prevention is important. Handwashing is the most effective intervention against nosocomial infection. Nurses play a key role in minimizing environmental sources by cleaning equipment, disposing of soiled linens and dressings

properly, and adhering to proper aseptic technique with all invasive procedures. Follow your institution's policies and use evidence-based practice guidelines for interventions such as invasive line dressing changes and intravenous tubing changes to reduce the risk of infection. Encourage immunization as recommended. To reduce group *B. streptococcus* infection in neonates, screen pregnant woman. If the results are positive, administer intrapartum antibiotics.

Take Note!
There has been a dramatic reduction in invasive *Haemophilus influenzae* type B diseases since the widespread use of the Hib vaccine (Infectious Diseases and Immunization Committee, 2017).

EDUCATING THE CHILD AND FAMILY

Early recognition of the signs of sepsis is essential in preventing morbidity and mortality. Educate parents about the significance of fever, especially in neonates and infants younger than 3 months old. Instruct parents to contact their physician or nurse practitioner if their infant or neonate has a fever. A physician or nurse practitioner should see any child with a fever accompanied by lethargy, poor responsiveness, or lack of facial expressions. Signs and symptoms of sepsis can be vague and vary from child to child. Encourage parents to contact their physician or nurse practitioner if they feel their febrile child is "just not acting right."

BACTERIAL INFECTIONS

Bacteria are one-celled organisms that can live, grow, and reproduce. They exist everywhere. Most are completely harmless and some are very useful. Others can lead to disease either because they are in the wrong place in the body or they are designed to invade and cause disease in humans and animals. Children are at a high risk of developing bacterial infections, which can result in life-threatening illness. Fortunately, many bacterial diseases, such as diphtheria, pertussis, and tetanus, can be prevented by immunization.

Community-Acquired Methicillin-Resistant *Staphylococcus aureus*

Community-acquired MRSA (CAMRSA) is a staphylococcal infection that is resistant to certain antibiotics; in Canada, the prevalence of this pathogen has increased in the 21st century (Leifso, Gravel, Mounchili, Kaldas, & Le Saux, 2013). These infections range from minor skin rashes to abscesses to serious, complicated, life-threatening infections. Serious and invasive infections, such as bacteremia, pneumonia with empyema, meningitis, and osteomyelitis, often are secondary to a skin or soft tissue infection.

Transmission occurs through direct person-to-person contact, respiratory droplets, blood, or sharing personal items, such as hair brushes, towels, and sports equipment, and touching surfaces or items contaminated with MRSA. Clusters of MRSA have been found in day care centres, among athletic teams, youth who experience homelessness as well as higher rates in Indigenous communities (Canadian Paediatric Society, 2017). *Staphylococci* are resistant to heat and drying and can be found on environmental surfaces months after contamination. Intact skin and mucous membranes, along with proper hand hygiene, are the best barriers to MRSA.

Nursing Assessment

In the child, skin and tissue infections are common infections caused by CAMRSA. Symptoms include a bump or skin area that is red, swollen, painful, and warm to touch. It may also include fever, fluctuance, and purulent drainage. The lesion may have appeared suddenly and be red and raised, resembling an insect bite. Necrotic areas may develop. Abscesses, especially abscessed hair follicles, and pimples are common presentations. Assessment needs to include a thorough past medical history to determine history of recurrent skin infections with or without complete resolution along with assessment for risk factors. Risk factors include frequent skin-to-skin contact; openings in the skin/skin trauma, such as abrasions and cuts; contact with potentially contaminated personal items, equipment and surfaces; poor hygiene; limited access to health care; frequent exposure to antimicrobial agents and crowded living conditions (Kaplan, 2015).

Diagnosis is determined through culture. Diagnostic tests include incision and drainage (I&D), aspiration of the abscess, and culturing the fluid or tissue. Antimicrobial susceptibility along with culture is critical.

Nursing Management

Care of the child with CAMRSA will typically occur at home. Antibiotics with microbial susceptibility will often be prescribed. Comprehensive wound care, which may include I&D, may occur. Follow-up for reassessment is key. Child and family education is crucial. Include the following in the teaching plan:

- Educate the family on the importance of taking the antibiotics as directed and finishing all the medicine. Emphasize that this will help slow the creation of antimicrobial-resistant organisms.
- Teach the child and parents proper hand hygiene and handwashing.
- Discourage family members from sharing personal items.
- Explain the risk factors involved in transmission.

- Explain the importance of keeping cuts and scrapes cleaned and covered.
- Review the signs of MRSA and emphasize the importance of early recognition and treatment.

Scarlet Fever

Scarlet fever is an infection resulting from group A streptococci. It usually occurs with a group A streptococci throat infection (i.e., strep throat) or rarely streptococcal skin infection. However, in the case of scarlet fever, the bacteria produce a toxin that causes a rash. Not all children with a group A streptococci infection will develop the rash of scarlet fever. Only children who are infected with streptococci that produce pyrogenic exotoxins and do not have antitoxin antibodies, making them sensitive to the bacterial toxin, will develop scarlet fever (Gerber, 2011). Scarlet fever is usually seen in children 5 to 12 years of age and is rare in children younger than 2 years old (Zabawski, 2014). Transmission is through droplets and follows contact with respiratory tract secretions. Transmission is facilitated by the type of close contact that occurs in schools and child care centres.

Statistics Canada (2015) reports zero mortality rate from scarlet fever (Statistics Canada, 2015). Rare but serious complications such as rheumatic fever, glomerulonephritis, skin infections, abscesses of the throat, pneumonia, and arthritis can still occur, and therefore prompt recognition and proper treatment are important (Government of Canada, 2013).

Nursing Assessment

Symptoms of scarlet fever begin abruptly. The health history may reveal a fever greater than 38.5°C, chills, body aches, sore throat and difficulty swallowing as well as loss of appetite, and nausea (Healthwise Staff, 2016). Inspect the pharynx, which is usually very red and swollen. The tonsils may have yellow or white specks of pus, and cervical lymph nodes may be swollen. Inspect the skin for the most striking symptom of scarlet fever, which is an erythematous rash appearing on the face, trunk, and extremities. The rash is typically absent from the palms and soles of the feet. It looks like a sunburn but feels like sandpaper (Fig. 37.1A). The rash lasts approximately 5 days and is followed by desquamation, typically on the fingers and toes. Early in the illness the tongue develops a thick coat with a strawberry appearance. The tongue will later lose the coating and become bright red (Fig. 37.1B).

Diagnosis is made by identification of group A streptococcus on throat culture. Several rapid tests for group A streptococcal pharyngitis are available. The accuracy of these tests depends on the quality of the specimen. It is important that the secretions obtained are pharyngeal

FIGURE 37.1 **A.** Rash of scarlet fever. **B.** Strawberry tongue.

or tonsillar (see Common Medical Treatments 37.1 for more information on throat cultures).

Nursing Management

Children with scarlet fever are usually cared for at home. Penicillin V is the antibiotic of choice (Healthwise Staff, 2016). In those sensitive to penicillin, erythromycin may be used. Educate the family on the importance of taking the antibiotic as directed and finishing all the medicine.

Encourage fluid intake to maintain adequate hydration due to fever. Teach parents ways to provide comfort for the child. A cool mist humidifier can soothe the child's sore throat. Soft foods, warm liquids like soup, or cold foods like popsicles may also be helpful. If the child is hospitalized, droplet precautions, along with standard precautions, are necessary.

Diphtheria

Diphtheria is caused by infection with *Corynebacterium diphtheriae* and may affect the nose, larynx, tonsils, or pharynx. Tonsillar and pharyngeal infections are the most common and will be the focus of this discussion. A pseudomembrane forms over the pharynx, uvula, tonsils, and soft palate (Fig. 37.2). The neck becomes edematous and lymphadenopathy develops. The pseudomembrane causes airway obstruction and suffocation. Diphtheria is rare in the developed countries but is reappearing in some regions and continues to be a serious disease worldwide due to lack of routine immunization (Public Health Agency of Canada, 2014a, 2014b, 2014c, 2014d). Risk factors include

children and adults who are unimmunized or under-immunized, living in crowded or unsanitary living conditions, having a compromised immune system, and travelling to developing countries where diphtheria remains endemic (Public Health Agency of Canada, 2014a, 2014b, 2014c, 2014d). Routine infant immunization can prevent the disease. Therapeutic management involves administration of antibiotics and antitoxin, as well as airway management.

FIGURE 37.2 In diphtheria, a pseudomembrane forms over the pharynx, uvula, tonsils, and soft palate.

Nursing Assessment

Children at risk for diphtheria are those who are unimmunized. Note history of sore throat and fever, usually less than 38.9°C. As the pseudomembrane forms, swallowing becomes difficult and signs of airway obstruction become apparent. A specimen of the membrane may be cultured for *C. diphtheriae*.

Nursing Management

Close observation of respiratory status is of utmost importance. Administration of antibiotics and the antitoxin is critical to encourage sloughing of the membrane. The child should remain on strict droplet precautions in addition to standard precautions and should maintain bed rest.

Pertussis

Pertussis is an acute respiratory disorder characterized by paroxysmal cough (whooping cough) and copious secretions. The highest incidence is seen in children younger than 1 year of age, and children younger than 3 months of age are at the greatest risk for severe disease and death (Public Health Agency of Canada, 2014a, 2014b, 2014c, 2014d). The disease is caused by *Bordetella pertussis*. The incubation period is 6 to 21 days, usually 7 to 10 days. Pertussis usually starts with 7 to 10 days of cold symptoms. The paroxysmal coughing spells then begin and can last 1 to 4 weeks. Convalescence occurs over the course of several weeks to months. Initially, immunization decreased the incidence of pertussis, but there was a gradual increase until the 1990s likely related to low efficacy of the whole-cell vaccine introduce in the early to mid-1980s and the implementation of the adolescent immunization program in 2005 to 2011. As a result, all provinces have reported a steady decline in the incidence of pertussis (Smith, Rotondo, Desai, & Deehan, 2014). However, in 2012, there was an increase in pertussis cases across the nation in all age groups, with the highest incidence in infants less than 1 year (Smith et al., 2014). Complications of pertussis include hypoxia, apnea, pneumonia, seizures, encephalopathy, and death. Mortality reported in the 2009 communicable disease report indicated a total of 6 deaths in Canada from 2000 to 2009 in which were attributed pertussis and 78% of those deaths occurred in infants less than 2 months of age (Smith et al., 2014).

Therapeutic Management

Therapeutic management of pertussis focuses on eradicating the bacterial infection and providing respiratory support. CDC guidelines recommend antimicrobial treatment (CDC, 2012a). For infants older than 1 month of age, macrolide drugs, including erythromycin, clarithromycin, and azithromycin, are the drugs of choice (CDC, 2015a). For younger infants, azithromycin should be used and erythromycin and clarithromycin avoided (CDC, 2015a). An alternative to macrolides in children older than 2 months is trimethoprim–sulfamethoxazole (TMP-SMZ) (CDC, 2015a). A course of macrolide antibiotics is also recommended to treat all close contacts regardless of age or immunization status (CDC, 2012a, 2015b). Also, all close contacts who are younger than 7 years of age and who are unimmunized or underimmunized should have pertussis immunization initiated or the series completed according to the recommended dosing schedule (CDC, 2012a).

> **Take Note!**
>
> In 2013, Health Canada issued a warning that azithromycin may cause potentially fatal heart rhythm in some patients because it can lead to abnormal changes in the electrical activity of the heart (Government of Canada, 2013). Therefore, when treating pertussis in children at risk for cardiovascular events, such as children with prolonged QT interval, alternative drugs should be considered.

Nursing Assessment

The most important risk factor for the development of pertussis is lack of immunization. The history may reveal cold and cough symptoms, progressing to paroxysmal coughing spells. During the paroxysms, the child might cough 10 to 30 times in a row, followed by a whooping sound. This might be accompanied by redness in the face, progressive cyanosis, and protrusion of the tongue. Saliva, mucus, and tears flow from the mouth, nose, and eyes. Between the paroxysmal episodes, the child might rest well and appear relatively unaffected. Auscultate the lungs to assess air exchange. The diagnosis may be confirmed by a variety of laboratory tests accompanied by clinical history. Culture is considered the gold standard, but polymerase chain reaction (PCR) is now used by many laboratories due to its increased sensitivity and faster results (CDC, 2012a).

Nursing Management

Nursing care will focus on providing a high-humidity environment and frequent suctioning to mobilize secretions. Observe for signs of airway obstruction. Encourage fluids to keep secretions thin and maintain adequate hydration. Offer reassurance to the child and family; the coughing episodes can be very frightening. Droplet precautions along with standard precautions are necessary for the hospitalized child.

Tetanus

Tetanus is an acute, often fatal neurologic disease caused by the toxins produced by *Clostridium tetani*. Tetanus is rare in Canada but continues to be significant worldwide due to lack of routine immunization (Public Health Agency of Canada, 2014a, 2014b, 2014c, 2014d). It is characterized by increased muscle tone and spasm. *C. tetani* spores can live anywhere but are found most commonly in soil, dust, and feces from humans or animals, such as sheep, cattle, chickens, dogs, cats, and rats. The spores can enter the body through a wound that is contaminated, through a burn, or by injecting contaminated street drugs. Once it enters the body, an anaerobic environment allows it to multiply and a poisonous toxin is released.

There are four forms of tetanus. Neonatal tetanus is the most common worldwide, affecting newborns in the first week of life secondary to an infected umbilical stump or unsterile surgical technique during circumcision in infants whose mothers were poorly immunized (Arnon, 2011). Most women have been immunized and will pass the immunity to their fetus. Also, proper hygiene during delivery and adequate cord care make this type rare, but in underdeveloped countries, it remains a significant problem (Sexton, 2015). The second form is local tetanus. This rare form is characterized by local muscle spasms within the area of the wound. The third type is cephalic tetanus, which is associated with recurrent otitis media or head trauma. It is also rare and affects the cranial nerves, especially facial nerves. Generalized tetanus is the most common and severe form and in half of patients will present with trismus (masseter muscle spasm or lockjaw) (Sexton, 2015). Symptoms then progress in a descending fashion with tonic contraction of the skeletal muscles and intermittent intense, painful muscular spasms. The most profoundly affected muscles are those of the neck and back.

In Canada, the fatality rate associated with tetanus has declined and cases are rare, but 10% to 80% of cases will result in death in unvaccinated individuals, with the highest rates in infants and the elderly (Public Health Agency of Canada, 2014a, 2014b, 2014c, 2014d). The general incubation period is 3 to 21 days, with an average of 8 days. Recovery can be long and difficult, and children with tetanus may have to spend several weeks in the hospital in an intensive care setting. Complications associated with tetanus include breathing problems, fractures, elevated blood pressure, dysrhythmias, clotting in the blood vessels of the lung, pneumonia, and coma.

Therapeutic Management

Therapeutic management is directed toward supporting respiratory and cardiovascular function, stopping toxin production, neutralizing unbound toxins, and controlling muscle spasms. Tetanus immunoglobulin may be given as well as the tetanus vaccine. Removal of the offending organism, by debridement of the wound, may occur, and intravenous antibiotics such as metronidazole may be initiated. In severe cases, the child may require intensive nursing care with mechanical ventilation.

Nursing Assessment

Note history of initial signs such as headache, spasms, crankiness, and cramping of the jaw (lockjaw), which are followed by difficulty swallowing and a stiff neck. Teta-

nus progresses in a descending fashion to other muscle groups, causing spasms of the neck, arms, legs, and stomach; seizures may result. Document the presence of fever along with an elevated blood pressure and tachycardia. Opisthotonos may be noted due to severe spasms of the neck and back. The spasms or muscle contractions in children may be strong enough to result in fractures. The diagnosis of tetanus is based on the clinical findings of the history and physical examination. There is no laboratory test to confirm tetanus.

Nursing Management

Nursing management focuses on observing for signs of respiratory distress. Provide a quiet environment with reduced external stimuli to decrease the incidence of spasms. Appropriately manage pain. Encourage adequate nutrition and hydration. Administer sedatives and muscle relaxants as ordered to reduce the pain associated with the muscle spasms and to prevent seizures. Encourage the parents to stay with their child. The child's mental status is unaffected by the disease, and therefore he or she is aware of what is happening. Efforts need to be made to reduce the child's anxiety and to provide reassuring, sympathetic care to the child and family. Tetanus is not contagious from person to person; therefore, standard precautions are sufficient.

Tetanus is a preventable but potentially fatal disease. Education is essential regarding the importance of receiving this routine immunization, as well as a booster every 10 years. Instructing parents on proper wound care can also help prevent tetanus. All wounds should be cleaned thoroughly and a proper antiseptic used. If a wound is deep and contamination is suspected, the child should be seen by a physician or nurse practitioner. If it has been more than 5 years since the last tetanus dose, a booster may be needed. This can help to neutralize the poison and prevent it from entering the nervous system.

Botulism

Botulism is a disease that is caused by a toxin produced in the immature intestines of young children resulting from infection with the bacterium *Clostridium botulinum*. It is rare but can cause serious paralytic illness. There are several types of botulism. Food-borne botulism results from ingestion of food contaminated with botulinum toxin. Wound botulism results from wounds infected with *C. botulinum*. Infant botulism is the most common in Canada and results from the ingestion of *C. botulinum* spores, most often from environmental dust. *C. botulinum* is common in soil and can also be found in a variety of foods, such as improperly preserved home-canned foods. It has been associated with feeding honey and corn syrup to infants; thus, these should be avoided in children younger than 1 year of age (Public

Health Agency of Canada, 2012a, 2012b). The disease is not infectious; to become infected, the child must ingest the bacterial spores. These spores then multiply in the intestinal tract and produce the toxin, which is absorbed in the immature intestines of the infant. It is generally not a problem for older children because the bacteria do not grow well in mature intestines due to the presence of the normal intestinal flora. Prognosis is good, but if treatment is not initiated, paralysis of the arms, legs, trunk, and respiratory system can develop. Therapeutic management is usually supportive but may involve administration of botulinum immune globulin or botulism antitoxin.

Nursing Assessment

For a full description of the assessment phase of the nursing process, refer to the assessment section of the Nursing Process Overview earlier in this chapter. Assessment findings pertinent to botulism are discussed below.

HEALTH HISTORY

Elicit a description of the present illness and chief complaint. Signs and symptoms usually occur soon after ingestion of the bacteria. Common signs and symptoms in infants reported during the health history might include:
- Constipation
- Poor feeding
- Listlessness
- Generalized weakness
- Weak cry

Common signs and symptoms in older children reported during the health history might include:
- Double vision
- Blurred vision
- Drooping eyelids
- Difficulty swallowing
- Slurred speech
- Muscle weakness

PHYSICAL EXAMINATION AND LABORATORY AND DIAGNOSTIC TESTS

Assess for a diminished gag reflex, which is indicative of botulism. Diagnostic tests include cultures of stool and serum. Botulism is a rare disease and is difficult to diagnose since its symptoms are similar to those of other neuromuscular diseases. Therefore, assessment may include diagnostic tests to help rule out other diseases, such as Guillain–Barré syndrome, stroke, and myasthenia gravis.

Nursing Management

Treatment is mainly supportive and focuses on maintaining respiratory status and nutritional status. If ordered, administer botulinum immune globulin early in the disease to reduce its severity and progression. Two botulism

antitoxins are available in Canada either at a provincial depot or through the Public Health Agency of Canada's National Emergency Stockpile System (NESS). Prevention is the focus in illuminating botulism through proper hygiene and safe food processing such as inspecting canned food for any risks, best before dates, refrigeration, and not feeding honey to infants under 1 year of age (Public Health Agency of Canada, 2012a, 2012b).

Osteomyelitis

Osteomyelitis is a bacterial infection of the bone and soft tissue surrounding the bone. The long bone metaphysis is the most common location (Haut, 2014). *S. aureus* is the most common infecting organism with methicillin-resistant *S. aureus* (MRSA) infections on the rise (Haut, 2014). Additional causes in infants and children include group A and B streptococcus, *E. coli*, *S. pneumoniae*, *Kingella kingae*, and *Haemophilus influenzae* (which is now rare due to improvements in immunizations) (Haut, 2014; Krogstad, 2014b). Children usually present for evaluation within a few days to a week of onset of symptoms, though some may present later.

Osteomyelitis is acquired hematogenously (spread through the blood). Bacteria from the bloodstream mainly invade the most rapidly growing portion of the bone. The invading bacteria trigger an inflammatory response, formation of pus and edema, and vascular congestion. Small blood vessels thrombose and the infection extends into the metaphyseal marrow cavity. As the infection progresses, the inflammation extends throughout the bone and blood supply is disrupted, resulting in death of the bone tissues (Fig. 37.3).

Therapeutic Management

Aspiration is necessary to confirm diagnosis and identify specific microorganisms. Treatment includes a 4- to 6-week course of antibiotics. Some children may receive 1 to 2 weeks of intravenous antibiotics and then be switched to oral antibiotics for the remainder of the course. Surgical debridement is rarely necessary. Early treatment may prevent the complications of bone destruction, fracture, and growth arrest. Additional complications include recurrent infection, septic arthritis, and systemic infection.

Nursing Assessment

For a full description of the assessment phase of the nursing process, refer to the assessment section of the Nursing Process Overview earlier in this chapter. Assessment findings pertinent to osteomyelitis are discussed here.

Explore the health history for risk factors and symptoms. Risk factors include impetigo, infected varicella lesions, furunculosis, recent trauma, infected burns, and prolonged intravenous line use. Obtain history of current

FIGURE 37.3 In osteomyelitis, bacterial invasion leads to infection within the bone.

or recent antibiotic therapy and response. Note history of irritability, lethargy, possible fever, and onset of pain or change in activity level. The child usually refuses to walk and demonstrates decreased range of motion in the affected extremity. Inspect the affected extremity for swelling. Palpate for local warmth and tenderness. Note point tenderness over affected bone.

Laboratory and diagnostic testing may reveal:
- Elevated white blood cell count, erythrocyte sedimentation rate, and C-reactive protein level
- Positive blood cultures
- Deep soft tissue swelling on radiography
- Changes on ultrasound, CT scan, or MRI

Nursing Management

Nursing management of the child with osteomyelitis focuses on assessment, pain management, and maintenance of intravenous access for administration of antibiotics. Individualize care based on the child's and family's response to the illness; see Nursing Care Plan 37.1 at the end of the chapter. Maintain bed rest initially to prevent injury and promote comfort. Administer antipyretics as ordered if the child is febrile in the initial stage of the illness. Encourage the use of unaffected extremities by providing developmentally appropriate toys and games. Instruct the child and family on safe and proper use of crutches or walker if prescribed. Some children will be discharged home on intravenous antibiotics, while others will finish an oral antibiotic course. Teach parents proper administration of medications and maintenance of a peripherally inserted central

catheter or central line at home if the child is finishing the antibiotic course intravenously.

Septic Arthritis

Acute septic arthritis is a condition in which bacteria invade the joint space, most often the hip or knee. It can occur at any age but usually occurs in children younger than 3 years old (Krogstad, 2014a). Usually, bacteria gain access to the joint through the bloodstream but can be due to direct puncture from injections, venipuncture, wound infection, surgery, or injury.

S. aureus is the most common causative organism with CAMRSA on the rise (Krogstad, 2014a). Various streptococci species, *K. kingae, N. meningitidis* (with or without an associated meningitis), *H. influenzae* (in unvaccinated children), and *Neisseria gonorrhoeae* are also responsible organisms (Krogstad, 2014a). Sepsis of the hip joint may cause avascular necrosis of the femoral head due to pressure on blood vessels and cartilage within the joint space. Septic arthritis is considered a medical emergency, as destruction of the joint cartilage may occur within just a few days. Additional complications of septic arthritis include permanent deformity, leg-length discrepancy, and long-term decreased range of motion and disability.

The goals of treatment of septic arthritis are to prevent destruction of the joint cartilage and maintain function, motion, and strength. Septic arthritis is treated rapidly with joint aspiration or arthrotomy, followed by intravenous antibiotic therapy while in the hospital and oral antibiotics at home.

Nursing Assessment

Note a history of predisposing factors such as respiratory infection or otitis media, skin or soft tissue infections, or, in the neonate, traumatic puncture wounds and femoral venipunctures. The history is usually significant for sudden onset of fever and moderate-to-severe pain.

Upon physical examination, the infant or child appears ill. Note extent of fever, reports of pain, refusal to bear weight or straighten the joint, and limited range of motion (the child usually maintains the joint in flexion and will not allow the leg to be straightened). The child will generally hold the joint in a position of comfort and the child or infant will appear without pain as long as the joint is immobile. Any attempt at passive range of motion will reveal pain. Palpate the affected joint for warmth and swelling.

Laboratory findings may include:
- White blood cell count normal or elevated with elevated neutrophil counts
- Elevated erythrocyte sedimentation rate and C-reactive protein levels
- Fluid from joint aspiration demonstrates elevated white blood cell count; culture determines responsible organism.

- Joint x-ray may show subtle soft tissue changes or increase in the joint space.
- Positive blood culture for the causative organism (15% of cases)

Nursing Management

Refer to Nursing Care Plan 37.1 at the end of the chapter for interventions related to musculoskeletal disorders. Assess aspiration wound for signs of infection. Monitor vital signs for resolution of fever. Pain management with ibuprofen or acetaminophen will be sufficient for some children; others may initially require opioid analgesia. Assess the affected joint for a decrease in swelling, increasing range of motion, and decreasing or absence of pain. The child may be discharged after 72 hours of intravenous antibiotics following joint aspiration if he or she is improving and can tolerate oral antibiotics. At discharge, if the child cannot ambulate, physical therapy may be consulted for short-term use of crutches or a wheelchair. Teach families how to assess for signs and symptoms of wound infection, how to administer oral antibiotics and pain medication, and how to assist their child with crutch walking.

VIRAL INFECTIONS

Viruses are very small particles that infect cells. They cannot multiply on their own and require a living host, such as humans, animals, or plants. They can reproduce only by invading and taking over the host cells. Young children are highly sensitive to viruses; their resistance is low and exposure is high. Viruses are hard to destroy without damaging or killing the living cells they infect. Therefore, drugs are not used to control them. However, many viral diseases can be prevented by immunization, such as measles, rubella, varicella, mumps, and poliomyelitis.

Viral Exanthems

Many viral infections of the skin in childhood are called viral exanthems. **Exanthem** means rash or skin eruption. Viral exanthems of childhood often present with a distinct rash pattern that assists in the diagnosis of the virus. Table 37.4 discusses common childhood exanthems. Immunizations have led to a decrease in the incidence of certain viral exanthems, such as measles, rubella, and varicella.

TABLE 37.4	COMMON VIRAL EXANTHEMS OF CHILDHOOD
Disease	**Clinical Manifestations**
Rubella (German measles) • Caused by rubella virus • Transmission: by direct or indirect contact with droplets, primarily by naso-pharyngeal secretions, but also in blood, stool, and urine. Also transmitted from mother to fetus • Peak incidence: late winter and early spring • Incubation period: 12–21 days (usually 14) • Communicable: 7 days before to 7 days after onset of rash Rubella rash. (Courtesy of CDC. [1966]. Obtained at http://phil.cdc.gov/PHIL_Images/03052002/00002/PHIL_712_lores.jpg)	• Rash usually first sign. Maculopapular rash that begins on face and spreads head to foot; disappears in the same order it spread, usually by the third day. On the second day, the rash may appear pinpoint. Desquamation is minimal • In older children: lymphadenopathy (retroauricular, posterior cervical, postoccipital) 24 hours before the onset of the rash; lasting up to 1 week; low-grade fever, malaise, upper respiratory symptoms • Mild pruritus • Polyarthralgia and polyarthritis (rare in children but common in adolescents)

Typically, children with viral exanthems are cared for at home, but there are times when a child may be hospitalized or may develop the disease while being hospitalized. Appropriate transmission-based precautions must be taken. Therapeutic management of the viral exanthems focuses on fever management and relief of discomfort.

Nursing Assessment

Obtain the history of the present illness, noting the onset of rash in relation to the onset of fever. Note accompanying symptoms such as respiratory complaints. Document known exposure to childhood diseases. Note immunization status. Inspect the skin for rash, noting the distribution, type, and extent of lesions. Table 37.4 describes the rash as well as accompanying symptoms for each of the viral exanthems.

Nursing Management

Nursing management of viral exanthems focuses on fever reduction, relief of discomfort, and protection of skin integrity. Encourage hydration. Administer antipyretics and antipruritics as needed (refer to

Drug Guide 37.1). Nonpharmacologic interventions to reduce fever, such as tepid sponging and cool compresses, may be used. Refer to Nursing Care Plan 37.1 at the end of the chapter for additional information. Care should be individualized based on the child's and family's response to the illness.

Take Note!

Trim the child's fingernails or cover hands with mitts, gloves, or socks (which work well with younger infants and children) if the rash itches to help prevent breaks in the skin, which can lead to discomfort and infection.

Mumps

Mumps, a contagious disease caused by Paramyxovirus, is characterized by fever and parotitis (inflammation and swelling of the parotid gland). Mumps is spread via contact with infected droplets. Infected individuals are contagious for up to 7 days prior to the onset of symptoms and from onset of symptoms to 9 days after parotid swelling begins (Public Health Agency of Canada, 2014a, 2014b, 2014c,

(*text continues on page 1360*)

Management/Complications	Nursing Implications
• Usually mild and self-limiting • Treatment is mainly supportive • Complications: encephalitis and thrombocytopenia (rare) • Maternal rubella during pregnancy can result in miscarriage, fetal death, or congenital malformations	• Comfort measures such as antipyretics, antipruritics, and analgesics for joint pain

TABLE 37.4	COMMON VIRAL EXANTHEMS OF CHILDHOOD (continued)

Disease	Clinical Manifestations
Rubeola (measles) • Caused by measles virus • Transmission: direct or indirect contact with droplets, primarily by nasopharyngeal secretions, but also blood and urine. Highly contagious • Peak incidence: late winter and spring • Incubation period: 7–18 days • Communicable 1 day before the onset of symptoms (4 days before onset of rash) until 4 days after rash has appeared 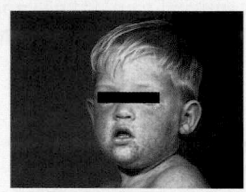 Koplik spots. (Courtesy of CDC/Dr. Heinz F. Eichenwald. [1958]. Obtained at http://phil.cdc.gov/phil/details.asp?pid=3187); Ruboela. (Courtesy of CDC [1963]; Obtained at http://phil.cdc.gov/phil/details.asp?pid=1150)	• Symptoms begin 7–18 days after the infection, consisting of fever, cough, coryza, conjunctivitis • Followed by Koplik spots (white spots on the inner lining of the mouth) • Erythematous maculopapular rash appears 14 days after the infection. Rash usually lasts 4–7 days, gradually proceeds from head downward and outward
Varicella zoster (chickenpox) • Caused by varicella zoster virus, human herpes virus 3 • Transmission: direct contact with infected persons' nasopharyngeal secretions or via airborne spread, to a lesser degree by contact with unscabbed lesions. Highly contagious. Also transmitted from mother to fetus • Peak incidence: late fall, winter, and spring • Incubation period: 10–21 days, usually 14–16 days • Most contagious 1–2 days before the onset of rash and shortly after the rash appears; however, the disease is communicable 1–2 days before until all vesicles have crusted over (about 3–7 days after the onset of rash) Varicella. (Courtesy of CDC/Dr. John Noble, Jr. [1968]. Obtained at http://phil.cdc.gov/phil/details.asp)	• Prodromal symptoms (fever, malaise, anorexia, headache, mild abdominal pain) may be present 24–48 hours before the onset of the rash. In children, rash is often the first sign of disease • Lesions often appear first on scalp, face, trunk, then extremities; initially intensely pruritic erythematous macules that evolve to papules and then form clear, fluid-filled vesicles • Vesicles eventually erupt, and then lesions scab and crust. A variety of lesions are present at one time • More severe in adolescents and adults than in young children
Exanthem subitum (roseola infantum or sixth disease) • Caused by human herpes virus 6 (HHV-6); two major strains of this virus, A and B with B being causative organism causing the primary infection in children • Transmission: little is known but suspected to be from saliva of infected person and enters the host through the oral, nasal, or conjunctival mucosa • Most cases present in the first 2 years of life and peak incidence: age 7–13 months • Incubation period: 5–15 days, average of 9 days • Most common in spring and fall • Communicability is unknown, but most likely contagious before symptoms appear 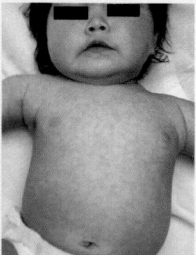 Exanthem subitum (roseola infantum)	• Prodromal phase: usually asymptomatic but may be listless and irritable • Clinical illness: high fever ranging from 37.9–40°C (101–106°F) for 3–5 days; resolves abruptly; diarrhea; rash appears 12–24 hours later, lasting about 2 days. Rash is maculopapular or erythematous lesions that blanch when touched. Rash is typically on the trunk and may spread to extremities

Management/Complications	Nursing Implications
• Treatment is mainly supportive, including antipyretics, bed rest, and adequate fluid intake • Possible vitamin A supplementation in children 6 months to 2 years hospitalized for measles or its complications or those with immunodeficiency[a] • Complications: diarrhea, otitis media, and pneumonia, common in young children; acute encephalitis; measles during pregnancy results in higher risk of premature labour, spontaneous abortion and low–birth-weight infants • Healthcare workers and other patients exposed to measles should have their immune status reviewed	• Comfort measures, such as antipyretics and antipruritics • Clean eyes with warm, moist cloth to remove secretions • Cool mist humidification to alleviate coryza and cough • Airborne precautions until 4 days after the onset of rash
• Usually self-limiting; treatment is mainly supportive: fever reduction, antipruritics, and skin care to prevent infection of lesions • Antiviral therapy and varicella zoster immune globulin may be used in those considered to be at high risk (immunocompromised, pregnant women, and newborns exposed to maternal varicella). Routine antiviral therapy is not recommended for the treatment of uncomplicated varicella infection in otherwise healthy children • Complications: bacterial superinfection of skin lesions, thrombocytopenia, arthritis, hepatitis, cerebellar ataxia, encephalitis, meningitis, pneumonia, glomerulonephritis, congenital infection, and life-threatening perinatal infection • Lifelong latent infection occurs; reactivation results in herpes zoster (shingles), uncommon in childhood	• Comfort measures, such as antipyretics and antipruritics • Airborne and contact precautions in the hospitalized child for a minimum of 5 days after the onset of rash and as long as vesicular lesions are present • For those with exposure to susceptible persons, airborne and contact precautions, from 8 to 21 days after exposure • Children may return to school or child care once lesions have crusted
• Course is generally benign • In children who are uncomfortable or irritable or have a history of febrile seizures, antipyretics may be warranted • Complications: HSV-6 may be responsible for some febrile seizures, encephalitis, and both meningoencephalitis and hepatitis (extremely rare)	• Comfort measures, such as antipyretics and antipruritics • Standard precautions are sufficient in the hospitalized child

(continued)

TABLE 37.4	COMMON VIRAL EXANTHEMS OF CHILDHOOD (continued)

Disease	Clinical Manifestations
Erythema infectiosum (fifth disease) • Caused by human parvovirus B19 • Transmitted by large droplet spread from nasopharyngeal viral shedding or percutaneous exposure to blood and blood products. Also transmitted from mother to fetus • Peak incidence late winter and early spring • Incubation period: 4–28 days, average 16–17 days • Communicability is uncertain, but most children are no longer infectious by the time the rash appears and diagnosis is made, so isolation or exclusion from school, once the child is diagnosed, is unnecessary (those with aplastic crisis may be communicable up to 1 week after the onset of symptoms and those who are immunosuppressed with chronic infection and severe anemia may be communicable for months to years) Erythema infectiosum (fifth disease)	• Prodromal phase: mild symptoms, low-grade fever, headache, mild upper respiratory infection • Characteristic rash occurs in three stages: • Begins with erythematous flushing often described as "slapped-cheek" appearance, often with circumoral pallor • Spreads to trunk • Moves peripherally, appearing as a maculopapular, lace-like appearance; often pruritic • Palms and soles are usually spared. Rash fluctuates in intensity and will disappear and reappear with environmental changes such as exposure to sunlight • Resolves spontaneously over 1–3 weeks • Pain or swelling in joints may be present • Children with pre-existing anemias may develop aplastic crisis (will have fever, malaise, myalgia, but usually no rash)
Hand, foot, and mouth disease, or herpangina (if only mouth involvement) • Caused by viruses belonging to enterovirus genus. Coxsackie A viruses (especially A16) is the most common. Transmitted by direct contact with infected fecal, oral secretions; spread mostly through saliva • Peak incidence during spring and summer, particularly in children who wear diapers (1- to 4-year olds) • Incubation period: 3–6 days • Communicable from time of infection until fever resolves; virus is shed for several weeks after the infection begins	• High fever usually occurs first • Vesicles on tongue and oral mucosa erode to shallow ulcers; vesicles on hands and feet are football shaped, with erythematous rims • Extensive mouth lesions may lead to anorexia, dehydration, and drooling

Adapted from Government of Canada (2015, 2016); Public Health Agency of Canada (2012a, 2012b); Government of Canada (2013).

Management/Complications	Nursing Implications
• Usually benign and self-limited; supportive treatment is all that is needed • Blood transfusion may be necessary in children with aplastic crisis • Complications: arthritis and arthralgia • May result in fetal loss, hydrops fetalis in pregnant woman	• Comfort measures, such as antipyretics and antipruritics • Droplet precautions are required in the hospitalized child • Inform pregnant women (including healthcare workers) of the potential risks to the fetus and preventive measures to decrease these risks (strict infection control practices, not caring for those likely to be contagious). The CDC does not recommended routine exclusion from a workplace where an outbreak is occurring
• Usually mild and self-limiting, resolving within 1 week • Treatment is mainly supportive • Complications: dehydration, meningitis, encephalitis, and pulmonary edema	• Standard precautions and good hand hygiene are necessary • Encourage oral fluids of preference, such as popsicles • Provide analgesics as needed

2014d). Although generally mild, complications such as viral meningitis, orchitis (inflammation of the testicles) in males and oophoritis (inflammation of the ovaries) in females can result in complications; because involvement of the reproductive organs is commonly unilateral, sterility is rare (Public Health Agency of Canada, 2014a, 2014b, 2014c, 2014d). Up to half of people with mumps will have nonspecific or mild respiratory symptoms or no symptoms at all (Public Health Agency of Canada, 2014a, 2014b, 2014c, 2014d). Complications of mumps include meningitis with or without encephalitis with seizures, pancreatitis, and auditory neuritis, which can result in hearing loss. Therapeutic management is supportive.

Since the recommendation of the two-dose MMR (measles, mumps, rubella) vaccine, the incidence of mumps has declined in Canada. Thanks to vaccination programs throughout Canada, mumps is no longer a common childhood disease. In fact, there has been a 99% reduction in the number of cases reported since the introduction of routine vaccinations against mumps (Butler-Jones, 2013).

However, several provinces are reporting an increase in mumps with Toronto Public Health (TPH, 2017) confirming cases, mostly in 18 to 35 year olds who perhaps did not receive two doses of vaccine in childhood. It is recommended that all children be immunized against mumps (Public Health Agency of Canada, 2014a, 2014b, 2014c, 2014d). Current recommendations include first mumps immunization between 12 and 15 months of age (or before their second birthday), followed by a second vaccine between 4 and 6 years of age (TPH, 2017). According to the CDC (2015c), research shows that one dose of MMR prevents 78% of cases and two doses prevent approximately 88% of cases.

Nursing Assessment

Note history of exposure to infected individuals as well as immunization status. Determine history of low-grade fever and onset and progression of parotid swelling. History may also include malaise, anorexia, headache, and abdominal pain. The parotid swelling is easily observed as swelling of the neck either bilaterally or unilaterally (Fig. 37.4). In boys, note orchitis. The diagnosis is usually based on the history and clinical presentation, but serum may be tested for the presence of mumps IgG or IgM antibody.

Nursing Management

Nursing management of mumps is primarily supportive. Acetaminophen or ibuprofen is used for fever management, and occasionally narcotic analgesics are required for pain management. Oral fluids are encouraged to prevent dehydration. If orchitis is present, ice packs to

FIGURE 37.4 **Parotitis associated with mumps.**

the testicles and gentle testicular support may be helpful. Hospitalized children should be on droplet precautions to prevent spread of the disease. Infected children are considered no longer contagious 9 days following the onset of parotid swelling (Public Health Agency, 2014).

Take Note!

In recent years, mumps outbreaks have occurred, mainly in settings where prolonged close contact with other people occurs, such as college campuses and camps. The mumps vaccine is not 100% effective, and mumps infection can occur in vaccinated individuals (Butler-Jones, 2013). During an outbreak, it is essential to define the population at risk and transmission setting, identify and isolate suspected cases, and identify and vaccinate susceptible individuals.

ZOONOTIC INFECTIONS

Zoonotic and **vector-borne** infections are diseases caused by infectious agents that are transmitted directly or indirectly from animals or vectors, such as ticks, mosquitos, or other insect vectors to humans. Zoonotic infections are responsible for about 75% of emerging infectious diseases, and often these diseases are transmitted by mosquitos and ticks. It is believed that environmental change is leading to the increased incidence of these diseases in Canada (Health Canada and the Public Health Agency of Canada, 2016).

Children are at a particular risk for contracting zoonotic or vector-borne diseases. Young children are unaware of the health risks around them and cannot take protective measures. Their immature immune system leads to a decreased capacity to resist zoonotic or vector-borne diseases. These diseases can be severe and even fatal, although most are treatable if identified early. Often the child presents initially with nonspecific symptoms which delay diagnosis. Coupled with the fact that there are few definitive diagnostic tests available, this can lead to difficulty in promptly recognizing and treating these diseases. Tick-borne diseases are common vector-borne illnesses in Canada. Determining the incidence of zoonotic and vector-borne diseases is difficult due to the complexity of the transmission cycle and geographic climate variability. Table 37.5 discusses other zoonotic and vector-borne diseases. Nurses need to be aware of zoonotic and vector borne diseases common in the area they are practicing as well as the impact of patient travel and the risk of these diseases. Nurses need to tap into provincial and local resources as well as national and international resources, such as Health Canada, the CDC, and WHO.

Take Note!

The Public Health Agency of Canada issues health notices of the current infectious disease outbreaks that are being reported at http://www.phac-aspc.gc.ca/phn-asp/index-eng.php.

Rabies

Rabies is a preventable viral infection of the central nervous system. It is transmitted to other animals and humans through close contact with the saliva of a rabid animal, usually by a bite. It is rare in Canada due to routine vaccination of domestic animals, such as dogs, and the availability of effective postexposure prophylaxis (PEP). Now most cases of rabies in Canada are due to wild animals such as raccoons and artic fox (Curry et al., 2016; Stevenson, Goltz, & Masse, 2016). Rabies continues to be a major health problem in other parts of the world, especially in areas where dogs are not controlled.

Most cases of rabies occur in children younger than 15 years of age, and most human deaths occur in Asia and Africa (World Health Organization [WHO], 2015). Children have an increased susceptibility to rabies due to their fearlessness around animals, eagerness to play with animals, shorter stature, and inability to protect themselves. The incubation period for rabies is extremely variable. Typically, it is 1 to 3 months but can range from days to years. The incubation period tends to be shorter in children. Once symptoms of rabies have developed, the prognosis is poor. Death usually occurs within days of the onset of symptoms. Prevention is of paramount importance, and eliminating infection in animal vectors is essential. Successful animal vaccination and animal

control campaigns in Canada have led to a very low rate of human rabies cases. Recently, rabies transmitted from other animals, such as bats, raccoons, and artic foxes, has become a cause for concern (Filejski, 2016; Willoughby, 2011; WHO, 2014).

It is important to contact the local health department whenever there is an exposure, or suspected exposure, to rabies. Several factors need to be considered when deciding to provide PEP, such as local epidemiology, type of animal involved, availability of the responsible animal for testing or quarantine, and the circumstances of the exposure, such as a provoked versus an unprovoked attack. Algorithms are available to help healthcare providers decide if PEP is warranted (Willoughby, 2011). In a previously unvaccinated child, PEP should begin with a thorough cleansing of all wounds with soap and water or a virucidal agent, such as povidone–iodine solution. In Canada, concurrent use of passive and active immunoprophylaxis is then recommended. It consists of a regimen of one dose of immune globulin and four doses of human rabies vaccine. Rabies immune globulin and the first dose of rabies vaccine should be given as soon as possible after exposure, ideally within 24 hours. Additional doses of rabies vaccine should be given on days 3, 7, and 14 after the first vaccination. Rabies immune globulin is infiltrated into and around the wound, with any remaining volume administered intramuscularly at a site distant from the vaccine inoculation. Human rabies vaccine is administered intramuscularly into the anterolateral thigh or deltoid, depending on the age and size of the child. Administration into the gluteus muscle should be avoided, since this site has been associated with vaccine failure (Rupprecht et al., 2010; Willoughby, 2011). Pre-exposure vaccination can be given to prevent rabies in people at high risk, such as veterinarians, laboratory technicians working with the virus, and people exposed to wild animals (Willoughby, 2011).

Nursing Assessment

Note the history of an animal bite, especially if it was unprovoked, and exposure to bats. Document history of early symptoms of rabies infection, which are nonspecific and flu-like, such as fever, headache, and general malaise. The child may complain of pain, pruritus, and paresthesia at the bite site. As the virus spreads to the central nervous system, encephalitis develops. The disease will have progressive neurologic manifestations, which may include insomnia, confusion, anxiety, changes in behaviour, agitation or excitation, hallucinations, hypersalivation, dysphagia, and hydrophobia, which result from aspiration when swallowing liquid or saliva. In some cases, progressive paralysis may be present. The child may have periods of lucidity alternating with these neurologic changes.

TABLE 37.5		OTHER ZOONOTIC AND VECTOR-BORNE ILLNESSES		
Disease	**Causative Organism**	**Geographic Distribution**	**Vector of Transmission**	**Manifestations**
West Nile virus	*Flavivirus*	Throughout Canada with higher incidence in British Columbia, Alberta, Saskatchewan, Manitoba, Ontario, and Quebec; seasonal epidemic from summer to fall	Mosquito bites Rare cases spread through blood transfusions, transplants, and mother to baby during pregnancy and breastfeeding	• Symptoms include febrile illness, meningitis, encephalitis, or acute flaccid paralysis • Children more likely to be asymptomatic or have milder form of disease than adults but children manifest as meningitis more often than adults[a]
Dengue	*Aedes aegypti, Aedes albopictus*	Tropics and subtropics Asia, the Pacific, the Americas, Africa, the Caribbean	Mosquito	• Sudden onset high fever, headache, severe pain behind eyes, joint, muscle and bone pain, rash, mild bleeding such as nose or gums bleeding and bruising easily, leukopenia, thrombocytopenia, and hemorrhagic manifestations
Anaplasmosis	*Anaplasma phagocytophilum*	Mostly upper Midwest and northeast United States	Tick	• Headache, fever, malaise, chills, muscle aches, nausea, abdominal pain, cough, and confusion • Rash is rarely seen • Symptoms appear 1–2 weeks after infected tick bite
Ehrlichiosis	Three pathogens: *Ehrlichia chaffeensis, Ehrlichia ewingii, Ehrlichia canis*	Mostly in southeastern and south-central United States	Tick	• Fever, headaches, fatigue, muscle aches, chills, nausea, vomiting, diarrhea, confusion, red eyes. Clinical signs similar to Rocky Mountain spotted fever. Rash is less commonly associated but is seen in up to 60% of children • May also present with leukopenia, anemia, and hepatitis
Zika Virus (Robinson, 2017)	*Flavivirus*	South America, Caribbean, Mexico in the USA (Florida and Texas only)	Bites of the *Aedes aegypti* mosquito and less commonly the *Aedes albopictus* (neither of which is known to be established in Canada) transmission occurs via blood and sexual transmission	• 75–80% are asymptomatic; however, symptomatic infections include: maculopapular rash proximally and spreading to limbs, low-grade fever, arthralgias of the small joints, headache, and non-purulent conjunctivitis • Congenital Zika Syndrome can be transmitted during pregnancy and commonly cause severe microcephaly, cerebral atrophy, abnormal cortical development in fetal development

TABLE 37.5	OTHER ZOONOTIC AND VECTOR-BORNE ILLNESSES (continued)			
Disease	**Causative Organism**	**Geographic Distribution**	**Vector of Transmission**	**Manifestations**
Malaria	*Plasmodium* (five species exist that infect humans: *P. falciparum, P. vivax, P. ovale, P. malariae, P. knowlesi*)	Endemic in tropical areas of the world Highest incidence in Africa, Asia, and South America. Cases in Canada are usually in travellers and immigrants returning from countries where malaria transmission occurs	Bite of *Anopheles* species of mosquito	• High fever with chills, rigours, sweats, and headache, which may be paroxysmal • Nausea, vomiting, diarrhea, cough, arthralgia, and abdominal and back pain may also occur • Anemia and thrombocytopenia with pallor and jaundice may be seen • May occur in a cyclic pattern, and depending on the species, fever may occur every other day or every third day

*Centers for Disease Control and Prevention. (2013a). *Anaplasmosis*. Retrieved from http://www.cdc.gov/anaplasmosis/; Centers for Disease Control and Prevention. (2013b). *Ehrlichiosis*. Retrieved from http://www.cdc.gov/ehrlichiosis/; Centers for Disease Control and Prevention. (2015e). *Dengue*. Retrieved from http://www.cdc.gov/Dengue/; Centers for Disease Control and Prevention. (2015f). *West Nile virus*. Retrieved from http://www.cdc.gov/westnile/index.html; and John, C. C., & Krause, P. J. (2011). Chapter 280: Malaria (plasmodium). In R. M. Kleigman, B. F. Stanton, J. W. St. Geme III, N. F. Schor, & R. E. Behrman (Eds.). *Nelson textbook of pediatrics* (19th ed., pp. 1198–1207). Philadelphia, PA: Saunders; Health Canada and the Public Health Agency of Canada (2016).

Laboratory testing may include hair and saliva specimens from which the virus may be isolated. Serum and cerebrospinal fluid can be tested for antibodies to the rabies virus. Direct fluorescent antibody testing can be done to diagnose rabies in a suspected animal. The test can only be done postmortem and requires brain tissue from the potentially rabid animal.

Nursing Management

Few people survive once symptomatic rabies infection develops. Intensive supportive care is required, but recovery is extremely rare. Therefore, it is vital to educate children and families about the importance of seeking medical care after any animal bite to prevent death from rabies infection. Also, teach children to avoid wild animals, stray animals, and any animal with unusual behaviour. Teach children not to provoke or attempt to capture wild or stray animals.

Take Note!

The North American Rabies Management Plan, signed in 2008 by Canada, the US, Mexico, and the Navajo Nations is a collaborative strategy that coordinates control measures to stop the spread and hopefully the elimination of raccoon rabies (Stevenson et al., 2016).

Regardless of whether immunoprophylaxis is initiated, appropriate wound management is necessary in all victims of a bite from a potentially rabid animal. This includes a thorough cleansing of all wounds with soap and water. Irrigation of wounds with large volumes of a virucidal agent, such as povidone–iodine solution, along with avoiding closure of the wound, is recommended (Willoughby, 2011).

When caring for a child requiring PEP, provide support and education to the child and family. Due to the seriousness and urgency surrounding this disease and treatment, the child and family are often very frightened. Consider comfort measures, such as EMLA (eutectic mixture of local anesthetics) cream and positioning, when giving immunization.

Lyme Disease

Lyme disease is caused by the spirochete *Borrelia burgdorferi* (CDC, 2012b). It is transmitted to humans via the bite of an infected black-legged (deer) tick. The number of cases reported in Canada is rapidly rising and has more than quadrupled in 5 years. In 2016, 987 cases (including cases classified as probable and confirmed according to the case definition) were reported by 9 provinces (British Columbia, Alberta, Manitoba, Ontario, Quebec, New-Brunswick, Nova Scotia, Prince Edward Island, and Newfoundland and Labrador) (Government of Canada, 2017a, 2017b). Note that pets (dogs) can carry ticks on fur into family homes.

Lyme disease can affect any age group, but among children 7 years of age was the median age for those age ranges between 4 months and 15 years based on surveillance studies in 2015 (Canadian Paediatric Society, 2015). The prognosis for recovery in children who are treated is excellent.

Therapeutic Management

In most cases, Lyme disease can be cured by antibiotics, especially if they are started early in the illness. Doxycycline is the drug of choice for children older than 8 years (Onyett & Canadian Paediatric Society, 2014). Because of the risk that it can cause permanent discoloration of the teeth, children younger than 8 years should be treated with amoxicillin (Onyett & Canadian Paediatric Society, 2014). For children allergic to penicillin, cefuroxime can be used. Duration of treatment is usually 14 to 28 days, depending on the stage of disease.

Nursing Assessment

The clinical signs of Lyme disease are divided into three stages—early localized, early disseminated, and late disease. Untreated children may progress through the three stages or may present with early disseminated or late disease without having any symptoms of the earlier stages. If children are treated in the early stage, it is uncommon to see them with late disease. Nursing assessment for Lyme disease includes an accurate health history as well as physical examination.

HEALTH HISTORY

Explore the health history for a tick bite. Document onset of rash. In early localized disease, the rash usually occurs 7 to 14 days after the tick bite (though it can appear 3 to 32 days after the bite). In early disseminated disease, the rash usually begins 3 to 5 weeks after the tick bite. Note complaints of fever, malaise, mild neck stiffness, headache, fatigue, myalgia, and arthralgia or pain in the joints. In late disease, note recurrent arthritis of the large joints, such as the knees, beginning weeks to months after the tick bite. The child with late disease may or may not have a history of earlier stages of the disease, including erythema migrans.

PHYSICAL EXAMINATION

Observe for a rash. A ring-like rash at the site of the tick bite (erythema migrans) characterizes early local disease (Fig. 37.5). If untreated, the rash gradually expands and will remain for 1 to 2 weeks. Suspect early disseminated disease if multiple areas of erythema migrans are found. The multiple lesions are usually smaller than the primary lesions. Note cranial nerve palsies (especially cranial nerve VII—facial), conjunctivitis, or signs of meningeal irritation, which occur in early disseminated disease.

FIGURE 37.5 Erythema migrans, a ring-like rash at the site of the tick bite, occurs in Lyme disease. (Courtesy of CDC/James Gathany. [2007]. Obtained at http://phil.cdc.gov/phil/details.asp?pid=9875.)

LABORATORY AND DIAGNOSTIC TESTING

Immunoglobulin-specific antibody tests may not be positive in the early stage of the disease but may be useful in the later stages. The CDC recommends a two-step test—an enzyme immunoassay (EIA) if positive, followed by a Western immunoblot (Government of Canada, 2017a, 2017b). If these are negative, no further testing is indicated.

Nursing Management

Administer antibiotics as ordered. In the hospitalized child, no transmission-based precautions are necessary. Educate the child and family on the importance of taking the antibiotic as directed and finishing all the medicine. Another important nursing function is educating the child, family, and community on prevention measures (Box 37.5). For infection to occur, typically the tick must be attached for >36 hours (Onyett & Canadian Paediatric Society, 2014). Therefore, prompt removal of ticks is essential to the prevention of Lyme disease. Teaching Guidelines 37.2 gives information on tick removal.

Teaching Guidelines 37.2
TICK REMOVAL

- Use fine-tipped tweezers.
- Protect fingers with a tissue, paper towel, or latex gloves.
- Grasp tick as close to the skin as possible and pull upward with steady, even pressure.

PREVENTION OF TICK-BORNE ILLNESSES

- Wear appropriate protective clothing when entering tick-infested areas. Clothing should fit tightly around wrists, waists, and ankles. Tuck pants into socks if possible
  - After leaving the area, do a full body check for ticks and remove them promptly
- Examine gear, clothes, and pets for ticks. Tumble dry clothes and appropriate gear on high heat for 10 minutes
- Insect repellent may provide temporary relief but may produce toxicity, especially in children, if used frequently or in large doses

- Do not twist or jerk the tick.
- Once the tick is removed, clean site with soap and water, rubbing alcohol, or iodine scrub and wash your hands.
- Save the tick for identification in case the child becomes sick. Place in a sealable plastic bag and put it in your freezer. Write date of bite on the bag.

Rocky Mountain Spotted Fever

Rocky Mountain spotted fever (RMSF) is the most severe and frequently reported rickettsial illness in the United States and is also reported in Western Canada (Reller & Dumler, 2011). RMSF is caused by the bacteria *Rickettsia rickettsii*. In Canada, the *Dermacentor andersoni* tick species is the primary vector (PHAC, 2011). RMSF can be fatal without prompt and appropriate treatment (Reller & Dumler, 2011). Most cases occur between April and September (Reller & Dumler, 2011). Its name is derived from the fact that it was discovered in the Rocky Mountain region. It occurs in all age groups but most frequently in children, with the peak incidence in children greater than 5 years of age (Reller & Dumler, 2011).

Complications of RMSF include noncardiogenic pulmonary edema, cerebral edema, and multiorgan damage. Long-term neurologic involvement, such as partial paralysis of the lower extremities, hearing loss, loss of bladder and bowel control, movement disorders, and language disorders, may be seen, especially in children with severe illness who require long hospital stays.

Therapeutic Management

The fatality rate from RMSF has decreased with the widespread use of antimicrobial therapy (Reller & Dumler, 2011). However, delays in diagnosis and therapy are significant factors associated with severity of disease and death. In most cases, RMSF resolves rapidly with appropriate antibiotic therapy, especially if it is started early.

Treatments of choice are tetracyclines, such as doxycycline. Doxycycline and other tetracyclines are not normally used in children younger than 8 years due to the risk of teeth staining. However, due to the life-threatening nature of RMSF and the limited course of antibiotic therapy, the American Academy of Pediatrics Committee on Infectious Diseases revised its recommendations and has identified doxycycline as the drug of choice for treating presumed or confirmed RMSF in children of any age (Centers for Disease Control and Prevention, 2013f). Length of treatment is typically 7 to 14 days (Centers for Disease Control and Prevention, 2016; CanLyme, 2016).

Nursing Assessment

Note history of early signs of RMSF, such as sudden onset of fever, headache, malaise, nausea and vomiting, muscle pain, and anorexia. The incubation period varies from 2 to 14 days, with the average being around 7 days after the tick bite (Reller & Dumler, 2011). Late signs include a rash, usually seen 2 to 5 days after the onset of the fever, abdominal pain, joint pain, and diarrhea. Inspect the skin for a rash, which starts as small, pink, macular, nonitchy, blanchable spots on the wrists, forearms, and ankles. The rash then spreads rapidly over the entire body, including the soles and palms. After several days, the rash will appear red, spotted, and petechial or hemorrhagic (Fig. 37.6). Approximately 5% of children with RMSF do not have a rash (Reller & Dumler, 2011). Laboratory findings may include a low leukocyte count, low or decreasing platelet count, and hyponatremia. Biopsy of the rash with immunofluorescent assay and serologic tests may also be used.

FIGURE 37.6 **Rash associated with Rocky Mountain spotted fever.**

TABLE 37.6	COMMON PARASITIC INFECTIONS IN CHILDREN		

Infection/Causative Organism	Transmission	Clinical Manifestations
Pediculosis capitis (head lice) Caused by *Pediculus humanus capitis* (head louse)	Direct contact with hair of infested people, less commonly with personal belongings, such as combs and hats, of those infested Incubation period from laying of eggs to hatching of nymph is 6–10 days; adult lice will appear 2–3 weeks later	Extreme pruritus is the most common symptom Adult eggs (nits) or lice may be seen, especially behind the ears and at the nape of the neck
Scabies Caused by *Sarcoptes scabiei* Scabies	Incubation period from laying of eggs to hatching of nymph is 3–4 days; adult lice will appear 2–4 weeks later Incubation period in those without previous exposure is 4–6 weeks. Usually, no symptoms are present during this time but transmission to others can occur People who were previously infested can develop symptoms in 1–4 days Transmission usually occurs through prolonged, close personal contact	Intense pruritus (especially at night) with the presence of erythematous, papular rash with excoriations. The lesions are generally distributed but often are concentrated on the hands and feet and in body folds. May be found on head and neck In infants and young children, the rash is often heavy on palms, soles, and fingers, and it may include vesicles, pustules, or bullous lesions

Goldstein, B. G., & Goldstein, A. O. (2015b). Scabies. Retrieved from http://www.uptodate.com/contents/scabies and Siegel, J. D., Rhinehart, E., Jackson, M., Chiarello, L.; The Healthcare Infection Control Practices Advisory Committee. (2007). Guideline for isolation precautions: Preventing transmission of infectious agents in healthcare settings. Retrieved from http://www.cdc.gov/hicpac/pdf/isolation/Isolation2007.pdf.

Nursing Management

Nursing management is similar to that for Lyme disease. Educate the family about completing the antibiotic course, preventing tick bites, and appropriate tick removal (refer to Box 37.5 and Teaching Guidelines 37.2).

Take Note!

Many folklore remedies exist for tick removal such as use of petroleum jelly or hot matches. These often do little to get the tick to detach and may actually irritate the tick and stimulate it to release more saliva or gut contents, therefore increasing the chance of disease. The goal of tick removal is to detach it as quickly as possible (CDC, 2015d).

PARASITIC AND HELMINTHIC INFECTION

Parasites are organisms larger than yeast or bacteria that can cause infection. They live in or on a host. Parasites receive nourishment from the host without benefiting or killing the host. Parasites frequently seen in children are scabies and head lice. A helminth is a parasitic intestinal worm. Helminthic infections seen in children include pinworms, roundworms, and hookworms. Children are at an increased risk for parasitic or helminthic infections due to poor hygiene practices. For example, children typically are more careless about handwashing and they tend to put things in their mouths and share toys and objects with other children.

Diagnosis/Treatment	Isolation/Control Measures/Concerns
Diagnosis by identification of eggs, nymph, and lice with the naked eye is possible; adult lice are rarely seen Treatment: washing hair with a pediculicide such as permethrin, pyrethrins, lindane, malathion Careful instructions on proper use of any product should be given and strict adherence to application instructions encouraged. Retreatment is usually recommended 9 days after first treatment, depending on treatment used Detection of living lice 24 hours after treatment suggests incorrect use, a very heavy infestation, reinfestation, or resistance to treatment	Contact precautions After treatment, check hair and comb nits and lice from hair shafts every 2–3 days to prevent reinfestation Control measures: Household and other close contacts should be examined and if infested treated. Bedmates should be treated prophylactically Head lice do not survive long once they have fallen off. Most children can be treated effectively without treating their clothing and bedding. But to help avoid reinfestation, disinfection of clothing, headgear, pillowcases, towels, and other items used by the individual within the past 2 days by washing in hot water and drying on the hot cycle may be helpful Dry-cleaning nonwashable items or simply sealing them in a plastic bag for 10 days is effective Soaking combs and hairbrushes in pediculicide, shampoo, or hot water Lice infestation is not a sign of poor hygiene; all socioeconomic groups are affected
Diagnosis can be made by a history of itching (especially at night), classic rash, and reports of itching in household or sexual contacts Mites can be seen on microscopic examination of skin scrapings to confirm diagnosis Treatment: A scabicide, such as permethrin or lindane, should be applied to the entire body below the head. Treatment of infants and young children should include the head, neck, and body. The cream is left on for a specified time (usually 8–14 hours) depending on the type of scabicide Careful instructions on proper use of any product should be given and strict adherence to application instructions should be urged Itching may not subside for several weeks, even after successful treatment	Contact precautions Prophylactic therapy for household members and sexual contacts Bedding and clothing used by infested person or household, sexual, or close contacts within 4 days before treatment should be laundered in hot water and dried on the hot cycle (mites do not survive more than 3–4 days without skin contact) Avoid direct skin-to-skin contact with person or items used by those infested Room used by an infected person, especially if he or she had crusted scabies, should be thoroughly cleaned and vacuumed

Nursing Assessment and Management

Parents are often embarrassed when they find out that their child has a parasitic or helminthic infection. Reassure them that these infections can occur in any child. Tables 37.6 and 37.7 give nursing assessment and management information related to specific common parasitic and helminthic infections in children.

Take Note!

The head louse becoming resistant to pediculicides is a growing concern (Goldstein & Goldstien, 2015a). This may lead parents to resort to home remedies, such as covering the head with real mayonnaise or Vaseline. Inform parents that these remedies have not been proven to be effective (Gupta, 2015).

Consider This!

After cheerleading practice, I noticed my head was itchy. When I got home I told my mom. She looked at my head and said she found lice. What am I going to do? Am I going to have to cut off all my hair? I love my hair! What are the girls on my cheerleading squad going to say if they find out? How could this happen to me?

Thoughts: Why is this girl so upset?

How does her developmental age affect her reaction to this discover?

How would you respond to her concerns?

TABLE 37.7   COMMON HELMINTHIC INFECTIONS IN CHILDREN

Infection/Causative Organism	Clinical Manifestations	Transmission
Ascariasis Caused by *Ascaris lumbricoides*, common in temperate and tropical areas, especially in areas with unsanitary conditions	Most people are asymptomatic, may demonstrate slower growth and weight gain In more severe infections, loss of appetite, nausea, vomiting, and abdominal pain may be seen. Cough and difficulty breathing may be present as immature worms migrate through the lungs In significant infestation, partial or complete intestinal obstruction may occur. The more worms, the worse the symptoms	Human feces are the major source of infected eggs Hand to mouth is the usual route of transmission. The eggs are swallowed due to unclean hands or contaminated food or water. They pass into the intestine; larvae then hatch, penetrate the intestinal wall, enter the circulatory system, and migrate to other body tissues, primarily the lungs first
Hookworm Caused by *Ancylostoma duodenale* (roundworm) and *Necator americanus* (roundworm); common in tropics and subtropics especially in areas with unsanitary conditions; rare in areas with <40 in of annual rain fall	Most often people are asymptomatic until significant worms are established May see pruritic erythematous papular rash at entry site (referred to as ground itch) or pulmonary symptoms as the larvae migrate One of the greatest concerns in chronic infection is anemia (microcytic hypochromic anemia) secondary to blood loss as the worms suck blood and juices from the intestines This can lead to hypoproteinemia, edema, pica, and wasting. The infection may result in physical or intellectual disability in children	Hookworms are found in soil and enter the host through pores, hair follicles, and even intact skin (hands and feet are major sites of entry) The maturing larvae travel through the circulatory system into the lungs and then up the bronchial tree and are swallowed with secretions. They then migrate into the intestinal tract and attach to the wall of the small intestines, where they feed and reproduce
Pinworm Caused by *Enterobius vermicularis* (roundworm); found in temperate climates	Some people are asymptomatic. May cause anal itching (pruritus ani), especially at night Other clinical findings may include restlessness and teeth grinding at night, weight loss, and enuresis	Fecal–oral route directly, indirectly, or inadvertently by contaminated hands or shared toys, bedding, clothing, toilet seats Incubation period is 1–2 months or longer

Adapted from Centers for Disease Control and Prevention. (2013c). Parasites—ascariasis. Retrieved from http://www.cdc.gov/parasites/ascariasis/; Centers for Disease Control and Prevention. (2013d). Parasites—enterobiasis (also known as pinworm infection). Retrieved from http://www.cdc.gov/parasites/pinworm/; Centers for Disease Control and Prevention. (2013e). Parasites—hookworm. Retrieved from http://www.cdc.gov/parasites/hookworm/; and Siegel, J. D., Rhinehart, E., Jackson, M., Chiarello, L.; The Healthcare Infection Control Practices Advisory Committee. (2007). Guideline for isolation precautions: Preventing transmission of infectious agents in healthcare settings. Retrieved from http://www.cdc.gov/hicpac/pdf/isolation/Isolation2007.pdf

Take Note!

In recent years, Health Canada has approved new topical noninsecticidal products for the treatment of head lice. However, permethrin 1% and pyrethrins remain the first line of treatment but the new medications may be helpful with difficult to get rid of cases or cases of resistant lice (CPS, 2016). All of these medications are available over-the-counter.

Take Note!

Several tropical diseases including soil-transmitted helminths (hookworm, Ascaris, and whipworm) are often treated through mass drug administrations. The same drug is used to treat several infections and these drugs are safe and inexpensive or donated. Entire risk groups are offered preventive treatment periodically (often yearly) (CDC, 2013c, 2013e).

Diagnosis/Treatment	Isolation/Control Measures
Diagnosis: once female worms are in the intestine, eggs can be visualized by microscopic evaluation of the stool Occasionally a worm may be coughed up and visualized or seen in vomit, stool, or urine Imaging can also be used Treatment is with mebendazole, albendazole, or pyrantel pamoate	Standard precautions are sufficient Sanitary disposal of feces Proper hand hygiene
Diagnosis: through microscopic examination of feces that reveals hookworm eggs Treatment is with albendazole, mebendazole, and pyrantel pamoate Iron supplementation and possible blood transfusion in severe cases	Standard precautions are sufficient Proper sanitation and disposal of feces Treatment of all known infested people Screening of high-risk individuals Encourage the wearing of shoes and avoiding going barefoot
Diagnosis: when adult worms are visualized in the perianal region; they are best viewed when the child is sleeping. Very few ova are present in stool, so examination of stool is not recommended Transparent tape pressed to perianal area and then viewed under a microscope may reveal eggs. Three consecutive specimens should be obtained when the child first awakens in the morning Treatment of choice is mebendazole, pyrantel pamoate, and albendazole, usually single doses and repeated in 2 weeks	Standard precautions are sufficient Reinfection occurs easily Infected people should bathe, preferably in a shower, in the morning, which will remove a large portion of the eggs Frequent changing of underclothes and bedding Personal hygiene measures such as keeping fingernails short, avoiding scratching of perianal area, and nail biting Good hand hygiene is the most effective preventive measure, especially after using the bathroom and before eating. All family members should be treated since transmission from person to person is very easy

NURSING CARE PLAN 37.1

Overview for the Child With an Infectious or Communicable Disorder

NURSING DIAGNOSIS: Risk for ineffective thermoregulation: fever related to infectious disease process as evidenced by rectal temperature greater than 38°C or 100.4°F

Outcome Identification and Evaluation

Child will maintain temperature within adaptive levels and be comfortable and remain hydrated. Temperature will be 38°C or 100.4°F or less. Child will verbalize or exhibit signs of comfort during febrile episode; child will demonstrate adequate signs of hydration.

Interventions: *Managing Fever*

- Assess temperature at least every 4 to 6 hours, 30 to 60 minutes after antipyretic is given and with any change in condition: *recognizing the pattern of fever may help identify source.*
- Use the same site and device for temperature measurement *to reflect a more accurate trend in temperature, since different sites can result in significant differences in temperature reading.*
- Administer antipyretics per physician or nurse practitioner order when the child is experiencing discomfort or cannot keep up with the metabolic demands of the fever. *Fever is a protective response of the body to fight infection. Antipyretics provide symptomatic relief but do not change the course of the infection. The major benefits to decreasing fever are increasing comfort in the child and decreasing fluid requirements, helping to prevent dehydration.*

- Notify physician or nurse practitioner of temperature per institution or specific order guidelines: *increases in temperature may indicate worsening infection and relevant changes in condition.*
- Assess fluid intake and encourage oral intake or administer intravenous fluids per physician order: *increased metabolic rate and diaphoresis related to fever can cause fluid loss and lead to fluid volume deficit.*
- Keep linens and clothing clean and dry: *diaphoresis can leave clothing and linen soaked, increasing discomfort for the child.*
- Use of nonpharmacologic measures such as tepid bath and removal of clothing and blankets is controversial. If used, discontinue if shivering begins.

NURSING DIAGNOSIS: Impaired comfort related to infectious and/or inflammatory process as evidenced by hyperthermia, pruritus, rash or skin lesions, sore throat, or joint pain

Outcome Identification and Evaluation

Pain or discomfort will be reduced to level acceptable to child. Child will verbalize absence or decrease of pain using a pain scale (e.g., FLACC, FACES, or linear pain scale), will verbalize decrease in uncomfortable sensations such as itching and aches; infants will exhibit decreased crying and ability to rest quietly.

Interventions: *Improving Comfort*

- Assess pain and response to interventions frequently with use of pain scales or other pain measurement tools: *provides baseline of pain and allows for evaluation of effectiveness of interventions.*
- Administer analgesics and antipruritics as ordered to *relieve pain via interruption of central nervous system (CNS) pathways and to decrease discomfort related to itching.*
- Apply cool compresses to areas of pruritus or provide a cool bath *to decrease inflammation and soothe pruritus.*
- Keep child's fingernails short (use mitts, gloves, or socks over hands if necessary) to prevent injury *to the skin, which leads to increased pain.*

Overview for the Child With an Infectious or Communicable Disorder (continued)

- Encourage child to press on rather than scratch the area of pruritus: *pressing on the area that itches can soothe the itching and prevent scratching, which can lead to skin injury.*
- Provide fluids frequently and offer warm fluids such as soup or cold foods such as popsicles *to ease the discomfort of a sore throat.*
- Provide cool mist humidification *to ease the discomfort of a sore throat.*
- Dress the child in light clothing: *restrictive clothing and diaphoresis can lead to increased pruritus.*
- Use diversional activities and distraction appropriate to developmental level: *distraction from pain can reduce the need for pharmacologic agents, and distraction from pruritus can minimize scratching.*

NURSING DIAGNOSIS: Impaired skin integrity related to mechanical trauma secondary to infectious disease process as evidenced by rash, pruritus, and scratching

Outcome Identification and Evaluation

Child will maintain or regain skin integrity. Child will not demonstrate increased skin breakdown. Child or parent will be able to describe or demonstrate measures to protect and heal skin and proper care for any lesions.

Interventions: *Promoting Skin Integrity*

- Monitor skin for colour changes, temperature, redness, swelling, warmth, pain, signs of infection, or changes in rash lesions, distribution, or size *to help identify problems early and allow for prevention of infection; can also provide information regarding the course of the illness.*
- Encourage fluid intake and proper nutrition *to promote wound healing.*
- Keep child's fingernails short (use mitts, gloves, or socks over hands if necessary) *to prevent injury to the skin, which leads to increased pain.*
- Encourage child to press on rather than scratch the area of pruritus; *pressing on the area that itches can soothe the itching and prevent scratching, which can lead to skin injury.*
- Use antipruritics and topical ointments or creams as ordered *to minimize scratching to prevent injury to skin; can aid in healing.*

NURSING DIAGNOSIS: Risk for infection related to insufficient knowledge regarding measures to avoid exposure to pathogens, increased environmental exposure to pathogens, transmission to others secondary to contagious organism, or presence of infectious organisms

Outcome Identification and Evaluation

Child will exhibit no signs or symptoms of local or systemic infection. Child will not spread infection to others. Symptoms of infection will decrease over time; others will remain free of infection. Child and family will demonstrate appropriate hygiene measures using proper technique, such as handwashing, to prevent the spread of infection.

Interventions: *Preventing and Controlling Infection*

- Monitor vital signs: *elevation in temperature may indicate infection.*
- Monitor skin lesions for signs of local infection: redness, warmth, drainage, swelling, and pain at lesions: *can indicate infection.*
- Maintain aseptic technique and practice good handwashing: *to prevent introduction of further infectious agents and prevent transmission to others.*
- Administer antibiotics as prescribed: *to prevent or treat bacterial infection.*

(continued)

NURSING CARE PLAN 37.1

Overview for the Child With an Infectious or Communicable Disorder (continued)

- Encourage nutritious diet and proper hydration according to child's preferences and ability to feed orally: *to assist body's natural defences against infection.*
- Isolate child as required based on transmission-based precautions: *to prevent nosocomial spread of infection.*

- Teach child and family preventive measures such as good handwashing, covering mouth and nose with cough or sneeze, and proper disposal of used tissues: *to prevent nosocomial or community spread of infection.*

NURSING DIAGNOSIS: Risk for deficient fluid volume, related to increased metabolic demands and insensible loss due to fever, vomiting, poor feeding, or intake

Outcome Identification and Evaluation

Fluid volume will be maintained and balanced. Oral mucosa is moist and pink, skin turgor is elastic, urine output is at least 1 to 2 mL/kg/h.

Interventions: *Promoting Adequate Fluid Balance*

- Administer IV fluids if ordered *to maintain adequate hydration in children who are NPO (nothing by mouth), unable to tolerate oral intake, or unable to keep up with fluid losses.*
- When oral intake is allowed and tolerated, encourage oral fluids *to promote intake and maintain hydration.*
- Assess for signs of adequate hydration such as pink and moist oral mucosa, elastic skin turgor, and adequate urine output *to detect fluid imbalance.*
- Monitor intake and output *to identify fluid imbalance.*
- Assess urine specific gravity, urine and serum electrolytes, blood urea nitrogen, creatinine, and osmolality and daily weights *to monitor fluid status.*

NURSING DIAGNOSIS: Social isolation related to required isolation from peers secondary to transmission-based precautions, as evidenced by disruption in usual play secondary to inability to leave hospital room, activity intolerance, and fatigue

Outcome Identification and Evaluation

Child will participate in stimulating activities. Child is able to verbalize reason for isolation and length of isolation (if developmentally appropriate); child verbalizes interest in activities.

Interventions: *Preventing Social Isolation*

- Explain reasons for transmission-based precautions and length of time: *this helps increase understanding and decrease anxiety about isolation. Children sometimes mistake isolation as punishment. Explaining length of time gives child an endpoint he or she can work toward.*
- Visit child frequently, at least every hour, and try to spend some uninterrupted time to play and allow child time to verbalize feelings about separation from others: *helps establish a therapeutic relationship and demonstrates caring.*

- Let child see caregiver's face before applying mask if appropriate: *to help child identify and relate to those caring for him or her and minimize anxiety about strangers and the unknown.*
- Consult child life specialist to arrange for stimulating activities child enjoys: *can help child to understand reasons for isolation and minimize feelings of social isolation.*
- Contact volunteers to spend time with child, if appropriate: *gives child attention and support, which will help child to cope and decrease stress.*

NURSING CARE PLAN 37.1

Overview for the Child With an Infectious or Communicable Disorder (continued)

NURSING DIAGNOSIS: Deficient knowledge related to lack of information regarding medical condition, prognosis, and medical needs as evidenced by verbalization, questions, or actions demonstrating lack of understanding regarding child's condition or care

Outcome Identification and Evaluation

Child and family will verbalize accurate information and understanding about condition, prognosis, and medical needs. Child and family demonstrate knowledge of condition and prognosis and medical needs, including possible causes, contributing factors, and treatment measures.

Interventions: *Providing Child and Family Teaching*

- Assess child's and family's willingness to learn: *child and family must be willing to learn in order for teaching to be effective.*
- Provide family with time to adjust to diagnosis: *to facilitate adjustment and ability to learn and participate in child's care.*
- Repeat information: *to give family and child time to learn and understand.*
- Teach in short sessions: *many short sessions are more helpful and facilitate learning compared to one long session.*

- Gear teaching to level of understanding of the child and family (depends on age of child, physical condition, memory) *to ensure understanding.*
- Provide reinforcement and rewards: *to facilitate the teaching/learning process.*
- Use multiple modes of learning involving many senses (provide written, verbal, demonstration, and videos) when possible: *the child and family are more likely to retain information when it is presented in different ways using many senses.*

KEY CONCEPTS

- Infants and young children are more susceptible to infection due to their immature immune system. Young children continue to have an increased risk for infections and communicable disorders because disease protection from immunizations is not complete.

- Healthcare providers need to remember to educate parents that fever is a protective mechanism the body uses to fight infection.

- When obtaining blood cultures, follow aseptic technique and hospital protocol to prevent contamination. Obtain the specimen before administering antibiotics.

- When administering antipyretics, proper education must be given to caregivers on appropriate dosing, concentration, dosing interval, and use of proper measuring device.

- Promoting proper fluid balance and reducing temperature in a febrile child are important nursing interventions when caring for a child with an infection or communicable illness.

- Many childhood infectious and communicable diseases involve a rash. Rashes can be difficult to identify, so a thorough description and history from the caregiver is important.

- Sepsis, a systemic overresponse to infection, resulting from bacteria, fungi, viruses, or parasites, can lead to septic shock. Any infant younger than 3 months old with a fever or any child with a fever accompanied by extreme lethargy, unresponsiveness, or lack of facial expressions should be seen by a physician or nurse practitioner.

- Many bacterial and viral infections, such as diphtheria, tetanus, pertussis, mumps, measles, rubella, varicella, and poliomyelitis, can be prevented by vaccination.

- Viral exanthems of childhood often present with a distinct rash pattern that assists in the diagnosis of the virus. Common childhood exanthems include exanthem subitum (roseola infantum), rubella (German measles), rubeola (measles), varicella (chickenpox), and erythema infectiosum (fifth disease).

- Nurses play a key role in educating the public on the importance of immunizations.

- Zoonotic infections are diseases caused by infectious agents that are transmitted directly or indirectly from animals to humans. Rabies is a type of zoonotic infections.

- Children are at a particular risk for contracting vector-borne diseases, which are diseases transmitted by ticks, mosquitoes, or other insect vectors. One of the most commonly seen is Lyme disease.

- Parasites frequently seen in children are scabies and head lice. Helminthic infections seen in children include pinworms, roundworms, and hookworms.

REFERENCES AND RECOMMENDED READINGS

Arnon, S. S. (2011). Tetanus (Clostridium tetani). In R. M. Kleigman, B. F. Stanton, J. W. St. Geme III, N. F. Schor, & R. E. Behrman (Eds.). *Nelson textbook of pediatrics* (19th ed., pp. 991–994). Philadelphia, PA: Saunders.

Butler-Jones, D. (2013). *The Chief Public Health Officers Report on the state of public health in Canada*. Ottawa: Public Health Agency of Canada.

Canadian Paediatric Society. (2015). *2015 Results Canadian Paediatric Surveillance Program*. Ottawa: Public Health Agency of Canada. Retrieved from https://www.cpsp.cps.ca/uploads/publications/Results-2015.pdf

Canadian Paediatric Society. (2016). Head lice infestations: A clinical update. Retrieved from http://www.cps.ca/documents/position/head-lice

Canadian Paediatric Society. (2017). *Management of community-associated methicillin-resistant Staphylococcus aureus skin abscesses in children*. Retrieved from http://www.cps.ca/documents/position/methicillin-resistant-Staphylococcus-aureus-skin-abscesses

CanLyme (2016). Canadian Lyme Disease Foundation. Retrieved from https://canlyme.com/tag/rocky-mountain-spotted-fever/

Carpenito, L. J. (2013). *Nursing diagnosis: Application to clinical practice* (14th ed.). Philadelphia, PA: Lippincott Williams & Wilkins.

Centers for Disease Control and Prevention. (2012a). In W. Atkinson, S. Wolfe, & J. Hamborsky (Eds.). *Epidemiology and prevention of vaccine-preventable diseases* (12th ed., second printing). Washington, DC: Public Health Foundation.

Centers for Disease Control and Prevention. (2012b). *Workplace safety and health topics: Tick-borne diseases*. Retrieved from http://www.cdc.gov/niosh/topics/tick-borne/

Centers for Disease Control and Prevention. (2013a). *Anaplasmosis*. Retrieved from http://www.cdc.gov/anaplasmosis/

Centers for Disease Control and Prevention. (2013b). *Ehrlichiosis*. Retrieved from http://www.cdc.gov/ehrlichiosis/

Centers for Disease Control and Prevention. (2013c). *Parasites—ascariasis*. Retrieved from http://www.cdc.gov/parasites/ascariasis/

Centers for Disease Control and Prevention. (2013d). *Parasites—enterobiasis (also known as pinworm infection)*. Retrieved from http://www.cdc.gov/parasites/pinworm/

Centres for Disease Control and Prevention. (2013e). *Parasites—hookworm*. Retrieved from http://www.cdc.gov/parasites/hookworm/

Centers for Disease Control and Prevention. (2015a). *Pertussis (whooping cough): Treatment*. Retrieved from http://www.cdc.gov/pertussis/clinical/treatment.html

Centers for Disease Control and Prevention. (2015b). *Pertussis (whooping cough): Postexposure antimicrobial prophylaxis*. Retrieved from http://www.cdc.gov/pertussis/outbreaks/pep.html

Centers for Disease Control and Prevention. (2015c). *Mumps cases and outbreaks*. Retrieved from http://www.cdc.gov/mumps/outbreaks.html

Centers for Disease Control and Prevention. (2015d). *Ticks. Tick removal*. Retrieved from http://www.cdc.gov/ticks/removing_a_tick.html

Centers for Disease Control and Prevention. (2015e). *Dengue*. Retrieved from http://www.cdc.gov/Dengue/; Centers for Disease Control and Prevention.

Centers for Disease Control and Prevention. (2015f). *West Nile virus*. Retrieved from http://www.cdc.gov/westnile/index.html

Centres for Disease Control and Prevention. (2016). Recommendations and Reports. Diagnosis and management of Tickborne Rickettsial Diseases: Rockey Mountain Spotted Fever and other Spotted *Fever Group Rickettsioses, Ehrlichiosis, and Anaplasmosis—United States*. 65(2). Retrieved from https://www.cdc.gov/mmwr/volumes/65/rr/pdfs/rr6502.pdf

Centre for Communicable Diseases and Infection Control. (2012). *Routine practices and additional precautions for preventing the transmission of infection in healthcare settings*. Ottawa: Public Health Agency of Canada.

Child Health BC. (2015). *Patient screening for sepsis*. Retrieved from http://www.childhealthbc.ca/sites/default/files/CHBC%20PEWS%20Modified%20Sepsis%20Screening%20Tool%20Sept%202015.pdf

CHILD Study. (n.d.). *Canadian Healthy Infant Longitudinal Development Study (CHILD)*. Retrieved from http://www.canadianchildstudy.ca/org.html#ap31_4

Curry, P. S., Kostiuk, D., Werker, D. H., Baikie, M., Ntiamoah, W., Atherton, F., … Mema, S. (2016). Translocated dogs from Nunavut and the spread of rabies. *Canadian Communicable Disease Report, 42*, 121–124.

Elkon-Tamir, E., Rimon, A., Scolnik, D., & Glatstein, M. (2017). Fever phobia as a reason for Pediatric Emergency Department visits: Does the primary care physician make a difference? *Rambam Maimonides Medical Journal, 8*(1). Retrieved from https://www.ncbi.nlm.nih.gov/pmc/articles/PMC5298368/

Enarson, M. C., Ali, S., Vandermeer, B., Wright, R. B., Klassen, T. P., & Spiers, J. A. (2012). Beliefs and expectations of Canadian parents who bring febrile children for medical care. *Pediatrics, 130*(4), e905–e912. Retrieved from www.pediatrics.org/cgi/doi/10.1542/peds.2011-2140

Filejski, C. (2016). The changing face of rabies in Canada. *Canada Communicable Disease Report, 42*(6), 118–121. Retrieved from http://www.phac-aspc.gc.ca/publicat/ccdr-rmtc/16vol42/dr-rm42-6/assets/pdf/16vol42_6-ar-01-eng.pdf

Fischbach, F. T., & Dunning III, M. B. (2015). *A manual of laboratory and diagnostic tests* (9th ed.). Philadelphia, PA: Wolters Kluwer Health/Lippincott Williams & Wilkins.

Gerber, M. A. (2011). Chapter 176: Group A streptococcus. In R. M. Kleigman, B. F. Stanton, J. W. St. Geme III, N. F. Schor, & R. E. Behrman (Eds.). *Nelson textbook of pediatrics* (19th ed., pp. 914–925). Philadelphia, PA: Saunders.

Goldstein, A. O., & Goldstein, B. G. (2015a). *Pediculosis capitis*. Retrieved from http://www.uptodate.com/contents/pediculosis-capitis

Goldstein, B. G., & Goldstein, A. O. (2015b). *Scabies*. Retrieved from http://www.uptodate.com/contents/scabies

Government of Canada. (n.d.). *List of nationally notifiable diseases*. Retrieved from http://diseases.canada.ca/notifiable/diseases-list

Government of Canada. (2013). Pediatric and Adolescent care—Chapter 18—Communicable diseases. Retrieved from www.Canada.ca: https://www.canada.ca/en/health-canada/services/first-nations-inuit-health/health-care-services/nursing/clinical-practice-guidelines-nurses-primary-care/pediatric-adolescent-care/chapter-18-communicable-diseases.html#a18

Government of Canada. (2015). *For health professionals: Rubella*. Retrieved from https://www.canada.ca/en/public-health/services/diseases/rubella/information-health-professionals-rubella.html

Government of Canada. (2016). *For health professionals: Measles*. Retrieved from https://www.canada.ca/en/public-health/services/diseases/measles/health-professionals-measles.html

Government of Canada. (2017a). *For health professionals: Lyme disease*. Retrieved from https://www.canada.ca/en/public-health/services/diseases/lyme-disease.html

Government of Canada. (2017b). *Surveillance of Lyme disease*. Retrieved from https://www.canada.ca/en/public-health/servises/diseases/lyme-disease/surveillance-lyme-disease.html#a2

Grossman, S. (2014). Chapter 25: Blood cells and the hematopoietic system. In S. Grossman & C. M. Porth (Eds.). *Porth's pathophysiology: Concepts of altered health states* (9th ed., pp. 638–664). Philadelphia, PA: Wolters Kluwer Health/Lippincott Williams & Wilkins.

Gupta, R. C. (2015). *Head lice*. Retrieved from http://kidshealth.org/parent/infections/common/head_lice.html

Hatfield, L. A., Chang, K., Bittle, M., Deluca, J., & Polomano, R. C. (2011). The analgesic properties of intraoral sucrose: An integrative review. *Advances in Neonatal Care*, 11(2), 83–92.

Haut, C. M. (2014). Chapter 54: Pediatric orthopedic problems. In S. M. Nettina (Ed.). *Lippincott manual of nursing practice* (10th ed., pp. 1743–1769). Philadelphia, PA: Wolters/Kluwer Health: Lippincott Williams & Wilkins.

Health Canada and the Public Health Agency of Canada. (2016). *Audit of the management of non-enteric zoonotic infectious disease activities at the public health agency of Canada—Final report*. Ottawa: Government of Canada—Audit and Accountability Bureau. Retrieved from phac-aspc.gc.ca

Healthwise Staff. (2016). *Scarlet fever*. Retrieved from https://www.healthlinkbc.ca/health-topics/tv7012spec

Infectious Diseases and Immunization Committee. (2017). *Guidelines for the management of suspected and confirmed bacterial meningitis in Canadian children older than one month of age*. Canadian Paediatric Society. Retrieved from https://www.cps.ca/en/documents/authors-auteurs/infectious-diseases-and-immunization-committee

InterAction. (2013). *Global health briefing book*. Retrieved from http://www.globalhealth.org/wp-content/uploads/GlobalHealthBriefingBook_FINAL_web.pdf

John, C. C., & Krause, P. J. (2011). Chapter 280: Malaria (Plasmodium). In R. M. Kleigman, B. F. Stanton, J. W. St. Geme III, N. F. Schor, & R. E. Behrman (Eds.). *Nelson textbook of pediatrics* (19th ed., pp. 1198–1207). Philadelphia, PA: Saunders.

Kaplan, S. L. (2015). *Methicillin-resistant Staphylococcus aureus infections in children: Epidemiology and clinical spectrum*. UpToDate. Retrieved from http://www.uptodate.com/contents/methicillin-resistant-staphylococcus-aureus-infections-in-children-epidemiology-and-clinical-spectrum

Kelly, M., Sahm, L. J., Shiely, F., O'Sullivan, R., de Bont, E. G., Mc Gillicuddy, A., … McCarthy, S. (2017). Parental knowledge, attitudes and beliefs on fever: A cross-sectional study in Ireland. *BMJ Open*, 7(7), e015684. Retrieved from http://creativecommons.org/licenses/by-nc/4.0/

Krogstad, P. (2014a). *Bacterial arthritis: Epidemiology, pathogenesis, and microbiology in infants and children*. UpToDate. Retrieved from http://www.uptodate.com/contents/bacterial-arthritis-epidemiology-pathogenesis-and-microbiology-in-infants-and-children

Krogstad, P. (2014b). Hematogenous osteomyelitis in children: Epidemiology, pathogenesis, and microbiology. Retrieved from http://www.uptodate.com/contents/hematogenous-osteomyelitis-in-children-epidemiology-pathogenesis-and-microbiology

Leifso, K. R., Gravel, D., Mounchili, A., Kaldas, S., & Le Saux, N. (2013). Clinical characteristics of pediatric patients hospitalized with methicillin-resistant Staphylococcus aureus in Canadian hospitals from 2008–2010. *Canadian Journal of Infectious Diseases and Medical Microbiology*, 24(3), e53–e56.

Merle, N. S., Noe, R., Halbwachs-Mecarelli, L., Fremeaux-Bacchi, V., & Roumenina, L. T. (2015). Complement system part II: Role in immunity. *Frontiers in Immunology*, 6:257. Retrieved from https://www.ncbi.nlm.nih.gov/pmc/articles/PMC4443744/

Naughton, K. A., & Ikuta, L. (2013). The combined use of sucrose and nonnutritive sucking for procedural pain in both term and preterm neonates: An integrative review of the literature. *Advances in Neonatal Care*, 13(1), 9–19.

Nield, L. S., & Kamat, D. (2011). Chapter 170: Fever without a focus. In R. M. Kleigman, B. F. Stanton, J. W. St. Geme III, N. F. Schor, & R. E. Behrman (Eds.). *Nelson textbook of pediatrics* (19th ed., pp. 896–902). Philadelphia, PA: Saunders.

Onyett, H.; Canadian Pediatric Society. (2014). Lyme disease in Canada: Focus on children. *Paediatric Child Health*, 19(7), 379–383. Retrieved from http://www.cps.ca/en/documents/position/lyme-disease-children

Pomerantz, W. J., & Weiss, S. L. (2015). *Systemic inflammatory response syndrome (SIRS) and sepsis in children: Definitions, epidemiology, clinical manifestations, and diagnosis*. UpToDate. Retrieved from http://www.uptodate.com/contents/systemic-inflammatory-response-syndrome-sirs-and-sepsis-in-children-definitions-epidemiology-clinical-manifestations-and-diagnosis

Public Health Agency of Canada. (2011). *Rickettsia rickettsii*. Retrieved from http://www.phac-aspc.gc.ca/lab-bio/res/psds-ftss/rickettsia-rickettsii-eng.php

Public Health Agency of Canada. (2012a). Botulism. Retrieved from www.publichealth.gc.ca; http://www.phac-aspc.gc.ca/fs-sa/fs-fi/botulism-eng.php

Public Health Agency of Canada. (2012b). Varicella (Chicken pox). Retrieved from www.publichealth.gc.ca; http://www.phac-aspc.gc.ca/im/vpd-mev/varicella-eng.php#amdat

Public Health Agency of Canada. (2014a). Diphtheria for health professionals. Retrieved from www.publichealth.gc.ca; www.phac-aspc.gc.ca/im/vpd-mev/diphtheria-diphterie/professionals-professionnels-eng.php

Public Health Agency of Canada. (2014b). Mumps for health professionals. Retrieved from www.publichealth.gc.ca; http://www.phac-aspc.gc.ca/im/vpd-mev/mumps-oreillons/professionals-professionnels-eng.php

Public Health Agency of Canada. (2014c). Pertussis for health care professionals. Retrieved from www.publichealth.gc.ca; http://www.phac-aspc.gc.ca/im/vpd-mev/pertussis/professionals-professionnels-eng.php

Public Health Agency of Canada. (2014d). Tetanus for health professionals. Retrieved from www.publichealth.gc.ca; http://www.phac-aspc.gc.ca/im/vpd-mev/tetanus-tetanos/professionals-professionnels-eng.php

Public Health Agency of Canada. (2017). *Notifiable diseases*. Canada: Government of Canada. Retrieved from http://diseases.canada.ca/notifiable/diseases-list. Accessed June 21, 2017,

Purssell, E., & Collin, J. (2016). Fever phobia: The impact of time and mortality—a systematic review and meta-analysis. *International Journal of Nursing Studies, 56*, 81–89.

Reller, M. E., & Dumler, J. S. (2011). Chapter 220: Spotted fever and transitional group rickettsioses. In R. M. Kleigman, B. F. Stanton, J. W. St. Geme III, N. F. Schor, & R. E. Behrman (Eds.). *Nelson textbook of pediatrics* (19th ed., pp. 1038–1045). Philadelphia, PA: Saunders.

Robinson, J. L. (2017). Zika virus: What does a physician caring for children in Canada need to know. *Paediatric Child Health, 22*(1), 48–51.

Rupprecht, C. E., Briggs, D., Brown, C. M., Franka R., Katz, S. L., Kerr, H. D., & Cieslak, P. R. (2010). Use of a reduced (4-dose) vaccine schedule for postexposure prophylaxis to prevent human rabies. *Morbidity and Mortality Weekly Report (MMWR), 59*(02), 1–9.

Santhanam, S. (2015). *Pediatric sepsis*. Retrieved from http://emedicine.medscape.com/article/972559-overview#a1

Sexton, D. J. (2015). *Tetanus*. UpToDate. Retrieved from http://www.uptodate.com/contents/tetanus; http://www.uptodate.com/contents/evaluation-and-management-of-the-febrile-young-infant-7-to-90-days-of-age

SickKids. (2014). *Infection control at SickKids*. Retrieved from www.sickkids.ca; http://www.sickkids.ca/nursing/education-and-learning/nursing-student-orientation/module-one-safety/infection-control-at-sickkids/index.html

Siegel, J. D., Rhinehart, E., Jackson, M., Chiarello, L.; The Healthcare Infection Control Practices Advisory Committee. (2007). *Guideline for isolation precautions: Preventing transmission of infectious agents in healthcare settings*. Retrieved from http://www.cdc.gov/hicpac/pdf/isolation/Isolation2007.pdf

Simon, A. K., Hollander, G. A., & McMichael, A. (2015). Evolution of the immune system in humans from infancy to old age. In *Proceedings of the Royal Society B*. (Vol. *282*, No. 1821, p. 20143085). The Royal Society. Retrieved from http://rspb.royalsocietypublishing.org/content/282/1821/20143085

Smith, T., Rotondo, J., Desai, S., & Deehan, H. (2014). *Pertussis surveillance in Canada: Trends to 2012*. Ottawa: Public Health Agency of Canada. Retrieved from http://www.phac-aspc.gc.ca/publicat/ccdr-rmtc/14vol40/dr-rm40-03/dr-rm40-03-per-eng.php

Smitherman, H. F., & Macias, C. G. (2015). *Evaluation and management of the febrile young infant (7 to 90 days of age)*. UpToDate. Retrieved from http://www.uptodate.com/contents/evaluation-and-management-of-the-febrile-young-infant-7-to-90-days-of-age

Statistics Canada. (2015). *Canadian vital statistics*. Retrieved from Deaths and morality rate, by selected grouped causes, sex and geography—Canada; www.statcan.gc.ca/pub/84f0209x/2009000/t001-eng.htm

Stevenson, B., Goltz, J., & Masse, A. (2016). Preparing for and responding to recent incursions of raccoon rabies variant into Canada. *Canadian Communicable Disease Report, 42*, 125–129.

Sullivan, J. E., Farrar, H. C.; The AAP's Section on Clinical Pharmacology and Therapeutics, and Committee on Drugs. (2011). Clinical report: Fever and antipyretic use in children. *Pediatrics, 127*(3), 580–587.

Taketokmo, C. K., Hodding, J. H., & Kraus, D. M. (2013). *Lexi-comp's drug reference handbook: Pediatric & neonatal dosage handbook* (20th ed.). Hudson, OH: Lexi-comp, Inc.

Thompson, G. C., & Kissoon, N. (2014). Sepsis in Canadian children: A national analysis using administrative data. *Clinical Epidemiology, 6*, 461. Retrieved from https://www.ncbi.nlm.nih.gov/pmc/articles/PMC4266244/

Toronto Public Health. (2017). *Mumps outbreak investigation*. Retrieved from https://www.toronto.ca/community-people/health-wellness-care/diseases-medications-vaccines/mumps-fact-sheet/mumps-outbreak-investigation/

Ward, M. A. (2015a). *Fever in infants and children: Pathophysiology and management*. UpToDate. Retrieved from http://www.uptodate.com/contents/fever-in-infants-and-children-pathophysiology-and-management

Ward, M. A. (2015b). *Patient information: Fever in children (beyond the basics)*. UpToDate. Retrieved from http://www.uptodate.com/contents/fever-in-children-beyond-the-basics

Willoughby, R. E, Jr. (2011). Chapter 266: Rabies. In R. M. Kleigman, B. F. Stanton, J. W. St. Geme III, N. F. Schor, & R. E. Behrman (Eds.). *Nelson textbook of pediatrics* (19th ed., pp. 1154–1157). Philadelphia, PA: Saunders.

Wong, T., Stang, A. S., Ganshorn, H., Hartling, L., Maconochie, I. K., Thomsen, A. M., & Johnson, D. W. (2013). Combined and alternating paracetamol and ibuprofen therapy for febrile children. *Cochrane Database of Systematic Reviews*, (10), CD009572.

World Health Organization. (2009). WHO guidelines on hand hygiene in healthcare. Retrieved from http://whqlibdoc.who.int/publications/2009/9789241597906_eng.pdf

World Health Organization. (2015). Rabies. Retrieved from http://www.who.int/mediacentre/factsheets/fs099/en/

Zabawski, E. J, Jr. (2014). Scarlet fever. Retrieved from http://emedicine.medscape.com/article/1053253-overview

MULTIPLE CHOICE QUESTIONS

1. Compared with adults, why are infants and children at an increased risk for infection and communicable diseases?
   a. The infant has had limited exposure to disease and is losing the passive immunity acquired from maternal antibodies.
   b. The infant demonstrates an increased inflammatory response.
   c. Cellular immunity is not functional at birth.
   d. Infants have an increased risk for infection until they receive their first set of immunizations.

2. A mother calls the clinic because her 2-year-old daughter has a rectal temperature of 37.8°C (100°F). She wonders how high a fever should be before she should give medications to reduce it. What is the best response by the nurse?
   a. "All fevers should be treated to prevent seizures."
   b. "Antipyretics should be used with any rise in temperature. They can help change the course of the infection."
   c. "Give your child aspirin when her fever is above 38°C (100.4°F)."
   d. "In a normal healthy child, if your child is not uncomfortable, fevers less than 39°C (102.2°F) do not require medication."

3. A neonate should be evaluated by a physician if which signs and symptoms are present?
   a. Acting fussier than normal
   b. Refusing the pacifier
   c. Rectal temperature above 38°C
   d. Mottling that is present during bathing

4. The public health nurse has been asked to provide information to local child care centres on controlling the spread of infectious diseases. What is the best information the nurse can provide?
   a. The etiology of common infectious diseases
   b. Proper handwashing techniques
   c. The physiology of the immune system
   d. Why children are at a higher risk of infection than adults

DOSAGE CALCULATION QUESTIONS

The nurse is caring for a child who has a rash and is complaining of feeling itchy and is continually scratching. The child weighs 14.5 kg (32 lb). The medication order reads: Diphenhydramine 6.25 mg PO every 4 to 6 hours as needed for itching. Diphenhydramine is supplied as 12.5 mg/5 mL. How many milliliters will the nurse administer. Round to the nearest tenth.

CRITICAL THINKING EXERCISES

1. A 12-year-old boy presents with a very sore throat and fever. On assessment, you find an erythematous rash on his face that feels like sandpaper. You obtain a throat culture, which is positive for group A streptococcus. What instructions would you give the parents regarding his care at home?

2. A 1-month-old infant is admitted to the hospital to rule out sepsis. What would be your priority nursing interventions?

3. A 4-year-old child presents with a fever and rash. What three of the following items should the nurse obtain during the health history?
   _____ a. Immunization history
   _____ b. Any exposure to communicable or infectious diseases
   _____ c. Whether the child takes a daily vitamin
   _____ d. Thorough description and history of the rash
   _____ e. Mother's immunization history

STUDY ACTIVITIES

1. The 4-year-old presented in Question 3 above was diagnosed with varicella zoster virus. Write a nursing care plan for a child with varicella.

2. A child is brought to the school nurse with intense itching. Upon assessment, the nurse finds an erythematous, papular rash with excoriations on the child's hands and feet. As suspected, the diagnosis of scabies is confirmed. What teaching is necessary for the parents, family, and classmates of the child?

BRINGING IT ALL TOGETHER: A CASE STUDY

As the nurse in a pediatric clinic, you see a child who comes in because she is having extreme itching, especially at night. The child is diagnosed with scabies. The mother is upset and says to you, "We are clean people! I don't understand how this could happen!"

Go to thePoint **to find questions to consider about this case.**

38

Nursing Care of the Child With a Neurologic Disorder

Learning Objectives

Upon completion of the chapter, you will be able to:

1. Compare how the anatomy and physiology of the neurologic system in children differs from adults.

2. Identify various factors associated with neurologic disease in infants and children.

3. Discuss common laboratory and other diagnostic tests useful in the diagnosis of neurologic conditions.

4. Discuss common medications and other treatments used for treatment and palliation of neurologic conditions.

5. Recognize risk factors associated with various neurologic disorders.

6. Distinguish among different neurologic illnesses based on the signs and symptoms associated with them.

7. Discuss nursing interventions commonly used for neurologic illnesses.

8. Devise an individualized nursing care plan for the child with a neurologic disorder.

9. Develop child and family teaching plans for the child with a neurologic disorder.

10. Describe the psychosocial impact of chronic neurologic disorders on children.

Antonio Chapman, **3 months old, has had increased irritability, poor sucking and feeding, and a fever for the past 24 hours. Today he is lethargic with a weak cry and is vomiting his feeds.**

Neurologic disorders in children can have a devastating and lasting impact. Neurologic function relies on several factors including structural integrity to maintain equilibrium of the central nervous system (Gooley, Gooley, Moniz, & Hunter, 2016). Neurologic disorders can be divided into several categories, including structural disorders, seizure disorders, infectious disorders, trauma to the neurologic system, blood flow disruption disorders, and chronic disorders.

Nurses must be familiar with neurologic conditions affecting children in order to provide prevention, prompt treatment, guidance, and support to families. Neurologic disorders require acute interventions, but many times have long-lasting implications on the child's health and development. Due to the potentially devastating effects that neurologic disorders can have on children and their families, nurses need to be skilled in assessment and interventions in this area and must be able to provide support throughout the course of the illness and beyond.

VARIATIONS IN PEDIATRIC ANATOMY AND PHYSIOLOGY

Neurologic disorders can result from congenital problems as well as from infections or traumas. Certain neurologic conditions occur in children more often than in adults and these conditions will affect their growth and development. In addition, children are at an increased risk for different neurologic problems compared with adults due to anatomic and physiologic differences.

Brain and Spinal Cord Development

The brain and spinal cord make up the **central nervous system (CNS)**. Development of these structures occurs in the first 3 to 4 weeks of gestation from the **neural tube**. Infection, trauma, **teratogens** (any environmental substance that can cause physical defects in the developing embryo and fetus), and malnutrition during this period can result in malformations in brain and spinal cord development and may affect normal CNS development.

At birth, the cranial bones are not well developed and are not fused. Therefore, there is an increased risk for fracture. The brain is highly vascular, leading to an increased risk for hemorrhage. Premature infants are at greater risk for brain damage; the more premature the infant, the greater the risk. The premature infant has more capillaries in the periventricular area, which is the brain tissue that lines the outside of the lateral ventricles. These capillaries are fragile

and at greater risk for rupture, leading to intracranial bleeding. Also, because the cranium is very soft in the preterm infant, external pressure can change its shape and cause increased pressure in areas of the brain and possible hemorrhage.

The sutures and fontanels present in the newborn help make the skull more flexible and help to accommodate for brain growth that continues after birth. Closure of the fontanels too early or too late can be indicative of problems with brain growth. The child's spine is very mobile, especially the cervical spine region, resulting in a high risk for cervical spine injury.

Nervous System

The development of the nervous system is complete but immature at birth. The infant is born with all the nerve cells that he or she will have throughout life. However, **myelinization**, the formation of myelin, which covers and protects the nerves, is incomplete. The speed and accuracy of nerve impulses increases as myelinization increases. This process accounts for the acquisition of fine and gross motor movements and coordination in early childhood. Myelinization proceeds in the cephalocaudal direction. For example, infants are able to control the head and neck before the trunk and extremities.

The immaturity of the CNS in preterm infants can result in delayed development of motor skills. Premature infants may have difficulty coordinating sucking and swallowing, leading to feeding and growth issues. Also, episodes of apnea can be problematic in the preterm infant due to the underdevelopment of the nervous system.

Head Size

The head of the infant and young child is large in proportion to the body. The head of an infant accounts for a quarter of the body height; in adults, it accounts for one eighth of the body height (Fig. 38.1). In addition, the infant's and child's neck muscles are not well developed. Both of these differences lead to an increased incidence of head injury from falls. The head is the fastest growing body part during infancy and continues to grow until the child is 5 years old.

COMMON MEDICAL TREATMENTS

A variety of interventions, including medical treatments and medications, are used to treat neurologic illness in children. The most common treatments and medications used for neurologic disorders are listed in Common Medical Treatments 38.1 and Drug Guide 38.1.

Newborn   6 years   25 years

FIGURE 38.1 Proportion of head-to-body height in the newborn, child, and adult.

NURSING PROCESS OVERVIEW FOR THE CHILD WITH A NEUROLOGIC DISORDER

Care of the child with a neurologic disorder includes assessment, nursing diagnosis, planning, intervention, and evaluation. There are a number of general concepts related to the nursing process that can be applied to the management of neurologic disorders. From a general understanding of the care involved for a child with neurologic dysfunction, the nurse can then individualize the care based on the particular child's specifics.

> Remember Antonio, the 3-month-old with lethargy, a weak cry, and vomiting? What additional health history and physical examination assessment information should the nurse obtain?

Assessment

Assessment of neurologic dysfunction in children includes health history, physical examination, and laboratory and diagnostic testing.

Take Note!

Neurologic assessment should proceed from least invasive to most invasive. The use of toys and familiar objects, as well as incorporating play, will help promote cooperation from the child.

Health History

The health history consists of past medical history, including the mother's pregnancy history, family history, and history of present illness (when the symptoms started and how they have progressed) as well as treatments used at home. The past medical history might be significant for prematurity, difficult birth, infection during pregnancy, nausea, vomiting, headaches, changes in gait, falls, visual disturbances, or recent trauma. Family history might be significant for genetic disorders with neurologic manifestations, seizure disorders, or headaches. When eliciting the history of the present illness, inquire about the following:

- Nausea
- Vomiting
- Changes in gait
- Visual disturbances
- Complaints of headaches
- Recent trauma
- Changes in cognition
- Change in consciousness, including any loss of consciousness
- Poor feeding
- Lethargy
- Increased irritability
- Fever
- Pain
- Altered muscle tonicity
- Delays in growth and development
- Ingestion or inhalation of neurotoxic substances or chemicals

COMMON MEDICAL TREATMENTS 38.1

Treatment	Explanation	Indications	Nursing Implications
Shunt placement	A catheter is placed in the ventricle to pass the CSF to the peritoneal cavity, atrium of the heart, or pleural spaces. (Ventriculoperitoneal shunts are commonly used)	Hydrocephalus, increased ICP	Monitor: • For signs and symptoms of increased ICP • Neurologic status closely • Level of consciousness and vital signs • For signs and symptoms of infection
Ventilation	Hyperventilation to decrease $PaCO_2$, which will result in vasoconstriction and therefore decrease ICP Adequate oxygenation to prevent hypoxia and further damage to the brain	Increased ICP	Monitor: • Arterial blood gases • For signs and symptoms of increased ICP • Pulse oximetry • Calculate Pediatric Early Warning Score (PEWS) as per local hospital guidelines
PT/OT/ST	Therapies are used to improve motor function and ability of children with neurologic disorders	Head injury, intellectual disability	Ensure adequate communication exists within the interdisciplinary team
External ventricular drainage (EVD)	A catheter is temporarily placed in the ventricle and CSF is drained in a closed system to an external reservoir	Most commonly used with shunt infections until CSF is sterile and shunt can be replaced; treats acute-onset hydrocephalus, meningitis, encephalitis, tumours that cause blockage of CSF, closed head injury, subarachnoid hemorrhage, increased ICP; also can be used to monitor ICP	Monitor: • For signs and symptoms of increased ICP • Neurologic status closely • Level of consciousness and vital signs • For signs and symptoms of infection • Level of collection container when drain is unclamped
Ventricular tap	To reduce accumulation of CSF and decrease ICP	Increased ICP	Monitor: • Level of consciousness • Neurologic status
Vagal nerve stimulator	A nerve stimulator is implanted and a lead wire running under the skin is wrapped around the vagus nerve. The stimulator is programmed to provide the appropriate dose of stimulation at preset intervals; additional stimulation can be administered	Short- and long-term seizure management in children older than 12 years of age	Monitor: • For signs and symptoms of infection • For seizure activity
Ketogenic diet	Diet involving high intake of fats, adequate protein, and a very low intake of carbohydrates, resulting in a ketosis state. Child is kept in a mild state of dehydration	Prevention, control, and reduction of seizures, in particular for children with difficult-to-control seizures	Monitor: • Input and output closely • For seizure activity • Growth and nutritional status • The diet is time-consuming and many children find it unpalatable; therefore, not all families and children accept it • Recommended for a minimum of 3 months, maximum of 2 years • Alternative diets include: the medium-chain triglyceride diet, modified Atkins diet, and a low glycemic index diet

The multi-disciplinary team is often involved with this group of children and young people, and can include occupational therapy (OT), physical therapy (PT), and speech therapy (ST).

DRUG GUIDE 38.1

Medication	Actions/Indications	Nursing Implications
Antibiotics (oral, parenteral, intrathecal)	Treatment of bacterial meningitis and shunt infections; kill and prevent the growth of bacteria	Check for antibiotic allergies. Monitor serum levels to ensure therapeutic dosing, if indicated. Give as prescribed for the length of time prescribed
Anticonvulsants (oral, parenteral)	Decrease hyperexcitability of nerves Treatment and prevention of seizures	Maintain seizure precautions. Monitor for drug interactions and long-term adverse effects Monitor and document all seizure activity Many are used in combination, but need to be aware of interactions and long-term adverse effects Stopping drug abruptly may precipitate seizures or even status epilepticus
Benzodiazepines Diazepam (oral, rectal, or parenteral) Lorazepam (parenteral or oral) Midazolam (IV, IM nasally, buccally)	Minor sedative that prevents or stops seizures by slowing down the CNS, making abnormal electrical activity unlikely. (Not recommended as first-line agent in status epilepticus) Treatment for status epilepticus Treatment for status epilepticus	Monitor IV administration closely as hypotension and respiratory depression can occur Diazepam is available in rectal form to stop prolonged seizures in children (safety not established in infants and children 6 months to 2 years). Useful for home management; nurses must educate family members on administration and when to call physician or nurse practitioner Monitor sedation level and for cessation of seizure activity Least effective when given peripherally, monitor sedation level and for cessation of seizure activity
Analgesics (acetaminophen, ibuprofen, ketorolac, morphine)	Block pain impulse in response to inhibition of prostaglandin synthesis Narcotic analgesics (i.e., morphine) act on receptors in the brain to alter perception of pain. Used to treat pain. Used to help avoid increase in ICP	Monitor for improvements in pain Monitor sedation and respiratory status with narcotics Monitor neurologic status closely Used cautiously because loss of accurate neurologic evaluation can occur
Osmotic diuretics (i.e., mannitol)	Increase plasma osmolality, therefore inducing diffusion back into plasma and extravascular space/reduces ICP	Monitor electrolytes Monitor I/O closely Monitor vital signs Monitor for signs and symptoms of increased ICP
Corticosteroids (i.e., dexamethasone)	Suppress inflammation and normal immune response/reduce cerebral edema	Give oral doses with food. Dosage must be tapered before discontinuing

I/O, intake/output.
Adapted from Taketokmo, C. K., Hodding, J. H., & Kraus, D. M. (2017). *Lexi-comp's drug reference handbook: Pediatric & neonatal dosage handbook* (20th ed.). Hudson, OH: Lexi-comp, Inc.

Physical Examination

Physical examination of the nervous system consists of inspection and observation, palpation, and auscultation.

INSPECTION AND OBSERVATION

Specific areas to inspect and observe include:
- Level of consciousness (LOC)
- Vital signs
- Head, face, and neck
- Cranial nerve function
- Motor function
- Reflexes
- Sensory function
- Increased **intracranial pressure (ICP)** (a rise in the normal pressure within the skull)

Level of Consciousness. Begin the physical examination with inspection and observation. Observe the child's LOC, noting a decrease or significant changes. LOC is the earliest indicator of improvement or deterioration of neurologic status. Extreme irritability or lethargy is considered an abnormal finding.

Consciousness consists of alertness, which is a wakeful state and includes the ability to respond to stimuli, and cognition, which includes the ability to process stimuli and demonstrate a verbal or motor response. Five different states constitute the levels of consciousness:

1. *Full consciousness* is defined as a state in which the child is awake and alert; is oriented to time, place, and person; and exhibits age-appropriate behaviours.

2. *Confusion* is defined as a state in which disorientation exists. The child may be alert but responds inappropriately to questions.

3. *Obtunded* is defined as a state in which the child has limited responses to the environment and falls asleep unless stimulation is provided.

4. *Stupor* exists when the child only responds to vigorous stimulation.

5. *Coma* defines a state in which the child cannot be aroused, even with painful stimuli.

Take Note!

Lack of response to painful stimuli is abnormal and can indicate a life-threatening condition. Report this finding immediately.

The Pediatric Glasgow Coma Scale (GCS) is a popular scale used to standardize degree of consciousness. It consists of three parts: eye opening, verbal response, and motor response (Fig. 38.2). When assessing LOC in children, consider that the infant or child may not respond to unfamiliar voices in an unfamiliar environment. Therefore, it may be helpful to have a parent present to elicit the response.

Take Note!

Parents will often be the first to notice changes in their child's LOC. Listen to parents and respond to their concerns.

Vital Signs. Assessment of vital signs can provide probable underlying causes for altered LOC as well as reveal the adequacy of oxygenation and circulation. Certain neurologic conditions like cerebral infections, increased ICP, coma, brain stem injury, or head injuries can cause alterations in the child's vital signs. Calculate Paediatric Early Warning (PEW) score as per local hospital and provincial guidelines and policies.

Head, Face, and Neck. Inspect and observe the head for size and shape. Abnormal skull shape can result from premature closure or widening of sutures. Inspect and observe the face for symmetry. Asymmetry may occur due to paralysis of certain cranial nerves, position in utero, or swelling caused by

FIGURE 38.2 Pediatric Glasgow Coma Scale (GCS). The Pediatric GCS provides for developmentally appropriate cues to assess level of consciousness (LOC) in infants and children. Numeric values are assigned to the levels of response and the sum provides an overall picture, as well as an objective measure, of the child's LOC. The lower the score, the less responsive the child.

trauma. Assess range of motion of the neck. Alterations in range of motion can indicate CNS infections such as meningitis.

The most dramatic increase in brain volume occurs during the last 3 months of fetal development and the first 2 years of life. The relationship between head and brain growth explains why head circumference is a standard assessment made in children younger than 3 years of age. All children younger than 3 years old, and any child whose head size is questionable, should have their head circumference

TABLE 38.1	ASSESSMENT OF CRANIAL NERVES IN INFANTS AND CHILDREN	

Cranial Nerve	Function	Assessment Procedure
I (olfactory)	Sense of smell	Not evaluated in infants and young children. In children, assess child's ability to recognize common smells (i.e., an orange) while eyes are closed.
II (optic), III (oculomotor), IV (trochlear), VI (abducens)	Vision, motor control, and sensation of eye muscles, movement of major eye muscles	Assess oculomotor ability by having child follow object (toy or brightly coloured object). Assess vision fields and visual acuity in older child. Assess pupil reaction same as adult. May need to talk to child or have parent in visual field while applying light stimulus.
V (trigeminal)	Mastication muscles and facial sensation	Note strength of infant's suck on pacifier, examiner's thumb, or bottle. In children, assess strength of bite and ability to discern light touch on face.
VII (facial)	Facial muscles, salivation, and taste	Note symmetry of facial expressions; in infant, monitor during spontaneous cries or smiles. In older child, test as in adults. Assess taste by asking to discern certain common tastes (salt, sugar).
VIII (acoustic)	Hearing	In infant, note response to voice. In children, use whisper test or Weber or Rinne test.
IX (glossopharyngeal), X (vagus)	Motor impulses to heart and other organs, swallowing, and gag reflex	Gag reflex and swallowing tested as in adults. Check time of last feeding, especially in the infant, to avoid vomiting when gag reflex is tested.
XI (accessory)	Impulses to muscles of shoulders and pharynx	In infants, note symmetry of head position when placed in the sitting position. In children, same as adults.
XII (hypoglossal)	Motor impulses to tongue and skeletal muscles	In infants, note spontaneous tongue movements. In children, same as adults.

measured and plotted on a growth chart (See thePoint for links to growth charts.).

Assessment of the growth trend of the head is important in detecting potential neurologic conditions. Report and investigate any variation in head circumference percentiles over time because variations may indicate abnormal brain or skull growth. A smaller than normal **head circumference**, which measures around the child's head at the largest area, may indicate microcephaly, and a larger than normal head circumference may indicate hydrocephalus.

Take Note!

Do not attempt any assessment that involves movement of the head and neck in cases of trauma or suspected trauma until cervical injury is ruled out. Maintain complete immobilization of the cervical spine until that time.

Cranial Nerve Function. Techniques of assessment of cranial nerve function are similar to techniques for adult assessment. The method of obtaining responses may vary based on age and developmental level of the child. Certain elements of the adult assessment may be omitted. Alterations in cranial nerve function can be the result of compression of a specific nerve, infection, or

trauma leading to brain injury. Refer to Table 38.1 for an explanation of cranial nerve assessment in children.

Use the doll's eyes manoeuvre to evaluate cranial nerves III, IV, and VI. This manoeuvre can be helpful when assessing an infant, uncooperative child, or comatose child. It examines horizontal and vertical eye movements by turning the head in one direction and assessing if the eyes move symmetrically in the other direction. For example, if you suddenly turn the child's head to the right, the child's eyes should look to the left symmetrically. Assess vertical eye movements in a similar manner by flexing or extending the neck. Absence of expected eye movements may indicate increased ICP.

When assessing oculomotor function, be sure to note nystagmus or sunset appearance of the eyes. Observe for nystagmus by looking for involuntary, rapid, rhythmic eye movements that may be present at rest or with eye movement. Horizontal nystagmus may occur with lesions in the brain stem and can be the result of certain medications (phenytoin in particular). Vertical nystagmus indicates brain stem dysfunction. Sunsetting is when the sclera of the eyes is showing over the top of the iris (Fig. 38.3). Sunset eyes may indicate increased ICP as seen in hydrocephalus. Pupillary response is often abnormal when a neurologic disorder

FIGURE 38.3 Sunsetting of the eyes is a sign of increased intracranial pressure.

is present. Refer to Figure 38.4 for illustrations of varied pupillary responses.

Take Note!

Immediately report the sudden presence of fixed and dilated pupils.

Motor Function. Observe muscle strength, size, and tone in the infant or child. Assess bilaterally and compare. Observe spontaneous activity, posture, and balance, and assess for asymmetric movements. In the infant, observe resting posture, which will normally

FIGURE 38.4 Assessing pupil size and reaction. **A.** *Pinpoint* is commonly observed in poisonings, brain stem dysfunction, and opiate use. **B.** *Dilated but reactive* is seen after seizures. *Fixed and dilated* is associated with brain stem herniation secondary to increased intracranial pressure. **C.** *One dilated but reactive* is associated with intracranial mass.

Decorticate   Extremities flexed

A

Decerebrate   Extremities extended and pronated

B

FIGURE 38.5 **A.** Decorticate posturing occurs with damage of the cerebral cortex and includes adduction of the arms, flexion at the elbows with arms held over chest, and flexion of the wrists with hands fisted. Lower extremities are adducted and extended. **B.** Decerebrate posturing occurs with damage to the midbrain and includes extension and pronation of the arms and legs.

be a slightly flexed posture. The infant should be able to extend extremities to a normal stretch. Alterations in motor function, like changes in gait, muscle tone, or strength, may indicate certain neurologic problems such as increased ICP, head injury, and cerebral infections. Because cortical control of motor function is lost in certain neurologic disorders, postural reflexes re-emerge and are directly related to the area of the brain that is damaged. Therefore, it is important to assess for two distinct types of posturing that may occur. **Decorticate posturing** occurs with damage of the cerebral cortex (Fig. 38.5A). **Decerebrate posturing** occurs with damage at the level of the brain stem (Fig. 38.5B). Both types of posturing are characterized by extremely rigid muscle tone.

Reflexes. Testing of deep tendon reflexes is part of the neurologic assessment, just as it is in adults. Testing of primitive and protective reflexes in the infant is important because infants cannot perform tasks on command. The Moro, tonic neck, and withdrawal reflexes are important in assessing neurologic health in infants. Refer to Chapter 25 for a further explanation of primitive and protective reflexes in infants (see Chapter 25, Table 25.1). Absence of certain reflexes, persistence of primitive reflexes after age of normal disappearance, or increases in reflexes may be present in specific neurologic conditions.

Sensory Function. When assessing the child, use techniques similar to those used in the adult assessment. Make sure to explain what you are doing to the child, especially before the pinprick test, to gain continued cooperation. When assessing sensory function,

COMPARISON CHART 38.1 — EARLY VERSUS LATE SIGNS OF INCREASED INTRACRANIAL PRESSURE

Early Signs	Late Signs

• Headache
• Vomiting, possibly projectile
• Blurred vision, double vision (diplopia)
• Dizziness
• Decreased pulse and respirations
• Increased blood pressure or pulse pressure
• Pupil reaction time decreased and unequal
• Sunset eyes
• Changes in level of consciousness, irritability
• Seizure activity
• In infant will also see:
  • Bulging, tense fontanel
  • Wide sutures and increased head circumference
  • Dilated scalp veins
  • High-pitched cry
	• Lowered level of consciousness
	• Decreased motor and sensory responses
	• Bradycardia
	• Irregular respirations
	• Cheyne–Stokes respirations
	• Decerebrate or decorticate posturing
	• Fixed and dilated pupils

the child should be able to distinguish between light touch, pain, vibration, heat, and cold. When assessing an infant, limit the examination to responses to touch or pain. The normal response in a 4-month-old infant will be movement away from the stimulus. Alterations in sensory function can result from brain or spinal cord lesions.

Increased Intracranial Pressure. Observe for signs and symptoms associated with increased ICP while caring for a child with a potential or suspected neurologic disorder. Refer to Comparison Chart 38.1 for early versus late signs and symptoms of increased ICP. Increased ICP is a sign that may occur with many neurologic disorders. It may result from head trauma, birth trauma, hydrocephalus, infection, and brain tumours. As ICP increases, LOC decreases and the signs and symptoms will become more pronounced. It is essential to recognize early signs and symptoms of increased ICP and intervene immediately to prevent long-term damage and possible death.

PALPATION

Palpation of the newborn and infant skull and fontanels is an important function of the neurologic examination. Changes in size or fullness of the fontanels may exist in certain neurologic conditions and must be noted. A bulging fontanel can be a sign of increased ICP and is seen in neurologic disorders such as hydrocephalus and head traumas. It is normal for the fontanels to be full or bulging during crying; take this into consideration during assessment.

Note any premature closure of fontanels, which can indicate skull deformities such as craniosynostosis. The posterior fontanel normally closes by 2 months of age and the anterior fontanel normally closes by 12

to 18 months of age. In children with hydrocephalus, widening of the fontanels may be noted, along with a tense appearance and a resulting increase in head circumference.

AUSCULTATION

Physicians or nurse practitioners may perform auscultation of the skull. Soft, symmetric bruits may be found in children younger than 4 years of age or in children with acute febrile illness. A finding of a loud or localized bruit is usually significant and requires immediate further investigation. Increased ICP, resulting from conditions such as hydrocephalus, tumour, or meningitis, frequently produces intracranial bruits. Arterial venous malformations may also produce large bruits.

Laboratory and Diagnostic Testing

Common Laboratory and Diagnostic Tests 38.1 offers an explanation of the most commonly used laboratory and diagnostic tests utilized when considering neurologic disorders. The tests can assist the physician or nurse practitioner in diagnosing the disorder and/or serve as guidelines in determining ongoing treatment. Laboratory or nonnursing personnel obtain some of the tests, while the nurse might obtain others. In either instance, it is important to be familiar with how the tests are obtained, what they are used for, and normal versus abnormal results. This knowledge will also be necessary when providing child and family education related to the testing. Many of these tests, such as lumbar puncture (LP) (Fig. 38.6), can be frightening to parents and the child. Prepare the family and the child and provide support and reassurance during and after the test or procedure.

(text continues on page 1390)

COMMON LABORATORY AND DIAGNOSTIC TESTS 38.1

Test	Explanation	Indications	Nursing Implications
Lumbar puncture (LP)	Withdrawal of cerebrospinal fluid (CSF) from the subarachnoid space for analysis	To diagnose hemorrhage, infection, or obstruction Can obtain measurement of spinal fluid pressure	Assess child status during procedure Assist with proper positioning (Fig. 38.6; (Hanson, Schunk, Corneli, & Soprano, 2016). Help child maintain position and remain still Maintain strict asepsis Assist with collection and transport of specimen Encourage fluids after procedure, if not contraindicated Keep child flat for 1 hour if ordered Apply topical anesthetic cream to puncture site 30 to 60 minutes before procedure to reduce pain, if ordered
Head and neck x-ray	Radiographic image of the head and neck will show skull and spine structures	Detects skull and spinal fractures; shows location and course of ventricular catheters; reveals information about increased intracranial pressure (ICP) and skull defects	Children may be afraid. Allow a parent or family member to accompany the child. If the child is unable or unwilling to stay still for the x-ray, restraint may be necessary. The time of restraint should be limited to the amount of time needed for the x-ray
Fluoroscopy	Radiographic examination that uses continuous x-rays to show live up-to-date images	Can assess cervical spine for instability during movement	Same as head and neck x-rays. Child will need to cooperate with flexion and extension of neck
Cerebral angiography	X-ray study of cerebral blood vessels. Involves injection of a contrast medium and use of fluoroscopy	Can assess for vessel defects or space-occupying lesions	Same as head and neck x-rays. Assess for allergy to contrast medium Push fluids following procedure, if not contraindicated, to help flush out contrast medium
Ultrasound	Use of sound waves to locate the depth and structure within soft tissues and fluid	Used to assess intracranial hemorrhage in newborns, and ventricular size	Better tolerated by nonsedated children than CT or MRI Can be performed portably at bedside
Computed tomography (CT)	Noninvasive x-ray study that looks at tissue density and structures. Images a "slice" of child's tissue	To diagnose congenital abnormalities, such as neural tube defects, hemorrhage, tumours, fractures	Machine is large and can be frightening to children Procedure can be lengthy, and the child must remain still. If unable to do so, sedation may be necessary Can be performed with or without use of contrast medium; if used, assess for allergy Encourage fluids post-procedure, if not contraindicated
Electroencephalogram (EEG)	Measures electrical activity of the brain	To diagnose seizures and brain death	Must remain still. If unable to do so, sedation may be necessary, but should be avoided if possible because sedatives can alter the EEG reading Inform technician of what anticonvulsants the child is taking. Morning anticonvulsants may need to be held

(continued)

COMMON LABORATORY AND DIAGNOSTIC TESTS 38.1 (continued)

Test	Explanation	Indications	Nursing Implications
Magnetic resonance imaging (MRI)	Use of magnetic field to show different tissue compositions	Used to assess tumours and inflammation; used to diagnose congenital abnormalities, such as neural tube defects; shows normal versus abnormal brain tissue	Child may not have any metal devices, internal or external, while undergoing MRI (ensure hospital gown does not have metal snaps). Procedure can be lengthy, and the child must remain still. Child is placed in long narrow tube and the machine makes a booming noise when it is turned on and off during the procedure, and therefore, can be difficult to gain cooperation. If the child is unable to remain still, sedation may be necessary Can be performed with or without use of a contrast medium. If contrast medium is used, assess for allergy. Encourage fluids post-procedure, if not contraindicated
Positron emission tomography (PET)	Similar to CT or MRI, but radioisotope is added. Measures physiologic function	Provides information on brain functional development. Can assist in identifying seizure foci. Can assess tumours and brain metabolism	Procedure can be lengthy, and the child must remain still. If unable to do so, sedation may be necessary Intravenous access will be needed for the procedure. Encourage fluids post-procedure, if not contraindicated, to help body eliminate radioisotopes
Single-photon emission computed tomography (SPECT)	Use of radiopharmaceuticals to provide three-dimensional splices; less expensive and more available than PET	Used to detect brain death, presence of encephalitis, hydrocephalus, to localize epileptic foci, assess metabolic activity, evaluate brain tumours, assessment of childhood development disorders	Similar to PET In uncooperative children, do not use sedation until after injection because it may affect brain activity Secure child's head Sudden distractions or loud noises can alter the distribution of radionuclide
Cisternography	Radiopharmaceuticals injected intrathecally during a lumbar puncture to assess flow and reabsorption of CSF	Can assist in selection of type of shunt and pathway to use in treating hydrocephalus	Sterile LP performed and radionuclide injected into cerebrospinal circulation Imaging performed at specified times Child must lie flat after puncture
Intracranial pressure (ICP) monitoring (intraventricular catheter, subarachnoid screw or bolt, epidural sensor, anterior fontanel pressure monitor)	A sensing device is placed in the head that monitors the pressure intracranially	Used to monitor ICP resulting from hydrocephalus, acute head trauma, and brain tumours. Ventricular catheter also allows for draining of CSF to help reduce ICP	Usually monitored in critical care setting Monitor for signs and symptoms of increased ICP Monitor for infection Keep head of bed elevated 15 to 30 degrees Alarms for monitoring device should remain on at all times Reduce stimulation and avoid interventions that may cause pain or stress and result in an increased ICP

COMMON LABORATORY AND DIAGNOSTIC TESTS 38.1 (continued)

Test	Explanation	Indications	Nursing Implications
Video EEG	Measures electrical activity of the brain continuously along with recorded video of actions and behaviours	Can help determine precise localization of seizure area before surgery. Assists in diagnosis and management of seizures by correlating behaviours with abnormal EEG activity	Ensure that seizure precautions are in place Parent or caregiver must be with child at all times The child's mobility is often limited and usually confined to the room. When the child changes position, ensure that he or she is still seen by video camera. Boredom can be a problem. Must notify nurse if seizure activity occurs; push the alert button to highlight attack on EEG recoding Nurse must immediately go to the room, expose as much of the child as possible (remove covers; if at night, turn on light), and avoid blocking the camera. Ask questions (I.e., what is your name, can you raise your left arm, remember the word banana) to help assess responsiveness more accurately. Stay with the child until a full recovery has occurred. Ask the child what word you asked him or her to remember and document all findings and time of the event

Adapted from Fischbach, F. T., & Dunning III, M. B., III. (2015). *A manual of laboratory and diagnostic tests* (9th ed.). Philadelphia, PA: Wolters Kluwer Health/Lippincott Williams & Wilkins.

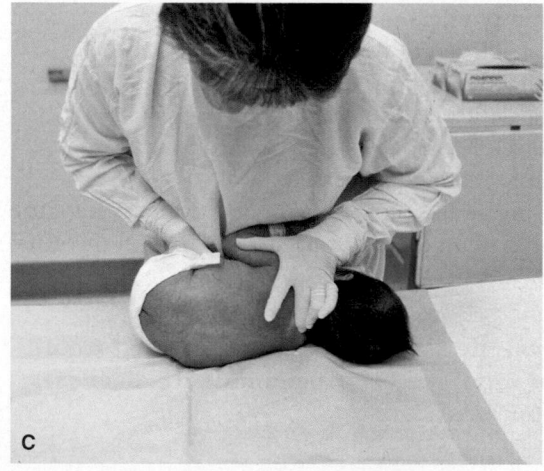

FIGURE 38.6 Proper positioning for a lumbar puncture. **A**. The newborn is positioned upright with head flexed forward. **B**. Child or older infant is positioned on the side with head flexed forward and knees flexed to abdomen. **C**. The infant in a knee chest position.

Atraumatic Care

During an LP, use distraction techniques that will allow the child to remain in the proper position, such as storytelling or music. Encourage parental involvement and enlist the help of a child life specialist, if possible. Oral sucrose may be helpful for infants during the LP.

> After completing an assessment of Antonio, the nurse noted the following: a full anterior fontanel; when being held, Antonio was inconsolable; when lying still, he was calmer and in the opisthotonic position.

Nursing Diagnoses and Related Interventions

Upon completion of a thorough assessment, the nurse might identify several nursing diagnoses, including:
- Decreased intracranial adaptive capacity
- Risk for ineffective tissue perfusion: cerebral
- Risk for injury
- Risk for complications of neurologic/sensory dysfunction
- Risk for infection
- Pain
- Self-care deficit (specify)
- Impaired physical mobility
- Risk for delayed development
- Imbalanced nutrition: less than body requirements
- Risk for deficient fluid volume
- Deficient knowledge (specify)
- Interrupted family processes

Nursing goals, interventions, and evaluation for the child with a neurologic disorder are based on the nursing diagnoses.

> Based on the assessment findings, what would be your top three prioritized nursing diagnoses for Antonio?

Nursing Care Plan 38.1, found at the end of the chapter, may be used as a guide in planning nursing care for the child with a neurologic disorder. It should be individualized based on the child's symptoms and needs. Additional information will be included later in this chapter related to specific disorders.

> Based on your top three nursing diagnoses for Antonio, describe appropriate nursing interventions.

SEIZURE DISORDERS

Seizures occur in approximately 4% to 10% of children, with a lifetime incidence of epilepsy being 3%, with half of these starting in childhood (Mikati, 2011). Most seizures are caused by disorders that originate outside of the brain such as a high fever, infection, head trauma, hypoxia, toxins, or cardiac arrhythmias. Seizure disorders discussed below include epilepsy, febrile seizures, and neonatal seizures.

Epilepsy

Epilepsy is a condition in which seizures are triggered recurrently from within the brain. Epilepsy is a common chronic neurologic disorder discovered in childhood, although brain injury or infection can cause epilepsy at any age. In Canada, 4.03 to 5.26 per 1,000 children are affected by epilepsy (Prasad, Corbett, & Prasad, 2014). The International League Against Epilepsy (ILAE, 2014) updated the classification of epilepsy which is now defined by the presence of any of the following conditions:
- Two or more unprovoked (or reflex) seizures, which occur more than 24 hours apart
- One unprovoked (or reflex) seizure and a chance of further seizures the same as the general recurrence risk (at least 60%) after two unprovoked seizures, happening over the next 10 years
- Diagnosis of an epilepsy syndrome (Fisher et al., 2014)

The prognosis for most children with seizures associated with epilepsy is good. Many children will outgrow epilepsy, but some children will have persistent seizures that are difficult to manage and may be unresponsive to pharmacologic interventions. Living with a seizure disorder may have a devastating impact on the quality of life of the child and family.

Pathophysiology

Epilepsy is a complex disorder of the CNS in which brain function is affected. Recurrent or unprovoked seizures are the clinical manifestation of epilepsy and result from a disruption of electrical communication among the neurons of the brain. This disruption results from an imbalance between the excitatory and inhibitory mechanisms in the brain, causing the neurons to either fire when they are not supposed to or not fire when they should. Epilepsy has numerous causes. It may be acquired and related to brain injury or it may be a familial tendency, but in many cases the cause is unknown (Fisher et al., 2014).

The International League Against Epilepsies classification was originally developed as a result of technologic and scientific advances, such as improved imaging and genomics, that have led to improved understanding of seizures and epilepsy (Scheffer et al., 2017). ILAE

Seizure type and signs
- Generalized (absence, tonic-clonic)
- Focal simple, complex, secondary generalized
- Unknown

Epilepsy type
- Focal (or partial) linked to one hemisphere site or focus - child can retain awareness or experience loss of awareness
- Generalized (wide spread activity left and right hemisphere)
- Combined (focal and generalized)

Additional seizure types
- Infantile spasm
- Psychogenic Non-epileptic Seizures (PNES)

FIGURE 38.7 Adapted framework for Epilepsies Classifications. The etiology of epilepsy is complex and influenced by various factors that can affect the brain such as injury, infection, developmental anomaly, genetic cause, metabolic processes, immune responses, circulatory difficulties (such as tumours), or venous malformations. (Classifications of Epilepsy as adapted from Scheffer, I. E., Berkovic, S., Capovilla, G., Connolly, M. B., French, J., Guilhoto, L.,… Zuberi, S. M. (2017). ILAE classification of the epilepsies: Position paper of the ILAE Commission for Classification and Terminology. *Epilepsia*, 58(4), 512–521. doi: 10.1111/epi.13709 and; and Epilepsy Ontario: http://epilepsyontario.org/about-epilepsy/types-of-seizures/.)

classifications of epileptic seizures are used by most neurologists to classify seizure types. There are three categories of seizures—focal (previously known as partial), generalized, and unknown seizures (i.e., epileptic spasms). In focal seizures, only one hemisphere of the brain is involved, while general seizures involve the entire brain. Focal seizures are seen in 60% of those with epilepsy and are described based on impairment of consciousness, localization, and progression of the seizure (Scheffer et al., 2017). Generalized seizures include absence seizures, tonic, clonic, tonic–clonic seizures, myoclonic seizures, and atonic seizures. Unknown is used for epileptic spasms where it is unclear whether the mode of onset is generalized or focal (Scheffer et al., 2017). There are many different types of seizures, and the classification of the type of seizure is crucial in assisting with the management and control of seizures. Figure 38.7 highlights the various classification of epilepsy recognizing that not all cases are easily classified. The most common seizure types are discussed in Table 38.2.

Therapeutic Management

Management of epilepsy focuses on controlling seizures or reducing their frequency. Another focus of epilepsy management involves helping the child who has recurrent seizures and his or her family to learn to live with the seizures. The primary mode of treatment is the use of anticonvulsants. The goal for every child should be the use of the fewest drugs with the fewest possible

side effects for the control of seizures. There have been significant advances in the treatment of epilepsy due to the many new anticonvulsant medications that have become available in recent years (Table 38.3). Most anticonvulsants are taken orally and are often used in combination. Different medications control different types of seizures, which may be due to individual variation. It can take time to find the right combination to best control an individual's seizures.

If seizures remain uncontrolled, surgery (corpus callosotomy) may be considered. Depending on the area of the brain that is affected, it may be possible to remove the area responsible for the seizure activity or to interrupt the impulses from spreading, and therefore stop or reduce the seizures. The adverse effects of surgery range from mild to severe, depending on the area of the brain that is affected. Other nonpharmacologic treatments that may be considered as second-line treatments in children with intractable seizures, such as those with Dravet syndrome, include a ketogenic diet or placement of a vagal nerve stimulator (Wirrell et al., 2017). Refer to Common Medical Treatments 38.1.

Nursing Assessment

For a full description of the assessment phase of the nursing process, refer to the Assessment section of the Nursing Process Overview earlier in the chapter. Assessment findings pertinent to epilepsy are discussed below.

(text continues on page 1394)

TABLE 38.2	COMMON TYPES OF SEIZURES	
Type	**Description**	**Characteristics**
Epileptic spasm such as infantile spasms	Mode of seizure onset unknown, whether focal or generalized Type of epileptic spasm seen in infancy Usually seen between 3 and 12 months of age, peak incidence 3–7 months and rarely seen after the age of 18 months	Occurs in series or clusters Presents as symmetrical flexing or extending, in variant clinical patterns, of the neck, arms, legs, and trunk May see: • Extension of neck, trunk, arms, and legs • Flexion of neck, trunk, and extremities with contracting of abdominal muscles (may cause body to bend forward, often referred to as "jackknife seizures") • Cry may precede or follow Majority of infants have some brain disorder before seizures begin The infant seems to stop developing and may lose skills that he or she has already attained after the onset of infantile spasms Hormonal therapy (mainly corticotropin) and anticonvulsants (most commonly, vigabatrin) are common forms of treatment
Absence (formerly *petit mal*)	Type of generalized seizure; uncommon before age 5	Abrupt onset and offset Sudden cessation of motor activity or speech with a blank facial expression or rhythmic twitching of the mouth, eyebrows, chin, eyelids, or other parts of the face Child may experience countless seizures in a day Not associated with a postictal (after seizure) state May go unrecognized or mistaken for inattentiveness because of subtle change in child's behaviour Myoclonic absence seizure consists of jerks of the shoulder and arms may result in lifting of the arms Eyelid myoclonia, brief (6 seconds) jerking of the eyelids with eyeballs rolling back; multiple seizures occur daily
Clonic	Type of generalized seizure that presents with repeated jerking movements	Muscles will spasm, jerk, then relax Spasm/jerking cannot be stopped by restraining or repositioning Clonic seizures alone are rare; may precede a tonic–clonic seizure
Tonic	Type of generalized seizures that present with stiffening of the muscles, typically the back, legs, arms	Consciousness usually preserved Tightening of chest muscles may lead to cyanosis; seen in children with Lennox–Gastaut syndrome
Tonic–clonic (formerly *grand mal*)	Extremely common generalized seizures. Most dramatic seizure type	Associated with an aura Loss of consciousness occurs and may be preceded by a piercing cry Presents with the entire body experiencing tonic contractions followed by rhythmic clonic contractions alternating with relaxation of all muscle groups Cyanosis may be noted due to apnea Saliva may collect in the mouth due to inability to swallow Child may bite tongue Loss of sphincter control, especially the bladder, is common Postictal phase: child will be semicomatose or in a deep sleep for approximately 30 min to 2 h; usually responds only to painful stimuli Child will have no memory of the seizure; may complain of headache and feeling fatigue Safety of the child is a primary concern See Teaching Guidelines 38.1

TABLE 38.2	COMMON TYPES OF SEIZURES (continued)	
Type	**Description**	**Characteristics**
Myoclonic	Type of generalized seizure that involves the motor cortex of the brain. May occur along with other seizure forms	Sudden, brief, massive muscle jerks that may involve the whole body or one body part Child may or may not lose consciousness
Atonic	Type of generalized seizure often referred to as "drop attacks" Seen in children with Lennox-Gastaut syndrome	Sudden loss of muscle tone. In children, may only be a sudden drop of the head. Child will regain consciousness within a few seconds to a minute Can result in injury related to violent fall
Focal seizure without impairment of consciousness (previously referred to as simple partial seizure)	Type of partial seizure that occurs in one part of the brain. The symptoms seen will depend on which area of the brain is affected	Motor activity characterized by clonic or tonic movements involving the face, neck, and extremities Can include sensory signs such as numbness, tingling, paresthesia, changes in vision and hearing, possible hallucinations, or pain Can include autonomic symptoms such as changes in blood pressure, heart rhythm, bowel function Can include psychic symptoms such as triggering emotions of fear, anxiety, joy, sadness Child remains conscious and may verbalize during the seizure No postictal state
Focal seizure with impaired consciousness (dyscognitive) previously known as complex partial seizure	Common type of partial seizure May begin with a focal seizure without impaired consciousness, then progress	May or may not have a preceding aura Consciousness will be impaired Automatisms and complex purposeful movements are common features in infants and children Infants will present with behaviours such as lip smacking, chewing, swallowing, and excessive salivation; can be difficult to distinguish from normal infant behaviour In older children, will see picking or pulling at bed sheets or clothing, rubbing objects, or running or walking in a nondirective and repetitive fashion These seizures can be difficult to control
Status epilepticus	Common neurologic emergency in children. Can occur with any seizure activity. Febrile seizures are the most common type. In children with epilepsy, it commonly occurs early in the course of epilepsy. Can be life-threatening	Prolonged or clustered seizures where consciousness does not return between seizures The age of the child, cause of the seizures, and duration of status epilepticus influence prognosis Prompt medical intervention is essential to reduce morbidity and mortality Treatment: • Basic life support—ABCs (airway, breathing, circulation) • Administration of anticonvulsants to cease seizures is crucial. Common medications include benzodiazepines such as lorazepam and diazepam, and fosphenytoin (see Drug Guide 38.1 and Table 38.3) • Blood glucose levels and electrolytes along with evaluation of the underlying cause should be initiated

Adapted from Mikati, M. A. (2011). Chapter 586. Seizures in childhood. In R. M. Kleigman, B. F. Stanton, J. W. St. Geme III, N. F. Schor, & R. E. Behrman (Eds.). *Nelson textbook of pediatrics* (19th ed., pp. 2013–2039). Philadelphia, PA: Saunders; Zak, M., & Chan, V. W. (2014). Chapter 46: Pediatric neurologic disorders. In S. M. Nettina (Ed.). *Lippincott manual of nursing practice* (10th ed., pp. 1545–1575). Philadelphia, PA: Wolters/Kluwer Health: Lippincott Williams & Wilkins.

TABLE 38.3	COMMON ANTICONVULSANT MEDICATIONS
Medication	**Nursing Implications**
Phenytoin (IV and PO; IM administration is contraindicated)	Monitor serum levels to ensure therapeutic dosing. Be aware that gingival hyperplasia appears most commonly in children and adolescents. If on prolonged therapy, ensure adequate intake of vitamin D–containing foods. Monitor serum calcium and magnesium levels. IV form given in normal saline to prevent precipitation.
Fosphenytoin (IM or IV only)	Adverse effects are said to be less common than with phenytoin. It does not cause local irritation, but it is a more expensive drug than phenytoin. It is water soluble, therefore allowing faster and easier administration than phenytoin. All dosing is in phenytoin sodium equivalents. It does not precipitate in commonly used IV diluents.
Phenobarbital	Assess for excessive sedation. Monitor serum levels to ensure therapeutic dosing. Monitor for drug interactions. Increase vitamin D–fortified foods or administer supplement, if prescribed. Withdrawal symptoms will occur if drug is stopped abruptly. Valproic acid interferes with this drug, causing increased phenobarbital levels.
Felbamate	Monitor for drug interactions, especially if child is taking phenytoin or carbamazepine.
Valproic acid (divalproex sodium, sodium valproate)	Monitor serum levels to ensure therapeutic dosing. Depakote sprinkles are available and useful for children who are unable to tolerate valproate suspension, tablets, or capsules. The contents can be sprinkled on food that does not require chewing.
Carbamazepine	Monitor serum levels to ensure therapeutic dosing; toxicity can occur even with levels slightly above therapeutic range. Plasma concentration decreased by phenytoin, phenobarbital, and valproic acid.
Gabapentin	Do not administer within 2 hours of antacids. Rapidly absorbed in the gastrointestinal tract. Primarily secreted in urine, may need to be adjusted in renal impairment.
Topiramate	Dilantin, Tegretol, and valproic acid decrease concentration of topiramate. May interact with oral contraceptives.
Oxcarbazepine	Monitor phenytoin levels, if administering concurrently. Monitor serum sodium.
Lamotrigine	Valproate inhibits metabolism; therefore, monitor serum blood values and decrease the dose, if necessary.
Levetiracetam	Monitor phenytoin levels, if administering concurrently. Monitor for difficulty with gait or coordination. B-complex vitamin supplementation can help manage side effects.
Ethosuximide	Give with food if GI upset occurs. Monitor closely during periods of dosage adjustment or addition of new medications.

GI, gastrointestinal; IM, intramuscular; IV, intravenous; PO, by mouth.

Adapted from Mikati, M. A. (2011). Chapter 586. Seizures in childhood. In R. M. Kleigman, B. F. Stanton, J. W. St. Geme III, N. F. Schor, & R. E. Behrman (Eds.). *Nelson textbook of pediatrics* (19th ed., pp. 2013–2039). Philadelphia, PA: Saunders; and Zak, M., & Chan, V. W. (2014). Chapter 46: Pediatric neurologic disorders. In S. M. Nettina (Ed.). *Lippincott manual of nursing practice* (10th ed., pp. 1545–1575). Philadelphia, PA: Wolters/Kluwer Health: Lippincott Williams & Wilkins.

HEALTH HISTORY

Elicit a description of the present illness and chief complaint, which will usually involve a seizure episode. Ask questions that help to characterize the episode as a seizure or as a nonepileptic event (see Box 38.1 for a list of nonepileptic events). A complete, accurate, and detailed history from a reliable source is essential. Questions should include:

- Where did the event occur—while sleeping, eating, playing, or just after waking?
- Description of child's behaviour during the event—what types of movements, progression, length, respiratory status, apnea?

BOX 38.1
NONEPILEPTIC EVENTS
- Syncope
- Breath holding
- Jitteriness
- Apnea
- Gastroesophageal reflux
- Cardiac conduction abnormalities
- Migraines
- Tics
- Night terrors
- Benign sleep movements

- How did the child act after the event?
- Have the episodes been recurrent? If so, how frequent?
- Any precipitating factors such as a fever, fall, activity, anxiety, infection, or exposure to strong stimuli such as flashing lights or loud noises?

Explore the child's current and past medical history for risk factors such as:

- Family history of seizures or epilepsy
- Any complications during the prenatal, perinatal, or postnatal periods
- Changes in developmental status or delays in developmental milestones
- Any recent illness, fever, trauma, or toxin exposure

Children known to have epilepsy are often admitted to the hospital for other health-related issues or complications and treatment of their seizure disorder. The health history should include questions related to:

- Age of onset of seizures
- Seizure control—what medications are the child taking, and has he or she been able to take them; when was his or her last seizure?
- Description and classification of seizures—does the child lose consciousness; does the child become apneic?
- Precipitating factors that may contribute to onset of seizures
- Adverse effects related to anticonvulsant medications
- Compliance with medication regimen

PHYSICAL EXAMINATION

Perform a complete neurologic examination. Careful assessment of the child's mental status, language, learning, behaviour, and motor abilities can help provide information about any neurologic deficits. If you observe seizure activity directly, provide a thorough and accurate description of the event. This description needs to include:

- Time of onset and length of seizure activity
- Alterations in behaviour such as a cry or changes in facial expression such as staring or blank expression, motor abilities, or sensory alterations before the seizure that may indicate an aura
- Precipitating factors such as fever, anxiety, just waking, or eating
- Description of movements and any progression
- Description of respiratory effort and any apnea noted
- Changes in colour (pallor or cyanosis) noted
- Position of mouth, any injury to mouth or tongue, inability to swallow, or excessive salivation
- Loss of bladder or bowel control
- State of consciousness during seizure and **postictal** (after seizure) state—during the seizure, the nurse may

ask the child to remember a word; after the seizure, assess if child is able to recall it, to help accurately establish current mental state

- Assess orientation to person, place, and time; motor abilities; speech; behaviour; alterations in sensation postictally
- Duration of postictal state (in minutes)

LABORATORY AND DIAGNOSTIC TESTS

Laboratory and diagnostic tests are used to evaluate the cause of, and also aid in identifying the type of, seizure activity (refer to Common Laboratory and Diagnostic Tests 38.1). Common laboratory and diagnostic studies ordered for the diagnosis and assessment of epilepsy include:

- Serum glucose, electrolytes, and calcium—to rule out metabolic causes such as hypoglycemia and hypocalcemia
- LP—to analyze cerebrospinal fluid (CSF) to rule out meningitis or encephalitis
- Skull x-ray examinations—to evaluate for the presence of fracture or trauma
- Computed tomography (CT) and magnetic resonance imaging (MRI) studies—to identify abnormalities and intracranial bleeds and rule out tumours
- Electroencephalographs (EEGs)—EEG findings may be noted with certain seizure types, but a normal EEG does not rule out epilepsy because seizure activity rarely occurs during the actual testing time. EEGs are useful in evaluating seizure type and assisting in medication selection. They can be useful in differentiating seizures from nonepileptic activity
- Video EEGs—provide the opportunity to see the child's actual behaviour on video, accompanied with EEG changes; can improve the chance of catching a seizure because the monitoring is done over a period of time

Nursing Management

Nursing management focuses on preventing injury during seizures, administering appropriate medication and treatments to prevent or reduce seizures, and providing education and support to the child and family to help them cope with the challenges of living with a chronic seizure disorder. See Box 38.2 for a list of basic seizure precautions. In addition to the nursing diagnoses and related interventions discussed in Nursing Care Plan 38.1 at the end of the chapter, interventions common to epilepsy follow.

 Dosage Calculation

Child's weight: 9.98 kg
Medication order: Phenobarbital 50 mg PO twice a day
As per the *Pediatric Dosage Handbook*, the recommended dose is 6 to 8 mg/kg/day in one to two divided doses. Is the ordered dose safe?

SEIZURE PRECAUTIONS

- Padding of side rails and other hard objects
- Side rails raised on bed at all times when child is in bed
- Oxygen and suction at bedside
- Supervision, especially during bathing, ambulation, or other potentially hazardous activities
- Use of a protective helmet during activity may be appropriate
- Child should wear a medical alert bracelet

Relieving Anxiety

Seizures produce fear and anxiety due to their unpredictable nature along with their uncontrolled, forceful, and, at times, violent appearance. Instruct parents and family members, along with those in the community who may care for the child, on how to respond in case of a seizure (see Teaching Guidelines 38.1). This will help to empower the parents, family, and other caregivers, and, in turn, alleviate some of the anxiety that they may feel.

Teaching Guidelines 38.1
HOW TO RESPOND WHEN YOUR CHILD HAS A SEIZURE

- Instruct parents and caregivers:
  - Remain calm
  - If child is standing or sitting, ease child to the ground, if possible
  - Time seizure episode
  - Tight clothing and jewellery around the neck should be loosened, if possible
  - Place child on one side and open airway, if possible
  - Do not restrain the child
  - Remove hazards in the area
  - Do not forcibly open jaw with a tongue blade or fingers
  - Document length of seizure and movements noted, also cyanosis or loss of bladder or bowel control and any other characteristics
  - Remain with child until fully conscious
- Call emergency services if:
  - The child stops breathing
  - Any injury has occurred
  - Seizure lasts for more than 5 minutes
  - This is the child's first seizure
  - Child is unresponsive to painful stimuli after seizure

MANAGING TREATMENT

Provide child and family teaching and instruction regarding the administration of anticonvulsant therapy and its importance. Included in this discussion should be common adverse effects, the need to continue the medication unless instructed otherwise by the physician or nurse practitioner, and the need to call the physician or nurse practitioner if the child is vomiting and unable to take his or her medication. Encourage parents to discuss unwanted adverse effects with the physician or nurse practitioner in order to maximize medication management. A common cause of breakthrough seizures is medication noncompliance.

PROVIDING FAMILY SUPPORT AND EDUCATION

Having a child with a chronic seizure disorder can place stress and anxiety on the family. This stress and anxiety is often due to fears and misconceptions they may have. An important nursing function is to educate not only the child and family but also the community, including the child's teachers and caregivers, on the reality and facts of the disorder. Encourage parents to be involved in the management of their child's seizures at the same time as encouraging the child to learn about their disorder and its management as soon as he or she is old enough. Support parents to treat the child with epilepsy just as they would treat a child without this disorder. Children who are brought up no differently than children without epilepsy will be more likely to develop a positive self-image and have increased self-esteem. Any activity restrictions, such as limiting swimming or participation in sports, will be based on the type, frequency, and severity of the seizures the child has. Educate parents and children on any restrictions and encourage parents to place only the necessary restrictions on the child.

The needs of the child and family will change as the child grows and develops. The nurse needs to recognize these changes and provide appropriate education and support. Referral to support groups is appropriate. Links to helpful information about epilepsy including educational resources can be found on thePoint.

Consider This

I am so worried about having a seizure at school. I think the other kids will tease me and not play with me if they see me having a seizure. I just don't want to go to school.
Thoughts: How would you respond to his concerns? How can you work with the school, family, and child to help ease his concerns?

Febrile Seizures

Febrile seizures are commonly reported in about 2% to 5% of children between the ages of 6 months and 5 years. These seizures are usually associated with fever often as a result of a viral infection (Public Health Agency of Canada [PHAC], 2016a). Usually, generalized febrile seizures are short-lived (<15 minutes), not repeated in a 24-hour period and thought to be benign (PHAC, 2016a). Febrile seizures are more commonly seen in boys, and there is an increased risk for children who have a family history of febrile seizures (Mikati, 2011). They can be very frightening for both the child and family. While in most cases the prognosis is excellent febrile, seizures may be a sign of a dangerous underlying infection, such as meningitis or sepsis. Though very rare, complications associated with febrile seizures include status epilepticus, motor coordination deficits, intellectual disability, and behavioural problems.

Therapeutic Management

Therapeutic management includes determination and treatment of the cause of the fever and interventions to control the fever. Due to the benign nature of febrile seizures, the risks of side effects from the antiepileptic agents usually outweigh the benefits (Millichap & Millichap, 2015). However, rectal diazepam has been shown to be safe and effective in terminating febrile seizures and may be used in children at high risk for febrile seizures. Buccal and intranasal midazolam, if available, has also been found to be effective and may be superior (Millichap & Millichap, 2015). Intranasal lorazepam is also an additional option.

Nursing Assessment

A febrile seizure is usually associated with a rapid rise in core temperature to 39°C (102.2°F) or higher. A simple febrile seizure is defined as a generalized seizure lasting less than 15 minutes (usually a few seconds to 10 minutes) that occurs once in a 24-hour period and is accompanied by fever without any CNS infection present (Mikati, 2011; Millichap & Millichap, 2015; Sullivan & Farrar, 2011). A brief postictal period is often seen when the child appears drowsy. The seizure is likely to have stopped by the time a child receives medical attention. Diagnosis is made based on a thorough history and physical examination, accompanied by a determination of the source of the fever. In some cases, an LP and/or neuroimaging may be performed to rule out meningitis or encephalitis. This will be based on the age and the clinical presentation of the child.

Risk factors for recurrence of a febrile seizure include young age at first febrile seizure and family history of febrile seizures and high fever. Children who experience one or more simple febrile seizures have a slightly greater risk of developing epilepsy than the general population (Holmes, 2013; Sullivan & Farrar, 2011). No evidence exists that febrile seizures cause structural damage or cognitive declines (Holmes, 2013; Sullivan & Farrar, 2011; Takasu et al., 2017).

Nursing Management

Provide parental support and education regarding febrile seizures. Reassure parents of the benign nature of febrile seizures. Counsel parents on controlling fever, discuss how to keep a child safe during a seizure, and provide instruction and demonstration in the administration of rectal diazepam at the onset of a seizure (if applicable). Instruct parents when to call their physician or nurse practitioner and when to take their child to the emergency room. Reinforce that any recurrent seizure activity will require prompt medical attention.

Neonatal Seizures

There is a high incidence of seizures during the neonatal period. Neonates, with the gestation age of 32 to 36 weeks, have twice the chance of being born with neurodevelopmental impairments (Johnson et al., 2015). The immature brain is more prone to seizure activity and metabolic, infectious, structural, and toxic diseases are more likely to be seen in this age group. Neonatal seizures are seizures that occur within the first 4 weeks of life and are most commonly seen within the first 10 days. The majority of seizures in newborns are associated with a specific underlying cause such as hypoxic ischemic encephalopathy (most common), metabolic disorders (hypoglycemia and hypocalcemia), neonatal infection (meningitis and encephalitis), cerebral infarction, and intracranial hemorrhage. The prognosis depends mainly on the underlying cause of the seizures and the severity of the insult. There is evidence that neonatal seizures have an adverse effect on neurodevelopment and may predispose the infant to cognitive, behavioural, or epileptic complications later in life (Johnson et al., 2015). About 20% to 30% of neonates with seizures will go on to develop postnatal epilepsy. Neonatal epileptic syndromes are rare but are a well-recognized cause of neonatal seizures and include benign myoclonic, neonatal convulsions, benign neonatal familial convulsions, early myoclonic encephalopathy, and early infantile epileptic encephalopathy. Our discussion below will focus on the more common symptomatic neonatal seizure related to a specific underlying cause.

Therapeutic Management

Although treatment of neonatal seizures has developed over the last few decades, there remains no consensus as to which medications offer optimal treatment (Slaughter, Patel, & Slaughter, 2013). However, acute neonatal seizures should be treated aggressively since repeated seizure activity may result in injury to the brain. Treatment focuses on addressing the underlying cause, such as correcting metabolic disturbances, treating CNS infections, ensuring adequate ventilation and cardiovascular support, and possibly administering anticonvulsant therapy. Phenobarbital is often used in the initial management of neonatal seizures, but long-term efficacy remains uncertain (Slaughter et al., 2013). Anti-epileptic medications may not be effective if the underlying cause is not treated (Slaughter et al., 2013).

Nursing Assessment

Neonatal seizures may be hard to recognize clinically and may be accompanied by a normal EEG, and in some cases, there may be no clinical signs, but only EEG changes (Mikati, 2011). Neonatal seizures have to be distinguished from nonseizure behaviours seen in newborns, such as stretching, sudden random movements, and random sucking movements, coughing, or gagging (Shellhaas, 2015). Therefore, clinical recognition of newborn seizures is critical. Assessment of neonatal seizures will include a detailed clinical characterization of the seizure activity, including appearance of the neonate; location and involvement of arms, legs, trunk, and face; sequence of clinical changes, and duration and frequency of seizure activity. If seizure activity is not witnessed by a health care provider, a detailed history is essential. Once identified, the seizure activity can be classified. To prioritize assessment, the ILAE proposes that neonatal seizures be classified not as a separate entity, but within the proposed categories (Table 38.2; Berg et al., 2010).

Laboratory and diagnostic tests, including serum testing (e.g., serum glucose, electrolytes, calcium), LP (to analyze CSF), cranial ultrasound, CT, and MRI may be performed to help determine the cause of the seizures. EEGs and video EEGs may assist in the characterization of neonatal seizures and thereby direct medical management.

Nursing Management

Nursing management will focus on carrying out interventions to cease seizure activity, monitoring neurologic status closely, recognizing the seizures, preventing injury during seizure activity, and providing support and education to the parents and family.

STRUCTURAL DEFECTS

Due to the sensitivity of the development of the neurologic system in the first weeks of embryonic life, there exists a potential for defects to occur. These structural defects include neural tube defects (NTDs), microcephaly, Chiari malformation, hydrocephalus, intracranial arteriovenous malformation (AVM), and craniosynostosis.

Neural Tube Defects

NTDs account for the majority of congenital anomalies of the CNS (Kinsman & Johnston, 2011). They are the second most common birth defect (the first being cardiac malformations) contributing to infant mortality and disability (Hochberg & Stone, 2015). The incidence in Canada has declined significantly from 1998 to 2007 from 5.5 to 4.1 per 10,000 births (Nelson, Leon, & Evans, 2014). NTDs are serious birth defects of the spine and the brain and include disorders such as spina bifida occulta, myelomeningocele, meningocele, anencephaly, and encephalocele. The neural tube closes between the third and fourth week in utero. The cause of NTDs is not known, but many factors such as drugs, malnutrition, chemicals, and genetics can adversely affect normal CNS development. Evidence supports the need for maternal preconception supplementation of folic acid since this can decrease the incidence of NTDs in pregnancies (Canadian Paediatric Society [CPS], 2016). Currently, Health Canada recommends that all women of childbearing age who are capable of becoming pregnant take a minimum of 400 μg (0.4 mg) of folic acid daily. Pregnant women with a history of pregnancies affected by NTDs are recommended to take a higher dosage. Prenatal screening of maternal serum for α-fetoprotein (AFP) and ultrasound examination can help identify antenatal NTD. Anencephaly and encephalocele are discussed below. Refer to Chapter 44 for information on spina bifida occulta, meningocele, and myelomeningocele.

Consider This

It wasn't until 1998 that Canada made it mandatory for all flour and grain products to be fortified with 150 mcg/100 g folic acid (CPS, 2016).

Anencephaly

Anencephaly is a defect in brain development resulting in small or missing brain hemispheres, skull, and scalp. It occurs when the cephalic or upper end of the neural tube fails to close during the third to fourth week of gestation. These infants are born without a forebrain, a cerebrum, and complete skull and scalp. The condition is usually incompatible with life.

NURSING ASSESSMENT

Anencephalic infants have a distinctive appearance, with a large defect noted in the vault of the skull (Fig. 38.8). The

FIGURE 38.8 Anencephalic infant.

mother may have had a difficult labour due to the malformation of the head not allowing it to engage in the cervix. The majority of infants will be stillborn. If not, most anencephalic infants die within hours to several days of birth (Tomita & Ogiwara, 2015). There have been a few cases in which the infant has lived for several months. The infant is usually blind, deaf, unconscious, and unable to feel pain. Some infants born with anencephaly may be born with a brain stem, but due to the lack of a cerebrum, there is no possibility of gaining consciousness. Reflex actions such as respirations, reactions to sound and touch, and ability to suck may be present.

NURSING MANAGEMENT

The prognosis is extremely poor. Nursing management is supportive in nature and focuses on comfort measures for the dying infant. Some parents may have been aware of the diagnosis prenatally due to screening tests such as AFP and ultrasounds. Parents and family will need support and understanding from all health care professionals during this difficult time. Fear of what the child will look like may be overwhelming. Use of an infant cap can be helpful and allow parents to feel more comfortable holding and comforting their infant. Assisting with anticipatory grieving and decision-making related to end-of-life care will also be key nursing interventions.

Encephalocele

Encephalocele is a protrusion of the brain and meninges through a skull defect. It results from failure of the anterior portion of the neural tube to close. The prognosis, including the extent of complications and cognitive deficits, will depend on the size and location of the encephalocele and involvement of other brain structures. Encephaloceles are often accompanied by craniofacial and other abnormalities such as hydrocephalus, microcephaly, spastic quadriplegia, ataxia, visual problems, developmental delay, mental and growth retardation, and seizures. Some children who are affected may display normal intelligence.

Therapeutic management consists of surgical repair, including placement of tissues back into the skull and removal of the sac; possible shunt placement to correct associated hydrocephalus; and corrective repair of any craniofacial abnormalities.

NURSING ASSESSMENT

Initial assessment after delivery will reveal a visible external sac protruding from the skull area. It occurs most commonly in the occipital region, but can occur elsewhere, such as frontally or nasofrontally. Generally, the lesion is covered by skin, but it may also be open. Therefore, assessment to ensure that the sac covering is intact remains important. Assess neurologic status carefully. Before surgical correction, the infant will be examined thoroughly to determine brain tissue involvement or associated anomalies. Diagnostic procedures such as CT, MRI, and ultrasound may be performed.

NURSING MANAGEMENT

Nursing management will consist of preoperative and postoperative care, along with symptomatic and supportive care. Preoperative and postoperative care will be similar to that for the child with myelomeningocele (refer to Chapter 44), with a focus on preventing rupture of the sac, preventing infection, and providing adequate nutrition and hydration. Infants with an encephalocele are at an increased risk for developing hydrocephalus. Therefore, monitor for signs and symptoms of increased ICP and head circumference.

Microcephaly

Microcephaly is defined as a head circumference that is more than three standard deviations below the mean for the age and sex of the infant (Kinsman & Johnston, 2011). It may be congenital or it may be acquired and develop in the first few years of life. It generally results in intellectual disability due to the lack of functioning brain tissue. There are many causes. Microcephaly can be caused by abnormal development during gestation or follow intrauterine infections such as Zika virus, rubella, toxoplasmosis, and cytomegalovirus (PHAC, 2016b). It can also be caused by chromosomal abnormalities or be associated with other syndromes. Acquired microcephaly may occur due to severe malnutrition, perinatal infections, or anoxia in early infancy.

Nursing Assessment

Microcephalic infants will present at birth with a normal or reduced head size. As the child ages, head growth will fail while the face will continue to grow at a normal rate. This results in a small head, a large face, and a loose, often wrinkled, scalp. As the child grows older, this smallness of the skull becomes more pronounced. Development of motor functions and speech may be delayed. The degree of intellectual disability varies, but it is a common occurrence. Convulsions may be present, and motor deficit ranges from clumsiness to spastic quadriplegia.

Nursing Management

There is no treatment. Nursing care will be supportive and focus on determining the extent of neurologic and cognitive deficits, as well as teaching parents how to care for a child with such impairments.

Chiari Malformation

Chiari malformations are classified into different groups and subgroups based on anatomic anomalies of the craniocervical junction along with downward displacement of the cerebellar structures (Khoury, 2015). The most common are type I and type II and are the types discussed here. Type I is usually not associated with hydrocephalus and is the more benign form. The deformity is a result of the cerebellar tonsils displacing into the upper cervical canal (Kinsman & Johnston, 2011). Type II (also referred to as Arnold–Chiari) is the most common and is usually associated with hydrocephalus and myelomeningocele. The deformity results from the cerebellum, the medulla oblongata, and the fourth ventricle displacing into the cervical canal, resulting in an obstruction of the CSF and causing hydrocephalus. The prognosis depends on the extent of the defect. Therapeutic management of the type II Chiari malformation includes surgical decompression.

Nursing Assessment

In type I, symptoms are typically seen in adolescence and adulthood. The client will usually complain of neck pain; recurrent headaches that increase with physical activity or with Valsalva manoeuvres such as coughing, laughing, or sneezing; lower extremity spasticity; and urinary frequency (Khoury, 2015). Type II is almost always associated with myelomeningocele; therefore, it is typically detected prenatally or at birth. Symptoms seen in infancy include a weak cry, stridor, and apnea (Kinsman & Johnston, 2011). These symptoms require prompt medical

treatment to reduce mortality. Gastrointestinal disturbances along with a history of chronic aspiration, choking, gagging, prolonged feeding times, and weight loss may also be present. In later infancy and childhood, progressive hydrocephalus is a common problem (Khoury, 2015). Assessment of shunt function is extremely important in the infant and older child presenting with type II Chiari malformation and associated hydrocephalus (refer to Hydrocephalus section). An MRI may be performed to help evaluate and diagnose Chiari malformations.

Nursing Management

Nursing management will focus on preoperative and postoperative care, prevention of infection, monitoring of blood loss, improvement of preoperative symptoms in the postoperative period, identification of any signs and symptoms of increased ICP, and identification of any resultant CNS injury.

Hydrocephalus

Hydrocephalus is not a specific illness, but results from underlying brain disorders. It is a frequently seen disorder of the nervous system occurring in 0.5 to 4 per 1,000 live births (Zak & Chan, 2014). It results from an imbalance in the production and absorption of CSF. In hydrocephalus, CSF accumulates within the ventricular system and causes the ventricles to enlarge and increases in ICP to occur.

Hydrocephalus may be congenital or acquired. Congenital hydrocephalus is present at birth and is often due to a genetic disposition or environmental influences during fetal development. Causes of congenital hydrocephalus include abnormal intrauterine development, as is the case with myelomeningocele or other NTDs or intrauterine infections. Acquired hydrocephalus develops at the time of birth or at some point after. It can occur at any age and can result from injury or disease. Acquired hydrocephalus can result from intentional or nonintentional trauma, intraventricular hemorrhage (IVH) in premature infants, neoplasms (e.g., posterior fossa brain tumour), infections (e.g., meningitis), or malformations (e.g., Chiari malformations).

Prognosis for the child with hydrocephalus depends mainly on the cause and whether or not brain damage has occurred prior to recognition and treatment. Children with hydrocephalus are at increased risk for developmental disabilities, visual problems, abnormalities in memory, and reduced intelligence. Long-term follow-up and multidisciplinary care are necessary.

Pathophysiology

CSF is formed primarily in the ventricular system by the choroid plexus. It flows as a result of the pressure gradient that exists between the ventricular system and the venous channels. CSF is absorbed primarily by the arachnoid villi. Hydrocephalus results when there is an obstruction in the ventricular system or obliteration or malfunction of the arachnoid villi. This results in impaired absorption or circulation of the CSF.

There are two types of hydrocephalus-noncommunicating (obstructive) or communicating. Noncommunicating hydrocephalus occurs when the flow of CSF is blocked within the ventricular system (Douglas, Drake, Rowe, & Vachhrajani, 2017). This type is more common than communicating hydrocephalus (Zak & Chan, 2014). NTDs, neonatal meningitis, trauma, tumours, or Chiari malformations usually result in this type of hydrocephalus. One of the most common causes of obstructive or noncommunicating hydrocephalus in children is aqueductal stenosis, which results from the narrowing of the aqueduct of Sylvius (a passageway between the third and fourth ventricles in the middle brain) (Kinsman & Johnston, 2011). Communicating hydrocephalus occurs when the flow of CSF is blocked after it exits from the ventricles. This form of hydrocephalus, in which the CSF can still flow between the ventricles, is most often caused by defective absorption of CSF. Examples include hydrocephalus that results from subarachnoid hemorrhage (most common), certain types of meningitis, and leukemia infiltrates (Kinsman & Johnston, 2011).

Therapeutic Management

Hydrocephalus must be identified early. Treatment needs to be initiated in order to prevent brain tissue damage that can result from the increased ICP that hydrocephalus creates. Specific treatment will depend on the underlying etiology. The goals of treatment include relieving hydrocephalus and managing complications associated with the disorder, such as growth and developmental delay. Most cases of hydrocephalus are treated with the surgical placement of an extracranial shunt. Most often, a ventriculoperitoneal (VP) shunt is placed. See Figure 38.9 for an illustration of a shunt. The shunt may need to be replaced as the child grows. Therefore, the child may undergo shunt revision surgery at various times during his or her life. It is important for health care professionals and parents to be able to recognize when a shunt needs replacing or when complications are occurring, to decrease the possibility of death or disability that may occur due to increased ICP.

Though shunts have been the mainstay of treatment for hydrocephalus, they are not without complications such as infection, obstruction, mechanical failure, or breakage resulting in the need for revision. Endoscopic third ventriculostomy is an alternative to shunt placement to treat obstructive hydrocephalus in select children. A small perforation is made in the thinned floor of the third ventricle, which allows for egress of CSF from

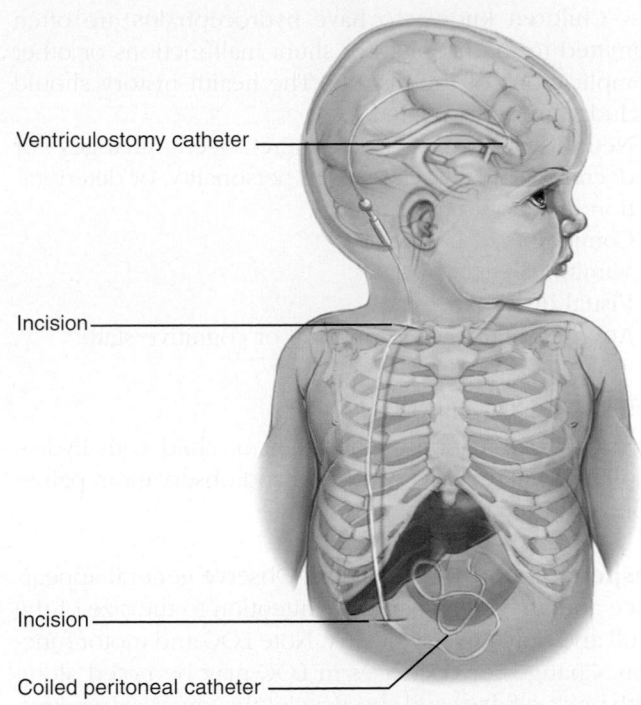

FIGURE 38.9 To treat hydrocephalus, a ventriculoperitoneal (VP) shunt catheter is placed in an enlarged ventricle. The shunt diverts the flow of cerebrospinal fluid (CSF) within the central nervous system to the peritoneum, where CSF is now absorbed across the peritoneal membrane into the body's circulation.

the ventricle to the subarachnoid space. No permanently implanted hardware is needed.

Nursing Assessment

For a full description of the assessment phase of the nursing process, refer to the assessment section of the Nursing Process Overview earlier in the chapter. Assessment findings pertinent to hydrocephalus are discussed below.

HEALTH HISTORY
Explore the pregnancy history and past medical history for:
• Intrauterine infections
• Prematurity with intracranial hemorrhage
• Meningitis
• Mumps encephalitis

Elicit a description of the present illness and chief complaint. Common signs and symptoms reported during the health history of the undiagnosed child might include:
• Irritability
• Lethargy
• Poor feeding
• Vomiting
• Complaints of headache in older children
• Altered, diminished, or changes in LOC

Children known to have hydrocephalus are often admitted to the hospital for shunt malfunctions or other complications of the disease. The health history should include questions related to:

• Neurologic status—have there been changes or decreases in LOC, changes in personality, or deterioration in school performance?
• Complaints of headache
• Vomiting
• Visual disturbances
• Any other changes in physical or cognitive state

PHYSICAL EXAMINATION

Physical examination of the infant or child with hydrocephalus will include inspection and observation, palpation, and percussion.

Inspection and Observation. Observe general appearance and affect. Pay particular attention to the size of the skull and note any asymmetry. Note LOC and motor function. Changes or decreases in LOC may be noted along with brisk reflexes and spasticity of the lower extremities. Symptoms seen vary by age, primarily due to the fact that the infant's skull is able to accommodate the build-up of CSF as the sutures have not closed. In the infant, the most obvious indication is often a rapid increase in head circumference (Fig. 38.10). In the older child, loss of development and changes in personality may be seen. Signs and symptoms associated with increased ICP may be seen (refer to Comparison Chart 38.1).

Palpation. In the infant, palpation of the fontanels may reveal wide-open, bulging fontanels. They will be non-pulsatile and feel tense and full.

Percussion. Upon percussion of the skull, by physicians or nurse practitioners, a positive Macewen sign may be noted. This is when a "cracked pot" sound is heard during percussion and can indicate separation of the sutures.

LABORATORY AND DIAGNOSTIC TESTS

Common laboratory and diagnostic tests ordered for the diagnosis and assessment of hydrocephalus include:

• Skull x-ray studies (may reveal separation of sutures)
• CT
• MRI

CT and MRI are used to evaluate for the presence of hydrocephalus and can also aid in identifying the cause of hydrocephalus. Refer to Common Laboratory and Diagnostic Tests 38.1.

Nursing Management

Nursing management of the child with hydrocephalus will focus on maintaining cerebral perfusion, minimizing neurologic complications, maintaining adequate nutrition, promoting growth and development, and supporting and educating the child and family. In addition to the nursing diagnoses and related interventions discussed in Nursing Care Plan 38.1 at the end of the chapter, interventions common to hydrocephalus are discussed below.

PREVENTING AND RECOGNIZING SHUNT INFECTION AND MALFUNCTION

The major complications associated with shunts are infection and malfunction. Due to the serious nature and potentially devastating effects of shunt infection or malfunction, parents and health professionals need to be aware of the signs and symptoms to provide early recognition and prompt treatment. Signs and symptoms of a shunt infection include elevated vital signs, poor feeding, vomiting, decreased responsiveness, seizure activity, and signs of local inflammation along the shunt tract. Signs and symptoms of shunt malfunction include vomiting, drowsiness, and headache. Signs and symptoms of increased ICP, as listed in Comparison Chart 38.1, can also be indicative of shunt complications.

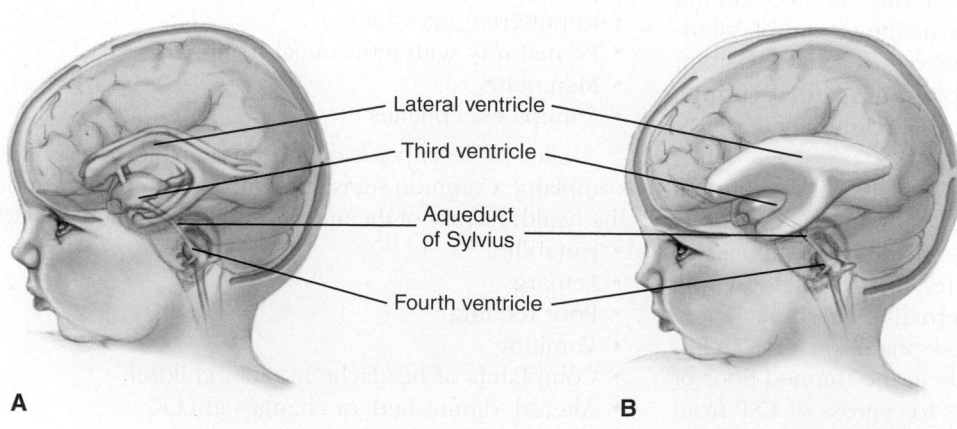

A   B

FIGURE 38.10 **A**. Infant without hydrocephalus. **B**. Infant with hydrocephalus. Note broadening of the forehead, bulging fontanel, and large head size.

Lateral ventricle
Third ventricle
Aqueduct of Sylvius
Fourth ventricle

Infection can occur at any time, but is more common 1 to 2 months after placement. Infection is treated with intravenous antibiotics and, if the infection is persistent, the shunt will be removed and an external ventricular drainage (EVD) system will be put into place until the CSF is sterile (refer to Common Medical Treatments 38.1 and Box 38.3).

Take Note!

Rapid drainage of CSF, which may occur if the child sits up without the EVD system being clamped, will decrease ICP and can lead to extreme headache, collapse of the ventricles, formation of subdural hematomas, and neurologic deterioration.

A new shunt will be placed after the infection has cleared. Intrathecal administration of antibiotics may be performed by the physician or nurse practitioner. Keeping the peritoneal surgical incision free of feces and urine can help prevent infection. In addition, inspect surgical incisions after shunt placement for signs and symptoms of infection and any signs of leaking CSF. Malfunction of the shunt can occur due to kinking, clogging, or separation of the tubing. Blockage is the most common reported complication. Early recognition and operative intervention are essential to prevent neurologic deficits or possible death from occurring.

BOX 38.3

NURSING MANAGEMENT OF EXTERNAL VENTRICULAR DRAINAGE (EVD) DEVICE

- Ensure all connections are secure and label line as EVD
- Regularly check that drip chamber of manometer is set at the height prescribed in relation to the child (i.e., zero at clavicle)
- Clamp the drain in the event of child movement or movement anticipated with care. Rezero and open clamps when done
- Accurately document volume and colour of cerebrospinal fluid (CSF) every hour (CSF is normally clear and colourless; cloudiness indicates infection). Notify physician, nurse practitioner, or charge nurse of any significant increase in amount of drainage (if exceeds 10 mL more than previous volumes)
- If minimal or no drainage, check tubing for kinks, blockage, or closed clamps. Check to see if CSF is oscillating in tubing. If blockage is suspected, notify neurosurgery department immediately
- Dress the entry site into the skull with a sterile occlusive dressing; change the dressing if it is soiled or nonocclusive
- Routine CSF samples may be sent for culture and analysis
- Child may be taking prophylactic antibiotics due to increased risk of infection from the drain

---

SUPPORTING AND EDUCATING THE CHILD AND FAMILY

Hydrocephalus is a serious and chronic illness. It will require lifelong follow-up and regular evaluations. It requires early recognition of complications to prevent neurologic damage. Children will require future surgeries and hospitalizations, which can place a strain on the family and its finances. Potential growth and developmental disabilities are an additional strain. The support of the family in establishing realistic goals and helping the child to achieve his or her developmental and educational potential is important.

The family should be involved in the child's care from the time of diagnosis. Initially, parents may be frightened because shunt placement involves entering the brain. Provide parents with accurate information regarding the procedure. Be available to listen to parents' concerns and to answer questions that arise before and after surgery, and at routine follow-up appointments. Ongoing education about the illness and its treatment is important, including signs and symptoms of shunt complications. As the family becomes more comfortable with the diagnosis, treatment, and signs and symptoms of complications, they will become experts on the child's care and will often recognize subtle changes in him or her that may be indicative of shunt complications. Referral to support groups can be helpful for both the family and the child. Links for helpful information about hydrocephalus are provided on thePoint.

Intracranial Arteriovenous Malformation

Intracranial AVM is a rare congenital disorder. It is caused by an abnormal development of blood vessels and can occur in the brain, brain stem, or spinal cord. AVMs that hemorrhage can lead to serious neurologic deficits and even death. However, some cases of AVMs never cause problems.

Therapeutic Management

More aggressive treatment strategies are used in children. Treatment options used include surgical excision; endovascular embolization, which involves closing off the vessels of the AVM by injecting glue into them; and radiosurgery, which involves focusing radiation on the AVM. The therapeutic management approach will be based on the age of the child and size and location of the malformation in the brain. The child will usually require at least 24 hours of intensive care monitoring following surgery.

Nursing Assessment

The most common symptoms seen include intracranial hemorrhage (children are more likely to present with hemorrhage than adults), seizures, headaches, and progressive neurologic deficits such as vision problems, loss of speech, problems with memory, and paralysis. In children younger than 2 years of age, presentation may include cardiac failure due to arteriovenous shunting in neonates and infants; a large head secondary to hydrocephalus; and seizure activity. Diagnosis is made using diagnostic imaging procedures such as MRI, CT, and arteriography.

Nursing Management

Nursing management for these children is aimed at supportive care. Monitor for changes in neurologic status, noting any seizure activity, signs or symptoms of increased ICP, or signs and symptoms of intracranial hemorrhage. Hydrocephalus may occur as a result of intracranial hemorrhage secondary to the AVM. An EVD and eventual shunt placement may be necessary (refer to Hydrocephalus section).

Craniosynostosis

Craniosynostosis is premature closure of the cranial sutures (Fig. 38.11). Complete closure of all sutures does not normally occur until late in childhood. Premature closure can inhibit brain growth and a distorted skull appearance will be evident. In cases where only one suture is fused, neurologic impairments are rarely seen. When two or more sutures are fused, neurologic complications such as hydrocephalus with increased ICP are more likely to occur. The incidence of craniosynostosis is approximately 1 in 2,500 births (Craniofacial

Program, 2017). The cause is unknown, but in 10% to 20% of cases, a genetic disorder such as Carpenter syndrome or Apert, Crouzon, or Pfeiffer disease is present (Kinsman & Johnston, 2011). There are numerous different types of craniosynostosis; they are listed and illustrated in Table 38.4. The prognosis is good for the majority of infants presenting with craniosynostosis, and normal brain development will occur. Exceptions to this are the infant or child who has associated genetic disorders that involve brain function and development.

Surgical correction may be done and allows for normal expansion of the brain and acceptable appearance of the head and skull. If one suture is fused, the surgical intervention is done mainly for cosmetic reasons. If more than one suture is fused, operative intervention is essential to prevent neurologic complications.

Nursing Assessment

Most cases of craniosynostosis are present at birth. Skull deformity is evident as well as a prominent bony ridge that can be palpated. X-ray studies can confirm fusion of the sutures. It is important that craniosynostosis be detected early if it is not evident at birth because premature closure of the suture lines will inhibit brain development. Therefore, measure head circumference in all children younger than 3 years old and compare findings with normal head circumference parameters as well as past measurements of the infant or child.

Nursing Management

Nursing management focuses on postoperative care. This includes observing hemoglobin and hematocrit levels due to large volumes of blood loss that can occur, and observing for pain, hemorrhage, fever, infection, and swelling. Due to the location of the surgery and incision line, large amounts of facial swelling may be present. This can result in an inability of the child to open his or her eyes for a few days postoperatively. Make sure that parents are aware of this. Encourage the parents to talk to, hold, and comfort their child during this time. Provide support and education to the parents before, during, and after the procedure.

Positional Plagiocephaly

Since the inception of the "back to sleep" program, which recommends placing all infants supine to sleep to decrease the risk of sudden infant death syndrome (SIDS), there has been a dramatic increase in the incidence of positional plagiocephaly (Community Paediatrics Committee, 2017). Positional plagiocephaly refers to asymmetry in head shape without fused sutures. It results from gravitational force exertion on the developing cranium. Torticollis, which is when the neck muscles

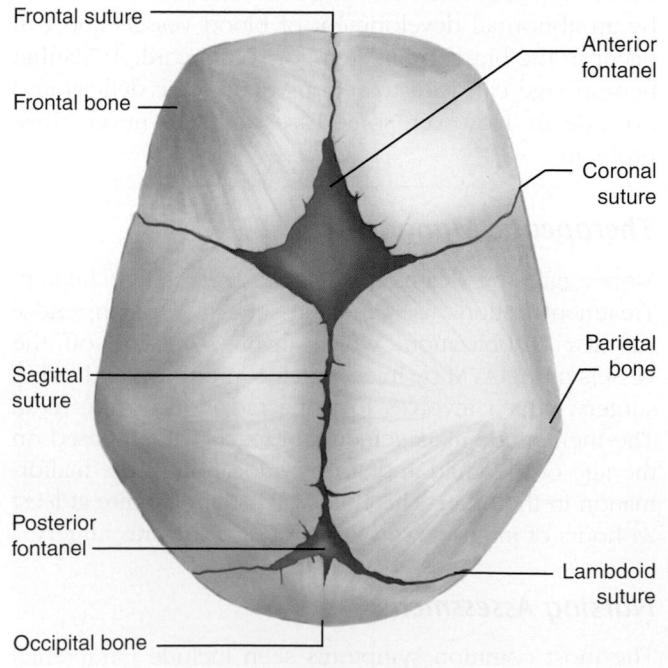

Frontal suture

Frontal bone

Sagittal suture

Posterior fontanel

Occipital bone

Anterior fontanel

Coronal suture

Parietal bone

Lambdoid suture

FIGURE 38.11 **Skull sutures in the infant.**

TABLE 38.4	TYPES OF CRANIOSYNOSTOSIS	
Types	**Description**	**Illustration**
Sagittal synostosis (scaphocephaly)	Sagittal suture is closed Head grows long and narrow in anterior–posterior direction Broad forehead and a prominent occiput are present Most common form	
Metopic synostosis (trigonocephaly)	Metopic suture is closed Usually a ridge down the forehead can be seen or felt Triangular-shaped forehead Eyebrows may appear "pinched" on either side Eyes may also appear close together	
Unilateral coronal synostosis (anterior plagiocephaly)	Early closure of one side of the coronal suture Forehead and orbital rim (eyebrow) have a flattened appearance on that side Eye on affected side has a different shape	
Bicoronal synostosis (brachycephaly)	Very flat, tall, recessed forehead Skull is shortened in the anterior–posterior direction Wide-shaped head Commonly seen in Apert and Crouzon disease	
Lambdoid (posterior plagiocephaly)	Early closure of one lambdoid suture Flattening of back of head. Similar to shape found in positional moulding or positional plagiocephaly	

FIGURE 38.12 Moulding helmet for positional plagiocephaly.

FIGURE 38.13 Note flattening of the right posterior parietal and occipital regions of the skull in this infant with positional plagiocephaly.

are too tight, have inadequate tone, or are shorter on one side, can contribute to plagiocephaly. Each condition, plagiocephaly and torticollis, exacerbates the other. Refer to Chapter 44 for further information on torticollis.

Therapeutic management for positional plagiocephaly is generally conservative, such as changing the infant's position, encouraging "tummy time," and avoiding excessive use of the car seat for infant seating outside of the automobile. Some infants may benefit from the use of a moulding helmet (Fig. 38.12).

Nursing Assessment

View the infant's head from the top, noting asymmetry ranging from flattening on one side posteriorly to posterior flattening associated with anterior bulging (Fig. 38.13). Assess neck range of motion to determine if torticollis is also present. Palpate the cranial sutures, which will not feel overlapped as they do when they are fused. Skull x-ray examination or head CT scan will rule out craniosynostosis by demonstrating evidence of open sutures.

Nursing Management

Nursing management is directed toward repositioning the infant to decrease time spent with the flattened area in the dependent position. Position the infant so that turning away from the affected side is necessary for him or her to view objects of interest. Place the infant on the abdomen when awake and supervised. Discourage use of the car seat outside of the automobile. Place a rolled washcloth along the affected side of the head to discourage turning the head in that direction. Following these recommendations may

prevent positional plagiocephaly in the infant without congenital torticollis.

INFECTIOUS DISORDERS

Infectious disorders of the neurologic system include bacterial meningitis, aseptic meningitis, encephalitis, and Reye syndrome.

Bacterial Meningitis

Bacterial meningitis is an infection of the meninges, the lining that surrounds the brain and spinal cord. It is a serious illness in children and can lead to brain damage, nerve damage, deafness, stroke, and even death. It requires rapid assessment and treatment. See Table 38.5 for the most common types of meningitis seen in different age groups. In developed countries, disease resulting from *Haemophilus influenzae* type B, once the most common cause of meningitis in children, has decreased dramatically since 1998 with the introduction of the Hib vaccine. However, disease due to non-b serogroups increased in all parts of Canada. Therefore, the Canadian immunization program has, as of 2011, been converted to a 13-valent pneumococcal conjugate vaccine and, according to preliminary studies, a number of these serotypes are on the decline. An emerging trend in many developed countries in relation to other seroforms of meningitis is a decreased susceptibility to penicillin. In the United States, ciprofloxacin resistant of *Neisseria meningitidis* strains have been

TABLE 38.5	COMMON CAUSES OF MENINGITIS IN DIFFERENT AGE GROUPS
Age Affected	**Causative Organism**
Newborns and infants (birth to 3 months)	*Escherichia coli*; *Streptococcus* group B; *Listeria monocytogenes*; *Pseudomonas aeruginosa*; *Staphylococcus* species
Infants and children (3 months to 6 years)	*Streptococcus pneumonia*; *Neisseria meningitidis (meningococcal meningitis)*; *Haemophilus influenzae* type B
Older children and adolescents (6–16 years)	*Streptococcus pneumonia*; *N. meningitidis (meningococcal meningitis)*; *Mycobacterium tuberculosis*

Adapted from Zak, M., & Chan, V. W. (2014). Chapter 46: Pediatric neurologic disorders. In: S. M. Nettina (Ed.). *Lippincott manual of nursing practice* (10th ed., pp. 1545–1575). Philadelphia, PA: Wolters/Kluwer Health: Lippincott Williams & Wilkins; and Centers for Disease Control and Prevention. (2014). *Meningitis: Bacterial meningitis*. Retrieved from http://www.cdc.gov/meningitis/bacterial.html

identified. Meningitic strains that have increased resistance to penicillin but no resistance to ciprofloxacin have been identified in Canada (Infectious Diseases and Immunization Committee, 2017).

Pathophysiology

Bacterial meningitis causes inflammation, swelling, purulent exudates, and tissue damage to the brain. It can occur as a secondary infection to upper respiratory infections, sinus infections, or ear infections, and can also be the result of direct introduction through LP; skull fracture or severe head injury; neurosurgical intervention; congenital structural abnormalities, such as spina bifida; or the presence of foreign bodies, such as a ventricular shunt or cochlear implants.

Therapeutic Management

Bacterial meningitis is a medical emergency and requires prompt hospitalization and treatment. Deterioration may be rapid and occur in less than 24 hours, leading to long-term neurologic damage and even death. Intravenous antibiotics will be started immediately after the LP and blood cultures have been obtained if bacterial meningitis is suspected. The length of therapy and specific antibiotic will be determined based on the analysis and the culture and sensitivity of the CSF. The role of corticosteroids is controversial; however, in cases of Hib meningitis, they may be ordered to help decrease hearing loss (Infectious Diseases and Immunization Committee, 2017). Specific medical treatment varies based on the suspected causative organism and will be determined by the physician or nurse practitioner.

Nursing Assessment

For a full description of the assessment phase of the nursing process, refer to the Assessment section of the Nursing Process Overview earlier in the chapter. Assessment

findings pertinent to bacterial meningitis are discussed below.

HEALTH HISTORY
Elicit a description of the present illness and chief complaint. Common signs and symptoms reported during the health history might include:
- Sudden onset of symptoms
- Preceding respiratory illness or sore throat
- Presence of fever, chills
- Headache
- Vomiting
- Photophobia
- Stiff neck
- Rash
- Irritability
- Drowsiness
- Lethargy
- Muscle rigidity
- Seizures

Symptoms in infants can be more subtle and atypical, but the history may reveal:
- Poor sucking and feeding
- Weak cry
- Lethargy
- Vomiting

Explore the child's current and past medical history for risk factors such as:
- Young age: 1 month to 5 years, with most cases in children younger than 1 year of age and young adults 15 to 24 years of age
- Any fever or illness during pregnancy or around delivery (for infants younger than 3 months of age)
- Exposure to ill persons
- Exposure to tuberculosis
- Travel history
- History of maternal illness
- Recent neurosurgical procedure or head trauma
- Presence of a foreign body, such as a shunt or a cochlear implant

- Immunocompromised status
- Close-contact living spaces such as dormitories or military bases
- Day care attendance

PHYSICAL EXAMINATION

Observe the general appearance of the child. The infant with bacterial meningitis may rest in the opisthotonic position (Fig. 38.14), and the older child may complain of neck pain. In the infant, a bulging fontanel may be present, which is often a late sign, and the infant may be consolable when lying still as opposed to being held. Presence of positive Kernig and Brudzinski signs can indicate irritation of the meninges (Fig. 38.15). Inspect the child for presence of a rash; a petechial, vesicular, or macular rash may be seen.

Take Note!

Abrupt eruption of a petechial or purplish rash can be indicative of meningococcemia (infection with *N. meningitidis*). Immediate medical attention is warranted.

FIGURE 38.14 Infant in **opisthotonic** position: head and neck are hyperextended to relieve discomfort.

LABORATORY AND DIAGNOSTIC TESTS

Common laboratory and diagnostic studies ordered for the assessment of bacterial meningitis include:

- LP—Fluid pressure will be measured and a sample is obtained for analysis and culture. CSF will be elevated and CSF will reveal increased white blood cells (WBCs)

FIGURE 38.15 **A.** Kernig sign is tested by flexing legs at the hip and knee (**A1**), then extending the knee (**A2**). A positive report of pain along the vertebral column and/or inability to extend knee is a positive sign and indicates irritation of meninges. **B.** Brudzinski sign is tested by the child lying supine with the neck flexed (**B1**). A positive sign occurs if resistance or pain is met. The child may also passively flex hip and knees in reaction, indicating meningeal irritation (**B2**).

and protein and low glucose (the bacteria present feed on the glucose).

- Complete blood count (CBC)—WBCs will be elevated.
- Blood, urine, and nasopharyngeal culture—Performed to look for source of infection and to rule out sepsis. Blood culture will be positive in cases of septicemia.

Nursing Management

Administer prescribed antibiotics as soon as possible after obtaining cultures. Quickly initiate supportive measures to ensure proper ventilation, reduce the inflammatory response, and help prevent injury to the brain. Interventions are aimed at reducing ICP and maintaining cerebral perfusion along with treating fluid volume deficit, controlling seizures, and preventing injury that may result from altered LOC or seizure activity. Initiate appropriate isolation precautions. In addition to standard precautions, infants and children diagnosed with bacterial meningitis will be placed on droplet isolation until 24 hours of antibiotics have been received to help prevent transmission to others. Refer to Nursing Care Plan 38.1 at the end of the chapter for nursing diagnoses and related interventions. In addition to those diagnoses and interventions, note any measures taken to reduce fever and prevent bacterial meningitis.

REDUCING FEVER

Hyperthermia related to infectious process, increased metabolic rate, and dehydration as evidenced by increased body temperature; warm, flushed skin; and tachycardia may be present. Reducing fever is important to help maintain optimal cerebral perfusion by reducing the metabolic needs of the brain. Administer antipyretics such as acetaminophen and nonsteroidal anti-inflammatory drugs (NSAIDs) such as ibuprofen, per order. Institute nonpharmacologic measures, if needed. Reduce environmental temperature and use cooling blankets, fans, cold compresses, and tepid baths to help reduce fever. Avoid measures that cause shivering because it increases heat production and is therefore counterproductive as well as uncomfortable for the child.

PREVENTING BACTERIAL MENINGITIS

Bacterial meningitis is a serious illness and prevention is important. It is transmitted by direct close contact with respiratory droplets from the nose or throat. Most at risk are those living with the child or anyone with whom the child played or was in close contact. Postexposure prophylaxis and postexposure immunization may be effective. Control measures should be initiated in environments where risk exists. Disinfect toys and other shared objects to decrease transmission of the microorganisms to others.

To reduce group B streptococcus infection in neonates, screen pregnant women. If the screening results are positive, discuss with the mother and offer treatment with intrapartum antibiotics. Vaccines are available for some specific causative organisms, but complete vaccination prevention is not possible at this time. The Hib vaccine is routine starting at 2 months of age and all children should be immunized to continue the reduction of bacterial meningitis caused by *H. influenzae* type B. The pneumococcal vaccine is also routine for all children starting at 2 months of age and should be considered for pre-schoolers who are at risk. Children at risk include those with immune deficiency; sickle cell disease; asplenia; chronic pulmonary, cardiac, or renal disease; diabetes mellitus; cochlear implants; cerebrospinal leaks; and organ transplants.

In Canada, prior to 2001, when pneumococcal conjugate and meningococcal C conjugate vaccines were not nationally approved, meningococcal meningitis was responsible for 36% of the reported cases of meningitis (PHAC, 2005). Living in close quarters, sleeping less than usual, and sharing personal items such as drinking glasses and lip balm contribute to the increase in disease. For these reasons, the CPS advise meningococcal vaccination (MCV-C) for all children at 12 months of age; MCV-4 should be given to children 2 years of age and older who are at increased risk of meningococcal infection and adolescents should get a booster of either MCV-C or MCV-4 at 12 years of age (CPS, 2017a; MacNeil & Cohn, 2011).

Take Note!

Three main serogroups of meningococcal bacteria cause disease, B, C, W, and Y. With improved vaccinations, meningococcal disease is still endemic to Canada while significant decreases have occurred. The PHAC is hopeful that with improvements to the immunization programs, there will be continued reductions in the incidence of meningococcal infections (Li, Tsang, Desai, & Deehan, 2014).

Aseptic Meningitis

Aseptic meningitis is the most common type of meningitis, and the majority of children affected are younger than 5 years of age. If the causative organism can be identified, it is usually a virus. Enteroviruses, such as echovirus and coxsackievirus, account for the majority of cases of aseptic meningitis (Lee et al., 2006). Less common causes include mumps, herpesvirus, HIV, measles, varicella, influenza, and vector-borne viruses.

Therapeutic Management

Prompt diagnosis and treatment are essential to improve outcomes. The child is treated aggressively as if he or she has bacterial meningitis until the diagnosis is confirmed. Antibiotics are administered and continued until the causative organism is recognized. If the cause is viral, antibiotics may be discontinued and antiviral agents may be started at this time. After diagnosis is confirmed, treatment is mainly supportive in nature and the illness is usually self-limiting, lasting 3 to 10 days.

Nursing Assessment

Elicit a description of the present illness and chief complaint. Common signs and symptoms reported during the health history might include:
- Fever
- General malaise
- Headache
- Photophobia
- Poor feeding
- Nausea
- Vomiting
- Irritability
- Lethargy
- Neck pain
- Positive Kernig and Brudzinski signs

The onset of symptoms may be abrupt or gradual. Assessment is similar to that of the child with bacterial meningitis. Signs and symptoms are similar to those seen in bacterial meningitis, but the child is usually less ill.

Nursing Management

Nursing management is similar to the nursing care of the child with bacterial meningitis and will focus on comfort measures to reduce pain and fever. Aseptic meningitis can be managed successfully at home if the child's neurologic status is stable and he or she is tolerating oral intake.

Encephalitis

Encephalitis is an inflammation of the brain that may also include an inflammation of the meninges. It is a rare complication and can be caused by protozoan, bacterial, fungal, or viral invasion. Viral illness and autoimmune disorders are the most commonly diagnosed cause in children, although in the majority of cases the cause remains unknown (Hardarson, 2015).

Common causative organisms include enteroviruses, such as poliovirus and coxsackievirus; herpes simplex virus 1 and 2; and vector-borne viruses. Recovery from encephalitis can occur in a few days or may be complicated and involve severe neurologic damage with residual effects. Prognosis depends on the age of the child and the causative organism. Prompt diagnosis and treatment are essential. The child suspected of having encephalitis should be hospitalized. Therapeutic management is mainly supportive in nature and focuses on maintaining optimal cerebral perfusion; hydration and nutrition; and injury prevention.

Nursing Assessment

For a full description of the assessment phase of the nursing process, refer to the Assessment section of the Nursing Process Overview earlier in the chapter. Assessment findings pertinent to encephalitis are discussed below.

HEALTH HISTORY

Elicit a description of the present illness and chief complaint. Common signs and symptoms reported during the health history might include:
- Fever
- Flu-like symptoms
- Altered LOC
- Headache
- Lethargy
- Drowsiness
- Generalized weakness
- Seizure activity

Explore the child's current history for risk factors such as:
- Recent travel
- Recreational activities, such as hiking and camping
- Animal contacts

PHYSICAL EXAMINATION

Perform a neurologic examination to distinguish between encephalitis and viral meningitis. In encephalitis, a neurologic examination will reveal changes in sensorium and focal neurologic changes. Neurologic findings vary and reflect the areas of the brain that are involved.

LABORATORY AND DIAGNOSTIC TESTS

An LP may be performed and the CSF may show an elevated leukocyte count and elevated protein and glucose levels. However, in some cases, levels may be normal. MRI, CT, and EEG procedures may be performed to help identify early changes and provide useful clues in developing a diagnosis.

Nursing Management

Nursing management is similar to nursing care for the child with meningitis. Specific antiviral therapy may be used for diseases caused by the herpes simplex virus. Teach children and their families how to prevent encephalitis. Avoiding exposure to viruses that cause encephalitis is one of the best ways to prevent it; avoidance can be accomplished by practicing good hand hygiene, eliminating sharing of eating utensils, and not kissing others (CPS, 2017a). Encephalitis can also result from complications of childhood illnesses such as measles, mumps, or chickenpox. Explain the importance of keeping children up to date in their immunizations. Effective vaccines are available for a few viral pathogens that cause encephalitis (such as rabies virus and Japanese encephalitis virus), but these vaccines are not routine; they are recommended for those at high risk. For example, postexposure rabies vaccines can be administered to a child who was bitten by a suspected rabid animal. Also, those traveling to areas where Japanese encephalitis is endemic, such as India and China, and planning a prolonged stay or extreme outdoor activity should receive the appropriate vaccine.

Vector control and avoiding mosquito and tick bites are the best prevention of vector-borne infection. Preventative measures include:

- Using insect repellents (repellents containing DEET should be used cautiously in children younger than 12 years of age and not at all in children younger than 1 year of age)
- Wearing clothing that covers the arms and legs
- Controlling mosquito populations by eliminating areas of standing water where mosquitoes can breed
- Using insect traps and public measures such as sprayed insecticides to reduce the mosquito population

Reye Syndrome

Reye syndrome is an extremely rare disease that primarily affects children younger than 15 years of age who are recovering from a viral illness. The exact cause of Reye syndrome is unknown. It has been found that Reye syndrome is a reaction that is triggered by the use of salicylates or salicylate-containing products to treat a viral infection. This reaction causes brain swelling, liver failure, and death in hours, if treatment in not initiated. In the 1980s, the adverse effects of salicylates used to treat viral illnesses began to be publicized and required warning labels to be placed on all salicylate-containing products, such as aspirin. Since then, there has been a dramatic decrease in the occurrence of Reye syndrome.

Early recognition and treatment are the most important aspects of managing this illness. Nursing management is aimed at maintaining cerebral perfusion, managing and preventing increased ICP, providing safety measures due to changes in LOC and risk for seizures, and monitoring fluid status to prevent dehydration and overhydration.

Education is an important aspect of preventing this disease. Salicylates are found in many products, including many over-the-counter products such as Alka-Seltzer and Pepto-Bismol. A complete list can be found on thePoint. Recovery from Reye syndrome is dependent on the severity of swelling of the brain. Some children will make a full recovery, while others may suffer long-term neurologic damage.

Take Note!

- Common signs and symptoms of Reye Syndrome include:
- Severe and continual vomiting
- Changes in mental status
- Lethargy
- Irritability
- Confusion
- Hyperreflexia
- Current and past medical history risk factors may include:
  - A prodromal viral illness, like chickenpox, croup, flu, or an upper respiratory infection
  - Ingestion of salicylate-containing products within 3 weeks of the start of the viral illness
  - Elevated liver function tests and elevated serum ammonia levels can confirm diagnosis

LEUKODYSTROPHY

Leukodystrophies are a group of progressive genetic disorders of the central and peripheral nervous system that affect the growth and/or maintenance of the myelin. Although they are considered rare, research suggests that with better diagnostics and definition, the incidence might be higher than previously identified (Vanderver, Hussey, Schmidt, Pastor, & Hoffman, 2012). While leukodystrophy types vary, they are often divided into two etiologies, inherited or spontaneous. While they do share some common characteristics with multiple sclerosis (MS), also associated with loss of myelin, the difference is that the loss of myelin in leukodystrophies is an autosomal recessive condition (United Leukodystrophy Foundation, 2017; Helman, Van Haren, Escolar, & Vanderver, 2015a; Helman et al., 2015b). Cree leukodystrophy (CLD), a form specific to Canada, affects infants of Cree and Chippawayan descent; it progresses rapidly and is always fatal. In most cases, a previously healthy 3- to 9-month-old infant experiences onset of symptoms, similar to that of Vanishing White Matter disease, following a viral infection or trauma.

Nursing Assessment

Elicit a description of the present illness and chief complaint. Common signs and symptoms reported during the health history may include:

- Febrile episodes
- Seizures (usually later in the illness)
- Spasticity or abnormally stiff muscle tone
- Loss of muscle coordination—including feeding and swallowing issues
- Lethargy
- Mental impairment
- Coma

The health history may indicate the infant was generally developing as expected with perhaps slow onset of the above symptoms; however, following an infection or trauma, there may be episodes of rapid deterioration which can lead to coma and death (Harder et al., 2010).

LABORATORY AND DIAGNOSTIC TESTS

The diagnosis is made based on clinical findings in combination with MRI, which shows abnormal signals in the white matter of the brain. On occasion, the specific genetic defect is known by the family; however, DNA analysis for genetic mutations is conclusive (Harder et al., 2010; United Leukodystrophy Foundation, 2017).

Nursing Management

A diagnosis of CLD is a devastating disorder that affects the entire family; the prognosis is dismal for children; however, therapeutic management is paramount (Dewan & Cohen, 2013). A multidisciplinary approach is required as care is aimed at symptomatic management. A multidisciplinary approach focuses on improvement in quality of life by managing seizures and safety measures, promoting mobility, nutrition, and providing family support. Refer to Nursing Care Plan 38.1 and the end of the chapter for nursing diagnoses and related interventions. Interventions common to CLD are discussed below.

PREVENTING INFECTION

CLD is noted to deteriorate significantly during periods of acute stress such as febrile illness. Medical strategies include timely and complete vaccinations, liberal antibiotic use, as well as regular dental care and hygiene. Attention to infection control measures such as handwashing can reduce infection which directly improves quality of life for these children. Often the child will require tube feeds to meet the nutritional requirement, specifically if swallowing issues arise (Helman et al., 2015a, 2015b).

SUPPORTING AND EDUCATING THE CHILD AND FAMILY

Families caring for children with CLD may experience high levels of stress since this complex condition is life-limiting. Additional burdens include family time spent in hospital settings as well as the financial burden of attending appointments. See Chapter 34 for more information on supporting the child with a chronic, life-limiting condition and their caregivers.

Supportive education and access to support groups is complicated by the rarity of the condition and lack of formal support groups. The goals of treatment focus on anticipatory care, risk management, and symptom treatment (Helman et al., 2015b).

TRAUMA

Trauma, or unintentional injury, is the leading cause of Canadian childhood morbidity and mortality (Farrell, 2016). Indigenous children and youth have disproportionality higher rates of unintentional injuries (CPS, 2017b). It has been estimated that the unintentional death rates for Indigenous children is 3 to 4 times higher than the rates for non-indigenous Canadian children (Canadian Institute of Child Health, 2000). However, unintentional injury rates differ across Canada. For example, Manitoba, Saskatchewan, and British Columbia have an Indigenous death rates 6.5 times higher than the death rates for non-Indigenous Canadian children in these provinces (Canadian Institute of Child Health, 2000). These higher rates may reflect Indigenous children and youth living in remote communities with limited access to health care services (CPS, 2017b).

Any child that is exposed to trauma or unintentional injuries faces significant risk to his or her developing neurologic system, often leading to neurologic disorders with life-threatening and lasting effects. Neurologic trauma may include head trauma, non-accidental head trauma, birth injuries, and near-drowning.

Head Trauma

In Canada, injury causes more death in children than disease (CICH, 2000; CPS, 2017b; Yanchar, Warda, & Fuselli, 2012). Head trauma causing brain injury is one of the most prevalent reasons pediatric patients seek medical attention (Farrell, 2016). Common causes of head trauma in children include falls, drowning, motor vehicle accidents, pedestrian and bicycle accidents, sports-related injuries, and child abuse (CPS, 2007). Many factors make children more susceptible to head trauma than adults. Larger head size in relation to the body, coupled with a higher center of gravity, causes the child to hit his or her head more readily when involved in motor vehicle accidents, bicycle accidents, and falls. Children are also at risk for injury related to psychosocial factors such as their high activity level, curiosity, incomplete motor development, and lack of knowledge and judgment skills.

Head trauma is a broad term that can include specific patterns of injury. Traumatic brain injury (TBI) occurs when a head trauma results in a disruption of the normal function of the brain. Not all head traumas result in a TBI. See Table 38.6 for descriptions of common head injuries seen in children. Head trauma in children is serious because it can cause an immediate threat to the child's life as well as a number of complications that can lead to lifelong impairment of an individual's physical, cognitive, and psychosocial functioning. Prognosis for the child who has suffered a head trauma depends on the extent and severity of the injury as well as any complications

TABLE 38.6	COMMON HEAD INJURIES SEEN IN CHILDREN	
Types	**Description**	**Characteristics**
Skull fractures	A break in the bone surrounding the brain	In infants and children younger than 2 years, a great deal of force is needed to produce a skull fracture. Due to the flexibility of the immature skull, it is able to withstand a great degree of deformation before a fracture will occur. Can result in little or no brain damage, but may have serious consequences if the underlying brain tissue is injured.
Linear skull fracture	A simple break in the skull that follows a relatively straight line	Most common skull fracture. Can result from minor head injuries such as being struck by a rock, stick, or other object; falls; or motor vehicle accidents. Not usually serious unless there is additional injury to the brain.
Depressed skull fractures	The bone is locally broken and pushed inward, causing pressure on the brain	Can result from forceful impact from a blunt object, such as a hammer or another heavy but fairly small object. Surgery is often required to elevate the bony pieces and inspect the brain for evidence of injury.
Diastatic skull fracture	A fracture through the skull sutures	Most commonly occurs in the lambdoid sutures (refer to Fig. 38.10 for location of sutures). Usually, treatment is not required, but observation will be necessary.
Compound skull fracture	A laceration of the skin and splintering of the bone	The fracture can be linear or depressed. Generally, it is the result of blunt force. Usually requires medical intervention and surgery may be necessary.
Basilar skull fracture	A fracture of the bones that form the base of the skull	Can result from severe blunt head trauma with significant force. Due to the proximity to the brain stem, this is a serious head injury. Findings include CSF rhinorrhea and otorrhea, bleeding from the ear, and orbital or postauricular ecchymosis (bruising behind ear is referred to as Battle sign), and these children are at increased risk for infection because the fracture may allow a portal of entry into the central nervous system.
Concussion	A type of traumatic brain injury that is caused by a bump, blow, jolt, jarring, or shaking and results in disruption or malfunction of the electrical activities of the brain	Most common head injury. Results from a blow or jolt to the head caused by sports injuries, motor vehicle accidents, and falls. Confusion and amnesia, after the head injury, are seen. Loss of consciousness may or may not occur. Noted symptoms may include increased distractibility and difficulty with concentration. Treatment includes rest and monitoring for neurologic changes that could indicate a more severe injury, such as increased sleepiness, worsening headache, increased vomiting, worsening confusion, difficulty walking or talking, changes in LOC, and seizures.
Contusion	Bruising of cerebral tissue	Results from a blow to the head from incidents such as a motor vehicle accident, falls, or abuse such as shaken baby syndrome. May cause focal disturbances in vision, strength, and sensation. The signs and symptoms will vary based on the extent of vascular injury and can range from mild weakness to prolonged unconsciousness and paralysis. Treatment includes close monitoring for neurologic changes. Surgery is usually not necessary.
Subdural hematoma	Collection of blood between the dura and cerebrum	Low incidence of fracture. Most common in children younger than 2 years old, especially infants. Results from birth trauma, falls, bicycle injuries, and abuse such as shaken baby syndrome. Usually consists of venous bleeding. Symptoms may occur within 3 days of trauma or as late as 20 days. Symptoms include vomiting, failure to thrive, changes in LOC, seizures, and retinal hemorrhage. Treatment depends on clinical symptoms, size of clot, and area of the brain involved. In some cases, the bleed may be closely monitored for resolution. In other cases, treatment may include subdural taps in infants and surgical evacuation in older children. Close monitoring of neurologic status and for signs of increased ICP is indicated.

(continued)

TABLE 38.6	COMMON HEAD INJURIES SEEN IN CHILDREN (continued)	
Types	Description	Characteristics
Epidural hematoma	Collection of blood located outside the dura but within the skull	Relatively uncommon. Often results from skull fracture. Seen when head trauma is severe. Usually arterial bleeding, therefore brain compression occurs rapidly and can result in impairment of the brain stem and respiratory or cardiovascular function. Symptoms include vomiting, headache, and lethargy. Treatment depends on clinical symptoms, the size of the clot, and the area of the brain involved. Treatment includes prompt surgical evacuation and cauterization of the artery. The earlier the bleed is recognized and treated, the more favorable the outcome. Close monitoring of neurologic status is indicated.

Nursing Assessment

For a full description of the assessment phase of the nursing process, refer to the Assessment section of the Nursing Process Overview earlier in the chapter. Assessment findings pertinent to head trauma are discussed below.

HEALTH HISTORY

Take a detailed history, including past medical history along with details of the events surrounding the injury such as mental status at the time of the injury, any loss of consciousness, irritability, lethargy, abnormal behaviour, vomiting (if so, how many times), any seizure activity, mechanism of injury, and any complaints of headache, visual changes, or neck pain.

Mechanism of injury is important to know as how, where, and why a child has experienced a head trauma will influence their injury pattern (Ibrahim, Wood, Margulies, & Christian, 2012). For example, studies have shown that fall height and injury acquired from a fall will differ in infants and toddlers. Ibrahim et al. (2012) found that infants were more likely to fall <3 ft while toddlers were more likely to fall from >10 ft heights. The likely fall heights can be explained through understanding the developmental differences found in infants versus toddlers discussed earlier. Additionally, infants that fell down stairs were more likely to experience intracranial injuries due to the repetitive nature of tumbling down stairs or being accidently crushed from the adult falling onto the infant (Ibrahim et al., 2012). Therefore, asking detailed questions regarding the mechanism of injury is important to inform assessment and be mindful of possible injuries.

PHYSICAL EXAMINATION

Perform a thorough physical examination. Initial physical assessment will focus on the ABCs (airway, breathing, and circulation) (refer to Chapter 51 for further information on emergency management). Children pose a special challenge as their developmental stages can make neurologic assessments difficult, especially in the pre-verbal stage. However, all children who experience head trauma need an assessment of their neurologic function as soon as they are seen. This includes GCS, LOC, pupillary response, and any seizure activity. Fixed and dilated pupils, fixed and constricted pupils, or sluggish pupillary reaction to light will warrant prompt intervention. First priority is to stabilize vitals and avoid secondary injury to the brain such as hypoxia, hypotension, hyperthermia, and ICP (Farrell, 2016).

Take Note!

A child's spine must remain stabilized after a head injury until spinal cord injury is ruled out.

LABORATORY AND DIAGNOSTIC TESTS

Diagnostic tests that may be utilized include x-ray examinations of the head and neck and CT and MRI scans. These procedures can assist in providing a more definitive diagnosis of the severity and type of trauma. The need for sedation should be medically led since there is heightened risk for respiratory repression. Be aware of local policy when escorting sedated children to investigative radiology.

Take Note!

If clear liquid fluid is noted draining from the ears or nose, notify physician or advanced nurse practitioner. If the fluid tests positive for glucose, this is indicative of leaking CSF.

Nursing Management

Nursing management of the child with head trauma depends on the seriousness of the injury. For all head trauma, however, the nurse provides support and education to the family and provides teaching on ways to prevent future head injuries.

CARING FOR THE CHILD WITH MILD-TO-MODERATE HEAD INJURY

Mild to moderate closed head injury is defined as brain injury without any penetrating injury to the brain, no loss of consciousness, no other injury to the head or body, normal behaviour after the injury, and healthy status before the injury. Most children with this type of injury can be cared for and observed at home. Provide parents and caregivers with clear instructions regarding the care of their child at home. Explain that they must seek medical attention if the child's condition worsens at any time during the first several days after injury. See Teaching Guidelines 38.2.

Teaching Guidelines 38.2
MONITORING THE CHILD WITH CLOSED HEAD INJURY AT HOME

Instruct parents and caregivers:

- Stay with the child for the first 24 hours and be ready to take the child to the hospital, if necessary.
- Wake the child every 2 hours to ensure that he or she moves normally, wakes enough to recognize the caregiver, and responds to the caregiver appropriately.
- Closely observe the child for a few days.
- Call the medical provider or bring child to the emergency room if the child exhibits any of the following:
  - Constant headache that gets worse
  - Slurred speech
  - Dizziness that does not go away or happens repeatedly
  - Extreme irritability or other abnormal behaviour
  - Vomiting more than two times
  - Clumsiness or difficulty walking
  - Oozing blood or watery fluid from ears or nose
  - Difficulty waking up
  - Unequal-sized pupils
  - Unusual paleness that lasts longer than 1 hour
  - Seizures
  - Review signs and symptoms of increased intracranial pressure and provide parents with a number they can call if they have questions or concerns.

Children with mild closed head injury may exhibit some cognitive and behavioural symptoms, such as difficulty paying attention, problems making sense of what has been seen or heard, and forgetting things, in the early days after the injury. The majority make a full recovery. However, some may experience ongoing cognitive and behavioural difficulties, including slow information processing and attention difficulties.

Thinking About Development

Antonio Blackman is an 11-year-old boy who suffered a concussion during his hockey game. Based on his developmental stage, how will you instruct him and his caregivers on managing his head injury at home? How would your instructions change if the child was 5 years old?

CARING FOR THE CHILD WITH SEVERE HEAD INJURY

Severe head injuries can range from a temporary unconsciousness that resolves quickly to children who may remain in a comatose state for a prolonged period. Nursing management of the comatose child is similar to nursing care of the comatose adult.

Children with more severe head injury may require intensive care initially until stabilized. Focus will be on maintaining the child's airway; monitoring breathing, circulation, and neurologic status closely; preventing and ceasing any seizure activity; and treating any other injuries that may have occurred as a result of the trauma. Nursing management will continue to focus on evaluation of neurologic status and assessing for changes in LOC and signs and symptoms of increased ICP. Initiate seizure precautions as ordered.

Individualize care to the specific needs of the child. Maintain a quiet environment to help reduce restlessness and irritability. Manage pain and administer sedation as ordered. Observe the level of sedation closely to ensure that LOC will not become altered, which would hinder the ability to assess adequately for neurologic changes. Monitor for the development of complications, which include hemorrhage, infection, cerebral edema, and herniation.

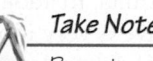

Take Note!

Parents are extremely helpful resources in evaluating a child's behaviour for changes or abnormalities. They can provide insight into whether a behaviour seen is normal or abnormal for this child. Examples include the ease at which a child is normally aroused, how much the child normally sleeps during the day, child's personality and developmental abilities, and what is the child's normal visual and hearing acuity.

PROVIDING SUPPORT AND EDUCATION

Provide support and education for the family of a child who has suffered a head trauma. Encourage involvement in the child's care. The extent of residual neurologic damage and recovery may be unclear for the child with a head injury. This can be frustrating and stressful for parents and family. Encourage verbalization of their feelings and concerns. Rehabilitation of the child with permanent brain damage is an essential component of his or her care. It should begin as soon as possible in the hospital setting and may continue for months to years. This can place a strain on the family and its finances. Families need to be involved in the rehabilitation process. The nurse will be a key member in ensuring the parents and family are involved with the interdisciplinary team.

PREVENTING HEAD INJURIES

Prevention of head injuries provides the greatest benefit to children and the community. Nurses play a key role in educating the public on topics such as helmet use with certain sports; bicycle and motorcycle safety; car seat and seat belt use; and providing adequate supervision of children to help prevent injuries and accidents—and resultant head trauma—from occurring.

Take Note!

Sports-related traumatic brain injuries, including concussions, in children and adolescents are a growing concern, particularly related to the long-term effects of these injuries. Increasing education, awareness, and research about concussions will help to improve prevention, recognition, and treatment to this injury among school professionals, parents, coaches, and children and adolescents. Some evidence-based concussion resources can be found at thePoint.

Nonaccidental Head Trauma

In Canada, inflicted or nonaccidental head trauma is the leading cause of traumatic death and morbidity during infancy (Yanchar et al., 2012). Children's dependence on others to care for them places them at a high risk for injuries caused by child abuse.

The infant's large head size and weak neck muscles place him or her at an increased risk for head trauma due to cranial impacts compared with adults. In addition, children younger than 3 years of age have a very mobile spine, especially in the cervical region, along with immature neck muscles. This places them at a higher risk for injury from acceleration/deceleration injuries, which occur when the head receives a blow or is shaken. The sudden acceleration causes deformation of the skull and movement of the brain, allowing brain contents to strike parts of the skull. Bruising of the brain can occur at the point of impact or at that point distant from the impact where the brain collides with the skull. Another result of brain movement is hemorrhages in the brain, which are caused by the shearing forces that may tear small arteries. The child's thin skull places him or her at increased risk for skull fractures and penetrating injuries resulting from head trauma.

Causes of non-accidental head trauma include violent shaking, referred to as shaken baby syndrome (SBS); blows to the head; and intentional cranial impacts against

the wall, furniture, or the floor. The average age of SBS in infants is <9 months. SBS is a form of child abuse. However, it differs from other forms of child abuse in that frequently there was no intent to harm the child. Shaking happens when the parent or caregiver becomes frustrated or angry with the infant.

The full scope of neurologic deficits resulting from non-accidental head trauma may take several years to recognize depending on the severity of the injury, and therefore recovery can be slow. Long-term outcomes are not known, but many of these infants and children may suffer neurologic defects such as profound intellectual disability, spastic quadriplegia, severe motor dysfunction, and blindness. The majority of children with inflicted head injuries have some impairment of motor and cognitive abilities, language, vision, and behaviour. These injuries may also contribute to later problems with education and social attainment.

Nursing Assessment

The infant who has been a victim of non-accidental trauma can present in various ways. Symptoms and physical findings may be similar to those seen in children with accidental head trauma or increased ICP related to infection. Therefore, many non-accidental traumas remain unidentified. Early recognition of suspected child abuse is essential to prevent death and disability from repetitive inflicted head trauma. Nurses are mandatory reporters of abuse; know and follow local policy.

HEALTH HISTORY

It is important to review the child's history closely and pay particular attention to the caregivers' explanation of the child's injury. Be alert to any discrepancies between the physical injuries and the history of injury given by the parent, especially if the stories are conflicting, or if the caregivers are unable to give an explanation for the injury. Also, note any previous intracranial or skeletal injuries that cannot be explained.

In less severe cases, common signs and symptoms may include:
- Poor feeding or sucking
- Vomiting
- Lethargy or irritability
- Failure to thrive
- Increased sleeping
- Difficulty arousing

In more severe cases, the symptoms will be more acute and may consist of:
- Seizure activity
- Apnea
- Bradycardia
- Decreased LOC
- Bulging fontanel

PHYSICAL EXAMINATION

External bruising of the head and face may be evident in some inflicted head traumas. However, no evidence of external trauma, but the presence of intracranial or intra-ocular hemorrhages, is the classic presentation of SBS. Retinal hemorrhages are seen in the majority of cases, which is a rare finding in accidental or non-traumatic events.

LABORATORY AND DIAGNOSTIC TESTS

Diagnostic tests including CT, MRI, and ophthalmologic examination to rule out retinal hemorrhages, and skeletal survey x-rays to rule out or confirm other injuries, may be performed to help determine the extent and type of injury.

Nursing Management

Treatment and nursing management will be similar to that for the child with accidental head trauma (see earlier section, Head Trauma). Prevention of non-accidental head trauma, including SBS, is a major concern for all health care professionals. Be aware of risk factors related to the potential for SBS to occur. Recognizing these risk factors will allow appropriate intervention and protection of the child to take place. See Box 38.4 for risk factors related to SBS.

Educating parents and caregivers on appropriate ways to handle stress and ways to cope with a crying infant can help to prevent non-accidental head trauma (see Teaching Guidelines 38.3). Many parents and caregivers may perceive shaking a child as a less violent way to react than other means of enforcing discipline. They need to be aware that shaking a baby, even for only a few seconds, can cause serious brain damage and death. Decreasing mortality and morbidity associated with SBS and non-accidental injury through early preventive education is an essential nursing concern. Information about the dangers of shaking a baby should be a part of prenatal care and standard discharge teaching on postpartum units and at scheduled child review.

BOX 38.4

RISK FACTORS ASSOCIATED WITH SHAKEN BABY SYNDROME

- Single parent
- Young parent
- Substance abuse by a parent
- Any external factors present such as financial, social, or physical burdens that place stress on the parent
- Premature or sick infant
- Infant with colic

Teaching Guidelines 38.3
TIPS TO CALM A CRYING BABY

Instruct parents and caregivers:
- Try to figure out what is upsetting the baby.
- Is the baby hungry?
- Is the baby's diaper dry?
- Is the baby cold or hot?
- Is the baby overtired or overstimulated?
- Is the baby in pain?
- Is the baby sick or running a fever?
- Try to help the baby relax.
- Turn down the lights.
- Swaddle the baby.
- Walk the baby.
- Rock the baby.
- Give the baby a breast, bottle, or pacifier.
- Shhh, talk to, or sing to the baby.
- Take the baby for a stroller or car ride.
- Sometimes the baby may continue to cry after all your efforts. If you feel overwhelmed, frustrated, or angry, focus on keeping the baby safe.
- Stop what you are doing, take a deep breath, and count to 10.
- Place the baby in a safe place, such as the crib or playpen.
- Leave the room, shut the door, and find a quiet place for yourself.
- Check on the baby every 5 to 15 minutes.
- Do not be afraid to call for help; call a friend, relative, or neighbour.

Near-Drowning

Drowning is the second leading cause of unintentional injury-related death for children between 1 and 14 years (Yanchar et al., 2012). Drowning death rates, generally across Canada, occur in rural and urban areas, increase over weekends and the summer months, are linked to recreational activities, and while reduced over the last two decades, numbers are generally static (Canadian Drowning Report, 2016). The death rate for children aged 5 years and younger is approximately 1.1 per 100,000; these deaths are considered preventable fatalities (Canadian Drowning Report, 2016). Major risk factors for drowning in young children and adolescents includes lack of supervision, not wearing personal floatation devices, teen alcohol consumption, and being around or in the water at night-time; males are at a higher risk (Canadian Drowning Report, 2016). Drowning fatalities for Indigenous people were reported to be six times higher when compared with non-Indigenous people (CPS, 2017b). This is an important statistic when only 5% of the Canadian population identify themselves as Indigenous (Canadian Drowning Report, 2016; CPS, 2017b).

Near-drowning is described as an incident in which a child has suffered a submersion injury and has survived for at least 24 hours. Near-drowning events can result in long-term neurologic deficits. For children <1 year old, most often near-drowning events occur in bathtubs, buckets, or toilets. For children between ages 1 and 5 years, near-drowning risks are linked to social leisure activities, for example, residential swimming pools (Canadian Drowning Report, 2016). In children older than 15 years of age, natural water settings, such as oceans or lakes, are risk factors (CPS, 2017b).

Nursing Assessment

Hypoxia is the primary problem resulting from near-drowning. Nursing assessment needs to begin with resuscitative measures. The child may be comatose, be hypothermic, lack spontaneous respirations, and present with hypoxia and hypercapnia. Gain information about the site of submersion (was it fresh or salt water?), the water temperature, the time of submersion, and how long it was until the child received interventions such as cardiopulmonary resuscitation (CPR) and emergency medical services (EMS).

Nursing Management

Resuscitative measures should be started as soon as the child is pulled from the water, and the child should be transported to a hospital immediately. Management will be based on the degree of cerebral insult that has occurred. The child who has been successfully resuscitated will usually require intensive nursing care and monitoring. Promotion of oxygenation and monitoring for infection related to aspiration of water are primary nursing concerns. Chronic neurologic damage occurs in many near-drownings secondary to hypoxia. The child may need rehabilitation and long-term follow-up. Provide parents with support and education relating to their child's condition. Educating children, families, and the community is an important nursing intervention to help prevent drowning (see Teaching Guidelines 38.4).

Teaching Guidelines 38.4
TEACHING TO PREVENT DROWNING

Instruct parents and caregivers:
- Install proper four-sided child-resistant pool fencing that is greater than 1.5 m tall and ensure pool fencing has self-closing gates with safety latches (Parachute Canada, 2011).
- Start water safety training at a young age.

- Never leave an infant or child without close adult supervision in or near water (this includes bathtubs).
- Empty water from all containers, such as 5-gallon buckets, immediately after use.
- Use proper-fitting, Coast Guard–approved personal flotation devices at all times when near water
- Never allow children to walk, skate, or ride on thinning or thawing ice.
- Learn CPR and keep emergency numbers handy (make sure babysitters are CPR qualified).
- Know the depth of water before permitting a child to jump or dive.

BLOOD FLOW DISRUPTION

Pediatric cerebral vascular disorders occur less often than in adults, but they are still an important cause of mortality and chronic morbidity in children (Smith & Fox, 2015). Many children will develop lifelong cognitive and motor impairments. Childhood cerebral vascular disorders (stroke) are usually seen after the first month of life. Periventricular/intraventricular hemorrhage occurs in preterm infants and in infants up to 1 month of age (see Chapter 24).

Cerebral Vascular Disorders (Stroke)

A cerebral vascular disorder is a sudden disruption of the blood supply to the brain. It affects neurologic functioning, such as movement and speech. Two major types of adult cerebral vascular disorders are seen in children—ischemic stroke and hemorrhagic stroke. Ischemic stroke is more common than hemorrhagic stroke in children. In children, there are a wide array of risk factors and causes as compared to adults (see Comparison Chart 38.2), but in many cases, the cause remains unidentified. The outcomes reported for cerebral vascular disorders in children vary, but many children will develop some neurologic or cognitive deficit.

Take Note!
Strokes in Children
Children are more likely to experience an ischemic stroke than a hemorrhagic stroke. If a child experiences a stroke, the symptoms are similar to those that an adult experiences.

Historically, children have been excluded from adult stroke studies. Therefore, many treatments used in children have had to be adapted from adult studies. Acute treatment is supportive and requires intensive care. The exact treatment will depend on the underlying cause.

COMPARISON CHART 38.2	RISK FACTORS AND CAUSES OF STROKE IN CHILDREN AND ADULTS	
	Risk Factors and Causes in Children	**Risk Factors and Causes in Adults**
Ischemic stroke	Cardiac disorders and intracardiac defects (congenital such as ventricular septal defect, atrial septal defect, and aortic stenosis, or acquired such as rheumatic heart disease) Coagulation abnormalities that lead to thrombosis Sickle cell disease Infection, such as meningitis Arterial dissection Genetic disorders	Cardiac disease, including atherosclerosis Diabetes mellitus Hyperlipidemia Hypercoagulability states Polycythemia Sickle cell disease Smoking Increased age Male gender Obesity Excessive alcohol consumption
Hemorrhagic stroke	Vascular malformations such as intracranial arteriovenous malformation (AVM) Aneurysms Warfarin therapy Cavernous malformations Malignancy Trauma Coagulation disorders such as hemophilia Thrombocytopenia Liver failure Leukemia Intracranial tumours such as medulloblastomas	Hypertension Aneurysms Use of anticoagulant medications Smoking Increased age Male gender Obesity Excessive alcohol consumption

Nursing Assessment

The clinical presentation will vary according to age, the underlying cause, and the location of the stroke. Signs and symptoms of acute stroke are similar to those seen in the adult and depend on the area of the brain that has been affected. Common signs include:

- Weakness on one side or hemiplegia
- Facial droop
- Slurred speech
- Speech deficits
- Seizures
- Headaches
- Lethargy

Strokes in children are diagnosed in the same manner as strokes in adults. However, further tests may need to be run in the child, such as metabolic studies, coagulation tests, echocardiogram, and LP to help identify the cause of the stroke.

Nursing Management

Nursing management will be similar to that for the adult patient who has suffered a stroke. Care will focus on assessing neurologic status, increasing mobility, providing adequate nutrition and hydration, and encouraging self-care. Rehabilitative care may be initiated, depending on the long-term deficits, to help the child attain optimal function. Parental support and education will be essential in helping them care for a child who has new disabilities.

CHRONIC DISORDERS

Chronic disorders in children necessitate multidisciplinary care. Parents and children are in need of both education and support from the health care team. Chronic neurologic disorders commonly seen in children include acute and chronic headaches.

Headaches

Acute and chronic headaches, including migraines, are common reasons why children miss school, visit their physician or nurse practitioner, and receive subsequent referrals to neurologists. Children reporting or presenting with symptoms of headaches need to be examined thoroughly. Headaches may result from sinusitis or eyestrain or can be indicative of more serious conditions such as brain tumours, acute meningitis, or increased ICP. Migraines are a specific type of headache. They are benign, recurrent, throbbing headaches often accompanied by nausea, vomiting, and photophobia. Acute migraines can occur in children as young as 3 to 4 years old. The cause of migraine headaches is not well understood.

After other acute or chronic conditions are ruled out, management will focus on treating the child's pain. Pharmacologic measures may be utilized in the treatment of chronic headaches and migraines. Medications used in children to treat and prevent headaches are similar to the medications used to treat adults. Recent attention has been paid to headaches caused by medication overuse. The child may have a primary headache disorder that is exacerbated by the frequent use of medications. Although medication overuse headaches are common in children, they are frequently underrecognized and underdiagnosed.

Nursing Assessment

Elicit a description of the present illness and chief complaint. Important health history information to obtain is onset of the pain, aggravating and alleviating factors, frequency and duration of the pain, time of day the pain usually occurs, location of the pain, and quality and intensity of the pain.

In young children, symptoms of headache may be hard to recognize. However, common signs and symptoms may include:

- Irritability
- Lethargy
- Head holding
- Head banging
- Sensitivity to sound or light

Assessment also includes a thorough physical examination to rule out any life-threatening illness, such as a brain tumour or increased ICP. A detailed neurologic examination is warranted. Neuroimaging may be performed based on the child's history and physical examination, if needed, to rule out a brain tumour or mass as the cause of the headaches.

| BOX 38.5 |

POTENTIAL HEADACHE TRIGGERS

- Foods, such as chocolate, caffeine, or monosodium glutamate (MSG)-containing foods
- Changes in hormone levels, around menses and ovulation
- Changes in:
  - Weather
  - Season
  - Sleep patterns
  - Meal schedule
- Stress
- Intense activity
- Bright or flickering lights
- Odours, such as strong perfumes

Nursing Management

Nursing measures will focus on support and education. After serious illness has been ruled out, reassure the child and family that no serious medical or neurologic disease is present. Because headaches are recurring and the cause may be unknown, pain management can be difficult. Provide education to help the child and parents gain control over the headaches. Teach the child and family to keep very accurate record of headaches and activities surrounding the headaches to help establish a pattern of occurrence and identify triggering factors. Encourage parents and the child to recognize the triggering factors and to avoid them (Box 38.5). Teach the child and family about pain medications and how to use them. Teach other management techniques, which may include exercise, sleep regulation, proper diet with regularly spaced meals, avoiding caffeine, avoiding inadequate hydration, regular attendance at school, use of biofeedback, stress reduction techniques, and possible psychiatric assessment.

NURSING CARE PLAN 38.1

Overview for the Child With a Neurologic Disorder

NURSING DIAGNOSIS: Decreased intracranial adaptive capacity related to compression of brain tissue due to increased CSF or cerebral edema secondary to increased ICP resulting from brain injury, congenital structural defects, brain tumour, decreased reabsorption of CSF, or shunt malfunction as evidenced by vomiting, headache, complaints of visual disturbances, decreased pulse and respirations, elevated blood pressure or pulse pressure, changes in level of consciousness, increased head circumference, or bulging fontanel

Outcome Identification and Evaluation

Child will remain free of signs and symptoms of increased ICP as evidenced by remaining free of headache, vomiting, vision disturbances, vital signs within parameters for age, no signs of altered levels of consciousness, able to maintain effective breathing pattern, free of excessive irritability or lethargy, head circumference within parameters for age.

NURSING CARE PLAN 38.1

Overview for the Child With a Neurologic Disorder (continued)

Interventions: *Promoting Adequate Intracranial Adaptive Capacity*

- Assess neurologic status closely, collect GCS, and monitor for signs and symptoms of increased ICP: *changes in level of consciousness, signs of irritability or lethargy, and changes in pupillary reaction can indicate changes in ICP.*
- Monitor vital signs and calculate Pediatric Early Warning Score (PEWS): *decreased pulse and respiratory rate and increased blood pressure or pulse pressure can indicate increased ICP.*
- Measure head circumference in children younger than 3 years of age: *increases in head circumference outside parameters for age can indicate increased ICP.*

- Elevate head of bed 15 to 30 degrees: *to facilitate venous return and help to reduce ICP.*
- Minimize environmental stimuli and noise, and avoid pain-producing procedures, if possible: *all can increase ICP.*
- Have emergency equipment ready and available: *increased ICP can result in respiratory or cardiac failure.*
- Notify physician or nurse practitioner immediately if changes in assessment are noted: *early intervention is critical to prevent neurologic damage and death.*

NURSING DIAGNOSIS: Risk for ineffective cerebral tissue perfusion related to increased ICP, alteration in blood flow secondary to hemorrhage, vessel malformation, cerebral edema

Outcome Identification and Evaluation

Child will exhibit adequate cerebral tissue perfusion through course of illness and childhood: child will remain alert and oriented with no signs of altered level of consciousness; vital signs will be within parameters for age; PEWS as per hospital guidelines; motor, sensory, and cognitive function will be within parameters for age; head circumference will remain within parameters for age.

Interventions: *Promoting Adequate Tissue Perfusion*

- Assess neurologic status closely and monitor for signs and symptoms of increased ICP: *changes in level of consciousness, signs of irritability or lethargy, and changes in pupillary reaction can indicate decreased cerebral tissue perfusion.*
- Monitor vital signs: *decreased pulse and respiratory rate and increased blood pressure or pulse pressure can indicate increased ICP, which can lead to decreased cerebral perfusion.*
- Have emergency equipment ready and available: *decreased cerebral perfusion can result in respiratory or cardiac failure.*
- Notify physician or nurse practitioner immediately if changes in assessment are noted: *early intervention is critical to prevent neurologic damage and death.*

NURSING DIAGNOSIS: Risk for injury related to altered level of consciousness, weakness, dizziness, ataxia, loss of muscle coordination secondary to seizure activity

Outcome Identification and Evaluation

Child will remain free of injury as evidenced by *no signs of aspiration or traumatic injury.*

Interventions: *Preventing Injury*

- Ensure child has patent airway and adequate oxygenation (have suction, oxygen available at bedside) and place child in side-lying position, if possible: *a child with altered level of consciousness may not be able to manage his or her secretions and is at risk for aspiration*

(continued)

Overview for the Child With a Neurologic Disorder (continued)

and ineffective airway clearance; providing suction and oxygenation can help ensure an open airway and the side-lying position can help secretions drain and prevent obstruction of airway or aspiration.

- Protect child from hurting self during seizures or changes in level of consciousness by removing environmental obstacles, easing child to lying position, and padding side rails: *helps to keep environment safe.*
- Institute seizure precautions for any child at risk for seizure activity (see Box 38.2) *to help prevent injury that can result from acute seizure activity.*
- With seizure activity, do not insert a tongue blade or restrain child: *can lead to injury to caregiver and child.*
- Administer anticonvulsant medications as ordered: *will help to promote cessation and prevention of seizure activity.*
- Assist child with ambulation: *to help prevent injury in child with weakness, dizziness, or ataxia.*
- Allow for periods of rest: *to prevent fatigue and decrease risk of injury.*

NURSING DIAGNOSIS: Risk for complications of neurologic/sensory dysfunction related to presence of neurologic lesion or pressure on sensory or motor nerves secondary to increased ICP, presence of tumour, swelling postoperatively as evidenced by visual disturbances (i.e., reports of double vision), pupillary changes, nystagmus, ataxia, balance disturbances, or loss of response to stimuli

Outcome Identification and Evaluation

Child will be free of changes in sensory perception or will remain at baseline as evidenced by no complaints of double vision, PERRLA (Pupils Equal, Round, Reactive to Light and Accommodation), no disturbances of gait or balance noted, and no increase in loss of responses to stimuli.

Interventions: *Managing Disturbed Sensory Perception*

- Assess for changes in sensory perception: *provides baseline data and allows nurse to recognize change in sensory perception early.*
- Monitor child for risk of injury secondary to changes in sensory perception: *visual changes and disturbances of gait or balance increase child's risk for injury.*
- Notify physician or nurse practitioner of changes in sensory perception: *can indicate increased ICP and medical emergency.*
- Assist child to learn to use adaptive methods to live with permanent changes in sensory perception (i.e., use of eyeglasses) and maximize the use of intact senses: *adaptive devices can enhance sensory input and intact senses can often compensate for impaired senses.*
- Provide familiar sounds (voices, music): *can help relieve anxiety related to changes in sensory perception, especially visual changes.*

NURSING DIAGNOSIS: Risk for infection related to surgical interventions, presence of foreign body (i.e., shunt), trauma to skull, nutritional deficiencies, dental caries, stasis of pulmonary secretions and urine, presence of infectious organisms as evidenced by fever, poor feeding, decreased responsiveness, and presence of virus or bacteria on laboratory screening

NURSING CARE PLAN 38.1

Overview for the Child With a Neurologic Disorder (continued)

Outcome Identification and Evaluation

Child will exhibit no signs or symptoms of local or systemic infection and will not spread infection to others: *symptoms of infection will decrease over time; others will remain free of infection.*

Interventions: *Preventing Infection*

- Monitor vital signs, PEWS scores and follow hospital Sepsis guidelines for detecting and reporting suspected septic patients: *elevation in temperature can indicate presence of infection.*
- Monitor incision sites for signs of local infection: *redness, warmth, drainage, swelling, and pain at incision site can indicate presence of infection.*
- Maintain aseptic technique—practice good handwashing and use proper technique when managing postoperative incisions and external shunts: *to prevent introduction of further infectious agents.*
- Administer antibiotics as prescribed: *to prevent or treat bacterial infection.*
- Encourage nutritious diet and proper hydration according to child's preferences and ability to feed orally: *to assist body's natural defences against infection.*
- Isolate the child as required: *to prevent nosocomial spread of infection.*
- Teach child and family preventive measures such as good handwashing, covering mouth and nose upon cough or sneeze, and adequate disposal of used tissues: *to prevent nosocomial or community spread of infection.*

NURSING DIAGNOSIS: Bathing, dressing, feeding, and toileting self-care deficit related to neuromuscular impairments; cognitive deficits as evidenced by an inability to perform hygiene care and transfer self independently

Outcome Identification and Evaluation

Child will demonstrate ability to care for self within age parameters and limits of disease: *child is able to feed, dress, and manage elimination within limits of disease and age.*

Interventions: *Maximizing Self-Care*

- Introduce child and family to self-help methods as soon as possible: *promotes independence from the beginning.*
- Encourage family and staff to allow child to do as much as possible: *allows child to gain confidence and independence.*
- Teach specific measures for bowel and urinary elimination as needed: *promotes independence and increases self-care abilities and self-esteem.*
- Collaborate with physical therapy, occupational therapy, speech therapy, and child life departments to provide child and family with appropriate tools to modify environment and methods to promote transferring and self-care: *allows for maximum functioning.*
- Praise accomplishments and emphasize child's abilities: *helps improve self-esteem and encourages feeling of confidence and competence.*
- Balance activity with periods to rest *to reduce fatigue and increase energy for self-care.*

NURSING DIAGNOSIS: Impaired physical mobility related to muscle weakness, hypertonicity, impaired coordination, loss of muscle function or control as evidenced by an inability to move extremities, to ambulate without assistance, to move without limitations

(continued)

Overview for the Child With a Neurologic Disorder (continued)

Outcome Identification and Evaluation

Child will be able to engage in activities within age parameters and limits of disease: child is able to move extremities, move about environment, and participate in exercise programs within limits of age and disease.

Interventions: *Maximizing Physical Mobility*

- Encourage gross and fine motor activities: *facilitates motor development.*
- Collaborate with physical therapy, occupational therapy, and speech therapy departments to strengthen muscles and promote optimal mobility: *facilitates motor development.*
- Utilize passive and active range of motion (ROM) and teach child and family how to perform: *prevents contractures and facilitates joint mobility and muscle development (active ROM) to help increase mobility.*
- Praise accomplishments and emphasize child's abilities: *helps improve self-esteem and encourages feeling of confidence and competence.*

NURSING DIAGNOSIS: Risk for delayed development related to physical disability, cognitive deficits, activity restrictions

Outcome Identification and Evaluation

Child will demonstrate developmental milestones within age parameters and limits of disease: child expresses interest in the environment and people around him or her and interacts with environment age appropriately.

Interventions: *Maximizing Development*

- Use therapeutic play and adaptive toys: *helps facilitate developmental functioning.*
- Provide stimulating environment when possible *to maximize potential for growth and development.*
- Praise accomplishments and emphasize child's abilities: *helps improve self-esteem and encourages feeling of confidence and competence.*

NURSING DIAGNOSIS: Imbalanced nutrition: less than body requirements related to vomiting and difficulty feeding secondary to increased ICP; difficulty sucking, swallowing, or chewing; surgical incision pain or difficulty assuming normal feeding position; inability to feed self as evidenced by decreased oral intake, impaired swallowing, weight loss

Outcome Identification and Evaluation

Child will exhibit signs of adequate nutrition: weight will remain within parameters for age, skin turgor will be good, intake/output (I/O) will be within normal limits, adequate calories will be ingested, and vomiting will cease or decrease.

Interventions: *Promoting Adequate Nutrition*

- Monitor height and weight: *insufficient intake will lead to impaired growth and weight gain.*
- Monitor hydration status (moist mucous membranes, elastic skin turgor, adequate urine output): *insufficient intake can lead to dehydration.*

NURSING CARE PLAN 38.1

Overview for the Child With a Neurologic Disorder (continued)

- Use techniques to promote caloric and nutritional intake and teach family (i.e., positioning, modified utensils, soft or blended foods, allow extra time): *these techniques can facilitate intake.*
- Assess respiratory system frequently *to assess for aspiration.*
- Monitor for nausea and vomiting and medicate, if ordered, *to help reduce vomiting and increase intake.*
- Monitor for pain and medicate, if ordered, *to help reduce pain related to surgical incisions and trauma, and increase intake.*
- Assist family to assume as normal a feeding position as possible *to help increase oral intake.*

NURSING DIAGNOSIS: Risk for deficient fluid volume related to vomiting, altered level of consciousness, poor feeding or intake, insensible loss due to fever, failure of regulatory mechanisms (as in diabetes insipidus) as evidenced by dry oral mucosa, decreased skin turgor, sudden weight loss, hypotension, and tachycardia

Outcome Identification and Evaluation

Fluid volume will be maintained and balanced: oral mucosa moist and pink, skin turgor elastic, urine output at least 1 to 2 mL/kg/hr.

Interventions: *Promoting Adequate Fluid Balance*

- Administer intravenous (IV) fluids, if ordered: *to maintain adequate hydration in children who are nothing by mouth (NPO) or unable to tolerate oral intake.*
- When oral intake is allowed and tolerated, encourage oral (PO) fluids: *to promote intake and maintain hydration.*
- Strict intake and output monitoring: can help identify fluid imbalance and also detect signs of abnormal pituitary secretions resulting in conditions like syndrome of inappropriate antidiuretic hormone secretion (SIADH) and diabetes insipidus (DI) (see Chapter 48 for further information).
- Maintain minimum hydration and avoid overhydration in children where cerebral edema is a concern: fluid overload can contribute to cerebral edema.
- Monitor urine specific gravity, urine and serum electrolytes (especially serum sodium), blood urea nitrogen, creatinine and osmolality, and daily weights as ordered reliable indicators of fluid status and can also detect signs of abnormal pituitary secretions resulting in conditions like SIADH and DI.

NURSING DIAGNOSIS: Deficient knowledge related to lack of information regarding complex medical condition, prognosis, and medical needs as evidenced by verbalization, questions, or actions demonstrating lack of understanding regarding child's condition or care

Outcome Identification and Evaluation

Child and family will verbalize accurate information and understanding about condition, prognosis, and medical needs: child and family demonstrate knowledge of condition and prognosis and medical needs including possible causes, contributing factors, and treatment measures.

(continued)

Overview for the Child With a Neurologic Disorder (continued)

Interventions: *Providing Child and Family Teaching*

- Assess child's and family's willingness to learn: *child and family must be willing to learn for teaching to be effective.*
- Provide family with time to adjust to diagnosis: *will help facilitate adjustment and ability to learn and participate in child's care.*
- Repeat information: *allows family and child time to learn and understand.*
- Teach in short sessions: *many short sessions are found to be more helpful than one long session.*
- Gear teaching to a level of understanding of the child and also the family (depends on age of child, physical condition, memory): *to ensure understanding.*
- Provide reinforcement and rewards: *helps facilitate the teaching–learning process.*
- Use multiple modes of learning involving many senses (provide written, verbal, demonstration, and videos) when possible: *child and family more likely to retain information when presented in different ways using many senses.*

NURSING DIAGNOSIS: Interrupted family processes, related to child's illness, hospitalization, diagnosis of chronic illness in child, and potential long-term effects of illness as evidenced by family's presence in hospital, missed work, demonstration of inadequate coping

Outcome Identification and Evaluation

Family will maintain functional system of support and demonstrate adequate coping, adaptation of roles and functions, and decreased anxiety: *parents are involved in child's care, ask appropriate questions, express fears and concerns, and are able to discuss child's care and condition calmly.*

Interventions: *Promoting Adequate Family Processes*

- Encourage parents and family members to verbalize concerns related to child's illness, diagnosis, and prognosis: *allows the nurse to identify concerns and areas where further education may be needed; demonstrates family-centered care.*
- Explain therapies, procedures, child's behaviours, and plan of care to parents: *understanding the child's current status and plan of care helps decrease anxiety.*
- Encourage parental involvement in care: *allows parents to feel needed and valued with a sense of control over their child's health.*
- Identify support system for family and child: *helps nurse identify needs and resources available for coping.*
- Educate family and child on additional resources available: *to help them develop a wide base of support.*

KEY CONCEPTS

- Development of the brain and spinal cord occurs early in gestation, in the first 3 to 4 weeks. Infection, trauma, teratogens, and malnutrition during this period can result in malformations and may affect normal CNS development.

- The brain of the newborn is highly vascular, leading to an increased risk for hemorrhage.

- The head of the infant and young child is large in proportion to the body, and the neck muscles are not well developed, which places the infant at an increased risk of head injury from falls and accidents.

- Neurologic disorders in children can result from congenital problems as well as infections or trauma.

- LP and CSF analysis can be useful in the diagnosis of hemorrhage, infection, or obstruction.

- CT and MRI studies can be useful in diagnosing congenital abnormalities such as neural tube defects, hemorrhage, tumours, fractures, demyelination, or inflammation.

- EEGs measure the electrical activity of the brain and can be used in diagnosing seizures or brain death.

- Antibiotics are utilized in the treatment of bacterial meningitis and shunt infections.

- Anticonvulsants are used in the treatment and prevention of seizures and are often used in combination.

- Corticosteroids are used to reduce cerebral edema and must be tapered before discontinuing.

- Risk factors associated with neurologic disorders include prematurity, difficult birth, infection during pregnancy, family history of genetic disorders with a neurologic manifestation, seizure disorders, and headaches.

- Alterations in motor function, such as changes in gait or muscle tone or strength, may indicate certain neurologic problems such as increased ICP, head injury, and cerebral infections.

- Increased ICP is a sign that may occur with many neurologic disorders. It may result from head trauma, birth trauma, hydrocephalus, infection, and brain tumours. It is essential that the nurse observes for signs and symptoms associated with increased ICP while caring for a child with a potential or suspected neurologic disorder.

- Sunset eyes may indicate increased ICP as seen in hydrocephalus.

- A bulging fontanel can be a sign of increased ICP and is seen in such neurologic disorders as hydrocephalus and head traumas.

- Cortical control of motor function is lost in certain neurologic disorders; postural reflexes re-emerge and are directly related to the area of the brain that is damaged. Decorticate posturing (child is stiff with bent arms; wrists and fingers are clenched and held on chest) occurs with damage of the cerebral cortex and/or cord. Decerebrate posturing (arms and legs held straight out, toes pointed downwards, arched head and neck) occurs with damage at the level of the brain stem.

- Nursing management of seizures focuses on preventing injury during seizures, instituting seizure precautions, maintaining a patent airway, administering appropriate medication and treatments to prevent or reduce seizures, and providing education and support to the child and family to help them cope with the challenges of living with a chronic seizure disorder.

- Hydrocephalus results from an imbalance in the production and absorption of CSF. Key assessment findings include a rapid increase in head circumference seen in the infant, or loss of development and changes in personality in the older child. Signs and symptoms associated with increased ICP may be seen.

- Nursing management of the child with hydrocephalus will focus on maintaining cerebral perfusion, minimizing neurologic complications, recognizing and preventing shunt infection and malfunction, maintaining adequate nutrition, promoting growth and development, and supporting and educating the child and family.

- Bacterial meningitis requires rapid assessment and treatment. On assessment, the nurse may find the infant with bacterial meningitis resting in the opisthotonic position (spasticity with hyperextension—seen as arching), and the older child may complain of neck pain.

- Nursing management of the child with bacterial meningitis will include administration of intravenous antibiotics, reducing ICP, and maintaining cerebral perfusion along with treating fluid volume deficit, controlling seizures, and preventing injury that may result from altered LOC or seizure activity.

- Nursing implications for leukodystrophy patients require use of collaborative approach to care since the needs are medically complex (i.e., a medical home model with its multidisciplinary approach). While this disease is considered incurable, nursing plays a key role in prevention of and management of symptoms related to improving quality of life.

- Nurses play a key role in educating the public on topics such as helmet use with certain sports, bicycle and motorcycle safety, car seat and seat belt use, and providing adequate supervision of children to help prevent injuries and accidents and resultant head trauma from occurring.

- Many neurologic disorders affect multiple body systems with lifelong deficits that require long-term rehabilitation. Adjusting to the demands this condition places on the child and family is difficult. Parents may need time to accept their child's condition but as soon as possible they should be involved in the child's care.

- Children with neurologic disorders and their families often need large amounts of education and support throughout the child's lifetime. As the child grows, the needs of the family and child will change. The nurse needs to provide ongoing education and support.

○ Some neurologic disorders require complete intensive daily care. Adjusting to these demands can be difficult for the family. Encourage respite care and provide meaningful education programs that emphasize independence for the child in the least restrictive educational environment. Refer caregivers to local resources, including education services and support groups.

REFERENCES AND RECOMMENDED READINGS

Berg, A. T., Berkovic, S. F., Brodie, M. J., Buchhalter, J., Cross, J. H., van Emde Boas, W., ... Scheffer, I. E. (2010). Revised terminology and concepts for organization of seizures and epilepsies: Report of the ILAE Commission on Classification and Terminology, 2005–2009. *Epilepsia, 51*(4), 676–685.

Canadian Drowning Report. (2016). Retrieved from http://www.lifesavingsociety.com/media/241812/canadiandrowningreport_english_web.pdf

Canadian Institute of Child Health. (2000). *The health of Canada's children: A CICH profile, 3rd ed. Chapter 6: Aboriginal children and youth*. Retrieved from http://www.cich.ca/PDFFiles/Profile/CICH%20Profile_06%20Aboriginal.pdf

Canadian Paediatric Society (CPS). (2007). *Multidisciplinary guidelines on the identification investigation and management of suspected abusive head trauma*. Retrieved from http://www.cps.ca/documents/position/multidisciplinary-guidelines-abusive-head-trauma

Canadian Paediatric Society (CPS). (2016). Folate and neural tube defects: The role of supplements and food fortification. *Paediatrics and Child Health, 21*(3), 145–149.

Canadian Pediatric Society (CPS). (2017a). *Position statement: Meningococcal vaccines in Canada: An update*. Retrieved from www.cps.ca/en/documents/position/meningococcal-vaccine

Canadian Paediatric Society (CPS). (2017b). *Position statement: Preventing unintentional injuries in Indigenous children and youth in Canada*. Retrieved from http://webcache.googleusercontent.com/search?q=cache:cU2SRll4c6sJ:www.cps.ca/assets/pdfreactor/pdf.php%3Flang%3Den%26paper%3Dunintentional-injuries-indigenous-children-youth+&cd=2&hl=en&ct=clnk&gl=ca

Community Paediatrics Committee. (2017). *Positional plagiocephaly*. Retrieved from Canadian Paediatric Society: http://www.cps.ca/documents/position/positional-plagiocephaly

Craniofacial Program. (2017). Retrieved from SickKids: http://www.sickkids.ca/craniofacial/what-we-do/craniofacial-conditions/craniosynostosis/index.html

Dewan, T., & Cohen, E. (2013). Children with medical complexity in Canada. *Paediatrics and Child Health, 18*(10), 518–522.

Douglas, M., Drake, J., Rowe, P., & Vachhrajani, S. (2017). aboutkidshealth. Retrieved from SickKids: http://www.aboutkidshealth.ca/En/HealthAZ/ConditionsandDiseases/BrainandNervousSystemDisorders/Pages/Hydrocephalus-and-Treatment-Shunts-andEndoscopic-Third-Ventriculostomy.aspx

Farrell, C. A. (2016). Position statement: Management of the paediatric patient with acute head trauma. *Paediatrics and Child Health, 18*(5), 253–258.

Fischbach, F. T., & Dunning, M. B. III. (2015). *A manual of laboratory and diagnostic tests* (9th ed.). Philadelphia, PA: Wolters Kluwer Health/Lippincott Williams & Wilkins.

Fisher, R. S., Acevedo, C., Arzimanoglou, A., Bogacz, A., Cross, J. H., Elger, C. E., ... Wiebe, S. (2014). ILAE Official Report: A practical clinical definition of epilepsy. *Epilepsia, 55*(4), 475–482.

Gooley, A. M., Gooley, N. M., Moniz, N. M., & Hunter, J. (2016). Management of patients with neurologic dysfunction. In P. Paul, R. A. Day, & B. Williams (Eds.). *Canadian textbook of medical-surgical nursing* (3rd ed., p. 2004). Philadelphia, PA: Wolters Kluwer.

Guidelines for Paediatric Concussions. (2014). Retrieved from http://concussionsontario.org/resources/guidelines-for-pediatric-concussion

Hanson, A. L., Schunk, J. E., Corneli, H. M., & Soprano, J. V. (2016). A randomized controlled trial of positioning for lumbar puncture in young infants. *Pediatric Emergency Care, 32*, 504–507.

Hardarson, H. S. (2015). *Acute viral encephalitis in children and adolescents: Clinical manifestations and diagnosis*. UpToDate. Retrieved from http://www.uptodate.com/contents/acute-viral-encephalitis-in-children-and-adolescents-clinical-manifestations-and-diagnosis

Harder, S., Gourgaris, A., Frangou, E., Hopp, K., Huntsman, R., Lowry, N., ... Tynan, J. (2010). Clinical and neuroimaging findings of Cree leukodystrophy: A retrospective case series. *American Journal of Neuroradiology, 31*, 1418–1423.

Helman, G., Van Haren, K., Escolar, M. L., & Vanderver, A. (2015a). Emerging treatment for pediatric leukodystrophies. *Pediatric Clinics of North America, 62*(3), 649–666.

Helman, G., Van Haren, K., Bonkowsky, J. L., Bernard, G., Pizzino, A., Braverman, N., ... Vanderver, A. (2015b). Disease specific therapies in leukodystrophies and leukoencephalopathies. *Molecular Genetics and Metabolism, 114*, 527–536.

Hochberg, L., & Stone, J. (2015). *Prenatal screening and diagnosis of neural tube defects*. UpToDate. Retrieved from http://www.uptodate.com/contents/prenatal-screening-and-diagnosis-of-neural-tube-defects

Holmes, G. L. (2013). *Who get's febrile seizures. Epilepsy Foundation*. Retrieved from http://www.epilepsy.com/learn/types-seizures/febrile-seizures

Ibrahim, N. G., Wood, J., Margulies, S. S., & Christian, C. W. (2012). Influence of age and fall type on head injuries in infants and toddlers. *International Journal of Developmental Neuroscience, 30*(3), 201–206.

Infectious Diseases and Immunization Committee. (2017). *Guidelines for the management of suspected and confirmed bacterial meningitis in Canadian children older than one month of age*. Canadian Paediatric Society. Retrieved from https://www.cps.ca/en/documents/authors-auteurs/infectious-diseases-and-immunization-committee

International League Against Epilepsy (ILAE). (2014). *Seizure classification*. Retrieved from https://www.epilepsydiagnosis.org/seizure/seizure-classification-groupoverview.html

Johnson S., Evans T. A., Draper E. S., Field D. J., Manktelow B. N., Marlow N., ... Boyle E. M. (2015). Neurodevelopmental outcomes following late and moderate prematurity: A population-based cohort study. *Archives of Disease in Childhood-Fetal and Neonatal Edition, 100*, F301–F308.

Johnston, M. V. (2011). Chapter 591: Encephalopathies. In: R. M. Kleigman, B. F. Stanton, J. W. St. Geme III, N. F. Schor, & R. E. Behrman (Eds.). *Nelson textbook of pediatrics* (19th ed., pp. 2061–2068). Philadelphia, PA: Saunders.

Khoury, C. (2015). *Chiari malformations.* UpToDate. Retrieved from http://www.uptodate.com/contents/chiari-malformations

Kinsman, S. L., & Johnston, M. V. (2011). Chapter 585: Congenital anomalies of the central nervous system. In R. M. Kleigman, B. F. Stanton, J. W. St. Geme III, N. F. Schor, & R. E. Behrman (Eds.). *Nelson textbook of pediatrics* (19th ed., pp. 1998–2013). Philadelphia, PA: Saunders.

Kohlschutter, A., & Eichler, F. (2011). Childhood leukodystrophies: a clinical perspective. *Expert Review of Neurotherapeutics, 11*(10), 1485–1496.

Lee, B. E., Chawla, R., Langley, J. M., Forgie, S. E., Al-Hosni, M., Baerg, K., ... Law, B. J. (2006). Paediatric Investigators Collaborative Network on Infections in Canada (PICNIC) study of aseptic meningitis. *BMC Infectious Diseases, 6*(1), 68. Retrieved from https://bmcinfectdis.biomedcentral.com/articles/10.1186/1471-2334-6-68

Li, Y. A., Tsang, R., Desai, S., & Deehan, H. (2014). *Enhanced surveillance of invasive meningococcal disease in Canada, 2006–2011.* Public Health Agency of Canada. Winnipeg, Manitoba: Canada Communicable Disease Report. Retrieved from http://www.phac-aspc.gc.ca/publicat/ccdr-rmtc/14vol40/dr-rm40-09/dr-rm40-09-surv-eng.php

MacNeil, J., & Cohn, A. (2011). Chapter 8: Meningococcal disease. In Centers for Disease Control and Prevention (Ed.). *Manual for the surveillance of vaccine-preventable diseases.* Atlanta, GA: Centers for Disease Control and Prevention.

Mikati, M. A. (2011). Chapter 586. Seizures in childhood. In R. M. Kleigman, B. F. Stanton, J. W. St. Geme III, N. F. Schor, & R. E. Behrman (Eds.). *Nelson textbook of pediatrics* (19th ed., pp. 2013–2039). Philadelphia, PA: Saunders.

Millichap, J. J., & Millichap, J. G. (2015). *Treatment and prognosis of febrile seizures.* UpToDate. Retrieved from http://www.uptodate.com/contents/treatment-and-prognosis-of-febrile-seizures

National Institute of Neurological Disorders and Stroke. (2015). The epilepsies and seizures: Hope through research. Retrieved from http://www.ninds.nih.gov/disorders/epilepsy/detail_epilepsy.htm

Nelson, C. R., Leon, J. A., & Evans, J. (2014). The relationship between awareness and supplementation: Which Canadian women know about folic acid and how does that translate into use? *Canadian Public Health Association, 105*(1), 40–46.

Parachute Canada. (2011). *Preventing drowning: Safer pool fencing legislation chart.* Retrieved from http://www.parachutecanada.org/downloads/policy/Pool_Fencing_Legislation_Chart.pdf

Parachute Canada. (2015). *The cost of injury in Canada. Parachute: Toronto, ON.* Retrieved from http://www.parachute-canada.org/downloads/research/Cost_of_Injury-2015.pdf

Prasad, C., Corbett, B. A., & Prasad, A. N. (2014). Epilepsy, school readiness in Canadian children: Data from National Longitudinal Study of Children and Youth. *Seizure, 23,* 435–438.

Public Health Agency of Canada (PHAC). (2005). *Bacterial meningitis in Canada: Hospitalizations (1994–2001). Ottawa, Ontario, Canada.* Retrieved from www.phac-aspc.gc.ca/publicat/ccdr-rmtc/05vol31/dr3123a-eng.php

Public Health Agency of Canada (PHAC). (2016a). *An advisory committee statement (ACS) National Advisory Committee on Immunization (NACL).* Ottawa: Government of Canada. Retrieved from http://healthycanadians.gc.ca/publications/healthy-living-vie-saine/vaccine-measles-mumps-rubella-varicella-seizures-2016-vaccin-rougeole-rubeole-oreillons-varicelle-convulsions/alt/pub1-eng.pdf. Accessed June 28, 2017.

Public Health Agency of Canada (PHAC). (2016b). *Canadian recommendations on the prevention and treatment of Zika virus: Update Canadian Communicable Disease Report. Volume 42–5,101–111.* Retrieved from http://www.phac-aspc.gc.ca/publicat/ccdr-rmtc/16vol42/dr-rm42-5/ar-01-eng.php

Roach, E. S., deVeber, G., Riela, A. R., & Wiznitzer, M. (2011). Recognition and treatment of stroke in children. Retrieved from http://www.ninds.nih.gov/news_and_events/proceedings/stroke_proceedings/childneurology.htm

Scheffer, I. E., Berkovic, S., Capovilla, G., Connolly, M. B., French, J., Guilhoto, L., ... Zuberi, S. M. (2017). ILAE classification of the epilepsies: Position paper of the ILAE Commission for Classification and Terminology. *Epilepsia, 58*(4), 512–521.

Shellhaas, R. (2015). Etiology and prognosis of neonatal seizures. Retrieved from http://www.uptodate.com/contents/etiology-and-prognosis-of-neonatal-seizures

Slaughter, L. A., Patel, A. D., & Slaughter, J. L. (2013). Pharmacological treatment of neonatal seizures: A systematic review. *Journal of Child Neurology, 28*(3), 351–362.

Smith, S. E., & Fox, C. (2015). *Ischemic stroke in children and young adults: Etiology and clinical features.* UpToDate. Retrieved from http://www.uptodate.com/contents/ischemic-stroke-in-children-and-young-adults-etiology-and-clinical-features

Sullivan, J. E., Farrar, H. C.; The Section on Clinical Pharmacology and Therapeutics and Committee on Drugs. (2011). Clinical report: Fever and antipyretic use in children. *Pediatrics, 127,* 580–587.

Takasu, M., Kubota, T., Tsuji, T., Kurahashi, H., Numoto, S., Watanabe, K., & Okumura, A. (2017). The semiology of febrile seizures: Focal features are frequent. *Epilepsy and Behavior, 73,* 59–63.

Taketokmo, C. K., Hodding, J. H., & Kraus, D. M. (2017). *Lexi-comp's drug reference handbook: Pediatric & neonatal dosage handbook* (20th ed.). Hudson, OH: Lexi-comp, Inc.

Tomita, T., & Ogiwara, H. (2015). *Anencephaly.* UpToDate. Retrieved from http://www.uptodate.com/contents/anencephaly?source=search_result&search=neural±tube±defects&selectedTitle=3~150

United Leukodystrophy Foundation. (2017). What is *leukodystrophy.* Retrieved from United Leukodystrophy Foundation: http://ulf.org/what-is-leukodystrophy/

Vanderver, A., Hussey, H., Schmidt, J. L., Pastor, W., & Hoffman, H. J. (2012). Relative incidence of inherited white matter disorders in childhood to acquired pediatric demyelinating disorders. *Seminars in Pediatric Neurology, 19,* 219–223.

Wirrell, E. C., Laux, L., Donner, E., Jette, N., Knupp, K., Meskis, M. A., … Berg, A. T. (2017). Optimizing the diagnosis and management of Dravet Syndrome: Recommendations from a North American consensus panel. *Pediatric Neurology, 68,* 18–34.

Yanchar, N. L., Warda L. J., & Fuselli. P. (2012). Child and youth injury prevention: A public health approach. *Paediatrics and Child Health,17*(9), 511–520. Retrieved from http://www.cps.ca/documents/position/child-and-youth-injury-prevention

Zak, M., & Chan, V. W. (2014). Chapter 46: Pediatric neurologic disorders. In S. M. Nettina (Ed.). *Lippincott manual of nursing practice* (10th ed., pp. 1545–1575). Philadelphia, PA: Wolters/Kluwer Health: Lippincott Williams & Wilkins.

Zemek, R., Duval, S., Dematteo, C., Solomon, B., Keightley, M., & Osmond, M. (2014). *Guidelines for diagnosing and managing pediatric concussion.* Toronto, ON: Ontario Neurotrauma Foundation

CHAPTER **WORKSHEET**

MULTIPLE CHOICE QUESTIONS

1. When compared with adults, why are infants and children at an increased risk of head trauma?
   a. The head of the infant and young child is large in proportion to the body and the neck muscles are not well developed.
   b. The development of the nervous system is complete at birth but remains immature.
   c. The spine is very immobile in infants and young children.
   d. The skull is more flexible due to the presence of sutures and fontanels.

2. At a well-child visit, hydrocephalus may be suspected in an infant if upon assessment the nurse finds
   a. narrow sutures
   b. sunken fontanels
   c. a rapid increase in head circumference
   d. increase in weight since last visit

3. A 10-year-old child is admitted to the hospital due to history of seizure activity. As his nurse, you are called into the room by his mother, who states he is having a seizure. What would be the priority nursing intervention related to prevention of injury?
   a. Remove the child from his bed.
   b. Place a tongue blade in the child's mouth.
   c. Restrain the child.
   d. Place the child on his side and opening his airway.

4. A 6-month-old infant is admitted to the hospital with suspected bacterial meningitis. She is crying, irritable, and lying in the opisthotonic position. The priority nursing intervention would be:
   a. Educate the family on ways to prevent bacterial meningitis.
   b. Initiate appropriate isolation precautions and begin intravenous antibiotics.
   c. Assess the infant's fontanels.
   d. Encourage the mother to hold the infant and feed her.

DOSAGE CALCULATION QUESTION

The nurse is caring for a child who is in status epilepticus. The child weighs 14.97 kg (33 lb). The medication order reads: Diazepam 3 mg IV push now. Per the Pediatric Dosage Handbook, the recommended dose is 0.1 to 0.3 mg/kg/dose. Diazepam is supplied as 5 mg/mL.

How many milliliters will the nurse administer? Round to the nearest tenth.

CRITICAL THINKING EXERCISES

1. A child is seen in the doctor's office after hitting his head while skateboarding. The child suffered no loss of consciousness, and has no external injuries and no significant past medical history. He is acting appropriately at this time. His only complaint is a dull headache. What instructions would you give the parents regarding his care at home? Include when they should seek further medical care.

2. A 10-year-old child is admitted to the pediatric unit after experiencing a seizure. A complete, accurate, and detailed history from a reliable source is essential. What information would you ask for while obtaining the history?

3. A 6-year-old child is admitted to the hospital because of a possible seizure. The child's mother calls the nurse to the room because the child is "jerking all over" and won't respond when she calls the child's name. List appropriate nursing interventions for this child. Prioritize the list of interventions.

4. Describe the impact of a cerebral vascular accident in the child as compared with the adult. How does it affect the child's future? How will the nurse provide care differently for the child stroke victim as compared with the adult?

STUDY ACTIVITIES

1. A 4-month-old child with a history of hydrocephalus has undergone surgery for placement of a VP shunt. What information would you include in the teaching plan?

2. Develop an example of a "headache log" that could be used by the family for chronicling the child's headaches, including triggers, relieving factors, and precipitating events. Ensure that the log is developed at a sixth-grade reading level to make it practical for low-literacy parents.

3. In the clinical setting, interview the parent of a child who has suffered significant brain trauma or injury (such as head trauma, IVH, or stroke). Talk with the family about the types of care the child requires. Reflect upon this interview in your clinical journal, and compare how the ongoing care for this child compares with that for a typical child.

BRINGING IT ALL TOGETHER: A CASE STUDY

Sandra and Michael Graham have brought their 6-month-old son, Thomas, to the pediatric unit for observation. Thomas' head circumference has increased from the 25th percentile at the 4-month check-up to the 75th percentile at the 6-month check-up. Upon assessment, the nurse notes a bulging anterior fontanel and persistent primitive reflexes.

Go to thePoint **to find questions to consider about this case.**

39

Nursing Care of the Child With an Alteration in Sensory Perception/ Disorder of the Eyes or Ears

Learning Objectives

Upon completion of the chapter, you will be able to:

1. Differentiate between the anatomic and physiologic differences of the eyes and ears in children as compared with adults.
2. Identify various factors associated with disorders of the eyes and ears in infants and children.
3. Discuss common laboratory and other diagnostic tests useful in the diagnosis of disorders of the eyes and ears.
4. Discuss common medications and other treatments used for treatment and palliation of conditions affecting the eyes and ears.
5. Recognize risk factors associated with various disorders of the eyes and ears.
6. Distinguish between different disorders of the eyes and ears based on the signs and symptoms associated with them.
7. Discuss nursing interventions commonly used in regard to disorders of the eyes and ears.
8. Devise an individualized nursing care plan for the child with a sensory impairment or other disorder of the eyes or ears.
9. Develop child/family teaching plans for the child with a disorder of the eyes or ears.
10. Describe the psychosocial impact of sensory impairments on children.

Alex John, a 9-month-old, is brought to the clinic by his mother. His mother tells you, "Alex has been fussy and not eating or sleeping well for the past 2 days."

Sensory perception refers to receiving and interpreting stimuli. Disorders of the eyes or ears may lead to alterations in sensory perception. It is important for nurses to understand how to appropriately intervene for sensory perception alterations as well as other eye and ear disorders.

Children commonly suffer from disorders related to the eyes and ears. Conjunctivitis and otitis media are two very common infectious and inflammatory disorders that affect the child's eyes or ears. Various alterations such as refractive error, strabismus, and amblyopia affect the development of visual **acuity** in children. Up to 20% of Canadian children have a vision-related disorder. Therefore, it is important for children to have an eye exam within the first 6 months and vision checked by an optometrist within the first 3 years (Canadian Association of Optometrists, n.d.). Any alteration in the ear that contributes to hearing loss may have a significant impact on the child's language acquisition. Hearing loss can go undetected, especially if it occurs gradually, so many Provinces provide audiology clinics (e.g., through Canadian Hearing Society) and access to speech and language pathologists (Speech-language & Audiology Canada). (See thePoint for links.)

It is important for the nurse to understand the impact of eye and ear disorders on the child's development. Some children may be born with anomalies of the eyes or ears that will have a significant impact on vision and hearing, as well as psychomotor development. On the other hand, disorders affecting the eyes or ears, particularly if chronic or recurrent, can have a significant impact on the development of visual acuity or may cause **hearing impairment**.

In addition, the nurse may be caring for a child with other health issues or conditions as well as being either visually or hearing impaired. The nurse must take these developmental differences into account when planning care for these children.

VARIATIONS IN PEDIATRIC ANATOMY AND PHYSIOLOGY

The anatomy of children's eyes and ears differs somewhat from that of adults. In addition, visual acuity develops from birth throughout early childhood. Hearing is intact at birth, but recurrent ear disorders may adversely affect the child's hearing.

Eyes

Light-skinned children are often born with blue eyes. The iris becomes pigmented over time and eye colour is determined by 6 to 12 months of age. The newborn's sclera may be slightly bluish tinged but becomes white within weeks. The eyeball of the infant and young child occupies a relatively larger space within the orbit than the adult's does, making it more susceptible to injury (Fig. 39.1).

The spherical shape of the newborn's lens does not allow for distance accommodation, so the newborn sees best at a distance of about 20 to 25 cm and the decreased number of cones further contributes to neonatal blurry vision (Bremond-Gignac, Copin, Lapillone, & Milazzo, 2011). The optic nerve is not completely myelinated, so colour discrimination is incomplete. Visual acuity develops over the first few years of the child's life. At birth, acuity ranges from 20/100 to 20/400. Visual acuity improves over the first few years of the child's life, with 20/20 achieved by ages 6 to 7 years (Weber & Kelley, 2014). The rectus muscles are uncoordinated at birth and mature over time so that binocular vision (the ability to focus with both eyes simultaneously) may be achieved by 4 months of age (Weber & Kelley, 2014). In the very preterm infant, retinal as well as neurovascular dysfunction in both the outer and inner immature retina result in complex issues that can impact on visual acuity (Rivera, Madaan, Zhou, & Chemtob, 2016).

Ears

Congenital deformities of the ear are often associated with other body system anomalies and genetic syndromes. The presence of ear anomalies may lead to the search for, and subsequent diagnosis of, the other anomalies or syndromes. The infant's relatively short, wide, and horizontally placed Eustachian tubes allow

FIGURE 39.1 The relatively larger space that the infant's and young child's eyeball occupies within the orbit makes it more susceptible to injury as compared with the adult's eye.

A   Eustachian tube (adult)

B   Eustachian tube (child)

FIGURE 39.2 Note the child's relatively shorter, wider Eustachian tubes and their horizontal positioning (**B**) as compared with the adult's (**A**).

bacteria and viruses to gain access to the middle ear easily, resulting in increased numbers of ear infections as compared to the adult (Friedman, Scholes, & Yoon, 2014). As the child matures, the tubes assume a more slanted position. Therefore, older children and adults generally have fewer cases of middle ear effusion and infection (Fig. 39.2). Sometimes, enlargement of the adenoids contributes to obstruction of the Eustachian tubes, leading to infection.

COMMON MEDICAL TREATMENTS

A variety of interventions are used to treat disorders of the eyes and ears in children. The treatments listed in Common Medical Treatments 39.1 and Drug Guide 39.1 usually require a physician's order when a child is hospitalized.

NURSING PROCESS OVERVIEW FOR THE CHILD WITH A DISORDER OF THE EYES OR EARS

Care of the child with a disorder of the eyes and ears includes assessment, nursing diagnosis, planning, interventions, and evaluation. There are a number of general concepts related to the nursing process that can be applied to disorders of the eyes and ears. From a general understanding of the care involved for a child with alterations in the eyes or ears, the nurse can then individualize the care based on child specifics.

Assessment

Assessment of disorders of the eyes and ears in children includes health history, physical assessment, and laboratory or diagnostic testing.

> Remember Alex, the 9-month-old with fussiness and poor feeding who was not sleeping well? What additional health history and physical examination assessment information should you obtain?

Health History

The health history consists of past medical history, family history, history of present illness, and treatments used at home. The past medical history may be significant for prematurity, genetic defect, eye or ear deformities, visual acuity deficit or blindness, hearing impairment or **deafness**, recurrent ear infections, or ear surgeries. Family history might be significant for eye or ear deformities or vision or hearing impairment or may reveal contacts for infectious exposure.

When eliciting the history of the present illness, inquire about its onset and progression and the presence of fever, nasal congestion, eye or ear pain, eye rubbing, ear pulling, headache, lethargy, or behavioural changes. Determine if the child has accessed assessment services or treatment as there is growing evidence that, despite service provision, attendance can be influenced by family socioeconomic status, ability to travel, and weather conditions when needing to travel to more specialist services, for example, amblyopia services (Sharma, Wong, Colpa, Chow, & Jin, 2016). As ear, nose, and throat issues have the potential to lead to obstructive sleep apnea, be mindful to ask about sleep disturbance at all health contacts (CPS, 2016d; Urquhart & Tan, 2016). Document if the child has corrective lenses or hearing aids prescribed and to what extent these devices are actually used.

COMMON MEDICAL TREATMENTS 39.1

Treatment	Explanation	Indications	Nursing Implications
Warm compress	Warm, moist washcloth	Conjunctivitis	• Use very warm water from the tap (to avoid risk of burning, do not microwave)
Corrective lenses	In eyeglass form or as contact lenses	Correction of astigmatism, refractive error, strabismus	• Use a safety strap to help young children wear their eyeglasses
Patching	An adhesive patch is applied to the healthier eye for several hours each day	Strabismus, amblyopia, any other eye condition that results in one eye being weaker than the other	• Inform parents that though difficult to obtain, compliance with patching is critical • A "pirate patch" may coax preschoolers into compliance
Eye muscle surgery	Surgical alignment of the eyes	Strabismus	• Protect the operative site with patching • Use elbow restraints if necessary
Pressure-equalizing (PE) tubes (tympanostomy tubes)	Tiny plastic tubes inserted in the tympanic membrane	Chronic otitis media with effusion	• Teach parents dry ears precautions if prescribed or preferred by the surgeon. Dry ears can be achieved by placing a cotton ball coated in petroleum jelly over the ear canal, in order to create a watertight seal
Hearing aids	Amplification device worn in the ear	Hearing impairment	• Ensure appropriate fit and adequate amplification • Direct families to outfitters that provide loaner aids of various brands and styles to determine best fit and amplification for the child
Cochlear implants	Surgically inserted electronic prosthetic device	Sensorineural hearing loss	• Inform families that the usual minimum age for this procedure is 12 months

Adapted from National Institute on Deafness and Other Communication Disorders. (2016). *Cochlear implants*. Retrieved from https://www.nidcd.nih.gov/health/cochlear-implants; and Friedman, N. R., Scholes, M. A., & Yoon, P. J. (2014). Ear, nose, & throat. In W. W. Hay, M. J. Levin, R. R. Deterding, & M. J. Abzug (Eds.). *Current pediatric diagnosis and treatment* (22nd ed.). New York: McGraw-Hill.

DRUG GUIDE 39.1 COMMON DRUGS FOR EAR AND EYE DISORDERS

Medication	Actions	Indications	Nursing Implications
Antibiotics (oral, otic, ophthalmic)	Treatment of bacterial infections of the eyes and ears	Acute otitis media, otitis externa, conjunctivitis	Teach families to complete the entire course as prescribed Check for drug allergies prior to administration
Antihistamines	Block histamine reaction	Allergic conjunctivitis	Topical drops used Oral agents usually prescribed if allergic rhinitis accompanies conjunctivitis
Analgesics	Pain relief	Otitis media, otitis externa, after eye or ear surgery	Narcotic analgesics may be necessary in some instances

Adapted from Taketomo, C. K., Hodding, J. H., & Kraus, D. M. (2013). *Pediatric & neonatal dosage handbook* (20th ed.). Hudson, OH: Lexicomp.

Physical Examination

When assessing the eyes and ears, begin with inspection and observation. In addition, testing of visual activity and hearing should be performed by an appropriately trained professional. The Canadian Paediatric Society (2016a) highlights the importance of childhood vision screening since 5% to 10% of pre-school-aged children may have difficulties. If left untreated, they are likely to impact on later visual development.

INSPECTION AND OBSERVATION

Begin the physical examination with inspection and observation. Note whether the child uses eyeglasses, corrective lenses, or a hearing aid. Observe the eyes: note their positioning and symmetry and the presence of strabismus, nystagmus, and squinting. The eyelids should open equally (failure to open fully is termed **ptosis**). Note variations in eye slant and the presence of epicanthal folds. Assess the eyes for the presence of eyelid edema, sclera colour, discharge, tearing, and pupillary equality, as well as the size and shape of the pupils. Make note of any evidence of trichotillomania (pulling out of hair which includes eyelashes and eyebrows); this is an impulse control behaviour often linked to anxiety disorders.

Take Note!

Though the sclerae are bluish in newborns, they become white in the first few weeks of life. Blue sclerae that persist beyond a few weeks of life may be an indicator of osteogenesis imperfecta type I, an inherited connective tissue disorder (Weber & Kelley, 2014).

Evert the eyelid to inspect the palpebral conjunctivae for redness. Test for extraocular movements and pupillary light response and accommodation. Note the symmetry of the corneal light reflex. In addition, note any symptoms that may indicate the child has a vision problem, such as sensitivity to light, squinting, covering or closing one eye, holding objects close, avoiding looking at books or television, challenges to concentration, or limited attention span. Refer the child to an optometrist or physician if you have any concerns.

Take Note!

Attempts to inspect the palpebral conjunctivae may be frightening to children. Ask the older, cooperative child to evert the eyelid himself or herself while the nurse inspects the conjunctivae.

Inspect the ears: note their size and shape, position, and the presence of skin tags, dimples, or other anomalies (Fig. 39.3). If skilled in undertaking otoscopic examination, note the presence of cerumen, discharge, inflammation, or a foreign body in the ear canal. Visualize the tympanic membrane and observe its colour, landmarks, and light reflex, as well as the presence of perforation, scars, bulging, or retraction. Tympanic membrane mobility may be tested with pneumatic otoscopy by someone with these skills. Check with the parents or caregiver if the infant/child had otoacoustic emission (OAE) screening as a newborn (CPS, 2016b). If OAE was not completed and there are concerns linked to the child's auditory development, refer the child to the physician, nurse practitioner, or audiologist.

PALPATION

Usually, the eyes are not palpated. In the case of injury, the upper eyelid may be everted for examination purposes. Palpate the ear for tenderness over the tragus or pinna. Note the presence of tenderness over the mastoid area (tenderness may be present when otitis media progresses to mastoiditis). Palpate for enlarged cervical lymph nodes (this occurs when the eyes or ears are infected).

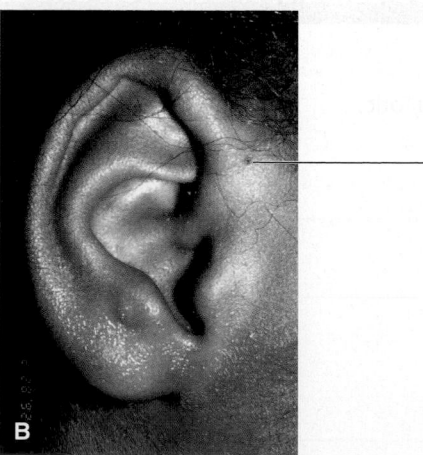

FIGURE 39.3 Note the skin tag (**A**) and preauricular pit (**B**) (in front of the ear).

COMMON LABORATORY AND DIAGNOSTIC TESTS 39.1

Test	Explanation	Indications	Nursing Implications
Culture of eye or ear discharge	Fluid draining from the eye or ear is cultured	To determine specific bacteria present and appropriate antibiotic coverage	Easy to collect, relatively pain-free. If drainage must be removed from within the ear canal, more likely to be painful
Tympanic fluid culture	Culture of fluid aspirated from the middle ear	To determine specific bacteria present and appropriate antibiotic coverage	Painful; usually performed only by specially trained physicians
Tympanometry	Probe in ear canal measures movement of the eardrum	Determines extent of effusion of the middle ear	Quick and easy to perform (seconds). Requires accurate-sized probe for adequate seal of the ear canal

Adapted from Friedman, N. R., Scholes, M. A., & Yoon, P. J. (2014). Ear, nose, & throat. In W. W. Hay, M. J. Levin, R. R. Deterding, & M. J. Abzug (Eds.). *Current pediatric diagnosis and treatment* (22nd ed.). New York: McGraw-Hill.

Laboratory and Diagnostic Testing

Common Laboratory and Diagnostic Tests 39.1 offers an explanation of the laboratory and diagnostic tests most commonly used for disorders of the eyes and ears. These tests can assist the physician or nurse practitioner in diagnosing the disorder and/or can be used as guidelines in determining ongoing treatment. Laboratory or nonnursing personnel obtain some of the tests, while the nurse may obtain others. In either instance, be familiar with how the tests are obtained, what they are used for, and normal versus abnormal results. This knowledge will also be necessary when providing child and family education related to the testing.

Nursing Diagnoses and Related Interventions

Upon completion of a thorough assessment, the nurse might identify several nursing diagnoses, including:

- Disturbed sensory perception
- Risk for infection
- Pain
- Delayed growth and development
- Impaired verbal communication
- Deficient knowledge
- Interrupted family processes
- Risk for injury

After completing an assessment of Alex, the nurse noted the following: fever, tugging at his ears, and increased crying when lying down. Based on the assessment findings, what would your top three nursing diagnoses be for Alex?

Nursing goals, interventions, and evaluation for the child with an eye or ear disorder are based on the nursing diagnoses. Nursing Care Plan 39.1, at the end of the chapter, may be used as a guide in planning nursing care for the child with an eye or ear disorder, but it should be individualized based on the child's symptoms and needs. Refer to Chapter 36 for the nursing care plan for pain management. Additional information will be included later in the chapter as it relates to specific disorders.

Based on your top three nursing diagnoses for Alex, describe appropriate nursing interventions.

INFECTIOUS AND INFLAMMATORY DISORDERS OF THE EYES

Infectious and inflammatory disorders of the eyes include conjunctivitis, nasolacrimal duct obstruction, eyelid lesions, and periorbital cellulitis.

Conjunctivitis

Inflammation of the bulbar or palpebral conjunctiva is referred to as conjunctivitis. It can be infectious, allergic, or chemical in nature. Viruses or bacteria may cause infectious conjunctivitis. Adenoviruses and influenza account for the bulk of cases of viral conjunctivitis. The most common bacterial cause is *Staphylococcus aureus*, but many cases are also caused by *Streptococcus pneumoniae*, *Haemophilus influenzae*, and other bacteria (Friedman et al., 2014). In the newborn, *Chlamydia*

TABLE 39.1	TYPES OF CONJUNCTIVITIS				
Type of Conjunctivitis	Conjunctivae	Discharge	Additional Findings	Eyelid Edema	Treatment
Bacterial	Inflamed	Purulent, mucoid	Mild pain	Occasional	Antibiotic drops or ointment
Viral	Inflamed	Watery, mucoid	Lymphadenopathy, photophobia, tearing	Usually present	Symptom relief; antiherpetic agent if cause is herpes
Allergic	Inflamed	Watery or stringy	Itching	Usually present	Antihistamine and/or mast cell stabilizer drops

Adapted from Braverman, R. S. (2014). Eye. In W. W. Hay, M. J. Levin, R. R. Deterding, & M. J. Abzug (Eds.). *Current pediatric diagnosis and treatment* (22nd ed.). New York: McGraw-Hill.

trachomatis and *Neisseria gonorrhoeae* are more common causes. Prevention treatment protocols (prophylaxis) for opthalmia neonatorum vary with Mulholland and Gardiner (2015) requesting a review of the CPS position statement (2015) in order to develop comprehensive approaches to management. Infectious conjunctivitis is very contagious, so epidemics are common, particularly in young children. Risk factors for acute infectious conjunctivitis include age younger than 2 weeks; day care, preschool, or school attendance; concomitant viral upper respiratory infection; pharyngitis; or otitis media. Concurrent acute otitis media (AOM) may occur depending on the bacterial cause. Complications from simple infectious conjunctivitis are uncommon. Neonates with chlamydial conjunctivitis may be at risk for the development of chlamydial pneumonia.

Allergic conjunctivitis results from exposure to particular allergens. Allergic conjunctivitis may be a seasonal or year-round complaint. A genetic predisposition to allergic conjunctivitis exists, just as it does for asthma, allergic rhinitis, and atopic dermatitis. Allergic conjunctivitis occurs more frequently in school-age children and adolescents than it does in infants and young children because of repeat exposure to allergens over time. In the case of seasonal allergic conjunctivitis, the severity of symptoms and the number of children affected are directly related to the pollen count in the area.

Pathophysiology

When bacteria or viruses come in contact with the bulbar or palpebral conjunctiva, they are recognized as foreign antigens and an antigen–antibody immune reaction occurs, resulting in inflammation. Allergic conjunctivitis occurs through a different mechanism. Contact with the allergen results in an allergic response (overreaction of the immune response). The mast cell and histamine mediators are then activated, resulting in inflammation.

Therapeutic Management

Therapeutic management of conjunctivitis is prescribed depending on the cause. Bacterial conjunctivitis is generally treated with an ophthalmic antibiotic preparation (drops or ointment). Viral conjunctivitis is a self-limiting disease and does not require topical medication. Eye drops with an antihistamine or mast cell stabilization effect may be helpful in alleviating symptoms of allergic conjunctivitis. If other allergy signs and symptoms are also present, an oral antihistamine may also be prescribed. Table 39.1 compares bacterial, viral, and allergic conjunctivitis.

Nursing Assessment

Nursing assessment of the child with conjunctivitis, regardless of the cause, is similar. It includes health history, physical examination, and, in rare instances, laboratory testing.

HEALTH HISTORY

Elicit a description of the present illness and chief complaint. Common signs and symptoms reported during the health history might include:

- Redness
- Edema
- Tearing
- Discharge
- Eye pain
- Itching of the eyes (usually with allergic conjunctivitis)

Determine the onset of symptoms and their progression as well as response to treatments used at home. Assess for risk factors for infectious conjunctivitis, such as day care or school attendance. Note any history of an upper respiratory infection, sore throat, or earache. Question parents about possible infectious exposure. Review the health history for risk factors for allergic conjunctivitis, such as a family history and a history of asthma, allergic rhinitis, or atopic dermatitis. Determine

FIGURE 39.4 **Note redness of conjunctiva.**

seasonality related to the symptoms and whether the symptoms occur after exposure to particular allergens, such as pollen, hay, or animals.

PHYSICAL EXAMINATION

Observe for eyelid swelling or redness. Inspect the conjunctivae for redness (Fig. 39.4). Note quantity, colour, and consistency of discharge. Bacterial infections generally result in a thick, coloured discharge, whereas a clear or white discharge is generally seen with viral conjunctivitis. Allergic conjunctivitis often results in a watery discharge, sometimes profuse, which is usually present bilaterally. Contact with an allergen rubbed into one of the eyes may result in unilateral symptoms. Observe the child for other signs of allergic or atopic disease, and document the presence of a runny nose or cough as well.

LABORATORY AND DIAGNOSTIC TESTS

Cases of bacterial, viral, and allergic conjunctivitis are generally diagnosed based on history and clinical presentation. Cases of viral and allergic conjunctivitis do not warrant laboratory testing. If bacterial conjunctivitis is suspected, then a bacterial culture of the eye drainage may be performed to determine the exact causative organism, thus allowing the most appropriate antibiotic to be prescribed.

Nursing Management

Nursing management of the various types of conjunctivitis focuses on alleviating symptoms and, for infectious causes, preventing spread.

ALLEVIATING SYMPTOMS

Teach parents how to apply eye drops or ointment (antibiotic for bacterial causes and antihistamine or mast cell stabilizer for allergic). Warm compresses may be used to help loosen the crust that accumulates on the eyelids overnight when drainage is copious, particularly with bacterial conjunctivitis.

The child with allergic conjunctivitis may experience perennial or seasonal allergies (or both). Encourage the child to avoid perennial allergens once the offending allergen is determined. Seasonal allergies may include tree pollen in the winter or spring, grass pollen in the summer, and ragweed or flower pollen in the fall.

It is impossible to completely eliminate seasonal allergic responses, partly because it is important for children to participate in physical activity outdoors. Teach families to minimize seasonal allergens on the child's skin and hair. Educate families to:

• Encourage the child not to rub or touch the eyes.
• Rinse the child's eyelids periodically with a clean washcloth and cool water.
• When the child comes in from outdoors, wash the child's face and hands.
• Ensure that the child showers and shampoos before bedtime.

Take Note!

The itching of allergic conjunctivitis may be relieved with cool compresses. An easy way to accomplish this is to have the child hold a tube of yogurt over the affected eye.

PREVENTING INFECTIOUS SPREAD

Because infectious conjunctivitis is extremely contagious, the parent must wash hands diligently after caring for the child. Teach parents and children about appropriate handwashing and discourage them from sharing towels and washcloths. Children with viral conjunctivitis may return to school or day care when symptoms lessen. When mucopurulent drainage is no longer present (usually after 24 to 48 hours of treatment with a topical antibiotic), the child with bacterial conjunctivitis may safely return to day care or school (Blosser, Brady, & Royal, 2013).

Take Note!

Avoid the use of vasoconstricting eye drops such as Visine to rid the eyes of redness. Rebound vasodilation may occur, and with it the redness returns. This leads to repeated frequent use of the drops to keep the eyes from being red but does not treat the actual cause of the redness (Taketomo, Hodding, & Kraus, 2013).

Talking About Development

Raisa Jordan is a 3-year-old girl who has been diagnosed with bacterial conjunctivitis and prescribed antibiotic eye drops. Based on her developmental stage, how will you assist her caregivers to administer the eye drops? How would this assistance change if the child was 12 years old?

Nasolacrimal Duct Obstruction

Stenosis or simple obstruction of the nasolacrimal duct is a common congenital disorder of infancy, occurring in about 6% to 30% of newborns, infants, and young children (Isaza & Arora, 2013). It is unilateral in about 65% of cases. Chronic tearing occurs and build-up in the lacrimal sac causes a mucoid or mucopurulent drainage. Over 90% of all cases resolve spontaneously by 1 year of age. No apparent risk factors exist for the development of nasolacrimal duct obstruction or stenosis. Therapeutic management involves a watchful waiting approach. Massage may be prescribed, and if secondary bacterial infection is suspected or confirmed, antibiotic ointment or drops may be ordered. If the obstruction does not resolve by 12 months of age, then the pediatric ophthalmologist may probe the duct to relieve the obstruction (a brief outpatient procedure that over the age of 1 year does not need fluorescein irrigation) (Isaza & Arora, 2013).

Nursing Assessment

Tearing or discharge from one or both eyes is often first noted at the 2-week checkup. Obtain a thorough history about the eye drainage to distinguish it from neonatal conjunctivitis. Determine the onset and progression of symptoms, as well as the newborn's response to any interventions attempted so far. Upon physical examination, note redness of the lower lid of the affected eye. If drainage is present, note its consistency, colour, and quantity. Nasolacrimal duct obstruction is usually a diagnosis based on clinical presentation, but culture of the eye drainage may be used to rule out conjunctivitis or secondary bacterial infection (Fig. 39.5).

FIGURE 39.5 Mild eyelid redness and crusting are present in the infant with nasolacrimal duct stenosis.

Nursing Management

As previously stated, the majority of cases of nasolacrimal duct stenosis resolve spontaneously by 12 months of age (CAPOS, 2016). Nevertheless, the continual tearing and discharge is quite upsetting to the parents. Teach parents to clean the eye area frequently with a moist cloth. In addition, teach parents to massage the nasolacrimal duct, which may change the pressure and cause it to open, allowing drainage to occur. Refer to Teaching Guidelines 39.1 for appropriate nasolacrimal duct massage technique. Ensure that parents are educated about when and how to administer antibiotic eye drops if ordered.

 Teaching Guidelines 39.1
NASOLACRIMAL DUCT MASSAGE

- Using the forefinger or little finger, push on top of the bone (the puncta must be blocked).

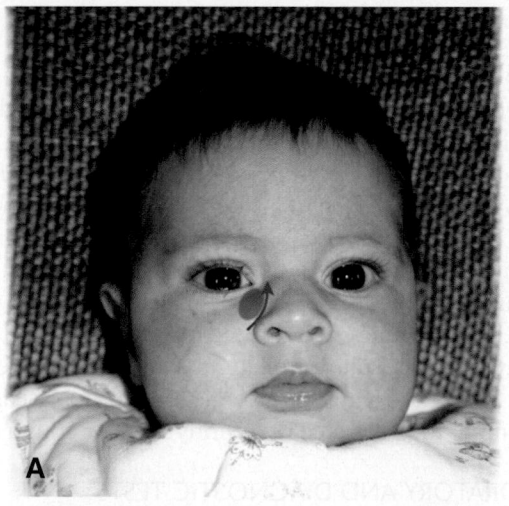

A

- Gently push in and up.

B

• Then, gently push downward along the side of the nose.

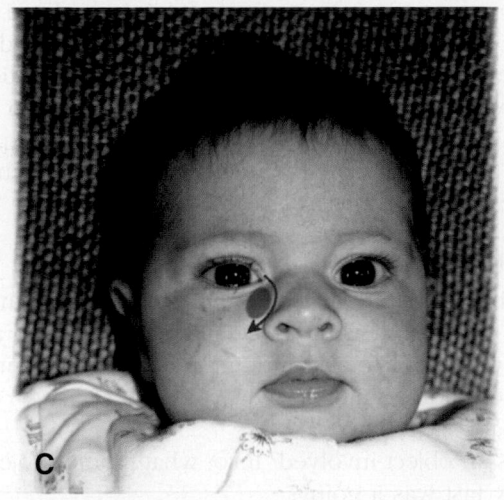

Eyelid Disorders

Disorders of the eyelid include hordeolum (stye, usually painful), chalazion, and blepharitis. Hordeolum is a localized infection of the sebaceous gland of the eyelid follicle, usually caused by bacterial invasion. Chalazion is a chronic painless infection of the meibomian (oil) gland resulting in a lump of swelling often on the eye lid. Blepharitis refers to chronic scaling and discharge along the eyelid margin. Chalazion may resolve spontaneously. Therapeutic management of hordeolum and blepharitis usually involves the use of antibiotic ointment.

Nursing Assessment

Determine the child's health history, noting onset of symptoms, extent and character of eye discharge, and presence of pain (hordeolum is usually painful). Inspect the eyelids, noting redness along the eyelid margin and presence of eyelid edema (hordeolum, blepharitis). Hordeolum may also be quite visible as an enlarged lesion along the lid margin, with purulent drainage present (Fig. 39.6). Chalazion may be visible as a small nodule

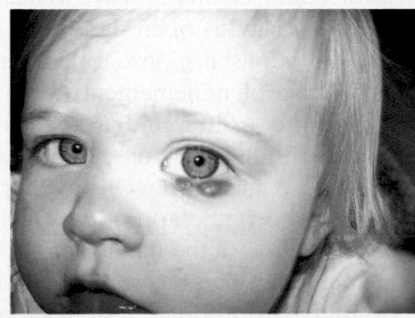

FIGURE 39.6 Hordeolum.

on the lid margin. The conjunctivae remain clear with all three of these disorders.

Nursing Management

For hordeolum and blepharitis, instruct parents how to administer antibiotic ointment. Encourage the use of warm, moist compresses. Inform parents that the stye may require several weeks to resolve completely. Also, inform parents that chalazion will usually resolve spontaneously; if it does not, it may require minor surgical drainage.

Periorbital Cellulitis

Periorbital cellulitis is a bacterial infection of the eyelids and tissue surrounding the eye. The bacteria may gain entry to the skin via an abrasion, laceration, insect bite, foreign body, or impetiginous lesion. Periorbital cellulitis may also result from a nearby bacterial infection, such as sinusitis. *S. aureus, Streptococcus pyogenes,* and *S. pneumoniae* are the most commonly implicated bacteria. The bacteria produce either an enzyme or endotoxins that initiate the inflammatory response. Redness, swelling, and infiltration of the skin by the inflammatory mediators occur.

Therapeutic management of periorbital cellulitis focuses on intravenous antibiotic administration during the acute phase followed by completion of the course with oral antibiotics. Complications of periorbital cellulitis include bacteremia and progression to orbital cellulitis, which is a more extensive infection involving the orbit of the eye.

Nursing Assessment

Note the onset and duration of symptoms, as well as any treatment used so far. Document any history of fever. The child may complain of pain around the eye as well as restricted movement of the eye area. Inspect the eye, noting marked eyelid edema as well as a purplish or red colour of the eyelid (Fig. 39.7). Usually, the conjunctivae are clear and no discharge is present. If the extent of the edema allows the child to open the eye, assess visual acuity, which should be normal.

> **Take Note!**
>
> Notify the physician or nurse practitioner immediately if any of these signs of progression to orbital cellulitis occur: conjunctival redness, change in vision, pain with eye movement, eye muscle weakness or paralysis, or proptosis.

Nursing Management

Apply warm soaks to the eye area for 20 minutes every 2 to 4 hours. Administer intravenous antibiotics as

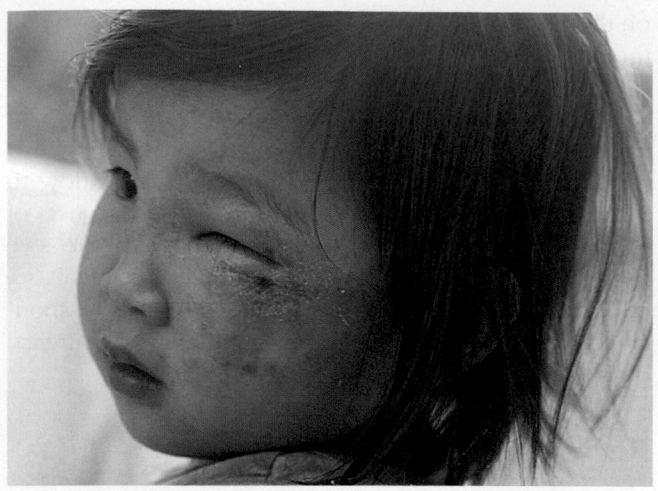

FIGURE 39.7 Periorbital cellulitis.

prescribed. Teach families the importance of completing the entire course of oral antibiotic treatment at home. Instruct parents to call the physician or nurse practitioner or have the child evaluated again if:

- The child is not improving.
- The child reports inability to move the eye.
- Visual acuity changes.
- Proptosis occurs.

EYE INJURIES

As mentioned earlier, infants and young children are more susceptible to eye injuries than adults since the eyeball is relatively larger in relation to the space within the orbit. Developmental maturity may also play a part in eye injuries. For example, as infants and toddlers learn to walk and run, they do not have the awareness and maturity to avert disaster. Older children involved in sports and school science experiments are also at risk for eye injuries. A few of the more common eye injuries are eyelid injuries, contusion, scleral hemorrhage, corneal abrasion, a foreign body in the eye, sports injuries, and chemical injury (Braverman, 2014).

Therapeutic management depends on the type of injury. Eyelid lacerations may require suturing. Deep lacerations may result in ptosis at a later date, so these children should be referred to an ophthalmologist. Simple contusions (black eye) usually need only observation, ice, and analgesics. Scleral hemorrhages resolve gradually without intervention over a few weeks. Corneal abrasions may be allowed to self-heal, or antibiotic ointment may be prescribed. Foreign bodies in the eye require removal to prevent further irritation or abrasion. Chemical injuries require irrigation and vision evaluation. Vision-threatening injuries are rare in Canadian children but require prompt assessment and management by specialist teams (Podbielski, Surkont, Tehrani, & Ratnapalan, 2009).

Nursing Assessment

When a child presents with an eye injury, it is very important to obtain an accurate history related to the injury. Follow the history by performing a focused physical examination, which consists mostly of inspection and observation. It is important to determine whether an eye injury is nonemergent or emergent in order to provide rapid and appropriate treatment in the case of an emergency so that vision may be preserved.

HEALTH HISTORY

Obtain an accurate history. Determine the mechanism of injury and obtain as much detail about the injury as possible. Questions to ask during the health history include:

- When did the injury occur?
- What exactly happened?
- Was an object involved? If so, what type of object, and how fast was it going?
- Was it a splash injury?
- Was the child wearing eye protective gear or eyeglasses when the injury occurred?

Determine the extent of pain. Document photosensitivity, sensation of a foreign body in the eye, blurry vision, and changes to or loss of vision. Inquire about past medical history, including previous eye injury or surgery or vision problems. Determine the child's immunization status.

PHYSICAL EXAMINATION

Regardless of the type of eye injury, the examination of the child's eye can be quite difficult. The nurse plays an important role in assisting the child and family to cope with the examination. Children with an eye injury often are in acute pain. The area surrounding the eye swells quickly after blunt trauma. Edema and tearing make the eye examination more difficult. Children are very frightened because of the pain and difficulty seeing. Approach the child in a calm and gentle manner. Support the child emotionally as the eye is examined. Younger children may need to be held firmly by a parent or caregiver briefly in order for the examination to proceed safely. Consider the need for sedation as necessary in order to minimize traumatic care.

Note the eyelid placement and look for signs of trauma such as bleeding, edema, and eyelid malformation. Evaluate the child's ability to open the eyes. Use a penlight to evaluate the pupils' response to light and accommodation (in the case of nonemergent eye trauma, the pupils should remain equally round and reactive to light and accommodation [PERRLA]). Note redness or irritation of the sclerae and/or conjunctivae. Observe for excessive tearing. Figure 39.8 shows the appropriate technique for eversion and examination of the interior of the eyelid.

In a nonemergent situation, evaluate visual acuity via the use of an age-appropriate vision-screening tool. Generally, radiologic testing is used only in emergency

FIGURE 39.8 Eversion of the eyelid for examination. Place a cotton-tipped applicator over the eyelid. Pull the eyelid outward and up over the applicator.

Twist cotton-tipped swab upward

Look downward

situations (Augsburger & Correa, 2011). Table 39.2 provides assessment information specific to eyelid laceration, simple contusion, scleral hemorrhage, corneal abrasion, and foreign body in the eye.

Take Note!

If pupillary reaction is abnormal, vision is affected (decreased acuity from the child's norm, diplopia, or blurriness), or extraocular movements are affected, the child should be immediately referred to an ophthalmologist for further evaluation (Braverman, 2014).

Nursing Management

Children with urgent or emergent conditions must be referred to an ophthalmologist immediately to preserve vision. Urgent and emergent conditions include:

- Traumatic hyphema
- Blowout fracture
- Ruptured globe
- Thermal/chemical injury
- Extensive animal bite
- Lid laceration with underlying structural involvement
- Corneal abrasion in which corneal penetration is suspected
- Foreign body embedded in the globe (Augsburger & Correa, 2011; Braverman, 2014)

MANAGING NONEMERGENT EYE INJURIES

Nonemergent eye injuries usually need only simple management. Assist the physician or nurse practitioner with positioning and distraction of the child for eyelid laceration suturing. The child will require sedation and pain medication for this procedure.

TABLE 39.2	ASSESSMENT OF EYE INJURIES
Description of Injury	**Nursing Assessment**
Eyelid Injuries: May occur as laceration to the eyelid	• Laceration is noted at any point along the lid • Vision is unaffected
Simple Contusion (Black Eye): Occurs as a result of blunt trauma to the eye area	• Bruising and edema of lids or area surrounding eye • PERRLA • Extraocular movements intact • Visual acuity intact • No diplopia or blurred vision • Pain surrounding eye but not within the eye
Scleral Hemorrhage: Caused by blunt trauma or increased pressure such as with coughing	• Painless • Appears as erythema in the sclera; can be quite large initially • Vision unaffected
Corneal Abrasion: Results from foreign body such as sand, grit, or other small object scratching the cornea	• May have tearing • Eye pain • PERRLA • Vision may be blurry • Photophobia may be present
Foreign Body: May be dirt, glass, or other small particle	• Tearing • Complaint of "something in the eye" • PERRLA • Vision may be blurry

Adapted from Augsburger, J. J., & Correa, C. M. (2011). Ophthalmic trauma. In P. Riordan-Eva, & E. T. Cunningham (Eds.). *Vaughan & Asbury's general ophthalmology* (18th ed.). New York: McGraw-Hill; and Braverman, R. S. (2014). Eye. In W. W. Hay, M. J. Levin, R. R. Deterding, & M. J. Abzug (Eds.). *Current pediatric diagnosis and treatment* (22nd ed.). New York: McGraw-Hill.

EVIDENCE-BASED PRACTICE 39.1

THE EFFECT OF PATCHING FOR CORNEAL ABRASION ON HEALING AND DECREASED PAIN

STUDY

Simple corneal abrasions are a common eye complaint. Eye patching with or without antibiotic ointment has often been used despite a lack of evidence for its use. In addition, patches are difficult to keep on young children and may be associated with corneal erosion. The authors included quasi-randomized and randomized studies evaluating patching versus no patching for treatment of simple corneal abrasion. Eleven trials with a total of 1,014 participants were included in the review.

Findings

The authors found that patching for simple corneal abrasions did not improve healing on day 1, nor did it decrease

the amount of pain experienced. In addition, binocular vision is lost when one eye is patched. Based on these results, it is not recommended that patching be used for treatment of simple corneal abrasions.

Nursing Implications

Parents worry significantly when their child experiences even a very mild eye injury. Teach parents about the ability of the cornea to heal quickly from a minor abrasion. Emphasize that nonpatched corneal abrasions have been shown to heal more rapidly than those that are patched.

Adapted from Turner, A., & Rabiu, M. (2007). Patching for corneal abrasion. *The Cochrane Library.* doi: 10.1002/14651858.CD004764.pub2

To decrease edema in the child with a black eye (simple contusion), instruct the parent to apply an ice pack to the area for 20 minutes, then remove it for 20 minutes, and continue to repeat the cycle as often as possible during the first 24 hours. Tell the parents and child that bruising of the surrounding eye area may take up to 3 weeks to resolve.

The appearance of a scleral hemorrhage may be frightening. Instruct the parents and child about the benign nature of the hemorrhage and its natural history of resolution without intervention over a period of a few weeks.

If the child with a corneal abrasion has pain, analgesics may be helpful. Tell parents that most corneal abrasions heal on their own. If an antibiotic ointment is prescribed, instruct the parents how to administer the ointment appropriately.

> **Take Note!**
>
> Patching of the eye with a small, uncomplicated corneal abrasion or abrasion from a contact lens is not recommended. Patching does not result in decreased pain nor promote faster healing. In addition, it may place the child at risk for injury due to visual field loss while patched (Jacobs, 2015).

Foreign bodies may be removed from the eye by gently everting the eyelid and wiping the foreign body away with a sterile cotton-tipped applicator. Irrigation with normal saline may also wash the foreign body away.

For chemical injury, irrigate the eye with copious amounts of water. Consult ophthalmology for further evaluation and management.

> **Take Note!**
>
> Refer the child with a large foreign body in the eye or one that is embedded in the globe of the eye to the ophthalmologist for appropriate, safe removal.

Eye injuries can be prevented, and nurses play a vital role in educating the public about prevention of eye injuries and use of appropriate safety equipment. See Evidence-Based Practice 39.1.

VISUAL DISORDERS

Adequate visual development requires appropriate sensory stimulation to both eyes over the first few years of life (Bremond-Gignac et al., 2011). When one or both eyes are deprived of this stimulation, visual development does not progress appropriately, and visual impairment or **blindness** may result. This may occur when the eyes are not aligned properly, visual acuity between the eyes is disparate, or other problems with the eyes exist (Bremond-Gignac et al., 2011). If vision disorders are diagnosed at an early age and treatment is begun, then vision may progress normally. However, when these disorders go untreated, the young child's developing vision may be reduced significantly. Therefore, it is important to appropriately screen children for these disorders.

Common visual disorders in childhood include refractive errors, astigmatism, strabismus, amblyopia, nystagmus, glaucoma, and cataracts.

Refractive Errors

The most common cause of visual difficulties in children is refractive errors. When the light that enters the lens does not bend appropriately to allow it to fall directly on the retina, then a refractive error occurs. Young children naturally have hyperopia (farsightedness) because the depth of the eye globe is not fully developed until about 5 years of age (Braverman, 2014). These children may have blurriness at close range, but by school age this blurriness usually resolves.

When the light entering the eye focuses in front of the retina, it results in myopia (nearsightedness). Children who are nearsighted may see well at close range but have difficulty focusing on the blackboard or other objects at a distance.

Therapeutic management for both hyperopia and myopia is prescription eyeglasses or contact lenses. Generally, a child of 12 years of age can demonstrate the responsibility necessary to wear and care for contact lenses. Contact lenses may be used in younger children but are lost or damaged more readily. Because of the continuing refractive development in the child's vision through adolescence, laser surgery for vision correction is not recommended until 18 to 21 years of age, though it may be done experimentally in some children (Lusby & Zieve, 2016).

Nursing Assessment

Elicit the health history, noting blurred vision, complaints of eye fatigue with reading, or complaints of eye strain (headache, pulling sensation, or eye burning). Note complaints of difficulty concentrating on or maintaining a clear focus on objects up close, avoidance of up-close work, or poor work performance (hyperopia). Note the risk factor of family history of myopia. Observe for squinting when the child looks at objects at a distance. Observe the hyperopic child for the presence of esotropia. Readily observable physical findings are not noted in the myopic child. Hyperopia is usually not identified with visual acuity screening alone; it usually requires a retinal examination by an ophthalmologist.

Nursing Management

Nursing management of the child with a refractive error focuses on providing education about corrective lens use and monitoring for the need for new eyeglasses or contact lenses.

EDUCATING ABOUT EYEGLASS USE

Children may or may not be compliant with wearing eyeglasses. Glasses may carry a stigma, and the child may be teased or bullied. However, many children enjoy the improved vision they achieve when wearing their eyeglasses and this can help them overcome the teasing they might suffer. Encourage the child with newly prescribed eyeglasses to wear them by having the parent spend "special time" with the child doing an activity that

requires the glasses (such as reading or drawing). Teach the parent and child to remove eyeglasses with both hands and to lay them on their side (not directly on the lens on any surface). Instruct the child and family about cleaning the glasses daily with mild soap and water or a commercial cleansing agent provided by the optometrist. Use a soft cloth to clean the glasses, not paper towels, tissues, or toilet paper.

Consider This

I can't believe I have to start wearing glasses! I have heard the other kids mock my classmates and call them 4-eyes. I'm old enough now to start wearing makeup and how will that look with glasses? I'll look like a nerd . . .

Thoughts: *How will you respond to her worries? With this preteen girl, what will your approach be to insure she wears her glasses as prescribed?*

EDUCATING ABOUT CONTACT LENS USE

Teach the older child or adolescent how to care for the contact lenses properly, including lens hygiene and lens insertion and removal. Inform the child and parents that protective eyewear should be worn when the child is participating in contact sports. If the eye becomes inflamed, remove the contact lens and wear eyeglasses until the eye is improved. Consult with the child's eye care provider to determine if medications prescribed for an eye problem can be used while the contact lens is in.

MONITORING FOR FIT AND VISUAL CORRECTION

Encourage the family to complete visual assessments as scheduled. Since the child's vision is continuing to develop and refraction is not stable, the corrective lens prescription may change more frequently than it does in an adult. As the young child in particular is continuing to grow at a rapid rate, the head size is also changing. Eyeglass frames may hurt or pinch the child as the child's head becomes larger. Teach families to check the fit of the glasses monthly. Monitor for signs of ill-fit, such as constant removal of the glasses in an older child or rubbing at the glasses or eyes in the very young child. Monitor for squinting, eye fatigue or strain, and complaints of headache or dizziness, which may indicate the need for a change in the lens prescription.

Astigmatism

In astigmatism, the cornea's curvature is uneven, which results in an irregular quality of vision because the light rays are refracted unevenly. Sometimes, the lens is irregularly shaped, having the same result.

Nursing Assessment

Explore the health history for symptoms of astigmatism. Children with astigmatism often have blurry vision and difficulty seeing letters as a whole, so their ability to read is affected. They may have headaches or dizziness. Older children may complain of eye fatigue or strain. Children with astigmatism often learn to tilt their heads slightly so that they can focus more effectively. This may lead to "normal" vision screenings, but the headache and dizziness still warrant further examination by an eye specialist (Braverman, 2014). The diagnosis of astigmatism requires not only a visual acuity test but also a refractive error evaluation by an optometrist or ophthalmologist.

Nursing Management

Corrective lenses can help to, in effect, smooth out the curvature of the cornea, making the light ray refraction occur smoothly. As with refractive errors, encourage the child who requires corrective lenses for astigmatism to wear the eyeglasses or contact lenses regularly.

Strabismus

Strabismus refers to misalignment of the eyes. It is common and occurs in up to 4% of the population (Coats & Paysse, 2016). The most common types of strabismus are exotropia and esotropia. In exotropia, the eyes turn outward; in esotropia, they turn inward (cross eye). Because of this unequal alignment, visual development in each eye may proceed at different rates. Diplopia (double vision) may result, so vision in one eye may be "turned off" by the brain to avoid diplopia. Many infants have strabismus intermittently, but this usually resolves by 3 to 6 months of age. Persistent esotropia that persists past 4 months of age or constant strabismus at any age warrants referral to an ophthalmologist for further evaluation (Coats & Paysse, 2016).

Therapeutic management of strabismus may include patching of the stronger eye or eye muscle surgery. Corrective lenses are also used for strabismus. Complications of strabismus include amblyopia and visual deficits.

Nursing Assessment

Parents may be the first persons to notice that the child's eyes do not face in the same direction. Question parents about the onset of the problem and whether it is continuous or intermittent. If intermittent, does it occur more often when the child is tired? Elicit the health history, noting complaints of blurred vision, tired eyes, squinting or closing one eye in bright sunlight, tilting the head to focus on an object, or a history of bumping into objects (depth perception may be limited).

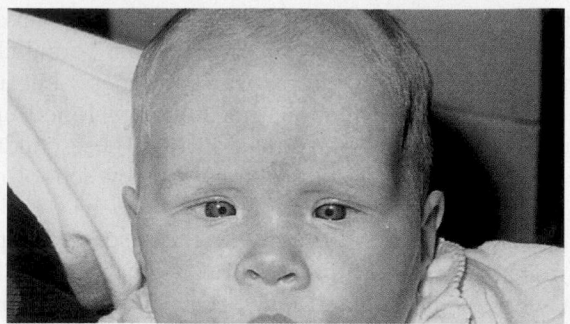

FIGURE 39.9 Esotropia. Test for strabismus by observing symmetry of the corneal light reflex. The reflex falls to the left of one pupil and to the right of the other.

Observe the child's eyes for obvious exotropia or esotropia. In the absence of an obvious finding, assessment of the symmetry of the corneal light reflex is extremely helpful (Fig. 39.9). The "cover test" is also a useful tool for the identification of strabismus.

True strabismus should not be confused with pseudostrabismus. In pseudostrabismus, the eyes may appear slightly crossed (as in the child with a wide nasal bridge and epicanthal folds), but the corneal light reflex remains symmetric (Weber & Kelley, 2014).

Nursing Management

It is extremely important to treat strabismus appropriately in the developing years so that equal visual acuity may be achieved in both eyes. When patching is prescribed, encourage the family to comply with this modality. Encourage eyeglass wearing if prescribed. Provide appropriate postoperative care by protecting the operative site with eye patching.

Amblyopia

Amblyopia refers to poor visual development in the otherwise structurally normal eye. It develops within the first decade of life and, if left untreated, it is the most common cause of vision loss in children and young adults (Coats & Paysse, 2016). Amblyopia occurs in about 1% to 4% of children (Coats & Paysse, 2016). The vision in one eye is reduced because the eye and the brain are not working together properly. While the eyes are fighting to focus differently because of their differences in visual acuity, one eye is stronger than the other. This is why amblyopia is often referred to as "lazy eye."

Amblyopia may be caused by any disorder that affects normal visual development, including strabismus and differences in visual acuity or astigmatism between the two eyes. It may also result from eye trauma, ptosis, or cataract. If untreated, children with amblyopia will have worsening acuity of the poorer eye and strain in the better eye, which may also lead to worsening of acuity in that eye. Eventually, blindness will result in one or both eyes.

Therapeutic management of amblyopia focuses on strengthening the weaker eye. This may be achieved through patching for several hours per day, using atropine drops in the better eye (once daily), vision therapy, or eye muscle surgery if the cause is strabismus.

Nursing Assessment

One of the most important functions of the nurse is to identify on screening the preschool child with amblyopia. Begin visual acuity testing using an age-appropriate tool by 3 years of age. Observe for asymmetry of the corneal light reflex in the child of any age. This may be the only sign in the preverbal child.

Nursing Management

It is very important for children with amblyopia to receive appropriate treatment during the early years of visual development. Patching the better eye for several hours each day encourages the eye with poorer vision to be used appropriately and promotes visual development in that eye. The once-daily use of atropine drops in the better eye results in blurring in that eye, similarly encouraging use and development of the weaker eye (Coats & Paysse, 2016). Support and encourage children and parents to comply with the patching protocol or atropine drop use.

Promoting eye safety is extremely important for the child with amblyopia; if the better eye suffers a serious injury, both eyes may become blind.

Nystagmus

Nystagmus refers to a very rapid, irregular eye movement. It is described by some as "bouncing" of the eyes. It may occur in children with congenital cataracts, but the most common cause is a neurologic problem. It is difficult for the brain and eyes to communicate when the eyes are in continuous motion; thus, visual development may be affected. Children with nystagmus must receive further evaluation by an ophthalmologist and possibly a neurologist.

Infantile Glaucoma

Infantile glaucoma is an autosomal recessive disorder that is more common in interrelated marriages or relationships. It is often associated with other genetic disorders. It occurs in about 1 of 10,000 live births (Yeung & Walton, 2012). Infantile glaucoma is characterized by obstruction of aqueous humor flow and increased intraocular pressure that results in large, prominent eyes. Vision loss may occur as a result of corneal scarring, optic nerve damage, or, most commonly, amblyopia.

Unlike adult glaucoma, in which medical management is the first step, therapeutic management of infantile glaucoma is focused on surgical intervention. Infantile glaucoma is treated surgically via goniotomy (removal of obstruction of the aqueous humor). Laser surgery is being used as well. Sometimes, several surgeries may be necessary to correct the problem. Ongoing medication therapy may also be required.

Nursing Assessment

Note any family history of infantile glaucoma or other genetic disorders. Elicit the health history, noting history of the infant keeping the eyes closed most of the time or rubbing the eyes. Observe the eye for corneal enlargement and clouding; the eye may appear enlarged. Photophobia may occur, so bright light may bother the infant. Tearing or conjunctivitis and eyelid squeezing or spasm may also occur. The pediatric ophthalmologist may use a tonometer to measure the intraocular pressure during the diagnostic phase.

Nursing Management

The main goal of nursing care for the infant with glaucoma is postoperative care. Family education will also be important.

Providing Postoperative Care

Postoperatively, the eye will be patched and the child should be maintained on bed rest. Nursing care focuses on protection of the surgical site. Infants and toddlers may require elbow restraints to prevent them from bending their elbows to rub the affected eye. These children may be quite anxious with one or both eyes patched, since their ability to see will be affected. Use a calm and soothing approach with these children, as well as distraction and developmentally appropriate play activities.

EDUCATING THE FAMILY

Instruct parents and children to make sure the child avoids rough play and contact sports for at least 2 weeks after surgery. Before the first surgery occurs, prepare parents for the possibility that three or four operations may be necessary. Teach families how to administer postoperative medications. Encourage parents to comply with ongoing recommended visual assessments.

Congenital Cataract

A congenital cataract is an opacity of the lens of the eye that is present at birth. Sensory amblyopia will result if the infant goes untreated. Complications include visual developmental delay related to amblyopia. In children younger than 5 years of age, congenital cataract causes more than 10% of the cases of legal blindness (International Council of Ophthalmology [ICP], 2016). Bilateral cataracts may be associated with metabolic or genetic syndromes. Surgery to remove the opaque lens can be done as early as 2 weeks of age. The infant is then fitted with a contact lens. Intraocular lens implants are also being used (Lin & Buckley, 2010). The best visual outcomes occur when cataracts are removed prior to 3 months of age. Glaucoma may occur as a complication after cataract surgery.

Nursing Assessment

Note history of lack of visual awareness. Observe the eyes for apparent cloudiness of the cornea (not always visible). Upon ophthalmoscopic examination, the red reflex will not be observed in the affected eye.

Nursing Management

Postoperative care focuses on protecting the operative site and providing developmentally appropriate activities. Ensure that the protective eye patch is secure. Elbow restraints may be necessary in the older infant to prevent accidental injury to the operative site. Teach families how to administer antibiotic or corticosteroid ophthalmic drops if prescribed for postoperative use. Once the surgical site is healed, the healthy eye may be patched for several hours a day to promote visual development in the eye with the contact or intraocular lens. Regular visual assessments are critical for determining the adequacy of visual development after cataract removal. Instruct parents about the importance of using sunglasses that block ultraviolet rays in the child who has had a lens removed.

Retinopathy of Prematurity

Retinopathy of prematurity (ROP) is a disorder characterized by rapid growth of retinal blood vessels in the premature infant. In the fetus, retinal vascularization begins at 4 months and progresses until completion at 9 months or shortly after birth. The premature infant is born with incomplete retinal vascularization, yet new vessels continue to grow between the vascularized and nonvascularized retina. Risk factors include low birthweight, early gestational age, sepsis, high light intensity, and hypothermia. Changes in oxygen tension resulting from hypoxia, oxyhemoglobin dissociation curve changes that occur when adult blood is transfused to the premature infant, and the duration/concentration of supplemental oxygen are thought to play an important role in the development of ROP.

Premature infants should have serial examinations by an ophthalmologist until the ROP has regressed and normal vascularization is seen. If ROP continues to progress, laser surgery may be necessary to prevent blindness. Complications of ROP include myopia, glaucoma,

and blindness. Strabismus may occur even in cases of regressed (resolved) ROP. Refractive errors and amblyopia may occur as early as 3 months corrected age. In the first year of life, ophthalmologic examinations should occur frequently so that if corrective lenses are needed, they may be prescribed at the earliest possible time. After 1-year corrected age, former premature infants should continue to have yearly ophthalmologic examinations to detect and treat visual deficits early (CAO, n.d.).

Nursing Assessment

Ensure that all former premature infants are routinely screened for visual deficits. Discuss developmental progress with the parents. Observe for the development of strabismus, manifested by an asymmetric corneal light reflex.

Nursing Management

Nursing management of infants with ROP mainly focuses on ensuring that the family is compliant with the ophthalmologist's follow-up recommendations. Recurrent illness or rehospitalization of premature infants may interfere with scheduled eye follow-up appointments. Ensure that these appointments are rescheduled and that the family understands the importance of them. Many children who have regressed ROP or who require cryotherapy have refractive errors, so even when the ROP is considered resolved, these children should still maintain appropriate ophthalmology follow-up.

Visual Impairment

Vision impairment in children refers to acuity between 20/60 and 20/200 in the better eye on examination. "Legal blindness" is a term used to refer to vision of less than 20/200 or peripheral vision less than 20 degrees. In most cases, vision may be augmented with corrective lenses. Some blind children can differentiate light versus dark, while others live in total darkness.

Visual impairment in children may result from a number of different causes. In the United States and likely Canada, visual impairment and blindness are most often caused by refractive error, astigmatism, strabismus, amblyopia, nystagmus, infantile glaucoma, congenital cataract, ROP, and retinoblastoma (ICP, 2016). Factors that increase the risk for developing visual impairment include prematurity, developmental delay, genetic syndrome, family history of eye disease, African-American heritage, previous serious eye injury, diabetes, HIV, and chronic corticosteroid use. Trauma is also an important cause of blindness in children. Visual impairments may also be associated with genetic syndromes.

Children with visual impairments often exhibit motor and cognitive delays as well (Carter, 2015). With one less sense with which to experience their environment, these children may lag behind in developmental milestones.

Take Note!

Laser pointers pose a risk of retinal damage in infants and young children. Damage occurs if the child stares at the red light for longer than 10 seconds. They should not be used as toys (Xu et al., 2016).

Nursing Assessment

Nursing assessment for visual impairment includes a careful health history, physical examination, and visual acuity testing.

HEALTH HISTORY
Parents and nurses alike should be alert to signs of potential visual impairment. One of the most important functions of the nurse is to recognize signs of visual impairment as early as possible. These signs may include:
- At any age:
  - Dull, vacant stare
- Infants:
  - Do not "fix and follow"
  - Do not make eye contact
  - Unaffected by bright light
  - Do not imitate facial expression
- Toddlers and older children:
  - Rub, shut, and cover eyes
  - Squinting
  - Frequent blinking
  - Hold objects close or sit close to television
  - Bumping into objects
  - Head tilt or forward thrust

PHYSICAL EXAMINATION
Assess for symmetry or asymmetry of the corneal light reflex. Perform the "cover test." Use an age-appropriate visual acuity screening tool (refer to Chapter 31 for additional information on visual acuity screening).

Nursing Management

Important nursing functions in relation to visual impairment and blindness are supporting the child and family and promoting socialization, development, and education. In addition, when the child with a visual impairment is hospitalized for any reason, the nurse must plan appropriate care for that child, taking into consideration the child's level of disability. Box 39.1 provides tips on working with the visually impaired child. It is important to teach these tips to families.

SUPPORTING THE CHILD AND FAMILY
Provide emotional support to the family with a visually impaired child. Ensure that the child's environment

---

BOX 39.1

TIPS FOR INTERACTING WITH THE VISUALLY IMPAIRED CHILD
- Use the child's name to gain attention.
- Identify yourself and let the child know you are there before you touch the child.
- Encourage the child to be independent while maintaining safety.
- Name and describe people/objects to make the child more aware of what is happening.
- Discuss upcoming activities with the child.
- Explain what other children or individuals are doing.
- Make directions simple and specific.
- Allow the child additional time to think about the response to a question or statement.
- Use touch and tone of voice appropriate to the situation.
- Use parts of the child's body as reference points for the location of items.
- Encourage exploration of objects through touch.
- Describe unfamiliar environments and provide reference points.
- Use the sighted-guide technique when walking with a visually impaired child.

Adapted from Delta Gamma Center for Children with Visual Impairments. (2011). *Interacting with visually impaired.* Retrieved from http://dgckids.org/resources/interacting-with-visually-impaired/

---

provides familiarity and security. Encourage activities that stimulate development; these activities will vary from child to child depending on whether the child also demonstrates impairment in other areas, such as hearing or motor skills. The blind infant will not provide the eye contact that parents are looking for, so educate the parents about other indicators that the infant is acknowledging the parents' presence, such as:
- Increased motor activity
- Eyelid movement
- Changes in breathing pattern
- Making sounds

Encourage the family of a visually impaired child to display affection through touch and tone of voice. Refer families to support networks and other resources for the blind and visually impaired such as CNIB (www.cnib.ca). Several online resources for families of children who are visually impaired or blind can be found on thePoint.

PROMOTING SOCIALIZATION, DEVELOPMENT, AND EDUCATION
Blind children, since they lack the visual stimulation that children usually receive, may develop self-stimulatory actions in compensation, often called blindisms. Examples of blindisms are eye pressing, rocking, spinning, bouncing, and head banging. These repetitive behaviours may indicate an effort to communicate or alternatively they may interfere with the child's ability to socialize (Hammer, n.d.).

Work with the parents to determine whether a strategy for the development of alternative behaviours specific to the individual child would be helpful.

Refer the blind or visually impaired child to the local child development centre or early childhood program to establish case management services for the child's developmental needs. An individualized education plan (IEP) should be developed to maximize the child's learning ability. Nurses may be one of the professionals involved in the development of the IEP.

The severely visually impaired or blind child will need to learn to read Braille and will also need to learn to navigate the environment with the use of a cane or via another method.

INFECTIOUS AND INFLAMMATORY DISORDERS OF THE EARS

Infectious and inflammatory disorders of the ears include otitis externa and types of otitis media. Otitis media is defined as inflammation of the middle ear with the presence of fluid. It can be subdivided into two categories: AOM and otitis media with effusion (OME). AOM refers to an acute infectious process of the middle ear that may produce a rapid onset of ear pain and possibly fever. OME refers to a collection of fluid in the middle ear space without signs and symptoms of infection. Chronic OME is defined as OME lasting longer than 3 months. Otitis externa refers to inflammation of the external ear canal.

Acute Otitis Media

AOM is a common illness in children, resulting from infection (bacterial or viral) of fluid in the middle ear. Increased susceptibility in infants and young children may be partly explained by the short length and horizontal positioning of the Eustachian tube, limited response to antigens, and lack of previous exposure to common pathogens (Friedman et al., 2014). AOM occurs mostly in the fall through spring, with the highest incidence in the winter. AOM often recurs in infants and young children when the fluid in the middle ear becomes reinfected. The most significant risk factors for otitis media are Eustachian tube dysfunction and susceptibility to recurrent upper respiratory infections.

Pathophysiology

An upper respiratory infection frequently precedes AOM. Fluid and pathogens travel upward from the nasopharyngeal area, invading the middle ear space. Fluid behind the eardrum has difficulty draining back out toward the nasopharyngeal area because of the horizontal positioning of the Eustachian tube. A viral upper respiratory infection may cause AOM or may place the child at risk for bacterial invasion. Pathogens gain access to

the Eustachian tube, where they proliferate and invade the mucosa. Fever and pain occur acutely. Increased pressure behind the tympanic membrane may result in perforation. This may result in decreased pain and yield drainage in the ear canal. Most perforations heal spontaneously and are completely benign.

AOM is most commonly caused by viral pathogens, *S. pneumoniae, Haemophilus influenzae,* and *Moraxella catarrhalis.* Viral causes of AOM resolve spontaneously.

After clearance of the infection, fluid remains in the middle ear space behind the tympanic membrane, sometimes for several months (OME). This may occur because of the positioning of the Eustachian tubes, resulting in difficulty in draining fluid back to the nasopharyngeal area. OME may also occur because of the high frequency of upper respiratory infections in infants and young children, which again result in back-up of fluid from the nasopharyngeal area.

The most common complications of AOM include:
- Hearing loss
- Expressive speech delay
- Tympanosclerosis (scarring of the tympanic membrane; usually has no effect on hearing)
- Tympanic membrane perforation (acute with resolution or chronic)
- Chronic suppurative otitis media (chronic drainage via perforation or **tympanostomy** tubes)
- Acute mastoiditis (infection of the mastoid process)
- Intracranial infections, including bacterial meningitis and abscesses

Therapeutic Management

Viral causes of AOM usually resolve spontaneously, but bacterial causes may require treatment with an antibiotic. It is unreasonable to obtain a culture of middle ear fluid with every episode of AOM to determine the specific cause. Scientific studies of fluid obtained via tympanostomy in children with AOM have been performed, and clinical decision-making is based on this research. Antibiotic resistance develops due to the overuse of antibiotics (CPS, 2016c). For this reason, clinical practice guidelines have been developed for a number of disorders based on large quantities of research.

Certain diagnosis of AOM is based on:
- Signs of middle ear fluid: moderate to severe bulging of the tympanic membrane, or mild bulging of the tympanic membrane,
  AND
- Acute onset of symptoms (otalgia or suspected otalgia).
  AND
- Signs or symptoms of inflammation in the middle ear: complaint of ear pain or intense erythema of the tympanic membrane
  OR
- Perforated tympanic membrane with purulent drainage (CPS, 2016c).

The choice of antibiotic will depend on the timing, the child's age, and whether the episode is a first or subsequent infection. The current recommendations by the CPS allow for a period of observation or watchful waiting in certain children. This allows for natural resolution of AOM related to viral causes and decreases the overuse of antibiotics in the pediatric population (CPS, 2016c; see Dosage Calculation Box 39.1).

Dosage Calculation Box 39.1

Child's weight: 5.5 kg (12 lb, 4 oz)
Medication order: cefuroxime 100 mg PO twice a day.
Per the *Pediatric Dosage Handbook*, the recommended dose is 20 to 30 mg/kg/day in two divided doses.
Is the ordered dose safe?

Recommendations for AOM treatment in previously healthy children are found in Table 39.3. Pain management is also an important component of AOM treatment, as is appropriate follow-up to ensure disease resolution.

Nursing Assessment

Nursing assessment of the child with AOM consists of health history and physical examination.

HEALTH HISTORY

Elicit a description of the present illness and chief complaint. Note acute, abrupt onset of signs and symptoms. Common signs and symptoms reported during the health history might include:
- Fever (may be low grade or higher)
- Complaints of otalgia (ear pain)

- Fussiness or irritability
- Crying inconsolably, particularly when lying down
- Batting or tugging at the ears (may also occur with teething or OME, or may be a habit)
- Rolling the head from side to side
- Poor feeding or loss of appetite
- Lethargy
- Difficulty sleeping or awakening crying in the night
- Fluid draining from the ear

Determine the child's response to any treatments used thus far. Explore the child's current and past medical history for risk factors such as:
- Young age
- Day care attendance
- Previous history of AOM or OME
- Antecedent or concurrent upper respiratory infection
- Other risk factors (Box 39.2)

Take Note!

Assessment of Otitis Media

Assessment findings in a child with AOM are typically a recent upper respiratory infection fever, loss of appetite, and a dull, opaque, bulging, or red tympanic membrane.

PHYSICAL EXAMINATION AND DIAGNOSTIC TESTING

The child may complain of pain when the ear is examined. On otoscopic examination, the tympanic membrane will have a dull or opaque appearance and is bulging and/or red (Fig. 39.10). Sometimes, pus (greenish or yellowish) may be visible behind the eardrum. Upon pneumatic otoscopy, the eardrum will be immobile. (A physician or nurse practitioner usually performs

TABLE 39.3	TREATMENT RECOMMENDATIONS FOR ACUTE OTITIS MEDIA			
Age	Unilateral or Bilateral AOM?	Severe Signs and Symptoms?[a]	Otorrhea Present?	Treatment
6 months–2 years	Either		Yes	Antibiotics
6 months–2 years	Either	Yes		Antibiotics
6 months–2 years	Bilateral	No	No	Antibiotics
6 months–2 years	Unilateral	No	No	Antibiotics or observation[b]
>2 years	Either		Yes	Antibiotics
>2 years	Either	Yes		Antibiotics
>2 years	Bilateral	No	No	Antibiotics or observation[b]
>2 years	Unilateral	No	No	Antibiotics or observation[b]

[a]Severe illness is defined as temperature 39°C (102.2°F) or higher or moderate to severe otalgia or otalgia for at least 48 hours. Nonsevere illness is defined as mild otalgia for less than 48 hours and fever less than 39°C (102.2°F).

[b]Observation is appropriate when follow-up can be ensured in order that antibiotic therapy may begin if the child fails to improve or worsens within 24–48 hours.

Adapted from CPS. (2016c). *Management of acute otitis media in children 6 months of age and older*. Retrieved from http://www.cps.ca/documents/position/acute-otitis-media

BOX 39.2

RISK FACTORS FOR ACUTE OTITIS MEDIA

- Eustachian tube dysfunction
- Recurrent upper respiratory infection
- First episode of acute otitis media (AOM) before 3 months of age
- Day care attendance (increases exposure to viruses causing upper respiratory infections)
- Previous episodes of AOM
- Family history
- Passive smoking
- Crowding in the home or large family size
- Aboriginal, Inuit, or Australian aborigine ethnicity
- Absence of infant breastfeeding
- Immunocompromise
- Poor nutrition
- Craniofacial anomalies
- Presence of allergies (possibly)

Adapted from American Academy of Pediatrics. (2013a). Clinical practice guideline: The diagnosis and management of acute otitis media. *Pediatrics*, *131*, e964–e999 and Friedman, N. R., Scholes, M. A., & Yoon, P. J. (2014). Ear, nose, & throat. In W. W. Hay, M. J. Levin, R. R. Deterding, & M. J. Abzug (Eds.). *Current pediatric diagnosis and treatment* (22nd ed.). New York: McGraw-Hill.

the otoscopic examination.) If the tympanic membrane has become perforated, drainage may be present in the ear canal, but the canal will otherwise appear normal. Palpate for possible cervical lymphadenopathy. **Tympanometry** is used to determine the presence of middle ear effusion.

Nursing Management

Nursing management of the child with AOM is mainly supportive in nature. It focuses on pain management, family education, and prevention of AOM.

MANAGING PAIN ASSOCIATED WITH ACUTE OTITIS MEDIA

Analgesics such as acetaminophen and ibuprofen have been shown to be effective at managing mild to moderate pain associated with AOM. They have the added benefit of reducing fever. Occasionally, narcotic analgesics may be prescribed for severe pain. Application of heat or a cool compress may also be helpful. Instruct the family to have the child lie on the affected side with the heating pad or covered ice pack in place to that ear. Numbing eardrops such as benzocaine (Auralgan) may be helpful in the event of acute, severe pain. They should be used in conjunction with analgesics, though, because of the short duration of action (Kenna, 2016).

EDUCATING THE FAMILY

If the treatment selected for AOM is observation or watchful waiting, explain the rationale for this to the family. Ensure that the family understands the importance of returning for re-evaluation if the child is not improving within 24 to 48 hours or if the AOM progresses to severe illness. When antibiotics are prescribed, the family must understand the importance of completing the entire course of antibiotics. Families are tempted to stop giving the antibiotic because the child is usually vastly improved after taking the medication for 24 to 48 hours. Follow-up for resolution of AOM is necessary for all children and the physician or nurse practitioner will determine the timing of that follow-up. Emphasize the importance of follow-up to the parents. Educating them about OME and its potential impact on hearing and speech can improve treatment and outcomes for children (Meherali, Scott, & Hartling, 2017). Evidence of risk within various Indigenous groups varies with possibly lower associated ear infection as a result of longer breast feeding (>3 months) (Karunanayake et al., 2016).

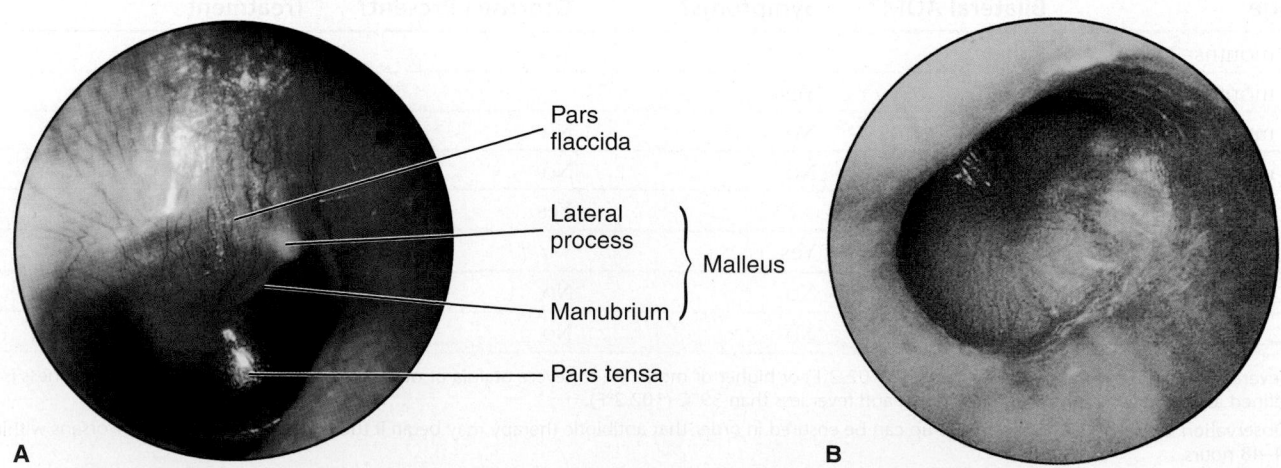

Pars flaccida

Lateral process

Manubrium

} Malleus

Pars tensa

A

B

FIGURE 39.10 **A.** Normal tympanic membrane. **B.** Acute otitis media: note opacity of the tympanic membrane.

PREVENTING ACUTE OTITIS MEDIA

Breastfed infants have a lower incidence of AOM than formula-fed infants, and breast milk's immunologic benefits are well known (Friedman et al., 2014). Therefore, encourage mothers to breastfeed for at least 6 to 12 months. Instruct families to avoid excess exposure to individuals with upper respiratory infections to decrease the incidence of these infections in their child. Infants and children should not be exposed to second-hand smoke. Encourage parents to stop smoking. If quitting smoking is not possible, then instruct parents not to smoke inside the house or automobile. Encourage the parents to have the child immunized with Prevnar and the influenza vaccine.

Xylitol syrup, a sucrose substitute, may also be protective (Klein & Pelton, 2015). Children who are old enough may chew xylitol-containing gum. Younger children and infants may be given xylitol syrup. Clinical studies are under way to validate the protective effects of xylitol. Care should be taken to avoid excessive dosing, as xylitol can cause diarrhea.

Otitis Media With Effusion

OME refers to the presence of fluid within the middle ear space, without signs or symptoms of infection. It may occur independent of AOM or may persist after the infectious process of AOM has resolved. Risk factors for OME include passive smoking, absence of breastfeeding, frequent viral upper respiratory infections, allergy, young age, male sex, adenoid hypertrophy, Eustachian tube dysfunction, and certain congenital disorders (Friedman et al., 2014). Complications of OME include AOM, hearing loss, and deafness.

Nursing Assessment

Nursing assessment of the child with OME includes health history, physical examination, and diagnostic testing.

HEALTH HISTORY

Determine the extent of symptoms. Children may be asymptomatic or may experience a popping sensation or fullness behind the eardrum. Explore the health history for risk factors such as passive smoking, absence of breastfeeding, frequent viral upper respiratory infections, allergy, or recent history of AOM.

PHYSICAL EXAMINATION

Otoscopic examination may reveal a dull, opaque tympanic membrane that may be white, grey, or bluish (Fig. 39.11). If the tympanic membrane is not opaque, a fluid level or air bubble may be visualized. Mobility may be absent or diminished upon pneumatic otoscopy. Tympanometry may be used to confirm the diagnosis of OME.

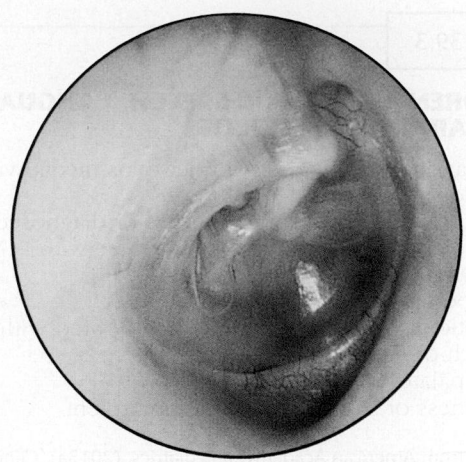

FIGURE 39.11 Otitis media with effusion; note dull white tympanic membrane.

Nursing Management

OME may take several months to resolve. Nursing management during the resolution phase focuses on education and monitoring for hearing loss.

EDUCATING THE FAMILY

Educate the family about the natural history of OME and the anatomic differences in young children that contribute to OME. Inform parents that antihistamines, decongestants, antibiotics, and corticosteroids have not been proven to hasten the resolution of OME and thus are not recommended. OME usually resolves spontaneously, but children should be rechecked every 4 weeks while this resolution is occurring. Teach parents not to feed infants in a supine position and to avoid bottle propping.

MONITORING FOR HEARING LOSS

When OME persists, the primary concern is its effect on hearing. In the infant or toddler who should be experiencing rapid language development, impaired hearing can depress language acquisition significantly (Klein & Pelton, 2016). Children with OME who are at risk for speech, language, or learning problems may be referred for evaluation of hearing earlier than a child with OME who is not at risk (Box 39.3). Children with chronic OME (persistent OME of 3 months' duration or longer) should be referred to a specialist for hearing evaluation (Klein & Pelton, 2016). Children who are not already at risk for speech concerns and are not experiencing difficulty with language acquisition may be reassessed every 3 to 6 months as long as hearing loss is not identified. At-risk children may require treatment earlier.

To communicate more effectively with children with OME who have hearing loss:

• Turn off music or television.
• Position yourself within 3 ft of the child before speaking.

BOX 39.3

CHILDREN AT RISK FOR SPEECH, LANGUAGE, OR LEARNING DIFFICULTIES

• Permanent hearing loss (without otitis media with effusion)
• Speech/language delay (suspected or diagnosed)
• Craniofacial disorder that may interfere with speech
• Any pervasive developmental disorder
• Genetic disorders or syndromes associated with speech or learning problems
• Cleft palate
• Blindness or significant visual impairment

Adapted from American Academy of Pediatrics. (2013a). Clinical practice guideline: The diagnosis and management of acute otitis media. *Pediatrics, 131*, e964–e999.

• Face the child while speaking.
• Use visual cues.
• Increase the volume of your speech only slightly.
• Speak clearly.
• Request preferential classroom seating.

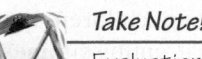 *Take Note!*

Evaluation of hearing is recommended when OME lasts 3 months or more if language delay, hearing loss, or a learning problem is suspected (Klein & Pelton, 2016).

PROVIDING POSTOPERATIVE CARE FOR THE CHILD WITH PRESSURE-EQUALIZING TUBES

The standard treatment for persistent or problematic OME is surgical insertion of **pressure-equalizing (PE) tubes** into the tympanic membrane (via myringotomy). The tubes stay in place for at least several months and generally fall out on their own (Fig. 39.12). The procedure is usually done as an outpatient surgery and the child returns home in the evening. Teach the parents to administer ear drops postoperatively if prescribed. After PE tube placement, the surgeon may recommend avoiding water entry into the ears. If recommended, advise parents to have the child wear earplugs in the bathtub or while swimming.

Placement of the PE tubes allows for adequate hearing, which in turn encourages appropriate speech development. Placement of PE tubes does not prevent middle ear infection. If the middle ear becomes infected with PE tubes in place, the tubes allow infected fluid to drain from the ear. Tell parents to contact their physician or nurse practitioner if drainage from the ear is noted. After PE tubes are placed, young children often have rapid increases in language acquisition, and parents should observe for this (O'Reilly, 2014).

FIGURE 39.12 Pressure-equalizing tube in place in the tympanic membrane.

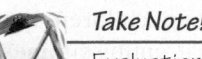 *Take Note!*

Children with PE tubes who swim in a lake must wear earplugs, as lake water is contaminated with bacteria and entry of that water into the middle ear should be avoided (Rosenfeld et al., 2013).

Otitis Externa

Otitis externa is defined as an infection and inflammation of the skin of the external ear canal. *Pseudomonas aeruginosa* and *S. aureus* are typical causative agents, though fungi such as *Aspergillus* and other bacteria also may be implicated. Moisture in the canal contributes to pathogen growth (Friedman et al., 2014). Otitis externa is commonly known as "swimmer's ear" since it occurs more frequently in those who swim often (and thus have wet ear canals). Changing the pH in the ear canal contributes to the inflammatory process.

Nursing Assessment

Nursing assessment of the child with otitis externa focuses on the health history and physical examination.

HEALTH HISTORY

Elicit a description of the present illness and chief complaint. Note history of ear itching or pain, ear drainage, or a feeling of fullness in the ear canal, with possible difficulty hearing. Note onset and progression of symptoms, as well as the child's response to treatments. Explore the child's current and past medical history for risk factors such as previous episodes of otitis externa or history of recent swimming in a pool, lake, or ocean.

FIGURE 39.13 Note edema and erythema of the ear canal as well as purulent discharge in the child with otitis externa.

Take Note!

The child with otitis externa usually has significant ear pain. Pressure on the tragus should be avoided, as it can worsen the pain.

PHYSICAL EXAMINATION

Typically, a white or coloured discharge can be seen in the ear canal or running from the ear. On otoscopy, the canal is red and edematous, often too swollen for insertion of the speculum and viewing of the tympanic membrane (Fig. 39.13). Diagnosis is based on clinical findings. Occasionally, the ear drainage is cultured for bacteria or fungus, particularly if otitis externa is not improving with treatment.

Nursing Management

The primary goals of nursing management are pain relief, treatment of the infection, and prevention of recurrence.

MANAGING PAIN

Analgesics (often narcotics) may be administered to manage the pain. A warm compress or heating pad to the affected ear is helpful in some children.

TREATING THE INFECTION

Administer antibiotic or antifungal eardrops as prescribed. In some cases, a wick is placed in the ear canal. The wick keeps the antibiotic drops in contact with the skin of the ear canal and promotes healing. Wick insertion can be extremely painful, and younger children will need to be restrained during insertion for their safety.

Atraumatic Care

When instilling ear drops in the young child, use distraction (a song, a favourite toy) to decrease perceived trauma to the child.

PREVENTING REINFECTION

Teach children and their parents about prevention of further episodes once the infection has resolved. Since moisture contributes to otitis externa, explain the importance of keeping the ear canals dry. Encourage the child and parents to use one of the methods described in Teaching Guidelines 39.2 after swimming or showering.

Teaching Guidelines 39.2
PREVENTING OTITIS EXTERNA

1. Avoid the use of cotton swabs, headphones, and earphones.
2. Wear earplugs, swimming cap, or band when swimming.
3. Promote ear canal dryness and alternate pH. Use one or more of the following methods:
   - Dry the ear canals using a hair dryer set on a lower setting.
   - Administer solutions that have a drying effect on the auditory canal skin and change the pH of the canal to discourage organism growth in susceptible children. The following solutions can be used:
   - A few drops of Domeboro solution can be placed in the canal, and then allowed to run out.
   - A mixture of half rubbing alcohol and half vinegar (squirted into the canal and then allowed to run out). The alcohol solution should be used only when the ear canals are healthy. Using it while the canals are inflamed will cause stinging and increased pain.

Adapted from Cook, S. P., & Gupta, R. C. (2016). *Swimmer's ear.* Retrieved from http://kidshealth.org/kid/ill_injure/aches/swimmers_ear.html

---

HEARING LOSS AND DEAFNESS

Infants are ordinarily born with the sense of hearing fully developed. Language development in infancy and early childhood is dependent upon adequate hearing, and even the fluctuating hearing loss associated with intermittent bouts of AOM can hinder language development (Klein & Pelton, 2015). Hearing loss may be unilateral (involving one ear) or bilateral (involving both ears). The extent of hearing loss is defined based on the softest intensity of sound that is perceived, described in **decibels** (dB). Levels of hearing loss are:

- 0 to 20 dB: normal
- 20 to 40 dB: mild loss
- 40 to 60 dB: moderate loss
- 60 to 80 dB: severe loss
- Greater than 80 dB: profound loss (American Speech-Language-Hearing Association [ASHA], 2016)

Hearing loss may be congenital or acquired. Congenital hearing loss affects 1 to 3 infants per 1,000 live births (CPS, 2016b). Most congenital hearing loss is inherited through a recessive gene, with only about 15% of cases resulting from an autosomal dominant trait (ASHA, 2016). Congenital hearing loss accounts for about one half of all the cases of hearing impairment; the remainder are acquired. Premature infants and those with persistent pulmonary hypertension of the newborn are at increased risk for hearing loss compared with other infants. Hearing loss commonly occurs with a large number of congenital or genetic syndromes, as well as in association with anomalies of the head and face. Unfortunately, in Canada, despite evidence supporting it, many infants are not offered universal newborn hearing screening. This results in delayed diagnosis of hearing loss which leads to significant harm for children and their families (CPS, 2016b).

Delayed-onset (acquired) hearing loss may be conductive, sensorineural, or mixed. **Conductive hearing loss** results when transmission of sound through the middle ear is disrupted, as in the case of OME. When fluid fills the middle ear, the tympanic membrane is unable to move properly, and partial or complete hearing loss occurs. **Sensorineural hearing loss** is caused by damage to the hair cells in the cochlea or along the auditory pathway. This may result from kernicterus, use of ototoxic medication, intrauterine infection with cytomegalovirus or rubella, neonatal or postnatal infection such as meningitis, severe neonatal respiratory depression, or exposure to excess noise. Mixed hearing loss occurs when the cause may be attributed to both conductive and sensorineural problems.

Regardless of the cause of hearing loss, early intervention can make a difference in the child's ability to communicate. Once the hearing loss has been determined, intervention can begin. Hearing aids, cochlear implants, communication devices, and speech education may enable these children to communicate verbally. Improved communication beginning in infancy and early childhood may also improve the child's school achievement.

Take Note!

Ear covers used to block ambient noise in premature infants in the neonatal intensive care may improve their physiologic state and protect future hearing potential (Khalesi, Khosravi, Ranjbar, Godarzi, & Karimi, 2017).

Nursing Assessment

Nursing assessment of the child with hearing loss or impairment focuses on the health history, physical examination, and diagnostic hearing testing.

HEALTH HISTORY

Common signs and symptoms reported during the health history might include:

- Infant:
  - Wakes only to touch, not environmental noises
  - Does not startle to loud noises
  - Does not turn to sound by 4 months of age
  - Does not babble at 6 months of age
- Younger child:
  - Does not progress with speech development
  - Does not speak by 2 years of age
  - Communicates needs through gestures
  - Does not speak distinctly, as appropriate for his or her age
  - Displays developmental (cognitive) delays
  - Prefers solitary play
  - Displays immature emotional behaviour
  - Does not respond to ringing of the telephone or doorbell
  - Focuses on facial expressions when communicating
- Older child:
  - Often asks for statements to be repeated
  - Is inattentive or daydreams
  - Performs poorly at school
  - Displays monotone or other abnormal speech
  - Gives inappropriate answers to questions except when able to view face of speaker
- At any age:
  - Speaks loudly
  - Sits very close to the TV or radio or turns volume up too loud
  - Responds only to moderate or loud voices

Investigate signs of hearing loss as early as possible in order for appropriate intervention to begin.

Explore the child's current and past medical history for risk factors such as congenital anomalies, genetic syndrome, infection, family history, kernicterus, neonatal ventilator use, ototoxic medication, or exposure to excess noise. Note whether newborn hearing screening was done and, if so, what the results were.

PHYSICAL EXAMINATION AND LABORATORY AND DIAGNOSTIC TESTS

Determine the child's level of interaction with the environment. For preschoolers and older children, administer the whisper test, keeping in mind that this is a gross screening test only. Perform the Weber and Rinne tests (refer to Chapter 31 for further explanation). If further evaluation is needed, the nurse may be responsible for administering an OAE test or auditory brain stem–evoked response test, either in the hospital or outpatient office.

Nursing Management

The primary goal of nursing care for the child with a hearing impairment is to provide education and support to the family and child. Individualize care for the child with a hearing impairment and the family based on their specific responses to the hearing impairment.

AUGMENTING HEARING

Compliance with hearing aids and communication curriculums is critical so that the child can develop hearing and speech. Teach the child and family that hearing aids should be cleaned daily with a damp cloth. In addition, it is important to change batteries weekly. When inserting the aid, the volume should be turned down, and then adjusted to the appropriate level after insertion. As the infant or child grows, the hearing aid will need to be reassessed for proper fit. Many schools for deaf children and other organizations provide loaner hearing aids so that the best fit and amplification may be determined prior to purchase. Assist the family to explore this type of option in the local community.

When cochlear implants are used, the nurse focuses on postoperative care of the incision site and pain management.

PROMOTING COMMUNICATION AND EDUCATION

Families and children need to learn how to communicate effectively with one another. If the child learns Sign Language, for instance, the parents and siblings should as well. Table 39.4 provides information on communication options for hearing-impaired children and their families. Communication may also be enhanced by the use of text telephone service in the home and closed-caption television. Bells and alarms in the home may use lights rather than sound to alert the child. Provide a sign language interpreter for the child at health care visits if the parent is not present for interpretation.

ENCOURAGING EDUCATION

Refer the child to the local child development centre or early childhood program. An IEP should be developed to maximize the child's learning ability. Nurses may be involved in the development of the IEP.

Some children attend schools specifically geared toward deaf students. The choice of school will depend on the family's preferences and resources.

PROVIDING SUPPORT

The diagnosis of a significant disability can be extremely stressful for the family. Encourage families to express their feelings and provide emotional support. Ensure that the needs of any siblings are also attended to. When the family is ready, encourage them to network with other families who have children with similar needs. Educate the family about the child's prescribed plan of care. Refer families to resources and support groups. Several helpful resources are listed on thePoint.

TABLE 39.4	COMPARING COMMUNICATION OPTIONS FOR THE HEARING IMPAIRED
Spoken Language	
Oral deaf education (auditory-verbal therapy)	Uses technology to boost auditory potential; teaches children to notice sound and give it meaning. Develops oral speech
Cued speech	A system using hand signs to clarify lip-reading; gives the person clues about the sounds the speaker is making
Signed Language	
American Sign Language (ASL)	Entirely communicated through hand signs, gestures, and facial expressions. Has its own grammar and syntax
Combination: Total communication	Combines auditory training and teaching of spoken language with SEE ("signing exact English"; corresponds to the words and syntax of English)
Augmentative and Alternative Communication (AAC)	
May use gestural communication	Can also include physical devices such as notebooks, communication boards, charts, or computers. Ranges from very low tech to technologically complex

Adapted from American Speech-Language-Hearing Association. (2016). *Augmentative and alternative communication (AAC)*. Retrieved from http://www.asha.org/public/speech/disorders/AAC.htm

NURSING CARE PLAN 39.1

Overview for the Child With a Disorder of Eyes or Ears

NURSING DIAGNOSIS: Disturbed sensory perception (visual) related to visual impairment squinting, holding items close, verbalization of inability to see clearly

Outcome Identification and Evaluation

Child will reach maximal vision potential: *Child uses corrective lenses appropriately and is able to participate in play and schoolwork.*

Intervention: *Improving Vision*

- Encourage corrective lens use *for enhancement of vision.*
- Support the family's efforts at vision therapy and other habilitation programs *to promote vision enhancement.*

- Encourage parents to comply with vision screening appointments *in order to determine visual acuity progression or problems.*

NURSING DIAGNOSIS: Fear related to severe visual impairment or blindness as evidenced by child's behaviours or verbalization

Outcome Identification and Evaluation

Child will experience decreased fear: *Child will verbalize comfort with environment or react calmly to interventions.*

Intervention: *Improving Vision*

- Allow verbal child to share his feelings *to promote coping in the child.*
- For the severely impaired or blind child, identify yourself via voice and name items in environment for the child *so that the child is aware of his or her surroundings.*
- Engage the parents in bedside caregiving *because the parents' voice and presence are reassuring to the child.*

NURSING DIAGNOSIS: Disturbed sensory perception (auditory) related to hearing loss as evidenced by lack of reaction to verbal stimuli, delayed attainment of language milestones

Outcome Identification and Evaluation

Child will reach maximal hearing and speech potential: *child uses aids appropriately and communicates effectively.*

Intervention: *Improving Hearing*

- Assess hearing ability frequently *because early detection of hearing loss allows for earlier intervention and correction.*
- Assess language development at each visit *to allow for early detection of hearing loss (earlier intervention and correction).*
- Encourage hearing aid use *for amplification of sound.*
- Teach about hearing aid battery safety *to avoid aspiration of battery.*
- Assist child with focusing on sounds in the environment *to encourage listening skills.*
- Refer for and encourage attendance at communication habilitation program *to maximize communication potential.*

NURSING CARE PLAN 39.1

Overview for the Child With a Disorder of Eyes or Ears (continued)

NURSING DIAGNOSIS: Risk for infection related to presence of infectious organisms

Outcome Identification and Evaluation

Child will exhibit no signs of secondary infection and will not spread infection to others: *symptoms of infection decrease over time, and others remain free from infection.*

Intervention: *Reducing Infection Risk*

• Maintain aseptic technique and practice good handwashing *to prevent introduction of further infectious agents.*
• Limit number of visitors, and screen for recent illness, *to prevent further infection.*
• Administer antibiotics if prescribed *to prevent or treat bacterial infection.*
• Encourage nutritious diet according to child's preferences *to assist body's natural infection-fighting mechanisms.*

• Isolate the child as required *to prevent nosocomial spread of infection.*
• Teach child and family preventive measures such as good handwashing, covering mouth and nose when coughing or sneezing, and adequate disposal of used tissues *to prevent nosocomial or community spread of infection.*

NURSING DIAGNOSIS: Risk for delayed development related to sensory impairment as evidenced by delay in attainment of developmental milestones

Outcome Identification and Evaluation

Child will achieve optimum independence for age: *child participates in age-appropriate developmental activities.*

Intervention: *Encouraging Growth and Development*

• Encourage attainment of developmental milestones with use of assistive devices as needed *for timely developmental achievements.*
• Foster independence in activities of daily living (ADLs) *to promote sense of accomplishment.*
• Encourage participation in play with another child or within a group *to promote socialization.*

• Assist family to set limits and apply discipline *because structure and routine provide a secure environment in which the developing child can grow.*
• Encourage friendships with other children with a sensory impairment *to promote socialization and let the child know that he or she is not the only one with these challenges.*

NURSING DIAGNOSIS: Impaired verbal communication related to hearing loss as evidenced by lack of or inarticulate speech, lack of alternate communication channel

Outcome Identification and Evaluation

The child will communicate effectively with the method chosen by the family (this may be sign language, oral/deaf speech, cued speech, or augmentative alternative communication device).

Intervention: *Improving Communication*

• Encourage choice of and attendance at communication habilitation program *to promote continued learning.*
• Provide consistency between home and hospital in regard to communication style/devices *to promote continued learning.*

• Support the child's efforts at correct speech *to promote speech development through reinforcement and praise.*
• Encourage family to use spoken language and read books at home *to continue to promote appropriate language development.*

(continued)

Overview for the Child With a Disorder of Eyes or Ears (continued)

NURSING DIAGNOSIS: Deficient knowledge related to sensory impairment (vision or hearing) as evidenced by new diagnosis and parents' questions

Outcome Identification and Evaluation

Parents express understanding of diagnosis and care of child: *parents verbalize understanding, demonstrate use of assistive devices, or independently perform medical treatments.*

Intervention: *Educating the Family*

- Review diagnosis and plan of care with the parents *to promote understanding of the disease process.*
- Refer family to resources available for sensory-impaired children *to provide further education and support to the parents.*
- Demonstrate medical treatments prescribed or use of assistive devices, requiring a return demonstra-

tion, *which shows the parents' ability to provide the prescribed care for the child.*
- Encourage exploration of different communication and learning modes available for the sensory-impaired child *to allow the child and family to find the right educational and communication style fit.*

NURSING DIAGNOSIS: Interrupted family processes, related to child's sensory impairment as evidenced by parent verbalization, nonverbal communication, altered coping

Outcome Identification and Evaluation

Parents demonstrate adequate coping and decreased anxiety: *parents are involved in child's care, ask appropriate questions, and are able to discuss child's care and condition calmly.*

Intervention: *Encouraging Appropriate Family Interactions*

- Encourage parents' verbalization of grief if child is hearing or vision impaired. *Parents must deal with their own feelings of loss to successfully care for the child with an impairment.*
- Encourage parents' verbalization of concerns related to child's illness: *allows for identification of concerns and demonstrates to the family that the nurse also cares about them, not just the child.*
- Explain therapy, procedures, and child's behaviour to parents: *developing an understanding of the child's current status helps decrease anxiety.*
- Encourage parental involvement in care *so that parents may continue to feel needed and valued.*

NURSING DIAGNOSIS: Risk for injury related to vision loss

Outcome Identification and Evaluation

The infant or child will remain free from injury.

Intervention: *Preventing Injury*

- Orient the child to hospital surroundings *because awareness is the first step to preventing injury.*
- Encourage parent to be at bedside *so that the child feels more comfortable.*
- Encourage use of assistive device *to promote safety.*

KEY CONCEPTS

○ Though hearing is fully developed at birth, visual development continues to progress until about age 7 years.

○ Binocular vision develops by age 4 months; visual acuity progresses to 20/50 by age 3 years and usually reaches 20/20 by age 7 years.

○ The relatively short and horizontally positioned Eustachian tubes of infants and young children make them more susceptible to otitis media than adults.

○ To maximize speech and language development, hearing loss should be identified early and intervention begun immediately.

○ Children with genetic syndromes or family history are at increased risk of visual and hearing impairments.

○ The corneal light reflex test and cover test are useful tools for identifying strabismus and amblyopia.

○ Tympanometry is used to determine the presence of fluid behind the eardrum (such as with otitis media with effusion).

○ Topical ophthalmic medications are used to treat certain infectious eye disorders.

○ Appropriate handwashing is the single most important factor to reduce the spread of acute viral or bacterial conjunctivitis.

○ Systemic antibiotics are used for the treatment of periorbital cellulitis.

○ Strabismus, glaucoma, and cataracts may all lead to visual impairment if left untreated.

○ Asymmetry of the corneal light reflex occurs with true strabismus.

○ Amblyopia must be identified early and treated with patching, corrective lenses, or surgery to prevent visual deterioration and promote appropriate vision development.

○ A cloudy cornea indicates the presence of cataract.

○ Very premature infants are at high risk of developing visual deficits related to retinopathy of prematurity and are also at increased risk of hearing impairment compared with other infants.

○ Eye strain, eye rubbing, and headaches may indicate a visual deficit.

○ Children with visual disorders should be encouraged to use prescribed corrective lenses.

○ Recurrent episodes of acute otitis media may negatively affect the child's hearing.

○ Recurrent or constant nasal congestion contributes to otitis media with effusion.

○ Otitis externa can be prevented by keeping the ear canal dry and altering canal pH.

○ The fluctuating hearing loss associated with recurrent otitis media and the hearing loss associated with chronic otitis media with effusion can significantly hinder language development in both the infant and the toddler.

○ The child with hearing loss should receive early intervention with hearing aids or other augmentative devices.

REFERENCES AND RECOMMENDED READINGS

American Speech-Language-Hearing Association. (2016). *Augmentative and alternative communication (AAC)*. Retrieved from http://www.asha.org/public/speech/disorders/AAC.htm.

Augsburger, J. J., & Correa, C. M. (2011). Ophthalmic trauma. In P. Riordan-Eva & E. T. Cunningham (Eds.). *Vaughan & Asbury's general ophthalmology* (18th ed.). New York: McGraw-Hill.

Blosser, C. G., Brady, M. A., & Royal, R. B. (2013). Infectious diseases & immunizations. In C. E. Burns, A. M. Dunn, M. A. Brady, N. B. Starr, & C. G. Blosser (Eds.). *Pediatric primary care* (5th ed.). Philadelphia, PA: Saunders.

Braverman, R. S. (2014). Eye. In W. W. Hay, M. J. Levin, R. R. Deterding, & M. J. Abzug (Eds.). *Current pediatric diagnosis and treatment* (22nd ed.). New York: McGraw-Hill.

Bremond-Gignac, D., Copin, H., Lapillone, A., & Milazzo, S. (2011). Visual development in infants: Physiological and pathological mechanisms. *Current Opinion in Ophthalmology, 22*(1), S1–S8.

Canadian Association for Pediatric Ophthalmology and Strabismus (CAPOS). (2016). *Screening*. Retrieved from http://www.capos.ca

Canadian Association of Optometrists. (n.d.). *Health Library*. Retrieved from https://opto.ca/health-library

Canadian Paediaric Society. (2015). *Preventing opthalmia neonatorum*. Retrieved from http://www.cps.ca/en/documents/position/ophthalmia-neonatorum

Canadian Paediatric Society. (2016a). *Vision screening in infants, children and youth*. Retrieved from http://www.cps.ca/documents/position/children-vision-screening

Canadian Paediatric Society. (2016b). *Universal newborn hearing screening*. Retrieved from http://www.cps.ca/en/documents/position/universal-hearing-screening-newborns

Canadian Paediatric Society. (2016c). *Management of acute otitis media in children 6 months of age and older*. Retrieved from http://www.cps.ca/documents/position/acute-otitis-media

Canadian Paediatric Society. (2016d). *Greig Health Record.* Retrieved from http://www.cps.ca/tools-outils/greig-health-record

Carpenito-Moyet, L. J. (2013). *Nursing diagnosis: Application to clinical practice* (14th ed.). Philadelphia, PA: Lippincott Williams & Wilkins.

Carter, S. L. (2015). *Sensory impairment.* Retrieved from http://www.pediatrics.emory.edu/divisions/neonatology/dpc/sensory.html

Coats, D. K., & Paysse, E. A. (2016). *Overview of amblyopia.* Retrieved from http://www.uptodate.com/contents/overview-of-amblyopia?source=search_result&search=amblyopia&selectedTitle=1~150

Cook, S. P., & Gupta, R. C. (2016). *Swimmer's ear.* Retrieved from http://kidshealth.org/kid/ill_injure/aches/swimmers_ear.html

Friedman, N. R., Scholes, M. A., & Yoon, P. J. (2014). Ear, nose, & throat. In W. W. Hay, M. J. Levin, R. R. Deterding, & M. J. Abzug (Eds.). *Current pediatric diagnosis and treatment* (22nd ed.). New York: McGraw-Hill.

Hammer, E. (n.d.). *Self-stimulation: Dr. Hammer responds.* Retrieved from http://www.nfb.org/images/nfb/Publications/fr/fr17/Issue3/F170308.htm

International Council of Ophthalmology (ICP). (2016). *Childhood blindness.* Retrieved from http://www.icoph.org/dynamic/attachments/resources/childhood-blindness.pdf

Isaza, G., & Arora, S. (2013). Probing without irrigation in children with congenital nasolacrimal duct obstruction. *Clinical and Investigative Medicine, 36*(3), 158–162.

Jacobs, D. S. (2015). *Corneal abrasions and corneal foreign bodies: Management.* Retrieved from http://www.uptodate.com/contents/corneal-abrasions-and-corneal-foreign-bodies-management

Karunanayake, C. P., Albritton, W., Rennie, D. C., Lawson, J. A., McCallum, L., Gardipy, P. J., ... Ramsden, V. (2016). Ear infection and its associated risk factors in first nations and rural school-aged Canadian children. *International Journal of Pediatrics, 2016,* 1523897.

Kenna, M. A. (2016). Acute otitis media—The long and the short of it. *New England Journal of Medicine, 375,* 2492–2493.

Khalesi, N., Khosravi, N., Ranjbar, A., Godarzi, Z., & Karimi, A. (2017). The effectiveness of earmuffs on the physiologic and behavioral stability in preterm infants. *International Journal of Pediatric Otorhinolaryngology, 98,* 43–47.

Klein, J. O., & Pelton, S. (2015). *Acute otitis media: Prevention of recurrence.* Retrieved from http://www.uptodate.com/contents/acute-otitis-media-in-children-prevention-of-recurrence

Klein, J. O., & Pelton, S. (2016). *Otitis media with effusion (serous otitis media) in children: Management.* Retrieved from http://www.uptodate.com/contents/otitis-media-with-effusion-serous-otitis-media-in-children-management

Lin, A. A., & Buckley, E. G. (2010). Update on pediatric cataract surgery and intraocular lens implantation. *Current Opinion in Ophthalmology, 21*(1), 55–59.

Lusby, F. W., & Zieve, D. (2016). *LASIK eye surgery.* Retrieved from http://umm.edu/health/medical/ency/articles/lasik-eye-surgery

Meherali, S., Scott, S. D., & Hartling, L. (2017). Parent information needs and experience regarding acute otitis media in children: A systematic review. Retrieved from https://doi.org/10.7939/R3RN30K8V

Mulholland, C., & Gardiner, J. (2015). Opthalmia neonatorum prophylaxis. *Canadian Journal of Ophthalmology, 50*(4), 328–329.

National Institute on Deafness and Other Communication Disorders. (2016). Cochlear implants. Retrieved from https://www.nidcd.nih.gov/health/cochlear-implants

Optometrists Network. (2016). *Strabismus.* Retrieved from http://www.strabismus.org/

O'Reilly, R. C. (2014). *Middle ear infections and ear tube surgery.* Retrieved from http://kidshealth.org/en/parents/ear-infections.html

Paysse, E. A., Coats, D. K., & Cassidy, M. (2015). *Nasolacrimal duct obstruction (dacryostenosis) in children and dacrocystocele.* Retrieved from http://www.uptodate.com/contents/congenital-nasolacrimal-duct-obstruction-dacryostenosis-and-dacryocystocele

Podbielski, D. W., Surkont, M., Tehrani, N. N., & Ratnapalan, R. S. (2009). Pediatric eye injuries in a Canadian emergency department. *Canadian Journal of Ophthalmology/Journal Canadien d'Ophtalmologie, 44*(5), 519–522.

Rivera, J. C., Madaan, A., Zhou, T. E., & Chemtob, S. (2016). Review of the mechanisms and therapeutic avenues for retinal and choroidal vascular dysfunctions in retinopathy of prematurity. *Acta Paediatrica, 105*(12), 1421–1433.

Rosenfeld, R. M., Schwartz, S. R., Pynnonen, M. A., Tunkel, D. E., Hussey, H. M., Fichera, J. S., ... Haynes, D. S. (2013). Clinical practice guideline: Tympanostomy tubes in children. *Otolaryngology—Head and Neck Surgery, 149*(1 Suppl), S1–S35.

Sharma, A., Wong, A. M., Colpa, L., Chow, A. H., & Jin, Y. P. (2016). Socioeconomic status and utilization of amblyopia services at a tertiary pediatric hospital in Canada. *Canadian Journal of Ophthalmology/Journal Canadien d'Ophtalmologie, 51*(6), 452–458.

Taketomo, C. K., Hodding, J. H., & Kraus, D. M. (2013). *Pediatric & neonatal dosage handbook* (20th ed.). Hudson, OH: Lexicomp.

Turner, A., & Rabiu, M. (2007). Patching for corneal abrasion. *The Cochrane Library.* doi: 10.1002/14 August 19, 2015, 651858.CD004764.pub2

Urquhart, D. S., & Tan, H. L. (2016). Sleep disordered breathing at the extremes of age: Infancy. *Breathe, 12*(1), e1.

Weber, J., & Kelley, J. H. (2014). *Health assessment in nursing* (5th ed.). Philadelphia, PA: Lippincott Williams & Wilkins.

Xu, K., Chin, E. K., Quiram, P. A., Davies, J. B., Parke, D. W., & Almeida, D. R. (2016). Retinal injury secondary to laser pointers in pediatric patients. *Pediatrics, 138*(4), e20161188. Retrieved from http://pediatrics.aappublications.org/content/138/4/e20161188

Yeung, H., & Walton, D. S. (2012). Recognizing childhood glaucoma in the primary pediatric setting. *Contemporary Pediatrics, 29*(5), 32–40.

CHAPTER **WORKSHEET**

MULTIPLE CHOICE QUESTIONS

1. Which situation would cause the nurse to become concerned about possible hearing loss?
   a. A 12-month-old who babbles incessantly, making no sense
   b. An 8-month-old who says only "da"
   c. A 3-month-old who startles easily to sound
   d. A 3-year-old who drops the letter "s"

2. A 4-year-old complains of extreme pain when the tragus is touched. Though not diagnostic, this sign is most indicative of which disorder?
   a. Acute otitis media
   b. Acute tympanic effusion
   c. Otitis interna
   d. Otitis externa

3. The nurse is caring for an infant who has undergone surgery for infantile glaucoma. What is the priority nursing intervention?
   a. Place the child prone postoperatively for comfort.
   b. Teach the family use of the contact lens.
   c. Place elbow restraints on the infant.
   d. Provide a mobile for optical stimulation.

4. A 2-year-old has been prescribed eye patching for strabismus 6 hours per day. What teaching does the nurse provide for the mother?
   a. Try to patch 6 hours per day, but if you miss some it is OK.
   b. Patching is necessary to strengthen vision in the weaker eye.
   c. Patching will keep the eye from turning in.
   d. Since the child is so young, patching can be delayed until school age.

DOSAGE CALCULATION QUESTION

1. The nurse is caring for a child with acute otitis media. The child weighs 22 lb. The medication order reads: amoxicillin 160 mg PO every 8 hours. Amoxicillin is supplied as 200 mg/5 mL. How many millilitres will the nurse administer? Round to the nearest whole number.

CRITICAL THINKING EXERCISES

1. A 16-month-old toddler is being seen for his sixth ear infection. What particular information about his growth and development must the nurse ask about? Be specific about the questions you would ask.

2. How would you distinguish allergic conjunctivitis from acute bacterial conjunctivitis?

3. A 13-month-old has been diagnosed with severe visual impairment. Develop a list of sample nursing diagnoses for this situation.

STUDY ACTIVITIES

1. Develop a sample plan for teaching a low-literacy parent about the etiology, treatment, and complications of recurrent acute otitis media.

2. While in the pediatric clinical setting, compare the play styles of a sighted child with those of a visually impaired child.

3. Research hearing and vision resources in your local community.

BRINGING IT ALL TOGETHER: A CASE STUDY

Bryn Carle, a 6-year-old, is brought to the clinic by her mother. She presents with redness of the left eye, edema, and drainage. What other assessment information would be helpful? Based on the history and clinical presentation, Bryn is diagnosed with conjunctivitis. What education will be necessary for the family to assist in alleviating symptoms and preventing infectious spread?

Go to thePoint **to find questions to consider about this case.**

40

Nursing Care of the Child With an Alteration in Gas Exchange/ Respiratory Disorder

Learning Objectives

Upon completion of the chapter, you will be able to:

1. Distinguish differences between the anatomy and physiology of the respiratory system in children versus adults.

2. Identify various factors associated with respiratory illness in infants and children.

3. Discuss common laboratory and other diagnostic tests useful in the diagnosis of respiratory conditions.

4. Describe nursing care related to common medications and other treatments used for management and palliation of respiratory conditions.

5. Recognize risk factors associated with various respiratory disorders.

6. Distinguish different respiratory disorders based on their signs and symptoms.

7. Discuss nursing interventions commonly used for respiratory illnesses.

8. Devise an individualized nursing care plan for the child with a respiratory disorder.

9. Develop child/family teaching plans for the child with a respiratory disorder.

10. Describe the psychosocial impact of chronic respiratory disorders on children.

Alexander Roberts, **4 months old, is brought to the clinic by his mother. He has a cold and has been coughing a great deal for 2 days. Today he has had difficulty taking his bottle and is breathing very quickly. Mrs. Roberts says he seems tired.**

Gas exchange refers to the process by which oxygen is transported to cells and carbon dioxide is transported from cells (Giddens, 2013). Nurses encounter potential and actual alterations in gas exchange in all types of clients and must detect problems and intervene early to prevent life-threatening complications.

Alterations in gas exchange (respiratory disorders) are the most common causes of illness and hospitalization in children. These illnesses range from mild, non-acute disorders (such as the common cold or sore throat) to serious life-threatening conditions (such as epiglottitis). Chronic disorders, such as allergic rhinitis or asthma, can affect quality of life, but frequent acute or recurrent infections also can interfere significantly with the well-being of some children.

Respiratory infections account for the majority of acute illnesses in children (Federico et al., 2014). The child's age, socioeconomic status, and general health status can influence both the development of respiratory disorders and the course of the illness. The incidence of respiratory infections is significantly higher in some social groups for various reasons linked to the determinants of health. For example, Indigenous children may experience increased respiratory risk as a result of housing issues, second-hand tobacco smoke exposure, and in some cases malnutrition (Kovesi, 2012). Pre-existing medical condition, infectious diseases, and malnutrition can also impact Immigrant and Refugee children (Canadian Paediatric Society, 2019). Infants and younger children are more likely to deteriorate quickly from a respiratory illness, and children with chronic disorders such as diabetes, congenital heart disease, sickle cell anemia, cystic fibrosis (CF), and cerebral palsy tend to be more severely affected with respiratory disorders.

In addition, the season of the year can influence the development of respiratory disorders and the course of the illness. For example, certain viruses are more prevalent in the winter, whereas allergen-related respiratory diseases are more prevalent in the spring and fall.

Nurses must be familiar with respiratory conditions affecting children so that they can provide guidance and support to families. Difficulty with breathing can be very frightening for both the child and their parents. Nurses must be able to ask questions that can help establish the severity of the child's illness and determine whether the family should seek care at a health care facility.

Since respiratory illnesses account for the majority of pediatric admissions to general hospitals, nurses caring for children need to have expert assessment and intervention skills in this area. Early detection of worsening respiratory status allows for timely treatment and the chance to prevent a minor problem from becoming a critical illness. Nurses are also in a unique position to provide education about respiratory illnesses and to promote efforts to prevent these illnesses.

VARIATIONS IN PEDIATRIC ANATOMY AND PHYSIOLOGY

Alterations in gas exchange/respiratory conditions often affect both the upper and lower respiratory tract, though some affect primarily one or the other. Respiratory dysfunction in children tends to be more severe than in adults, and several differences in the infant's or child's respiratory system account for this increased severity.

Nose

In newborns, nasal breathing is preferred over mouth breathing. This route allows for warming, humidifying, cleaning, and regulation of air entering the lungs. While newborns are often described as "obligate nose breathers," mouth breathing can be seen in instances of severe obstruction. However, this route is ineffective and can lead to apneic periods, respiratory distress, and oxygen desaturations (Bergeson & Shaw, 2001). Thus, nares must be patent to allow for proper ventilation and gas exchange, and to facilitate breathing while feeding.

The upper respiratory mucus serves as a cleansing agent, yet newborns produce very little mucus, making them more susceptible to infection. However, the newborn and young infant have very small nasal passages, so when excess mucus is present, airway obstruction is more likely.

Infants are born with maxillary and ethmoid sinuses present. The frontal sinuses (most often associated with sinus infection) and the sphenoid sinuses develop by age 6 to 8 years. Therefore, younger children are less likely to acquire sinus infections when compared with adults.

Throat

The tongue of the infant relative to the oropharynx is larger than in adults. Posterior displacement of the tongue can quickly lead to severe airway obstruction. Through early school age, children tend to have enlarged tonsillar and adenoidal tissue even in the absence of illness. This can contribute to an increased incidence of airway obstruction.

Trachea

The airway lumen is smaller in infants and children than in adults. The infant's trachea is approximately 4 mm wide compared with the adult width of 20 mm. When edema, mucus, or bronchospasm is present, the capacity for air passage is greatly diminished. A small reduction in the diameter of a child's airway, resulting from the presence of edema or mucus, will result in an exponential increase in resistance to airflow (Fig. 40.1). Increased **work of breathing** (effort or labour associated with respiration) then occurs.

In teenagers and adults, the larynx is cylindrical and uniform in width. In infants and children younger than

1 mm circumferential edema causes 50% reduction of diameter and radius, increasing pulmonary resistance by a factor of 16.

1 mm circumferential edema causes 20% reduction of diameter and radius, increasing pulmonary resistance by a factor of 2.4.

FIGURE 40.1 **A.** Note the smaller diameter of the child's airway under normal circumstances. **B.** With 1 mm of edema present, note the exponential decrease in airway lumen diameter as compared with the adult.

10 years old, the cricoid cartilage is underdeveloped, resulting in laryngeal narrowing in a funnel shape (Tewfik & Alghonaim, 2015). In addition, the larynx and glottis are located higher in the neck, increasing the chance of aspiration of foreign material into the lower airways. Congenital laryngomalacia occurs in some infants and results in the laryngeal structure being weaker than normal, yielding greater collapse on inspiration. Box 40.1 discusses congenital laryngomalacia.

The child's airway is highly compliant, making it quite susceptible to dynamic collapse in the presence of airway

---

BOX 40.1

CONGENITAL LARYNGOMALACIA

- Inspiratory stridor is present and is intensified with certain positions.
- Suprasternal retractions may be present, but the infant exhibits no other signs of respiratory distress.
- Congenital laryngomalacia is generally a benign condition that improves as the cartilage in the larynx matures. It usually disappears by age 1 year.
- The crowing noise heard with breathing can make parents very anxious. Reassure parents that the condition will improve with time.
- Parents become very familiar with the "normal" sound their infant makes and are often able to identify intensification or change in the stridor. Airway obstruction may occur earlier in infants with this condition, so intensification of stridor or symptoms of respiratory illness should be evaluated early by the physician or nurse practitioner.

---

obstruction (American Heart Association [AHA], 2011). The muscles supporting the airway are less functional than those in the adult. Children have a large amount of soft tissue surrounding the trachea, and the mucus membranes lining the airway are less securely attached when compared with adults. This increases the risk for airway edema and obstruction. Upper airway obstruction resulting from a foreign body, croup, or epiglottitis can result in tracheal collapse during inspiration.

Lower Respiratory Structures

The bifurcation of the trachea occurs at the level of the third thoracic vertebra in children, compared with the level of the sixth thoracic vertebra in adults (Tewfik & Alghonaim, 2015). This anatomic difference is important when suctioning children and when endotracheal intubation is required. This difference in placement also contributes to risk for foreign material aspiration. The bronchi and bronchioles of infants and children are narrower in diameter than the adult's, placing them at increased risk for lower airway obstruction (see Fig. 40.1). Lower airway obstruction during exhalation often results from bronchiolitis and asthma or is caused by foreign body aspiration into the lower airway.

Alveoli develop at approximately 24 weeks' gestation. Term infants are born with about 50 million alveoli. After birth, alveolar growth slows until 3 months of age and then progresses until the child reaches 7 or 8 years of age, at which time the alveoli reach the adult number of around 300 million (Moore, Persaud, & Torchia, 2013). Alveoli make up most of the lung tissue and are the major sites for gas exchange. Oxygen moves from the alveolar air to the blood, while carbon dioxide moves from the blood into the alveolar air. Smaller numbers of alveoli, particularly in the premature and/or young infant, place the child at a higher risk of **hypoxemia** (deficiency in the concentration of oxygen in arterial blood) and carbon dioxide retention.

Chest Wall

In older children and adults, the ribs and sternum support the lungs and help keep them well expanded. The movement of the diaphragm and intercostal muscles alters volume and pressure within the chest cavity, resulting in air movement into the lungs. Infants' chest walls are highly compliant (pliable) and fail to support the lungs adequately. Functional residual capacity can be greatly reduced if respiratory effort is diminished. This lack of lung support also makes the tidal volume of infants and toddlers almost completely dependent upon movement of the diaphragm. If diaphragm movement is impaired (as in states of hyperinflation, such as asthma), the intercostal muscles cannot lift the chest wall and respiration is further compromised.

Metabolic Rate and Oxygen Need

Children have a significantly higher metabolic rate than adults. Their resting respiratory rates are faster and their demand for oxygen is higher. Adult oxygen consumption is 3 to 4 L/min, while infants consume 6 to 8 L/min. In any situation of respiratory distress, infants and children will develop hypoxemia more rapidly than adults (AHA, 2011). This may be attributed not only to the child's increased oxygen requirement but also to the effect that certain conditions have on the oxyhemoglobin dissociation curve.

Normal oxygen transport relies on binding of oxygen to hemoglobin in areas of high partial pressure of oxygen (pO_2) (pulmonary arterial beds) and release of oxygen from hemoglobin when the pO_2 is low (peripheral tissues). Normally, a pO_2 of 95 mm Hg results in an oxygen saturation of 97%. A decrease in oxygen saturation results in a disproportionate (much larger) decrease in pO_2 (Fig. 40.2). Thus, a small decrease in oxygen saturation reflects a larger decrease in pO_2. Conditions such as alkalosis, hypothermia, hypocarbia, anemia, and fetal hemoglobin cause oxygen to become more tightly bound to hemoglobin, resulting in the curve shifting to the left. Common pediatric conditions, such as acidosis, hyperthermia, and hypercarbia, cause hemoglobin to decrease its affinity for oxygen, further shifting the curve to the right.

COMMON MEDICAL TREATMENTS

A variety of interventions are used to treat respiratory illness in children. The treatments listed in Common Medical Treatments 40.1 and Drug Guide 40.1 usually require a physician or nurse practitioner's order when a child is hospitalized.

FIGURE 40.2 Normal hemoglobin dissociation curve (*green*), shift to the right (*red*), and shift to the left (*blue*).

NURSING PROCESS OVERVIEW FOR THE CHILD WITH A RESPIRATORY DISORDER

Care of the child with a respiratory disorder includes assessment, nursing diagnosis, planning, interventions, and evaluation. A number of general concepts related to the nursing process can be applied to respiratory disorders. From a general understanding of the care involved for a child with an alteration in gas exchange, the nurse can individualize the care based on specifics for each child.

Assessment

Assessment of respiratory dysfunction in children includes health history, physical examination, and laboratory or diagnostic testing.

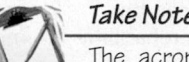

Take Note!

The acronyms OLDCARTSp or LOTARPS can be helpful in obtaining the child's history of present illness. These acronyms can be especially useful for symptoms such as cough, fever, and pain.

OLDCARTS: Onset, Location and Radiation, Duration, Characteristics, Associated/Aggravating and Alleviating factors, Relieving factors, Timing, Severity, and any Prior episodes.

LOTARPS: Location, Onset, Type, Associated and Alleviating symptoms, Radiation and Recurrence, Precipitating events, and Severity.

Remember Alexander, the 4-month old with the cold, cough, fatigue, feeding difficulty, and fast breathing? What additional health history and physical examination assessment information should the nurse obtain?

Health History

The health history consists of the history of present illness (when the symptoms started and how they have progressed), past medical history, family history, social and environmental history, as well as treatments used at home, current medications, and allergies to foods, medication, or environment. Ascertain immunization history. The past medical history might be significant for recurrent colds or sore throats, **atopy** (such as asthma, atopic dermatitis, or allergic rhinitis), prematurity, respiratory dysfunction at birth, poor weight gain, or history of recurrent respiratory illnesses or chronic lung disease. Family history might be significant for chronic respiratory disorders such as asthma or might reveal contacts for infectious exposure. When eliciting the history of the present illness, enquire about onset and progression; fever; nasal

COMMON MEDICAL TREATMENTS 40.1 RESPIRATORY DISORDERS

Treatment	Explanation	Indications	Nursing Implications
Oxygen	Administer via mask, nasal cannula, hood, tent, or endotracheal or nasotracheal tube	Hypoxemia, respiratory distress	Monitor response via work of breathing and pulse oximetry
High humidity	Addition of moisture to inspired air	Common cold, tonsillectomy	Infant may require extra blankets with cool mist, and frequent changes of bedclothes under oxygen hood or tent as they become damp
Suctioning	Removal of secretions via bulb syringe, Neosucker or suction catheter, the latter two of which are hospital interventions	Excessive airway secretions (common cold, flu, bronchiolitis, pertussis)	Deep suction should be done carefully and only as far as recommended for age or tracheostomy tube size, or until cough or gag occurs. Inline or closed suction units should be premeasured
Respiratory physiotherapy	A group of treatment strategies used to promote secretion clearance, increased lung volumes, and/or reduced work of breathing. They can be used acutely or in a rehabilitative nature	Increased work of breathing, retained secretions, poor lung volumes, ineffective cough, and altered breathing mechanics	Usually prescribed and performed by a Physiotherapist, but can be taught to parents and other health care professionals. Care should be taken as some techniques are contraindicated in certain conditions. Percussions can exacerbate bronchospasm and increase mucus production and should therefore be used with caution in certain conditions (e.g., asthma, bronchiolitis)
Saline gargles	Relieves throat pain via salt water gargle	Pharyngitis, tonsillitis	Recommended for children old enough to understand the concept of gargling (to avoid choking)
Honey	Cough suppressant. Promotes sleep by reducing cough	Upper respiratory tract infections	Only for children 1 year of age and over. 2.5 to 10 mL by mouth at bedtime (Allen & Arroll, 2014)
Saline lavage	Normal saline introduced into the airway, followed by suctioning	Common cold, flu, bronchiolitis, any condition resulting in increased mucus production in the upper airway	Very helpful for loosening thick mucus; child may need to be in semi-upright position to avoid aspiration
Chest tube	Insertion of a drainage tube into the pleural cavity to facilitate removal of air or fluid and allow full lung expansion	Pneumothorax, empyema	Should tube become dislodged from container, the chest tube must be clamped immediately, or the open end placed into a container of sterile water to avoid further air entry into the chest cavity
Bronchoscopy	Introduction of a bronchoscope into the bronchial tree for diagnostic purposes. Also allows for bronchiolar lavage	Removal of foreign body, cleansing of bronchial tree	Watch for postprocedural airway swelling, complaints of sore throat

congestion; noisy breathing; presence and description of cough; rapid respirations; increased work of breathing; activity intolerance; ear, nose, sinus, or throat pain; ear pulling; headache; vomiting with coughing; poor feeding; cyanosis; and lethargy. Also enquire about exposure to second-hand smoke. Children exposed to environmental smoke have an increased incidence of respiratory illnesses such as asthma, bronchitis, and pneumonia (World Health Organization [WHO], n. d.).

Physical Examination

Physical examination of the respiratory system includes inspection and observation, auscultation, percussion, and palpation.

INSPECTION AND OBSERVATION

Colour. Observe the child's skin colour, noting pallor or cyanosis (circumoral or central). Pallor (pale

DRUG GUIDE 40.1 COMMON DRUGS FOR RESPIRATORY DISORDERS

Medication	Actions/Indications	Nursing Implications
Cough and cold medications (expectorants, cough suppressants, decongestants, and combinations)	Symptomatic relief of mucus build-up, cough, and congestion	Effectiveness of most cough and cold medications has not been established in children, and most are potential for harm. Should not be given to children under the age of 6 (Health Canada, 2016a)
Antihistamines	Treatment of allergic conditions such as allergic rhinitis and asthma	May cause drowsiness or dry mouth
Antibiotics (oral, parenteral)	Treatment of bacterial infections of the respiratory tract such as Group A streptococcal pharyngitis, tonsillitis, acute bacterial sinusitis, bacterial pneumonia, cystic fibrosis, empyema, abscess, tuberculosis	Check for antibiotic allergies. Should be given as prescribed for the length of time prescribed
Antibiotics (inhaled)	Treatment of bacterial infections of the respiratory tract in children with cystic fibrosis	Can be given via nebulizer
β_2-Adrenergic agonists (short acting) (i.e., salbutamol, levalbuterol, pirbuterol)	Relax airway smooth muscle, resulting in bronchodilation Used for acute and chronic treatment of wheezing and bronchospasm in asthma, cystic fibrosis, chronic lung disease. Also, used to prevent wheezing in exercise-induced asthma	Administered via inhalation Can be used for acute relief of bronchospasm May cause nervousness, tachycardia, and jitteriness Inhaled agents result in fewer systemic side effects
β_2-Adrenergic agonists (long acting) (i.e., formoterol, salmeterol)	Long-acting bronchodilator used in chronic asthma management and for prevention of exercise-induced asthma Long-term control in chronic asthma Prevention of exercise-induced asthma	Administered via inhalation Used only for long-term control or for exercise-induced asthma. Not for relief of bronchospasm in an acute wheezing episode
Nebulized L-epinephrine	Produces bronchodilation Indicated for croup	Assess lung sounds and work of breathing Observe for rebound bronchospasm
Anticholinergic (ipratropium)	Produces bronchodilation in asthma or chronic lung disease	In children, generally used as an adjunct to β_2-adrenergic agonists for treatment of acute bronchospasm
Antiviral agents (oral: amantadine, oseltamivir; inhaled zanamivir)	Treatment and prevention of influenza A	Amantadine: monitor for confusion, nervousness, and jitteriness Oseltamivir, zanamivir: well tolerated but expensive
Antiviral (specific to respiratory syncytial virus [RSV]) (Ribavirin)	Treatment of severe lower respiratory tract infection with RSV. Not recommended for routine use; occasionally used for ventilated children and those with or at risk for severe disease (Canadian Paediatric Society, 2017a)	Administer via aerosol with the small-particle aerosol generator (SPAG). Suction children on assisted ventilation every 2 hours; monitor pulmonary pressures every 2 to –4 hours. May cause blurred vision and photosensitivity. Pregnant women should not be exposed to drug due to teratogenic effects

(continued)

DRUG GUIDE 40.1 COMMON DRUGS FOR RESPIRATORY DISORDERS (continued)

Medication	Actions/Indications	Nursing Implications
Corticosteroids (inhaled) (beclomethasone, budesonide, fluticasone, mometasone, ciclesonide)	Exert a potent, locally acting anti-inflammatory effect to decrease the frequency and severity of asthma attacks. May also delay pulmonary damage that occurs with chronic asthma. Also, used for chronic lung disease and croup syndromes	Not for treatment of acute wheezing. Rinse mouth after inhalation to decrease incidence of fungal infections, dry mouth, and hoarseness. Minimal systemic absorption makes inhaled steroids the treatment of choice for asthma maintenance program
Corticosteroids (oral, parenteral) (dexamethasone, prednisolone, prednisone)	Suppress inflammation and normal immune response. Used for acute asthma exacerbations, wheezing with chronic lung disease, and croup	May cause hyperglycemia. May suppress reaction to allergy tests. Consult physician or nurse practitioner if vaccinations are ordered during course of systemic corticosteroid therapy. Short courses of therapy are generally safe. Very effective, but long-term or chronic use can result in peptic ulceration, altered growth, and numerous other side effects. Children on long-term dosing should have growth assessed
Leukotriene receptor antagonists (montelukast, zafirlukast)	Decrease inflammatory response by antagonizing the effects of leukotrienes to control asthma in children age 1 year and older. Montelukast: for allergic rhinitis in children 6 months and older	Given once daily, in the evening. Not for relief of bronchospasm during an acute wheezing episode, but may be continued during the episode
Respiratory stimulants (methylxanthines: theophylline, aminophylline, caffeine)	To provide for continuous airway relaxation to achieve long-term control (methylxanthines)	Administered orally or intravenously. Sustained-release oral preparation can be used to prevent nocturnal symptoms. Monitor drug levels routinely. Report signs of toxicity immediately: tachycardia, nausea, vomiting, diarrhea, stomach cramps, anorexia, confusion, headache, restlessness, flushing, increased urination, seizures, arrhythmias, insomnia
Inhaled pulmonary enzyme (dornase alfa)	Enzyme that hydrolyzes the DNA in sputum, reducing sputum viscosity in children with cystic fibrosis	Administered via nebulizer. Monitor for dysphonia and pharyngitis
Monoclonal antibody (palivizumab)	Used to prevent serious lower respiratory RSV disease in certain high-risk groups of children	Should be administered monthly during the RSV season. Given intramuscularly only

Adapted from Taketomo, C. K., Hodding, J. H., & Kraus, D. M. (2013). *Pediatric & neonatal dosage handbook* (20th ed.). Hudson, OH: Lexi-comp.

appearance) occurs as a result of peripheral vasoconstriction in an effort to conserve oxygen for vital functions. **Cyanosis**, a bluish tinge to the skin and mucus membranes, occurs as a result of **hypoxia** (oxygen deficiency). It might first present circumorally (just around the mouth) and progress to central cyanosis. Newborns might have blue hands and feet (acrocyanosis), a normal finding. The infant might have pale hands and feet when cold or when ill, as peripheral circulation is not well developed in early infancy. It is important, then, to note if the cyanosis is central (involving the midline), as this is a true sign of hypoxia. Children with low red blood cell counts might not demonstrate cyanosis as early during hypoxemia as children with normal hemoglobin levels. Therefore, absence of cyanosis or the degree of cyanosis present is not always an accurate indication of the severity of respiratory involvement.

Note the rate and depth of respiration as well as work of breathing. Often the first sign of respiratory illness in infants and children is **tachypnea** (increased respiratory rate).

Take Note!

A slow or irregular respiratory rate in an acutely ill infant or child is an ominous sign (AHA, 2011). See Chapter 51. Many hospitals have implemented tools to assist frontline providers in recognizing and preventing decompensation in children. The Pediatric Early Warning System (PEWS) is an example; this tool varies slightly among sites, but generally provides a score derived from the assessment findings, with an algorithm to follow based on the score (Duncan, Hutchison, & Parshuram, 2006).

Take Note!

Often five key indicators are used when assessing the severity of respiratory illness in children. These are the child's behaviour, tachypnea, signs of work of breathing (WOB), heart rate, and blood pressure. During assessment and reporting, the nurse determines if the child's symptoms are mild, moderate, or severe. PEWS scoring documentation provide detailed information to aid in nursing assessment and diagnosis (Royal Children's Hospital Melbourne [n.d.]; Child Health BC [2016]).

Nose and Oral Cavity. Inspect the nose and oral cavity. Note nasal drainage and redness or swelling in the nose. Note the colour of the pharynx, presence of exudate, tonsil size, and status and presence of lesions anywhere in the oral cavity.

Cough and Other Airway Noises. Note the sound of the cough (Is it wet or productive, dry and hacking, barky, tight? When does the cough occur? Is it only or mainly at night?). Also note if noises associated with breathing are present (e.g., grunting, stridor, or audible wheeze). Grunting occurs on expiration and is produced by premature glottic closure. It is an attempt to preserve or increase functional residual capacity. Grunting might occur with alveolar collapse or loss of lung volume, such as in **atelectasis** (a collapsed or airless portion of the lung), pneumonia, and pulmonary edema. **Stridor**, a high-pitched, readily audible inspiratory noise, is a sign of upper airway obstruction. Sometimes wheezes can be heard with the naked ear; these are referred to as audible wheezes.

Respiratory Effort. Assess respiratory effort for depth and quality. Is breathing laboured? Infants and children with significant nasal congestion may have tachypnea, which usually resolves when the nose is cleared of mucus. Mouth breathing may occur when a large amount of nasal congestion is present. Increased work of breathing, particularly if associated with restlessness and anxiety, usually indicates lower respiratory involvement. Assess for the presence of nasal flaring, retractions, or bobbing of the head with each breath.

FIGURE 40.3 **Location of retractions.**

Nasal flaring can occur early during respiratory illness and is an effort to inhale greater amounts of oxygen.

Retractions. The inward pulling of soft tissues with respiration can occur in the intercostal, subcostal, substernal, supraclavicular, or suprasternal regions (Fig. 40.3). Document the severity of the retractions: mild, moderate, or severe. Also note the use of accessory neck muscles and nasal flaring. (Note the presence of paradoxical breathing, lack of simultaneous chest and abdominal rise with the inspiratory phase.)

Take Note!

Seesaw (or paradoxical) respirations are very ineffective for ventilation and oxygenation (binding of oxygen). The chest falls on inspiration and rises on expiration.

Anxiety and Restlessness. Is the child anxious or restless? Restlessness, irritability, and anxiety result from difficulty in securing adequate oxygen. These might be very early signs of respiratory distress, especially if accompanied by tachypnea. Restlessness might progress to listlessness and lethargy if the respiratory dysfunction is not corrected.

Clubbing. Inspect the fingertips for the presence of clubbing, an enlargement of the terminal phalanx of the finger, resulting in a change in the angle of the nail to the fingertip (Fig. 40.4). Clubbing might occur in children with a chronic respiratory illness. It is the result of increased capillary growth as the body attempts to supply more oxygen to distal body cells.

Hydration Status. Note the child's hydration status. Palpate the infant's anterior and posterior fontanelles

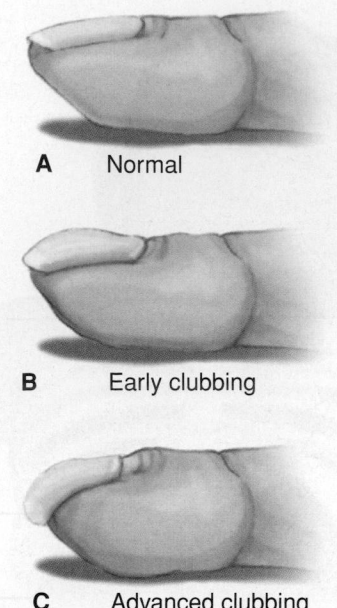

A Normal

B Early clubbing

C Advanced clubbing

FIGURE 40.4 **A.** Normal fingertip. Early clubbing (**B**) may progress eventually to advanced clubbing (**C**) as a result of chronic hypoxemia.

to determine if sunken. Assess the oral mucosa for colour and moisture. Note skin turgor, presence of tears, any weight changes, and adequacy of urine output. The child with a respiratory illness is at risk for dehydration. Pain related to sore throat or mouth lesions may prevent the child from drinking properly. Nasal congestion interferes with the infant's ability to suck effectively at the breast or bottle. Tachypnea and increased work of breathing interfere with the ability to safely ingest fluids.

Auscultation

Assess lung sounds via auscultation. Evaluate breath sounds over the anterior and posterior chest, as well as in the axillary areas. Note the adequacy of aeration. Breath sounds should be equal bilaterally. The intensity and pitch should be equal throughout the lungs; document diminished breath sounds. In the absence of concurrent lower respiratory illness, the breath sounds should be clear throughout all lung fields. During normal respiration, the inspiratory phase is usually softer and longer than the expiratory phase. Prolonged expiration is a sign of bronchial or bronchiolar obstruction. Bronchiolitis, asthma, pulmonary edema, and an intrathoracic foreign body can cause prolonged expiratory phases.

Infants and young children have thin chest walls. When the upper airway is congested (as in a severe cold), the noise produced in the upper airway might be transmitted throughout the lung fields. When upper airway congestion is transmitted to the lung fields, the congested sounding noise heard over the trachea is the same type of noise heard over the lungs but is much louder and more intense. To ascertain if these sounds are truly adventitious lung sounds or if they are transmitted from the upper airway, auscultate again after the child coughs or his or her nose has been suctioned. Another way to discern the difference is to compare auscultatory findings over the trachea to the lung fields to determine if the abnormal sound is truly from within the lung or is actually a sound transmitted from the upper airway.

Note adventitious sounds heard on auscultation. **Wheezing**, a high-pitched sound that usually occurs on expiration, results from obstruction in the lower trachea or bronchioles. Wheezing that occurs on inspiration and clears with coughing is most likely a result of secretions in the lower trachea. Wheezing resulting from obstruction of the bronchioles, as in bronchiolitis, asthma, chronic lung disease, or CF, does not clear with coughing. **Rales** (crackling sounds) result when the alveoli become fluid filled, such as in pneumonia. Note the location of the adventitious sounds as well as the timing (on inspiration, expiration, or both). Tachycardia might also be present. An increase in heart rate often initially accompanies hypoxemia. There are numerous online resources available offering audio clips of lung auscultation sounds. For example, see the MedEdu (2016) website at www.easyauscultation.com.

Percussion

When percussing, note sounds that are not resonant in nature. Flat or dull sounds might be percussed over partially consolidated lung tissue, as in pneumonia. Tympany might be percussed with a pneumothorax. Note the presence of hyperresonance (as might be apparent with asthma).

Palpation

Palpate the sinuses for tenderness in the older child. Assess for enlargement or tenderness of the lymph nodes of the head and neck. Document alterations in tactile fremitus detected on palpation. Increased tactile fremitus might occur in a case of pneumonia or pleural effusion. Fremitus might be decreased in the case of barrel chest, as with CF. Absent fremitus might be noted with pneumothorax or atelectasis. Palpate for crepitus as this might be noted with pneumothorax or occluded chest tube. Observe and palpate the chest wall for symmetry of movement, as this indicates decreased air flow into one lung.

Compare central and peripheral pulses. Note the quality of the pulse as well as the rate. With significant respiratory distress, perfusion often becomes compromised. Poor perfusion might be reflected in weaker peripheral pulses (radial, pedal) when compared with central pulses.

Laboratory and Diagnostic Testing

Common Laboratory and Diagnostic Tests 40.1 explains the laboratory and diagnostic tests most

COMMON LABORATORY AND DIAGNOSTIC TESTS 40.1 ALTERATIONS IN GAS EXCHANGE/ RESPIRATORY DISORDERS

Test	Explanation	Indications	Nursing Implications
Allergy skin testing	Suggested allergen is applied to skin via scratch, pin, or prick. A wheal response indicates allergy to the substance	Allergic rhinitis, asthma	Antihistamines must be discontinued 72 hours before testing, as they inhibit the test Close observation for anaphylaxis is necessary. Epinephrine and emergency equipment should be readily available Some children react to the skin test almost immediately; others take several minutes
Arterial blood gases	Invasive method (requires blood sampling) of measuring arterial pH, partial pressure of oxygen and carbon dioxide, and base excess in blood	Usually reserved for severe illness, the intubated child, or suspected carbon dioxide retention	Hold pressure for several minutes after a peripheral arterial stick to avoid bleeding Radial arterial sticks are common and can be very painful Note if the child is crying excessively during the blood draw, as this affects the carbon dioxide level
Chest x-ray	Radiographic image of the expanded lungs: can show hyperinflation, atelectasis, pneumonia, foreign body, pleural effusion, abnormal heart or lung size	Bronchiolitis, pneumonia, tuberculosis, asthma, cystic fibrosis, bronchopulmonary dysplasia	Children may be afraid of the x-ray equipment. If a parent or familiar adult can accompany the child, often the child is less afraid. If the child is unable or unwilling to hold still for the x-ray, restraint may be necessary. Restraint should be limited to the amount of time needed for the x-ray
Fluorescent antibody testing	Determines presence of respiratory syncytial virus (RSV), adenovirus, influenza, parainfluenza, or *Chlamydia* in nasopharyngeal secretions	Bronchiolitis, pneumonia	To obtain a nasopharyngeal specimen, use appropriate swab or obtain wash by instilling 1 to 3 mL of sterile normal saline into one nostril, aspirate the contents using a small sterile bulb syringe, place the contents in sterile container, and immediately send them to the lab
Fluoroscopy	Radiographic examination that uses a fluorescent screen "real-time" imaging	Identification of masses, abscesses	Requires the child to lie still. Equipment can be frightening. Children may respond to presence of parent or familiar adult
Gastric washings for acid-fast bacilli (AFB)	Determines presence of AFB in stomach (children often swallow sputum)	Tuberculosis	Nasogastric tube is inserted and saline is instilled and suctioned out of the stomach to obtain the specimen
Peak expiratory flow	Measures the maximum flow of air (in L/s) that can be forcefully exhaled in 1 second	Daily use can indicate adequacy of asthma control	It is important to establish the child's "personal best" by taking twice-daily readings over a 2-week period while well. The average of these is termed "personal best." Charts based on height and age are also available to determine expected peak expiratory flow
Pulmonary function tests	Measure respiratory flow and lung volumes	Asthma, cystic fibrosis, chronic lung disease	Usually performed by a respiratory therapist trained to do the full spectrum of tests. Spirometry can be obtained by the trained health provider in the outpatient setting
Pulse oximetry	Non-invasive method of continuously (or intermittently) measuring oxygen saturation	Can be useful in any situation in which a child is experiencing respiratory distress	Probe must be applied correctly to finger, toe, foot, hand, forehead, or ear for the machine to appropriately pick up the pulse and oxygen saturation. Check skin integrity under probe and adhesive

(continued)

COMMON LABORATORY AND DIAGNOSTIC TESTS 40.1 ALTERATIONS IN GAS EXCHANGE/ RESPIRATORY DISORDERS (continued)

Test	Explanation	Indications	Nursing Implications
Culture or rapid pertussis test via polymerase chain reaction	Determines presence of *Bordetella pertussis* in nasopharyngeal secretions	Pertussis or "whooping cough"	Collected via nasopharyngeal swab or washings. Many laboratories facilitate the use of a single nasopharyngeal specimen for multiple tests (e.g., fluorescent antibody tests and pertussis)
Rapid flu test	Rapid test for detection of influenza A or B	Influenza	Should be done in first 24 hours of illness so that medication administration can begin Have the child gargle with sterile normal saline and then spit into a sterile container. Send immediately to the lab
Rapid strep test	Instant test for presence of streptococcus A antibody in pharyngeal secretions	Pharyngitis, tonsillitis	Results in 5 to 10 minutes. Negative tests should be backed up with throat culture
RAST (radioallergo-sorbent test)	Measures minute quantities of immunoglobulin E in the blood Carries no risk of anaphylaxis but is not as sensitive as skin testing	Asthma (food allergies)	Blood test that is usually sent out to a reference laboratory
Sinus x-rays, computed tomography (CT), or magnetic resonance imaging (MRI)	Radiologic tests that may show sinus involvement	Sinusitis, recurrent colds	X-ray results are usually received more quickly than CT or MRI results
Sputum culture	Bacterial culture of invasive organisms in the sputum	Pneumonia, cystic fibrosis, tuberculosis	Must be true sputum, not mucus from the mouth or nose. Child can deep breathe, cough, and spit, or specimen may be obtained via suctioning of the artificial airway
Sweat chloride test	Collection of sweat on filter paper after stimulation of skin with pilocarpine Measures concentration of chloride in the sweat	Cystic fibrosis	May be difficult to obtain sweat in a young infant
Throat culture	Bacterial culture (minimum of 24 to 48 hours required) to determine presence of streptococcus A or other bacteria	Pharyngitis, tonsillitis	Can be obtained on separate swab at same time as rapid strep test to decrease trauma to the child (swab both applicators at once) Do not perform immediately after the child has had medication or something to eat or drink
Tuberculin skin test	Mantoux test (intradermal injection of purified protein derivative)	Tuberculosis, chronic cough	Must be given intradermally; not a valid test if injected incorrectly Must be read between 48 and 72 hours after administration by a trained health care provider

Adapted from Beckton Dickinson and Company. (2016). *Product center*. Retrieved from http://www.bd.com/ds/productCenter/index.asp; Corbett, J. A., & Banks, A. D. (2013). *Laboratory tests and diagnostic procedures with nursing diagnoses* (8th ed.). Upper Saddle River, NJ: Pearson Education Inc., and Fouzas, S., Priftis, K. N., & Anthracopoulos, M. B. (2011). Pulse oximetry in pediatric practice. *Pediatrics, 128*, 740–752.

commonly used for a child with a respiratory disorder. The tests can assist the physician or nurse practitioner in diagnosing the disorder and/or be used as guidelines in determining ongoing treatment. Laboratory or non-nursing personnel obtain some of the tests, while the nurse might obtain others. In either instance, it is important for the nurse to be familiar with how the tests are obtained, what they are used for, and normal versus abnormal results. This knowledge will also be necessary when providing child and family education related to the testing.

Take Note!

Ambient light may interfere with pulse oximetry readings. When the pulse oximeter probe is placed on the infant's foot or the young child's toe, covering the probe and foot with a sock may help to ensure an accurate measurement (Fouzas, Priftis, & Anthracopoulos, 2011).

Nursing Diagnoses, Goals, Interventions, and Evaluation

Upon completion of a thorough assessment, the nurse might identify several nursing diagnoses, including:
- Ineffective airway clearance
- Ineffective breathing pattern
- Impaired gas exchange
- Risk for infection
- Pain
- Risk for fluid volume deficit
- Altered nutrition, less than body requirements
- Activity intolerance
- Fear
- Altered family processes

After completing an assessment of Alexander, the nurse notes the following: lots of clear secretions in the airway, child appears pale, respiratory rate 68, retractions, nasal flaring, wheezing, and diminished breath sounds. Based on these assessment findings, what would your top three nursing diagnoses be for Alexander?

Nursing goals, interventions, and evaluation for the child with a respiratory disorder are based on the nursing diagnoses. Nursing Care Plan 40.1 (at the end of the chapter) can be used as a guide in planning nursing care for the child with a respiratory disorder. The nursing care plan should be individualized based on the child's symptoms and needs; refer to Chapter 36 for detailed information on pain management. Additional information will be included later in the chapter as it relates to specific disorders.

Based on your top three nursing diagnoses for Alexander, describe appropriate nursing interventions.

Providing Oxygen Supplementation

Oxygen may be delivered to the child by a variety of methods (Fig. 40.5). Since oxygen is considered a drug, it requires a physician or nurse practitioner's order, except when following emergency protocols outlined in a health care facility's policies and procedures. Many health care settings develop specific guidelines for oxygen administration that are often coordinated by respiratory therapists, yet the nurse remains responsible for ensuring that oxygen is administered properly.

Oxygen sources include wall-mounted systems as well as cylinders. The supply of oxygen available from a wall-mounted source is limitless, but use of a wall-mounted source restricts the child to the hospital room. Cylinders are portable oxygen tanks and are useful for the child on low-flow oxygen because it allows for mobility. The tank empties relatively quickly if the child requires a high flow of oxygen, so this is not the best oxygen source in an emergency.

Take Note!

Oxygen is highly flammable, so use safety precautions. Post signs ("Oxygen in Use"); inform the family to avoid matches, lighters, and flammable or volatile materials; and use only facility-approved equipment.

The efficiency of oxygen delivery systems is affected by several variables, including the child's respiratory effort, the litre flow of oxygen delivered, and whether the equipment is being used appropriately. In general, oxygen facemasks come in infant, child, and adult sizes. Select the mask that best fits the child. In addition, ensure that the mask is sealed properly to decrease the amount of oxygen that escapes from the mask. Ensure that the litre flow is set according to the manufacturer's recommendations for use with that delivery method. The oxygen flow rate or concentration is usually determined by the physician or nurse practitioner's order. There is inconclusive evidence in the literature regarding the use of humidification during oxygen delivery, though it is generally deemed unnecessary when flow rate is less than 4 L/min (WHO, 2016). Table 40.1 provides details on oxygen delivery methods.

Take Note!

Monitor vital signs, colour, respiratory effort, pulse oximetry, and level of consciousness before, during, and after oxygen therapy to evaluate its effectiveness.

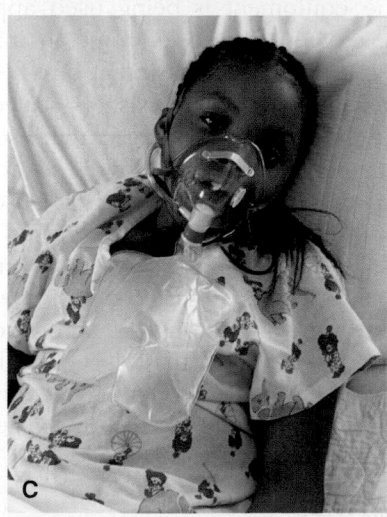

FIGURE 40.5 **A.** Simple oxygen mask provides about 40% oxygen. **B.** The nasal cannula provides an additional 4% oxygen per 1 L of oxygen flow (i.e., 1 L will deliver 25% oxygen). **C.** The nonrebreather mask provides 80% to 100% oxygen.

ACUTE INFECTIOUS DISORDERS

Acute infectious disorders include, but are not limited to, the common cold, sinusitis, influenza, pharyngitis, tonsillitis, laryngitis, croup syndromes, bronchiolitis, pneumonia, and bronchitis.

Common Cold

The common cold is also referred to as a viral upper respiratory infection (URI) or nasopharyngitis. Colds can be caused by rhinoviruses, parainfluenza, respiratory syncytial virus (RSV), enteroviruses, adenoviruses, and human metapneumovirus. Viral particles spread through the air or from person-to-person contact. Colds occur more frequently in the winter months, however can occur all year around. They affect children of all ages and have a higher incidence among children who attend day care and school-age children (Yoon, Scholes, & Friedman, 2014). It is not unusual for a child to have six to nine colds per year. Spontaneous resolution of the common cold occurs after about 7 to 10 days. Potential complications include dehydration and secondary bacterial infections of the ears, throat, sinuses, or lungs.

Therapeutic management of the common cold is directed toward symptom relief. Nasal congestion may be relieved via humidity and use of normal saline nasal wash or spray followed by **suctioning**. Antihistamines are not indicated, as they dry secretions further.

Take Note!

In 2009, over-the-counter cough and cold preparations intended for use in children under 6 years of age were removed from the market. Several research studies have not shown the preparations to be effective and they are known to have potentially serious side effects (Health Canada, 2016a; Yust & Slattery, 2012).

Nursing Assessment

The child with a common cold may have either a stuffy or runny nose. Nasal discharge is usually thin and watery at first but may become thicker and discoloured. The colour of nasal discharge is not an accurate indicator of viral versus bacterial infection. The child may be hoarse and complain of a sore throat. Cough usually produces very little sputum. Fever, fatigue, watery eyes, and appetite loss may also occur. Symptoms are generally at their worst over the first few days and then decrease over the course of the illness.

Assess for risk factors such as day-care or school attendance. Inspect for edema and vasodilation of the mucosa. Diagnosis is based on clinical presentation rather than laboratory or x-ray studies.

Nursing Management

Nursing management of the child with a common cold consists of promoting comfort, providing family education, and preventing spread of the cold.

TABLE 40.1	OXYGEN DELIVERY METHODS	
Delivery Method	**Description**	**Nursing Implications**
Simple mask	Provides 35–60% oxygen with a flow rate of 6–10 L/min. Oxygen delivery percentage is affected by respiratory rate, inspiratory flow, and adequacy of mask fit	• Must maintain oxygen flow rate of at least 6 L/min to maintain inspired oxygen concentration and prevent rebreathing of carbon dioxide • Mask must fit snugly to be effective but should not be so tight as to irritate the face
Venturi mask	Provides 24–50% oxygen by using a special gauge at the base of the mask that allows mixing of room air with oxygen flow	• Set oxygen flow rate according to percentage of oxygen desired as indicated on the gauge/dial • As with simple mask, must fit snugly
Nasal cannula	Provides low oxygen concentration (22–44%)	• Can provide very small amounts of oxygen (as low as 25 mL/min) • Maximum recommended litre flow in children is 4 L/min • Children can eat or talk while on oxygen • Inspired oxygen concentration affected by mouth breathing • Requires patent nasal passages
Partial rebreathing mask	Simple facemask with an oxygen reservoir bag. Provides 50–60% oxygen concentration	• Must set litre flow rate at 10–12 L/min to prevent rebreathing of carbon dioxide • The reservoir bag does not completely empty when child inspires if flow rate is set properly
Nonrebreathing mask	Simple facemask with valves at the exhalation ports and an oxygen reservoir bag with a valve to prevent exhaled air from entering the reservoir. Provides 95% oxygen concentration	• Must set litre flow rate at 10–12 L/min to prevent rebreathing of carbon dioxide • The reservoir bag does not completely empty when child inspires if flow rate is set properly

Adapted from American Heart Association. (2011). *Pediatric advanced life support provider manual*. Dallas, TX: Author; and Bowden, V. R., & Greenberg, C. S. (2012). *Pediatric nursing procedures* (3rd ed.). Philadelphia, PA: Lippincott Williams & Wilkins.

PROMOTING COMFORT

Nursing care of the common cold is aimed at supportive measures. Nasal congestion may be relieved with the use of normal saline nose drops, followed by bulb syringe suctioning in infants and toddlers. Older children may use a normal saline nose spray to mobilize secretions. A cool mist humidifier also helps with nasal congestion. Generally, other over-the-counter nose sprays are not recommended for use in children, but they are sometimes prescribed by a Physician or Nurse Practitioner for very short-term use. Promotion of adequate oral fluid intake is important to loosen secretions.

Educate parents about the use of cold and cough medications. Although they may offer some symptomatic relief, they have not been proven to shorten the length of cold symptoms. Counsel parents to use the appropriate product depending on the symptom relief desired, rather than a combination product. Products containing acetaminophen combined with other "cold symptom" medications may mask a fever in the child who is developing a secondary bacterial infection. As with all viral infections in children, teach parents that aspirin use should be avoided because of its association with Reye syndrome (Clute, 2014).

PROVIDING FAMILY EDUCATION

Currently, there are no medications available to treat the viruses that cause the common cold, so symptomatic treatment is all that is necessary. Antibiotics do not reduce symptoms or the incidence of complications from the common cold and are associated with adverse effects in children (Kenealy & Arroll, 2013). See Evidence-Based Practice 40.1. Explain to parents the importance of reserving antibiotic use for appropriate illnesses. Provide education about the use of normal saline nose drops and **bulb suctioning** to clear the infant's nose of secretions. Normal saline nasal wash using a bulb syringe to instil the solution is also helpful for children of all ages with nasal congestion. Though normal saline for nasal administration is available commercially, parents can also make it at home (Box 40.2). Teaching Guidelines 40.1 gives instructions on use of the bulb syringe.

Counsel parents about how to recognize complications of the common cold, which includes:
• Prolonged fever (37.5°C axillary or higher for 3 days or more, or any fever over 37.5°C axillary or 38°C rectally in an infant under 3 months of age [Canadian Paediatric Society, 2017b]).

BOX 40.2

HOMEMADE SALT WATER NOSE DROPS

Mix 250-mL distilled water, a half-teaspoon sea salt, and a quarter-teaspoon baking soda. Keep for 24 hours in the refrigerator, but should be allowed to come to room temperature prior to use.

- Increased throat pain or enlarged, painful lymph nodes
- Increased or worsening cough, cough lasting longer than 10 days, chest pain, difficulty breathing
- Earache, headache, tooth or sinus pain
- Unusual irritability or lethargy
- Skin rash
- Dehydration

Teaching Guidelines 40.1

USING THE BULB SYRINGE TO SUCTION NASAL SECRETIONS

1. Hold the infant on your lap or on the bed with the head tilted slightly back.

2. If using saline, instil several drops of saline solution in one of the infant's nostrils.

3. Compress the sides of the bulb syringe completely. Use only a rubber-tipped bulb syringe. Place the rubber tip in the infant's nose.

4. Release pressure on the bulb.

5. Remove the syringe and squeeze bulb over tissue or the sink to empty it of secretions.

6. Repeat on other nostril if necessary. Using a bulb syringe prior to bottle-feeding or breastfeeding may relieve congestion enough to allow the infant to suck more efficiently.
7. Clean the bulb syringe thoroughly with warm water after each use and allow to air dry.

EVIDENCE-BASED PRACTICE 40.1 — ANTIBIOTICS FOR THE COMMON COLD AND ACUTE PURULENT RHINITIS

STUDY

Though the common cold is known to be viral in origin, antibiotics continue to be prescribed for colds and purulent rhinitis as treatment or for prophylaxis against development of a bacterial infection. Overuse of antibiotics is known to contribute to the problem of antibiotic resistance. The review included 11 randomized controlled trials evaluating the effectiveness of antibiotics versus placebo in the common cold or acute purulent rhinitis.

Findings

Use of antibiotics for the common cold and acute purulent rhinitis is not effective. In the studies reviewed, use of antibiotics did not contribute to cure, nor did it decrease persistence of symptoms as compared with placebo.

Nursing Implications

Nurses should consider the results of this review. With antibiotic resistance continuing to rise, it is important to support non-use of antibiotics in the instance of viral infections. Teach families about the difference between viral and bacterial illness. Provide support and ensure that families understand the natural history of the common cold and that when symptoms persist rather than improve over time, they should reconnect with their physician or nurse practitioner.

Adapted from Kenealy, T., & Arroll, B. (2013). Antibiotics for the common cold and acute purulent rhinitis. *Cochrane Database of Systematic Reviews,* *6*, CD000247. doi: 10.1002/14651858.CD000247.pub3.

If complications do occur, tell parents to seek medical advice. Depending on the severity, this may involve calling a health provider, attending a primary care or walk-in clinic, or seeking emergency services. Most provinces have 24-hour health information lines where parents can speak to a health professional prior to seeking emergency or after hours' care.

PREVENTING THE COMMON COLD

Teaching about ways to prevent the common cold is a vital nursing intervention. Explain that frequent handwashing helps to decrease the spread of viruses that cause the common cold. Teach parents and family to avoid second-hand smoke as well as crowded places, especially during the winter. Avoid close contact with individuals known to have a cold. Encourage parents and families to consume a healthy diet and get enough rest.

Consider This

Corey Davis, a 3-year old, is brought to the clinic by her mother. She presents with a runny nose, congestion, and a non-productive cough. Her mother says, "She's miserable." "I just don't know what to do." "Ever since I put her in day care she gets sick every few weeks." "This is all my fault."

How should the nurse respond? How would you feel if your child was healthy until entering day care? What type of support can the nurse provide to Corey's mother?

Sinusitis

Sinusitis, or rhinosinusitis, refers to inflammation of the paranasal sinuses, and can be a result of allergic, viral, bacterial, or environmental causes (Brook, 2013; Fryters & Blondell-Hill, 2014). Approximately 2% to 10% of URIs are a result of dental disease, and 6% to 13% of cases are complicated with acute bacterial sinusitis (Fryters & Blondell-Hill, 2014). In young children, the maxillary and ethmoid sinuses are the main sites of infection. After age 10 years, the frontal sinuses may be more commonly involved (Yoon et al., 2014). Mucosal swelling, decreased ciliary movement, and thickened nasal discharge all contribute to bacterial invasion of the nose. Nasal polyps also place the child at risk for bacterial sinusitis. Complications include orbital cellulitis and intracranial infections, such as subdural empyemas.

Symptoms lasting less than 30 days generally indicate acute sinusitis, whereas symptoms persisting longer than 4 to 6 weeks usually indicate chronic sinusitis. Bacterial sinusitis is managed with antibiotic treatment. The therapeutic management approach varies with chronicity. The course of treatment is usually 14 days. Naturally, chronic sinusitis requires a longer course of treatment than acute bacterial sinusitis. Surgical therapy may be indicated for children with chronic sinusitis, particularly if it is recurrent or if nasal polyps are present.

Nursing Assessment

The most common presentation of bacterial sinusitis is persistent signs and symptoms of a cold. Rather than improving after 7 to 10 days, nasal discharge persists. Explore the history for:

- Cough
- Fever
- In pre-schoolers or older children, halitosis (bad breath)
- Facial pain may or may not be present, so is not a reliable indicator of disease

- Eyelid edema (in the case of ethmoid sinus involvement)
- Irritability
- Poor appetite

Assess for risk factors such as a history of recurrent cold symptoms or a history of nasal polyps.

On physical examination, note eyelid swelling, extent of nasal drainage, and halitosis. Inspect the throat for postnasal drainage. Inspect the nasal mucosa for erythema. Palpate the sinuses, noting pain with mild pressure. The diagnosis may be made based on the history and clinical presentation. The use of x-ray, computed tomography scan, or magnetic resonance imaging is not necessary as they are not specific and do not distinguish viral from bacterial infection (Brook, 2013).

Nursing Management

Normal saline nose drops or spray, cool mist humidifiers, and adequate oral fluid intake are recommended for children with sinusitis. Teach families the importance of continuing the full course of antibiotics to eradicate the cause of infection. Also educate the family that the use of decongestants, antihistamines, and intranasal steroids as adjuncts in the treatment of sinusitis has not been shown to be beneficial (Brook, 2013). Normal saline nose spray or nasal washes may promote drainage.

Influenza

Influenza viral infection (known commonly as the "flu") occurs primarily during the winter. It is spread through inhalation of droplets or contact with fine-particle aerosols. Infected children shed the virus for 1 to 2 days before symptoms begin and may continue shedding the virus in increased amounts (as compared with adults) for as long as 2 weeks. Average annual infection rates in children range from 20% to 30% (Pubic Health Agency of Canada, 2016). Influenza viruses primarily affect the upper respiratory epithelium but can cause systemic effects as well. Children with chronic heart or lung conditions, diabetes, chronic renal disease, or immune deficiency are at higher risk for more severe influenza infection compared with other children.

Bacterial infections of the respiratory system commonly occur as complications of influenza infection, severe pneumococcal pneumonia in particular. Otitis media occurs in 18% to 40% of all influenza cases (Wright, 2011). Less common complications include Reye syndrome and acute myositis. Reye syndrome is an acute encephalopathy that has been associated with aspirin use in the influenza-infected child (Clute, 2014). Acute myositis is particular to children. A sudden onset of severe pain and tenderness in both calves causes the child to refuse to walk. Due to the potential for complications, a prolonged fever or a fever that returns during convalescence should be investigated.

Take Note!

Current recommendations are for all children older than 6 months of age to be immunized yearly against influenza (Government of Canada, 2017).

Nursing Assessment

Children who attend day care or school are at higher risk for influenza infection than those who are routinely at home. Note the presence of risk factors for severe disease, such as low socioeconomic scores, chronic heart, lung, or renal disease, diabetes, immune deficiency, or children with cancer receiving chemotherapy. School-age children and adolescents experience the illness similarly to adults. Abrupt onset of fever, facial flushing, chills, headache, myalgia, and malaise are accompanied by cough and **coryza** (nasal discharge). About half of infected individuals have a dry or sore throat. Ocular symptoms such as photophobia, tearing, burning, and eye pain are common.

Infants and young children exhibit symptoms like other respiratory illnesses. Fever greater than 39.5°C is common. Infants may be mildly toxic in appearance, irritable, have a cough, coryza, and pharyngitis. Wheezing may occur, as influenza also can cause bronchiolitis. An erythematous rash may be present and diarrhea may also occur. The diagnosis may be confirmed by a rapid assay test.

Nursing Management

Nursing management of influenza is mainly supportive. Symptomatic treatment of cough and fever and maintenance of hydration are the focus of care. Antiviral drugs can reduce the symptoms associated with influenza if they are started within the first 12 to 48 hours of the illness (Allen, 2018; Wright, 2011).

Pharyngitis

Inflammation of the throat mucosa (pharynx) is referred to as pharyngitis. A sore throat may accompany nasal congestion and is often viral in nature. Bacterial pharyngitis most often occurs without nasal symptoms or cough. Group A streptococci account for 15% to 30% of cases, are most common in school-aged children and teenagers, and rare in children under 3 years of age. The remainder are caused by other viruses or bacteria (John & Brady, 2013b; Schulman et al., 2012).

Suppurative complications of group A streptococcal infection include peritonsillar or retropharyngeal abscess. Peritonsillar abscess may be noted by asymmetric swelling of the tonsils, shifting of the uvula to one side, and palatal edema. Retropharyngeal abscess may progress to the point of airway obstruction, hence requiring careful evaluation and appropriate treatment. Additional complications include acute rheumatic fever (see Chapter 41) and acute glomerulonephritis (see Chapter 43).

Viral pharyngitis is usually self-limited and does not require therapy beyond symptomatic relief. Group A streptococcal pharyngitis requires antibiotic therapy. If either the rapid diagnostic test or throat culture (described below) is positive for group A streptococci, penicillin is generally prescribed. Appropriate alternative antibiotics include amoxicillin, mainly for those allergic to penicillin, macrolides, and cephalosporins.

Take Note!

A "strep carrier" is a child who has a positive throat culture for streptococci when asymptomatic. Strep carriers are not at risk for complications from streptococci, as are those who are acutely infected with streptococci and are symptomatic (Hayden & Turner, 2011).

Nursing Assessment

Onset of pharyngitis is often quite abrupt. The history may include a fever, sore throat and difficulty swallowing, headache, and abdominal pain. Enquire about recent incidence of viral or strep throat in the family, day care centre, or school.

Inspect the pharynx and tonsils, which may demonstrate varying degrees of inflammation (Fig. 40.6). Exudate may be present but is not diagnostic of bacterial infection. Note the presence of petechiae on the palate. Inspect the tongue for a strawberry appearance. Palpate for enlargement and tenderness of the anterior cervical nodes. Inspect the skin for a fine, red, sandpaper-like rash (called scarlatiniform), particularly on the trunk or abdomen, a common finding with streptococcus A infection. The nurse may obtain a throat swab for rapid diagnostic testing and throat culture. The rapid strep test is a sensitive and reliable measure, rarely resulting in false-positive readings (John & Brady, 2013b). If the rapid strep test is negative, the second swab may be sent for a throat culture.

Atraumatic Care 40.1

When obtaining two swabs for rapid strep testing and throat culture, swab the applicators simultaneously to decrease perceived trauma to the child.

Nursing Management

Nursing management of the child with pharyngitis focuses on promoting comfort and providing family education (Atraumatic Care 40.1).

PROMOTING COMFORT

Saline gargles (made with 250 mL of warm water and a half teaspoon of table salt) or honey and warm water are soothing for children old enough to cooperate. Analgesics such as acetaminophen and ibuprofen may ease pain and reduce fever. Sucking on throat lozenges or hard candy may also ease pain. Cool mist humidity helps to keep the mucosa moist in the event of mouth breathing. Encourage the child to ingest popsicles, cool liquids, and ice chips to maintain hydration.

PROVIDING FAMILY EDUCATION

Parents may be accustomed to "sore throats" being treated with antibiotics. However, in the case of a viral cause, antibiotics will not be necessary and may be harmful and the pharyngitis will resolve in a few days. For the child with streptococcal pharyngitis, urge parents to have the child complete the entire prescribed course of antibiotics. After 24 hours of antibiotic therapy, instruct the parents to discard the child's toothbrush to avoid reinfection. Children may return to day care or school after they have been receiving antibiotics for 24 hours.

Tonsillitis

Inflammation of the tonsils often occurs with pharyngitis and, thus, may also be viral or bacterial in nature. Viral infections require only symptomatic treatment. Treatment for bacterial tonsillitis is the same as for bacterial pharyngitis. Occasionally surgical intervention is warranted. Tonsillectomy (surgical removal of the palatine

FIGURE 40.6 Note the redness of the pharynx, tonsillar exudate, and white strawberry tongue coating.

tonsils) may be indicated for the child with recurrent streptococcal tonsillitis, massive tonsillar hypertrophy, or for other reasons. When hypertrophied adenoids obstruct breathing, then adenoidectomy (surgical removal of the adenoids) may be indicated.

Nursing Assessment

Note whether fever is present currently or by history. Enquire about the history of recurrent pharyngitis or tonsillitis. Note if the child's voice sounds muffled or hoarse. Inspect the pharynx for redness and enlargement of the tonsils. As the tonsils enlarge, the child may experience difficulty breathing and swallowing. When tonsils touch at the midline ("kissing tonsils" or 4+ in size), the airway may become obstructed. Also, if the adenoids are enlarged, the posterior nares become obstructed. The child may breathe through the mouth and may snore. Palpate the anterior cervical nodes for enlargement and tenderness. Rapid test or culture may be positive for streptococcus A.

Nursing Management

Tonsillitis that is medically treated requires the same nursing management as pharyngitis. Nursing care for the child after tonsillectomy is described below.

PROMOTING AIRWAY CLEARANCE

Until fully awake, place the child in a side-lying or prone position to facilitate safe drainage of secretions. Once alert, the child may prefer to sit up or have the head of the bed elevated. Suctioning, if necessary, should be done carefully to avoid trauma to the surgical site. Dried blood may be present on the teeth and the nares, with old blood present in emesis. Since the presence of blood can be very frightening to parents, alert them to this possibility.

MAINTAINING FLUID VOLUME

Hemorrhage is unusual postoperatively but may occur any time from the immediate postoperative period to as late as 10 days after surgery. Inspect the throat for bleeding. Mucus tinged with blood may be expected, but fresh blood in the secretions indicates bleeding. Early bleeding may be identified by continuous swallowing of small amounts of blood while awake or sleeping. Other signs of hemorrhage include tachycardia, pallor, restlessness, frequent throat clearing or rapid swallowing, and emesis of bright red blood.

To avoid trauma to the surgical site, discourage the child from coughing, clearing the throat, blowing the nose, and using straws. Upon discharge, instruct the parents to immediately report any sign of bleeding to the physician or nurse practitioner. To maintain fluid volume postoperatively, encourage children to take any fluids they desire; popsicles and ice chips are particularly soothing. Citrus juice and brown or red fluids should be avoided: the acid in citrus juice may irritate the throat, and red or brown fluids may be confused with blood if vomiting occurs.

RELIEVING PAIN

For the first 24 hours after surgery, the throat is very sore. Adequate pain relief is essential to establish adequate oral fluid intake. An ice collar may be prescribed, as well as analgesics with or without narcotics. Note that codeine is no longer indicated in children under 18 years of age for postoperative pain management following tonsillectomy or adenoidectomy due to risk of serious respiratory complications. Codeine is also contraindicated in children under 12 for all indications (Health Canada, 2016b). Counsel parents to maintain pain control upon discharge from the facility, not only for comfort, but to promote oral intake.

Infectious Mononucleosis

Infectious mononucleosis is a self-limited illness most commonly caused by the Epstein–Barr virus (EBV). It is characterized by fever, malaise, sore throat, and lymphadenopathy. Mononucleosis is commonly called the "kissing disease" since it is transmitted by oropharyngeal secretions. It can occur at any age but is most often diagnosed in adolescents and young adults (Blosser, Brady, & Royal, 2013). Some infected individuals may have concomitant streptococcal pharyngitis. Complications include splenic rupture, Guillain–Barré syndrome, and aseptic meningitis.

Nursing Assessment

Note any history of exposure to infected individuals. Determine history of fever and onset and progression of sore throat, malaise, and other complaints. Observe for periorbital edema. Inspect the pharynx and tonsils for inflammation and patches of grey exudate. Petechiae may be present on the palate. Palpate for bilateral nontender enlargement of the posterior cervical lymph nodes. After 3 to 5 days of illness, the pharynx may become edematous and the tonsillar exudate more extensive. Lymphadenopathy may progress to include the anterior cervical nodes, which may become tender. Palpate and/or percuss the abdomen for splenomegaly or hepatomegaly. An erythematous maculopapular rash may appear as the illness progresses. Monospot or EBV titers can assist with confirming diagnosis.

Take Note!

The Monospot is usually negative if obtained within the first 7 to 10 days of illness with infectious mononucleosis since it can produce both false positive and false negative results (Centers for Disease Control and Prevention [CDC], 2016). EBV titer is reliable at any point in the illness for EBV mononucleosis (Blosser et al., 2013).

Nursing Management

Nursing management of mononucleosis is primarily symptomatic. The throat may be very sore, so analgesics and salt-water gargles are recommended. Bed rest should be encouraged while the child is febrile. Frequent rest periods may be necessary for several weeks after the onset of illness, as fatigue may persist for up to 6 weeks. During the acute phase, if tonsillar or pharyngeal edema threatens to obstruct the airway, then corticosteroids may be given to decrease the inflammation. In the presence of splenomegaly or hepatomegaly, strenuous activity and contact sports should be avoided for approximately 3 weeks following illness, or as determined by the physician or nurse practitioner based on the individual case (Becker & Smith, 2014). Appearance of rash or jaundice should be reported to the physician or nurse practitioner.

Laryngitis

Inflammation of the larynx is termed laryngitis. It may occur alone or in conjunction with other respiratory symptoms. It is characterized by a hoarse voice or loss of the voice (so soft as to make it difficult to hear). Oral fluids might offer relief, but resting the voice for 24 hours will allow the inflammation to subside. Laryngitis alone requires no further intervention.

Croup

Children between 3 months and 3 years of age are most frequently affected with croup, though it can occur in all ages (John & Brady, 2013b). Croup is also referred to as laryngotracheobronchitis because inflammation and edema of the larynx, trachea, and bronchi occur as a result of viral infection. Parainfluenza is responsible for the majority of cases of croup (John & Brady, 2013b). Other causes include adenovirus, influenza virus

A and B, RSV, and rarely measles virus or *Mycoplasma pneumoniae*. The inflammation and edema obstruct the airway, resulting in symptoms. Mucus production also occurs, further contributing to obstruction of the airway. Narrowing of the subglottic area of the trachea results in audible inspiratory stridor. Edema of the larynx causes hoarseness. Inflammation in the larynx and trachea causes the characteristic barking cough of croup.

Symptoms occur most often at night, presenting suddenly, with resolution of symptoms in the morning. Croup is usually self-limited, lasting only about 3 to 5 days. Complications of croup are rare but may include worsening respiratory distress, hypoxia, or bacterial superinfection (as in the case of bacterial tracheitis).

Croup is usually managed on an outpatient basis, with affected children rarely requiring hospitalization. Corticosteroids (usually a single dose) are used to decrease inflammation, and nebulized epinephrine demonstrates the α-adrenergic effect of mucosal vasoconstriction, helping to decrease edema (Canadian Paediatric Society, 2017c). Children with croup may be hospitalized if they have significant stridor at rest or severe retractions after several hours of observation. Comparison Chart 40.1 compares croup to epiglottitis.

Nursing Assessment

Note the age of the child; children between 3 months and 3 years of age are most likely to present with viral croup. History may reveal a cough that developed during the night (most common presentation) and that sounds like barking (or a seal). Inspect for the presence of mild URI symptoms. Temperature may be normal or elevated mildly. Listen for inspiratory stridor and observe for suprasternal retractions. Auscultate the lungs for adequacy of breath sounds. Croup is usually diagnosed based on history and clinical presentation, but a lateral neck x-ray may be obtained to rule out epiglottitis.

COMPARISON CHART 40.1	CROUP VERSUS EPIGLOTTITIS	
	Spasmodic Croup	**Epiglottitis**
Preceding illness	None or minimal coryza	None or mild URI
Age group usually affected	3 months to 3 years	1–8 years
Onset	Usually sudden, often at night	Rapid (within hours)
Fever	Variable	High
Barking cough, hoarseness	Yes	No
Dysphagia	No	Yes
Toxic appearance	No	Yes
Drooling	No	Yes
Cause	Viral	*Haemophilus influenzae* type B

Take Note!

The child with fever, a toxic appearance, and increasing respiratory distress despite appropriate croup treatment may have bacterial tracheitis. Notify the physician or nurse practitioner of these findings in a child with croup (John & Brady, 2013b).

Nursing Management

If the child's care is being managed at home, advise parents about the symptoms of respiratory distress and instruct them to seek treatment if the child's respiratory condition worsens. Teach parents to expose their child to humidified air (via a cool mist humidifier or steamy bathroom). Though not clinically proven, use of humidified air has long been recommended for alleviating paroxysmal coughing, and has been anecdotally reported as helpful (particularly exposure to cooler air). Administer dexamethasone if ordered or teach parents about home administration. Explain to parents that the effects of epinephrine last about 2 hours and the child must be observed closely, as occasionally a child will worsen again, requiring another aerosol. Teaching Guidelines 40.2 provides information about home care of croup.

Teaching Guidelines 40.2
HOME CARE OF CROUP

- Encourage quiet activities and avoid crying that triggers as much as possible.
- Allow the child to sit up (in your arms).
- Encourage rest and fluid intake.
- If stridor occurs, take the child into a steamy bathroom for 10 minutes, or expose to cold air (e.g., outside or near open freezer).
- Administer medication (corticosteroid) as directed.
- Watch the child closely. Go to the emergency department if:
  - The child breathes faster, has retractions, or has any other difficulty breathing
  - The nostrils flare or the lips or nails have a bluish tint
  - The cough or stridor does not improve with exposure to moist air
  - Restlessness increases or the child is confused or lethargic
  - The child begins to drool or cannot swallow

Adapted from Durani, Y. (2012). *Croup*. Retrieved from http://kidshealth.org/parent/infections/lung/croup.html

---

Epiglottitis

Epiglottitis (inflammation and swelling of the epiglottis) is most often caused by *Haemophilus influenzae* type b.

Extensive use of the Hib vaccine since the 1980s has resulted in a significant decrease in the incidence of epiglottitis (John & Brady, 2013b). Though now rare, epiglottitis most often occurs in children between the ages of 2 and 7 years and can be life-threatening (John & Brady, 2013b). Respiratory arrest and death may occur if the airway becomes completely occluded. Additional complications include pneumothorax and pulmonary edema. Therapeutic management focuses on airway maintenance and support. Intravenous antibiotic therapy is necessary. The child will be managed in the intensive care unit. See Comparison Chart 40.1 for information comparing croup to epiglottitis.

Nursing Assessment

Carefully assess the child with suspected epiglottitis. Note sudden onset of symptoms, high fever, and if the child has an overall toxic appearance. He or she may refuse to speak or may speak only with a very soft voice. The child may refuse to lie down and may assume the characteristic position: sitting forward with the neck extended. Drooling may be present. Note anxiety or a frightened appearance. Note the child's colour. Cough is usually absent. A lateral neck x-ray may be performed to determine whether epiglottitis is present. This is done cautiously, so as not to induce airway obstruction with changes in position of the child's neck.

Take Note!

Do not under any circumstance attempt to visualize the throat: reflex laryngospasm may occur, precipitating immediate airway occlusion (John & Brady, 2013b).

Nursing Management

Do not leave the child unattended. Keep the child and parents as calm as possible. Allow the child to assume a position of comfort. Do not place the child in a supine position, as airway occlusion may occur. Provide 100% oxygen in the least invasive manner that is acceptable to the child. If the child with epiglottitis experiences complete airway occlusion, an emergency tracheostomy may be necessary. Ensure that emergency equipment is available and that personnel trained in intubation of the pediatric occluded airway and percutaneous tracheostomy are notified of the child's presence in the facility.

Bronchiolitis

Bronchiolitis is an acute inflammatory process of the bronchioles and small bronchi. Nearly always caused by a viral pathogen, RSV accounts for the majority of cases of bronchiolitis, with adenovirus, parainfluenza, and human meta-pneumovirus also being important causative agents. This discussion will focus on RSV bronchiolitis.

RSV season in Canada generally begins in November and continues through March, with the exception of northern communities where RSV begins in December and lasts until April (Canadian Paediatric Society, 2015). Virtually all children will contract RSV infection within the first few years of life. RSV bronchiolitis occurs most often in infants and toddlers, with a peak incidence around 6 months of age (DeNicola, Maraqa, Udeani, & Custodio, 2016). Infants residing in remote Inuit communities are more likely to progress to severe RSV and require hospitalization (Robinson & Le Saux, 2018). The severity of disease is also related inversely to the age of the child; decreasing with age. Repeated RSV infections occur throughout life but are usually localized to the upper respiratory tract after toddlerhood. Children at high risk for complication with RSV may qualify for immunization against this virus. See local/provincial qualifications for this vaccine.

Pathophysiology

RSV is a highly contagious virus and may be contracted through direct contact with respiratory secretions or from particles on objects contaminated with the virus. RSV invades the nasopharynx, where it replicates and then spreads down to the lower airway via aspiration of upper airway secretions. RSV infection causes necrosis of the respiratory epithelium of the small airways, peribronchiolar mononuclear infiltration, and plugging of the lumens with mucus and exudate. The small airways become variably obstructed; this allows adequate inspiratory volume but prevents full expiration. This leads to hyperinflation and atelectasis. Serious alterations in gas exchange occur, with arterial hypoxemia and carbon dioxide retention resulting from mismatching of pulmonary **ventilation** (gas exchange within the lungs) and perfusion. Hypoventilation occurs secondary to markedly increased work of breathing.

Therapeutic Management

Management of RSV focuses on supportive treatment. Supplemental oxygen, nasal and/or nasopharyngeal suctioning, oral or intravenous hydration, and inhaled bronchodilator therapy (epinephrine or albuterol/levalbuterol) may be used, depending on the child and their medical risk factors. Many infants are managed at home with close observation and adequate hydration. Hospitalization is required for children with more severe disease. The infant with tachypnea, significant retractions, poor oral intake, or lethargy can deteriorate quickly, to the point of requiring ventilatory support. Children with an impaired neuromuscular system may benefit from some secretions clearance techniques. However, care should be taken so as not to worsen bronchospasm, and advice sought from a Physiotherapist.

Nursing Assessment

For a full description of the assessment phase of the nursing process, refer to Nursing Process Overview section earlier in the chapter. Assessment findings pertinent to RSV bronchiolitis are discussed below.

HEALTH HISTORY

Elicit a description of the present illness and chief complaint. Common signs and symptoms reported during the health history might include:
- Onset of illness with a clear runny nose (sometimes profuse)
- Pharyngitis
- Low-grade fever
- Development of cough 1 to 3 days into the illness, followed by a wheeze shortly thereafter
- Poor feeding

Explore the child's current and past medical history for risk factors such as:
- Young age (younger than 2 years old), more severe disease in a child younger than 6 months old
- Prematurity
- Multiple births
- Birth during April to September
- History of chronic lung disease (bronchopulmonary disease)
- Cyanotic or complicated congenital heart disease
- Immunocompromise
- Male gender
- Exposure to passive tobacco smoke and wood burning stoves
- Crowded living conditions, including some Indigenous communities
- Day care attendance
- School-age siblings
- Low socioeconomic status
- Lack of breastfeeding

PHYSICAL EXAMINATION

Examination of the child with RSV involves inspection, observation, and auscultation.

Inspection and Observation. Observe the child's general appearance and colour centrally and peripherally. The infant with RSV bronchiolitis might appear air-hungry, exhibiting various degrees of cyanosis and respiratory distress, including tachypnea, retractions, accessory muscle use, grunting, nasal flaring, head bobbing, and periods of apnea. Cough and audible wheeze might be heard. The infant might appear listless and uninterested in feeding, surroundings, or parents.

Auscultation. Auscultate the lungs, noting adventitious sounds and determining the quality of aeration of the lung fields. Earlier in the illness, expiratory wheezes might be heard scattered throughout the lung fields. In more serious cases, the chest might sound quiet and without wheeze. This is due to significant hyperexpansion with very poor air exchange, and possible mucus plugging leading to atelectasis.

LABORATORY AND DIAGNOSTIC TESTS

Common laboratory and diagnostic studies ordered for the assessment of RSV bronchiolitis include:

- Pulse oximetry: oxygen saturation might be decreased significantly
- Chest x-ray: might reveal hyperinflation and patchy areas of atelectasis or infiltration
- Blood gases: might show carbon dioxide retention and hypoxemia
- Nasal-pharyngeal washings or swabs: positive identification of RSV can be made via enzyme-linked immunosorbent assay (ELISA) or immunofluorescent antibody (IFA) testing

Nursing Management

RSV infection is usually self-limited, and nursing diagnoses, goals, and interventions for the child with bronchiolitis are aimed at supportive care. Children with less severe disease might require only antipyretics, adequate hydration, and close observation. They can often be successfully managed at home, provided the primary caregiver is reliable and comfortable with close observation. Teach parents or caregivers to watch for signs of worsening, and to seek care quickly should the child's condition deteriorate.

Hospitalization is required for children with more severe disease, and children admitted with RSV bronchiolitis warrant close observation. In addition to the nursing diagnoses and related interventions discussed in Nursing Care Plan 40.1 at the end of the chapter for respiratory disorders, interventions common to bronchiolitis follow.

Take Note!

Currently, no safe and effective antiviral drug is available for definitive treatment of RSV. Aerosolized ribavirin is recommended only for the highest risk, most severely ill children. Routine antibiotic use is discouraged in RSV bronchiolitis treatment because secondary bacterial infection rate is very low (DeNicola et al., 2016).

MAINTAINING PATENT AIRWAY

Infants and young children with RSV tend to have copious secretions. Position the child with the head of the bed elevated to facilitate an open airway. These children often require frequent assessment and suctioning to maintain a patent airway. Use a Yankauer or tonsil-tip suction catheter to suction the mouth or pharynx of older infants or children, rinsing the catheter after

---

NURSING PROCEDURE 40.1

Nasopharyngeal or Artificial Airway Suction Technique

1. Make sure the suction equipment works properly before starting.
2. After washing your hands, assemble the equipment needed:
    - Appropriate-size sterile suction catheter
    - Sterile gloves
    - Supplemental oxygen
    - Sterile water-based lubricant
    - Sterile normal saline if indicated
3. Don sterile gloves, keeping dominant hand sterile and nondominant hand clean.
4. Preoxygenate the infant or child if indicated.
5. Apply lubricant to the end of the suction catheter.
6. If indicated for loosening of secretions, instil sterile saline.
7. Maintaining sterile technique, insert the suction catheter into the child's nostril or airway.
    - Insert only to the point of gagging if inserting via the nostril.
    - Insert only 0.5 cm further than the length of the artificial airway.
8. Intermittently apply suction for no longer than 10 seconds while twisting and removing the catheter.
9. Supplement with oxygen after suctioning.

---

each suctioning. Nasal bulb suctioning may be sufficient to clear the airway in some infants, while others will require nasopharyngeal suctioning with a suction catheter. Nursing Procedure 40.1 gives further information. Adjust the pressure ranges for suctioning infants and children between 60 and 100 mm Hg (40 and 60 mm Hg for premature infants).

PROMOTING ADEQUATE GAS EXCHANGE

Infants and children with RSV bronchiolitis might deteriorate quickly as the disease progresses. In the child ill enough to require oxygen, the risk is even greater. Assessment should include work of breathing, respiratory rate, capillary refill, oxygen saturation, heart rate, and blood pressure. The percentage of inspired oxygen (FiO_2) should be adjusted as needed to maintain oxygen saturation within the desired range. Positioning the infant with the head of the bed elevated may also improve gas exchange. Frequent assessment is necessary for the hospitalized child with bronchiolitis.

Take Note!

In the tachypneic infant, slowing of the respiratory rate does not necessarily indicate improvement: often, a slower respiratory rate is an indication of tiring, and carbon dioxide retention may soon be followed by apnea (AHA, 2011).

REDUCING RISK FOR INFECTION

Since RSV is easily spread through contact with droplets, isolate inpatients according to hospital policy to decrease the risk of nosocomial spread to other children. Children with RSV can be safely cohorted. Attention to handwashing is necessary, as droplets might enter the eyes, nose, or mouth via the hands.

PROVIDING FAMILY EDUCATION

Educate parents so they can recognize signs of worsening distress. If the child's breathing becomes rapid or more difficult or if the child cannot eat secondary to tachypnea, the child should be assessed by a medical provider. Children who are younger than 1 year of age or who are at higher risk (those who were born prematurely or who have chronic heart or lung conditions) might have a longer course of illness. Instruct parents that cough can persist for several days to weeks after resolution of the disease, but infants usually act well otherwise.

PREVENTING RESPIRATORY SYNCYTIAL VIRUS DISEASE

Strict adherence to handwashing policies in day care centres and when exposed to individuals with cold symptoms is important for all age groups. Though generally benign in healthy older children, RSV can be devastating in young infants or children with preexisting risk factors. Palivizumab (Synagis) is a monoclonal antibody that can prevent severe RSV disease in those who are most susceptible (Ohler & Pham, 2013). It is given as an intramuscular injection once a month throughout the RSV season. As Palivizumab is expensive, provincial and territorial guidelines determine eligibility requirements (Robinson & Le Saux, 2018). Although eligibility may vary, general qualifying factors include:
- Prematurity
- Chronic lung disease (bronchopulmonary dysplasia) requiring medication or oxygen
- Certain congenital heart diseases
- Indigenous Canadian children, those with social risk factors, and those with certain neuromuscular, genetic, or immunocompromising disorders may also qualify.

Pneumonia

Pneumonia is an inflammation of the lung parenchyma. It can be caused by a virus, bacteria, *Mycoplasma*, or a

fungus. Respiratory viruses are the most common cause of pneumonia in younger children and the least common cause in older children. Viral pneumonia is usually better tolerated in children of all ages. Children with bacterial pneumonia are more apt to present with a toxic appearance, but they generally recover rapidly if appropriate antibiotic treatment is instituted early. *Streptococcus pneumoniae* is a common cause of bacterial pneumonia in all ages of children, and *M. pneumoniae* and *Chlamydophila pneumoniae* are common causative agents in the school-age child and adolescent. Fungal infection may also result in pneumonia. Aspiration pneumonia may result from aspiration of foreign material into the lower respiratory tract. Pneumonia occurs more often in winter and early spring. It is common in children but is seen most frequently in infants and young toddlers.

Take Note!

Community-acquired pneumonia (CAP) refers to pneumonia in a previously healthy person that is contracted outside of the hospital setting (Barson, 2016).

Pneumonia is usually a self-limited disease. A child who presents with recurrent pneumonia should be evaluated for chronic lung disease such as asthma or CF. Potential complications of pneumonia include bacteremia, pleural effusion, empyema, lung abscess, and pneumothorax. Excluding bacteremia, these complications are often treated with thoracentesis and/or chest tubes as well as antibiotics if appropriate. Pneumatoceles (thin-walled cavities developing in the lung) might occur with certain bacterial pneumonias and usually resolve spontaneously over time.

Therapeutic management of children with less severe disease includes antipyretics, adequate hydration, and close observation. Even bacterial pneumonia can be successfully managed at home if the work of breathing is not severe and oxygen saturation is within normal limits. However, hospitalization is required for children with more severe disease. The child with tachypnea, significant retractions, poor oral intake, or lethargy might require hospital admission for the administration of supplemental oxygen, intravenous hydration, and antibiotics.

Nursing Assessment

For a full description of the assessment phase of the nursing process, refer to the earlier section. Assessment findings pertinent to pneumonia are discussed below.

HEALTH HISTORY

Elicit a description of the present illness and chief complaint. Note onset and progression of symptoms.

Common signs and symptoms reported during the health history include:
- Antecedent viral URI
- Fever
- Cough (note type and whether productive or not)
- Increased respiratory rate
- History of lethargy, poor feeding, vomiting, or diarrhea in infants
- Chills, headache, dyspnea, chest pain, abdominal pain, and nausea or vomiting in older children

Explore the child's past and current medical history for risk factors known to be associated with an increase in the severity of pneumonia, such as:
- Prematurity
- Malnutrition
- Passive smoke exposure
- Low socioeconomic status
- Day care attendance
- Recent entry into Canada history of Refugee
- Underlying cardiopulmonary, immune, or nervous system disease (John & Brady, 2013a)

PHYSICAL EXAMINATION
Physical examination consists of inspection, auscultation, percussion, and palpation.

Inspection. Observe the child's general appearance and colour (centrally and peripherally). Cyanosis might accompany coughing spells. The child with bacterial pneumonia may appear ill. Assess work of breathing. Children with pneumonia might exhibit scalene, suprasternal (tracheal tug), substernal, subcostal, or intercostal retractions. Tachypnea and nasal flaring may be present. Describe cough and quality of sputum if produced.

Auscultation. Auscultation of the lungs might reveal wheezes or rales in the younger child. Local or diffuse rales may be present in the older child. Document diminished or bronchial breath sounds, vocal fremitus or bronchophony.

Percussion and Palpation. In the older child, percussion might yield local dullness over a consolidated area. Percussion is much less valuable in the infant or younger child. Tactile fremitus felt upon palpation may be increased with pneumonia.

LABORATORY AND DIAGNOSTIC TESTS
Common laboratory and diagnostic studies ordered for the assessment of pneumonia include:
- Pulse oximetry: oxygen saturation might be decreased significantly or within normal range
- Chest x-ray: varies according to child's age and causative agent. In infants and young children, bilateral air trapping and perihilar **infiltrates** (collection of

inflammatory cells, cellular debris, and foreign organisms) are the most common findings. Patchy areas of consolidation might also be present. In older children, lobar consolidation is seen more frequently
- Sputum culture: may be useful in determining causative bacteria in older children and adolescents
- White blood cell count and C-reactive protein: might be elevated in the case of bacterial pneumonia

Nursing Management

Nursing diagnoses, goals, and interventions for the child with pneumonia are primarily aimed at providing supportive care and education about the illness and its treatment. Prevention of pneumococcal infection is also important. Children with more severe disease will require hospitalization. Refer to Nursing Care Plan 40.1 at the end of the chapter for nursing diagnoses and related interventions. In addition to the interventions listed there, the following should be noted.

PROVIDING SUPPORTIVE CARE
Ensure adequate hydration and assist in thinning of secretions by encouraging oral fluid intake in the child whose respiratory status is stable. In children with increased work of breathing, intravenous fluids may be necessary to maintain hydration. Allow and encourage the child to assume a position of comfort, usually with the head of the bed elevated to promote aeration of the lungs. If pain due to coughing or pneumonia itself is severe, administer analgesics as prescribed. Provide supplemental oxygen to the child with respiratory distress or hypoxia as needed.

PROVIDING FAMILY EDUCATION
Educate the family about the importance of adhering to the prescribed antibiotic regimen. Antibiotics may be given intravenously if the child is hospitalized. Oral antibiotics are used upon discharge or if the child is managed on an outpatient basis.

Teach the parents or caregivers that following resolution of the acute illness, the child might continue to tire easily for 1 to 2 weeks, and the infant might continue to need small, frequent feedings. Cough may also persist after the acute recovery period but should lessen over time.

If the child is diagnosed with viral pneumonia, parents might not understand that their child does not require an antibiotic. Pneumonia is often perceived by the public as a bacterial infection, so most parents will need an explanation related to treatment of viral infections.

The young child is at risk for the development of aspiration pneumonia. Parents need to understand that the child might be at risk for injury related to his or her age and developmental stage. To prevent recurrent or further aspiration, teach the parents the safety measures in Teaching Guidelines 40.3.

Teaching Guidelines 40.3
PREVENTING ASPIRATION

- Keep toxic substances such as lighter fluid, solvents, and hydrocarbons out of reach of young children. Toddlers and pre-schoolers cannot distinguish safe from unsafe fluids due to their developmental stage.
- Avoid oily nose drops and oil-based vitamins or home remedies to avoid lipid aspiration into the lungs.
- Avoid oral feedings if the infant's respiratory rate is 60 or greater to minimize the risk of aspiration of the feeding.
- Discourage parents from "force-feeding" in the event of poor oral intake or severe illness to minimize the risk of aspiration of the feeding.
- Position upright after feeding to minimize the risk of acid reflux, aspirating emesis, or regurgitated feeding.

PREVENTING PNEUMOCOCCAL INFECTION

Immunization against pneumococcal infection is included in standard childhood immunizations across Canada. Standard schedules vary slightly between provinces, with doses being provided in a three- or four-dose series between 2 and 18 months of age (Government of Canada, 2017). For additional information on immunization, refer to Chapter 31.

Bronchitis

Bronchitis is an inflammation of the trachea and major bronchi. It is often associated with a URI. Bronchitis is usually viral in nature, though *M. pneumoniae* and other bacterial organisms are causative in about 10% of cases (Carolan & Bye, 2015). Recovery usually occurs within 5 to 10 days. Therapeutic management involves mainly supportive care. Expectorant administration and adequate hydration are important. If bacterial infection is the cause, antibiotics are indicated.

Nursing Assessment

The illness might begin with a mild URI. Fever develops, followed by a dry, hacking cough that might become productive in older children. The cough might wake the child at night. Auscultation of the lungs might reveal coarse rales. Respirations remain unlaboured. The chest x-ray might show diffuse alveolar hyperinflation and perihilar markings.

Nursing Management

Nursing management is aimed at providing supportive care. Teach parents that antipyretics will help reduce the fever, making the child more comfortable. Encourage adequate hydration. Antibiotics are prescribed only in cases believed to be bacterial in nature. Discourage the use of cough suppressants: it is important for accumulated sputum to be expectorated.

Tuberculosis

Tuberculosis (TB) is a highly contagious disease caused by inhalation of droplets of *Mycobacterium tuberculosis* or *Mycobacterium bovis*. Children usually contract the disease from an immediate household member. Homeless and impoverished children are at higher risk, as are those exposed to an adult with TB infection (Batra & Ang, 2015). In Canada, Canadian-born Indigenous and foreign-born children (and adults) continue to experience disproportionately high rates of this disease (Canadian Thoracic Society & Public Health Agency of Canada [CTS & PHAC], 2014). After exposure to an infected individual, the incubation period is 2 to 10 weeks. The inhaled tubercle bacilli multiply in the alveoli and alveolar ducts, forming an inflammatory exudate. The bacilli are spread by the bloodstream and lymphatic system to various parts of the body. Though pulmonary tuberculosis is the most common, children may also have infection in other parts of the body, such as the gastrointestinal tract or central nervous system. Young children, especially infants, are at particularly high risk of progression from latent to active TB, and severe disease (CTS & PHAC, 2014).

In the case of drug-sensitive, active tuberculosis, the CTS and PHAC (2014) recommend a minimum 6-month course of oral therapy. The first 2 months consist of isoniazid, rifampin, and pyrazinamide given daily. In special circumstances, three times weekly regimens may be considered, however are considered sub-optimal. This is followed by 4 months of daily isoniazid and rifampin, or twice-weekly dosing in cases of mild disease and high adherence history. In the case of multidrug resistant TB, ethambutol and fluoroquinolones may be used alongside first-line drugs. Direct observed therapy is strongly advised for the full duration of treatment. Many areas in Canada have specialized teams and clinics for the care of tuberculosis.

Nursing Assessment

Routine screening for children considered to be high risk for contracting tuberculosis should be completed using the Mantoux/tuberculin skin test. This includes children who:

- Are close contacts of an active case of pulmonary TB
- Are infected with HIV
- Are injection drug-users
- Are homeless, incarcerated, or institutionalized
- Have a positive recent history of latent tuberculosis infection

- Are immigrants from or have a history of travel to endemic countries
- Are of Canadian-born Indigenous descent
- Are exposed at home to HIV-infected or homeless persons, illicit drug users, persons recently incarcerated, and migrant farm workers

The presentation of tuberculosis in children is quite varied. Children can be asymptomatic (especially those under 5 years of age) or exhibit a broad range of symptoms. Symptoms may include fever, malaise, weight loss, anorexia, pain and tightness in the chest, and rarely hemoptysis. Cough may or may not be present and usually progresses slowly over several weeks to months. As tuberculosis progresses, the respiratory rate increases and the lung on the affected side is poorly expanded. Dullness to percussion might be present, as well as diminished breath sounds and crackles. Fever persists and pallor, anemia, weakness, and weight loss are present. Diagnosis is confirmed with a positive Mantoux/tuberculin skin test, positive gastric washings for acid-fast bacillus, interferon-gamma release assay (IGRA), and/or a chest x-ray.

Nursing Management

Hospitalization of children with tuberculosis is necessary only for the most serious cases. Nursing management is aimed at providing supportive care and encouraging adherence to the treatment regimen. Most nursing care for childhood tuberculosis is provided in outpatient clinics, schools, or a public health setting. Supportive care includes ensuring adequate nutrition and adequate rest, providing comfort measures such as fever reduction, preventing exposure to other infectious diseases, and preventing reinfection. Providing education and support to the family is an equally important part of promoting overall health and well-being, and preventing further spread of the disease.

PROVIDING CARE FOR THE CHILD WITH LATENT TUBERCULOSIS INFECTION
Children who test positive for tuberculosis but who do not have symptoms or radiographic/laboratory evidence of disease are considered to have latent infection. These children should be treated with isoniazid for 9 months to prevent progression to active disease. Follow-up and appropriate monitoring can be achieved via the child's physician or nurse practitioner or local health department.

PREVENTING INFECTION
Tuberculosis infection is prevented by avoiding contact with the tubercle bacillus. Thus, hospitalized children with tuberculosis must be isolated according to hospital policy to prevent nosocomial spread of the infection. Promotion of natural resistance through nutrition, rest, and avoidance of serious infections does not prevent

infection. Pasteurization of milk has helped to decrease the transmission of *M. bovis*. Due to incomplete and variable tuberculosis protection, the Bacille Calmette–Guérin (BCG) vaccine is not widely used in Canada (CTS & PHAC, 2014).

ACUTE NONINFECTIOUS DISORDERS

Acute non-infectious disorders include epistaxis, foreign body aspiration, acute respiratory distress syndrome (ARDS), and pneumothorax.

Epistaxis

Epistaxis (a nosebleed) occurs most frequently in children before adolescence. Bleeding of the nasal mucosa occurs most often from the anterior portion of the septum. Epistaxis may be recurrent and idiopathic (meaning there is no cause). Most cases are benign, but in children with bleeding disorders or other hematologic concerns, epistaxis should be further investigated and treated. Furthermore, the child with recurrent epistaxis or epistaxis that is difficult to control should be evaluated for underlying bleeding or platelet concerns.

Nursing Assessment

Explore the child's history for initiating factors such as local inflammation, mucosal drying, or local trauma (usually nose picking). Inspect the nasal cavity for blood.

Nursing Management

The presence of blood often frightens children and their parents. The nurse and parents should remain calm. The child should sit up and lean forward (lying down may allow aspiration of the blood). Apply continuous pressure to the anterior portion of the nose by pinching it closed. Encourage the child to breathe through the mouth during this portion of the treatment. Ice or a cold cloth applied to the bridge of the nose may also be helpful. The bleeding usually stops within 10 to 15 minutes. Apply water-soluble gel to the nasal mucosa with a cotton-tipped applicator to moisten the mucosa and prevent recurrence.

Foreign Body Aspiration

Foreign body aspiration occurs when any solid or liquid substance is inhaled into the respiratory tract. It is common in infants and young children and can present in a life-threatening manner. The object may lodge in the upper or lower airway, causing varying degrees of respiratory difficulty. Small, smooth objects such as peanuts are the most frequently aspirated, but any small toy, article, or piece of food smaller than the diameter of the young child's airway can be aspirated.

> **Take Note!**
>
> Items smaller than 1.25 in (3.2 cm) can be aspirated easily. A simple way for parents to estimate the safe size of a small item or toy piece is to gauge its size against a standard toilet paper roll, which is generally about 1.5 in in diameter (Safe Kids, 2016).

Foreign body aspiration occurs most frequently in children between 6 months and 4 years of age (John & Brady, 2013b). Children of this age are growing and developing rapidly, and tend to explore things with their mouths.

The child often coughs out foreign bodies from the upper airway. If the foreign body reaches the bronchus, then it may need to be removed via bronchoscopy. Postoperative antibiotics are used if an infection is also present. Complications of foreign body aspiration include pneumonia or abscess formation, hypoxia, respiratory failure, and death.

Nursing Assessment

The infant or young child might present with a history of sudden onset of cough, wheeze, stridor, and drooling. Stridor suggests that the foreign body is lodged in the upper airway. Sometimes the onset of respiratory symptoms is much more gradual. When the item has travelled down one of the bronchi, then wheezing, rhonchi, and decreased aeration can be heard on the affected side. A chest x-ray will demonstrate the foreign body only if it is radiopaque (Fig. 40.7).

Nursing Management

The most important nursing intervention related to foreign body aspiration is prevention. Anticipatory guidance for families with 6-month olds should include a discussion of aspiration avoidance. Repeat this information at each subsequent well-child visit through age 5. Tell parents to avoid letting their child play with toys with small parts and to keep coins and other small objects out of the reach of children. Teach parents not to feed peanuts and popcorn to their child until at least 3 years of age and to chop all foods so that they are small enough to pass down the trachea in case the child neglects to chew them up thoroughly (Gavin, 2013). Carrots, grapes, and hot dogs should be cut into small pieces and children supervised at meal times.

> **Take Note!**
>
> Prevent young children from playing with latex balloons. When popped, small pieces pose an aspiration danger (Gavin, 2013).

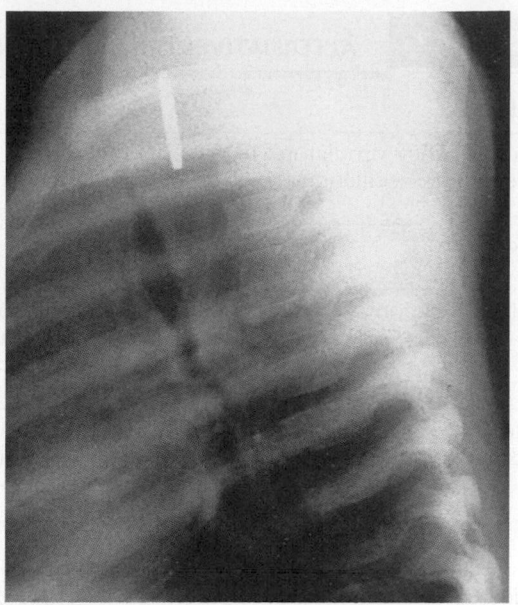

FIGURE 40.7 Foreign body is noted in the bronchus on a chest x-ray.

Respiratory Distress Syndrome

Respiratory distress syndrome (RDS) is a respiratory disorder that is specific to neonates. It results from lung immaturity and a deficiency in surfactant, so it is seen most often in premature infants. Other infants who might experience RDS include infants of diabetic mothers, those delivered via cesarean section without preceding labour, and those experiencing perinatal asphyxia (Aldana-Aguirre, Pinto, Featherstone, & Kumar, 2017). It is believed that each of these conditions has an impact on surfactant production, thus resulting in RDS in the term infant.

Pathophysiology

The lack of surfactant in the affected newborn's lungs results in stiff, poorly compliant lungs with poor gas exchange. Right-to-left shunting and hypoxemia result. As the disease progresses, fluid and fibrin leak from the pulmonary capillaries, causing a hyaline membrane to form in the bronchioles, alveolar ducts, and alveoli. Presence of the membrane further decreases gas exchange.

Acute Respiratory Distress Syndrome

ARDS occurs following a primary insult such as sepsis, viral pneumonia, smoke inhalation, or near-drowning. Respiratory distress and hypoxemia occur acutely within 72 hours of the insult in infants and children with previously healthy lungs (Cornfield, 2013). The alveolar–capillary membrane becomes more permeable and pulmonary edema develops. Hyaline membrane formation over the alveolar surfaces

TABLE 40.2	ALTERNATIVES TO TRADITIONAL MECHANICAL VENTILATION	
Mode	**Description**	**Additional Information**
High-frequency ventilators (high-frequency, oscillating, or jet)	Provide very high respiratory rates (up to 1,200 breaths/min) and very low tidal volumes	May decrease risk of barotrauma associated with ventilator pressures
Nitric oxide	Causes pulmonary vasodilation, helping to increase blood flow to alveoli	Safe; no long-term developmental risks
Liquid ventilation	Perfluorocarbon liquid acts as a surfactant. Provides an effective medium for gas exchange and increases pulmonary function	Virtually no reported physiologic sequelae
Extracorporeal membrane oxygenation (ECMO)	Blood is removed from body via catheter, warmed and oxygenated in the ECMO machine, and then returned to infant	Labour-intensive. Risk of bleeding is great

and decreased surfactant production cause lung stiffness. Mucosal swelling and cellular debris lead to atelectasis. Gas diffusion is impaired significantly. Some children have residual lung disease and some recover completely. However, ARDS can progress to respiratory failure and death.

Therapeutic management is aimed at improving oxygenation and ventilation. Mechanical ventilation is used, with special attention to lung volumes and positive end-expiratory pressure (PEEP). Newer treatment modalities show promise for improving outcomes of ARDS (see Table 40.2 for additional information on alternative methods of mechanical ventilation).

Nursing Assessment

Tachycardia and tachypnea occur over the first few hours of the illness. Significantly increased work of breathing with nasal flaring and retractions develops. Auscultate the breath sounds, which might range from normal to high-pitched crackles throughout the lung fields. Hypoxemia develops. Bilateral infiltrates can be seen on a chest x-ray.

Nursing Management

Nursing care of the child with ARDS is mainly supportive and occurs in the intensive care unit. Closely monitor respiratory and cardiovascular status. Comfort measures such as hygiene and positioning as well as pain and anxiety management, maintenance of nutrition, and prevention of infection are also key nursing interventions. The acute phase of worsening respiratory distress can be frightening for a child of any age, and the nurse can be instrumental in soothing the child's fears. As the disease worsens and progresses, especially when ventilatory support is required, it is especially important to provide psychological support for the family as well as education about the intensive care unit procedures.

Take Note!

Consult your Physiotherapist for guidance on positioning for VQ match.

Pneumothorax

A collection of air in the pleural space is called a pneumothorax. It can occur spontaneously in an otherwise healthy child or as a result of chronic lung disease, cardiopulmonary resuscitation, surgery, or trauma. Trapped air consumes space within the pleural cavity, and the affected lung suffers at least partial collapse. Needle aspiration and/or placement of a chest tube are used to evacuate the air from the chest. Some small pneumothoraces resolve independently, without intervention.

Nursing Assessment

Primary pneumothorax (spontaneous) occurs most often in adolescence (Winnie & Lossef, 2011). Tall, thin males are at greatest risk. The infant or child with a pneumothorax might have a sudden or gradual onset of symptoms. Chest pain might be present as well as signs of respiratory distress such as tachypnea, retractions, nasal flaring, or grunting. Assess risk factors for acquiring a pneumothorax, including chest trauma or surgery, intubation and mechanical ventilation, or a history of chronic lung disease such as CF. Inspect the child for a pale or cyanotic appearance. Auscultate for increased heart rate (tachycardia) and absent or diminished breath sounds on the affected side. The x-ray reveals air within the thoracic cavity (Fig. 40.8).

Nursing Management

The child with a pneumothorax requires frequent respiratory assessments. Pulse oximetry might be used as an adjunct, but clinical evaluation of respiratory status

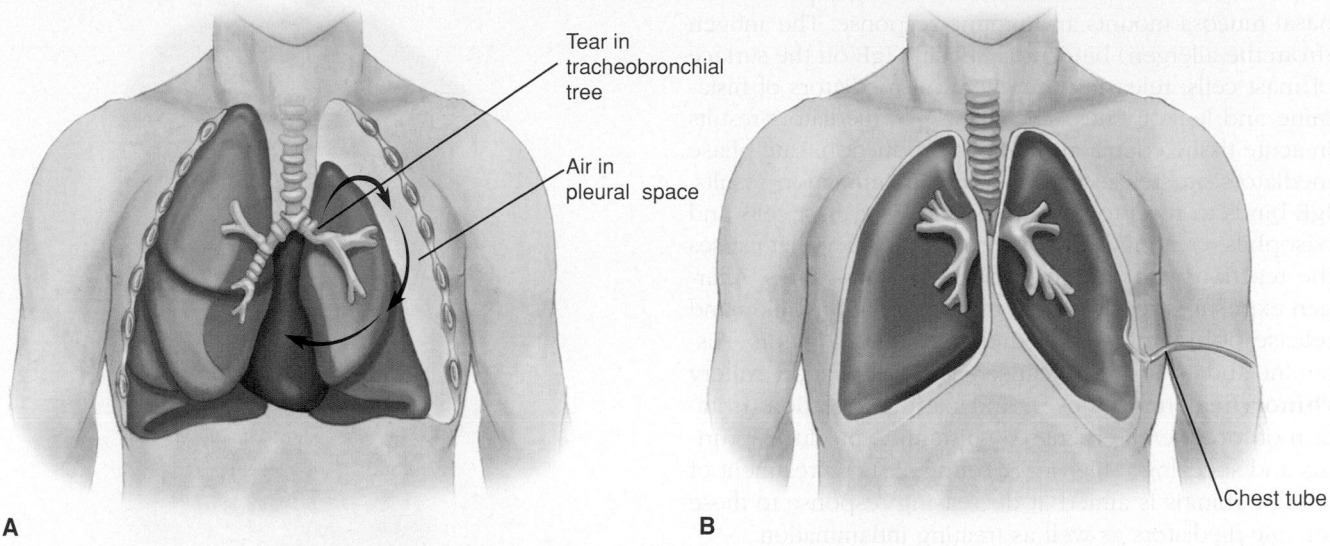

Tear in tracheobronchial tree

Air in pleural space

Chest tube

A

B

FIGURE 40.8 **A.** Pneumothorax. **B.** Note reinflation of the lung when the chest tube is present.

is most useful. In some cases, administration of 100% oxygen hastens the reabsorption of air, but it is generally used only for a few hours (Winnie & Lossef, 2011). If a chest tube is connected to a dry suction or water seal apparatus, provide care of the drainage apparatus as appropriate (Fig. 40.9). A pair of hemostats should be kept at the bedside to clamp the tube should it become dislodged from the drainage container or the open end may be placed in a container of sterile water. The dressing around the chest tube is occlusive and is not routinely changed. If the tube becomes dislodged from the child's chest, apply Vaseline gauze and an occlusive dressing, immediately perform appropriate respiratory assessment, and notify the physician or nurse practitioner. See your specific organization policies, procedures, and guidelines on chest tubes.

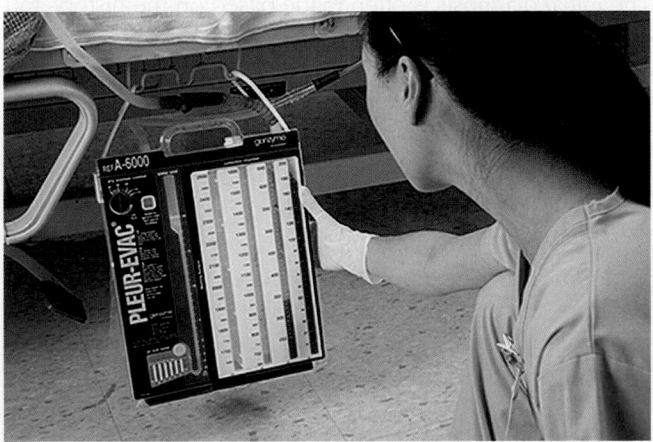

FIGURE 40.9 The chest tube is connected to a suction or water seal via a drainage container.

Take Note!

Use of Oxygen with a Pneumothorax

In a child with a pneumothorax, the nurse would administer 100% oxygen to hasten air reabsorption. This treatment is only used for a short period of time early in the course of treatment. Although it does help to prevent hypoxemia during administration, this is not the primary reason it is administered, and there is a risk of toxicity

CHRONIC RESPIRATORY DISORDERS

Chronic respiratory disorders include allergic rhinitis, asthma, chronic lung disease (bronchopulmonary dysplasia), CF, and apnea.

Allergic Rhinitis

Allergic rhinitis is a common chronic condition in childhood, affecting a significant number of children. Allergic rhinitis is associated with atopic dermatitis and asthma. Perennial allergic rhinitis occurs year-round and is associated with indoor environments. Allergens commonly implicated in perennial allergic rhinitis include dust mites, pet dander, cockroach antigens, and moulds. Seasonal allergic rhinitis is caused by elevations in outdoor levels of allergens. It is typically caused by certain pollens, trees, weeds, fungi, and moulds. Complications from allergic rhinitis include exacerbation of asthma symptoms, recurrent sinusitis and otitis media, and dental malocclusion.

Pathophysiology

Allergic rhinitis is an intermittent or persistent inflammatory state that is mediated by immunoglobulin E (IgE). In response to contact with an airborne allergen protein, the nasal mucosa mounts an immune response. The antigen (from the allergen) binds to a specific IgE on the surface of mast cells, releasing the chemical mediators of histamine and leukotrienes. The release of mediators results in acute tissue edema and mucus production. Late-phase mediators are released and more inflammation results. IgE binds to receptors on the surfaces of mast cells and basophils, creating the sensitization memory that causes the reaction with subsequent allergen exposures. Allergen exposure then results in mast cell degranulation and release of histamine and other chemotactic factors. Histamine and other factors cause nasal vasodilation, watery **rhinorrhea** (runny nose), and nasal congestion. Irritation of local nerve endings by histamine produces pruritus and sneezing (Milgrom & Leung, 2011). Treatment of allergic rhinitis is aimed at decreasing response to these allergic mediators as well as treating inflammation.

Nursing Assessment

For a full description of the assessment phase of the nursing process, refer to the Nursing Process Overview section earlier in the chapter. Assessment findings pertinent to allergic rhinitis are discussed below.

HEALTH HISTORY

Elicit a description of the present illness and chief complaint. Common signs and symptoms reported during the health history might include:

- Mild, intermittent to chronic nasal stuffiness
- Thin, runny nasal discharge
- Sneezing
- Itching of nose, eyes, palate
- Mouth breathing and snoring

Determine the seasonality of symptoms. Are they perennial (year-round) or do they occur during certain seasons only? What types of medications or other treatments have been used, and what was the child's response?

Explore the history for the presence of risk factors such as:

- Family history of atopic disease (asthma, allergic rhinitis, or atopic dermatitis)
- Known allergy to dust mites, pet dander, cockroach antigens, pollens, or moulds
- Early childhood exposure to indoor allergens
- Early introduction to foods or formula in infancy
- Exposure to tobacco smoke
- Environmental air pollution
- Recurrent viral infections (Milgrom & Leung, 2011)
- Various ethnic backgrounds and higher socioeconomic status have also been noted as risk factors.

PHYSICAL EXAMINATION

Physical examination of the child with allergic rhinitis includes inspection, observation, and auscultation.

FIGURE 40.10 Allergic shiners beneath the eyes and allergic salute across the nose.

Inspection and Observation. Observe the child's facies for red-rimmed eyes or tearing, mild eyelid edema, "allergic shiners" (bluish or greyish cast beneath the eyes), and "allergic salute" (a transverse nasal crease between the lower and middle thirds of the nose that results from repeated nose rubbing) (Fig. 40.10). Inspect the nasal cavity. The turbinates may be swollen and grey/blue. Clear mucoid nasal drainage may be observed. Inspect the skin for rash. Listen for nasal phonation with speech.

Auscultation. Auscultate the lungs for adequate aeration and clarity of breath sounds. In the child who also has asthma, exacerbation with wheezing often occurs with allergic rhinitis.

LABORATORY AND DIAGNOSTIC TESTS

The initial diagnosis is often made based on the history and clinical findings. Common laboratory and diagnostic studies ordered for the assessment of allergic rhinitis may include:

- Nasal smear (positive for eosinophilia)
- Positive allergy skin test
- Positive radioallergosorbent test (RAST)

Nursing Management

In addition to the nursing diagnoses and related interventions discussed in Nursing Care Plan 40.1 at the end of the chapter for disorders of the nose, mouth, and throat, interventions common to allergic rhinitis follow.

MAINTAINING PATENT AIRWAY

The constant nasal obstruction that occurs with allergic rhinitis can be very problematic for some children.

Performing nasal washes with normal saline may keep the nasal mucus from becoming thickened. Thickened, immobile secretions often lead to a secondary bacterial infection. The nasal wash also decongests the nose, allowing for improved nasal airflow. Anti-inflammatory (corticosteroid) nasal sprays can decrease the inflammatory response to allergens but are not recommended for long-term use. A mast cell stabilizing nasal spray such as cromolyn sodium may decrease the intensity and frequency of allergic responses. Oral antihistamines are now available in once-daily dosing, providing convenience for the family. Some children may benefit from a combined antihistamine/nasal decongestant if nasal congestion is significant. Leukotriene modifiers such as montelukast may also be beneficial for some children. See Dosage Calculation Box 40.1.

Dosage Calculation Box 40.1

Child's weight: 30 lb
Medication order: cetirizine 2.5 mg PO every morning
Cetirizine is supplied as 5 mg/5 mL
How many millilitres will the nurse administer? Round to the nearest tenth

PROVIDING FAMILY EDUCATION

One of the most important tools in the treatment of allergic rhinitis is learning to avoid known allergens. Teaching Guidelines 40.4 gives information on educating families about avoidance of allergens. Children may be referred to a specialist for allergen desensitization (allergy shots).

Teaching Guidelines 40.4
CONTROLLING EXPOSURE TO ALLERGENS

Tobacco
- Avoid all exposure to tobacco smoke, including second and third hand (e.g., on clothing).
- No parental smoking inside the home or car.

Dust Mites
- Use pillow and mattress covers.
- Wash bed linens once a week in 130°F water.
- Use blinds rather than curtains in bedroom.
- Remove stuffed animals from bedroom or minimize number and wash weekly.
- Reduce indoor humidity to <50%.
- Remove carpet from bedroom.
- Clean solid-surface floors with wet mop each week.

Pet Dander
- Remove pets from home permanently.
- If unable to remove them, keep them out of bedroom and off carpet and upholstered furniture.

Cockroaches
- Keep kitchen very clean.
- Avoiding leaving food or drinks out.
- Use pesticides if necessary but ensure that the asthmatic child is not inside the home when the pesticide is sprayed.

Indoor Moulds
- Repair water leaks.
- Use dehumidifier to keep basement dry.
- Reduce indoor humidity to <50%.
- Remove indoor plants from warm, moist places in the home i.e., the bathroom.

Outdoor Moulds, Pollen, and Air Pollution
- Avoid going outdoors when mould and pollen counts are high, and/or consider medications as prophylactic treatment.
- Avoid outdoor activity when pollution levels are high.

Adapted from National Asthma Education and Prevention Program. (2007). *Expert panel report 3: Guidelines for the diagnosis and management of asthma* (NIH Publication No. 07–4051). Bethesda, MD: National Institutes of Health, National Heart, Lung and Blood Institute; and Ratcliffe, M. M., & Kieckhefer, G. M. (2010). Asthma. In P. J. Allen, J. A. Vessey, & N. A. Schapiro (Eds.). *Primary care of the child with a chronic condition* (5th ed.). St. Louis, MO: Mosby.

 Asthma

Asthma is a chronic inflammatory airway disorder characterized by airway hyper-responsiveness, airway edema, and mucus production. Airway obstruction resulting from asthma might be partially or completely reversed. Severity ranges from long periods of control with infrequent acute exacerbations in some children to the presence of persistent daily symptoms in others. It is the most common chronic illness of childhood, affecting 14% of children globally (Global Asthma Network, 2014), 10% of children ages 2 to 7 in Canada, and 8.5% of the population ages 12 and over (Statistics Canada, 2010). A small percentage of children with asthma account for a large percentage of health care use and expense. In Canada, asthma is the leading cause of hospitalization in children (Ortiz-Alvarez & Mikrogianakis, 2012), and is estimated to cost over 1 billion dollars annually in combined direct and indirect expenses (Asthma Society of Canada, 2014). The incidence and severity of asthma are increasing; this might be attributed to increased urbanization, increased air pollution, and more accurate diagnosis.

Severity ranges from symptoms associated only with vigorous activity (exercise-induced bronchospasm) to daily symptoms that interfere with quality of life. Table 40.3 discusses classification of asthma severity. Though uncommon, childhood death related to asthma is also on the rise worldwide. Air pollution, allergens, family history, and viral infections might all play a role in asthma (John & Brady, 2013a). Many children with asthma also

TABLE 40.3	ASTHMA SEVERITY CLASSIFICATION IN CHILDREN NOT TAKING LONG-TERM CONTROL MEDICATIONS			
Classification	**Symptoms**	**Lung Function**	**Interference With Normal Activity**	**Short-Acting β₂-Agonist Use for Symptom Control**
Intermittent	1 or 2 times a week Night-time symptoms 1 or 2 times a month	FEV 80% or more of predicted	None	1 or 2 days per week
Mild persistent	Symptoms more than twice a week but less than once a day Night-time symptoms 3 or 4 times a month	FEV 80% or more of predicted, variability	Minor limitation	Greater than twice per week, but not more than once a day
Moderate persistent	Daily symptoms Night-time symptoms >1 time a week, but not nightly	FEV 60–80% of predicted	Some limitation	Daily
Severe persistent	Throughout the day Night-time symptoms often 7 times per week	FEV <60% of predicted	Extremely limited	Several times per day

FEV, forced expiratory volume.

Adapted from National Asthma Education and Prevention Program. (2007). *Expert panel report 3: Guidelines for the diagnosis and management of asthma* (NIH Publication No. 07–4051). Bethesda, MD: National Institutes of Health, National Heart, Lung and Blood Institute.

have gastroesophageal disease, though the relationship between the two diseases is not clearly understood.

A significant long-term complication, chronic airway remodelling, may result from recurrent asthma exacerbation and inflammation. Children with asthma are more susceptible to serious bacterial and viral respiratory infections (John & Brady, 2013a). Acute complications also include status asthmaticus and respiratory failure. Childhood asthma can lead to significant family and social stressors. For example, frequent exacerbations can lead to missed school for the child, missed work for the caregiver, as well as the psychological stress of having a sick child.

Pathophysiology

In asthma, the inflammatory process contributes to increased airway activity. Thus, control or prevention of inflammation is the core of asthma management. Asthma results from a complex variety of responses in relation to a trigger. When the process begins, mast cells, T lymphocytes, macrophages, and epithelial cells are involved in the release of inflammatory mediators. Eosinophils and neutrophils migrate to the airway, causing injury. Chemical mediators such as leukotrienes, bradykinin, histamine, and platelet-activating factor also contribute to the inflammatory response. The presence of leukotrienes contributes to prolonged airway constriction. Autonomic neural control of airway tone is affected, airway mucus secretion is increased, mucociliary function

changes, and airway smooth muscle responsiveness increases. As a result, acute bronchoconstriction, airway edema, and mucus plugging occur (Fig. 40.11).

In most children, this process is considered reversible and until recently it was not considered to have long-standing effects on lung function. Current research and scientific thought, however, recognize the concept of airway remodelling (Sirivimonpan, 2013). Airway remodelling occurs as a result of chronic inflammation of the airway. Following the acute response to a trigger, continued allergen response results in a chronic phase. During this phase, the epithelial cells are denuded and the influx of inflammatory cells into the airway continues. This results in structural changes of the airway that are irreversible, and further loss of pulmonary function might occur. The irreversible changes include thickening of the sub-basement membrane, subepithelial fibrosis, airway smooth muscle hypertrophy and hyperplasia, blood vessel proliferation and dilation, and mucus gland hyperplasia and hypersecretion (Sirivimonpan, 2013). In some individuals with poorly controlled asthma, these changes may be permanent, resulting in decreased responsiveness to therapy.

Therapeutic Management

Current goals of medical therapy are avoidance of asthma triggers and reduction or control of inflammatory episodes. The most recent recommendations by the Canadian Thoracic Society (Canadian Respiratory Guidelines, 2018)

FIGURE 40.11 Note airway edema, mucus production, and bronchospasm occurring with asthma.

Normal airway

Airway with inflammation

Airway with inflammation, bronchospasm, and mucus production

suggest a stepwise approach to medication management as well as control of environmental factors (allergens) and comorbid conditions that affect asthma. The CTS guidelines stress periodic assessment of asthma control. Treatment decisions may then be made based on the individual's level of asthma control, rather than on the severity at diagnosis.

The stepwise approach to asthma treatment involves increasing medications as the child's condition worsens, then backing off treatment as he or she improves (Fig. 40.12). The Canadian Paediatric Society offer ongoing updated diagnostic and management algorithms which can be sources via their website (Ducharme et al., 2015).

Short-acting bronchodilators may be used in the acute treatment of bronchoconstriction and long-acting forms may be used to prevent bronchospasm. Exercise-induced bronchospasm may occur in any child with asthma or as the only symptom in the child with mild intermittent

asthma. Most children may avoid exercise-induced bronchospasm by using a longer warm-up period prior to vigorous exercise and, if necessary, inhaling a short-acting bronchodilator just prior to exercise. Long-term prevention usually involves inhaled steroids. Leukotriene modifiers may be used as an alternative but are not preferred for mild persistent asthma (National Asthma Education and Prevention Program [NAEPP], 2007).

Nursing Assessment

For a full description of the assessment phase of the nursing process, refer to the Nursing Process Overview section earlier in the chapter. Assessment findings pertinent to asthma are discussed below.

HEALTH HISTORY

Elicit a description of the present illness and chief complaint. Common signs and symptoms reported during the health history might include:

- Cough, particularly at night: hacking cough that is initially non-productive, becoming productive of frothy sputum
- Difficulty breathing: shortness of breath, chest tightness or pain, dyspnea with exercise
- Wheezing

Explore the child's current and past medical history for risk factors such as:

- History of allergic rhinitis or atopic dermatitis
- Family history of atopy (asthma, allergic rhinitis, atopic dermatitis)
- Recurrent episodes diagnosed as wheezing, bronchiolitis, or bronchitis
- History of GERD
- Known allergies
- Seasonal response to environmental pollen
- Tobacco smoke exposure
- Poverty

FIGURE 40.12 Children with asthma benefit from patient education, including instruction on treatment methods (Shutterstock/Levent Konuk).

Take Note!
Inquire about any bronchodilator use with activity, throughout the day, and at night.

PHYSICAL EXAMINATION

Physical examination of the child with asthma includes inspection, auscultation, and percussion.

Inspection. Observe the child's general appearance and colour. During mild exacerbations, the child's colour might remain pink, but as the child worsens, cyanosis might result. Work of breathing is variable. Some children present with mild retractions, while others demonstrate significant accessory muscle use and eventually head bobbing if not treated effectively. The child may appear anxious and fearful or may be lethargic and irritable. An audible wheeze might be present. Children with persistent severe asthma may have a barrel chest and routinely demonstrate mildly increased work of breathing.

Auscultation and Percussion. A thorough assessment of lung fields is necessary. Wheezing is the hallmark of airway obstruction and might vary throughout the lung fields. Coarseness might also be present. Assess the adequacy of aeration. Breath sounds might be diminished in the bases or throughout. A quiet chest in an asthmatic child can be an ominous sign. With severe airway obstruction, air movement can be so poor that wheezes might not be heard upon auscultation. Percussion may yield hyperresonance.

The Pediatric Respiratory Assessment Measure (PRAM) (Ducharme et al., 2015) for asthma exacerbation severity is a tool that can be used during nursing assessment. The age range for use is between 3 and 17 years and the tool can be used pre- and post-treatment (see thePoint for online tool and application).

LABORATORY AND DIAGNOSTIC TESTS

Laboratory and diagnostic studies commonly ordered for the assessment of asthma include:

- Pulse oximetry: oxygen saturation may be decreased significantly or normal during a mild exacerbation
- Chest x-ray: usually reveals hyperinflation
- Blood gases: might show carbon dioxide retention and hypoxemia
- Pulmonary function tests (PFTs): can be very useful in determining the degree of disease but are not useful during an acute attack. Children as young as 5 or 6 years might be able to comply with spirometry.
- Peak expiratory flow rate (PEFR): is decreased during an exacerbation
- Allergy testing: skin test or RAST can determine allergic triggers for the asthmatic child

Atraumatic Care 40.2

When caring for a young child who must receive a nebulizer treatment by mask, play make-believe about the mask and utilize other distraction techniques such as reading a book. Making activities into games, and utilizing distraction both help to minimize trauma when providing necessary care to young children. It should be noted, however, that nebulizers are rarely indicated and whenever possible, a metered-dose inhaler with a spacer device should be used.

Nursing Management

Initial nursing management of the child with an acute exacerbation of asthma is aimed at restoring a clear airway and effective breathing pattern as well as promoting adequate oxygenation and ventilation (gas exchange). Refer to Nursing Care Plan 40.1 at the end of the chapter. Additional considerations are reviewed below.

EDUCATING THE CHILD AND FAMILY

Asthma is a chronic illness and needs to be understood as such. Teach families of children with asthma, and the children themselves, how to care for the disease (Atraumatic Care 40.2). Symptom-free periods (often very long) are interspersed with episodes of exacerbation. Parents and children often do not understand the importance of maintenance medications for long-term control. They may view the episodes of exacerbation (sometimes requiring hospitalization or emergency room visits) as an acute illness and are simply relieved when they are over. Frequently during the periods between acute episodes, children are viewed as disease-free and long-term maintenance schedules are abandoned. The prolonged inflammatory process occurring in the absence of symptoms, primarily in children with moderate to severe asthma, can lead to airway remodelling and eventual irreversible disease.

Each child should have a management plan in place to determine when to step up or step down treatment. Figure 40.13 provides an example of an action plan that may be helpful to families in the management of asthma. The action plan should also be kept on file at the child's school, and relief medication should be available to the child at all times. The action plan should be reviewed at every follow-up appointment and updated as needed. Children who experience exercise-induced bronchospasm may still participate in physical education or athletics, but may need to be allowed to use their medicine before the activity. Provide appropriate education to the child and family based on the child's individualized stepwise treatment plan. Stress the concept of maintenance medications for the prevention of future serious disease in addition to controlling or preventing current symptoms.

AAAAI
AMERICAN ACADEMY OF ALLERGY
ASTHMA & IMMUNOLOGY
www.aaaai.org

ASTHMA ACTION PLAN

Name: _____   Date: _____
Emergency Contact: _____   Relationship: _____
Cell phone: _____   Work phone: _____
Health Care Provider: _____   Phone number: _____
Personal Best Peak Flow: _____

GREEN ZONE:
Doing Well
✓ No coughing, wheezing, chest tightness, or difficulty breathing
✓ Can work, play, exercise, perform usual activities without symptoms
OR
✓ Peak flow ____ to ____ (80% to 100% of personal best)

Take these medicines every day for control and maintenance:

Medicine	How much to take	When and how often

YELLOW ZONE:
Caution/Getting Worse
✓ Coughing, wheezing, chest tightness, or difficulty breathing
✓ Symptoms with daily activities, work, play, and exercise
✓ Nighttime awakenings with symptoms
OR
✓ Peak flow ____ to ____ (50% to 80% of personal best)

CONTINUE your Green Zone medicines PLUS take these quick-relief medicines:

Medicine	How much to take	When and how often

Call your doctor if you have been in the Yellow Zone for more than 24 hours.

Also call your doctor if: _____

RED ZONE:
Alert!
✓ Difficulty breathing, coughing, wheezing not helped with medications
✓ Trouble walking or talking due to asthma symptoms
✓ Not responding to quick relief medication
OR
✓ Peak flow is less than ____ (50% of personal best)

FOR EXTREME TROUBLE BREATHING/SHORTNESS OF BREATH GET IMMEDIATE HELP!
Take these quick-relief medicines:

Medicine	How much to take	When and how often

CALL your doctor NOW.
GO to the hospital/emergency department or CALL for an ambulance NOW!

This information is for general purposes and is not intended to replace the advice of a qualified health professional. For more information on asthma, visit www.aaaai.org. © 2009 American Academy of Allergy, Asthma & Immunology

FIGURE 40.13 Asthma action plan. (Used with permission from American Academy of Allergy, Asthma and Immunology, http://www.aaaai.org/professionals/asthma-action-plan.pdf)

Educate families and children on the appropriate use of medication delivery devices as well as the purposes, functions, and side effects of the medications. Require return demonstrations of equipment use to ensure that children and families can use the equipment properly (Teaching Guidelines 40.5).

Take Note!
The NAEPP (2007) recommends use of a spacer or holding chamber with metered-dose inhalers to increase the bioavailability of medication in the lungs (John & Brady, 2013a).

In children who have more severe asthma, the NAEPP (2007) recommends the use of the PEFR to determine daily control. PEFR measurements obtained via a home peak flow meter can be very helpful as long as the meter is used appropriately (John & Brady, 2013a); Teaching Guidelines 40.6 gives instructions on peak flow meter use. The child's "personal best" is determined

collaboratively with the physician or nurse practitioner during a symptom-free period. PEFR is measured daily at home using the peak flow meter. The asthma management plan then gives specific instructions based on the PEFR measurement (Table 40.4).

Take Note!
Young children with asthma receiving inhaled medications via a nebulizer should use a snugly fitting mask to ensure accurate deposition of medication to the lungs. Discourage "blow-by" via nebulizer, as medication delivery is variable and unreliable (NAEPP, 2007).

Avoidance of allergens is another key component of asthma management. Avoiding known triggers helps to prevent exacerbations as well as long-term inflammatory changes. This can be a difficult task for most families, particularly if the affected child suffers from several allergies. Refer to Teaching Guidelines 40.4 for strategies of allergen avoidance.

Teaching Guidelines 40.5
USING COMMON ASTHMA MEDICATION DELIVERY DEVICES

Nebulizer

1. Plug in the nebulizer and connect the air compressor tubing.

2. Add the medication to the medicine cup.

3. Attach the mask or the mouthpiece and hose to the medicine cup.

4. Place the mask on the child or (see step 5).

5. Instruct the child to close the lips around the mouthpiece and breathe through the mouth.

6. After use, wash the mouthpiece and medicine cup with water and allow to air dry.

Metered-Dose Inhaler

1. Shake the inhaler and take off the cap.

2. Attach the inhaler to the spacer or holding chamber.

3. Breathe out completely.

4. Put the spacer mouthpiece in the mouth (or place the mask over the child's nose and mouth, ensuring a good seal).

5. Compress the inhaler and inhale slowly and deeply. Hold the breath for a count of 10.

6. Wait 1 full minute before second inhalation, if prescribed.

Turbuhaler

1. Hold the Turbuhaler upright. Load the dose by twisting the brown grip fully to the right.

4. Holding the Turbuhaler horizontally, place the mouth firmly around the mouthpiece and inhale deeply and forcefully.

2. Then twist it to the left until you hear it click.

3. Breathe out fully.

5. Remove the Turbuhaler from the mouth and then breathe out.

Teaching Guidelines 40.6
USING A PEAK FLOW METER

- Slide the arrow down to "zero."
- Stand up straight.
- Take a deep breath and close the lips tightly around the mouthpiece.
- Blow out hard and fast (like blowing out a candle).
- Note the number the arrow moves to.
- Repeat three times and record the highest reading.
- Keep a record of daily readings, being sure to measure peak flow at the same time each day.

Adapted from John, R. M., & Brady, M. A. (2013a). Atopic and rheumatic disorders. In C. E. Burns, A. M. Dunn, M. A. Brady, N. B. Starr, & C. G. Blosser (Eds.). *Pediatric primary care* (5th ed.). Philadelphia, PA: Elsevier Saunders.

Take Note!

Teach the child and family that exposure to cigarette smoke increases the need for medications in children with asthma as well as the frequency of asthma exacerbations. Both indoor air quality and environmental pollution contribute to asthma in children (John & Brady, 2013a).

Asthma education is a critical component for ensuring optimal health in children with asthma. This education is not limited to the hospital or clinic setting. Nurses and other health providers can become involved in community asthma education: community-centred education in schools, churches, and day care centres or through peer educators has been shown to be effective. Furthermore, technology is improving access to health visits; telephone and video conferencing can facilitate education for families in rural and isolated areas. Education should include pathophysiology, asthma triggers,

TABLE 40.4	ASSESSMENT OF PEAK EXPIRATORY FLOW RATE (PEFR)		
Zone[a]	PEFR	Symptoms	Action
Green: Good control	>80% personal best	None	Take usual medications
Yellow: Caution	50–80% personal best	Possibly present	Take short-acting inhaled β_2-agonist right away. Talk to your physician or nurse practitioner
Red: Medical alert	<50% personal best	Usually present	Take short-acting inhaled β_2-agonist right away. Go to office or emergency department

[a]The National Asthma Education and Prevention Program recommended the "traffic light" approach for educating individuals on PEFRs and management plans.

Adapted from National Asthma Education and Prevention Program. (2007). *Expert panel report 3: Guidelines for the diagnosis and management of asthma* (NIH Publication No. 07–4051). Bethesda, MD: National Institutes of Health, National Heart, Lung and Blood Institute.

and prevention and treatment strategies. With such a large number of children affected with this chronic disease, community education has the potential to make a broad impact.

PROMOTING THE CHILD'S SELF-ESTEEM

Fear of an exacerbation and feeling "different" from other children can harm a child's self-esteem. In qualitative research studies, children have made such statements as "my body shuts down" and "I feel like I'm going to die" (Yoos, Kitzman, McMullen, Sidora-Arcoleo, & Anson, 2005). The fatigue and fear associated with chronic asthma may reduce the child's confidence and sense of control over his or her body and life. In addition to coping with a chronic illness, the asthmatic child often also has to cope with school-related issues. Moodiness, acting out, and withdrawal correlate with increases in school absence, which can contribute to poor school performance. To live in fear of an exacerbation or to be unable to participate in activities affects the child's self-esteem (Yoos et al., 2005).

Through education and support, the child can gain a sense of control. Children need to learn to master their disease. Accurate evaluation of asthma symptoms and improvement of self-esteem may help the child to experience less panic with an acute episode. Improved self-esteem might also help the child cope with the disease in general and with feeling different from his or her peers. The school-age child has the cognitive ability to begin taking responsibility for asthma management, with continued involvement on the part of the parents. Transferring control of asthma care to the child is an important developmental process that will increase the child's feeling of control over the illness.

PROMOTING FAMILY COPING

Caregiver fear and denial occurs in many families. The family, through education and encouragement, can become the experts on the child's illness as well as advocates for the child's well-being. The resilient child is better able to cope with the challenges facing him or her, including asthma. Cohesiveness and warmth in the family environment can improve a child's resiliency as well as contribute to family hardiness. Parents need to be allowed to ask questions and voice their concerns. A nurse who understands the family's issues and concerns is better able to plan for support and education. Tools are available to assess and monitor how a family is coping, and the effect the child's asthma is having on their lives. The Pediatric Asthma Caregiver Quality of Life Questionnaire (PACQLQ) (Juniper et al., 1996) is an example of a screening tool that can contribute to family-centred care in practice. Provide culturally sensitive education and interventions that focus on increasing the family's commitment to, and control of, asthma management. As the child and parents become confident in their ability to recognize asthma symptoms and cope with asthma and its periodic episodes, the family's ability to cope will improve.

Thinking About Development

Ryan Jennings is a 13-year-old male with a history of moderate asthma. He has been prescribed a long-term control medication to be taken routinely and a rescue medicine to be used as needed and before exercise. He is a talented pitcher and would like to participate with his school's baseball team.

How will Ryan's developmental stage affect self-care related to his asthma? What is the most appropriate approach for the nurse to take to educate Ryan about his medications and disease process?

How will the nurse foster compliance in Ryan?

Chronic Lung Disease

Chronic lung disease (formerly termed bronchopulmonary dysplasia) is often diagnosed in infants who have experienced RDS and continue to require oxygen at 28 days of age. It is a chronic respiratory condition seen most commonly in premature infants. It results from a variety of factors, including pulmonary immaturity, acute lung injury, barotrauma, inflammatory mediators, and volutrauma. Epithelial stretching, macrophage and polymorphonuclear cell invasion, and airway edema affect the growth and development of lung structures. Cilia loss and airway lining denudation reduce the normal cleansing abilities of the lung. The number of normal alveoli is reduced by one third to one half. Lower birth weights, white race, and male gender pose increased risk for development of chronic lung disease. Complications include pulmonary artery hypertension, cor pulmonale, congestive heart failure, and severe bacterial or viral pneumonia.

Anti-inflammatory inhaled medications are used for maintenance, and short-acting bronchodilators are used as needed for wheezing episodes. Supplemental long-term oxygen therapy may be required in some infants.

Nursing Assessment

Tachypnea and increased work of breathing are characteristic of chronic lung disease. After discharge from the neonatal intensive care unit (NICU), these symptoms can continue. Exertion such as activity or oral feeding can cause dyspnea to worsen. Failure to thrive might also be evident. Auscultation might reveal breath sounds that are diminished in the bases. These infants have reactive airway episodes, so wheezing might be present during times of exacerbation. If fluid overload develops, rales may be heard.

Nursing Management

If the infant is oxygen dependent, provide education to the parents about oxygen tanks, nasal cannula use, pulse oximetry use, and nebulizer treatments. Often these children require increased calorie formulas to grow adequately. Fluid restrictions and/or diuretics are necessary in some infants. Follow-up echocardiograms might be used to determine resolution of pulmonary artery hypertension prior to weaning from oxygen. Encourage developmentally appropriate activities. It might be difficult for the oxygen-dependent infant or toddler to reach gross motor milestones or explore the environment because the length of the oxygen tubing limits him or her.

Parental support is also a key nursing intervention. After a long and trying period of ups and downs with their newborn in the intensive care unit, parents find themselves exhausted caring for their medically fragile infant at home.

Cystic Fibrosis

Cystic fibrosis (CF) is an autosomal recessive disorder that affects 1 in 3,600 children born in Canada (Cystic Fibrosis Canada, 2017). A deletion occurring on the long arm of chromosome 7 at the cystic fibrosis transmembrane regulator (CFTR) is the responsible gene mutation. DNA testing can be used prenatally and in newborns to identify the presence of the mutation. In Canada, screening for CF is a part of routine newborn screening panels. Pre-conception genetic screening may be indicated for couples deemed high-risk.

CF is the most common debilitating disease of childhood among those of European descent. Medical advances in recent years have greatly increased the length and quality of life for affected children, with median age for survival being 50.9 years (Cystic Fibrosis Canada, 2015). Complications include hemoptysis, pneumothorax, bacterial colonization, cor pulmonale, volvulus, intussusception, intestinal obstruction, rectal prolapse, gastroesophageal reflux disease (GERD), diabetes, portal hypertension, liver failure, gallstones, and decreased fertility.

Pathophysiology

In CF, the CFTR mutation causes alterations in epithelial ion transport on mucosal surfaces, resulting in generalized dysfunction of the exocrine glands. The epithelial cells fail to conduct chloride, and water transport abnormalities occur. This results in thickened, tenacious secretions in the sweat glands, gastrointestinal tract, pancreas, respiratory tract, and other exocrine tissues. The increased viscosity of these secretions makes them difficult to clear. The sweat glands produce a larger amount of chloride, leading to a salty taste of the skin and alterations in electrolyte balance and dehydration. The pancreas, intrahepatic bile ducts, intestinal glands, gallbladder, and submaxillary glands become obstructed by viscous mucus and eosinophilic material. Pancreatic enzyme activity is lost and malabsorption of fats, proteins, and carbohydrates occurs, resulting in poor growth and large, malodorous stools. Excess mucus is produced by the tracheobronchial glands. Abnormally thick mucus plugs the small airways, and then bronchiolitis and further plugging of the airways occur. Secondary bacterial infection with *Staphylococcus aureus*, *Pseudomonas aeruginosa*, and *Burkholderia cepacia* often occurs. This contributes to obstruction and inflammation, leading to chronic infection, tissue damage, and respiratory failure. Nasal polyps and recurrent sinusitis are common. Boys have tenacious seminal fluid and experience blocking of the vas deferens, often making them infertile (Hazle, 2010). In girls, thick cervical secretions might limit penetration of sperm. Table 40.5 gives further details of the pathophysiology and resulting respiratory and gastrointestinal clinical manifestations of CF.

TABLE 40.5	PATHOPHYSIOLOGY OF CYSTIC FIBROSIS AND RESULTANT RESPIRATORY AND GASTROINTESTINAL CLINICAL MANIFESTATIONS	
Defect in the CFTR Gene Effects	**Pathophysiology**	**Clinical Manifestations**
Respiratory tract	• Infection leads to neutrophilic inflammation • Cleavage of complement receptors and immunoglobin G leads to opsono-phagocytosis failure • Chemoattractant interleukin-8 and elastin degradase contribute to inflammatory response • Thick, tenacious sputum that is chronically colonized with bacteria results • Air trapping related to airway obstruction occurs • Pulmonary parenchyma is eventually destroyed	• Airway obstruction • Difficulty clearing secretions • Respiratory distress and impaired gas exchange • Chronic cough • Barrel-shaped chest • Decreased pulmonary function • Clubbing • Recurrent pneumonia • Hemoptysis • Pneumothorax • Chronic sinusitis • Nasal polyps • Cor pulmonale (right-sided heart failure)
Gastrointestinal tract	• Decreased chloride and water secretion into the intestine (causing dehydration of the intestinal material) and into the bile ducts (causing increased bile viscosity) • Reduced pancreatic bicarbonate secretion • Hypersecretion of gastric acid • Insufficiency of pancreatic enzymes (amylase, lipase, pancrease) necessary for digestion and absorption • Pancreas secretes thick mucus	• Meconium ileus • Retention of fecal matter in distal intestine, resulting in vomiting, abdominal distention and cramping, anorexia, right lower quadrant pain • Sludging of intestinal contents may lead to fecal impaction, rectal prolapse, bowel obstruction, and intussusception. • Obstructive cirrhosis with esophageal varices, and splenomegaly • Gallstones • Gastroesophageal reflux disease (compounded by postural drainage with chest physiotherapy) • Inadequate protein absorption • Altered absorption of iron and vitamins A, D, E, and K • Failure to thrive • Hyperglycemia and development of diabetes later in life

Adapted from Federico, M. J., Halbower, S., Kerby, G. S., Sagel, S. D., Stillwell, P., Zemanick, E. T., . . . Deterding, R. R. (2014). *Respiratory tract & mediastinum.* In W. W. Hay, M. J. Levin, R. R. Deterding, M. J. Abzug, & J. M. Sondheimer (Eds.). *Current pediatric diagnosis and treatment* (21st ed.). New York: McGraw-Hill; and Hazle, L. A. (2010). Cystic fibrosis. In P. J. Allen, J. A. Vessey, & N. A. Schapiro (Eds.). *Primary care of the child with a chronic condition* (5th ed.). St. Louis, MO: Mosby.

Therapeutic Management

Therapeutic management of CF is aimed toward minimizing pulmonary complications, maximizing lung function, preventing infection, and facilitating growth. All children with CF who have pulmonary involvement require chest physiotherapy daily to mobilize secretions from the lungs. Depending on the child's age, this regime will differ. The regional Cystic Fibrosis Clinics throughout Canada often guide this treatment. In younger children, postural drainage, percussion, and vibrations along with a forced expiratory breathing technique tend to be the treatment of choice. However, positive expiratory pressure mask treatments and autogenic drainage are routinely used for older children to promote independence in respiratory hygiene. Other adjuncts have been researched such as the high oscillating vest, but their effectiveness has

not been proven more beneficial than current treatment strategies (McIlwaine et al., 2013). Physical exercise is encouraged. Recombinant human DNase (Pulmozyme) may be given daily using a nebulizer to decrease sputum viscosity and help clear secretions. Nebulized hypertonic saline (available in different strengths) is also used in some children, prior to their secretion clearance regime, in order to assist with secretion clearance. Inhaled bronchodilators and anti-inflammatory agents are prescribed for some children. Aerosolized antibiotics are often prescribed and may be given at home as well as in the hospital. Choice of antibiotic is determined by sputum culture and sensitivity results. Pancreatic enzymes and supplemental fat-soluble vitamins are prescribed to promote adequate digestion and absorption of nutrients and optimize nutritional status. Increased-calorie, high-protein diets are recommended, and sometimes supplemental high-calorie formula, either orally or via feeding tube, is needed. Some children require total parenteral nutrition to maintain or gain weight. Lung transplantation has been successful in some children with CF.

Nursing Assessment

For a full description of the assessment phase of the nursing process, refer to the Nursing Process Overview section earlier in the chapter. Assessment findings pertinent to CF are discussed below.

HEALTH HISTORY

Elicit a description of the present illness and chief complaint. Common signs and symptoms reported during the health history in the undiagnosed child might include:

- A salty taste to the child's skin (resulting from excess chloride loss via perspiration)
- Meconium ileus or late, difficult passage of meconium stool in the newborn period
- Abdominal pain or difficulty passing stool (infants or toddlers might present with intestinal obstruction or intussusception at the time of diagnosis)
- Bulky, greasy stools
- Poor weight gain and growth despite good appetite
- Chronic or recurrent cough and/or upper or lower respiratory infections

Children known to have CF are often admitted to the hospital for pulmonary exacerbations or other complications of the disease. The health history should include questions related to:

- Respiratory status: has cough, sputum production, or work of breathing increased?
- Appetite and weight gain
- Activity tolerance
- Increased need for pulmonary or pancreatic medications
- Presence of fever
- Presence of bone pain
- Any other changes in physical state or medication regimen

PHYSICAL EXAMINATION

The physical examination includes inspection, auscultation, percussion, and palpation.

Inspection. Observe the child's general appearance and colour. Check the nasal passages for polyps. Note respiratory rate, work of breathing, use of accessory muscles, position of comfort, frequency and severity of cough, and quality and quantity of sputum produced. The child with CF often has a barrel chest (anterior–posterior diameter approximates transverse diameter) (Fig. 40.14). Clubbing of the nail beds might also be present. Note whether rectal prolapse is present. Does the child appear small or thin for his or her age? The child might have a protuberant abdomen and thin extremities, with decreased amounts

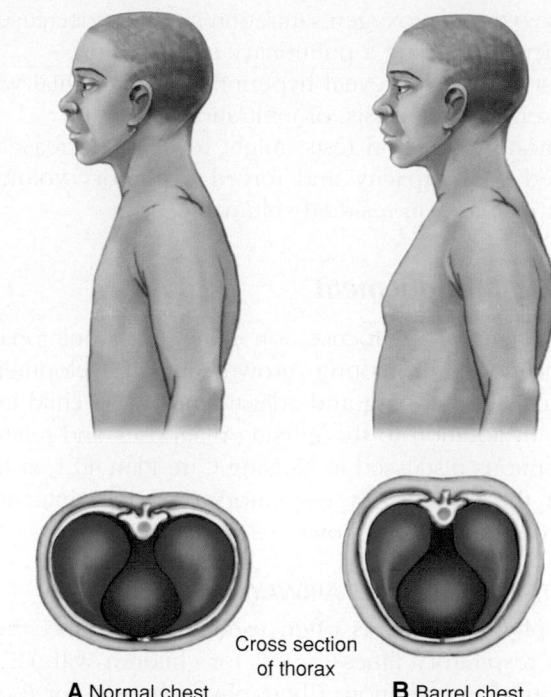

Cross section of thorax

A Normal chest   **B** Barrel chest

FIGURE 40.14 **A.** Normal chest shape—transverse diameter is greater than anterior–posterior diameter. **B.** Barrel chest—transverse diameter equals anterior–posterior diameter.

of subcutaneous fat. Observe for the presence of edema (sign of cardiac or liver failure). Note distended neck veins or the presence of a heave (signs of cor pulmonale).

Auscultation. Auscultation may reveal a variety of adventitious breath sounds. Fine or coarse crackles and scattered or localized wheezing might be present. With progressive obstructive pulmonary involvement, breath sounds might be diminished. Tachycardia might be present. Note the presence of a gallop (might occur with cor pulmonale). Note the adequacy of bowel sounds.

Percussion. Percussion over the lung fields usually yields hyperresonance due to air trapping. Diaphragmatic excursion might be decreased. Percussion of the abdomen might reveal dullness over an enlarged liver or mass related to intestinal obstruction.

Palpation. Palpation might yield a finding of asymmetric chest excursion if atelectasis is present. Tactile fremitus may be decreased over areas of atelectasis. Note if tenderness is present over the liver (might be an early sign of cor pulmonale).

LABORATORY AND DIAGNOSTIC TESTS

Common laboratory and diagnostic studies ordered for the diagnosis and assessment of CF include:

- Sweat chloride test: considered suspicious if the level of chloride in collected sweat is above 50 mEq/L and diagnostic if the level is above 60 mEq/L

- Pulse oximetry: oxygen saturation might be decreased, particularly during a pulmonary exacerbation
- Chest x-ray: may reveal hyperinflation, bronchial wall thickening, atelectasis, or infiltration
- Pulmonary function tests: might reveal a decrease in forced vital capacity and forced expiratory volume, with increases in residual volume

Nursing Management

Management of CF focuses on minimizing pulmonary complications, promoting growth and development, and facilitating coping and adjustment by the child and family. In addition to the nursing diagnoses and related interventions discussed in Nursing Care Plan 40.1, at the end of the chapter, for respiratory disorders, interventions common to CF follow.

MAINTAINING PATENT AIRWAY

Chest physiotherapy is often used as an adjunct therapy in respiratory illnesses, but for children with CF, it is a critical intervention. Chest physiotherapy for these patients must be performed several times a day to assist with mobilization of secretions. Their routine will be tailored to them specifically by the Regional Cystic Fibrosis Clinic. Nursing Procedure 40.2 provides education on performance of postural drainage, percussion, and vibration treatments. Routines may be changed based on the child's need and local management approach; the Cystic Fibrosis Canada provides a provincial list; further information can be found at thePoint.

For older children and adolescents, the flutter-valve device, positive expiratory pressure therapy, or a high-frequency chest compression vest may also be used. The flutter valve device provides high-frequency oscillation to the airway as the child exhales into a mouthpiece that contains a steel ball. Positive expiratory pressure therapy involves exhaling through a flow resistor, which creates positive expiratory pressure. The cycles of exhalation are repeated until coughing yields expectoration of secretions. The vest airway clearance system provides high-frequency chest wall oscillation to increase airflow velocity to create repetitive cough-like shear forces and to decrease the viscosity of secretions. Breathing exercises are also helpful in promoting mucus clearance. Encourage physical exercise, as it helps to promote mucus secretion as well as provides cardiopulmonary conditioning. Ensure that Pulmozyme is administered, as well as inhaled bronchodilators and anti-inflammatory agents if prescribed.

PREVENTING INFECTION

Vigorous pulmonary hygiene for mobilization of secretions is critical to prevent infection. Aerosolized antibiotics can be given at home as well as in the hospital. Children with frequent or severe respiratory exacerbations might require lengthy courses of intravenous antibiotics.

MAINTAINING GROWTH

Pancreatic enzyme supplements (pancrelipase) must be administered with all meals and snacks to promote adequate digestion and absorption of nutrients. The number of capsules required depends on the extent of pancreatic insufficiency and the amount of food being ingested. The dosage can be adjusted until an adequate growth pattern is established and the number of stools is consistent at one or two per day. Children will need additional enzyme capsules when high-fat foods are being eaten. In the infant or young child, the enzyme capsule can be opened and sprinkled on cereal or applesauce. A well-balanced, high-calorie, high-protein diet is necessary to ensure adequate growth. Some children require up to one and a half times the recommended daily allowance of calories for children of their age. A number of commercially available nutritional formulas and shakes are available for diet supplementation.

In infants, breastfeeding should be continued with enzyme administration. Some infants will require fortification of breast milk or supplementation with high-calorie formulas. Commercially available infant formulas can continue to be used for the formula-fed infant and can be mixed to provide a larger number of calories if necessary. Supplementation with vitamins A, D, E, and K is necessary. Administer gavage feedings or total parenteral nutrition as prescribed to provide for adequate growth.

PROMOTING FAMILY COPING

CF is a serious chronic illness that requires daily interventions. It can be hard to maintain a schedule that requires pulmonary hygiene several times daily as well as close attention to appropriate diet and enzyme supplementation. Adjusting to the demands that the illness places on the child and family is difficult. Continual adjustments within the family must occur. Children are frequently hospitalized, and this may place an additional strain on the family and its finances. Children with CF may express fear or feelings of isolation, and siblings may be worried or jealous. Encourage the family to lead a normal life through involvement in activities and school attendance during periods of wellness.

Take Note!

Children aged 6 and older who have the G551D, G1244E, G1349D, G178R, G551 S, S1251 N, S1255P, S549 N, or S549R mutation of the cystic fibrosis gene may be prescribed ivacaftor. Use of ivacaftor results in thinning of lung mucus, resulting in easier airway clearance via coughing. It is the first drug to act directly on the defective gene (Vertex Pharmaceuticals, 2015).

Starting at the time of diagnosis, families often demonstrate significant stress as the severity of the diagnosis and the significance of disease chronicity become real

NURSING PROCEDURE 40.2

Performing Chest Percussions and Vibrations

May be preceded by an inhalation treatment; should not be performed after eating.

1. Provide percussion via a cupped hand or an infant percussion device. Appropriate percussion yields a hollow sound, not a slapping sound.

2. Percuss each segment of the lung for 1 to 2 minutes.

POSITION #1
UPPER LOBES, Apical segments

POSITION #1, for infants
UPPER LOBES, Apical segments

POSITION #2
UPPER LOBES, Posterior segments

POSITION #3
UPPER LOBES, Anterior segments

(continued)

NURSING PROCEDURE 40.2

Performing Chest Percussions and Vibrations (continued)

POSITION #4
LINGULA

POSITION #5
MIDDLE LOBE

POSITION #6
LOWER LOBES, Anterior basal segments

POSITION #7
LOWER LOBES, Posterior basal segments

POSITION #8 & 9
LOWER LOBES, Lateral basal segments

POSITION #10
LOWER LOBES, Superior segments

3. Place the ball of the hand on the lung segment, keeping the arm and shoulder straight. Vibrate by tensing and relaxing your arms during the child's exhalation. Vibrate each lung segment for at least five exhalations.

4. Encourage the child to deep breathe and cough.

5. Change drainage positions and repeat percussion and vibration.

for them. The family should be involved in the child's care from the time of diagnosis, whether in the outpatient setting or in the hospital. Ongoing education about the illness and its treatments is necessary. Once the initial shock of diagnosis has passed and the family has adjusted to initial care, the family usually learns how to manage the requirements of care. Powerlessness gives way to adaptation. As family members become more comfortable with their understanding of the illness and the required treatments, they will eventually become the experts on the child's care. It is important for the nurse to recognize and respect the family's changing needs over time.

Providing daily intense care can be tiring, and noncompliance on the part of the family or child might occur as a result of this fatigue. Hypervigilance may also occur as parents attempt to control the difficult situation and protect the child. Families welcome support and encouragement. Most families eventually progress past the stages of fear, guilt, and powerlessness to a way of living that is different than what they anticipated but is something that they can manage.

Refer parents to a local support group for families of children with CF. Cystic Fibrosis Canada has chapters and events throughout Canada. Further information can be found at http://www.cysticfibrosis.ca/.

Parents of children with a terminal illness might face the death of their child at an earlier age than expected. Assisting with anticipatory grieving and making decisions related to end-of-life care are other important nursing interventions.

PREPARING THE CHILD AND FAMILY FOR ADULTHOOD WITH CYSTIC FIBROSIS

With current technologic and medication advances, many more children with CF are surviving to adulthood and beyond their 50s (Cystic Fibrosis Canada, 2015). Lung transplantation is now being used in some children with success, thus prolonging life expectancy (barring transplant complications) (Hazle, 2010). Children with CF should have the goal of independent living as an adult, as other children do. Making the transition from a pediatric medical home to an adult medical home should be viewed as a normal part of growing up, similar to completing school or finding a first job. Pediatric clinics are focused on family-centred care that heavily involves the child's parents, but adults with CF need a different focus, one that views them as independent adults.

Those with CF can make the transition from pediatric to adult care with thoughtful preparation and coordination. They desire and deserve a smooth transition in care that will result in appropriate ongoing medical management of CF in an environment that is geared toward adults rather than children.

Adults with CF are able to find rewarding work and pursue relationships. Most men with CF are capable of sexual intercourse. While the vas deference is blocked or absent, most men with CF will have sperm present in their testicles. Therefore, men with CF will need to access assisted reproductive technology (ART) to have biologic children. Females might have difficulty conceiving, for example, linked to cervical mucus and nutritional status. If a female with CF becomes pregnant, she should be cautioned about the additional respiratory strain that pregnancy causes. All children of parents with CF will be carriers of the gene.

Apnea

Apnea is defined as absence of breathing for longer than 20 seconds; it might be accompanied by bradycardia. Sometimes apnea presents in the form of an acute life-threatening event (ALTE), an event in which the infant or child exhibits some combination of apnea, colour change, muscle tone alteration, coughing, or gagging. Apnea may also occur acutely at any age as a result of respiratory distress. This discussion will focus on apnea that is chronic or recurrent in nature or that occurs as part of an ALTE.

Apnea in infants may be central (unrelated to any other cause) or may occur with other illnesses such as sepsis and respiratory infection. Apnea in newborns might be associated with hypothermia, hypoglycemia, infection, or hyperbilirubinemia. Apnea of prematurity occurs secondary to an immature respiratory system. Apnea should not be considered a predecessor to sudden infant death syndrome (SIDS). Current research has not proven this theory, and SIDS generally occurs in otherwise healthy young infants (American Academy of Pediatrics [AAP], 2011). Box 40.3 gives more information about SIDS and its prevention.

Therapeutic management of apnea varies depending on the cause. When apnea occurs as a result of another disorder or infection, treatment is directed toward that cause. In the event of apnea, stimulation may trigger the infant to take a breath. If breathing does not resume, rescue breathing or bag-valve-mask ventilation is necessary. Infants and children who have experienced an ALTE or who have chronic apnea may require ongoing cardiac/apnea monitoring. Caffeine or theophylline is sometimes administered, primarily in premature infants, to stimulate respirations (Kelly, 2010).

Nursing Assessment

Question about the infant's position and activities preceding the apneic episode. Did the infant experience a colour change? Did the infant self-stimulate (breathe again on his or her own), or did he or she require stimulation from the caretaker? Assess risk factors for apnea, which may include prematurity, anemia, and history of metabolic disorders. Apnea may occur in association with cardiac or neurologic disturbances, respiratory infection, sepsis, child abuse, or poisoning.

SUDDEN INFANT DEATH SYNDROME (SIDS)

Definition

Sudden death of a previously healthy infant younger than 1 year of age

Prevention

- Place all infants in the supine position to sleep (even side-lying is not as safe and is not recommended by the AAP).
- Provide a firm sleep surface and avoid soft bedding, excess covers, pillows, bumper pads, and stuffed animals in the crib.
- Avoid maternal prenatal smoking and exposure of the infant to second-hand smoke.
- Ensure the infant sleeps separately from the parents.
- Avoid overbundling or overdressing the infant.
- Encourage pacifier use during naps and at bedtime if the infant is receptive to it (Canadian Paediatric Society, 2016).

Support and Information

- Association for SIDS and Infant Mortality Program: www.asip1.org
- National Sudden Infant Death Resource Center: www.sidscenter.org
- SIDS Alliance: www.sidsalliance.org
- Sudden Infant Death Syndrome Network, Inc.: http://sids-network.org/

FIGURE 40.15 The home apnea monitor uses a soft belt with a Velcro attachment to hold two leads in the appropriate position on the chest.

often experience disrupted sleep and some may display negative coping patterns (Scollan-Koliopoulos & Koliopoulos, 2010). Providing appropriate education to the parents about the nature of the child's disorder as well as action to take in the event of apnea may give the family a sense of mastery over the situation, thus decreasing their anxiety. Refer families to local support groups.

TRACHEOSTOMY

A **tracheostomy** is an artificial opening in the airway; usually, a plastic tracheostomy tube is in place to form a patent airway. Tracheostomies are performed to relieve airway obstruction, such as with subglottic stenosis (narrowing of the airway sometimes resulting from long-term intubation). They are also used for pulmonary hygiene and in the child who requires chronic mechanical ventilation. The tracheostomy facilitates secretion removal, reduces work of breathing, and increases the child's comfort. In some cases, the tracheostomy facilitates mechanical ventilation weaning. It may be permanent or temporary, depending on the indication. The tracheostomy tube varies in size and type depending on the child's airway size and health and the length of time the child will require the tracheostomy. Silastic tracheostomy tubes are soft and flexible; they are available with a single lumen or may have an outer and inner lumen. Both types have an obturator (the guide used during tube changes). Uncuffed tubes are used more often in the pediatric population (Deutsch, 2010). Figure 40.16 shows various types of tracheostomy tubes.

Complications immediately after surgery include hemorrhage, air entry, pulmonary edema, anatomic damage, and respiratory arrest. At any point in time the tracheostomy tube may become occluded, which compromises ventilation. Complications of chronic tracheostomy include infection, cellulitis, and formation of granulation tissue around the insertion site.

In the hospitalized infant, note absence of respiration, position, colour, and other associated findings, such as emesis on the bedclothes.

Nursing Management

If an infant who is apneic fails to be stimulated and does not breathe again, pulselessness will result. When an infant is noted to be apneic, gently stimulate him or her to take a breath again. If gentle stimulation is unsuccessful, then rescue breathing or bag-valve-mask ventilation must be started.

To avoid apnea in the newborn, maintain a neutral thermal environment. Avoid excessive vagal stimulation and taking rectal temperatures (the vagal response can cause bradycardia, resulting in apnea) (Jarvis, 2012). Administer caffeine or theophylline if prescribed and teach families about the use of these medications.

Infants with recurrent apnea or ALTE may be discharged on a home apnea monitor (Fig. 40.15). Provide education on use of the monitor, guidance about when to notify the physician or nurse practitioner or monitor service about alarms, and training in infant cardiopulmonary resuscitation (CPR). The monitor is usually discontinued after 3 months without a significant event of apnea or bradycardia. In some ways, the monitor gives parents peace of mind, but in others it can make them more nervous about the well-being of their child. Parents

FIGURE 40.16 Note smaller size and absence of inner cannula on particular brands of pediatric tracheostomy tubes.

FIGURE 40.17 The trach collar allows for humidification of inspired air or supplemental oxygen.

Nursing Assessment

When obtaining the history for a child with a tracheostomy, note the reason for the tracheostomy, as well as the size and type of tracheostomy tube. Inspect the site. The stoma should appear pink and without bleeding or drainage. The tube itself should be clean and free from secretions. The tracheostomy ties should fit securely, allowing one finger to slide beneath the ties. Inspect the skin under the ties for rash or redness. Observe work of breathing.

When caring for the infant or child with a tracheostomy, whether in the hospital, home, or community setting, a thorough respiratory assessment is necessary. Note the presence of secretions and their colour, thickness, and amount. Auscultate for breath sounds, which should be clear and equal throughout all lung fields. Measure pulse oximetry. When infection is suspected or secretions are discoloured or have a foul odour, a sputum culture may be obtained.

Take Note!

Keep small toys (risk of aspiration), plastic bibs or bedding (risk of airway occlusion), and talcum powder (risk of inhalation injury) out of reach of the child with a tracheostomy.

Nursing Management

In the immediate postoperative period, the infant or child may require restraints to avoid accidental dislodgment of the tracheostomy tube. Infants and children who have had a tracheostomy for a period of time become accustomed to it and usually do not attempt to remove the tube. Since air inspired via the tracheostomy tube bypasses the upper airway, it lacks humidification, and this lack of humidity can lead to a mucus plug in the tracheostomy and resultant hypoxia. Provide humidity to either room air or oxygen via a tracheostomy collar or ventilator, depending on the child's need (Fig. 40.17). Box 40.4 lists the equipment that should be available at the bedside of any child who has a tracheostomy.

Tracheostomies require frequent suctioning to maintain patency. The appropriate length for insertion of the suction catheter depends on the size of the tracheostomy and the child's needs. Place a sign at the head of the child's bed indicating the suction catheter size and the length (in centimetres) that it should be inserted for suctioning. Keep an extra tracheostomy tube of the same size and one size smaller at the bedside in the event of an emergency.

Many pediatric tracheostomy tubes do not have an inner cannula that requires periodic removal and cleaning, so periodic removal and replacement of the chronic tracheostomy tube is required. Clean the removed tracheostomy tube with half-strength hydrogen peroxide and pipe cleaners. Rinse with distilled water and allow it to dry. The tracheostomy tube can be reused many times if adequately cleaned between uses.

Perform tracheostomy care every 8 hours or per institution protocol. Change the tracheostomy tube only as needed or per institution protocol. Nursing Procedure 40.3 gives information about tracheostomy care. Always change tracheostomy ties with an assistant to avoid accidental dislodgement of the tube.

BOX 40.4

EMERGENCY EQUIPMENT (AVAILABLE AT BEDSIDE)

- Two spare tracheostomy tubes (one the same size and one a size smaller)
- Suction equipment
- Stitch cutter (new tracheostomy)
- Spare tracheostomy ties
- Lubricating jelly
- Bag-valve-mask device
- Call bell within child's/parent's reach

NURSING PROCEDURE 40.3

Tracheostomy Care

1. Gather the necessary equipment:
   - Cleaning solution
   - Gloves
   - Pre-cut gauze pad
   - Cotton-tipped applicators
   - Clean tracheostomy ties
   - Extra tracheostomy tube in case of accidental dislodgement
2. Position the infant/child supine with a blanket or towel roll to extend the neck.
3. Open all packaging and cut tracheostomy ties to appropriate length if necessary.
4. Cleanse around the tracheostomy site with pre-scribed solution (half-strength hydrogen peroxide or acetic acid, normal saline or soap and water if at home) and cotton-tipped applicators, working from just around the tracheostomy tube outward.
5. Rinse with sterile water and cotton-tipped applicator in a similar fashion.
6. Place the pre-cut sterile gauze under the tracheostomy tube.
7. With the assistant holding the tube in place, cut the ties and remove from the tube.
8. Attach the clean ties to the tube and tie or secure in place with Velcro (Fig. 40.18).

FIGURE 40.18 Trach ties are attached to the tube and secured in place with Velcro.

If the older child or teen has a tracheostomy tube with an inner cannula, care of the inner cannula is similar to that of an adult. Involve parents in care of the tracheostomy and begin education about caring for the tracheostomy tube at home as soon as the child is stable. The child with a tracheostomy may qualify for home nursing care. Refer the family to local support groups.

NURSING CARE PLAN 40.1

Overview for the Child With a Respiratory Disorder

NURSING DIAGNOSIS: Ineffective airway clearance related to inflammation, increased secretions, mechanical obstruction, or pain as evidenced by presence of secretions, productive cough, tachypnea, and increased work of breathing

Outcome Identification and Evaluation

Child will maintain patent airway, *free from secretions or obstruction, easy work of breathing, respiratory rate within parameters for age.*

Interventions with rationale: *Maintaining a Patent Airway*

- Position with airway open (sniffing position if supine) and/or elevate head of bed *to allow for adequate ventilation.*
- Humidify oxygen or room air and ensure adequate fluid intake (intravenous or oral) *to liquefy secretions for ease in clearance.*
- Suction with bulb syringe, nasal suction catheter, or via nasopharyngeal catheter as needed, particularly prior to bottle-feeding, *to promote clearance of secretions.*

- If tachypneic, maintain nothing by mouth (NPO) status *to avoid aspiration.*
- In older child, encourage expectoration of sputum with coughing *to promote airway clearance.*
- Perform secretion clearance techniques if ordered *to mobilize secretions.*
- Ensure emergency equipment is readily available *to avoid delay should airway become at-risk.*

NURSING CARE PLAN 40.1

Overview for the Child With a Respiratory Disorder (continued)

NURSING DIAGNOSIS: Ineffective breathing pattern related to inflammatory or infectious process as evidenced by tachypnea, increased work of breathing, nasal flaring, retractions, diminished breath sounds

Outcome Identification and Evaluation

Child will exhibit adequate ventilation: *respiratory rate within parameters for age, easy work of breathing (absence of retractions, accessory muscle use, grunting), clear breath sounds with adequate aeration, oxygen saturation within prescribed parameters.*

Interventions with rationale: *Promoting Effective Breathing Patterns*

- Assess respiratory rate, breath sounds, and work of breathing frequently to ensure progress with treatment and so that deterioration can be noted early.
- Use pulse oximetry to monitor oxygen saturation in the least invasive manner to note adequacy of oxygenation and ensure early detection of hypoxemia.
- Position for comfort with open airway and room for lung expansion (usually with head of bed elevated). Use pillows or padding if necessary to maintain position to ensure optimal ventilation via maximum lung expansion.

- Administer supplemental oxygen and/or humidity as ordered to improve oxygenation.
- Allow for adequate sleep and rest periods to conserve energy.
- Administer antibiotics as ordered: may be indicated in the case of bacterial respiratory infection.
- Encourage coughing with deep breathing (can be accomplished through play) to maximize ventilation (play enhances the child's participation). If incentive spirometry is ordered, it is important to review proper technique with the child and family.

NURSING DIAGNOSIS: Impaired gas exchange, related to airway plugging, hyperinflation, atelectasis, as evidenced by cyanosis, decreased oxygen saturation, and alterations in arterial blood gases

Outcome Identification and Evaluation

Gas exchange will be adequate: *pulse oximetry reading on room air is within normal parameters for age, blood gases within normal limits, absence of cyanosis.*

Interventions with rationale: *Promoting Adequate Gas Exchange*

- Administer oxygen as ordered *to improve oxygenation.*
- Monitor oxygen saturation via pulse oximetry *to detect alterations in oxygenation.*
- Encourage clearance of secretions via coughing, expectoration, manual secretion clearance techniques, and suctioning *to improve gas exchange.*
- Administer bronchodilators if ordered (salbutamol, levalbuterol, and racemic epinephrine) *to treat bronchospasm and improve gas exchange.*

- Provide frequent contact and support to the child and family *to decrease anxiety, which increases the child's oxygen demands.*
- Assess and monitor mental status (confusion, lethargy, restlessness, combativeness): *hypoxemia and hypercarbia can lead to changes in mental status.*

NURSING DIAGNOSIS: Risk for infection related to presence of infectious organisms

Outcome Identification and Evaluation

Child will exhibit no signs of secondary infection and will not spread infection to others: *symptoms of infection decrease over time; others remain free from infection.*

(continued)

NURSING CARE PLAN 40.1

Overview for the Child With a Respiratory Disorder (continued)

Interventions with rationale: *Preventing Infection*

- Maintain aseptic technique, practice good handwashing, and use disposable suction catheters *to prevent introduction of further infectious agents.*
- Limit number of visitors and screen them for recent illness *to prevent further infection.*
- Administer antibiotics if prescribed *to prevent or treat bacterial infection.*
- Encourage nutritious diet according to child's preferences and ability to feed orally *to assist body's natural infection-fighting mechanisms.*

- Isolate the child as required *to prevent nosocomial spread of infection.*
- Teach child and family preventive measures such as good handwashing, covering mouth and nose when coughing or sneezing, and proper disposal of used tissues *to prevent nosocomial or community spread of infection.*

NURSING DIAGNOSIS: Risk for deficient fluid volume, related to decreased oral intake, insensible losses via fever, tachypnea, or diaphoresis

Outcome Identification and Evaluation

Fluid volume will be maintained: oral mucosa moist and pink, skin turgor elastic, urine output at least 1–2 mL/kg/h.

Interventions with rationale: *Maintaining Adequate Fluid Volume*

- Administer intravenous fluids if ordered *to maintain adequate hydration in NPO state.*
- When allowed oral intake, encourage oral fluids. Popsicles, favourite fluids, and games can be used *to promote intake.*
- Assess for signs of adequate hydration (flat fontanels, elastic skin turgor, moist mucosa, adequate urine output).

- Monitor intake and output *to identify fluid imbalance.*
- Monitor urine specific gravity, urine and serum electrolytes, blood urea, nitrogen, creatinine, and osmolality *to determine fluid status.*

NURSING DIAGNOSIS: Imbalanced nutrition: less than body requirements related to difficulty feeding as evidenced by poor oral intake, tiring with feeding

Outcome Identification and Evaluation

Child will maintain adequate nutritional intake: *weight is gained or maintained. Child consumes adequate diet for age.*

Interventions with rationale: *Promoting Adequate Nutritional Intake*

- Weigh on same scale at same time daily *so that measurements are consistent.*
- Perform calorie counts over a 3-day period *to determine whether caloric intake is sufficient.*
- Encourage child to choose high-calorie, protein-rich foods *to optimize growth potential.*
- Encourage young children to eat better by playing games and offering favourite foods *to improve intake.*
- Assess for risk of aspiration and possible need for alternative feeding routes. Refer to Occupational Therapist, Physical Therapist, Dietician, and/or Speech and Language Pathologist as needed.

NURSING CARE PLAN 40.1

Overview for the Child With a Respiratory Disorder (continued)

NURSING DIAGNOSIS: Activity intolerance related to high respiratory demand as evidenced by increased work of breathing and need for frequent rest when playing

Outcome Identification and Evaluation

Child will resume normal activity level: *activity is tolerated without difficulty breathing. Pulse oximetry readings and vital signs are within parameters for age and activity level.*

Interventions with rationale: *Increasing Activity Tolerance*

- Provide rest periods balanced with periods of activity, and group nursing activities and visits *to allow for sufficient rest.*
- Provide small, frequent meals *to prevent overtiring (energy is expended while eating).*

- Encourage quiet activities that do not require exertion *to prevent boredom.*
- Allow gradual increase in activity as tolerated, keeping pulse oximetry reading within normal parameters, *to minimize risk for further respiratory compromise.*

NURSING DIAGNOSIS: Fear related to difficulty breathing, unfamiliar personnel, procedures, and environment (hospital), as evidenced by clinging, crying, fussing, verbalization, or lack of cooperation

Outcome Identification and Evaluation

Fear/anxiety will be reduced: *decreased episodes of crying or fussing, happy and playful at times.*

Interventions with rationale: *Relieving Fear*

- Establish trusting relationship with child and family *to decrease anxiety and fear.*
- Utilize play *to gain child's cooperation and trust.*
- Explain procedures to child at developmentally appropriate level *to decrease fear of unknown.*
- Provide favourite blanket or soft toy/stuffy as well as comfort measures preferred by child such as rocking or music *for added security.*
- Promote family-centred care by involving parents/caregivers *to give child reassurance and decrease fear.*

NURSING DIAGNOSIS: Family processes, altered, related to child's illness or hospitalization as evidenced by family's presence in hospital, missed work, demonstration of inadequate coping

Outcome Identification and Evaluation

Parents demonstrate adequate coping and decreased anxiety: *parents are involved in child's care, ask appropriate questions, and are able to discuss child's care and condition calmly.*

Interventions with rationale: *Promoting Adequate Family Processes*

- Encourage parents to discuss their concerns related to child's illness to identify concerns and show parents that the nurse also cares about them, not just the child.
- Explain therapy, procedures, and child's behaviour to parents to decrease their anxiety.
- Encourage parents to be involved in care so they feel needed and valued.

KEY CONCEPTS

- Respiratory infections account for the majority of acute illnesses in children.

- The upper and lower airways are smaller in children than adults, making them more susceptible to obstruction in the presence of mucus, debris, or edema.

- Newborns are obligatory nose breathers.

- The child's highly compliant airway is quite susceptible to dynamic collapse in the presence of airway obstruction.

- Because they have fewer alveoli, children have a higher risk for hypoxemia than adults.

- Generally, disorders of the nose and throat do not result in increased work of breathing or affect the lungs. Thus, if the lungs are involved, lower respiratory disease must be considered.

- Wheezing may be associated with a variety of lower respiratory disorders, such as asthma, bronchiolitis, and cystic fibrosis.

- Pulse oximetry is a useful tool for determining the extent of hypoxia. Findings should be correlated with the child's clinical presentation.

- Rapid streptococcus and rapid influenza tests are very useful for the quick diagnosis of strep throat or influenza so that appropriate treatment may be instituted early in the illness.

- Supplemental oxygen is often necessary in the child who is hospitalized (particularly with lower respiratory disease). Oxygen should be humidified to prevent drying of secretions.

- Suctioning, whether with a bulb syringe or suction catheter, is very effective at maintaining airway patency, especially in the younger child or infant.

- Normal saline nasal wash is an inexpensive, simple, and safe method for decongesting the nose in the case of the common cold, allergic rhinitis, and sinusitis.

- Infants who were born prematurely; children with a chronic illness such as diabetes, congenital heart disease, sickle cell anemia, or cystic fibrosis; and children with developmental disorders such as cerebral palsy tend to be more severely affected with respiratory disorders.

- Passive cigarette smoke exposure increases the infant's and child's risk for respiratory disease.

- Continual swallowing while awake or asleep is an indication of bleeding in the postoperative tonsillectomy child.

- Positioning to ease work of breathing and maintaining a patent airway are priorities for the child with a respiratory disorder.

- To avoid Reye syndrome, aspirin should not be given to treat fever or pain in the infant or child with a viral infection.

- Infants and children at high risk for serious RSV disease should be immunized with palivizumab each RSV season. Children older than 6 months of age should be immunized against influenza yearly.

- Children at high risk for exposure to tuberculosis should be screened for infection.

- Promoting airway clearance and maintenance, effective breathing patterns, and adequate gas exchange is the priority focus of nursing intervention in pediatric respiratory disease.

- Children with any degree of respiratory distress require frequent assessment and early intervention to prevent progression to respiratory failure.

- Avoidance of allergens is critical in the treatment plan for the child with allergic rhinitis.

- Avoidance of triggers, control of the inflammatory process, and education of the child and family are the focus of asthma management.

- Respiratory physiotherapy is useful in promoting secretion clearance, increasing lung volumes, and reducing work of breathing in compromised respiratory systems.

- Children with chronic respiratory disorders and their families often need large amounts of education and psychosocial support: children often experience fear and isolation, while families must learn to balance care of the chronically ill child with other family life.

REFERENCES AND RECOMMENDED READINGS

Aldana-Aguirre, J. C., Pinto, M., Featherstone, R. M., & Kumar, M. (2017). Less invasive surfactant administration versus intubation for surfactant delivery in preterm infants with respiratory distress syndrome: A systematic review and meta-analysis. *Archives of Disease in Childhood-Fetal and Neonatal Edition*, *102*(1), F17–F23.

Allan, G. M., & Arroll, B. (2014). Prevention and treatment of the common cold: making sense of the evidence. *Canadian Medical Association Journal*, *186*(3), 190–199.

Allen, U. D.; Canadian Paediatric Society , Infectious Diseases & Immunization Committee. (2018). *The use of antiviral drugs for influenza: Guidance for practitioners*. Retrieved from https://www.cps.ca/en/documents/position/antiviral-drugs-for-influenza

Allergy and Asthma Network Mothers of Asthmatics. (2014). *Indoor AIRepair at home, school, and play.* Vienna, VA: Author.

American Academy of Allergy, Asthma and Immunology. (2011). *Asthma action plan.* Retrieved from http://www.aaaai.org/Aaaai/media/MediaLibrary/PDF%20Documents/Libraries/NEW-WEBSITE-LOGO-asthma-action-plan_HI.pdf

American Academy of Pediatrics, Task Force on Sudden Infant Death Syndrome. (2011). Policy statement: SIDS and other sleep-related deaths: Expansion of recommendations for a safe infant sleeping environment. *Pediatrics, 128*(5), 1030–1039.

American Heart Association (AHA). (2011). *Pediatric advanced life support provider manual.* Dallas, TX: Author.

Asthma Society of Canada. (2014). *Severe asthma: The Canadian patient journey.* Retrieved from https://www.asthma.ca/wp-content/uploads/2017/06/SAstudyES.pdf

Barson, W. J. (2016). *Outpatient treatment of community-acquired pneumonia in children.* Retrieved from http://www.uptodate.com/contents/outpatient-treatment-of-community-acquired-pneumonia-in-children

Batra, V., & Ang, J. Y. (2015). *Pediatric tuberculosis.* Retrieved from emedicine.medscape.com/article/969401-overview

Becker, J. A., & Smith, J. A. (2014). Return to play after infectious mononucleosis. *Sports Health, 6*(3), 232–238.

Beckton Dickinson and Company. (2016). *Product center.* Retrieved from http://www.bd.com/ds/productCenter/index.asp

Bergeson, P. S., & Shaw, J. C. (2001). Are infants really obligatory nasal breathers? *Clinical Pediatrics, 40*(10), 567–569.

Bichara, M. D., & Goldman, R. D. (2009). Magnesium for treatment of asthma in children. *Canadian Family Physician, 55*(9), 887–889.

Blosser, C. G., Brady, M. A., & Royal, R. B. (2013). Infectious diseases and immunizations. In C. A. Burns, A. M. Dunn, M. A. Brady, N. B. Starr, & C. G. Blosser (Eds.). *Pediatric primary care* (5th ed.). Philadelphia, PA: Elsevier Saunders.

Bowden, V. R., & Greenberg, C. S. (2012). *Pediatric nursing procedures* (3rd ed.). Philadelphia, PA: Lippincott Williams & Wilkins.

Brook, I. (2013). Acute sinusitis in children. *Pediatric Clinics of North America, 60,* 409–424.

Canadian Paediatric Society. (2015). *Preventing hospitalizations for respiratory syncytial virus infection.* Retrieved from http://www.cps.ca/en/documents/position/preventing-hospitalizations-for-rsv-infections

Canadian Paediatric Society. (2016). *Recommendations for the use of pacifiers.* Retrieved from http://www.cps.ca/documents/position/pacifiers (2016)

Canadian Paediatric Society. (2017a). *Bronchiolitis: Recommendations for diagnosis, monitoring, and management of children one to 24 months of age.* Retrieved from http://www.cps.ca/en/documents/position/bronchiolitis

Canadian Paediatric Society. (2017b). *Temperature measurement in paediatrics.* Retrieved from http://www.cps.ca/documents/position/temperature-measurement

Canadian Paediatric Society. (2017c). *Acute management of croup in the emergency department.* Retrieved from http://www.cps.ca/en/documents/position/acute-management-of-croup

Canadian Paediatric Society. (2019). *Caring for Kids New to Canada.* Retrieved from https://www.kidsnewtocanada.ca

Canadian Respiratory Guidelines. (2018). *Guidelines library.* Retrieved from https://cts-sct.ca/guideline-library/

Canadian Thoracic Society & Public Health Agency of Canada. (2014). *Canadian tuberculosis standards* (7th ed.). Retrieved from https://www.canada.ca/en/public-health/services/infectious-diseases/canadian-tuberculosis-standards-7th-edition/edition-22.html

Carolan, P. L., & Bye, M. R. (2015). *Pediatric bronchitis.* Retrieved from http://emedicine.medscape.com/article/1001332-overview#aw2aab6b2b3aa

Carpenito-Moyet, L. J. (2013). *Nursing diagnosis: Application to clinical practice* (14th ed.). Philadelphia, PA: Lippincott Williams & Wilkins.

Centers for Disease Control and Prevention (CDC). (2016). *Epstein-Barr virus and infectious mononucleosis.* Retrieved from https://www.cdc.gov/epstein-barr/laboratory-testing.html

Child Health BC. (2016). *Pediatric Early Warning System (PEWS).* Retrieved from http://www.childhealthbc.ca/initiatives/pediatric-early-warning-system-pews

Clute, J. L. (2014). *Reye syndrome.* Retrieved from http://kidshealth.org/parent/infections/bacterial_viral/reye.html#

Corbett, J. A., & Banks, A. D. (2013). *Laboratory tests and diagnostic procedures with nursing diagnoses* (8th ed.). Upper Saddle River, NJ: Pearson Education Inc.

Cornfield, D. N. (2013). Acute respiratory distress syndrome in children: Physiology and management. *Current Opinion in Pediatrics, 25*(3), 338–343.

Cystic Fibrosis Canada. (2015). *The Canadian Cystic Fibrosis Registry: 2013 annual report.* Retrieved from www.cysticfibrosis.ca/uploads/cf%20care/Canadian-CF-Registry-2013-FINAL.pdf

Cystic Fibrosis Canada. (2017). *What is cystic fibrosis?* Retrieved from http://www.cysticfibrosis.ca/about-cf/what-is-cystic-fibrosis

DeNicola, L. K., Maraqa, N. F., Udeani, J., & Custodio, H. T. (2016). *Bronchiolitis.* Retrieved from http://emedicine.medscape.com/article/961963-overview

Deutsch, E. S. (2010). Tracheostomy: Pediatric considerations. *Respiratory Care, 55*(8), 1082–1090. Retrieved from http://www.rcjournal.com/contents/08.10/08.10.1082.pdf

Ducharme, F. M., Bell, S. D., Radhakrishnan, D., Grad, R. M., Watson, W. T., Yang, C. L., & Zelman, M. (2015). Diagnosis and management of asthma in preschoolers: A Canadian Thoracic Society position paper. *Canadian Respiratory Journal, 22*(3), 135–143. Retrieved from https://www.cps.ca/en/documents/position/asthma-in-preschoolers

Duncan, H., Hutchinson, J., & Parshuram, C. S. (2006). The pediatric early warning system score: A severity of illness score to predict urgent medical need in hospitalized children. *Journal of Critical Care, 21*(3), 271–278.

Durani, Y. (2012). *Croup.* Retrieved from http://kidshealth.org/parent/infections/lung/croup.html

Environmental Protection Agency. (2016). *Healthy schools, healthy kids.* Retrieved from http://www2.epa.gov/schools

Federico, M. J., Baker, C. D., Balasubramaniam, V., Deboer, E. M., Deterding, R. R., Halbower, S., & Zemanick, E. T. (2014). Respiratory tract & mediastinum. In W. W. Hay, M. J. Levin, R. R. Deterding, & M. J. Abzug (Eds.). *Current pediatric diagnosis and treatment* (22nd ed.). New York: McGraw-Hill.

Fouzas, S., Priftis, K. N., & Anthracopoulos, M. B. (2011). Pulse oximetry in pediatric practice. *Pediatrics, 128*, 740–752.

Fryters, S. R., & Blondel-Hill, E. M. (2014). Sinusitis. In *Compendium of therapeutic choices* (7th ed., pp. 1489–1504). Ottawa, ON: Canadian Pharmacists Association.

Gavin, M. L. (2013). *Preventing choking*. Retrieved from http://kidshealth.org/parent/firstaid_safe/home/safety_choking.html

Giddens, J. F. (2013). *Concepts for nursing practice*. St. Louis, MO: Elsevier.

Global Asthma Network. (2014). *The Global Asthma Report 2014: Global burden of disease due to asthma*. Retrieved from http://www.globalasthmareport.org/2014/about/executive.php

Government of Canada. (2012). *Strong foundation, renewed focus: An overview of Canada's federal tobacco control strategy 2012–2017*. Retrieved from https://www.canada.ca/en/health-canada/services/publications/healthy-living/strong-foundation-renewed-focus-overview-canada-federal-tobacco-control-strategy-2012-17.html

Government of Canada. (2017). *Canada's provincial and territorial routine (and catch-up) vaccination programs for infants and children*. Retrieved from https://www.canada.ca/en/public-health/services/provincial-territorial-immunization-information/provincial-territorial-routine-vaccination-programs-infants-children.html

Hayden, G. F., & Turner, R. B. (2011). Acute pharyngitis. In R. M. Kliegman, B. M. D. Stanton, J. St. Geme, N. F. Schor, & R. E. Behrman (Eds.). *Nelson textbook of pediatrics* (19th ed.). Philadelphia, PA: Elsevier Saunders.

Hazle, L. A. (2010). Cystic fibrosis. In P. J. Allen, J. A. Vessey, & N. A. Schapiro (Eds.). *Primary care of the child with a chronic condition* (5th ed.). St. Louis, MO: Mosby.

Health Canada. (2016a). *Recalls and safety alerts: Health Canada reminds parents not to give cough and cold medication to children under 6 years old*. Retrieved from http://healthycanadians.gc.ca/recall-alert-rappel-avis/hc-sc/2016/57622a-eng.php

Health Canada. (2016b). *Recalls and safety alerts: New safety measure for prescription codeine and hydrocodone to further restrict use in children and adolescents*. Retrieved from http://healthycanadians.gc.ca/recall-alert-rappel-avis/hc-sc/2016/59584a-eng.php

Hill-Rom, Inc. (2016). *The Visi-Vest system™*. Retrieved from https://respiratorycare.hill-rom.com/en/patients/products/the-visivest-system/

Isaacson, G. (2012). Tonsillectomy care for the pediatrician. *Pediatrics, 130*(2), 324–334.

Jarvis, C. (2012). *Physical examination and health assessment* (6th ed.). St. Louis, MO: Saunders.

John, R. M., & Brady, M. A. (2013a). Atopic and rheumatic disorders. In C. E. Burns, A. M. Dunn, M. A. Brady, N. B. Starr, & C. G. Blosser (Eds.). *Pediatric primary care* (5th ed.). Philadelphia, PA: Elsevier Saunders.

John, R. M., & Brady, M. A. (2013b). Respiratory disorders. In C. E. Burns, A. M. Dunn, M. A. Brady, N. B. Starr, & C. G. Blosser (Eds.). *Pediatric primary care* (5th ed.). Philadelphia, PA: Elsevier Saunders.

Juniper, E. F., Guyett, G. H., Feeny, D. H., Ferrie, P. J., Griffith, L. E., & Townsend, M. (1996). Measuring quality of life in the parents of children with asthma. *Quality of Life Research, 5*(1), 27–34.

Kelly, M. M. (2010). Prematurity. In P. J. Allen, J. A. Vessey, & N. A. Schapiro (Eds.). *Primary care of the child with a chronic condition* (5th ed.). St. Louis, MO: Mosby.

Kenealy, T., & Arroll, B. (2013). Antibiotics for the common cold and acute purulent rhinitis. *Cochrane Database of Systematic Reviews*, (6), CD000247. doi: 10.1002/14651858.CD000247.pub3

Kovesi, T. (2012). Respiratory disease in Canadian First Nations and Inuit Children. *Paediatrics & Child Health, 17*(7), 376–380.

Lannefors, L., Button, B. M., & McIlwaine, M. P. (2004). Physiotherapy in infants and young children with cystic fibrosis: Current practice and future developments. *Journal of the Royal Society of Medicine, 97*(44), 8–25.

Lougheed, M. D., Lemiere, C., Ducharme, F. M., Licskai, C., Dell, S. D., Rowe, B. H., … Boulet, L. P. (2012). *Canadian Thoracic Society 2012 guideline update: Diagnosis and management of asthma in preschoolers, children, and adults*. Retrieved from https://cts-sct.ca/guideline-library/

McIlwaine, M. (2007). Chest physical therapy, breathing techniques and exercise in children with CF. *Paediatric Respiratory Reviews, 8*, 8–16.

McIlwaine, M. P., Alarie, N., Davidson G. F., Lands L. C., Ratjen, F., Milner, R., … Agnew, J. L. (2013). Long-term multicentre randomised controlled study of high frequency chest wall oscillation versus positive expiratory pressure mask in cystic fibrosis. *Thorax, 68*(8), 746–751.

MedEdu. (2016). *Easy auscultation: Lessons, quizzes & guides*. Retrieved from www.easyauscultation.com

Milgrom, H., & Leung, D. Y. M. (2011). Allergic rhinitis. In R. M. Kliegman, B. M. D. Stanton, J. St. Geme, N. F. Schor, & R. E. Behrman (Eds.). *Nelson textbook of pediatrics* (19th ed.). Philadelphia, PA: Elsevier Saunders.

Moore, K. L., Persaud, T. V. N., & Torchia, M. G. (2013). *The developing human: Clinically oriented embryology*. Philadelphia, PA: Elsevier Saunders.

National Asthma Education and Prevention Program. (2007). *Expert panel report 3: Guidelines for the diagnosis and management of asthma (NIH Publication No. 07–4051)*. Bethesda, MD: National Institutes of Health, National Heart, Lung and Blood Institute.

Ohler, K. H., & Pham, J. T. (2013). Comparison of the timing of initial prophylactic palivizumab dosing on hospitalization of neonates for respiratory syncytial virus. *American Journal of Health-System Pharmacy, 70*, 1342–1346.

Ortiz-Alvarez, O., & Mikrogianakis, A. (2012). Managing the paediatric patient with an acute asthma exacerbation. *Paediatrics & Child Health, 17*(5), 251–255.

Public Health Agency of Canada. (2015). *Federal action plan on antimicrobial resistance and use in Canada*. Retrieved from http://healthycanadians.gc.ca/alt/pdf/publications/drugs-products-medicaments-produits/antibiotic-resistance-antibiotique/action-plan-daction-eng.pdf

Public Health Agency of Canada. (2016). *Canadian immunization guide chapter on influenza and statement on seasonal influenza for 2016–2017*. Retrieved from http://www.phac-aspc.gc.ca/naci-ccni/flu-2016-grippe-eng.php

Ratcliffe, M. M., & Kieckhefer, G. M. (2010). Asthma. In P. J. Allen, J. A. Vessey, & N. A. Schapiro (Eds.). *Primary care of the child with a chronic condition* (5th ed.). St. Louis, MO: Mosby.

Royal Children's Hospital Melbourne. (n.d). *Clinical practice guidelines: Assessment of severity of respiratory conditions.* Retrieved from http://www.rch.org.au/clinicalguide/guideline_index/Assessment_of_severity_of_respiratory_conditions/

Robinson, J. L., & Le Saux, N. (2018). Preventing hospitalization for respiratory syncytial virus infection. *Paediatric Child Health, 20*(6), 321–326. Retrieved from https://www.cps.ca/en/documents/position/preventing-hospitalizations-for-rsv-infections

Safe Kids. (2016). *Choking and strangulation.* Retrieved from https://www.safekids.org/safetytips/field_risks/choking-and-strangulation

Schechter, M. S. (2007). Airway clearance applications in infants and children. *Respiratory Care, 52*(10), 1382–1391.

Schulman, S. T., Bisno, A. L., Clegg, H. W., Gerber, M. A., Kaplan, E. L., Lee, G., … Van Beneden, C. (2012). Clinical practice guideline for the diagnosis and management of Group A Streptococcal Pharyngitis: 2012 update by the Infectious Diseases Society of America. *Clinical Infectious Diseases, 55*(10), 86–102.

Scollan-Koliopoulos, M., & Koliopoulos, J. S. (2010). Evaluation and management of apparent life-threatening events in infants. *Pediatric Nursing, 36*(2), 77–83.

Sirivimonpan, S. (2013). *Airway remodelling in asthma.* Retrieved from http://www.slideshare.net/AllergyChula/airway-remodeling-in-asthma

Statistics Canada. (2010). *Study: Recent trends in upper respiratory infections, ear infections and asthma in children.* Retrieved from http://www.statcan.gc.ca/daily-quotidien/101117/dq101117b-eng.htm

Taketomo, C. K., Hodding, J. H., & Kraus, D. M. (2013). *Pediatric & neonatal dosage handbook* (20th ed.). Hudson, OH: Lexicomp.

Tewfik, T. L., & Alghonaim, Y. (2015). *Trachea anatomy.* Retrieved from http://emedicine.medscape.com/article/1949391-overview

Vertex Pharmaceuticals. (2015). *Kalydeco.* Retrieved from http://www.kalydeco.com

Winnie, G. B., & Lossef, S. V. (2011). Pneumothorax. In R. M. Kliegman, B. M. D. Stanton, J. St. Geme, N. F. Schor, & R. E. Behrman (Eds.). *Nelson textbook of pediatrics* (19th ed.). Philadelphia, PA: Elsevier Saunders.

World Health Organization (WHO). (n.d.). *Passive smoking.* Retrieved from http://www.who.int/tobacco/en/atlas10.pdf

World Health Organization (WHO). (2016). *Oxygen therapy for children.* Retrieved from http://apps.who.int/iris/bitstream/10665/204584/1/9789241549554_eng.pdf

Wright, P. F. (2011). Influenza viruses. In R. M. Kliegman, B. M. D. Stanton, J. St. Geme, N. F. Schor, & R. E. Behrman (Eds.). *Nelson textbook of pediatrics* (19th ed.). Philadelphia, PA: Elsevier Saunders.

Yoon, P. J., Kelley, P. E., & Friedman, N. R. (2012). Ear, nose, & throat. In W. W. Hay, M. J. Levin, J. R. R. Deterding, M. J. Abzug, & M. Sondheimer (Eds.). *Current pediatric diagnosis and treatment* (21st ed.). New York: McGraw-Hill.

Yoon, P. J., Scholes, A., & Friedman, N. R. (2014). Ear Nose and Throat. In W. W. Hay, M. J. Levin, J. R. R. Deterding, M. J. Abzug, & M. Sondheimer (Eds.), *Current Diagnosis & Treatment Pediatrics* (24th ed.). New York, NY: McGraw-Hill.

Yoos, H. L., Kitzman, H., McMullen, A., Sidora-Arcoleo, K., & Anson, E. (2005). The language of breathlessness: Do families and health care providers speak the same language when describing asthma symptoms? *Journal of Pediatric Health Care, 19*(4), 197–205.

Yust, E., & Slattery, A. (2012). Cold and cough medications for children. *Clinical Pediatric Emergency Medicine, 13*(4), 292–299.

CHAPTER **WORKSHEET**

MULTIPLE CHOICE QUESTIONS

1. A 5-month-old infant with RSV bronchiolitis is in respiratory distress. The baby has copious secretions, increased work of breathing, cyanosis, and a respiratory rate of 78. What is the most appropriate initial nursing intervention?
   a. Attempt to calm the infant by placing him in his mother's lap and offering him a bottle.
   b. Alert the physician or nurse practitioner to the situation and ask for an order for a stat chest x-ray.
   c. Suction secretions, provide 100% oxygen via mask, and anticipate respiratory failure.
   d. Bring the emergency equipment to the room and begin bag-valve-mask ventilation.

2. A toddler has moderate respiratory distress, is mildly cyanotic, and has increased work of breathing, with a respiratory rate of 40. What is the priority nursing intervention?
   a. Airway maintenance and 100% oxygen by mask
   b. 100% oxygen and pulse oximetry monitoring
   c. Airway maintenance and continued reassessment
   d. 100% oxygen and provision of comfort

3. A nurse is caring for a 6-year old with suspected pulmonary tuberculosis, which of the statements is false?
   a. Hemoptysis is common in young children
   b. Prevalence is higher in children of Canadian-born Indigenous descent and foreign-born children
   c. Signs and symptoms can vary in children, and children can be asymptomatic, especially under age 5
   d. Young children (especially infants) are at risk of more severe disease

4. Which of these factors contributes to infants' and children's increased risk for upper airway obstruction as compared with adults?
   a. Underdeveloped cricoid cartilage and narrow nasal passages
   b. Small tonsils and narrow nasal passages
   c. Cylinder-shaped larynx and underdeveloped sinuses
   d. Underdeveloped cricoid cartilage and smaller tongue

5. Which is the most appropriate treatment for epistaxis?
   a. With the child lying down and breathing through the mouth, apply pressure to the bridge of the nose.
   b. With the child lying down and breathing through the mouth, pinch the lower third of the nose closed.
   c. With the child sitting up and leaning forward, apply pressure to the bridge of the nose.
   d. With the child sitting up and leaning forward, pinch the lower third of the nose closed.

DOSAGE CALCULATION QUESTION

1. The nurse is caring for a child with allergic acute asthma. The child weighs 17 kg (37½ lb). The medication order reads: methylprednisolone 20 mg IV twice a day. The Pediatric Dosage Handbook provides a recommended dose for acute asthma of 1 to 2 mg/kg/day in two divided doses. Is the ordered dose safe?

CRITICAL THINKING EXERCISES

1. A 10-month-old girl is admitted to the pediatric unit with a history of recurrent pneumonia and failure to thrive. Her sweat chloride test confirms the diagnosis of cystic fibrosis. She is a frail-appearing infant with thin extremities and a slightly protuberant abdomen. She is tachypneic, has retractions, and coughs frequently. Based on the limited information given here and your knowledge of cystic fibrosis, choose three of the categories below as priorities to focus on when planning her care:
   a. Prevention of bronchospasm
   b. Promotion of adequate nutrition
   c. Education of the child and family
   d. Prevention of pulmonary infection
   e. Balancing fluid and electrolytes
   f. Management of excess weight gain
   g. Prevention of spread of infection
   h. Promoting adequate sleep and rest

2. A boy with asthma is admitted to the pediatric unit for the fourth time this year. The mother expresses frustration that he is getting sick so often. Besides information about onset of symptoms and events leading up to this present episode, what other types of information would you ask for while obtaining the history?

3. The mother of the boy in the previous question tells you that she smokes (but never around the boy), the family has a cat that comes inside sometimes, and she always gives her son the medication prescribed. She gives salmeterol and budesonide as soon as he starts to cough. When he is not having an episode, she gives him albuterol before his baseball games. Diphenhydramine helps his runny nose in the springtime. Based on this new information, what advice/instructions would you give the mother?

4. A 7-year old presents with a history of recurrent nasal discharge. He sneezes every time he visits his cousins, who have pets. He lives in an older home that is carpeted. Tobacco smokers live in the home. His mother reports that he snores and is a mouth breather. She says he has symptoms nearly year-round, but they are worse in the fall and the spring. She reports that diphenhydramine is somewhat helpful with his symptoms, but she doesn't like to give it to him on school days because it makes him drowsy. Based on the history above, develop a teaching plan for this child.

5. The nurse is caring for a 4-year-old girl who returned from the recovery room after a tonsillectomy 3 hours ago. She has cried off and on over the past 2 hours and is now sleeping. What areas should the nurse assess and focus on for this child?

STUDY ACTIVITIES

1. While caring for children in the pediatric setting, compare the signs and symptoms of a child with asthma to those of an infant with bronchiolitis. What are the most notable differences? How does the history of the two children differ?

2. A child with asthma has been prescribed Advair (fluticasone and salmeterol), albuterol, and prednisone. Develop a sample teaching plan for the child and family. Include appropriate use of the devices used to deliver the medications, as well as important information about the medications (uses and adverse effects).

3. While caring for children in the pediatric setting, compare the signs and symptoms and presentation of a child with the common cold to those of a child with either sinusitis or allergic rhinitis.

4.
   a. While caring for children in the pediatric setting, review the census of children and identify those at risk for severe influenza.
   b. Identify children in the pediatric setting at risk for more severe RSV bronchiolitis.

5. Compare the differences in oxygen administration between a young infant and an older child.

BRINGING IT ALL TOGETHER: A CASE STUDY

Bradley is a 5-year old with a history of moderate asthma who was started on oral steroids yesterday after visiting his pediatrician for an asthma exacerbation. In addition, he has been receiving aerosol treatments every 4 hours since yesterday. He received his last levalbuterol nebulizer treatment 3 hours ago. His mother has brought him back to the office because she is concerned that he does not seem to be getting any better.

41

Nursing Care of the Child With an Alteration in Perfusion/Cardiovascular Disorder

Learning Objectives

Upon completion of the chapter, you will be able to:

1. Compare anatomic and physiologic differences of the cardiovascular system in infants and children versus adults.

2. Describe nursing care related to common laboratory and diagnostic tests used in the medical diagnosis of pediatric cardiovascular conditions.

3. Distinguish cardiovascular disorders common in infants, children, and adolescents.

4. Identify appropriate nursing assessments and interventions related to medications and treatments for pediatric cardiovascular disorders.

5. Develop an individualized nursing care plan for the child with a cardiovascular disorder.

6. Describe the psychosocial impact of chronic cardiovascular disorders on children.

7. Devise a nutrition plan for the child with cardiovascular disease.

8. Develop child/family teaching plans for the child with a cardiovascular disorder.

Logan Bernstein, **6 weeks old, is brought to the clinic by his mother. He presents with poor feeding. His mother states, "Logan falls asleep while feeding, and he's always very sweaty during feedings."**

🌀 **Perfusion** refers to the mechanisms that facilitate blood through tissue. Nurses may encounter alterations in perfusion in children and should be familiar with various cardiovascular disorders that children experience. Alterations in perfusion, or cardiovascular disease is a significant cause of chronic illness and death in children. Typically cardiovascular disorders in children are divided into two major categories—congenital heart disease (CHD) and acquired heart disease.

CHD is defined as structural anomalies that are present at birth, though they may not be diagnosed until later in life (Kantor et al., 2013). CHD accounts for the largest percentage of all birth defects. In Canada there are approximately 8 per 1,000 live births that are born with CHD (Canadian Congenital Heart Alliance, 2016). Over 100 genes have been identified that may be involved in the development of CHD (Cunningham et al., 2014). Additional noncardiac anomalies occur in about 28% of children with CHD. CHD is also commonly associated with chromosomal abnormalities (Marian, Brugada, & Roberts, 2011).

Acquired heart disease includes disorders that occur after birth. These disorders develop from a wide range of causes, for example Kawasaki disease is the leading cause of acquired heart disease in Canadian children (Kawasaki Disease Canada, n.d.). Rheumatic fever caused by streptococcal bacteria can cause mitral valve damage.

The diagnosis of a CHD for both child and parent can feel overwhelming. Nurses need to have a good understanding of cardiac disease and the medical and surgical management options available. Surgeries and interventions improve every year. Most of the straightforward children with CHD needing surgical repair, such as ASD, have a complication rate of less than 1%. Nurses also become the family's main resource: for cardiac care and monitoring both in hospital and in the community, education and knowledge of available support. Families may need some or all of the following supports: nutrition, psychology, genetics, medication teaching and special authority coverage, social worker, accommodation and travel arrangements, at home nursing and ongoing education.

VARIATIONS IN PEDIATRIC ANATOMY AND PHYSIOLOGY

The cardiovascular system undergoes numerous changes at birth. Structures that were vital to the fetus are no longer needed. Circulation via the umbilical arteries and vein is replaced with the child's own closed independent circulation. Changes in the size of the heart, pulse rate, and blood pressure (BP) also occur.

Circulatory Changes From Gestation to Birth

The fetal heart rate is present on about postconceptual day 17. The four chambers of the heart and arteries are formed during gestational weeks 2 through 8, with maturation of the structures occurring throughout the remainder of gestation. During fetal development, oxygenation of the fetus occurs via the placenta; the lungs, though perfused, do not perform oxygenation and ventilation. The foramen ovale, an opening between the atria, allows blood flow from the right to the left atrium. The ductus arteriosus allows blood flow between the pulmonary artery and the aorta, shunting blood away from the pulmonary circulation (Cunningham et al., 2014). Figure 41.1 illustrates fetal circulation.

With the newborn's first breath, several changes occur in the cardiopulmonary system that enable the newborn to make the transition from fetal circulation to normal circulation. As the newborn breathes for the first time, the lungs inflate, reducing pulmonary vascular resistance to blood flow. As a result, pulmonary artery pressure drops. Subsequently, pressure in the right atrium decreases. Blood flow to the left side of the heart increases the pressure in the left atrium. This change in pressure leads to closure of the foramen ovale. The drop in pressure of the pulmonary artery promotes closure of the ductus arteriosus, which is located between the aorta and pulmonary artery. The ductus venosus, located between the left umbilical vein and the inferior vena cava, closes because of a lack of blood flow and vasoconstriction. The closed ductus arteriosus and ductus venosus eventually become ligaments. With the lack of blood flow to the umbilical arteries and vein, these structures atrophy (Cunningham et al., 2014).

Structural and Functional Differences

The structure and function of the infant's and child's cardiovascular system differ from those of adults, depending on age. In infants and children younger than 7 years of age, the heart lies more horizontally, resulting in the apex lying higher in the chest, below the fourth intercostal space. As the lungs grow over time, the heart is displaced downward. Between ages 1 and 6 years, the heart is four times the birth size. Between 6 and 12 years of age, the child's heart is 10 times the size it was at birth. However, the heart is smaller proportionally at this time than at any other stage in life. During the school-age years, the heart grows more vertically within the thoracic cavity. During adolescence, the heart continues to grow in relation to the youth's rapid growth.

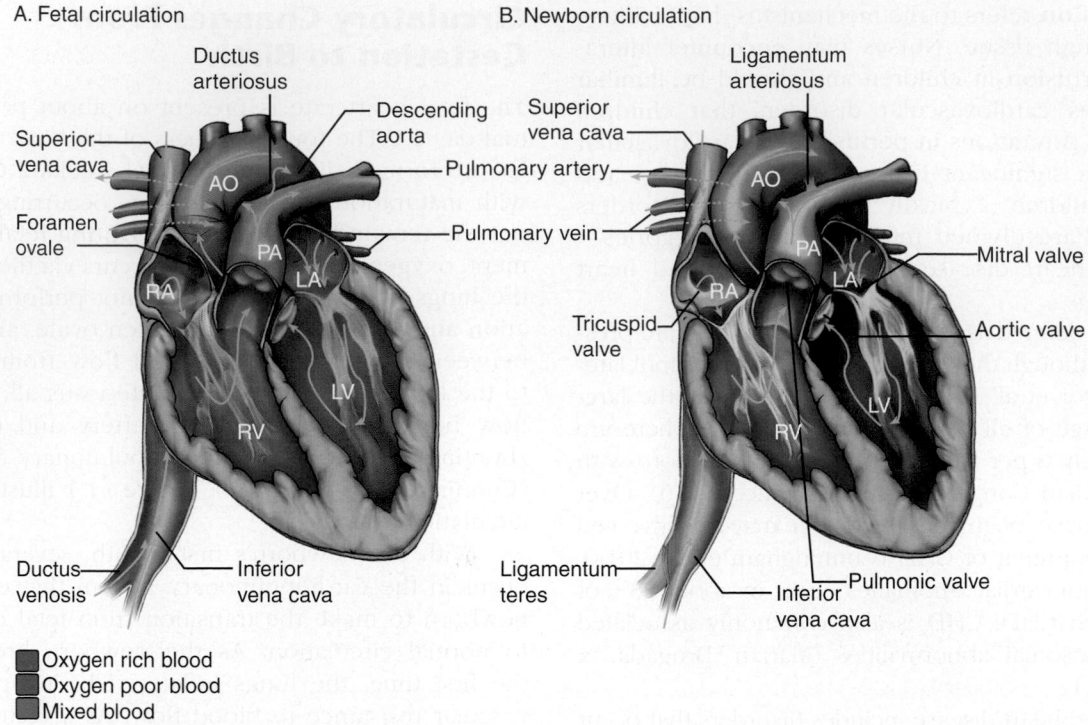

A. Fetal circulation

B. Newborn circulation

FIGURE 41.1 Fetal and newborn circulation.

At birth, the ventricle walls are similar in thickness, but with time the left ventricular wall thickens. The immature myocytes of the infant's heart are thinner and less compliant than those of the adult. Right ventricular function dominates at birth, and over the first few months of life, left ventricular function becomes dominant. The infant's heart at rest exhibits a greater resting tension than the adult's, so volume loading or increased stretch may actually lead to decreased cardiac output. The infant's sarcoplasmic reticulum is less well organized than the adult's, making the infant dependent on serum calcium for contraction. Inotropic response to calcium in the actin and myosin (contractile proteins) increases with age.

The normal heart rate is higher in infancy than in adulthood, limiting the infant's ability to increase cardiac output by increasing the heart rate. The heart's efficiency increases as the child ages and the heart rate drops over time. The normal infant heart rate ranges from 90 to 160 beats per minute (bpm), the toddler's or preschooler's is 80 to 115 bpm, the school-age child's and the adolescent's ranges from 60 to 100 bpm. Innocent murmurs and physiologic splitting of heart sounds may be noted in infancy or childhood. These findings are related to the change in the size of the heart in relation to the thoracic cavity. The infant's and child's blood vessels widen and increase in length over time. The average infant's BP is about 80/55 mm Hg; BP is usually lower in the younger infant, and can be slightly higher in the older infant. The

BP increases over time to the adult level. The toddler's or preschooler's BP averages 90 to 110/55 to 75 mm Hg, the school-age child's 100 to 120/60 to 75 mm Hg, and the adolescent's 100 to 120/70 to 80 mm Hg (Engorn & Flerlage, 2015).

COMMON MEDICAL TREATMENTS

A variety of medications as well as other medical treatments and surgical procedures are used to treat cardiovascular problems in children. Most of these treatments will require a physician's order when the child is in the hospital. The most common treatments include the need for oxygen therapy, respiratory physiotherapy, or care of a chest tube (drain). Oxygen use may be indicated when an infant of child experiences hypoxemia, respiratory distress or heart failure. Administration is via mask, nasal cannula, hood, tent or endotracheal/nasotracheal tube. Nursing care includes monitoring the work of breathing (WOB) and pulse oximetry. Respiratory physiotherapy aims to aid secretion clearance thereby increasing lung volumes. Nurses should work with physical/respiratory therapists and offer supportive teaching to parents. Care should be taken as some of these techniques can be contraindicated in certain conditions, for example, percussions can exacerbate bronchospasm and increase mucous production. A chest tube is a drainage tube inserted into the pleural cavity to facilitate removal or air (pneumothorax), drainage of fluid (hemothorax, pleural effusion) thereby allowing lung inflation and expansion. Immediate clamping of the tube is necessary should it become dislodged. Local policy and guidelines should be reviewed prior to caring for a child with a chest tube. The nurse caring for the child with a cardiovascular disorder should be familiar with what medications are commonly prescribed, how they work as well as common nursing implications related to use of these modalities; see Drug Guide 41.1.

Take Note!

Give digoxin at regular intervals, every 12 hours, such as at 8 AM and 8 PM, 1 hour before or 2 hours after a feeding. If a digoxin dose is missed and more than 4 hours have elapsed, withhold the dose and give the dose at the regular time; if less than 4 hours have elapsed, give the missed dose. If the child vomits digoxin, do not give a second dose. Monitor potassium levels, as a decrease enhances the effects of digitalis, causing toxicity (Taketomo, Hodding, & Kraus, 2013).

DRUG GUIDE 41.1

Medication	Actions/Indications	Nursing Implications
Alprostadil (prostaglandin, PGE)	Direct vasodilation of the ductus arteriosus smooth muscle Indicated for temporary maintenance of ductus arteriosus patency in infants with ductal-dependent congenital heart defects	• Apnea occurs in 10–20% of neonates within first hour of infusion. • Monitor arterial BP, respiratory rate, heart rate, ECG, temperature, and pO₂; watch for abdominal distention. • Fresh IV solution required every 24 hours. • Reposition catheter if facial or arm flushing occurs. • Use with caution in neonate with bleeding tendency. • Contraindicated in respiratory distress syndrome or persistent fetal circulation.
Digoxin (cardiac glycoside, antiarrhythmic agent)	Increases contractility of the heart muscle by decreasing conduction and increasing force Used for heart failure, atrial fibrillation, atrial flutter, supraventricular tachycardia	• Prior to administering each dose, count apical pulse for 1 full minute, noting rate, rhythm, and quality. Withhold if apical pulse is <60 in an adolescent, <90 in an infant. • Administer 1 hour before or 2 hours after feed, don't mix with food. Home care instructions for parents are important and need to be comprehensive education about missed dose management/child vomiting/overdose etc. • Monitor serum digoxin levels (therapeutic range: 0.8–2 ng/mL). Half-life 36 hours. • Notes signs of toxicity: nausea, vomiting, diarrhea, lethargy, dysrhythmias and bradycardia. • Ginseng, hawthorn, and liquorice intake increases risk for drug toxicity. • Note contraindications (ventricular fibrillation and hypersensitivity to digitalis). • Avoid rapid IV administration, as this may lead to systemic and coronary artery vasoconstriction.
Furosemide (Lasix) (loop diuretic)	Inhibits resorption of sodium and chloride Used to manage edema associated with heart failure, and hypertension in combination with antihypertensive (e.g. spironolactone)	• Administer with food or milk to decrease GI upset. • Monitor BP, renal function, electrolytes (particularly potassium—hypokalemia), and hearing. • May cause photosensitivity. • Monitor for muscle weakness, cramping, confusion, irritability, restlessness and inverted T waves or prominent U waves on ECG

(continued)

DRUG GUIDE 41.1 (continued)

Medication	Actions/Indications	Nursing Implications
Heparin (anticoagulant) Low–Molecular-Weight Heparin, Warfarin, ASA (common pediatric medication)	Interferes with conversion of pro-thrombin to thrombin, preventing clot formation Indicated for the prophylaxis and treatment of thromboembolic disorders, especially after cardiac surgery and low–molecular-weight heparin used in conjunction with commonly prescribed pediatric cardiac drugs	• Administer SQ, not IM. • Dose is adjusted according to coagulation test results. • Monitor for signs of bleeding, platelet counts. • Ensure that the antidote, protamine sulfate, is available. • Do not administer with uncontrolled bleeding or if subacute bacterial endocarditis is suspected.
Indomethacin (nonsteroidal anti-inflammatory agent)	Inhibits prostaglandin synthesis in order to close patent ductus arteriosus	• Monitor heart rate, BP, ECG, and urine output; monitor for murmur. • Monitor serum sodium, glucose, platelet count, BUN, creatinine, potassium, and liver enzymes. • May mask signs of infection. • Note development of edema.
Spironolactone (potassium sparing diuretic)	Competes with aldosterone to result in increased water and sodium excretion (spares potassium) Used to manage edema due to heart failure and for treatment of hypertension	• Administer with food. • Monitor serum potassium, sodium, and renal function. • May cause drowsiness, headache, and arrhythmia. • May cause false elevations in digitalis level. • Teach children to avoid high-potassium diets, salt substitutes, and natural liquorice. • Contraindicated in hyperkalemia, renal failure, and anuria.
Antibiotics		
Penicillin G benzathine Penicillin V potassium	Inhibits bacterial wall synthesis in susceptible organisms Indicated in mild to moderate infections, for prophylaxis of endocarditis and rheumatic fever	• Contraindications include hypersensitivity to penicillins. • Report hypersensitivity reactions (chills, fever, wheezing, pruritus, anaphylaxis) immediately. • PCN-G: administer IM. • Pen-VK: administer orally on empty stomach 1 hour prior to or 2 hours after a meal.
Erythromycin (macrolide)	Inhibits RNA transcription in susceptible organisms Used in children with penicillin allergy, mild to moderate infections, or endocarditis, and for rheumatic fever prophylaxis	• Contraindicated in pre-existing liver disease. • IV administration may result in CV abnormalities. • Abdominal distress common with oral use. • Fever, dizziness, and rash may occur.
Antihypertensive Drugs		
Angiotensin-converting enzyme (ACE) inhibitors (captopril, enalapril)	Competitive inhibition of ACE for management of hypertension Heart failure management in conjunction with digitalis and diuretics	• Monitor BP (hypotension), renal function, WBC count, and serum potassium, serum protein, urine output. • Discontinue if angioedema occurs. • Captopril: administer orally on empty stomach 1 hour before or 2 hours after meals. • Enalapril: may administer orally without regard to food.

DRUG GUIDE 41.1 (continued)

Medication	Actions/Indications	Nursing Implications
β-Adrenergic blockers (propranolol, atenolol, sotalol)	Competitively block response to β-adrenergic stimulation, decreasing heart rate and force of contraction Used for management of hypertension, arrhythmias, and prevention of myocardial infarction	• Monitor ECG and BP. • Propranolol: administer with food. • Atenolol, sotalol: administer without regard to food. Do not stop drug abruptly. • May result in bradycardia, dizziness, nausea and vomiting, dyspnea, and hypoglycemia (propranolol). • Contraindications: heart block, uncompensated heart failure, cardiogenic shock, asthma, or hypersensitivity. • **Note:** Children with tetralogy of Fallot may be prescribed propranolol to prevent spasms underneath the pulmonary valve. Most of the time, cardiologists prefer to continue propranolol before a cardiac catheterization to prevent a "tet spell" during the procedure.
Hydralazine (vasodilator)	Direct vasodilation of arterioles to manage moderate to severe hypertension, heart failure	• Monitor heart rate and BP. • Closely monitor BP with IV use. • Administer oral dose with food. • May cause palpitations, flushing, tachycardia, dizziness, nausea, and vomiting. • Notify physician or nurse practitioner if flu-like symptoms occur. • Contraindicated in rheumatic valvular disease.

BUN, blood urea nitrogen; CV, cardiovascular; GI, gastrointestinal; IM, intramuscularly; pO₂, partial pressure of oxygen; SQ, subcutaneously; WBC, white blood cell.
Adapted from Taketomo, C. K., Hodding, J. H., & Kraus, D. M. (2013). *Pediatric & neonatal dosage handbook* (20th ed.). Hudson, OH: Lexicomp.

Dosage Calculation Box 41.1

Child's weight: 5.54 kg
Medication order: digoxin 60 mcg by mouth every 12 hours.
Per the *Pediatric Dosage Handbook*, the recommended dose is 10–15 mcg/kg/day in 2 divided doses.
Is the ordered dose safe?

NURSING PROCESS OVERVIEW FOR THE CHILD WITH A CARDIOVASCULAR DISORDER

Care of the child with a cardiovascular disorder includes all steps of the nursing process: assessment, nursing diagnosis, planning, interventions, and evaluation. There are a number of general concepts related to the nursing process that may be applied to any child with a cardiovascular disorder. The nurse should be knowledgeable about the procedures, treatments, and medications as well as familiar with the nursing

implications related to these interventions. With an understanding of these concepts, the nurse can individualize the care based on the child's and family's needs.

Remember Logan, the 6-week-old with poor feeding? What additional health history and physical examination assessment information should the nurse obtain?

Assessment

When assessing a child with a cardiovascular disorder, expect to obtain a health history, perform a physical examination, and prepare the child for laboratory and diagnostic testing.

Health History

The health history consists of a history of the present illness, past medical history, and family history.

TABLE 41.1	EXAMPLES OF QUESTIONS FOR OBTAINING A CHILD'S HEALTH HISTORY

Questions	Provides Information About
• What types and amounts (dosages) of medications has the child received? What were they used for?	• Possible underlying conditions that may be related to the child's current status
• Who prescribed them?	• Other health care personnel involved in the child's care as well as the parents' health care beliefs and patterns
• Were they effective? Did the child experience any adverse effects?	• How the medications may be affecting the child's health
• To whom does the child go for medical evaluation? How often? Were the visits for regular health check-ups or for situational problems? Were there previous hospitalizations? What for?	• The child's health status and the parents' health care knowledge, practices, and beliefs
• Has the child experienced any growth delay? Does the child have any problems with activity and coordination?	• Problems that may result from impaired cardiac output, adequacy of tissue oxygenation, and concomitant disorders associated with heart disease
• Does the child's skin colour change when crying? If so, what colour do you see?	• Effectiveness of tissue oxygenation. A blue or grey skin colour may be due to cyanosis
• Does the child stop frequently during play to sit or squat?	• The child's exercise tolerance and tissue oxygenation
• Does the child have feeding difficulty? Does the child tire easily or sleep excessively?	• The child's energy expenditure, ability to tolerate activity, and tissue oxygenation
• Does the child frequently develop strep throat?	• The child's risk for developing rheumatic fever and heart disease

Adapted from Park, M. K. (2014). *Park's pediatric cardiology for practitioners* (6th ed.). Philadelphia, PA: Saunders.

Depending on his or her age, the child should be included in the health history interview; the child's age will determine the degree of involvement and the terminology used. Table 41.1 gives examples of typical questions that can be used when obtaining the child's health history.

HISTORY OF PRESENT ILLNESS

Elicit the history of the present illness: when the symptoms started and how they have progressed. Inquire about any treatments and medications used at home. Ask parents about history of **orthopnea**, dyspnea, syncope, easy fatigability, growth delays, squatting, edema, dizziness, wheezing, chest pain, exercise intolerance and/or frequent occurrences of pneumonia, which can be significant signs of pediatric heart disease. The history of present illness may reveal a history of poor feeding, including fatigue, lethargy, and/or vomiting, or failure to thrive, even with adequate caloric intake. The parents may report diaphoresis, which is often seen in early heart failure. The parent or caregiver may also report delays in gross motor development, cyanosis (possibly reported by the parents as more of a grey colour than blue centrally, that is, lips, tongue, and core rather than peripherally), and tachypnea (indicative of heart failure).

PAST MEDICAL HISTORY

The past medical history includes information about the child as well as the mother's pregnancy history. Assess the child's past medical history for:
• Problems occurring after birth (history of the child's condition after birth may reveal evidence of an associated congenital malformation or other disorder)
• Frequent infections
• Chromosomal abnormalities
• Prematurity
• Autoimmune disorders
• Use of medications, such as corticosteroids, for example, Prednisone

Review the mother's pregnancy, labour, and delivery history. Be sure to include information about the status of the neonate at birth. Also inquire about maternal use of medications, including illicit or over-the-counter drugs and alcohol; exposure to radiation; presence of hypertension; and maternal viral illnesses such as coxsackievirus, cytomegalovirus, influenza, mumps, or rubella. A history of significant problems related to labour and delivery is also important: stress or asphyxia at birth may be related to cardiac dysfunction and pulmonary hypertension in the newborn.

Assess for additional risk factors such as:
- Family history of heart disease or CHD (investigate the history further if heart disease occurred in a first-degree relative)
- Hyperlipidemia
- Diabetes mellitus
- Family history of stroke, aneurism, arrhythmias
- Family history of sudden and unexplained death <50-year-old relative
- Obesity, inactivity, stress
- High-cholesterol diet
- Sudden infant death syndrome (SIDS)

Physical Examination

Physical examination of the child with a cardiovascular condition consists of inspection, palpation, and auscultation. In addition, obtain the child's vital signs and measure the child's length (in the neonate), height and weight. Plot this information on a standard growth chart to evaluate nutritional status and growth. If the child is younger than 3 years of age, measure and plot the head circumference.

INSPECTION

Assess the child's overall appearance and complete a general systems assessment including signs of fatigue and irritability. Inspect the colour of the skin, noting cyanosis (acrocyanosis maybe normal in infants <1 month). Inspect the skin for edema (less frequent in infants but can be present in older children) and if found to be present record the degree and site of edema. Note any profuse scalp diaphoresis especially in infants which increases with feeding.

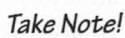

Take Note!

Suspect CHD in the cyanotic newborn who does not improve with oxygen administration (Canadian Congenital Heart Alliance, 2017).

Inspect the fingers and toes for **clubbing**. Clubbing (which usually does not appear until after 1 year of age) implies chronic hypoxia due to severe CHD. The first sign of clubbing is softening of the nail beds, followed by rounding of the fingernails, followed by shininess and thickening of the nail ends (see Fig. 40.4 in Chapter 40).

Obtain the child's temperature; fever would suggest infection. Assess respirations, including rate, rhythm, and effort at rest and slight exertion as well as any audible noise such as grunting. Note location and severity of retractions if present. Inspect the chest configuration, noting any prominence of the precordial chest wall, which is often seen in infants and children with **cardiomegaly** (abnormal heart enlargement). Note visible pulsations, which may indicate increased heart activity. Also

inspect the neck veins for engorgement or abnormal pulsations (jugular vein distention in older children or adolescents not a reliable indicator in infants). Inspect the abdomen for any easily noticeable liver/spleen distention (hepatosplenomegaly).

Take Note!

Children with cardiac conditions resulting in cyanosis will often have baseline oxygen saturations that are relatively low because of the mixing of oxygenated with deoxygenated blood.

PALPATION

Palpate the right and left radial or brachial pulse to assess cardiac rate and rhythm. Throughout infancy and childhood, the rate may vary. Palpate the femoral pulse; it should be readily palpable and equal in amplitude and strength to the brachial or radial pulse. A femoral pulse that is weak or absent in comparison to the brachial pulse is associated with coarctation of the aorta. Significant variations in pulse occur with activity, so the most accurate heart rate may be determined during sleep. In older children, exercise and emotional factors may influence the heart rate. A bounding pulse is characteristic of patent ductus arteriosus (PDA) or aortic regurgitation. Narrow or thready pulses may occur in children with heart failure or severe aortic stenosis (Cassidy, Allen, & Phillips, 2013). Note tachycardia, bradycardia, rhythm irregularities, diminished peripheral pulses, or thready pulse. Palpate the child's abdomen for hepatomegaly, a sign of right-sided heart failure in the infant and child.

AUSCULTATION

Auscultate the apical pulse for a full minute to determine heart rate and rhythm. Note irregularities in rhythm, tachycardia, or bradycardia. Auscultate the heart for murmurs. Many children have functional or innocent murmurs, but all murmurs must be evaluated on the basis of the following characteristics:
- Location
- Relation to the heart cycle and duration
- Intensity: grade I, soft and hard to hear; grade II, soft and easily heard; grade III, loud without thrill; grade IV, loud with a precordial thrill; grade V, loud, with a precordial thrill, audible with a stethoscope partially off chest; grade VI, very loud, audible with a stethoscope or with the naked ear
- Quality: harsh, musical, or rough; high, medium, or low pitch
- Variation with position (sitting, lying, standing) (Cassidy et al., 2013)

Auscultate for the character of heart sounds. Note distinct, muffled, or distant heart sounds. Abnormal splitting or intensifying of S_2 sounds occurs in children with major heart problems. Ejection clicks, which are high pitched, are related to problems with dilated vessels and/or valve abnormalities. Heard throughout systole, they can be early, moderate, or late. Clicks on the upper left sternal border are related to the pulmonary area. Aortic clicks are best heard at the apex and can be mitral or aortic in origin. A mild to late ejection click at the apex is typical of a mitral valve prolapse. The S_3 heart sound may be heard in children and is associated with cardiac abnormalities. The S_4 heart sound is not normally heard and is always associated with cardiac abnormalities (Lorts, Krawczeski, & Marino, 2013).

Auscultate the BP in the upper extremities and lower extremities and compare the findings; there should be no major differences between the upper and lower extremities. Determine the pulse pressure by subtracting the diastolic pressure from the systolic pressure. The pulse pressure is less than 50 mm Hg, or less than half the systolic pressure. A widened pulse pressure, which usually is accompanied by a bounding pulse, is associated with PDA, aortic insufficiency, fever, anemia, or complete heart block. A narrowed pulse pressure is associated with aortic stenosis. Note hypotension or hypertension.

Take Note!

Alert health care provider (physician/nurse practitioner) if noted and discuss with the children and parents if a heart murmur diagnosis is detected, even if it is benign.

Laboratory and Diagnostic Testing

Common Laboratory and Diagnostic Tests 41.1 explains the laboratory and diagnostic tests most commonly used when considering cardiovascular disorders in children. The tests can assist the physician in diagnosing the disorder or can be used as guidelines in determining ongoing treatment. Laboratory or non-nursing personnel obtain some of the tests, while the nurse might obtain others. In either instance the nurse should be familiar with how the tests are obtained, what they are used for, and normal versus abnormal results. This knowledge will also be necessary when providing child and family education related to the testing.

CARDIAC CATHETERIZATION

Cardiac catheterization is the definitive study for infants and children with cardiac disease and thus deserves special attention in this section on assessment of cardiovascular disorders. Cardiac catheterization has become almost a routine diagnostic procedure and may be performed on an outpatient basis. However, it is highly invasive and not without risks, especially in sick

infants and children. Indications for cardiac catheterization include:

- Cardiovascular disease causing cyanosis in infants: these infants need to be catheterized as soon as they are in a reasonably stable condition
- Severe heart failure or progressive problems such as pulmonary edema
- Questionable anatomic or physiologic abnormalities
- Planned cardiac surgery
- Progressive monitoring related to pulmonary hypertension
- Periodic assessment after repair of a cardiac defect
- Therapeutic interventions such as septostomy or balloon valvotomy

Cardiac catheterization may be categorized as diagnostic, interventional, or electrophysiologic. Diagnostic cardiac catheterization typically is used to identify structural defects. Interventional cardiac catheterization is used as a treatment measure to dilate occluded or stenotic structures or vessels or close some defects. Electrophysiologic cardiac catheterization involves the use of electrodes to identify abnormal rhythms and destroy sites of abnormal electrical conduction. The type of catheterization performed varies based on the individual needs of the child. The procedure lasts from 1 to 3 hours (Park, 2014).

PERFORMING CARDIAC CATHETERIZATION

In cardiac catheterization, a radiopaque catheter is inserted into a blood vessel and is then guided through the vessel to the heart with the aid of fluoroscopy. For a right-sided catheterization, the catheter is threaded to the right atrium via a major vein such as the femoral vein. With a left-sided catheterization, the catheter is threaded to the aorta and heart via an artery. Once the tip of the catheter is in the heart, contrast material is injected via the catheter and radiographic images are taken.

While the catheter is in the heart, several procedures can be performed. The BPs, changes in cardiac output or stroke volume, and oxygen saturation in each heart chamber and major blood vessels are recorded. With the injection of contrast material, information is revealed about the heart anatomy, ventricular wall motion and ejection fraction, intracardiac pressures and hemodynamic parameters, cardiac valve function, and structural abnormalities. The movement of the contrast material is filmed so that the details of the cardiac procedure are recorded. Samples of heart tissue to evaluate for infection, muscular dysfunction, or rejection after a transplant may also be obtained (Park, 2014).

NURSING MANAGEMENT OF CARDIAC CATHETERIZATION

For children and parents or guardians, cardiac catheterization can be a source of much anxiety. Therefore,

COMMON LABORATORY AND DIAGNOSTIC TESTS 41.1

Test	Explanation	Indications	Nursing Implications
Arteriogram (angiogram: visualization of arteries or veins)	Radiopaque contrast solution is injected through a catheter and into the circulation. X-rays are then taken to visualize the structure of the heart and blood vessels	To observe blood flow to parts of body and detect lesions; to confirm a diagnosis. Catheters can be used to remove plaques	• Make sure the parent signs a consent form. • Administer premedication as ordered. • Obtain child's weight to determine amount of dye needed. • Keep the child NPO before the procedure according to institutional protocol. • After the procedure, maintain the child on bed rest. • Observe the puncture site for bleeding. • Monitor vital signs frequently and check the pulse distal to the site.
Ambulatory electrocardiographic monitoring (Holter)	Monitoring of the heart's electrical patterns for 24 hours using a portable compact unit	To identify and quantify arrhythmias in a 24-hour period during normal daily activities	• Instruct the child and parent to push the "event button" whenever chest pain, syncope, or palpitations occur. • Normal daily activities should be carried out during the testing period. • Having the child wear a snug undershirt over the leads helps to keep them in place.
Chest x-ray	A radiographic film of the chest area; will determine size of the heart and its chambers and pulmonary blood flow	Serves as a baseline for comparison with films taken after surgery; used to identify abnormalities of the lungs, heart, and other structures in the chest	• Instruct child not to wear jewellery or any metal around neck or on the hospital gown. • Explain to the child and family that no pain or discomfort should result. • If a portable x-ray at bedside is done, remove electrodes temporarily.
Echocardiogram	Noninvasive ultrasound procedure used to assess heart wall thickness, size of heart chambers, motion of valves and septa, and relationship of great vessels to other cardiac structures	Specific diagnosis of structural defects; determines hemodynamics and detects valvular defects	• Assure the child that the echo does not hurt. • Instruct the child about ECG lead placement and use of gel on the scope's wand during the procedure. • Encourage the child to lie still throughout the test.
Electrocardiogram (ECG)	A graphic record produced by an electrocardiograph (device used to record the electrical activity of the myocardium to detect transmission of the cardiac impulse through the conductive tissues of the muscle). Facilitates evaluation of the heart rate, rhythm, conduction, and musculature	To detect heart rhythm and chamber overload; also serves as a baseline for measuring postoperative complications	• Assure the child that monitoring is a painless procedure. • Place electrodes in the appropriate location. • The child must lie still during the ECG recording period (usually about 5 minutes). • Wipe electrode paste or jelly off after procedure.

(continued)

COMMON LABORATORY AND DIAGNOSTIC TESTS 41.1 (continued)

Test	Explanation	Indications	Nursing Implications
Exercise stress test	Monitoring of heart rate, blood pressure, ECG, and oxygen consumption at rest and during exercise	Quantifies exercise tolerance; can be used to provoke symptoms or arrhythmias	• Child should be NPO for 4 hours prior to test. • Obtain baseline ECG and vital signs. • Instruct child to verbalize symptoms during testing. • Usually takes about 45 minutes.
Hemoglobin (Hgb) and hematocrit (Hct)	Measures the total amount of hemoglobin in the blood and indirectly measures the red blood cell number and volume	To detect anemia or polycythemia (may occur with CHD resulting in cyanosis)	• False elevations occur with dehydration. • May be obtained quickly via capillary puncture. • Normal values vary with age.
Partial pressure of oxygen (pO$_2$)	Measures the amount of oxygen in the blood	To determine the presence and degree of hypoxia	• Most accurate result is with arterial specimen (venous and capillary specimens demonstrate lower levels). • Observe child for cyanosis. • Supplement with oxygen per protocol.

Adapted from Abdallah, H. (2016). *About the Children's Heart Institute*. Retrieved from www.childrenheartinstitute.org/testing/testhome.htm; and Corbett, J. A., & Banks, A. D. (2013). *Laboratory tests and diagnostic procedures with nursing diagnoses* (8th ed.). Upper Saddle River, NJ: Pearson Education Inc.

the nurse needs to educate the parents and, if appropriate for age, the child about all aspects of the procedure. The procedure is commonly performed on an outpatient basis, but some physicians or nurse practitioners require the child to be admitted for an overnight stay for observation. Nursing management of the child undergoing cardiac catheterization includes preprocedure nursing assessment and preparation of the child and family, postprocedural nursing care, and discharge teaching.

Before the Procedure. A thorough history and physical examination are necessary to establish a baseline. Obtain vital signs. Note fever or other signs and symptoms of infection, which may necessitate rescheduling the procedure. Obtain the child's height and weight to aid in determining medication dosages. Assess the child for any allergies, especially to iodine and shellfish, because some contrast materials contain iodine as a base. Review the child's medications: medications such as anticoagulants are typically withheld for several days or longer prior to the procedure to reduce the child's risk for bleeding. Check the results of any laboratory tests, such as hemoglobin and hematocrit levels.

Perform a complete physical examination. Pay particular attention to assessing the child's peripheral pulses, including pedal pulses. Use an indelible pen to

mark the location of the child's pedal pulses so they can be easily assessed after the procedure. Document the location and quality in the child's medical record.

Teach the parents and child, if appropriate, about the procedure. Include information about what the procedure involves, how long it will take, and any special instructions from the physician or nurse practitioner. Use a variety of teaching methods as appropriate, such as videotapes, books, and pamphlets. Adapt these teaching methods to the child's developmental stage. For example, introduce the younger child to equipment through play therapy. For school-age and older children and their parents, offer a tour of the cardiac catheterization laboratory. Mention sounds and sights they may experience during the procedure. Explain the use of intravenous fluid therapy, sedation, and, or anesthesia to the child and parents. Tell the child that he or she may feel a sensation of the heart racing when the catheter is inserted if this is performed without a general anesthetic (yet most centres will suggest a GA). Also warn the older child or adolescent that he or she may experience a feeling of warmth or stinging when the contrast material is injected. Encourage the child to use familiar ways to help him or her relax. If necessary, teach the child simple relaxation measures.

Typically, food and fluid are withheld for 4 to 6 hours before the procedure. Prescribed medications may be taken with a sip of water. On the day of the procedure, check to ensure that a signed informed consent form is on the child's medical record and that all necessary assessment data have been included. Just before the procedure, ask the child to void and administer a sedative, as ordered. If appropriate and permitted, allow the parents to accompany the child to the catheterization area.

Teach the child and family what to expect after the procedure is completed. Inform the parents of the possible complications that might occur, such as bleeding, low-grade fever, loss of pulse in the extremity used for the catheterization, and development of **arrhythmia** (abnormal heart rhythm). Explain to the child that he or she will have a dressing over the catheter site and that he or she will need to keep the leg straight for several hours after the procedure. Teach the child and parent that frequent monitoring will be required after the procedure.

Take Note!

In order to decrease the risk for catheterization-induced arrhythmia, an order for digitalis to be held the night before and morning of the catheterization may be written (Park, 2014). Children with tetralogy of Fallot (TOF) who have narrowing below the pulmonary valve are often prescribed a beta blocker such as propranolol to relax the narrowing. Usually, the Cardiologist wants this medication continued and not held before catheterization.

After the Procedure. Closely monitor the child for complications of bleeding, arrhythmia, hematoma, and thrombus formation and infection. After the procedure, evaluate the child's vital signs, the neurovascular status of the lower extremities, and the pressure dressing over the catheterization site every 15 minutes for the first hour and then every 30 minutes for 1 hour. Vital signs should remain within acceptable parameters. Hypotension may signify hemorrhage due to perforation of the heart muscle or bleeding from the insertion site. Expect to monitor cardiac rhythm and oxygen saturation levels via pulse oximetry for the first few hours after the procedure to help identify possible complications.

Assess the child's distal pulses bilaterally for presence and quality. The pulse of the affected extremity may be slightly less than that of the other extremity in the initial postprocedure period, but it should gradually return to baseline. Also assess the colour and temperature of the extremity; pallor or blanching would indicate an obstruction in blood flow. Check capillary refill and sensation to evaluate blood flow to the area.

Maintain bed rest in the immediate postprocedure period. Ensure that the child maintains the extremity in a straight position for approximately 4 to 8 hours, depending on the approach used and the facility's policy. Inspect the pressure dressing in all children frequently, checking under any diaper. Check to make sure that it is dry and intact, without evidence of bleeding. Reinforce the dressing as necessary and report any evidence of drainage on the dressing. If there is a risk of the dressing becoming soiled or wet, cover it with plastic. If bleeding occurs it will usually happen at the puncture site. Assess abdomen to ensure it is soft as there are rare occurrences of retroperitoneal bleeding (BC Children's Hospital, 2015). Parents are given instructions to monitor for bleeding, decreased circulation to the affected leg and signs of infection. For infants post catheterization, check under the diaper area for bleeding and keep area very clean and dry.

Take Note!

If bleeding occurs after a cardiac catheterization, apply pressure 2 cm above the site to create pressure over the vessel, thereby reducing the blood flow to the area.

Monitor the child's intake and output closely to ensure adequate hydration. The contrast material has a diuretic effect, so assess the child for signs and symptoms of dehydration and hypovolemia. Typically, the child resumes oral intake as tolerated, beginning with sips of clear liquids and progressing to his or her preprocedure diet. Continue intravenous fluids as ordered and encourage oral fluid intake as allowed and ordered to promote elimination of the contrast material.

Allow the child to talk about the experience and how and what he or she felt. Provide positive reinforcement for the child's actions.

Provide child and family education before the child is discharged home (see Teaching Guidelines 41.1). Areas to address include site care, signs and symptoms of complications (especially within 24 hours after the catheterization, such as fever, bleeding or bruising at the catheterization site, or changes in colour, temperature, or sensation in the extremity used), diet, and activity level.

Teaching Guidelines 41.1
PROVIDING CARE AFTER A CARDIAC CATHETERIZATION

- Change the pressure dressing on the day after the procedure. Apply a dry sterile dressing or adhesive bandage for the next several days. Keep the dressing dry; cover it with plastic if there is a chance that the dressing could become wet or soiled.
- When changing the dressing, inspect the insertion site for redness, irritation, swelling, drainage, and bleeding. Report any of these to the physician or nurse practitioner.

- Check the temperature, colour, sensation, and pulses on the child's extremities and compare. Report any changes to the physician or nurse practitioner.
- Resume the child's usual diet after the procedure; report any nausea or vomiting.
- Check the child's temperature at least once a day for approximately 3 days after the procedure. Report any temperature elevation of 38.0°C or greater.
- Avoid giving the child a tub bath for approximately 3 days after the procedure; use sponge baths or showers instead.
- Discourage strenuous exercise or activity for approximately 3 days after the procedure.
- Watch for changes in the child's appearance, such as changes in skin colour (cool, mottled, swollen or cyanotic), reports of the heart "fluttering" or "skipping a beat," fever, or difficulty breathing.
- Give acetaminophen (Tylenol) or ibuprofen (Motrin) for complaints of pain.
- Schedule a follow-up appointment with the physician or nurse practitioner in the time specified.

Adapted from Children's Healthcare of Atlanta. (2010). *Your child's heart catheterization.* Retrieved from www.choa.org/Childrens-Hospital-Services/Cardiac/Testing-and-Treatments/Heart-Testing/~/media/CHOA/Documents/Services/Cardiac/Your-Childs-Heart-Cath.pdf; and The University of Chicago Medicine Comer Children's Hospital. (2016). *Heart catheterization in children.* Retrieved from www.uchicagokidshospital.org/specialties/heart/patient-education/cath-guide.html

Thinking About Development

Jeremy Titus is a 2-year-old male with congenital heart disease. He is having a cardiac catheterization today. How will the nurse encourage Jeremy to stay in bed and keep his leg straight for several hours following the catheterization? What types of activities would be appropriate for occupying Jeremy while he is confined to bed? How would the nurse's approach differ if Jeremy were an older child? Remember that children often want to sit cross-legged or kneeling, however the catheter puncture site is often sore and children prefer to keep the affected leg straight.

Nursing Diagnoses and Related Interventions

Upon completion of a thorough assessment, the nurse might identify several nursing diagnoses. These may include but are not limited to:

- Decreased cardiac output
- Ineffective tissue perfusion
- Imbalanced nutrition, less than body requirements
- Risk for delayed growth and development
- Risk for infection
- Excess fluid volume
- Interrupted family processes
- Activity intolerance
- Pain

After completing Logan's assessment, the nurse noted the following: poor weight gain, tachypnea with occasional nasal flaring, crackles heard on auscultation, and edema noted in the face, presacral area, and extremities. Based on these assessment findings, what would your top three nursing diagnoses be for Logan?

Nursing goals, interventions, and evaluation for the child with a cardiovascular disorder are based on the nursing diagnoses. Nursing Care Plan 41.1, at the end of the chapter, can be used as a guide in planning nursing care for the child with a cardiovascular disorder. The nursing care plan overview should be individualized based on the child's symptoms and needs. Refer to Chapter 36 for detailed information about pain assessment and management. Additional information will be included later in the chapter as it relates to specific disorders.

Based on your top three nursing diagnoses for Logan, describe appropriate nursing interventions.

CONGENITAL HEART DISEASE

In North America, more than 1% of newborn infants have CHD resulting from numerous causes. The prevalence of CHD ranges from 6 to 13 per 1,000 live births; premature infants have a higher rate (Altman, 2015). Many chromosome defects are associated with CHD, including Down syndrome, velocardiofacial syndrome, Turner syndrome, trisomy 13, trisomy 18, Williams syndrome, Prader–Willi syndrome, and cri-du-chat (Marian et al., 2011). About one third of infants with CHD will have disease serious enough to result in death or will require cardiac catheterization or cardiac surgery within the first year of life. Complications of CHD include heart failure, hypoxemia, growth retardation, developmental delay, and pulmonary vascular disease. Children with severe anomalies frequently experience failure to thrive.

With advances in palliative and corrective surgery in the past 20 years, many more children are now able to survive into adulthood. As many as 85% of children with

CHD grow to be adults, yet many have problems related to education, insurance, and employment (Abdoulhosn & Child, 2011). Hypothermia, cardiopulmonary bypass required during cardiac surgery for CHD, and episodes of hypoxemia may have a long-term impact on the child's cognitive ability and academic function (Brown & Fulton, 2011). Due to the potential long-term effects that CHD may have on these children, nurses must be expertly equipped to care for them.

Pathophysiology

The exact cause of CHD is unknown. Most of the time it is unknown what caused the CHD and parents usually feel very guilty. Mothers frequently think they have done something which caused the heart defect. Sharing with parents that we don't know the reason for the CHD can reassure them (if there are no identified causes such as maternal lupus or use of nonsteroidal anti-inflammatory drugs [NSAIDs] during pregnancy). While there may be complex factors leading to CHD such as genetics (e.g., chromosomal alterations) and maternal exposure to environmental factors (e.g., toxins, infections) in detail discussion when there is uncertainty can be troubling for parents and this needs to be managed with sensitivity and compassion.

Congenital heart defects result from some interference in the development of the heart structure during fetal life. Subsequently, the septal walls or valves may fail to develop completely, or vessels or valves may be stenotic, narrowed, or transposed. Structures that formed to allow fetal circulation may fail to close after birth, altering the pressures necessary to maintain adequate blood flow.

After birth, with the change from fetal to newborn circulation, pressures within the chambers of the right side of the heart are less than those of the left side and pulmonary vascular resistance is less than that for the systemic circulation. These normal pressure gradients are necessary for adequate circulation to the lungs and the rest of the body. However, these pressure gradients become disrupted if a structure has failed to develop, a fetal structure has failed to close, or a narrowing, stenosis, or transposition of a vessel has occurred. For example, blood typically flows from an area of higher pressure to lower pressure. If the ductus arteriosus fails to close, blood will move from the aorta to the pulmonary artery, ultimately increasing right atrial pressure. With this shunting of blood, highly oxygenated blood can mix with less oxygenated blood, interfering with the amount available to the tissues via the systemic circulation. Some of the defects may result in significant hypoxemia, the sequelae of which include clubbing, polycythemia, exercise intolerance, hypercyanotic spells, brain abscess, and cerebrovascular accident (CVA) (Brown & Fulton, 2011).

Congenital heart defects are categorized based on hemodynamic characteristics (blood flow patterns in the heart):
- Disorders with decreased pulmonary blood flow: TOF and tricuspid atresia
- Disorders with increased pulmonary blood flow: PDA, atrial septal defect (ASD), and ventricular septal defect (VSD)
- Obstructive disorders: coarctation of the aorta, aortic stenosis, and pulmonary stenosis
- Mixed disorders: transposition of the great vessels (TGA), total anomalous pulmonary venous return (TAPVR), truncus arteriosus, and hypoplastic left heart syndrome (HLHS)

Therapeutic Management

Prenatal education about avoiding certain substances or preventing infection is essential to promote optimal outcomes for the fetus. Encourage parents of children with CHD to receive genetic counselling because of the probability of having subsequent children with a congenital heart defect. Children with small septal defects are urged to lead a normal life and often require no medical intervention. In the newborn a prostaglandin infusion will maintain patency of the ductus arteriosus, improving pulmonary blood flow. Prevention of secondary infection in this population is important therefore Synagia, an immunoglobulin is given by injection every month during the cold and flu winter months to prevent RSV (see local hospital and public health guidelines for updates). In premature or fragile infants or infants with CHD, the RSV virus can make the child extremely ill. Definitive correction of structural disorders requires surgical intervention. Table 41.2 describes the surgical procedures used for the various congenital heart defects and the relevant nursing measures.

Nursing management for the child with CHD will be provided following the disorders section. See Evidence-Based Practice 41.1.

Disorders With Decreased Pulmonary Blood Flow

Defects involving decreased pulmonary blood flow occur when there is some obstruction of blood flow to the lungs. As a result of the obstruction, pressure in the right side of the heart increases and becomes greater than that of the left side of the heart. Blood from the higher-pressure right side of the heart then shunts to the lower-pressure left side through a structural defect. Subsequently, deoxygenated blood mixes with oxygenated blood on the left side of the heart. This mixed blood, which is low in oxygen, is pumped via the systemic circulation to the body tissues.

TABLE 41.2	COMMON SURGICAL PROCEDURES AND NURSING MEASURES FOR CONGENITAL HEART DEFECTS	
Disorder	**Surgical Procedure**	**Nursing Measures**
Tetralogy of Fallot	Palliation with systemic-to-pulmonary anastomoses: • Blalock–Taussig shunt: an end-to-side anastomosis (or connection with a small Gore-Tex tube) of the subclavian artery and the pulmonary artery. • Waterston shunt: anastomosis of the ascending aorta and the pulmonary artery. • Definitive correction involves patch closure of the ventricular septal defect and repair of the pulmonary valve and right ventricular outflow tract.	• Avoid BP measurements and venipunctures in the affected arm after a Blalock–Taussig shunt. Pulse will not be palpable in that arm because of use of the subclavian artery for the shunt. • Monitor for ventricular arrhythmias after corrective repair.
Tricuspid atresia	• Palliation with Blalock–Taussig shunt or pulmonary artery banding may be performed. • At 3–6 months of age, the superior vena cava is detached from the heart and connected to the pulmonary artery (Glenn procedure). • By age 2–5 years, a modified Fontan procedure may be performed. Systemic venous return is redirected to the pulmonary artery directly.	• Monitor for atrial arrhythmias, left ventricular dysfunction, and protein-losing enteropathy. • Some children may eventually require a pacemaker.
Atrial septal defect (ASD)	• If small, the defect may be sutured closed. Larger defects may require a patch of pericardium or synthetic material. • Ostium secundum ASD may be repaired percutaneously via cardiac catheterization with a Gore Helex septal occluder (other brands are also available).	• Monitor for atrial arrhythmias (lifelong) after surgical closure. • With the Gore Helex device, strenuous activity should be avoided for 2 weeks after the procedure.[a]
Ventricular septal defect (VSD)	• If surgical closure is required, it should be performed before permanent pulmonary vascular changes develop. • Surgical closure may be in the form of suture closure of the VSD, transcatheter placement of a device in the defect, or Dacron patch closure.	• Monitor for ventricular dysrhythmias or AV block. • With the clamshell occluding or Amplatzer device, strenuous activity should be avoided for 1 month after the procedure.[b]
Atrioventricular canal defect	• Pulmonary artery banding as palliation in very young infants. • Surgical correction by 3–18 months of age • Patch closure of the septal defects and suturing of the valve leaflets or valve reconstruction are performed.	• Monitor for complete heart block postoperatively. • Teach parents that mitral regurgitation is a long-term complication and may require valve replacement.
Patent ductus arteriosus (PDA)	• PDA is closed by coil embolization or device via cardiac catheterization. • May also be surgically ligated.	• Monitor for bleeding and laryngeal nerve damage.
Coarctation of the aorta	• Balloon angioplasty via cardiac catheterization is possible in some children. • Most common surgical repair is resection of the narrowed portion of the aorta, followed by end-to-end reanastomosis.	• Preoperatively, administer prostaglandin medications as ordered to relax the ductal tissue. • Postoperatively, measure and compare BP in all four extremities and quality of upper vs. lower pulses.
Aortic stenosis	• Balloon dilatation is accomplished via the umbilical artery in the newborn or the femoral artery via cardiac catheterization in the older child.	• Provide routine postcatheterization care. • Teach parents that long-term aortic regurgitation requiring valve replacement may occur.

TABLE 41.2	COMMON SURGICAL PROCEDURES AND NURSING MEASURES FOR CONGENITAL HEART DEFECTS (continued)	
Disorder	**Surgical Procedure**	**Nursing Measures**
Pulmonary stenosis	• Balloon dilation valvuloplasty is performed via cardiac catheterization to dilate the valve. This is effective in all but the most severe of cases, which will require surgical valvotomy.	• Provide routine postcatheterization care for balloon dilation. • Explain to parents that prognosis is excellent.
Transposition of the great vessels (arteries)	• Balloon atrial septotomy is usually done as soon as the diagnosis is made. A balloon-tipped catheter is passed through the atrial septum to enlarge the atrial septum. • Surgical correction involves switching the arteries into their normal anatomic positions.	• Administer prostaglandin to maintain the open state of the ductus arteriosus, which will allow the mixing of poorly oxygenated blood with well-oxygenated blood. • Monitor for rapid respirations and cyanosis. • Administer oxygen as needed preoperatively.
Total anomalous pulmonary venous return	The pulmonary vein is repositioned to the back of the left atrium and the ASD is closed.	• Monitor for dysrhythmias, heart block, and persistent heart failure.
Truncus arteriosus	VSD repair, separation of the pulmonary arteries from the aorta, with subsequent connection to the right ventricle with a valve conduit.	• Preoperatively, administer prostaglandin infusion to prevent closing of the ductus arteriosus.
Hypoplastic left heart syndrome	• Heart transplantation is the treatment of choice. • Palliative staged treatment. First: Norwood procedure, reconstruction of the aorta and pulmonary arteries includes a cardiac transplant. Second: bidirectional Glenn procedure, connection of the superior vena cava to the right pulmonary artery to increase the blood flow to the lungs. Third: modified Fontan procedure	• Preoperatively, administer prostaglandin infusion to prevent closing of the ductus arteriosus. • After palliative repairs, monitor for dysrhythmias or worsening ventricular function.
Valve disorders	• The incompetent valve is replaced with valve prosthesis.	• Lifelong anticoagulation therapy is necessary with prosthetic valves. • Monitor prothrombin times. • Monitor heart sounds for alterations.

*a*W. L. Gore & Associates, Inc. (2010). Instructions for use: Gore® Helex septal occluder. Retrieved from www.fda.gov/ucm/groups/fdagov-public/@ fdagov-afda-adcom/documents/document/ucm304933.pdf
*b*AGA Medical Corporation. (2014). *Amplatzer™ muscular VSD occluder: Instructions for use.* Plymouth, MN: Author.
Adapted from Brown, D. W., & Fulton, D. R. (2011). Congenital heart disease in children and adolescents. In V. Fuster, R. A. Walsh, & R. A. Harrington (Eds.). *Hurst's the heart* (13th ed.). New York: McGraw-Hill Companies, Inc.; and Darst, J. R., Collins, K. K., & Miyamoto, S. D. (2014). Cardiovascular diseases. In W. W. Hay, M. J. Levin, R. R. Deterding, & M. J. Abzug (Eds.). *Current pediatric diagnosis and treatment* (22nd ed.). New York: McGraw-Hill.

Defects with decreased pulmonary blood flow are characterized by mild to severe oxygen desaturation. Typically, the child exhibits oxygen saturation levels ranging from 50% to 90%, which can produce severe cyanosis. To compensate for low blood oxygen levels, the kidneys produce the hormone erythropoietin to stimulate the bone marrow to produce more red blood cells (RBCs). This increase in RBCs is called **polycythemia**. Polycythemia can lead to an increase in blood volume and possibly blood viscosity, further taxing the workload of the heart. Although the number of RBCs increases, there is no change in the amount of blood that reaches

the lungs for oxygenation. Disorders within this classification include TOF and tricuspid atresia.

Tetralogy of Fallot

TOF is a congenital heart defect composed of four heart defects: pulmonary stenosis (a narrowing of the pulmonary valve and outflow tract, creating an obstruction of blood flow from the right ventricle to the pulmonary artery), VSD, overriding aorta (enlargement of the aortic valve to the extent that it appears to arise from the right and left ventricles rather than the anatomically correct

EVIDENCE-BASED PRACTICE 41.1   **EFFECTS OF CHRONIC OR INTERMITTENT HYPOXIA ON COGNITION IN CHILDREN**

STUDY

It is well known that significant hypoxia demonstrates an adverse effect on cognition, yet little is known about the effects of chronic or intermittent hypoxia on cognition in children. Many children with congenital heart disease (CHD) suffer either chronic or intermittent hypoxia. The authors performed a systematic literature review to study this question. Fifty-five studies were included, and a significant proportion of them addressed hypoxia with CHD.

Findings

About 80% of the studies reported adverse effects on cognition in children who suffered chronic or intermittent hypoxia, including developmental and academic achievement. Adverse effects were noted at all childhood age levels except premature infants. The effects were noted even with mild oxygen desaturation. Keep in mind the unborn fetus has saturation levels of between 30% and 70%. Babies born with cyanotic defects will adapt better than a healthy infant who has a sudden and sustained saturation drop to the 70's.

Nursing Implications

It is critical that the developing child be afforded the opportunity to develop optimal cognition. Know the child's normal oxygen saturation so that decreases may be quickly acted upon. Use supplemental oxygen judiciously and within the physician order parameters. Since many children experience improved oxygenation after CHD repair, encourage adequate nutrition so that, in turn, the infant or child will demonstrate growth adequate for safe surgical intervention.

Adapted from Bass, J. L., Corwin, M., Gozal, D., Moore, C., Nishida, H., Parker, S., . . . Kinane, T. B. (2004). The effect of chronic or intermittent hypoxia on cognition in childhood: A review of the evidence. *Pediatrics, 114*(3), 805–816.

---

left ventricle), and right ventricular hypertrophy (the muscle walls of the right ventricle increase in size due to continued overuse as the right ventricle attempts to overcome a high-pressure gradient). Surgical intervention is usually required during the first year of life (Brown & Fulton, 2011; Darst, Collins, & Miyamoto, 2014).

PATHOPHYSIOLOGY

With pulmonary stenosis, the blood flow from the right ventricle is obstructed and slowed, resulting in a decrease in blood flow to the lungs for oxygenation and a decrease in the amount of oxygenated blood returning to the left atrium from the lungs. The obstructed flow also increases the pressure in the right ventricle. This blood, which is poorly oxygenated, is then shunted across the VSD into the left atrium. Poorly oxygenated blood also travels through the overriding aorta (if it extends to both ventricles). In some cases when the VSD is large, the pressure in the right ventricle may be equal to that of the left ventricle. In this case, the path of blood shunting depends on which circulation is exerting the higher pressure, pulmonary or systemic.

Knowledge of what shunts are and how they work in CHD are critical concepts. Shunts are simply abnormal paths that blood takes. Shunts can be described as:

- From the right to the left side of the heart or pulmonary to systemic (TGA, tricuspid atresia, TOF, TAPVR, truncus)
- Left to right or systemic to pulmonary (VSD, ASD, AVSD, PDA)
- Bidirectional

Shunts can also be surgically or as part of a heart catheterization procedure, removed, corrected or created.

Examples of these are a PDA coil embolization, a BT shunt, a Fontan surgery, an RV to PA conduit.

Regardless of which way shunting occurs, a mixing of oxygenated and poorly oxygenated blood occurs, with this blood ultimately being pumped into the systemic circulation. The oxygen saturation of the blood in the systemic circulation is reduced, leading to cyanosis. The degree of cyanosis depends on the extent of the pulmonary stenosis, the size of the VSD, and the vascular resistance of the pulmonary and systemic circulations.

TOF is usually diagnosed during the first weeks of life due to the presence of a murmur and/or cyanosis. Some newborns may be acutely cyanotic, while others may exhibit only mild cyanosis that gradually becomes more severe, particularly during times of stress as the child grows older. Most often, infants with TOF have a PDA at birth, providing additional pulmonary blood flow and thereby decreasing the severity of the initial cyanosis. Later, as the ductus arteriosus closes, such as within the first days of life, more severe cyanosis can occur (Fig. 41.2) (Brown & Fulton, 2011; Darst et al., 2014).

NURSING ASSESSMENT

Nursing assessment consists of the health history, physical examination, and laboratory and diagnostic tests.

Health History and Physical Examination

Obtain the health history, noting a history of colour changes associated with feeding, activity, or crying. Determine if the infant or child is demonstrating hypercyanotic spells. Hypercyanosis develops suddenly and is manifested as increased cyanosis, hypoxemia, dyspnea,

To body

From body

To lungs

To lungs

From lungs

From lungs

AO

LA

PA

RA

Aorta overrides
septal defect

LV

RV

From body

Pulmonary stenosis
(Narrowing in the
pulmonary valve area)

Thickened right
ventricle wall

To body

Ventricular septal defect

FIGURE 41.2 **Tetralogy of Fallot.**

and agitation. If the infant's oxygen demand is greater than the supply, such as with crying or during feeding, then the spell progresses to anoxia. When the degree of cyanosis is severe and persistent, the infant may become unresponsive. In a younger child presenting with a late diagnosis he or she may use specific postures, such as bending at the knees or assuming the fetal position, to relieve a hypercyanotic spell. The walking infant or toddler may squat periodically. These positions improve pulmonary blood flow by increasing systemic vascular resistance. Ask the parents if they have noticed any of these unusual positions. Note history of irritability, sleepiness, or difficulty breathing.

During the physical examination, observe the skin colour and note any evidence of cyanosis. Also observe for changes in skin colour with positional changes, and inspect the fingers for clubbing. Note if the child has a hypercyanotic spell during the assessment or intervention; this can be linked to crying. While the nurse observes for signs of the child becoming dusky, laboured breathing, irritability, or lethargy he or she should also teach parents to watch and manage these symptoms in their child. Remember to teach parents the knee-chest position (if parent is holding the infant and tucks the knees up to the infant's chest). This position increases

systemic vascular resistance and decreases the shunting of blood right to left across the VSD. Spasms under the pulmonary valve which restricts blood flow to the lungs are called infundibular spasms, which result in the changes in the child's colour and respiratory rate. During an acute episode the aims are to decrease pulmonary vascular resistance, increase systemic vascular resistance, and treat hypoxia. This can be achieved by reducing infant stress, giving blow by O_2, placing child in knee-chest position, administer medication such as Propranolol to relax the infundibular spasm, or treat acidosis. Count the child's respiratory rate and observe work of breathing, noting retractions, shortness of breath, or noisy breathing. Document oxygen saturation via pulse oximetry; it will likely be decreased. Auscultate the chest for adventitious breath sounds, which may suggest the development of heart failure. Auscultate the heart, noting a loud, harsh murmur characteristic of this disorder.

Laboratory and Diagnostic Tests

Note increased hematocrit, hemoglobin, and RBC count associated with polycythemia. Additional testing may include:

- **Echocardiography** (ultrasound study of structure and motion of heart), possibly revealing right ventricular hypertrophy, decreased pulmonary blood flow, and reduced size of the pulmonary artery (Lai, Mertens, Cohen, & Geva, 2015).
- Electrocardiogram (ECG), indicating right ventricular hypertrophy
- Cardiac catheterization and angiography, which reveal the extent of the structural defects

Consider This!

Ava Gardener, 2 weeks old, is brought to the clinic by her mother. She presents with trouble feeding. Her mother states, "When Ava eats, she seems to have trouble breathing, and a couple of times she has looked a little bluish." As the nurse takes Ava into her arms, Ava has a hypercyanotic spell.

Ava is to be admitted to the hospital secondary to suspected TOF. Ava's mother is very upset about the diagnosis. She says "my poor baby; she'll never ever be able to run and play like a normal child."

How should the nurse respond? How would you feel if your young baby was diagnosed with a serious disorder? What type of support can the nurse provide to Ava's mother? Think about the importance of communication, health literacy, and social connections to wider support groups.

Tricuspid Atresia

Tricuspid atresia is a congenital heart defect in which the valve between the right atrium and right ventricle fails to develop. As a result, there is no opening to allow blood to flow from the right atrium to the right ventricle and subsequently through the pulmonary artery into the lungs (Brown & Fulton, 2011; Darst et al., 2014).

Pathophysiology

In tricuspid atresia, blood returning from the systemic circulation to the right atrium cannot directly enter the right ventricle due to agenesis of the tricuspid valve. Subsequently, deoxygenated blood may pass through an opening in the atrial septum (patent foramen ovale) into the left atrium, never entering the pulmonary vasculature. Thus, deoxygenated blood mixes with oxygenated blood in the left atrium. The blood then travels to the lungs through a PDA. Most cases of tricuspid atresia are associated with a VSD and the newborn receives inadequately oxygenated blood (Fig. 41.3) (Darst et al., 2014).

Nursing Assessment

Nursing assessment consists of the health history, physical examination, and laboratory and diagnostic tests.

Oxygen rich blood
Oxygen poor blood
Mixed blood

FIGURE 41.3 Tricuspid atresia.

Health History and Physical Examination

Note the infant's history since birth. Document history of cyanosis either at birth or a few days later when the ductus arteriosus closed. Note history of rapid respirations and difficulty with feeding. Inspect the skin for cyanosis or a pale grey colour. Observe the apical impulse, noting overactivity. Evaluate the baby's sucking strength (will usually have a weak or poor suck). Count the respiratory rate, noting tachypnea. Note increased work of breathing. Auscultate the lungs, noting crackles or wheezes if heart failure is beginning to develop. Auscultate the heart, noting a murmur. Palpate the skin, noting coolness and clamminess of the extremities. Document the presence of clubbing in the older infant or child.

Laboratory and Diagnostic Testing

Laboratory and diagnostic testing is similar to that for TOF. A complete blood cell (CBC) count is needed to assess compensatory increases in hematocrit, hemoglobin, and erythrocyte count (RBC) indicating the development of polycythemia. Pulse oximetry or arterial blood gas tests may be used to determine oxygen saturation levels (typically reduced). Additional testing may include:
- Echocardiography, revealing absence of tricuspid valve or underdeveloped right ventricle
- ECG, indicating possible heart failure

- Cardiac catheterization and angiography, which reveal the extent of the structural defects

Disorders With Increased Pulmonary Flow

Most congenital heart defects involve increased pulmonary blood flow. Normally, the left side of the heart has a higher pressure than the right side. Defects with connections involving the left and right sides will shunt blood from the higher-pressure left side to the lower-pressure right side. Even a small pressure gradient such as a 1- to 3-mm difference between the left and right sides will produce a movement of blood from the left to the right. In turn, the increase of blood on the right side of the heart will cause a greater amount of blood to move through the heart. If the amount of blood flowing to the lungs is large, the child may develop heart failure early in life. In addition, right ventricular hypertrophy may result. Sometimes with ventricular hypertrophy the right side of the heart pumps so forcefully that left-to-right shunting is reversed to right-to-left shunting. If this occurs, deoxygenated blood mixes with oxygenated blood, thereby lowering the overall blood oxygen saturation level.

Excessive blood flow to the lungs can produce a compensatory response such as tachypnea or tachycardia. Tachypnea increases caloric expenditure; poor cellular nutrition from decreased peripheral blood flow leads to feeding problems. Subsequently, the infant experiences poor weight gain, which retards overall growth and development. Increased pulmonary blood flow results in decreased systemic blood flow, so sodium and fluid retention may occur. Increased pulmonary blood flow also places the child at higher risk for pulmonary infections. As the child grows, the continuous increased pulmonary blood flow will cause vasoconstriction of the pulmonary vessels, actually decreasing the pulmonary blood flow. This may lead to pulmonary hypertension. For children with congenital defects with increased pulmonary blood flow, oxygen supplementation is not helpful. Oxygen acts as a pulmonary vasodilator. If pulmonary dilation occurs, pulmonary blood flow is even greater, causing tachypnea, increasing lung fluid retention, and eventually causing a much greater problem

with oxygenation. Over time, continuous increased pulmonary blood flow may cause pulmonary vasoconstriction and pulmonary hypertension. Therefore, preventing the development of pulmonary disease via early surgical correction is essential.

Examples of defects with increased pulmonary blood flow are ASD, VSD, atrioventricular canal defect, and PDA.

Atrial Septal Defect

An ASD is a passageway or hole in the wall (septum) that divides the right atrium from the left atrium (Fig. 41.4). Three types of ASDs are identified based on the location of the opening:

- Ostium primum (ASD1): the opening is at the lower portion of the septum.
- Ostium secundum (ASD2): the opening is near the centre of the septum.
- Sinus venosus defect: the opening is near the junction of the superior vena cava and the right atrium.

When the ASD is small, as many as 80% of infants may have a spontaneous closure within the first 18 months of life. If it does not spontaneously close by age 3, the child will most likely need corrective surgery (Brown & Fulton, 2011; Darst et al., 2014). Some ASD's can be closed, where there is enough tissue available, with a transcatheter device such as, such as an Amplatzer (Wan,

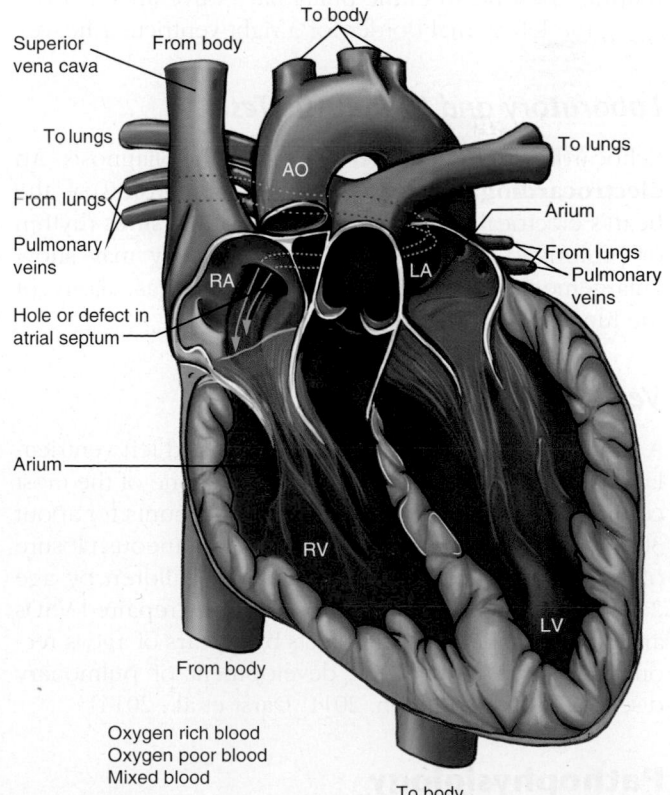

FIGURE 41.4 Atrial septal defect; note the opening between the two atria.

Vijarnsorn and Rutledge, 2014). This is usually done when the child is around 4 to 5 years of age through a heart catheterization procedure.

Pathophysiology

With ASD, blood flows through the opening from the left atrium to the right atrium due to pressure differences. The shunting increases the blood volume entering the right atrium. This, in turn, leads to increased blood flow into the lungs. If untreated, the defect can cause problems such as pulmonary hypertension, heart failure, atrial arrhythmias, or stroke (Brown & Fulton, 2011; Darst et al., 2014).

Nursing Assessment

Most children with ASDs are asymptomatic. However, a very large defect can cause increased blood flow, leading to heart failure, which results in shortness of breath, easy fatigability, or poor growth.

Health History and Physical Examination

Obtain the health history, noting poor feeding as an infant, decreased ability to keep up with peers, or history of difficulty growing. Observe the child's chest, noting a hyperdynamic precordium. Auscultate the heart, noting a fixed split second heart sound and a systolic ejection murmur, best heard in the pulmonary valve area. Palpate along the left sternal border for a right ventricular heave.

Laboratory and Diagnostic Tests

Echocardiography is done to confirm the diagnosis. An **electrocardiogram (ECG)** (graphic recording of the heart's electrical activity) may show normal sinus rhythm or prolonged PR intervals. The chest x-ray may show enlargement of the heart and increased vascularity of the lungs.

Ventricular Septal Defect

A VSD is an opening between the right and left ventricular chambers of the heart (Fig. 41.5). It is one of the most common congenital heart defects and accounts for about 30% of all congenital heart defects. Spontaneous closure of small VSDs occurs in about half of children by age 2 years. Long-term outcomes for surgically repaired VSDs are good. Repair of larger defects by 2 years of age is recommended to prevent the development of pulmonary disease (Brown & Fulton, 2011; Darst et al., 2014).

Pathophysiology

In VSD, there is an abnormal opening between the right and left ventricles. The opening varies in size, from as

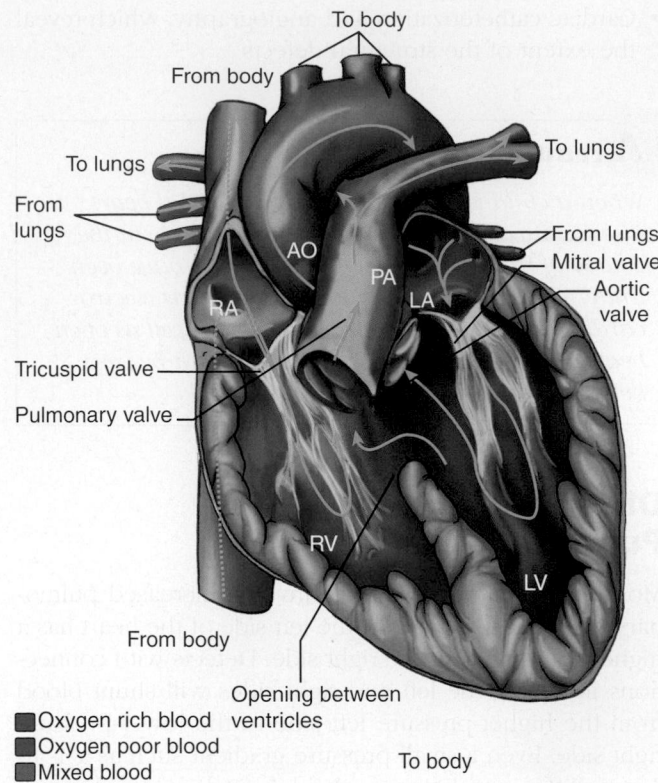

Oxygen rich blood
Oxygen poor blood
Mixed blood

FIGURE 41.5 Ventricular septal defect; note the opening between the ventricles.

small as a pinhole to a complete opening between the ventricles so that the right and left sides are as one. Children with small VSDs may remain asymptomatic. In other children, blood shunts across the opening in the septum. Pulmonary vascular resistance and systemic vascular resistance determine the direction of blood flow. A left-to-right shunt results when pulmonary vascular resistance is low. Increased amounts of blood flowing into the right ventricle are then pumped to the pulmonary circulation, eventually causing an increase in pulmonary vascular resistance. Increased pulmonary vascular resistance leads to increased pulmonary artery pressure (pulmonary hypertension) and right ventricular hypertrophy. When the pulmonary vascular resistance exceeds the systemic vascular resistance, right-to-left shunting of blood across the VSD occurs, resulting in Eisenmenger syndrome (pulmonary hypertension and cyanosis). Heart failure commonly occurs in children with moderate to severe unrepaired VSDs. Children with VSDs are also at risk for the development of aortic valve regurgitation as well as infective endocarditis (Brown & Fulton, 2011; Darst et al., 2014).

Nursing Assessment

Initially, the newborn may not exhibit any signs and symptoms at birth because left-to-right shunting is most likely minimal due to the high pulmonary resistance common after birth.

Health History and Physical Examination

Determine the health history, which commonly reveals signs of heart failure around 4 to 8 weeks of age. Note history of tiring easily, particularly with exertion or feeding. Document the child's growth history, noting difficulty thriving. Ask the parent about colour change or diaphoresis with nipple feeding in the infant. Note history of frequent pulmonary infections, shortness of breath, and possibly edema. Inspect the extremities for edema, noting whether pitting is present. Note mild tachypnea.

Auscultate the heart, noting a characteristic holosystolic harsh murmur along the left sternal border. In some instances, a murmur may be noted only with excessive blood flow across the opening. Adventitious lung sounds may be auscultated if the child is experiencing heart failure. Palpate the chest for a thrill.

Laboratory and Diagnostic Tests

Magnetic resonance imaging (MRI) or echocardiogram with colour flow Doppler may reveal the opening as well as the extent of left-to-right shunting. These studies also may identify right ventricular hypertrophy and dilation of the pulmonary artery resulting from the increased blood flow. Cardiac catheterization may be used to evaluate the extent of blood flow being pumped to the pulmonary circulation and to evaluate hemodynamic pressures.

Atrioventricular Canal Defect

Atrioventricular canal defect (atrioventricular septal defect [AVSD], AV canal, or endocardial cushion defect) accounts for 3.5% of CHD. Forty-five percent of children with Down syndrome and CHD have this defect (Brown & Fulton, 2011).

Pathophysiology

AV canal defect occurs as a result of failure of the endocardial cushions to fuse (Fig. 41.6). These cushions are needed to separate the central parts of the heart near the tricuspid and mitral (AV) valves. The complete AV canal defect involves ASDs and VSDs as well as a common AV orifice and a common AV valve. Partial and transitional forms of AV canal defect also occur, involving variations of the complete form.

The complete AV canal defect permits oxygenated blood from the lungs to enter the left atrium and ventricle, crossing over the atrial or ventricular septum and returning to the lungs via the pulmonary artery. This recirculation problem, which typically involves a left-to-right shunt, is inefficient because the left ventricle must

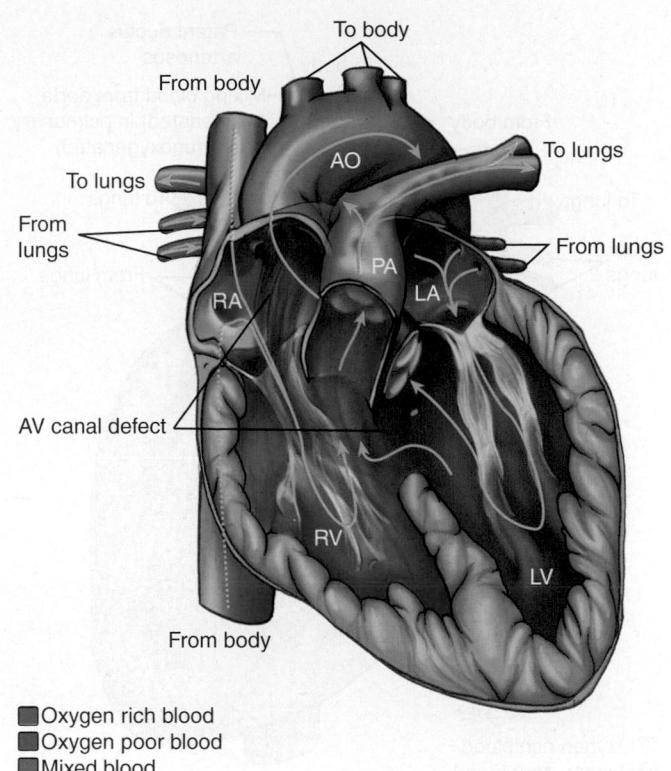

■ Oxygen rich blood
■ Oxygen poor blood
■ Mixed blood

FIGURE 41.6 Atrioventricular canal defect.

pump blood back to the lungs and also meet the body's peripheral demand for oxygenated blood. Subsequently, the left ventricle must pump two to three times more blood than in a normal heart. Therefore, this specific type of cardiac defect causes a large left-to-right shunt; an increased workload of the left ventricle; and high pulmonary arterial pressure, resulting in an increased amount of blood in the lungs causing pulmonary edema (Brown & Fulton, 2011; Darst et al., 2014).

Nursing Assessment

The infant with a complete AV canal defect commonly exhibits moderate to severe signs and symptoms of heart failure. However, for infants with partial or transitional AV canal defects, the signs and symptoms will be subtler.

Health History and Physical Examination

Obtain the health history, noting frequent respiratory infections and difficulty gaining weight. Ask the parent if the infant has been experiencing difficulty feeding or increased work of breathing.

Inspect the skin, fingernails, and lips for cyanosis. Observe for retractions, tachypnea, and nasal flaring. Auscultate the lungs and heart, noting rales and a loud murmur. The murmur is commonly noted within the first 2 weeks of life. Infants with partial or transitional AV canal defects may display more subtle signs.

FIGURE 41.7 Patent ductus arteriosus.

*Labels in figure:*
- Patent ductus arteriosus
- To body
- From body
- Mixing blood from aorta (oxygenated) in pulmonary artery (unoxygenated)
- To lungs
- From lungs
- To lungs
- From lungs
- AO
- PA
- RA
- LA
- RV
- LV
- From body
- To body
- ■ Oxygen rich blood
- ■ Oxygen poor blood
- ■ Mixed blood

Laboratory and Diagnostic Tests

Echocardiography will reveal the extent of the defect and shunting as well as right ventricular hypertrophy. ECG may indicate right ventricular hypertrophy and possible first-degree heart block due to impulse blocking before reaching the AV node.

Patent Ductus Arteriosus

PDA is failure of the ductus arteriosus, a fetal circulatory structure, to close within the first weeks of life (Fig. 41.7). As a result, there is a connection between the aorta and pulmonary artery. PDA is the second most common congenital heart defect and accounts for 10% of CHD cases (Darst et al., 2014). PDA occurs much more frequently in premature than in term infants and in infants born at high altitudes compared with those born at sea level. Infants with other CHDs that result in right-to-left shunting of blood and cyanosis may additionally display a PDA. In these infants, the PDA allows for some level of oxygenated blood to reach the systemic circulation (Brown & Fulton, 2011; Darst et al., 2014).

Pathophysiology

Failure of the ductus arteriosus to close leads to continued blood flow from the aorta to the pulmonary artery. Blood returning to the left atrium passes to the left ventricle, enters the aorta, and then travels to the pulmonary artery via the PDA instead of entering the systemic circulation. This altered blood flow pattern increases the workload of the left side of the heart. Pulmonary vascular congestion occurs, causing an increase in pressure. Right ventricular pressure increases in an attempt to overcome this increase in pulmonary pressure. Eventually, right ventricular hypertrophy occurs (Brown & Fulton, 2011; Darst et al., 2014).

Nursing Assessment

The symptoms of PDA depend on the size of the ductus arteriosus and the amount of blood flow it carries. If it is small, the infant may be asymptomatic. Some infants demonstrate signs and symptoms of heart failure.

Health History and Physical Examination

Determine the health history, which may reveal frequent respiratory infections, fatigue, and poor growth and development. On physical examination, note tachycardia, tachypnea, bounding peripheral pulses, and a widened pulse pressure. The diastolic BP typically is low due to the shunting. Auscultate the lungs and heart, noting rales if heart failure is present. Note a harsh, continuous, machine-like murmur, usually loudest under the left clavicle at the first and second intercostal spaces.

Laboratory and Diagnostic Tests

Echocardiogram reveals the extent of the defective opening and confirms the diagnosis. ECG may be normal or it may indicate ventricular hypertrophy, especially if the defect is large. Chest radiography demonstrates cardiomegaly.

Obstructive Disorders

Another group of congenital heart defects is classified as obstructive disorders. These disorders involve some type of narrowing of a major vessel, interfering with the ability of the blood to flow freely through the vessel. As a result, peripheral circulation or blood flow to the lungs is affected. Increased pressure backing up toward the heart causes an increased workload on the heart. Examples of defects in this group include coarctation of the aorta, aortic stenosis, and pulmonic stenosis.

Coarctation of the Aorta

Coarctation of the aorta is narrowing of the aorta, the major blood vessel carrying highly oxygenated blood from the left ventricle of the heart to the rest of the body (Fig. 41.8). It accounts for 4.2% to 6% of congenital heart defects and occurs three times more often in males than in females (Brown & Fulton, 2011; Darst et al., 2014).

To body — Narrowed aorta

From body

To lungs

To lungs

From lungs

AO

PA

LA

RA

From lungs

RV

LV

From body

■ Oxygen rich blood
■ Oxygen poor blood
■ Mixed blood

To body

FIGURE 41.8 **Coarctation of the aorta.**

Pathophysiology

Coarctation of the aorta occurs most often in the area near the ductus arteriosus. The narrowing can be preductal (between the subclavian artery and ductus arteriosus) or postductal (after the ductus arteriosus). As a result of the narrowing, blood flow is impeded, causing pressure to increase in the area proximal to the defect and to decrease in the area distal to it. Thus, BP is increased in the heart and upper portions of the body and decreased in the lower portions of the body. Left ventricular afterload is increased, and in some children this may lead to heart failure. Collateral circulation also may develop as the body attempts to ensure adequate blood flow to the descending aorta. Due to the elevation in BP, the child is also at risk for aortic rupture, aortic aneurysm, and CVA (Brown & Fulton, 2011; Darst et al., 2014).

Nursing Assessment

The extent of the symptoms depends on the severity of the coarctation. Some children with coarctation of the aorta grow well into the school-age years before the defect is discovered.

Health History and Physical Examination

Determine the health history, noting problems with irritability and frequent epistaxis. In older children, there also

may be reports of leg pain with activity, dizziness, fainting, and headaches. Assess pulses throughout, noting full, bounding pulses in the upper extremities with weak or absent pulses in the lower extremities. Determine BP in all four extremities. BP in the upper extremities may be 20 mm Hg or higher than that in the lower extremities. Inspect the school-age child's chest, noting notching of the ribs. Auscultate the heart for a soft or moderately loud systolic murmur, most often heard at the base of the heart (on the back or in the left axilla) (Darst et al., 2014).

Laboratory and Diagnostic Tests

Diagnosis of coarctation of the aorta is based primarily on the history and physical examination. In addition, an echocardiogram may disclose the extent of narrowing and evidence of collateral circulation. Chest radiography may reveal left-sided cardiac enlargement and rib notching indicative of collateral arterial enlargement. Other tests, such as ECG, computed tomography, or MRI, may be done to provide additional evidence about the extent of the coarctation and subsequent effects.

Aortic Stenosis

Aortic stenosis is a condition causing obstruction of the blood flow between the left ventricle and the aorta. The occurrence of aortic stenosis is 3.8 per 1,000 live births, with more than 75% of cases occurring in males (Brown & Fulton, 2011).

Pathophysiology

Aortic stenosis can be caused by a muscle obstruction below the aortic valve, an obstruction at the valve itself, or an aortic narrowing just above the valve (Fig. 41.9). The most common type is an obstruction of the valve itself, called aortic valve stenosis. The aortic valve consists of three very pliable leaflets. Normally the leaflets of the aortic valve spread open easily when the left ventricle ejects blood into the aorta. Aortic stenosis occurs when the aortic valve narrows, causing an obstruction between the left ventricle and the aorta. As a result, cardiac output decreases. When the aortic valve does not function properly, the left ventricle must work harder to pump blood into the aorta. Because of the increased workload, the left ventricular muscle hypertrophies. If this continues, left ventricular failure can occur, leading to a backup of pressure in the pulmonary circulation and pulmonary edema. Heart failure may occur, but this is more commonly seen in the infant (Brown & Fulton, 2011).

Nursing Assessment

Typically, the child with aortic stenosis is asymptomatic. However, it is important to obtain an accurate health history and perform a physical examination.

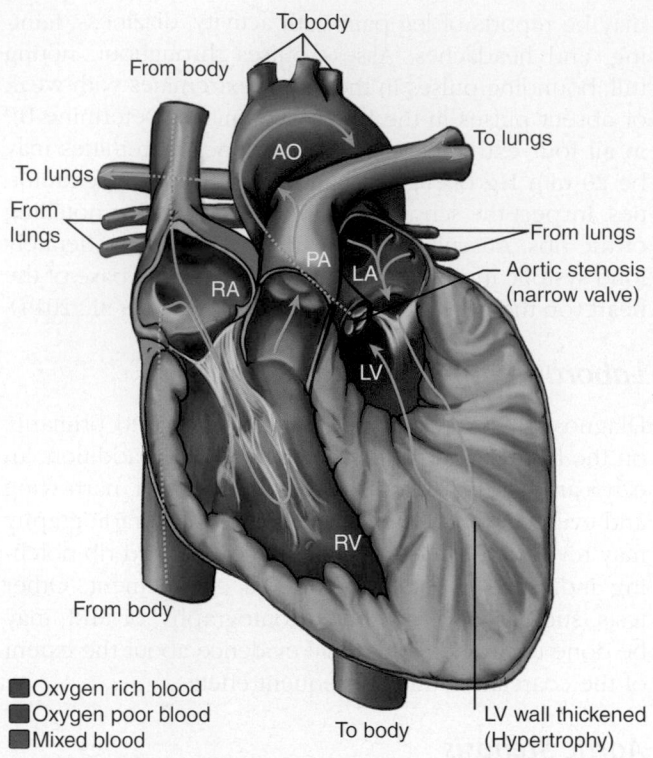

■ Oxygen rich blood
■ Oxygen poor blood
■ Mixed blood

LV wall thickened
(Hypertrophy)

FIGURE 41.9 Aortic stenosis.

Health History and Physical Examination

Obtain the child's health history, noting easy fatigability or complaints of chest pain similar to anginal pain when active. Dizziness with prolonged standing also may be reported. In the infant, note difficulty with feeding. Palpate the child's pulse; if aortic stenosis is severe, the pulses may be faint. Palpate the child's chest, noting a thrill at the base of the heart. Auscultate the heart, noting a systolic murmur best heard along the left sternal border with radiation to the right upper sternal border.

Laboratory and Diagnostic Tests

The echocardiogram is the most important noninvasive test to identify aortic stenosis. An ECG may be normal in children with mild to moderate forms of aortic stenosis. For children with severe aortic stenosis, left ventricular hypertrophy may be determined from the ECG. For children experiencing easy fatigability and chest pain, an exercise stress test may be done to evaluate the degree of cardiac compromise.

Pulmonary Stenosis

Pulmonary stenosis is a condition that causes an obstruction in blood flow between the right ventricle and the pulmonary arteries. Pulmonary stenosis occurs in 0.6 to 0.8 per 1,000 live births (Peng & Perry, 2016). It is often

associated with other heart anomalies and with genetic syndromes. Children may be asymptomatic, although some children with severe stenosis may exhibit dyspnea and fatigue with exertion (demonstrating hypercyanotic spells similar to those in children with TOF) (Peng & Perry, 2016).

Pathophysiology

Pulmonary stenosis may occur as a muscular obstruction below the pulmonary valve, an obstruction at the valve, or a narrowing of the pulmonary artery above the valve (Fig. 41.10). Valve obstruction is the most common form of pulmonary stenosis. Normally the pulmonary valve is constructed with three thin and pliable valve leaflets; they spread apart easily, allowing the right ventricle to eject blood freely into the pulmonary artery. The most common problem causing pulmonary stenosis is that the pulmonary valve leaflets are thickened and fused together along their separation lines, causing the obstruction to blood flow. The right ventricle has an additional workload, causing the muscle to thicken, resulting in right ventricular hypertrophy and decreased pulmonary blood flow. When the pulmonary valve is severely obstructed, the right ventricle cannot eject sufficient blood into the pulmonary artery. As a result, pressure in the right atrium increases, which could lead to a reopening of the foramen ovale. If this occurs, deoxygenated blood would

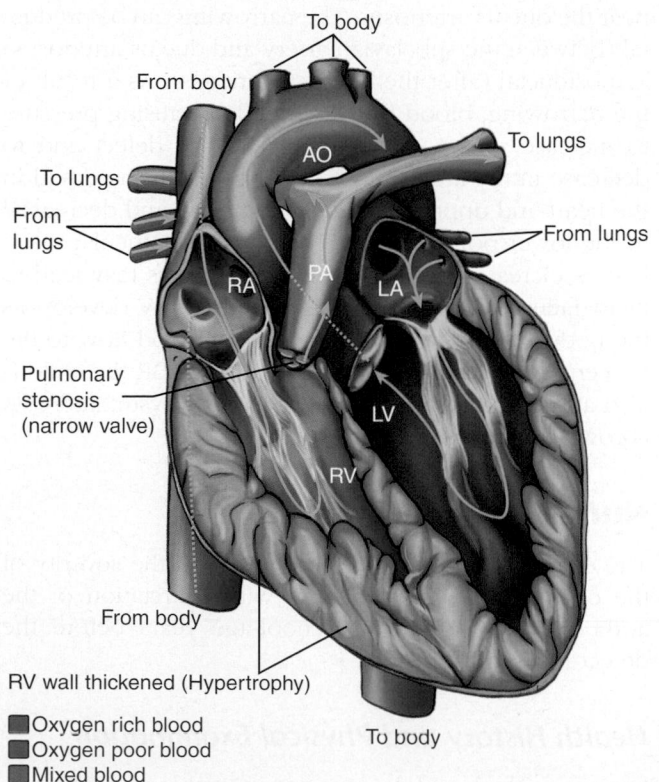

■ Oxygen rich blood
■ Oxygen poor blood
■ Mixed blood

RV wall thickened (Hypertrophy)

FIGURE 41.10 Pulmonary stenosis.

pass through the foramen ovale into the left side of the heart and would then be pumped to the systemic circulation. In some cases, a PDA may be present, thus allowing for some compensation by shunting blood from the aorta to the pulmonary circulation for oxygenation (Brown & Fulton, 2011; Peng & Perry, 2016).

Nursing Assessment

The child with pulmonary stenosis may be asymptomatic or may exhibit signs and symptoms of mild heart failure. If the stenosis is severe, the child may demonstrate cyanosis. Therefore, it is important for the nurse to obtain an accurate health history and physical examination.

Health History and Physical Examination

Elicit the health history, noting mild dyspnea or cyanosis with exertion. Document the child's growth history, which is typically normal. Carefully palpate the sternal border for a thrill (not always present). Auscultate the heart, noting a high-pitched click following the second heart sound and a systolic ejection murmur loudest at the upper left sternal border.

Laboratory and Diagnostic Tests

An echocardiogram reveals the extent of obstruction present at the valve, as well as right ventricular hypertrophy. An ECG also helps to detect right ventricular hypertrophy.

Mixed Defects

Mixed defects are congenital heart defects that involve a mixing of well-oxygenated blood with poorly oxygenated blood. As a result, systemic blood flow contains a lower oxygen content. Cardiac output is decreased, and heart failure occurs. Examples of mixed defects include TGA, total anomalous pulmonary venous connection (TAPVC), truncus arteriosus, and HLHS.

Transposition of the Great Arteries (Vessels)

TGA is a congenital heart defect in which the pulmonary artery and the aorta are transposed from their normal positions. The aorta arises from the right ventricle instead of the left ventricle and the pulmonary artery arises from the left ventricle instead of the right ventricle. TGA accounts for 3.4% to 5% of all CHD cases (Brown & Fulton, 2011; Darst et al., 2014). It is most often diagnosed in the first few days of life when the infant manifests cyanosis, which indicates decreased oxygenation. As the ductus arteriosus closes, the symptoms will worsen. Corrective surgery is usually performed by age 4 to 7 days.

■ Oxygen rich blood
■ Oxygen poor blood
■ Mixed blood

FIGURE 41.11 Transposition of the great vessels.

Pathophysiology

TGA creates a situation in which poorly oxygenated blood returning to the right atrium and ventricle is then pumped out to the aorta and back to the body (Fig. 41.11). Oxygenated blood returning from the lungs to the left atrium and ventricle is then sent back to the lungs through the pulmonary artery. Unless there is a connection somewhere in the circulation where the oxygen-rich and oxygen-poor blood can mix, all the organs of the body will be poorly oxygenated. Often the ductus arteriosus remains patent, allowing for some mixing of blood. Similarly, if a VSD is also present, mixing of blood may occur and cyanosis will be delayed. However, these associated defects can lead to increased pulmonary blood flow that increases pressure in the pulmonary circulation. This predisposes the child to heart failure (Brown & Fulton, 2011; Darst et al., 2014).

Nursing Assessment

Significant cyanosis without a murmur in the newborn period is highly indicative of TGA. In some infants, cyanosis will not develop until several days of age as the PDA closes. In infants with septal defects, cyanosis may be further delayed.

Health History and Physical Examination

Elicit the health history, noting onset of cyanosis with feeding or crying. Observe the infant for cyanosis while active and at rest. Observe the chest, noting a prominent ventricular impulse. Auscultate the heart, noting a loud second heart sound. A murmur may be heard if the ductus remains open or a septal defect is present. If heart failure is present, note edema, tachypnea, and adventitious lung sounds.

Laboratory and Diagnostic Tests

Echocardiography clearly reveals evidence of the transposition. Cardiac catheterization may be performed to determine whether oxygen saturation levels are low due to the mixing of the blood.

Anomalous Pulmonary Venous Return (Connection) Total (TAPVR) or Partial (PAPVR)

TAPVR or PAPVR are rare congenital heart defects in which the pulmonary veins do not connect normally to the left atrium. Instead, they connect to the right atrium, often by way of the superior vena cava. Relatively rare, it occurs in about 1 in 17,000 live births (Brown & Fulton, 2011).

Pathophysiology

Oxygenated blood that would normally enter the left atrium now enters the right atrium and passes to the right ventricle. As a result, the pressure on the right side of the heart increases, leading to hypertrophy. TAPVR is incompatible with life unless there is an associated defect present that allows for shunting of blood from the highly pressured right side of the heart. A patent foramen ovale or an ASD is usually present. Since none of the pulmonary veins connect normally to the left atrium, the only source of blood to the left atrium is blood that is shunted from the right atrium across the defect to the left side of the heart (Fig. 41.12). The highly oxygenated blood from the lungs completely mixes with the poorly oxygenated blood returning from the systemic circulation. This causes an overload of the right atrium and right ventricle. The increased blood volume going into the lungs can lead to pulmonary hypertension and pulmonary edema (Brown & Fulton, 2011; Darst et al., 2014).

Nursing Assessment

The degree of cyanosis present with TAPVR depends on the extent of the associated defects. For example, if the foramen ovale closes or the ASD is small, significant cyanosis will be present. The physical examination findings will vary depending on the type of TAPVR the infant has, whether obstruction is present, and whether other associated cardiac anomalies are present.

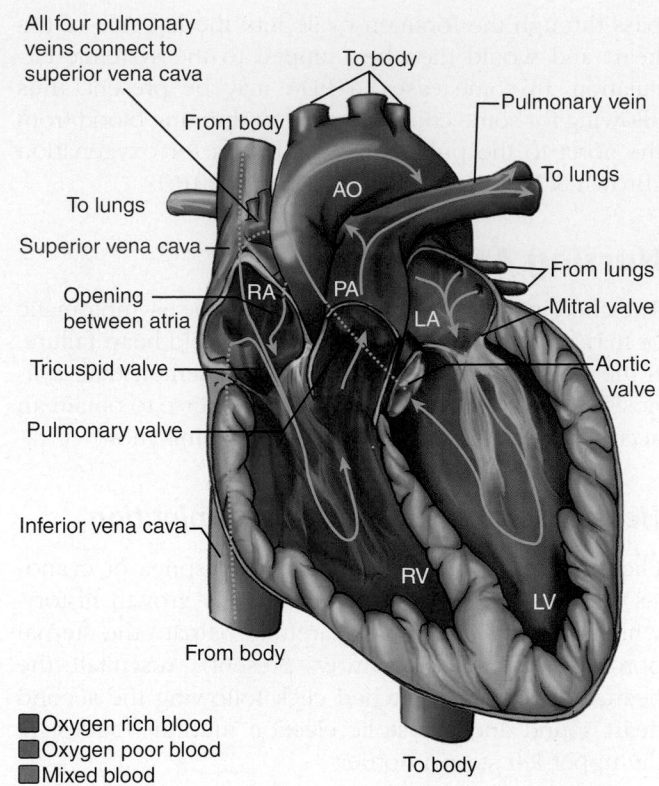

All four pulmonary veins connect to superior vena cava

To body

Pulmonary vein

From body

AO

To lungs

To lungs

Superior vena cava

From lungs

Opening between atria

RA

PA

LA

Mitral valve

Tricuspid valve

Aortic valve

Pulmonary valve

Inferior vena cava

RV

LV

From body

■ Oxygen rich blood
■ Oxygen poor blood
■ Mixed blood

To body

FIGURE 41.12 Total anomalous pulmonary venous connection.

Health History and Physical Examination

Note history of cyanosis, tiring easily, and difficulty feeding. Observe the chest for prominence of the right ventricular impulse and retractions with tachypnea. Auscultate the heart, noting fixed splitting of the second heart sound and a murmur. Palpate the abdomen for hepatomegaly.

Laboratory and Diagnostic Tests

An echocardiogram will reveal the abnormal connection of the pulmonary veins, enlargement of the right atrium and right ventricle, and an ASD if present. The chest x-ray will demonstrate an enlarged heart and pulmonary edema. Cardiac catheterization can also be useful to visualize the abnormal connection of the pulmonary veins, particularly if an obstruction is present.

Truncus Arteriosus

Truncus arteriosus is a congenital heart defect in which only one major artery leaves the heart and supplies blood to the pulmonary and systemic circulations. It affects males and females equally and accounts for less than 1% all CHD cases (Darst et al., 2014). A VSD may also be present.

Pathophysiology

The one great vessel contains one valve. This valve consists of two to five leaflets and is positioned over both the left and right ventricles (Fig. 41.13). Due to the location of the valve, blood from the left ventricle mixes with blood from the right ventricle. Pressure in the pulmonary circulation typically is less than that of the systemic circulation, leading to increased blood flow to the lungs. As a result, systemic blood flow is decreased. Over time, the increased pulmonary blood flow can lead to pulmonary vascular disease (Brown & Fulton, 2011; Darst et al., 2014).

Nursing Assessment

Typically, the infant demonstrates cyanosis in varying degrees, depending on the extent of compromise in the systemic circulation. Obtain an accurate health history and perform a physical examination.

Health History and Physical Examination

Elicit the health history, noting history of cyanosis that increases with periods of activity such as feeding. Also note history of tiring easily, difficulty in feeding, and poor growth. Count the respiratory rate, which may be elevated. Observe for nasal flaring, grunting or noisy breathing, retractions, and restlessness. Auscultate the lungs, noting adventitious breath sounds, and the heart, noting a murmur associated with a VSD.

Laboratory and Diagnostic Tests

An echocardiogram will confirm the presence of truncus arteriosus as the anatomy of the great vessels, the single truncal valve, and the VSD will be seen. On rare occasions a cardiac catheterization may be done to determine pressures in the pulmonary arteries.

Hypoplastic Left Heart Syndrome

HLHS is a congenital heart defect in which all of the structures on the left side of the heart are severely underdeveloped (Fig. 41.14). The mitral and aortic valves are completely closed or very small. The left ventricle is nonfunctional. Thus, the left side of the heart is completely unable to supply blood to the systemic circulation. HLHS is the fourth most common congenital heart defect. It appears to have a multifactorial and autosomal recessive inheritance pattern and occurs in 1.4% to 3.8% of cases of CHD (Darst et al., 2014). The options for treatment include palliative care, cardiac transplantation within the first few weeks of life, or palliative reconstructive surgery consisting of three stages, beginning within days to weeks of birth.

FIGURE 41.13 Truncus arteriosus.

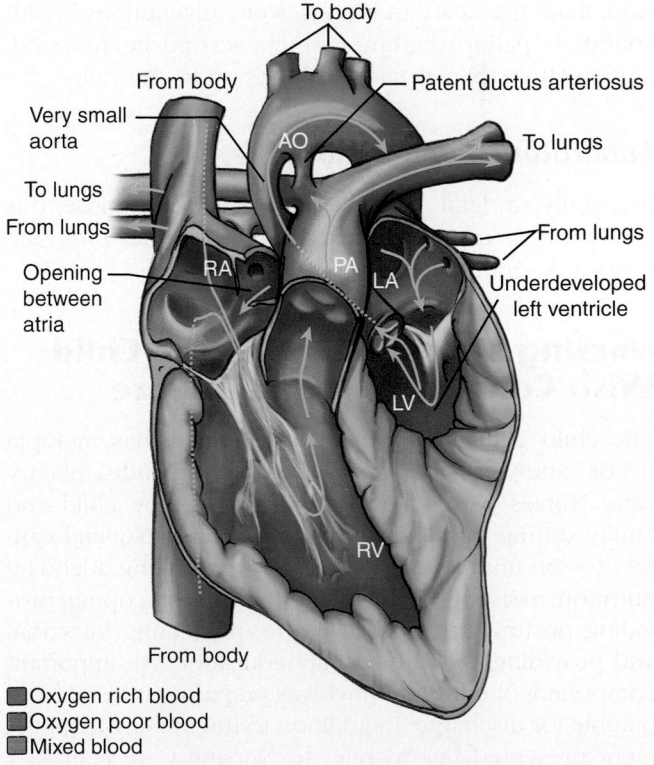

FIGURE 41.14 Hypoplastic left heart syndrome.

Pathophysiology

With HLHS, the right side of the heart is the main working part of the heart. Blood returning from the lungs into the left atrium must pass through an ASD to the right side of the heart. The right ventricle must then pump blood to the lungs and also to the systemic circulation through the PDA. A few days after birth, when the ductus arteriosus closes, the heart cannot pump blood into the systemic circulation, causing poor perfusion of the vital organs and shock. Death will occur rapidly without intervention (Brown & Fulton, 2011; Darst et al., 2014).

Nursing Assessment

Initially after birth, the newborn may be asymptomatic because the ductus arteriosus is still patent. However, as the ductus begins to close at a few days of age, the newborn will begin to exhibit cyanosis. Some infants may present with circulatory collapse (shock) and must be resuscitated emergently.

Health History and Physical Examination

Obtain the health history, noting onset of cyanosis. Note poor feeding and history of tiring easily. Evaluate the vital signs, noting tachycardia, tachypnea, and hypothermia. Observe for increased work of breathing and gradually increasing cyanosis. Note pallor of the extremities and decreased oxygen saturation via pulse oximetry. Auscultate the heart and lungs. Note adventitious breath sounds, a gallop rhythm, a single second heart sound, and a soft systolic ejection or holosystolic murmur.

Laboratory and Diagnostic Tests

Prenatally, a fetal echocardiogram can diagnose this syndrome, as can a maternal ultrasound. After birth, the echocardiogram illustrates the defect.

Nursing Management of the Child With Congenital Heart Disease

The child with a congenital heart defect has multiple needs and requires comprehensive, multidisciplinary care. Nurses play a key role in helping the child and family during this intensely stressful time. Nursing care focuses on improving oxygenation, promoting adequate nutrition, assisting the child and family with coping, providing postoperative nursing care, preventing infection, and providing child and family education. An important component of education involves preparing the child and parents for discharge. In addition to the nursing management presented below, refer to Nursing Care Plan 41.1 for additional interventions appropriate for the child with

CHD. Individualize nursing care specific to the child's needs.

Improving Oxygenation

Due to the hemodynamic changes accompanying the underlying structural defect, oxygenation is key. Provide frequent ongoing assessment of the child's cardiopulmonary status. Assess airway patency and suction as needed. Position the child in the Fowler or semi-Fowler position to facilitate lung expansion. Monitor vital signs, especially heart and respiratory rates. Monitor the child's colour and oxygen saturation levels closely, using these to guide oxygen administration. Observe for tachypnea and other signs of respiratory distress, such as nasal flaring, grunting, and retractions. Auscultate the lungs for adventitious sounds. Provide humidified supplemental oxygen as ordered, warming it to prevent wide temperature fluctuations. Anticipate the need for assisted ventilation if the child has difficulty maintaining the airway or experiences deterioration in oxygenation capacity. Box 41.1 lists interventions related to relief of hypercyanotic spells. The child may also require monitoring for arrhythmias with telemetry.

Promoting Adequate Nutrition

Adequate nutrition is critical to foster growth and development as well as to reduce the risk for infection. Children with congenital heart defects typically have increased nutritional needs due to the increased energy expenditure associated with increased cardiac and respiratory workloads. In addition, many of the defects lead to heart failure, which may affect the child's fluid balance status, further increasing the child's energy expenditure.

Nutrition may be provided orally, enterally, or parenterally. For example, for the newborn or infant, nutrition via breast milk or formula may be provided orally or via gavage (nasogastric/orogastric) feedings. Breastfeeding

---

> ### BOX 41.1
>
> **RELIEVING HYPERCYANOTIC SPELLS**
> - Use a calm, comforting approach.
> - Place the infant or child in a knee-to-chest position.
> - Provide supplemental oxygen.
> - Administer morphine sulfate (0.1 mg/kg IV, IM, or SQ).
> - Supply IV fluids.
> - Administer propranolol (0.1 mg/kg IV).
>
> IM, intramuscularly; SQ, subcutaneously.
> Adapted from Doyle, T., Kavanaugh-McHugh, A., & Fish, F. A. (2016). *Management and outcome of tetralogy of Fallot*. Retrieved from www.uptodate.com/contents/management-and-outcome-of-tetralogy-of-fallot

is usually associated with decreased energy expenditure during the act of feeding, yet some infants in intensive care are not stable enough to breastfeed. Gavage feeds with expressed breast milk is possible, and the use of human milk fortifier added to the gavage feed, adds additional calories that the infant requires. Formula-fed infants may also require increased-calorie formula, which may be achieved by more concentrated mixing of the formula or through the use of additives such as Polycose or vegetable oil. Consult the nutritionist to determine the individual infant's caloric needs and prescription of appropriate feeding.

Cutting a large hole in the nipple or "cross-cutting" the nipple decreases the work of feeding for some infants. Generally, nipple feedings should be limited to a 20-minute duration, as feeding for longer periods results in excess caloric expenditure. Many infants may feed orally for 20 minutes, receiving the remainder of that feeding via gavage feed. Offer older children small, frequent feedings to reduce the amount of energy required to feed or eat and to prevent overtiring the child. When needed, administer and monitor total parenteral nutrition as prescribed.

Take Note!

Breastfeeding a child before and after cardiac surgery may boost the infant's immune system, which can help fight postoperative infection. If breastfeeding is not possible, mothers can pump milk and the breast milk may be given via bottle, dropper, or gavage feed.

Assisting the Child and Family to Cope

The diagnosis of CHD is especially overwhelming for the child and the parents. The numerous examinations, diagnostic tests, and procedures are sources of stress for the infant or child regardless of age and for the parents (Rempel, Ravindran, Rogers, & Magill-Evans, 2013). The parents may fear long-term disability or death or may worry that allowing the child to engage in any activity will worsen his or her status. Allow the parents to voice their feelings, concerns, or questions providing ample time to address these. Assist the parents to be involved in their infants care, connecting to their infant through touch (Jackson, Frydenberg, Liang, Higgins, & Murphy, 2015). Be mindful of parents beliefs and spiritual needs as well as cultural practice. Parents of a sick infant may be overprotective of the child. It is important for the parents to continue parenting the child, even when the child requires extended hospitalizations or intensive care. Provide developmentally appropriate honest explanations to the child. Encourage play therapy to help the child understand what is happening. If the child is older, offer suggestions as to how the parents can meet the child's emotional needs.

Preventing Infection

Teach parents proper hand hygiene: wash hands with soap and water scrubbing front and backs of hands, or using an alcohol-based sanitizer if water is not available (CPS, 2012). Provide appropriate dental care: begin brushing teeth with the appearance of the first tooth, using nonfluorinated toothpaste until 3 years of age, and ensuring first dental check-up at 12 months of age. Make sure the child receives prophylaxis for infective endocarditis as needed. Ensure that children 24 months or younger who have hemodynamically significant heart defects receive respiratory syncytial virus (RSV) prophylaxis as recommended during RSV season (Ralston et al., 2014).

Providing Care for the Child Undergoing Cardiac Surgery

Cardiac surgery may be necessary to correct a congenital defect or to provide symptomatic relief. The surgery may be planned as an elective procedure or done as an emergency. Open heart surgery involves an incision of the heart muscle to repair the internal structures. This may require cardiopulmonary bypass. Closed heart surgery involves structures related to the heart but not the heart muscle itself and may be performed with or without cardiopulmonary bypass.

PROVIDING PREOPERATIVE CARE

The preoperative nursing assessment complements the history and physical examination and provides important baseline information for comparison during the postoperative period. Establish a relationship with the child and parents. Identify problems that may require particular nursing interventions during the postoperative period. Before cardiac surgery, interview the parents and, if age appropriate, the child. Focus the interview on the history of the present illness, cardiac risk factors, the child's present physical and functional status, additional medical problems, current medications and drug allergies, the child's and family's understanding of the illness and planned procedure, and the family support system.

The preoperative physical assessment includes:
- Temperature and weight measurements
- Examination of extremities for peripheral edema, clubbing, and evaluation of peripheral pulses
- Auscultation of the heart (rate, rhythm, heart sounds, murmurs, clicks, and rubs)
- Respiratory assessment, including respiratory rate, work of breathing, and auscultation of the lungs for breath sounds

Obtain any necessary laboratory and diagnostic tests to establish a baseline. In addition, review the results of any tests done previously. Testing may include CBC count, electrolyte levels, clotting studies, urinalysis, cultures of blood and other body secretions, renal and hepatic function tests, chest radiography, ECG, echocardiogram, and cardiac catheterization.

In most nonemergent cases, preoperative assessment is performed in an outpatient setting and the child is admitted to the hospital on the day of surgery. Nursing care during this phase focuses on thorough child and parent education. If the surgery is an emergency, teaching must be done quickly, emphasizing the most important elements of the child's care.

Child and parent education typically includes the following topics:

• Heart anatomy and its function, including what area is involved with the defect that is to be corrected
• Events before surgery, including any testing or preparation such as a skin scrub
• Location of the child after surgery, such as a pediatric intensive care unit, which may include a visit to the unit if appropriate and explanation of the sights and sounds that may be present
• Appearance of the child after surgery (equipment or devices used for monitoring, such as oxygen administration, ECG leads, pulse oximeter, chest tubes, mechanical ventilation, or intravenous lines)
• Approximate location of the incision and coverage with dressings
• Postoperative activity level, including measures to reduce the risk of complications, such as coughing and deep-breathing exercises, incentive spirometry, early ambulation, and leg exercises
• Nutritional restrictions, such as nothing by mouth for a specified time before surgery and use of intravenous fluids
• Medications, such as anesthesia, sedation, and analgesics as well as medications the child is taking now that need to be continued or withheld (Beke, Braudis, & Lincoln, 2005)

Prepare and educate the child at an age and developmentally appropriate level. Advise parents to read books with their child about hospitalization as well as those linked to specific heart conditions. The Heart and Stroke Foundation of Canada offers the *Heart and Soul Binder* which is accessible via the BC Children's Hospital website and found in thePoint. Honest, age-appropriate information about the surgery should be communicated with the patient (DeMaso & Snell, 2013). Child life specialists can facilitate this process and can help promote strong coping mechanisms for the child and decrease anxiety. Hospital tours are appropriate for school-age children and older children and teens may benefit from an intensive care unit tour before surgery. Parents will be instructed when to arrive at the hospital, when to stop food and liquids prior to the operation, and which medications to administer. Some medications, such as anticoagulants, aspirin, and NSAIDs should be withheld prior to surgery

to mitigate bleeding risks. This decision is ultimately up to the surgeon once risk of bleeding is evaluated based on the procedure (McKenzie, Douglas, & Bazargan, 2013). When it is time for the child to be transported to the surgical area, allow the parents to accompany the child as far as possible, depending on the institution's policy. Also reinforce with the child that his or her parents will be present at the bedside when he or she awakens from surgery.

PROVIDING POSTOPERATIVE CARE

The child will usually be transported from the operating room to the intensive care unit. Depending on the child's age, postoperative stability, and type of surgery, the child may stay in the intensive care unit for several hours up to several days.

During the postoperative period the nurse should do the following:

• Assess vital signs frequently, as often as every 1 hour, until stable.
• Assess the colour of the skin and mucous membranes, check capillary refill, and palpate peripheral pulses.
• Observe cardiac rate and rhythm via electronic telemetry monitoring and auscultate heart rate, rhythm, and heart sounds frequently.
• Monitor hemodynamic status via arterial and/or central venous lines (left and right atrial and pulmonary artery pressures, pulmonary artery oxygen saturation).
• Provide site care and tubing changes according to the institution's policy.
• Auscultate lungs for adventitious, diminished, or absent breath sounds.
• Assess oxygen saturation levels via pulse oximetry and arterial blood gases as well as work of breathing and level of consciousness frequently.
• Administer supplemental oxygen as needed.
• Monitor mechanical ventilation and suction as ordered.
• Inspect chest tube functioning, noting amount, colour, and character of drainage. Strip or milk the tube every 1 to 2 hours to promote drainage.
• Inspect the dressing (incision and chest tube) for drainage and intactness. Reinforce or change the dressing as ordered.
• Assess the incision for redness, drainage, edema, or separation.
• Assess the sternum for stability.
• Monitor intake and output hourly.
• Maintain accurate intravenous infusion rate; restrict fluids as ordered to prevent hypervolemia.
• Assess for changes in level of consciousness. Report restlessness, irritability, or seizures.
• Obtain ordered laboratory tests, such as CBC count, coagulation studies, cardiac enzyme levels, BUN, creatinine, lactate, and electrolyte levels. Report abnormal results.

- Administer medications, such as digoxin or inotropic or vasopressor agents, as ordered, watching the child closely for possible adverse effects (Strehlow, 2015; Trinh & Palmer, 2012; Ziff & Kotecha, 2016).
  - Digoxin may cause adverse effects including nausea, vomiting, visual changes, and possibly arrhythmias.
  - Inotropic agents may cause adverse effects including ischemia, ventricular ectopy, arrhythmias, myocyte necrosis.
  - Vasopressor agents may cause adverse effects including arrhythmias and myocardial ischemia.
- Encourage the child to turn, cough, deep breathe, use the incentive spirometer, and splint the incisional area with pillows.
- Assess the child's pain level and administer analgesics as ordered. Allow time for the child to rest and sleep.
- Assist the child to get out of bed as soon as possible and as ordered.
- Assess daily weights.
- Administer small, frequent feedings or meals when oral intake is allowed.
- Position the child in a comfortable position, one that maximizes chest expansion. Change position frequently.
- Assess the child for complications (Box 41.2).
- Provide emotional and physical support to the child and family, making appropriate referrals such as to social services for assistance.
- Prepare the child and family for discharge (Beke et al., 2005).

BOX 41.2

POSSIBLE COMPLICATIONS AFTER CARDIAC SURGERY

- Atelectasis
- Bacterial endocarditis
- Cardiac arrhythmias
- Cardiac tamponade
- Cerebrovascular accident
- Heart failure
- Hemorrhage
- Pleural effusion
- Pneumonia
- Pneumothorax
- Postperfusion syndrome
- Postcardiac surgery syndrome
- Pulmonary edema
- Seizures
- Wound infection

Adapted from Bacha, E. A., Cooper, D., Thiagarajan, R., Franklin, R. C., Krogmann, O., Deal, B., . . . Colan, S. D. (2008). Cardiac complications associated with the treatment of patients with congenital cardiac disease: Consensus definitions from the Multi-Societal Database Committee for Pediatric and Congenital Heart Disease. *Cardiology in the Young, 18*(Suppl 2), 196–201.

Take Note!

Abrupt cessation of chest tube output accompanied by an increase in heart rate and increased filling pressure (right atrial) may indicate cardiac tamponade (Beke et al., 2005).

Safety Check

GOAL 3: Improve the Safety of Using Medications (Use Medicines Safely)

NPSG 03.05.01 Reduce the likelihood of patient harm associated with the use of anticoagulant therapy

Steps: Follow the facility's protocol for starting and continuing anticoagulant therapy, including assessment of laboratory tests. For children, use pre-filled syringes ONLY if specifically designed for pediatric use. Provide family education related to compliance, follow-up monitoring, drug–food interactions, drug–drug interactions, and adverse drug reactions.

Joint Commission. (2015). *National patient safety goals effective January 1, 2015.* Retrieved from www.jointcommission.org/assets/1/6/2015_NPSG_HAP.pdf

---

Providing Child and Family Education

Provide child and family education throughout the child's stay. Initially, teaching focuses on the underlying defect and measures to treat or control the problem. If the child requires surgery, teaching shifts to preoperative and postoperative events. Emphasize discharge teaching for each admission. Teaching Guidelines 41.2 highlights the major areas to be addressed in child and family education.

 Teaching Guidelines 41.2

CARING FOR THE CHILD WITH A CONGENITAL HEART DISEASE

- Give medications, if ordered, exactly as prescribed.
- Weigh the child at least once a week or as ordered, at approximately the same time of the day with the same scale, and wearing the same amount of clothing.
- Allow the child to engage in activity as directed. Provide time for the child to rest frequently throughout the day to prevent overexertion.
- Provide a nutritious diet, taking into account any restrictions for fluids or foods.
- Use measures to prevent infection, such as frequent hand washing, prophylactic antibiotics, and skin care.
- Adhere to schedule for follow-up diagnostic tests and procedures.
- Support the child's growth and development needs.
- Use available community support services.

• Notify the physician or nurse practitioner if the child has increasing episodes of respiratory distress, cyanosis, or difficulty breathing; fever; increased edema of the hands, feet, or face; decreased urinary output; weight loss or difficulty eating or drinking; increased fatigue or irritability; decreased level of alertness; or vomiting or diarrhea.

Adapted from Cook, E. H., & Higgins, S. S. (2010). Congenital heart disease. In P. J. Allen, J. A. Vessey, & N. A. Schapiro (Eds.). *Primary care of the child with a chronic condition* (5th ed.). St. Louis, MO: Mosby.

ACQUIRED CARDIOVASCULAR DISORDERS

Acquired cardiovascular disorders occur in children as a result of an underlying cardiovascular problem or may refer to other cardiac disorders that are not congenital. The most common type of acquired cardiovascular disorder in children is heart failure. Other acquired disorders include rheumatic fever, cardiomyopathy, infective endocarditis, hyperlipidemia, hypertension, and Kawasaki disease.

Heart Failure

Heart failure occurs most often in children with CHD and is the most common reason for admission to the hospital for children with CHD. Most cases of heart failure in children with CHD occur by 6 months of age (Darst et al., 2014). Heart failure also occurs secondary to other conditions such as myocardial dysfunction following surgical intervention for CHD, cardiomyopathy, myocarditis, fluid volume overload, hypertension, anemia, or sepsis or as a toxic effect of certain chemotherapeutic agents used in the treatment of cancer. **Heart failure** refers to a set of clinical signs and symptoms that reflect the heart's inability to pump effectively to provide adequate blood, oxygen, and nutrients to the body organs and tissues (Francis, Wilson Tang, & Walsh, 2011; Darst et al., 2014). The child experiencing heart failure requires a multidisciplinary approach to care including physicians, nurses, dieticians, physiotherapists, and in some cases, respiratory therapists. Collaboration is necessary to achieve improved cardiac function, restored fluid balance, decreased cardiac workload, and improved oxygen delivery to the tissues.

Pathophysiology

Cardiac output is controlled by preload (diastolic volume), afterload (ventricular wall tension), myocardial contractility (inotropic state), and heart rate. Protracted alterations in any of these factors may lead to heart failure. In the event of reduced cardiac output, multiple compensatory mechanisms are activated. When the ventricular contraction is impaired (systolic dysfunction), reduced ejection of blood occurs, and therefore cardiac output is reduced. Diminished ability to receive venous return (diastolic dysfunction) occurs when high venous pressures are required to support ventricular function. As a result of decreased cardiac output, the renin–angiotensin–aldosterone system is activated as a compensatory mechanism. Fluid and sodium retention as well as improved contractility and vasoconstriction then occur. Initially BP is supported and organ perfusion is maintained, but increased afterload worsens systolic dysfunction. As the heart chambers dilate, myocardial oxygen consumption increases and cardiac output is limited by excessive wall stretch. Over time, the capacity of the heart to respond to these compensatory mechanisms fails, and cardiac output is further decreased (Darst et al., 2014; Francis et al., 2011). Figure 41.15 shows the clinical manifestations that occur related to the mechanisms of heart failure.

Therapeutic Management

Management of heart failure is supportive. Promotion of oxygenation and ventilation is of utmost importance. Digitalis, diuretics, inotropic agents, vasodilators, antiarrhythmics, and antithrombotics have been widely used in children for palliation of symptoms. Many children with heart failure require management in the intensive care unit until they are stabilized. Augmenting nutrition and ensuring adequate rest are also key components of management.

Nursing Assessment

For a full description of the assessment phase of the nursing process, refer to the Assessment section of the Nursing Process Overview earlier in the chapter. Specific assessment findings related to heart failure are discussed below.

Health History

When obtaining the health history, elicit a description of the present illness and chief complaint. Common complaints reported during the health history might include:
• Failure to gain weight or rapid weight gain
• Failure to thrive seen as slowed or stalled weight gain
• Difficulty or taking long time to feed (often >20 minutes)
• Feeding intolerance (vomiting) or aversion
• Fatigue
• Shortness of breath
• Syncope
• Decreased number of wet diapers
• Tachypnea
• Diaphoresis
• Exercise intolerance
• Dizziness, irritability

FIGURE 41.15 **Pathophysiology of heart failure.** (Adapted from Francis, G. S., Wilson Tang, W. H., & Walsh, R. A. [2011]. Pathophysiology of heart failure. In V. Fuster, R. A. Walsh, & R. A. Harrington [Eds.]. *Hurst's the heart* [13th ed.]. New York: McGraw-Hill Companies, Inc.)

Infants with heart failure often display subtle signs such as difficulty feeding and tiring easily. Pay close attention for reports of these problems from the parents. Also be alert for statements such as "The baby drinks a small amount of breast milk (or formula) and stops, but then wants feeding again very soon afterwards"; "The baby seems to perspire a lot during feedings"; or "The baby seems to be more comfortable when he's sitting up or on my shoulder than when he's lying flat." In addition, the parents may report episodes of rapid breathing and grunting.

The child's current and past medical history also provide additional clues. Question the parents about any history of congenital heart defects and treatments such as surgery to repair the defect. Determine the current medication regimen. Also ask about any recent or past infections, such as streptococcal infections or fever.

Physical Examination

Weigh the child and note recent rapid weight gain or lack of weight gain. Obtain the child's vital signs, noting tachycardia or tachypnea. These findings are often the first indicators of heart failure in an infant or older child. Measure the BP in the upper and lower extremities, comparing the findings for differences. Note decreased BP, which may be due to impaired cardiac muscle function. Inspect the skin colour, noting pallor or cyanosis. Also observe for diaphoresis (profuse sweating). Inspect the face, hands, and lower extremities for edema. Observe for increased work of breathing, such as nasal flaring or retractions. Note the presence of a cough, which may be productive with bloody sputum. Auscultate the apical pulse, noting its location and character. Listen for a murmur, which may suggest a congenital heart defect, a gallop rhythm, or an accentuated third heart sound, suggesting sudden ventricular distention. Auscultate the lungs, noting crackles or wheezes suggestive of pulmonary congestion. Palpate the peripheral pulses, noting weak or thready pulses. Note the temperature and colour of the extremities; they may be cool, clammy, and pale.

Assess the child's abdomen, looking for distention indicative of ascites. Gently palpate the abdomen to identify hepatomegaly or splenomegaly.

Laboratory and Diagnostic Tests

The diagnosis of heart failure is based on the child's signs and symptoms and is confirmed with several laboratory and diagnostic tests. These include:

- Chest x-ray, revealing an enlarged heart and/or pulmonary edema
- Electrocardiogram, indicating ventricular hypertrophy and possibly arrhythmias
- Echocardiogram, revealing the underlying cause of heart failure, such as a congenital heart defect

Other tests may be done to support the diagnosis. For example, the CBC count may show evidence of anemia or infection. Electrolyte levels may reveal hyponatremia secondary to fluid retention and hyperkalemia secondary to tissue destruction or impaired renal function. Arterial blood gas results may demonstrate respiratory alkalosis in mild heart failure or metabolic acidosis. Tissue hypoxia may be evidenced by increased lactic acid and decreased bicarbonate levels. A BNP level can also help identify heart failure and distinguish from other causes of respiratory congestion.

Nursing Management

Nursing management of the child with heart failure focuses on promoting oxygenation, supporting cardiac function, providing adequate nutrition, and promoting rest.

Promoting Oxygenation

Position the infant or child in a semi-upright position to decrease work of breathing and lessen pulmonary congestion. Suction as needed. Chest physiotherapy and postural drainage may also be beneficial. Administer supplemental oxygen as ordered and monitor oxygen saturation via pulse oximetry. Oxygen also serves the function of vasodilator and decreases pulmonary vascular resistance. Occasionally, the infant or child with heart failure may require intubation and positive pressure ventilation to normalize blood gas tension.

Take Note!

In a child with a large left-to-right shunt, oxygen will decrease pulmonary vascular resistance while increasing the systemic vascular resistance, which leads to increased left-to-right shunting. Monitor the child carefully and use oxygen only as prescribed.

Supporting Cardiac Function

Administer digitalis, angiotensin-converting enzyme (ACE) inhibitors, beta blockers, aldosterone antagonists, and diuretics as prescribed. IV inotropic support may also be necessary. Digoxin therapy begins with a digitalizing dose divided into several doses (oral or intravenous [IV]) over a 24-hour period to reach maximum cardiac effect. During digitalization, monitor the ECG for a prolonged PR interval and decreased ventricular rate. Doses are then administered every 12 hours. Monitor the child for signs of digoxin toxicity. Measure BP before and after administration of ACE inhibitors, holding the dose and notifying the physician if the BP falls more than 15 mm Hg. Observe for signs of hypotension such as lightheadedness, dizziness, or fainting. Weigh the child daily to determine fluid loss. Maintain accurate records of intake and output, restricting fluid intake if ordered. Carefully monitor potassium levels, administering potassium supplements if prescribed. Sodium intake is not usually restricted in the child with heart failure.

Providing Adequate Nutrition

Due to the increased metabolic rate associated with heart failure, the infant may require as much as 150 calories/kg/day. Older children will also require higher caloric intake than typical children. Offer small, frequent feedings if the child can tolerate them. During the acute phase of heart failure, many infants in particular will require continuous or intermittent gavage feeding to maintain or gain weight. Concentrate infant formula to 24 to 28 calories/ounce as instructed by the dietician since breast milk or formula contains 20 kcal/oz.

Promoting Rest

Minimize metabolic needs to decrease cardiac demand. The infant or older child with heart failure will usually limit activities based on energy level. Ensure adequate time for sleep and attempt to limit disturbing interventions. Provide age-appropriate activities that can be performed quietly or in bed, such as books, colouring or drawing, and video or board games. The older child or adolescent with significant heart failure may require home schooling. As the child improves, a rehabilitation program may be helpful for maximizing activity within the child's cardiovascular status limits.

INFECTIVE ENDOCARDITIS

Infective endocarditis is a microbial infection of the endothelial surfaces of the heart's chambers, septum, or valves (most common). Children with congenital heart defects (septum or valve defects) or prosthetic valves are at increased risk of acquiring bacterial endocarditis, which is potentially fatal in these children. Cyanotic heart disease particularly raises this risk. Other risk factors for endocarditis include central venous catheters and intravenous drug use. Infective endocarditis occurs when bacteria or fungi gain access to a damaged epithelium. Turbulence in blood flow associated with narrowed or incompetent valves or with a communication between the systemic and pulmonary circulation leads to damage of the endothelium. Thrombi and platelets then adhere to the endothelium, forming vegetations. When a microbe gains access to the bloodstream, it colonizes the vegetation, using the thrombi as a breeding ground. Clumps may separate from the vegetative patch and travel to other organs of the body, causing significant damage (septic emboli). Fungi or more commonly bacteria (particularly α-hemolytic streptococcus or *Staphylococcus aureus*) are frequently implicated in infective endocarditis (Brusch & Bronze, 2015; Darst et al., 2014).

Complete antibiotic or antifungal treatment of the causative organism is necessary, and treatment generally lasts 4 to 6 weeks. Prevention of infective endocarditis in the susceptible child with CHD or a valvular disorder is of the utmost importance (Brusch & Bronze, 2015; Darst et al., 2014).

Nursing Assessment

For a full description of the assessment phase of the nursing process, see earlier in the chapter. Assessment findings related to endocarditis are discussed below.

Health History

Obtain the health history, noting intermittent, unexplained low-grade fever. Document history of fatigue, anorexia, weight loss, or flu-like symptoms (e.g., arthralgia, myalgia, chills, night sweats). Note history of CHD, valve disorder, or heart failure.

Physical Examination

Measure the child's temperature, noting low-grade fever. Observe for edema if heart failure is also present. Note petechiae on the palpebral conjunctiva, the oral mucosa, or the extremities. Inspect for signs of extracardiac emboli:
- Roth spots: splinter hemorrhages with pale centres on sclerae, palate, buccal mucosa, chest, fingers, or toes
- Janeway lesions: painless, flat, red or blue hemorrhagic lesions on the palms or the soles
- Osler nodes: small, tender nodules on the pads of the toes or fingers
- Black lines (splinter hemorrhages) under the nails (Brusch & Bronze, 2015; Darst et al., 2014)

Evaluate the ECG for a prolonged PR interval or dysrhythmias. Auscultate the heart for a new or changing murmur. Auscultate the lungs for adventitious breath sounds. Palpate the abdomen for splenomegaly.

Laboratory and Diagnostic Tests

Diagnosis is usually based on the clinical presentation. Laboratory tests may reveal:

- Blood culture: bacteria or fungus
- CBC count: anemia, leukocytosis
- Urinalysis: microscopic hematuria
- Echocardiogram: cardiomegaly, abnormal valve function, area of vegetation

Nursing Management

Nursing management focuses on maintaining IV access for at least 4 weeks to appropriately administer the antibiotic or antifungal course of therapy. Monitor the child's temperature and subsequent blood culture results.

Ideally, infective endocarditis in children should be prevented. Children at increased risk for the development of infective endocarditis include those with:
- Prosthetic cardiac valve or prosthetic material used for cardiac valve repair
- Previous endocarditis
- Unrepaired cyanotic CHD
- Completely repaired congenital heart defect with prosthetic material or device within the first 6 months after the procedure
- Repaired CHD with residual defects at the site or adjacent to the site of a prosthetic patch or prosthetic device
- Cardiac transplantation recipients who develop cardiac valve abnormalities (Brusch & Bronze, 2015)

Children at high risk should practice good oral hygiene, including regular tooth brushing and flossing. Instruct parents or the older child to carry emergency medical identification at all times. Advise parents to use a health App on their cell phone. Instruct the parents to notify the primary care provider or cardiologist if the child develops flu-like symptoms or a fever.

High-risk children (as noted above) who are undergoing dental procedures should receive prophylaxis. Antibiotics typically used for prophylaxis may include ampicillin, amoxicillin, gentamicin, or vancomycin.

ACUTE RHEUMATIC FEVER

Acute rheumatic fever (ARF) is a delayed sequela of group A streptococcal pharyngeal infection. In Canada there have been reports of ARF incidence at 21.3% per 100,000 which is 75 times greater than overall Canadian figures. These reports from Ontario were from populations with poor social determinants of health, namely Indigenous communities (Gordon et al., 2015). ARF occurs most often in school-age children between 5 and 15 years of age in areas where streptococcal pharyngitis is more prevalent, especially during the colder months. It usually develops 2 to 4 weeks after the initial streptococcal infection. Current understanding of the disease process of ARF is that the child develops an antibody response to surface proteins of the bacteria. The antibodies then

---

BOX 41.3

**MODIFIED JONES CRITERIA
(AMERICAN HEART ASSOCIATION)**

Diagnosis of acute rheumatic fever requires the presence of either two major criteria or one major plus two minor criteria.

Major Criteria

- Carditis
- Migratory polyarthritis
- Subcutaneous nodules
- Erythema marginatum
- Sydenham chorea

Minor Criteria

- Arthralgia
- Fever
- Elevated erythrocyte sedimentation rate or C-reactive protein
- Prolonged PR interval

Adapted from Darst, J. R., Collins, K. K., & Miyamoto, S. D. (2014). Cardiovascular diseases. In W. W. Hay, M. J. Levin, R. R. Deterding, & M. J. Abzug (Eds.). *Current pediatric diagnosis and treatment* (22nd ed.). New York: McGraw-Hill.

cross-react with antigens in cardiac muscle and neuronal and synovial tissues, causing carditis, arthritis, and chorea (involuntary random, jerking movements). ARF affects the joints, central nervous system, skin, and subcutaneous tissue and causes chronic, progressive damage to the heart and valves. Most attacks of ARF last 6 to 12 weeks and then are resolved, but rheumatic fever may recur with subsequent streptococcal infections (Gibofsky, 2015).

Diagnosis of ARF is based on the modified Jones criteria (Box 41.3). Therapeutic management is directed toward managing inflammation and fever, eradicating the bacteria, preventing permanent heart damage, and preventing recurrences. A full 10-day course of penicillin therapy (or equivalent) is used along with corticosteroids and NSAIDs. Children without valvular disease will receive continued prophylaxis with monthly intramuscular injections of penicillin G benzathine or daily oral doses of penicillin or erythromycin following the initial illness in order to prevent a new streptococcal infection and recurrent ARF. Prophylaxis is continued until adulthood (Gibofsky, 2015).

Nursing Assessment

Elicit a description of the present illness and chief complaint, noting fever and joint pain. Explore the child's recent medical history for risk factors such as documented streptococcal infection or sore throat within the past 2 to 3 weeks, or for past history of ARF. Observe the child for Sydenham chorea, a movement disorder of the face and upper extremities. Inspect the skin for evidence of the classic rash, erythema marginatum, a maculopapular red rash with central clearing and elevated edges. Auscultate the heart, noting a murmur. Palpate the surfaces of the wrist, elbows, and knees for firm, painless, subcutaneous nodules. Note prolonged PR interval on the ECG. Throat culture will provide definitive diagnosis of current streptococcal infection, while streptococcal antibody tests may yield evidence of recent infection. Echocardiogram is required to determine if carditis is present.

Nursing Management

Nursing management of the child with ARF focuses on ensuring compliance with the acute course of antibiotics as well as prophylaxis following initial recovery from ARF. Allow the child to verbalize the frustration he or she may be feeling in relation to chorea symptoms. Offer support for dealing with the abnormal movements. Educate the child and others that the sudden jerky movements of chorea will eventually disappear, though they may last as long as several months. Some children may require a neuroleptic agent such as haloperidol (Haldol) for management of chorea. Administer corticosteroids or nonsteroidal anti-inflammatory agents for control of joint pain and swelling.

CARDIOMYOPATHY

Cardiomyopathy is a condition in which the myocardium cannot contract properly. Cardiomyopathy may occur in children with genetic disorders or congenital heart defects, as a result of an inflammatory or infectious process or hypertension, or after cardiac transplantation or surgery, but most commonly it is idiopathic. Cardiomyopathy occurs predominately in clusters in infancy and adolescence. Three types of cardiomyopathy exist—restrictive, dilated, and hypertrophic. Restrictive cardiomyopathy is rare in children and results in atrial relaxation. Dilated cardiomyopathy is the most common type in childhood and may result in heart failure because of ventricular dilatation with decreased contractility (Kantor, Abraham, Dipchand, Benson, & Redington, 2010). There is some familial tendency toward dilated cardiomyopathy, and it is also associated with Duchenne and Becker muscular dystrophy (Marian et al., 2011). Children with dilated cardiomyopathy may present with heart failure (Kantor et al., 2010). Hypertrophic cardiomyopathy is more common in adolescence and results in hypertrophy of the heart muscle, particularly the left ventricle, affecting the heart's ability to fill. About two thirds of all cases of hypertrophic cardiomyopathy are familial, with some inherited in an autosomal dominant fashion (Marian et al., 2011).

There is no cure for cardiomyopathy, meaning that, currently, heart muscle function cannot be restored. Therapeutic management is directed toward improving heart function and BP. Mechanical ventilation and vasoactive medications are needed in many children. ACE inhibitors, beta blockers, or calcium channel blockers may be used. Pacemakers or surgery is helpful in some children. For severely affected children, heart transplantation is the only viable long-term treatment option (Kantor et al., 2010).

Nursing Assessment

Explore the health history for risk factors such as:
- Congenital heart defect, cardiac transplantation, or surgery
- Duchenne or Becker muscular dystrophy
- History of myocarditis, HIV infection, or Kawasaki disease
- Hypertension
- Drugs, alcohol, or radiation exposure
- Connective tissue, autoimmune, or endocrine disease
- Maternal diabetes
- Familial history of sudden death

Inquire about a history of respiratory distress, fatigue, poor growth (dilated), chest pain, dizziness, or syncope (hypertrophic). Observe the child for extremity edema and abdominal distention. Note increased work of breathing. Auscultate the heart, noting tachycardia and irregular rhythm. Evaluate heart rhythm via ECG, noting dysrhythmias or indications of left ventricular hypertrophy.

Chest radiography may reveal cardiomegaly or congested lungs. Echocardiogram demonstrates increased heart size, poor contractility, decreased ejection fraction, or asymmetric septal hypertrophy. Cardiac catheterization is usually performed to aid in the diagnosis.

Nursing Management

Many children with cardiomyopathy require intensive care initially. Monitor for complications such as blood clots or arrhythmias, which could lead to cardiac arrest. Refer to the previous section on heart failure for nursing interventions related to heart failure, which may be present with dilated cardiomyopathy. Administer vasoactive and other medications as prescribed, monitoring the child closely for response to these therapies as well as for complications. Support the child in choosing activities that fit within the prescribed restrictions. Provide extensive emotional support to the child and family, who may experience significant stress as they realize the severity of this illness.

HYPERTENSION

Hypertension has seen a rise in prevalence among children and adolescents. It has been found to be independently associated with body mass index and waist circumference. Childhood/adolescent hypertension often leads to long-term health consequences such as cardiovascular disease and left ventricular hypertrophy (Mattoo, 2016a). In children, acceptable BP values are based on gender, age, and height. Hypertension is defined as BP persistently greater than the 95th percentile for gender, age, and height. Prehypertension refers to BP that is persistently between the 90th and 95th percentiles. BP is considered normal when the systolic and diastolic values are less than the 90th percentile for gender, age, and height (Mattoo, 2016a).

Childhood hypertension may be further defined as primary or secondary. Primary hypertension in children is found more commonly in postpubertal children, African Americans, and children who are overweight or obese (Mattoo, 2016a). Secondary hypertension in children most frequently occurs with an underlying medical problem such as renal or cardiac disease (Mattoo, 2016a). Mild to moderate hypertension in childhood is usually asymptomatic and usually is determined only upon BP screening during a well-child visit or during follow-up for known risk factors. Refer to Table 31.5 in Chapter 31, for a synopsis of childhood hypertension guidelines.

It is important to screen for and treat prehypertension and hypertension in children and adolescents, as they are more likely to experience hypertension as adults progressing to further cardiovascular disease (Mattoo, 2016b). Therapeutic management depends on the extent of the hypertension and the length of time it has existed. Weight reduction, appropriate diet (including sodium restriction in some children), and increased physical activity are important components of management of prehypertensive and asymptomatic hypertensive children. Some children are candidates for, and require, antihypertensive medications or diuretics (Mattoo, 2016b).

Pathophysiology

The balance between cardiac output and vascular resistance determines the BP. An increase in either of these variables, in the absence of a compensatory decrease in the other, increases the mean BP. Factors regulating cardiac output and vascular resistance include changes in electrolyte balance, particularly sodium, calcium, and potassium.

Nursing Assessment

Nursing assessment consists of the health history, physical examination, and laboratory and diagnostic tests.

Health History

Elicit the health history, determining the presence of risk factors for hypertension such as:
- Family history
- History of sleep apnea
- Obesity
- Hyperlipidemia
- Renal disease (including frequent urinary tract infections)
- Systemic lupus erythematosus
- CHD
- Neurofibromatosis, Turner syndrome, and other genetic disorders
- Prematurity
- Prolonged neonatal ventilation
- Umbilical artery catheterization
- Diabetes mellitus
- Increased intracranial pressure
- Malignancy
- Solid organ transplant
- Medications known to raise BP

Signs and symptoms reported during the health history might include:
- Growth retardation (with certain chronic medical conditions)
- Obesity
- Signs and symptoms seen particularly in older children
- Headache
- Subtle behavioural or school performance changes
- Fatigue
- Blurred vision
- Nosebleed
- Bell palsy

Physical Examination

Determine the child's weight and height/length. Plot these growth parameters on the gender-appropriate chart for the child's age. Note the percentile for height/length, as it will be used to determine the BP percentile (see Appendix F: Blood Pressure Charts for Children and Adolescents). Measure the BP in all four extremities (to rule out coarctation of the aorta). Ensure that the child is relaxed and sitting or reclined. Refer to Chapter 32 for specific information related to accurate BP measurement in children.

Inspect the skin for:
- Acne, hirsutism, or striae (associated with anabolic steroid use)
- Café-au-lait spots (associated with neurofibromatosis)
- Malar rash (associated with lupus)
- Pallor, diaphoresis, or flushing (associated with pheochromocytoma)

Observe the extremities for edema (renal disease) or joint swelling (lupus). Inspect the chest for apical heave (ventricular hypertrophy) or wide-spaced nipples (Turner syndrome). Auscultate heart sounds, noting tachycardia (associated with primary hypertension) or murmur (associated with coarctation of the aorta). Palpate the abdomen for a mass or enlarged kidney.

Laboratory and Diagnostic Testing

Though diagnosis of hypertension is based on BP measurements, additional laboratory or diagnostic tests may be used to evaluate the underlying cause of secondary hypertension, including:
- Urinalysis, blood urea nitrogen, and serum creatinine: may determine the presence of renal disease
- Renal ultrasound or angiography: may reveal kidney or genitourinary tract abnormalities
- Echocardiogram: may show left ventricular hypertrophy
- Lipid profile: determines the presence of hyperlipidemia

Nursing Management

Salt restriction and potassium or calcium supplements have not been scientifically shown to decrease BP in children. However, obese children may benefit from salt restriction, as those children seem to be sensitive to salt intake. Assist the child and family to develop a plan for weight reduction if the child is overweight or obese. Encourage the child and family to control portion sizes, decrease the intake of sugary beverages and snacks, eat more fresh fruits and vegetables, eat a healthy breakfast, and consume more home-cooked meals. Consult the nutritionist for additional assistance with meal planning. To increase physical activity, encourage the child to find a sport or type of exercise in which he or she is interested. Aerobic activities involving running, walking, or cycling are particularly helpful. When a child requires antihypertensive therapy, teach the child and family how to administer the medication. Caution the parents about side effects related to antihypertensives. Teach the parent to measure the child's BP as determined by the physician or nurse practitioner, as well as to keep appointments for BP follow-up.

KAWASAKI DISEASE

Kawasaki disease is an acute systemic vasculitis occurring mostly in children 6 months to 5 years of age. It is the leading cause of acquired heart disease among children and occurs more often in the winter and summer, affecting 20 per 100,000 children (Sundel, 2016b). Although Kawasaki disease affects all ethnic groups, it occurs more frequently in those of Asian or Pacific descent. It is a self-limited syndrome but can cause cardiovascular complications such as coronary artery aneurysm and cardiomyopathy, among others (Sundel, 2016a).

Therapeutic management of acute Kawasaki disease focuses on reducing inflammation in the walls of the coronary arteries and preventing coronary thrombosis. Chronic management of children developing aneurysms during the initial phase is directed toward preventing myocardial ischemia. In the acute phase, high-dose aspirin in four divided doses daily and a single infusion of intravenous immunoglobulin (IVIG) are used. It appears that the best response occurs if IVIG is given within the first 7 to 10 days of the illness (Sundel, 2016c).

Pathophysiology

Though the etiology is still unknown, current thought is that some infectious organism (as yet unidentified) causes disease in genetically susceptible people. Kawasaki disease appears to be an autoimmune response mediated by cytokine-induced endothelial cell surface antigens that leads to vasculitis. Neutrophils, followed by mononuclear cells, T lymphocytes, and immunoglobulin A–producing plasma cells, infiltrate the vessels. Then elastin and collagen fibres' fragment and the structural integrity of the vessel wall are impaired. Generalized systemic vasculitis occurs in the blood vessels throughout the body due to the inflammation and edema and can lead to coronary dilatation or aneurysm. Some children never develop coronary artery changes, while others develop an aneurysm in either the acute phase or as a long-term sequela (Sundel, 2016a).

Nursing Assessment

Nursing assessment consists of determining the health history, physical examination, and laboratory and diagnostic testing.

Health History

Elicit the health history, noting any of the following:
- Fever
- Chills
- Headache
- Malaise
- Extreme irritability
- Vomiting
- Diarrhea
- Abdominal pain
- Joint pain

Of particular note is a history of high fever (39.9°C) of at least 5 days' duration that is unresponsive to antibiotics.

Physical Examination

Observe for significant bilateral conjunctivitis without exudate. Inspect the mouth and throat for dry, fissured lips; strawberry (cracked and reddened) tongue; and pharyngeal and oral mucosa erythema. Note hyperdynamic precordium. Evaluate the skin for:
- Diffuse, erythematous, polymorphous rash
- Edema of the hands and feet
- Erythema and painful induration of the palms and soles
- Desquamation (peeling) of the perineal region, fingers, and toes, extending to the palms and soles
- Possible jaundice

Palpate the neck for cervical lymphadenopathy (usually unilateral) and the joints for tenderness. Palpate the abdomen for liver enlargement. Auscultate the heart, noting tachycardia, gallop, or murmur.

Laboratory and Diagnostic Testing

The CBC count may reveal mild to moderate anemia, an elevated white blood cell count during the acute phase, and significant thrombocytosis (elevated platelet count [500,000 to 1 million]) in the later phase. The erythrocyte sedimentation rate (ESR) and the C-reactive protein (CRP) level are elevated. Echocardiogram is performed as soon as possible after the diagnosis is confirmed to provide a baseline of a healthy heart or to evaluate for coronary artery involvement. Echocardiograms may be repeated during the illness and as part of long-term follow-up. Occasionally cardiac involvement warrants cardiac catheterization.

Nursing Management

In addition to the administration of aspirin and immunoglobulin, nursing management of the child with Kawasaki disease focuses on monitoring cardiac status, promoting comfort, and providing family education.

Monitoring Cardiac Status

Administer intravenous and oral fluids as ordered, evaluating intake and output carefully. Prepare the child for the echocardiogram. Assess frequently for signs of developing heart failure such as tachycardia, gallop, decreased urine output, or respiratory distress. Evaluate quality and strength of pulses. Provide cardiac monitoring as ordered, reporting arrhythmias.

Promoting Comfort

Provide acetaminophen for fever management and apply cool cloths as tolerated. Keep the environment quiet and cluster nursing care activities to decrease stimulation and hence irritability. Teach parents that irritability is a prominent feature of Kawasaki disease, and support their efforts to console the child. Apply petrolatum jelly or another lubricating ointment to the lips. Encourage the older child to suck on ice chips; the younger child may suck on a cool, moist washcloth. Popsicles are also soothing. Provide comfortable positioning, particularly if the child has joint pain or arthritis.

Providing Child and Family Education

Teach parents to continue to monitor the child's temperature after discharge until the child has been afebrile for several days. Children with prolonged or recurrent fever may require a second dose of IVIG. Inform parents that irritability may last for up to 2 months after initial diagnosis with Kawasaki disease. Report any toxic effects of aspirin therapy, such as headache, confusion, dizziness, or tinnitus to the physician or nurse practitioner. It is important to avoid nonsteroidal anti-inflammatory agents while aspirin therapy is ongoing. For children with continued arthritis (which resolves in several weeks), range-of-motion exercises with a morning bath may help to decrease stiffness. Instruct parents to avoid measles and varicella vaccination for 11 months after high-dose IVIG administration. It is critical that the family comply with regularly scheduled cardiology follow-up appointments to determine development or progression of coronary artery ectasia or aneurysm. If the child has severe cardiac involvement, teach the parents about infant and/or child cardiopulmonary resuscitation before discharge from the hospital.

HYPERLIPIDEMIA

Hyperlipidemia refers to high levels of lipids (fats/cholesterol) in the blood. High lipid levels are a risk factor for the development of atherosclerosis, which can result in coronary artery disease, a serious cardiovascular disorder occurring in adults. Children with high lipid levels, though remaining asymptomatic, are likely to have high levels as adults, which increases their risk for coronary artery disease. Therefore, detection, screening, and early intervention are important, especially if there is a family tendency toward heart disease (Schuman, 2013).

Pathophysiology

Cholesterol is a building block for hormones and cell membranes. It occurs naturally in foods derived from animals such as eggs, dairy products, meat, poultry, and seafood. Cholesterol is also manufactured in the body. Together, cholesterol and triglycerides are known as lipids. Very low–density lipoprotein (VLDL) is a lipoprotein composed mainly of triglycerides with only small amounts of cholesterol, phospholipid, and protein. VLDLs are easily converted to low-density lipoproteins (LDLs). Cholesterol is expressed in terms of LDL cholesterol or high-density lipoprotein (HDL) cholesterol. LDLs

contain relatively more cholesterol and triglycerides than they do protein. HDLs contain about 50% protein, with the rest being cholesterol, triglyceride, and phospholipid. High levels of cholesterol and triglycerides place a person at risk for atherosclerosis. Elevated VLDL and LDL levels and decreased HDL levels produce a particular increase in the risk for atherosclerosis (Darst et al., 2014).

Therapeutic Management

Screening children for hyperlipidemia is of prime importance for early detection, intervention, and subsequent prevention of adult atherosclerosis. The Greig Health Record recommends screening overweight or obese children over 10 years for fasting plasma glucose and a lipid profile (Canadian Paediatric Society, 2016). Selectively screening of children at high risk for hyperlipidemia can reduce their lifelong risk of coronary artery disease with further information being found from the Bright Futures Guidelines at the Point. The risk assessment focuses on the child's family history. Screen if parents, grandparents, aunts and uncles, or siblings, have or have had documented:
- Coronary atherosclerosis
- Myocardial infarction
- Angina pectoris
- Peripheral vascular disease
- Cerebrovascular disease/stroke
- Coronary artery bypass graft/stent/angioplasty at less than 55 years of age in males and less than 65 years in females
- Sudden cardiac death
- Blood cholesterol level of 240 mg/dL or higher

The child should be screened at the health care provider's discretion if the parental history is unobtainable, the child has diabetes or hypertension, or if the child has any lifestyle risk factors (cigarette smoking, obesity, sedentary lifestyle, or high-fat dietary intake) (National Heart, Lung, and Blood Institute, 2012).

All children should eat a diet with the appropriate amount of fats (see the section on nursing management below) and should participate in physical activity. When diet and exercise are not enough to lower cholesterol to appropriate levels, medications such as resins, fibric acid derivatives, statins, or niacin may be used (Gauthier et al., 2009; Schuman, 2013).

Nursing Assessment

Elicit the health history, noting risk factors such as family history of hyperlipidemia, early heart disease, hypertension, diabetes or other endocrine abnormality, cerebral vascular accident, or sudden death. Note prior lipid levels if available. Measure the child's height and weight, plotting them on standardized growth charts. Note if the child is overweight or obese, as these are risk factors associated with hyperlipidemia. Typically, there are no

TABLE 41.3	INTERPRETATION OF CHOLESTEROL LEVELS FOR CHILDREN AGE 2–19 YEARS		
Total Cholesterol (mg/dL)	LDL (mg/dL)	Interpretation	
<170	<110	Acceptable	
170–199	100–129	Borderline	
≥200	≥130	Elevated	

Adapted from National Heart, Lung, and Blood Institute. (2012). *Expert Panel on Integrated Guidelines for Cardiovascular Health and Risk Reduction in Children and Adolescents.* SUMMARY REPORT (NIH Publication No. 12–7486). Washington, DC: U.S. Department of Health and Human Services.

other particular physical findings associated with hyperlipidemia. Table 41.3 gives details about the interpretation of cholesterol levels.

Nursing Management

Instruct families that the child must fast for 12 hours before lipid screening (initially and on follow-up samples). Dietary management is the first step in the prevention and management of hyperlipidemia in children older than 2 years of age. The diet should consist primarily of fruits, vegetables, low-fat dairy products, whole grains, beans, lean meat, poultry, and fish. As in adults, fat should account for no more than 30% of daily caloric intake. Fat intake may vary over a period of days, as many young children are picky eaters. Limit saturated fats by choosing lean meats, removing skin from poultry before cooking, and avoiding palm, palm kernel, and coconut oils as well as hydrogenated fats. Teach families to read nutrition labels to determine the content of the food. Limit intake of processed or refined foods as well as high-sugar drinks; these products provide minimal nutrition and significant calories. Refer parents to Canada Food guide for information. Developmentally appropriate physical activity is recommended and the Canadian Paediatric Society (2012) offers recommendations linked to age.

If medications are required, teach the child and family about the dose, administration, and possible adverse effects. Assist the family to develop a medication-dosing plan that is compatible with school and work schedules to increase compliance.

HEART TRANSPLANTATION

Heart transplantation is indicated in children with end-stage heart disease related to cardiomyopathy or inoperable CHD. Over 500 children receive a heart transplant each year (Chinnock & Ohye, 2014). The 1-year survival rate is 80% to 90%, 5-year survival rate is 70% to 80%, and although 20-year survival has been achieved, many children require a second transplantation (Chinnock & Ohye, 2014). While awaiting transplantation, about 30% of young infants and 20% of children over 6 months of age die (Lankin, 2012).

A comprehensive evaluation is performed to determine whether the child is a candidate for heart transplant. The evaluation includes:
- Chest x-ray, ECG, echocardiogram, exercise stress test, cardiac catheterization, and pulmonary function tests
- CBC count with differential, prothrombin and partial thromboplastin time, serum chemistries and electrolytes, blood urea nitrogen, and creatinine
- Urinalysis and urine creatinine clearance
- Blood, throat, urine, stool, and sputum cultures for bacteria, viruses, fungi, and parasites
- Epstein–Barr virus, cytomegalovirus, varicella, herpes, hepatitis, and HIV titers
- HLA typing and panel reactive antibody typing and titer
- Computed tomography or MRI scan and electroencephalogram
- Consults with neurology, psychology, genetics, social work, nutritionist, physical and occupational therapy, and financial coordinator or case manager (Dipchand, Bastardi, & Dupuis, 2013)

Children with irreversible lung, liver, kidney, or central nervous system disease; recent malignancy (past 5 years); or chronic viral infection may be excluded as candidates.

Once candidacy is determined, the transplant centre registers the child as a potential recipient with the particular province's organ transplant centre. Blood type, body size, length of time on the waiting list, and medical urgency are used to evaluate compatibility. Children awaiting transplantation may need continuous or intermittent hospitalization. Coordination of organ procurement and the transplantation procedure is essential.

Surgical Procedure and Postoperative Therapeutic Management

Most transplantation procedures are **orthotopic**, which means that the recipient's heart is removed and the donor heart is implanted in its place in the normal anatomic position. Cardiopulmonary bypass and hypothermia are used to maintain circulation, protect the brain, and oxygenate the recipient during the procedure. Postoperatively, the child may have near-normal heart function and capacity for exercise and may be able to return to school.

Immunosuppressive therapy is necessary for the rest of the child's life to avoid rejection of the transplanted heart. Usually a three-drug regimen is used that includes calcineurin inhibitors (cyclosporine, tacrolimus), cell

Overview for the Child With a Cardiovascular Disorder (continued)

NURSING DIAGNOSIS: Ineffective peripheral tissue perfusion, related to inadequate cardiac function or cardiac surgery as evidenced by pallor, cyanosis, edema, changes in mental status, prolonged capillary refill, clubbing, or diminished pulses

Outcome Identification and Evaluation

Child will demonstrate adequate tissue perfusion: child will be alert, not restless or lethargic, will have pink colour, decrease in edema, normal perfusion, and strong pulses.

Interventions: *Promoting Tissue Perfusion*

- Assess level of consciousness, pulse, BP, peripheral perfusion, and skin colour frequently *to determine baseline and ongoing improvement.*
- Administer cardiac glycosides or vasodilators as ordered *to promote cardiac output necessary for proper perfusion.*
- Monitor pulse oximetry and arterial blood gas results *to assess ability to appropriately oxygenate.*
- Supplement oxygen as needed *to provide oxygen to organs for proper functioning.*

- Monitor hemoglobin and hematocrit *to identify blood loss.*
- Strictly assess intake and output *to determine adequacy of renal perfusion.*
- Position with head of bed elevated *to decrease blood volume returning to heart.*
- Change position every 2 to 4 hours *to promote circulation and avoid skin breakdown in areas of poor perfusion.*

NURSING DIAGNOSIS: Risk for delayed development related to effects of cardiac disease and necessary treatments, inadequate nutrition, or frequent separation from caregivers secondary to illness

Outcome Identification and Evaluation

Child will display development appropriate for age: will display evidence of cognitive and motor function within normal limits (individualized for each child).

Interventions: *Promoting Appropriate Development*

- Promote adequate caloric intake to stimulate growth and provide adequate energy.
- Provide age-appropriate developmental activities to stimulate development.
- Consult with the physical or occupational therapist or child life specialist to determine activities most appropriate for the child within the constraints of the child's illness.

- Schedule daily activities to allow for essential rest periods for energy conservation.
- Encourage parents, teachers, and playmates to be sensitive to child's self-image, using positive comments, to improve the child's self-concept.
- As energy allows, encourage participation in all activities as feasible to allow the child to feel normal.

NURSING DIAGNOSIS: Risk for infection related to need for multiple invasive procedures or cardiac surgery

Outcome Identification and Evaluation

Child will remain free from infection: vital signs will be within normal limits, white blood cell count normal, and cultures negative. Child will exhibit no signs or symptoms of infection.

NURSING CARE PLAN 41.1

Overview for the Child With a Cardiovascular Disorder (continued)

Interventions: *Preventing Infection*

- Maintain strict hand hygiene to prevent spread of infectious organisms to the child.
- Assess temperature to detect elevation early in course of infection.
- Avoid contact with persons with known infections to prevent risk of becoming ill.
- Ensure appropriate immunization, including pneumococcal and influenza vaccinations, to prevent development of common childhood illness. Influenza vaccination is recommended for all children greater than 6 months with chronic health issues such as cardiac disorders.
- Administer prophylactic antibiotics prior to all dental procedures, surgery, and many invasive procedures to prevent subacute bacterial endocarditis.
- Encourage good dental hygiene to reduce the risk of endocarditis.

NURSING DIAGNOSIS: Interrupted family processes related to crisis associated with heart disease, frequent need for testing and hospitalizations, or stresses associated with care demands, as evidenced by inadequate parental coping, frequent separations of parent and child, or inadequate support

Outcome Identification and Evaluation

Family will maintain functional system of support and will demonstrate adequate coping, adaptation of roles and functions, and decreased anxiety: *parents are involved in child's care, ask appropriate questions, express fears and concerns, and can discuss child's care and condition calmly.*

Interventions: *Promoting Family Processes*

- Provide ongoing support to the child and family *to help them cope.*
- Encourage parents and family members to verbalize concerns related to child's illness, diagnosis, and prognosis: *allows the nurse to identify concerns and areas where further education may be needed and demonstrates family-centred care.*
- Allow families to grieve over the loss of a "perfect" child: *parents must work through those grief feelings so they can be fully "present" for this chronically ill child.*
- Explain therapies, procedures, child's behaviours, and plan of care to parents: *understanding the child's current status and plan of care helps decrease anxiety.*
- Encourage parents to be involved in care: *allows parents to feel needed and valued and gives them a sense of control over their child's health.*
- Identify support system for family and child: *helps nurse identify needs and resources available for coping.*
- Educate family and child on additional resources available *to help them develop a wide base of support.*
- Encourage parents to seek genetic counselling *to provide them with the information required to make an informed decision about having another child.*

NURSING DIAGNOSIS: Activity intolerance related to ineffective cardiac muscle function, increased energy expenditure, or inability to meet increased oxygen or metabolic demands as evidenced by squatting positions, shortness of breath, cyanosis, or fatigue

Outcome Identification and Evaluation

Child will increase activity level as tolerated: child participates in play and activities (specify particular activities and level as individualized for each child).

(continued)

NURSING CARE PLAN 41.1

Overview for the Child With a Cardiovascular Disorder (continued)

Interventions: *Promoting Activity*

- Assess level of fatigue and activity tolerance *to determine baseline for comparison.*
- Note extent of dyspnea, oxygen requirement, or colour change with exertion *to provide baseline for comparison.*
- Cluster care activities, allowing rest periods in between, *to conserve child's energy.*
- Work with the parent and child to determine a mutually satisfactory daily schedule *to allow adequate rest and energy conservation.*

- Instruct family and child in prescribed activity restrictions *to prevent fatigue while allowing some activity.*
- In the infant, avoid long periods of crying or prolonged nipple feeding: *expends excessive calories.*
- Provide neutral thermal environment *to avoid increased oxygen and energy needs associated with excessive heat or cold.*

KEY CONCEPTS

- ○ At birth, when the umbilical cord is cut and the neonate's first breath occurs, the ductus venosus closes with the foramen ovale and the ductus arteriosus closes shortly thereafter. Pulmonary vascular resistance decreases and systemic vascular resistance increases.

- ○ The infant's heart rate averages 120 to 130 bpm and decreases throughout childhood, reaching the adult rate in adolescence. Conversely, the infant's and child's BP is significantly lower than the adult's, increasing as the child ages.

- ○ Check the infant's apical pulse prior to digoxin administration and hold the dose if the heart rate is less than 90.

- ○ Poor weight gain, failure to thrive, and increased fatigability commonly occur with congestive heart failure.

- ○ Clubbing of the fingernails occurs as a result of chronic hypoxia in the child with severe CHD.

- ○ Children with cardiac conditions resulting in cyanosis often have baseline oxygen saturations that are relatively low, because of the mixing of oxygenated with deoxygenated blood.

- ○ Document the presence of a murmur by grading its intensity (I through IV), describing where it occurs within the cardiac cycle, and noting the location where the murmur is best heard.

- ○ CHD should be suspected in the cyanotic newborn who does not improve with oxygen administration.

- ○ Cardiac catheterization postprocedure care focuses on evaluation of the child's vital signs and condition of the pressure dressing, as well as assessment of the distal pulses bilaterally for presence and quality.

- ○ Congenital heart disorders resulting in decreased pulmonary blood flow (TOF, tricuspid atresia) result in cyanosis.

- ○ Disorders with increased pulmonary blood flow (PDA, ASD, and VSD) may result in pulmonary edema if the defect is severe.

- ○ A decrease in the lower extremity pulses or BP as compared with the upper extremities may be indicative of coarctation of the aorta.

- ○ It is important to remain calm when an infant or child demonstrates a hypercyanotic spell. Place the child in a knee-chest position, administer oxygen and/or morphine or propranolol, and supply intravenous fluids.

- ○ Children with certain congenital heart defects and/ or heart failure require additional calories in order to display adequate growth.

- ○ Children with hypertrophic cardiomyopathy, certain congenital heart defects, valve dysfunction, or prosthetic valves require prophylaxis for infective endocarditis when undergoing procedures or invasive dental work.

- ○ Hypertension in the child or adolescent often leads to long-term health consequences such as cardiovascular disease and left ventricular hypertrophy.

- Kawasaki disease may result in severe cardiac sequelae, so these children need ongoing cardiac follow-up to screen for development of problems.

- It is important to screen for hyperlipidemia in high-risk children.

- Abrupt cessation of chest tube output, accompanied by an increase in the heart rate and increased filling pressure, may indicate cardiac tamponade.

REFERENCES AND RECOMMENDED READINGS

Abdallah, H. (2016). *About the Children's Heart Institute.* Retrieved from www.childrenheartinstitute.org/testing/testhome.htm.

Abdoulhosn, J. A., & Child, J. S. (2011). Congenital heart disease in adults. In V. Fuster, R. A. Walsh, & R. A. Harrington (Eds.). *Hurst's the heart* (13th ed.). New York: McGraw Hill Companies, Inc.

AGA Medical Corporation. (2014). *Amplatzer™ muscular VSD occluder: Instructions for use.* Plymouth, MN: Author.

Altman, C. A. (2015). *Identifying newborns with critical congenital heart disease.* Retrieved from www.uptodate.com/contents/identifying-newborns-with-critical-congenital-heart-disease.

Canadian Congenital Heart Alliance. (2017). *CHD Information* Retrieved from https://www.cchaforlife.org/about-us

Bacha, E. A., Cooper, D., Thiagarajan, R., Franklin, R. C., Krogmann, O., Deal, B., . . . Colan, S. D. (2008). Cardiac complications associated with the treatment of patients with congenital cardiac disease: Consensus definitions from the Multi-Societal Database Committee for Pediatric and Congenital Heart Disease. *Cardiology in the Young, 18*(Suppl 2), 196–201.

Baltimore, R., Gewitz, M., Baddour, L. M., Beerman, L. B., Jackson, M. A., Lockhart, P. B., . . . Willoughby, R. (2015). Infective endocarditis in childhood: 2015 Update. *Circulation, 132*(15), 1487–1515.

Bass, J. L., Corwin, M., Gozal, D., Moore, C., Nishida, H., Parker, S., . . . Kinane, T. B. (2004). The effect of chronic or intermittent hypoxia on cognition in childhood: A review of the evidence. *Pediatrics, 114*(3), 805–816.

BC Children's Hospital. (2015). *Post cardiac catheterization procedure (Including diagnostic and interventional catherizations).* Retrieved from http://policyandorders.cw.bc.ca/resource-gallery/Documents/BC%20Children's%20Hospital/RCP_cardiac_catheterization_Revised_Jan_12_2015.pdf.

Beke, D. M., Braudis, N. J., & Lincoln, P. (2005). Management of the pediatric postoperative cardiac surgery patient. *Critical Care Nursing Clinics of North America, 17*(4), 405–416.

Brown, D. W., & Fulton, D. R. (2011). Congenital heart disease in children and adolescents. In V. Fuster, R. A. Walsh, & R. A. Harrington (Eds.). *Hurst's the heart* (13th ed.). New York: McGraw-Hill Companies, Inc.

Brusch, J. L., & Bronze, M. S. (2015). *Infective endocarditis.* Retrieved from http://emedicine.medscape.com/article/216650-overview.

Canadian Congenital Heart Alliance. (2016). *Facts and issues.* Retrieved from: www.cchaforlife.org.

Canadian Paediatric Society. (2012). *Health active living: Physical activity guideline for children and adolescents.* Retrieved from http://www.cps.ca/documents/position/physical-activity-guidelines.

Canadian Paediatric Society. (2016). *Greig Health Record.* Retrieved from https://www.cps.ca/en/tools-outils/greig-health-record

CPS: Caring for Kids. (2012). *Handwashing for parents and children.* Retrieved from http://www.caringforkids.cps.ca/handouts/handwashing.

CPS: Caring for Kids. (2013). *Healthy teeth for children.* Retrieved from http://www.caringforkids.cps.ca/handouts/healthy_teeth_for_children.

Carpenito-Moyet, L. J. (2013). *Nursing diagnosis: Application to clinical practice* (14th ed.). Philadelphia, PA: Lippincott Williams & Wilkins.

Cassidy, S. C., Allen, H. D., & Phillips, J. R. (2013). History and physical examination. In H. D. Allen, D. J. Driscoll, R. E. Shaddy, & T. F. Feltes (Eds.). *Moss and Adams' heart disease in infants, children, and adolescents. Including the fetus and young adult.* Philadelphia, PA: Lippincott Williams & Wilkins.

Centers for Disease Control and Prevention. (2016). *Who should not get vaccinated with these vaccines?* Retrieved from www.cdc.gov/vaccines/vpd-vac/should-not-vacc.htm#mmr.

Children's Healthcare of Atlanta. (2010). *Your child's heart catheterization.* Retrieved from www.choa.org/Childrens-Hospital-Services/Cardiac/Testing-and-Treatments/Heart-Testing/~/media/CHOA/Documents/Services/Cardiac/Your-Childs-Heart-Cath.pdf.

Chinnock, R. E., & Ohye, R. G. (2014). *Pediatric heart transplantation.* Retrieved from http://emedicine.medscape.com/article/1011927-overview.

Cook, E. H., & Higgins, S. S. (2010). Congenital heart disease. In P. J. Allen, J. A. Vessey, & N. A. Schapiro (Eds.). *Primary care of the child with a chronic condition* (5th ed.). St. Louis, MO: Mosby.

Corbett, J. A., & Banks, A. D. (2013). *Laboratory tests and diagnostic procedures with nursing diagnoses* (8th ed.). Upper Saddle River, NJ: Pearson Education Inc.

Cunningham, F. G., Leveno, K. J., Bloom, S. L., Spong, C. Y., Dashe, J. S., Hoffman, B. L., . . . Sheffield, J. S. (2014). *Williams obstetrics* (24th ed.). New York: McGraw-Hill Education.

Darst, J. R., Collins, K. K., & Miyamoto, S. D. (2014). Cardiovascular diseases. In W. W. Hay, M. J. Levin, R. R. Deterding, & M. J. Abzug (Eds.). *Current pediatric diagnosis and treatment* (22nd ed.). New York: McGraw-Hill.

DeMaso, D., & Snell, C. (2013). Promoting coping in children facing pediatric surgery. *Seminars in Pediatric Surgery, 22*(3): 134–138.

Dipchand, A. I., Bastardi, H., & Dupuis, J. (2013). *Pediatric heart transplants: A guide for patients and families.* Birmingham, AL: Pediatric Heart Transplant Study Foundation.

Doyle, T., Kavanaugh-McHugh, A., & Fish, F. A. (2016). *Management and outcome of tetralogy of Fallot.* Retrieved from www.uptodate.com/contents/management-and-outcome-of-tetralogy-of-fallot.

Engorn, B., & Flerlage, J. (2015). *The Harriet Lane handbook* (20th ed.). Philadelphia, PA: Saunders.

Francis, G. S., Wilson Tang, W. H., & Walsh, R. A. (2011). Pathophysiology of heart failure. In V. Fuster, R. A. Walsh, & R. A. Harrington (Eds.). *Hurst's the heart* (13th ed.). New York: McGraw-Hill Companies, Inc.

Gauthier, M., Issenman, R. M., Wilson, I., Canadian Paediatric Society, & Paediatric Human Resources Planning Committee. (2009). A model of paediatrics: Rethinking health care for children and youth. *Paediatr Child Health, 14*(5), 319–332.

Gibofsky, A. (2015). *Clinical manifestations and diagnosis of acute rheumatic fever.* Retrieved from www.uptodate.com/contents/clinical-manifestations-and-diagnosis-of-acute-rheumatic-fever.

Gordon, J., Kirlew, M., Schreiber, Y., Saginur, R., Bocking, N., Blakelock, B., . . . Kelly, L. (2015). Acute rheumatic fever in First Nations communities in northwestern Ontario Social determinants of health "bite the heart". *Canadian Family Physician, 61*(10), 881–886. Retrieved from http://www.cfp.ca/content/61/10/881.

Health Canada (n.d.). *Canada's Food Guide.* Retrieved from http://www.hc-sc.gc.ca/fn-an/food-guide-aliment/index-eng.php.

Horne, R. S., Yang, J. S., Walter, L. M., Richardsion, H. L., O'Driscoll, D. M., Foster, A. M., . . . Davey, M. J. (2011). Elevated blood pressure during sleep and wake in children with sleep-disordered breathing. *Pediatrics, 128*(1), 85–92.

Jackson, A. C., Frydenberg, E., Liang, R. P. T., Higgins, R. O., & Murphy, B. M. (2015). Familial impact and coping with child heart disease: a systematic review. *Pediatric Cardiology, 36*(4), 695–712.

Kantor, P. F., Abraham, J. R., Dipchand, A. I., Benson, L. N., & Redington, A. N. (2010). The impact of changing medical therapy on transplantation-free survival in pediatric dilated cardiomyopathy. *Journal of the American College of Cardiology, 55*(13), 1377–1384.

Kantor, P. F., Lougheed, J., Dancea, A., McGillion, M., Barbosa, N., Chan, C., . . . Wong, K. (2013). Presentation, diagnosis, and medical management of heart failure in children: Canadian Cardiovascular Society Guidelines. *Canadian Journal of Cardiology, 29*(12), 1535–1552.

Kawasaki Disease Canada. (n.d.). Retrieved from http://kdcanada.org.

Lai, W. W., Mertens, L. L., Cohen, M. S., & Geva, T. (2015). *Echocardiography in pediatric and congenital heart disease: from fetus to adult.* John Wiley & Sons.

Lankin, K. (2012). Pediatric heart transplantation. In: Hazinski, M. F. (Ed.). *Nursing care of the critically ill child* (3rd ed.). St. Louis, MO: Elsevier, Mosby.

Lorts, A., Krawczeski, C. D., & Marino, B. S. (2013). Cardiology. In B. S. Marino & K. S. Fine (Eds.). *Blueprints: Pediatrics* (6th ed.). Philadelphia, PA: Lippincott Williams & Wilkins.

Marian, A. J., Brugada, R., & Roberts, R. (2011). Cardiovascular disease due to genetic abnormalities. In V. Fuster, R. A. Walsh, & R. A. Harrington (Eds.). *Hurst's the heart* (13th ed.). New York: McGraw-Hill Companies, Inc.

Mattoo, T. K. (2016a). *Epidemiology, risk factors, and etiology of hypertension in children and adolescents.* Retrieved from www.uptodate.com/contents/epidemiology-risk-factors-and-etiology-of-hypertension-in-children-and-adolescents.

Mattoo, T. K. (2016b). *Treatment of hypertension in children and adolescents.* Retrieved from www.uptodate.com/contents/treatment-of-hypertension-in-children-and-adolescents.

McKenzie, J., Douglas, G., & Bazargan, A. (2013). Perioperative management of anticoagulation in elective surgery. *ANZ Journal of Surgery, 83*(11):814–820.

National Heart, Lung, and Blood Institute. (2012). *Expert Panel on Integrated Guidelines for Cardiovascular Health and Risk Reduction in Children and Adolescents.* SUMMARY REPORT (NIH Publication No. 12–7486). Washington, DC: U.S. Department of Health and Human Services.

Park, M. K. (2014). *Park's pediatric cardiology for practitioners* (6th ed.). Philadelphia, PA: Saunders.

Peng, L. F., & Perry, S. (2016). *Pulmonic stenosis (PS) in neonates, infants, and children.* Retrieved from www.uptodate.com/contents/pulmonic-stenosis-ps-in-neonates-infants-and-children.

Ralston, S. L., Lieberthal, A. S., Meissner, C., Alverson, B. K., Baley, J. E., Gadomski, A. M., . . . Hernandez-Cancio, S. (2014). Clinical practice guideline: The diagnosis, management, and prevention of bronchiolitis. *Pediatrics, 134*(5), e1474–e1502.

Rempel, G. R., Ravindran, V., Rogers, L. G., Magill-Evans, J. (2013). Parenting under pressure: a grounded theory of parenting young children with life-threatening congenital heart disease. *Journal of Advanced Nursing, 69*(3), 619–630.

Schuman, A. J. (2013). Making a difference. *Contemporary Pediatrics, 30*(4), 38–41.

Strehlow, M. (2015). Vasopressors and Inotropes. In J. Arbo, S. Ruoss, G. Lighthall, M. Jones, & G. Sternbach (Eds.). *Decision Making in Emergency Critical Care* (pp. 404–412). Philadelphia, PA: Wolters Kluwer.

Sundel, R. (2016a). *Kawasaki disease: Clinical features and diagnosis.* Retrieved from www.uptodate.com/contents/kawasaki-disease-clinical-features-and-diagnosis.

Sundel, R. (2016b). *Kawasaki disease: Epidemiology and etiology.* Retrieved from www.uptodate.com/contents/kawasaki-disease-epidemiology-and-etiology.

Sundel, R. (2016c). *Kawasaki disease: Initial treatment and prognosis.* Retrieved from www.uptodate.com/contents/kawasaki-disease-initial-treatment-and-prognosis.

Taketomo, C. K., Hodding, J. H., & Kraus, D. M. (2013). *Pediatric & neonatal dosage handbook* (20th ed.). Hudson, OH: Lexicomp.

The University of Chicago Medicine Comer Children's Hospital. (2016). *Heart catheterization in children.* Retrieved from www.uchicagokidshospital.org/specialties/heart/patient-education/cath-guide.html.

Trinh, J., & Palmer, K. (2012). Inotropes. *Anaesthesia & Intensive Care Medicine, 13*(10):492–498.

Wan, A., Vijarnsorn, C., & Rutledge, J. (2014). Initial experience with the GORE® septal occlude for atrial septal defect closure in children. *Canadian Journal of Cardiology, 30*(10), S170–S171. Retrieved from http://www.onlinecjc.ca/article/S0828-282X(14)00743-0/abstract

W. L. Gore & Associates, Inc. (2010). *Instructions for use: Gore Helex septal occluder.* Retrieved fromwww.fda.gov/ucm/groups/fdagov-public/@fdagov-afda-adcom/documents/document/ucm304933.pdf.

Ziff, O., & Kotecha, D. (2016). Digoxin: The good and the bad. *Trends in Cardiovascular Medicine, 26*(7):585–595.

CHAPTER **WORKSHEET**

MULTIPLE CHOICE QUESTIONS

1. The nurse is caring for a 5-year-old child with a congenital heart anomaly causing chronic cyanosis. When performing the history and physical examination, what is the nurse least likely to assess?
   a. Obesity from overeating
   b. Clubbing of the nail beds
   c. Squatting during play activities
   d. Exercise intolerance

2. A 2-day-old infant was just diagnosed with aortic stenosis. What is the most likely nursing assessment finding?
   a. Gallop and rales
   b. Blood pressure discrepancies in the extremities
   c. Right ventricular hypertrophy on ECG
   d. Heart murmur

3. Sam, age 11, has a diagnosis of rheumatic fever. What is the most likely cause of this problem?
   a. Previous streptococcal throat infection
   b. History of open heart surgery at 5 years of age
   c. Playing too much soccer and not getting enough rest
   d. Exposure to a sibling with pneumonia

4. The nurse is caring for a child after a cardiac catheterization. What is the nursing priority?
   a. Allow early ambulation to encourage activity participation.
   b. Check pulses above the catheter insertion site for strength and quality.
   c. Assess extremity distal to the insertion site for temperature and colour.
   d. Change the dressing to evaluate the site for infection.

5. While assessing a 4-month-old infant, the nurse notes that the baby experiences a hypercyanotic spell. What is the priority nursing action?
   a. Provide supplemental oxygen by face mask.
   b. Administer a dose of IV morphine sulfate.
   c. Begin cardiopulmonary resuscitation.
   d. Place the infant in a knee-to-chest position.

DOSAGE CALCULATION QUESTION

The nurse is caring for an infant with a ventricular septal defect who has heart failure. The infant weighs 5 kg (11 lb). The medication order reads: spironolactone 5 mg PO every 12 hours. Spironolactone is provided by the pharmacy in a solution of 2.5 mg/1 mL. How many millilitres will the nurse administer? Round to the nearest whole number.

CRITICAL THINKING EXERCISES

1. A baby boy was born at 26 weeks' gestation to 15-year-old unmarried parents who abuse drugs. The infant weighed 1.5 kg at birth and was diagnosed with AV canal defect and Down syndrome. Discuss some of the major issues in planning for care. Include a care plan and a list of teaching needs for the family.

2. A 4-year-old boy has parents with little education, limited social support living in a rural community. Another child is 7 years old and has well-educated parents with good social networks, living close to an urban centre. Both of these children need a heart transplant, and a heart is available that is a very good match for both children. Discuss some of the issues involved in deciding which child should receive the heart.

3. A 13-year-old boy was diagnosed with hypertension over 2 years ago. He is noncompliant with his antihypertensive medication regimen. He is 5 ft tall and weighs 170 lb. His favourite activity is video games. Develop a teaching plan for this teen, providing creative approaches at the appropriate developmental level.

STUDY ACTIVITIES

1. Teach a class of sixth graders about healthy activities to prevent high cholesterol levels, hypertension, and heart disease. Use visual materials.

2. Spend the day with a nurse practitioner in the pediatric cardiology clinic. Report to the clinical group your observations about the children's quality of life, growth, and development.

3. Observe in the pediatric cardiothoracic intensive care unit or telemetry unit. Note the different cardiac rhythms displayed by children with a variety of cardiovascular disorders.

BRINGING IT ALL TOGETHER: A CASE STUDY

Mitchell Ryder, 4 months old, is brought to the hospital by his mother. He presents with difficulty gaining weight. His mother states, "He just gets so tired when he eats, and sometimes when he is nursing he has a bluish colour around his lips."

Go to thePoint **to find questions to consider about this case.**

42

Nursing Care of the Child With an Alteration in Bowel Elimination/ Gastrointestinal Disorder

Learning Objectives

Upon completion of the chapter, you will be able to:

1. Compare the differences in the anatomy and physiology of the gastrointestinal system between children and adults.

2. Discuss common medical treatments for infants and children with alterations in bowel elimination (gastrointestinal disorders).

3. Discuss common laboratory and diagnostic tests used to identify disorders of the gastrointestinal tract.

4. Discuss medication therapy used in infants and children with alterations in bowel elimination (gastrointestinal disorders).

5. Recognize risk factors associated with various gastrointestinal illnesses.

6. Differentiate between acute and chronic gastrointestinal disorders.

7. Distinguish common gastrointestinal illnesses of childhood.

8. Discuss nursing interventions commonly used for gastrointestinal illnesses.

9. Devise an individualized nursing care plan for infants/children with an alteration in bowel elimination/gastrointestinal disorder.

10. Develop teaching plans for family/child education for children with gastrointestinal illnesses.

11. Describe the psychosocial impact that chronic gastrointestinal illnesses have on children.

Ethan Richardson, 2 months old, is brought to the clinic by his mother. He has been vomiting for the past 3 days. His mother states that she switched formula to see if that would help, but the vomiting worsened. Since last night she has attempted to feed him only Pedialyte. Mrs. Roberts says, "He can't keep anything down and he's very irritable." His weight at birth was 8 lb 9 oz, length 21 in, and head circumference 37 cm. At his 2-month check-up last week, he weighed 13 lb.

INTRODUCTION

Bowel elimination refers to the secretion and excretion of body waste through the intestinal system. Since nurses encounter children with alterations in bowel elimination, they should be familiar with the various gastrointestinal disorders or disturbances that children may experience. Alterations in bowel elimination, or gastrointestinal (GI) disorders, affect children of all ages. GI illnesses range from acute to chronic and from non–life-threatening to life-threatening problems. However, even acute, non–life-threatening illnesses (e.g., diarrhea or vomiting) can become life-threatening without appropriate nursing assessment and interventions. The most common result of a GI illness is dehydration, requiring fluid therapy at home or, in more extreme cases, in a hospital setting. It is important to take all GI disorders seriously until symptoms are well controlled.

Child and family education related to the treatment of GI disturbance is key to preventing the illness from progressing to an emergency situation. Therefore, the nurse's knowledge of the disorders that affect the GI system is crucial. Most often, the parents or child, if the child is older, will contact the physician or nurse practitioner to seek help. The nurse is usually the person to triage the phone call to determine the next step in the situation, which may be determining whether the child should be managed at home, brought to the office for assessment, or sent directly to an emergency room for evaluation. The majority of GI disorders can be handled in an outpatient setting to avoid unnecessary hospitalizations. However, some life-threatening problems (e.g., bowel obstruction) require emergency care in the hospital. Again, the knowledge base of the nurse is instrumental in obtaining the proper information by taking a thorough and accurate health history from the parents or child (if the child is older).

VARIATIONS IN PEDIATRIC ANATOMY AND PHYSIOLOGY

The GI tract includes all of the structures from the mouth to the anus. The primary functions of the GI system are the digestion and absorption of nutrients and water, elimination of waste products, and secretion of various substances required for digestion. Babies are born with immature GI tracts that are not fully mature until age 2. Due to this immaturity, there are many differences between the digestive tract of the young child and that of the older child or adult.

Mouth

The mouth is highly vascular, making it a common entry point for infectious invaders. In addition, the infant and young child repeatedly bring objects to their mouths and explore them in that fashion. This behaviour increases the infant's and young child's risk for contracting infectious agents via the mouth.

Esophagus

The esophagus provides a passageway from the mouth to the stomach for food. The lower esophageal sphincter (LES) prevents **regurgitation** (backflow) of stomach contents up into the esophagus and/or oral cavity. The muscle tone of the LES is not fully developed until age 1 month, so infants younger than 1 month of age frequently regurgitate after feedings. Many children younger than 1 year of age continue to regurgitate for several months, but this usually disappears with age. If edema or narrowing of the esophagus occurs in a child with undeveloped esophageal muscle tone, **dysphagia** (difficult or painful swallowing) may occur.

Stomach

Newborns have a stomach capacity of only 10 to 20 mL. At 2 months of age, an infant has the capacity to hold up to 200 mL, though most young infants cannot tolerate 200-mL feedings. By age 16, the stomach capacity is 1,500 mL; by adulthood, it is 2,000 to 3,000 mL. Hydrochloric acid, which is found in gastric contents to aid in digestion, reaches the adult level by the time the child is 6 months old.

Intestines

The small intestine is not functionally mature at birth. A full-term infant has approximately 250 cm of small intestine; an adult has up to 600 cm. Infants who have small bowel loss during early infancy have more problems with absorption and diarrhea than adults who have the same amount of small bowel loss.

Biliary System

The liver is relatively large at birth, allowing for the smooth edge of the liver to be easily palpated in infancy, as much as 2 cm below the costal margin. The pancreatic enzymes continue to develop postnatally, reaching adult levels around 2 years of age.

Fluid Balance and Losses

Compared with adults, children exhibit differences in how fluid volume is maintained. These differences are evident in body fluid balance and insensible fluid losses.

Body Fluid Balance

Infants and children have a proportionately greater amount of body water than do adults. Infants and young children require a larger relative fluid intake than adults and excrete a relatively greater amount of fluid. This places them at increased risk for fluid loss with illness compared to adults. Until age 2 years, the extracellular fluid, with its larger proportion of sodium and chloride, makes up about half of the child's total body water. Therefore, when potential fluid-loss states occur, water loss occurs more rapidly and in larger amounts than in adults.

Insensible Fluid Losses

Fever increases fluid loss at a rate of about 7 mL/kg/24-hr period for every sustained 1°C rise in temperature. Since children become febrile with illness more readily and their fevers are higher than those of adults, infants and young children are more apt than adults to experience insensible fluid loss with fever when ill.

Fluid loss via the skin accounts for about two thirds of insensible fluid loss. Infants have a relatively larger body surface area (BSA) relative to their body mass as compared to older children and adults. The newborn's BSA ratio to body mass is about two or three times greater than the adult's, and the preterm infant's is about five times greater than the adult's. This places infants, especially young infants, at increased risk of insensible fluid loss as compared to older children and adults.

The basal metabolic rate in infants and children is higher than that of adults in order to support growth. This higher metabolic rate, even in states of wellness, accounts for increased insensible fluid losses and increased need for water for excretory functions. The young infant's renal immaturity does not allow the kidneys to concentrate urine as well as in older children and adults. This puts infants at particular risk for dehydration or overhydration, depending on the circumstances.

COMMON MEDICAL TREATMENTS

There are many different forms of medical treatment for GI disorders. In the hospital setting, most medical treatments will require a physician's order. The most common treatments and medications used for GI disorders are listed in Common Medical Treatments 42.1 and Drug Guide 42.1. Both tables provide essential information about medical treatments and medications used in pediatric GI disorders. Refer to these tables as needed while completing the remainder of the chapter.

NURSING PROCESS OVERVIEW FOR THE CHILD WITH AN ALTERATION IN BOWEL ELIMINATION OR GASTROINTESTINAL DISORDER

Nursing care of the child with a GI disorder or alteration in bowel elimination includes nursing assessment, nursing diagnosis, planning, interventions, and evaluation. It is important to individualize each step of this process for each child. A general understanding of the GI tract and the most common disorders can help the nurse to individualize the nursing care plan.

> **Remember Ethan, the 2-month-old with vomiting and irritability? What additional health history and physical examination assessment information should you obtain?**

Assessment

The assessment of the child with a GI disorder includes a health history, physical examination, and laboratory and diagnostic testing.

Health History

A thorough health history is very important in the assessment of a child with a GI disorder. The health history includes past history (previous illnesses/surgeries), past family history, present illness (when the symptoms began and how this differs from the child's normal status), and how the child's symptoms have been managed up to this point (relevant medical records/home treatments). Detailed knowledge of the past medical and surgical history of the child may reveal bowel resection, previous intestinal infections, and dietary issues and problems.

The child's growth patterns can also be an instrumental part of the health history and may help to generate a timeline for when the current problems appeared. The family history is also extremely important in identifying common genetic or familial GI symptoms or disorders such as irritable bowel syndrome (IBS), inflammatory bowel disease, or food allergies. The history of the present illness and symptoms can often distinguish chronic problems from acute disorders. All of these pieces of the health history require descriptive questions and answers from both the nurse and the child, or the child's family. The person providing the history must be able to provide accurate details of the health history.

Physical Examination

Perform the physical examination of the child from the least invasive part of the examination to the most invasive. It is important for the child to remain as relaxed as possible during this part of the assessment.

INSPECTION AND OBSERVATION

Inspect and observe the child's colour, hydration status, abdominal size and shape, and mental status.

Colour. First observe the child's skin, eye, and lip colour. Pale skin or lips in a child with a GI disorder

COMMON MEDICAL TREATMENTS 42.1 GASTROINTESTINAL DISORDERS

Treatment	Explanation	Indications	Nursing Implications
Cleansing enema	Insertion of fluid into the rectum to soften the stool and stimulate bowel activity	Fecal impaction, severe constipation	Explain procedure to child prior to enema. With sodium phosphate enemas, observe for electrolyte imbalances (hypocalcemia or hyperphosphatemia) and discuss with the physician if no or little result in 24 hours. Only give as prescribed
Bowel preparation	Use of highly osmotic fluids to induce frequent diarrhea to cleanse the entire bowel	Preparation for colonoscopy or bowel surgery	Some children may need to have a nasogastric tube placed so they can consume the needed amounts of fluids. Observe for signs and symptoms of dehydration/electrolyte imbalance.
Feeding tubes	Flexible tubes used for enteral feeding when the infant or child is incapable of swallowing safely or for augmenting nutrition. May be orogastric, nasogastric, gastrostomy, or jejunostomy	Feeding difficulties, failure to thrive, chronic illness	Orogastric and nasogastric tubes must be checked for placement prior to each use. If required long term, use a softer, flexible tube intended for long-term use. Stomahesive or Duoderm applied to the cheek may decrease risk of skin breakdown from tape. Gastrostomy and jejunostomy tubes vary in type. Keep insertion site clean and dry
Intravenous therapy	Administration of fluids via a catheter that delivers electrolytes and fluids into the venous system	Dehydration, bowel rest, NPO status	Monitor intravenous site for redness, swelling, and pain. Assess urine output to evaluate hydration status
Ostomy	A portion of the intestine is brought to the level of the skin to allow passage of stool	Imperforate anus, gastroschisis, omphalocele, Hirschsprung disease, necrotizing enterocolitis, Crohn disease, ulcerative colitis	Ostomy contents may be acidic and irritate the skin. Use Stomahesive or Duoderm under the pouch to avoid tape irritation to the skin. Pouch should fit the stoma correctly. Assess stoma for pinkness and moist appearance
Oral rehydration therapy	Administration by mouth of fluids that contain certain amounts of electrolytes and glucose to prevent dehydration and/or promote rehydration	Diarrhea, acute gastroenteritis, vomiting	Fluid administration should begin prior to the onset of dehydration. Urine output should be monitored to evaluate hydration status
Probiotics (*Lactobacillus acidophilus*)	Food supplement containing dormant bacteria that when activated may alter the intestinal microflora	Treatment/prevention of diarrhea	Particularly helpful in prevention of or decreasing incidence of antibiotic-induced diarrhea
Total parenteral nutrition (TPN)	Intravenous complete nutrition. Provides glucose, protein, lipids, vitamins, and minerals	Long-term NPO status, swallowing difficulties, difficulties tolerating enteral feeding (short bowel syndrome, necrotizing enterocolitis)	Higher glucose and protein concentrations and solutions containing calcium require central venous access. Monitor blood glucose levels with initiation, rate changes, and discontinuation. Blood chemistries should be monitored on a regular basis

DRUG GUIDE 42.1 COMMON DRUGS FOR GI DISORDERS

Classification	Actions/Indications	Nursing Implications
Histamine-2 blockers (ranitidine, famotidine, cimetidine, nizatidine)	Decrease histamine production, thereby reducing gastric acid secretion Used for heartburn, esophagitis, GER	May cause drowsiness or dizziness
Proton pump inhibitors (omeprazole, lansoprazole, esomeprazole, pantoprazole, rabeprazole)	Block the pump that produces gastric acids Indicated for erosive esophagitis, GERD, *Helicobacter pylori* eradication	Adverse effects include headache, nausea, abdominal pain, or diarrhea
Prokinetics side effects and ADRs present in up to 40% patients (domperidone, metoclopramide, cisapride). Used very rarely in children	Stimulate GI motility to help empty the stomach faster and promote intestinal motility	Metoclopramide may have serious central nervous system adverse effects such as involuntary movements (tardive dyskinesia). Cisapride available only in limited-access protocol studies May require ECG as increased risk of cardiac adverse effects
Antibacterials/antibiotics (metronidazole, vancomycin)	Treatment of bacterial infections of the GI tract Used for suspected or proven bacterial infections of the GI tract, such as *Clostridium difficile* or parasitic infections	May cause GI upset, diarrhea. Take metronidazole with food. Very important to finish entire course of treatment
Immunosuppressants (6-mercaptopurine, azathioprine)	Suppress the immune system to keep autoimmune disorders such as Crohn disease, ulcerative colitis, autoimmune hepatitis in remission	Drug enzyme activity levels (TPMT) should be checked to determine risk for potential hepatotoxicity or bone marrow suppression prior to starting drug
Stimulants (senna)	Stimulate peristalsis in the large intestine to produce a bowel movement Used to relieve constipation	May cause cramping or diarrhea. Stool patterns should be assessed daily. Long-term use not recommended
Laxatives (polyethylene glycol, milk of magnesia, lactulose, docusate sodium)	Soften the stool to allow for easier passage through the colon Used to relieve constipation	Stool patterns should be monitored. Doses may need to be readjusted to find the correct dose for the child
Antidiarrheals (loperamide, diphenoxylate/atropine)	Decrease peristalsis, thus prolonging transit time of stool through the intestines Indicated to treat diarrhea related to short bowel syndrome, chronic nonspecific diarrhea, irritable bowel syndrome	May cause drowsiness or constipation. Should be used with caution when bowel inflammation is suspected
Corticosteroids (prednisone)	Act systemically to reduce inflammation and suppress the immune response Used in inflammatory bowel disease, autoimmune disorders	Systemic adverse effects include increased appetite, weight gain, insomnia, increased acne, hirsutism, GI upset, cushingoid appearance. Some children may exhibit mood swings. Long-term use may cause growth failure, increased intraocular pressure, hypertension, and osteoporosis. Should be taken as directed. Stopping the medication suddenly may cause illness due to drug-induced adrenal insufficiency
Antiemetics (promethazine, metoclopramide)	Act on the central nervous system transmitters to prevent nausea and vomiting	Can cause drowsiness and irritability. With long-term use may have serious central nervous system adverse effects, such as tardive dyskinesia

DRUG GUIDE 42.1   COMMON DRUGS FOR GI DISORDERS (continued)

Classification	Actions/Indications	Nursing Implications
Anticholinergic/antispasmodics (hyoscyamine, mebeverine dicyclomine, glycopyrrolate)	Used to control abdominal spasms and cramping associated with irritable bowel syndrome, functional bowel disorders	May cause excessive thirst or dizziness, nausea, insomnia Encourage plenty of fluids while taking these medications
Anti-inflammatories (5-aminosalicylic acid: mesalamine, sulfasalazine)	Work topically to reduce inflammation in the colon associated with ulcerative colitis, proctitis. Can be given orally or rectally	Stool output should be monitored to assess for presence of oral medications (indicating poor absorption)

Adapted from Taketomo, C. K., Hodding, J. H., & Kraus, D. M. (2013). *Pediatric & neonatal dosage handbook* (20th ed.). Hudson, OH: Lexicomp.

may be a sign of anemia or dehydration. During liver dysfunction, the bilirubin levels can rise, causing the skin to look jaundiced (yellow). The sclerae can also become **icteric** (yellowed in colour), further indicating that the liver is not functioning correctly. Inspect the abdomen for distended veins, which can indicate abdominal or vascular obstruction or distention. As in any part of a physical assessment, watch for areas of ecchymosis (bruising), which may suggest disordered blood clotting or can be a sign of non-accidental injury.

Hydration Status. The child's hydration status often indicates how severe the current GI illness is. Dehydration can occur rapidly in children, especially in infants and young children. The oral mucosa should be pink and moist. Skin turgor should be elastic. Decreased turgor and tenting indicate dehydration. During crying, especially in infants, the absence of tears may indicate dehydration. Watch for depressed fontanel in infants. Assess the amount of urine output the child has had in the past 24 hours.

Abdominal Size and Shape. Inspect the size and shape of the abdomen while the child is standing and while the child is lying supine. The abdomen should be flat when the child is supine. An especially **protuberant** (bulging outward) abdomen suggests the presence of ascites, fluid retention, gaseous distention, or even a tumour. However, many children (toddlers in particular) have a prominent "pot-bellied" abdomen as a normal variation of their anatomy (Weber & Kelley, 2014). A depressed or concave abdomen could indicate malnutrition and/or dehydration. Inspect the umbilicus for colour, odour, discharge, inflammation, and herniation.

Mental Status. Perform a brief mental status examination of all children with GI complaints. Mental status changes can occur in many instances, such as during severe dehydration, with anaphylactic reactions to foods or medicines, when ammonia levels are elevated with severe liver disease, and with other metabolic disorders. Irritability and restlessness are usually the early signs of mental status changes. **Lethargy** (sluggishness or abnormal drowsiness) and listlessness can occur much more rapidly in children than in adults. It is important to identify this promptly and treat it emergently.

AUSCULTATION

As with all children, auscultate bowel sounds in all four quadrants. Hyperactive bowel sounds may be noted in children with diarrhea or gastroenteritis. Hypoactive or absent bowel sounds may signify an obstructive process. The nurse can determine absence of bowel sounds after a 5-minute period of auscultation. This can be extremely difficult to perform with children and infants, who may be uncooperative during the examination. Immediately report hypoactive or absent bowel sound findings to the physician or nurse practitioner.

PERCUSSION

Dullness or flatness is normally found along the right costal margin and 1 to 3 cm below the costal margin of the liver. The area above the symphysis pubis may be dull in young children with full bladders, which is a normal finding. Percussion of the remainder of the abdomen should reveal tympany. Note abnormal findings.

PALPATION

Reserve palpation for last in the sequence of abdominal examination. First, lightly palpate the abdomen to assess for areas of tenderness, lesions, muscle tone, turgor, and cutaneous hyperesthesia (a finding in acute peritonitis). Then perform deep palpation from the lower quadrants upward to best feel the liver edge, which should be firm and smooth. In infants and children, palpate the liver during inspiration below the right costal margin. The tip of the spleen may be palpated also during inspiration; it should be 1 to 2 cm below the left costal margin. Palpable kidneys, except in neonates, may indicate tumour or hydronephrosis. The sigmoid colon can be palpated in the left lower quadrant. The cecum may be felt in the right lower quadrant as a soft mass. Areas of firmness or masses may indicate tumour or stool in the abdomen.

Tenderness in the abdomen is not a normal physical finding. Right lower quadrant pain, including **rebound tenderness** (pain upon release of pressure during palpation), can be a warning sign of appendicitis; immediately report any positive findings to a physician. Palpate the external inguinal canals for the presence of inguinal hernias.

Laboratory and Diagnostic Testing

Common Laboratory and Diagnostic Tests 42.1 gives information about the tests most often ordered by physicians for children with GI illnesses. Some of these tests are ordered in the hospital setting; others are done on an outpatient basis. Typically, the nurse is involved directly in specimen collection while a specifically trained person performs the diagnostic tests. For any tests that involve x-ray, the nurse must follow local procedure to enquire re-pregnancy in young women who have started their periods. Regardless of who performs the test, nurses must be familiar with preparation guidelines for the child, how each test is performed, and normal and abnormal findings and their significance in order to provide appropriate child and family education. Teaching Guidelines 42.1 gives tips on collecting stool specimens.

COMMON LABORATORY AND DIAGNOSTIC TESTS 42.1

Test	Explanation	Indications	Nursing Implications
Abdominal ultrasonography	Visualizes abdominal organs and related vessels	Abdominal pain, vomiting, pregnancy, abnormal liver tests, abdominal mass, enlarged organs on palpation	Some studies require fasting. Barium decreases visualization of organs on ultrasound
Abdominal x-ray (KUB)	Plain x-ray of the abdomen without contrast media	Gastrointestinal transit studies, abdominal pain, abdominal distention, ascites, foreign body, palpable mass	Usually ordered as flat and upright to allow for free air and fluid levels in the bowel to be detected
Amylase (serum)	An enzyme that changes starch to sugar, which enters the blood with inflammation of the pancreas	Acute pancreatitis, pancreatic trauma, acute cholecystitis	Increased levels are seen after 3 to 6 hours of the onset of abdominal pain
Barium enema	After instillation of barium, fluoroscopy allows visualization of the colon	Suspected lower intestinal obstruction such as long-segment Hirschsprung disease, suspected intussusception	Bowel preparation prior to examination may be ordered. Stool will be light coloured due to barium for a few days
Anorectal manometry	Catheter with a balloon passed in to rectum that has a pressure sensor is connected to a device to measure rectal pressure	Constipation or fecal incontinence, assessment of anal sphincter muscle/rectal sensation	Enema may be used a day before study and invasive as involves passing a catheter PR
Electrolytes (serum)	Sodium, potassium, CO_2, chloride, blood urea nitrogen (BUN), creatinine	To determine hydration status	BUN and creatinine may be elevated with dehydration. Sodium, potassium, chloride, and CO_2 levels can be greatly affected with dehydration
Barium swallow/ upper GI series	Visualizes the form, position, mucosal folds, peristaltic activity, and motility of the esophagus, stomach, and upper GI tract	Foreign body ingestion, abdominal pain, vomiting, dysphagia, malrotation	Infants may need to be given barium via syringe

COMMON LABORATORY AND DIAGNOSTIC TESTS 42.1 (continued)

Test	Explanation	Indications	Nursing Implications
Small bowel series	Done in conjunction with upper GI series to visualize the small intestine contour, position, and motility	Suspected inflammatory bowel disease (bowel wall thickening), intussusception	Contraindicated if pregnant. Encourage large amounts of water/fluids after test to avoid barium-induced constipation
Endoscopic retrograde cholangio-pancreatography (ERCP)	Under sedation, a fibre-optic endoscope is used to view the hepatobiliary system by instilling contrast to outline the pancreatic and common bile ducts	Pancreatitis, jaundice, pancreatic tumours, common duct stones, biliary tract disease	Monitor for infection, cholangitis, or pancreatitis after the procedure. Done only occasionally in children
Esophageal manometry	Tests the esophagus for normal contractile activity and effectiveness of swallowing by measurement of intraluminal pressures	Abnormal esophageal muscle function, dysphagia, esophagitis, vomiting	Often done in conjunction with pH probe. The manometric catheter is placed through the nose into the esophagus. May cause nasal irritation/sore throat
Esophageal pH probe	A single- or double-channelled probe placed into the esophagus to monitor the pH of the contents that are regurgitated into the esophagus from the stomach	Vomiting, gastroesophageal reflux, correlation of symptoms to gastroesophageal reflux events and problems, such as recurrent apnoea, or choking/gagging episodes	24-hour study is most accurate. Accurate diary of symptoms and feedings during the study is essential. May cause nasal irritation/sore throat
Gastric emptying scan	Assesses the rate at which the stomach empties food into the small intestine by adding isotopes to food and visualizing with scans	Unexplained nausea, vomiting, bloating, early satiety, abdominal cramping	Medications may alter gastric emptying times. This study takes several hours
Hemoccult	Checks for occult blood in the stool	Crohn disease, ulcerative colitis, malabsorption syndromes, abdominal pain	Indicates bleeding in the GI tract
Hepatobiliary scan (HIDA scan)	Visualizes the gallbladder and determines patency of the biliary system by use of a radionuclide. The amount of radionuclide ejected from the gallbladder (ejection fraction) is calculated	Differentiate between biliary atresia and neonatal hepatitis; assess liver trauma, right upper quadrant pain, and congenital malformations	Intravenous line will be established to give radionuclide. Often require 5 days of oral phenobarbital prior to scan to optimize biliary drainage
Lactose breath test	After ingesting lactose, this tests the hydrogen levels in the breath, which will increase with lactose build-up in the intestines	Postprandial diarrhea, gassiness, bloating, abdominal pain	May produce similar symptoms during the test itself. A positive test will require diet modification and education regarding lactose intolerance
Lipase (serum)	An enzyme that changes fat to fatty acids and glycerol appearing in the blood with pancreatic change	Pancreatitis, pancreatic carcinoma, cholecystitis	Lipase levels stay elevated longer with acute pancreatitis
Liver biopsy	A test done to evaluate the microscopic hepatic structures	Hyperbilirubinemia, jaundice, chronic liver disease, hepatitis	Assess blood clotting prior to biopsy and correct if required. Monitor after procedure for bleeding complications; must maintain strict bed rest for up to 8 hours.

(continued)

COMMON LABORATORY AND DIAGNOSTIC TESTS 42.1 (continued)

Test	Explanation	Indications	Nursing Implications
Liver function tests (LFTs) (AST/ALT/GGT)	Transaminases are present in liver and in usually low levels in the blood. When the liver is injured more leak from the liver cells into the blood stream	Elevations indicate liver damage	May be affected by drugs or viral illnesses
Lower endoscopy (colonoscopy)	Allows visualization and biopsies of the lining of the lower GI tract from the anus to the terminal ileum with a fibre-optic instrument	Rectal bleeding, lower abdominal pain, suspected tumours or strictures, foreign body removal	The child must undergo a bowel cleansing prior to the examination. Encourage fluids to prevent dehydration. Conscious sedation or anaesthesia care; post-procedure monitor for possible complications of perforation or bleeding
Meckel scan	A Nuclear Medicine imaging test used to identify the presence of ectopic gastric mucosa in the large bowel	Painless rectal or GI bleeding, anemia	Requires IV to deliver radiopharmaceuticals. Gloves are worn by nurse during and after scan
Oropharyngeal motility study (OPMS)	A swallowing study done giving the child different textures to evaluate the dynamics of swallowing and reveal transient abnormalities	Dysphagia, recurrent aspiration, gagging, choking	Usually done in combination with occupational or speech therapists and nutritionist
Rectal suction biopsy	Biopsy is taken of the rectum at different levels to assess for the presence of ganglion cells	Absence of ganglion cells indicates Hirschsprung disease	Infants/children should be assessed for rectal bleeding after examination
Stool culture	Stool sent to lab where a sample is cultured to assess for pathogenic bacteria	To determine bacterial cause of diarrhea	Requires minimum of 48 hours for growth, several days to weeks in some cases. Can be done with a small amount of stool
Stool for ova and parasites (O&P)	Checks for the presence of parasites or their eggs in the stool	To determine cause of diarrhea or abdominal pain	Collection bottle has special preservative—keep away from children
Upper endoscopy (EGD)	Allows visualization and biopsies of the upper GI tract (mouth to duodenum) with a fibre-optic instrument	Dysphagia, foreign body removal, epigastric/abdominal pain, suspected celiac disease	Conscious sedation or anaesthesia care; post-procedure monitor for complications of perforation/bleeding
Urea breath test	Measures exhaled carbon dioxide after drinking preparation of urea. Used to detect the presence of *H. pylori* in the exhaled breath	*To assess for presence of H. pylori infection*	Child must be fasting before this test, follow test instructions about stopping H_2 blockers, proton pump inhibitors, antibiotics, and bismuth prior to examination

Adapted from Corbett, J. A., & Banks, A. D. (2013). *Laboratory tests and diagnostic procedures with nursing diagnoses* (8th ed.). Upper Saddle River, NJ: Pearson Education Inc.; and Dowshen, S. (2014). *Stool tests.* Retrieved from http://www.kidshealth.org/parent/general/sick/labtest8.html

Teaching Guidelines 42.1
STOOL SPECIMEN COLLECTION VARIATIONS

- If the child is in diapers, use a tongue blade to scrape a specimen into the collection container.
- If the child has runny stool, a piece of plastic wrap in the diaper may catch the stool specimen. Very liquid stool may require application of a urine bag to the anal area to collect the stool.
- The older ambulatory child may first urinate in the toilet, and then the stool specimen may be retrieved from the new or clean collection container that fits under the seat at the back of the toilet.
- For the bedridden child, collect the stool specimen from a clean bedpan (do not allow urine to contaminate the stool specimen).
- Send the specimen to the laboratory immediately for accuracy of results.

Nursing Diagnoses, Goals, Interventions, and Evaluation

Upon completion of a thorough assessment, the nurse might identify several nursing diagnoses, including:

- Risk for deficient fluid volume
- Diarrhea
- Constipation
- Risk for impaired skin integrity
- Imbalanced nutrition: less than body requirements
- Pain
- Ineffective breathing pattern
- Risk for caregiver role strain
- Disturbed body image

After completing an assessment on Ethan, you note the following: weight 10 lb, length 23.5 in, head circumference 40.75 cm. Head is round with sunken anterior fontanel, eyes appear sunken, mucous membranes are dry, heart rate 158, breath sounds clear with respiratory rate of 42, positive bowel sounds in all four quadrants, difficulty palpating abdomen due to crying. Based on these assessment findings, what would your top three nursing diagnoses be for Ethan?

Nursing goals, interventions, and evaluation for the child with a GI disorder are based on the nursing diagnoses. Nursing Care Plan 42.1, at the end of the chapter, can be used as a guide in planning nursing care for the child with a GI disorder. Individualize the nursing care plan based on the child's symptoms and needs. Refer to Chapter 36 for detailed information about pain management. Additional information will be included later in the chapter as it relates to specific disorders.

Based on your top three nursing diagnoses for Ethan, describe appropriate nursing interventions.

Stool Diversions

Children may undergo stool diversions for a variety of GI disorders. Surgical procedures involve the creation of an ostomy, primarily an *ileostomy* or *colostomy*, by bringing a portion of the small or large intestine to the surface of the abdomen (Fig. 42.1).

Ostomy pouches are worn over the ostomy site to collect stool. The pouch must be of an appropriate size

FIGURE 42.1 **A.** A colostomy is a stoma from the colon. **B.** An ileostomy is a stoma from the ileum.   **A**   **B**

FIGURE 42.2 Ensure that the ostomy pouch fits closely around the stoma to prevent irritation of the surrounding skin.

FIGURE 42.3 The healthy stoma is pink and moist.

and it should fit around the stoma properly (Fig. 42.2). The pouch may be tucked inside the diaper or underwear or angled to fit outside of the diaper/underwear. Contemporary pouches cannot be seen under most clothing because they are designed to lie flat against the body. Avoid tight or constricting clothing around the stoma site. Teach families to store ostomy supplies in a cool, dry place. Children with ostomies require increased oral fluids due to increased fluid losses in the ostomy. Educate parents to inform school staff that the child should be allowed to use the water fountain or keep a water bottle at their desk. The child should be allowed to use the bathroom without restriction, and the school should have extra ostomy supplies available.

Ostomy care for a child can be challenging due to the child's normal growth and development as well as activity. Post-surgery, empty the ostomy pouch and measure for stool output several times per day. The stool may be semisolid to very liquid in consistency depending on the location of the stoma. Liquid stool output can be acidic, causing irritation and severe burn-like areas on the surrounding skin, so special attention to skin care around the ostomy site is essential. Products such as powders and pastes are available to help protect the skin.

The stoma should be moist and pink or red, demonstrating proper circulation to the intestine (Fig. 42.3). Immediately notify the provider if the stoma is not moist and pink or red. Also notify the provider if the volume of stool output is greatly increased, or if the stoma is prolapsed or retracted or any new lesions are noted on the stoma.

Perform ostomy care as needed; pouches usually need to be changed every 1 to 4 days. Refer to Nursing Procedure 42.1 for an explanation of the steps for changing an ostomy pouch.

STRUCTURAL ANOMALIES OF THE GASTROINTESTINAL TRACT

Structural anomalies of the GI tract include cleft lip and palate, omphalocele and gastroschisis, hernias (inguinal and umbilical), and anorectal malformations. Omphalocele, gastroschisis, and anorectal malformations are discussed in Chapter 24.

NURSING PROCEDURE 42.1

Performing Ostomy Care

1. Set up the equipment:
   • Warm, wet washcloths or paper towels
   • Clean pouch and clamp
   • Skin barrier powder, paste, and/or sealant
   • Pencil or pen
   • Scissors
   • Pattern to measure stoma size

2. Take off the pouch (may need to use adhesive remover or wet washcloth to ease pouch removal).

3. Observe the stoma and surrounding skin. Clean the stoma and skin as needed, allowing it to dry thoroughly.

4. Measure the stoma, mark the new pouch backing, and cut the new backing to size.

5. Apply the new pouch.

Adapted from University of California, San Francisco. (2016). *Colostomy*. Retrieved from http://pedsurg.ucsf.edu/conditions–procedures/colostomy.aspx

Cleft Lip and Palate

Cleft lip and palate (Fig. 42.4) is the most common congenital craniofacial anomaly, affecting about 400 to 500 newborns every year in Canada (Health Canada, 2002). The prevalence rate (1998 to 2007) appears to be stable (Mathews, Oddone-Paolucci, & Harrop, 2015) with Indigenous populations having higher rates of orofacial clefts (Vrouwe, Lowry, Olson, & Wilkes, 2013). There are 21 clinics across Canada that provide specialist services (Batsos, 2009). It occurs frequently in association with other anomalies and has been identified in more than 350 syndromes (Curtin & Boekelheide, 2010). The most common anomalies associated with cleft lip and cleft palate include heart defects, ear malformations, skeletal deformities, and genitourinary abnormality.

Complications of cleft lip and palate include feeding difficulties, altered dentition, delayed or altered speech development, and otitis media. The infant with cleft lip may have difficulty forming an adequate seal around a nipple in order to create the necessary suction for feeding and may also experience excessive air intake. Gagging, choking, and nasal regurgitation of milk may occur in babies with cleft palate. Excessive feeding time, inadequate intake, and fatigue contribute to insufficient growth. Primary or permanent teeth may be missing, malformed, or unusually positioned. Children with cleft palate may have a nasal quality to the speech as well as delays in speech development. Optimally, speech articulation should be clear by 4 years of age, or additional surgical intervention may be necessary (Curtin & Boekelheide, 2010). The opening in the cleft palate contributes to build-up of fluid in the middle ear (otitis media with effusion), which can lead to an acute infection (acute otitis media). Long-lasting otitis media with effusion leads to temporary and sometimes permanent hearing loss (Curtin & Boekelheide, 2010).

Pathophysiology

Development of the **cleft** occurs early in pregnancy. The tissue that forms the lip ordinarily fuses by 5 to 6 weeks' gestation, and the palate closes between 7 and 9 weeks' gestation. Therefore, if either the lip or palate does not fuse, then the infant is born with a cleft. Cleft lip or cleft palate may occur in isolation from one another, but 50% of infants born with cleft lip also have cleft palate (Curtin & Boekelheide, 2010). The cleft may be unilateral (the left side is affected more often) or bilateral.

Therapeutic Management

Babies with cleft lip and cleft palate are usually managed by a specialized team that may include a plastic surgeon or craniofacial specialist, oral surgeon, dentist or orthodontist, prosthodontist, psychologist, otolaryngologist, nurse, social worker, audiologist, and speech-language pathologist. Many children's hospitals offer these services in one location, such as a craniofacial specialty centre (see CleftSmile.org). Historically, cleft lip has been repaired surgically around the age of 2 to 3 months and cleft palate at 6 to 9 months. Early repair of the cleft lip influences appearance to the child's face and may improve parent–infant bonding. Regardless of the timing of the surgical repair, however, surgical revision of the palate may be required as the child grows.

Nursing Assessment

For a full description of the assessment phase of the nursing process, refer to the Assessment section of the Nursing Process Overview earlier in the chapter. Assessment findings pertinent to cleft lip and palate are discussed below.

FIGURE 42.4 **The cleft lip may extend all the way through the vermilion border and up into the nostril, or it may be significantly smaller. The cleft palate may be a small opening or may involve the entire palate.**

FIGURE 42.5 Cleft lip.

HEALTH HISTORY

For the newborn, explore pregnancy history for risk factors for development of cleft lip and cleft palate, which include:

- Maternal smoking
- Prenatal infection
- Advanced maternal age
- Use of anticonvulsants, steroids, and other medications during early pregnancy

When an infant or child with cleft lip or palate returns for a clinic visit or hospitalization, inquire about feeding difficulties, respiratory difficulties, speech development, and otitis media.

PHYSICAL EXAMINATION

Observe the infant for the presence of the characteristic physical appearance of cleft lip. The cleft may involve the lip only or extend up into the nostril (Fig. 42.5). Cleft palate may be visualized on examination of the mouth. Palpate with a gloved finger to discover mild clefts.

LABORATORY AND DIAGNOSTIC TESTS

Cleft lip may be diagnosed by prenatal ultrasound, but it is diagnosed most commonly at birth by the classic physical appearance.

Consider This

The nurse is caring for a 2-week-old infant with a cleft lip who presents for a well-child check. The mother states, "I can't believe she looks like this; I always wanted a perfect baby girl. I feel like I can't go anywhere with her, other people will look at her like she's a monster. And after her surgery she's going to have an ugly scar over her lip." She then begins crying.

How will you respond as the nurse? Are you concerned about anything other than the mother's feelings in the situation? What would it feel like if you had a baby with a facial deformity? Think about the best ways to respond to this mother in a therapeutic manner.

Nursing Management

Refer to Nursing Care Plan 42.1 at the end of the chapter for nursing diagnoses and interventions related to airway maintenance, fluid balance promotion, and restoration of family processes, and to Chapter 36 for pain management. These should be individualized for the particular situation. In addition to the nursing diagnoses and related interventions discussed in Nursing Care Plan 42.1, interventions common to cleft lip and cleft palate follow.

PREVENTING INJURY TO THE SUTURE LINE

It is critical to prevent injury to the facial suture line or to the palatal operative sites. Do not allow the infant to rub the facial suture line. To prevent this, position the infant in a supine or side-lying position. It may be necessary to use arm restraints to stop the hands from touching the face or entering the mouth. Clean the suture line as ordered by the surgeon. Possible care options include using petroleum jelly on the facial suture line or a lip-protective device such as a Logan bow (curved thin metal apparatus) or a butterfly adhesive, both of which protect and maintain the suture line. Protect the palate operative site. Avoid putting items in the mouth that might disrupt the sutures (e.g., suction catheter, spoon, straw, pacifier, or plastic syringe).

Prevent vigorous or sustained crying in the infant, because this may cause tension on either suture line. Ways to prevent crying include administering medications as needed for pain and providing other comfort or distraction measures, such as cuddling, rocking, and anticipation of needs.

PROMOTING ADEQUATE NUTRITION

Preoperatively, the baby with a cleft lip may demonstrate enhanced growth patterns if breastfed. The contour and softness of the breast against the lip may allow for a better seal to be maintained for adequate sucking in some infants (Donovan, 2012). Some infants will be fed with a special cleft lip nipple (Fig. 42.6). Parent and surgeon preference will determine the method of feeding. Burp the infant well to expel excess air taken in during difficulty with sucking.

The infant with unrepaired cleft palate is at risk for aspiration with oral feeding. In some instances, a

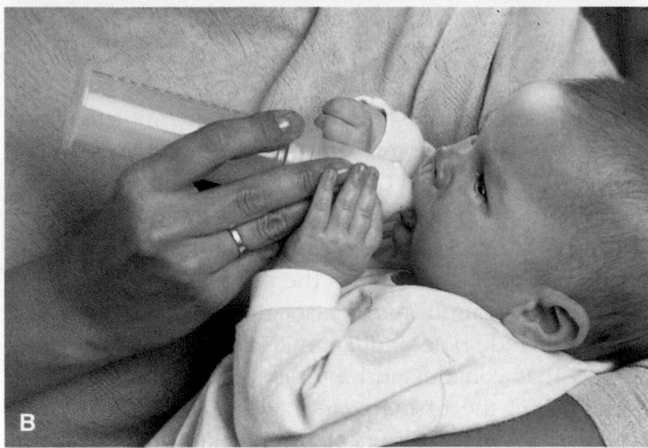

FIGURE 42.6 **A.** Specialty feeding devices used for infants with cleft lip and cleft palate. **B.** An infant uses a Haberman feeder.

prosthodontic device may be created to form a false palate covering. This device may prevent breast milk or formula from being aspirated. Breastfeeding may be effective in the infant with cleft palate due to the pliability of the breast and the fact that soft breast tissue may cover the opening in the palate. Postoperatively, some surgeons allow breastfeeding to be resumed almost immediately (Donovan, 2012). In the bottle-fed infant, special nipples or feeders may have to be used. When the suture line is healed, ordinary feeding may resume.

ENCOURAGING INFANT–PARENT BONDING

For some parents, the appearance of a cleft lip is bothersome (Curtin & Boekelheide, 2010). Encourage parents to hold the medically stable infant immediately after delivery to encourage bonding. Acknowledge normal feelings of guilt, anger, and sadness. Support the parents in providing care for the infant, particularly feeding, which is viewed as a significant nurturing function. Provide education about the anticipated surgical procedure and eventual normal appearance of the infant's lip.

PROVIDING EMOTIONAL SUPPORT

Many families will benefit from support in addition to that received from the craniofacial team. Refer parents to a parent-to-parent support network. National organizations like Cleftsmile.org provide resources for families of children with Cleft lip/Cleft palate.

Esophageal Atresia and Tracheoesophageal Fistula

Congenital malformations that result in the esophagus ending before it reaches the stomach or a fistula between the esophagus and trachea are rare malformations that result from a failure of separation around 4 weeks' gestation. Esophageal atresia (EA) with or without tracheoesophageal fistula (TEF) can occur at the same stage of embryonic development as anorectal malformations; see box 42.1 for associated anomalies. As a result of the condition, either oral intake enters the lungs or air in the stomach, presenting risk of coughing, choking, or severe abdominal distention. Aspiration pneumonia and severe respiratory distress occur with EA, which are life-threatening. Surgical repair is required, chest tubes will be necessary, and care is often within an intensive care setting. Following surgery gastrostomy, feeding can be common place until healing allows for commencement of oral feeding.

Nursing Assessment

Observe the newborn for frothy oral secretions around the mouth and nose. If feeding has been trailed, observe for coughing, choking, and cyanosis. Monitor respiratory rate and effort closely. Abdominal distention is an indicator of TEF with increased respiratory distress following feeding.

Nursing Management

Nurse the infant in an incubator and provide humidified oxygen as instructed. Mechanical ventilation may be necessary and the parents will need support as this emergency

---

BOX 42.1

ANOMALIES ASSOCIATED WITH ANORECTAL MALFORMATIONS

- VACTERL syndrome: vertebral, anorectal, cardiovascular, tracheoesophageal, renal, and limb
- Esophageal atresia
- Intestinal atresia
- Malrotation
- Renal agenesis
- Hypospadias
- Vesicoureteral reflux
- Bladder exstrophy
- Cardiac anomalies
- Skeletal anomalies

situation can be a frightening experience. Maintain NPO and IV fluids as prescribed. Suction secretions from the oral/nasal passageways and the pharynx/pouch and look to position infant at 30 degrees to minimize the risk of aspiration. Regular review will be necessary into childhood, as will assessment of feeding, dysphagia, and regurgitation; involve speech and language therapist in ongoing care.

Anorectal Malformations

Imperforate anus is a congenital malformation with either incomplete development or absence of the anus. Refer to Chapter 24 for information related to the incidence and etiology of anorectal malformations, as well as nursing care in the neonatal period. Other congenital anomalies may be associated with imperforate anus in 50% of cases (Hoffenberg et al., 2014) (Box 42.1). Surgical intervention is needed for all types of imperforate anus; high, intermediate, or low. Surgery for a high type of defect involves a colostomy in the newborn period, with corrective anoplasty and pull-through surgery performed in stages. Surgery for the low type of anomaly involves closure of the fistula creation of an anal opening, and repositioning of the rectal pouch into the anal opening. After repair, only about 30% with a high defect will achieve continence (Hoffenberg et al., 2014). A major challenge for either type of surgical repair is finding, using, or creating adequate nerve and muscle structures around the rectum to provide for normal evacuation.

Nursing Assessment

In the newborn, observe for an appropriate anal opening. If the anal opening exists, observe for passage of meconium stool within the first 24 hours of life (generally not passed in the infant with imperforate anus). Assess urine output to identify accompanying genitourinary problems. Assess for signs of intestinal obstruction, which may occur as a result of the malformation. These include abdominal distention and bilious vomiting. Refer to Chapter 24 for information related to nursing assessment in the newborn period. In the older infant, noted condition of the stoma, as well as quantity and quality of stoma output.

Nursing Management

Nursing management focuses on preparing the infant for surgery and providing postoperative care. It is important to provide the parents with a full explanation of the typical postoperative course, and long-term care needed. Postoperative care includes pain management, maintaining NPO status and gastric decompression until normal bowel function is restored, and providing colostomy care, if applicable. Following anoplasty surgery, dilatation is often necessary. The nurse will need to instruct parents to use the dilators supplied by the surgical team,

which can be an upsetting time for parents. In addition, after the intestinal pull-through procedure is completed, it will be the first time that stool has passed through the anal sphincter. The stool may be quite loose depending on the severity of the imperforate anus. The perianal skin is at significant risk for breakdown. Therefore, use a barrier cream on the area and clean it once daily with soap and water. Otherwise, wipe liquid stool off the barrier cream with mineral oil and cotton balls. Most of the barrier cream will remain intact, protecting the infant's perianal area.

Take Note!

To decrease the drying associated with frequent cleaning, avoid baby wipes and frequent use of soap and water.

Meckel Diverticulum

Meckel diverticulum is the result of an incomplete fusion of the omphalomesenteric duct during embryonic development. This causes a fibrous band to connect the small intestine to the umbilicus, known as a Meckel diverticulum. It is the most common congenital anomaly of the GI tract, occurring in 1.5% of the population (Hoffenberg et al., 2014). Complications associated with Meckel diverticulum include bleeding, anemia, and intestinal obstruction such as volvulus and intussusception, half of which occur within the first 2 years of life (Hoffenberg et al., 2014). Surgical correction of the Meckel diverticulum is necessary in children who have complications. The surgery is usually done to remove the diverticulum itself. At times, ileal resection is necessary.

Nursing Assessment

For a full description of the assessment phase of the nursing process, refer to the earlier assessment section. Assessment findings pertinent to Meckel diverticulum are discussed below.

HEALTH HISTORY

Elicit a description of the present illness and chief complaint. Common signs and symptoms reported during the health history might include:

- Bleeding (painless)
- Anemia
- Severe colicky abdominal pain (in children with associated intestinal obstruction)

PHYSICAL EXAMINATION

Assess the child for an acute abdomen. Observe for abdominal distention, auscultate for hypoactive bowel sounds, and then palpate for an abdominal mass, **guarding** (tensing of the abdominal wall muscles), and rebound tenderness. Assess for rectal bleeding and signs of low hemoglobin.

LABORATORY AND DIAGNOSTIC TESTS

Common laboratory and diagnostic tests ordered for assessment of Meckel diverticulum include:

- Abdominal x-rays to rule out an acute obstructive process
- Meckel scan (conclusive)
- Stool tests for colour, consistency, and frank or occult blood (usually positive in Meckel diverticulum)
- Complete blood count (CBC) to assess for anemia

Nursing Management

If anemia is significant, administer ordered blood products (packed red blood cells) to stabilize the child before surgery. Administer intravenous fluids and maintain NPO status for symptomatic children while further evaluation is being performed. Immediately report an acute abdomen to a physician or nurse practitioner. Postoperative care will vary depending on the surgery that was performed. Provide child and family education as necessary to relieve anxiety related to the diagnosis and surgical intervention. Refer to Nursing Care Plan 42.1 at the end of the chapter for additional information.

Inguinal and Umbilical Hernias

Inguinal and umbilical hernias are defects that occur during fetal development. Either may be visible at birth, and inguinal hernias may be noted later in life (Hoffenberg et al., 2014).

Inguinal Hernia

When the processus vaginalis fails to close completely during embryonal development, an inguinal hernia may occur. This allows the abdominal or pelvic viscera to travel through the internal inguinal ring into the inguinal canal. The hernia sacs that develop most often contain bowel in males and fallopian tubes or ovaries in females. Boys are more likely than girls to develop inguinal hernia and premature infants demonstrate an increased incidence overall (Hoffenberg et al., 2014). In boys, a hydrocele is the presence of abdominal fluid in the scrotal sac. This can be either a noncommunicating or communicating hydrocele. The noncommunicating results from residual peritoneal fluid being trapped and often disappears by 1 year of age. A communicating hydrocele is associated with a hernia. Surgical correction of the inguinal hernia is usually performed when the infant is several weeks old and has been thriving.

NURSING ASSESSMENT

Assess infants and children with an inguinal hernia for the presence of a bulging mass in the lower abdomen

FIGURE 42.7 **A.** Inguinal hernia: note the bulge in the inguinal (groin) area. **B.** Umbilical hernia: note the protrusion in the umbilical area.

or groin area (Fig. 42.7). It may be possible to visualize the mass, but often the mass is seen only during crying or straining, making it difficult to actually identify in the clinic setting.

NURSING MANAGEMENT

If a mass is felt upon palpation, the physician or nurse practitioner may attempt to reduce the hernia by pushing it back through the external inguinal ring. The physician or nurse practitioner may ask the nurse to assist in a reduction, most likely helping to hold the child in a position that will allow the physician or nurse practitioner to reduce the hernia. If reduction is not possible even with sedation, the hernia could be incarcerated (Hoffenberg et al., 2014). An incarcerated hernia could eventually lead to bowel strangulation.

Reduction is only a temporary method of managing inguinal hernias; they must be corrected surgically. The hernia should be manually reduced as needed until the time of the surgery, so teach the family how to reduce the hernia. Instruct the family to contact the surgeon immediately if the hernia becomes irreducible. Provide routine pre- and postoperative care during inguinal hernia surgical repair, including child and family education to relieve anxiety.

> **Take Note!**
>
> Tell the parents that if the child's inguinal hernia becomes hard, discoloured, or painful (evidenced by inconsolable crying), they should immediately call the physician or nurse practitioner to determine the next course of action (usually attendance at emergency department).

Umbilical Hernia

Umbilical hernia occurs commonly in preterm infants (Hoffenberg et al., 2014). An umbilical hernia is caused by an incomplete closure of the umbilical ring, allowing intestinal contents to herniate through the opening. Unlike inguinal hernias, most umbilical hernias are not corrected surgically. Most children will have spontaneous closure of the umbilical hernia by 4 years of age (Hoffenberg et al., 2014). Surgical correction is necessary only for the largest umbilical hernias that have failed to close by the time the child is 4 years old.

NURSING ASSESSMENT

Assess whether the hernia can be reduced. Notify the surgeon if the hernia will not reduce. Incarceration is extremely rare, but when it does occur, the child will report abdominal pain, tenderness, or redness at the umbilicus (Fig. 42.7).

NURSING MANAGEMENT

Since operative repair is not as likely with umbilical hernias as with inguinal hernias, the aim of nursing management is education. Teach the child and family how to reduce the hernia. The child may have some self-esteem issues related to the large protrusion of the unrepaired umbilical hernia. Teach the child coping skills to help relieve anxiety.

> **Take Note!**
>
> The use of home remedies to reduce an umbilical hernia should be discouraged because of the risk of bowel strangulation. This includes taping a quarter over a reduced umbilical hernia and the use of "belly bands" (American Academy of Pediatrics, 2015).

ACUTE GASTROINTESTINAL DISORDERS

Acute GI disorders include dehydration, vomiting, diarrhea, oral candidiasis, oral lesions, hypertrophic pyloric stenosis, necrotizing enterocolitis, intussusception, malrotation and volvulus, and appendicitis.

Dehydration

Dehydration occurs more readily in infants and young children than it does in adults. The risk is increased in infants and young children because they have an increased extracellular fluid percentage and a relative increase in body water compared with adults. Increased basal metabolic rate, increased ratio of BSA to body mass, immature renal function, and increased insensible fluid loss through temperature elevation also contribute to the increased risk for dehydration in infants and young children as compared with adults. Dehydration left unchecked leads to shock, so early recognition and treatment of dehydration is critical to prevent progression to hypovolemic shock. The goals of therapeutic management of dehydration are to restore appropriate fluid balance and to prevent complications.

Nursing Assessment

For a full description of the assessment phase of the nursing process, refer to the earlier assessment section. Assessment findings pertinent to dehydration are discussed below.

HEALTH HISTORY

Elicit a description of the present illness and chief complaint. Common signs and symptoms reported during the health history are included in Comparison Chart 42.1, which compares the clinical manifestations of mild, moderate, and severe dehydration.

Explore the child's current and past medical history for risk factors for dehydration such as:

- Diarrhea
- Vomiting
- Decreased oral intake
- Sustained high fever
- Diabetic ketoacidosis
- Extensive burns

> **Take Note!**
>
> Nurses must be able to assess a child's hydration status accurately and intervene quickly. Children are at higher risk than adults for hypovolemic shock. Dehydrated children may deteriorate very quickly and experience shock.

PHYSICAL EXAMINATION AND LABORATORY AND DIAGNOSTIC TESTS

Assess the child's hydration status, including heart rate, blood pressure, skin turgor, fontanels, oral mucosa, eyes, temperature and colour of extremities, mental status, and urine output. Children usually compensate well initially; their heart rate increases in moderate dehydration, but blood pressure remains normal until it decreases in severe dehydration.

COMPARISON CHART 42.1	DEHYDRATION		
	Mild	**Moderate**	**Severe**
Mental status/behaviour	Alert	Alert to irritable to listless	Hyperirritable to lethargic to comatose
Fontanels	Soft and flat	Sunken	Sunken
Eyes/tears	Normal	Mildly sunken orbits and decreased tears	Deeply sunken orbits and no tears
Oral mucosa	Pink and moist	Pale and slightly dry	Dry
Skin turgor	Elastic	Decreased	Tenting
Heart rate (pulse)	Normal	May be increased	Increased, progressing to bradycardia
Blood pressure	Normal	Normal to orthostatic > 10 mm Hg change	Normal, progressing to hypotension (shock)
Extremities	Warm, pink, brisk capillary refill	Delayed capillary refill	Cool, mottled, or dusky, significantly delayed capillary refill
Urine output and specific gravity	May be slightly decreased: SG > 1.020	<1 mL/kg/hr SG > 1.020 and oliguria	Significantly <1 mL/kg/hr; oliguria to anuria

Adapted from Engorn, B., & Flerlage, J. (2015). *The Harriet Lane handbook* (20th ed.). Philadelphia, PA: Saunders; and Ford, D. M. (2014). Fluid, electrolyte, and acid-base disorders & therapy. In W. W. Hay, M. J. Levin, R. R. Deterding, & M. J. Abzug (Eds.). *Current pediatric diagnosis and treatment* (22nd ed.). New York: McGraw-Hill.

Nursing Management

Nursing goals for the infant or child with dehydration are aimed at restoring fluid volume and preventing progression to hypovolemia. Provide oral rehydration to children for mild to moderate states of dehydration (see Teaching Guidelines 42.2). Children with severe dehydration should receive intravenous fluids.

Teaching Guidelines 42.2
ORAL REHYDRATION THERAPY

- Oral rehydration solution (ORS) should contain 75 mmol/L sodium chloride and 13.5 g/L glucose (standard ORS solutions include Pedialyte, Infalyte, and Ricelyte).
- Tap water, milk, undiluted fruit juice, soup, and broth are NOT appropriate for oral rehydration.
- Children with mild to moderate dehydration require 50 to 100 mL/kg of ORS over 4 hours.
- After re-evaluation, oral rehydration may need to be continued if the child is still dehydrated.
- When rehydrated, the child can resume a regular diet.

Adapted from Freedman, S. (2016). *Oral rehydration therapy.* Retrieved from http://www.uptodate.com/contents/oral-rehydration-therapy

Once initial fluid balance is restored, the physician or nurse practitioner may order intravenous fluids at the maintenance rate or as much as 1.5 times maintenance.

Maintenance fluid requirements refer to the amount needed under conditions of normal hydration. Maintenance fluid requirements may be determined with the use of the formula found in Box 42.2. In the example provided in Box 42.2, a 23-kg child will need maintenance fluid equivalent to 65 mL/hr.

The same anatomic and physiologic differences that make infants and young children susceptible to dehydration also make them susceptible to overhydration. Thus, continuously evaluate hydration status and be aware of the appropriateness of intravenous fluid orders.

BOX 42.2

FORMULA FOR FLUID MAINTENANCE

- 100 mL/kg for first 10 kg
- 50 mL/kg for next 11 to 20 kg
- 20 mL/kg for each additional kg > 20 kg
- Add together for total mL needed per 24-hour period
- Divide by 24 for mL/hr fluid requirement

Thus, for a 23-kg child:
- 100 × 10 = 1,000
- 50 × 10 = 500
- 20 × 3 = 60
- 1,000 + 500 + 60 = 1,560
  1,560/24 = 65 mL/hr

Adapted from Engorn, B., & Flerlage, J. (2015). *The Harriet Lane handbook* (20th ed.). Philadelphia, PA: Saunders.

Vomiting

Vomiting is the forceful expulsion of gastric contents through the mouth. It occurs as a reflex with three different phases:

- Prodromal period: nausea and signs of autonomic nervous system stimulation
- Retching
- Vomiting

Vomiting in infants and children has many different causes and is considered to be a symptom of some other condition. Table 42.1 lists common causes of vomiting.

Therapeutic management of vomiting most often involves slow oral rehydration and at times may require administration of antiemetics. The major concern with acute persistent vomiting is dehydration, loss of fluid, and the development of metabolic alkalosis.

Nursing Assessment

For a full description of the assessment phase of the nursing process, refer to the earlier assessment section. Assessment findings pertinent to vomiting are discussed below.

HEALTH HISTORY

Elicit a description of the present illness and chief complaint. Note onset and progression of symptoms. The assessment of an infant or child with vomiting should include a history of the vomiting events, including:

- Contents/character of the emesis
- Effort and force of vomiting episodes
- Timing (in relation to meals, as well as time of day)

Contents and character of the vomitus may give clues to the cause of vomiting. Bilious vomiting is never considered normal and suggests an obstruction, whereas bloody emesis can signify esophageal or GI bleeding (Hoffenberg et al., 2014). Assess the effort and force of vomiting to identify whether the episodes are projectile, as with pyloric stenosis, or effortless, as is often seen in gastroesophageal reflux (GER). The timing of the vomiting also is helpful in determining the cause. Vomiting that occurs several hours past meals could signify delayed gastric emptying. When vomiting occurs upon waking or in the middle of the night, particularly if it is associated with headaches, an intracranial lesion or tumour may be suspected.

Note any events associated with the vomiting, such as diarrhea or pain. Diarrhea may occur with viral gastroenteritis or food poisoning. Pain in the epigastric area could signify peptic ulcer disease (PUD), pancreatitis, or cholecystitis.

Assess the child's past medical history to identify pre-existing illnesses, drug abuse, trauma, prescribed medications, and previous abdominal surgery. Risk factors for vomiting include exposure to viruses, certain medication use, and overfeeding in an infant.

PHYSICAL EXAMINATION

Perform a physical examination, noting the child's general appearance. Note hydration status, as well as mental status changes. Note the quality of bowel sounds upon auscultation. Palpate the abdomen for the presence of abdominal masses, tenderness, or signs of trauma.

TABLE 42.1	CAUSES OF VOMITING BY TEMPORAL PATTERN		
Category	Acute	Chronic	Cyclic
Infectious	Gastroenteritis, otitis media, pharyngitis, sinusitis (acute), hepatitis, pyelonephritis, meningitis	*H. pylori*, *Giardia*, sinusitis (chronic)	Chronic sinusitis
GI	Intussusception, malrotation with volvulus, appendicitis, cholecystitis, pancreatitis	GERD, gastritis, peptic ulcer disease Inflammatory bowel disease	GERD, malrotation with volvulus
Genitourinary	Ureteropelvic junction obstruction, pyelonephritis	Pregnancy, pyelonephritis	Hydronephrosis
Endocrine (metabolic)	Diabetic ketoacidosis	Adrenal hyperplasia	Diabetic ketoacidosis, Addison disease, acute intermittent porphyria
Neurologic (raised intercranial pressure)	Concussion, subdural hematoma, brain tumour	Brain tumour, Arnold–Chiari malformation	Migraines, Arnold–Chiari malformation, brain tumour
Other	Food poisoning, toxic ingestion, food intolerance, or psychogenic disorders	Bulimia, rumination	Cyclic vomiting syndrome

LABORATORY AND DIAGNOSTIC TESTS

Laboratory studies may be ordered to assess the child's hydration status or to rule out certain causes of vomiting, such as urinary tract infection, pancreatitis, or an acute infectious process. Common laboratory and diagnostic tests ordered for assessment of the cause of vomiting include:

- Abdominal ultrasound
- Upper GI series
- Plain abdominal x-rays

Nursing Management

Nursing management focuses on promoting fluid and electrolyte balance. Oral rehydration is accomplished successfully in most outpatient cases of simple vomiting. Teach the primary caregiver about oral rehydration (refer to Teaching Guidelines 42.2). In the child with mild to moderate dehydration resulting from vomiting, withhold oral feeding for 1 to 2 hours after emesis, after which time oral rehydration can begin. Give the infant or child 15 to 60 mL (0.5 to 2 oz) of oral rehydration solution every 15 minutes, depending on the child's age and size. Most infants and children can retain this small amount of fluid if fed the restricted amount every 15 minutes. As the child improves, larger amounts will be tolerated.

Take Note!

Homemade oral rehydration solution can be made by combining 1 quart of water (can be water poured from cooking rice if desired), 8 teaspoons sugar, and 1 teaspoon salt.

If oral rehydration is not possible due to continued nausea and vomiting, intravenous fluids will likely be ordered. In some cases, antiemetics may be used to help control the vomiting. Some antiemetics can cause drowsiness or other side effects and should not be used until a definitive diagnosis is made or severe pathologic processes can be excluded (Hoffenberg et al., 2014).

Take Note!

Ginger capsules, ginger tea, and candied ginger are generally useful in reducing nausea, are safe for use in children over age 2 years, and usually produce no side effects (University of Maryland Medical Center, 2016).

Diarrhea

Diarrhea is either an increase in the frequency or a decrease in the consistency of stool. Diarrhea in children can either be acute or chronic. In the developed world, viruses account for most diarrhea cases leading to more than 1.5 million office visits and 200,000 hospitalizations each year (Fleisher, 2014). Foodborne illnesses are most common in Indigenous Canadian children, especially those from more rural communities, which can result in diarrhea and illness (Jung & Skinner, 2017).

Pathophysiology

Acute diarrhea in children is most commonly caused by viruses, but it may also be related to bacterial or parasitic enteropathogens. Viruses injure the absorptive surface of mature villous cells, resulting in decreased fluid absorption and disaccharidase deficiency. Bacteria produce intestinal injury by directly invading the mucosa, damaging the villous surface, or releasing toxins. Acute diarrhea may be bloody or nonbloody. The viral, bacterial, and parasitic causes of acute infectious diarrhea are discussed in Box 42.3. Diarrhea may also occur in relation to antibiotic use. Risk factors for acute diarrhea include recent ingestion of undercooked meats, raw food or fermented food (Jung & Skinner, 2017), foreign travel, day care attendance, and drinking contaminated water.

Since most cases of diarrhea are acute and viral in nature, therapeutic management of diarrhea is usually supportive (maintaining fluid balance and nutrition). Probiotic supplementation may decrease the length and extent of diarrhea in otherwise healthy children (Hoffenberg et al., 2014).

Chronic diarrhea is defined as increased water content in stool as well as increased frequency lasting for more than 2 weeks. This type of diarrhea is not usually caused by serious illnesses but by chronic conditions such as malabsorption syndromes, inflammatory bowel disease (IBD), and food allergy. The causes of chronic diarrhea are listed according to age groups in Box 42.4.

Nursing Assessment

For a full description of the assessment phase of the nursing process, refer to the Assessment section of the Nursing Process Overview earlier in the chapter. Assessment findings pertinent to diarrhea are discussed below.

HEALTH HISTORY

Elicit a description of the present illness and chief complaint. Important information related to the course of the diarrhea includes:

- Number and frequency of stools
- Duration of symptoms
- Stool volume
- Associated symptoms (abdominal pain, cramping, nausea, vomiting, fever)
- Presence of blood or mucus in the stool

Explore the child's current and past medical history for risk factors such as:

- Likelihood of exposure to infectious agents (well water, farm animals, day care attendance)

BOX 42.3

ACUTE INFECTIOUS DIARRHEA

Causes	Manifestations	Distinguishing Features	Treatment
Viruses: rotavirus, adenovirus, norovirus, parvovirus, pestivirus, calicivirus, astrovirus, cytomegalovirus	Loose, watery stools, fever, vomiting	Rotavirus most common, especially in young children Norovirus more common in older children	Supportive care: oral rehydration, electrolyte replacement in some cases, early refeeding of diet. Antidiarrheals are not effective
Bacteria: *Salmonella, Shigella,* *Escherichia coli* 0157:H7, *Campylobacter,* *Clostridium difficile,* *Yersinia enterocolitica*	Stools may be bloody or mucousy	*Salmonella* may be shed for a year *E. coli* 0157:H7 causes hemolytic anemia *Clostridium difficile* results from antibiotic use	Rehydration, early refeeding of diet. Some but not all cases require antibiotic therapy
Parasites: *Giardia lamblia,* *Entamoeba histolytica,* *Cryptosporidium*	Fever, watery stools	Oral–fecal transmission, *Cryptosporidium* spread by farm animals	Some cases require antiparasitic therapy

Adapted from Hoffenberg, E., Brumbaugh, D., Furuta, G. T., Kobak, G., Liu, E., Soden, J., & Kramer, R. (2014). Gastrointestinal tract. In W. W. Hay, M. J. Levin, R. R. Deterding, & M. J. Abzug (Eds.). *Current pediatric diagnosis and treatment* (22nd ed.). New York: McGraw-Hill; and Gilger, M. A. (2016). *Pathogenesis of acute diarrhea in children*. Retrieved from http://www.uptodate.com/contents/pathogenesis-of-acute-diarrhea-in-children

- Dietary history
- Family history of similar symptoms
- Recent travel
- Child's age (to identify common etiology for that age group)

PHYSICAL EXAMINATION

Inspection. Assess the child with diarrhea for dehydration. Observe the child's general appearance and colour. Review the signs of dehydration (see Comparison Chart 42.1) and also consider the child's weight loss. Generally, in infants and children, weight loss can indicate mild dehydration (loss between 3% and 5%), moderate (loss 6% and 9%), and severe >10%. Abdominal distention or concavity may be present. Stool output may be available to assess for colour and consistency. Inspect the anal area for presence of redness or rash related to increased stool volumes and increased frequency.

Auscultation. Auscultate bowel sounds to assess for the presence of hypoactive or hyperactive bowel sounds. Hypoactive bowel sounds may indicate obstruction or peritonitis. Hyperactive bowel sounds may indicate diarrhea/gastroenteritis.

Percussion. Percuss the abdomen. Note any abnormalities. The presence of abnormalities on examination for a diagnosis of acute or chronic diarrhea would indicate a pathologic process.

Palpation. Tenderness in the lower quadrants may be related to gastroenteritis. Rebound tenderness or pain should not be found on palpation. If found, it could indicate appendicitis or peritonitis.

BOX 42.4

CAUSES OF CHRONIC DIARRHEA BY AGE

Infants	Toddlers	School-Age Children
Intractable diarrhea of infancy	Chronic nonspecific diarrhea	Inflammatory bowel disease
Milk and soy protein intolerance	Viral enteritis	Appendiceal abscess
Infectious enteritis	*Giardia*	Lactase deficiency
Hirschsprung disease	Tumours (secretory diarrhea)	Constipation with encopresis
Nutrient malabsorption syndromes	Inflammatory bowel disease	
Immunodeficiency	Celiac disease	

LABORATORY AND DIAGNOSTIC TESTS

Common laboratory and diagnostic studies ordered for the assessment of diarrhea include:

- Stool culture: may indicate presence of bacteria
- Stool for ova and parasites (O&P): may indicate the presence of parasites
- Stool viral panel or culture: to determine the presence of rotavirus or other viruses
- Stool for occult blood: may be positive if inflammation or ulceration is present in the GI tract
- Stool for leukocytes: may be positive in cases of inflammation or infection
- Stool pH/reducing substances: to see if the diarrhea is caused by carbohydrate intolerance
- Electrolyte panel: may indicate dehydration
- Abdominal x-rays (KUB): presence of stool in colon may indicate constipation or **fecal impaction** (hardened immobile bulk of stool); air–fluid levels may indicate intestinal obstruction

Nursing Management

Nursing management of the child with diarrhea focuses on restoring fluid and electrolyte balance and providing family education.

RESTORING FLUID AND ELECTROLYTE BALANCE

Continue the child's regular diet if the child is not dehydrated. Initial nursing management of the dehydrated child with diarrhea is focused on fluid and electrolyte balance restoration. Refer to Nursing Care Plan 42.1. Probiotic supplementation while a child is taking antibiotics for other disorders may reduce the incidence of antibiotic-related diarrhea (Hoffenberg et al., 2014) (see Common Medical Treatments 42.1 and Evidence-Based Practice 42.1). After rehydration is achieved, it is important to encourage the child to consume a regular diet to maintain energy and growth.

Take Note!

Avoid prolonged use of clear liquids in the child with diarrhea because "starvation stools" may result. Also avoid fluids high in glucose, such as fruit juice, gelatin, and soda, which may worsen diarrhea (Fleisher, 2014).

PROVIDING FAMILY EDUCATION

Teach the parents the importance of oral rehydration therapy (see Teaching Guidelines 42.2). The physician may order medication therapy. In such instances, teach the importance of finishing all prescribed antibiotic therapy. After the cause of the diarrhea is known, teach the child and family how to prevent further occurrences. As most cases of acute diarrhea are infectious, provide education about proper handwashing techniques and transmission route.

Oral Candidiasis (Thrush)

Oral candidiasis (thrush) is a fungal infection of the oral mucosa. It is most common in newborns and infants. Children at risk for thrush include those with immune disorders, those using corticosteroid inhalers, and those receiving therapy that suppresses the immune system (e.g., chemotherapy for cancer). Antibiotic use may also contribute to thrush. In addition, fungal infection may be transmitted between the infant and the breastfeeding mother. Therapeutic management includes treatment with oral antifungal agents such as nystatin or fluconazole.

Nursing Assessment

Assess for risk factors for oral candidiasis such as young age, immune suppression, antibiotic use, use of corticosteroid inhalers, or presence of fungal infection in the mother. Inspect the oral mucosa. Thrush appears as thick

---

EVIDENCE-BASED PRACTICE 42.1   PROBIOTICS FOR TREATING ACUTE INFECTIOUS DIARRHEA

STUDY

Diarrhea (more than three loose, watery stools in a 24-hour period) occurs frequently in children, and can result in dehydration. Most cases of diarrhea are caused by viruses, thereby warranting symptomatic management. The authors reviewed 63 RCTs with >8,000 pooled participants, most of which were infants and young children. The studies evaluated the use of probiotics as compared with placebo or no treatment in relation to the severity and length of diarrhea.

Findings

A variety of probiotics were noted to reduce stool frequency in infants and children as well as adults, as well as shortening the course of diarrhea. The results were statistically significant, leading the authors to determine that probiotic therapy during acute diarrhea may be beneficial.

Nursing Implications

Probiotics are available as supplements: capsules or powder that may be sprinkled on food. In addition, live culture yogurt contains probiotics. Recommend these additions to the diet of older infants or children with acute diarrhea.

Adapted from Allen, S. J., Martinez, E. G., Gregorio, G. V., & Dans, L. F. (2010). *Probiotics for treating acute infectious diarrhoea (review). The Cochrane Library 2007, 12.* Indianapolis, IN: John Wiley & Sons.

FIGURE 42.8 Thick white patches in the infant with oral candidiasis (thrush). Diagnosis is usually based on clinical presentation. However, a careful scraping of the lesions can be sent out for fungal culture.

white patches on the tongue, mucosa, or palate, resembling curdled milk (Fig. 42.8). Unlike milk retained in the mouth, the patches do not easily wipe off with a swab or washcloth. Also assess for the presence of candida diaper rash (beefy-red rash with satellite lesions). Determine the extent to which the presence of the lesions is interfering with the infant's ability to feed. The lesions may cause significant discomfort.

Nursing Management

Nursing management of the child with thrush includes administering medications and providing family education.

ADMINISTERING MEDICATIONS

Ensure appropriate administration of oral antifungal agents. Administer nystatin suspension four times per day following feeding to allow the medication to remain in contact with the lesions. In the younger infant, apply nystatin to the lesions with a cotton-tipped applicator. The older infant or child can easily swallow the pleasantly flavoured suspension. An advantage of fluconazole is its once-daily dosing, but monitor infants and children receiving it for hepatotoxicity. Unlike nystatin, it is important to administer fluconazole with food to decrease the side effects of nausea and vomiting.

EDUCATING THE FAMILY

If the mother is also infected, she must receive antifungal treatment as well. Fungal infection of the breast can cause the mother a great deal of pain, but if appropriately treated breastfeeding can continue without interruption. Stress appropriate handwashing. It is important to keep bottle nipples and pacifiers clean. Infants and young children often mouth their toys, so it is important to clean them appropriately. Explain to parents of infants with thrush the importance of reporting diaper rash because fungal infections in the diaper area often occur concomitantly with thrush and also need to be treated.

Take Note!

Geographic tongue is a benign, noncontagious condition. A reduction in the filiform papillae (bumps on the tongue) occurs in patches that migrate periodically, thus giving a map-like appearance to the tongue, with darker and lighter, higher and lower patches. Do not confuse the lighter patches of geographic tongue with the thick white plaques that form on the tongue with thrush.

Oral Lesions

A number of oral lesions may affect infants and children. A few of the most common are aphthous ulcers, gingivostomatitis (from herpes simplex virus [HSV]), and herpangina. Table 42.2 lists the causes of common oral lesions. Regardless of type, oral lesions are often painful and can interfere with the child's ability to eat. Therapeutic management of oral lesions varies depending on the cause.

Nursing Assessment

Explore the health history for the presence of risk factors such as immune deficiency, cancer chemotherapy treatment, exposure to infectious agents, trauma, stress, or celiac or Crohn disease. Note the onset of the lesion(s) and progression over time. Question the parent or child about the presence of sore throat or dysphagia (occurs with herpangina). Inspect the oral cavity, including the tongue, buccal mucosa, palate, and hypoglossal area. Note the presence of lesions and their distribution. Refer to Table 42.2 for descriptions and illustrations of various oral lesions. Inspect the pharynx, which may be red with herpangina. Generally, the diagnosis is based on the history and clinical presentation, but occasionally oral lesions are cultured for HSV.

Nursing Management

The primary concerns with oral lesions are pain management and maintenance of hydration. A corticosteroid-containing dental paste used for aphthous ulcers is formulated to "stick" to mucous membranes, so the lesion area should be as dry as possible prior to application of the paste. Children do not care for having the paste applied and will often resist. Older children with herpangina or stomatitis can "swish and spit" various formulations of "magic mouthwash" (typically a combination of liquid diphenhydramine, liquid acetaminophen,

TABLE 42.2	ORAL LESIONS		
	Aphthous Ulcers	**Gingivostomatitis**	**Herpangina**
Cause	Trauma, vitamin deficiency, celiac disease, Crohn disease	Herpes simplex virus	Enterovirus (Coxsackie)
Appearance	Erythematous border, often yellow appearance to the ulcer, anywhere on oral mucosa or lips	Vesicular lesions on erythematous base, anywhere in oral cavity, including lips	Bright-red ulcers, generally in posterior oral cavity
Fever	Generally absent	May have high fever with initial outbreak	Abrupt onset of high fever (up to 39.4–40.6°C), lasting 1–4 days
Length of illness	Generally heal within 7–14 days; may recur	10–12 days initially; may recur with stress, febrile illness, or intense sunlight exposure (as virus lies dormant in system)	Generally resolves within 5–7 days
Therapeutic management	Topical corticosteroid in dental paste may help	Acyclovir	Supportive treatment only

Adapted from Ben-Joseph, E. P. (2013). *Canker sores.* Retrieved from http://kidshealth.org/parent/general/aches/canker.html#; Keels, M. A., & Clements, D. A. (2015). *Herpetic gingivostomatitis in young children.* Retrieved from http://www.uptodate.com/contents/herpetic-gingivostomatitis-in-young-children; and Romero, J. R. (2015). *Hand, foot, and mouth disease and herpangina: An overview.* Retrieved from http://www.uptodate.com/contents/hand-foot-and-mouth-disease-and-herpangina-an-overview

and milk of magnesia); they may offer some pain relief. Common over-the-counter medications often contain benzocaine. Caution and advice needs to be given to parents to be alert to any side effects.

The child with herpangina is typically an infant or young child (Romero, 2015). It may be very difficult to coach a young child to drink fluids when his or her mouth is hurting. Playing games and offering favourite fluids and popsicles may encourage adequate oral intake. It is important to avoid carbonated beverages and citrus juices when oral lesions are present as they can cause further stinging and burning. Fluids that are lukewarm are usually better tolerated than hot or cold fluids.

Take Note!

Viscous lidocaine should be used with caution in younger children as a topical treatment for numbing the lesions or as a swish-and-spit treatment because they may swallow the lidocaine (Taketomo, Hodding, & Kraus, 2013).

Hypertrophic Pyloric Stenosis

In hypertrophic pyloric stenosis, the circular muscle of the pylorus becomes hypertrophied, causing thickness in the luminal side of the pyloric canal (Fig. 42.9). This thickness creates a gastric outlet obstruction, causing nonbilious vomiting that presents between weeks 3 and 6 of life. The vomiting becomes more frequent and forceful as time goes on and is often projectile. The incidence

is 2 to 3.5 per 1,000 live births, occurring more often in males than females, with 30% to 40% being in first-born infants (Olivé & Endom, 2016). The cause of pyloric stenosis is probably multifactorial.

Pyloric stenosis requires surgical intervention. A pyloromyotomy is performed to cut the muscle of the pylorus and relieve the gastric outlet obstruction (Fig. 42.9). Postoperative complications are rare.

A

B

FIGURE 42.9 **A.** Hypertrophied pylorus muscle and narrowed stomach outlet. **B.** In pyloromyotomy, the pylorus is incised, thus increasing the diameter of the pyloric outlet.

Nursing Assessment

For a full description of the assessment phase of the nursing process, refer to the Assessment section in the Nursing Process Overview earlier in the chapter. Assessment findings pertinent to hypertrophic pyloric stenosis are discussed below.

HEALTH HISTORY

Elicit a description of the present illness and chief complaint. Common signs and symptoms reported during the health history might include:

- Forceful, nonbilious vomiting, unrelated to feeding position
- Hunger soon after vomiting episode
- Weight loss due to vomiting
- Progressive dehydration with subsequent lethargy
- Possible positive family history

PHYSICAL EXAMINATION AND LABORATORY AND DIAGNOSTIC TESTS

Palpate for a hard, moveable "olive" in the right upper quadrant (hypertrophied pylorus). If an easily palpable mass is felt, no further testing is necessary and a surgical consult is called. If no mass is identified, a pyloric ultrasound may be ordered to identify a thickened hypoechoic ring in the region of the pylorus. An upper GI series may identify pyloric stenosis as well, but an ultrasound is less invasive and is considered more diagnostic of pyloric stenosis. Assess laboratory values to determine if the infant has metabolic alkalosis resulting from dehydration.

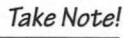

Take Note!

It may be difficult to examine the infant's abdomen when pyloric stenosis is suspected because of the infant's extreme irritability. A pacifier or nipple dipped in glucose water may soothe the infant long enough to perform the abdominal examination.

Nursing Management

Preoperative management of infants with pyloric stenosis is aimed at fluid management and correcting abnormal electrolyte values. Family anxiety is high during this time because of the impending surgery for an otherwise healthy infant. Provide emotional support to the family. Teach them about the surgical procedure and what to expect postoperatively. After surgery, infants usually resume oral feedings after 1 to 2 days.

Intussusception

Intussusception is a process that occurs when a proximal segment of bowel "telescopes" into a more distal

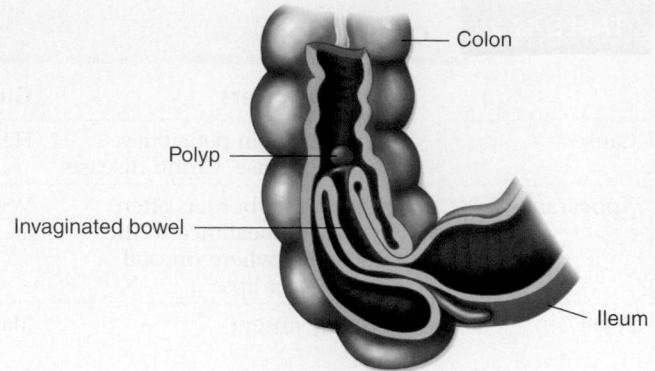

FIGURE 42.10 In intussusception, the intestine telescopes upon itself.

segment, causing edema, vascular compromise, and, ultimately, partial or total bowel obstruction (Fig. 42.10). In children younger than 2 years of age, intussusception is the most common cause of intestinal obstruction (Galloway & Seguias, 2013). A lead point (i.e., pathologic point) may cause the telescoping. Examples of lead points are Meckel diverticulum, duplication cysts, polyps, hemangiomas, tumours, or the appendix.

A barium or air enema can be successful at reducing a large percentage of intussusception cases; other cases are reduced surgically. If surgical reduction is unsuccessful or bowel necrosis has occurred, a portion of the bowel must be resected.

Nursing Assessment

For a full description of the assessment phase of the nursing process, refer to the Assessment section in the Nursing Process Overview earlier in the chapter. Assessment findings pertinent to intussusception are discussed below.

HEALTH HISTORY

Elicit a description of the present illness and chief complaint. Common signs and symptoms reported during the health history might include:

- Sudden onset of intermittent, crampy abdominal pain
- Severe pain (children usually draw up their knees and scream)
- Vomiting
- Diarrhea
- Currant-jelly stools, gross blood, or hemoccult-positive stools
- Lethargy

Typically, symptoms flare and then regress. Between episodes, children may have no symptoms of intussusception. This return to a normal state is due to the intussusception reducing on its own. The child may be asymptomatic and may appear well when presenting to the physician or nurse practitioner or emergency room.

Again, this may be a sign that the bowel has reduced spontaneously. Assess the severity of pain, length of time the symptoms have been present, presence of vomiting, and stool patterns and colour. Immediately report the presence of bilious vomiting, which occurs only in an obstructive situation. Also, assess for signs and symptoms of acute peritonitis. Explore the child's current and past medical history for risk factors, such as cystic fibrosis or celiac disease.

PHYSICAL EXAMINATION
Palpate the abdomen for the presence of a sausage-shaped mass in the upper midabdomen; this is a hallmark sign of intussusception. Note any mental status changes.

LABORATORY AND DIAGNOSTIC TESTS
Intussusception is usually diagnosed with an air or barium enema. Use of an enema may show the intussusception and also may reduce it, making the enema therapeutic. A pediatric surgeon should be available at the time the enema is given in case the enema is unsuccessful or perforation (rare) occurs. White blood cell elevation may occur and electrolytes may show signs of dehydration.

Nursing Management

Administer intravenous fluids and antibiotics before the diagnostic laboratory and x-ray studies are performed. Refer to Nursing Care Plan 42.1, at the end of the chapter, for nursing management of the postoperative child.

The parents may be very fatigued after dealing with a crying infant. They are often quite anxious about surgery in an otherwise healthy child. Offer emotional support and provide appropriate preoperative and postoperative education to the family.

Malrotation and Volvulus

Intestinal malrotation results from a disruption in embryonic development. When malrotation occurs, the intestine is abnormally attached and the mesentery narrows, twisting on itself (volvulus). If the volvulus involves the entire small bowel, it is termed a midgut volvulus.

The main symptom of malrotation is bilious vomiting. Many children also have abdominal pain, shock symptoms, abdominal distention, tachycardia, and bloody stools. Most cases of malrotation will present in the first few weeks of life, but symptoms may occur in the older infant, child, or adult (Brandt, 2014).

Therapeutic management of malrotation and volvulus is accomplished surgically. A Ladd procedure is performed, during which the intestine is straightened out and bands contributing to the misalignment are divided. If bowel necrosis has occurred (rare), then an ostomy may be necessary.

Nursing Assessment

For a full description of the assessment phase of the nursing process, refer to the Assessment section in the Nursing Process Overview earlier in the chapter. Assessment findings pertinent to malrotation and volvulus are discussed below.

HEALTH HISTORY
Elicit a description of the present illness and chief complaint. Common signs and symptoms reported during the health history might include vomiting and abdominal pain. Since obstruction can occur with resulting necrosis of the bowel, immediately inform the physician if obstruction is suspected.

PHYSICAL EXAMINATION AND DIAGNOSTIC AND LABORATORY TESTS
Observe for severity of pain, auscultate for hypoactive bowel sounds, and palpate for abdominal guarding or rebound tenderness. Common laboratory and diagnostic studies ordered for the assessment of malrotation and volvulus include:
- KUB to reveal obstruction
- Upper GI series to identify the location of the duodenojejunal junction and corkscrew appearance of the twisted bowel

Nursing Management

When diagnostic testing reveals malrotation/volvulus, administer ordered intravenous fluids and intravenous antibiotics. Often a nasogastric tube is placed to decompress the stomach. Surgery is performed as soon as possible. After surgery, provide postoperative care of the child (see Nursing Care Plan 42.1 at the end of the chapter). Provide continuous emotional support and family education.

Appendicitis

Appendicitis, an acute inflammation of the appendix, is the most common cause of emergent abdominal surgery in children (Hoffenberg et al., 2014). It occurs in all age groups; the median age in the pediatric population is 4 to 15 years (Wall & Albanese, 2015). Outcomes in Canadian children can be influenced by age and treatment level factors while rurality and socioeconomic factors do not affect outcome (Cheong & Emil, 2014).

Pathophysiology

Appendicitis is due to a closed-loop obstruction of the appendix (Fig. 42.11). It is thought that the obstruction is due to fecal material impacted into the relatively narrow appendix, though other causes such as

FIGURE 42.11 **A.** In appendicitis, the lumen of the appendix is obstructed, resulting in edema and compressed blood vessels. **B.** As appendicitis progresses, pain may become localized at McBurney's point.

ingested foreign bodies may exist. This causes a subsequent increase in the intraluminal pressure of the appendix, resulting in mucosal edema, bacterial overgrowth, and eventual perforation. The rate of perforation is high in children, especially those under 2 years old (Hoffenberg et al., 2014). Due to the fecal material in the appendix, perforation causes inflammatory fluid and bacterial contents to leak into the abdominal cavity, resulting in peritonitis. Diffuse peritonitis is more likely in younger children. Older children and adolescents have a more developed omentum, which walls off the inflamed or perforated appendix, often causing a focal abscess.

Therapeutic Management

Appendicitis is considered an emergency because if left uninvestigated or uncorrected, the appendix may perforate. Surgical removal of the appendix may be necessary and is often accomplished via a minimally invasive laparoscopic technique. In the case of perforation, an open surgical procedure is usually required, and lavage of the abdominal cavity may be performed to cleanse it of the infected fluid released from the appendix.

Nursing Assessment

Early diagnosis and intervention are the key elements to avoid perforation. For a full description of the assessment phase of the nursing process, refer to the Assessment section in the Nursing Process Overview earlier in the chapter. Assessment findings pertinent to appendicitis are discussed below.

HEALTH HISTORY

Elicit a description of the present illness and chief complaint. Appendicitis may be gradual, but symptoms usually do not come and go; they remain persistent and intensify. Common signs and symptoms reported during the health history might include:

- Vague abdominal pain in the initial stages, maybe periumbilical pain at first descending to the right lower quadrant. Abdominal pain that is most intense at McBurney's point (one third distance from anterior superior iliac spine to the umbilicus). Referred pain may indicate the presence of peritoneal irritation.
- Side lying position, maybe difficulty walking, and pain in the right hip. Rebound tenderness and abdominal rigidity.

- Anorexia, nausea, and vomiting (which usually develop after the onset of pain)
- Small-volume, frequent, soft stools, often confused with diarrhea
- Fever (usually low grade unless perforation occurs, which results in high fever) with elevated white cell count.

Thinking About Development

As many as 40% of children with appendicitis experience referred pain (Hoffenberg et al., 2014). How will you accurately assess pain location in a school-age child, as compared with a toddler?

PHYSICAL EXAMINATION

Children with appendicitis often appear anorexic and ill. They often cannot walk or climb up onto the examination table without assistance. Upon palpation, maximal tenderness occurs over the McBurney's point in the right lower quadrant (Fig. 42.11).

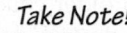

Take Note!

If the child's abdominal pain is suddenly relieved without intervention, suspect perforation and notify the physician immediately.

Assess the abdomen for acute peritonitis, as indicated by diffuse abdominal tenderness or distention. Immediately report positive findings to a physician or nurse practitioner.

LABORATORY AND DIAGNOSTIC TESTS

Common laboratory and diagnostic studies ordered for the assessment of appendicitis include:

- Abdominal computed tomography (CT) scan: performed to visualize the appendix for further evaluation
- Laboratory testing: may reveal an elevated white blood cell count
- C-reactive protein: may be elevated

Nursing Management

Provide preoperative and postoperative care and child and family education (see Nursing Care Plan 42.1 at the end of the chapter). Care depends on what was found during surgical exploration. A nonruptured, nongangrenous appendix usually requires no antibiotic therapy, so provide routine surgical care.

In addition to routine surgical care, administer 48 to 72 hours of ordered antibiotics to the child with a suppurative or gangrenous (nonperforated) appendix to decrease the risk of postoperative infection. The child

with a perforated appendix will require 7 to 14 days of intravenous antibiotic therapy in addition to normal postoperative care. Provide family teaching, because the child is often discharged home while still receiving intravenous antibiotic therapy.

Atraumatic Care

For the child requiring a postsurgical dressing change, make sure to administer prescribed analgesia. Use distractions techniques appropriate for age and/or personal preference. Work with the child life specialist to plan for interventions to maximize child/youth control and to be respectful of their wishes.

CHRONIC GASTROINTESTINAL DISORDERS

Chronic GI disorders include GER, PUD, constipation/encopresis, Hirschsprung disease, short bowel syndrome, IBD, celiac disease, functional abdominal pain, failure to thrive, and chronic feeding problems.

Gastroesophageal Reflux

GER is passage of gastric contents into the esophagus. It is considered a normal physiologic process that occurs in healthy infants and children. However, when complications develop from the reflux of gastric contents back into the esophagus or oropharynx, it becomes more of a pathologic process known as gastroesophageal reflux disease (GERD). GER occurs frequently during the first year of life, is considered benign, and usually resolves by 12 to 18 months of age (Hoffenberg et al., 2014). GER is particularly common in premature infants. Other possible diagnoses that can be mistaken for GER include food allergies, formula enteropathies, gastric outlet obstruction, malrotation, cyclic vomiting, and central nervous system lesions.

Pathophysiology

The process of GER occurs during episodes of transient relaxation of the LES, which can occur during swallowing, crying, or other Valsalva manoeuvres that increase intra-abdominal pressure. Delayed esophageal clearance and gastric emptying, highly acidic gastric contents, hiatal hernia (protrusion of the stomach upward into the mediastinal cavity through the esophageal hiatus of the diaphragm), or neurologic disease may also be contributing factors associated with reflux.

The signs and symptoms of GERD are often seen as a result of the damaging components of the refluxate (the pH of the gastric contents, bile acids, and pepsin). The longer the pH of the refluxate is below 4, the higher the suspicion of GERD, but results must be correlated with the child's clinical presentation (Winter, 2015). Symptoms of GERD in infants and children are listed below in the Health History section.

GERD may cause esophagitis, esophageal stricture, Barrett esophagus (a precancerous condition), or anemia from chronic esophageal erosion. In addition, complications such as laryngitis, recurrent pneumonia, or worsening asthma may occur.

Therapeutic Management

Conservative medical management begins with appropriate positioning, such as elevating the head of the bed and keeping the infant or child upright for 30 minutes after feeding. Smaller, more frequent feedings may be helpful. If reflux does not improve with these measures, medications are prescribed to decrease acid production and stabilize the pH of the gastric contents. Also, prokinetic agents may be used to help empty the stomach more quickly, minimizing the amount of gastric contents in the stomach that the child can reflux (Winter, 2016a, 2016b; Dosage Calculation Box 42.1).

Dosage Calculation Box 42.1

Infant's weight: 5.216 kg (11 lbs 8 oz)
Medication order: omeprazole 4 mg PO once a day
Per the Pediatric Dosage Handbook, the recommended dose is 0.7 mg/kg/dose
Is the ordered dose safe?

If the GERD cannot be medically managed effectively or requires long-term medication therapy, surgical intervention may be necessary. A Nissen fundoplication is the most common surgical procedure performed for antireflux therapy. The gastric fundus is wrapped around the lower 2 to 3 cm of the esophagus (Fig. 42.12). Laparoscopic fundoplications are being performed as a way to minimize the recovery period and reduce potential complications.

Nursing Assessment

For a full description of the assessment phase of the nursing process, refer to the Assessment section in the Nursing Process Overview earlier in the chapter. Assessment findings pertinent to GER are discussed below.

HEALTH HISTORY

Elicit a description of the present illness and chief complaint. Note onset and progression of symptoms. Common signs and symptoms reported during the health history include:

FIGURE 42.12 In the Nissen fundoplication, the fundus (upper portion of the stomach) is wrapped around the lower segment of the esophagus.

- Recurrent vomiting or regurgitation
- Weight loss or poor weight gain, dysphagia or feeding refusal
- Irritability in infants
- Respiratory symptoms (chronic cough, wheezing, stridor, asthma, apnea)
- Hoarseness/sore throat, otitis media
- Chronic sinusitis, halitosis (mostly in older children)
- Heartburn or chest pain or abdominal pain
- Abnormal neck posturing (Sandifer syndrome)
- Hematemesis
- Poor dentition (caused by acid erosion)

Explore the child's current and past medical history for risk factors such as:
- Prematurity, noting prolonged ventilator use or chronic lung disease, feeding positions and patterns (especially important in infants)
- Dietary habits (e.g., chocolate, coffee, spicy or fatty foods, caffeine, formula-fed or breastfed, overeating or overfeeding)
- Current medications
- Smoking/alcohol use (older children)
- Food allergies
- Other GI disorders (gastric outlet dysfunction/hiatal hernia) or congenital abnormalities
- Sleeping positions/patterns
- Other medical history, such as asthma or recurrent infections/pneumonia

PHYSICAL EXAMINATION

The physical examination consists of inspection, auscultation, percussion, and palpation.

Inspection. Observe the child's general appearance and colour. Infants and children with uncontrolled GER for a period of time may appear underweight or malnourished. Infants may be irritable due to painful regurgitation/reflux events. Note breathing patterns, because reflux-induced asthma may have developed. Acute life-threatening events (ALTEs) and apnea have been associated with severe GERD (Hoffenberg et al., 2014). Observe the child for dusky skin colour, altered mental status, and alterations in tone. Inspect emesis for blood or bile.

Auscultation. Evaluate the lung fields for the presence of complications related to GERD, such as wheezing or pneumonia. No further pathologic findings related to GERD should be auscultated on examination.

Percussion. Perform routine abdominal percussion, noting any abnormalities. No specific findings should be noted.

Palpation. Use caution when palpating the abdomen, especially with infants with GERD, because it may induce vomiting. No abnormalities should be palpated.

Take Note!

Not all infants with GERD actually vomit. Some may only demonstrate irritability associated with feeding or posturing (arching back during or after feeding [termed Sandifer syndrome]) and grimacing. Episodes of GERD often cause bradycardia, so if the above signs occur, they should be reported to the physician or nurse practitioner, even if the baby is not vomiting (Winter, 2016b). GI events may also contribute to apparent life-threatening (ALTE) or Brief Resolved Unexplained Events (BRUEs) event in infancy < 6 months of age (Zwemer, Claudius, & Tieder, 2017).

LABORATORY AND DIAGNOSTIC TESTS

Common laboratory and diagnostic studies ordered for the assessment of GER include:

- Upper GI series: though not sensitive or specific to GER, may show some reflux; studies are used to narrow down the differential diagnosis
- Esophageal pH probe study: quantifies GER episodes as they correlate to symptoms
- Esophagogastroduodenoscopy (EGD): shows esophageal and gastric tissue damage from GERD
- CBC: may demonstrate anemia if chronic esophagitis or hematemesis is present
- Hemoccult: may be positive if chronic esophagitis is present

Nursing Management

As with most GI disorders, initial nursing management is aimed at restoring proper fluid balance and nutrition. Refer to Nursing Care Plan 42.1 at the end of the chapter. Additional considerations are reviewed below.

PROMOTING SAFE FEEDING TECHNIQUES AND POSITIONING

Feeding adjustments are an essential part of reflux management. Give infants smaller, more frequent feedings using a nipple that controls flow well. Frequently burp the infant during feeds to control reflux. Thickening of the formula with products such as rice or oatmeal cereal can significantly help keep the formula and gastric contents down. Positioning after feedings is important. Keep infants upright for 30 to 45 minutes after feeding by holding them and/or elevating the head of the crib 30 degrees. Placing in infant seats or swings is not recommended as this increases intra-abdominal pressure (Winter, 2016a). For older children, elevate the head of the bed as much as possible and restrict meals for several hours before bedtime.

MAINTAINING A PATENT AIRWAY

GER symptoms often involve the airway. Maximize reflux precautions to keep the risk of airway involvement to a minimum. In rare instances, GERD causes apnea or an ALTE (Hoffenberg et al., 2014). In these cases, use an apnea or bradycardia monitor to detect such episodes. The monitor requires a physician's order and can be ordered through a home health company. Teach parents how to deal with these episodes, as their anxiety is very high. Provide cardiopulmonary resuscitation (CPR) instruction to all parents whose infant is high-risk (Zwemer et al., 2017).

EDUCATING THE FAMILY AND CHILD

The goals for the infant and child with GER are a decrease in symptoms, a decrease in the frequency and duration of reflux episodes, healing of the injured mucosa, and prevention of further complications of GERD. Teach the parents the signs and symptoms of complications. Explain that reflux is usually limited to the first year of life, though in some cases it persists. If medications are prescribed, thoroughly explain their use and their side effects (see Drug Guide 42.1).

PROVIDING POSTOPERATIVE CARE

If the child requires fundoplication, a gastrostomy tube is often placed for use in the immediate postoperative period or for long-term feeding. In the immediate postoperative period, assess for pain, abdominal distention, and return of bowel sounds. If a gastrostomy tube is placed, it is often open to straight drain for a period of time postoperatively to keep the stomach empty and allow for the internal incision to heal. When bowel sounds have returned and the infant or child is stable, introduce feedings slowly (typically via the gastrostomy tube). Assess for tolerance of feedings (absence of abdominal distention or pain, minimal residual, and passage of stool). If the abdomen does become distended or the child has discomfort, open the gastrostomy tube to air to decompress the stomach. Assess the insertion site of the gastrostomy tube for redness, edema, or drainage. Keep the site clean and dry per surgeon or hospital protocol. Teach the parents how to care for the gastrostomy tube and insertion site and how to use the tube for feeding.

PROMOTING FAMILY AND CHILD COPING

Parents may experience a great deal of anxiety. Teach the family about all aspects of GERD to help promote coping. School-age children often have reflux episodes exhibited by postprandial vomiting, which can be very embarrassing for the children. Provide education to school (if possible) or work with community nursing team.

Peptic Ulcer Disease

PUD is a term used to describe a variety of disorders of the upper GI tract that result from the action of gastric secretions (Fig. 42.13). Mucosal inflammation and subsequent ulceration occur as a result of either a primary or a secondary factor. In children, duodenal ulcers are more common than gastric ulcers (Hoffenberg et al., 2014). Primary peptic ulcers are usually associated with *Helicobacter pylori*, a Gram-negative organism that causes mucosal inflammation and in some cases more severe disease (Hoffenberg et al., 2014). *H. pylori* is found mostly in the duodenum.

Secondary peptic ulcers may occur as a result of an identifiable factor, such as excess acid production, stress, medications, or the presence of other underlying conditions. Secondary ulcers tend to be gastric in location as opposed to duodenal.

> **Take Note!**
>
> Severe stress, such as burns or another illness necessitating critical care, can contribute to the development of a peptic ulcer in children (Hoffenberg et al., 2014).

FIGURE 42.13 **Peptic ulcer disease.**

Therapeutic Management

PUD may be treated with antibiotics (if *H. pylori* is verified), histamine agonists, and/or proton pump inhibitors. If the child presents with a severe esophageal or gastric hemorrhage, a nasogastric tube may be placed to decompress the stomach. The child may require intravenous infusion of a histamine-2 receptor antagonist or a proton pump inhibitor initially until the bleeding has stopped and the disease is stabilized.

Nursing Assessment

For a full description of the assessment phase of the nursing process, refer to the Assessment section in the Nursing Process Overview earlier in the chapter. Assessment findings pertinent to PUD are discussed below.

HEALTH HISTORY

Elicit a description of the present illness and chief complaint. Common signs and symptoms reported during the health history might include:

- Abdominal pain
- GI bleeding
- Vomiting

Abdominal pain is the most common complaint of children with PUD. It is important to characterize the abdominal pain, as many other digestive disorders may mimic PUD. The pain can be mostly epigastric or periumbilical and characterized as burning pain. However, sometimes children will complain of dull and vague abdominal pain. Most often, children with PUD have pain that worsens after meals, and the pain may wake them at night. Vomiting may be noted. Explore the child's current and past medical history for risk factors such as a family history of PUD or other GI diseases, or chronic NSAID or prednisone use.

> **Take Note!**
>
> Adolescents at increased risk for the development of PUD include those who smoke, and/or use alcohol (Vakil, 2014).

PHYSICAL EXAMINATION AND LABORATORY AND DIAGNOSTIC TESTS

Palpate the abdomen for the location of the pain, which is usually epigastric or periumbilical. Note the presence of blood in emesis or stools, as GI bleeding may occur. Blood in emesis can be brown from contact with stomach acid and may look like coffee grounds. Blood from stomach that is excreted in stool may make the stool look shiny tarry black. Common laboratory and diagnostic studies ordered for the assessment of PUD include the following:

- Laboratory studies: to identify anemia
- Urea breath test: to identify active *H. pylori*
- Upper GI series: to detect presence of ulcerations

- Upper endoscopy: the definitive diagnostic test to look for ulceration and nodularity in the upper GI tract
- Biopsies: to assess for *H. pylori*, granulomas or eosinophils

Nursing Management

Hemodynamic stabilization should be the focus of nursing management if significant GI bleeding occurs. Once children are stabilized and tolerating oral feeds, they may be discharged to home. Provide discharge instructions on the following topics:
- Medications and importance of adherence
- Signs of rebleeding—when to seek medical attention
- Stress importance of medical follow-up

Constipation and Encopresis

Constipation is a very common problem among children, affecting about 30% of the pediatric population, and accounting for 3% to 5% of all pediatric outpatient visits (Sood, 2016). It may be defined as failure to achieve complete evacuation of the lower colon. Term newborns should pass a meconium stool within the first 24 hours of life. If this does not occur, the newborn may have an underlying GI disorder. Breastfed infants may produce a stool with each feeding, though some will skip a few days between stools. Most bottle-fed babies will produce a stool one or two times per day, but they may go 2 to 3 days without producing a stool. The bowel habits of both infants and children vary widely, so assess and treat each child on an individual basis.

Functional constipation occurs commonly in preschool-age children (Sood, 2016). It may be defined by the presence of at least two of the following over the course of 2 months:
- Less than three bowel movements weekly
- At least one episode of fecal incontinence weekly
- Stool-withholding behaviour (retentive posturing)
- Hard or painful bowel movements
- Large fecal rectal mass
- Stool passage of a volume to clog the toilet (Dunn, 2013; Sood, 2016)

Encopresis is a term used to describe soiling of fecal contents into the underwear beyond the age of expected toilet training (4 to 5 years of age). Encopresis is often seen as a result of chronic constipation and withholding of stool. As stool is withheld in the rectum, the rectal muscle can stretch over time, and this stretching of the rectum causes fecal impactions. Children who have a stretched rectal vault may experience liquid stool leakage around a fecal mass. This is often an embarrassing issue that occurs with school-age children, and the child may hide his or her underwear to avoid punishment. Many psychological issues arise from chronic

constipation and encopresis as the child may experience ridicule and shame (Dunn, 2013).

Pathophysiology

As stool passes through the colon, water is reabsorbed into the colon, resulting in a formed stool by the time it reaches the rectum. At this point, the anal sphincter relaxes to allow the passage of stool from the anus. In constipation, however, this relaxation does not occur.

Most causes of constipation are functional in nature (inorganic) (Sood, 2016). Children with functional constipation usually present with this problem during the toilet-training years. Children have a painful experience during defecation, which in turn creates a fear of defecation, resulting in further withholding of stool. Organic causes of constipation rarely occur in children. When they do occur, they may be a sign of a disease such as spina bifida or sacral agenesis. The causes of pediatric constipation are discussed in Table 42.3.

Therapeutic Management

Once any organic process is ruled out as a cause, constipation may initially be managed with dietary manipulation such as increasing fibre and fluids. However, behaviour modification is necessary for most children. Children need to relearn to allow bowel evacuation when stool is present. Children with severe constipation and withholding behaviours may not benefit from dietary management and may require laxative therapy. Sometimes, mechanical disimpaction is required initially, followed by the above measures.

Nursing Assessment

For a full description of the assessment phase of the nursing process, refer to the Assessment section in the Nursing Process Overview earlier in the chapter. Assessment findings pertinent to constipation/encopresis are discussed below.

HEALTH HISTORY

Elicit a description of the present illness and chief complaint. Note the onset of symptoms as described by the parent/child. Common signs and symptoms reported during the health history may include:
- Altered stooling patterns (size, frequency, amount, and colour)—using a stool chart, such as the Bristol Stool Chart, to help with descriptions provides child-friendly pictures
- Pain with defecation
- Withholding behaviours (postures to try to withhold the stool, such as crossing the legs, squatting or hiding in a corner, or "dancing")

TABLE 42.3	CAUSES OF PEDIATRIC CONSTIPATION BY AGE			

Newborn/Infant	Toddler and Ages 2–4 Years	School Age	Adolescent	Any Age
• Meconium plug • Hirschsprung disease • Cystic fibrosis • Congenital anorectal malformations • Congenital pseudo-obstruction • Endocrine: hypothyroidism • Metabolic: diabetes insipidus, renal tubular acidosis • Withholding • Dietary changes	• Anal fissures • Withholding • Toilet refusal • Short-segment Hirschsprung disease • Neurologic disorders • Spinal cord: meningomyelocele, tumours, tethered cord	• Toilet or bathroom access limited or unavailable • Limited ability to recognize physiologic cues, preoccupation with other activities • Tethered cord • Withholding	• Spinal cord injury (accidents, trauma) • Dieting • Anorexia • Pregnancy • Idiopathic slow transit constipation, particularly in females • Laxative abuse • Irritable bowel syndrome, constipation variant	• Medication side effect, dietary, postoperative state • Previous anorectal surgery • Withholding and overflow from chronic rectal distention • Relatively rapid change to sedentary state, dehydration • Hypothyroidism

Adapted from Dunn, A. (2013). Elimination patterns. In C. Burns, A. Dunn, M. Brady, N. B. Starr, & C. Blosser (Eds.). *Pediatric primary care* (5th ed.). Philadelphia, PA: Saunders; and Hoffenberg, E., Brumbaugh, D., Furuta, G. T., Kobak, G., Liu, E., Soden, J., & Kramer, R. (2014). Gastrointestinal tract. In W. W. Hay, M. J. Levin, R. R. Deterding, & M. J. Abzug (Eds.). *Current pediatric diagnosis and treatment* (22nd ed.). New York: McGraw-Hill.

• Complaints of abdominal pain and cramping and poor appetite
• Diarrhea leakage (overflow) possibly with soiling of undergarments

It is important to note the duration of the symptoms to determine an acute onset versus a chronic disorder. Explore the child's past and current medical history for risk factors such as:
• Family history of GI disorders
• History of rectal bleeding or anal fissures
• Report of first meconium stool after 24 hours of age
• History of sexual abuse

It is important to take an accurate dietary history as well as a history of fluid intake. Also, explore current medication or laxative use.

PHYSICAL EXAMINATION

Physical examination of the child with constipation consists of inspection, auscultation, percussion, and palpation.

Inspection. Observe the child's general appearance. Note whether the abdomen appears distended or rounded. Observe the lower back for a deep pilonidal dimple with hair tuft, which is suggestive of spina bifida occulta. Flat buttocks may be suggestive of sacral agenesis. Inspect the anus for signs of fissures or soiling. Inspect the child's underwear for stains or smears, which are indicative of soiling.

Auscultation. Auscultate bowel sounds to determine the possibility of an obstruction (hypoactive or absent bowel sounds) in the child with an acute case of constipation.

Percussion. Percuss the abdomen to reveal dullness, which would indicate a fecal mass.

Palpation. Palpate the abdomen for any tenderness or masses. The nurse may assist the physician or nurse practitioner with the performance of a rectal examination to assess for rectal tone and rectal vault size.

LABORATORY AND DIAGNOSTIC TESTS

Laboratory and diagnostic tests are not routine with the diagnosis of functional constipation, but if an organic cause is suspected, the following laboratory and diagnostic tests would be ordered:
• Stool for occult blood: the presence of blood could indicate some other disease process
• Abdominal x-ray: large quantities of stool may be seen in the colon
• Sitz marker study: to detect colonic dysmotility
• Barium enema: to rule out a stricture or Hirschsprung disease
• Rectal manometry: to evaluate rectal musculature dysfunction
• Rectal suction biopsy: to rule out Hirschsprung disease

Nursing Management

Nursing management for the infant or child with constipation is aimed at educating the child and family and promoting child and family coping. Refer to Nursing Care Plan 42.1 at the end of the chapter. Additional considerations are reviewed below.

EDUCATING THE FAMILY AND CHILD

Teach parents how to assess for signs of constipation and withholding behaviours. Also, provide guidelines on scheduling and supervising bowel habits in reconditioning the child to use the toilet regularly. Teach parents to use positive reinforcement techniques. For example, when the child engages in positive toilet habits, produces an adequate-volume bowel movement, reward him or her with stickers, extra playtime or an agreed incentive. Changes to diet coupled with increased fluid intake may aid in bringing extra water into the bowel, thereby softening the stool. Infants and toddlers with constipation may be experiencing constipation from formula or milk changes. Therefore, manipulating the formula or milk may result in better bowel habits.

Educate families about the importance of compliance with medication use, if medication is ordered. Parents often are very anxious about the use of these medications, but stress to them that compliance is essential and stopping too early can result in a return of symptoms.

Nursing Procedure 42.2 gives instructions on enema administration in children. Explain the procedure to the child in developmentally appropriate terms. Enema administration can be uncomfortable, but calming measures, such as distraction and praise, provide a comforting environment. After the impaction is removed, promote regular bowel habits to keep the impaction from recurring.

PROMOTING CHILD AND FAMILY COPING

Childhood constipation can be a very stressful process for both the child and family. Behaviour modification is necessary for many children. To facilitate daily bowel evacuation, the child should sit on the toilet twice a day (after breakfast and dinner) for 5 to 8 minutes. A stool by the toilet should be used to allow the child to have their feet supported. Instruct the family to keep a "star" or reward chart to encourage compliance. Parents should award the star for compliance with time sitting on the toilet and should not reserve rewards for successful bowel movements only. Weeks to months may be required to change the stooling pattern (Dunn, 2013).

Many parents seek counsellors to help the entire family deal with the issues. Counselling is geared toward allaying the fears of a child who is afraid to defecate due to pain. Also, children who are older may have behavioural issues that need to be addressed. Psychological evaluation and possible behavioural therapy may need to be implemented if constipation becomes a power struggle.

Hirschsprung Disease (Congenital Aganglionic Megacolon)

Hirschsprung disease is a movement disorder of the intestinal track resulting in obstruction (Wesson, 2015; Fig. 42.14). The disease is most commonly characterized by failure to pass a stool (meconium) within the first 24 hours of life. This is due to a lack of ganglion cells in a segment of the bowel, which causes inadequate motility in part of the intestine. These ganglion cells can be absent from the rectosigmoid colon all the way into the small intestine. Hirschsprung disease occurs in 1 of every 5,000 live births, being about four times more common in boys than in girls (Hoffenberg et al., 2014; Wesson, 2015).

NURSING PROCEDURE 42.2

Administering an Enema

1. Gather supplies (enema bag, lubricant, enema solution).

2. Wash hands and apply gloves.

3. Position the child:
   - Infant or toddler on abdomen with knees bent
   - Child or adolescent on left side with right leg flexed toward chest

4. Clamp the enema tubing, remove the cap, and apply lubricant to the tip.

5. Insert the tube into the rectum:
   - 2.5 to 4 cm (1 to 1.5 in) in the infant
   - 5 to 7.5 cm (2 to 3 in) in the child

6. Unclamp the tubing and administer the prescribed volume of enema solution at a rate of about 100 mL per minute. Recommended volumes:
   - 250 mL or less for the infant
   - 250 to 500 mL for the toddler or preschooler
   - 500 to 1,000 mL for the school-age child

7. Hold the child's buttocks together if needed to encourage retention of the enema for 5 to 10 minutes.

Adapted from Cincinnati Children's. (2016). *Enema administration.* Retrieved from http://www.cincinnatichildrens.org/health/e/enema/

FIGURE 42.14 Enlarged megacolon of Hirschsprung disease.

Distended sigmoid colon
Aganglionic portion
Rectum

Therapeutic Management

Surgical resection of the aganglionic bowel and reanastomosis of the remaining intestine are necessary to promote proper bowel function. There are several types of surgical procedures to correct this, usually performed in stages. The surgical resection requires the child to have an ostomy to divert the stool through a stoma on the abdomen. This allows the area of the resected bowel and anastomosis to heal before it is used. The ostomy is closed at a later date.

Nursing Assessment

For a full description of the assessment phase of the nursing process, refer to the Assessment section in the Nursing Process Overview earlier in the chapter. Assessment findings pertinent to Hirschsprung disease are discussed below.

HEALTH HISTORY

Elicit a description of the present illness and chief complaint. Newborn stool patterns are a key element in recognizing this diagnosis. Assess whether the newborn passed a meconium stool; most children with Hirschsprung disease do not pass a meconium stool within the first 24 to 48 hours of life. Also, newborns who required rectal stimulation to pass their first meconium stool or who passed ribbon-like stools or a meconium plug should be evaluated for Hirschsprung disease. Explore the child's current and past medical history for risk factors such as a family history of Hirschsprung disease or Down syndrome, or intestinal **atresia** (lack of a normal opening) (Wesson, 2015).

PHYSICAL EXAMINATION

Inspect and palpate the abdomen. The abdomen is typically distended, and, often, it is possible to palpate stool masses in the abdomen. Perform a rectal examination to assess for rectal tone and the presence of stool in the rectum. Often with Hirschsprung disease, no stool is present in the rectum. However, at the end of the rectal examination, when the finger is being withdrawn, a child with Hirschsprung disease may have a forceful expulsion of fecal material.

LABORATORY AND DIAGNOSTIC TESTS

Common laboratory and diagnostic studies ordered for the assessment of Hirschsprung disease include:
- Barium enema: to look for a narrowing of the intestine
- Rectal suction biopsy: to demonstrate an absence of ganglion cells (definitive diagnosis)

Nursing Management

Nursing management includes providing postoperative care, performing ostomy care, and providing child and family education.

PROVIDING POSTOPERATIVE AND OSTOMY CARE

Prior to surgery, observe for the possible complication of enterocolitis (see Nursing Care Plan 42.1 at the end of the chapter), and post-surgery, provide routine postoperative care.

Observe for the following signs and symptoms of enterocolitis:
- Fever
- Abdominal distention
- Chronic diarrhea
- Explosive stools
- Rectal bleeding

If any of the above symptoms are noted, immediately notify the physician or nurse practitioner, maintain bowel rest, and administer intravenous fluids and antibiotics to prevent the development of shock and possibly death. The child with Hirschsprung disease may have either a colostomy or ileostomy, depending on the extent of disease in the intestine. In either case, perform proper ostomy care to avoid skin breakdown. Accurately measure stool output to assess the child's fluid volume status.

PROVIDING CHILD AND FAMILY EDUCATION

The family may be anxious and fearful about upcoming surgeries and possible complications. Help to relieve their anxiety by providing information about the diagnosis and the stages of surgical procedures the child will undergo. Provide postoperative teaching to educate parents on proper stoma care as well as medication management (to avoid dehydration, children with Hirschsprung disease may be prescribed medications to slow stool output). Arrange for the family to consult with a stoma nurse to help them deal with the anxieties and care of newly placed stomas. Provide education about possible postsurgical problems, emphasizing the importance of prompt medical treatment for signs of enterocolitis.

Short Bowel Syndrome

Short bowel syndrome is a clinical syndrome of nutrient malabsorption and excessive intestinal fluid and electrolyte losses that occurs following massive small intestinal loss or surgical resection. The degree of malabsorption is usually related to the extent of resection of small bowel (Hoffenberg et al., 2014). The most common causes of short bowel syndrome are necrotizing enterocolitis, small intestinal atresia, gastroschisis, malrotation with volvulus, cloacal exstrophy, and trauma to the small intestine. The extent of malabsorption experienced by an individual child is dependent upon the extent of duodenal, ileal, and/or jejunal loss and the length of small intestine lost, as well as the type. If the terminal ileum is lost, vitamin B_{12} deficiency and bile salt malabsorption may occur. If the ileocecal valve is lost, small bowel bacterial overgrowth is likely to occur, as well as poor intestinal motility.

Therapeutic Management

The child with short bowel syndrome is at risk for chronic complications. The goals of therapeutic management are to minimize bacterial overgrowth and to maximize the child's nutritional status. Antibiotics may be used to control bacterial overgrowth. Vitamin and mineral supplementation is necessary because the small intestine is usually where fat-soluble vitamins, calcium, magnesium, and zinc are absorbed. Antidiarrheal agents such as loperamide and gastric acid–suppressive medications may be used to decrease stool output. Many children with short bowel syndrome require TPN for extended periods to achieve adequate growth. Progression to enteral feeding may occur extremely slowly, depending on the intestine's response. Despite a markedly improved prognosis for these children, some will not do as well and may ultimately require intestinal and liver transplantation due to irreversible liver damage from long-term use of TPN.

Nursing Assessment

Elicit the health history, noting diarrhea, which is the primary symptom of short bowel syndrome. Note past history of bowel loss or resection as noted above. Assess the child's hydration state. Inspect the stool for consistency, colour, odour, and volume. Review laboratory results, particularly chemistries, to evaluate hydration status, and liver function tests, which may reveal evolving **cholestasis** (impairment of bile flow) secondary to long-term TPN use.

Nursing Management

Nursing management focuses on encouraging adequate nutrition and promoting effective family coping.

ENCOURAGING ADEQUATE NUTRITION

Treatment for short bowel syndrome can be a slow and tedious process. Most children will require TPN until they can tolerate enteral feeds without significant malabsorption. TPN is usually required for a lengthy time, so most children will require long-term intravenous access. Long-term intravenous access places the child at high risk for infection and resulting sepsis. Therefore, closely monitor for signs and symptoms of infection. Immediately report to the physician or nurse practitioner any fevers or redness or drainage at the intravenous site.

When started, enteral feeding must be administered very slowly to avoid further malabsorption. Usually the feeding is started continuously, 24 hours per day, via a feeding pump. Most children have long-term feeding tubes, usually gastrostomy tubes. Most of these children will require special formulas to promote absorption. Assess for abdominal distention or discomfort. Strictly monitor intake and output to avoid dehydration.

Assess the stool for signs of carbohydrate malabsorption. Administer vitamin and mineral supplementation, antidiarrheals, and antibiotics as ordered. Teach the family about use of enteral feeding tubes, feeding pumps, and medication administration.

PROMOTING EFFECTIVE FAMILY COPING

Children with short bowel syndrome are considered to be medically fragile for a lengthy period. There is much anxiety related to the initial bowel resection that resulted in short bowel. Long-term hospitalization is almost always required, causing parents to miss work and cutting down on the time they have to spend with other children. This can lead to even more anxiety about finances and relationships. Encourage families to become the experts on their child's needs and condition via education and participation in care. Provide teaching so that the family is better able to care for the child in an outpatient setting. Education focuses on information about TPN and central line care, enteral feedings, assessing for hydration status, and managing medications.

> **Take Note!**
> Maintaining long-term central venous access for TPN in infants can present a challenge. One-piece clothing with the central venous line (CVL) tubing exiting and secured on the back of the outfit can help discourage the infant from pulling on (and subsequently dislodging) the line.

Inflammatory Bowel Disease

Inflammatory bowel disease (IBD) in children can be divided into Crohn's disease or ulcerative colitis. The causes are unknown. However, these conditions may be due to an abnormal or uncontrolled genetically determined immunologic or inflammatory response to an environmental antigenic trigger, possibly a virus or bacterium (Judge, Giordano, & English, 2014). The features of Crohn disease and ulcerative colitis are listed in Comparison Chart 42.2.

Therapeutic Management

Medication is used to control inflammation and symptoms. Medications commonly used include 5-aminosalicylates, antibiotics, immunomodulators, immunosuppressives, and anti–tumour necrosis antibody therapy. Sometimes, a specialized fluid diet (exclusive enteral nutrition) is used to induce remission.

Failure to respond to medical therapy may result in surgical intervention. Many children with ulcerative colitis eventually undergo a subtotal colectomy, with resulting ostomy, as a curative measure. Children or adolescents with Crohn disease may require surgery to relieve obstruction from a strictured piece of bowel, drain an abscess, or relieve intractable symptoms.

COMPARISON CHART 42.2 FEATURES OF CROHN DISEASE AND ULCERATIVE COLITIS

Feature	Crohn Disease	Ulcerative Colitis
Usual age at onset	10 to 20 years	10 to 20 years
Incidence	4 to 6 per 100,000	3 to 15 per 100,000
Area of bowel affected	Oropharynx, esophagus, and stomach, rare: small bowel only, 25% to 30%; colon and anus only, 25%; ileocolitis, 40%; diffuse disease, 5%	Total colon, 90%; proctitis, 10%
Distribution	Segmental; disease-free skip areas common	Continuous; distal to proximal
Pathology	Full-thickness, acute, and chronic inflammation; non-caseating granulomas (50%), extraintestinal fistulas, abscesses, stricture, and fibrosis may be present	Superficial, acute inflammation of mucosa with microscopic crypt abscess
Radiography findings	Segmental lesions; thickened, circular folds; cobblestone appearance of bowel wall secondary to longitudinal ulcers and transverse fissures; fixation and separation of loops; narrowed lumen; "sting sign"; fistulas	Superficial colitis; loss of haustra; shortened colon; and pseudopolyps (islands of normal tissue surrounded by denuded mucosa) are late findings
Intestinal symptoms	Abdominal pain, diarrhea (usually loose with blood if colon involved), perianal disease, enteroenteric or enterocutaneous fistula, abscess, anorexia	Abdominal pain, bloody diarrhea, urgency, tenesmus
Extraintestinal symptoms		
Arthritis/arthralgia	15%	9%
Fever	40% to 50%	40% to 50%
Stomatitis	9%	2%
Weight loss	90% (mean 5.7 kg)	68% (mean 4.1 kg)
Delayed growth and sexual development	30%	5% to 10%
Uveitis, conjunctivitis	15% (in Crohn colitis)	4%
Sclerosing cholangitis	–	4%
Renal stones	6% (oxalate)	6% (urate)
Pyoderma gangrenosum	1% to 3%	5%
Erythema nodosum	8% to 15%	4%
Laboratory findings	High erythrocyte sedimentation rate; microcytic anemia; low serum iron and total iron-binding capacity; increased fecal protein loss; low serum albumin; antineutrophil cytoplasmic antibodies present in 10% to 20%; *Saccharomyces cerevisiae* antibodies positive in 60%	High erythrocyte sedimentation rate; microcytic anemia; high white blood cell count with left shift; antineutrophil cytoplasmic antibodies present in 80%

Adapted from Haas-Beckert, B., & Heyman, M. B. (2010). Inflammatory bowel disease. In P. J. Allen, J. A. Vessey, & N. A. Schapiro (Eds.). *Primary care of the child with a chronic condition* (5th ed.). St. Louis, MO: Mosby; and Hoffenberg, E., Brumbaugh, D., Furuta, G. T., Kobak, G., Liu, E., Soden, J., & Kramer, R. (2014). Gastrointestinal tract. In W. W. Hay, M. J. Levin, R. R. Deterding, & M. J. Abzug (Eds.). *Current pediatric diagnosis and treatment* (22nd ed.). New York: McGraw-Hill.

Nursing Assessment

For a full description of the assessment phase of the nursing process, refer to the Assessment section in the Nursing Process Overview earlier in the chapter. Assessment findings pertinent to Crohn disease and ulcerative colitis are discussed below.

HEALTH HISTORY

Elicit a description of the present illness and chief complaint. Common signs and symptoms reported during the health history include:
- Abdominal cramping, frequent/loose stools, urgency to defecate
- Blood with stools
- Night-time symptoms, including waking, due to abdominal pain or need to defecate
- Fever
- Weight loss
- Poor growth
- Delayed sexual development
- Joint pain (arthralgia)
- Unexplained rashes or bruising

Children may be reluctant or unwilling to talk about their bowel movements, so explain the importance of doing so. Assess stool pattern history, including frequency, presence of blood or mucus, and duration of symptoms.

Explore the child's current and past medical history for risk factors, such as:
- Family history of IBD, colon cancer, or immunologic disorders

PHYSICAL EXAMINATION

Assess the child's growth using growth charts to identify any poor growth patterns. Assess for mouth ulcers, red or painful eyes, unexplained rashes or sores especially on lower limbs, joint pain, or arthralgia. Perform a full abdominal examination, noting tenderness, masses, or fullness. Inspect the perianal area to look for skin tags or fissures, which would be highly suspicious for Crohn disease. Assist the physician in performing a rectal examination to further assess the rectal area for blood or other lesions.

LABORATORY AND DIAGNOSTIC TESTS

Laboratory test results may be normal. Results for children with Crohn disease and ulcerative colitis are found in Comparison Chart 42.2. Common laboratory and diagnostic studies ordered for the assessment of IBD include:
- Radiologic studies such as upper GI series with small bowel series: may identify evidence of intestinal inflammation, estimate distribution and extent of disease, and help distinguish between Crohn disease and ulcerative colitis. Many centres use abdominal MRI (MRE) to do this assessment as there is no radiation exposure
- CT scan or MRI: to rule out suspected abscess or assess for fistula and perianal disease
- Colonoscopy: to assess for inflammation of the mucosa of the colon and the terminal ileum
- Upper endoscopy: to assess for inflammation of mucosa between the mouth and the duodenum

Nursing Management

Nursing management focuses on teaching about disease management, teaching about nutritional management, teaching about medication therapy, and promoting family and child coping.

TEACHING ABOUT DISEASE MANAGEMENT

The diagnosis of Crohn disease or ulcerative colitis can be very difficult for the child and family to comprehend. Provide teaching about the disease process and medication/nutritional therapy to help the child and family understand the disease. Encourage families to write down their questions. Provide educational materials for them to read or reputable websites for them to review. The physician may discuss surgical options in some circumstances. Often the nurse is the person to whom the family members or children address their questions. Provide the family with information to help answer some of their questions and allay fears.

TEACHING ABOUT NUTRITIONAL MANAGEMENT

Teach the child and family about nutritional management of the disease. For example, adequate nutrition with a high-protein and high-carbohydrate diet may be recommended. When the disease is active, lactose may be tolerated poorly, and vitamin and iron supplements may be recommended. Exclusive enteral nutrition (a formula-only diet taken orally or via nasogastric tube for 6 to 12 weeks) is often used to induce remission for children diagnosed with Crohn disease.

TEACHING ABOUT MEDICATION THERAPY

Medications are extremely important in controlling IBD. Provide information about the following common medications used to control the disease:
- 5-Aminosalicylates (5-ASA): topical anti-inflammatory therapy given by oral and or rectal route. Most often used to treat mild to moderate colitis
- Antibiotics (usually metronidazole and ciprofloxacin): typically used in children who have perianal Crohn disease.
- Immunomodulators (6-mercaptopurine [6-MP], azathioprine, or methotrexate): used to help maintain remission. Monitor children for neutropenia and hepatotoxicity. While on these medications, children should not have any live vaccines.
- Prednisone (oral or via IV and then oral): systemic anti-inflammatory/immune suppression medication used to treat both Crohn disease and ulcerative colitis. While on this medication, children should not have any live vaccines.

• Biologic therapy/anti-TNF (Infliximab and Adalimumab): used to treat moderate to severe IBD

PROMOTING FAMILY AND CHILD COPING

IBD is a chronic and often debilitating illness. Many children with this diagnosis can lead normal lives, but frequent illnesses can cause school absences, which in turn add stress to the situation. Because schools have become much less tolerant of absences and tardiness, it may be necessary to write letters to the school explaining the frequent absences or in-school needs. Bathroom privileges should be very flexible for children during flare-ups. Children tend to be of small stature due to the illness itself and steroid use, which stunts growth; this may cause psychological issues, especially for older boys (Haas-Beckert & Heyman, 2010). Children with ostomies as a result of surgical resection may have self-esteem issues related to the presence and care of the ostomy. Arrange for counselling for both the child and family to discuss fears and anxiety related to a chronic disease.

Celiac Disease

Celiac disease, also known as celiac sprue, is an immunologic disorder in which gluten, a protein most commonly found in grains, causes damage to the small intestine. The villi of the small intestine are damaged due to the body's immunologic response to the digestion of gluten. As the function of the villi is to absorb nutrients into the bloodstream, when they are blunted or damaged, malnutrition can occur.

Celiac disease is one of the most common chronic disorders in Europe and North America, affecting about 1% of the general population and up to 2% of Caucasians (Swanson & John, 2013). Increased incidence occurs in those with a family history of celiac disease and in persons with autoimmune or genetic disorders (Swanson & John, 2013).

The only current treatment for celiac disease is a strict gluten-free diet. Eliminating gluten will cause the villi of the intestines to heal and function normally, with subsequent improvement of symptoms. Even very small amounts of gluten introduced back into the diet can cause damage to the villi, so the child must adhere to the diet throughout life (Swanson & John, 2013).

Nursing Assessment

For a full description of the assessment phase of the nursing process, refer to the Assessment section in the Nursing Process Overview earlier in the chapter. Assessment findings pertinent to celiac disease are discussed below.

HEALTH HISTORY

Elicit a description of the present illness and chief complaint. The symptoms of celiac disease are very broad and are easily confused with other GI disorders. The classic symptoms of children with celiac disease are:

• Diarrhea
• **Steatorrhea** (fatty stools)
• Constipation
• Failure to thrive or weight loss
• Abdominal distention or bloating
• Poor muscle tone
• Irritability and listlessness
• Dental disorders
• Anemia
• Delayed onset of puberty or amenorrhea
• Nutritional deficiencies

Explore the child's current and past medical history for risk factors.

PHYSICAL EXAMINATION

Assess for the typical appearance of children with celiac disease: distended abdomen, wasted buttocks, and very thin extremities (Fig. 42.15).

FIGURE 42.15 The child with celiac disease typically displays a distended abdomen and wasted extremities.

LABORATORY AND DIAGNOSTIC TESTS

Common laboratory and diagnostic studies ordered for the assessment of celiac disease include autotissue transglutaminase IgA (TTG), intestinal biopsy, and genetic testing. Autotissue transglutaminase IgA (TTG) is a first-line test, and the most sensitive, but if the child is IgA-deficient, the test is not useful, in which case the antiendomysium IgA test is a more useful test (Swanson & John, 2013). One positive blood test does not necessarily indicate that the child has celiac disease. The most definitive test is a small bowel biopsy that reveals partial or subtotal villous atrophy or blunting of the villi of the small intestine. This diagnostic testing requires the child remain in a regular gluten-containing diet. Genetic testing for celiac disease includes DQ2 and/or DQ8 human leukocyte antigen (HLA) haplotypes (Denham, 2014).

Nursing Management

Providing child and family education is the key nursing role in managing children with celiac disease. After diagnosis, the child must adhere to a strict gluten-free diet for his or her entire life. This is often very challenging, because gluten is found in most wheat products, rye, barley, and possibly oats. Encourage the parents and child to learn how to maintain this gluten-free diet. There are many resources available about the celiac diet at the public library and on the internet. Often, families consult a dietitian to learn about the gluten-free diet (Teaching Guidelines 42.3).

Provide educational materials and resources to the parents. Many resources are available today about celiac disease. These resources can offer information on all aspects of celiac disease, including dietary guidelines and resources for food shopping and eating in restaurants. A reading source appropriate for school-age children is *Gluten-free Friends: An Activity Book for Kids* by Nancy Patin Falini.

Functional Abdominal Pain

Functional abdominal pain is a common GI complaint of children and adolescents. It affects children of all ages, and about 2% to 4% of all pediatric outpatient visits are related to functional abdominal pain (Hoffenberg et al., 2014). The etiology remains unclear. The Rome Committee is a group of specialists who are focusing on the identification, management, and treatment of both adults and children with functional GI disorders. Functional abdominal pain in children should not be confused with IBS. Box 42.5 outlines the Rome Committee's criteria for IBS and information on treatment of IBS.

Pathophysiology

The etiology of functional abdominal pain is likely multifactorial (Starr et al., 2013). It is thought that the autonomic nervous system, which controls the body's response to emotions and stress, and intestinal motility are the two mechanisms. Symptoms may result from an

---

 Teaching Guidelines 42.3
DIETARY CONSIDERATIONS IN A GLUTEN-FREE DIET

Foods Allowed	Foods to Avoid
Potato, soy, rice, or bean flour; rice bran, cornmeal, arrowroot, corn or potato starch, sago, tapioca, buckwheat, millet, flax, teff, sorghum, amaranth, quinoa	All wheat products; rye, triticale, barley, oats, or oat bran; graham, spelt, or durum flour, bulgur, farina, or kamut; malt extract; hydrolyzed vegetable protein
Plain, fresh, frozen, or canned vegetables made with allowed ingredients	Any creamed or breaded vegetables, canned baked beans, some French fries
All fruits and fruit juices	Some commercial fruit pie fillings and dried fruit
All milk and milk products except those made with gluten additives, aged cheese	Malted milk, flavoured or frozen yogurt
All meat, poultry, fish, and shellfish; dried peas and beans, nuts; peanut butter; soybean; cold cuts, frankfurters or sausage without fillers	Any meats or poultry prepared with wheat, rye, oats, barley, gluten stabilizers, or fillers for meats; canned meats; self-basting turkey; some egg substitutes
Butter, margarine, salad dressings, sauces, soups, and desserts with allowable ingredients; sugar, honey, jelly, jam, hard candy, plain chocolate, coconut, molasses, marshmallows, meringues, pure instant or ground coffee, tea, carbonated drinks, wine (from the United States)	Commercial salad dressings, prepared soups, condiments, sauces, and seasonings made with avoided products; nondairy cream substitutes, flavoured instant coffee, alcohol distilled from cereals, licorice

Adapted from Celiac Disease Foundation. (2016). *Gluten-free diet*. Retrieved from http://celiac.org/live-gluten-free/glutenfreediet/

BOX 42.5

ROME COMMITTEE CRITERIA FOR IRRITABLE BOWEL SYNDROME

All of the following occur at least once per week minimum for at least 2 months before diagnosis:
- Abdominal pain relieved 25% of the time by defecation
- Onset of discomfort associated with a change in frequency of stool
- Onset of discomfort associated with a change in appearance of the stool
- No structural, neoplastic, inflammatory, or metabolic explanation for this abdominal pain

TREATMENT OF IBS

For some children, dietary manipulation or medications may help to control diarrhea.

Adapted from Starr, N. B., Blosser, C. G., Brady, M. A., Burns, C. E., Dunn, A. M., & Petersen-Smith, A. M. (2013). Gastrointestinal disorders. In C. Burns, A. Dunn, M. Brady, N. B. Starr, & C. Blosser (Eds.). *Pediatric primary care* (5th ed.). Philadelphia, PA: Saunders.

alteration in the transmission of messages between the enteric nervous system and the central nervous system, leading to visceral hypersensitivity. Information from the GI tract is transmitted through bidirectional nerve pathways to the brain. Most neurotransmitters are found in both the brain and the gut, suggesting the potential for integrated effects of pain modulation. As different possibilities exist for the pathophysiology of functional abdominal pain, it is clear that there are no structural or biochemical abnormalities that are identifiable. Therapeutic management most often focuses on increasing the child's coping skills (Starr et al., 2013).

Nursing Assessment

For a full description of the assessment phase of the nursing process, refer to the Assessment section of the Nursing Process Overview earlier in the chapter. Assessment findings pertinent to functional abdominal pain are discussed below.

HEALTH HISTORY

The diagnosis of functional abdominal pain is made on a symptom-based approach. Elicit a description of the present illness and chief complaint. The symptom reported mostly commonly during the health history is abdominal pain. The child may have difficulty providing a good description of the pain. It is usually periumbilical and is usually described as attacks of pain. It is uncommon for the child to wake up in the middle of the night with this type of pain. Because diet may play a large role in the symptoms, obtain a dietary history. Take a detailed medication history, because abdominal pain may be an adverse effect of some medications. Identifying social and school stressors is essential.

PHYSICAL EXAMINATION

Note the child's body positioning and facial expressions. Interactions with family members during the interview may provide more details regarding social stressors. Palpate the abdomen for tenderness.

LABORATORY AND DIAGNOSTIC TESTS

Common laboratory and diagnostic studies ordered for the assessment of functional abdominal pain include:
- CBC: to rule out organic causes of abdominal pain
- Erythrocyte sedimentation rate or C-reactive protein: to rule out organic causes of abdominal pain
- Urinalysis: to rule out organic causes of abdominal pain
- Stool studies: to assess for routine pathogens that can contribute to abdominal pain

Nursing Management

Once the diagnosis of functional abdominal pain with no organic cause is made, the majority of the nursing management is focused on promoting coping skills. Often the physician or nurse practitioner performs a battery of tests to rule out organic causes, especially when child and family anxiety is high. After these tests are complete, teach the family about the factors that exacerbate the pain and how to deal with these factors.

Diet changes may need to be implemented. High-fibre diets help with bowel regulation by keeping motility regular. Medications may be used to relieve abdominal cramps. Occasionally, pain modulators and antidepressants are used to help block the neurotransmitters in the brain–gut connection that cause pain. Encourage compliance with the medication regimen; compliance is needed to achieve beneficial results with many of these medications (Almadhoun, 2012).

Arrange for counselling, if necessary, for children with social stressors. Children with functional abdominal pain may become so debilitated that they cannot function in school, possibly requiring homebound instruction. Provide education to the school, with parental permission, regarding the child's illness and how to best deal with it. Explain that this recurrent abdominal pain is a true pain that children feel and is not "in their minds."

HEPATOBILIARY DISORDERS

Hepatobiliary disorders include pancreatitis, gallbladder disease, biliary atresia, infectious and non-infectious hepatitis, cirrhosis, and portal hypertension.

Pancreatitis

Pancreatitis is increasingly being recognized as a childhood problem (Sokol, Narkewicz, Sundaram, & Mack, 2014). It is classified into two categories—acute and chronic. Acute pancreatitis is an acute inflammatory process that occurs within the pancreas, with variable involvement of localized tissues and remote organ systems. Most common causes of acute pancreatitis include abdominal trauma, drugs and alcohol (though probably rare in children), multisystem disease (such as IBD or systemic lupus erythematosus), infections (usually viruses such as cytomegalovirus or hepatitis), congenital anomalies (ductal or pancreatic malformations), obstruction (most likely gallstones or tumours in children), or metabolic disorders. Chronic pancreatitis is defined based on the structural and/or functional permanent changes that occur in the pancreas.

When pancreatitis is suspected, the child is placed on immediate bowel rest (NPO). Often, a nasogastric tube placed for suction will be needed to keep the stomach decompressed. Serial monitoring of serum amylase levels will determine when oral feeding may be restarted.

Nursing Assessment

For a full description of the assessment phase of the nursing process, refer to the Assessment section of the Nursing Process Overview earlier in the chapter. Assessment findings pertinent to pancreatitis are discussed below.

HEALTH HISTORY

Elicit a description of the present illness and chief complaint. Common signs and symptoms reported during the health history include:
- Acute onset of persistent midepigastric and periumbilical abdominal pain, often with radiation to the back or chest
- Nausea and vomiting, especially after meals
- Fever

Explore the child's current and past medical history for risk factors such as:
- Cystic fibrosis
- History of gallstones
- Traumatic injury
- Family history of hereditary pancreatitis

PHYSICAL EXAMINATION

On abdominal assessment, the bowel sounds may be diminished, suggesting peritonitis. The abdomen may be tender, and distention may occur in younger children and infants. In severe cases, jaundice, ascites, or pleural effusions may occur. Bluish discolouration around the umbilicus or flanks is seen in the most severe cases of pancreatitis when hemorrhage is present.

LABORATORY AND DIAGNOSTIC TESTS

Common laboratory and diagnostic studies ordered for the assessment and monitoring of pancreatitis include:
- Serum amylase and/or lipase: levels three times the normal values are indicative of pancreatitis
- Liver profile: often done to check for increased liver enzymes, and/or elevated bilirubin levels
- CBC and chemistry: leukocytosis is common with acute pancreatitis. Hyperglycemia and hypocalcemia may also be noted.
- C-reactive protein: levels may be elevated

Diagnostic imaging studies performed to identify malformations or cysts on the pancreas include:
- Plain abdominal x-ray: may show a localized ileus
- Ultrasound: allows direct visualization of the pancreas and the surrounding structures. This is used most frequently with children, as it is less invasive than a CT scan. A CT scan is usually used when there is difficulty in determining the cause of the pancreatitis during ultrasonography. Magnetic resonance cholangiopancreatography (MRCP) is also used as it does not expose the child to radiation.
- Endoscopic retrograde cholangiopancreatography (ERCP): used in some children who may have ductal anomalies, usually with chronic pancreatitis, though complications from this procedure may occur

Nursing Management

Maintain NPO status and nasogastric tube suction and patency. Administer intravenous fluids to keep the child hydrated and correct any alterations in fluid and electrolyte balance. Pain management is crucial in children with pancreatitis. If hemorrhagic pancreatitis has occurred, blood products and/or intravenous antibiotics may be needed. Oral feedings are restarted only after the serum amylase level has returned to normal (usually in 2 to 4 days). Often, pancreatic enzymes are given with oral feedings if pain occurs after oral feeds are restarted. A low fat diet is recommended.

Surgery is rarely needed in children with pancreatitis, except in those with severe abdominal trauma or major ductal abnormalities.

Though chronic pancreatitis is rare in children, provide child and family education regarding the signs and symptoms of recurrence and complications.

Gallbladder Disease

Cholelithiasis is the presence of stones in the gallbladder. Cholesterol stones are usually associated with hyperlipidemia, obesity, pregnancy, birth control pill use, or cystic fibrosis (Schwarz & Hebra, 2015). They are seen more often in females than males, and increased risk occurs with age and onset of puberty (Schwarz & Hebra, 2015). These stones occur in the gallbladder and may be found in the common bile duct. Pigment stones are found in prepubertal children and occur about equally in males and females. They are usually found in the common bile duct (associated with bacterial or parasitic infections) or the gallbladder itself (associated with hemolytic anemia or liver cirrhosis).

Cholecystitis is an inflammation of the gallbladder that is caused by the chemical irritation due to the obstruction of bile flow from the gallbladder into the cystic ducts. This inflammation is typically associated with gallstones in children. The most common complication in children with gallstone disease is pancreatitis.

If cholelithiasis results in symptomatic cholecystitis, then surgical removal of the gallbladder (cholecystectomy) will be necessary. This is often accomplished laparoscopically.

Nursing Assessment

For a full description of the assessment phase of the nursing process, refer to the Assessment section of the Nursing Process Overview earlier in the chapter. Assessment findings pertinent to gallbladder disease are discussed below.

HEALTH HISTORY

Elicit a description of the present illness and chief complaint. Common signs and symptoms reported during the health history include:

- Right upper quadrant pain, often radiating substernally or to the right shoulder
- Nausea and vomiting
- Jaundice and fever (with cholecystitis)

Document a detailed diet history as it relates to the presenting symptoms. Pain episodes usually occur after meals (postprandially), especially after the ingestion of fatty or greasy foods. Younger children may present with more nonspecific symptoms, most often due to their lack of ability to communicate their symptoms to others. Explore the child's current and past medical history for risk factors such as chronic TPN use or sickle cell disease.

PHYSICAL EXAMINATION

Palpate the abdomen for tenderness. If cholecystitis is present, the gallbladder becomes inflamed, often to the point of causing localized tenderness upon palpation. Assess skin and sclerae colour for jaundice. Note presence of fever.

LABORATORY AND DIAGNOSTIC TESTS

Common laboratory and diagnostic studies ordered for the assessment of cholecystitis include:

- Liver function tests, bilirubin, and C-reactive protein: values may be elevated if ductal stones are present
- CBC: may reveal leukocytosis
- Amylase and lipase: may be elevated if pancreatitis is also present

- Plain abdominal x-rays: may reveal radiopaque stones
- Ultrasound of the gallbladder and surrounding structures: to assess the intraluminal contents of the gallbladder as well as any anatomic alterations
- ERCP: to rule out ductal stones
- Hepatobiliary iminodiacetic acid (HIDA) scan: to evaluate the function of the gallbladder

Nursing Management

The child with symptomatic cholecystitis will usually be hospitalized. Administer intravenous fluids, maintain NPO status and gastric decompression, and administer pain medications. If ordered, administer intravenous antibiotics to treat clinically worsening symptoms of cholecystitis, such as persistent fever. Provide routine postoperative care after cholecystectomy is performed. Provide pre- and postoperative teaching for families of children undergoing gallbladder removal.

Biliary Atresia

Biliary atresia is an absence of some or all of the major biliary ducts, resulting in obstruction of bile flow. The ensuing obstruction to bile flow from the liver causes cholestasis resulting in jaundice and eventual progressive liver fibrosis with end-stage cirrhosis of the liver. Biliary atresia affects 1 in 12,000 infants (Sokol et al., 2014). The etiology of biliary atresia is unknown, but there are several theories, including infectious, autoimmune, or ischemic causes.

Therapeutic Management

If there is a high suspicion of biliary atresia, the infant will undergo an intraoperative cholangiogram which will identify bile drainage from the liver. If biliary atresia is found, a Kasai procedure (hepatoportoenterostomy) is performed to connect the bowel lumen to the bile duct remnants found at the porta hepatis. This procedure is most successful for infants up to 45 days of age, as bile flow restoration after this age is minimal (Sokol et al., 2014). Infants who are not identified early enough or those who have failed to respond to the Kasai procedure will likely need to undergo liver transplantation (Sokol et al., 2014).

Nursing Assessment

For a full description of the assessment phase of the nursing process, refer to the Assessment section of the Nursing Process Overview earlier in the chapter. Assessment findings pertinent to biliary atresia are discussed below.

HEALTH HISTORY

Elicit a description of the present illness and chief complaint. Persistent or recurring jaundice is the most common symptom reported during the health history.

PHYSICAL EXAMINATION

In the initial assessment of an infant with cholestasis of unknown origin, assess the stool character. In biliary atresia, stools will be acholic (chalky and white due to the lack of bile pigment). Note jaundice of the skin and sclerae (yellow discolouration caused by bile pigment deposition). Palpate the abdomen; the liver will feel enlarged and hardened. Splenomegaly may occur. In the absence of other congenital malformations, the infant will otherwise appear healthy.

LABORATORY AND DIAGNOSTIC STUDIES

Common laboratory and diagnostic studies ordered for the assessment of biliary atresia include:
- Serum bilirubin, alkaline phosphatase, liver enzymes, γ-glutamyl transferase (GGT): elevated
- Ultrasound: to identify anomalies
- HIDA scan: to distinguish whether the cholestasis is intrahepatic or extrahepatic
- Liver biopsy: to confirm the diagnosis

Nursing Management

Nursing management of infants who have biliary atresia will focus on vitamin and caloric support. Administer fat-soluble vitamins A, D, E, and K. Special formulas containing medium-chain triglycerides are used because significant fat malabsorption occurs when cholestasis is present. Administer feedings via nasogastric tube as needed to ensure increased caloric intake. Identify infections as quickly as possible and administer intravenous antibiotics as ordered. Manage ascites with diuretics and dietary restrictions. Preoperative management before a Kasai procedure is focused on preparation for surgery; infants who have suspected biliary atresia require surgery to optimize outcomes.

Parents and family members of these infants will have extreme anxiety due to the implications of the diagnosis and outcomes. Focus education on the diagnosis and postoperative care. Nursing Care Plan 42.1, at the end of the chapter, gives information about routine postoperative care.

Hepatitis

Hepatitis is an inflammation of the liver that is caused by a variety of agents, including viral infections, bacterial invasion, metabolic disorders, chemical toxicity, autoimmune disorder, and trauma. The most common viral causes of hepatitis are listed in Table 42.4. Other viruses that may cause hepatitis are cytomegalovirus (CMV), Epstein–Barr virus (EBV), and adenovirus. Autoimmune hepatitis is a chronic disorder, affecting mostly adolescents. The clinical presentation of a child with autoimmune hepatitis includes hepatosplenomegaly, jaundice, fever, fatigue, and right upper quadrant pain.

Children who present with fulminant hepatitis (severe liver injury) have acute massive hepatic necrosis. The disease progresses rapidly to severe jaundice, coagulopathy, elevated ammonia levels, significantly elevated liver enzyme levels (aspartate aminotransferase [AST] and alanine aminotransferase [ALT]), and progressive coma, resulting in death without liver transplantation.

Therapeutic Management

Acute hepatitis is treated with rest, hydration, and nutrition. Control of bleeding may also be necessary. Chronic hepatitis often eventually requires liver transplantation. Corticosteroids and immunosuppressants may be used for autoimmune hepatitis. The child with fulminant hepatitis usually requires intensive care with cardiorespiratory support.

Nursing Assessment

For a full description of the assessment phase of the nursing process, refer to the Assessment section of the Nursing Process Overview earlier in the chapter. Assessment findings pertinent to hepatitis are discussed below. The nursing assessment for any child who presents with suspected hepatitis should be the same.

HEALTH HISTORY

Elicit a description of the present illness and the chief complaint. Common signs and symptoms reported during the health history include:
- Jaundice
- Fever
- Fatigue
- Abdominal pain

Explore the child's current and past medical history for risk factors such as:
- Recent foreign travel
- Sick contacts
- Medication use (assess for acetaminophen ingestion and complete assessment and ongoing mental health assessments if taken as an over dose, using local protocols)
- Abdominal trauma
- Sexual activity
- Intravenous drug use
- Blood product transfusion

Document onset of symptoms as well as all signs and symptoms the child has been experiencing.

PHYSICAL EXAMINATION

Observe the skin for jaundice and the sclerae for icterus. Urine may be dark, tea-like colour. Stools may be pale. Palpate the abdomen to reveal abnormal liver and spleen size or tenderness.

TABLE 42.4 HEPATITIS VIRUSES A–E

	Hepatitis A (HAV)	Hepatitis B (HBV)	Hepatitis C (HCV)	Hepatitis D (HDV)	Hepatitis E (HEV)
Transmission route	Oral–fecal route, poor sanitation, waterborne	Sexual, intravenous drug use, blood transfusion, perinatally transmitted from mother to infant	Sexual, blood product transfusion, intravenous drug use, perinatally transmitted from mother to infant	Same as HBV; HBV markers in serum must be present	Oral–fecal
Incubation period	15–30 days	50–150 days	30–160 days	50–150 days	15–65 days
Signs and symptoms	Flu-like symptoms Preicteric phase: headache, fatigue, fever, anorexia Icteric phase: jaundice, dark urine, tender liver (right upper quadrant pain)	Some cases are asymptomatic; others present with anorexia, abdominal pain, and fatigue, rash, slight fever, visible jaundice, enlarged liver	Chronic cases usually present asymptomatically; others with flu-like symptoms, jaundice, hepatosplenomegaly	Same as HBV	Same as HAV, more severe in pregnant women
Prognosis	Rarely develops into fulminant liver failure; 95% of children recover without sequelae	Chronic disease state likely; increased risk of hepatic cancer	Many will develop chronic hepatitis and cirrhosis	Same as HBV, but increased likelihood of chronic active hepatitis and cirrhosis	Same as HAV; high mortality in pregnant women

Adapted from Sokol, R. J., Narkewicz, M. R., Sundaram, S. S., & Mack, C. L. (2014). Liver & pancreas. In W. W. Hay, M. J. Levin, R. R. Deterding, & M. J. Abzug (Eds.). *Current pediatric diagnosis and treatment* (22nd ed.). New York: McGraw-Hill.

LABORATORY AND DIAGNOSTIC STUDIES

Common laboratory and diagnostic studies ordered for the assessment of hepatitis include:

- Liver enzymes, GGT: elevated
- Prothrombin time (PT)/partial thromboplastin time (PTT): prolonged
- Ammonia: elevated in the presence of encephalopathy
- Autoimmune studies, such as antinuclear antibodies, anti–smooth muscle antibodies, and liver–kidney microsomal antibodies: may be used to diagnose autoimmune hepatitis
- Viral studies: to identify viral causes of hepatitis, such as hepatitis A to E antigens and antibodies, CMV, and EBV
- Ultrasound: to assess liver or spleen abnormalities
- Liver biopsy: to determine the type of hepatitis and to assess for damage that has already been done to the liver

Nursing Management

Acute hepatitis requires rest, hydration, and nutrition. If the child develops vomiting, dehydration, elevated bleeding times (PT/PTT), or mental status changes (encephalopathy), hospitalization may be required. When caring for children with infectious hepatitis, provide education about transmission and prevention, including proper hygiene, safe sexual activity, careful handwashing techniques, and blood/bodily fluid precautions.

Fulminant hepatitis treatment is aggressive and will require NPO status, nasogastric tube administration of lactulose to decrease ammonia levels that lead to encephalopathic conditions, TPN administration, vitamin K injections to help with coagulopathies, and, ultimately, liver transplantation. Fear and anxiety of the child and parents will likely be very high. Teach the child and family about the diagnosis and what to expect during treatment. Provide immunoglobulin therapy and vaccinations to close contacts of children with infectious hepatitis.

Cirrhosis and Portal Hypertension

Cirrhosis of the liver occurs as a result of the destructive processes that occur during liver damage, leading to the formation of nodules. These nodules can be small (micronodular [less than 3 mm]) or large (macronodular [greater than 3 mm]) and distort the vasculature of the liver, leading to further complications. Causes of cirrhosis in children include biliary malformations, α_1-antitrypsin deficiency, Wilson disease, galactosemia, tyrosinemia, chronic active hepatitis, and prolonged TPN use (Sokol et al., 2014).

Major complications may exist due to cirrhosis of the liver, including portal hypertension. In portal hypertension, the blood flow to, through, or from the liver meets resistance, causing portal blood flow pressures to rise. As these pressures rise, collateral veins form between the portal and systemic venous circulations. The most significant complication of portal hypertension is GI bleeding, from shunting to submucosal veins (varices) in the stomach and esophagus. Esophageal varices may be treated with sclerotherapy or variceal banding during endoscopy to stop acute bleeding. Often blood product administration and vasopressive drugs are needed. In the long term, the only cure for cirrhosis is liver transplantation.

Nursing Assessment

For a full description of the assessment phase of the nursing process, refer to the Assessment section of the Nursing Process Overview earlier in the chapter. Assessment findings pertinent to cirrhosis and portal hypertension are discussed below.

HEALTH HISTORY

Elicit a description of the present illness and chief complaint. Common signs and symptoms reported during the health history include:

- Nausea and vomiting
- Jaundice
- Weakness
- Swelling
- Weight loss

Explore the child's current and past medical history for risk factors such as hepatitis, cystic fibrosis, Wilson disease, hematochromatosis, and biliary atresia. Assess the past medical history to identify possible causes for liver disease.

PHYSICAL EXAMINATION

Inspect for jaundice, ascites, spider angiomas, and palmar erythema. Gynecomastia is often seen in males. Palpate the liver; typically it is enlarged and hard, but occasionally it is small and shrunken. Evaluate mental status to determine the presence of hepatic encephalopathy.

LABORATORY AND DIAGNOSTIC STUDIES

Laboratory and diagnostic testing will be similar to that of a child with hepatitis. Common laboratory and diagnostic studies ordered for the assessment of cirrhosis or portal hypertension include:

- Liver biopsy: reveals regenerating nodules and surrounding fibrosis
- Upper endoscopy: reveals varices and bleeding risk

Nursing Management

Nursing management is very similar to the care of the child with hepatitis. In cases of cirrhosis causing portal hypertension and bleeding varices, GI bleeding must be controlled. This is usually done by replacing blood loss and providing vasopressive therapy to constrict the shunted blood flow. As with all liver disorders and GI bleeding, address and manage family and child anxiety. Be honest about the child's treatment plan and prognosis.

Involve the family in the care of the child and educate them as needed.

Liver Transplantation

Hepatobiliary disorders that result in failure of the liver to function result in the need for liver transplantation. Liver transplantation in children has become increasingly successful in the past several years due to advances in immunosuppression, better selection of transplant candidates, and improvements in surgical techniques and postoperative care (Sokol et al., 2014). Transplant centres now offer both cadaveric and living-related liver transplants for children. Rejection of the transplanted liver is the most significant complication. Most children will require immunosuppressive therapy for a lifetime, putting them at risk for infections.

Nursing Assessment

Many children will be admitted to a transplant centre for a preoperative workup to determine the best possible tissue and blood match for the child. There is much anxiety among family members when a cadaveric transplant is the only possibility for survival. This puts a child on a waiting list that is prioritized based on several criteria. Because

there are a limited number of pediatric liver transplant centres throughout the country, there may be many issues regarding transportation, finances, job loss, and lodging. Assess the need for social work intervention; a social worker is almost always involved with these children. A liver transplant coordinator will assist with coordinating the care for pre- and post-transplant children.

Nursing Management

Preoperatively, assist with the transplant workup and teach the child and family what to expect during and after the liver transplantation. Postoperatively, the child will be in the intensive care unit for several days until he or she is stabilized from the actual surgery (see Nursing Care Plan 42.1 at the end of the chapter). After the child is sent to a regular unit in the hospital, monitor the child for several days to weeks for signs and symptoms of rejection and infection, including fever, increasing liver function test results and GGT, and increasing pain, redness, and swelling at the incision site.

Child and family education is an important element of nursing management in the post-transplant child. Assess and reassess medication knowledge throughout the entire hospitalization, as these children usually require medications for a lifetime.

NURSING CARE PLAN 42.1

Overview for the Child With a Gastrointestinal Disorder

NURSING DIAGNOSIS: Risk for deficient fluid volume: risk factors may include excessive losses through vomiting or diarrhea, inadequate oral intake, possible NPO status (particularly in the surgical child)

Outcome Identification and Evaluation

Child will maintain adequate fluid volume as evidenced by elastic skin turgor; moist, pink oral mucosa; presence of tears; urine output 1 mL/kg/hr or more.

Interventions: *Maintaining Fluid Balance*

- Maintain IV line and administer IV fluid as ordered *to maintain fluid volume.*
- Offer small amounts of oral rehydration solution frequently *to maintain fluid volume. Small amounts are usually well tolerated by children with diarrhea and vomiting.*
- When symptoms have lessened or resolved, reintroduce regular diet *to reduce number of stools, provide adequate nutrition, and shorten duration of effects of illness.*
- Avoid high-carbohydrate fluids such as Kool-aid and fruit juice, *as they are low in electrolytes, and increased simple carbohydrate consumption can decrease stool transit time.*

- Assess hydration status (skin turgor, oral mucosa, presence of tears) every 4 to 8 hours *to evaluate maintenance of adequate fluid volume.*
- Assess adequacy of urine output *to assess end-organ perfusion.*
- Maintain strict intake and output record and weigh child daily *to evaluate effectiveness of rehydration.*
- Weigh child daily: *accurate weight is one of the best indicators of fluid volume status in children.*
- Discourage milk products and fluids that contain high levels of sugar during the acute phase of illness, *as these products may worsen diarrhea.*

NURSING CARE PLAN 42.1

Overview for the Child With a Gastrointestinal Disorder (continued)

NURSING DIAGNOSIS: Diarrhea; may be related to inflammation of small intestines, presence of infectious agents or toxins, possibly evidenced by loose liquid stools, hyperactive bowel sounds, or abdominal cramping

Outcome Identification and Evaluation

Child will experience decrease in diarrhea: *will have bulkier stool as per normal routine.*

Interventions: *Relieving Diarrhea*

- Maintain clear liquid diet no longer than 24 hours, as prolonged clear liquids will result in continued liquid (starvation) stools.
- Avoid milk products until diarrhea improves: temporary poor absorption from villus injury follows viral diarrhea.

- Encourage complex carbohydrate foods to bulk up the stools.
- Add fat to carbohydrates to increase intestinal transit time to encourage water absorption (bulks up stool).

NURSING DIAGNOSIS: Constipation, related to GI obstructive lesions, pain on defecation, diagnostic procedures, inadequate toileting, or behavioural stool holding, possibly evidenced by change in character or frequency of stools, feeling of abdominal or rectal fullness or pressure, changes in bowel sounds, and abdominal distention

Outcome Identification and Evaluation

Child will experience improvement in constipation by passing daily soft bowel movement without pain or straining.

Intervention: *Relieving Constipation*

- Palpate for abdominal distention, percuss for dullness, and auscultate for bowel sounds *to assess for signs of constipation.*
- Encourage adequate fluid intake *to soften the stool.*
- Administer medications as ordered *to keep stool moving on daily basis.*
- Encourage activity as tolerated: *immobility contributes to constipation.*

- The child with stool withholding should sit on the toilet twice daily, preferably after breakfast and dinner, *to maximize chances for successful stool passage by taking advantage of the gastrocolic reflex.*
- For behavioural stool holding, use rewards or stickers *to encourage appropriate toileting.*

NURSING DIAGNOSIS: Risk for impaired skin integrity: risk factors include frequent loose stools, poor nutritional status, presence of stoma, acidic gastric contents contact with skin if gastrostomy present

Outcome Identification and Evaluation

Infant's skin will remain intact: *buttocks skin will be free from rash, excoriation.* In the child with an ostomy: skin surrounding stoma will remain intact: *free from redness, rash, excoriation.*

(continued)

Overview for the Child With a Gastrointestinal Disorder (continued)

Intervention: *Maintaining Skin Integrity*

- Change diapers frequently to limit acidic stool content contact with skin.
- Use barrier diaper cream to protect skin.
- Assess skin integrity at every diaper change to recognize skin changes early so that corrective measures can begin.
- Leave diaper area open to air several times a day if redness is present so that air can circulate and skin healing can be facilitated.
- Use plain water or only mild soap to cleanse the skin with diaper changes to avoid pH changes that contribute to diaper area skin breakdown.
- Avoid diaper wipes that contain fragrance or alcohol if the skin is red or has a rash, as both alcohol and

perfume cause stinging if used on nonintact skin and can worsen skin breakdown.

For the child with an ostomy:
- Ensure proper fit of the ostomy appliance/pouch *to avoid acidic stool contact with skin.*
- Use a barrier wafer (e.g., Stomahesive or Duoderm) to attach appliance: *avoids repeated pulling of adhesive tape from skin.*
- If redness occurs, use barrier/healing cream or paste on skin around stoma *to promote healing and prevent further skin breakdown.*
- Consult enterostomal therapy nurse as needed *to provide additional support.*

NURSING DIAGNOSIS: Imbalanced nutrition: less than body requirements; may be related to inability to ingest, digest, or absorb nutrients; intestinal pain after eating; decreased transit time through bowel; or psychosocial factors, possibly evidenced by lack of appropriate weight gain or growth, weight loss, aversion to eating, poor muscle tone, or observed lack of intake

Outcome Identification and Evaluation

Nutritional status will be maximized: child will maintain or gain weight appropriately.

Intervention: *Maintaining Appropriate Nutrition*

- Encourage favourite foods (within prescribed diet restrictions if present) *to maximize oral intake.*
- Administer enteral tube feedings as ordered *to maximize caloric intake.*
- Add butter, gravy, or cheese as appropriate to foods (if allowed within diet restrictions) *to increase caloric intake.*
- Encourage high-quality, high-calorie snacks between meals, *so as not to interfere with meal intake.*
- Document response to feeding *to determine feeding tolerance.*
- Limit intake of calorie-free beverages: *beverages should contain nutrients and calories.*
- Consult nutritionist *for appropriate diet supplementation recommendations.*

NURSING DIAGNOSIS: Ineffective breathing pattern, related to postoperative immobility, abdominal pain interfering with breathing, use of narcotic analgesics as evidenced by increased work of or shallow breathing, tachypnea, decreased lung aeration

Outcome Identification and Evaluation

Child will demonstrate effective breathing pattern: respiratory rate normal for age, absence of accessory muscle use, adequate aeration with clear breath sounds throughout all lung fields.

NURSING CARE PLAN 42.1

Overview for the Child With a Gastrointestinal Disorder (continued)

Intervention: *Promoting Effective Breathing Patterns*

- Turn, cough, and deep breathe every 2 hours *to encourage adequate aeration and discourage fluid pooling in lungs.* In the infant or toddler, turn every 2 hours and use percussor or chest physiotherapy *to prevent pooling of secretions.*
- Play games to encourage deep breathing (blow out penlight, blow cotton ball across bedside table with straw, etc.): *children are more likely to cooperate with interventions if play is involved.*
- In the developmentally able child, encourage incentive spirometer use every 2 hours *to improve lung aeration.*
- Demonstrate/encourage use of pillow splinting with coughing *to decrease abdominal pain and stress on incision.*

NURSING DIAGNOSIS: Risk for caregiver role strain: risk factors may include infant with congenital defect, child with chronic illness, marginal caregiver coping patterns, long-term stress, complexity and quantity of care child requires

Outcome Identification and Evaluation

Caregiver will exhibit emotional health: verbalizes concerns calmly, participates in child's care, and demonstrates knowledge of resources.

Intervention: *Easing Caregiver Role Strain*

- Assess parental behaviour *to identify role strain.*
- Provide emotional support and encourage talking about feelings, fears, and concerns *to promote trust in nurse as a source of emotional support.*
- Arrange for and/or encourage respite care for child: *provides parent with time away from continual care.*
- Consult social services *to identify community resources available for caregiver support (home health, support group, etc.).*
- Encourage parent to meet own needs and find personal time *to increase energy level and self-esteem, ultimately enhancing the quality of care given.*

NURSING DIAGNOSIS: Disturbed body image; may be related to presence of stoma, loss of control of bowel elimination, scars from multiple surgical procedures, or effects of treatment regimen, possibly evidenced by verbalization of negative feelings about body, refusal to look at stoma, or participate in care

Outcome Identification and Evaluation

Child or teen will demonstrate acceptance of change in body image by verbalization of adjustment; looking at, touching, and caring for body; and returning to previous social involvement.

Intervention: *Promoting Proper Body Image*

- Observe child's coping mechanisms to reinforce their use in times of stress.
- Acknowledge denial, anger, and other feelings as normal to support child/teen through difficult transition.
- Allow child gradual introduction to stoma to ease transition.
- Encourage child/teen to participate in care, as this sense of control will contribute to positive self-esteem.

KEY CONCEPTS

● The esophagus of the young child exhibits under-developed muscle tone compared with the adult.

● A major difference between children and adults is the reduced stomach capacity in the child and the significantly shorter length of the small intestine (250 cm in the child vs. 600 cm in the adult).

● Infants and children have a proportionately greater amount of body water than adults, resulting in a relatively greater fluid intake requirement than adults and placing infants and children at higher risk for fluid loss as compared with adults.

● The most common result of GI illnesses in infants and children is dehydration.

● The mildly or moderately dehydrated child must be identified and receive rehydration therapy to prevent progression to hypovolemic shock.

● Rehydration is a key medical treatment for dehydration as a result of many different GI disorders. Oral rehydration is most common, but in cases requiring hospitalization intravenous fluid therapy is key.

● Promotion of adequate nutrition is another significant treatment component. The child with a chronic GI disorder may require intravenous TPN or enteral tube feedings to exhibit appropriate growth.

● Surgical intervention is necessary for many acute or congenital GI disorders, such as pyloric stenosis, cleft lip and palate, appendicitis, Hirschsprung disease, and intestinal malrotation.

● Monitoring the blood count, electrolyte levels, and liver function tests is necessary in many pediatric GI disorders.

● Histamine-2 blockers, proton pump inhibitors, and prokinetic agents are used to treat disorders in which gastric acid is a problem, such as esophagitis, GERD, and ulcers.

● Close monitoring for infection is important in children with inflammatory bowel disease, autoimmune hepatitis, or liver transplant who are being treated with immunosuppressants and/or corticosteroids.

● GI stimulants and laxatives may be necessary for treating constipation and encopresis.

● Diarrhea, vomiting, decreased oral intake, sustained high fever, diabetic ketoacidosis, and extensive burns place the infant or child at risk for the development of dehydration.

● Risk factors for vomiting include exposure to viruses, use of certain medications, and overfeeding in the infant.

● Risk factors for acute diarrhea include recent ingestion of undercooked meats, foreign travel, day care attendance, and well water ingestion.

● Vomiting is a symptom and should be characterized in terms of volume, colour, relation to meals, duration, and associated symptoms.

● Bleeding may occur as a result of a GI disorder, particularly from the intestine with Meckel diverticulum and from esophageal varices with portal hypertension.

● Acute GI disorders are those that usually have a rapid onset and a short course, which at times may be severe. Examples include dehydration, vomiting, diarrhea, hypertrophic pyloric stenosis, and appendicitis.

● Chronic GI disorders are those that are long-lasting or recur over time. Examples include constipation, GER, inflammatory bowel disease, functional abdominal pain, and failure to thrive.

● Right lower quadrant pain and rebound tenderness of the abdomen found on physical examination are telltale signs of appendicitis, which is considered a surgical emergency.

● Bilious vomiting is the main symptom of conditions resulting in bowel obstruction, such as malrotation with volvulus.

● The focus of nursing management of the child with diarrhea or vomiting is restoring proper fluid and electrolyte balance through oral rehydration therapy or intravenous fluids if necessary.

● Reduction of inguinal and umbilical hernias should be attempted; if reduction of the hernia is impossible, immediately notify the physician.

● Small, frequent, and thickened feedings and proper positioning after feedings are key elements in the treatment of GER.

● A crucial nursing intervention related to cleft lip and palate repair is protection of the surgical site while it is healing.

● Palpation of the abdomen should be the last part of the physical examination of an infant or a child.

● A key element of nursing care for the child with a GI disorder is promotion of appropriate bowel elimination.

- Maximizing nutritional status is a critical nursing function for the child with a GI disorder.

- For the child who has undergone surgical repair for correction of a GI disorder, promoting effective breathing patterns and managing pain are important nursing goals.

- Counselling families about how to manage the child with vomiting or diarrhea at home, including oral rehydration therapy, is a key component of child/family education.

- Education of the child and family regarding the importance of medication compliance for management of inflammatory bowel disease is critical.

- Behavioural therapy and counselling may be necessary for children who have functional constipation and stool withholding.

- The child or adolescent with ineffective bowel control, poor growth, or an ostomy may have poor self-esteem and body image.

REFERENCES AND RECOMMENDED READINGS

Allen, S. J., Martinez, E. G., Gregorio, G. V, & Dans, L. F. (2010). *Probiotics for treating acute infectious diarrhoea (review). The Cochrane Library 2007, 12.* Indianapolis, IN: John Wiley & Sons.

Almadhoun, O. (2012). Managing chronic abdominal pain in children: Understanding physical and behavioral components of functional abdominal pain. *Contemporary Pediatrics, 29*(3), 18–23.

American Academy of Pediatrics. (2015). *Umbilical cord care.* Retrieved from http://www.healthychildren.org/English/ages-stages/baby/bathing-skin-care/Pages/Umbilical-Cord-Care.aspx

Batsos, C. (2009). *An environmental scan of cleft lip and palate clinics and dental benefits programs in Canada.* Retrieved from http://www.caphd.ca/sites/default/files/1008-CleftLipAndPalateScan.pdf

Ben-Joseph, E. P. (2013). *Canker sores.* Retrieved from http://kidshealth.org/en/parents/canker.html#

Brandt, M. (2014). *Intestinal malrotation.* Retrieved from http://www.uptodate.com/contents/intestinal-malrotation

Celiac Disease Foundation. (2016). *Gluten-free diet.* Retrieved from http://celiac.org/live-gluten-free/glutenfreediet/

Cheong, L. H. A., & Emil, S. (2014). Determinants of appendicitis outcomes in Canadian children. *Journal of Pediatric Surgery, 49*(5), 777–781. doi: http://dx.doi.org/10.1016/j.jpedsurg.2014.02.074

Cincinnati Children's. (2016). *Enema administration.* Retrieved from http://www.cincinnatichildrens.org/health/e/enema/

Corbett, J. A., & Banks, A. D. (2013). *Laboratory tests and diagnostic procedures with nursing diagnoses* (8th ed.). Upper Saddle River, NJ: Pearson Education Inc.

Curtin, G., & Boekelheide, A. (2010). Cleft lip and cleft palate. In P. J. Allen, J. A. Vessey, & N. A. Schapiro (Eds.). *Primary care of the child with a chronic condition* (5th ed.). St. Louis, MO: Mosby.

Denham, J. M. (2014). Non-celiac gluten sensitivity. *Presented at meeting of the Florida Chapter of the National Association of Pediatric Nurse Practitioners, Orlando, FL.*

Donovan, K. (2012). Breastfeeding the infant with cleft lip and palate. *ICAN: Infant, Child, & Adolescent Nutrition, 4*(4), 194–198.

Dowshen, S. (2014). *Stool tests.* Retrieved from http://www.kidshealth.org/parent/general/sick/labtest8.html

Dunn, A. (2013). Elimination patterns. In C. Burns, A. Dunn, M. Brady, N. B. Starr, & C. Blosser (Eds.). *Pediatric primary care* (5th ed.). Philadelphia, PA: Saunders.

Engorn, B., & Flerlage, J. (2015). *The Harriet Lane handbook* (20th ed.). Philadelphia, PA: Saunders.

Fleisher, G. R. (2014). *Evaluation of diarrhea in children.* Retrieved from http://www.uptodate.com/contents/evaluation-of-diarrhea-in-children

Ford, D. M. (2014). Fluid, electrolyte, and acid-base disorders & therapy. In W. W. Hay, M. J. Levin, R. R. Deterding, & M. J. Abzug (Eds.). *Current pediatric diagnosis and treatment* (22nd ed.). New York: McGraw-Hill.

Freedman, S. (2016). *Oral rehydration therapy.* Retrieved from http://www.uptodate.com/contents/oral-rehydration-therapy

Galloway, A., & Seguias, L. (2013). A 7-year-old Hispanic boy with acute onset of abdominal pain. *Pediatric Annals, 42*(12), 491–493.

Gilger, M. A. (2016). *Pathogenesis of acute diarrhea in children.* Retrieved from http://www.uptodate.com/contents/pathogenesis-of-acute-diarrhea-in-children

Haas-Beckert, B., & Heyman, M. B. (2010). Inflammatory bowel disease. In P. J. Allen, J. A. Vessey, & N. A. Schapiro (Eds.). *Primary care of the child with a chronic condition* (5th ed.). St. Louis, MO: Mosby.

Health Canada. (2002). *Congenital Anomalies in Canada—A Perinatal Health Report, 2002.* Ottawa: Minister of Public Works and Government Services Canada. Retrieved from http://www.hc-sc.gc.ca/pphb-dgspsp/rhs-ssg/index.html

Hoffenberg, E., Brumbaugh, D., Furuta, G. T., Kobak, G., Liu, E., Soden, J., & Kramer, R. (2014). Gastrointestinal tract. In W. W. Hay, M. J. Levin, R. R. Deterding, & M. J. Abzug (Eds.). *Current pediatric diagnosis and treatment* (22nd ed.). New York: McGraw-Hill.

Judge, J., Giordano, B. P., & English, J. (2014). Crohn's disease masquerading as an acute abdomen. *Journal of Pediatric Health Care, 28*(5), 444–450.

Jung, J. K. H., & Skinner, K. (2017). Foodborne and water-borne illness among Canadian Indigenous populations: a scoping review. *Canada Communicable Disease Report, 43*(1), 7–13.

Keels, M. A., & Clements, D. A. (2015). *Herpetic gingivostomatitis in young children.* Retrieved from http://www.uptodate.com/contents/herpetic-gingivostomatitis-in young-children

Matthews, J. L., Oddone-Paolucci, E., & Harrop, R. A. (2015). The epidemiology of cleft lip and palate in Canada, 1998 to 2007. *The Cleft Palate-Craniofacial Journal, 52*(4), 417–424. doi: http://dx.doi.org/10.1597/14-047

Olivé, A. P., & Endom, E. E. (2016). *Infantile hypertrophic pyloric stenosis.* Retrieved from http://www.uptodate.com/contents/infantile-hypertrophic-pyloric-stenosis.

43

KEY TERMS

amenorrhea
anasarca
anuria
bacteriuria
dysmenorrhea
dysuria
enuresis
hematuria
menorrhagia
neuropathic/
  neurogenic
  bladder
oliguria
proteinuria
urgency
urinary frequency

Nursing Care of the Child With an Alteration in Urinary Elimination/ Genitourinary Disorder

Learning Objectives

Upon completion of the chapter, you will be able to:

1. Compare anatomic and physiologic differences of the genitourinary system in infants and children versus adults.

2. Describe nursing care related to common laboratory and diagnostic testing used in the medical diagnosis of pediatric genitourinary conditions.

3. Distinguish alterations in urinary elimination and genitourinary disorders common in infants, children, and adolescents.

4. Identify appropriate nursing assessments and interventions related to medications and treatments for alterations in urinary elimination and pediatric genitourinary disorders.

5. Develop an individualized nursing care plan for the child with an alteration in urinary elimination or genitourinary disorder.

6. Describe the psychosocial impact of chronic genitourinary disorders on children.

7. Devise a nutrition plan for the child with renal insufficiency.

8. Develop child/family teaching plans for the child with an alteration in urinary elimination or genitourinary disorder.

Corey Bond, **5 years old, is brought to the clinic by her mother. She presents with fever and lethargy for the past 24 hours. Her mother states, "Corey has had a few accidents in her pants over the past few days, which is unusual for her. She also has been getting up at night more often to use the bathroom."**

🌀 **Urinary** elimination refers to the secretion and excretion of body waste through the urinary/renal system. Nurses may encounter children with alterations in urinary elimination and should be familiar with various genitourinary (GU) disorders that children experience. Alterations in urinary elimination, or GU disorders in children and adolescents may occur as a result of abnormalities in fetal development, infectious processes, trauma, neurologic deficit, genetic influences, or other causes.

Congenital disorders account for a large proportion of GU disorders in infants. External GU malformations are easily identified at birth, but internal structural defects may not be identified until later in infancy or childhood when symptoms or complications arise. Enuresis and urinary tract infection (UTI) also occur in a significant number of children.

Some alterations in urinary elimination directly involve the kidney from the outset, while others involve other parts of the urinary tract and may have a long-term effect on the kidneys and renal function, particularly if left untreated or treated inadequately.

Disorders affecting the reproductive organs often require early diagnosis and management to preserve future reproductive capabilities.

Nurses must be knowledgeable about pediatric GU conditions to provide prompt recognition, nursing care, education, and support to children and their families. Though some disorders are acute and resolve quickly, many have a long-term effect on quality of life and will require more intense, extended support.

Management of acute or common pediatric GU disorders may be provided in the pediatric or family practice outpatient setting, while specialists such as pediatric nephrologists or urologists usually manage chronic or involved GU disorders.

VARIATIONS IN PEDIATRIC ANATOMY AND PHYSIOLOGY

Though all of the urinary tract and reproductive organs are present at birth, their functioning is immature initially. The infant or child is at increased risk for the development of certain urinary elimination alterations because of the anatomic and physiologic differences between children and adults.

Structural Differences

The kidney is large in relation to the size of the abdomen until the child reaches adolescence. Due to this increased size, the kidneys of the child are less well protected from injury by the ribs and fat padding than they are in the adult. The urethra is naturally shorter in all ages of females compared with males, placing them at increased risk for the entrance of bacteria into the bladder via the urethra. In the female infant or young child,

this risk is compounded by the physical proximity of the urethral opening to the rectum.

Urinary Concentration

Blood flow through the kidneys (glomerular filtration rate [GFR]) is slower in the infant and young toddler compared with the adult (Lum, 2014). The kidney is less able to concentrate urine and reabsorb amino acids, placing the infant and young toddler at increased risk for dehydration during times when fluid loss or decreased fluid intake occurs. The normal range for serum blood urea nitrogen (BUN) and creatinine of the healthy infant or young toddler is usually less than the older child's or adult's. The renal system usually reaches functional maturity at around 2 years of age.

Urine Output

Bladder capacity is approximately 15 to 30 mL in the newborn with an interrupted voiding pattern (Guerra, Leonard, & Castagnetti, 2014). While bladder storage capacity increases over time, how to best estimate the amount of urine in infant remains challenging (Costa, Lavallée, Dubois, Leonard, & Guerra, 2014). The infant and toddler may void as often as 9 or 10 times per day. The expected urine output in the infant and child is 0.5 to 2 mL/kg/h, with the average 1-year old voiding about 400 to 500 mL per day. By 5 years of age, the average number of voids per day is the same as the adult's (three to eight). Adult bladder capacity (300 to 400 mL) is usually achieved around 12 to 14 years of age.

Reproductive Organ Maturity

The reproductive organs are also immature at birth. The gonads are not mature until adolescence in most children. The hormonal changes that occur with puberty account for some of the reproductive concerns, particularly for female adolescents.

COMMON MEDICAL TREATMENTS

A variety of medications as well as other medical treatments and surgical procedures are used to treat urinary elimination alterations and GU problems in children. These treatments will require a physician's or nurse practitioner's order. The most common treatments and medications are listed in Common Medical Treatments 43.1 and Drug Guide 43.1. The nurse caring for the child with a GU disorder should be familiar with what the procedures are, how the treatments and medications work, and common nursing implications related to use of these modalities.

COMMON MEDICAL TREATMENTS 43.1 GENITOURINARY DISORDERS

Treatment	Explanation	Indications	Nursing Implications
Urinary diversion	Surgical diversion of ureters to the abdominal wall. Continent diversion uses a piece of intestine to create a bladder that can be catheterized. Noncontinent diversion involves a stoma on the abdominal wall that requires use of an ostomy pouch	Any situation in which the bladder needs to be removed or does not function correctly (bladder exstrophy or prune belly, neurogenic bladder, e.g., spina bifida)	Meticulous skin care is necessary to prevent breakdown around stoma. Teach families how to care for ostomy pouch or how to catheterize continent stoma. Expect mucus in urine if intestine is used for urinary reservoir. Monitor for signs of urinary tract infection.
Foley catheter	An indwelling urinary catheter stays in place by means of an inflated balloon	Usually used only during the postoperative period	Monitor for urethral drainage or irritation. Keep area clean and dry. Monitor colour, consistency, clarity, and amount of urine in drainage bag. Monitor for infection, checking results of urinalysis and urine cultures.
Ureteral stent	A thin catheter temporarily placed in the ureter to drain urine. Removed via cystoscopy when it is time for discontinuation	Urinary tract anomalies	Monitor urine output carefully. Check for bleeding postoperatively.
Nephrostomy tube	Tube placed directly into the rena pelvis to drain urine externally to a bag	Urinary tract anomalies	Monitor urine output carefully, change dressings ensuring that the tube does not become dislodged.
Suprapubic tube	Catheter placed in the bladder via the abdominal wall above the symphysis pubis	Postoperative urine drainage with reconstructive surgeries	Monitor for blood in urine, adequate urine output. Minimize manipulation of suprapubic tube to avoid triggering bladder spasms.
Vesicostomy	Stoma in the abdominal wall to the bladder	Urinary tract anomalies, neurogenic bladder	Constant urine drainage requires diaper use. Monitor urine output. Assess skin around stoma for breakdown.
Appendicovesicostomy (Mitrofanoff procedure)	Uses appendix or a Monti (tubularization of a segment of the GI tract) to create a stoma on the abdominal wall that allows for catheterization of the bladder	Urinary tract anomalies, neurogenic bladder	Allows for urinary drainage when the child cannot catherize urethrally. Teach family and child how to catheterize stoma.
Bladder augmentation	Uses a piece of intestine (usually ileum) to enlarge bladder capacity, reduce bladder pressures	Decreased bladder capacity and function (usually neurogenic but can been used with chronic cystitis)	Since a portion of the GI tract is used, urine is often mucus-like.

NURSING PROCESS OVERVIEW FOR THE CHILD WITH AN ALTERATION IN URINARY ELIMINATION OR GENITOURINARY DISORDER

Care of the child with an alteration in urinary elimination or GU disorder includes assessment, nursing diagnosis, planning, interventions, and evaluation. There are a number of general concepts related to the nursing process that may be applied to GU disorders.

From a general understanding of the care involved for a child with urinary, renal, or reproductive dysfunction, the nurse can then individualize the care based on specifics for that child.

Assessment

Assessment of urinary tract, renal, or reproductive dysfunction includes health history, physical examination, and laboratory and diagnostic testing.

DRUG GUIDE 43.1 COMMON DRUGS FOR GU DISORDERS

Medication	Actions/Indications	Nursing Implications
Anticholinergic agents (oxybutynin, propantheline bromide, tolerodine, etc.)	Cause smooth muscle relaxation of the bladder, used for urinary tract spasms or contractions related to surgical procedure or use of catheters. Can be used in management nocturnal enuresis	Increase daily fluids; assess for constipation, dry mouth (which may increase risk for cavities due to < production of saliva) Avoid use in febrile child Sun exposure caution (photosensitivity)
Antibiotics (oral, parenteral)	Kill bacteria or arrest their growth. Used for urinary tract infection	Check for antibiotic allergies Should be given as prescribed for the length of time indicated
Desmopressin	Antidiuretic hormone effects by causing renal tubule to absorb more water, decreasing volume of urine in children with nocturnal enuresis	Sublingual medications available—no longer nasal preparations for this group Restrict fluid before sleep and during the night
Human chorionic gonadotropin (hCG)	Stimulates production of gonadal steroids to precipitate testicular descent	Monitor for signs of precocious puberty if used long term
Corticosteroids	Anti-inflammatory and immunosuppressive action to induce remission and promote diuresis in nephrotic syndrome. High-dose intravenous therapy used when nephrotic syndrome is resistant to conventional doses	Administer with food to decrease GI irritation May mask signs of infection Do not stop treatment abruptly, or acute adrenal insufficiency may occur Monitor for Cushing syndrome
Cytotoxic drugs (cyclophosphamide and chlorambucil)	Interfere with normal function of DNA by alkylation. Used to induce prolonged remission in nephrotic syndrome	Doses may be tapered over time Monitor for hypertension during infusion Causes bone marrow suppression Monitor for signs of infection Cyclophosphamide: administer in the morning; provide adequate hydration; have child void frequently during and after infusion to decrease risk of hemorrhagic cystitis Chlorambucil: administer with nonspicy, nonacidic foods; rarely seizures occur
Immunosuppressant drugs (cyclosporine A [CyA], azathioprine, tacrolimus, mycophenolate)	Cause immune suppression to prevent rejection of renal transplants. CyA and tacrolimus may be used for steroid-dependent nephrotic syndrome	Monitor complete blood count, serum creatinine, potassium, and magnesium Monitor blood pressure and observe for signs of infection Blood levels should be drawn prior to morning dose CyA: do not give with grapefruit juice Azathioprine and mycophenolate: give on empty stomach; do not open capsule or crush tablet Tacrolimus: give on empty stomach; assess for development of hyperglycemia Relapse of nephrotic syndrome may occur after withdrawal of CyA or tacrolimus therapy
Muromonab-CD3	Removal of all CD3 molecules from T-lymphocyte surface so it has inability to act. Used for treatment of acute renal transplant rejection	Monitor for development of pulmonary edema First-dose effect may cause fever, chills, chest tightness, wheezing, nausea, and vomiting

(continued)

DRUG GUIDE 43.1 COMMON DRUGS FOR GU DISORDERS (continued)

Medication	Actions/Indications	Nursing Implications
Angiotensin-converting enzyme (ACE) inhibitors (captopril, enalapril)	Potent vasoconstrictor, prevent conversion of angiotensin I to angiotensin II. Used to treat renal causes of hypertension	Monitor blood pressure frequently. May cause cough, hyperkalemia Captopril: administer on empty stomach Enalapril: administer without food
Imipramine (tricyclic antidepressant)	Increases the synaptic concentration of serotonin and/or norepinephrine. Treatment of nocturnal enuresis	Monitor for urinary retention. May cause decreased appetite Used infrequently as risk of accidental fatal poisoning
Diuretics: furosemide, hydrochlorothiazide	Inhibit resorption of sodium and chloride leading to increased excretion of water and electrolytes. Used in nephrotic syndrome, acute glomerulonephritis, hemolytic-uremic syndrome, or other instances of fluid overload with renal sufficiency	Administer with food or milk to decrease GI irritation Monitor blood pressure, renal function, and electrolytes (particularly potassium) May cause photosensitivity
Vasodilators: hydralazine, minoxidil	Direct vasodilation of arterioles, resulting in decreased systemic resistance. Used to treat renal causes of hypertension	May cause fluid retention Hydralazine: administer with food. Monitor heart rate and blood pressure (closely with intravenous use) Minoxidil: may be administered without regard to food. May cause dizziness
Calcium channel blocker: nifedipine	Prevents calcium from entering voltage-sensitive channels, resulting in coronary vasodilation. Used to treat renal causes of hypertension	Administer with food; avoid grapefruit juice Insoluble shell of extended-release tablet may pass in stool Use caution when administering liquid-filled capsule sublingually or by bite-and-swallow method, as significant hypotension may occur
Albumin (intravenous)	Increases intravascular oncotic pressure, resulting in movement of fluid from interstitial to intravascular space. Indicated for fluid volume excess associated with nephrotic syndrome	May require a filter depending on brand used Rapid infusion can result in vascular overload Monitor vital signs; observe for pulmonary edema and cardiac failure

Adapted from Taketomo, C. K., Hodding, J. H., & Kraus, D. M. (2013). *Pediatric & neonatal dosage handbook* (20th ed.). Hudson, OH: Lexicomp.

Remember Corey, the 5-year-old with fever and lethargy? What additional health history and physical examination assessment information should you obtain?

Health History

The health history consists of the past medical history, including the mother's pregnancy history; family history; and history of present illness (when the symptoms started and how they have progressed), as well as medications and treatments used at home. The past medical history may be significant for maternal polyhydramnios, oligohydramnios, diabetes, hypertension, or alcohol or cocaine ingestion. Neonatal history may include the presence of a single umbilical artery or an abdominal mass, chromosome abnormality, or congenital malformation. Document past medical history of UTI or other problems with the GU tract. Family history may be significant for renal disease or uropathology, chronic UTIs, renal calculi, polycystic kidney disease, vesico-urinary reflux (VUR), or a history of parental enuresis. Determine age of successful toilet training, pattern of incontinent episodes (having "accidents"), and self-care routines related to toileting hygiene. Note myelomeningocele or other spinal disorders that may affect the child's ability to urinate. Note previous urologic surgeries or ongoing renal interventions (e.g., dialysis). For the adolescent girl, obtain a thorough menstrual history, including sexual behaviour and pregnancy history.

When determining the history of the present illness, inquire about the following:
- Burning on urination
- Changes in voiding patterns
- Foul-smelling urine
- Vaginal or urethral discharge
- Genital pain, irritation, or discomfort
- Blood in the urine
- Edema
- Masses in the groin, scrotum, or abdomen
- Flank or abdominal pain
- Cramps
- Nausea and/or vomiting
- Poor growth
- Weight gain
- Fever
- Infectious exposure (particularly *Streptococcus* A or *Escherichia coli*)
- Trauma

Record medications used for acute or chronic conditions, or for contraception.

Physical Examination

Physical examination of the GU system includes inspection and observation, auscultation, percussion, and palpation.

INSPECTION AND OBSERVATION

Observe the child's general appearance, noting growth retardation or unusual weight gain. Inspect the skin for the presence of pruritus, edema (generalized or periorbital), or bruising. Note pallor of the skin or dysmorphic features (associated with genetic conditions). Document the presence of lethargy, fatigue, rapid respirations, confusion, or developmental delay. Observe the external genitalia area for infant diaper rash, constant urine dribble, displaced urethral opening, reddened urethral opening, or discharge. In females, note vaginal irritation or labial fusion. In males, observe the scrotal sac for enlargement or discolouration. Note the condition of a urinary stoma or diversion if present. With the child lying flat, observe the abdomen for distention, ascites, or slack abdominal musculature.

AUSCULTATION

Listen carefully to heart sounds, as a flow murmur may be present in the anemic child with a renal disorder (Klein, 2010). Note elevated heart rate. Auscultate blood pressure with the appropriate-size cuff, noting elevation or depression. In the edematous child, carefully auscultate the lungs, noting the presence of adventitious sounds. Note the absence of bowel sounds, as this may indicate peritonitis. In the child who receives chronic hemodialysis, auscultate the fistula for the presence of a bruit (desired normal finding).

Take Note!

Use the bell of the stethoscope when auscultating the infant's or child's blood pressure so that you can hear the softer Korotkoff sounds more accurately.

PERCUSSION

Percuss the abdomen. Note unusual dullness or flatness (dullness is usually heard over the spleen at the right costal margin, over the kidneys, and 1 to 3 cm below the left costal margin). A full bladder may yield dullness above the symphysis pubis.

PALPATION

Palpate the abdomen. Note the presence of palpable kidneys (indicating enlargement or mass, as they are usually difficult to palpate in the older infant or child). Note the presence of abdominal masses or a distended bladder. Document tenderness to palpation or along the costovertebral angle. Palpate the scrotum for the presence of descended testicles, masses, or other abnormalities. Note whether the foreskin, if present, can be retracted and if any scarring or inflammation noted. In the child who receives chronic hemodialysis, palpate the fistula or graft for the presence of a thrill (desired normal finding).

Laboratory and Diagnostic Testing

Common Laboratory and Diagnostic Tests 43.1 offers an explanation of the most commonly used laboratory and diagnostic tests for a child suspected of having a GU disorder. The test results can help the physician or nurse practitioner to diagnose the disorder or to determine treatment. Laboratory or nonnursing personnel obtain some of the tests, while the nurse might obtain others. In either instance, the nurse should be familiar with how the tests are obtained, what they are used for, and normal versus abnormal results. This knowledge will also be necessary when providing child and family education related to the tests and results.

Urine specimens may be collected using a variety of different methods in infants and children. The Canadian Paediatric Society (2014) suggests urethral catheterization or suprapubic aspiration, if a clean catch cannot be obtained. Urine bag collections are not recommended for culture as a result of contamination (CPS, 2014). Sterile urinary catheterization is performed like that in adults. The size of the catheter varies depending on the size of the child. General size recommendations are:
- 6 French: Birth to 2 years old
- 6 to 8 French: 2 to 5 years old
- 8 to 10 French: 5 to 10 years old
- 10 to 12 French: 10 to 16 years old (Bowden & Greenberg, 2012)

(text continues on page 1634)

COMMON LABORATORY AND DIAGNOSTIC TESTS 43.1 GENITOURINARY DISORDERS (continued)

Test	Explanation	Indications	Nursing Implications
Radioisotope imaging	Contrast medium injected IV; computer analysis uptake, washout to assess for scaring and function	DTPA—GFR, differential renal function, visualize obstruction Dimercaptosuccinic acid (DMSA)—renal scar(s) differential function (cannot visualize ureters or bladder) MAG3—combines DTPA and DMSA—obstruction, duplex, etc.	IV for administration isotope, wait for screening (approx. 2 hours after injection). May require catheterization when using DTPA depending on rationale for test.
Computer tomography (CT) ± contrast	Narrow beam x-rays can give detail of renal system	Assess physiology/tumour and cysts	No contrast noninvasive. Contrast requires IV and use with caution in patients with CKD as contrast-induced nephropathy can occur.
Renal ultrasound	Reflected sound waves allow visualization of the kidneys, ureters, and bladder	Useful in determining kidney size (as with hydronephrosis and polycystic kidney), presence of cysts or tumours, or rejection of kidney transplant	No fasting is required prior to the procedure. Does not require contrast material. The child should feel no discomfort during the ultrasound.

Adapted from Corbett, J. A., & Banks, A. D. (2013). *Laboratory tests and diagnostic procedures with nursing diagnoses* (8th ed.). Upper Saddle River, NJ: Pearson Education Inc.

Nursing Diagnoses and Related Interventions

Upon completion of a thorough assessment, the nurse might identify several nursing diagnoses, such as:

- Impaired urinary elimination
- Fluid volume excess
- Imbalanced nutrition, less (or more) than body requirements
- Risk for infection
- Deficient knowledge of the child or family
- Urinary retention
- Activity intolerance
- Interrupted family processes
- Disturbed body image

After completing an assessment of Corey, you note the following: foul-smelling urine, abdominal tenderness, redness in her perineal area, and slightly blood-tinged, cloudy urine. Based on these assessment findings, what would your top three nursing diagnoses be for Corey?

Nursing goals, interventions, and evaluation for the child with a GU disorder are based on the nursing

diagnoses. Nursing Care Plan 43.1, at the end of the chapter, can be used as a guide in planning nursing care for the child with a GU disorder. The care plan overview includes nursing diagnoses and interventions for urinary tract disorders as well as genital (or reproductive system) disorders. It is important to individualize it based on the child's symptoms and needs. Refer to Chapter 36 for detailed information about pain management. Additional information will be included later in the chapter as it relates to specific disorders.

Based on your top three nursing diagnoses for Corey, describe appropriate nursing interventions.

URINARY TRACT AND RENAL DISORDERS

The urinary tract and renal disorders discussed below include structural disorders, UTI, enuresis, and acquired disorders that result in altered renal function and/or neurogenic bladder.

Structural Disorders

Numerous urologic conditions are congenital (present at birth) and occur as a result of altered fetal development. Many of these defects are apparent at birth such as bladder exstrophy, cloaca, prune belly, or neurogenic bladder as a result of neurologic defect such as spina bifida. However, some are not recognized until later in infancy or childhood when symptoms and complications arise, or illnesses arise, for example, neurogenic bladder as a result of a lipomyelomeningocele. Both epispadias and hypospadias are urethral anomalies usually noted at birth.

Bladder Exstrophy

Bladder exstrophy is a congenital defect resulting in the bladder being open and exposed outside of the abdomen. Refer to Chapter 24 for additional information as well as nursing assessment. Nursing management consists of preventing infection and skin breakdown (covered in Chapter 24) as well as providing postoperative care and catheterizing the stoma.

Providing Postoperative Care. Nursing management in the postoperative period focuses on preventing infection and maintaining urinary drainage. Repairs are complex, can be staged and surgical approach and outcome vary globally (Alsowayan, Capolicchio, Jednak, & El-Sherbiny, 2016). Ensure urinary catheters drain freely and do not become kinked. Sometimes tubes or catheters used in the postoperative period require irrigation. Refer to the institution's policy and the surgeon's orders for specifics related to urinary catheter irrigation. Manage bladder spasms with medication and be aware of side effects such as constipation. Note blood-tinged urine upon return from surgery, with clearing of urine within hours to days.

Bladder Reconstruction (Augmentation). If bladder tissue is insufficient for repair, then the bladder is removed or augmented with a view to creating a continent urinary reservoir. Reconstruction can involve various approaches, including repositioning of the ureters and ileum pouch, and bladder neck repair to limit incontinence. Often, a stoma (Mitrofanoff) is created on the abdominal wall; it provides access to the urinary reservoir (Fig. 43.1). The stoma is catheterized at least four to six times per day and the bladder may require overnight drainage. Urine from an intestine-based urinary reservoir tends to be mucus-like and is often cloudier than urine from a urinary bladder, with an increased risk of bladder stone formation. Teach parents the procedure for catheterizing the urinary reservoir which is likely to include bladder washouts and be mindful of long-term outcome and surgical risk (i.e., perforation, tumour risk) (Hoen et al., 2017). Instruct the family to call the child's urologist or physician or nurse practitioner if signs or symptoms of

FIGURE 43.1 The abdominal stoma allows for urinary continence and requires catheterization.

UTI occur or attend ED if they have any cause for concern that could be suggestive of perforation (i.e., sudden onset abdominal pain, vomiting).

> **Take Note!**
> Children with congenital urologic malformations are at high risk for the development of latex allergy (Hamilton, 2015). Latex allergy can result in anaphylaxis. Primary prevention of latex allergy is warranted in all children with urologic malformations, so use latex-free gloves, tubes, and catheters in these children.

NEUROGENIC BLADDER

Neurogenic bladder refers to the failure of the bladder to either store urine or empty itself of urine as a result of nerve damage. Children with neurogenic bladder have loss of control over voiding. The spastic type of neurogenic bladder is hyperreflexive resulting in frequent urinary incontinence with expulsion of urine (under pressure from the hyperreflexive detrusor bladder muscle) and usually associated with incomplete emptying. The hypotonic neurogenic bladder is flaccid and weak and becomes stretched out; it can hold very large amounts of urine, resulting in continuous dribbling of urine from the urethra. Urinary stasis and retention occur in both types, placing the child at risk for UTI as well as reflux of bladder contents back up into the ureters and kidneys, resulting in renal scarring and insufficiency.

The goals of neurogenic bladder management are to promote optimal urinary continence and prevent renal complications. Interventions for neurogenic bladder include clean intermittent catheterization to promote bladder emptying; medications such as oxybutynin chloride (Ditropan) to improve bladder capacity; prompt recognition and treatment of infections; and in some children surgical interventions such as a urinary diversion

Educating the Family. If the child is to be discharged with the urinary catheter in place (which is common), teach the parents how to care for the catheter and drainage system. Tub baths are generally prohibited until it is time to remove the penile dressing. Ride-on toys, or any activity involving straddling, are not allowed for 2 to 3 weeks after surgery.

Obstructive Uropathy

Obstructive uropathy is an obstruction at any level along the upper or lower urinary tract. This discussion will focus on congenital structural defects, though obstruction can also occur as a result of other disease processes (acquired obstructive uropathy). The most common sites of obstruction are listed in Table 43.1. The defect may be unilateral or bilateral and can cause partial or complete obstruction of urine flow, resulting in dilation of the affected kidney (hydronephrosis). Complications include recurrent UTI, renal insufficiency, and for some children progressive damage to the kidney resulting in renal failure.

NURSING ASSESSMENT

For a full description of the assessment phase of the nursing process, refer to the Assessment section of the Nursing Process Overview earlier in the chapter. Assessment findings pertinent to obstructive uropathy are discussed below.

Health History. Elicit a description of the present illness and chief complaint. Common signs and symptoms reported during the health history might include:
- Recurrent UTI
- Incontinence
- Fever
- Foul-smelling urine
- Flank pain
- Abdominal pain
- Urinary frequency (needing to void often)
- Urinary urgency (urge to void immediately)
- Dysuria (difficulty or pain with voiding)
- Hematuria (blood in the urine)

Explore the child's current and past medical history for risk factors such as:
- "Prune belly" syndrome
- Chromosome abnormalities
- Anorectal malformations
- Ear defects

Physical Examination and Laboratory and Diagnostic Tests. Palpate the abdomen for the presence of an abdominal mass (hydronephrotic kidney). Assess the blood pressure; elevation may occur if renal insufficiency is present. Many cases of obstructive uropathy may be diagnosed with prenatal ultrasound if the obstruction has been significant enough to cause hydronephrosis or dilatation elsewhere along the urinary tract.

NURSING MANAGEMENT

Surgical correction is specific to the type of obstruction and generally consists of removal of the obstruction, reimplantation of the ureters as necessary, and, occasionally, creation of a urinary diversion. Postoperatively, assess urine output via vesicostomy, nephrostomy, suprapubic tube, or urethral catheter for colour, clots, clarity, and amount. Encourage fluids once the child can tolerate them orally. Administer analgesics and/or antispasmodics as needed for bladder spasms. Teach parents care of vesicostomy or drainage tubes, with which the child may be discharged.

> **Take Note!**
>
> Upon return from surgery, most children have intravenous fluids without added potassium infusion. Potassium is withheld from the intravenous fluid until adequate urine output is established postoperatively to avoid the development of hyperkalemia as the kidneys fail to function properly (Browne, Flanigan, McComiskey, & Pieper, 2013).

Hydronephrosis

Hydronephrosis is a condition in which the pelvis and calyces of the kidney are dilated (Fig. 43.3). Hydronephrosis may occur as a congenital defect, as a result of obstructive uropathy, or secondary to vesicoureteral reflux (VUR). Congenital hydronephrosis may be revealed on prenatal ultrasound. Complications of hydronephrosis include renal insufficiency, hypertension, and possible future renal failure.

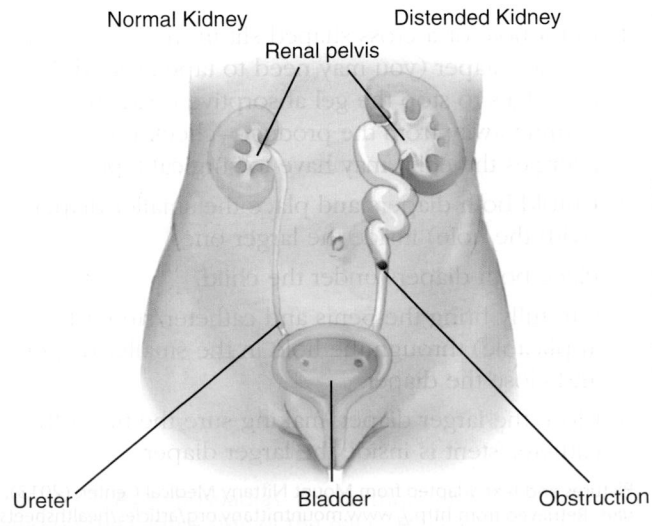

FIGURE 43.3 Hydronephrosis.

TABLE 43.1	COMMON SITES OF OBSTRUCTIVE UROPATHY	
Disorder	**Site**	**Illustration**
Ureteropelvic junction (UPJ) obstruction	Junction of the upper ureter with the pelvis of the kidney	Urinary tract with unilateral hydronephrosis and narrowing of the UPJ on that side
Ureterovesical junction (UVJ) obstruction	Junction of the lower ureter and the bladder	Urinary tract with unilateral hydronephrosis and dilated ureters with narrowing of the UVJ on that side
Ureterocele	Ureter swells into the bladder	Bladder with cystic pouch where ureters insert (unilateral)
Posterior urethral valves (males only)	Flaps of tissue in the proximal urethra	Distended proximal urethra, bladder, ureters, and hydronephrosis

Adapted from Gaylord, N. M., & Petersen-Smith, A. M. (2013). Genitourinary disorders. In C. Burns, A. Dunn, M. Brady, N. B. Starr, & C. Blosser (Eds.). *Pediatric primary care* (5th ed.). Philadelphia, PA: Saunders; and Lum, G. M. (2014). Kidney & urinary tract. In W. W. Hay, M. J. Levin, R. R. Deterding, & M. J. Abzug (Eds.). *Current pediatric diagnosis and treatment* (22nd ed.). New York: McGraw-Hill.

NURSING ASSESSMENT

For a full description of the assessment phase of the nursing process, refer to the Assessment section of the Nursing Process Overview earlier in the chapter. Assessment findings pertinent to hydronephrosis are discussed below.

Health History. Elicit a description of the present illness and chief complaint. The infant may be asymptomatic, but signs and symptoms reported during the health history might include:

- Failure to thrive
- Intermittent hematuria
- Presence of an abdominal mass
- Signs and symptoms associated with a UTI such as fever, vomiting, poor feeding, and irritability

Explore the child's current and past medical history for risk factors such as:

- Maternal oligohydramnios or polyhydramnios (congenital hydronephrosis)
- Elevated levels of serum α-fetoprotein (congenital hydronephrosis)

Physical Examination and Diagnostic and Laboratory Tests. Monitor the blood pressure of infants and children suspected of having hydronephrosis. Palpation of the abdomen may reveal enlarged kidney(s) or a distended bladder. A renal ultrasound as well as a voiding cystourethrogram (VCUG) will be performed to determine the presence of a structural defect that may be causing the hydronephrosis. Other diagnostic tests may be ordered to look for renal duplications or obstruction that could be associated with horseshoe kidney.

NURSING MANAGEMENT

Teach the parents signs and symptoms of UTI and sepsis, as these complications may occur. Explain to the parents that they should observe the child for adequacy of urine output and hydration status. Teach the parents to perform appropriate perineal hygiene and to avoid using irritants in the genital area. The infant or child with hydronephrosis will need follow-up with a pediatric nephrologist or urologist.

Vesicoureteral Reflux

VUR is a condition in which urine from the bladder flows back up the ureters and is graded from I to V (Mattoo, Mathews, & Gupta, 2014). Reflux of urine occurs during bladder filling and/or with voiding (Fig. 43.4). While reflux may occur in one or both ureters, prevalence in a healthy population of children is unknown (Mattoo et al., 2014). If reflux occurs when the urine is infected, the kidney is exposed to bacteria which may result in pyelonephritis. Renal scarring associated with VUR is referred to as reflux neuropathy and can result

FIGURE 43.4 Note retrograde flow of urine up the ureter upon bladder contraction.

in proteinuria, hypertension, and end-stage renal failure (Mattoo et al., 2014).

Primary VUR results from a congenital abnormality at the vesicoureteral junction that results in incompetence of the valve. Secondary VUR is related to other structural or functional problems such as neurogenic bladder, bladder dysfunction, or bladder outlet obstruction. As many as 70% of all children diagnosed with UTI have VUR (Nelson & Koo, 2014).

VUR grading is based on severity with grade I characterized by minor dilatation of the proximal ureter, to grade V, which is characterized by severe dilatation of the ureter and pelvis of the kidney. Grade I and II and 50% grade III VUR cases usually resolve spontaneously (Blais, Bolduc, & Moore, 2017) while unresolved grade III through V cases are generally associated with recurrent UTIs, hydronephrosis, and progressive renal damage (Nelson & Koo, 2014).

The goal of therapeutic management of VUR is prevention of pyelonephritis. Management continues to include antibiotic prophylaxis, though evidence is nonconclusive as to whether prophylaxis is actually beneficial (Easterbrook, Capolicchio, & Braga, 2017). Additionally, hygiene, bladder and bowel training, and voiding practices are used to assist with prevention of UTI and promote bladder emptying (Blais et al., 2017). Serial urine cultures can be used to determine recurrence of UTI. Biannual, annual, or biennial radionuclide VCUGs may be performed to determine the status of VUR.

Grade III, IV, and V cases with ongoing symptoms usually warrant varying surgical interventions (Blais et al., 2017). Endoscopic management with injection at VUR using a cystoscope is often performed as day case surgery. Multiple surgical approaches have been used to re-implant refluxing ureters into a bladder. The ureters are resected from the bladder and reimplanted elsewhere in the bladder via open or laparoscopic approaches (Blais et al., 2017).

Take Note!

The keys to prevention of long-term sequelae such as hypertension in children with urologic conditions are early diagnosis and intervention, prevention of infection, and close clinical follow-up. Nurses play a key role in monitoring and education.

NURSING ASSESSMENT

For a full description of the assessment phase of the nursing process, refer to the Assessment section of the Nursing Process Overview earlier in the chapter. Assessment findings pertinent to VUR are discussed below.

Health History. Elicit a description of the present illness and chief complaint. Common signs and symptoms reported during the health history might include:

- Fever
- Dysuria
- Frequency or urgency, incontinence
- Nocturia
- Hematuria
- Pain in the back, abdomen, or flank

Explore the child's current and past medical history for risk factors such as:

- Recurrent UTI in the female
- Single episode of UTI in the male
- Congenital defect
- Family history of VUR

For the child who is receiving ongoing follow-up for VUR, determine whether UTIs have occurred since the last visit, as well as the name and dose of prophylactic antibiotic.

Physical Examination. Monitor the blood pressure for elevation. Palpate the abdomen for presence of a mass (if hydronephrosis is present). VCUG may be used to diagnose VUR.

NURSING MANAGEMENT

Nursing management for the child with VUR includes preventing infection and providing postoperative care.

Preventing Infection. When VUR is present, the goal is to avoid urine infection so that infected urine cannot gain access to the kidneys. Initially, most cases of VUR are managed medically. Teach the importance of good oral fluid intake and teach the child to empty the bladder completely as well as treating any underlying constipation. Teach the child and parents appropriate perineal hygiene as well as toileting hygiene to prevent recurrence of UTI. Teach parents about the antibiotic therapy prescribed; the child will be maintained on a low daily dose to prevent UTI. The drug is most effective when given at bedtime because of urinary stasis overnight. Inform parents of the schedule for serial urine cultures and follow-up VCUG.

Providing Postoperative Care. If VUR is severe or if UTI is recurrent, surgical correction will be necessary. In the first 24 to 48 hours after surgery, maintain the intravenous fluid rate at 1.5 times maintenance to encourage a high urinary output. Monitor urine output via the Foley or SP catheter; urine should be bloody initially, clearing within 2 to 3 days. If ureteral stents are present, monitor urine output. Administer analgesics for incisional pain relief and antispasmodics as needed for bladder spasms. Encourage ambulation and advancement of diet as ordered to promote return of appropriate bowel function. Teach parents that prophylactic antibiotics will be given until 1 to 2 months after surgery, when the VCUG demonstrates absence of reflux.

Safety Check

GOAL: Reduce the Risk of Health care-Associated Infections (Prevent Infection)

In neonates, underestimation of UTI is probable. Use proven guidelines to prevent infections of the urinary tract that are caused by catheters

Steps: Ensure aseptic technique utilized for indwelling catheter insertion and ongoing catheter care provided according to facility policy. Maintain urine drainage by providing unobstructed flow and securing catheter; remove as soon as indicated.

Canadian Patient Safety Institute. (2016). *Hospital harm improvement resources.* Retrieved from http://www.patientsafetyinstitute.ca/en/toolsResources/Hospital-Harm-Measure/Documents/Resource-Library/HHIR%20UTI.pdf

Take Note!

When caring for the child who has undergone urologic surgery, avoid manipulating the Foley or suprapubic catheter: catheter manipulation contributes to bladder spasms.

Urinary Tract Infection

UTI is an infection of the urinary tract, most commonly affecting the bladder. UTI occurs most often as a result of bacteria ascending to the bladder via the urethra. About 8% of girls and 2% of boys will experience at least one UTI during childhood (Lum, 2014). One explanation for the more common occurrence in females is that the female's shorter urethra allows bacteria to have easier access to the bladder. The urethra is also located quite close to the vagina and anus in females, allowing spread of bacteria from those areas. The sexually active female adolescent is at risk for the development of UTI, as bacteria may be forced into the urethra by pressure from intercourse. The adolescent male may be somewhat protected from UTI by the antibacterial properties of prostate secretions.

UTI presents differently in infants than it does in children. Infants may exhibit fever, irritability, vomiting, failure to thrive, or jaundice. Children may also experience fever and vomiting, but also may have dysuria, frequency, hesitancy, urgency, and/or pain.

PATHOPHYSIOLOGY

E. coli most commonly causes UTI, as it is usually found in the perineal and anal region, close to the urethral opening. Other organisms include *Klebsiella, Staphylococcus aureus, Proteus, Pseudomonas,* and *Haemophilus.* Numerous factors may contribute to bacterial proliferation. Urinary stasis contributes to the development of a UTI once the bacteria have gained entry. Urine that remains in the bladder after voiding allows bacteria to grow rapidly. A decreased fluid intake also contributes to bacterial growth, as the bacteria become more concentrated. If the urine is alkaline, bacteria are better able to flourish. Untreated bladder infection may allow reflux of infected urine up the ureters to the kidneys and result in pyelonephritis, a more serious infection.

THERAPEUTIC MANAGEMENT

UTIs are treated with either oral or intravenous antibiotics, depending on the severity of the infection. Urine culture and sensitivity determines the appropriate antibiotic. A 7- to 14-day course of antibiotics is often prescribed, though 2- to 5-day courses may be as effective. Adequate fluid intake is necessary to flush the bacteria from the bladder. Fever management may also be needed.

NURSING ASSESSMENT

For a full description of the assessment phase of the nursing process, refer to the Assessment section of the Nursing Process Overview earlier in the chapter. Assessment findings pertinent to UTI are discussed below.

Health History. Elicit a description of the present illness and chief complaint. Common signs and symptoms reported during the health history might include:
- Fever
- Nausea or vomiting
- Chills
- Abdomen, back, or flank pain
- Lethargy
- Jaundice (in the neonate)
- Poor feeding or "just not acting right" (in the infant)
- Urinary urgency or frequency
- Burning or stinging with urination (the infant may cry with urination, the toddler may grab the diaper)
- Foul-smelling urine
- Poor appetite (child)
- Enuresis or incontinence in a previously toilet-trained child
- Blood in the urine

Explore the child's current and past medical history for risk factors such as:
- Previous UTI
- Obstructive uropathy
- Inadequate toileting hygiene (often occurs with preschool girls)
- VUR
- Constipation
- Urine holding or dysfunctional voiding
- Neurogenic bladder
- Sexual intercourse
- Pregnancy
- Chronic illness

Physical Examination. In the neonate or young infant, observe for jaundice or increased respiratory rate. In infants and children, inspect the perineal area for redness or irritation. Observe the urine for visible blood, cloudiness, dark colour, sediment, mucus, or foul odour. Note pallor, edema, or elevated blood pressure. Palpate the abdomen. Note distended bladder, abdominal mass, or tenderness, particularly in the flank area.

Laboratory and Diagnostic Tests. Common laboratory and diagnostic studies ordered for the assessment of UTI include:
- Urinalysis (clean-catch, suprapubic, or catheterized): may be positive for blood, nitrites, leukocyte esterase, white blood cells, or bacteria (**bacteriuria**)
- Urine culture: will be positive for infecting organism
- Renal ultrasound: may show hydronephrosis if child also has a structural defect
- VCUG performed once the urine has regained sterility may be positive for VUR.

Renal ultrasound, or VCUG, may be indicated in certain populations. The physician or nurse practitioner will determine the need for radiologic testing.

NURSING MANAGEMENT

Goals for nursing management include eradicating infection, promoting comfort, and preventing recurrence of infection.

Eradicating Infection. The child who can tolerate oral intake will be prescribed an oral antibiotic. The child who has protracted vomiting related to the UTI or who has suspected pyelonephritis will require hospitalization and intravenous antibiotics. Children younger than 3 months, and those with dehydration, a toxic appearance, or sepsis should also be hospitalized for administration of intravenous antibiotics (Lum, 2014). Administer oral or intravenous antibiotics as prescribed. Urge the parent to complete the entire course of oral antibiotic at home, even though the child is feeling better. Administer intravenous fluids as ordered or encourage generous oral fluid intake to help flush the bacteria from the bladder.

Promoting Comfort. Administer antipyretics such as acetaminophen or ibuprofen to reduce fever. A heating pad or warm compress may help relieve abdomen or flank pain. If the child is afraid to urinate due to burning or stinging (dysuria), encourage voiding in a warm sitz or tub bath.

Preventing Recurrence of Infection. Encourage the parents to return as ordered for a repeat urine culture after completion of the antibiotic course to ensure eradication of bacteria. Teaching Guidelines 43.1 gives further information on preventing UTI.

Teaching Guidelines 43.1
PREVENTING URINARY TRACT INFECTION IN FEMALES

- Drink enough fluid (to keep urine flushed through bladder).
- Drink cranberry juice to acidify the urine.
- Avoid carbonated and caffeine drinks, which irritate the bladder.
- Urinate frequently and do not "hold" urine (to discourage urinary stasis).
- Avoid bubble baths (they contribute to vulvar and perineal irritation).
- Wipe from front to back after voiding (to avoid contaminating the urethra with rectal material).
- Wear cotton underwear (to decrease the incidence of perineal irritation).
- Avoid wearing tight jeans or pants.
- Wash the perineal area daily with non-scented soap and water.
- While menstruating, change sanitary pads frequently to discourage bacterial growth.
- Void immediately after sexual intercourse.

Enuresis

Enuresis is continued incontinence of urine past the age of toilet training. Box 43.1 gives further definitions related to enuresis. Nocturnal enuresis generally subsides by 6 years of age; if it does not, further investigation and treatment may be warranted. Occasional daytime wetting or dribbling of urine is usually not a cause for concern, but frequent daytime wetting concerns both the child and the parents. Nocturnal enuresis may persist in some children into late childhood and adolescence, causing significant distress for the affected child and family.

In some children, enuresis may occur secondary to a physical disorder such as diabetes mellitus or insipidus,

---

> **BOX 43.1**
>
> ### DEFINITIONS RELATED TO ENURESIS
> - **Primary enuresis:** enuresis in the child who has never achieved voluntary bladder control
> - **Secondary enuresis:** urinary incontinence in the child who previously demonstrated bladder control over a period of at least 3 to 6 consecutive months
> - **Daytime wetting (previously diurnal enuresis):** can be primary or secondary—daytime loss of urinary control
> - **Nocturnal enuresis:** night-time bedwetting

---

sickle cell anemia, ectopic ureter, or urethral obstruction. Other causes common to both diurnal and nocturnal enuresis include a urine-concentrating defect, UTI, constipation, and emotional distress (sometimes serious). The most frequent cause of daytime enuresis is dysfunctional voiding or holding of urine, though giggle incontinence and stress incontinence can occur. Nocturnal enuresis may be related to a high fluid intake in the evening, obstructive sleep apnea, sexual abuse, a family history of enuresis, failure for the child to be producing sufficient antidiuretic hormone (ADH) at night, or inappropriate family expectations. Physical causes of enuresis must be treated; further management of the disorder focuses on behavioural training, which may be augmented with the use of enuresis alarms or medications.

NURSING ASSESSMENT

Elicit a description of the present illness and chief complaint. Determine the age of toilet training and when or if the child achieved successful daytime and night-time dryness. Enquire about urine-holding behaviours such as squatting, dancing, or staring as well as rushing to the bathroom (diurnal enuresis). Ask about the amount and types of fluid the child typically consumes before bedtime (nocturnal enuresis). Assess for risk factors such as:

- Family disruption or other stressors
- Chronic constipation (carefully assess bowel movement patterns)
- Excessive family demands related to toileting patterns
- History of being difficult to arouse from sleep
- Family history of enuresis

Assess the child's cognitive status: developmentally delayed children may take significantly longer to achieve urine continence than their typical same-age peers. Assess for short stature or elevated blood pressure, as these may occur when renal abnormalities are present.

NURSING MANAGEMENT

For the child with diurnal enuresis, encourage him or her to increase the amount of fluid consumed during the day in order to increase the frequency of the urge to

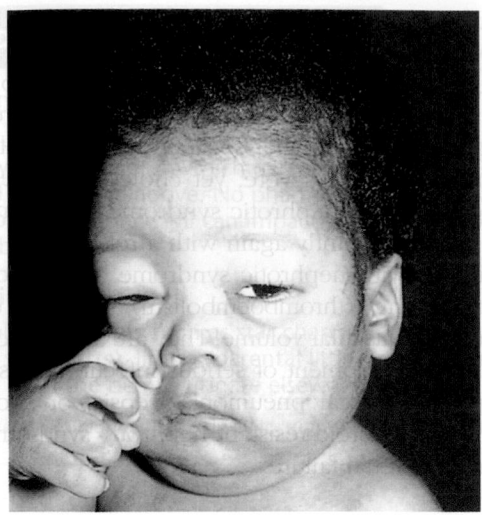

FIGURE 43.6 Note marked edema associated with nephrotic syndrome.

Observe the child for edema (periorbital, generalized [**anasarca**], or abdominal ascites). As the disease progresses, the edema also progresses to become more generalized, eventually becoming severe. Inspect the skin for a stretched, tight appearance; pallor; or skin breakdown related to significant edema (Fig. 43.6). Document height (or length) and weight. Note increased respiratory rate or increased work of breathing related to ascites and edema.

Note the blood pressure; it may be elevated in the child with nephrotic syndrome, though it is most often either normal or decreased unless the child is progressing to renal failure. Auscultate heart and lung sounds, noting abnormalities related to fluid overload. Palpate the skin, noting tautness. Palpate the abdomen and document the presence of ascites.

Laboratory and Diagnostic Tests. Urine dipstick will reveal marked proteinuria. Infrequently, mild hematuria is also present. Serum protein and albumin levels will be low (often markedly so). Serum cholesterol and triglyceride levels are elevated. With continued nephrotic syndrome, creatinine and BUN may become elevated.

NURSING MANAGEMENT

Goals for nursing management include promoting diuresis, preventing infection, promoting adequate nutrition, and educating the parents about ongoing care at home. As with other chronic disorders, provide ongoing emotional support to the child and family.

Promoting Diuresis. Administer corticosteroids as ordered. Tapering or weaning doses are required when the time comes to stop corticosteroid therapy. Administer diuretics if ordered, usually furosemide. Children

may develop hypokalemia because of potassium loss as an adverse effect of furosemide. Those children may require potassium supplementation or a diet higher in potassium-containing foods. Monitor urine output and the amount of protein in the urine (by dipstick). Weigh the child daily on the same scale either naked or wearing the same amount of clothing. Assess for resolution of edema. Measure pulse rate and blood pressure every 4 hours to detect hypovolemia resulting from excessive fluid shifts. Enforce oral fluid restrictions if ordered.

In cases of severe hypoalbuminemia, intravenous albumin may be administered. Increases in the serum albumin level cause fluid to shift from the subcutaneous spaces back into the bloodstream. A diuretic such as furosemide administered immediately after the albumin infusion allows for optimal diuresis and prevents fluid overload. Refer to Drug Guide 43.1 for the nursing implications related to use of these medications.

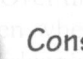

Consider This

Thirteen-year-old Jimmy Sanderson has a history of steroid-responsive nephrotic syndrome. In the clinic, today he tells you, "I am not going to take those steroids any more!" "I am shorter than everyone in my class, my 11-year-old brother is taller than me." "It's just not fair, I'll never get a girlfriend, if I'm a shorty."

Think back to when you were an adolescent. How would you have felt if you had a chronic illness and your necessary medications stunted your growth? As the nurse, how can you help Jimmy in this situation?

Preventing Infection. Monitor the child's temperature. Administer pneumococcal vaccine as prescribed (see Chapter 31 for information on immunizations). Administer prophylactic antibiotics, if prescribed. Delay administering live vaccines until at least 2 weeks after corticosteroid or other immunosuppressive medication therapy ceases. Teach parents that if the child is unimmunized and is exposed to chickenpox, the parents should notify the child's pediatrician, nurse practitioner, or nephrologist immediately so that the child may receive varicella zoster immunoglobulin.

Encouraging Adequate Nutrition and Growth. Encourage a nutrient-rich diet within prescribed restrictions. Fluid restriction is reserved for children with massive edema. Sodium intake may be restricted in the edematous child in an effort to prevent further fluid retention. Consultation with the dietitian is often helpful in meal planning because many of the foods that children like are high in sodium. Encourage protein-rich snacks. Consult with the child and family in planning meals and snacks that the child likes and will be likely to consume. Use of nutritional supplement shakes may be helpful for some children.

Educating the Family. Teach parents how to give medications and monitor for adverse effects. Demonstrate the urine dipstick technique for detecting protein, and encourage the family to keep a chart of dipstick results. The child may return to school but should avoid contact with sick playmates. If the child is exposed to another child with an infectious illness, explain to the parents that they should monitor temperature and urine dipstick results more frequently to identify a relapse in nephrotic syndrome early so that treatment can begin.

Providing Emotional Support. Nephrotic syndrome is often a chronic condition, and children who are responsive to steroid treatment may enter remission only to experience relapse. This cycle of relapse and remission takes an emotional toll on the child and family. Frequent hospitalizations require the child to miss school and the parents to miss work; this creates further stress for the family. The child may experience social isolation because he or she must avoid exposure to infections or because of self-esteem problems. The child may be dissatisfied with his or her appearance because of edema and weight gain, short stature, and the classic "moon face" associated with chronic steroid use.

Provide emotional support to the child and family. Encourage them in their efforts to maintain the treatment plan. Introduce the child to other youngsters with chronic renal conditions. Refer families to The Kidney Foundation of Canada, a link to which can be found on thePoint, for information about local support groups and resources.

Acute Post-Streptococcal Glomerulonephritis

Acute post-streptococcal glomerulonephritis (APSGN) is a condition in which immune processes injure the glomeruli. Immune mechanisms cause inflammation, which results in altered glomerular structure and function in both kidneys. It often occurs following an infection, usually an upper respiratory or skin infection. APSGN is caused by an antibody–antigen reaction secondary to an infection with a nephritogenic strain of group A β-hemolytic streptococcus. APSGN occurs more frequently in males than females and more frequently between the ages of 5 and 12 years (Gaylord & Petersen-Smith, 2013). The most serious complication is progression to uremia and renal failure (either acute or chronic).

There is no specific medical treatment for APSGN. Treatment is aimed at maintaining fluid volume and

managing hypertension. If there is evidence of a current streptococcal infection, antibiotic therapy will be necessary.

NURSING ASSESSMENT

For a full description of the assessment phase of the nursing process, refer to the Assessment section of the Nursing Process Overview earlier in the chapter. Assessment findings pertinent to acute glomerulonephritis are discussed below.

Health History. Elicit a description of the present illness and chief complaint. Common signs and symptoms reported during the health history might include:
- Fever
- Lethargy
- Headache
- Decreased urine output
- Abdominal pain
- Vomiting
- Anorexia

Assess the child's current and past medical history for risk factors such as a recent episode of pharyngitis or other streptococcal infection, age older than 2 years, or male sex.

Physical Examination and Laboratory and Diagnostic Tests. Assess the child's blood pressure for elevation, which is common. Note the presence of mild edema. Observe for signs of cardiopulmonary congestion such as increased work of breathing or cough. Auscultate the lungs for crackles and the heart for gallop. The urine dipstick test will reveal proteinuria as well as hematuria. Inspect the urine for gross hematuria, which will cause the urine to appear tea coloured, cola coloured, or even a dirty green colour. Serum creatinine and BUN may be normal or elevated, the serum complement level is depressed, and the erythrocyte sedimentation rate is elevated. Laboratory findings specific to streptococcus include an elevated antistreptolysin O (ASO) titer and an elevated DNAase B antigen titer.

NURSING MANAGEMENT

Administer antihypertensives such as labetalol or nifedipine and diuretics as ordered. Monitor blood pressure frequently. Maintain sodium and fluid restrictions as prescribed during the initial edematous phase. Weigh the child daily on the same scale wearing the same amount of clothing. Monitor increasing urine output and note improvement in the urine colour. Document resolution of edema. Provide a careful neurologic evaluation, as hypertension may cause encephalopathy and seizures. Children with APSGN generally are fatigued and choose bed rest during the acute phase. Provide the child with age-appropriate activities and cluster care to allow rest periods.

Some children may be managed at home if edema is mild and they are not hypertensive. Teach the family to monitor urine output and colour, take blood pressure measurements, and restrict the diet as prescribed. The child cared for at home should not participate in strenuous activity until proteinuria and hematuria are resolved. If renal involvement progresses, dialysis may become necessary.

Take Note!
Avoid use of nonsteroidal anti-inflammatory drugs (NSAIDs) in children with questionable renal function, as the antiprostaglandin action of NSAIDs may cause a further decrease in the glomerular filtration rate (Solomon, 2015).

Hemolytic-Uremic Syndrome

Hemolytic-uremic syndrome (HUS) is defined by three features—hemolytic anemia, thrombocytopenia, and acute renal failure. Typical HUS features an antecedent diarrheal illness. Other causes of HUS include idiopathic, inherited, drug-related, association with malignancies, transplantation, and malignant hypertension. This discussion will focus on typical HUS, the type preceded by a diarrheal illness. Watery diarrhea progresses to hemorrhagic colitis, then to the triad of HUS. The features of HUS, as well as effects on other organs, are caused primarily by microthrombi and ischemic changes within the organs. The thrombotic events in the small blood vessels of the glomerulus lead to occlusion of the glomerular capillary loops and glomerulosclerosis, resulting in renal failure.

A verotoxin-producing strain of *E. coli*, O157:H7, causes the majority of cases, though *Streptococcus pneumoniae*, *Shigella dysenteriae*, and other bacteria may also be the cause (Tan & Silverberg, 2015). It is thought that antibiotic treatment for the bacteria may contribute to release of the verotoxin. Undercooked ground beef accounts for most cases of *E. coli* O157:H7 infection, but it is also transmitted via the feces of numerous animals as well as unpasteurized dairy and fruit products. Transmission also occurs via human feces, and cases have been linked to public swimming pools. HUS occurs most often in children aged 6 months to 4 years (Tan & Silverberg, 2015). Complications include chronic renal failure, seizures and coma, pancreatitis, intussusception, rectal prolapse, cardiomyopathy, congestive heart failure, and acute respiratory distress syndrome.

Therapeutic management of HUS is directed toward maintaining fluid balance; correcting hypertension, acidosis, and electrolyte abnormalities; replenishing circulating red blood cells; and providing dialysis if needed.

NURSING ASSESSMENT

For a full description of the assessment phase of the nursing process, refer to the Assessment section of the Nursing Process Overview earlier in the chapter. Assessment findings pertinent to HUS are discussed below.

Health History. Elicit a description of the present illness and chief complaint. Common signs and symptoms reported during the health history might include watery diarrhea accompanied by cramping and sometimes vomiting. After several days, the diarrhea becomes bloody and eventually improves.

Explore the child's current and past medical history for risk factors such as ingestion of ground beef, visits to a water park or to a petting zoo before the onset of the diarrheal illness, or use of antidiarrheal medications or antibiotics.

Physical Examination. Observe the child for pallor, toxic appearance, edema, **oliguria** (decreased urine output), or **anuria** (absent urine output). Assess for elevated blood pressure and tenderness in the abdomen. Assess the child for neurologic involvement, which may include irritability, altered level of consciousness, seizures, posturing, or coma.

Laboratory and Diagnostic Tests. Urinalysis may reveal the presence of blood, protein, pus, and/or casts. Serum laboratory abnormalities are numerous and may include:
- Elevated BUN and creatinine
- Moderate to severe anemia (with the presence of Burr cells, schistocytes, spherocytes, or helmet cells), mild to severe thrombocytopenia
- Increased reticulocyte count
- Increased bilirubin and lactic dehydrogenase (LDH) levels
- Negative Coombs test (except in cases of *Streptococcus pneumoniae* infection)
- Leukocytosis with left shift
- Hyponatremia
- Hyperkalemia
- Hyperphosphatemia
- Metabolic acidosis

NURSING MANAGEMENT

Nursing management of the child with HUS focuses on close observation and monitoring of the child's status. Institute and maintain contact precautions to prevent spread of *E. coli* O157:H7 to other children (bacteria are shed for up to 17 days after resolution of the diarrhea). Close attention must be paid to fluid volume status. Prevention of HUS is also an important nursing function.

Maintaining Appropriate Fluid Volume Balance. Maintain strict intake and output monitoring and recording to evaluate the progression toward renal failure. Carefully monitor intravenous infusions and blood chemistries. Administer diuretics as ordered. Assess blood pressure frequently and report elevations to the physician or nurse practitioner. Administer antihypertensives as ordered and monitor their effectiveness. Encourage adequate nutritional intake within the constraints of prescribed dietary restrictions. Monitor for bleeding as well as for fatigue and pallor. Follow the institutional protocol for transfusion of packed red blood cells and/or platelets (platelets are usually transfused only if active bleeding or severe thrombocytopenia occurs). Report progressive deterioration in laboratory findings to the physician or nurse practitioner. Some children with HUS will require dialysis for at least several days.

Preventing Hemolytic-Uremic Syndrome. Proper handwashing is necessary. Teach children to wash their hands after using the bathroom, before eating, and after petting farm animals. Encourage the use of "swim diapers," which contain feces, for children who are not toilet trained. Teach parents to thoroughly cook all meats to a core temperature of 155°F, or until the meat is grey or brown throughout and the juices from the meat are clear rather than pink. Wash all fruits and vegetables thoroughly. Ensure that drinking water and water used for recreation are treated appropriately. Avoid unpasteurized dairy products and fruit juices (including cider).

Renal Failure

Renal failure is a condition in which the kidneys cannot concentrate urine, conserve electrolytes, or excrete waste products. As in adults, renal failure in children may occur as an acute or chronic condition. Some cases of acute renal failure resolve without further complications, while dialysis is necessary in other children. When acute renal failure continues to progress, it becomes chronic (also known as end-stage renal disease [ESRD]). Dialysis and kidney transplantation are treatment modalities used for ESRD.

Safety Check

GOAL: Improve the Effectiveness of Communication Among Caregivers (Improve Staff Communication)

Report critical results of tests and diagnostic procedures on a timely basis.

Steps: When caring for a child with a renal disorder, notify appropriate health care provider with critical lab values (oftentimes potassium), and critical changes to other laboratory values.

Joint Commission. (2015). *National patient safety goals effective January 1, 2015.* Retrieved from http://www.jointcommission.org/assets/1/6/2015_NPSG_HAP.pdf

Acute Renal Failure

Acute renal failure is defined as a sudden, often reversible, decline in renal function that results in the accumulation of metabolic toxins (particularly nitrogenous wastes) as well as fluid and electrolyte imbalance. Fluid overload may lead to hypertension, pulmonary edema, and congestive heart failure. Additional complications include hyperkalemia, metabolic acidosis, hyperphosphatemia, and uremia. In children, acute renal failure most commonly occurs as a result of decreased renal perfusion, as occurs in hypovolemic or septic shock. It may also occur in children with hemolytic anemia or as a result of nephrotoxicity from medications. Complications include anemia, hyperkalemia, hypertension, pulmonary edema, cardiac failure, and altered level of consciousness or seizures. In addition, acute renal failure may also progress to a chronic state.

Therapeutic management is aimed at treating the underlying cause, managing the fluid and electrolyte disturbances, and decreasing blood pressure.

Take Note!
Medications commonly used in children can reduce renal function. Cephalosporins may cause a transient increase in BUN and creatinine. Truly nephrotoxic drugs often used in children include aminoglycosides, sulphonamides, vancomycin, and NSAIDs. Make sure that potentially nephrotoxic drugs are administered according to published safe guidelines (dosage, frequency, rate of administration) (Taketomo, Hodding, & Kraus, 2013).

NURSING ASSESSMENT

For a full description of the assessment phase of the nursing process, refer to the Assessment section of the Nursing Process Overview earlier in the chapter. Assessment findings pertinent to acute renal failure are discussed below.

Health History. Elicit a description of the present illness and chief complaint. Common signs and symptoms reported during the health history might include:
- Nausea
- Vomiting
- Diarrhea
- Lethargy
- Fever
- Decreased urine output

Assess the child's current and past medical history for risk factors such as history of shock, trauma, burns, urologic abnormalities, renal disease, use of nephrotoxic medications, or severe blood transfusion reaction.

Physical Examination and Laboratory and Diagnostic Tests. Note decreased skin elasticity, dry mucus membranes, or edema. Auscultate the lungs for crackles, which may occur with pulmonary edema. Document tachypnea. Note cardiac rhythm disturbances. Evaluate the child's level of consciousness. Laboratory tests will reveal increased serum creatinine levels and possible electrolyte disturbances, such as hyperkalemia or hypocalcemia. Urinalysis may reveal proteinuria or hematuria.

Take Note!

Monitor the infant or child with renal failure carefully for signs of congestive heart failure, such as edema accompanied by bounding pulse, presence of an S_3 heart sound, adventitious lung sounds, and shortness of breath.

NURSING MANAGEMENT

Nursing care focuses on managing hypertension, restoring fluid and electrolyte balance, and educating the family.

Managing Hypertension. Carefully monitor the child's blood pressure. Administer antihypertensive as prescribed. When a fast-acting drug such as nifedipine (Procardia) sublingually or labetalol intravenously is used, stay with the child and frequently monitor blood pressure. Immediately notify the physician or nurse practitioner if high blood pressure is resistant to medication and the blood pressure remains elevated.

Restoring Fluid and Electrolyte Balance. Monitor vital signs frequently and assess urine specific gravity. Maintain strict records of intake and output. Administer diuretics as ordered. When urine output is restored, diuresis may be significant. Monitor for signs of hyperkalemia (weak, irregular pulse; muscle weakness; abdominal cramping) and hypocalcemia (muscle twitching or tetany). Administer polystyrene sulphonate as ordered orally, rectally, or through a nasogastric tube to decrease potassium levels. Polystyrene sulphonate removes potassium primarily by exchanging sodium for it, which is then eliminated in the feces. Administer packed red blood cell transfusions as ordered (may need to be followed by a dose of diuretic). Dialysis may become necessary if oliguria is sustained and leads to significant fluid overload, the electrolyte imbalance reaches dangerous levels, or uremia results in depression of the central nervous system.

Providing Family Education. Educate the family about the plan of care and the need for fluid restriction, if ordered. Instruct the family to save all voids for observation and measurement by the nurse. Provide education about the use of dialysis if relevant.

End-Stage Renal Disease

ESRD is chronic renal failure requiring long-term dialysis or renal transplantation. Chronic renal failure in children most often results from congenital structural defects such as obstructive uropathy (Klein, 2010). It may also be caused by an inherited condition such as familial nephritis or may result from an acquired problem such as glomerulonephritis; it may follow an infectious process such as pyelonephritis or HUS (Klein, 2010). This is in contrast to chronic renal failure in adults, which primarily results from diabetes or hypertension.

Uremia, hypocalcemia, hyperkalemia, and metabolic acidosis occur. Complications of ESRD are many. Uremic toxins deplete erythrocytes and the failing kidneys cannot produce erythropoietin, so severe anemia results. Hypertension is common and heart failure may occur. Hypocalcemia results in renal rickets (brittle bones). Growth is retarded and sexual maturation may be delayed or absent. Many children with ESRD experience depression, anxiety, impaired social interaction, and poor self-esteem (Klein, 2010).

NURSING ASSESSMENT

For a full description of the assessment phase of the nursing process, refer to the Assessment section of the Nursing Process Overview earlier in the chapter. Assessment findings pertinent to ESRD are discussed below.

Health History. Explore the health history for low birthweight (associated with kidney dysfunction and anatomic alterations), poor growth (weight, length/height, and head circumference), and regimen of dialysis. Note decreased appetite or energy level, dry or itchy skin, or bone or joint pain.

Physical Examination and Laboratory and Diagnostic Tests. Perform a thorough physical assessment, noting any abnormalities (may vary from child to child). If present, assess the peritoneal catheter site for absence of drainage, bleeding, or redness. If the child undergoes hemodialysis, assess the fistula or graft site for the presence of a bruit and a thrill. Laboratory tests may reveal low hemoglobin and hematocrit, increased serum phosphorus and potassium levels, and decreased sodium, calcium, and bicarbonate levels. BUN, uric acid, and creatinine levels will be elevated. A 24-hour urine creatinine clearance test will show increased amounts of creatinine in the urine, reflecting decreasing kidney function.

Take Note!

Carefully assess children with ESRD for worsening uremia or metabolic acidosis. Uremia may result in central nervous system symptoms such as headache or coma, or gastrointestinal or neuromuscular disturbances. Metabolic acidosis causes lethargy, dull headache, and confusion.

TABLE 43.2	MEDICATIONS AND SUPPLEMENTS COMMONLY USED TO TREAT ESRD COMPLICATIONS
Medication or Supplement	**Purpose**
Vitamin D and calcium	Correction of hypocalcemia and hyperphosphatemia
Ferrous sulphate	Treatment of anemia
Bicitra or sodium bicarbonate tablets	Correction of acidosis
Multivitamin	Augment nutritional status
Erythropoietin injections	Stimulate red blood cell growth
Growth hormone injections	Stimulate growth in stature

Adapted from Klein, M. S. (2010). Kidney disease, chronic. In P. J. Allen, J. A. Vessey, & N. A. Schapiro (Eds.). *Primary care of the child with a chronic condition* (5th ed.). St. Louis, MO: Mosby.

NURSING MANAGEMENT

Nursing goals for the child with ESRD include promoting growth and development, removing waste products and maintaining fluid balance via dialysis, encouraging psychosocial well-being, and supporting and educating the family.

Promoting Growth and Development. Encourage the child to choose foods he or she likes that are within the imposed dietary restrictions. Daily protein requirements for adequate growth range from 0.9 to 1.5 g of protein per kilogram of weight. Sodium and/or potassium restrictions may also be necessary. Enforce fluid restrictions if prescribed. Administer medications such as erythropoietin, growth hormone, and vitamin and mineral supplements to augment nutritional status and promote growth. Table 43.2 lists medications and supplements used to support growth.

Encouraging Psychosocial Well-Being. The child with chronic renal failure and particularly ESRD often suffers from depression and anxiety. Refer children and their families to the hospital social worker or counsellor as needed for depression or anxiety issues. The chronic need for dialysis (daily with peritoneal dialysis or three or four times per week with hemodialysis) confers long-term stress on the child and family. The child usually demonstrates poor growth and often suffers from body image disturbance. Frequent medical appointments and hospitalizations interfere with the child's scholastic achievements. Introduce the child to other children with ESRD (this often happens anyway at the hemodialysis centre).

Ensure that the family is aware of financial and support resources within the community and refer them to The Kidney Foundation of Canada. Such organizations can provide financial aid and access to summer camps for children with renal problems. Camp is an excellent way for children to demonstrate that they have mastered some of the loss-of-control issues related to their disease.

Several links are available in the website of The Kidney Foundation of Canada which provide forums for children and teens with kidney failure or transplantation so they can learn about their disease, access resources, and/or communicate with other children (peer support).

Dialysis and Transplantation

Peritoneal dialysis or hemodialysis is required on a long-term basis for children with chronic renal failure or ESRD. Once the child has progressed to ESRD, kidney transplantation is needed in order for the child to progress with normal growth and development.

Peritoneal Dialysis

Peritoneal dialysis uses the child's abdominal cavity as a semipermeable membrane to help remove excess fluid and waste products (Figs. 43.7 and 43.8). The parent or caregiver performs peritoneal dialysis at home after completing a training course. The process is either completed overnight with the use of a machine (continuous cyclic peritoneal dialysis) or in increments throughout the day for a total of 4 to 8 hours (continuous ambulatory peritoneal dialysis). Comparison Chart 43.1 compares these two methods of peritoneal dialysis.

The advantages of peritoneal dialysis over hemodialysis include improved growth as a result of more dietary freedom, increased independence in daily activities, and a steadier state of electrolyte balance. However, the risk for infection (peritonitis and sepsis) is a continual concern with peritoneal dialysis (Klein, 2010). Dialysate exchange protocols, care of the catheter in the abdomen, and dressing changes must all be performed using sterile technique to avoid introducing microorganisms into the peritoneal cavity. Box 43.2 lists additional risks associated with peritoneal dialysis.

FIGURE 43.7 The peritoneal dialysis catheter is tunnelled under the skin into the peritoneal cavity.

Hemodialysis

Hemodialysis removes toxins and excess fluid from the blood by pumping the child's blood through a hemodialysis machine and then reinfusing the blood into the child. Needles to remove and reinfuse the blood are inserted into an arteriovenous fistula or graft, usually located in the child's arm (Figs. 43.9 and 43.10).

Hemodialysis frees the parent from the need to perform daily dialysis, but the procedure, which takes 3 to 6 hours, must be done two to four times per week (usually three) at a pediatric hemodialysis centre. This requires time away from school and other activities for the child and from work and other family responsibilities for the parent. Since hemodialysis is usually performed only every other day, larger amounts of waste products

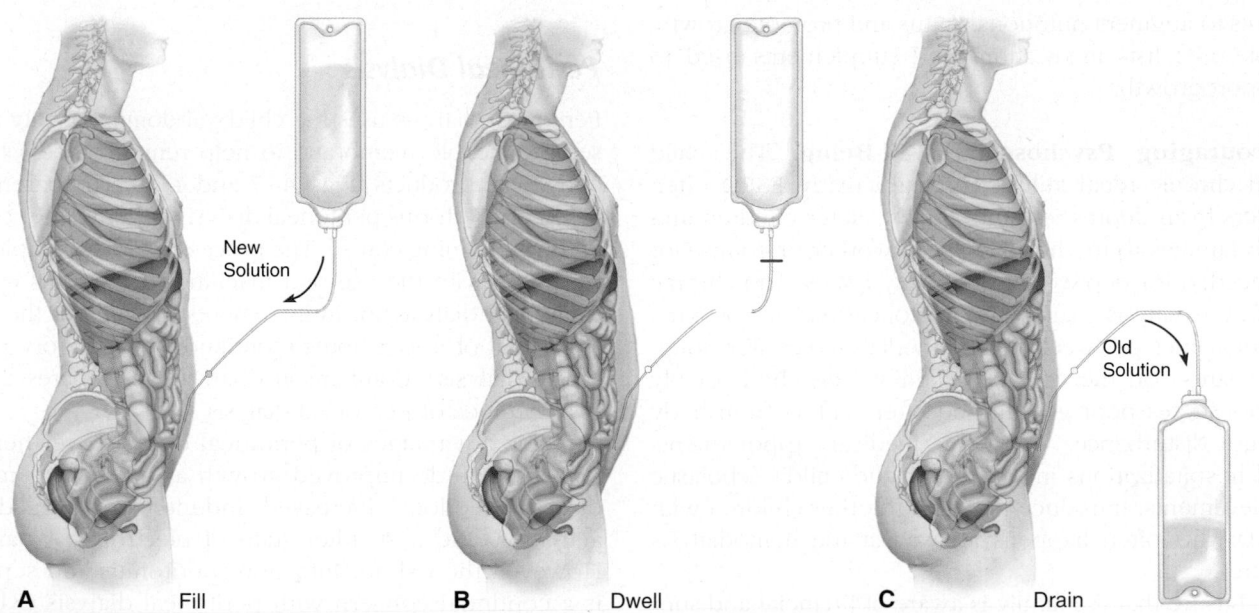

FIGURE 43.8 **A.** During the "fill" phase of peritoneal dialysis, dialysate fluid is instilled into the peritoneal cavity. **B.** During the "dwell" phase, the child may be up out of bed with the empty dialysate bag folded up with the tubing under his clothing. **C.** During the "drain" phase, the old dialysate is drained from the peritoneum by gravity, bringing with it waste products and excess fluid. The dialysate bags are weighed prior to filling and after draining to determine the amount of fluid removed from the child.

COMPARISON CHART 43.1	METHODS OF PERITONEAL DIALYSIS	
	Continuous Ambulatory Peritoneal Dialysis (CAPD)	**Continuous Cyclic Peritoneal Dialysis (CCPD)**
When performed	Throughout the day, with exchanges every 3 to 6 hours. Fluid is usually allowed to dwell overnight to allow child to sleep	Usually overnight while child is sleeping
Method	Manual instillation and draining and changing of dialysate bags with each exchange	Automated via CCPD machine; bags and tubing are attached when started, then disconnected in the morning
Dwell time	3 to 6 hours	Usually 30 minutes to 1 hour
Mobility	Allows for mobility and permits child to participate in activities between exchanges	Child is confined to bed during the night while CCPD is ongoing but completely mobile while off CCPD during the day

build up in the child's blood (uremia), placing the child at higher risk for seizures. The access site may become infected, and occlusion is also possible. The child must follow a stricter diet between hemodialysis treatments, though dietary restrictions are usually lifted while the child is actually undergoing the treatment.

NURSING ASSESSMENT

Refer to the section on nursing assessment of the child with chronic renal failure/ESRD, as it is similar to assessment of the child undergoing dialysis. Assess for alterations in blood pressure and laboratory values following dialysis. Monitor for signs and symptoms of infection.

Assess the child receiving peritoneal dialysis for toleration of the fluid volume instilled within the peritoneum. The abdomen will remain distended while the fluid is indwelling and will be significantly flatter when the fluid is drained. Assess the Tenckhoff catheter site for signs of infection. Monitor the child's temperature. Inspect the dialysate effluent for fibrin or cloudiness, which may indicate infection. Weigh the child daily (in the drain phase if on peritoneal dialysis).

A

B

FIGURE 43.9 **A.** Arteriovenous fistula. **B.** Arteriovenous graft.

BOX 43.2

RISKS ASSOCIATED WITH PERITONEAL DIALYSIS

- Hypertension and other cardiac complications
- Seizures
- Obstructed catheter
- Dialysate leakage
- Hyperglycemia
- Increased triglyceride levels
- Increased protein loss
- Parental stress and burnout related to repetitive nature of daily intervention

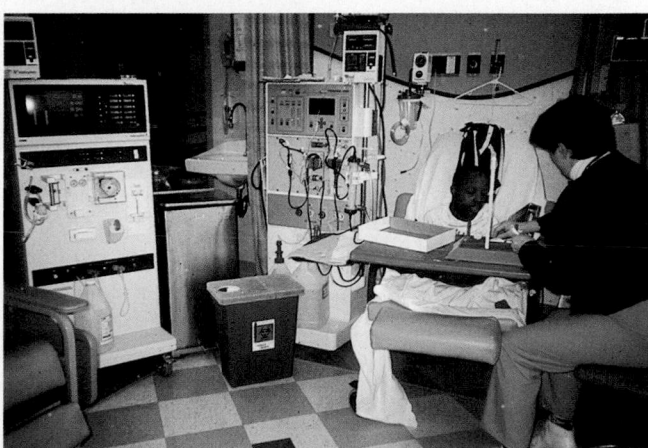

FIGURE 43.10 Pediatric hemodialysis.

For the child who receives hemodialysis, assess the arteriovenous fistula or graft site with each set of vital signs. Auscultate the site for the presence of a bruit and palpate for the presence of a thrill. Notify the physician or nurse practitioner immediately if either is absent.

Take Note!

Avoid taking blood pressure, performing venipuncture, or using a tourniquet in the extremity with the arteriovenous fistula or graft; these procedures may cause occlusion and subsequent malfunction of the fistula or graft. Teach parents and children to inform all health care providers they come in contact with about the presence of the fistula or graft.

NURSING MANAGEMENT

Specially trained and certified nurses perform both peritoneal dialysis and hemodialysis. The general pediatric nurse's role is related to the ongoing care of the child. The child undergoing peritoneal dialysis usually is allowed a more liberal diet and intake of fluid than the child undergoing hemodialysis. Peritoneal dialysis removes waste and excess fluids on a daily basis, whereas hemodialysis occurs about every other day. Most routine medications are withheld on the morning that hemodialysis is scheduled, since they would be filtered out through the dialysis process anyway. Administer these medications as soon as the child returns from the dialysis unit.

Thinking About Development

Trevon Smith is a 17-year-old male football player who was on track for a college scholarship. Following an episode of acute glomerulonephritis, Trevon has progressed to chronic renal failure and is dependent upon hemodialysis. He is listed for a kidney transplant.

How will Trevon's developmental stage affect his desire to comply with the medical regimen? What types of psychosocial issues might Trevon be experiencing and how can the nurse best support Trevon at this time?

How will the nurse educate Trevon about self-care?

Renal Transplantation

Renal transplantation is the optimal treatment for ESRD and offers the best opportunity for the child to live a normal life. Vigilant medication administration is necessary after the transplant to prevent organ rejection. The child achieves improved renal function with the transplant and may demonstrate improved growth, enhanced cognitive development, and improved psychosocial development and quality of life.

Kidneys are obtained from a cadaver (a patient declared brain-dead who had previously given consent to organ donation) or from a blood relative (living-related). The transplanted kidney must match the child's blood type and the child's human leukocyte antigens (HLAs). The cadaver kidney or living-related kidney is implanted surgically in the abdomen and the blood vessels are anastomosed to the aorta and superior vena cava.

Generally, living-related transplants have a decreased rejection rate compared with cadaver transplants (Klein & Martin, 2010). Living-related kidney donation and subsequent transplantation can be planned ahead and scheduled in advance. In contrast, cadaver kidneys become available suddenly, leaving less time for preoperative preparation. For either type, last-minute blood tissue typing is required before the final decision is made to move forward with transplantation. Often the child's native kidneys are removed before or at the time of the renal transplant because of their association with hypertension in the child (Klein & Martin, 2010).

Take Note!

Cadaver kidneys are allocated to potential recipients based on the age of the child with renal failure, the time that he or she has been awaiting a transplant, blood type, HLA antibody matching, panel reactive antibodies, and region of the country (so that the donated kidney can be received expeditiously).

Nursing Assessment

A thorough physical assessment is warranted for any child undergoing renal transplant, whether in the initial postoperative period, at a clinic visit, or when admitted to the hospital, to rule out transplant rejection. Note recent health history, medications and their doses, and any symptoms the child has been having. In the initial postoperative period, assess the incision for redness, edema, or drainage. If any of these signs of infection or rejection occur, notify the transplant surgeon and nephrologist immediately. Monitor blood pressure and other vital signs closely. Document resolution of edema. Record intake and output accurately. Assess for signs and symptoms of transplant rejection such as malaise, fever, unexplained weight gain, or pain over the transplant area.

NURSING MANAGEMENT

Postoperative care focuses on preventing rejection, monitoring renal function, maintaining fluid and electrolyte balance, and educating the child and family.

Take Note!

Encourage the child with a renal transplant to wear a medical alert necklace or bracelet, and urge the parents to inform community emergency services of the child's transplant status.

Preventing Rejection and Promoting Renal Function. Administer immunosuppressants accurately and in a timely fashion. Obtain and monitor serum levels of these medications per protocol. Immediately report significant alterations in vital signs or edema at the surgical site, as they may indicate transplant rejection. Maintain strict documentation of intake and output. Once adequate urine output is established, intake is usually liberalized.

Educating the Child and Family. Develop a schedule to cluster care so that the child may receive the rest needed for recovery despite the many and frequent assessments and interventions. With the family, develop a medication schedule that will be compatible with the family's life at home as well as the restrictions related to some medications. Begin teaching with the family as soon as the child's condition is stable. Accurate medication administration and home monitoring are necessary to prevent rejection. The child may return to school when discharged from the hospital, but the family will need to communicate closely with the school nurse about the child's immunosuppressed status. The Hospital for Sick Children (SickKids) has developed a renal transplant fact sheet that can be shared with the school nurse. A link to the website is located on the**Point**.

> **Take Note!**
> Tell the parents to inform their child's physician or nurse practitioner about the child's long-term corticosteroid use and/or immunosuppressed status, as the child should not receive any live vaccines.

REPRODUCTIVE ORGAN DISORDERS

A number of disorders may occur within the female or male genitalia and internal reproductive organs in children. These problems may be structural or infectious.

Female Disorders

Disorders of the female reproductive organs that occur in children and adolescents include structural disorders, infectious disorders, and menstrual disorders.

Labial Adhesions

Labial adhesion or labial fusion is partial or almost complete adherence of the labia minora (Fig. 43.11). UTI may result from urinary stasis behind the labia. Collecting of urine behind the adhesion can also result in post-void dribbling which may result in perineal soreness. Generally, adhesions do not cause problems for most infants or children and will resolve spontaneously.

FIGURE 43.11 Labial adhesions. Note fusion of the labia minora. (From Baskin, L. S., Kogan, B. A., & Stock, J. A. [2019]. *Handbook of pediatric urology*. Philadelphia, PA: Wolters Kluwer.)

NURSING ASSESSMENT

Younger girls have a higher risk of adhesions (3 months to 6 years) (Gerlt & Starr, 2013). Assess the history for dysuria or urinary frequency. Inspect the genitalia for fusion or adherence of the labia minora.

NURSING MANAGEMENT

If treatment has been indicated apply small amounts of topical estrogen cream as prescribed, usually once or twice daily. Teach the parents to continue cream application until the labia separate (maximum use 2 to 3 months, then suggest review). Be mindful that this is hormone treatment and parents may notice fine pubic hair growth. Treatment success varies with more than a third having no change noted or reoccurrence of adhesions. If adhesions do separate, encourage use of petroleum jelly daily for 1 month following labial separation to prevent recurrence of adhesion.

Vulvovaginitis (VV)

Vulvovaginitis is inflammation of the vulva and vagina. Inflammation may occur as a result of bacterial or yeast overgrowth or from chemical factors such as bubble bath, soaps, or perfumes found in personal care products. Poor hygiene may also cause vulvovaginitis. Tight clothing may cause a heat rash in the perineal area. Persistent scratching of the irritated area may result in the complication of superficial skin infection.

NURSING ASSESSMENT

Elicit a description of the present illness and chief complaint. Common signs and symptoms reported during the health history may include itching or burning in the perineal area. Explore the child's current and past medical history for risk factors, which may include:
• Young age (toilet-trained preschooler)
• Poor hygiene

- Sexual activity
- Immune disorders
- Diabetes mellitus
- Ask about thread/pin worms

Inspect the perineum for redness, edema, irritation, rash, or vaginal discharge (note colour, consistency, and odour).

Lichen Sclerosus et Atrophicus (LSA) is a skin condition that can affect girls and boys (as well as men and women) noted at examination for VV. In girls, it can be noted before puberty, is diagnosed with history, and examination rarely needing biopsy. LSA causes itching, soreness, and bleeding or vaginal discharge. The skin outside and around the vagina, labia, or clitoris can appear whitish or there may be areas of thickening, bruised, or broken skin. If the condition is mild, no treatment may be needed, but if symptoms are present, steroid cream can be prescribed and applied usually twice daily for 2 to 3 weeks.

NURSING MANAGEMENT

Teach appropriate hygiene (daily and toileting). Girls (or their parents) should wash the genital area thoroughly on a daily basis with mild soap and water. Rinse the area well. Encourage girls to wipe after urinating and after bowel movements to wipe in a front-to-back motion. The girl should wear cotton underwear and should change it at least once a day. Administer topical or oral medications as ordered. Table 43.3 lists treatments related to specific types of vulvovaginitis.

Inflammatory Disease

Pelvic inflammatory disease (PID) is an inflammation of the upper female genital tract and nearby structures. The fallopian tubes, ovaries, or peritoneum may be involved, and endometriosis may also be present. PID results from bacterial invasion through the cervix and vagina, ascending into the uterus and fallopian tubes. The most common causes of PID are *Chlamydia trachomatis* and *Neisseria gonorrhoeae*, although other bacteria and normal vaginal flora may be implicated. PID may result in fever, abdominal pain, pain with intercourse, **dysmenorrhea** (painful menstrual cycles), and abnormal uterine bleeding. Long-term complications include chronic pelvic pain, ectopic pregnancy, and infertility related to scarring.

NURSING ASSESSMENT

For a full description of the assessment phase of the nursing process, refer to the Assessment section of the Nursing Process Overview earlier in the chapter.

When discussing any problem related to the reproductive organs or menstruation with the preteen or teen, it is necessary to discuss sexuality. The girl may be reluctant to share this information with the nurse. Approaches to discussing sexuality with the adolescent that may increase the likelihood of obtaining a truthful history include:

- Discuss the girl's general health, menarche, and menstrual cycle first, and then work toward discussing sexual behaviour.
- Start with questions about the girl's friends and social life, moving the conversation toward sexual behaviour.
- Always discuss sexual behaviour one on one with the adolescent (without the parent present), and then ask the adolescent's permission to discuss concerns with the parent. If the adolescent does not consent to parental involvement, then confidentiality must be maintained.

TABLE 43.3	**VULVOVAGINITIS: TYPES AND TREATMENTS**	
Cause	**Assessment Findings**	**Treatment**
Unhygienic practices	Irritation of labia and vaginal opening. May have foul brownish-green discharge if infected with bacteria from rectum	Good hygiene. Sometimes a mild anti-inflammatory cream is prescribed. Assess for signs and symptoms of UTI, which may occur as a complication
Candida albicans	Red bumpy perineal rash in infants. White cottage-cheese–like discharge. Intense itching	Antifungal cream or vaginal suppository. Prevent by ingesting probiotics (found in yogurt and kefir) daily and supplementing with a probiotic such as Lactinex when taking antibiotics
Bordetella, Gardnerella	Thin grey vaginal discharge with fishy odour	Metronidazole orally
Trichomonas vaginalis	Foul yellow-grey or green vaginal discharge	Metronidazole orally. Sexually transmitted, so can be prevented with the use of condoms

Adapted from Neinstein, L. S., Gordon, C. M., Katzman, D. K., Rosen, D. S., & Woods, E. R. (2009). *Handbook of adolescent health care*. Philadelphia, PA: Lippincott Williams & Wilkins.

Assessment findings pertinent to PID are discussed below.

Health History. Elicit a description of the present illness and chief complaint. Common signs and symptoms reported during the health history might include:
- Abdominal pain (ranging from mild to severe)
- Prolonged or increased menstrual bleeding
- Dysmenorrhea
- Dysuria
- Painful sexual intercourse
- Nausea
- Vomiting

Explore the girl's current and past medical health history for risk factors such as:
- Multiple sexual partners
- Lack of consistent condom use
- Lack of contraceptive use
- History of prior sexually transmitted infection
- Douching
- Prostitution
- Alcohol or drug use (particularly if associated with sexual activity)

Physical Examination. Inspect for fever (usually over 101°F) or vaginal discharge. Palpate the abdomen, noting tenderness over the uterus or ovaries. An elevated C-reactive protein level and an elevated erythrocyte sedimentation rate indicate an inflammatory process. Cervical culture reveals the causative bacterial organism.

NURSING MANAGEMENT

PID is often treated in the outpatient setting with intramuscular or oral antibiotic regimens. If the adolescent is severely ill or has a very high fever or protracted vomiting, then she may be hospitalized. Antibiotics are needed to eradicate the infection. Maintain hydration via intravenous fluids if necessary and administer analgesics as needed for pain. Semi-Fowler positioning promotes pelvic drainage. A key element to treatment of PID is education to prevent recurrence (see Teaching Guideline 43.2).

Teaching Guidelines 43.2
PREVENTING PELVIC INFLAMMATORY DISEASE
- Insist that sexual partners use condoms.
- Do not use a vaginal douche routinely, as this may lead to bacterial overgrowth.
- Get screened regularly for sexually transmitted infections.
- Make sure that each sexual partner also receives antibiotic treatment.

Menstrual Disorders

Menstruation begins in most girls about 2 years after breast development starts, around the time of Tanner stage 4 breast and pubic hair development, and on average at around 12 to 13 years of age. Menstruation has many effects on girls and women, including emotional and self-image issues. Adolescents may suffer from a variety of menstrual disorders, including premenstrual syndrome and several different disorders related to menstrual bleeding and cramping (Table 43.4).

In healthy girls, the menstrual period varies in the heaviness of flow. Periods may occur irregularly for up to 2 years after menarche (the onset of menstruation), but after that the regular menstrual cycle should be established. The normal cycle can vary from 21 to 35 days in length, with the period usually lasting 2 to 7 days. Girls who take oral contraceptives usually have very regular 28-day cycles, with lighter bleeding than those who do not take contraceptives.

PATHOPHYSIOLOGY

Premenstrual syndrome is a collection of physical and/or affective symptoms that occur predictably during the luteal phase of the menstrual cycle. Symptoms begin 5 to 10 days before each period and usually resolve by the time the period begins or shortly thereafter (the timing may vary by adolescent but is consistent with each cycle). Disorders of bleeding and cramping are summarized in Table 43.4.

NURSING ASSESSMENT

For a full description of the assessment phase of the nursing process, refer to the Assessment section of the Nursing Process Overview earlier in the chapter. When girls present for evaluation of menstrual concerns, a focused yet thorough nursing assessment is necessary.

Health History. Obtain a thorough and accurate menstrual history; determine age at menarche, usual length of menstrual period, usual menstrual flow, number of pads or tampons used per day, date of last normal menstrual period, premenstrual symptoms, and any pain related to the menstrual cycle. Obtain a description of the pain, what relief measures have been tried, and what the success of those measures has been. If pain occurs with menstrual periods, assess for associated symptoms such as nausea, vomiting, dizziness, or loose stools. Explore the history for symptoms of bloating, water retention, weight gain, headache, muscle aches, abdominal pain, food cravings, or breast tenderness. Determine the extent of emotional symptoms related to the menstrual cycle, such as anxiety, insomnia, mood swings, tension, crying spells, or irritability. Note the timing of these symptoms within the menstrual cycle.

incision to release the foreskin. Circumcision may be used to treat either condition.

NURSING ASSESSMENT

Elicit a description of the present illness and chief complaint. Common signs and symptoms reported during the health history might include:

- Irritation or bleeding from the opening of the prepuce (phimosis)
- Dysuria (phimosis)
- Pain (paraphimosis)
- Swollen penis (paraphimosis)

Determine the onset of symptoms and inspect the penis for irritation, erythema, edema, or discharge.

Take Note!

A swollen, reddened penis (paraphimosis) is a medical emergency and can quickly result in necrosis of the tip of the penis if left untreated.

NURSING MANAGEMENT

Apply topical steroid medication as prescribed for phimosis, following gentle retraction to stretch the foreskin back. When surgical intervention is necessary, provide routine postprocedural care and pain management (refer to the section on circumcision below). Teach the parents and uncircumcised boy proper hygiene, which will help to prevent phimosis and paraphimosis (Teaching Guidelines 43.3).

Teaching Guidelines 43.3
HYGIENE IN THE UNCIRCUMCISED MALE

- The foreskin does not normally retract in the newborn boy, so do not force it to do so.
- Change the diaper frequently and wash the penis daily with water and mild soap.
- When the infant is older and the foreskin easily retracts, gently retract the foreskin and clean around the glans with water and mild soap once a week.
- Dry the area prior to replacing the foreskin.
- Always replace the foreskin after retraction.
- Teach the preschool-age boy to retract the foreskin and clean the penis during each bath or shower.

Circumcision

Circumcision is the removal of the excess foreskin of the penis. Some newborn boys are circumcised shortly after birth before going home from the hospital. Some parents elect not to have their newborn boy circumcised at that time but may desire it later. Circumcision is indicated later for the conditions of phimosis and paraphimosis. Circumcision done after the newborn period usually requires general anesthesia.

The benefits of circumcision may include a decreased incidence of UTI and penile cancer. Complications of circumcision are rare and include bleeding, penile adhesions, imperfect amount of foreskin removal, and meatal stenosis (Canadian Paediatric Society [CPS], 2014). There are a growing number of men globally who are unhappy with the surgical decision made on their behalf for circumcision in childhood. Whether to circumcise or not is a personal decision taken by parents, often based on religious beliefs or social or cultural customs. Nurses should support and educate the parents in either case.

NURSING ASSESSMENT

Prior to the procedure, assess for normal placement of the urinary meatus on the glans penis (in boys with hypospadias, circumcision should be delayed until evaluation by the pediatric urologist). After the circumcision, assess for redness, edema, or active bleeding. Note signs of infection, such as purulent drainage. Assess pain level.

NURSING MANAGEMENT

Nursing care of the boy undergoing circumcision focuses on managing pain, providing postprocedural care, and educating the parents.

Managing Pain. Whether circumcision is performed in the obstetric area of the hospital before newborn discharge or in the outpatient setting at a few days of age, pain management during the procedure must not be neglected. Advocate for appropriate pain management for the infant undergoing circumcision. The Canadian Paediatric Society recommends using a subcutaneous ring block with lidocaine, local anesthetic with lidocaine/prilocaine, or a dorsal nerve block to the penis (CPS, 2014). Playing calming music during the procedure may also help to soothe the infant, providing distraction. A sucrose-dipped pacifier may also be used as adjuvant therapy for pain management.

Atraumatic Care

Restrain the infant in a padded circumcision chair with blankets covering the legs and upper body to provide a sense of comfort. If a padded restraint chair is not available, provide atraumatic care by padding the circumcision board and covering the infant as previously described.

Providing Postprocedural Care. Usual care after circumcision depends on the type of appliance used (Gomco or Mogen clamp or Plastibell apparatus). Cleanse the penis with clear water for the first few days and avoid using alcohol-containing wipes. To avoid irritation to the penis, fasten diapers loosely. Notify the physician or nurse practitioner if excessive redness, active bleeding, or purulent discharge occurs. Assess for the first void following the procedure, or if performed in the outpatient setting, instruct parents to call the physician or nurse practitioner if the infant has not voided by 6 to 8 hours after the circumcision. Apply antibiotic ointment or petroleum jelly to the penile head with each diaper change as prescribed, based on the circumcision method used and the preference of the physician or nurse practitioner.

> **Take Note!**
> If excess bleeding occurs after the circumcision, apply direct pressure and notify the physician or nurse practitioner immediately.

Educating the Parents. Instruct parents to give sponge baths until the circumcision is healed. Describe the normal granulation tissue that will be present during the healing process. Teach parents to apply ointment or petroleum jelly if indicated. Instruct the parents to call the physician or nurse practitioner if any of the following occur:

- The infant does not urinate within 6 to 8 hours after the procedure.
- Heavy bleeding occurs (more than small spots on the diaper or bleeding that requires direct pressure to stop it).
- There is purulent or serous drainage from the circumcised area.
- There is redness or swelling of the penile shaft.

> **Take Note!**
> If the Plastibell is used, teach parents NOT to use petroleum jelly, as it may cause the ring to be dislodged. A yellowish crust may form that should be allowed to fall off on its own after several days.

Cryptorchidism

Cryptorchidism (also known as undescended testicles) occurs when one or both testicles do not descend into the scrotal sac. Ordinarily the testes, which in the fetus develop in the abdomen, make their descent into the scrotal sac during the seventh month of gestation. The cause for this failure to descend may be mechanical, hormonal, chromosomal, or enzymatic. The disorder may occur unilaterally or bilaterally. Up to 3% of term male infants exhibit cryptorchidism (Fantasia, Aidlen, Lathrop, & Ellsworth, 2015).

Complications associated with cryptorchidism that is allowed to progress into the school-age years include sterility and an increased risk for testicular cancer in adolescence or the young adult years. Therapeutic management is surgical. An orchiopexy is performed to release the spermatic cord, and the testes are then pulled into the scrotum and tacked into place.

NURSING ASSESSMENT
Explore the health history for risk factors such as:
- Prematurity
- First-born child
- Cesarean birth
- Low birthweight
- Hypospadias

Palpate for the presence (or absence) of both testes in the scrotal sac.

> **Take Note!**
> A retractile testis is one that may be brought into the scrotum, remains for a time, and then retracts back up the inguinal canal. This should not be confused with true cryptorchidism.

NURSING MANAGEMENT
If the testes are not descended by 6 months of age, the infant should be referred for surgical repair (Fantasia et al., 2015). Postoperatively, observe the incision for signs of bleeding or infection.

Hydrocele and Varicocele

Hydrocele (fluid in the scrotal sac) is usually a benign and self-limiting disorder. It is usually noted early in infancy and often resolves spontaneously by 1 year of age. Varicocele (a venous varicosity along the spermatic cord) is often noted as a swelling of the scrotal sac. Complications of varicocele include low sperm count or reduced sperm motility, which can result in infertility.

NURSING ASSESSMENT
Elicit a description of the present illness and chief complaint. The boy with hydrocele will have an enlarged scrotum that may decrease in size when he is lying down. Inspect the scrotum for a fluid-filled appearance.

The boy with varicocele will have a mass on one or both sides of the scrotum and bluish discolouration. Inspect the scrotum for masses; the spermatic vein feels worm-like on palpation. The boy with varicocele may have pain.

NURSING MANAGEMENT
Both hydrocele and painless varicocele require watchful waiting, as these conditions will usually resolve spontaneously. If they do not resolve, or if the difference in testicular volume is marked in the boy with varicocele, refer the child to a urologist, as surgery may be indicated. Reassure parents that hydrocele is not associated with the development of infertility. Varicocele may lead to infertility if left untreated, so instruct parents to seek care if pain occurs or if there is a large difference in testicular size. Either condition may be surgically corrected on an outpatient basis. Provide routine postoperative care following either surgery.

Testicular Torsion

In testicular torsion, a testicle is abnormally attached to the scrotum and twisted. It requires immediate attention because ischemia can result if the torsion is left untreated, leading to infertility. Testicular torsion may occur at any age but most commonly occurs in boys aged 12 to 18 years (Brenner & Ojo, 2015).

NURSING ASSESSMENT

Elicit a description of the present illness and chief complaint. Signs and symptoms of testicular torsion include sudden, severe scrotal pain. Inspect the affected side for significant swelling, which may appear hemorrhagic or blue-black.

NURSING MANAGEMENT

Surgical correction is necessary immediately. Administer pain medication prior to surgery. Reassure the child and family that surgery will alleviate the problem and is performed to restore adequate blood flow to the testicle. After surgical repair, provide routine postoperative care.

Take Note!

Testicular torsion is considered a surgical emergency, as necrosis of the testis may occur and gangrene may set in.

Epididymitis

Epididymitis (inflammation of the epididymis) is caused by infection with bacteria. It is the most common cause of pain in the scrotum. It rarely occurs before puberty,

but if it does it may occur as a result of a urethral or bladder infection related to a urogenital anomaly. Therapeutic management is directed toward eradicating the bacteria. If left untreated, a scrotal abscess, testicular infarction, or infertility may occur.

NURSING ASSESSMENT

Note history of painful swelling of the scrotum, which may be gradual or acute. If the boy is sexually active, explore history of sexual encounters prior to the onset of symptoms. Document history of dysuria or urethral discharge. Note fever, which may last from days to weeks. On inspection, note edema and erythema of the scrotum. Gently palpate the scrotum for a hardened and tender epididymis. Note urethral discharge if present. Palpate the inguinal lymph nodes for enlargement. Urinalysis may be positive for bacteria and white blood cells. The culture of urethral discharge may be positive for a sexually transmitted infection such as gonorrhea or *Chlamydia*. The complete blood count may reveal an elevated white blood cell count.

NURSING MANAGEMENT

Encourage the boy to rest in bed with the scrotum elevated. Ice packs to the scrotum may help with pain relief. Administer pain medications such as NSAIDs or other analgesics as needed.

Administer antibiotics as prescribed. Educate the boy and his family to complete the entire course of antibiotics as prescribed to eradicate the infection. Advise the child and family to notify the physician or nurse practitioner if the condition is not improving or if the pain and swelling worsen.

NURSING CARE PLAN 43.1

Overview for the Child With a Genitourinary Disorder

NURSING DIAGNOSIS: Activity intolerance related to generalized edema, anemia, or generalized weakness as evidenced by verbalization of weakness or fatigue; elevated heart rate, respiratory rate, or blood pressure with activity; complaint of shortness of breath with play or activity

Outcome Identification and Evaluation

Child will display increased activity tolerance, desire to play without developing symptoms of exertion.

Intervention: *Promoting Activity*

• Encourage activity or ambulation per physician's or nurse practitioner's orders: *early mobilization results in better outcomes.*
• Observe child for symptoms of activity intolerance such as pallor, nausea, lightheadedness, or dizziness or changes in vital signs *to determine level of tolerance.*
• If child is on bed rest, perform range-of-motion exercises and frequent position changes, *as negative changes to the musculoskeletal system occur quickly with inactivity and immobility.*

Overview for the Child With a Genitourinary Disorder (continued)

- Cluster nursing care activities and plan for periods of rest before and after exertional activities *to decrease oxygen need and consumption.*
- Refer the child to physical therapy *for exercise prescription to increase skeletal muscle strength.*

NURSING DIAGNOSIS: Excess fluid volume related to decreased protein in the bloodstream, decreased urine output, sodium retention, possible inappropriate fluid intake, or altered hormone levels inducing fluid retention as evidenced by edema, bloating, weight gain, oliguria, azotemia, or changes in heart and lung sounds

Outcome Identification and Evaluation

Child will attain appropriate fluid balance, will lose weight (fluid), edema or bloating will decrease, lung sounds will be clear and heart sounds normal.

Intervention: *Encouraging Fluid Loss*

- Weigh child daily on same scale in similar amount of clothing: *in children, weight is the best indicator of changes in fluid status.*
- Monitor location and extent of edema (measure abdominal girth daily if ascites present): *decrease in edema indicates positive increase in oncotic pressure.*
- Auscultate lungs carefully to determine presence of crackles *(indicating pulmonary edema).*
- Assess work of breathing and respiratory rate: *increased work of breathing is associated with pulmonary edema.*
- Assess heart sounds for presence or absence of gallop: *presence of S_3 may indicate fluid overload.*

- Maintain fluid restriction as ordered *to decrease intravascular volume and workload on the heart.*
- Strictly monitor intake and output *to quickly note discrepancies and provide intervention.*
- Provide sodium-restricted diet as ordered: *restricting sodium in the diet allows for better renal excretion of extra fluid.*
- Administer diuretics as ordered and monitor for side effects of those medications. *Diuretics encourage excretion of fluid and elimination of edema, reduce cardiac filling pressures, and increase renal blood flow. Side effects include electrolyte imbalance as well as orthostatic hypotension.*

NURSING DIAGNOSIS: Imbalanced nutrition: less than body requirements related to anorexia and protein loss as evidenced by weight, length/height, and/or BMI below average for age

Outcome Identification and Evaluation

Child will improve nutritional intake, resulting in steady increase in weight and length/height.

Intervention: *Promoting Adequate Nutrition*

- Determine body weight and length/height norm for age *to determine goal to work toward.*
- Assess child for food preferences that fall within dietary restrictions, *as the child will be more likely to consume adequate amounts of foods that he or she likes.*
- Weigh daily or weekly (according to physician's or nurse practitioner's order or institutional standard) and measure length/height weekly *to monitor for increased growth.*
- Offer highest-calorie meals at the time of day when the child's appetite is the greatest *to increase likelihood of increased caloric intake.*
- Provide increased-calorie shakes or puddings within diet restriction: *high-calorie foods increase weight gain.*
- Administer vitamin and mineral supplements as prescribed *to attain/maintain vitamin and mineral balance in the body.*

(continued)

Overview for the Child With a Genitourinary Disorder (continued)

NURSING DIAGNOSIS: Overweight related to increased appetite secondary to steroid therapy as evidenced by weight greater than 95th percentile for age or recent increase in weight

Outcome Identification and Evaluation

Child will demonstrate balanced nutritional intake, will maintain current weight or steadily lose excess weight.

Intervention: *Encouraging Appropriate Nutritional Intake*

- Determine ideal body weight and body mass index for age *to determine goal to work toward.*
- Consult dietitian *for guidance in planning nutrient-rich diet in context of restrictions.*
- Evaluate for emotional/psychological reasons for overeating *to address these concerns.*
- Formulate a contract with the child *to involve him or her in the planning process and encourage compliance with the plan.*

- With the child, plan for daily exercise/activity to expend excess calories: *it is important to involve the child in planning, in order to increase compliance.*
- Instruct the child/parent about appropriate nutrient-rich foods to choose within the constraints of diet and fluid restrictions *to provide basis for ongoing diet management at home.*
- Weigh child twice weekly on same scale *to determine progress toward goal.*

NURSING DIAGNOSIS: Impaired urinary elimination related to urinary tract infection, anatomic obstruction, sensory motor impairment, or dysfunctional voiding as evidenced by urinary retention or incontinence, dribbling, urgency, or dysuria

Child's bladder will empty adequately, according to pre-established quantities and frequencies individualized for the child (usual urine output is 0.5 to 2 mL/kg/hr).

Intervention: *Promoting Adequate Urinary Elimination and Successful Bladder Emptying*

- Assess the child's usual voiding pattern and success within that pattern *to determine baseline.*
- Assess child's ability to adequately empty bladder via history focused on character and duration of lower urinary symptoms *to determine baseline.*
- Develop a schedule for bladder emptying *to decrease bladder overdistention and to encourage voiding in the toilet.*
- Maintain adequate hydration, *to avoid irritating effects of dehydration on the bladder.*
- Avoid constipation, encopresis, or fecal impaction *as alterations in bowel elimination may have a negative impact on urinary elimination.*
- Assess for bladder distention by palpation or urinary retention by postvoid residual obtained via catheterization or bladder ultrasound *to determine extent of retention.*
- Teach parents to restrict child's fluid intake after dinner *to avoid bedwetting.*
- Ensure child voids prior to going to bed *to avoid bedwetting.*
- Teach bladder-stretching exercises as prescribed per physician or nurse practitioner *to increase bladder capacity.*
- In the child with significant urinary retention, teach parents/child the technique of clean intermittent catheterization, *which allows for regular complete bladder emptying.*

NURSING CARE PLAN 43.1

Overview for the Child With a Genitourinary Disorder (continued)

NURSING DIAGNOSIS: Disturbed body image related to anatomic differences, short stature, or effects of long-term corticosteroid use as evidenced by verbalization of dissatisfaction with the child's or adolescent's looks

Outcome Identification and Evaluation

Child or adolescent will display appropriate body image, will look at self in mirror and participate in social activities.

Intervention: *Promoting Body Image*

- Acknowledge feelings of anger over body changes and illness: *venting feelings is associated with less body image disturbance.*
- Support the child's or teen's choices of comfortable, fashionable clothing *that may disguise anatomic abnormalities and dialysis tubing.*
- Involve the child and especially the teen in the decision-making process, *as a sense of control of his or her own body will improve body image.*
- Encourage children or teens to spend time with others of their own age who have short stature or other effects of renal disorders: *a peer's opinions are often better accepted than those of persons in authority, such as parents or health care professionals.*

NURSING DIAGNOSIS: Deficient knowledge related to lack of information regarding complex medical condition, prognosis, and medical needs as evidenced by verbalization, questions, or actions demonstrating lack of understanding regarding child's condition or care

Outcome Identification and Evaluation

Child and parents will verbalize accurate information and understanding about condition, prognosis, and medical needs: *child and parents demonstrate knowledge of condition and medications and will demonstrate therapeutic procedures the child requires.*

Intervention: *Educating the Child and Parents*

- Assess child's and parents' willingness to learn: *child and parents must be open to learning for teaching to be effective.*
- Provide parents with time to adjust to diagnosis: *will facilitate adjustment and ability to learn and participate in child's care.*
- Teach in short sessions: *many short sessions are found to be more helpful than one long session.*
- Repeat information: *allows parents and child time to learn and understand.*
- Individualize teaching to the parents' and child's level of understanding (depends on age of child, physical condition, memory) *to ensure understanding.*
- Provide reinforcement and rewards *to facilitate the teaching/learning process.*
- Use multiple modes of learning involving many senses (written, verbal, demonstration, and videos) when possible: *child and parents are more likely to retain information when it is presented in different ways using many senses.*

KEY CONCEPTS

- Though present at birth, the reproductive organs do not reach functional maturity until puberty.

- The short length of the urethra in girls and its proximity to the vagina and anus place the young girl at higher risk for the development of urinary tract infections compared with the adult.

- The urinary tract is immature in infants and young children, with a slower glomerular filtration rate and a decreased ability to concentrate urine and reabsorb amino acids compared with the adult.

- The expected urine output in the infant and child is 0.5 to 2 mL/kg/hr.

- Obtaining a clean or sterile urine specimen is necessary for accurate urine culture results.

- A urinary catheter must be inserted just prior to the voiding cystourethrogram.

- Close monitoring of serum blood counts and electrolytes is a critical component of nursing care related to renal disorders.

- Certain congenital urologic anomalies may require multiple surgeries as well as urinary diversion; urine drains through a stoma on the abdominal wall that is either pouched or catheterized.

- The treatment for nocturnal enuresis may include the use of desmopressin nasal spray and/or an enuresis alarm to train the child to awaken to the sensation of a filling bladder.

- Nephrotic syndrome results in significant proteinuria and edema.

- Acute glomerulonephritis most often follows a group A streptococcal infection and commonly results in hematuria, proteinuria, and hypertension.

- The most common cause of hemolytic-uremic syndrome is infection with *E. coli* O157:H7. It can be prevented by adequately cooking ground meat, washing hands and produce well, and making sure that an appropriate chemical balance is maintained in public recreational water sources such as swimming pools and water parks.

- Corticosteroids can cause gastrointestinal upset. If used on a long-term basis, they should be tapered rather than discontinued abruptly to avoid adrenal crisis.

- In children, chronic kidney disease is most often the result of congenital structural defects, or infectious, inflammatory, or immune processes that damage the kidney, whereas in adults it usually results from hypertension or diabetes.

- Children taking immunosuppressants for nephrotic syndrome or for renal transplant are at increased risk for the development of overwhelming infection.

- Peritoneal dialysis may be accomplished at home by the parent. Close attention to sterile technique is needed.

- Hemodialysis requires an arteriovenous fistula or graft that is accessed with needles three or four times per week at a hemodialysis centre. This is disruptive to the child's academic, social, and family lives.

- Renal transplantation is the best option for the treatment of end-stage renal disease in children, but vigilant medication administration is needed to prevent organ rejection.

- Children with renal failure experience anemia, poor growth, depression, anxiety, and low self-esteem.

- The diet for a child with a renal disorder must be individualized according to prescribed sodium, fluid, and/or protein restrictions.

- Postoperative care for the child undergoing urologic surgery includes pain management, avoidance or treatment of bladder spasms, and monitoring of urine output.

REFERENCES AND RECOMMENDED READINGS

Alsowayan, O., Capolicchio, J. P., Jednak, R., & El-Sherbiny, M. (2016). Long-term functional outcomes after bladder exstrophy repair: A single, low-volume centre experience. *Canadian Urological Association Journal, 10*(3-4), E94–E98.

American Nephrology Nurses' Association. (2013). *Pediatric ESRD renal transplant fact sheet*. Pitman, NJ: Author.

Blais, A. S., Bolduc, S., & Moore, K. (2017). Vesicoureteral reflux: From prophylaxis to surgery. *Canadian Urological Association Journal, 11*(1–2 Suppl 1), S13–S18.

Bowden, V. R., & Greenberg, C. S. (2012). *Pediatric nursing procedures* (3rd ed.). Philadelphia, PA: Lippincott Williams & Wilkins.

Brenner, J. S., & Ojo, A. (2015). *Causes of scrotal pain in children and adolescents*. Retrieved from http://www.uptodate.com/contents/causes-of-scrotal-pain-in-children-and-adolescents

Browne, N. T., Flanigan, L. M., McComiskey, C. A., & Pieper, P. (2013). *Nursing care of the pediatric surgical patient* (3rd ed.). Burlington, MA: Jones & Bartlett Learning.

Canadian Paediatric Society. (2014). *Urinary tract infection in infants and children: Diagnosis and management*. Retrieved from http://www.cps.ca/documents/position/urinary-tract-infections-in-children

Canadian Urological Association. (2014). *Foreskin care for boys*. Retrieved from https://www.cua.org/themes/web/assets/files/patient_info/secured/en/15e-foreskin_boys_s.pdf

Carpenito-Moyet, L. J. (2013). *Nursing diagnosis: Application to clinical practice* (14th ed.). Philadelphia, PA: Lippincott Williams & Wilkins.

Centers for Disease Control and Prevention (CDC). (2016). *Pelvic inflammatory disease (PID)—CDC fact sheet*. Retrieved from http://www.cdc.gov/std/PID/STDFact-PID.htm

Corbett, J. A., & Banks, A. D. (2013). *Laboratory tests and diagnostic procedures with nursing diagnoses* (8th ed.). Upper Saddle River, NJ: Pearson Education Inc.

Costa, D. F., Lavallée, L. T., Dubois, C., Leonard, M., & Guerra, L. (2014). Are we accurately predicting bladder capacity in infants? *Canadian Urological Association Journal, 8*(9–10), 329–332.

Dunn, A. (2013). Elimination patterns. In C. Burns, A. Dunn, M. Brady, N. B. Starr, & C. Blosser (Eds.). *Pediatric primary care* (5th ed.). Philadelphia, PA: Saunders.

Easterbrook, B., Capolicchio, J.-P., & Braga, L. H. (2017). Antibiotic prophylaxis for prevention of urinary tract infections in prenatal hydronephrosis: An updated systematic review. *Canadian Urological Association Journal, 11*(1–2 Suppl 1), S3–S11.

Fantasia, J., Aidlen, J., Lathrop, W., & Ellsworth, P. (2015). Undescended testes: A clinical and surgical review. *Urologic Nursing, 35*(3), 117–126.

Gaylord, N. M., & Petersen-Smith, A. M. (2013). Genitourinary disorders. In C. Burns, A. Dunn, M. Brady, N. B. Starr, & C. Blosser (Eds.). *Pediatric primary care* (5th ed.). Philadelphia, PA: Saunders.

Gerlt, T., & Starr, N. B. (2013). Gynecologic disorders. In C. Burns, A. Dunn, M. Brady, N. B. Starr, & C. Blosser (Eds.). *Pediatric primary care* (5th ed.). Philadelphia, PA: Saunders.

Guerra, L., Leonard, M., & Castagnetti, M. (2014). Best practice in the assessment of bladder function in infants. *Therapeutic advances in urology, 6*(4), 148–164.

Hamilton, R. G. (2015). *Latex allergy: Epidemiology, clinical manifestations, and diagnosis*. Retrieved from http://www.uptodate.com/contents/latex-allergy-epidemiology-clinical-manifestations-and-diagnosis

Hoen, L. T., Ecclestone, H., Blok, B. F., Karsenty, G., Phé, V., Bossier, R., . . . Hamid, R. (2017). Long-term effectiveness and complication rates of bladder augmentation in patients with neurogenic bladder dysfunction: A systematic review. *Neurourology and Urodynamics, 36*(7), 1685–1702.

Keays, M. A., & Dave, S. (2017). Current hypospadias management: Diagnosis, surgical management, and long-term patient-centred outcomes. *Canadian Urological Association Journal, 11*(1–2 Suppl 1), S48–S53. Retrieved from http://doi.org/10.5489/cuaj.4386.

Kiddoo, D. (2015). Nocturnal enuresis: Non-pharmacological treatments. *BMJ Clinical Evidence, 2015*, 0305. Retrieved from https://www.ncbi.nlm.nih.gov/pmc/articles/PMC4292411/

Kidney Foundation of Canada. (n.d.). *Kidney disease and management*. Retrieved from https://www.kidney.ca

Klein, M. S. (2010). Kidney disease, chronic. In P. J. Allen, J. A. Vessey, & N. A. Schapiro (Eds.). *Primary care of the child with a chronic condition* (5th ed.). St. Louis, MO: Mosby.

Klein, M. S., & Martin, K. (2010). Organ transplantation. In P. J. Allen, J. A. Vessey, & N. A. Schapiro (Eds.). *Primary care of*

the child with a chronic condition (5th ed.). St. Louis, MO: Mosby.

Lum, G. M. (2014). Kidney & urinary tract. In W. W. Hay, M. J. Levin, R. R. Deterding, & M. J. Abzug (Eds.). *Current pediatric diagnosis and treatment* (22nd ed.). New York: McGraw-Hill.

Mattoo, T. K. (2016). *Treatment of hypertension in children and adolescents*. Retrieved from http://www.uptodate.com/contents/treatment-of-hypertension-in-children-and-adolescents?source=see_link

Mattoo, T. K., Mathews, R., & Gupta, I. R. (2014). Vesicoureteral reflux and renal scarring in children. *Pediatric Nephrology*, 1–40.

Moreno, M. A., Giesel, A. E., Rogers, C. B., & Clark, L. R. (2015). *Premenstrual syndrome*. Retrieved from http://emedicine.medscape.com/article/953696-overview

Mount Nittany Medical Center. (2013). *When your son needs surgery for hypospadias*. Retrieved from http://www.mount-nittany.org/articles/healthsheets/11970

Neinstein, L. S., Gordon, C. M., Katzman, D. K., Rosen, D. S., & Woods, E. R. (2009). *Handbook of adolescent health care*. Philadelphia, PA: Lippincott Williams & Wilkins.

Nelson, C. P., & Koo, H. P. (2014). *Pediatric vesicoureteral reflux*. Retrieved from http://emedicine.medscape.com/article/1016439-overview

Robinson, J. L., Finlay, J. C., Lang, M. E., Bortolussi, R., & Canadian Paediatric Society, Infectious Diseases and Immunization Committee, Community Paediatrics Committee. (2014). Urinary tract infections in infants and children: Diagnosis and management. *Paediatrics & Child Health, 19*(6), 315–319.

Sass, A. E., & Kaplan, D. W. (2014). Adolescence. In W. W. Hay, M. J. Levin, R. R. Deterding, & M. J. Abzug (Eds.). *Current pediatric diagnosis and treatment* (22nd ed.). New York: McGraw-Hill.

Solomon, D. H. (2015). *Patient information: Nonsteroidal anti-inflammatory drugs (NSAIDs) (beyond the basics)*. Retrieved from http://www.uptodate.com/contents/nonsteroidal-antiinflammatory-drugs-nsaids-beyond-the-basics

Sorokan, S. T., Finlay, J. C., Jefferies A. L.; Canadian Paediatric Society Fetus and Newborn Committee, Infectious Diseases and Immunization Committee. (2015). Newborn male circumcision. *Paediatric Child Health, 20*(6), 311–315. Retrieved from https://www.cps.ca/en/documents/position/circumcision

Springer, A., & Baskin, L. S. (2014). Timing of hypospadias repair in patients with disorders of sex development. In O. Hiort, S. F. Ahmed (Eds.). *Understanding Differences and Disorders of Sex Development (DSD)* (Vol. 27, pp. 197–202). Karger Publishers.

Taketomo, C. K., Hodding, J. H., & Kraus, D. M. (2013). *Pediatric & neonatal dosage handbook* (20th ed.). Hudson, OH: Lexicomp.

Tan, A. J., & Silverberg, M. A. (2015). *Hemolytic uremic syndrome in emergency medicine*. Retrieved from http://emedicine.medscape.com/article/779218-overview

Tews, M., & Singer, J. I. (2014). *Paraphimosis: Definition, pathophysiology, and clinical features*. Retrieved from http://www.uptodate.com/contents/paraphimosis-definition-pathophysiology-and-clinical-features

CHAPTER **WORKSHEET**

MULTIPLE CHOICE QUESTIONS

1. The nurse is performing education for the parents of an infant with bladder exstrophy. Which statement by the parents would indicate an understanding of the child's future care?
   a. "Care will be no different than that of any other infant."
   b. "My infant will only need this one surgery."
   c. "My child will wear diapers all his life."
   d. "We will need to care for the urinary diversion."

2. A 4-year-old girl presents with recurrent urinary tract infection. A prior workup did not reveal any urinary tract abnormalities. What is the priority nursing action?
   a. Obtain a sterile urine sample after completion of antibiotics.
   b. Teach appropriate toileting hygiene.
   c. Prepare the child for surgery to reimplant the ureters.
   d. Administer antibiotics intramuscularly.

3. A 5-year-old who had a renal transplant 9 months ago and has no history of chickenpox presents to the pediatric clinic for his vaccinations. Which is the most appropriate set to give?
   a. DTaP, IPV
   b. DTaP, IPV, MMR, varicella
   c. DTaP, IPV, varicella
   d. IPV only

4. When the nurse is caring for a child with hemolytic-uremic syndrome or acute glomerulonephritis and the child is not yet toilet trained, which action by the nurse would best determine fluid retention?
   a. Test urine for specific gravity.
   b. Weigh child daily.
   c. Weigh the wet diapers.
   d. Measure abdominal girth daily.

DOSAGE CALCULATION QUESTION

1. The nurse is caring for a child who has had a renal transplant. The child weighs 47 lb. The medication order reads: cyclosporine 96 mg PO every 12 hours. Cyclosporine is supplied as 100 mg/mL. How many millilitres will the nurse administer? Round to the nearest whole number.

CRITICAL THINKING EXERCISES

1. Devise a meal plan for a 5-year-old child with a renal disorder that requires a 2-g sodium restriction per day. Keep in mind the child's developmental level and feeding idiosyncrasies at this age.

2. Develop a discharge teaching plan for a 3-year-old with nephrotic syndrome who will be taking cortico-steroids long term.

3. Devise a developmental stimulation plan for an 11-month-old who has had significant urinary tract reconstruction surgery and is facing a prolonged period of confinement to the crib.

STUDY ACTIVITIES

1. In the clinical setting, compare the growth and development of two children of the same age, one with chronic renal failure and one who has been healthy.

2. While caring for children in the clinical setting, compare and contrast the medical history, signs and symptoms of illness, and prescribed treatments for a child with nephrotic syndrome and one with acute glomerulonephritis.

3. Observe peritoneal dialysis in the hospital or hemodialysis in a hospital or outpatient centre. Record observations about the children's psychosocial and developmental status.

BRINGING IT ALL TOGETHER: A CASE STUDY

Antonio Cruise, a 7-year-old boy, is brought to the clinic by his mother for his annual examination. During your assessment, the mother brings up concerns that Antonio continues to wet the bed at night. She states, "I was hoping this would end on its own, but now I'm concerned that there is a problem."

Go to thePoint **to find questions to consider about this case.**

44

Nursing Care of the Child With an Alteration in Mobility/Neuromuscular or Musculoskeletal Disorder

Learning Objectives

Upon completion of the chapter, you will be able to:

1. Compare differences between the anatomy and physiology of the neuromuscular and musculoskeletal systems in children versus adults.
2. Identify nursing interventions related to common laboratory and diagnostic tests used in the diagnosis and management of neuromuscular and musculoskeletal conditions.
3. Identify appropriate nursing assessments and interventions related to medications and treatments used for childhood neuromuscular and musculoskeletal conditions.
4. Distinguish various neuromuscular and musculoskeletal disorders occurring in childhood.
5. Devise an individualized nursing care plan for the child with a neuromuscular and musculoskeletal disorder.
6. Develop child/family teaching plans for the child with a neuromuscular and musculoskeletal disorder, in conjunction with family centred care.
7. Describe the psychosocial impact of chronic neuromuscular and musculoskeletal disorders on the growth and development of children.

Frederick Stevens, **4 years old, seems to be falling often and has started to have difficulty climbing the stairs on his own. His mother states, "Recently he hasn't been able to keep up with his 6-year-old sister when we're playing at the park. He usually ends up sitting on the bench with me." She is concerned about the changes she has seen in her son.**

Mobility refers to mechanisms (physical, biologic, and environmental) that assist or impair a person's ability to move. Nurses encounter potential or actual alterations in mobility in all types of clients and must provide health promotion to minimize risk and screen for and detect problems, thereby intervening early to prevent complications. Infants and young children have resilient soft tissue, so sprains and strains are less common in this age group. Older school-age children and adolescents often participate in athletics, and therefore sports injuries, sprains, fractures, and torn ligaments are common complaints (Statistics Canada, n.d.). A variety of alterations in mobility (neuromuscular or musculoskeletal disorders) may affect children, resulting in muscular and/or skeletal functional limitation. Some of the disorders result from a neurologic insult such as trauma or hypoxia to the brain or spinal cord or non-accidental injury. Others occur as a result of congenital anomalies (e.g., spina bifida), genetic dysfunction (e.g., osteogenesis imperfecta), structural abnormality present from birth (e.g., limb absence [Amelia]), inborn or developmental problems (e.g., hip and foot anomalies), or degenerative conditions that may not be identified until later in childhood or adolescence (e.g., muscular dystrophy). Acute infection (osteomyelitis), or inflammation of the nervous system (e.g., transverse myelitis), cancers (e.g., osteosarcoma), and chronic conditions such as metabolic conditions, inflammatory bowel disease, juvenile idiopathic arthritis, and connective tissues disorders, such as Marfan syndrome, can all impact on the musculoskeletal system. The immobility associated with most neuromuscular and musculoskeletal disorders may affect the child's development and acquisition of motor skills, leading to motor dysfunction, lifelong limited mobility, acute and/or chronic pain, and challenges related to self-esteem and quality of life.

The nurse caring for a child with altered mobility plays an important role in the management of these disorders. Not only must the nurse provide direct intervention in response to health alterations, within a patient- and family-centred model, but is often part of the larger interdisciplinary team and may serve as the coordinator of many specialists or interventions. Understanding the most common responses to these disorders gives the nurse the foundation required to plan care for any child or youth with a neuromuscular or musculoskeletal disorder.

VARIATIONS IN PEDIATRIC ANATOMY AND PHYSIOLOGY

The neuromuscular system is the combination of the nervous system and the muscles working together to create movement. The musculoskeletal system provides the body with form, support, stability, protection, and the ability to move. It is made up of bones, muscles, cartilage, tendons, ligaments, joints, and connective tissue. Anatomic and physiologic differences in infants and children, such as the immaturity of the neurologic and musculoskeletal systems, place them at increased risk for the development of a neuromuscular and musculoskeletal disorder and may hinder the child's growth and movement.

Brain and Spinal Cord Development

Early in gestation, around 3 to 4 weeks, the neural tube of the embryo begins to differentiate into the brain and spinal cord. If the fetus suffers infection, trauma, malnutrition, or teratogen exposure during this critical period of growth and differentiation, brain or spinal cord development may be altered. The premature infant is also at risk since the central nervous system is less mature than the term infant. Prematurity places the infant at a higher risk of central nervous insult within the neonatal period, which may result in delayed motor skill attainment or cerebral palsy (CP). Compared with the adult, the child's spine is very mobile, especially the cervical spine region, resulting in a higher risk for cervical spine injury.

Myelinization

Though development of the structures of the nervous system is complete at birth, myelinization is incomplete. Myelinization continues to progress and is complete by about 2 years of age. Myelinization proceeds in a cephalocaudal and proximodistal fashion, allowing the infant to gain head and neck control before becoming able to control the trunk and the extremities. As myelinization proceeds, the speed and accuracy of nerve impulses increase. Primitive reflexes are replaced with voluntary movement.

Muscular Development

The muscular system, including tendons, ligaments, and cartilage, arises from the mesoderm in early embryonic development. At birth (term or preterm), the muscles, tendons, ligaments, and cartilage are all present and functional. The newborn infant is capable of spontaneous movement but lacks purposeful control, yet there is motor symmetry in movement and posture. A full range of motion is present at birth; any persistent asymmetry may be a sign of neurologic disease (Esposito & Venuti, 2009). Healthy infants and children demonstrate normal muscle tone; **hypertonia** (increased muscle tone) or **hypotonia** (low muscle tone) is an abnormal finding. Deep tendon reflexes are present at birth and are initially brisk in the newborn and progress to average over the first few months. Sluggish deep tendon reflexes indicate an abnormality. As the infant matures and becomes mobile, the muscles develop further and become stronger. The infant's muscles account for approximately 25% of total body weight, as compared with the adult's muscle mass, which accounts for about 40% of total body weight (Carroll & Kerr, 2013). Muscles grow rapidly in adolescence; this contributes to clumsiness, which places the teen at increased risk for injury. In response to testosterone release, the adolescent boy experiences a growth spurt, particularly in the trunk and legs, and develops bulkier muscles. Female infants tend to have laxer ligaments than male infants, possibly due to the presence of female hormones, placing them at increased risk for developmental dysplasia of the hip (DDH) (Sankar, Horn, Wells, & Dormans, 2011).

Skeletal Development

Around the 4th week of gestation, the skeletal system starts to develop but is not fully ossified at birth. The infant and young child's bones are more flexible, more porous, and have a lower mineral content than the adult's. These structural differences of a young child's bones allow for greater shock absorption, so the bones will often bend rather than break when an injury occurs. The thick, strong periosteum of the child's bones allows for a greater absorption of force than is seen in adults. As a result, the cortex of the bone does not always break, sometimes buckling or bending only. The skeleton contains increased amounts of cartilage compared with adolescents and adults. **Ossification**, the conversion of cartilage to bone, continues throughout childhood and is complete at adolescence.

During fetal development, the spine displays **kyphosis**, an outward curvature. Cervical **lordosis**, inward curvature, develops as the infant starts to hold the head up. When the infant or toddler assumes an upright position, the primary and secondary curves of the spine begin to develop. The balance of the curves allows the head to be centred over the pelvis. During the toddler years, the period of early walking, lumbar lordosis may be significant (also termed toddler lordosis), and the toddler appears quite swaybacked and potbellied. As the child develops, the spine takes on more adult-like curves. Scoliosis (structural) can be noted in childhood and usually involves lateral curvature, rotation of the vertebrae, and thoracic hypokyphosis. It can be congenital, infantile (up to 3 years), childhood (juvenile) 4 to 10 years, or develop in adolescence (Bazner-Chandler & Brady, 2013).

Growth Plate

The ends of the bones in young children are composed of the **epiphysis**, the end of a long bone, and the physis, together called the epiphyseal growth plate. In infants, the epiphyses are cartilaginous and ossify over time. In children, the epiphysis is the secondary ossification centre at the end of the bone. The physis is a cartilaginous area between the epiphysis and the metaphysis. Growth of the bones occurs primarily in the epiphyseal region.

FIGURE 44.1 Anatomic areas of growing bone.

This area is vulnerable and structurally weak. Traumatic force applied to the epiphysis during injury may result in fracture in that area of the bone. Classification of growth plates fractures using the Salter–Harris type (Table 44.7) is useful in diagnosis and management of childhood growth plate fractures (Boutis et al., 2016). Epiphyseal injury may result in early, incomplete, or partial closure of the growth plate, leading to deformity or shortening of the bone. Epiphyseal growth continues until skeletal maturity is reached during adolescence. Production of androgens in adolescence gradually causes the growth plates to fuse, and thus long bone growth is complete (Fig. 44.1).

Bone Healing

The child's bones have a thick, strong periosteum with an abundant blood supply. Bone healing occurs in the same fashion as in the adult, but because of the rich nutrient supply to the periosteum, it occurs more quickly in children. Children's bones produce callus more rapidly and in larger quantities than do adults. As new bone cells quickly form, a bulge of new bone growth occurs at the site of the fracture. The younger the child, the more quickly the bone heals. Also, the closer the fracture is to the growth plate (epiphysis), the more quickly the fracture heals. The capacity for remodelling (the process of breaking down and forming new bone) is increased in children as compared with adults. This means that straightening of the bone over time occurs more easily in children.

Positional Alterations

The lower extremities of the infant tend to have a bowed appearance, attributed to in utero positioning (or uterine packing). In utero, the fetus' hips are usually flexed, abducted, and externally rotated, with the knees also

FIGURE 44.2 Internal tibial torsion with metatarsus adductus—normal findings in the infant.

flexed and the lower limbs inwardly rotated. This normal developmental variation is termed internal tibial torsion. The legs straighten with passive motion, and internal tibial torsion should not be confused with "bowlegs" (Fig. 44.2). Internal tibial torsion usually resolves independently sometime in the second or third year of life as the toddler bears weight and the lower extremity muscles and bones mature. The bowlegged appearance is sometimes also referred to as genu varum. As internal tibial torsion or genu varum resolves, physiologic genu valgum occurs. Children usually demonstrate symmetric genu valgum (knock-knees) by the age of 2 to 3 years. In genu valgum, when the knees are touching, the ankles

FIGURE 44.3 Genu valgum (knock-knees): note knees touching at midline and outward angle of the lower half of the legs.

are significantly separated, with the lower portion of the legs angled outward (Fig. 44.3). By age 7 or 8 years, genu valgum gradually resolves in most children.

The newborn's feet also display in-toeing (metatarsus adductus) as a result of in utero positioning (see Fig. 44.2). The feet remain flexible and may be passively moved to midline and in a straight position. This also resolves as the infant's musculoskeletal system matures. Pes planus (flat feet) is noted in infants when they begin to walk. The long arch of the foot is not yet developed and makes contact with the floor, resulting in a medial bulge. As the child grows and the muscles become less lax, the arch generally develops. Some children may continue with flexible flat feet, and this is considered a normal variation.

Take Note!

Fractures are uncommon in children younger than 1 year of age. Carefully evaluate the infant who presents with a fracture for child abuse or an underlying musculoskeletal disorder (Haut, 2014).

COMMON MEDICAL TREATMENTS

A variety of medications as well as other medical treatments are used to treat neuromuscular and musculoskeletal disorders in children. Most of these treatments will require a physician's or nurse practitioner's order when the child is in the hospital. The most common treatments and medications are listed in Common Medical Treatments 44.1 and Drug Guide 44.1. The nurse caring for the child with a neuromuscular or musculoskeletal disorder should become familiar with what these procedures are and how they work as well as common nursing implications related to use of these modalities. The treatment of musculoskeletal disorders often involves immobilization via casting, bracing, splinting, surgical fixation, or traction to allow healing with the bones in appropriate alignment. The length of treatment with these immobilization methods varies from weeks to months depending on the type of disorder being treated and its severity. Complications related to casting and traction include neurovascular compromise, skin integrity impairment, soft tissue injury, compartment syndrome, and, with skeletal traction, pin site infection or osteomyelitis.

Casts

Casts are used to immobilize a bone that has been injured or a diseased joint. When a fracture has occurred, a cast serves to hold the bone in reduction, thus preventing deformity as the fracture heals. Casts are constructed of a hard material, traditionally plaster but now more commonly fibreglass or polyurethane resin, both of which are lighter in weight than plaster of Paris. The

COMMON MEDICAL TREATMENTS 44.1

Treatment	Explanation	Indications	Nursing Implications
Casting	Application of plaster or fibreglass material to form a rigid apparatus to immobilize a body part	Fracture reduction, dislocations, correction of deformities	Assess frequently for neurovascular compromise, skin impairment at cast edges. Protect cast from moisture (including urine/stool if a hip spica). Teach family how to care for cast at home.
Splinting	Temporary stiff support of injured area	Temporary fracture reduction, immobilization, and support of sprains	Similar to cast care. Some splints are removable and are replaced when the child is up out of bed. Teach family appropriate use of splints. Ensure review with prosthetics/orthotic service if splints are to be used longer term as the child grows.
Fixation	Surgical reduction of a fracture or skeletal deformity with an internal or external pin or fixation device	Fractures, skeletal deformities	No additional care for internal fixation, wound care. External fixation: perform pin care as prescribed by the surgeon (24 to 48 hours post-surgery) assess for blood clot, compartment syndrome, nerve impairment. Ongoing check for erythema, signs of infection pin sites. Assess for excess drainage or pin slippage, notifying physician or nurse practitioner if this occurs. Velcro or snaps on sleeves and pant legs help with dressing.
Cold therapy	Application of ice bags, commercial cold packs, or cold compresses	Most often used in acute injuries to cause vasoconstriction, followed by vasodilation, thereby decreasing pain and swelling	Ensure skin sensation is intact to hot and cold in order to prevent an ice burn. Document this response. Apply for 10 to 20 minutes, then remove for 1 hour, and then reapply for 10 to 20 minutes. Discontinue when numbness occurs. Place a towel between the cold pack and the skin to prevent thermal injury.
Gait aids	Ambulatory devices that transfer body weight from lower to upper extremities	Used whenever weight-bearing is restricted or contraindicated	When measuring axilla crutches, the top of the crutch should reach 2 to 3 fingerbreadths below the axillae to prevent nerve palsy. The hand-hold should be measured to the wrist crease. With elbow crutches, walkers, or canes, the handle should be measured to the wrist crease. Teach child appropriate ambulation (including stairs) with gait aid or reinforce teaching if performed by physical therapist.
Skeletal or cervical, skin traction	Traction is an application of a pulling force on an extremity or body part	To minimize or prevent trauma to the spinal cord; fracture reduction, dislocations, correction of deformities	To maintain even, constant traction: • Ensure weights hang free at all times and ropes remain in the pulley grooves. • Keep weights out of child's reach. • Maintain prescribed weight to promote alignment. • Elevate head or foot of bed only with physician order. • Replace nonadhesive straps or elastic bandage on skin, assess applied and intact, skin integrity (allergy risk). Monitor for complications: • Perform neurovascular checks at least every 4 hours. • Monitor neurologic status closely. • Assess for signs and symptoms of infection or impaired skin integrity. • Provide appropriate pin site care.

(continued)

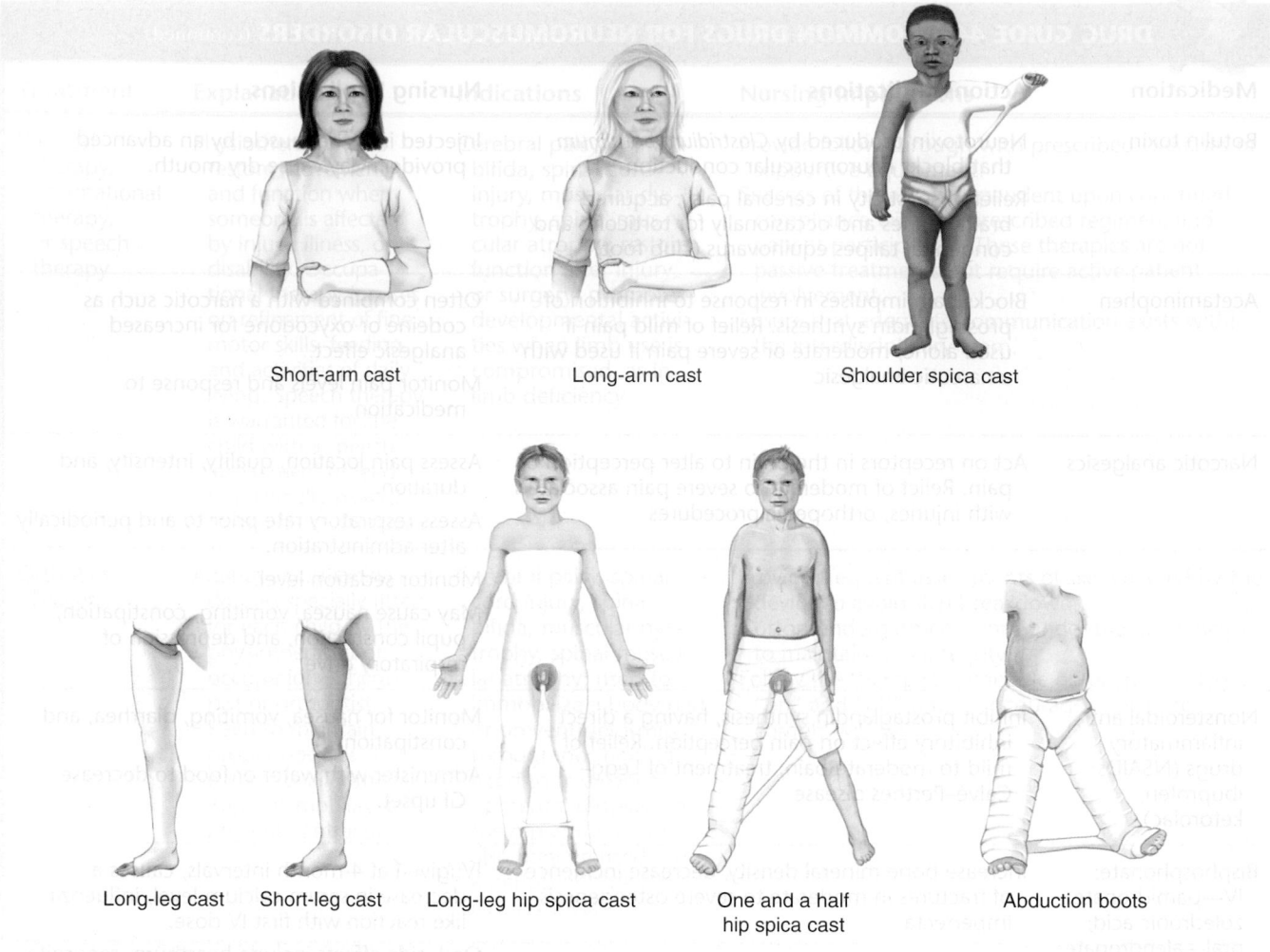

Short-arm cast   Long-arm cast   Shoulder spica cast

Long-leg cast   Short-leg cast   Long-leg hip spica cast   One and a half hip spica cast   Abduction boots

FIGURE 44.4 Selected casts used in children.

External Fixation

External fixation may be used for complicated fractures, especially open fractures with soft tissue damage. A series of pins or wires are inserted into bone and then attached to an external frame. The fixator apparatus may be adjusted as needed by the physician or nurse practitioner. Once the desired level of correction is achieved, no further adjustment occurs and the bone is allowed to heal. Advantages of external fixation include increased comfort for the injured child and improved function of muscles and joints when complicated fracture occurs. External and internal fixators can be used for limb lengthening and correction of deformity (see Table 44.1).

COMPARISON CHART 44.1	SKIN VERSUS SKELETAL TRACTION	
	Skin Traction	**Skeletal Traction**
Application of force	To the skin via strips or tapes secured with Ace bandages or traction boots	To the body part directly by fixation into or through the bone
Length of treatment	Usually limited	Allows for longer periods of traction
Amount of force	Less	More

TABLE 44.1	TYPES OF TRACTION AND NURSING IMPLICATIONS	
Type of Traction	**Description**	**Nursing Implications**
Bryant traction	Both legs are extended vertically, with child's weight serving as countertraction. Skin traction is applied to both legs. Used to reduce femur fracture in children younger than 2 years or with developmental dysplasia of the hip	Maintain appropriate position. Ensure heels and ankles are free from pressure. Assess condition and position of elastic bandages every shift and rewrap elastic bandages as ordered
Russell traction	Skin traction for femur fracture, hip, and specific types of knee injuries or contractures. Uses a knee sling. In split Russell traction, a portion of the traction weight may be redistributed via a pulley from the sling to the head of the bed (used for femur fracture, Legg–Calvé–Perthes disease, slipped capital femoral epiphysis)	Wrap bandages from ankle to thigh on children younger than age 2 years, from ankle to knee on children older than 2 years. Use a foot support to prevent foot drop. Ensure heel is free from bed. Assess popliteal region for skin breakdown from the sling. Mark leg to ensure proper replacement of sling
Buck traction	Skin traction for hip and knee contractures, Legg–Calvé–Perthes disease, slipped capital femoral epiphysis. Used to rest an injured limb or to prevent spasms of injured muscles or joints. Traction force delivered in straight line	Remove traction boot every 8 hours to assess skin. Leg may be slightly abducted
Cervical skin traction	Skin traction applied with a skin strap (head halter). Used for neck sprains/strains, torticollis, or nerve trauma	Ensure that head halter or skin strap does not place pressure on ears or throat. Limit of 5–7 lb of weight
Side-arm 90–90	Skin traction for humerus fractures and injuries in or around the shoulder girdle	Maintain elbow flexed at 90 degrees. Fingers and hand may feel cool because of elevation. Child may turn to affected side only

(continued)

INSPECTION AND OBSERVATION

Observe the infant or child playing with toys, crawling, or walking to obtain significant information about cranial nerve, cerebellar, and motor function. Observe the child's general appearance, noting any asymmetry in facial muscle development. Inspect the extremities for: symmetry in appearance and movement, absence or duplication, or webbing of any digits or limb-length discrepancy. When extremities are not used, muscular atrophy develops, so a shortened limb may indicate chronic hemiparesis. Observe gait in the child who has achieved the developmental skill of walking. Note refusal to walk, limping, in-toeing, out-toeing, or foot slap. Inspect injured joints for ecchymosis (spontaneous reddish or bluish discolouration of the skin greater than 10 mm) or swelling. In the injured extremity, note the colour of the fingertips or toes and range of spontaneous motion. Inspect the skin for redness, warmth, bruises, and puncture sites. Inspect the spine for cutaneous abnormalities such as dimples or hair tufts, which may be associated with spinal cord abnormalities. Observe the child's posture and alignment of the trunk. Perform scoliosis screening to determine spinal alignment, positive Trendelenburg's sign, or gait if child is weightbearing. Note symmetry of thigh folds. Observe the child's level of consciousness (LOC), noting a decrease or significant changes. Note the presence of lethargy.

Motor Function. Observe spontaneous activity, posture, and balance, and assess for asymmetric movements. In the infant, observe resting posture, which will normally be a slight flexion of the limbs until approximately 2 months of age. The infant should be able to extend extremities to a normal stretch. Note position of comfort of the infant's or child's neck.

Reflexes. Note sluggish or brisk deep tendon reflexes. Note persistence of primitive reflexes in the older infant or child, such as Moro or tonic neck, and palmar and plantar grasp responses. Assess for development of protective reflexes, which is often delayed in infants with motor disorders.

Sensory Function. Alterations in sensory function accompany many neuromuscular disorders. Assess sensory function in a similar fashion to that used in the adult. The sensory functions of light touch, pain, vibration, heat, and cold are distinguishable by a child. In the infant, assess for response to light touch or pain. The usual response to pain will be withdrawal from the stimulus. Always prepare the child for the sensory examination in order to gain cooperation. The pinprick test may be particularly frightening, but most children will cooperate if educated appropriately.

FIGURE 44.5 Assessing neck tone in an infant.

PALPATION

Assess muscle strength and tone in the infant or child. Compare strength and tone bilaterally. Evaluate neck tone by pulling the infant from a supine position to a sitting position (Fig. 44.5). By 4 to 5 months, the infant should be able to maintain the head in a neutral position. Perform passive range of motion of the neck. Alterations in range of motion may indicate a neuromuscular disorder or torticollis. Note trunk tone in the infant by holding the infant under the axillae and palpating for trunk tone. The hypotonic infant will feel as though he or she is slipping through the examiner's hands. Generalized hypotonia is a common sign of neuromuscular disease in the infant and young child (Sarant, 2011a). The hypertonic infant will feel rigid, extending the trunk and legs. Assess leg tone in the infant by placing the infant in the vertical position with the feet on a flat surface; the 4-month-old infant should be able to momentarily support his or her weight (Fig. 44.6). Assess the strength of the infant or young child by noting ability to move the muscles against gravity. In older children, have the child push against the examiner's hand with the sole of the foot to determine muscle strength (Fig. 44.7). Note any hypertonia or **spasticity**, which is involuntary muscle contractions that are not coordinated with other muscles (e.g., when you stretch out your forearm, the triceps contract and the biceps stretch; in spasticity, they both contract at the same time). These may be an early indication of CP or another neuromuscular disorder.

Take Note!

In cases of trauma or suspected trauma, do not perform any assessment that involves movement of the head and neck until cervical injury is ruled out. Maintain complete immobilization of the cervical spine until that time.

Infant fractures can occur after a stressful childbirth and can be difficult to detect. Clavicle fractures are the most common. Note crying when affected area

FIGURE 44.6 Assessing leg tone in an infant.

is touched (dressing infant); limited movement; slight droop when compared with unaffected side; and a lump in the affected area, usually a few weeks after the injury. Perform active range of motion to determine if a joint position is fixed or flexible. Palpate the affected joint or extremity to detect warmth or tenderness. In the injured child or the child with a cast or splint, thoroughly assess the neurovascular status of the affected extremities.

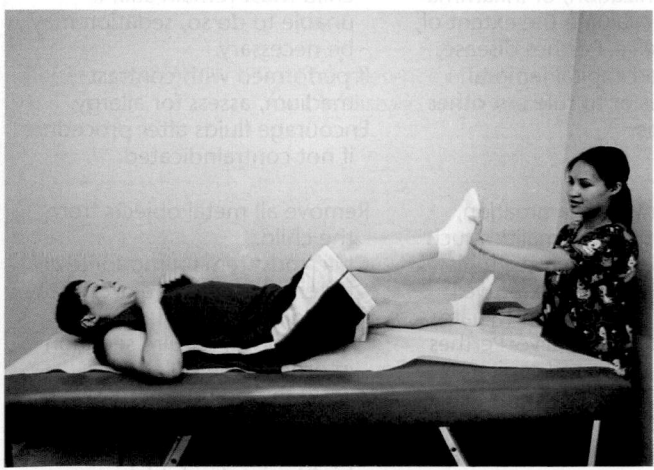

FIGURE 44.7 Assessing leg strength of the child.

Palpate the fingers or toes for warmth. Determine the capillary refill time. Note the presence of sensation or motion. Evaluate muscle strength. Palpate pulses distal to the injury, noting their strength and quality. The Ortolani and Barlow manoeuvres must be performed by an experienced professional to prevent further damage to the hip (see section on Developmental Dysplasia of the Hip later in this chapter) to assess for DDH.

Take Note!

Assess the injured site last, and do so gently.

AUSCULTATION

Auscultate the child's lungs; adventitious sounds may be present when respiratory muscle function is impaired. However, if the child has impaired neuromuscular system, there may not be enough turbulence to create adventitious sound and the chest may sound clear or quiet to the novice ear.

Laboratory and Diagnostic Testing

Common Laboratory and Diagnostic Tests 44.1 offers an explanation of the laboratory and diagnostic tests most commonly used in neuromuscular and musculoskeletal disorders. The tests can assist the physician or nurse practitioner in diagnosing the disorder and/or be used as guidelines in determining ongoing treatment. Laboratory or nonnursing personnel perform some of the tests, while the nurse might perform others. In either instance, the nurse should be familiar with how the tests are performed, what they are used for, and normal versus abnormal results. This knowledge will also be necessary when providing child and family education related to the testing.

Nursing Diagnoses, Goals, Interventions, and Evaluations

Upon completion of a thorough assessment, the nurse might identify several nursing diagnoses, including:
- Pain (see Chapter 36)
- Impaired physical mobility
- Imbalanced nutrition: less than body requirements
- Urinary retention
- Risk for constipation
- Self-care deficit (specify)
- Risk for impaired skin integrity
- Dysthymia (mood disorder with long-lasting symptoms)
- Risk for injury
- Deficient knowledge (specify)
- Family processes, interrupted

(text continues on page 1684)

After completing an assessment of Fredrick, the nurse noted the following: he started walking at 2 years of age, he has difficulty jumping, his gait has a waddling appearance, and he does not rise from the floor in the usual fashion. Based on these assessment findings, what would your top three nursing diagnoses be for Fredrick?

Nursing goals, interventions, and evaluation for the child with neuromuscular and musculoskeletal dysfunction are based on the nursing diagnoses (see Nursing Care Plan 44.1 at the end of the chapter). The nursing care plan may be used as a guide in planning nursing care for the child with a neuromuscular or musculoskeletal disorder. The care plan includes many nursing diagnoses that are applicable to the child or adolescent. Children's responses to neuromuscular or musculoskeletal dysfunction and its treatment will vary, and nursing care should be individualized based on the child's and family's responses to illness. The nursing care of immobilized children is similar to that of adults, but developmental and age-appropriate effects must be taken into account. Prevention of complications is a key nursing function. Additional information about nursing care related to certain disorders will be included later in the chapter as it relates to specific disorders. Particular care related to casts, traction, and external fixation is discussed below.

Based on your top three nursing diagnoses for Fredrick, describe appropriate nursing interventions.

Assisting With Cast Application

Before cast or splint application, perform baseline neurovascular assessment for comparison after immobilization. This includes:
• Colour (note cyanosis or other discolouration)
• Movement (note inability to move fingers or toes)
• Sensation (note whether loss of sensation is present)
• Edema
• Quality of pulses

Enlist the cooperation of the child and reduce his or her fear by showing the child the cast materials and using an age-appropriate approach to describe cast application. Remember pre-schoolers and younger children may worry about having a cast because of their difficulty with defining body boundaries. Administer analgesia as prescribed to reduce pain prior to any intervention (e.g., manual traction to align the bone). Use distraction throughout cast application and assist with application of the cast or splint (Fig. 44.8).

FIGURE 44.8 Assist with cast application by distracting or comforting the child.

> **Take Note!**
> Modern fibreglass cast materials are available in a variety of colours, as well as a few patterns. Allowing the child to choose the colour may increase the child's cooperation with the procedure.

After the cast or splint is applied, drying time will vary based on the type of material used. Splints and fibreglass casts usually take only a few minutes to dry and will cause a very warm feeling inside the cast, so prepare the child for this. Plaster requires 24 to 48 hours to dry. Take care not to cause depressions in the plaster cast while drying, as those may cause skin pressure and breakdown. Instruct the child and family to keep the cast still, positioning it with pillows as needed.

Caring for the Child With a Cast

Perform frequent neurovascular checks of the casted extremity to identify early signs of compromise. These signs include:
• Increased pain
• Increased edema
• Pale or blue colour
• Skin coolness
• Numbness or tingling
• Prolonged capillary refill
• Decreased pulse strength (or absence of pulse)

Notify the physician or nurse practitioner of changes in neurovascular status or odour or drainage from the cast.

Fibreglass casts usually have a soft fabric edge, so they usually do not cause skin rubbing at the edges of the cast. On the other hand, plaster casts require special treatment of the cast edge to prevent skin rubbing. This may be accomplished through a technique called

To petal a cast:

1. Cut several strips of adhesive tape or moleskin three to four inches in length. Use one inch tape for smaller areas (e.g., infant's foot) and two inch tape for larger areas (e.g., adolescent's waist).

2. Round one end of each strip to keep the corners from rolling.

3. Apply the first strip by tucking the straight end inside the cast and by bringing the rounded end over the cast edge to the outside.

4. Repeat the procedure, overlapping each additional strip, until all rough edges are completely covered.

FIGURE 44.9 **Petaling the cast.**

petaling (which can also be used on fibreglass casts that come into contact with urine or stool, e.g., hip spica). Petaling is an important nursing intervention and involves cutting rounded-edge strips of moleskin or another soft material with an adhesive backing and applying them to the edge of cast, as shown in Figure 44.9.

Position the child with the casted extremity elevated on pillows. Ice may be applied during the first 24 to 48 hours after casting if needed, but be careful to avoid ice burn. Teaching the child to use gait aids (e.g., crutches) is an important nursing intervention for any child with lower extremity immobilization so that the child can maintain mobility (Fig. 44.10). Refer to the physical therapist if any concerns or when caring for children with complex comorbidities that

impact on mobility. Provide home care instructions to the family about cast care (see Teaching Guidelines 44.1).

 Teaching Guidelines 44.1
HOME CAST CARE

• For the first 48 hours, elevate the extremity above the level of the heart and apply cold therapy for 20 to 30 minutes, then off 1 to 2 hours, and repeat.
• Take your prescribed pain medication.
• Assess for swelling, and have the child wiggle the fingers or toes hourly when awake and inspect during the night as instructed.
• For itching inside the cast:
  • Never insert anything into the cast for the purposes of scratching.
  • Blow cool air in from a hair dryer set on the lowest setting or tap lightly on the cast.
  • Do not use lotions or powders.
• Do not pull padding out from the inside of the cast.
• Protect the cast from wetness.
  • Apply a plastic bag around cast and tape securely for bathing or showering. Continue to avoid placing the cast directly in water (unless it is Gore-Tex lined).
  • If a cast becomes soiled, it can be wiped clean with a slightly damp clean cloth.
  • If the cast gets wet, dry it with a blow dryer on the cold setting (if warm setting is used, the child could get burned). Use of a vacuum cleaner with a hose attachment to pull air through may speed drying—be careful to avoid skin.
• If the child has a large cast, change position every 2 hours during the day and while sleeping change position as often as possible. Assess pressure areas as per local risk management tools.
• Check the skin for irritation.
  • Press the skin back around edges of the cast.
  • Use a flashlight to look for reddened or irritated areas.
  • Feel for blisters or sores.
• Call the physician or nurse practitioner if:
  • The casted extremity is cool to the touch, pale, blue, or very swollen.
  • The child cannot move the fingers or toes.
  • Severe pain occurs when the child attempts to move the fingers or toes.
  • Persistent numbness or tingling occurs.
  • Drainage or a foul smell comes from under the cast.
  • Severe itching occurs inside the cast.
  • The child runs a fever greater than 101.5°F for longer than 24 hours.

FIGURE 44.10 Reinforce appropriate crutch walking for children with lower extremity immobilization.

- Skin edges are red and swollen or exhibit breakdown.
- Child complains of rubbing or burning under cast.
- The cast gets wet and does not dry or is cracked, split, or softened.

Adapted from Bowden, V. R., & Greenberg, C. S. (2012). *Pediatric nursing procedures* (3rd ed.). Philadelphia, PA: Lippincott Williams & Wilkins; Schweich, P. (2017). *Patient information: Cast and splint care (Beyond the basics).* UpToDate. Retrieved from http://www.uptodate.com/contents/cast-and-splint-care-beyond-the-basics

Take Note!

Persistent complaints of pain may indicate compromised skin integrity under the cast.

Assisting With Cast Removal

Children may be frightened by cast removal. Prepare the child using age-appropriate terminology:
- The cast cutter will make a loud noise (Fig. 44.11).
- The skin or extremity will not be injured (demonstrate by touching the cast cutter lightly to your palm).
- The child will feel warmth or vibration during cast removal.

Teaching Guidelines 44.2 gives instructions related to skin care after cast removal.

FIGURE 44.11 The loud noise of the cast saw may frighten the child.

Teaching Guidelines 44.2
SKIN CARE AFTER CAST REMOVAL

- Brown, flaky skin is normal and occurs as dead skin and secretions accumulate under the cast.
- New skin may be tender.
- Soak with warm water daily.
- Wash with warm soapy water, avoiding excessive rubbing, which may traumatize the skin.
- Discourage the child from scratching the dry skin.
- Apply moisturizing lotion to relieve dry skin.
- Encourage activity to regain strength and motion of extremity.

Caring for the Child in Traction

Nursing care of the child in any type of traction focuses not only on appropriate application and maintenance of traction but also on promoting normal growth and development and preventing complications (see Table 44.1). Apply skin traction over intact skin only so that the pull of the traction is effective. Prepare the skin with an appropriate adhesive before applying the traction tapes to ensure that the tapes adhere well, preventing skin friction. After application of the traction tapes, apply the elastic bandage or use the foam boot. Attach the traction spreader block and then apply the prescribed amount of weight via a rope attached to the spreader block. Ensure that the rope moves without obstruction and that the weights hang freely without touching the floor.

In skeletal traction, apply weight via ropes attached to the skeletal pins. Treat the pin sites as surgical wounds (see section on pin site care). Protect the exposed ends of the pins to avoid injury. Whether skin or skeletal traction is used, be sure that constant and even traction is maintained.

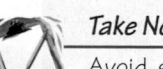

Take Note!

Avoid sudden bumping or movement of the bed: this can disturb traction alignment and cause additional pain to the child as the weights are jostled.

Preventing Complications

Refer to Nursing Care Plan 36.1 for interventions related to pain management and refer to Nursing Care Plan 44.1 for interventions related to prevention of complications of immobility such as skin integrity impairment. To prevent contractures and atrophy that may result from disuse of muscles, ensure that unaffected extremities are exercised. Assist the child to exercise the unaffected joints and to use the unaffected extremity if

FIGURE 44.12 Provide age-appropriate diversional activities and schoolwork for children confined to bed in traction.

this does not disrupt traction alignment. Promote use of a trapeze if not contraindicated to involve the child in repositioning and assist with movement. Encourage deep-breathing exercises to prevent the pulmonary complications of long-term immobilization.

Promote normal growth and development by:
- Placing age-appropriate toys within the child's reach
- Encouraging visits from friends
- Providing diversional activities such as drawing, colouring, or video games (Fig. 44.12)

Take Note!

Ongoing, careful neurovascular assessments are critical in the child with a cast or in skeletal traction. Notify the physician or nurse practitioner immediately if these signs of compartment syndrome occur: extreme pain (out of proportion to the situation), pain with passive range of motion of digits, distal extremity pallor, inability to move digits, or loss of pulses.

Caring for the Child With an External Fixator

Care of an external fixator involves maintaining skin integrity, preventing infection, and preventing injury. Routine neurovascular and skin assessment is essential. Skin care is similar to a child in skeletal traction and includes pin care daily. Elevation of the extremity can help prevent swelling. The fixator may be moved by gently grasping the frame, as the fixator can tolerate ordinary movement. Encourage weightbearing as prescribed. Provide appropriate education to the child and family. Encourage the child to look at the apparatus. Teach the child not to pick or manipulate the pins. Baggy or loose clothing can be worn over the device. Velcro sewn into the seams can be helpful and allows clothes to slip over the device.

Providing Pin Care

Whether pins are inserted for skeletal traction or as part of an external fixator (see section on fractures), keeping the pin sites clean is important to prevent infection. Cleaning of the pin sites prevents infection by promoting comfort and preventing healing skin from adhering to the metal pin. Notify the orthopedic surgeon if signs of pin site infection are present or if pin slippage occurs.

Thus far, there is insufficient evidence that supports a particular strategy of pin care. More randomized trials are needed. The National Association of Orthopaedic Nurses and the Royal College of Nursing have published minimal guidelines, which include:
- Perform pin care weekly after the first 48 to 72 hours. Perform earlier if large amounts of drainage are present, dressing becomes wet, or infection is suspected.
- The most effective solution for pin site care may be chlorhexidine 2 mg/mL in alcohol. If child has sensitivity to this, use normal saline.
- Use a nonshedding material for cleaning.
- Cover pin sites with a nonshedding dressing.
- Teach children and their families pin site care along with instructions on the signs and symptoms of infection before discharge (Timms, Vincent, Santy-Tomlinson, & Hertz, 2011).

Since the research available is minimal, these recommendations are made tentatively (Lethaby, Temple, & Santy-Tomlinson, 2013). Therefore, interventions for pin care need to be individualized based on the child's condition and response to treatment and according to institutional policy or the physician's or nurse practitioner's orders. Certain physicians or nurse practitioners prefer the site to be cleaned with normal saline; others choose a solution with antibacterial properties. Some institutions recommend removal of all crusts formed on the skin around the pin; others do not. The rationale for crust removal is to promote free drainage and prevent the surrounding skin from adhering to the pin. A keyhole dressing may be necessary around the pin if drainage is present. No matter which procedure is ordered or preferred, perform pin care as necessary to prevent infection at the pin site. The Ilizarov fixator uses wires that are thinner than ordinary pins, so simply cleansing by showering is usually sufficient to keep the pin site clean. If drainage is present, cleanse the skin around the wires with a dry gauze pad.

When caring for children in the hospital, particularly those with complex medical needs, follow their home care routines as much as possible.

CONGENITAL AND DEVELOPMENTAL DISORDERS

Several disorders with neuromuscular and musculoskeletal effects are congenital in nature. These include neural tube defects and genetic neuromuscular disorders. The structural disorders related to malformation of the spinal cord are complex and are broadly grouped under the term spinal dysraphism, which includes closed bony anomalies (spina bifida occulta), closed neural tube defects (meningocele and lipomyelomeningocele), or open lesions (myelomeningocele). Caudal regression syndrome, or sacral agenesis, is a congenital disorder resulting in abnormal development of the lower spine. Congenital anomalies of the musculoskeletal system are usually readily identified at birth. Congenital structural anomalies involving the skeleton include, but are not limited to, pectus excavatum, pectus carinatum, limb deficiencies, polydactyly or syndactyly, metatarsus adductus, congenital clubfoot, and osteogenesis imperfecta. A developmental anomaly that may be diagnosed at birth or later in life is DDH. A muscular condition, torticollis, most often presents as a congenital condition but may also develop after birth. Tibia vara is a developmental disorder affecting young children. Rarely, a developmental positional alteration such as genu varum, genu valgum, or pes planus will persist past the usual age of resolution or cause the child pain. If those situations occur, bracing, orthotics, or surgical correction may become necessary. The genetic neuromuscular disorders include the various types of muscular dystrophy and spinal muscular atrophy (SMA). These disorders are not always recognized at birth because signs and symptoms are not evident until months or even years after birth. However, they are still considered to be congenital as they have a genetic basis.

Neural Tube Defects

Neural tube defects account for the majority of congenital anomalies of the central nervous system. The neural tube closes between the third and fourth weeks of gestation. The cause of neural tube defects is complex and influenced by many factors, including malnutrition, environmental factors, and genetics, since all can hinder normal central nervous system development. Strong evidence exists that maternal preconception supplementation of folic acid can decrease the incidence of neural tube defects in pregnancies by 50% or more (Canadian Paediatric Society [CPS], 2016a). The Public Health Agency of Canada, CPS, and the Society of Obstetricians and Gynaecologists of Canada recommend that women of childbearing age who could conceive take 0.4 mg (400 mcg) of folic acid daily. Pregnant women who had a previous pregnancy or child with a neural tube defect are recommended to take a higher dosage and should consult with their physician or nurse practitioner. Prenatal screening of maternal serum for α-fetoprotein (AFP) and ultrasound examination can help identify fetuses at risk. Neural tube defects primarily affecting spinal cord development include spina bifida occulta, meningocele, and myelomeningocele (MMC; Fig. 44.13). Neural tube defects primarily affecting brain development are discussed in Chapter 38.

Spina Bifida Occulta

Spina bifida is a term that is often used to refer to all neural tube disorders that affect the spinal cord. This can be confusing and a cause of concern for parents. There are well-defined degrees of spinal cord involvement, and it is important for health care professionals to use the correct terminology.

FIGURE 44.13 **A.** Normal spine. **B.** Spina bifida occulta. **C.** Meningocele. **D.** Myelomeningocele.

Spina bifida occulta is a defect of the vertebral bodies without protrusion of the spinal cord or meninges. This defect is not visible externally and in most cases has no adverse effects (see Fig. 44.13). Spina bifida occulta is a common anomaly. It is estimated that it affects 10% to 20% of otherwise healthy people (National Institute of Neurological Disorders and Stroke [NINDS], 2015a). Children with spina bifida occulta need no immediate medical intervention. Complications are rare, but may include more significant abnormalities of the spinal cord such as tethered cord, syringomyelia, or diastematomyelia.

NURSING ASSESSMENT

In most cases, spina bifida occulta is benign and asymptomatic and produces no neurologic signs. The defect, which is usually present in the lumbosacral area, often goes undetected. However, there may be noticeable dimpling, abnormal patches of hair, or discolouration of skin at the defect site. If so, further investigation, including magnetic resonance imaging (MRI), may be warranted.

NURSING MANAGEMENT

Nursing care will focus on educating the family. Inform parents of its presence and what the diagnosis means. Occasionally, children with spina bifida occulta need surgical intervention due to degenerative changes or involvement of the spine and nerve roots resulting in complications such as tethered cord, syringomyelia, or diastematomyelia. When these associated problems occur, the condition is often termed "occult spinal dysraphism" to avoid confusion.

Meningocele and Lipomyelomeningocele

Meningocele occurs when the meninges herniate through a defect in the vertebrae. The spinal cord is usually normal and there are typically minor or no associated neurologic deficits. Treatment for meningocele involves surgical correction of the lesion (see Fig. 44.13). Lipomyelomeningocele (LMMC) is a closed lesion (comprising fatty tissue attached to the spinal cord and membranes) that may be visible as a soft lump on the spine following birth or as the child grows. While it may not cause symptoms, the fat deposits can result in tethered cord. With the child's growth and development, the LMMC will grow and could further impact the spinal cord. Symptoms of an LMMC can include bladder and bowel problems, spasticity, leg and back pain, sensory loss and/or leg weakness, foot or leg anomalies, neuromuscular scoliosis, and impaired mobility (Spina Bifida & Hydrocephalus Association of Canada, 2019).

NURSING ASSESSMENT

Initial assessment after delivery will reveal a visible external sac (meningocele) protruding from the spinal area. It is most often seen in the lumbar region but can be anywhere along the spinal canal. Most are covered with skin. However, assessment to ensure that the sac covering is intact remains important. Assess neurologic status carefully. Before surgical correction, the infant will be thoroughly examined to determine whether there is any neural involvement or associated anomalies. Diagnostic procedures such as computed tomography (CT), MRI, and ultrasound may be performed.

NURSING MANAGEMENT

If the skin covering the sac is intact and the child has normal neurologic functioning, surgical correction may be delayed (Kinsman & Johnston, 2011). However, as in a child with MMC, immediately report any evidence of leaking cerebrospinal fluid (CSF) to ensure prompt intervention to prevent infection. Nursing management will be supportive. Provide preoperative and postoperative care similar to the child with MMC to prevent rupture of the sac, to prevent infection, and to provide adequate nutrition and hydration. Monitor for symptoms of constipation or bladder dysfunction that may result due to increasing size of the lesion. Resulting hydrocephalus has been associated with some cases of meningocele (Kinsman & Johnston, 2011). Therefore, monitor head circumference and watch for signs and symptoms of increased intracranial pressure (ICP).

Myelomeningocele

Myelomeningocele (MMC), also often called "spina bifida," is the most severe form of neural tube defect. While figures are unclear, in Canada, it is estimated that approximately 120 to 250 children per year are born with a form of spina bifida (Public Health Agency Canada, 2011). It may be diagnosed in utero via ultrasound. Otherwise, it is visually obvious at birth. The newborn with MMC is at increased risk for meningitis, hypoxia, and hemorrhage.

In MMC, the spinal cord often ends at the point of the defect, resulting in absent motor and sensory function beyond that point (see Fig. 44.14). Therefore,

FIGURE 44.14 Usually a sac covers the deformity of myelomeningocele and is visible at birth.

wall deformities (Boas, 2011). The remainder are mixed deformities. Male predominance is evident in both types (Boas, 2011).

Pectus excavatum does not resolve as the child grows; rather, it progresses with growth. The chest depression may be minimal or marked. When the pectus is more pronounced, cardiac and pulmonary compression occurs. Symptoms of this compression most often present during puberty, when the pectus quickly worsens, which can have implications for body image. Children may complain of shortness of breath, chest pain, and decreased exercise tolerance.

Therapeutic Management

Therapeutic management of pectus excavatum is based on the severity and physiologic compromise. Options vary depending on degree of severity and include observation, use of physical therapy to work on musculoskeletal compromise, and surgical correction, preferably before puberty, when the skeleton is more pliable. Various surgical techniques may be used and generally involve either the placement of a surgical steel bar or using a piece of bone in the rib cage to lift the depression. This discussion will focus on care of the child who undergoes surgical steel bar placement for pectus correction. Consider the impact of hospitalization on the child and family and the role of atraumatic interventions (see Chapter 30).

Nursing Assessment

Elicit the health history, noting progression of the defect and effects on the child's cardiopulmonary function. Note shortness of breath, exercise intolerance, or chest pain. Observe the child's chest for anterior wall deformity, noting depth and severity. Auscultate the lungs to determine the adequacy of aeration. Various investigations such as x-rays, CT, or MRI and pulmonary function testing may be used to determine the extent of the anomaly and compression of inner structures. ECG can be used and is important in youth with evidence of Marfan syndrome (Box 44.1). Explore issues of self-image and worries or concerns the youth may have about postoperative appearance.

BOX 44.1

MARFAN SYNDROME

Marfan syndrome (MFS) is an autosomal dominant genetic (fibrillin-1 gene) connective tissue disorder that affects the skeletal system, cardiovascular system, skin, and eyes. Skeletal deformities can include thoracolumbar scoliosis, pectus excavatum, and thoracic lordosis. MFS patients are tall, with a thin body structure, abnormally long digits (arachnodactyly), and long limbs (dolichostenomelia).

Nursing Management

Postoperatively, nursing management focuses on assessment, protection of the surgical site, and pain management. Auscultate lung sounds frequently to determine the adequacy of aeration and to monitor for development of the complication of pneumothorax. Assess for signs of wound infection that would necessitate removal of the curved bar. During the first few postoperative days, positioning is challenging; do not allow the child to roll in bed, lie on either side, or rotate or flex the spine (these positions may disrupt the bar's position). Administer analgesics as needed either intravenously or via the epidural catheter. Teach families that the child will not be allowed to lie on his or her side at home for 4 weeks after the surgery to ensure that the band does not shift. Encourage aerobic activity at home after being cleared by the surgeon (this will increase the child's vital capacity, previously hindered by the pectus). The bar will be removed 2 to 4 years after the initial placement.

Limb Deficiencies

Limb deficiencies, either complete absence of a limb or a portion of it or deformity, occur as the fetus is developing. The limb either fails to form normally or does not form at all. The cause is unknown. Certain behaviours and exposures can increase the risk of limb deficiencies such as exposure to certain chemicals, viruses, medications, and possible maternal exposure to tobacco smoke (Centers for Disease Control and Prevention, 2014). These defects can be attributed to an amniotic band constricting the limb, resulting in either incomplete development or amputation of the limb. Many children born with limb deformities also have congenital anomalies such as craniofacial abnormalities, cardiac, and abdominal wall defects (Centers for Disease Control and Prevention, 2014).

Therapeutic management is aimed at improving the child's functional ability. Physical therapy and occupational therapy are helpful. Adaptive equipment such as a prosthesis may also be prescribed.

Nursing Assessment

Note the extent of limb deformity, providing an accurate description of the presence or absence of a portion of the arm or leg, or missing fingers or toes. Assess the child's ability to use the extremity as a helper (arms) or in ambulation (legs). Determine status of acquisition of developmental skills.

Nursing Management

Reinforce prescribed activities that are meant to improve the child's function. Provide activities in which the child is capable of participating. Discuss referral to the local Child Development Centre or early intervention service provider as soon as possible after birth. Early intervention is designed to promote development from birth to age 5 years. Absence of a limb or a significant portion of a limb will have a considerable impact on the child's ability to meet developmental milestones as expected.

Polydactyly/Syndactyly

Polydactyly is the presence of extra digits on the hand or foot (Fig. 44.16). One third of the time, polydactyly occurs in both the hand and foot (Hosalkar, Spiegel, & Davidson, 2011). It usually involves digits at the border of the hand or foot, but can also occur by a central digit (Hosalkar et al., 2011). Syndactyly is webbing of the fingers and toes. Both polydactyly and syndactyly can be normal variants in the newborn and can also be inherited and associated with other genetic syndromes (Hosalkar et al., 2011).

Therapeutic management includes surgical removal of the digit. No treatment is usually required for syndactyly, though surgical repair is sometimes performed for cosmetic reasons.

Nursing Assessment

Inspect the hands and feet for the presence of extra digits. Note whether the additional digits are soft (without bone) or are full or partial digits with bone present. Note location of webbing.

Nursing Management

When surgical removal is necessary, provide routine pre- and postoperative care as appropriate.

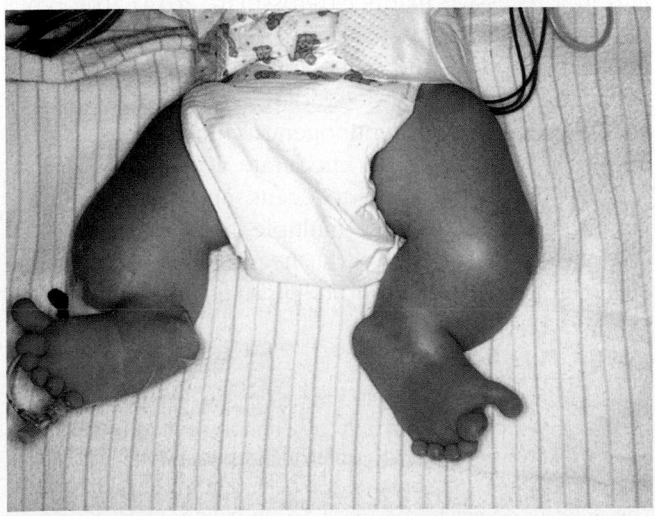

FIGURE 44.16 Note additional digits (toes) of polydactyly.

FIGURE 44.17 Metatarsus adductus: note medial deviation of the forefoot.

Metatarsus Adductus

Metatarsus adductus, a medial deviation of the forefoot, is one of the most common foot deformities of childhood (Fig. 44.17). It occurs most commonly as a result of in utero positioning (Hosalkar et al., 2011). Half of all cases occur bilaterally (Hosalkar et al., 2011). The degree of flexibility is important and determines treatment. Use of a "v" sign with your fingers, and placing baby's foot between your fingers, gives a good indication of severity. If the forefoot is flexible past neutral manipulation passively, observation is often sufficient. If the forefoot is flexible only to neutral manipulation, stretching exercises may be beneficial. If the forefoot is rigid and is not flexible to neutral manipulation, serial casting, preferably before the age of 8 months, may be required (Hosalkar et al., 2011). Surgical intervention is rarely needed.

Nursing Assessment

The deformity is usually noted at birth. Note inward deviation of the forefoot with the hindfoot remaining in normal position. The great and second toes might be separated. Determine forefoot flexibility. Range of motion of the ankle, hindfoot, and midfoot is normal.

Nursing Management

Most cases will resolve without treatment and nursing care is aimed at education and reassurance of the parents. Nursing care for the child with severe metatarsus adductus is similar to that of the child with clubfoot (see below).

Congenital Clubfoot

Congenital clubfoot (also termed congenital talipes equinovarus) is a congenital anomaly that occurs in about 1 of 1,000 live births (Hosalkar et al., 2011). Clubfoot consists of:

- Talipes varus (inversion of the heel)
- Talipes equinus (plantarflexion of the foot; the heel is raised and would not strike the ground in a standing position)
- Cavus (plantarflexion of the forefoot on the hindfoot)
- Forefoot adduction with supination (the forefoot is inverted and turned slightly upward)

The foot resembles the head of a golf club with increased skin creases on medial lower extremity (Fig. 44.18). Half of all cases occur bilaterally and males are affected more frequently than females (Hosalkar et al., 2011). The exact etiology of clubfoot is unknown.

Clubfoot may be classified into four categories: postural, neurogenic, syndromic, and idiopathic. Postural clubfoot often resolves with a short series of manipulative casting. Neurogenic clubfoot occurs in infants with MMC. Clubfoot in association with other syndromes (syndromic) is often resistant to treatment. Idiopathic clubfoot occurs in otherwise normal healthy infants. The approach to treatment is similar regardless of the classification.

Therapeutic Management

The goal of therapeutic management of clubfoot is achievement of a functional foot; treatment starts as soon after birth as possible. Weekly manipulation with serial cast changes is performed; later, cast changes occur every 2 weeks. Other infants require corrective shoes or bracing. In some infants, surgical release of soft tissue may be necessary. Following surgery, the foot is immobilized with a cast for up to 12 weeks, and then ankle–foot

FIGURE 44.18 Note inverted heel, ankle equinus, and forefoot adduction in this infant with bilateral clubfoot.

orthoses (AFOs) or corrective shoes are used for several years. Botulinum Toxin A (Botox) has also been used to treat club foot without the need for surgery (BCCH, n.d.).

Complications of clubfoot and its treatment include residual deformity, rocker-bottom foot, awkward gait, weightbearing on the lateral portion of the foot if uncorrected, and disturbance to the epiphysis.

Nursing Assessment

Note family history of foot deformities and obstetric history of breech position. Inspect the foot for position at rest. Perform active range of motion, noting inability to move foot into normal positioning at midline.

Nursing Management

Perform neurovascular assessment and cast care for infants requiring casting and monitor for signs of pain. Provide emotional support, as treatment often begins in the newborn period and families may have a difficult time adjusting to the diagnosis and treatment required for their new baby (Canadian Orthopaedic Foundation, n.d.). Teach families cast care and about the use of orthotics or braces as prescribed.

Osteogenesis Imperfecta

Osteogenesis imperfecta is a genetic bone disorder that results in low bone mass, increased fragility of the bones, and other connective tissue problems such as joint hypermobility, resulting in instability of the joints. All of these contribute to fracture occurrence. Dentinogenesis imperfecta may also occur. This is characterized by the tooth enamel wearing easily and brittle and discoloured teeth.

The disorder usually occurs as a result of a defect in the collagen type 1 gene, usually through an autosomal dominant inheritance pattern but some types are inherited in a recessive manner (Grossman, 2014). The types of osteogenesis imperfecta range from mild to severe connective tissue and bone involvement (Table 44.2). Subtypes A and B exist depending on (A) the absence or (B) the presence of dentinogenesis imperfecta (Marini, 2011). In children with moderate to severe disease, fractures are more likely to occur, and short stature is common. In addition to multiple fractures, additional complications include early hearing loss, acute and chronic pain, scoliosis, and respiratory problems.

> **Take Note!**
>
> Blue/grey sclera is not diagnostic of osteogenesis imperfecta, but it is a common finding (Grossman, 2014). However, there are some individuals with blue sclerae who do not have osteogenesis imperfecta. Keep in mind that the sclerae of newborns tend to be bluish, progressing to white over the first few weeks of life.

TABLE 44.2	CLASSIFICATION OF OSTEOGENESIS IMPERFECTA
Classification	**Characteristics**
I	Mild Accounts for 50% of OI cases[a] Blue sclera Hearing loss Frequent shoulder and elbow dislocations Recurrent fractures in childhood After growth is complete, incidence of fractures diminishes dramatically. Average or slightly shorter stature compared with family members Gross motor development delays
II	Most severe form Lethal in perinatal period or die within first year of life Low birthweight, very short limbs, small chest, and soft skull Intrauterine fractures evident Very dark blue/grey sclera
III	Most severe nonlethal form Sclera ranges from white to blue Fractures in utero and at birth with progressive deformity Bone fragility and fracture rate vary Results in significant disability Marked short stature
IV	Moderately severe Sclera may be light blue in infancy and lighten to white during childhood Fragile bones May present at birth with in utero fractures or bowing of lower long bones Height may be less than average for age
V and VI	Clinically within type IV but microscopic studies reveal distinct bone patterns; do not involve deficits of type I collagen Moderate in severity Similar to type IV in degree of fractures and skeletal deformity Type VI is extremely rare
VII and VIII	Recessive inheritance patterns Type VII resembles type IV or III, except infants have white sclera; stature is short Type VIII resembles type II or III, except for white sclera; growth deficiency is severe

[a]Osteogenesis Imperfecta Foundation. (2015). *Types of OI*. Retrieved from http://www.oif.org/site/PageServer?pagename=AOI_Types
Adapted from Marini, J. C. (2011). Chapter 692: Osteogenesis imperfecta. Osteogenesis imperfecta. In R. M. Kleigman, B. F. Stanton, J. W. St. Geme III, N. F. Schor, & R. E. Behrman (Eds.). *Nelson textbook of pediatrics* (19th ed., pp. 2437–2440). Philadelphia, PA: Saunders.

Therapeutic Management

The goal of medical and surgical management is to decrease the incidence of fractures, positional contractures, muscle weakness, and misalignment, thereby sustaining weightbearing and maximizing mobility. Bisphosphonate therapy is used for moderate to severe disease to increase bone density. Physical therapy and occupational therapy prevent contractures and maximize mobility. Standing with bracing is encouraged. Lightweight splints or braces may allow the child to bear weight earlier. Severe cases may require surgical insertion of rods into the long bones. Fracture care is often required.

Nursing Assessment

Elicit a health history, which may reveal a family history of osteogenesis imperfecta, a pattern of frequent fractures, or screaming associated with routine care and handling of the newborn. Inspect the eyes for sclerae that have a blue, purple, or grey tint. Note abnormalities of the primary teeth. Inspect skin for bruising and note joint hypermobility with active range of motion. Laboratory tests may include a skin biopsy (which reveals abnormalities in type 1 collagen) or DNA testing (locating the genetic mutation).

Nursing Management

Handle the child carefully and teach the family to avoid trauma (Teaching Guidelines 44.3). Refer families to the Osteogenesis Imperfecta Foundation (a link to which can be found on thePoint), which provides access to multiple resources as well as clinical trials. The site includes an online store with excellent books and booklets.

Teaching Guidelines 44.3

PREVENTING INJURY IN CHILDREN WITH OSTEOGENESIS IMPERFECTA

- Never push or pull on an arm or leg.
- Do not bend an arm or leg into an awkward position.
- Lift a baby by placing one hand under the legs and buttocks and the other hand under the shoulders, head, and neck.
- Do not lift a baby's legs by the ankles to change the diaper.
- Do not lift a baby or small child from under the armpits.
- Provide supported positioning.
- If fracture is suspected, handle the limb minimally.

FIGURE 44.19 Developmental dysplasia of the hip.

Encourage safe mobility. Reinforce physical and occupational therapists' recommendations for promotion of fine motor skills and independence in activities of daily living, as well as use of adaptive equipment and appropriate promotion of mobility. Adapted physical education is important to promote mobility and maintain bone and muscle mass. If the child is ambulatory, even with adaptive equipment use, walking is a good form of exercise. Swimming and water therapies are appropriate, allowing independent movement with little fracture risk.

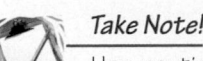

Take Note!

Use caution when inserting an intravenous line or taking a blood pressure measurement, as pressure on the arm or leg can lead to bruising and fractures.

Developmental Dysplasia of the Hip (DDH)

DDH refers to abnormalities of the developing hip that include dislocation, subluxation, and dysplasia of the hip joint. In DDH, the femoral head has an abnormal relationship to the acetabulum. Frank dislocation of the hip may occur, in which there is no contact between the femoral head and acetabulum. Subluxation is a partial dislocation, meaning that the head of the femur is not fully seated within the acetabulum. Dysplasia refers to an acetabulum that is shallow or sloping instead of cup shaped. DDH may affect just one or both hips. The dysplastic hip may be prone to subluxation or dislocated and then reduced again (Fig. 44.19).

Pathophysiology

While dislocation may occur during a growth period in utero, the laxity of the newborn's hip allows dislocation and relocation of the hip to occur. The hip can develop normally only if the femoral head is appropriately and deeply seated within the acetabulum. If subluxation and periodic or continued dislocation occur, then structural changes in the hip's anatomy occur. Continued dysplasia of the hip leads to limited abduction of the hip and contracture of muscles. DDH is more common in females, probably due to the greater susceptibility of the female newborn to maternal hormones that contribute to laxity of the ligaments (Sankar et al., 2011). Mechanical factors such as breech positioning or the presence of oligohydramnios also contribute to the development of DDH. Complications of DDH include avascular necrosis of the femoral head, loss of range of motion, recurrently unstable hip, femoral nerve palsy, leg-length discrepancy, and early osteoarthritis.

Therapeutic Management

The goal of therapeutic management is to maintain the hip joint in reduction so that the femoral head and acetabulum can develop properly.

Treatment varies based on the child's age and the severity of DDH. Infants younger than 6 months of age may be treated with a Pavlik harness, which reduces and stabilizes the hip by preventing hip extension and adduction and maintaining the hip in flexion and abduction (Grossman, 2014; Sankar et al., 2011). The Pavlik harness is successful in the treatment of DDH in the majority of infants younger than 6 months of age if it is used on a full-time basis and applied properly (Sankar et al., 2011). Children from 4 months to 2 years of age often require closed reduction (Sankar et al., 2011). Skin or skeletal traction may be used first to gradually stretch the associated soft tissue structures. Closed reduction occurs under general anesthesia, with the hip being gently manoeuvred back into the acetabulum. A spica cast worn for 12 weeks maintains reduction of the hip. After the cast is removed, the child may wear an abduction brace full time (except for baths) (Sankar et al., 2011). Then, the brace is worn at night and during naps until development of the acetabulum is normal. Children older than 2 years of age or those who have failed to respond to prior treatment require an open surgical reduction followed by a period of casting (Sankar et al., 2011). Follow-up continues until the age of skeletal maturity.

Nursing Assessment

Nursing assessment of children with DDH includes obtaining a health history and inspecting, observing, and palpating for findings common to DDH.

HEALTH HISTORY

Assess the health history for risk factors such as:

- Family history of DDH
- Female gender
- Oligohydramnios or breech birth
- Associated lower limb deformity, metatarsus adductus, hip asymmetry, torticollis, or other congenital musculoskeletal deformity

Previously undiagnosed older children may complain of hip pain.

PHYSICAL ASSESSMENT

The physical examination for DDH includes inspection, observation, and palpation. Since DDH is a developmental process, ongoing screening assessments are required throughout at least the first several months of the infant's life.

Inspection and Observation. Ensure that the infant is on a flat surface and is relaxed. Note asymmetry of thigh or gluteal folds with the infant in a prone position. Document shortening of the affected femur observed as limb-length discrepancy. Older children may exhibit **Trendelenburg gait**; due to the weakness of the hip abductors, the child's trunk is shifted over the affected hip during ambulation. Figure 44.20 illustrates these assessments.

Palpation. Note limited hip abduction while performing passive range of motion. Abduction should ordinarily occur to 75 degrees and adduction to within 30 degrees with the infant's pelvis stabilized. Perform Barlow and Ortolani tests, feeling for, or noting, a "clunk" as the femoral head dislocates (positive Barlow) or reduces (positive Ortolani) back into the acetabulum. Force is not necessary when performing the Barlow and Ortolani manoeuvres (Fig. 44.20 and Nursing Procedure 44.1).

FIGURE 44.20 Assessment techniques for developmental dysplasia of the hip. **A.** Assess for asymmetry of thigh and gluteal folds. **B.** Assess for unequal knee height related to femur shortening. **C.** Note limitation in hip abduction. **D.** Positive Trendelenburg sign: note pelvis/hip drops when leg is raised. **E.** Feel for "clunk" when adduction and depression of femur dislocates hip (Barlow test). Assess for "clunk" when the dislocated hip is abducted and relocated (Ortolani sign).

FIGURE 44.24 The Gower sign.
A. First, the child must roll onto his hands and knees. **B.** Then, he must bear weight by using his hands to support some of his weight, while raising his posterior. **C–E.** The boy then uses his hands to "walk" up his legs to assume an upright position.

need respite from continual caregiving duties. Therefore, working with social care providers and charitable organizations (e.g., Muscular Dystrophy Canada; see thePoint) is important to help families access available local supports (CPS, 2016b). Positive academic and social engagement is a protective factor for long-term health (CPS, 2016b). Therefore, assess educational opportunity (home school) and/or school involvement, care plan, and integration approaches.

Spinal Muscular Atrophy (SMA)

SMA is a genetic motor neuron disease that affects the spinal nerves' ability to communicate with the muscles. It is inherited via an autosomal recessive mechanism. The motor neuron protein survival of motor neurons (SMNs) is deficient as a result of a faulty gene on chromosome 5. The motor neurons are located mostly in the spinal cord. Without adequate SMN, the signals from the neurons to the muscles instructing them to contract are ineffective, so the muscles lose function and over time atrophy results. The proximal muscles, those closer to the body's centre, are usually more affected than the distal muscles. The heart, emotional, and mental development, as well as sensation are unaffected by the disease (Sarant, 2011c).

There are several types of SMA, including type 1 (Werdnig–Hoffmann disease, infantile SMA), type 2 (intermediate), and type 3 (Kugelberg-Welander disease or juvenile SMA). Their usual progression and prognosis are compared in Table 44.4.

Respiratory muscle weakness may occur with all types of SMA and is usually the cause of death in type 1 SMA. Upper respiratory tract infections and aspiration related to dysphagia or gastroesophageal reflux often develop into pneumonia and eventual respiratory failure, as the affected child cannot effectively cough independently in order to clear the airway. Many children with severe type 1 SMA are ventilator dependent. Pectus excavatum develops in children with type 1 and type 2 SMA who exhibit paradoxical breathing (use of the diaphragm without intercostal muscle support). The chest becomes funnel shaped and the xiphoid process is retracted (pectus excavatum), further restricting respiratory development. Inability to appropriately suck and swallow leads to difficulty feeding in the child with type 1 SMA. Weak back muscles affect the developing spine, resulting in the complication of scoliosis, kyphosis, or both.

Therapeutic management of SMA is supportive, aimed at promoting mobility, maintaining adequate nutrition and pulmonary function, and preventing complications. Spinal fusion may be performed in older children with significant scoliosis. Since the discovery of the disease-causing gene for SMA, further research and improved diagnostic techniques have occurred. The

TABLE 44.4	FEATURES OF SPINAL MUSCULAR ATROPHY		
Features	Type 1 SMA (Werdnig–Hoffman Disease, Infantile SMA)	Type 2 SMA (Intermediate SMA)	Type 3 SMA (Kugelberg-Welander Disease or Juvenile SMA)
Onset	Before birth to 6 months of age	6–18 months of age	After 18 months of age; child has started walking or has taken at least five independent steps
Symptoms	• Generalized weakness; cannot sit without support • Weak cry • Difficulty sucking, swallowing, and breathing	• Proximal muscles are more affected; that is, thighs are weaker than lower legs; legs tend to be weaker than arms • Respiratory muscles may be involved • Scoliosis may occur	• Weakness that is most severe in the shoulders, hips, thighs, and upper back • Respiratory muscles may be involved • Scoliosis may occur
Progression	Rapidly progresses to early childhood death. Use of ventilators and gastrostomy feeding tubes may prolong life expectancy but typically death occurring by age 2	Slower progression. Life expectancy related to age of onset (the younger the onset, the more severe the disease and the shorter the life expectancy). Survival into adulthood common if respiratory status maintained appropriately	Slow progression. Life span usually unaffected. Walking ability maintained until at least adolescence; may need wheelchair later in life

Adapted from Muscular Dystrophy Association. (2009). *Facts about spinal muscular atrophy (SMA)*. Retrieved from http://www.mda.org/publications/PDFs/FA-SMA.pdf; National Institute of Neurological Disorders and Stroke. (2015b). *NINDS spinal muscular atrophy information page*. Retrieved from http://www.ninds.nih.gov/disorders/sma/sma.htm

in infants, children, and adolescents (Misra, 2015). Rickets may also occur if the body cannot regulate calcium and phosphorus in the appropriate balance, such as in chronic renal disease. Gastrointestinal disorders in which fat absorption is altered (e.g., Crohn disease, celiac disease, and cystic fibrosis) may lead to rickets, as vitamin D is a fat-soluble vitamin.

Calcium is primarily laid down in the bones of the fetus during the third trimester. Premature infants miss this period of calcium accumulation and also suffer from inadequate calcium intake in the neonatal period. Thus, premature infants often demonstrate rickets of prematurity. Regardless of the underlying cause, rickets is most likely to occur during periods of rapid growth.

Vitamin D regulates calcium absorption from the small intestine and levels of calcium and phosphate in the bones. When calcium and phosphate levels in the blood are imbalanced, then calcium is released from the bones into the blood, resulting in loss of the supportive bony matrix.

Therapeutic Management

Treatment of rickets is aimed at correcting the calcium imbalance so that the skeleton may develop properly and without deformity. Calcium and phosphorus supplements are given, and some children also require vitamin D supplements. If rickets is not corrected while the child is still growing, permanent skeletal deformities and short stature may result.

> **Take Note!**
> Health Canada's daily recommendation for vitamin D are 400 IU for infants, while for infants living in the north, levels of supplementation can range between 400 and 800 IU/day (CPS, 2017).

Nursing Assessment

Obtain a health history, determining risk factors such as:
- Limited exposure to sunlight
- Strict vegetarian diet or lactose intolerance (either one without milk product ingestion)
- Exclusive breastfeeding by a mother who has a vitamin D deficiency
- Dark-pigmented skin
- Prematurity
- Malabsorptive gastrointestinal disorder
- Chronic renal disease

Note history of fractures or bone pain. Observe for dental deformities and bowlegs. Decreased muscle tone may also be present. Note low serum calcium and phosphate levels and high alkaline phosphatase levels. X-rays may show changes in the shape and structure of the bone.

Nursing Management

Administer calcium and phosphorus supplements at alternate times to promote proper absorption of both of these supplements. Encourage exposure to moderate amounts of sunlight and administer vitamin D supplements as prescribed. Teach families that good dietary sources of vitamin D are fish, liver, and processed milk.

Slipped Capital Femoral Epiphysis (SCFE)

SCFE is a condition in which the femoral head dislocates from the neck and shaft of the femur at the level of the epiphyseal plate. The epiphysis slips downward and backward. The left hip is more often affected (Haut, 2014). The exact cause is unknown, but it is thought that during the teenage growth spurt, the femoral growth plate weakens and becomes less resistant to stressors. Hormonal alterations during this period may also play a role.

SCFE is classified based on its severity and whether the slip is acute or chronic. Chronic SCFE may lead to shortening of the affected leg and thigh atrophy.

Therapeutic Management

Promptly refer the child with SCFE to an orthopedic surgeon, as early surgical intervention will decrease the risk of long-term deformity. The goals of therapeutic management are to prevent further slippage, minimize deformity, and avoid the complications of cartilage necrosis (chondrolysis) and avascular necrosis of the femoral head. Surgical intervention may include in situ pinning, in which a pin or screw is inserted percutaneously into the femoral head to hold it in place. Osteotomy may be used for more severe cases. Osteoarthritis may be a long-term complication of SCFE.

Nursing Assessment

Elicit a health history, determining the onset and extent of pain. In acute SCFE, the pain is usually sudden in onset and results in inability to bear weight. Chronic SCFE may present with an insidious onset of pain and limp. Note risk factors for SCFE, including ages 9 to 16 years, African-American or Polynesian race, sedentary lifestyle, rapid growth spurt, and being overweight or obese (Haut, 2014; Sankar et al., 2011). Observe ambulation, noting Trendelenburg gait. Assess for pain that is in the hip or that is referred to the groin, medial thigh, or knee. Note decreased range of motion in the affected hip with external rotation. X-rays will be obtained to confirm the diagnosis (anteroposterior and lateral frog-leg views of hips). Bone scan can rule out avascular necrosis, and CT scan helps define the extent of slippage.

> ### Take Note!
> Do not attempt to perform passive range of motion to determine the extent of limitation in the child with SCFE; this may cause worsening of the condition.

Nursing Management

Enforce bed rest and activity restriction (i.e., non-weightbearing). If surgery is performed, provide routine preoperative and postoperative care. Assess pain and administer analgesics as needed. After in situ pinning, assist the child with crutch walking. Teach the family that weightbearing can be resumed according to local protocol (range 1 to 6 weeks depending on severity and activities). Prolonged immobility may isolate the adolescent from usual peer interactions, so encourage phone calls and visits with friends. Provide books, games, electronic devices, and magazines for distraction during the period of immobility. Provide education and support to the child and family.

Legg–Calvé–Perthes Disease

Legg–Calvé–Perthes disease is a self-limiting condition that involves avascular necrosis of the femoral head. It most often affects children between 4 and 8 years of age, but it can occur as early as 18 months and up until skeletal maturity (Haut, 2014; Sankar et al., 2011). The disease affects males more often (Haut, 2014). The etiology is unknown, but interruption of the blood supply to the femoral head results in bone death, and the spherical shape of the femoral head may be lost. Swelling of the soft tissues around the hip may occur. As new blood vessels develop, the area is supplied with circulation, allowing bone resorption and deposition to take place. During this period of revascularization, which takes 18 to 24 months, the bone is soft and more likely to fracture. Over time, the femoral head reforms.

Therapeutic Management

The goal of therapeutic management is to maintain normal femoral head shape and to restore appropriate motion. Treatment of Legg–Calvé–Perthes disease includes anti-inflammatory medication to decrease muscle spasms around the hip joint and to relieve pain. Activity limitation may be prescribed, and sometimes bracing, casting, or traction is recommended to contain the femoral head. Serial x-ray follow-up determines progress of the disease. If surgery becomes warranted, which is rarely done, then osteotomy may be performed. Complications include joint deformity, early degenerative joint disease, persistent pain, loss of hip motion or function, and gait disturbance.

Nursing Assessment

Explore the health history for short stature, delayed bone maturation, related trauma, or a family history of Legg–Calvé–Perthes disease. Note painless limp, which may be intermittent over a period of months. Mild hip pain may result and may be referred to the knee or the thigh. Pain may be aggravated by exercise. Observe the child walking and note Trendelenburg gait. Perform range of motion, noting internal rotation of the hip and limited abduction. Muscle spasm may result with hip extension and rotation. Hip x-rays are obtained to evaluate the extent of epiphyseal involvement. MRI or bone scan may also be used to differentiate Legg–Calvé–Perthes disease from other disorders. Ultrasound and arthrograms may also be useful.

Nursing Management

Nursing care of Legg–Calvé–Perthes disease is highly variable and depends on the stage of the disease and its severity. Administer anti-inflammatory medications, noting their effect on pain. If activities are restricted, exercise the unaffected body parts. Assist families with use of the brace if prescribed. The brace may be wiped with a damp cloth if it becomes dirty. Some children will be prescribed no treatment other than avoidance of contact or high-impact sports. Swimming and bicycle riding help to maintain range of motion with little risk. If mobility equipment is needed, educate the child and family on its use. If osteotomy is performed, provide routine postoperative care, including education and support of the child and family.

Transient Synovitis of the Hip

Transient synovitis of the hip (also termed toxic synovitis) is a common cause of acute hip pain and limping in children (Goldman, 2013). It typically occurs in children (greater number of boys) between 3 and 8 years old (Nigrovic, 2017). The exact cause is unclear, but it is thought to be associated with recent or active infection, trauma, or allergic hypersensitivity (Nigrovic, 2017). It is a self-limiting disease and most cases resolve within a week, but it may last as long as 4 weeks. Usually, septic arthritis and osteomyelitis must be excluded before diagnosis can be confirmed.

Therapeutic management involves nonsteroidal anti-inflammatory medications, analgesics, and bed rest to relieve weight bearing on the affected hip joint.

Nursing Assessment

Explore the health history for risk factors such as antecedent trauma, concurrent or recent upper respiratory tract infection, pharyngitis, or otitis media. Note sudden acute onset of moderate to severe pain of one hip. Sometimes, pain is referred to the anterior thigh or knee. Pain is usually the worst upon arising in the morning, and the child refuses to walk; pain then decreases throughout the day. Temperature usually will be normal or low grade (less than 38°C). Observe for a limp or for refusal to bear weight. Observe position of the affected hip: it will be held in a flexed and externally rotated position. Note restricted range of motion for abduction and internal rotation.

Nursing Management

Nursing care focuses on educating the family, including instructions on administering nonsteroidal anti-inflammatory medications, analgesics, and bed rest. Parents are very concerned when their child refuses to walk; therefore, provide significant support and reassure the child and family of the self-limiting nature of the disease.

Scoliosis

Scoliosis is a lateral curvature of the spine that exceeds 10 degrees. It may be congenital, associated with other disorders, or idiopathic. Table 44.6 explains the types of scoliosis. Idiopathic scoliosis, with the majority of cases occurring during adolescence, is the most common scoliosis (Spiegel & Dormans, 2011b). Hence, this discussion will focus on adolescent idiopathic scoliosis. The etiology of idiopathic scoliosis is not known, but genetic factors, growth abnormalities, and bone, muscle, disc, or central nervous system disorders may contribute to its development. Routine screening varies globally and is not currently recommended by the CPS (Labelle et al., 2013).

TABLE 44.6	TYPES OF SCOLIOSIS
Type	**Associated Factors**
Idiopathic	Unknown cause Infantile: occurs in the first 3 years of life Juvenile: diagnosed between age 4 and 10 years, or prior to adolescence Adolescent: age 11–17 years
Neuromuscular	Associated with neurologic or muscular disease such as cerebral palsy, myelomeningocele, spinal cord tumours, spinal muscular atrophy, muscular dystrophies
Congenital	Results from anomalous vertebral development

Pathophysiology

In the rapidly growing adolescent, the involved vertebrae rotate around a vertical axis, resulting in lateral curvature. The vertebrae rotate to the convex side of the curve, with the spinous processes rotating toward the concave side. Wedge-shaped vertebral bodies and discs develop because growth is suppressed on the concave side of the curve (Haut, 2014). Predicting whether a curve will progress into a more serious condition that will require treatment or surgery can be difficult in children. As the curve progresses, the shape of the thoracic cage changes and respiratory and cardiovascular compromise may occur (the main complications of severe scoliosis).

Therapeutic Management

Treatment of scoliosis is aimed at preventing progression of the curve and decreasing the impact on pulmonary and cardiac function. Treatment is based on the age of the child, expected future growth, and severity of the curve. Observation with serial examinations and spine x-rays is used to monitor curve progression. A curve of less than 10 degrees is considered a postural variation while curves of 20 degree that are non-progressive are considered mild. For curves of 25 to 40 degrees, bracing may be sufficient to decrease progression of the curve (Haut, 2014). Box 44.3 describes the types of scoliosis braces and Figure 44.28 shows examples of braces. The choice of brace will depend on the location and severity of the curve. Some curves will progress despite appropriate bracing and compliance.

Surgical correction is often required for curves greater than 45 to 50 degrees; it is achieved with rod placement and bone grafting (Spiegel & Dormans, 2011b). Partial spinal fusion accompanies many of the corrective surgeries. Multiple surgical approaches and techniques with various instrumentation methods exist for fusion and rod placement. The surgical approach may be anterior, posterior, or both. Traditional rod placement (Harrington rod) involves a single rod fused to the vertebrae, resulting in curve correction but also

---

BOX 44.3

TYPES OF BRACES USED TO TREAT SCOLIOSIS

- Underarm (thoracolumbosacral orthosis [TLSO], Boston, Wilmington): for low thoracic and thoracolumbar curves; less conspicuous, no visible neckpiece
- Milwaukee: for thoracic or major double curves; traditional, standard, has a visible neckpiece with chin rest
- Nighttime bending (Charleston): creates a curve so severe that walking is not possible, so can be worn only at night

FIGURE 44.28 **A.** Boston brace. **B.** Milwaukee brace. **C.** Nighttime bending brace.

a flat-backed appearance. Newer rod instrumentations allow for scoliosis curve correction with maintenance of normal back curvature. The rods are shorter, and several are wired or grafted to the appropriate vertebrae to achieve correction.

Nursing Assessment

For a full description of the assessment phase of the nursing process, refer to the Assessment section of the Nursing Process Overview earlier in the chapter. Assessment findings pertinent to scoliosis are discussed below.

HEALTH HISTORY

Determine why the child is presenting for evaluation of scoliosis. Commonly the child or adolescent will not report back pain; only mild discomfort is associated with idiopathic scoliosis until the curve becomes severe. Often the family recognizes asymmetry in the hips or shoulders or the child is screened for scoliosis at school and determined to be at risk. Explore the child's current and past medical history for risk factors such as:
- Family history of scoliosis
- Recent growth spurt
- Physical changes related to puberty

Determine the age of development of secondary sex characteristics and the age of menarche, as these signs of pubertal development indicate the expected velocity and length of remaining growth.

PHYSICAL EXAMINATION

The physical assessment of a child with possible or actual scoliosis involves mainly inspection and observation.

Auscultate the heart and lungs to determine compromise related to severe curvature.

Observe the child at rest, sitting, and standing for evidence of poor posture. Inspect the child's back in a standing position. Note asymmetries such as shoulder elevation, prominence of one scapula, uneven curve at the waistline, rib positioning, and hip height. Asymmetry of the ribs and flank should be noted when the child bends as far forward as possible from the waist and hangs the arms downwards towards the feet (Adam's test). A scoliometer is often used to measure truncal rotation. Figure 44.29 shows scoliosis noted upon visual inspection. Note leg-length discrepancy if present. During the neurologic examination, balance, motor strength, sensation, and reflexes should all be normal.

LABORATORY AND DIAGNOSTIC TESTS

Full-spine x-rays are necessary to determine the degree of curvature. The radiologist will determine the extent of the curve based on specific formulas and techniques of measurement (e.g., the Risser scale).

Nursing Management

Nursing Care Plan 44.1, at the end of the chapter, lists general interventions. Tailor nursing care based on the adolescent's response to the disease and its treatment. Additional nursing interventions specific to scoliosis are discussed here.

ENCOURAGING COMPLIANCE WITH BRACING

Bracing is intended to prevent progression of the curve but does not correct the current curve. Although modern treatment (Wells, Sehgal, & Dormans, 2011). Midclavicular, humerus, or femur fractures can occur as a result of birth trauma. They typically heal well but may require limiting mobility or splinting. In addition, feeding may be altered as a result of positioning and the infant's weight gain should be monitored.

Fractures in children result most frequently from accidental trauma (Haut, 2014). Non-accidental trauma (child abuse) and other disease processes are the other causes of fractures. In children younger than 2 years, most fractures that occur are the result of another person causing the injury (Haut, 2014).

> **Take Note!**
> Fracture in the newborn (with the exception of birth trauma) or infant should raise a high index of suspicion for abuse, as fractures are very unusual in children who are not mobile.

Pathophysiology

The growth plate is the most vulnerable portion of the child's bone and is frequently the site of injury. The Salter–Harris classification system is used to describe fractures involving the growth plate (Table 44.7). The thicker, more elastic periosteum in children yields to the force encountered with trauma, resulting more frequently in nondisplaced fractures in children. The increased vascularity and decreased mineral content make the child's bones more flexible. Plastic or bowing deformities and buckle and greenstick fractures are the result. Complete fractures do occur in children, but they tend to be more stable than in the adult, resulting in improved healing and function. Spiral, pelvic, and hip fractures are rare in children. Table 44.8 explains common types of fractures in children.

Fractures in children heal more rapidly and result in less disability and deformity than adults. The younger the child, the more quickly the bone heals. However, plastic deformity and Salter–Harris type IV fractures may result in an angular deformity. Though healing of fractures is usually quick and without incident in children, delayed union, nonunion, or malunion can occur. Additional complications include infection, avascular necrosis, bone shortening from epiphyseal arrest, vascular or nerve injuries, fat embolism, reflex sympathetic dystrophy, and compartment syndrome, which is an orthopedic emergency. Later in life, osteoarthritis may occur as a long-term complication from childhood fracture (Haut, 2014).

> **Take Note!**
> Any type of fracture can be the result of child abuse but spiral femur fractures, rib fractures, and humerus fractures, particularly in the child younger than 2 years of age, should always be thoroughly investigated to rule out the possibility of abuse (Wells et al., 2011).

Therapeutic Management

The vast majority of childhood fractures could heal well with splinting only, but casting of these fractures is performed to provide further comfort to the child and to allow for increased activity while the fracture is healing. Displaced fractures require manual traction to align the bones, followed by casting. More severe fractures may require traction for a period of time, usually followed by casting. Severe or complicated fractures may alternatively require open reduction and internal fixation for healing to occur.

> **Take Note!**
> Significant swelling may occur initially after immobilization with a splint. Delaying casting for a few days provides time for some of the swelling to subside, allowing for successful casting a few days after the injury.

Nursing Assessment

For a full description of the assessment phase of the nursing process, refer to the Assessment section of the Nursing Process Overview earlier in the chapter. Assessment findings pertinent to fractures are discussed below.

HEALTH HISTORY

Elicit a description of the presenting issue or illness. Common signs and symptoms reported during the health history might include recent injury, trauma, or fall; complaint of pain; difficulty bearing weight; limp; or refusal to use an extremity. Young children often demonstrate sudden onset of irritability and refusal to bear weight. Ask about the mechanism of injury and obtain a description of the traumatic event. Be alert to inconsistencies between the history and the clinical picture or mechanism of injury; inconsistency may be an indicator of child abuse. Explore the child's current and past medical history for risk factors such as:

- Rickets
- Renal osteodystrophy (can be noted in patients with renal disease and dialysis when kidneys fail to maintain adequate levels of calcium and phosphorous)
- Osteogenesis imperfecta
- Participation in sports, particularly contact sports
- Failure to use protective equipment as recommended for various physical activities and sports (e.g., wrist guards while rollerblading)

PHYSICAL EXAMINATION

Perform the physical examination of the child with a potential fracture carefully, so as not to cause further pain or trauma. The physical examination particular to fractures includes inspection, observation, and palpation.

> **Take Note!**
>
> Do not attempt to straighten or manipulate an injured limb.

TABLE 44.7	THE SALTER–HARRIS CLASSIFICATION SYSTEM	
Type	**Description**	**Illustration**
I	Fracture is through the physis, widening it	
II	Fracture is partially through the physis, extending into the metaphysis	
III	Fracture is partially through the epiphysis, extending into the epiphysis	

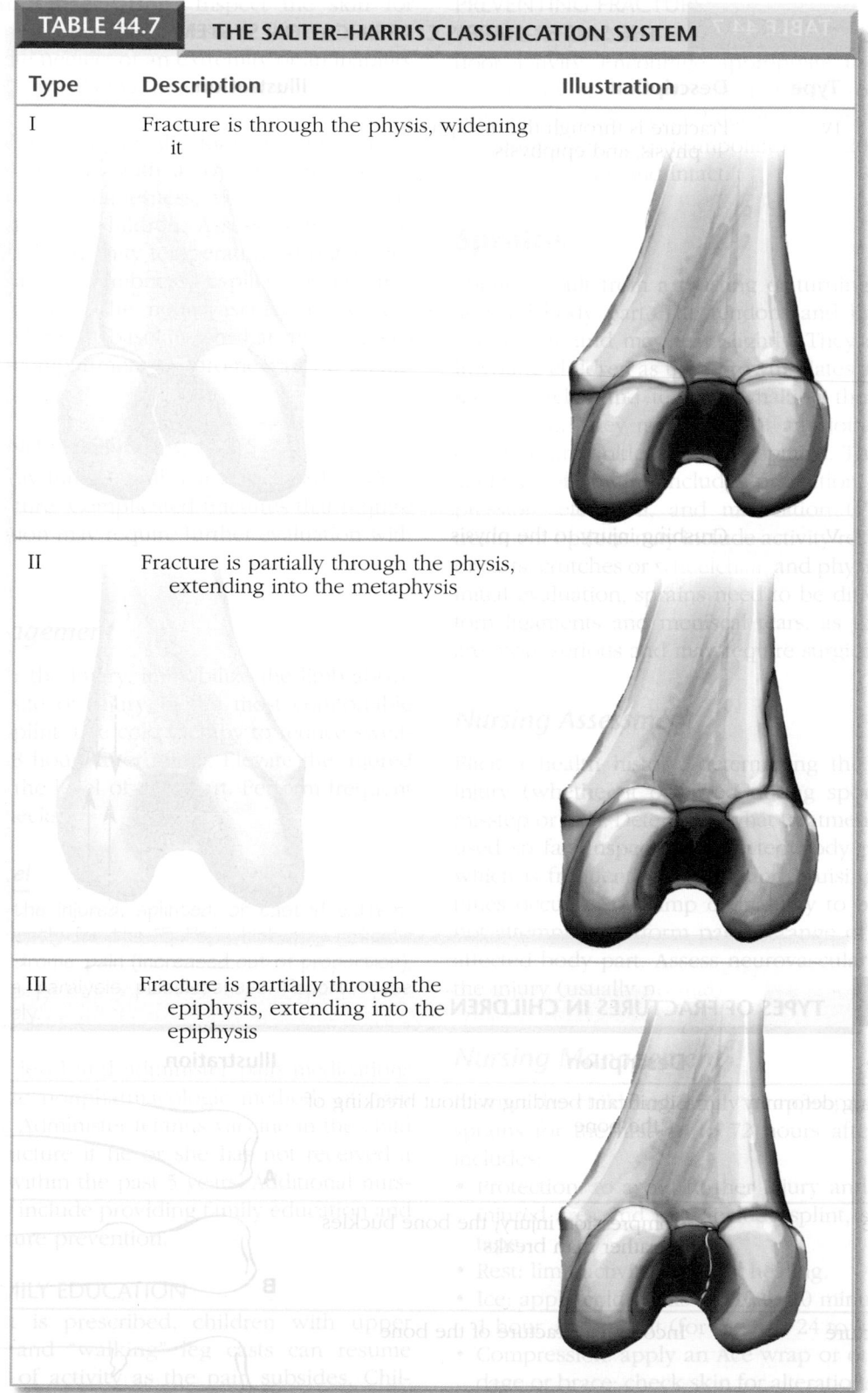

(continued)

NURSING CARE PLAN 44.1

Overview for the Child With a Neuromuscular or Musculoskeletal Disorder (continued)

- Repeat information to allow family and child time to learn and understand.
- Teach in short sessions: many short sessions are more helpful than one long session.
- Gear teaching to the level of understanding of the child and family (depends on age of child, physical condition, memory) to ensure understanding.

- Provide reinforcement and rewards to facilitate the teaching/learning process.
- Use multiple modes of learning involving many senses (provide written, verbal, demonstration, and videos) when possible: child and family are more likely to retain information when it is presented in different ways using many senses.

NURSING DIAGNOSIS: Family processes, interrupted, related to child's illness, hospitalization, and diagnosis of chronic illness in child, and potential long-term effects of illness as evidenced by family's presence in hospital, missed work, and demonstration of inadequate coping

Outcome Identification and Evaluation

Family will maintain functional system of support and demonstrate adequate coping and adaptation of roles: parents are involved in child's care, ask appropriate questions, express fears and concerns, and are able to discuss child's care and condition calmly.

Intervention: *Promoting Appropriate Family Functioning*

- Encourage parents and family to verbalize concerns related to child's illness, diagnosis, and prognosis: allows the nurse to identify concerns and areas where further education may be needed; demonstrates family-centred care.
- Explain therapies, procedures, child's behaviours, and plan of care to parents: understanding of the child's current status and plan of care helps decrease anxiety.

- Encourage parental involvement in care to allow parents to feel needed and valued and to have a sense of control over their child's health.
- Identify support system for family and child: support system is often needed by stressed families to assist with coping.
- Educate family and child on additional resources available to help them develop a wide base of support.

NURSING DIAGNOSIS: Risk for delayed development related to immobility, alterations in extremities

Outcome Identification and Evaluation

Development will be enhanced: child will make continued progress toward developmental milestones and will not show regression in abilities.

Intervention: *Promoting Development*

- Screen for developmental capabilities to determine child's current level of functioning.
- Offer age-appropriate toys, play, and activities (including gross motor) to encourage further development. Refer to a Child Life or Play Specialist.
- Perform exercises or interventions as prescribed by physical or occupational therapist: repeat participation in those activities helps to promote function and acquisition of developmental skills.
- Provide support to child and families: immobility and extremity deficits may lead to slow progress in achieving developmental milestones, so ongoing motivation is needed.

KEY CONCEPTS

- Muscles, tendons, ligaments, and cartilage are all present and functional at birth, though intentional, purposeful movement develops only as the infant matures.

- The spine is very mobile in the newborn and infant, especially the cervical spine region, resulting in a high risk for cervical spine injury.

- Rapid muscle growth in the adolescent years places the teenager at increased risk for injury compared with other age groups.

- The bones of the infant and young child are more flexible and have a thicker periosteum and more abundant blood supply than the adult's; as a result, bending occurs more frequently than breaking of the bone, and the fractured bone heals more quickly.

- The epiphysis of long bones is the growth centre of the bones in children. Injury to this area may result in long-term extremity deformity.

- The nurse's role in laboratory and diagnostic testing for neuromuscular or musculoskeletal disorders is mainly that of educating the child and family about and preparing the child for the test or procedure.

- Plain x-rays are usually sufficient for diagnosing injuries in children. If CT or MRI scans are required, the nurse may need to help the child stay calm and still during the procedure.

- Apply a pressure dressing following joint aspiration to prevent hematoma formation or fluid recollection.

- Perform frequent assessments of pain status and the effect of pain medication in the child with a musculoskeletal disorder.

- Diazepam (Valium) may be helpful in relieving muscle spasm associated with traction.

- Maintain traction and the appropriate amount of weight as ordered.

- The bulk of cast care occurs in the home. Teach the family of a child with a cast to perform neurovascular assessments, prevent the cast from getting wet, and care for the skin appropriately.

- Assessment of range of motion and muscle tone is critical in the child with a neuromuscular disorder. Hypertonia or hypotonia is an abnormal finding in the infant or child.

- Assessment of neurovascular status is an essential component of care for a child with a musculoskeletal disorder.

- Determining attainment of developmental milestones and subsequent progression or loss of those milestones is useful in distinguishing various neuromuscular disorders.

- The nurse reinforces and carries out the exercise plans and adaptive equipment use as prescribed by the physical or occupational therapist in order to maintain neuromuscular and musculoskeletal function and to prevent complications.

- Nursing management of a child with myelomeningocele focuses on preventing infection, promoting bowel and urinary elimination, promoting adequate nutrition, preventing latex allergy reaction, maintaining skin integrity, providing education and support to the family, and recognizing complications, such as hydrocephalus or increased ICP, associated with the disorder.

- Cerebral palsy may result in significant motor impairment. Children with cerebral palsy require ongoing physiotherapy, occupational therapy, and speech therapy, as well as nutritional intervention.

- Boys with Duchenne muscular dystrophy initially learn to walk but later lose this ability.

- Respiratory compromise occurs in muscular dystrophy and spinal muscular atrophy and eventually leads to death.

- Children with chronic disorders such as osteogenesis imperfecta may demonstrate slower or lesser growth than other children and may also be unable to participate in certain activities because of bone fragility.

- Congenital or developmental disorders such as DDH or clubfoot require bracing or casting for correction and to prevent deformity later in life.

- Torticollis may be treated by teaching the family to perform daily neck muscle stretching exercises.

- To prevent complications after a spinal fusion for scoliosis correction, use the log-roll method for turning the child so that back flexion is avoided.

- Children with spinal cord injury require intense nursing management and lengthy rehabilitation to maintain or regain function.

- Children with neuromuscular disorders often suffer depression related to the chronic nature of the disorder.

- School attendance and participation in activities such as the Special Olympics are important for children with neuromuscular dysfunction.

- Fractures may occur as a result of unintentional or intentional injury, or because the bones are fragile, as in rickets or osteogenesis imperfecta.

- Sprains, fractures, and overuse syndromes occur frequently in young athletes. Appropriate warm-up and stretching may help prevent some of these injuries.

- Rest, ice, compression, and elevation is the appropriate treatment for sprains.

REFERENCES AND RECOMMENDED READINGS

Aboutkidshealth. (n.d.). *Baclofen (Intrathecal)*. Retrieved from http://www.aboutkidshealth.ca/En/HealthAZ/Drugs/Pages/Baclofen-Intrathecal.aspx

Bazner-Chandler, J., & Brady, M. A. (2013). Musculoskeletal disorders. In C. E. Burns, A. M. Dunn, M. A. Brady, N. B. Starr, C. G. Blosser, & D. L. Garzon. (2012). *Pediatric primary care*. Philadelphia, PA. Elsevier Health Sciences.

BCCH. (n.d.). *Clubfoot program and clinic*. Retrieved from http://www.bcchildrens.ca/Orthopaedics-Site/Documents/clubfootclinic.pdf

Boas, S. R. (2011). Chapter 411: Skeletal diseases influencing pulmonary function. In R. M. Kleigman, B. F. Stanton, J. W. St. Geme III, N. F. Schor, & R. E. Behrman (Eds.). *Nelson textbook of pediatrics* (19th ed., pp. 1516–1519). Philadelphia, PA: Saunders.

Boutis, K., Plint, A., Stimec, J., Miller, E., Babyn, P., Schuh, S., … Narayanan, UG. (2016). Radiograph-negative lateral ankle injuries in children. Occult growth plate fracture or sprain. *JAMA Pediatrics, 170*(1), e154115.

Bowden, V. R., & Greenberg, C. S. (2012). *Pediatric nursing procedures* (3rd ed.). Philadelphia, PA: Lippincott Williams & Wilkins.

Brenner, J. S., & The Council on Sports Medicine and Fitness. (2014). Overuse injuries, overtraining, and burnout in child and adolescent athletes. *Pediatrics, 119*(6), 1242–1245.

Canadian Orthopaedic Foundation. (n.d.). *A parent's guide to clubfoot*. Retrieved from http://whenithurtstomove.org/wp-content/uploads/Clubfoot-Booklet_2015-EN.pdf

Canadian Paediatric Society (CPS). (2007). *Trampoline use in homes and playgrounds*. Retrieved from http://www.cps.ca/documents/position/trampoline-home-use

Canadian Paediatric Society (CPS). (2010). *Physical activity recommendations for children with specific chronic health conditions: Juvenile idiopathic arthritis, hemaophilia, asthma and cystic fibrosis*. Retrieved from http://www.cps.ca/documents/position/physical-activity-chronic-condition

Canadian Paediatric Society (CPS). (2012a). *Biologic response modifiers to decrease inflammation: Focus on infection risks*. Retrieved from http://www.cps.ca/documents/position/biologic-response-modifiers

Canadian Paediatric Society (CPS). (2012b). *Child and youth injury prevention: A public health approach*. Retrieved from http://www.cps.ca/documents/position/child-and-youth-injury-prevention

Canadian Paediatric Society (CPS). (2016a). Folate and neural tube defects: The role of supplements and food fortification. Retrieved from http://www.cps.ca/en/documents/position/folate

Canadian Paediatric Society (CPS). (2016b). *Mental health problems in children with neuromotor disabilities*. Retrieved from http://www.cps.ca/en/documents/position/mental-health-problems-neuromotor-disabilities

Canadian Paediatric Society (CPS). (2017). *Vitamin D supplementation: Recommendations for Canadian mothers and infants*. Retrieved from http://www.cps.ca/documents/position/vitamin-d

Carrigan, R. B. (2011). Chapter 673: The upper limb. In R. M. Kleigman, B. F. Stanton, J. W. St. Geme III, N. F. Schor, & R. E. Behrman (Eds.). *Nelson textbook of pediatrics* (19th ed., pp. 2383–2387). Philadelphia, PA: Saunders.

Carroll, K. L., & Kerr, L. M. (2013). Chapter 45: Alterations in musculoskeletal function in children. In K. L. McCance & S. E. Huether (Eds.). *Pathophysiology: The biologic basis for disease in adults and children* (7th ed., pp. 1591–1615). St Louis, MO: Elsevier/Mosby.

Cellucci, T., Guzman, J., Petty, R. E., Batthish, M., Benseler, S. M., Ellsworth, J. E., … & Schmeling, H. (2016). Management of Juvenile Idiopathic Arthritis 2015: a position statement from the pediatric Committee of the Canadian Rheumatology Association. Retrieved from http://www.jrheum.org/content/43/10/1773.short

Centers for Disease Control and Prevention. (2014). *Facts about upper and lower limb reduction defects*. Retrieved from http://www.cdc.gov/ncbddd/birthdefects/UL-LimbReductionDefects.html

Cervasio, K. (2011). Lower extremity orthoses in children with spastic quadriplegic cerebral palsy: Implications for nurses, parents, and caregivers. *Orthopaedic Nursing, 30*(3), 155–159.

Cincinnati's Children's. (2013). *Cast care*. Retrieved from http://www.cincinnatichildrens.org/health/c/cast-care/

Danzer, E., Thomas, N. H., Thomas, A., Friedman, K. B., Gerdes, M., Koh, J., … Johnson, M. P. (2016). Long-term neurofunctional outcome, executive functioning, and behavioral adaptive skills following fetal myelomeningocele surgery. *American Journal of Obstetrics and Gynecology, 214*(2), 269.e1–269.e8.

Espositio, G., & Venuti, P. (2009). Symmetry in infancy: Analysis of motor development in autism spectrum disorders. *Symmetry,1*, 215–225.

Fairhurst, C. B., & Cockerill, H. (2011). Management of drooling in children. *Archives of Diseases in Childhood Education & Practice, 96*(1), 25–30.

Fischbach, F. T., & Dunning, M. B. III. (2015). *A manual of laboratory and diagnostic tests* (9th ed.). Philadelphia, PA: Wolters Kluwer Health/Lippincott Williams & Wilkins.

Golman, R. (2013). Acute limping child. Retrieved from http://thischangedmypractice.com/acute-limping-in-children/

Grossman, S. (2014). Chapter 58: Disorders of musculoskeletal function: Developmental and metabolic disorders. In S. Grossman, & C. M. Porth (Eds.). *Porth's pathophysiology: Concepts of altered health states* (9th ed., pp. 489–574). Philadelphia, PA: Wolters Kluwer Health/Lippincott Williams & Wilkins.

Hamdy, R. C. (2016). Evolution in long bone deformity correction in the post-Ilizarov era: External to internal devices.

Journal of Limb Lengthening and Reconstruction [Serial Online], *2*, 61–67. Retrieved from http://www.jlimblengthre-con.org/text.asp?2016/2/2/61/190703

Haut, C. M. (2014). Chapter 54: Pediatric orthopedic disorders. In S. M. Nettina (Ed.). *Lippincott manual of nursing practice* (10th ed., pp. 1743–1769). Philadelphia, PA: Wolters Kluwer Health/Lippincott Williams & Wilkins.

Health Charities Coalition of Canada. (2016). The How to Health Guide 2016 Ed. Retrieved from http://www.muscle.ca/living-with-muscular-dystrophy/how-to-health-guide/

Hosalkar, H. S., Spiegel, D. A., & Davidson, R. S. (2011). Chapter 666: The foot and toes. In R. M. Kleigman, B. F. Stanton, J. W. St. Geme III, N. F. Schor, & R. E. Behrman (Eds.). *Nelson textbook of pediatrics* (19th ed., pp. 2335–2344). Philadelphia, PA: Saunders.

Kane, K. J., Lanovaz, J., Bisaro, D., Oates, A., & Musselman, K. E. (2016). Preliminary study of novel, timed walking tests for children with spina bifida or cerebral palsy. *SAGE Open Medicine*, *4*, 2050312116658908.

Kiddoo, D., Sawatzky, B., Bascu, C. D., Dharamsi, N., Afshar, K., & Moore, K. N. (2015). Randomized crossover trial of single use hydrophilic coated vs multiple use polyvinylchloride catheters for intermittent catheterization to determine incidence of urinary infection. *The Journal of Urology*, *194*(1), 174–179.

Kienstra, A. J., & Macias, C. G. (2014). Osgood-Schlatter disease (tibial tuberosity avulsion). UpToDate. Retrieved from http://www.uptodate.com/contents/osgood-schlatter-disease-tibial-tuberosity-avulsion

Kinsman, S. L., & Johnston, M. V. (2011). Chapter 585: Congenital anomalies of the central nervous system. In R. M. Kleigman, B. F. Stanton, J. W. St. Geme III, N. F. Schor, & R. E. Behrman (Eds.). *Nelson textbook of pediatrics* (19th ed., pp. 1998–2013). Philadelphia, PA: Saunders.

Labelle, H., Richards, S. B., De Kleuver, M., Grivas, T. B., Luk, K. D. K., Wong, H. K., ... Fong D. Y. T. (2013). Screening for adolescent idiopathic scoliosis: An information statement by the Scoliosis Research Society International Task Force. *Scoliosis*, *8*, 17. Retrieved fromhttps://scoliosisjournal.biomedcentral.com/articles/10.1186/1748-7161-8-17

Law, M., Hanna, S., Anaby, D., Kertoy, M., King, G., & Xu, L. (2014). Health-related quality of life of children with physical disabilities: A longitudinal study. *BMC Pediatrics*, *14*(1), 26.

Lethaby, A., Temple, J., & Santy-Tomlinson, J. (2013). Pin site care for preventing infections associated with external bone fixators and pins. *Cochrane Database of Systematic Reviews*, *12*, CD004551. Retrieved from http://onlinelibrary.wiley.com/doi/10.1002/14651858.CD004551.pub3/epdf

Marini, J. C. (2011). Chapter 692: Osteogenesis imperfecta. In R. M. Kleigman, B. F. Stanton, J. W. St. Geme III, N. F. Schor, & R. E. Behrman (Eds.). *Nelson textbook of pediatrics* (19th ed., pp. 2437–2440). Philadelphia, PA: Saunders.

McPherson, A. C., Leo, J., Church, P., Lyons, J., Chen, L., & Swift, J. (2014). An environmental scan of weight assessment and management practices in paediatric spina bifida clinics across Canada. *Journal of Pediatric Rehabilitation Medicine*, *7*(3), 207–217.

Miller, G. (2015). Management and prognosis of cerebral palsy. UpToDate. Retrieved from http://www.uptodate.com/contents/management-and-prognosis-of-cerebral-palsy

Misra, M. (2015). Vitamin D insufficiency and deficiency in children and adolescents. UpToDate. Retrieved from http://www.uptodate.com/contents/vitamin-d-insufficiency-and-deficiency-in-children-and-adolescents

Muscular Dystrophy Association. (2009). *Facts about spinal muscular atrophy (SMA)*. Retrieved from http://www.mda.org/publications/PDFs/FA-SMA.pdf

Muscular Dystrophy Association. (2011). *Facts about Duchenne and Becker muscular dystrophies*. Retrieved from http://www.mda.org/publications/PDFs/FA-DMD.pdf

National Institute of Neurological Disorders and Stroke. (2015a). *Spina bifida fact sheet*. Retrieved from http://www.ninds.nih.gov/disorders/spina_bifida/detail_spina_bifida.htm

National Institute of Neurological Disorders and Stroke. (2015b). *NINDS spinal muscular atrophy information page*. Retrieved from http://www.ninds.nih.gov/disorders/sma/sma.htm

Nigrovic, P. A. (2017). *Overview of hip pain in childhood*. UpToDate. Retrieved from http://www.uptodate.com/contents/overview-of-hip-pain-in-childhood

Noonan, V. K., Fingas, M., Farry, A., Baxter, D., Singh, A., Fehlings, M. G., & Dvorak, M. F. (2012). Incidence and prevalence of spinal cord injury in Canada: a national perspective. *Neuroepidemiology*, *38*(4), 219–226.

Oskoui, M., Joseph, L., Dagenais, L., & Shevell, M. (2013). Prevalence of cerebral palsy in Quebec: Alternative approaches. *Neuroepidemiology*, *40*, 264–268.

Osteogenesis Imperfecta Foundation. (2015). *Types of OI*. Retrieved from http://www.oif.org/site/PageServer?pagename=AOI_Types

Passamano, L., Taglia, A., Palladino, A., Viggiano, E., D'Ambrosio, P., Scutifero, M., ... Politano, L. (2012). Improvement of survival in Duchenne muscular dystrophy: Retrospective analysis of 835 patients. *Acta Myologica*, *31*(2), 121–125.

Pollet, V., Percy, V., & Prior, H. J. (2017). Relative risk and incidence for developmental dysplasia of the hip. *The Journal of Pediatrics*, *181*, 202–207.

Public Health Agency Canada. (n.d.). *Leading causes of death and hospitalization in Canada*. Retrieved from http://www.phac-aspc.gc.ca/publicat/lcd-pcd97/index-eng.php

Public Health Agency Canada. (2011). *Mapping Connections: An understanding of neurological conditions in Canada*. Retrieved from http://www.phac-aspc.gc.ca/publicat/cd-mc/mc-ec/section-3-eng.php#t3-1-ft5

Sankar, W. N., Horn, B. D., Wells, L., & Dormans, J. P. (2011). Chapter 670: The hip. In R. M. Kleigman, B. F. Stanton, J. W. St. Geme III, N. F. Schor, & R. E. Behrman (Eds.). *Nelson textbook of pediatrics* (19th ed., pp. 2355–2365). Philadelphia, PA: Saunders.

Sarant, H. B. (2011a). Chapter 599. Neuromuscular disorders. In R. M. Kleigman, B. F. Stanton, J. W. St. Geme III, N. F. Schor, & R. E. Behrman (Eds.). *Nelson textbook of pediatrics* (19th ed., pp. 2109–2122). Philadelphia, PA: Saunders.

Sarant, H. B. (2011b). Chapter 601: Muscular dystrophies. In R. M. Kleigman, B. F. Stanton, J. W. St. Geme III, N. F. Schor, & R. E. Behrman (Eds.), *Nelson textbook of pediatrics* (19th ed., pp. 2119–2129). Philadelphia, PA: Saunders.

Sarant, H. B. (2011c). Chapter 604: Disorders of neuromuscular transmission and of motor neuron. In R. M. Kleigman, B. F. Stanton, J. W. St. Geme III, N. F. Schor, & R. E. Behrman (Eds.). *Nelson textbook of pediatrics* (19th ed., pp. 2132–2138). Philadelphia, PA: Saunders.

Schweich, P. (2014). Patient information: Cast and splint care (Beyond the basics). UpToDate. Retrieved from http://www.uptodate.com/contents/cast-and-splint-care-beyond-the-basics

Spiegel, D. A., & Dormans, J. P. (2011a). Chapter 672.1 Torticollis. In R. M. Kleigman, B. F. Stanton, J. W. St. Geme III, N. F. Schor, & R. E. Behrman (Eds.). *Nelson textbook of pediatrics* (19th ed., pp. 2377–2379). Philadelphia, PA: Saunders.

Spiegel, D. A., & Dormans, J. P. (2011b). Chapter 671: The spine. In R. M. Kleigman, B. F. Stanton, J. W. St. Geme III, N. F. Schor, & R. E. Behrman (Eds.). *Nelson textbook of pediatrics* (19th ed., pp. 2365–2377). Philadelphia, PA: Saunders.

Spina Bifida Association. (2015). *Latex in the hospital environment.* Retrieved from http://spinabifidaassociation.org/infosheets/latex-hospital/

Spina Bifida & Hydrochephalus Association of Canada. (2019). *Information and Library.* Retrieved from http://sbhac.ca/information/

Statistics Canada. (n.d.). *Health at a glance. Injuries in Canada: Insight from Canadian Community Health Survey.* Retrieved from http://www.statcan.gc.ca/pub/82-624-x/2011001/article/11506-eng.htm

Taketokmo, C. K., Hodding, J. H., & Kraus, D. M. (2013). *Lexi-comp's drug reference handbook: Pediatric & neonatal dosage handbook* (20th ed.). Hudson, OH: Lexi-comp, Inc.

Timms, A., Vincent, M., Santy-Tomlinson, J., & Hertz, K. (2011). *Guidance on Pin Site Care. A Report and Recommendations From the 2010 Consensus Project on Pin Site Care.* London: Royal College of Nursing.

Wajchendler, A., Anderson, P., & Koyle, M. A. (2017). The transition process of spina bifida patients to adult-centred care: An assessment of the Canadian urology landscape. *Canadian Urological Association Journal, 11*(1–2 Suppl 1), S88.

Wang, C. H., Finkel, R. S., Bertini, E. S., Schroth, M., Simonds, A., Wong, B., … Trela, A. (2007). Consensus statement for standard of care in spinal muscular atrophy. *Journal of Child Neurology, 22*(8), 1027–1049.

Wells, L., & Sehgal, K. (2011). Chapter 667.4: Coronal plane deformities. In R. M. Kleigman, B. F. Stanton, J. W. St. Geme III, N. F. Schor, & R. E. Behrman (Eds.). *Nelson textbook of pediatrics* (19th ed., pp. 2348–2351). Philadelphia, PA: Saunders.

Wells, L., Sehgal, K., & Dormans, J. P. (2011). Chapter 675: Common fractures. In R. M. Kleigman, R. E. Behrman, H. B. Jenson, & B. F. Stanton (Eds.). *Nelson's textbook of pediatrics* (19th ed., pp. 2387–2394). Philadelphia, PA: Saunders.

Yoshihara, H., & Yoneoka, D. (2014). National trends in spinal fusion for pediatric patients with idiopathic scoliosis: Demographics, blood transfusions, and in-hospital outcomes. *Spine, 39*(14), 1144–1150.

Zak, M., & Chan, V. W. (2014). Chapter 46: Pediatric neurologic disorders. In S. M. Nettina (Ed.). *Lippincott manual of nursing practice* (10th ed., pp. 1545–1575). Philadelphia, PA: Wolters/Kluwer Health: Lippincott Williams & Wilkins.

CHAPTER **WORKSHEET**

MULTIPLE CHOICE QUESTIONS

1. A boy with Duchenne muscular dystrophy is admitted to the pediatric unit. He has an ineffective cough. Lung auscultation reveals diminished breath sounds. What is the priority nursing intervention?
   a. Apply supplemental oxygen.
   b. Notify the respiratory therapist.
   c. Monitor pulse oximetry.
   d. Position for adequate airway clearance.

2. A 7-year-old child with cerebral palsy has been admitted to the hospital. Which information is most important for the nurse to obtain in the history?
   a. Age that the child learned to walk
   b. Parents' expectations of the child's development
   c. Functional status related to eating and mobility
   d. Birth history to identify cause of cerebral palsy

3. The nurse is caring for a 2-year-old with myelomeningocele. When teaching about care related to neurogenic bladder, what response by the parent would indicate that additional teaching is required?
   a. "Routine catheterization will decrease the risk of infection from urine staying in the bladder."
   b. "I know it will be important for me to catheterize my child for the rest of her life."
   c. "I will make sure that I always use latex-free catheters."
   d. "I will wash the catheter with warm soapy water after each use."

4. The nurse is caring for a child with cerebral palsy who requires a wheelchair to attain mobility. Which intervention would help the child achieve a sense of normality?
   a. Encourage follow-through with physical therapy exercises.
   b. Restrict the child to a special needs classroom.
   c. Encourage after-school activities within the limits of the child's abilities.
   d. Ensure the school is aware of the child's capabilities.

5. The nurse is caring for orthopedic children who are in the postoperative period following spinal fusion. What is the most appropriate activity to delegate to unlicensed assistive personnel?
   a. Ambulate the children twice daily to promote mobility.
   b. Encourage commode use to promote bowel function.
   c. Provide diversionary activities, as the children must stay flat on their backs.
   d. Assist with log-rolling the children every 2 hours.

DOSAGE CALCULATION EXERCISE

The nurse is caring for a child who is experiencing painful spasms. The child is 6 years old and weighs 42 lb. The medication order reads: Baclofen 25 mg per GT every 8 hours. Baclofen is supplied as 5 mg/mL.

How many millilitres will the nurse administer? Round to the nearest tenth.

CRITICAL THINKING EXERCISES

1. A 5-year-old girl, diagnosed with myelomeningocele, is admitted to the hospital for a corrective surgical procedure. Choose four questions from below that the nurse should ask when obtaining the health history that would assist in planning the child's care.
   a. What is the child's current mobility status?
   b. Is there a family history of myelomeningocele?
   c. What is the child's genitourinary and bowel function and regimen?
   d. Does this child have a history of hydrocephalus with presence of shunt?
   e. Does she have known latex sensitivity?
   f. Were there any complications during the pregnancy or birth of this child?
   g. Did the mother take prenatal folic acid supplementation?

2. Based on the case in the above question, develop a nursing care plan for the child with myelomeningocele.

3. A 5-year-old child is admitted to the pediatric unit with a history of cerebral palsy sustained at birth. The child is admitted for a scheduled tendon lengthening procedure. Based on your knowledge about the effects of cerebral palsy, list three priorities to focus on when planning her care. Compare this to a child admitted for surgical correction of a broken femur with no significant past medical history.

4. Develop a discharge teaching plan for a 2-year old who will be in a hip spica cast for 10 more weeks at home.

5. Devise a developmental/education plan for a child who will be confined to traction for 6 weeks. Choose a child in the clinical area whom you have cared for or choose a particular age group and develop the plan.

1733

Tissue integrity refers to the body's ability to maintain epidermal and dermal integrity to promote normal tissue's physiologic processes (Moorhead, Johnson, Maas, & Swanson, 2013). Alterations in tissue integrity or integumentary disorders occur often in children and are caused by exposure to infectious microorganisms, hypersensitivity reactions, hormonal influences, and injuries. Some integumentary disorders are mild and self-limited, such as a minor abrasion. Others, such as atopic dermatitis (AD), are chronic and must be managed consistently. Finally, some tissue integrity alterations can be severe and even life-threatening, such as full-thickness burns. If the integumentary disorders are chronic or severe, they can have a major impact on the child's physiologic or psychological status, and on the family (Bakker, Koen, Van Son, & Van Loey, 2013; Filanovsky et al., 2016; Magin, Adams, Heading, Pond, & Smith, 2008). Nurses who care for children need to be familiar with common skin disorders and related psychosocial impacts of infancy, childhood, and adolescence so they can effectively support children and their families.

VARIATIONS IN PEDIATRIC ANATOMY AND PHYSIOLOGY

Skin is the largest organ of the body and serves to protect the underlying tissues from trauma, loss of body fluid, and invasion by microorganisms. The skin's health reflects the internal well-being of the body (Vernon, Brady, Starr, & Petersen-Smith, 2013). The skin is also important for the perception of pain, heat, and cold, the regulation of body temperature, and activation of vitamin D (Martini, Timmons, & Tallitsch, 2012).

Differences in the Skin Between Children and Adults

The infant's epidermis is thinner than the adult's, and the blood vessels lie closer to the surface as a result of decreased subcutaneous fat. Thus, the infant loses heat more readily through the skin's surface than the older child or adult. The thinness of the infant's skin also allows topical substances to be readily absorbed through the skin. Bacteria on infant's skin can be superficial resulting in localized skin infection or access the circulatory system if skin integrity is lost. The infant's skin contains more water than the adult's, and the epidermis is loosely bound to the dermis. This means that friction may easily cause separation of the layers, resulting in blistering or skin breakdown. The infant's skin is also less pigmented than that of the adult (in all races), placing the infant at increased risk of skin damage from ultraviolet radiation. Over time, the infant's skin toughens and becomes less hydrated and thus is less susceptible to microorganism invasion. The skin thickness and characteristics reach adult levels in the late teenage years.

Differences in Dark-Skinned Children

Children with dark skin tend to have more pronounced cutaneous reactions compared to children with lighter

FIGURE 45.1 Keloid formation is more common in dark-skinned than light-skinned children.

skin. Hypopigmentation or hyperpigmentation in the affected area following healing of a dermatologic condition is common in dark-skinned children. This change in pigmentation may be temporary (a few months following a superficial skin disorder) or permanent (following a more involved skin condition). Dark-skinned children tend to have more prominent **papules** (rounded, nonpustular elevation on the skin), follicular responses, lichenification, and vesicular or bullous reactions than lighter skinned children with the same disorder. Hypertrophic scarring and keloid formation (Fig. 45.1) occur more often in dark-skinned children (Vernon et al., 2013).

Sebaceous and Sweat Glands

Sebaceous glands function immaturely at birth. The sebum secreted serves to lubricate the skin and hair. Sebum production increases in the preadolescent and adolescent years, which is why acne develops at that time. The infant's eccrine sweat glands (cover the body, open on to surface of the skin, greatest proliferation hands, feet, head) are somewhat functional and will produce sweat as a response to emotional stimuli and heat. They become fully functional in the middle childhood years. Until that time, temperature regulation is less effective compared with older children and adults. The apocrine sweat glands (associated with hair follicles) are small and nonfunctional in the infant. They mature during puberty, at which time body odour develops in response to the fluid secreted by these glands.

COMMON MEDICAL TREATMENTS

A variety of medications as well as other medical treatments are used to treat integumentary disorders in children. Most of these treatments will require a physician's or nurse practitioner's order. The most common treatments and medications are listed in Common Medical Treatments 45.1 and Drug Guide 45.1. The nurse caring for the child with an integumentary disorder should be familiar

COMMON MEDICAL TREATMENTS 45.1

Treatment	Explanation	Indications	Nursing Implications
Wet dressing	Dressing moistened with lukewarm water (sterile water may be required in certain cases)	In the presence of itching, crusting, or oozing—helps to remove crusts	May use Burow, Domeboro, or saline solutions in certain cases Provide atraumatic care by giving premedication before dressing change
Sunscreen	Lotion, gel, or cream with a sun-protective factor (SPF)	All children older than 6 months of age	Use a fragrance-free, para-aminobenzoic acid (PABA)– free preparation with an SPF of 30 or higher Apply at least 30 minutes prior to sun exposure. Reapply at least every 2 hours while exposed (every 60 to 80 minutes while in the water) Sweat- and water-resistant preparations are available yet still require reapplication as noted above Use daily in summer and in warm climates, even on overcast and cloudy days
Bathing	Use of lukewarm water (with or without soap) to bathe	Itchy and irritating skin conditions	Recommend fragrance-free, dye-free soaps Colloid oatmeal baths are especially helpful Pat the child dry; do not rub the skin. Leave the child moist before applying medication, dressing, or moisturizer

DRUG GUIDE 45.1 COMMON DRUGS FOR INTEGUMENTARY DISORDERS

Medication	Actions/Indications	Nursing Implications
Antibiotics (topical)	Decrease skin colonization with bacteria Indicated for mild acne vulgaris, impetigo, folliculitis	Apply as prescribed to clean skin or a cleansed wound Be alert for neomycin allergy
Antibiotics (systemic)	Bactericidal or bacteriostatic against a variety of organisms, depending on the preparation Used for moderate to severe acne vulgaris, extensive impetigo, cellulitis, scalded skin syndrome	Check for medication allergies prior to administration Teach families to finish entire course of antibiotics
Corticosteroids (topical)	Anti-inflammatory effect in atopic dermatitis and certain kinds of contact dermatitis	Do not use moderate- or high-potency corticosteroid preparations on the face or genitals (without specific specialist physician direction) Do not cover with an occlusive dressing Absorption is increased in the young infant
Antifungals (topical)	Fungicidal used to treat tinea, candida diaper rash	Apply a thin layer as prescribed Comply with length of treatment as prescribed to prevent re-emergence of the rash
Antifungals (systemic): griseofulvin, ketoconazole	Kill fungus; bind to human keratin, making it resistant to fungus Indicated for tinea capitis and severe or widespread fungal skin infections	Griseofulvin: give with fatty food to increase absorption. Requires minimum 4-week course Monitor liver function tests and CBC. May cause photosensitivity Ketoconazole: administer with food to decrease GI upset
Benzoyl peroxide	Decreases colonization of *P. acnes* in mild acne vulgaris	Available in combination with topical antibiotics Apply sparingly. Shake before application Avoid contact with eyes and mucous membranes

(continued)

DRUG GUIDE 45.1 COMMON DRUGS FOR INTEGUMENTARY DISORDERS (continued)

Medication	Actions/Indications	Nursing Implications
Retinoids (topical): tretinoin, adapalene, tazarotene	Anti-comedogenic activity in moderate to severe acne vulgaris	Adverse effects: dryness, burning, photosensitivity Instruct child to use SPF 15 or higher sunscreen
Topical immune modulators (tacrolimus, pimecrolimus)	Inhibit T-lymphocyte action at the skin level Used for moderate to severe atopic dermatitis, or in conditions resistant to topical steroids	Use only in children older than 2 years Avoid sunlight exposure May cause burning, pruritus, flu-like symptoms, or headache
Antihistamines (diphenhydramine, chlorpheniramine, hydroxyzine)	Antihistaminic effect, results in sedation Indicated for hypersensitivity reactions, atopic dermatitis, or contact dermatitis that is severely pruritic	May give three or four times a day unless sedation effect interferes with activities of daily living or school
Systemic corticosteroids (prednisone, dexamethasone, methylprednisolone)	Anti-inflammatory and immunosuppressive action Used in severe contact dermatitis	Administer with food to decrease GI upset May mask signs of infection Monitor blood pressure, urine for glucose Do not stop treatment abruptly or acute adrenal insufficiency may occur Monitor for Cushing syndrome Doses may be tapered over time
Isotretinoin	Reduces sebaceous gland size, decreases sebum production, and regulates cell proliferation and differentiation Indicated for cystic acne or severe acne that is resistant to 3 months of treatment with oral antibiotics	Ensure that the adolescent girl is not pregnant and does not become pregnant Monitor CBC, lipid profiles, liver function tests, and β-human chorionic gonadotropin monthly Monitor for suicide risk
Coal tar preparations	Antipruritic and anti-inflammatory effect Useful in psoriasis, atopic dermatitis	May stain fabrics; strong and unpleasant odour Apply at bedtime and rinse off in the morning to improve compliance
Silver sulfadiazine 1%	Bactericidal against gram-positive and gram-negative bacteria and yeasts Indicated for burns	Cover with occlusive dressing Apply twice daily Do not use in children with sulfa allergy Forms a gel on the burn that is painful to remove May cause transient neutropenia Do not use on the child's face or on an infant younger than 2 months of age

CBC, complete blood count; GI, gastrointestinal.

Adapted from Taketomo, C. K., Hodding, J. H., & Kraus, D. M. (2013). *Pediatric & neonatal dosage handbook* (20th ed.). Hudson, OH: Lexi-comp.

with the procedures and medications, how they work, and common nursing implications related to their use.

NURSING PROCESS OVERVIEW FOR THE CHILD WITH AN INTEGUMENTARY DISORDER

Nursing management of the child with an alteration in tissue integrity/integumentary disorder requires astute assessment skills, development of accurate nursing diagnoses and expected outcomes, implementation of appropriate interventions, and comprehensive evaluation. Many

skin rashes may be associated with other, often serious illnesses. Therefore, the nurse must pay close attention to assessing for possible systemic infection when evaluating rashes in children. Certain integumentary conditions are chronic and require ongoing care related to health maintenance, education, and psychosocial needs.

Assessment

Nursing assessment of the child with an integumentary disorder/tissue integrity alteration includes obtaining the health history and performing a physical examination. Assisting with or obtaining laboratory tests may also be necessary.

> Remember Eva, the 1-year-old with the dry patches, itching, and trouble sleeping? What additional health history and physical examination assessment information should the nurse obtain?

Health History

Determine the child's or parent's chief complaint, which is most often related to pruritus, **scaling** (dry, flaky skin), or a cosmetic disruption. Document the history of the present illness, noting onset, location, duration, characteristics, other symptoms, and relieving factors, particularly if related to a rash or lesion. Also, ask about the quantity and quality of any discharge from the rash or lesions. Document accompanying symptoms. Note the child's general state of health, history of chronic medical conditions, recent surgeries, hospitalizations, medications, or immunizations. Has there been a recent change in the child's food intake or environment? Is there a family history of chronic or acute skin conditions? Does anyone in the home have a similar concern at this time? Does the family have pets that go outdoors? Does the child play in the woods or garden? Note usual skin care routines, as well as types of soaps, cosmetics, or other skin care products used. Determine the amount of daily sun exposure and whether the child regularly uses sunscreen.

Physical Examination

Perform a complete physical examination, noting any abnormalities. Perform a focused and thorough examination of the skin. The best lighting for examination of the skin is natural daylight. Look at the skin in general, noting distribution of any obvious rashes or lesions. Inspect the mucous membranes, noting and describing lesions if present. Examine all surfaces of the skin and scalp carefully. Note temperature, moisture, texture, and fragility of the skin. If a rash or lesions are present, note their location and provide a detailed description of them. Describe whether a rash is macular, papular, pustular, or vesicular.

Provide a description of vascular lesions if present. If lesions are present on the scalp, has hair loss in that region occurred? Describe lesions according to the following criteria:
- Linear: in a line
- Shape: are the lesions round, oval, or **annular** (ring around central clearing)?
- Morbilliform: a rosy, maculopapular rash
- Target lesions: like a bull's eye

If drainage is present, describe it as clear, purulent, honey coloured, or otherwise. Note scaling or lichenification of the skin. Palpate for regional lymphadenopathy.

Laboratory and Diagnostic Testing

Common Laboratory and Diagnostic Tests 45.1 details the laboratory and diagnostic tests most commonly used when considering integumentary disorders. The tests can assist the physician or nurse practitioner in diagnosing the disorder or can be used as guidelines in determining ongoing treatment. Some of the tests are obtained by laboratory or nonnursing personnel, while others might be obtained by the nurse. In either instance, the nurse should be familiar with how the tests are obtained, what they are used for, and normal versus abnormal results. This knowledge will also be necessary when providing child and family education related to the testing.

Nursing Diagnoses and Related Interventions

Upon completion of a thorough assessment, the nurse might identify several nursing diagnoses, such as:
- Impaired skin integrity
- Pain
- Risk for infection
- Disturbed body image
- Risk for fluid volume deficit
- Altered nutrition

> After completing an assessment of Eva, the nurse noted the following: hypopigmentation of the skin behind her knees, dry patches on her wrists and face, and slight wheezing heard bilaterally on auscultation. Based on these assessment findings, what would your top three nursing diagnoses be for Eva?

Desired outcomes and interventions are based on the nursing diagnoses. Nursing Care Plan 45.1, found at the end of the chapter, can be used as a guide in planning nursing care for the child with an integumentary disorder. Individualize the plan of care based on the child's and family's responses to the health alteration. See Chapter 36 for information about pain management. Additional information will be included later in the chapter as it relates to specific disorders.

> Based on your top three nursing diagnoses for Eva, describe appropriate nursing interventions.

COMMON LABORATORY AND DIAGNOSTIC TESTS 45.1

Test	Explanation	Indications	Nursing Implications
Complete blood count (CBC) with differential	Evaluate hemoglobin and hematocrit, WBC count (particularly the percentage of individual WBCs), and platelet count	Infection or inflammatory process	Normal values vary according to age and gender WBC differential is helpful in evaluating source of infection May be affected by myelosuppressive drugs Eosinophils may be elevated in the child with atopic dermatitis
Erythrocyte sedimentation rate (ESR)	Nonspecific test used to detect presence of infection or inflammation	Infection or inflammatory process	Send sample to laboratory immediately; if allowed to stand for longer than 3 hours, may result in falsely low result
Potassium hydroxide (KOH) prep	Reveals branching hyphae (fungus) when viewed under microscope	To identify fungal infection	Place skin scrapings on a microscope slide and add KOH 20% drop
Culture of wound or skin drainage	Allows for microbial growth and organism identification	Identification of specific organism	Note sensitivities
Immunoglobulin E (IgE)	Measurement of serum IgE	Atopic dermatitis	Often elevated in allergic or atopic disease, though this is a nonspecific finding. May be increased if the child takes systemic corticosteroids
Patch or skin testing	Needle prick testing with allergens	Atopic or contact dermatitis	Have emergency equipment available in the event of anaphylaxis (rare)

Adapted from Corbett, J. A., & Banks, A. D. (2013). *Laboratory tests and diagnostic procedures with nursing diagnoses* (8th ed.). Upper Saddle River, NJ: Pearson Education Inc.

INFECTIOUS DISORDERS

Infectious disorders of the skin include those caused by viral, bacterial, or fungal infection. The viral exanthems are discussed in Chapter 37. Bacterial and fungal infections of the skin are discussed below.

Bacterial Infections

Bacterial infections of the skin include bullous and nonbullous impetigo, folliculitis, cellulitis, and staphylococcal scalded skin syndrome. These bacterial skin infections are often caused by *Staphylococcus aureus* (*S. aureus*) and group A β-hemolytic streptococcus, which are ordinarily normal flora on the skin. Impetigo, folliculitis, and cellulitis are usually self-limited disorders that rarely become severe.

Impetigo is a readily recognizable skin rash (Fig. 45.2) and is the most common bacterial skin infection in children 2 to 5 years of age. *S. aureus* or *Streptococcus pyogenes* cause nonbullous impetigo generally following skin trauma or may arise as a secondary bacterial infection of another skin disorder, such as AD. It is characterized by honey-coloured crusts on the face and extremities. Bullous impetigo is caused exclusively by *S. aureus*, with

toxin production by the bacteria resulting in large, soft bullae (Hartman-Adams, Banvard, & Juckett, 2014).

Folliculitis, infection of the hair follicle, most often results from occlusion of the hair follicle. It may occur as

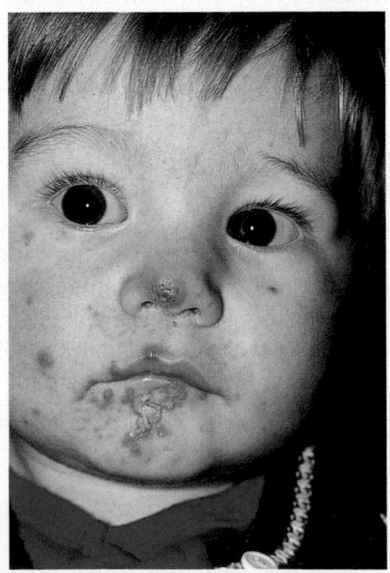

FIGURE 45.2 Note honey-coloured crusting with impetigo.

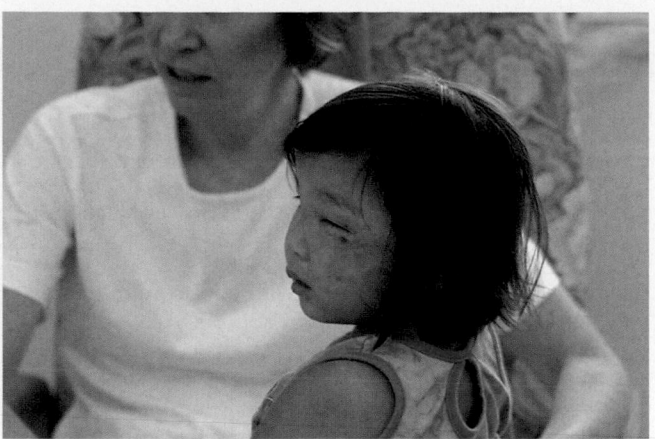

FIGURE 45.3 Note erythema and edema associated with cellulitis.

a result of poor hygiene, prolonged contact with contaminated water, maceration, a moist environment, or use of occlusive emollient products.

Cellulitis is a localized infection and inflammation of the skin and subcutaneous tissues and is usually preceded by skin trauma of some sort (Fig. 45.3).

Staphylococcal scalded skin syndrome results from infection with *S. aureus* that produces a toxin, which then causes exfoliation. It has an abrupt onset and results in diffuse **erythema** (reddening of the skin) and skin tenderness (Fig. 45.4). Blisters and bullae may form, which then slough off, exposing the dermis. The skin should be treated in the same manner as a severe burn, with aseptic technique and pain management. Scalded skin syndrome is the most serious staphylococcal infection that affects the skin and is most common in infancy and rare beyond 5 years of age (Handler & Schwartz, 2014). Of particular concern are community-acquired

FIGURE 45.4 Staphylococcal scalded skin syndrome (SSSS) with ruptured bullae. (Used with permission from Goodheart, H. P. (2009). *Goodheart's photoguide to common skin disorders: Diagnosis and management* (3rd ed.). Philadelphia, PA: Lippincott Williams & Wilkins.)

bacterial skin infections caused by methicillin-resistant *S. aureus* (CA-MRSA) (Loewen et al., 2017). CA-MRSA most commonly occurs as a skin or soft tissue infection, such as cellulitis or an abscess. Risk factors for CA-MRSA are turf burns, towel sharing, participation in team sports, or attendance at day care or outdoor camps. If the child presents with a moderate to severe skin infection or with an infection that is not responding as expected to therapy, it is important to culture the infected area for MRSA. Furthermore, CA-MRSA infections can be common in some Indigenous communities (Canadian Paediatric Society [CPS], 2017a); education about transmission as well as the impact of overcrowding and in-home portable water supply must be considered when implementing health-promoting strategies. In addition, street-involved youth (SIY) experiencing homelessness are at increased risk of CA-MRSA (CPS, 2016a). This is difficult to treat due to delayed presentation, poor nutritional status, and likely associated illness or disease (CPS, 2016a).

Therapeutic management of bacterial skin infections includes topical or systemic antibiotics and appropriate hygiene (see Table 45.1).

Nursing Assessment

Obtain the history as noted in the Nursing Process Overview section. Note history of skin disruption such as a cut, scrape, or insect or spider bite (nonbullous impetigo and cellulitis). Note body piercing in the adolescent, which can lead to impetigo or cellulitis. Measure the child's temperature. Fever may occur with bullous impetigo or cellulitis and is common with scalded skin syndrome. Inspect the skin, noting abnormalities, documenting their location and distribution, and describing drainage if present. Table 45.1 gives specific clinical manifestations of the various bacterial skin infections. Palpate for regional lymphadenopathy, which may be present with impetigo or cellulitis. Blood cultures are indicated in the child with cellulitis with lymphangitic streaking and in all cases of periorbital or orbital cellulitis. Consider the broader social aspects of care and look to working in collaboration with public health, social care providers, and other community teams as necessary.

Nursing Management

Administer antibiotics topically or systemically as prescribed. Teach the family about antibiotic administration and care of the lesions or rash. Soak impetiginous lesions with cool compresses or Burow solution to remove crusts before applying topical antibiotics. Though impetigo is considered a contagious disorder among vulnerable populations, removal from school or day care is not necessary unless the condition is widespread or actively weeping. Prevent transmission of nosocomial MRSA by

TABLE 45.1	BACTERIAL SKIN INFECTIONS	
Disorder	**Skin Findings**	**Usual Treatment**
Nonbullous impetigo	• **Papules** progressing to vesicles, then painless pustules with a narrow erythematous border • Honey-coloured exudate when the vesicles or pustules rupture, which forms a crust on the ulcer-like base (see Fig. 45.2)	• Limited amount: treat topically with mupirocin ointment • If numerous lesions, oral first-generation cephalosporin is indicated • Clindamycin may be needed for MRSA • Remove honey-coloured crust with cool compresses twice daily
Bullous impetigo	• Red macules and bullous eruptions on an erythematous base • Size may be from a few millimetres to several centimetres	• Oral first-generation cephalosporin • Good hygiene
Folliculitis	• Red, raised hair follicles	• Treat with aggressive hygiene: warm compresses after washing with soap and water several times a day • Topical mupirocin is indicated; occasionally, oral antibiotics are required
Cellulitis	• Localized reaction: **erythema**, pain, edema, warmth at site of skin disruption (see Fig. 45.3)	• Mild cases are usually treated with cephalexin or amoxicillin/clavulanic acid • More severe cases and periorbital or orbital cellulitis require IV cephalosporins
Staphylococcal scalded skin syndrome	• Flattish bullae that rupture within hours • Red, weeping surface is left, most commonly on face, groin, neck, and axillary region (see Fig. 45.4)	• Mild to moderate cases are treated with oral cephalexin, dicloxacillin, or amoxicillin/clavulanic acid • Severe cases are managed similar to burns with aggressive fluid management and IV oxacillin or clindamycin

Adapted from Hartman-Adams, H., Banvard, C., & Juckett, G. (2014). Impetigo: diagnosis and treatment. *American Family Physician, 90*(4), 229–235.

appropriately isolating children according to the institution's policy when the child is hospitalized. In children with scalded skin syndrome, reduce the risk of scarring by minimal handling, avoiding corticosteroids, and applying soothing ointments as the skin heals.

Educate the family about prevention of bacterial skin infections. Stress the importance of cleanliness and hygiene. Teach the family to keep the child's fingernails cut short and to clean the nails with a nail brush at bath time. When a skin disruption, such as a cut, scrape, or insect bite, occurs, teach the family to clean the area well to prevent the development of cellulitis. Folliculitis may be prevented with diligent hygiene and avoidance of occlusive emollients. Table 45.1 gives additional information about specific treatments for bacterial skin infections. See Dosage Calculation Box 45.1.

Dosage Calculation Box 45.1

Child's weight: 6 kg (approx. 13 lb, 3 oz)
Medication order: cephalexin 125 mg/5 mL, 4 mL PO every 6 hours
Per the *Pediatric Dosage Handbook*, the recommended dose is 25 to 50 mg/kg/day divided every 6 to 8 hours daily
Is the ordered dose safe?

Fungal Infections

Fungi also cause infections on children's skin. *Tinea* is a fungal disease of the skin occurring on any part of the body. The part of the body affected determines the second word in the name. Examples of tinea infections occurring on various parts of the body include:
• Tinea pedis: fungal infection on the feet
• Tinea corporis: fungal infection on the arms or legs
• Tinea versicolour: fungal infection on the trunk and extremities
• Tinea capitis: fungal infection on the scalp, eyebrows, or eyelashes
• Tinea cruris: fungal infection on the groin

The three organisms most often responsible for tinea are *Epidermophyton*, *Microsporum*, and *Trichophyton*, though *Malassezia furfur* causes tinea versicolour. *Candida albicans* may cause an infection of the skin, particularly in a warm, moist area such as the diaper area. Fungal skin infections may occur year-round, but tinea versicolour is more common in warm weather.

Therapeutic management of fungal infections involves appropriate hygiene and administration of an antifungal agent. Table 45.2 gives further information about treatment.

TABLE 45.2	MANAGEMENT OF FUNGAL INFECTIONS	
Disorder	**Skin Findings**	**Usual Treatment**
Tinea corporis (ringworm)	• Annular lesion with raised peripheral scaling and central clearing (looks like a ring; Fig. 45.5)	• Topical antifungal cream is required for at least 4 weeks
Tinea capitis	• Patches of scaling in the scalp with central hair loss • Risk of kerion development (inflamed, boggy mass that is filled with pustules; Fig. 45.6)	• Oral griseofulvin for 4–6 weeks • Selenium sulphide shampoo may be used to decrease contagiousness (adjunct only) • No school or day care for 1 week after treatment initiated
Tinea versicolour	• Superficial tan or hypopigmented oval scaly lesions, especially on upper back and chest and proximal arms • More noticeable in the summer with tanning of unaffected areas (Fig. 45.7)	• Apply selenium sulphide shampoo all over body (from face to knees) and allow to stay on skin overnight, rinsing in the morning, once a week for 4 weeks (this may cause skin irritation) • Topical antifungals in the imidazole family may be used instead
Tinea pedis (athlete's foot)	• Red, scaling rash on soles and between the toes (Fig. 45.8)	• Topical antifungal cream, powder, or spray • Appropriate foot hygiene
Tinea cruris	• Erythema, scaling, maceration in the inguinal creases and inner thighs (penis/scrotum spared)	• Topical antifungal preparation for 4–6 weeks
Diaper candidiasis (also called monilial diaper rash)	• Fiery red lesions, scaling in the skin folds, and satellite lesions (located further out from the main rash; Fig. 45.9)	• Topical nystatin with diaper changes for several days • See section on diaper dermatitis for additional information

Adapted from Ely, J. W., Rosenfield, S., & Seabury Stone, M. (2014). Diagnosis and management of tinea infections. *American Family Physician*, *90*(10), 702–711; Coughlin, C. C., Eichenfield, L. F., & Frieden, I. J. (2014). Diaper dermatitis: Clinical characteristics and differential diagnosis. *Pediatric Dermatology*, *31*, 19–24.

Nursing Assessment

Elicit the health history, noting exposure to another person with a fungal infection or exposure to a pet (fungi are often carried by pets). Note onset of the rash and whether it is itchy. Determine if the child has recently visited the barber (tinea capitis). Note contact with damp areas such as locker rooms and swimming pools, use of nylon socks or nonbreathable shoes, or minor trauma to the feet (tinea pedis). Document a history of wearing tight clothing or participating in a contact sport such as wrestling (tinea cruris). Inspect the skin and scalp, noting the location, description, and distribution of the rash or lesions (Figs. 45.5 to 45.9). Table 45.2 describes the clinical findings associated with various types of tinea.

Skin, hair or nail scrapings are covered with a potassium hydroxide preparation (KOH) which allows the viewer to visualize dematophytes under the microscope, identifying branching hyphae. For tinea capitis, the Wood lamp will fluoresce yellow-green if it is caused by *Microsporum*, but not with *Trichophyton*, which limits its use as a diagnostic as *Trichophyton is common*; therefore, a fungal culture of a plucked hair is more reliable for diagnosis of tinea capitis (Ely, Rosenfield, & Seabury Stone, 2014).

Nursing Management

Maintain appropriate hygiene and administer antifungal agents as prescribed (see Table 45.2). Additional specifics related to the individual fungal disorders are as follows:

FIGURE 45.5 **Tinea corporis: note raised scaly border with clearing in centre.**

Pathophysiology

AD is a chronic disorder characterized by extreme itching and inflamed, reddened, and swollen skin. It has a relapsing and remitting nature. The skin reaction occurs in response to specific allergens, usually food (especially eggs, wheat, milk, and peanuts) or environmental triggers (e.g., molds, dust mites, and cat dander). Other factors, such as high or low ambient temperatures, perspiring, scratching, skin irritants, or stress, may contribute to flare-ups. When the child encounters a triggering antigen, antigen-presenting cells stimulate interleukins to begin the inflammatory process. The skin begins to feel pruritic and the child starts to scratch. The sensation of itchiness comes first, and then the rash becomes apparent. The scratching causes the rash to appear. Sweating causes AD to worsen, as does excessively humid or dry environments.

FIGURE 45.11 Atopic dermatitis rash is red, dry, and scaly.

Nursing Assessment

For a full description of the assessment phase of the nursing process, refer to the Assessment section of the Nursing Process Overview earlier in the chapter. Assessment findings pertinent to AD are discussed below.

HEALTH HISTORY

Elicit a description of the present illness and chief complaint. Common signs and symptoms reported during the health history might include:
• Wiggling or scratching
• Dry skin
• Scratch marks noticed by the parents
• Disrupted sleep
• Irritability

Explore the child's current and past medical history for risk factors such as:
• Family history of AD, allergic rhinitis, or asthma
• Child's history of asthma or allergic rhinitis
• Food or environmental allergies

Determine the onset of the rash; its location, progression, and severity; and response to treatments used so far. Note medications used to treat the rash, as well as other medications the child may be taking.

PHYSICAL EXAMINATION

Physical examination consists of inspection and observation and auscultation.

Inspection and Observation. Observe whether the infant is wiggling or the child is actively scratching. Carefully inspect the skin. Document dry, scaly, or flaky skin, as well as hypertrophy and lichenification (Fig. 45.11). If lesions are present, they may be dry lesions or weepy papules or **vesicles** (fluid-filled lesions). In children younger than 2 years old, the rash is most likely to occur on the face, scalp, wrists, and extensor surfaces of the arms or legs. In older children, the rash can occur anywhere, but tends to be found on the flexor areas and hands and feet. Note erythema or warmth, which may indicate associated secondary bacterial infection. Document areas of hyperpigmentation or hypopigmentation, which may have resulted from a prior exacerbation of AD or its treatment. Inspect the eyes, nose, and throat for symptoms of allergic rhinitis.

Auscultation. Auscultate the lungs for wheezing (commonly found in the associated condition of asthma).

LABORATORY AND DIAGNOSTIC TESTS

Serum immunoglobulin E (IgE) levels may be elevated in the child with AD. Skin prick allergy testing may determine the food or environmental allergen to which the child is sensitive.

Nursing Management

Nursing management of the child with AD focuses on promoting skin hydration, maintaining skin integrity, and preventing infection.

PROMOTING SKIN HYDRATION

First and foremost, avoid hot water and any skin or hair product containing perfumes, preservatives, dyes, or fragrance. Bathe the child twice daily in warm (not hot) water for 5 to 15 minutes to hydrate the skin, and remove scales, crusts, irritants, and allergens. Use a mild soap to clean only the dirty areas. Recommended mild soaps or cleansing agents include:
• Mustela®
• Kiss of Nature
• Aveeno®
• MD Moms®
• Cetaphil
• Spectro®
• Exederm®

(Adapted from Eczema Products, National Eczema Association; Skincare Products, Eczema Society of Canada.)

Slightly pat the child dry after the bath, but do not rub the skin with the towel. Leave the child moist. Moisturize immediately after bathing to seal in moisture. Apply prescribed topical ointments or creams to the affected area. Apply fragrance-free moisturizer over the prescribed topical medication and all over the child's body. Recommended moisturizers include:

- Exederm®
- Mustela®
- CeraVe®
- Cetaphil®
- Vaseline
- Dermakalm®

(Adapted from Eczema Products, National Eczema Association; Skincare Products, Eczema Society of Canada.)

 Take Note!

Vaseline or generic petrolatum is an inexpensive, readily available moisturizer.

Apply moisturizer multiple times throughout the day. Avoid clothing made of synthetic fabrics or wool. Avoid triggers known to exacerbate AD. There are studies examining the efficacy and safety for paediatric use of homeopathic oral supplements, such as evening primrose, but to date, there is no sufficient research to currently recommend routine use for the treatment of AD. Encourage parents or caregivers to seek support from community pharmacists since this group are well positioned to support both patients and advice prescribers when treating AD (Wong, Tsuyuki, Cresswell-Melville, Doiron, & Drucker, 2017). Phototherapy and systemic medications may be considered for more complex and severe cases of AD by paediatric dermatologists.

MAINTAINING SKIN INTEGRITY AND PREVENTING INFECTION

Cut the child's fingernails short and keep them clean. Avoid tight clothing and heat. While current guidance suggests use of 100% cotton bed sheets, ongoing studies are examining the impact of silk therapeutic clothing in the management of AD (Harrison et al., 2015). In addition to keeping the child's skin well moisturized, it is extremely important to prevent the child from scratching. Scratching causes the rash to appear and further scratching may lead to secondary infection. Antihistamines given at bedtime may sedate the child enough to allow him or her to sleep without awakening because of itching.

During the waking hours, behaviour modification may help to keep the child from scratching. Have the parent keep a diary for 1 week to determine the pattern of scratching. Help the parent to determine specific strategies that may raise the child's awareness of scratching. A handheld clicker or counter may help to identify the scratching episode for the child, thus raising awareness. The use of diversion, imagination, and play may help to distract the child from scratching. The parent and child may create a game together that results in the child participating in a behaviour rather than scratching. Pressing the skin or clenching the fist may replace scratching. It is important for the child to stay active to distract his or her mind from the itching. It is important for the parent to positively reinforce and reward the desired behaviours.

Contact Dermatitis

Contact dermatitis is a cell-mediated response to an antigenic substance exposure. The first exposure is the sensitization phase. The antigen attaches to cells that migrate to regional lymph nodes and have contact with T-lymphocytes, where recognition of antigen is developed. During the second phase, elicitation, contact with the antigen results in T-lymphocyte proliferation and release of inflammatory mediators. An allergic response occurs within 24 to 48 hours after contact with the substance.

Contact dermatitis may occur because of allergy to nickel or cobalt found in clothing hardware and dyes, and chemicals found in many hygiene products and cosmetics. One of the more common causes of contact dermatitis in children results from exposure to highly allergenic plants such as *Toxicodendron radicans* (poison ivy; common across Canada), *Toxicodendron quercifolium* (Eastern poison oak), *Toxicodendron diversilobum* (Western poison oak), and *Toxicodendron vernix* (poison sumac) (HealthLink BC, 2016).

Direct or indirect contact with the plant's oleoresin found in the leaves, stems, and roots results in an allergic reaction (Government of Canada, 2016). Even contact with dormant plants or plants perceived to be dead may cause an allergic response. The rash is extremely pruritic and may last for 2 to 4 weeks; lesions continue to appear during the illness. Contact dermatitis is not contagious and does not spread either to other parts of the affected child's skin or to other people. Scratching does not spread the rash, but it may cause skin damage or secondary infection. Complications of contact dermatitis include secondary bacterial skin infections and lichenification or hyperpigmentation, particularly in people with dark skin.

Therapeutic management is directed toward management of itching and the use of topical corticosteroids. Moderate-potency topical glucocorticoid cream or ointment is used for mild to moderate contact dermatitis, and high-potency preparations are used for more severe cases. Some severe cases of contact dermatitis may require the use of systemic steroids.

Nursing Management

Identify and remove the offending trigger. Discontinue antibiotics. Administer antihistamines, corticosteroids, and topical antipruritics as prescribed. Inform the child and family that the episode should resolve within a few days. If it lasts up to 6 weeks, the child should be reevaluated (Vernon et al., 2013). Advise the family to obtain a medical alert bracelet for the child if the reaction is severe.

> **Take Note!**
>
> In an emergency situation when airway and breathing are compromised, subcutaneous epinephrine followed by intravenous (IV) diphenhydramine and corticosteroids is necessary.

Seborrhea

Seborrhea is a chronic inflammatory dermatitis that may occur on the skin or scalp. In infants, it occurs most often on the scalp and is commonly referred to as cradle cap. Infants may also manifest seborrhea on the nose or eyebrows, behind the ears, or in the diaper area. It usually resolves over a period of weeks to months (Sasseville, 2015). Adolescents manifest seborrhea on the scalp (dandruff) and on the eyebrows and eyelashes, behind the ears, and between the shoulder blades.

It is thought that seborrhea is an inflammatory reaction to the fungus *Pityrosporum ovale* and is worsened by sebaceous involvement related to maternal hormones in the infant and androgens in the adolescent.

Therapeutic management includes treating the skin lesions with corticosteroid creams or lotions. Antidandruff shampoos containing selenium sulphide, ketoconazole, or tar are used to treat the scalp.

Nursing Assessment

Elicit the health history, determining onset and progression of skin and scalp changes. Note response to treatment used so far. In the infant, inspect the scalp and forehead, behind the ears, and the neck, trunk, and diaper area for thick or flaky greasy yellow scales (Fig. 45.15). In the adolescent, note mild flakes in the hair with yellow greasy scales on the scalp, forehead, and eyebrows; behind the ears; or between the scapulae.

Nursing Management

Wash or shampoo the affected areas with a mild soap. Apply anti-inflammatory cream to skin lesions if prescribed. In the infant, apply mineral oil to the scalp, massage it well with a washcloth, and then shampoo 10 to 15 minutes later, using a brush to gently lift the crusts;

FIGURE 45.15 Severe cradle cap (yellow, greasy-appearing plaques).

do not forcibly remove the crusts. If needed, selenium sulphide shampoo may safely be used on the infant, following the aforementioned procedure. The adolescent may require daily shampooing with an antidandruff shampoo.

Psoriasis

Psoriasis is a chronic inflammatory skin disease with periods of remission and exacerbation; control is possible with conscientious therapy. It is an immune-mediated disorder occurring in persons with a genetic predisposition. Approximately 30% to 50% of adults with psoriasis develop it before the age of 20 (Bronckers, Paller, van Geel, van der Kerkhof, & Seyger, 2015).

Hyperproliferation of the epidermis occurs, with a rash developing at sites of mechanical, thermal, or physical trauma. Therapeutic management includes skin hydration with emollient creams, use of tar preparations, topical steroids, and ultraviolet light, among others. Narrow-band ultraviolet light has been used with some success in children with severe psoriasis.

Nursing Assessment

Note family history of psoriasis. Determine onset and progression of rash, as well as treatments used and the response to treatment. Question the child about pruritus, which is usually absent with psoriasis. Inspect the skin for erythematous papules that coalesce to form plaques, most frequently found on the scalp, elbows, genital area, and knees (Fig. 45.16). Facial plaques may also occur and are more common in children than adults. The plaques have a silvery or yellow-white scale and

FIGURE 45.16 Psoriasis. (Used with permission from Goodheart, H. P. (2009). *Goodheart's photoguide to common skin disorders: Diagnosis and management* (3rd ed.). Philadelphia, PA: Lippincott Williams & Wilkins.)

sharply demarcated borders. Layers of scale may be present, which, when removed, result in pinpoint bleeding (referred to as the Auspitz sign). Plaques on the scalp may result in alopecia. Examine the palms and soles, noting fissures and scaling. Skin biopsy, though rarely needed for diagnosis, will show hyperplastic epidermis, with thinning of the papillary dermis.

Nursing Management

Exposure to sunlight may promote healing, but take care not to allow the child to become sunburned. Apply skin moisturizers or emollients daily to prevent dry skin and flare-ups. Apply topical anti-inflammatory creams as prescribed during flare-ups. Apply tar shampoos or skin preparations. Use mineral oil and warm towels to soak and remove thick plaques.

Thinking About Development

Emily Wilson is a 15-year-old female with a history of moderate psoriasis. She experiences significant scaling along her hairline, forehead, scalp, and arms. Hypopigmentation and striae are beginning to occur on her arms as a result of topical medication use. She is a talented ballerina but expresses increasing concerns about her skin alterations showing while she is performing.

How does Emily's developmental stage affect self-care related to her psoriasis?

What is the most appropriate approach for the nurse to take to educate Emily about control of her psoriasis?

How will the nurse best promote an appropriate body image for Emily?

ACNE

Acne, the most common skin condition occurring in childhood (Lynn, Umari, Dunnick, & Dellavalle, 2016), is a disorder that affects the pilosebaceous unit. It affects males and females, as well as all ethnic groups. Overall, males tend to have more severe disease than females, probably because of the androgen influence (Lynn et al., 2016). Acne that persists past the usual course of time for infantile or adolescent acne may be caused by endocrine abnormalities. It may also occur in response to the use of certain types of drugs such as corticosteroids, androgens, phenytoin, and others. The usual presentation and nursing management of acne neonatorum and acne vulgaris is presented below.

Acne Neonatorum

Acne neonatorum occurs as a response to the presence of maternal androgens or to transient androgen production in the newborn. It affects about 20% of newborns (Vernon et al., 2013). Usually no treatment is necessary, but in severe cases there is a risk of scarring, so a topical preparation may be prescribed.

Nursing Assessment

Note oily face or scalp. Examine the face (especially the cheeks), upper chest, and back for inflammatory papules and pustules. Document absence of fever.

Nursing Management

Instruct parents to avoid picking or squeezing the pimples; to do so places the infant at risk for secondary bacterial infection and cellulitis. Teach parents to wash the affected areas daily with clear water. Avoid using fragranced soaps or lotions on the area with acne. Inform the parents that as the newborn's hormones stabilize over time, the acne usually resolves without additional intervention.

Acne Vulgaris

Acne vulgaris affects 50% to 85% of adolescents between the ages of 12 and 16 years, and endogenous androgens play a role in its development (Lynn et al., 2016). It occurs most frequently on the face, chest, and back. Risk factors for the development of acne vulgaris include preadolescent or adolescent age, male gender (due to the presence of androgens), an oily complexion, Cushing syndrome, or another disease process resulting in increased androgen production.

Pathophysiology

The sebaceous gland produces sebum and is connected by a duct to the follicular canal that opens on the skin's surface. Androgenous hormones stimulate sebaceous gland proliferation and production of sebum. These hormones exhibit increased activity during the pubertal years. Abnormal shedding of the outermost layer of the skin (the stratum corneum) occurs at the level of the follicular opening, resulting in a keratin plug that fills the follicle. The sebaceous glands increase sebum production. Bacterial overgrowth of *Propionibacterium acnes* occurs because the presence of sebum and keratin in the follicular canal creates an excellent environment for growth. Inflammation occurs as the follicular wall perforates, allowing the contents to leak into nearby tissue.

Therapeutic Management

Therapeutic management focuses on reducing *P. acnes*, decreasing sebum production, normalizing skin shedding, and eliminating inflammation. Teach the adolescent to cleanse the skin gently twice a day. Medication therapy may include a combination of benzoyl peroxide, salicylic acid, retinoids, and topical or oral antibiotics. Isotretinoin may be used in severe cases. Drug Guide 45.1 gives further information on these medications. In girls, oral contraceptives may help lessen acne by decreasing the effects of androgens on the sebaceous glands. Diode laser or blue ultraviolet light therapy may also be used. CO_2 lasers and dermabrasion may be used to treat pitted scarring.

Nursing Assessment

Note history of onset of acne lesions, as well as family history of acne. Determine medication use; certain medications may hasten the onset of acne or worsen it when already present. In particular, note use of corticosteroids, androgens, lithium, phenytoin, and isoniazid. Document history of an endocrine disorder, particularly one that results in hyperandrogenism. In girls, note worsening of acne 2 to 7 days before the start of her menstrual period. Ask and note if her cycle is irregular referring to physician or nurse practitioner if there is a suspicion of polycystic ovary syndrome. Inspect the skin for lesions (particularly on the face and upper chest and back, which are the areas of highest sebaceous activity). Note presence, distribution, and extent of noninflammatory lesions, such as open and closed comedones, as well as inflammatory lesions such as papules, pustules, nodules, or cysts (open comedones are commonly referred to as blackheads and closed comedones as whiteheads; see Fig. 45.17). Examine the skin for hypertrophic scarring resulting from inflammatory lesions. Table 45.3 explains the acne classification. Note oily skin and oily hair, which result from increased sebum production. Determine remedies that have been used and the extent of success of those treatments. Assess the child's or teen's feelings about the disorder.

FIGURE 45.17 Acne vulgaris.

Nursing Management

Avoid oil-based cosmetics and hair products, as their use may block pores, contributing to noninflammatory lesions. Look for cosmetic products labelled as noncomedogenic. Headbands, helmets, and hats may exacerbate the lesions by causing friction. Dryness and peeling may occur with acne treatment, so encourage the child to use a humectant moisturizer. Mild cleansing with soap and water twice daily is appropriate. Avoid excessive scrubbing and harsh chemical or alcohol-based cleansers. Avoid picking or squeezing the lesions. Using a noncomedogenic sunscreen with an SPF of 30 or higher may reduce the risk of postinflammatory discolouration from acne lesions (Zaenglein et al., 2016). Teach adolescents that the prescribed topical medications must be used daily and that it may take 4 to 6 weeks to see results. Avoid the use of over-the-counter preparations because they are irritating and aggravate the drying effect of prescription acne treatments. Instruct boys to shave gently

TABLE 45.3	CLASSIFICATION OF ACNE
Classification	**Manifestations**
Mild acne	Primarily noninflammatory lesions (comedones)
Moderate acne	Comedones plus inflammatory lesions such as papules or pustules (localized to face or back)
Severe acne	Lesions similar to moderate acne, but more widespread, and/or presence of cysts or nodules. Associated more frequently with scarring

Adapted from Zaenglein, A. L., Pathy, A. L., Schlosser, B. J., Alikhan, A., Baldwin, H. E., Berson, D. S., . . . Bhushan, R. (2016). Guidelines of care for the management of acne vulgaris. *American Academy of Dermatology, 74*(5), 945–973.e33. Retrieved from http://dx.doi.org/10.1016/j.jaad.2015.12.037

and avoid using dull razors, so as not to further irritate the condition. While in the U.S. adolescent girls taking isotretinoin are opted on to the iPLEADGE SMART program (Zaenglein et al., 2016) requiring monthly pregnancy testing, Health Canada's Scientific Advisory Panel rejected a similar registry in Canada (Choi, Koren, & Nulman, 2013).

Adolescents interested in complementary medicine approaches may try topical use of a tea tree oil preparation. However, there is little conclusive evidence for its effectiveness (Cao et al., 2015).

If the acne is severe, depression may occur as a result of body image disturbances. Provide emotional support to adolescents undergoing acne therapy. Refer teens for counselling if necessary.

Take Note!

Chocolate, skim milk, and French fries have not been proven to contribute to the incidence or severity of acne. However, advise teens to wash their hands after eating greasy finger foods to avoid spreading additional oil and bacteria to the surface of the face (Zaenglein et al., 2016).

Consider This

Paul Herman, age 16, comes to the clinic with complaints of acne on his face and back. He states, "I hate the way my face looks." "I'll never get a date looking like this." "I don't even want to take my shirt off at the beach, because there's bumps on my back."

Think back to when you were an adolescent. How would you have felt if you had a skin condition that altered the way your face looked? As the nurse, how can you help Paul in this situation?

INJURIES

Children, by their inquisitive natures, developmental immaturity, and skin's properties, are prone to experience a variety of skin injuries. Pressure injuries are most likely to occur in hospitalized, immobile children or those who require daily use of mobility aid, braces, or splints. Typical healthy, active children are likely to suffer cuts, abrasions, foreign body penetration, burns or other thermal injuries, bites, and stings.

Pressure Injuries

Skin breakdown involves changes in intact skin, which may range from blanchable erythema to deep pressure ulcers. The term pressure injury refers to damage to the skin resulting in skin loss and development of a crater that may range from mild to deep (Wounds Canada,

2018). The incidence of pressure injuries in critically ill children is 18% to 27% (Schindler et al., 2011). Pressure injuries develop from a combination of factors, including immobility or decreased activity, decreased sensory perception, increased moisture, impaired nutritional status, inadequate tissue perfusion, and the forces of friction and shear. Common sites of pressure injuries in hospitalized children include the occiput and toes, while children who require wheelchairs for mobility have pressure injuries in the sacral or hip area more frequently.

Nursing Assessment

Use a paediatric risk assessment tool (e.g., Braden Q, Glamorgan Scale, and Neonatal Risk Assessment Scale [NSRAS]) to identify and document the risk for skin breakdown. Note history of immobility (chronic, related to a condition such as paralysis) or lengthy hospitalization, particularly in intensive care. Inspect the skin for areas of erythema or warmth. Note and record pressure injuries to any areas of the skin in accordance with Pediatric Early Warning Tools (PEWS) since these include a comprehensive space to record skin integrity. Use the local providers wound assessment scale to document the extent of the pressure injury or ulcer. Consider taking a photo of the ulcer if possible in accordance with local consent procedures.

Nursing Management

Position the child to alleviate pressure on the area of the injury. Use specialized beds, devices, or mattresses to prevent further pressure areas from developing. Perform prescribed wound care meticulously, noting the formation of granulation tissue as the ulcer begins to heal. Prevent pressure injuries in the child who is hospitalized for long periods of time by turning the child frequently, assessing the entire surface of the child's skin at least every shift, using pressure-alleviating beds and mattresses. Assess tubes and drains, ensuring devices are not placing stress/pressure on the child's skin, maintaining the child's nutritional status, and ensuring sufficient pain management. See Evidence-Based Practice 45.1.

Minor Injuries

Children suffer minor injuries frequently. Because of their developmental immaturity and inquisitive nature, children often attempt tasks they are not yet capable of or take risks that an adult would not, often resulting in a fall or other accident. Minor injuries include minor cuts and abrasions, as well as skin penetration of foreign bodies such as splinters or glass fragments. The break in the skin allows an entry point for bacteria, and the complication

EVIDENCE-BASED PRACTICE 45.1   PAEDIATRIC SKIN INTEGRITY PRACTICE GUIDELINE

STUDY

Immobility in the paediatric critical care unit places the child at increased risk of the development of pressure ulcers or other alterations in tissue integrity. About ¾ of children in critical care units have a Braden Q score of 16 or less, indicating increased risk for skin breakdown. The researchers undertook a study to determine the effect of implementation of a paediatric skin integrity practice guideline on skin breakdown in intubated children. Over a 6-month period, 200 charts were reviewed.

Findings

Children admitted to the unit prior to implementation of the guideline were 1.35 times more likely to develop alterations in skin integrity, than those cared for after the paediatric skin integrity practice guideline implementation.

Nursing Implications

Following practice guidelines that address assessment and interventions related to skin, device use, and pressure relief, such as the guideline used in this study, may result in decreased tissue integrity alterations such as skin breakdown and pressure ulcers in immobile children. The study was small, involving one institution only, so should be replicated for further demonstration of effectiveness. Nurse should pay close attention to skin assessments and interventions designed to decrease the incidence of tissue integrity alteration, in order to best preserve immobile children's skin integrity.

Adapted from Kiss, E. A., & Heiler, M. (2014). Pediatric skin integrity practice guideline for institutional use: A quality improvement project. *Journal of Pediatric Nursing, 29*, 362–367.

---

of cellulitis may occur. Treatment is directed at cleaning the wound and preventing infection.

Nursing Assessment

Obtain the history from the child or caregiver to determine whether dirt or a foreign object may be present in the wound. Inspect the wound, noting depth of injury, a foreign body, and bleeding.

Nursing Management

Before any intervention, ensure the child has received adequate pain relief. Use distraction techniques involving a child life specialist if available. The routine practice of using gauze to scrub the wound surface is discouraged. The recommended method to clean the wound is by running water over it. A wound irrigation tip (or 18-gauge catheter tip) can be used with a 35 cc syringe to irrigate the wound. Cleanse the area around the wound with mild soap and water or with an antibacterial cleanser to remove debris (Orsted et al., 2018). Remove pieces of loose skin with sterile scissors, foreign particles with sterile forceps, and road tar with petrolatum. Small abrasions and minor, well-approximated cuts may be left open to the air. Apply a small amount of antibacterial ointment and cover large abrasions with a loose dressing. Be aware of the growing body of literature about antimicrobial stewardship and ensure that the appropriate selection, dose, and duration of treatment are followed both in practice and by the parents or caregivers (CPS, 2017b). Change the dressing as necessary (should it become soaked/loose) or as per the wound management approach being used.

Assess the wound daily for signs of infection, which include purulence, warmth, edema, increasing pain, and erythema that extends past the margin of the cut or abrasion.

Burns

Burns are a common preventable mechanism of injury among children and adolescents, and are caused by exposure to hot liquids (scalds), hot solids (such as household appliances), or flames. Injuries due to exposure to radiation, radioactivity, electricity, or some chemicals are less common. Young children are at highest risk for burns and the mortality rate from burns is highest in children younger than 5 years of age (Statistics Canada, 2017 [Table 102-0551]). In children, scalds represent the most common mechanism for burn injuries, representing 50% of all hospitalizations (Spinks Wasiak, Cleland, Beben, & Macpherson, 2008). In Canada, burns are the third leading cause for hospital admissions due to injury for those aged 0 to 4 years. Three hundred and forty-six children aged 0 to 4 years and fifty-nine children aged 5 to 9 years were admitted to hospital as a result of a burn in 2010/11 (Fuselli & Rothman, 2015). These admissions do not reflect the true number of paediatric burn injuries as most children sustaining burns are only seen in the emergency room or at a clinic, and are not admitted to hospital (Parachute, 2015). Most paediatric burn-related injuries do not result in death, but injuries from burns often cause extreme pain and extensive burns can result in serious disfigurement. Fires in the home are often related to cooking, cigarette or other smoking materials (Egilson, 2016). Carbon monoxide poisoning often occurs in conjunction with burns as a result of smoke inhalation, and infants and children are at greater risk for carbon monoxide poisoning than adults (Etzel & Balk, 2011).

> **Take Note!**
>
> Rural, First Nations Communities, and people of lower socioeconomic status are at increased risk of burn injuries, have less access to preventative resources such as smoke detectors, and have higher rates of morbidity and mortality related to burn injuries.

Conventional wisdom is that children with severe burns should be transferred to a specialized burn unit. Based on the American Burn Association criteria, Critical Care Services Ontario (2014) uses the following criteria for referral of paediatric burn cases to a specialized burn unit:

- ≥20% total body surface area (TBSA) partial and/or full thickness at any age
- Partial thickness burns greater than 10% of total body surface area for ≤10 years of age
- Burns that involve the face, the hands and feet, genitalia, perineum, or major joints
- Full-thickness burns of any size
- Chemical or electrical burns (including lightning injury)
- Inhalation injury
- Burn injury in children who have pre-existing conditions that might affect their care
- Persons with burns and traumatic injuries
- Persons who will require special social, emotional, or long-term rehabilitative care
- Burned children in a hospital without qualified personnel or equipment for the care of children

The old terms used to describe the depth of burns as first, second, and third degree have been replaced by contemporary terminology. Burns are now classified according to the extent of injury and the terminology used to describe each type includes superficial, superficial partial thickness, deep partial thickness, and full thickness (Krishnamoorthy, Ramaiah, & Bhananker, 2012). Superficial burns involve only epidermal injury and usually heal without scarring or other sequelae within 4 to 5 days. In superficial partial-thickness burns, the epidermis is destroyed and the upper layers of the dermis are injured. These burns usually heal within 2 to 3 weeks and carry a minimal risk of scar formation. Deep partial-thickness burns involve injury to the deep portions of the dermis, take longer to heal, may scar, and result in changes in nail and hair appearance as well as sebaceous gland function in the affected area. They may require surgical intervention. Full-thickness burns result in significant tissue damage as they extend through the epidermis, dermis, and hypodermis. Extensive scarring results, as hair follicles and sweat glands are destroyed. Full-thickness burns require a significant time to heal. If underlying tendons, muscles, and/or bone are involved, the burn may be termed fourth degree. Contractures and limited function may occur as a complication of full-thickness burns. Skin grafting is usually necessary. Full or partially circumferential burns may result in ischemia from loss of blood flow related to progressive swelling of the area.

Pathophysiology

Burned tissue begins to coagulate after the injury, and direct coagulation and microvascular reactions in the adjacent dermis may extend the burn. The blood vessels demonstrate increased capillary permeability, resulting in vasodilatation. This leads to increased hydrostatic pressure in the capillaries, causing water, electrolytes, and protein to leak out of the vasculature and result in significant edema. Edema forms very rapidly in the first 18 hours after the burn, peaking at around 48 hours. Capillary permeability then returns to normal between 48 and 72 hours after the burn and the lymphatics can reabsorb the edema fluid. Diuresis occurs, ridding the body of the excess fluid. Fluid loss from burned skin occurs at an amount that is 5 to 10 times greater than that from undamaged skin, and this fluid loss continues until the damaged surface is healed or grafted (Krishnamoorthy et al., 2012).

Initially, the severely burned child experiences a decrease in cardiac output, with a subsequent hypermetabolic response during which cardiac output increases dramatically. During this heightened metabolic state, the child is at risk for insulin resistance and increased protein catabolism. Children who are burned during an indoor or chemical fire are at an increased risk of respiratory injury. Children who have aspirated hot liquids are particularly at risk for airway-altering edema.

Therapeutic Management

Therapeutic management of burns focuses on fluid resuscitation, wound care, prevention of infection, and restoration of function. Burn infections are treated with antibiotics specific to the causative organism. If invasive burn damage occurs, surgery may be necessary.

Nursing Assessment

For a full description of the assessment phase of the nursing process, refer to the Assessment section of the Nursing Process Overview earlier in the chapter. Upon arrival, evaluate the child with burns to determine if he or she will require intensive management. Remove any smoldering clothing. Obtain a brief history of the burn circumstances while you are assessing the child and providing care.

HEALTH HISTORY

If the burn is severe or there is a potential for respiratory compromise, obtain a brief history while simultaneously evaluating the child and providing emergency care. If the burn does not appear to pose an immediate life-threatening risk, obtain an in-depth history. Elicit a description of how the burn occurred, noting date, time, and cause. Determine if smoke inhalation or an associated fall may have occurred. Document treatment that the parent or caregiver has provided to the child's burn so far. Note the child's recent health status, current medications, recent or chronic illness, and immunization status, in particular noting the date of the most recent tetanus vaccination.

EXAMPLE

Calculating TBSA By Age
(Total Body Surface Area)

Color Code
Red - 3° (full thickness)
Blue - 2° (partial thickness)

Area	Birth 1 yr	1-4 yrs	5-9 yrs	10-14 yrs	15 yrs	Adult	2	3	Total
Head	19	17	13	11	9	7	—	8	8.0
Neck	2	2	2	2	2	2	—	1	1.0
Ant. Trunk	13	13	13	13	13	13	1	12	13.0
Post. Trunk	13	13	13	13	13	13	—	—	—
R. Buttock	2 1/2	2 1/2	2 1/2	2 1/2	2 1/2	2 1/2	—	—	—
L. Buttock	2 1/2	2 1/2	2 1/2	2 1/2	2 1/2	2 1/2	—	—	—
Genitalia	1	1	1	1	1	1	—	—	—
R.U. Arm	4	4	4	4	4	4	—	3.5	3.5
L.U. Arm	4	4	4	4	4	4	1	2.5	3.5
R.L. Arm	3	3	3	3	3	3	—	3	3
L.L. Arm	3	3	3	3	3	3	—	3	3
R. Hand	2 1/2	2 1/2	2 1/2	2 1/2	2 1/2	2 1/2	—	2.5	2.5
L. Hand	2 1/2	2 1/2	2 1/2	2 1/2	2 1/2	2 1/2	—	2.5	2.5
R. Thigh	5 1/2	6 1/2	8	8 1/2	9	9 1/2	1	2	3
L. Thigh	5 1/2	6 1/2	8	8 1/2	9	9 1/2	—	2	2
R. Leg	5	5	5 1/2	6	6 1/2	7	—	—	—
L. Leg	5	5	5 1/2	6	6 1/2	7	—	—	—
R. Foot	3 1/2	3 1/2	3 1/2	3 1/2	3 1/2	3 1/2	—	—	—
L. Foot	3 1/2	3 1/2	3 1/2	3 1/2	3 1/2	3 1/2	—	—	—
						Total	3%	42%	45%

FIGURE 45.21 Calculate total body surface area (TBSA) affected by using the child's age and the area affected, as well as whether the burned area is second degree (partial thickness) or third degree (full thickness).

- Administration of most of the volume during the first 8 hours (amounts and timing of fluid volume resuscitation will vary from child to child).
- Reassessment of the child and adjustment of the fluid rate accordingly; fluid requirements greatly decrease after 24 hours and should be adjusted to reflect this.
- Administration of a colloid fluid later in therapy once capillary permeability is less of a concern.
- Monitoring of the child's urine output as part of ongoing assessment of response to therapy, expecting at least 1 mL/kg/hr.
- Daily weights obtained at the same time each day (the best indicator of fluid volume status).
- Monitoring of electrolyte levels (particularly sodium and potassium) for their return to normal levels.

PREVENTING HYPOTHERMIA

Due to the loss of the protective dermis, children who are burned are at high risk for hypothermia and secondary infection. Therefore, take care to keep the child warm. Warm intravenous fluids before administration. Maintain a neutral thermal environment and monitor the child's temperature frequently.

CLEANSING THE BURN

Initially, it is very important to stop the burning. Therefore, remove charred clothing. Wash and rinse the burn thoroughly with mild soap and cool water from the tap. Never apply ice. Children who are burned with tar require special care. Remove tar with cool water and mineral oil. Do not routinely remove blisters because they provide a protective barrier; however, debridement is recommended in certain cases where large blisters impede wound care. Wounds that are open require debridement. Debridement involves the removal of loose skin and eschar (dead, charred skin). This procedure is usually performed with sterile scissors and a pair of forceps. Gently cleanse the burned area; there is no advantage to aggressive scrubbing, and this technique only makes the pain more intense for the child. Wear a gown, mask, head covering, and gloves during dressing changes. Debridement is a necessary, but often excruciatingly painful, procedure. Thus, pain management needs of the child are of utmost importance (refer to the pain management section below).

When children return for evaluation of a wound that was previously seen in your facility, remove the dressing. Soak the dressing in lukewarm tap water to ease the removal of gauze, which may be stuck to the wound. The nurse plays an important role in ensuring that the dressing change goes smoothly. Be sure to:

- Have all dressing supplies ready.
- Provide pain medication as ordered.
- Promote good infection control technique among your colleagues.
- Assist with restraining young children, using the positions of comfort previously discussed in relation to atraumatic care.
- Encourage participation by the child's parents.
- Talk soothingly to the child, explain what you are going to do, and provide distraction during the procedure.

PREVENTING INFECTION

Prevention of infection is critical to successful outcomes for burned children. If the child's immunization status is unknown or if it has been 5 years or longer since the last tetanus vaccine, administer the tetanus vaccine (Krishnamoorthy et al., 2012). If the child has never received tetanus vaccination, also give 250 units tetanus human immunoglobulin intravenously. Apply antibiotic ointment in conjunction with burn dressing changes. Refer to Drug Guide 45.1 for information about topical antibiotics. Membrane dressings such as biosynthetic, hydrocolloid, and antibiotic-impregnated foam dressings are alternatives to topical antibiotics and sterile dressings. Evaluate the child's wound during dressing changes, looking for wound redness, swelling, odour, or drainage. Strictly adhere to infection control procedures and hand hygiene to decrease the risk of burn infection. Maximize the child's nutritional status to decrease his or her susceptibility to a burn infection. Monitor the child's temperature for the development of fever. Upon discharge, instruct the parents about the signs of a wound infection.

MANAGING PAIN

Pain management is of the utmost importance, and several options are available for the treatment of burn-related pain. Local anesthesia, sedatives, and systemic analgesics are commonly used. Children who have less severe burns that are managed at home or outpatient/clinic setting can be given oral medications such as acetaminophen in combination with opioids 30 to 45 minutes before dressing changes. In burns that result in more severe pain, the child should be hospitalized and given intravenous pain control with medications such as morphine sulphate, Remifentanil, or Gabapentin, during both assessment and management phases of care (Ali, Kircher, Meyers, MacLellan, & Ali, 2015). Midazolam (a sedative) or nitrous oxide/oxygen mixture may be used in conjunction with pain medication for pain reduction during dressing changes.

Pain may also occur at any time of the day or night, not just in relation to dressing changes. Assess the child's pain status frequently using an age-appropriate pain assessment scale. Administer pain medications as prescribed and/or use nonpharmacologic techniques to alleviate or decrease the child's perception of pain.

Atraumatic Care

Immersion in virtual reality computer games before and during burn dressing changes provides an exceptionally powerful form of cognitive distraction (Li, Montano, Chen, & Gold, 2011).

TREATING INFECTED BURNS

The potential for burn infection increases if the child has a large, open burn wound and if there are other sources of infection, such as multiple intravenous lines. In addition, children who are immunocompromised have an increased risk of burn infection. In burn wound cellulitis, the area around the burn becomes increasingly red, swollen, and painful early in the course of burn management. With invasive burn cellulitis, the burn develops a dark brown, black, or purplish colour, with a discharge and foul odour. Burn impetigo is characterized by multifocal small superficial abscesses. Burn impetigo causes marked destruction of skin-grafted areas. Extensive infected burns may also become infected with a fungus.

When an infection is suspected, antibiotics are usually started, pending wound culture results. Administer antibiotics as prescribed or antifungals if necessary.

PROVIDING BURN REHABILITATION

Children who have suffered a significant burn injury face many physical and psychological challenges that extend well beyond the acute injury phase. Burned children most often exhibit anxiety and attention or behavioural problems (Bakker et al., 2013). Skin grafting or special burn dressings are required for some children (Box 45.4).

TABLE 45.4		BURN TIMES FOR HOT WATER	
Water/Liquid Temperature		**Time in Which a Young Child Can Suffer a Full-Thickness Burn**[a] **(or Injury)**	**This Is As Hot As …**
212°F	100°C	Less than 1 second	Just-boiled water from a kettle
160°F	70°C	Less than 1–2 seconds	Maximum setting on home hot water heaters. Freshly poured tea and coffee (approx. 70–85°C or 160–175°F)
148°F	64°C	Less than 1 second	
140°F	60°C	1 second (younger child) – 5 seconds (older child)	Factory setting for Canadian hot water heaters
130°F	55°C	6–10 seconds	Hot water from a kettle approx. 5 to 10 minutes after boiling
124°F	51°C	2–10 minute (older child)	
120°F	49°C	5–10 minutes (average estimated at 8 minutes older child)	Recommended safe setting for home hot water heaters
110–112°F	43.3–44.4°C	20–25 minutes child up to 60–120 minutes young adult	Skin injury vs. full thickness burns possible even at this temperature
100°F	37°C	Safe temperature for bathing children	Body temperature—bath will feel "just warm" to adults, fine for children

[a]Times in this table are offered as estimates to indicate the time required to produce a serious burn in children to adolescents.
Adapted from Fuselli and Rothman (2015).

Teaching Guidelines 45.4
PROVIDING BURN CARE AT HOME

For First-Degree (Superficial) Burns
- Run cool water over the burned area until the pain lessens.
- Do not apply ice to the skin.
- Do not apply butter, ointment, or cream.
- Cover the burn lightly with a clean, nonadhesive bandage.
- Administer acetaminophen or ibuprofen for pain.
- Have the child seen by the physician or nurse practitioner within 24 hours.
- Ongoing care: clean in tub or shower with fragrance-free mild soap; pat or air-dry.
  - Apply a thin layer of antibiotic ointment.
  - Cover with a nonadherent dressing such as Adaptic, and then cover with dry gauze.

For More Extensive Burns
- Remove clothing only if it comes off easily or if it is still smoldering.
- Check the child's ABCs (airway, breathing, and circulation) and perform cardiopulmonary resuscitation (CPR) if necessary.
- Do not apply butter, ointment, or any other type of cream.
- Cover the burn with a clean, lint-free bandage or sheet.
- Avoid applying large, wet sheets, as this can cause the child to become too cold.

- Do not attempt to break any blisters.
- If the child appears to be in shock, elevate the legs while protecting the burn and call 911.

Sunburn

Sunburn occurs as a result of overexposure to the ultraviolet (UV) rays of the sun (see Box 45.5 for sunburn prevention tips). The erythema and eventual blisters occur as a result of the skin's blood flow changes as well as alterations in cell kinetics and pigment products in response to UV exposures. Erythema may occur within 4 hours and blisters within 6 hours. Excessive sun exposure has been linked to the development of skin cancer later in life (Leiter, Eigentler, & Garbe, 2014). Sunburn is usually treated with cool compresses, cooling lotions, and oral nonsteroidal anti-inflammatory agents.

Nursing Assessment

Obtain the health history, noting recent sun exposure. Determine length of exposure and whether any type of sunscreen or sun block product was used. Note redness of the skin on the exposed areas. More severe areas will have a darker red, slightly purple hue. Blisters may be noted with more severe sunburn.

Nursing Management

Cool compresses may help to cool the burn. Aloe vera gel applied topically may provide significant soothing.

BOX 45.5

WORLD HEALTH ORGANIZATION'S STEPS FOR SUN PROTECTION

- Limit time in the midday sun. The sun's UV rays are the strongest between 10 AM and 4 PM. Take particular care when in the sun during these hours.
- Watch for the UV index. This important resource helps you plan your outdoor activities in ways that prevent overexposure to the sun's rays. When the UV Index is moderate, i.e., a UVI of 3 or above, sun protection is required.
- Use shade wisely. Seek shade when UV rays are the most intense, but keep in mind that shade structures such as trees, umbrellas, or canopies do not offer complete sun protection.
- Wear protective clothing. A hat with a wide brim offers good sun protection for your eyes, ears, face, and the back or your neck. Sunglasses that provide 99% to 100% UV-A and UV-B protection will greatly reduce eye damage from sun exposure. Tightly woven, loose fitting clothes that cover as much of the body as possible will provide additional protection from the sun.
- Use sunscreen. Apply a broad-spectrum sunscreen of SPF 30+ liberally to exposed skin and re-apply every 2 hours, or after working, swimming, playing, or exercising outdoors.
- Encourage use of sunscreen in all children older than 6 months of age to encourage a lifelong habit.
- Avoid sunlamps and tanning parlours. Sunbeds and sunlamps increase the risk of skin cancer and can damage unprotected eyes. They should be avoided entirely.
- Protect children. Children are generally more susceptible to environmental hazards than adults. During outdoor activities, they should be protected from high UV exposure as above, and babies should always remain in the shade.

Adapted from WHO INTERSUN Programme (2014).

Rarely are adverse effects reported with the use of aloe vera gel. Administer a nonsteroidal anti-inflammatory such as ibuprofen. Discourage hot showers or baths. Instruct the child to wear loose clothing and to ensure that burned areas are covered when going outside (until they are healed). If skin flaking occurs, discourage the child from "peeling" the flaked skin in order to prevent further injury. Refer to Chapter 31 for further information about safe sun exposure.

Cold Injury

The term "frostbite" implies freezing of the tissues. It is described on a continuum from first to fourth degree. When a child is exposed to an extremely cold environment, changes in cutaneous circulation help to maintain the core body temperature. Because circulation is shunted to the core, the most peripheral body parts are those at the highest risk for frostbite. Local damage occurs when the tissue temperature drops to 0°C (32°F). Initially skin

sensation is lost, the vasculature constricts, and plasma leakage occurs. Ice crystals develop in the extracellular fluid, and eventually vascular stasis leads to endothelial cell damage, necrosis, and sloughing of dead tissue.

Nursing Assessment

Note history of cold exposure. Inquire about pain or numbness. Examine the skin for indications of frostbite. First-degree frostbite results in superficial white plaques with surrounding erythema. Second-degree frostbite demonstrates blistering with erythema and edema. In third-degree frostbite, hemorrhagic blisters occur, progressing to tissue necrosis and sloughing in fourth-degree frostbite.

Nursing Management

Remove wet or tight clothing. Avoid vigorous massage to decrease the chance of damaging the skin further. Immerse the affected part in 37°C to 39°C water for 15 to 60 minutes (Sachs, Lehnhardt, Daigeler, & Goertz, 2015). Thawing may cause significant pain, so administer analgesics. Keep the thawed part loosely covered, warm, and dry. Splinting may be used to help decrease associated edema. Consult the wound care specialist or plastic surgeon for further management.

Prevent frostbite by:
- Dressing warmly in non-cotton layers, and keeping warm and dry
- Avoiding exertion
- Not playing outside when wind chill advisories are in effect, and locking doors with high locks to prevent toddlers from going outside

Human and Animal Bites

Yearly, significant emergency room visits occur as a result of bites from mammals. Dog bites account for the majority of injuries, but children may be bitten by other children, cats, or rodents (Hansen & Ahmed, 2010). The hand and face are common locations for animal bites. A dog is most often provoked to bite a child when the child is playing with the dog or when the child hits, kicks, hugs, grabs, or chases the dog.

Therapeutic management involves cleansing and irrigating the wound, wound suturing or stapling if necessary, and administering topical and/or systemic antibiotic therapy. Rabies prophylaxis is indicated if the rabies status of the dog is unknown. Secondary bacterial infection of the bite wound with streptococci, staphylococci, or *Pasteurella multocida* may occur. Cat and human bites are the most likely to become infected (Hansen & Ahmed, 2010). Human bites can occur during play or fighting in home, school, or day care setting. The CPS (2016b) offers advice regarding management and supporting parents who may be anxious about transmission of disease.

Cao, H., Yang, G., Wang, Y., Liu, J. P., Smith, C. A., Luo, H., & Liu, Y. (2015). Complementary therapies for acne vulgaris. *Cochrane Database System Review, 1*, CD009436. doi:10.1002/14651858.CD009436.pub2.

Choi, J. S., Koren, G., & Nulman, I. (2013). Pregnancy and isotretinoin therapy. *Canadian Medical Association Journal, 185*(5), 411–413. http://doi.org/10.1503/cmaj.120729

Corbett, J. A., & Banks, A. D. (2013). *Laboratory tests and diagnostic procedures with nursing diagnoses* (8th ed.). Upper Saddle River, NJ: Pearson Education Inc.

Coughlin, C. C., Eichenfield, L. F., & Frieden, I. J. (2014). Diaper dermatitis: Clinical characteristics and differential diagnosis. *Pediatric Dermatology, 31*, 19–24. doi:10.1111/pde.12500

Diamond, J. S., Abdoo, D. C., Brady, M. A., & Dunn, A. M. (2013). Role relationships. In C. Burns, A. Dunn, M. Brady, N. B. Starr, & C. Blosser (Eds.). *Pediatric primary care* (5th ed.). Philadelphia, PA: Saunders.

Eczema Society of Canada. (2017). *Skincare products*. Retrieved from the Eczema Society of Canada website: https://eczemahelp.ca/get-support/email-a-volunteer/#section=products

Egilson, M. (2016). *British Columbia coroners service child death review panel: A review of fire-related deaths in children and youth 2005–2014*. Burnaby, BC: Canadian Electronic Library (Firm); British Columbia Coroners Service.

Eichenfield, L. F., Tom, W. L., Berger, T. G., Krol, A., Paller, A. S., Schwarzenberger, K., ... Sidbury, R. (2014). Guidelines for care for the management of atopic dermatitis: Part 1: Diagnosis and assessment of atopic dermatitis. *Journal of the American Academy of Dermatology, 70*(2), 338–351. doi: 10.1016/j.jaad.2013.10.010

Ely, J. W., Rosenfield, S., & Seabury Stone, M. (2014). Diagnosis and management of tinea infections. *American Family Physician, 90*(10), 702–711. Retrieved from http://www.aafp.org/afp/2014/1115/p702.html

Etzel, R. A., & Balk, S. J. (Eds.). (2011). *Handbook of pediatric environmental health* (3rd ed.). Chicago: American Academy of Pediatrics.

Filanovsky, M. G., Pootongkam, S., Tamburro, J. E., Smith, M. C., Ganocy, S. J., & Nederost, S. T. (2016). The financial and emotional impact of atopic dermatitis on children and their families. *The Journal of Pediatrics, 169*, 284–290.e5. Retrieved from https://doi.org/10.1016/j.jpeds.2015.10.077

Fuselli, P., & Rothman, L. (2015). Burns. In I. Pike, S. Richmond, L. Rothman, & A. Macpherson (Eds.). *Canadian injury prevention resource* (pp. 467–474). Toronto, ON: Parachute.

Garlich, F. M., & Nelson, L. S. (2011). Inhalation of baby powder. *Emergency Medicine, 43*(1), 17–20.

Government of Canada. (2016). *Poison ivy*. Retrieved from https://www.canada.ca/en/health-canada/services/home-garden-safety/poison-ivy.html

Handler, M. Z., & Schwartz, R. A. (2014). Staphylococcal scalded skin syndrome: Diagnosis and management in children and adults. *Journal of the European Academy of Dermatology and Venereology, 28*(11), 1418–1423. doi: 10.1111/jdv.12541

Hansen, J. J., & Ahmed, A. (2010). Emergent management of bite wounds. *Emergency Medicine, 42*(6), 6–11.

Harrison, E. F., Haines, R. H., Cowdell, F., Sach, T. H., Dean, T., Pollock, I., ... Lawton, S. (2015). A multi-centre, parallel group superiority trial of silk therapeutic clothing compared to standard care for the management of eczema in children (CLOTHES Trial): Study protocol for a randomised controlled trial. *Trials, 16*(1), 390. doi: 10.1186/s13063-015-0921-9

Hartman-Adams, H., Banvard, C., & Juckett, G. (2014). Impetigo: Diagnosis and treatment. *American Family Physician, 90*(4), 229–235. Retrieved from http://www.aafp.org/afp/2014/0815/p229.html

HealthLink BC. (2016). *Poison ivy, oak and sumac*. Retrieved from https://www.healthlinkbc.ca/health-topics/hw75039

Insect Repellent. (2016). Retrieved from the Government of Canada, https://www.canada.ca/en/health-canada/services/about-pesticides/insect-repellents.html

Joffe, M. D. (2015). *Emergency care of moderate and severe thermal burns in children*. Retrieved from http://www.uptodate.com/contents/emergency-care-of-moderate-and-severe-thermal-burns-in-children

Kiss, E. A., & Heiler, M. (2014). Pediatric skin integrity practice guideline for institutional use: A quality improvement project. *Journal of Pediatric Nursing, 29*, 362–357.

Krishnamoorthy, V., Ramaiah, R., & Bhananker, S. M. (2012). Pediatric burn injuries. *International Journal of Critical Illness and Injury Science, 2*(3), 128–134. doi: 10.4103/2229-5151.100889

Leiter, U., Eigentler, T., & Garbe, C. (2014). Epidemiology of skin cancer. In J. Reichrath (Ed.). *Sunlight, vitamin D and skin cancer*. New York: Springer-Verlag.

Li, A., Montano, Z., Chen, V. J., & Gold, J. I. (2011). Virtual reality and pain management: Current trends and future directions. *Pain Management, 1*(2), 147–157.

Loewen, K., Schreiber, Y., Kirlew, M., Bocking, N., & Kelly, L. (2017). Community-associated methicillin-resistant Staphylococcus aureus infection: Literature review and clinical update. *Canadian Family Physician, 63*(7), 512–520.

Lynn, D. D., Umari, T., Dunnick, C. A., & Dellavalle, R. P. (2016). The epidemiology of acne vulgaris in late adolescence. *Adolescent Health, Medicine and Therapeutics, 7*, 13–25. Retrieved from https://www.ncbi.nlm.nih.gov/pmc/articles/PMC4769025/pdf/ahmt-7-013.pdf

Magin, P., Adams, J., Heading, G., Pond, D., & Smith, W. (2008). Experiences of appearance-related teasing and bullying in skin disease and their psychological sequelae: Results of a qualitative study. *Scandinavian Journal of Caring Sciences, 22*(3), 430–435.

Martini, F. H., Timmons, M. J., & Tallitsch, R. B. (2012). *Human anatomy* (7th ed.). Toronto, ON: Pearson Benjamin Cummings.

Mechem, C. C. (2016). *Pulse oximetry in adults*. Retrieved from http://www.uptodate.com/contents/pulse-oximetry

Moorhead, S., Johnson, M., Maas, M., & Swanson, E. (2013). *Nursing outcomes classification (NOC): Measurement of health outcomes* (5th ed.). St. Louis, MO: Mosby.

Myers, T. (2011). When to treat or refer a burn-injured patient. *Clinical Advisor, 14*(7), 31–36.

National Eczema Association. (n.d.). *Eczema products*. Retrieved from https://nationaleczema.org/

National Health Service. (2016). *Animal and human bites.* Retrieved from http://www.nhs.uk/Conditions/Bites-human-and-animal/Pages/Introduction.aspx

Nirken, M. H., High, W. A., & Roujeau, J. C. (2015). *Stevens-Johnson syndrome and toxic epidermal necrolysis: Pathogenesis, clinical manifestations, and diagnosis.* Retrieved from http://www.uptodate.com/contents/stevens-johnson-syndrome-and-toxic-epidermal-necrolysis-pathogenesis-clinical-manifestations-and-diagnosis

Orsted, H. L., Keast, D. H., Forest-Lalande, L., Kuhnke, J. L., O'Sullivan-Drombolis, D., Jin, S., Haley, J., & Evans, R. (2018). *Best practice recommendations for the prevention and management of wounds.* Retrieved from https://www.woundscanada.ca/docman/public/health-care-professional/bpr-workshop/165-wc-bpr-prevention-and-management-of-wounds/file.

Parachute. (2015). *Burns and scalds prevention, 0–6 years.* Retrieved from http://www.parachutecanada.org/child-injury-prevention/item/burns-and-scalds-prevention

Pite, H., Wedi, B., Borrego, L. M., Kapp, A., & Raap, U. (2013). Management of childhood urticaria: Current knowledge and practical recommendations. *Acto Dermato-Venereologica, 93,* 500–508. doi: 10.2340/00015555-1573

Sachs, C., Lehnhardt, M., Daigeler, A., & Goertz, O. (2015). The triaging and treatment of cold-induced injuries. *Deutsches Ärzteblatt International, 112*(44), 741–747. doi: 10.3238/arztebl.2015.0741

Sasseville, D. (2015). *Cradle cap and seborrheic dermatitis in infants.* Retrieved from http://www.uptodate.com/contents/cradle-cap-and-seborrheic-dermatitis-in-infants

Schindler, C. A., Mikhailov, T. A., Kuhn, E. M., Christopher, J., Conway, P., Ridling, D., . . . Simpson, V. S. (2011). Protecting fragile skin: Nursing interventions to decrease development of pressure ulcers in pediatric intensive care. *American Journal of Critical Care, 20*(1), 26–35.

Spinks, A., Wasiak, J., Cleland, H., Beben, N., & Macpherson, A. K. (2008). Ten-year epidemiological study of pediatric burns in Canada. *Journal of Burn Care and Research, 29*(3), 482–488. doi: 10.1097/BCR.0b013e3181776ed9

Statistics Canada. (2017). *Table 102–0551—Deaths and mortality rate, by selected grouped causes, age group and sex, Canada, annual, CANSIM (database).* Retrieved from Statistics Canada website: http://www.statcan.gc.ca

Taketomo, C. K., Hodding, J. H., & Kraus, D. M. (2013). *Pediatric & neonatal dosage handbook* (20th ed.). Hudson, OH: Lexi-comp.

Vernon, P., Brady, M. A., Starr, N. B., & Petersen-Smith, A. M. (2013). Dermatologic disorders. In C. Burns, A. Dunn, M. Brady, N. B. Starr, & C. Blosser (Eds.). *Pediatric primary care* (5th ed.). Philadelphia, PA: Saunders.

Watson, W., & Kapur, S. (2011). Practical guide for allergy and immunology in Canada. *Allergy, Asthma & Clinical Immunology, 7*(Suppl 1), S4. doi: 10.1186/1710-1492-7-S1-S4

Wong, I. T., Tsuyuki, R. T., Cresswell-Melville, A., Doiron, P., & Drucker, A. M. (2017). Guidelines for the management of atopic dermatitis (eczema) for pharmacists. *Canadian Pharmacists Journal/Revue des Pharmaciens du Canada, 150,* 285–297.

World Health Organization (WHO). (2014). *Ultraviolet radiation and the INTERSUN.* Geneva: WHO.

Wounds Canada. (2018). *Best practice recommendations for the prevention and management of pressure injuries.* Retrieved from https://www.woundscanada.ca/docman/public/health-care-professional/bpr-workshop/172-bpr-prevention-and-management-of-pressure-injuries-2/file

Zaenglein, A. L., Pathy, A. L., Schlosser, B. J., Alikhan, A., Baldwin, H. E., Berson, D. S., . . . Bhushan, R. (2016). Guidelines of care for the management of acne vulgaris. *American Academy of Dermatology, 74*(5), 945–973.e33. Retrieved from http://dx.doi.org/10.1016/j.jaad.2015.12.037

Cellular regulation is the process by which cells replicate, proliferate, and grow. The hematologic system is integrally involved in the process of cellular regulation. The hematologic system consists of the blood and blood-forming tissues of the body. These typically function together in a balance that affects the metabolism of the body. The three categories of cells are erythrocytes, or **red blood cells (RBCs)**; thrombocytes, or platelets; and leukocytes, or **white blood cells (WBCs)**. RBCs are responsible for transporting nutrients and oxygen to the body tissues and waste products from the tissues. The platelets are responsible for clotting. WBCs are responsible for fighting infection. WBCs are further divided into granulocytes (neutrophils, eosinophils, and basophils) and agranulocytes (lymphocytes and monocytes).

All blood cells originate from a single type of cell called a multipotent stem cell, which goes on to differentiate into the various types of blood cells. Thrombopoietin (TPO) and interleukin-7 (IL-7) act on the cell and differentiate the cell into either myeloid or lymphoid progenitor cells. The lymphoid cells either, under the influence of IL-6, become B lymphocytes or change directly into T lymphocytes. The myeloid cells are differentiated in one of two ways, by the action of either erythropoietin (EPO) or granulocyte–monocyte colony-stimulating factor (GM-CSF). When the cell is acted upon by EPO, which is produced by the kidneys, the cell becomes the megakaryocyte, also

known as the erythroid progenitor cell. The megakaryocyte is acted on by either EPO, to become the RBC, or TPO and IL-11, to become a megakaryocyte that goes on to form platelets. GM-CSF influences the cell to become the granulocyte, also known as the macrophage progenitor cell. These cells further differentiate under various influences to become the WBCs (Fig. 46.1).

Certain conditions may cause problems to develop within this system resulting in an alteration in blood cellular regulation. These problems are related to either the production of the blood cells (too much or too little) or loss and destruction of these cells. Many factors are involved in the development of hematologic disorders, ranging from genetic causes to disorders resulting from injury, infection, or nutritional deficit.

Neoplastic (referring to cells that abnormally proliferate) disorders are also alterations in cellular regulation. **Cancer** results from an alteration in cellular regulation resulting in out-of-control cell growth. Cancer accounts for the majority of deaths from disease in children between 6 months of age to young adulthood with the incidence of cancer being highest between 0 and 5 years of age (Kids Cancer Care, n.d.). Cure has been achieved in some children with childhood leukemia and other cancers, but there is no universal long-term cure available for any of the childhood cancers. The combined 5-year survival rate for all cancers in children younger than 20 years of age at diagnosis is 81% (Kids Cancer Care, n.d.).

FIGURE 46.1 Process of blood cell formation.

Cancer is a life-threatening illness that involves emotional distress, fear of the unknown, and changes in life priorities for the child and family. Initial and ongoing diagnostic testing and the adverse effects of treatment for cancer, including chemotherapy, radiation, surgery, or other treatments, are often painful. Management of cancer also has a significant psychosocial impact on the child or adolescent. Children with cancer are at risk for distress because they have a life-threatening illness and must undergo frequent, stressful tests, and treatments (National Cancer Institute, 2016). In addition, the child often feels isolated from his or her peers, and the adolescent may have difficulty achieving independence, which is the core developmental task of the teenage years. Children and teens with cancer often demonstrate poorer school performance compared with healthy peers.

Increasing numbers of children diagnosed with cancer are surviving into adulthood (Health Canada, 2017). As a result of their treatments, late effects are increasingly common into adulthood. Often, systems impacted by the effect of cancer treatment in childhood include neurocognitive difficulties (following brain tumour treatment), cardiac effects depending on treatment medication and location of radiation, and endocrine effects on growth, puberty, thyroid function, and fertility. See thePoint for additional information and link to resources.

Nursing care for the child with a hematologic disorder is often multifaceted. A child who has iron-deficiency anemia requires adequate oxygenation and may require packed red blood cells (PRBCs); a child with hemophilia requires factor replacement and monitoring for safety. Nursing care for the child with cancer is also complex. Nurses caring for children with cellular regulation alterations such as cancer and hematologic disorders need not only be knowledgeable about the medical treatment of the disease (including adverse effects) but must also be able to effectively intervene with these children. Nurses need to be particularly aware of the psychosocial and emotional impact of cancer or a chronic hematologic disorder on the child, parents (Moules, Estefan, McCaffrey, Tapp, & Strother, 2016) and extended family, such as grandparents (Scheinemann, 2017).

VARIATIONS IN PEDIATRIC ANATOMY AND PHYSIOLOGY

In the absence of a congenital defect, the hematologic system is intact and functional at birth. RBC and hemoglobin production as well as iron stores undergo changes in the first few months of life; after this time, hematologic function is stable.

Red Blood Cell Production

The production of blood cells in the embryo begins by 8 weeks' gestation. In the embryo, blood cells primarily form in the liver; this continues until a few weeks before delivery. Some cell production, lymphoid cells in particular, takes place in the spleen of the embryo, and the thymus is a site for some transient lymphocyte production. EPO, the hormone that regulates RBC production, is derived primarily from the liver in the fetus, and after birth the kidneys take over this production.

Hemoglobin

Three types of normal **hemoglobin (Hgb)** are present at any given time in the blood: Hgb A, Hgb F or fetal, and Hgb A_2. After 6 months of age, Hgb A is the predominant type. In the neonatal period, the largest difference is with the RBCs. Fetal hemoglobin, which has a much shorter cell life, is present in higher quantities, putting the infant at risk for anemia and leading to problems with the oxygen-carrying capacity of the blood. As the production of the cells transfers from the liver to the bone marrow of the long and flat bones, the balance between oxygenation and production is affected.

Iron

The fetus receives iron through the placenta from the mother. The preterm infant misses out on the final weeks or months of transplacental iron transfer, putting him or her at increased risk for anemia. In the term infant, a period of physiologic anemia occurs between the age of 2 and 6 months. This is due to the fact that the infant demonstrates rapid growth and an increase in blood volume over the first several months of life, and maternally derived iron stores are depleted by 4 to 6 months of age. Sufficient iron intake is critical for the appropriate development of hemoglobin and RBCs. Therefore, the infant must ingest adequate quantities of iron either from breast milk or from iron-fortified formula in early infancy and other food sources in later infancy (Alberta Health Services, 2016). Iron intake is important at all ages. Review developmental chapters for additional information.

CHILDHOOD CANCER VERSUS ADULT CANCER

Infant, childhood, and adolescent cancers vary from adult cancer resulting in unique needs both biologically and in their cancer care journey (Canadian Partnership Against Cancer, 2017). Pediatric cancers most often arise from primitive embryonal (mesodermal) and neuroectodermal tissues, resulting in leukemia's, lymphomas, sarcomas, or central nervous system (CNS) tumours (American Cancer Society, 2015). This is in direct contrast to adult cancers, which mostly arise from epithelial cells, resulting in carcinomas. The most common childhood

COMPARISON CHART 46.1   CHILDHOOD CANCER VERSUS ADULT CANCER

	Childhood Cancer	Adult Cancer
Cancer usually affects	Tissues	Organs
Histologic type	Embryonal, leukemia, lymphoma	Epithelial in origin
Most common sites	Blood, lymph, brain, bone, kidney, muscle	Breast, lung, prostate, bowel, bladder
Environmental and lifestyle factors	Only a small amount of environmental influence proven	Strong influence on cancer development
Cancer prevention	Little known	80% preventable
Detection	Usually incidental or accidental	Very early detection possible if screening recommendations followed
Latent period	Relatively short	Can be very long (20 years or greater)
Extent of disease	Metastasis often present at diagnosis	Metastasis less often present at diagnosis
Response to treatment	Very responsive	Less responsive

Adapted from American Cancer Society. (2015). *Cancer in children.* Retrieved from http://www.cancer.org/acs/groups/cid/documents/webcontent/002287-pdf.pdf

cancers, in order of frequency, are leukemia, CNS tumours, lymphoma, neuroblastoma, rhabdomyosarcoma, Wilms tumour, bone tumours, and retinoblastoma. Comparison Chart 46.1 explains how cancer is different in children versus adults.

In children, warning signs of cancer are most often related to changes in blood cell production or as a result of compression, infiltration, or obstruction caused by the tumour. Changes in blood cell production may result in fatigue, pallor, frequent or severe infection, or easy bruising. Infiltration, obstruction, or compression by a tumour may result in bone or abdominal pain, pain in other parts of the body, swelling, or unusual discharge.

COMMON MEDICAL TREATMENTS

Various medications as well as other medical treatments are used to treat hematologic and neoplastic disorders in children. Most of these treatments will require a physician's or nurse practitioner's order when the child is in the hospital. Deciding on a course of medical treatment for cancer in a developing child is complicated. Some of the treatments can impair the child's growth and development. Many pediatric oncologists and cancer treatment centres are active members of the Children's Oncology Group (COG) with links in British Columbia, Alberta, Saskatchewan, Manitoba, Ontario Quebec Nova Scotia, New Foundland and Labrador (Childhood Oncology Group [n.d.]). This International Cancer Institute–supported group approves and administers clinical trials devoted exclusively to childhood and adolescent cancer research. A **clinical trial** is a carefully designed research study

that assesses the effectiveness of a treatment as well as its acute and long-term effects on the child. Current cancer care in children is a result of the knowledge gained through clinical trials. A clinical trial may include existing medications or treatments in combination with new drugs or may involve a different approach to sequencing or dosing of medications and treatment (Gilger, 2014).

To provide optimal outcomes, the child with cancer should be treated at an institution with multidisciplinary cancer care specialists that can provide the most advanced care available. Each case of pediatric cancer should be considered individually, with the oncology health care team and the family reaching treatment decisions together, whether the treatment plan is standard or involves enrolment in a clinical trial.

In the child with cancer, particularly advanced disease, the decision to provide treatment ("let's do everything we can") or to withhold treatment in the event of an extremely poor prognosis is extraordinarily challenging in an ethical sense. A mature older child or adolescent may have a strong desire to continue or discontinue treatment, and sometimes this desire conflicts with the parents' desires or choices. The Canadian Paediatric Society (CPS) Bioethics Committee (2016) recommends that children and adolescents who have the ability and desire to make medical decisions should be included in the decision-making process. This can be achieved through the concept of assent whereby children are given both developmentally appropriate information and some choice in their treatment (Box 46.1).

Hospice or palliative care may be needed for the child with cancer. Children facing the end of life experience

CANADIAN PAEDIATRIC SOCIETY BIOETHICS COMMITTEE RECOMMENDATIONS REGARDING TREATMENT DECISIONS FOR INFANTS, CHILDREN, AND ADOLESCENTS

- Appropriate Information—Give truthful and clear information. Help each child/family to achieve a developmentally appropriate understanding of the illness to make an informed decision.
- Decision-making Capacity—Assess the child/families understanding of the situation, the purpose of the intervention, consequences of refusal, alternatives, and possibilities of harm vs. benefits.
- Involving children in decision-making is linked to children's agency. Understand that children have the ability, capacity, and capability to make choices and decisions that will impact on their life, social world, and family, is a focus in oncology care. Often, childhood agency is linked to daily decision-making choices and linked to promoting independence. For the child with cancer developmental outcomes and future reproductive potential can change, and metastatic disease can result in relapse (Health Canada, 2017).
- Voluntariness—Tell the child/family what they can expect regarding testing procedures and treatments. Note if there is inappropriate pressure to assent to testing or treatment. Seriously solicit the child's expression of willingness to accept the proposed plan of care.

Adapted from Canadian Paediatric Society, Committee on Bioethics. (2016). *Position statement: Treatment decisions regarding infants, children and adolescents.* Retrieved from http://www.cps.ca/documents/position/treatment-decisions

the same symptoms that adults do, including pain, fatigue, nausea, and dyspnea. Standards for end-of-life care are still in development, but all dying children have the right to die comfortably and with palliation of symptoms, as has been well established in adult hospice programs. Canadian Hospice Palliative Care Association (CHPCA, 2006) has created guiding principles and norms of practice for pediatric hospice palliative care. The guiding principles of pediatric hospice palliative care are to provide child/family focused care; to value the therapeutic relationship; to deliver interdisciplinary continuity of care from illness, to dying, to bereavement; to provide collaborative communication throughout palliative care; and to ensure pediatric hospice palliative care is accessible to all children and their families (CHPCA, 2006). For further information related to nursing care of the dying child, refer to Chapter 34.

Commonly, chemotherapy and radiation therapy are used to treat childhood cancers. In some instances, hematopoietic stem cell transplantation (HSCT) is used. The nurse caring for the child with cancer should be familiar with the procedures, how the treatments and medications work, and common nursing implications related to use of these modalities. The most common treatments and medications are listed in Common Medical Treatments 46.1 and Drug Guide 46.1. The nurse caring for the child with a hematologic disorder or cancer should be familiar with the procedures used, how the medications work, and common nursing implications related to their use.

(text continues on page 1782)

COMMON MEDICAL TREATMENTS 46.1

Treatment	Explanation	Indications	Nursing Implications
Blood product transfusion	Intravenous administration of whole blood, packed red blood cells (PRBCs), platelets, or plasma	PRBCs: severe anemia, thalassemia, sickle cell disease Whole blood: acute hemorrhage or trauma Fresh-frozen plasma: hemophilia Platelets: thrombocytopenia	Follow institution's transfusion protocol Double-check blood type and product label with a second nurse Use only leukodepleted, CMV-negative blood products in the child with a hemoglobinopathy or cancer Monitor vital signs and assess child frequently to detect adverse reaction to blood transfusion If adverse reaction is suspected, immediately discontinue transfusion, run normal saline IV, reassess the child, and notify the physician Some children require premedication with diphenhydramine and/or acetaminophen before receiving blood products
Leukapheresis	Whole blood is removed from the body, the WBCs are extracted, and then the blood is retransfused into the child	Hyperviscosity with leukemia (WBC >100,000)	Performed by specially trained personnel Monitor blood pressure and other vital signs

(continued)

Chemotherapy

To understand how **chemotherapy** works to destroy cancer cells, it is necessary to review the normal cell cycle, through which all cells progress (Fig. 46.2). The cell cycle consists of five phases:

- G0 phase: the resting phase; lasts from a few hours to a few years; cells have not started to divide
- G1 phase: cell makes more protein in preparation for dividing; lasts 18 to 30 hours
- S phase: chromosomes are copied so that newly formed cells have the appropriate DNA; lasts 18 to 20 hours
- G2 phase: just before the cell splits into two cells; lasts 2 to 10 hours
- M phase: mitosis, the actual splitting of the cell into two new cells; lasts 30 minutes to 1 hour

Chemotherapy drugs work in two different ways in relation to the cell cycle. Cell-cycle-specific agents exert their actions during a specific phase of the cell cycle. Cell-cycle-nonspecific drugs exert their effect on the cells

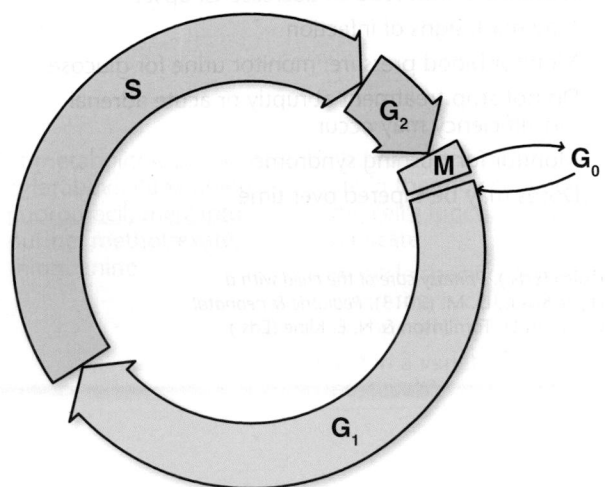
FIGURE 46.2 Phases of the cell cycle.

regardless of which phase the cell is in. Chemotherapy protocols often call for a combination of drugs that act on different phases of the cell cycle, thus maximizing the destruction of cancer cells.

Chemotherapy drugs are divided into classes that exert slightly different actions and have an effect on different portions of the cell cycle. Drug Guide 46.1 gives further explanation about the different classes of chemotherapy drugs.

Unfortunately, chemotherapeutic medications disrupt the cell cycle of not only cancer cells but also normal rapidly dividing cells. This results in a significant number of adverse effects. The cells most likely to be affected by chemotherapy are those in the bone marrow, the digestive tract (especially the mouth), the reproductive system, and hair follicles.

Adverse effects common to chemotherapeutic drugs include immunosuppression, infection, myelosuppression, nausea, vomiting, constipation, oral mucositis, alopecia, and pain. Long-term complications include microdontia and missing teeth as a result of damage to developing permanent teeth; hearing and vision changes; hematopoietic, immunologic, or gonadal dysfunction; endocrine dysfunction, including altered growth and precocious or delayed puberty; various alterations of the cardiorespiratory, gastrointestinal, and genitourinary systems; and development of a second cancer as an adolescent or adult (Toomey, 2014).

Take Note!
Acupuncture as an adjunct therapy may help to decrease nausea, vomiting, and aversion to chemotherapy.

Radiation Therapy

Radiation therapy uses high-energy radiation to damage or kill cancer cells. Radiant energy in either a gamma or particle form is emitted during the treatment. Radiation affects not only cancer cells but also any rapidly growing cells with which they are in contact. It may be used as a curative, adjuvant, or palliative treatment, either alone or in combination with chemotherapy. Radiation therapy is also used to shrink a tumour prior to surgical resection. The area to be treated is marked carefully to minimize damage to normal cells.

Adverse effects of radiation therapy include fatigue, nausea, vomiting, oral mucositis, myelosuppression, and alterations in skin integrity at the site of irradiation. Long-term complications are related to the area of the body that was irradiated and include alterations in growth; hormone dysfunction; hearing and vision alterations; learning problems; cardiac dysfunction; pulmonary fibrosis; hepatic, sexual, or renal dysfunction; osteoporosis; and development of secondary cancer (particularly at the site of irradiation) (Hesselgrave & Chordas, 2014).

Hematopoietic Stem Cell Transplantation

HSCT, also called bone marrow transplantation, is a procedure in which healthy hematopoietic progenitor cells (HPCs) are infused intravenously into the child to replace diseased or damaged cells (Norville & Staton, 2014). This follows a period of purging of abnormal cells in the child that is accomplished through high-dose chemotherapy or irradiation. The use of high-dose chemotherapy and total body irradiation kills the tumour cells but also destroys the child's bone marrow. The transplanted cells migrate to the empty spaces in the child's bone marrow and re-establish normal hematopoiesis in the child.

HSCT is used for a variety of childhood cancers, including leukemia, lymphoma, brain tumours, neuroblastoma, and other solid tumours. For most pediatric cancers, it is not the first line of treatment but is used for refractory or advanced disease.

Autologous HSCT is used in the treatment of solid tumours to provide an HPC rescue after large doses of chemotherapy or radiation. This process includes the harvest of the child's own HPC, cells purged to remove residual tumour cells, and the HPC re-infused into the child (Norville & Staton, 2014). Children have no graft-versus-host disease (GVHD) with autologous HSCT; however, risk for relapse of the original disease is highest in this type of HSCT. Allogenic HSCT refers to transplantation using stem cells from another individual that are harvested from the bone marrow, peripheral blood, or umbilical cord blood. Allogenic HSCT requires human leukocyte antibody (HLA) matching for antigen-specific sites on the leukocytes. Closely matched HLA donors may be difficult to find from a donor listing, and sibling donors are often the closest match. The degree of match is inversely related to the risk for graft rejection and the development of GVHD. In other words, the lesser the degree of HLA matching in the donor, the higher the risk for graft rejection and GVHD. GVHD occurs to at least some extent in 11% to 85% of all allogenic HSCT recipients (Kristovich & Callard, 2010). In addition, chronic GVHD has a complex immunopathology which results in late, nonrelapse mortality and disability which impacts on children's short- to long-term outcomes (Cooke et al., 2017).

In addition to graft rejection and GVHD, additional initial complications of HSCT are infection, electrolyte imbalance, bleeding, and organ, skin, and mucous membrane toxicities. Long-term complications include impaired growth and fertility related to endocrine dysfunction, developmental delay, cataracts, pulmonary and cardiac disease, avascular necrosis of the bone, and development of secondary cancers.

NURSING PROCESS OVERVIEW FOR THE CHILD WITH AN ALTERATION IN CELLULAR REGULATION (HEMATOLOGIC DISORDER OR CANCER)

Care of the child with a hematologic disorder or cancer includes assessment, nursing diagnosis, planning, interventions, and evaluation. There are a number of general concepts related to the nursing process that may be applied to hematologic dysfunction and neoplasia in children.

Development of a plan of care will depend on which component of the blood is altered in the hematologic disorder. A decrease in hemoglobin will necessitate evaluation of oxygen-carrying capacity and effects of hypoxia on the tissues. A reduction in platelet production will lead the nurse to evaluate for prolonged bleeding, hemorrhage, and shock. An elevation in WBCs would require an evaluation for infection.

From a general understanding of the care involved for a child with cancer, the nurse can then individualize the care based on specifics for the particular child. Children with cancer often suffer many physical effects as a result of the disease and its treatment. The nurse must be diligent when assessing for these effects and should involve the parents as a reliable source for reporting the child's physical symptoms.

Remember Shaun, the 10-month-old with the laceration and prolonged bleeding? What additional health history and physical examination assessment information should you obtain?

Assessment

Signs of changes in the hematologic system are often insidious and overlooked. Children with cancer often demonstrate similar signs. Skin colour changes such as pallor, bruising, and flushing are often the first signs that a problem is developing. Changes in mental status such as lethargy can indicate a decrease in Hgb and a decreased amount of oxygen being delivered to the brain. Nursing assessment must include a thorough approach.

Health History

Elicit the birth and maternal history, noting low birth weight or gestational diabetes and ascertaining whether vitamin K was given after birth. The past medical history might be significant for recent illnesses that may contribute to a change in blood cell distribution.

TABLE 46.1　NORMAL HEMOGRAM VALUES

Age	WBC (×10³/mm³)	RBC (×10⁶/mm³)	Hgb (g/dL)	Hct (%)	MCV (fL)	MCH (pg/cell)	MCHC (g/dL)	Platelets (×10³/mm³)	RDW (%)	MPV (fL)
Birth–2 weeks	9.0–30.0	4.1–6.1	14.5–24.5	44–54	98–112	34–40	33–37	150–450	–	–
2–8 weeks	5.0–21.0	4.0–6.0	12.5–20.5	39–59	98–112	30–36	32–36	–	–	–
2–6 months	5.0–19.0	3.8–5.6	10.7–17.3	35–49	83–97	27–33	31–35	–	–	–
6 months–1 year	5.0–19.0	3.8–5.2	9.9–14.5	29–43	73–87	24–30	32–36	–	–	–
1–6 years	5.0–19.0	3.9–5.3	9.5–14.1	30–40	70–84	23–29	31–35	–	–	–
6–16 years	4.8–10.8	4.0–5.2	10.3–14.9	32–42	73–87	24–30	32–36	–	–	–
16–18 years	4.8–10.8	4.2–5.4	11.1–15.7	34–44	75–89	25–31	32–36	–	–	–
>18 years (males)	5.0–10.0	4.5–5.5	14.0–17.4	42–52	84–96	28–34	32–36	140–400	11.5–14.5	7.4–10.4
>18 years (females)	5.0–10.0	4.0–5.0	12.0–16.0	36–48	84–96	28–34	32–36	140–400	11.5–14.5	7.4–10.4

Adapted from Fischbach, F. T., & Dunning, M. B. (2014). *A manual of laboratory and diagnostic tests* (9th ed.). Philadelphia, PA: Lippincott Williams & Wilkins. Various facilities may report using different SI units; a conversion chart is found at http://unitslab.com/node/8 to alternatively review local lab reporting values.

TABLE 46.2		NORMAL DIFFERENTIAL FOR LEUKOCYTES (WHITE BLOOD CELL DIFFERENTIAL)					
Age	Bands/Stab (%)	Segs/Polys (%)	Eos (%)	Basos (%)	Lymphs (%)	Monos (%)
Birth–1 week	10–18	32–62	0–2	0–1	26–36	0–6
1–2 weeks	8–16	19–49	0–4	0	38–46	0–9
2–4 weeks	7–15	14–34	0–3	0	43–53	0–9
4–8 weeks	7–13	15–35	0–3	0–1	41–71	0–7
2–6 months	5–11	15–35	0–3	0–1	42–72	0–6
6 months–1 year	6–12	13–33	0–3	0	46–76	0–5
1–6 years	5–11	13–33	0–3	0	46–76	0–5
6–16 years	5–11	32–54	0–3	0–1	27–57	0–5
16–18 years	5–11	34–64	0–3	0–1	25–45	0–5
>18 years	3–6	50–62	0–3	0–1	25–40	3–7

Adapted from Fischbach, F. T., & Dunning, M. B. (2014). *A manual of laboratory and diagnostic tests* (9th ed.). Philadelphia, PA: Lippincott Williams & Wilkins. Various facilities may report using different SI units; a conversion chart is found at http://unitslab.com/node/8 to alternatively review local lab reporting values.

COMMON LABORATORY AND DIAGNOSTIC TESTS 46.1

Test	Explanation	Indications	Nursing Implications
α-Fetoprotein (AFP)	Produced by the fetal liver and yolk sac; normally decreases to very low levels by 1 year of age	May be elevated in Hodgkin disease and other cancers. Used to determine tumour burden	No food or fluid restriction required
Blood type and cross-match	Determines ABO blood type as well as presence of antigens. Cross-match is performed on RBC-containing products to avoid transfusion reaction	Trauma victim or any person in whom blood loss is suspected, in preparation for transfusion	Avoid hemolysis of specimen Appropriately sign and date specimen. Apply "type and cross" or "blood band" to child at the time of blood draw if indicated by the institution Most type and cross-match specimens expire after 48 to 72 hours
Bone marrow aspiration and biopsy	A needle is inserted through the cortex of the bone into the bone marrow (most often the iliac spine), bone marrow is aspirated, and the cells are evaluated	Evaluation for leukemia or metastasis of other cancers to bone marrow	Use topical anesthetic, i.e., with lidocaine to decrease pain with procedure Often performed under conscious sedation Apply a pressure dressing to arrest bleeding Assess for tenderness or erythema May require mild analgesia for post-procedure pain
Bone scan	Administration of IV radionuclide material, which is taken up by the bone and is visible on the scans	Identify metastasis to bone	Requires patent IV for injection Encourage fluid intake after injection to increase uptake of injected radionuclide Scan will be performed 1 to 3 hours after injection

(continued)

COMMON LABORATORY AND DIAGNOSTIC TESTS 46.1 (continued)

Test	Explanation	Indications	Nursing Implications
Chest radiography	X-ray of the chest	Identify tumour or metastasis in the thorax	Chest must be held stationary for a brief time
Clotting studies	Prothrombin time (PT), partial thromboplastin time (PTT), activated partial thromboplastin time (aPTT), international normalized ratio (INR)	Evaluation of common pathway in clotting mechanism PT, INR: evaluation of extrinsic system PTT, aPTT: evaluation of intrinsic system	Apply pressure to venipuncture site Assess for bleeding (gums, bruising, blood in urine or stool)
Coagulating factor concentration	Measures concentration of specific coagulating factors in the blood	Hemophilia, DIC	Apply pressure to venipuncture site Assess for bleeding (gums, bruising, blood in urine or stool) Deliver specimen to laboratory as soon as possible (unstable at room temperature)
Complete blood count (CBC) with differential	Evaluates hemoglobin and hematocrit, WBC count (particularly the percentage of individual WBCs), and platelet count	Anemia, infection, bleeding disorder, clotting disorder, immunosuppression, to determine neutropenia in myelosuppression	Normal values vary according to age and gender WBC differential is helpful in evaluating source of infection May be affected by certain medications
Computed tomography (CT) scan	Multiple films taken in successive layers to provide a 3D view of the body part being scanned	Identify tumour location or metastasis	Some CT scans are done with oral or IV contrast (notify physician if child has iodine or shellfish allergy) May require a several-hour period of NPO if contrast is used (contrast may cause nausea). Encourage fluid intake after scan to facilitate excretion of contrast dye
Hemoglobin electrophoresis	Measures percentage of normal and abnormal hemoglobin in the blood	Sickle cell anemia, thalassemia	Blood transfusions within the previous 12 weeks may alter test results
Iron	Evaluates iron metabolism	Iron-deficiency anemia, hemosiderosis with chronic transfusion or hemoglobinopathies	Recent blood transfusions increase level Child should fast for 12 hours before the test Avoid hemolysis (will falsely elevate result)
Lead	Measures level of lead in blood	Lead poisoning	Normal amount in blood is zero
Lumbar puncture (LP)	A needle is placed in the subarachnoid space of the spinal column, below the base of the cord, and cerebrospinal fluid is withdrawn for analysis	Evaluation of tumour or metastasis to brain or spinal cord. Also used to administer intrathecal medications	Use topical anesthetic before the procedure to decrease pain. May be performed under conscious sedation. Position child appropriately Use distraction techniques in the older child or teen Encourage child to recline for up to 12 hours after LP

COMMON LABORATORY AND DIAGNOSTIC TESTS 46.1 (continued)

Test	Explanation	Indications	Nursing Implications
Magnetic resonance imaging (MRI)	Based on how hydrogen atoms behave in a magnetic field when disturbed by radiofrequency signals. Does not require ionizing radiation. Provides a 3D view of the body part being scanned	Identify extent of tumour or metastatic spread	Remove all metal objects from the child Child must remain motionless for entire scan; parent can stay in room with child. Younger children will require sedation to keep still A loud thumping sound occurs inside the machine during the scan procedure; this can be frightening to children
Reticulocyte count	Measures the amount of reticulocytes (immature RBCs) in the blood	Indicates bone marrow's ability to respond to anemia with production of RBCs	Rises quickly in response to iron supplementation in the iron-deficient child
Serum ferritin	Measures the level of ferritin (the major iron storage protein) in the blood	Most sensitive test for determining iron-deficiency anemia	Elevated in hemolytic disease and if transfused recently Iron supplementation increases ferritin levels
Urine catechol amines (VMA, HVA)	Catabolism of catecholamines causes elevated levels in urine	Diagnosis of neuroblastoma (produces catecholamines)	24-hour urine collection Levels may be altered with certain foods and drugs or vigorous exercise
Ultrasound	High-frequency sound waves are directed at internal organs and structures, and an image is made of the waves as they are reflected back through the tissues	Identify tumour presence, especially in abdomen or on kidney	Fasting for a few hours may be required when certain organs are to be visualized

Adapted from Corbett, J. A., & Banks, A. D. (2013). *Laboratory tests and diagnostic procedures with nursing diagnoses* (8th ed.). Upper Saddle River, NJ: Pearson Education Inc.

on the nursing diagnoses. Nursing Care Plan 46.1, found at the end of the chapter, may be used as a guide in planning nursing care for the child with a hematologic disorder. Refer to Chapter 36 for additional information related to pain management. Children's responses to alterations in cellular regulation and their treatments will vary, and nursing care should be individualized based on the child's and family's responses to illness. Other conditions may contribute to these nursing diagnoses and must also be considered when prioritizing care. Additional information about nursing management will be included later in the chapter as it relates to specific disorders.

Based on your top three nursing diagnoses for Shaun, describe appropriate nursing interventions.

CARING FOR THE CHILD WITH CANCER

Providing Education

Provide education to families of all children with cancer as outlined in Teaching Guidelines 46.1.

Teaching Guidelines 46.1

EDUCATION FOR FAMILIES OF CHILDREN WITH CANCER

- Obtain a printed or written copy of the child's treatment plan
- Keep a calendar of all appointment times, blood count lab draw days, and phone numbers of all physicians and nurse practitioners, home care companies, the laboratory, and the hospital

- Seek medical care IMMEDIATELY if the child's temperature is 38.3°C (101°F) or higher
- Call the oncologist or seek medical care if any of the following occur:
  - Cough or rapid breathing
  - Increased bruising, bleeding or petechiae, pallor, or increased levels of fatigue
  - Earache, sore throat, nuchal rigidity
  - Blisters, rashes, ulcers
  - Red, irritated skin on the child's buttocks
  - Abdominal pain, difficulty or pain with eating, drinking, or swallowing
  - Constipation or diarrhea
  - For children with central venous catheters:
    - Pus, redness, or swelling at the site
    - Breakage of the catheter
- Do not give the child aspirin

Mosadegh, S. (2014). Patient and family education: Family education. In N. Kline (Ed.). *Essentials of pediatric hematology/oncology nursing: A core curriculum* (4th ed., pp. 353–356). Chicago, IL: Association of Pediatric Hematology/Oncology Nurses.

Administering Chemotherapy

All chemotherapy medications have the potential to cause toxicities in the child as well as the persons handling or preparing the medication. General guidelines related to the preparation and administration of chemotherapy include:

- Chemotherapy should be prepared and administered only by specially trained personnel.
- Personal protective equipment (PPE) in the form of double gloves and nonpermeable gowns should be worn when preparing or administering chemotherapy. If splashing is possible or a spill occurs, then a face shield and/or mask may also be necessary.
- Dispose of all equipment used in chemotherapy preparation and administration in a puncture-resistant container (Brewster Conley, 2014).

It is critical to calculate the chemotherapy dose correctly. Chemotherapy medication doses in children are based on body surface area (BSA). A nomogram is a commonly used device for determining BSA. To use the nomogram, draw a straight line between the child's height on the left and the child's weight on the right. The point at which the straight line crosses the centre is the child's BSA expressed in metres squared (Fig. 46.3).

An alternative to using the nomogram is to use the following formula: BSA (m₂) = the square root of (height [in centimetres] × weight [in kilograms] divided by 3,600) (Colby-Graham & Chordas, 2003). For example, for a child 140 cm tall and weighing 30 kg: 140 × 30 = 4,200; 4,200/3,600 = 1.167; and the square root of 1.167 is 1.08. The BSA would be 1.08.

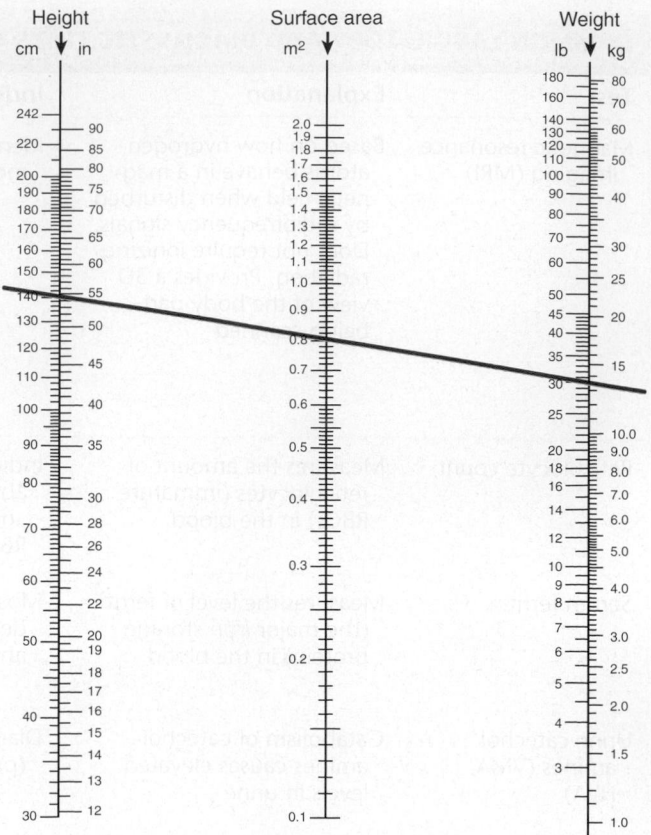

FIGURE 46.3 A child who weighs 13.2 kg and is 140 cm tall has a body surface area (BSA) of 0.80 m².

Managing Adverse Effects of Chemotherapy

Chemotherapy can result in multiple adverse effects. Myelosuppression leads to low blood counts in all cell lines, placing the child at risk for infection, hemorrhage, and anemia. Nausea, vomiting, and anorexia may hinder the child's growth. Alopecia and facial changes may affect the child's self-esteem (Fig. 46.4). Nursing interventions

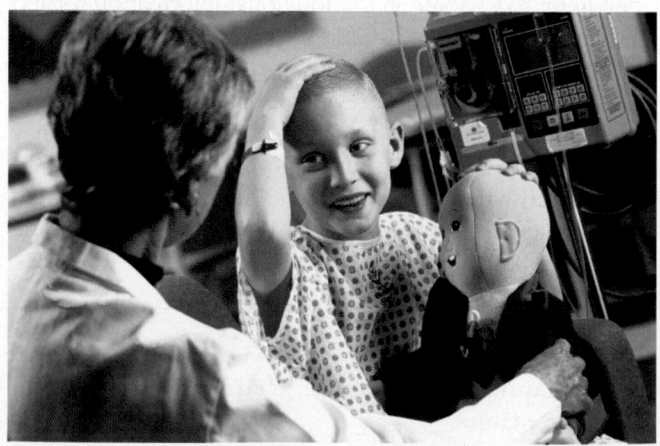

FIGURE 46.4 Chemotherapy often causes alopecia.

related to the effects of myelosuppression, nausea, vomiting, and anorexia are discussed below. Refer to Nursing Care Plan 46.1, at the end of the chapter, for nursing interventions related to altered body image.

Preventing Infection

Many chemotherapeutic drugs cause significant bone marrow suppression and decreased amounts of circulating mature neutrophils ("segs," or segmented neutrophils). Administer granulocyte colony–stimulating factor (GCSF) as ordered to promote neutrophil growth and maturation (Hill Dansereau, 2014). Administer varicella zoster immunoglobulin (VZIG) within 72 hours of exposure to active chickenpox. If the child is actively infected with chickenpox, administer intravenous acyclovir as ordered. Children receiving treatment for acute lymphoblastic leukemia (ALL) are at risk for opportunistic infection with *Pneumocystis jirovecii*, as most children are colonized with this fungus. Administer prophylactic antibiotics as ordered and teach the parents to administer them at home (Morrissey, 2014). Teaching Guidelines 46.2 gives further information about infection prevention at home.

Teaching Guidelines 46.2
PREVENTING INFECTION IN CHILDREN RECEIVING CHEMOTHERAPY FOR CANCER

- Practice meticulous hygiene (oral, body, perianal).
- Avoid known ill contacts, especially persons with chickenpox.
- Immediately notify the physician or nurse practitioner if exposed to chickenpox.
- Avoid crowded areas.
- Do not let the child receive live vaccines.
- Do not take the child's temperature rectally or give medications by the rectal route.
- Administer trimethoprim–sulfamethoxazole twice daily for 3 consecutive days each week as ordered for prevention of *Pneumocystis* pneumonia.

Adapted from Baggott, C. (2010). Cancer. In P. J. Allen, J. A. Vessey, & N. A. Schapiro (Eds.). *Primary care of the child with a chronic condition* (5th ed.). St. Louis, MO: Mosby; and Bryant, R. (2010). Anemias. In D. Tomlinson & N. E. Kline (Eds.). *Pediatric oncology nursing*. New York: Springer.

As neutrophils are the primary means of fighting bacterial infection, when the neutrophil count is low, the chance for developing an overwhelming bacterial infection is high. Each drug that causes bone marrow suppression has a point of nadir. *Nadir* is the time after administration of the drug when bone marrow

---

BOX 46.2

CALCULATING THE ABSOLUTE NEUTROPHIL COUNT (ANC)

- Add together the percentage of banded and segmented neutrophils reported on the complete blood count with differential (CBC with diff).
- Multiply the total number of white blood cells reported on the CBC by the sum above. This yields the ANC (total number of neutrophils present).

Example: Bands 5%, Segs 15%, WBCs 2,500

5% + 15% = 20% (0.20)

2,500 × 0.20 = 500

ANC = 500

Adapted from Brundige, K. (2010). Neutropenia. In D. Tomlinson & N. E. Kline (Eds.). *Pediatric oncology nursing*. New York: Springer.

---

suppression is expected to be at its greatest and the neutrophil count is expected to be at its lowest (neutropenia). Nadir is individual for each drug and ranges from 7 to 28 days after dosing. An absolute neutrophil count (ANC) below 500×10^6/L places the child at greatest risk, although an ANC below $1,500 \times 10^6$/L usually warrants evaluation (Brundige, 2010). Refer to Box 46.2 for information related to calculating the ANC.

Depending on institutional policy, precautions for neutropenia will be followed if the ANC is depressed. Precautions related to neutropenia generally include:

- Place the child in a private room.
- Perform hand hygiene before and after contact with each child.
- Monitor vital signs every 4 hours.
- Assess for signs and symptoms of infection at least every 8 hours.
- Avoid rectal suppositories, enemas, or examinations; urinary catheterization; and invasive procedures.
- Restrict visitors with fever, cough, or other signs/symptoms of infection.
- Do not permit raw fruits or vegetables or fresh flowers or live plants in the room.
- Place a mask on the child when he or she is being transported outside of the room.
- Perform dental care with a soft toothbrush if the platelet count is adequate.

Children with neutropenia and fever must be started on intravenous broad-spectrum antibiotics without delay to avoid overwhelming sepsis (Werther, 2014).

Preventing Hemorrhage

Assess for petechiae, purpura, bruising, or bleeding. Determine changes from baseline that warrant intervention. Encourage quiet activities or play to avoid trauma.

Avoid rectal temperatures and examinations to avoid rectal mucosal damage that results in bleeding. Post a sign at the head of the bed stating "no rectal temperatures or medications." Avoid intramuscular injections and lumbar puncture if possible to decrease the risk of bleeding from a puncture site. If bone marrow aspiration must be performed, apply a pressure dressing to the site to prevent bleeding. For active or uncontrolled bleeding, transfuse platelets as ordered to control bleeding.

Preventing Anemia

To maintain blood volume, limit blood draws to the minimum volume required. Encourage the child to eat an appropriate diet that includes adequate iron. Administer EPO injections as ordered. Teach families to give the injections at home if prescribed.

Managing Nausea, Vomiting, and Anorexia

Many chemotherapeutic drugs produce the adverse effect of nausea and vomiting, which often leads to anorexia. The cycle of nausea, vomiting, and anorexia is difficult to break once it begins. In addition, taste alterations are common in children who have received chemotherapy. During or after chemotherapy, children may develop an aversion to a food that was previously their favourite. Provide foods the child desires or asks for in order to increase the likelihood of eating.

Prevent nausea by administering antiemetic medications prior to the administration of chemotherapy and on a routine schedule around the clock for the first 1 to 2 days rather than on an as-needed (PRN) basis. Herbal or complementary therapies may provide another option for management of nausea.

Bright lights and noise may worsen nausea. Therefore, keep the child's environment dimly lit and calm. Relaxation therapy and guided imagery may also be helpful in preventing or treating nausea and vomiting. Refer to Nursing Care Plan 46.1 at the end of the chapter for additional interventions.

Monitoring the Child Receiving Radiation Therapy

Radiation causes damage to the cells in a localized area, which may include normal cells in addition to the cancerous ones. Assess the child's skin daily, particularly at the treatment site. Provide good hygiene, but perform this care gently. Encourage moisture retention in the skin by applying aqueous creams or moisturizers. Do not apply deodorants or perfumed lotions on the radiation treatment site. Avoid the use of heat or ice packs at the site. Instruct the child and family that clothing should fit loosely so as not to irritate the site (Hesselgrave &

Chordas, 2014). During, and for 8 weeks after, the radiation treatment, the skin will be more photosensitive. Explain the importance of protecting the skin with a high-SPF (30 or above) sunscreen.

Providing Care to the Child Undergoing Hematopoietic Stem Cell Transplantation

Stem cell transplantation is performed at limited specialty medical centres in Canada. In addition, special training is required for all personnel caring for the child who undergoes a stem cell transplant. The intent of this discussion is to provide only a brief introduction to, and overview of, nursing management related to HSCT.

Care for the child undergoing HSCT may be divided into three phases—the pre-transplant phase, the post-transplant phase, and the lengthy supportive care phase. Nursing management of each phase is briefly discussed below.

Pre-Transplant Phase

In the pre-transplant phase, the child is being prepared to receive the transplant. The child's own bone marrow cells are eradicated through high-dose chemotherapy and total body irradiation. This phase usually occurs over 7 to 10 days. The child will be hospitalized because he or she is at extreme risk for serious infection. Maintain protective isolation in a positive-pressure room and limit visitors. Administer gamma-globulin, acyclovir, or antibiotics as ordered to prevent or treat infection. Lymphohematopoietic rescue occurs with infusion of the donor or autologous cells (Norville & Tomlinson, 2010).

Post-Transplant Phase

The post-transplant phase is also a time of high risk for the child. Monitor closely for symptoms of GVHD such as severe diarrhea and maculopapular rash progressing to redness or desquamation of the skin (especially palms or soles) (Fig. 46.5). If GVHD occurs, administer immunosuppressive drugs such as cyclosporine, tacrolimus, or mycophenolate (which place the child at further risk for infection) (Norville & Tomlinson, 2010).

Supportive Care

During the supportive care phase, which lasts several months after the transplant, continue to monitor for and prevent infection. Administer PRBCs or platelets and granulocyte colony-stimulating factor as needed.

Families and children who undergo HSCT need prolonged and extensive emotional and psychosocial support. A medical social worker and psychologist or

FIGURE 46.5 The first sign of graft-versus-host disease (GVHD) may be a maculopapular rash. (Courtesy of Mary L. Brandt, MD.)

counsellor are usually members of the transplant team and are excellent resources for these families' needs (Norville & Tomlinson, 2010).

Promoting a Normal Life

Children and youth want to be normal and to experience the things that other children of their age do (Laing & Moules, 2016). The child should attend school when he or she is well enough and the WBC counts are not dangerously low. Children, their families, and their teachers should be aware that cancer and its treatment can affect scholarly activity and achievements. Learning disabilities, difficulty with memory, attention disorders, and cognitive deficits can occur as a result of the cancer and its treatment.

Maintain other activities if the child is able and if platelet counts are within normal limits. Special camps are available for children with cancer, such as those offered by Kids Cancer Care. These camps offer an opportunity for children and adolescents to experience a variety of activities safely and to network with other children who are experiencing similar physical and emotional challenges (Laing & Moules, 2016).

Promoting Growth

Promote growth in children with cancer by encouraging an appropriate diet and preventing nausea and vomiting and also by addressing concerns such as diarrhea and constipation. Chronic diarrhea related to radiation therapy may prevent the child from gaining weight and growing properly (see Nursing Care Plan 46.1 at the end of the chapter). The use of vinca alkaloids and opioids, as well as the decreased activity level of the child with cancer, may contribute to constipation. Constipation increases the pain experience, contributes to the child's malaise, and decreases quality of life. It directly affects the child's ability to grow by increasing anorexia, nausea,

and vomiting. Nursing Care Plan 46.1 details interventions related to preventing and managing constipation.

Preventing and Treating Oncologic Emergencies

Oncologic emergencies may occur as an effect of the disease process itself or from cancer treatment. As progress is made in chemotherapy and radiation treatment, children with cancer have an increased survival rate, but they still face the risk of developing an oncologic emergency. Nurses caring for children with cancer need to be familiar with signs and symptoms of oncologic emergencies as well as with their treatment. All of these problems warrant careful, frequent monitoring of respiratory, cardiovascular, neurologic, and renal status. Table 46.3 provides information about oncologic emergencies.

Caring for the Dying Child

On average, from those Canadian children (0 to 14 years of age) diagnosed with cancer, 119 will die from the disease each year. Additionally, an average of 290 adolescents and young adults (15 to 29 years of age) will die of cancer each year (Canadian Cancer Society, 2017). A "do not resuscitate" (DNR) order for the child with progressive cancer is obtained in many situations. This order helps to optimize care in the terminal phase of cancer. Nurses serve as child and family advocates, clarifying terminology and providing support as needed during the discussion of DNR orders and throughout the rest of the terminal phase.

Children with terminal cancer can often experience a great deal of pain, particularly when death is imminent. Pain is often accompanied by agitation and dyspnea, which further contribute to the child's discomfort. Regardless of the child's treatment plan (active or DNR), pain management is central to the nursing care of the child who is dying from cancer. Pain is one of the most distressing symptoms to manage in children who are terminally ill (Kline, 2014a). Prevention and alleviation of pain is a primary goal of care. Pain management needs to be a family-centred, interdisciplinary, and collaborative approach. Specific actions must be taken to provide the most effective pain management for the terminally ill child:

- develop a plan with the child/family which includes measurable goals.
- consider adjuvant and nonpharmaceutical therapy when creating a plan.
- educate the family about pain and implementation of the treatment plan.
- utilize consistent pain assessment tools for rapid assessment, intervention, and reassessment of the child's pain.
- work to minimize side effects associated with pain management (Nuuhiwa, 2014).

| TABLE 46.3 | ONCOLOGIC EMERGENCIES | | | |

Emergency	Associated With	Signs and Symptoms	Laboratory or Diagnostic Test Findings	Management
Sepsis	Neutropenia resulting from bone marrow suppression due to chemotherapy	• Fever or low temperature • Respiratory distress • Poor perfusion • Altered level of consciousness	• ANC <500 • Positive blood culture • Increased BUN, creatinine, potassium, clotting times • Decreased platelet count • Metabolic acidosis	• Airway and ventilation maintenance • Fluid volume resuscitation • Inotropic support • Broad-spectrum antibiotics and antifungals • Dialysis if needed
Tumour lysis syndrome	ALL, lymphoma, neuroblastoma	• Nausea, vomiting, diarrhea, anorexia • Lethargy • Increased heart rate and blood pressure • Decreased or absent urine output • Altered level of consciousness	• Hyperuricemia • Hyperkalemia • Hyperphosphatemia • Hypocalcemia • Hypoxia	• Prevent by giving allopurinol for several days prior to chemotherapy (also treat with allopurinol) • Double IV fluid maintenance • Sodium bicarbonate
Typhlitis (neutropenic enterocolitis)	Inflammatory process of GI tract occurring with induction phase of leukemia chemotherapy	• Acute abdominal pain • Nausea, vomiting • Bloody diarrhea and emesis • Fever • Anorexia	• KUB: scarcity of bowel gas, possibly ileus • CT (abdominal): inflammation, bowel wall thickening, peritoneal fluid	• Bowel rest (NPO status) • IV nutrition • Assess for bowel perforation/shock • Broad-spectrum antibiotics and antifungals • Comfort measures
Superior vena cava (SVC) syndrome	Compression on the SVC by NHL or other mediastinal mass, such as neuroblastoma	• Dyspnea and cyanosis • Large cervical lymph nodes • Wheezing, diminished breath sounds	• Chest x-ray or CT shows mediastinal mass • Pleural effusion	• Intubation and ventilation • Comfort measures • Treat cause (usually surgical removal of mass)
Spinal cord compression	Tumour or metastasis compresses spinal cord	• Back, neck, or leg pain • Sensory or autonomic dysfunction • Extremity weakness or paralysis	• MRI reveals location of tumour or metastasis to epidural space	• Dexamethasone • Careful assessment • Radiation therapy • Comfort measures
Increased intracranial pressure	Brain tumour or metastasis to brain causing compression of brain; may result in herniation	• Headache, visual disturbances • Morning vomiting • Infants: increased head circumference • Altered level of consciousness • Cushing triad • Seizure activity	• Head CT or MRI reveals extent of mass	• Frequent, careful neurologic assessment • Limit fluids • Dexamethasone • Anticonvulsants • Tumour resection, radiation, or chemotherapy • Comfort measures

TABLE 46.3	ONCOLOGIC EMERGENCIES (continued)			
Emergency	**Associated With**	**Signs and Symptoms**	**Laboratory or Diagnostic Test Findings**	**Management**
Massive hepatomegaly	Obstruction caused by neuroblastoma filling a large portion of the abdominal cavity	• Distended, enlarged abdomen • Respiratory distress, hypoxia • Poor perfusion • Tachycardia, hypotension	• Abdominal CT reveals extent of tumour • Coagulopathy	• Tumour resection or debulking • Mechanical ventilation, inotropic support • Nasogastric decompression • Position to minimize abdominal pressure • Blood transfusions • Comfort measures

GI, gastrointestinal; KUB, kidney, ureters, and bladder scan; NPO, nothing by mouth.

Adapted from Graham, D. K., Craddock, J. A., Quinones, R. R., Keating, A. K., Maloney, K., & Foreman, N. K. (2014). Neoplastic disease. In W. W. Hay, M. J. Levin, R. R. Deterding, & M. J. Abzug (Eds.). *Current pediatric diagnosis and treatment* (22nd ed.). New York: McGraw-Hill; and Bryant, R. (2010). Anemias. In D. Tomlinson & N. E. Kline (Eds.). *Pediatric oncology nursing*. New York: Springer.

Interventions related to pain management may be found in Nursing Care Plan 46.1, at the end of the chapter. Further discussion related to care of the dying child is found in Chapter 34.

ANEMIA

Anemia is a condition in which levels of RBCs and Hgb are lower than normal. Hgb levels vary throughout childhood. Therefore, it is important to monitor them to ensure that adequate growth and development will be achieved. Anemia may develop as a result of decreased production of RBCs or loss and destruction of RBCs. The loss of production can be related to lack of dietary intake of the nutrients needed to produce the cells, alterations in the cell structure, or malfunctioning tissues (e.g., bone marrow). Anemia related to nutritional deficiency includes iron deficiency, folic acid deficiency, and pernicious anemia. Anemia may also result from toxin exposure (lead poisoning) or as an adverse reaction to a medication (aplastic anemia). Blood loss may result from surgery or trauma. Alteration or destruction of cells occurs in certain genetic and cellular development disorders (Bryant, 2010).

Anemia caused by the alteration or destruction of the RBCs is termed hemolytic anemia. There are several types of hemolytic anemia, such as sickle cell disease and thalassemia; these two disorders are discussed under the section on Hemoglobinopathies.

Anemia related to insufficient intake of specific nutrients is the most common type of anemia in children. Nutrient intake may be reduced in children due to food dislikes or conditions that produce malabsorption.

Iron-Deficiency Anemia

Iron-deficiency anemia occurs when the body does not have enough iron to produce Hgb. In Canada, universal screening for iron deficiency is not done; as a result, national prevalence rates are not available (Alberta Health Services, 2016). However, in the United States, iron-deficiency anemia has a peak prevalence in children between the ages of 6 and 24 months, and again at the age of puberty (Ambruso, Nuss, & Wang, 2014). Cow's milk consumption contributes to iron-deficiency anemia in older infants and young children due to its poor iron availability and may displace iron-rich foods (Alberta Health Services, 2016). It is recommended that children are not introduced to 3.25% milk before the age of 9 to 12 months.

The heme portion of Hgb consists of iron surrounded by protoporphyrin. When not enough iron is available to the bone marrow, Hgb production is reduced. Adequate dietary intake of iron is required for the body to make enough Hgb. As Hgb levels decrease, the oxygen-carrying capacity of the blood is decreased, resulting in weakness and fatigue. In addition to delayed growth, iron-deficiency anemia has been associated with cognitive delays and behavioural changes.

> **Take Note!**
>
> For appropriate growth to occur in infants, children, and adolescence, increased amounts of iron must be consumed and absorbed. See additional information on healthy eating resources and nutritional education materials from Alberta Health Services retrieved from http://www.albertahealthservices.ca/nutrition/Page11115.aspx

mouths, and immaturity of the renal system to excrete lead (Wachtel, McKee, Harding, Suthermaraj, & Kosatsky, 2017). The presence of lead in the bloodstream interferes with the enzymatic processes of the biosynthesis of heme. The process results in hypochromic, microcytic anemia, and children may exhibit classic signs of anemia. Risk factors for lead poisoning are related to lead exposure in the home, school, or local environment. Sources of lead include:

- Paint in homes built before 1978, at which time lead was banned as an additive to paint used in houses
- Glazed pottery
- Stained glass products
- Lead pipes supplying water to the home
- On the clothing of parents who work in certain manufacturing jobs (battery makers, cable makers)
- Certain folk remedies, such as *greta or arzacon*
- Old painted toys or furniture (Lee & Hurwitz, 2016)

Complications of lead poisoning include behavioural problems and learning difficulties and, with higher lead levels, encephalopathy, seizures, and brain damage.

Therapeutic management for high blood levels of lead involves **chelation therapy** (removal of heavy metals from the body via chelating agents), either orally or intravenously. Drug Guide 46.1 gives further information on chelating agents.

Nursing Assessment

Explore the health history for subtle signs such as anorexia, fatigue, or abdominal pain. Determine whether behavioural problems, irritability, hyperactivity, or lack of ability to meet developmental milestones have occurred in recent months. Screen children for risk of exposure to lead in the home. Blood levels of lead should be <0.48 μmol/L (10 μg/dL). Note pallor of the skin.

Nursing Management

Prevention of elevated lead levels is critical. Screen children for lead exposure risk. Blood lead levels in Canadians have reduced in the last three decades (Wachtel, Mckee, Harding, Suthermaraj, & Kosatsky, 2017); however, recommendations for treatment based on blood lead levels are outlined in Table 46.4. Removing old paint is the best way to eliminate the most significant source of lead exposure for a large number of children. Educate families about how to prevent exposure to lead, particularly in young children.

If the child is undergoing chelation therapy, ensure adequate fluid intake and monitor intake and output closely. Refer children with elevated lead levels and developmental or cognitive deficits to developmental centres. These children may need an early intervention program for further evaluation and treatment of developmental delays.

Aplastic Anemia

Aplastic anemia (failure of the bone marrow to produce cells) is characterized by bone marrow aplasia and pancytopenia (decreased numbers of all blood cells). Most cases are acquired, but there are a few rare types of inherited aplastic anemias (O'Brien Shea, 2014). The inherited types present as congenital bone marrow failure; the best known is Fanconi anemia, an autosomal recessive disorder. Acquired aplastic anemia is thought to be an immune-mediated response. Most cases are idiopathic,

TABLE 46.4	INTERVENTIONS BASED ON BLOOD LEAD LEVEL
Blood Lead Level (in mcg/dL) with μmol/L in brackets	**Recommended Action**
<5 (0.2 μmol/L)	Repeat test annually or sooner if <2 years old.
5–14 (0.2–0.7 μmol/L)	Confirm with repeat test in 1 month and educate parents to decrease lead exposure. Repeat test within 3 months.
15–19 (0.7–0.9 μmol/L)	Confirm with repeat test in 1 month and educate parents to decrease lead exposure. Report to local health authorities for surveillance. Repeat test within 2 months.
20–44 (1.0–2.1 μmol/L)	Confirm with repeat test within 1 week and educate parents to decrease lead exposure. Refer to local health department for investigation of home for lead reduction, with referrals for support services.
45–69 (2.2–3.3 μmol/L)	Confirm with repeat test within 2 days and educate parents to decrease lead exposure. Begin chelation therapy and refer to health department as above.
>70 (>3.4 μmol/L)	Hospitalize child and begin chelation therapy. Ensure lead is removed from the home.

Adapted from Hurwitz, R. L., & Lee, D. A. (2016). *Childhood lead poisoning: Management.* Retrieved from http://www.uptodate.com/contents/childhood-lead-poisoning-management

meaning the trigger remains unidentified. Other causes include exposure to environmental toxins, viruses, myelosuppressive drugs, or radiation.

Aplastic anemia may be classified as severe or nonsevere. In the severe form, the granulocyte count is less than 500 µL (<0.5 × 10⁹/L), the platelet count is less than 20,000 µL (<20 × 10⁹/L), and the reticulocyte count is less than 1%. In nonsevere aplastic anemia, the granulocyte count is about 500 µL, the platelet count is over 20,000 µL, and the reticulocyte count is over 1% (Ambruso et al., 2014). Complications of aplastic anemia include severe overwhelming infection, hemorrhage, and death. Therapeutic management of aplastic anemia in children involves hematopoietic stem cell transplantation from a human leukocyte antigen (HLA)–matched sibling donor; if one is not available, immunosuppressive therapy or high-dose cyclophosphamide can be given.

Nursing Assessment

Determine history of exposure to myelosuppressive medications or radiation therapy. Obtain a detailed family, environmental, and infectious disease history. Note history of epistaxis, gingival oozing, or increased bleeding with menstruation. Anemia may lead to headache and fatigue. On physical examination, note ecchymoses, petechiae or purpura, oral ulcerations, tachycardia, or tachypnea. In addition to suppression of all blood cells, laboratory and diagnostic testing may reveal:

- Guaiac-positive stool
- Blood in the urine
- Severe decrease in or the absence of hematopoietic cells on bone marrow aspiration

Nursing Management

Safety is of the utmost concern in children with aplastic anemia. It is important to prevent injury in order to avoid hemorrhage. Stool softeners may be used to prevent anal fissures associated with constipation. Administer only irradiated and leukocyte-depleted PRBCs or platelet transfusions as necessary. This limits exposure to HLA antigens should the child require bone marrow transplantation in the future. If the child requires hematopoietic stem cell transplantation, refer to the section earlier in this chapter for additional nursing management information.

Refer families whose child has only mild or moderate disease to the Aplastic Anemia and Myelodysplastic Syndrome International Foundation, a link to which can be found on thePoint.

Hemoglobinopathies

Hemoglobinopathy is a condition in which abnormal hemoglobin is present. A large percentage of the newborn's hemoglobin is fetal hemoglobin (Hgb F). Hgb F can exchange oxygen molecules at lower oxygen tensions compared with adult hemoglobin. Over the first several months of life, Hgb F levels fall as it is replaced with Hgb A (adult hemoglobin). The healthy older infant then displays Hgb AA. In hemoglobinopathies, this normal hemoglobin configuration is disturbed. Causes of hemoglobinopathies are genetic and include sickle cell (SC) anemia, hemoglobin SC disease, α-thalassemia, and β-thalassemia. This discussion will focus on sickle cell disease and β-thalassemia (Cooley anemia).

Sickle Cell Disease

Sickle cell disease is a group of inherited hemoglobinopathies in which the RBCs do not carry the normal adult hemoglobin, but instead carry a less effective type. In Canada and the United States, the most common types of sickle cell disease are hemoglobin SS disease (sickle cell anemia), hemoglobin SC disease, and hemoglobin sickle–β-thalassemia. Among the sickle cell diseases, sickle cell anemia is the most common and will be the focus of this discussion (Bryant, 2014a). It is most common in individuals of African, Mediterranean, Middle Eastern, and Indian decent. One in 400 African Americans has sickle cell anemia (Ambruso et al., 2014). Instead of Hgb AA, individuals with sickle cell anemia have Hgb SS. In hemoglobin S, glutamic acid is replaced with valine in the hemoglobin molecule. This results in an elongated RBC with a shortened life span. The elongated cell is more rigid than a normal cell and sickle shaped (Fig. 46.7). Persons with heterozygous representation (Hgb AS) are said to have sickle cell trait and are carriers for the disorder; about 8% of African Americans have sickle cell trait (Ambruso et al., 2014). Generally, persons with sickle cell trait have only minimal health problems.

FIGURE 46.7 This peripheral blood smear demonstrates the elongated sickle-shaped red blood cell seen in sickle cell disease.

FIGURE 46.12 Iron overload related to thalassemia leads to bony changes such as frontal bossing and maxillary prominence.

taken at home and any concerns that have arisen since the last visit. Inspect the skin, oral mucosa, conjunctivae, soles, and/or palms for pallor. Note icteric sclerae or jaundice of the skin. Measure weight and height (or length) and plot on an appropriate growth chart. Observe the child for bony deformities and frontal bossing (prominent forehead) (Fig. 46.12). Measure oxygen saturation via pulse oximetry. Evaluate neurologic status, determining level of consciousness and developmental abilities.

Laboratory testing may reveal the following:
- Hemoglobin and hematocrit are significantly decreased.
- Peripheral blood smear shows prominence of target cells, hypochromia, microcytosis, and extensive **anisocytosis** and **poikilocytosis** (variation in the size and shape of the RBCs, respectively).
- Bilirubin levels are elevated.
- Hgb electrophoresis shows the presence of Hgb F and Hgb A_2 only.
- Iron level is elevated.

NURSING MANAGEMENT

The nursing care of the child with thalassemia is primarily aimed at supporting and teaching the family to help minimizing the effects of the illness. This includes educating the family on transfusion therapy, vitamin supplementation, and medication therapy such as hydroxyurea and chelation therapy to prevent complications such as iron overload (Bryant, 2014b).

Administering Packed Red Blood Cell Transfusions.
Administer PRBC transfusions as prescribed to maintain an adequate level of hemoglobin for oxygen delivery to the tissues and to suppress erythrocytosis in the bone marrow. Monitor for reactions to the transfusions.

Excess iron (hemosiderosis) is removed by chelation therapy. Administer the chelating agent deferoxamine with the transfusion (Bryant, 2014b). Deferoxamine binds to the iron and allows it to be removed through the stool or urine. Oral deferasirox may also be prescribed and is generally well tolerated, with minimal gastrointestinal side effects.

Safety Check

GOAL: Improve the Accuracy of Patient Identification (Identify Patients Correctly)

Eliminate transfusion errors related to patient misidentification.

Steps: Always match the blood component to the order. Use a two-person independent verification process as determined by facility policy to match the patient to the blood component.

Educating the Family. Educate the child and family about the recommended regimen. Ensure that families understand that adhering to the prescribed blood transfusion and chelation therapy schedule is essential to the child's survival. Chelation therapy must be maintained at home to continuously decrease the iron levels in the body. Teach family members to administer deferoxamine exactly as their doctor or nurse practitioner prescribed (SickKids, 2017).

Refer the family for genetic counselling and family support as needed. A good resource for families of children with thalassemia is the Cooley's Anemia Foundation, a link to which can be found on thePoint. A group of young adults with Cooley anemia started the Thalassemia Action Group (TAG) (a subgroup of the Cooley's Anemia Foundation) to provide a forum for communication and information, promote a positive outlook on living with the disease, and raise awareness of the importance of continuing therapy for the disease.

Atraumatic Care

When a child is receiving blood transfusion every few weeks, he or she must experience at least two venipunctures each time, one for the type and cross-match and other relevant laboratory tests on the day before transfusion, and the intravenous (IV) insertion for the actual transfusion. Minimize trauma by teaching the parent to apply EMLA (eutectic mixture of local anesthetic) cream at home just before leaving for the blood draw or transfusion appointment.

Glucose-6-Phosphate Dehydrogenase Deficiency

Glucose-6-phosphate dehydrogenase (G6PD) is an enzyme that is responsible for maintaining the integrity of RBCs by protecting them from oxidative substances. G6PD deficiency is an X-linked recessive disorder that occurs when the RBCs have insufficient G6PD, or the enzyme is abnormal and does not function properly. The RBCs are then affected by oxidative stress more easily. Triggers that may result in oxidative stress and hemolysis include bacterial or viral illness or exposure to certain substances such as medications (e.g., sulphonamides, sulphones, malaria-fighting drugs [such as quinine], or methylene blue [for treating urinary tract infections]), naphthalene (an agent in mothballs), or fava beans.

G6PD deficiency occurs most commonly in children of African, Mediterranean, or Asian descent (Ambruso et al., 2014). Complications include prolonged neonatal jaundice and life-threatening acute episodes of hemolysis. Therapeutic management is primarily aimed at avoiding triggers that cause oxidative stress.

NURSING ASSESSMENT

Note health history, including fatigue. Determine the parents' understanding of the disorder and the medications and foods to avoid. Inspect the skin for pallor or jaundice. Evaluate neurologic status, which may also be affected. Measure heart rate and respiratory rate, noting elevations. Determine oxygen saturation via pulse oximeter or blood gas analysis. Note tea-coloured urine. Palpate the abdomen for splenomegaly. Laboratory studies will reveal anemia.

NURSING MANAGEMENT

Administer oxygen and treat the symptoms. Once the triggering agent is removed or the child recovers from an illness, the child will improve. Provide further education to the child and family about triggers and advise them that the child should avoid contact with these agents.

CLOTTING DISORDERS

Clotting of blood is a process that occurs after injury. The blood clotting system requires certain factors in the blood and platelets to perform adequately. Individuals with deficiencies of these factors or platelets tend to bleed; they do not bleed more easily than people without these conditions, but it is just more difficult for the clot to form, and bleeding cannot be stopped easily. Factors that are most often involved in problems with clotting include factor VIII, factor IX, and factor XI. Each plays a role in clot formation. Platelets also play a role in the clotting cascade and are necessary for clot formation. Some processes can lead to destruction of the platelets and may lead to a reduction in clotting. Bleeding

TABLE 46.5	CLOTTING STUDIES
Test	**Measure**
Prothrombin time (PT)	11.0–13.0 seconds (may vary by laboratory)
Partial thromboplastin time (PTT), activated partial thromboplastin time (aPTT)	21–35 seconds
International normalized ratio (INR) (used to evaluate coagulation)	2.0–3.0 usual target in thromboembolic conditions

Adapted from Fischbach, F. T., & Dunning, M. B. (2014). *A manual of laboratory and diagnostic tests* (9th ed.). Philadelphia, PA: Lippincott Williams & Wilkins.

times are prolonged when a clotting disorder is present. Table 46.5 provides usual values for clotting studies.

Conditions affecting clotting include idiopathic thrombocytopenia purpura (ITP), Henoch–Schönlein purpura, disseminated intravascular coagulation (DIC), and factor deficiencies such as hemophilia A (factor VIII deficiency), von Willebrand disease (vWD), hemophilia B (Christmas disease, factor IX deficiency), and hemophilia C (factor XI deficiency). Table 46.6 reviews the proteins involved in coagulation.

Idiopathic Thrombocytopenia Purpura

ITP is thought to be an immune response following a viral infection (e.g., chicken pox/upper respiratory tract infection) that produces antiplatelet antibodies. These antibodies destroy platelets, which then lead to the development of petechiae, purpura, and excessive bruising. **Petechiae** are pinpoint hemorrhages that occur anywhere on the body and do not blanch to pressure (Fig. 46.13). **Purpura** are larger areas of hemorrhage in which blood collects under the tissues; they are purplish (see Fig. 46.13). ITP usually develops a few weeks after a viral infection and is most common in young children (Ambruso et al., 2014). Within a few months, most children will recover spontaneously (Ambruso et al., 2014). Complications include severe hemorrhage and bleeding into vital organs and intracranial hemorrhage, although these rarely occur.

For children with platelet counts below 10,000 µL (10×10^9/L), corticosteroids may be administered for 2 to 3 weeks. In acute or chronic ITP, intravenous immunoglobulin (IVIG) may be used as an adjunct and is infused for 1 to 2 doses over 4 to 6 hours each (Ambruso et al., 2014), repeating platelet count after 24 hours to repeat dose if no improvement (Breakey, Kassam, Thampi, & Kirby, 2009).

parents that chemotherapy will be necessary. Monitor for side effects of chemotherapy (see the Nursing Process Overview section). Follow-up will include eye examinations every 3 to 6 months until age 6 and then annually to check for further tumour development. If the eye is enucleated, a prosthetic eye will be fitted several weeks after removal. Teach families use of the prosthetic eye; it does not require daily removal.

Provide parents with support and encouragement. Refer the family for genetic counselling. Children with a family history of retinoblastoma need ophthalmologic examination shortly after birth and routinely until ages 5 to 6 years (Kaufman, Kim, & Berry, 2016). Children with the heritable form of retinoblastoma should have genetic counselling as they reach puberty because of the risk of bilateral disease in their offspring (Kaufman et al., 2016).

 Take Note!

Educate parents about protecting vision in the remaining eye: routine eye check-ups, protection from accidental injury, use of safety goggles during sports, and prompt treatment of eye infections. Generally, children with one eye should not participate in contact sports.

SCREENING FOR REPRODUCTIVE CANCERS IN ADOLESCENTS

Increasingly, reproductive cancers are being diagnosed in adolescents. Cervical cancer and testicular cancer may be discovered early with appropriate screening, and earlier discovery leads to better outcomes. Starting screening in the teenage years may also instil a lifelong healthy habit in the adolescent.

Cervical Cancer

Risk factors for cervical cancer include young age at first intercourse, infection with a sexually transmitted disease, and a history of multiple sex partners. More and more teenagers are presenting with these risk factors.

Cervical cancer is most commonly attributed to human papillomavirus (HPV) (AAP, 2016). HPV vaccine (Gardasil) is recommended to be given as a three-vaccine series to all girls and boys beginning at ages 11 to 12 years (AAP, 2016). Despite the availability of the vaccine, not all girls and boys will receive it. Counsel all sexually active adolescents to seek reproductive care, which is available without parental consent in most states. The screening Papanicolaou (Pap) smear is efficient and reliable at determining abnormal cervical cells and is a key part of screening for cervical cancer (if cancer is present, the parent will have to be notified). Cervical cancer has a very high response to therapy and rate of cure if treated in its early stages. Therefore, encourage teenage girls to be responsible for their sexual health by seeking appropriate examination and screening.

Testicular Cancer

Although uncommon in teens, testicular cancer is the most frequently diagnosed cancer in males between 20 and 34 years of age (National Cancer Institute, n. d.). It is one of the most curable cancers if diagnosed early. To get into the habit of screening for testicular lumps, encourage adolescent boys to begin performing testicular self-examinations monthly (Teaching Guidelines 46.5).

Teaching Guidelines 46.5
TESTICULAR SELF-EXAMINATION

- Perform the examination once a month, after a shower.
- Be familiar with the size and weight of your testicles.
- Roll the testicle between your fingers. The small rope-like structure is the epididymis; this is normal.
- Report any lump, swelling, or heaviness of one testicle to your physician or nurse practitioner.

Adapted from Figueroa, T. E. (2012). *How to perform a testicular self-examination.* Retrieved from http://kidshealth.org/teen/sexual_health/guys/tse.html

---

NURSING CARE PLAN 46.1

Overview for the Child With an Alteration in Cellular Regulation

NURSING DIAGNOSIS: Fatigue related to decreased oxygen supply in the body as evidenced by lack of energy, increased sleep requirements, or decreased interest in play

Outcome Identification and Evaluation

Child will display increased endurance, desire to play without developing symptoms of exertion.

Overview for the Child With an Alteration in Cellular Regulation (continued)

Intervention: *Decreasing Fatigue*

- Cluster nursing care activities and plan for periods of rest before and after exertion *to decrease oxygen need and consumption.*
- Encourage activity or ambulation per physician's orders: *early mobilization results in better outcomes.*
- Observe child for signs of activity intolerance such as pallor, nausea, lightheadedness, or dizziness or changes in vital signs *to determine level of tolerance.*
- If child is on bed rest, perform range-of-motion exercises and frequent position changes: *negative changes to the musculoskeletal system occur quickly with inactivity and immobility.*
- Refer the child to physical therapy *for exercise prescription to increase skeletal muscle strength.*

NURSING DIAGNOSIS: Impaired physical mobility related to pain from sickle cell crisis or acute bleeds or imposed activity restrictions, as evidenced by guarding of painful extremity, resistance to activity

Outcome Identification and Evaluation

Child will be able to engage in activities within age parameters and limits of disease: child is able to move extremities, move about environment, and participate in exercise programs within limits of age and disease.

Interventions: *Promoting Physical Mobility*

- Encourage gross and fine motor activities as able within constraints of pain/bleed *to facilitate motor development.*
- Collaborate with physical therapy to strengthen muscles and promote mobility *to facilitate motor development.*
- Use passive and active range-of-motion (ROM) exercises and teach the child and family how to perform

them *to prevent contractures and facilitate joint mobility and muscle development (active ROM) to help increase mobility.*
- Praise accomplishments and emphasize child's abilities *to improve self-esteem and encourage feelings of confidence and competence.*

NURSING DIAGNOSIS: Ineffective health management related to knowledge and skill acquisition regarding nutritional and medical treatment of anemia, prevention of infection, home administration of intravenous clotting factors, or protection from injury as evidenced by new diagnosis and inability to verbalize appropriate treatment regimen or demonstrate medication administration skills

Outcome Identification and Evaluation

Child's health will be maintained: child will receive supplements, medications as prescribed, and will eat an appropriate diet.

Intervention: *Educating Parents About Effective Health Maintenance*

- Educate the family about iron-rich foods to be promoted in the child with iron-deficiency anemia and limited in the child with thalassemia.
- Limit cow's milk intake in the child with iron-deficiency anemia *to decrease risk of microscopic gastrointestinal (GI) bleeding and increase appetite for other foods.*

(continued)

NURSING CARE PLAN 46.1

Overview for the Child With an Alteration in Cellular Regulation (continued)

- Provide ongoing evaluation of nutritional intake *to ensure that appropriate dietary restrictions are followed.*
- Ensure that parents can verbalize understanding of home medication regimen: iron or folic acid supplementation for anemia, prophylactic antibiotics for sickle cell anemia, chelation for thalassemia, and factor replacement for hemophilia.
- Have parents provide return demonstration of subcutaneous infusion of deferoxamine or intravenous factor as appropriate *to ensure accuracy and independence in the home environment.*
- Educate families about when to call or visit physician or nurse practitioner *to ensure timely intervention when signs and symptoms develop.*

NURSING DIAGNOSIS: Anxiety related to diagnostic testing as evidenced by parent verbalization, child resistance, or crying with procedures

Outcome Identification and Evaluation

Child's anxiety will be minimized: child will verbalize less fear, experience less pain with procedures.

Intervention: *Relieving Anxiety*

- Use topical anesthetic creams or agents for nonemergency laboratory draws to decrease stress related *to needlesticks or venipunctures.*
- Maintain a quiet and calm environment *to reduce the child's stress.*
- Educate the child, as appropriate, and the family regarding the need for laboratory specimens *to alleviate anxiety related to the unknown.*

- Identify the need for the specific test and explain the procedure before obtaining the specimen *to decrease the anxiety and time required for the procedure.*
- Provide developmentally appropriate activities for the child: *activities can reduce stress and also provide stimulus for children; serves as a model for the family.*

NURSING DIAGNOSIS: Compromised family coping related to hospitalization of child or chronic, possibly life-threatening genetic disorder as evidenced by excessive tearfulness or denial statements, withdrawal, or verbalization of inadequate coping skills

Outcome Identification and Evaluation

Child and/or family will demonstrate adequate coping skills, will verbalize feeling supported and demonstrate healthy family interactions.

Intervention: *Promoting Effective Family Coping*

- Provide emotional support to the child and family *to improve coping abilities.*
- Actively listen to the child's and family's concerns *to validate their feelings and establish trust.*
- Encourage parents to talk about their child and the illness *to bring feelings out in the open.*
- Validate feelings of guilt, shock, frustration, resentment, or depression *to promote trust and begin appropriate coping.*

- Provide open communication with the child and siblings: *children appreciate honesty about their illness, and coping is improved.*
- Refer families to community resources such as parent support groups and grief counselling *to improve coping abilities.*
- Encourage role-playing and play activities *to identify the child's fears and work through feelings.*

NURSING CARE PLAN 46.1

Overview for the Child With an Alteration in Cellular Regulation (continued)

NURSING DIAGNOSIS: Risk for injury related to alteration in peripheral sensory perception, decreased platelet count, deficient coagulation factor, or excessive iron load

Outcome Identification and Evaluation

Child will not experience hemorrhage: will experience decreased bruising or episodes of prolonged bleeding.

Intervention: *Preventing Injury*

- Assess for petechiae, purpura, bruising, or bleeding to provide baseline data for comparison; if present, may warrant intervention.
- Encourage quiet activities or play to avoid trauma with active play.
- Avoid rectal temperatures and examinations. Post sign at head of bed "no rectal temperatures or medications" to avoid rectal mucosa damage resulting in bleeding.

- Avoid intramuscular injections and lumbar puncture if possible to decrease risk of bleeding from a puncture site.
- If bone marrow aspiration must be performed, apply pressure dressing to site to prevent bleeding.
- Teach families about preferred physical activities for the child with idiopathic thrombocytopenia purpura (ITP) or hemophilia to provide safe physical activities and decrease risk for injury.

NURSING DIAGNOSIS: Risk for infection related to neutropenia and immunosuppression

Outcome Identification and Evaluation

Child will not experience overwhelming infection: *will be free from infection or able to recover if he or she becomes infected.*

Interventions: *Preventing Infection*

- Assess for fever, pain, cough, tachypnea, adventitious breath sounds, skin ulceration, stomatitis, and perirectal fissures *to identify potential infection.*
- Administer antibiotics for temperature greater than 38.4°C *to decrease likelihood of overwhelming sepsis.*
- Maintain meticulous handwashing procedures (including family, visitors, staff) *to minimize spread of infectious organisms.*
- Maintain isolation as prescribed *to minimize exposure to infectious organisms.*
- Avoid rectal temperatures and examinations, intramuscular injections, and urinary catheterization when child is neutropenic *to decrease the possibility of introducing microorganisms.*
- Educate family and visitors that child should be restricted from contact with known infectious exposures (in hospital and at home) *to encourage cooperation with infection control.*
- Strictly observe medical asepsis *to avoid unintentional introduction of microorganisms.*
- Promote nutrition and appropriate rest *to maximize body's potential to heal.*
- Inform family to contact the physician or nurse practitioner if child has known exposure to chickenpox or measles *so that preventive measures (e.g., varicella zoster immunoglobulin [VZIG]) can be taken.*
- Administer vaccines (not live) as prescribed (after clearance with oncologist) *to prevent common childhood communicable diseases.*
- Teach family to monitor for fever at home and report temperature elevations to oncologist immediately *so that antibiotic therapy may be instituted as soon as possible.*

(continued)

Overview for the Child With an Alteration in Cellular Regulation (continued)

NURSING DIAGNOSIS: Acute pain related to invasive diagnostic testing, surgical procedure, neuropathy, disease progression, or adverse effects of treatment as evidenced by verbalization of pain, elevated pain scale ratings, guarding, withdrawal from play or refusal to participate in activities of daily living, or physiologic indicators such as elevated heart rate, diaphoresis, muscle tension, or rigidity

Outcome Identification and Evaluation

Child will demonstrate pain relief *in amount sufficient to allow participation in play, activities of daily living, or therapeutic interventions. Use the age-appropriate pain scale to set the goal and set a time frame for achievement of the goal.*

Interventions: *Promoting Comfort*

- Determine level of pain using child interview, pain scale, and assessment of physiologic variables *to determine baseline.*
- Document location, intensity, and description of pain to *determine baseline.*
- Discuss with the child and parent techniques that have helped alleviate pain in the past *to incorporate successful interventions into the plan of care.*
- Administer acetaminophen for mild pain: *avoid salicylate and NSAIDs due to increased risk for bleeding.*
- Administer medications as ordered using the least invasive method possible *to avoid pain (intramuscular, subcutaneous, and rectal route should be avoided in the child with thrombocytopenia).*
- Monitor frequently for adverse effects (particularly respiratory effects) of opioid analgesics, *as opioids*

- *reduce responsiveness of carbon dioxide receptors in the brain's respiratory centre.*
- Use nonpharmacologic measures such as play therapy, games, TV, guided breathing, imagery, hypnosis, or meditation as appropriate: *distracts child's attention from the pain.*
- Use massage, positioning, or heat *to relieve pain in a particular area.*
- Use EMLA before needlesticks and conscious sedation with lumbar puncture and bone marrow aspiration *to reduce recurrent acute painful episodes associated with frequent blood draws and diagnostic/treatment procedures.*
- Have the child lie flat for 30 minutes after a lumbar puncture and increase fluid intake for 24 hours after the procedure *to decrease incidence of headache.*

NURSING DIAGNOSIS: Impaired oral mucous membrane integrity related to chemotherapy, radiation therapy, immunocompromise, decreased platelet count, malnutrition, or dehydration as evidenced by oral lesions, ulcers, plaques, hyperemia or bleeding, difficulty eating or swallowing, or complaint of oral discomfort

Outcome Identification and Evaluation

Child will maintain intact, moist mucosa *free from redness, ulceration, or debris.*

Interventions: *Restoring Healthy Oral Mucosa*

- Frequently assess oral cavity for redness, lesions, ulcers, plaques, or bleeding *to provide baseline for comparison and identify alterations early.*
- Offer ice chips frequently while child is NPO *to maintain hydration of mucosa.*
- Use only a soft toothbrush or toothette for dental care, avoiding excessive pressure with brushing, *to decrease incidence of bleeding with mouth care.*
- Keep lips lubricated with petroleum jelly or fragrance-free lip balm *to maintain moist, hydrated lips.*
- Rinse with salt solution or mouthwash every 1 to 2 hours *to keep oral cavity clean and moist.*

- Administer glutamine and/or β-carotene supplements, *which have been shown to decrease the incidence and severity of mucositis.*
- Have child swish and spit 1:1 Benadryl/Maalox solution *to decrease pain.*
- Administer antifungal solution *to prevent or treat oral candidiasis.*
- Avoid spicy, acidic, or very hot or very cold foods *to decrease pain.*
- Administer pain medication (usually acetaminophen or codeine) as ordered *to decrease pain.*

Overview for the Child With an Alteration in Cellular Regulation (continued)

NURSING DIAGNOSIS: Nausea related to adverse effects of chemotherapy or radiation therapy as evidenced by verbalization of nausea, increased salivation, swallowing movements, or vomiting

Outcome Identification and Evaluation

Child will experience decreased nausea: *will verbalize symptom relief and will be free from vomiting.*

Interventions: *Alleviating Nausea and Vomiting*

- Administer antiemetics prior to chemotherapy and as needed thereafter *to decrease frequency of nausea.*
- Assess frequency of vomiting and level of hydration *to provide baseline data and recognize alterations early.*
- Offer frequent, smaller meals or snacks: *smaller amounts are less likely to be vomited.*
- Avoid spicy foods *to avoid stomach upset.*

- Allow bubbles to dissipate from carbonated beverages before they are ingested: *carbonation may contribute to nausea.*
- Remove cover from meal tray before entering child's room: *this will allow the food odour to dissipate outside of the room; food odours may trigger nausea and vomiting.*

NURSING DIAGNOSIS: Imbalanced nutrition: less than body requirements related to anorexia, nausea, vomiting, or mucosal irritation associated with chemotherapy or radiation as evidenced by decreased oral intake and weight, length/height, and/or body mass index (BMI) below average for age or individual child's usual measures

Outcome Identification and Evaluation

Child will improve nutritional intake, resulting in *steady increase in weight and length/height.*

Interventions: *Promoting Adequate Nutrition*

- Determine body weight and length/height norm for age or find out what the child's pretreatment measurements were *to determine goal to work toward.*
- Determine child's food preferences and provide favourite foods as able *to increase the likelihood that the child will consume adequate amounts of foods.*
- Administer antiemetics as ordered *to increase the likelihood that the child will retain the food he or she ingests.*
- Weigh child daily or weekly (according to physician order or institutional standard) and measure length/height weekly *to monitor for growth.*

- Offer highest-calorie meals at the time of day when the child's appetite is the greatest *to increase likelihood of increased caloric intake.*
- Provide increased-calorie shakes or puddings within diet restriction: *high-calorie foods increase weight gain.*
- Administer vitamin and mineral supplements as prescribed *to attain/maintain vitamin and mineral balance in the body.*
- Administer total parenteral nutrition and intravenous lipids as ordered *to provide adequate nutrition for healing.*

NURSING DIAGNOSIS: Constipation related to effects of vinca alkaloids, opioid use, decreased activity, and dietary changes as evidenced by hard stool or stool that is difficult to pass

Outcome Identification and Evaluation

Child's bowel function will return to usual pattern: *child will pass a formed, soft stool every day (or modify this criterion according to child's usual pattern).*

(continued)

NURSING CARE PLAN 46.1

Overview for the Child With an Alteration in Cellular Regulation (continued)

Interventions: *Preventing or Managing Constipation*

- Ensure that child increases fluid intake to provide enough water in the intestines for soft stool formation.
- Increase fibre in the diet to provide bulk for stool formation.
- Administer stool softeners such as mineral oil or docusate sodium: these help soften the stool, aiding in passage.

- Provide motivator laxatives such as magnesium hydroxide, lactulose, or sorbitol to stimulate stool passage.
- Use stimulant laxatives such as senna or bisacodyl only intermittently rather than on a daily basis to avoid dependency and diarrhea.

NURSING DIAGNOSIS: Diarrhea related to effects of radiation therapy as evidenced by loose or watery stools, possibly frequent

Child's bowel function will return to usual pattern: child will pass a formed, soft stool daily (or modify this criterion according to child's usual pattern).

Interventions: *Managing Diarrhea*

- Assess frequency of diarrhea and level of hydration *to provide data about severity.*
- Obtain weight daily on same scale *to determine extent of fluid loss.*
- Maintain accurate intake and output records *to determine extent of fluid loss.*
- Administer oral rehydration solutions or intravenous fluids as ordered *to maintain or restore adequate hydration.*
- Restrict roughage and residue in diet *to decrease likelihood of diarrhea.*
- Avoid milk products during acute diarrheal phase: *lactose often worsens diarrhea.*
- Provide an elemental diet to relieve symptoms: *absorbed in the upper small bowel.*
- Provide meticulous perineal care *to avoid skin breakdown related to frequent or loose stools.*
- Administer antidiarrheal medications if ordered *to decrease frequency of stools.*
- If severe and related to radiation therapy, a 3- to 4-day rest period from radiation may be required *to begin recovery of normal absorptive capabilities of bowel.*

NURSING DIAGNOSIS: Risk for impaired skin integrity related to radiation therapy

Outcome Identification and Evaluation

Child's skin will remain intact: *areas of redness in radiation field will not progress to desquamation.*

Interventions: *Promoting Skin Integrity*

- Assess skin frequently for erythema, erosions, ulcers, or blisters *to provide baseline data and intervene early if skin is impaired.*
- Use a mild soap for cleansing and pat dry rather than rubbing *to avoid skin irritation.*
- Use aloe vera lotion *to moisturize the skin.*
- Avoid perfumed lotions, soaps, heat, cold, or sun, *as these will further irritate the skin in the irradiated area.*

- Do not scrub ink from marked radiation field, and avoid adhesive tape in that area, *to avoid further skin irritation.*
- Administer diphenhydramine or apply hydrocortisone 1% cream *to reduce itching and urge to scratch.*
- For areas of desquamation related to radiation, apply Silvadene cream once or twice a day *to hasten skin repair.*

NURSING CARE PLAN 46.1

Overview for the Child With an Alteration in Cellular Regulation (continued)

NURSING DIAGNOSIS: Activity intolerance related to treatment adverse effects, anemia, or generalized weakness as evidenced by verbalization of weakness or fatigue; elevation of heart rate, respiratory rate, or blood pressure with activity; complaint of shortness of breath with play or activity

Outcome Identification and Evaluation

Child will display increased activity tolerance: desire to play without developing symptoms of exertion.

Interventions: *Promoting Activity*

- Encourage activity or ambulation per physician's orders: *early mobilization results in better outcomes.*
- Observe child for symptoms of activity intolerance such as pallor, nausea, lightheadedness or dizziness, or changes in vital signs *to determine level of tolerance.*
- If child is on bed rest, perform range-of-motion exercises and frequent position changes: *negative changes to the musculoskeletal system occur quickly with inactivity and immobility.*
- Cluster nursing care activities and plan for periods of rest before and after exertion *to decrease oxygen need and consumption.*
- Refer the child to physical therapy *for exercise prescription to increase skeletal muscle strength.*

NURSING DIAGNOSIS: Disturbed body image related to hair loss as evidenced by verbalization of dissatisfaction with appearance

Outcome Identification and Evaluation

Child or adolescent will display appropriate body image: *will look at self in mirror and participate in social activities.*

Interventions: *Promoting Body Image*

- Acknowledge the child's feelings of anger over body changes and illness: *venting feelings is associated with less body image disturbance.*
- Encourage the child or teen to choose a wig or hats and scarves *to involve the child in making decisions about appearance.*
- Support the child's or teen's choices of comfortable, fashionable clothing *to disguise weight loss or scarring while promoting self-esteem.*
- Involve the child in the decision-making process, *as a sense of control will improve body image.*
- Encourage the child to spend time with peers who have experienced hair, limb, or weight loss, *as peers' opinions are often better accepted than those of persons in authority, such as parents or health care professionals.*

NURSING DIAGNOSIS: Risk for situational low self-esteem related to loss of control and inability to progress with quest for independence (adolescents)

Outcome Identification and Evaluation

Adolescent will maintain or increase self-esteem: *will display increased coping responses and verbalize control as appropriate as well as discuss plans for future.*

(continued)

Overview for the Child With an Alteration in Cellular Regulation (continued)

Interventions: *Promoting Self-Esteem*

- Identify the adolescent's positive abilities *to promote self-esteem.*
- Give genuine and honest positive feedback, *as the child or adolescent desires honesty.*
- Explore strengths and weaknesses with the adolescent: *helps the teen to see similarities and differences with healthy peers of the same age.*
- Encourage the teen to perform self-care as possible *to promote independence.*

- Offer emotional support: *reduces psychological distress and increases coping abilities.*
- Encourage participation in a support group *to allow teens to discuss body changes and the reactions they perceive in others.*
- When the adolescent is physically able, encourage attendance at camp or an adventure/wilderness event: *these programs have been shown to improve mental health and coping skills.*

NURSING DIAGNOSIS: Compromised family coping related to potentially life-threatening illness and stressors involved with cancer treatment

Outcome Identification and Evaluation

Child and/or family will demonstrate adequate coping skills: will verbalize feeling supported and demonstrate healthy family interactions.

Interventions: *Promoting Child and Family Coping*

- Provide emotional support to the child and family: *improves coping abilities.*
- Actively listen to the child's and family's concerns: *validates their feelings and establishes trust.*
- Provide open communication with the child and siblings: *children appreciate honesty about their illness, and coping is improved.*
- Refer families to community resources such as parent support groups and grief counselling: *such support improves coping abilities.*
- Give terminally ill children permission to discuss their feelings about their illness, *allowing them to conquer fears and express love for their family and friends.*
- Encourage families to be honest with siblings about the treatment and prognosis of the child with cancer: *children often sense what is going on and cope better when they are prepared and are given an honest explanation of events.*
- Prepare siblings for the death of the child with cancer, using the child life specialist and chaplain as necessary: *the bereavement period is eased when siblings are prepared.*

NURSING DIAGNOSIS: Grief related to diagnosis of cancer in a child and impending loss of child as evidenced by crying, disbelief of diagnosis, and expressions of grief

Outcome Identification and Evaluation

Family will express feelings of grief: *seek help in dealing with feelings, plan for future one day at the time.*

Intervention: *Supporting the Grieving Family*

- Use therapeutic communication with open-ended questions to encourage an open and trusting relationship for better communication.
- Actively listen to the family's expression of grief: *just being present and listening conveys support.*

NURSING CARE PLAN 46.1

Overview for the Child With an Alteration in Cellular Regulation (continued)

- Encourage the family to cry and express feelings away from the child to work through feelings, but also be mindful that not all families will adopt or wish to use this approach.
- Assess for spiritual distress, spiritualist as a protective factor and refer the family to their support network. Consider how an elder and community may wish to be involved to support the child and family.
- Educate the family about the child's condition honestly: knowing what is going on, what is to be expected, and what the treatment plan is gives the family a sense of control.
- Support the family through discussions with the child about anticipated death when the illness is deemed terminal.

KEY CONCEPTS

- The major forms of anemia affecting children are iron-deficiency anemia, lead poisoning, folic acid deficiency, pernicious anemia, sickle cell anemia, thalassemia, and G6PD deficiency.

- The major bleeding disorders affecting children are idiopathic thrombocytopenic purpura, Henoch–Schönlein purpura, DIC, and hemophilia and vWD.

- Childhood cancer tends to develop from embryonal tissue; in general, it is more responsive to therapy than adult cancers, which tend to be derived from epithelial tissue.

- In adults, cancer is influenced to a large extent by environmental factors. Cancer in children is most often not attributed to environmental factors, so generally there are no routine screening measures or prevention strategies for childhood cancer.

- The pain associated with lumbar puncture or bone marrow aspiration may be minimized with the use of topical anesthetics or conscious sedation.

- CT scans and MRI are used extensively in the diagnosis and follow-up of childhood cancer. The young child may have difficulty holding still for these scans and may need short-term sedation.

- Assess for hypoxia, fatigue, and pallor in the child with anemia.

- Nursing assessment for the child with a bleeding disorder focuses on determining its extent and severity.

- Supplementation with iron is the key intervention for the child with iron-deficiency anemia.

- All young children should be screened for lead exposure.

- Prevention of infection and vaso-occlusive episodes takes priority in children with sickle cell anemia.

- Multimodal pain management and astute physical assessment for serious complications are critical in the nursing care of the child having a sickle cell crisis.

- The priority intervention for management of thalassemia is chronic transfusion of PRBCs and chelation of iron.

- Idiopathic thrombocytopenic purpura and Henoch–Schönlein purpura are usually self-limiting diseases.

- Administration of factor VII or desmopressin is the key nursing intervention when a bleeding episode occurs in the child with hemophilia or vWD.

- Significant anemia may result in hypoxia to the tissues.

- Prolonged bleeding times place the child at risk for hemorrhage.

- Prevention of injury is key for all children with hematologic disorders. Leukemia often presents in children with a history of fever, infection, and fatigue. Bone pain or CNS symptoms may be present if metastasis to the bone or brain has occurred.

- Lymphomas in children present similarly to those in adults, often with an enlarged, nontender lymph node.

- Symptoms of brain tumours depend on the location of the tumour; commonly they present with signs and symptoms of increased intracranial pressure, such as headache, nausea, and vomiting.

Kaufman, P. L., Kim, J., & Berry, J. L. (2016). *Overview of retinoblastoma*. Retrieved from http://www.uptodate.com/contents/overview-of-retinoblastoma

Kids Cancer Care (n.d.). *Childhood cancer care*. Retrieved from http://www.kidscancercare.ab.ca/childhood-cancer/stats

Kline, N. (2011). General cancer overview: Cancer cell characteristics. In N. E. Kline (Ed.). *The pediatric chemotherapy and biotherapy curriculum* (3rd ed.). Glenview, IL: Association of Pediatric Hematology/Oncology Nurses.

Kline, N. (2014a). *Essentials of pediatric oncology nursing: A core curriculum* (4th ed.). Chicago, IL: Association of Pediatric Hematology/Oncology Nurses.

Kline, N. (2014b). Hematology: Von Willebrand disease. In N. E. Kline & R. Bryant (Eds.). *Essentials of pediatric hematology/oncology nursing: A core curriculum* (4th ed., pp. 516–521). Chicago, IL: Association of Pediatric Hematology/Oncology Nurses.

Kristovich, K. M., & Callard, E. (2010). Bone marrow transplantation. In P. J. Allen, J. A. Vessey, & N. A. Schapiro (Eds.). *Primary care of the child with a chronic condition* (5th ed.). St. Louis, MO: Mosby.

Lahl, M. (2014). Pediatric cancers: Hodgkin lymphoma. In N. E. Kline (Ed.). *Essentials of pediatric hematology/oncology nursing: A core curriculum* (4th ed., pp. 39–44). Chicago, IL: Association of Pediatric Hematology/Oncology Nurses.

Laing, C. M., & Moules, N. J. (2016). "It's not Just Camp!" Understanding the meaning of children's Cancer Camps for Children and Families. *Journal of Pediatric Oncology Nursing, 33*(1), 33–44. doi: 10.1177/1043454214563934

Lee, D. A., & Hurwitz, R. L. (2016). *Childhood lead poisoning: Exposure and prevention*. Retrieved from http://www.uptodate.com/contents/childhood-lead-poisoning-exposure-and-prevention

Mahoney, D. H. (2015). *Iron deficiency in infants and young children: Treatment*. Retrieved from http://www.uptodate.com/contents/iron-deficiency-in-infants-and-young-children-treatment

Mahoney, D. H. (2016). Iron deficiency in infants and young children: Screening, prevention, clinical manifestations, and diagnosis. Retrieved from http://www.uptodate.com/contents/iron-deficiency-in-infants-andyoung-children-screening-prevention-clinical-manifestations-and-diagnosis

McCarthy, K. (2014). Pediatric cancers: Leukemia. In N. E. Kline (Ed.). *Essentials of pediatric hematology/oncology nursing: A core curriculum* (4th ed., pp. 25–32). Chicago, IL: Association of Pediatric Hematology/Oncology Nurses.

Morrissey, L. (2014). Side effects of treatment: Impairment of the immune system. In N. E. Kline & C. Nixon (Eds.). *Essentials of pediatric hematology/oncology nursing: A core curriculum* (4th ed., pp. 203–207). Chicago, IL: Association of Pediatric Hematology/Oncology Nurses.

Mosadegh, S. (2014). Patient and family education: Family education. In N. Kline (Ed.). *Essentials of pediatric hematology/oncology nursing: A core curriculum* (4th ed., pp. 353–356). Chicago, IL: Association of Pediatric Hematology/Oncology Nurses.

Moules, N. J., Estefan, A., McCaffrey, G., Tapp, D. M., & Strother, D. (2016). Differences and trading: Examining the effects of childhood cancer on the parental subsystem-Part 1. *Journal of Family Nursing, 22*(4), 515–539. doi: 10.1177/1074840716668102

National Cancer Institute. (n.d.). *SEER stat fact sheets: Testis cancer*. Retrieved from http://seer.cancer.gov/statfacts/html/testis.html

National Cancer Institute. (2016). *Pediatric supportive care (PDQ®)—health professional version*. Retrieved from http://www.cancer.gov/types/childhood-cancers/pediatric-care-hp-pdq#section/all

National Heart, Lung, and Blood Institute. (2014). *Evidence-based management of sickle cell disease: Expert panel report, 2014*. Bethesda, MD: Author.

National Heart, Lung, and Blood Institute. (2015). *Living with sickle cell disease*. Retrieved from https://www.nhlbi.nih.gov/health/health-topics/topics/sca/livingwith

Norville, R., & Staton, S. (2014). Childhood cancer treatment: Hematopoietic stem-cell transplantation. In N. E. Kline & C. Nixon (Eds.). *Essentials of pediatric hematology/oncology nursing: A core curriculum* (4th ed., pp. 160–180). Chicago, IL: Association of Pediatric Hematology/Oncology Nurses.

Norville, R., & Tomlinson, D. (2010). Hematopoietic stem cell transplantation. In D. Tomlinson & N. E. Kline (Eds.). *Pediatric oncology nursing*. New York: Springer.

Nuuhiwa, J. (2014). Care of the terminally ill child and the family: Physical care of the terminally ill child. In N. E. Kline (Ed.). *Essentials of pediatric hematology/oncology nursing: A core curriculum* (4th ed., pp. 368–374). Chicago, IL: Association of Pediatric Hematology/Oncology Nurses.

O'Brien Shea, J. (2014). Hematology: Bone-marrow-failure syndromes. In N. E. Kline & R. Bryant (Eds.). *Essentials of pediatric hematology/oncology nursing: A core curriculum* (4th ed., pp. 476–484). Chicago, IL: Association of Pediatric Hematology/Oncology Nurses.

Pitts, R. H., & Record, E. O. (2010). Sickle cell disease. In P. J. Allen, J. A. Vessey, & N. A. Schapiro (Eds.). *Primary care of the child with a chronic condition* (5th ed.). St. Louis, MO: Mosby.

Scheinemann, K. (2017). Grandparents: A hardly recognized part of the childhood cancer family. *Pediatric Blood and Cancer, 64*(1), 9–10. doi: 10.1002/pbc.26229.

Shields, C. L. (2008). Forget-me-nots in the care of children with retinoblastoma. *Seminars in Ophthalmology, 23*(5), 324–334.

SickKids. (2017). *Aboutkidshealth: Deferoxamine*. Retrieved from http://www.aboutkidshealth.ca/En/HealthAZ/Drugs/Pages/Deferoxamine.aspx

Taketomo, C. K., Hodding, J. H., & Kraus, D. M. (2013). *Pediatric & neonatal dosage handbook* (20th ed.). Hudson, OH: Lexicomp.

Toomey, C. (2014). Childhood cancer treatment: Chemotherapy. In N. E. Kline & C. Nixon (Eds.). *Essentials of pediatric hematology/oncology nursing: A core curriculum* (4th ed., pp. 109–111). Chicago, IL: Association of Paediatric Hematology/Oncology Nurses.

Verhovsek, M., & Simpson, E. (2015). *Consensus statement on the care of patients with sickle cell disease in Canada*. Retrieved from http://www.sicklecelldisease.ca/pdf/CAN-HAEM-Consensus-Statement-for-SCD-Guide2015_v10.pdf

Wachtel, S., Mckee, G., Harding, J., Suthermaraj, G., & Kosatsky, T. (2017). *Managing risks to children's health from lead in drinking water in British Columbia's day-*

cares and school. BC Centre for Disease Control. Retrieved from http://www.bccdc.ca/resource-gallery/Documents/Guidelines%20and%20Forms/Guidelines%20and%20Manuals/Health-Environment/Lead%20in%20BC%20schools%20and%20daycares.pdf

Watral, M. A. (2014a). Pediatric cancers: Central nervous system tumors. In N. E. Kline (Ed.). *Essentials of pediatric hematology/oncology nursing: A core curriculum* (4th ed., pp. 44–50). Chicago, IL: Association of Pediatric Hematology/Oncology Nurses.

Watral, M. A. (2014b). Pediatric cancers: Neuroblastoma. In N. E. Kline (Ed.). *Essentials of pediatric hematology/oncology nursing: A core curriculum* (4th ed., pp. 50–58).

Chicago, IL: Association of Pediatric Hematology/Oncology Nurses.

Werther, N. (2014). Side effects of treatment: Bone-marrow suppression. In N. E. Kline & C. Nixon (Eds.). *Essentials of pediatric hematology/oncology nursing: A core curriculum* (4th ed., pp. 200–203). Chicago, IL: Association of Pediatric Hematology/Oncology Nurses.

Zupanec, S. (2010). *Lymphoma.* In D. Tomlinson & N. E. Kline (Eds.). *Pediatric oncology nursing.* New York: Springer.

Zupanec, S., & Tomlinson, D. (2010). Leukemia. In D. Tomlinson & N. E. Kline (Eds.). *Pediatric oncology nursing.* New York: Springer.

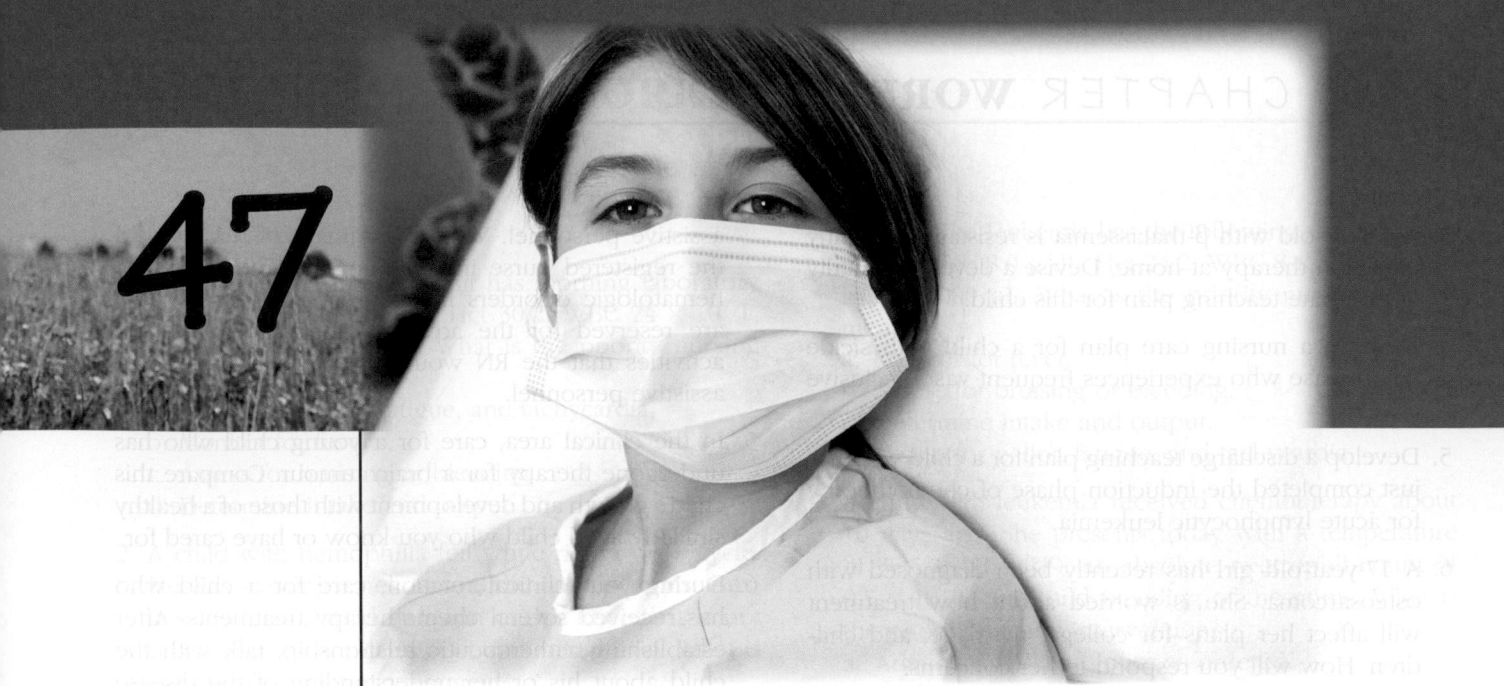

47

Nursing Care of the Child With an Alteration in Immunity or Immunologic Disorder

KEY TERMS

antibodies
antigen
autoantibodies
cellular immunity
chemotaxis
graft-versus-host
  disease
humoral immunity
immunodeficiency
immunoglobulins
immunosuppressive
opsonization
phagocytosis

Learning Objectives

Upon completion of the chapter, the learner will be able to:

1. Explain anatomic and physiologic differences of the immune system in infants and children versus adults.

2. Describe nursing care related to common laboratory and diagnostic testing used in the medical diagnosis of pediatric immune and autoimmune disorders.

3. Distinguish immune, autoimmune, and allergic disorders common in infants, children, and adolescents.

4. Identify appropriate nursing assessments and interventions related to medications and treatments for pediatric immune, autoimmune, and allergic disorders.

5. Develop an individualized nursing care plan for the child with an immune or autoimmune disorder.

6. Describe the psychosocial impact of chronic immune disorders on children.

7. Devise a nutrition plan for the child with immunodeficiency.

8. Develop child/family teaching plans for the child with an immune or autoimmune disorder.

Lakeisha Harris, 15 years old, is brought to the clinic by her mother. She presents with complaints of pain and swelling in her joints, weight gain, and fatigue. Lakeisha states, "I'm just very tired all the time, and my knees and ankles ache."

🔆 **Immunity** refers to natural or induced resistance to infection. Nurses may encounter children with alterations in immunity and should be familiar with various immunologic disorders that children experience. **Immunodeficiency** (incapacity to mount an appropriate immune response), autoimmune, and allergic disorders have a significant impact on the lives of affected children. Infants and children are exposed to many infectious microorganisms and allergens and thus need a functional immune system to protect themselves. Temporary immune deficiencies may follow a common viral infection, surgery, or blood transfusion, and may also be caused by malnutrition or the use of certain medications (Atkinson, Wolfe, & Hamborsky, 2012). In addition, an emerging area of study is the impact of maternal prenatal stress on the foetus. For example, stress plays a role in lowering infant fecal sIgA levels, which are important for immune maturation in early life (Kang, 2017). Temporary immune depression resolves over a period of time. Primary and secondary immune deficiencies are the focus of this chapter, along with allergy and anaphylaxis. These immune disorders are chronic, and affected children have more infections compared with healthy children. Recurrent viral or bacterial infections may cause the child to miss significant amounts of school or playtime with other children. Many immunodeficiencies require chronic and frequent clinic visits as well as daily medications. This can be a stress on the family as well. Autoimmune disorders are also chronic, causing significant disruption to the child's and family's life. Allergic disorders in some children may cause significant stress for the child and family. Nurses who care for children need to be familiar with common immunodeficiencies, autoimmune disorders, and allergies to intervene effectively with children and their families.

VARIATIONS IN PEDIATRIC ANATOMY AND PHYSIOLOGY

Normal immune function is a complex process involving **phagocytosis** (process by which phagocytes swallow up and break down microorganisms), **humoral immunity** (immunity mediated by antibodies secreted by B-cells), **cellular immunity** (cell-mediated immunity controlled by T-cells), and activation of the complement system. The lymphatic system and the white blood cells (WBCs) are the primary players in the immune response. Though these structures and cells are present at birth, the healthy full-term infant's immune system is still immature. The newborn exhibits a decreased inflammatory response to invading organisms, and this increases his or her susceptibility to infection. Cellular immunity is generally functional at birth, and as the infant is exposed to various substances over time, humoral immunity develops. Comparison Chart 47.1 provides more information on humoral and cellular immunity.

Lymph System

Lymph nodes in the newborn are widely distributed, relatively small, soft, and difficult to palpate. As the infant is exposed to various germs or illnesses, the lymph system passively filters plasma for bacteria or other foreign material before returning it to the bloodstream and back to the heart. As WBCs infiltrate the lymph nodes to attack the foreign substance, the nodes enlarge. Young children have frequent episodes of localized enlarged lymph nodes because of their repeated exposure to viral illnesses (Tosi, 2014). The spleen is functional at birth and also filters the blood for foreign cells. The thymus, responsible for the production of lymphocyte T-cells as well as for the development and maturation of peripheral lymphoid tissue, is quite enlarged at birth and remains so until about 10 years of age. It then involutes slowly throughout adulthood. The tonsils are also often enlarged throughout early childhood. The bone marrow is functional at birth, producing stem cells capable of differentiating into various blood cells.

Phagocytosis

Under conditions of stress, the newborn and infant exhibit decreased phagocytic activity. The complement system, which is responsible for **opsonization** (process

COMPARISON CHART 47.1	HUMORAL VERSUS CELLULAR IMMUNITY
Humoral Immunity (Antibody Protection)	**Cellular Immunity (Cell-Mediated Immune Response)**
• Lymphocytes: B-cells	• Lymphocytes: T-cells
• Secrete antibodies to viruses and bacteria	• Do not recognize antigens
• Recognize antigens	• Direct and regulate immune response (helper T-cells)
• Antibodies mark the antigen cell for destruction	• Attack infected or foreign cells (killer T-cells and natural killer cells)
• Do not destroy the foreign cell	• Do not cross the placenta
• Crosses the placenta in the form of IgG	

of making microorganisms more susceptible to phagocytosis) and **chemotaxis** (movement of neutrophils toward microorganisms), is immature in the newborn but reaches adult levels of activity by 3 to 6 months of age. The infant's phagocytic cells (neutrophils and monocytes) demonstrate decreased chemotaxis, reaching adult levels when the child is several years old. With complement levels being only 50% to 75% of adult levels in the full-term infant, decreased opsonization may be responsible for decreased phagocytic activity compared with adults.

Cellular Immunity

Maternal lymphocytes do not normally cross the placenta; therefore T-cell–mediated immunity is not passed to the infant (Marchant & Goldman, 2005). The infant has a higher WBC (leukocytosis) compared to adults and high turnover rate, possibly up to 2 to 5 years of age (Marchant & Goldman, 2005). Breastfeeding may bolster the immature immune system since breast milk contains various levels of immunological factors including lactoferrin, lysozyme, cytokines, and maternal leukocytes (Hassiotou & Geddes, 2015). Elevated lymphocytosis in infancy is likely a consequence of infection, dehydration, excessive thyroid hormone, or associated with an underlying syndrome (Zafar et al., 2017). Viral infection, hyperbilirubinemia, bone marrow failure, and drugs taken by the mother late in pregnancy may contribute to depressed T-cell function in the newborn. Since delayed hypersensitivity reactions are mediated by T-cells rather than antibodies, skin test responses (such as purified protein derivative [PPD] for tuberculosis detection) are diminished until about 1 year of age, probably due to the infant's decreased ability to mount an inflammatory response. Reference ranges for lymphocyte counts in neonates support early identification of neonates at higher risk (Christensen et al., 2012).

Humoral Immunity

The newborn's B-cells do not respond as well to infection as do adults. B-cells are responsible for the production of **antibodies** (specific immunity). The antibodies bind to the **antigen** (substance stimulating an immune response), thus disabling the specific toxin. The fetus is normally in an antigen-free environment and so produces only trace amounts of **immunoglobulins** (Ig; gammaglobulin antibody proteins), specifically IgM. Most of the newborn's IgG is acquired transplacentally from the mother. Hence, the newborn exhibits passive immunity to antigens to which the mother had developed antibodies. These antibodies wane over the first months of life as the transplacental IgG is catabolized, having a half-life of only about 25 days.

The newborn begins to make IgG but ordinarily experiences a physiologic hypogammaglobulinemia between 2 and 6 months of age until self-production of IgG reaches higher levels. The infant that takes human milk (breast or expressed) will acquire passive transfer of maternal immunity via the human milk and will be better protected during the physiologic hypogammaglobulinemia phase. By 1 year of age IgG is 50% of the adult level, and by 7 years of age it reaches the average adult level.

IgA, IgD, IgE, and IgM do not cross the placenta; they require an antigenic challenge for production. IgD and IgE constitute a very small percentage of the immunoglobulins in all ages. Immunoglobulins G, A, and M do not reach adult levels until around 12 years of age.

Hypersensitivity Reactions

Hypersensitivity is an altered or inappropriate response by the immune system to an antigen. Hypersensitivity reactions include allergy, autoimmunity or alloimmunity (isoimmunity) and can be immediate or delayed. Reactions occurring within minutes to a few hours after re-exposure to an antigen are classified as immediate hypersensitivity reactions. The most rapid and severe type of immediate reaction is anaphylaxis, discussed later in the chapter. With delayed hypersensitivity reactions, symptoms may take several hours to appear with the reaction at maximum severity days after the re-exposure to the antigen (Rote & McCance, 2015).

COMMON MEDICAL TREATMENTS

A variety of medications and other medical treatments are used to treat immune deficiencies and autoimmune problems in children. Most of these treatments will require a physician's or nurse practitioner's order when the child is in the hospital. The most common treatments and medications are listed in Common Medical Treatments 47.1 and Drug Guide 47.1. The nurse caring for the child with an immune deficiency or autoimmune disorder should be familiar with what the procedures and medications are, how they work, and common nursing implications related to use of these modalities.

Atraumatic Care

When a child requires repeat injections related to an immune or allergic disorder, use a local anesthetic such as Maxilene or eutectic mixture of local anesthetic (EMLA) cream or a numbing spray to reduce the amount of associated pain.

COMMON MEDICAL TREATMENTS 47.1

Treatment	Explanation	Indications	Nursing Implications
Immunizations	Killed or modified microorganisms, or components of them, cause the immune system to develop antibodies to the microorganism without developing a disease	Prevention of certain viral and bacterial infections	Do not administer live vaccines to immunosuppressed persons Refer to the individual vaccine for method of administration and contraindications Report adverse reactions via the vaccine adverse reaction (VAR) reporting system
Bone marrow or stem cell transplantation	Bone marrow transplant: transfer of healthy bone marrow into the bones of a person with immune malfunction; the transplanted cells can then develop into functional B- and T-cells Stem cell transplant: peripheral stem cells are removed from the donor via apheresis or stem cells are retrieved from the umbilical cord and placenta. The stem cells are then transplanted into the recipient	Wiskott–Aldrich syndrome, severe combined immune deficiency (SCID)	Administer immunosuppressive medications as ordered Maintain medical asepsis and protective isolation to prevent infection Monitor closely for graft-versus-host disease Provide meticulous oral care. Avoid rectal temperatures and suppositories Encourage appropriate nutrition

DRUG GUIDE 47.1 COMMON DRUGS FOR IMMUNOLOGIC DISORDERS

Medication	Actions/Indications	Nursing Implications
Intravenous immune globulin (IVIG)	Provides exogenous IgG antibodies Indicated for primary immune deficiencies, HIV infection, myasthenia gravis	Do not mix with IV medications or with other IV fluids Do not give IM or SQ Monitor vital signs and watch for adverse reactions frequently during infusion May require antipyretic or antihistamine to prevent chills and fever during infusion Have epinephrine available during infusion
Nucleoside analogue reverse transcriptase inhibitors (NRTIs): abacavir, lamivudine, zidovudine	Inhibit reverse transcription of the viral DNA chain For the treatment of HIV-1 infection as part of a three-drug regimen. Zidovudine is also used to prevent perinatal transmission of HIV	Notify physician of muscle weakness, shortness of breath, headache, insomnia, rash, or unusual bleeding. Give IV zidovudine over 1 hour. Fatal hypersensitivity reaction may occur with abacavir
Nonnucleoside analogue reverse transcriptase inhibitors (NNRTIs): efavirenz, nevirapine	Bind to HIV-1 reverse transcriptase, blocking DNA polymerase activity and disrupting the virus life cycle. Used for the treatment of HIV-1 infection as part of a three-drug regimen	*Nevirapine:* Avoid St. John's wort Shake suspension gently before administration Observe for symptoms of Stevens–Johnson syndrome *Efavirenz:* May cause drowsiness
Protease inhibitors: amprenavir, atazanavir, indinavir, lopinavir, nelfinavir, ritonavir, saquinavir	Inhibit protease activity in the HIV-1 cell, resulting in immature, noninfectious viral particles. Used for the treatment of HIV-1 infection as part of a three-drug regimen	Multiple drug interactions. Review specific medication for adverse effects and administration implications

(continued)

Nursing goals, interventions, and evaluation for the child with an immunologic disorder are based on the nursing diagnoses. Nursing Care Plan 47.1 can be used as a guide in planning nursing care for the child with an immunologic disorder, autoimmune disorder, or allergic response. It should be individualized based on the child's symptoms and needs. Refer to Chapter 36 for thorough information related to pain management.

Additional information will be included later in the chapter as it relates to specific disorders.

Based on your top three nursing diagnoses for Lakeisha, describe appropriate nursing interventions.

COMMON LABORATORY AND DIAGNOSTIC TESTS 47.1

Test	Explanation	Indications	Nursing Implications
Complete blood count (CBC) with differential	Evaluates hemoglobin and hematocrit, WBC count (particularly the percentage of individual WBCs), and platelet count	Infection, inflammatory process, immunosuppression	Normal values vary according to the age and gender. WBC count differential is helpful in evaluating the source of infection. May be affected by myelosuppressive drugs
Immunoglobulin electrophoresis	Determines the level of individual immunoglobulins (IgA, IgD, IgE, IgG, IgM) in the blood	Immune deficiency, autoimmune disorders	Normal levels vary with age. IVIG administration and steroids alter levels
IgG subclasses	Measure the levels of the four subclasses of IgG (1, 2, 3, and 4)	Determine immune deficiency	Normal levels vary with age. IVIG administration and steroids alter levels
Lymphocyte immunophenotyping T-cell quantification	Measures level of T-cells (T-helper [CD4], T-suppressor [CD8]), B-cells, and natural killer cells in the blood	Ongoing monitoring of progressive depletion of CD4 T-lymphocytes in HIV disease	Do not refrigerate the specimen. Steroids may elevate and immunosuppressive drugs may depress lymphocyte levels
Delayed hypersensitivity skin test	Measures the presence of activated T-cells that recognize certain substances	Immune disorders	Administered intradermally. Read and document the size of reaction at 48 to 72 hours (tuberculosis, mumps, Candida, tetanus)
HIV antibodies	Used to detect antibodies to HIV	Determining HIV infection when suspected	The ELISA method detects only antibodies, so may remain negative for several weeks up to 6 months (false negative). False-positive may result with autoimmune disease. Requires serial testing. HIV test results are confidential.
Virologic assay (HIV RNA and DNA nucleic acid and polymerase chain reaction tests)	Used to detect HIV RNA and DNA	Diagnosis of HIV infection in children older than 2 weeks of age and ongoing monitoring of viral load	Sensitive and specific for presence of HIV in the blood. Sequential testing needed to determine perinatal transmission
CD4 count	Measures the number of CD4 T-lymphocytes in the blood	Used in HIV-infected persons to determine response to antiretroviral therapy	Normal (immune category 1) is ≥1,500/mm^3 in the infant, ≥1,000/mm^3 in the 1–5-year-old, ≥500/mm^3 in children 6–12 years
Complement assay (C3 and C4)	Measures the level of total complement in the blood, as well as levels of C3 and C4	Monitor SLE. Determine complement deficiency	Send to laboratory immediately (unstable at room temperature). Usually sent out to a reference laboratory

COMMON LABORATORY AND DIAGNOSTIC TESTS 47.1 (continued)

Test	Explanation	Indications	Nursing Implications
Erythrocyte sedimentation rate (ESR)	Nonspecific test used to determine the presence of infection or inflammation	Immune disorder initial workup, ongoing monitoring of autoimmune disease	Send to laboratory immediately; if allowed to stand >3 hours, falsely low result may occur
Rheumatoid factor (RF)	Determines the presence of RF in the blood	Juvenile idiopathic arthritis, SLE	Positive RF is also sometimes seen in chronic infectious disorders
Antinuclear antibody (ANA)	Tests for presence of autoantibodies that react against cellular nuclear material	SLE	Check for signs of infection at venipuncture site Steroid use can cause false-negative result May be weakly positive in about 20% of healthy individuals
RAST (radioallergosorbent test)	Measures minute quantities of IgE in the blood Carries no risk of anaphylaxis but is not as sensitive as skin testing	Asthma (food allergies)	Blood test that is usually sent out to a reference laboratory
Allergy skin testing	Suggested allergen is applied to skin via scratch, pin, or prick. A wheal response indicates allergy to the substance. Carries risk of anaphylaxis. (Nursing note: Antihistamines must be discontinued before testing, as they inhibit the test.)	Allergic rhinitis, asthma	Close observation for anaphylaxis is necessary. Epinephrine and emergency equipment should be readily available Some children react to the skin test almost immediately; others take several minutes
Food-specific IgE antibody testing	Measures IgE antibody to specific food allergens	Accurately determine specific food allergy	IVIG administration and steroids alter levels

Adapted from Corbett, J. A., & Banks, A. D. (2013). *Laboratory tests and diagnostic procedures with nursing diagnoses* (8th ed.). Upper Saddle River, NJ: Pearson Education Inc.

PRIMARY IMMUNODEFICIENCIES

Many primary immunodeficiencies have been identified. They are mostly hereditary or congenital. Primary immunodeficiencies may be related to humoral deficiencies, cellular immunity deficiencies, or a combination of the two; phagocytic system defects; or complement deficiencies. This discussion will focus on a few of the more common and/or severe primary immunodeficiencies in children. Box 47.1 lists 10 warning signs that a child may need further evaluation for the possibility of primary immunodeficiency.

Hypogammaglobulinemia

Hypogammaglobulinemia refers to a variety of conditions in which the child does not form antibodies appropriately. It results in low or absent levels of one or more of the immunoglobulin classes or subclasses. Table 47.1

provides an overview of several types of hypogammaglobulinemia. Therapeutic management of most types of hypogammaglobulinemia is periodic administration of intravenous immunoglobulin (IVIG).

Nursing Assessment

Note the history of recurrent respiratory, gastrointestinal, or genitourinary infections. Palpate for enlarged lymph nodes and spleen in the child with X-linked hyper-IgM syndrome. In children presenting for routine administration of IVIG, determine whether any infections have occurred since the previous infusion.

Nursing Management

Nursing management of hypogammaglobulinemia can involve IVIG administration and the provision of education

FIGURE 47.2 **Boys with the Wiskott–Aldrich syndrome often have worsening of eczema over time.**

only cure is hematopoietic cell transplantation, though gene therapy is currently under investigation.

Nursing Assessment

Note the history of petechiae, bloody diarrhea, or bleeding episode in the first 6 months of life. Note any history of hematemesis or intracranial or conjunctival hemorrhages. Observe the skin for eczema, which usually worsens with time and tends to become secondarily infected (Fig. 47.2). Laboratory findings include low IgM concentration, elevated IgA and IgE concentrations, and normal IgG concentrations.

Take Note!

An episode of prolonged bleeding, such as at the umbilical stump or after circumcision, may be the first sign of the Wiskott–Aldrich syndrome in the newborn (Ochs, 2015).

Nursing Management

Administer IVIG as ordered to help decrease the frequency of bacterial infections. Perform good skin care and frequently assess eczematous areas to detect secondary infection (refer to Chapter 45 for care of eczema). If the child undergoes splenectomy, in addition to providing routine postoperative care, be aware of the additional risk for development of infection in the asplenic child. Refer to Chapter 46 for information related to hematopoietic cell transplantation.

Severe Combined Immune Deficiency

Severe combined immune deficiency (SCID) is a rare X-linked or autosomal recessive disorder; it can occur in girls or boys. SCID is characterized by absent T-cell and B-cell functions. There are at least five types of SCID, classified according to the exact genetic defect. SCID is a potentially fatal disorder requiring emergency intervention at the time of diagnosis. Gene therapy provides some promise for the future treatment of SCID, but until then hematopoietic cell transplantation is necessary (Bonilla, 2015).

Take Note!

Use only cytomegalovirus (CMV)-negative, irradiated blood or platelets if transfusion is necessary in the infant with SCID. CMV-positive blood could cause an infection in the infant, and T-lymphocytes in blood products may cause fatal graft-versus-host disease to occur (Norville & Tomlinson, 2010).

IVIG infusions may help decrease the number of infections until bone marrow or stem cell transplantation can be done (Bonilla, 2015). Children with SCID resulting from adenosine deaminase enzyme deficiency may benefit from lifelong subcutaneous adenosine deaminase enzyme replacement; these children are deficient in T- and B-cells as well as natural killer cells (Rote & McCance, 2015). In addition, long-term antibiotic therapy helps to contain chronic infections in some children with SCID.

Nursing Assessment

Note the history of chronic diarrhea and failure to thrive. Note the history of severe infections beginning early in infancy. Inspect the mouth for persistent thrush. Auscultate the lungs, noting adventitious sounds related to pneumonia. Laboratory findings include very low levels of all of the immunoglobulins.

Nursing Management

Preventing infection is critical. Teach the family to practice good hand washing. Because humoral and cell-mediated immunity is absent, exposure to persons outside the family, particularly young children, must be minimized as much as possible. Instruct families to administer prophylactic antibiotics if prescribed. Educate families that the child should not receive live vaccines. Encourage adequate nutrition; supplemental enteral feedings may be necessary in the child with poor appetite. Administer IVIG infusions as prescribed and monitor for adverse reactions (refer to the nursing management section for hypogammaglobulinemia for further information related to IVIG administration). If the child receives a bone marrow transplant (human leukocyte antigen [HLA]–matched sibling is preferred), provide posttransplant care as outlined in Chapter 46. Teach the family that severe cutaneous human papillomavirus infection may occur after stem cell transplantation (even years later). Refer the family for genetic counselling. Provide ongoing support; this is a difficult disease for families to cope with and the therapy required is lifelong.

Take Note!

Monitor the child who had a bone marrow or stem cell transplant closely for a maculopapular rash that usually starts on the palms and soles; this is an indication that **graft-versus-host disease** (GVHD) is developing. GVHD is a life-threatening condition in which donor cells attack host cells (Norville & Tomlinson, 2010).

SECONDARY IMMUNODEFICIENCIES

Secondary immunodeficiency may occur as a result of chronic illness, malignancy, use of **immunosuppressive** (lowering the immune response) medication, malnutrition or protein-losing state, prematurity, or HIV infection. This discussion will focus on HIV infection.

HIV Infection

Worldwide, 3.2 million children younger than 18 years old are living with HIV infection and about 650 become infected with HIV each day (UNAIDS, 2014). Children acquire HIV either vertically or horizontally. Vertical transmission refers to perinatal (in utero or during birth) transmission or via breast milk. Vertical transmission may also be referred to as mother to child transmission. Horizontal transmission refers to transmission via nonsterile needles (as in intravenous drug use or tattooing) or via intimate sexual contact. With nationwide screening of blood products, HIV transmission via

transfused blood products has become rare (Fahrner & Romano, 2010; McFarland, 2014). HIV infection in children may be further classified depending on the severity of immune suppression. This classification may serve to guide healthcare planning.

Infants primarily become infected through their mothers, whereas adolescents primarily contract HIV infection through sexual activity or intravenous drug use (Fahrner & Romano, 2010). In 2014, the number of HIV cases reported in Canada for less than 15 years of age is nine, with four cases under 5 years of age and five cases between the ages of 10 to 14. Moreover, between the ages 15 to 19, there were 37 cases reported for the same year (Public Health Agency Canada (Government of Canada, 2016; 2017)). Since 2008, the number of reported HIV cases each year has gradually declined. However, it should be noted that different HIV and AIDS reporting requirements do vary across the country (PHAC). The Canadian Paediatric Society (CPS) reaffirmed the recommendation for physicians to refer to the US National Institute of Health guidelines for providing care to HIV-exposed or HIV-infected children (2016). Currently, there is no cure for HIV infection, though survival has improved since the advent of highly active antiretroviral therapy (HAART) (see Evidence-Based Practice 47.1). In addition to improved survival, improved growth, neurodevelopment, and immune function occur with HAART (Fahrner & Romano, 2010).

Pathophysiology

HIV affects immune function via alterations mainly in T-cell function, but it also affects B-cells, natural killer cells, and monocyte/macrophage function. HIV infects the CD4 (T-helper) cells. The virus replicates itself via the CD4 cell and renders the cell dysfunctional. Immune deficiency results as the number of normal, functioning CD4 cells drops. Initially, as CD4 counts decrease, the T-suppressor (CD8) counts increase, but as the disease

---

EVIDENCE-BASED PRACTICE 47.1   DOES TEXT MESSAGING PROMOTE ADHERENCE TO ANTIRETROVIRAL THERAPY FOR HIV INFECTION?

STUDY

The key determinant of the degree and length of viral suppression in HIV infection is high adherence to antiretroviral therapy. Conversely, poor adherence leads to treatment failure. Children potentially have a significant number of years of life for which they will need to remain compliant with antiretroviral therapy. The authors evaluated 17 randomized controlled trials that examined the effect of text messaging on improving antiretroviral adherence.

Findings

Weekly text messaging reminders to patients and/or their caregivers (of infants and children) were found to be effective in improving antiretroviral adherence.

Nursing Implications

Antiretroviral adherence is critical to the potential life of an HIV-infected child. Implementing a weekly text-message reminder system related to antiretroviral therapy has the potential to improve adherence.

Adapted from Horvath, T., Azman, H., Kennedy, G. E., & Rutherford, G. W. (2012). *Mobile phone text messaging for promoting adherence to antiretroviral therapy in patients with HIV infection. The Cochrane Library 2012, 3*. Indianapolis, IN: John Wiley & Sons.

progresses, CD8 counts also fall. The helper T-cell function declines even in asymptomatic infants and children who have not experienced significant decreases in the CD4 cell count. The T-cells lose response to recall antigens, and this loss is associated with an increased risk of serious bacterial infection (McFarland, 2014).

B-cell defects also occur in HIV-infected children, contributing to high rates of serious bacterial infections. The B-cells demonstrate impaired response to mitogens and antigens. They also exhibit defective antibody production in response to antigen exposure or vaccination. Also, infants lack a pool of memory B-cells for recall antigens (simply from lack of exposure). Natural killer cells also are affected by HIV infection, as they are dependant on cytokines secreted by the CD4 cells for development of functionality. Functional killer cells play a role in fighting viruses and are critical to immunity in the newborn while the T-cell line develops. Decreased function of the natural killer cells then contributes to increased severity of viral infection in the HIV-infected child or infant. Though the virus does not destroy monocytes and macrophages, their function is affected. Macrophages in the HIV-infected child exhibit decreased chemotaxis and the antigen-presenting capability of the monocytes is defective.

Without appropriate T-cell, B-cell, natural killer cell, monocyte, and macrophage function, the infant's or child's immune system cannot fight infections it ordinarily could. Recurrent infection with ordinary organisms occurs more frequently in children with HIV infection, and the infections are more severe than in noninfected children. Opportunistic infections also occur in HIV-infected children, similar to those in adults with HIV infection. Current guidelines related to opportunistic infection prevention emphasize antiretroviral therapy for prevention as well as insuring appropriate immunization and antibiotic prophylaxis for certain organisms (Siberry, Abzug, & Nachman, 2013).

HIV rapidly invades the central nervous system in infants and children and is responsible for progressive HIV encephalopathy. As a result of encephalopathy, acquired microcephaly, motor deficits, or loss of previously achieved developmental milestones may occur. In children with progressive HIV encephalopathy, neurologic symptoms may present before immune suppression.

Therapeutic Management

Current recommendations for the treatment of HIV infection in children include the use of a combination of antiretroviral drugs (McFarland, 2014). Medication therapy ranges from single-drug therapy in the asymptomatic HIV-exposed newborn to HAART, consisting of a combination of antiretroviral drugs. Medications are prescribed based on the severity of the child's illness. One of the goals of HAART is to prevent or arrest progressive HIV encephalopathy (Fahrner & Romano, 2010).

Nursing Assessment

For a full description of the assessment phase of the nursing process, refer to the Assessment section of the Nursing Process Overview earlier in the chapter. Assessment findings pertinent to HIV infection in children are discussed below.

HEALTH HISTORY

Elicit a description of the present illness and chief complaint. Common signs and symptoms reported during the health history might include:

- Failure to thrive
- Recurrent bacterial infections
- Opportunistic infections
- Chronic or recurrent diarrhea
- Recurrent or persistent fever
- Developmental delay
- Prolonged candidiasis

These signs and symptoms may be present in either the child who is undergoing initial diagnosis or the child with known HIV infection. Explore the child's current and past medical history for risk factors such as maternal HIV infection or AIDS, receipt of blood transfusions in a developing country (without adequate screening measures), adolescent or childhood sexual abuse, substance use or abuse (including intravenous drug use), or participation in vaginal or anal sex without the use of a condom. Document who the primary caregiver is, as many children with HIV have lost their parents to the disease. In addition, for the child with known HIV infection, determine the child's medications and dosages as well as the outcome of any recent healthcare visits or hospitalizations.

PHYSICAL EXAMINATION

Perform a thorough and complete physical examination on the child with suspected or known HIV infection.

Inspection and Observation. Note the presence of fever. Measure the weight, height or length, and head circumference (in children younger than 3 years old) and plot this information on standard growth charts, noting whether the measurements fall within the average or below the lower percentiles. Perform a developmental screening test to detect developmental delay. Inspect the oral cavity for candidiasis. Observe work of breathing (may be increased if pneumonitis or pneumonia is present). Determine the level of consciousness (may be depressed if HIV encephalopathy is present).

Auscultation and Palpation. Auscultate the lungs, noting adventitious breath sounds associated with pneumonia or pneumonitis. Palpate for the presence of enlarged lymph nodes (lymphadenopathy) or swollen parotid glands. Palpate the abdomen, noting hepatosplenomegaly.

BOX 47.2

VIROLOGIC ASSAY TESTING FOR HIV-EXPOSED INFANTS

- 14 to 21 days of age
- 1 to 2 months of age
- 4 to 6 months of age
- In the nonbreastfed infant, two or more negative tests (one at ≥1 month of age and one at ≥4 months of age) determine the absence of HIV infection

From Panel on Antiretroviral Therapy and Medical Management of HIV-Infected Children. (2016). *Guidelines for the use of antiretroviral agents in pediatric HIV infection.* Retrieved from http://aidsinfo.nih.gov/contentfiles/lvguidelines/pediatricguidelines.pdf

LABORATORY AND DIAGNOSTIC TESTS

Common laboratory and diagnostic studies ordered for the assessment of HIV infection include:

- Reverse transcriptase polymerase chain reaction (RT-PCR) test: positive in infected infants older than 1 month of age. RT-PCR is the preferred test to determine HIV infection in infants and to exclude HIV infection as early as possible. Box 47.2 gives information on testing.
- Enzyme-linked immunosorbent assay (ELISA) test: positive in infants of HIV-infected mothers because of transplacentally received antibodies. These antibodies may persist and remain detectable up to 24 months of age, making the ELISA test less accurate at detecting HIV infection in infants and toddlers than the PCR.
- CD4 counts (low in HIV infection)

Nursing Management

Nursing care of the child with HIV infection is directed at avoiding infection, promoting compliance with the medication regimen, promoting nutrition, providing pain management and comfort measures, educating the child and caregivers, and providing ongoing psychosocial support. The Public Health Agency of Canada's *HIV and Hepatitis C Community Action Fund* supports community programming to address priority public health issues. The Agency is investing $26.4 million per year in community-based programs across the country to address HIV/AIDS, hepatitis C, and other sexually transmitted and blood-borne infections (PHAC, n.d.). Organizations from the provinces and territories have the opportunity to apply for assistance from this fund. Nursing Care Plan 47.1, found at the end of the chapter, lists appropriate nursing diagnoses and interventions. In addition, nursing management specific to HIV infection is covered below.

PREVENTING HIV INFECTION IN CHILDREN

It is important to offer all pregnant women routine HIV counselling and voluntary testing (See Box 47.3.). Depending on the stage of pregnancy, the mother should be treated with an antiretroviral drug if she is HIV positive. Children born to HIV-positive mothers should receive a 6-week course of zidovudine (ZDV) therapy (McFarland, 2014). Discourage breastfeeding in the HIV-infected mother and instruct her about safe alternatives to breastfeeding. Early recognition of infection is crucial so that the treatment can begin, HIV encephalopathy may be prevented, and progression to acquired immune deficiency syndrome can be prevented. Educate sexually active adolescents about HIV transmission and urge them to use condoms. Counsel teens about the increased risk of HIV transmission with all forms of sexual activity, explaining that vaginal and anal sex are even riskier than oral sex. Urge teens to limit the number of sexual partners. Discourage substance use, as the effects of drugs and alcohol often impair the teen's ability to make wise choices about sexual conduct. Warn teens of the risk of contracting HIV infection via shared needles (as with intravenous drug use or via unclean needles used in tattooing).

The CPS has issued a position statement, which was reaffirmed in 2017, regarding testing for HIV infection in pregnancy (2017). Refer to Recommendations from the CPS (Robinson, 2008).

BOX 47.3

TESTING FOR HIV INFECTION IN PREGNANCY—ADAPTED FROM POSITION STATEMENT FROM THE CANADIAN PAEDIATRIC SOCIETY

- HIV testing should be offered both early and routinely to all women during pregnancy. Repeat testing if risk of exposure to HIV while the woman is pregnant.
- Confidential counselling should be available to any woman or child undergoing HIV testing.
- Testing in the perinatal period should be program based and include others at risk such as the father and siblings.
- Information regarding HIV-positive status must be shared with the team caring for the woman in order to decrease the risk of neonatal HIV acquisition.
- If the mother has not been tested at any stage during pregnancy or has risk factors for acquiring HIV (drug use, multiple sexual partners, and sexual partner with HIV) collection of samples while in labour must be considered.
- If the mother refuses testing, this should be documented. Offer testing later in the pregnancy and referral to counselling services.
- HIV-positive pregnant women should be given information on factors that reduce perinatal HIV transmission, which includes antiretroviral therapy, obstetrical options, and resources for formula feeding.
- An expert in managing HIV care should be included in the care of the women or children with HIV.
- All provinces and territories must ensure that they have comprehensive, accessible testing and follow-up programs for HIV.

Complete table and detailed information of rapid testing for HIV in pregnancy is accessed via the Position Statement Canadian Paediatric Society (2017) Retrieved from http://www.cps.ca/documents/position/testing-for-hiv-infection-in-pregnancy

PROMOTING COMPLIANCE WITH ANTIRETROVIRAL THERAPY

Before HAART was available as a treatment option, progressive HIV encephalopathy was inevitably fatal, usually within 2 years of diagnosis (Fahrner & Romano, 2010). To prevent progression of HIV disease and prevent encephalopathy, compliance with the HAART regimen is required. Educate the family about the importance of complying with the medication regimen. Help the caregivers develop a schedule for medication administration that is compatible with the family's home routine.

REDUCING RISK FOR INFECTION

In the newborn whose mother is infected with tuberculosis, syphilis, toxoplasmosis, CMV, hepatitis B or C, or herpes simplex virus, provide testing and treatment. To prevent infection with *Pneumocystis jirovecii,* administer prophylactic antibiotics as prescribed in any HIV-exposed infant in whom HIV infection has not yet been excluded. Provide tuberculosis screening and childhood immunization in accordance with national guidelines.

Thinking About Development

Jasmine Smith is a 5-year-old female with HIV infection. She fights taking her antiretroviral medications because of the nausea and vomiting associated with them. Lucy Panco is a 15-year-old female also with HIV infection. She is noncompliant with her antiretroviral medications, also because of the associated nausea and vomiting.

How will the nurse teach Jasmine about the medications? How will she foster compliance in Jasmine?

What is the most appropriate approach for the nurse to take to educate Lucy about compliance with medications?

How will the approaches to education and encouragement of compliance be different for these two children? How will they be similar?

Take Note!

Do not administer live vaccines to the immunocompromised child without the express consent of the infectious disease or immunology specialist. Immunosuppression is a contraindication to vaccination with live vaccines (Atkinson et al., 2012).

PROMOTING NUTRITION

For the infant, provide increased-calorie formula as tolerated. For the child, provide high-calorie, high-protein meals and snacks. Supplements may be added to milk-shakes to increase the protein intake. Ensure that the child is able to choose foods that he or she prefers from the hospital menu. Document growth through weekly measurements of weight and height/length.

PROMOTING COMFORT

Children with HIV infection experience pain from infections, encephalopathy, adverse effects of medications, and the numerous procedures and treatments that are required, such as venipuncture, biopsy, or lumbar puncture. Refer to Chapter 36 for detailed information about pain assessment and management.

Take Note!

Family-centred care of the HIV-exposed child and HIV-infected mother may involve a multidisciplinary approach and can result in improved outcomes for both the mother and the child (Fahrner & Romano, 2010).

PROVIDING FAMILY EDUCATION AND SUPPORT

Educate caregivers about the medication regimen, the ongoing followup that is needed, and when to call the infectious disease provider. Families of HIV-infected children experience a significant amount of stress from many sources: the diagnosis of an incurable disease, financial difficulties, multiple family members with HIV, HIV-associated stigmas, desire to keep HIV infection confidential, and multiple medical appointments and hospitalizations. Parents of HIV-infected children often die of AIDS themselves, leaving care of the child to another relative or foster parent. The daycare centre or school that the child attends will need education about HIV, which can be provided only if the parent or caretaker consents to divulging the child's diagnosis to that agency. Provide education to the school or daycare centre about how the infection is transmitted (i.e., not through casual contact).

Disclosure of the diagnosis of HIV to the child is another source of stress for the family. The timing of this disclosure will vary considerably depending on the child's and family's situation. Generally, children older than 6 years of age will eventually need to have their diagnosis disclosed to them in an age-appropriate manner. They begin to ask questions and often seem to sense that something is going on other than what they've been told so far. When made aware of the diagnosis and educated about the disease, the child may exhibit a variety of reactions. Anger, depression, or school problems may occur. The child may experience a spiritual dilemma. Adolescents with perinatal HIV infection reported that disclosure of the diagnosis resulted in significant stress in their lives (De Santis, Garcia, Chaparro, & Beltran, 2014). The nurse should continue to provide emotional support to the child and family. If the disclosure results in significant emotional turmoil, refer the child and caregivers to a counsellor, social worker, or psychologist. Anticipatory grieving also may occur. Parents or caregivers may express guilt or anger over the diagnosis of HIV infection. At the other end of the spectrum, families may use denial as their method for coping. Use therapeutic communication with open-ended questions to discover the family's thoughts and fears. Provide emotional support and allow for crying and verbalization. If needed, refer the caregivers to the appropriate professional for additional psychological and emotional intervention.

Many children with HIV have psychosocial, emotional, and cognitive problems. These contribute to a lower quality of life. They are affected by the stigma of their diagnosis and often by the social isolation associated with it. Adolescents with HIV infection note that this stigma has a profound impact on their coping abilities (De Santis et al., 2014). They may suffer multiple losses within the family related to deaths caused by HIV infection. Children with HIV infection need significant psychosocial support and intervention. Resources for families of HIV-infected children are listed in Box 47.4.

AUTOIMMUNE DISORDERS

Autoimmune disorders result from the immune system's malfunction. The body manufactures T-cells and antibodies against its own cells and organs **(autoantibodies)**. The development of an autoimmune disorder is thought to be multifactorial. Potential influencing factors include heredity, hormones, self-marker molecules, and environmental influences such as viruses and certain drugs.

Systemic Lupus Erythematosus

Systemic lupus erythematosus (SLE) is a multisystem autoimmune disorder that affects both humoral and cellular immunity. SLE can affect any organ system, so the onset and course of the disease are quite variable. SLE is usually diagnosed after age 5 years (usually between 15 and 45 years of age), but onset can occur at any age. The peak incidence for diagnosis is in the preadolescent years (Mattingly, 2011). The female-to-male ratio for persons affected by SLE is 4:1 in childhood and 8:1 in adolescence (Lehman, 2015). SLE is more common in non-Caucasians, and typically African-American and Hispanic children and adolescents experience more severe effects from SLE than other racial or ethnic groups (Lehman, 2015).

Pathophysiology

In SLE, autoantibodies react with the child's self-antigens to form immune complexes. The immune complexes accumulate in the tissues and organs, causing an inflammatory response resulting in vasculitis. Injury to the tissues and pain occur. Since SLE may affect any organ system, the potential for alterations or damage to tissues anywhere in the body is significant. In some cases, the autoimmune response may be preceded by a drug reaction, an infection, or excessive sun exposure. In children, the most common initial symptoms are hematologic, cutaneous, and musculoskeletal in origin. The disease is chronic, with periods of remission and exacerbation (flares). Common complications of SLE include ocular or visual changes, cerebrovascular accident (CVA), transverse myelitis, immune complex–mediated glomerulonephritis, pericarditis, valvular heart disease, coronary artery disease, seizures, and psychosis.

Therapeutic Management

Therapeutic management focuses on treating the inflammatory response. Nonsteroidal anti-inflammatory drugs (NSAIDs), corticosteroids, and antimalarial agents are often prescribed for the child with mild to moderate SLE. The child with severe SLE or frequent flare-ups of symptoms may require high-dose (pulse) corticosteroid therapy or immunosuppressive drugs. When end-stage renal failure develops as a result of glomerulonephritis, dialysis becomes necessary.

Nursing Assessment

For a full description of the assessment phase of the nursing process, refer to the Assessment section of the Nursing Process Overview earlier in the chapter. Assessment findings pertinent to SLE in children are discussed below.

HEALTH HISTORY

Elicit a description of the present illness and chief complaint. Common signs and symptoms reported during the health history are history of fatigue, fever, weight changes, pain or swelling in the joints, numbness, tingling or coolness of extremities, or prolonged bleeding. Assess for risk factors, which include female sex; family history; African, Native American, or Asian descent; recent infection; drug reaction; or excessive sun exposure.

PHYSICAL EXAMINATION

Measure temperature and document the presence of fever. Observe the skin for malar rash (a butterfly-shaped rash over the cheeks); discoid lesions on the face, scalp, or neck; changes in skin pigmentation; or scarring (Fig. 47.3). Document alopecia. Inspect the oral cavity for painless ulcerations and the joints for edema.

FIGURE 47.3 The malar or butterfly rash (erythema over the cheeks in the shape of a butterfly) is typical in systemic lupus erythematosus (SLE).

Measure the blood pressure, as hypertension may occur with renal involvement. Auscultate the lungs; adventitious breath sounds may be present if the pulmonary system is involved. Palpate the joints, noting tenderness. Palpate the abdomen and note areas of tenderness (abdominal involvement is more common in children with SLE than in adults). Box 47.5 lists common clinical findings in SLE.

LABORATORY AND DIAGNOSTIC FINDINGS

Laboratory findings may include decreased hemoglobin and hematocrit, decreased platelet count, and low WBC count. Complement levels, C3 and C4, will also be decreased. Though not specific to SLE, the antinuclear antibody (ANA) is usually positive in children with SLE.

Nursing Management

Nursing management of the child or adolescent with SLE is long term and supportive. Management focuses on preventing and monitoring for complications. Educate the child and family about the importance of a healthy diet, regular exercise, and adequate sleep and rest. Administer NSAIDs, corticosteroids, and antimalarial agents as ordered for the child with mild to moderate SLE and pulse corticosteroid therapy or immunomodulators to the child with severe SLE or frequent flare-ups. Dealing with a chronic illness can be difficult for the child and family. In addition, adolescents struggle with body image and independence (Mattingly, 2011). Refer families to support services such as Lupus Canada and the Kidney Foundation of Canada, links to which can be found on thePoint.

> **Take Note!**
> Counsel adolescents with SLE about the risk of autoantibody transmission to the fetus should they become pregnant. This antibody transmission can result in lupus in the newborn (Johnson, 2014).

PREVENTING AND MONITORING FOR COMPLICATIONS

Teach families to apply sunscreen (minimum SPF 15) to their child's skin daily to prevent rashes resulting from photosensitivity. Instruct the child and family to protect against cold weather by layering warm socks and wearing gloves when outdoors in the winter. If the child is outside for extended periods during the winter months, inspect the fingers and toes for discolouration. Watch for the development of nephritis by evaluating the blood pressure, serum BUN and creatinine levels, and urine output and monitoring for hematuria or proteinuria. Ensure that yearly vision screening and ophthalmic examinations are performed to preserve visual function should changes occur.

> **Take Note!**
> Avascular necrosis (lack of blood supply to a joint, resulting in tissue damage) may occur as an adverse effect of long-term or high-dose corticosteroid use. Teach families to report new onset of joint pain, particularly with weight bearing, or limited range of motion to their physician or nurse practitioner (Tofferi, 2015).

Juvenile Idiopathic Arthritis

Juvenile idiopathic arthritis is an autoimmune disorder in which the autoantibodies mainly target the joints. Inflammatory changes in the joints cause pain, redness, warmth, stiffness, and swelling. Stiffness usually occurs after inactivity (as in the morning, after sleep). Some forms also affect the eyes or other organs. Table 47.2 explains the three types. Juvenile idiopathic arthritis is a chronic disease; the child may experience healthy periods alternating with flare-ups. In some children the disease resolves as they approach adolescence or adulthood, while others

---

BOX 47.5

MOST COMMON CLINICAL MANIFESTATIONS OF SYSTEMIC LUPUS ERYTHEMATOSUS

- Alopecia
- Anemia
- Arthralgia
- Arthritis
- Fatigue
- Lupus nephritis
- Photosensitivity
- Pleurisy
- Raynaud phenomenon
- Seizures
- Skin rashes, including malar rash
- Stomatitis
- Thrombocytopenia

TABLE 47.2	TYPES OF JUVENILE IDIOPATHIC ARTHRITIS		
Type	Definition	Nonjoint Manifestations	Complications
Pauciarticular (oligoarticular)	Involvement of four or fewer joints; quite often the knee is involved. Most common type	Eye inflammation, malaise, poor appetite, poor weight gain	Iritis, uveitis, uneven leg bone growth
Polyarticular	Involvement of five or more joints; frequently involves small joints and often affects the body symmetrically	Malaise, lymphadenopathy, organomegaly, poor growth	Often a severe form of arthritis; rapidly progressing joint damage, rheumatoid nodules
Systemic	In addition to joint involvement, fever and rash may be present at diagnosis	Enlarged spleen, liver, and lymph nodes; myalgia; severe anemia	Pericarditis, pericardial effusion, pleuritis, pulmonary fibrosis

Adapted from Jones, K. B., & Higgins, G. C. (2010). Juvenile rheumatoid arthritis. In P. J. Allen, J. A. Vessey, & N. A. Schapiro (Eds.). *Primary care of the child with a chronic condition* (5th ed.). St. Louis, MO: Mosby and Stanley, L. C., & Ward-Smith, P. (2011). The diagnosis and management of juvenile idiopathic arthritis. *Journal of Pediatric Health Care, 25*(3), 191–194.

will have more severe disease that continues throughout the adult years (Jones & Higgins, 2010). Juvenile idiopathic arthritis was formerly termed "juvenile rheumatoid arthritis," but unlike adult rheumatoid arthritis, few types of juvenile arthritis actually demonstrate a positive rheumatoid factor.

Therapeutic management focuses on inflammation control, pain relief, promotion of remission, and maintenance of mobility. NSAIDs, corticosteroids, and antirheumatic drugs such as methotrexate and etanercept are prescribed, depending on the type and severity of the disease. NSAIDs are helpful with pain relief, but disease-modifying (antirheumatic) drugs are necessary to prevent disease progression.

Take Note!

Juvenile Idiopathic Arthritis

Prednisone is used to decrease the inflammatory process in children with juvenile idiopathic arthritis. Methotrexate is used to prevent disease progression.

Nursing Assessment

Note the history of irritability or fussiness, which may be the first sign of this disease in the infant or very young child. Note complaints of pain, though children do not always communicate this. Document the history of withdrawal from play or difficulty getting the child out of bed in the morning (joint stiffness after inactivity). Inquire about history of fever (above 39.5°C for 2 weeks or more in systemic disease).

Measure temperature (fever is present with systemic disease). Inspect the skin for evanescent, pale red, nonpruritic macular rash, which may be present at the diagnosis of systemic disease. Observe the gait, noting limping or guarding of a joint or extremity. Document growth, which may be delayed. Inspect and palpate

each joint for edema, redness, warmth, and tenderness (Fig. 47.4). Note positioning of joints (usually flexed in position of comfort). Mild to moderate anemia and an elevated erythrocyte sedimentation rate are common. Young children with the pauciarticular form may demonstrate a positive ANA, and adolescents with polyarticular disease may have a positive rheumatoid factor.

Nursing Management

Nursing management focuses on managing pain, maintaining mobility, and promoting a normal life. Refer the child to a pediatric rheumatologist to ensure that he or she receives the most up-to-date treatment. Disease-modifying medications approved for use in children may produce better long-term outcomes than were possible in the past. Encourage regular eye examinations and vision screening to allow for early treatment of visual changes and to prevent blindness. Check out thePoint for an example of a Canadian clinical research trial.

FIGURE 47.4 Note the swollen, reddened joints of this child with juvenile arthritis.

MANAGING PAIN AND MAINTAINING MOBILITY

Administer medications as prescribed to control inflammation and prevent disease progression. Refer to Drug Guide 47.1 for information related to NSAIDs, corticosteroids, and disease-modifying antirheumatic drugs. Maintain joint range of motion and muscle strength via exercise (physical or occupational therapy). Swimming is a particularly useful exercise to maintain joint mobility without placing pressure on the joints. Teach families the appropriate use of splints prescribed to prevent joint contractures. Monitor for pressure areas or skin breakdown with splint or orthotic use.

PROMOTING NORMAL LIFE

Chronic pain and decreased mobility may impact the child's psychological and emotional status significantly, during both childhood and adulthood. Providing adequate pain relief and promoting compliance with the disease-modifying medication regimen may allow the child to have a more normal life in the present as well as in the future. In addition to measures described in the previous section, encourage adequate sleep. Sleep disturbance contributes to daytime sleepiness and fatigue which interferes with the child's ability to cope with symptoms and with school function (Ward et al., 2014). Sleep may be promoted by a warm bath at bedtime and warm compresses to affected joints or massage. To prevent social isolation, encourage the child to attend school and ensure that teachers, the school nurse, and classmates are educated about the child's disease and any limitations on activity. Involve the staff and faculty at the school to devise strategies to assist with the logistics of attending school without too many interruptions. Some suggestions are: having two sets of books (one at school and one at home) allows the child to do homework without having to carry heavy books home. Modifications such as allowing the child to leave the classroom early in order to get to the next class on time may seem small but can have a significant impact on the child's life.

Encourage children and families to become involved with local support groups so they can see that they are not alone. Assist children to set and achieve goals to increase their sense of hopefulness. Special summer camps for children with juvenile arthritis allow the child to socialize and belong to a group and have been shown to promote self-esteem in the child with chronic illness. Encourage appropriate family functioning and refer the family to support groups such as those sponsored by the American Juvenile Arthritis Organization.

Guillain–Barré Syndrome

Guillain–Barré syndrome (GBS) (also called acute immune-mediated polyneuropathies) is a diverse group of syndromes with several forms. The disorder occurring most often is the one in which an immune response within the body attacks the peripheral nervous system but does not usually affect the brain or spinal cord. GBS results in inflammation and demyelination of the peripheral nerves. Weakness and paralysis occur in a progressive fashion. Progression is usually complete in 2 to 4 weeks, followed by a stable period leading to the recovery phase, which lasts for a few weeks to months in most cases but can take years. Severity of the disorder ranges from mild weakness to total paralysis.

Though not fully understood, it is believed to be an autoimmune condition that most commonly is triggered by a previous viral or bacterial infection, usually described as an upper respiratory tract infection or an acute gastroenteritis with fever. In rare cases it has occurred after the child has had an immunization or surgery. GBS is more commonly seen in adults than in children (Cruse, 2014).

Therapeutic Management

The treatment of GBS is symptomatic and focuses on lessening the severity and speeding recovery. Management may include plasma exchange and administration of IVIGs, especially in severe cases (van Doorn et al., 2008; van Doorn et al., 2010). The goal of treatment is to keep the body functioning until the nervous system recovers. GBS is a life-threatening condition, and some children will die during the acute phase due to respiratory failure. Most children will make a full recovery, but a few may have residual damage.

Nursing Assessment

Early diagnosis and prompt treatment are essential since the disorder can quickly lead to respiratory failure and death from muscle paralysis. For a full description of the assessment phase of the nursing process, refer to the Assessment section of the Nursing Process Overview earlier in the chapter. Assessment findings pertinent to GBS are discussed below.

HEALTH HISTORY

Elicit a description of the present illness and chief complaint. The clinical presentation of GBS is fairly similar in children and adults. Note the onset of symptoms within a few days or weeks after the causative infection or event. Determine the presence of muscle weakness and paresthesias such as numbness and tingling which have a quick onset. Classically GBS initially affects the legs and progresses in an ascending manner, but occasionally it affects the arms or face first and proceeds in a descending manner. Note paralysis if present.

In children, pain, especially of the lower extremities, as the initial presentation preceding motor involvement has been reported. Other symptoms which may be present during the course of the illness ataxia and sensory disturbances.

PHYSICAL EXAMINATION AND LABORATORY AND DIAGNOSTIC TESTS

Physical examination findings may include decreased or absent tendon reflexes. Facial weakness or difficulty swallowing may be noted. Diagnosis is usually based on clinical findings of paralysis. Cerebrospinal fluid (CSF) analysis may reveal an increased level of protein, but this may not be evident until after the first week of the illness. Electrodiagnostic studies, such as electromyelogram (EMG) and nerve conduction velocity, can assist in the diagnosis of GBS.

Take Note!

Tickling may be a successful technique for assessing the level of paralysis in the child with GBS, either initially or in the recovery phase.

Nursing Management

Nursing management is supportive. In severe cases the child may require intensive nursing care along with mechanical ventilation. Observe the child closely for the extent of paralysis and monitor for respiratory involvement. Nursing care focuses on the same concerns as in any child with extreme immobility or paralysis.

Prevention of complications associated with immobility is a central concern and involves maintaining skin integrity, preventing respiratory complications and contractures, maintaining adequate nutrition, and managing pain. Interventions include turning and repositioning every 2 hours, assessing the skin for redness or breakdown, performing range-of-motion exercises, keeping the skin clean and dry, encouraging intake of fluids to maintain hydration status, and encouraging coughing and deep breathing every 2 hours and as needed. Enteral feeding or parenteral nutrition may be indicated if swallowing becomes impaired. Physical therapy may be helpful in preventing complications and promoting motor skill recovery. Provide support and education to the parent and child. The rapid onset and long recovery can be difficult and can cause strain on the family and its finances. If residual disability occurs, the family will need help adjusting and caring for their child.

Take Note!

Serial measurement of tidal volumes may reveal respiratory deterioration in the child with GBS.

Myasthenia Gravis

Myasthenia gravis is an autoimmune disease that may be inherited as a rare genetic disease (congenital), may be acquired by infants born to mothers with myasthenia gravis (neonatal), or may develop later in childhood (juvenile). The most common form seen is juvenile myasthenia gravis and will be covered here. See Comparison Chart 47.2 for further information on the less common forms, neonatal myasthenia gravis and congenital myasthenia gravis. Juvenile myasthenia gravis is a relatively rare autoimmune disorder (Liew & Kang, 2013). The child's antibodies attack the acetylcholine receptor (AchR) and other proteins at the neuromuscular junction, inhibiting normal neuromuscular transmission. The result is progressive weakness and fatigue of the skeletal muscles.

There is no cure for myasthenia gravis. Symptoms can be controlled, but it is a lifelong condition, with early detection being the key to managing the disorder successfully. The disease may be aggravated by stress, exposure to extreme temperatures, and infections, resulting in a myasthenic crisis. Myasthenic crisis is a medical emergency with symptoms including sudden respiratory distress, dysphagia, dysarthria, ptosis, diplopia, tachycardia, anxiety, and rapidly increasing weakness.

Therapeutic management generally involves the use of anticholinesterase medications such as pyridostigmine, which blocks the breakdown of acetylcholine at the neuromuscular junction and enhances neuromuscular transmission. If weakness is not controlled, additional medications may include corticosteroids and other immunosuppressants. Other treatments include plasmapheresis, which removes antibodies from the blood, IVIG, and thymectomy. The thymectomy procedure has resulted in quicker remission and improvement in symptoms for some individuals, but the effects are not consistent. Consequently, surgical removal of the thymus continues to be questioned, despite it being an accepted treatment of myasthenia gravis (Aydin et al., 2017; Gronseth & Barohn, 2002).

Nursing Assessment

Note the history of fatigue and weakness; difficulty chewing, swallowing, or holding up the head; or pain with muscle fatigue. In the verbal child, note complaints of double vision. Observe the child for ptosis (droopy eyelids) or altered eye movements from partial paralysis. Note increased work of breathing. Laboratory testing may involve the edrophonium (Tensilon) test, in which a short-acting cholinesterase inhibitor is used. AchR antibodies may be present in elevated quantities in the serum.

Nursing Management

The goals of nursing management include prevention of respiratory problems and providing adequate nutrition. Administer anticholinergic or other medications as ordered, teaching children and families about the use of these drugs. Anticholinergic drugs should be given 30 to 45 minutes before meals, on time and

COMPARISON CHART 47.2   **TYPES OF MYASTHENIA GRAVIS**

	Neonatal Myasthenia Gravis	Congenital Myasthenia Gravis
Definition	Transient form resulting from transplacental transfer of maternal antibodies that interfere with the neuromuscular junction	A group of disorders resulting from a genetic mutation of components of the neuromuscular junction resulting in neuromuscular junction failure
Characteristics	Present within a few hours after birth. Generalized weakness and hypotonia. Bulbar and respiratory weakness leads to poor suck and swallow, weak cry, and possible respiratory failure. Neonate will be very ill. Prompt diagnosis and treatment is essential. Recovery usually within a few weeks	Apparent at birth. Frequently have ptosis, ophthalmoplegia, bulbar, and respiratory muscle weakness. Fluctuating generalized weakness and hypotonia, life-threatening apnea. Typically improves with age but spontaneous exacerbations seen. Exacerbations also during periods of stress, increased activity, or febrile illness are seen. Management depends on specific type

exactly as ordered. Encourage families to seek prompt medical treatment for suspected infections. Encourage appropriate stress management and avoidance of extreme temperatures. Teach families that physical activities should be performed during times of peak energy; rest periods are needed for energy conservation. Teach families to call their neurologist immediately if signs and symptoms of myasthenic crisis or cholinergic crisis, which results from overmedication with anticholinergic medications, appear. Myasthenic crisis and cholinergic crisis have a similar presentation: rapidly increasing muscle weakness with resultant respiratory distress. Encourage children to wear a medical alert bracelet.

Take Note!

Signs and symptoms of myasthenic crisis include severe muscle weakness, respiratory difficulty, tachycardia, and dysphagia. Signs and symptoms of cholinergic crisis include severe muscle weakness, sweating, increased salivation, bradycardia, and hypotension.

Dermatomyositis

Juvenile dermatomyositis is an autoimmune disease that results in inflammation of the muscles or associated tissues. It occurs more often in girls and is generally diagnosed between the ages of 5 and 10 years (Hutchinson & Feldman, 2016a). The cause remains unclear but it may be an autoimmune response triggered by exposure to a virus or to certain medications (Hutchinson & Feldman, 2016a). As with other autoimmune diseases, a genetic predisposition is present. The inflammatory cells of the immune system cause a vasculitis that affects the skin, muscles, kidneys, retinas, and gastrointestinal tract.

Therapeutic management involving the use of high-dose glucocorticoid or other immunosuppressants is necessary to prevent the complications of painful calcium deposits under the skin, as well as joint contractures. Methotrexate, IVIG, and cyclosporine may also be used. With appropriate treatment, children may recover completely, though some children experience relapses (Hutchinson & Feldman, 2016b).

Nursing Assessment

Elicit a health history, which commonly includes fever, fatigue, and rash, usually followed by muscle pain and weakness. Determine the onset and progression of muscle weakness. Inspect the skin for the presence of rash involving the upper eyelids and extensor surfaces of the knuckles, elbows, and knees. The rash is initially a reddish-purple colour, and then progresses to scaling with resulting roughness of the skin. Test muscle strength, particularly noting weakness in the pelvic and shoulder girdles. Laboratory and diagnostic testing may include muscle enzyme levels, a positive ANA test, and an EMG to distinguish muscular weakness from other causes.

Nursing Management

Administer medications as ordered and teach families about their use; instruct them to monitor for side effects. Educate the family about the importance of maintaining the medication regimen in order to prevent calcinosis (calcium deposits) and joint deformity in the future. Encourage compliance with physical therapy regimens. Ensure that children are excused from physical education classes while the disease is active.

ALLERGY AND ANAPHYLAXIS

Allergy is an immune-mediated response resulting in an adverse physiologic event or reaction and affects up to 25% of population in developed countries (Covar,

Fleischer, Cho, & Boguniewicz, 2014). The extent of the allergic response is determined by the duration, rate, and amount of exposure to the allergen as well as environmental and host factors. IgE-mediated allergy will be the focus of this discussion. This type of allergic response is mediated by antigen-specific IgE antibodies. When the antibody is exposed to the antigen (allergen), rapid cell activation occurs and potent mediators and cytokines are released, resulting in changes in the blood vessels, bronchi, and mucus-secreting glands. In addition to the atopic diseases (asthma, allergic rhinitis, and atopic dermatitis), urticaria, digestive allergy, and systemic anaphylaxis are also IgE mediated. Though any allergen has the potential to trigger an anaphylactic response, food and insect-sting allergies are most common (Sloand & Caschera, 2010; Rote & McCance, 2015).

Food Allergies

A true food hypersensitivity or allergy is defined as an immunologic reaction resulting from the ingestion of a food or food additive. This type of reaction is an IgE-mediated response to a particular food. Food allergy affects approximately 8% of children and can lead to significant medical complications (Covar et al., 2014). During the first few years of life, the most common food allergens are milk, eggs, peanuts, tree nuts, fish and shellfish, wheat, and soy. Typically, allergies to these foods are acquired in childhood. For most children only allergies to peanuts, tree nuts, and fish and shellfish persist into adulthood (Covar et al., 2014). Most reactions occur within minutes of exposure, but they may occur up to 2 hours after ingestion. Signs and symptoms of a food allergy reaction include hives, flushing, facial swelling, mouth and throat itching, and runny nose. Many children also have a gastrointestinal reaction, including vomiting, abdominal pain, and diarrhea. In extreme cases, swelling of the tongue, uvula, pharynx, or upper airway may occur. Wheezing can be an ominous sign that the airway is edematous. Rarely, cardiovascular collapse occurs. Though the risk for anaphylaxis is small, parents, caregivers, and physicians and nurse practitioners should be vigilant when caring for children with food allergies.

Therapeutic Management

Therapeutic management involves verifying the food allergy, avoiding the allergen, and treating the reaction with medications, including antihistamines and epinephrine (in the case of an anaphylactic reaction).

Discerning a true food allergy from intolerance to certain foods is an important part of therapeutic management. "Food intolerance" is a general term that describes an abnormal physiologic response to an ingested food or food additive that has not been proven to be immunologic. Often a milk allergy is confused with lactose intolerance. Therefore, a detailed dietary history is important when distinguishing a true allergy versus intolerance. To prevent the development of food allergies, infants should be breastfed for at least the first 6 months of life.

Nursing Assessment

It is important to accurately assess children with food allergy reactions. In the initial nursing assessment, immediately assess the child for airway, breathing, or circulation problems (see Chapter 51). If the child's condition is stable, finish the assessment. Make sure that the health history includes a detailed food history and documentation of the reaction, including the food suspected of causing the reaction, the quantity of food ingested, the length of time between ingestion and development of symptoms, the symptoms, what treatment has been administered, and the subsequent response. Note gastrointestinal symptoms such as:

- Burning in the mouth or throat
- Bloating
- Nausea
- Diarrhea

Assess for risk factors such as previous exposure to the food, history of poorly controlled asthma, or an increase in atopic dermatitis flare-ups in relation to food intake.

Inspect the skin for colour, rash, hives, or edema. Auscultate the heart and lungs to determine the heart rate and to assess for wheezing.

Allergy skin-prick tests and radioallergosorbent blood tests (RASTs) are used widely by physicians and nurse practitioners to look for allergic reactions. However, these tests may have false-positive results, and children may need to avoid many foods unnecessarily (Sloand & Caschera, 2010). Food-specific IgE testing is recommended if the child has a history of food allergy. If the child has episodic symptoms, an oral challenge in a controlled setting may be appropriate. For an oral challenge, the child slowly eats a serving of the offending food over the period of 1 hour. Record vital signs and note the presence or absence of allergic symptoms.

If symptoms are chronic, a trial elimination diet may be indicated. If symptoms resolve without the food, true allergy may be present. On an elimination diet, the child should stop eating all suspicious foods for 1 to 2 weeks and then retry the foods one at a time, over a period of several days, to see whether a similar reaction occurs. Oral challenge testing and retrying of foods after an elimination diet are often done in the physician's or nurse practitioner's office or hospital setting if severe reactions have occurred in the past. If a similar reaction to a previous reaction to a certain food or foods occurs with the oral challenge or elimination diet testing, it is very

NURSING CARE PLAN 47.1

Overview for the Child With an Immunologic Disorder (continued)

NURSING DIAGNOSIS: Impaired skin integrity related to disease process or photosensitivity as evidenced by skin rash or alopecia

Outcome Identification and Evaluation

Skin integrity will be maintained: *secondary infection will not occur, rash will not increase.*

Intervention: *Preventing Skin Impairment*

- Assess and monitor the extent and location of rash to provide baseline information and evaluate success of interventions.
- Keep the skin clean and dry to prevent secondary infection.
- For the child with eczema, apply topical medications as ordered to decrease inflammatory response.
- For the child with limited mobility, turn frequently and use specialty mattress or bed to prevent pressure ulcers.

- Implement a written plan of care directed toward topical treatment of skin integrity impairment to provide consistency of care and documentation.
- Educate the child and family to limit direct sun exposure and use sunscreen to prevent sun damage.

NURSING DIAGNOSIS: Activity intolerance related to joint pain, fatigue or weakness, concurrent illness as evidenced by dyspnea, lack of desire to participate in play, inability to maintain usual routine

Outcome Identification and Evaluation

Child will participate in activities: *will demonstrate easy work of breathing and participate in daily routine and play.*

Intervention: *Promoting Activity*

- Cluster care to decrease disturbances and allow for longer uninterrupted rest periods.
- Pace activities and encourage regular rest periods to conserve energy.
- Administer early morning warm bath to ease a.m. stiffness (juvenile arthritis).
- Use assistive devices such as splints and orthotics to improve physical function.

- Plan developmentally appropriate activities that the child can participate in while in bed to encourage play and continued development.
- Schedule activities for the time of day the child usually has the most energy to encourage successful participation.

NURSING DIAGNOSIS: Risk for delayed development related to physical effects of chronic illness, or physical disability (juvenile arthritis) as evidenced by the delay in meeting expected milestones

Outcome Identification and Evaluation

Development will be enhanced: *child will make continued progress toward expected developmental milestones.*

NURSING CARE PLAN 47.1

Overview for the Child With an Immunologic Disorder (continued)

Intervention: *Enhancing Growth and Development*

- Screen for developmental capabilities to determine the child's current level of functioning.
- Offer age-appropriate toys, play, and activities (including gross motor) to encourage further development.
- Encourage peer contact through telephone, e-mail, or letters to promote/continue socialization.
- Perform interventions as prescribed by physical or occupational therapist: repeat participation in those activities helps the child improve function and acquire developmental skills.

- Provide support to families of children with developmental delay: progress in achieving developmental milestones can be slow, and ongoing motivation is needed.
- Encourage the child to continue schoolwork so that child will not fall behind.
- Reinforce positive attributes in the child to maintain motivation.

KEY CONCEPTS

- Waning of maternal antibodies in early infancy while humoral immunity is developing leads to physiologic hypogammaglobulinemia, placing the young infant at risk for overwhelming infection.

- Infants and young children have large lymph nodes, tonsils, and thymus compared with adults.

- Infants have decreased phagocytic activity, placing them at higher risk for serious infection.

- Children with immune disorders often show a decreased or absent response to delayed hypersensitivity skin testing (e.g., the tuberculosis test).

- The ELISA test for HIV detects only antibodies to HIV (which in the infant may be maternal in origin), whereas the PCR test for HIV tests for HIV genetic material, making it the more accurate test for HIV infection in infants and young children.

- Primary immune deficiencies such as the SCID and Wiskott–Aldrich syndrome are congenital and serious; they can be cured only by bone marrow or stem cell transplantation.

- SLE is a chronic autoimmune disorder that can affect any organ system, primarily causing vasculitis.

- Juvenile idiopathic arthritis results in chronic pain and affects growth and development as well as school performance.

- Nasal, palatal, or throat pruritus and difficulty breathing may indicate an anaphylactic reaction.

- Various forms of hypogammaglobulinemia may be treated with exogenous immunoglobulin

administered intravenously every several weeks, allowing children to lead a healthier life with fewer infections.

- Children with severe allergy or previous anaphylactic episodes must avoid contact with allergens.

- Nursing management of lupus focuses on preventing flare-ups and complications.

- Managing pain, maintaining mobility, and administering disease-modifying medications are key nursing interventions in the management of juvenile idiopathic arthritis.

- HIV infection may be prevented in infants by prenatal screening and maternal treatment, as well as postnatal treatment with zidovudine.

- HIV infection in children often results in encephalopathy and developmental delay.

- Spread of HIV infection can be prevented in adolescence by avoiding high-risk behaviours.

- For children with immune deficiency or autoimmune disease, prevention of infection is a primary nursing concern.

- A chronic illness such as immune deficiency, SLE, or juvenile arthritis has a significant impact on the family as well as the child.

- When planning care for the child with an immune deficiency or autoimmune disorder, the nurse should include the child and the family.

- To promote proper growth, encourage the child with an immune or autoimmune disorder to eat a balanced diet.

○ Teach families of children with immune deficiencies about infection prevention.

○ Teach the family of the child with juvenile arthritis about ways to decrease pain while increasing or maintaining the child's mobility.

○ Teach families of children with severe allergy how to avoid allergens and how to use the EpiPen. Make sure that the staff at the child's school or daycare centre are aware of the allergy.

○ Explain to the child with severe allergy the importance of wearing a medical ID alert bracelet or necklace.

REFERENCES AND RECOMMENDED READINGS

Atkinson, W., Wolfe, S., & Hamborsky, J. (Eds.). (2012). *Epidemiology and prevention of vaccine-preventable diseases* (12th ed.). Washington, DC: Public Health Foundation.

Atlantic SCIG Working Group. (2016). *Atlantic Guideline for Subcutaneous Immune Globulin Home Administration Programs*. Retrieved from https://novascotia.ca/dhw/nspbcp/docs/Atlantic-Guideline-for-Subcutaneous-Immune-Globulin-Home-Administration-Programs-September-2016.pdf.

Aydin, Y., Ulas, A. B., Mutlu, V., Corlak, A., & Eroglu, A. (2017). Thymectomy in myasthenia gravis. *Eurasian Journal of Medicine, 49*(1), 48–52.

Blaese, R. M., Bonilla, F. A., Stiehm, E. R., & Younger, M. E. (Eds.). (2013). *Patient and family handbook for primary immune deficiency diseases* (5th ed.). Towson, MD: Immune Deficiency Foundation.

Bonilla, F. A. (2015). *Severe combined immunodeficiency (SCID): An overview*. Retrieved from http://www.uptodate.com/contents/severe-combined-immunodeficiency-scid-an-overview.

Canadian Paediatric Society. (2018). *Emergency treatment of anaphylaxis in infants and children*. Retrieved from https://www.cps.ca/en/documents/position/emergency-treatment-anaphylaxis.

Carpenito-Moyet, L. J. (2013). *Nursing diagnosis: Application to clinical practice* (14th ed.). Philadelphia, PA: Lippincott Williams & Wilkins.

Centers for Disease Control and Prevention. (2015). *HIV surveillance report, 2013. Vol. 25*. Atlanta, GA: Author.

Christensen, R. D., Baer, V. L., Gordon, P. V., Henry, E., Whitaker, C., Andres, R. L., & Bennett, S. T. (2012). Reference ranges for lymphocyte counts of neonates: associations between abnormal counts and outcomes. *Pediatrics, 129*(5), e1165–e1172. doi: 10.1542/peds.2011-2661.

Corbett, J. A., & Banks, A. D. (2013). *Laboratory tests and diagnostic procedures with nursing diagnoses* (8th ed.). Upper Saddle River, NJ: Pearson Education Inc.

Covar, R. A., Fleischer, D. M., Cho, C., & Boguniewicz, M. (2014). Allergic disorders. In W. W. Hay, M. J. Levin, R. R. Deterding, & M. J. Abzug (Eds.). *Current pediatric diagnosis and treatment* (22nd ed.). New York, NY: McGraw-Hill.

Cruse, R. P. (2014). *Epidemiology, clinical features, and diagnosis of Guillain-Barré syndrome in children*. Retrieved from http://www.uptodate.com/contents/epidemiology-clinical-features-and-diagnosis-of-guillain-barre-syndrome-in-children.

De Santis, J. P., Garcia, A., Chaparro, A., & Beltran, O. (2014). Integration versus disintegration: A grounded theory study of adolescent and young adult development in the context of perinatally-acquired HIV infection. *Journal of Pediatric Nursing, 29*(5), 422–435.

Durani, Y., Egan, M., Baffa, J., Selbst, S. M., & Nager, A. L. (2009). Pediatric myocarditis: presenting clinical characteristics. *The American Journal of Emergency Medicine, 27*(8), 942–947.

Fahrner, R., & Romano, S. (2010). HIV infection and AIDS. In P. J. Allen, J. A. Vessey, & N. A. Schapiro (Eds.). *Primary care of the child with a chronic condition* (5th ed.). St. Louis, MO: Mosby.

Freedman, S. B., Haladyn, J. K., Floh, A., Kirsh, J. A., Taylor, G., & Thull-Freedman, J. (2007). Pediatric myocarditis: emergency department clinical findings and diagnostic evaluation. *Pediatrics, 120*(6), 1278–1285.

Government of Canada. (2016). HIV in Canada: Surveillance summary tables, 2014-2015. Retrieved from https://www.canada.ca/en/public-health/services/publications/diseases-conditions/hiv-in-canada-surveillance-summary-tables-2014-2015.html

Government of Canada. (2017). HIV in Canada: 2016. HIV in Canada—Surveillance Report, 2016. 43-12. Retrieved from https://www.canada.ca/en/public-health/services/reports-publications/canada-communicable-disease-report-ccdr/monthly-issue/2017-43/ccdr-volume-43-12-december-7-2017/hiv-canada-2016.html

Gronseth, G. S., & Barohn, R. J. (2002). Thymectomy for myasthenia gravis. *Current Treatment Options in Neurology, 4*(3), 203–209.

Hassiotou, F., & Geddes, D. T. (2015). Immune cell–mediated protection of the mammary gland and the infant during breastfeeding. *Advances in Nutrition: An International Review Journal, 6*(3), 267–275. doi: 10.3945/an.114.007377.

Hauk, P. J., Johnston, R. B., & Liu, A. H. (2014). Immunodeficiency. In W. W. Hay, M. J. Levin, R. R. Deterding, & M. J. Abzug (Eds.). *Current pediatric diagnosis and treatment* (22nd ed.). New York, NY: McGraw-Hill.

Horvath, T., Azman, H., Kennedy, G. E., & Rutherford, G. W. (2012). *Mobile phone text messaging for promoting adherence to antiretroviral therapy in patients with HIV infection. The Cochrane Library 2012, 3*. Indianapolis, IN: John Wiley & Sons.

Hutchinson, C., & Feldman, B. M. (2016a). *Juvenile dermatomyositis and polymyositis: Epidemiology, pathogenesis, and clinical manifestations*. Retrieved from http://www.uptodate.com/contents/juvenile-dermatomyositis-and-polymyositis-epidemiology-pathogenesis-and-clinical-manifestations.

Hutchinson, C., & Feldman, B. M. (2016b). *Juvenile dermatomyositis and polymyositis: Treatment, complications, and prognosis*. Retrieved from http://www.uptodate.com/contents/juvenile-dermatomyositis-and-polymyositis-treatment-complications-and-prognosis.

Jeffrey Modell Foundation. (2013). *10 warning signs of primary immunodeficiency*. Retrieved from http://downloads.info4pi.org/pdfs/General10WarningSignsFINAL.pdf.

Johnson, B. (2014). Overview of neonatal lupus. *Journal of Pediatric Health Care, 28*(4), 331–341.

Jones, K. B., & Higgins, G. C. (2010). Juvenile rheumatoid arthritis. In P. J. Allen, J. A. Vessey, & N. A. Schapiro (Eds.). *Primary care of the child with a chronic condition* (5th ed.). St. Louis, MO: Mosby.

Kang, L. J. (2017). *Pre and postnatal maternal distress and infant gut immunity in the Canadian Healthy Infant Longitudinal Development (CHILD) birth cohort.* (Doctoral dissertation, University of Alberta). Retrieved from https://era.library.ualberta.ca/files/ccz30pt01p#.WWgs1TPMzMI.

Kids with Food Allergies. (2016). *Allergen avoidance lists.* Retrieved from http://www.kidswithfoodallergies.org/page/top-food-allergens.aspx.

Lehman, T. J. A. (2015). *Systemic lupus erythematosus (SLE) in children: Clinical manifestations and diagnosis.* Retrieved from http://www.uptodate.com/contents/systemic-lupus-erythematosus-sle-in-children-clinical-manifestations-and-diagnosis.

Lierl, M. B. (2011). Allergen immunotherapy: Shots for asthma, wheezing, and bee sting. *Pediatric Annals, 40*(4), 192–199.

Liew, W. K., & Kang, P. B. (2013). Update on juvenile myasthenia gravis. *Current Opinion in Pediatrics, 25*(6), 694–700.

Marchant, A., & Goldman, M. (2005). T cell-mediated immune responses in human newborns: ready to learn?. *Clinical & Experimental Immunology, 141*(1), 10–18. doi:10.1111/j.1365-2249.2005.02799.x.

Mattingly, E. (2011). Lupus in adolescents. *Advance for NPs & PAs, 2*(4), 27–32.

McFarland, E. J. (2014). Human immunodeficiency virus infection. In W. W. Hay, M. J. Levin, R. R. Deterding, & M. J. Abzug (Eds.). *Current pediatric diagnosis and treatment* (22nd ed.). New York: McGraw-Hill.

Mylan Specialty. (2016). *How to use your EpiPen® (epinephrine injection) autoinjector.* Retrieved from http://www.epipen.com/how-to-use-epipen.

Norville, R., & Tomlinson, D. (2010). Hematopoietic stem cell transplantation. In D. Tomlinson & N. E. Kline (Eds.). *Pediatric oncology nursing: Advanced clinical handbook* (2nd ed.). New York: Springer.

Ochs, H. D. (2015). *Wiskott-Aldrich syndrome.* Retrieved from http://www.uptodate.com/contents/wiskott-aldrich-syndrome.

Pagana, K. D., Pagana, T. J., & Pike-MacDonald, S. A. (2012). *Mosby's Canadian Manual of Diagnostic and Laboratory Tests* (1st Canadian ed.). Toronto: Elsevier Canada.

Panel on Antiretroviral Therapy and Medical Management of HIV-Infected Children. (2016). *Guidelines for the use of antiretroviral agents in pediatric HIV infection.* Retrieved from http://aidsinfo.nih.gov/contentfiles/lvguidelines/pediatricguidelines.pdf.

Public Health Agency of Canada. (2015). *HIV and AIDS in Canada: Surveillance Report to December 31, 2014.* Ottawa: Minister of Public Works and Government Services Canada.

Robinson, J. L. (2008). Testing for HIV infection in pregnancy. *Paediatric Child Health, 13*(3), 221–224. Retrieved from https://www.cps.ca/en/documents/position/testing-for-hiv-infection-in-pregnancy

Rote, N. S., & McCance, K. L. (2015). Alterations in immunity and inflammation. In K. McCance & S. Huether (Eds.). *Pathophysiology: The biologic basis for disease in adults and children* (7th ed.). St. Louis, MO: Elsevier.

Schwartz, A., & Rote, N. S. (2015). Alterations of leukocyte, lymphoid, and hemostatic Function. In K. McCance & S. Huether (Eds.). *Pathophysiology: The biologic basis for disease in adults and children.* St. Louis, MO: Elsevier.

Siberry, G. K., Abzug, M. J., & Nachman, S. (2013). Executive summary: 2013 update of the guidelines for the prevention and treatment of opportunistic infections in HIV-exposed and HIV-infected children. *Pediatric Infectious Disease Journal, 32*(12), 1303–1307.

Sloand, E., & Caschera, J. (2010). Allergies. In P. J. Allen, J. A. Vessey, & N. A. Schapiro (Eds.). *Primary care of the child with a chronic condition* (5th ed.). St. Louis, MO: Mosby.

Soep, J. B. (2014). Rheumatic diseases. In W. W. Hay, M. J. Levin, R. R. Deterding, & M. J. Abzug (Eds.). *Current pediatric diagnosis and treatment* (22nd ed.). New York: McGraw-Hill.

Stanley, L. C., & Ward-Smith, P. (2011). The diagnosis and management of juvenile idiopathic arthritis. *Journal of Pediatric Health Care, 25*(3), 191–194.

Taketomo, C. K., Hodding, J. H., & Kraus, D. M. (2013). *Pediatric & neonatal dosage handbook* (20th ed.). Hudson, OH: Lexicomp.

Tofferi, J. K. (2015). *Avascular necrosis.* Retrieved from http://emedicine.medscape.com/article/333364-overview

Tosi, M. F. (2014). Normal and impaired immunologic responses to infection. In J. Cherry, G. J. Demmler-Harrison, S. L. Kaplan, W. J. Steinbach, & P. Hotez (Eds.). *Feigin & Cherry's textbook of pediatric infectious disease* (7th ed.). Philadelphia, PA: Saunders.

UNAIDS. (2014). *Children and HIV fact sheet.* Geneva, Switzerland: World Health Organization.

van Doorn, P. A., Ruts, L., & Jacobs, B. C. (2008). Clinical features, pathogenesis, and treatment of Guillain-Barré syndrome. *The Lancet Neurology, 7*(10), 939–950.

van Doorn, P. A., Kuitwaard, K., Walgaard, C., van Koningsveld, R., Ruts, L., & Jacobs, B. C. (2010). IVIG treatment and prognosis in Guillain–Barre syndrome. *Journal of Clinical Immunology, 30*(Suppl 1), 74–78.

Varadhi, A., Hageman, J. R., & Yu, K. O. A. (2013). The "five fingers" of the diagnostic evaluation for suspected immunodeficiency. *Pediatric Annals, 42*(5), 210–215.

Wagner, C. W. (2013). Anaphylaxis in the pediatric patient: Optimizing management and prevention. *Journal of Pediatric Health Care, 27*(2S), S5–S17.

Ward, T. M., Sonney, J., Ringold, S., Stockfish, S., Wallace, C. A., & Landis, C. A. (2014). Sleep disturbances and behavior problems in children with and without arthritis. *Journal of Pediatric Nursing, 29*(4), 321–328.

Winkels, K. (2015). *Allergy-free substitutes.* Retrieved from http://www.eatingwithfoodallergies.com/allergyfreesubstitutes.html

Woo, C. K., & Bahna, S. L. (2011). Evaluation of the child with immunodeficiency disorder. *Pediatric Annals, 40*(4), 205–211.

Zafar, R., Ver Heul, A., Beigelman, A., Bednarski, J. J., Bayliss, S. J., Dehner, L. P., … & Coughlin, C. C. (2017). Omenn Syndrome Presenting with Striking Erythroderma and Extreme Lymphocytosis in a Newborn. *Pediatric Dermatology, 34*(1), e37–e39. doi: 10.1111/pde.13023

48

Nursing Care of the Child With an Alteration in Metabolism/Endocrine Disorder

Learning Objectives

Upon completion of the chapter, the learner will be able to:

1. Describe the major components and functions of a child's endocrine system.

2. Differentiate between the anatomic and physiologic differences of the endocrine system in children versus adults.

3. Identify the essential assessment elements, common diagnostic procedures, and laboratory tests associated with the diagnosis of endocrine disorders in children.

4. Identify the common medications and treatment modalities used for palliation of endocrine disorders in children.

5. Distinguish specific disorders of the endocrine system affecting children.

6. Link the clinical manifestations of specific disorders in the endocrine system of a child with the appropriate nursing diagnoses.

7. Establish the nursing outcomes, evaluative criteria, and interventions for a child with specific disorders in the endocrine system.

8. Develop child/family teaching plans for the child with an endocrine disorder.

Carlos Rodriguez, **12 years old, is seen in the clinic today with complaints of weakness, fatigue, blurred vision, and headaches. His mother states, "Carlos' teacher has noticed mood changes and is concerned about his behaviour at school. He's always been a good boy. I'm not sure what's going on."**

Metabolism refers to all physical and chemical reaction occurring in the body's cells that are necessary to sustain life (Herzing University–Orlando, 2014). Nurses encounter potential and actual alterations in metabolism in all types of clients and must detect problems and intervene early to prevent life-threatening or long-term complications. The endocrine system consists of various glands, tissues, or clusters of cells that produce and release hormones. **Hormones** are chemical messengers that stimulate and/or regulate the actions of other tissues, organs, or other endocrine glands that have specific receptors to a hormone. Along with the nervous system, the endocrine system regulates physiologic effects such as growth and development, metabolic processes related to fluid and electrolyte balance and energy production, sexual maturation and reproduction, and the body's response to stress. While the timing and release patterns of the hormones vary, levels in the body are maintained to support homeostasis.

Alterations in metabolism develop when there is an imbalance in the endocrine system, either as a deficiency **(hypofunction)** or excess **(hyperfunction)** of a specific hormone. In children, alterations in hormone production influence the neuroendocrine system as well as metabolism. If the problem is not diagnosed and treated early, neurologic symptoms may arise or there may be a delay in growth and development, or even death. Generally, the treatment plan involves correction of the underlying reason for the dysfunction, such as surgical removal of a tumour, and supplementation of missing hormones or adjustment of specific hormone levels.

VARIATIONS IN ANATOMY AND PHYSIOLOGY

The organs or tissues of the endocrine system include the hypothalamus, pituitary gland, thyroid gland, parathyroid glands, adrenal glands, gonads, and islets of Langerhans located in the pancreas. Figure 48.1 shows the location of the organs or tissues involved in the endocrine system. Typically, most endocrine glands begin to develop during the first trimester of gestation, but their development is incomplete at birth. Thus, complete hormonal control is lacking during the early years of life, and the infant cannot appropriately balance fluid concentration, electrolytes, amino acids, glucose, and trace substances.

Hormone Production and Secretion

The hypothalamic–pituitary axis produces a number of releasing and inhibiting hormones that regulate the function of many of the other endocrine glands, including the thyroid gland, the adrenal glands, and the male and female gonads. Some glands regulate their function in connection with the nervous system, such as the islets of Langerhans in the pancreas and the parathyroid glands. Many other cells in the body secrete hormones such as the pineal gland, the scattered epithelial cells in the gastrointestinal (GI) tract, and the thymus. Disorders related to these other cells are discussed in other chapters in this textbook.

Figure 48.1 shows the major glands, the hormones produced by the glands, and the effect each hormone has on the target cell, tissue, or organ. The process of hormone production and secretion involves the principle of feedback control. One gland produces a hormone that affects another endocrine gland. Once the physiologic effect is achieved, this gland, known as the target organ, inhibits the further release of the original hormone. The reverse occurs when the first gland detects low levels of the target gland hormone. If the original gland does not release enough of the hormone, the inhibition process stops so that the gland increases the production of the hormone. The endocrine system and the nervous system work closely together to maintain an optimal internal environment for the body, known as homeostasis.

COMMON MEDICAL TREATMENTS

Primarily, the treatment of endocrine disorders involves decreasing hormone production (in cases of hypersecretion) or replacing the hormones (in cases of hypofunction). The first step in treating many of these disorders is to screen for potential problems, especially when familial patterns are present. Since the proper functioning of the endocrine system is critical to growth and development, the child's growth is affected by endocrine dysfunction and lack of treatment may lead to serious problems, such as intellectual disability or even death. Early treatment is often associated with better prognosis and prevention of long-term problems. The next step in treatment involves identifying underlying causes for the dysfunction (e.g., a tumour or growth that requires surgical removal or irradiation). The use of supplemental hormone in cases of hypofunction is generally successful in children, as is the use of inhibiting substances in cases of hyperfunction.

Common Medical Treatments 48.1 describes the common treatments used in children with endocrine disorders. The table explains and gives indications for each treatment as well as relevant nursing implications. Advances in technology and our understanding of molecular biology (i.e., genetics and immunologic influences) and environmental factors continue to increase our knowledge of these disorders and the modalities needed to prevent them or improve quality of life for affected children.

Hypothalamus—stimulates pituitary gland
to release or withhold hormones

Pituitary—anterior:
releases growth,
thyroid-stimulating,
adrenocorticotropic,
follicle-stimulating,
luteinizing,
melanocyte-producing
hormones, and prolactin.
Posterior: releases
antidiuretic hormone and
oxytocin

Thymus—produces humoral factors key
to the development of immunity

Pancreas—releases insulin,
glucagon, and somatostatin
for regulation of
blood glucose levels

Ovary—releases estrogen
and progesterone

Testes—release
testosterone

Adrenal—releases aldosterone,
mineralocorticoids, androgens,
epinephrine, and norepinephrine

Parathyroid—regulates calcium
and phosphorus concentrations

Thyroid—releases thyroid hormone for regulation of metabolism
and growth, and thyrocalcitonin for bone development

FIGURE 48.1 Location of the endocrine glands in the body, with the major effects of the
glands listed.

Drug Guide 48.1 lists the medications most commonly used to treat endocrine disorders. The table gives
the actions and indications of each drug, as well as pertinent nursing implications. Many of the medications
are synthetic preparations of the actual hormones. It is
important to maintain specific blood levels of the drugs
to mimic the actual hormone in the body. Nurses must
monitor for side effects of too little or too much of the
hormone in the child's system. Most endocrine disorders
in children require treatment and follow-up with a pediatric endocrinologist as well as a multidisciplinary team
that includes a registered nurse who specializes in this
area.

NURSING PROCESS OVERVIEW FOR THE CHILD WITH AN ENDOCRINE DISORDER

The nursing care of the child with an endocrine
disorder requires astute assessment skills, accurate nursing diagnoses and expected outcomes, skilled interventions, and evaluation of the entire process. Children,
especially very young ones, easily develop imbalances
such as fluid and electrolyte disturbances that can cause
further problems. Most of the endocrine disorders are
chronic conditions that require ongoing care related to
health maintenance, education, developmental issues,

COMMON MEDICAL TREATMENTS 48.1

Interventions	Explanation	Indications	Nursing Implications
Surgery	Surgical removal of tumours or cysts	Any endocrine malfunction caused by the presence of a mass	• Provide routine preoperative and postoperative care, depending on location and extent of surgery. • Keep family informed of choices.
Irradiation/radioactive iodine	Radiation is used to influence the hormone secretion of a gland; it is less invasive than surgery	Hyperfunction of an endocrine gland; may be used when surgery is not possible	• Prepare child for specific procedures following protocols. • Explain the procedure. • Check to ensure child has no sensitivity to iodine preparations.
Glucose monitoring	Fingerstick blood sample several times per day	Monitoring of glucose control	• Teach family appropriate procedure. • Refer family to sources for equipment and supplies. • Assist family to develop a system of record keeping that works for them.
Dietary interventions (medical nutrition therapy)	Restriction or manipulation of dietary intake	Diabetes mellitus (DM)	• Refer family to a dietitian specializing in pediatric diabetes mellitus. • Reinforce teaching related to special diets.

DRUG GUIDE 48.1 COMMON DRUGS FOR ENDOCRINE DISORDERS

Medication	Actions/Indications	Nursing Implications
Insulin	Used for DM to replace body's natural insulin, which is necessary for proper glucose use. Indicated for DM type 1 and, sometimes, DM type 2	• Monitor vital signs and blood glucose levels. • Educate child and family on proper techniques, actions, and adverse effects. • Rotate site of injections to prevent adipose hypertrophy.
Oral hypoglycemic drugs (sulfonylureas, biguanides)	Assist body's production of insulin by stimulating β cells to secrete more insulin Indicated for DM type 2	• Monitor vital signs and glucose levels. • Administer with food to minimize gastric upset. • Instruct child and family on use of drug and adverse effects. • Warn family that some over-the-counter or other drugs may increase hypoglycemic effect.
Growth hormone (GH)/ somatropin	Stimulates linear bone, skeletal muscle, and organ growth Used for GH deficiency, growth failure related to inadequate pituitary hormone	• Monitor blood sugar and electrolyte levels. • Administer before epiphyses are fused. • Monitor growth with accurate measurements. • Instruct child and family on appropriate route and method of administration. • Periodic thyroid function tests will be needed. • May interact with glucocorticoid therapy. • Monitor for limping or complaints in knee or hip related to slipped epiphysis.
Octreotide acetate	Suppresses GH release Indicated for acromegaly	• Monitor for biliary tract abnormalities, glucose tolerance, and hypothyroidism. • Give subcutaneous injections between meals to decrease gastric effects.

(continued)

DRUG GUIDE 48.1 COMMON DRUGS FOR ENDOCRINE DISORDERS (continued)

Medication	Actions/Indications	Nursing Implications
Corticosteroids (dexamethasone hydrocortisone or prednisone)	Cortisol replacement in congenital adrenal hyperplasia, absence or insufficiency of adrenal glands. Also used to close epiphyseal plates in hyperpituitarism	• Give with milk or food. • Teach need to increase dose if child is ill or runs fever. • Teach use of injectable hydrocortisone. • Monitor for edema, weight gain, glycosuria, signs of infection, and symptoms of peptic ulcer development. • Do not decrease dose or abruptly stop drug to avoid adrenal crisis.
Desmopressin acetate	Synthetic antidiuretic hormone that promotes reabsorption of water by action on renal tubules Used to control diabetes insipidus	• Monitor for water intoxication, signs and symptoms of hyponatremia, and adverse effects such as nasal irritation, headache, nausea, and increased blood pressure. • Record fluid intake and output and weigh child daily. • Titrate dose until appropriate fluid output is obtained. • Instruct child and family in proper intranasal administration. • Avoid over-the-counter cough/hay fever preparations, as they may decrease the drug response. • Store in refrigerator.
Levothyroxine	Thyroid hormone replacement for hypothyroidism	• Check blood pressure and pulse before each dose. • Monitor fluid intake and output, daily weights, and thyroid function tests. • Watch for thyroid storm. • Report irritability or anxiety. • Instruct child and family to avoid over-the-counter preparations with iodine or foods such as soybeans, iodized salt, tofu, and turnips. • Administer at same time each day.
Methimazole	Antithyroid drug; blocks synthesis of T_3 and T_4 Indicated for hyperthyroidism	• Check pulse and blood pressure before each dose. • Monitor input and output, daily weights, serum T_3 and T_4 levels; watch for edema, leukopenia, thrombocytopenia, or agranulocytosis. • Administer with meals to decrease gastric upset. • Give at the same time each day. • Store in light-resistant container. • Instruct child and family to report sore throat, mouth lesions, unusual bleeding, or bruising. • Signs of overdose: periorbital edema, cold intolerance, mental depression • Signs of inadequate dose: tachycardia, diarrhea, fever, or irritability
Mineralocorticoid (fludrocortisone)	Promotes reabsorption of Na and K, water from distal renal tubules Used in adrenal insufficiency	• Monitor daily weights, blood pressure, and intake and output. • Observe for potassium depletion. • Titrate dose to lowest effective dose. • Adverse effects include flushing, sweating, headache, and increased blood pressure.

Adapted from Taketokmo, C. K., Hodding, J. H., & Kraus, D. M. (2013). *Lexi-comp's drug reference handbook: Pediatric & neonatal dosage handbook* (20th ed.). Hudson, OH: Lexi-comp, Inc.

and psychosocial needs. These conditions are sometimes complex and range from mild to profound. Early diagnosis and treatment can improve the long-term outcomes for these children.

> **Remember Carlos, the 12-year-old with weakness, fatigue, blurred vision, headaches, and mood changes? What additional health history and physical examination assessment information should the nurse obtain?**

Assessment

Nursing assessment of a child with endocrine dysfunction includes obtaining a thorough health history, performing a physical assessment, and assisting with or obtaining laboratory and diagnostic tests. The clinical manifestations of endocrine disorders occur as a result of the altered control of the bodily processes normally regulated by the gland or hormone. These manifestations present in many areas of the body because of the diverse functions associated with the endocrine system.

Health History

The health history should include questions regarding any family history of an endocrine disorder or growth and development difficulties. Use a genogram or family tree to detail the information about the family history in a clear and concise manner.

Discuss prenatal history, including any maternal factors that may affect growth and development such as substance abuse, use of tobacco or alcohol, and Graves disease; birth history, such as trauma during delivery, birth size, feeding difficulties, and neonatal screening and results; past medical history, such as any chronic childhood disease, treatment for any endocrine problems, recent gastroenteritis or viral syndrome, or exposures to exogenous steroids or gonadotropins; and growth and development patterns, including presence of any delays, learning disabilities, and early or late development of secondary sexual characteristics.

Discuss present complaints or illness. Note onset of symptoms, whether gradual or sudden. Endocrine disorders often cause problems in normal growth and development as well as behavioural changes. Question the parent or caregiver about prior growth patterns, achievement of developmental milestones, and the child's behaviour. Inquire about recent increases or decreases in weight and height, changes in physical appearance, sleep patterns, muscle weakness, cramps, twitching, or headaches. Have the child and family describe the child's activities on a typical day, including school performance, to identify subtle variations in the

child's behaviour or moods. For example, a child who is typically quiet might ordinarily be less active than average children of that age, and the child with decreased endocrine function also often displays inactivity and fatigue. By having the family and child describe a typical day, the nurse can distinguish between what is appropriate for that child and what may be a change related to endocrine dysfunction.

In addition, obtain a history of dietary and elimination habits. Note extreme thirst, excessive appetite, vomiting, or frequent voiding. Children with endocrine disorders may have some of these symptoms.

Physical Examination

Physical examination of the child with an endocrine disorder includes inspection and observation, auscultation, percussion, and palpation. Table 48.1 lists key physical examination findings that may be present in the child with endocrine dysfunction.

INSPECTION AND OBSERVATION

Note a fatigued appearance, poor muscle tone, sweatiness, faintness, nervousness, or confusion. Inspect the head and face, and note hair texture and growth, a protuberant tongue, drooping eyelids, or **exophthalmos** (protrusion of the eyeballs). Plot the child's height and weight on growth charts to determine abnormal growth velocity, which occurs in many of these disorders.

AUSCULTATION

Auscultate the heart and lungs. Note heart rate and rhythm. During auscultation of the lungs, note laboured respiratory effort, such as Kussmaul breathing, which occurs in diabetic ketoacidosis. Document blood pressure.

PERCUSSION AND PALPATION

Percuss and then palpate the abdomen. Dull (nontympanic) sounds or the presence of masses may indicate constipation or a tumour of the ovaries.

Laboratory and Diagnostic Testing

Common Laboratory and Diagnostic Tests 48.1 describes the diagnostic tests and procedures frequently used in identifying and monitoring endocrine disorders in children. Serum and urine hormone and other levels are used to determine whether amounts are adequate, deficient, or excessive. Radiographic studies are used to evaluate bone maturation and growth potential as well as density or tissue calcification. Genetic studies may be used to determine enzyme deficiencies or chromosome defects. Stimulation studies provide a more accurate or definitive test for identifying the disorder after preliminary serum levels are abnormal. Serial blood sampling

(text continues on page 1883)

TABLE 48.1	KEY PHYSICAL EXAMINATION FINDINGS RELATED TO ENDOCRINE PROBLEMS
Height and weight	Below 3rd percentile or above 90th percentile (pituitary, thyroid, adrenal, or diabetes mellitus)
Hair	Coarse, brittle, excessive (hypothyroidism) Abnormal distribution (adrenal disorders)
Face	Round with hair growth (Cushing syndrome) Deformities or abnormal features (hypoparathyroidism)
Eyes	Blurred or changes in vision (diabetes mellitus, pituitary tumours, precocious puberty)
Mouth	Delayed dentition (hypocalcemia, hypopituitarism) Fruity breath (ketoacidosis)
Neck	Goitre (hyperthyroidism)
Skin	Cool to touch, dry (hypothyroidism) Changes in colour or texture (pituitary disorders) Easy bruising, striae (Cushing syndrome)
Chest	Tachycardia (hyperthyroidism) Palpitations, sweating (thyroid disorders) Deep, laboured breathing (ketoacidosis), hypertension (Cushing syndrome)
Abdomen	Extreme weight loss (diabetes mellitus) Extreme fat (Cushing syndrome) Changes in bowel habits (SIADH, diabetes insipidus, diabetes mellitus)
Fingers	Trembling (hyperthyroidism, parathyroid disorders)
Genitals	Excessive growth (adrenogenital syndrome) Early growth (precocious puberty) Delayed growth (hypopituitarism)

COMMON LABORATORY AND DIAGNOSTIC TESTS 48.1

Diagnostic Test or Procedure	Explanation	Indications	Nursing Implications
Newborn metabolic screening programs (refer to Chapter 31 for further information)	Newborn blood testing to identify certain harmful or potentially fatal disorders that are otherwise not apparent at birth. Disorders tested vary by province	Identify newborns so that treatment can begin early to prevent impact of disorder, such as severe cognitive impairment or death	• Refer to each province's protocol for fetal/newborn screening for endocrine disorders. • Explain to family the rationale and procedure. • Collect blood sample accurately. • Collect prior to blood transfusion if possible. • Ensure screening is done for early discharges. • Screening typically between 24 and 48 hours[a] after birth. • If collected before 24 hours of age, a repeat test is needed within 14 days.
Random serum hormone levels	Serum levels of various hormones; immunoassay measures levels with very small amounts of blood	High or low levels are used to evaluate the function of the specific gland	• May need to draw specimens at specific times. • Keep child NPO after midnight before test if ordered. • Diurnal variations and episodic secretion of many hormones may require special directions or further testing.

COMMON LABORATORY AND DIAGNOSTIC TESTS 48.1 (continued)

Diagnostic Test or Procedure	Explanation	Indications	Nursing Implications
Self-monitoring blood glucose (SMBG)	Fingerstick (monitors that utilize alternative sites, such as the forearm, are available); blood sample several times per day Noninvasive methods are being developed.[c]	Monitor glucose level and effectiveness of treatment	• Teach family appropriate procedure. • Refer family to sources for equipment and supplies. • Assist family to develop a system of record keeping that works for them. • Refer to Teaching Guideline 48.2.
Fasting plasma glucose	Fasting forces the body to produce glucagon, which causes the release of glucose. In a healthy child, the body will respond by releasing insulin, therefore lowering blood glucose and preventing hyperglycemia	Detect hyperglycemia related to diabetes or other conditions such as Cushing syndrome or liver or kidney disease Can detect prediabetes May detect hypoglycemia	• Child may not have had any caloric intake for at least 8 hours. • Draw sample prior to insulin or oral diabetic medications. • Normal value in children 2 to 18 years of age 3.5 to 5.6 mmol/L; in children 0 to 2 yrs of age 3.3 to 6.1 mmol/L; impaired fasting glucose or prediabetes is between 5.6 and 7 mmol/L; diabetes is considered with a result greater than or equal to 7 mmol/L on two separate occasions.
2-h plasma glucose test (2-h PG)	Oral glucose tolerance test Oral glucose is ingested, and in a healthy child, insulin will respond and return blood glucose to normal levels.	Usually performed to detect diabetes, often gestational diabetes Can also detect prediabetes	• Child should not have taken any insulin or oral diabetic medication before the test. • Time of oral glucose ingestion needs to be noted. • Specimen to be drawn at specified time interval from ingestion. • May have limited value in diagnosing children.[c]
Urine or serum ketone testing	Ketones are the result of the metabolism of fat and in a healthy child are present in insignificant amounts	Screening for ketones in urine is regularly performed in children, people with diabetes, hospitalized patients, preoperatively, and in pregnant women In children, ketones found in urine during routine urinalysis can detect undiagnosed diabetes In children with diabetes, the presence of ketones in serum or urine is a sign that their diabetes is not well controlled and can be an early sign of diabetic ketoacidosis (DKA)	• Urine ketone testing can be performed using dipsticks at the bedside and at home (follow manufacturer's directions; time reaction accurately and compare the strip to the control chart on the bottle). • Encourage testing for ketones when blood glucose is elevated, when therapy regimen is changing, or during times of stress or illness.

(*continued*)

COMMON LABORATORY AND DIAGNOSTIC TESTS 48.1 (continued)

Diagnostic Test or Procedure	Explanation	Indications	Nursing Implications
Hemoglobin A1c (glycated hemoglobin)	Glycated hemoglobin reflects the percentage of hemoglobin to which glucose is attached. In the case of hyperglycemia, an increase in glycohemoglobin leads to an increase in hemoglobin A1c. This test shows the average blood glucose level for the past 2 to 3 months.	Diagnose diabetes Indicated for children with diabetes. Provides information regarding long-term glycemic control and effectiveness of therapy	• Elevated levels seen in newly diagnosed diabetes or poorly controlled diabetes. • Levels can be elevated in nondiabetic children with certain conditions such as blood loss, hemolysis, iron-deficiency anemia, sickle cell disease, and lead toxicity.
Genetic testing	Tests for the presence of the gene for disease or carrier status	Determine genetic involvement of any disorder	• Explain procedure and the expense involved. • Refer for genetic counselling if needed.
Serum chemistry levels	Serum blood urea nitrogen (BUN), creatinine, sodium, potassium, glucose, calcium, phosphorus, alkaline phosphatase, etc.	Rule out chronic renal failure or other chronic illnesses; monitor effects of treatment	• BUN levels may be elevated with high-protein diet or dehydration, and may be decreased with overhydration or malnutrition. • A diet high in meat may cause a transient but not pronounced increase in creatinine. There are also slight diurnal variations in levels. • Avoid hemolysis of specimen, as this may cause elevation in potassium levels. • Calcium and phosphorus: avoid prolonged tourniquet use during blood draw, as this may falsely increase levels. Child should be NPO past midnight prior to the morning of the blood draw.
Growth hormone stimulation	Stimulate release of GH in response to administration of insulin, arginine, clonidine, or glucagon	Evaluate and diagnose GH deficiency	• Keep child NPO for specified time. • Limit stress and physical activity at least 30 minutes before test. • Obtain serial blood samples at specific times. • Monitor blood glucose levels during study. • Observe for signs of hypoglycemia, diaphoresis, and somnolence. • Provide a snack, such as cookies and juice at end of test.
Water deprivation study	Child is deprived of fluids for several hours, and serum sodium and urine osmolality are monitored	Diagnose diabetes insipidus (DI) and distinguish between types of DI	• Stop test if child exhibits extreme weight loss or changes in vital signs or neurologic status. • Weigh child before, during, and after test. • Rehydrate child after test. • Monitor for orthostatic hypotension.

COMMON LABORATORY AND DIAGNOSTIC TESTS 48.1 (continued)

Diagnostic Test or Procedure	Explanation	Indications	Nursing Implications
Bone age x-ray	Radiographic study of wrist or hand to determine bone maturation compared with national standards	Determine if bone age is consistent with chronologic age to rule out GH deficiency or excess or hypothyroidism	• Explain procedure to child because child must hold still for the x-ray. • Allow family to accompany child. Enlist the family's help if needed to calm child during radiography.
Other nuclear medicine studies	Contrast media uptake is assessed with serial x-rays	Visualize an ectopic, enlarged, absent, or nodular gland	• Assess child for allergy to iodine or shellfish. • Explain procedure to child.
Computed tomography (CT)	Noninvasive x-ray study that looks at tissue density and structures. Images a "slice" of tissue	Evaluate presence of tumours, cysts, or structural abnormalities that may affect specific gland or structure	• Machine is large and can be frightening to children. • Scan may be lengthy and the child must remain still, so sedation may be necessary. • If contrast medium is to be used, assess for allergy. • Encourage fluids after procedure if not contraindicated.
Magnetic resonance imaging (MRI)	Based on how hydrogen atoms behave in a magnetic field when disturbed by radiofrequency signals. Does not require ionizing radiation. Provides a 3D view of the body part being scanned	Evaluate presence of tumours, cysts, or structural abnormalities that may affect specific gland or structure	• Remove all metal objects from the child. • Child must remain motionless for entire scan; parent can stay in room with child. Younger children will require sedation in order to be still. • A loud thumping sound occurs inside the machine during the procedure, which can be frightening to children.
Ultrasonography	Noninvasive sound waves are used to visualize structures such as thyroid or pelvic region	Evaluate presence of tumours or cysts in specific gland, such as the adrenal glands or ovaries, to rule out disorders	• Requires full bladder if in pelvic region. • Better tolerated by nonsedated children than CT or MRI. • Can be performed with a portable unit at bedside.

[a]March of Dimes. (2012). *Newborn screening.* Retrieved from http://www.marchofdimes.org/baby/newborn-screening-tests-for-your-baby.aspx

[b]Centers for Disease Control and Prevention (2014a). *Newborn Screening: Importance of Newborn Screening.* Retrieved from http://www.cdc.gov/ncbddd/newbornscreening/

[c]Fischbach, F. T., & Dunning III, M. B. (2015). *A manual of laboratory and diagnostic tests* (9th ed.). Philadelphia, PA: Wolters Kluwer Health/Lippincott Williams & Wilkins.

Adapted from Fischbach, F. T., & Dunning III, M. B. (2015). *A manual of laboratory and diagnostic tests* (9th ed.). Philadelphia, PA: Wolters Kluwer Health/Lippincott Williams & Wilkins.

identifies peak or trough levels of hormones. Computed tomography (CT) scans, magnetic resonance imaging (MRI), nuclear medicine studies, and ultrasonography are used to look for tumours, cysts, or structural defects.

Nursing Diagnoses, Goals, Interventions, and Evaluation

After completing the assessment, the nurse identifies nursing diagnoses with related goals/outcomes, interventions, and evaluations. The nursing diagnoses for a child with endocrine dysfunction may include:
• Delayed growth and development
• Disturbed body image
• Deficient knowledge (specify)
• Interrupted family processes
• Imbalanced nutrition: less than or more than body requirements
• Deficient or excess fluid volume
• Noncompliance

After completing an assessment of Carlos, the nurse noted the following: history reveals Carlos has had episodes of bedwetting over the past month and has had polydipsia and polyphagia. His weight continues to be greater than the 95th percentile on the growth chart. Based on these assessment findings, what would your top three nursing diagnoses be for Carlos?

Because of the gradual, insidious onset of many of these disorders, the child may first be seen in an acute situation. It may be easier for the child and family to work with short-term goals until they accept the chronic situation. A major goal will be to achieve compliance with medical management. The goals for the child with a disorder of the endocrine system generally include re-establishing homeostasis, promoting adequate growth and development, establishing appropriate body image, promoting health-seeking behaviours, and providing education so the family can manage the condition.

Nursing Care Plan 48.1, found at the end of the chapter, can be used as a guide in planning care for the child with a disorder of the endocrine system. Of course, this plan will need to be individualized based on the child's symptoms, needs, and disorder as well as the family's requirements. A key element to include in any care plan for the child with an endocrine disorder involves preparing the child, based on his or her developmental needs, for invasive procedures and tests. Provide an opportunity for the family and child to express their concerns and fears during diagnosis and treatment. Reinforce realistic expectations for treatment and prospects for improvement with the family and child. The care plan also needs to address developmental, acute, chronic, and home care issues as well as child and family education. Families will need assistance with managing the condition from a multidisciplinary team.

Based on your top three nursing diagnoses for Carlos, describe appropriate nursing interventions.

PITUITARY DISORDERS

Because of the close anatomic and functional relationships between the hypothalamus and pituitary gland, we will discuss them together. The hypothalamus affects the pituitary by releasing and inhibiting hormones and may be the cause of pituitary disorders. In general, disorders of the pituitary fall into two major groups: the anterior pituitary hormones and the posterior pituitary hormones. Anterior pituitary primary disorders in children include growth hormone (GH) deficiency, hyperpituitarism, hypopituitarism, and precocious puberty. Posterior pituitary disorders include diabetes insipidus (DI) and syndrome of inappropriate antidiuretic hormone (ADH) secretion.

Take Note!

Infants with congenital defects of the pituitary gland or hypothalamus may present as a neonatal emergency. The symptoms include apnea, cyanosis, severe hypoglycemia with possible seizures, and prolonged jaundice (Parks & Felner, 2011).

Growth Hormone Deficiency

GH deficiency is characterized by poor growth and short stature. GH is vital for postnatal growth. It is released throughout the day, with most secreted during sleep. GH stimulates linear growth, bone mineral density, and growth in all body tissues.

GH deficiency occurs in approximately 1 in 4,000 children (Nelson-Tuttle, 2014) and can be linked to an underlying condition such as chronic renal failure or disorder such as Noonan syndrome (Cohen, 2016). Often idiopathic GH deficiency is first identified when the physician or nurse practitioner assesses growth patterns. Children may start with a normal birth weight and length, but within a few years the child is less than the third percentile on the growth chart.

Possible complications related to GH deficiency and its treatment include altered carbohydrate, protein, and fat metabolism; hypoglycemia; glucose intolerance/diabetes; slipped capital femoral epiphysis; pseudotumour cerebri; leukemia; recurrence of central nervous system (CNS) tumours; infection at the injection site; edema; and sodium retention.

Pathophysiology

GH deficiency is generally a result of the failure of the anterior pituitary or hypothalamic stimulation on the pituitary to produce sufficient GH. This lack of GH impairs the body's ability to metabolize protein, fat, and carbohydrates.

Primary causes of GH deficiency include injury to, or destruction of, the anterior pituitary gland or hypothalamus. Causes include a tumour (e.g., craniopharyngioma), infection, infarction, CNS irradiation, abnormal formation of these organs in utero, or damage or trauma during birth or after.

In some cases, the cause may be idiopathic, or due to nutritional deprivation or psychosocial issues, and reversible. Psychosocial short stature (PSS) results in growth failure and is linked to extreme emotional deprivation that causes suppression of production of the pituitary hormones, resulting in decreased growth hormone (Kumaran & Kershaw, 2014). The treatment involves removing the child from the dysfunctional environment and providing normal dietary intake. With normalized eating and behavioural habits, pituitary secretion is restored and the child dramatically catches up in growth parameters.

Therapeutic Management

Treatment of primary GH deficiency involves the use of supplemental GH. Secondary GH deficiency requires removal of any tumours that might be the underlying problem, followed by GH therapy. Biosynthetic GH, derived from recombinant DNA, is given by subcutaneous injection. The weekly dosage is 0.18 to 0.3 mg/kg, divided into equal doses given daily for best growth (Nelson-Tuttle, 2014). Treatment continues until near final height is achieved. This can be determined by the child deciding he or she is tall enough, a growth rate of less than 2.5 cm (1 in) year, or bone age greater than 16 years in boys and greater than 14 years in girls (Parks & Felner, 2011).

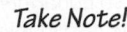 **Take Note!**

Reports have found no evidence linking GH therapy to higher risk of leukemias or brain tumours (Parks & Felner, 2011).

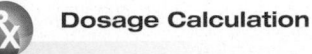 **Dosage Calculation Box 48.1**

Child's weight: 13.6 kg (30 lb).

Medication order: Somatropin 0.5 mg subcutaneously once a day.

Per the *Pediatric Dosage Handbook*, the recommended dose is 0.18 to 0.3 mg/kg weekly divided into 6 to 7 doses.

Is the ordered dose safe?

Nursing Assessment

The focus of the evaluation for GH deficiency is to rule out chronic illnesses such as renal failure, liver disorders, and thyroid dysfunction. For a full description of the assessment phase of the nursing process, refer to the Assessment section of the Nursing Process Overview earlier in the chapter. Assessment findings pertinent to GH deficiency are discussed below.

HEALTH HISTORY

The health history may reveal a familial pattern of short stature or a prenatal history of maternal disorders such as malnutrition. The past history may be significant for birth history of intrauterine growth retardation or past history of severe head trauma or a brain tumour such as craniopharyngioma. Evaluate previous and current growth patterns.

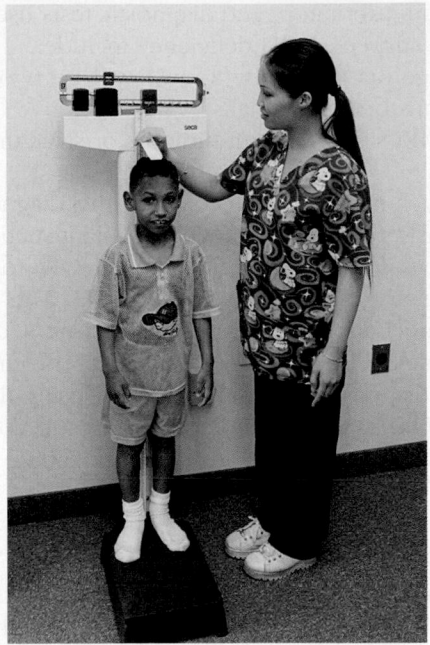

FIGURE 48.2 The child with growth hormone deficiency displays short stature.

Note history of chronic illness such as cardiac, kidney, or intestinal disorders that may contribute to a decreased growth pattern. Assess the child's feelings about being short.

PHYSICAL EXAMINATION

In addition to the linear height being at or below the third percentile on standard growth charts, the physical assessment findings may show that the child has a higher weight-to-height ratio (Fig. 48.2). Other physical findings may include prominent subcutaneous deposits of abdominal fat; a child-like face with a large, prominent forehead; a high-pitched voice; delayed sexual maturation (e.g., micropenis and undescended testes in boys); delayed dentition; delayed skeletal maturation; and decreased muscle mass.

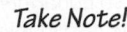 **Take Note!**

Growth measurements are often inaccurate and unreliable in children. Improved accuracy, especially in performing linear measurements, could yield earlier detection and diagnosis of growth disorders (Foote et al., 2011). Evidence-based clinical practice guidelines on linear growth measurement of children have been developed and have been endorsed by the Pediatric Endocrinology Nursing Society (PENS, 2014). A link to these and other helpful resources are provided on thePoint.

LABORATORY AND DIAGNOSTIC TESTING

The child will undergo laboratory tests to rule out chronic illnesses such as renal failure or liver and thyroid dysfunction. Laboratory and diagnostic tests used in children with suspected GH deficiency include:

- Bone age (as shown by x-rays) will be two or more deviations below normal.
- CT or MRI scans rule out tumours or structural abnormalities.
- Pituitary function testing confirms the diagnosis. This test consists of providing a GH stimulant such as glucagon, clonidine, insulin, arginine, or L-DOPA to stimulate the pituitary to release a burst of GH. The Canadian Paediatric Endocrine group has reached a consensus that peak GH levels below 8.0 ng/mL is the cut-off level for the diagnosis of GHD in children using the Immulite 2000 assayin, with at least two tests to confirm the diagnosis (Amed, Delvin, & Hamilton, 2008).

Nursing Management

Nursing management for the child with GH deficiency focuses on promoting growth, enhancing the child's self-esteem related to short stature, and providing appropriate education about the disorder.

PROMOTING GROWTH

The goal of growth promotion is for the child to demonstrate an improved growth rate, as evidenced by at least 7.6 to 12.7 cm (3 to 5 in) in linear growth in the first year of treatment without complications. With early diagnosis and treatment, the child has a better prognosis for reaching a normal adult height. Growth is usually excellent in the first year of therapy compared with later years (Parks & Felner, 2011). Treatment stops when the epiphyseal growth plates fuse.

At the beginning of treatment, monitor for height increase and possible side effects related to the medications. Measure the child's height at least every 3 to 6 months and plot growth over time on standardized growth charts. Provide information to the child and family about normal development and growth rates, bone age, and growth potential. Explore with the family and child the expectations and their understanding of what is normal so they will have realistic expectations of treatment. Consult a dietitian if the child and family need assistance in providing adequate nutrition for growth and development.

ENHANCING THE CHILD'S SELF-ESTEEM

The child with GH deficiency often has younger looking features and is shorter than his or her peers. Encourage the child to express positive feelings about his or her self-image, as shown by comments during health care visits as well as involvement with peers. Encourage the child to voice concerns. Emphasize the child's strengths and assets. Provide information about community support groups or websites related to GH deficiency. Evaluate

for long-term learning problems that may develop if the child had a tumour and surgery or irradiation to remove it. Unidentified learning problems can have a negative impact on the child's self-esteem. Treat and communicate with the child in an age-appropriate manner even though he or she may appear younger.

EDUCATING THE FAMILY

GH is available as a powder that is mixed with packaged diluents. Recently, pen delivery systems and auto-injectors have become available, with some systems not requiring reconstitution (Kremidas et al., 2013). Explain how to prepare the medication and give the correct dosage. Encourage rotation of sites in the subcutaneous tissue to prevent skin irritation. Have the family provide a return demonstration to make sure they understand correct dilution and administration of GH. Continue to provide periodic evaluation and ongoing support.

Take Note!
A recent study found that suboptimal treatment outcomes remain a concern due to nonadherence to the treatment plan, and they can often be attributed to the administration burden of the medication, such as the need for refrigeration storage, reconstitution, and discomfort and bruising from injection of the medication. Providing the child and caregivers with choices regarding medication delivery systems may lead to increased adherence to treatment plan and better clinical outcomes (Kremidas et al., 2013).

Instruct the family to report headaches, rapid weight gain, increased thirst or urination, or painful hip or knee joints as possible adverse reactions. Explain to the family that the child will need to visit the pediatric endocrinologist every 3 to 6 months to monitor for growth, for potential adverse effects, and for compliance with therapy. Stress the importance of complying with the GH replacement therapy and frequent supervision by a pediatric endocrinologist. Educate the family about the financial costs of therapy, which may be high; the family may need help in obtaining assistance and require referral to social services.

Guide the family and child in setting realistic goals and expectations based on age, personal abilities and strengths, and the effectiveness of the GH replacement therapy. For example, the family may want to encourage the child to choose sports that are not dependent on height. Encourage the family to dress the child according to age, not size. Refer the child and family to counselling if indicated. Inform families about support groups such as the Short Stature Foundation, and the Human Growth Foundation. The Magic Foundation-Canada provides provincial links to federal and provincial health information sites. Links and additional information about these groups are provided on thePoint.

Precocious Puberty

In precocious puberty, the child develops sexual characteristics before the usual age of pubertal onset. Puberty, also known as sexual maturation, occurs when the gonads produce increased amounts of sex hormones. Typically, this occurs around 10 to 12 years of age for girls and 11 to 14 years of age for boys. In precocious puberty, secondary sex characteristics develop in girls before the age of 8 years and in boys younger than 9 years (Saenger, 2013). The disorder is more common in females and the majority of the time the cause is unknown in females, while in males the majority of the time a structural CNS abnormality is present (Garibaldi & Chemaitilly, 2011). Other causes include benign hypothalamic tumour, brain injury or radiation, a history of infectious encephalitis, meningitis, congenital adrenal hyperplasia (CAH), and tumours of the ovary, adrenal gland, pituitary gland, or testes.

Pathophysiology

Central precocious puberty, the most common form, develops as a result of premature activation of the hypothalamic–pituitary–gonadal axis that results in the production of gonadotropin-releasing hormone (GnRH), which stimulates the pituitary to produce luteinizing hormone (LH) and follicle-stimulating hormone (FSH). These hormones in turn stimulate the gonads to secrete the sex hormones (estrogen or testosterone). The child develops sexual characteristics, shows increased growth and skeletal maturation, and has reproductive capability.

Peripheral precocious puberty presents with no early secretion of gonadotropin or maturation of gonads but rather early overproduction of sex hormones, caused by tumour (in adrenal or pituitary gland) or as part of an underlying syndrome such as McCune–Albright syndrome. The condition results in increased end-organ sensitivity to low levels of circulating sex hormones and leads to premature pubic hair and breast development. If left untreated, the child may become fertile. In addition, the hormones stimulate rapid growth. Therefore, the child may appear taller than peers but will reach skeletal maturity and closure of the epiphyseal plates early, which results in overall short stature.

Therapeutic Management

The clinical treatment for precocious puberty first involves determining the cause. For example, if the etiology is a tumour of the CNS, the child undergoes surgery, radiation, or chemotherapy. The treatment for central precocious puberty involves administering a GnRH analogue. This is available as a depot injection given every 3 to 4 weeks or a depot injection given quarterly. This analogue stimulates gonadotropin release initially but when given on a long-term basis will suppress gonadotropin release.

With this treatment, the growth rate slows and secondary sexual development stabilizes or regresses. Medroxyprogesterone injections reduce secretion of gonadotropins and prevent menstruation. When treatment is discontinued, puberty resumes according to appropriate developmental stages. The overall aim of treatment is to halt sexual development and rapid growth as well as promote psychosocial well-being.

Nursing Assessment

For a full description of the assessment phase of the nursing process, refer to the Assessment section of the Nursing Process Overview earlier in the chapter. Pertinent assessment findings related to precocious puberty are discussed below.

HEALTH HISTORY

The health history may reveal complaints of headaches, nausea, vomiting, and visual difficulties due to the circulating hormones. The psychosocial development is typical for the child's age, but the child may show emotional lability, aggressive behaviour, and mood swings. Information from the child and family may also reveal risk factors such as exposure to exogenous hormones, history of CNS trauma or infection, or a family history of early puberty.

PHYSICAL EXAMINATION

Physical examination may reveal acne and an adult-like body odour. The child will present with an accelerated rate of growth. The Tanner staging of breasts, pubic hair, and genitalia reveals advanced maturation for the child's age, but the child does not typically display sexual behaviour.

LABORATORY AND DIAGNOSTIC TESTING

Radiologic examinations and pelvic ultrasound identify advanced bone age, increased uterus size, and development of ovaries consistent with the diagnosis of precocious puberty. Laboratory studies include screening radioimmunoassays for LH, FSH, estradiol, or testosterone. The child's response to GnRH stimulation confirms the diagnosis of central precocious puberty versus gonadotropin-independent puberty. This test involves administering synthetic GnRH intravenously and drawing serial blood levels of LH, FSH, and estrogen or testosterone. A positive result is defined as pubertal or adult levels of these hormones in response to the GnRH administration. CT, MRI, or skull radiography reveals any lesions in the CNS or tumours or cysts present in the abdomen, pelvic area, or testes.

Nursing Management

In general, nursing management of the child with precocious puberty focuses on educating the child and family about the physical changes the child is experiencing and how to correctly use the prescribed medications and helping the child to deal with self-esteem issues related to the accelerated growth and development of secondary sexual characteristics. Goals of nursing management include appropriate physical development and pubertal progression appropriate for age. Refer to Nursing Care Plan 48.1, at the end of the chapter, and individualize care based on the child's and family's response to this condition.

PROVIDING EDUCATION

Nursing care involves assessing and documenting the physical changes the child is experiencing and administering medications. Demonstrate correct administration of medication and observe for potential adverse effects (teach this information to the family as well). Encourage the family to comply with follow-up appointments, which typically occur every 6 months and include scheduled stimulation tests. Inform families that pharmacologic intervention stops when the child reaches the age appropriate for pubertal development. Provide appropriate sex education. Reassure parents that precocious puberty does not always involve precocious sexual behaviour, but that it may be seen, especially in boys (Kaplowitz, 2013).

DEALING WITH SELF-ESTEEM ISSUES

Often these children develop self-esteem issues and anxiety related to body image disturbances and impaired social interactions (Kaplowitz, 2013). The goal is for the child to exhibit normal psychosocial development and understand the physical and emotional changes that occur with early onset of puberty. Communicate with the child on an age-appropriate level, even when physical characteristics make the child appear older. Maintain a calm, supportive atmosphere and provide for privacy during examinations. Refer the child and family for counselling as needed. Since the child may have issues with self-image and may be self-conscious, encourage him or her to express his or her feelings about the changes, and use role-playing to show the child how to handle teasing from other children. Let the child know that everyone develops sexual characteristics in time.

Delayed Puberty

Delayed puberty is a condition of delayed secondary sexual development. In girls, it exists if the breasts have not developed by age 12, pubic hair has not appeared by age 14, or **menarche** (first menstrual period) has not occurred by age 15 (Nelson-Tuttle, 2014). In boys, it exists when no testicular enlargement or scrotal changes have occurred by age 14 or pubic hair has not appeared by age 15 followed by testicular enlargement (Nelson-Tuttle, 2014).

The most common cause for delayed puberty is a hereditary pattern of growth and development known as **constitutional delay** (or a "late bloomer") (Kaplowitz, 2014). In these cases, there is a family pattern of late-onset puberty. These teens will usually develop normally, just at a later time than their peers. Hypogonadism also may result when there is decreased stimulation of the gonads due to dysfunction or tumours in the hypothalamus or pituitary gland. Other causes include irradiation, infection, trauma, or genetic syndromes such as Turner or Klinefelter syndrome or Complete Androgen Insensitivity Syndrome (absence of periods, with 46, XY karyotype).

Another common cause is a chronic condition such as anorexia or cystic fibrosis or an underlying condition such as primary ovarian failure or Mayer Rokitansky Küster Hauser syndrome (a congenital abnormality often of the uterus which can result in puberty but no periods).

Therapeutic management varies depending on the reason for delay but may involve administering testosterone (males) or estradiol conjugated estrogen (females) in low dosages if there is no underlying situation to address. For those with constitutional delay, this is usually necessary for only a short time to get puberty started; for those with an absence of hormone, therapy can continue into adult life.

Nursing Assessment

Assessment involves obtaining a health history to identify the indications for this condition. Assessment of the growth pattern using correct techniques and standards for comparison is essential. On physical assessment, note absence of secondary sex characteristics as noted above. Laboratory and diagnostic testing rules out other causes for delayed puberty. Blood levels of reproductive hormones may also be evaluated.

Nursing Management

In addition to the general interventions presented in Nursing Care Plan 48.1 (at the end of the chapter), instruct the child and family about the medication therapy. Educate the child and family about the different stages of puberty. Help the family develop a home management schedule for the administration of medication. Answer the family's questions about the condition or potential complications (e.g., infertility), depending on the cause of the condition.

Diabetes Insipidus

DI can be classified into two types—nephrogenic DI and central DI. Nephrogenic DI can be transmitted genetically (e.g., sex-linked, autosomal dominant, or autosomal recessive forms) or be acquired due to chronic renal disease, hypercalcemia, hypokalemia, or use of certain drugs such as lithium, amphotericin, methicillin, and rifampin (Breault & Majzoub, 2011a). This variant of DI is not associated with the pituitary gland and is related to decreased renal sensitivity to ADH. Therapeutic management for nephrogenic DI involves diuretics, high fluid intake, restricted sodium intake, and a high-protein diet. Desmopressin acetate is usually ineffective in the treatment of nephrogenic DI.

Central DI is a disorder of the posterior pituitary gland and is the most common form of DI (Children's Hospital of Boston, 2012). Therefore, central DI will be the focus of the remainder of this discussion. Central DI is characterized by excessive thirst **(polydipsia)** and excessive urination **(polyuria)** that is not affected by decreasing fluid intake. Typically, this disorder occurs in children as a result of complications from head trauma or after cranial surgery to remove hypothalamic–pituitary tumours such as craniopharyngioma. Other causes include genetic mutations, granulomatous disease, infections such as meningitis or encephalitis, vascular anomalies, congenital malformations, infiltrative disease such as leukemia, or administration of certain drugs that are associated with inhibition of vasopressin release, such as phenytoin (Breault & Majzoub, 2011a). However, 10% of central DI cases in children are idiopathic (Breault & Majzoub, 2011a). Some cases can be hereditary.

DI is usually permanent and requires treatment throughout life.

Pathophysiology

Central DI results from a deficiency in the secretion of ADH. This hormone, also known as vasopressin, is produced in the hypothalamus and stored in the pituitary gland. ADH is involved in concentrating the urine from the kidneys by stimulating reabsorption of water in the renal collecting tubules through increased membrane permeability. This conserves water and maintains normal osmolality. With a deficiency in ADH, the kidney loses massive amounts of water and retains sodium in the serum.

Therapeutic Management

Unless a tumour is present (in which case it is removed by surgery), the usual treatment of central DI involves a low-solute diet (low sodium and low protein), daily replacement of ADH, and/or use of a thiazide diuretic (Bichet, 2013a). The drug of choice for home treatment is Desmopressin acetate, a long-acting vasopressin analogue (Breault & Majzoub, 2011a; Nelson-Tuttle, 2014). In children, it is typically given intranasally. However, it can also be administered subcutaneously or orally. The drug is given every 8 to 12 hours. The dose depends on the child's age, urine output, and urine-specific gravity. Treatment of

DI using Desmopressin acetate in infants and small children is challenging and complicated due to their inability to access fluids and articulate thirst (Bichet, 2013a). In neonates and young infants, the treatment is often solely fluid therapy due to their large volume requirements of nutritive fluid (i.e., the drive behind an infant's fluid intake is hunger rather than thirst) (Breault & Majzoub, 2011a). However, research has shown that subcutaneously administered Desmopressin acetate may be more effective than oral or intranasal therapy in infants and small children related to variable absorption and the challenge of administering accurate doses via these routes (Bichet, 2013a).

In the hospital, the child may receive aqueous vasopressin, 8-arginine vasopressin (Pitressin), intravenously (Breault & Majzoub, 2011a). This is a short-acting drug, so the dosage can be adjusted quickly.

Both the long-acting and short-acting forms of the medication decrease urinary output and thirst, and the dosages of both forms of these drugs need to be titrated to achieve the desired effect.

Take Note!
A metered nasal spray form of Desmopressin acetate is available, but the prescribed dose must be greater than 10 μg/0.1 mL in order for the child to use the spray (Bichet, 2013a).

Nursing Assessment

For a full description of the assessment phase of the nursing process, refer to the Assessment section of the Nursing Process Overview earlier in the chapter. Assessment findings pertinent to DI are discussed below.

HEALTH HISTORY
Nursing assessment involves obtaining a history of any conditions that led to the development of the disorder. This review includes information about the neonatal period as well as a current history of infections such as meningitis, diseases such as leukemia, or familial patterns. Although most symptoms of endocrine disorders develop slowly, the onset of this disorder is abrupt. The health history usually elicits the cardinal symptoms as well as complaints representing the early signs of dehydration.

The most common initial symptoms reported are polyuria and polydipsia (Bichet, 2013b; Breault & Majzoub, 2011a). Except for children who cannot access water on their own or do not sense thirst, the child typically maintains adequate perfusion by drinking water. The parent or child may report frequent trips to the bathroom, nocturia, or enuresis. When the child cannot compensate for the excessive loss of water by increasing fluid intake, other symptoms will be reported, such as weight loss or signs of dehydration. For example, irritability may be due to the early signs of dehydration or the frustration the child feels at being unable to quench his or her thirst. Other signs may be intermittent fever, vomiting, and constipation and in serious cases seizures and loss of consciousness.

PHYSICAL EXAMINATION

Observation and inspection may reveal weight loss or failure to thrive in the young infant. Inspection may also reveal signs of dehydration, such as dry mucous membranes or decreased tears. The child may excrete greater than 3 L/m² of urine per day. On auscultation, tachycardia or increased respiratory rate may be signs of compensation for the decrease in fluid volume. Palpation reveals slightly depressed fontanels or decreased skin turgor.

LABORATORY AND DIAGNOSTIC TESTING

Diagnostic tests used to evaluate DI include:
- Radiographic studies such as CT scan, MRI, or ultrasound of the skull and kidneys can determine whether a lesion or tumour is present.
- Urinalysis: urine is dilute, osmolarity is less than 3,000 mOsm/L (SI: 300 to 900 mmol/kg/24 hr average fluid intake or 50 to 1,200 mmol/kg random urine depending on fluid intake—expected range), specific gravity is less than 1.005, and sodium is decreased.
- Serum osmolarity is greater than 300 mOsm/L (SI: 282 to 300 mmol/kg expected range).
- Serum sodium is elevated.
- Fluid deprivation test measures vasopressin release from the pituitary in response to water deprivation. Normal results will show decreased urine output, increased urine-specific gravity, and no change in serum sodium.

Take Note!
During a fluid deprivation test, the child may be irritable and frustrated because fluid is being withheld. Don't drink in front of the child.

Nursing Management

Refer to Nursing Care Plan 48.1 at the end of the chapter and individualize the plan of care based on the child's and family's response to the illness. Specific interventions related to nursing care of the child with DI are discussed below.

PROMOTING HYDRATION

The goal of treatment is to achieve hourly urine output of 1 to 2 mL/kg and urine-specific gravity of at least 1.010.

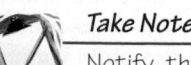
Take Note!
Notify the physician or nurse practitioner if the urine output is greater than 1,000 mL per hour for two consecutive voids.

Maintain fluid intake regimens as ordered. Monitor fluid status by measuring vital signs, fluid intake and output, and daily weights (using the same scale at the same time of day). If fluids are stopped too soon, the child may become hypernatremic, which can lead to seizures. Feed infants more frequently, since they excrete more dilute urine, consume larger volumes of free water, and secrete lower amounts of vasopressin than older children. Monitor for signs and symptoms of dehydration during the fluid deprivation test as well as when starting the treatment regimen.

Take Note!
Monitor blood pressure closely when initiating vasopressin.

If the child is unconscious or has brain injury, maintain hydration and nutrition with nasogastric or gastrostomy feedings.

PROMOTING ACTIVITY

Establish appropriate activity for the child, and allow time for him or her to regain strength and the desire to increase level of activity. Assess the child's abilities daily, schedule frequent bathroom breaks, keep fluids available at all times, and fit the treatment plan to the child's daily activities.

EDUCATING THE FAMILY

Involve the family in development of the fluid intake regimens. A journal or daily log is essential in maintaining the fluid regimen and identifying problems. Children with intact thirst centres can self-regulate their need for fluids, but if this is not the situation, help the family develop a plan for 24-hour fluid replacement. This may require instruction on nasogastric or gastrostomy feedings. Infants will need fluid intake at night. Educate the family about "breakthrough" (signs that the medication has worn off), the symptoms of water intoxication (drowsiness, listlessness, headache, confusion, sudden weight gain, and anuria), and dehydration. Help the family develop a plan to inform the school and other individuals in the child's life about the need for liberal bathroom privileges and extra fluids to prevent accidents or dehydration. Teaching Guidelines 48.1 gives tips on educating the family about the medication regimen. Recommend that the family obtain a medical ID alert bracelet or necklace for the child. Encourage compliance with follow-up appointments, which will probably be every 6 months.

Teaching Guidelines 48.1
DESMOPRESSIN ACETATE INTRANASAL ADMINISTRATION
- Keep DDAVP in the refrigerator at all times (if directed, some products no longer require refrigeration; refer to product insert).

- Ensure the child has had a void before giving the next dose.
- Clear the nostrils (the medication may be poorly absorbed if the child has nasal congestion).
- Insert the measuring tube into the bottle.
- Fill to proper dosage and hold the top of the tube closed while inserting the medication-filled end into the nostril.
- Blow the liquid out of the tubing into the nostril.
- When using metered nasal spray, spray must be primed before first use.
- If the child sneezes, repeat the dosage.
- Measure urine-specific gravity to monitor effectiveness of the drug.
- Monitor for signs and symptoms of overdosage such as confusion, headache, drowsiness, and rapid weight gain due to fluid retention.

Syndrome of Inappropriate Antidiuretic Hormone

Syndrome of inappropriate antidiuretic hormone (SIADH) occurs when ADH (vasopressin) is secreted in the presence of low serum osmolality because the feedback mechanism that regulates ADH does not function properly. ADH continues to be released, and this leads to water retention, decreased serum sodium due to hemodilution, and extracellular fluid volume expansion. SIADH can be caused by CNS infections such as meningitis, head trauma, brain tumours, intracranial surgery, and certain medications such as analgesics, barbiturates, or chemotherapy. SIADH is rare in children (Breault & Majzoub, 2011b). However, when seen, it is often related to excessive administration of vasopressin during the treatment of DI (Breault & Majzoub, 2011b).

Therapeutic management of SIADH includes correcting the underlying disorder in addition to fluid restriction and intravenous sodium chloride administration to correct hyponatremia and increase serum osmolality.

Nursing Assessment

Obtain a health history, noting history of a CNS infection or tumour, intracranial surgery, head trauma, use of the above-mentioned medications, or a history of DI. Note symptoms such as decreased urine output and weight gain, or GI symptoms such as anorexia, nausea, and vomiting. Assess neurologic status, noting lethargy, behavioural changes, headache, altered level of consciousness, seizure, or coma. Neurologic signs develop as the sodium level decreases. Diagnostic tests reveal low serum sodium and osmolality, as well as decreased urea, creatinine, uric acid, and albumin levels. Urine samples demonstrate elevated osmolality, high sodium concentrations, and specific gravity greater than 1.030. Adrenal, thyroid, and renal function studies may be used to rule out other causes of hyponatremia.

Comparison Chart 48.1 lists the differences between DI and SIADH.

Nursing Management

Nursing goals focus on restoring fluid balance and preventing injury. Institute safety precautions if altered levels of consciousness, confusion, or seizures are present. Notify the physician or nurse practitioner if headache or irritability is present. Monitor fluid intake and output and weigh the child daily. An indwelling urinary catheter may be needed to allow for hourly monitoring of urine volume and specific gravity. Help the child cope with fluid restriction by offering sugarless candy, a wet washcloth, or, perhaps, ice chips. Administer electrolyte replacement as necessary to correct imbalances.

DISORDERS OF THYROID FUNCTION

Disorders of the thyroid gland are seen in infancy and childhood and are broadly classified as hypothyroidism and hyperthyroidism (Nelson-Tuttle, 2014). These disorders

COMPARISON CHART 48.1	DIABETES INSIPIDUS VERSUS SIADH
Diabetes Insipidus	**Syndrome of Inappropriate Antidiuretic Hormone**
• "High and dry"	• "Low and wet"
• Increased urination	• Decreased urination
• Hypernatremia	• Hyponatremia
• Serum osmolality >300 mOsm/kg	• Serum osmolality <280 mOsm/kg
• Urine-specific gravity <1.005	• Urine-specific gravity >1.030
• Decreased urine osmolality	• Increased urine osmolality
• Dehydration, thirst	• Fluid retention, weight gain, and hypertension

can be serious because thyroid hormones are important for growth and development; they regulate metabolism of nutrients and energy production.

Congenital Hypothyroidism

Congenital hypothyroidism usually results from failure of the thyroid gland to migrate during fetal development (LaFranchi, 2011). This results in malformation or malfunction of the thyroid gland, which leads to insufficient production of the thyroid hormones that are required to meet the body's metabolic and growth and development needs. Congenital hypothyroidism leads to low concentrations of circulating thyroid hormones (triiodothyronine [T_3] and thyroxine [T_4]).

Congenital hypothyroidism occurs in 1 in 4,000 live births (Nelson-Tuttle, 2014). It occurs over a wide range of ethnic groups, though less among African Americans, and is more common in girls than boys (LaFranchi, 2011). Complications include intellectual disability if untreated, short stature, growth failure, and delayed physical maturation and development (Nelson-Tuttle, 2014). Congenital hypothyroidism (previously referred to as cretinism) is one of the most common preventable causes of intellectual disability. The later it is diagnosed, the greater the disability is (LaFranchi, 2014a). Most newborns have few if any symptoms and the occurrence is sporadic not typically hereditary; therefore, most cases of congenital hypothyroidism are detected via newborn screening programs.

Pathophysiology

Congenital hypothyroidism is due to a defect in the development of the thyroid gland in the fetus due to a spontaneous gene mutation, an inborn error of thyroid hormone synthesis resulting from an autosomal recessive trait, pituitary dysfunction, or failure of the CNS–thyroid feedback mechanism to develop. Transient primary hypothyroidism may also occur; it results from transplacental transfer of maternal medications, maternal thyroid-blocking antibodies, iodine deficiency, and fetal or neonatal exposure to excessive iodines (such as use of iodine antiseptics during delivery or procedures or excess ingestion of iodine by the mother) (LaFranchi, 2014a).

Therapeutic Management

To prevent intellectual disability and restore normal growth and motor development, thyroid hormone replacement with sodium L-thyroxin is given. The recommended starting dosage is 10 to 15 µg/kg per day; infants and younger children typically require a higher dosage per unit of body weight (American Academy of Pediatrics, 2011). There are no adverse effects with physiologic doses, but thyroid function tests are performed initially every 2 weeks to closely monitor for effects and to ensure proper dosing. Since thyroid hormone is vital to the infant's developing CNS, the goal is to normalize thyroid function as quickly as possible. This treatment will be needed lifelong to maintain normal metabolism and promote normal physical and mental growth and development.

Nursing Assessment

Nursing assessment of the child with congenital hypothyroidism includes health history, physical examination, and laboratory testing.

HEALTH HISTORY

Inquire whether the neonatal metabolic screening test was performed and results obtained. Determine if the test was done less than 24 to 48 hours after birth. If so, a repeat test may be warranted (see Laboratory and Diagnostic Testing below). Inquire about maternal history that may indicate a connection to hypothyroidism, such as maternal exposure to iodine. Additional history findings may include sensitivity to cold, constipation, feeding problems, or lethargy. Since parents like babies to sleep well, the parents may not complain that the baby is sleeping too much; rather, they may remark that it is difficult to keep the baby awake.

PHYSICAL EXAMINATION

Most infants are asymptomatic until the first month, when they begin to develop clinical signs. Inspection and observation reveal a lethargic baby or a child with hypotonia, hypoactivity, and a dull expression. A combination of lethargy and irritability may exist, with an overall delayed mental responsiveness. Measurements of weight and height may reveal delayed growth. Other findings may include a persistent open posterior fontanel, coarse facies with short neck and limbs, periorbital puffiness, enlarged tongue, and poor sucking response (Fig. 48.3). The skin may appear pale with mottling or yellow from prolonged jaundice, or it may be cool, dry, and scaly to the touch, with sparse hair development on the older child. Auscultation of the chest might reveal bradycardia. Signs of respiratory distress and decreased pulse pressure may also be present. On palpation of the abdomen, there may be evidence of an umbilical hernia or a mass due to constipation.

LABORATORY AND DIAGNOSTIC TESTING

Every infant should have a newborn screen for thyroid hormone levels before discharge from the hospital or 2 to 4 days after birth (American Academy of Pediatrics, 2011). When the test is performed within the first 24 to 48 hours along with other metabolic screenings, the result may be inaccurate because of the immediate increase in thyroid-stimulating hormone (TSH) shortly after birth

FIGURE 48.3 **Younger child with hypothyroidism.** (From Rosdahl, C. B., & Kowalski, M. T. [2012]. *Textbook of basic nursing*. Philadelphia, PA: Lippincott Williams & Wilkins.)

(American Academy of Pediatrics, 2011; Nelson-Tuttle, 2014). Radioimmunoassay is used to measure levels of T_4, which accurately reflects the child's thyroid status. If the T_4 level is low, then a second confirming laboratory test is performed, as well as determining whether the TSH is elevated. A thyroid scan may also be used to check for the absence or ectopic placement of the gland. In addition to serum measurement of T_4, other diagnostic tests include serum T_3, radioiodine uptake, thyroid-bound globulin, and ultrasonography.

Nursing Management

The overall goal of nursing management of the infant or child with congenital hypothyroidism is to establish a normal growth pattern without complications such as intellectual disability or failure to thrive. Individualize the nursing care plan based on the infant's responses to the illness.

PROMOTING APPROPRIATE GROWTH

Measure and record growth at regular intervals. Thyroid levels are measured at recommended intervals, such as every 2 weeks until the target range is reached on a stabilized dose of medication, then every 1 to 3 months until the child is 1 year old, every 2 to 3 months until the child is 3 years old, and becoming less frequent as the child gets

older (LaFranchi, 2014b). A trial off the medication may be performed around the age of 3, under physician or nurse practitioner supervision, to confirm the diagnosis (Nelson-Tuttle, 2014). Monitor for signs of hypo- or hyperfunction, including changes in vital signs, thermoregulation, and activity level. Provide adequate rest periods and meet thermoregulation needs. If the infant's tongue is unusually large, observe feeding ability, prevent airway obstruction, and position the infant on the side. Fluid restrictions or a low-salt diet may be ordered.

Take Note!

Observe for signs of thyroid hormone overdose (irritability, rapid pulse, dyspnea, sweating, and fever) or ineffective treatment (fatigue, constipation, and decreased appetite).

EDUCATING THE FAMILY

Since many infants are asymptomatic, the diagnosis may be unexpected, so reassure and convey realistic expectations to the family. Developmental screening may be required if the child showed any symptoms initially or as the child gets older to ensure that drug therapy is appropriate. Educate the family about the disorder, the medication and method of administration, and adverse effects such as increased pulse rate (which may indicate an overdose of thyroid hormone).

L-Thyroxine is an oral medication and is not available in a liquid form. The pill form must be crushed for infants and young children. It can be mixed with a small amount of formula or breastmilk and placed in the nipple, but it should not be placed in a full bottle of formula or breastmilk because the infant will not ingest all the medication if he or she does not finish the bottle. The medication can also be mixed with a small amount of liquid and given with a dropper. Medication absorption is affected by soy-based formulas, fibre, and iron preparations (American Academy of Pediatrics, 2011; LaFranchi, 2014b). Therefore, carefully evaluate the formula the infant is on before administering L-thyroxine.

Inform the family that this medication will be needed throughout the child's life. Explain that missed doses may lead to developmental delays and poor growth. Tell them that frequent blood tests will be needed to evaluate thyroid function and the child's growth rate; genetic counselling may be needed. Clinical examination, including growth and development assessment, should occur every few months until the child is 3 years old. Serum T_4 and TSH should be evaluated often, and more frequent monitoring may be needed if noncompliance occurs, if abnormal values occur, or with any changes in medication dosage or treatment regimen. The nurse may need to help the family to find a laboratory nearby or to handle financial issues related to the therapy. Educate the family about infant stimulation programs if the child shows cognitive problems, retarded physical growth, or slow intellectual development. Some information may need to be reinforced during school-age or adolescent stages of development. Finally, encourage the family to obtain a medical ID bracelet or necklace for the child.

Consider This

Asha Virani, 1 week old, is brought to the clinic. Her newborn screening test was positive for hypothyroidism. Her parents are shocked and upset by the news. Her mother states, "My daughter's been doing so well since she came home from the hospital. She seems to be doing everything she should be. I just can't believe anything's wrong with her. I felt so blessed to have a baby that slept so much but she could have died. What kind of mother will I be?"

Thoughts: How would you respond to this mother?

Acquired Hypothyroidism

Hypothyroidism also occurs as an acquired condition. This disorder most commonly results from an autoimmune chronic lymphocytic thyroiditis (LaFranchi, 2011, 2013). As a genetic condition, antibodies develop against the thyroid gland, causing the gland to become inflamed, infiltrated, and progressively destroyed. It occurs more often in girls during childhood and adolescence (LaFranchi, 2011, 2013). Less common etiologies include hypothyroidism associated with pituitary or hypothalamic dysfunction or exposure to drugs or substances such as lithium and amiodarone that interfere with thyroid hormone synthesis, radiation, thyroidectomy, hemiangiomas, and iodine deficiency (LaFranchi, 2011, 2013).

Therapeutic management is the same as for congenital hypothyroidism. Management involves oral sodium L-thyroxine, which is given at 2 to 5 µg/kg per day to maintain T_4 in the upper half of the normal range and to suppress TSH.

Nursing Assessment

Interview the family and child to determine activity tolerance and behaviour changes. The symptoms may develop over a period of time and may be subtle. Note vague complaints of fatigue, weakness, weight gain, cold intolerance, constipation, and dry skin. The severity of symptoms depends on the length of time that the hormone deficiency has existed and its extent. Reviewing the growth pattern may reveal a slowed or arrested growth rate (height) and increased weight.

Physical examination may reveal a **goitre** (enlargement of the thyroid gland). Deep tendon reflexes may be sluggish and the face, eyes, and hands may be edematous.

Note thinning or coarse hair, muscle hypertrophy with muscle weakness, and signs of delayed or precocious puberty. The diagnostic evaluation involves serum thyroid function studies (TSH, T_3, and T_4) as well as serum thyroid antibodies to confirm autoimmune thyroiditis. MRI and a thyroid uptake test and scan may also be necessary.

Nursing Management

Work with the family to establish a daily schedule for administering L-thyroxine, which should be taken 30 to 60 minutes before a meal for optimal absorption. Explain to the family that growth is related to the child's response to the treatment, and there are no specific strategies to aid in this growth. The family should understand the diagnosis, should be able to recognize signs and symptoms of thyroid hypo- and hyperfunction, and should know when to notify the physician or nurse practitioner. The family and child may need assistance in accepting the therapy as well as the experience of catch-up growth that may occur at the beginning of therapy. The child with chronic or severe hypothyroidism may be at risk for adverse effects such as restlessness, insomnia, or irritability. The child's thyroid levels should be evaluated at recommended intervals such as every 3 to 6 months by a pediatric endocrinologist.

Hyperthyroidism

Hyperthyroidism is the result of hyperfunction of the thyroid gland. This leads to excessive levels of circulating thyroid hormones. This condition is uncommon in children. The peak incidence in children occurs in adolescence as a result of Graves disease (LaFranchi, 2011). Graves disease is an autoimmune disorder that causes excessive amounts of thyroid hormone to be released in response to human thyroid stimulator immunoglobulin (TSI). It occurs five times more often in girls than in boys (LaFranchi, 2011). A goitre usually develops in this condition. There is a genetic marker in individuals affected by Graves disease, with the majority of children having a positive family history of autoimmune thyroid problems (LaFranchi, 2011). A congenital form of hyperthyroidism, neonatal thyrotoxicosis, occurs in infants of mothers with Graves disease. This neonatal condition, which can be life-threatening, is a self-limiting disorder lasting 2 to 4 months. Less common causes of hyperthyroidism are thyroiditis, thyroid hormone–producing tumours, and pituitary adenomas.

Therapeutic management is aimed at decreasing thyroid hormone levels. Current treatment involves antithyroid medication, radioactive iodine therapy, and subtotal thyroidectomy. First-line treatment involves methimazole, which blocks the production of T_3 and T_4. Adjunct therapy with β-adrenergic blockers (such as propranolol or atenolol) may also be used if the child has marked symptoms. Radioactive iodine therapy is becoming acceptable for children greater than 10 years as a long-term therapy (LaFranchi, 2011). This therapy is administered orally and results in tissue damage and destruction of the thyroid gland within 6 to 18 weeks, but it can result in hypothyroidism. Subtotal thyroidectomy is used when drug therapy is not possible or other treatments have failed. Risks include hypothyroidism, hypoparathyroidism, or laryngeal nerve damage.

Nursing Assessment

Initially, symptoms of hyperthyroidism are mild and often overlooked. Many children with hyperthyroidism are first seen in the outpatient setting with a history of a problem with sleep, school performance, and distractibility. They become easily frustrated, overheated, and fatigued during physical education class. The child may complain of diarrhea, excessive perspiration, and muscle weakness. The history may also reveal hyperactivity, heat intolerance, emotional lability, and insomnia.

Physical examination of the older child may reveal an increased rate of growth; weight loss despite an excellent appetite; hyperactivity; warm, moist skin; tachycardia; fine tremors; an enlarged thyroid gland or goitre; and ophthalmic changes (exophthalmos, which is less pronounced in children; proptosis; lid lag and retraction; staring expression; periorbital edema; and diplopia) (Fig. 48.4). Elevated pulse and blood pressure may also be noted. Laboratory and diagnostic tests reveal that serum T_4 and T_3 levels are markedly elevated while TSH levels are suppressed.

FIGURE 48.4 **Adolescent with Graves disease.**

Take Note!

The sudden release of high levels of thyroid hormones results in thyroid storm, which progresses to heart failure and shock. Immediately report the signs of thyroid storm, which include sudden onset of severe restlessness and irritability, fever, diaphoresis, and severe tachycardia (LaFranchi, 2011).

Nursing Management

Once the treatment plan is initiated, educate the family and child about the medication and potential adverse effects, the goals of treatment, and possible complications. Monitor for adverse drug effects such as rash, mild leukopenia, loss of taste, sore throat, GI disturbances, and arthralgia. If the medication is given two or three times a day, teach the family to use a pill dispenser and alarm clock. Inform the family of the need for routine blood tests and follow-up visits with the pediatric endocrinologist every 2 to 4 months until normal levels are reached; then visits may be decreased to once or twice a year. Instruct the parents to contact the physician or nurse practitioner if the child has tachycardia or extreme fatigue.

Help the child and family to cope with symptoms such as heat intolerance, emotional lability, or eye problems. Explain these symptoms to the school or day care personnel and make sure that they understand that the child should take more frequent rest breaks in a cool environment, and should avoid physical education classes until normal hormone levels are attained. Encourage the family to have the child consume a healthy diet with an appropriate level of calories; the child may need to eat five or six meals a day. Provide community referrals such as the National Graves' Disease Foundation and the Thyroid Foundation of Canada, links to which can be found on thePoint. Encourage the family to obtain a medical ID bracelet or necklace.

If surgical intervention is chosen, provide appropriate preoperative teaching and postoperative care. Provide supportive measures such as fluid maintenance, nutritional support, and electrolyte correction. Monitor red blood cell count and liver function tests. Close monitoring for signs and symptoms of hypothyroidism is important.

Comparison Chart 48.2 compares hypothyroidism and hyperthyroidism.

DISORDERS RELATED TO PARATHYROID GLAND FUNCTION

The parathyroid glands secrete parathyroid hormone (PTH). This hormone, along with vitamin D and calcitonin, regulates calcium/phosphate homeostasis by increasing osteoclastic activity, absorption of calcium and

COMPARISON CHART 48.2   **HYPERTHYROIDISM VERSUS HYPOTHYROIDISM**

Hyperthyroidism	Hypothyroidism
• Nervousness/anxiety	• Tiredness/fatigue
• Diarrhea	• Constipation
• Heat intolerance	• Cold intolerance
• Weight loss	• Weight gain
• Smooth, velvety skin	• Dry, thick skin; edema of face, eyes, and hands
	• Decreased growth

excretion of phosphate by the kidneys, and absorption of calcium in the GI tract. The two disorders associated with parathyroid gland dysfunction are hypoparathyroidism and hyperparathyroidism. Both of these disorders are rare in children. Refer to Table 48.2.

DISORDERS RELATED TO ADRENAL GLAND FUNCTION

Disorders of the adrenal gland include acute and chronic adrenal insufficiency (hypofunction) and disorders of hyperfunction, such as Cushing syndrome. The adrenal cortex is the site of production of glucocorticoids (for blood glucose regulation), mineralocorticoids (for sodium retention), and androgenic and estrogenic steroid compounds (for phallic and secondary sex development). The adrenal medulla is the site of production of the catecholamines (dopamine, norepinephrine, and epinephrine) and is under neuroendocrine control. When production of these compounds is altered, disease results. Pediatric adrenocortical insufficiency is similar to adults with the exception of CAH, which will be discussed below. Refer to Table 48.3 for an overview of other disorders of the adrenal gland.

Congenital Adrenal Hyperplasia

CAH is a group of autosomal recessive inherited disorders in which there is an insufficient supply of the enzymes required for the synthesis of cortisol and aldosterone. It is the most common type of adrenocortical insufficiency seen in children with an incidence of about 1 in 15,000 to 20,000 live births (White, 2011). More than 90% of the cases of CAH are caused by a deficiency of 21-hydroxylase (21-OH) enzyme (Nelson-Tuttle, 2014; White, 2011). Therefore, our discussion will focus on this type. This condition can be life-threatening and requires prompt diagnosis and treatment after birth (Nelson-Tuttle, 2014). Complications of CAH include hyponatremia, hypoglycemia, hypotension, and hyperkalemia metabolic acidosis leading to shock and adrenal crisis. Developmental

challenges can vary depending on the CAH genetic profile of the child; however, more common challenges include failure to thrive, short adult stature, altered fertility, and adult testicular adrenal rest tumour in males.

Pathophysiology

21-OH enzyme deficiency results in blocking the production of adrenal mineralocorticoids and glucocorticoids. A reduction of cortisol occurs, which leads to increased adrenocorticotropic hormone (ACTH) production by the anterior pituitary to stimulate adrenal gland production. Prolonged oversecretion of ACTH causes enlargement or hyperplasia of the adrenal glands and excess production of androgens, leading to male characteristics appearing early or inappropriately.

In males, the enzyme deficiency of 21-OH with excessive androgen secretion leads to a slightly enlarged penis, which may become adult-sized by school age, and a hyperpigmented scrotum. Males do not have obvious signs at birth but may enter puberty by 2 to 3 years of age. The female fetus develops male secondary sexual characteristics; thus, CAH can cause atypical genitalia in girls (Nelson-Tuttle, 2014). The clitoris is enlarged and may resemble the penis, the labia have a rugated appearance, and the labial folds are fused, but the internal reproductive organs, including the ovaries, fallopian tubes, and uterus, are normal. In some females with CAH, virilization can result in a urogenital sinus (UGS). Surgical management of atypical genitalia remains controversial and decision-making is complex (Fleming, Van Riper, & Knafl, 2017).

A milder form of 21-OH deficiency becomes evident later (genitals are normal at birth), in the toddler or preschool years, with premature **adrenarche** (early sexual maturation), pubic hair development, accelerated growth velocity, advanced bone age, early closure of the epiphyseal plates resulting in short stature as an adult, acne, and **hirsutism** (excessive body hair growth). Fertility in males with CAH can be altered but often to a lesser degree than females who have lower fertility as well as an altered menstrual cycle.

TABLE 48.2	PARATHYROID DISORDERS

Parathyroid Disorder	Cause	Nursing Assessment	Nursing Management
Hypoparathyroidism (deficiency of PTH)	Most common is accidental removal or destruction of the parathyroid gland during thyroidectomy or radial neck dissection; may also be congenital (result of aplasia or hypoplasia of the parathyroid gland)	Hypocalcemia Hyperphosphatemia Hyperexcitability of neuromuscular function, uncontrolled spasms, and hypocalcemic tetany (general muscular hypertonia); positive Chvostek sign (facial muscle spasm elicited by tapping the facial nerve); positive Trousseau sign (carpopedal spasm that results from oxygen deficiency) Laryngeal spasm, stridor Poor eating Lethargy	• Administer intravenous calcium gluconate for acute or severe tetany, then intramuscular or oral calcium as prescribed. • Monitor the child for the development of cardiac arrhythmias. Ensure that the intravenous site is patent; if extravasation occurs, tissue damage or cardiac arrhythmias may result. • Monitor fluid and electrolyte status, weigh the child daily, and measure urinary calcium excretion to prevent nephrocalcinosis. • Institute seizure precautions and reduce environmental stimuli (e.g., loud or sudden noises, bright lights, or stimulating activities). • Observe for signs and symptoms of laryngospasm (e.g., stridor, hoarseness, or a feeling of tightness in the throat). Teach the child and family about the need for continuous daily administration of calcium salts and vitamin D. Have the family observe for vitamin D toxicity by observing for signs such as weakness, fatigue, lassitude, headache, nausea and vomiting, and diarrhea.
Hyperparathyroidism (hypersecretion of PTH)	Parathyroid adenoma is the most common cause; secondary hyperparathyroidism is primarily due to renal failure	Hypercalcemia Hypophosphatemia Depression of neuromuscular function, child may trip and drop objects, general fatigue, failure to thrive, headaches, poor school performance, and irritability, somnolence, stupor, or difficulty concentrating. Irregular heart rate, possibly related to cardiac dysrhythmias. Skeletal pain, fractures, formation of bone tumours, or flank pain related to renal calculi	• Administer IV fluids and diuretics as prescribed to increase urinary excretion of calcium in children not in renal failure. • Administer prescribed medication to treat hypercalcemia, such as oral phosphate (antihypercalcemic agent), pamidronate, calcitonin, or etidronate disodium (by inhibiting bone resorption of calcium). • Increase the child's fluid intake to minimize renal calculi formation. Provide fruit juices to maintain low urinary pH, acidity of body fluids, and calcium absorption. Strain the urine for renal casts. • Dietary calcium is restricted. • Monitor for safety by assessing the child's level of muscular weakness, preventing falls or injury, and checking for fractures. • If the child develops renal rickets (osteodystrophy), long-term braces may be required, so provide family education and encourage compliance. • Surgery may be performed to remove abnormal parathyroid tumour. • Keep the diet low in phosphorus and watch for hypocalcemia and onset of tetany after surgery.

TABLE 48.3	OTHER DISORDERS OF THE ADRENAL GLAND		
Disorder	**Cause**	**Nursing Assessment**	**Nursing Management**
Addison disease (deficiency in the adrenal steroids, glucocorticoids [cortisol], and mineralocorticoids [aldosterone])	It results from damage or destruction of the adrenal glands caused by infections such as tuberculosis, fungal infections, or HIV-related infections; hemorrhage or surgical removal of both glands; or dysfunction of the hypothalamus or pituitary gland. Generally, the etiology in children is an autoimmune process that is familial or sporadic[a]	Hyponatremia Hyperkalemia Water loss, dehydration, muscular weakness, fatigue, weight loss, anorexia, syncope, nausea, vomiting, and diarrhea Hypoglycemia Hypotension Hyperpigmentation of skin Adrenal crisis, also referred to as addisonian crisis, can occur (refer to section on CAH for more information)	• Similar to that of congenital adrenal insufficiency
Cushing syndrome (excess levels of one or all the hormones [glucocorticoids, mineralocorticoids, and adrenal androgens] but most commonly glucocorticoid excess)	Usually this condition is due to a small ACTH-producing pituitary adenoma. The most common cause in older children is prolonged or excessive use of corticosteroid therapy[a]	Note history of rapid weight gain, decreased velocity of linear growth, muscle weakness, fatigue, irritability, sleep disturbance, and hypertension History of long-term corticosteroid use, water retention, poor wound healing, frequent infections, and in teenage girls, missed menstrual periods Refer to Figure 48.5 Skin may be thin and fragile; acne may be present	• Management varies depending on the cause. • The goal is to restore hormone balance and reverse Cushing syndrome. • If the cause is an adrenal or pituitary tumour, then surgical removal of the tumour alone or the entire adrenal gland is performed. • If the cause is long-term steroid therapy, then the corticosteroid dose is reduced to the lowest dose that is effective in treating the underlying disorder. • Cortisol synthesis–inhibiting medications may be used. • Counsel the family that the cushingoid appearance is reversible with appropriate treatment. • Be alert for signs of adrenal insufficiency if the child has surgery or if corticosteroid withdrawal occurs quickly.

[a]White, P. C. (2011). Section 4: Disorders of the adrenal glands. In R. M. Kleigman, B. F. Stanton, J. W. St. Geme III, N. F. Schor, & R. E. Behrman (Eds.). *Nelson textbook of pediatrics* (19th ed., pp. 1923–1943). Philadelphia, PA: Saunders.

Aldosterone insufficiency also leads to fluid and electrolyte imbalances, such as hyponatremia, hyperkalemia, and hypotension due to depletion of extracellular fluid. Cortisol insufficiency leads to hypoglycemia.

Therapeutic Management

The goal of treatment is to stop excessive adrenal secretion of androgens while maintaining normal growth and development and later cardiovascular health. Most children with 21-OH deficiency will take a glucocorticoid such as hydrocortisone and the mineralocorticoid fludrocortisone (Florinef) for life. Infants may also require sodium supplementation. When the medications are taken at physiologic doses, there are no adverse effects, but if the drug levels become elevated, hypertension, growth impairment, and acne become a problem. Regular follow-up care and appropriate titration maintain the

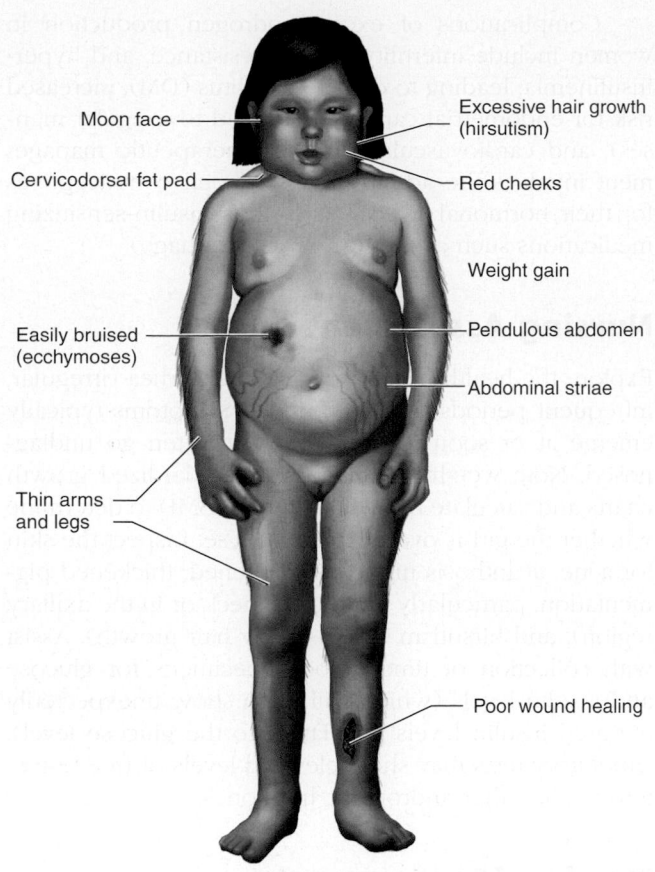

Moon face

Cervicodorsal fat pad

Excessive hair growth (hirsutism)

Red cheeks

Weight gain

Easily bruised (ecchymoses)

Pendulous abdomen

Abdominal striae

Thin arms and legs

Poor wound healing

FIGURE 48.5 Cushing syndrome.

dose at appropriate levels to allow normal growth and development.

When girls are born with atypical genitalia, sex can be determined by karyotyping chromosomes and also pelvic ultrasound. Historically, surgical treatment involved clitoral surgery to alter the appearance in infancy and correction of the UGS to permit future vaginal intercourse at puberty. More recently, some argue that surgery should be delayed until the child is old enough to decide what kind of correction (if any) should be performed (Meyer-Bahlburg, Khuri, Reyes-Portillo, Ehrhardt, & New, 2017). The decision to intervene immediately or to delay treatment is a complex one that raises many concerns for the family. Therefore, parents can be supported by both professionals and support groups. Further long-term follow-up research is needed to determine risks and benefits of early versus delayed treatment (White, 2011).

Nursing Assessment

Nursing assessment of the child with CAH includes health history, physical examination, and laboratory and diagnostic testing. Specific findings related to CAH are presented below.

HEALTH HISTORY AND PHYSICAL EXAMINATION

Obtain the health history, noting history of atypical genitalia at birth in the infant. In the toddler or preschooler, note history of accelerated growth velocity and signs of premature adrenarche. Upon inspection of the infant's genitalia, note a large penis in the boy and atypical genitalia in the girl. When observing the toddler or preschooler, note pubic hair development, acne, and hirsutism.

LABORATORY AND DIAGNOSTIC TESTING

The most common type of CAH, 21-OH enzyme deficiency, is detected by newborn metabolic screening. If this test has not been done or the results are unavailable, obtain random hormone levels or levels associated with ACTH stimulation. X-rays reveal advanced bone age and premature closure of epiphyseal plates of the long bones.

Nursing Management

In addition to the common interventions associated with endocrine disorders in childhood (see Nursing Care Plan 48.1 at the end of the chapter), nursing management of the infant or child with CAH focuses on preventing and monitoring for acute adrenal crisis, helping the family to understand the disease, providing education to the child and family about the importance of maintaining hormone supplementation, and providing emotional support to the family.

PREVENTING AND MONITORING FOR ACUTE ADRENAL CRISIS

Providing ongoing assessment of the ill or hospitalized child with a history of CAH is crucial in order to recognize the development of life-threatening acute adrenal crisis. Signs and symptoms of acute adrenal crisis include persistent vomiting, dehydration, hyponatremia, hyperkalemia, hypotension, tachycardia, and shock. Monitor children with CAH closely and notify the physician or nurse practitioner if adrenal crisis is suspected. If signs and symptoms of adrenal crisis develop, the child will receive intravenous steroids, such as hydrocortisone, and aggressive fluid resuscitation, often using 5% dextrose in normal saline (D5NS), to correct electrolyte imbalances.

Take Note!

Adrenal crisis in the newborn is often unrecognized. It presents within the first few days to weeks of life with vomiting, lethargy, and feeding difficulties.

EDUCATING THE FAMILY ABOUT THE MEDICATION REGIMEN

Medication will be required throughout the child's life because cortisone is necessary to sustain life. Teach the family the appropriate oral dosages of hydrocortisone and fludrocortisone. It is critical to maintain tight control over the levels of these medications in the bloodstream. Either underdosing or overdosing may lead to short adult stature. Low levels of the hormones may also result in adrenal crisis (as discussed above). These drugs are usually given orally but in some instances will need to be given via intramuscular injections. Teach families how to give hydrocortisone intramuscularly if the child is vomiting and cannot keep down oral medication. If the child becomes ill, is under stress, or needs surgery, additional doses of medications may be required. Encourage the family to obtain a medical ID bracelet or necklace for the child.

Take Note!

Families must keep extra steroids in an injectable form, such as Solu-Cortef or Decadron, at home to give during an emergency.

PROVIDING FAMILY SUPPORT

Make sure the family of a newborn with atypical genitalia feels able to ask questions and exploring their feelings. The birth certificate may pose a problem if the province requires identification of sex and there is a delay in making this decision. Cultural attitudes, the parents' expectations, and the extent of family support may influence the family's response to the child and the decision-making process related to sex of rearing and the possibility of surgical correction.

In general, laypeople do not understand adrenal function and what this diagnosis may mean to the family. Provide families with privacy to discuss these issues, and offer emotional and spiritual support. When referring to the infant, use terms such as "your baby" instead of the pronouns "he," "she," or "it," and describe the genitals as "sex organs" instead of "penis" or "clitoris." Refer families to the CARES Foundation (Congenital Adrenal Hyperplasia Research, Education, and Support) and the Magic Foundation for additional support and resources. Links to these resources are provided on thePoint.

POLYCYSTIC OVARY SYNDROME

Polycystic ovary syndrome (PCOS), also referred to as functional ovarian hyperandrogenism or ovarian androgen excess, is an endocrine disorder that produces a variety of symptoms in adolescent girls and women. The exact cause is unknown. Testosterone production by the ovaries and adrenal cells is excessive, causing hirsutism, balding, acne, increased muscle mass, and decreased breast size. Polycystic ovaries may or may not be present. There is a genetic predisposition for PCOS along with nonhereditary factors, the most common being insulin resistance and obesity (Rosenfield, 2014).

Complications of excess androgen production in women include infertility, insulin resistance, and hyperinsulinemia, leading to diabetes mellitus (DM), increased risk for endometrial carcinoma (linked to irregular menses), and cardiovascular disease. Therapeutic management involves the administration of oral contraceptives for their hormonal effects, as well as insulin-sensitizing medications such as metformin (Glucophage).

Nursing Assessment

Explore the health history for oligomenorrhea (irregular, infrequent periods) or amenorrhea. Symptoms typically emerge at or soon after puberty but often go undiagnosed. Note weight in relation to standardized growth charts and calculate body mass index (BMI) to determine whether the girl is overweight or obese. Inspect the skin for acne, acanthosis nigricans (darkened, thickened pigmentation, particularly around the neck or in the axillary region), and hirsutism (excess body hair growth). Assist with collection of timed blood specimens for glucose and insulin levels (which will often show unexpectedly elevated insulin levels in relation to the glucose level). Laboratory tests may show elevated levels of free testosterone and other androgenic hormones.

Nursing Management

One of the most important functions of the nurse in relation to PCOS is to assist with early recognition and treatment. Educate the adolescent girl about the use of oral contraceptives to normalize hormone levels, which will decrease androgenic effects. Support the teen in her efforts to diet and exercise to lose weight. Oral insulin-sensitizing drugs such as metformin (Glucophage) may be prescribed. Encourage the teen to comply with the medication regimen. Routinely measure weight to determine progress with weight loss. Measure blood pressure to screen for hypertension, which may develop as a complication of PCOS. Online support groups and education are available. Links to several resources are provided on thePoint.

DIABETES MELLITUS

DM is a common chronic disease seen in children and adolescents. In DM, carbohydrate, protein, and lipid metabolism are impaired. The key feature of DM is hyperglycemia. The major forms of diabetes are classified as:

- Type 1, which is caused by a deficiency of insulin secretion due to pancreatic β-cell damage
- Type 2, which is a consequence of insulin resistance that occurs at the level of skeletal muscle, liver, and adipose tissue with different degrees of β-cell impairment (Alemzadeh & Ali, 2011)

- Other types of diabetes secondary to certain conditions such as cystic fibrosis, glucocorticoid use (as in Cushing syndrome), infections, and certain genetic syndromes such as Down syndrome, Klinefelter syndrome, and Turner syndrome (Alemzadeh & Ali, 2011)
- Gestational diabetes (diabetes during pregnancy)

The discussion for this chapter will focus on type 1 and type 2 diabetes as these are the most common types seen in children. However, clinical presentation and disease progression of DM can vary considerably. Therefore, in some cases, children cannot be clearly defined as having type 1 or type 2 (American Diabetes Association, 2014).

While diabetes is a common chronic condition in children and youth, current Canadian population-based surveillance data after 2008/09 is unavailable (Public Health Agency Canada, 2011). It is estimated that by 2018, 3.7 million Canadians will be affected by diabetes (Thibault et al., 2016). A percentage of these, likely higher than the 0.3% prevalence rate offered by the Provincial Health Service Authority in 2008/09, will be children and youth. Historically, childhood DM was assumed to be type 1, while type 2 DM occurred mostly in adults. However, in recent years, type 2 DM has been reported in US children and adolescents at an increasing rate (Dabelea et al., 2014). Some studies report that between 20% and 50% of American children with newly diagnosed diabetes have type 2 DM (Dabelea et al., 2014). This increase in incidence of type 2 DM among children and adolescents may be attributed to the rise in obesity and decreased physical activity in young people along with exposure to diabetes in utero (Dabelea et al., 2014). Many children with type 2 DM have a relative with type 2 DM and/or are overweight. Certain minority ethnic groups, such as Hispanic, Asian, South Asian, Indigenous, and African-American children, have a higher rate of type 2 DM (Canadian Paediatric Society, 2016).

Care of children with diabetes differs from that of adults due to physiologic and developmental differences. In children, insulin sensitivity varies as the child grows and goes through sexual maturation. Children are dependent on others for their care, and self-management ability varies among children based on age, developmental level, and individual differences. Care will be needed in a variety of settings such as school, day care, and extracurricular activities (CPS, 2015). Therefore, teaching and education will need to involve parents and other caregivers throughout childhood and adolescence. Refer to Table 48.4, which discusses developmental issues related to DM.

Pathophysiology

Type 1 DM is an autoimmune disorder that occurs in genetically susceptible individuals who may also be exposed to one of several environmental or acquired factors, such as chemicals, viruses, or other toxic agents implicated in the development process. As the genetically susceptible individual is exposed to environmental factors, the immune system begins a T-lymphocyte–mediated process that damages and destroys the β cells of the pancreas, resulting in inadequate insulin secretion. This deficiency of insulin leads to an inability of cells to take up glucose. The end result is hyperglycemia, glucose accumulation in the blood, and the body's inability to use its main source of fuel efficiently. The kidneys try to lower blood glucose, resulting in glycosuria and polyuria, and protein and fat are broken down for energy. The metabolism of fat leads to a build-up of ketones and acidosis (see discussion of diabetic ketoacidosis [DKA] below).

In type 2 DM, the pancreas usually produces insulin but the body is resistant to the insulin or there is an inadequate insulin secretion response (the body can produce insulin but not enough to meet the body's needs). Eventually, insulin production decreases (resulting from the pancreas working overtime to produce insulin), with a result similar to type 1 DM.

If DM goes unrecognized or is inadequately treated (especially type 1 DM), **diabetic ketoacidosis (DKA)** or fat catabolism develops (a deficiency or ineffectiveness of insulin results in the body using fat instead of glucose for energy), resulting in anorexia, nausea and vomiting, lethargy, stupor, altered level of consciousness, confusion, decreased skin turgor, abdominal pain, Kussmaul respirations and air hunger, fruity (sweet-smelling) or acetone breath odour, presence of ketones in urine and blood, tachycardia, and, if left untreated, coma and death.

Take Note!

DKA is a medical emergency. It requires early recognition and prompt intervention. Be alert to the increased chance of DKA during times of stress such as illness, infection, and surgery, as hormones produced by the body in times of stress result in decreased insulin sensitivity and increased glucose production.

Prolonged exposure to high blood glucose levels results in damage to blood vessels and nerves. Long-term complications of DM include failure to grow, delayed sexual maturation, poor wound healing, recurrent infections (especially of the skin), retinopathy, neuropathy, vascular complications, nephropathy, cerebrovascular disease, peripheral vascular disease, and cardiovascular disease. Consistent, well-controlled blood glucose levels can prevent these complications from developing for many years. On the other hand, poorly controlled DM can lead to complications much earlier.

Therapeutic Management

Treatment for DM must occur as part of a multidisciplinary health care team, with the family and child as a central part of that team. In the past, the child would be

TABLE 48.4	DEVELOPMENTAL ISSUES RELATED TO DIABETES MELLITUS	
Age Group	**Child and Family Implications**	**Nursing Implications**
Infants	Management falls on parents/caretakers. Infant is unable to communicate hypo-/hyperglycemic symptoms; signs and symptoms are sometimes difficult to assess. Increased risk of hypoglycemia due to inconsistent feeding times and amounts. Developing brain may experience adverse consequences to severe hypo-/hyperglycemia	Prevent extreme fluctuations in blood glucose. Prevent hypoglycemia and, if present, treat promptly. Attempt to achieve consistent dietary intake. Establish rituals/routines with home management. Provide support for parents and caregivers
Toddlers	Management falls on parents/caretakers. Increased risk of hypoglycemia due to inconsistent food intake (picky eaters). Developing brain may experience adverse consequences to severe hypo-/hyperglycemia. Discipline and temper tantrums common in this age group; may be hard to distinguish between normal toddler behaviour and hypoglycemia symptoms Parents may be overcautious and hinder child's ability to explore and develop normally	Prevent hypoglycemia and if present treat promptly. Assist parents in managing a picky eater. Let toddler choose foods. Get toddler to find a word or phrase to use to describe feelings when hypoglycemic Help parents to provide appropriate discipline and protection while continuing to promote normal development Establish rituals/routines with home management
Preschoolers	Increased motor maturity. Widening social circle, so the child will notice that he or she is "different." Magical thinking presents some issues. Developing brain may experience more adverse consequences to severe hypo-/hyperglycemia than older children. Preschooler wants to be an active participant in diabetes care but may lack some of the developmental skills (such as fine motor and cognitive skills). Some children can begin to perform blood glucose testing with the newer devices. Increased risk of hypoglycemia due to varied food intake and activity	Prevent hypoglycemia and if present treat promptly. Use simple explanations and play therapy when instructing or preparing for a procedure. Encourage child's participation as appropriate
School-age children	Can begin to participate in more of the daily diabetes care; may be able to perform self-monitoring blood glucose testing, record glucose levels, choose injection sites and give injections, perform ketone testing, count carbohydrates, recognize need to eat, and treat for hypoglycemia. Beginning to rely on others (such as school nurse, child care provider, teacher) to provide diabetes care. Children may feel different from their peers and struggle socially. Must incorporate management into school day, and plan for field trips	Use concise and concrete terms when instructing. Allow child to proceed at his or her own rate. Assist family to incorporate the testing and injections into school day and plan for field trips. Involve the school nurse in helping with the school plan Encourage the child's participation but emphasize importance of continued adult supervision Encourage regular attendance at school and participation in extracurricular activities Assist in the development of a care schedule that is flexible enough to allow for participation in school activities Assist with education of other care providers as needed
Adolescents	Undergoing rapid physical, emotional, and cognitive growth. Working toward separate identity from parents and the demands of diabetic care can hinder this. This struggle for independence can lead to nonadherence of diabetic care regimen. Conflicts develop with self-management, body image, and peer group acceptance. They acquire the skills to perform tasks related to diabetic care but may lack decision-making skills needed to adjust treatment plan. Teens do not always foresee the consequences of their activity	Slowly care is turned over to the adolescent with minor supervision from the family Encourage parents and teen to find the right balance of shared management. Encourage parents to continue to provide guidance and supervision and be actively involved in the plan of care. Assess adherence to diabetic care regimen Assess for signs/symptoms of depression, eating disorders, or evidence of risky behaviours In later adolescence, assist teen in transitioning to independent self-management and adult diabetes physician or nurse practitioner

admitted to the hospital for 3 to 5 days for stabilization and education, but today the trend is toward treating children on an outpatient basis. Established glucose control is essential in reducing the risk of long-term complications associated with DM. Therefore, general goals for therapeutic management include:

- Achieving normal growth and development
- Promoting optimal serum glucose control, including fluid and electrolyte levels and near-normal **hemoglobin A1c** (HbA1c) or glycosylated hemoglobin (which is hemoglobin that glucose is bound to and it monitors long-term control of blood sugars and diabetes) levels
- Preventing complications
- Promoting positive adjustment to the disease, with ability to self-manage in the home

The key to success is to educate the child and family so they can self-manage this chronic condition. Therapeutic management involves blood glucose monitoring; daily injections or infusion of insulin and/or administration of oral hypoglycemic medications; a realistic and well-balanced diet; an exercise program; and self-management and decision-making skills.

Research is ongoing to develop alternative medications, including alternative routes for insulin administration and therapies to monitor and treat diabetes, such as inhaled insulin before meals.

Monitoring Glycemic Control

Consistent glycemic control leads to fewer long-term diabetes-related complications. Three important methods for monitoring glycemic control include blood glucose monitoring, continuous glucose monitoring (CGM) and monitoring hemoglobin A1c levels.

BLOOD GLUCOSE MONITORING

Blood glucose monitoring evaluates short-term glycemic control. It allows for tight glucose control because supplemental insulin can be used to correct or prevent hyperglycemia; it also enables children and their parents and their physicians or nurse practitioners to provide better management of the disease. (Refer to Common Laboratory and Diagnostic Tests 48.1.) The frequency of blood glucose monitoring is based on the goals for each particular child. Children who are in the hospital for management of their DM or are on insulin therapy require blood glucose monitoring before meals and at bedtime if not more frequently. Additional glucose checks may be necessary if glycemic control has not occurred, during times of illness, during episodes of hypoglycemic or hyperglycemic symptoms, or when there are changes in therapy. Children receiving noninsulin therapy may check their blood glucose less frequently but it can remain a useful guide to their therapy and its effectiveness. The procedure for glucose monitoring will vary based on equipment used but often involves a fingerstick, a reagent strip, and a glucometer.

Self-monitoring of blood glucose (SMBG) at home is essential to improve glycemic control, to provide self-management of this disease, and to help to prevent complications such as severe hypo-/hyperglycemia. The child and caregiver need to be aware of the importance of checking blood glucose regularly and more frequently when needed. Documenting blood glucose values is necessary to provide information on glucose control. This allows their physician or nurse practitioner to evaluate the effectiveness of their treatment regimen. Accuracy of SMBG is dependent on proper user technique; therefore, assessment of technique and education reinforcement are important at each visit (see Teaching Guidelines 48.2).

Teaching Guidelines 48.2
BLOOD GLUCOSE MONITORING

- Obtain glucose levels before meals and bedtime snacks.
- Perform monitoring more often during prolonged exercise, if you are ill, if you have eaten more food than usual, or if you suspect nighttime hypoglycemia.
- Use the manufacturer's recommendations and perform quality control measures as directed.
- Look for patterns. For example, 3 to 4 days of a consistent pattern of glucose values above 11.1 mmol/L (200 mg/dL) before dinner indicates a need to adjust the insulin dose.
- Blood glucose measurements are the best way to determine daily insulin dosages.
- Normal levels are as follows: nondiabetics >12 years: 3.3 to 6.1 mmol/L (60 to 110 mg/dL); toddlers and children with type 1 DM younger than 6 years old: before meals 5.5 to 10 mmol/L (100 to 180 mg/dL), at bedtime 6.1 to 11.1 mmol/L (110 to 200 mg/dL); children with type 1 DM aged 6 to 12: before meals 5.0 to 10 mmol/L (90 to 180 mg/dL), at bedtime 5.5 to 10 mmol/L (100 to 180 mg/dL); adolescents 13 to 19 years of age, before meals 5.0 to 7.2 mmol/L (90 to 130 mg/dL), at bedtime 5 to 8.3 mmol/L (90 to 150 mg/dL) (Diabetes Canada CPG guidelines, 2013).

CGM is available in Canada; many provinces have access to information. See for example, HealthLink BC (2017).

MONITORING HEMOGLOBIN A1c LEVELS

Hemoglobin A1c (HbA1c) provides the physician or nurse practitioner with information regarding the long-term control of glucose levels (refer to Common Laboratory and Diagnostic Tests 48.1). In adults, the goal is to achieve a near-normal HbA1c. However, in children, especially infants and children younger than 3 years, hypoglycemia poses some unique risks and can be hard to recognize. Therefore, the HbA1c goals in children need to take into account the risks of severe hypoglycemia and glycemic control goals need to be individualized (Diabetes Canada CPG guidelines, 2013; refer to Table 48.1). The Diabetes Canada CPG guidelines (2013) suggest HbA1c goals in children with type 1 diabetes. These include:

- Infants and young children 0 to 6 years: HbA1c less than 8.5% and less than 8.0% if this can be achieved without excessive hypoglycemia
- Children 6 to 12 years: less than 7.5%
- Children and adolescents 13 to 19 years: less than 7.0%

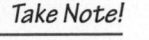

Take Note!

HbA1c levels may vary in different races/ethnicities. Recent studies have questioned the validity of HbA1c in the pediatric population, especially ethnic minorities. Further research is needed to investigate these issues. At the current time, the American Diabetes Association continues to recommend its use in the pediatric population (American Diabetes Association, 2014).

Insulin Replacement Therapy

Insulin replacement therapy is the cornerstone of management of type 1 DM. Insulin is administered daily by subcutaneous injections into adipose tissue over large muscle masses using a traditional insulin syringe or a subcutaneous injector (also known as insulin pen) (Fig. 48.6). U-100 insulin may also be administered using a portable insulin pump (see discussion below). The frequency, dose, and type of insulin are based on how much the child needs to achieve a normal, average blood glucose concentration and to prevent hypoglycemia. Typically, two to four daily injections are commonly used, with dosage depending on the needs of the child. The dose may need to be increased during the pubertal growth spurt as well as during times of illness or stress.

An insulin pump is a device that administers a continuous infusion of rapid-acting insulin. These devices have been increasing in usage and studies have found them to be a safe and effective way to improve glycemic control and reduce episodes of severe hypoglycemia in young people (Johnson, Cooper, Jones, & Davis, 2013). See Evidence-Based Practice 48.1. It consists of a computer, a reservoir of rapid-acting insulin, thin tubing through which the insulin is delivered, and a small guide needle inserted into the abdomen. Insulin pumps attempt to mimic the physiologic insulin release by delivering small, continuous infusions of insulin with additional bolus units administered at mealtimes, for planned carbohydrate intake, and if glucose testing

FIGURE 48.6 The subcutaneous injector uses pressure jets to deliver insulin safely and accurately.

results show it is needed. Advantages of this kind of therapy include:

- There are fewer injections and less trauma.
- Children's food intake can be unpredictable, so insulin delivery can occur after a meal and be adjusted based on actual intake.
- Children can be sensitive to insulin and require only minute doses, which the pump can deliver with precision.
- The pumps can store different basal rates for different times during the day and days of the week. For example, a higher basal rate may be needed in the morning when the child is sitting at his or her desk and a lower rate may be necessary during the afternoon when the child is more active with recess and physical education classes. In addition, rates can be programmed differently for school days versus weekend days, when the child may sleep later and have differing activity levels.

The use of an insulin pump does require a commitment from the child and caregiver in order to achieve success and improved glycemic control. The child and caregiver must be able to count carbohydrates, monitor glucose levels frequently, and work closely with the physician or nurse practitioner.

Take Note!

Some insulin pumps have a built-in sensor technology to monitor interstitial or sensor glucose continuously. These more accurate CGM technologies also show the value of the CGM in both MDI (multiple daily injections) and insulin pump users (McAdams & Rizvi, 2016).

Types of insulin include rapid acting, short acting, intermediate acting, and long acting (Table 48.5). Each type works at a different pace and most children will use more than one type. In some cases, premixed combinations of intermediate and short or rapid acting, such as 70% NPH and 30% regular, may be used. Again, this

EVIDENCE-BASED PRACTICE 48.1

WHAT IS THE LONG-TERM IMPACT OF INSULIN PUMP THERAPY IN CHILDREN?

STUDY

A case–control design study was performed to assess the impact insulin pump therapy has on long-term glycemic control, BMI, rate of severe hypoglycemia, and diabetes ketoacidosis. Three hundred and forty-five children on pump therapy were matched with 345 children on injection therapy. The average age was 11.4 years (±3.5), average duration of diabetes at the time pump was started was 4.1 years (±3.0), and the average duration of follow-up was 3.5 years (±2.5).

Findings

The mean hemoglobin A1c in the pump group decreased by 0.6% and remained significant throughout the 7-year follow-up. No significant change in BMI was found between the two groups. Severe hypoglycemia was reduced in the pump group and was increased in the injection group. The rate of hospitalization due to diabetic ketoacidosis was lower in the pump group versus the injection group.

Nursing Implications

The use of insulin pump therapy improves glycemic control over a sustained period of time and was accomplished with a reduction in severe hypoglycemia and diabetic ketoacidosis and without an increase in BMI. Children with poor glycemic control were found to have the biggest improvements in hemoglobin A1c levels with the use of insulin pump therapy. Nurses need to recognize the success of insulin pump therapy use in children as evidenced by this long-term study.

Adapted from Johnson, S. R., Cooper, M. N., Jones, T. W., & Davis, E. A. (2013). Long-term outcome of insulin pump therapy in children with type 1 diabetes assessed in a large population-based case–control study. *Diabetologia, 56*(11), 2392–2400.

depends on the needs of the child. Insulin can be kept at room temperature (insulin that is administered cold may increase discomfort with injection) but should be discarded 1 month after opening even if refrigerated. Any extra, unopened vials should be stored in the refrigerator.

Take Note!

Lantus is usually given in a single dose at bedtime. Do not mix Lantus with other insulins.

Oral Diabetic Medications

Oral diabetic medications, also referred to as hypoglycemic, antidiabetic, or antihyperglycemic medications, are used in DM type 2 if glycemic control cannot be achieved by diet and exercise. Oral diabetic medications work in a variety of ways. Sulfonylureas (such as glipizide

[Glucotrol] and glyburide [DiaBeta]), meglitinides (such as repaglinide [Prandin]), and nateglinide (Starlix) stimulate insulin secretion by increasing the response of β cells to glucose. Another group, the biguanides, reduces glucose production from the liver. Metformin is an example of a biguanide and is an effective initial therapy unless significant liver or kidney impairment is present. Insulin sensitizers are used to help decrease insulin resistance and improve the body's ability to use insulin in the liver and skeletal tissues. α-Glucosidase inhibitors are used to slow digestion of starch in the small intestines so that glucose from the starch enters the bloodstream more slowly and can be matched more effectively with the impaired insulin response of the body. Combination agents are also available.

Common adverse effects of these oral diabetic medications include headache, dizziness, flatulence and GI

TABLE 48.5	INSULIN TYPE, ACTION, AND DURATION			
Type	**Generic (Brand) Name**	**Onset**	**Peak**	**Duration (hours)**
Rapid acting	Aspart/(NovoLog) Lispro/(Humalog) Glulisine/(Apidra)	Within 15 minutes	30–90 minutes	3–5
Short acting	Regular (Humulin R, Novolin R)	30–60 minutes	2–4 hours	5–8
Intermediate acting	NPH (Humulin N, Novolin N)	1–3 hours	4–10 hours	10–16
Long acting	Glargine (Lantus) Detemir (Levemir)	1–2 hours	No clear peak, offer continuously steady coverage	6–24

Adapted from National Diabetes Information Clearinghouse (NDIC). (2012). *What I need to know about diabetes medicines: Types of insulin.* Retrieved from http://diabetes.niddk.nih.gov/dm/pubs/medicines_ez/insert_C.aspx

distress, edema, and liver enzyme elevation. If the oral hypoglycemics fail to maintain a normal glucose level, then insulin injections will be required to manage type 2 DM.

Diet and Exercise

Other therapies involve diet and exercise protocols. Medical nutrition therapy (MNT) can be initiated to prevent type 2 diabetes in children showing signs of prediabetes, to help glycemic control in existing diabetes, and to help slow the development of complications associated with diabetes (Gerard, 2014). MNT can be complex and must be individualized to each child incorporating the child's food preferences, activity level, cultural preferences, and family habits and schedule. Enlisting the help of a registered dietitian who has expertise in diabetic management is recommended (American Diabetes Association, 2014).

The appropriate diet for a child or adolescent with diabetes is a balanced, healthy diet that meets the child's growth and development needs just like any other child. The child and family need to understand the effect that food has on the child's glucose levels. Monitoring carbohydrate intake is an important component of diet management and assists with glycemic control. Nutritional recommendations for a child with or without diabetes or prediabetes include the following: limit sweets, ensure consistent food intake (eat often and try to avoid skipping meals), monitor carbohydrate intake, eat whole grains and plenty of fruits and vegetables, and limit saturated fat.

It has been shown that regular exercise can improve glycemic control and can help delay or prevent the development of type 2 diabetes (American Diabetes Association, 2014). Also, exercise has an important influence on the hypoglycemic effects of insulin (by causing the release of glucagon, which will result in increased blood glucose). Therefore, it is important for the child to maintain or increase his or her activity levels. If the child is taking insulin, the family must know how to change the medication dosage or add food to maintain blood glucose control. Children with type 2 DM are often overweight, so the exercise plan is very important in helping the child to lose weight as well as assisting with the hypoglycemic effects of the medications.

Thinking About Development

Jayda Jones is a 12-year-old girl recently diagnosed with type 2 diabetes.

Based on her developmental age, how will you instruct her and her caregivers on ways to manage her diabetes at home?

How would your instructions change if she was 16 years old?

Management of Complications

Another important aspect of therapeutic management includes monitoring and managing complications. The American Diabetes Association (2014) has developed recommendations for standards of medical care to help monitor complications and reduce risk. These include:

- Retinopathy:
  - Type 1 diabetes: eye examination by ophthalmologist (with expertise in diabetes) once child is 10 and has had diabetes for 3 to 5 years; annual examinations unless different recommendation by professional
  - Type 2 diabetes: eye examination by ophthalmologist (with expertise in diabetes) shortly after diagnosis; annual examinations unless different recommendation by professional
- Nephropathy:
  - Type 1 diabetes: annual screening for microalbuminuria (which occurs when the kidneys leak small amounts of albumin into the urine) once child is 10 and has had diabetes for 5 years
  - Type 2 diabetes: annual screening for microalbuminuria shortly after diagnosis
  - Dyslipidemia: in children older than 2 years with a family history of high cholesterol or cardiovascular disease or unknown family history, obtain a lipid profile at time of diagnosis (once glucose level has been stabilized); otherwise, obtain lipid panel at puberty
  - Hypertension: blood pressure measured at each routine visit
- In addition, children with type 1 diabetes should be screened for celiac disease and hypothyroidism every 1 to 2 years (once glucose levels are stabilized) since both are commonly associated with diabetes

Nursing Assessment

Assessment involves understanding the ever-changing needs of children as they grow and develop. The first phase of assessment involves identifying the child who may have DM. The second phase involves identifying problems that might develop in the child with DM. It is important to always be aware of this when observing the child for possible complications or management problems. In addition, always be alert for opportunities to provide education that will expand the understanding and skills related to management of DM of the child and family.

Health History and Physical Examination

During the initial diagnosis of DM, obtain a detailed history of family patterns and problems in school related to some of the mental and behaviour changes that may occur in a hyperglycemic state (e.g., weakness, fatigue, and mood changes). The child or parent may report unusual or excessive thirst (polydipsia) coupled with

COMPARISON CHART 48.3	TYPE 1 VERSUS TYPE 2 DIABETES MELLITUS	
History and Physical Findings Usually Present at Diagnosis	**Type 1**	**Type 2**
Family history	Less tendency than type 2	Yes
Prone ethnic groups	All	Native American, African American, Hispanic/ Latino, Asian/Pacific Island descent
Polydipsia, polyuria, polyphagia	Yes	Yes, may be mild or absent
Weight	Possibly weight loss	Usually obese
Age of onset	Usually younger children	Usually pubertal children
Incidental finding on screening urinalysis	Rare	Common
Antecedent flu-like illness/symptoms	Common	Possible
Autoimmune antibodies	Yes	No
Diabetic ketoacidosis	Common	Possible
Hypertension	No	Common
Acanthosis nigricans	No	Common
Dyslipidemia	No	Common

Adapted from Alemzadeh, R., & Ali, O. (2011). Section 6: Diabetes mellitus in children. In R. M. Kleigman, B. F. Stanton, J. W. St. Geme III, N. F. Schor, & R. E. Behrman (Eds.). *Nelson textbook of pediatrics* (19th ed., pp. 1968–1997). Philadelphia, PA: Saunders.

frequent urination (polyuria). The child may also complain of blurred vision, headaches, or bedwetting. The child with type 1 DM may have a history of poor growth. Comparison Chart 48.3 gives information about common history and physical examination findings in children with type 1 DM versus type 2 DM. Type 1 DM typically presents with acute symptoms and hyperglycemia, while type 2 DM can frequently go undiagnosed until complications appear (American Diabetes Association, 2014).

In the child who is known to have DM, the health history includes any problems with hyperglycemia or hypoglycemia, diet, activity and exercise patterns, types of medications (insulin or oral diabetes medications) and dose and times of administration, ability to monitor blood glucose levels, ability to manage sick days, and ability to administer insulin. Perform a thorough physical examination, noting any abnormal findings.

Laboratory and Diagnostic Testing

The American Diabetes Association (2014) currently recommends the use of fasting plasma glucose levels, 2-hour postprandial glucose levels, and/or hemoglobin A1c as reliable sources to diagnose diabetes (refer to Common Laboratory and Diagnostic Tests 48.1). A fasting glucose level greater than or equal to 7.0 mmol/L (126 mg/dL), a 2-hour plasma glucose level greater than or equal to 11.0 mmol/L (200 mg/dL) during an oral

glucose tolerance test, a random glucose level greater than or equal to 11.0 mmol/L (200 mg/dL) (accompanied by typical symptoms of diabetes), or a hemoglobin A1c greater than 6.5% are laboratory criteria for the diagnosis of DM (American Diabetes Association, 2014). With each of these tests, if hyperglycemia is not explicit, the results should be confirmed with a repeat test on a different day (American Diabetes Association, 2014). Other laboratory and diagnostic tests include serum measurements of islet cell antibodies. Serum levels of urea nitrogen, creatinine, calcium, magnesium, phosphate, and electrolytes such as potassium and sodium may be drawn. Additional tests include a complete blood count, urinalysis, and immunoassay to measure levels of C peptides after a glucose challenge to verify endogenous insulin secretion.

The American Diabetes Association (2014) recommends screening for type 2 DM if a child presents with being overweight or obese and also has any two of the following risk factors:

- Family history: a parent or relative with type 2 DM
- Ethnic background: Native American, African American, Latino, Asian American, or Pacific Islander
- Conditions associated with insulin resistance such as acanthosis nigricans, hypertension, dyslipidemia, or PCOS
- History of maternal diabetes or mother with gestational diabetes when child was in utero
- Age older than 10 years or onset of puberty before age 10 (American Diabetes Association, 2014)

Nursing Management

Individualize the general nursing care discussed in Nursing Care Plan 48.1, at the end of the chapter, based on the child's and family's response to illness. Additional nursing care topics related to DM are discussed below, including regulating glucose control, monitoring for complications, providing education to the child and family, and supporting the child and family.

Regulating Glucose Control

Consistent and established glucose control can reduce the risk of long-term complications associated with diabetes. Therefore, regulating glucose is a very important nursing function.

Typically, in children with type 1 DM and sometimes in cases of type 2 DM, glucose is regulated by subcutaneous injections of insulin. Often, the regimen consists of two injections of intermediate-acting insulin, with the addition of rapid-acting insulin before breakfast and dinner or three injections of a short-acting (rapid) insulin with a long-acting injection at bedtime. Insulin doses are typically ordered on a sliding scale related to the serum glucose level and how the insulin works. Insulin doses and frequency are based on the needs of the child utilizing information gained from blood glucose testing. Regulating glucose can be challenging in children due to continual growth, onset of puberty, varying activity levels with unpredictable schedules, unpredictable eating habits, and the inability to always verbalize the way they are feeling. Thus, close monitoring of changing glucose levels through SMBG is essential in determining adjustments needed in insulin therapy, food intake, and activity level. Adjustment of insulin dosing based on carbohydrate intake is essential to manage blood sugar levels. The use of carbohydrate counting can help children enjoy more freedom to choose their type or amount of food and can allow them to vary their meal and snack times. It allows them to predict the rise in blood sugar that will occur after eating a specific amount or type of carbohydrate and allows them to take into account recent or expected activity level. It requires knowledge of carbohydrate amounts and calculations with each dose of short-acting insulin. Each scale will vary per child as the insulin per carbohydrate serving is calculated on an individual basis. See the Dosage Calculation Question on the Chapter Worksheet for an example. Parents will need extensive education and continual follow-up in order to ensure successful use of this method.

Take Note!

Blood sugar level should never be the only factor considered when calculating insulin dosing. Food intake and recent or expected activity/exercise must be factored.

FIGURE 48.7 Insulin injection sites. (From Silbert-Flagg, J., Pillitteri, A., & Pillitteri, A. [2018]. *Maternal & child health nursing: Care of the childbearing & childrearing family.* Philadelphia, PA: Wolters Kluwer.)

Teach the child and family to use proper subcutaneous injection techniques to avoid injecting into muscle or vascular spaces. Figure 48.7 shows appropriate sites for subcutaneous injection of insulin. Teach the child and family to rotate sites to avoid adipose hypertrophy (fatty lumps that absorb insulin poorly). If the child is using an insulin pump, additional education will be needed.

Atraumatic Care

Children with diabetes experience numerous fingerpricks and injections. Providing atraumatic care remains important. Allow the child to choose the prick or injection site when possible. Use positioning that is comforting to the child. Encourage participation in care as developmentally appropriate.

Take Note!

When giving a combination of short- and long-acting insulin, draw up the clear (short-acting) insulin first to prevent contamination with the long-acting insulin.

In children with type 2 diabetes, glucose levels can be controlled by the use of oral diabetic medications, diet, and exercise or a combination of all three.

COMPARISON CHART 48.4	HYPOGLYCEMIA VERSUS HYPERGLYCEMIA
Hypoglycemia	**Hyperglycemia**
Behavioural changes (tearfulness, irritability, naughtiness), confusion, slurred speech, belligerence	Mental status changes, fatigue, weakness
Diaphoresis	Dry, flushed skin
Tremors	Blurred vision
Palpitations, tachycardia	Abdominal cramping, nausea, vomiting, fruity breath odour

Monitoring for and Managing Complications

While the child is in the hospital, monitor for signs of complications such as acidosis, coma, hyperkalemia or hypokalemia, hypocalcemia, cerebral edema, or hyponatremia. Assess for the development of hypoglycemia or hyperglycemia every 2 hours (Comparison Chart 48.4). Monitor the child's status closely during peak times of insulin action. Perform blood glucose testing as ordered or as needed if the child develops symptoms.

Take Note!

Manifestations of Hypoglycemia Versus Hyperglycemia

Manifestations of hypoglycemia include behavioural changes, confusion, slurred speech, diaphoresis, tremors, palpitations, and tachycardia. In contrast, manifestations of hyperglycemia are blurred vision; dry, flushed skin; and a fruity odour to the breath.

If the child has a severe hypoglycemic reaction, administer glucagon (a hormone produced by the pancreas and stored in the liver) either subcutaneously or intramuscularly. Children under 20 kg receive 0.5 mg; children over 20 kg receive 1 mg (Alemzadeh & Ali, 2011). Dextrose (50%) may be given intravenously if needed. If the child is not having a severe reaction and is coherent, glucose paste or tablets may be used. Offer 10 to 15 g of a simple carbohydrate such as orange juice if the child feels some symptoms of low blood glucose and glucose monitoring indicates a drop in blood glucose level. Follow this with a more complex carbohydrate such as peanut butter and crackers to maintain the glucose level.

The child with severe hyperglycemia resulting in DKA is usually treated in the pediatric intensive care unit. In the case of a child presenting with DKA to the hospital, monitor the glucose level hourly to prevent it from falling more than 5.5 mmol/L (100 mg/dL) per hour. A too-rapid decline in blood glucose predisposes the child to cerebral edema. Fluid therapy is given to treat dehydration, correct electrolyte imbalances (sodium and potassium due to osmotic diuresis), and improve peripheral perfusion. Administration of regular insulin, given intravenously, is preferred during DKA (only regular insulin may be given intravenously [IV]). A bolus dose of 0.1 unit/kg is given, followed by a continuous infusion of 0.1 unit/kg per hour (Nelson-Tuttle, 2014).

Any child exhibiting signs and symptoms of hyperglycemia requires insulin. The dosage is usually based on a sliding scale or determined after consultation with the physician or nurse practitioner.

Take Note!

Double check all insulin doses against the order sheet and with another nurse to ensure accuracy.

Educating the Family

Education is the priority intervention for DM because it will enable the child and family to self-manage this chronic condition. Allow the child and family time to adjust to the diagnosis of a chronic illness that will require self-management. DM is a lifelong condition that requires regular follow-up visits (three or four times a year) to a diabetes specialty clinic. Daily management of the child with DM is complex and dynamic. It will require frequent monitoring of blood glucose levels, medications (including oral diabetic medications and insulin injections), and individual meal plans, including snacks, while the child is at school. The school nurse or community care nurse will be a principal contact person for both staff and family. With appropriate management, involvement of the community, and confidence and compliance by the family, the child can maintain a happy, productive life.

Challenges related to educating children with DM include:

- Children lack the maturity to understand the long-term consequences of this serious chronic illness.
- Children do not want to be different from their peers; having to make lifestyle changes may result in anger or depression.
- Poor families may not be able to afford appropriate food, medication, transportation, and telephone service.

- Families may demonstrate unhealthy behaviours, making it difficult for the child to initiate change because of the lack of supervision or role modelling.
- Family dynamics are affected because management of diabetes must occur all day, every day.

> **Take Note!**
>
> Children with DM have higher rates of depression and may have other comorbid conditions, such as eating disorders, adjustment disorders, or anxiety disorders (Alemzadeh & Ali, 2011).

The initial goal of education is for the family to develop basic management and decision-making skills. Assess the family's ability to learn the basic concepts and offer psychological support. Teach about specific topics in sessions lasting 15 to 20 minutes for the children and 45 to 60 minutes for the caregivers. Teaching must be geared toward the child's level of development and understanding (refer to Table 48.4).

Among the topics to include when teaching children and their families about diabetes management are:
- Self-measurement of blood glucose (Fig. 48.8)
- Urine ketone testing
- Medication use (Fig. 48.9)
- Oral diabetic agents
- Subcutaneous insulin injection or insulin pump use
- Subcutaneous site selection and rotation
- When to alter insulin dosages
- Use of glucagon to treat severe hypoglycemia
- Signs and symptoms of hypoglycemia and hyperglycemia (refer to Comparison Chart 48.4)
- Treatment for hypoglycemia and hyperglycemia at home or other setting such as school
- Monitoring for and managing complications (see above)
- Sick-day instructions

FIGURE 48.8 The school-age child has developed the psychomotor skills needed for blood glucose monitoring and insulin injection sites.

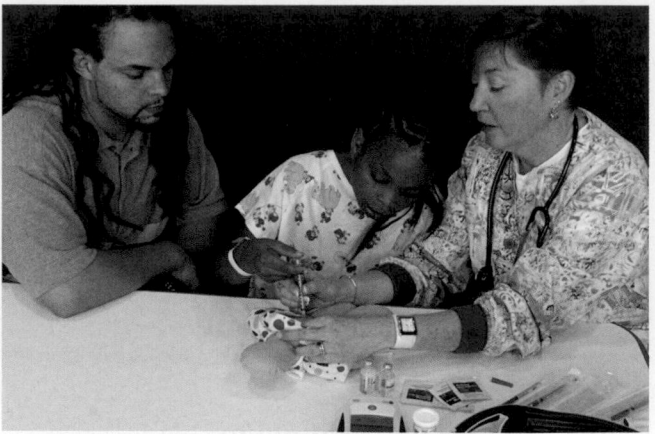

FIGURE 48.9 The school-age child may first practice insulin injections on a doll.

- Laboratory testing and follow-up care
- Diet and exercise as part of DM management (see above)
- Psychosocial aspects of DM

Teaching Guidelines 48.2 presents information for the family about self-monitoring of blood glucose. Teach families how to give insulin, how to use the insulin pump, and how to rotate injection sites (see above).

Good glucose control is dependent on accurate monitoring and medication administration by the child or caregiver. Assessment of the child's or parent's technique and review of procedure and instructions should occur with each visit. Treatment of hypoglycemia and hyperglycemia may have to occur at home or in another setting such as school. In either case, someone who is trained and able to check the child's blood glucose level needs to be available. In the case of hypoglycemia, early recognition is key. Therefore, all caregivers need to be educated on the causes of hypoglycemia (such as increased physical activity, delayed meals or snacks, insulin, oral diabetic medication, illness, stress, and hormonal fluctuations) along with the signs and symptoms. The child also needs access to glucose tablets or a rapidly absorbing carbohydrate such as orange juice as well as a snack with complex carbohydrates and protein within 30 to 60 minutes of the hypoglycemic episode. Injectable glucagon needs to be available in the case that the hypoglycemia is severe and the child is unconscious. In the event of hyperglycemia, the child needs immediate access to rapid-acting insulin injection.

Sick-day instructions may include the following:
- Contact the physician or nurse practitioner.
- Perform SMBG more often.
- Check for ketones in the urine, especially if blood glucose is elevated.
- Use a sliding scale to calculate the insulin dosage.
- Stay hydrated.

A dietitian can help the family with detailed meal planning and dietary guidelines. Review basic nutritional information with the child and family and provide sample meals. Encourage the child and family to keep a food diary. For the child who needs to lose weight, suggest low-carbohydrate snacks. Encourage all children with DM to incorporate physical activity daily (Teaching Guidelines 48.3).

Teaching Guidelines 48.3
DIET AND EXERCISE FOR CHILDREN WITH DIABETES MELLITUS

- Provide sufficient calories and good nutrition for normal growth and development. The diet should be low in saturated fats and concentrated carbohydrates.
- Learn to identify carbohydrate, protein, and fat foods.
- Make adjustments during periods of rapid growth and for issues such as travel, school parties, and holidays.
- Consult a dietitian with expertise in diabetes education as needed.
- Provide three meals per day and midafternoon and bedtime snacks. Consistency of intake can help prevent complications and maintain near-normal blood glucose levels.
- Encourage the child to exercise routinely to help the body use insulin efficiently, thus reducing the insulin requirement.

- Encourage the child to participate in age-appropriate sports.
- When exercising, monitor insulin dose and nutritional and fluid intake, and observe for hypoglycemic reactions. Add an extra snack containing 15 to 30 g carbohydrate for each 45 to 60 minutes of exercise. Avoid exercising excessively when insulin is peaking.

Supporting the Child and Family

Children with DM and their families may have difficulty coping if they lack confidence in their self-management skills. Assess the ability of the child and family to handle situations. Role-play specific situations related to symptoms or complications to help them see different ways to solve problems. Work with the child and family to enhance their conflict resolution skills. Provide opportunities for them to express their feelings. Observe for signs of depression, especially in adolescents.

To enhance the child's confidence and promote feelings of mastery and inclusion, refer him or her to a special camp for children with DM. Also refer families to local support groups, parent-to-parent networks, or one of many national support resources and foundations. Links to camps for children as well as support groups, parent-to-parent networks, and national foundations are provided on the Point.

NURSING CARE PLAN 48.1

Overview for the Child With an Endocrine Disorder

NURSING DIAGNOSIS: Risk for delayed development related to hypo- or hyperfunction of gland/hormone as evidenced by weight and/or height less than expected for age, failure to meet expected age-appropriate developmental milestones

Outcome Identification and Evaluation

Nutritional status will be maximized and development will be enhanced: *child will maintain or gain weight appropriately and will make continued progress toward expected developmental milestones.*

Interventions: *Enhancing Growth and Development*

- Monitor growth parameters using standard growth charts: *to establish baseline and monitor growth trend.*
- Encourage favourite foods (within prescribed diet restrictions if present) *to maximize oral intake.*
- Consult dietitian *for appropriate diet supplementation recommendations.*
- Encourage compliance with hormone supplementation *to enhance ability to achieve appropriate growth.*

- Provide care related to any complications of dysfunction *such as correcting fluid and electrolyte imbalances or diarrhea.*
- Screen for developmental capabilities *to determine child's current level of functioning.*
- Offer age-appropriate toys, play, and activities (including gross motor) *to encourage further development.*

(continued)

Overview for the Child With an Endocrine Disorder (continued)

- Provide support to families of children with developmental delay: *progress in achieving developmental milestones can be slow and ongoing motivation is needed.*
- Reinforce positive attributes in the child *to maintain motivation.*

For the child with diabetes mellitus:
- Provide a calorie-appropriate, nonrestricted, well-balanced diet *to maintain appropriate growth.*
- Encourage three meals with two or three snacks with consistent carbohydrates *to maintain appropriate blood glucose levels and promote growth.*

NURSING DIAGNOSIS: Disturbed body image related to abnormal growth and development/ changes in physical appearance due to hormone dysfunction as evidenced by verbalization of dissatisfaction with the child's or adolescent's looks

Outcome Identification and Evaluation

Child demonstrates appropriate self-esteem in relation to body image: *expresses positive feelings about self and participates in social activities.*

Interventions: *Promoting Healthy Body Image*

- Provide opportunities for child to explore feelings related to appearance: *venting feelings is associated with less body image disturbance.*
- Relate to child on age level, not appearance level: *"babying" a child who looks younger due to his or her small size reduces self-image.*
- Involve the child and especially the teen in the decision-making process: *a sense of control will improve body image.*

- Encourage the child to spend time with peers who have similar endocrine disorders: *peers' opinions are often better accepted than those of persons in authority, such as parents or health care professionals.*
- Refer to counselling or support groups *to further support the child.*

NURSING DIAGNOSIS: Deficient knowledge related to therapeutic regimen as evidenced by questions about endocrine disorder and self-management

Outcome Identification and Evaluation

Child and family will demonstrate sufficient understanding and skills for self-management: *verbalize information about disorder, complications/adverse effects, home care regimen, and long-term needs, and provide return demonstrations of medication administration or other procedures.*

Interventions: *Promoting Knowledge Required for Self-Management*

- Assess child's developmental level and family's ability to absorb instruction *to determine how to approach teaching sessions.*
- Establish teaching plan with child and family *to gain cooperation and involvement.*
- Teach and give printed instructions on disorder, complications, home care, and follow-up requirements *so family has a source to refer to at home.*
- Evaluate teaching with return demonstrations *to determine whether child/family is skilled enough for home management of the disorder.*

For the child with diabetes mellitus:
- First teach "survival skills" (e.g., glucose and urine testing, administering insulin, record keeping, food guidelines, when to call physician) *to provide initial base of knowledge for self-management.*
- Implement second-phase home management program with more extensive instruction: *providing additional teaching over time is necessary for management of a significant chronic illness.*
- Monitor outcomes of teaching with every contact *to ensure progress with child/family education.*

Overview for the Child With an Endocrine Disorder (continued)

NURSING DIAGNOSIS: Interrupted family processes or adjustment issues related to lifestyle changes required to manage chronic illness and possible lifestyle changes as evidenced by family's presence in the hospital, missed work, demonstration of inadequate coping

Outcome Identification and Evaluation

Family will maintain functional system of support; demonstrate adequate coping, adaptation of roles and functions, and decreased anxiety: *parents are involved in child's care, ask appropriate questions, express fears and concerns, identify needs, seek appropriate resources and support, can discuss child's care and condition calmly.*

Interventions: *Encouraging Healthy Family Processes*

- Encourage parents and family members to verbalize concerns related to child's illness, diagnosis, and prognosis: *allows the nurse to identify concerns and areas where further education may be needed.*
- Explain treatments, medications, procedures, child's behaviours, and plan of care to parents: *understanding of the child's current status and plan of care helps decrease anxiety.*
- Identify support system for family and child: *helps nurse identify needs and resources available for coping.*

- Provide family with information about support groups, financial resources, and special clinics in the area for the particular type of disorder *to provide family with a wide base of support.*
- Encourage parents to become involved in care: *allows parents to feel needed and valued and gives them a sense of control over their child's health.*
- Evaluate coping processes on follow-up visits *to determine restoration of family processes.*

NURSING DIAGNOSIS: Imbalanced nutrition: less than or more than body requirements related to pathophysiology of dysfunction as evidenced by growth parameters significantly less or more than expected for age

Outcome Identification and Evaluation

Child's nutritional status is balanced: *child adheres to nutritional guidelines, demonstrates adequate growth (weight and height) pattern within normal range for age and gender or, in the child who has difficulty growing, a progressive increase over time.*

Interventions: *Maintaining Adequate Nutrition*

- Determine body weight and length/height norm for age or what the child's pretreatment measurements were *to determine goal to work toward.*
- Weigh daily or weekly (according to physician order or institutional standard) and measure length/height weekly *to monitor for appropriate growth.*
- Determine child's food preferences and provide favourite foods as able *to increase the likelihood that the child will consume appropriate amounts of foods.*
- Instruct child and family about nutritional requirements *so that they are involved and are prepared for home care.*
- Refer to dietitian *for more detailed information and assistance.*

For the child who needs to gain weight:

- Offer highest-calorie meals at the time of day when the child's appetite is the greatest *to increase likelihood of increased caloric intake.*
- Provide increased-calorie shakes or puddings within dietary restrictions: *high-calorie foods increase weight gain.*
- Administer vitamin and mineral supplements as prescribed *to attain/maintain vitamin and mineral balance in the body.*

(continued)

NURSING CARE PLAN 48.1

Overview for the Child With an Endocrine Disorder (continued)

NURSING DIAGNOSIS: Deficient or excess fluid volume related to pathophysiology of endocrine dysfunction as evidenced by signs and symptoms of dehydration (deficient fluid volume) or edema and excessive urine output (excess fluid volume)

Outcome Identification and Evaluation

Child will maintain adequate fluid volume *as evidenced by elastic skin turgor; absence of edema; moist, pink oral mucosa; presence of tears; urine output 1 mL/kg/h or more; vital signs within normal range for age; and normal electrolyte/hormone serum levels.*

Interventions: *Maintaining Adequate Fluid Volume*

- Assess hydration status (skin turgor, oral mucosa, presence of tears) every 4 to 8 hours *to evaluate maintenance of adequate fluid volume.*
- Assess adequacy of urine output *to evaluate end-organ perfusion.*
- Maintain strict intake and output record *to evaluate effectiveness of rehydration.*
- Weigh child daily: *accurate weight is one of the best indicators of fluid volume status in children.*

- Administer specific hormone, fluid, and electrolyte requirements as ordered *to aid in fluid balance.*

Fluid volume deficit:
- Maintain IV line and administer IV fluid as ordered *to maintain fluid volume.*

Fluid volume excess:
- Maintain fluid restriction as ordered *to restore homeostasis.*

NURSING DIAGNOSIS: Noncompliance related to long-term/complex management of some disorders as evidenced by failure to keep appointments, development of complications or exacerbation of symptoms, or child/family verbalization of inability to maintain treatment plan

Outcome Identification and Evaluation

Child and family will comply with treatment regimen: *child and family will list treatment expectations and agree to follow through.*

Interventions: *Encouraging Compliance*

- Listen nonjudgmentally while the child and family describe reasons for noncompliance: *assessment of problem should begin with nonthreatening discussion.*
- Help the child and family develop a schedule for medication administration and other home regimens that work best for them: *involving child and family in planning care will increase compliance by making them feel respected and valued.*
- Work with the child and family to develop a written treatment plan or schedule that best suits their

needs *to provide support for maintenance of treatment plan.*
- Establish follow-up visits to fit family's situation *to promote compliance.*
- Encourage monitoring with pediatric endocrinologist and specialists: *multidisciplinary involvement has been shown to increase compliance.*
- Recognize that behavioural change comes slowly: *allows time for child and family to adjust to chronic nature of illness.*

KEY CONCEPTS

- The endocrine system consists of cells, tissues, and glands that produce and/or secrete hormones (chemical messengers) in response to a negative

feedback system involving the hypothalamus and nervous system.

- Hormones (chemical messengers), along with the nervous system, play an intricate role in reproduction, growth and development, energy production and use, and maintenance of the internal homeostasis.

- The pituitary, along with the hypothalamus connection, is considered the "control centre," producing hormones that stimulate many glands to produce other hormones or to inhibit the process.

- Hormonal control is immature at birth; this is partly why the infant has trouble maintaining an appropriate balance of fluid concentration, electrolytes, amino acids, glucose, and trace substances.

- Linear growth and cognitive development may be impaired by untreated endocrine dysfunction in the infant or child.

- A thorough health history of the child with a known or potential endocrine disorder often reveals poor growth, school or learning problems, and inactivity or fatigue.

- Serial measurement of growth parameters is a key part of the physical assessment for children with endocrine dysfunction.

- Close monitoring of the child's status is critical during a hormone stimulation test or water deprivation study.

- Hormone supplementation is required lifelong for many of the endocrine disorders.

- The key nursing functions related to hormone supplementation are educating the child and family about medication use and monitoring for therapeutic results and adverse effects.

- Children with adrenocortical dysfunction will require additional hormone supplementation during times of stress such as fever, infection, or surgery.

- GH deficiency is characterized by poor growth and short stature as a result of failure of the anterior pituitary to produce sufficient growth hormone. Early treatment enables the child to reach normal growth.

- Precocious puberty involves early development of secondary sex characteristics as a result of premature activation of the hypothalamic–pituitary–gonadal axis.

- DI is characterized by water intoxication as a result of a deficiency in the antidiuretic hormone that leads to the cardinal signs of polyuria and polydipsia, resulting in hypernatremic dehydration.

- Key findings in congenital hypothyroidism are a thickened protuberant tongue, an enlarged posterior fontanel, feeding difficulties, hypotonia, and lethargy.

- Early diagnosis and treatment of hypothyroidism can prevent impaired growth and severe cognitive impairment.

- CAH results from a genetic defect that causes a breakdown in steroid synthesis and an overproduction of androgens that can lead to ambiguous genitalia in females.

- DM is the most common endocrine disorder now seen in children.

- Type 1 DM is an autoimmune disorder resulting from damage and destruction of the β cells in the islets of Langerhans in the pancreas; the end result is insulin insufficiency. Peak onset occurs in childhood.

- Type 2 DM results in an insensitivity or resistance to insulin. The incidence of type 2 DM has risen dramatically. It is occurring at an alarming rate in children, especially in those who are obese and from certain ethnic groups.

- DKA is a medical emergency. The child will usually be admitted to a pediatric intensive care unit.

- The focus of DM management is regulation of glucose control, which is accomplished by medications, diet, and exercise.

- DM education involves instruction in glucose monitoring, administration of insulin or oral hypoglycemics, meal planning, and promotion of a healthy lifestyle.

- Critical areas in the nursing management of children with endocrine dysfunction include maintaining appropriate nutrition and fluid balance and promoting growth and development.

- The nurse provides ongoing assessment and education of the child and family, imparting to them the knowledge and skills required for self-management.

- Encouraging the child to have a healthy body image and working with the family in establishing healthy family processes are also key nursing functions.

REFERENCES AND RECOMMENDED READINGS

Alemzadeh, R., & Ali, O. (2011). Section 6: Diabetes mellitus in children. In R. M. Kleigman, B. F. Stanton, J. W. St. Geme III, N. F. Schor, & R. E. Behrman (Eds.). *Nelson textbook of pediatrics* (19th ed., pp. 1968–1997). Philadelphia, PA: Saunders.

Amed, S., Delvin, E., & Hamilton, J. (2008). Variation in growth hormone immunoassay in clinical practice in Canada. *Hormone Research*, 69(5):290–294.

American Academy of Pediatrics. (2011). Update of newborn screening and therapy for congenital hypothyroidism. *Pediatric, 117*(6). Retrieved from http://pediatrics.aappublications.org/cgi/content/full/pediatrics;117/6/2290

American Diabetes Association. (2014). Standards of medical care in diabetes—2014. *Diabetes Care, 37*(Suppl 1), S14–S80. Retrieved from http://care.diabetesjournals.org/content/37/Supplement_1/S14.full.pdf+html

Bichet, D. G. (2013a). *Treatment of central diabetes insipidus.* UpToDate. Retrieved from http://www.uptodate.com/contents/treatment-of-central-diabetes-insipidus

Bichet, D. G. (2013b). *Clinical manifestations and causes of central diabetes insipidus.* UpToDate. Retrieved from http://www.uptodate.com/contents/clinical-manifestations-and-causes-of-central-diabetes-insipidus

Breault, D. T., & Majzoub, J. A. (2011a). Chapter 552: Diabetes insipidus. In R. M. Kleigman, B. F. Stanton, J. W. St. Geme III, N. F. Schor, & R. E. Behrman (Eds.). *Nelson textbook of pediatrics* (19th ed., pp. 1881–1884). Philadelphia, PA: Saunders.

Breault, D. T., & Majzoub, J. A. (2011b). Chapter 553: Other abnormalities of arginine vasopressin metabolism and action. In R. M. Kleigman, B. F. Stanton, J. W. St. Geme III, N. F. Schor, & R. E. Behrman (Eds.). *Nelson textbook of pediatrics* (19th ed., pp. 1884–1886). Philadelphia, PA: Saunders.

Canadian Paediatric Society. (2015). *Managing type 1 diabetes in school: Recommendations for policy and practice.* Retrieved from http://www.cps.ca/en/documents/position/type-1-diabetes-in-school

Canadian Paediatric Society. (2016). *Risk reduction for type 2 diabetes in Aboriginal children in Canada.* Retrieved from http://www.cps.ca/documents/position/risk-reduction-type-two-diabetes-aboriginal-children

Carpenito, L. J. (2013). *Nursing diagnosis: Application to clinical practice* (14th ed.). Philadelphia, PA: Lippincott Williams & Wilkins.

Centers for Disease Control and Prevention. (2014a). *Newborn screening: Importance of newborn screening.* Retrieved from http://www.cdc.gov/ncbddd/newbornscreening/

Centers for Disease Control and Prevention. (2014b). *National diabetes statistics report: Estimates of diabetes and its burden in the United States, 2014.* Atlanta, GA: U.S. Department of Health and Human. Retrieved from https://www.cdc.gov/diabetes/pdfs/data/2014-report-estimates-of-diabetes-and-its-burden-in-the-united-states.pdf

Children's Hospital of Boston. (2012). *Diabetes insipidus: Disease information.* Retrieved from http://www.childrenshospital.org/conditions-and-treatments/conditions/d/diabetes-insipidus

Cohen, L. E. (Ed.). (2016). *Growth hormone deficiency: Physiology and clinical management.* Springer. Retrieved from https://books.google.ca/books?hl=en&lr=&id=xjqlDAAAQBAJ&oi=fnd&pg=PR5&dq=Growth+Hormone+Deficiency++Physiology+and+Clinical+Management++Editors:+Cohen,+Laurie+E.+(Ed.)&ots=VgwCGjyzco&sig=hLYkJrmHK0bPHRTs_9WFS3nkE1o#v=onepage&q=Growth%20Hormone%20Deficiency%20%20Physiology%20and%20Clinical%20Management%20%20Editors%3A%20Cohen%2C%20Laurie%20E.%20(Ed.)&f=false

Dabelea, D., Mayer-Davis, E. J., Sharon Saydah, S., Imperatore, G., Linder, B., Divers, J., ... SEARCH for Diabetes in Youth Study. (2014). Prevalence of type 1 and type 2 diabetes among children and adolescents from 2001 to 2009. *Journal of the American Medical Association, 311*(17), 1778–1786.

Diabetes Canada. (n.d.). *Children and type 2 diabetes.* Retrieved from https://www.diabetes.ca/diabetes-and-you/kids-teens-diabetes/children-type-2-diabetes

Diabetes Canada CPG Guidelines. (2013). *Monitoring glycemic control.* Retrieved from http://guidelines.diabetes.ca/

Doyle, D. A. (2011). Section 3: Disorders of the parathyroid. In R. M. Kleigman, B. F. Stanton, J. W. St. Geme III, N. F. Schor, & R. E. Behrman (Eds.). *Nelson textbook of pediatrics* (19th ed., pp. 11916–11923). Philadelphia, PA: Saunders.

Fischbach, F. T., & Dunning III, M. B. (2015). *A manual of laboratory and diagnostic tests* (9th ed.). Philadelphia, PA: Wolters Kluwer Health/Lippincott Williams & Wilkins.

Fleming, L., Van Riper, M., & Knafl, K. (2017). Management of childhood congenital adrenal hyperplasia—An integrative review of the literature. *Journal of Pediatric Health Care, 31*(5), 560–577.

Foote, J. M., Brady, L. H., Burke, A. L., Cook, J. S., Dutcher, M. E., Gradoville, K. M., ... Phillips, K. T. (2011). Development of an evidence-based clinical practice guideline on linear growth measurement of children. *Journal of Pediatric Nursing, 26*(4), 312–324.

Garibaldi, L., & Chemaitilly, W. (2011). Chapter 556: Disorders of pubertal development. In R. M. Kleigman, B. F. Stanton, J. W. St. Geme III, N. F. Schor, & R. E. Behrman (Eds.). *Nelson textbook of pediatrics* (19th ed., pp. 1886–1895). Philadelphia, PA: Saunders.

Gerard, S. (2014). Chapter 50: Diabetes mellitus and the metabolic syndrome. In S. Grossman & C. M. Porth (Eds.). *Porth's pathophysiology: Concepts of altered health states* (9th ed., pp. 1303–1332). Philadelphia, PA: Wolters Kluwer Health/Lippincott Williams & Wilkins.

HealthLink BC. (2017). *Continuous glucose monitoring.* Retrieved from https://www.healthlinkbc.ca/health-topics/abk4683

Herzing University–Orlando. (2014). *ASN/BSN concept definitions.* Winter Park, FL: Author.

Hofman, P. L., Derraik, J. G., Pinto, T. E., Tregurtha, S., Faherty, A., Peart, J. M., ... Cutfield, W. S. (2010). Defining the ideal injection techniques when using 5-mm needles in children and adults. *Diabetes Care, 33*(9), 1940–1944.

Hosono, H., & Cohen, P. (2011). Chapter 554: Hyperpituitarism, tall stature, and overgrowth syndromes. In R. M. Kleigman, B. F. Stanton, J. W. St. Geme III, N. F. Schor, & R. E. Behrman (Eds.). *Nelson textbook of pediatrics* (19th ed., p. 1886). Philadelphia, PA: Saunders.

Johnson, S. R., Cooper, M. N., Jones, T. W., & Davis, E. A. (2013). Long-term outcome of insulin pump therapy in children with type 1 diabetes assessed in a large population-based case–control study. *Diabetologia, 56*(11), 2392–2400.

Kaplowitz, P. B. (2013). Chapter 15: Precious puberty. In P. J. Hillard (Ed.). *Practical pediatric adolescent gynaecology.* Oxford, UK: Blackwell Publishing Ltd.

Kaplowitz, P. B. (2014). *Delayed puberty in girls: A guide for families. Pediatric Endocrinology Fact Sheet.* Retrieved from https://www.uthsc.edu/pediatrics/clerkship/documents/electives/delayed-puberty.pdf

Kremidas, D., Wisniewski, T., Divino, V. M., Bala, K., Olsen, M., Germak, J., ... Lee, W. C. (2013). Administration burden associated with recombinant human growth hormone treatment: Perspectives of patients and caregivers. *Journal of Pediatric Nursing, 28*(1), 55–63.

Kumaran, A., & Kershaw, M. (2014). Hyperphagic psychosocial short stature—a clinical review. *Paediatrics and Child Health, 24*(12), 567–571.

LaFranchi, S. (2011). Section 2: Disorders of the thyroid gland. In R. M. Kleigman, B. F. Stanton, J. W. St. Geme III, N. F. Schor, & R. E. Behrman (Eds.). *Nelson textbook of pediatrics* (19th ed., pp. 1894–1916). Philadelphia, PA: Saunders.

LaFranchi, S. (2013). *Acquired hypothyroidism in childhood and adolescence.* UpToDate. Retrieved from http://www.uptodate.com/contents/acquired-hypothyroidism-in-childhood-and-adolescence

LaFranchi, S. (2014a). *Clinical features and detection of congenital hypothyroidism.* UpToDate. Retrieved from http://www.uptodate.com/contents/clinical-features-and-detection-of-congenital-hypothyroidism

LaFranchi, S. (2014b). *Treatment and prognosis of congenital hypothyroidism.* UpToDate. Retrieved from http://www.uptodate.com/contents/treatment-and-prognosis-of-congenital-hypothyroidism

LaFranchi, S. (2014c). *Treatment and prognosis of Graves' disease in children and adolescents.* UpToDate. Retrieved from http://www.uptodate.com/contents/treatment-and-prognosis-of-graves-disease-in-children-and-adolescents

March of Dimes. (2012). *Newborn screening.* Retrieved from http://www.marchofdimes.org/baby/newborn-screening-tests-for-your-baby.aspx

McAdams, B. H., & Rizvi, A. A. (2016). An overview of insulin pumps and glucose sensors for the generalist. *Journal of Clinical Medicine, 5*(1), E5. Retrieved from https://www.ncbi.nlm.nih.gov/pmc/articles/PMC4730130/

Meyer-Bahlburg, H. F., Khuri, J., Reyes-Portillo, J., Ehrhardt, A. A., & New, M. I. (2017). Stigma associated with classical congenital adrenal hyperplasia in women's sexual lives. *Archives of Sexual Behavior, 47*(4), 1–9.

National Diabetes Education Program. (2014). *Overview of diabetes in children and adolescents.* Retrieved from http://ndep.nih.gov/media/Overview-of-Diabetes-Children-508_2014.pdf

National Diabetes Information Clearinghouse (NDIC). (2012). *What I need to know about diabetes medicines: Types of Insulin.* Retrieved from http://diabetes.niddk.nih.gov/dm/pubs/medicines_ez/insert_C.aspx

Nelson-Tuttle, C. (2014). Chapter 50: Pediatric metabolic and endocrine disorders. In S. M. Nettina (Ed.). *Lippincott manual of nursing practice* (10th ed., pp. 1657–1678). Philadelphia, PA: Wolters/Kluwer Health: Lippincott Williams & Wilkins.

Parks, J. S., & Felner, E. I. (2011). Hypopituitarism. In R. M. Kleigman, B. F. Stanton, J. W. St. Geme III, N. F. Schor, & R. E. Behrman (Eds.). *Nelson textbook of pediatrics* (19th ed., pp. 1876–1881). Philadelphia, PA: Saunders.

Pediatric Endocrinology Nursing Society. (2014). *PENS position statement on linear growth measurement of children.* Retrieved from http://www.pens.org/Pages/default.aspx

Public Health Agency Canada. (2011). *Diabetes in Canada: Facts and figures from a public health perspective.* Retrieved from http://www.phac-aspc.gc.ca/cd-mc/publications/diabetes-diabete/facts-figures-faits-chiffres-2011/chap5-eng.php

Rosenfield, R. L. (2014). *Definition, clinical features and differential diagnosis of polycystic ovary syndrome in adolescents.* UpToDate. Retrieved from http://www.uptodate.com/contents/definition-clinical-features-and-differential-diagnosis-of-polycystic-ovary-syndrome-in-adolescents

Saenger, P. (2013). *Definition, etiology, and evaluation of precocious puberty.* UpToDate. Retrieved from http://www.uptodate.com/contents/definition-etiology-and-evaluation-of-precocious-puberty

Taketokmo, C. K., Hodding, J. H., & Kraus, D. M. (2013). *Lexi-comp's drug reference handbook: Pediatric & neonatal dosage handbook* (20th ed.). Hudson, OH: Lexi-comp, Inc.

Thibault, V., Bélanger, M., LeBlanc, E., Babin, L., Halpine, S., Greene, B., & Mancuso, M. (2016). Factors that could explain the increasing prevalence of type 2 diabetes among adults in a Canadian province: A critical review and analysis. *Diabetology & Metabolic Syndrome, 8*(1), 71.

White, P. C. (2011). Section 4: Disorders of the adrenal glands. In R. M. Kleigman, B. F. Stanton, J. W. St. Geme III, N. F. Schor, & R. E. Behrman (Eds.). *Nelson textbook of pediatrics* (19th ed., pp. 1923–1943). Philadelphia, PA: Saunders.

CHAPTER **WORKSHEET**

MULTIPLE CHOICE QUESTIONS

1. A young mother brings her new baby, diagnosed with congenital hypothyroidism, to the clinic so she can learn how to administer levothyroxine. The nurse should include which of the following instructions?
   a. Crush the medication and place it in a full bottle of formula to disguise the taste.
   b. Administer the medication every other day.
   c. Use an oral dispenser syringe or nipple to give the crushed medication mixed with a small amount of formula.
   d. Tell the mother that the medication will not be needed after the age of 7.

2. During a well-child examination, which of the following comments made by the parent would indicate the possibility of a growth hormone deficiency?
   a. "I have to buy my child new clothes every 2 to 3 months."
   b. "I have to buy my child much larger shirts than pants but then the sleeves are too long."
   c. "My child wears out his clothes before he outgrows them."
   d. "I can hand down my child's clothes to his younger brother."

3. The nurse is caring for a 14-year-old boy with type 1 DM. He takes NPH insulin every morning at 7:30 AM. Which assessment data will the nurse use to evaluate the therapeutic effectiveness of the medication?
   a. Presence of signs and symptoms of hypoglycemia or hyperglycemia during the morning physical assessment
   b. Blood glucose level at 1630
   c. Appetite and food intake at lunch
   d. Blood glucose level before breakfast

4. When monitoring the blood glucose level of a 12-year-old child with type 2 DM, your reading is 2.8 mmol/L (50 mg/dL). Which is the most appropriate action?
   a. Encourage the child to get out of bed and increase activity.
   b. Take the child's vital signs.
   c. Ask the child about frequent urine output.
   d. Give the child 4 oz of orange juice.

DOSAGE CALCULATION QUESTION

The school nurse is caring for a child with type 1 diabetes. The child weighs 25.4 kg (56 lb). The sliding scale corrective dose order reads: Insulin aspart before meals: (blood sugar − 120 divided by 70) + (total carbohydrate expected intake divided by 13 carbohydrates per unit). This is the corrective dose + carbohydrate consumption correction. Her blood sugar before lunch is 7.8 mmol/L (139 mg/dl) with an expected intake of 47 carbohydrates at lunch and regular activity level the rest of the day.

Calculate the insulin dose to be administered. Round to the nearest unit.

CRITICAL THINKING EXERCISES

1. A 12-year-old boy with type 1 DM has the flu. His mother calls the diabetes clinic to report that he stayed home from school and does not have an appetite, so he is not eating. The mother asks the nurse how much insulin the boy should take. He is currently taking three injections daily with regular and NPH in the morning before breakfast, regular and NPH in the evening after dinner, and regular before bedtime. What questions should the nurse ask before answering the mother's question? Based on the answers to these questions, how would you instruct the mother?

2. The mother of Robin, a 5-year-old girl, reports that Robin has a body odour. She is developing breasts and some pubic hair and was teased when she had a sleepover with friends. The review of her growth charts reveals that Robin went from the 50th percentile to the 93rd percentile in the past 6 months. Based on this information, what are the three major nursing diagnoses to begin establishing a plan of care for the child and family? What are the expected outcomes and major interventions associated with the nursing diagnosis of knowledge deficit?

3. A mother brings her baby to the clinic after receiving a phone message from the clinic saying there was a problem with the baby's thyroid test. She says the trip on the bus took a long time, but the infant slept the entire way. She says that the baby is sleeping much of the time and does not want to eat very much. The baby was discharged from the hospital 2 weeks ago. The birth was without difficulty and there were no problems during labour. Why is this visit urgent? What would the test show if the disorder was due to a pituitary gland problem and not the thyroid gland?

STUDY ACTIVITIES

1. During your clinical experiences, ask to be on an inpatient unit that provides care for children with alterations in endocrine function. Compare and contrast the health histories, assessments, laboratory tests, diagnostic procedures, and plans of care for these children with those for the care of children on other units. Participate in the teaching plan for these children and their families.

2. Attend an outpatient clinic that provides care to children with endocrine disorders. Identify the role of the registered nurse in providing coordination of care, health teaching, and referrals for these children and their families.

3. Shadow a diabetes nurse educator to observe the teaching methods and strategies he or she uses to provide an education plan for a child with DM. Observe how the nurse educator includes the family in the plan. Are there any differences between the teaching plans for type 1 DM and type 2 DM?

4. Conduct a literature review for one of the common endocrine disorders to research current management practices. Are there evidence-based practice guidelines for nursing interventions?

5. Conduct an Internet search to research the information that is available to children and their families related to DM.

BRINGING IT ALL TOGETHER: A CASE STUDY

Paige is a 5-year-old recently diagnosed with type 1 diabetes. She is currently in kindergarten at a local elementary school. Her mother is very concerned about learning all her care. She states "How can I send her to school if I am still learning how to take care of her?"

Go to thePoint **to find questions to consider about this case**.

49

Nursing Care of the Child With a Genetic Variation

Learning Objectives

Upon completion of the chapter, the learner will be able to:

1. Discuss the nurse's role and responsibilities when caring for a child diagnosed with a genetic condition and his or her family.

2. Identify nursing interventions related to the diagnosis and management of genetic conditions.

3. Distinguish various genetic conditions occurring in childhood.

4. Devise an individualized nursing care plan for the child with a genetic condition.

5. Develop child/family teaching plans for the child with a genetic condition.

Julie Woods, a 5-year-old, is brought to the clinic for her annual examination. Her mother states, "She's so much smaller than all of the other kindergartners."

Genetics refers to the principles and mechanics of heredity—its transmission, and its variation and includes the areas of **gene testing** and screening within health programs (Government of Canada, n.d.; Genetics Education Canada, n.d.). Nurses encounter potential or actual alterations in genetics in all types of clients and must detect problems and intervene early to prevent complications. A genetic condition is a disease caused by a difference in an individual's genetic material or genome. Some genetic conditions occur in multiple family members (via inheritance of abnormal genes). Other conditions may occur in only a single family member (via spontaneous mutation).

A genetic condition is caused by completely or partially altered genetic material. In contrast, a familial condition is more common in relatives of the affected individual but may be caused by environmental influences, not genetic alterations.

Many chronic conditions of childhood have a genetic or inherited cause. Common conditions suspected to be caused or influenced by genetic factors include birth defects, chromosomal abnormalities, **neurocutaneous conditions,** intellectual disability, many types of short stature conditions, connective tissue conditions, and **inborn errors of metabolism.** Genetic conditions can present at any age; testing can be appropriate as part of medical care with an aim to enhance medical monitoring (Canadian Paediatric Society, 2017; Boycott et al., 2015).

Our ability to diagnose genetic conditions is far superior to our ability to cure or treat them. However, accurate diagnosis does lead to improved management and outcomes. Nurses should have a basic knowledge of genetics, common genetic conditions in children, genetic testing, and genetic counselling so that they can provide support and information to families and can promote an improved quality of life. Refer to Chapter 10 for information on advances in genetics, inheritance, and genetic counselling and evaluation.

NURSE'S ROLE AND RESPONSIBILITIES

Pediatric nurses will encounter children with genetic conditions in every clinical specialty area. This includes clinics, hospitals, schools, and community-based centers. Talking with families who have recently been diagnosed with a genetic condition or who have had a child born with congenital anomalies maybe challenging. Many times the nurse is the one who has first contact with these parents and will be the one to provide follow-up care. Genetic conditions can be significant, life-changing, and possibly life-threatening situations. The information can be highly technical, and the field is still evolving. Therefore, it is important to refer the family to a physician or nurse practitioner who specializes in genetics. The nurse should understand who will benefit from genetic counselling and should be able to discuss the role of the genetic counsellor with families. Inform families at increased risk that, if they desire, genetic counselling is available before they attempt to have another baby.

The nurse is in an ideal position to help families review what has been discussed during the genetic counselling sessions. Nurses play an essential role in providing emotional support to the family throughout this often challenging time. In addition, some families may benefit from referral to appropriate agencies, support groups, and resources, such as a social worker, a spiritual or religious leader, or a bioethicist.

COMMON MEDICAL TREATMENTS

A variety of medications and other medical treatments may be used to treat the symptoms of genetic conditions in children. Most genetic conditions do not have specific treatments or cure, so treatment focuses on the specific symptoms of each condition. Genetic conditions often involve multiple organ systems and children with these conditions often have complex medical needs. Thus, a multidisciplinary approach and good communication are imperative. See below for a discussion on common genetic conditions and their management.

NURSING PROCESS OVERVIEW FOR THE CHILD WITH A GENETIC CONDITION

Care of the child with a genetic condition includes assessment, nursing diagnosis, planning, interventions, and evaluation. There are a number of general concepts related to the nursing process that may be applied to the care of children with genetic conditions. From a general understanding of the care involved for a child with a genetic condition, the nurse can then individualize the care based on specifics for the particular child, including the care preferences of the child and their family.

Assessment

Assessment of the child with a genetic condition includes health history, physical examination, and laboratory and diagnostic testing.

> Remember Julie, the 5-year-old brought in for her annual examination? What additional health history and physical examination information should you obtain?

Health History

The health history consists of past medical history, including the mother's pregnancy history; family history;

neonatal history; and history of present illness (when the symptoms started and how they have progressed), as well as treatments used at home. Explore the child's current and past medical history for risk factors such as:

- Family history of genetic conditions
- Any complications during the prenatal, perinatal, or postnatal periods
- Changes in developmental status or delays in developmental milestones

The pregnancy history can be extremely relevant when identifying a genetic condition. The pregnancy history may be significant for maternal age older than 35 years or paternal age older than 50 years, repeated premature births, breech delivery, congenital hip dysplasia, abnormalities found on ultrasound, abnormalities in prenatal blood screening tests (e.g., triple/quadruple screen, α-fetoprotein [AFP]), amniotic fluid abnormalities (polyhydramnios, oligohydramnios), multiple births, exposure to medications and known teratogens, and decreased fetal movement. Nurses should be aware that there are disparities in the number of conditions for which infants are screened, depending on the province in which infants are born (Etchegary et al., 2016). See Chapter 10 for discussion of the laboratory and diagnostic tests used most commonly to detect genetic disorders.

A focused neonatal history can also help identify a genetic problem. The neonatal history may be significant for symmetric intrauterine growth restriction, large for gestational age without known cause, hearing impaired, persistent hyperbilirubinemia, poor adaptation to the extrauterine environment (demonstrated by temperature and heart rate instability and poor feeding), hypotonia or hypertonia, seizures, and abnormal **newborn screening** results.

The family history plays a critical role in identifying genetic conditions. Gather data for three generations. If there is a positive family history, the likelihood of a genetic condition in the child is increased. It is helpful to create a family pedigree (refer to Chapter 10 for genetic evaluation and counselling). The family history may be significant for major congenital anomalies, intellectual disability, genetic diseases, metabolic conditions, multiple miscarriages or stillbirths, developmental delays, significant learning disabilities, psychiatric problems, consanguinity, and chronic serious illness (e.g., diabetes, hypertension, renal disease, hearing impairment, blindness, asthma, seizures, and unexplained death).

When eliciting the history of the present illness, inquire about:

- Developmental delay
- Seizures
- Hypotonia or hypertonia
- Feeding problems
- Lethargy
- Failure to thrive

- Septic appearance
- Vomiting

Children known to have a genetic condition are often admitted to the hospital for other health-related issues, or for complications and management of the genetic condition. The health history should include questions related to:

- Age when the condition was diagnosed
- Developmental delay
- Complications of the condition (e.g., thyroid problems, cardiac problems, respiratory problems, leukemia, seizures, cognitive impairment)
- Medications the child takes for complications associated with the condition
- Dietary restrictions
- Compliance with management regimen

Once complications have been identified, further investigation into their severity, frequency, and management is essential to the care of this child while in the hospital.

Physical Examination

Physical examination of the child with a genetic condition includes inspection and observation, palpation, and auscultation.

INSPECTION AND OBSERVATION

Inspect and observe for congenital anomalies, either major or minor. A major anomaly is a **chromosome difference**, irregularity or malformation that creates significant medical problems and requires surgical or medical management (Bacino, 2014) (Box 49.1). Minor anomalies are features that vary from those seen in the general population but do not cause an increase in morbidity in and of themselves (Bacino, 2014) (Box 49.2).

BOX 49.1

EXAMPLES OF MAJOR CONGENITAL ANOMALIES

- Cleft lip
- Cleft palate
- Congenital heart disease, structural and conduction conditions
- Neural tube defects, such as myelomeningocele
- Chromosomal difference
- Omphalocele; gastrochisis
- Renal agenesis/hypoplasia
- Limb reduction defects
- Generalized dysmorphism
- Ambiguous genitalia

Adapted from Bacino, C. A. (2014). *Approach to congenital malformations.* UpToDate. Retrieved from http://www.uptodate.com/contents/approach-to-congenital-malformations.

BOX 49.2

EXAMPLES OF MINOR CONGENITAL ANOMALIES

- Flat occiput
- Prominent occiput
- Triple hair whorl
- Flat-bridged nose
- Nostrils anteverted
- Ear lobe crease
- Ear lobe notched
- Cup-shaped ears
- Small ears
- Cleft uvula
- Webbed neck
- Short neck
- Extra nipples
- Sacral dimple
- Tapered fingers
- Overlapping digits
- Syndactyly
- Hemangioma
- Nevi

Adapted from Bacino, C. A. (2014). *Approach to congenital malformations.* UpToDate. Retrieved from http://www.uptodate.com/contents/approach-to-congenital-malformations

 Take Note!

Low-set ears are a minor anomaly that is associated with several genetic syndromes. If noted, assess thoroughly for other abnormalities, but be mindful that this observation as a screening approach can result in no genetic variation being found.

As the number of minor anomalies present increases, the probability of the presence of a major anomaly increases. In fact, when three or more minor anomalies are present, the risk for a major anomaly or intellectual disability is approximately 19% to 26% (Bacino, 2014). Assess for a recognized pattern of anomalies that may be associated with certain syndromes.

Take Note!

Cleft lip and cleft palate are associated with many syndromes. If noted, assess for other anomalies.

Inspect and observe for an abnormal or foul odour of the child's excretions. Certain metabolic conditions or inborn errors of metabolism are associated with specific odours (Table 49.1).

AUSCULTATION

Physical examination includes auscultation of the heart. Murmurs or dysrhythmias may have a genetic cause. In a child with a congenital heart problem (e.g., ventricular septal defect) and a strong family history of cardiac structural problems, a genetic cause needs to be considered.

TABLE 49.1	INBORN ERRORS OF METABOLISM AND ASSOCIATED ODOUR
Inborn Error of Metabolism	**Associated Odour**
Phenylketonuria	Mousy or musty
Maple syrup urine disease	Maple syrup, burnt sugar, or curry
Tyrosinemia	Cabbage-like, rancid butter
Trimethylaminuria	Rotting fish

Adapted from Rezvani, I., & Rezvani, G. (2011). An approach to inborn errors of metabolism. In R. M. Kleigman, B. F. Stanton, J. W. St. Geme III, N. F. Schor, & R. E. Behrman (Eds.). *Nelson textbook of pediatrics* (19th ed., pp. 416–418). Philadelphia, PA: Saunders.

PALPATION

Palpation can be used to detect hepatosplenomegaly (an enlarged spleen and liver). However, physicians or nurse practitioners usually perform this assessment because it requires skill and experience. Hepatosplenomegaly may indicate a metabolic condition.

Nursing Diagnoses, Goals, Interventions, and Evaluation

Upon completion of an assessment, the nurse might identify several nursing diagnoses, including:
- Deficient knowledge (specify)
- Decisional conflict
- Risk for delayed growth and development
- Fear
- Interrupted family processes

After completing an assessment of Julie, the nurse noted the following: short stature for age and a low posterior hairline. Based on these assessment findings, what would your top three nursing diagnoses be for Julie?

Nursing goals, interventions, and evaluation for the child with a genetic condition are based on the nursing diagnoses. Nursing Care Plan 49.1, found at the end of the chapter, provides a general guide for planning care for a child with a genetic condition. Additional information about nursing management will be included later in the chapter as it relates to specific conditions.

When providing support and education to families of children with serious genetic abnormalities, use these guiding principles:
- Build a trusting relationship;
- Stress the authenticity of the parents' feelings;
- Reject your own personal biases;

- Recognize that individuals cope in various ways; the family's behaviour may not be what you would expect;
- Help the family to identify their own strengths and supports, building on those as able;
- Know that the family's emotions may exhaust and disorganize them;
- Assist the family members to maintain open communication among themselves;
- Provide referrals to local parent groups or other families with a child with a similar condition;
- Allow the family to verbalize their emotions and ask questions;
- Always ask the parents how *they* are doing, acknowledging they may have chosen to continue with a pregnancy after prenatal diagnosis (Guon, Wilfond, Farlow, Brazg, & Janvier, 2015).

Based on your top three nursing diagnoses for Julie, describe appropriate nursing interventions.

COMMON CHROMOSOMAL ABNORMALITIES

Genetic disorders are thought to impact on the lives of approximately 500,000 children in Canada (Genome BC, n.d.). Many children with chromosomal abnormalities, linked to genetic disorders, have associated intellectual disabilities, learning disabilities, behavioural challenges, and distinct features, including physical birth differences. The likelihood of autosomal trisomies increases with advanced maternal age (Government of Canada, 2017). The most common chromosomal abnormalities will be discussed below. New and improved techniques in chromosome analysis allow for the identification of tiny and more complex abnormalities that could not be seen before (Searl, 2014). Therefore, more chromosomal abnormalities are being identified in children (Table 49.2).

TABLE 49.2	LESS COMMON CHROMOSOMAL ABNORMALITIES
Chromosomal Difference	**Features**
Prader–Willi syndrome (difference on chromosome 15)	Affects 1 in 16,000 to 25,000 babies[a] Severe hypotonia—with poor feeding, obesity, short stature, small hands and feet, hypogonadism, hyperphagia, and intellectual disability (varies from mild to severe)
Angelman syndrome (difference on chromosome 15)	Affects 1 in 12,000 to 20,000 babies[b] Microcephaly with flatness on the back of the head, fair skin and light hair, large mouth with tongue protrusion, seizures, jerky ataxic movements (resembling a puppet gait), uncontrolled bouts of laughter/smiling, happy demeanour, easily excitable personality, developmental delay and speech impairment, and severe intellectual disability
Cri-du-chat syndrome (difference on chromosome 5)	Affects 1 in 20,000 to 50,000 babies[c] Hypotonia; short stature; slow growth; low birth weight; failure to thrive; characteristic weak, cat-like cry during infancy; microcephaly with protruding metopic suture; moon-like round face; bilateral epicanthal folds (folds of skin over the eyelids); high-arched palate; wide and flat nasal bridge; micrognathia (small receding chin); wide set eyes (hypertelorism); low-set malformed ears; simian crease; intellectual disability and developmental delay
Wolf–Hirschhorn syndrome (difference on chromosome 4)	Affects 1 in 50,000 babies[d] Hypotonia, intellectual disability, delayed growth and development, seizures, and characteristic facial features (broad, flat nose bridge; high forehead; widely spaced, protruding eyes; microcephaly)
Williams syndrome (difference on chromosome 4)	Affects 1 in 7,500 to 10,000 children[e] Affects multiple systems. Cardiovascular disease (supravalvular aortic stenosis most common, hypertension also seen); distinct facial features often described as elphin like, such as broad forehead, flat nasal bridge, short nose with broad tip, full cheeks, and a wide mouth with full lips; small, wide-spaced teeth with occlusal abnormalities; hypercalcemia; early puberty for both males and females; structural abnormalities of the kidneys, delayed bladder training and urinary frequency, hypotonia, and joint laxity; learning disabilities and intellectual disability, attention deficit condition, problems with anxiety and phobias such as fears of sounds and tactile issues; unique personality characteristics, such as outgoing and engaging personality; other medical problems involving eyes and vision and digestive tract

TABLE 49.2	LESS COMMON CHROMOSOMAL ABNORMALITIES (continued)

Chromosomal Difference	Features
Beckwith–Wiedemann syndrome (difference on chromosome 11)	Affects 1 in 13,700 babies[f] Infants can be considerably larger than normal and grow at an unusual rate in childhood, growth slows in later childhood with adults not unusually tall, specific parts of the body may grow larger leading to asymmetric appearance; abdominal wall defects such as omphalocele, umbilical hernia; infants present with abnormally large tongue that may interfere with breathing, swallowing, and speaking; abnormally large abdominal organs; crease or pits in skin near ears, hypoglycemia, and kidney abnormalities; increased risk of developing cancerous and noncancerous tumours, such as Wilms tumour, neuroblastoma
22q11 deletion syndrome (Velocardiofacial/DiGeorge syndrome) (difference of chromosome 22)	Affects 1 in 4,000 babies[g] Hypoplasia or agenesis of the thymus and parathyroid glands, hypocalcemia, hypoplasia of auricle and external auditory canal, cardiac anomalies, immune system abnormalities, cleft palate, short stature, distinctive facial appearance (elongated face, almond-shaped eyes, wide nose, small ears), and developmental delays, learning, speech, feeding, and behavioural problems http://www.vcfsfa.org.au/pages/home.php:Velo-Cardio-Facial Syndrome Educational Foundation, Inc.

Helpful links related to the chromosomal abnormalities and features outlined here are provided on thePoint.

[a]Ann O Scheimann, A. O. (2014). *Epidemiology and genetics of Prader-Willi syndrome.* UpToDate. Retrieved from http://www.uptodate.com/contents/epidemiology-and-genetics-of-prader-willi-syndrome.

[b]Genetics Home Reference. (2015a). *Angelman syndrome.* Retrieved from http://ghr.nlm.nih.gov/condition/angelman-syndrome.

[c]Genetics Home Reference. (2015b). *Cri-Du-Chat syndrome.* Retrieved from http://ghr.nlm.nih.gov/condition/cri-du-chat-syndrome.

[d]Genetics Home Reference. (2015c). *Wolf-Hirschhorn syndrome.* Retrieved from http://ghr.nlm.nih.gov/condition/wolf-hirschhorn-syndrome.

[e]Genetics Home Reference. (2015d). *Williams syndrome.* Retrieved from http://ghr.nlm.nih.gov/condition/williams-syndrome.

[f]Hon-Yin, B. C., Shuman, C., Choufani, S., & Weksberg, R. (2014). *Beckwith-Wiedemann syndrome.* UpToDate. Retrieved from http://www.uptodate.com/contents/beckwith-wiedemann-syndrome.

[g]Genetics Home Reference. (2015e). *22q11.2 deletion syndrome.* Retrieved from http://ghr.nlm.nih.gov/condition/22q112-deletion-syndrome.

Trisomy 21 (Down Syndrome)

Trisomy 21 (Down syndrome) is a genetic condition caused by the presence of all or part of an extra 21st chromosome. It is the most common chromosomal difference associated with intellectual disability (Ostermaier, 2015). Canada reports 13.5 infants per 10,000 live births with trisomy 21 (which equates to 1 in 750 live born babies) while approximately 31.2 per 1,000 stillbirths are noted to have Down syndrome (Government of Canada, 2017). Trisomy 21 is seen in all ages, races, and socioeconomic levels, but a higher incidence can be found with increased maternal age older than 35 years. However, more than half the infants born in Canada are to mothers under 35 years (Government of Canada, 2017).

Trisomy 21 is associated with a range of functionality levels (see Table 49.3), characteristic facial features (e.g., slanted eyes and depressed nasal bridge), and other health problems (e.g., cardiac defects, visual and hearing impairment, intestinal malformations, and an increased susceptibility to infections). The severity of these problems varies.

The prognosis has been improving over the past few decades. Fundamental changes in the care of these children have resulted in longer life expectancy (around 55 to 56 years of age) and an improved quality of life (Ostermaier, 2014).

Pathophysiology

Trisomy 21 is a condition caused by nondisjunction or translocation before, at, or after conception. Each egg and sperm cell normally contain 23 chromosomes. When they join, this results in 23 pairs or 46 chromosomes. Sometimes an extra chromosome originates in the development of either the egg or the sperm, resulting in an embryo with three chromosomes 21s in *all* cells (Fig. 49.1). This results in the characteristic features and birth defects of Down syndrome. This type and timing of nondisjunction, resulting in the presence of three chromosome 21s in all cells, is responsible for 95% of cases of Down syndrome (Bull & the Committee on Genetics, 2011).

In approximately 1% to 2% of cases of Down syndrome, the nondisjunction occurs *after* fertilization and a mixture of two cell types is seen (Bull & the Committee on Genetics, 2011). In these cases some cells have

TABLE 49.3	AVERAGE AGE OF SKILL ACQUISITION IN CHILDREN WITH DOWN SYNDROME	
Developmental Milestone	Average Age of Acquisition, Children With Down Syndrome (Months)	Average Age of Acquisition, Typical Children (Months)
Smile	2	1
Roll over	6	4
Sit alone	9	7
Crawl	11	9
Walk	21	13
Speak words	14	10
Speak in sentences	24	21
Feed self with fingers	12	8
Use spoon	20	13
Bladder training	48	32
Bowel training	42	29
Undress	40	32
Put on clothes	58	47

Adapted from Pueschel, S. M. (2011). *A parent's guide to Down syndrome: Toward a brighter future* (rev. ed.). Baltimore, MD: Paul H. Brookes Publishing Company, Inc.

47 chromosomes (due to three chromosome 21s), while others have the normal 46 chromosomes (with the normal two chromosome 21s present). This is referred to as the mosaic form of Down syndrome. Children with mosaic Down syndrome may have a milder form of the condition, but this is not a definitive finding.

About 3% to 4% of Down syndrome cases involve a translocation, in which part of the number 21 chromosome breaks off during cell division *before or at* conception and attaches (or translocates) to another chromosome (usually chromosome 14) (Bull & the Committee on Genetics, 2011). The cells will remain with

46 chromosomes, but this extra portion of the number 21 chromosome results in the clinical findings of Down syndrome. Cases of translocation are not associated with advanced maternal age, as is the situation with nondisjunction errors (Weremowicz, 2014).

Therapeutic Management

Management of Down syndrome will involve multiple disciplines, including a primary physician; specialty physicians such as a cardiologist, ophthalmologist, and gastroenterologist; nurses; physical therapists; occupational therapists; speech therapists; dietitians; psychologists; counsellors; teachers; and, of course, the parents. There is no standard treatment for all children, and there is no prevention or cure. Treatment is mainly symptomatic and supportive. The overall focus of therapeutic management will be to promote the child's optimal growth and development and function within the limits of the disease.

MANAGING COMPLICATIONS

Children with Down syndrome need the usual immunizations, well-child care, and screening recommended by the American Academy of Pediatrics. In addition, medical management will focus on complications associated with Down syndrome.

Congenital heart disease occurs in 40% to 50% of children with Down syndrome (Bull & the Committee

FIGURE 49.1 Down syndrome karyotype. Note the third chromosome located at chromosome 21.

on Genetics, 2011). Cardiac problems vary from minor defects that respond to medication therapy to major defects that require surgical intervention. Children with Down syndrome also have an increased incidence of gastrointestinal conditions (Bull & the Committee on Genetics, 2011). These conditions vary from those that can be managed by dietary manipulation, such as celiac disease and constipation, to intestinal malformations such as Hirschsprung disease and imperforate anus, which require surgical intervention.

Hearing and vision impairments are also common. More than 75% of children with Down syndrome have hearing loss (Bull & the Committee on Genetics, 2011). Otitis media is a common problem, affecting 50% to 70% of children with Down syndrome and is often the cause of hearing loss (Ostermaier, 2015). Sixty percent of children with Down syndrome have an eye disease (Bull & the Committee on Genetics, 2011). Therefore, regular evaluation of vision and hearing is essential.

Sleep disordered breathing, which includes obstructive sleep apnea (OSA), is 10 times more prevalent in children with Down syndrome. Investigation with polysomnography (PSG) is recommended for children by age 4 years, especially in those who snore (Katz et al., 2016).

Children with Down syndrome have a higher incidence of thyroid disease, which can affect growth and cognitive function (King, O'Gorman, & Gallagher, 2013). Most of these children have hypothyroidism (an underactive thyroid), but sometimes hyperthyroidism (an overactive thyroid) occurs. Periodic thyroid testing may be warranted. Children with Down syndrome are also at a higher risk for obesity and delayed dental eruptions or hypodontia (King et al., 2013). Some studies have found an increased risk of type 1 diabetes in children with Down syndrome (Ostermaier, 2015).

Children with Down syndrome may demonstrate atlantoaxial instability (increased mobility of the cervical spine at the first and second vertebrae) (Bull & the Committee on Genetics, 2011). In most cases these children are asymptomatic, but symptoms may appear if spinal cord compression occurs, noted below. Screening for atlantoaxial instability may be appropriate, especially if the child is involved in sports.

Take Note!

If neck pain, unusual posturing of the head and neck (torticollis), change in gait, loss of upper body strength, abnormal reflexes, or change in bowel or bladder functioning is noted in the child with Down syndrome, immediate attention is required.

Children with Down syndrome are at a higher risk for certain hematologic problems, such as anemia, transient leukemia (mostly during the newborn period), leukemia (later onset) and polycythemia during infancy (Hitzler

et al., 2014). Children with Down syndrome also have a higher susceptibility to infection and a higher mortality rate from infectious diseases. Precautions to prevent and monitor for infection are needed. Other potential complications include alopecia, communication conditions, and seizures.

EARLY INTERVENTION THERAPY

Early intervention refers to a variety of programs and resources available to young children with developmental delay or other impairment. These programs may involve an array of healthcare professionals such as physical, occupational, and speech therapists; special educators; and social workers. The programs focus on providing stimulation and encouragement to children with Down syndrome. The programs are individualized to meet the specific needs of each child. Some families find these programs helpful, other may prefer less involvement with structured approaches.

Refer to Table 49.3 for the average age of skill acquisition in children with Down syndrome. For example, the average child with Down syndrome walks at 24 months (vs. 12 months for a child without Down syndrome). Conditions such as hypotonia, ligament laxity, decreased strength, enlarged tongue, and short arms and legs are common in children with Down syndrome, and early intervention may help in the development of gross and fine motor skills, language, and social and self-care skills.

Some parents benefit from early intervention programs in terms of support, encouragement, and information.

Nursing Assessment

For a full description of the assessment phase of the nursing process, refer to the Nursing Process section at the beginning of this chapter. Assessment findings pertinent to Down syndrome are discussed below.

HEALTH HISTORY

Down syndrome is often diagnosed prenatally using perinatal screening and diagnostic tests. If not diagnosed prenatally, most cases are diagnosed in the first few days of life based on the physical characteristics associated with Down syndrome. Identify high-risk deliveries. Explore the pregnancy history and past medical history for risk factors such as:

- Lack of prenatal care or screening
- Abnormal prenatal screening or diagnostic tests for Down syndrome (e.g., fetal nuchal translucency, triple/quadruple screen, ultrasound, amniocentesis)
- Maternal age older than 35 years

The older infant or child known to have Down syndrome is often admitted to the hospital for surgeries or other complications of the disease, such as infections.

Elicit a description of the present illness and chief complaint. In an infant or child returning for a clinic visit or hospitalization, the health history should include questions related to:

- Cardiac defects or disease (treatment regimen, surgical repair)
- Hearing or vision impairment (last hearing and vision evaluation, any corrective measures)
- Developmental delays (speech, gross and fine motor skills)
- Sucking or feeding problems
- Cognitive abilities (degree of intellectual disability)
- Gastrointestinal conditions such as vomiting or absence of stools (special dietary management, surgical interventions)
- Thyroid disease
- Hematologic problems, such as anemia, leukemia
- Atlantoaxial instability
- Seizures
- Infections such as recurrent or chronic respiratory infections, otitis media
- Growth (height and weight changes, feeding problems, unexplained weight gain)
- Signs and symptoms of sleep apnea, such as snoring, restlessness during sleep, daytime sleepiness
- Any other changes in physical state or medication regimen

PHYSICAL EXAMINATION

The initial assessment after birth may reveal certain physical features characteristic of Down syndrome (Box 49.3 and Fig. 49.2).

Observe the child's general appearance. Note lack of muscle tone and loose joints; this is usually more pronounced in infancy, and the infant has a floppy appearance. Observe growth and development. Plot growth on appropriate growth charts. Because children with Down syndrome grow at a slower rate, special growth charts have been developed (see thePoint for an example).

Perform a subjective assessment of hearing and refer the child for further evaluation if indicated. Assess vision, especially for cataracts. Assess respiratory status and cardiac status. Auscultate for murmurs and pulmonary changes, which can indicate congenital heart disease. Chronic or recurrent respiratory infections, such as pneumonia and otitis media, may be found.

LABORATORY AND DIAGNOSTIC TESTS

Down syndrome risk screening can be calculated incorporating maternal age prenatally between 11 and 14 weeks using ultrasound and blood tests (nuchal translucency and pregnancy-associated plasma protein A [PAPP-A] and human chorionic gonadotropin [hCG]), and around 16 and 18 weeks using triple/quadruple blood tests to detect AFP, hCG, estriol, and/or inhibin A levels

---

BOX 49.3

COMMON CLINICAL MANIFESTATIONS OF DOWN SYNDROME

- Hypotonia
- Short stature
- Flattened occiput
- Small (brachycephalic) head
- Flat facial profile
- Depressed nasal bridge and small nose
- Oblique palpebral fissures (an upward slant to the eyes)
- Brushfield spots (white spots on the iris of the eye)
- Low-set ears
- Abnormally shaped ears
- Small mouth
- Protrusion of tongue; tongue is large compared to mouth size
- Arched palate
- Hands with broad, short fingers
- A single deep transverse crease on the palm of the hand
- Congenital heart defect
- Short neck, with excessive skin at the nape
- Hyperflexibility and looseness of joints (excessive ability to extend the joints)
- Dysplastic middle phalanx of fifth finger (one flexion furrow instead of two)
- Epicanthal folds (small skin folds on the inner corner of the eyes)
- Excessive space between large and second toe

Adapted from Summar, K., & Lee, B. (2011). Chapter 76.2: Down syndrome and other abnormalities of chromosome number. In R. M. Kleigman, B. F. Stanton, J. W. St. Geme III, N. F. Schor, & R. E. Behrman (Eds.), *Nelson textbook of pediatrics* (19th ed., pp. 399–403). Philadelphia, PA: Saunders; and Bull, M. J., & Committee on Genetics. (2011). From the American Academy of Pediatrics: Clinical report: Health supervision for children with Down syndrome. *Pediatrics*, *128*(2), 393–406. Retrieved from http://pediatrics.aappublications.org/content/128/2/393.full.

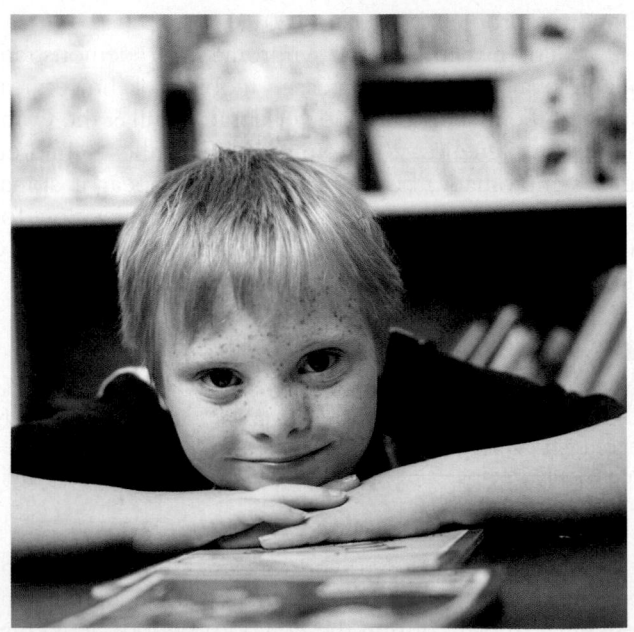

FIGURE 49.2 Child with Down syndrome.

(Bull & the Committee on Genetics, 2011). Ultrasound and amniocentesis or chorionic villi sampling (CVS) to detect chromosomal abnormalities can also occur prenatally. Down syndrome can be confirmed after birth using chromosome analysis.

Common laboratory and diagnostic studies ordered for the diagnosis and assessment of complications associated with Down syndrome include:

- Echocardiogram: to detect cardiac defects
- Vision and hearing screening: to detect vision and hearing impairments
- Thyroid hormone level: to detect thyroid disease
- Cervical x-rays: to assess for atlantoaxial instability
- Ultrasound: to assess for gastrointestinal malformations

These tests will be important in evaluating manifestations of the syndrome.

Nursing Management

Due to the high incidence of Down syndrome and the complex medical needs of these children, most pediatric nurses are likely to care for these children in their practice. Nursing management focuses on providing supportive measures such as promoting growth and development, preventing complications, promoting nutrition, and providing support and education to the child and family. In addition to the nursing diagnoses and related interventions discussed in Nursing Care Plan 49.1, additional considerations are reviewed below.

Atraumatic Care

When planning atraumatic care interventions when caring for a child with Down syndrome, be sure to individualize interventions based on the child's developmental level.

PROMOTING GROWTH AND DEVELOPMENT

Children with Down syndrome tend to grow more slowly, learn more slowly, have shorter attention spans, and have trouble with reasoning and judgment. They exhibit a full range of personalities and behaviours but commonly children with Down syndrome are described as warm and cheerful, patient, gentle, and having a natural spontaneity.

Thinking About Development

As a nurse in a primary care team, how will your education on safety differ when caring for an infant with Down syndrome compared to a toddler or adolescent?

PREVENTING COMPLICATIONS

Children with Down syndrome are at risk for certain health problems (see above). Even though most nurses will encounter a child with Down syndrome in their practice, only a few nurses will become experts in their care. The needs of these children are complex, and the American Academy of Pediatrics has developed guidelines that can help the nurse care for these children and their families. Nurses play a key role in educating parents and caregivers about how to prevent the complications of Down syndrome (see Teaching Guidelines 49.1).

Teaching Guidelines 49.1
HEALTH GUIDELINES FOR CHILDREN WITH DOWN SYNDROME

- Have your child evaluated by a pediatric cardiologist, including an echocardiogram.
- Take your child for routine vision and hearing tests. By 6 months have your child seen by a pediatric ophthalmologist.
- Make sure your child gets regular medical care, including recommended immunizations and a thyroid test at 6 and 12 months and then yearly.
- Have your child follow a regular diet and exercise routine.
- Make sure all family members perform proper hand hygiene to prevent infection.
- Monitor for signs and symptoms of respiratory infections, such as pneumonia and otitis media.
- Discuss with your physician the use of pneumococcal, respiratory syncytial virus, and influenza vaccines.
- Begin early interventions, therapy, and education as soon as possible.
- Make sure you brush your child's teeth regularly. He or she should visit the dentist every 6 months.
- Make sure the child gets a cervical x-ray between 3 and 5 years of age to screen for atlantoaxial instability. Report any changes in gait or use of arms and hands, weakness, changes in bowel or bladder function, complaints of neck pain or stiffness, head tilt, torticollis, or generalized changes in function. Ensure cervical spine positioning precautions (to avoid over extending or flexing of the neck) are utilized during procedures, such as those involving anesthetic, surgery, or x-rays.

Adapted from Bull, M. J., & Committee on Genetics. (2011). From the American Academy of Pediatrics: Clinical Report: Health supervision for children with Down syndrome. *Pediatrics, 128*(2), 393–406. Retrieved from http://pediatrics.aappublications.org/content/128/2/393.full.

PROMOTING NUTRITION

Children with Down syndrome may have difficulty sucking and feeding due to lack of muscle tone. They tend to have small mouths; a smooth, flat, large tongue; and, due to the underdeveloped nasal bone, chronically stuffy noses. This may lead to poor nutritional intake and problems with growth. These problems usually improve as the child gains tongue control. Use of a bulb syringe, humidification, and changing the infant's position can lessen the problem. Breastfeeding a baby with Down syndrome is usually possible, and the antibodies in breast milk can help the infant fight infections. The caregiver's hand can be used to provide additional support of the chin and throat. Speech or occupational therapists can work on strengthening muscles and assisting in feeding accommodations. Other feeding problems and failure to thrive can be related to cardiac defects and usually improve after medical management is initiated or corrective surgery performed.

Children with Down syndrome do not need a special diet unless underlying gastrointestinal disease is present, such as celiac disease. A balanced, high-fibre diet and regular exercise are important. Research has suggested that children with Down syndrome have lower basal metabolic rates, which can lead to problems with obesity, so it is important in the early years to develop appropriate eating habits and a regular exercise routine. Exercise can be challenging as a result of MSK issues, motor skills, and associated respiratory health problems. Therefore, variations in exercise routines should be explored (Pitetti, Baynard, & Agiovlasitis, 2012).

PROVIDING SUPPORT AND EDUCATION FOR THE CHILD AND FAMILY

Down syndrome is a lifelong condition that can result in health problems and cognitive disability. The diagnosis is usually made prenatally or shortly after birth. Parents and caregivers will need support and education during this time. Some families may see having a child with Down syndrome as a lifelong tragedy; others may view it as a positive growing experience. Evaluate how the family defines and manages this experience. Base the plan of care on each individual family's values, beliefs, strengths, and resources.

Family members may have trouble meeting the demands of caring for a child with Down syndrome. Some of these children have complex medical and caregiving needs, which can place strains on the family's resources, including their finances. From the time of diagnosis, the family should be involved in the child's care. Include parents in planning interventions and care for the child. In most cases, they are the primary caregivers and will provide daily care as well as assisting the child in the development of functioning and skills. They can provide essential information to the healthcare team and will be advocates for their child throughout his or her life.

As the child grows, the needs of the family and child will change. Recognize and respect these needs and provide ongoing education and support for the child and

family. Children with Down syndrome will need meaningful education programs. Many children with Down syndrome begin formal education in infancy and continue through high school.

The outlook is brighter than it once was for children with Down syndrome. Some go on in adulthood to obtain jobs, to receive secondary education, and to live on their own or in semi-independent housing. Be familiar with local and national resources for families of children with Down syndrome so that you can help these children fulfill their potential. An extensive list of helpful resources is provided on the**Point**.

Consider This

"The day after my son was born I was told they suspected he had Down syndrome. Once the diagnosis was confirmed I felt devastated. I grieved the loss of all the dreams I had for him and felt alone and scared. I wonder why us?"

"I could see the features of Down syndrome when my daughter was born, I felt acceptance and love. I wanted everyone to congratulate and celebrate her birth with me, the way they would have if she did not have Down syndrome."

Thoughts: How will you respond to these mothers?

Trisomy 18 and Trisomy 13

Trisomy 18 (also known as Edwards syndrome) and trisomy 13 (also known as Patau syndrome) are two other common trisomies. These trisomies are much more severe and debilitating than trisomy 21. The incidence of trisomy 18 (the presence of three number 18 chromosomes) is 1 in 6,000 births; the incidence of trisomy 13 (the presence of three number 13 chromosomes) is 1 in 10,000 births (Bacino & Lee, 2011). Like Down syndrome, trisomy 13 and trisomy 18 usually result from nondisjunction during cell division. Trisomy 18 and trisomy 13 can be present in all cells or may occur in mosaic forms. Both are associated with a characteristic set of anomalies and severe intellectual disability. Increased surgical experiences and lower survival rates are reported with 10% to 13% surviving for 10 years (Nelson, Rosella, Mahant, & Guttmann, 2016).

Nursing Assessment

Nursing assessment will include a general observation for characteristic anomalies.

Prenatal screening and diagnostic tests for trisomy 18 (Figs. 49.3A & B) and trisomy 13 exist (Figs. 49.4A & B). If not diagnosed during the prenatal period, most cases

TABLE 49.4	CLINICAL MANIFESTATIONS OF TRISOMY 18 AND TRISOMY 13
Chromosomal Difference	**Clinical Manifestations**
Trisomy 18	Prominent occiput, low-set ears, short eyelid fissures, severe intellectual disability, severe hypotonia, webbing, clenched fist with index finger over third digit and fifth digit overlapping the fourth, hypoplasia of fingernails, narrow hips with limited abduction, short sternum, congenital cardiac defects
Trisomy 13	Microcephalic head, wide sagittal suture and fontanels, malformed ears, small eyes, extra digits, severe hypotonia, severe intellectual disability, congenital heart defects, cleft lip, cleft palate

FIGURE 49.4 Trisomy 13.

are diagnosed in the first few days of life based on the physical characteristics associated with the conditions.

Nursing Management

Nursing management will be mainly supportive. This will be a difficult time for the family, so providing support and resources for the family will be an important nursing function. Canadian Organization for Rare Disorders can provide supportive information to professionals and families (visit thePoint for a link to this resource).

Turner Syndrome

Turner syndrome is a common difference of the sex chromosome and a chronic health condition (CPS, 2016).

The phenotype is female. It occurs in about 1 in 2,500 live female births (Bacino, 2015). The difference is due to a loss of all or part of one of the sex chromosomes. About half of the affected individuals have only one X chromosome; the other half have a variety of abnormalities of one of their sex chromosomes and may present with the mosaic form.

There is no cure for Turner syndrome. Therapeutic management will focus on managing the health issues associated with the syndrome. Children with Turner syndrome are more prone to cardiovascular problems, kidney and thyroid problems, skeletal conditions such as scoliosis and osteoporosis, hearing and eye disturbances,

FIGURE 49.3 Trisomy 18.

FIGURE 49.5 Note the webbed neck of the child with Turner syndrome.

learning disabilities, and obesity (Saenger, 2014). Infertility is usually present, but a few spontaneous pregnancies have been reported (Kansra & Donohoue, 2011; Nelson-Tuttle, 2014). Management may include growth hormone and/or hormone replacement therapy (etc).

Nursing Assessment

On assessment, note patterns of growth; short stature and slow growth are often characteristic findings. Other physical characteristics include a webbed neck, low posterior hairline, wide-spaced nipples, edema of the hands and feet, amenorrhea, no development of secondary sex characteristics, sterility, and perceptual and social skill difficulties (Fig. 49.5).

Turner syndrome can be suspected prenatally by ultrasound findings such as fetal edema or redundant nuchal skin (Conley, 2014). It can be diagnosed by chromosomal analysis, either prenatally or after birth. Most children are diagnosed at birth or in early childhood when slow growth or growth failure is noted. Some cases will not be diagnosed until the pubertal growth spurt does not occur.

Nursing Management

Nursing management is mainly supportive. Provide education and support to the family; they need to understand that short stature and infertility are likely.

Explain that intellectual disability is unlikely, but some learning disabilities may be present. Emphasize that with medical supervision and support, girls with Turner syndrome may lead healthy, satisfying lives. Counselling about infertility is important at appropriate ages and stages of development. Parents may be upset that their daughter will not be able to reproduce, so explain that many alternatives for reproduction, such as in vitro fertilization may be possible and adoption is a choice into adulthood.

Providing resources for the family is an important nursing function. The Turner Syndrome Society of Canada provides assistance, support, and education to individuals with Turner syndrome and their families. A link to resources is provided on thePoint.

Klinefelter Syndrome

Klinefelter syndrome is the most common sex chromosomal difference (Bacino & Lee, 2011). The karyotype and phenotype are male, two X chromosomes are present. The difference is usually caused by nondisjunction during meiosis, but mosaic forms do present. The incidence of Klinefelter syndrome is 1 in 500 to 1,000 males (Bacino, 2015). Males present with some physical features that are caused by testosterone deficiency.

There is no cure for Klinefelter syndrome. Therapeutic management will focus on interventions such as testosterone replacement. Early recognition and hormonal treatment improve quality of life. Any cosmetic surgery should be an informed choice, for example gynecomastia (increased breast size).

Nursing Assessment

Due to nonspecific findings during childhood, the diagnosis is not usually made until adolescence or adulthood. Prenatal diagnosis is rare unless amniocentesis was performed for genetic testing. Many males with Klinefelter syndrome reach adulthood without being diagnosed (Bacino & Lee, 2011). The diagnosis is confirmed by chromosomal analysis.

On assessment, under development of secondary sex characteristics may be found. The individual may have decreased facial hair, gynecomastia, decreased pubic hair, and hypogonadism or underdeveloped testes, which leads to infertility. The individual may be taller than average by 5 years of age, with long legs and a short torso (Fig. 49.6). Intellectual disability is not present, but motor delay, speech or language difficulties, attention deficits, and learning disabilities, may be found.

Nursing Management

Nursing management will be mainly supportive. Provide education and support to the family. Links to The Klinefelter Support Association of Canada Group can be found on thePoint.

FIGURE 49.6 **Klinefelter syndrome.**

Counselling about infertility is important at the appropriate time and context. Educate children and families that marriage and sexual relations are possible. Parents may be upset so explain that many alternatives for reproduction are available and technology is advancing in the field of infertility and can provide help in some cases.

Fragile X Syndrome

Fragile X syndrome is the most common inherited cause of intellectual disability (Van Esch, 2014). It is the outcome of a mutation of a gene (fragile X mental retardation [FMR1]) on the X chromosome. This mutation essentially "turns off" the gene, triggering fragile X syndrome. Males and females are both affected, but it is more commonly seen in males, and affected females usually have milder symptoms (Genetics Home Reference, 2012a). The incidence is approximately 1 in 8,000 females and 1 in 4,000 males (Genetics Home Reference, 2012a). The inheritance of fragile X is complex and is less straightforward than single-gene or mendelian inheritance. Some carrier females are affected, and not all males with the gene difference show symptoms. Males and females are both fertile and can transmit the condition to their offspring, so genetic counselling is appropriate.

There is no cure for fragile X syndrome. Therapeutic management will be multidisciplinary and aimed at interventions to improve cognitive, emotional, and behavioural impairments.

Nursing Assessment

During childhood, clinical manifestations are subtle, with minor dysmorphic features and developmental delay. Problems with sensation, emotion, and behaviour often are the first signs. A delay in attaining developmental milestones will most likely be the first clue found on assessment. Intellectual impairment can range from subtle learning disabilities to severe intellectual disability and autistic-like behaviours. In adolescence, boys tend to present with characteristic features such as an elongated face; prominent jaw; large, protruding ears; large size; macroorchidism (large testes); and a range of behavioural abnormalities and cognitive deficits (Fig. 49.7). There is a characteristic pattern to the cognitive deficits, with problems in abstract reasoning, sequential processing, and mathematics. Typical behaviour problems include attention deficits, hand flapping and biting, hyperactivity, shyness, social isolation, low self-esteem, and gaze aversion. In females the clinical manifestations are similar but are more varied and often present in a milder form.

Diagnosis is confirmed by molecular genetic testing. Fragile X can be diagnosed prenatally in pregnancies at increased risk.

FIGURE 49.7 Fragile X syndrome.

Nursing Management

Nursing management will be mainly supportive. Early diagnosis and intervention with developmental therapies and an individualized education plan are ideal (see Chapter 50 for further information on intellectual disability).

Provide education and support to the family. The National Fragile X Foundation provides education and emotional support and works to increase awareness and advance research for fragile X. Links to resources are provided on thePoint.

NEUROCUTANEOUS CONDITIONS

Neurocutaneous conditions, also referred to as hamartoses, are a group of conditions characterized by abnormalities of both the skin and the central nervous system. Many neurologic conditions are associated with cutaneous manifestations, since the skin and the nervous system share a common embryologic origin. They are complex conditions and most also affect other organs or systems such as eyes, bones, heart, and kidneys. Most are hereditary and follow an autosomal dominant inheritance pattern or sporadic occurrence. Neurofibromatosis is a common neurocutaneous syndrome and will be discussed in detail below. Table 49.5 provides information on other neurocutaneous syndromes.

Neurofibromatosis

Neurofibromatoses are neurocutaneous genetic conditions of the nervous system that primarily affect the development and growth of neural cell tissues. There are distinct types: neurofibromatosis 1, neurofibromatosis 2, and schwannomatosis (which used to be considered a variation of neurofibromatosis 2) (Korf, 2014).

Neurofibromatosis 1 (von Recklinghausen disease) is the more common type and is discussed here (Korf, 2014). This condition causes tumours to grow on nerves and produce other abnormalities such as skin changes and bone deformities. Although many affected persons inherit the condition, nearly 30% to 50% of the cases are due to a new mutation (National Institute of Neurological Conditions and Stroke, 2015; Korf, 2014). The inheritance pattern is autosomal dominant; therefore, offspring of affected individuals have a 50% chance of inheriting the altered gene. Neurofibromatoses are due to a mutation of the neurofibromin gene on chromosome 17. The estimated prevalence is 1 in 2,600 to 3,000 live births (Korf, 2014).

Complications associated with neurofibromatosis include headaches; hydrocephalus; scoliosis; cardiac defects; hypertension; seizures; vision and hearing loss; neurocognitive deficits, including learning disabilities, attention deficit condition, fine and gross motor delays, autism spectrum condition, and behaviour and psychosocial issues; abnormalities of speech; and a higher risk for neoplasms.

TABLE 49.5	OTHER NEUROCUTANEOUS SYNDROMES		
Condition	**Incidence**	**Clinical Manifestations**	**Nursing Considerations**
Tuberous sclerosis	1 in 6,000[a]	Benign tumours present in the brain and skin. Presents most often as a generalized seizure condition. Tumours can also involve heart, kidney, eyes, lung, and bones. Developmental delay and behavioural problems may be noted. Usually evident in early childhood. Wide clinical spectrum from severe intellectual disability with incapacitating seizures to normal intelligence and no seizures	Treatment will be mainly symptomatic with goal to prevent and treat associated complications Seizure control will be a primary concern Provide support and education to the family Referral for genetic counselling (it follows an autosomal dominant inheritance pattern and half the cases are due to a new mutation) and appropriate resources www.tsalliance.org: Tuberous Sclerosis Alliance
Sturge–Weber syndrome	1 in 50,000[a]	Facial nevus (port wine stain) most often seen on the forehead and on one side of the face, seizures, hemiparesis, intracranial calcifications. In many cases intellectual disability, behavioural and emotional problems, and learning disabilities are present. Seizures usually begin in infancy and may worsen with age. Convulsions are usually noted on the side of the body opposite the facial nevus. Muscle weakness may be present on the same side. Affected individuals can have glaucoma at birth or will develop it later in life	Treatment will be mainly symptomatic. Seizure control will be a primary concern (use of anticonvulsants or surgery). Seizures due to Sturge–Weber are often difficult to control Laser treatment may be used to lighten or remove the facial nevus Surgery may be performed on more serious cases of glaucoma Physical therapy should be considered for infants and children with muscle weakness Educational therapy is often prescribed for those with intellectual disability or developmental delays Provide support and education to the family Refer to appropriate resources Genetic counselling may be appropriate (inheritance is unclear and sporadic) www.sturge-weber.org: Sturge-Weber Foundation

[a]Sahin, M. (2011). Chapter 589: Neurocutaneous syndromes. In R. M. Kleigman, B. F. Stanton, J. W. St. Geme III, N. F. Schor, & R. E. Behrman (Eds.). *Nelson textbook of pediatrics* (19th ed., pp. 2046–2053). Philadelphia, PA: Saunders.

There is no cure for neurofibromatosis. Therapeutic management is aimed at controlling symptoms and managing complications. Surgical intervention can help reduce some of the bone malformations and remove painful or disfiguring tumours. These children should have a yearly physical, including blood pressure and cardiovascular examination, scoliosis screening, ophthalmology examination, developmental screening, and a neurologic examination.

The disease is progressive and symptoms usually worsen over time, but it is difficult to predict the course. Most affected individuals develop mild to moderate symptoms, with non–life-threatening complications, and live a normal life.

Nursing Assessment

On assessment the nurse may find café-au-lait spots (light brown macules), which are the hallmark of neurofibromatosis (Sahin, 2011) (Fig. 49.8). These are usually present at birth but can appear during the 1st year of life and usually increase in size, number, and pigmentation. They are present all over the body, particularly the trunk and extremities, while usually sparing the

FIGURE 49.8 Café-au-lait spots associated with neurofibromatosis.

CLINICAL SIGNS OF NEUROFIBROMATOSIS

Diagnosis is made if two or more of the following are present:
- Six or more café-au-lait macules (light-brown spots) >5 mm in diameter in children and >15 mm in diameter in adolescents and adults
- Two or more neurofibromas (benign tumours) or one plexiform neurofibroma (tumour that involves many nerves)
- Freckling in the armpit or groin
- Presence of an optic glioma (a tumour on the optic nerve)
- Two or more growths on the iris of the eye (Lisch nodules or iris hamartomas)
- Abnormal development of the spine (scoliosis), the temple bone of the skull, or the tibia
- A first-degree relative (parent, sibling, or child) with neurofibromatosis

Adapted from National Institute of Neurological Conditions and Stroke. (2015). *Neurofibromatosis fact sheet*. Retrieved from http://www.ninds.nih.gov/conditions/neurofibromatosis/detail_neurofibromatosis.htm; Sahin, M. (2011). Chapter 589: Neurocutaneous syndromes. In R. M. Kleigman, B. F. Stanton, J. W. St. Geme III, N. F. Schor, & R. E. Behrman (Eds.). *Nelson textbook of pediatrics* (19th ed., pp. 2046–2053). Philadelphia, PA: Saunders.

---

face. Pigmented nevi, axillary freckling, and slow-growing cutaneous, subcutaneous, or dermal neurofibromas, which are benign tumours, are other signs of neurofibromatosis. Many children with neurofibromatosis have larger than normal head circumference and are shorter than average. The severity of symptoms varies greatly, but the diagnosis is made if two or more of the clinical signs in Box 49.4 are present.

Take Note!

If more than six café-au-lait spots are present, neurofibromatosis should be suspected.

Nursing Management

Nursing management will be mainly supportive. Early detection of treatable conditions and complications is a priority. Provide support and education to the child and family. Discuss genetic counselling with the family. Referral to appropriate resources is essential. Links to resources for neurofibromatosis are found on thePoint.

OSTEOGENESIS IMPERFECTA

Osteogenesis imperfecta (OI), a genetic connective tissue condition of childhood onset, causes bone fragility and frequent fractures after minimal physical stress

(Glorieux, 2008). It may lead to hearing impairments, blue sclera, dental brittleness, spinal deformities, and/or shortened limbs (Dogba et al., 2013). These phenotypic variations are due to mutations in *COL1A1* and *COL1A2* that encode collagen, the most prevalent extracellular matrix protein in bone and skin (Cheung & Glorieux, 2008). There is nothing inherent about OI that affects cognition. A clinical classification system distinguishes several types of OI with varying severity and inheritance patterns (Van Dijk & Sillence, 2014). There is no cure for OI although bisphosphonates are widely used to improve bone strength (Brizola, Staub, & Félix, 2014). Children with OI may experience symptoms such as acute and chronic pain, fear, fatigue, and physical limitations. These may hinder participation in daily activities and peer acceptance resulting in social isolation (Fegran, Hall, Uhrenfeldt, Aagaard, & Ludvigsen, 2014; Shapiro & Germain-Lee, 2012). Additional resources can be found in thePoint.

If a child presents with a history of fractures and any combination of the signs and symptoms above, make sure to take a thorough family history, and be mindful of the deleterious ramifications associated with falsely accusing a family of child abuse. Has anyone in the family been diagnosed with OI? Genetic counselling may be recommended as a potential resource (Marr, Seasman, & Bishop, 2017). Nursing priorities will include preventing fractures, managing pain, managing side effects of treatment, and fostering inter- and independence as the child develops (Hartman, 2003). An important responsibility will be to refer children and families to local or national supportive resources.

OTHER GENETIC CONDITIONS

Thousands of genetic conditions are known, and new ones are being discovered, but most of them are rare. Table 49.6 lists other genetic conditions that the pediatric nurse may encounter. Nursing management of these conditions will be mainly supportive and will focus on providing support and education to the family and child, with an emphasis on developmental and educational needs. Referral to genetic counselling and appropriate resources is an important nursing function.

INBORN ERRORS OF METABOLISM

Inborn errors of metabolism are a group of genetic disorders. They are collectively common, but individually rare with most having an incidence of less than 1 in 100,000 (Sutton, 2014). Most follow an autosomal recessive inheritance pattern. They are caused by gene mutations that result in abnormalities in the synthesis or catabolism of proteins, carbohydrates, or fats. The

TABLE 49.6	OTHER GENETIC CONDITIONS, SYNDROMES, AND ASSOCIATIONS

Condition	Inheritance/Cause	Signs and Symptoms	Management
CHARGE syndrome (a recognizable pattern of congenital anomalies seen) **C: C**oloboma **H: H**eart disease **A: A**tresia (choanal) **R: R**etarded growth and development and/or CNS anomalies **G: G**enital anomalies, hypogonadism **E: E**ar anomalies and deafness Incidence is 0.1–1.2 in 10,000 live births[a]	Autosomal dominant inheritance possible, but most cases are due to new mutation of the gene. Mutations in the gene CDH7 have been indicated in most cases. Occurs during fetal development and affects multiple organ systems	Coloboma is a lesion or defect of the eye, usually a fissure or cleft in the iris, ciliary, or choroid; can also see microphthalmos (small eyes) and cryptophthalmos (absent eye). Can lead to vision impairments Heart anomaly can include any type but most common are aortic arch anomalies and Tetralogy of Fallot Atresia (choanal) is blocked or narrowed passages from the nose to the throat, which can lead to aspiration Retarded growth or cognitive development can range from mild to severe Genital anomaly may include micropenis, undescended testes, and hypoplastic labia Ear anomalies include short, wide ears with little or no lobe, prominent inner fold, floppy appearance, asymmetry; can have hearing impairment Each feature occurs in a spectrum from absent to severe; no single feature is present in all individuals	Focus is on identifying and treating all defects; early diagnosis is important www.chargesyndrome. org: CHARGE Syndrome Foundation
Marfan syndrome: condition of connective tissue incidence is 1 in 3,000 to 5,000[b]	Autosomal dominant inheritance; caused by a mutation in the gene fibrillin-1, which results in changes in connective tissue	Primarily involves the skeletal, cardiovascular, and ocular systems. Tall stature with long slim limbs, minimal subcutaneous fat, muscle hypotonia, loose joints, long and narrow face, abnormalities of skeletal system (e.g., pectus excavatum [funnel chest] or pectus carinatum [pigeon breast]), ocular system (e.g., enlarged cornea or lens subluxation), and cardiovascular system (e.g., dilation of the aorta or mitral valve prolapse) Delayed achievement of gross and fine motor milestones may occur	Focus is on preventing complications www.marfan.org: National Marfan Foundation www.marfan.ca: Canadian Marfan Association

(continued)

TABLE 49.6	OTHER GENETIC CONDITIONS, SYNDROMES, AND ASSOCIATIONS (continued)		
Condition	**Inheritance/Cause**	**Signs and Symptoms**	**Management**
VATER association (not a diagnosis, but refers to a nonrandom association of defects found to occur together) **V: V**ertebral defects **A: A**nal atresia **TE: T**racheo**E**sophageal fistula with esophageal atresia **R**adial and **R**enal dysplasia May also occur as VACTERL association, with **C: C**ardiac anomalies **L: L**imb abnormalities added	Sporadic inheritance. Cause is unknown Can occur with other chromosomal abnormalities such as trisomy 18 Frequently seen in the offspring of diabetic mothers	Three or more anomalies are present. Anomalies seen include hypoplastic (small) vertebrae or hemivertebra (only half the bones are formed). These anomalies lead to an increased risk of scoliosis With imperforate anus or anal atresia, the anus does not open to the outside of the body Tracheoesophageal fistula and/or esophageal atresia leads to increased risk for aspiration, feeding and swallowing problems Incomplete formation of one or more kidneys, obstruction of urine flow out of kidneys, or severe reflux back into kidneys can all lead to kidney failure later in life Cardiac anomalies: most common are ventricular septal defects, atrial septal defects, and Tetralogy of Fallot Absent or displaced thumb, polydactyly (extra digits), syndactyly (fusion of digits) A single umbilical artery at birth is often present Failure to thrive and slow development in early infancy due to anomalies Usually normal intelligence	Focus is on identifying and treating all defects. www.tefvater.org: TEF VATER National Support Network Take Note! Children with VATER syndrome who have only one kidney may need to consider the types of sports they engage in
Apert syndrome (named for the French physician who described the syndrome) Incidence is 6 to 15.5 out of 1 million live births[c]	Autosomal dominant inheritance. Cases are sporadic	Craniosynostosis and maxillary hypoplasia resulting in a flat recessed forehead and flat midface, bilateral symmetric syndactyly, and craniofacial anomalies such as high-arched palate and associated clefting, short anteroposterior diameter, protruding eyes, down-slanting eyelids, and low-set ears Small nasopharynx can lead to upper airway obstruction and sleep apnea Acne vulgaris, strabismus, and hearing loss Learning disabilities and mental deficiency	Early surgery for craniosynostosis when increased intracranial pressure is noted. Vigorous early management should occur with a multidisciplinary approach to address multiple anomalies. www.aboutfaceusa.org: About Face USA www.ccakids.com: Children's Craniofacial Association www.faces-cranio.org:

TABLE 49.6	OTHER GENETIC CONDITIONS, SYNDROMES, AND ASSOCIATIONS (continued)

Condition	Inheritance/Cause	Signs and Symptoms	Management
Achondroplasia (most common chondrodysplasia [diseases resulting in conditioned growth]) Incidence is 1 in 15,000 to 40,000[d,e]	Autosomal dominant inheritance pattern. Caused by mutations in fibroblast growth factor receptor 3 (FGFR3). 80% new gene mutation[d]	Characterized by abnormal body proportion Small stature (average adult height is 4 ft for both men and women), short limbs with normal-size torso, low nasal bridge with prominent forehead. Midface hypoplasia, caudal narrowing of spinal canal, megalocephaly, small foramen magnum; hands are short and stubby with separation between middle and ring fingers ("trident hand"). Delayed motor skills, problems with persistent middle ear dysfunction and infections, and bowing of lower legs. Less common complications include hydrocephalus, craniocervical junction compression, upper airway obstruction, and thoracolumbar kyphosis Usually present with normal intelligence and lead independent, productive lives	Medical management of symptoms Monitor height, weight, and head circumference Manage and prevent complications (careful and thorough neurologic examination, assessment for sleep apnea) Growth hormone therapy is controversial and still experimental Limb-lengthening surgeries may be performed http://www.lpaonline.org/: Little People of America

[a]NORD. (2012a). *Charge syndrome.* Retrieved from https://www.rarediseases.org/rare-disease-information/rare-diseases/byID/550/viewFullReport.
[b]Wright, M. J., & Connolly, H. M. (2014). *Genetics, clinical features, and diagnosis of Marfan syndrome and related conditions.* UpToDate. Retrieved from http://www.uptodate.com/contents/genetics-clinical-features-and-diagnosis-of-marfan-syndrome-and-related-conditions.
[c]Hollier, L. H. (2014). *Craniosynostosis syndromes.* UpToDate. Retrieved from http://www.uptodate.com/contents/craniosynostosis-syndromes.
[d]Genetics Home Reference. (2012b). *Achondroplasia.* Retrieved from http://ghr.nlm.nih.gov/condition/achondroplasia.
[e]March of Dimes. (2013). *Achondroplasia.* Retrieved from http://www.marchofdimes.org/baby/achondroplasia.aspx#.

body cannot convert food into energy as it normally would. Most inborn errors are due to a defect in an enzyme or transport protein that results in a block in the metabolic pathway. The blocked metabolic pathway allows for accumulation of the damaging by-product of the impaired metabolic process or may be responsible for a deficiency or absence of a necessary product. Presentation can occur at any time, even in adulthood, but many affected individuals exhibit signs in the newborn period or shortly after. Most inborn errors of metabolism presenting in the neonatal period are lethal if specific treatment is not initiated immediately.

Newborn screening is used to detect these conditions before symptoms develop. During the 1990s, developments in screening techniques (tandem mass spectrometry) now allow dozens of metabolic conditions to be detected from a single drop of blood (Wheeler, 2012). A child who tests positive will require additional testing to confirm the diagnosis (see Chapter 31 for more

information on newborn screening for inborn errors of metabolism).

Therapeutic management of these conditions varies depending on the cause of the error of metabolism, but dietary management is often a key component.

Nursing Assessment

Clinical signs and symptoms vary with each condition. Table 49.7 gives information on some common inborn errors of metabolism seen in children. See Evidence-Based Practice 49.1.

Take Note!

If the blood sample for the newborn screening was obtained within the first 24 hours after birth, check with local provincial recommendations to determine if this should be repeated (CORD, 2015).

(text continues on page 1942)

TABLE 49.7	INBORN ERRORS OF METABOLISM		
Condition/Explanation	**Incidence (estimates)**[a]	**Clinical Manifestations**	**Management**
Phenylketonuria (PKU): deficiency in a liver enzyme leading to inability to process the essential amino acid phenylalanine properly. Phenylalanine accumulation can lead to brain damage unless PKU is detected soon after birth and treated.	1 in 13,500 to 1 in 19,000	No symptoms at birth. If untreated intellectual disability develops [common sign is vomiting, irritability, eczema-like rash, mousy odour to urine]	Low-phenylalanine diet Phenylalanine is found mostly in protein-containing foods such as meat and milk (including breast milk and formula) www.pkunetwork.org: Children's PKU Network www.pkunews.org: National PKU News
Galactosemia: deficiency in the liver enzyme needed to convert galactose, the breakdown product of lactose, which is commonly found in dairy products, into glucose. Galactose accumulation leads to damage to vital organs	1 in 47,000	No symptoms at birth. If undiagnosed, newborn can have jaundice, feeding intolerance, diarrhea, and vomiting and will not gain weight. Signs and symptoms of sepsis and cataracts are often seen. If untreated, can lead to liver disease, blindness, severe intellectual disability, and death	Ingestion of galactose can produce sepsis in an affected child; therefore, septic workup and antibiotics may be necessary in a child if galactose ingestion has occurred Elimination of galactose and lactose from the diet is the only treatment. Therefore, milk and dairy products will be eliminated for life www.galactosemia.org: Parents of Galactosemic Children
Maple sugar urine disease: affects the metabolism of amino acids. A deficiency in the enzyme that metabolizes leucine, isoleucine, and valine, which are components of protein often referred to as the branch chain amino acids. These amino acids then accumulate in the blood and cause damage to the brain	1 in 185,000	No symptoms at birth, but if untreated newborns soon begin to show neurologic signs, vomiting, poor feeding, increased reflex action, and seizures. Lower intake of protein (as occurs with breastfeeding) may delay presentation of symptoms. If untreated, can lead to life-threatening neurologic damage	Special low-protein diet, will vary based on severity of symptoms; limited natural protein requires medical food product supplements such as BCAA free Thiamine supplements may be given Diet must be continued throughout life www.msud-support.org: Maple Syrup Urine Disease Family Support Group
Biotinidase deficiency: lack of the enzyme biotinidase results in biotin deficiency	1 in 129,000	Typically no symptoms at birth; in first weeks or months of life, symptoms such as hypotonia, uncoordinated movement, seizures, developmental delay, alopecia, seborrheic dermatitis, hearing loss, optic nerve atrophy, and intellectual disability develop. Metabolic acidosis can lead to death	Daily oral free biotin http://biotinidasedeficiency. 20m.com/: Biotinidase Deficiency Family Support Group

| TABLE 49.7 | INBORN ERRORS OF METABOLISM (continued) | | |

Condition/Explanation	Incidence (estimates)[a]	Clinical Manifestations	Management
Medium-chain acyl-CoA dehydrogenase deficiency (MCAD): lack of an enzyme required to metabolize fatty acids	1 in 46,000 to 1 in 6,400	Classic presentation is a child 3 to 15 months old with vomiting and lethargy after a period of not eating (fasting typically associated with a viral illness) Recurrent episodes of metabolic acidosis and hypoglycemia, lethargy, seizures, liver failure, brain damage, coma, and cardiac arrest. Can lead to serious and fatal illness in children not eating well	Avoid fasting; have frequent meals. L-carnitine supplementation particularly when ill. Special considerations during illness. If unable to tolerate food, IV dextrose is required www.fodsupport.org: Fatty Oxidation Conditions (FOD) Family Support Group
Homocystinuria: deficiency in the enzyme needed to digest a component of food called methionine (an amino acid)	1 in 250,000	If undetected and untreated can lead to intellectual disability, psychiatric disturbances, developmental delays, displacement of the lens of the eye, abnormal thinning and weakness of bones, and formation of thrombi in veins and arteries that can lead to life-threatening complications such as stroke	Vitamin B_6 and B_{12} supplements and possibly other supplements, such as betaine and folic acid; Methionine-restricted diet and cystine supplements; Aspirin and dipyridamole to decrease thromboembolic events www.rarediseases.org: National Organization for Rare Conditions
Tyrosinemia: deficiency in an enzyme essential in the metabolism of tyrosine; accumulation of the by-products results in liver and kidney damage	1 in 12,000 to 1 in 100,000 (typically northern European descent)	Symptoms usually appear in the first months of life: fever, failure to thrive, poor weight gain, vomiting, diarrhea, cabbage-like odour, enlarged liver and spleen, increased bleeding tendency, distended abdomen, jaundice, cirrhosis, and liver failure	Diet low in phenylalanine, methionine, and tyrosine www.liverfoundation.org: American Liver Foundation
Tay–Sachs: caused by insufficient activity of an enzyme called hexosaminidase A, which is necessary for the breakdown of certain fatty substances in brain and nerve cells	Occurs more frequently among persons of Central and Eastern European and Ashkenazi Jewish descent. ~1 in every 27 Jews is a carrier, whereas in the general population 1 in 250 people is a carrier.[b] Non-Jewish French Canadians from the East St. Lawrence River Valley of Quebec and members of the Cajun population in Louisiana are also at an increased risk	Infants appear normal and healthy for the first few months of life. Then, as harmful quantities of the fatty substances (called gangliosides) build up in tissues and nerve cells and cause damage, mental and physical deterioration occur. The child becomes blind, deaf, and unable to swallow; muscles begin to atrophy; and paralysis sets in. Dementia, seizures, and an increased startle reflex may be seen. There is a late-onset type of Tay–Sachs seen in persons in their 20s and early 30s, but this is much rarer	No treatment or cure. Medical management will focus on managing symptoms and maintaining comfort Anticonvulsants may be given to control seizures Death usually occurs in early childhood, by age 4 or 5 Carriers can be identified by a blood test and prenatal testing is available www.ntsad.org: National Tay-Sachs & Allied Diseases Association

[a]Kaye, C. I., & The Committee on Genetics (2011a). From the American Academy of Pediatrics: Newborn screening fact sheets. *Pediatrics, 118*(3), e934–e963. Retrieved from http://pediatrics.aappublications.org/content/118/3/e934.full.

[b]National Human Genome Research Institute. (2011). *Learning about Tay-Sachs disease.* Retrieved from http://www.genome.gov/10001220.

Adapted from Kaye, C. I., & the Committee on Genetics. (2011a). From the American Academy of Pediatrics: Newborn screening fact sheets. *Pediatrics, 118*(3), e934–e963. Retrieved from http://pediatrics.aappublications.org/content/118/3/e934.full.

EVIDENCE-BASED PRACTICE 49.1   **EFFECTS OF A NEW COLLECTION PROTOCOL ON FALSE-POSITIVE NEWBORN SCREENING RATES**

Newborn screening tests have improved outcomes and the health of infants and children. However, the rates of false-positive results are a concern. False-positive newborn screening results have been found to be higher among infants in the neonatal intensive care unit leading to increased testing and family stress. Higher rates of false positives have been contributed to the use of medical therapies, such as total parenteral nutrition (TPN), and the liver immaturity of preterm infants. What are the effects of a new sample collection protocol on false-positive results?

STUDY

A 2-year retrospective cohort study was conducted at the Children's Hospital of Orange County. Infants were grouped into pre- and postprotocol groups and further categorized by birth weight. Preprotocol newborn screen samples were collected regardless of TPN administration. Postprotocol newborn screen samples, in neonates receiving TPN, were collected 3 hours after TPN was replaced with 10% Dextrose in water (D10W).

Findings

A total of 539 neonates were screened during the study period. The new protocol was found to decrease false positives in each birth weight group by at least 50% with an overall decrease of 74%. An estimated reduction in cost >80% was also found.

Nursing Implications

TPN is an important medical therapy for many preterm infants. This protocol allows for the benefits of TPN to be maintained while decreasing the negative consequences of false-positive newborn screen results, such as increased testing, increased family stress and anxiety, and increased healthcare costs. Further investigation with a larger sample is needed. Further study investigating the need for different laboratory cutoff values for term versus preterm infants and for infants receiving TPN is warranted. Obtaining repeat samples at different ages may help guard against the occurrence of false negatives.

Adapted from Morris, M., Fischer, K., Leydiker, K., Elliott, L., Newby, J., & Abdenur, J. N. (2014). Reduction in newborn screening metabolic false-positive results following a new collection protocol. *Genetics in Medicine, 16*(6), 477–483.

Because of newborn screening and early identification and management, it is rare to see an untreated newborn with clinical signs and symptoms of disease caused by one of the inborn error of metabolism conditions. If seen, a newborn who was healthy at birth will often present with lethargy, poor feeding, apnea or tachypnea, recurrent vomiting, altered consciousness, failure to thrive, seizures, septic appearance, or developmental delay. Physical changes that may be seen include dysmorphology, cardiomegaly, rashes, cataracts, retinitis, optic atrophy, corneal opacity, deafness, skeletal dysplasia, macrocephaly, hepatomegaly, jaundice, or cirrhosis.

Take Note!

When a previously healthy newborn presents with a history of deterioration, suspect an inborn error of metabolism.

The diagnostic workup usually requires a variety of specific laboratory studies and may include:
- Glucose: may be elevated
- Ammonia: may be elevated
- Blood gases: may have low bicarbonate and low pH, metabolic acidosis (respiratory alkalosis may also be seen, especially when high ammonia levels are present)

Early diagnosis is the key to saving and improving the lives of these children.

Take Note!

If an inborn error of metabolism is suspected, feedings may be altered or stopped until the test results are received.

When a child who has previously been diagnosed with an inborn error of metabolism is hospitalized, the nurse must determine the prescribed diet and medications so these may be continued while in the hospital setting.

Nursing Management

Ensure that the diet prescribed for the infant or child is followed. For amino acid conditions (e.g., phenylketonuria [PKU]), urea cycle defects (e.g., tyrosinemia type I), and organic acidemia (e.g., maple syrup urine disease), nutritional therapy is the major intervention. Dietary intake of specific amino acids is restricted according to the condition. Ensure that overall protein and calorie needs are still met, as children need sufficient calories for proper growth. In children with urea cycle defects and organic acidemia, anorexia is common and severe, and the child may need gastrostomy tube feeding supplementation. In fatty acid oxidation conditions (e.g., medium-chain acyl-coenzyme A [CoA] dehydrogenase deficiency), the goal is to avoid prolonged periods of fasting and to provide frequent feeds when the child is sick. Supplementation with specific vitamins may also be important in the treatment of these conditions. Strict adherence to the diet is necessary and will require close supervision by registered dietitians, physicians, and nurses and the cooperation of both the parent and child.

Nursing management will focus on education and support for the family, who will need thorough knowledge about the child's disease and management. Refer the child and family to a dietitian and appropriate resources, including support groups. In addition, monitor the child's developmental progress and begin therapies as soon as a concern arises.

NURSING CARE PLAN 49.1

Overview for the Child With a Genetic Condition

NURSING DIAGNOSIS: Deficient knowledge related to lack of information regarding complex, technical medical condition; prognosis; and medical needs as evidenced by verbalization, questions, or actions demonstrating lack of understanding about child's condition or care

Outcome Identification and Evaluation

Child and family will verbalize accurate information and understanding about condition, prognosis, and medical needs: *child and family demonstrate knowledge of condition, prognosis, and medical needs, including possible causes, contributing factors, and treatment measures.*

Intervention: *Providing Child and Family Teaching*

- Assess child's and family's willingness to learn: child and family must be willing to learn for teaching to be effective. Genetic syndromes can be complex and sometimes it may be inappropriate to provide too much information too quickly. Attend carefully to what the individual and family are expressing as current needs. Pay attention to privacy of the affected individual.
- Provide family with time to adjust to diagnosis: will facilitate adjustment and ability to learn and participate in child's care.
- Repeat information: allows family and child time to learn and understand.
- Teach in short sessions: many short sessions are more helpful than one long session.
- Gear teaching to the child and family's level of understanding (depends on age of child, physical condition, memory) to ensure understanding.

- Provide reinforcement and rewards: facilitates the teaching/learning process.
- Use multiple modes of learning involving many senses (written, verbal, demonstration, and videos) when possible: child and family are more likely to retain information when it is presented in different ways using many senses.
- Refer child and family to a genetics specialist: genetic information is highly technical; the field is advancing at a rapid pace, and information needs to be the most current and accurate. Be aware that families may be seeking information online from resources that are not necessarily accurate. A genetic specialist can provide this along with expertise, support, and resources.

NURSING DIAGNOSIS: Decisional conflict related to treatment options, conflicting values, and ethical, legal, and social issues surrounding genetic testing as evidenced by verbalization of uncertainty about choices, verbalization of undesired consequences of alternative actions being considered, delayed decision making, physical signs of stress

Outcome Identification and Evaluation

Family will state they are able to make an informed decision: family will state advantages and disadvantages of choices and share fears and concerns regarding choices.

Intervention: *Providing Decision-Making Support*

- Give family time and encourage them to express their feelings associated with decision making: *the decision-making process becomes more difficult if feelings are not expressed.*
- Encourage family to list advantages and disadvantages of each alternative: *aids in problem solving and helps family recognize all alternatives.*
- Initiate health teaching and referral to genetic specialist when needed: *genetic testing information is often*

technical and complex. Families need accurate and up-to-date information to aid in decision making.
- Maintain a nondirective manner: *this is a difficult decision that the family must make for themselves; the nurse should provide all the necessary information while maintaining an unobtrusive role.*
- Validate the family's feelings regarding the decisional conflict: *validation is a therapeutic communication technique that promotes the nurse–family relationship.*

(continued)

Overview for the Child With a Genetic Condition (continued)

NURSING DIAGNOSIS: Risk for delayed development related to physical disability, cognitive deficits, activity restrictions secondary to genetic condition

Outcome Identification and Evaluation

Child's growth and development will be enhanced: *child will demonstrate adequate growth patterns and optimal developmental course within parameters of their condition.*

Intervention: *Promoting Growth and Development*

• Screen for developmental capabilities to determine child's current level of functioning.
• Offer age-appropriate toys, play, and activities (including gross motor) to encourage further development.
• Perform exercises or interventions as prescribed by physical or occupational therapist: these activities promote function and developmental skills.
• Provide support to families: due to disability and deficits, the child's progress toward developmental milestones may be slow.
• Use therapeutic play and adaptive toys to facilitate developmental functioning.
• Provide stimulating environment when possible to maximize potential for growth and development.
• Praise accomplishments and emphasize child's abilities to improve self-esteem and encourage feeling of confidence and competence.
• Monitor height and weight and plot on growth chart to identify growth patterns and deviations in these patterns.
• Be sensitive to the wider family, and the fact that offers of developmental coaching and support can sometimes be stressful and unwelcome by parents.

NURSING DIAGNOSIS: Fear related to outcome of genetic testing as evidenced by reports of apprehension and increased tension

Outcome Identification and Evaluation

Family will state they can cope with the results of the genetic testing or demonstrate reduced fear: *family accurately discusses chances of offspring having genetic disease, demonstrates positive coping, and asks questions about genetic testing and meaning of results.*

Intervention: *Managing Fear*

• Empathize with the family and avoid false reassurances; be truthful: allows family to recognize that fear is a reasonable response. Giving false information or reassurance will actually increase fear.
• Explore coping skills used previously by the family to cope with fear. Reinforce these skills and explore other outlets, such as relaxation, breathing, and physical activity: encourages use of coping mechanisms that help control fear.
• Encourage verbalization of feelings and concerns about genetic testing. Allow time for questions: provides a safe outlet to express feelings and encourages open communication between the family members.
• Explain all procedures and review results as available: knowledge deficit contributes to fear.
• Refer to appropriate support groups and genetic counselling: talking with families who have gone through similar situations can help decrease fear and provide methods of coping. Genetic counselling provides information along with support and additional resources.

NURSING CARE PLAN 49.1

Overview for the Child With a Genetic Condition (continued)

NURSING DIAGNOSIS: Interrupted family processes, related to child's illness, hospitalization, diagnosis of genetic illness in child, and potential long-term effects of illness as evidenced by family's presence in hospital and clinic, missed work, demonstration of inadequate coping

Outcome Identification and Evaluation

Family will maintain functional system of support and demonstrate adequate coping, adaptation of roles and functions, and decreased anxiety: *parents are involved in child's care, ask appropriate questions, express fears and concerns, and can discuss child's care and condition calmly.*

Intervention: *Promoting Family Coping*

- Encourage family to verbalize concerns about child's illness, diagnosis, and prognosis: allows the nurse to identify concerns and areas where further education may be needed and demonstrates family-centered care.
- Explain therapies, procedures, child's behaviours, and plan of care to parents: understanding the child's current status and plan of care helps decrease anxiety.
- Encourage parental involvement in care: allows parents to feel needed and valued and gives them a sense of control over their child's health.
- Identify support system for family and child: helps nurse identify needs and resources available for coping.
- Educate family about resources available to help them develop a wide base of support.

KEY CONCEPTS

- Nurses play an important role in the counselling process. Many times the nurse is the one who has first contact with these parents and is the one to provide follow-up care.

- Nurses play an essential role in providing emotional support and referrals to appropriate agencies, support groups, and resources when caring for families with suspected or diagnosed genetic conditions.

- Referral for genetic counselling prior to genetic testing may be appropriate.

- Many children with chromosomal abnormalities have intellectual disability, learning disabilities, behavioural problems, and distinct features, including birth defects.

- In Turner syndrome, short stature and slow growth are characteristic findings.

- Klinefelter syndrome is usually diagnosed in adolescence or adulthood due to a lack of development of secondary sex characteristics.

- Fragile X syndrome's clinical manifestations are subtle during childhood, with minor dysmorphic features and developmental delay. Problems with sensation, emotion, and behaviour often are the first signs.

- Café-au-lait spots (light brown macules) are the hallmark of neurofibromatosis (Sahin, 2011).

- In osteogenesis imperfecta (OI), frequent fractures, short stature, blue sclera, dentinogenese imperfecta (hypoplastic discolored teeth), and hearing impairments are characteristic clinical features.

- Inborn errors of metabolism are caused by gene mutations that result in abnormalities in the synthesis or catabolism of proteins, carbohydrates, or fats. Most inborn errors of metabolism presenting in the neonatal period are lethal if specific treatment is not initiated immediately.

- Nurses should have a basic knowledge of genetics, common genetic conditions in children, genetic testing, and genetic counselling so they can provide support and information to families and can help improve their quality of life.

○ Genetic conditions usually result in a lifelong complex medical condition. Nurses must provide ongoing education and support for the child and family about the condition, treatment, and management as well as available resources.

REFERENCES AND RECOMMENDED READINGS

Bacino, C. A. (2014). *Approach to congenital malformations*. UpToDate. Retrieved from http://www.uptodate.com/contents/approach-to-congenital-malformations.

Bacino, C. A. (2015). *Sex chromosome abnormalities*. UpToDate. Retrieved from http://www.uptodate.com/contents/sex-chromosome-abnormalities.

Bacino, C. A., & Lee, B. (2011). Chapter 76: Cytogenetics. In R. M. Kleigman, B. F. Stanton, J. W. St. Geme III, N. F. Schor, & R. E. Behrman (Eds.). *Nelson textbook of pediatrics* (19th ed., p. 383). Philadelphia, PA: Saunders.

Basel, D., & Steiner, R. D. (2009). Osteogenesis imperfecta: Recent findings shed new light on this once well-understood condition. *Genetics in Medicine, 11*(6), 375–385.

Boycott, K., Hartley, T., Adam, S., Bernier, F., Chong, K., Fernandez, B. A., . . . & Laberge, A. M. (2015). The clinical application of genome-wide sequencing for monogenic diseases in Canada: Position Statement of the Canadian College of Medical Geneticists. *Journal of medical genetics, 52*(7), 431–437.

Brizola, E., Staub, A. L., & Félix, T. M. (2014). Muscle strength, joint range of motion, and gait in children and adolescents with osteogenesis imperfecta. *Pediatric Physical Therapy, 26*(2), 245–252.

Bull, M. J., & the Committee on Genetics. (2011). From the American Academy of Pediatrics: Clinical Report: Health supervision for children with Down syndrome. *Pediatrics, 128*(2), 393–406.

Canadian Organisation for Rare Disorders. (2015). *Newborn Screening in Canada Status Report*. Retrieved from https://www.raredisorders.ca/content/uploads/Canada-NBS-status-updated-Sept.-3-2015.pdf.

Canadian Paediatric Society. (2016). *Care of adolescents with chronic conditions*. Retrieved from http://www.cps.ca/documents/position/care-of-youth-chronic-conditions.

Canadian Paediatric Society. (2017). *Guidelines for genetic testing of healthy children*. Retrieved from http://www.cps.ca/en/documents/position/guidelines-for-genetic-testing-of-healthy-children.

Carpenito-Moyet, L. J. (2013). *Nursing diagnosis: Application to clinical practice* (14th ed.). Philadelphia, PA: Lippincott Williams & Wilkins.

Cheung, M. S., & Glorieux, F. H. (2008). Osteogenesis imperfecta: Update on presentation and management. *Reviews in Endocrine & Metabolic Conditions, 9*(2), 153–160.

Conley, Y. P. (2014). Chapter 4: Genetics and health applications. In S. M. Nettina (Ed.). *Lippincott manual of nursing practice* (10th ed., pp. 33–44). Philadelphia, PA: Wolters Kluwer Health/Lippincott Williams & Wilkins.

Dogba, M. J., Bedos, C., Durigova, M., Montpetit, K., Wong, T., Glorieux, F. H., & Rauch, F. (2013). The impact of severe osteogenesis imperfecta on the lives of young patients and their parents—A qualitative analysis. *BMC Pediatrics, 13*(1), 153.

Etchegary, H., Nicholls, S. G., Tessier, L., Simmonds, C., Potter, B. K., Brehaut, J. C., . . . & Milburn, J. (2016). Consent for newborn screening: Parents' and health-care professionals' experiences of consent in practice. *European Journal of Human Genetics, 24*(11), 1530–1534.

Fegran, L., Hall, E. O., Uhrenfeldt, L., Aagaard, H., & Ludvigsen, M. S. (2014). Adolescents' and young adults' transition experiences when transferring from paediatric to adult care: A qualitative metasynthesis. *International Journal of Nursing Studies, 51*(1), 123–135.

Fischbach, F. T., & Dunning, M. B. (2015). *A manual of laboratory and diagnostic tests* (9th ed.). Philadelphia, PA: Wolters Kluwer Health/Lippincott Williams & Wilkins.

Gemone, BC. (n.d.). *Findings of rare disease genes in Canada*. Retrieved from https://www.genomebc.ca/research-programs/projects/health/finding-of-rare-disease-genes-in-canada-forge-canada/.

Genetic Education Canada—Knowledge Organization. (n.d.). *Newborn genetics*. Retrieved from http://geneticseducation.ca/public-resources/newborn-genetics/.

Genetics Home Reference. (2012a). *Fragile X syndrome*. Retrieved from http://ghr.nlm.nih.gov/condition/fragile-x-syndrome.

Genetics Home Reference. (2012b). *Achondroplasia*. Retrieved from http://ghr.nlm.nih.gov/condition/achondroplasia.

Genetics Home Reference. (2015a). *Angelman syndrome*. Retrieved from http://ghr.nlm.nih.gov/condition/angelman-syndrome.

Genetics Home Reference. (2015b). *Cri-Du-Chat syndrome*. Retrieved from http://ghr.nlm.nih.gov/condition/cri-du-chat-syndrome.

Genetics Home Reference. (2015c). *Wolf-Hirschhorn syndrome*. Retrieved from http://ghr.nlm.nih.gov/condition/wolf-hirschhorn-syndrome.

Genetics Home Reference. (2015d). *Williams syndrome*. Retrieved from http://ghr.nlm.nih.gov/condition/williams-syndrome.

Genetics Home Reference. (2015e). *22q11.2 deletion syndrome*. Retrieved from http://ghr.nlm.nih.gov/condition/22q112-deletion-syndrome.

Glorieux, F. H. (2008). Osteogenesis imperfecta. *Best Practice & Research Clinical Rheumatology, 22*(1), 85–100.

Government of Canada. (n.d.). *Genetic testing and screening*. Retrieved from https://www.canada.ca/en/public-health/services/fertility/genetic-testing-screening.html.

Government of Canada. (2017). *Down syndrome surveillance in Canada 2005–2013*. Retrieved from https://www.canada.ca/en/public-health/services/publications/healthy-living/down-syndrome-surveillance-2005-2013.html.

Guon, J., Wilfond, B. S., Farlow, B., Brazg, T., & Janvier, A. (2014). Our children are not a diagnosis: The experience of parents who continue their pregnancy after a prenatal diagnosis of trisomy 13 or 18. *American Journal of Medical Genetics Part A, 164*(2), 308–318.

Hartman A. (2003). *Osteogenesis imperfecta: A guide for nurses*. Retrieved from http://www.oif.org/site/DocServer?docID=181.

Hitzler, J. K., He, W., Doyle, J., Cairo, M., Camitta, B. M., Chan, K. W., . . . & Kennedy-Nasser, A. A. (2014). Outcome of transplantation for acute lymphoblastic leukemia in children with Down syndrome. *Pediatric Blood & Cancer, 61*(6), 1126–1128.

Hon-Yin, B. C., Shuman, C., Choufani, S., & Weksberg, R. (2014). *Beckwith-Wiedemann syndrome.* UpToDate. Retrieved from http://www.uptodate.com/contents/beckwith-wiedemann-syndrome.

Kansra, A. R., & Donohoue, P. A. (2011). Chapter 580: Hypofunction of the ovaries. In R. M. Kleigman, B. F. Stanton, J. W. St. Geme III, N. F. Schor, & R. E. Behrman (Eds.). *Nelson textbook of pediatrics* (19th ed., pp. 1951–1957). Philadelphia, PA: Saunders.

Katz, S. L., Nehme, J., LaBerge, R., Barrowman, N., Hoey, L., Monsour, A., … & Pothos, M. (2016). Predicting presence of sleep disordered breathing in children with down syndrome. In *A27. ADVANCES IN PEDIATRIC SLEEP* (pp. A1220–A1220). American Thoracic Society 2016 International Conference, May 13-18 San Francisco, New York. Retrieved from https://www.atsjournals.org/doi/book/10.1164/ajrccm-conference.2016

Kaye, C. I., & the Committee on Genetics. (Reaffirmed 2011a). From the American Academy of Pediatrics: Newborn screening fact sheets. *Pediatrics, 118*(3), e934–e963. Retrieved from http://pediatrics.aappublications.org/content/118/3/e934.full

Kaye, C. I., & the Committee on Genetics. (Reaffirmed 2011b). From the American Academy of Pediatrics: Introduction to the newborn screening fact sheets. *Pediatrics, 118*(3), 1304–1312. Retrieved from htttp://pediatrics.aappublications.org/content/118/3/1304.full.

King, K., O'Gorman, C., & Gallagher, S. (2014). Thyroid dysfunction in children with Down syndrome: A literature review. *Irish Journal of Medical Science, 183*(1), 1–6.

Korf, B. R. (2014). *Neurofibromatosis type 1 (NF1): Pathogenesis, clinical features, and diagnosis.* UpToDate. Retrieved from http://www.uptodate.com/contents/neurofibromatosis-type-1-nf1-pathogenesis-clinical-features-and-diagnosis.

Lashley, F. R. (2005). *Clinical genetics in nursing practice.* New York: Springer Publishing.

Marr, C., Seasman, A., & Bishop, N. (2017). Managing the patient with osteogenesis imperfecta: A multidisciplinary approach. *Journal of Multidisciplinary Healthcare, 10,* 145–155.

Morris, M., Fischer, K., Leydiker, K., Elliott, L., Newby, J., & Abdenur, J. E. (2014). Reduction in newborn screening metabolic false-positive results following a new collection protocol. *Genetics in Medicine, 16*(6), 477–483.

National Human Genome Research Institute. (2011). *Learning about Tay-Sachs disease.* Retrieved from http://www.genome.gov/10001220.

National Institute of Neurological Conditions and Stroke. (2015). *Neurofibromatosis fact sheet.* Retrieved from http://www.ninds.nih.gov/conditions/neurofibromatosis/detail_neurofibromatosis.htm.

Nelson, K. E., Rosella, L. C., Mahant, S., & Guttmann, A. (2016). Survival and surgical interventions for children with trisomy 13 and 18. *JAMA, 316*(4), 420–428.

Nelson-Tuttle, C. (2014). Chapter 56: Developmental disabilities. In S. M. Nettina (Ed.), *Lippincott manual of nursing practice* (10th ed., pp. 1791–1807). Philadelphia, PA: Wolters Kluwer Health/Lippincott Williams & Wilkins.

NORD. (2012a). *Charge syndrome.* Retrieved from https://www.rarediseases.org/rare-disease-information/rare-diseases/byID/550/viewFullReport.

NORD. (2012b). *Vacterl association.* Retrieved from https://www.rarediseases.org/rare-disease-information/rare-diseases/byID/486/viewFullReport.

[Oi World]. (2014). *Me, Myself, and OI: The extraordinary adventures of a breakable girl [video file].* Retrieved from https://www.youtube.com/watch?v=IAhs-piej1o.

Ostermaier, K. K. (2014). *Down syndrome: Management.* UpToDate. Retrieved from http://www.uptodate.com/contents/down-syndrome-management.

Ostermaier, K. K. (2015). *Down syndrome: Clinical features and diagnosis.* UpToDate. Retrieved from http://www.uptodate.com/contents/down-syndrome-clinical-features-and-diagnosis.

Pitetti, K., Baynard, T., & Agiovlasitis, S. (2013). Children and adolescents with Down syndrome, physical fitness and physical activity. *Journal of Sport and Health Science, 2*(1), 47–57. https://doi.org/10.1016/j.jshs.2012.10.004.

Pueschel, S. M. (2011). *A parent's guide to Down syndrome: Toward a brighter future* (rev. ed.). Baltimore, MD: Paul H. Brookes Publishing Company, Inc.

Rezvani, I., & Rezvani, G. (2011). An approach to inborn errors of metabolism. In R. M. Kleigman, B. F. Stanton, J. W. St. Geme III, N. F. Schor, & R. E. Behrman (Eds.). *Nelson textbook of pediatrics* (19th ed., pp. 416–418). Philadelphia, PA: Saunders.

Saenger, P. (2014). *Clinical manifestations and diagnosis of Turner syndrome (gonadal dysgenesis).* UpToDate. Retrieved from http://www.uptodate.com/contents/clinical-manifestations-and-diagnosis-of-turner-syndrome-gonadal-dysgenesis.

Sahin, M. (2011). Chapter 589: Neurocutaneous syndromes. In R. M. Kleigman, B. F. Stanton, J. W. St. Geme III, N. F. Schor, & R. E. Behrman (Eds.). *Nelson textbook of pediatrics* (19th ed., pp. 2046–2053). Philadelphia, PA: Saunders.

Scheimann, A. O. (2014). *Epidemiology and genetics of Prader-Willi syndrome.* UpToDate. Retrieved from http://www.uptodate.com/contents/epidemiology-and-genetics-of-prader-willi-syndrome.

Schrijver, I., Zehnder, J. L., & Cherry, A. M. (2014). *Chromosomal translocations, deletions, and inversions.* UpToDate. Retrieved from http://www.uptodate.com/contents/chromosomal-translocations-deletions-and-inversions.

Scott, D. A., & Lee, B. (2011a). Chapter 73: The genetic approach in pediatric medicine. In R. M. Kleigman, B. F. Stanton, J. W. St. Geme III, N. F. Schor, & R. E. Behrman (Eds.). *Nelson textbook of pediatrics* (19th ed., pp. 380–383). Philadelphia, PA: Saunders.

Searl, B. (2014). *Chromosomes and rare chromosome conditions in general.* Retrieved from http://www.rarechromo.org/html/chromosomesandconditions.asp.

Shapiro, J. R., & Germain-Lee, E. L. (2012). Osteogenesis imperfecta: Effecting the transition from adolescent to adult medical care. *Journal Musculoskeletal and Neuronal Interactions, 12*(1), 24–27.

Slaughter, J. L., Meinzen-Derr, J., Rose, S. R., Leslie, N. D., Chandrasekar, R., Linard, S. M., & Akinbi, H. T. (2010). The effects of gestational age and birth weight on false-positive newborn-screening rates. *Pediatrics, 126*(5), 910–916.

Summar, K., & Lee, B. (2011). Chapter 76.2: Down syndrome and other abnormalities of chromosome number. In R. M. Kleigman, B. F. Stanton, J. W. St. Geme III, N. F. Schor, & R. E. Behrman (Eds.). *Nelson textbook of pediatrics* (19th ed., pp. 399–403). Philadelphia, PA: Saunders.

Sutton, V. R. (2014). *Inborn errors of metabolism: Epidemiology, pathogenesis, and clinical features.* UpToDate. Retrieved from http://www.uptodate.com/contents/inborn-errors-of-metabolism-epidemiology-pathogenesis-and-clinical-features.

The American College of Obstetricians and Gynecologists Committee on Genetics & The Society for Maternal-Fetal Medicine Publications Committee. (2012). Committee opinion no. 545: Noninvasive prenatal testing for fetal aneuploidy. *American College of Obstetricians and Gynecologists, 120,* 1532–1534.

Van Dijk, F. S., & Sillence, D. O. (2014). Osteogenesis imperfecta: Clinical diagnosis, nomenclature and severity assessment. *American Journal of Medical Genetics Part A, 164*(6), 1470–1481.

Van Esch, H. (2014). *Fragile X syndrome: Clinical features and diagnosis in children and adolescents.* UpToDate. Retrieved from http://www.uptodate.com/contents/fragile-x-syndrome-clinical-features-and-diagnosis-in-children-and-adolescents.

Weremowicz, S. (2014). *Congenital cytogenetic abnormalities.* UpToDate. Retrieved from http://www.uptodate.com/contents/congenital-cytogenetic-abnormalities.

Wheeler, P. G. (2012). *Newborn screening testing. kids health.* Retrieved from http://kidshealth.org/parent/system/medical/newborn_screening_tests.html#.

Wright, M. J., & Connolly, H. M. (2014). *Genetics, clinical features, and diagnosis of Marfan syndrome and related conditions.* UpToDate. Retrieved from http://www.uptodate.com/contents/genetics-clinical-features-and-diagnosis-of-marfan-syndrome-and-related-conditions.

CHAPTER **WORKSHEET**

MULTIPLE CHOICE QUESTIONS

1. A child born with a single transverse palmar crease, a short neck with excessive skin at the nape, a depressed nasal bridge, and cardiac defects is most likely to have which autosomal difference?
   a. Trisomy 21
   b. Trisomy 18
   c. Trisomy 14
   d. Trisomy 13

2. A mother brings her 4-day-old infant to the clinic with vomiting and poor feeding. The newborn was healthy at birth. The nurse should suspect:
   a. Sturge–Weber syndrome
   b. An inborn error of metabolism
   c. Trisomy 18
   d. Turner syndrome

3. The nurse is caring for a child with Down syndrome. What should the nurse's focus be?
   a. Teaching hygiene skills to the child in order to increase self-esteem
   b. Screening for anomalies and teaching about prevention of respiratory infection
   c. Finding opportunities to increase socialization for the child and family
   d. Expecting walking at age 1 year and toilet training completion at age 2 years

4. The nurse is caring for a child with Turner syndrome admitted to the unit for treatment of a kidney infection. What characteristics associated with this syndrome may the nurse expect to find upon assessment?
   a. Microcephaly, polydactyly
   b. Low-set ears, cleft lip
   c. Short stature, webbed neck
   d. Gynecomastia, taller than average

DOSAGE CALCULATION QUESTION

1. The nurse is caring for a child with Down syndrome. The child weighs 11.7 kg (26 lbs). The physician orders intravenous maintenance fluids. What would be the expected maintenance IV fluid rate? (round to the nearest mL)

CRITICAL THINKING EXERCISES

1. An 8-month-old is seen in the clinic. On assessment the nurse finds eight café-au-lait spots on the child's trunk and extremities. What other assessment findings may be pertinent?

2. A child's newborn screen came back positive for phenylketonuria. After further testing, the diagnosis is confirmed. What instructions would you give the parents regarding care of their child?

3. A 6-year-old boy with Down syndrome is admitted to the hospital with pneumonia. Choose three pieces of information that the nurse should seek when obtaining the health history:
   a. Presence of cardiac defects or disease
   b. Last hearing and vision evaluation
   c. Mother's pregnancy history
   d. Presence of thyroid disease
   e. Mother's immunization history

STUDY ACTIVITIES

1. Develop a nursing care plan for a child with Down syndrome.

2. Shadow a genetic counsellor. Identify ways he or she helps families understand and cope with genetic conditions.

3. Attend a meeting of an ethics committee at a local hospital. Identify some of the ethical, legal, and social issues in health care that they discuss, particularly related to genetic testing and genetic conditions.

BRINGING IT ALL TOGETHER: A CASE STUDY

Charles Faust, a 10-month-old with Down syndrome, is seen in the clinic for a well-child examination. The parents have questions about his growth and development. They want to discuss the developmental aspects of the syndrome. They explain they were aware there would be difference but these are only now becoming apparent in comparison to his peers.

Go to thePoint **to find questions to consider about this case.**

50

Nursing Care of the Child With an Alteration in Behaviour, Cognition, or Development

Learning Objectives

Upon completion of the chapter, you will be able to:

1. Discuss the impact of alterations in mental health on the growth and development of infants, children, and adolescents.

2. Describe techniques used to evaluate the status of mental health in children.

3. Identify appropriate nursing assessments and interventions related to therapy and medications for the treatment of childhood and adolescent mental health disorders.

4. Distinguish mental health disorders common in infants, children, and adolescents.

5. Develop an individualized nursing care plan for the child with a mental health disorder.

6. Develop child/family teaching plans for the child with a mental health disorder.

John Howard, age 6 years, is brought to the clinic for his annual examination. His father states, "John has frequent emotional outbursts and his mood seems to switch from happy to sad rather quickly. His teachers have said his performance at school has been poor."

✿ **Mental** health issues make up the bulk of the "new morbidity" of children. Such issues include developmental and behavioural disorders, eating disorders, mood disorders, anxiety disorders, and abuse and **violence** (acts of aggression) directed toward children. As many as 14% to 20% of children may be suffering from mental health–related problems, yet only 2% are seen by mental health care providers (Burstein, Talmi, Stafford, & Kelsay, 2014). Failure to receive appropriate treatment may lead to further academic and social difficulties (Burstein et al., 2014). Mental illness manifested in the early years increases the risk of adolescent emotional issues, use of firearms, reckless driving, substance abuse, and promiscuous sexual activity. Some cognitive or neurobehavioural disorders may have a genetic or physiologic cause, whereas others result from family or environmental stressors. In addition, **PANDAs** (pediatric autoimmune neuropsychiatric disorders associated with streptococcal infections) have an abrupt onset. Presentation may include: obsessive-compulsive disorder (OCD), tic disorder, ADHD type behaviours, or oppositional behaviour (Sigra, Hesselmark, & Bejerot, 2018).

Usually children with cognitive or mental health disorders are treated in the community or on an outpatient basis, but sometimes the disorder has such a significant impact on the child and family that hospitalization is required. Many hospitalized children also suffer from cognitive or mental health disorders. When a child is diagnosed with a cognitive or mental health disorder, the family may become overwhelmed by the multifaceted services that he or she requires.

The scope of mental health issues and the impact mental health illness has during infancy, childhood into adolescence, and later adult life are a growing concern for Canada (Canadian Paediatric Society [CPS], 2015a). The Mental Health Commission Canada (MHCC, n.d.) suggest that 1.2 million, or 1 in 12 (Canadian Institute Health Information [CIHI], n.d.) children and youth are affected by mental illness with only 20% receiving treatment. Similar to other health providers, universal goals include:

1. Promoting public awareness of infant, childhood, and youth mental health issues in order to reduce the stigma associated with mental illness.
2. Continuing to develop, disseminate, and implement scientifically proven prevention and treatment services in the field of children's mental health in rural and remote communities.
3. Improving the assessment of and recognition of mental health needs in all children, for all background including focus on key areas such as Indigenous youth.
4. Eliminating racial/ethnic and socioeconomic inequities in service provision, access, and waiting times.
5. Improving the infrastructure for children's mental health services, including support for scientifically proven interventions across professions.

6. Providing or recommending on-going education to those in public, private, and voluntary settings caring for this population, across all partnerships such as health, education, social care, etc.
7. Embedding and sustaining health promotion strategies focused on evaluation and measurable outcomes.

Mental health problems in children are real and painful and can be severe. For affected children to have a chance at a healthy future, nurses must participate in the early identification and referral of children with potential cognitive deficits or other mental health issues. For some mental health problems, nurses can play an important role in assessing and identifying precursors to illness and prevention of worsening of disease.

EFFECTS OF MENTAL HEALTH ISSUES ON HEALTH AND DEVELOPMENT

Children's behaviour, as well as their ability to develop resilience, is influenced by biologic or genetic characteristics, nutrition, physical health, developmental ability, environmental and family interactions, the child's individual temperament, and the parents' or caregivers' responses to the child's behaviour. The transitions that occur with normal growth and development are often a source of stress for children, and in some children, they may result in altered function. Children progress at very different rates, so it is often difficult to identify subtle abnormalities. When stress, fatigue, pain, or trauma occurs in children, they may quickly regress to earlier patterns of behaviour. These regressive behaviours may continue if a mental health concern is present. It is possible that early childhood stress and trauma influences developing neurons which leads to decreased coping abilities later in life (Shaffer, Smith, & Ornstein, 2018). Children learn through their experiences, which can hold an intergenerational legacy (Rose, 2018). Therefore, individuals may develop maladaptive behaviours through life interactions as a consequence of early trauma (Burstein et al., 2014; Shaffer et al., 2018).

The concept of resilience is important for nurses to understand when taking care of children with mental health issues. It is important for the nurse to not only focus on aspects or behaviours of the child that can diagnosed and treated, but also to foster early those characteristics or protective factors that are integral to coping (CPS, 2015b). Resilience refers to the ability to "bounce-back" when living in adverse circumstances. It involves doing well against the odds and having an ability to cope well and recover from adverse circumstances. It is essentially successful adaptation. Individual factors associated with resilience include having an internal locus of control, empathy with others, and an ability to reflect. Family and community factors include nurturance and trust, peer contact, and positive role models. The nurse can play an integral role in fostering these factors or prioritizing them when developing a plan of care.

COMMON MEDICAL TREATMENTS

A variety of medications and other medical and psychological treatments are used to treat mental health disorders in children. The most common medications are listed in Drug Guide 50.1. The nurse caring for the child with a

mental health disorder should become familiar with how the medications work, as well as medication adverse effects to monitor for. Many mental health disorders are treated with some type of therapy, including behavioural, play, family, and cognitive therapies. Table 50.1 reviews the types of therapies commonly used. These therapies are generally carried out only by specially trained personnel.

Behaviour management techniques can be used with these therapies to support children to develop new

DRUG GUIDE 50.1 DRUGS USED FOR PEDIATRIC MENTAL HEALTH DISORDERS

Medication	Actions	Indications	Nursing Implications
Psychostimulants: methylphenidate, dextroamphetamine, lisdexamfetamine, pemoline, long-acting methylphenidate, long-acting dextroamphetamine	Increase synaptic levels of dopamine and norepinephrine	ADHD	• Methylphenidate has a short half-life; give TID (AM, midday at school, at home after school). • Long-acting preparations are given once daily in the AM. • Adverse effects: decreased appetite, headache, abdominal pain, difficulty sleeping, irritability, social withdrawal, motor tics. If dose is too high, child may have flat affect. • lisdexamfetamine—if chest pain and fainting occur notify physician at once. • Pemoline is only rarely used because of hepatotoxicity.
Antianxiety agent: buspirone	Highly blocks reuptake of dopamine	Anxiety, rage, mania, psychosis, depression, Tourette syndrome	• Administer in consistent relation to food (either with or without). • May cause drowsiness • Monitor for disinhibition, agitation, confusion, depression.
Antimanic agent: lithium	Influences reuptake of serotonin and/or norepinephrine	Bipolar disorder, depression, hyperaggression	• Monitor closely. • May cause polyuria, polydipsia, tremor, nausea, weight gain, diarrhea
Selective serotonin reuptake inhibitors: fluoxetine, paroxetine, sertraline	Potentiate serotonin activity in the brain	Depression, obsessive-compulsive disorder, anxiety	• Observe for irritability, insomnia, GI distress, nausea, headache. • Monitor BP for increase.
Atypical antidepressants: trazodone	Inhibit reuptake of serotonin	Depression	• Monitor BP for postural hypotension. • Observe for sedation and drowsiness; avoid alcohol use. • Administer after meals or with a snack.
Nonstimulant norepinephrine reuptake inhibitors: atomoxetine	Enhance norepinephrine activity	ADHD	• Administer without regard to food once or twice daily. • Monitor weight, height, BP, heart rate. • May cause dizziness, dry mouth
α-Agonist antihypertensive agents: clonidine, guanfacine	Activate inhibitory neurons in the brain stem	ADHD, Tourette syndrome, self-abuse, aggression	• Clonidine is strongly sedating. • Monitor BP and pulse. • Observe for dry mouth, confusion, depression, urinary retention, constipation.

DRUG GUIDE 50.1 DRUGS USED FOR PEDIATRIC MENTAL HEALTH DISORDERS (continued)

Medication	Actions	Indications	Nursing Implications
Antipsychotic agents: thioridazine, chlorpromazine, haloperidol	Reversibly block type 2 dopamine receptors in the central nervous system	Psychosis, mania, self-harm, violent or destructive behaviour	• May cause drowsiness • Monitor for anticholinergic effects, drowsiness and dystonia (extrapyramidal effects), dizziness. • Evaluate for the development of orthostatic hypotension, tachycardia. • Observe closely for the development of tardive dyskinesia, particularly early in treatment.
Atypical antipsychotics: risperidone, clozapine, olanzapine	Reversibly block type 2 dopamine receptors in the central nervous system	Psychosis, bipolar disorder, autism spectrum disorder, Tourette syndrome	• Monitor for seizures, agitation, headache, nausea, sedation. • Olanzapine may cause weight gain. • Note WBC count.
Tricyclic antidepressants: amitriptyline, desipramine, imipramine, nortriptyline	Enhance synaptic concentration of serotonin and/or norepinephrine	Depression, ADHD, tics, anxiety	• Monitor for anticholinergic effects, weight loss. • Check blood levels. • Monitor ECG for arrhythmias.

BP, blood pressure; ECG, electrocardiogram; GI, gastrointestinal; WBC, white blood cell.

Adapted from Preston, J., O'Neal, J. H., & Talaga, M. C. (2015). *Child and adolescent clinical psychopharmacology made simple.* Oakland, CA: New Harbinger Publications, Inc.; Taketomo, C. K., Hodding, J. H., & Kraus, D. M. (2013). *Pediatric & neonatal dosage handbook* (20th ed.). Hudson, OH: Lexicomp; and Varcarolis, E. M. (2011). *Manual of psychiatric nursing care planning: Assessment guides, diagnoses, and psychopharmacology* (4th ed.). St. Louis, MO: Saunders.

TABLE 50.1   TYPES OF THERAPY

Treatment	Explanation
Behavioural therapy	Uses stimulus and response conditioning to manage or alter behaviour. Reinforces desired behaviours, replacing the inappropriate ones. Consistency is of utmost importance.
Play therapy	Designed to change emotional status. Encourages the child to act out feelings of sadness, fear, hostility, or anger.
Cognitive behavioural therapy	Teaches children to change reactions so that automatic negative thought patterns are replaced with alternative ones.
Dialectical behavioural therapy	Group and individual sessions to treat chronic suicidal thoughts in borderline personality disorder. Individuals learn responsibility for their problems and better deal with negative emotions.
Family therapy	Exploration of the child's emotional issue and its effect on family members. Helps the family to focus in more constructive ways.
Group therapy	May be conducted in a school, hospital, treatment facility, or neighbourhood centre. Feelings are expressed and participants gain hope, feel a part of something, and benefit from role modelling. Takes advantage of peer relationships as developmental focus in preteen and teen groups.
Milieu therapy	A specially structured setting designed to promote the child's adaptive and social skills. A safe and supportive environment for those at risk for self-harm or those who are very ill or very aggressive.
Individual therapy	The child and therapist work together to resolve the conflicts, emotions, or behaviour problems. Trust is central. Structured based on the child's developmental level (e.g., may use play therapy for a younger child).
Hypnosis	Deep relaxation with suggestibility remarks.

Adapted from American Academy of Child and Adolescent Psychiatry. (2013). *Fast facts for families no. 86: Psychotherapies for children and adolescents.* Washington, DC: Author; Varcarolis, E. M. (2011). *Manual of psychiatric nursing care planning: Assessment guides, diagnoses, and psychopharmacology* (4th ed.). St. Louis, MO: Saunders.

behaviours and management strategies. The methods may be used outside of therapy sessions, in the hospital, clinic, classroom, or home. Behaviour management techniques include the following:

- Identify and assess child for current coping strategies and patterns of behaviours.
- Understand the child's baseline functioning (what is their presentation when they are safe and settled) and identify stressors and triggers for altered or unsafe behaviour patterns.
- Include patient, family, and health care team in the risk assessment process.
- Plan with the child and family specific interventions that will support the child in practicing new coping strategies.
- Set the child up for success by creating plans that are achievable and responsive to the child's developmental needs.
- Provide consistent caregivers (unlicensed assistive personnel and nurses for the hospitalized child) and establish a predictable daily routine.
- Use a calm approach and low tone of voice.
- Redirect the child by reminding them of expectations and support them to achieve.
- Recognize that unwanted behaviours are a communication for an unmet need.
- Provide positive feedback to the child and family in a way that is meaningful to them.
- Restraint should never be used to change or punish behaviour. Restraint use is traumatic to the child, family, and health care provider. Canada has adopted the stance of least restraint (Clinical Best Practice Guidelines, 2012) which embeds the concepts of trauma informed care, ethical decision making, therapeutic relationships, and legal and legislative requirements.

NURSING PROCESS OVERVIEW FOR THE CHILD WITH A MENTAL HEALTH DISORDER

Care of the child with a mental health disorder includes assessment, nursing diagnosis, planning, interventions, and evaluation. There are several concepts related to the nursing process that may be applied to mental health concerns in children. From a general understanding of the care involved for a child with a mental health disorder, the nurse can then individualize the care based on specifics for each child.

Assessment

A careful and thorough health history forms the basis of the nursing assessment of a child with a mental health or cognitive disorder. The physical examination

may yield clues to the type of disorder, but the physical examination is often completely normal (except in cases of physical or sexual abuse).

Take Note!

Observe a child's play or drawings; if the manner or theme of play or content of the drawings leads you to suspect cognitive or psychological issues, refer the child for further mental health evaluation.

Health History

Elicit the health history, noting the child's prenatal and birth history, past medical history (including previously diagnosed cognitive or mental health disorders), history of neurologic injury or disease, and family history of mental health disorder. Perform a developmental history, noting age of attainment (or loss) of milestones. Question the child and/or parent about behaviour changes such as:

- Altered sleep
- Difference in eating patterns, weight loss or gain, change in appetite
- Functioning at school
- Participation in risk-taking behaviours
- Alterations in friendships
- Changes in extracurricular activity participation

A number of tools are available for screening for mental health disorders in children and adolescents (CPS, 2015c). Screening for risk of suicide in children over the age of 10 and youth should be part of the pediatric nurse's assessment. The CPS (2015c) has a comprehensive practice point document that covers general and specific issues which include: mental illness, prior suicide attempt, impulsivity, precipitating factors, family factors, lack of connections and support and plan formulation. During the health interview ask child and family about any altered milestones and completed developmental testing. Note strengths as well as impairments, delay or regression. Determine if child and family have experienced any recent stress, trauma, illness, or change in family structure. Ask if any family members are chronically ill. Note medications the child takes routinely, and ask about any allergies to food, drugs, medications, or environmental agents.

Interview the child at an age-appropriate level to determine his or her self-perception, future plans, and stressors and how he or she copes with them. Determine the child's perception of his or her relationship with parents, siblings, friends, peers, pets, inanimate objects, and transitional or security objects. Ask the child about his/her daily mood? How does the child or youth view him/herself and present situation? Ask questions such as, "What do you like most about yourself?"

and "What would you change about your situation?" Does the child and family acknowledge their accomplishments and are they future-orientated? What are the family values?

Assess the child or youth for the following during the health interview:

- Hallucinations/Delusions
- Aggression/Emotional Intelligence
- Depression/Suicidality
- Affect/Mood
- Impulsivity/Distractibility
- Inhibition/Disinhibition
- Potential cognitive or learning disabilities
- Unusual motor activities

Note history of physical complaints that may be associated with physical abuse such as burns or other injuries or with sexual abuse situations, such as sore throat, difficulty swallowing, or genital burning or itching.

> **Remember John, the 6-year-old brought in for his annual examination? What additional health history and physical examination assessment information should the nurse obtain?**

Physical Examination

Observe the child's (or youth's) appearance, noting cleanliness, clothing, and appropriateness for environment. It is important for the nurse to remain nonjudgmental, for example, if it is summer do they have on winter clothes do not judge their choice or pass comment. Note the child's facial expression and response to their parent or caretaker, and the nurse. Does he or she make eye contact? Determine the child's level of consciousness and extent of interest in and interaction with surroundings. Note the child's posture, **affect** (facial emotional display), and mood (subjective experience of child or youth). Are the emotional reactions congruent to situation? How does the child communicate?

Measure the child's weight and height/length, as well as head circumference for children under 3 years old. Perform a thorough physical examination, noting any physical abnormalities or signs of other physical health disorders. Note abnormal findings that may be associated with particular mental health disorders. For example, in youth with eating disorders you may see increased bruising, soft/sparse body hair, eroded tooth enamel, reddened gums, and split fingernails. Children and youth at risk for self-harm and abuse may have burns, contusions, cuts, abrasions, unusual skin marks, inflamed oropharynx, or genitourinary discharge, bleeding perhaps as a result of cutting.

Laboratory and Diagnostic Testing

Mental health disorders are generally diagnosed based on clinical features. However, brain imaging such as computed tomography (CT) or magnetic resonance imaging (MRI) may be used to determine if there is evidence of congenital abnormality or alterations in the brain tissue that may lead to developmental delay. A blood or urine toxicology panel is useful in the diagnosis of substance misuse (drug) or overdose, or instances of bizarre behaviour related to ketoacidosis.

Nursing Diagnoses and Related Interventions

The overall goal of nursing management of cognitive and mental health disorders in children is to help the child and family reach an optimal level of functioning. This may be achieved through interventions designed to decrease the impact of stressors on the child's life. Upon completion of a thorough assessment of the child and family, the nurse might identify several nursing diagnoses, including:

- Impaired social interaction
- Delayed growth and development
- Ineffective individual coping
- Hopelessness/Suicidality
- Imbalanced nutrition, less than body requirements
- Disturbed thought processes
- Caregiver role strain

> **After completing an assessment of John, the nurse noted the following: difficulty sitting still for the examination, easily distracted and frustrated, labile mood. Based on the assessment findings, what would your top three nursing diagnoses be for John?**

Nursing goals, interventions, and evaluation for the child with a mental health disorder are based on the nursing diagnoses. Nursing Care Plan 50.1, found at the end of the chapter, provides a general guide for planning care for a child with a mental health disorder. Children's responses to a mental health issue and its treatment will vary, and nursing care should be individualized based on the child's and family's responses. Additional information about nursing management will be included later in the chapter as it relates to specific disorders.

> **Based on your top three nursing diagnoses for John, describe appropriate nursing interventions.**

DEVELOPMENTAL AND BEHAVIOURAL DISORDERS

Developmental and behavioural disorders make up a large proportion of mental health disorders in children. They include learning disabilities, intellectual disability (ID), autism spectrum disorder, and attention-deficit/hyperactivity disorder (ADHD).

Learning Disabilities

About 10% of children and adolescents have learning disabilities (von Hahn, 2015a). Early identification of learning disabilities may improve health and education outcome for children and youth (CPS, 2012). In children with chronic illness, learning disabilities are two times more common than in the general population (von Hahn, 2015a). The essential characteristic of learning disability is an innate cognitive difficulty resulting in lower academic achievement than would be expected for the child's intellectual potential (von Hahn, 2015a). Learning disabilities become evident when a child of average intelligence has difficulty mastering basic academic skills. Learning disabilities can affect the child's ability to listen, speak, read, write, and perform mathematics. For example:

- Children with dyslexia have difficulty with reading, writing, and spelling.
- Children with dyscalculia have problems with mathematics and computation.
- Children with dyspraxia have problems with manual dexterity and coordination.
- Children with dysgraphia have difficulty producing the written word (composition, spelling, and writing).

Take Note!

Sensory processing disorder may be mistaken for a learning disability, but it is not and should be treated differently (Box 50.1).

BOX 50.1

SENSORY PROCESSING DISORDER (ALSO CALLED SENSORY INTEGRATION DYSFUNCTION)

- A neurologic disorder in which the child cannot organize sensory input used in daily living
- Hyposensitivity or hypersensitivity to sensory input
- Results in overreaction to different textures, decreasing the child's ability to participate in the world
- Preterm and low–birth-weight infants are at increased risk compared with typical infants.
- Occupational and other therapies may increase the child's ability to function.

Adapted from Sensory Processing Disorder Foundation. (2016). *About SPD*. Retrieved from http://www.spdfoundation.net/about-sensory-processing-disorder/

Therapeutic Management

Therapeutic management may involve remedial or compensatory approaches or may use interventions directed toward social-emotional problems. The focus of the remedial approach is to improve specific skills. The compensatory approach helps the child to compensate for the disability, rather than attempting to directly correct it. Social-emotional problems may result from frustration or low self-esteem related to capabilities. These may respond to strength based interventions and support.

Consider This

Victor Johnson, a third grader with learning disabilities, tells the nurse, "I get made fun of at school." He begins to sniffle and says, "Everybody calls me stupid. It hurts my feelings." Victor's mother adds "I really just don't know how to help him. . ." How should the nurse reply? What would be the most therapeutic response?

Nursing Assessment

Elicit the health history, noting risk factors such as a family history of learning disability, problems during pregnancy or birth, prenatal alcohol or drug use, low birth weight, premature or prolonged labour, head injury, poor nutritional status or failure to thrive, or lead poisoning. Obtain detailed information about the educational difficulties the child is experiencing (e.g., he or she seems to do fine in math but always reverses letters when reading). A thorough physical examination may reveal clues to comorbid conditions. Ensure that the child has undergone a comprehensive education evaluation with assessment testing to diagnose the specific learning disability. Testing may be performed by a school, educational, developmental, or clinical psychologist; occupational therapist; speech and language therapist; or other developmental specialist, depending on the areas of learning with which the child is experiencing difficulty.

Nursing Management

Each child will need an individualized education plan (IEP) that reflects his or her particular needs, which then must be provided for through the school system. Offer encouragement and support to families as they advocate for their child. Follow up at subsequent health care visits to determine that the child is receiving the services he or she needs to optimize his or her potential for success. The nurse could help advocate for a learning disability designation, by referring the child to their school-based team for designation through the ministry of education in each Canadian province.

Ensure that families are aware of their child's rights under the Canadian Charter of Rights and Freedoms and the Canadian Human Rights Act (Government of Canada, 2016a). However, a recent United Nations review of Canada's actions focusing on children with disabilities and their rights highlighted the lack of data collection in Canada since 2006 (United Nations Convention on the Rights of persons with Disabilities, 2017). Nurses must be aware of provincial and territory disability benefits programs. Information can often be accessed via social and health service networks, for example, the chronic disease program, Yukon Health and Social Services.

Intellectual Disability

ID refers to a functional state in which significant limitations in intellectual status and adaptive behaviour (functioning in daily life) develop before the age of 18 years. ID occurs in about 1% of the population (Pivalizza & Lalani, 2016). Although ID includes the definition of intellectual quotient (IQ) less than 70 to 75, the range of impairments associated with the low IQ are variable. Impairments in the adaptive domains of conceptual, social, or practical assist with determining the severity of ID (from mild to profound) (Pivalizza & Lalani, 2016). Historically, children with ID were labelled with more negative language, however a shift in social norms has resulted in a change to more socially acceptable terms. For example the Diagnostic and Statistical Manual for Mental Disorders (DSM-5) (American Psychiatric Association [APA], 2013) has changed *mental retardation* to *ID* (mild, moderate, or severe). The new nomenclature used in practice is neurodevelopmental disorder which includes a range of conditions such as ID, learning disability, global developmental delay, communications disorders (APA, 2013).

Pathophysiology

For those children with ID the exact cause may remain undiscovered. Often genetic anomalies, prenatal errors in central nervous system development, or exposure of the prenatal developing brain to harmful substances (such as drugs, toxins, alcohol, or tobacco) may be responsible. Infants, children, and youth with ID may also experience associated difficulties including; developmental coordination disorder or ataxia (lack of voluntary coordination of muscle movements). In addition, capacity and capability may be further limited in children with ID if there is an associated sensory processing impairment. ID may be categorized according to severity of impairment across domains. See Table 50.2.

Therapeutic Management

The goal of therapeutic management of children with ID is to provide appropriate educational and social experiences that allow the child an opportunity to reach their full potential. In addition, goals may include exploring how youth may be able to live either independently or with support, engage with community life, and experience leisure and vocational opportunities. A multidisciplinary approach may be used and the child's conceptual, social, practical, and intellectual abilities may drive school placement as well as focus on strategies for optimal learning. The majority of individuals with ID require only minimal support in the school or home setting, and these individuals are able to achieve some level of independence. Only a few children and adults with

TABLE 50.2	SEVERITY OF INTELLECTUAL DISABILITY			
Classification Percentage Affected	IQ (generally)	Conceptual	Social	Practical
Mild 85%	Between 50–55 and 70	Requires academic supports	Immature social skills and personal judgment	Usually independent in activities of daily living
Moderate 10%	Between 35–40 and 50–55	Complex tasks require substantial support	Social cues, judgment and life decisions need regular support	Independent self-care with moderate supports
Severe 3–4%	Between 20–25 and 35–40	Little understanding of written language, time; require extensive supports	Benefit from healthy supportive interactions	Require significant and ongoing supervision for activities of daily living
Profound 1–2%	Less than 20–25	May use objects in a goal-directed fashion	May understand gestures and emotional cues; use nonverbal expression	Dependent upon support for all activities of daily living

ID require extensive support and require long-term care or supervision.

Nursing Assessment

Perform developmental screening at health care checks when there is indication of developmental delays early (CPS, 2012). Obtain a detailed pregnancy and birth history, being sure to note any mental health issues for the mother such as depression and bipolar (can be associated with the odds of having a child with ID; Wang, McDermott, Mann, & Hardin, 2016) as well as ensuring that metabolic screening was completed per province provision. Document sequence and age of attainment of developmental milestones. Note history of motor, visual, and language development and delays or difficulties. Assess the child's health history for risk factors such as preterm or post-term birth, low birth weight, birth injury, prenatal or neonatal infection, prenatal alcohol or drug exposure, genetic syndrome, chromosomal alteration, metabolic disease, exposure to toxins (e.g., lead), head injury or other trauma, nutritional deficiency, cerebral malformation, and other brain disease or mental health disorder. Note history of or concomitant seizure disorder, orthopedic problems, speech problems, or vision or hearing deficit.

For the child with known ID, assess language, sensory, and psychomotor functioning. Determine the child's ability to toilet, dress, and feed himself or herself. Ask the parents about involvement with school and community services and support.

On physical examination note dysmorphic features (possibly very mild) consistent with certain syndromes (e.g., fetal alcohol syndrome; see Box 50.2). Be mindful that fetal alcohol effects can result in a child with behavioural challenges and delay but without a change in physical appearance.

If the history indicates (e.g., birth trauma) a CT or MRI of the head may be performed to evaluate the brain structure. Thyroid function tests may be ordered to rule out thyroid problems (in the child or history in the mother) since these can be linked to behaviour and intellectual development (Andersen, Carlé, Karmisholt, Pedersen, & Andersen, 2017).

Take Note!
Due to the extent of cognition required to understand and produce speech, the most sensitive early indicator of ID is delayed language development.

Nursing Management

When children with ID are admitted to the hospital, usually for some other physical or medical condition such as a chronic condition or dental care (Dunn, Hughes-McCormack, & Cooper, 2017), it is important for the nurse to include the family in care. Working in a family-centred way can support the child, promote continuity of home routines, and ensure the child's dietary needs are met if any special feeding support is required. Maintaining patient safety is critical. Be mindful of any mobility needs, communication needs or limitations, supervision, or environmental or equipment needs the child may have. Provide parents or caregivers with time to explore any worries or concerns and ensure that they can access support and have the opportunity for rest during the child's admission.

Autism Spectrum Disorder

Autism spectrum disorder (ASD), also termed pervasive developmental disorder, is a group of neurodevelopmental disorders with a range of severity. The number of children with ASD in Canada is increasing, with occurrence ranging from approximately one child in 63 to one in 106 being diagnosed with ASD, depending on province (Government of Canada, 2016b; Ng, Montigny, Ofner, & Do, 2017). The spectrum of autism disorder ranges from mild (e.g., Asperger syndrome) to severe. Autistic behaviours may first be noticed in infancy as developmental delays or between the age of 12 and 36 months when the child regresses or loses previously acquired skills. Parental concerns about development may be sensitive indicators of the development of autism. However, diagnosis can be delayed as a result of various factors, including a lack of primary care provider education; resources have been developed to support ongoing education for both families and physicians (Autism Physician Handbook, n.d.).

Pathophysiology

The exact etiology of autism remains unclear, but it may be due to physiological factors (e.g., genetic factors, brain abnormalities, altered chemistry, or disease), chemical factors (e.g., heavy metals, medications), nutritional factors (e.g., vitamin D, socioeconomic barriers), and social

---

BOX 50.2

FETAL ALCOHOL SYNDROME
- Results from in utero alcohol exposure
- Typical facial features include low nasal bridge with short upturned nose, flattened midface, long philtrum with narrow upper lip
- Poor coordination, skeletal abnormalities
- Microcephaly
- Failure to thrive
- Hearing loss

Adapted from Goldson, E., & Reynolds, A. (2014). Child development and behaviour. In W. W. Hay, Jr., M. J. Levin, R. R. Deterding, & M. J. Abzug (Eds.). *Current diagnosis and treatment: Pediatrics* (22nd ed.). New York: McGraw-Hill Education.

factors (i.e., ethnicity, stress, immigration status) (Ng et al., 2017). Children with ASD display impaired social interactions and communication as well as perseverative or stereotypic behaviours. They may fail to develop interpersonal relationships and experience social isolation. Many children with autism are intellectually disabled, requiring lifelong supervision, though some are gifted (Starr, Fookson, Burns, & Bowman-Harvey, 2013).

Therapeutic Management

There are no medications or treatments available to cure autism. The goal of therapeutic management is for the child to reach optimal functioning within the limitations of the disorder. Each child's treatment is individualized; behavioural and communication therapies are very important. Children with ASD respond very well to highly structured educational environments. Be mindful of sensory sensitivities, for example, dislike of noise, tactile dislikes such as avoidance of specific textured surfaces or clothing, or strong odours. Stimulant medication may be used to control hyperactivity, and antipsychotic medications are sometimes helpful in children with repetitive and aggressive behaviours.

Many families use complementary and alternative therapies to support their autistic child such as vitamins, nutritional and herbal supplements, restrictive diets, music therapy, art therapy, and sensory integration techniques. It is important to assess all therapeutic interventions for safety and support families when they must add medical choices in the care of their child which they may view as intrusive or scary.

Nursing Assessment

Elicit the health history, noting delay or regression in developmental skills, particularly speech and language abilities. Failure to point at objects and to gaze at an object jointly with another by 18 months are concerning signs (Goldson & Reynolds, 2014). The child may be mute, utter only sounds (not words), or repeat words or phrases over and over. The parent may report that the infant or toddler spends hours in repetitive activity and demonstrates bizarre motor and stereotypic behaviours. The infant may resist cuddling, lack eye contact, be indifferent to touch or affection, and have little change in facial expression. Toddlers may display hyperactivity, aggression, temper tantrums, or self-injury behaviours, such as head banging or hand biting. The history may also reveal hypersensitivity to touch or hyposensitivity to pain or noise. Assess the child's functional status, including behaviour, nutrition, sleep, speech and language, education needs, and developmental or neurologic limitations. Assist with screening, using an approved autism screening tool such as the Modified Checklist for Autism in Toddlers-Revised (M-CHAT-R), which is recommended for administration at 18 months of age, and then again at 24 to 30 months of age. Additional screening tools include the Social Communication Questionnaire (SCQ) and the Pervasive Developmental Disorders Screening Test-II (PDDST-II).

Perform a thorough physical examination. Observe the infant or toddler for lack of eye contact, failure to look at objects pointed to by the examiner, failure to point to himself or herself, failure to let his or her needs be known, perseverative play activities, and unusual behaviour such as hand flapping or spinning. Measure growth parameters, such as head circumference (macrocephaly or microcephaly may be associated with ASD). Note the presence of large, prominent, or posteriorly rotated ears. Examine the skin for hypo- or hyperpigmented lesions. Note asymmetry of nerve function or palsy, hypertonia, hypotonia, alterations in deep tendon reflexes, toe-walking, loose gait, or poor coordination. Obtain hearing screening results and ascertain that lead screening has been performed.

> **Take Note!**
>
> Screen all infants and toddlers for warning signs of autism:
> - Not babbling by 12 months
> - Not pointing or using gestures by 12 months
> - No single words by 16 months
> - No two-word utterances by 24 months
> - Losing language or social skills at any age (Starr et al., 2013)

Nursing Management

When children are initially diagnosed with autism, provide parents with emotional support, professional guidance, and education about the disorder while they are attempting to adjust to the diagnosis. Assess the fit between the child's developmental needs and the treatment plan. Help parents overcome barriers to obtain appropriate education, developmental, and behavioural treatment programs. Ensure that the child younger than 36 months of age receives services via the local early intervention program and children 3 years and older have an IEP in place if enrolled in preschool. Stress the importance of consistent and predictable routines, as children with ASD often act out when their routine changes (which is likely to occur if the child must be hospitalized for another condition). Assess the parents' need for respite care or autism support groups and make referrals accordingly.

Atraumatic Care

Provide family-centred care, being sure to treat the family not just the child. Minimize parent–child separation.

COMPARISON CHART 50.1	OPPOSITIONAL DEFIANT DISORDER VERSUS CONDUCT DISORDER	
Oppositional Defiant Disorder	**Conduct Disorder**	
• Excessive arguing with adults • Frequent temper tantrums • Active defiance • Revenge-seeking behaviours • Frequent resentment or anger • Touchiness; easily annoyed. • Noncompliance with adult requests or limits • Blaming of others for misbehaviour or mistakes	• Bullying and threatening of others • Initiation of physical fights • Weapon use to cause others harm • Physical cruelty to animals or people • Destruction of property or arson • Lying and stealing • Serious violation of rules: staying out past curfew, truancy, running away • Use of force in sexual activity	

Adapted from Burstein, A., Talmi, A., Stafford, B., & Kelsay, K. (2014). *Child & adolescent psychiatric disorders & psychosocial aspects of pediatrics.* In W. W. Hay, M. J. Levin, R. R. Deterding, & M. J. Abzug (Eds.). *Current pediatric diagnosis and treatment* (22nd ed.). New York: McGraw-Hill.

Attention-Deficit/ Hyperactivity Disorder

ADHD is the most common neurodevelopmental disorder of childhood, affecting nearly 10% of school-age children aged 4 to 17 years (Starr et al., 2013). ADHD is characterized by inattention, impulsivity, distractibility, and hyperactivity. Three subtypes of ADHD exist: hyperactive–impulsive, inattentive, and combined. The child with ADHD has a disruption in learning ability, socialization, and compliance, placing significant demands on the child, parents, teachers, and community. Children with ADHD often have a **comorbidity** (disorder accompanying the primary illness) such as oppositional defiant disorder, conduct disorder, an anxiety disorder, depression, a less severe developmental disorder, an auditory processing disorder, or learning or reading disabilities (Krull, 2016). Comparison Chart 50.1 gives information about oppositional defiant disorder and conduct disorder to distinguish them from ADHD.

Pathophysiology

Though the exact cause of ADHD remains unidentified, current thought includes as its etiology an alteration in the dopamine and norepinephrine neurotransmitter system. The symptoms of impulsivity, hyperactivity, and inattention begin before 7 years of age and persist longer than 6 months. Symptoms exist in the school and home settings, impairing family and social interactions. Children and teens with ADHD experience frustration, labile moods, emotional outbursts, peer rejection, poor school performance, and low self-esteem. They may also have poor metacognitive abilities such as organization, time management, and the ability to break a project down into a series of smaller tasks. They are not lazy or unmotivated, but simply have poor skills in these areas. Box 50.3 provides criteria for the diagnosis of ADHD (Starr et al., 2013).

BOX 50.3

DIAGNOSIS OF ATTENTION-DEFICIT/ HYPERACTIVITY DISORDER

Presence of six or more of the following in the child 17 years of age and younger:
• Failure to pay close attention
• Careless mistakes on schoolwork
• Difficulty paying attention to tasks or play
• Doesn't listen
• Doesn't follow through
• Doesn't complete tasks
• Doesn't understand instructions
• Poorly organized
• Avoids, dislikes, or fails to engage in activities requiring mental effort
• Loses things needed for task completion
• Easily distracted
• Forgetful
• Fidgety or squirmy
• Often out of seat
• Activity inappropriate to the situation
• Cannot engage in quiet play
• Always on the go
• Talks excessively
• Blurts out answers
• Has difficulty waiting his or her turn
• Often interrupts or intrudes on others

Additionally, symptoms have been present in two or more settings, at least two of the symptoms occurred prior to age 12, persistence of symptoms beyond 6 months and to a degree inconsistent with developmental level or negatively interferes with social or academic performance, and symptoms are not associated with purely oppositional behaviour or as a component of a psychotic disorder, and cannot be explained by the diagnosis of a different mental health disorder.

Adapted from French, W. P. (2015). Assessment and treatment of attention-deficit/hyperactivity disorder: Part 1. *Pediatric Annals,* *44*(3), 114–120.

Therapeutic Management

Medication management of ADHD includes the use of psychostimulants, nonstimulant norepinephrine reuptake inhibitors, and/or α-agonist antihypertensive agents. These medications are not a cure for ADHD, but help to increase the child's ability to pay attention and decrease the level of impulsive behaviour. The child's activity level is not usually affected. Behaviour therapy and classroom restructuring may be useful as part of the therapeutic management plan. Since about 50% of ADHD cases persist into adulthood, management should continue throughout adolescence and beyond as needed (Solanto, 2015). Concomitant disorders, such as anxiety, should also be treated (see discussion of anxiety disorders below).

Nursing Assessment

For a full description of the assessment phase of the nursing process, refer to the Assessment section of the Nursing Process Overview. Assessment findings pertinent to ADHD are discussed below.

HEALTH HISTORY

Elicit a description of the maladaptive behaviour or school performance problem. Explore the child's history for risk factors such as head trauma, lead exposure, cigarette smoke exposure, prematurity, or low birth weight. The past history may also reveal a larger than usual number of accidents. Determine if there is a family history of ADHD. Question the parent about school behaviour. The school-age child may be unable to stay on task, talks out of turn, leaves his or her desk frequently, and either neglects to complete in-class and homework assignments or forgets to turn them in. The adolescent may be inattentive in school, poorly organized, and forgetful.

Several behavioural checklists are available that may assist in the diagnosis of ADHD. These may be completed by the child's teacher and/or parent and focus on behaviour patterns related to conduct or learning problems, social competence, anxiety, activity level, and attention. Obtain the completed behavioural checklists (usually one from the parent and one from the teacher) as well as any school records or testing performed examples and advice can be found at HealthLink BC (n.d.) all provinces will have their own resources.

PHYSICAL EXAMINATION

Perform vision and hearing screening to rule out vision or hearing impairment as the cause of poor school performance. Observe the preschool child's behaviour, noting quickness, agility, fearlessness, and the desire to touch or explore everything in the room. The older child or adolescent may have difficulty staying on task during the examination or change the subject frequently while conversing.

LABORATORY AND DIAGNOSTIC TESTS

No definitive laboratory or diagnostic test is available for the identification of ADHD. A complete blood count may be performed to rule out anemia, and thyroid hormone levels may be drawn to determine whether they are normal.

Nursing Management

Having a child with ADHD can be frustrating as the child's inattention, high activity level, impulsivity, and distractibility are often very difficult to deal with. Parents may doubt their ability to be effective parents or may view their child as somehow defective. Children with ADHD may also feel they are bad, faulty, stupid, or intellectually challenged. Provide emotional support, allowing enough time for the family to air their concerns. Work with the child and family to develop goals such as completion of homework, improved communication, or increasing independence in self-care.

Assist the family to advocate for their child's needs through the public school system. The child is entitled to a developmentally appropriate education via an IEP as necessary. The IEP should be updated as needed. Ensure coordination of health and school services and schedule systematic communication with the family and school. Teach families and school personnel to use calming techniques such as snack/water/walk breaks and positive reinforcement. Focus on strengths based independent education plans and incorporate strength building exercises within manageable time frames to attention span. Refer families and youth to local support groups and resource centres.

Explain that stimulant medications should be taken in the morning to decrease the adverse effect of insomnia. Some children may experience decreased appetite, so giving the medication with or after the meal may be beneficial. The child may feel "different" from his or her peers if he or she must visit the school nurse for a lunchtime dose of ADHD medication; this may lead to noncompliance and a subsequent increase in ADHD symptoms, with deterioration in schoolwork. In this situation, encourage the family to explore with their physician or nurse practitioner the option of one of the newer extended-release or once-daily ADHD medications. See Dosage Calculation Box 50.1.

Dosage Calculation Box 50.1

Child's weight: 50 lb
Medication order: start methylphenidate 10 mg PO now.
Per the *Pediatric Dosage Handbook*, for initial dosing, the recommended dose is 0.3 mg/kg/dose.
Is the ordered dose safe?

PANDAS

Pediatric autoimmune neuropsychiatric disorders associated with streptococcal infection (PANDAs) were first described in the late 1990s (Swedo, et al., 1998) as a subset of PANs (pediatric acute-onset neuropsychiatry).

Diagnosis

Since no definitive blood test for PANs or PANDAs exists, collection of a detailed clinical history and in-depth assessment are essential. If there is concern of ongoing strep infection, a throat culture should be ordered. An anti-streptococcal antibody titer may be collected, and if elevated, provides evidence that a child has had a strep infection sometime within the past few months, and they have antibodies (National Institute of Mental Health, 2016). Clinical diagnostic criteria are:

- Signs of OCD or tic disorder
- Onset somewhere between age 3 and puberty
- Episodic course of symptoms
- Association with neurologic abnormalities such as jerky nonpurposeful movements or physical hyperactivity
- Onset or exacerbation is abrupt
- Association with group A β-hemolytic streptococcus (for PANDAs only)
- Other, related symptoms may include: ADHD symptoms, separation anxiety, mood changes, sleep problems, changes in urinary habits or motor skills, or joint pain (National Institute of Mental Health, 2016)

Nursing Assessment

Nurses must elicit a recent health history, taking note, of risk factors such as recent sore throat or throat infection. Any parent or patient reports of changes in motor activity, onset or exacerbation of tics or obsessive-compulsive thoughts or activities, or jerky movements should be noted. The nurse should also examine and observe the child documenting any signs and symptoms linked to PANDAs.

Therapeutic Management

Since PANs and PANDAs are relatively newly identified phenomena, treatment regimens and diagnostic investigation continue to develop. Traditional pharmacologic treatment of tics and OCD, as well as cognitive behavioural therapy can be helpful, depending on the individual presentation (O'Connor & Speros, 2008). Therapies including antibiotics, IVIG, plasma exchange, tonsillectomy, NSAIDs, and corticosteroids may be considered (Sigra et al., 2018).

Nursing Management

Depending on the therapeutic management received, the nurse will need to educate the patient and family about the prescribed medications, such as SSRIs (including signs of adverse effects), or cognitive behavioural therapy (CBT) (O'Connor & Speros, 2008). The nurse provides education about the episodic nature of the diagnosis and the patient or family role in recognizing and reporting changes in symptoms. Follow-up is typically 2 to 4 weeks after initiation of SSRI or CBT.

TOURETTE SYNDROME

Tourette syndrome consists of multiple motor tics and one or more vocal tics occurring either simultaneously or at different times. Children are not tic-free for longer than 3 months. Tics are defined as sudden rapid recurrent stereotypical movements and/or sounds over which the child appears to have no control. Tourette syndrome is estimated to affect up to 1% to 2% of children (Garzon, 2013). Its onset is before 18 years of age.

Comorbid conditions such as ADHD, OCD, and others may occur in up to 60% of children with Tourette syndrome (incidence depending upon the comorbid condition) (Jankovic, 2015). The exact pathophysiologic mechanism of Tourette syndrome has yet to be identified, though genetics does seem to play a part. Therapeutic management is highly individualized and involves psychopharmacology and behavioural therapies. Habit reversal training may help in some children.

Nursing Assessment

Evaluate the health history for the occurrence of tics. The child may be embarrassed or ashamed about the tics and the parents may feel fearful, angry, or guilty. Determine the presence of symptoms of comorbid conditions. Elicit the child's past health history, noting a family history of tics. Assess the child's psychosocial history to determine the extent to which the tics interfere with friendship, school performance, and self-esteem. Observe the child for simple or complex motor tics. Vocal tics such as sniffling, grunting, clicking, or word utterance may occur. Perform a thorough physical examination, which is usually normal.

Nursing Management

Inform families that the tics become more noticeable or severe during times of stress and less pronounced when the child is focused on an activity such as watching TV, reading, or playing a video game. Help the family to build on the child's functional behaviours and adaptive skills to improve the child's self-esteem. Encourage the family to pursue classroom accommodations such as allowing for "tic breaks," taking untimed tests or tests in another room, or using note takers or tape recording. Support the family's decisions related to medication use and therapy and provide appropriate education about the particular drugs and therapies. "Teaching the Tiger" by M. P. Dornbush and S. K. Pruitt (Hope Press) is useful for teachers of the child with Tourette syndrome. For additional support, refer families to Tourette Syndrome Association, Tourette Syndrome Foundation of Canada, or Tourette Syndrome Plus (links to these resources are provided on thePoint).

EATING DISORDERS

Eating disorders include pica, rumination, anorexia nervosa, bulimia and avoidant/restrictive food intake disorder (ARFID). These disorders affect a significant number of children, especially adolescents. Pica, which occurs most frequently in 2- to 3-year olds, is an eating disorder in which the child ingests (over at least a 1-month period) a nonnutritive material such as paint, clay, or sand. Rumination is an eating disorder occurring in infants in which the baby regurgitates partially digested food or formula and expels or swallows it. The numbers of children affected by pica and rumination is not known. ARFID is a complex and a new diagnostic category in the DSM-5. It is characterised by failure to eat to allow for nutritional and/or energy needs resulting in nutritional deficiency, altered growth, and altered psychosocial functioning since there is an inability to eat in the company of others (Katzman and Norris, 2017). This discussion will focus on anorexia nervosa and bulimia, as they are more commonly encountered.

Anorexia nervosa and bulimia are common eating disorders affecting primarily adolescents, though younger children may also be affected. In North America being thin is highly valued, which compounds the problem. The lifetime prevalence rate for anorexia nervosa and bulimia is about 1% each, yet these problems often arise in childhood, particularly adolescence (Garzon, 2013). Anorexia nervosa is characterized by dramatic weight loss because of decreased food intake and sharply increased physical exercise. Bulimia refers to a cycle of normal food intake, followed by binge-eating and then purging. Typically, the adolescent with bulimia remains at a near-normal weight. Complications of anorexia and bulimia include fluid and electrolyte imbalance, decreased blood volume, cardiac arrhythmias, esophagitis, rupture of the esophagus or stomach, tooth loss, and menstrual problems. The 5-year mortality rate for anorexia nervosa is 15% to 20% (Garzon, 2013).

Therapeutic management may occur in either the inpatient or outpatient setting. In either case, a multidisciplinary approach including individual and family therapy and nutritional therapy is needed for the best chance at successful treatment. Atypical antipsychotics or antidepressants may be used, but their effectiveness remains controversial (Garzon, 2013).

Nursing Assessment

Determine the health history, noting risk factors such as family history, female gender, race, preoccupation with appearance, obsessive traits, or low self-esteem. Adolescents with anorexia may have a history of constipation, syncope, secondary amenorrhea, abdominal pain, and periodic episodes of cold hands and feet. Parents usually note the chief complaint as weight loss. Note history of depression in the child with bulimia. Evaluate the child's self-concept, noting multiple fears, high need for acceptance, disordered body image, and perfectionism.

Perform a thorough physical examination. The child or youth with anorexia is usually severely underweight, with a body mass index (BMI) of less than 17. Note cachectic appearance, dry sallow skin, thinning scalp hair, soft sparse body hair, and nail pitting. Measure vital signs, noting low temperature, bradycardia, or hypotension. Auscultate the heart, noting murmur as a result of mitral valve prolapse (occurs in about one third of adolescents with anorexia).

The adolescent with bulimia will be of normal weight or slightly overweight. Inspect the hands for calluses on the backs of the knuckles and split fingernails. Inspect the mouth and oropharynx for eroded dental enamel, red gums, and inflamed throat from self-induced vomiting.

Careful laboratory and diagnostic evaluation of serum electrolytes and an electrocardiogram are needed in adolescents with anorexia because severe electrolyte disturbances and cardiac arrhythmias often occur.

Take Note!

An adolescent with anorexia nervosa would most likely experience amenorrhea, hypothermia, low blood pressure, and bradycardia. The nurse would also note soft hair on the individual's back and arms.

Nursing Management

Most children with eating disorders can be treated successfully on an outpatient basis, though this treatment may require many months. Those with anorexia who display severe weight loss, unstable vital signs, food refusal, or arrested pubertal development or who require enteral nutrition will need to be hospitalized. Refeeding syndrome (cardiovascular, hematologic, and neurologic complications) may occur in the severely malnourished adolescent with anorexia if rapid nutritional replacement is given. Therefore, slow refeeding is essential to avoid complications. Give phosphorus supplements as ordered. Assess vital signs frequently for orthostatic hypotension, irregular and decreased pulse, or hypothermia.

Consult the nutritionist for assistance with calculating caloric needs and determining an appropriate diet.

Aim for a weight gain goal of 0.2 to 1 kg (0.5 to 2 lb) per week. Instruct the child and family to keep a daily journal of intake, **bingeing** (excessive consumption) and **purging** (forced vomiting) behaviours, mood, and exercise. The journal may be used as an assessment tool as well as to document progress toward recovery. Assist the child and family to plan a suitably structured routine for the child that includes meals, snacks, and appropriate physical activity.

Use the physical findings associated with anorexia to educate the child about the consequences of malnutrition and how they can be remedied with adequate nutrient intake. Refer the adolescent, as appropriate, to individual or group therapy. Assess the child's need for medical intervention for concomitant depression or anxiety (they may require psychotropic medications). Provide emotional support and positive reinforcement to the child and family. Refer the family to local support groups or online resources such as the Academy for Eating Disorders or the National Eating Disorders Association (links to these resources are provided on thePoint).

MOOD DISORDERS

Mood disorders in children include depressive disorders and bipolar disorder. It is difficult to quantify the incidence of depression in children under age 5 years, due to lack of sophistication of communication skills. Up to 3% of school-age children and 5% of adolescents may suffer from depression (Garzon, 2013). Children may experience major depressive disorder or dysthymic disorder. Girls are twice as likely to be affected as boys, particularly during the teenage years. Bipolar disorder refers to a condition of alternating manic and depressive episodes and affects about 2.6% of children (Garzon, 2013). During the manic episode, mood is significantly elevated and the child displays excess energy.

Depression may cause significant alterations in school performance and social relationships. Family traumas and social situations may contribute to the development of depression because of the ongoing psychological impact of circumstance and perceptions of hopelessness. Be aware that youth may also have comorbidities such as concurrent substance use, anxiety disorders, and other maladaptive behaviours. The Canadian Mental Health Association suggests that approximately 3.2 million 12- to -19-year olds are at risk of depression (CMHA, n.d.).

Children and adolescents experiencing depressive episodes may harm themselves purposefully (without intent to kill themselves). They may hit, cut, or burn themselves (Goldson & Reynolds, 2014). Additionally, depressed children are at risk for suicide. Across Canada suicide rates vary by province, with higher numbers in some Indigenous communities (CPS, 2015c).

Pathophysiology

Both norepinephrine and dopamine play a role in mood. Norepinephrine is important in the areas of energy and alertness, while dopamine is important in the areas of pleasure and motivation. When alterations in the neurotransmission of norepinephrine and dopamine occur, the symptoms of depression (apathy, loss of interest, and pleasure) result. Decreased levels of serotonin have also been implicated in depressive symptoms. Development of a depressive disorder may be related to genetics, cognitive function, situation, and trauma. Children of parents with a depressive disorder are at an increased risk for developing one themselves. Maladaptive cognitive functions or lack of social skills resulting in negative feelings may also play a role (Garzon, 2013).

Therapeutic Management

Children with mood disorders may benefit from functional goal setting psychotherapy. How the child is coping within his or her environment and having clear goals that are reasonable to work toward can provide the framework for a successful treatment plan. For example, a child with depression may have difficulty with peer relationships from the depression simply as a result of fatigue. Exploring how important this is to the child and how it is affecting his/her ability to perform in school or develop healthy relationships is integral to the treatment plan. A plan of care could then include developing stronger relationships with a few peers rather than expect healthy relationships with numerous different peers to minimize fatigue. Setting small and achievable goals with reasonable expectations often prevents further deterioration in function.

Crisis management, parental counselling, and individual, group, or family therapy may be useful. Major depressive disorder warrants the use of pharmacologic antidepressants. Bipolar disorder may be treated with mood stabilizers or atypical antipsychotics, best combined with psychotherapy (Garzon, 2013).

Take Note!

Closely observe children taking antidepressants for the development of presuicidal behaviour.

Nursing Assessment

Children with untreated depression are at high risk for suicide as well as the development of comorbid disorders such as anxiety disorders, substance abuse, eating disorders, self-harm, and disruptive behavioural disorders (such as conduct disorder) (Burstein et al., 2014). The nurse must screen all children for the development of depression. Assess the child/youth for any sadness or irritability or loss of interest in activities and determine the duration and frequency they report these feelings.

HEALTH HISTORY

Obtain a health history from the child and separately from the parents or caregivers. Evaluate the child for history of recent changes in behaviour, changes in peer relationships, alterations in school performance, withdrawal from previously enjoyed activities, sleep disturbances, changes in eating behaviours, increase in accidents, or sexual promiscuity. If possible, use a standardized depression screening questionnaire; check which tool is used in your local area.

Ask about potential stressors such as school concerns, conflicts with parents, dating issues, and **abuse** (physical or sexual). When bipolar disorder is suspected, the history may reveal rapid, pressured speech; increased energy/mania; decreased sleep; grandiose thoughts; and irritability.

Note history of weight loss, failure to thrive, or increased incidence of infections in the infant. For the toddler, note delay or regression in developmental skills, increase in nightmares, or parental reports of clinginess. The preschooler may have a history of loss of interest in newly acquired skills; manifest encopresis, enuresis, anorexia, or binge-eating; or make frequent negative self-statements. The parents of a school-age child may report that he or she has a depressed, irritable, or aggressive mood.

Assess risk factors and warning signs for suicide, which include:

- Previous suicide attempt of self/family member or member of peer group
- Change in school performance, sleep, or appetite
- Loss of interest in activities/increased risk taking behaviour
- Feelings of hopelessness or depression
- Statements/writings/drawings about suicide
- Trauma history (sexual, physical, emotional, intergenerational, neglect, loss, medical illness)
- Suicidal thoughts—assess if child has a plan

Nursing Management

Nursing management of children and adolescents with mood disorders focuses on education and support, as well as involvement with programs such as functional goal setting and prevention of depression and suicide.

EDUCATING AND SUPPORTING THE CHILD AND FAMILY

Teach families that mood disorders are biologic conditions, not personality flaws. Comparing depression to other biologic disorders such as diabetes and asthma is often a good way to help parents understand this. Teach families how to administer antidepressant medication and

---

> **BOX 50.4**
>
> ### SCREENING TOOLS FOR DEPRESSION
>
> The following tools are used to screen for depression. Links to each of these screening tools are provided on thePoint.
> - Children's Depression Rating Scale-Revised (CDRS-R)
> - Center for Epidemiological Studies Depression Scale Modified for Children (CES-DC)
> - Weinberg Depression Scale for Children and Adolescents (WDSCA)
> - Children's Depression Inventory (CDI)
> - Beck Depression Inventory for Youth (BDI-Y)

to monitor for adverse effects. Encourage the child's and family's efforts at following through with cognitive and behavioural therapies. Support the family throughout the process, as sometimes treatment may be lengthy. Refer parents to local support resources or to the Depression and Bipolar Support Alliance or the Child and Adolescent Bipolar Foundation.

traumatic Care

Promote a family's sense of control through effective communication and teaching and providing the family with appropriate resources and referrals.

PREVENTING DEPRESSION AND SUICIDE

Build a trusting relationship with the children and adolescents with whom you interact. Be consistent and provide safety during all interactions. Screen all healthy and chronically ill preteens and teens for the development of depression (Burstein et al., 2014). Use standardized screening tools such as those listed in Box 50.4. When a potential problem is identified, refer the child for mental health assessment and intervention immediately. It is important to identify depression early so that treatment can start. When a grief-inducing event is impending (such as the death of a family member), begin preventive intervention to help the child cope with the loss. Manage suicidal ideation as per facility guidelines.

ANXIETY DISORDERS

Anxiety disorders are the most commonly diagnosed psychiatric conditions among children and adolescents with prevalence ranging from 10% to 30% (Bennett & Walkup, 2016). Anxiety often occurs together with other mental health disorders, especially depression. Normal children experience fear, worry, and shyness. Infants fear loud noises, being startled, and strangers. Toddlers are afraid of the dark and of separation. Preschoolers fear imaginary creatures and body mutilation. School-age children worry about injury and natural events, whereas adolescents are anxious about bodily appearance, school and social performance. These normal fears produce a certain level of anxiety that is tolerated by most children, but it is important to distinguish normal developmentally appropriate anxiety from an anxiety disorder.

Anxiety is a reaction to a perceived or actual threat. Regardless, the emotional distress leads to a neurochemical response known as "fight-or-flight." The fight response results in tachycardia, increased blood pressure, sweating, enhanced arousal and reactivity, tremors, and increased blood flow to the muscles, and the flight response can be complete dissociation (Garzon, 2013). Anxiety that affects day-to-day functioning of the child such as refusal to attend school or get out of bed in the morning is a concern. How the child responds and handles the anxious thoughts are also areas that need to be explored.

Thinking About Development

Consider the issue of military deployment of a parent. How might a toddler or preschooler react to the parent's absence and return as contrasted to the response of an adolescent? What types of mental health concerns might be manifested in either group?

Types of Anxiety Disorders

Generalized anxiety disorder (GAD) is characterized by unrealistic concerns over past behaviour, future events, and personal competence. Social phobia is a disorder characterized by the child or teen demonstrating a persistent fear of speaking or eating in front of others, using public restrooms, or speaking to authorities. Selective mutism refers to a persistent failure to speak. Separation anxiety is more common in children than adolescents. In this disorder, the child may need to remain close to the parents, and the child's worries focus on separation themes. OCD is characterized by compulsions (repetitive behaviours such as cleaning, washing, or checking something), which the child performs to reduce anxiety about obsessions (unwanted and intrusive thoughts). Posttraumatic stress disorder (PTSD) is an anxiety disorder that occurs after a child experiences a traumatic event, later experiencing physiologic arousal when a stimulus triggers memories of the event.

Pathophysiology

Anxiety disorders are thought to occur because of disrupted modulation within the central nervous system. Underactivation of the serotonergic system and overactivation of the noradrenergic system are thought to be responsible for dysregulation of physiologic arousal and the resulting emotional experience. Disruption of the γ-aminobutyric acid (GABA) system may also play a role. Genetic factors may also play a role in the development of anxiety disorders, as may family and environmental influences. Additionally, abnormal thoughts or behaviours may have been learned through observation or conditioning (Bennett & Walkup, 2016; Garzon, 2013).

Therapeutic Management

Therapeutic management of anxiety disorders generally involves the use of pharmacologic agents and psychological therapies. Anxiolytics or antidepressants are the most common pharmacologic approaches. Cognitive-behavioural therapy; individual, family, or group psychotherapy; and other stress reducing techniques may also be useful.

Nursing Assessment

Children and adolescents do not usually express anxiety directly. Therefore, it is very important for the nurse to evaluate somatic complaints and perform a careful health history.

HEALTH HISTORY

Explore the child's current and past medical history for risk factors such as depression, anxious temperament, family history of anxiety disorders, certain environmental or life experiences (such as parental dysfunction or significant stressful event or trauma), or unstable parental attachment. Elicit the health history, noting history of social inhibition, panic, or "heart racing." Young children may display overactivity, acting out, sleep difficulties, or separation issues. Older children may describe feelings of nervousness, anger, fear, or tension and may display disruptive behaviour. Ask the child to choose a number on a scale from 0 to 10 to describe how much he or she worries about things. Have the parent rank the child's worry in the same fashion, and ask the parent what the child worries about most. Determine frequency of headaches and stomachaches. Use a standardized screening tool such as the Multidimensional Anxiety Scale for Children (MASC), Spence Children's Anxiety Scale (SACS), Preschool Anxiety Scale, and Beck Anxiety Inventory for Youth.

PHYSICAL EXAMINATION

Perform a complete physical examination to rule out physiologic causes of the child's symptoms. Note patches of hair loss that occur with repetitive hair twisting or pulling associated with anxiety. Evaluate for evidence of nail biting, sucking blisters, or skin erosion from finger rubbing. Inspect the entire body for signs of self-injury, which may or may not be present.

Nursing Management

Screen children at health care visits, as well as upon admission to the hospital, for anxiety symptoms. If an anxiety disorder is suspected, refer the child to the appropriate mental health provider for further evaluation. When the child is diagnosed with an anxiety disorder and medication is prescribed, teach families about medication administration and adverse effects. Encourage follow-through with supportive therapies, and provide emotional support and healthy attachment between the child and family. Assess for parental anxiety through a strengths based and nonjudgmental approach.

ABUSE AND VIOLENCE

Abuse and violence contribute significantly to mental illness in children. Children may suffer from child maltreatment, Munchausen syndrome (fabricated illness or factitious disorder), or substance use disorder (SUD).

Child Maltreatment

Child maltreatment includes physical abuse, sexual abuse, emotional abuse, and neglect with some provinces including exposure to domestic violence as a fifth risk (Canadian Child Welfare, n.d.). Physical abuse refers to injuries that are intentionally inflicted on a child and result in morbidity or mortality. Sexual abuse refers to involvement of the child in any activity meant to provide sexual gratification to an adult and includes female genital mutilation. Emotional abuse may be verbal denigration of the child or occur because of the child witnessing domestic violence. **Neglect** is defined as failure to provide a child with appropriate food, clothing, shelter, medical care, and schooling (Chiesa & Sirotnak, 2014).

Statistics related to family violence as well as child physical and sexual abuse is difficult to determine, as the perpetrator usually forces the victim into silence. Children usually do not want to admit that their parent or relative has hurt them, partly from feelings of guilt and partly because they do not want to lose that parent. In 2011, 3.4 million referrals to child protective services were made alleging child maltreatment in 6.2 million children, yet this may be an underestimate of the prevalence of child abuse (Chiesa & Sirotnak, 2014). Abuse and violence occur across all socioeconomic levels but are more prevalent among the poor, and the largest percentage of those affected are under 3 years of age. Despite the lack of adequate statistics, it is well known that the problem of abuse and violence is widespread. Parents or caregivers are the most frequent perpetrators of abuse against children (Chiesa & Sirotnak, 2014).

A history of childhood abuse is associated with the development of depressive disorders, suicidal ideation and attempts (Martin, Dykxhoorn, Afifi, & Colman, 2016), anxiety disorders, and alcohol and drug use. Abuse may result in significant physical injury, poor physical health, and, in some cases, impaired brain development. Being a victim of abuse places children at risk for low self-esteem, poor academic achievement, poor emotional health, and social difficulties. Additional long-term consequences include juvenile delinquency and perpetuation of the violence cycle (Lindert et al., 2014).

Therapeutic management of victims of abuse and violence involves physical treatment of the injury, palliative care in some cases, and intervention to preserve or restore the child's mental well-being as well as family functioning. To protect children, all provinces require by law that health care professionals report suspected cases of child abuse or neglect (Child and Family Services Act, 1990).

Nursing Assessment

Elicit the health history, noting the chief complaint and timing of onset. Assess for appropriateness of the parent–child attachment (often altered in the case of neglect). Pay attention to statements made by the child's parent or caretaker. Is the history given consistent with the child's injury? Identify abuse and violence by screening all children and families using these questions:
- Questions for children:
  - Are you afraid of anyone at home?
  - Who could you tell if someone hurt you or touched you in a way that made you uncomfortable?
  - Has anyone hurt you or touched you in that way?
- Questions for parents:
  - Are you afraid of anyone at home?
  - Do you ever feel like you may hit or hurt your child when frustrated?

Assess for risk factors in children and parents or caretakers. Risk factors for abuse in children include poverty, prematurity, cerebral palsy, chronic illness, or ID. Risk factors for being abusers in parents or caretakers include a history of being abused themselves, alcohol or substance abuse, or extreme stress.

Determine if the child has a history of hurting self or others (e.g., cutting), running away, attempting **suicide** (taking one's own life), or being involved in high-risk behaviours. Note inappropriate sexual behaviour for developmental age, such as seductiveness, as this may indicate sexual abuse. Note history of chronic sore throat or difficulty swallowing, which may occur with forced oral sex or sexually transmitted infections. Document history of genital burning or itching or smearing (associated with sexual abuse). Note nonspecific symptoms of emotional abuse such as low self-confidence, sleep disturbance, hypervigilance, headaches, or stomachaches.

Take Note!

A delay in seeking medical treatment, a history that changes over time, or a history of trauma that is inconsistent with the observed injury all suggest child abuse.

PHYSICAL EXAMINATION

When conducting the physical examination (following sexual assault or rape) follow local policy and have forensic examination training and skills. Samples and images are likely to be collected for later prosecution where any form of physical or sexual abuse is investigated (Caring for Kids New to Canada, n.d.). Observe the parent–child interaction, noting fear or an excessive desire to please. Note the infant's level of consciousness. Vigorous shaking in the infant leads to intracranial hemorrhage and shaken baby syndrome. Inspect the skin for bruises, burns, cuts, abrasions, contusions, scars, and any other unusual or suspicious marks. Current or healed scratches or cuts may be found on parts of the body ordinarily covered by clothing in the child who self-mutilates. Burns that occur in a stocking or glove pattern, or only to the soles or palms, are highly suspicious for inflicted burns. Injuries in various stages of healing are also indicative of abuse. Bruises on the chest, head, neck, or abdomen are suspicious for abuse. Nonambulatory children infrequently experience bruises or fractures. Figure 50.1 shows injury sites usually indicative of abuse; Figure 50.2 is a photograph of a child who was beaten with an electric cord. Observe for inflammation of the oropharynx (may occur with forced oral sex).

FIGURE 50.2 Note the mark left from a looped electric cord.

LABORATORY AND DIAGNOSTIC TESTS

Common laboratory and diagnostic studies ordered for the assessment of abuse include:

- Radiographic skeletal survey or bone scan may reveal current or past fractures.
- CT scan of the head may reveal intracranial hemorrhage.
- Rectal, oral, vaginal, or urethral specimens may reveal sexually transmitted infections such as gonorrhea or chlamydia.

Nursing Management

Refer suspected cases of neglect or abuse to the local child protection agency. When abusive activity is identified in the hospital, notify the social services and risk management departments. In addition to physical or palliative care needed for the injuries, abused children need to redevelop a sense of trust in adults. Provide consistent care to the abused child by assigning a core group of nurses. Child abuse requires a multidisciplinary approach that may include psychological therapy for the child and family.

Role model appropriate caretaking activities to the parent or caregiver. Call attention to normal growth and development activities noted in the infant or child, as sometimes parents have expectations of child behaviour that may be unrealistic based on the child's age, leading to the abuse. Praise parents and caretakers for taking appropriate steps toward getting help and for providing appropriate care to the child. Refer parents to Parents Anonymous, an organization dedicated to the prevention of child abuse through strengthening of the family.

When it is determined by the child protective team that the child would be in danger to continue living in the current situation, the child may be removed from the

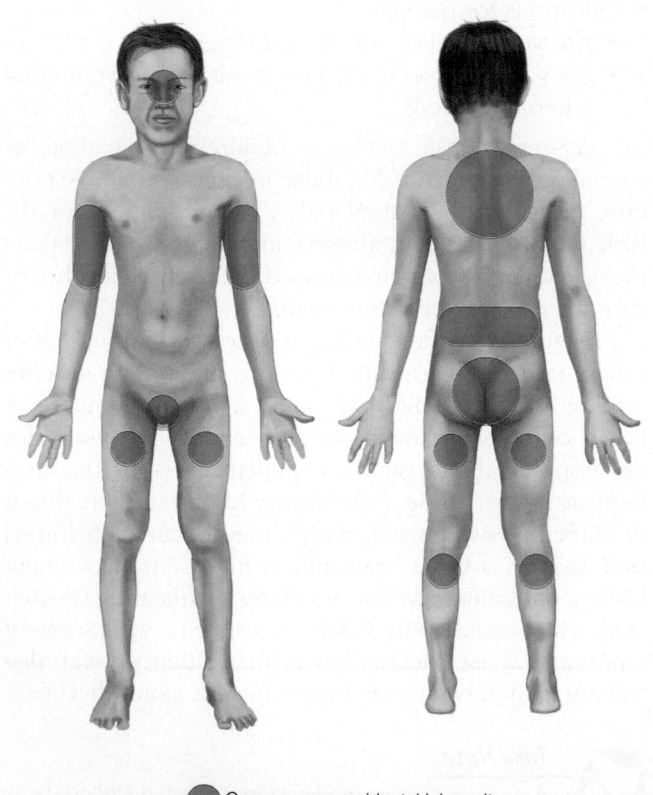

● Common nonaccidental injury sites

FIGURE 50.1 Injury sites that are suspicious for abuse.

EVIDENCE-BASED PRACTICE 50.1 | **CARE BY RELATIVES FOR CHILDREN REMOVED FROM HOME FOR MALTREATMENT**

STUDY

Annually, large numbers of children are removed from their homes due to maltreatment. Child protection agencies are tasked with attempting to ensure the well-being and safety of these children, and in many cases, a sense of permanency. Usually, children removed from their home display an increased prevalence of educational, behavioural, and psychological problems than their peers.

The authors reviewed 102 controlled experimental and quasi-experimental studies involving over 660,000 children. The studies compared child welfare outcomes related to well-being, safety, or permanency in children placed in kinship foster as opposed to those placed in non-kinship care.

Findings

Results from this review demonstrate that children placed in kinship foster care demonstrated fewer behavioural problems, fewer mental health disorders, less placement disruption, better well-being, and less use of mental health services, than those placed in non-kinship care.

Nursing Implications

Encourage families to explore the possibility of adding BT/CBT to the treatment plan. Assist families with finding an appropriate provider of BT/CBT in their local area. Praise children and families for ongoing dedication to BT/CBT. Continue to offer emotional support to all members of the family throughout the treatment process.

Adapted from Winokur, M., Holtan, A., & Valentine, D. (2014). *Kinship care for the safety, permanency, and well-being of children removed from the home for maltreatment. The Cochrane Library 2014, 1.* Indianapolis, IN: John Wiley & Sons.

---

home. If the child is removed from the family temporarily or permanently, provide the foster or adoptive family with education necessary to assume the child's care. See Evidence-Based Practice 50.1.

Medical Child Abuse (Munchausen Syndrome)

Medical child abuse has historically been termed Munchausen syndrome by proxy (MSBP) but depending on country or area it is also termed fabricated illness or factitious disorder. It is a type of child abuse in which the parent (or sometimes the child) creates physical and/or psychological symptoms of illness or impairment in the child. The adult meets his or her own psychological needs by having an ill child. Medical child abuse is difficult to detect and may remain hidden for years. In most cases, the biologic mother is the perpetrator (Roesler & Jenny, 2016). Therapeutic management focuses on ensuring the safety and well-being of the child, as well providing psychotherapy for the perpetrator.

Nursing Assessment

Take a thorough and detailed health history of the child's illness or illnesses. Use quotations to document the parent's responses. Warning signs of medical child abuse include:

- Child with one or more illnesses that do not respond to treatment or that follow a puzzling course; a similar history in siblings
- Symptoms that do not make sense or that disappear when the perpetrator is removed or not present; the symptoms are witnessed only by the caregiver (e.g., cyanosis, apnea, seizure)

- Physical and laboratory findings that do not fit with the reported history
- Repeated hospitalizations failing to produce a medical diagnosis, transfers to other hospitals, discharges against medical advice
- Parent who refuses to accept that the diagnosis is not medical (Chiesa & Sirotnak, 2014; Roesler & Jenny, 2016)

Observe the mother's behaviour with the child, spouse or partner, and staff. Use of covert video surveillance has been reported in some countries and remains controversial. Perform a thorough physical examination, noting where the physical examination findings differ from the reported health history.

Nursing Management

Management of medical child abuse is complex. When abusive activity is identified, notify the social services and risk management departments of the hospital. Ensure that the local child protection team and the caregiver's family or support system is present when the caregiver is confronted. Inform the caregiver of the plan of care for the child and of the availability of psychiatric assistance for the caregiver.

Substance Abuse

Substance use most often begins before age 20. The 2013 Canadian Alcohol and Drug Use Monitoring Survey indicated that young people aged 15 to 24 years reported the highest self-reported use of illicit substances in the population (Canadian Centre on Substance Use and Addiction, n.d.). In addition to alcohol (regularly and binge drinking), youth also use cocaine, heroin, methamphetamines, inhalants, ecstasy, nonprescribed steroids, and prescription drugs not intended for them such as fentanyl (Government of Canada, 2017).

Nursing Assessment

Note risk factors for substance abuse, such as family history of substance abuse, current parental substance use, dysfunctional family relationships, concurrent mental health disorder, aggressive behaviours, low self-esteem or poor academic performance, negative life events, poor social skills, or peers who use substances. Determine the child's history, noting altered school performance or attendance, changes in peer group participation, frequent mood swings, changes in physical appearance, or an altered relationship with or perception of parents. Document history of insomnia, appetite loss, excessive itching, sleepiness or extreme fatigue, dry mouth, or shakiness. Note violent behaviour, drunkenness, stupor, blank expression, drowsiness, lack of coordination, confusion, incoherent speech, extremes in emotions, aggressive behaviour, silly behaviour, or rapid speech. Perform a complete physical examination. Observe for an odour of alcohol. Assess the eyes, noting wateriness or dilated pupils. Inspect the nares, noting rhinorrhea or absence of nasal hair. Inspect the fingers for glue smears or discolouration and the skin for needle marks or tracks. Palpate the hands and feet for coolness.

Laboratory and diagnostic tests include toxicology studies, such as urine screening, to determine the presence of stimulants, sedative–hypnotics, barbiturates, hallucinogens, opiates, cocaine, and marijuana.

Nursing Management

Help the adolescent to acknowledge that he or she has a problem. Explain the negative consequences of substance use and raise the teen's awareness of risks. Remain empathetic, yet leave responsibility with the adolescent. Key nursing interventions include promoting participation in treatment programs and preventing substance abuse.

PROMOTING PARTICIPATION IN TREATMENT PROGRAMS

Refer the adolescent to an SUD program. Outpatient or day treatment programs are useful in most situations. Family-based programs produce the highest level of recovery. Serious addiction, the presence of one or more comorbid psychiatric conditions, or suicidal ideation requires residential treatment or hospitalization.

PREVENTING SUBSTANCE ABUSE

Establish a trusting relationship with children and adolescents in order to improve acceptance of education about substance use and to provide a safe environment for confiding about their problems. Screen all children and adolescents for risk factors. During routine psychosocial screening, be alert to alterations as noted earlier. Teach all children, beginning at the elementary school level (or earlier in some high-risk communities), that all chemicals have the potential to be harmful to the body, including tobacco, alcohol, and illicit drugs. Educate children and adolescents that no matter which administration route is used, the drug still enters the body and affects it (negatively). Help children to learn problem-solving skills that they can call upon in the future rather than relying on drugs or other substances to avoid their problems. Teach children to "just say no." Reinforce that they are the ones who have control over their body and what they expose it to. Encourage children to participate in the local community DARE program (Drug Abuse Resistance Education) and praise them for completing it. Teach parents that being involved in their child's social life and knowing where they are and with whom when they are outside of the home is an important step toward limiting substance exposure.

NURSING CARE PLAN 50.1

Overview for the Child With a Mental Health Disorder

NURSING DIAGNOSIS: Impaired social interaction related to altered social skills as evidenced by impulsivity, intrusive behaviour, inability to follow through, anxiety, depressed mood, feelings of unattractiveness or unworthiness

Outcome Identification and Evaluation

The child will demonstrate socially acceptable skills, interacting successfully with peers and in the educational setting, completing tasks as required.

NURSING CARE PLAN 50.1

Overview for the Child With a Mental Health Disorder (continued)

Interventions: *Promoting Appropriate Social Interaction*

- Identify factors that may aggravate the child's performance to minimize stimuli that exacerbate the child's undesired behaviours.
- Modify the environment to decrease distracting stimuli as the child's ability to deal with external stimuli may be impaired.
- Ensure that the child hears his or her name and makes eye contact prior to conversing or instructions so that the child is engaged and has increased ability to follow through.
- State expectations for tasks or behaviours clearly as understanding is necessary to ensure completion.
- Provide positive feedback for appropriate behaviours or task completion, encouraging the child to adopt expectations into his behaviours and routine.

NURSING DIAGNOSIS: Ineffective coping related to inability to deal with life stressors as evidenced by few or no meaningful friendships, inability to empathize or give/receive affection, low self-esteem, or maladaptive coping behaviours such as substance abuse

Outcome Identification and Evaluation

The child will demonstrate improved coping, *verbalize feelings, socially engage, demonstrate problem-solving skills.*

Interventions: *Promoting Coping Skills*

- Encourage discussion of thoughts and feelings, as this is an initial step toward learning to deal with them appropriately.
- Provide positive feedback for appropriate discussion, as this increases the likelihood of continuing performance.
- Demonstrate unconditional acceptance of the child as a person to increase self-esteem in the child who has been feeling rejection.
- Set clear limits on behaviour as needed so the child has a structure to adhere to.
- Teach the child problem-solving skills as an alternative to acting-out behaviours.
- Role model appropriate social and conversation skills so the child can see what is expected in a nonthreatening manner.

NURSING DIAGNOSIS: Imbalanced nutrition, less than body requirements, related to intake insufficient to meet metabolic needs as evidenced by weight loss, failure to gain weight, less-than-expected increases in stature and weight, loss of appetite, or refusal to eat

Outcome Identification and Evaluation

The child or adolescent will demonstrate appropriate growth, *making gains in weight and stature as appropriate.*

Interventions: *Improving Nutritional Intake*

- Provide favourite foods to encourage the child with poor appetite to eat more.
- Assist families to choose nutrient-rich foods so that the food the child does eat is most beneficial.

For the child with an eating disorder:

- Mutually establish a contract related to treatment *to promote the child's sense of control.*
- Provide mealtime structure, *as clear limits let the child know what the expectations are.*
- Encourage the child to choose foods and timing of meals *to develop independence in eating habits.*
- Ensure the eating environment is pleasant and relaxed, with minimal distractions, *to minimize the child's anxiety and guilt about not eating.*
- Withdraw attention if the child refuses to eat: *secondary gain is minimized if refusal to eat is ignored.*
- Provide continuous supervision during the meal and for 30 minutes following it so that the child cannot conceal or dispose of food or induce vomiting.

(continued)

Overview for the Child With a Mental Health Disorder (continued)

NURSING DIAGNOSIS: Risk for delayed development related to disability, behavioural disorder, or altered nutrition

Outcome Identification and Evaluation

Child will demonstrate progress toward developmental milestones: *child expresses interest in the environment and people around him or her, interacts with environment in an age-appropriate way.*

Interventions: *Promoting Development*

- Use therapeutic play and adaptive toys *to facilitate developmental functioning.*
- Provide stimulating environment when possible *to maximize potential for growth and development.*
- Praise accomplishments and emphasize the child's abilities *to improve self-esteem and encourage feelings of confidence and competence.*

- Follow through with physical, occupational, and speech therapists' recommendations *to maximize exposure to exercises designed to increase the child's skills.*
- Determine parents' expectations of the child's future achievement *to help them work toward these goals.*

NURSING DIAGNOSIS: Acute or chronic confusion related to behavioural disorder, depression, anxiety, abusive situation, or substance abuse as evidenced by distractibility, non–reality-based thinking, hypervigilance, or inaccurate interpretation of interactions of others

Outcome Identification and Evaluation

Child's consciousness, attention, cognition, and perception will improve: *child will demonstrate appropriate orientation, remain free from physical harm, and perform activities of daily living as able.*

Interventions: *Reducing Confusion*

- Observe for causes of altered thought processes to provide a baseline for assessment and intervention.
- Perform an age-appropriate mental status examination to determine extent of altered thinking.
- Adjust communication style based on the child's cues to improve communication.

- Listen carefully and seek clarification to determine basis for the child's agitation or other behaviours.
- Provide validation of the child's thoughts and feelings to improve trust in the relationship.
- Establish a daily routine to provide the child with a sense of security.

NURSING DIAGNOSIS: Hopelessness related to child's perception of his or her life situation, negative life view, or alteration in mental well-being as evidenced by passivity, verbalization, alterations in sleep, or lack of initiative

Outcome Identification and Evaluation

Child will display a sense of hope: will verbalize feelings, participate in care, make positive statements.

NURSING CARE PLAN 50.1

Overview for the Child With a Mental Health Disorder (continued)

Interventions: *Promoting Hope*

- Monitor and document potential for suicide, as hopelessness often leads to suicidal ideation.
- Assist the child to identify reasons for hope and for living, so the nurse is aware of the child's values.
- Help the child to set goals that are important to him or her to allow the child to see possibilities.
- Encourage simple decision making on a daily basis, as hopelessness often occurs as a response to loss of control.

- Assist the child to identify positive qualities in himself or herself and his or her life to facilitate the development of hope.
- Involve parents or others the child loves in the child's care as social support is critical to the development of hope.

NURSING DIAGNOSIS: Caregiver role strain related to long-term care of the child with a chronic mental health disorder as evidenced by fatigue, inattention to own needs, conflict, or ambivalence

Outcome Identification and Evaluation

The child's caregiver will participate in the child's care, *verbalizing the child's needs and treatment plan and demonstrating skills necessary for care.*

Interventions: *Decreasing Role Strain*

- Teach the parent or caregiver about the child's illness, treatments, and medications *to clarify expectations for the child and parent.*
- Role model appropriate interaction behaviours with the child *so the parent can learn these techniques by watching.*
- Encourage structure in daily routines *to allow the parent to meet his or her own needs and allow for adequate rest.*

- Gradually increase the parent's responsibility related to care of the child *to help the parent feel less overwhelmed.*
- Allow the parent to move at his or her own pace in assuming care *to enhance the chances for success.*
- Help the parent to identify a back-up caregiver *so the parent has times of respite from constant involvement with the child.*

KEY CONCEPTS

- Mental health and behavioural disorders account for the bulk of the "new morbidity" among children and adolescents.
- The child with behavioural problems or mental health issues often has difficulty in the areas of school, peer relationships, and the family, all of which may worsen the child's self-concept, further hindering his or her emotional health.
- Developmental screening is a key component in the evaluation of a child's mental health.
- Various screening tools are available for depression, ADHD, and anxiety.

- Children with autism spectrum disorder often have impaired social interactions as well as altered communication.
- Learning disabilities and ADHD have a significant negative impact on the child's potential for appropriate education.
- Individualized education plans help children with learning disabilities, intellectual disability, and ADHD receive the educational support they require to optimize their educational capacity.
- Provide support and education to children with mood or anxiety disorders and their families.

- Educating parents about medication administration and its adverse effects is a critical aspect of nursing management of the child with a mental health disorder.

- Provide nutritional replacement at the appropriate pace in the child with anorexia nervosa. Monitor the child closely for the development of refeeding syndrome.

- A key nursing function is screening all children and their families for abuse and violence.

- Report suspected cases of child abuse to the appropriate authorities.

- Educate children about the dangers associated with substance abuse. Reward and praise children and adolescents who do not experiment with or use alcohol or illicit drugs.

REFERENCES AND RECOMMENDED READINGS

American Psychiatric Association (APA). (2013). *Diagnostic and statistical manual of mental disorders* (5th ed.). Retrieved from https://www.psychiatry.org/psychiatrists/practice/dsm

Andersen, S. L., Carlé, A., Karmisholt, J., Pedersen, I. B., & Andersen, S. (2017). MECHANISMS IN ENDOCRINOLOGY: Neurodevelopmental disorders in children born to mothers with thyroid dysfunction: evidence of fetal programming?. *European Journal of Endocrinology, 177*(1), R27–R36.

Autism Physician Handbook. (n.d.) Autism Canada. Retrieved from http://autismcanada.org/wp-content/uploads/2016/05/PhyHandbook_Eng051116-2.pdf

Bennett, S., & Walkup, J. T. (2016). Anxiety disorders in children: Epidemiology, pathogenesis, clinical manifestations, and course. Retrieved from http://www.uptodate.com/contents/anxiety-disorders-in-children-and-adolescents-epidemiology-pathogenesis-clinical-manifestations-and-course

Burstein, A., Talmi, A., Stafford, B., & Kelsay, K. (2014). Child & adolescent psychiatric disorders & psychosocial aspects of pediatrics. In W. W. Hay, M. J. Levin, R. R. Deterding, & M. J. Abzug (Eds.). *Current pediatric diagnosis and treatment* (22nd ed.). New York: McGraw-Hill.

Canadian Centre on Substance use and Addiction. (n.d.). Children and youth. Retrieved from http://www.cclt.ca/Eng/topics/Children-and-Youth/Pages/default.aspx

Canadian Child Welfare, Research Portal. (n.d.). Child abuse and neglect. Retrieved from http://cwrp.ca/child-abuse-neglect

Canadian Institute Health Information (CIHI). (n.d.). *Child and Youth mental health in Canada*. Retrieved from https://www.cihi.ca/en/child-and-youth-mental-health-in-canada-infographic

Canadian Mental health Association. (n.d.). *Children, youth and depression*. Retrieved from http://www.cmha.ca/mental_health/children-and-depression/#.WW7-YjPMzMI

Canadian Paediatric Society (CPS). (2012). *Getting help sooner: New book helps doctors diagnose and treat children with learning problems*. Retrieved from https://www.cps.ca/en/media/book-helps-doctors-diagnose-and-treat-children-with-learning-problems

Canadian Paediatric Society (CPS). (2015a). *Mental health: Screening tools and rating scales*. Retrieved from http://www.cps.ca/en/tools-outils/mental-health-screening-tools-and-rating-scales

Canadian Paediatric Society (CPS). (2015b). *Early childhood development: First years first*. Retrieved from http://www.cps.ca/first-debut

Canadian Paediatric Society (CPS). (2015c). *Suicidal ideation and behaviour*. Retrieved from http://www.cps.ca/documents/position/suicidal-ideation-and-behaviour

Caring for Kids New to Canada. (n.d.). *A mindful approach: Assessing child maltreatments in a multicultural setting*. Retrieved from http://www.kidsnewtocanada.ca/screening/maltreatment

Chiesa, A., & Sirotnak, A. P. (2014). Child abuse & neglect. In W. W. Hay, M. J. Levin, R. R. Deterding, & M. J. Abzug (Eds.). *Current pediatric diagnosis and treatment* (22nd ed.). New York: McGraw-Hill.

Child and family Services Act. (1990). *Version e-Laws*. Retrieved from https://www.ncjrs.gov/pdffiles1/Digitization/128329NCJRS.pdf

Chronic Disease Program. (n.d.). Yukon health and social services. Retrieved from http://www.hss.gov.yk.ca/chronicdisease.php

Clinical Best Practice Guidelines. (2012). *Promoting Safety: Alternative approaches to the use of restraints*. Retrieved from http://rnao.ca/sites/rnao-ca/files/Promoting_Safety_-_Alternative_Approaches_to_the_Use_of_Restraints_0.pdf

Diamond, J. S., Abdoo, D. C., Brady, M. A., & Dunn, A. M. (2013). Role relationships. In C. E. Burns, A. M. Dunn, M. A. Brady, N. B. Starr, & C. G. Blosser (Eds.). *Pediatric primary care* (5th ed.). Philadelphia, PA: Saunders.

Dunn, K., Hughes-McCormack, L., & Cooper, S. A. (2018). Hospital admissions for physical health conditions for people with intellectual disabilities: Systematic review. *Journal of Applied Research in Intellectual Disabilities, 31*, 1–10.

Forman, S. F. (2016). Eating disorders: Overview of epidemiology, diagnosis, and course of illness. Retrieved from http://www.uptodate.com/contents/eating-disorders-overview-of-epidemiology-diagnosis-and-course-of-illness

French, W. P. (2015). Assessment and treatment of attention-deficit/hyperactivity disorder: Part 1. *Pediatric Annals, 44*(3), 114–120.

Garzon, D. L. (2013). Coping and stress tolerance: Mental health and illness. In C. E. Burns, A. M. Dunn, M. A. Brady, N. B. Starr, & C. G. Blosser (Eds.). *Pediatric primary care* (5th ed.). Philadelphia, PA: Saunders.

Goldson, E., & Reynolds, A. (2014). Child development and behaviour. In W. W. Hay, Jr., M. J. Levin, R. R. Deterding, & M. J. Abzug (Eds.). *Current diagnosis and treatment: Pediatrics* (22nd ed.). New York: McGraw-Hill Education.

Government of Canada. (2016a). *Rights of people with disabilities*. Retrieved from http://www.canada.pch.gc.ca/eng/1448633334025#a1

Government of Canada. (2016b). *Surveillance of autism spectrum disorder (ASD)*. Retrieved from https://www.canada.ca/en/public-health/services/diseases/autism-spectrum-disorder-asd/surveillance-autism-spectrum-disorder-asd.html

Government of Canada. (2017). *Controlled and illegal drugs.* Retrieved from https://www.canada.ca/en/health-canada/services/substance-abuse/controlled-illegal-drugs.html

HealthLink BC. (n.d.). *Attention deficit hyperactivity disorder (ADHD).* Retrieved from https://www.healthlinkbc.ca/health-topics/hw166083

Herdman, T. H., & Kamitsuru, S. (Eds.). (2014). *NANDA International nursing diagnoses: Definitions & classifications 2015–2017* (10th ed.). West Sussex, UK: John Wiley & Sons, Ltd.

Jankovic, J. (2015). Tourette syndrome. Retrieved from http://www.uptodate.com/contents/tourette-syndrome

Katzman, D., & Norris, M. L. (2017) *Avoidant/restrictive food intake disorder. Canadian Paediatric Surveillance Program.* Retrieved from http://www.cpsp.cps.ca/surveillance/study-etude/avoidant-restrictive-food-intake-disorder

Krull, K. R. (2016). Attention deficit hyperactivity disorder in children and adolescents: Epidemiology and pathogenesis. Retrieved from http://www.uptodate.com/contents/attention-deficit-hyperactivity-disorder-in-children-and-adolescents-epidemiology-and-pathogenesis

Lindert, J., von Ehrenstein, O. S., Grashow, R., Gal, G., Braehler, E., & Weisskopf, M. G. (2014). Sexual and physical abuse in childhood is associated with depression and anxiety over the life course: systematic review and meta-analysis. *International Journal of Public Health, 59*(2), 359–372. Retrieved from https://link.springer.com/article/10.1007/s00038-013-0519-5

Martin, M. S., Dykxhoorn, J., Afifi, T. O., & Colman, I. (2016). Child abuse and the prevalence of suicide attempts among those reporting suicide ideation. *Social psychiatry and psychiatric epidemiology, 51*(11), 1477–1484. Retrieved from http://dx.doi.org/10.1007/s00127-016-1250-3

Mental Health Commission Canada (MHCC). (n.d.). *Children and youth.* Retrieved from https://www.mentalhealthcommission.ca/English/focus-areas/children-and-youth

National Institute of Mental Health, Office of Science Policy, Planning and Communications. (2016). *PANDAS—Questions and Answers.* Bethesda, MD: Author.

Ng, M., Montigny, J. G., Ofner, M., & Do, M. T. (2017). *Environmental factors associated with autism spectrum disorder: a scoping review for the years 2003–2013.* Retrieved from http://www.phac-aspc.gc.ca/publicat/hpcdp-pspmc/37-1/ar-01-eng.php

O'Connor, K. M., & Speros, C. I. (2008). PANDAS in primary care: A pediatric case study. *The American Journal for Nurse Practitioners, 12*(3), 21–31.

Pivalizza, P., & Lalani, S. R. (2016). Intellectual disability (mental retardation) in children: Definition; diagnosis; and assessment of needs. Retrieved from http://www.uptodate.com/contents/intellectual-disability-mental-retardation-in-children-definition-diagnosis-and-assessment-of-needs

Preston, J., O'Neal, J. H., & Talaga, M. C. (2015). *Child and adolescent clinical psychopharmacology made simple.* Oakland, CA: New Harbinger Publications, Inc.

Roesler, T. A., & Jenny, C. (2016). Medical child abuse (Munchausen syndrome by proxy). Retrieved from http://www.uptodate.com/contents/medical-child-abuse-munchausen-syndrome-by-proxy

Rose, H. A. (2018). "I Didn't Get to Say Good-Bye. . . Didn't Get to Pet My Dogs or Nothing": Bioecological Theory and the Indian Residential School Experience in Canada. *Journal of Family Theory & Review, 10*(2), 348–366. Retrieved from https://doi.org/10.1111/jftr.12261

Sensory Processing Disorder Foundation. (2016). About SPD. Retrieved from http://www.spdfoundation.net/about-sensory-processing-disorder/

Shaffer, C. L., Smith, T. D., & Ornstein, A. E. (2018). Child and youth advocacy centres: A change in practice that can change a lifetime. *Paediatrics & Child Health, 23*(2), 116–118. Retrieved from https://doi.org/10.1093/pch/pxy008

Sigra, S., Hesselmark, E., & Bejerot, S. (2018). Treatment of PANDAS and PANS: a systematic review. *Neuroscience & Biobehavioral Reviews. 86*, 51–65. Retrieved from https://doi.org/10.1016/j.neubiorev.2018.01.001

Solanto, M. V. (2015). Psychotherapy for adult ADHD. Retrieved from http://www.uptodate.com/contents/psychotherapy-for-adult-adhd?

Starr, N. B., Fookson, M., Burns, C. D., & Bowman-Harvey, C. A. (2013). Cognitive perceptual Disorders. In C. E. Burns, A. M. Dunn, M. A. Brady, N. B. Starr, & C. G. Blosser (Eds.). *Pediatric primary care* (5th ed.). Philadelphia, PA: Saunders.

Swedo, S. E., Leonard, H. L., Garvey, M., Mittleman, B., Allen, A. J., Perlmutter, S., . . . Dubbert, B. K. (1998). Pediatric autoimmune neuropsychiatric disorders associated with streptococcal infections: clinical description of the first 50 cases. *American Journal of Psychiatry, 155*(4), 264–271.

Taketomo, C. K., Hodding, J. H., & Kraus, D. M. (2013). *Pediatric & neonatal dosage handbook* (20th ed.). Hudson, OH: Lexicomp.

United Nations Convention on the Rights of persons with Disabilities. (2017). *Concluding observations on the initial report of Canada.* Retrieved from http://rightsofchildren.ca/uncategorized/children-with-disabilities-recommendations-for-canada/attachment/disabilities-canada-concluding-observations/

Varcarolis, E. M. (2011). *Manual of psychiatric nursing care planning: Assessment guides, diagnoses, and psychopharmacology* (4th ed.). St. Louis, MO: Saunders.

von Hahn, L. E. (2015a). Specific learning disabilities in children: Clinical features. Retrieved from http://www.uptodate.com/contents/specific-learning-disabilitiesin-children-clinical-features

von Hahn, L. E. (2015b). Specific learning disabilities in children: Role of the primary care provider. Retrieved from http://www.uptodate.com/contents/specific-learning-disabilities-in-children-role-of-the-primary-care-provider

Wang, Y., McDermott, S., Mann, J. R., & Hardin, J. W. (2016). Preventing intellectual disability during pregnancy: what are the potentially high yield targets?. *Journal of Perinatal Medicine, 44*(4), 421–432. doi: https://doi.org/10.1515/jpm-2015-0059

Winokur, M., Holtan, A., & Valentine, D. (2014). *Kinship care for the safety, permanency, and well-being of children removed from the home for maltreatment. The Cochrane Library 2014, 1.* Indianapolis, IN: John Wiley & Sons.

MULTIPLE CHOICE QUESTIONS

1. The nurse is caring for a child with ADHD. Which behaviour would the nurse *not* expect the child to display?
   a. Moody, morose behaviour with pouting
   b. Interruption and inability to take turns
   c. Forgetfulness and easy distractibility
   d. Excessive motor activities and fidgeting

2. An adolescent girl who has been receiving treatment for anorexia nervosa has failed to gain weight over the past week despite eating all of her meals and snacks. What is the priority nursing intervention?
   a. Increase the teen's daily caloric intake by at least 500 calories.
   b. Ensure that the teen's entire fluid intake includes calories.
   c. Supervise the teen for 2 hours after all meals and snacks.
   d. Assess the teen's anxiety level to determine need for medication.

3. A 15-year-old girl has been making demands all day, exaggerating her every need. She is now crying, saying she has nothing to live for and threatening to kill herself. What is the priority nursing action?
   a. Ignore her continued exaggerated and melodramatic behaviour.
   b. Consult with the physician or nurse practitioner to increase her antidepressant dose.
   c. Leave the girl alone for a little while until she composes herself.
   d. Take the girl's suicidal threat seriously and provide close supervision.

4. When trying to manage aggressive or impulsive behaviours in children or adolescents, what is the best nursing intervention?
   a. Train the child to be assertive.
   b. Provide consistency and limit setting.
   c. Allow the child to negotiate the rules.
   d. Encourage the child to express feelings.

5. The nurse is caring for an adolescent who says, "I'm sick of this. I wish I weren't alive anymore." What is the best response by the nurse?
   a. "I often feel sad and sick of things."
   b. "Have you thought about hurting yourself?"
   c. "Are you trying to escape your problems?"
   d. "Do your parents know about this feeling?"

DOSAGE CALCULATION QUESTION

1. The nurse is caring for a 10-year-old diagnosed with depression. The child weighs 32.6 kg (72 lb). The medication order reads: fluoxetine 10 mg PO daily. The child refuses to swallow pills. Fluoxetine is supplied as 20 mg/5 mL. How many millilitres will the nurse administer? Round to the nearest tenth. Would you consider this a low dose and for what reason?

CRITICAL THINKING EXERCISES

1. A mother tells you that her son's behaviour is unmanageable, and she is having difficulty coping with it. The boy is argumentative and is bullying others. He is struggling with his schoolwork because he has difficulty staying on task, gets out of his chair often, and frequently distracts others. What additional assessments should you obtain? What interventions would be helpful in managing the boy's behaviour?

2. A 14-year-old boy with moderate intellectual disability is able to feed himself but is incontinent. Discuss the issues with which his family must deal.

STUDY ACTIVITIES

1. Explore several of the websites related to child abuse prevention listed on thePoint. Develop a list of resources for families in your local area.

2. Attend a group therapy session during your pediatric clinical rotation. Observe the children's verbal and nonverbal communication, noting inconsistencies or other interesting observations.

3. Visit a school for autistic children. Spend time with the various specialists who work with children with ASD, determining their roles and the effect the treatment they are providing has on the children. Report your findings to your classmates.

4. Attend a local CHADD meeting. Talk to parents about having a child with ADHD.

BRINGING IT ALL TOGETHER: A CASE STUDY

Nicole Ashton, 16 years old, is seen in your clinic due to weight loss. Her mother states that she has lost noticeable weight over the past few months and has stopped menstruating.

Go to thePoint **to find questions to consider about this case.**

51

Nursing Care During a Pediatric Emergency

Learning Objectives

Upon completion of the chapter, the learner will be able to:

1. Identify various factors contributing to emergency situations among infants and children.

2. Discuss common treatments and medications used during pediatric emergencies.

3. Conduct a health history of a child in an emergency situation, specific to the emergency.

4. Perform a rapid cardiopulmonary assessment.

5. Discuss common laboratory and other diagnostic tests used during pediatric emergencies.

6. Integrate the principles of the American Heart Association (AHA) and Pediatric Advanced Life Support (PALS) in the comprehensive management of pediatric emergencies, such as respiratory arrest, shock, cardiac arrest, near-drowning, poisoning, and trauma.

Alma Anderson, **age 8 years, has been admitted to the pediatric unit. Her mother calls the nurse into the room, stating, "Alma's having trouble breathing!"**

Children are uniquely vulnerable to a range of emergency situations. These situations are often life-threatening if not treated emergently and effectively. On account of their developmental level, children are at greater risk for near-drowning, poisoning, and traumatic injury compared with adults. Most pediatric cardiopulmonary arrests result from respiratory failure or shock. Data suggest that children who have a cardiopulmonary arrest requiring resuscitative measures have poor outcomes. For these reasons, the AHA has delineated two distinct chains of survival, one for adults and one for children, which should become familiar to all health care providers who may encounter life-threatening situations.

The pediatric chain of survival is:
- Rapid recognition and prevention of arrest
- Early cardiopulmonary resuscitation (CPR)
- Activation of emergency medical system (EMS)
- Rapid advanced pediatric life support (PALS)
- Integrated post–cardiac arrest care (AHA, 2016b)

Considering the special risks that threaten children, the AHA has developed specific guidelines for PALS. Courses in PALS are offered for health care professionals so that they can provide expert care for children in emergencies. This chapter emphasizes the principles of PALS and their application in relation to the nurse's role in the management of pediatric emergencies.

Take Note!

The current pediatric basic life support guidelines define an infant as between 0 and 12 months of age, and a child as age 1 year up until puberty. Children in this range should be managed using the PALS guidelines rather than those for adults (Berg et al., 2010).

COMMON MEDICAL TREATMENTS

A variety of medications and other medical treatments are used in pediatric emergencies. Most of these treatments will require a physician's order in the hospital; some emergency departments and pediatric units may have standing orders for pediatric emergencies. The most common medical treatments and medications used in pediatric emergencies are listed in Common Medical Treatments 51.1 and Drug Guide 51.1. The nurse should be familiar with these procedures and medications, how they work, and nursing implications.

Certain emergency medications for children may be given via a **tracheal (endotracheal) tube**, an advanced airway tube inserted into the trachea that can be connected to a ventilator to maintain the airway and facilitate artificial respirations. Tracheal drug administration is reserved for cases in which intravenous (IV) or intraosseous (IO) access cannot be obtained. Although the AHA (2016b) continues to have tracheal administration of rescue drugs in their guidelines, they suggest more

research is needed to understand their effectiveness. Use the mnemonic LEAN (lidocaine, epinephrine, atropine, and naloxone) to remember which medications may be given by the tracheal tube. In certain cases, when an emergency medication is given by a tracheal tube, the dosage must be increased. All medications given by the tracheal tube should be followed by 5 mL of sterile saline and five consecutive multiple positive-pressure ventilations to ensure that the drugs are delivered (Kleinman et al., 2010a).

NURSING PROCESS OVERVIEW FOR THE CHILD IN AN EMERGENCY SITUATION

The nurse may encounter a pediatric emergency in a variety of settings. As a member of an emergency team, the nurse must be prepared to participate in the stabilization of a child who has suffered a near-drowning, motor vehicle crash, trauma from a fall, sport's accident, poisoning, or other emergency. In an inpatient unit, a child with asthma may suffer respiratory distress or stop breathing or demonstrate shock for a variety of reasons. Regardless of the setting or how the emergency developed, the principles for managing pediatric emergencies are the same.

Care of the child in an emergency includes all components of the nursing process: assessment, nursing diagnosis, planning, interventions, and evaluation. In an emergency, the nurse must act quickly, intervening immediately when an abnormality is determined during assessment. When evaluating a child who presents emergently, always follow the AHA's guidelines for basic life support (Berg et al., 2010), which includes evaluating the child's:
- Airway
- Breathing
- Circulation

After you have assessed the child's airway, breathing, and circulation, provide care as necessary, including cardiac compressions and rescue breathing as necessary. Once the child has return of spontaneous circulation (ROSC), assessment and management will vary depending on the cause of the emergency.

Assessment

Assessment begins with the Pediatric Assessment Triangle (PAT) while the nurse approaches the child. PAT is a non-invasive and non-threatening assessment tool used to identify a child that is critically ill and needs immediate intervention. The nurse does not need to touch the child to use this tool and it can be used as the nurse approaches the child from a distance.

(text continues on page 1982)

COMMON MEDICAL TREATMENTS 51.1 PEDIATRIC EMERGENCIES

Treatment	Explanation	Indications	Nursing Implications
Suctioning oral/ airway (oropharyngeal, nasopharyngeal, tracheal, or tracheostomy)	Removal of secretions using a bulb syringe or suction catheter	Excessive airway secretions affecting airway patency	Use caution and suction only as far as recommended for age, tracheal tube size, or tracheostomy tube size or until coughing or gagging occurs
Oxygen	Supplementation via nasal cannula, hood, face mask, tent or tracheal/ nasotracheal tube	Hypoxemia, respiratory distress, shock, trauma	Monitor response via skin colour, work of breathing, respiratory rate, oxygen saturation levels, and level of consciousness
Bag-valve-mask ventilation	Provision of manual ventilation using a bag-valve-mask device	Apnea, ineffective ventilation, and oxygenation with spontaneous breaths, extremely slow respiratory rate	Ensure adequate chest rise with ventilation Use appropriate-sized bag Be careful not to overventilate or bag aggressively to avoid barotrauma Maintain a mask seal around the child's nose and mouth with the appropriate-sized mask Ensure the oxygen supply tubing is connected to 100% oxygen
Intubation	Insertion of tracheal tube into the trachea by a skilled practitioner to provide artificial ventilation.	Apnea An unprotected airway Airway that cannot be maintained Need for prolonged assisted ventilation	Determine adequacy of breath sounds with bagging immediately upon insertion of the tracheal tube Assess for symmetric chest rise Secure tube in place and note number marking on the tube at the child's lips Connect to ventilator when available Confirm placement with x-ray
Needle thoracotomy (decompression)	Insertion of a needle between the rib intercostal spaces into the pleural space to remove air from the affected lung	Tension pneumothorax	There should be a rush of air as the needle reaches the air space Often followed by a chest tube insertion Monitor breath sounds, work of breathing, pulse oximetry Ensure patency of needle
IV fluid therapy	Administration of crystalloid or colloid solutions to provide hydration and improve perfusion	Altered perfusion states such as respiratory distress, shock, trauma, cardiac disturbances	Use intraosseous (IO) route if a peripheral IV cannot be obtained quickly in shock Reassess respiratory and circulatory status immediately after each fluid bolus and during continuous infusion
Blood product transfusion	Administration of whole blood, packed red blood cells, platelets, or plasma intravenously	Trauma, hemorrhage	Follow institution's transfusion protocol Double-check blood type and product label with a second nurse Monitor vital signs and assess child frequently to identify adverse reaction to blood transfusion If adverse reaction is suspected, immediately discontinue transfusion, infuse normal saline IV, reassess the child, notify the physician, and following your institution's transfusion adverse event protocol
Cervical stabilization	Maintenance of the cervical spine in an immobile position being aware of patient's inability to protect their airway with vomiting	Trauma, near-drowning	Use the jaw-thrust manoeuvre without head tilt to open the airway Maintain cervical stabilization until the cervical spine is cleared after x-rays and physical examination are by the physician and/or radiologist

(continued)

COMMON MEDICAL TREATMENTS 51.1 PEDIATRIC EMERGENCIES (continued)

Treatment	Explanation	Indications	Nursing Implications
Defibrillation and synchronized cardioversion	Provision of electrical current to alter the heart's electrical rhythm	Defibrillation: ventricular fibrillation and pulseless ventricular tachycardia Synchronized cardioversion: supraventricular tachycardia and ventricular tachycardia with a pulse	In the pulseless child, always ensure quality CPR is ongoing while the defibrillator is being readied Ensure adequate oxygenation Provide epinephrine every 3 min For synchronized cardioversion, sedate the child if time allows. Ensure your defibrillator has been set to synchronize on the R wave

DRUG GUIDE 51.1 COMMON MEDICATIONS USED IN PEDIATRIC EMERGENCIES

Medication	Actions/Indications	Nursing Implications
Adenosine (antiarrhythmic)	Temporary block of conduction through AV node, restoring normal sinus rhythm Treatment of supraventricular tachycardia (SVT)	• Administer first dose IV or IO push at 0.05 mg/kg for neonates, and 0.1 mg/kg (max 6 mg) for all other children • Half-life is <10 seconds, and therefore requires rapid administration followed by a rapid, generous saline flush • Repeat up to three doses every 1 to 2 minutes, remaining doses are 0.2 mg/kg with a maximum dose of 12 mg • Monitor for shortness of breath, dyspnea, worsening of asthma • A brief sinus pause will be noted when the AV node resets, warn caregivers and the patient
Amiodarone (antiarrhythmic)	Prolongs repolarization of action potential, thus slowing the heart rate Used with ventricular tachycardia, ventricular fibrillation	• Administer 5 mg/kg (maximum single dose 300 mg) IV or IO push in arrest, may repeat up to 15 mg/kg or 2.2 g in 24 hours • Infuse over 20 to 60 minutes with perfusing rhythm • Avoid use with procainamide and other medications that can prolong QT segment • Monitor for prolonged QT segments with infusions
Atropine (anticholinergic)	Increases heart rate, dries secretions, and inhibits serotonin and histamine Used with sinus bradycardia, asystole, pulseless electrical activity (PEA)	• Administer 0.02 mg/kg undiluted IV or IO (maximum single dose 0.5 mg, 1 mg for adolescent). • Dose per ET, 0.04 to 0.06 mg/kg, dilute with 3 to 5 mL normal saline, follow with five positive pressure ventilations • May repeat once
Dobutamine (adrenergic agent)	β-Adrenergic agent primarily affecting β-1 receptors; increases myocardial contractility and heart rate Ongoing short-term management of shock (hypovolemic and cardiogenic)	• Administer at 2 to 20 µg/kg/min IV or IO continuous infusion • Monitor for development of ventricular arrhythmias • Expect to titrate infusion rate based on cardiac output and central venous pressure (CVP) • Administer through a central line if possible, due to risk of extravasation • Monitor child closely, preferably in an ICU setting with CVP monitoring
Dopamine (inotropic)	Increases cardiac output, BP, and renal perfusion (β-adrenergic agonist) Bradycardia, hypotension, and poor cardiac output	• Administer 10 to 20 µg/kg/min IV or IO continuous infusion with hypotensive shock • Administer 2 to 20 µg/kg/min IV or IO for normotensive shock • Ensure that child has received adequate fluid resuscitation prior to administration • Administer through a central venous line if possible, due to risk of extravasation • Monitor child closely, preferably in an ICU setting with CVP monitoring • Monitor for ventricular arrhythmias

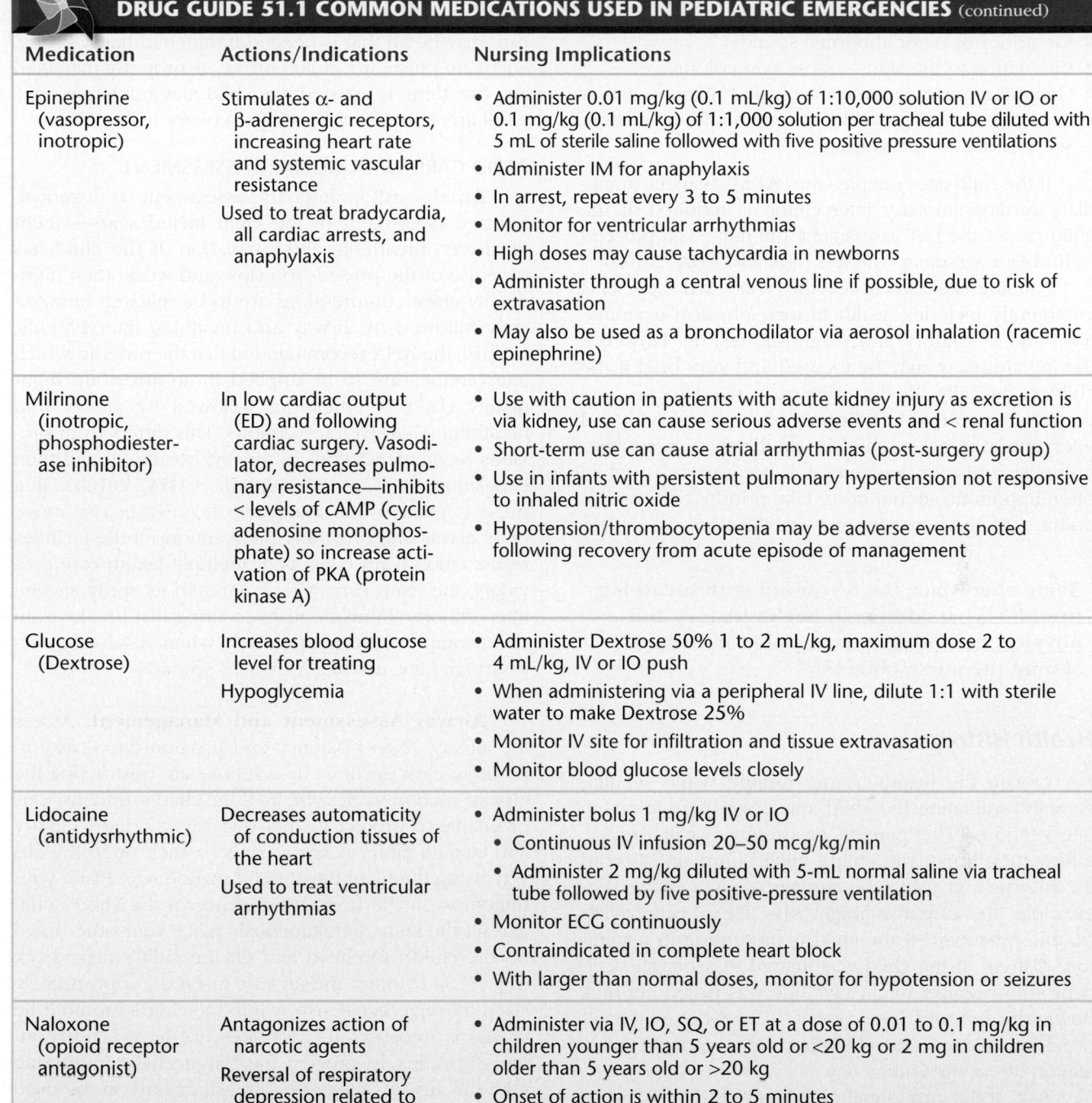

DRUG GUIDE 51.1 COMMON MEDICATIONS USED IN PEDIATRIC EMERGENCIES (continued)

Medication	Actions/Indications	Nursing Implications
Epinephrine (vasopressor, inotropic)	Stimulates α- and β-adrenergic receptors, increasing heart rate and systemic vascular resistance Used to treat bradycardia, all cardiac arrests, and anaphylaxis	• Administer 0.01 mg/kg (0.1 mL/kg) of 1:10,000 solution IV or IO or 0.1 mg/kg (0.1 mL/kg) of 1:1,000 solution per tracheal tube diluted with 5 mL of sterile saline followed with five positive pressure ventilations • Administer IM for anaphylaxis • In arrest, repeat every 3 to 5 minutes • Monitor for ventricular arrhythmias • High doses may cause tachycardia in newborns • Administer through a central venous line if possible, due to risk of extravasation • May also be used as a bronchodilator via aerosol inhalation (racemic epinephrine)
Milrinone (inotropic, phosphodiesterase inhibitor)	In low cardiac output (ED) and following cardiac surgery. Vasodilator, decreases pulmonary resistance—inhibits < levels of cAMP (cyclic adenosine monophosphate) so increase activation of PKA (protein kinase A)	• Use with caution in patients with acute kidney injury as excretion is via kidney, use can cause serious adverse events and < renal function • Short-term use can cause atrial arrhythmias (post-surgery group) • Use in infants with persistent pulmonary hypertension not responsive to inhaled nitric oxide • Hypotension/thrombocytopenia may be adverse events noted following recovery from acute episode of management
Glucose (Dextrose)	Increases blood glucose level for treating Hypoglycemia	• Administer Dextrose 50% 1 to 2 mL/kg, maximum dose 2 to 4 mL/kg, IV or IO push • When administering via a peripheral IV line, dilute 1:1 with sterile water to make Dextrose 25% • Monitor IV site for infiltration and tissue extravasation • Monitor blood glucose levels closely

Lidocaine (antidysrhythmic)	Decreases automaticity of conduction tissues of the heart
	
	Used to treat ventricular arrhythmias
		• Administer bolus 1 mg/kg IV or IO
		  • Continuous IV infusion 20–50 mcg/kg/min
		  • Administer 2 mg/kg diluted with 5-mL normal saline via tracheal tube followed by five positive-pressure ventilation
		• Monitor ECG continuously
		• Contraindicated in complete heart block
		• With larger than normal doses, monitor for hypotension or seizures

Naloxone (opioid receptor antagonist)	Antagonizes action of narcotic agents Reversal of respiratory depression related to narcotic effects	• Administer via IV, IO, SQ, or ET at a dose of 0.01 to 0.1 mg/kg in children younger than 5 years old or <20 kg or 2 mg in children older than 5 years old or >20 kg • Onset of action is within 2 to 5 minutes • May repeat dose as necessary; narcotic effects outlast therapeutic effects of naloxone, frequent reassessment is necessary

AV, atrioventricular; ET, endotracheal; IO, intraosseous; SQ, subcutaneous; IM, intramuscular.

Adapted from American Heart Association. (2015). *Pediatric advanced life support provider manual*. Dallas, TX: Author; Field, J. M., Hazinski, M. F., Sayre, M. R., Chameides, L., Schexnayder, S. M., Hemphill, R., . . . & Cave, D. M. (2010). Part 1: executive summary: 2010 American Heart Association guidelines for cardiopulmonary resuscitation and emergency cardiovascular care. *Circulation, 122*(18_suppl_3), S640–S656. Taketomo, C. K., Hodding, J. H., & Kraus, D. M. (2013). *Pediatric & neonatal dosage handbook* (20th ed.). Hudson, OH: Lexicomp; Samiee-Zafarghandy, S., Raman, S. R., van den Anker, J. N., McHutchison, K., Hornik, C. P., Clark, R. H., . . . Best Pharmaceuticals for Children Act—Pediatric Trials Network Administrative Core Committee. (2015). Safety of milrinone use in neonatal intensive care units. *Early Human Development, 91*(1), 31–35.

There are three elements to PAT:

* Work of breathing—assess respiratory effort listening for stridor or other abnormal sounds
* Circulation to the skin—assess skin colour
* General appearance for neurologic function—assess level of consciousness, attentiveness and interaction; see thePoint for infographic

If the child does not pass the PAT assessment, immediate cardiopulmonary intervention is required. If the child passes the PAT assessment, the nurse can proceed to further assessment with less urgency (AHA, 2016b).

Nursing assessment of the child who presents emergently includes health history, physical examination, and laboratory and diagnostic testing. However, the initial history may be focused and very brief if the child is critically ill; the nurse may need to proceed immediately to rapid cardiopulmonary assessment and intervention. Once a child is stabilized, a more comprehensive history is obtained. Laboratory tests, while often important, should never take priority over cardiopulmonary and hemodynamic stabilization.

> **Remember Alma, the 8-year-old with breathing trouble? What additional health history and physical examination assessment information should the nurse obtain?**

Health History

Obtain the health history rapidly while simultaneously evaluating the child and providing life-saving interventions. The parents or caregiver will provide information about the child's chief complaint. Record the information using the caregiver's own words. For example, the caregiver might say, "He's been having trouble breathing" if the child is presenting in respiratory distress. If the child was injured in a bicycle accident, the caregiver might say, "She was riding her bike down the hill and lost control." This brief statement provides guidance for obtaining more in-depth information about the emergency.

Ask about any significant past history that may affect the care of the child. For example, children who are medically complex, who were born prematurely, or who have a significant genetically linked disease (e.g., sickle cell anemia) may require special consideration when planning and implementing care.

Physical Examination

In an emergency, the nurse must perform a rapid assessment to identify cardiopulmonary emergencies and intervene immediately if alterations are noted. Identifying early warning signs and intervening can prevent a full cardiac arrest. Most pediatric arrests are related primarily to airway and breathing, and usually only secondarily to the heart. Supported respiratory care may be all that is needed if the child has a strong, adequate pulse. If a child's airway is properly managed and breathing is assisted, the child may not experience a full arrest requiring cardiopulmonary resuscitation.

RAPID CARDIOPULMONARY ASSESSMENT

Rapid cardiopulmonary assessment is essential. Primary assessment of the child includes assessment of airway, breathing, and circulation. If the child has no pulse or the pulse is too slow and weak, then high-quality chest compressions are to be initiated immediately followed by airway and breathing interventions. In 2010, the AHA recommended that the order in which interventions are to be applied in an arrest are high-quality chest compressions followed by airway and breathing (C–A–B) interventions. This differs from previous recommendations of airway, breathing, and then circulation (A–B–C) interventions (AHA, 2016b). If a pulse is present and adequate, the rescuer can move onto airway and breathing interventions. If the facilities resuscitation team consists of multiple health care providers, the team can work in tandem to apply several interventions simultaneously ensuring that breaks from chest compressions happen only when absolutely necessary and are no longer than 10 seconds.

Airway Assessment and Management. Assess the airway. Assess patency and position the airway to promote clear air flow. If secretions are obstructing the airway, suction to clear them. If the child is unconscious or unable to protect his/her own airway due to injury and c-spine injury is not a concern, then open the airway using the head tilt–chin lift manoeuvre. Place your fingertips on the bony prominence of the child's chin and lift the chin. Simultaneously place your other hand on the child's forehead and tilt the child's head back (Fig. 51.1) to open the airway. Insert an appropriately sized oropharyngeal airway into the child's mouth if he or she is unconscious and does not have a functioning gag reflex to prevent the tongue from interfering with the airway. A nasopharyngeal airway can be used in the absence of a suspected basilar skull fracture. If required, place the child on oxygen at 100% and apply a pulse oximeter to monitor oxygen saturation levels.

> *Take Note!*
>
> If cervical spine injury is suspected, do not use the head tilt–chin lift manoeuvre. Use only the jaw-thrust technique for opening the airway (see trauma section for explanation and illustration).

Breathing Assessment and Management. After establishing an open airway, assess breathing. Turn your head and place your ear over the child's mouth to "look,

FIGURE 51.1 **Head tilt–chin lift manoeuvre in a child.**

listen, and feel" for spontaneous respirations. Look to see if the child's chest is rising, listen for air escaping, and note if you feel any exhaled air from the child's nose or mouth. If the child is breathing, evaluate the quality of the respirations: is ventilation effective, or is the child gasping ineffectively for air? Count the respiratory rate. Observe the child's colour for cyanosis. Note depth of respirations, chest rise and symmetry of the rise, auscultate for adequacy of air flow in all lung fields, and presence of adventitious sounds. Assess for increased work of breathing and the use of accessory muscles.

When signs of respiratory distress are identified, place the child on oxygen at 100% and apply a pulse oximeter to monitor oxygen saturation levels. For the child receiving 100% oxygen who does not improve with repositioning, begin assisted ventilation with a bag-valve-mask (BVM) device in conjunction with an appropriately sized oropharyngeal airway. A need for ongoing BVM ventilation may require airway **intubation**, a process by which a breathing tube, such as a tracheal tube, is inserted into a child's trachea to assist with breathing; see the section on Respiratory Arrest for information on assisting with ventilation using the BVM device and airway intubation.

Circulation Assessment and Management. Next, evaluate circulation. During this phase, assess the heart rate, pulses, perfusion, skin colour and temperature, blood pressure, cardiac rhythm, and level of consciousness. Determine the heart rate by auscultation or palpation of central pulses. Radial and brachial pulses are difficult to palpate, especially in infants and young children. In the young infant, assess the brachial artery for a pulse. In the child and adolescent, assess the

carotid pulse. If perfusion is poor, as with shock or cardiac arrest, the child may have a weak pulse or no pulse.

Take Note!

ALWAYS evaluate the presence of a heart rate by auscultation of the heart or by palpation of central pulses. NEVER use the cardiac monitor to determine if the child has a perfusing pulse. The presence of a cardiac rhythm is not a reliable method for assessment of perfusion to the body. In certain circumstances, electrical activity continues but there is no pulse; this is called pulseless electrical activity (PEA).

If the child's pulse is inadequate or absent, begin cardiac compressions. See below for information on performing CPR. High-quality chest compressions of adequate rate and depth are essential (Kleinman et al., 2010a).

If there is a pulse, note its quality: Is it strong, bounding, or weak? Compare the strength and quality of central and peripheral pulses. Assess capillary refill time. Assess for active bleeding including internal bleeding. Assess the child's perfusion by noting skin temperature and colour. Is the skin pink? Is it warm to the touch? Is child's skin cool? Is the child's skin pale, mottled, ashen, or cyanotic? As the child's condition worsens with progressing shock and cardiovascular compromise, the nurse may note a line of demarcation of skin temperature change; the distal extremities will feel cooler than the proximal regions of the body. Measure the child's blood pressure (BP) and place the child on a cardiac monitor to evaluate the cardiac rhythm. Note the child's level of consciousness; if circulation is poor, the child will demonstrate an altered level of consciousness as perfusion to the brain is compromised.

Take Note!

According to PALS, the minimum acceptable systolic BP is 60 for the neonate, 70 for the infant aged 1 to 12 months, and 70+ twice the age in years for children aged 1 to 10 years (e.g., a 4-year old should have a minimal systolic BP of 78: 70 + [2 × 4] = 78). For children older than age 10, the minimum acceptable systolic BP is 90 (Kleinman et al., 2010a).

If the child's circulation or perfusion is compromised, then fluid resuscitation is necessary. Establish large-bore intravenous (IV) access immediately and bolus isotonic fluid; attempt to establish two lines. Bolus 20 mL/kg of normal saline (NS) or lactated Ringer's (LR) IV, administer 10 mL/kg if the infant is younger than 1 month old. Follow with immediate reassessment and repeat as necessary. If peripheral IV access cannot be obtained in the child with altered perfusion within three attempts or 90 seconds, assist with insertion of an intraosseous (IO) needle for fluid administration (refer to Shock section for further information about IO access). Central venous or cutdown access may also be used, but these interventions may take longer to accomplish.

ADDITIONAL PHYSICAL EXAMINATION COMPONENTS

In addition to assessing and stabilizing the child's airway, breathing, and circulation, perform a thorough physical examination and assess pain.

Neurologic Assessment. Quickly evaluate the sensorium in an older child. Ask the child to state his or her name. Ask what happened to the child. Does the child know what day it is? Is the child aware of where he or she is?

If the child is an infant, evaluate his or her interest in the environment and interaction with parents and surroundings. An infant who is not interested in the environment or seems unable to recognize his or her parents is a cause for concern. In contrast, an infant who enjoys sucking on a finger and making eye contact with the nurse during the assessment is reassuring. Assess serum glucose for hypoglycemia when an altered level of consciousness is identified.

Assess the infant or young toddler's fontanel, palpate the anterior fontanel to determine if it is normal (soft and flat), depressed, or full. A sunken fontanel is associated with volume depletion from dehydration or blood loss. If the fontanel is full, note if it is bulging or tense, which may indicate increased intracranial pressure (ICP). Next assess the eyes. Are they open or closed? If closed, do they open spontaneously, to voice, to pain? Does the child focus on and follow the nurse's movements? Evaluate the pupils for equality and reactivity. Sluggish pupillary reaction may occur with increased ICP or presence of narcotics.

Take Note!
A nonreactive pupil is an ominous sign indicating a need for immediate relief of increased ICP.

Assess the child's face. Does the child smile or cry? Does the child react to playfulness with a laugh? Does the young infant cry vigorously? Are facial movements symmetrical? In a child, a normal or near-normal neurologic examination can be a reassuring sign. Conversely, obtunded or muted responses to environmental stimuli are a cause for concern.

Assess for spontaneous movement of the extremities. Young infants cannot walk, so assess their ability to move their arms and legs and assess the tone of their extremities. Does the infant vigorously and equally move the arms and legs? Is their muscle tone normal, or are they floppy or flaccid? When assessing the older child, note whether he or she is ambulatory alone, with assistance, or unable to ambulate. Note whether the child has use of the upper extremities. In the case of trauma, the child may arrive immobilized for c-spine stabilization. In this scenario, assess the child's motor responsiveness and sensation in each extremity, comparing findings bilaterally while the child is in the supine position. Ask the child if he or she feels you touching each extremity. Ask the child to squeeze your fingers and to wiggle their toes. This will provide information about cerebral integrity and perfusion, cerebellar health, and spinal cord integrity.

The pediatric Glasgow Coma Scale (GCS) is useful in determining neurologic status in children (AHA, 2016b). Chapter 38 provides a more in-depth discussion of this scale.

Skin and Extremity Assessment. Remove the child's clothing and thoroughly examine the skin for bruising, lesions, or rashes. If the child has a rash, note the size, shape, colour, configuration, and location. Apply pressure to the rash with your fingertips to assess for blanching. Inspect the trunk, abdomen, and extremities for abrasions or deformities.

Take Note!
Rashes that do not blanch may be classified as petechiae or purpura. This type of rash may be associated with certain serious conditions, such as meningococcemia. Report this finding to the physician or nurse practitioner immediately.

Pain Assessment. In emergencies, children may experience pain as a direct result of their injury or disease; life-saving interventions such as resuscitation, insertion of IV lines, and administration of medications may cause further pain. The child's pain may also be exaggerated by light, noise, movement of the stretcher or bed, and sensations of cold or heat. Nurses play a key role in minimizing the child's pain, and this may decrease the child's distress (Stanley & Pollard, 2013). If the child is awake and verbal, use an age-appropriate pain assessment scale to determine the child's pain level. If the child is sedated or unconscious, assess pain with a standardized scale that relies on physiologic measurements as well as behavioural parameters. Refer to Chapter 36 for additional information on pain assessment in children.

Laboratory and Diagnostic Testing

A number of laboratory and diagnostic tests may be ordered in a pediatric emergency. Laboratory tests can help distinguish the cause of the emergency and additional problems that need to be treated. Standard laboratory tests obtained in most emergency departments include:

- Arterial blood gases (ABGs), obtained initially and then serially to assess for changes
- Electrolytes and glucose levels

- Complete blood count (CBC)
- Blood cultures
- Urinalysis
- Pregnancy test with age-appropriate females

If toxic ingestion is suspected, a toxicology panel will be obtained. In suspected sepsis, erythrocyte sedimentation rate (ESR), C-reactive protein (CRP), lactate (BCPSQC, 2017), along with urine, wound, and spinal fluid cultures, as well as cultures from any attached medical devices, may be obtained. The pediatric trauma victim may have additional laboratory tests performed, including amylase, liver enzymes, and blood type and cross-match.

Diagnostic tests may include radiologic tests, computed tomography (CT) scanning, and magnetic resonance imaging (MRI). One advantage of radiologic diagnostic testing is that the tests are relatively non-invasive. A disadvantage of CT and MRI scans is that before they can be performed, the child must be stabilized. Bedside ultrasound, focused assessment sonogram in trauma (FAST), is becoming common in facilities that have trained operators, most commonly the physician. Common Laboratory and Diagnostic Tests 51.1 discusses the tests most commonly used in pediatric emergencies.

> After completing an assessment of Alma, the nurse noted the following: a patent airway, anxious but able to speak in short sentences, and skin temperature cool on the extremities. Based on these assessment findings, what would your top three nursing diagnoses be for Alma? Describe appropriate nursing interventions.

COMMON LABORATORY AND DIAGNOSTIC TESTS 51.1 PEDIATRIC EMERGENCIES

Test	Explanation	Indications	Nursing Implications
Chest x-ray	X-ray used to evaluate heart and lung structures	To identify: • Chest infections • Foreign body • Injury • Tracheal tube placement • Central line placement • Pneumothorax • Re-evaluation of lungs after chest tube placement	• Portable x-ray machines allow x-rays to be obtained quickly during resuscitation. • Assist the child to lie still if necessary.
Computed tomography (CT)	Use of high radiation (equivalent to about 100 to 150 chest x-rays) with computer processing targeting specific body areas	Rapid evaluation of tissues and skeletal areas Superior test for the evaluation of internal bleeding	• Expect the child to be transported out of the area for the study. • Accompany the child to provide continued emotional support, observation, and management, especially if child's condition is unstable. • Sedation may be required. The child must be still for the duration of the test.
Magnetic resonance imaging (MRI)	Incorporation of responses of hydrogen protons to a dynamic magnetic field	Superior test for the evaluation of the spinal cord and the cerebrospinal fluid spaces; less useful in emergency situations	• Administer sedation as ordered as the child must remain still for the duration of the test. • Assist the conscious child to deal with fear related to the loud banging noise of the machine.
Arterial blood gases (ABGs)	Evaluation of blood pH and arterial blood levels of oxygen and carbon dioxide	Evaluation of quality of respiration and evaluation of acid–base balance	• Anticipate serial ABGs to assess for status changes. • Never delay resuscitation efforts pending blood gas results.
Serum electrolytes	Evaluation of electrolyte levels, such as sodium, potassium, and chloride, in the blood	Useful for determining baseline and if dehydration is hypertonic or isotonic	• Hemolysis of specimen may lead to falsely elevated potassium levels.

(continued)

COMMON LABORATORY AND DIAGNOSTIC TESTS 51.1 PEDIATRIC EMERGENCIES (continued)

Test	Explanation	Indications	Nursing Implications
Glucose	Evaluation of glucose level in the blood	Valuable for determining need for supplementation, as in the case of hypoglycemia	• Use a rapid glucose test at the bedside or obtain serum blood specimen. • Elevated glucose levels can be associated with stress or with use of corticosteroids.
Toxicology panel (blood and/or urine)	Determination of most commonly abused mood-altering medications, as well as commonly ingested drugs	Drug abuse, overdose, or poisoning	• Standard toxicology panel varies with the agency. • Follow agency protocol; may require special handling or labelling of specimen.
Complete blood count (CBC)	Evaluation of hemoglobin and hematocrit, white blood cell count, and platelet count	Any condition in which anemia, infection, or thrombocytopenia is suspected Trauma if blood loss is suspected	• Be aware of normal values and how they vary with age and gender. • Hemoglobin and hematocrit may be elevated secondary to hemoconcentration in the case of hypovolemia.
Blood type and cross-match	Determination of ABO blood typing as well as presence of antigens to avoid transfusion reaction	Trauma victim or any person with suspected blood loss as preparation for transfusion	• Handle specimen gently to avoid hemolysis. • Ensure that specimen request and label are appropriately signed and dated. • Apply "type and cross" or "blood band" to child at time of specimen collection as required by agency. • Most type and cross-match specimens expire after 48 to 72 hours.
Urinalysis	Evaluation of colour, pH, specific gravity, and odour of urine Assessment for protein, glucose, ketones, blood, leukocyte esterase, RBCs, WBCs, bacteria, crystals, and casts	Children with fever, dysuria, flank pain, urgency, or hematuria or those who have experienced trauma to provide information about the urinary tract and renal contusion	• Many medications can affect urine colour; notify the laboratory if the child is taking one. • Notify the laboratory and document on the laboratory form if the female child or adolescent is menstruating. • Refrigerate the specimen if it is not processed promptly. • Specimen may be obtained by catheterization, clean-catch voiding sample, or a U-bag.

RBCs, red blood cells; WBCs, white blood cells.

Adapted from Corbett, J. A., & Banks, A. D. (2013). *Laboratory tests and diagnostic procedures with nursing diagnoses* (8th ed.). Upper Saddle River, NJ: Pearson Education Inc.

Nursing Diagnoses and Related Interventions

After completing a thorough assessment and initial stabilization of the child, the nurse might identify several nursing diagnoses, including:
• Ineffective airway clearance
• Ineffective breathing pattern
• Impaired gas exchange
• Deficient fluid volume
• Decreased cardiac output
• Ineffective tissue perfusion (cardiopulmonary, peripheral cerebral, or renal)
• Deficient knowledge
• Fear
• Interrupted family processes

Specific nursing goals, interventions, and evaluation for the child in an emergency are based on the nursing diagnoses. Additional information about nursing management will be included later in this chapter as it relates to specific disorders.

Providing Cardiopulmonary Resuscitation

High-quality chest compression takes priority (AHA, 2016b). Assess for a pulse. In the child, the carotid or femoral pulses are the easiest to assess; in the infant, the femoral pulse is the easiest to assess. Carefully assess for signs of a pulse, being careful not to exceed 10 seconds to ensure you do not delay chest compressions. If the pulse is absent or inadequate (less than 60 beats per minute), begin high-quality chest compressions. Call for help and for someone to obtain the automatic external defibrillator (AED) and rescue cart (crash cart). Open the airway and assess for adequate breathing. If the child is not breathing, begin rescue breathing.

Take Note!

When a cardiac arrest or sudden collapse occurs in a child out of the hospital and is a witnessed, initial management is slightly different than that for in-patient arrests. In these sudden, witnessed events, call 9-1-1 or the local emergency number first, get the AED, and return to start CPR (Berg et al., 2010). When more than one responder is present, these steps can be done simultaneously.

Table 51.1 presents the AHA's most recent recommendations (2015) for ratios of breaths and compressions. These recommendations stress the importance of high-quality chest compressions.

- Rescuers must provide compressions of adequate rate, 100 to 120 compressions per minute for infants and children ensuring adequate depth, depressing the chest one third of the anteroposterior diameter of the chest, approximately 4 cm in infants and 5 cm in children and adolescence.
- Chest recoil must be allowed.
- Minimal interruption of chest compressions, no more than 10 seconds and only when absolutely necessary.
- For infant two-person CPR, chest compressions can be performed by encircling the chest with two thumbs and simultaneously using the hands to provide a thoracic squeeze.
- Chest compression providers should trade off every 2 minutes to maintain quality.
- For two-person CPR, no pauses should occur for ventilation, with the compressing health care provider giving continuous compressions (Berg et al., 2010).

Providing Defibrillation or Synchronized Cardioversion

In some cases, the child has an abnormal life-threatening cardiac rhythm or an arrhythmia that does not respond to pharmacologic therapy and leads to hemodynamic instability. In these cases, electrical therapy, in the form of defibrillation or synchronized cardioversion, may be required.

Defibrillation is the use of electrical energy to depolarize the cells of the myocardium to terminate an abnormal life-threatening cardiac rhythm, such as pulseless ventricular tachycardia or ventricular fibrillation. Defibrillation is used in conjunction with oxygen, chest compressions, and medications. The effects of defibrillation are enhanced in an oxygen-rich environment coupled with high-quality chest compressions.

Cardioversion, another means of applying electrical current to the heart, is used when the child has supraventricular tachycardia (SVT) or ventricular tachycardia with a pulse. Cardioversion may also be enhanced with medications. Cardioversion is delivered

TABLE 51.1	RATIOS OF BREATHS TO COMPRESSIONS	
Age	One-Person CPR	Two-Person CPR
Infant	• 30 compressions to 2 breaths • Hand placement: two fingers, placed one fingerbreadth below the nipple line	• 15 compressions to 2 breaths • Hand placement: two thumbs encircling the chest at the nipple line
Child	• 30 compressions to 2 breaths • Hand placement: heel of hand or two hands (adult position in larger child), pressing on the sternum at the nipple line	• 15 compressions to 2 breaths • Hand placement: heel of one hand or two hands (adult position in larger child), pressing on the sternum at the nipple line

Adapted from Berg, M. D., Schexnayder, S. M., Chameides, L., Terry, M., Donoghue, A., Hickey, R. W., . . . Hazinski, M. F. (2010). Part 13: Pediatric basic life support: 2010 American Heart Association guidelines for cardiopulmonary resuscitation and emergency cardiovascular care. *Circulation*, *122*(18 Suppl 3), S862–S875.

EVIDENCE-BASED PRACTICE 51.1 THE ROLE OF AUTOMATED EXTERNAL DEFIBRILLATORS (AEDS) IN CARDIAC RESUSCITATION OF CHILDREN

Primary cardiac arrest resulting from arrhythmia or commotio cordis is rare in children and adolescents but often has very poor outcomes. Sudden death during sporting events has occurred in children and adolescents. Traditionally, manual defibrillation has been the only form of defibrillation used in children. With newer technology available in AEDs, the question arose as to whether they could be used effectively to treat arrhythmias in children.

STUDY

Cecchin et al. (2001) performed a study of over 600 children to determine the specificity and sensitivity of automated external defibrillation in children.

Findings

The researchers found that AEDs can be sensitive and specific for detecting and treating arrhythmia by defibrillation

in children older than 1 year of age. Salib, Cyran, Cilley, Maron, and Thomas (2005) report a positive and healthy outcome after an AED was used at the scene on a 13-year-old who suffered a baseball blow to the chest resulting in commotio cordis. As a result of these and many other studies, in 2005, the American Heart Association recommended changes in the pediatric basic life support guidelines to include the use of AEDs in sudden witnessed collapse in children.

Nursing Implications

For nurses working in hospitals, ensure that witnessed collapse in children includes assessing for the need for defibrillation. Outside the hospital, nurses should advocate for AEDs to be placed in all high school gymnasiums and at all parks and ball fields.

Adapted from Cecchin, F., Jorgenson, D. B., Berul, C. I., Perry, J. C., Zimmerman, A. A., Duncan, B. W., . . . Atkins, D. L. (2001). Is arrhythmia detection by automatic external defibrillator accurate for children? Sensitivity and specificity of an automatic external defibrillator algorithm in 696 pediatric arrhythmias. *Circulation, 103,* 2438–2483; and Salib, E. A., Cyran, S. E., Cilley, R. E., Maron, B. J., & Thomas, N. J. (2005). Efficacy of bystander cardiopulmonary resuscitation and out-of-hospital automated external defibrillation as life-saving therapy in commotio cordis. *Journal of Pediatrics, 147,* 863–866.

synchronized—that is, the electrical current is applied on the R wave of the electrocardiogram (ECG).

The basic defibrillator is equipped with adult- and pediatric-sized paddles or pads. A power button turns the machine on and controls are used to select the amount of energy (joules) to be delivered. Typically, the initial energy amount is 2 J/kg; it can be increased up to 4 J/kg for defibrillation. Energy for cardioversion is delivered at 0.5 to 1 J/kg.

When the defibrillator is being used in an acute care setting, a code team member will take charge of defibrillator operations. He or she is responsible for ensuring that only the child receives the energy from the defibrillator. The operator will verbalize a warning and do a visual check before delivering electricity to the child to ensure that all personnel and other equipment are clear of the bed to avoid accidental shock.

Using Automated External Defibrillation

In cases of sudden, witnessed, out-of-hospital collapse, an arrhythmia is often the cause. Therefore, the AHA has revised its recommendations about the use of an AED in children (Berg et al., 2010). An AED is an alternative to manually defibrillating an individual. The AED device consists of chest pads that act as both electrodes and conduction pads. These electrodes are used to monitor the heart rhythm and deliver the electrical current. AED devices are readily available in a variety of locations, such as airports, sports facilities, and businesses. Traditionally, the AED was designed for

use in adults, but newer AEDs with smaller pads and the ability to adjust energy (joules) delivery are now more available. Therefore, the AHA has recommended that an AED be used for children who are older than age 1 year who have no pulse and have suffered a sudden, witnessed collapse (Berg et al., 2010).

The AED is designed for persons to use in prehospital settings. Once the AED is turned on, the machine uses auditory commands to guide laypersons and health care professionals alike through the correct placement of the pads and the administration of energy. The AED periodically evaluates the victim's cardiac rhythm and instructs the user to check for a pulse, continuing CPR, and delivering electricity when appropriate. Nurses who care for children should be able to operate an AED. See Evidence-Based Practice 51.1.

Determining Medication Doses and Equipment Sizes

Many pediatric acute care facilities prepare code reference sheets when a child is admitted. This sheet uses the child's actual weight to determine emergency medication doses and equipment sizes. It is important for the nurse to understand where these are located in the each facility when caring for children.

Ambulatory care providers often use the Broselow tape to estimate the child's weight based on the child's length (Fig. 51.2). The tape is colour coded and emergency equipment for a child of that size is stored in corresponding colour-coded packages or in colour-

A

B

FIGURE 51.2 **A.** Broselow tape. **B.** Measure the child's length with the Broselow tape to determine medication doses and tracheal tube size.

coded drawers on the pediatric emergency cart. Medication doses and equipment sizes are also located on the tape. The most accurate calculation for code medications is based on the child's weight, but use of the Broselow tape for estimating the weight has been shown to be successful in children weighing less than 25 kg (Jones, 2016).

Managing Pain

Depending on the child's status and pain level, individualize pain management interventions. For the alert child, nonpharmacologic measures may be used in addition to medications. Provide atraumatic care for procedures and use pharmacologic treatments to manage pain as the child's condition allows. Refer to Chapter 36 for additional information on pain management strategies.

Ensuring Stabilization

After a child has been resuscitated, the nurse plays a key role in stabilization and transport. Thoroughly document the interventions that were performed as well as the ongoing assessment of the child's response to the interventions. Provide continued monitoring of the child while awaiting transport. Copy and assemble any pertinent documentation, such as the resuscitation record, nurse's notes, and laboratory test results, to be given to the receiving institution. Ensure that all lines are taped securely and that vascular access sites are dressed and labelled with the date and time of insertion. As soon as possible, bring the child's family in to visit the child. Provide explanations about the IV lines, monitoring equipment, and other medical equipment and devices. Encourage the family to talk to and touch the child.

Providing Support and Education to the Child and Family

The experience of respiratory distress, oxygen deprivation, and an emergency situation is frightening for persons of all ages. The life-saving interventions that take place during an emergency can be especially intimidating and upsetting to children. Infants and young children cannot understand explanations about interventions, and older children and adolescents may feel frightened and angry about their loss of control. The caregivers may feel fear, anger, guilt, and sadness. They may be concerned about the very real possibility that their child might die.

Resuscitation of a child is often a perplexing and frightening event for laypersons to observe. Traditionally family members have been excluded during the resuscitation of children. Recently, however, there has been a trend to allow family members to be present during pediatric resuscitation. Studies have shown that family presence during resuscitation may assist with family coping (McAlvin & Carew-Lyons, 2014).

Considering the highly technical nature of resuscitation, the rapidity with which interventions occur, and the fear associated with a life-threatening event, nurses can play a crucial role in providing understandable explanations to families, with empathic support. During the acute phase, the nurse should give brief explanations as life-saving interventions are being provided. Examples of these types of explanations include:
• When applying the pulse oximeter sensor: "This light will check your child's oxygen level; it won't hurt."

- When connecting the child to the cardiac monitor: "We're going to put these sticky patches on your child and connect the patches to the leads so we can monitor his heart rate on this screen."
- When preparing for intubation and ventilation: "Your child can't breathe on his own right now, so we are going to give him some extra help with this tube. This tube will go into his breathing passage and this machine will help him to breathe."

The nurse plays a key role in providing empathy and support. Do not provide false reassurance and say, for example, "He's going to be all right." The outcome is never certain. Rather, communicate empathically. For example, say, "This must be very difficult for you. We are doing everything we can to help your child." Provide honest answers in a reassuring manner. Respect each family's diversity and observe their strengths and weaknesses. Be nonjudgmental in all interactions with families, even when the child's emergency situation may have resulted from family neglect.

Parents often feel helpless when their child is in a medical environment. Suddenly overwhelmed with the equipment and monitoring devices, they no longer are the persons who are the most skilled in caring for their child. Integrate the child's parents into the health care team. Suggest ways the parents can make the hospital experience more normal for their child. For example, allow a parent to read a story to their child or encouraging a parent to hold their child's hand is therapeutic both for the child and the parents. Be aware of this dramatic change and how it affects the parents. Always ensure that they feel like they are a welcome part of their child's care.

Providing the child with familiar comfort objects helps to decrease anxiety. Once the intubated child is alert and stabilized, assist them with communication. Some children can lift one finger for yes and two fingers for no. If the child is old enough to write, provide paper and pencil. Play is essential to the work of the child, and even if he or she is immobile, play is still possible. Puppets at the bedside and books help normalize experience in a scary situation. Teenagers may enjoy listening to music through headphones. Even children who are comatose should be talked to and allowed to listen to familiar music.

Even if the outcomes are serious, the nurse can provide critical support to children and families. Whether hugging a crying mother or playing "peek-a-boo" with an intubated child, the nurse can make a difference during a frightening experience.

Atraumatic Care

In the conscious child, ensure proximity of the caregiver during the post-resuscitation phase to provide security and assist with keeping the child calm.

NURSING MANAGEMENT OF CHILDREN IN EMERGENCIES

Nurses must be adept at identifying the early warning signs of an emergency so they can quickly and appropriately intervene to prevent deterioration to cardiopulmonary arrest. Assessment and management of the most common types of emergencies in children are discussed below. The topics covered include respiratory arrest, shock, cardiac arrhythmias and arrest, near-drowning, poisoning, and traumatic injury.

Respiratory Arrest

Respiratory emergencies may lead to respiratory failure and eventual cardiopulmonary arrest in children. Infants and young children are at greater risk for respiratory emergencies than adolescents and adults because they have smaller airways and underdeveloped immune systems, resulting in a diminished ability to combat serious respiratory illnesses. Young children often lack coordination, making them susceptible to choking on foods and small objects, which may also lead to cardiopulmonary arrest. In addition, sudden infant death syndrome (SIDS) is a leading cause of cardiopulmonary arrest in young infants and thus is the leading cause of post-neonatal mortality (Canadian Paediatric Society, 2016). For these reasons, nurses must be skilled at recognizing the early warning signs of pediatric respiratory distress in order to prevent progression to cardiopulmonary arrest. Table 51.2 lists some of the more common causes of pediatric respiratory arrest.

Nursing Assessment

If the child has severe respiratory compromise, obtain a brief history while simultaneously providing respiratory interventions. To obtain the history, use the following questions as a guide:
- When did the symptoms begin and when do they occur?
- Did the symptoms have a sudden onset (as with a foreign-body aspiration)?
- How have the symptoms progressed?
- Is the cough continual, intermittent, or worse at night or with exercise?
- Has there been any stridor? (Stridor is heard upon inhalation and may be associated with swelling of the trachea, as with croup or a foreign body in the upper airway.)
- Is there wheezing? If so, is the wheezing on inspiration or on expiration, or both?
- What makes the symptoms better or worse?
- Does drinking from a bottle induce the symptoms (as with gastroesophageal reflux–induced aspiration)?
- Is the child taking any medication for the symptoms?
- Does the child or do any members of the immediate family have a history of chronic respiratory disease, such as asthma?

TABLE 51.2	CAUSES OF RESPIRATORY ARREST IN CHILDREN
Condition	**Cause**
Upper airway	Burns Croup Epiglottitis Foreign-body aspiration Reflux Strangulation or near strangulation Tracheomalacia Vascular ring
Lower airway	Asthma Bronchiolitis Burns Foreign-body aspiration Pertussis infection Pneumonia Pneumothorax Reflux
Nonrespiratory origins	Septic shock HIV
Neurologic	CNS infection Guillain–Barré syndrome Poliomyelitis Seizures Sleep apnea Spinal cord trauma Sudden infant death
Chronic illness	Complications of severe prematurity Cystic fibrosis Bone marrow transplant Neutropenia
Metabolic/ endocrine disorders	Diabetic ketoacidosis Mitochondrial disorders
Cardiac conditions	Arrhythmia Congenital cardiac problems Acquired cardiac problems
Traumatic/ unintentional/ intentional injury	Asphyxia Child abuse/"shaken baby syndrome" Drowning Electrocution Gunshot wound Toxic ingestion Vehicular-related trauma

CNS, central nervous system.

Adapted from Fleisher, G. R., & Ludwig, S. (2010). *Textbook of pediatric emergency medicine* (6th ed.). Philadelphia, PA: Lippincott Williams & Wilkins.

- Are the child's immunizations up to date?
- Was the child born prematurely? Or require mechanical ventilation? For how long?
- Were there any respiratory problems during the first few days of life?
- When did the child last eat? This question is important because a recent meal will increase the child's risk of

aspiration in the event of a respiratory arrest or during tracheal intubation.

If the child can communicate, ask how they are feeling? Are they short of breath? Does their chest hurt? Observe the child while speaking. Children who are in respiratory distress may speak in short sentences with gasping between words.

PHYSICAL EXAMINATION

In an emergency, physical examination is often limited to inspection, observation, and auscultation. First, survey the respiratory status. Determine if the child is breathing.

Inspection and Observation. Establish if the airway is patent, maintainable, or at risk of obstruction. If required, open the airway with interventions such as a towel roll under an infant's neck and insert an appropriately sized oropharyngeal or nasopharyngeal airway. The airway at risk requires aggressive intervention and the insertion of a tracheal tube may be required.

Observe the child's posture. Is the child sitting up, leaning forward (tripoding), and drooling, as with epiglottitis? Observe the child's face: does he or she appear anxious or relaxed? Children in respiratory distress often appear anxious. Look at the nose and mouth. Are the nares patent? Is there noticeable nasal congestion or mucous? Note nasal flaring or mouth breathing. Observe for head bobbing. Listen for audible expiratory grunting or inspiratory stridor. Note the child's colour. Does the child appear pale, mottled, dusky, ashen, or cyanotic? Children may appear mottled in response to poor oxygenation, hypothermia, or stress. Children with severe respiratory compromise may appear dusky or ashen. Look for cyanosis around the mouth or on the trunk. Cyanosis is a late and often ominous sign of respiratory distress. Central cyanosis is most likely to be associated with respiratory or cardiac compromise. In contrast, peripheral cyanosis is most likely to be associated with circulatory alteration.

Take Note!

Closely inspect the colour of the skin around the mouth. Circumoral pallor is a sign of poor oxygenation.

Evaluate the pattern and quality of respiration, noting the respiratory rate. **Tachypnea** (increased respiratory rate) is often noted in respiratory distress. However, seriously ill children grunt and may have normal or subnormal respiratory rates. **Hypoventilation**, a decrease in the depth and rate of respirations, is noted in very ill children or children who have central respiratory depression possibly secondary to narcotics. In premature or young infants (younger than 2 months), periodic breathing may occur. **Periodic breathing** is regular breathing with occasional short pauses of apnea. After the apneic pause, the infant will breathe rapidly (up to 60 breaths per minute) for a short period and will then resume a normal respiratory rate. In general, the infant who has periodic breathing looks pink and has a normal heart rate (HR). Observe for the use of accessory muscles in the neck or retractions in the chest, determining the extent and severity of the retractions.

Auscultation. Auscultate the lungs with the diaphragm of the stethoscope. Breath sounds over the tracheal region are higher pitched and are described as vesicular, while breath sounds over the peripheral lung fields tend to be lower pitched, described as bronchial. Instruct the child to take deep breaths with an open mouth. To encourage the young child to exhale strongly, instruct him or her to "blow out" the penlight (as with a candle) or to blow on a tissue. Encourage the child not to breathe more rapidly than normal to prevent **hyperventilation** (increased depth and rate of respirations) and to avoid making any noises with the mouth.

> **Take Note!**
> Significant upper respiratory congestion often interferes with assessment of the lower airways because the sound is easily transmitted throughout the chest. Differentiate between the upper and lower airway noises by listening with the stethoscope over the noise to assist with determining whether the noise is nasal or bronchial.

Auscultate the child's chest systematically. Listen in all anterior, axillary, and posterior regions, comparing the left to the right sides. Note any decreased or absent breath sounds, which may be the result of bronchial obstruction (as with mucous infection) or air trapping (as in children with asthma). Unilateral absent breath sounds are associated with foreign-body aspiration and pneumothorax.

> **Take Note!**
> Sometimes a child's respiratory status is so severely compromised that little or no air movement is noted. This commonly occurs during a severe asthma exacerbation. Minimal or no air movement requires immediate intervention.

Note the presence and location of adventitious breath sounds such as crackles, wheezes, rhonchi, or pleural friction rub (a low-pitched, grating sound resulting from inflammation of the pleura).

Palpation. Palpate the chest for any abnormalities. In the more cooperative child, assess for tactile fremitus, using the palm of the hand palpate over the lung regions in the same manner as for auscultation and percussion while the child says "ninety-nine." Increased vibrations elicited during this manoeuvre are associated with consolidating conditions, such as pneumonia.

Percussion. Percuss the intercostal spaces between the ribs in the same systematic fashion as with auscultation. Normally, percussion over an air-filled lung reveals resonant sounds. Note the presence of hyperresonance, which may indicate an acute problem such as a pneumothorax or a chronic disease such as asthma. In contrast, percussion sounds will be dull over a lobe of the lung that is consolidated with fluid, infectious organisms, and blood cells, as in the case of pneumonia.

LABORATORY AND DIAGNOSTIC TESTING

Use continuous pulse oximetry if respiratory status is a concern. Note and report oxygen saturation levels below 95%. (See Chapter 40 for additional information about use of the pulse oximeter.)

Additional tests may reveal:
- Arterial or capillary blood gases: hypoxemia, hypercarbia, altered pH
- Chest x-ray: alterations in normal anatomy or lung expansion, or evidence of pneumonia, tumour, or foreign body
- Metal detector: evidence of metallic foreign body, in particular coins (Gilger, Jain, & McOmber, 2015).

> **Take Note!**
> Children with cardiac conditions resulting in cyanosis often have baseline oxygen saturations that are relatively low because of the mixing of oxygenated with deoxygenated blood.

Nursing Management

The basic principle of pediatric emergency care and PALS is prevention of cardiopulmonary arrest (Kleinman et al., 2010a). Therefore, the nurse must rapidly assess and appropriately manage children who have signs of respiratory distress. Nursing management of the child in respiratory distress involves maintaining a patent airway, providing supplemental oxygen, monitoring for changes in status, and in some cases assisting ventilation. In addition to providing these life-saving measures and monitoring the child's progress, offer support and education to the child and family.

MAINTAINING A PATENT AIRWAY

When a child exhibits signs of respiratory distress, make a quick decision about whether it will be safe to allow the child to stay with the parent or whether the child must be placed on the examination table or bed. For example, in the case of croup, the child will often breathe more comfortably and experience less stridor while in the comfort of the parent's lap. Many children in respiratory distress are often most comfortable sitting upright, as this position helps to decrease the work of breathing by allowing appropriate diaphragmatic movement. In contrast, a child with a decreasing level of consciousness may need to be placed in the supine position to facilitate positioning of the airway.

The infant may benefit from a small towel folded under the shoulders or neck (Fig. 51.3). Avoid neck flexion or hyperextension, which may completely occlude

FIGURE 51.4 Jaw-thrust technique for opening the airway.

FIGURE 51.3 **A.** The infant and young child's prominent occiput encourages flexion of the neck and may result in airway occlusion. **B.** Putting a towel roll under the shoulders or neck helps to open the infant's or young child's airway by placing it in the neutral or "sniff" position.

the infant's airway. In children older than 1 year, without suspected cervical spine injury, use the head tilt–chin lift technique to open the airway. If the child has suffered head or neck trauma and cervical spine instability is a concern, use the jaw-thrust manoeuvre by placing three fingers under both sides of the child's lower jaw and lift the jaw upward and outward (Fig. 51.4). In either case, never place the hand under the neck to open the airway.

Often the nurse encounters an acutely ill child who cannot maintain their airway independently but may be able to do so with some assistance. Often simply opening the airway by moving the tongue away from the tracheal opening is all that is required to regain airway patency. In certain conditions, an appropriately sized nasopharyngeal or oropharyngeal airway may be necessary for airway maintenance. Comparison Chart 51.1 provides additional information about these types of airways.

COMPARISON CHART 51.1	OROPHARYNGEAL VERSUS NASOPHARYNGEAL AIRWAYS
Oropharyngeal airway (used only in unconscious children with absent gag reflex)	• Consists of a simple plastic curved device that has a central air channel to allow for aeration • Is used when an unconscious child has difficulty maintaining airway patency due to upper airway obstruction, from the tongue • Allows for oral suction • Determine the correct size of the airway by placing it next to the child's cheek from the corner of their mouth to the tragus of their ear with the tip pointing down. An airway that is too large will extend past the angle of the child's mandible and can obstruct the glottic opening when inserted • Choose the airway that best fits the child to decrease the risk of injury to the structures of the mouth
Nasopharyngeal airway (may be used in conscious children and children who have an intact gag reflex)	• Consists of a flexible curved tube that is inserted nasally • Is used when the child has difficulty maintaining airway patency due to tongue obstruction or palate problems, when neurologic impairment causes poor pharyngeal tone, or in the child with impaired consciousness • Allows for nasopharyngeal suction • The diameter of the airway should not be so large that it puts too much pressure on the internal nasal tissue. There are two steps for measuring this airway: (1) measure the distance from the opening of the child's nare to the tragus of their ear; (2) match the diameter of the child's fifth digit, the approximate diameter of their nasopharyngeal passage to the diameter of the nasopharyngeal airway • Monitor for mucosal irritation, nasal septum swelling, and laceration of the adenoids • Do not use this type of airway in children with a history of bleeding disorders and basilar skull fractures • This airway's small diameter can easily become obstructed with secretions and blood

TABLE 51.3	AIRWAY AND VENTILATION METHODS	
Method	**Description**	**Comments**
Anesthesia bag or flow-inflating ventilation systems	A small, collapsible bag that consists of a reservoir bag, an overflow port, and a fresh gas inflow port	• Adjustment of the oxygen flow and of the outlet control valve is necessary • Useful in providing positive end-expiratory pressure (PEEP) or continuous positive airway pressure (CPAP) • Adequate training and significant skill are needed to properly operate this device • Hypercapnia and barotrauma may result with improper use • Used more commonly in the postanesthesia care unit (PACU) and in the neonatal intensive care unit
Bag-valve-mask device or manual resuscitator	A self-inflating oxygen delivery bag that does not require an oxygen source for resuscitation and ventilation. The bag can be connected to oxygen to provide higher oxygen levels than room air. When the child exhales, the non-rebreathing valve closes, allowing exhaled, deoxygenated air to escape	• Effective in providing oxygen to a child who is in severe respiratory distress or who has suffered a respiratory arrest • A more efficient method of respiratory resuscitation than mouth-to-mouth resuscitation; decreased rescuer exposure to communicable disease • Most medical personnel can be trained to perform resuscitation with this method • Possibly tiring for the rescuer when used to ventilate a child for long periods of time (see discussion on bag-mask ventilation)
Laryngeal mask airway	An inflatable silicone mask and rubber connecting tube that is inserted blindly into the airway, forming a seal	• The airway is introduced into the pharynx and advanced until it meets resistance; balloon cuff is then inflated • Easier insertion than a tracheal tube • Usually used in the unconscious child who benefits from bag-valve-mask ventilation but does not require intubation • Improvement in child comfort
Tracheal intubation	A plastic tube inserted in the trachea to establish and maintain an airway when the airway cannot be maintained effectively using other measures (e.g., nasal trumpet or bag-valve-mask ventilation)	• Skilled medical professional (physician, nurse practitioner, respiratory specialist, emergency medical technician, or physician's assistant) necessary for insertion • The nurse acts as a valuable assistant during the intubation procedure

ASSISTING VENTILATION USING A BAG-VALVE-MASK

The child in respiratory distress may ventilate poorly, hypoventilate, or tire and become apneic. In this case, the child may require assistance with ventilation through bag-valve-mask (BVM) ventilation (see Table 51.3 for methods in assisting with ventilation using tracheal intubation [discussed in detail below]), an anesthesia bag or flow-inflating ventilation system, and a laryngeal mask airway.

BVM ventilation is used in the management of children who cannot ventilate or oxygenate effectively on their own. This technique can improve efficiency of ventilation and is superior to mouth-to-mouth resuscitation as it provides higher oxygen concentrations, increases tidal volume, and protects the nurse from exposure to oral secretions (Berg et al., 2010). However, this technique requires proper training and practice and requires a patent airway and appropriate use of the BVM.

Ventilation with the BVM may be performed with one or two rescuers. First, choose an appropriate-sized bag and a corresponding face mask that fits the infant or child. Self-inflating bags and masks are available in neonatal, infant, child, and adult sizes. Choose a face mask that fits the child's face appropriately providing a seal over the nose and mouth and excludes the eyes to prevent pressure on the eyes (Fig. 51.5).

Take Note!

Face masks should be clear so that the rescuer can see the child's lip colour and identify any emesis during resuscitation.

FIGURE 51.5 The mask should form a seal over the nose and mouth, across the chin and nose bridge.

FIGURE 51.6 Proper hand placement for maintaining airway and adequate mask seal using one-rescuer technique.

Connect the BVM via the tubing to the oxygen source and turn on the oxygen. When resuscitating infants and children, set the flow rate at 10 L/min. For an adolescent who is adult sized, set the flow rate at 15 L/min or higher to compensate for the larger volume bag. Check to make sure that the oxygen is flowing through the tubing to the bag. Self-inflating bags do not provide free-flow oxygen out of the face mask; manual pumping of the bag is necessary. However, the bags have a corrugated plastic tail that allows oxygen to flow freely. Therefore, check over the tail for oxygen flow through the bag.

After opening the airway appropriately (see above), place the mask over the child's face. When one rescuer is providing ventilation (commonly referred to as "bagging"), the person must provide a seal with the mask over the child's nose and mouth with one hand and use the other hand to manipulate the resuscitator bag. The hand used to provide the mask seal will simultaneously maintain the airway in an open position. Generally, use the left thumb and index finger to hold the mask on the child's face. While maintaining a good seal with the mask, use upward pressure on the jaw angle to lift the chin to keep the mouth and airway open while pressing downward on the mask (Fig. 51.6). Take care not to put pressure on the trachea with the fourth and fifth fingers.

If adequate personnel are available, a more desirable situation involves one person standing behind the child's head to maintain an open airway and to provide a seal of the mask over the nose and mouth with a hand on each side of the mask using the thumbs and second fingers. A second rescuer stands on one side of the child and compresses the bag to ventilate the child using both hands. If the child is difficult to ventilate, the two-rescuer method allows the ventilating rescuer to provide better ventilation than with the one-rescuer method. In addition, the two-rescuer method ensures the best possible mask seal, as the rescuer holding the mask can use both hands to maintain the seal.

Regardless of the number of persons present, proper placement and fit of the face mask is critical, and a good seal must be maintained throughout the resuscitation. During ventilation, use only the force and tidal volume necessary to cause the chest to rise, no more. If a good chest rise is not observed, attempt to open the airway by repositioning. It may be necessary to adjust the position of the airway a few times to achieve a patency conducive to ventilation.

Compress the bag to deliver breaths at the amount recommended in infants and children. Initially, provide two rescue breaths observing for the chest to rise. Rescue breaths should not overinflate the lungs. Breaths should be delivered over 1 second. After the first two rescue ventilations, perform rescue breathing at a rate of one breath every 3 to 5 seconds, about 12 to 20 breaths per minute. Delivering each breath should be a steady, one-inhalation-to-one-exhalation ratio ensuring that the amount of time delivering the inspiratory ventilation is equal to the amount of time that expiratory is allowed. While ventilating the infant or child, work with, not against, any spontaneous respiratory effort; in other words, if the child is breathing out, do not attempt to force air in at the same time.

Monitoring Effectiveness of Ventilation. During the resuscitation, continually reassess the child's response to the resuscitative efforts, noting:

- Adequacy of chest rise
- Absence or minimal presence of abdominal distention
- Improved HR and pulse oximetry readings
- Improved colour
- Capillary refill less than 3 seconds with strengthening pulses

If the child's status deteriorates and he or she becomes pulseless, then chest compressions must be initiated. In addition, periodically and briefly stop ventilating to evaluate for spontaneous respirations.

Preventing Complications Related to Bag-Valve-Mask Ventilation. During resuscitation, health care personnel usually exhibit high-energy levels, a normal physiologic response that facilitates resuscitative efforts as the rescuers act quickly. However, this heightened state can lead to overzealousness while ventilating an infant or child. Health care providers may inadvertently hyperventilate the child by ventilating too rapidly using too much tidal volume, leading to excessive ventilation volume and increased airway pressure. Poor technique can be detrimental to the child, resulting in:

- Reduced cardiac output (CO) as a result increased intrathoracic pressure and increased cardiac afterload
- Air trapping
- **Barotrauma** resulting from changes in pressure
- Air leak from poor seal around nose and mouth resulting in decreased oxygen

In addition, children with head injuries who receive excessive ventilation volumes at high rates are at risk for:

- Decreased cerebral blood flow
- Cerebral edema
- Further neurologic damage (AHA, 2016b)

For these reasons, nurses must be mindful of their technique during bagging. Ventilate the child in a controlled and uniform manner, providing just enough volume to result in the chest rising, being careful to not exceed the recommended respiratory rate or provide too much tidal volume to the child.

ASSISTING WITH VENTILATION USING TRACHEAL INTUBATION

Tracheal intubation is required when the infant or child cannot maintain their own airway or requires artificial ventilation for a prolonged time (see Table 51.3). Intubation of infants and children is a procedure that requires great skill and therefore should be performed by only the most qualified and experienced personnel. In acute situations, children are most commonly intubated orally, rather than nasally.

Nurses are an essential part of the intubation team in assisting a physician, nurse practitioner, respiratory therapist, or physician's assistant during the intubation

---

NURSING PROCEDURE 51.1

Assisting With Tracheal Intubation

1. Prepare equipment and supplies.
2. Prepare medications (for rapid sequence intubation).
3. Turn up the volume on the cardiac monitor so that members of the team can easily hear the audible QRS indication of the child's heart rate in order to alert them to bradycardia during the procedure.
4. Turn on and test the suction.
5. Continue to ventilate the child with the bag-valve-mask (BVM) and 100% oxygen as the team prepares to intubate the child.
6. When there is no suspected cervical spine injury, in the child older than age 2 years, place a small pillow under the child's head to facilitate opening of the airway; this is not necessary in children younger than 2 years due to the prominence of their occiput.
7. Preoxygenate the child before the initial intubation attempt with several inhalations of 100% oxygen using the BVM.
8. Administer premedication and medications for sedation.
9. Administer paralyzing medication.
10. When assisting with the intubation, stand beside the child's head and prepare to assist with suctioning oral secretions, providing BVM ventilation, and assisting with securing the tube with an approved securing device.
11. After each intubation attempt, provide several inhalations of 100% oxygen using the BVM.
12. Observe as the health care professional who is intubating the child follows the recommended procedure for intubation using the laryngoscope to visualize the vocal cords.

---

procedure (Nursing Procedure 51.1). The nurse may set up the equipment, prepare and administer intubation medications, and assist with suctioning oral secretions and preparing the securing device to secure the tracheal tube. When a child is in full arrest, the nurse might be responsible for performing ongoing chest compressions while other team members manage the child's airway.

Preparing Equipment. Appropriate setup and preparation of equipment is essential (Table 51.4). The tracheal

TABLE 51.4	EQUIPMENT AND SUPPLIES FOR TRACHEAL INTUBATION
Laryngoscope blades	Straight blades (Miller) are often used for infants and young children. A curved-blade laryngoscope (Macintosh) may be used for older children and adolescents. The blade has a little light bulb attached to it for visualization of the trachea. The light bulb should be bright and must be attached securely.
Tracheal tubes	Three sizes should be readily available: the estimated size, a size smaller, and a size larger. A stylet may be used to guide the tube through the child's vocal cords.
Oxygen	100% oxygen is provided using a bag-valve-mask before intubation and after unsuccessful intubation attempts.
Suction	Properly working wall or portable suction with appropriate-sized suction catheters (that fit the tracheal tube) should be prepared; the package is opened, leaving the sterile-tipped end inside the package and connecting the other end to the suction tubing. A Yankauer suction catheter (large, stiff catheter) should also be available to clear secretions that interfere with the ability to visualize the airway.
Monitors	Pulse oximeter and cardiac monitor with an audible tone indicating the QRS complex should be in place. Exhaled end-tidal CO_2 device is needed to detect increased CO_2 levels after the intubation to assist in confirmation of placement.
Nasogastric tube	Inserting a nasogastric (NG) tube will help to mitigate abdominal distention. Children who are manually ventilated typically have some abdominal distention as some air passes into the stomach.
Personal protective equipment	Gloves, goggles, and a mask are necessary to protect health care workers. In the case of copious bleeding, health care workers should also wear gowns.
Approved securing device	Approved securing device should be prepared for securing the tube. For children who have had multiple intubations, a protective barrier may be applied under the securing device to protect the skin.

tube size depends on the child's size. To calculate tracheal tube size, divide the child's age by 4 and add 4. The resulting number will indicate the size of the tracheal tube in millimetres. For example, if the child is 2 years old, the proper-sized tube would be 4.5 ([2/4] + 4 = 4.5). Always have one size smaller on hand, so have a 4.0 and a 4.5 tracheal tube for this child.

Administering Medications. Several medications are often given to facilitate intubation of children. Premedicating a child before passing a tracheal tube aids in the following:

- Reducing pain and anxiety (consistent with the concept of atraumatic care)
- Minimizing the adverse effects of passing the tracheal tube in to the airway (vagal stimulation leading to **bradycardia**, a decrease in HR)
- Preventing hypoxia
- Reducing intracranial pressure
- Preventing airway trauma and aspiration of stomach contents

The use of medications for sedation and paralyzation during the intubation process is known as rapid sequence intubation (Table 51.5). Typically, these medications are used in controlled settings such as the emergency department or the intensive care unit (ICU). Rapid sequence intubation is done only in children who are not experiencing

cardiac arrest. If the intubation is expected to be particularly difficult, paralyzing medications should not be used.

The nurse must be aware of the differences in the various medication classes, their advantages, their disadvantages, and adverse effects. The nurse must also be able to distinguish between medications that produce sedation and ones that produce analgesia. Children who are paralyzed and sedated may be suffering severe pain and not be able to communicate it. Pain control needs of children who are acutely ill are of paramount importance and cannot be overstated. Do not mistake a child who is immobilized as a result of sedative and paralytic medications for a child who is pain-free.

Take Note!

Each attempt to insert a tracheal tube should last no longer than 20 to 30 seconds. After each attempt, the child should receive multiple ventilations using the BVM method with 100% oxygen (AHA, 2016b).

Ensuring and Maintaining Correct Tube Placement. To assess for correct placement once the tracheal tube is inserted, observe for symmetric rise of the chest and auscultate over the lung fields for equal breath sounds. Inspect the tracheal tube for the presence of water vapour on the inside, indicating that the tube is in the trachea. To rule out accidental esophageal intubation, auscultate

TABLE 51.5	MEDICATIONS FOR RAPID SEQUENCE INTUBATION	
Medications	**Desired Effects**	**Undesirable Effects**
Sedatives: barbiturates—thiopental (short-acting barbiturate)	Has very rapid onset and short duration of action; reduces intracranial pressure and oxygen demand	Hypotensive effects of this drug are more severe in the dehydrated child When given in combination with narcotics, respiratory depression is potentiated
Sedatives: benzodiazepines—midazolam	Has a slightly slower onset than thiopental but is associated with fewer adverse effects Causes amnesia Can be titrated: at lower doses, it causes conscious sedation; at higher doses, it can induce anesthesia	When given in combination with narcotics, respiratory depression is potentiated
Anesthetic agent: ketamine	Has a rapid onset with sedative, amnesic, and analgesic affects. Can be dissociative (child is awake but unaware). May improve BP and cause bronchodilation (helpful for children with status asthmaticus)	Ketamine can cause increased intracranial pressure and increased ocular pressure. Therefore, children who have suffered head trauma or globe injury should not receive this medication Because of ketamine's sympathetic effects, hypertension can result from its use Ketamine tends to cause increased secretions, often necessitating the concomitant use of atropine to counteract this adverse effect May cause hallucinations and is therefore contraindicated in children with psychiatric problems
Anesthetic agent: lidocaine	Can decrease intracranial pressure at higher doses Advantageous in the management of hypovolemia as it is less likely to cause hypotension	Lidocaine can cause adverse cardiac effects such as bradycardia, hypotension, and dysrhythmias in high doses May be associated with CNS depression and seizures
Narcotic analgesic: fentanyl citrate	A highly concentrated opioid that causes fewer adverse effects (e.g., pruritus) than other opioids, with less hypotensive effect	Constipation and urinary retention (common with opioids) may occur Increases risk for respiratory depression, increased intracranial pressure, and hypotension Chest wall rigidity is common with this drug and may cause difficulty with ventilation
Paralyzing or neuromuscular blocking agents: Rocuronium, Succinylcholine, Vecuronium	Used for short-term paralysis during the intubation process. May be used for extended paralysis in ICU for children in whom movement would be detrimental. For example, a child with epiglottitis has a very precarious airway and must remain intubated until the epiglottis decreases in size. In certain respiratory conditions, spontaneous respiratory effort would interfere with the ventilation of a child and therefore prolonged paralysis is desirable	Succinylcholine (a depolarizing agent) has always been the gold standard for paralysis because it has a relatively rapid onset and is short-acting. However, it has a greater risk of adverse effects (bradycardia, hyperkalemia, hypertension, increased intracranial, and ocular pressure) and is contraindicated in a variety of clinical conditions. The contemporary approach to paralysis involves the use of longer acting agents, such as Rocuronium and Vecuronium, because children have fewer adverse effects with these medications. In addition, Rocuronium and Vecuronium may be used for extended paralysis (not an option with Succinylcholine)

CNS, central nervous system.

Adapted from Kleinman, M. E., Chameides, L., Schexnayder, S. M., Samson, R. A., Hazinski, M. F., Atkins, D. L., . . . Zaritsky, A. L. (2010a). Part 14: Pediatric advanced life support—2010 American Heart Association guidelines for cardiopulmonary resuscitation and emergency cardiovascular care. *Circulation, 122*(18 Suppl 3), S876–S908; and Taketomo, C. K., Hodding, J. H., & Kraus, D. M. (2013). *Pediatric & neonatal dosage handbook* (20th ed.). Hudson, OH: Lexicomp.

BOX 51.1

EXHALED CO₂ MONITORING OR END-TIDAL CO₂ MONITORING

- Device that connects to the child's ventilator circuit to detect CO_2 in the tubing. CO_2 should be noted in the tubing after six ventilations.
- End-tidal CO_2 devices that do not connect to a monitor are colour coded. Their change in colour confirms presence of CO_2, confirming tracheal tube placement.
- NOTE: end-tidal CO_2 devices may at times fail to detect the presence of exhaled carbon dioxide, continue to rely upon visualization of tube placement, symmetric chest rise, and bilateral breath sounds (AHA, 2016a, 2016b)
- Waveform capnography

over the abdomen while the child is being ventilated: there should not be breath sounds in the abdomen. Note improvement in the oxygen saturation level via pulse oximetry and assess skin colour.

Once tracheal tube placement is verified, mark the tube with indelible ink at the level of the child's lip and secure it with a securing device. Document the number on the tracheal tube at the level of the child's lips. Anticipate a chest x-ray to confirm correct placement of the tracheal tube.

After placement is confirmed, the tracheal tube is connected to the ventilator by respiratory personnel. The ventilator will provide continuous artificial ventilation and oxygenation. Exhaled CO_2 monitoring is recommended as it provides an indication of appropriate ventilation and tracheal tube placement (Box 51.1). If an exhaled CO_2 monitor is being used, the exhaled CO_2 should be yellow.

The nurse plays a key role in ensuring that the tracheal tube remains securely in place by doing the following:

- Using soft wrist restraints if necessary to prevent the child from removing the tracheal tube
- Providing sedative and/or paralyzing medications as required and ordered
- Using caution when moving the child for diagnostic imaging, personal care, changing linens, and performing other procedures

Monitoring the Child Who Is Intubated. Provide ongoing and frequent monitoring of the intubated child to determine adequacy of oxygenation and ventilation as noted earlier. Once the child is intubated, the ventilatory support being provided should result in improvement in oxygen saturation, skin colour, and vital signs. If the child begins to exhibit signs of poor oxygenation, assess the airway and breathing. Auscultate the lungs for equal air entry and determine the HR. Are the breath sounds

equal? Is the HR normal for age? Perform a quick survey of the equipment and look for any kinked or disconnected tubes. Determine oxygen saturation levels using a pulse oximeter and evaluate the end-tidal CO_2 using an exhaled device or a calibrated monitor (see Box 51.1). Use the mnemonic "DOPE" for troubleshooting when the status of a child who is intubated deteriorates:

D = Displacement, displacement of the tracheal tube from the trachea.

O = Obstruction, of the tracheal tube (e.g., with a mucous plug).

P = Pneumothorax which can result in a sudden change in the child's assessment. The signs of a pneumothorax include decreased breath sounds and decreased chest expansion on the side of the pneumothorax. Subcutaneous emphysema may be noted over the chest. In the case of tension pneumothorax, there may be a sudden drop in HR and blood pressure, and tracheal deviation may be observed.

E = Equipment failure, disconnected oxygen supply, a leak in the ventilator circuit, or a loss of power can cause the child to deteriorate (Kleinman et al., 2010a).

Make sure all equipment is appropriately connected and functional. When obstruction with secretions is suspected, suction the tracheal tube. If the tracheal tube is displaced from the trachea, remove the tube if it remains in the child's mouth and begin BVM ventilation. In the case of pneumothorax, prepare to assist with needle thoracotomy and/or chest tube insertion.

Preparing the Intubated Child for Transport. Once the child is stabilized with a secure tracheal tube in place, prepare to transport the child. The child will be moved by stretcher to an ICU in the same acute care facility or by air or land ambulance to another facility that specializes in the care of acutely ill children. Make sure that all tubes are secured appropriately. During transport, use portable oxygen and ventilate manually with the BVM. Some transport teams may have portable transport ventilators. As the sending nurse, ensure that all laboratory results are obtained and provided to the receiving nurse. If the child is going to another facility, complete a detailed summary of the resuscitation and provide a copy of the nurse's and physician's progress notes. Complete the appropriate transfer forms as determined by the institution.

If the child is being transported by ambulance, the parents may not be able to accompany their child. In this case, find out as much as possible about the transport and assist the parents by giving directions to the receiving institution.

SHOCK

Shock is caused by an inability for blood flow and oxygen delivery to meet the metabolic demands of tissue (Kleinman et al., 2010b). If shock is left untreated, cardiopulmonary arrest will result. Shock, which may be classified as compensated or decompensated, is due to a variety of clinical problems. Compensated shock occurs when poor perfusion exists without a decrease in BP. In decompensated shock, inadequate perfusion is accompanied by a decrease in BP (hypotension). Uncorrected decompensated shock leads to cardiac arrest and may become irreversible, thus leading to death. The principles of PALS stress early assessment and management of children in compensated shock with the goal of preventing decompensated shock (Kleinman et al., 2010b). Once the child in shock is hypotensive, organ perfusion is dramatically impaired and a dire clinical scenario ensues.

Pathophysiology

Shock is the result of dramatic respiratory or hemodynamic compromise. Impaired CO, impaired systemic vascular resistance (SVR), or a combination of both causes shock. CO is equal to HR times ventricular stroke volume (SV) (CO = HR × SV). Stroke volume is how much blood is ejected from the heart with each beat. Stroke volume is affected by left ventricular filling pressure (preload), the impedance to ventricular filling (afterload), and myocardial contractility. Young children and infants have relatively small stroke volumes compared with older children and adults. Therefore, infants and young children differ from their adult counterparts in that their CO depends on their HR as they cannot alter their stroke volume. In cases of circulatory compromise and compensated shock in infants and children, their HR is increased. The exception to this is a paradoxical phenomenon in neonates, who may have bradycardia rather than tachycardia.

SVR or afterload is the impediment to the heart's ventricular ejection. Increased SVR will result in a decrease in blood flow unless the ventricular pressure increases. Increased vascular resistance is a common problem in shock. In children who have shock-related increased SVR, CO will fall unless the ventricle can compensate by increasing pressure. In cardiac insufficiency, the child's heart will have impaired ability to compensate for the increased afterload.

Altered microcirculatory status is common in all types of shock. Compensatory mechanisms are activated in response to decreased blood flow. Sympathetic nervous system response results in marked contraction of larger vessel sphincters and arterioles, resulting in dramatically impaired capillary blood flow. Blood is redirected away from less important body systems, such as the skin and the kidneys, to the vital organs such as the heart and brain.

During compensated shock, the body can maintain some level of blood flow to the vital organs. Peripheral vasoconstriction, the body's compensatory response to diminished blood flow, often results in the child's ability to maintain a normal or near-normal BP. As shock continues, capillary beds become obstructed by cellular debris while platelets and white blood cells aggregate. Endothelial damage occurs as a result of capillary congestion. Poor blood flow to the capillaries results in anaerobic metabolism producing lactic acid that can lead to acidosis. In addition, children with septic shock sustain marked endothelial damage as a result of exposure to bacterial toxins further increasing lactic acid production.

The cumulative effect of capillary obstruction and dramatically impaired blood flow is tissue ischemia. As tissue ischemia progresses, the child will show signs of altered perfusion to vital organs. As blood flow to the brain is diminished, the child will demonstrate an altered level of consciousness. Altered blood flow to the kidneys will result in decreased urine output or absence of urine output (oliguria). Commonly, the HR will increase in the early stages of shock, but as the heart becomes compromised from poor perfusion, the child will become bradycardic. The child will demonstrate an increased respiratory rate in the initial phase of shock. Tachypnea is often seen in septic shock. In fact, the child may demonstrate marked hyperventilation in an effort to blow off carbon dioxide in response to the acidosis that is associated with septic shock.

Types of Shock

The types of shock are hypovolemic, septic, cardiogenic, and distributive. Hypovolemic shock, the most common type of shock in children, occurs when systemic perfusion decreases as a result of inadequate vascular volume (Kleinman et al., 2010b). Children commonly have hypovolemic shock associated with fluid loss. Hypovolemic shock may occur with gastroenteritis resulting in vomiting and diarrhea, medications such as diuretics, and heat stroke. Other causes of hypovolemia in children include blood loss from a major injury, and third spacing of fluid, as with burns.

Septic shock is related to a systemic inflammatory response in which there may be increased CO with a low SVR, known as warm shock. More commonly in children, septic shock results in a decrease in CO with an increase in SVR, known as cold shock.

Cardiogenic shock results from an ineffective pump, the heart, with a resultant decrease in stroke volume. Children with structural heart disease and resultant arrhythmia are at risk for cardiogenic shock (Pomerantz & Roback, 2014).

Distributive shock is the result of a loss in the SVR. A relative hypovolemia occurs, most often with neurogenic injury–related shock and anaphylaxis. In relative hypovolemia, the vascular compartment expands due to systemic vasodilation. This results in a relatively larger vasculature requiring more fluid to maintain CO despite no actual loss of fluid.

Finally, toxic drug ingestions may also lead to shock.

Nursing Assessment

Nursing assessment of the child in shock includes the health history and physical examination as well as laboratory and diagnostic testing. The nursing assessment must be performed quickly and accurately so that resuscitation can be expedited.

HEALTH HISTORY

In shock, the health history is based on the child's presentation. Children with shock are critically ill and require emergent intervention. Therefore, the history is obtained as life-saving interventions are provided. Determine when the child first became ill and treatments that have been given thus far. Inquire about sources of volume loss, such as:

- Vomiting
- Diarrhea
- Decreased oral intake
- Blood loss

Ask when the child last urinated. Investigate for other related symptoms such as behavioural changes or lethargy. Has the child had a fever or rash, complained of headache, or been exposed to anyone with similar symptoms? Inquire about day care attendance and whether the family has recently travelled outside of the country. Determine if the child has a history of a congenital heart defect or other heart condition or if the child has severe allergies. Ask the parent about accidental ingestion of medications or other substances and, for the older child or adolescent, about the possibility of illicit substance use.

PHYSICAL EXAMINATION

The key to successful shock management is early recognition of the signs and symptoms. Obtain vital signs, noting any alterations. Measure BP, although this is not a reliable method of evaluating for shock in children, as children maintain a normal or slightly less than normal BP in compensated shock while sacrificing tissue perfusion until the child suffers a cardiopulmonary arrest. Therefore, other components of the circulatory evaluation are more reliable when assessing a child.

Take Note!

Bradycardia is a serious sign in neonates and may occur with respiratory compromise, circulatory compromise, or overwhelming sepsis (Kattwinkel et al., 2010).

As with any emergency, evaluate the airway and assess for a pulse. Is the child's airway patent? Is there a pulse and is it perfusing? Determine if the child is breathing. The child in shock will often demonstrate signs of respiratory distress, such as grunting, gasping, nasal flaring, tachypnea, and increased work of breathing. Auscultate breath sounds to determine the adequacy of air entry. If the child shows signs of respiratory distress, manage the airway and breathing problem, as discussed earlier in this chapter.

Assess skin colour, palpate skin temperature, and determine quality of pulses. Except in special cases, such as distributive shock, the child in shock will generally have paler and cooler extremities with delayed capillary refill. Note the line of demarcation if present. This refers to the point on the distal extremity where cool temperature begins (the proximal portion of the extremity may continue to be warm). In distributive shock, the initial assessment may reveal full and bounding pulses and warm, erythemic skin. Evaluate the pulse quality. Distal pulses will likely be weaker than central pulses.

Evaluate the child's hydration state and check skin turgor. Decreased elasticity is associated with hypovolemic states, though this is usually a late sign. Observe the child's face; in compensated shock, the child may be awake but obtunded and demonstrate signs of distress. The child in decompensated shock may have his or her eyes closed and may be responsive only to voice or other stimulation. Evaluate pupillary responses. Determine urinary output, which will be decreased in the child with shock.

After having evaluated and provided initial life-saving management for airway, breathing, and circulation, evaluate the child's entire body for other disabilities. Injuries warrant vigilant evaluation for ongoing blood loss as they may result in internal blood loss (e.g., a femur fracture). Signs of malformation, swelling, redness, or pain of the extremities may suggest internal blood loss. Inspect for any open wounds and active sites of bleeding. Children with abdominal injuries may lose large amounts of blood internally. Inspect the abdomen for redness, skin discolouration, or distention. Auscultate for bowel sounds in all four quadrants.

LABORATORY AND DIAGNOSTIC TESTING

As the child is being resuscitated, laboratory tests and x-rays will be ordered and obtained. However, no diagnostic test should replace the priority of respiratory support, vascular access, and fluid administration. Laboratory results will guide ongoing management. Common laboratory and diagnostic tests used for children with shock include:

- Blood glucose levels: usually performed at the bedside using a glucose meter to obtain a rapid result
- Electrolytes: to evaluate for electrolyte abnormalities
- CBC with differential: to assess for viral or bacterial infection (septic shock) and to evaluate for anemia and platelet abnormalities
- Blood culture: to evaluate for sepsis; preliminary results will not be available for 1 to 2 days
- C-reactive protein: to evaluate for infection
- Arterial blood gases: to assess oxygen and carbon dioxide levels and to provide information about acid–base balance

- Toxicology panel when ingestion is suspected
- Lumbar puncture: to evaluate cerebrospinal fluid for meningitis
- Urinalysis: to evaluate for glucose, ketones, and protein; concentration (specific gravity) is increased in dehydration states
- Urine culture: to evaluate for urinary tract or kidney infection
- Serum lactate to determine sepsis
- Cultures of any wounds or indwelling medical devices for infection
- Blood type and cross-match to prepare for blood transfusion
- Chest x-ray: to evaluate heart size, to evaluate the lungs for pneumonia or pulmonary edema in cardiogenic shock

Nursing Management

Signs of shock in children warrant an emergent response.

MANAGING THE CHILD'S ABCs

Always evaluate and manage the airway, breathing, and circulation. Initiate chest compressions if the child is pulseless until the pulse is sufficient. All children who have signs and symptoms of shock should receive 100% oxygen via mask. If the child has poor respiratory effort or is apneic, administer 100% oxygen via BVM or tracheal tube, as discussed previously in this chapter. As part of ongoing monitoring, initiate cardiac and apnea monitoring and assess oxygen saturation levels using pulse oximetry.

OBTAINING VASCULAR ACCESS

Once the airway and breathing are addressed, nursing management of shock focuses on obtaining vascular access and restoring fluid volume. Children with signs of shock should receive generous amounts of isotonic IV fluids rapidly. However, obtaining vascular access in critically ill children can be challenging. Vascular access must be obtained using the quickest route possible in children whose condition is deteriorating to decompensated shock.

Various forms of vascular access available for the management of the critically ill child include:
- Peripheral IV access: a large-bore catheter used to give large amounts of fluid rapidly. This route may not be feasible in children with significant vascular compromise.
- Central venous access: central lines can be inserted into the jugular vein and threaded into the superior vena cava. The femoral route is best for obtaining central venous access while CPR is in progress because the insertion procedure will not interfere with lifesaving interventions involving the airway and chest compressions. The subclavian vein, located under the clavicle, is an alternative route for central access.

- Saphenous vein: the saphenous vein (found in the ankle) is an alternative route for venous access that is obtained using a surgical incision.
- IO access: IO access, obtained by cannulating the bone marrow, is recommended in cases of decompensated shock or cardiac arrest if IV access cannot be attained rapidly. The preferred site is the anterior tibia. Special IO needles are used (generally, a 15-gauge needle for older children, 18-gauge for younger children). The needle is inserted using a firm twisting motion slightly away from the growth plate. Any medications or fluids that can be administered using an IV site can be given using this route. Alternative sites include the femur, the iliac crest, and the distal tibia; utilizing a pressure bag can assist with infusion success.

RESTORING FLUID VOLUME

Administer IV isotonic fluids, such as Ringer's lactate (RL) or normal saline (NS), rapidly. Administer 20 mL/kg of the prescribed fluid as a bolus, infusing the fluid as rapidly as possible. A large-bore syringe, such as a 35- to 60-mL syringe attached to a three-way stopcock, is the preferred method for rapid fluid delivery in children. Infusing the fluid via gravity is often too slow. Repeat the fluid bolus if required; administration of blood products may be required.

> **Take Note!**
> Dextrose solutions are contraindicated in shock because of the risk of complications such as osmotic diuresis, hypokalemia, hyperglycemia, and worsening of ischemic brain injury (AHA, 2016b).

Children in septic shock will often require larger volumes of fluid as a result of their increased capillary permeability. Children in shock due to trauma will usually receive a colloid, such as blood, when there is an inadequate response to crystalloid isotonic fluid. After each fluid bolus, reassess the child for signs of positive response to the fluid administration.

Insert an indwelling urinary catheter to allow for accurate and frequent measurement of urine output.

Indicators of improvement include:
- Improved cardiovascular status: the central and peripheral pulses become stronger. The line of demarcation of extremity coolness diminishes, capillary refill improves (time is decreased), and BP improves.
- Improved mental status: the child is more alert, his or her eyes are open and watching personnel, and the younger child may pull at any lines.
- Improved urine output: the goal is 1 to 2 mL/kg/hr.

Fluid resuscitation involves giving the fluid, assessing and reassessing the child, and documenting findings. Children in shock may require as much as 100 to 200 mL/kg of resuscitative fluid during the initial hours of shock management. Most children in shock need and can tolerate this large volume of fluid. Continued reassessment will determine if the child is beginning to experience fluid overload in the form of pulmonary edema; this is rare but may occur in children with pre-existing cardiac conditions or severe chronic pulmonary disease (Pasman & Watson, 2015).

Take Note!
Do not focus solely on the child's circulatory status; you may overlook signs and symptoms of respiratory deterioration.

ADMINISTERING MEDICATIONS

In some circumstances, such as septic shock or distributive shock, fluid alone does not adequately improve the child's status and adjunctive medications may be ordered. Vasoactive medications are used either alone or in combination to improve CO, increase SVR, or decrease SVR. The selection of medications is dictated by the child's cardiac and vascular status. These medications may be administered as a loading dose, followed by a continuous infusion. When vasoactive drugs are administered, continuous monitoring of HR, BP, and urine output is necessary in order to titrate the medications appropriately for improvement.

Some of the medications used are:
- Dobutamine: a significant β-adrenergic affecting cardiac contractility
- Epinephrine: affects the heart muscle, and is a powerful vasoconstrictor
- Dopamine affects the heart at lower doses. Increased doses act on the vasculature.

Dosage Calculation Box 51.1

Child's weight: 55 lb
Medication order: epinephrine 100 mg IV STAT. Per the *Pediatric Dosage Handbook*, the recommended dose is 0.01 mg/kg (0.1 mL/kg of 1:10,000 solution) per dose. Is the ordered dose safe?

CARDIAC ARRHYTHMIAS AND ARREST

Unlike adults, in whom cardiopulmonary arrest is most often caused by a primary cardiac event, children typically have healthy hearts and thus rarely experience primary cardiac arrest. More commonly they experience cardiopulmonary arrest from gradual deterioration of respiration and/or circulation (Kleinman et al., 2010a). In particular, children experiencing a respiratory emergency or shock may deteriorate and eventually demonstrate

cardiopulmonary arrest. Thus, the standard of care for managing a child in this situation is vastly different from that for an adult.

Nurses should be skilled in assessing and managing respiratory alterations and shock in children, as discussed in previous sections. Overwhelming evidence suggests that if primary respiratory compromise or shock is identified and treated early in the critically ill child, a secondary cardiac arrest can be prevented.

Rare exceptions do exist. Causes of sudden cardiac arrest without gradual deterioration include:
- History of a serious primary congenital or acquired cardiac defect
- Electrolyte abnormalities
- Toxic drug ingestions
- Potentially lethal arrhythmias, such as prolonged QT syndrome
- Hyper- or hypotrophic cardiomyopathy
- Traumatic cardiac injury from a sharp blow of high-velocity (blunt trauma) to the chest, known as "commotio cordis."

Children rarely experience cardiac arrhythmias, so it is beyond the scope of this chapter to discuss the myriad of possible complex rhythm disturbances. Therefore, this discussion will be limited to the management of emergent cardiac conditions that are more typically found in children.

Pathophysiology

The AHA (2016b) has simplified the nomenclature used to describe pediatric cardiac compromise and has established three major categories of cardiac rhythm disturbances:
- Slow: bradyarrhythmias
- Fast: tachyarrhythmias
- Absent: pulseless, cardiovascular collapse

The pathophysiology, causes, and therapeutic management of each of the categories of rhythm disturbances are discussed below.

BRADYARRHYTHMIAS

Bradycardia is an HR significantly slower than the normal HR for age. Bradycardia in children is most commonly sinus bradycardia. No cardiac nodal abnormality is associated with a sinus bradycardia. In sinus bradycardia, the P waves and QRS complexes remain normal on the ECG. Brief dips in HRs can be normal, often seen when the child sleeps and with vagal stimulation. Passing an orogastric tube down the esophagus or a tracheal tube into the trachea of a young infant may induce a temporary bradycardic effect in response to vagal stimulation. These normal decreases in the child's HR should be self-limiting with the child recovering with or without stimulation and are not normally associated with signs of altered perfusion.

COMPARISON CHART 51.2	CAUSES OF SINUS BRADYCARDIA VERSUS HEART BLOCK	
	Sinus Bradycardia	**Heart Block**
Causes	• Pathologic: medications such as digoxin, hypoxia, hypothermia, head injury • Nonpathologic: well-conditioned athlete	• Congenital: associated with cardiac anomalies • Acquired: endocarditis, rheumatic fever, Kawasaki disease

Less commonly, children manifest bradycardia as a result of cardiac abnormalities and heart block. Infants with bradycardia related to heart block may exhibit poor feeding and tachypnea, whereas older children may demonstrate fatigue, dizziness, and syncope. Comparison Chart 51.2 compares the causes of sinus bradycardia and heart block in children.

In contrast, the child with a serious and possibly life-threatening bradyarrhythmia will have an HR below 60 bpm, with signs of altered perfusion. The most common causes of profound bradycardia in children are respiratory compromise, hypoxia, and shock. Sustained bradycardia is commonly associated with arrest. It is an ominous sign and should receive emergent intervention.

TACHYARRHYTHMIAS

Children have faster HRs than adults. Fever, fear, and pain are common explanations for significant increases in the HR (**tachycardia**) of a child. This normal elevation in HR is known as sinus tachycardia. Once the fever is reduced, the child is comforted, or the pain is managed, the HR should return close to the child's normal baseline. Hypoxia and hypovolemia are pathologic reasons for tachycardia in the child. The signs, symptoms, and management of these concerns were discussed in previous sections. If the child has sinus tachycardia that results from any of these causes, the focus is on the underlying cause. It is inappropriate and dangerous to treat sinus tachycardia with medications aimed at decreasing the HR or with a defibrillation device.

Tachyarrhythmias in children that are associated with cardiac compromise have unique characteristics that present differently from sinus tachycardia. These rhythms include supraventricular tachycardia (SVT) and ventricular tachycardia. SVT is a cardiac conduction problem in which the HR is extremely rapid, the rhythm remains regular, and it is often described as "no beat-to-beat variability." Comparison Chart 51.3 explains the differences between SVT and sinus tachycardia. The most common cause of SVT is a re-entry problem in the cardiac conduction system. Commonly, SVT is the result of a genetic cardiac conduction problem such as Wolff–Parkinson–White syndrome. SVT may also be associated with stimulating medications such as caffeine and theophylline. Children can tolerate the characteristically higher HR that is associated with SVT for short periods of time. However, untreated, the increased demand that is placed on the cardiovascular system eventually overtakes the child and results in congestive heart failure.

Ventricular tachycardia is a rhythm involving an elevation of the HR and a wide QRS (greater than 0.08 s) that is the result of an abnormal, rapid firing of one or both of the ventricles. Ventricular tachycardia is a rare arrhythmia in children and is usually associated with a congenital or acquired cardiac abnormality. Prolonged QT syndrome is a conduction abnormality that can result in ventricular tachycardia and sudden death in children. Less commonly, ingestion of medications and toxins, acidosis, hypocalcemia, abnormalities of potassium, and hypoxemia have been associated with the development of ventricular tachycardia in children.

COMPARISON CHART 51.3	DISTINGUISHING SUPRAVENTRICULAR TACHYCARDIA (SVT) FROM SINUS TACHYCARDIA	
	SVT	**Sinus Tachycardia**
Rate (bpm)	Infants >220, children >180	Infants <220, children <180
Rhythm	Abrupt onset and termination	Beat-to-beat variability
P waves	Flattened	Present and normal
QRS	Narrow (<0.08 seconds)	Normal
History	Usually no significant history	Fever, fluid loss, hypoxia, pain, fear

COLLAPSED RHYTHMS (PULSELESS RHYTHMS)

A collapsed rhythm, as defined by PALS, is one that produces cardiac arrest with no palpable pulse and no signs of perfusion (cardiac arrest) (AHA, 2016b). Typically, the most common pulseless arrest rhythms in children are asystole or pulseless electrical activity (PEA). **Asystole** occurs when there is no cardiac electrical activity, commonly referred to as a "straight line" or "flat line" on the ECG. The child with PEA has an appreciable rhythm on the ECG but no palpable pulses or CO. PEA may be caused by hypoxemia, hypovolemia, hypothermia, electrolyte imbalance, tamponade, toxic ingestion, tension pneumothorax, or thromboembolism. Ventricular tachycardia may also present as pulseless. Ventricular fibrillation (VF), once thought to be rare in children, occurs in serious cardiac conditions in which the ventricle is not pumping effectively and may develop from ventricular tachycardia. VF is characterized by variable waveforms of either high-amplitude (coarse VF) or finer, lower amplitude (fine VF) with no discernible cardiac rhythm. In either case, CO is insufficient.

Nursing Assessment

Nursing assessment of the child with a cardiac emergency includes the health history and physical examination as well as laboratory and diagnostic testing. The nursing assessment must be performed quickly and accurately so that resuscitation can be initiated emergently.

HEALTH HISTORY

Obtain a brief health history of the child with a cardiac emergency while simultaneously assessing the child and providing life-saving interventions. Key areas to inquire about include:

- History of cardiac problems, asthma, chromosomal anomaly, delayed growth
- Symptoms such as syncope, dizziness, palpitations or racing heart, chest pain, coughing, wheezing, increased work of breathing
- Activity tolerance with play or feeding:
  - Does the child get out of breath, turn blue, or squat during play?
  - Can the child keep up with playmates?
  - Does the infant tire with feedings?
- Precipitating illness, fever, unexplained joint pains
- Ingested medications
- Participation in a sport before the cardiac event occurred
- Injury to the chest
- Family history of cardiac problems:
  - Sudden death from a cardiac condition
  - Heart attacks at a young age
  - Chromosomal abnormalities
- Treatment measures performed at the scene:
  - Was CPR initiated?
  - Was an AED used?

PHYSICAL EXAMINATION

Quickly establish the child's status. A child who is obviously in distress or in cardiac arrest must receive emergent life-saving interventions. Briefly perform the assessment while simultaneously providing life-saving interventions.

Inspection and Observation. Assess the child's airway patency and efficiency of breathing. Observe the child's colour, noting circumoral pallor or duskiness or central pallor, mottling, duskiness, or cyanosis. Note any increased work of breathing, grunting, head bobbing, or apnea. Inspect the chest for barrel shape, which may be associated with chronic pulmonary or cardiac disease. Observe the pericardium for the presence of lifts or heaves. Note diaphoresis, anxious appearance, or dysmorphic features (almost 50% of children with Down syndrome also have a congenital cardiac defect [Chen, 2016]). Determine if neck vein distention is present. Inspect the fingertips for clubbing, which is indicative of chronic tissue hypoxemia.

Auscultation

Auscultate the breath sounds, noting any crackles or wheezes. Auscultate the HR. If the child does not have an adequate pulse, initiate chest compressions. If the child has a strong, perfusing pulse, complete the cardiac assessment. Auscultate with the diaphragm of the stethoscope first and then listen with the bell. Evaluate all of the auscultatory areas, listening first over the second right intercostal space, the aortic valve, and then over the second left intercostal space, the pulmonic valve; next move to the left lower sternal border, the tricuspid area; and finally auscultate over the fifth interspace, midclavicular line, mitral area. Evaluate the rate and rhythm of the heart. Listen for any extra sounds or murmurs. Note and describe the quality, intensity, and location of any cardiac murmurs.

Take Note!

Murmurs are most often systolic and can be benign or associated with pathology.

Percussion and Palpation. Percuss between the intercostal spaces and note the heart's size. Palpate the heart to find the point of maximal impulse (PMI) and to evaluate for an associated thrill. A thrill feels like a fluttering under the fingers and is associated with cardiac pathology. Palpate and note the quality of the pulses. Evaluate each of the pulses bilaterally and note whether they are absent, faint, normal, or bounding. Compare the quality of pulses on each side of the body and also those of the upper and lower body. Note the skin temperature and evaluate capillary refill.

LABORATORY AND DIAGNOSTIC TESTING

The major diagnostic test used in cardiac investigation is the electrocardiogram (ECG), used to identify the cardiac rhythm and to assess for arrhythmias (see Fig. 51.7).

A

B

C

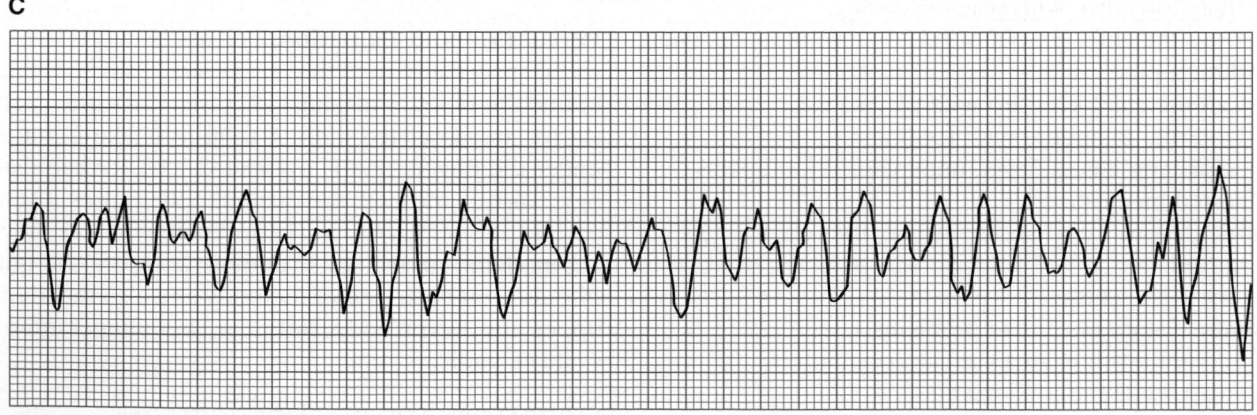

D

FIGURE 51.7 Arrhythmias. **A.** Sinus tachycardia: normal QRS and P waves, mild beat-to-beat variability.
B. Supraventricular tachycardia: note rate above 220, abnormal P waves, no beat-to-beat variability.
C. Ventricular tachycardia: rapid and regular rhythm, wide QRS without P waves. **D.** Coarse ventricular
fibrillation: chaotic electrical activity.

Nursing Management

Provide oxygen at 100%. Initiate cardiac monitoring and pulse oximetry to assess oxygen saturation levels. Obtain the child's pre-printed code drug sheet or use the Broselow tape to obtain the child's height to estimate the tracheal tube sizes and medication dosages that are appropriate for the child. The remainder of this discussion will assume that the nurse has initiated interventions for airway, breathing, and circulation, as discussed earlier in the chapter.

Take Note!
Pay attention to the rhythm on the monitor, but continually monitor the child's pulse. If the child does not have a pulse or has an inadequate pulse of less than 60 bpm, perform cardiac compressions despite the monitor reading (AHA, 2016b).

MANAGING BRADYARRHYTHMIAS

The management of sinus bradycardia is focused on remedying the underlying cause of the slow HR. Since hypoxia is the most common cause of sustained bradycardia, oxygenation and ventilation are necessary. The newborn is particularly susceptible to bradycardia in relation to hypoxemia. Continue to reassess the child to determine if the bradycardia improves with adequate oxygenation and ventilation. If bradycardia persists, administer epinephrine and/or atropine as ordered. Epinephrine is the drug of choice for the treatment of persistent bradycardia.

Other causes of bradycardia such as hypothermia, head injury, and toxic ingestion are managed by addressing the underlying condition. Warming the hypothermic child may restore a normal sinus rhythm. Children with head injuries may have bradycardia without any cardiac involvement that resolves with successful management of the head injury. Antidotes to toxins may be necessary in children whose bradycardia is the result of a toxic ingestion.

MANAGING TACHYARRHYTHMIAS

Tachyarrhythmias include SVT (stable or unstable) and ventricular tachycardia with a pulse. Examine the ECG to determine if the child is experiencing ventricular tachycardia or SVT. Clinically, determine whether the child in SVT is stable or unstable, showing signs that require emergent intervention. In compensated SVT, the child will appear to be alert, breathing comfortably, and well perfused. The child who is demonstrating signs of compromise, such as an altered level of consciousness, respiratory distress, and poor perfusion, is considered to be in uncompensated SVT. Uncompensated SVT requires emergent intervention. The child who has ventricular tachycardia with a pulse will have poor perfusion and also requires immediate intervention. The assessment and interventions to the tachyarrhythmias are discussed in Table 51.6.

Take Note!
Adenosine has a rapid onset of action and an extremely short half-life. Administer it extremely rapidly with a generous amount of IV flush; otherwise, it will be ineffective (Kleinman et al., 2010a).

MANAGING COLLAPSED RHYTHMS

As in any pediatric emergency, support the airway, breathing, and circulation. Manage the airway, provide oxygen, and give fluids. In addition, if the child is pulseless or has

TABLE 51.6	CHARACTERISTICS AND MANAGEMENT OF TACHYARRHYTHMIAS	
Tachyarrhythmia	**Signs and Symptoms**	**Management**
Compensated SVT	• Tachycardia, heart rate >220 • Abnormal P waves • Alert, well-perfused child • Possible complaints of headache and dizziness in older children	• Vagal manoeuvres such as ice to face or blowing through a straw that is obstructed • Adenosine if vagal manoeuvres fail
Uncompensated SVT	• Tachycardia, heart rate >220 • Abnormal P waves • Signs of shock: altered level of consciousness, poor perfusion, weak pulses	• Adenosine or synchronized cardioversion
Ventricular tachycardia	• Rate may range from normal to 200 bpm • Wide QRS • No P waves • Pulse present, poor perfusion	• Synchronized cardioversion • IV Amiodarone • Treatment of underlying causes

Adapted from Kleinman, M. E., Chameides, L., Schexnayder, S. M., Samson, R. A., Hazinski, M. F., Atkins, D. L., . . . American Heart Association. (2010b). Pediatric advanced life support: 2010 American Heart Association guidelines for cardiopulmonary resuscitation and emergency cardiovascular care. *Pediatrics, 126*(5), e1361–e1399.

TABLE 51.7	ECG CHARACTERISTICS AND MANAGEMENT OF PULSELESS RHYTHMS	
Pulseless Arrhythmia	**ECG Characteristics**	**Management**
Ventricular tachycardia	Wide QRS, no P waves	• CPR • Defibrillation • Epinephrine; also, possibly amiodarone, lidocaine, or magnesium • Treat underlying causes
Ventricular fibrillation	• Chaotic ventricular activity • No P waves, no QRS, no T waves	• CPR • Defibrillation • Epinephrine; possibly amiodarone, lidocaine, or magnesium • Treat underlying causes
Asystole	Flat line	• Check lead placement • CPR if no pulse • Epinephrine
Pulseless electrical activity	Electrical activity that is not consistent with ventricular tachycardia or ventricular fibrillation	• Check lead placement • CPR • Treat underlying cause • Epinephrine

Adapted from Kleinman, M. E., Chameides, L., Schexnayder, S. M., Samson, R. A., Hazinski, M. F., Atkins, D. L., . . . American Heart Association. (2010b). Pediatric advanced life support: 2010 American Heart Association guidelines for cardiopulmonary resuscitation and emergency cardiovascular care. *Pediatrics, 126*(5), e1361–e1399.

an HR less than 60 bpm, initiate cardiac compressions (see the section on providing CPR earlier in the chapter). In addition, some children may require medications and/or defibrillation or synchronized cardioversion. The pulseless rhythms include ventricular tachycardia, VF, asystole, and PEA. ECG characteristics and management of these rhythms are summarized in Table 51.7. Whenever possible, treat the underlying cause of the arrhythmia. The AHA emphasizes the importance of cardiac compressions in pulseless individuals with arrhythmias (Kleinman et al., 2010a). Give compressions before and immediately after defibrillation (see Defibrillation section earlier in the chapter). Administer medications such as epinephrine, lidocaine, or amiodarone as ordered. In the past, it was recommended that individuals who required defibrillation be given three rapid "stacked" shocks in a row, but recent research findings have shown that the individual should receive five cycles of CPR immediately following each defibrillation to be most effective. Cardiac compressions must be performed effectively with minimal interruptions (Kleinman et al., 2010a).

DROWNING (SUBMERSION INJURY)

Water can be a great source of fun and exercise for children and adolescents; however, drowning is the second leading cause of preventable death in children and adolescents worldwide (CPS, 2012; World Health Organization, 2014).

Survival and neurologic outcome of drowning depend on early and appropriate resuscitation. In recent years, with appropriate resuscitation efforts and treatment, children have demonstrated better neurologic outcomes (Chandy & Weinhouse, 2015).

Pathophysiology

Typically, a child who is drowning will struggle to breathe eventually aspirating water. Aspiration of relatively small amounts of water leads to poor oxygenation, and retention of carbon dioxide. Alveolar surfactant is depleted and pulmonary edema commonly occurs. Hypoxemia results in increased capillary permeability and resultant hypovolemia. Even small amounts of aspirated water may lead to pulmonary edema within an 8-hour period after the drowning episode (Chandy & Weinhouse, 2015). A drowning survivor is at risk for renal complications resulting from renal hypoperfusion during the hypoxemic state.

Nursing Assessment

Nursing assessment of the drowning survivor is crucial and must take place quickly and accurately.

HEALTH HISTORY

Obtain the history rapidly while providing life-saving interventions. Ask about the circumstances of the event:
• Where did the incident occur?
• Was the child in a lake, river, ocean, or swimming pool?

- Was the child submerged in a toilet, bucket, or bathtub?
- Did someone witness the child's entry into the water?
- Was the water fresh, salty, or contaminated? Cold or warm?
- Were there any extenuating circumstances, such as a diving or automobile accident, associated with the near-drowning?
- What was the approximate length of time of the submersion?
- Was the child conscious or unconscious when rescued?
- What was done at the scene?
- Was CPR initiated? If so, when?
- Was an AED used?
- If a cervical spine injury was suspected, was the cervical spine immobilized?
- When did the child last eat in preparation for intubation?

PHYSICAL EXAMINATION

Evaluate airway patency and breathing. Auscultate all lung fields for signs of pulmonary edema, such as coarseness or crackles. Evaluate the HR, pulses, and perfusion. Note the cardiac rhythm on the monitor and report arrhythmias. Evaluate the child's neurologic status. Use a pen light to determine pupillary reaction. Use the pediatric Glasgow Coma Score to further assess the neurologic status. Does the child open the eyes spontaneously, to stimuli, or not at all? Is there any spontaneous movement? Is the younger child crying? Can the older child speak? Measure the child's temperature, as hypothermia is common with near-drowning.

LABORATORY AND DIAGNOSTIC TESTING

While awaiting laboratory and diagnostic testing results, continue resuscitative efforts as addressed below. Laboratory and diagnostic tests typically include the following:

- Arterial blood gases: hypoxemia, acidosis
- ECG: cardiac arrhythmias
- Chest radiography: pulmonary edema, infiltrates
- Serum electrolytes: imbalance related to the development of shock

Nursing Management

Because of the potentially devastating effects that drowning-related hypoxia has on the child's brain, airway interventions must be initiated immediately after retrieving a child from the water. Every second counts. Initial interventions for a drowning victim are always focused on the airway, breathing, and circulation commonly; resuscitative efforts should begin before the child arrives at the acute care facility.

If a cervical spine injury is suspected (as in the case of a diving accident), provide c-spine stabilization and immobilization manually or with an appropriately sized cervical collar. As with any suspected neck injury, do not remove the cervical collar until injury to the cervical spine has been ruled out with radiology imagining (x-ray or CT scan) and physical assessment. Suction the airway, if required, to ensure airway patency. Aspiration of particles from a contaminated water source or emesis is a common complication associated with drowning. A large-bore suction catheter (e.g., Yankauer) is an effective tool for clearing the upper airway. Administer supplemental oxygen at 100%. Children who have poor or absent respiratory effort will likely require intubation. Insert an orogastric or nasogastric tube to decompress the stomach and prevent aspiration of stomach contents. Initiate cardiac compressions if a pulse is not present or not perfused.

Usually, the child exhibits some degree of hypothermia and will require warming. The core body temperature should be raised slowly, as warming a drowning victim too quickly may have deleterious effects. Remove any wet clothing, dry the child, and cover him or her with warmed blankets. Warm IV fluids and use other warming methods as prescribed.

Consider This

A father says to you, "I can't believe my toddler almost drowned. I turned away for a few minutes to check the hamburgers on the grill. I feel terrible. I'll never be able to let her go near a swimming pool again."

Thoughts: What will your response be to this father? How can you best support him and assist him to work through his emotions?

POISONING

Emergency care of the pediatric poisoning victim consists of rapid nursing assessment and prompt management.

Take Note!

If a normally healthy child (particularly a young child) suddenly *deteriorates* without a known cause, suspect a toxic ingestion.

Nursing Assessment

Nursing assessment of the poisoning victim focuses on a thorough health history, followed by physical examination and laboratory and diagnostic testing.

Health History

Obtain the health history from the parents or caregiver or, in the case of an older child or teenager, directly from the child.

- Inquire about the approximate time and amount of poisoning.

- The nature of the toxin and the amount ingested?
- Was the toxin ingested, inhaled, or applied to the skin?
- In the case of pill ingestion, does the caregiver have the medication bottle?
- Did the child experience nausea, vomiting, anorexia, abdominal pain, or neurologic changes such as disorientation, slurred speech, or altered gait?
- Determine the progression of the symptoms.
- Did the parent or caregiver call the Provincial Poison Control Center Hotline?
- Has any treatment been given?
- In the case of older children and teens, inquire about any history of depression or threatened suicide, and determine if the ingestion was intentional self-harm.

Take Note!

The Canadian Association of Poison Control Centres (2017) provides the contact information for each provincial poison control centre in Canada at: http://www.capcc.ca/en/content/provincial-centres

Physical Examination

Ingestion of medications or chemicals may result in a wide variety of clinical manifestations. Perform a thorough physical examination, noting alterations that may occur with particular ingestions, such as:

- Hyper- or hypotension
- Hyper- or hypothermia
- Respiratory depression or hyperventilation (note decreased CO_2 (**hypocapnia**))
- Miosis (pupillary contraction) or mydriasis (pupillary dilatation)
- Cardiac arrhythmias including prolonged QT segments

Pay particular attention to the child's mental status, skin moisture and colour, and bowel sounds (Velez, Shepherd, & Goto, 2016).

Laboratory and Diagnostic Testing

The suspected poison will direct the laboratory and diagnostic testing. A variety of blood tests may be performed:

- Chemistry panel: to detect hypoglycemia or metabolic acidosis and assess renal function
- ECG: to identify arrhythmias or conduction delays
- Liver function tests: to assess for liver injury
- Urine and blood toxicology screens (available for a limited number of medications; may vary per institution)
- Specific drug levels if the substance ingested is known or highly suspected

Nursing Management

When poisoning occurs, give priority to the child's airway, breathing, and circulation. Treat alterations as discussed earlier in this chapter. Monitor vital signs frequently and

provide supportive care. A few specific antidotes are available for medications or other toxins. Activated charcoal may be administered to bind with the chemical substance in the bowel. Alternatively, whole bowel irrigation with polyethylene glycol electrolyte solutions may be necessary. Occasionally, dialysis is required to lower the level of the toxin in the bloodstream. The intervention is based on the toxin. For example, activated charcoal is an effective method for preventing the absorption of many medications but is not effective in the case of an iron overdose.

If opiate or other narcotic ingestion is suspected, administer naloxone to reverse the respiratory depression or altered level of consciousness. Treatment of seizures and alterations in thermoregulation may also be needed.

Specific treatment of the poisoning will be determined when the toxin is identified and poison control is queried. Maintain ongoing assessment of the poisoned child because many toxins exhibit very late effects.

Take Note!

Syrup of ipecac is no longer recommended for home treatment to induce vomiting after an accidental ingestion (AAP, 2019).

TRAUMA

The leading cause of death in children and youth in Canada is unintentional injuries (Public Health Agency of Canada [PHAC], 2016). Falls are the most common cause of injury leading to hospitalization, and motor vehicle accidents continue to be the leading cause of death in children 1 to 19 years of age (PHAC, 2016). Childhood trauma also results from pedestrian accidents, sporting, bicycling, and blunt and penetrating injures. Children of varying ages are susceptible to various forms of injury related to their developmental level as well as their environmental exposure. Young children rely on their caregivers to promote their safety. Young children are not developmentally equipped to recognize dangerous situations. Because pediatric injury is so common, nurses must become adept at assessment and intervention in the pediatric trauma victim.

Nursing Assessment

The trauma survey includes a brief health history as the child is being assessed and life-saving measures are being instituted.

Health History

Obtain the health history by asking:
- When the injury happened.
- If the child sustained a motor vehicle–related injury, ask how fast the vehicle was going.

- Determine if the child was appropriately restrained in the automobile.
- If the child was riding a bicycle, skateboarding, or using in-line skates, was he or she wearing a helmet, knee pads, and wrist guards?
- Determine what interventions were performed at the scene.
- Was the child's c-spine immobilized?
- If the child is bleeding, ask the person who transported the child to estimate the amount of blood lost.
- If the child experienced a fall, ask if the fall was witnessed and the height from which the child fell.
- Did the child fall onto a hard surface such as concrete?
- How did the child land: on their head or back, or did the child catch themselves with their hands?
- Did the child lose consciousness at the scene? Younger children and boys are at higher risk for injuring their head.
- What kind of behaviour did the child exhibit after the fall? Since the fall, has the child complained of a headache or vomited?

While obtaining a detailed history about the fall, think about the child's developmental stage considering the possibility of child abuse. Does it seem plausible that a toddler might fall down the stairs? In contrast, what is the likelihood that a 2-month-old would suffer a fractured femur from a fall? Critically evaluate the reported circumstances and try to determine if the history, developmental stage of the child, and type of injury sustained match. In addition, evaluate the type of injury that the child sustained and the history given by the caregiver. For example, children who fall from significant heights often suffer skeletal fractures, but abdominal and chest injuries rarely result from falling from significant heights.

Physical Examination

Physical examination of the child with a traumatic injury should be approached with a primary assessment of their ABCs. Assess the patency of the airway and establish the effectiveness of breathing (as discussed earlier in this chapter). Examine the child's respiratory effort, breath sounds, and colour. Assess the pulse rate and quality. Observe their skin colour, temperature, and perfusion. Observe for active bleeding.

After assessing and intervening for the child's ABCs, proceed to the secondary survey. Assess for disability (D) assessing neurologic function. Determine the level of consciousness, pupillary reaction, and best verbal and motor responses to auditory and painful stimuli. If the child is a young infant, palpate the anterior fontanel: a full and bulging fontanel signals increased intracranial pressure. The traumatized child's neurologic status may range from completely normal to comatose.

Take Note!

Unequal pupils or a fixed and dilated pupil is considered a neurosurgical emergency. Immediately report this finding.

Following the ABCs and D (disability) is E (exposure). Expose the child to observe the entire body for signs of blunt or penetrating injury. Perform a systematic, thorough inspection of the child's body. Note active bleeding and extremity deformity, as well as any lacerations and abrasions. Observe for movement and immobility noting strength or pain with movement. Inspect the abdomen for redness, skin discolouration, or distention. Auscultate for bowel sounds in all four quadrants. If the child is verbal, ask if he or she has any abdominal pain. If the child is younger, ask, "Do you have a tummy ache?" If the child reports abdominal pain, ask the child to point to where it hurts. Note any guarding of the abdomen, which is an indication of abdominal pain. If bowel injury is a possibility, only light palpation is acceptable. Always assess the least tender areas first and palpate the more sensitive areas last.

Laboratory and Diagnostic Testing

As in other pediatric emergencies, never delay life-saving measures to wait for laboratory or diagnostic test results. In addition to routine laboratory tests, common laboratory and diagnostic tests for the pediatric trauma victim include:

- Type and cross-match: to assess the child's blood type before blood products are given
- Prothrombin time (PT) and partial thromboplastin time (PTT): to evaluate for clotting dysfunction
- Amylase and lipase: to identify pancreatic injury
- Liver function tests: to assess for liver injury
- Pregnancy test in females who have reached puberty
- CT scan, ultrasound, or MRI of the head, abdomen, c-spine or extremities: to evaluate the extent of injuries

Nursing Management

Nursing management of the pediatric trauma victim focuses initially on the ABCs.

Providing Immediate Care

Assess the strength of the child's central pulse. If the child has no pulse, initiate chest compressions immediately.

If head or c-spine injury is suspected, open the airway using the jaw-thrust manoeuvre with cervical spine stabilization (see Fig. 51.4). The guidelines for basic life support recommend that if the airway cannot be opened using the jaw-thrust manoeuvre, it may be opened using the head tilt–chin lift manoeuvre since opening the airway is a priority (Berg et al., 2010). The head and neck of a trauma victim should be stabilized manually.

> **Take Note!**
>
> Infants and young children require unique cervical spine management because they have prominent occiputs that result in flexion of the neck in the supine position. To maintain the optimal neutral spinal position in the young child, use a special pediatric backboard with a head indentation, or use a folded towel to elevate the child's torso.

Clear the airway of obstruction using a large-bore suction device such as a Yankauer; insert an oropharyngeal airway if the child is unconscious. If the child is breathing on their own, give oxygen at the highest flow possible with a non-rebreathing mask. If the child is not breathing independently, intervene with basic life support discussed earlier in this chapter (Berg et al., 2010).

If a BVM device is available, connect it to the oxygen source and use the bag to ventilate the child with altered respiratory effort. Observe the chest rise and be careful not to overventilate, as this results in abdominal distention and barotrauma. Deliver breaths at a rate of one breath every 3 seconds (Berg et al., 2010). Hyperventilation may be used initially and briefly if the child is showing signs of a possible brain stem herniation. This differs from the past when most head injuries where hyperventilated. Assess the strength of the child's central pulse. If the child has no pulse, initiate chest compressions immediately. When perfusion is compromised, administer IV fluid resuscitation as discussed earlier in this chapter. Trauma victims are likely to require colloids or blood products due to blood loss from the injury.

> **Take Note!**
>
> Children with head injuries who have signs of shock such as poor perfusion and bradycardia should receive fluid volume resuscitation (Kleinman et al., 2010b).

KEY CONCEPTS

- Young children's smaller airways and immature respiratory and immune systems place them at higher risk for respiratory distress than older children and adults.

- Children generally have healthy hearts and cardiovascular systems and thus rarely present with primary cardiac arrest.

- Younger children and adolescents are at higher risk for injury due to normal development at those ages.

- Children present with a variety of emergencies and injuries and must be evaluated and treated in an appropriate and timely fashion to achieve a positive outcome. The health history is obtained rapidly while life-saving measures are performed simultaneously.

- Assess the airway, then breathing, then circulation, providing interventions for alterations before moving on to the next assessment. Provide continuous reassessment, as children respond quickly to interventions and deteriorate quickly as well.

- Pulse oximetry and capnometry can be useful tools for evaluating respiratory status.

- **Never** delay intervention pending laboratory results if the child's clinical status warrants immediate action.

- Provide support and education to the child and family involved in an emergency. Teach families and children why certain procedures are being done, explaining technical medical interventions in simple terms at appropriate developmental levels.

- Small amounts of edema or secretions can contribute to significant respiratory distress in infants and young children.

- Children dehydrate quicker than adults and experience alterations in perfusion related to hypovolemia.

- Children in respiratory distress and shock require supplemental oxygen. Intubation is necessary for the apneic child or the child who cannot protect their own airway.

- Accurate assessment of perfusion status and appropriate fluid resuscitation are critical in the prevention and treatment of shock in children.

- Life-threatening arrhythmias in children, though uncommon, must be treated emergently with defibrillation or synchronized cardioversion in addition to CPR.

- In the case of near-drowning, maintain ongoing assessment and intervention of pulmonary status.

- Maintain airway, breathing, and circulation in the child who has experienced an accidental ingestion and prepare for administration of activated charcoal and possible antidotes.

- In addition to intervening for airway, breathing, and circulation problems in the pediatric trauma victim, assess for altered neurologic status and extent of bleeding or injury.

REFERENCES AND RECOMMENDED READINGS

American Academy of Pediatrics. (2019). *Ipecac*. Retrieved from https://www.aap.org/en-us/about-the-aap/aap-press-room/aap-press-room-media-center/Pages/Ipecac.aspx

American Heart Association. (2016a). *Advanced cardiac life support provider manual*. Dallas, TX: Author.

American Heart Association. (2016b). *Pediatric advanced life support provider manual*. Dallas, TX: Author.

BC Patient Safety and Quality Council. (2017). *BC sepsis network: emergency department sepsis guidelines*. Retrieved from https://bcpsqc.ca/improve-care/bc-sepsis-network/

Berg, M. D., Schexnayder, S. M., Chameides, L., Terry, M., Donoghue, A., Hickey, R. W., . . . Hazinski, M. F. (2010). Part 13: Pediatric basic life support: 2010 American Heart Association guidelines for cardiopulmonary resuscitation and emergency cardiovascular care. *Circulation, 122*(18 Suppl 3), S862–S875.

Bowden, V. R., & Greenberg, C. S. (2012). *Pediatric nursing procedures* (3rd ed.). Philadelphia, PA: Lippincott Williams & Wilkins.

Canadian Association of Poison Control Centres. (2017). *Provincial centres*. Retrieved from http://www.capcc.ca/en/content/provincial-centres

Canadian Paediatric Society. (2012). *Child and youth injury prevention: A public health approach*. Retrieved from http://www.cps.ca/documents/position/child-and-youth-injury-prevention

Canadian Paediatric Society. (2016). *Neonatal resuscitation program*. Retrieved from http://www.cps.ca/nrp-prn

Carpenito-Moyet, L. J. (2013). *Nursing diagnosis: Application to clinical practice* (14th ed.). Philadelphia, PA: Lippincott Williams & Wilkins.

Cecchin, F., Jorgenson, D. B., Berul, C. I., Perry, J. C., Zimmerman, A. A., Duncan, B. W., . . . Atkins, D. L. (2001). Is arrhythmia detection by automatic external defibrillator accurate for children?: Sensitivity and specificity of an automatic external defibrillator algorithm in 696 pediatric arrhythmias. *Circulation, 103*(20), 2438–2483.

Chandy, D., & Weinhouse, G. L. (2015). *Drowning (submersion injuries)*. Retrieved from http://www.uptodate.com/contents/drowning-submersion-injuries

Chen, H. (2016). *Down syndrome*. Retrieved from http://emedicine.medscape.com/article/943216-overview

Corbett, J. A., & Banks, A. D. (2013). *Laboratory tests and diagnostic procedures with nursing diagnoses* (8th ed.). Upper Saddle River, NJ: Pearson Education Inc.

Diaz, M. C. (2013). Early use of AEDs can save kids' lives. *Contemporary Pediatrics, 30*(3), 12–20.

Fleisher, G. R., & Ludwig, S. (2010). *Textbook of pediatric emergency medicine* (6th ed.). Philadelphia, PA: Lippincott Williams & Wilkins.

Field, J. M., Hazinski, M. F., Sayre, M. R., Chameides, L., Schexnayder, S. M., Hemphill, R., ... & Cave, D. M. (2010). Part 1: executive summary: 2010 American Heart Association guidelines for cardiopulmonary resuscitation and emergency cardiovascular care. *Circulation, 122*(18_suppl_3), S640–S656.

Gilger, M. A., Jain, A. K., & McOmber, M. E. (2015). *Foreign bodies of the esophagus and gastrointestinal tract in children*. Retrieved from http://www.uptodate.com/contents/foreign-bodies-of-the-esophagus-and-gastrointestinal-tract-in-children

Jones, M. A. (2016). *Preparing an office practice for pediatric emergencies*. Retrieved from http://www.uptodate.com/contents/preparing-an-office-practice-for-pediatric-emergencies

Kattwinkel, J., Perlman, J. M., Aziz, K., Colby, C., Fairchild, K., Gallagher, J., . . . Zaichkin, J. (2010). Part 15: Neonatal resuscitation: 2010 American Heart Association guidelines for cardiopulmonary resuscitation and emergency cardiovascular care. *Circulation, 122*(18 Suppl 3), S909–S919.

Kleinman, M. E., Chameides, L., Schexnayder, S. M., Samson, R. A., Hazinski, M. F., Atkins, D. L., . . . Zaritsky, A. L. (2010a). Part 14: Pediatric advanced life support—2010 American Heart Association guidelines for cardiopulmonary resuscitation and emergency cardiovascular care. *Circulation, 122*(18 Suppl 3), S876–S908.

Kleinman, M. E., Chameides, L., Schexnayder, S. M., Samson, R. A., Hazinski, M. F., Atkins, D. L., . . . American Heart Association. (2010b). Pediatric advanced life support: 2010 American Heart Association guidelines for cardiopulmonary resuscitation and emergency cardiovascular care. *Pediatrics, 126*(5), e1361–e1399.

McAlvin, S. S., & Carew-Lyons, A. (2014). Family presence during resuscitation and invasive procedures in pediatric critical care: A systematic review. *American Journal of Critical Care, 23*(6), 477–484.

Pasman, E. A., & Watson, C. M. (2015). *Shock in pediatrics*. Retrieved from http://emedicine.medscape.com/article/1833578-overview

Pomerantz, W. J., & Roback, M. G. (2014). *Physiology and classification of shock in children*. Retrieved from http://www.uptodate.com/contents/physiology-and-classification-of-shock-in-children

Public Health Agency of Canada. (2016). *Injuries*. Retrieved from http://cbpp-pcpe.phac-aspc.gc.ca/public-health-topics/injuries/

Salib, E. A., Cyran, S. E., Cilley, R. E., Maron, B. J., & Thomas, N. J. (2005). Efficacy of bystander cardiopulmonary resuscitation and out-of-hospital automated external defibrillation as life-saving therapy in commotio cordis. *Journal of Pediatrics, 147*(6), 863–866.

Samiee-Zafarghandy, S., Raman, S. R., van den Anker, J. N., McHutchison, K., Hornik, C. P., Clark, R. H., . . . Best Pharmaceuticals for Children Act—Pediatric Trials Network Administrative Core Committee. (2015). Safety of milrinone use in neonatal intensive care units. *Early Human Development, 91*(1), 31–35.

Stanley, M., & Pollard, D. (2013). Relationship between knowledge, attitudes, and self-efficacy of nurses in the management of pediatric pain. *Pediatric Nursing, 39*(4), 165–171.

Taketomo, C. K., Hodding, J. H., & Kraus, D. M. (2013). *Pediatric & neonatal dosage handbook* (20th ed.). Hudson, OH: Lexicomp.

Velez, L. I., Shepherd, J. G., & Goto, C. S. (2016). *Approach to the child with occult toxic exposure*. Retrieved from http://www.uptodate.com/contents/approach-to-the-child-with-occult-toxic-exposure

World Health Organization. (2014). *Drowning*. Retrieved from http://www.who.int/mediacentre/factsheets/fs347/en/

MULTIPLE CHOICE QUESTIONS

1. An unresponsive toddler is brought to the emergency department. Assessment reveals mottled skin colour, respiratory rate of 10 breaths per minute, and a brachial pulse of 52 bpm. What is the priority nursing action?
   a. Prepare the defibrillator and prepare rescue medications.
   b. Provide 100% oxygen with a bag-valve-mask and start chest compressions.
   c. Start chest compressions and provide 100% oxygen via non-rebreather mask.
   d. Begin an IV fluid infusion and administer epinephrine IV.

2. A 10-year-old child in respiratory distress requires intubation. Which sizes of tracheal tubes will the nurse prepare?
   a. 9.5 mm and 10.0 mm
   b. 8.5 mm and 9.0 mm
   c. 6.0 mm and 6.5 mm
   d. 6.5 mm and 7.0 mm

3. A preschooler presents to the emergency department with a history of vomiting, diarrhea, and fever over the past few days. She is receiving 100% oxygen via non-rebreather mask. Vital signs: temperature 40°C, pulse 144 bpm, respiratory rate 22 breaths per minute, and BP 70/50 mm Hg. She is listless and difficult to arouse with weak peripheral pulses and prolonged capillary refill. What nursing intervention takes priority?
   a. Administering acetaminophen rectally for the high fever.
   b. Administering IV antibiotics for the infection.
   c. Preparing the child for tracheal intubation.
   d. Administering an IV bolus of normal saline 20 mL/kg.

4. Assessment of a 12-year-old who crashed his bicycle without a helmet reveals the following: temperature 37.0°C, pulse 100 bpm, respiratory rate 24 breaths per minute with easy work of breathing, and BP 102/70 mm Hg. What is the priority action by the nurse?
   a. Assess neurologic status while observing for obvious injuries.
   b. Administer IV fluid bolus of normal saline at 20 mL/kg.
   c. Remove the cervical collar if he complains that it bothers him.
   d. Listen for bowel sounds while assessing for pain.

5. An 18-month-old child is brought to the emergency department via ambulance after an accidental ingestion. What is the priority nursing action?
   a. Take the child's vital signs.
   b. Give oral syrup of ipecac.
   c. Insert a nasogastric tube.
   d. Start an IV line.

DOSAGE CALCULATION QUESTION

1. The nurse is caring for an infant with supraventricular tachycardia who is symptomatic and has an IV line in place. The infant weighs 7.5 kg. The medication order reads: adenosine 0.01 mg/kg IV STAT followed by rapid flush. Adenosine is supplied as 6 mg/2 mL. How many millilitres will the nurse administer? Round to the nearest hundredth.

CRITICAL THINKING EXERCISES

1. A school-age child presents to the emergency department for evaluation. He had been feeling faint off and on and today he fainted at school. On the cardiac monitor, an abnormal cardiac rhythm is noted. At present, the child is stable. What questions would be most appropriate for the nurse to ask when obtaining the child's health history? What objective assessments should the nurse make?

2. Charlie is a 2-year-old who is admitted to the hospital after accidentally ingesting a medication. His accompanying mother is upset and crying. How does Charlie's age and stage of development affect his risk for accidental ingestion? How should the nurse respond to the mother's distress? Develop a discharge teaching plan for Charlie and his family related to poison prevention.

3. A 7-month-old is brought to the hospital with a chief complaint of difficulty breathing. The infant's mother says that his cold has gotten worse and he won't eat. What additional questions should the nurse ask about the infant's health history? How would the nurse appropriately manage this infant's airway?

CHAPTER **WORKSHEET**

STUDY ACTIVITIES

1. Spend a day in the pediatric emergency department or urgent care centre and document the role of the triage nurse.

2. Observe the pediatric emergency medical team at work or observe a pediatric code in the hospital. Compare and contrast the measures performed for the child with those performed for an adult in a similar emergency situation.

3. Develop a teaching project related to injury prevention and present it at a local elementary, middle, or high school. Ensure that the education is appropriate to the children's developmental level.

4. Interview the parents of a child who has experienced an emergency situation about how they felt during and after the emergency. Present the information to your classmates.

5. When providing care to a child in an emergency, the nurse performs the following assessments. Place them in the proper sequence.
   a. Pupillary reaction
   b. Presence of cough or sputum
   c. HR and capillary refill
   d. Presence of bruises and abrasions
   e. Work of breathing

BRINGING IT ALL TOGETHER: A CASE STUDY

Teva Dawson, a 2-year-old girl, is admitted to the emergency department by ambulance after experiencing a near-drowning in the family swimming pool. Teva was resuscitated at the scene and is now breathing spontaneously. She is lethargic and coughs occasionally.

Go to thePoint **to find questions to consider about this case.**

Appendix **A**

Standard Laboratory Values

PREGNANT AND NONPREGNANT INDIVIDUALS

Values	Nonpregnant	Pregnant
Hematologic		
Complete blood count (CBC)		
Hemoglobin, g/dL	12–16[a]	11.5–14[a]
Hematocrit, PCV, %	37–47	32–42
Red cell volume, mL	1,600	1,900
Plasma volume, mL	2,400	3,700
Red blood cell count, million/mm³	4–5.5	3.75–5.0
White blood cells, total per mm³	4,500–10,000	5,000–15,000
Polymorphonuclear cells, %	54–62	60–85
Lymphocytes, %	38–46	15–40
Erythrocyte sedimentation rate, mm/h	≤	30–90
MCHC, g/dL packed RBCs (mean corpuscular hemoglobin concentration)	30–36	No change
MCH (mean corpuscular hemoglobin per picogram)	29–32	No change
MCV/μm³ (mean corpuscular volume per cubic micrometer)	82–96	No change
Blood coagulation and fibrinolytic activity[b]		
Factors VII, VIII, IX, X		Increase in pregnancy, return to normal in early puerperium; factor VIII increases during and immediately after delivery
Factors XI, XIII		Decrease in pregnancy
Prothrombin time (protime), seconds	60–70	Slight decrease in pregnancy
Partial thromboplastin time (PTT), seconds	12–14	Slight decrease in pregnancy and again during second and third stages of labour (indicates clotting at placental site)
Bleeding time, minutes	1–3 (Duke) 2–4 (Ivy)	No appreciable change
Coagulation time, minutes	6–10 (Lee/White)	No appreciable change
Platelets	150,000–350,000/mm³	No significant change until 3–5 days after delivery, then marked increase (may predispose woman to thrombosis) and gradual return to normal
Fibrinolytic activity		Decreases in pregnancy, then abrupt return to normal (protection against thromboembolism)
Fibrinogen, mg/dL	250	400

PREGNANT AND NONPREGNANT INDIVIDUALS (continued)

Values	Nonpregnant	Pregnant
Mineral and vitamin Concentrations		
Serum iron, mcg	75–150	65–120
Total iron-binding capacity, mcg	250–450	300–500
Iron saturation, %	30–40	15–30
Vitamin B_{12}, folic acid, ascorbic acid	Normal	Moderate decrease
Serum protein		
Total, g/dL	6.7–8.3	5.5–7.5
Albumin, g/dL	3.5–5.5	3.0–5.0
Globulin, total, g/dL	2.3–3.5	3.0–4.0
Blood sugar		
Fasting, mg/dL	70–80	65
2-hour postprandial, mg/dL	60–110	Under 140 after a 100-g carbohydrate meal is considered normal
Cardiovascular		
Blood pressure, mm Hg	120/80[c]	114/65
Peripheral resistance, dyne/s · cm^{-5}	120	100
Venous pressure, cm H_2O		
Femoral	9	24
Antecubital	8	8
Pulse, rate/min	70	80
Stroke volume, mL	65	75
Cardiac output, L/min	4.5	6
Circulation time (arm-tongue), sec	15–16	12–14
Blood volume, mL		
Whole blood	4,000	5,600
Plasma	2,400	3,700
Red blood cells	1,600	1,900
Plasma renin, units/L	3–10	10–80
Chest x-ray studies		
Transverse diameter of heart	–	1–2-cm increase
Left border of heart	–	Straightened
Cardiac volume	–	70-mL increase

(continued)

PREGNANT AND NONPREGNANT INDIVIDUALS (continued)

Values	Nonpregnant	Pregnant
Electrocardiogram	–	15-degree left axis deviation
V_1 and V_2	–	Inverted T-wave
kV_4	–	Low T
III	–	Q + inverted T
aVr	–	Small Q
Hepatic		
Bilirubin total	Not more than 1 mg/dL	Unchanged
Cephalin flocculation	Up to 2+ in 48 hr	Positive in 10%
Serum cholesterol, mg/dL	110–300	↑ 60% from 16–32 weeks of pregnancy; remains at this level until after delivery
Thymol turbidity	0–4 units	Positive in 15%
Serum alkaline phosphatase	2–4.5 units (Bodansky)	↑ from week 12 of pregnancy to 6 weeks after childbirth
Serum lactate dehydrogenase		Unchanged
Serum glutamic-oxaloacetic transaminase		Unchanged
Serum globulin albumin, g/dL	1.5–3.0	↑ slight
	4.5–5.3	↓ 3.0 g by late pregnancy
A/G ratio		Decreased
α_2-globulin		Increased
β-globulin		Increased
Serum cholinesterase		Decreased
Leucine aminopeptidase		Increased
Sulfobromophthalein (5 mg/kg)	5% dye or less in 45 minutes	Somewhat decreased
Renal		
Bladder capacity, mL	1,300	1,500
Renal plasma flow (RPF), mL/min	490–700	Increase by 25%, to 612–875
Glomerular filtration rate (GFR), mL/min	105–132	Increase by 50%, to 160–198
Nonprotein nitrogen (NPN), mg/dL	25–40	Decreases
Blood urea nitrogen (BUN), mg/dL	20–25	Decreases
Serum creatinine, mg/kg/24 hr	20–22	Decreases
Serum uric acid, mg/kg/24 hr	257–750	Decreases
Urine glucose	Negative	Present in 20% of gravidas

PREGNANT AND NONPREGNANT INDIVIDUALS (continued)

Values	Nonpregnant	Pregnant
Intravenous pyelogram (IVP)	Normal	Slight to moderate hydroureter and hydronephrosis; right kidney larger than left kidney
Miscellaneous		
Total thyroxine concentration	5–12 mcg/dL thyroxine	↑ 9–16 mcg/dL thyroxine (however, unbound thyroxine not greatly increased)
Ionized calcium		Relatively unchanged
Aldosterone		↑ 1 mg/24 hr by third trimester
Dehydroisoandrosterone	Plasma clearance 6–8 L/24 hr	↑ plasma clearance 10–20-fold

Adapted from Cunningham, F. G. (2018). Normal reference ranges for laboratory values in pregnancy. *UpToDate*. Retrieved from http://www.uptodate.com/contents/normal-reference-ranges-for-laboratory-values-in-pregnancy; and Van Leeuwen, A. M., & Bladh, M. L. (2015). *Davis's comprehensive handbook of laboratory & diagnostic tests with nursing implications*. (6th ed.), Philadelphia, PA: F. A. Davis.

[a]At sea level. Permanent residents of higher levels require higher levels of hemoglobin.
[b]Pregnancy represents a hypercoagulable state.
[c]For the woman about 20 years of age.
10 years of age: 103/70.
30 years of age: 123/82.
40 years of age: 126/84.

Appendix B

Clinical Paths

LABOUR AND DELIVERY CLINICAL PATH—LABOUR: EXPECTED OUTCOMES

	Active Phase	Expulsion/Pushing	Recovery First Hour Postpartum
CLIENT	Client coping with labour support Client utilizing appropriate labour options Client verbalizes satisfaction with plan Management interventions	Client demonstrates effective pushing technique Client coping effectively with pushing Support person coping effectively with labour	Bonding with baby Initiation of first breastfeed within the first 30 minutes to 1 hour of life
CLIENT'S STATUS	Cervix dilated 5 cm—complete Contraction regularly with progressive cervical change Client/fetal well-being maintained Hydration maintained If indicated: FSE and/or IUPC placed • Pitocin IV started • Epidural placed/WE encouraged • Medicate with PRN pain meds	Vaginal birth	Placenta delivered Fundus firm Lochia small–moderate Without clots Perineum intact/repaired Hemodynamically stable EBL <500 mL
CONTINUUM OF CARE	Prenatal record available after 32 weeks Prenatal labs WNL Preregistered to hospital/birthing centre Pregnancy care provider identified Support after hospitalization identified Discharge plan discussed with client/family Communicates understanding of hospital and community resources		
ASSESSMENT/TREATMENT	Assess: Continuous EFM or intermittent auscultation Q 15 of 30 min as indicated Vital signs hourly/temp Q 4 hr if intact membranes/Q 2 hr if membranes ruptured Uterine by monitor or palpation Bladder for distention Hydration status Cervical dilation, effacement, station	Assess: Q 5 min monitoring of fetal well-being Vital signs hourly/temp. Q 2–4 hr depending on membrane status Bladder for distention Hydration status Pushing effectiveness Descent of presenting part Caput	Assess: Uterine fundus Vital signs Lochia Bladder Perineum Placenta
CLIENT EDUCATION	Reinforce comfort measures Encourage use of labour options Inform client/support person of plan of care	Teaching of upright pushing positions Discourage prolonged breath-holding Encourage to assume position of choice Inform client of progress	Baby status Breastfeeding

LABOUR AND DELIVERY CLINICAL PATH—LABOUR: EXPECTED OUTCOMES (continued)

	Interventions		
TESTS/ PROCEDURES	Hgb or Hct (if not done recently) T & S (if ordered) VE as indicated IV therapy AROM by MD or midwife: assess for colour, amount, and odour, as appropriate FSE/IUPC placement if indicated	AROM: assess for colour, amount, and odour, as appropriate	Cord blood or RhoGAM workup if appropriate
THERAPIES	Comfort measures/birthing ball/ ambulate/telemetry/shower IV therapy If indicated: Amnioinfusion for variable decelerations If appropriate, pain management reviewed	Perineal massage Warm soaks to perineal area Allow to rest until feels the urge to push Frequent position changes Cool cloth/ice chips	Ice pack to perineum Warm blankets
MEDS	Antibiotics as indicated for + GBS Pitocin if indicated PRN pain medication if indicated	Pitocin if indicated	Pitocin IV if indicated
ACTIVITY/ SAFETY	Labour option usage Position changes	Provide wedge if supine Promote effective position for pushing: i.e., squatting, side lying, upright Breathing technique client most comfortable with	Assist with ambulate to bathroom Infant care Assist with positioning for breastfeeding Infant ID bands applied
NUTRITION	Clear liquids Ice chips Others	Clear liquids Ice chips	Return to previous diet
UNIQUE CLIENT NEEDS			

INTEGRATED PLAN OF CARE FOR CESAREAN DELIVERY

	Expected Client Outcomes			
	Phase 1 Preadmission (Cesarean Delivery)	**Phase 2 Surgery/ Immediate Postop/ Day of Surgery**	**Phase 3 Postop Day 1**	
Usual time in phase assessment/ potential complications	**N/A Date Started:** VS WNL for client Hgb or Hct/values within normal SLH antepartum range	Up to 23 hours VS WNL for client Systems assessment: Skin warm, dry Clear ⇒ Alert and oriented ⇒ Breast soft/nipples intact ⇒ Lungs clear ⇒ Bowel sounds present ⇒ Fundus firm u/u or u 1–2 (–/+) Lochia sm—mod Dsg dry and intact No signs infiltration IV site Verbalizes comfort using pain rating scale 0–10	1 day VS WNL for client Afebrile Voiding without Foley ⇒ Passing flatus Incision without redness or drainage Lochia small amount Fundus firm u/1–2 Verbalizes comfort using pain scale 0–10 on oral pain meds	1–2 days Incision well approximated, without drainage or redness Passing flatus Lochia sm/mod amt Fundus firm u/1–2 Verbalizes comfort using pain medication as described
Client/family knowledge	**Date All Above Met** Verbalizes understanding of condition and need for surgery Verbalizes understanding of all preop teaching	**Date All Above Met** Verbalizes correct use of PCA/fentanyl pump and when to request pain medication Turn, cough, and deep breathe appropriately	**Date All Above Met** Can state criteria for when to call doctor for problems postdischarge ⇒ ↑ Bleeding ↑ Temperature ⇒ Incision redness, odour, or drainage ⇒	**Date All Above Met** Verbalizes follow-up appointment date and time Verbalizes proper dosing of pain medication
ADLs/activity	**Date All Above Met** Verbalizes understanding of NPO status	**Date All Above Met** Able to ambulate with minimal assistance Tolerating clear/full liquid diet Bonding observed with newborn—taking-in phase ⇒	**Date All Above Met** Ambulating without assistance Tolerating soft to regular diet	**Date All Above Met** Ambulating in hall
	Date All Above Met	**Date All Above Met**	**Date All Above Met**	**Date All Above Met**
Unique client needs	**Date All Above Met Entire Phase Outcomes met; progress client to next phase**	**Date All Above Met Entire Phase Outcomes met; progress client to next phase**	**Date All Above Met Entire Phase Outcomes met; progress client to next phase**	**Date All Above Met Entire Phase Outcomes met; progress client to next phase**

INTEGRATED PLAN OF CARE FOR CESAREAN DELIVERY (continued)

	Plan of Care			
	#1 Preadmission	**#2 Surgery/ Immediate Postop/ Day of Surgery**	**#3 Postop Day 1**	**#4 Postop Day 2/ Discharge**
Assessments	Vital signs Fetal status immediately prior to surgery	VS per PACU then Q 4 hr Systems assessment: • Skin, LOC, FROM • Breasts, lungs, fundus, incision • Lochia, bladder, bowel sounds, IV, and site • I & O Q shift • Assess pain control 0–10 scale • Assess RhoGAM status • Assess Rubella titer status • ID band on parent(s)	VS Q 6 hr Assess pain control 0–10 scale Incision Foley-voiding Fundus/lochia IV site Breasts ID band on parent(s) Activity	Assess pain control 0–10 scale Incision Voiding Fundus lochia Homans sign IV site as needed ID band on parent(s) Activity
Consults	Anesthesia	Social work as needed, anesthesia, lactation, dietitian as needed	Social work, lactation, dietitian as needed	Social work, lactation, dietitian as needed
Client/family education discharge planning	Need for surgery Review cesarean birth Review procedure, postop expectations Demonstrate/discuss equipment—PCA, fentanyl pump	Review postop expectations Review equipment use PRN Instruct client on: Hospital/infant security systems Unity orientation Newborn orientation/ care/feeding (if breastfeeding challenges, see decision trees)	Review dietary needs postsurgery Review bleeding/ lochia Precautions post– cesarean birth Review follow-up care and doctor Appointments Review incision care, pericare Infant care Infant feeding	Verify follow-up appointment date and time Activity restrictions Follow-up for staple removal as needed Offer home follow-up care Discuss birth control
Tests and procedures	PAT; Hgb and Hct (if not done recently— within 1 mo) T & S (if ordered)			
Pharmacologic needs		IV fluids as ordered Pain control: PCA, fentanyl pump, IM to PO	IV lock PO pain meds Give RhoGAM if indicated Give rubella vaccine if indicated	DC IV lock as ordered

(continued)

INTEGRATED PLAN OF CARE FOR CESAREAN DELIVERY (continued)

	Plan of Care			
	#1 Preadmission	#2 Surgery/ Immediate Postop/ Day of Surgery	#3 Postop Day 1	#4 Postop Day 2/ Discharge
Activity/ rehabilitation	Client's usual	Change position Q 2 hr while in bed, OOB stand at bedside postop night/dangle and transfer to chair Progress to client endurance Observe bonding with infant Observe family support system (if concerns identified, consult SW)	Progress endurance/ begin Ambulation in hall OOB in AM May shower	Ambulate in halls without assistance
Nutrition/ elimination		NPO then clear liquids to DAT Foley empty Q shift	DAT to regular or previous diet at home Foley discontinued	
Miscellaneous interventions		TCDB Q 2 hr while awake	Dressing removed by MD or RN with MD request	
Unique client needs				

Appendix C

Cervical Dilation Chart

Appendix D

Weight Conversion Charts

CONVERSION OF POUNDS TO KILOGRAMS

Pounds	0	1	2	3	4	5	6	7	8	9
0	—	0.45	0.90	1.36	1.81	2.26	2.72	3.17	3.62	4.08
10	4.53	4.98	5.44	5.89	6.35	6.80	7.25	7.71	8.16	8.61
20	9.07	9.52	9.97	10.43	10.88	11.34	11.79	12.24	12.70	13.15
30	13.60	14.06	14.51	14.96	15.42	15.87	16.32	16.78	17.23	17.69
40	18.14	18.59	19.05	19.50	19.95	20.41	20.86	21.31	21.77	22.22
50	22.68	23.13	23.58	24.04	24.49	24.94	25.40	25.85	26.30	26.76
60	27.21	27.66	28.12	28.57	29.03	29.48	29.93	30.39	30.84	31.29
70	31.75	32.20	32.65	33.11	33.56	34.02	34.47	34.92	35.38	35.83
80	36.28	36.74	37.19	37.64	38.10	38.55	39.00	39.46	39.91	40.37
90	40.82	41.27	41.73	42.18	42.63	43.09	43.54	43.99	44.45	44.90
100	45.36	45.81	46.26	46.72	47.17	47.62	48.08	48.53	48.98	49.44
110	49.89	50.34	50.80	51.25	51.71	52.16	52.61	53.07	53.52	53.97
120	54.43	54.88	55.33	55.79	56.24	56.70	57.15	57.60	58.06	58.51
130	58.96	59.42	59.87	60.32	60.78	61.23	61.68	62.14	62.59	63.05
140	63.50	63.95	64.41	64.86	65.31	65.77	66.22	66.67	67.13	67.58
150	68.04	68.49	68.94	69.40	69.85	70.30	70.76	71.21	71.66	72.12
160	72.57	73.02	73.48	73.93	74.39	74.84	75.29	75.75	76.20	76.65
170	77.11	77.56	78.01	78.47	78.92	79.38	79.83	80.28	80.74	81.19
180	81.64	82.10	82.55	83.00	83.46	83.91	84.36	84.82	85.27	85.73
190	86.18	86.68	87.09	87.54	87.99	88.45	88.90	89.35	89.81	90.26
200	90.72	91.17	91.62	92.08	92.53	92.98	93.44	93.89	94.34	94.80

CONVERSION OF POUNDS AND OUNCES TO GRAMS FOR NEWBORN WEIGHTS

Pounds	Ounces															
	0	1	2	3	4	5	6	7	8	9	10	11	12	13	14	15
0	—	28	57	85	113	142	170	198	227	255	283	312	340	369	397	425
1	454	482	510	539	567	595	624	652	680	709	737	765	794	822	850	879
2	907	936	964	992	1,021	1,049	1,077	1,106	1,134	1,162	1,191	1,219	1,247	1,276	1,304	1,332
3	1,361	1,389	1,417	1,446	1,474	1,503	1,531	1,559	1,588	1,616	1,644	1,673	1,701	1,729	1,758	1,786
4	1,814	1,843	1,871	1,899	1,928	1,956	1,984	2,013	2,041	2,070	2,098	2,126	2,155	2,183	2,211	2,240
5	2,268	2,296	2,325	2,353	2,381	2,410	2,438	2,466	2,495	2,523	2,551	2,580	2,608	2,637	2,665	2,693
6	2,722	2,750	2,778	2,807	2,835	2,863	2,892	2,920	2,948	2,977	3,005	3,033	3,062	3,090	3,118	3,147
7	3,175	3,203	3,232	3,260	3,289	3,317	3,345	3,374	3,402	3,430	3,459	3,487	3,515	3,544	3,572	3,600
8	3,629	3,657	3,685	3,714	3,742	3,770	3,799	3,827	3,856	3,884	3,912	3,941	3,969	3,997	4,026	4,054
9	4,082	4,111	4,139	4,167	4,196	4,224	4,252	4,281	4,309	4,337	4,366	4,394	4,423	4,451	4,479	4,508
10	4,536	4,564	4,593	4,621	4,649	4,678	4,706	4,734	4,763	4,791	4,819	4,848	4,876	4,904	4,933	4,961
11	4,990	5,018	5,046	5,075	5,103	5,131	5,160	5,188	5,216	5,245	5,273	5,301	5,330	5,358	5,386	5,415
12	5,443	5,471	5,500	5,528	5,557	5,585	5,613	5,642	5,670	5,698	5,727	5,755	5,783	5,812	5,840	5,868
13	5,897	5,925	5,953	5,982	6,010	6,038	6,067	6,095	6,123	6,152	6,180	6,209	6,237	6,265	6,294	6,322
14	6,350	6,379	6,407	6,435	6,464	6,492	6,520	6,549	6,577	6,605	6,634	6,662	6,690	6,719	6,747	6,776
15	6,804	6,832	6,860	6,889	6,917	6,945	6,973	7,002	7,030	7,059	7,087	7,115	7,144	7,172	7,201	7,228

Appendix E

Breastfeeding and Medication Use

GENERAL CONSIDERATIONS

- Most medications are safe to use while breastfeeding; however, the parent should always check with the pediatrician, physician, nurse practitioner, pharmacist, or lactation specialist before taking any medications, including over-the-counter and herbal products.
- Inform clients about their right to seek a second opinion if their primary care provider does not perform a thoughtful risk-versus-benefit assessment before prescribing medications or advising against breastfeeding.
- Most medications pass from the breastfeeding parent's bloodstream into the breastmilk. However, the amount is usually very small and unlikely to harm the baby.
- A preterm or other special needs neonate is more susceptible to the adverse effects of medications in breastmilk. A person who is taking medications and whose baby is in the neonatal intensive care unit or special care nursery should consult with the pediatrician or neonatologist before feeding breastmilk to the baby.
- A parent who is taking a prescribed medication should ideally take the medication just after breastfeeding. This practice helps ensure that the lowest possible dose of medication reaches the baby through the breastmilk.
- Some medications can cause changes in the amount of milk an individual will produce. Encourage the parent to report any changes in milk production.

LACTATION RISK CATEGORIES (LRC)

Lactation Category	Risk	Rationale
L1	Compatible	Clinical research or long-term observation of use in many breastfeeding parents has not demonstrated risk to the infant.
L2	Probably compatible	Limited clinical research has not demonstrated an increase in adverse effects in the infant.
L3	Probably compatible	There is possible risk to the infant; however, the risks are minimal or nonthreatening in nature. These medications should be given only when the potential benefit outweighs the risk to the infant.

Lactation Category	Risk	Rationale
L4	Possibly hazardous	There is positive evidence of risk to the infant; however, in life-threatening situations or for serious diseases, the benefit might outweigh the risk.
L5	No data: Hazardous	The risk of using the medication clearly outweighs any possible benefit from breastfeeding.

POTENTIAL EFFECTS OF SELECTED MEDICATION CATEGORIES ON THE BREASTFED INFANT

Narcotic Analgesics

- Codeine and hydrocodone appear to be safe in moderate doses. Rarely the neonate may experience sedation and/or apnea. (LRC: L3)
- Meperidine (Demerol) can lead to sedation of the neonate. (LRC: L3)
- Low to moderate doses of morphine appear to be safe. (LRC: L2)
- Trace-to-negligible amounts of fentanyl are found in human milk. (LRC: L2)

Nonnarcotic Analgesics and NSAIDs

- Acetaminophen and ibuprofen are approved for use. (LRC: L1)
- Naproxen may cause neonatal hemorrhage and anemia if used for prolonged periods. (LRC: L3 for short-term use and L4 for long-term use)
- The newer COX2 inhibitors, such as celecoxib (Celebrex), appear to be safe for use. (LRC: L2)

Antibiotics

- Levels in breastmilk are usually very low.
- The penicillins and cephalosporins are generally considered safe to use. (LRC: L1 and L2)
- Tetracyclines can be safely used for short periods but are not suitable for long-term therapy (e.g., for treatment of acne). (LRC: L2)
- Sulfonamides should not be used during the neonatal stage (the first month of life). (LRC: L3)

Antihypertensives

- A high degree of caution is advised when antihypertensives are used during breastfeeding.
- Some beta blockers can be used.
- Hydralazine and methyldopa are considered to be safe. (LRC: L2)
- Angiotensin-converting enzyme (ACE) inhibitors are not recommended in the early postpartum period.

Sedatives and Hypnotics

- Neonatal withdrawal can occur when antianxiety medications, such as lorazepam, are taken. Fortunately withdrawal is generally mild.
- Phenothiazines, such as Phenergan and Thorazine, may lead to sleep apnea and increase the risk for sudden infant death syndrome.

Antidepressants

- The risk to the baby is often higher if the breastfeeding parent is depressed and remains untreated, rather than taking the medication.
- The older tricyclics are considered to be safe; however, they cause many bothersome side effects, such as weight gain and dry mouth, which may lead to noncompliance on the part of the woman.
- The selective serotonin uptake inhibitors (SSRIs) are also considered to be safe and have a lower side effect profile, which makes them more palatable to the client. (LRC: L2 and L3)

Mood Stabilizers (Antimanic Medication)

- Lithium is found in breastmilk and is best not used while breastfeeding. (LRC: L4)

- Valproic acid seems to be a more appropriate choice for the client with bipolar disorder. The infant will need periodic lab studies to check platelets and liver function.

Corticosteroids

- Corticosteroids do not pass into the milk in large quantities.
- Inhaled steroids are safe to use because they do not accumulate in the bloodstream.

Thyroid Medication

- Thyroid medications, such as levothyroxine (Synthroid), can be taken while breastfeeding.
- Most are in LRC category L1.

MEDICATIONS THAT USUALLY ARE CONTRAINDICATED FOR BREASTFEEDING

- Amiodarone
- Antineoplastic agents
- Chloramphenicol
- Doxepin
- Ergotamine and other ergot derivatives
- Iodides
- Methotrexate and immunosuppressants
- Lithium
- Radiopharmaceuticals
- Ribavirin
- Tetracycline (prolonged use—more than 3 weeks)
- Pseudoephedrine (found in many over-the-counter medications)

Material in this appendix was adapted from information found in the following sources:
Brucker, M. C., & King, T. L. (2017). *Pharmacology for women's health* (2nd ed.). Burlington, MA: Jones & Bartlett Learning.
Lauwers, J., & Swisher, A. (2016). *Counseling the nursing mother: A lactation consultant's guide* (6th ed.). Burlington, MA: Jones & Bartlett Learning.
Wamback, K., & Riordan, J. (2015). *Breastfeeding and human lactation* (5th ed.). Burlington, MA: Jones & Bartlett Learning.

Appendix F

Blood Pressure Charts for Children and Adolescents

TABLE F.1	BLOOD PRESSURE LEVELS FOR BOYS BY AGE AND HEIGHT PERCENTILE

Age (Year)	BP Percentile	SBP (mmHg) Height Percentile or Measured Height							DBP (mmHg) Height Percentile or Measured Height						
		5%	10%	25%	50%	75%	90%	95%	5%	10%	25%	50%	75%	90%	95%
1	Height (in)	30.4	30.8	31.6	32.4	33.3	34.1	34.6	30.4	30.8	31.6	32.4	33.3	34.1	34.6
	Height (cm)	77.2	78.3	80.2	82.4	84.6	86.7	87.9	77.2	78.3	80.2	82.4	84.6	86.7	87.9
	50th	85	85	86	86	87	88	88	40	40	40	41	41	42	42
	90th	98	99	99	100	100	101	101	52	52	53	53	54	54	54
	95th	102	102	103	103	104	105	105	54	54	55	55	56	57	57
	95th + 12 mmHg	114	114	115	115	116	117	117	66	66	67	67	68	69	69
2	Height (in)	33.9	34.4	35.3	36.3	37.3	38.2	38.8	33.9	34.4	35.3	36.3	37.3	38.2	38.8
	Height (cm)	86.1	87.4	89.6	92.1	94.7	97.1	98.5	86.1	87.4	89.6	92.1	94.7	97.1	98.5
	50th	87	87	88	89	89	90	91	43	43	44	44	45	46	46
	90th	100	100	101	102	103	103	104	55	55	56	56	57	58	58
	95th	104	105	105	106	107	107	108	57	58	58	59	60	61	61
	95th + 12 mmHg	116	117	117	118	119	119	120	69	70	70	71	72	73	73
3	Height (in)	36.4	37	37.9	39	40.1	41.1	41.7	36.4	37	37.9	39	40.1	41.1	41.7
	Height (cm)	92.5	93.9	96.3	99	101.8	104.3	105.8	92.5	93.9	96.3	99	101.8	104.3	105.8
	50th	88	89	89	90	91	92	92	45	46	46	47	48	49	49
	90th	101	102	102	103	104	105	105	58	58	59	59	60	61	61
	95th	106	106	107	107	108	109	109	60	61	61	62	63	64	64
	95th + 12 mmHg	118	118	119	119	120	121	121	72	73	73	74	75	76	76
4	Height (in)	38.8	39.4	40.5	41.7	42.9	43.9	44.5	38.8	39.4	40.5	41.7	42.9	43.9	44.5
	Height (cm)	98.5	100.2	102.9	105.9	108.9	111.5	113.2	98.5	100.2	102.9	105.9	108.9	111.5	113.2
	50th	90	90	91	92	93	94	94	48	49	49	50	51	52	52
	90th	102	103	104	105	105	106	107	60	61	62	62	63	64	64
	95th	107	107	108	108	109	110	110	63	64	65	66	67	67	68
	95th + 12 mmHg	119	119	120	120	121	122	122	75	76	77	78	79	79	80
5	Height (in)	41.1	41.8	43.0	44.3	45.5	46.7	47.4	41.1	41.8	43.0	44.3	45.5	46.7	47.4
	Height (cm)	104.4	106.2	109.1	112.4	115.7	118.6	120.3	104.4	106.2	109.1	112.4	115.7	118.6	120.3
	50th	91	92	93	94	95	96	96	51	51	52	53	54	55	55
	90th	103	104	105	106	107	108	108	63	64	65	65	66	67	67
	95th	107	108	109	109	110	111	112	66	67	68	69	70	70	71
	95th + 12 mmHg	119	120	121	121	122	123	124	78	79	80	81	82	82	83
6	Height (in)	43.4	44.2	45.4	46.8	48.2	49.4	50.2	43.4	44.2	45.4	46.8	48.2	49.4	50.2
	Height (cm)	110.3	112.2	115.3	118.9	122.4	125.6	127.5	110.3	112.2	115.3	118.9	122.4	125.6	127.5
	50th	93	93	94	95	96	97	98	54	54	55	56	57	57	58
	90th	105	105	106	107	109	110	110	66	66	67	68	68	69	69
	95th	108	109	110	111	112	113	114	69	70	70	71	72	72	73
	95th + 12 mmHg	120	121	122	123	124	125	126	81	82	82	83	84	84	85
7	Height (in)	45.7	46.5	47.8	49.3	50.8	52.1	52.9	45.7	46.5	47.8	49.3	50.8	52.1	52.9
	Height (cm)	116.1	118	121.4	125.1	128.9	132.4	134.5	116.1	118	121.4	125.1	128.9	132.4	134.5
	50th	94	94	95	97	98	98	99	56	56	57	58	58	59	59
	90th	106	107	108	109	110	111	111	68	68	69	70	70	71	71
	95th	110	110	111	112	114	115	116	71	71	72	73	73	74	74
	95th + 12 mmHg	122	122	123	124	126	127	128	83	83	84	85	85	86	86
8	Height (in)	47.8	48.6	50	51.6	53.2	54.6	55.5	47.8	48.6	50	51.6	53.2	54.6	55.5
	Height (cm)	121.4	123.5	127	131	135.1	138.8	141	121.4	123.5	127	131	135.1	138.8	141
	50th	95	96	97	98	99	99	100	57	57	58	59	59	60	60
	90th	107	108	109	110	111	112	112	69	70	70	71	72	72	73
	95th	111	112	112	114	115	116	117	72	73	73	74	75	75	75
	95th + 12 mmHg	123	124	124	126	127	128	129	84	85	85	86	87	87	87
9	Height (in)	49.6	50.5	52	53.7	55.4	56.9	57.9	49.6	50.5	52	53.7	55.4	56.9	57.9
	Height (cm)	126	128.3	132.1	136.3	140.7	144.7	147.1	126	128.3	132.1	136.3	140.7	144.7	147.1
	50th	96	97	98	99	100	101	101	57	58	59	60	61	62	62
	90th	107	108	109	110	112	113	114	70	71	72	73	74	74	74
	95th	112	112	113	115	116	118	119	74	74	75	76	76	77	77
	95th + 12 mmHg	124	124	125	127	128	130	131	86	86	87	88	88	89	89

TABLE F.1 — BLOOD PRESSURE LEVELS FOR BOYS BY AGE AND HEIGHT PERCENTILE (continued)

Age (Year)	BP Percentile	SBP (mmHg) Height Percentile or Measured Height							DBP (mmHg) Height Percentile or Measured Height						
		5%	10%	25%	50%	75%	90%	95%	5%	10%	25%	50%	75%	90%	95%
10	Height (in)	51.3	52.2	53.8	55.6	57.4	59.1	60.1	51.3	52.2	53.8	55.6	57.4	59.1	60.1
	Height (cm)	130.2	132.7	136.7	141.3	145.9	150.1	152.7	130.2	132.7	136.7	141.3	145.9	150.1	152.7
	50th	97	98	99	100	101	102	103	59	60	61	62	63	63	64
	90th	108	109	111	112	113	115	116	72	73	74	74	75	75	76
	95th	112	113	114	116	118	120	121	76	76	77	77	78	78	78
	95th + 12 mmHg	124	125	126	128	130	132	133	88	88	89	89	90	90	90
11	Height (in)	53	54	55.7	57.6	59.6	61.3	62.4	53	54	55.7	57.6	59.6	61.3	62.4
	Height (cm)	134.7	137.3	141.5	146.4	151.3	155.8	158.6	134.7	137.3	141.5	146.4	151.3	155.8	158.6
	50th	99	99	101	102	103	104	106	61	61	62	63	63	63	63
	90th	110	111	112	114	116	117	118	74	74	75	75	75	76	76
	95th	114	114	116	118	120	123	124	77	78	78	78	78	78	78
	95th + 12 mmHg	126	126	128	130	132	135	136	89	90	90	90	90	90	90
12	Height (in)	55.2	56.3	58.1	60.1	62.2	64	65.2	55.2	56.3	58.1	60.1	62.2	64	65.2
	Height (cm)	140.3	143	147.5	152.7	157.9	162.6	165.5	140.3	143	147.5	152.7	157.9	162.6	165.5
	50th	101	101	102	104	106	108	109	61	62	62	62	62	63	63
	90th	113	114	115	117	119	121	122	75	75	75	75	75	76	76
	95th	116	117	118	121	124	126	128	78	78	78	78	78	79	79
	95th + 12 mmHg	128	129	130	133	136	138	140	90	90	90	90	90	91	91
13	Height (in)	57.9	59.1	61	63.1	65.2	67.1	68.3	57.9	59.1	61	63.1	65.2	67.1	68.3
	Height (cm)	147	150	154.9	160.3	165.7	170.5	173.4	147	150	154.9	160.3	165.7	170.5	173.4
	50th	103	104	105	108	110	111	112	61	60	61	62	63	64	65
	90th	115	116	118	121	124	126	126	74	74	74	75	76	77	77
	95th	119	120	122	125	128	130	131	78	78	78	78	80	81	81
	95th and 12 mmHg	131	132	134	137	140	142	143	90	90	90	90	92	93	93
14	Height (in)	60.6	61.8	63.8	65.9	68.0	69.8	70.9	60.6	61.8	63.8	65.9	68.0	69.8	70.9
	Height (cm)	153.8	156.9	162	167.5	172.7	177.4	180.1	153.8	156.9	162	167.5	172.7	177.4	180.1
	50th	105	106	109	111	112	113	113	60	60	62	64	65	66	67
	90th	119	120	123	126	127	128	129	74	74	75	77	78	79	80
	95th	123	125	127	130	132	133	134	77	78	79	81	82	83	84
	95th and 12 mmHg	135	137	139	142	144	145	146	89	90	91	93	94	95	96
15	Height (in)	62.6	63.8	65.7	67.8	69.8	71.5	72.5	62.6	63.8	65.7	67.8	69.8	71.5	72.5
	Height (cm)	159	162	166.9	172.2	177.2	181.6	184.2	159	162	166.9	172.2	177.2	181.6	184.2
	50th	108	110	112	113	114	114	114	61	62	64	65	66	67	68
	90th	123	124	126	128	129	130	130	75	76	78	79	80	81	81
	95th	127	129	131	132	134	135	135	78	79	81	83	84	85	85
	95th and 12 mmHg	139	141	143	144	146	147	147	90	91	93	95	96	97	97
16	Height (in)	63.8	64.9	66.8	68.8	70.7	72.4	73.4	63.8	64.9	66.8	68.8	70.7	72.4	73.4
	Height (cm)	162.1	165	169.6	174.6	179.5	183.8	186.4	162.1	165	169.6	174.6	179.5	183.8	186.4
	50th	111	112	114	115	115	116	116	63	64	66	67	68	69	69
	90th	126	127	128	129	131	131	132	77	78	79	80	81	82	82
	95th	130	131	133	134	135	136	137	80	81	83	84	85	86	86
	95th and 12 mmHg	142	143	145	146	147	148	149	92	93	95	96	97	98	98
17	Height (in)	64.5	65.5	67.3	69.2	71.1	72.8	73.8	64.5	65.5	67.3	69.2	71.1	72.8	73.8
	Height (cm)	163.8	166.5	170.9	175.8	180.7	184.9	187.5	163.8	166.5	170.9	175.8	180.7	184.9	187.5
	50th	114	115	116	117	117	118	118	65	66	67	68	69	70	70
	90th	128	129	130	131	132	133	134	78	79	80	81	82	82	83
	95th	132	133	134	135	137	138	138	81	82	84	85	86	86	87
	95th and 12 mmHg	144	145	146	147	149	150	150	93	94	96	97	98	98	99

Elevated BP, ≥90th percentile; stage 1 HTN, ≥95th percentile; stage 2 HTN, ≥95th percentile + 12 mmHg. The 50th, 90th, and 95th percentiles were derived by using quantile regression on the basis of normal-weight children (BMI <85th percentile).
From Flynn, J. T., Kaelber, D. C., Baker-Smith, C. M., et al. (2017). Clinical Practice Guideline for Screening and Management of High Blood Pressure in Children and Adolescents. *Pediatrics*, *140*(3):e20171904. Retrieved from https://pediatrics.aappublications.org/content/140/3/e20171904.

TABLE F.2 **BLOOD PRESSURE LEVELS FOR GIRLS BY AGE AND HEIGHT PERCENTILE**

Age (Year)	BP Percentile	SBP (mm Hg) Height Percentile or Measured Height							DBP (mm Hg) Height Percentile or Measured Height						
		5%	10%	25%	50%	75%	90%	95%	5%	10%	25%	50%	75%	90%	95%
1	Height (in)	29.7	30.2	30.9	31.8	32.7	33.4	33.9	29.7	30.2	30.9	31.8	32.7	33.4	33.9
	Height (cm)	75.4	76.6	78.6	80.8	83	84.9	86.1	75.4	76.6	78.6	80.8	83	84.9	86.1
	50th	84	85	86	86	87	88	88	41	42	42	43	44	45	46
	90th	98	99	99	100	101	102	102	54	55	56	56	57	58	58
	95th	101	102	102	103	104	105	105	59	59	60	60	61	62	62
	95th + 12 mm Hg	113	114	114	115	116	117	117	71	71	72	72	73	74	74
2	Height (in)	33.4	34	34.9	35.9	36.9	37.8	38.4	33.4	34	34.9	35.9	36.9	37.8	38.4
	Height (cm)	84.9	86.3	88.6	91.1	93.7	96	97.4	84.9	86.3	88.6	91.1	93.7	96	97.4
	50th	87	87	88	89	90	91	91	45	46	47	48	49	50	51
	90th	101	101	102	103	104	105	106	58	58	59	60	61	62	62
	95th	104	105	106	106	107	108	109	62	63	63	64	65	66	66
	95th + 12 mm Hg	116	117	118	118	119	120	121	74	75	75	76	77	78	78
3	Height (in)	35.8	36.4	37.3	38.4	39.6	40.6	41.2	35.8	36.4	37.3	38.4	39.6	40.6	41.2
	Height (cm)	91	92.4	94.9	97.6	100.5	103.1	104.6	91	92.4	94.9	97.6	100.5	103.1	104.6
	50th	88	89	89	90	91	92	93	48	48	49	50	51	53	53
	90th	102	103	104	104	105	106	107	60	61	61	62	63	64	65
	95th	106	106	107	108	109	110	110	64	65	65	66	67	68	69
	95th + 12 mm Hg	118	118	119	120	121	122	122	76	77	77	78	79	80	81
4	Height (in)	38.3	38.9	39.9	41.1	42.4	43.5	44.2	38.3	38.9	39.9	41.1	42.4	43.5	44.2
	Height (cm)	97.2	98.8	101.4	104.5	107.6	110.5	112.2	97.2	98.8	101.4	104.5	107.6	110.5	112.2
	50th	89	90	91	92	93	94	94	50	51	51	53	54	55	55
	90th	103	104	105	106	107	108	108	62	63	64	65	66	67	67
	95th	107	108	109	109	110	111	112	66	67	68	69	70	70	71
	95th + 12 mm Hg	119	120	121	121	122	123	124	78	79	80	81	82	82	83
5	Height (in)	40.8	41.5	42.6	43.9	45.2	46.5	47.3	40.8	41.5	42.6	43.9	45.2	46.5	47.3
	Height (cm)	103.6	105.3	108.2	111.5	114.9	118.1	120	103.6	105.3	108.2	111.5	114.9	118.1	120
	50th	90	91	92	93	94	95	96	52	52	53	55	56	57	57
	90th	104	105	106	107	108	109	110	64	65	66	67	68	69	70
	95th	108	109	109	110	111	112	113	68	69	70	71	72	73	73
	95th + 12 mm Hg	120	121	121	122	123	124	125	80	81	82	83	84	85	85
6	Height (in)	43.3	44	45.2	46.6	48.1	49.4	50.3	43.3	44	45.2	46.6	48.1	49.4	50.3
	Height (cm)	110	111.8	114.9	118.4	122.1	125.6	127.7	110	111.8	114.9	118.4	122.1	125.6	127.7
	50th	92	92	93	94	96	97	97	54	54	55	56	57	58	59
	90th	105	106	107	108	109	110	111	67	67	68	69	70	71	71
	95th	109	109	110	111	112	113	114	70	71	72	72	73	74	74
	95th + 12 mm Hg	121	121	122	123	124	125	126	82	83	84	84	85	86	86
7	Height (in)	45.6	46.4	47.7	49.2	50.7	52.1	53	45.6	46.4	47.7	49.2	50.7	52.1	53
	Height (cm)	115.9	117.8	121.1	124.9	128.8	132.5	134.7	115.9	117.8	121.1	124.9	128.8	132.5	134.7
	50th	92	93	94	95	97	98	99	55	55	56	57	58	59	60
	90th	106	106	107	109	110	111	112	68	68	69	70	71	72	72
	95th	109	110	111	112	113	114	115	72	72	73	73	74	74	75
	95th + 12 mm Hg	121	122	123	124	125	126	127	84	84	85	85	86	86	87
8	Height (in)	47.6	48.4	49.8	51.4	53	54.5	55.5	47.6	48.4	49.8	51.4	53	54.5	55.5
	Height (cm)	121	123	126.5	130.6	134.7	138.5	140.9	121	123	126.5	130.6	134.7	138.5	140.9
	50th	93	94	95	97	98	99	100	56	56	57	59	60	61	61
	90th	107	107	108	110	111	112	113	69	70	71	72	72	73	73
	95th	110	111	112	113	115	116	117	72	73	74	74	75	75	75
	95th + 12 mm Hg	122	123	124	125	127	128	129	84	85	86	86	87	87	87

TABLE F.2															

BLOOD PRESSURE LEVELS FOR GIRLS BY AGE AND HEIGHT PERCENTILE (continued)

Age (Year)	BP Percentile	SBP (mm Hg) Height Percentile or Measured Height							DBP (mm Hg) Height Percentile or Measured Height						
		5%	10%	25%	50%	75%	90%	95%	5%	10%	25%	50%	75%	90%	95%
9	Height (in)	49.3	50.2	51.7	53.4	55.1	56.7	57.7	49.3	50.2	51.7	53.4	55.1	56.7	57.7
	Height (cm)	125.3	127.6	131.3	135.6	140.1	144.1	146.6	125.3	127.6	131.3	135.6	140.1	144.1	146.6
	50th	95	95	97	98	99	100	101	57	58	59	60	60	61	61
	90th	108	108	109	111	112	113	114	71	71	72	73	73	73	73
	95th	112	112	113	114	116	117	118	74	74	75	75	75	75	75
	95th + 12 mm Hg	124	124	125	126	128	129	130	86	86	87	87	87	87	87
10	Height (in)	51.1	52	53.7	55.5	57.4	59.1	60.2	51.1	52	53.7	55.5	57.4	59.1	60.2
	Height (cm)	129.7	132.2	136.3	141	145.8	150.2	152.8	129.7	132.2	136.3	141	145.8	150.2	152.8
	50th	96	97	98	99	101	102	103	58	59	59	60	61	61	62
	90th	109	110	111	112	113	115	116	72	73	73	73	73	73	73
	95th	113	114	114	116	117	119	120	75	75	76	76	76	76	76
	95th + 12 mm Hg	125	126	126	128	129	131	132	87	87	88	88	88	88	88
11	Height (in)	53.4	54.5	56.2	58.2	60.2	61.9	63	53.4	54.5	56.2	58.2	60.2	61.9	63
	Height (cm)	135.6	138.3	142.8	147.8	152.8	157.3	160	135.6	138.3	142.8	147.8	152.8	157.3	160
	50th	98	99	101	102	104	105	106	60	60	60	61	62	63	64
	90th	111	112	113	114	116	118	120	74	74	74	74	74	75	75
	95th	115	116	117	118	120	123	124	76	77	77	77	77	77	77
	95th + 12 mm Hg	127	128	129	130	132	135	136	88	89	89	89	89	89	89
12	Height (in)	56.2	57.3	59	60.9	62.8	64.5	65.5	56.2	57.3	59	60.9	62.8	64.5	65.5
	Height (cm)	142.8	145.5	149.9	154.8	159.6	163.8	166.4	142.8	145.5	149.9	154.8	159.6	163.8	166.4
	50th	102	102	104	105	107	108	108	61	61	61	62	64	65	65
	90th	114	115	116	118	120	122	122	75	75	75	75	76	76	76
	95th	118	119	120	122	124	125	126	78	78	78	78	79	79	79
	95th and 12 mm Hg	130	131	132	134	136	137	138	90	90	90	90	91	91	91
13	Height (in)	58.3	59.3	60.9	62.7	64.5	66.1	67	58.3	59.3	60.9	62.7	64.5	66.1	67
	Height (cm)	148.1	150.6	154.7	159.2	163.7	167.8	170.2	148.1	150.6	154.7	159.2	163.7	167.8	170.2
	50th	104	105	106	107	108	108	109	62	62	63	64	65	65	66
	90th	116	117	119	121	122	123	123	75	75	75	76	76	76	76
	95th	121	122	123	124	126	126	127	79	79	79	79	80	80	81
	95th + 12 mm Hg	133	134	135	136	138	138	139	91	91	91	91	92	92	93
14	Height (in)	59.3	60.2	61.8	63.5	65.2	66.8	67.7	59.3	60.2	61.8	63.5	65.2	66.8	67.7
	Height (cm)	150.6	153	156.9	161.3	165.7	169.7	172.1	150.6	153	156.9	161.3	165.7	169.7	172.1
	50th	105	106	107	108	109	109	109	63	63	64	65	66	66	66
	90th	118	118	120	122	123	123	123	76	76	76	76	77	77	77
	95th	123	123	124	125	126	127	127	80	80	80	80	81	81	82
	95th + 12 mm Hg	135	135	136	137	138	139	139	92	92	92	92	93	93	94
15	Height (in)	59.7	60.6	62.2	63.9	65.6	67.2	68.1	59.7	60.6	62.2	63.9	65.6	67.2	68.1
	Height (cm)	151.7	154	157.9	162.3	166.7	170.6	173	151.7	154	157.9	162.3	166.7	170.6	173
	50th	105	106	107	108	109	109	109	64	64	64	65	66	67	67
	90th	118	119	121	122	123	123	124	76	76	76	77	77	78	78
	95th	124	124	125	126	127	127	128	80	80	80	81	82	82	82
	95th + 12 mm Hg	136	136	137	138	139	139	140	92	92	92	93	94	94	94
16	Height (in)	59.9	60.8	62.4	64.1	65.8	67.3	68.3	59.9	60.8	62.4	64.1	65.8	67.3	68.3
	Height (cm)	152.1	154.5	158.4	162.8	167.1	171.1	173.4	152.1	154.5	158.4	162.8	167.1	171.1	173.4
	50th	106	107	108	109	109	110	110	64	64	65	66	66	67	67
	90th	119	120	122	123	124	124	124	76	76	76	77	78	78	78
	95th	124	125	125	127	127	128	128	80	80	80	81	82	82	82
	95th + 12 mm Hg	136	137	137	139	139	140	140	92	92	92	93	94	94	94

(continued)

TABLE F.2	BLOOD PRESSURE LEVELS FOR GIRLS BY AGE AND HEIGHT PERCENTILE (continued)

Age (Year)	BP Percentile	SBP (mm Hg) Height Percentile or Measured Height							DBP (mm Hg) Height Percentile or Measured Height						
		5%	10%	25%	50%	75%	90%	95%	5%	10%	25%	50%	75%	90%	95%
17	Height (in)	60.0	60.9	62.5	64.2	65.9	67.4	68.4	60.0	60.9	62.5	64.2	65.9	67.4	68.4
	Height (cm)	152.4	154.7	158.7	163.0	167.4	171.3	173.7	152.4	154.7	158.7	163.0	167.4	171.3	173.7
	50th	107	108	109	110	110	110	111	64	64	65	66	66	66	67
	90th	120	121	123	124	124	125	125	76	76	77	77	78	78	78
	95th	125	125	126	127	128	128	128	80	80	80	81	82	82	82
	95th + 12 mm Hg	137	137	138	139	140	140	140	92	92	92	93	94	94	94

Elevated BP, ≥90th percentile; stage 1 HTN, ≥95th percentile; stage 2 HTN, ≥95th percentile + 12 mm Hg. The 50th, 90th, and 95th percentiles were derived by using quantile regression on the basis of normal-weight children (BMI <85th percentile).
From Flynn, J. T., Kaelber, D. C., Baker-Smith, C. M., et al. (2017). Clinical Practice Guideline for Screening and Management of High Blood Pressure in Children and Adolescents. *Pediatrics, 140*(3):e20171904. Retrieved from https://pediatrics.aappublications.org/content/140/3/e20171904.

Appendix G

Select NANDA-I Nursing Diagnoses

The following nursing diagnoses, each of which is referenced in the preceding pages, come from:

T. Heather Herdman/Shigemi Kamitsuru (Eds.), NANDA International, Inc. Nursing Diagnoses: Definitions and Classification 2018–2020, Eleventh Edition © 2017 NANDA International, ISBN 978-1-62623-929-6. Used by arrangement with the Thieme Group, Stuttgart/New York.

ACTIVITY INTOLERANCE

Definition: Insufficient physiologic or psychological energy to endure or complete required or desired daily activities.

Defining characteristics: Abnormal blood pressure response to activity; Abnormal heart rate response to activity; Electrocardiogram (ECG) change; Exertional discomfort; Exertional dyspnea; Fatigue; Generalized weakness

ACUTE CONFUSION

Definition: Reversible disturbances of consciousness, attention, cognition, and perception that develop over a short period of time, and which last less than 3 months.

Defining characteristics: Agitation; Alteration in cognitive functioning; Alteration in level of consciousness; Alteration in psychomotor functioning; Hallucinations; Inability to initiate goal-directed behavior; Inability to initiate purposeful behavior; Insufficient follow-through with goal-directed behavior; Insufficient follow-through with purposeful behavior; Misperception; Restlessness

ACUTE PAIN

Definition: Unpleasant sensory and emotional experience associated with actual or potential tissue damage, or described in terms of such damage (International Association for the Study of Pain); sudden or slow onset of any intensity from mild to severe with an anticipated or predictable end, and with a duration of less than 3 months.

Defining characteristics: Appetite change; Change in physiologic parameter; Diaphoresis; Distraction behavior; Evidence of pain using standardized pain behavior checklist for those unable to communicate verbally; Expressive behavior; Facial expression of pain; Guarding behavior; Hopelessness; Narrowed Focus; Positioning to ease pain; Protective behavior; Proxy report of pain behavior/activity changes; Pupil dilation; Self-focused; Self-report of intensity using standardized pain scale; Self-report of pain characteristics using standardized pain instrument

ANXIETY

Definition: Vague, uneasy feeling of discomfort or dread accompanied by an autonomic response (the source is often nonspecific or unknown to the individual); a feeling of apprehension caused by anticipation of danger. It is an alerting sign that warns of impending danger and enables the individual to take measures to deal with that threat.

Defining characteristics: Decrease in productivity; Extraneous movement; Fidgeting; Glancing about; Hypervigilance; Insomnia; Poor eye contact; Restlessness; Scanning behavior; Worried about changes in life event

BATHING SELF-CARE DEFICIT

Definition: Inability to independently complete cleansing activities.

Defining characteristics: Impaired ability to access bathroom; Impaired ability to access water; Impaired ability to dry body; Impaired ability to gather bathing supplies; Impaired ability to regulate bath water; Impaired ability to wash body

CAREGIVER ROLE STRAIN

Definition: Difficulty in fulfilling care responsibilities, expectations, and/or behaviors for family or significant others.

Defining characteristics: Apprehensiveness about future ability to provide care; Apprehensiveness about future health of care receiver; Apprehensiveness about potential institutionalization of care receiver; Apprehensiveness about well-being of care receiver if unable to provide care; Difficulty completing required tasks; Difficulty performing required tasks; Dysfunctional change in caregiving activities; Preoccupation with care routine

CHRONIC CONFUSION

Definition: Irreversible, progressive, insidious, and long-term alteration of intellect, behavior and personality, manifested by impairment in cognitive functions (memory, speech, language, decision making, and executive function), and dependency in execution of daily activities.

Defining characteristics: Adequate alertness to surroundings; Alteration in at least one cognitive function other than memory; Alteration in behavior; Alteration in long-term memory; Alteration in personality; Alteration in short-term memory; Alteration in social functioning; Inability to perform at least one daily activity; Insidious and irreversible onset in cognitive impairment; Long-term cognitive impairment; Progressive impairment in cognitive functioning

CHRONIC PAIN

Definition: Unpleasant sensory and emotional experience associated with actual or potential tissue damage, or described in terms of such damage (International Association for the Study of Pain); sudden or slow onset of any intensity from mild to severe, constant or recurring with an anticipated or predictable end, and with a duration of great than 3 months.

Defining characteristics: Alteration in ability to continue previous activities; Alteration in sleep pattern; Anorexia; Evidence of pain using standardized pain behavior checklist for those unable to communicate verbally; Facial expressions of pain; Proxy report of pain behavior/activity changes; Self-focused; Self-report of intensity using standardized pain scale; Self-report of pain characteristics using standardized pain instrument

CHRONIC SORROW

Definition: Cyclical, recurring, and potentially progressive pattern of pervasive sadness experienced (by a parent, caregiver, individual with chronic illness or disability) in response to continual loss, throughout the trajectory of an illness or disability.

Defining characteristics: Feeling that interferes with well-being; Overwhelming negative feelings; Sadness

COMPROMISED FAMILY COPING

Definition: A usually supportive primary person (family member, significant other, or close friend) provides insufficient, ineffective, or compromised support, comfort, assistance, or encouragement that may be needed by the client to manage or master adaptive tasks related to his or her health challenge.

Defining characteristics: Assistive behaviors by support person produce unsatisfactory results; Client complaint about support person's response to health problem; Client concern about support person's response to health problem; Limitation in communication between support person and client; Protective behavior by support person incongruent with client's abilities; Protective behavior by support person incongruent with client's need for autonomy; Support person reports inadequate understanding that interferes with effective behaviors; Support person reports insufficient knowledge that interferes with effective behaviors; Support person reports preoccupation with own reaction to client's need; Support person withdraws from client

CONSTIPATION

Definition: Decrease in normal frequency of defecation accompanied by difficult or incomplete passage of stool and/or passage of excessively hard, dry stool.

Defining characteristics: Abdominal pain; Abdominal tenderness with palpable muscle resistance; Abdominal tenderness without palpable muscle resistance; Anorexia;

Atypical presentations in older adults; Borborygmi; Bright red blood with stool; Change in bowel pattern; Decrease in stool frequency; Decrease in stool volume; Distended abdomen; fatigue; Hard, formed stool; Headache; Hyperactive bowel sounds; Hypoactive bowel sounds; Inability to defecate; Increase in intra-abdominal pressure; Indigestion; Liquid stool; Pain with defecation; Palpable abdominal mass; Palpable rectal mass; Percussed abdominal dullness; Rectal fullness; Rectal pressure; Severe flatus; Soft, paste-like stool in rectum; Straining with defecation; Vomiting

DECISIONAL CONFLICT

Definition: Uncertainty about course of action to be taken when choice among competing actions involves risk, loss, or challenge to values and beliefs.

Defining characteristics: Delay in decision-making; Distress while attempting a decision; Physical sign of distress; Physical sign of tension; Questioning of moral principle while attempting a decision; Questioning of moral rule while attempting a decision; Questioning of moral values while attempting a decision; Questioning of personal beliefs while attempting a decision; Questioning of personal values while attempting a decision; Recognizes undesired consequences of actions being considered; Self-focused; Uncertainty about choices; Vacillating among choices

DECREASED CARDIAC OUTPUT

Definition: Inadequate blood pumped by the heart to meet the metabolic demands of the body.

Defining characteristics: Altered Heart Rate/Rhythm: Bradycardia; Electrocardiogram (ECG) change; Heart palpitations; Tachycardia

Altered Preload: Decrease in central venous pressure (CVP); Decrease in pulmonary artery wedge pressure (PAWP); Edema; Fatigue; Heart Murmur; Increase in central venous pressure (CVP); Increase in pulmonary artery wedge pressure (PAWP); Jugular vein distention; Weight gain

Altered Afterload: Abnormal skin color; Alteration in blood pressure; Clammy skin; Decrease in peripheral pulses; Decrease in pulmonary vascular resistance (PVR); Decrease in systemic vascular resistance (SVR); Dyspnea; Increase in pulmonary vascular resistance (PVR); Increase in systemic vascular resistance (SVR); Oliguria; Prolonged capillary refill

Altered Contractility: Adventitious breath sounds; Coughing; Decrease in cardiac index; Decrease in ejection fraction; Decrease in left ventricular stroke work index (LVSWI); Decrease in stoke volume index (SVI); Orthopnea; Paroxysmal nocturnal dyspnea; Presence of S3 heart sound; Presence of S4 heart sound

Behavioral/Emotional: Anxiety; Restlessness

DECREASED DIVERSIONAL ACTIVITY ENGAGEMENT

Definition: Reduced stimulation, interest, or participation in recreational or leisure activities.

Defining characteristics: Alteration in mood; Boredom; Discontent with situation; Flat affect; Frequent naps; Physical deconditioning

DECREASED INTRACRANIAL ADAPTIVE CAPACITY

Definition: Compromise in intracranial fluid dynamic, mechanisms that normally compensate for increases in intracranial volumes, resulting in repeated disproportionate increases in intracranial pressure (ICP) in response to a variety of noxious and non-noxious stimuli.

Defining characteristics: Baseline intracranial pressure (ICP) ≥10 mm Hg; Disproportionate increase in intracranial pressure (ICP) following stimuli; Elevated tidal wave intracranial pressure (P2 ICP) waveform; Repeated increase in intracranial pressure (ICP) ≥10 mm Hg for ≥5 minutes following external stimuli; Volume–pressure response test variation (volume:pressure ratio 2, pressure–volume index <10); Wide-amplitude intracranial pressure (ICP) waveform

DEFICIENT FLUID VOLUME

Definition: Decreased intravascular, interstitial, and/or intracellular fluid. This refers to dehydration, water loss alone without change in sodium.

Defining characteristics: Alteration in mental status; Alteration in skin turgor; Decrease in blood pressure; Decrease in pulse pressure; Decrease in pulse volume; Decrease in tongue turgor; Decrease in urine output; Decrease in venous filling; Dry mucous membranes; Dry skin; Increase in body temperature; Increase in heart rate; Increase in hematocrit; Increase in urine concentration; Sudden weight loss; Thirst; Weakness

DEFICIENT KNOWLEDGE

Definition: Absence of cognitive information related to a specific topic, or its acquisition.

Defining characteristics: Inaccurate follow-through of instruction; Inaccurate performance on a test; Inappropriate behavior; Insufficient knowledge

DIARRHEA

Definition: Passage of loose, unformed stools.

Defining characteristics: Abdominal pain; Bowel urgency; Cramping; Hyperactive bowel sounds; Loose liquid stools, >3 in 24 hours

DISTURBED BODY IMAGE

Definition: Confusion in mental picture of one's physical self.

Defining characteristics: Absence of body part; Alteration in body function; Alteration in body structure; Alteration in view of one's body; Avoids looking at one's body; Avoids touching one's body; Behavior of acknowledging one's body; Behavior of monitoring one's body; Change in ability to estimate spatial relationship of body to environment; Change in lifestyle; Change in social involvement; Depersonalization of body part by use of impersonal pronouns; Depersonalization of loss by use of impersonal pronouns; Emphasis on remaining strengths; Extension of body boundary; Fear of reaction by others; Focus on past appearance; Focus on past function; Focus on previous strength; Heightened achievement; Hiding of body part; Negative feeling about body; Nonverbal response to change in body; Nonverbal response to perceived change in body; Overexposure of body part; Perceptions that reflect an altered view of one's body appearance; Personalization of body part by name; Personalization of loss by name; Preoccupation with change; Preoccupation with loss; Refusal to acknowledge change; Trauma to nonfunctioning body part

DRESSING SELF-CARE DEFICIT

Definition: Inability to independently put on or remove clothing.

Defining characteristics: Impaired ability to choose clothing; Impaired ability to fasten clothing; Impaired ability to gather clothing; Impaired ability to maintain appearance; Impaired ability to pick up clothing; Impaired ability to put clothing on lower body; Impaired ability to put clothing on upper body; Impaired ability to put on various items of clothing; Impaired ability to remove clothing item; Impaired ability to use assistive device; Impaired ability to use zipper

EXCESS FLUID VOLUME

Definition: Surplus intake and/or retention of fluid.

Defining characteristics: Adventitious breath sounds; Alteration in blood pressure; Alteration in mental status; Alteration in pulmonary artery pressure (PAP); Alteration in respiratory pattern; Alteration in urine specific gravity; Anasarca; Anxiety; Azotemia; Decrease in hematocrit; Decrease in hemoglobin; Dyspnea; Edema; Electrolyte imbalance; Hepatomegaly; Increase in central venous pressure (CVP); Intake exceeds output; Jugular vein distention; Oliguria; Orthopnea; Paroxysmal nocturnal dyspnea; Pleural effusion; Positive hepatojugular reflex; Presence of S3 heart sound; Pulmonary congestion; Restlessness; Weight gain over short period of time

FATIGUE

Definition: An overwhelming sustained sense of exhaustion and decreased capacity for physical and mental work at the usual level.

Defining characteristics: Alteration in concentration; Alteration in libido; Apathy; Disinterest in surroundings; Drowsiness; Guilt about difficulty maintaining responsibilities; Impaired ability to maintain usual physical activity; Impaired ability to maintain usual routines; Increase in physical symptoms; Increase in rest requirement; Ineffective role performance; Insufficient energy; Introspection; Lethargy; Nonrestorative sleep pattern; Tiredness

FEAR

Definition: Response to perceived threat that is consciously recognized as a danger.

Defining characteristics: Apprehensive; Decrease in self-assurance; Excitedness; Feeling of Alarm; Feeling of dread; Feeling of fear; Feeling of panic; Feeling of terror; Fidgeting; Increase in blood pressure; Increase in tension; Muscle tension; Nausea; Pallor; Pupil dilation; Vomiting

FEEDING SELF-CARE DEFICIT

Definition: Inability to eat independently.

Defining characteristics: Impaired ability to bring food to mouth; Impaired ability to chew food; Impaired ability to get food onto utensil; Impaired ability to handle utensils; Impaired ability to manipulate food in mouth; Impaired ability to open containers; Impaired ability to pick up cup; Impaired ability to prepare food; Impaired ability to self-feed a complete meal; Impaired ability to self-feed in an acceptable manner; Impaired ability to swallow food; Impaired ability to swallow sufficient amount of food; Impaired ability to use assistive device

GRIEVING

Definition: A normal, complex process that includes emotional, physical, spiritual, social, and intellectual responses and behaviors by which individuals, families, and communities incorporate an actual, anticipated, or perceived loss into their daily lives.

Defining characteristics: Alteration in activity level; Alteration in dream pattern; Alteration in immune functioning; Alteration in neuroendocrine functioning; Alteration in sleep pattern; Anger; Blaming; Despair; Detachment; Disorganization; Distress; Finding meaning in a loss; Guilt about feeling relieved; Maintaining a connection to the deceased; Pain; Panic behavior; Personal growth; Psychological distress

HOPELESSNESS

Definition: Subjective state in which an individual sees limited or no alternatives or personal choices available and is unable to mobilize energy on own behalf.

Defining characteristics: Alteration in sleep pattern; Decrease in affect; Decrease in appetite; Decrease in initiative; Decrease in response to stimuli; Decrease in verbalization; Despondent verbal cues; Inadequate involvement in care; Passivity; Poor eye contact; Shrugging in response to speaker; Turning away from speaker

HYPERTHERMIA

Definition: Core body temperature above the normal diurnal range due to failure of thermoregulation.

Defining characteristics: Abnormal posturing; Apnea; Coma; Flushed skin; Hypotension; Infant does not maintain suck; Irritability; Lethargy; Seizure; Skin warm to touch; Stupor; Tachycardia; Tachypnea; Vasodilation

IMBALANCED NUTRITION: LESS THAN BODY REQUIREMENTS

Definition: Intake of nutrition insufficient to meet metabolic needs.

Defining characteristics: Abdominal cramping; Abdominal pain; Alteration in taste sensation; Body weight 20% or more below ideal weight range; Capillary fragility; Diarrhea; Excessive hair loss; Food aversion; Food intake less than recommended daily allowance (RDA); Hyperactive bowel sounds; Insufficient information; Insufficient interest in food; Insufficient muscle tone; Misinformation; Misperception; Pale mucous membranes; Perceived inability to ingest food; Satiety immediately upon ingesting food; Sore buccal cavity; Weakness of muscles required for mastication; Weakness of muscles required for swallowing; Weight loss with adequate food intake

IMPAIRED COMFORT

Definition: Perceived lack of ease, relief, and transcendence in physical, psychospiritual, environmental, cultural, and/or social dimensions.

Defining characteristics: Alteration in sleep pattern; Anxiety; Crying; Discontent with situation; Distressing symptoms; Fear; Feeling cold; Feeling of discomfort; Feeling of hunger; Feeling warm; Inability to relax; Irritability; Itching; Moaning; Restlessness; Sighing; Uneasy in situation

IMPAIRED GAS EXCHANGE

Definition: Excess or deficit in oxygenation and/or carbon dioxide elimination at the alveolar–capillary membrane.

Defining characteristics: Abnormal arterial blood gases; Abnormal arterial pH; Abnormal breathing pattern; Abnormal skin color; Confusion; Decrease in carbon dioxide (CO₂) level; Diaphoresis; Dyspnea; Headache upon awakening; Hypercapnia; Hypoxemia; Hypoxia; Irritability; Nasal flaring; Restlessness; Somnolence; Tachycardia; Visual disturbance

IMPAIRED ORAL MUCOUS MEMBRANE INTEGRITY

Definition: Injury to the lips, soft tissue, buccal cavity, and/or oropharynx.

Defining characteristics: Bad taste in mouth; Bleeding; Cheilitis; Coated tongue; Decrease in taste sensation; Desquamation; Difficulty eating; Difficulty speaking; Enlarged tonsils; Exposure to pathogen; Geographic tongue; Gingival hyperplasia; Gingival pallor; Gingival pocketing deeper than 4 mm; Gingival recession; Halitosis; Hyperemia; Impaired ability to swallow; Macroplasia; Mucosal denudation; Oral discomfort; Oral edema; Oral fissure; Oral lesion; Oral mucosal pallor; Oral nodule; Oral pain; Oral papule; Oral ulcer; Oral vesicles; Presence of mass; Purulent oral–nasal drainage; Purulent oral–nasal exudates; Smooth atrophic tongue; Spongy patches in mouth; Stomatitis; White patches in mouth; White plaque in mouth; White, curd-like oral exudate; Xerostomia

IMPAIRED PHYSICAL MOBILITY

Definition: Limitation in independent. Purposeful movement of the body or of one or more extremities.

Defining characteristics: Alteration in gait; Decrease in fine motor skills; Decrease in gross motor skills; Decrease in range of motion; Decrease in reaction time; Difficulty turning; Discomfort; Engages in substitutions for movement; Exertional dyspnea; Movement-induced tremor; Postural instability; Slowed movement; Spastic movement; Uncoordinated movement

IMPAIRED SKIN INTEGRITY

Definition: Altered epidermis and/or dermis.

Defining characteristics: Acute pain; Alteration in skin integrity; Bleeding; Foreign matter piercing skin; Hematoma; Localized area hot to touch; Redness

IMPAIRED SOCIAL INTERACTION

Definition: Insufficient or excessive quantity or ineffective quality of social exchange.

Defining characteristics: Discomfort in social situations; Dissatisfaction with social engagement; Dysfunctional interaction with others; Family reports change in interaction; Impaired social functioning

IMPAIRED TISSUE INTEGRITY

Definition: Damage to the mucous membrane, cornea, integumentary system, muscular fascia, muscle, tendon, done, cartilage, joint capsule, and/or ligament

Defining characteristics: Acute pain; Bleeding; Destroyed tissue; Hematoma; Localized area hot to touch; Redness; Tissue damage

IMPAIRED URINARY ELIMINATION

Definition: Dysfunction in urine elimination.

Defining characteristics: Dysuria; Frequent voiding; Hesitancy; Nocturia; Urinary incontinence; Urinary retention; Urinary urgency

IMPAIRED VERBAL COMMUNICATION

Definition: Decreased delayed, or absent ability to receive, process, transmit, and/or use a system of symbols.

Defining characteristics: Absence of eye contact; Difficulty comprehending communication; Difficulty expressing thoughts verbally; Difficulty forming sentences; Difficulty forming words; Difficulty in selective attending; Difficulty in use of body expressions; Difficulty in use of facial expressions; Difficulty maintaining communication; Difficulty speaking; Difficulty verbalizing; Disoriented to person; Disoriented to place; Disoriented to time; Dyspnea; Inability to speak; Inability to speak language of caregiver; Inability to use body expressions; Inability to use facial expressions; Inappropriate verbalization; Partial visual deficit; Slurred speech; Stuttering; Total visual deficit

INEFFECTIVE ADOLESCENT EATING DYNAMICS

Definition: Altered eating attitudes and behaviors resulting in over- or undereating patterns that compromise nutritional health.

Defining characteristics: Avoids participation in regular mealtimes; Complains of hunger between meals; Food refusal; Frequent snacking; Frequently eating from fast food restaurants; Frequently eating poor-quality food; Frequently eating processed food; Overeating; Poor appetite; Undereating

INEFFECTIVE AIRWAY CLEARANCE

Definition: Inability to clear secretions or obstructions from the respiratory tract to maintain a clear airway.

Defining characteristics: Absence of cough; Adventitious breath sounds; Alteration in respiratory pattern; Alteration in respiratory rate; Cyanosis; Difficulty verbalizing Diminished breath sounds; Dyspnea; Excessive sputum; Ineffective cough; Orthopnea; Restlessness; Wide-eyed look

INEFFECTIVE BREASTFEEDING

Definition: Difficulty feeding milk from the breasts, which may compromise nutritional status of the infant/child.

Defining characteristics: Inadequate infant stooling; Infant arching at breast; Infant crying at the breast; Infant crying within the first hour after breastfeeding; Infant fussing within 1 hour of breastfeeding; Infant inability to latch on to maternal breast correctly; Infant resisting latching onto breast; Infant unresponsive to other comfort measures; Insufficient emptying of each breast per feeding; Insufficient infant weight gain; Insufficient signs of oxytocin release; Perceived inadequate milk supply; Sore nipples persisting beyond first week; Sustained infant weight loss; Unsustained suckling at the breast

INEFFECTIVE BREATHING PATTERN

Definition: Inspiration and/or expiration that does not provide adequate ventilation.

Defining characteristics: Abnormal breathing pattern; Altered chest excursion; Bradypnea; Decrease in expiratory pressure; Decrease in inspiratory pressure; Decrease in minute ventilation; Decrease in vital capacity; Dyspnea; Increase in anterior-posterior chest diameter; Nasal flaring; Orthopnea; Prolonged expiration phase; Pursed-lip breathing; Tachypnea; Use of accessory muscles to breathe; Use of three-point position

INEFFECTIVE COPING

Definition: A pattern of invalid appraisal of stressors, with cognitive and/or behavioral efforts, that fails to manage demands related to well-being.

Defining characteristics: Alteration in concentration; Alteration in sleep pattern; Change in communication pattern; Destructive behavior toward others; Difficulty organizing information; Fatigue; Frequent illness; Inability to ask for help; Inability to attend to information; Inability with a situation; Inability to meet basic needs; Inability to meet role expectation; Ineffective coping strategies; Insufficient access of social support; Insufficient goal-directed behavior; Insufficient problem resolution; Insufficient problem-solving skills; Risk-taking behavior; Substance misuse

INEFFECTIVE HEALTH MAINTENANCE

Definition: Inability to identify, manage, and/or seek out help to maintain well-being.

Defining characteristics: Absence of adaptive behaviors to environmental changes; Absence of interest in improving health behaviors; Inability to take responsibility for meeting basic health practices; Insufficient knowledge about basic health practices; Insufficient social support; Pattern of health-seeking behavior

INEFFECTIVE HEALTH MANAGEMENT

Definition: Pattern of regulating and integrating into daily living a therapeutic regimen for the treatment of illness and its sequelae that is unsatisfactory for meeting specific health goals.

Defining characteristics: Difficulty with prescribed regimen; Failure to include treatment regimen in daily living; Failure to take action to reduce risk factor; Ineffective choices in daily living for meeting health goal

INEFFECTIVE PERIPHERAL TISSUE PERFUSION

Definition: Decrease in blood circulation to the periphery, which may compromise health.

Defining characteristics: Absence of peripheral pulses; Alteration in motor function; Alteration in skin characteristic; Ankle–brachial index <0.90; Capillary refill time >3 seconds; Color does not return to lowered limb after 1-minute leg elevation; Decrease in blood pressure in extremities; Decrease in pain-free distances during a 6-minute walk test; Decrease in peripheral pulses; Delay in peripheral wound healing; Distance in the 6-minute walk test below normal range; Edema; Extremity pain; Femoral bruit; Intermittent claudication; Paresthesia; Skin color pales with limb elevation

INEFFECTIVE PROTECTION

Definition: Decrease in the ability to guard self from internal or external threats such as illness or injury.

Defining characteristics: Alteration in clotting; Alteration in perspiration; Anorexia; Chilling; Coughing; Deficient immunity; Disorientation; Dyspnea; Fatigue; Immobility; Insomnia; Itching; Maladaptive stress response; Neurosensory impairment; Pressure ulcer; Restlessness; Weakness

INEFFECTIVE THERMOREGULATION

Definition: Temperature fluctuation between hypothermia and hyperthermia.

Defining characteristics: Cyanotic nail beds; Flushed skin; Hypertension; Increase in body temperature above normal range; Increase in respiratory rate; Mild shivering; Moderate pallor; Piloerection; Reduction in body temperature below normal range; Seizure; Skin cool to touch; Skin warm to touch; Slow capillary refill; Tachycardia

INTERRUPTED FAMILY PROCESSES

Definition: Break in the continuity of family functioning which fails to support the well-being of its members.

Defining characteristics: Change in availability for affective responsiveness; Change in family conflict resolution; Change in family satisfaction; Change in intimacy; Change in participation for problem-solving; Assigned tasks change; Change in communication pattern; Change in somatization; Change in stress-reduction behavior; Changes in expression of conflict with community resources; Changes in expressions of isolation from community resources; Changes in participation for decision making; Changes in relationship pattern; Decrease in available emotional support; Ineffective task completion; Power alliance chance; Ritual change

NAUSEA

Definition: A subjective phenomenon of an unpleasant feeling in the back of the throat and stomach, which may or may not result in vomiting.

Defining characteristics: Aversion toward food; Gagging sensation; Increase in salivation; Increase in swallowing; Sour taste

OVERWEIGHT

Definition: A condition in which an individual accumulates excessive fat for age and gender.

Defining characteristics: ADULT: Body mass index (BMI) >25 kg/m^2; CHILD <2 years: Weight-for-length >95th percentile; CHILD 2 to 19 years: Body mass index (BMI) >85th percentile or 25 kg/m^2 but <95th percentile or 30 kg/m^2 for age and gender

RAPE-TRAUMA SYNDROME

Definition: Sustained maladaptive response to a forced, violent, sexual penetration against the victim's will and consent.

Defining characteristics: Aggression; Agitation; Alteration in sleep pattern; Anger; Anxiety; Change in relationship(s); Confusion; Denial; Dependency; Depression; Disorganization; Dissociative identity disorder; Embarrassment; Fear; Guilt; Helplessness; History of suicide attempt; Hyperalertness; Impaired decision-making; Low self-esteem; Mood swings; Muscle spasm; Muscle tension; Nightmares; Paranoia; Perceived vulnerability; Phobias; Physical trauma; Powerlessness; Self-blame; Sexual dysfunction; Shame; Shock; Substance misuse; Thoughts of revenge

READINESS FOR ENHANCED PARENTING

Definition: A pattern of providing an environment for children to nurture growth and development, which can be strengthened.

Defining characteristics: Children express desire

RISK FOR CAREGIVER ROLE STRAIN

Definition: Susceptible to difficulty in fulfilling care responsibilities, expectations, and/or behaviors for family or significant others, which may compromise health

RISK FOR CONSTIPATION

Definition: Susceptible to a decrease in normal frequency of defecation accompanied by difficult or incomplete passage of stool, which may compromise health.

RISK FOR DEFICIENT FLUID VOLUME

Definition: Susceptible to experiencing decreased intravascular, interstitial, and/or intracellular fluid volumes, which may compromise health.

RISK FOR DELAYED DEVELOPMENT

Definition: Susceptible to delay of 25% or more in one or more of the areas of social of self-regulatory behavior, or in cognitive, language, gross, or fine motor skills, which may compromise health.

RISK FOR IMPAIRED ATTACHMENT

Definition: Susceptible to disruption of the interactive process between parent or significant other and child that fosters the development of a protective and nurturing reciprocal relationship.

RISK FOR IMPAIRED PARENTING

Definition: Susceptible to primary caretaker difficulty in creating, maintaining, or regaining an environment that promotes the optimum growth and development of the child, which may compromise the well-being of the child.

RISK FOR IMPAIRED SKIN INTEGRITY

Definition: Susceptible to alteration in epidermis and/or dermis, which may compromise health.

RISK FOR INEFFECTIVE CEREBRAL TISSUE PERFUSION

Definition: Susceptible to a decrease in cerebral tissue circulation, which may compromise health.

RISK FOR INEFFECTIVE THERMOREGULATION

Definition: Susceptible to a decrease in cerebral tissue circulation, which may compromise health.

RISK FOR INFECTION

Definition: Susceptible to invasion and multiplication of pathogenic organisms, which may compromise health.

RISK FOR INJURY

Definition: Susceptible to physical damage due to environmental conditions, interacting with the individual's adaptive and defensive resources, which may compromise health.

RISK FOR OVERWEIGHT

Definition: Susceptible to excessive fat accumulation for age and gender, which may compromise health.

RISK FOR POWERLESSNESS

Definition: Susceptible to the lived experience of lack of control over a situation, including apperception that one's actions do not significantly affect the outcome, which may compromise health.

RISK FOR SITUATIONAL LOW SELF-ESTEEM

Definition: Susceptible to developing a negative perception of self-worth in response to a current situation, which may compromise health.

RISK FOR UNSTABLE BLOOD GLUCOSE LEVEL

Definition: Susceptible to variation in serum levels of glucose from the normal range, which may compromise health.

SLEEP DEPRIVATION

Definition: Prolonged periods of time without sustained natural, periodic, suspension of relative consciousness that provides rest.

   Defining characteristics: Agitation; Alteration in concentration; Anxiety; Apathy; Combativeness; Confusion; Decrease in functional ability; Decrease in reaction time; Drowsiness; Fatigue; Fleeting nystagmus; Hallucinations; Hand tremors; Heightened sensitivity to pain; Irritability; Lethargy; Malaise; Perceptual disorders; Restlessness; Transient paranoia

SOCIAL ISOLATION

Definition: Aloneness experienced by the individual and perceived as imposed by others and as a negative or threatening state.

   Defining characteristics: Absence of support system; Aloneness imposed by others; Cultural incongruence; Desire to be alone; Developmental delay; Disabling condition; Feeling different from others; Flat affect; History of rejection; Hostility; Illness; Inability to meet expectations of others; Insecurity in public; Meaningless actions; Member of a subculture; Poor eye contact; Preoccupation with own thoughts; Purposelessness; Repetitive actions; Sad affect; Values incongruent with cultural norms; Withdrawn

URINARY RETENTION

Definition: Inability to empty bladder completely.

   Defining characteristics: Absence of urinary output; Bladder distention; Dribbling of urine; Dysuria; Frequent voiding; Overflow incontinence; Residual urine; Sensation of bladder fullness; Small voiding

Note: Page numbers followed by b, f and t indicate text in box, figure, and table respectively.